SELF-STUDY PROGRAM INSTRUCTIONS

System Requirements

A PC compatible computer with an Intel 386 or better processor. Windows 3.1 or later.

4 Megabytes of RAM (minimum); but recommend 8 MB RAM on Windows 3.1; or 8 Megabytes of RAM (minimum); but recommend 12 MB RAM minimum on Windows 95; and 3 Megabytes of available hard disk space.

Installation

Installing the Medical-Surgical Nursing Self-Study program

1. Start up Windows.
2. Insert the disk into the floppy drive. From the Program Manager's File Menu, choose the RUN command.
3. When the RUN dialog appears, type a:\setup (or b:\setup if you are using b: as your disk drive) in the command line box. Click OK or press the "Enter" button.
4. The installation process will begin. A dialog proposing the directory **"MSNSG"** on the drive containing Windows will appear. If the name and location are correct, click OK. If you want to change this information, type over the existing data, then click OK.
5. When the setup routine is complete, a new group called **"MEDICAL SURGICAL NURSING"** will appear on your desktop.
6. Start the self-study program by double clicking on its icon.

The *Medical-Surgical Nursing* Self-Study Program

This self-study program contains questions that review the content covered in Medical-Surgical Nursing.

This is not a timed test. Take your time; consider the questions and the possible answers carefully. The Main Menu screen allows you to select which unit you would like to review. To begin a unit test, choose Start Test for that unit. To continue a test that you have already begun, choose Resume test. To re-start the test and erase your results from a previous test, choose Restart test. To review the answers you have given and compare them to the correct answers, choose Answers.

When you choose Start test, Resume test, Restart test, or Answers, the test and the program's Toolbar will appear.

Medical-Surgical Nursing Toolbar

The Toolbar contains a series of buttons that provide direc cess to all test program functions. When you move the c over a button, an explanation of its function displays i Status Bar immediately above the Toolbar.

To get help at any time during the test, choose the Pro Help button. Program Help reviews basic functions o program.

Answer each question by clicking on the oval to the left of an answer selection or by selecting the appropriate letter on the keyboard (e.g. A, B, C, D, etc.). When an answer is selected, its oval will darken. If you change your mind about an answer, simply select that choice, by mouse or keyboard, again.

To register your answer selection and proceed to the next question, click on the Right Arrow button or press Return.

After taking the test and receiving your score, you may review your answers by clicking on the Answers button on the Main Menu screen.

If you are unsure about an answer to a particular question, the program allows you to mark it for later review. Flag the question by clicking on the Mark button. To review all marked questions for a test, click on the Table of Contents button, which is immediately to the right of the Mark button.

The Table of Contents window lists every question included on the test and summarizes whether it has been answered, left unanswered, or marked for later review. Click on an item in the Table of Contents window and the program will move to that question. Use the Arrow buttons to move to the first, previous, next, or last question.

At any time during the test or when you are finished tak the test, click on the Stop button. If you wish, you may ret to the session at a later time without erasing your existin swers by clicking on the Resume Test button on the M Menu.

After taking the test, view the correct answer for each question by using the Answers button on the Main Menu. will take you back to the test, but you will not be able to m ify the answers you have given. Click on the Q/A butto the right of the Stop button), and a window pops up plaining the correct answer to the question. The Q/A bu will only appear when you are in the Answer section of the You may also wish to use the Table of Contents button to s you which questions you would like to review.

To exit the **MEDICAL-SURGICAL NURSING** self-s program, press the Quit button on the Main Menu.

BRUNNER & SUDDARTH'S
Textbook of
MEDICAL-
SURGICAL
NURSING

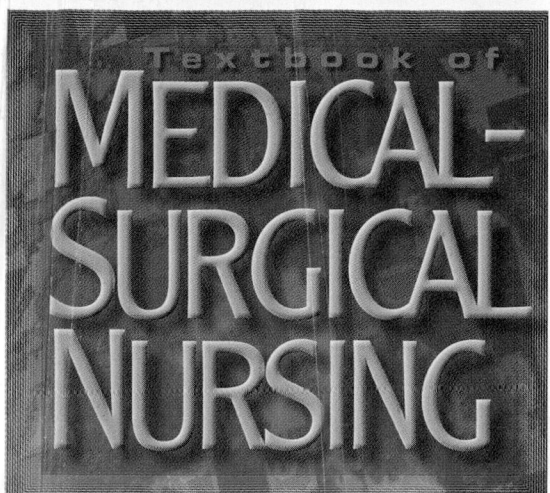

BRUNNER & SUDDARTH'S

Textbook of MEDICAL-SURGICAL NURSING

Suzanne C. Smeltzer, RN, EdD, FAAN

Associate Professor and Coordinator, Nursing Research
Villanova University College of Nursing
Villanova, Pennsylvania

Brenda G. Bare, RN, MSN

Associate Administrator Patient Care Services/Chief Nurse Executive
Inova Mount Vernon Hospital
Alexandria, Virginia

With 50 Contributors

9th edition

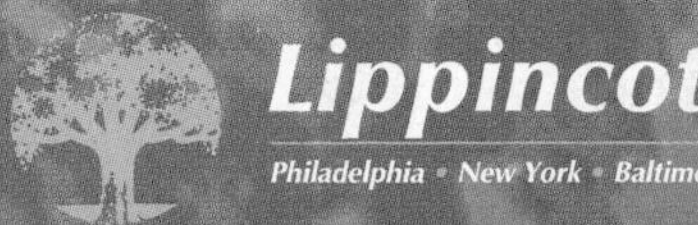

Acquisitions Editor: Lisa Stead
Developmental Editor: Deedie McMahon
Editorial Assistant: Claudia Vaughn
Senior Project Editor: Erika Kors
Senior Production Manager: Helen Ewan
Senior Production Coordinator: Nannette Winski
Design Coordinator: Doug Smock
Cover Designer: Larry Didona
Indexer: Ann Cassar/Alexandria Nickerson/Maria Coughlin
Compositor: Circle Graphics
Prepress: Jays
Printer/Binder: World Color
Cover Printer: Lehigh Press, Inc.

9th Edition

9 8 7 6 5 4 3 2 1

Library of Congress Cataloging-in-Publication Data

Brunner and Suddarth's textbook of medical-surgical nursing. — 9th ed. / [edited by] Suzanne C. Smeltzer, Brenda G. Bare.
p. cm.
Includes bibliographical references and index.
ISBN 0-7817-1575-X [one-vol. ed.]
ISBN 0-7817-2191-1 [two-vol. ed.]
1. Nursing. 2. Surgical nursing. I. Brunner, Lillian Sholtis. II. Suddarth, Doris Smith. III. Smeltzer, Suzanne C. O'Connell. IV. Bare, Brenda G. V. Title: Textbook of medical-surgical nursing.
[DNLM: 1. Nursing Care. 2. Perioperative Nursing. WY 150 B8972 2000]
RT41.T46 1999
610.73—dc21
DNLM/DLC
for Library of Congress 99-16398
CIP

Care has been taken to confirm the accuracy of the information presented and to describe generally accepted practices. However, the authors, editors, and publisher are not responsible for errors or omissions or for any consequences from application of the information in this book and make no warranty, express or implied, with respect to the contents of the publication.

The authors, editors and publisher have exerted every effort to ensure that drug selection and dosage set forth in this text are in accordance with current recommendations and practice at the time of publication. However, in view of ongoing research, changes in government regulations, and the constant flow of information relating to drug therapy and drug reactions, the reader is urged to check the package insert for each drug for any change in indications and dosage and for added warnings and precautions. This is particularly important when the recommended agent is a new or infrequently employed drug.

Some drugs and medical devices presented in this publication have Food and Drug Administration (FDA) clearance for limited use in restricted research settings. It is the responsibility of the health care provider to ascertain the FDA status of each drug or device planned for use in their clinical practice.

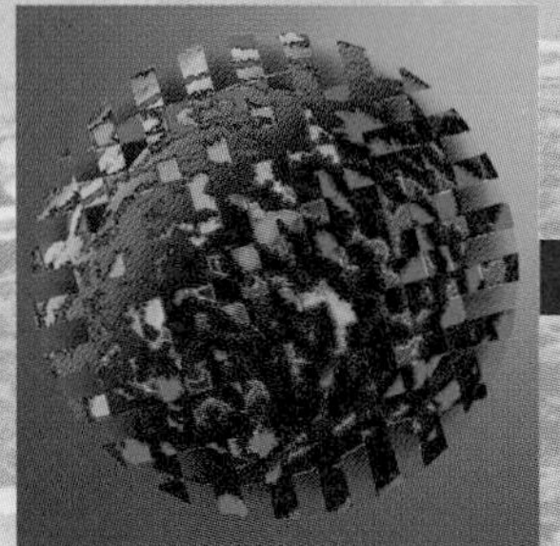

Consultants and Reviewers

CONSULTANTS ON HOME CARE

Elise R. Pizzi, RN, MSN, CRNP
Assistant Professor
College of Nursing
Villanova University
Villanova, Pennsylvania

Karen McKenna, RN, MSN
Clinical Assistant Professor
College of Nursing
Villanova University
Villanova, Pennsylvania

REVIEWERS

Susan Appling, RN, MS, CRNP
Assistant Professor
The Johns Hopkins University School of Nursing
Nurse Practitioner, Breast Center
The Johns Hopkins Hospital
Baltimore, Maryland

Diane S. Aschenbrenner, RN, MS, CS
Undergraduate Faculty
The Johns Hopkins University School of Nursing
Baltimore, Maryland

Abbie Bailey, RN, C MSN
Nursing Instructor
Carl Albert State College
Poteau, Oklahoma

Karen Tipton Bailey, RN, MSN, C-FNP
Assistant Professor of Nursing
Marshall University
Huntington, West Virginia

Jean Krajicek Bartek, RN, PhD, CCRN
Associate Professor
University of Nebraska Medical Center School of Nursing
Omaha, Nebraska

Verla Beck, RN, MSN
Program Director and Instructor
Department of Vocational Nursing
Long Beach City College
Long Beach, California

Janice E. Beeken, RN, PhD
Assistant Professor of Nursing
University of Wyoming, School of Nursing
Laramie, Wyoming

Patricia C. Birchfield, RN, DSN
Associate Professor
Department of Baccalaureate and Graduate Nursing
Eastern Kentucky University
Richmond, Kentucky

Emily Bond, RN, PhD
Associate Professor
Southeastern Louisiana University, School of Nursing
Hammond, Louisiana

Karen Burger, RN, PhD
Professor
Department of Nursing Technology
Columbus State Community College
Columbus, Ohio

Mary Ellen Cahoon, BSN, MSN
Coordinator, Curriculum/Evaluation
Nurse Educator, Level II Nursing
Sisters School of Nursing
Buffalo, New York

Mary E. Calkins, RN, PhD, CNN
Assistant Professor
University of Wyoming School of Nursing
Cheyenne, Wyoming

David S. Castelán, RN, BS, CCRN
Instructor
Department of Nursing
East Los Angeles College
Monterey Park, California
Lead Nurse
Critical Care Unit
Alhambra Hospital
Temple City, California

Joan W. Conklin, RN, C, EdD
Professor of Nursing
Bloomfield College, Division of Nursing
Bloomfield, New Jersey

Robert Contino, RN, BSN, MSN, EdD
Associate Professor of Nursing
Wesley College
Dover, Delaware

Gloria Coschigano, RN, MSN, CS
Assistant Professor of Nursing
Westchester Community College
Valhalla, New York

Christy L. Crowther, RN, BSN, MS, CRNP
Clinical Instructor
University of Maryland School of Nursing, Department of Family Medicine
Baltimore, Maryland
Nurse Practitioner
Chesapeake Orthopedic and Sports Medicine Center
Baltimore, Maryland

Dolly Daniel, RNC, BSN, CDE
Diabetes Nurse Specialist
Inova Alexandria Hospital
Alexandria, Virginia

Sherri C. Daniels, RN, DSN
Chair, Adult Health Department
University of South Alabama
Mobile, Alabama

Bernice Daugherty, RN, MSN, CS, FNP
Assistant Professor
Lauder University School of Nursing
Greenwood, South Carolina

Marie Amos Dobyns, MD
Private Practice Internal Medicine and Geriatrics
Laurel and Glenelg, Maryland

Chris Eaton, RN, MS, CETN
Interim Director of Nursing and Health Services
Nursing Instructor
Hartnell College
Salinas, California

Laurel Eisenhauer, RN, MS, PhD, FAAN
Professor of Nursing
Boston College School of Nursing
Chestnut Hill, Massachusetts

Peggy A. Ellis, RNCS, PhD, ANP, FNP
Clinical Associate Professor
Barnes College of Nursing
University of Missouri, St. Louis
St. Louis, Missouri

Betty Farrell, RN, PhD, FAAN
Research Scientist
City of Hope National Medical Center and Beekman Research Institute
Duarte, California

Michelle C. Foley, RN, C, MA
Senior Nursing Instructor
Charles E. Gregory School of Nursing
Perth Amboy, New Jersey

Lillian Goodman, RN, MEd
Director, Vocational Nursing
Consultant, Health Careers
Los Angeles Unified School District
Los Angeles, California

Janet L. Gysi, RN, MA, CCRN
Instructor, Division of Nursing
Iowa Wesleyan College
Burlington, Iowa
Staff Registered Nurse
Emergency Treatment Center
Burlington Medical Center
Burlington, Iowa

Elaine Hagerty, RN, MSN
Clinical Instructor
Department of Nursing
Franciscan University
Steubenville, Ohio
Staff Nurse
Emergency Room
Wheeling Medical Park Hospital
Wheeling, West Virginia

Susan J. W. Hsia, RN, PhD
Associate Professor
Washburn University School of Nursing
Topeka, Kansas

Linda M. Janelli, RN, C, EdD
Associate Professor
Department of Nursing
Nazareth College of Rochester
Rochester, New York

Joyce Young Johnson, RN, PhD, CCRN
Adjunct Faculty
School of Nursing
Georgia State University
Atlanta, Georgia

Mary Jayne Johnson, MS, APRN, FNP-C
Clinical Instructor
College of Nursing
Brigham Young University
Provo, Utah

Kathy Lauer, RN, PhD
Assistant Professor and Associate Chairperson
Department of Adult Health Nursing
Rush University College of Nursing
Chicago, Illinois

Patricia Lange-Otsuka, RN, MSN, CS, CCRN, EdD
Academic Coordinator and Assistant Professor of Nursing
Hawaii Pacific University
Kaeohe, Hawaii

Elizabeth Matheny Long, RN, MSN, CNS
Instructor
Department of Nursing
Lamar University
Beaumont, Texas

Lynda A. Mackin, RN, C, MS, ANP
Assistant Clinical Professor
Department of Physiological Nursing
University of California, San Francisco, School of Nursing
San Francisco, California

Josephine D. Marick, RN, MA, MSN, EdD
Professor
Department of Nursing
Fort Hays State University
Hays, Kansas

Jane V. McCloskey, RN, MSN
Faculty
Carolinas College of Health Science, School of Nursing
Charlotte, North Carolina

Valerie H. Michaelson, RN, C, MS
Assistant Professor of Nursing
Long Island University
Brooklyn, New York

Barbara Moffett, RN, PhD
Associate Professor of Nursing
Southeast Louisiana University
Hammond, Louisiana

Patti J. Moss, RN, MSN
Assistant Professor
Department of Nursing
Lamar University
Beaumont, Texas

Donna Ann Nayduch, RN, MSN, CCRN
Trauma Network Director
Western Plains Health Network
Greeley, Colorado

Bonnie J. Nesbit, RN, CS, PhD
Associate Professor of Nursing
Viterbo College
LaCrosse, Wisconsin

Sandra M. Nettina, MSN, RN, CS, ANP
Nurse Practitioner
Glenelg, Maryland
Adjunct Faculty
George Washington University
Washington, District of Columbia
Adjunct Faculty
George Mason University
Fairfax, Virginia

Dorothy Obester, BSNE, MSN, PhD
Professor of Nursing
St. Francis College
Loretto, Pennsylvania

Janet Rhorer, RN, CS, EdD
Assistant Professor
College of Nursing and Health Sciences
University of Texas at El Paso
El Paso, Texas

Leslie Rice, BSN, MSN, PhD
Assistant Professor
Division of Professional Nursing
The College of New Jersey
Ewing, New Jersey

Lee W. Richard, RN, PhD, CNAA
Assistant Professor
School of Nursing and
Graduate School of Biomedical Sciences
University of Texas Health Sciences Center at San Antonio
San Antonio, Texas

Isabel Romena, RN, BSN, MSN, CCRN
Nursing Instructor
San Joaquin Delta College
Stockton, CA 95207

Otto Sanchez-Sweatman, MS, MD, PhD
Assistant Professor
School of Nursing
McMaster University
Toronto, Canada

Carolyn Sigmund Shields, RN, C, MSN
Adjunct Faculty
Widener University School of Nursing
Chester, Pennsylvania
Coordinator of Nursing Education
Education Services
Bryn Mawr Rehabilitation Center and Hospital
Malvern, Pennsylvania

Jane C. Shivnan, RN, MSN
Nurse Manager
Bone Marrow Transplant
The Johns Hopkins Oncology Center
Baltimore, Maryland

Lynne M. Simko, RN, MSN, MPH, CCRN
Assistant Professor
School of Nursing
Duquesne University
Pittsburgh, Pennsylvania

Gwendolynne Skinner, RN, MA
Assistant Professor of Nursing
University of Texas, PanAmerican
Edinburg, Texas

Carol A. Stephenson, RNC, EdD, CRNH
Associate Professor
Harris College of Nursing
Texas Christian University
Fort Worth, Texas

M. Margaret Rayman Stinner, RN, C, MS
Instructor of Nursing
Mt. Carmel College of Nursing
Columbus, Ohio

Patricia Stockert, RN, MS, PS
Assistant Professor
St Francis Medical College of Nursing
Peoria, Illinois

Alison Stull, RN, MSN
Assistant Professor
Department of Nursing
Dickinson State University
Dickinson, North Dakota

Cheryl L. Szenasi, BSN, MSN
Senior Instructor
The Charles E. Gregory School of Nursing
Perth Amboy, New Jersey

Rosalena Thorpe, RN, PhD
Professor and Chairperson
Nursing Department
Community College of Allegheny County,
Allegheny Campus
Pittsburgh, Pennsylvania

Linda Ulak, RN, CCRN, CS, EdD
Associate Professor
College of Nursing
Seton Hall University
South Orange, New Jersey

Catherine Ultrino, MSN, RN, OCN
Nurse Manager, Outpatient Oncology Clinic
Inpatient Surgical Oncology
Boston Regional Medical Center
Stoneham, Massachusetts

Elise Vernarsky, RNCS, MSN
Instructor in Nursing
Pennsylvania State University at Altoona
Altoona, Pennsylvania

Laura Jean Waight, RN, MSN
Instructor of Nursing
West Texas A&M University
Canyon, Texas

Myrtle Ruth Welch, RN, MS
Instructor of Nursing
Angelina College
Lufkin, Texas

Deborah F. Wilson, RN, CS, MSN
Assistant Lecturer
University of Wyoming School of Nursing
Laramie, Wyoming

Sherry B. Wilson, RN, MSN
Nursing Instructor
Durham Technical Community College
Durham, North Carolina

Karen Thomas Yehle, RN, CS, MS
Clinical Assistant Professor of Nursing
Purdue University
School of Nursing
West Lafayette, Indiana

Contributors

Margaret Ahearn-Spera, RN, CS, MSN, CANP
Nurse Practitioner
Family Medical
Ridgefield, Connecticut
Chapter 56: Assessment of Neurologic Function

Debra A. Bancroft, RN, MSN, FNP
Nurse Practitioner
Rheumatic Disease Center
Milwaukee, Wisconsin
Chapter 50: Management of Patients With Rheumatic Disorders

Jo Ann Brooks-Brunn, DNS, RN, FAAN, FCCP
Assistant Professor
Pulmonary and Critical Care Medicine
Indiana University School of Medicine
Indianapolis, Indiana
Chapter 21: Management of Patients With Chest and Lower Respiratory Tract Disorders

Jaqueline Fowler Byers, RN, PhD
Associate Professor
School of Nursing/College of Health and Public Affairs
University of Central Florida
Orlando, Florida
Chapter 19: Assessment of Respiratory Function
Chapter 22: Respiratory Care Modalities
Chapter 53: Management of Patients With Burn Injury

Kim Cantwell-Gab, BSN, RN, CVN, RVT, RDMS
Vascular Surgery Nurse Coordinator
Department of Surgery, Division of Vascular Surgery
University of Washington School of Medicine
Seattle, Washington
Chapter 28: Assessment and Management of Patients with Vascular Disorders and Problems of Peripheral Circulation

Patricia E. Casey, RN, MSN
Medical Cardiac Clinical Nurse Specialist
Washington Adventist Hospital
Takoma Park, Maryland
Chapter 24: Management of Patients With Dysrhythmias and Conduction Problems
Chapter 25: Management of Patients With Coronary Vascular Disorders
Chapter 27: Management of Patients With Complications From Heart Disease

Linda Carman Copel, PhD, RN, CS, CGP, DAPA
Associate Professor
Villanova University College of Nursing
Villanova, Pennsylvania
Chapter 4: Health Education and Promotion
Chapter 6: Homeostasis, Stress, and Adaptation
Chapter 7: Individual and Family Considerations Related to Illness

Juliet Corbin, RNC, DNS, FNP
Lecturer, School of Nursing
San Jose State University
San Jose, California
Chapter 9: Chronic Illness

Susanna G. Cunningham, RN, PhD, FAAN
Professor
Department of Biobehavioral Nursing and Health Systems
University of Washington School of Nursing
Seattle, Washington
Chapter 29: Assessment and Management of Patients With Hypertension

Margaret A. Degler, RN, MSN, CRNP, CUNP
Geriatric/Urologic Nurse Practitioner
University of Pennsylvania School of Nursing
Philadelphia, Pennsylvania
Consultant
Gerontological Nursing Consultation Service
Philadelphia, Pennsylvania
Chapter 11: Health Care of the Older Adult

Ann S. Dellaira, RN, CS, PhD
Director, Nurse Wellness Clinic
Northgate II
Camden, New Jersey
Chapter 46: Assessment of Immune Function
Chapter 47: Management of Patients With Immunodeficiency
Chapter 48: Management of Patients With HIV Infection and AIDS
Chapter 49: Management of Patients With Allergic Disorders

Nancy E. Donegan, RN, MPH
Director, Infection Control
Washington Hospital Center
Washington, DC
Chapter 64: Management of Patients With Infectious Diseases

Joan Webb Dresh, RN, MSN
Instructor, College of Nursing
Widener University
Chester, Pennsylvania
Chapter 38: Assessment and Management of Patients With Endocrine Disorders

Constance B. Easterling, MSN, ARNP, CCRN
Clinical Coordinator
Orlando Regional Multiple Sclerosis Center
Orlando, Florida
Chapter 59: Management of Patients With Neurologic Disorders

Eleanor Fitzpatrick, RN, MSN
Clinical Nurse Specialist
Thomas Jefferson University Hospital
Philadelphia, Pennsylvania
Chapter 36: Assessment and Management of Patients With Hepatic and Biliary Disorders

Mary Beth Flynn, RN, MS, CCRN
Critical Care Clinical Nurse Educator
University Hospital
Denver, Colorado
Chapter 14: Shock and Multisystem Failure

Kathleen K. Furniss, RN,C, MSN
Women's Health Nurse Practitioner
Associates in Women's Health Care and Women's Health Initiative

University of Medicine and Dentistry of New Jersey
Newark, New Jersey
Chapter 42: Assessment and Management of Problems Related to Female Physiologic Processes
Chapter 43: Management of Patients With Female Reproductive Disorders

Maureen Giuffre, RN, PhD
Clinical Research Consultant
Salisbury, Maryland
Chapter 12: Pain Management

Janet Goshorn, ARNP, MSN, CCRN
Nurse Practitioner
Division of Nephrology
Nemours Children's Clinic
Orlando, Florida
Chapter 39: Assessment of Urinary and Renal Function
Chapter 40: Management of Patients With Urinary and Renal Dysfunction
Chapter 41: Management of Patients With Urinary and Renal Disorders

Randolph E. Gross, RN, MS, CS, AOCN
Clinical Nurse IV
Ambulatory Care Nursing
Memorial Sloan-Kettering Cancer Center
New York, New York
Chapter 44: Assessment and Management of Patients With Breast Disorders

Doreen Chaffinch Grzelak, RN, MSN, AOCN
Director, Medical/Oncology Unit
Reston Hospital Center
Reston, Virginia
Chapter 32: Management of Patients With Oral and Esophageal Disorders
Chapter 34: Management of Patients With Gastric and Duodenal Disorders

Shelby Hixson, RN, MSN, CCRN
Clinical Outcomes Manager, Medical Critical Care
Orlando Regional Healthcare System
Orlando, Florida
Chapter 58: Management of Patients With Neurologic Trauma

Ryan R. Iwamoto, ARNP, MS, CS, AOCN
Clinical Nurse Specialist
Department of Radiation Oncology
Virginia Mason Medical Center
Seattle, Washington
Clinical Instructor
University of Washington, School of Nursing
Seattle, Washington
Chapter 45: Assessment and Management of Problems Related to Male Reproductive Processes

Joyce Young Johnson, RN, PhD, CCRN
Adjunct Faculty
School of Nursing
Georgia State University
Atlanta, Georgia
Chapter 1: Health Care Delivery and Nursing Practice
Chapter 2: Community-Based Nursing Practice
Chapter 3: Critical Thinking, Ethical Decision-Making, and the Nursing Process
Chapter 8: Perspectives in Transcultural Nursing

H. Lynn Kane, RN, MSN, CCRN
Clinician, Acute Pain Management Service
Thomas Jefferson University Hospital
Philadelphia, Pennsylvania
Chapter 16: Preoperative Nursing Management
Chapter 17: Intraoperative Nursing Management
Chapter 18: Postoperative Nursing Management

M. Jan Keffer, PhD, RN, CS, ANP
Associate Professor Family Health Nursing
School of Nursing
Consultant, Health Care Ethics
Indiana University
Indianapolis, Indiana
Ethics Related Issues

Rhonda Kyanko, RN, MS, CRRN
Nursing Education Coordinator
National Rehabilitation Hospital
Washington, DC
Chapter 10: Principles and Practices of Rehabilitation

Pamela J. LaBorde, RN, MSN
Clinical Nurse Specialist, Burn Unit
Quality Management Department
Orlando Regional Medical Center
Orlando, Florida
Chapter 53: Management of Patients With Burn Injury

Dorothy B. Liddel, RN, MSN, ONC
Assistant Professor
Columbia Union College
Takoma Park, Maryland
Chapter 60: Assessment of Musculoskeletal Function
Chapter 61: Musculoskeletal Care Modalities
Chapter 62: Management of Patients With Musculoskeletal Disorders
Chapter 63: Management of Patients With Musculoskeletal Trauma

Martha V. Manning, RN, MSN
Wellness Nurse Coordinator
Sunrise/Inova Assisted Living Center
Fairfax, Virginia
Chapter 31: Assessment of Digestive and Gastrointestinal Function
Chapter 35: Management of Patients With Intestinal and Rectal Disorders

Barbara J. Maschak-Carey, RN, MSN, CDE
Diabetes Clinical Nurse Specialist
EDIC Study Coordinator
Department of Medicine
Hospital of the University of Pennsylvania
Philadelphia, Pennsylvania
Chapter 37: Assessment and Management of Patients With Diabetes Mellitus

Shawn M. McCabe, RN, MSN, CCRN, CNSC
Clinical Nurse Specialist, Trauma
Department of Education and Special Projects
University of Medicine and Dentistry of New Jersey-University Hospital
Newark, New Jersey
Chapter 57: Management of Patients With Neurologic Dysfunction

Nancy A. Morrissey, RN,C, PhD
Patient Care Director
Inova Alexandria Hospital
Alexandria, Virginia
Chapter 33: Gastrointestinal Intubation and Special Nutritional Modalities

Martha A. Mulvey, RN, MS, CNS
Nurse Clinician, Epilepsy Program
University of Medicine and Dentistry of New Jersey
Newark, New Jersey
Chapter 13: Fluid and Electrolytes: Balance and Disturbances

Victoria B. Navarro, RN, MAS, MSN
Director of Clinical Services
Wilmer Eye Institute
The Johns Hopkins Medical Institutions
Baltimore, Maryland
Chapter 54: Assessment and Management of Patients With Eye and Vision Disorders

Donna Nayduch, RN, MSN, CCRN
Trauma Network Director
Western Plains Health Network
Greeley, Colorado
Chapter 65: Emergency Nursing

Lily P. Oriticio, RN, MSN, MBA
Nurse Manager/Supervisor
Bascom Palmer Eye Institute
Anne Bates Leach Eye Hospital
University of Miami School of Medicine, Department of Ophthalmology
Miami, Florida
Chapter 54: Assessment and Management of Patients With Eye and Vision Disorders

Janet A. Parkosewich, RN, MSN, CCRN
Cardiac Clinic Nurse Specialist
Yale-New Haven Hospital
New Haven, Connecticut
Chapter 23: Assessment of Cardiovascular Function

Ann Gallagher Peach, RN, MSN
Executive Director
Orlando Regional Sand Lake Hospital
Orlando, Florida
Chapter 20: Management of Patients With Upper Respiratory Tract Disorders

Janice Smith Pigg, RN, BSN, MS
Nurse Consultant, Rheumatology
Smith-Pigg Consultants
Cedarburg, Wisconsin
Chapter 50: Management of Patients With Rheumatic Disorders

Karen M. Reining, RN, MSN, CCRN, CPAN
Nurse Manager, PACU and SPU
Presbyterian Medical Center
University of Pennsylvania Health System
Philadelphia, Pennsylvania
Chapter 16: Preoperative Nursing Management
Chapter 17: Intraoperative Nursing Management
Chapter 18: Postoperative Nursing Management

Susan A. Rokita, RN, MS
Oncology Clinical Nurse Specialist
Nurse Coordinator, Cancer Center
M.S. Hershey Medical Center
Hershey, Pennsylvania
Chapter 15: Oncology: Nursing Management in Cancer Care

Catherine S. Sackett, RN, BS, CANP
Ophthalmic Research Nurse Practitioner
Wilmer Eye Institute
Retinal Vascular Center
The Johns Hopkins Medical Institutions
Baltimore, Maryland
Chapter 54: Assessment and Management of Patients With Eye and Vision Disorders

Linda H. Schakenbach, RN, MSN, CNS, CCRN, CETN, CS
Clinical Nurse Specialist, Critical Care
Inova Mount Vernon Hospital
Alexandria, Virginia
Chapter 25: Management of Patients With Coronary Vascular Disorders
Chapter 26: Management of Patients With Structural, Infectious, or Inflammatory Cardiac Disorders
Chapter 27: Management of Patients With Complications From Heart Disease

Linda Traxler Schuring, RN, MSN
Clinical Nurse Specialist
Director of Balance Clinics
Warren Otologic Group
Warren, Ohio
Mt. Sinai Hearing and Balance Center
Cleveland, Ohio
Chapter 55: Assessment and Management of Patients With Hearing and Balance Disorders

Daun A. Smith, RN, MS
Staff Nurse
Emergency Department
Dartmouth Hitchcock Medical Center
Lebanon, New Hampshire
Adjunct Professor
Colby-Sawyer College and New Hampshire Community Technical College
Lebanon, New Hampshire
Chapter 12: Pain Management

Cindy Stern, RN, MSN
Cancer Network Coordinator
University of Pennsylvania Cancer Center
University of Pennsylvania Health System
Philadelphia, Pennsylvania
Chapter 15: Oncology: Nursing Management in Cancer Care

Mary Laudon Thomas, RN, MS, AOCN
Hematology Clinical Nurse Specialist
Veterans' Administration Palo Alto Health Care System
Palo Alto, California
Chapter 30: Assessment and Management of Patients With Hematologic Disorders

Iris Woodard, BSN, RN-CS, ANP
Nurse Practitioner
Department of Dermatology
Kaiser Permanente
Springfield, Virginia
Chapter 51: Assessment of Integumentary Function
Chapter 52: Management of Patients with Dermatologic Problems

Linda B. Wilson, RN, MSN, CPAN, CAPA, C
Education Specialist
Nursing Continuing Education and Perianesthesia
Thomas Jefferson University Hospital
Philadelphia, Pennsylvania
Chapter 16: Preoperative Nursing Management
Chapter 17: Intraoperative Nursing Management
Chapter 18: Postoperative Nursing Management

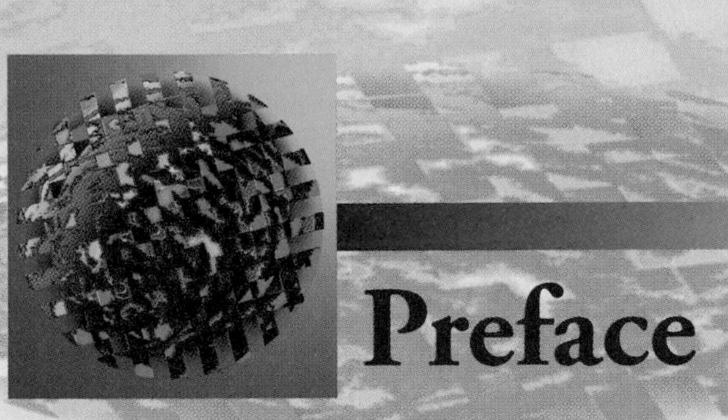

Preface

The past century was shaped by a multitude of changes resulting from economic, demographic, sociological, and technological forces that were greater and more influential than in any previous era. The century was characterized by wars, epidemics, social and civil upheaval, space travel, human rights victories, and a host of technological and scientific advances. Additional changes included migration of groups and individuals far from their families of origin, often resulting in less availability of family resources. This also resulted in greater ethnic and cultural diversity of patients and clients as well as in the health care professions. These and other forces and factors had a profound effect on health care and the profession of nursing.

Health care was also affected by changes in the nature of major diseases. Early in the century, the primary concern was infectious disease. Soon, however, scientists and health care professionals gained control of many infectious diseases through immunization, improved sanitation, and advances in treatments. Later, diseases of lifestyle became the major cause of morbidity and mortality. Of critical concern at the close of the twentieth century was the phenomenon of increasing bacterial resistance to antibiotics ("drug resistance") and growing worldwide concern about new and emerging infections, particularly those related to lifestyles and risky behaviors.

Advances in genetics knowledge have enabled individuals to learn about their likelihood of developing certain diseases and to make decisions based on information that was unavailable or unimaginable a few years ago. Advances in pharmacology have turned diseases that were considered inevitably fatal within a few years of diagnosis into chronic illnesses.

Worldwide, changes in modes of communication have given people almost instantaneous and unlimited access to information related to health as well as to other issues. At the same time, expectations about health have increased—with an emphasis on quality health care at a reasonable cost.

Health care in the twenty-first century is propelled by the health care legacy of the twentieth century, evolving from hospital-based treatment to care provided in a wide variety of settings such as acute care, the community, or the home. Attempts to reduce the cost of health care focus on providing care outside the hospital setting whenever and for as long as possible. As a result, patients admitted to hospitals are significantly sicker than they were in the past. Likewise, patients are discharged as early as possible. Many return to a home or community setting with complex health care needs.

Because of these changes, nurses and the profession of nursing are faced with the need to respond to an array of demands and challenges to ensure a seamless continuum of care. Education and specialization can enable nurses to meet these demands and challenges. Today, nurses are providing care in an environment that focuses on evidence-based practice and that encourages collaborative, interdisciplinary health care with patients taking an increasingly active role in decisions related to their own health care.

Past and future changes and challenges make it essential for today's nurses to be knowledgeable about the problems faced by patients and their families. It is essential for nurses in the twenty-first century to have well-developed critical thinking skills that allow examination of the issues encountered in the course of providing care. An understanding of all of the influences that affect the patient—cultural, ethnic, socioeconomic, and ethical—is crucial if the nurse is to provide the high-quality care that is expected by the public.

ABOUT THE NINTH EDITION

This edition of *Brunner and Suddarth's Textbook of Medical-Surgical Nursing* was written with today's health care challenges as a key focus on a background of a traditionally comprehensive and solid facts on which to build a skillful, up-to-date, culturally sensitive "med-surg" nursing practice.

QUALITY CONTENT—BASIC TO COMPLEX

The ninth edition of *Brunner and Suddarth's Textbook of Medical-Surgical Nursing* is an encyclopedic textbook–reference resource arranged in 16 units. Units 1 through 4 present the core concepts to be mastered by nurses entering practice. Units 5 through 16 focus on the assessment and management concepts and skills needed to provide care for patients with specific diseases and disorders of the various body systems. The entire text is presented in full color for emphasis and reader stimulation.

UNIT 1

The five chapters in this unit focus on Basic Concepts in Nursing Practice as they apply to current Health Care Delivery and Nursing Practice; Community-Based Nursing Practice; Critical Thinking, Ethical Decision Making and the Nursing Process; Health Education and Promotion (along with illness prevention); and Health Assessment.

UNIT 2

The six chapters in Unit 2 highlight Biophysical and Psychosocial Concepts in Nursing Practice. Complete coverage starts with Homeostasis, Stress, and Adaptation and Individual and

Family Considerations Related to Illness. Then coverage continues with Perspectives in Transcultural Nursing and concludes with Chronic Illness, Principles and Practices of Rehabilitation, and Health Care of the Older Adult.

UNIT 3

The four chapters in this unit present complex Concepts and Challenges in Patient Management, including Pain Management, Fluid and Electrolytes: Balance and Disturbances, Shock and Multisystem Failure, and Oncology: Nursing Management in Cancer Care.

UNIT 4

The student learns about Preoperative, Intraoperative, and Postoperative Nursing Management from beginning to end in the three well-rounded chapters of this unit.

UNITS 5–16

Key nursing concepts, responsibilities, activities, and rationales are advanced throughout the heart of the text from the extensive chapters dealing with Gas Exchange and Respiratory Function in Unit 5 to the inclusive information on Musculoskeletal Function in Unit 15. Each chapter is formatted to accent normal and abnormal physiology, treatment modalities, and nursing process in acute and community health care settings.

NEW EMPHASES, UPBEAT DESIGN

To help students learn, the text features full color and all-new or significantly updated features. For example, the presentation and discussion of clinical pathways in *Chapter 1* is supplemented in *Appendix A,* with examples of actual clinical pathways currently used in various health care settings.

The focus on critical thinking in *Chapter 3* includes an introduction to nursing outcome and nursing intervention classifications (NOC and NIC), which are further identified in *Appendix B.*

To illustrate the new full-text focus on preventive health care, health promotion, home and community-based nursing, content has been revised and expanded throughout including those chapters that present Health Education and Promotion (4); Individual and Family Considerations Related to Illness (7); and Principles and Practices of Rehabilitation (10). The importance of nursing care for patients recently discharged from acute care has been highlighted in all clinical chapters.

The text is composed of new chapters and newly organized chapters, and up-to-date, research-based information to address health care changes that affect nursing care in the twenty-first century.

NEW TEACHING–LEARNING DEVICES

Reliable Formats

To speed the reader's journey, the text consistently highlights specific concepts. Selected topics include

- Physiology and pathophysiology
- Clinical manifestations
- Assessment and diagnostic findings
- Gerontologic considerations
- Medical management (surgical, pharmacologic, nutritional)
- Nursing management (process, interventions, and rationale)
- Home and community-based care with emphasis on patient teaching and continuing care

Information about major and often-encountered disorders appears in Nursing Process sections that detail strategies and rationale for acute and continuing care—from assessment to planning and outcomes to collaborative problems, to interventions, evaluations, and the continuum of health care and teaching in the home and community.

CONSISTENT AND LIVELY TEACHING TOOLS

Every chapter begins with a set of learning objectives that highlight important concepts and guide the reader through the text. Every clinically focused chapter begins with a glossary of special terms the reader will encounter when studying. Every chapter ends with pertinent and provocative critical thinking exercises followed by an extensive updated list of references, and additional resources, such as support groups, national and community agencies, and pertinent web sites.

Interspersed throughout each chapter are well-marked discussions about

- Gerontologic considerations
- Nursing alerts
- Home and community-based care.

WEALTH OF FULL-COLOR TEACHING AND LEARNING TOOLS

Colorful figures, tables, and charts are positioned in the text to enhance the reader's understanding. Readily recognized by individual icons, or symbols, special learning tables and charts include the following titles:

- **Risk Factors**—spotlights factors or behaviors that jeopardize health
- **Physiology/Pathophysiology**—explains normal or abnormal physiologic processes or both in regard to health and illness
- **Assessment**—describes activities, circumstances, signs and other features of nursing assessment related to patients' conditions
- **Health Promotion and Illness Prevention**—presents strategies for health promotion and illness prevention
- **Gerontologic Considerations**—introduces need-to-know data about age-related variations in physical and mental processes and their implications for nursing care both in acute and long-term health care settings as well as in the community or home.
- **Pharmacology**—identifies important points about medications and their administration from dosages and delivery modes to side effects and safety concerns
- **Nutrition**—provides information on diet and related strategies for use in patient education
- **Plan of Nursing Care**—illustrates application of the nursing process to a particularly complex or common disease or disorder

- **Guidelines**—offer step-by-step instructions and rationale for nursing interventions and collaborative procedures
- **Nursing Research**—summarizes current nursing research findings and interprets their implications
- **Ethics and Related Issues**—presents ethical dilemmas and poses questions, and offers thought-provoking discussions
- **Patient Education and Home Care**—speaks directly to patients from a nursing perspective, teaching patients how to perform self-care and explaining the rationale
- **Home Care Teaching Checklist**—lists key topics and skills for nurses to teach patients and their caregivers for home care

ANCILLARY TEACHING–LEARNING PACKAGE

Supplemental teaching/learning products available with *Brunner and Suddarth's Textbook of Medical-Surgical Nursing, Ninth Edition,* consist of materials for students and instructors alike. A printed study guide, a student self-study disk, and a clinical handbook offer effective help to students while the combined instructor's manual and printed testbank, images on disk, overhead transparencies, and a computerized testing program offer state-of-the-art assistance to busy instructors.

ESPECIALLY FOR STUDENTS

- The **Student Study Guide** contains questions and exercises designed to help the student correlate and apply the content covered in the textbook. Knowledge-based and critical analysis questions enrich the student's ability to interpret information as well as to develop problem-solving skills. Labeling exercises are also included.
- A **Self-Study Disk** located inside the text offers further practice in evaluating knowledge and thinking skills. The disk presents several different ways to enhance self-evaluation and provides rationale for use in assessing the appropriateness of the student's responses.
- A **Clinical Handbook** accompanies this edition and covers the most frequent disorders encountered in medical-surgical nursing. The content is organized alphabetically in outline form making this an easy-to-use reference for clinical settings.

ESPECIALLY FOR INSTRUCTORS

- For this edition of *Brunner and Suddarth's Textbook of Medical-Surgical Nursing* the **Instructor's Manual and Printed Testbank** were combined into a convenient and comprehensive package. Additional learning exercises, key terms, and collaborative learning and critical thinking activities are included for use in classroom and clinical settings. The manual–testbank also suggests take-home assignments and offers instructional improvement tools that give students the opportunity to evaluate classroom presentations.
- **Images on Disk** allow instructors to manipulate and customize textbook figures in accord with individual specifications. Files are in a generic format that can be downloaded into Power Point, Excel, or any other art-file programs in use.
- A set of about 60 selected **Overhead Transparencies** are prepared for instructors who may not have access to computers or who may not wish to use the images on disk to alter figures used in the text.
- A **Computerized Testing Program** includes approximately 1500 NCLEX-style, multiple-choice test questions in an automatic test-generating program. The program enables the instructor to sort and select questions by computer and then generate a test complete with instructions and an answer key.

GOING FORWARD

Brunner and Suddarth's Textbook of Medical-Surgical Nursing, Ninth Edition, continues the tradition of addressing current issues and promoting the skills necessary to provide effective, safe, and professional care in an evolving workplace. Preventive health care, chronic illness, gerontologic concerns, patient education, and home and community care receive special emphasis because of their increasing prominence in today's health care environment.

We feel confident that this textbook retains the focus on patients' needs and the caring values that characterized previous editions. We also feel confident that this textbook prepares the nursing student to adapt to changes in the provision of health care in the new millennium.

Suzanne C. O'Connell Smeltzer
Brenda G. Bare

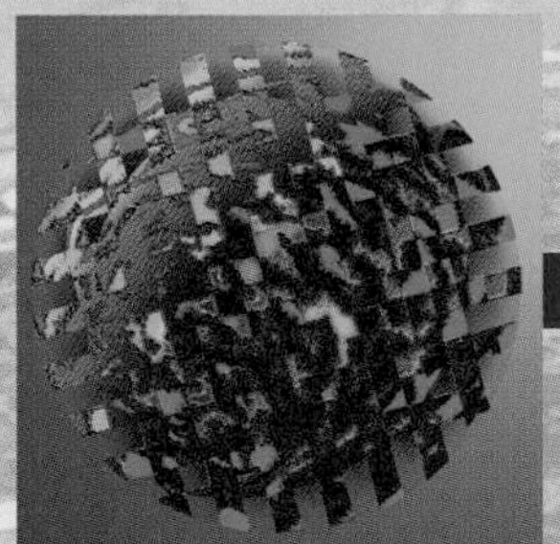

Acknowledgments

The authors and publisher wish to thank the following people for their hard work and dedication to this project.

Linda Ardini
Monitor Technician
Inova Fairfax Hospital
Falls Church, Virginia

Catherine Berkmeyer
Monitor Technician
Inova Fairfax Hospital
Falls Church, Virginia

Kathleen M. Bury, RN
Coordinator IV Services, Infection Control
Inova Alexandria Hospital
Alexandria, Virginia

Nicole Celona-Jacobs, MS, RD, CDE
Clinical Dietitian
Children's Hospital of Pennsylvania
Philadelphia, Pennsylvania

Sue Erickson
Assistant Hospital Director
Vanderbilt University Medical Center
Nashville, Tennessee

Debra Gordon, RN, MS
Senior Clinical Nurse Specialist, Pain Management
University of Wisconsin Hospital and Clinics
Madison, Wisconsin

Tracey Hopkins, BSN, RN,C
Consultant
Ardmore, Pennsylvania

Sande Gracia Jones, ARNP, ACRN, CS, C, MSN, MEd
Mount Sinai Medical Center
Miami Beach, Florida

Nina S. McClesky, MLS
Director, Medical Library
Inova Alexandria Hospital
Alexandria, Virginia

Lisa Mandeville
Assistant Hospital Director
Vanderbilt University Medical Center
Nashville, Tennessee

Kathy Sengner
Supervisor, Laboratory Services
Washington Adventist Hospital
Takoma Park, Maryland

Ronald K. Smeltzer, PhD

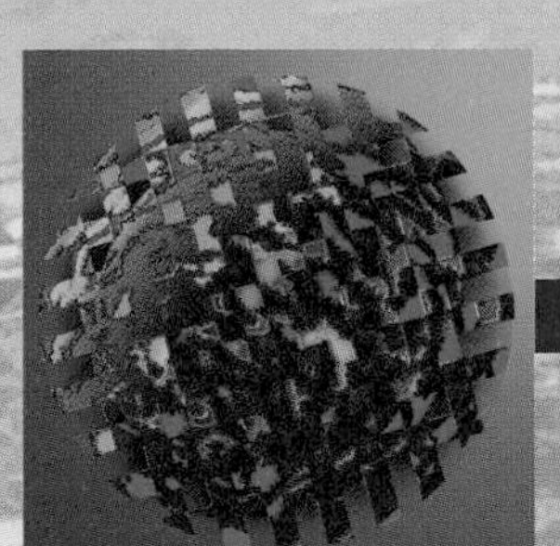

Contents

UNIT 1

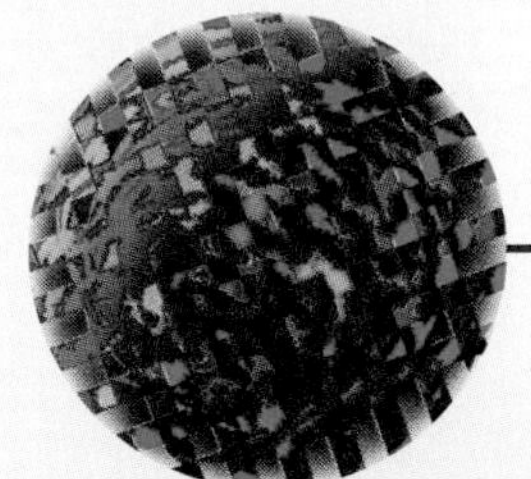

Basic Concepts in Nursing Practice

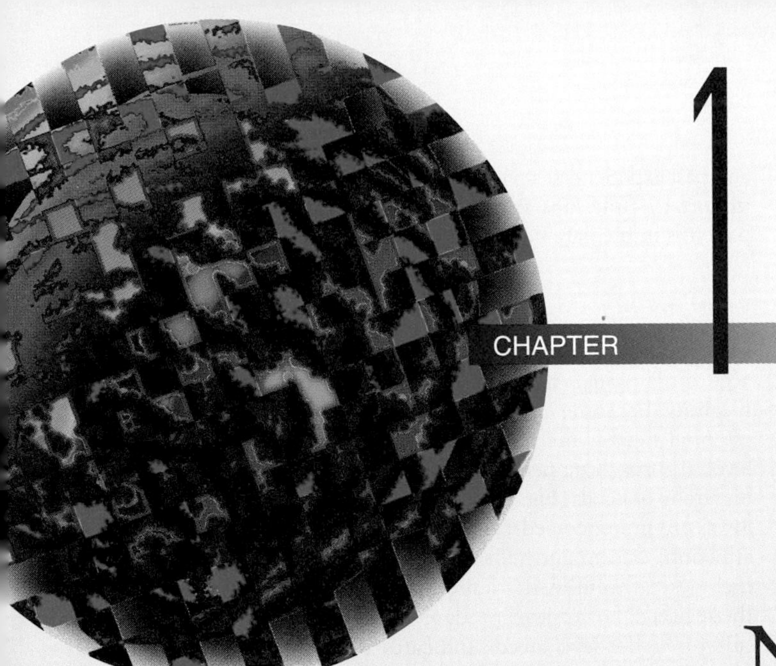

Health Care Delivery and Nursing Practice

Learning Objectives

On completion of the chapter, the learner will be able to:

1. Define health and wellness.
2. Describe factors causing significant changes in the health care delivery system.
3. Discuss the impact of changes in the health care field on the profession of nursing.
4. Describe the practitioner, leadership, and research roles of the nurse.
5. Describe primary nursing, case management, and collaborative practice.
6. Specify the expanded roles of the nurse.

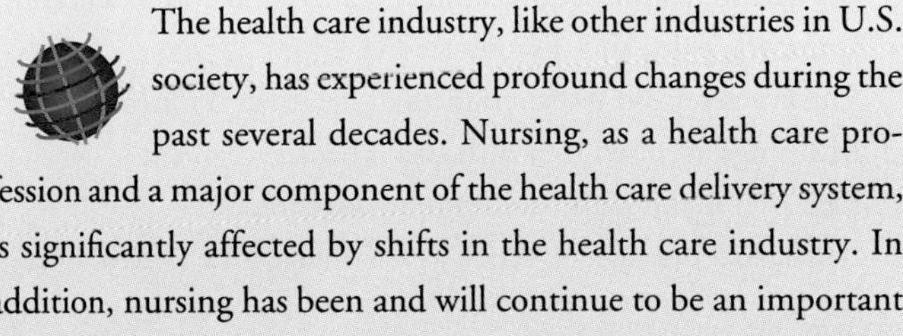

The health care industry, like other industries in U.S. society, has experienced profound changes during the past several decades. Nursing, as a health care profession and a major component of the health care delivery system, is significantly affected by shifts in the health care industry. In addition, nursing has been and will continue to be an important force in shaping the future of the health care system.

THE HEALTH CARE INDUSTRY AND THE NURSING PROFESSION

While the delivery of nursing care has obviously been affected by the changes occurring in the health care system, the purpose of nursing care has continued to be directed toward achieving the goals inherent in the definition of nursing.

Nursing Defined

Since the time of Florence Nightingale, who wrote in 1858 that the goal of nursing was "to put the patient in the best condition for nature to act upon him," nursing leaders have described nursing as both an art and a science. However, the definition of nursing has evolved over time. The American Nurses Association (ANA), in its *Social Policy Statement* (ANA, 1995), defines nursing as "the diagnosis and treatment of human responses to health and illness" and provides the following illustrative list of phenomena that are the focus for nursing care and research:

- Self-care processes
- Physiologic and pathophysiologic processes in areas such as rest, sleep, respiration, circulation, reproduction, activity, nutrition, elimination, skin, sexuality, and communication
- Comfort, pain, and discomfort
- Emotions related to experiences of health and illness
- Meanings ascribed to health and illnesses
- Decision making and ability to make choices
- Perceptual orientations such as self-image and control over one's body and environments
- Transitions across the life span, such as birth, growth, development, and death
- Affiliative relationships, including freedom from oppression and abuse
- Environmental systems

Nurses have a responsibility to carry out their role, as defined in the *Social Policy Statement*, to comply with the nurse practice act of the state where they practice and to comply with the code for nurses as spelled out by the International Council of Nurses and the ANA. Understanding the needs of health care consumers *and* the health care delivery system, including understanding forces affecting *both* this system and nursing, will provide a foundation for examining the delivery of nursing care.

The Patient/Client: Consumer of Nursing and Health Care

The central figure in health care services is, of course, the patient. The term *patient*, which is derived from the Latin verb meaning "to suffer," has traditionally been used to describe those who are recipients of care. The connotation commonly attached to the word is one of dependence. For this reason, many nurses prefer to use the term *client*, which is derived from the Latin verb meaning "to lean" and which connotes alliance and interdependence. For the purposes of this book, the term *patient* will be used throughout, but with the understanding that either term is acceptable.

The patient who seeks care for a health problem or problems (increasing numbers of people have multiple health problems) is also an individual, a member of a family, and a citizen of the community. Depending on the problem, associated circumstances, and past experiences, a patient's needs will vary. One of the nurse's important functions in health care delivery is to identify the patient's immediate needs and take measures to alleviate them.

The Patient's Basic Needs

Certain needs are basic to all people and require satisfaction accordingly. Such needs are addressed on the basis of priority, meaning that some needs are more pressing than others. Once an essential need is met, a person experiences a need on a higher level. Approaching needs according to priority reflects Maslow's hierarchy of needs (Fig. 1-1). Maslow ranked human needs as follows: physiologic needs; safety and security; belongingness and affection; esteem and self-respect; and self-actualization, which includes self-fulfillment, desire to know and understand, and aesthetic needs. Lower-level needs always remain, but a person's pursuit of higher-level needs indicates that he or she is moving toward psychological health and well-being. Such a hierarchy of needs is a useful organizational framework that can be applied to the various nursing models for assessment of a patient's strengths, limitations, and need for nursing interventions.

Health Care in Transition

Changes occurring in health care delivery and nursing are a result of societal, economic, technological, scientific, and political forces that have evolved throughout the 20th century. Among the most significant changes are shifts in population demographics, particularly the increase in the aging population and the cultural diversity of the population; changing patterns of diseases; increased technology; increased consumer expectations; the high costs of health care and changes in health care financing; and other health care reform efforts. These changes have led to institutional restructur-

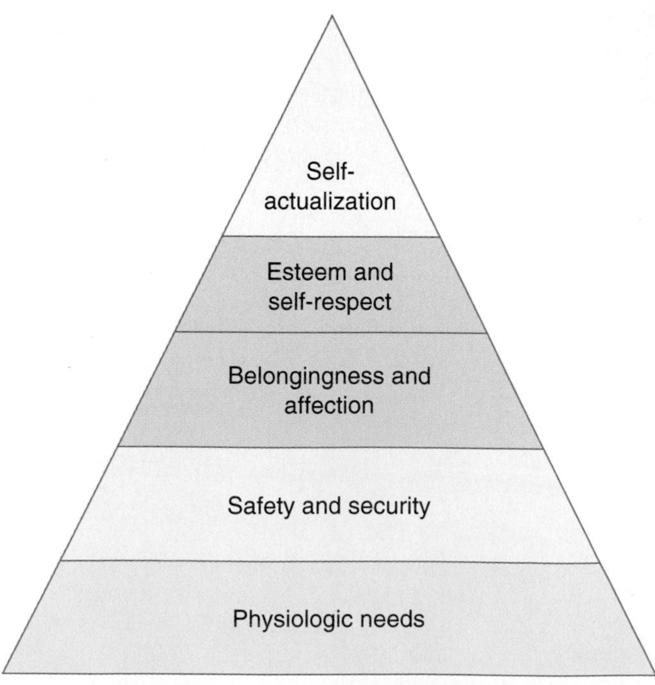

FIGURE 1•1 This scheme of Maslow's hierarchy of human needs shows how a person moves from fulfillment of basic needs to higher levels of needs, with the ultimate goal being integrated human functioning and health.

ing, staff downsizing, increased outpatient care services, decreased length of hospital stays, and more care being provided in the community and in the home. Such changes are having a dramatic influence on where nurses practice, with an increasing trend for nurses to provide health care in community and home settings. Indeed, these changes have a dynamic influence on our view of health and illness and, thus, affect the focus of nursing and health care.

As an increasing proportion of the population reaches age 65 and older, and as disease patterns shift from acute illnesses to chronic illnesses, the traditional disease management and care focus of the health care professions has expanded to include a greater focus on prevention, health promotion, and management of chronic conditions. This shift in focus coincides with a nationwide emphasis on cost control and resource management directed toward providing cost-efficient and cost-effective health care services to the population as a whole.

Health and Health Promotion

The health care system of the United States, which traditionally has been disease-oriented, is currently placing greater emphasis on health and its promotion. Similarly, a significant portion of nursing's workforce formerly was focused on the care of patients with acute conditions. Now much of nursing's workforce is directing its efforts toward health promotion and disease prevention.

Health

How health is perceived depends on how health is defined. In the preamble to its constitution, the World Health Organization (WHO) defines health as a "state of complete physical, mental, and social well being and not merely the absence of disease and infirmity." Such a definition of health does not allow for any variation in the degrees of wellness or illness. On the other hand, the concept of a health–illness continuum allows for a greater range in describing a person's health status. By viewing health and illness on a continuum, it is possible to consider a person as having neither complete health nor complete illness. Instead, a person's state of health is ever-changing and has the potential to range from high-level wellness to extremely poor health and imminent death. The model of the health–illness continuum makes it possible to view a person as simultaneously possessing degrees of both health and illness.

The limitations of the WHO definition of health are clear in relation to chronic illness. A chronically ill person cannot meet the standards of health as established by the WHO definition. However, when viewed from the perspective of the health–illness continuum, people with chronic illness can be understood as having the potential to attain a high level of wellness, if they are successful in meeting their health potential within the limits of their chronic illness.

Wellness

Wellness has been defined as being equivalent to health. Cookfair (1996) indicates that wellness "includes a conscious and deliberate approach to an advanced state of physical, psychological, and spiritual health and is a dynamic, fluctuating state of being" (p. 149). Leddy and Pepper (1998) contend that wellness is indicated by (1) the capacity of the person to perform to the best of his ability, (2) the ability to adjust and adapt to varying situations, (3) a reported feeling of well-being, and (4) a feeling that 'everything is together' and 'harmonious.' With this in mind, it becomes evident that the goal of health care providers is to promote positive changes that are directed toward health and well-being. The fact that the sense of wellness has a subjective aspect emphasizes the importance of recognizing and responding to patient individuality and diversity in health care and nursing.

Health Promotion

Today, increasing emphasis is placed on health, health promotion, wellness, and self-care. Health is seen as resulting from a lifestyle that is oriented toward wellness. The result has been the evolution of a wide range of health promotion strategies, including multiphasic screening, genetic testing, lifetime health monitoring programs, environmental and mental health programs, risk reduction, and nutrition and health education. A growing interest in self-care skills is evidenced by the large number of health-related publications, conferences, and workshops designed for the lay public.

Individuals are increasingly knowledgeable about their health and are encouraged to take more interest in and responsibility for their health and well-being. Organized self-care education programs emphasize health promotion, disease prevention, management of illness, self-medication, and judicious use of the professional health care system. In addition, well over 500,000 self-help groups exist for the purpose of sharing experiences and information about self-care with others who have similar chronic diseases or disabilities.

Special efforts are being made by health care professionals to reach and motivate members of various cultural and socioeconomic groups concerning lifestyle and health practices. Stress, improper diet, lack of exercise, smoking, drugs, high-risk behaviors, including sexual practices, and poor hygiene are all lifestyle behaviors known to have a negative effect on health. Health care professionals are concerned with encouraging behavior that promotes health. The goal is to motivate people to make improvements in the way they live, to modify risky behaviors, and to adopt healthy behaviors.

FORCES INFLUENCING HEALTH CARE

The health care delivery system is rapidly changing as the population and its health care needs and expectations change. The shifting demographics of the population, the increase in chronic illnesses, the greater emphasis on economics, and technological advances have resulted in changing emphases in health care delivery and in nursing.

Population Demographics

Changes in the population in general are affecting the need for and the delivery of health care. It is estimated that by the year 2000, there will be close to 300 million people in the United States (U.S. Department of Commerce, Economics, and Statistics Administration, 1997). This population expansion has been attributed in part to improved public health services and improved nutrition.

Not only is the population increasing, but the composition of the population is also changing. The decline in birth rate and the increase in life span attributed to improved health care have resulted in fewer school-age children and more senior citizens, the majority of whom are women. Much of the population resides in highly congested urban areas, with a steady migration of minority groups to the inner cities and a migration of middle-class people to suburban areas. The number of homeless people, including entire families, has increased significantly. The population has become more culturally diverse as increasing numbers of people from different national backgrounds enter the country. Because of such population changes, the need for health care for specific age groups, for women, and for people within specific geographic locations is altering the effectiveness of traditional means of providing health care and is necessitating far-reaching changes in the overall health care delivery system.

Aging Population

The elderly population in the United States has increased significantly and will continue to grow in future years. In 1995, the nation's 34 million older adults constituted 13% of the population. The number of people in the United States over the age of 65 is expected to reach 20% of the population by the year 2050. Those 85 and older constitute one of the fastest-growing segments of the population. According to the U.S. Department of Commerce, Economics, and Statistics Administration (1997), by the year 2050 the population of people age 85 and older is expected to triple to 4.6% of the population, from the 1.4% noted in 1995.

Many elderly people suffer from multiple chronic conditions that are exacerbated by acute episodes. Elderly women, whose conditions are frequently underdiagnosed and undertreated, are of particular concern. There are three women for every two men in the older population, and elderly women are expected to continue to outnumber elderly men. The health care needs of older adults are complex and demand significant investments, both professional and financial, by the health care industry.

Cultural Diversity

An appreciation for the diverse characteristics and needs of individuals from varied ethnic and cultural backgrounds is important in health care and nursing. Some demographers predict that in the twenty-first century, up to half of the population of the United States will be other than Euro-Caucasian (Ketefian & Redman, 1997). As the cultural composition of the population changes, it becomes increasingly important to address cultural considerations in the delivery of health care. Patients from diverse sociocultural groups bring to the health care setting different health care beliefs, values, and practices. These factors significantly affect the way an individual responds to health care problems or illness, to those who provide the care, and to the care itself. Unless these factors are understood and respected by health care providers, the care delivered may be ineffective and health care outcomes may be negatively affected.

Culture is defined as learned patterns of behavior, beliefs, and values that can be attributed to a particular group of people. Included among the many characteristics that distinguish cultural groups are the manner of dress, language spoken, values, rules or norms of behavior, economics, politics, law and social control, artifacts, technology, dietary practices, and health beliefs and practices.

Health promotion, illness prevention, causes of sickness, treatment, coping, caring, dying, and death are part of the health component of every culture. Every person has a unique belief and value system that has been shaped at least in part by his or her cultural environment. This belief and value system is very important and guides the individual's thinking, decisions, and actions. It provides direction for interpreting and responding to illness and to health care.

To promote an effective nurse–patient relationship and positive outcomes of care, nursing care must be culturally competent—appropriate and sensitive to cultural differences. All attempts should be made to help the individual retain his or her unique cultural characteristics. Providing special foods that have significance and arranging for special religious observances may enable the patient to maintain a feeling of wholeness at a time when he or she may feel isolated from family and community.

It is important to know the cultural and social significance that particular situations have for each patient and to avoid imposing one's own value system when the patient has a different point of view. In most cases, cooperation with the plan of care is greatest when communication among the nurse, the patient, and the patient's family is directed toward understanding the situation or the problem and respecting each other's goals.

Changing Patterns of Disease

During the past 50 years, the health problems of the American people have changed significantly. Many infectious diseases have been controlled or eradicated; others (eg, tuberculosis, AIDS, sexually transmitted diseases) are on the rise. An increasing number of infectious agents are becoming resistant to antibiotic therapy as a result of widespread inappropriate use of antibiotics. Thus, conditions that were once easily treated have become complex and more life-threatening than ever before.

The chronicity of illnesses is increasing because of the lengthening life span of Americans and the expansion of successful treatment options for conditions such as cancer and HIV infection; many people with these diseases live decades longer than in prior years. Since the majority of health problems seen today are chronic in nature, many people are learning to protect and maximize their health within the constraints of chronic illness. Almost 50% of the U.S. population has one or more chronic conditions (National Center for Health Statistics, 1996).

As chronic conditions increase, health care broadens from a focus on cure and eradication of disease to include the prevention or rapid treatment of exacerbations of chronic conditions. Nursing, which has always encouraged patients to take control of their conditions, plays a prominent role in the current focus on management of chronic illness.

Technology

Technological advances have occurred with greater frequency during the past several decades than in all other periods of civilization. Sophisticated techniques and devices have revolutionized surgery and diagnostic testing making it possible to perform many procedures and tests on an outpatient basis. This is also an era of sophisticated communication systems that connect most parts of the world, rapidly storing, retrieving, and disseminating information. Such scientific and technological advances are themselves stimulating brisk change as well as swift obsolescence in health care delivery strategies.

Economic Changes

The philosophy that comprehensive, quality health care should be provided for all citizens has prompted governmental concern about spiraling health care costs and wide variations in charges among providers. These concerns led to the Medicare prospective payment system and the use of diagnosis-related groups.

In 1983, the U.S. Congress enacted the most significant health legislation since the Medicare program in 1965. The government was no longer able to afford to reimburse hospitals for patient care that was delivered without any defined limits or costs. Therefore, it approved a prospective payment system for hospital inpatient services. This system of reimbursement, referred to as diagnosis-related groups (DRGs), set the rates for Medicare payments for hospital services. Hospitals receive payment at a fixed rate for patients with diagnoses that fall into specific DRGs. A fixed payment has been predetermined for over 470 possible diagnostic categories, covering the majority of medical diagnoses of all patients admitted to the hospital. Hospitals receive the same payment for every patient with a given diagnosis or DRG. If the cost of the patient's care is lower than the payment, the hospital gains a profit; if the cost is higher, the hospital incurs a loss. As a result, hospitals now place greater emphasis on reducing costs, utilization of services, and lengths of patient stay.

To qualify for Medicare reimbursement, hospitals must contract with peer review organizations (PROs) to perform quality and utilization review. The PROs monitor admission patterns, lengths of stay, transfers, and the quality of services and validate DRG coding.

The DRG system has provided hospitals with an incentive to cut costs and discharge patients as quickly as possible. Consequently, nurses in hospitals are caring for patients who are older and sicker and require more nursing services; nurses in the community are caring for patients who have been discharged earlier and need acute care services with high-technology and long-term care. The importance of an effective discharge planning program, along with utilization review and a quality improvement program, is unquestionable. Nurses must assume responsibility with other health care team members for maintaining quality care while facing pressures to discharge patients and decrease staffing costs.

Demand for Quality Care

The general public has become increasingly interested in and knowledgeable about health care and health promotion. This awareness has been stimulated by television, newspapers, magazines, and other communications media and by political debate. The public has become more health-conscious and has in general begun to subscribe strongly to the belief that health and quality health care constitute a basic right, rather than a privilege for a chosen few.

Patients' Rights to Quality Care

Health care providers have become increasingly aware of the public's beliefs about health and health care. One indication of such awareness is the time-honored Patient's Bill of Rights (Chart 1-1). Prepared by the American Hospital Association, the Patient's Bill of Rights is directed toward the promotion of more effective patient care and patient satisfaction.

In 1977, the National League for Nursing (NLN) issued a statement on nurses' responsibility to uphold patients' rights. The statement addressed patients' rights to privacy, confidentiality, informed participation, self-determination, and access to health records. This statement also indicated ways in which respect for patients' rights and a commitment to safeguarding them could be incorporated into nursing education programs and upheld and reinforced by those in nursing service. Nurses can directly involve themselves in ensuring specific rights or can make their influence felt indirectly (NLN, 1977).

The ANA has worked diligently to promote the delivery of quality health and nursing care. Efforts by the ANA range from assessing the quality of health care provided to the public in these changing times to lobbying legislators to pass bills related to issues such as health insurance or length of hospital stay for new mothers.

Legislative changes have promoted both delivery of quality health care and increased access by the public to this care. The National Health Planning and Resources Act of 1974 emphasized the need for planning and providing quality health care for all Americans through coordinated health services, staffing, and facilities at the national, state, and local levels. Medically underserved populations were the target for the primary care services provided for by this act. Passage of bills supporting health insurance reform, barring discrimination against individuals with preexisting conditions, and expanding portability of health care coverage acknowledges the needs of consumers for adequate health insurance in this time of longer life spans and chronic illnesses. Efforts in some states to provide full health care coverage for citizens represent measures by state governments to promote access to health care. In addition, passage of legislative bills supporting funding of nursing education shows recognition of the contribution of nursing to the health of consumers (Gonzalez & Reed, 1997).

Quality Improvement Programs

In the 1980s, hospitals and other health care agencies implemented ongoing quality assurance (QA) programs. These programs were required for reimbursement for services and for accreditation by the Joint Commission on Accreditation of Healthcare Organizations (JCAHO). QA programs sought to establish accountability on the part of the health professions to society for the quality, appropriateness, and cost of health services provided.

The JCAHO developed a generic model that required monitoring and evaluating quality and appropriateness of care. The model was implemented in health care institutions and agencies through organization-wide QA programs and reporting systems. Many aspects of the programs were centralized in a QA department. In addition, each patient care and patient services department was responsible for developing its own plan for monitoring and evaluation. Objective and measurable indicators were used to monitor, evaluate, and communicate the quality and appropriateness of care delivered.

In the early 1990s, QA received intense scrutiny. It was recognized that quality of care as defined by regulatory agencies continued to be difficult to measure. QA criteria were identified as measures to ensure minimal expectations only; they did not provide mechanisms for identifying causes of problems or for determining systems or processes that need improvement. Continuous quality improvement (CQI) was identified as a more effective mechanism for improving the quality of health care. In 1992, the revised standards of the JCAHO mandated that health care organizations implement a CQI program.

Unlike QA, which focuses on individual incidents or errors and minimal expectations, CQI focuses on the processes used to provide care, with the aim of improving quality by assessing and improving those interrelated processes that most affect patient care outcomes and patient satisfaction. CQI involves analyzing, understanding, and improving clinical, financial, or operational processes. Problems identified as more than isolated events are analyzed, and all issues that may affect the outcome are studied. The main focus is on the processes that affect quality.

As health care agencies continue to implement CQI, nurses have many opportunities to be involved in quality improvement.

CHART 1•1 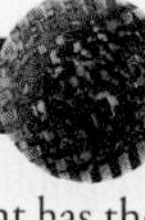 **AHA's Patient's Bill of Rights**

1. The patient has the right to considerate and respectful care.
2. The patient has the right to and is encouraged to obtain from physicians and other direct caregivers relevant, current, and understandable information concerning diagnosis, treatment, and prognosis.

   Except in emergencies when the patient lacks decision-making capacity and the need for treatment is urgent, the patient is entitled to the opportunity to discuss and request information related to the specific procedures and/or treatments, the risks involved, the possible length of recuperation, and the medically reasonable alternatives and their accompanying risks and benefits.

   Patients have the right to know the identity of physicians, nurses, and others involved in their care, as well as when those involved are students, residents, or other trainees. The patient also has the right to know the immediate and long-term financial implications of treatment choices, insofar as they are known.
3. The patient has the right to make decisions about the plan of care prior to and during the course of treatment and to refuse a recommended treatment or plan of care to the extent permitted by law and hospital policy and to be informed of the medical consequences of this action. In case of such refusal, the patient is entitled to other appropriate care and services that the hospital provides or transfer to another hospital. The hospital should notify patients of any policy that might affect patient choice within the institution.
4. The patient has the right to have an advance directive (such as a living will, health care proxy, or durable power of attorney for health care) concerning treatment or designating a surrogate decision maker with the expectation that the hospital will honor the intent of that directive to the extent permitted by law and hospital policy.

   Health care institutions must advise patients of their rights under state law and hospital policy to make informed medical choices, ask if the patient has an advance directive, and include that information in patient records. The patient has the right to timely information about hospital policy that may limit its ability to implement fully a legally valid advance directive.
5. The patient has the right to every consideration of his privacy. Case discussion, consultation, examination, and treatment should be conducted so as to protect each patient's privacy.
6. The patient has the right to expect that all communications and records pertaining to his care will be treated as confidential by the hospital, except in cases such as suspected abuse and public health hazards when reporting is permitted or required by law. The patient has the right to expect that the hospital will emphasize the confidentiality of this information when it releases it to any other parties entitled to review information in these records.
7. The patient has the right to review the records pertaining to his/her medical care and to have the information explained or interpreted as necessary, except when restricted by law.
8. The patient has the right to expect that, within its capacity and policies, a hospital will make reasonable response to the request of a patient for appropriate and medically indicated care and services. The hospital must provide evaluation, service, and/or referral as indicated by the urgency of the case. When medically appropriate and legally permissible, or when a patient has so requested, a patient may be transferred to another facility. The institution to which the patient is to be transferred must first have accepted the patient for transfer. The patient must also have the benefit of complete information and explanation concerning the need for, risks, benefits, and alternatives to such a transfer.
9. The patient has the right to ask and be informed of the existence of business relationships among the hospital, educational institutions, other health care providers, or payors that may influence the patient's treatment and care.
10. The patient has the right to consent to or decline to participate in proposed research studies or human experimentation affecting care and treatment or requiring direct patient involvement, and to have those studies fully explained prior to consent. A patient who declines to participate in research or experimentation is entitled to the most effective care that the hospital can otherwise provide.
11. The patient has the right to expect reasonable continuity of care when appropriate and to be informed by physicians and other caregivers of available and realistic patient care options when hospital care is no longer appropriate.
12. The patient has the right to be informed of hospital policies and practices that relate to patient care, treatment, and responsibilities. The patient has the right to be informed of available resources for resolving disputes, grievances, and conflicts, such as ethics committees, patient representatives, and other mechanisms available at the institution. The patient has the right to be informed of the hospital's charges for services and available payment methods.

These rights can be exercised on the patient's behalf by designated surrogate or proxy decision maker if the patient lacks decision-making capacity, is legally incompetent, or is a minor.

Note: The American Hospital Association encourages health care institutions to tailor this bill of rights to their patient community by translating and/or simplifying the language of this bill of rights as may be necessary to ensure that patients and their families understand their rights and responsibilities.

Reprinted with permission from the AHA, 840 North Lake Shore Drive, Chicago, IL, 1992.

Nurse managers as well as nurses directly involved in the delivery of care are engaged in analyzing the processes that are being evaluated. Their knowledge of the processes and conditions that affect patient care is critical in designing changes to improve the quality of the care provided.

Alternative Health Care Delivery Systems

The rising cost of health care over the last few decades has led to alternative health care delivery systems, including health maintenance organizations, preferred provider organizations, and managed health care.

Health Maintenance Organizations

Health maintenance organizations (HMOs) are prepaid, group health practice systems designed to deliver comprehensive health care services to a defined group of voluntarily enrolled individuals. Members pay premiums as well as designated copayments for services and medications. Individuals receive care from a preselected group of physicians, nurse practitioners, or other care provider members of the HMO, although some programs allow selection of outside providers for a higher fee. HMOs are based on the holistic concept of care—providing outpatient (ambulatory) and preventive teaching and health care, and inpatient care that meets the health care needs of the whole person. The goal of HMOs is to give comprehensive health care that is of the best quality and quantity for the money available, while eliminating fragmentation and duplication of services. As HMOs have grown, they have expanded to include specialist services and programs for Medicare and Medicaid populations. Some studies show that HMOs are cost-effective and that the quality of care provided by these health care delivery systems is comparable to the care provided elsewhere in the same communities. However, concerns have surfaced regarding the limitations on choice of health care provider, diagnostic testing, or length of hospitalization that might be imposed by some HMOs (Silver, 1997).

Preferred Provider Organizations

HMOs have paved the way and served as the model for preferred provider organizations (PPOs). In contrast to the HMO, the PPO is not a distinct entity; rather, it is a business arrangement between a group of providers, usually hospitals and physicians, who contract to provide health care to subscribers, usually businesses, for a negotiated fee that often is discounted. PPOs allow businesses to decrease their expenses for employee health care benefits and hospitals and physicians to market their services to employers.

Some nurses serve as preferred providers through nursing centers. Nursing centers represent a model of health care delivery that is unique, client-based, and holistic. These centers often provide care to vulnerable populations, allowing direct access to nursing services. Nurses provide the majority of services, control the budget, and function as chief executive officers. Nursing centers emphasize primary care with collaborative, interdisciplinary models of practice (Hoffman, 1997).

Managed Care

HMOs and PPOs have given rise to a much broader pattern of reimbursement and cost control—managed health care. Managed care is an important trend in health care. The failure of the regulatory efforts of past decades to cut costs and the escalation of health care costs to 15% to 22% of the gross domestic product have prompted business, labor, and government to assume greater control over the financing and delivery of health care. The result is significant expansion of managed health care to the point that distinctions among HMOs, PPOs, exclusive provider arrangements, managed indemnity plans, and self-insured managed care are blurring. The common features that characterize managed care include prenegotiated payment rates, mandatory precertification, utilization review, limited choice of provider, and fixed-price reimbursement. The scope of managed care has expanded from in-hospital services to ambulatory, long-term, and home care services, as well as related diagnostic and therapeutic services.

The results of managed care include a dramatic reduction in inpatient hospital days, continuing expansion of ambulatory care, fierce competition, and marketing strategies that appeal to consumers as well as to insurers and regulators. Hospitals are faced with declining revenues, a declining number of patients, more severely ill patients, and shorter lengths of stay. As patients return to the community, they have more health care needs, many of which are complex. The demand for home care and community-based services is escalating. Despite their successes, managed care organizations are faced with the challenge of providing quality services under even greater resource constraints.

Case and Care Management

Case management, more broadly termed care management, has become a prominent method for coordinating health care services to ensure cost-effectiveness, accountability, and quality care. The case management process dates back to the public health programs of the early 1900s, in which public health nursing always played a dominant role. Over the years, the process has varied in form and function, but the basic theme has remained: responsibility for meeting patient needs rests with one individual or team whose goals are to provide the patient and family with access to required services, to ensure coordination of these services, and to evaluate how effectively these services are delivered.

The reasons case management has gained such prominence can be traced to the decreased cost of care associated with decreased length of hospital stay, coupled with rapid and frequent interunit transfers from specialty to standard care units. The case manager role, instead of focusing on direct patient care, focuses on managing the care of an entire caseload of patients and collaborating with the nurses and other health care personnel who care for the patients. In most instances, the caseload is limited in scope to patients with similar diagnoses, needs, and therapies, and the case managers function across units. They are experts in their specialty areas and coordinate the inpatient and outpatient services needed by patients. The goals of this coordination include quality, appropriateness, and timeliness of services as well as cost reduction. The case manager follows the patient throughout hospitalization and at home after discharge in an effort to promote coordination of health care services that will avert or delay rehospitalization.

Clinical Pathways and Care Mapping

Many managed care facilities nationwide use clinical pathways or care mapping to coordinate care for a caseload of patients (Forkner, 1996). Clinical pathways serve as the interdisciplinary care plan and the tool for tracking a patient's progress toward achieving positive outcomes within specified time frames. Clinical pathways have been developed for certain DRGs (eg, open heart surgery, pneumonia with comorbidity, fractured hip), for high-risk patients (eg, patients receiving chemotherapy), and for patients with certain common health problems (eg, patients with diabetes or patients with chronic pain). They identify key events such as diagnostic tests, treatments, activities, medications, consultation, and education that must occur within specified times for the patient to achieve the desired and timely outcomes. The case manager facilitates and coordinates interventions to ensure that the patient progresses through the key events and achieves the desired outcomes (Forkner, 1996; Smith, 1997). Nurses providing direct care have an important role in clinical pathway development and use through their participation in developing, piloting, implementing, and revising clinical pathways. In addition, nurses monitor outcome achievement, and document and analyze variances. Figure 1-2 presents an example of a clinical pathway. Other examples of clinical pathways can be found in Appendix A.

☐ Please ✓ when physician has signed "Physician's Orders: Post Total Knee Replacement"

TOTAL KNEE REPLACEMENT	PREADMISSION DATE______	PERI-OP DATE______________	POST-OP NURSING UNIT
KEY PATIENT OUTCOMES	Pt will verbalize understanding of pre-op teaching plan, clinical pathway & discharge plan.	AM Admissions: All pre-op requirements met. PACU: D/C criteria met	Tolerates liquids Pain @ level acceptable to pt with meds. NV status intact Vital signs per baseline Use IS with assistance
DIAGNOSTICS (all = ✓)	✓CBC, ✓UA, ✓PT, ✓PTT, ✓EKG ✓Type & Screen, ✓18 Chan, ✓CXR	SSU: Check lytes OR: Chart—labs, x-ray PACU: ✓H&H, ✓Hip X-ray	
ASSESSMENT	Pt Serv; comm fin info Schedule app'ts Nursing pre-admit	SSU: Nursing assess. Doc allergies OR: ✓Pre-op SAO_2, Periph pulses PACU: Per protocol, ✓Con't SAO_2	Nursing assessment per unit protocol NV & VS q4h Foot dorsiflexion
MEDICATIONS (all = ✓)	✓Hematinic agent	OR: ✓Antibiotic IV & ✓wound irrigation PACU: ✓Pain, ✓Anxiety pm	✓Antibiotic IV ✓Pain, ✓Anxiety pm ✓Anticoagulant ✓Stool softener
TREATMENTS (all = ✓)		OR: ✓TEDS, Sequential compression device ✓Reinfusion/drainage PACU: ✓Knee immobilizer ✓CPM ≥ 8 hours per order	✓ISx2/q2h ✓O2, ✓TEDS, ✓SCD, ✓Hemovac ✓Reinfusion/drainage ✓Knee immobilizer, ✓CPM ≥ 8 hours per order ✓Air mattress ✓Dressing reinforced PRN
NUTRITION/ FLUIDS	✓NPO after midnight	✓NPO	✓DAT/Enc po fluids IV
INFLAMMATION			✓I & O ✓Foley
SKIN / SAFETY ACTIVITY	PT evaluation OT evaluation		✓Turn q2h, Reposition PRN ✓PT: Bedside- evaluation, exercises, dangle
PSYCHO SOCIAL	Team assessment Advance directives Pt/fam support	S.O. with pt Chaplain PRN Advance directive	Team Assess/support
ED: PATIENT FAMILY	PT/OT: Pre-op plan Nursing: Assess of needs & pre-op ed Lovenox self-administration Orient: Hosp, unit, clinical path	Explain all procedures	Incentive spirometry, total knee precautions, Explain all procedures/equip/Tx, Pain/Anx mgt, Meds
CONSULTS	Dietitian	Per assessments	Per assessments
D/C PLAN: PATIENT FAMILY	SW assessment Ref:ECF/HH/etc., Lovenox PT/OT home envir, equipment needs Nursing: Assess spec needs		
SIGNATURE/DATE: Please record signature & date under each day. Signature denotes that the pathway is followed as the Plan of Care. Clinical variances are documented as a VAR notation on the Patient Progress Record or per discipline's protocol. Washington Adventist Hospital			

✓ Interventions must have a signed physician's order before implementation!
CLINICAL PATHWAY: TOTAL KNEE REPLACEMENT
WAH601-399 18/96

FIGURE 1•2 A portion of a clinical pathway. This section of the pathway indicates the type of clinical treatment or patient care activities to be carried out before admission and during and after surgery for a patient undergoing total knee replacement. Clinical pathway reproduced with permission of Washington Adventist Hospital, Takoma Park, Maryland.

Care mapping is a broader interdisciplinary process of moving patients toward predetermined outcome markers using phases and stages of the disease or condition. Coordination of care and education through hospitalization and after discharge remains a key factor. Care mapping is used for conditions in which the patient's progression often defies prediction; thus, specific time frames for achieving outcomes are excluded. Patients with highly complex conditions or multiple underlying illnesses may benefit more from care mapping than from clinical pathways because the use of outcome markers, not specific time frames, is more realistic (Burns, Daly, & Tice, 1997).

Through case management and the use of clinical paths or care mapping, patients and the care they receive are continually assessed from preadmission to discharge—and in many cases after discharge in the home care and community settings. The resultant continuity of care, effective utilization of services, and cost containment are expected to be major benefits for society and for the health care system.

NURSING DELIVERY SYSTEMS

As stated earlier, nursing is the diagnosis and treatment of human responses to health and illness, and therefore focuses on a broad array of phenomena. There are three major roles assumed by the nurse when caring for patients. These roles are often used in concert with one another to provide comprehensive care.

Roles of the Nurse

The professional nurse in both institutional and community health care settings has three major roles: the practitioner role, which includes teaching and collaborating; the leadership role; and the research role. Although each role carries specific responsibilities, these roles relate to one another and are found in all nursing positions. These roles are designed to meet the immediate and future health care and nursing needs of consumers who are the recipients of nursing care.

Practitioner Role

The practitioner role of the nurse involves those actions that the nurse takes when assuming responsibility for meeting the health care and nursing needs of individual patients, their families, and significant others. This role is the dominant role of nurses in primary, secondary, and tertiary health care settings and in home care and community nursing. It is a role that can be achieved only through use of the nursing process, the basis for all nursing practice. The nurse helps patients meet their needs through direct intervention, by teaching patients and family members to perform care, and by coordinating and collaborating with other disciplines to provide needed services.

Leadership Role

The leadership role of the nurse has traditionally been perceived as a specialized role assumed only by those nurses who have titles that suggest leadership and who are the leaders of large groups of nurses or related health care professionals. However, the definition of nursing leadership developed by Yura, Ozimek, and Walsh (1981) gives a broader scope to the concept and identifies leadership as a role that is inherent within all nursing positions. The leadership role of the nurse involves those actions the nurse executes when assuming responsibility for the actions of others that are directed toward determining and achieving patient care goals.

Nursing leadership is a process involving four components: decision making, relating, influencing, and facilitating. Each of these components promotes change and the ultimate outcome of goal achievement. Basic to the entire process is effective communication, which determines the accomplishment of the process. Leadership in nursing is a process in which the nurse uses interpersonal skills to effect change in the behavior of others. The components of the leadership process are appropriate during all phases of the nursing process and in all settings.

Research Role

The research role of the nurse was traditionally viewed as one being carried out only by academicians, nurse scientists, and graduate nursing students. Today, participation in the research process is also considered to be a responsibility of nurses in clinical practice.

The primary task of nursing research is to contribute to the scientific base of nursing practice. Studies are needed to determine the effectiveness of nursing interventions and nursing care. Through such research efforts, the science of nursing will grow and a scientifically based rationale for making changes in nursing practice and patient care will be generated.

Nurses who have preparation in research methods can use their research knowledge and skills to initiate and implement timely, relevant studies. This is not to say that nurses who do not initiate and implement nursing research studies do not play a significant role in nursing research. Every nurse has valuable contributions to make to nursing research and a responsibility to make these contributions. All nurses must constantly be alert for nursing problems and important issues related to patient care that can serve as the basis for the identification of researchable questions.

Those nurses directly involved in patient care are often in the best position to identify potential research problems and questions. Their clinical insights are invaluable. Nurses also have a responsibility to become actively involved in ongoing research studies. This participation may involve facilitating the data collection process, or it may include actual collection of data. Explaining the study to other health care professionals or to patients and their families is often of invaluable assistance to the nurse who is conducting the study.

Above all, nurses must use research findings in their nursing practice. Research for the sake of research alone is meaningless. Only with the use and evaluation of research findings in nursing practice will the science of nursing be furthered. Research findings can be substantiated only through use, validation, replication, and dissemination. Nurses must continually be aware of studies that are directly related to their own area of clinical practice and critically analyze these studies to determine the applicability of their conclusions and implications to specific patient populations. Relevant conclusions and implications can be used to improve patient care.

Nursing Care Delivery

Nursing care can be carried out through a variety of organizational methods. The model of nursing care used varies greatly from one facility to another and from one set of patient circumstances to another. A review of past and current models used provides a background for understanding the nursing models and methods needed for the changing health care delivery system.

Team Nursing

Team nursing, which had its origins in the 1950s and 1960s, involved using a team leader and team members to provide various aspects of nursing care to a group of patients. In team nursing, medications may be given by one nurse while baths and physical care are given by a nursing assistant under the supervision of a nurse team leader. Skill mixes include registered nurses (RNs), often as team leaders; licensed practical nurses; and nursing assistants or unlicensed assistive personnel (UAP). With the current emphasis on cost containment in health care agencies, variations of team nursing are being used, with increased use of UAPs as team members. There has been little substantiation, however, that team nursing is cost-effective. The quality of patient care with this system is questionable, and fragmentation of care is of concern.

Primary Nursing

Primary nursing (not to be confused with primary health care, which pertains to first-contact general health care) refers to comprehensive, individualized care provided by the same nurse throughout the period of care. This type of nursing care allows the nurse to give direct patient care rather than manage and supervise the functions of others who provide direct care for the patient. This care method is rejected by many institutions as too costly; the patient–nurse ratio is small and a larger professional staff is needed, because the primary nurse is usually an RN. However, primary nursing may provide a foundation for transition to case management in some institutions.

The primary nurse accepts total 24-hour responsibility for quality nursing care for the patient. Thus, nursing care is directed toward meeting total, individualized patient needs. The primary nurse is responsible and accountable for involving the patient and family directly in all facets of care and has autonomy in making decisions in this regard. Communications with other members of the health care team regarding the patient's health care are made by the primary nurse, thereby providing continuity of care and promoting collaborative efforts directed toward quality patient care.

During times when the primary nurse is not scheduled to work, an associate nurse or co-nurse assists in overseeing the delivery of care. The associate nurse implements the nursing care plan and provides feedback to the primary nurse for evaluating the plan of care. The primary nurse assumes the responsibility for making appropriate referrals and for ensuring that all relevant information is provided to those who will be involved in the patient's continuing care, including the family.

The long-term survival of primary nursing as it is currently designed is uncertain. As cost-containment measures continue and patient acuity increases, staffing ratios of patients to nurses are increasing. Many nursing service departments and agencies are meeting the increased workload demands by making modifications in their approach to primary nursing or by reverting to team or functional systems for delivering care. Others are changing their staffing mix and redesigning their models of practice to accommodate nurse-extender roles. Still others are changing to more innovative systems such as case management.

Community-Based Nursing

Community-based care is not a new concept for nursing. Nursing has played a vital role in the community since the mid- to late 1800s, as visiting nurses provided care to the sick and poor in their homes and communities and educated patients and family members. The central idea of community-based nursing is that nursing intervention could reduce the spread of illness and improve the health status of groups of citizens.

Community and home health care nursing, which have traditionally focused on health promotion, maternal and child health, and chronic care, now are expanding to meet the needs of many other groups of patients with a variety of problems and needs. Although community nursing and home health nursing may be discussed together, and aspects of care overlap, there is a distinction between the terms. Community health nursing practice is concerned with the general and comprehensive care of the community at large, with emphasis on primary, secondary, and tertiary prevention. Home health care is directed chiefly toward specific patient groups with identified needs, usually related to illness, injury, or debilitation resulting from advanced age or chronic illness. As such, home health care will be a major aspect of community-based care discussed throughout this text. Home health care services are provided by community-based programs or agencies for specific populations (eg, the elderly or ventilator-dependent patient), as well as by hospital-based home health care agencies, hospices, independent professional nursing practices, and freestanding health care agencies.

As trends continue toward shortened hospital stays and increased use of outpatient health care services, the need for nursing care in the home and community setting has increased dramatically. Because nursing services are being provided outside as well as within the hospital, nurses have a choice of practicing in a variety of health care delivery settings: acute medical centers, ambulatory care settings, clinics, urgent care centers, outpatient departments, neighborhood health centers, home health care agencies, independent or group nursing centers, and managed care agencies.

Community nursing centers, which have emerged over the past two decades with the advent of nurse practitioners, are nurse-managed and provide primary care services that include ambulatory and outpatient care, immunizations, health assessment and screening services, and patient and family education and counseling. The populations that these centers serve are varied, but most typically include a high proportion of patients who are rural, very young, very old, poor, or racial minorities—groups that are generally underserved.

The numbers and kinds of agencies that provide care in the home and community have expanded because of the expanding needs of patients requiring care. Home health care nurses are challenged because patients are discharged from acute care institutions to their homes and communities early in the recovery process and at more acute levels of illness. Many are elderly, and many have multiple medical and nursing diagnoses and multisystem health problems that require acute and intensive nursing care. Medical technologies, such as ventilatory support, and intravenous and total parenteral nutrition therapy, once limited to acute care settings, have been adapted to the home care setting.

As a result, the community-based care setting is becoming one of the largest practice areas for nursing. Home care nursing is now a specialty area that requires advanced knowledge and skills in general nursing practice, with emphasis on community health and acute medical-surgical nursing. Also required are high-level assessment skills, critical thinking, and decision-making skills in a setting where other health care professionals are not available to validate observations, conclusions, and decisions.

Home care nurses often function as acute care nurses in the home, providing "high-tech, high-touch" services to patients with acute health care needs. In addition, they are responsible for patient and family teaching and for contacting community resources and coordinating the continuing care of the patient. For these reasons, the scope of medical-surgical nursing encompasses not only the acute care setting within hospitals, but also the acute care setting as it expands into the community and the home. Throughout this textbook, emphasis is placed on the home health care needs of patients, with particular attention given to the teaching, self-care management, and health maintenance needs of patients and their families.

ADVANCED PRACTICE NURSING

Professional nursing is adapting to meet changing health needs and expectations. One such adaptation is through the expanded role of the nurse, which has developed in response to the need to improve the distribution of health care services and to decrease the cost of health care. The nurse who functions in an advanced practice role provides direct care to patients through independent practice, practice within a health care agency, or collaboration with a physician. Specialization has evolved within the expanded roles of nursing, a result of the recent explosion of technology and knowledge.

Nurses receive advanced education in such specialties as critical care, coronary care, respiratory care, oncologic care, maternal/child, neonatal intensive care, rehabilitation, trauma, rural health, and gerontologic nursing, to name just a few. With the expanded role of the nurse, various titles have emerged that attempt to specify the functions as well as the educational preparation of nurses, although functions are less distinct than in previous years. In medical-surgical nursing, the most significant of these titles are nurse practitioner and clinical nurse specialist, and the more recent title of advanced practice nurse, which encompasses both nurse practitioners and clinical specialists.

Although initially the educational preparation for nurse practitioners was in certificate programs, in most states both nurse practitioners and clinical nurse specialists require graduate-level education. The two programs, which originally differed significantly in scope and in the definition of the role component, now have many similarities and areas of overlap. Nurse practitioners and clinical nurse specialists (along with certified nurse-midwives and certified registered nurse anesthetists) are identified as advanced practice nurses.

Nurse practitioners are, for the most part, prepared as generalists (eg, pediatric nurse practitioner, geriatric nurse practitioner). They define their role in terms of the direct provision of a broad range of primary health care services to patients and families. The focus is on providing primary health care to patients and collaborating with other health professionals. They practice in both acute and nonacute care settings. New federal legislation has provided for nurse practitioners to receive direct Medicare reimbursement (Hemlinger, 1997). In addition, in some states—and with new legislation possibly nationwide—nurse practitioners have prescriptive authority.

Clinical nurse specialists, on the other hand, are prepared as specialists who practice within a circumscribed area of care (eg, cardiovascular clinical nurse specialist, oncology clinical nurse specialist). They define their role as having five major components: clinical practice, education, management, consultation, and research. Studies have shown that in reality the focus is often on the education and consultation roles: education and counseling of patients and families and education, counseling, and consultation with nursing staff. They practice in a variety of settings, including the community and home, although most practice in acute care settings. Recently, clinical nurse specialists have been identified by many nursing leaders as ideal case managers. They have the educational background and the clinical expertise to organize and coordinate services and resources to meet the patient's health care needs in a cost-effective and efficient manner.

With advanced practice roles has come a continuing effort by professional nursing organizations to define more clearly the practice of nursing. Nurse practice acts have been amended to give nurses the authority to perform functions that were previously restricted to the practice of medicine. These functions include diagnosis (nursing), treatment, performance of selected invasive procedures, and prescription of medications and treatments. Regulations regarding these functions are stipulated by the board of nursing in each state. The board defines the education and experience required and determines the clinical situations in which a nurse may perform these functions.

In general, initial care, ambulatory health care, and anticipatory guidance are all becoming increasingly important in nursing practice. The advanced practice roles enable nurses to function interdependently with other health care professionals and to establish a more collegial relationship with physicians. As changes in health care continue, the role of advanced practice nurses, especially in primary care settings, is expected to increase in terms of scope, responsibility, and recognition.

COLLABORATIVE PRACTICE

Throughout this chapter we have explored the changing role of nursing. Many references have been made to the significance of the nurse as a member of the health care team. As the unique competencies of nurses are becoming more clearly articulated, there is increasing evidence that nurses provide certain health care services distinctive to the profession. However, nursing continues to recognize the importance of collaboration with other health care disciplines in meeting the needs of patients.

Some institutions use the nurse–physician collaborative practice model. Within a decentralized organizational structure, nurses and physicians function collaboratively in making clinical decisions. A joint practice committee, with equal representation from both professions, may function at the unit level to monitor, support, and foster collaboration. Collaborative practice is further enhanced with integration of the clinical record and with joint patient care record reviews. Figure 1-3 compares the traditional with the collaborative practice model.

The collaborative model, or a variation of it, should be a primary goal for nursing—a venture that would promote shared participation, responsibility, and accountability in a health care environment that is striving to meet the complex health care needs of the public.

Critical Thinking Exercises

1. Your clinical assignment is on a medical-surgical unit in an acute care hospital. Identify a patient care issue (eg, patient education) that could be improved. Describe the mechanism that is available within the hospital to address such quality improvement issues.

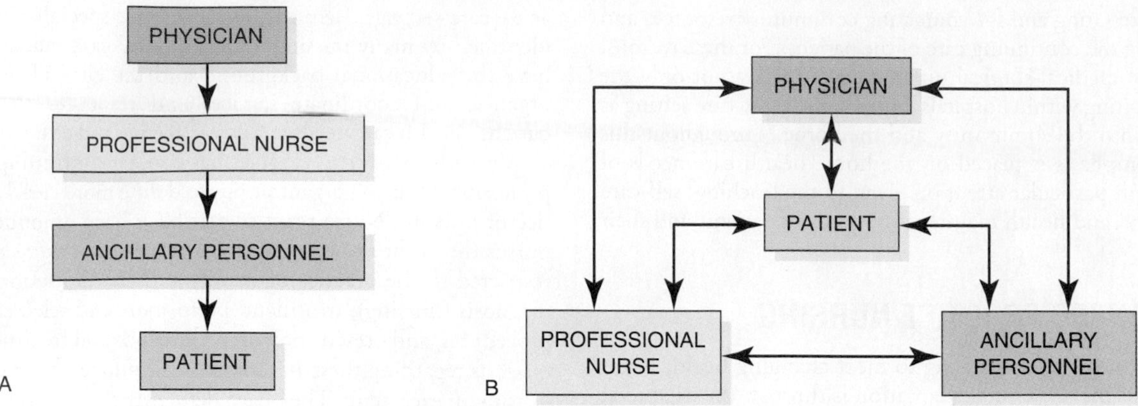

FIGURE 1•3 Comparison of traditional practice model (**A**) and collaborative practice model (**B**).

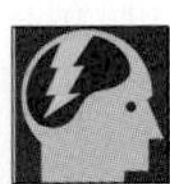

Critical Thinking Exercises *continued*

2.
You are caring for an elderly patient who has several chronic medical conditions and is soon to be discharged. A case manager has been assigned to this patient. How would you explain the role of the case manager to the patient and her daughter?

3.
You are assigned to care for a patient whose health care is covered by a managed health care plan. How have managed health care plans affected nursing care delivery in acute care hospitals and outpatient settings? How might this specific patient's care be affected?

References and Selected Readings

BOOKS

American Nurses Association. (1995). *Nursing's social policy statement.* Washington, DC: Author.

American Nurses Association. (1991). *Nursing's agenda for health care reform.* Kansas City, MO: Author.

Cookfair, J. M. (1996). *Nursing care in the community.* St. Louis: Mosby–Year Book.

Giger, J. N., & Davidhizer, R. (1995). *Transcultural nursing: Assessment and intervention* (2nd ed.). St. Louis: C. V. Mosby.

Leddy, S., & Pepper, J. M. (1998). *Conceptual bases of professional nursing.* Philadelphia: Lippincott-Raven.

National Center for Health Statistics. (1996). *Vital and health statistics.* Hyattsville, MD: U.S. Department of Health and Human Services.

National League for Nursing. (1977). *Nursing's role in patients' rights.* New York: Author.

U.S. Department of Commerce, Economics, and Statistics Administration. Bureau of the Census. (1997). *How we're changing: Demographic state of the nation.* Current Population Reports Special Studies (Series P23-193). Washington, DC: Author.

U.S. Public Health Service. (1990). *Healthy people 2000: National health promotion and disease prevention objectives.* Washington, DC: U.S. Government Printing Office.

Yura, H., Ozimek, D., & Walsh, M. B. (1981). *Nursing leadership: Theory and process.* New York: Appleton-Century-Crofts.

JOURNALS

Boyd, M. L., Fisher, B., Davidson, A. W., & Neilsen, C. A. (1996). Community-based case management for chronically ill older adults. *Nursing Management, 27*(11), 31–32.

Brown, L., Deckers, C., Magallanes, A., Quiamas, D., & Deschner, S. (1996). Clinical case management—what works, what doesn't. *Nursing Management, 27*(11), 28–30.

Burns, S. M., Daly, B., & Tice, P. (1997). Being led down the critical pathway: A perspective on the importance of care managers vs. critical pathways for patients requiring prolonged mechanical ventilation. *Critical Care Nurse, 17*(6), 70–75.

Forkner, D. J. (1996). Clinical pathways—benefits and liabilities. *Nursing Management, 27*(11), 35–37.

Gonzalez, R., & Reed, S. (1997). Washington watch. *American Journal of Nursing, 97*(11), 16.

Hemlinger, C. (1997). ANA hails passage of Medicare reimbursement. *The American Nurse,* (Sept./Oct.), 1,10.

Hoffman, S. E. (1997). Nursing centers—models of professional practice. *Journal of Professional Nursing, 13*(6), 335.

Ketefian, S., & Redman, R. W. (1997). Nursing science in the global community. *Image: Journal of Nursing Scholarship, 29*(1), 11–15.

Naish, J. (1997). Future shock. *Nursing Times, 93*(6), 34–36.

Reed, S., & Peterson, C. (1996). Washington Watch. *American Journal of Nursing, 96*(12), 19–20.

Silver, G. (1997). Editorial: The road from managed care. *American Journal of Public Health, 87*(1), 8–9.

Smith, P. (1997). Issues and interventions. *Nursing Case Management, 2*(3), 127–129.

Stahl, D. A. (1996). Disease management: A challenge to subacute care. *Nursing Management, 27*(11), 25–26.

Stahl, D. A. (1997). Five pitfalls of work redesign in acute care. *Nursing Management, 28*(10), 49–50.

Trofino, J. (1997). The courage to change—reshaping health care delivery. *Nursing Management, 28*(11), 50–53.

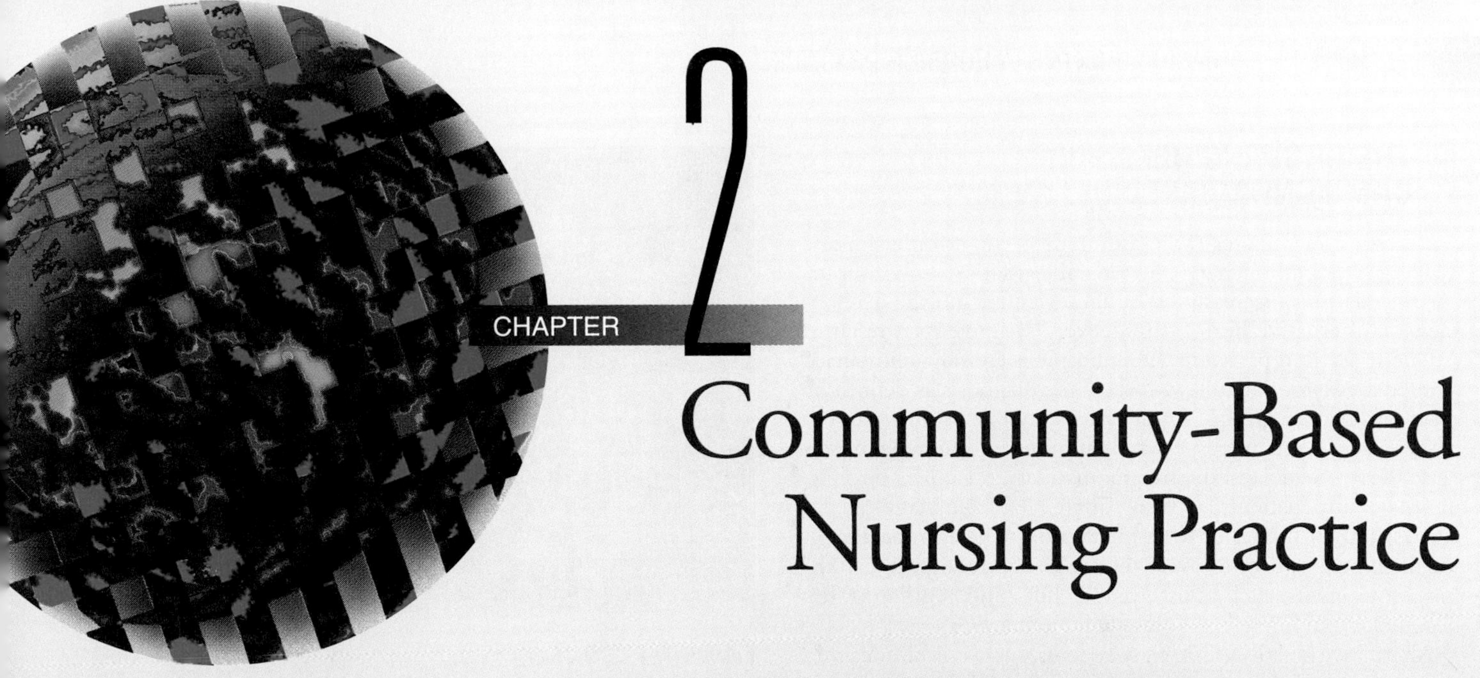

Community-Based Nursing Practice

Learning Objectives

On completion of the chapter, the learner will be able to:

1. Discuss the changes in the health care system that have increased the need for medical-surgical nurses to practice in community-based settings.
2. Compare the differences and similarities between community-based and hospital nursing.
3. Describe the discharge planning process in relation to home care preparation.
4. Explain methods for identifying community resources and making referrals.
5. Discuss how to prepare for a home health care visit and how to conduct the visit.
6. Identify personal safety precautions a home care nurse should take when making home visits.
7. Describe the various types of nursing functions carried out in ambulatory care facilities, school nursing programs, and primary care clinics.
8. Describe barriers to providing health care services to the homeless.

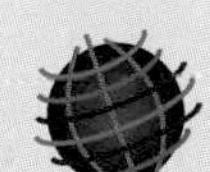

The changes that have occurred in the health care system for almost two decades have increased the need for care in ambulatory settings and in the home. These changes have created a demand for highly skilled and well-prepared nurses to provide community-based care.

THE GROWING NEED FOR COMMUNITY-BASED HEALTH CARE

As described in Chapter 1, the shift in the settings for health care delivery is a result of changes in federal legislation, tighter insurance regulations, decreasing hospital revenues, and the development of alternative health care delivery systems. As a result of federal legislation passed in 1983, hospitals are now reimbursed at a fixed rate for patients with the same diagnosis as defined by diagnosis-related groups. Under this system, hospitals can cut costs and earn income by carefully monitoring the types of services they provide and discharging patients as soon as possible. Consequently, patients are being discharged from acute care facilities to their homes or to residential or long-term facilities at much earlier stages of recovery than in the past. High-level technical equipment, such as intravenous lines and ventilators, has become part of home health care (McNeal, 1996).

Alternative health care delivery systems, such as health maintenance organizations, preferred provider organizations, and managed health care systems, have contributed to the drive to control costs and the availability of health care services. These regulations have dramatically reduced the length of hospital stays and have led to patients being treated more frequently in ambulatory care settings and at home. Chapter 1 provides a more thorough discussion of alternative health care delivery systems.

As more health care delivery shifts into the community, more nurses are working in a variety of community-based settings, such as public health departments, ambulatory health clinics, long-term care facilities, prenatal and well-baby clinics, hospice agencies, industrial settings (as occupational nurses), homeless shelters and clinics, nursing centers, home health agencies, and patients' homes.

Nurses in these settings often deliver care without direct on-site supervision or backup by other hospital personnel. They must be self-directed, flexible, adaptable, and tolerant of various lifestyles and living conditions. Expertise in independent decision making, critical thinking, assessment, and health education and competence in basic nursing care are essential to function effectively in the community-based setting.

Community-based nursing encompasses various kinds of services provided outside of hospitals. Although the phrase "community-based nursing" is often interchanged with "community health nursing," a distinction should be made. Some believe that community-based nursing is not a nursing specialty but an umbrella philosophy guiding nursing care given to individuals and families in the setting in which they live, work, play, and go to school (Zotti, Brown, & Stotts, 1996). It includes community health nursing as well as home health nursing, school health nursing, and a host of other nursing services provided to individuals and groups in the community (Fig. 2-1).

COMMUNITY/PUBLIC HEALTH CARE

Community/public health nursing practice focuses on promoting and maintaining the health of populations and on preventing and minimizing the progression of disease (Cookfair, 1996). Although nursing interventions used by public health nurses might involve individuals, families, or small groups, the central focus remains promoting health and preventing disease in the entire community. The actions of community health nurses may include provision of direct care to patients and families as well as political advocacy to secure resources for aggregate populations such as the aged population (Zotti, Brown, & Stotts, 1996).

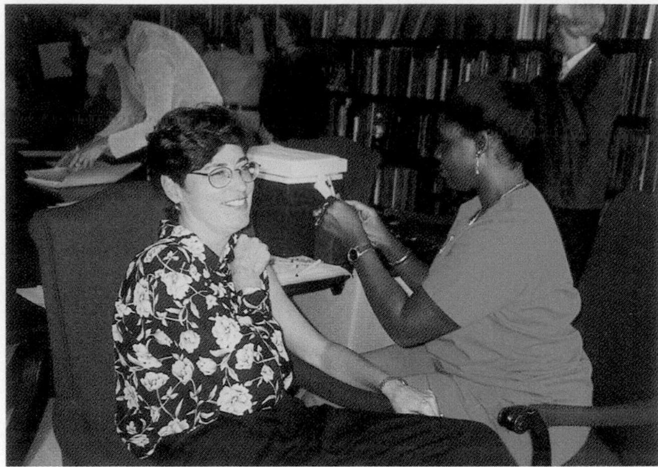

FIGURE 2•1 Community-based nursing takes many forms and focuses. Here the nursing focus is on wellness and the nursing setting is industry. When enlightened employers offer flu vaccines or other health services, the whole community benefits.

Primary, secondary, and tertiary levels of preventive care are used by community health nurses. Primary prevention centers on health promotion and protection from health problems, and includes interventions such as health teaching regarding healthy lifestyles. Secondary prevention centers on health maintenance and is aimed at early detection and intervention to minimize loss of function and independence; it includes interventions such as health screening and health risk appraisal. Tertiary prevention focuses on rehabilitation to assist patients in achieving their maximum potential, working through their physical or psychological challenge (Cookfair, 1996).

Community health nursing services may include functioning as an epidemiologist, a case manager for a group of patients, a coordinator of services provided to an aggregate of patients, an occupational health nurse, a school nurse, or a visiting nurse. The commonality of these various roles is that the nurse maintains a focus on community needs as well as on the needs of the individual patient (Abraham & Fallon, 1997). Some community health nurse practice areas have become specialties in their own right.

HOME HEALTH CARE

Home health care is becoming one of the biggest practice areas for nurses. Because of the high acuity level of patients, nurses with acute care and high-technology experience are in demand in this field. Tertiary preventive nursing care, focusing on rehabilitation and restoring maximum health function, is a major goal for home care nurses, although primary and secondary prevention are also included in care.

Home care nursing is a unique aspect of community-based nursing. Home care visits are made by nurses who work for home care and public health agencies and visiting nurse associations, or by nurses who are employed by hospitals. Such visits can also be part of the responsibilities of school nurses, clinic nurses, or occupational health nurses. The type of nursing services provided to patients in their homes varies from agency to agency. Nurses working for home care or hospice agencies make home visits to provide skilled nursing care, follow-up care, and teaching to promote health and prevent complications (Cookfair, 1996). Clinic nurses conduct home visits as part of patient follow-up. Public health and school nurses may make visits to provide anticipatory guidance to high-risk families and follow-up care to patients with communicable diseases. Many home care patients are acutely ill, and many have chronic health problems, requiring nurses to provide more education to the patient and family (Buerhaus & Staiger, 1997).

A multidisciplinary team that includes professional nurses, home health aides, social workers, and physical, speech, and occupational therapists provides health and social services. The patient's medical care is under the direction of a physician, with oversight of the total health care plan by a case manager, clinical nurse specialist, or nurse practitioner. Health care visits are intermittent or periodic.

Health care services are provided by official, publicly funded agencies, nonprofit agencies, private businesses, proprietary chains, and hospital-based agencies. Some agencies specialize in high-technology services. Most agencies are reimbursed from a variety of sources, including Medicare and Medicaid programs, private insurance, and direct payments by patients. Each funding source has its own requirements for services rendered, the number of visits allowed, and the amount of reimbursement the agency will receive. However, over one half of home health care expenditures are funded by Medicare.

The elderly are the most frequent users of home care services. To be eligible for service, the patient must be acutely ill, homebound, and in need of skilled nursing services. Nursing care includes skilled assessment of the patient's physical, psychological, social, and environmental status. Nursing interventions include intravenous therapy and injections (Fig. 2-2), total parenteral nutrition, venipuncture, catheter insertion, pressure ulcer treatment, wound care, ostomy care, and patient and family teaching. The nurse instructs the patient and family in skills and self-care strategies as well as in health maintenance and promotion activities, such as nutritional counseling, exercise programs, and stress management.

Medicare allows nurses to manage and evaluate patient care for seriously ill patients who have complex, labile conditions and are at high risk for rehospitalization. The nurse serves as a case manager and monitors the delivery of care provided to patients in their homes.

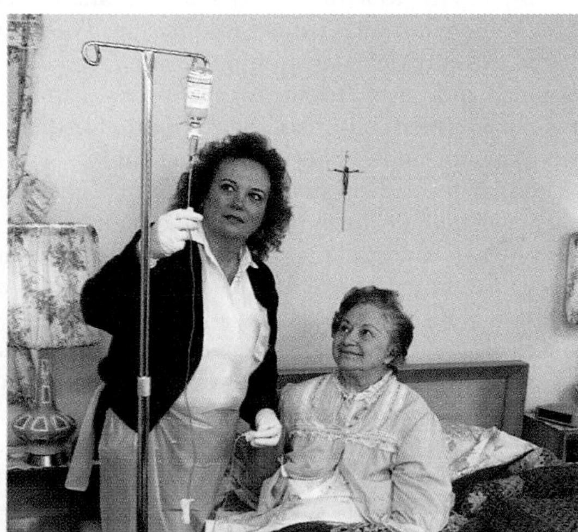

FIGURE 2•2 Intravenous therapy is one of the types of skilled nursing care that may be provided in the home. Courtesy Good Samaritan Certified Home Health Agency, Babylon, New York.

Hospital Versus Community-Based Nursing Care

Giving nursing care in a patient's home is different from providing care in a hospital. Patients must sign a release form to stay and receive treatment in a hospital. They have little control over what happens to them, and they are expected to comply with the hospital's rules, regulations, and schedule of activities. They sleep in the hospital's beds and wear hospital gowns or similar-looking sleeping clothes. They are given their treatments, care, baths, and medications at a time that is usually determined by institutional schedules rather than at a time that is convenient for them. Although they may select meals from a daily menu, there is a limited choice in the type of food they are offered. Family members and friends are allowed to visit at the hospital's discretion.

In contrast, the home care nurse is considered a guest in the patient's home and needs permission to visit and give care. The nurse has minimal control over the lifestyle, living situation, and health practices of the patients he or she visits (Johnson, Smith-Temple, & Carr, 1998). The lack of full decision-making authority can create a conflict for the nurse and lead to problems in the nurse–patient relationship. To work successfully with patients, no matter what the setting, it is important for the nurse to be nonjudgmental and convey respect for the patient's beliefs, even when they differ sharply from the nurse's. This can be difficult when a patient's lifestyle involves activities that the nurse considers harmful or unacceptable, such as alcohol or drug abuse.

The cleanliness of a patient's home may not meet the standards of a hospital. Although the nurse can provide teaching points about maintaining clean surroundings, the patient and family determine whether or not to implement the nurse's suggestions. The nurse must accept the reality of the situation and deliver the care required regardless of the sanitary conditions of the surroundings.

The kind of equipment and supplies or resources usually available in acute care settings are often unavailable in the patient's home. The nurse has to learn to improvise when providing care, such as when changing a dressing or catheterizing a patient in a regular bed that is not adjustable and lacks a bedside stand (Johnson, Smith-Temple, & Carr, 1998).

Infection control is as important in the home as it is in the hospital but can be more challenging and require creative approaches. As in any situation, it is important to cleanse one's hands before and after giving direct patient care, even in a home that does not have running water. If aseptic technique is required, the nurse must have a plan for implementing this before going to the home. This applies also to the use of standard precautions, transmission-based precautions, and disposal of bodily secretions and excretions (Centers for Disease Control & Prevention, 1996).

If injections are given, the nurse should use a closed container to dispose of syringes. Injectable and other medications need to be kept out of the reach of children during visits and stored in a safe place if they are to remain in the house. Nurses performing invasive procedures need to be up-to-date with their immunizations, including hepatitis B and tetanus.

The home environment often has more distractions than a hospital. The home can be filled with background noise and crowded with people and objects. A nurse may have to request that the television be turned down during the visit or that the patient move to a more private place to be interviewed.

Friends, neighbors, or family members may ask the nurse about the patient's condition. A patient has a right to confidentiality, and information should be shared only with the patient's permission. If the nurse carries the patient's chart into the house, it must be put in a secure place to prevent it from being picked up by others or misplaced.

Discharge Planning for Home Care

To prepare for early hospital discharge and the possible need for follow-up care in the home, discharge planning begins with the patient's admission. Several different personnel or agencies may be involved in the planning process. In hospitals, social workers or nurses may serve as the discharge planners. Some home care agencies have liaison nurses who work with the discharge planners to ensure the patient's needs are met when he or she is released from the hospital. Professionals in ambulatory health care settings may refer sick patients for home care services to prevent hospitalization. Public health nurses have patients referred for anticipatory guidance for high-risk families, for case finding, and for follow-up treatment (for patients with communicable diseases).

The development of a comprehensive discharge plan requires collaboration with professionals both at the referring agency and at the home care or public health agency. The process involves identifying the patient's needs and developing a thorough plan to meet them. Communication with and cooperation of the patient and family are essential.

Community Resources and Referrals

Home health nurses and public health nurses act as case managers. After assessing the patient's needs, they might make referrals to other team members, such as home health aides and social workers. They work collaboratively with the health team and the agency or person who referred the patient for service. Continuous coordinated care among all health care providers involved in the patient's care is essential to avoid duplication of effort by the various personnel caring for the patient.

Home care and public health nurses are responsible for providing the patient and family with information about other available community resources to meet their needs. During the initial and subsequent visits, they help patients identify these community services and encourage the patient and family to contact the appropriate agencies. On occasion the nurse may need to make the initial contact if the patient or family is unable to do so (Cookfair, 1996; Zotti, Brown, & Stotts, 1996).

A community-based nurse needs to be knowledgeable about community resources available to patients and the services the agencies provide, eligibility requirements, and any possible charges for the services. Most communities have directories of health and social service agencies that the nurse can consult. These directories need to be continually updated as resources change. If a community does not have a resource booklet, the agency may develop one for its staff. It should include the commonly used community resources that patients need, the cost of the services, and eligibility requirements. The telephone book is also a good resource for helping patients identify the locations of grocery and drug stores, banks, health care facilities, ambulances, physicians, dentists, pharmacists, social service agencies, and senior citizen programs.

Preparing for a Home Visit

Most agencies have a policy manual that states their philosophy and procedures and defines the services they provide. Becoming familiar with these policies is an essential step before initiating a home visit. It is also important to know the agency's policies and the state law regarding what action to take if the nurse finds a patient dead, encounters an abusive situation in the family, or determines that a patient cannot remain safely at home.

Before making a home visit, the nurse should review the patient's referral form and other pertinent data concerning the patient. It may be necessary to contact the referring agency if the purpose for the referral is unclear or if important information is missing.

The first step is to call the patient to obtain permission to visit, schedule a time for the visit, and verify the address. This initial phone conversation provides an opportunity to introduce oneself, identify the agency, and explain the reason for the visit.

If a patient does not have a telephone, the nurse should see if those who made the referral have a number where a phone message can be left for the patient. If an unannounced visit must be made to a patient's home, the nurse should ask permission to come in before entering the house. Explaining the purpose of the referral at the outset and setting up the time for future visits before leaving are also recommended approaches.

Most agencies provide nurses with bags that contain standard supplies and equipment needed during home visits. It is important to keep the bag properly supplied and to bring any additional items that might be needed for the visit. Patients usually do not have the medical supplies needed for treatment.

Personal Safety Precautions

Whenever a nurse makes a home visit, the agency should know the nurse's schedule and the locations of the visits. The nurse should learn about the neighborhood and obtain directions for reaching the expected destination. A plan of action should always be established in case of emergencies.

Nurses are not expected to disregard their personal safety in an effort to make or complete home visits. If nurses encounter dangerous situations during visits, they should return to their agencies and contact their supervisors and/or law enforcement officials. A list of suggested precautions to take when making a home visit is presented in Chart 2-1.

Conducting a Home Visit

The first visit sets the tone for subsequent visits and is a crucial step in establishing the nurse–patient relationship. The situations encountered can vary depending on numerous factors. Patients may be in pain and unable to care for themselves. Families may be overwhelmed and doubt their ability to care for their loved one. They may not understand why the patient was sent home from the hospital before being totally rehabilitated. They may not comprehend what home care is or why they cannot have 24-hour nursing services. It is critical that the nurse try to convey an understanding of what the patient and family are experiencing and how the illness is affecting their lives.

During the initial home visit, which usually lasts less than an hour, the patient is evaluated and a plan of care established that is followed or modified on subsequent visits. The nurse informs the patient of the agency's practices and policies and hours of operation. If the agency is to be reimbursed for the visit, the nurse will ask for insurance information, such as a Medicare card or Medicaid stickers.

The initial assessment includes evaluating the patient, the home environment, the patient's self-care abilities or the family's ability to provide care, and the patient's need for additional re-

CHART 2•1 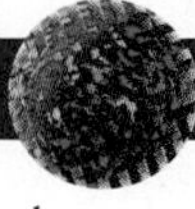 **Safety Precautions in Home Health Care**

- Know the phone number of the agency, police, and emergency services.
- Let the agency know your daily schedule and the phone numbers of your patients so that you can be located if you do not return when expected.
- Know where the patient lives before leaving to make the visit and carry a map for quick referral.
- Keep your car in good working order and have sufficient gas in the tank.
- Park the car near the patient's home and lock it during the visit.
- Do not drive an expensive car or wear expensive jewelry when making visits.
- Know the regular bus schedule and know the routes when using public transportation or walking to the patient's house.
- Carry agency identification and have enough change to make phone calls in case you get lost or have problems. (Some agencies provide cellular phones for their nurses to enable them to contact the agency in case of an emergency or if unexpected situations arise.)
- When making visits in high-crime areas, visit with another person rather than alone.
- Schedule visits only during daylight hours.
- Never walk into a patient's home uninvited.
- If you do not feel safe entering a patient's home, leave the area.
- Become familiar with the layout of the house, including exits from the house.
- If a patient or family member is intoxicated, hostile, or obnoxious, reschedule the visit and leave.
- If a family is having a serious argument or abusing the patient, reschedule the visit and contact your supervisor and report the abuse to the appropriate authorities.

sources. Identifying possible hazards such as cluttered walk areas, potential fire risks, pollution (air, water), or inadequate sanitation facilities is also part of the initial assessment.

Documentation considerations for home visits follow fairly specific regulations. The patient's needs and the nursing care given are documented accurately to ensure that the agency will qualify for payment for the visit. Medicare, Medicaid, and third-party payers require documentation of the patient's homebound status and the need for skilled professional nursing care. The medical diagnosis and specific detailed information on the functional limitations of the patient are usually part of the documentation. The goals and the actions appropriate for attaining them need to be identified. Expected outcomes of the nursing interventions must be stated in terms of the patient's behaviors and must be realistic and measurable. They must reflect the nursing diagnosis or the patient's problems and specify those actions that are expected to solve the patient's problems. If the documentation is not done correctly, the agency may not be paid for the visit (Johnson, Smith-Temple, & Carr, 1998).

Determining the Need for Future Visits

While conducting an assessment of the patient's situation, the nurse evaluates the need for future visits and the frequency with which those visits may need to be made. To make these judgments, the nurse may find it helpful to consider the following factors:

- *Current health status:* How well is the patient progressing? How serious are the present signs and symptoms? Has the patient shown signs of progressing as expected, or does it seem that recovery will be delayed?
- *Home environment:* Are worrisome safety factors apparent? Are family or friends available to provide care, or is the patient alone?
- *Level of self-care abilities:* Is the patient capable of self-care? What is the patient's level of independence? Is the patient ambulatory or bedridden? Does the patient have sufficient energy or is he or she frail and easily fatigued?
- *Level of nursing care needed:* What level of nursing care does the patient require? Does the care require basic skills or more complex interventions?
- *Prognosis:* What is the expectation of recovery in this particular instance? What are the chances that complications may develop if nursing care is not provided?
- *Patient education needs:* How well has the patient or family grasped the teaching points made? Is there a need for further follow-up and retraining? What level of proficiency does the patient or family show in carrying out the necessary care?
- *Mental status:* How alert is the patient? Are there signs of confusion or thinking difficulties? Does the patient tend to be forgetful or have a limited attention span?
- *Level of adherence:* Is the patient following the instructions provided? Does the patient seem capable of doing so? Are the family members helpful in this regard, or are they unwilling or unable to assist in caring for the patient as expected?

With each subsequent visit, these factors are evaluated to determine the continuing health needs of the patient. As progress is made and the patient, with or without the help of significant others, becomes more capable of self-care and more independent, the need for home visits may decline.

Closing the Visit

As the visit comes to a close, it is important to summarize the main points of the visit for the patient and family and identify expectations for future visits or patient achievements.

The following points should be considered at the end of each visit:

- What are the main points the patient or family should remember from the visit?
- What positive attributes have been noted about the patient and the family that will give them a sense of accomplishment?
- What were the main points of the teaching plan or the treatments needed to ensure that the patient and family understand what they must do? A written set of instructions should be left with the patient or family, provided they can read.
- Whom should the patient or family call in case they need to contact someone immediately? Are current emergency phone numbers readily available?

- What signs of complications should be reported immediately?
- What is the day and time of the next visit? Will a different nurse make the visit? How frequently will visits be made, and for how long, if determinable at this time?

OTHER COMMUNITY-BASED HEALTH CARE SETTINGS

Ambulatory Settings

Ambulatory health care is provided for patients in community or hospital-based settings. The types of agencies that provide ambulatory health care are medical clinics, ambulatory care units, urgent care centers, cardiac rehabilitation programs, mental health centers, student health centers, community outreach programs, and nursing centers. Some ambulatory centers provide care to a specific population, such as migrant workers or Native Americans. Neighborhood health centers provide services to patients who live in a geographically defined area. The centers may operate in freestanding buildings, storefronts, or mobile units. Agencies can provide ambulatory health care in addition to other services, such as offering an adult day care or health program. The kinds of services offered and the patients served depend on the agency's mission.

Nursing responsibilities in ambulatory health care settings include providing direct patient care, conducting patient intake screenings, treating patients with acute or chronic illnesses or emergent conditions, referring patients to other agencies for additional services, teaching patients self-care activities, and offering health education programs that promote health maintenance. A useful tool for the community-based nurse might be the classification scheme developed by the Visiting Nurses Association of Omaha, which contains patient-focused problems that are in one of four domains: environmental, psychosocial, physiologic, and health-related behaviors (Cookfair, 1996).

Nurses also work as the clinic managers, direct the operation of the clinic, and supervise other health team members. Nurse practitioners, educated in primary care, often practice in ambulatory care settings with a focus on gerontology, pediatrics, family or adult health, or women's health.

Occupational Health Programs

Federal legislation, especially the Occupational Safety and Health Act (OSHA), has had a major impact on health conditions in the workplace. The law is directed at creating safer and healthier work conditions. It is in an employer's interest to try to provide a safe working environment, because the result is reduced costs associated with employee absenteeism, hospitalization, and disability.

Occupational nurses can work in solo units in an industrial setting, may serve as consultants on a limited or part-time basis, or may be members of an interdisciplinary team composed of a variety of health care workers such as nurses, physicians, exercise physiologists, health educators, counselors, nutritionists, safety engineers, and industrial hygienists.

The occupational health nurse functions in several ways and may provide direct care to employees who become ill, conduct health education programs for company staff members, or set up health programs aimed at establishing specific health behaviors, such as eating properly and getting enough exercise. The nurse must also be knowledgeable about federal regulations pertaining to occupational health and be familiar with other pertinent legislation, such as the Americans with Disabilities Act.

School Health Programs

School-age children and adolescents with health problems are at major risk for underachieving or failing in school. The leading health problems of elementary-school children are injuries, infections (including influenza and pneumonia), malnutrition, dental disease, and cancer. The leading problems for high-school students are alcohol and drug abuse, injuries, homicide, pregnancy, sexually transmitted disease, sports injuries, dental disease, and mental and emotional problems.

An ideal school health program would have an interdisciplinary health team consisting of physicians, nurses, dentists, social workers, counselors, school administrators, and parents and students. The school would serve as the site for a family health clinic, which would offer primary health and mental health services to children and adolescents as well as to all family members in the community.

Advanced practice nurses are ideally suited to provide the primary care in these settings, and several schools have established school nurse programs to provide care in the community (Abraham & Fallon, 1997). The advanced practice nurse performs physical examinations and diagnoses and treats students and families for acute and chronic illnesses. These clinics are cost-effective and are especially beneficial for students from low-income families who lack access to health care or have no health insurance.

The roles of the school nurse are care provider, health educator, consultant, and counselor. The school nurse collaborates with students, parents, administrators, and other health and social service professionals regarding a student's health problems. Nurses perform health screenings, give basic care for minor injuries and complaints, administer medications, monitor students' and families' immunization status, and identify children with health problems. They need to be knowledgeable about state and local regulations affecting school-age children, such as ordinances for excluding students from school because of communicable diseases and lice, scabies, or other parasites.

The school nurse is also a health education consultant for teachers. In addition to providing information on health practices, teaching health classes, or helping with the development of the health education curriculum, the school nurse educates the teacher and class when one of the students has a special problem, a disability, or a disease such as hemophilia or AIDS. The school nurse can train volunteers to perform basic health screenings, interpret the results to the parents, make referrals, and follow up to ensure that the student has received adequate care.

Care for the Homeless

No exact figures exist on the number of homeless people in the United States. It is a growing problem and includes increasing numbers of women with children (often abuse victims) and elderly people. The homeless are a heterogeneous group that includes the chronically mentally ill, people who abuse alcohol and other drugs, members of dysfunctional families, the unemployed, and those who cannot find affordable housing. Some are temporarily homeless as a result of catastrophic natural disasters.

The homeless often have difficulty affording or gaining access to health care. Because of numerous obstacles, they seek health care late in the course of the disease and deteriorate more quickly than other patients. Many of the health problems they experience are related in large part to their living situations. Street life exposes the homeless to the extremes of hot and cold environments and compounds their health risks.

The homeless have high rates of trauma, tuberculosis, upper respiratory infection, poor nutrition and anemia, lice, scabies, peripheral vascular problems, sexually transmitted diseases, dental problems, arthritis, hypothermia, and foot problems. Common chronic health problems of the homeless include diabetes, hypertension, heart disease, AIDS, and mental illness. These problems are made more difficult by living on the street and being discharged to a transitory, homeless situation in which follow-up is unlikely (Hunter, Crosby, Ventura, & Warkentin, 1997). The homeless who live in shelters frequently encounter overcrowded, unventilated quarters that provide an ideal environment for the spread of communicable diseases such as tuberculosis.

Community-based nurses who work with the homeless must be nonjudgmental, patient, and understanding. They must be proficient in dealing with many different kinds of people with a wide variety of health problems and needs. Nursing interventions are aimed at attempting to obtain health care services for the homeless and evaluating the health care needs of those who reside in the shelters. A national data networking system would facilitate continuity of care among the homeless and optimal provision of services (Hunter, Crosby, Ventura, & Warkentin, 1997). However, unless the social problems that underlie homelessness are resolved, the plight of the homeless will continue to be a major problem in this country.

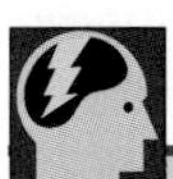

Critical Thinking Exercises

1.
Identify several discharge planning situations in which you have been involved. Evaluate the effectiveness of the processes used to accomplish the goals. What changes could have been made that would have improved the processes and the outcomes?

2.
An elderly man was referred for home care after discharge from the hospital. During the initial visit, the patient's daughter asks how often home care visits will be made and for how long. What assessment criteria will you use to develop answers to these questions? What factors affect the patient's eligibility for home care services versus ambulatory health services?

References and Selected Readings

BOOKS

Cookfair, J. M. (1996). *Nursing care in the community* (2nd ed.). St. Louis: Mosby–Year Book.

Johnson, J. Y., Smith-Temple, A.J., & Carr, P. (1998). *Nurses' guide to home health procedures.* Philadelphia: Lippincott-Raven.

Rice, R. (1995). *Home health nursing procedures.* St Louis: Mosby–Year Book.

JOURNALS

Abraham, T., & Fallon, P. J. (1997). Caring for the community: Development of the advanced practice nurse role. *Clinical Nurse Specialist, 11*(5), 224–229.

Allison, D. M. (1997). The nurse practitioner and culturally diverse populations. *Nurse Practitioner Forum, 8*(1), 4.

Buerhaus, P. I., & Staiger, D. O. (1997). Future of the nurse labor market according to health executives in high managed-care areas of the United States. *Image: Journal of Nursing Scholarship, 29*(4), 313–318.

Centers for Disease Control and Prevention, Hospital Infection Control Practices Advisory Committee, Public Health Service, U.S. Department of Health and Human Services. (1996). Guidelines for isolation precautions in hospitals—Part II: Recommendations for isolation precautions in hospitals. *American Journal of Infection Control, 24*(1), 32–52.

Hunter, J. K., Crosby, F., Ventura, M. R., & Warkentin, L. (1997). Factors limiting evaluation of health care programs for the homeless. *Nursing Outlook, 45*(2), 224–228.

McNeal, G. J. (1996). High-tech home care: An expanding critical care frontier. *Critical Care Nurse, 16*(5), 51–58.

Nugent, K. E., & Lambert, V. A. (1996). The advanced practice nurse in collaborative practice. *Nursing Connections, 9*(1), 5–16.

Porter-O'Grady, T. (1997). Over the horizon: The future and the advanced practice nurse. *Nursing Administration Quarterly, 21*(4), 1–11.

Zotti, M. E., Brown, P., & Stotts, R. C. (1996). Community-based nursing versus community health nursing: What does it all mean? *Nursing Outlook, 44*(5), 211–217.

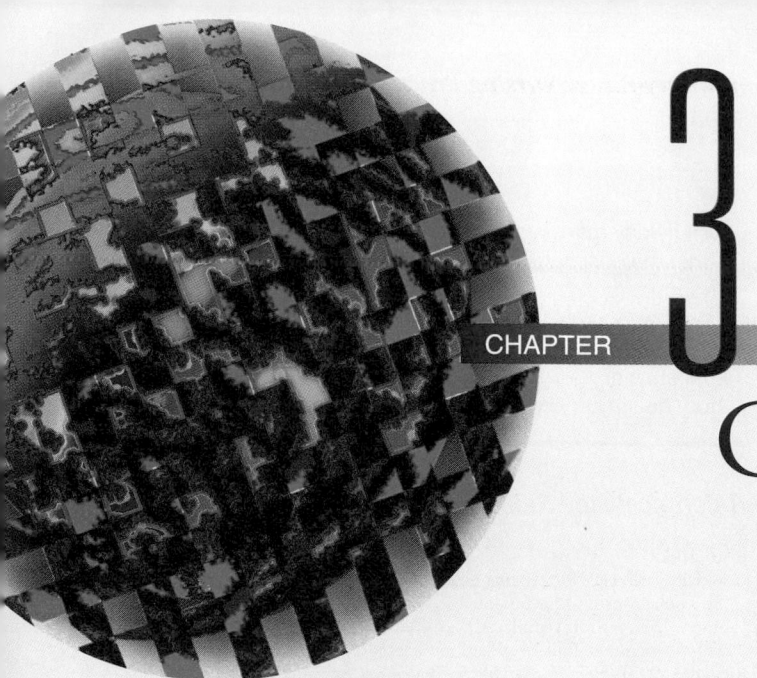

CHAPTER 3

Critical Thinking, Ethical Decision Making, and the Nursing Process

Learning Objectives

On completion of the chapter, the learner will be able to:

1. Define the characteristics of critical thinking and critical thinkers.
2. Describe strategies for and skills of critical thinking.
3. Define ethics and nursing ethics.
4. Identify several ethical dilemmas common to the medical-surgical area of nursing practice.
5. Specify strategies that can be helpful to nurses in ethical decision making.
6. Describe the components of the nursing process.
7. Describe the process of identifying nursing diagnoses, collaborative problems, expected outcomes, and outcome criteria.
8. Identify the purposes and essential components of the plan of nursing care.
9. Develop a plan of nursing care for a patient using strategies of critical thinking.

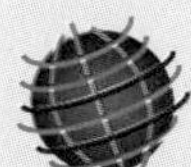

In today's health care arena, the nurse is faced with increasingly complex issues and situations resulting from advanced technology, greater acuity of patients in hospital and community settings, an aging population, complex disease processes, and continually changing ethical and cultural factors. Traditionally, nurses have used a problem-solving approach in planning and providing nursing care. Today the decision-making part of problem solving has become increasingly complex and requires critical thinking.

CRITICAL THINKING

Critical thinking is a cognitive or mental process that involves conscious, systematic, reflective, rational, and goal-oriented examination and analysis of all available information and ideas, and the formulation of conclusions and the most appropriate, often creative, decisions (Alfaro-LeFevre, 1997; Kennison & Brace, 1997).

Critical thinking includes metacognition, examining one's own reasoning or thought process while thinking, a process that helps to strengthen and refine thinking skills (Miller & Babcock, 1996). Independent judgments and decisions evolve from a sound knowledge base and the ability to synthesize information within the context in which it is presented. Nursing practice in today's society mandates the use of high-level critical thinking skills within the nursing process. Critical thinking enhances clinical decision making, helping to identify patient needs and to determine the best nursing actions that will assist the patient in meeting those needs.

Characteristics of Critical Thinking and Critical Thinkers

Critical thinking and critical thinkers have distinctive characteristics. As indicated in the above definition, critical thinking is a conscious, goal-oriented activity; it is purposeful and intentional. The critical thinker is an inquisitive truth-seeker with an open-mindedness to the alternative solutions that might surface.

Rationality and Insight

Critical thinking is also systematic and organized. The critical thinker has a cognitive maturity and an analytic nature (Fonteyn, 1998). Critical thinking is rational, indicating the use of reality-based deliberation with validation of the accuracy of data and the reliability of sources, including monitoring for, recognizing, and questioning inconsistencies. Critical thinking is also reflective, involving metacognition and active evaluation and refinement of the thinking process. Consideration is given to the possibility of personal bias in interpretation of data and determination of appropriate actions. The critical thinker must be insightful, have a sense of fairness and integrity, and have the courage to question personal ethics and the perseverance to strive continuously to minimize the effects of egocentricity, ethnocentricity, and other biases on the decision-making process (Alfaro-LeFevre, 1997; Fonteyn, 1998).

Components of Critical Thinking

Certain cognitive or mental activities can be identified as key components of critical thinking. When thinking critically, a person will:

- Ask questions to determine the reason why certain developments have occurred and to see if more information is needed to understand the situation accurately.
- Gather as much relevant information as possible to consider all factors involved.
- Validate the information presented to make sure that it is accurate, not just supposition or opinion, and that it makes sense and is based on fact and evidence.
- Analyze the information to determine what it means and to see if it forms clusters or patterns that point to certain conclusions.
- Draw on past clinical experience and knowledge to explain what is happening and to anticipate what might happen next, acknowledging personal bias and cultural influences.
- Maintain a flexible attitude that allows the facts to guide the thinking and takes into account all possibilities.
- Consider available options and examine each in terms of its advantages and disadvantages.
- Formulate decisions that reflect creativity and independent decision making.

Critical thinking requires going beyond basic problem solving into a realm of inquisitive exploration, looking for all relevant factors that have an impact on the issue. It includes questioning all findings until a comprehensive picture emerges that explains the phenomenon, possible solutions, and creative methods for proceeding (Kennison & Brace, 1997). Critical thinking in nursing practice results in a comprehensive plan of care with maximized potential for success.

Critical Thinking in Nursing Practice

Using critical thinking to develop a plan of nursing care requires considering the human factors that might have an impact on the plan. The nurse interacts with the patient and numerous other people in the process of providing appropriate, individualized nursing care.

The attitude and thought processes of the nurse, patient, and others will have an impact on the critical thinking process from the data-gathering stage through the decision-making stage; thus, aspects of the nurse–patient interaction must be considered (Miller & Babcock, 1996).

Nurses must use critical thinking skills in all practice settings: acute care, ambulatory, and extended care settings, as well as in the home and community. Regardless of the setting, each patient situation is viewed as unique and dynamic. The unique factors that the patient and nurse bring to the health care situation are considered, studied, analyzed, and interpreted. Interpretation of the information presented then allows the nurse to focus on those factors that are most relevant and most significant to the clinical situation. Decisions about what to do and how to do it are then developed into a plan of action.

Fonteyn (1998) identified 12 predominant thinking strategies used by nurses, regardless of their area of clinical practice. These strategies are recognizing a pattern, setting priorities, searching for information, generating hypotheses, making predictions, forming relationships, stating a proposition (if___then), asserting a practice rule, making choices (alternative actions), judging the value, drawing conclusions, and providing explanations. Fonteyn further identified other less prominent thinking strategies the nurse might use: pondering, posing a question, making assumptions (supposing), qualifying, and making generalizations. These thought processes are consistent with the characteristics of critical thinking and cognitive activities discussed above. Fonteyn asserted that exploring how these thinking strategies are used in varied clinical situations, and practicing using the strategies, might assist the nurse-learner in examining and refining his or her own thinking skills.

The critical thinking skills necessary for making decisions in nursing are used in all steps of the nursing process. Developing the skill of critical thinking takes time and practice (Jacobs et al., 1997). Throughout this text, critical thinking exercises are offered as a means of practicing one's ability to think critically. Additional exercises can be found in the Study Guide that accompanies the text. The questions listed in Chart 3-1 can serve as a guide in working through the exercises, although it is important to remember that each situation is unique and calls for an approach that fits the particular circumstances being described.

ETHICAL NURSING CARE

In the complex world in which we live, we are surrounded by ethical issues in all facets of our lives. Consequently, there has been a heightened interest in the field of ethics in an attempt to gain a better understanding of how these issues influence us. Specifically, in health care the focus on ethics has intensified in response to controversial developments, including increased technological advances and diminished health care and financial resources. Both of these areas have an impact on the role of the professional nurse.

CHART 3•1 The Inquiring Mind: Critical Thinking in Action

Throughout the critical thinking process, a continuous flow of questions evolves in the thinker's mind. Although the questions will vary according to the particular clinical situation, certain general inquiries can serve as a basis for reaching conclusions and determining a course of action.

When faced with a patient situation, it is often helpful to seek answers to some or all of the following questions in an attempt to determine those actions that are most appropriate:

- What relevant assessment information do I need, and how do I interpret this information? What does this information tell me?
- What problems does this information point to? Have I identified the most important ones? Does the information point to any other problems that I should consider?
- Have I gathered all the information I need (signs/symptoms, laboratory values, medication history, emotional factors, mental status)? Is anything missing?
- Is there anything that needs to be reported immediately? Do I need to seek additional assistance?
- Does this patient have any special risk factors? Which ones are most significant? What must I do to minimize these risks?
- What possible complications must I watch for?
- What are the most important problems that we are facing in this situation? Do the patient and the patient's family see the same problems?
- What are the desired outcomes for this patient? Which have the highest priority? Do the patient and I see eye to eye on these points?
- What is going to be my first action in this situation?
- How can I construct a plan of care to achieve the goals?
- Are there any age-related factors involved, and will they require some special approach? Will I need to make some change in the plan of care to take these factors into account?
- How do the family dynamics affect this situation, and will this have an impact on my actions or plan of care?
- Are there cultural factors that I must address and consider?
- Am I dealing with an ethical problem here? If so, how am I going to resolve it?
- Has any nursing research been conducted on this subject?

Today, sophisticated technology can prolong life well beyond the time when death would have occurred in the past. Expensive experimental procedures and medications are available for use in attempting to preserve life, even when such attempts are likely to fail. The development of technological support has had an influence on all stages of life. For example, the prenatal period has been influenced by genetic screening, *in vitro* fertilization, the harvesting and freezing of embryos, and prenatal surgery. In the early stages of life, premature infants are given a chance for survival as a result of technical support. Children and adults who would have died as a result of organ failure are living longer because of organ transplants. Technological advances have also contributed to an increase in the average life expectancy. However, these advances in technology have been a mixed blessing. Questions have been raised about whether, and under what circumstances, it is appropriate to use this technology. Although many individuals are afforded a better quality of life, others face extended suffering as a result of efforts to prolong life, usually at great expense. Ethical issues surround those practices or policies that seem to allocate health care resources unjustly on the basis of age, race, gender, or social mores.

DOMAIN OF NURSING ETHICS

The ethical dilemmas a nurse may encounter in the medical-surgical arena are numerous and diverse. An awareness of the underlying philosophical concepts will help the nurse to reason through these dilemmas. Basic concepts related to moral philosophy, such as ethics terminology, theories, and approaches, are included in this chapter. Understanding the role of the professional nurse in ethical decision making will assist nurses in articulating their ethical positions and in developing the skills needed to make ethical decisions.

Ethics Versus Morality

The terms ethics and morality are used in relation to beliefs about right and wrong and to appropriate guidelines for action. In essence, ethics is the formal, systematic study of moral beliefs, whereas morality is the adherence to informal personal values. Because the distinction between the two is slight, they are often used interchangeably.

Ethics Theories

One classic theory in ethics is teleological or consequentialism theory, which focuses on the ends or consequences of actions. The most well-known form of this theory, utilitarian theory, is based on the concept of "the greatest good for the greatest number." The choice of action is clear under this theory, since the action that maximizes good over bad is the correct one. The difficulty with this theory comes when one has to judge intrinsic values and determine whose good is the greatest. Additionally, the question must be asked whether good consequences can justify any amoral actions that might be used to achieve them.

Another theory in ethics is deontological or formalist theory, which argues that moral standards or principles exist independently of the ends or consequences. In a given situation, one or more moral principles may apply. The nurse has a duty to act based on the one primary, or the most primary of several, moral principles.

CHART 3•2 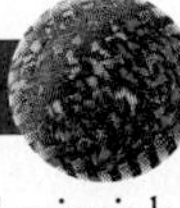 **Common Ethical Principles**

Common ethical principles one may use to validate moral claims:

Autonomy

Derived from the Greek words *autos* ("self") and *nomos* ("rule" or "law"), and thus refers to self-rule. In contemporary discourse it has broad meanings, including individual rights, privacy, and choice. Autonomy entails the ability to make a choice free from external constraints.

Beneficence

The duty to do good and the active promotion of benevolent acts (eg, goodness, kindness, and charity). May also include the injunction not to inflict harm (see *Nonmaleficence*).

Confidentiality

This principle relates to the concept of privacy. Information obtained from an individual will not be disclosed to another unless it will benefit the person or there is a direct threat to the social good.

Double Effect

A principle that may morally justify some actions that may produce both good and evil effects. All four of the following criteria must be fulfilled:

1. The action itself is good or morally neutral.
2. The agent sincerely intends the good and not the evil effect (the evil effect may be foreseen but not intended).
3. The good effect is not achieved by means of the evil effect.
4. There is proportionate or favorable balance of good over evil.

Fidelity

Promise keeping; the duty to be faithful to one's commitments. It includes both explicit and implicit promises to another.

Justice

From a broad perspective, justice states that like cases should be treated alike. A more restricted version of justice is distributive justice, which refers to the distribution of social benefits and burdens. Various theories of distributive justice may include the following notions: That each person receive

1. Equally
2. According to need
3. According to effort
4. According to societal contribution
5. According to merit
6. According to legal entitlement

Retributive justice is concerned with the distribution of punishment.

Nonmaleficence

The duty not to inflict as well as to prevent and remove harm. Nonmaleficence may be included within the principle of beneficence, in which case nonmaleficence would be more binding.

Paternalism

The intentional limitation of another's autonomy, justified by an appeal to beneficence or the welfare or needs of another. Thus, the prevention of any evils or harm is greater than any potential evils caused by the interference of the individual's autonomy or liberty.

Respect for Persons

Frequently used synonymously with autonomy. However, it goes beyond accepting the notion or attitude that people have autonomous choice to treat others in such a way that enables them to make the choice.

Sanctity of Life

The perspective that life is the highest good. Thus, all forms of life, including mere biologic existence, should take precedence over external criteria for judging quality of life.

Veracity

The obligation to tell the truth and not to lie or deceive others.

Approaches to Ethics

Two approaches to ethics are metaethics and applied ethics. An example of metaethics (understanding the concepts and linguistic terminology used in ethics) in the health care environment would be analysis of the concept of informed consent. Nurses are aware that patients must give consent before surgery, but sometimes a question arises as to whether the patient is truly informed. Delving deeper into the concept of informed consent would be a metaethical inquiry.

Applied ethics is the term used when questions are asked of a specific discipline to identify ethical problems within that discipline's practice. Various disciplines use the frameworks of general ethical theories and moral principles and apply them to specific problems within their domain.

Common ethical principles that apply in nursing include autonomy, beneficence, confidentiality, double effect, fidelity, justice, nonmaleficence, paternalism, respect for people, sanctity of life, and veracity. Brief definitions of these important principles can be found in Chart 3-2.

Nursing ethics may be considered a distinct form of applied ethics because it addresses many moral situations that are specific to the nursing profession. Some ethical problems that affect nursing may also apply to the broader area of health care ethics. However, because the nursing profession is a "caring" rather than a predominantly "curing" profession, with its own professional code of ethics, it is *imperative* that one not equate nursing ethics solely with medical ethics.

Moral Situations

Many situations exist in which ethical analysis is needed. Some are moral dilemmas, situations in which a clear conflict exists between two or more moral principles or competing moral claims, and the nurse must choose the lesser of two evils. Other situations represent moral problems, in which there may be competing moral claims or principles but one claim or principle is clearly dominant. Some situations result in moral uncertainty, when one cannot accurately define what the moral situation is or what moral principles apply, but has a strong feeling that something is not right. Still other situations may result in moral distress, in which the nurse is aware of the correct course of action, but institutional constraints stand in the way of pursuing the correct action (Jameton, 1984).

For example, a patient tells a nurse that if he is dying he wants everything possible done. The surgeon and family have made the decision not to tell the patient he is terminally ill and not to resuscitate him if he stops breathing. From an ethical perspective, patients should be told the truth about their diagnoses and should have the opportunity to make decisions about treatments. Ideally, this information should come from the physician, with the nurse present to assist the patient in understanding the terminology and to provide further support, if necessary. A moral problem exists because of the competing moral claims of the family and physician, who wish to spare the patient distress, and the nurse, who wishes to be truthful with the patient *as the patient has requested.* If the patient's competency were questionable, a moral dilemma would exist because no dominant principle would be evident. The nurse could experience moral distress if the hospital threatens disciplinary action or job termination if the information is disclosed without the agreement of the physician and/or the family.

It is essential that nurses freely engage in dialogue concerning moral situations, even though such dialogue is difficult for everyone involved. Improved interdisciplinary communication is supported when all members of the health care team can voice their concerns and come to an understanding of the moral situation (Heitman & Robinson, 1997).

Types of Ethical Problems in Nursing

As a profession, nursing is accountable to society. This accountability is spelled out in the American Hospital Association's Patient's Bill of Rights (see Chap. 1), which reflects social beliefs about health and health care. In addition to accepting this document as one measure of accountability, nursing has further defined its standards of accountability through a formal code of ethics that explicitly states nursing's values and goals. The code (Chart 3-3), established by the American Nurses Association (1985), consists of ethical standards, each with its own interpretive statements. A revision of the code is pending publication; however, the current code offers interpretive statements amplified to incorporate universal moral principles (Daly, 1997). The code is an ideal framework for nurses to use in ethical decision making.

Ethical issues have always had an impact on the role of the professional nurse. The accepted definition of professional nursing has inspired a new advocacy role for nurses. The American Nurses Association, in its publication *Nursing's Social Policy Statement* (1995), defines nursing as "the diagnosis and treatment of human responses to health and illness." This definition supports the claim that nurses must be actively involved in the decision-making process regarding ethical concerns surrounding health care and human responses. This belief, however, may come into conflict in health care settings in which the traditional roles of the nurse are delineated within a bureaucratic structure (Heitman & Robinson, 1997). Health care settings in which nurses are valued members of the team promote interdisciplinary communication and may enhance patient care. To practice effectively in these settings, nurses must be aware of ethical issues and assist patients in voicing their moral concerns.

This perspective underscores the basic ethical framework of the nursing profession: the phenomenon of human caring. Nursing theories that incorporate the biopsychosocial–spiritual dimensions portray a holistic viewpoint with humanism or caring as the core. As the nursing profession strives to delineate its own theory of ethics, *caring* is often cited as the *moral* foundation. For nurses to embrace this professional ethos, it is necessary to be aware not only of major ethical dilemmas but also of those daily interactions with health care consumers that frequently give rise to ethical challenges that are not as easily identified (Erlen, 1997). Although technological advances and diminished resources have been instrumental in raising numerous ethical questions and controversies, including life-and-death issues, nurses should not ignore the many routine situations that involve ethical considerations. Some of the primary issues faced by nurses today include confidentiality, use of restraints, trust, refusing care, and end-of-life issues.

Confidentiality

We all need to be aware of the confidential nature of information obtained in daily practice. If information is not pertinent to a case, the nurse should question if it is prudent to record it in the patient's chart. In the practice setting, discussion of the patient with other members of the health care team is often necessary. However, these discussions should occur in a private area where it is unlikely that the conversation can be overheard.

Another threat to keeping information confidential is the widespread use of computers and the easy access people have to them. This can increase the potential for misuse of information that may have negative social consequences. For example, laboratory results regarding AIDS testing or genetic screening may lead to loss of employment or insurance if the information is disclosed. Because of these possibilities, sensitivity to the principle of confidentiality is essential (Scanlon & Fibison, 1995).

Restraints

The use of restraints is another area that carries ethical overtones. It is important to weigh carefully the risks of limiting a person's autonomy by using restraints (including physical and pharmacologic measures) against the safety risks involved in not using restraints (Constantino, Boneysteele, Gesmond, & Nelson, 1997).

CHART 3•3 American Nurses Association Code for Nurses

1. The nurse provides services with respect for human dignity and the uniqueness of the client, unrestricted by considerations of social or economic status, personal attributes, or the nature of the health problems.
2. The nurse safeguards the client's right to privacy by judiciously protecting information of a confidential nature.
3. The nurse acts to safeguard the client and the public when health care and safety are affected by the incompetent, unethical, or illegal practice of any person.
4. The nurse assumes responsibility and accountability for individual nursing judgments and actions.
5. The nurse maintains competence in nursing.
6. The nurse exercises informed judgment and uses individual competence and qualifications as criteria in seeking consultation, accepting responsibilities, and delegating nursing activities to others.
7. The nurse participates in activities that contribute to the ongoing development of the profession's body of knowledge.
8. The nurse participates in the profession's efforts to implement and improve standards of nursing.
9. The nurse participates in the profession's efforts to establish and maintain conditions of employment conducive to high-quality nursing care.
10. The nurse participates in the profession's effort to protect the public from misinformation and misrepresentation and to maintain the integrity of nursing.
11. The nurse collaborates with members of the health professions and other citizens in promoting community and national efforts to meet the health needs of the public.

Before restraints are used, other strategies, such as asking family to sit with the patient, should be tried.

Trust Issues

Telling the truth is one of the basic principles in our cultural mores. Two ethical dilemmas in clinical practice that can come in direct conflict with this principle of veracity are the use of placebos (nonactive drugs) and not revealing a diagnosis to the patient. Both involve the issue of trust, which is an essential element in the nurse–patient relationship. The use of a placebo (other than in experimental research in which the patient is involved in the decision-making process and is aware that placebos are being used in the treatment regimen) as a substitute for an active drug to show that a patient does not have real pain is deceptive. This practice may severely undermine the nurse–patient relationship.

Informing patients of their diagnoses when the family and physician have chosen to withhold information is a common ethical situation in nursing practice. The nursing staff often use evasive comments with the patient as a means to maintain professional relationships with other health practitioners. This area is indeed complex because it challenges the nurse's integrity (Ballinger, 1997). Some strategies the nurse could consider in this situation include:

- Not lying to the patient
- Providing all information related to nursing procedures and diagnoses
- Communicating to the family and physician the patient's requests for information

Families often are unaware of the patient's repeated questions to the nurse. With a better understanding of the situation, families may change their perspective. Finally, although providing the information may be the morally appropriate behavior, the manner in which the patient is told is important. Nurses must be compassionate and caring while informing patients; disclosure of information merely for the sake of patient autonomy does not convey respect for others.

Refusing Care

Any nurse who feels compelled to refuse to provide care for a particular type of patient faces an ethical dilemma. The reasons given for refusal range from a conflict of personal values to fear of personal risk of injury (Sherman, 1996). Such instances have increased with the advent of AIDS as a major health problem.

The ethical obligation to care for all patients is clearly identified in Statement One of the Nursing Code of Ethics. However, to avoid facing these moral situations, a nurse can follow certain strategies. For example, when applying for a job, one should ask questions regarding the patient population. If one is uncomfortable with a particular situation, then a choice would be not to accept the position. The denial of care, or providing substandard nursing care to some members of our society, is not acceptable nursing practice.

End-of Life Issues

Dilemmas that revolve around death and dying are prevalent in medical-surgical practice and frequently initiate moral discussion. The dilemmas are compounded by the fact that the idea of curing is paramount in health care. With advanced technology, it may be difficult to accept the fact that nothing more can be done, or that technology may prolong life, but at the expense of comfort and quality of life. Focusing on the caring as well as the curing role may assist nurses in dealing with these difficult moral situations.

PAIN CONTROL

The use of narcotics to alleviate a patient's pain may present a dilemma for nurses. Patients with excruciating pain may require large doses of analgesics. Fear of respiratory depression or unwarranted fear of addiction should not prevent nurses from attempting to alleviate pain for the dying patient or a patient experiencing an acute pain episode. In the case of the terminally ill patient, for example, the actions may be justified by the principle of double effect (see definition in Chart 3-2). The intent or goal of nursing interventions is to alleviate pain and suffering while promoting comfort. The risk of respiratory depression is not the intent of the actions and should not be used as an excuse for withholding analgesia. However, the patient's respiratory status should be carefully monitored and any signs of respiratory depression reported to the physician. The administration of analgesia should be governed by the patient's needs without unethical judgment by the nurse.

DNR ORDERS

The "do-not-resuscitate" (DNR) order is frequently a controversial issue. When a patient is competent to make decisions, his or her choice for a DNR order should be honored, according to the principles of autonomy or respect for the individual (Mason, 1997). However, a DNR order is at times interpreted to mean that the patient requires less nursing care, when these patients actually have significant medical and nursing needs, all of which demand attention. Ethically, all patients deserve and should receive appropriate nursing interventions, regardless of their resuscitation status.

LIFE SUPPORT

In contrast to the previous situations are those in which the decision not to resuscitate has not been made for a dying patient. The nurse may be put in the uncomfortable position of initiating life-support measures when, because of the patient's status, they appear futile. This frequently occurs when the patient is not competent to make the decision and the family (or surrogate decision maker) refuses DNR as an option. The nurse may be told to perform a "slow code" (ie, not to rush to resuscitate the patient) or given a verbal order not to resuscitate the patient. Both are unacceptable medical orders. The best recourse for nurses in these situations is to open communication. Discussing the matter with the physician may lead to further communication with the family and to a reconsideration of their decision, especially if they are afraid to let a loved one die with no further efforts to resuscitate. Finally, when working with colleagues who are confronting such difficult situations, it helps to talk and listen to their concerns as a way of providing support.

FOOD AND FLUID

In addition to requesting that no heroic measures be taken to prolong life, a dying patient may request that no more food or fluid be administered. Many individuals think that food and hydration are basic human needs, not "invasive measures"; thus, they should always be maintained. However, some consider food and hydration as means of prolonging suffering. In evaluating this issue, nurses must take into consideration the potential harm as well as the benefit to the patient of either administering or withdrawing sustenance. Research has not supported the belief that withholding fluids results in painful death due to thirst (Smith, 1997; Zerwekh, 1997).

Evaluation of harm necessitates a careful review of the reasons the person has requested the withdrawal of food and hydration. Although the principle of autonomy has considerable merit and is supported by the ethics code for nurses, there may be situations when the request for withdrawal of food and hydration cannot be upheld. For patients who are not competent, the issues are more complex. Some of these cases have reached courts of law, and different states have different case law precedents forbidding withdrawal of sustenance. At present, there are no firm guidelines to assist nurses in this area.

PREVENTIVE ETHICS

As previously mentioned, a dilemma refers to a conflict between two alternatives. In such instances, one's moral decision is to choose the lesser evil of the two. However, there are various strategies available to assist nurses in ethical decision making. These strategies are referred to as "preventive" because they may be helpful in anticipating and avoiding certain kinds of ethical dilemmas.

Frequently, dilemmas occur when the health care practitioners are unsure of the patient's wishes because the person is unconscious or too cognitively impaired to communicate directly. One famous court case in this area of clinical ethics is that of Nancy Cruzan. Nancy Cruzan was a young woman involved in a single-car crash, after which she remained in a persistent vegetative state. Her family endured a 3-year legal battle to have her feeding tube removed so that she could be allowed to die. The U.S. Supreme Court decided that a state may require "clear and convincing evidence" of the patient's wishes before withdrawing life support. This ruling and the public response to it served as an impetus to legislation on advance directives, entitled the Patient Self-Determination Act, that became effective in December 1991. The intent of this legislation is to encourage people to prepare advance directives in which they indicate their wishes concerning the degree of supportive care to be provided if they become incapacitated. The regulatory language is quite broad and allows for different institutions to have latitude in implementing the person's directives. This legislation does not require a patient to have an advance directive, but it does require that the patient be informed about them. Consequently, this is an area where nursing can play a significant role in patient education.

Advance Directives

Advance directives provide valuable information and may assist health care providers in decision making. Advance directives are legal documents that specify the patient's wishes before hospitalization. A living will is one type of advance directive. In most situations, living wills are limited to situations where the patient's medical condition is deemed terminal. Because it is difficult to define "terminal" accurately, the living will is not always honored. Another potential drawback to the living will is that these documents are frequently written when the person is in good health. It is not unusual for people to change their minds as their illness progresses. Therefore, the patient retains the option to nullify the document.

Another type of advance directive is the durable power of attorney. With the power of attorney, the patient has identified another individual to make decisions on his or her behalf. In this type of decision making, the patient may have clarified his or her wishes concerning a variety of medical situations. As such, the power of attorney is a less restrictive type of advance directive. These advance directives vary among state jurisdictions. However, even in states where these documents are not legally binding, they provide helpful information. They assist health care practitioners in determining the patient's prior expressed wishes in situations where this information can no longer be obtained directly.

Another type of preventive ethics is available through institutional ethics committees, which exist in many hospitals to assist practitioners with ethical dilemmas. The purpose of these multidisciplinary committees may vary among institutions. In some hospitals, the committee exists solely for the purpose of developing policies; others may have a strong education or consultation focus. Because these committees usually comprise individuals with some advanced background in ethical decision making, nurses can consult the committee members. Nurses with a particular interest or expertise in the area of ethics are valuable members of ethics committees and can serve as valuable resources for staff nurses (Heitman & Robinson, 1997).

The heightened interest in ethical decision making has resulted in many continuing education programs, ranging from small seminars or workshops to full-semester courses offered by local colleges or professional organizations. In addition, nursing and medical journals contain articles on ethical issues, and numerous textbooks on clinical ethics or nursing ethics are available. These are valuable resources because they cover the ethical theory and dilemmas of practice in greater depth. The American Nurses Association also has publications available to assist nurses in this field of inquiry.

Ethical Decision Making

As noted in the preceding discussions, ethical dilemmas are common and diverse in nursing practice. Although the situations vary, the fundamental philosophical principles remain. Experience indicates that there are no clear solutions to these dilemmas. The process of moral reflection will help nurses to justify their actions.

The approach to ethical decision making can follow the steps of the nursing process. Chart 3-4 outlines the steps of an ethical analysis.

STEPS OF THE NURSING PROCESS

The nursing process is a deliberate problem-solving approach for meeting a person's health care and nursing needs. Although the steps of the nursing process have been stated in various ways by different writers, the common components cited are assessment, diagnosis, planning, implementation, and evaluation. The ANA's *Standards of Clinical Nursing Practice* (1998) include an additional component entitled outcome identification and established the sequence of steps in the following order: assessment, diagnosis, outcome identification, planning, implementation, and evaluation. For the purposes of this text, the nursing process will be based on the traditional five steps and will delineate two components in the diagnosis step: nursing diagnoses and collaborative problems. The steps are defined as follows:

1. *Assessment*—the systematic collection of data to determine the patient's health status and identify any actual or potential health problems. (Analysis of data is included as part of the assessment. For those who wish to emphasize its importance, analysis may be identified as a separate step of the nursing process.)
2. *Diagnosis*—identification of the following two types of patient problems:

CHART 3•4 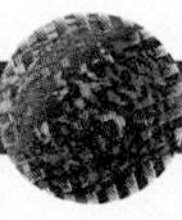 **Steps of an Ethical Analysis**

The following are guidelines to assist nurses in ethical decision making. These guidelines reflect an active process in decision making, similar to the nursing process detailed in this chapter.

Assessment

1. Assess the ethical/moral situations of the problem. This step entails the recognition of the ethical, legal, and professional dimensions of the situation.
   a. Does the situation entail *substantive* moral problems (conflicts among ethical principles or professional obligations)?
   b. Are there *procedural* conflicts? (For example, who should make the decisions? Any conflicts among the health care providers, family, guardians, and patient?)
   c. Identify the significant people involved and those affected by the decision.

Planning

2. Collect information.
   a. Include the following information: the medical facts, treatment options, nursing diagnoses, legal data, and the values, beliefs, and religious components.
   b. Make a distinction between the factual and the values/beliefs.
   c. Validate the patient's capacity, or lack of capacity, to make decisions.
   d. Identify any other relevant information that should be elicited.
   e. Identify the ethical/moral issues and the competing claims.

Implementation

3. List the alternatives. Compare alternatives with applicable ethical principles and professional code of ethics. May choose either framework below, or other frameworks, and compare outcomes.

Utilitarian Approach

   a. Predict the consequences of the alternatives.
   b. Assign a positive or negative value to each consequence.
   c. Choose the consequence that predicts the highest positive value or "the greatest good for the greatest number."

Deontological Approach

   a. Identify the relevant moral principles.
   b. Compare alternatives with moral principles.
   c. Appeal to the "higher-level" moral principle if there is a conflict.

Evaluation

4. Decide and evaluate the decision.
   a. What is the best or morally correct action?
   b. Give the ethical reasons for your decision.
   c. What are the ethical reasons against your decision?
   d. How do you respond to the reasons against your decision?

---

   a. *Nursing diagnoses*—actual or potential health problems that can be managed by independent nursing interventions
   b. *Collaborative problems*—"certain physiologic complications that nurses monitor to detect onset or changes in status. Nurses manage collaborative problems using physician-prescribed and nursing-prescribed interventions to minimize the complications of the events" (Carpenito, 1999, p. 7).
3. *Planning*—development of goals and a plan of care designed to assist the patient in resolving the diagnosed problems and achieving the identified goals
4. *Implementation*—actualization of the plan of care through nursing interventions
5. *Evaluation*—determination of the patient's responses to the nursing interventions and the extent to which the outcomes have been achieved

Dividing the nursing process into five distinct steps serves to emphasize the essential nursing actions that must be taken to resolve the patient's nursing diagnoses and manage any collaborative problems or complications. However, dividing the process into separate steps is artificial: the process functions as an integrated whole, with the steps being interrelated, interdependent, and recurrent (Fig. 3-1). Chart 3-5 presents an overview of the nursing activities involved in applying the nursing process.

ASSESSMENT

Assessment data are gathered through the health history and the health assessment. In addition, ongoing monitoring is crucial to remain aware of patient needs and the effectiveness of the nursing care that the patient receives.

Health History

The health history is conducted to determine the individual's state of wellness or illness and is best accomplished as part of a planned interview. The interview is a dialogue between the patient and the nurse and involves the sensitive direction of conversation in order to obtain information. The nurse's approach to the person will largely determine the amount and quality of information that are received. Achieving a relationship of mutual trust and respect

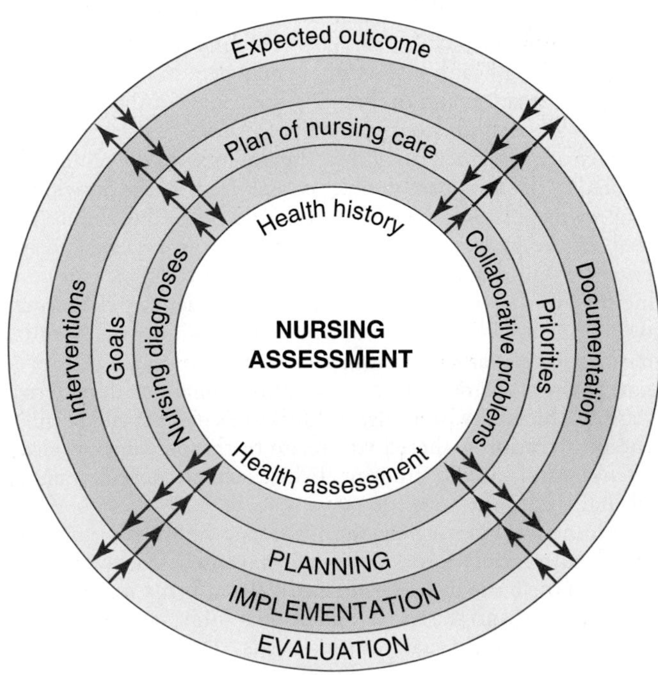

FIGURE 3•1 The nursing process is depicted schematically in this circle. Starting from the innermost circle, nursing assessment, the process moves outward through the formulation of nursing diagnoses and collaborative problems, planning, the setting of goals and priorities, establishing the nursing care plan, and actual implementation and documentation, and arrives at the ongoing process of evaluation and expected outcomes.

CHART 3•5 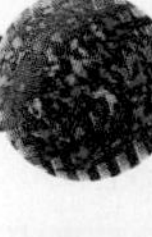 **Steps of the Nursing Process**

Assessment

1. Conduct the health history.
2. Perform the health assessment.
3. Interview the patient's family or significant others.
4. Study the health record.
5. Organize, analyze, synthesize, and summarize the collected data.

Diagnosis

Nursing Diagnosis

1. Identify the patient's nursing problems.
2. Identify the defining characteristics of the nursing problems.
3. Identify the etiology of the nursing problems.
4. State nursing diagnoses concisely and precisely.

Collaborative Problems

1. Identify potential problems or complications that require collaborative interventions.
2. Identify health team members with whom collaboration is essential.

Planning

1. Assign priority to the nursing diagnoses.
2. Specify the goals.
   a. Develop immediate, intermediate, and long-term goals.
   b. State the goals in realistic and measurable terms.
3. Identify nursing interventions appropriate for goal attainment.
4. Establish expected outcomes.
   a. Make sure that the outcomes are realistic and measurable.
   b. Identify critical times for the attainment of outcomes.
5. Develop the written plan of nursing care.
   a. Include nursing diagnoses, goals, nursing interventions, expected outcomes, and critical times.
   b. Write all entries precisely, concisely, and systematically.
   c. Keep the plan current and flexible to meet the patient's changing problems and needs.
6. Involve the patient, family or significant others, nursing team members, and other health team members in all aspects of planning.

Implementation

1. Put the plan of nursing care into action.
2. Coordinate the activities of the patient, family or significant others, nursing team members, and other health team members.
3. Record the patient's responses to the nursing actions.

Evaluation

1. Collect objective data.
2. Compare the patient's behavioral outcomes with the expected outcomes. Determine the extent to which the goals were achieved.
3. Include the patient, family or significant others, nursing team members, and other health care team members in the evaluation.
4. Identify alterations that need to be made in the nursing diagnoses, collaborative problems, goals, nursing interventions, and expected outcomes.
5. Continue all steps of the nursing process: assessment, diagnosis, planning, implementation, and evaluation.

requires the ability to communicate a sincere interest in the person. Examples of effective therapeutic communication techniques that can be used to achieve this goal are found in Table 3-1.

The use of a health history guide may help in obtaining pertinent information and in directing the course of the interview. A variety of health history formats are available. Although these formats are designed to guide the interview, they must be adapted to the responses, problems, and needs of the individual. If a previous history is available, it should be used to reduce the need for the patient to repeat information. An experienced interviewer will develop a comfortable style and format for conducting an interview and will be flexible in adapting the format to suit the individual situation, while still obtaining the essential information. A variety of models can serve as frameworks for acquiring the assessment data, such as functional health patterns, Maslow's hierarchy of needs, and Erikson's eight stages of man. The information gathered will relate to the person's physical, psychological, social, emotional, intellectual, developmental, cultural, and spiritual needs.

In some instances it may be appropriate for the patient to fill out a health history form. When a form is used, it is the responsibility of the nurse to verify and clarify the information provided by the patient and to seek any additional information necessary to identify the individual's nursing needs.

Physical Assessment

A physical assessment may be carried out before, during, or after the health history, depending on the patient's physical and emotional state and the immediate priorities of the situation.

The purpose of the health assessment is to identify those aspects of the person's physical, psychological, and emotional state that indicate the existence of a nursing need. It requires the use of sight, hearing, touch, and smell as well as the appropriate interview skills and techniques. Physical examination techniques as well as techniques and strategies for assessing behaviors and role changes are discussed in Chapters 5 and 7.

Other Components of the Database

Additional relevant information should be obtained from the person's family or significant others, from other members of the health team, and from the person's health record or chart. Depending on the person's immediate illness needs, this information may have been obtained before the health history and the physical assessment. Whatever the sequence of events, it is important to use all available sources of pertinent data to complete the nursing assessment.

Recording the Database

After the health history and health assessment are completed, the information obtained is recorded in the patient's permanent record. The record provides a means of communication between the members of the health care team and facilitates coordinated planning and continuity of care. The record fulfills other functions as well:

- It serves as the business and legal record for the health care agency and for the professional staff responsible for the person's care.
- It serves as a basis for evaluating the quality and appropriateness of care as well as for reviewing the effective use of patient care services.
- It provides data useful in research, education, and short- and long-range planning.

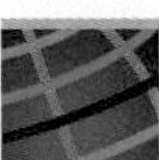

TABLE 3•1 **Summary of Therapeutic Communication Techniques**

Technique	Definition	Therapeutic Value
Listening	An active process of receiving information and examining one's reaction to the messages received	Nonverbally communicates nurse's interest in patient
Silence	Periods of no verbal communication among participants	Nonverbally communicates nurse's acceptance of patient
Establishing guidelines	Statements regarding roles, purpose, and limitations for a particular interaction	Helps patient to know what is expected of him/her
Open-ended comments	General comments asking the patient to determine the direction the interaction should take	Allows patient to decide what material is most relevant and encourages him/her to continue
Reducing distance	Diminishing physical space between the nurse and patient	Nonverbally communicates that nurse wants to be involved with patient
Acknowledgment	Recognition given to a patient for contribution to an interaction	Demonstrates the importance of the patient's role within the relationship
Restating	Repeating to the patient what the nurse believes is the main thought or idea expressed	Asks for validation of nurse's interpretation of the message
Reflecting	Directing back to the patient his ideas, feelings, questions, or content	Attempts to show patient the importance of his/her own ideas, feelings, and interpretations
Seeking clarification	Asking for additional inputs to understand the message received	Demonstrates nurse's desire to understand patient's communication
Seeking consensual validation	Attempts to reach a mutual denotative and connotative meaning of specific words	Demonstrates nurse's desire to understand patient's communication
Focusing	Questions or statements to help the patient develop or expand an idea	Directs conversation toward topics of importance
Summarizing	Statement of main areas discussed during interaction	Helps patient to separate relevant from irrelevant material; serves as a review and closing for the interaction
Planning	Mutual decision making regarding the goals, direction, and so on, of future interactions	Reiterates patient's role within relationship

Reprinted with permission from Sundeen, S. J. et al. (1994). *Nurse-client interaction: Interpreting the nursing process.* St. Louis: Mosby–Year Book.

There are a variety of systems used for documenting patient care. Each health care agency selects the system that best meets its needs. The types of systems available include the problem-oriented health record system or more simplified charting processes such as focus charting, patient outcome charting, problem intervention evaluation (PIE) charting, and charting by exception (CBE). In addition, many health care agencies have moved toward computerized documentation systems; these appear to save time, improve the monitoring of quality improvement issues, and make it easier to gain access to patient information.

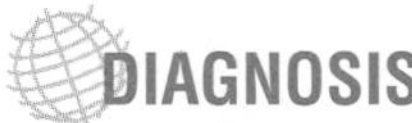

DIAGNOSIS

The assessment component of the nursing process serves as the basis for identifying nursing diagnoses and collaborative problems. Soon after the completion of the health history and the physical assessment, the nurse organizes, analyzes, synthesizes, and summarizes the data collected and determines the patient's need for nursing care.

Nursing Diagnosis

Nursing, unlike medicine, does not yet have a complete taxonomy of diagnostic labels that convey the same meaning to all nurses. A taxonomy is a classification system. Classifying discrete items into meaningful categories organizes components of knowledge into coherent units of related information. Some reasons for establishing taxonomies are to help identify what is known about a field of study, to discover what gaps in knowledge exist, to provide a common language that enhances communication among colleagues, and to facilitate the coding of standardized information for use in databases. Nursing diagnoses, the first taxonomy created in nursing, have fostered the development of autonomy and accountability in nursing and have helped to delineate the scope of practice. Many state nurse practice acts include nursing diagnosis as a nursing function, and nursing diagnosis is included in the American Nurses Association's standards of nursing practice and those of many nursing specialty organizations.

The official organization that has assumed responsibility for developing the taxonomy of nursing diagnoses and formulating nursing diagnoses acceptable for study is the North American Nursing Diagnosis Association (NANDA). NANDA has grouped diagnoses according to patterns of human responses (Chart 3-6). The diagnostic labels identified by NANDA have been generally accepted but require further validation and expansion based on clinical use and research; they are not yet complete or mutually exclusive, and more investigation is needed to determine their validity and clinical applicability.

Choosing a Nursing Diagnosis

When choosing the nursing diagnoses for a particular patient, the nurse must first identify the commonalities among the assessment data collected. These common features lead to the categorization of

CHART 3•6 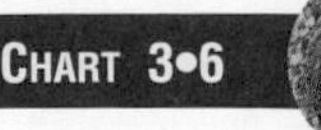 **NANDA-Approved Nursing Diagnoses — 1999–2000**

This list represents the NANDA-approved nursing diagnoses for clinical use and testing.

Pattern 1: Exchanging

- Altered Nutrition: More Than Body Requirements
- Altered Nutrition: Less Than Body Requirements
- Altered Nutrition: Risk for More Than Body Requirements
- Risk for Infection
- Risk for Altered Body Temperature
- Hypothermia
- Hyperthermia
- Ineffective Thermoregulation
- Dysreflexia
- Risk for Autonomic Dysreflexia
- Constipation
- Perceived Constipation
- Colonic Constipation (deleted in 1998)
- Diarrhea
- Bowel Incontinence
- Risk for Constipation
- Altered Urinary Elimination
- Stress Incontinence
- Reflex Urinary Incontinence
- Urge Incontinence
- Functional Urinary Incontinence
- Total Incontinence
- Risk for Urinary Urge Incontinence
- Urinary Retention
- Altered Tissue Perfusion (Specify type: Renal, Cerebral, Cardiopulmonary, Gastrointestinal, Peripheral)
- Risk for Fluid Volume Imbalance
- Fluid Volume Excess
- Fluid Volume Deficit
- Risk for Fluid Volume Deficit
- Decreased Cardiac Output
- Impaired Gas Exchange
- Ineffective Airway Clearance
- Ineffective Breathing Pattern
- Inability to Sustain Spontaneous Ventilation
- Dysfunctional Ventilatory Weaning Response
- Risk for Injury
- Risk for Suffocation
- Risk for Poisoning
- Risk for Trauma
- Risk for Aspiration
- Risk for Disuse Syndrome
- Latex Allergy Response
- Risk for Latex Allergy Response
- Altered Protection
- Impaired Tissue Integrity
- Altered Oral Mucous Membrane
- Impaired Skin Integrity
- Risk for Impaired Skin Integrity
- Altered Dentition
- Decreased Adaptive Capacity: Intracranial
- Energy Field Disturbance

Pattern 2: Communicating

- Impaired Verbal Communication

Pattern 3: Relating

- Impaired Social Interaction
- Social Isolation
- Risk for Loneliness
- Altered Role Performance
- Altered Parenting
- Risk for Altered Parenting
- Risk for Altered Parent/Infant/Child Attachment
- Sexual Dysfunction
- Altered Family Processes
- Caregiver Role Strain
- Risk for Caregiver Role Strain
- Altered Family Processes: Alcoholism
- Parental Role Conflict
- Altered Sexuality Patterns

Pattern 4: Valuing

- Spiritual Distress (Distress of the Human Spirit)
- Risk for Spiritual Distress
- Potential for Enhanced Spiritual Well-Being

Pattern 5: Choosing

- Ineffective Individual Coping
- Impaired Adjustment
- Defensive Coping
- Ineffective Denial
- Ineffective Family Coping: Disabling
- Ineffective Family Coping: Compromised
- Family Coping: Potential for Growth
- Potential for Enhanced Community Coping
- Ineffective Community Coping
- Ineffective Management of Therapeutic Regimen: Individuals
- Noncompliance (specify)
- Ineffective Management of Therapeutic Regimen: Families
- Ineffective Management of Therapeutic Regimen: Community
- Effective Management of Therapeutic Regimen: Individual
- Decisional Conflict (specify)
- Health-Seeking Behaviors (specify)

Pattern 6: Moving

- Impaired Physical Mobility
- Risk for Peripheral Neurovascular Dysfunction
- Risk for Perioperative Positioning Injury
- Impaired Walking
- Impaired Wheelchair Mobility
- Impaired Transfer Ability
- Impaired Bed Mobility
- Activity Intolerance
- Fatigue
- Risk for Activity Intolerance
- Sleep Pattern Disturbance
- Sleep Deprivation
- Diversional Activity Deficit

(continued)

CHART 3•6 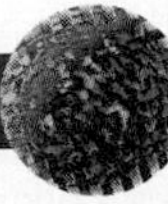 **NANDA-Approved Nursing Diagnoses — 1999–2000 (*continued*)**

Impaired Home Maintenance Management
Altered Health Maintenance
Delayed Surgical Recovery
Adult Failure to Thrive
Feeding Self-Care Deficit
Impaired Swallowing
Ineffective Breastfeeding
Interrupted Breastfeeding
Effective Breastfeeding
Ineffective Infant Feeding Pattern
Bathing/Hygiene Self-Care Deficit
Dressing/Grooming Self-Care Deficit
Toileting Self-Care Deficit
Altered Growth and Development
Risk for Altered Development
Risk for Altered Growth
Relocation Stress Syndrome
Risk for Disorganized Infant Behavior
Disorganized Infant Behavior
Potential for Enhanced Organized Infant Behavior

Pattern 7: Perceiving

Body Image Disturbance
Self-Esteem Disturbance
Chronic Low Self-Esteem
Situational Low Self-Esteem
Personal Identity Disturbance
Sensory/Perceptual Alterations (Specify: Visual, Auditory, Kinesthetic, Gustatory, Tactile, Olfactory)
Unilateral Neglect
Hopelessness
Powerlessness

Pattern 8: Knowing

Knowledge Deficit (Specify)
Impaired Environmental Interpretation Syndrome
Acute Confusion
Chronic Confusion
Altered Thought Processes
Impaired Memory

Pattern 9: Feeling

Pain
Chronic Pain
Nausea
Dysfunctional Grieving
Anticipatory Grieving
Chronic Sorrow
Risk for Violence: Directed at Others
Risk for Self-Mutilation
Risk for Violence: Self-Directed
Post-Trauma Syndrome
Rape-Trauma Syndrome
Rape-Trauma Syndrome: Compound Reaction
Rape-Trauma Syndrome: Silent Reaction
Risk for Post-Trauma Syndrome
Anxiety
Death Anxiety
Fear

North American Nursing Diagnosis Association (1999). *Nursing diagnoses: Definitions and classification 1999–2000.* Philadelphia: Author.

related data that reveal the existence of a problem and the need for nursing intervention. The patient's identified problems are then defined in the nursing diagnosis. The most commonly selected nursing diagnoses are compiled and categorized by NANDA in a taxonomy that is updated at least every 2 years. It is important to remember that nursing diagnoses are *not* medical diagnoses; they are *not* medical treatments prescribed by the physician; they are *not* diagnostic studies; they are *not* the equipment used to implement medical therapy; and they are *not* the problems that the nurse experiences while caring for the patient. They *are* the patient's actual or potential health problems that are amenable to resolution by independent nursing actions. Nursing diagnoses that are succinctly stated in terms of the specific problems of the patient will guide the nurse in the development of the nursing plan of care.

To give additional meaning to the diagnosis, the characteristics and the etiology of the problem must be identified and included as part of the diagnosis. For example, the nursing diagnoses and their defining characteristics and etiology for a patient who has rheumatoid arthritis may include:

- Impaired physical mobility related to pain and stiffness with joint movement
- Self-care deficits (feeding, bathing, dressing, toileting) related to fatigue and joint stiffness
- Self-esteem disturbance related to loss of independence
- Altered nutrition (less than body requirements) related to fatigue and inadequate food intake

Collaborative Problems

In addition to nursing diagnoses and their related nursing interventions, nursing practice encompasses certain situations and interventions that do not fall within the definition of nursing diagnoses. These activities pertain to potential problems or complications that are medical in origin and require collaborative interventions with the physician and other members of the health care team. The term "collaborative problem" is used to identify these situations.

> Collaborative problems are certain physiologic complications that nurses monitor to detect onset or changes in status. Nurses manage collaborative problems using physician-prescribed and nursing-prescribed interventions to minimize the complications of the events (Carpenito, 1999, p. 7).

Thus, a primary focus of the nurse when treating collaborative problems is monitoring the patient for the onset of complications or changes in the status of existing complications. The complications are usually related to the patient's disease process or to treatments, medications, or diagnostic studies. The nurse prescribes nursing interventions that are appropriate for managing the complications and implements the treatments prescribed by the physician. Figure 3-2 depicts the differences between nursing diagnoses and collaborative problems. After the nursing diagnoses and collaborative problems have been identified, they are recorded on the plan of nursing care.

PLANNING

Once the nursing diagnoses have been identified, the planning component of the nursing process begins. This phase entails:

1. Assigning priorities to the nursing diagnoses and collaborative problems
2. Specifying the immediate, intermediate, and long-term goals of nursing action
3. Identifying specific nursing interventions appropriate for attaining the goals
4. Identifying interdependent interventions
5. Specifying expected outcomes
6. Documenting the nursing diagnoses, collaborative problems, goals, nursing interventions, and expected outcomes on the plan of nursing care
7. Communicating to appropriate personnel any assessment data that point to health needs that can best be met by other members of the health care team

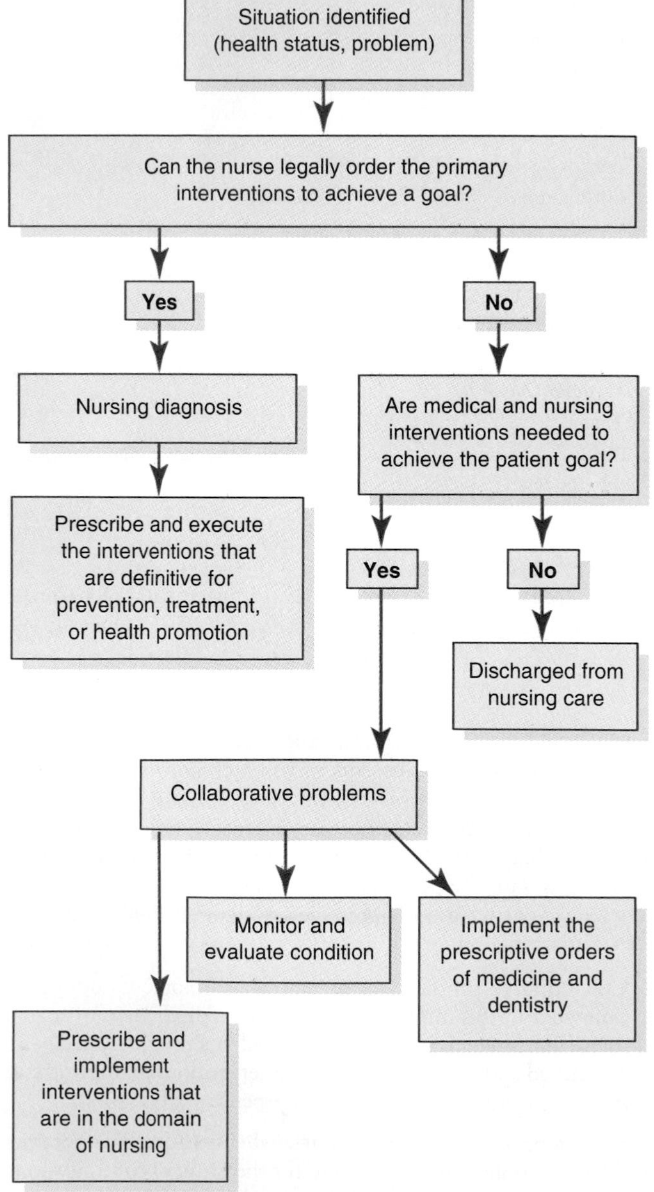

FIGURE 3•2 Differentiating nursing diagnoses from collaborative problems. Source: Carpenito, L. J. (1997). *Nursing diagnosis: Application to clinical practice* (7th ed). Philadelphia; Lippincott-Raven.

Setting Priorities

Assigning priorities to the nursing diagnoses and collaborative problems is a joint effort by the nurse and the patient or the family members. Any disagreement about priorities is resolved in a way that is mutually acceptable. Consideration must be given to the urgency of the problems, the most critical problems receiving the highest priority. Maslow's hierarchy of needs provides a useful framework for prioritizing problems, with importance being given first to physical needs; once these lower-level needs are met, higher-level needs can be addressed.

Establishing Goals

After the priorities of the nursing diagnoses have been established, the immediate, intermediate, and long-term goals and the nursing actions appropriate for attaining the goals are identified. The patient and his or her family are included in establishing goals for the nursing actions. The immediate goals are those that can be reached in a short period of time. The intermediate and long-term goals require a longer period of time to be achieved, and usually involve preventing complications and other health problems and promoting self-care and rehabilitation. For example, goals for a diabetic patient with a nursing diagnosis of knowledge deficit related to the prescribed diet may be stated as follows:

Immediate goal: Demonstrates oral intake and tolerance of 1500-calorie diabetic diet spaced in three meals and one snack.

Intermediate goal: Plans meals for 1 week based on diabetic exchange list.

Long-term goal: Adheres to prescribed diabetic diet.

Establishing Expected Outcomes

Expected outcomes of the nursing interventions are stated in terms of the patient's behaviors and the time period in which they are to be achieved, as well as any special circumstances related to achieving the outcome (Smith-Temple & Johnson, 1998). These outcomes must be realistic and measurable. The Nursing-Sensitive Outcomes Classification (NOC) (Chart 3-7) and standard outcome criteria for people with specific health problems established by health care agencies are resources for identifying appropriate expected outcomes. These outcomes should be used whenever possible, although they may need to be adapted to establish realistic criteria for the specific person involved.

The expected outcomes that define the desired behavior of the patient will be used to measure to what extent progress toward resolving the problem has been made. The expected outcomes also serve as the basis for evaluating the effectiveness of the nursing interventions and deciding whether additional nursing care is needed or whether the plan of care needs to be adjusted.

CHART 3•7 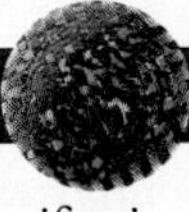 **Nursing-Sensitive Outcomes Classification (NOC)**

The NOC is a classification of patient outcomes sensitive to nursing interventions. Each outcome is a neutral statement about a variable patient condition, behavior, or perception coupled with a rating scale. The outcome statement and scale can be used to identify baseline functioning, expected outcomes, and actual outcomes for individual patients.

Nutritional Status: Body Mass

Definition: Congruence of body weight, muscle, and fat to height, frame, and gender

Nutritional Status: Body Mass	Extreme deviation from expected range **1**	Substantial deviation from expected range **2**	Moderate deviation from expected range **3**	Mild deviation from expected range **4**	No deviation from expected range **5**
Indicators:					
Weight	1	2	3	4	5
Triceps skinfold thickness	1	2	3	4	5
Subscapular skinfold thickness	1	2	3	4	5
Waist/hip circumference ratio (women)	1	2	3	4	5
Neck/waist circumference ratio (men)	1	2	3	4	5
Body fat percentage	1	2	3	4	5
Head circumference percentile (child)	1	2	3	4	5
Height percentile (child)	1	2	3	4	5
Weight percentile (child)	1	2	3	4	5
Other ________ Specify	1	2	3	4	5

An example of nursing-sensitive outcome. With permission from Johnson, M. & Maas, M. (Eds.). (1997). *Nursing outcomes classification (NOC): Iowa Outcomes Project.* St. Louis: Mosby–Year Book.

Determining Nursing Actions

In planning appropriate nursing actions to achieve the desired goals and outcomes, the nurse, with input from the patient and significant others, identifies individualized interventions based on the patient's circumstances and preferences that will address each outcome. Interventions should identify the activities needed and who should carry out those activities. Determination of interdisciplinary activities is made in collaboration with other health care workers as needed.

The nurse identifies and plans patient teaching and return demonstrations as needed to assist the patient in learning self-care activities to be performed. Planned interventions should be ethical and appropriate to the patient's culture, age, and gender. Standardized interventions, such as those found on institutional care plans or in the Nursing Interventions Classification (NIC; McCloskey & Bulechek, 1996) can be used. Chart 3-8 describes the NIC system and provides an example of an NIC system intervention. It is important to individualize prewritten interventions to promote optimal effectiveness for each patient.

IMPLEMENTATION

The implementation phase of the nursing process follows the formulation of the plan of nursing care. Implementation refers to carrying out the proposed plan of care. The nurse assumes responsibility for the implementation; however, performance of interventions may be carried out by the patient and the family, other members of the nursing team, or other members of the health care team as appropriate. The activities of all those involved in implementation are coordinated by the nurse so that the schedule of activities facilitates the patient's recovery.

- The plan of nursing care serves as the basis for implementation.
- The immediate, intermediate, and long-term goals are used as a focus for the implementation of the designated nursing interventions.
- While implementing nursing care, the nurse continually assesses the patient and his or her response to the nursing care.
- Alterations are made in the plan of care as the patient's condition, problems, and responses change and when reassignment of priorities is required.

Implementation includes direct or indirect execution of the planned interventions. It is focused on resolving the patient's nursing diagnoses and collaborative problems and achieving expected outcomes, thus meeting the patient's health needs.

Included among nursing interventions are assisting with hygienic care; promoting physical and psychological comfort; supporting respiratory and elimination functions; facilitating the ingestion of food, fluids, and nutrients; managing the patient's

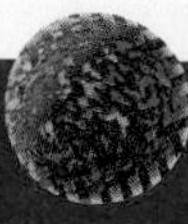

CHART 3•8 The Nursing Interventions Classification (NIC)

The NIC is a standardized classification of nursing treatments (interventions) that includes independent and collaborative interventions. Intervention labels are terms such as hemorrhage control, medication administration, or pain management. Listed under each intervention are multiple discrete nursing actions that together constitute a comprehensive approach to treatment of a particular condition. Not all actions will be applicable to every patient; nursing judgment will determine which actions to implement.

Weight Management

Definition: Facilitating maintenance of optimal body weight and percent body fat

Activities:

Discuss with the patient the relationship between food intake, exercise, weight gain, and weight loss

Discuss with patient the medical conditions that may affect weight

Discuss with patient the habits and customs and cultural and heredity factors that influence weight

Discuss risks associated with being over- and underweight

Determine patient motivation for changing eating habits

Determine patient's ideal body weight

Determine patient's ideal percent body fat

Develop with the patient a method to keep a daily record of intake

Encourage patient to write down realistic weekly goals for food intake and exercise and to display them in a location where they can be reviewed daily

Encourage patient to chart weekly weights, as appropriate

Inform patient about whether support groups are available for assistance

Assist in developing well-balanced meal plans consistent with level of energy expenditure

An example of nursing intervention. With permission from McCloskey, J. C. & Bulechek, G. M. (Eds.). (1996). *Nursing interventions classification (NIC): Iowa Interventions Project.* St. Louis: Mosby–Year Book.

immediate surroundings; providing health teaching; promoting a therapeutic relationship; and carrying out a variety of therapeutic nursing activities. Judgment, critical thinking, sound principles, and good decision-making skills are essential in the selection of appropriate and scientifically and ethically based nursing interventions. All nursing interventions are patient-focused and outcome-directed. They are based on scientific principles and are implemented with compassion, confidence, and a willingness to accept and understand the patient's responses.

Many nursing actions are independent. Others are interdependent, such as carrying out prescribed treatments, administering medications and therapies, and collaborating with other health care team members to accomplish specific expected outcomes and to monitor and manage potential complications. Such interdependent functioning is just that—interdependent. Requests or orders from other health care team members should not be followed blindly but should be assessed critically and questioned as necessary. The implementation phase of the nursing process is concluded when the nursing interventions have been completed.

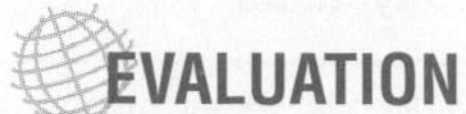

EVALUATION

Evaluation, the final step of the nursing process, allows the nurse to determine the patient's response to the nursing interventions and the extent to which the objectives have been achieved. The plan of nursing care is the basis for evaluation. The nursing diagnoses, collaborative problems, goals, nursing interventions, and expected outcomes provide the specific guidelines that dictate the focus of the evaluation. Through evaluation, the nurse can answer the following questions:

- Were the nursing diagnoses and collaborative problems accurate?
- Did the patient achieve the expected outcomes within the critical time periods?
- Have the patient's nursing diagnoses been resolved?
- Have the collaborative problems been resolved?
- Have the patient's nursing needs been met?
- Should the nursing interventions be continued, altered, or discontinued?
- Have new problems evolved for which nursing interventions have not been planned or implemented?
- What factors influenced the achievement or lack of achievement of the objectives?
- Do priorities need to be reassigned?
- Should changes be made in the expected outcomes and outcome criteria?

Objective data that provide answers to these questions must be collected from all available sources (ie, patient, family or significant others, nursing and other health care team members). These data should be available in the patient's record and must be substantiated by direct observation of the patient before recording the outcomes.

Outcomes

Outcomes are documented concisely and objectively. Documentation should show how the outcomes relate to the nursing diagnoses and collaborative problems, describe the patient's responses to the interventions, indicate whether or not the goals were met, and include any additional pertinent data.

The plan of care is subject to change as the patient's problems change, as the priorities of the problems shift, as problems are resolved, and as additional information about the patient's state of health is collected. As the nursing interventions are implemented, the patient's responses are evaluated and documented and the plan of care is modified accordingly. A well-developed, continuously updated plan of care is the greatest assurance that the patient's nursing diagnoses and collaborative problems will be addressed and his or her basic needs will be met. See Plan of Nursing Care 3-1 for an example of a plan based on a case study.

3•1

PLAN OF NURSING CARE 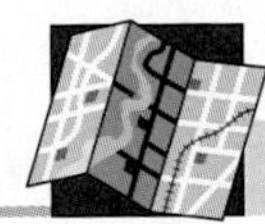

Example of an Individualized Plan of Nursing Care

Mr. John Lee, a 50-year-old management consultant, was admitted to the nursing unit from his physician's office. A routine physical examination 3 months previously had revealed essential hypertension with BP 170/110 and decreased urine creatinine clearance. During the subsequent 3 months the blood pressure elevation did not respond to diet therapy. Mr. Lee admitted that he had not been successful in adhering to the low-sodium, low-cholesterol weight-reduction diet that had been prescribed for him. He stated, "My life is just too busy—I work all hours of the day and night." He indicated that in addition to his work he and his wife share the responsibility for raising their two teenage daughters. He drinks five to seven cups of coffee daily and drinks alcohol only at social occasions. Admission physical examination revealed BP 162/112, P 96, R 20, T 37°C (98.6°F), height 5′10″, weight 210 lbs, and slight edema of the ankles and feet. Mr. Lee stated that his feet are "always puffy at night." There were several darkened areas (2 cm in diameter) on the anterior lower legs bilaterally. A brief hospitalization was planned for thorough evaluation and initiation of therapy. The physician's orders on admission included: activity as desired; Lasix, 40 mg bid; monitor vital signs every 4 hours while awake; 1500 calorie, 1 g sodium, low-cholesterol diet.

Nursing Diagnosis

- Altered health maintenance related to hypertension, stress, obesity, and caffeine
- Ineffective individual coping related to role responsibilities at work and home
- Noncompliance with dietary regimen related to knowledge deficit and lifestyle

Collaborative Problems

1. Ischemic ulcers of lower legs

Goals

Immediate: Gradual decrease in blood pressure

Intermediate: Initiation of lifestyle alterations to decrease stress

Long-term: Alteration of lifestyle to reduce emotional and environmental stressors
Compliance with dietary regimen
Absence of ischemic leg ulcers

Nursing Interventions	Expected Outcomes	Outcomes
Monitor BP lying, sitting, and standing every 4 h	Experiences no further increase in BP	BP range of 162/112–138/98 since admission No variation greater than 5 mm Hg in systolic or diastolic pressures with position changes No variation between right and left arms Maximum BP from 24 h after admission to time of discharge: 138/98
Monitor fluid status:		
I&O	Urinary output adequate in relation to oral intake	Intake: 1850 mL Output: 1685 mL
Peripheral edema	No evidence of peripheral edema	Minimal edema of feet late in evening
Promote atmosphere conducive to physical and mental rest:		
Encourage alternation of rest and activity	Alternates periods of rest and activity	Rests in bed 1 h in morning and 2 h in afternoon; disconnects phone during rest periods Awake at intervals during night: 8 h of uninterrupted sleep at night after initiation of 30 mg Dalmane at bedtime
Encourage limitation of visitors and interactions that are stress-producing	Limits visitors to family in the evenings	Wife and daughters visit 2 h in evening; patient calm and relaxed after visits
	Avoids stress-producing interactions	Wife and daughters aware of need to decrease stress: they consult with patient about regular family activities
Assist patient to alter lifestyle to decrease stress	Describes stress as a precursor to alteration in physiologic functioning	Accurately described relationship between stress and hypertension
Discuss relationship between emotional stress and physiologic functioning		

(continued)

3•1 PLAN OF NURSING CARE

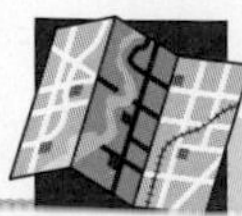

Example of an Individualized Plan of Nursing Care (*continued*)

Nursing Interventions	Expected Outcomes	Outcomes
Encourage patient to identify stress-producing stimuli	Identifies lifestyle factors that produce stress	Identified the following stressors: Self-imposed demands of job; unwillingness to refer clients; Excessive involvement in daughters' school and recreational activities
Encourage patient to identify adjustments necessary to reduce stress	Identifies lifestyle adjustments necessary to reduce stress	Verbalized plans to make more referrals; Identified need to decrease work hours to maximum of 8 h per day
	Discusses lifestyle adjustments with family	Consulted with wife and daughters; will alternate with wife in attending daughters' activities; all family members supportive
Encourage patient to identify obesity and caffeine as stressors and aggravators of hypertension; request consultation with dietitian and reinforce instructions given	Identifies harmful effects of obesity and caffeine	Accurately described effects of obesity and caffeine on blood pressure
	Makes plans for losing weight	Plans to go to Weight Watchers; has had success with this program in the past
	Makes plans for decreasing caffeine intake	Drinks 1 cup of coffee for breakfast; uses decaffeinated coffee at midmorning, lunch, and dinner; expressed satisfaction with this plan
Assess for ischemic leg ulcers; report changes in darkened spots on legs to physician	Absence of changes in skin integrity on lower extremities	No changes noted in characteristics of skin of lower legs on days 2 and 3
Teach foot care: daily inspection and washing, nail care, avoidance of caustic solutions, lubrication of dry skin, avoidance of heat to feet, well-fitting shoes and socks, avoidance of crossing legs	Describes principles and techniques of proper foot care	Discussed importance of proper foot care; demonstrated proper technique of foot care; shoes and socks fit well; does not cross legs when sitting

Critical Thinking Exercises

1. How does the approach to critical thinking differ among nursing practice settings (ie, acute care, ambulatory, extended care, home, and community settings)?

2. You have just completed the physical assessment of your assigned patient. How would you identify the patient's nursing diagnoses? Describe the kind of resources that are available to help you with identifying these diagnoses.

3. You have developed a plan of nursing care for your assigned patient, who is terminally ill. The next day you noted a "do not resuscitate" order on the chart. Describe how you used critical thinking skills to develop the plan of care. How did you integrate your critical thinking into the nursing process? What changes might you make in your plan of care considering the DNR order? What ethical problems or dilemmas might you anticipate?

4. A family member of your patient tells you information about the patient that the patient has not revealed. How would you determine if you should communicate this information to the patient's primary nurse?

References and Selected Readings

BOOKS

American Nurses Association. (1985). *Code for nurses with interpretive statements.* Kansas City, MO: Author.

American Nurses Association. (1995). *Nursing's social policy statement.* Washington, DC: Author.

American Nurses Association. (1998). *Standards of clinical nursing practice (2nd ed).* Washington, DC: Author.

Bickley, L. S. & Hoekelman, R. A. (1999). *Bates' guide to physical examination and history taking* (7th ed.). Philadelphia: Lippincott Williams & Wilkins.

Carnevali, D. L., & Thomas, M. D. (1993). *Diagnostic reasoning and treatment decision making in nursing.* Philadelphia: J. B. Lippincott.

Carpenito, L. J. (1997). *Nursing diagnosis: Application to clinical practice* (7th ed.). Philadelphia: Lippincott-Raven.

Carpenito, L. J. (1999). *Nursing care plan and documentation.* Philadelphia: Lippincott Williams & Wilkins.

Fonteyn, M. E. (1998). *Thinking strategies for nursing practice.* Philadelphia: Lippincott-Raven.

Jameton, A. (1984). *Nursing practice: The ethical issues.* Englewood Cliffs, NJ: Prentice-Hall.

Johnson, M., & Maas, M. (Eds.). (1997). *Nursing outcomes classification (NOC): Iowa Outcomes Project.* St. Louis: Mosby–Year Book.

McCloskey, J. C., & Bulechek, G. M. (Eds.). (1996). *Nursing interventions classification (NIC): Iowa Interventions Project.* St. Louis: Mosby–Year Book.

Miller, M. A., & Babcock, D. E. (1996). *Critical thinking applied to nursing.* St. Louis: C. V. Mosby.

Scanlon, C., & Fibison, W. (1995). *Managing genetic information: Implications for nursing practice.* Washington, DC: American Nurses Association.

Smith-Temple, J., & Johnson, J. Y. (1998). *Nurses' guide to clinical procedures* (3rd ed.). Philadelphia: Lippincott-Raven.

JOURNALS

Alfaro-LeFevre, R. (1997). Critical thinking. *The Nursing Spectrum,* (April 7), p. 4.

Ballinger, D. (1997). Is it ever acceptable to deceive a patient? *Nursing Times, 93*(35), 44–45.

Brown, J., Moore, D. E., Potter, D., & Stewart, R. (1997). Placebos and the need for good communication: The case of George Hunter. *Orthopaedic Nursing, 16*(3), 61–65.

Cameron, M. E. (1997) Ethical distress in nursing. *Journal of Professional Nursing, 13*(5), 280.

Constantino, R. E., Boneysteele, G., Gesmond, S.A., & Nelson, B. (1997). Restraining an aggressive suicidal, paraplegic patient: A look at the ethical and legal issues. *Dimensions in Critical Care Nursing, 16*(3), 144–151.

Daly, B. (1997). Nursing ethical code reflects changing times. *American Nurse,* (Sept.–Oct.), p. 9.

Daly, J. M., et al. (1996). A care planning tool that proves what we do. *RN, 59*(6), 26–30.

Erlen, J. A. (1997). Everyday ethics. *Orthopaedic Nursing, 16*(4), 60–63.

Gordon, S. (1997). Life support. *MedSurg Nursing, 6*(3), 162–165.

Heitman, L. K., & Robinson, B. E. S. (1997). Developing a nursing ethics roundtable. *American Journal of Nursing, 97*(1), 36–38.

Jacobs, P. M., Ott, B., Sullivan, B., Ulrich, Y., & Short, L. (1997). An approach to defining and operationalizing critical thinking. *Journal of Nursing Education, 36*(1), 19–22.

Kennison, M., & Brace, J. (1997). Critical thinking—digging deeper for creative solutions. *Nursing, 27*(9), 52–54.

Mason, S. (1997). The ethical dilemma of the do not resuscitate order. *British Journal of Nursing, 6*(11), 646–649.

Sherman, D. W. (1996). Taking the fear out of AIDS nursing: Voices from the field. *Journal of New York State Nurses Association, 27*(1), 4–8.

Shultz, L. (1997). Not for resuscitation: Two decades of challenge for nursing ethics and practice. *Nursing Ethics, 4*(3), 227–238.

Smith, S. A. (1997). Controversies in hydrating the terminally ill patient. *Journal of Intravenous Nursing, 20*(4), 193–200.

Ulsenheimer, J. H., Bailey, D. W., McCollough, E. M., Thornton, S. E., & Warden, E. W. (1997). Thinking about thinking. *Journal of Continuing Education Nursing, 28*(4), 150–156.

Zerwekh, J. V. (1997). Do dying patients really need IV fluids? *American Journal of Nursing, 97*(3), 26–31.

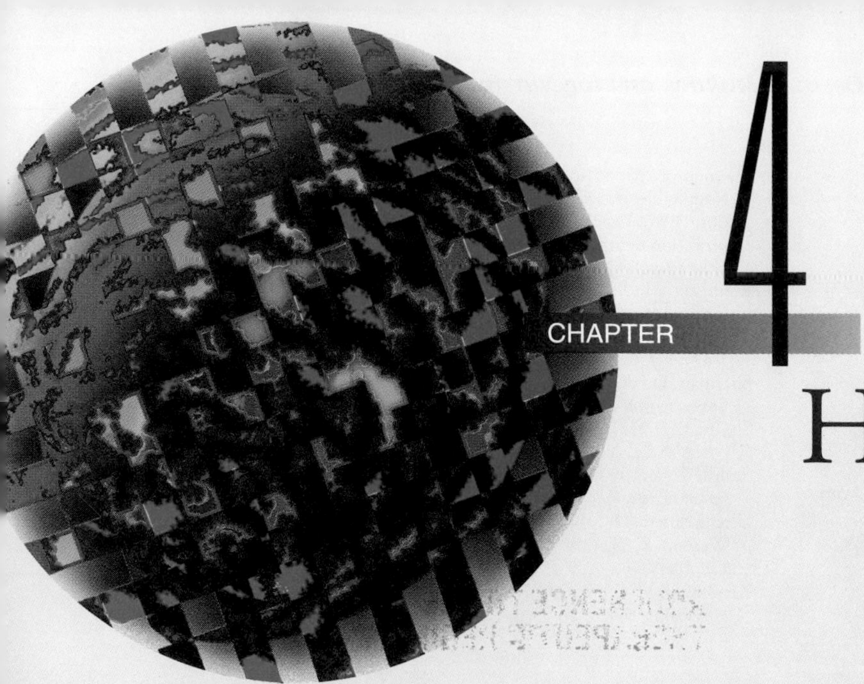

4 Health Education and Promotion

Learning Objectives

On completion of this chapter, the learner will be able to:

1. Describe the purposes and significance of health education.
2. Describe the concept of adherence to a therapeutic regimen.
3. Identify variables influencing the elderly person's adherence to a therapeutic regimen.
4. Distinguish the variables that affect learning readiness.
5. Describe strategies that facilitate elderly adults' learning abilities.
6. Describe the relationship of the teaching–learning process to the nursing process.
7. Develop a teaching plan for a patient.
8. Define the concepts of health, wellness, and health promotion.
9. Discuss major health promotion theories.
10. Describe the health promotion principles of self-responsibility, nutrition, stress management, and exercise.
11. Specify the variables that affect health promotion activities for children, young and middle-aged adults, and elderly adults.
12. Describe the role of the nurse in health promotion.

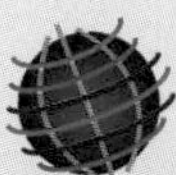

Effective health education lays a solid foundation for individual and community wellness. Teaching is an integral tool that all nurses use to assist patients and families in developing effective health behaviors and altering lifestyle patterns that predispose people to health risks. Health education is a direct link to successful patient care outcomes in all clinical settings (O'Halloran, 1997).

HEALTH EDUCATION TODAY

The changes in today's health care environment mandate the use of an organized approach to health education so that patients can meet their specific health care needs. Significant factors for the nurse to consider when planning patient education include the availability of health care outside the conventional hospital setting, the employment of diverse health care providers to accomplish care management goals, and the increased use of alternative strategies rather than traditional approaches to care. These trends can result in fragmentation of care and highlight the need to provide patients with the comprehensive information essential to informed decision making. Further, the demands from consumers for comprehensive information about their health issues throughout the life cycle accentuate the need for health education to occur in every patient–nurse encounter.

The nurse as a teacher is challenged not only to provide specific patient and family education, but also to focus on the educational needs of society. Health education is important to nursing care, since it can determine how well individuals and families are able to perform behaviors conducive to optimal self-care.

Teaching, as a function of nursing, is included in all state nurse practice acts and in the American Nurses Association's *Standards of Clinical Nursing Practice* (ANA, 1992). Health education is an independent function of nursing practice and a primary responsibility of the nursing profession. All nursing care is directed toward promoting, maintaining, and restoring health; preventing illness; and assisting people to adapt to the residual effects of illness. These nursing activities are accomplished through health education or patient teaching.

Every contact a nurse has with a health care consumer, whether that person is ill or not, should be considered an opportunity for health teaching. Although the person has a right to decide whether or not to learn, the nurse has the responsibility to present information that will motivate the person to recognize the need to learn. Therefore, the nurse must seize opportunities both inside and outside of health care settings to facilitate wellness. Educational environments can include homes, hospitals, community health centers, places of business, service organizations, shelters, and consumer action or support groups.

The Purpose of Health Education

The emphasis on health education stems in part from the public's right to comprehensive health care, which includes health education. The emphasis on health education also reflects the emergence of an informed public that is asking more significant questions about health and the health care services it receives. Because of the importance American society places on health and the responsibility each of us has to maintain and promote our own health, it is the obligation of the members of the health care team, and specifically nurses, to make health education consistently available. Without adequate knowledge and training in self-care skills, consumers cannot make effective decisions about their health.

People with chronic illnesses are among those most in need of health education today. As the life span of our population continues to increase, the number of people with such illnesses will also increase. People with chronic illness need health care information to participate actively in and assume responsibility for much of their own care. Health education can aid these individuals to adapt to illness, prevent complications, carry out prescribed therapy, and solve problems when confronted with new situations. It can also prevent rehospitalization resulting from inadequate information about self-care. The goal of health education is to teach people to live life to its healthiest—that is, to strive toward achieving their maximum health potential.

In addition to the public's right to and desire for health education, patient education is also a strategy for reducing health care costs by preventing illness, avoiding expensive medical treatment, decreasing lengthy hospital stays, and facilitating earlier discharge. For hospitals, offering community wellness programs is a public relations tool for increasing patient satisfaction and developing a positive image of the institution. Patient education is also a cost-avoidance strategy for those who believe that positive staff–patient relationships avert malpractice suits.

ADHERENCE TO THE THERAPEUTIC REGIMEN

One of the goals of patient education is to encourage people to adhere to their therapeutic regimen. Adherence to a therapeutic regimen requires that the person make one or more lifestyle changes to carry out specific activities that promote and maintain health. Common examples of behaviors facilitating health include taking prescribed medications, maintaining a diet, restricting activities, self-monitoring for signs and symptoms of illness, practicing specific hygienic measures, seeking periodic health evaluations, and performing other therapeutic and preventive measures. The fact that many people do not adhere to their prescribed regimens cannot be ignored or minimized; rates of adherence are generally very low, especially when the regimens are complex or of long duration.

Nonadherence to prescribed therapy has been the subject of many studies. For the most part, the findings have been inconclusive, and no one predominant causative factor has been found. Instead, a wide range of variables appear to influence the degree of adherence:

- Demographic variables, such as age, gender, race, socioeconomic status, and education
- Illness variables, such as the severity of the illness and the relief of symptoms afforded by the therapy
- Therapeutic regimen variables, such as the complexity of the regimen and uncomfortable side effects
- Psychosocial variables, such as intelligence, attitudes toward health professionals, acceptance or denial of illness, and religious or cultural beliefs
- Financial variables, especially the direct and indirect costs associated with a prescribed regimen.

The nurse's success with health education is determined by ongoing assessment of the variables affecting the patient's capacity to adopt specific behaviors, to obtain resources, and to maintain a helpful social environment (Green & Kreuter, 1991). Teaching programs are more likely to succeed if the variables affecting the person's adherence are identified and considered in the teaching plan.

The problem of nonadherence to therapeutic regimens is a substantial one that must be remedied before patients can achieve their maximum self-care capabilities and health potential. Interestingly, a patient's need for knowledge has not been found to be a sufficient stimulus for acquiring knowledge and thus enabling complete adherence to a health regimen. Teaching programs directed toward stimulating patient motivation produce varying degrees of adherence. The variables of choice, establishment of mutual goals, and the quality of the patient–provider relationship directly influence the behavioral changes that can occur from patient education (Rankin & Stallings, 1995). These factors are directly linked to motivation for learning.

Using a learning contract can also be a motivator for learning. Such a contract is based on the assessment of patient needs, health care data, and specific, measurable goals (Redman, 1996). A well-designed learning contract is realistic and positive; it includes measurable goals, with a specific time frame and reward system for goal achievement. The learning contract is recorded in writing and contains methods for ongoing evaluation.

The value of the contract lies in its clarity, specific delineation of what is to be accomplished, and usefulness for evaluating behavioral change. In a typical learning contract, a series of goals are established, beginning with small, easily attainable objectives and progressing to more advanced goals. Frequent, positive reinforcement is provided as the person moves from one goal to the next. An example of incremental goals would be a weight reduction program based on losing 1 to 2 pounds per week rather than one that merely identifies a general goal of losing 30 pounds.

Gerontologic Considerations

Nonadherence to therapeutic regimens is a significant problem for elderly people, leading to increased morbidity and mortality and increased cost of treatment (U.S. Public Health Service, 1990). Many nursing home admissions and hospital admissions are linked to nonadherence.

Elderly people frequently have one or more chronic illnesses that are managed with numerous medications and complicated by periodic acute episodes. Elderly people also may have other problems that affect adherence to therapeutic regimens, such as increased sensitivity to medications and their side effects, difficulty in adjusting to change and stress, financial constraints, forgetfulness, inadequate support systems, lifetime habits of self-treatment with over-the-counter medications, visual and hearing impairments, and mobility limitations. To promote adherence among the elderly, time and effort must be taken to assess all variables that may affect health behavior (Fig. 4-1). The nurse must consider that cognitive deficiencies can be manifested by the elderly person's inability to draw inferences, apply information, or understand the major teaching points (Eliopoulos, 1997). The person's strengths and limitations must be assessed in order to use current strengths to compensate for limitations. Above all, health care professionals must work together to provide continuous, coordinated care; otherwise, the efforts of one health care professional may be negated by those of another.

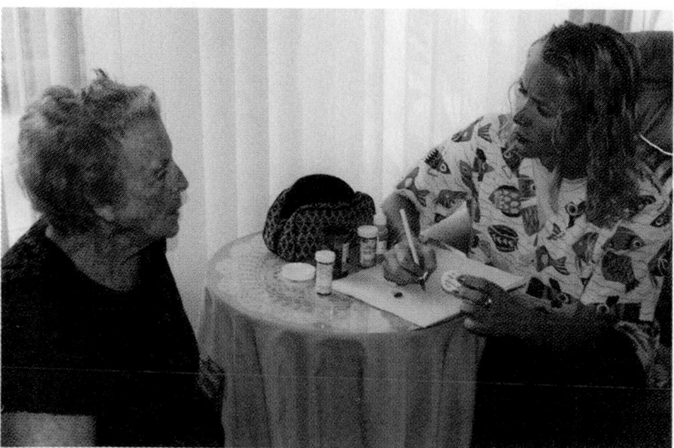

FIGURE 4•1 Taking time to teach patients about their medication and treatment program promotes interest and cooperation. Older adults who are actively involved in learning about their medication and treatment program and the expected effects may be more likely to adhere to the therapeutic regimen.

THE NATURE OF TEACHING AND LEARNING

Learning can be defined as acquiring knowledge, attitudes, or skills. Teaching is defined as helping another person to learn. These definitions indicate that the teaching–learning process is an active one, requiring the involvement of both teacher and learner in the effort to reach the desired outcome, a change in behavior. The teacher does not simply give knowledge to the learner, but instead serves as a facilitator of learning.

In general, there is no definitive theory about how learning occurs and how it is affected by teaching. However, studies indicate that learning can be affected by factors such as readiness to learn, the learning environment, and the teaching techniques employed.

Learning Readiness

One of the most significant factors influencing learning is the person's readiness to learn. For adults, readiness is based on culture, personal values, physical and emotional status, and past experiences in learning. The teachable moment for an adult occurs when the content and skills being taught are congruent with the task to be accomplished (Redman, 1996).

Culture encompasses values, ideals, and behaviors. The traditions within each culture are the framework for solving the issues and concerns of daily living. Since people with different cultural backgrounds hold different values, lifestyles and choices about health care vary. Culture is a major variable influencing readiness to learn because it affects how a person learns and what information gets learned. Sometimes people will not accept health teaching because it conflicts with culturally mediated values. Before beginning health teaching, the nurse must perform an individual cultural assessment instead of simply relying on generalized assumptions about a particular culture. A patient's social and cultural patterns must be appropriately incorporated into the teaching–learning interaction.

Values are an individual's perceptions about what is desirable and undesirable behavior. The nurse must know what value the patient places on health and health care. In clinical situations, values are expressed through the actions performed and the level of knowledge a patient pursues (Andrews & Boyle, 1995). When the nurse lacks knowledge about the cultural values of the patient being instructed, misunderstanding, lack of cooperation, and negative health outcomes may occur (Leininger, 1991). Each person's values and behaviors can be either an asset or a deficit to the readiness to learn. Therefore, no amount of health education will be accepted by patients unless their values and beliefs about health and illness are respected (Giger & Davidhizar, 1991).

Physical readiness is of vital importance, because until a person is physically capable of learning, attempts at teaching and learning may be both futile and frustrating. Someone in acute pain will be unable to focus attention away from the pain long enough to concentrate on learning. Likewise, a person who is short of breath will concentrate on breathing rather than on learning.

Emotional readiness has an impact on the motivation to learn. A person who has not accepted an existing illness or the threat of illness will not be motivated to learn. People who do not accept a therapeutic regimen, or view it as conflicting with their present lifestyle, may consciously avoid learning. Until a person recognizes the need to learn and acknowledges an ability to learn, teaching efforts may be thwarted. However, it is not always wise to wait for a patient to become emotionally ready to learn, because this time may never come unless efforts are made by the nurse to stimulate the individual's motivation.

Illness and the threat of illness are usually accompanied by anxiety and stress. The nurse who recognizes such reactions can use simple explanations and instructions to alleviate these anxieties and provide further motivation to learn. Because learning involves changes in behavior, it normally produces mild anxiety, which can often be a useful motivating factor.

Emotional readiness can be promoted by creating a warm, accepting, positive atmosphere and by establishing realistic learning goals. When the learners realize success and a feeling of accomplishment, they will experience further motivation for participating in additional learning opportunities.

Feedback about progress also motivates learning. Such feedback should be presented in the form of positive reinforcement when learners are successful and in the form of constructive suggestions for improvement when they are unsuccessful.

Experiential readiness refers to past experiences that influence a person's ability to learn. Previous educational experiences and life experiences in general are significant determinants of an individual's approach to learning. A person who has had little or no formal education may not be able to understand the instructional materials presented. A person who has had difficulty learning in the past may be hesitant to try again. Many behaviors required for reaching maximum health potential demand a rather extensive background of knowledge, physical skills, and attitudes. Without this background on which to build, learning may be very difficult and very slow. For example, someone who does not understand the basics of normal nutrition may not be able to understand the restrictions of a specific diet. A person who does not view the desired learning as personally meaningful may reject teaching efforts. Also, a person who is not future-oriented may be unable to appreciate many aspects of preventive health teaching. Thus, experiential readiness is closely related to emotional readiness, because motivation tends to be stimulated by an appreciation for the need to learn and by those learning tasks that are familiar, interesting, and meaningful.

Before initiating a teaching–learning program, it is important to assess the learner's physical and emotional readiness to learn, as well as his or her ability to learn what is being taught. This information then becomes the basis for establishing goals that can motivate the person to learn. Involving the learner in the establishment of mutually acceptable goals serves the purpose of encouraging active involvement in the learning process and a willingness to share responsibility for learning.

The Learning Environment

Although learning can take place without a teacher, most people who are attempting to learn new or altered health behaviors will need the services of a nurse at least part of the time. The interpersonal interaction between the learner and the nurse who is attempting to meet the individual's learning needs may be formal or informal, depending on the method and techniques of teaching that are found to be most appropriate.

Learning can be optimized by minimizing external variables that interfere with the learning process. For example, the room temperature, lighting, noise levels, and other environmental conditions should be appropriate to the learning situation. Also, the time selected for teaching should be suited to the individual's needs. Scheduling a teaching session at a time of day when the patient is fatigued, uncomfortable, or anxious about a pending diagnostic or therapeutic procedure, or when visitors are present does not provide an environment conducive to learning. However, if family members are to participate in providing care, the sessions should be timed to take place when the family is present so they can learn any necessary skills or techniques.

Teaching Techniques

Teaching techniques and methods will enhance learning if they are appropriate to the individual's needs. Numerous techniques are available, including lectures, group teaching, and demonstrations, all of which can be enhanced with specially prepared teaching materials. The lecture or explanation method of teaching is commonly used but should always be accompanied by discussion. The discussion is important because it affords the learner an opportunity to express feelings and concerns, to ask questions, and to receive clarification.

Group teaching is appropriate for some people because it allows them not only to receive needed information, but also to feel secure as members of the group. Those with similar problems or learning needs have the opportunity to identify with each other and gain moral support and encouragement. However, not everyone relates or learns well in groups; therefore, some people may not benefit from such experiences. Also, if group teaching is used, assessment and follow-up of each individual are imperative to ensure that each has gained sufficient knowledge and skills.

Demonstration and practice are essential ingredients of a teaching program, especially when skills are to be learned. It is best to demonstrate the skill and then allow the learner ample opportunity for practice. When special equipment is involved, such as insulin syringes, colostomy bags, or dressings, it is important to teach with the same equipment that will be used in the home setting. Learning to perform a skill with one kind of equipment and then having to change to a different kind can lead to confusion and mistakes.

Teaching aids available to enhance learning include materials such as books, pamphlets, pictures, films, slides, audio and video tapes, models, programmed instruction, and computer-assisted learning modules. Such teaching aids are invaluable when used appropriately and can save a significant amount of personnel time and related cost. However, all such aids should be reviewed before use to ensure they meet the individual's learning needs.

Reinforcement and follow-up are important because learning takes time. Allowing ample time to learn and reinforcing what is learned are successful teaching strategies; a single teaching session is never adequate. Follow-up sessions are imperative to promote the learners' confidence in their abilities and to plan for additional teaching sessions. For the hospitalized patient who may not be able to transfer what has been learned in the hospital to the home setting, follow-up after discharge is essential to ensure that the full benefits of a teaching program have been realized.

Gerontologic Considerations

Nurses caring for elderly people must be aware of how the normal changes that occur with aging affect learning abilities and how an elderly person can be assisted to adjust to these changes. Above all, it is most important to recognize that just because a person is elderly does not mean he or she cannot learn. Studies have shown that older adults can learn and remember if information is paced appropriately, is relevant, and is followed by appropriate feedback strategies that apply to all learners (Rankin & Stallings, 1995). Because changes associated with aging vary significantly among elderly people, a thorough assessment of each person's level of physiologic and psychological functioning should be conducted before teaching begins.

Changes in cognition with age may include slowed mental functioning; decreased short-term memory, abstract thinking, and concentration; and slowed reaction time. These changes are often accentuated by the health problems that cause the elderly to seek health care in the first place. Effective teaching strategies include a slow-paced presentation of small amounts of material at a time, frequent repetition of information, and the use of reinforcement techniques, such as audiovisual and written materials, and repeated practice sessions. The teaching environment must be one in which distracting stimuli are minimized as much as possible.

Sensory changes associated with aging also affect teaching and learning. Teaching strategies to accommodate decreased visual acuity include large-print and easy-to-read materials printed on nonglare paper. Because color discrimination is often impaired, the use of color-coded or highlighted teaching materials may not be effective. To maximize hearing, the teacher must speak distinctly with a normal or lowered pitch, facing the person so lip reading can occur as needed. Visual cues are often helpful to reinforce verbal teaching.

Family members should be involved in teaching sessions when possible. They provide another source for reinforcement of material and can help the learner to recall instructions later. They can also provide valuable assessment information about the person's living situation and related learning needs.

When the nurse, the family, and other involved health care professionals work collaboratively to facilitate an elderly person's learning, the chances of success will be maximized. Successful learning for the elderly should result in improved self-care management skills, enhanced self-esteem, and a willingness to learn in future sessions.

THE NURSING PROCESS IN PATIENT TEACHING

The steps of the nursing process—assessment, diagnosis, planning, implementation, and evaluation—are used when constructing a teaching plan to meet an individual's teaching and learning needs (Chart 4-1).

Assessment

Assessment in the teaching–learning process is directed toward the systematic collection of data about the person's learning needs, the person's readiness to learn, and the family's learning needs. All internal and external variables that affect the patient's readiness to learn are identified. A learning assessment guide may be used for this purpose. Some of the guides available are very general and are directed toward the collection of general health information. Others are specific to common medication regimens or disease processes. Such guides facilitate the assessment but must be adapted to the individual's responses, problems, and needs.

As soon as possible after completing the assessment, the nurse organizes, analyzes, synthesizes, and summarizes the data collected and determines the patient's need for teaching.

Nursing Diagnosis

Formulating nursing diagnoses makes educational goals and evaluation of progress more specific and meaningful. Teaching is an integral intervention implied by all nursing diagnoses; however, for some diagnoses, education is the primary intervention. Risk for ineffective management of therapeutic regimen, risk for impaired home management, health-seeking behaviors, and decisional conflict are examples of nursing diagnoses that direct planning for educational needs. The diagnosis knowledge deficit should be used cautiously because knowledge deficit is not a human response but a factor relating to or causing the diagnosis (risk for ineffective management of therapeutic regimen related to knowledge deficit about wound care) (Carpenito, 1997). Choosing a nursing diagnosis that relates specifically to the patient's and family's learning needs will serve as a guide in the development of the teaching plan.

Planning

Once the nursing diagnoses have been identified, the planning component of the teaching–learning process is established in accordance with the steps of the nursing process:

1. Assigning priorities to the diagnoses
2. Specifying the immediate, intermediate, and long-term goals of learning
3. Identifying specific teaching strategies appropriate for attaining goals
4. Specifying the expected outcomes
5. Documenting the diagnoses, goals, teaching strategies, and expected outcomes on the teaching plan

As in the nursing process, the assignment of priorities to the diagnoses should be a joint effort by the nurse and the learner or family members. Consideration must be given to the urgency of the individual's learning needs, with the most critical needs receiving the highest priority.

After the priorities of the diagnoses have been established, the immediate and long-term goals and the teaching strategies appropriate for attaining the goals are identified. Studies have found that teaching is most effective when the objectives of both the learner and the nurse are in agreement. Learning begins with the establishment of goals that are appropriate to the situation and realistic in terms of the individual's ability and desire to achieve them. Involving the patient and family in establishing goals and the subsequent planning of teaching strategies promotes their cooperation in the implementation of the teaching plan.

Expected outcomes of teaching strategies can be stated in terms of behaviors of the person, the family, or both. Every effort is made to develop outcomes that are realistic and measurable. The critical time periods for attaining the outcomes are also identified. The desired outcomes and the critical time periods will serve as a basis for evaluating the effectiveness of the teaching strategies.

During the planning phase, the nurse must consider the sequence in which the subject matter will be presented in each of the teaching strategies. Critical information (such as survival skills for the person with diabetes) and material that the person or family identifies to be of particular importance receives high priority. An outline is often helpful for arranging subject matter and for ensuring that all necessary information is included. Also during this time, appropriate teaching aids to be used in implementing the teaching strategies are prepared or selected.

The entire planning phase of the teaching–learning process is concluded with the formulation of the teaching plan. This teach-

CHART 4•1 A Guide to Patient Education

Assessment

1. Assess the person's readiness for health education.
   a. What are the person's health beliefs and behaviors?
   b. What psychosocial adaptation is the person making?
   c. Is the learner ready to learn?
   d. Is the person able to learn these behaviors?
   e. What additional information about the person is needed?
   f. What are the person's expectations?
   g. What does the person want to learn?
2. Organize, analyze, synthesize, and summarize the collected data.

Nursing Diagnosis

1. Formulate the nursing diagnoses that relate to the person's learning needs.
2. Identify the learning needs, their characteristics, and etiology.
3. State nursing diagnoses concisely and precisely.

Planning and Goals

1. Assign priority to the nursing diagnoses that relate to the individual's learning needs.
2. Specify the immediate, intermediate, and long-term teacher–learner-established learning goals.
3. Identify teaching strategies appropriate for goal attainment.
4. Establish expected outcomes.
5. Develop the written teaching plan.
   a. Include diagnoses, goals, teaching strategies, and expected outcomes.
   b. Put the information to be taught in logical sequence.
   c. Write down the key points.
   d. Select appropriate teaching aids.
   e. Keep the plan current and flexible to meet the person's changing learning needs.
6. Involve the learner, family or significant others, nursing team members, and other health care team members in all aspects of planning.

Implementation

1. Put the teaching plan into action.
2. Use language the person can understand.
3. Use appropriate teaching aids.
4. Use the same equipment that the person will use after discharge.
5. Encourage the person to participate actively in learning.
6. Record the learner's responses to the teaching actions.
7. Provide feedback.

Evaluation

1. Collect objective data.
   a. Observe the person.
   b. Ask questions to determine if the person understands.
   c. Use rating scales, checklists, anecdotal notes, and written tests when appropriate.
2. Compare the person's behavioral responses with the expected outcomes. Determine the extent to which the goals were achieved.
3. Include the person, family or significant others, nursing team members, and other health care team members in the evaluation.
4. Identify alterations that need to be made in the teaching plan.
5. Make referrals to appropriate sources or agencies for reinforcement of learning after discharge.
6. Continue all steps of the teaching process: assessment, diagnosis, planning, implementation, and evaluation.

ing plan communicates the following information to all members of the nursing team:

1. The nursing diagnoses that specifically relate to the individual's learning needs and the priorities of these diagnoses
2. The goals of the teaching strategies
3. The teaching strategies, expressed in the form of teaching orders
4. The expected outcomes, which identify the desired behavioral responses of the learner
5. The critical time period within which each outcome is expected to be met
6. The individual's behavioral responses (which must be documented on the teaching plan)

The same rules that apply to writing and revising the plan of nursing care apply to the teaching plan.

Implementation

In the implementation phase of the teaching–learning process, the patient, the family, and other members of the nursing and health care teams carry out the activities outlined in the teaching plan. All activities are coordinated by the nurse.

Flexibility during the implementation phase of the teaching–learning process and ongoing assessment of the individual's responses to the teaching strategies support modification of the teaching plan as necessary. Creativity in promoting and sustaining the learner's motivation to learn is essential. Consideration should be given to new learning needs that may arise after discharge from the hospital or after home care visits have ended.

The implementation phase is concluded when the teaching strategies have been completed and when the individual's responses to the actions have been recorded. This record serves as the basis for evaluating how well the defined goals and expected outcomes have been achieved.

Evaluation

Evaluation of the teaching–learning process determines how effectively the person has responded to the teaching strategies and to what extent the goals have been achieved. An important part of the evaluation phase addresses the question, "What can be done to improve the teaching and enhance the learning?" Answers to this question will direct the changes to be made in the teaching plan.

An evaluation must be made of what was done well, and what needs to be changed or reinforced. It cannot be assumed that individuals have learned because they have been taught; learning does not automatically follow teaching. A variety of measurement techniques can be used to identify changes in behavior as evidence that learning has taken place. These techniques include directly observing the behavior; using rating scales, checklists, or anecdotal notes to document the behaviors; and indirectly measuring results through oral questioning and written tests. Measurement of actual behavior (direct measurement) is the most accurate and appropriate technique in many patient teaching situations. Nurses often do comparative analysis using patient admission data as the baseline:

selected data points observed during the period that nursing care is given and self-care initiated are compared to the patient's baseline.

Some examples of indirect measurements are patient satisfaction surveys, attitude surveys, and instruments that evaluate specific health status variables. All direct measurements should be supplemented with indirect measurements whenever possible. When more than one measurement technique is employed, the reliability of the resultant data is enhanced. The potential for error from a specific measurement strategy is decreased when data are obtained using multiple evaluation methods.

Using measurement techniques is only the beginning of evaluation. These must be followed by interpreting the data and making value judgments about the learning and teaching. Such evaluation should be done periodically throughout the teaching–learning program, at its conclusion, and at varying periods after the teaching has ended.

Evaluation of learning after hospitalization is highly desirable, since the analysis of teaching outcomes must extend into home care. With shortened lengths of hospital stay and with short-stay and same-day surgical procedures, there is a particular need for follow-up evaluation in the home. Coordination of efforts and sharing of information between hospital-based and community-based nursing personnel facilitate postteaching and home care evaluation.

Evaluation is not the end step in the teaching–learning process, but the beginning of a new patient assessment. The information gathered during evaluation should be used to redirect teaching actions, with the goal of improving the learner's responses and outcomes.

HEALTH PROMOTION

Health teaching and health promotion are linked by a common goal—to encourage people to achieve as high a level of wellness as possible so that they can live maximally healthy lives and avoid preventable illnesses. The call for health promotion has become a cornerstone in health policy because of the need to control costs and reduce unnecessary sickness and death.

The nation's first public health agenda was established in 1979 and set goals for improving the health of all Americans. Additional goals were defined in 1980 by a list referred to as the "1990 health objectives." These goals identified improvements to be made in health status, risk reduction, public awareness, health services, and protective measures.

The most recent national health goals have been specified in *Healthy People 2000*. The priorities identified include health promotion, health protection, and the use of preventive services (Chart 4-2). Increased emphasis has been placed on the following objectives: prevention of disability and morbidity, greater attention to improvements in the health status of specific groups at highest risk for premature death, and increased provision for early detection of asymptomatic disease conditions in an attempt to prevent disability and early death. These objectives are directed toward meeting the World Health Organization's goal of "health for all by the year 2000" (U.S. Department of Health & Human Services, 1990).

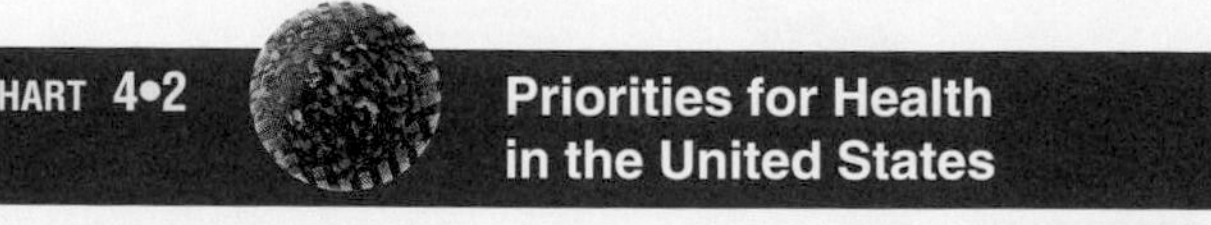

CHART 4•2
Priorities for Health in the United States

Health Promotion

1. Physical activity and fitness
2. Nutrition
3. Tobacco
4. Alcohol and other drugs
5. Family planning
6. Mental health and mental disorders
7. Violent and abusive behavior
8. Educational and community-based programs

Health Protection

9. Unintentional injuries
10. Occupational safety and health
11. Environmental health
12. Food and drug safety
13. Oral health

Preventive Services

14. Maternal and infant health
15. Heart disease and stroke
16. Cancer
17. Diabetes and chronic disabling conditions
18. HIV infection
19. Sexually transmitted diseases
20. Immunization and infectious diseases
21. Clinical preventive services

Surveillance and data systems

22. Surveillance and data systems

Age-Related Objectives

Children
Adolescents and young adults
Adults
Older adults

From U.S. Department of Health & Human Services (1995). *Healthy people 2000. Midcourse review and 1995 revisions.* Washington, DC: U.S. Government Printing Office.

Health and Wellness

The concept of health promotion has evolved because of a changing definition of health and an awareness that wellness exists at many levels of functioning. The definition of health as the mere absence of disease is no longer accepted. Today, health is viewed as a dynamic, ever-changing condition that enables a person to function at an optimum potential at any given time. The ideal health status is one in which people are successful in achieving their full potential regardless of any disabilities they might have.

Wellness, as a reflection of health, involves a conscious and deliberate attempt to maximize one's health. Wellness does not just happen; it requires planning and conscious commitment. It is the result of adopting lifestyle behaviors for the purpose of attaining one's highest potential for well-being. Wellness is not the same for every person. The person with a chronic illness or disability may still be able to achieve a desirable level of wellness. The key to wellness is to function at the highest potential within the limitations over which there is no control.

A significant amount of information has shown that people, by virtue of what they do or fail to do, influence their own health. Today, many of the major causes of illness are chronic diseases that have been closely related to lifestyle behaviors (eg, heart disease, lung and colon cancer, chronic obstructive pulmonary diseases, hypertension, cirrhosis, peptic ulcers, traumatic injury, HIV infection, and AIDS). Consequently, a person's health status to a large extent is reflective of lifestyle.

Health Promotion Models

Since the 1950s, many health-promotion models have been constructed to identify health-protecting behaviors and to help explain what makes people engage in these preventive behaviors. A health-protecting behavior is defined as any behavior performed by people, regardless of their actual or perceived health condition, for the purpose of promoting or maintaining their health, whether or not the behavior produces the desired outcome (Downie, Fyfe, & Tannahill, 1990). One framework, the health belief model, was devised to foster understanding of what made some healthy people choose actions to prevent illness while others refused to engage in these protective recommendations (Becker, 1974).

Another model, the resource model of preventive health behavior (Downie, Fyfe, & Tannahill, 1990), addresses the ways that people use resources to promote health. Nurse educators can use this model to assess how demographic variables, health behaviors, and social and health resources influence health promotion. LaLonde's (1977) health determinants model views human biology, environment, lifestyle, and the health care delivery system as the four determinants of a person's health.

A more recent model, the health promotion model developed by Pender (1996), is based on social learning theory and emphasizes the importance of motivational factors that influence the acquiring and sustaining of health-promotion behaviors. This model looks at how cognitive-perceptual factors affect one's view of the importance of health. It further examines perceived control of health, self-efficacy, health status, and the benefits and barriers to health promoting behaviors.

These models, along with other examples that can be found in the health promotion literature, can serve as an organizing framework for clinical work and research that supports the enhancement of health. In the future, efforts need to be made to advance understanding of the health promotion behaviors of families and communities.

Definition of Health Promotion

Health promotion can be defined as activities that assist a person to develop those resources that will maintain or enhance well-being and improve the quality of life. These activities refer to a person's actions to remain healthy in the absence of symptoms; such activities do not need the assistance of a member of the health care team.

The purpose of health promotion is to focus on a person's potential for wellness and to encourage appropriate alterations in personal habits, lifestyle, and environment in ways that will reduce risks and enhance health and well-being. Health promotion is an active process; that is, it is not something that can be prescribed or dictated. It is up to the individual to decide whether or not to make the changes that will promote a higher level of wellness. Choices must be made, and only the individual can make these choices.

Health Promotion Programs

The concepts of health, wellness, health promotion, and disease prevention have been extensively addressed in the lay literature and news media as well as in professional journals. The result has been a public demand for health information and a response by health care professionals and agencies to provide this information. Health-promotion programs that were once limited to hospital settings have now moved into community settings such as clinics, schools, churches, businesses, and industry. The workplace is quickly becoming an important site for health promotion programs, as employers strive to reduce costs associated with absenteeism, health insurance, hospitalization, disability, excessive turnover of personnel, and early death.

Health Promotion Principles

Certain principles underlie the concept of health promotion as an active process: self-responsibility, nutritional awareness, stress reduction and management, and physical fitness.

Self-Responsibility

Taking responsibility for oneself is the key to successful health promotion. This concept is based on the understanding that individuals control their lives. Each of us alone must make those choices that determine how healthy our lifestyle is. As more people recognize the significant effect that lifestyle and behavior have on health, they may assume responsibility for avoiding high-risk behaviors such as smoking, alcohol and drug abuse, overeating, driving while intoxicated, risky sexual practices, and other unhealthy habits. They may also assume responsibility for adopting routines that have been found to have a positive influence on health, such as engaging in regular exercise, wearing a seat belt, and eating a balanced diet.

A variety of different techniques have been used to encourage people to accept responsibility for their health. These methods have ranged from extensive educational programs to reward systems. Studies have not shown any one technique to be superior to any other. Instead, self-responsibility for health promotion is very individualized and depends on a person's desires and inner motivations. Health promotion programs are important tools for encouraging people to assume responsibility for their health and to develop behaviors that improve health.

Nutrition

Nutrition as a component of health promotion has become the focus of considerable attention and publicity. A vast array of books and magazine articles address the topics of special diets, natural foods, and the hazards of certain substances, such as sugar, salt, cholesterol, artificial colors, and food additives. Good nutrition has been suggested as the single most significant factor in determining health status and longevity.

Nutritional awareness involves an understanding of the importance of a properly balanced diet that supplies all of the essential nutrients. Understanding the relationship between diet and disease is an important facet of a person's self-care. Some clinicians believe that a healthy diet is one that substitutes "natural" foods for processed and refined ones; in addition, there must be a reduced intake of sugar, salt, fat, cholesterol, caffeine, alcohol, and food additives and preservatives.

Chapter 5 contains detailed information about assessment of an individual's nutritional status. Physical signs indicating nutritional status, anthropometric measurements, assessment of food intake (food record, 24-hour recall), comparison of food intake to the dietary guidelines outlined in the Food Guide Pyramid, and calculation of ideal body weight are covered in that chapter.

Stress Management

Stress management and stress reduction are important aspects of health promotion. Studies have shown the negative effects of stress on health and a cause-and-effect relationship between stress and infectious diseases, traumatic injuries (eg, motor vehicle crashes), and some chronic illnesses. Stress has become inevitable in contemporary urban societies in which demands for productivity have become excessive. More and more emphasis is placed on encouraging people to manage stress appropriately and to reduce stress that is counterproductive. Techniques such as relaxation training, exercise, and modification of stressful situations are often included in health-promotion programs that deal with stress. Further information on stress management, including health risk appraisal and stress reduction methods such as biofeedback and the relaxation response, can be found in Chapter 6.

Exercise

Physical fitness is another important component of health promotion. Studies examining the relationship between health and physical fitness have found that a regular exercise program can promote health by improving the function of the circulatory system and the lungs, decreasing cholesterol and low-density lipoproteins, lowering body weight by increasing calorie expenditure, delaying degenerative changes such as osteoporosis, and improving flexibility and overall muscle strength and endurance. On the other hand, exercise can be harmful if it is not started gradually and increased slowly in accordance with the individual's response. An exercise program should be designed specifically for the individual, with consideration given to age, physical condition, and any known cardiovascular or other risk factors. An appropriate exercise program can have a significant positive effect on the individual's performance capacity, appearance, and general state of physical and emotional health.

HEALTH PROMOTION THROUGHOUT THE LIFE SPAN

Health promotion as a concept and a process extends throughout the life span. Studies have shown that the health of a child can be affected either positively or negatively by the health practices of the mother during the prenatal period. Thus, health promotion starts before birth and extends through childhood, adulthood, and old age.

Health promotion includes health screening. The American Academy of Family Physicians has developed recommendations for periodic health examinations, identifying the age groups for whom specific screening interventions are appropriate. Table 4-1 presents the general population guidelines, and specific population standards and guidelines have also been recommended.

Children and Adolescents

Health screening has traditionally been an important aspect of childhood health care. The goal has been to detect health problems at an early age so that they can be treated early in a child's life. Today, health promotion goes beyond the mere screening of children for disabilities. Extensive efforts are made to promote positive health practices at a very young age. Since health habits and practices are formed early in life, children should be encouraged to develop positive health attitudes. For this reason, more and more programs are being offered to school-age children and to adolescents to help them develop good health habits. While the negative results of practices such as smoking, risky sexual activities, alcohol and drug abuse, and poor nutrition are explained in these educational programs, emphasis is also placed on values training, self-esteem, and healthy lifestyle practices. The projects are designed to appeal to a particular age group, with emphasis on learning experiences that are fun, interesting, and relevant.

Young and Middle-Aged Adults

Young and middle-aged adults represent an age group that not only expresses an interest in health and health promotion, but also responds enthusiastically to suggestions that show how lifestyle practices can improve health. Adults are frequently motivated to change their lifestyles in ways that are believed to enhance their health and wellness. Many adults who wish to improve their health turn to health-promotion programs to help them make the desired changes in their lifestyles. They respond in overwhelming numbers to programs that focus on topics such as general wellness, smoking cessation, exercise, physical conditioning, weight control, conflict resolution, and stress management. Because of the nationwide emphasis on health during the reproductive years, young adults actively seek programs that address prenatal health, parenting, family planning, and women's health issues.

Programs that provide health screening, such as those that screen for cancer, hypertension, diabetes, and hearing impairments, are quite popular with this age group. Programs that cover health promotion for people with specific chronic illnesses such as cancer, diabetes, heart disease, and pulmonary disease are also popular. It is becoming more evident that chronic disease does not preclude health and wellness; rather, positive health attitudes and practices can promote optimal health for people who must live with the limitations imposed by their chronic illnesses.

Health-promotion programs can be offered almost anywhere in the community. Common sites include local clinics, elementary schools, high schools, community colleges, recreation centers, churches, and even private homes. Health fairs are frequently held in civic centers and shopping malls. The outreach idea for health-promotion programs has served to meet the needs of many adults who otherwise would not avail themselves of opportunities to strive toward a healthier lifestyle.

The workplace has become a center for health-promotion activity. Employers are increasingly concerned about the rising costs of health care insurance to treat illnesses that are related to lifestyle behaviors. They are also concerned about increased absenteeism and lost productivity. For these reasons, many businesses have instituted health-promotion programs in the workplace. Some employ health-promotion specialists to develop and implement the program; others purchase packaged programs that have already been developed by health care agencies or private health-promotion corporations.

Programs offered at the workplace usually include employee health screening and counseling, physical fitness, nutritional awareness, work safety, and stress management and reduction. In addition, efforts are made to promote a safe and healthy work environment. Many large businesses provide exercise facilities for their employees and offer their health-promotion programs to retirees. If employers can show cost-containment benefits from such programs, their dollars will be considered well spent, and more businesses will provide health-promotion programs as a benefit of employment.

Elderly Adults

Health promotion is as important for the elderly as it is for other age groups. Despite the fact that 80% of people over the age of 65 have one or more chronic illnesses and about 50% of the

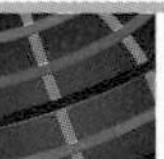

TABLE 4•1 **Routine Health Promotion Screening for Adults***

Type of Screening	Suggested Time Frame
Routine health exam	Yearly
Blood chemistry profile	Baseline at age 20, then as mutually determined by patient and clinician
Complete blood count	Baseline at age 20, then as mutually determined by patient and clinician
Lipid profile	Baseline at age 20, then as mutually determined by patient and clinician
Hemoccult screening	Yearly after age 50
Electrocardiogram	Baseline at age 40, then as mutually determined by patient and clinician
Blood pressure	Yearly, then as mutually determined by patient and clinician
Tuberculosis skin test	Every 2 years or as mutually determined by patient and clinician
Breast self-exam	Monthly
Mammogram	Yearly for women over 40
Clinical breast exam	Yearly
Gynecologic exam	Yearly
Pap test	Yearly
Bone density screening	Based on identification of primary and secondary risk factors and prior to initiation of menopause
Digital rectal exam	Yearly
Sigmoidoscopy	Every 3–5 years after age 50 or as mutually determined by patient and clinician
Prostate exam	Yearly
Prostate specific antigen	Every 1–2 years after age 50
Testicular exam	Monthly
Skin exam	Yearly or as mutually determined by patient and clinician
Vision screening	Every 2–3 years
Glaucoma	Baseline at age 40, then every 2–3 years until age 70, then yearly
Dental screening	Every 6 months
Hearing screening	As needed
Dietary profile	As needed
Health risk appraisal	As needed
Adult immunizations	
Tetanus	Boosters every 10 years
Diphtheria	Boosters every 10 years
Flu vaccine	Yearly

**Note:* Any of these screenings may be performed more frequently if deemed necessary by the patient or recommended by the health care provider.

elderly are limited in their activity, the elderly as a group experience significant gains from health promotion. Studies have shown that the elderly are very health-conscious and that most view their health positively and are willing to adopt practices that will improve their health and well-being. Although their chronic illnesses and disabilities cannot be eliminated, these adults can benefit from activities that help them maintain independence and achieve an optimal level of health.

Various health-promotion programs have been developed to meet the needs of older Americans. Many of these began within the Department of Health and Human Services. Both public and private organizations continue to be responsive to this initiative, and more programs that serve the elderly are emerging. Many of these are offered by health care agencies, churches, community centers, senior citizen residences, and a variety of other organizations. The activities directed toward health promotion for the elderly are the same as those for other age groups: physical fitness and exercise, nutrition, safety, and stress management.

IMPLICATIONS FOR NURSING

Nurses, by virtue of their expertise in health and health care and their long-established credibility with consumers, play a vital role in health promotion. In many instances they have initiated health-promotion programs or have participated with other health care personnel in developing and providing wellness services in a variety of settings (Fig. 4-2).

As health care professionals, nurses have a responsibility to promote activities that foster well-being, self-actualization, and personal fulfillment. Every interaction with consumers of health

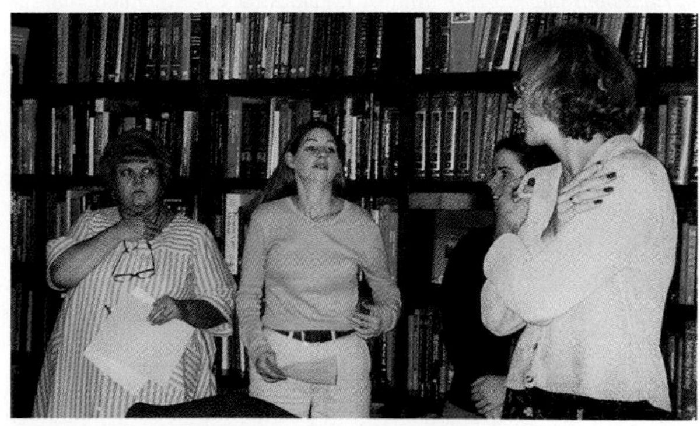

FIGURE 4•2 Teaching aids and demonstrations enhance learning. Here a nurse (*right*) instructs learners during a community health education program. Often generated and developed by nurses, these programs offer the public opportunities to obtain health information about topics ranging from diet, nutrition, and hypercholesterolemia to hypertension, diabetes, cardiopulmonary resuscitation, and others.

care must be viewed as an opportunity to promote positive health attitudes and behaviors.

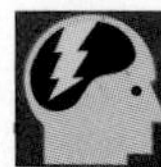

Critical Thinking Exercises

1. You are developing a patient teaching plan for a patient with diabetes mellitus. Describe the strategies you would develop for promoting adherence to the therapeutic regimen. Indicate the possible variables that could influence the patient's willingness or ability to follow the instructions.
2. You are assigned to teach an elderly patient about the medications that she will be taking at home. How would you assess this patient's condition and psychosocial situation to determine how best to instruct her about her medications?
3. A neighbor tells you that he has heard about a health fair that is being offered at a nearby civic center. He asks you if you think that he should attend. Describe the reasons you might give for why he should attend.

References and Selected Readings

BOOKS

American Nurses Association. (1998). *Standards of clinical nursing practice.* Washington DC: Author.

Andrews, M. M., & Boyle, J. S. (1995). *Transcultural concepts in nursing care* (2nd ed.). Philadelphia: J. B. Lippincott.

Becker, M. H. (Ed.). (1974). *The health belief model and personal health behavior.* Thorofare, NJ: Charles B. Slack.

Carpenito, L. J. (1997). *Nursing diagnosis: Application to clinical practice.* Philadelphia: Lippincott-Raven.

Dickey, L. L. (1994). *Clinician's handbook of preventive services: Put prevention into practice.* Waldorf, MD: American Nurses Publishing.

Downie, R. S., Fyfe, C., & Tannahill, A. (1990). *Health promotion: Models and values.* New York: Oxford University Press.

Edelman, C., & Mandle, C. L. (1998). *Health promotion throughout the lifespan* (4th ed.) St. Louis: C. V. Mosby.

Eliopoulos, C. (1997). *Gerontological nursing.* Philadelphia: Lippincott-Raven.

Giger, J. N., & Davidhizar, R. E. (1991). *Transcultural nursing.* St. Louis: C. V. Mosby.

Green, L., & Kreuter, M. (1991). *Health promotion planning: An educational and environmental approach* (2nd ed.). Palo Alto, CA: Mayfield Publishing.

Knollmueller, R. N. (1993). *Prevention across the life span: Healthy people for the twenty-first century.* Washington DC: American Nurses Publishing.

LaLonde, M. (1977). *New perspectives on the health of Canadians: A working document.* Ottawa, Canada: Minister of Supply and Services.

Leininger, M. M. (1991). *Culture care diversity and universality: A theory of nursing.* New York: National League of Nursing.

Murray, R. B., & Zentner, J. P. (1997). *Nursing assessment and health promotion through the life span* (6th ed.). Englewood Cliffs, NJ: Prentice-Hall.

Pender, N. J. (1996). *Health promotion in nursing practice* (3rd ed.) Norwalk, CT: Appleton & Lange.

Rankin, S. H., & Stallings, K. D. (1995). *Patient education: Issues, principles, practices* (3rd ed.). Philadelphia: J. B. Lippincott.

Redman, B. (1996). *The practice of patient education* (8th ed.). St. Louis: C. V. Mosby.

Simnett, I. (1995). *Managing health promotion: Developing healthy organizations and communities.* New York: Wiley.

U.S. Public Health Service. (1990). *Healthy people 2000.* Washington, DC: U.S. Government Printing Office.

U.S. Public Health Service. (1995). *Healthy people 2000: Midcourse review and 1995 revision.* Washington, DC: U.S. Government Printing Office.

Woolf, S. H., Jonas, S., & Lawrence, R. S. (1996). *Health promotion and disease prevention in clinical practice.* Baltimore: Williams & Wilkins.

JOURNALS

Asterisks indicate nursing research articles.

Appling, S. E. (1997). Advanced practice nursing: Wellness promotion and the elderly. *MedSurg Nursing, 6*(1), 45–46.

Barry, R., & Burggraf, V. (1996). Healthy people: Objective look at the elderly. *Journal of Gerontological Nursing, 22*(10), 9–11.

Bowman, M. A., Braly, P., Johnson, S., & Mikuta, J. J. (1996). Who are you screening for cancer—and when? *Patient Care, 30*(13), 54–64.

Drugay, M. (1997). Healthy People 2000: Breaking the silence: A health promotion approach to osteoporosis. *Journal of Gerontological Nursing, 23*(6), 36–43.

Herje, P. A. (1980). Hows and whys of patient contracting. *Journal of Nursing Education, 5*, 30–34.

Jones, J. M., & Jones, K. D. (1997). Healthy People 2000: Promoting physical activity in the senior years. *Journal of Gerontological Nursing, 23*(7), 41–48.

Keeling, A., Utz, S. W., Shuster, G. F., & Boyle, A. (1993). Noncompliance revisited: A disciplinary perspective on a nursing diagnosis. *Nursing Diagnosis, 4*(3), 91–98.

Kelleher, C. (1996). Education and training in health promotion: Theory and methods. *Health Promotion International, 11*(1), 47–53.

*Lev, E. L., & Owen, S. V. (1996). A measure of self-care self-efficacy: Strategies used by people to promote health. *Research in Nursing & Health, 19*(5), 421–429.

McQueen, D. V. (1996). The search for theory in health behavior and health promotion. *Health Promotion International, 11*(1), 27–32.

O'Halloran, V. E. (1997). Defining educational settings to improve client health teaching. *MedSurg Nursing, 6*(3), 130–136.

Powell, D. R., Sharp, S. L., Farnell, S. D., & Smith, P. T. (1997). Implementing a self-care program: Effect on employee health care utilization. *AAOHN Journal, 45*(5), 247–253.

Robinson, B. E. (1996). Progress in prevention: The Prevention for Elderly Persons (PEP) program: A model of municipal and academic partnership to meet the needs of older persons for preventive services. *Journal of the American Geriatrics Society, 44*(11), 1399.

Schneider, S. L., Richard, M., Huss, K., et al. (1997). Moving health care education into the community. *Nursing Management, 28*(9), 40–43.

Snow, E. B. (1997). The periodic health exam for older adults. *Journal of the American Academy of Physician Assistants, 10*(4), 89–104.

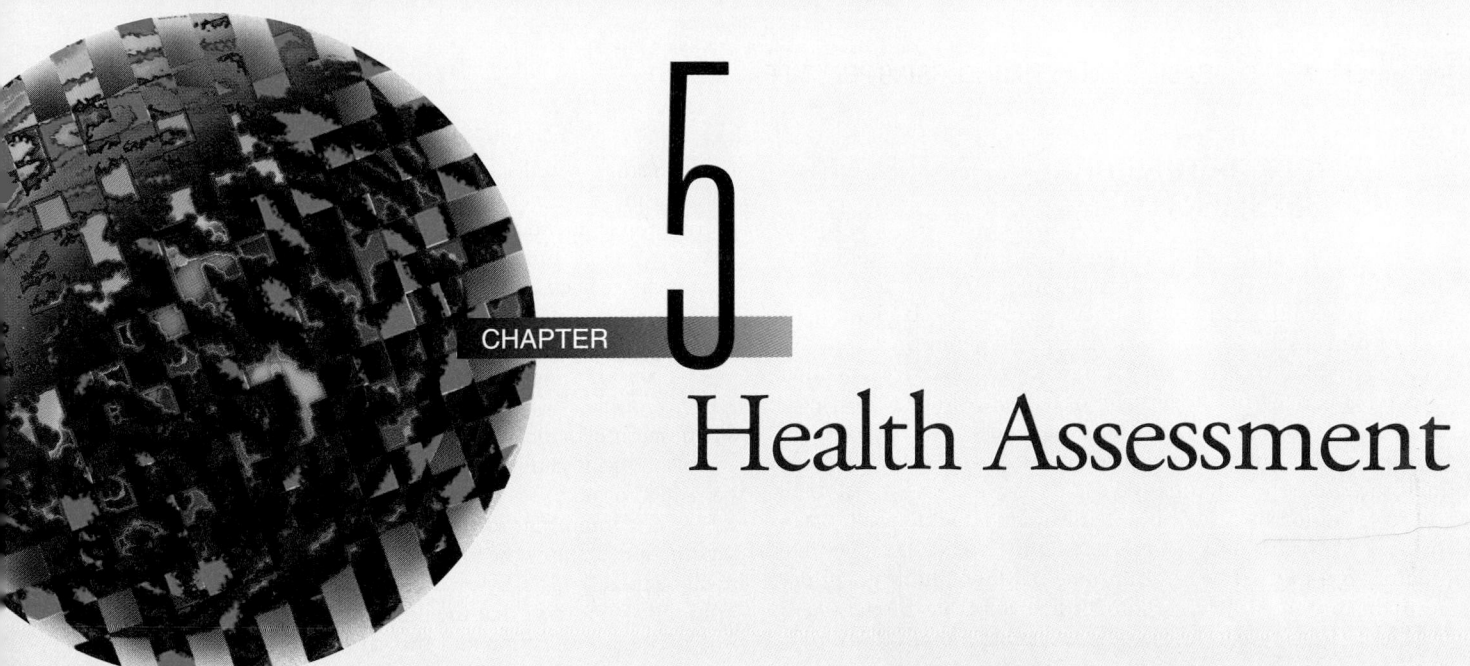

Health Assessment

Learning Objectives

On completion of this chapter, the learner will be able to:

1. Describe the components of the health history.
2. Identify ethical considerations necessary for protection of the individual's rights related to data collected in the health history or physical examination.
3. Use interviewing skills and techniques to conduct a successful interview.
4. Describe the physical examination techniques of inspection, palpation, percussion, and auscultation.
5. Use inspection, palpation, percussion, and auscultation to perform physical assessment of the major body systems.
6. Use clinical examination, anthropometric measurements, biochemical assessment, and assessment of food intake to assess a person's nutritional status.
7. Describe factors that may contribute to altered nutritional status in the elderly.
8. Conduct a health history and physical and nutritional assessment of the patient at home.

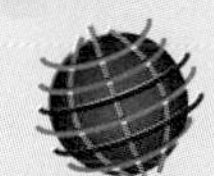

The ability to assess the patient is one of the most important skills of the nurse, regardless of the practice setting. In all settings where nurses provide care, eliciting a complete history and using appropriate assessment skills are critical to identifying physical and psychological problems and concerns experienced by the patient. Patient assessment is the first step in the nursing process and is necessary to obtain data that will enable the nurse to make a nursing diagnosis, identify and implement nursing interventions, and assess their effectiveness.

THE ROLE OF THE NURSE IN ASSESSMENT

The role of the nurse includes obtaining the patient's history and performing a physical assessment; this role can be carried out in a variety of settings, including the acute care setting, clinic or outpatient office, school, long-term care facility, and the home. A growing list of nursing diagnoses is used by nurses to identify and categorize patient problems that nurses have the knowledge, skills, and responsibility to treat. All members of the health care team, comprising physicians, nurses, nutritionists, social workers, and others, use their unique skills and knowledge to contribute to the resolution of patient problems by first obtaining a health history and physical examination. Because the focus of each member of the health care team may be different, a variety of health history and physical examination formats have been developed. Regardless of the format, the database obtained by the nurse is complementary to the databases obtained by other members of the health care team and focuses on nursing's unique concern for the patient.

BASIC GUIDELINES FOR CONDUCTING A HEALTH ASSESSMENT

People who seek health care for a specific problem are often anxious; this anxiety may be increased by fear about potential disruption of lifestyle and by other concerns. The examiner attempts to put the person at ease and to encourage honest communication. The examiner listens carefully to the person's responses to questions about health issues and makes eye contact (Fig. 5-1). When obtaining the health history or performing the physical examination, the interviewer is aware of his or her own nonverbal communication as well as that of the patient. The examiner takes into consideration the educational background and language proficiency of the patient. Questions and instructions to the patient are phrased in a way that is easily understandable, avoiding technical terms. In addition, the examiner is aware of the patient's disabilities or limitations (hearing, vision, cognitive and physical limitations) and takes these into consideration during the history as well as the physical examination. At the end of the assessment, the examiner may summarize and clarify the information obtained and ask if the person has any questions; this provides an opportunity to correct misinformation and add facts that may have been omitted.

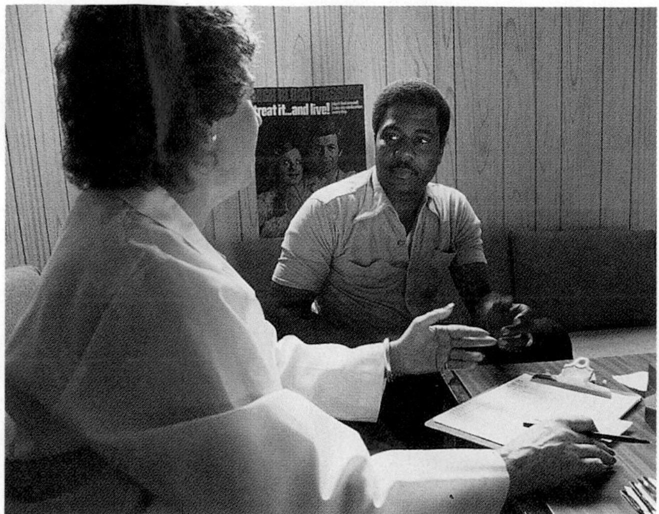

FIGURE 5•1 A comfortable, relaxed atmosphere and an attentive interviewer are essential for a successful clinical interview.

ETHICAL USE OF HISTORY OR PHYSICAL EXAMINATION DATA

Whenever information is elicited from a person through the history or physical examination, that person has the right to know why the information is sought and how it will be used. For this reason, it is important to explain what the history and physical examination are, how the information will be obtained, and how it will be used.

It is also important that the individual be informed about the process of data collection and that the decision to participate is voluntary. A private setting for the history interview and physical examination promotes trust and encourages open, honest communication. After the history and examination, the nurse selectively records the data pertinent to the patient's health status. The written record of the patient's history and physical examination findings is maintained in a secure place and made available only to those health professionals directly involved in the care of the patient. This protects confidentiality and promotes professional conduct.

THE HEALTH HISTORY

Throughout assessment, and particularly when obtaining the history, attention is focused on the impact of psychosocial, ethnic, and cultural patterns on the person's health, illness, and health-promotion behaviors. The interpersonal and physical environments, as well as the person's lifestyle and activities of daily living, are explored in depth. Many nurses are responsible for obtaining a detailed history of the person's current health problems, past medical history, and family history, and reviewing the functional status of body systems. This results in a total health profile that focuses on health as well as illness and is more appropriately called a health history rather than a medical or a nursing history.

The format of the health history has traditionally been a combination of the medical history and the nursing assessment, although formats based on nursing frameworks such as functional health patterns have also become a standard. Both the review of systems and patient profile are expanded to include individual and family relationships, lifestyle patterns, health practices, and coping strategies. These components of the health history are the basis of nursing assessment and can be easily adapted to address the needs of any patient population in any setting, institution, or agency.

Combining the information obtained by the physician and the nurse in one health history avoids duplication of information, minimizes efforts on the part of the person to provide this information, and encourages collaboration between members of the health care team who share in the collection and interpretation of the database.

The Informant

The informant, or the person providing the health history, may not always be the patient, as in the case of a child or a disoriented, confused, unconscious, or comatose patient. The interviewer assesses the reliability of the informant and the usefulness of the information provided. For example, a disoriented patient is often unable to provide a reliable database; people who abuse drugs and alcohol often deny using these substances. The interviewer must make a judgment about the reliability of the information (based on the context of the entire interview), and he or she includes this evaluation in the record.

Cultural Considerations

When obtaining the health history, the interviewer takes into account the person's cultural background. Cultural attitudes and beliefs about health, illness, health care, hospitalization, and the use of medications must be accepted at face value. These beliefs and attitudes are derived from each person's experiences, which vary according to the person's ethnic and cultural background. A person from another culture may have a different view of personal health practices than the practitioners providing care.

Similarly, people from some ethnic backgrounds will not complain of pain, even when it is severe, because their culture does not condone outward expressions of pain. In some instances they may refuse to take analgesics. Other cultures have their own folklore and beliefs about the treatment of illnesses. All such differences in outlook must be taken into account and accepted when caring for members of other cultures. Attitudes and beliefs about family relationships and the role of women and elderly members of a family must be respected even if those attitudes and beliefs conflict with those of the interviewer.

Content of the Health History

When the patient is seen for the first time by a member of the health team (except in emergency situations), the first requirement is a database. The sequence and format of obtaining data about the patient vary, but the content, regardless of format, usually addresses the same general topics. A traditional approach includes the following:

1. Biographical data
2. Chief complaint
3. Present illness (or present health concern)
4. Past history
5. Family history
6. Review of systems
7. Patient profile

Biographical Data

Biographical information puts the health history in context. This information includes the person's name, address, age, gender, marital status, occupation, and ethnic origins. Some interviewers prefer to ask more personal questions at this part of the interview, while others wait until more trust and confidence have been established or until the patient's immediate or urgent needs are first addressed. The patient in severe pain or with another urgent problem is unlikely to have a great deal of patience for an interviewer who is more concerned about marital or occupational status than with quickly addressing the problem at hand.

Chief Complaint

The chief complaint is the issue that brings the person to the attention of the health care provider. Questions such as, "Why have you come to the health center today?" or "Why have you been admitted to the hospital?" usually elicit the chief complaint. In the home setting, the initial question might be, "What is bothering you most today?" When a problem is identified, the person's exact words are usually recorded in quotation marks. However, a statement such as, "My doctor sent me" should be followed up with a question that identifies the probable reason why the person is seeking health care; this reason is then identified as the chief complaint.

Present Illness

The history of the present illness is the single most important factor in assisting the health professional in arriving at a diagnosis or determining the person's needs. The physical examination is helpful but often only validates the information obtained from the history. A careful history assists in correct selection of appropriate diagnostic tests. While diagnostic test results can be helpful, they often verify rather than establish the diagnosis.

If the present illness is only one episode in a series of episodes, the entire sequence of events is recorded. For example, a history from a patient whose chief complaint is an episode of insulin shock describes the entire course of the diabetes to put the current episode in context. The details of the present illness or health concern are described from onset until the time of contact with the health care team. These facts are recorded in chronological order, beginning with, for example, "The patient was in good health until . . ." or "The patient first experienced abdominal pain 2 months prior to seeking help."

The history of the present illness or problem includes such information as the date and manner (sudden, gradual) in which the problem occurred, the setting in which the problem developed (at home, at work, after an argument, after exercise), manifestations of the problem, and the course of the illness or problem. This includes self-treatment, medical interventions, progress and effects of treatment, and the patient's perceptions of the cause or meaning of the problem.

Specific symptoms (pain, headache, fever, change in bowel habits) are described in detail, along with the location and radiation (if pain), quality, severity, and duration. The interviewer also asks if the problem is persistent or intermittent, what factors aggravate or alleviate it, and if any associated manifestations exist.

Associated manifestations are symptoms that occur simultaneously with the chief complaint. The presence or absence of such symptoms may shed light on the origin or extent of the problem, as well as on the diagnosis. These symptoms are referred to as significant positive or negative findings and are obtained from a review of systems directly related to the chief complaint. For example, if the person reports a vague symptom, such as fatigue or weight loss, all body systems are reviewed and included in the history of the present illness. If, on the other hand, the person's chief complaint is chest pain, only the cardiopulmonary and gastrointestinal systems may be included in the history of the present illness. In either situation, both positive and negative findings are recorded to define the problem further.

Past Health History

A detailed summary of the person's past health is an important part of the database. After the general health status is determined, inquiries are made about immunization status and any known allergies to medications or other substances. The dates of immunization are recorded, along with the type of allergy and adverse reactions. The person is asked to provide information, if known, about his or her last physical examination, chest x-ray, electrocardiogram, eye examination, hearing tests, dental checkup, and Papanicolaou (Pap) smear (if female). Previous illnesses are then discussed. Negative as well as positive responses to a list of specific diseases are recorded. Dates, or the age of the patient at the time of illness, as well as the names of the primary care provider and hospital, the diagnosis, and the treatment are also recorded. A history of the following areas is elicited:

- Childhood illness—rubeola, rubella, polio, whooping cough, mumps, chickenpox, scarlet fever, rheumatic fever, strep throat
- Adult illnesses
- Psychiatric illnesses
- Injuries—burns, fractures, head injuries
- Hospitalizations
- Surgical and diagnostic procedures
- Current medications—prescription, over-the-counter, home remedies
- Use of alcohol and other drugs

If a particular hospitalization or major medical intervention is related to the present illness, it is not repeated; rather, the report refers to the appropriate part of the report, such as "see history of present illness" or "see HPI" on the data sheet.

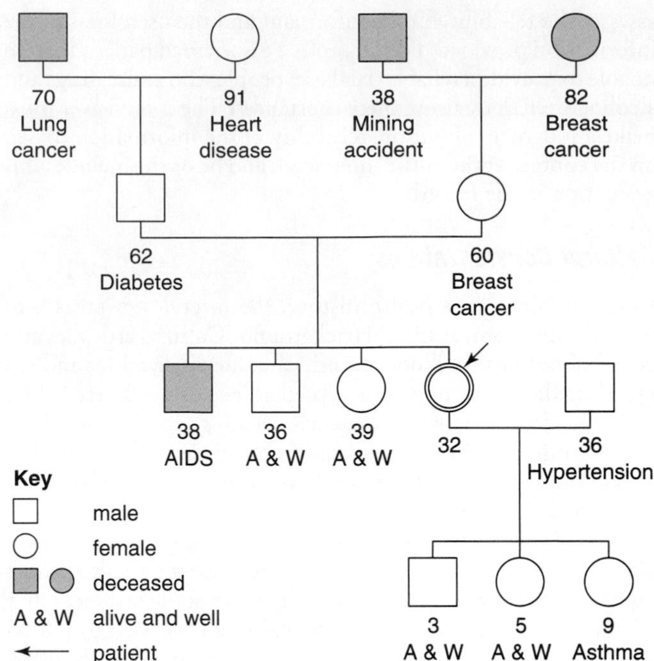

FIGURE 5•2 Diagram (called a genogram) used to record history of family members including their age and cause of death or, if living, their current health status.

Family History

The age and health status, or the age and cause of death, of first-order relatives (parents, siblings, spouse, children) and second-order relatives (grandparents, cousins) are elicited to identify diseases that may be genetic in origin, communicable, or possibly environmental in cause. The following diseases are generally covered: cancer, hypertension, heart disease, diabetes, epilepsy, mental illness, tuberculosis, kidney disease, arthritis, allergies, asthma, alcoholism, and obesity. One of the easiest methods of recording such data is by using the family tree or genogram (Fig. 5-2). The results of genetic testing or screening, if known, are recorded.

Review of Systems

The systems review includes an overview of general health as well as symptoms related to each body system. Questions are asked about each of the major body systems in terms of past or present symptoms. Reviewing each body system helps reveal any relevant data. Negative as well as positive answers are recorded. If the patient responds positively to questions about a particular system, the information is analyzed carefully. If any illnesses were previously mentioned or recorded, it is not necessary to repeat them in this part of the history. Instead, reference is made to the appropriate place in the history where the information can be found.

A review of systems can be organized in a formal checklist, which becomes a part of the health history. One advantage of a checklist is that it can be easily audited and is less subject to error than a system that relies heavily on the interviewer's memory.

Patient Profile

In the patient profile, more biographical information is gathered. A complete composite, or profile, of the patient is critical to an analysis of the chief complaint and of the person's ability to deal with the problem.

The information elicited at this point in the interview is highly personal and subjective. During this stage, the person is encouraged to express feelings honestly and to discuss personal experiences. It is best to begin with general, open-ended questions and to move to direct questioning when specific facts are needed. The patient is often less anxious when the interview progresses from information that is less personal (birthplace, occupation, education) to information that is more personal (sexuality, body image, coping abilities).

A general patient profile consists of the following content areas:

1. Past life events related to health
2. Education and occupation
3. Environment (physical, spiritual, cultural, interpersonal)
4. Lifestyle (patterns and habits)
5. Self-concept
6. Sexuality
7. Risk for abuse
8. Stress and coping response

The patient profile is summarized in Chart 5-1.

PAST LIFE EVENTS RELATED TO HEALTH

The patient profile begins with a brief life history. Questions about place of birth and past places of residence help focus attention on the earlier years of life. Personal experiences during childhood or adolescence that have special significance may be elicited by asking, "Was there anything that you experienced as a child or adolescent that would be helpful for me to know about?" The interviewer's intent is to encourage the person to make a quick review of his or her earlier life, highlighting information of particular significance. Although many patients may not recall anything significant, others may share information such as a personal achievement, a failure, a developmental crisis, or an instance of physical or emotional abuse.

EDUCATION AND OCCUPATION

Inquiring about current occupation can reveal much about a person's economic status and educational preparation. A statement such as, "Tell me about your job" often elicits information about

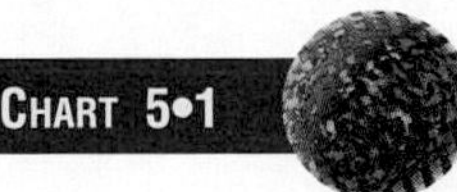

CHART 5•1 Patient Profile

Past Events Related to Health

Place of birth
Places lived
Significant childhood/adolescent experiences

Education and Occupation

Jobs held in past
Current position/job
Length of time at position
Educational preparation
Work satisfaction and career goals
Financial resources
Insurance coverage

Environment

Physical

Living arrangements (type of housing, neighborhood, presence of hazards)

Spiritual

Extent to which religion is a part of individual's life
Religious beliefs related to perception of health and illness
Religious practices

Interpersonal

Ethnic background (language spoken, customs and values held, folk practices used to maintain health or to cure illness)
Family relationships (family structure, roles, communication patterns, support system)
Friendships (quality of relationship)

Lifestyle Patterns

Sleep (time individual retires, hours per night, comfort measures, awakens rested)
Exercise (type, frequency, time spent)
Nutrition (24-hour diet recall, idiosyncrasies, restrictions)
Recreation (type of activity, time spent)
Caffeine (coffee, tea, cola, chocolate)—kind, amount
Smoking (cigarette, pipe, cigar, marijuana)—kind, amount per day, number of years, desire to quit
Alcohol—kind, amount, pattern over past year
Drugs—kind, amount, route of administration

Self-Concept

View of self in present
View of self in future
Body image (level of satisfaction, concerns)

Sexuality

Perception of self as a man or woman
Quality of sexual relationships
Concerns related to sexuality or sexual functioning

Risk for Abuse

Physical injury in past
Afraid of partner, caregiver, family

Stress and Coping Response

Major concerns or problems at present
Daily "hassles"
Past experiences with similar problems
Past coping patterns and outcomes
Present coping strategies and anticipated outcomes
Individual's expectations of family/friends and health care team in problem resolution

---

role, job tasks, and satisfaction with the position. Direct questions about past employment and career goals may be asked if the person does not provide this information.

Asking the person what kind of educational requirements were necessary to attain his or her present job is a more sensitive approach to educational background than asking whether he or she graduated from high school. Information about the patient's general financial status may be obtained by questions such as, "Do you have any financial concerns at this time?" or "Sometimes there just doesn't seem to be enough money to make ends meet. Are you finding this true?" Inquiry about the person's insurance coverage and plans for health care payment is also appropriate.

ENVIRONMENT

The person's physical environment and its potential hazards, spiritual awareness, cultural background, interpersonal relationships, and support system are included in the concept of environment.

Physical Environment. Information is elicited about the type of housing (apartment, duplex, single family) in which the person lives, its location, the level of safety and comfort within the home and neighborhood, and the presence of environmental hazards (eg, isolation, potential fire risks, inadequate sanitation). The patient's environment takes on special importance if the patient is homeless or living in a homeless shelter.

Spiritual Environment. The term spiritual environment refers to the degree to which a person is thoughtful or contemplative about his or her existence, accepts challenges in life, and seeks and finds answers to personal questions. Spirituality may be expressed through identification with a particular religion. Spiritual values and beliefs often direct a person's behavior and approach to health problems and can influence responses to sickness. Illness may create a spiritual crisis and can place considerable stress on a person's internal resources and beliefs. Inquiring about spirituality can identify possible support systems as well as beliefs and customs that need to be considered in planning care. Thus, information is gathered in the following three areas:

- The extent to which religion is a part of the person's life
- Religious beliefs related to the person's perception of health and illness
- Religious practices

The following questions can be used in a spiritual assessment:

- Is religion or God important to you?
- If yes, in what way?
- If no, what is the most important thing in your life?
- Are there any religious practices that are important to you?
- Do you have any spiritual concerns because of your present health problem?

Interpersonal and Cultural Environment. Cultural influences, relationships with family and friends, and the presence or absence of a support system are all a part of one's interpersonal environment. The beliefs and practices that have been shared from generation to generation are known as cultural or ethnic patterns. They are expressed through language, dress, dietary choices, and role behaviors, in perceptions of health and illness, and in health-related behaviors. The influence of these beliefs and customs on how a person reacts to health problems and interacts with health care providers cannot be underestimated. For this reason, the health history includes information on ethnic identity (cultural and social) and racial identity (biologic). The following questions may assist in obtaining relevant information:

- Where did your parents or ancestors come from? When?
- What language do you speak at home?
- Are there certain customs or values that are important to you?
- Is there anything special you do to keep in good health?
- Do you have any specific practices for treating illness?

Family Relationships and Support System. An assessment of family structure (members, ages, roles), patterns of communication, and the presence or absence of a support system is an integral part of the patient profile. Although the traditional family is recognized as a mother, a father, and children, many different types of living arrangements exist within our society. "Family" may mean two or more people bound by emotional ties or commitments. Live-in companions, roommates, and close friends can all play a significant role in an individual's support system.

LIFESTYLE

The lifestyle section of the patient profile provides information about health-related behaviors. These behaviors include patterns of sleep, exercise, nutrition, and recreation, as well as personal habits such as smoking and the use of drugs, alcohol, and caffeine. Although most people readily describe their exercise patterns or recreational activities, many are unwilling to report their smoking, alcohol use, and drug use; many deny or understate the degree to which they use such substances. Questions such as, "What kind of alcohol do you enjoy drinking at a party?" may elicit more accurate information than, "Do you drink?" The specific type of alcohol (eg, wine, liquor, beer) and the amount ingested per day or per week (eg, 1 pint of whiskey daily for 2 years) are described.

When alcohol abuse is suspected, additional information may be obtained by asking, "Has anyone ever said that drinking might be causing a problem for you?" or "Have you ever considered cutting down your alcohol intake?" The same approach can be used to elicit information about smoking and caffeine consumption. Questions about drug use follow naturally after questions about smoking, caffeine consumption, and alcohol use. A nonjudgmental approach will make it easier for the person to respond truthfully and factually. If street names or unfamiliar terms are used to describe drugs, the person is asked to define the terms used.

SELF-CONCEPT

Self-concept refers to one's view of oneself, an image that has developed over many years. To assess self-concept, the interviewer might ask the person how he or she views life: "How do you feel about your life in general?" A person's self-concept can be threatened very easily by changes in physical function or appearance or other threats to health. The impact of certain medical conditions or surgical interventions, such as a colostomy or a mastectomy, can threaten body image. Asking, "Do you have any particular concerns about your body?" may elicit useful information about self-image.

SEXUALITY

No area of assessment is more personal than the sexual history. Interviewers are frequently uncomfortable with such questions and ignore this area of the patient profile or conduct a very cursory interview at this point. Lack of knowledge about sexuality and anxiety about one's own sexuality may hamper the interviewer's effectiveness in dealing with this subject.

Sexual assessment can be approached at the end of the interview, at the time interpersonal or lifestyle factors are assessed, or it can be a part of the genitourinary history within the review of systems. For instance, it may be easier to approach a discussion of sexuality after a discussion of menstruation. A similar discussion with the male patient would follow questions related to the urinary system.

Obtaining the sexual history provides an opportunity to discuss sexual matters openly and gives the person permission to express sexual concerns to an informed professional. The interviewer must be nonjudgmental and must use language appropriate to the patient's age and background. It is advisable to begin the assessment with a general question concerning the person's developmental stage and the presence or absence of intimate relationships. Such questions may lead to a discussion of concerns related to sexual expression, to the quality of a relationship, or to questions about contraception, risky sexual behaviors, and safer sex practices.

Finding out whether a person is sexually active should precede any attempts to explore issues related to sexuality and sexual function. Questions are worded in such a way that the person feels free to discuss his or her sexuality regardless of marital status or sexual preference. Direct questions are usually less threatening when prefaced with such statements as, "Most people feel that . . ." or "Many people worry about . . . ." This suggests the normalcy of such feelings or behavior and encourages the person to share information that might otherwise be omitted from fear of seeming "different."

If the person answers abruptly or does not wish to carry the discussion any further, then the interviewer should move to the next topic. However, introducing the subject of sexuality indicates to the person that a discussion of sexual concerns is acceptable and can be approached again in the future if so desired. Further discussion of the sexual history is presented in Chapter 42.

RISK FOR ABUSE

A topic of growing importance in today's society is physical, sexual, and psychological abuse. Such abuse occurs at all ages, to men and women from all socioeconomic, ethnic, and cultural groups. Few patients, however, will discuss this topic unless they are asked specifically about it. Therefore, it is important to ask direct questions, such as:

- Is anyone physically hurting you?
- Has anyone ever hurt you physically or threatened to do so?
- Are you ever afraid of anyone close to you (your partner, caretaker, or other family members)?

If the person's response indicates that abuse is a risk, further assessment is called for and efforts are made to ensure the person's safety and provide access to appropriate community and professional resources and support systems.

STRESS AND COPING RESPONSES

Each person handles stress differently. How well we adapt depends on our ability to cope. During a health history, past coping patterns and perceptions of current stresses and anticipated outcomes are explored to identify the person's overall ability to handle stress. It is especially important to identify expectations that the person may have of family, friends, and caregivers in providing support.

Gerontologic Considerations

A health history from the elderly patient should be obtained in a calm, unrushed manner. Because of the increased incidence of impaired hearing and sight in the elderly, lighting should be adequate but not glaring, and distracting noises should be kept to a minimum. The interviewer should assume a position that enables the person to read lips and facial expressions. People who normally use a hearing aid are asked to use it during the interview.

Elderly people often assume that new physical problems are a result of age rather than a treatable illness. In addition, the signs and symptoms of illness in the elderly are often more subtle than those in younger people and may go unreported. Therefore, the interviewer inquires about subtle physical symptoms and recent changes in function and well-being. Special care is taken in obtaining a complete history of medications used, because many elderly people take many different kinds of medications. Although elderly people may experience a decline in mental function, it should not be assumed that an elderly person is unable to provide an adequate history. Including a member of the family in the interview process, however (ie, spouse, adult child, sibling, or caretaker), may validate information and provide missing details. Further details about assessment of the elderly are provided in Chapter 11.

Other Health History Formats

The health history format discussed in this chapter is only one possible format that is useful in obtaining and organizing information about a person's health status. Some consider this traditional format to be inappropriate for nurses because it does not focus exclusively on the assessment of human responses to actual or potential health problems. Several attempts have been made to develop an assessment format and database with this focus in mind. One example is the nursing database prototype based on the North American Nursing Diagnosis Association's (NANDA) Unitary Person Framework and its nine human response patterns: exchanging, communicating, relating, valuing, choosing, moving, perceiving, knowing, and feeling. Although there is some support in nursing for using this approach, no consensus for its use has been reached.

The National Center for Health Services Research of the U.S. Department of Health & Human Services and other groups from the public and private sectors have focused on assessing not only biologic health but other dimensions of health as well. These dimensions include physical, functional, emotional, mental, and social health. Modern efforts to assess health status have focused on the manner in which disease or disability affects the patient's functional status, that is, the ability of the person to function normally and perform his or her usual physical, mental, and social activities. An emphasis on functional assessment is viewed as more holistic than the traditional health or medical history. Instruments to assess health status in these ways may be used by nurses along with their own clinical assessment skills to determine the impact of illness, disease, disability, and health problems on functional status.

Health concerns that are not complex (earache, tonsillectomy) and can be resolved in a short period of time usually do not require the depth or detail that is required when a person is experiencing a major illness or health problem. Additional assessments that go beyond the general patient profile may be used when the patient's health problems are acute and complex or when the illness is chronic.

Regardless of the format used, the nurse's focus during data collection is different from that of the physician and other health team members; however, it complements these approaches and encourages collaboration among the health care providers, as each member brings his or her own expertise and focus to the situation.

PHYSICAL ASSESSMENT

Physical assessment, or the physical examination, is an integral part of nursing assessment. The basic techniques and tools used in performing a physical examination are described in general in this chapter. The examination of specific systems, including special maneuvers, is described in the appropriate chapters throughout the book. Because the patient's nutritional status is an important factor in health and well-being, a section on nutritional assessment is included in this chapter.

The physical examination is usually performed after the health history is obtained. It is carried out in a well-lighted, warm area. The patient is undressed and draped appropriately so that only the area to be examined is exposed. The person's physical and psychological comfort is considered at all times. Procedures and sensations to expect are described to the patient before each part of the examination. The examiner's hands are washed before and immediately after the examination. Fingernails are kept short to avoid injuring the patient. Gloves are worn by the examiner when there is a possibility of coming into contact with blood or other body secretions during the physical examination.

An organized and systematic examination is the key to obtaining appropriate data in the shortest time. Such an approach encourages cooperation and trust on the part of the patient.

The individual's health history provides the examiner with a health profile that guides all aspects of the physical examination.

Although the sequence of physical examination depends on the circumstances and on the patient's reason for seeking health care, the complete examination usually proceeds as follows:

1. Skin
2. Head and neck
3. Thorax and lungs
4. Breasts
5. Cardiovascular system
6. Abdomen
7. Rectum
8. Genitalia
9. Neurologic system
10. Musculoskeletal system

In clinical practice, all relevant body systems are tested throughout the physical examination, not necessarily in the sequence described. For example, when the face is examined, it is appropriate to check for facial asymmetry and, thus, for the integrity of the seventh cranial nerve; the examiner does not need to repeat this as part of a neurologic examination. When systems are combined in this manner, the patient does not need to change positions repeatedly, which can be exhausting and time-consuming.

A "complete" physical examination is not routine. Many of the body systems are selectively assessed on the basis of the individual's presenting problem. If, for example, a healthy 20-year-old college student requires an examination to play basketball and reports no history of neurologic abnormality, the neurologic assessment is brief. Conversely, a history of transient numbness and diplopia (double vision) usually necessitates a complete neurologic investigation. Similarly, a person with pleuritic chest pain receives a much more intensive examination of the chest than the person with a wrist fracture. In general, the individual's health history guides the examiner in obtaining additional data for a complete picture of the patient's health.

The process of learning physical examination requires repetition and reinforcement in a clinical setting. Only after basic physical assessment techniques are mastered can the examiner tailor the routine screening examination to include thorough assessments of a particular system, including special maneuvers.

The basic tools of the physical examination are vision, hearing, touch, and smell. These human senses may be augmented by special tools (eg, stethoscope, ophthalmoscope, reflex hammer) that are extensions of the human senses; they are simple tools that anyone can learn to use well. Expertise comes with practice, and sophistication comes with the interpretation of what is seen and heard. The four fundamental techniques used in the physical examination are inspection, palpation, percussion, and auscultation.

Inspection

The first fundamental technique is inspection or observation. General inspection begins with the first contact with the patient. Introducing oneself to the patient and shaking hands with him or her provide opportunities for making initial observations: Is the person old or young? How old? How young? Does the person appear to be his or her stated age? Is the person thin or obese? Does the person appear anxious or depressed? Is the person's body structure normal or abnormal? In what way, and how different from normal?

It is essential to pay attention to the details in observation. Vague, general statements are not a substitute for specific descriptions based on careful observation:

- *The person appears sick.* In what way does he or she appear sick? Is the skin clammy, pale, jaundiced, or cyanotic; is the person grimacing in pain; is breathing difficult; does he or she have edema? What specific physical features or behavioral manifestations indicate that the person is "sick?"
- *The person appears chronically ill.* In what way does he or she appear chronically ill? Does the person appear to have lost weight? People who lose weight secondary to muscle-wasting diseases (eg, AIDS, malignancy) have a different appearance than those who are merely thin; the distribution of their weight loss takes a different form. Does the skin have the appearance of chronic illness—that is, is it pale, or does it give the appearance of dehydration or loss of subcutaneous tissue? These important observations are documented in the patient's chart or health record.

Among general observations that should be noted in the initial examination of the patient are posture and stature, body movements, nutrition, speech pattern, and vital signs.

Posture and Stature

The posture that a person assumes often provides valuable information about the illness. Patients who have breathing difficulties (dyspnea) secondary to cardiac disease prefer to sit and may report feeling short of breath lying flat for even a brief time. People with emphysema not only sit upright but may also thrust their arms forward and laterally onto the edge of the bed (tripod position) to place accessory respiratory muscles at an optimal mechanical advantage. Those with abdominal pain due to peritonitis prefer to lie perfectly still; even slight jarring of the bed will cause agonizing pain. In contrast, patients with abdominal pain due to renal or biliary colic are often restless and may pace the room. Patients with meningeal irritation may experience head or neck pain on bending the head or flexing their knees.

Body Movements

Abnormalities of body movement may be of two general kinds: generalized disruption of voluntary or involuntary movement, and asymmetry of movement. The first category includes tremors of a wide variety; some tremors may occur at rest (Parkinson's disease), whereas others occur only on voluntary movement (cerebellar ataxia). Other tremors may exist during both rest and activity (alcohol withdrawal delirium, thyrotoxicosis). Some voluntary or involuntary movements are fine, others quite coarse. At the extreme are the convulsive movements of epilepsy or tetanus and the choreiform (involuntary and irregular) movements of patients with rheumatic fever or Huntington's disease.

Asymmetry of movement, in which only one side of the body is affected, may occur with disorders of the central nervous system (CNS), principally in those who have had cerebrovascular accidents (strokes). The patient may have drooping of one side of the face, weakness or paralysis of the extremities on one side of the body, and a foot-dragging gait.

Nutrition

Nutritional status is important to note. Obesity may be generalized as a result of excessive intake of calories or may be specifically localized to the trunk in those with endocrine disorders (Cushing's disease) or those who have been taking steroids for long periods of time. Loss of weight may be generalized as a result of inadequate caloric intake or may be seen in loss of muscle mass with disorders that affect protein synthesis. Nutritional assessment is discussed in more detail later in this chapter.

Speech Pattern

Speech may be slurred because of CNS disease or because of damage to cranial nerves. Recurrent damage to the laryngeal nerve will produce hoarseness, as will disorders that produce edema or swelling of the vocal cords. Speech may be halting, slurred, or interrupted in flow in some CNS disorders (eg, multiple sclerosis).

Vital Signs

The recording of vital signs is a part of every physical examination. Blood pressure, pulse, respiratory rate, and body temperature measurements are obtained and recorded. Acute changes and trends over time are documented; unexpected changes and values that deviate significantly from the patient's normal values are brought to the attention of the patient's primary health care provider.

Fever is an increase in body temperature above normal. A normal oral temperature for most people is an average of 37.0°C (98.6°F); however, some variation is normal. Some people's temperatures are quite normal at 36.6°C (98°F) and others at 37.3°C (99°F). There is a normal diurnal variation of a degree or two in body temperature throughout the day; it is usually lowest in the morning and rises during the day to between 37.3° and 37.5°C (99° to 99.5°F), decreasing again during the night.

Palpation

Palpation is a vital part of the physical examination. Many structures of the body, although not visible, may be assessed through touch (Fig. 5-3). Examples include superficial blood vessels, lymph nodes, the thyroid, the organs of the abdomen and pelvis, and the rectum. When the abdomen is examined, auscultation is performed *before* palpation and percussion to avoid altering bowel sounds.

Sounds generated within the body, if within specified frequency ranges, also may be detected through touch. Thus, certain murmurs generated in the heart or within blood vessels (thrills) may be detected. Thrills cause a sensation to the hand much like the purring of a cat. Voice sounds are transmitted along the bronchi to the periphery of the lung. These may be perceived by touch and may be altered by disorders affecting the lungs. The phenomenon is called *tactile fremitus* and is useful in assessing diseases of the chest. The significance of these findings is discussed in the relevant chapters of this book.

Percussion

The technique of percussion (Fig. 5-4) translates the application of physical force into sound. It is a skill requiring practice but one that yields much information about disease processes in the chest and abdomen. The principle is to set the chest wall or abdominal wall into vibration by striking it with a firm object. The sound produced reflects the density of the underlying structure. Certain densities produce sounds as percussion notes. These sounds, listed in a sequence that proceeds from the least to the most dense, are called *tympany, hyperresonance, resonance, dullness*, and *flatness*. Tympany is the drumlike sound produced by percussing the air-filled stomach. Hyperresonance is audible when one percusses over inflated lung tissue in someone with emphysema. Resonance is the sound elicited over air-filled lungs. Percussion of the liver produces a dull sound, whereas percussion of the thigh results in flatness.

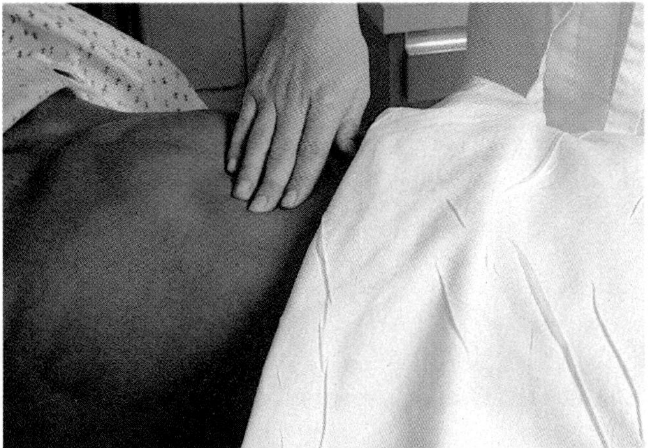

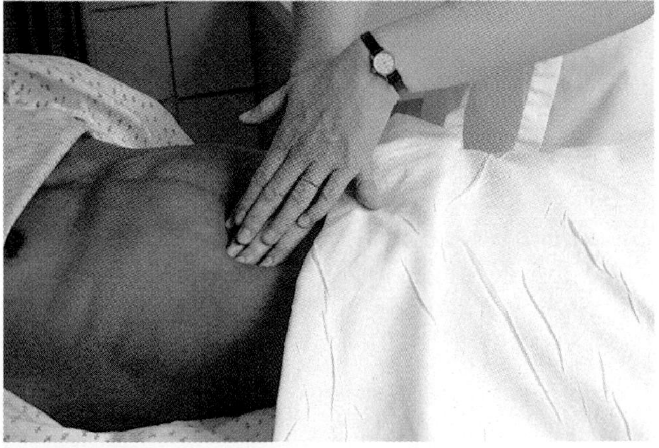

FIGURE 5•3 Light palpation technique (*top*) and deep palpation (*bottom*). Photo © Ken Kasper.

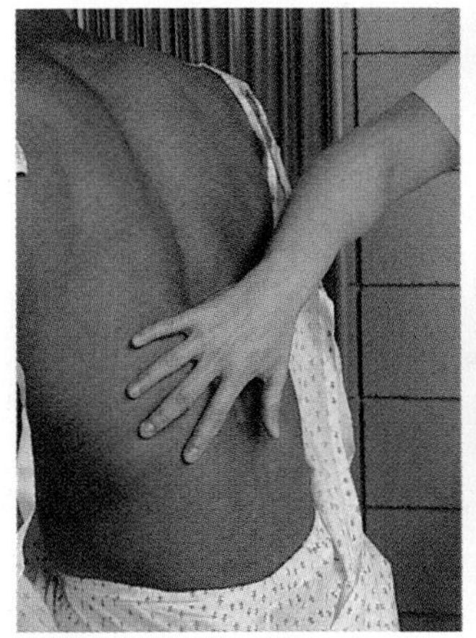

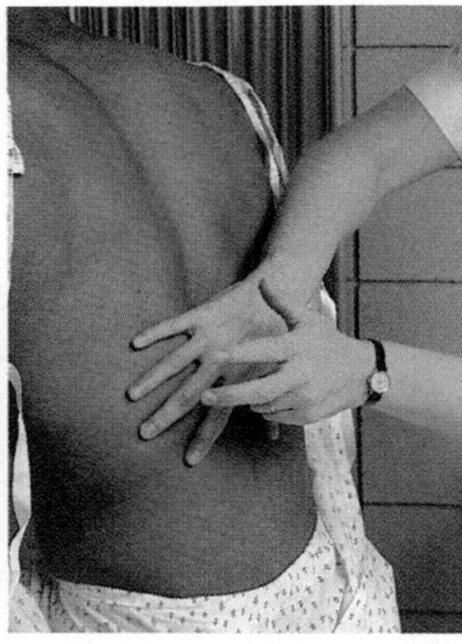

FIGURE 5•4 Percussion technique. The middle finger of one hand strikes the terminal phalanx of the middle finger of the other hand, which is placed firmly against the body. If the action is performed sharply, a brief resonant tone will be produced. The clarity of the tone depends on the brevity of the action. The intensity of the tone varies with the force used. Photo © Ken Kasper.

Percussion allows the examiner to assess such normal anatomic details as the borders of the heart and the movement of the diaphragm during inspiration. One may determine the level of pleural effusion (fluid in the pleural cavity) and the location of a consolidated area caused by pneumonia or atelectasis (collapse) of a lobe of the lung. The use of percussion is described further with disorders of the thorax and abdomen.

Auscultation

Auscultation is the skill of listening to sounds produced within the body created by the movement of air or fluid. Examples include breath sounds, the spoken voice, bowel sounds, cardiac murmurs, and heart sounds. Physiologic sounds may be normal (eg, first and second heart sounds) or pathologic (eg, heart murmurs in diastole, or crackles in the lung). Some normal sounds may be distorted by abnormalities of structures through which the sound must travel (eg, changes in the character of breath sounds as they travel through the consolidated lung of the patient with lobar pneumonia).

Sound produced within the body, if of sufficient amplitude, may be detected with the stethoscope, which functions as an extension of the human ear and channels sound. Two end pieces are available for the stethoscope: the bell and the diaphragm. The bell is used to assess very-low-frequency sounds such as diastolic heart murmurs. The entire surface of the bell's disc is placed lightly on the skin surface to avoid flattening the skin and reducing audible vibratory sensations. The diaphragm, the larger disc, is used to assess high-frequency sounds such as lung sounds and is held in firm contact with the skin surface (Fig. 5-5). Touching the tubing or rubbing other surfaces (hair, clothing) during auscultation is avoided to minimize extraneous noises.

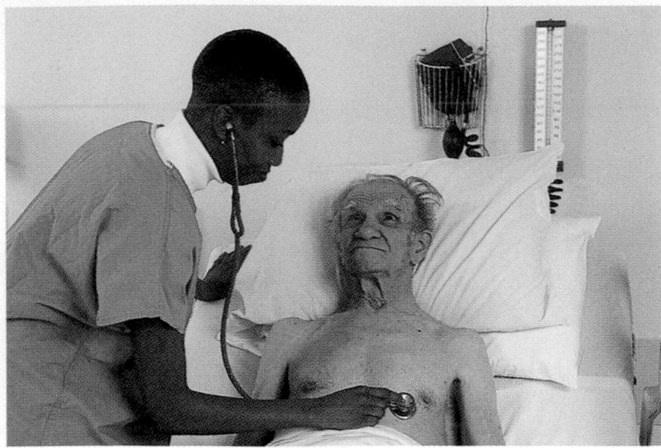

FIGURE 5•5 Technique for auscultating the heart. © B. Proud Photography.

Sound produced by the body, like any other sound, is characterized by intensity, frequency, and quality. *Intensity*, or loudness, associated with physiologic sound is low; thus, the use of the stethoscope is needed. *Frequency*, or pitch, of physiologic sound is in reality "noise," in that most sounds consist of a frequency spectrum as opposed to the single-frequency sounds that we associate with music or the tuning fork. The frequency spectrum may be quite low, yielding a rumbling noise, or comparatively high, producing a harsh or blowing sound. *Quality* of sound relates to overtones that allow one to distinguish between different sounds. Sound quality enables the examiner to distinguish between the musical quality of high-pitched wheezing and the low-pitched rumbling of a diastolic murmur.

THE NUTRITIONAL ASSESSMENT

Nutrition is important to maintain health and prevent disease. Disorders caused by nutritional deficiency, overeating, or eating poorly balanced meals are among the leading causes of illness and death in the United States today. Examples of health problems associated with poor nutrition include obesity, coronary artery disease, osteoporosis, cirrhosis, diverticulitis, and eating disorders. When illness or injury occurs, optimal nutrition is an essential factor in promoting healing and resisting infection. Assessment of a person's nutritional status provides information on obesity, undernutrition, weight loss, malnutrition, deficiencies in specific nutrients, metabolic abnormalities, the effects of medications on nutrition, and special problems of the hospitalized patient and the person who is cared for in the home and in other community settings.

Certain signs and symptoms that suggest possible nutritional deficiency are easy to note because they are specific. Other physical signs may be subtle and must be carefully assessed. A physical sign that suggests a nutritional abnormality should be pursued further. For example, certain signs that may appear to indicate nutritional deficiency may actually reflect other systemic conditions (eg, endocrine disorders, infectious disease). Others may result from impaired digestion, absorption, excretion, or storage of nutrients in the body.

The acronym ABCD may be used to identify the parameters of nutritional assessment. Although the sequence of assessment of these parameters may vary, evaluation of nutritional status includes one or more of the following methods:

1. **A**nthropometric measurement
   Weight/height and body mass index
   Triceps skinfold thickness, midarm and arm muscle circumferences
2. **B**iochemical measurements
   Albumin
   Transferrin
   Prealbumin
   Retinol-binding protein
   Total lymphocyte count
   Electrolyte levels
   Creatinine/height index
3. **C**linical examination findings
4. **D**ietary data

Anthropometric Measurements

The most common anthropometric measurements (measures of body size, weight, and proportions) include height, weight, and the circumferences of the upper arm and arm muscle. When anthropometric measurements are obtained, standardized equipment and procedures are used, as well as standard measurement guides. Although such measurements focus on undernutrition, they also detect obesity. Charts 5-2 and 5-3 provide guidelines for calculating ideal body weight (IBW) and for determining frame size. Current weight is then compared to IBW to determine how over or under IBW the patient's current weight is:

$$\% \text{ of IBW} = (\text{current body weight/IBW}) \times 100$$

Weight loss is extremely important because it reflects inadequate caloric intake. In someone who is malnourished, weight loss indicates an increased loss of protein from the body cell mass. Current weight does not provide information about recent changes in weight; therefore, the patient is asked about his or her usual body weight. This information is then used to compare current weight with usual body weight (UBW):

$$\% \text{ of UBW} = (\text{current body weight/UBW}) \times 100$$

CHART 5•2  **Guidelines for Calculating Ideal Body Weight**

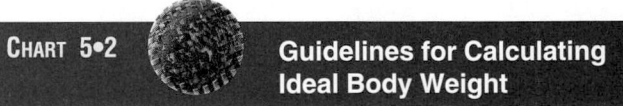

Women

- Allow 100 lb for 5 feet of height.
- Add 5 lb for each additional inch over 5 feet.
- Subtract 10% for small frame; add 10% for large frame.

Men

- Allow 106 lb for 5 feet of height.
- Add 6 lb for each additional inch over 5 feet.
- Subtract 10% for small frame, add 10% for large frame.

Example: Ideal body weight for a 5′6″ adult is

	Female	Male
5′ of height	100 lb	106 lb
Per additional inch	6″ × 5 lb/inch = 30 lb	6″ × 6 lb/inch = 36 lb
Ideal body weight	130 lb ± 13 lb depending on frame size	142 lb ± 14 lb depending on frame size

Dudek, S. G. (1997). *Nutrition handbook for nursing practice* (2nd ed.). Philadelphia: Lippincott-Raven.

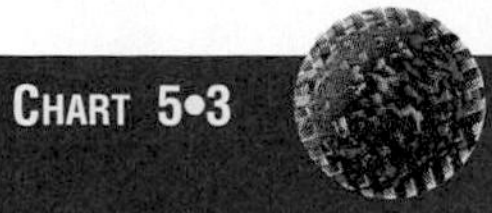

CHART 5•3 Guidelines for Calculating Frame Size

- Measure height in centimeters.
- Measure wrist circumference in centimeters by placing a tape measure around the wrist where it bends at the styloid process.
- Calculate the ratio of height to wrist circumference to estimate frame size.

Height (cm)/Wrist circumference (cm)

	Female	Male
Small frame	>11	>10.4
Medium frame	10.1–11	9.6–10.4
Large frame	<10.1	<9.6

Example: Height = 5′10″(178 cm) adult
Wrist circumference = 6.2″(15.4 cm)
178/15.4 = 11.6

Result: A ratio of 11.6 indicates a small frame for females and males.

Decreased height may be due to osteoporosis, an important problem related to nutrition, especially in postmenopausal women. A loss of 2″ or 3″ of height may indicate osteoporosis.

Measurement of skinfold thickness and arm and muscle circumference is described in Figures 5-6 and 5-7. Triceps skinfold thickness (TSF) indicates fat stores. Midarm muscle circumference (MAMC), calculated from midarm circumference (MAC) and TSF, indicates the state of muscle protein. Thus, these measures provide information about protein–calorie malnutrition. The calculation for MAMC is as follows:

$$\text{MAMC (cm)} = \text{MAC (cm)} - (0.314 \times \text{TSF [mm]})$$

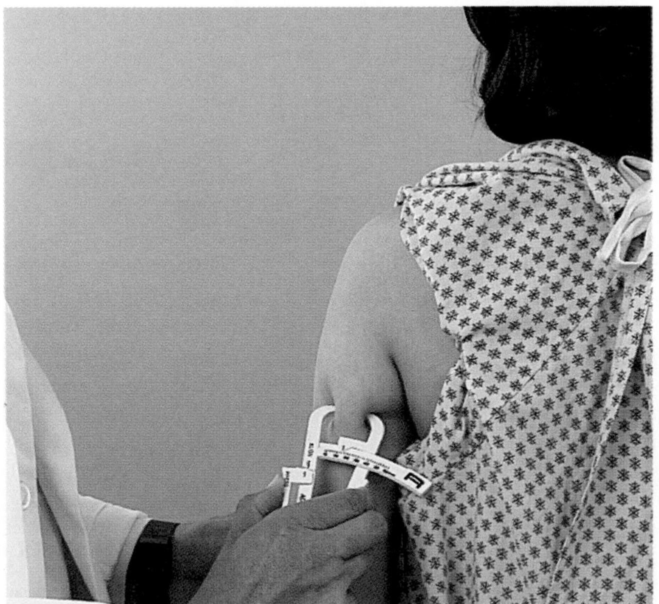

FIGURE 5•6 Measurement of triceps skinfold thickness. The nondominant arm is used for measurement. The midpoint of the arm is located; this is the midpoint between the acromial process of the scapula (at the top of the humerus) and the olecranon process of the ulna (elbow). With the arm hanging loosely at the side, a double fold of skin (not muscle) is grasped by the calipers. The measurement is recorded in millimeters. From Weber, J. W., & Kelley, J. (1998). *Health assessment in nursing.* Philadelphia: Lippincott-Raven.

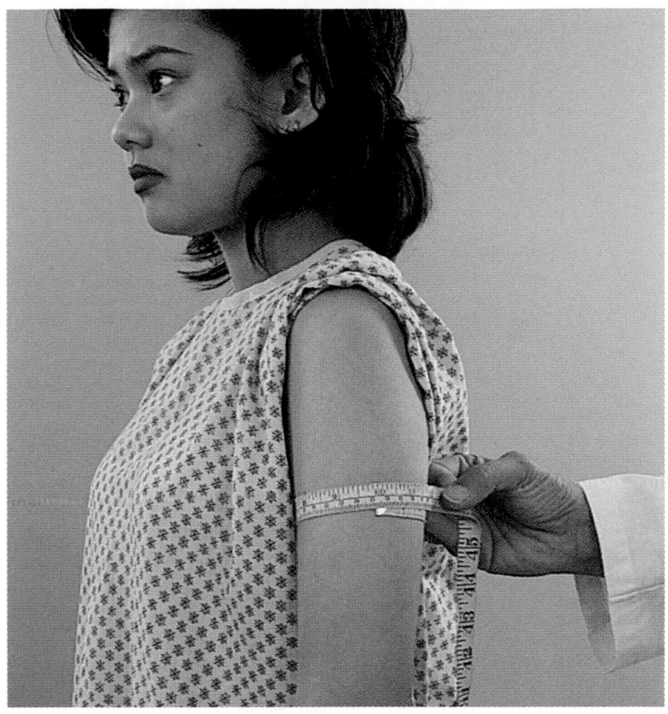

FIGURE 5•7 Measurement of midarm circumference. A flexible tape is placed midway between the top of the acromial process of the scapula and the olecranon process of the ulna; the tape is held firmly but gently to avoid compressing the soft tissue. The measurement is recorded in centimeters. From Weber, J. W., & Kelley, J. (1998). *Health assessment in nursing.* Philadelphia: Lippincott-Raven.

The TSF, MAC, and MAMC values obtained from these procedures (Table 5-1) are compared with the standards for anthropometric measurements to assess the person's nutritional status.

Body mass index (BMI) is a ratio based on body weight and height. The obtained value is then compared to the established standards; however, trends or changes in values over time are considered more useful than isolated or one-time measurements. The BMI (Fig. 5-8) is highly correlated with body fat, but increased lean body mass or a large body frame can also increase the BMI. Individuals who have a BMI below 24 (or who are 80% or less of their desirable body weight for height) are at increased risk for problems associated with poor nutritional status. Those who have a BMI of 25 or above are considered overweight; those with a BMI of 30 or above are considered obese and are at high risk for

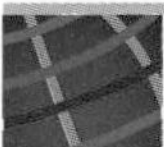

TABLE 5•1 Standard and Decreased Values for Anthropometric Measurements for Adults

	Standard	90% of Standard	70% of Standard
Triceps Skinfold Thickness (mm)			
Men	12.5	11.3	8.8
Women	16.5	14.9	11.6
Midarm Circumference (cm)			
Men	29.3	26.3	20.5
Women	28.5	25.7	20.0
Midarm Muscle Circumference (cm)			
Men	25.3	22.8	17.7
Women	23.2	20.9	16.2

Based on Dudek, S.G. (1997). *Nutrition handbook for nursing practice* (3rd ed.). Philadelphia: Lippincott-Raven.

Body Mass Index

The body mass index (BMI) is used to determine who is overweight.

$$\textbf{BMI} = \frac{703 \times \text{weight in pounds}}{(\text{height in inches})^2} \quad \text{OR} \quad \frac{\text{weight in kilograms}}{(\text{height in meters})^2}$$

BMI score is at the intersection of height and weight. A body mass index score of 25 or more is considered overweight and 30 or more is considered obese.

25 Overweight Limit   Overweight

Weight / Height	100	105	110	115	120	125	130	135	140	145	150	155	160	165	170	175	180	185	190	195	200	205
5′0″	20	21	21	22	23	24	**25**	26	27	28	29	30	31	32	33	34	35	36	37	38	39	40
5′1″	19	20	21	22	23	24	**25**	26	26	27	28	29	30	31	32	33	34	35	36	37	38	39
5′2″	18	19	20	21	22	23	24	**25**	26	27	27	28	29	30	31	32	33	34	35	36	37	37
5′3″	18	19	19	20	21	22	23	24	**25**	26	27	27	28	29	30	31	32	33	34	35	35	36
5′4″	17	18	19	20	21	21	22	23	24	**25**	26	27	27	28	29	30	31	32	33	33	34	35
5′5″	17	17	18	19	20	21	22	22	23	24	**25**	26	27	27	28	29	30	31	32	32	33	34
5′6″	16	17	18	19	19	20	21	22	23	23	24	**25**	26	27	27	28	29	30	31	31	32	33
5′7″	16	16	17	18	19	20	20	21	22	23	23	24	**25**	26	27	27	28	29	30	31	31	32
5′8″	15	16	17	17	18	19	20	21	21	22	23	24	24	**25**	26	27	27	28	29	30	30	31
5′9″	15	16	16	17	18	18	19	20	21	21	22	23	24	24	**25**	26	27	27	28	29	30	30
5′10″	14	15	16	17	17	18	19	19	20	21	22	22	23	24	24	**25**	26	27	27	28	29	29
5′11″	14	15	15	16	17	17	18	19	20	20	21	22	22	23	24	24	**25**	26	26	27	28	29
6′0″	14	14	15	16	16	17	18	18	19	20	20	21	22	22	23	24	24	**25**	26	26	27	28
6′1″	13	14	15	15	16	16	17	18	18	19	20	20	21	22	22	23	24	24	**25**	26	26	27
6′2″	13	13	14	15	15	16	17	17	18	19	19	20	21	21	22	22	23	24	24	**25**	26	26
6′3″	12	13	14	14	15	16	16	17	17	18	19	19	20	21	21	22	22	23	24	24	**25**	26
6′4″	12	13	13	14	15	15	16	16	17	18	18	19	19	20	21	21	22	23	23	24	24	**25**

Source: Shape Up America. National Institutes of Health

FIGURE 5•8 Body mass index.

hypertension, diabetes, osteoarthritis, and other problems associated with obesity.

Biochemical Assessment

Biochemical assessment reflects both the tissue level of a given nutrient and any abnormality of metabolism in the utilization of nutrients. These determinations are made from studies of serum (serum protein, serum albumin and globulin, transferrin, retinol-binding protein, hemoglobin, serum vitamin A, carotene, and vitamin C) and from urine (creatinine, thiamine, riboflavin, niacin, and iodine). Some of these tests, while reflecting recent intake of the elements detected, can also identify below-normal levels when there are no clinical symptoms of deficiency (see Table 5-2 for a description of serum protein measurement).

Low serum albumin and transferrin levels are often used as measures of protein deficits in adults and are expressed as percentages of normal values. Albumin synthesis depends on normal liver function and an adequate supply of amino acids. Because the body stores a large amount of albumin, the serum albumin level may not decrease until malnutrition is severe; thus, its usefulness in detecting recent protein depletion is limited. Decreased albumin levels may also occur with liver or renal disease, congestive heart failure, and excessive protein loss because of burns, major surgery, infection, and cancer. Transferrin is a protein that binds and carries iron from the intestine through the serum. Because of its short half-life, decreased transferrin levels respond more quickly to protein depletion than albumin. Serial measurements of these, as well as prealbumin levels, are used to assess the results of nutritional therapy.

Although not available from many laboratories, retinol-binding protein may be a useful means of monitoring acute, short-term changes in protein status.

Reduced numbers of lymphocytes in people who become acutely malnourished as a result of stress and low-calorie feeding are associated with impairment of cellular immunity. Anergy, the absence of an immune response to injection of small concentrations of recall antigen under the skin, may also indicate malnutrition because of delayed antibody synthesis and response.

Serum electrolyte levels provide information about fluid and electrolyte balance and kidney function. The creatinine/height index calculated over a 24-hour period assesses the metabolically

TABLE 5•2 Standard Serum Protein Indices

Serum Protein	Standard Range
Albumin	3.5–5.0 g/dL
Transferrin	>200 mg/dL
Prealbumin	20–50 mg/dL
Retinol-binding protein	3–7 mg/dL

From Dudek, S.G. (1997). *Nutrition handbook for nursing practice.* (3rd ed.). Philadelphia: Lippincott-Raven.

active tissue and indicates the degree of protein depletion, comparing expected body mass for height and actual body cell mass. A 24-hour urine sample is obtained and the amount of creatinine is measured and compared to normal ranges based on the patient's height and gender. Values less than normal may indicate loss of lean body mass and protein malnutrition.

Clinical Examination

The state of nutrition is often reflected in a person's appearance. Although the most obvious physical sign of good nutrition is a normal body weight with respect to height, body frame, and age, other tissues can serve as indicators of general nutritional status and adequate intake of specific nutrients; these include the hair, skin, teeth, gums, mucous membranes, mouth and tongue, skeletal muscles, abdomen, lower extremities, and thyroid gland (Table 5-3). Specific clinical examination parameters useful in identifying nutritional deficits include oral examination and assessment of skin for turgor, edema, elasticity, dryness, subcutaneous tone, poorly healing wounds and ulcers, purpura, and bruises. The musculoskeletal examination also provides information about muscle wasting and weakness.

Dietary Intake

The appraisal of food intake considers the quantity and quality of the diet and also the frequency with which certain food items and nutrients are consumed. Commonly used methods of determining individual eating patterns include the food record and the 24-hour food recall, which can help estimate if the food intake is adequate and appropriate. If these methods are used, instructions are given when the patient's diet history is obtained.

Food Record

The food record is used most often in nutritional status studies. The person is instructed to keep a record of food actually consumed over a period of time, varying from 3 to 7 days, and to accurately estimate and describe the specific foods consumed. Food records are fairly accurate if the person is willing to provide factual information and able to estimate food quantities.

24-Hour Recall

The 24-hour recall method is, as the name implies, a recall of food intake over a 24-hour period. The person is asked by the interviewer to recall all food eaten during the previous day and to estimate the quantities of the food consumed. Because information does not always represent usual intake, at the end of the interview the patient is asked if the previous day's food intake was a typical one. To obtain supplementary information about the typical diet, the interviewer also asks how frequently the person eats foods from the major food groups.

Conducting the Dietary Interview

The success of the interviewer in obtaining information for dietary assessment depends on effective communication, which requires that good rapport be established to promote respect and trust. The interviewer explains the purpose of the interview. It is conducted in a nondirective and exploratory way, allowing the respondent to express feelings and thoughts while encouraging him or her to answer specific questions. The manner in which questions are asked will influence the respondent's cooperation. Thus, the interviewer must be nonjudgmental and avoid expressing disapproval, either verbally or by facial expression.

Several questions may be necessary to elicit the information needed. When attempting to elicit information about the type and quantity of food eaten at a particular time, the interviewer avoids leading questions, such as, "Did you put sugar or cream in your coffee?" Also, assumptions are not made about the size of servings; instead, questions are phrased so that quantities are more clearly determined. For example, to help determine the size of one hamburger eaten, the patient may be asked, "How many servings were prepared with the pound of meat you bought?" Another approach to determining quantities is to use food models of known sizes in

TABLE 5•3 Physical Signs Indicative of Nutritional Status

	Signs of Good Nutrition	Signs of Poor Nutrition
General appearance	Alert, responsive	Listless, appears acutely or chronically ill
Hair	Shiny, lustrous; firm, healthy scalp	Dull and dry, brittle, depigmented, easily plucked; thin and sparse
Face	Skin color uniform; healthy appearance	Skin dark over cheeks and under eyes, skin flaky, face swollen or hollow/sunken cheeks
Eyes	Bright, clear, moist	Eye membranes pale, dry (xerophthalmia); increased vascularity, cornea soft (keratomalacia)
Lips	Good color (pink), smooth	Swollen and puffy; angular lesion at corners of mouth (cheilosis)
Tongue	Deep red in appearance; surface papillae present	Smooth appearance, swollen, beefy red, sores, atrophic papillae
Teeth	Straight, no crowding, no dental caries, bright	Dental caries, mottled appearance (fluorosis), malpositioned
Gums	Firm, good color (pink)	Spongy, bleed easily, marginal redness, recession
Glands	No enlargement of the thyroid	Thyroid enlargement (simple goiter)
Skin	Smooth, good color, moist	Rough, dry, flaky, swollen, pale, pigmented; lack of fat under skin
Nails	Firm, pink	Spoon-shaped, ridged, brittle
Skeleton	Good posture, no malformation	Poor posture, beading of ribs, bowed legs or knock knees
Muscles	Well developed, firm	Flaccid, poor tone, wasted, underdeveloped
Extremities	No tenderness	Weak and tender; edematous
Abdomen	Flat	Swollen
Nervous system	Normal reflexes	Decreased or absent ankle and knee reflexes
Weight	Normal for height, age, and body build	Overweight or underweight

estimating portions of meat, cake, or pie or to record quantities in common measurements, such as cups or spoonfuls (or according to the size of containers, when discussing intake of bottled beverages).

In recording a particular combination dish, such as a casserole, it is useful to ask for the ingredients in the recipe, recording the largest quantities first. When recording quantities of ingredients, one notes whether the food item was raw or cooked and the number of servings provided by the recipe. When the client lists the foods for the recall questionnaire, it may be helpful to read back the list of foods and ask if anything was forgotten, such as fruit, cake, candy, between-meal snacks, or alcoholic beverages.

Additional information obtained during the interview should include methods of preparing food, sources available for food (donated foods, food stamps), food-buying practices, vitamin and mineral supplements, and income range.

Cultural Considerations

An individual's culture determines to a large extent what foods are eaten and how they are prepared and served. Culture and religion together often determine if certain foods are prohibited and if certain foods and spices are eaten on certain holidays or at specific family gatherings. Because of the importance of culture and religious beliefs to many individuals, it is important to be sensitive to these factors when obtaining a dietary history. It is, however, equally important not to stereotype individuals and assume that because they are from a certain culture or religion that they adhere to specific dietary customs.

Evaluating the Dietary Information

After the dietary information has been obtained, the nurse evaluates the patient's dietary intake. If the goal is to determine if the person generally eats a healthful diet, the food intake may be compared to the dietary guidelines outlined in the USDA's Food Guide Pyramid (Fig. 5-9). The pyramid divides foods into five major groups and offers recommendations for variety in the diet, proportion of food from each food group, and moderation in eating fats, oils, and sweets. The person's food intake is compared with recommendations based on various food groups for various age levels.

If the nurse or dietitian is interested in knowing about the intake of specific nutrients, such as vitamin A, iron, or calcium, the patient's food intake would be analyzed by consulting a list of foods and their composition and nutrient content. The diet is then analyzed in terms of grams and milligrams of specific nutrients. The total nutritive value is then compared with the recommended dietary allowances, or RDAs (Table 5-4), and the nutritional evaluation is expressed in terms of percentage of adequacy for each nutrient.

The nurse frequently participates in the nutrition screening of patients and communicates the information to the dietitian and the rest of the team for more detailed assessment and for clinical nutrition intervention.

Factors Influencing Nutritional Status in Varied Situations

One sensitive indicator of the body's gain or loss of protein is its nitrogen balance. An adult is said to be in nitrogen equilibrium when the nitrogen intake (from food) equals the nitrogen output (in urine, feces, and perspiration); it is a sign of health. A positive nitrogen balance exists when nitrogen intake exceeds nitrogen output and indicates tissue growth, such as occurs during pregnancy, childhood, recovery from surgery, and rebuilding of wasted tissue. Negative nitrogen balance indicates that tissue is breaking down faster than it is being replaced. In the absence of an adequate intake of protein, the body converts protein to glucose for energy. This can occur with fever, starvation, surgery, burns, and debilitating diseases. Each gram of nitrogen loss in excess of intake represents the depletion of 6.25 g of protein or 25 g of muscle tissue. Therefore, a negative nitrogen balance of 10 g/day for 10 days could mean the wasting of 2.5 kg (5.5 lb) of muscle tissue as it is converted to glucose for energy.

When conditions that result in negative nitrogen balance are coupled with anorexia (loss of appetite), they can lead to malnutrition. Malnutrition interferes with wound healing, increases susceptibility to infection, and contributes to an increased incidence of complications, longer hospital stay, and prolonged confinement of the patient to bed.

The patient who is hospitalized may have an inadequate dietary intake because of the illness or disorder that necessitated the hospital stay or because the hospital's food is unfamiliar or unappealing. The person who is cared for at home may feel too sick or fatigued to shop and prepare food or may be unable to eat because of other physical problems or limitations. Limited or fixed incomes or the high costs of medications may result in insufficient money to buy nutritious foods. Patients with inadequate housing or inadequate cooking facilities are unlikely to have an adequate nutritional intake.

Because complex treatments (eg, ventilators, intravenous infusions, chemotherapy) once used only in the hospital setting are now being provided in the home and outpatient settings, nutritional assessment of the patient in these settings is an important aspect of home and community-based care as well as hospital-based care.

Many medications influence nutritional status by suppressing the appetite, irritating the mucosa, or causing nausea and vomiting. Others may influence bacterial flora in the intestine or directly affect nutrient absorption so that secondary malnutrition results. People who must take many medications in a single day often report feeling too full to eat. The person's use of prescription and over-the-counter medications and their effect on appetite and dietary intake are assessed. Many of the factors that contribute to poor nutritional status are identified in Table 5-5.

Analysis of Nutritional Status

Anthropometric, biochemical, clinical, and dietary data are used together to determine the patient's nutritional status. Often the anthropometric and biochemical measures and dietary data provide more information about the patient's nutritional status than the clinical examination; the clinical examination may not detect subclinical deficiencies unless such deficiencies become so advanced that overt signs develop. A low intake of nutrients over a period of time may lead to low biochemical levels and without nutritional intervention may result in characteristic and observable signs and symptoms (see Table 5-3). A plan of action for nutritional intervention is based on the results of the dietary assessment and the patient's profile. To be effective, the plan must meet the patient's need for a balanced diet, maintain or control weight, and compensate for increased nutritional needs.

Gerontologic Considerations

It has been estimated that one in four elderly people is malnourished. Elderly people who are malnourished tend to have longer and more expensive hospital stays than those who are adequately

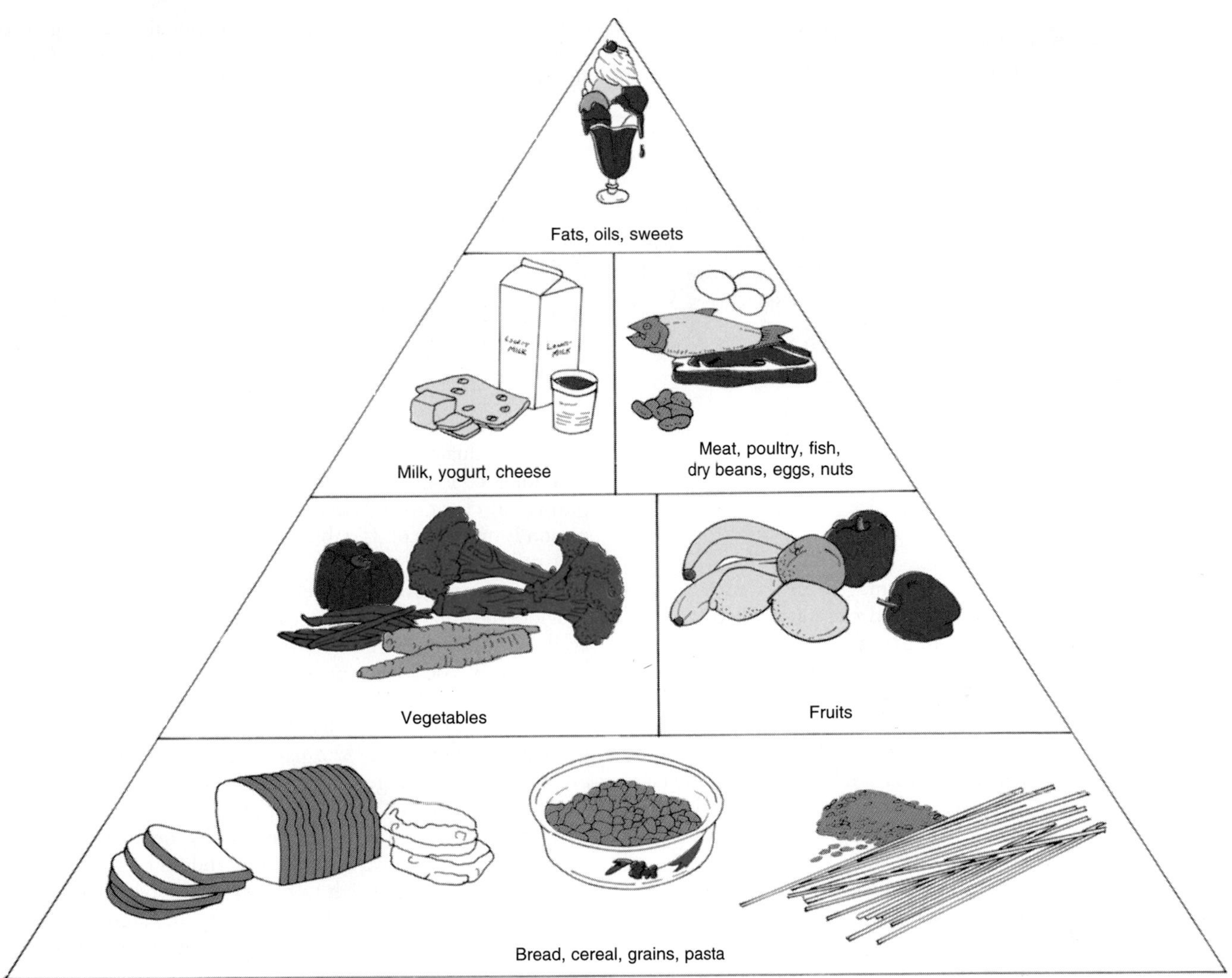

FIGURE 5•9 The Food Guide Pyramid emphasizes foods from the five major food groups shown in the three lower sections of the pyramid. Each of these food groups provides some, but not all, of the nutrients an adult needs. Foods in one group cannot replace those in another. No one of these major food groups is more important than another. To receive adequate vitamins, minerals, carbohydrates, and protein, an average adult should eat at least the lowest number of servings from the five major groups. Examples of 1 serving of a food group follow: **Fats and sweets:** use sparingly; **milk, yogurt, cheese *(dairy):*** 1 C milk or yogurt, 1½ oz natural cheese, 2 oz processed cheese; **meat, poultry, fish, dry beans, eggs, nuts *(proteins):*** ½ C cooked beans, 1 egg, 2 to 3 oz cooked lean meat, poultry or fish (2 T peanut butter = 1 oz cooked lean meat); **vegetables:** 1 C raw leafy vegetables, ½ C other vegetables (cooked or chopped, raw), ¾ C vegetable juice; **fruits:** 1 medium apple, banana, orange, ½ C chopped or cooked or canned fruit, ¾ C fruit juice; **bread, cereal, rice, pasta:** 1 slice bread, 1 oz ready-to-eat cereal, ½ C cooked cereal, rice or pasta. Source: U.S. Department of Agriculture/U.S. Department of Health and Human Services.

nourished; the risk of costly complications is also increased in those who are malnourished.

Inadequate dietary intake in the elderly may result from physiologic changes in the gastrointestinal tract, social and economic factors, drug interactions, disease, excessive use of alcohol, and poor dentition or missing teeth. Malnutrition is a common consequence of these factors and in turn leads to illness and frailty of the elderly. Important aspects of care of the elderly in the hospital, home, outpatient setting, or extended care facility include recognizing risk factors and identifying those at risk for inadequate nutrition.

Many elderly people take excessive and inappropriate medications; this is referred to as polypharmacy. The number of adverse reactions increases proportionately with the number of prescribed and over-the-counter medications taken. Age-related physiologic and pathophysiologic changes may alter the metabolism and elimination of many medications. Medications can influence food intake by producing side effects such as nausea, vomiting, decreased appetite, and changes in sensorium. They may also interfere with the distribution, utilization, and storage of nutrients. Disorders affecting any part of the gastrointestinal tract can alter nutritional requirements and health status in people of any age; however, they are likely to occur quickly and more frequently in the elderly.

Nutritional problems in the elderly often occur or are precipitated by such illnesses as pneumonia and urinary tract in-

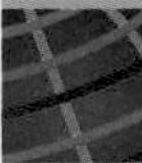

TABLE 5•4 Recommended Daily Dietary Allowances for Adults

Nutrient	Male	Female
Vitamin B_6	2.0 mg	1.6 mg
Vitamin B_{12}	2.0 μg	2.0 μg
Calcium (age 25 and older)	800 mg	800 mg
Calcium (11–24 years of age)	1200 mg	1200 mg
Vitamin C	60 mg	60 mg
Folate	200 μg	180 μg
Vitamin K	80 μg	65 μg
Iron	10 mg	15 mg
Magnesium	350 mg	280 mg
Selenium	70 μg	55 μg
Zinc	15 mg	12 mg

Source: Food and Nutrition Board, National Academy of Sciences: National Research Council.

fections. Acute and chronic diseases may affect the metabolism and utilization of nutrients, which already are altered by the aging process. Flu and pneumonia immunizations, prompt treatment of bacterial infections, and social programs such as Meals on Wheels may reduce the risk of illness-associated malnutrition.

Even the well elderly may be nutritionally at risk because of limited ability to shop and cook, financial hardship, and the fact that they often eat alone. Also, reduction in exercise with age without concomitant changes in carbohydrate intake places the elderly at risk for obesity.

The Nutrition Screening Initiative has developed easy-to-use tools for routine nutrition screening of the elderly to assist in identifying those at risk for poor nutrition. Information about the Nutrition Screening Initiative can be found in the list of references at the end of the chapter. Nutritional screening in the elderly is a first step in maintaining adequate nutrition and replacing nutrient losses to maintain the individual's health and well-being.

ASSESSMENT IN THE HOME AND COMMUNITY

Assessment of the person in community settings including the home consists of collecting information specific to existing health problems, including the patient's physiologic and emotional status, the community and home environment, the adequacy of support systems or care given by family and other care providers, and the availability of needed resources. In addition, the ability of the individual and family to cope with and address their respective needs is evaluated. The physical assessment in the community and home consists of the same techniques used in the hospital, outpatient clinic, or office setting. Privacy is provided and the person is made as comfortable as possible.

A call made to the patient's home before the first home visit lets the patient know when to expect the home care nurse and also provides the opportunity for the patient's primary caregiver to be available. During the home visit, the nurse's assessment is not limited to physical assessment of the patient. Other aspects of assessment include the home environment, safety factors (eg, smoke alarms, obstacles, safety bars in the bathroom), adequacy of facilities required for the patient's care and recovery, food preparation and storage facilities, bathroom facilities, access to a telephone, and the availability of family and community supports. Because patients may have no family members available to assist them and may live alone in substandard housing or homeless shelters, the nurse needs to be aware of resources available in the community and methods of obtaining those resources for the patient. Figure 5-10 provides an example of a checklist that may be useful in conducting assessment in the home.

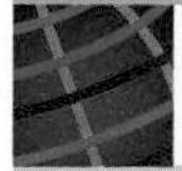

TABLE 5•5 Factors Associated With Potential Nutritional Deficits

Factors	Possible Consequences
Dental and oral problems (missing teeth, ill-fitting dentures, impaired swallowing or chewing)	Inadequate intake of high-fiber foods
NPO for diagnostic testing	Inadequate caloric and protein intake; dehydration
Prolonged use of glucose and saline IV fluids	Inadequate caloric and protein intake
Nausea and vomiting	Inadequate caloric and protein intake; loss of fluid, electrolytes, and minerals
Stress of illness, surgery, and/or hospitalization	Increased protein and caloric requirement; increased catabolism
Wound drainage	Loss of protein, fluid, electrolytes, and minerals
Pain	Loss of appetite; inability to shop, cook, eat
Fever	Increased caloric and fluid requirement; increased catabolism
Gastrointestinal intubation	Loss of protein, fluid, and minerals
Tube feedings	Inadequate amounts; various nutrients in each formula
Gastrointestinal disease	Inadequate intake and malabsorption of nutrients
Alcoholism	Inadequate intake of nutrients; increased consumption of calories without other nutrients; vitamin deficiencies
Depression	Loss of appetite; inability to shop, cook, eat
Eating disorders (anorexia, bulimia)	Inadequate caloric and protein intake; loss of fluid, electrolytes, and minerals
Medications	Inadequate intake due to medication side effects, such as dry mouth, loss of appetite, decreased taste perception, difficulty swallowing, nausea and vomiting, physical problems that limit shopping, cooking, eating; malabsorption of nutrients
Restricted ambulation or disability	Inability to help self to food, liquids, other nutrients

Physical Facilities (check all that apply)

Exterior

- ☐ steps____
- ☐ unsafe steps____
- ☐ porch____
- ☐ litter____
- ☐ noise____
- ☐ inadequate lighting____
- ☐ other____

Interior

- ☐ accessible bathroom____
- ☐ level, safe floor surface____
- ☐ number of rooms____
- ☐ privacy____
- ☐ sleeping arrangements____
- ☐ refrigeration____
- ☐ trash management____
- ☐ animals____
- ☐ adequate lighting____
- ☐ steps/stairs____
- ☐ other____

____

Safety Hazards found in the patient's current residence (check all that apply)

- ☐ none
- ☐ inadequate floor, roof, or windows
- ☐ inadequate lighting
- ☐ unsafe gas/electric appliances
- ☐ inadequate heating
- ☐ inadequate cooling
- ☐ lack of fire safety devices
- ☐ unsafe floor coverings
- ☐ inadequate stair rails
- ☐ lead-based paint
- ☐ improperly stored hazardous material
- ☐ improper wiring/electrical cords
- ☐ other____

____

Safety Factors (check all that apply)

- ☐ smoke/fire detectors____
- ☐ telephone____
- ☐ placement of electrical cords____
- ☐ emergency plan____

____

- ☐ emergency phone numbers displayed
- ☐ safe portable heaters____
- ☐ obstacle-free paths____
- ☐ other____

____

FIGURE 5•10 Home assessment checklist.

Critical Thinking Exercises

1.
Compare the approaches you would use in assessing a patient who is experiencing severe acute pain; is blind or hard of hearing; is mentally retarded; is from a culture with very different values from yours.

2.
Your nutritional assessment reveals that your patient has an inadequate protein intake. How would you develop dietary instructions for the patient who is a vegetarian? For the elderly patient on a fixed income? For the patient who has an intolerance for dairy foods?

3.
The findings of your physical and nutritional assessment of an 18-year-old college student suggest to you that she may have an eating disorder. How would you further assess this patient and develop a plan of management for her?

4.
You have received a referral for home care for a 72-year-old patient who lives in a single room on the third floor of a boarding house. He is malnourished and requires daily injections of antibiotics for the treatment of osteomyelitis. What factors would you include in your initial assessment on your first home visit?

References and Selected Readings

BOOKS

Barkauskas, V. H. (1998). *Health and physical assessment* (2nd ed.). St. Louis: C. V. Mosby.

Bickley, L. S. & Hoekelman, R. A. (1999). *Bates' guide to physical examination and history taking* (7th ed.). Philadelphia: Lippincott Williams & Wilkins.

Dudek, S. G. (1997). *Nutrition handbook for nursing practice* (2nd ed.). Philadelphia: Lippincott-Raven.

Gordon, M. (1994). *Nursing diagnosis: Process and application.* St. Louis: C. V. Mosby.

National Research Council. (1989). *Recommended dietary allowances* (10th ed.). Washington, DC: National Academy Press.

Nutrition Screening Initiative. (1992). *Nutrition interventions manual for professionals caring for older Americans.* Washington, DC: Author.

Seidel, H., et al. (1995). *Mosby's physical examination handbook.* St. Louis: C. V. Mosby.

Silverman, M. E., & Hurst, J. W. (1996). *Clinical skills for adult primary care.* Philadelphia: Lippincott-Raven.

U.S. Public Health Service. (1995). *Healthy people 2000: Midcourse review and 1995 revisions.* Washington, DC: U.S. Government Printing Office.

U.S. Department of Agriculture, and the United States Department of Health and Human Services. (1995). *Nutrition and your health: Guidelines for Americans* (4th ed.). Home & Garden Bulletin No. 232. Hyattsville, MD: Human Nutrition Information Service.

JOURNALS

General Assessment

Ball, R. (1997). Geriatric assessment: Special considerations of the over-65 patient. *Journal of Emergency Medical Services,* (March), 96–102.

Dubin, S. (1996). Geriatric assessment. *American Journal of Nursing,* May (5 Nurse Pract Extra Ed), 49–50.

Goodfellow, L. M. (1997). Physical assessment: A vital nursing tool in both developing and developed countries. *Critical Care Nursing Quarterly, 20*(2), 6–8.

Healy, L. F. (1997). Adult periodic health assessment guides. *Nurse Practitioner: American Journal of Primary Health Care, 22*(2), 171–177.

Jessop, J., Williamson, S., & Zinobar, B. (1995). An assessment tool for older patients. *Professional Nurse, 10*(12), 773–777.

Keleher, K. C. (1995). Primary care for women: Environmental assessment of the home, community and workplace. *Journal of Nurse Midwifery, 40*(2), 88–96.

Martin, K., Jarvis, L. A., & Beale, B. (1997). Healthy lifestyle check: A computerized health screening program. *Computers in Nursing, 15*(2), 77–81.

Nowazek, V., & Neeley, M. A. (1996). Health assessment of the older patient. *Critical Care Nursing Quarterly, 19*(2), 1–6.

Pressman, E., Zeidman, S., & Summers, L. (1995). Primary care for women: Comprehensive assessment of the neurologic system. *Journal of Nurse Midwifery, 40*(2), 216–219.

Quirk, M., & Casey, L. (1995). Primary care for women: The art of interviewing. *Journal of Nurse Midwifery, 40*(2), 97–103.

Smith, M., & Martin, F. (1995). Domestic violence: Recognition, intervention, and prevention. *MedSurg Nursing, 4*(1), 21–25.

Williams, G. D. (1997). Preoperative assessment and health history interview. *Nursing Clinics of North America, 32*(2), 395–416.

Nutritional Assessment

Barrocas, A., Belcher, D., Champagne, C., & Jastram, C. (1995). Nutrition assessment: Practical approaches. *Clinics in Geriatric Medicine, 11*(4), 675–713.

ACOG Educational Bulletin. (1997). Nutrition and women. *International Journal of Gynaecology and Obstetrics, 56,* 71–81.

Costello, M. C., & Todd-Magel, C. (1997). Bridging the gap: Hospital to home nutrition support. *MedSurg Nursing, 6*(6), 328–337.

Cotton, E., Zinobar, B., & Jessop, J. (1996). A nutritional assessment tool for older patients. *Professional Nurse, 11*(9), 609–612.

Edington, J., Kon, P., & Martyn, C. N. (1997). Prevalence of malnutrition after major surgery. *Journal of Human Nutrition and Dietetics, 10*(2), 111–116.

Evans-Stoner, N. (1997) Nutrition assessment: A practical approach. *Nursing Clinics of North America, 32*(4), 637–650.

Grindel, C. G., & Costello, M. C. (1996). Nutrition screening: An essential assessment parameter. *MedSurg Nursing, 5*(3), 145–154.

Hammond, K. (1997). Physical assessment: A nutritional perspective. *Nursing Clinics of North America, 32*(4), 779–790.

Howard, J. H. (1996). Nutritional parameters and assessment in the elderly. *Topics in Clinical Nutrition, 11*(3), 77–85.

Incalzi, R. A., Landi, F., Cipriani, L., et al. (1996). Nutritional assessment: A primary component of multidimensional geriatric assessment in the acute care setting. *Journal of the American Geriatrics Society, 44*(2), 166–174.

Keithley, J. K., Keller, A., & Vazquez, M. G. (1996). Promoting good nutrition: Using the food guide pyramid in clinical practice. *MedSurg Nursing, 5*(6), 397–403.

Manning, E. M. C., & Shenkin, A. (1995). Nutritional assessment in the critically ill. *Critical Care Clinics, 11*(3), 603–634.

Morrisson, S. G. (1997). Feeding the elderly population. *Nursing Clinics of North America, 32*(4), 791–812.

Phaneuf, C. (1996). Currents in practice. Screening elders for nutritional deficits. *American Journal of Nursing, 96*(3 Nurse Pract Extra Ed), 58–60.

Webber, C. B., & Splett, P. L. (1995). Nutrition risk factors in a home health population. *Home Health Care Services Quarterly, 15*(3), 97–110.

Weindruch, R., & Sohal, R. S. (1997). Caloric intake and aging. *New England Journal of Medicine, 337*(14) 986–993.

Wilson, J. M. (1996). Nutritional assessment and its application. *Journal of Intravenous Nursing, 19*(6), 307–314.

Resources

American Dietetic Association, 216 W. Jackson Blvd., Suite 800, Chicago, IL 60606; Consumer Nutrition Hotline: 800-366-1655; http://www.eatright.org.

American Heart Association, 7320 Greenville Ave., Dallas, TX 75231; National Center: 214-373-6300, Nutrition Information: 214-706-1179; http://www.americanheart.org.

National Cancer Institute, Cancer Information Service, 9000 Rockville Pike, Bldg. 31, Room 10A-24, Bethesda, MD 20892; 1-800-4-CANCER; http://www.nci.nih.gov, http://www.ncu.nih.gov/hpage/cis.htm.

Nutrition Screening Initiative, P.O. Box 753, Waldorf, MD 20604; 202-625-1662, http://www.fiu.edu/~nutreld/NSI.html.

Pennsylvania State Nutrition Center, The Pennsylvania State University, Ruth Building, 417 E. Calder Way, University Park, PA 16802; 814-865-6323.

UNIT

2

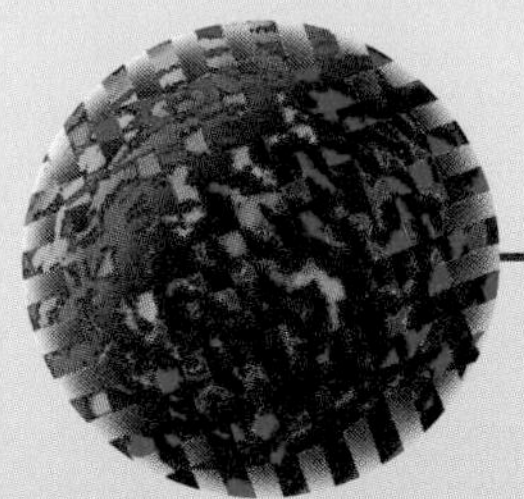

Biophysical and Psychosocial Concepts in Nursing Practice

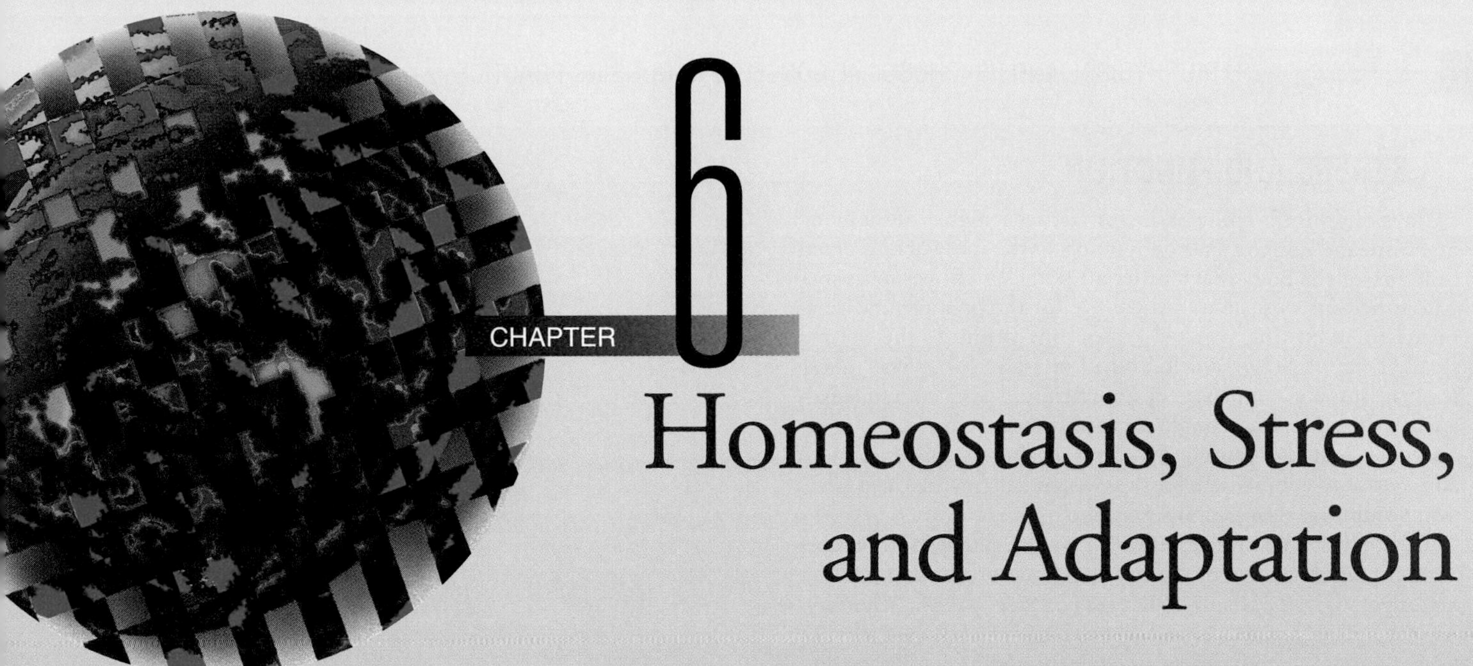

CHAPTER 6

Homeostasis, Stress, and Adaptation

Learning Objectives

On completion of the chapter, the learner will be able to:

1. Relate the principles of internal constancy, homeostasis, stress, and adaptation to the concept of steady state.
2. Identify the significance of the body's compensatory mechanisms in promoting adaptation and maintaining the steady state.
3. Identify physiologic and psychosocial stressors.
4. Compare the sympathetic–adrenal–medullary response to stress to the hypothalamic–pituitary response to stress.
5. Describe the general adaptation syndrome as a theory of adaptation to biologic stress.
6. Describe the relationship of the process of negative feedback to the maintenance of the steady state.
7. Compare the adaptive processes of hypertrophy, atrophy, hyperplasia, dysplasia, and metaplasia.
8. Describe the inflammatory and reparative processes.
9. Assess the health patterns of an individual and determine their effects on maintenance of the steady state.
10. Identify ways in which maladaptive responses to stress can increase the risk of illness and cause disease.
11. Identify measures that are useful in reducing stress.
12. Specify the functions of social networks and support groups in reducing stress.

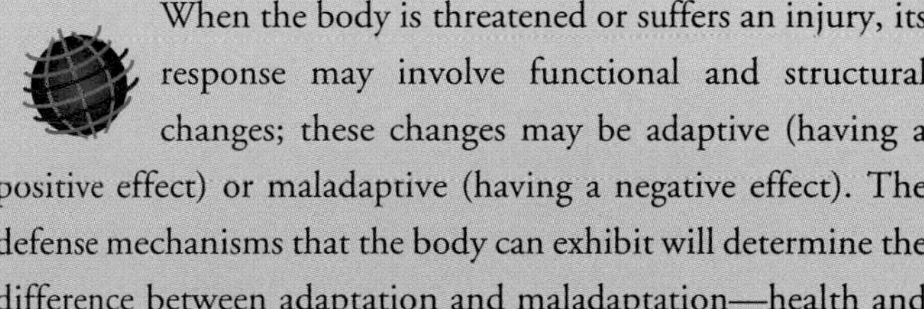

When the body is threatened or suffers an injury, its response may involve functional and structural changes; these changes may be adaptive (having a positive effect) or maladaptive (having a negative effect). The defense mechanisms that the body can exhibit will determine the difference between adaptation and maladaptation—health and disease.

STRESS AND FUNCTION

Physiology is the study of the functional activities of the living organism and its parts. Pathophysiology is the study of disordered function of the body. Each different body system performs specific functions to sustain optimal life for the organism. Mechanisms for adjusting internal conditions promote the normal steady state of the organism and ultimately its survival. These mechanisms are compensatory in nature and work to restore balance in the body. An example of this restorative effort is the development of rapid breathing (hyperpnea) after intense exercise in an attempt to compensate for the oxygen deficit and excess lactic acid accumulated in the muscle tissue.

Pathophysiologic processes result when cellular injury occurs at such a rapid rate that the body's compensatory mechanisms can no longer make the adaptive changes necessary to remain healthy. An example of a pathophysiologic change is the development of heart failure: the body reacts by retaining sodium and water and increasing venous pressure, which worsens the condition. These pathophysiologic mechanisms give rise to signs that are observed by the patient, nurse, or other health care provider, or symptoms that are reported by the patient. These observations, plus a sound knowledge of physiologic and pathophysiologic processes, can assist in determining the existence of a problem and can guide the nurse in planning the appropriate course of action.

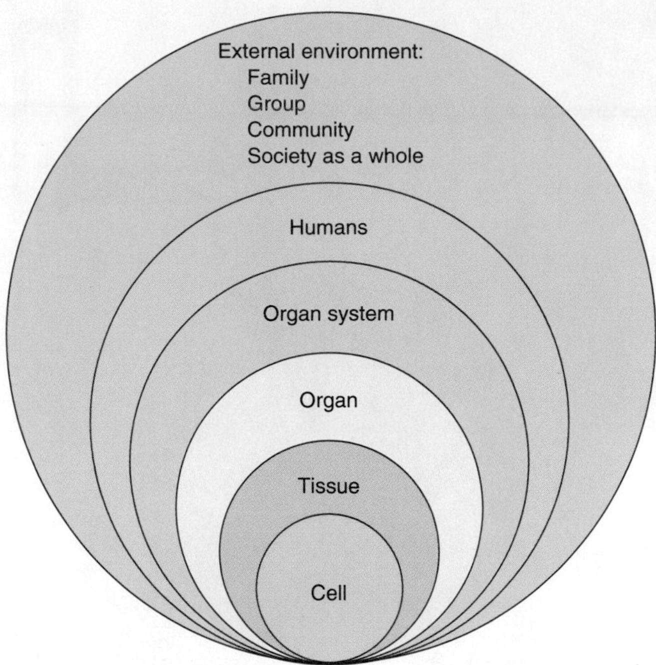

FIGURE 6•1 Constellation of systems. Each system is a subsystem of the larger system (suprasystem) of which it is a part. In this figure the cell is the smallest system, being a subsystem of all other systems.

DYNAMIC BALANCE: THE STEADY STATE

Physiologic mechanisms must be understood in the context of the body as a whole. The person, as a living system, has both an internal and an external environment. Information and matter are continuously exchanged between one environment and the other. Within the internal environment each organ, tissue, and cell is also a system or subsystem of the whole, each with its own internal and external environment, each exchanging information and matter (Fig. 6-1). The goal of the interaction of the body's subsystems is to produce a dynamic balance or steady state (even in the presence of change), so that all subsystems are in harmony with each other. The four concepts, constancy, homeostasis, stress, and adaptation, enhance the nurse's understanding of steady state.

Historical Theories of the Steady State

Claude Bernard, a 19th-century French physiologist, developed the biological principle that for life there must be a constancy or "fixity of the internal milieu" despite changes in the external environment. The internal milieu was the fluid that bathed the cells, and the constancy was the balanced internal state maintained by physiologic and biochemical processes. His principle implied a static process.

Later, Walter Cannon used the term *homeostasis* to describe the stability of the internal environment, which, he said, was coordinated by homeostatic or compensatory processes that responded to changes in the internal environment. Any change within the internal environment initiated a "righting" response to minimize the change. These biologic processes sought physiologic and chemical balance and were under involuntary control.

Dubos (1965) provided further insight into the dynamic nature of the internal environment. He stated that two complementary concepts, homeostasis and adaptation, were necessary for balance. Homeostatic processes occurred quickly in response to stress, rapidly making the adjustments necessary to maintain the internal environment. Adaptive processes resulted in structural or functional changes over time. Dubos also emphasized that acceptable ranges of response to stimuli existed and that these responses varied for different individuals: "absolute constancy is only a concept of the ideal." Homeostasis and adaptation were both necessary for survival in a changing world.

Homeostasis, then, refers to a steady state within the body. When a change or stress occurs that causes a body function to deviate from its stable range, processes are initiated to restore and maintain the dynamic balance. When these adjustment processes or compensatory mechanisms are not adequate, the steady state is threatened, function becomes disordered, and pathophysiologic mechanisms occur. The pathophysiologic processes can lead to disease and may be active during disease. Disease is a threat to the steady state. It is an abnormal variation in the structure or function of any part of the body. Disease disrupts function and therefore limits the person's freedom of action.

Stress and Adaptation

Stress is a state produced by a change in the environment that is perceived as challenging, threatening, or damaging to the person's dynamic balance or equilibrium. There is an actual or perceived imbalance in the person's ability to meet the demands of the new situation. The change or stimulus that evokes this state is the stressor. The nature of the stressor is variable; an event or change that will produce stress in one person may be neutral for another, and an event that may produce stress at one time and place for one person may not do so for the same person at another time and place. A person appraises and copes with changing situations. The desired goal is adaptation, or adjustment to the change so that the person is again in equilibrium and has the energy and ability to meet new demands. This is the stress-coping process, a compensatory process with physiologic and psychological components.

Adaptation is a constant, ongoing process that requires a change in structure, function, or behavior so that the person is better suited to the environment; it involves an interaction between the person and the environment. The outcome depends on the degree of "fit" between the skills and capacities of the person, the type of social support available, and the various challenges or stressors being confronted. As such, adaptation is an individual process: each individual has varying abilities to cope or respond. As new challenges are met, this ability to cope and adapt can change, thereby providing the individual with a wide range of adaptive ability. Adaptation occurs throughout the life span as the individual encounters many developmental and situational challenges, especially related to health and illness. The goal of these encounters is to promote adaptation. In situations of health and illness, this goal is realized by optimal wellness.

Because both stress and adaptation may exist at different levels of a system, it is possible to study these reactions at the cellular, tissue, and organ levels. The biologist's study is concerned mainly with subcellular components or with subsystems of the total body. Behavioral scientists, including nurse researchers, study stress and adaptation in individuals, families, groups, and societies; they focus on how a group's organizational features are modified to meet the requirements of the social and physical environment in which they exist. Adaptation is a continuous process of seeking harmony in an environment. The desired goals of adaptation for any system are survival, growth, and reproduction.

STRESSORS: THREATS TO THE STEADY STATE

Each person operates at a certain level of adaptation and regularly encounters a certain amount of change. Such change is expected; it contributes to growth, and it enhances life. Stressors, however, can upset this equilibrium. A stressor may be defined as an internal or external event or situation that creates the potential for physiologic, emotional, cognitive, or behavioral changes in an individual.

Types of Stressors

Stressors exist in many forms and categories. They may be described as physical, physiologic, or psychosocial. Physical stressors include cold, heat, or chemical agents; physiologic stressors include pain or fatigue; and psychosocial stressors include fear of failing an exam or losing a job. Stressors can also occur as normal life transitions that require some adjustment, such as going from childhood into puberty, getting married, or giving birth.

Stressors have also been classified as: (1) day-to-day frustrations or hassles; (2) major complex occurrences, involving large groups, even entire nations; and (3) stressors that occur less frequently and involve fewer people. The first group, the day-to-day stressors, includes such common occurrences as getting caught in a traffic jam, experiencing computer downtime, and having an argument with a spouse or roommate. These experiences vary in effect; for example, encountering a rainstorm while one is vacationing at the beach will most likely evoke a more negative response than it might at another time. These less dramatic, frustrating, and irritating events—daily hassles—have been shown to have a greater health impact than major life events because of the cumulative effect they have over time. They can lead to high blood pressure, palpitations, or other physiologic problems.

The second group of stressors influences larger groups of people, possibly even entire nations. These include events of history, such as terrorism and war, which are threatening situations when experienced either directly in the war zone, or indirectly, as through live news coverage. The demographic, economic, and technological changes occurring in society also serve as stressors. The tension produced by any stressor is sometimes a result not only of the change itself, but also of the speed with which the change occurs.

The third group of stressors has been studied most extensively and concerns relatively infrequent situations that directly affect the individual. This category includes the influence of life events, such as death, birth, marriage, divorce, and retirement. It includes the psychosocial crises described by Erikson as occurring in the life cycle stages of the human experience. More enduring chronic stressors have also been placed in this category and may include such things as having a permanent functional disability or coping with the difficulties of providing long-term care to a frail elderly parent.

A stressor can also be categorized according to duration. It may be:

- An acute, time-limited stressor, such as studying for final exams
- A stressor sequence—a series of stressful events that result from an initial event such as job loss or divorce
- A chronic intermittent stressor, such as daily hassles
- A chronic enduring stressor that persists over time, such as chronic illness or poverty

Stress as a Stimulus for Disease

Relating life events to illness (the theoretical approach that defines stress as a stimulus) has been a major focus of psychosocial studies. This can be traced to Adolph Meyer, who in the 1930s observed in "life charts" of his patients a linkage between illnesses and critical life events. Subsequent research revealed that people under constant stress have a high incidence of psychosomatic disease.

Holmes and Rahe (1967) developed life events scales that assign numerical values, called life-change units, to typical life events. Since the items reflect events that require a change in the person's life pattern, and stress is defined as an accumulation of changes in one's life that require psychological adaptation, one can theoretically predict the likelihood of illness by checking off the number of recent events and deriving a total score. The Recent Life Changes Questionnaire (Tausig, 1982) contains 118 items such as death, birth, marriage, divorce, promotions, serious arguments, and vacations. The events listed include both desirable and undesirable circumstances.

Sources of stress for hospitalized patients have also been researched. Ballard (1981) identified immobilization, isolation, disorientation, and sensory deprivation as stressful conditions in a study of patients in the surgical intensive care unit. She observed that nurses could alter many of the stressors. She also observed that not only are illness and major surgery stressors, but the resulting role changes and financial demands created by the illness are additional stressors.

Psychological Responses to Stress

After the recognition of a stressor, the individual will consciously or unconsciously react to manage the situation. This is called the mediating process. A theory developed by Lazarus emphasizes cognitive appraisal and coping as important mediators of stress. Appraisal and coping are influenced by antecedent variables that include the internal and external resources of the person.

Appraisal of the Stressful Event

Cognitive appraisal (Lazarus, 1991a; Lazarus & Folkman, 1984) is a process through which an event is evaluated with respect to what is at stake (primary appraisal) and what might and can be done (secondary appraisal). What individuals see as at stake is influenced by their personal goals, commitments, or motivations. For example, how important or how relevant is the event? Is it in conflict with what the person wants or desires? Does the situation threaten the person's own sense of strength and ego identity?

As an outcome of primary appraisal, the situation will be identified as either nonstressful or stressful. If nonstressful, the situation is irrelevant or benign/positive. A stressful situation may be one of three kinds: (1) those in which harm or loss has occurred; (2) those that are threatening, in that harm or loss is anticipated; and (3) those that are challenging, in that some opportunity or gain is anticipated.

Secondary appraisal is an evaluation of what might and can be done. This includes assigning blame to those responsible for a frustrating event, thinking about whether or not one can do something about the situation (one's coping potential), and determining future expectancy, or whether things are likely to change for better or worse (Lazarus, 1991a, 1991c). The degree of stress is determined by a comparison of what is at stake and what can be done about it (a type of risk–benefit analysis).

Reappraisal also occurs and refers to a changed appraisal based on new information. The appraisal process is not necessarily sequential; primary and secondary appraisal and reappraisal may occur simultaneously. Information learned from an adaptational encounter can be stored, so that when a similar situation is encountered again the whole process does not need to be repeated.

The appraisal process contributes to the development of an emotion. Negative emotions such as fear and anger accompany harm/loss appraisals, while positive emotions accompany challenge. Besides the subjective component or feeling that accompanies a particular emotion, each emotion also includes a tendency to act in a certain way. To illustrate this concept, an unexpected quiz in the classroom might be judged as threatening by the unprepared student, and fear, anger, and resentment might be felt. These emotions might be expressed by outwardly hostile behavior or comments.

Lazarus (1991a) expanded his former ideas about stress, appraisal, and coping into a more complex model relating emotion to adaptation. He called this a "cognitive-motivational-relational theory," with relational "standing for a focus on negotiation with a physical and social world" (p. 13). A theory of emotion was proposed as the bridge to connect psychology, physiology, and sociology. "More than any other arena of psychological thought, emotion is an integrative, organismic concept that subsumes psychological stress and coping within itself and unites motivation, cognition, and adaptation in a complex configuration" (p. 40).

Coping with the Stressful Event

Coping, according to Lazarus, consists of the cognitive and behavioral efforts made to manage the specific external or internal demands that tax a person's resources. Coping can be emotion-focused or problem-focused. Coping that is emotion-focused seeks to make the person feel better by lessening the emotional distress felt. Problem-focused coping aims to make direct changes in the environment so that the situation can be managed more effectively. Both types of coping usually occur in a stressful situation. Even when the situation is viewed as challenging or beneficial, coping efforts may be required to develop and sustain the challenge—that is, to maintain the positive benefits of the challenge and to ward off any threats. In harmful or threatening situations, successful coping will reduce or eliminate the source of stress and relieve the emotion it generated.

Appraisal and coping are affected by internal characteristics such as health, energy, personal belief systems, commitments or life goals, self-esteem, control, mastery, knowledge, problem-solving skills, and social skills. The characteristics that have been studied the most in nursing research are health-promoting lifestyles and hardiness. A health-promoting lifestyle buffers the effect of stressors. From a nursing practice standpoint, this outcome—buffering the effect of stressors—supports nursing's goal of promoting health. In many circumstances, promoting a healthy lifestyle is more achievable than altering the stressors.

Hardiness is the name given to a general quality that comes from rich, varied, and rewarding experiences. It is a personality characteristic composed of control, commitment, and challenge. Hardy people perceive stressors as something they can change and therefore control. Potentially stressful situations are interesting and meaningful; change and new situations are viewed as challenging opportunities for growth. Some positive support has been found for hardiness as a mediator of the psychosocial stress associated with chronic illness (Ruiz-Bueno, 1993).

Physiologic Response to Stress

The physiologic response to a stressor, whether it is a physical stressor or a psychological stressor, is a protective and adaptive mechanism to maintain the homeostatic balance of the body. The stress response is a "cascade of neural and hormonal events that have short- and long-lasting consequences for both brain and body . . . a stressor is an event that challenges homeostasis, with a disease outcome being looked upon as a failure of the normal process of adaptation to the stress" (McEwen & Mendelson, 1993, p. 101).

The General Adaptation Syndrome

Because of its profound influence on the scientific development of the study of stress, it is important to understand the theory of adaptation developed by Hans Selye. In 1936, Selye, experimenting with animals, first described a syndrome consisting of enlargement of the adrenal cortex; shrinkage of the thymus, spleen, lymph nodes, and other lymphatic structures; and the appearance of deep, bleeding ulcers in the stomach and duodenum. He identified this as a nonspecific response to diverse, noxious stimuli. From this beginning, he developed a theory of adaptation to biologic stress that he named the general adaptation syndrome.

PHASES OF THE GENERAL ADAPTATION SYNDROME

The general adaptation syndrome has three phases: alarm, resistance, and exhaustion. During the alarm phase, the sympathetic "fight-or-flight response" is activated with release of catecholamines and the onset of the adrenocorticotropic hormone

(ACTH)–adrenal cortical response. The alarm reaction is defensive and anti-inflammatory but self-limited. Because it is impossible to live in a continuous state of alarm (death would ensue), the person moves into the second stage, resistance. During this stage, adaptation to the noxious stressor occurs. Cortisol activity is still increased. If exposure to the stressor is prolonged, exhaustion sets in and endocrine activity increases. This produces deleterious effects on the body systems (especially circulatory, digestive, and immune) that can lead to death. Stages one and two of this syndrome are repeated, in different degrees, throughout life as the person encounters stressors.

Selye compared the general adaptation syndrome with the life process. During childhood, there are few encounters with stress to promote the development of adaptive functioning, and the child is vulnerable. During adulthood, the person encounters a number of life's stressful events and develops a resistance or adaptation. During the later years, the accumulation of life's stressors and the wear and tear on the organism again deplete the person's ability to adapt, resistance falls, and eventually death ensues.

LOCAL ADAPTATION SYNDROME

According to Selye's theory, there is also a local adaptation syndrome. This syndrome includes the inflammatory response and repair processes that occur at the local site of tissue injury. The local adaptation syndrome occurs in small, topical injuries, such as contact dermatitis. If the local injury is severe enough, the general adaptation syndrome is activated also.

Selye emphasized that stress is the nonspecific response common to all stressors, regardless of whether they are physiologic, psychological, or social. The fact that different demands are interpreted by different people as stressors is explained by the many conditioning factors in each person's environment. Conditioning factors also account for differences in the tolerance of different people for stress. Some people may develop diseases of adaptation, such as hypertension and migraine headaches, while others are unaffected.

Interpretation of Stressful Stimuli by the Brain

Physiologic responses to stress are mediated by the brain through a complex network of chemical and electrical messages. The neural and hormonal actions that maintain homeostatic balance are integrated by the hypothalamus. The hypothalamus is located in the center of the brain, surrounded by the limbic system and the cerebral hemispheres. It integrates autonomic nervous system mechanisms that maintain the chemical constancy of the internal environment of the body. The hypothalamus and the limbic system regulate emotions and many visceral behaviors necessary for survival (eg, eating, drinking, temperature control, reproduction, defense, and aggression). The hypothalamus is made up of a number of nuclei; the limbic system contains the amygdala, hippocampus, and septal nuclei, along with other structures.

Research supports the concept that each of these structures responds differently to stimuli, and each has its own characteristic response. The cerebral hemispheres are concerned with cognitive functions: thought processes, learning, and memory. The limbic system has connections with both the cerebral hemispheres and the brain stem. In addition, the reticular activating system, which is a network of cells that forms a two-way communication system, extends from the brain stem into the midbrain and limbic system. This network controls the alert or waking state of the body.

In the stress response, afferent impulses are carried from sensory organs (eye, ear, nose, skin) and internal sensors (baroreceptors, chemoreceptors) to nerve centers in the brain. The response to the perception of stress is integrated in the hypothalamus, which coordinates the adjustments necessary to return to homeostatic balance. The degree and duration of the response will vary; major stress evokes both sympathetic and pituitary adrenal responses.

Neural and neuroendocrine pathways under the control of the hypothalamus are activated in the stress response. First, there is a sympathetic nervous system discharge, followed by a sympathetic–adrenal–medullary discharge. If the stress persists, the hypothalamic–pituitary system is activated (Fig. 6-2).

SYMPATHETIC NERVOUS SYSTEM RESPONSE

The sympathetic nervous system response is rapid and short-lived. Norepinephrine is released at nerve endings in direct contact with their respective end organs to cause an increase in function of the vital organs and a state of general body arousal. The heart rate is increased. Peripheral vasoconstriction occurs, raising the blood pressure. Blood is also shunted away from abdominal organs. The purpose of these activities is to provide better perfusion of vital organs (brain, heart, skeletal muscles). Blood glucose is increased, supplying more readily available energy. The pupils are dilated, and mental activity is increased; a greater sense of awareness exists. Constriction of the blood vessels of the skin limits bleeding in the event of trauma. The person is likely to experience cold feet, clammy skin and hands, chills, palpitations, and a knot in the stomach. Typically, the person appears tense, with the muscles of the neck, upper back, and shoulders tightened; respirations may be rapid and shallow, with the diaphragm tense.

SYMPATHETIC–ADRENAL–MEDULLARY RESPONSE

In addition to its direct effect on major end organs, the sympathetic nervous system stimulates the medulla of the adrenal gland to release the hormones epinephrine and norepinephrine into the bloodstream. The action of these hormones is similar to that of the sympathetic nervous system and has the effect of sustaining and prolonging its actions. Epinephrine and norepinephrine are catecholamines that stimulate the nervous system and produce metabolic effects that increase the blood glucose level and increase the metabolic rate. The effect of the sympathetic and adrenal–medullary responses is summarized in Table 6-1. This effect is called the fight-or-flight reaction.

HYPOTHALAMIC–PITUITARY RESPONSE

The longest-acting phase of the physiologic response, which is more likely to occur in persistent stress, involves the hypothalamic–pituitary pathway. The hypothalamus secretes corticotropin-releasing factor, which stimulates the anterior pituitary to produce ACTH. ACTH in turn stimulates the adrenal cortex to produce glucocorticoids, primarily cortisol. Cortisol stimulates protein catabolism, releasing amino acids; stimulates liver uptake of amino acids and their conversion to glucose (gluconeogenesis); and inhibits glucose uptake (anti-insulin action) by many body cells but not those of the brain and heart. These cortisol-induced metabolic effects provide the body with a ready source of energy during a stressful situation. There are some important implications to this effect: a person with diabetes who is under stress, such as that caused by an infection, will need more insulin than usual. Any patient who is under stress (illness, surgery, prolonged psycholog-

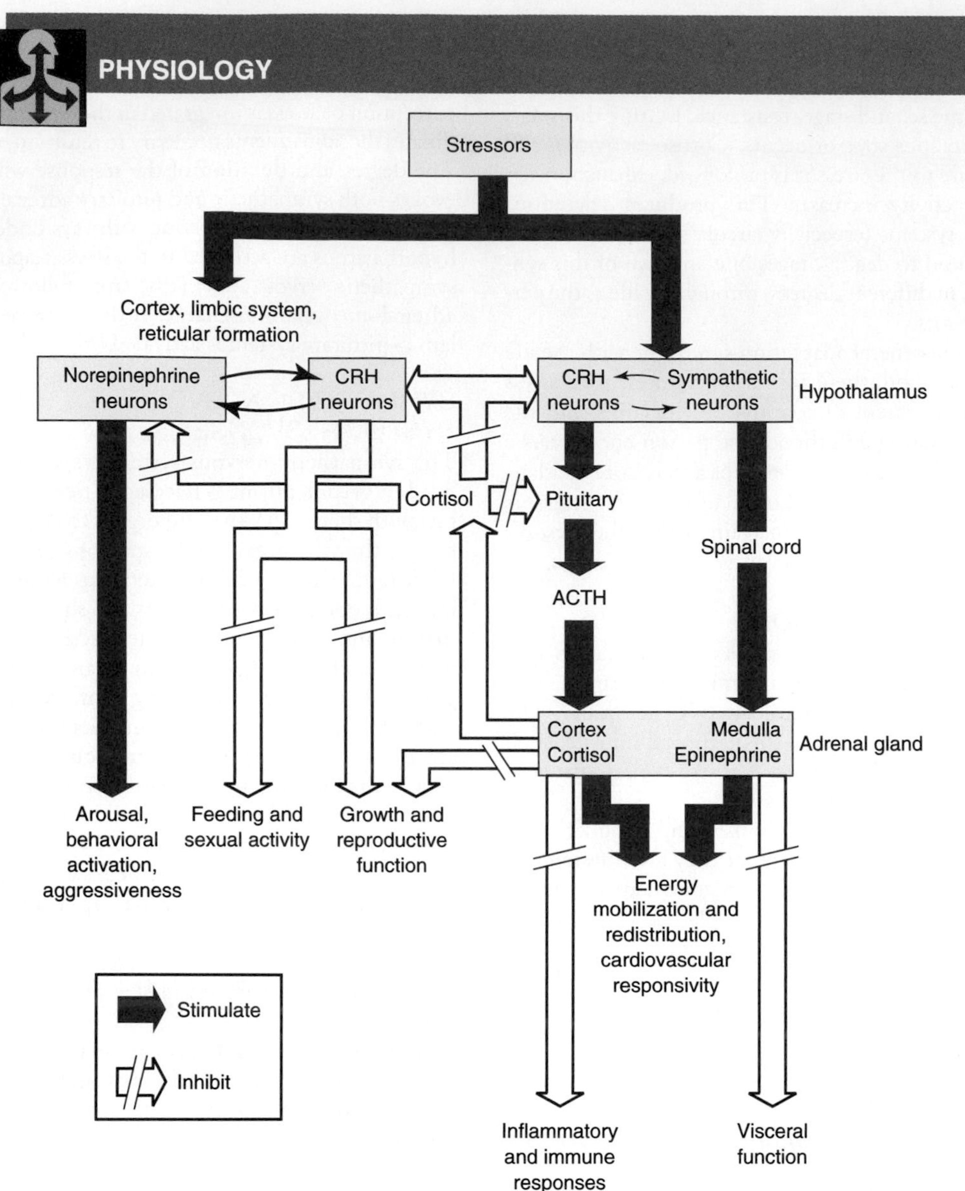

FIGURE 6•2 Integrated responses to stress mediated by the sympathetic nervous system and the hypothalamic–pituitary–adrenocortical axis. The responses are mutually reinforcing, both at the central and peripheral levels. Negative feedback by cortisol also can limit an overresponse that might be harmful to the individual. *Colored arrows,* stimulation; *open arrows,* inhibition; CRH, corticotropin-releasing hormone; ACTH, adrenocorticotropic hormone. Reproduced with permission from Berne, R. M., & Levy, M. N. (1993). *Physiology.* St. Louis: C. V. Mosby.

ical stress) will catabolize body protein and need supplements. Children subjected to severe stress will have retarded growth.

The actions of the catecholamines (epinephrine and norepinephrine) and cortisol are most important in the general response to stress. Other hormones released are antidiuretic hormone (ADH) from the posterior pituitary and aldosterone from the adrenal cortex. ADH and aldosterone promote sodium and water retention, which is an adaptive mechanism in the event of hemorrhage or loss of fluids through excessive perspiration. ADH has also been shown to influence learning and so may facilitate coping in new and threatening situations. Secretion of growth hormone and glucagon stimulate the uptake of amino acids by cells, helping to mobilize energy resources. Endorphins, an endogenous opiate, increase during stress and enhance the threshold for tolerance of painful stimuli. They may also affect mood and have been implicated in the so-called "high" that long-distance runners experience. The secretion of other hormones is also affected, but their adaptive function is less clear.

IMMUNOLOGIC RESPONSE

Research findings show that the immune system is connected to the neuroendocrine and autonomic systems. Lymphoid tissue is richly supplied by autonomic nerves capable of releasing a number of different neuropeptides that can have a direct effect on leukocyte regulation and the inflammatory response. Neuroendocrine hormones released by the central nervous system and endocrine tissues can inhibit or stimulate leukocyte function. The wide variety of stressors people experience may result in different alterations in

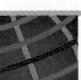

TABLE 6•1 **Sympathetic–Adrenal–Medullary Response to Stress**

Effect	Purpose	Mechanism
↑Heart rate ↑Blood pressure	Better perfusion of vital organs	Increased cardiac output due to increased myocardial contractility and heart rate; increased venous return (peripheral vasoconstriction)
↑Blood glucose	Increased available energy	Increased liver and muscle glycogen breakdown; increased breakdown of adipose tissue triglycerides
↑Mental activity	Alert state	Increase in amount of blood shunted to the brain from the abdominal viscera and skin
Dilated pupils	Increased awareness	Contraction of radial muscle of iris
↑Tension of skeletal muscles	Preparedness for activity, decreased fatigue	Excitation of muscles; increase in amount of blood shunted to the muscles from the abdominal viscera and skin
↑Ventilation (may be rapid and shallow)	Provision of oxygen for energy	Stimulation of respiratory center in medulla; bronchodilation
↑Coagulability of blood	Prevention of hemorrhage in event of trauma	Vasoconstriction of surface vessels

autonomic activity and subtle variations in neurohormone and neuropeptide synthesis. All of these possible autonomic and neuroendocrine responses can interact to initiate, weaken, enhance, or terminate an immune response (Watkins, 1996).

The study of the relationships among the neuroendocrine system, the central and autonomic nervous systems, and the immune system, and the effects of these relationships on overall health outcomes is called psychoneuroimmunology. Since our perception of events and our coping styles determine whether or not, and to what extent, an event activates the stress response system, and since the stress response affects immune activity, our perceptions, ideas, and thoughts can have profound neurochemical and immunologic consequences. Multiple studies have demonstrated alteration of immune function, as evidenced by a decrease in the number of leukocytes, impaired immune response to immunizations, and diminished cytotoxicity of natural killer cells in people under stress (Andersen et al., 1998; Biondi et al., 1994; Black, 1994; Glaser & Kiecolt-Glaser, 1997; Mills et al., 1996; Pike et al., 1997). Other studies have identified certain personality traits, such as optimism and active coping, as having positive effects on health or specific immune measures (Goodkin et al., 1996 Sergerstrom et al., 1998). As research continues, this new field of study will continue to uncover to what extent and by what mechanisms people can consciously influence our immunity.

Maladaptive Responses to Stress

As indicated earlier, the stress response facilitates adaptation to threatening situations. It has been retained from our evolutionary past. The fight-or-flight response, for example, is an anticipatory response that mobilized the bodily resources of our ancestors to deal with predators and other harsh factors in their environment. This same mobilization comes into play in response to emotional stimuli unrelated to danger. For example, a person may get an "adrenaline rush" when competing over a decisive point in a ball game, or when excited about attending a party.

When the responses to stress are ineffective, they are referred to as *maladaptive*. Maladaptive responses are chronic, recurrent responses or patterns of response over time that do not promote the goals of adaptation. The goals of adaptation are somatic or physical health, the goal being optimal wellness; psychological health or having a sense of well-being (happiness, satisfaction with life, morale); and enhanced social functioning, which includes work, social, and family relationships, with the goal being positive relationships. Maladaptive responses that threaten these goals include faulty appraisals and inappropriate coping (Lazarus, 1991a).

The frequency, intensity, and duration of stressful situations contribute to the development of negative emotions and subsequent patterns of neurochemical discharge. By appraising situations more adequately and by coping more appropriately, it is possible to anticipate and defuse some of these situations. For example, frequent potentially stressful encounters (eg, marital discord) might be avoided with better communication and problem solving, or a pattern of procrastination (eg, delaying work on tasks) can be corrected to reduce stress when deadlines approach.

Coping processes that include the use of alcohol or drugs to reduce stress increase the risk of illness. Other inappropriate coping patterns may increase the risk of illness less directly. For example, people who demonstrate "type A" personality behaviors such as impatience, competitiveness, and achievement orientation and have an underlying hostile approach to life are more prone than others to develop stress-related illnesses. Type A behaviors increase the output of catecholamines, the adrenal–medullary hormones, with their attendant effects on the body.

Other forms of inappropriate coping include denial, avoidance, and distancing. Denial may be illustrated by the woman who feels a lump in her breast but downplays its seriousness and delays seeking medical attention. The intent of denial is to control the threat, but it may endanger life.

Models of illness frequently cite stress and maladaptation as precursors to disease. A general model of illness, based on Selye's theory, basically suggests that any stressor elicits a state of disturbed physiologic equilibrium. If this state is prolonged or the response is excessive, it will increase the susceptibility of the person to illness. This susceptibility, coupled with a predisposition in the person (genetic traits, health, age), leads to illness. When the sympathetic adrenal–medullary response is prolonged or excessive, a state of chronic arousal develops that may lead to high blood pressure, arteriosclerotic changes, and cardiovascular disease.

When the production of the ACTH is prolonged or excessive, behavior patterns of withdrawal and depression are seen. In addition, the immune response is decreased, and infections and tumors may develop.

Selye (1976, pp. 169–170) proposed a list of disorders that he called diseases of maladaptation:

> High blood pressure, diseases of the heart and blood vessels, diseases of the kidney, eclampsia, rheumatic and rheumatoid arthritis, inflammatory diseases of the skin and eyes, infections, allergic and hypersensitivity diseases, nervous and mental diseases, sexual derangements, digestive diseases, metabolic diseases, cancer, and diseases of resistance in general.

Indicators of Stress

Indicators of stress and the stress response include subjective and objective measures. Chart 6-1 lists signs and symptoms that may be observed directly or reported by the person. They are psychological, physiologic, or behavioral and reflect social behaviors and thought processes. Some of these reactions may be coping behaviors. Over time, each person tends to develop a characteristic pattern of behavior during stress that is a warning that the system is out of balance.

Laboratory measurements of indicators of stress have helped in understanding this complex process. Among the measures, blood and urine analyses can be used to demonstrate changes in hormonal levels and hormonal breakdown products. Reliable measures of stress include blood levels of catecholamines, corticoids, ACTH, and eosinophils. The serum creatine/creatinine ratio and elevations of cholesterol and free fatty acids can also be measured. Immunoglobulin assays may be determined. With the growth of neuroimmunology, improved laboratory measures are likely to follow. Increases in blood pressure and heart rate can also be measured.

In addition to using laboratory tests, researchers have developed questionnaires to identify and assess stressors, stress, and coping. Many of these are discussed in the research monograph developed by Barnfather and Lyon (1993) based on a synthesis conference held by nurse scientists on the state of the science in stress and coping nursing research. Miller and Smith (1993) provided a stress audit and a stress profile measurement that is available in the popular literature.

CHART 6•1 Signs and Symptoms of Stress

General irritability, hyperexcitation, or depression
Dryness of the throat and mouth
Overpowering urge to cry, scream, or run and hide
Easily fatigued, loss of interest
"Floating anxiety"—do not know exactly why or what
Easily startled
Stuttering or other speech difficulties
Hypermotility: pacing, moving about, cannot sit still
Gastrointestinal signs and symptoms: "butterflies" in the stomach, diarrhea, vomiting
Change in menstrual cycle
Loss of or excessive appetite
Increased use of legally prescribed drugs, such as anxiolytics or antidepressants
Prone to injuries
Disturbed behavior
Pounding of the heart
Impulsive behavior, emotional instability
Inability to concentrate
Feelings of unreality, weakness, or dizziness
Tension, alertness
Trembling, nervous tics
Nervous laughter
Grinding of teeth
Insomnia, nightmares, or other sleep difficulties
Excessive perspiration
Increased frequency of urination
Muscle tension and migraine headaches
Pain in the neck or lower back
Increased smoking
Alcohol and drug addiction

Based on Selye, H. (1976). *Stress in health and disease.* Stoneham, MA: Butterworths. Reprinted with permission of the publisher.

Nursing Implications

It is important for the nurse to realize that the optimal point of intervention to promote health is during the stage when the individual's own compensatory processes are still functioning. Early identification of both physiologic and psychological stressors remains a major role of the nurse. Information on the interrelationships between physical and emotional health can be found in research journals. The nurse should be able to relate the presenting signs and symptoms of distress to the physiology they represent and identify the individual's position on the continuum of function, from health and compensation to pathophysiology and disease. Thus, if an anxious middle-aged woman presented for a checkup and was found to be overweight, with a blood pressure of 130/85 mm Hg, the nurse would most likely counsel her with respect to diet, stress management, and activity. The nurse would encourage weight loss and discuss the woman's intake of salt (which affects fluid balance) and caffeine (which provides a stimulant effect). The patient and the nurse would identify both individual and environmental stressors and discuss strategies to decrease the lifestyle stress. The ultimate goal would be to create a healthy lifestyle and prevent hypertension and its sequelae.

STRESS AT THE CELLULAR LEVEL

Pathologic processes may occur at all levels of the biologic organism. If the cell is considered the smallest unit or subsystem (tissues being aggregates of cells, organs aggregates of tissues, and so forth), the processes of health and disease or adaptation and maladaptation can all occur at the cellular level. Indeed, pathologic processes are often described by scientists at the subcellular or molecular level.

The cell exists on a continuum of function and structure, ranging from the normal cell, to the adapted cell, to the injured or diseased cell, to the dead cell (Fig. 6-3). Changes from one state to another may occur rapidly and may not be readily detectable because each state does not have discrete boundaries, and disease represents an extension and distortion of normal processes. The earliest changes occur at the molecular or subcellular level and are not perceptible until steady-state functions or structures are altered. With cell injury, some changes may be reversible; in other instances, the injuries are lethal. For example, tanning of the skin is an adaptive, morphologic response from exposure to the rays of the sun. If the exposure is continued, how-

PHYSIOLOGY

HEALTH		DISEASE	
Normal cell	Adapted cell	Injured or diseased cell	Dead cell

Compensatory mechanisms; Cell remains intact | Pathophysiologic mechanisms; Loss of cell integrity

FIGURE 6•3 The cell on a continuum of function and structure. Changes in the cell are not as easily discerned as the diagram depicts. The point at which compensation subsides and pathophysiology begins is not clearly defined.

ever, sunburn and injury occur, and some cells may die, as evidenced by desquamation ("peeling").

Different cells and tissues respond to stimuli with different patterns and rates of response; some cells are more vulnerable to one type of stimulus or stressor than others. The cell involved, its ability to adapt, and its physiologic state are determinants of the response. For example, cardiac muscle cells respond to hypoxia (inadequate oxygenation) more quickly than smooth muscle cells.

Other determinants of cellular response are the type or nature of the stimulus, its duration, and its severity. For example, neurons that control respiration can develop a tolerance to regular small amounts of a barbiturate, but one large dose may result in respiratory depression and death.

Control of the Steady State

The concept of the cell on a continuum of function and structure includes the relationship of the cell to compensatory mechanisms. These mechanisms occur continuously in the body to maintain the steady state. Compensatory processes are primarily regulated by the autonomic nervous system and the endocrine system, with control achieved through negative feedback.

Negative Feedback

Negative feedback mechanisms throughout the body monitor the internal environment and restore homeostasis when conditions shift out of the normal range. These mechanisms work by sensing deviations from a predetermined set point or range of adaptability and triggering a response aimed at offsetting the deviation. Blood pressure, acid–base balance, blood glucose level, body temperature, and fluid and electrolyte balance are examples of functions regulated through such compensatory mechanisms.

Most of the human body's control systems are integrated by the brain and effected through the nervous and endocrine systems. Control activities involve detecting deviations from the predetermined reference point and stimulating compensatory responses in the muscles and glands of the body. The major organs affected are the heart, lungs, kidneys, liver, gastrointestinal tract, and skin. When stimulated, these organs alter the rate of their activity or the amount of secretions they produce. They have been called the "organs of homeostasis or adjustment."

In addition to the responses controlled by the nervous and endocrine systems, local responses consisting of small feedback loops in a group of cells or tissues are possible. The cells detect a change in their immediate environment and initiate an action to counteract its effect. For example, the accumulation of lactic acid in an exercised muscle will stimulate dilation of blood vessels in the area to increase blood flow and improve the delivery of oxygen and removal of waste products.

The net result of the activities of feedback loops is homeostasis. A steady state is achieved by the continuous, variable action of the organs involved in making the adjustment and the continuous small exchanges of chemical substances among cells, interstitial fluid, and blood. For example, an increase in the carbon dioxide concentration of the extracellular fluid leads to increased pulmonary ventilation, which decreases the carbon dioxide level. On a cellular level, increased carbon dioxide raises the hydrogen ion concentration of the blood. This is detected by chemosensitive receptors in the respiratory control center of the medulla of the brain. The chemoreceptors stimulate an increase in the rate of discharge of the neurons, which innervates the diaphragm and intercostal muscles and increases the rate of respiration. Excess carbon dioxide is exhaled, the hydrogen ion concentration returns to normal, and the chemically sensitive neurons are no longer stimulated.

Positive Feedback

Another type of feedback, positive feedback, perpetuates the chain of events set in motion by the original disturbance. Compensation does not occur, and as the system becomes more unbalanced, disorder and disintegration occur. There are some exceptions to this; blood clotting in humans, for example, is an important positive feedback mechanism.

Cellular Adaptation

Cells are complex units dynamically responding to the changing demands and stresses of daily life. They possess a maintenance function and a specialized function. The maintenance function refers to the activities that the cell must perform with respect to itself; specialized functions are those that the cell performs in relation to the tissues and organs of which it is a part. Individual cells may cease to function without posing a threat to the organism; however, as the number of dead cells increases, the specialized functions of the tissues are altered and the individual's health is threatened.

Cells can adapt to environmental stress by structural and functional changes. Some of these adaptations are hypertrophy, atrophy, hyperplasia, dysplasia, and metaplasia (Table 6-2).

Hypertrophy and atrophy lead to changes in the size of cells and hence the size of the organs they form. Compensatory hypertrophy is the result of an enlarged muscle mass and commonly occurs in skeletal and cardiac muscle that experiences a prolonged, increased workload. The bulging muscles of the athlete who engages in body building is one example. Atrophy can be the consequence of a disease or of decreased use, decreased blood supply, loss of nerve supply, or inadequate nutrition. Disuse of a body part is often associated with the aging process. Cell size and organ size decrease; structures principally affected are the skeletal muscle, the secondary sex organs, the heart, and the brain.

Hyperplasia is an increase in the number of new cells in an organ or tissue. As cells multiply and are subjected to increased stimulation, tissue mass enlarges. It is a mitotic response (a change occurring with mitosis), but it is reversible when the stimulus is removed. This distinguishes it from neoplasia or malignant growth, which continues after the stimulus is removed. Hyperplasia may be hor-

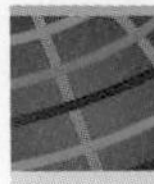

TABLE 6•2 Cellular Adaptation to Stressors

Adaptation	Stimulus	Example
Hypertrophy—increase in cell size leading to increase in organ size	Increased workload	Leg muscles of runner Arm muscles in tennis player Cardiac muscle in person with hypertension
Atrophy—shrinkage in size of cell, leading to decrease in organ size	Decrease in: Use Blood supply Nutrition Hormonal stimulation Innervation	Secondary sex organs in aging person Extremity immobilized in plaster cast
Hyperplasia—increase in number of new cells (increase in mitosis)	Hormonal influence	Breast changes of a girl in puberty or of a pregnant woman Regeneration of liver cells New red blood cells in blood loss
Dysplasia—change in the appearance of cells after they have been subjected to chronic irritation	Reproduction of cells that may be transformed into uncontrolled rapid multiplication	Alterations in epithelial cells of the skin or the cervix, producing irregular tissue changes that could be the precursors of a malignancy
Metaplasia—transformation of one adult cell type to another (reversible)	Stress applied to highly specialized cell	Changes in epithelial cells lining bronchi in response to smoke irritation (cells become less specialized)

monally induced. An example is the increase in the size of the thyroid gland by thyroid-stimulating hormone (secreted from the pituitary gland) when a deficit in thyroid hormone is detected.

Dysplasia is the change in the appearance of cells after they have been subjected to chronic irritation. Dysplastic cells have a tendency to become malignant; dysplasia is seen commonly in epithelial cells in the bronchi of smokers.

Metaplasia is a cell transformation in which a highly specialized cell changes to a less specialized cell. This serves a protective function because the less specialized cell is more resistant to the stress that stimulated the change. For example, the ciliated columnar epithelium lining the bronchi of smokers is replaced by squamous epithelium. The squamous cells can survive; however, loss of the cilia and protective mucus can have damaging consequences.

These adaptations allow the survival of the organism. They also reflect changes in the normal cell in response to stress. If the stress is unrelenting, the function of the adapted cell may succumb, and cell injury will occur.

Cellular Injury

Injury is defined as a disorder in steady-state regulation. Any stressor that alters the ability of the cell or system to maintain optimal balance of its adjustment processes will lead to injury. Structural and functional damage then occurs, which may be reversible (permitting recovery) or irreversible (leading to disability or death). Homeostatic adjustments are concerned with the small changes within the body's systems. With adaptive changes, compensation occurs and a steady state is achieved, although it may be at new levels. With injury, steady-state regulation is lost, and changes in functioning ensue.

Causes of disorder and injury in the system (cell, tissue, organ, body) may arise from the external or internal environment (Fig. 6-4) and include hypoxia, nutritional imbalance, physical agents, chemical agents, infectious agents, immune mechanisms, genetic defects, and psychogenic factors. The most common causes are hypoxia (oxygen deficiency), chemical injury, and infectious agents. In addition, the presence of one injury makes the system more susceptible to another injury. For example, inadequate oxygenation and nutritional deficiencies make the system vulnerable to infection. These agents act at the cellular level by damaging or destroying:

- The integrity of the cell membrane, necessary for ionic balance
- The ability of the cell to transform energy (aerobic respiration, production of adenosine triphosphate)
- The ability of the cell to synthesize enzymes and other necessary proteins
- The ability of the cell to grow and reproduce (genetic integrity)

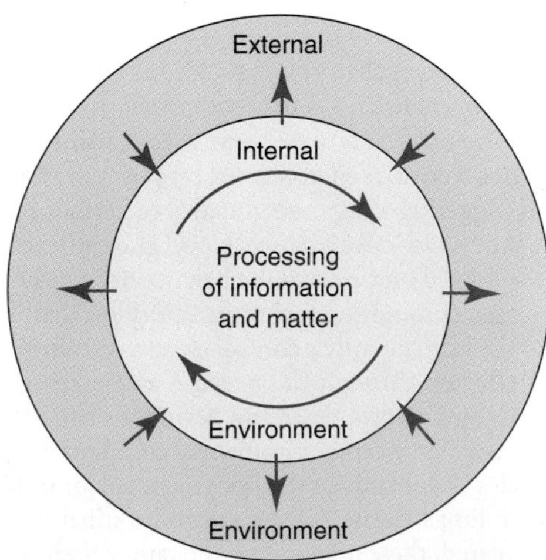

FIGURE 6•4 Influences leading to disorder may arise from the internal environment and the external environment of the system. Excesses or deficits of information and matter may occur, or there may be faulty regulation of processing.

Hypoxia

Inadequate cellular oxygenation (hypoxia) interferes with the cell's ability to transform energy. Hypoxia may be caused by:

- A decrease in blood supply to an area
- A decrease in the oxygen-carrying capacity of the blood (decreased hemoglobin)
- A ventilation/perfusion or respiratory problem, reducing the amount of oxygen available in the blood
- A problem in the cell's enzyme system, making it unable to use the oxygen delivered to it

The usual cause is ischemia, or deficient blood supply. Ischemia is commonly seen in myocardial cell injury in which arterial blood flow is decreased because of atherosclerotic narrowing of blood vessels. Ischemia also results from intravascular clots that may form and interfere with blood supply. Thrombi and emboli are common causes of cerebrovascular accidents (strokes). The length of time different tissues can survive without oxygen varies. For example, brain cells may succumb in 3 to 6 minutes, depending on the situation. If the condition leading to hypoxia is slow and progressive, collateral circulation may develop, whereby blood is supplied by other blood vessels in the area. However, this mechanism is not highly reliable.

Nutritional Imbalance

Nutritional imbalance refers to a relative or absolute deficiency or excess of one or more essential nutrients. This may be manifested as undernutrition (inadequate consumption of food or calories) or overnutrition (caloric excess). Caloric excess to the point of obesity overloads cells in the body with lipids. By requiring more energy to maintain the extra tissue, obesity places a strain on the body and has been associated with the development of disease, especially pulmonary and cardiovascular disease.

Specific deficiencies arise when an essential nutrient is deficient or when there is an imbalance of nutrients. Protein deficiencies and avitaminosis (deficiency of vitamins) are typical examples. An energy deficit leading to cell injury can occur when there is insufficient glucose, or insufficient oxygen to transform the glucose into energy. A lack of insulin, or the inability to use insulin, may also prevent glucose from entering the cell from the blood. This is the problem in diabetes mellitus, a metabolic disorder that can lead to nutritional deficiency.

Physical Agents

Physical agents, including temperature extremes, radiation, electrical shock, and mechanical trauma, can cause injury to the cells or the entire body. The duration of exposure and the intensity of the stressor determine the severity of damage.

EXTREMES OF HIGH TEMPERATURE

When a person's temperature is elevated, hypermetabolism occurs and the respiratory rate, heart rate, and basal metabolic rate increase. With fever induced by infections, the hypothalamic thermostat may be reset at a higher temperature. When the fever abates, the thermostat returns to normal. The increase in body temperature is achieved through physiologic mechanisms. Body temperatures above 41°C (106°F) suggest hyperthermia, since the physiologic function of the thermoregulatory center breaks down and the temperature soars. This physiologic condition occurs in people with heat stroke. Eventually, the high temperature causes coagulation of cell proteins, and the cells die. The body must be cooled rapidly to prevent brain damage.

The local response to thermal or burn injury is similar. There is an increase in metabolic activity, and as heat increases, protein is coagulated, enzyme systems are destroyed, and, in the extreme, charring or carbonization occurs. Burns of the epithelium are classified as partial-thickness burns if epithelializing elements remain to support healing. Full-thickness burns lack such elements and must be grafted for healing. The amount of body surface involved determines the prognosis for the patient. If the injury is severe, the entire body system becomes involved, and hypermetabolism will develop as a pathophysiologic response.

EXTREMES OF LOW TEMPERATURE

Extremes of low temperature or cold cause vasoconstriction, causing blood flow to become sluggish and clots to form, leading to ischemic damage in the involved tissues. With still lower temperatures, ice crystals may form, and the cells may burst.

RADIATION AND ELECTRICAL SHOCK

Radiation is used for diagnosis and treatment of diseases. Ionizing forms of radiation may cause injury by their destructive action. Radiation decreases the protective inflammatory response of the cell, creating a favorable environment for opportunistic infections. Electrical shock produces burns as a result of the heat generated when electric current travels through the body. It may also abnormally stimulate nerves, leading, for example, to fibrillation of the heart.

MECHANICAL TRAUMA

Mechanical trauma can result in wounds that disrupt the cells and tissues of the body. The severity of the wound, the amount of blood loss, and the extent of nerve damage are significant factors in the outcome.

Chemical Agents

Chemical injuries are caused by poisons, such as lye, which has a corrosive action on epithelial tissue, or by heavy metals, such as mercury, arsenic, and lead, each with its own specific destructive action. Many other chemicals are toxic in specific amounts, in certain people, and in distinctive tissues. Too much hydrochloric acid can damage the stomach lining; large amounts of glucose can cause osmotic shifts, affecting the fluid and electrolyte balance; and too much insulin can cause subnormal levels of sugar in the blood (hypoglycemia) and lead to coma.

Drugs, including prescribed medications, can cause chemical poisoning. Some individuals are less tolerant of medications than others and manifest toxic reactions at the usual or customary dosages. Aging tends to decrease tolerance to medications. Polypharmacy (taking many medications at one time) also occurs frequently in the aging population and is a problem because of the unpredictable effects of the resulting medication interactions.

Alcohol (ethanol) is a chemical irritant. In the body, alcohol is broken down into acetaldehyde, which has a direct toxic effect on liver cells that leads to a variety of liver abnormalities, including cirrhosis in susceptible individuals. Disordered liver cell function leads to complications in other organs of the body.

Infectious Agents

Biologic agents known to cause disease in humans are viruses, bacteria, rickettsiae, mycoplasmas, fungi, protozoa, and nematodes. The severity of the infectious disease depends on the number of microorganisms entering the body, their virulence, and the host's defenses, such as health, age, and immune defenses.

Some bacteria, such as those in tetanus and diphtheria, produce exotoxins that circulate and create cell damage. Others, such as the gram-negative bacteria, produce endotoxins when they are killed. The tubercle bacillus induces an immune reaction.

Viruses, as the smallest living organisms, survive as parasites of the living cells they invade. Viruses infect specific cells. Through a complex mechanism, they replicate within the cells and then invade other cells and continue to replicate. An immune response is mounted by the body to eliminate the viruses, and the cells harboring the viruses can be injured in the process. Typically, an inflammatory response and immune reaction are the physiologic responses of the body to the presence of infection.

Disordered Immune Responses

The immune system is an exceedingly complex system; its purpose is to defend the body from invasion by any foreign object or foreign cell type, such as cancerous cells. This is a steady-state mechanism, but like other adjustment processes it can become disordered, and cell injury will occur. Basically, the immune response detects foreign bodies by distinguishing non-self substances from self substances and destroying the non-self entities. The entrance of an antigen (foreign body) into the body evokes the production of antibodies that attack and destroy the antigen (antigen–antibody reaction).

The immune system can be hypoactive or hyperactive. When it is hypoactive, immunodeficiency diseases occur; when it is hyperactive, hypersensitivity disorders arise. A disorder of the immune system itself can result in damage to the body's own tissues. Such disorders are labeled autoimmune diseases (see Unit 11).

Genetic Disorders

Genetic defects as causes of disease are of intense interest as more of them and their effects on genetic structure are studied. Many of these defects produce mutations that have no recognizable effect, such as lack of a single enzyme; others contribute to more obvious congenital abnormalities, such as Down's syndrome. As a result of the Human Genome Project, patients can be genetically assessed for conditions such as sickle cell disease, cystic fibrosis, hemophilia A and B, breast cancer, obesity, cardiovascular disease, phenylketonuria, and Alzheimer's disease. The availability of genetic information and technology enables some health care providers to perform screening, testing, and counseling for patients with genetic concerns. Current knowledge obtained from the Human Genome Project has created opportunities for evaluating a person's genetic endowment and preventing or treating disease. Genetic diagnostics and gene therapy have the potential to identify a gene before it begins to express traits that would lead to disease or disability.

Cellular Response to Injury: Inflammation

Cells or tissues of the body may be injured or killed by any of the agents (physical, chemical, infectious) described earlier. When this happens, there is a naturally occurring response in the healthy tissues adjacent to the site of injury. This is called the inflammatory response, or inflammation. It is a defensive reaction intended to neutralize, control, or eliminate the offending agent and to prepare the site for repair. It is a nonspecific response (not dependent on a particular cause) meant to serve a protective function. For example, inflammation may be observed at the site of a bee sting, in a sore throat, in a surgical incision, and at a burn site. Inflammation also occurs in cell injury events, such as strokes and myocardial infarctions.

Inflammation is not the same as infection. An infectious agent is only one of several agents that may trigger an inflammatory response. An infection exists when the infectious agent is living, growing, and multiplying in the tissues and is able to overcome the body's normal defenses.

Regardless of the cause, a general sequence of events occurs in the local inflammatory response. This sequence involves changes in the microcirculation, including vasodilation, increased vascular permeability, and leukocytic cellular infiltration (Fig. 6-5). As these changes take place, five cardinal signs of inflammation are produced: redness, heat, swelling, pain, and loss of function.

The transient vasoconstriction that occurs immediately after injury is followed by vasodilation and an increased rate of blood flow through the microcirculation. Local heat and redness result. Next, vascular permeability increases, and plasma fluids (including proteins and solutes) leak into the inflamed tissues, producing swelling. The pain produced is attributed to the pressure of fluids or swelling on nerve endings, and to the irritation of nerve endings by chemical mediators released at the site. Bradykinin is one of the chemical mediators suspected of causing pain. Loss of function is most likely related to the pain and swelling, but the exact mechanism is not completely known.

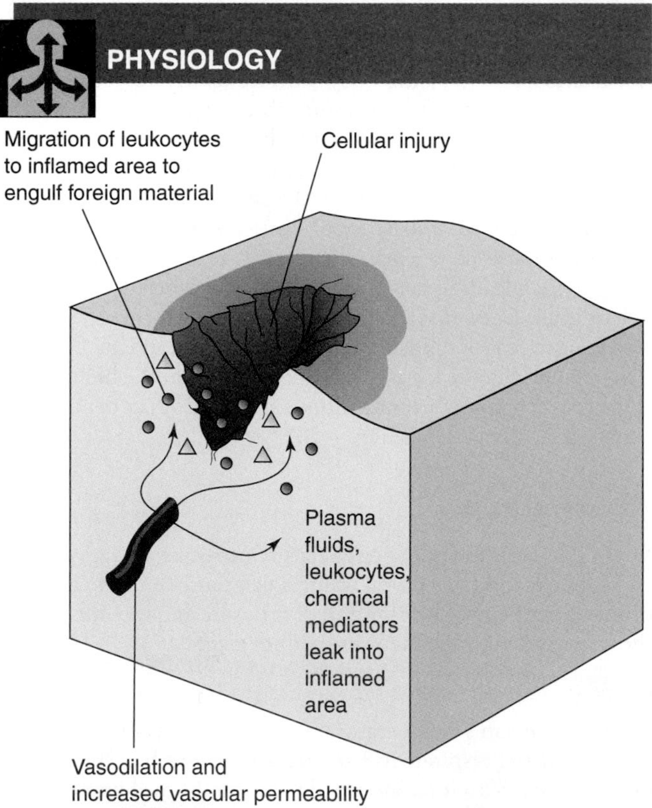

FIGURE 6•5 Inflammatory response. Chemical, physical, infectious, or other factors cause cellular injury. Vasodilation and release of chemical-mediators, leukocytes, and proteins occur. Leukocytes remove cellular debris. Fibrinogen and plasma coagulate to prevent spread of infection.

As the blood flow increases and fluid leaks into the surrounding tissues, the formed elements (red blood cells, white blood cells, and platelets) remain in the blood, causing it to become more viscous. Leukocytes (white blood cells) collect in the vessels, exit, and migrate to the site of injury to engulf offending organisms and to remove cellular debris in a process called phagocytosis. Fibrinogen in the leaked plasma fluid coagulates, forming fibrin for clot formation, which serves to wall off the injured area and prevent the spread of infection.

Chemical Mediators

Injury initiates the inflammatory response, but chemical substances released at the site induce the vascular changes. Foremost among these chemicals are histamine and the kinins. Histamine is present in many tissues of the body but is concentrated in the mast cells. It is released when injury occurs and is responsible for the early changes in vasodilation and vascular permeability. Kinins increase vasodilation and vascular permeability; they also attract neutrophils to the area. Prostaglandins, another group of chemical substances, are also suspected of causing increased permeability.

Systemic Response to Inflammation

The inflammatory response is often confined to the site, causing only local signs and symptoms. However, systemic responses can also occur. Fever is the most common sign of a systemic response to injury. It is most likely caused by endogenous pyrogens (internal substances that cause fever) released from neutrophils and macrophages (specialized forms of leukocytes). These substances reset the hypothalamic thermostat (which controls body temperature) and produce fever. Leukocytosis, an increase in the synthesis and release of neutrophils from bone marrow, may occur to provide the body with greater ability to fight infection. During this process, general, nonspecific symptoms develop, including malaise, loss of appetite, aching, and weakness.

Types of Inflammation

Inflammation is categorized primarily by its duration and the type of exudate produced. It may be acute, subacute, or chronic. Acute inflammation is characterized by the local vascular and exudative changes described above and usually lasts less than 2 weeks. An acute inflammatory response is immediate, and it serves a protective function. When the injurious agent is removed, the inflammation subsides, and healing takes place with the return of normal or near-normal structure and function.

Chronic inflammation develops when the injurious agent persists and the acute response is perpetuated. Symptoms appear for many months or years. Chronic inflammation may also begin insidiously and never have an acute phase. The chronic response does not serve a beneficial and protective function; on the contrary, it is debilitating and can produce long-lasting effects. As the inflammation becomes chronic, changes occur at the site of injury, and the nature of the exudate becomes proliferative. There is a continuing cycle of cellular infiltration, necrosis, and fibrosis (repair and breakdown occur simultaneously). Considerable scarring may occur, resulting in permanent tissue damage.

Subacute inflammation falls between acute and chronic inflammation. There are elements of the active exudative phase of the acute response as well as elements of repair, as in the chronic phase. The term subacute inflammation is not widely used.

Cellular Healing

The reparative process begins at approximately the same time as the injury and is interwoven with inflammation. Healing proceeds after the inflammatory debris is removed. Healing may be by regeneration, in which gradual repair of the defect occurs by proliferation of cells of the same type as those destroyed, or by replacement, in which cells of another type, usually connective tissue, fill in the tissue defect, resulting in scar formation.

Healing by Regeneration

The ability of cells to regenerate depends on whether they are labile, permanent, or stable. Labile cells multiply constantly to replace cells worn out by normal physiologic processes; these include epithelial cells of the skin and those lining the gastrointestinal tract. Permanent cells include neurons—the nerve cell bodies, not their axons. Destruction of a neuron is a permanent loss, but axons may regenerate. If normal activity is to return, tissue regeneration must occur in a functional pattern, especially in the growth of several axons. Stable cells have a latent ability to regenerate. Under normal physiologic processes, they are not shed and do not need replacement, but if they are damaged or destroyed, they are able to regenerate. These include functional cells of the kidney, liver and pancreas.

Healing by Replacement

Depending on the extent of damage, tissue healing may be by primary intention or secondary intention. In primary intention healing, the wound is clean and dry and the edges are approximated, as in a surgical wound. Little scar formation occurs, and the wound is usually healed in a week. In secondary intention healing, the wound or defect is larger and gaping and has necrotic or dead material. The wound fills from the bottom upward with granulation tissue. The process of repair takes longer and results in more scar formation, with loss of specialized function. People who have recovered from myocardial infarctions have abnormal electrocardiographic (ECG) tracings because the electrical signal cannot be conducted through the connective tissue that replaces the infarcted area.

The condition of the host, the environment, and the nature and severity of the injury affect the processes of inflammation and repair. However, any of the injuries discussed in the preceding pages can lead to death of the cell. Essentially, the cell membrane becomes impaired, resulting in a nonrestricted flow of ions. Sodium and calcium enter the cell, followed by water, which leads to edema, and energy transformation ceases. Nerve impulses are no longer transmitted; muscles no longer contract. As the cells rupture, lysosomal enzymes that destroy tissues escape, and cell death and necrosis occur.

Nursing Implications

In the assessment of the person who seeks health care, both objective signs and subjective symptoms are the primary indicators of the physiologic processes that are occurring. The following questions are addressed during the assessment:

- Are the heart rate, respiratory rate, and temperature normal?
- What emotional distress may be contributing to the patient's health problems?
- Are there other indicators of steady-state deviation?

- What is the person's blood pressure, height, and weight?
- Are there any problems in movement or sensation?
- Does the person demonstrate any problems with affect, behavior, speech, cognitive ability, orientation, or memory?
- Are there obvious impairments, lesions, or deformities?

Further signs of change are indicated in diagnostic studies such as computed tomography (CT) scans, magnetic resonance imaging (MRI), and positron emission tomography (PET) scans. Objective evidence can also be obtained from laboratory data, including electrolytes, blood urea nitrogen (BUN), blood glucose, and urinalysis.

In making a nursing diagnosis, the nurse must relate the symptoms or complaints expressed by the patient to the physical signs that are present. Management of specific biologic disorders is discussed in subsequent chapters; however, the nurse can assist any patient to respond to stress-inducing biologic or psychological disorders with stress-management interventions.

STRESS MANAGEMENT: NURSING INTERVENTIONS

Stress or the potential for stress is ubiquitous; that is, it is everywhere and anywhere at once. Anxiety, frustration, anger, and feelings of inadequacy, helplessness, or powerlessness are emotions often associated with stress. In the presence of these emotions, the customary activities of daily living may be disrupted; for example, a sleep disturbance may be present, eating and activity patterns may be altered, and family processes or role performance may be disrupted.

Many nursing diagnoses are possible for patients suffering from stress. One nursing diagnosis related to stress is anxiety, which is defined as a vague, uneasy feeling, the source of which may be nonspecific or not known to the person. Stress may also be manifested as ineffective coping patterns, impaired thought processes, and disrupted relationships. These human responses are reflected in the nursing diagnoses of impaired adjustment, ineffective individual coping, defensive coping, and ineffective denial, all of which indicate poor adaptive responses. Other possible nursing diagnoses include social isolation, risk for altered parenting, spiritual distress, ineffective denial, family coping: potential for growth, decisional conflict, self-esteem disturbance, powerlessness, and others. Since human responses to stress are varied, as are the sources of stress, arriving at an accurate diagnosis allows interventions and goals to be more specific and leads to improved outcomes.

Methods for stress management aim to reduce and control stress and improve coping. Nurses might use these methods not only with their patients but also in their own lives. The need to prevent illness, improve the quality of life, and decrease the cost of health care makes efforts to promote health crucial. Stress control is a significant health-promotion goal. Stress-reduction methods and coping enhancements can derive from either internal or external sources. For example, adopting healthy eating habits and practicing relaxation techniques are internal resources that help to reduce stress; developing a broad social network is an external resource that helps reduce stress. Goods and services that can be purchased are also external resources for stress management, and it is much easier for individuals with adequate financial resources to cope with constraints in the environment because their sense of vulnerability to threat is decreased.

Promoting a Healthy Lifestyle

An individual's personal resources that aid in coping include health and energy. A health-promoting lifestyle provides these resources and buffers or cushions the impact of stressors. Lifestyles or habits that contribute to the risk of developing illness can be identified through a health risk appraisal.

A health risk appraisal is an assessment method designed to promote health by examining the individual's personal habits and recommending changes when a health risk is identified. Health risk questionnaires estimate the likelihood that a person with a given set of characteristics will become ill. It is reasoned that if people are provided with this information, they will alter their activities (eg, stop smoking, have periodic screening examinations) to improve their health. Questionnaires typically determine the following information:

1. Demographic data: age, sex, race, ethnic background
2. Personal and family history of diseases and health problems
3. Lifestyle choices
    a. Eating, sleeping, exercise, smoking, drinking, and driving habits
    b. Stressors at home and on the job
    c. Role relationships and associated stressors
4. Physical measurements
    a. Blood pressure
    b. Height, weight
    c. Laboratory analyses of blood and urine
5. Participation in high-risk behaviors

The personal information is compared with average population risk data, and the risk factors are identified and weighted. From this analysis, the person's risks and major health hazards are identified. If a person makes the suggested changes, further comparisons with population data can estimate how many years will be added to one's life span. However, research so far has not demonstrated that providing people with such information ensures that they will change their habits. The single most important factor for determining health status is social class, and within a social class the research suggests that the major factor influencing health is level of education (Mickler, 1997).

Enhancing Coping Strategies

McCloskey and Bulechek (1996) identified "coping enhancement" as a nursing intervention and defined it as "assisting a patient to adapt to perceived stressors, changes, or threats which interfere with meeting life demands and roles" (Chart 6-2). The nurse can build on the patient's existing coping strategies, as identified in the health appraisal, or teach new strategies for coping if necessary.

The five predominant ways of coping with illness identified in a review of 57 nursing research studies were:

- Trying to be optimistic about the outcome
- Using social support
- Using spiritual resources
- Trying to maintain control either over the situation or over feelings
- Trying to accept the situation. (Jalowiec, 1993, p. 80)

Other ways of coping included seeking information, reprioritizing needs and roles, lowering expectations, making compromises, comparing oneself to others, planning activities to con-

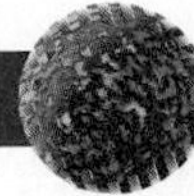

CHART 6•2 Coping Enhancement: Nursing Interventions

Definition: Assisting a patient to adapt to perceived stressors, changes, or threats that interfere with meeting life demands and roles

Activities

Appraise a patient's adjustment to changes in body image as indicated.
Appraise the impact of the patient's life situation on roles and relationships.
Encourage patient to identify a realistic description of change in role.
Appraise the patient's understanding of the disease process.
Appraise and discuss alternative responses to situation.
Use a calm, reassuring approach.
Provide an atmosphere of acceptance.
Assist the patient in developing an objective appraisal of the event.
Help the patient to identify the information he/she is most interested in obtaining.
Provide factual information concerning diagnosis, treatment, and prognosis.
Provide the patient with realistic choices about certain aspects of care.
Encourage an attitude of realistic hope as a way of dealing with feelings of helplessness.
Evaluate the patient's decision-making ability.
Seek to understand the patient's perspective of a stressful situation.
Discourage decision making when the patient is under severe stress.
Encourage gradual mastery of the situation.
Encourage patience in developing relationships.
Encourage relationships with persons who have common interests and goals.
Encourage social and community activities.
Encourage the acceptance of limitations of others.
Acknowledge the patient's spiritual/cultural background.
Encourage the use of spiritual resources if desired.
Explore patient's previous achievements of success.
Explore patient's reasons for self-criticism.
Confront patient's ambivalent (angry or depressed) feelings.
Foster constructive outlets for anger and hostility.
Arrange situations that encourage patient's autonomy.
Assist patient in identifying positive responses from others.
Encourage the identification of specific life values.
Explore with the patient previous methods of dealing with life problems.
Introduce patient to persons (or groups) who have successfully undergone the same experience.
Support the use of appropriate defense mechanisms.
Encourage verbalization of feelings, perceptions, and fears.
Discuss consequences of not dealing with guilt and shame.
Encourage the patient to identify own strengths and abilities.
Assist the patient in identifying appropriate short- and long-term goals.
Assist the patient in breaking down complex goals into small, manageable steps.
Assist the patient in examining available resources to meet the goals.
Reduce stimuli in the environment that could be misinterpreted as threatening.
Appraise patient needs/desires for social support.
Assist the patient to identify available support systems.
Determine the risk of the patient's inflicting self-harm.
Encourage family involvement as appropriate.
Encourage the family to verbalize feelings about ill family member.
Provide appropriate social skills training.
Assist the patient to identify positive strategies to deal with limitations and manage needed lifestyle or role changes.
Assist the patient to solve problems in a constructive manner.
Instruct the patient in the use of relaxation techniques as needed.
Assist the patient to grieve and to work through the losses of chronic illness and/or disability if appropriate.
Assist the patient to clarify misconceptions.
Encourage the patient to evaluate own behavior.

Reproduced with permission from McCloskey, J. C., & Bulechek, G. M. (1996). *Nursing intervention classification (NIC)* (2nd ed.) St. Louis: Mosby–Year Book.

serve energy, taking things one step at a time, listening to one's body, and using self-talk for encouragement.

The nurse can implement the coping enhancement interventions and explore methods for improving the person's coping abilities.

Teaching Relaxation Techniques

Relaxation techniques are a major method used to relieve stress. Commonly used techniques include progressive muscle relaxation, relaxation with guided imagery, and the Benson Relaxation Response. The goal of relaxation training is to produce a response that counters the stress response. When this goal is achieved, the action of the hypothalamus adjusts and decreases the activity of the sympathetic and parasympathetic nervous systems. The sequence of physiologic effects and their signs and symptoms are interrupted, and psychological stress is reduced. This is a learned response and requires practice to achieve.

The different relaxation techniques share four similar elements: (1) a quiet environment, (2) a comfortable position, (3) a passive attitude, and (4) a mental device (something on which to focus the attention, such as a word, phrase, or sound).

Progressive Muscle Relaxation

Progressive muscle relaxation involves tensing and releasing the muscles of the body in sequence and sensing the difference in feeling. It is best if the person lies on a soft cushion on the floor, in a quiet room, breathing easily. Someone usually reads the instructions in a low tone and a slow and relaxed manner, or a tape of the instructions can be played. The person tenses the muscles in the whole body, holds, senses the tension, and then relaxes. As the muscle groups are tensed, the person keeps the rest of the body relaxed. Each time the focus is on feeling the tension and relaxation. When completed, the whole body should be relaxed (Benson, 1993; Scandrett-Hibdon & Uecker, 1992).

Benson's Relaxation Response

Benson (1993) describes the following steps of the Benson Relaxation Response (pp. 106–117):

1. Pick a brief phrase or word that reflects your basic belief system.
2. Choose a comfortable position.
3. Close your eyes.
4. Relax your muscles.

5. Become aware of your breathing, and start using your selected focus word.
6. Maintain a passive attitude.
7. Continue for a set period of time.
8. Practice the technique twice daily.

This response combines meditation with relaxation. Along with the repeated word or phrase, a passive attitude is essential. Other thoughts or distractions (noises, the pain of an ailment) may occur; however, Benson recommends not fighting the distraction but simply continuing to repeat the focus phrase. The time of day is not important, but the exercise works best on an empty stomach.

Relaxation with Guided Imagery

Simple guided imagery is the "purposeful use of imagination to achieve relaxation or direct attention away from undesirable sensations" (McCloskey & Bulechek, 1996, p. 506). The nurse helps the person select a pleasant scene or experience, such as watching the ocean or dabbling the feet in a cool stream. This image serves as the mental device in this technique. As the person sits comfortably and quietly, the nurse guides the individual to review the scene, trying to feel and relive the imagery with all of the senses. A tape recording may be made of the description of the image, or commercial tape recordings for guided imagery and relaxation can be used.

Other relaxation techniques include meditation, breathing techniques, massage, music therapy, biofeedback, and the use of humor.

Educating

Two commonly prescribed nursing educational interventions—providing sensory and procedural information (eg, preoperative teaching)—have the goal of reducing stress and improving the patient's coping ability. This preparatory education includes giving structured content, such as a lesson in childbirth preparation to expectant parents, a review of cardiovascular anatomy to the cardiac patient, or a description of sensations the patient will experience during cardiac catheterization. These techniques may alter the person–environment relationship such that something that might have been viewed as a harm or threat is now perceived more positively. Giving patients information also reduces the emotional response so that they can concentrate and solve problems more effectively.

Major nursing research using these interventions was conducted by Leventhal and Johnson (1983). They tested the theory that people acquire a sense of control over events when they are given information that makes it possible for them to form a mental image of the event. For example, if people were provided with a description of the sensations they could expect to feel (eg, pulling, burning, pressure), if the routine of the procedure was described to them, and if they were given instructions about coping behaviors (deep breathing, coughing, turning, exercises), they would experience less distress and have better outcomes (less pain, better mood, fewer analgesics needed, more rapid recovery). These techniques were tested alone and in combination with different short-term and long-term threatening situations (diagnostic examinations and surgery). The outcomes were complex, illustrating that individual differences in the perception of stress and its management must be taken into consideration.

Among their findings, Leventhal and Johnson discovered that the combination of sensory information and postoperative exercise instruction was not consistently effective. If the instruction provided the patient with a way of coping where none had previously existed, it was more likely to be effective. If the patient already had an effective coping strategy, any new ones could be considered conflicting. In some instances, attempting to use the new strategy rather than relying on existing strategies was thought to delay recovery, particularly after the patient went home. Specific coping strategies were usually more effective in short-term than in long-term events. Individual differences were found to be significant. This research can help the nurse decide who will benefit from the information provided, which coping enhancement strategies to implement, the goal to be achieved, and the specific outcome criteria to be used in evaluating the interventions.

Enhancing Social Support

The nature of social support and its influence on coping have been studied extensively; social support has been demonstrated to be an effective moderator of life stress. Cobb (1976) found that social support provided the individual with different types of emotional information. The first type of information leads people to believe that they are cared for and loved. This emotional support appears most often in a relationship between two people in which mutual trust and attachment are expressed by helping one another meet their emotional needs. The second type of information leads people to believe that they are esteemed and valued. This is most effective when there is recognition that demonstrates the individual's favorable position in the group. It elevates the person's sense of self-worth. This is called esteem support. The third type of information leads people to believe that they belong to a network of communication and mutual obligation. Members of this network share information and make goods and services available to the members on demand.

Social support also facilitates the individual's coping behaviors; however, this depends on the nature of the social support. People can have extensive relationships and interact frequently, but the necessary support comes only when there is a deep level of involvement and concern, not when people merely touch the surface of each other's lives. The critical qualities within the social network are the exchange of intimate communications and the presence of solidarity and trust.

Emotional support from family and significant others provides a person with love and a sense of sharing the burden. The emotions that accompany stress are unpleasant and often increase in a spiraling fashion if relief is not provided. Being able to talk with someone and express feelings openly may help the person to gain mastery of the situation. Nurses can provide this support; however, it is important to identify the person's social support system and encourage its use. People who are loners or isolated, or who withdraw in times of stress have a high risk of coping failure.

Because anxiety may also distort a person's ability to process information, it helps to seek information and advice from others who can assist with analyzing the threat and developing a strategy to manage it. Again, this use of others helps the person to maintain mastery of a situation and to retain self-esteem.

Thus, social networks assist with management of stress by providing the individual with:

- A positive social identity
- Emotional support
- Material aid and tangible services
- Access to information
- Access to new social contacts and new social roles

Recommending Support and Therapy Groups

Support groups exist especially for people in similar stressful situations. Groups have been formed by parents of children with leukemia, people with ostomies, mastectomy patients, and those with other kinds of cancer or other serious diseases and chronic illnesses. There are groups for single parents, substance abusers and their family members, and victims of child abuse. Professional, civic, and religious support groups are active in many communities. There are also encounter groups, assertiveness training programs, and consciousness-raising groups to help people modify their usual behavior in their transactions with their environment. Being a member of a group with similar problems or goals has a releasing effect on the person that promotes freedom of expression and exchange of ideas.

As previously noted, a person's psychological and biologic health, internal and external sources of stress management, and relationship with the environment are predictors of health outcomes. These factors are directly related to the health patterns of the individual. The nurse has a significant role and responsibility in identifying the health patterns of the person receiving care. If those patterns are not achieving physiologic, psychological, and social balance, the nurse is obligated, with the assistance and agreement of the patient, to seek ways to promote balance.

While this chapter has analyzed some physiologic mechanisms and perspectives on health and disease, the way that one copes with stress, the way one relates to others, and the values and goals held are also interwoven into those physiologic patterns. To evaluate the patient's health patterns and to intervene if a problem exists requires a total assessment of the person. Specific problems and their nursing management are addressed in greater depth in other chapters.

Critical Thinking Exercises

1. Think back to a time when you had an acute illness. Describe the illness-related stressors you experienced. How did you cope with these stressors? What evidence was there that your coping ability was successful or unsuccessful?
2. Think back to a time when you had an injury. How was homeostasis maintained or disrupted, and what compensatory mechanisms were evident?
3. Select a patient to whom you are assigned who has an acute illness or injury. Describe the manner in which homeostasis has been maintained or disrupted and the compensatory mechanisms that are evident. How does the patient's medical treatment support the compensatory mechanisms? How do you determine the nursing interventions that are appropriate for promoting the healing process?
4. You are caring for a patient in his home. Describe how you would assess the patient's health status and lifestyle to determine health-promotion activities that should be explored with the patient and his family. How would your plans vary between a patient who is weak and debilitated versus a patient who is recuperating according to schedule; or has failing eyesight; or is alone most of the day?

References and Selected Readings

BOOKS

Aldwin, C. M. (1994). *Stress, coping, and development.* New York: Guilford Press.

Andreoli, T. E. (Ed.). (1997). *Cecil essentials of medicine* (4th ed.). Philadelphia: W. B. Saunders.

Barnfather, J. S., & Lyon, B. L. (Eds.). (1993). *Stress and coping: State of the science and implications for nursing theory, research and practice.* Indianapolis: Sigma Theta Tau International Inc.

Benson, H. (1993). The relaxation response. In D. Goleman & J. Gurin (Eds.), *Mind-body medicine: How to use your mind for better health.* Yonkers, NY: Consumer Reports Books.

Benson, H., & Proctor, W. (1984). *Beyond the relaxation response.* New York: Berkley Books.

Copel, L. C. (1996). *Nurse's clinical guide psychiatric and mental health care.* Springhouse, PA: Springhouse.

Dubos, R. (1965). *Man adapting.* New Haven, CT: Yale University Press.

Fauci, A. (Ed.). (1997). *Harrison's principles of internal medicine* (14th ed.). New York: McGraw-Hill.

Guyton, A. C. (1996). *Human physiology: Mechanisms of disease* (6th ed.). Philadelphia: W. B. Saunders.

Guyton, A. C. (1995). *Textbook of medical physiology* (9th ed.). Philadelphia: W. B. Saunders.

Jalowiec, A. (1993). Coping with illness: Synthesis and critique of the nursing literature from 1980–1990. In J. S. Barnfather & B. L. Lyon (Eds.), *Stress and coping: State of the science and implications for nursing theory, research and practice.* Indianapolis: Sigma Theta Tau International Inc.

Lazarus, R. S. (1993). Why we should think of stress as a subset of emotion. In L. Goldberger & S. Breznitz (Eds.), *Handbook of stress* (2nd ed.). New York: The Free Press.

Lazarus, R. S. (1991a). *Emotion and adaptation.* New York: Oxford University Press.

Lazarus, R. S., & Folkman, S. (1984). *Stress, appraisal, and coping.* New York: Springer Publishing Co.

Leventhal, H., & Johnson, J. E. (1983). Laboratory and field experimentation: Development of a theory of self-regulation. In P. J. Wooldridge, et al. (Eds.), *Behavioral science and nursing theory.* St. Louis: C. V. Mosby.

Lyon, B. L., & Werner, J. S. (1987). Stress. In J. Fitzpatrick & R. Taunton (Eds.), *Annual review of nursing research.* New York: Springer Publishing Co.

McCloskey, J. C., & Bulechek, G. M. (Eds.). (1996). *Nursing interventions classification (NIC).* St. Louis: Mosby–Year Book.

McEwen, B., & Mendelson, S. (1993). Effects of stress on the neurochemistry and morphology of the brain: Counterregulation versus damage. In I. Goldberger & S. Breznitz (Eds.), *Handbook of stress* (2nd ed.). New York: The Free Press.

Mickler, M. (1997). *Community organizing and community building for health.* New Brunswick, NJ: Rutgers University Press.

Miller, L. H., & Smith, A. D. (1993). *The stress solution.* New York: Pocket Books.

North American Nursing Diagnosis Association. (1996). *NANDA nursing diagnoses: Definitions and classifications.* Philadelphia: Author

Ruiz-Bueno, J. B. (1993). Commentary on resources as mediators of the stress-health outcome linkage. In J. S. Barnfather & B. L. Lyon (Eds.), *Stress and coping: State of the science and implications for nursing theory, research and practice.* Indianapolis: Sigma Theta Tau International Inc.

Scandrett-Hibdon, S., & Uecker, S. (1992). Relaxation training. In G. M. Bulechek & J. C. McCloskey (Eds.), *Nursing interventions: Essential nursing treatments.* Philadelphia: W. B. Saunders.

Selye, H. (1976). *The stress of life.* (Rev. ed.). New York: McGraw Hill.

Watkins, A. (Ed.). (1997). *Mind-body medicine: A clinician's guide to psychoneuroimmunology.* New York: Churchill Livingstone.

JOURNALS

Asterisks indicate nursing research articles.

*Almberg, B., Grafstrom, M., & Winblad, B. (1997). Major strain and coping strategies as reported by family members who care for aged demented relatives. *Journal of Advanced Nursing, 26*(4), 683–691.

Anderson, B. L., Farrar, W. B., Golden-Kreutz, D., et al. (1998). Stress and immune responses after surgical treatment for regional breast cancer. *Journal of National Cancer Institute, 90*(1), 30–36.

*Ballard, K. S. (1981). Identification of environmental stressors for patients in a surgical intensive care unit. *Issues in Mental Health Nursing,* (3), 89–108.

Biondi, M., Peronti, M., Pacitti, F., Pancheri, P., Pacifici, R., Altieri, I., Paris, L., & Zuccaro, P. (1994). Personality, endocrine and immune changes after eight months in healthy individuals under normal daily stress. *Psychotherapy and Psychosomatics, 62*(3–4), 176–184.

Black, P. H. (1994). Central nervous system-immune system interactions: Psychoneuroendocrinology of stress and its immune consequences. *Antimicrobial Agents and Chemotherapy, 38*(1), 1–6.

*Brillhart, B., & Johnson, K. (1997). Motivation and the coping process of adults with disabilities: a qualitative study. *Rehabilitation Nursing, 22*(5), 249–256.

Bryla, C. M. (1996). The relationship between stress and the development of breast cancer: a literature review. *Oncology Nursing Forum, 23*(3), 441–448.

Byers, J. F., & Smyth, K. A. (1997). Application of a transactional model of stress and coping with critically ill patients. *Dimensions in Critical Care Nursing, 16*(6), 292–300.

Cobb, S. (1976). Social support as a moderator of life stress. *Psychosomatic Medicine, 38*(5), 300–314.

*Collins, M. A. (1996). The relation of work stress, hardiness, and burnout among full-time hospital staff nurses. *Journal of Nursing Staff Development, 12*(2), 81–85.

*Cormier-Daigle, M., & Stewart, M. (1997). Support and coping of male hemodialysis-dependent patients. *International Journal of Nursing Studies, 34*(6), 420–430.

*Courtens, A. M., Stevens, F. C., Crebolder, H. F., & Philipsen, H. (1996). Longitudinal study on quality of life and social support in cancer patients. *Cancer Nursing, 19*(3), 162–169.

Engler, M. B., & Engler, M. M. (1995). Assessment of the cardiovascular effects of stress. *Journal of Cardiovascular Nursing, 10*(1), 51–63.

*Fallon, M., Gould, D., & Wainwright, S. P. (1997). Stress and quality of life in the renal transplant patient, a preliminary investigation. *Journal of Advanced Nursing, 25*(3), 562–570.

Glaser, R., & Kiecolt-Glaser, J. K. (1997). Chronic stress modulates the virus-specific immune response to latent herpes simplex virus type 1. *Annals Behavioral Medicine, 19*(2), 78–82.

Goodkin, K., Feaster, D. J., Tuttle, R., Blaney, N. T., Kumar, M., Baum, M. K., Shapshak, P., & Fletcher, M. A. (1996). Bereavement is associated with time-dependent decrements in cellular immune function in asymptomatic human immunodeficiency virus type 1-seropositive homosexual men. *Clinics in Diagnostic Laboratory Immunology, 3*(1), 109–180.

Hagerty, B. M., Williams, R. A., Coyne, J. C., & Early, M. R. (1996). Sense of belonging and indicators of social and psychological functioning. *Archives of Psychiatric Nursing, 10*(4), 235–244.

Holmes, T. H., & Rahe, R. H. (1967). The social readjustment rating scale. *Journal of Psychosomatic Research, 11*, 213–218.

Hostick, T., Newell, R., & Ward, T. (1997). Evaluation of stress prevention and management workshops in the community. *Journal of Clinical Nursing, 6*(2), 139–145.

Ingram, L. (1995). Roy's adaptation model and accident and emergency nursing. *Accident and Emergency Nursing, 3*(3), 150–153.

*Langford, C. P., Bowsher, J., Maloney, J. P., & Lillis, P. P. (1997). Social support, a conceptual analysis. *Journal of Advanced Nursing, 25*(1), 95–100.

Lazarus, R. S. (1991b). Cognition and motivation in emotion. *American Psychologist, 46*(4), 352–367.

Lazarus, R. S. (1991c). Progress on a cognitive-motivational-relational theory of emotion. *American Psychologist, 46*(8), 819–834.

*Mahat, G. (1997). Perceived stressors and coping strategies among individuals with rheumatoid arthritis. *Journal of Advanced Nursing, 25*(6), 1144–1150.

Matthews, K. A., Caggiula, A. R., McAllister, C. G., et al. (1995). Sympathetic reactivity to acute stress and immune response in women. *Psychosomatic Medicine, 57*(6), 564–571.

Mills, P. J., Dimsdale, J. E., Nelesen, R. A. , & Dillon, R. A. (1997). Psychologic characteristics associated with acute stressor-induced leukocyte subset redistribution. *Journal of Psychosomatic Research, 40*(4), 417–423.

*Morse, S. R., & Fife, B. (1998). Coping with a partner's cancer, adjustment at four stages of the illness trajectory. *Oncology Nursing Forum, 25*(4), 751–760.

Pike, J. L., Smith, T. L., Hauger, R. L., et al. (1997). Chronic life stress alters sympathetic, neuroendocrine, and immune responsivity to an acute psychological stressor in humans. *Psychosomatic Medicine, 59*(4), 447–457.

Post-White, J. (1996). The immune system. *Seminars in Oncology Nursing, 12*(2), 89–96.

*Rowe, M. A. (1996). The impact of internal and external resources on functional outcomes in chronic illness. *Research in Nursing & Health, 19*(6), 485–497.

*Ryan, M. C. (1996). Loneliness, social support and depression as interactive variables with cognitive status: testing Roy's model. *Nursing Science Quarterly, 9*(3), 107–114.

Sawatzky, J. A. (1998). Understanding nursing students' stress, a proposed framework. *Nurse Educator Today, 18*(2), 108–115.

Schrader, K. A. (1996). Stress and immunity after traumatic injury, the mind–body link. AACN Clinical Issues. *Advanced Practice in Acute & Critical Care, 7*(3), 351–358.

Seers, K., & Carrol, D. (1998). Relaxation techniques for acute pain management, a systematic review. *Journal of Advanced Nursing, 27*(3), 466–475.

Sergerstrom, S. C., Fahey, J. L., Kemeny, M. E., & Taylor, S. E. (1998). Optimism is associated with mood, coping, and immune change in response to stress. *Journal of Perspectives in Social Psychology, 74*(6), 1646–1655.

Shephard, R. J., & Shek, P. N. (1996). Physical activity and immune changes, a potential model of subclinical inflammation and sepsis. *Critical Reviews in Physical & Rehabilitation Medicine, 8*(3), 153–181.

Tausig, M. (1982). Measuring life events. *Journal of Health and Social Behavior, 23*(1), 52–64.

*Twibell, R. S., Wieseke, A. W., Marine, M., & Schoger, J. (1996). Spiritual and coping needs of critically ill patients, validation of nursing diagnoses. *Dimensions in Critical Care Nursing, 15*(5), 245–253.

Wells-Federman, C. (1996). Awakening the nurse healer within. *Holistic Nursing Practice, 10*(2), 13–29.

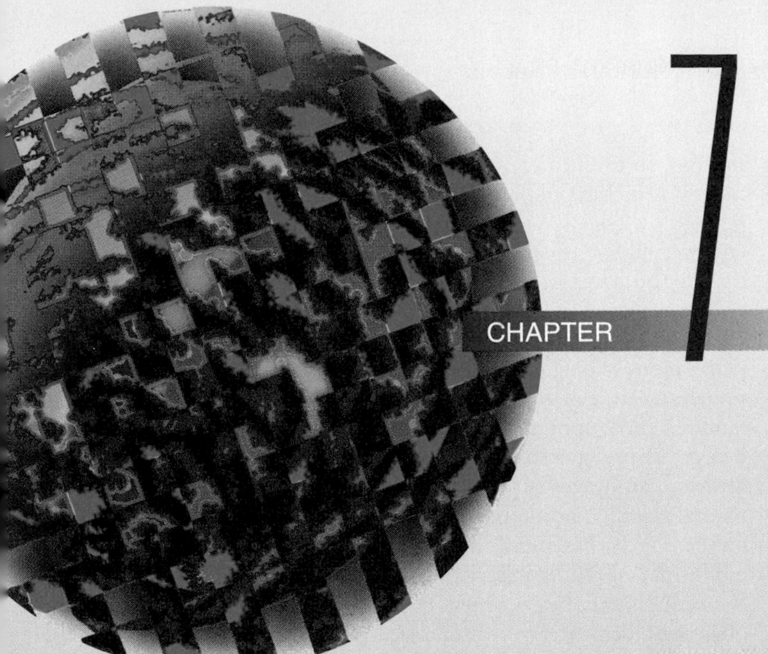

7

Individual and Family Considerations Related to Illness

Learning Objectives

On completion of the chapter, the learner will be able to:

1. Describe the holistic approach to sustaining health and well-being.
2. Discuss the concepts of emotional well-being and emotional distress.
3. Identify variables that influence the ability to cope with stress and that are antecedents to emotional disorders.
4. Explain the concepts of anxiety, posttraumatic stress disorder, depression, loss, and grief.
5. Describe a framework for understanding death and dying.
6. Assess the impact of illness on the patient's family and on family functioning.
7. Determine the role of the nurse in identifying substance abuse problems and in assisting the family to cope.
8. Describe the characteristics of the developmental phases of young adulthood, middle adulthood, and older adulthood.
9. Explore the concept of spirituality and address the spiritual needs of patients.
10. Identify nursing actions that promote effective coping for both the patient and family.

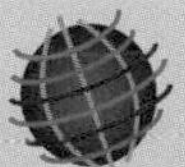

When people experience threats to their health, they seek out various care providers for the purpose of maintaining or restoring health. In recent years, both the patient and the family have become more involved participants in health care and health promotion activities. At the same time, recognition of the interconnectedness of the mind, body, and spirit in sustaining well-being and overcoming or coping with illness has been embraced by greater numbers of consumers and practitioners. This holistic approach to health and wellness and the increased consumer involvement reflect a renewed emphasis on the concepts of choice, healing, and patient–practitioner partnerships. The holistic perspective focuses not only on promoting well-being but also on understanding how one's emotional state contributes to health and illness. By using this knowledge, people are better able to prevent the reoccurrence or exacerbation of problems and to develop strategies to improve their future health status.

HOLISTIC APPROACH TO HEALTH AND HEALTH CARE

Since the 1980s, traditional health care has more frequently been accompanied by the use of holistic therapies. A survey on the use of holistic health practices reported that about 34% of the 1539 respondents in a national random sample of adults older than 18 years of age (732 female and 807 male respondents) had consulted with at least one holistic health care practitioner within the past year. The study further noted that although many of the people were also seeing a traditional health care provider, 72% did not inform the physician that they were obtaining holistic treatment (Eisenberg, Kessler, Foster, & Norlock et al., 1993).

For some people, the holistic approach is viewed as a way to capitalize on personal strengths and recultivate the values and beliefs about health that were common before the age of technological innovations and the sophistication of biomedical science. A lack of focus on the individual patient, the family, and the environment by some health care providers has created feelings of disillusionment and depersonalization in many patients. The cost of illness, especially chronic illness care, continues to escalate and accounts for an increasing percentage of health care dollars. At the same time, patient satisfaction with the health care received has decreased.

Active participation of the patient and family in promoting health supports the self-care model historically embraced by the nursing profession. This framework is congruent with the philosophy that seeks to balance and integrate the use of crisis medicine and advanced technology with the influence of the mind and spirit on healing. A holistic approach to health reconnects the traditionally separate approach to mind and body. Factors such as physical environment, economic conditions, sociocultural issues, emotional state, interpersonal relationships, and support systems can work together or alone to influence health. This connection among physical health, emotional health, and spiritual well-being must be understood and considered when providing health care. It is the nurse's conceptual integration of the physiologic health condition with the emotional and social context, along with the tasks and developments of the patient's life stage, that allows for the development of a holistic plan of nursing care.

THE BRAIN AND PHYSICAL AND EMOTIONAL HEALTH

Research into brain structure and function, neurochemical messenger systems (neurotransmitters), and brain–body connections suggests fundamental, delicate, two-way relationships between the brain's environment and mood, behavior, and resistance to disease (Cohen & Herbert, 1996). One focus of brain research has been to identify and integrate traditional medical and psychiatric knowledge with new psychobiologic and psychoneuroimmunologic data. Researchers in the field of psychobiology study the biologic basis of mental disturbances and have established some relationships between mental disorders and changes in the structure and function of the brain. Researchers in the field of psychoneuroimmunology study the connections between the emotions, the central nervous system, the neuroendocrine system, and the immune system and have established compelling evidence that psychosocial variables can affect the functioning of the immune system. As this neuroscientific research continues, data on neurotransmitters and the functioning of the brain will augment existing understanding of emotions, intelligence, memory, and many aspects of general body functioning. In the future, an accepted definition of mental illness may well include biologic information. By enhancing the biologic knowledge base about the brain and nervous system, scientists establish the foundation for breakthroughs in the treatment of both symptoms and illnesses.

As a result of this information, the health care community is challenged to place as much emphasis on emotional health as it places on physiologic health and to recognize how biologic, emotional, and societal problems combine to affect individual patients, families, and communities. Some problems that nurses and other health care providers must address include substance abuse, homelessness, family violence, eating disorders, trauma, and chronic mental health conditions such as depression. To focus attention on these and other mental health problems, the U.S. Department of Health and Human Services initiated the mental health agenda for the nation in the document entitled *Healthy People 2000*. The objectives identified are summarized in Chart 7-1. Nurses in all settings encounter patients with mental health problems and have an integral role in helping to achieve the national goals by recognizing and treating emotional distress and by promoting emotional health.

EMOTIONAL HEALTH AND EMOTIONAL DISTRESS

The concept of emotional health encompasses a person's ability to function as comfortably and productively as possible. Typically, people who are mentally healthy are satisfied with themselves and their life situations. In the usual course of living, emotionally healthy people focus on activities geared to meet their needs and attempt to accomplish personal goals while concurrently managing everyday challenges and problems. Often, people must work hard to balance their feelings, thoughts, and behaviors to alleviate emotional distress, and much energy is used to change, adapt, or manage the obstacles inherent in daily living. A mentally healthy person accepts reality and has a positive sense of self. Emotional health is also manifested by having moral and humanistic values and beliefs, having satisfying interpersonal relationships, doing productive work, and maintaining a realistic sense of hope (Chart 7-2).

When people have unmet emotional needs or distress, they experience an overall feeling of unhappiness. As tension escalates, security and survival are threatened. How different people respond to these troublesome situations reflects their level of coping and maturity. Emotionally healthy people endeavor to meet the demands of distressing situations while still facing the typical issues that emerge in their lives. The way people respond to uncomfortable stimuli reflects their exposure to various biologic, emotional, and sociocultural experiences.

When stress interferes with a person's ability to function comfortably and inhibits the effective management of personal needs, that person is at risk for emotional problems. The use of ineffective and unhealthy methods of coping is manifested by dysfunctional behaviors, thoughts, and feelings. These behaviors are aimed at relieving the overwhelming stress, even though they may cause further problems.

Coping ability is strongly influenced by biologic or genetic factors, physical and emotional growth and development, family and childhood experiences, and learning. Typically, a person reverts to the strategies observed early in life that were used by family members, caregivers, and others to solve conflict. If these strategies were not adaptive, the person exhibits a range of painful and nonproductive behaviors. Dysfunctional behavior in one person not only

CHART 7•1 Mental Health Objectives for Healthy People in the Year 2000

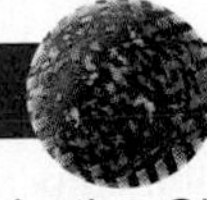

Incidence Reduction Objectives

1. The incidence of all suicides from 11.7 per 100,000 population to 10.5 per 100,000 population
2. The rate of injurious adolescent (aged 14 to 17 years) suicide attempts by 15%
3. The rate of child and adolescent mental disorders from 12% to less than 10%
4. The rate of mentally disordered adults in the community from 12.6% to less than 10.7%
5. The rate of negative effects of stress on adults from 42.6% to less than 35%

Risk Reduction Objectives

1. Increase to at least 30% (baseline, 15%) the rate at which community resources are used by adults with severe mental illness
2. Increase to at least 45% (baseline, 31%) the percentage of people with major depression who obtain treatment
3. Increase to at least 20% (baseline, 11.1%) the percentage of adults with emotional and personal problems who seek help
4. Decrease by 5% (baseline, 21%) the percentage of people who report experiencing high stress levels and do not initiate methods to control their stress

Services and Protection Objectives

1. Establish protocols in all 50 states for mental health, drug and alcohol, and public health services to provide interventions for preventing suicides by jail inmates (baseline, 39 states)
2. Increase the percentage of work-site programs on reducing stress in employment settings (that employ more than 50 people) to 40% (baseline, 26.6%)
3. Establish mutual help clearinghouses in at least 25 states (baseline, 9 states)
4. Increase the percentage of primary care providers who routinely assess the cognitive, emotional, and behavioral functioning of adults, and identify resources to handle difficulties, to 50% (baseline, 30%)
5. Increase the percentage of primary care providers who routinely assess children for cognitive, emotional, and behavioral functioning to 75% (no available baseline)

U.S. Department of Health and Human Services. (1995). *Healthy people 2000.* (DHHS Publication No. [PHS] 91-1679). Washington, DC: U.S. Government Printing Office.

seriously affects that person's emotional health but can also put others at risk of injury or death. As these destructive behaviors are repeated, a cyclical pattern becomes evident: impaired thinking, negative feelings, and more dysfunctional actions that prevent the person from meeting the demands of daily living (Chart 7-3).

There is no universally accepted definition of what constitutes an emotional disorder. The common theme of many views and theories is that a number of variables can interfere with emotional growth and development and impede successful adaptation to the environment. Most clinicians have adopted the statement from the American Psychiatric Association's (APA's) *Diagnostic and Statistical Manual of Mental Disorders* (DSM-IV) that defines the term **mental disorder** as a group of behavioral or psychological symptoms or a pattern that manifests itself in significant distress, impaired functioning, or accentuated risk of enduring severe suffering or possible death (American Psychiatric Association, 1994, p. xxi).

Patients seen in medical-surgical settings often struggle with psychosocial issues of anxiety, depression, loss, and grief. Health problems such as abuse, chemical dependency, body image disturbances, and eating disorders are a few examples of health situations that require extensive physical and emotional care to restore optimal functioning. The dual challenge for the health team is to understand how the patient's emotions influence current physiologic conditions and to identify the best care for any underlying emotional and spiritual distress.

CHART 7•2 Characteristics Associated With Mental Health

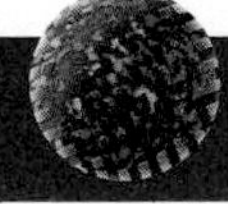

- Developing a positive sense of self
- Developing and sustaining satisfying interpersonal relationships
- Expressing a wide range of appropriate emotions
- Loving and caring for self and others
- Behaving in a realistic and responsible manner
- Coping effectively
- Negotiating and resolving conflict
- Cooperating and working interdependently with others
- Engaging in rewarding, productive work
- Adapting to the daily challenges of life
- Finding meaning and purpose in life
- Having hopes and dreams
- Knowing personal strengths and areas needing improvement
- Having a sense of humor
- Respecting the rights and differences of others

Risk Factors for MENTAL HEALTH PROBLEMS

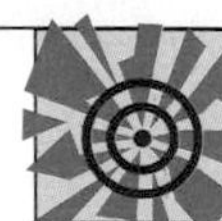

Risk Factors That Cannot Be Changed

Age
Gender
Genetic background
Family history

Risk Factors That Can Be Changed

Marital status
Family environment
Housing problems
Poverty or economic difficulties
Physical health
Nutritional status
Stress level
Social environment and activities
Exposure to trauma
Alcohol and drug use
Environmental toxins or other pollutants
Availability, accessibility, and cost of health services

CHART 7•3 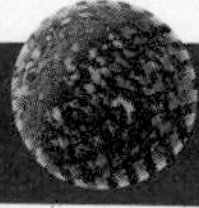 **Characteristics Associated With Mental Disorders**

- Severe anxiety
- Severe depression
- Ineffective coping mechanisms
- Extreme feelings of helplessness or powerlessness
- Maladaptive ways of dealing with stress
- Uncomfortable with self and others
- Lack of pleasure from living
- Extreme negative thoughts, feelings, and behaviors
- Disorganized or disturbed thoughts
- Inability to accept reality
- Personality traits that contribute to dysfunctional behaviors
- Desire to hurt self or others
- History of traumatic experience
- Inability to satisfy basic needs
- Lack of a support system
- Physiologic problems resulting from severe, unrelenting stress

FAMILY HEALTH AND DISTRESS

The family plays a central role in the life of the patient and is a major part of the context of the patient's life. It is within families that people grow, are nurtured, attain a sense of self, cultivate beliefs and values about life, and progress through life's developmental stages (Chart 7-4). The family is the first guide for socialization and teaching about health and illness. The family prepares the person with strategies for balancing closeness with separateness, and togetherness with individuality. A major role of the family is to provide physical and emotional resources to maintain health and a system of support in times of crises, such as in periods of illness. Educating families has been shown to add to their resiliency, adaptation, and adjustment to life stressors (McCubbin & McCubbin, 1993).

When a family member becomes ill, all members of the family are affected. Depending on the nature of the health problem, the family members may need to make several adaptations to their existing lifestyles, or they may need to restructure their lifestyles.

Health problems often have an impact on the family's ability to function. Five family functions described by Wright and Leahy (1994) are viewed as essential to the individual's and family's growth. The first function, management, addresses the use of power, decision making about resources, establishment of rules, provision of finances, and future planning. These responsibilities are assumed by the adults of the family. The second function, boundary setting, places clear distinctions between the generations and sets the stage for adults to be adults and children to be children. Communication is the third function important to individual and family growth; healthy families have a full range of clear, direct, and meaningful communication among their members. The fourth function is education and support. Education refers to modeling skills for living a physically, emotionally, and socially healthy life. Support is manifested by actions that tell family members they are cared about and loved. Family support promotes health and is seen as a critical factor in coping with crises and illness situations. The last function is socialization. Families transmit culture and the acceptable behaviors needed to perform adequately in the home and in the world.

CHART 7•4 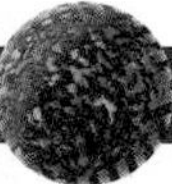 **Adult Developmental Tasks**

Developmental stage and associated tasks can have an impact on how individuals cope with illness.

Young Adult

Establish independence
Establish lifestyle
Develop career
Develop intimate relationships
Marry and start a family

Middle Adult

Establish financial security
Prepare for retirement
Launch children
Refocus on marital relationship
Support growing children and aging parents

Older Adult

Adapt to retirement and alteration in role
Adapt to declining physical stamina
Review life's accomplishments
Prepare for death

Nursing Implications

There are many degrees of family functioning. The nurse assesses the family functioning to determine whether the family can withstand the impact of the health condition. If the family is chaotic or disorganized, promoting coping skills becomes a priority in the plan of care. The family with preexisting problems may require additional aid before participating fully in the current health dilemma. In performing a family assessment, the nurse must completely evaluate the present family structure and function. Areas of appraisal include demographic data, developmental information (keeping in mind that a family can be in several developmental stages simultaneously), family structure, family functioning, and coping abilities. The role that the environment plays in family health is also assessed.

Interventions with family members are based on strengthening coping skills through direct care, communication skills, and education. Healthy family communication has a strong influence on the quality of family life. Effective communication can help the family to make appropriate choices, look at alternative strategies, or persevere through complex circumstances. It is entirely possible that within a family system, the identified patient is undergoing extensive surgery for cancer while the partner has cardiac disease, the adolescent has type 1 diabetes, and the child has a fractured wrist. In this situation, there are multiple health concerns along with competing developmental tasks and needs. Despite the obvious concerns of the family members both individually and collectively, a crisis may or may not be present. It is entirely possible that this family is coping effectively; alternatively, the family may be in crisis, or may manifest a chronic inability to handle the situation. The health team conducts a careful and comprehensive family assessment, develops interventions tailored to handle the stressors, implements the specified treatment protocols, and facilitates the construction of social support systems.

The use of existing family strengths, resources, and education is augmented by therapeutic family interventions. The nurse's primary goals are to maintain and improve the patient's present level of health and to prevent physical and emotional deterioration. Next, the nurse intervenes in the cycle that the illness creates: patient illness, stress for other family members, generation of potential for illness in family members, and additional stress for the identified patient.

Helping the family members handle the myriad stressors that bombard them on a daily basis involves working with family members to develop coping skills. In a study in 1994, Burr and associates identified seven traits that enhance coping of family members under stress. Communication skills and spirituality were the most useful traits, and cognitive abilities, emotional strengths, relationship capabilities, willingness to use community resources, and individual strengths and talents were also associated with effective coping. As nurses work with families, they must not underestimate the impact that their therapeutic interactions, educational information, positive role modeling, provision of direct care, and corrective teaching have on promoting health.

Without the active support of the family members and the health team, there is the potential for using maladaptive coping mechanisms. Often, denial and blaming of individuals occur. Sometimes, physiologic illness, emotional withdrawal, and physical distancing are the results of severe family conflict, violent behaviors, or addiction to drugs and alcohol. Substance abuse is sometimes the outcome for family members who view their ability to cope or solve problems as impossible. Often, it is in difficult or problematic situations that people engage in these dysfunctional behaviors.

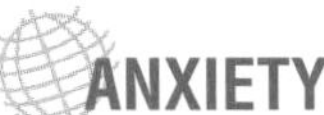

ANXIETY

All people experience some degree of anxiety as they face new, challenging, or threatening life situations. In clinical settings, fear of the unknown, unexpected news about one's health, and any impairment of bodily functions engenders anxiety. Although a mild level of anxiety can mobilize people to take a position, act on the task that needs to be done, or learn to alter lifestyle habits, a more severe level of anxiety can be almost paralyzing. Anxiety that escalates to a near panic state can be incapacitating (Varcarolis, 1998). When patients receive unwelcome news about results of diagnostic studies, they are sure to experience a tense emotional state known as anxiety. Different patients manifest the physiologic, emotional, and behavioral signs and symptoms of anxiety in various ways.

Nursing Implications

Early clinical observations of guilt or anxiety are an essential component of nursing care. When patients are anxious, it is likely that their high level of anxiety will exacerbate physiologic distress. For example, a postoperative patient in pain may discover that anxiety intensifies the sensation of pain. A patient newly diagnosed with type 1 diabetes mellitus may be worried and fearful and therefore unable to focus on or complete essential self-care activities. The possibility of developing somatic symptoms is high in any patient experiencing moderate to severe anxiety.

The APA's *Diagnostic and Statistical Manual of Mental Disorders* (1994, p. 238) presents general medical conditions that cause anxiety. These conditions include endocrine diseases, such as hypothyroidism, hyperthyroidism, hypoglycemia, and hyperadrenocorticism; cardiovascular conditions, such as cardiac dysrhythmia, congestive heart failure, and pulmonary emboli; respiratory problems, such as pneumonia and chronic obstructive pulmonary disease; and neurologic conditions, such as encephalitis and neoplasms.

Every nurse must be vigilant about the patient who worries excessively and demonstrates deterioration in emotional, social, or occupational functioning. If participation in the therapeutic regimen (eg, administration of insulin) becomes a problem because of extreme anxiety, nursing intervention must be imme-

ASSESSMENT
SIGNS AND SYMPTOMS OF ANXIETY

Physiologic Symptoms

Appetite change
Headaches
Muscle tension
Fatigue or lethargy
Weight change
Cold and flu symptoms
Digestive upsets
Grinding teeth
Palpitations
Hypertension
Restlessness
Difficulty sleeping
Skin irritations
Injury prone
Increased use of any drugs

Emotional Symptoms

Forgetfulness
Low productivity
Feeling dull
Poor concentration
Negative attitude
Confusion
Whirling mind
No new ideas
Boredom
Negative self-talk
Anxiety
Frustration
Depression
Crying periods
Irritability
Worrying
Feeling discouraged
Nervous laughter

Relational Symptoms

Isolation
Intolerance
Resentment
Loneliness
Lashing out
"Clamming up"
Nagging
Distrust
Few friends
No intimacy
Using people

Spiritual Symptoms

Emptiness
Loss of meaning
Doubt
Unforgiving
Martyrdom
Loss of direction
Cynicism
Apathy

diately initiated. Caring strategies emphasize ways for the patient to verbalize feelings and fears and to identify sources of anxiety. The need to teach and promote effective coping abilities and the use of relaxation techniques are the priorities of care. In some cases, antianxiety medication may be prescribed. Guideline 7-1 provides a list of basic nursing principles that are useful for assisting patients to manage severe anxiety. Refer to Chapter 6 for additional information about stress and the relaxation response.

POSTTRAUMATIC STRESS DISORDER

In medical-surgical settings, especially in emergency departments, burn units, and rehabilitation centers, nurses care for extremely anxious patients who have experienced devastating events that are typically considered to be outside the realm of normal human experience. Many of these patients suffer from **posttraumatic stress disorder** (PTSD). PTSD has been described as a condition generating waves of anxiety, anger, aggression, depression, and suspicion that threaten the person's sense of self and ability to heal (McCann & Pearlman, 1990). Specific examples of events that place a person at risk for PTSD are rape, domestic violence, torture, terrorism, fire, earthquake, or military combat. Patients who have suffered a traumatic event are often frequent users of the health care system by virtue of their extensive injuries, the various treatment modalities that they require, and the overall emotional and physical difficulties experienced.

The physiologic responses noted in people who have been severely traumatized include increased activity of the sympathetic nervous system, increased plasma catecholamine levels, and increased urinary epinephrine and norepinephrine levels. It is postulated that people with PTSD lose their ability to control their response to stimuli. The resulting excessive arousal can increase overall body metabolism and trigger emotional reactivity. In this situation, the nurse would observe that the patient has difficulty sleeping, has an exaggerated startle response, and is excessively vigilant.

Older people are more susceptible to the physical effects of trauma and the effects of PTSD, because of the increased neural inactivation associated with aging. It has been speculated that when people have a preexisting tendency to become extremely anxious, their vulnerability to PTSD increases.

Symptoms of PTSD can occur from hours to years after the trauma is experienced. Acute PTSD is defined as the experience of symptoms for less than a 3-month period. Chronic PTSD is defined as the experience of symptoms lasting longer than 3 months. In the case of delayed PTSD, there may be up to a 6-month period of time that elapses between the trauma and the manifestation of symptoms (American Psychiatric Association, 1994).

Nursing Implications

It is often thought that the incidence of PTSD is very low in the overall population; however, when high-risk groups are studied, the results indicate that more than 50% of study participants have PTSD (McCann & Pearlman, 1990). Therefore, it is important that nurses consider which of their patients are at risk for PTSD and be knowledgeable about the common symptoms associated with it.

It is the sensitivity and caring of the nurse that create the interpersonal relationship necessary to work with the patient who has PTSD. These patients are physically compromised and are struggling emotionally with situations that are beyond the realm of ordinary human experience–situations that violate the commonly held perceptions of human social justice. Treatment of patients with PTSD includes five essential components: establishing a trust relationship, providing education about recovery and self-care, teaching stress management techniques, helping the patient work through the trauma, and helping the patient integrate the trauma experience (Scurfield, 1985). The patient's progress can be influenced by the ability to cope with the various aspects of both the physical and emotional distress.

DEPRESSION

Depression is a common response to health problems and is an often underdiagnosed problem in the patient population. People may become depressed as a result of injury or illness, may be suffering from an earlier loss that is compounded by a new health problem, or may seek health care for somatic complaints that are bodily manifestations of depression.

Clinical depression is distinguished from everyday feelings of sadness by duration and severity. Most people occasionally feel down or depressed, but these feelings are short-lived and do not result in impaired functioning. Clinically depressed people usually have had signs of a depressed mood or a decreased interest in pleasurable activities for at least a 2-week period. For some peo-

7•1 Guidelines For Managing Anxiety

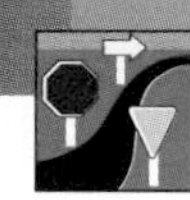

- Listen actively and focus on having the patient discuss personal feelings.
- Use positive remarks and focus on the positive aspects of life in the "here and now."
- Use appropriate touch (with patient permission) to demonstrate support.
- Discuss the importance of safety and the patient's overall sense of well-being.
- Explain all procedures, policies, diagnostic studies, medications, treatments, or protocols for care.
- Explore coping strategies and work with the patient to practice and use them effectively (eg, breathing, progressive relaxation, visualization, imagery).
- Use distraction as indicated to relax and prevent self from being overwhelmed.

ASSESSMENT
PHYSIOLOGIC AND PSYCHOLOGICAL INDICATORS OF POSTTRAUMATIC STRESS DISORDER

Physiologic Indicators

Dilated pupils
Headaches
Sleep pattern disturbances
Tremors
Elevated blood pressure
Tachycardia or palpitations
Diaphoresis with cold, clammy skin
Hyperventilation
Dyspnea
Smothering or choking sensation
Nausea, vomiting, or diarrhea
Stomach ulcers
Dry mouth
Abdominal pain
Muscle tension or soreness
Exhaustion

Psychological Indicators

Anxiety
Anger
Depression
Fears or phobias
Survivor guilt
Hypervigilance
Nightmares or flashbacks
Intrusive thoughts about the trauma
Impaired memory
Dissociative states
Restlessness or irritability
Strong startle response
Substance abuse
Self-hatred
Feelings of estrangement
Feelings of helplessness, hopelessness, or powerlessness
Lack of interest in life
Inability to concentrate
Difficulty communicating, caring, and expressing love
Problems with relationships
Sexual problems ranging from acting out to impotence
Difficulty with intimacy
Inability to trust
Lack of impulse control
Aggressive, abusive, or violent behavior, including suicide
Thrill-seeking behaviors

Copel, L. C. (1996). *Nurse's clinical guide: Psychiatric and mental health care.* Springhouse, PA: Springhouse.

ple, there is obvious impairment in social, occupational, and overall daily functioning. Others function appropriately in their interactions with the outside world by exerting much effort and forcing themselves to mask their distress. Sometimes, they are successful at camouflaging their depression for months or years and astonish family members and others when they finally succumb to the problem.

Many people experience depression but seek treatment for somatic complaints. The leading somatic complaints of patients struggling with depression are headache, backache, abdominal pain, fatigue, malaise, anxiety, and decreased desire or problems with sexual functioning (Stuart & Sundeen, 1995). These sensations are frequently manifestations of depression. The depression is undiagnosed about half of the time and masquerades as physical health problems (Haber, McMahon, Price-Hoskins, & Sideleau, 1992). People with depression also exhibit poor functioning and high rates of absenteeism.

Specific symptoms of clinical depression include feelings of sadness, worthlessness, fatigue, and guilt and difficulty concentrating or making decisions. Changes in appetite, weight gain or loss, sleep disturbances, and psychomotor retardation or agitation are common. Often, patients have recurrent thoughts about death or suicide, or have made suicide attempts (American Psychiatric Association, 1994). A diagnosis of clinical depression is made when a person presents with at least five of nine diagnostic criteria for depression. Chart 7-5 lists these criteria (American Psychiatric Association, 1994). Unfortunately, only one of three depressed people is properly diagnosed and appropriately treated.

In the United States, about 15% of severely depressed people commit suicide, and two thirds of patients who have committed suicide had been seen by health care practitioners during the 4-week period before their death (National Institute of Mental Health, 1992). When patients make statements that are self-deprecating, express feelings of failure, or are convinced that things are hopeless and will not improve, they may be at risk for suicide. Risk factors for suicide include the following:

- Age: younger than 20 or older than 45 years, especially older than 65 years
- Gender: women make more attempts, men are more successful
- Dysfunctional family: members have experienced cumulative multiple losses and possess limited coping skills
- Family history of suicide
- Severe depression
- Severe, intractable pain
- Chronic, debilitating medical problems
- Substance abuse
- Severe anxiety

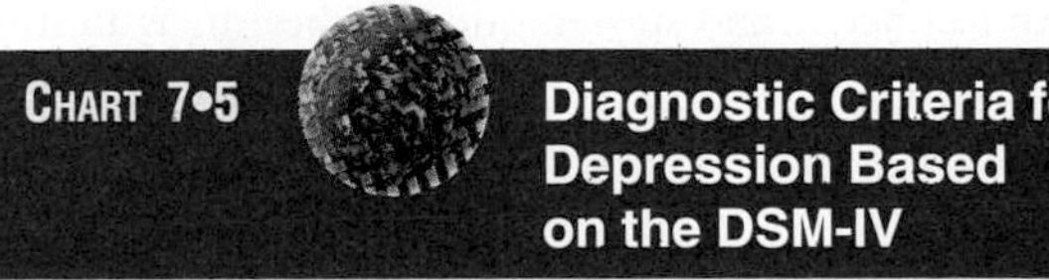

CHART 7•5 Diagnostic Criteria for Depression Based on the DSM-IV

A person experiences at least five out of nine characteristics with one of the first two symptoms present most of the time.

1. Depressed mood
2. Loss of pleasure or interest
3. Weight gain or loss
4. Sleeping difficulties
5. Psychomotor agitation or retardation
6. Fatigue
7. Feeling worthless
8. Inability to concentrate
9. Thoughts of suicide or death

American Psychiatric Association. (1994). *Diagnostic and statistical manual of mental disorders* (DSM IV) (4th ed.). Washington, DC: Author

- Overwhelming problems
- Severe alteration in self-esteem or body image
- Lethal suicide plan

Nursing Implications

Because any loss in function, change in role, or alteration in body image is a possible antecedent to depression, nurses in all settings encounter patients who are depressed or who have thought about suicide. Depression is suspected when changes in the patient's thoughts or feelings and a loss of self-esteem are noted.

It is important to recognize that depression can occur at any age, and that it is diagnosed more frequently in women than in men. For elderly patients, the nurse should be aware that decreased mental alertness and withdrawal-type responses may be indicative of depression. Consultation with the psychiatric liaison nurse to assess and differentiate between dementia-like symptoms and depression is often helpful.

For all patients, talking about their fears, frustration, anger, and despair can help alleviate a sense of helplessness and facilitate the process of obtaining the necessary treatment. Helping patients learn to cope effectively with conflict, interpersonal problems, and grief, and encouraging patients to discuss actual and potential losses may hasten their recovery from depression. Patients can be aided in identifying and decreasing negative self-talk and unrealistic expectations, and shown how negative thinking contributes to depression. Because physical health and self-care activities are adversely affected by depression, nurses can monitor patients for the onset of new problems. All patients with depression should be evaluated to determine whether they would benefit from antidepressant therapy.

In addition to the measures cited previously for helping patients manage depression, research studies indicate a reduction in distress when anxiety and depression are treated with psychoeducational programs, the establishment of support systems, and counseling (Devine & Westlake, 1995). Referrals to psychoeducational programs can be instrumental in helping patients and their families understand depression, treatment options, and coping strategies. (In crisis situations, it is better to refer the patient to a psychiatrist, psychiatric nurse specialist, or a crisis center.) Explaining to patients that depression is a medical illness and not a sign of personal weakness, and that effective treatment will allow them to feel better and stay emotionally healthy is an important aspect of care (Stuart & Sundeen, 1995).

Risk Factors for DEPRESSION

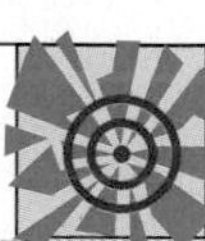

Family history
Stressful situations
Female gender
Prior episodes of depression
Onset before age 40 years
Medical comorbidity
Past suicide attempts
Lack of support systems
History of physical or sexual abuse
Current substance abuse

SUBSTANCE ABUSE

Some people use mood-altering substances in an attempt to cope with life's challenges. A person who abuses substances has an inability to make healthy decisions and to solve problems effectively. Typically, people who abuse substances are unable to identify and implement adaptive behaviors and use illegally obtained drugs, prescribed or over-the-counter medications, and alcohol alone or in combination with other drugs in an ineffective attempt to cope with the pressures, strains, and burdens of life. Over time, physiologic, emotional, cognitive, and behavioral problems develop as a result of continuous substance use. These problems cause distress for the individual, the family, and the community. Some people may respond to personal illness or the illness of a loved one by using substances to decrease emotional pain.

Nursing Implications

Substance abuse is encountered in all clinical settings. Intoxication and withdrawal are two common substance abuse problems. Often, the nurse sees patients who have experienced trauma as a result of inebriation. Other patients who are active substance abusers enter the primary care setting with a diagnosis other than that of substance abuse. Many do not disclose the extent of their substance use. The patient's use of denial or lack of knowledge about the devastating effects of psychoactive substances can be detected by the nurse who performs a substance use assessment. In addition, the nurse can incorporate tools into the assessment that enable information on drug use to be detected. Examples of such instruments are the CAGE Questions (Ewing, 1984), the Michigan Alcohol Screening Test (Selzer, 1971), and the Addiction Severity Index (McLellan, Kushner, Metzger, & Peters, 1992).

Health professionals are in pivotal positions for identifying the substance abuse problem, instituting treatment protocols, and making follow-up referrals. Because substance abuse severely affects the family, the nurse helps the family members confront the situation, decrease their enabling behaviors, and motivate the person to obtain treatment.

Caring for codependent family members is another nursing priority. A codependent person tends to manifest unhealthy patterns in relationships with others. Codependents struggle with a need to be needed, the urge to control others, and a willingness to remain involved and suffer with a person who has a drug problem.

The family may approach the health care team to help set limits on the dysfunctional behavior of a person who abuses substances. At these times, a therapeutic intervention is organized for the purpose of confronting the patient about substance use and the need for obtaining drug and alcohol treatment. The nurse or other knowledgeable addictions counselor helps the family present the addicted person with a realistic perspective about the problem, their concerns about and caring for the person, and a specific plan for treatment. This therapeutic intervention works on the premise that honest and caring confrontation can break through the person's denial of the addiction. If the person refuses to participate in the designed plan, the family members define the consequences and state their commitment to follow through with them. This intervention is empowering to the family and usually provides the structure needed to secure treatment.

Even with treatment, patients may experience relapse. Nurses work with patients and their families to prevent relapse and to

ASSESSMENT
SUBSTANCE ABUSE

- Past and recurrent use of the substance
- Patient's view of substance use as a problem
- Age when first used and last used substance
- Length and duration of use of substance
- Preferred method of use of substance
- Amount of substance used
- How substance is procured
- Effect of or reaction to substance
- All attempts to cease or decrease substance use

be prepared if relapse occurs. It is important to remember that relapse is considered a part of the illness process and therefore must be viewed and addressed in the same way that chronic illness is treated.

The nurse working with the patient and family struggling with an addiction must dispel the myth that addiction is a defect in character or a moral fault. Views on substance abuse vary within our society. Some of the answers to the questions about whether a person uses drugs, what drugs are used, and when drugs are used are found in that person's background (Copel, 1996). It is the combination of variables, such as values and beliefs, family and personal norms, spiritual convictions, and conditions of the current social environment, that predisposes a person to the possibility of drug use, motivation for treatment, and continual recovery (Copel, 1996). It has been said that a person's attitude, especially toward alcohol, reflects the overall beliefs and attitudes of that individual's culture (Frances & Miller, 1991).

LOSS AND GRIEF

Loss is a part of the life cycle. All people experience loss in the form of change, growth, and transition. The experience of loss is painful, frightening, and lonely, and it triggers an array of emotional responses. People may vacillate between denial, shock, disbelief, anger, inertia, intense yearning, loneliness, sadness, loss of control, depression, and spiritual despair (Carter, 1989; Hogan & Balk, 1990; Steele, 1990).

Superimposed on normal losses associated with life cycle stages are the potential losses of health, a body part, self-image, self-esteem, and even one's life. When loss is not acknowledged or is cumulative, anxiety, depression, and health problems may occur. Likewise, people with physical health problems, such as diabetes mellitus, acquired immunodeficiency syndrome (AIDS), cardiac conditions, gastrointestinal disorders, and neurologic impairments, tend to respond to these illnesses with feelings of grief.

People grieve in different ways, and there is no time line for completing the grief process. The time of grieving often depends on the significance of the loss, the length of time the person or object was known and loved, the anticipation of or preparation for the loss, the person's emotional stability and maturity, and the person's coping ability (Carson, 1995). Regardless of the duration of the grieving process, there are two basic goals: (1) healing the self, and (2) recovering from the loss (Gyulay, 1989). Other factors that influence grieving are the type of loss, life experiences with various changes and transitions, religious beliefs, cultural background, and personality type (Bright, 1996). Some patients may resort to abuse of prescription medications, illegal drugs, or alcohol if they find it difficult to cope with the loss; the grief process is then complicated by the use of addictive substances.

Nursing Implications

Nurses identify patients and family members who are grieving and work with them to accomplish the four major tasks of the grief process: (1) acceptance of the loss, (2) acknowledgment of the intensity of the pain, (3) adaptation to life after the loss, and (4) cultivation of new relationships and activities (Worden, 1982). Chart 7-6 outlines nursing care activities useful for those who are bereaved.

Another responsibility of the nurse is to assess and differentiate between grief and depression by knowing the common thoughts, feelings, physical or bodily reactions, and behaviors associated with grief in comparison with depression. A description of a physical response to grief is the sensation of somatic distress, a tightness in the throat followed by a choking sensation or shortness of breath, the need to sigh, an empty feeling inside the abdomen, lack of muscle power, and intense disabling distress. It is clear that grief can further debilitate an already compromised patient and have a strong impact on family functioning.

ASSESSMENT
SIGNS AND SYMPTOMS OF GRIEVING

Physiologic Signs and Symptoms

Heart rate changes
Blood pressure alterations
Gastrointestinal disturbances
Chest discomfort
Shortness of breath
Weakness
Appetite changes
Sleep problems
Vague, but distressing physical symptoms

Emotional Symptoms

Sadness
Depression
Anger
Social withdrawal
Loneliness
Apathy
Longing for who or what was lost
Blaming of self or others
Questions beliefs

Behavioral Symptoms

Slow movements
Forgetfulness
Purposeless activity
Crying
Sighing
Lack of interest
Easily distracted from tasks

CHART 7•6 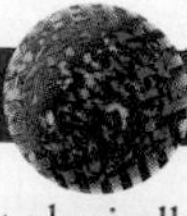 **Caring for the Bereaved**

- Have contact physically (with the patient's permission) and emotionally with the person.
- Assess where the person is in the grieving process.
- Demonstrate genuine compassion and caring.
- Give permission to grieve and normalize the grieving process.
- Mention the loss or the deceased person's name.
- Encourage the person to talk about the relationship he or she had with the deceased person.
- Understand that people need to talk about the events and feelings around the death and will repeat themselves.
- Tell the person to expect mood swings, pain, and various life changes.
- Focus on clarifying and using coping skills.
- Allow the person to take a break from grieving and focus on self-care.
- Encourage sources of comfort such as religion or nature.
- Identify secondary losses and unfinished business.
- Acknowledge that there will be eventual recovery.
- Discuss the anniversary phenomenon.
- Encourage medical or psychiatric care as needed.

DEATH AND DYING

Coping with death, one's own or a loved one's, is considered the ultimate challenge. The idea of death is threatening and anxiety provoking to many people. Kubler-Ross (1975, p. 1) stated, "The key to the question of death unlocks the door of life. . . . For those who seek to understand it, death is a highly creative force." Common fears of dying people are fear of the unknown, pain, suffering, loneliness, loss of the body, and loss of personal control.

In recent years, the process of dying has changed as advances have been made in the care of chronically and terminally ill patients. Technological innovations and modern therapeutic treatments have prolonged the life span, and many deaths are now the result of chronic illnesses that result in physiologic deterioration and subsequent multisystem failure.

Preparation for the impending death can precipitate the experience of anticipatory grieving. Although anticipatory grief can have positive effects on later grief, this sequence of events does not hold true for all people. For some family members, anticipatory grief is seen as a risk factor for poor early bereavement adjustment (Levy, 1991). The nurse must be aware of the uniqueness and individuality inherent in the grieving process and work to meet the needs of those involved in the best way possible.

Death and Dying Frameworks

Various frameworks for understanding the concept of grief and the stages of death and dying may be useful to the nurse. The stages of bereavement described by Bowlby (1961) are protest, disorganization, and reorganization. Kubler-Ross (1975) conceptualized five stages of grieving: denial, anger, bargaining, depression, and acceptance. Often, the dying person and the survivors do not experience these responses in an orderly or linear fashion; rather, there is random movement between all the stages for different periods of time. Another model for successful grieving, proposed by Engel (1964), is shock and disbelief, development of awareness, and restitution. The themes universal to almost all models of grieving are the periods of avoidance, confrontation, and acceptance (Cooley, 1992).

Another framework for understanding the individuality of the dying process is the patterns of living while dying described by Martocchio (1982). There are four identified patterns of living based on the clinical trajectories of dying people. The first is referred to as peaks and valleys or periods of hope and periods of depression. Despite the hopeful times, there is still an overall movement toward decline and death. The second pattern is one described as distinct, but descending plateaus. This course also reflects a downward trend with progressive debilitation and eventual death. The third pattern is a clear downward slope with many physiologic parameters indicating that death is imminent. This pattern is often observed in the critical care unit when people and families have no time to prepare for the death. The last pattern is a downward slant that reveals a crisis event, such as a severe cerebral hemorrhage with almost no hope of recovery. Often, a patient in this pattern is on life support systems. The nurse should recognize that a person may experience one or more of these living–dying patterns.

Nursing Implications

Nursing care involves providing comfort, maintaining safety, addressing physical and emotional needs, and teaching coping strategies to patients who are terminally ill and their families. More than ever, the nurse must explain what is happening to the patient and the family, and be a confidante who listens to the talk about dying. Hospice care, attention to family and individual psychosocial issues, and symptom and pain management are all part of the nurse's responsibilities. The nurse must also be concerned with ethical considerations and quality-of-life issues that affect dying people. Of utmost importance to the patient is assistance with the transition from living to dying, maintaining and sustaining relationships, finishing well with the family, and accomplishing what needs to be said and done

The nurse is the consistent link in promoting understanding of the disease and the dying process and in making the event more manageable for the patient and family. The patient and family require assistance to resolve problems and proceed through the grief work. Retaining as much control as possible during the process of dying allows the patient and family to make as much sense as possible out of an overwhelming situation. In the hospital, long-term care, and home settings, the nurse explores choices and end-of-life decisions with the patient and family. Referrals to home care and hospice services, as well as specific referrals appropriate for the management of the situation, are initiated. The nurse is an advocate for the dying person and works to uphold that person's rights. The use of living wills and advance directives allows the person to exercise the right to have a "good" death or to die with dignity.

SPIRITUALITY AND SPIRITUAL DISTRESS

Spirituality is defined as connectedness with self, others, a life force, or God that allows people to experience self-transcendence and find meaning in life. Spirituality helps people discover a purpose in life, understand the vicissitudes of life, and develop their relationships with God or a Higher Power. Within the framework of spirituality, a person discovers truths about self, the world, and concepts such as love, compassion, wisdom, honesty, commitment, imagination, reverence, and morality (Friedman, 1992). Often, spiritual behavior is expressed through sacrifice, self-discipline, and spending time in activities that focus on the inner self or the soul. Religion and nature are two vehicles that people use to connect themselves with God or a Higher Power; however, bonds to religious institutions, beliefs, or dogma are not required to experience the spiritual sense of self. **Faith,** considered the foundation of spirituality, is a belief in something that a person cannot see (Carson, 1992). The spiritual part of a person views life as a mystery that unfolds over the lifetime, encompassing questions about meaning, hope, relatedness to God, acceptance or forgiveness, and transcendence (Burkhardt, 1994; Sussman, Nezami, & Mishra, 1997).

A strong sense of spirituality or religious faith can have a positive impact on health (Idler & Kasl, 1992; Koenig et al., 1994; Matthews & Larson, 1995). Spirituality is also a component of hope, and especially during chronic, serious, or terminal illness, patients and their families often find comfort and emotional strength in their religious traditions or spiritual beliefs. At other times, illness and loss can cause a loss of faith or meaning in life, and a spiritual crisis. The nursing diagnosis of spiritual distress is applicable to those who have a disturbance in the belief or value system that provides strength, hope, and meaning in life.

Nursing Implications

Spiritually distressed patients (or family members) may show despair, discouragement, ambivalence, detachment, anger, resentment, or fear. They may question the meaning of suffering, life, and death, and express a sense of emptiness. The nurse assesses spiritual strength by inquiring about the person's sense of spiritual well-being, hope, and peacefulness. Have spiritual beliefs and values changed in response to illness or loss? The nurse assesses current and past participation in religious or spiritual practices and notes the patient's response to questions about spiritual needs–grief, anger, guilt, depression, doubt, anxiety, or calmness—to help determine the patient's need for spiritual care. Another simple assessment technique is to inquire about the patient's and family's desire for spiritual support.

For nurses to provide spiritual care, they must be open to being present and supportive when patients experience doubt, fearfulness, suffering, despair, or other difficult psychological states of being (Friedlander, 1976). Interventions that foster spiritual growth or reconciliation include being fully present; listening actively; conveying a sense of caring, respect, and acceptance; using therapeutic communication techniques to encourage expression; suggesting the use of prayer, meditation, or imagery; and facilitating contact with spiritual leaders or performance of spiritual rituals (Sumner, 1998).

Patients with serious, chronic, or terminal illnesses face physical and emotional losses that threaten their spiritual integrity. During acute and chronic illness, rehabilitation, or the dying process, spiritual support can stimulate patients to regain or strengthen their connections with their inner selves, their loved ones, and their God or Higher Power to transcend suffering and find meaning. Nurses can alleviate distress and suffering and enhance wellness by meeting their patients' spiritual needs.

Critical Thinking Exercises

1. The wife of a patient who is dying from bone cancer tells the nurse that she is prepared for the death of her partner. Her distress is based on family members who tell her that she is an "uncaring, cold person" because she is not openly crying and expressing other outward signs of being emotionally distraught. In counseling this family member what would you say to her? How could the wife's behavior be explained to other family members?
2. The nurse is working with a family to develop therapeutic interventions for a member who has a cocaine and alcohol addiction problem. One family member tells the nurse she will never be able to support the plan decided on by the rest of the family. How would you approach this person? What strategies would be useful for this person and for the entire family?
3. The nurse notices that a patient has pain and exacerbation of symptoms after the family visits. The patient tells the nurse that he is letting his family down and he feels like a failure because he can no longer provide for them in the way that he promised. During visits, his spouse and children complain to him about financial, social, and other problems. What strategies would be useful in talking to the patient? How could the nurse approach the entire family to tell them about the patient's distress and request that they change their behavior? What referrals could be helpful to this family?

References and Selected Readings

BOOKS

American Psychiatric Association. (1994). *Diagnostic and statistical manual of mental disorders* (DSM IV) (4th ed.). Washington, DC: Author.

Barry, P. D. (1998). *Mental health and mental illness* (6th ed.). Philadelphia: Lippincott-Raven.

Bates, B., & Brim, O. G. (1980). *Life-span development and behavior* (Vol. 3). New York: Academic Press.

Bowlby, J. (1961). *Attachment and loss* (Vol. I). New York: Basic Books.

Boyd-Franklin, N. (1989). *Black families in therapy: A multisystems approach.* New York: Guilford Press.

Bright, R. (1996). *Grief and powerlessness.* London: Jessica Kingsley Publishers.

Burnside, I. (1988). *Nursing and the aged: A self-care approach.* New York: McGraw-Hill.

Burr, W., Klein, S., Burr, R., Doxey, C., Haeker, B., Holman, T., Martin, P., McClure, R., Parrish, S., Stuart, D., Taylor, A., & White, M. (1994). *Reexamining family stress: New theory and research.* Thousand Oaks, CA: Sage.

Burr, W., et al. (1993). *Family science.* Pacific Grove, CA: Brooks/Cole.

Carson, V. (1995). Losses and endings in the nurse-patient relationship. In E. Arnold & K. Boggs (Eds.). *Interpersonal relationships: Professional communication skills for nurses* (2nd ed.). New York: W. B. Saunders.

Copel, L. C. (1996). *Nurse's clinical guide: Psychiatric and mental health care.* Springhouse, PA: Springhouse.

Frances, R. J., & Miller, S. I. (1991). *Clinical textbook of addictive disorders.* New York: Guilford Press.

Freeman, E. M. (Ed.). (1993). *Substance abuse treatment: A family perspective.* Newbury, CA: Sage.

Friedlander, A. H. (Ed.). (1976). *Out of the whirlwind.* New York: Schocken Books.

Giger, J. N., & Davidhizer, R. E. (1995). *Transcultural nursing: Assessment and intervention.* St. Louis: C. V. Mosby.

Haber, J., McMahon, A. L., Price-Hoskins, P., & Sideleau, B. F. (1992). *Comprehensive psychiatric nursing* (3rd ed.). St. Louis: C. V. Mosby.

Kubler-Ross, E. (1975). *Death: The final stage of growth.* Englewood Cliffs, NJ: Prentice-Hall.

Martocchio, B. C. (1982). *Living while dying.* Bowie, MD: Robert J. Brady.

Matthews D. A., & Larson D. B. (1995). *The faith factor: An annotated bibliography of clinical research on spiritual subjects* (Vol. III). Rockville, MD: National Institute for Health Care Research.

McCann, I. J., & Pearlman, L. A. (1990). *Psychological trauma and the adult survivor.* New York: Brunner/Mazel.

McCubbin, M. A., & McCubbin, H. I. (1993). Families coping with illness: The resiliency model of family stress, adjustment, & adaptation. In C. Danielson, B. Hamel-Bissell, & P. Winstead-Fry (Eds.). *Families, health, and illness: Perspectives on coping and intervention.* St. Louis: C. V. Mosby.

Papolos, D., & Papolos, J. (1997). *Overcoming depression.* New York: Harper Perennial.

Scurfield, R. (1985). Post-traumatic stress assessment and treatment: Overview and formulations. In C. R. Figley (Ed.). *Trauma and its wake.* New York: Brunner/Mazel.

Spector, R. E. (1996). *Cultural diversity in health and illness* (4th ed.). Norwalk, CT: Appleton & Lange.

Stanhope, M., & Lancaster, J. (1996). *Community health nursing: Promoting health of aggregates, families, and individuals* (5th ed.). St. Louis: C. V. Mosby.

Stuart, G. W., & Sundeen, S. J. (1995). *Principles and practice of psychiatric nursing* (5th ed.). St. Louis: C. V. Mosby.

U.S. Department of Health and Human Services. (1990). *Healthy people 2000.* (DHHS Publication No. (PHS) 91-1679). Washington, DC: U.S. Government Printing Office.

U.S. Department of Health and Human Services. (1995). *Healthy people 2000: Midcourse review and 1995 revisions.* Washington, DC: U.S. Government Printing Office.

Varcarolis, E. M. (1998). *Foundations of psychiatric mental health nursing.* Philadelphia: W. B. Saunders.

Worden, W. (1982). *Grief counseling and grief therapy: A handbook for the mental health practitioner.* New York: Springer Publishing.

Wright, L. M., & Leahy, M. (1994). *Families and psychosocial problems* (2nd ed.). Springhouse, PA: Springhouse.

Zerwekh, J. (1991). Supportive care of the dying patient. In S. B. Baird, R. McCorkle, & M. Grant (Eds.). *Cancer nursing.* Philadelphia: W. B. Saunders.

JOURNALS AND GOVERNMENT REPORTS

General

Cohen S., & Herbert T. (1996). Health psychology: psychological factors and physical disease from the perspective of human psychoneuroimmunology. *Annual Review of Psychology, 47,* 113–142.

Curtin, L. (1986). Nursing in the year 2000: Learning from the future. *Nursing Administration Quarterly, 11*(2), 1–8.

Devine, E. C., & Westlake, S. K. (1995). The effects of psychoeducational care provided to adults with cancer: Metaanalysis of 116 studies. *Oncology Nursing Forum, 22*(9), 1369–1376.

McBride, A. B. (1986). Present issues and future perspectives of psychosocial nursing: Theory and research. *Journal of Psychosocial Nursing and Mental Health Services, 24*(9), 27–32.

U.S. Department of Health & Human Services, Public Health Service, Agency for Health Care Policy and Research. (1993). *Depression in primary care: Vol. 1, Detection and diagnosis.* Clinical Practice Guideline. (AHCPR Publication No. 93-0550). Rockville, MD: U.S. Government Printing Office.

U.S. Department of Health & Human Services, Public Health Service, Agency for Health Care Policy and Research. (1993) *Depression in primary care: Vol. 2, Treatment of major depression.* Clinical Practice Guideline. (AHCPR Publication No. 93-0551). Rockville, MD: U.S. Government Printing Office.

Coping

King, K. B., Zewic J. J., Kimble L. P., & Rowe M. A. (1998). Optimism, coping, and long-term recovery from coronary artery surgery in women. *Research in Nursing & Health, 21*(1), 15–26.

Morse, S. R., & Fife B. (1998). Coping with a partner's cancer: Adjustment at four stages of the illness trajectory. *Oncology Nursing Forum, 25*(4), 751–760.

Twibell, R. S. (1998). Family coping during critical illness. *Dimensions in Critical Care Nursing, 17*(2), 100–112.

Depression

DeWester, J. N. (1996). Recognizing and treating the patient with somatic manifestations of depression. *Journal of Family Practice, 43*(6 Suppl), S3–15.

Doerfler, J. F., Pbert, L., & DeCosimo, D. (1997). Self-reported depression in patients with coronary heart disease. *Journal of Cardiopulmonary Rehabilitation, 17*(3): 163–170.

el-Mallakh, R. S., Lippmann S. B., Breen K. S., Wright J. C. (1996). Clues to depression in primary care practice. *Postgraduate Medicine, 100*(1), 85-8, 93-6.

National Institute of Mental Health. (1992). *Depression awareness, recognition, treatment fact sheet* (DHHS Publication No. [ADM] 92-1680). Rockville, MD: Government Printing Office.

U.S. Department of Health & Human Services (1993). *Clinical practice guidelines number 5. Depression in clinical care, Vol. 1: Detection and diagnosis.* Rockville, MD: U.S. Government Printing Office.

U.S. Department of Health & Human Services (1993). *Clinical practice guidelines number 5: Depression in primary care: Vol. 2: Treatment of major depression.* Rockville, MD: U.S. Government Printing Office.

Grief, Death, and Dying

Basile C. M. (1998). Advance directives and advocacy in end-of-life decisions. *Nurse Practitioner, 23*(5), 44–46, 54, 57–60.

Carter, S. (1989). Themes of grief. *Nursing Research, 38*(6), 354–358.

Conrad, N. L. (1985). Spiritual support for the dying. *Nursing Clinics of North America, 20*(2), 415–425.

Cooley, M. E. (1992). Bereavement care: A role for nurses. *Cancer Nursing, 15*(2): 125–129.

Engel, G. (1964). Grief and grieving. *American Journal of Nursing, 64*(7): 93–96.

Ferrell, B. R., Grant M., & Virani R. (1998). HOPE. Home care outreach for palliative care education. *Cancer Practitioner, 6*(2), 79–85.

Gyulay, J. E. (1989). Grief responses. *Issues in Comprehensive Pediatric Nursing, 12*(1), 1–31.

Hogan, N. S., & Balk, D. E. (1990). Adolescent reactions to sibling death: Perceptions of mothers, fathers, and teenagers. *Nursing Research, 39*(2), 103–106.

Kolcaba, K. Y., & Fisher E. M. (1996). A holistic perspective on comfort care as an advance directive. *Critical Care Nursing Quarterly, 18*(4), 66–67.

Levy, L. H. (1991). Anticipatory grief: Its measurement and proposed reconceptualization. *Hospice Journal, 7*(4), 1–28.

Lindemann, E. (1944). Symptomatology and management of acute grief. *American Journal of Psychiatry, 101,* 141–148.

Nishimoto, P. (1996). Venturing into the unknown: Cultural beliefs about death and dying. *Oncology Nursing Forum, 23*(6), 889–894.

Steele, L. L. (1990). The death surround: Factors influencing the grief experience of survivors. *Oncology Nursing Forum, 17*(2), 235–241.

Wheeler S. R. (1996). Helping families cope with death and dying. *Nursing, 26*(7), 25–30.

Posttraumatic Stress Disorder

Kolb, L. (1987). Neuropsychological hypothesis explaining posttraumatic stress disorder. *American Journal of Psychiatry, 144*(8), 989–995.

Norman, E. (1989). Analysis of the concept of posttraumatic stress disorder. *Journal of Advanced Medical Surgical Nursing, 1*(4), 55–64.

Spirituality

Burkhardt, M. A. (1994). Becoming and connecting: Elements of spirituality for women. *Holistic Nursing Practice, 8*(4), 12–21.

Dyom J., Forman D., & Cobb M. (1997). The meaning of spirituality: A literature review. *Journal of Advanced Nursing, 26*(6), 1183–1188.

Idler E. L., Kasl S. V. (1992). Religion, disability, depression, and the timing of death. *American Journal of Sociology, 97*(4):1052–1079.

Koenig, H. G., George L. K., Meador K. G., Blaazer D. G., & Dyck P. B. (1994). Religious affiliation and psychiatric disorder among Protestant baby boomers. *Hospital and Community Psychiatry, 45*(6), 586–596.

Leetun, M. C. (1996). Wellness spirituality in the older adult: Assessment and intervention protocol. *Nurse Practitioner, 21*(8), 60, 65–70.

Miller, M. A. (1995). Culture, spirituality, and women's health. *Journal of Obstetric, Gynecologic, and Neonatal Nursing, 24*(3), 257–263.

Ross, L. A. (1997). Elderly patients' perception of their spiritual needs and care: A pilot study. *Journal of Advanced Nursing, 26*(4), 710–715.

Sumner, C. H. (1998). Recognizing and responding to spiritual distress, *American Journal of Nursing, 98*(1):26–30.

Sussman, S., Nezami, E., & Mishra, S. (1997). On operationalizing spiritual experience for health promotion research and practice. *Alternative Therapies in Clinical Practice, 4*(4), 120–125.

Wright, K. B. (1998). Professional, ethical, and legal implications for spiritual care in nursing. *Image: Journal of Nursing Scholarship, 30*(1), 81–83.

Substance Abuse

Ewing, J. A. (1984). CAGE. *Journal of the American Medical Association, 252*(14), 1906.

McLellan, A. T., Kushner, H., Metzger, D., & Peters, R. (1992). The fifth edition of the addiction severity index. *Journal of Substance Abuse Treatment, 9*(3): 199–213.

Selzer, M. L. (1971). The Michigan alcoholism screening test: The quest for a new diagnostic instrument. *American Journal of Psychiatry, 127*, 1653–1658.

Resources

AGENCIES

Depression Awareness, Recognition, and Treatment Program, National Institute of Mental Health, D/ART Public Inquiries, 5600 Fishers Lane, Room 7C02, Rockville, MD 20857; 1-800-421-4211.
National Center for Post Traumatic Stress Disorder, VA Medical Center, White River Junction, VT 05009; 1-802-296-5132; www.dartmouth.edu/dms/ptsd.
National Hospice Organization (NHO), 1901 North Moore Street, Suite 901, Arlington, VA 22209; 1-703-243-5900.
Grief Recovery Institute Education Foundation, Inc. (GRIEF), 8306 Wilshire Boulevard, Suite 21A, Beverly Hills, CA 90211; 1-213-650-1234; 1-800-445-4808 (Hotline).
American Holistic Nurses Association (AHNA), P.O. Box 2130, Flagstaff, AZ 86003-2130; 1-800-278-AHNA.

Aging

National Council on the Aging, 409 3rd Street SW, Washington, DC 20024, 1-202-424-1200; 1-800-424-9046; info@ncoa.org.
American Association of Retired Persons (AARP), 601 'E' Street NW, Washington, DC 20049-0001; 1-202-434-227; 1-800-424-3410; www.aarp.org.
National Office of the Gray Panthers, 2025 Pennsylvania Avenue NW #821, Washington, DC 20006-1813; 1-202-466-3132; 1-800-280-5362; dixieh1064@aol.com.
National Association for Families Caring for their Elders—Eldercare America, 1141 Loxford Terrace, Silver Spring, MD 20901-1130; 1-301-593-1621.
Children of Aging Parents, 1609 Woodbourne Road #302A, Levittown, PA 19057-1511; 1-215-945-6900; 1-800-227-7294.

Anxiety

Anxiety Disorders Association of America, 11900 Parklawn Drive #100, Rockville, MD 20852-2624; 1-301-231-9350; anxdis@aol.com.

Bereavement

Compassionate Friends, P.O. Box 3696, Oak Brook, IL 60522-3696; 1-630-990-0010; tcf_nat'l@prodigy.com.
Grief Recovery Institute, 8306 Wilshire Boulevard #21A, Beverly Hills, CA 90211; 1-213-650-1231; 1-800-445-4808.
They Help Each Other Spiritually (THEOS), 322 Boulevard of the Allies #105, Pittsburgh, PA 15222-1919; 1-412-471-7779.
Widowed Persons Service, 601 'E' Street NW, Washington, DC 20049-0001; 1-202-434-2260.

Depression

Depression Awareness, Recognition, & Treatment (D/ART) NIMH, 5600 Fishers Lane Room 10-85, Rockville, MD 20857; 1-800-421-4211; 1-301-443-4140.
National Alliance for the Mentally Ill, 200 N. Grebe Road #1015, Arlington, VA 22201-3062; 1-703-524-7600; 1-800-950-NAMI; namioffC@aol.com.
National Mental Health Association, 1021 Prince Street, Alexandria, VA 22314-2971; 1-703-684-7722; 1-800-969-6642; 1-800-433-5959; nmhainfo@aol.com.

Eating Disorders

American Anorexia Bulimia Association Inc., 165 W. 46th Street, #1108, New York, NY 10036-2501; 1-212-575-6200.
National Eating Disorders Association (NEDO), 6655 S. Yale Avenue, Tulsa, OK 74136; 1-918-481-4044.

Holistic Nursing Association

American Holistic Nursing Association, P.O. Box 2130, Sedona, AR 86003-2130; 1-800-278-ahna (1-800-278-2462); www.ahna.org.

Posttraumatic Stress Disorder

National Center for PTSD, VA Medical Center (116D), White River Junction, VT 05009; 1-802-296-5132; ptsd@dartmouth.edu.

Substance Abuse

Alcoholics Anonymous, 475 Riverside, New York, NY 10115; 1-212-870-3400; www.alcoholics-anonymous.org.
Alanon and Alateen Family Group Headquarters Inc., 1600 Corporate Landing Parkway, Virginia Beach, VA 23454-5617; 1-888-4AL-ANON (888-425-2666); www.al-anon.org.
Children of Alcoholics Foundation, Box 4185, Grand Central Station, New York, NY 10115; 1-800-359-2623.
Adult Children of Alcoholics, P.O. Box 3216, Torrence, CA 90510; 1-310-534-1815; www.info@adultchildren.org.
Narcotics Anonymous, P.O. Box 9999, Van Nuys, CA 91409; 1-818-780-3951; www.na.org.
Cocaine Anonymous, 3740 Overland Avenue Suite G, Los Angeles, CA 90034; 1-800-347-8998; www.ca.org.
Co-Anon Family Groups, P.O. Box 64742-66, Los Angeles, CA 90064; 1-818-377-4317.
Dual Recovery Anonymous, 1617 16th Avenue South, Nashville, TN 37212; 1-888-869-9230; www.dualrecovery.base.org.
Rational Recovery Systems, Box 800, Lotus, CA 95651; 1-530-621-4374.
Secular Organizations for Sobriety (SOS), The Center for Inquiry, 5521 Grosvenor Boulevard, Los Angeles, CA 90066; 1-310-821-8430.

HOTLINE NUMBERS

Center for Substance Abuse Treatment, National Treatment Hotline 800-662-HELP (1-800-662-4357).
Center for Substance Abuse Prevention Workplace, Hotline 800-WORK-PLACE (1-800-967-5752).
National Alcohol Hotline, Helpline: 1-800-ALCOHOL (1-800-252-6465).
National Cocaine Hotline, 1-800-COCAINE (1-800-262-2463).

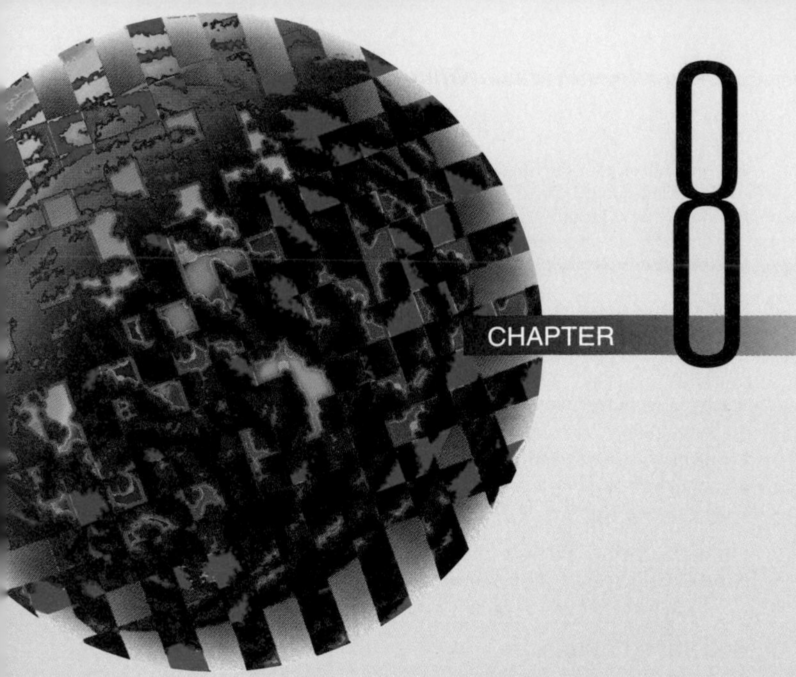

CHAPTER 8

Perspectives in Transcultural Nursing

Learning Objectives

On completion of this chapter, the learner will be able to:

1. Apply transcultural nursing principles, concepts, and theories when providing nursing care to patients (individuals, families, groups, and communities).
2. Identify key components of cultural assessment for self and patients.
3. Critically analyze the influence of culture on nursing care decisions and actions for patients.
4. Develop strategies for planning, providing, and evaluating culturally competent nursing care for patients from diverse backgrounds.

In the health care delivery system, as in society, the nurse interacts with people of similar and diverse cultural backgrounds. These people may have similar or different frames of reference and varied preferences regarding their health and health care needs. Acknowledging and adapting to the cultural needs of the patient and significant others is an important component of nursing care. To plan and deliver culturally competent care, the nurse must understand the definitions of culture and cultural competence and the various aspects of culture that should be explored for each patient.

DEFINITIONS OF CULTURE

The concept of culture and its relationship to the health care beliefs and practices of patients and their family and friends provides the foundation for transcultural nursing. This awareness of culture in the delivery of nursing care has been described in different ways, including respect for cultural diversity, culturally sensitive or culturally comprehensive care, culturally competent nursing care (American Association of Colleges of Nursing, 1996; Andrews & Boyle, 1998; Bond & Jones, 1997; Giger & Davidhizar, 1995; Habayeb, 1995; McGee, 1994; Villarruel, 1995), or culturally congruent nursing care (Leininger, 1991). Two commonly discussed concepts are cultural diversity and culturally competent care.

The term culture was initially defined by the British anthropologist Sir Edward Tylor in 1871 as including the knowledge, belief, art, morals, laws, customs, and any other capabilities and habits acquired by humans as members of society. During the past century, and especially during recent decades, culture has been defined in hundreds of ways with the themes stated by Tylor and with the theme of ethnic variations of a population based on race, nationality, religion, and geography (Habayeb, 1995) integrated into these definitions. Madeleine Leininger, founder of the specialty called transcultural nursing, indicates that culture involves learned and transmitted knowledge about values, beliefs, rules of behavior, and lifestyle practices that guide a designated group in their thinking and actions in patterned ways (1988). Giger and Davidhizar (1995) further state that culture develops over time as a result of "imprinting the mind through social and religious structures and intellectual and artistic manifestations" (p. 3).

Culture has four basic characteristics:

1. It is learned from birth through language and socialization.
2. It is shared by members of the same cultural group.
3. It is influenced by specific conditions related to environmental and technical factors and to the availability of resources.
4. It is dynamic and ever-changing.

Cultural diversity has similarly been defined in a number of ways. Often, color, religion, and geographic area are the only elements used to identify diversity, with ethnic minorities being considered the primary sources of cultural diversity. Habayeb states that "discrepancies in definitions arise when nurses do not visualize every person (themselves included) as having a culture, as having a cultural heritage, and as being culturally diverse" (1995, p. 224).

Culturally competent nursing care is defined as providing effective care in cross-cultural situations (Villarruel, 1995). Culturally competent care requires a comprehensive knowledge of culture-specific information and sensitivity to the effect that culture has on the care situation; it requires synthesis of knowledge of the culture and the individual's cultural perspectives into the plan of care (Bond & Jones, 1997; McGee, 1994). Understanding the diversity within cultures, such as subcultures, is also important.

Subcultures and Minorities

Although culture is a universal phenomenon, it takes on specific and distinctive features for a particular group, encompassing all of the knowledge, beliefs, customs, and skills acquired by the members of that group. When such groups function within a larger cultural group, they are referred to as subcultures.

The term subculture is used for relatively large groups of people who share characteristics that enable them to be identified as a distinct entity. Examples of American subcultures based on ethnicity (ie, subcultures with common traits such as physical characteristics, language, or ancestry) include African Americans, Hispanic Americans, and Native Americans. Each of the aforementioned subcultures may be further divided; for example, Native Americans consist of American Indians and Alaska Natives, who represent more than 500 federally and state-recognized tribes in addition to an unknown number of tribes that receive no official recognition.

Subcultures may also be based on religion (more than 1200 exist in the United States); occupation (including nurse, physician, and other members of the health care team); age (infants, children, adolescents, adults, older adults); gender (man or woman); sexual orientation (homosexual or bisexual men and women); or geographic location (Texans, Southerners, Appalachians).

The term minority refers to a group of people whose physical or cultural characteristics differ from the majority of people in a society. At times, minorities may be singled out or isolated from others in society or treated in different or unequal ways. Although there are four federally identified minority groups (blacks, Hispanics, Asian/Pacific Islanders, and Native Americans), the concept of minority varies widely and must be understood in a cultural context. For example, men may be considered minorities within the nursing profession, but they constitute a majority within the field of medicine. Because at times the term minority connotes inferiority, members of many racial and ethnic groups object to being identified as minorities.

TRANSCULTURAL NURSING

Transcultural nursing, a term sometimes used interchangeably with cross-cultural, intercultural, or multicultural nursing, refers to a formal area of study and practice that focuses on the cultural care (caring) values, beliefs, and practices of individuals and groups from a particular culture (Dreher, 1997; White, 1997). The underlying focus of transcultural nursing is to provide culture-specific and culture-universal care that promotes the well-being or health of individuals, families, groups, communities, and institutions (Giger & Davidhizar, 1995; Giger, Davidhizar, Johnson, & Poole, 1997; Leininger, 1991). When the care is delivered beyond the nurse's national boundaries, the term international or transnational nursing is often used.

Although many nurses, anthropologists, and others have written about the cultural aspects of nursing and health care, Leininger (1991) has developed a comprehensive research-based theory called Culture Care Diversity and Universality. The goal of the theory is to provide culturally congruent nursing care to improve care for people of different or similar cultures. This means promoting recovery from illness, preventing conditions that would limit the patient's health or well-being, or facilitating a peaceful death in ways that are culturally meaningful and appropriate. Nursing care needs to be tailored to fit the patient's cultural values, beliefs, and life-ways.

Leininger's theory includes providing culturally congruent care (meaningful, beneficial, and satisfying health care tailored to fit the patient's cultural values) through culture care accommodation and culture care restructuring. Culture care accommodation refers to those professional actions and decisions that help people of a designated culture achieve a beneficial or satisfying health

CHART 8•1 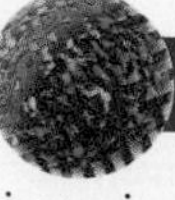 **Overcoming Language Barriers**

- Greet the patient using the last or complete name. Avoid being too casual or familiar. Point to yourself and say your name. Smile.
- Proceed in an unhurried manner. Pay attention to any effort by the patient or family to communicate.
- Speak in a low, moderate voice. Avoid talking loudly. Remember that there is a tendency to raise the volume and pitch of your voice when the listener appears not to understand. The listener may perceive that you are shouting and/or angry.
- Organize your thoughts. Repeat and summarize frequently. Use audiovisual aids when feasible.
- Use short, simple sentence structure and speak in the active voice.
- Use simple words, such as "pain" instead of "discomfort." Avoid medical jargon, idioms, and slang. Avoid using contractions, such as don't, can't, won't.
- Use nouns repeatedly instead of pronouns.
  Example:
  Do not say: "He has been taking his medicine, hasn't he?"
  Do say: "Does Juan take medicine?"
- Pantomime words and simple actions while verbalizing them.
- Give instructions in the proper sequence.
  Example:
  Do not say: "Before you rinse the bottle, sterilize it."
  Do say: "First wash the bottle. Second, rinse the bottle."
- Discuss one topic at a time and avoid giving too much information in a single conversation. Avoid using conjunctions.
  Example:
  Do not say: "Are you cold and in pain?"
  Do say: "Are you cold?" (while pantomiming) "Are you in pain?"
- Validate whether the person understands by having him or her repeat instructions, demonstrate the procedure, or act out the meaning.
- Use any words you know in the person's language. This indicates that you are aware of and respect the patient's primary means of communicating.
- Try a third language. Many Indo-Chinese speak French. Europeans often know three or four languages. Try Latin words or phrases, if you are familiar with the language.
- Ask who among the patient's family and friends could serve as an interpreter. Be aware of culturally based gender and age differences and diverse socioeconomic, educational, and tribal/regional differences when choosing an interpreter.
- Obtain phrase books from a library or bookstore, make or purchase flash cards, contact hospitals for a list of interpreters, and use both formal and informal networking to locate a suitable interpreter. Although costly, some telecommunication companies provide translation services.

outcome. Culture care restructuring or repatterning refers to those professional actions and decisions that help patients reorder, change, or modify their lifestyles toward new, different, or more beneficial health care patterns. At the same time, the patient's cultural values and beliefs are respected, and a better or healthier lifestyle is provided.

Other terms and definitions that provide further insight into culture and health care include the following:

- Acculturation is the process by which members of a cultural group adapt to or learn how to take on the behaviors of another group.
- Cultural blindness is the inability of a person to recognize his or her own values, beliefs, and practices and those of others because of strong ethnocentric tendencies.
- Cultural imposition is the tendency to impose one's cultural beliefs, values, and patterns of behavior on a person or persons from a different culture.
- Cultural taboos are those activities governed by rules of behavior that are avoided, forbidden, or prohibited by a particular cultural group.

CULTURALLY COMPETENT NURSING CARE

Culturally competent or congruent nursing care refers to a complex integration of attitudes, knowledge, and skills (including assessment, decision making, judgments, critical thinking, and evaluation) that enables the nurse to provide care in a culturally sensitive manner. Agency and institutional policies are important to achieve culturally competent care.

Policies that promote culturally congruent care establish flexible regulations pertaining to visitors (number, frequency, and length of visits); provide translation services for non–English-speaking patients; recognize special dietary needs of patients from selected cultural groups; and create an environment in which the traditional healing, spiritual, and religious practices of patients are respected and encouraged.

CROSS-CULTURAL COMMUNICATION

Establishing an environment of culturally congruent care and respect begins with effective communication. Communication occurs through words, body language, and other cues, such as voice, tone, and loudness. Nurse–patient interactions, as well as communications among members of a multicultural health care team, are dependent on the ability to understand and be understood.

About 150 different languages are spoken in the United States, with Spanish accounting for the largest percentage among minority groups. Obviously, nurses cannot become fluent in all languages, but certain strategies for fostering effective cross-cultural communication are necessary when providing care for patients who are not fluent in English. Care should be taken to consider cultural and ethical appropriateness when choosing an interpreter (Dibble, 1997). The interpreter's voice quality, pronunciation, use of silence, touch, and use of nonverbal communication should be assessed (Giger & Davidhizar, 1995).

During illness, patients of all ages tend to regress, and the regression often involves language skills. Chart 8-1 summarizes suggested strategies for overcoming language barriers. The nurse should also assess how well the patient and family have understood what has been said. The following cues may signal lack of effective communication:

Efforts to change the subject. This could indicate that the patient does not understand what you are saying and is attempting to talk about something more familiar.

Absence of questions. Paradoxically, this often means that the listener is not grasping the message and therefore has difficulty formulating questions to ask.

Inappropriate laughter. A self-conscious giggle may signal poor comprehension and may be an attempt to disguise embarrassment.

Nonverbal cues. Although a blank expression may signal poor understanding, among some Asian Americans, it may reflect a desire to avoid overt expression of emotion. Similarly, avoidance of eye contact may be a cultural expression of respect for the speaker (eg, some Native Americans and Asian Americans use this).

CULTURALLY MEDIATED CHARACTERISTICS

Because so many human behaviors and attitudes are shaped by cultural influences, nurses should be aware that patients act and behave in a variety of ways, based on their cultural background. However, although certain attributes and attitudes are frequently associated with particular cultural groups, as described in the following pages, it is important to realize that not all people from the same cultural background share the same behaviors and views. Although the nurse who fails to consider a patient's cultural preferences and beliefs is considered insensitive and possibly indifferent, the nurse who assumes that all members of any one culture act and behave in the same way runs the risk of stereotyping people. The best way to avoid stereotyping is to view each patient as an individual and to find out which cultural preferences the patient has.

Space and Distance

People tend to regard the space in their immediate vicinity as an extension of themselves. How much space they need between themselves and others to feel comfortable is a culturally determined phenomenon.

Because nurses and patients usually are not consciously aware of their personal space requirements, they frequently have difficulty understanding different behaviors in this regard. For example, positioning oneself close to another may be perceived as an expression of warmth and care by one person but as a threatening invasion of personal space by another. Research reveals that people from the United States, Canada, and Great Britain require the most personal space between themselves and others, whereas those from Latin America, Japan, and the Middle East need the least amount of space and feel comfortable standing close to others.

If patients appear to position themselves too close or too far away, the nurse should consider cultural preferences for space and distance. Ideally, patients should be permitted to assume a position that is comfortable to them in terms of personal space and distance. Because a significant amount of communication during nursing care requires close physical contact, the nurse should be aware of these important cultural differences and consider them when delivering care (Giger et al., 1997).

Eye Contact

Eye contact is also a culturally determined behavior. Although most nurses have been taught to maintain eye contact when speaking with patients, some people from culturally diverse backgrounds may interpret this behavior differently. Some Asians, Native Americans, Indo-Chinese, Arabs, and Appalachians may consider direct eye contact impolite or aggressive, and they may avert their own eyes when talking with nurses and others whom they perceive to be in positions of authority. Some Native Americans stare at the floor during conversations, a cultural behavior conveying respect and indicating that the listener is paying close attention to the speaker. Some Hispanic patients maintain downcast eyes as a sign of appropriate deferential behavior toward others on the basis of age, gender, social position, economic status, and position of authority. Being aware that eye contact carries certain meanings in such circumstances will help the nurse understand a patient's behavior and provide an atmosphere in which the patient can feel comfortable.

Time

Attitudes about time vary widely among cultures and can be a common barrier to effective communication between nurses and patients. Views about punctuality and the use of time are culturally determined, as is the concept of waiting. Symbols of time, such as watches, sunrises, and sunsets, represent methods for measuring the duration and passage of time (Andrews & Boyle, 1998; Giger & Davidhizar, 1995).

For most health care providers, time is extremely important, as is promptness. For example, nurses frequently expect patients to arrive at an exact time for an appointment, despite the fact that the patient is often kept waiting by health care providers who are running late. Health care providers are likely to function according to an appointment system in which there are short intervals of perhaps only a few minutes. For patients from some cultures, time is a relative phenomenon, with little attention paid to the *exact* hour or minute. Some Hispanic people, for example, consider time in a wider frame of reference and make the primary distinction between day and night. Time may also be determined according to traditional times for meals, sleep, and other activities or events. For people from some cultures, the present is of the greatest importance, and time is viewed in broad ranges rather than in terms of a fixed hour. Being flexible in regard to schedules is the norm.

Value differences also may influence a person's sense of priority when it comes to time. For example, responding to a family matter may be more important to a patient than a scheduled health care appointment. Allowing for these different views is essential in maintaining an effective nurse–patient relationship. Scolding a patient for being late or acting annoyed undermines the patient's confidence in the health care system and might result in further missed appointments or indifference to health care suggestions.

Touch

The meaning people associate with touching is culturally determined to a great degree. In some cultures (eg, Hispanic and Arab), male health care providers may be prohibited from touching or examining certain parts of the female body. Similarly, it may be inappropriate for females to care for males. Among many Asian Americans, it is impolite to touch a person's head because the spirit is believed to reside there. Thus, assessment of the head or evaluation of a head injury requires alternate approaches. The patient's culturally defined sense of modesty must also be considered when providing nursing care (eg, some Jewish and Islamic women believe that modesty requires covering their head, arms, and legs with clothing).

Observance of Holidays

All cultures celebrate civil and religious holidays. Nurses should familiarize themselves with major holidays for members of the cultural groups they serve. Information about these important celebrations is available from various sources, including religious organizations, hospital chaplains, and patients themselves. Routine health appointments, diagnostic tests, surgery, and other major procedures should be scheduled to avoid those holidays a patient identifies as significant.

Diet

The cultural meanings associated with food vary widely but usually include one or more of the following: relief of hunger; promotion of health and healing; prevention of disease or illness; expression of caring for another; promotion of interpersonal closeness among individuals, families, groups, communities, or nations; promotion of kinship and family alliances; solidification of social ties; celebration of life events (eg, birthdays, marriages, funerals); expression of gratitude or appreciation; recognition of achievement or accomplishment; validation of social, cultural, or religious ceremonial functions; facilitation of business negotiations; and expression of affluence, wealth, or social status.

Culture determines what foods are served and when they are served; the number and frequency of meals; who eats with whom; who is given the choicest portions; how foods are prepared, served, and eaten (eg, chop sticks, hands, fork-knife-spoon); and where people shop for their favorite food items (eg, ethnic grocery stores and specialty food markets).

Religious practice may include fasting (eg, Mormons, Catholics, Buddhists, Jews, Muslims, and others), abstaining from selected foods at particular times (eg, Catholics abstain from meat on Ash Wednesday and the Fridays of Lent), and the ritualistic use of food and beverages (eg, Passover dinner, consumption of bread and wine during religious ceremonies). Chart 8-2 summarizes some dietary practices of selected religious groups.

Many groups tend to feast, often in the company of family and friends, on selected holidays. For example, many Christians eat large dinners on Christmas and Easter and consume other traditional high-calorie, high-fat foods, such as seasonal cookies, pastries, and candies. These culturally based dietary practices are especially significant in the care of patients with diabetes, hypertension, gastrointestinal disorders, and other conditions in which diet plays a key role.

CHART 8•2 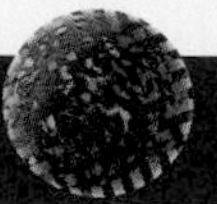 **Dietary Practices of Selected Religious Groups**

Prohibited Foods and Beverages

Hinduism
All meats
Animal shortenings

Islam
Pork
Alcoholic products and beverages (including extracts, such as vanilla and lemon)
Animal shortenings
Gelatin made with pork, marshmallow, and other confections made with gelatin

Judaism
Pork
Predatory fowl
Shellfish and scavenger fish (eg, shrimp, crab, lobster, escargot, catfish). Fish with fins and scales are permissible.
Mixing milk and meat dishes at same meal
Blood by ingestion (eg, blood sausage, raw meat). Blood by transfusion is acceptable.
Note: Packaged foods will contain labels identifying *kosher* ("properly preserved" or "fitting") and *pareve* (made without meat or milk) items.

Mormonism (Church of Jesus Christ of Latter-Day Saints)
Alcohol
Tobacco
Beverages containing caffeine stimulants (coffee, tea, colas, and selected carbonated soft drinks)

Seventh-Day Adventism
Pork
Certain seafood, including shellfish
Fermented beverages
Note: Optional vegetarianism is encouraged.

CAUSES OF ILLNESS

Three major views, or paradigms, attempt to explain the causes of disease and illness: the biomedical or scientific view, the naturalistic or holistic perspective, and the magico-religious view.

The biomedical or scientific world view prevails in most health care settings and is embraced by most nurses and other health care providers. The basic assumptions underlying the biomedical perspective are that all events in life have a cause and effect, that the human body functions much like a machine, and that all of reality can be observed and measured (eg, intelligence tests). One example of the biomedical or scientific view is the bacterial or viral explanation of communicable diseases.

The second way that some cultures attempt to explain the cause of illness is through the naturalistic or holistic perspective, a viewpoint that is found among many Native Americans, Asians, and others who believe that human life is only one aspect of nature. According to this view, the forces of nature must be kept in natural balance or harmony.

One naturalistic belief, held by many Asian groups, is the yin/yang theory, in which health is believed to exist when all aspects of a person are in perfect balance or harmony. Rooted in the ancient Chinese philosophy of Tao (The Way), the yin/yang theory proposes that all organisms and objects in the universe consist of yin and yang energy. The seat of the energy forces is within the autonomic nervous system, where balance between the opposing forces is maintained during health. Yin energy represents the female and negative forces, such as emptiness, darkness, and cold, whereas the yang forces are male and positive, emitting warmth and fullness. Foods are classified as hot and cold in this theory and are transformed into yin and yang energy when metabolized by the body. Yin foods are cold, and yang foods are hot. Cold foods are eaten when the person has a hot illness (eg, fever, rash, sore throat, ulcer, infection), and hot foods are eaten with a cold illness (eg, cancer, headache, stomach cramps, colds). The yin/yang theory is the basis for Eastern or Chinese medicine and is embraced by some Asian Americans.

Many Hispanic, African American, and Arab groups embrace the hot/cold theory of health and illness. The four humors of the body—blood, phlegm, black bile, and yellow bile—regulate basic bodily functions and are described in terms of temperature, dryness, and moisture. The treatment of disease consists of adding or subtracting cold, heat, dryness, or wetness to restore the balance of the humors. Beverages, foods, herbs, medicines, and diseases are classified as hot or cold according to their perceived effects on the body, not their physical characteristics. According to the hot/cold theory, the individual as a whole, not just a particular ailment, is significant. Those who embrace the hot/cold theory maintain that health consists of a positive state of total well-being, including physical, psychological, spiritual, and social aspects of the person.

According to the naturalistic world view, breaking the laws of nature creates imbalances, chaos, and disease. People who embrace the naturalistic paradigm use metaphors such as "the healing power of Nature." From the perspective of the Chinese, for example, illness is seen, not as an intruding agent, but as a part of life's rhythmic course and as an outward sign of disharmony within.

The third major way in which people view the world and explain the causes of illness is the magico-religious world view. The basic premise is that the world is seen as an arena in which supernatural forces dominate. The fate of the world and those in it depends on the action of supernatural forces for good or evil. Examples of magical causes of illness include belief in voodoo or witchcraft among some African Americans and others from Caribbean countries. Faith healing is based on religious beliefs and is most prevalent among selected Christian religions, including Christian Science, whereas various healing rituals may be found in many other religions, such as Roman Catholicism, Mormonism (Church of Jesus Christ of Latter-Day Saints), and others.

Of course, it is possible to hold a combination of world views, and many patients are likely to offer more than one explanation for the cause of their illness. As a profession, nursing largely embraces the scientific or biomedical world view, but some aspects of holism have begun to gain popularity, including a wide variety of techniques for managing chronic pain, such as hypnosis, therapeutic touch, and biofeedback. Belief in spiritual power is also held by many nurses who credit supernatural forces with various unexplained phenomena related to patients' health and illness states.

Regardless of the view held and whether the nurse agrees with the patient's beliefs in this regard, it is important to be aware of how people view their illness and their health and to work within this framework to promote the patient's care and well-being.

FOLK HEALERS

Several cultures believe in folk or indigenous healers. The nurse may find some Hispanic patients turning to a *curandero/a, espiritualista* (spiritualist), *yerbo* (herbalist), or *sabador* (healer who manipulates bones and muscles). Some African American patients may seek assistance from a *hougan* (voodoo priest or priestess), *spiritualist, root doctor* (usually a woman who uses magic rituals to treat diseases), or *"old lady"* (an older woman who has successfully raised a family and who specializes in child care and folk remedies). Native American patients may seek assistance from a *shaman* or *medicine man* or *woman.* Patients of Asian descent may mention that they have visited *herbalists, acupuncturists,* or *bone setters.* Several cultures have their own healers, most of whom speak the native tongue of the patient, make house calls, and cost significantly less than healers practicing in the biomedical or scientific health care system.

It is best not to disdain a patient's belief in a folk healer or try to undermine trust in the healer. To do so may alienate and drive the patient away from receiving the care prescribed. Efforts should be made to accommodate the patient's beliefs while advocating the treatment proposed by modern health science.

CULTURAL ASSESSMENT

Cultural nursing assessment refers to a systematic appraisal or examination of individuals, families, groups, and communities in terms of their cultural beliefs, values, and practices. The purpose of such an assessment is to provide culturally competent care (Andrews & Boyle, 1998; Calnins, 1997). In an effort to establish a database for determining a patient's cultural background, nurses have developed cultural assessment tools or have modified existing assessment tools (Andrews & Boyle, 1998; Leininger, 1991) to ensure that transcultural considerations are included in the plan of care. Giger and Davidhizar (1995) developed a model for assessing the needs of culturally diverse patients by examining six phenomena that are evident in all cultural groups: communication, space, social organization, time, environmental control, and biologic variations. This model has been used to design nursing care from health promotion to nursing skills activities (Giger et al., 1997; Smith-Temple & Johnson, 1998). The information presented in this chapter and the following general guidelines can be used to direct the nurse's assessment of culture and its influence on a patient's health beliefs and practices.

- What is the patient's country of origin? How long has the patient lived in this country? What is the primary language and literacy level?
- What is the patient's ethnic background? Does he or she identify strongly with others from the same cultural background?
- What is the patient's religion, and how important is it to his or her daily life?
- Does the patient participate in cultural activities such as dressing in traditional clothing and observing traditional holidays and festivals?
- Are there any food preferences or restrictions?
- What are the patient's communication styles? Is eye contact avoided? How much physical distance is maintained? Is the patient open and verbal about symptoms?
- Who is the head of the family, and is he or she involved in decision making about the patient?
- What does the patient do to maintain his or her health?
- What does the patient think caused the current problem?
- Has the the advice of traditional healers been sought?
- What kind of treatment does the patient think will help? What are the most important results he or she hopes to get from this treatment?
- Are there religious rituals related to sickness, death, or health that the patient observes?

ADDITIONAL CULTURAL CONSIDERATIONS: KNOW THYSELF

Because the nurse–patient interaction is the focal point of nursing, nurses should consider their own cultural orientation when conducting assessment of the patient and the patient's family and friends.

- Know your own cultural attitudes, values, beliefs, and practices.
- Regardless of "good intention," everyone has cultural "baggage" that ultimately results in ethnocentrism (the tendency to view one's own culture as superior to others).
- In general, it is easier to understand those whose cultural heritage is similar to our own, while viewing those who are unlike us as strange and different.
- Maintain a broad, open attitude. Expect the unexpected. Enjoy surprises.

- Avoid seeing all people as alike; that is, avoid cultural stereotypes, such as "all Chinese like rice" or "all Italians eat spaghetti."
- Try to understand the reasons for any behavior by discussing commonalities and differences.
- If a patient has said or done something that you do not understand, ask for clarification. Be a good listener. Most patients will respond positively to questions that arise from a genuine concern for and interest in them.
- If at all possible, speak the patient's language (even simple greetings and social courtesies will be appreciated). Avoid feigning an accent or using words that are ordinarily not part of your vocabulary.
- Be yourself. There are no right or wrong ways to learn about cultural diversity.

THE FUTURE OF TRANSCULTURAL NURSING CARE

By the middle of the 21st century, the average American patient will trace his or her ancestry to Africa, Asia, the Pacific Islands, or the Hispanic or Arab worlds, rather than to Europe (Giger et al., 1997). As indicated previously, the concept of culturally competent care applies to health care institutions, which must develop culturally sensitive policies and provide an atmosphere that fosters the provision of culturally competent care by nurses. Those nurses, who reflect the multicultural complexion of our society, must learn to acknowledge and adapt to diversity among their colleagues in the workplace. In addition, educational institutions must prepare nurses to deliver culturally competent care. Nursing programs, therefore, are exploring creative ways to promote cultural competence in nursing students (Bond & Jones, 1997).

With increasing frequency, nurses will be expected to provide culturally competent care for patients. Nurses must work effectively with patients, one another, and other health care team members whose ancestry reflects the multicultural complexion of contemporary society in increasing numbers. Cultural diversity remains one of the foremost issues in health care today.

Critical Thinking Exercises

1.
You are assigned to care for a hospitalized young adult whose cultural background is very different from yours. Describe how you would assess his cultural beliefs and practices in developing a nursing care plan. Explain why it is important to examine your own feelings about his cultural beliefs and practices.

2.
An elderly patient who does not speak English is hospitalized after elective surgery. Even though he is progressing well and his discharge has been planned, his family insists on staying with him for as many hours as possible, refusing to leave when visiting hours are over. How can you help the nursing staff to explore the meaning of the family's behavior and to understand their own feelings about this behavior? Devise a strategy that you think will help resolve this situation.

3.
You are preparing for a home visit to provide care for an elderly patient who is of foreign origin. The record indicates that she does not speak English and lives in a neighborhood where most of the residents are from the same ethnic background as herself. Describe how you would plan for this visit to ensure that you can communicate with the patient and family while providing the necessary nursing care. Explore other aspects of the patient's and family's background that you would want to assess before making the visit and while you are at the home.

References and Selected Readings

BOOKS

American Academy of Nursing. (1995). *Promoting cultural competence in and through nursing education.* Subpanel on Cultural Competence in Nursing Education. New York: Author.

American Association of Colleges of Nursing. (1996). *Diversity Task Force Report, October 1996.* Washington, D.C.: Author.

Andrews, M. M. & Boyle J. S. (1998). *Transcultural concepts in nursing care* (3rd ed.). Philadelphia: J. B. Lippincott.

Giger, J. N., & Davidhizar, R. E. (1995). *Transcultural nursing: Assessment and intervention.* St. Louis: C. V. Mosby.

Leininger, M. M. (1991). *Culture care diversity and universality: A theory of nursing.* New York: National League for Nursing Press.

Lipson, J. G., Dibble, S. L., & Minarik P. A. (1996). *Culture and nursing care: A pocket guide.* San Francisco: UCSF Nursing Press.

Smith-Temple, J., & Johnson J. Y. (1998). *Nurse's guide to clinical procedures.* Philadelphia: Lippincott-Raven.

JOURNALS

Bond, M. L. & Jones, M. E. (1997). Creating culturally competent professionals. *Reflections, 23*(2), 18–19.

Calnins, Z. P. (1997). The cultural and critical thinking connection. *Journal of Cultural Diversity, 4*(1):3–4.

Dibble, S. L. (1997). Celebrating diversity. *Reflections, 23*(2), 10–11.

Dreher, M. C. (1997). Global sharing among nurses. *Reflections, 23*(2), 5.

Giger, J. N., Davidhizar, R. E, Johnson, J. Y., & Poole, V. L. (1997). Health promotion among ethnic minorities: The importance of cultural phenomena. *Rehabilitation Nursing, 22*(6), 303–307.

Habayeb, G. L. (1995). Cultural diversity: A nursing concept not yet reliably defined. *Nursing Outlook, 43*(5), 224–227.

Leininger, M. M. (1988). Leininger's theory of nursing: Cultural care diversity and universality. *Nursing Science Quarterly, 1*(4), 152–159.

McGee, P. (1994). Culturally sensitive and culturally comprehensive care. *British Journal of Nursing, 3*(15), 789–793.

McSweeney J. C., Allan J. D., & Mayo K. (1997). Exploring the use of explanatory models in nursing research and practice. *Image: Journal of Nursing Scholarship, 29*(2), 243–248.

Taylor, R. (1998). Check your cultural competence. *Nursing Management, 29*(8): 30–32.

Villarruel, A. M. (1995). Culturally competent nursing research: Are we there yet? *Capsules and Comments in Pediatric Nursing, 1*(4), 18–25.

White, M. A. (1997). Global nursing collaborations. *Reflections, 23*(2), 22–23.

Resources

ORGANIZATIONS

Asian-Pacific Islander Nurses Association, c/o College of Mount Saint Vincent, 6301 Riverdale Avenue, Riverdale, NY 10471; 1-718-405-3354.

Council on Nursing and Anthropology, c/o Dr. Mildred Roberson, Nursing and Health Sciences, Salisbury State University, Salisbury, MD 21801

National Association of Hispanic Nurses, 1501 16th Street NW, Washington, DC 20036; 1-202-387-2477

National Black Nurses Association, P.O. Box 1823, Washington, DC 20012-1823; 1-202-393-6870

Native American Indian Association, 927 Treadale Lane, Cloquet, MN 55720; 1-218-879-1227

Office of Minority Health, U.S. Department of Health and Human Services, P.O. Box 37337, Washington, DC 20013-7337; 1-800-444-6472. No cost for accessing database, information specialists, resource network, and publications on major health problems affecting African Americans, Hispanics, Native Americans, and Asian/Pacific Islanders.

Transcultural Nursing Society, c/o Madonna University College of Nursing and Health, 36600 Schoolcraft Road, Livonia MI 48150-1173; 1-800-TCN-9995

TRANSLATION SERVICES

AT&T Language Line Services; 1-800-752-6096. Provides written and oral translation in 140 languages.

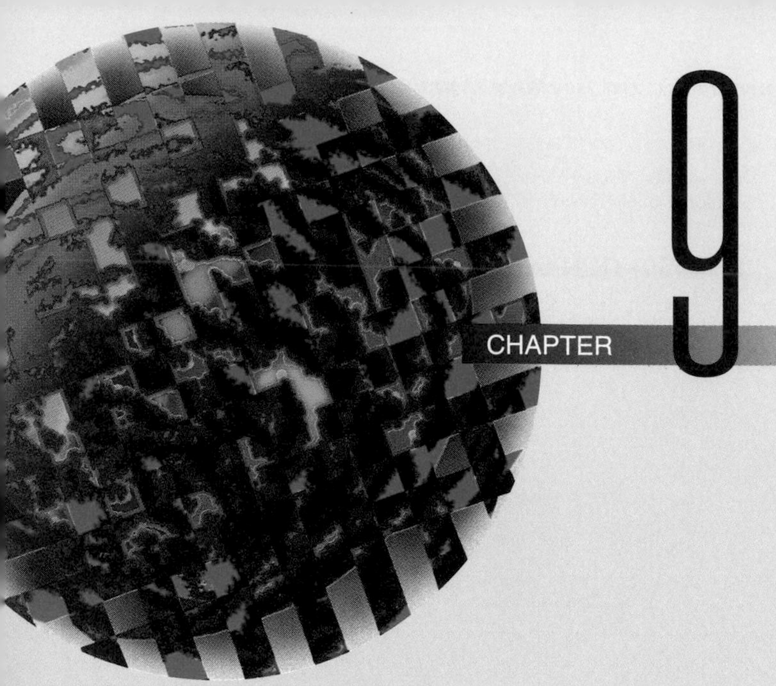

Chronic Illness

Learning Objectives

On completion of this chapter, the learner will be able to:

1. Define chronic conditions.
2. Identify factors related to the increasing incidence of chronic conditions.
3. Describe characteristics of chronic conditions and implications for people with chronic conditions and their family.
4. Describe the phases of chronic conditions.
5. Apply the nursing process to the care of the patient with chronic conditions.

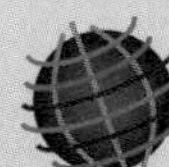

Chronic health problems affect people of all ages—they occur in the very young, the middle aged, and the very old (Hoffman, Rice, & Sung, 1996). Many chronic conditions are more common in one age group than another; however, chronic conditions increase in frequency with age, and elderly people often have multiple chronic illnesses (Wilkins & Park, 1996). Chronic illnesses are found in all socioeconomic, ethnic, cultural, and racial groups but are more common in people from lower socioeconomic groups (Kington & Smith, 1997). This is most likely a result of this population having suboptimal nutrition and less access to health care. Chronic conditions can have little if any effect on activity or lifestyle (as in a very mild skin condition or chronic sinusitis) or can lead to dependence on advanced technology for survival (as in advanced amyotrophic lateral sclerosis or end-stage renal disease). Some people with chronic health problems function independently and lead full lives with only minor disruption, whereas others require frequent and close monitoring or permanent placement in a long-term care facility.

THE PHENOMENON OF CHRONICITY

Each chronic condition has its own specific physiologic characteristics; however, chronic conditions also share common qualities. For example, many chronic conditions have pain and fatigue as associated symptoms. Some degree of disability is usually present in severe or advanced chronic illness, limiting the patient's participation in activities (Collins, 1997). Many chronic conditions require therapeutic regimens to keep them under control. Unlike the term *acute*, which implies a curable and relatively short disease course, *chronic* describes a long disease course and conditions that may be incurable (Murrow & Oglesby, 1996). It is this characteristic of duration that often makes managing chronic conditions so difficult for those who must live with them.

Psychological and emotional reactions of patients to acute and chronic conditions and changes in their health status are described in detail in Chapter 7. People who develop chronic conditions may react with shock and disbelief, depression, anger, resentment, or a number of other emotions. The ways that people react and cope with chronic conditions are often similar to their reactions to other events in their lives, depending, in part, on their understanding of the condition and their perceptions of its potential effect on their lives, their families, and their lifestyles.

Psychological, emotional, and cognitive reactions to chronic conditions are likely to occur at initial onset but tend to reoccur as symptoms reappear or worsen. Symptoms associated with chronic illnesses are often unpredictable, and some are perceived as crisis events by patients and their families, who must contend with both the uncertainty of chronic illness and the changes brought about in their lives. This chapter describes some of the problems of living with and managing chronic conditions and offers a guide to nursing assessment and intervention when providing care to people with chronic illness.

Definition of Chronic Conditions

Chronic conditions are defined as medical conditions or health problems with associated symptoms or disabilities that require long-term (3 months or longer) management (Robert Wood Johnson Foundation, 1996). The condition may be due to illness, congenital defect, or injury. Part of the management of such conditions includes learning to live with symptoms or disabilities and coming to terms with identity changes that might result from having a chronic condition. Another part of the management consists of carrying out the lifestyle changes and regimens that are designed to keep symptoms under control and to prevent complications. Although some people take on what might be called a "sick role" identity, most people with chronic conditions do not consider themselves sick or ill and try to live as normal a life as is possible (Robinson, 1993). Often it is only when complications develop or when severe symptoms interfere with performance of daily life activities that those who are chronically ill think of themselves as being "sick" (Nijhof, 1998).

Prevalence and Causes of Chronic Conditions

Chronic conditions occur in people of every age group, socioeconomic level, and culture. In 1995, an estimated 99 million people in the United States had chronic conditions. It has been projected that, by the year 2030, 150 million people will be affected (Robert Wood Johnson Foundation, 1996). Table 9-1 shows the projected increase in rates of people with chronic conditions by year, along with an estimation of the costs to be incurred in managing those conditions. As stated, not all chronic conditions are disabling. Some cause only minor inconveniences. Many, however, are severe enough to cause major activity limitations. Figures 9-1 and 9-2 present overviews of the projected number of people in millions with activity limitations and the five most disabling chronic conditions. People with activity limitations need assistance with their activities of daily living. Figure 9-3 indicates what happens to people with activity limitations whose needs for health care and personal services are not met for various reasons. They may be unable to carry out their therapeutic regimens as prescribed or have their prescriptions filled on time; they may miss physicians' appointments and office visits; and they may be unable to carry out the activities of daily living (Robert Wood Johnson Foundation, 1996). These figures provide an overview of the scope of the problem and are useful in planning health promotion and education programs as well as in allocating resources and services.

Chronic conditions have become the major cause of health-related problems in developed countries. Even developing countries are seeing an increase in chronic conditions, giving these countries the dual burden of trying to eradicate infectious diseases while learning to manage chronic conditions (Kickbusch, 1997). Some of the reasons that so many people are afflicted with chronic conditions include the following:

- A decrease in mortality rates from infectious diseases, such as smallpox and diphtheria, and other serious conditions

TABLE 9•1 Estimated Number of People and Direct Medical Costs for People With Chronic Conditions, Selected Years, 1995–2050

	1995	2000	2005	2010	2020	2030	2040	2050
People	99 million	105 million	112 million	120 million	134 million	148 million	158 million	167 million
Dollar costs	$470 billion	$503 billion	$539 billion	$582 billion	$685 billion	$798 billion	$864 billion	$906 billion

With permission from Robert Wood Johnson Foundation. (1996). *Chronic care in America: A 21st century challenge.* Princeton, NJ: Author.

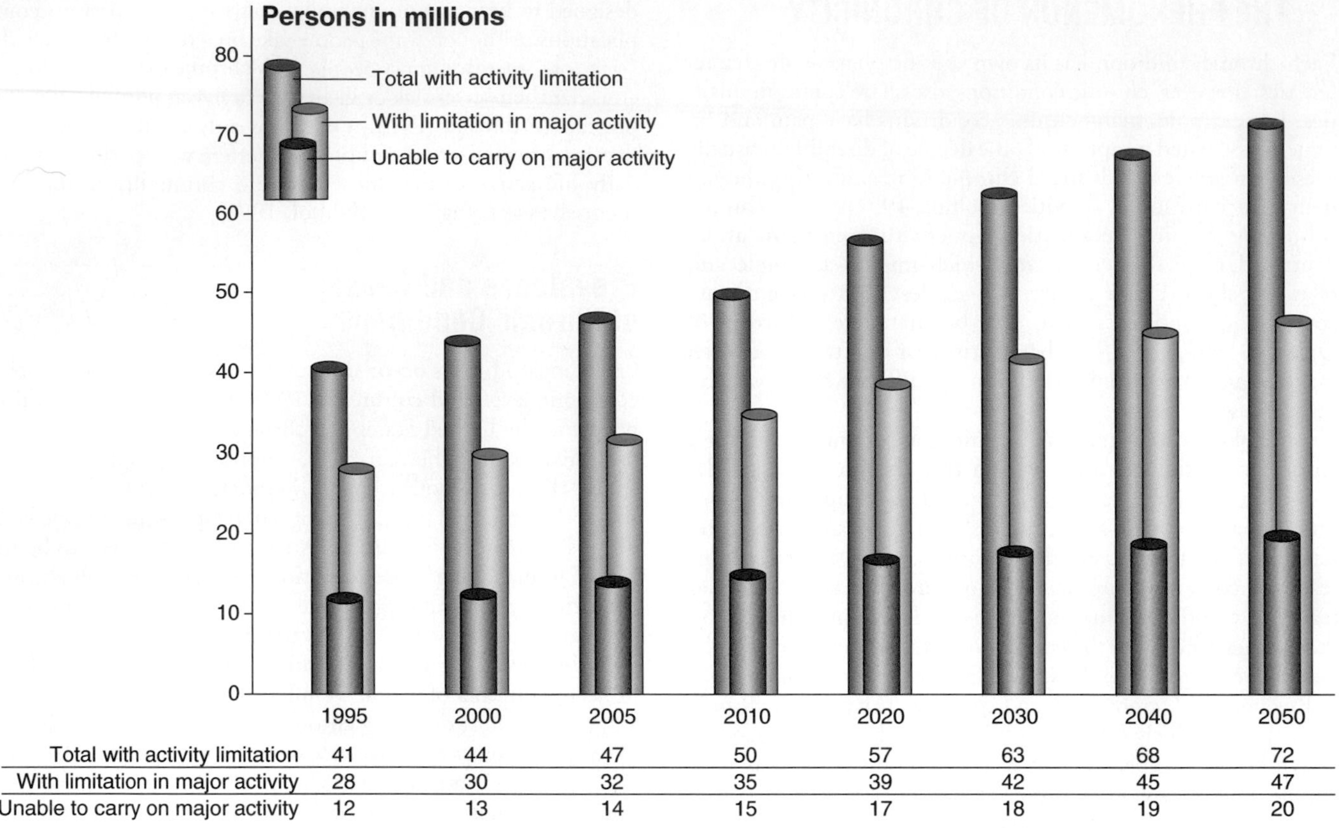

	1995	2000	2005	2010	2020	2030	2040	2050
Total with activity limitation	41	44	47	50	57	63	68	72
With limitation in major activity	28	30	32	35	39	42	45	47
Unable to carry on major activity	12	13	14	15	17	18	19	20

FIGURE 9•1 Projected number of persons by degree of activity limitation due to chronic condition, selected years, 1995–2050. The number of people who will be unable to go to school, to work, or to live independently because of a chronic condition is projected to reach 20 million by 2050. With permission from Robert Wood Johnson Foundation. (1996). *Chronic care in America: A 21st century challenge*. Princeton, NJ: Author.

- Longer life spans because of advances in technology and pharmacology, improved nutrition, safer working conditions, and greater access (for some people) to health care
- Improved screening and diagnostic procedures enabling early detection and treatment of diseases
- Prompt and aggressive management of acute conditions, such as myocardial infarction and AIDS-related infections
- The tendency to develop single and often multiple chronic illnesses with advancing age
- Modern living habits, such as smoking, that lead to increased risk of chronic illnesses such as chronic obstructive pulmonary disease and cardiovascular disease

A major problem with chronic conditions is that although the physiologic changes often begin early in life, symptoms and disability usually do not appear until later (De Flora et al., 1996). Greater emphasis has recently been placed on the promotion of healthy lifestyles (beginning in childhood); however, it will be

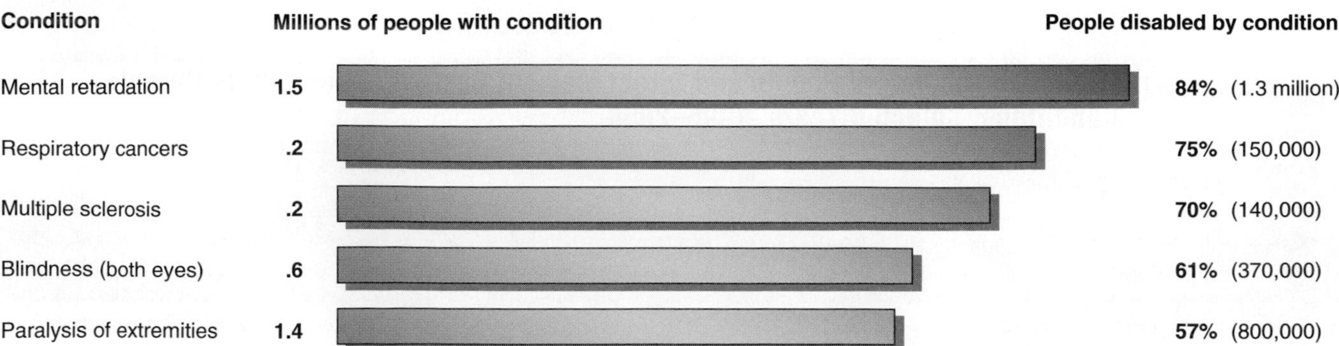

FIGURE 9•2 Five most disabling chronic conditions. With permission from Robert Wood Johnson Foundation. (1996). *Chronic care in America: A 21st century challenge.* Princeton, NJ: Author.

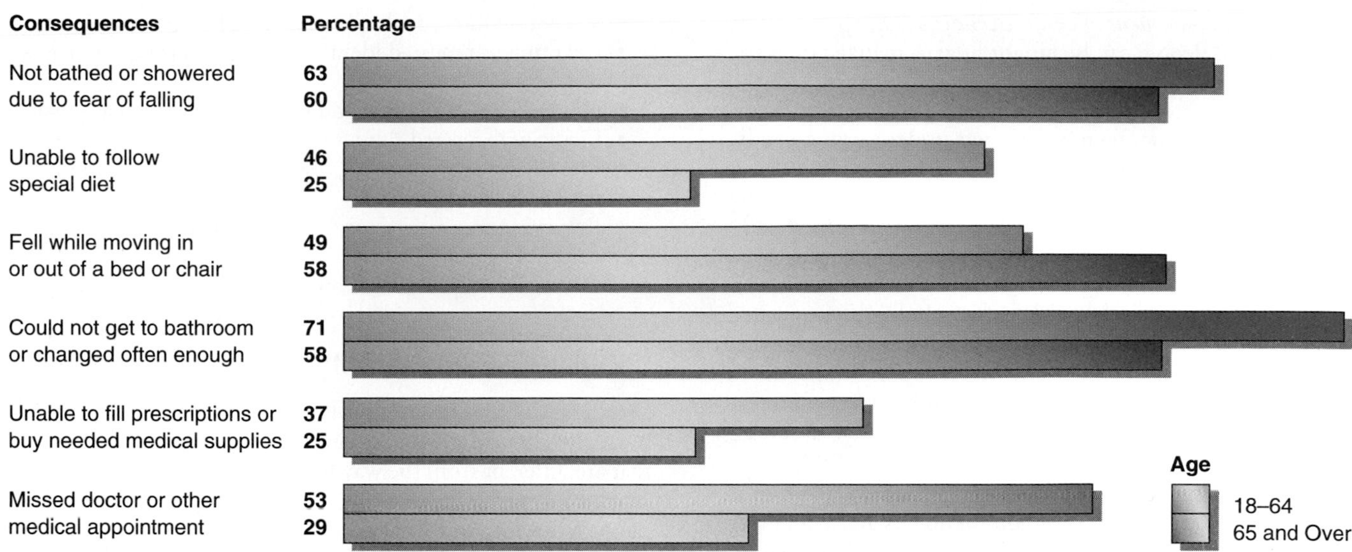

FIGURE 9•3 The consequences of unmet needs for help, by age group. With permission from Robert Wood Johnson Foundation. (1996). *Chronic care in America: A 21st century challenge.* Princeton, NJ: Author.

some time before this results in a measurable decrease in the incidence of chronic health problems.

THE IMPLICATIONS OF CHRONICITY

Chronic conditions affect the lives of many people in many ways, either directly or indirectly. At a time when so much emphasis is placed on youth and good health, it can be difficult to understand how lives are affected and often changed forever because of chronic illness. Only by developing sensitivity to these issues can nurses, other health care providers, and society begin to address these problems (Lubkin, 1997; Sidell, 1997). The implications of chronicity include the following:

1. *Managing chronic illness involves more than managing medical problems.* Associated psychological and social problems must also be addressed. Living permanently or for long periods of time with symptoms and disability may lead to identity adjustments, role changes, and the need to cope with an altered body image or lifestyle (Charmaz, 1994). Adaptation to illness and disability is a continuous process. Each major change or decrease in functional ability requires further physical, emotional, and social adaptation, for both the patient and the family (Bury, 1991; Lewis, 1998).
2. *Chronic conditions can pass through many different phases over the course of the disease* (Roland, 1987). There can be stable and unstable periods, flare-ups, and remissions. Each phase brings its own set of physical, psychological, and social problems, and each requires different regimens and types of management (Corbin & Strauss, 1988).
3. *Keeping chronic conditions under control requires persistent adherence to therapeutic regimens.* Failing to adhere to a treatment plan or to follow the regimen in a consistent manner can increase the risks of developing complications or accelerate the disease process. Yet, the realities of daily living, as well as culture, values, and socioeconomic factors, affect the degree to which a person will adhere to a treatment regimen. Managing a chronic illness takes time, requires knowledge and planning (Baker, 1998), and can be uncomfortable and inconvenient. It is not unusual for patients to discontinue taking medications or to alter dosages because the side effects are more disturbing or disruptive than illness symptoms. People frequently cut back on regimens they consider overly time-consuming, fatiguing, or costly (Cameron, 1996; Wiebe & Christensen, 1996).
4. *One chronic disease can lead to other chronic conditions.* For example, diabetes can eventually lead to neurologic and circulatory changes that may result in vision, cardiac, sexual, and kidney problems.
5. *Chronic illness affects the whole family.* Not only do family members become involved in managing chronic conditions, especially those affecting children and the elderly, but family life can be dramatically altered as a result of role reversals (Saiki-Craighill, 1997), unfilled roles, loss of income, time spent managing illness, decreases in family socialization activities, and the costs of treatment. There is often tension, stress, and fatigue within the family, especially among the caregivers. The effects of chronic conditions on the family can be profound, sometimes drawing members closer together, other times driving them apart (Graves & Hayes, 1996; Knafl, Breitmayer, Gallo, & Zoeller, 1996; Robert Wood Johnson Foundation, 1996).
6. *People with chronic conditions and their families must assume major responsibility for the day-to-day management of the condition.* With chronic conditions, the home, rather than the hospital, is the center of care. Settings such as hospitals, clinics, doctors' offices, nursing homes, nursing centers, and community agencies (visiting nurse services, social services, and disease-specific associations and societies) are adjuncts to that care, but the day-to-day work of following or managing the treatment regimens falls on the shoulders of the patient and family (Strauss & Corbin, 1988).

7. *The management of chronic conditions is a process of discovery.* People can be taught how to manage their condition. Teaching about symptoms, however, is not the same as experiencing them. Each person must discover how his or her own body reacts under varying conditions, for example, what it is like to be hypoglycemic, what activities are likely to bring on angina, and how either of these conditions can best be prevented and managed.
8. *Managing chronic conditions is a collaborative process.* Because the medical, social, and psychological problems associated with chronic problems tend to be so complex and interrelated, especially in severe conditions, the collaborative efforts of many different health care professionals are required to provide the full range of services that are often needed (Corbin & Cherry, 1997).
9. *The management of chronic conditions is expensive.* As indicated in Table 9-1, billions of dollars are spent every year on health care, including hospitalizations, and on the purchase of equipment, medications, and assistive services. These expenditures cause a drain on the individual, the family, and the national financial resources.
10. *Chronic conditions pose ethical dilemmas for the patient, health care professionals, and society.* There are no easy solutions to issues, such as when to terminate care, how to establish cost controls, how to allocate scarce resources (eg, transplantations), and how to evaluate quality of life. Ethical issues are moral ones, and each patient responds according to his or her own set of criteria and the constraints set by the situation (Wurzbach, 1996).
11. *Living with chronic illness means living with uncertainty* (Mishel, 1990; Yarcheski, 1988). Although health care professionals can identify the anticipated course of an illness, they cannot determine with certainty what that exact course will be for each patient. Even when a patient has been labeled as being "in remission" or "disease free," there is always that lingering doubt and dread that the illness will recur (Smeltzer, 1992).

The Problems of Managing Chronic Care Conditions

The implications of chronic conditions for people and society are profound. These implications can be translated into everyday problems, such as the difficulties and challenges of living with or managing chronic conditions on the part of patients, their families, and their health care providers. Initial efforts should be directed at preventing chronic conditions. Once a chronic condition occurs, however, the overall management problem shifts from prevention to managing symptoms and obtaining some control over the course of the condition, while maintaining an acceptable quality of life. The problems of chronicity are felt most acutely by the patient and family. These problems also present challenges to health care providers and other professionals who provide the supportive assistance and services that enable patients and their families to manage at home. Everyday problems associated with chronic conditions include the following:

- Preventing the occurrence of chronic conditions
- Alleviating and managing symptoms
- Preventing, adapting to, and managing disabilities
- Preventing and managing crises and complications
- Attaining, maintaining, and regaining illness stability
- Validating individual self-worth and family functioning
- Adapting to repeated identity threats and progressive loss of function
- Normalizing individual and family life as much as possible
- Living with altered time, social isolation, and loneliness
- Identifying and obtaining resources and establishing networks of support
- Returning to a satisfactory life after an acute phase of a chronic illness
- Dying with dignity and comfort

Implications for Nursing

Working with the chronically ill presents a set of challenges to the nurse. People living with an illness often act or respond in ways that are different from the way health care providers expect. Perception of quality of life is often the driving force behind a patient's behavior, and what is considered quality of life is determined by each patient individually. Although it may be difficult for nurses and other health care providers to stand by while patients make unwise decisions about their health, they must accept the fact that patients have the right to make their own choices about lifestyle and health care. Patients should be able to make such decisions and choices without fear of ridicule or refusal of treatment.

As stated previously, chronic conditions have a course, although that course might be uncertain. The course can be thought of as a trajectory, or as a path that can be directed or at least somewhat controlled through proper illness management strategies (Robinson et al., 1993; Strauss et al., 1984; Woog, 1992). The trajectory can be broken into phases. This enables more precise thinking about the condition, what is happening now, what came before, and what can be anticipated in the future. Each phase brings different problems and necessitates a specific approach to care. It is important to remember that not all chronic conditions are necessarily life-threatening, and not all people pass through each phase.

Phases of Chronic Illness

During the course of their trajectory, chronic conditions can pass through several different phases (Corbin & Strauss, 1991). Nine phases have been identified, as follows (Table 9-2):

1. The **pretrajectory phase** describes the stage at which the person is at risk for developing a chronic condition because of genetic factors or lifestyle behaviors that increase the person's susceptibility to chronic illness.
2. The **trajectory phase** is characterized by the onset of symptoms or disability associated with a chronic condition. This phase is often accompanied by uncertainty of the trajectory of the chronic condition as symptoms are being evaluated and diagnostic tests are performed.
3. The **stable phase** of the trajectory indicates that symptoms and disability are under control or managed.
4. The **unstable phase** is characterized by instability of the course because of recurrence of symptoms, development of complications, or reactivation of the illness. During this phase, the person's everyday activities may be disrupted by symptoms and the need to develop new regimens or strategies to manage the problems.
5. The **acute phase** is characterized by sudden onset of severe or unrelieved symptoms or complications that

TABLE 9•2 Phases in the Trajectory Model of Chronic Illness

Phase	Description
Pretrajectory	Genetic factors or lifestyle behaviors that place an individual or community at risk for the development of a chronic condition
Trajectory onset	Appearance of noticeable symptoms; includes period of diagnostic workup and announcement of diagnosis; may be accompanied by biographic limbo as patient begins to discover and cope with implications of diagnosis
Stable	Illness course and symptoms are under control; biography and everyday life activities are being managed within limitations of illness; illness management centered in the home
Unstable	Period of inability to keep symptoms under control or reactivation of illness; biographic disruption and difficulty in carrying out everyday life activities; adjustments being made in regimen with care usually taking place at home
Acute	Severe and unrelieved symptoms or the development of illness complications necessitating hospitalization or bed rest to bring illness course under control; biography and everyday life activities temporarily placed on hold or drastically cut back
Crisis	Critical or life-threatening situation requiring emergency treatment or care; biography and everyday life activities suspended until the crisis passes
Comeback	Gradual return to an acceptable way of life within limits imposed by disability or illness; involves physical healing, stretching limitations through rehabilitative procedures, psychosocial coming to terms, and biographic reengagement with adjustments in everyday life activities
Downward	Illness course characterized by rapid or gradual physical decline accompanied by increasing disability or difficulty in controlling symptoms; requires biographic adjustment and alterations in everyday life activity with each major downward step
Dying	Final days or weeks before death; characterized by gradual or rapid shutting down of body processes, biographic disengagement and closure, and relinquishment of everyday life interests and activities

necessitate hospitalization for their management. This phase may require major modification of the person's usual activities for a period of time.

6. The **crisis phase** is characterized by a critical or life-threatening situation that requires emergency treatment or care.
7. The **comeback phase** is the period in the trajectory marked by recovery after an acute period. It includes learning to live with or to overcome disabilities and a return to an acceptable way of living within the limitations imposed by the chronic condition.
8. The **downward phase** occurs when symptoms worsen or the disability progresses despite attempts to control the course through proper regimen management. A downward turn does not necessarily lead to death. The downward trend can be arrested and the trajectory restabilized at any point depending on the condition and the treatment.
9. The **dying phase** is characterized by the gradual or rapid decline in the trajectory despite efforts to halt the disorder or slow the decline through illness management; it is characterized by failure of life-maintaining body functions.

Nursing Management

Nursing care of patients with chronic conditions is varied and occurs in an assortment of settings from home to hospital, depending on the trajectory phase. It can include provision of direct care, such as the administration of medications or treatments either at home, in the clinic, or in the hospital. Because much of the responsibility for managing the condition lies with the patient (and family), the nurse often takes on a more supportive role; this includes helping patients and families to manage their conditions through teaching, counseling, serving as an advocate for the patient, making referrals, and case-managing. In fact, when it comes to chronic conditions, these latter roles are equal in importance to the provision of direct care. For example, a nurse might detect signs of an impending complication before it is noticeable to the patient and refer the patient for medical care, thereby preventing lengthy and costly hospitalization.

Care by Phase: Applying the Nursing Process

The focus of care of patients with chronic conditions is determined largely by trajectory phase and directed by the nursing process—assessment, diagnosis, planning, implementation, and evaluation.

Step 1: Identifying the Trajectory Phase

The first step is assessment of the patient to determine the specific phase (see Table 9-2). Assessment enables the nurse to identify the specific medical, social, and psychological problems likely to be encountered in a phase. For instance, the problems and subsequent care of a patient having an acute myocardial infarction (type of direct care, teaching needs, psychological needs) are different from those likely to be encountered in later stages of the disease, for example, when the patient is dying at home of heart failure or living at home with the disabilities of multiple sclerosis.

Step 2: Establishing Goals

Once the patient has been located within the trajectory and the specific medical, social, and psychological problems are identified, the second step involves establishing the goals of care with the patient and family. As an example, a patient may report that frequent angina or chest pain interferes with the ability to carry out activities of daily living. Related nursing diagnoses might include activity intolerance self-care deficit related to discomfort or pain (angina) secondary to cardiac disease. The goal of care might be to prevent or minimize these episodes. An example of a goal for a patient with impaired self-care related to fatigue associated with multiple sclerosis might be identifying strategies to improve self-care abilities. Goals for a patient at home with terminal cancer are likely to be relief of pain and dying with dignity.

Step 3: Establishing a Plan to Meet Goals

The third step consists of establishing a realistic and mutually agreed on plan for reaching the established goals. Specific criteria to be used to assess progress in meeting the goals would also be identified. For example, a plan of care for the patient with angina might include assisting the patient to identify which activities of daily living are likely to precipitate angina and developing symptom management or organizing self-care strategies that minimize the occurrence of such episodes. Criteria might include statements that indicate progress toward the goal, such as the following:

- At the end of the first nurse–patient session, the patient will be able to state four activities of daily living that usually precipitate angina and describe how those situations can be avoided or altered to minimize angina.
- Two weeks after discharge from the hospital, the patient will report fewer episodes of angina and a greater ability to engage in desired activities of daily living.
- One month after discharge, the patient will report the ability to anticipate which activities of daily living are likely to cause angina and will identify specific preventive actions.

The goal is to help the patient improve his or her quality of life through participating in activities while keeping the episodes of angina to a minimum.

Criteria for a patient who is unable to participate in self-care activities because of fatigue secondary to multiple sclerosis might include the following:

- The patient will identify those self-care activities of highest personal priority by the time the home care nurse has completed the first visit.
- Strategies to minimize nonessential activities will be identified by the patient at the beginning of the second visit by the nurse.
- By the third home care visit, the patient will report increased participation in those self-care activities that are personally important.

Step 4: Identifying Factors That Facilitate or Hinder Attainment of Goals

This step involves determining environmental, social, and psychological factors that may interfere with or facilitate achieving the goal. For example, in the case of the patient with angina, having to climb stairs several times a day may increase fatigue and precipitate symptoms. The nurse would also want to know if symptoms are associated with other activities, such as eating. Are there certain activities, such as sex, that the patient or spouse fears? Does the person carry nitroglycerin tablets at all times? How does the person use and store the tablets? Identifying barriers as well as factors that might enhance goal attainment is important. Nurses help patients and families to develop strategies to work around barriers to self-care and to make use of other factors in the environment, such as resources, that might enhance goal attainment.

In the example of the patient with multiple sclerosis, the nurse and patient might identify evening as the period when the patient is the most fatigued and therefore most likely to encounter difficulty carrying out activities of daily living, such as getting ready for bed. Obtaining help with these activities may be difficult because of lack of resources needed to hire help. The lack of resources is a barrier to self-care. In that case, the nurse and patient might work out a schedule for pacing activities throughout the day and planning for rest periods, so that the patient is not so tired at night. Additionally, the nurse would assist the patient to identify resources, such as neighbors or family members who might be called on when fatigue becomes overwhelming. The nurse might make a referral to social service personnel, who might work with the patient to find ways of financing additional help.

Step 5: Implementing Interventions

The fifth step is the intervention phase. Interventions include providing direct care, serving as advocate for the patient, teaching, counseling, making referrals, and case-managing—arranging for resources. For example, if it is determined in the previous step that one of the situations most likely to precipitate angina is showering and shaving after breakfast, the nurse might counsel the patient to shower and shave before eating breakfast or to shower the evening before retiring and shave the next morning, so that both activities do not occur together. If climbing the stairs precipitates angina, the nurse could counsel the patient to plan activities so that most activities of daily living were completed before going downstairs, minimizing the number of trips up or down. Also, counseling the patient to take prophylactic nitroglycerin before climbing the stairs and climbing stairs slowly and stopping to rest every few steps might be appropriate.

If the patient with multiple sclerosis attempts to carry out self-care activities when fatigue is at its highest level, such as at night, the nurse might suggest ways to reschedule and plan activities more efficiently. There are many different strategies that a patient might use to prevent or minimize episodes of angina or fatigue; the patient and nurse have to discover which work the best to control the symptoms and which fit best with the patient's and family's lifestyle.

Nursing Alert *Whereas the physician can prescribe appropriate medication and give advice on when and how to use it, it is the nurse who can best help patients develop the strategies needed to implement their regimens and carry out activities of daily living within the limits of a chronic condition. In fact, this is the most important role of the nurse working with patients with chronic conditions and their families.*

Step 6: Evaluating the Effectiveness of Interventions

The final step is evaluating the effectiveness of interventions. In chronic illness, ongoing management is the goal. In many situations, success is more a matter of making progress toward meeting the goals than of making drastic changes. Changing lifestyles, habits, and behaviors is difficult. Nurses cannot expect that sedentary patients are going to develop a sudden passion for exercise, or that others can easily rearrange their day to accommodate time-consuming regimens. Bringing about change takes time, patience, and a lot of encouragement on the part of the nurse. If no progress is made or progress toward goals is unduly slow, it may be necessary to redefine the goals. The patient may not be ready, or other conditions such as depression may be interfering with the ability to carry out regimens or accept lifestyle changes. This is why it is so important to identify barriers to change. Also, nurses must accept that there are people for whom change is not possible. For example, a person might be unwilling to give up smoking despite advanced chronic obstructive pulmonary disease. Nurses should not feel that this is a failure on their part. Patients share responsibility for management of their condition, and outcomes are as much related to the patient's ability to accommodate to the illness and carry out regimens as they are to nursing intervention.

PROMOTING HOME AND COMMUNITY-BASED CARE

Teaching Patients Self-Care

Chronic conditions are costly to individuals, families, and societies. The major focus of nursing as we move into the twenty-first century should be on the prevention of chronic conditions. This means promoting healthy lifestyles and encouraging the use of safety and disease prevention measures, such as wearing seat belts and obtaining immunizations. Prevention should begin early in the prenatal period, infancy, or childhood, and continue throughout the life span. The importance of patient and family teaching cannot be overemphasized. It is one of the most significant aspects of nursing care and may make the difference between a patient's success or failure at preventing chronic health conditions or at adapting to chronic health conditions. Well-informed, educated patients are more likely to be concerned about their health and what is necessary to maintain it. They are more likely to recognize symptoms and the onset of complications and to seek health care early. Knowledge is the key to making informed choices and decisions during any phase of the chronic illness trajectory.

Despite the importance of teaching the patient and family, the nurse must recognize that patients recently diagnosed with serious chronic conditions and their families need time to grasp the significance of their condition and its effect on their life. Teaching should be planned carefully so that it provides information that is important to the patient's well-being at the time without being overwhelming.

The nurse who cares for patients with chronic conditions in the hospital, clinic, or home needs to assess the patient's knowledge about the illness and its management. The nurse cannot assume that a patient who has had an illness for a number of years has all the knowledge needed. The patient's learning needs change as the trajectory phases and the patient's personal life change. The nurse must also realize that patients may have managed their own care at home for some time, and they know how their body responds under certain conditions and how best to manage their symptoms. Nevertheless, the nurse's contact with the patient in the hospital, clinic, or home is often an ideal time to reassess the patient's learning needs and ability to manage the health care problem and to provide additional information about its management.

Continuing Care

Chronic illness management is a collaborative process between patient, family, nurse, and other health care professionals (Graves & Hayes, 1996). Collaboration is not limited to hospital settings; rather, it should continue throughout the illness trajectory. Keeping an illness stable over time requires careful and continued monitoring of symptoms and attention to regimens. Detecting problems early and assisting patients to develop appropriate management strategies can make a significant difference in outcome.

Most chronic conditions are managed in the home. Therefore, care and teaching during hospitalization should focus on what the patient needs to know to manage the condition at home. Nurses in all settings should be aware of the resources and services available and facilitate without delay arrangements to secure those resources and services. When appropriate, home care services are contacted directly. The home care nurse will continue the plan of care and assess how well the patient and family are adapting to the chronic condition and its treatment. Finally, because chronic conditions occur worldwide and the world is becoming increasingly interconnected, nurses should think beyond the individual level to the community and global levels, especially in terms of prevention and health promotion.

Critical Thinking Exercises

1. A 24-year-old woman has just been diagnosed with lupus. She is very upset about the diagnosis, concerned about her potential for childbearing, and refusing to listen to teaching about illness management. How would you respond to her reaction to the diagnosis?
2. A 46-year-old man has developed complications from a chronic health problem that he has had but largely ignored for the past 20 years. Describe how you would determine what factors and psychological reactions to consider in developing a teaching plan to assist the patient in dealing with the complications.
3. How would the learning needs of a patient with a newly diagnosed chronic condition differ from those of a patient with a chronic condition that has been stable for many years, and from those of a patient who has experienced progressive deterioration in health status? Describe those factors that would be the focus of your assessment in these three patients to assess their needs for patient education.
4. A 55-year-old patient with continuous severe pain has been informed by his physician that he has cancer, that he is likely to survive for no longer than 6 months, and that no medical treatment is likely to increase the length of his survival. How would you address the patient's goals to maintain his quality of life and to "get his affairs in order" in the time he has remaining? What resources would you consider in helping him to accomplish his goals?

References and Selected Readings

BOOKS

Corbin, J., & Cherry, J. (1997). Caring for the chronically ill elderly in the community. In L. Swanson & T. Tripp-Reiner (Eds.). *Advances in gerontological nursing* (Vol. 2). New York: Springer.

Corbin, J., & Strauss, A. (1988). *Unending work and care.* San Francisco: Jossey-Bass.

Lubkin, I. M. (1997). *Chronic illness: Impact and interventions.* Boston: Jones & Bartlett.

Robert Wood Johnson Foundation. (1996). *Chronic care in America: A 21st century challenge.* Princeton, NJ: Author.

Roland, J. S. (1987). Chronic illness and the family: An overview. In L. Wright & M. Leahey (Eds.). *Families and chronic illness* (pp. 239–252). Springhouse, PA: Springhouse.

Smeltzer, S. C. (1992). Use of the trajectory model of nursing in multiple sclerosis. In P. Woog (Ed.). *The chronic illness trajectory framework* (pp. 73–88). New York: Springer.

Strauss, A., & Corbin, J. (1988). *Shaping a new health care system.* San Francisco: Jossey-Bass.

Strauss, A., et al. (1984). *Chronic illness and the quality of life* (2nd ed.). St. Louis: C.V. Mosby.

Woog, P. (Ed.). (1992). *The chronic illness trajectory framework.* New York: Springer.

JOURNALS

Asterisks indicate nursing research articles.

Baker, L. M. (1988). Sense making in multiple sclerosis: The information needs of people during an acute exacerbation. *Qualitative Health Journal, 8*(1), 106–120.

Bury, M. (1991). The sociology of chronic illness: A review of research and prospects. *Sociology of Health and Illness, 13*(4), 451–468.

Cameron, C. (1996). Patient compliance: Recognition of factors involved and suggestions for promoting compliance with therapeutic regimens. *Journal of Advanced Nursing, 24,* 244–250.

Charmaz, K. (1994). Identity dilemmas of chronically ill men. *Sociology Quarterly, 35*(2), 269–288.

Collins, J. G. (1997). Prevalence of selected chronic conditions: United States, 1990–1992. *Vital Health Statistics, 10*(194), 1–89.

Corbin, J., & Strauss, A. (1991). A nursing model for chronic illness management based upon the trajectory framework. *Scholarly Inquiry for Nursing Practice, 5*(3), 155–174.

*De Flora, S., et al. (1996). DNA adducts and chronic degenerative disease: Pathogenetic relevance and implications in preventive medicine. *Mutation Research, 366*(3), 197–238.

Forsyth, G., Delaney, K., & Gresham, L. (1984). Vying for a winning position: Management style of the chronically ill. *Research in Nursing & Health, 7,* 181–188.

Graves, C., & Hayes, V. (1996). Do nurses and parents of children with chronic conditions agree of parental needs? *Journal of Pediatric Nursing, 11*(5), 288–299.

Hoffman, C., Rice, D., & Sung, H. Y. (1996). Persons with chronic conditions: Their prevalence and costs. *Journal of the American Medical Association, 276*(18), 1473–1479.

Jillings, C. (1987). Is chronic illness a relevant topic for the critical care nurse? *Critical Care Nurse, 7*(3), 14–17.

Kickbusch, I. (1997). *Think health: What makes the difference?* Paper Presented at the Fourth International Conference on Health Promotion, World Health Organization, Jakarta, July.

Kington, R. S., & Smith, J. P. (1997). Socioeconomic status and racial and ethnic differences in functional status associated with chronic disease. *American Journal of Public Health, 87*(5), 805–810.

*Knafl, K., Breitmayer, B., Gallo, A., & Zoeller, L. (1996). Family response to childhood chronic illness: Description of management styles. *Journal of Pediatric Nursing, 11*(5), 315–326.

Lewis, K. S. (1998). Emotional adjustment to a chronic illness. *Lippincott's Primary Care Practice, 2*(1), 38–51.

*Michael, S. R. (1996). Integrating chronic illness into one's life: A phenomenological inquiry. *Journal of Holistic Nursing, 14*(3), 251–267.

*Mishel, M. H. (1990). Reconceptualization of the uncertainty in illness theory. *Image: Journal of Nursing Scholarship, 22*(4), 256–262.

Murrow, E. J., & Oglesby F. M. (1996). Acute and chronic illness: Similarities, differences and challenges. *Orthopaedic Nursing, 15*(5), 47–51.

Nijhof, G. (1998). Heterogeneity in the interpretation of epilepsy. *Qualitative Health Research, 8*(1), 95–105.

*Pollock, S. E. (1993). Adaptation to chronic illness: A program of research for testing nursing theory. *Nursing Science Quarterly, 6*(2), 86–92.

*Price, B. (1996). Illness careers: The chronic illness experience. *Journal of Advanced Nursing, 24*(2), 275–279.

*Robinson, C. A. (1993). Managing life with a chronic condition: The story of normalization. *Qualitative Health Research, 3*(1), 6–28.

Robinson, L., et al. (1993). Operationalizing the Corbin & Strauss Trajectory Model for elderly clients with chronic illness. *Scholarly Inquiry for Nursing Practice, 7*(4), 253–264.

Saiki-Craighill, S. (1997). The children's sentinels: Mothers and their relationships with health professionals in the context of Japanese health care. *Social Science and Medicine, 44*(3), 291–300.

Shaw, M. C., & Halliday P. H. (1992). The family, crisis and chronic illness: An evolutionary model. *Journal of Advanced Nursing, 17*(5), 537–543.

Sidell, N. L. (1997). Adult adjustment to chronic illness: A review of the literature. *Health and Social Work, 22*(1):5–11.

*Thorne, S., McCormick, J., & Carty, E. (1997). Deconstructing the gender neutrality of chronic illness and disability. *Health Care Women International, 18*(1), 1–16.

Wiebe, J. S., & Christensen, A. J. (1996). Patient adherence in chronic illness: Personality and coping in context. *Journal of Personality, 64*(4), 815–835.

*Wiener, C., & Dodd M. J. (1993). Coping amid uncertainty: An illness trajectory perspective. *Scholarly Inquiry for Nursing Practice, 7*(1), 17–31, 33–35.

Wilkins, K., & Park, E. (1996). Chronic conditions, physical limitations and dependency among seniors living in the community. *Health Reports, 8*(3), 7–15.

*Wurzbach, M. E. (1988). Comfort and nurses' moral choices. *Journal of Advanced Nursing, 24,* 260–264.

*Yarcheski, A. (1988). Uncertainty in illness and the future. *Western Journal of Nursing Research, 10*(4), 401–413.

Resources

ChronicNet: http//www.chronicnet.org/chronnet/project.htm. This website provides local and national data on chronic care issues and populations.

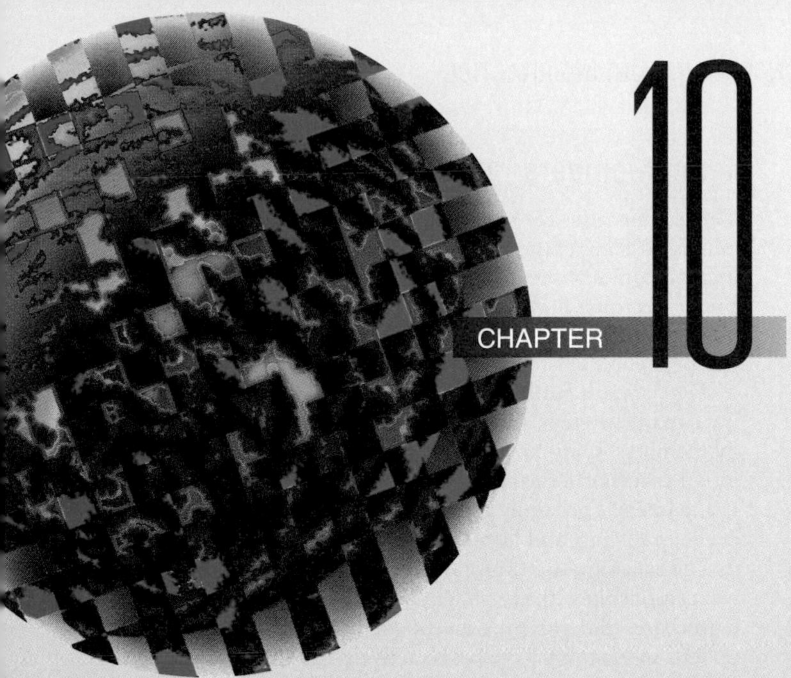

Principles and Practices of Rehabilitation

Learning Objectives

On completion of this chapter, the learner will be able to:

1. Describe the goals of rehabilitation.
2. Discuss the interdisciplinary approach to rehabilitation.
3. Identify emotional reactions exhibited by patients with disabilities.
4. Use the nursing process as a framework for care of patients with self-care deficits, impaired physical mobility, impaired skin integrity, and altered patterns of elimination.
5. Describe nursing strategies appropriate for promoting self-care through activities of daily living.
6. Describe nursing strategies appropriate for promoting mobility and ambulation and the use of assistive devices.
7. Describe risk factors and related nursing measures to prevent development of pressure ulcers.
8. Incorporate bladder training and bowel training into the plan of care for patients with bladder and bowel problems.
9. Describe the significance of continuity of care from the health care facility to the home or extended care facility for patients who need rehabilitative assistance and services.

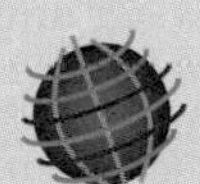

Rehabilitation is a dynamic, health-oriented process that assists an ill or disabled person to achieve the greatest possible level of physical, mental, spiritual, social and economic functioning. The rehabilitation process helps the patient achieve an acceptable quality of life with dignity, self-respect, and independence and is designed for people with physical, mental, or emotional disabilities. During rehabilitation, the patient adjusts to the disability by learning how to use resources and to focus on existing abilities. Abilities, not disabilities, are emphasized.

Rehabilitation is an integral part of nursing. Rehabilitation efforts should begin during the initial contact with the patient. Every major illness or injury carries with it the threat of disability. The principles of rehabilitation are basic to the care of all patients. The emphasis of rehabilitation is to restore the patient to independence or to the preillness or preinjury level of functioning in as short a time as possible. If this is not possible, the aims of rehabilitation are maximal independence and quality of life acceptable to the patient. Realistic goals based on individual patient assessment are established with the patient to guide the rehabilitation program.

Rehabilitation services are required by more people than ever before because of advances in technology that save the lives of seriously ill, injured, and disabled patients. Increasing numbers of patients who are recovering from serious illnesses or injuries are returning to their homes and communities with ongoing needs. Every patient, regardless of age, socioeconomic status, or diagnosis, has a right to rehabilitation services.

FOCUS OF REHABILITATION

Disability can occur at any age and may result from an acute incident, such as stroke or trauma, or from the progression of a chronic condition, such as arthritis or multiple sclerosis. The disabled person experiences many losses, including loss of function, independence, social role, status, and income. The patient and family members experience a range of emotional reactions to these losses. The reactions may progress from disorganization and confusion to denial of the disability, grief over the lost function or body part, depression, anger, and finally acceptance of the disability. Not all patients experience all the stages, although most exhibit grief, which is believed to be necessary to adapt to disability. Patients exhibiting grief should not be blithely encouraged to "cheer up." The nurse should show a willingness to listen to the patient talk about the disability and understand that grief, anger, regret, and resentment are part of the healing process.

The patient's preexisting coping abilities play an important role in the adaptation process. One patient may be particularly independent and determined, whereas another may be dependent and seem to lack personal power. A goal of rehabilitation is to help the patient gain a positive self-image through effective coping. The nurse must recognize different coping abilities and identify when the patient is not coping well or not adjusting to the disability. The patient and family may benefit from participating in a support group or talking with a mental health professional to achieve this goal. Refer to Chapter 6 for a detailed discussion of adaptive and maladaptive responses to illness.

THE REHABILITATION TEAM

Rehabilitation is a creative, dynamic process that requires a team of professionals working together with the patient and the family. The team members represent a variety of disciplines, with each health professional making a unique contribution. Each health professional assesses the patient and identifies patient needs within the discipline's domain. Rehabilitative goals are set. Team members meet in group sessions at frequent intervals to collaborate, evaluate progress, and modify goals as needed to facilitate rehabilitation.

GERONTOLOGIC CONSIDERATIONS

Concerns of Older Adults Facing Disability

- Loss of independence, which is a source of self-respect and dignity
- Increased potential for discrimination or abuse
- Increased social isolation
- Added burden on spouse who may also have impaired health
- Less access to community services and health care
- Less access to religious institutions
- Increased vulnerability to declining health secondary to other disorders, reduced physiologic reserve, or preexisting impairments of mobility and balance
- Fears and doubts about ability to learn or relearn self-care activities, exercises, and transfer and independent mobility techniques
- Inadequate support system for successful rehabilitation

Team Members

The patient is the key member of the rehabilitation team. The patient is the focus of the team effort and the one who determines the final outcomes of the process. The patient participates in goal setting, in learning to function using remaining abilities, and in adjusting to living with disabilities. The rehabilitation team promotes independence, self-respect, and an acceptable quality of life.

The patient's family is incorporated into the team. The family is a dynamic system. Disability of one member affects other family members. Only by incorporating the family into the rehabilitation process can the family system adapt to the change in one of its members. The family provides ongoing support, participates in problem solving, and learns to provide necessary ongoing care.

The rehabilitation nurse develops a therapeutic and supportive relationship with the patient and the family. The nurse always emphasizes the patient's assets and strengths. During nurse–patient interactions, the nurse actively listens, encourages, and shares the patient's successes. The patient is praised for efforts to improve self-concept and self-care abilities.

Through application of the nursing process, the nurse develops a plan of care designed to facilitate rehabilitation, to restore and maintain optimum health, and to prevent complications. The nurse helps the patient to identify strengths and past successes and to develop new goals. Frequently, coping with the disability, self-care, mobility, skin care, and bowel and bladder management are areas for nursing intervention. The nurse assumes roles of caregiver, teacher, counselor, patient advocate, and consultant. The nurse is often the case manager responsible for coordinating the total rehabilitative plan. The nurse collaborates with and coordinates the services provided by all members of the health care team, including the home care nurse, who is responsible for directing the patient's care after return to the home.

The rehabilitation team may also include a physician, nurse practitioner, physiatrist, physical therapist, occupational therapist, speech-language therapist, psychologist, psychiatric liaison nurse, social worker, vocational counselor, orthotist or prosthetist, rehabilitation engineer, and sex counselor or therapist.

AREAS OF SPECIALITY PRACTICE IN REHABILITATION

Although rehabilitation is a component of every patient's care, there are speciality rehabilitation programs established in general hospitals, free-standing rehabilitation hospitals, and outpatient facilities. The Commission for the Accreditation of Rehabilitation Facilities sets standards for these programs and monitors compliance.

Speciality rehabilitation programs often meet the needs of patients with neurologic disabilities. **Stroke recovery programs** and **traumatic brain injury rehabilitation** emphasize cognitive remediation, that is, assisting patients to compensate for memory, perceptual, judgment, and safety deficits as well as teaching self-care and mobility skills. Assisting patients to swallow food safely and communicate effectively are other goals. In addition to stroke and brain injury, other neurologic disorders treated include multiple sclerosis, Parkinson's disease, amyotrophic lateral sclerosis, and nervous system tumors.

Spinal cord injury rehabilitation programs have grown since World War II. Understanding the effects and complications of spinal cord injury; neurogenic bowel and bladder management; sexuality and male fertility enhancement; self-care, including prevention of skin breakdown; bed mobility and transfers; and driving with adaptive equipment are integral components of the program. Intense efforts are given to vocational assessment, training, and reentry into employment and the community.

Orthopedic rehabilitation programs provide comprehensive services to traumatic or nontraumatic amputee patients, patients undergoing joint replacements, and patients with arthritis. Learning to be independent with a prosthesis or new joint is a major goal of the program. Pain management, energy conservation, and joint protection are other focuses.

For patients who have had myocardial infarction, **cardiac rehabilitation** begins during the acute hospitalization and continues on an outpatient basis. Emphasis is placed on monitored, progressive exercise, nutritional counseling, stress management, and sexuality.

Patients with restrictive or chronic obstructive pulmonary disease or ventilator dependency may be admitted to **pulmonary rehabilitation programs**. The services of respiratory therapists are included to facilitate achievement of more effective breathing patterns. Energy conservation techniques, self-medication, and home ventilatory management are taught.

For sufferers of chronic pain, especially low back pain, comprehensive **pain management programs** are offered. These programs focus on alternative pain treatment modalities, exercise, supportive counseling, and vocational evaluation.

A comprehensive **burn rehabilitation program** may serve as a step-down unit from an intensive care burn unit. Although rehabilitation strategies are implemented immediately in acute care, a program focused on progressive joint mobility, self-care, and ongoing counseling are imperative for the burn patient.

Children are not exempt from the need for specialized rehabilitation. **Pediatric rehabilitation programs** meet the needs of children with developmental and acquired disabilities, including cerebral palsy, spina bifida, traumatic brain injuries, and spinal cord injuries.

All speciality areas of rehabilitation require implementation of the nursing process as described in this chapter.

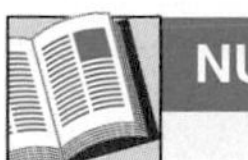

NURSING RESEARCH

Alterations in Self-Care

Ailinger, R., & Dear, M. (1977). An examination of the self-care needs of clients with rheumatoid arthritis. *Rehabilitation Nursing 22*(3), 135–140.

Purpose

Self-care is a strategy to improve the health status of patients with arthritis. Universal self-care requirements (USCRs) include the need for maintenance of sufficient air, food, water, and elimination; a balance between activity and rest; a balance between solitude and social interaction; prevention of hazards to life and well-being; and promotion of normalcy. The purpose of this study was to examine changes in USCRs reported by patients with rheumatoid arthritis (RA) and to examine the effects of age, gender, and changes in health state on patients' USCRs. The indicators of health state used in this study were disease severity, pain, functional status, and duration of illness.

Study Sample and Design

The study sample consisted of 47 women and 12 men between the ages of 27 and 79 years, with a mean age of 52.34 years. The mean number of years since the subjects had been diagnosed with RA was 14.17. A rheumatologist assessed disease severity on a 5-point scale in which 0 = asymptomatic, 1 = mild, 2 = moderate, 3 = severe, and 4 = very severe. The degree of difficulty that respondents experienced when performing activities of daily living (ADLs) was assessed using a portion of the Health Assessment Questionnaire. Scoring was based on a 4-point scale in which 0 = without difficulty, 1 = with some difficulty, 2 = with much difficulty, and 3 = unable to do. Pain was measured using a self-report visual analog scale. Patients marked their pain status ranging from 0 = no pain to 10 = severe pain. Personal interviews were conducted and tape-recorded. Subjects were asked, "Since you have had arthritis, in what ways do you care for yourself differently than before you had it?"

Findings

Most of the subjects had mild to moderate disease severity and experienced some to much difficulty performing ADLs. The mean pain score was 3.95 on the 10-point visual analog scale. They reported that the following USCRs were affected by RA: the need to maintain a balance between activity and rest (83%), promote normalcy (66%), prevent hazards (58%), maintain a sufficient intake of food (27%), and maintain a balance between solitude and social interaction (17%). No one reported a need to maintain a sufficient intake of air or water, and only 1% mentioned elimination. The researchers found that age was related to promotion of normalcy; older patients reported more changes associated with the USCR. Of the four indicators of health status, duration of illness was associated with the need to prevent hazards.

Nursing Implications

Nurses need to assess the patient's baseline activity and rest patterns and to provide education about balancing activity and rest. Ensuring adequate rest periods is an important strategy to facilitate self-care activities. For older RA patients, nurses must identify the patient's attitudes and feelings about normalcy. Interventions should be aimed at helping patients feel more positive about themselves and the activities that they are able to do. The rehabilitation plan of nursing care should also include education about safety, such as preventing falls and joint injuries.

ASSESSING FUNCTIONAL ABILITIES

Comprehensive assessment of functional capacity is the basis for developing the rehabilitation program. Functional capacity entails activities of daily living (ADLs) and instrumental activities of daily living (IADLs). ADLs include basic needs, such as personal hygiene, dressing, toileting, eating, and moving. IADLs include skills necessary for independent living, such as ability to shop for and prepare meals, use the telephone, clean, manage finances, and travel.

The nurse observes the patient performing specific activities (eg, eating, dressing) and notes the degree of independence; the time taken; the patient's mobility, coordination, and endurance; and the amount of assistance required. Functional ability depends on good joint motion, muscle strength, and cardiovascular reserve and an intact neurologic system, and these factors are also carefully assessed. Observations are recorded on a functional assessment tool. These tools provide a way to standardize assessment parameters and supply a scale or score against which improvements may be measured. They also clearly communicate the patient's level of functioning to all members of the rehabilitation team. Rehabilitation centers use these tools to form an initial assessment of the patient's abilities and to monitor the patient's progress in independence.

The PULSES profile is used to assess **p**hysical condition (eg, health/illness status), **u**pper extremity functions (eg, eating, bathing), **l**ower extremity functions (eg, transfer, ambulation), **s**ensory function (eg, vision, hearing, speech), **e**xcretory function (ie, control of bowel or bladder), and **s**ituational factors (eg, social and financial support). Each of these areas is rated on a scale from 1 (independent) to 4 (greatest dependency).

The Barthel Index is used to measure the patient's level of independence in ADLs (feeding, bathing, dressing, grooming), continence, toileting, transfers, and ambulation (or wheelchair mobility). This scale does not address communicative or cognitive abilities.

The Functional Independence Measure (FIM) is used to assess the patient's level of independence. The six areas assessed are self-care, sphincter management, mobility, locomotion, communication and cognitive ability, and social cognition.

The Patient Evaluation Conference System (PECS) contains 15 categories. This comprehensive assessment scale includes such areas as medications, pain, nutrition, use of assistive devices, psychological status, vocation, and recreation.

In addition to the detailed functional assessment, the nurse assesses the patient's physical, mental, emotional, spiritual, social, and economic status. Secondary problems related to the disability, such as muscle atrophy and deconditioning, are assessed, as are residual strengths unaffected by disease or disability. The nurse recognizes the patient as an individual and as a part of a family system, and because no two people react in the same way to a disability, the nurse determines the patient's and family's perceptions and coping patterns. Other areas that require nursing assessment include potential for altered skin integrity, altered bowel and bladder control, and sexual dysfunction.

NURSING PROCESS: THE PATIENT WITH SELF-CARE DEFICIT—ACTIVITIES OF DAILY LIVING

ADLs are those self-care activities that the patient must accomplish each day to meet personal needs. ADLs include personal hygiene/bathing, dressing/grooming, feeding, and toileting. Many patients are unable to perform these activities easily. An ADL program is started as soon as the rehabilitation process begins. The ability to perform ADLs is frequently the key to independence, return to the home, and reentry into the community.

Assessment

The nurse must observe and assess the patient's ability to perform ADLs to determine the level of independence in self-care and the need for nursing intervention. The activity of bathing requires obtaining bath water and utensils, undressing, washing, and drying the body after bathing. Dressing requires selecting, putting on, and taking off clothing; fastening the clothing; and combing the hair. Self-feeding requires selecting foods, using utensils to bring food to the mouth, and chewing and swallowing the food. The activity of toileting includes the ability to get to the toilet, remove clothing to use the toilet, get on and off the toilet, cleanse self, redress self, and perform hand hygiene. Patients who can sit up and raise their hands to their head probably can begin to bathe and feed themselves. Balance and some muscle strength and coordination are required for dressing. Toileting requires transfer and dressing abilities.

In addition, the nurse needs to be aware of the patient's medical conditions and the effect that they have on the ability to perform ADLs. Assessment of the family's involvement in the patient's ADLs is also important. This information is valuable in goal setting and development of the plan of care to maximize self-care.

Nursing Diagnosis

Based on the assessment data, major nursing diagnoses for the patient may include the following:

- Self-care deficit: bathing/hygiene, dressing/grooming, feeding, toileting

Planning and Goals

The major goals of the patient include bathing/hygiene independently or with assistance, using adaptive devices as appropriate; dressing/grooming independently or with assistance, using adaptive devices as appropriate; feeding independently or with assistance, using adaptive devices as appropriate; and toileting independently or with assistance, using adaptive devices as appropriate. Also, the patient with a self-care deficit expresses satisfaction with the extent of independence in self-care activities.

Nursing Interventions

Fostering Self-Care Abilities

To learn methods of self-care effectively, the patient must be motivated. An "I'd rather do it myself" attitude is encouraged. The nurse must also help the patient identify the safe limits of independent activity. Knowing when to ask for assistance is particularly important.

The nurse teaches, guides, and supports the patient who is learning how to perform self-care activities. Consistency in instructions and assistance given by the caregiver facilitates the learning process. Recording the patient's performance provides data for evaluating progress and may be used as a source of motivation and for morale building (Guideline 10-1).

Self-care techniques need to be adapted to accommodate the individual patient's lifestyle. Often, a simple maneuver requires concentration and the exertion of considerable effort on the part of the patient with a disability. Common sense and a little ingenuity may promote increased independence. It is important to remember that there is usually more than one way to accomplish a self-care activity. For example, a person who cannot quite reach his or her head may be able to do so by leaning forward. Encouraging the patient to participate in a support group may help the patient to discover inventive solutions to self-care problems.

Recommending Assistive Devices

If the patient has difficulty in performing an ADL, an adaptive/assistive device (self-help device) may be useful. A large variety of assistive devices are available commercially or can be fabricated by the nurse, the occupational therapist, the patient, or the family. The nurse should be alert to "gadgets" coming on the market that may be useful. At the same time, the nurse must exercise professional judgment and caution in recommending devices because unscrupulous vendors have marketed unnecessary, overly expensive, or useless items to patients in the past.

A wide selection of computerized assistive devices is available, or devices can be designed to help individual patients with severe disabilities to function more independently. The ABLEDATA project* offers a computerized listing of commercially available aids and equipment for patients with disabilities.

* National Rehabilitation Information Center, 8455 Colesville Rd., Silver Spring, MD 20910-3319. 1-800-346-2742 (voice/TDD).

10•1 GUIDELINES FOR TEACHING ACTIVITIES OF DAILY LIVING

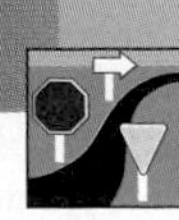

1. Define the goal of the activity with the patient. Be realistic. Set short-term goals that can be accomplished in the near future.
2. Identify several approaches to accomplish the task. (Example: There are several ways to put on a given garment.)
3. Select the approach most likely to succeed.
4. Specify the approach on the patient's care plan and the patient's level of accomplishment on the progress notes.
5. Identify the motions necessary to accomplish the activity. (Example: To pick up a glass, extend arm; place open hand next to glass; flex fingers around glass; move arm and hand holding glass vertically; flex arm toward body.)
6. Focus on gross functional movements initially, and gradually include activities that use finer motions (eg, buttoning clothes, eating with a fork).
7. Encourage the patient to perform the activity up to maximal capacity within the limitations of the disability.
8. Monitor the patient's tolerance.
9. Minimize frustration and fatigue.
10. Support the patient by giving appropriate praise for effort put forth and for acts accomplished.
11. Assist the patient to perform and practice the activity in real-life situations.

Helping the Patient Accept Limitations

When the patient has a severe disability, independent self-care may be an unrealistic goal. The rehabilitation nurse teaches the patient how to direct his or her own care. The patient may require a personal attendant to perform ADLs. Family members may not be appropriate for providing bathing/hygiene, dressing/grooming, feeding, and toileting assistance. A spouse may have difficulty providing bowel and bladder care for the patient and maintaining the role of sexual partner. If a personal caregiver is needed, the disabled person or family members must learn how to manage an employee effectively. The patient is assisted in accepting self-care dependency. Independence in other areas, such as social interaction, should be emphasized to promote positive self-concept.

Evaluation

Expected Outcomes

Expected outcomes may include:

1. Demonstrates independent self-care in bathing/hygiene or with assistance, using adaptive devices as appropriate
   a. Bathes self at maximal level of independence
   b. Uses adaptive devices effectively
   c. Reports satisfaction with level of independence in bathing/hygiene
2. Demonstrates independent self-care in dressing/grooming or with assistance, using adaptive devices as appropriate
   a. Dresses/grooms self at maximal level of independence
   b. Uses adaptive devices effectively
   c. Reports satisfaction with level of independence in dressing/grooming
   d. Demonstrates increased interest in appearance
3. Demonstrates independent self-care in feeding or with assistance, using adaptive devices as appropriate
   a. Feeds self at maximal level of independence
   b. Uses adaptive devices effectively
   c. Demonstrates increased interest in eating
   d. Maintains adequate nutritional intake
4. Demonstrates independent self-care in toileting or with assistance, using adaptive devices as appropriate
   a. Toilets self at maximal level of independence
   b. Uses adaptive devices effectively
   c. Indicates positive feelings regarding level of toileting independence
   d. Experiences adequate frequency of bowel and bladder elimination
   e. Does not experience incontinence, constipation, urinary tract infection, or other complications

NURSING PROCESS: THE PATIENT WITH IMPAIRED PHYSICAL MOBILITY

Patients who are ill or injured are frequently placed on bed rest or have their activities limited. Problems commonly associated with immobility include weakened muscles, joint contracture, and deformity. Each joint of the body has a normal range of motion. If the range is limited, the functions of the joint and of the muscles that move the joint are impaired, and painful deformities may develop. Nurses must identify patients at risk for such complications.

Another problem frequently seen in rehabilitation nursing is an altered ambulatory/mobility pattern. The patient with a disability may be unable either temporarily or permanently to walk independently and unaided. The nurse assesses the mobility of the patient and designs care that promotes independent mobility within the prescribed therapeutic limits.

When a person is not able to exercise and move joints through the full range of motion, contractures may develop. A **contracture** is a shortening of the muscle and tendon that leads to deformity. Contractures limit joint mobility. When the contracted joint is moved, the patient experiences pain. In addition, more energy is required to move when joints are contracted and deformed.

Assessment

At times, a patient's mobility is restricted because of pain, paralysis, loss of muscle strength, systemic disease, presence of an immobilizing device (eg, cast, brace), or prescribed limits to promote healing. Assessment of the patient's mobility includes positioning, ability to move, muscle strength and tone, joint function, and the prescribed mobility limits. The nurse may

NURSING RESEARCH

Patient Teaching and Pulmonary Rehabilitation

Scherer, Y., Schmieder, L. E., & Schimmel, S. (1998). The effects of education alone and in combination with pulmonary rehabilitation on self-efficacy in patients with COPD. *Rehabilitation Nursing 23*(2), 71–77.

Purpose

Self-efficacy expectation is a person's perception that he or she will be able to perform a given behavior successfully to produce a certain outcome. Because dyspnea is the most debilitating symptom of chronic obstructive pulmonary disease (COPD), the researchers compared the effects on the self-efficacy expectations of patients with COPD with regard to managing or avoiding breathing difficulty when they participated in a combined education and supervised exercise program or education program only.

Study Sample and Design

One group of 37 subjects participated in a pulmonary rehabilitation program conducted by a clinical nurse specialist for 1 hour, three times a week for 12 weeks. Their program included educational topics and 20 to 30 minutes of supervised exercise. A second group of 22 subjects participated in 2-hour sessions offered once a week over a 4-week period. They received the same educational component: pathophysiology of COPD, pursed-lip and diaphragmatic breathing, nutrition, self-care instruction, and stress management. However, they did not participate in supervised exercise. They were encouraged to practice breathing exercises taught in class and to walk moderately. They were also told to consult their physician about more strenuous exercise. During both programs, techniques to increase self-efficacy were incorporated. These techniques included having participants identify goals and breaking those goals down into achievable steps to ensure success; providing role models who had successfully mastered skills; verbally praising and encouraging efforts and achievements; and teaching stress management techniques to decrease emotional and physical arousal, which can increase breathing difficulty. Both groups completed the COPD Self-Efficacy Scale (CSES) before beginning their respective programs and at 1 and 6 month intervals after program completion. The CSES consists of five subscales: Negative Affect, Intense Emotional Arousal, Physical Exertion, Weather/Environment, and Behavioral Risk Factors.

The researchers calculated mean scores and standard deviations on the CSES before and after completion of the two programs. Paired t-test analyses were done to compare preprogram and 1-month postprogram scores and to compare 1-month and 6-month postprogram scores.

Results

The results showed that scores for the rehabilitation program group significantly improved and remained significantly improved 6 months later. The education-only group had significantly improved scores, but their scores 6 months later were not better than preprogram scores.

Nursing Implications

Nurses need to continue to refer COPD patients to comprehensive rehabilitation programs that can offer supervised exercise and education because a combined program may produce more lasting results than a program that does not have both components. In situations in which finances or geography do not permit participation, the nurse can provide valuable education about pursed-lip and diaphragmatic breathing, nutrition, and self-care techniques. In addition, assisting patients to identify goals and steps to achieve them, verbally praising their efforts and successes, teaching stress reduction techniques, and providing access to role models, when possible, help COPD patients to improve their confidence in managing breathing difficulties.

need to collaborate with the physical therapist or other team members to assess mobility.

During position change, transfer, and ambulation activities, the nurse assesses the patient's abilities, the extent of disability, and residual capacity for physiologic adaptation. The nurse observes for orthostatic hypotension, pallor, diaphoresis, nausea, tachycardia, and fatigue.

If a patient is not able to ambulate independently, without assistance, the nurse assesses ability to balance, transfer, and use assistive devices (eg, crutches, walker). Crutch walking requires a high-energy expenditure and produces considerable cardiovascular stress. Older people with reduced exercise capacity, decreased arm strength, and problems with balance because of old age and multiple diseases may be unable to use crutches. A walker is more stable and may be a better choice for these patients. The nurse assesses the patient's ability to use various devices that promote mobility.

If a patient uses an orthosis, the nurse monitors the patient for effective use and potential problems associated with its use.

Nursing Diagnosis

Based on the assessment data, major nursing diagnoses for the patient may include the following:

- Impaired physical mobility
- Activity intolerance
- Risk for injury
- Risk for disuse syndrome
- Impaired walking
- Impaired wheelchair transfer ability
- Impaired bed mobility

Planning and Goals

The major goals of the patient may include absence of contracture and deformity, maintenance of muscle strength and joint mobility, independent mobility, and increased activity tolerance.

Nursing Interventions

Positioning to Prevent Musculoskeletal Complications

Deformities and contractures can often be prevented by proper positioning. Maintaining correct body alignment while in bed is essential regardless of the position selected. During each contact with the patient, the nurse evaluates the patient's position. The nurse assists the patient to achieve proper positioning and alignment.

The most common positions that a patient assumes in bed are supine (dorsal), side-lying (lateral), and prone. The nurse helps the patient assume these positions and supports the body in correct alignment with pillows (Guideline 10-2). At times, a splint (eg, wrist or hand splint) may be fabricated by the occupational therapist to support a joint and prevent deformity. The nurse must ensure proper use of the splint and provide skin care.

PREVENTING EXTERNAL ROTATION OF THE HIP

Patients who are in bed for any period of time may develop external rotation deformity of the hip. The ball-and-socket joint of the hip has a tendency to rotate outward when the patient lies on his or her back. A trochanter roll extending from the crest of the ilium to the midthigh prevents this deformity. With correct

10•2
GUIDELINES FOR

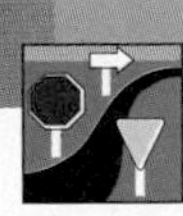

POSITIONING A PATIENT IN BED

Supine (Dorsal) Position

1. Align the head with the spine, both laterally and anteroposteriorly.
2. Position the trunk to minimize hip flexion.
3. Flex the arms at the elbow and rest the hands against the lateral abdomen.
4. Extend the legs with a small, firm support under the popliteal area.
5. Support the heels off the mattress with a small pillow or towel roll at the ankles.
6. Point the toes straight up using protective boots to prevent footdrop.
7. Place trochanter rolls under the greater trochanters to prevent external rotation of the hip.

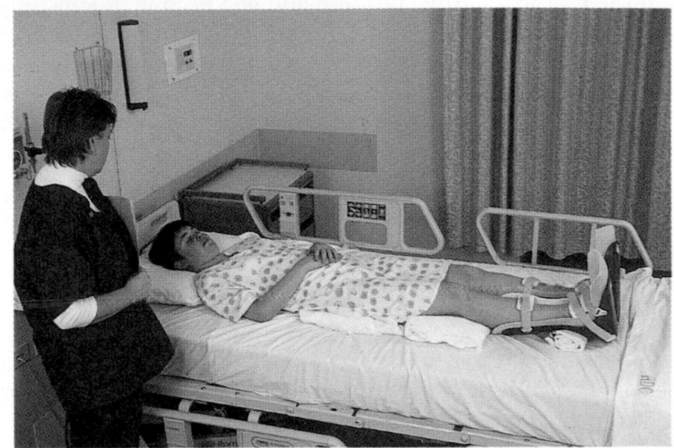

Side-Lying (Lateral Position)

1. Align the head with the spine, and support it with a pillow.
2. Properly align the body; avoid twisting at the shoulders, waist, or hips.
3. Flex shoulders and elbows and support the upper arm with a pillow.
4. Position the uppermost hip joint slightly forward and support the leg in a position of slight abduction by a pillow.
5. Place and support the feet in neutral dorsiflexion.
6. Support the back with a pillow.

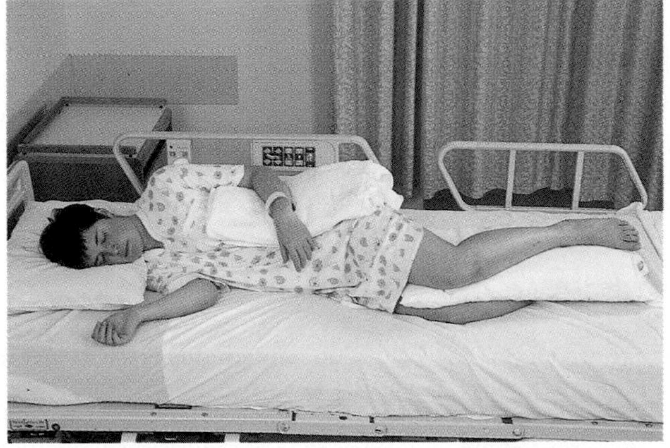

Prone (on Abdomen) Position

1. Turn the head laterally and align it with the rest of the body.
2. Abduct and externally rotate the arms at the shoulder joint; flex the elbows.
3. Place a small flat support under the pelvis, extending from the level of the umbilicus to the upper third of the thigh.
4. Maintain the lower extremities in a neutral position.
5. Suspend the toes over the edge of the mattress.

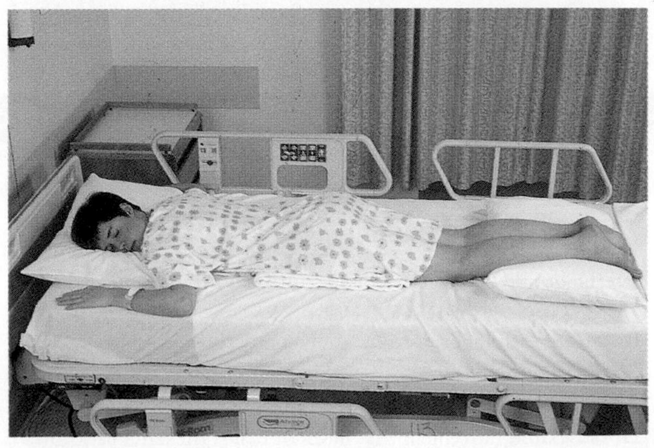

Note: Side rails of bed should remain raised if the patient is at risk for falling.

placement, the trochanter roll serves as a mechanical wedge under the projection of the greater trochanter.

PREVENTING FOOTDROP

Footdrop is a deformity in which the foot is plantar flexed (the ankle bends in the direction of the sole of the foot). If the condition continues without correction, the patient will not be able to hold the foot in a normal position and will be able to walk only on his or her toes without touching the ground with the heel of the foot. The deformity is caused by contracture of both the gastrocnemius and soleus muscles. Damage to the peroneal nerve may result in footdrop. It may also be produced by loss of flexibility of the Achilles tendon.

Nursing Alert *Prolonged bed rest, lack of exercise, incorrect positioning in bed, and the weight of the bedding forcing the toes into plantar flexion are factors that contribute to footdrop.*

To prevent this disabling deformity, pillows, splints, or protective boots are used to keep the feet at right angles to the legs when the patient is in a supine position. High-top athletic shoes may be used to maintain the 90-degree angle for short time periods. Frequent skin inspection of the feet must be performed to determine if positioning devices have created any unwanted pressure areas.

The patient is encouraged to perform ankle exercises several times each hour. These exercises include dorsiflexion and plantar flexion of the feet, flexion and extension (curl and stretch) of the toes, and eversion and inversion of the feet at the ankles.

Maintaining Muscle Strength and Joint Mobility

Optimal functioning depends on the strength of the muscles and joint motion. Active participation in ADLs promotes maintenance of muscle strength and joint mobility. Range-of-motion exercises and specific therapeutic exercises may be included in the nursing plan of care.

PERFORMING RANGE-OF-MOTION EXERCISES

Range of motion is movement of a joint through its full range in all appropriate planes (Chart 10-1).

To maintain or increase the motion of a joint, range-of-motion exercises are initiated as soon as the patient's condition permits. The exercises are planned for the individual to accommodate the wide variation in the degrees of motion that people of varying body build and age groups can attain (Guideline 10-3).

Range-of-motion exercises may be active (performed by the patient under supervision of the nurse), assisted (the nurse helps the patient if unable to do exercise independently), or passive (performed by the nurse). Unless prescribed otherwise, a joint should be moved through its range of motion three times, at least twice a day. The joint to be exercised is supported, the bones above the joint are stabilized, and the body part distal to the joint is moved through the range of motion of the joint. For example, when the elbow is taken through its range of motion, the humerus must be stabilized while the radius and ulna are moved through their range of motion at the elbow joint.

The joint should not be moved beyond its free range of motion. Therefore, the joint is moved to the point of resistance and stopped at the point of pain. If muscle spasms are present, move the joint slowly to the point of resistance, then apply gentle steady pressure until the muscle relaxes. Continue the motion to the joint's final point of resistance.

To perform assisted or passive range-of-motion exercises, the patient must be in a comfortable supine position with arms at the sides and knees extended. Good body posture is maintained during the exercises. The nurse also uses good body mechanics during the exercise session.

PERFORMING THERAPEUTIC EXERCISES

Therapeutic exercises are prescribed by the physician and performed with the assistance and guidance of a physical therapist or nurse.

The patient should have a clear understanding of the goal of the prescribed exercise. Written instructions about the frequency, duration, and number of repetitions, as well as simple line drawings of the exercise, help to ensure adherence to the exercise program.

Exercise, when performed correctly, assists in (1) maintaining and building muscle strength, (2) maintaining joint function, (3) preventing deformity, (4) stimulating circulation, (5) developing endurance, and (6) promoting relaxation. Exercise is also valuable in helping to restore motivation and well-being of the patient. There are five types of exercise: passive, active-assistive, active, resistive, and isometric. The description, purpose, and action of each of these exercises are summarized in Table 10-1.

Promoting Independent Mobility

When the patient's condition stabilizes and the physical condition permits, the patient is assisted to sit up on the side of the bed and then to stand. The patient's tolerance of this activity is assessed.

Orthostatic (postural) hypotension may develop when the patient assumes a vertical position. Because of inadequate vasomo-

(text continues on page 129)

CHART 10•1 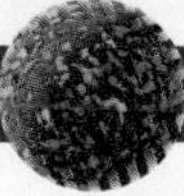 **Definition of Terms: Range of Motion**

Abduction: movement away from the midline of the body
Adduction: movement toward the midline of the body
Flexion: bending of a joint so that the angle of the joint diminishes
Extension: the return movement from flexion; the joint angle is increased
Rotation: turning or movement of a part around its axis
Internal: turning inward, toward the center
External: turning outward, away from the center
Dorsiflexion: movement that flexes or bends the hand back toward the body or foot toward the leg
Palmar flexion: movement that flexes or bends the hand in the direction of the palm
Plantar flexion: movement that flexes or bends the foot in the direction of the sole
Pronation: rotation of the forearm so that the palm of the hand is down
Supination: rotation of the forearm so that the palm of the hand is up
Opposition: touching thumb to each finger tip on same hand
Inversion: movement that turns the sole of the foot inward
Eversion: movement that turns the sole of the foot outward

10•3 GUIDELINES FOR PERFORMING RANGE-OF-MOTION EXERCISES

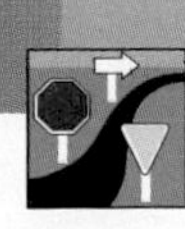

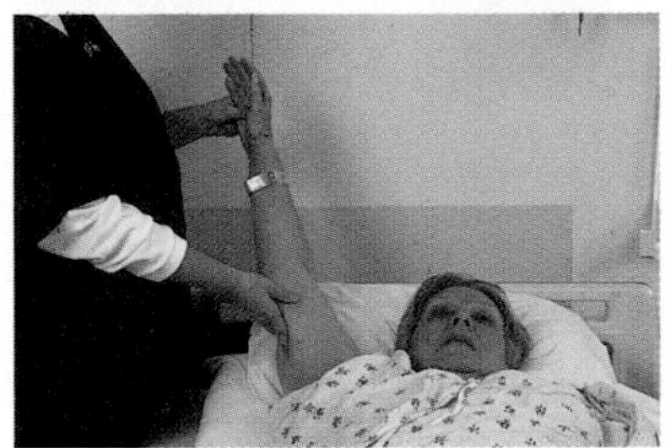

Abduction of shoulder. Move arm from side of body to above the head, then return arm to side of body or neutral position (adduction).

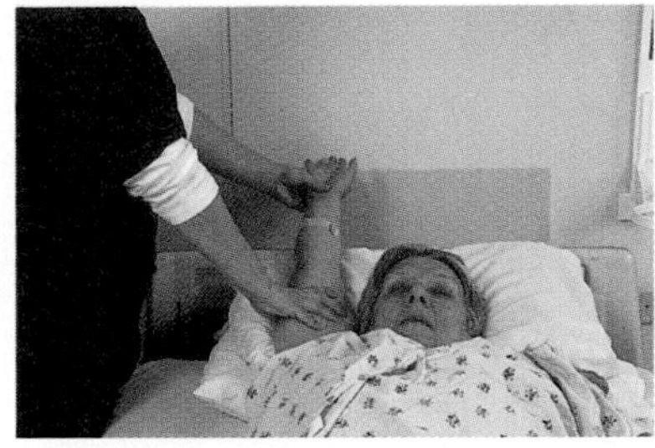

Forward flexion of shoulder. Move arm forward and upward until it is alongside of head.

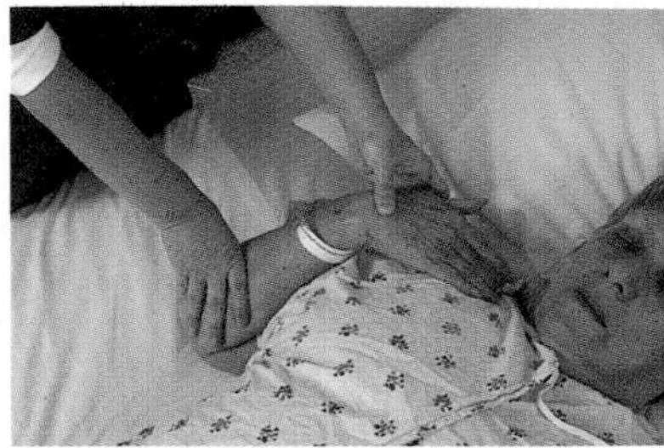

Flexion of elbow. Bend elbow, bringing forearm and hand toward shoulder, then return forearm and hand to neutral position (arm straight).

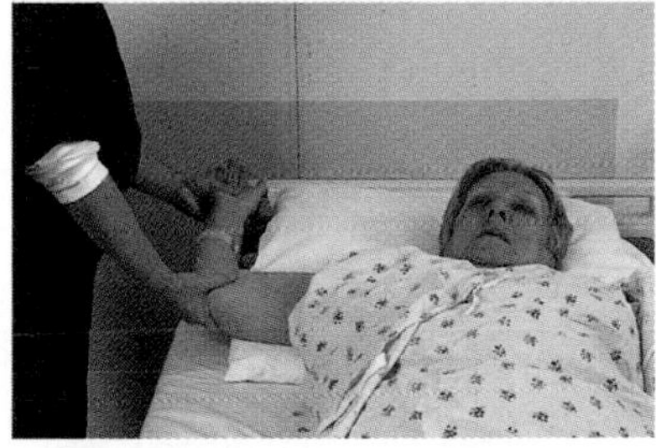

Internal rotation of shoulder. With arm at shoulder height, elbow bent at a 90-degree angle, and palm toward feet, turn upper arm until palm and forearm point backward.

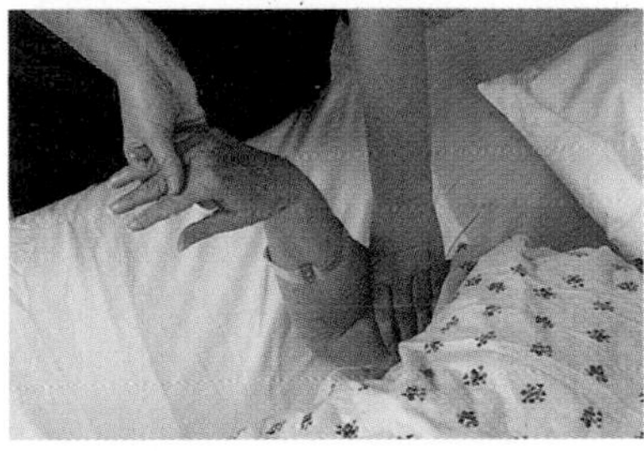

Pronation of forearm. With elbow at waist and bent at a 90-degree angle, turn hand so that palm is facing down.

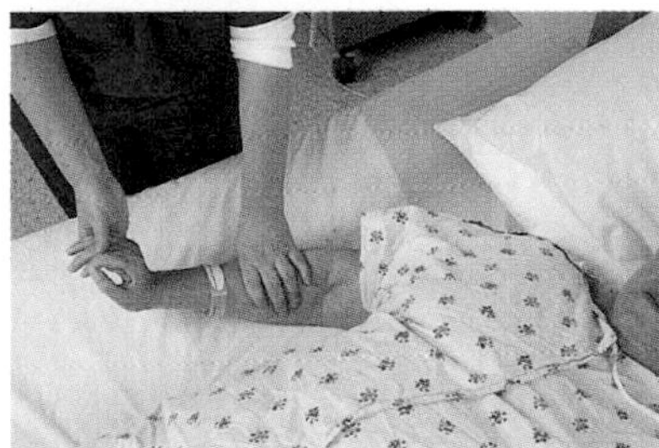

Wrist extension.

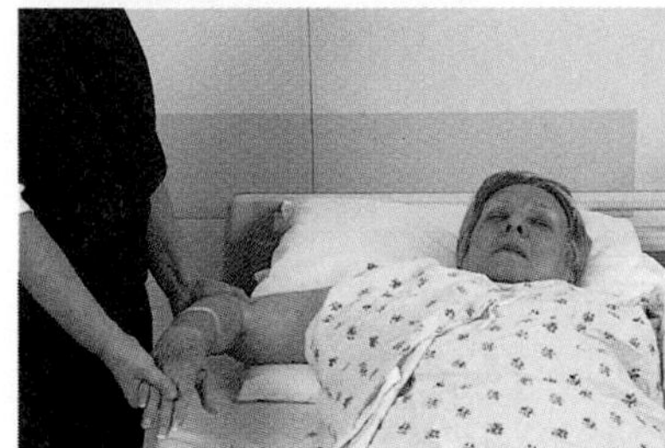

External rotation of shoulder. With arm at shoulder height, elbow bent at a 90-degree angle, and palm toward feet, turn upper arm until the palm and forearm point forward.

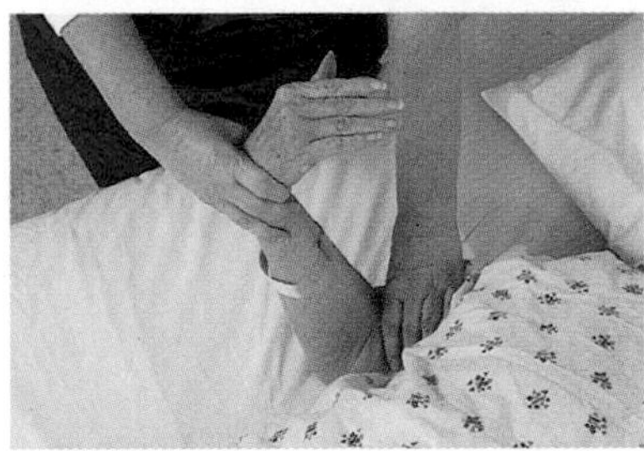

Supination of forearm. With elbow at waist and arm bent at a 90-degree angle, turn hand so that palm is facing up.

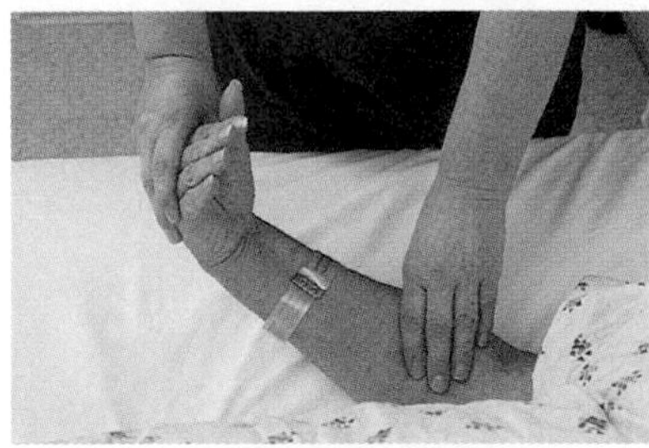

Flexion of wrist. Bend wrist so that palm is toward forearm. Straighten to a neutral position.

(*continued*)

10•3 GUIDELINES FOR

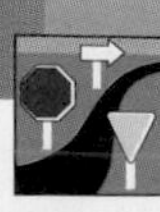

PERFORMING RANGE-OF-MOTION EXERCISES *(Continued)*

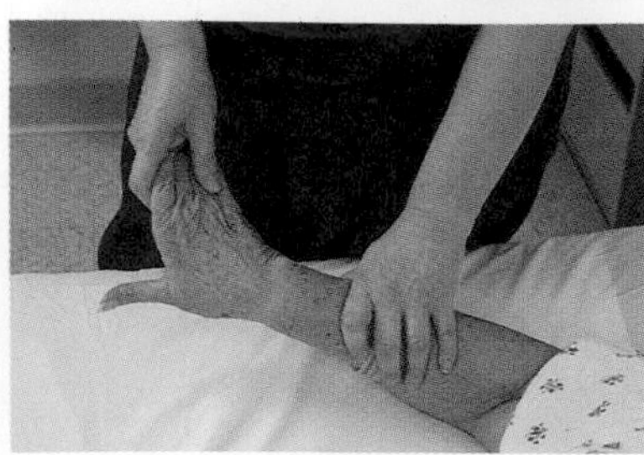

Ulnar deviation. Move hand sideways so that the side of hand on which the little finger is located moves toward forearm.

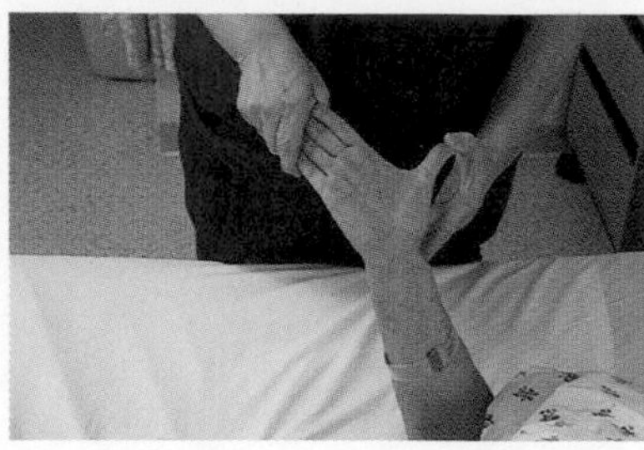

Extension of fingers.

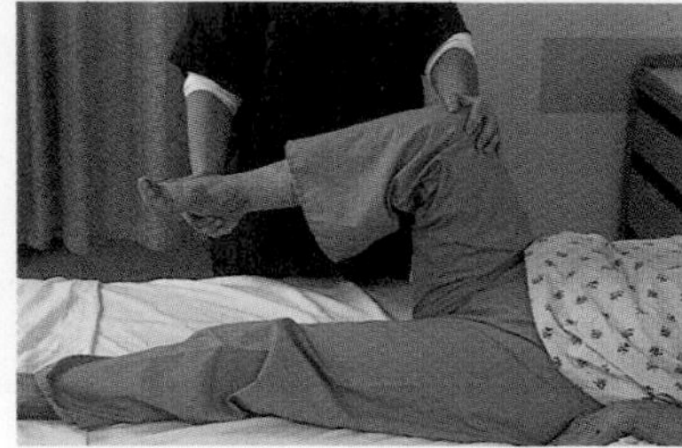

Internal-external rotation of hip. Turn leg in an inward motion so that toes point in. Turn leg in an outward motion so that toes point out.

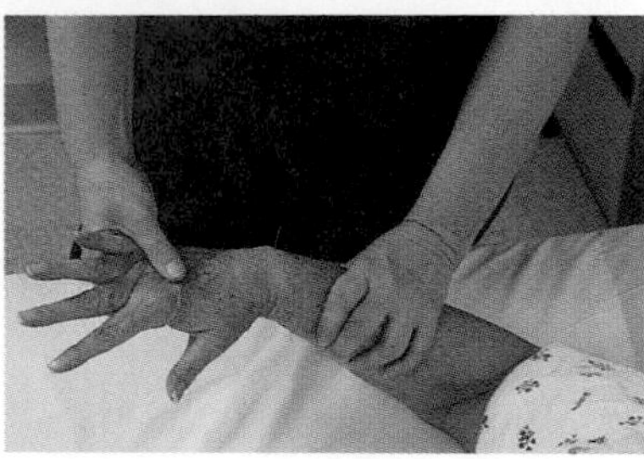

Radial deviation. Move hand sideways so that side of hand on which thumb is located moves toward forearm.

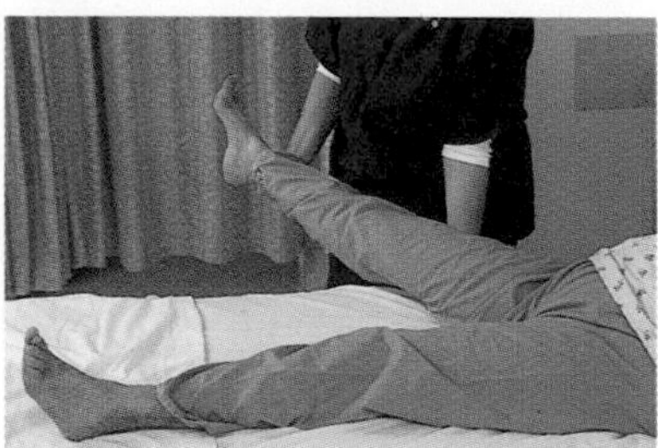

To perform abduction-adduction of hip, move leg outward from the body as far as possible, as shown. Return leg from abducted position to neutral position and across the other leg as far as possible.

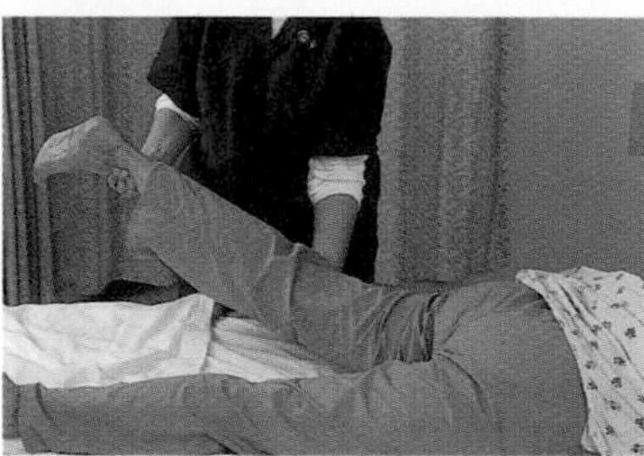

Hyperextension of hip. Place the patient in a prone position, and move leg backward from the body as far as possible.

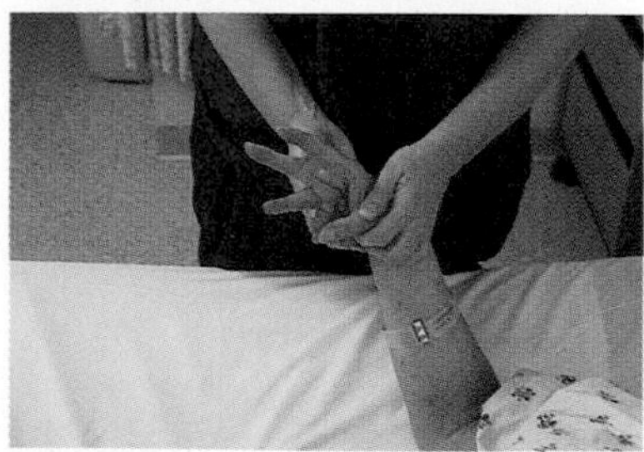

Thumb opposition. Move thumb out and around to touch little finger.

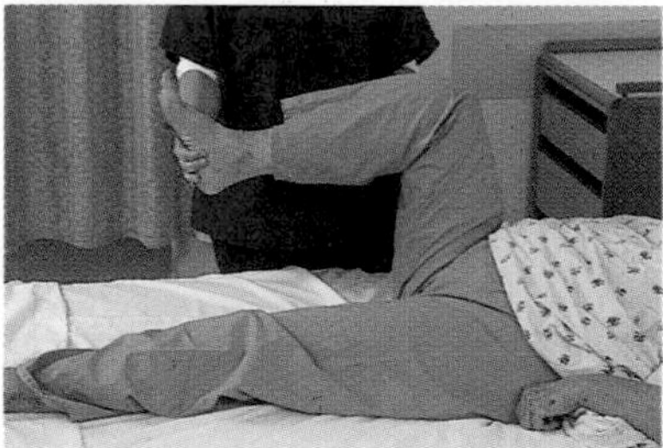

Flexion of the hip and the knee. Bend hip by moving the leg forward as far as possible. Return leg from the flexed position to the neutral position.

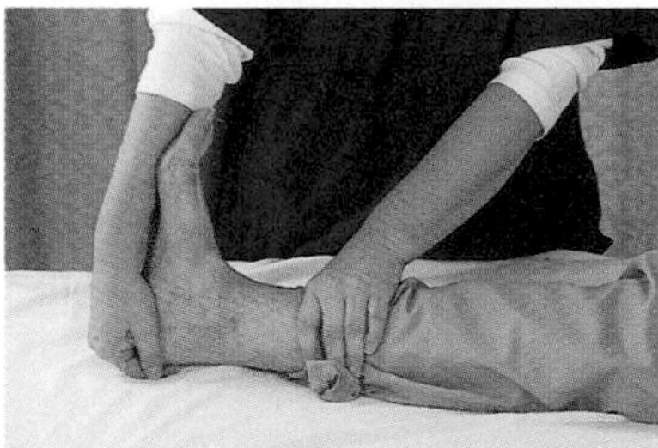

Dorsiflexion of foot. Move foot up and toward the leg. Then move the foot down and away from the leg (plantar flexion).

(continued)

10•3 GUIDELINES FOR PERFORMING RANGE-OF-MOTION EXERCISES *(Continued)*

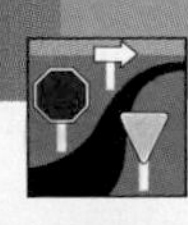

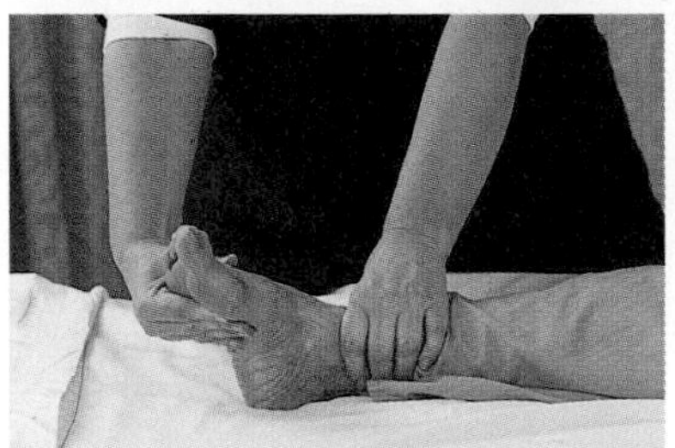

Inversion and eversion of foot. Move foot so that sole is facing outward (eversion). Then move foot so that sole is facing inward (inversion).

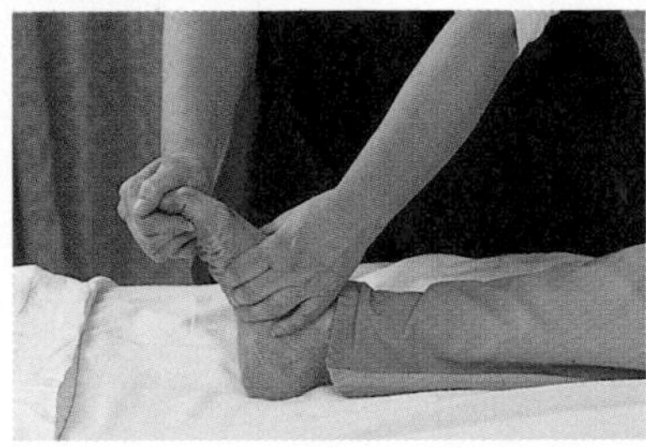

Flexion of toes. Bend the toes toward the ball of foot.

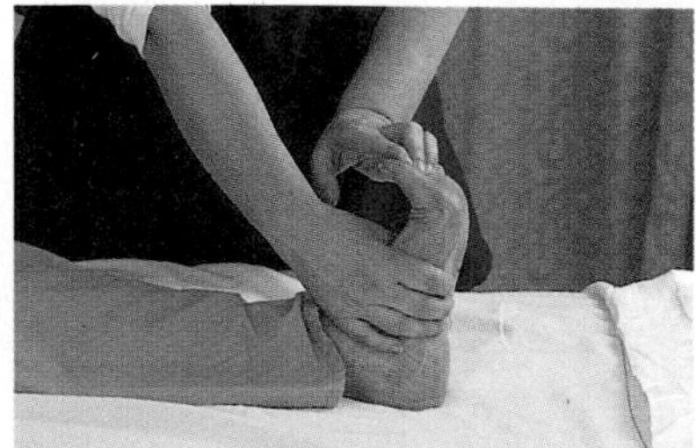

Extension of toes. Straighten toes and pull them toward the leg as far as possible.

tor reflexes, blood pools in the splanchnic (visceral) area and in the legs, resulting in inadequate cerebral circulation. If indicators of orthostatic hypotension (ie, drop in blood pressure, pallor, diaphoresis, nausea, tachycardia, dizziness) are present, the activity is stopped, and the patient is assisted to a supine position in bed.

Some disabilities, such as spinal cord injury, brain damage, and conditions that require extended periods in the recumbent position, prevent patients from assuming an upright position at the bedside. Several strategies can be used to assist a patient to assume a 90-degree sitting position. First, a reclining wheelchair with elevating leg rests allows a slow and controlled progression from a supine position to a 90-degree sitting position. Or, a tilt table, a board that can be tilted in 5- to 10-degree increments from a horizontal to a vertical position, may be used. The tilt table promotes vasomotor adjustment to positional changes and helps the patient with limited standing balance and weight-bearing activities to avoid decalcification of bones associated with disuse syndrome.

Elastic stockings are used to prevent venous stasis. At times, a compression leotard or snug-fitting abdominal binder and elastic compression bandaging of the legs are needed to prevent venous stasis and ensuing orthostatic hypotension. The nurse monitors the patient's blood pressure and pulse and observes for signs of orthostatic hypotension and cerebral insufficiency (ie, the patient reports feeling faint and weak), which suggest intolerance of the upright position. If the patient does not tolerate the upright position, the nurse should recline the patient and elevate the patient's legs. When the patient is standing, the feet are protected with a pair of properly fitted shoes. Extended periods of standing are avoided because of venous pooling and pressure on the soles of the feet.

ASSISTING THE PATIENT WITH TRANSFER

A **transfer** is the movement of the patient from one place to another (eg, bed to chair, chair to commode, wheelchair to tub). As soon as the patient is permitted out of bed, transfer activities are started. The nurse assesses the patient's ability to participate actively in the transfer and determines in conjunction with an occupational therapist or physical therapist the required adaptive equipment to promote independence and safety. A light-weight wheelchair with brake extensions, removable and detachable arm rests, and leg rests minimizes structural obstacles during the transfer. Tub seats or benches make transfers in and out of tubs easier and safer. Raised, padded commode seats may also be warranted for patients who must avoid flexing the hips greater than 90 degrees when transferring to a toilet.

It is important that the patient maintain muscle strength and, if possible, perform push-up exercises to strengthen the arm and shoulder extensor muscles. The push-up exercise requires the patient to sit upright in bed; a book is placed under each of the patient's hands to provide a hard surface, and the patient is instructed to push down on the book raising the body. It is desirable that the patient be able to raise and move the body in different directions by means of these push-up exercises.

The nurse teaches the patient how to transfer. There are several methods of transferring from the bed to the wheelchair when the patient is unable to stand. The technique chosen should be appropriate for the patient, considering the abilities and disabilities. It is helpful for the nurse to demonstrate the technique. If the physical therapist is involved in teaching the patient to transfer, the nurse and the physical therapist must collaborate so that consistent instructions are given to the patient. During transfer, the nurse assists and coaches the patient. Figure 10-1 shows weight-bearing and non–weight-bearing transfer.

If the patient's muscles are not strong enough to overcome the resistance of body weight, a polished light-weight board (transfer board, sliding board) may be used to bridge the gap between the bed and the chair. The patient slides across on the board with or without assistance from a caregiver. This board may also be used to transfer the patient from the chair to the toilet or bathtub bench. Care must be taken to ensure that the patient does not curl the fingers around the edge of the board during the transfer because the weight of the patient's body can crush the fingers as the patient moves across the board. Safety is a primary concern during a transfer.

- Wheelchairs and beds must be locked before the patient transfers.

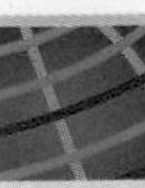

Table 10•1 Therapeutic Exercises

Exercise	Description	Purposes	Action
Passive	An exercise carried out by the therapist or the nurse without assistance from the patient	To retain as much joint range of motion as possible, to maintain circulation	Stabilize the proximal joint, and support the distal part. Move the joint smoothly, slowly, and gently through its full range of motion. Avoid producing pain.
Active-assistive	An exercise carried out by the patient with the assistance of the therapist or the nurse	To encourage normal muscle function	Support the distal part, and encourage the patient to take the joint actively through its range of motion. Give no more assistance than is necessary to accomplish the action. Short periods of activity should be followed by adequate rest periods.
Active	An exercise accomplished by the patient without assistance; activities include turning from side to side and from back to abdomen and moving up and down in bed	To increase muscle strength	When possible, active exercise should be performed against gravity. The joint is moved through full range of motion without assistance. (Make sure that the patient does not substitute another joint movement for the one intended.)
Resistive	An active exercise carried out by the patient working against resistance produced by either manual or mechanical means	To provide resistance to increase muscle power	The patient moves the joint through its range of motion while the therapist resists slightly at first and then with progressively increasing resistance. Sandbags and weights can be used and are applied at the distal point of the involved joint. The movements should be performed smoothly.
Isometric or muscle setting	Alternately contracting and relaxing a muscle while keeping the part in a fixed position; this exercise is performed by the patient	To maintain strength when a joint is immobilized	Contract or tighten the muscle as much as possible without moving the joint, hold for several seconds, then let go and relax. Breathe deeply.

- Detachable arm and foot rests are removed to make getting in and out of the chair easier.
- One end of the transfer board is placed under the patient's buttocks and the other end on the surface to which the transfer is being made (eg, the chair).
- The patient is instructed to lean forward, push up with his or her hands, and then slide across the board to the other surface.

The nurse frequently assists weak and incapacitated patients out of bed. The nurse supports and gently assists the patient during position changes, protecting the patient from injury. The nurse avoids pulling on the weak or paralyzed upper extremity, to prevent dislocation of the shoulder. The patient is assisted to move toward the stronger side (Guideline 10-4).

In the home setting, getting in and out of bed and performing chair, toilet, and tub transfers are difficult for patients with weak musculature and loss of hip, knee, and ankle motion. A rope attached to the headboard of the bed enables the patient to pull toward the center of the bed, and the use of a rope attached to the footboard facilitates getting in and out of bed. The height of a chair can be raised with cushions on the seat or with hollowed-out blocks placed under the chair legs. Grab bars can be attached to the wall near the toilet and tub to provide leverage and stability.

PREPARING FOR AMBULATION

Regaining the ability to walk is a prime morale builder. To be prepared for ambulation—whether with brace, walker, cane, or crutches—the patient must strengthen the muscles required. Exercise is the foundation of preparation. The nurse instructs and supervises the patient in these exercises.

For ambulation, the quadriceps muscles and the gluteal muscles are strengthened. The quadriceps muscles stabilize the knee joint. To perform quadricep-setting exercises, the patient contracts the quadriceps muscle by attempting to push the popliteal area against the mattress and at the same time raising the heel. The patient maintains the muscle contraction until a count of five and relaxes for a count of five. The exercise is repeated 10 to 15 times hourly. Exercising the quadriceps muscles prevents flexion contractures of the knee. In gluteal setting, the patient contracts or "pinches" the buttocks together to the count of five, relaxes for the count of five, and repeats 10 to 15 times hourly.

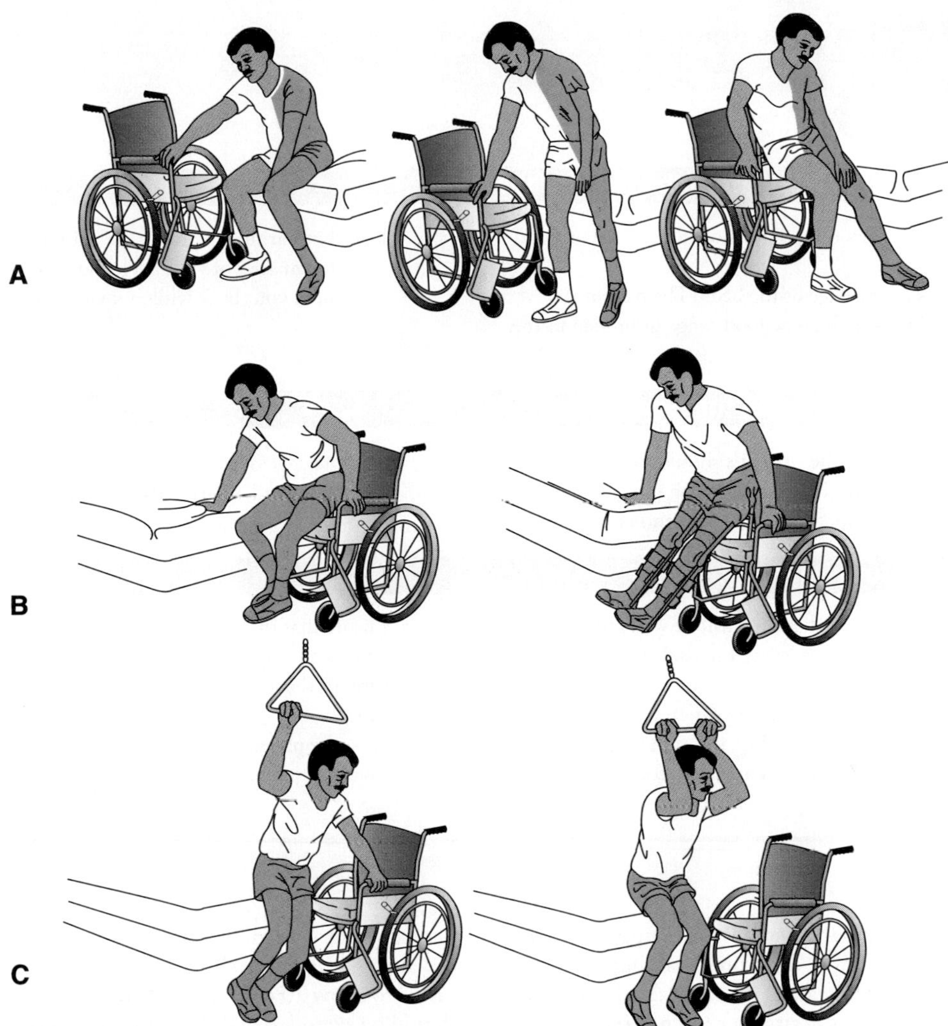

FIGURE 10•1 Methods of transferring the patient from the bed to a wheelchair. The wheelchair is in a locked position. Colored areas indicate non–weight-bearing body parts. (**A**) Weight-bearing transfer from bed to chair. The patient stands up, pivots until his back is opposite the new seat, and sits down. (**B**) (*Left*) Non–weight-bearing transfer from chair to bed. (*Right*) With legs braced. (**C**) (*Left*) Non–weight-bearing transfer, combined method. (*Right*) Non–weight-bearing transfer, pull-up method.

When ambulatory aids (ie, walker, cane, crutches) are used, the muscles of the upper extremities are exercised and strengthened. Push-up exercises are useful. While in a sitting position, the patient raises the body by pushing the hands against the chair seat or mattress. The patient should be encouraged to push-up exercises while in a prone position also. Pull-up exercises done on a trapeze while lifting the body are also effective conditioners. The patient is taught to raise the arms above the head and lower them in a slow, rhythmic manner while holding weights. Gradually, the weight is increased. The hands are strengthened by squeezing a rubber ball.

The physical therapist designs exercises to help the patient develop sitting and standing balance, stability, and coordination needed for ambulation. After sitting and standing balance are achieved, the patient uses parallel bars. Under the supervision of the physical therapist, the patient practices shifting weight from side to side, lifting one leg while supporting weight on the other, and then walking between the parallel bars.

A patient who is ready to begin ambulation must be fitted with the appropriate ambulatory aid, instructed about the prescribed weight-bearing limits (eg, non–weight-bearing, partial weight-bearing ambulation) and taught how to use the aid safely. The nurse continually assesses the patient for stability and adherence to weight-bearing precautions and protects the patient from falling. The nurse provides contact guarding by holding on to a gait belt that the patient wears around the waist. The patient should wear sturdy, well-fitting shoes and be advised of the dangers of wet and highly polished floors and throw rugs. The patient needs to learn how to ambulate on inclines, uneven surfaces, and stairs.

AMBULATING WITH CRUTCHES

Patients prescribed partial weight-bearing or non–weight-bearing ambulation may use crutches. The nurse or physical therapist determines if crutches are appropriate for the patient because good

10•4 GUIDELINES FOR ASSISTING THE PATIENT OUT OF BED

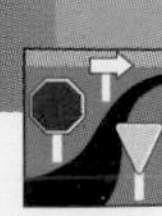

Technique for Moving the Patient to the Edge of the Bed

- Move head and shoulders of patient toward the edge of the bed.
- Move feet and legs to the edge of the bed. (The patient is now in a crescent position, which gives good range of motion to the lateral trunk muscles.)
- Place both arms well under the patient's hips. Next, tighten (set) the muscles of your back and abdomen.
- Straighten your back while moving the patient toward you.

Technique for Sitting Patient on the Edge of the Bed

- Place arm and hand under the patient's shoulders.
- Instruct the patient to push into the bed with the elbow while you lift the patient's shoulders with one arm and swing the legs over the edge of the bed with the other. (Gravity pulls the legs downward, which aids in raising the patient's trunk.)

Technique for Assisting Patient to Stand

- Position the patient's feet so that they will be well grounded.
- Face the patient while firmly grasping each side of the patient's rib cage with your hands.
- Push your knee against one knee of the patient.
- Rock the patient forward to a standing position. (Your knee is pushed against the patient's knee as he or she comes to the standing position.)
- Ensure that the patient's knees are "locked" (in full extension) while standing. (Locking the patient's knees is a safety measure for those who are weak or have been in bed for some time.)
- Give the patient enough time to establish balance.
- Pivot the patient into a sitting position in the chair.

balance, adequate cardiovascular reserve, strong upper extremities, and erect posture are essential for crutch walking.

Ambulating a functional distance (at least the length of a room or house) or maneuvering stairs on crutches requires sufficient arm strength because the arms bear the patient's weight. Muscle groups important for crutch walking include the following:

- Shoulder depressors—to stabilize the upper extremity and prevent shoulder hiking
- Shoulder adductors—to hold the crutch top against the chest wall
- Arm flexors, extensors, and abductors (at the shoulder)—to move crutches forward, backward, and sideways
- Forearm extensors—to prevent flexion or buckling; important in raising the body for swinging gait
- Wrist extensors—to enable weight bearing on hand pieces
- Finger and thumb flexors—to grasp the hand piece

Preparatory exercises are prescribed to strengthen the shoulder girdle and upper extremity muscles.

Before ambulating, the crutches must be adjusted to the patient. To determine the approximate crutch length, the patient may be measured standing or lying down. To measure a standing patient for crutches, the patient is positioned against the wall with the feet slightly apart and away from the wall. Five centimeters (2 inches) are marked out to the side from the tip of the toe. Fifteen centimeters (6 inches) are measured straight ahead from the first mark, and this point is marked. Five centimeters (2 inches) are measured below the axilla to the second mark for the approximate crutch length. If the patient has to be measured while lying down, he or she is measured from the anterior fold of the axilla to the sole of the foot, and then 5 cm (2 inches) are added. If the patient's height is used, 40 cm (16 inches) are subtracted to obtain the approximate crutch length. The hand piece should be adjusted to allow 20 to 30 degrees of flexion at the elbow. The wrist should be extended and the hand dorsiflexed. A foam rubber pad on the under arm piece is used to relieve pressure of the crutch on the upper arm and thoracic cage. For safety, crutches should have large rubber tips, and the patient should wear well-fitting shoes with firm soles.

Teaching Crutch Walking.

The patient is instructed to wear sturdy, well-fitting shoes. The nurse or physical therapist explains and demonstrates to the patient how to use the crutches. The patient learns standing balance by standing on the unaffected leg by a chair. To help the patient maintain balance, the nurse holds the patient near the waist or uses a transfer belt.

The patient is taught to support weight on the hand pieces. (For patients unable to support weight through the wrist and hand because of arthritis or fracture, platform crutches that support the forearm and allow the weight to be borne through the elbow are available.) If weight is borne on the axilla, the pressure of the crutch can damage the brachial plexus nerves, producing "crutch paralysis."

For maximum stability, the patient first assumes the tripod position by placing the crutches about 20 to 25 cm (8 to 10 inches) in front and to the side of his or her toes (Fig. 10-2). (This base of support is adjusted according to the height of the patient, ie, a tall person requires a broader base of support than a short person). In this position, the patient learns how to shift weight and maintain balance.

Before teaching crutch walking, the nurse or therapist determines which gait will be best for the patient. The selection of the crutch gait depends on the type and severity of the disability and on the patient's physical condition, arm and trunk strength, and body balance. The patient should be taught two gaits so he or she can change from one to another. Shifting crutch gaits relieves fatigue because each gait requires the use of a different combination of muscles. (If a muscle is forced to contract steadily without relaxing, the circulation of the blood to that part is reduced.) A faster gait can be used when walking an uninterrupted distance, and a slower gait can be used for short distances or in crowded places. The more common gaits are the four-point, the three-point, the two-point, and the swinging-to and swinging-through gaits. The sequence of movements for each of these gaits is depicted in Chart 10-2.

The nurse walks with the patient just learning how to ambulate with crutches, holding him or her at the waist as needed for balance. During this time, the nurse protects the patient from falls and continually assesses the patient's stability and stamina. Prolonged periods of bed rest and inactivity affect the patient's strength and endurance. Sweating and shortness of breath are indications that crutch walking practice should be stopped and the patient permitted to rest.

Teaching Other Crutch-Maneuvering Techniques.

Before a patient is considered independent in crutch walking, he or she needs to learn to sit in a chair, stand from sitting, and go up and down stairs.

- To sit down:
  1. Grasp the crutches at the hand pieces for control.
  2. Bend forward slightly while assuming a sitting position.
  3. Place the affected leg forward to prevent weight-bearing and flexion.
- To stand up:
  1. Move forward to the edge of the chair with the strong leg slightly under the seat.
  2. Place both crutches in the hand on the side of the affected extremity.
  3. Push down on the hand piece while raising the body to a standing position.
- To go down stairs:
  1. Walk forward as far as possible on the step.
  2. Advance crutches to the lower step. The weaker leg is advanced first and then the stronger one. In this way, the stronger extremity shares with the arms the work of raising and lowering the body weight.
- To go up stairs:
  1. Advance the stronger leg first up to the next step.
  2. Advance the crutches and the weaker extremity. Note that the strong leg goes up first and comes down last. A memory device for the patients is, "up with the good, down with the bad."

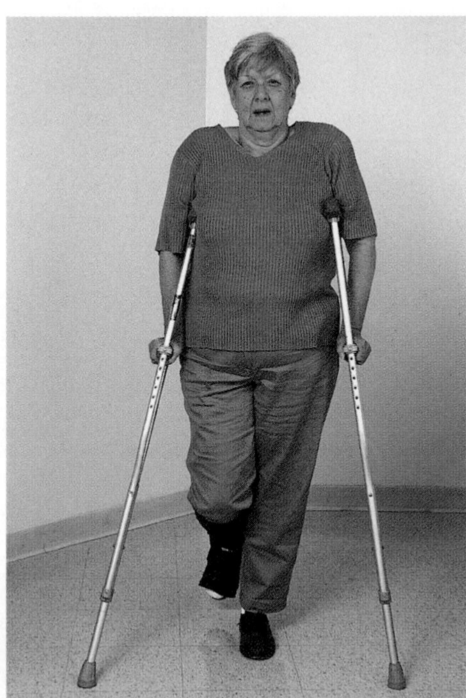

FIGURE 10•2 Crutch walking. The tripod position for basic crutch stance.

AMBULATING WITH A WALKER

A walker provides more support and stability than a cane or crutches. There are two types of walkers: pick-up walkers and rolling walkers. A pick-up walker (one that has to be picked up and moved with each step forward) does not permit a natural walking pattern. It is useful for patients who have poor balance or limited cardiovascular reserve, or who cannot use crutches. A rolling walker allows automatic walking and is used by patients who cannot lift or who inappropriately carry a pick-up walker. The height of the walker is adjusted to the patient. The patient's arms resting on the walker hand grips should exhibit 20 to 30 degrees of flexion at the elbows. The patient should wear sturdy, well-fitting shoes. The nurse walks with the patient, holds him or her at the waist as needed for balance, continually assessing the patient's stability, and protects the patient from falls.

The patient is taught to ambulate with a pick-up walker as follows:

1. Push off a chair or bed to come to a standing position. Never pull yourself up using the walker.
2. Hold the walker on the hand grips for stability.
3. Lift the walker, placing it in front of you while leaning your body slightly forward.
4. Walk into the walker, supporting your body weight on your hands when advancing your weaker leg, permitting partial weight bearing or non–weight bearing as prescribed.
5. Balance yourself on your feet.
6. Lift the walker, and place it in front of you again. Continue this pattern of walking.
7. Remember to look up as you walk.

AMBULATING WITH A CANE

A cane helps the patient walk with greater balance and support and relieves the pressure on weight-bearing joints by redistributing the weight. Quad canes (four-footed canes) provide more stability than straight canes. To fit the patient for a cane, the patient is instructed to flex the elbow at a 30-degree angle, hold the handle of the cane about level with the greater trochanter, and place the tip of the cane 15 cm (6 inches) lateral to the base of the fifth toe. Adjustable canes make individualization easy. The cane should be fitted with a gently flaring tip that has flexible, concentric rings; the tip with its concentric rings provides optimal stability, functions as a shock absorber, and enables the patient to walk with greater speed and less fatigue.

CHART 10•2 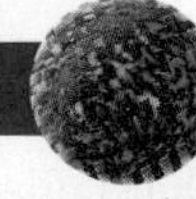 Crutch Gaits

Shaded areas are weight-bearing. Arrow indicates advance of foot or crutch.

4 POINT GAIT	2 POINT GAIT	3 POINT GAIT	SWING TO	SWING THROUGH
• Partial weight bearing both feet • Maximal support provided • Requires constant shift of weight	• Partial weight bearing both feet • Provides less support • Faster than a 4 point gait	• Non-weight bearing • Requires good balance • Requires arm strength • Faster gait • Can use with walker	• Weight bearing both feet • Provides stability • Requires arm strength • Can use with walker	• Weight bearing • Requires arm strength • Requires coordination/ balance • Most advanced gait
4. Advance right foot	4. Advance right foot and left crutch	4. Advance right foot	4. Lift both feet/swing forward/land feet next to crutches	4. Lift both feet/swing forward/land feet in front of crutches
3. Advance left crutch	3. Advance left foot and right crutch	3. Advance left foot and both crutches	3. Advance both crutches	3. Advance both crutches
2. Advance left foot	2. Advance right foot and left crutch	2. Advance right foot	2. Lift both feet/swing forward/land feet next to crutches	2. Lift both feet/swing forward/land feet in front of crutches
1. Advance right crutch	1. Advance left foot and right crutch	1. Advance left foot and both crutches	1. Advance both crutches	1. Advance both crutches
Beginning stance	Beginning stance	Beginning stance	Beginning stance	Beginning stance

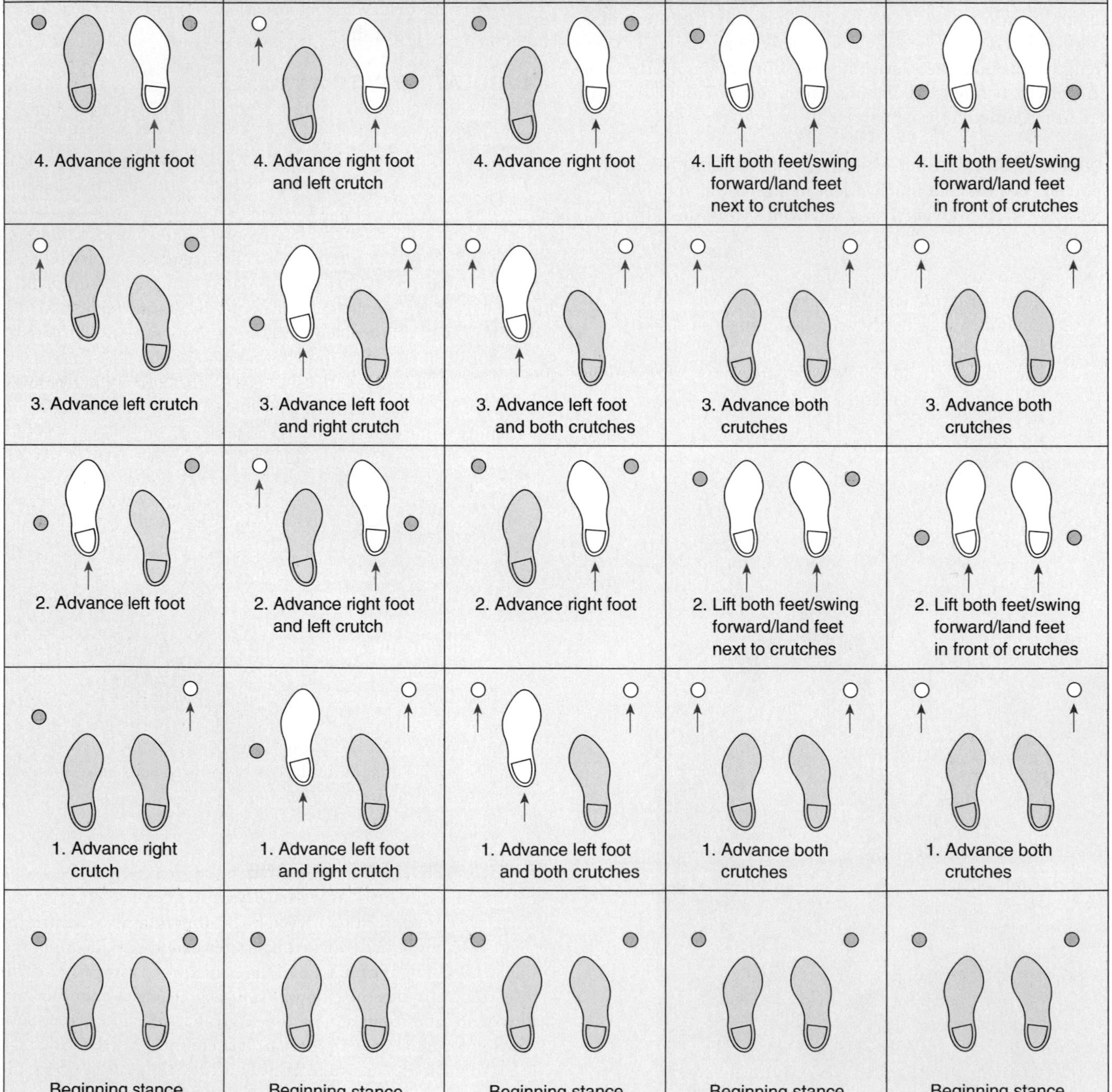

The cane is held in the hand opposite the affected extremity. In normal walking, the opposite leg and arm move together (reciprocal motion); and this motion is to be carried through in walking with a cane. The patient is taught to ambulate with a cane as follows:

- Cane–foot sequence:
  1. Hold the cane in the hand opposite the affected extremity to widen the base of support and to reduce the stress on the involved extremity. (If the patient for some reason is unable to use the cane in the opposite hand, the cane may be used on the same side.)
  2. Advance the cane at the same time the affected leg is moved forward.
  3. Keep the cane fairly close to the body to prevent leaning.
  4. Bear down on the cane when the unaffected extremity begins the swing phase.
- To go up and down stairs using the cane:
  1. Step up on the unaffected extremity.
  2. Place the cane and affected extremity up on the step.
  3. Reverse this procedure for descending steps ("up with the good, down with the bad").

As for all patients beginning ambulation with an ambulatory aid, the nurse continually assesses the patient's stability and protects the patient from falls. The nurse accompanies the patient, holding him or her at the waist as needed for balance. The patient is assessed for tolerance of walking, and rest periods are provided as needed.

ASSISTING THE PATIENT USING AN ORTHOSIS OR PROSTHESIS

Orthoses and prostheses are designed to facilitate mobilization and maximize the patient's quality of life. An orthosis is an external appliance that provides support, prevents or corrects deformities, and improves function. Orthoses include braces, splints, collars, corsets, or supports that are designed and fitted by an orthotist or prosthetist. Static orthoses (no moving parts) are used to stabilize joints and prevent contractures. Dynamic orthoses are flexible and are used to improve function by assisting weak muscles. A prosthesis is an artificial body part. Prostheses may be internal, such as an artificial knee or hip joint, or external, such as an artificial leg or arm.

In addition to learning how to apply and remove the orthosis and maneuver the affected body part correctly, rehabilitation patients must learn how to properly care for the skin that comes in contact with the appliance. Skin problems or pressure ulcers may develop if the device is applied too tightly or too loosely, or if it is adjusted improperly. The nurse instructs the patient to clean and inspect the skin daily, to make sure the brace fits snugly without being too tight, to check that the padding distributes pressure evenly, and to wear a cotton garment without seams between the orthosis and the skin.

If the patient has had an amputation, the nurse promotes tissue healing, uses compression dressings to promote residual limb shaping, and minimizes contracture formation. A permanent prosthetic limb cannot be fitted until the tissue has healed completely and the residual limb shape is stable and free of edema. The nurse also helps the patient cope with the emotional issues surrounding loss of a limb and encourages acceptance of the prosthesis. The prosthetist, the nurse, and the physician collaborate to provide instructions related to skin care and care of the prosthesis.

Evaluation

Expected Outcomes

Expected outcomes may include:

1. Demonstrates improved physical mobility
   a. Maintains muscle strength and joint mobility
   b. Does not develop contractures
   c. Participates in exercise program
2. Transfers safely
   a. Demonstrates assisted transfers
   b. Performs independent transfers
3. Ambulates with maximum independence
   a. Uses ambulatory aid safely
   b. Adheres to weight-bearing prescription
   c. Requests assistance as needed
4. Demonstrates increased activity tolerance
   a. Does not experience orthostatic hypotension episodes
   b. Reports absence of fatigue with ambulatory efforts
   c. Gradually increases distance and speed of ambulation

NURSING PROCESS: THE PATIENT WITH IMPAIRED SKIN INTEGRITY

Patients confined to bed for long periods, patients with motor or sensory dysfunction, and patients who experience muscular atrophy and reduction of padding between the overlying skin and the underlying bone are prone to pressure ulcers. Pressure ulcers are localized areas of infarcted soft tissue that occur when pressure applied to the skin over time is greater than normal capillary closure pressure, which is about 32 mm Hg. Critically ill patients have a lower capillary closure pressure and are at greater risk for pressure ulcers. The initial sign of pressure is erythema (redness of the skin) due to reactive hyperemia. Normally reactive hyperemia resolves in less than 1 hour. Unrelieved pressure results in tissue ischemia or anoxia. The cutaneous tissues become broken or destroyed, leading to progressive destruction and necrosis of underlying soft tissue. The resulting pressure ulcer is painful and slow to heal.

Assessment of Factors Contributing to Pressure Ulcers

Immobility, impaired sensory perception or cognition, decreased tissue perfusion, decreased nutritional status, friction and shear forces, increased moisture, and age-related skin changes all contribute to the development of pressure ulcers.

Immobility

When a person is immobile and inactive, pressure is exerted on the skin and subcutaneous tissue by objects on which the person rests, such as a mattress, chair seat, or cast. The development of pressure ulcers is directly related to the duration of immobility. If pressure continues long enough, small vessel thrombosis and tissue necrosis occur, resulting in a pressure ulcer. Weight-bearing bony prominences are most susceptible to pressure ulcer development. These prominences are covered by skin and small amounts of subcutaneous tissue. Susceptible areas include the sacrum and coccygeal areas, ischial tuberosities (especially in people who sit for prolonged periods), greater trochanter, heel, knee, malleolus, medial condyle of the tibia, fibular head, scapula, and elbow (Fig. 10-3).

Impaired Sensory Perception or Cognition

Patients with sensory loss, impaired levels of consciousness, or paralysis may not be aware of the discomfort associated with prolonged pressure on the skin. Therefore, they do not change position themselves to relieve the pressure. This prolonged pressure impedes blood flow, reducing nourishment of the skin. A pressure ulcer may develop in a short period.

Decreased Tissue Perfusion

Any condition that reduces the circulation and nourishment of the skin and subcutaneous tissue (altered peripheral tissue perfusion) increases the risk of pressure ulcer development. Patients with diabetes mellitus experience an alteration in microcirculation. Similarly, patients with edema have impaired circulation and poor nourishment of the skin tissue. Obese patients have large amounts of poorly vascularized adipose tissue, which is susceptible to breakdown.

Decreased Nutritional Status

Nutritional deficiencies, anemias, and metabolic disorders also contribute to pressure ulcer development. Anemia, regardless of its cause, decreases the blood's oxygen-carrying ability and predisposes to pressure ulcer formation. Patients who have low protein levels or who are in a negative nitrogen balance experience tissue wasting and inhibited tissue repair. Serum albumin is a sensitive indicator of protein deficiency. Albumin levels of less than 3 g/mL are associated with hypoalbuminemic tissue edema and increased risk of pressure ulcers. Specific nutrients, such as vitamin C and trace minerals, are needed for tissue maintenance and repair.

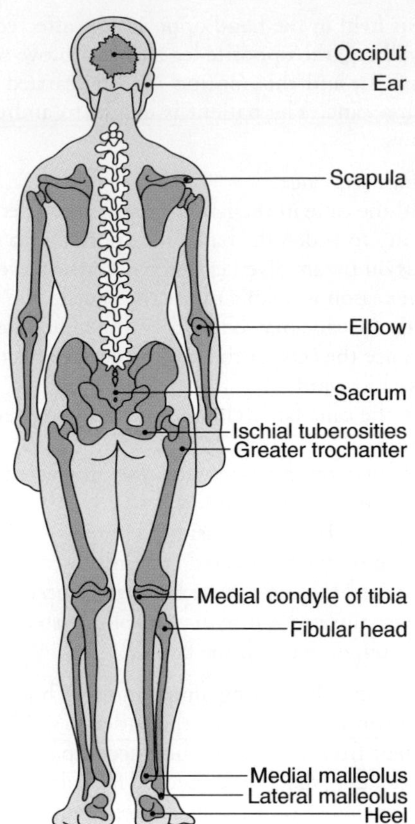

FIGURE 10•3 Areas susceptible to pressure ulcers.

Friction and Shear

Mechanical forces contribute to the development of pressure ulcers. Friction is the resistance to movement that occurs when two surfaces are moved across each other. Shear is created by the interplay of gravitational forces (forces that push the body down) and friction. With shear, tissue layers slide over one another, blood vessels stretch and twist, and the microcirculation of the skin and subcutaneous tissue is disrupted. Evidence of deep tissue damage may be slow to develop and may present through the development of a draining tract. The sacrum and heels are most susceptible to the effects of shear. Pressure ulcers from friction and shear occur when the patient slides down in bed (Fig. 10-4) or when the patient is moved or positioned improperly (eg, dragging the patient up in bed). Spastic muscles and paralysis increase the patient's vulnerability to pressure ulcers related to friction and shear.

Increased Moisture

Prolonged contact with moisture from perspiration, urine, feces, or drainage produces maceration (softening) of the skin. The skin reacts to the caustic substances in the excreta or drainage and becomes irritated. Moist, irritated skin is more vulnerable to pressure breakdown.

Once the skin is broken, the area is invaded by microorganisms (eg, streptococci and staphylococci, *Pseudomonas aeruginosa, Escherichia coli*), and infection occurs. Foul-smelling infectious drainage is present. The lesion may enlarge and allow a continuous loss of serum, which may further deplete the body of essential protein needed for tissue repair and maintenance. The lesion may continue to enlarge and extend deep into the fascia, muscle, and bone, with multiple sinus tracts radiating from the pressure ulcer.

With extensive pressure ulcers, systemic infections may develop, frequently from gram-negative organisms.

Gerontologic Considerations

In older adults, the skin has diminished epidermal thickness, dermal collagen, and tissue elasticity. The skin is drier as a result of diminished sebaceous and sweat gland activity. Cardiovascular changes result in decreased tissue perfusion. Muscles atrophy, and bone structures become prominent. Diminished sensory perception and reduced ability to reposition oneself contribute to prolonged pressure on the skin. Therefore, the older adult is more susceptible to pressure ulcers, which cause pain and suffering and reduce quality of life (Agency for Health Care Policy and Research [AHCPR], 1994).

An estimated 1.7 million patients develop pressure ulcers annually. Both prevention and treatment of pressure ulcers are costly in terms of health care dollars and quality of life for patients at risk. Because the cost in terms of pain and suffering for a person with a pressure ulcer cannot be quantified, the old saying, "an ounce of prevention is worth a pound of cure," is particularly applicable to pressure ulcers.

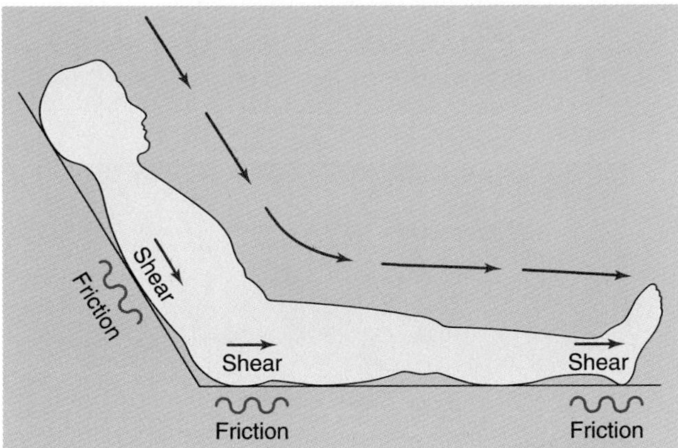

FIGURE 10•4 Mechanical forces contribute to pressure ulcer development. As the person slides down or is improperly pulled up in bed, *friction* resists this movement. *Shear* occurs when one layer of tissue slides over another, disrupting microcirculation of skin and subcutaneous tissue.

Additional Risk Factors

In assessing the patient for potential risk for pressure ulcer development, the nurse assesses the patient's mobility, sensory perception and cognitive abilities, tissue perfusion, nutritional status, friction and shear forces, sources of moisture on the skin, and age. The nurse undertakes the following:

- Assesses total skin condition at least twice a day
- Inspects each pressure site for erythema
- Assesses areas of erythema for blanching response
- Palpates the skin for increased warmth
- Inspects for dry skin, moist skin, breaks in skin
- Notes drainage and odor
- Evaluates level of mobility
- Notes restrictive devices (eg, restraints, splints)
- Evaluates circulatory status (eg, peripheral pulses, edema)
- Assesses neurologic status
- Determines presence of incontinence
- Evaluates nutritional and hydration status
- Reviews the patient's record for laboratory studies, including hematocrit, hemoglobin, electrolytes, albumin, transferrin, and creatinine
- Notes present health problems
- Reviews current medications

To facilitate systematic assessment and quantification of a patient's risk for pressure ulcer, scales such as the Braden or Norton scales may be used. The nurse needs to recognize that the reliability of these scales is not well established. They tend to overpredict those at risk and may promote unwarranted use of costly preventive equipment.

If a pressure area is noted, the nurse notes its size and location and may use a grading system to describe its severity.

Generally, a **stage I** pressure ulcer is an area of nonblanchable erythema, tissue swelling, and congestion, and the patient complains of discomfort. The skin temperature is elevated because of the increased vasodilation. The redness progresses to a dusky, cyanotic blue-gray appearance, which is the result of skin capillary occlusion and subcutaneous weakening.

Risk Factors for DEVELOPING PRESSURE ULCERS

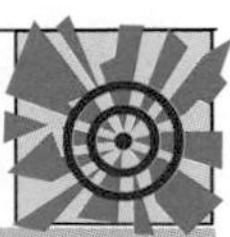

Prolonged pressure on tissue
Immobility, compromised mobility
Loss of protective reflexes, sensory deficit/loss
Poor skin perfusion, edema
Malnutrition, hypoproteinemia, anemia, vitamin deficiency
Friction, shearing forces, trauma
Incontinence of urine or feces
Altered skin moisture: excessively dry, excessively moist
Advanced age, debilitation
Equipment: casts, traction, restraints

A **stage II** pressure ulcer exhibits a break in the skin through the epidermis or the dermis. An abrasion, blister, or shallow crater may be seen. Necrosis occurs. There is venous sludging and thrombosis and edema with cellular extravasation and infiltration.

A **stage III** pressure ulcer extends into the subcutaneous tissues. Clinically, a deep crater with or without undermining of adjacent tissues is noted.

A **stage IV** pressure ulcer extends into the underlying structures, including the muscle and possibly the bone. The skin lesion may represent only the "tip of the iceberg" because a small surface ulcer may be present over a large undermined area.

The appearance of purulent drainage or foul odor suggests an infection. With an extensive pressure ulcer, deep pockets of infection are often present. Drying and crusting of exudate may be present. Infection of a pressure ulcer may advance to osteomyelitis, pyarthrosis (pus formation within a joint cavity), sepsis, and septic shock.

Nursing Diagnosis

Based on the assessment data, the nursing diagnoses include the following:

- Risk for impaired skin integrity
- Impaired skin integrity (related to immobility, decreased sensory perception, decreased tissue perfusion, decreased nutritional status, friction and shear forces, increased moisture, or advanced age)

Planning and Goals

The major goals of the patient may include relief of pressure, improved mobility, improved sensory perception, improved tissue perfusion, improved nutritional status, minimized friction and shear forces, dry surfaces in contact with skin, and healing of pressure ulcer, if present.

Nursing Interventions

Relieving Pressure

Frequent changes of position are needed to relieve and redistribute the pressure on the patient's skin and to prevent prolonged reduced blood flow to the skin and subcutaneous tissues. This can be accomplished by teaching the patient to change position or by turning and repositioning the patient. The patient's family mem-

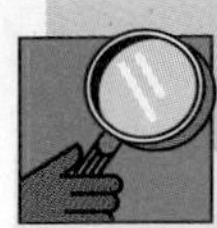

ASSESSMENT
PRESSURE ULCER STAGE

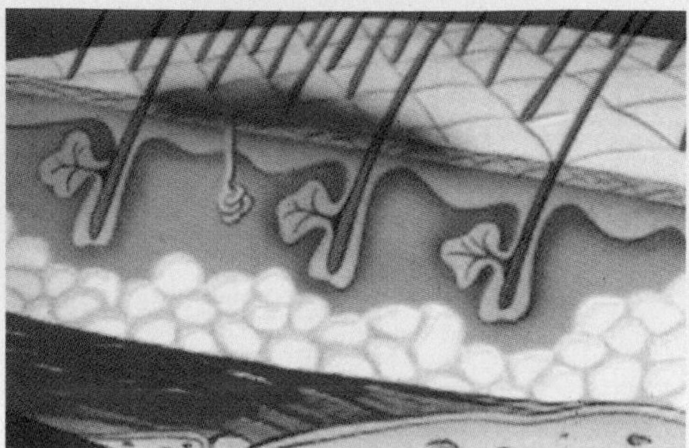

Stage I

- Area of erythema
- Erythema does not blanch with pressure
- Skin temperature elevated
- Tissue swollen and congested
- Patient complains of discomfort
- Erythema progresses to dusky blue-gray

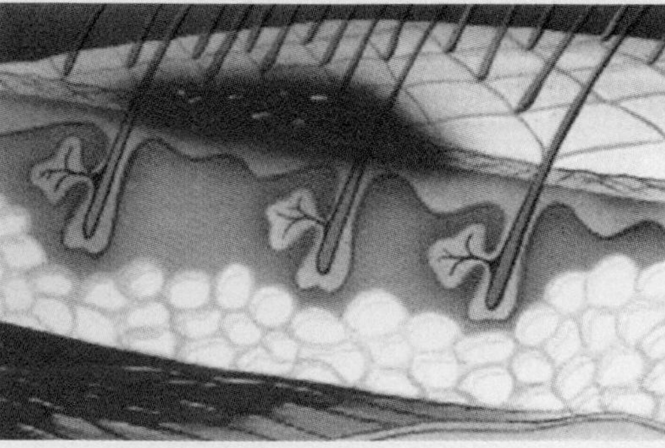

Stage II

- Skin breaks
- Abrasion, blister, or shallow crater
- Edema persists
- Ulcer drains
- Infection may develop

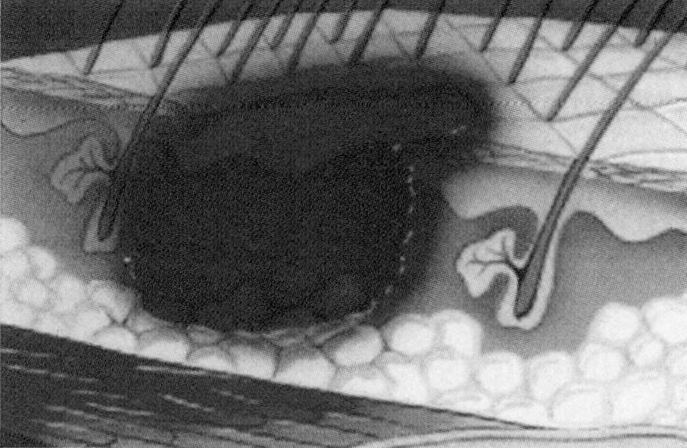

Stage III

- Ulcer extends into subcutaneous tissue
- Necrosis and drainage continue
- Infection develops

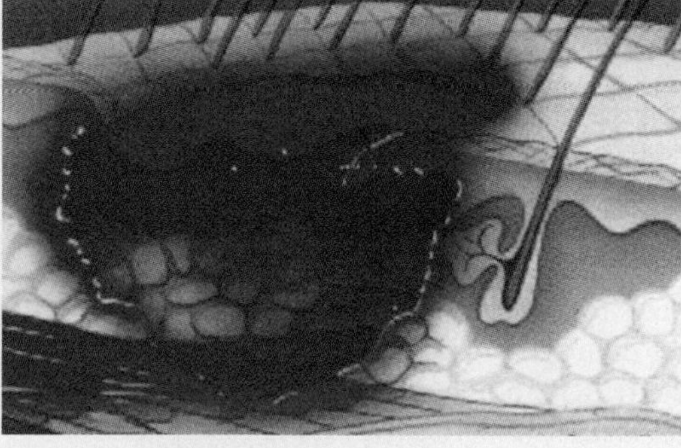

Stage IV

- Ulcer extends to underlying muscle and bone
- Deep pockets of infection develop
- Necrosis and drainage continue

From Weber, J. W., & Kelley, J. (1998). *Health assessment in nursing.* Philadelphia: Lippincott-Raven.

bers should be taught how to position and turn patients at home to prevent pressure ulcers. Shifting weight allows the blood to flow into the ischemic areas and helps the tissues recover from the effects of pressure. Thus, the patient should be cared for as follows:

- Turned and repositioned at 1-hour to 2-hour intervals
- Encouraged to shift weight actively every 15 minutes

POSITIONING

The patient should be positioned laterally, prone, and dorsally in sequence unless not tolerated or contraindicated. The recumbent position is preferred to the semi-Fowler's position because of increased supporting body surface area in this position. In addition to regular turning, there should be small shifts of body weight, such as repositioning an ankle, elbow, or shoulder. The skin is inspected at each position change and assessed for temperature elevation. If redness or heat is noted or if the patient complains of discomfort, pressure on the area must be relieved.

Another way to relieve pressure over bony prominences is the bridging technique, accomplished through the correct positioning of pillows. Just as a bridge is supported on pillars to allow traffic to move underneath, so can the body be supported by pillows to allow for space between bony prominences and the mattress.

A pillow or commercial heel protector may be used to support the heels off the bed when the patient is supine. Placing pillows superior and inferior to the sacrum relieves sacral pressure. Supporting the patient in a 30-degree side-lying position avoids pressure on the trochanter. In the aging patient, frequent small shifts of body weight may be effective. Placing a small rolled towel or sheepskin under a shoulder or hip will allow a return of blood flow to the skin on which the patient is sitting or lying. The towel or sheepskin is moved around the patient's pressure points in a clockwise fashion.

PRESSURE-RELIEVING DEVICES

At times, special equipment and beds may be needed to help relieve the pressure on the skin. These are designed to provide support for specific body areas or for distributing pressure evenly.

Patients sitting in wheelchairs for prolonged periods should have wheelchair cushions fitted and adjusted on an individualized basis, using pressure measurement techniques as a guide to selection and fitting. The aim is to redistribute pressure away from areas at risk for ulcers. However, no cushion is able to eliminate excessive pressure. The patient should be reminded to shift weight frequently and rise for a few seconds every 15 minutes while sitting in a chair (Fig. 10-5).

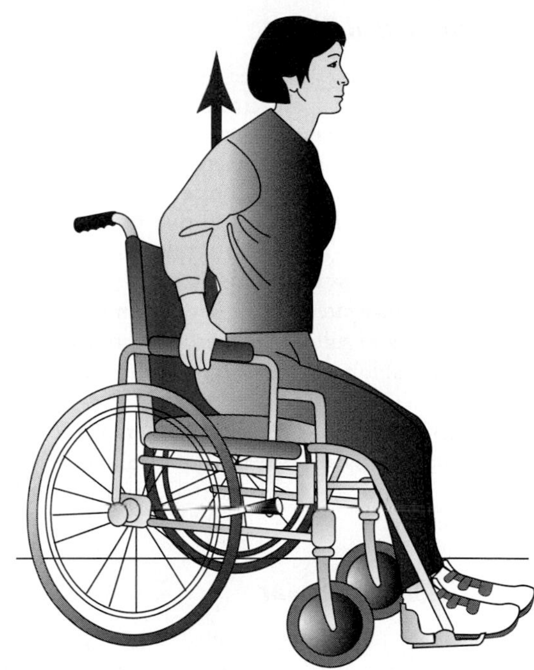

FIGURE 10•5 Wheelchair push-up to prevent ischial pressure ulcers. These push-ups should become an automatic routine (every 15 minutes) for the person with paraplegia. The person should stay up, out of contact with the seat for several seconds. The wheels are kept in the locked position during the exercise.

Static support devices (eg, high-density foam, air, or liquid mattress overlays) distribute pressure evenly by bringing more of the patient's body surface into contact with the supporting surface. The gel-type flotation pad and air-fluidized beds reduce pressure. As the patient's body sinks into the fluid, additional surface becomes available for weight bearing, thereby further decreasing body weight per unit area. (Pascal's law states that the weight of the body floating on a fluid system is evenly distributed over the entire supporting surface.) Thus, there is less pressure on the body parts.

Soft, moisture-absorbing padding is also useful because the softness and resilience of padding provides even distribution of pressure and the dissipation and absorption of moisture, along with freedom from wrinkles and friction. Bony prominences may be protected by gel pads, sheepskin padding, or soft foam rubber beneath the sacrum, the trochanters, heels, elbows, scapulae, and the back of the head when there is pressure on the sites.

Specialized beds have been designed to prevent pressure on the skin. Air-fluidized beds float the patient. Dynamic support surfaces, such as low air-loss pockets, alternately inflate and deflate sections to change support pressure for very high-risk patients who are critically ill and debilitated and cannot be repositioned to relieve pressure. Oscillating or kinetic beds change pressure by means of rocking movements of the bed. The constant movement redistributes the patient's weight and stimulates circulation. These beds are frequently used with patients who have experienced multiple trauma.

Improving Mobility

The patient is encouraged to remain active and is ambulated whenever possible. When sitting, the patient is reminded to change positions frequently to redistribute weight. Active and passive exercises increase muscular, skin, and vascular tone. Circulation is stimulated with activity, which relieves tissue ischemia, the forerunner of pressure ulcers. For the patient at risk for pressure ulcers, turning and exercise schedules are essential. Repositioning must occur around the clock.

Improving Sensory Perception

The nurse helps the patient recognize and compensate for altered sensory perception. Depending on the origin of the alteration (eg, decreased level of consciousness, spinal cord lesion), specific interventions are selected. Strategies to improve cognition and sensory perception may include stimulating the patient to increase awareness of self in the environment, encouraging the patient to participate in self-care, or supporting the patient's efforts toward active compensation for loss of sensation (eg, a paraplegic patient lifting up from the sitting position every 15 minutes). When decreased sensory perception exists, the patient and caregiver are taught to inspect potential pressure areas visually, using a mirror if needed, for evidence of pressure ulcer development every morning and evening.

Improving Tissue Perfusion

Exercise and repositioning improve tissue perfusion. Massage of erythematous areas is avoided because damage to the capillaries and deep tissue may occur.

Nursing Alert *Reddened areas are not massaged because this may increase the damage to already traumatized skin and tissue.*

In patients who have evidence of compromised peripheral circulation such as edema, positioning and elevation of the edematous body part to promote venous return and diminish congestion improve tissue perfusion. In addition, the nurse or family must be alert to environmental factors (eg, wrinkles in sheets, pressure of tubes) that may contribute to pressure on the skin and diminished circulation; the source of pressure must be removed.

Improving Nutritional Status

The patient's nutritional status must be adequate, and a positive nitrogen balance must be maintained. Pressure ulcers develop more quickly and are more resistant to treatment in patients suffering from nutritional disorders. A high-protein diet with protein supplements may be helpful. Iron preparations may be necessary to raise the hemoglobin level so that tissue oxygen levels can be maintained within acceptable limits. Ascorbic acid (vitamin C) is necessary for tissue healing.

Other nutrients associated with healthy skin include vitamin A, B vitamins, zinc, and sulfur. With balanced nutrition and hydration, the skin is able to remain healthy, and damaged tissues can be repaired.

To assess nutritional status response to therapeutic strategies, the nurse monitors the patient's hemoglobin, albumin, and body weight weekly. Nutritional assessment is described in further detail in Chapter 5.

Reducing Friction and Shear

Shear occurs when the patient is pulled, allowed to slump, or moves by digging heels or elbows into the mattress. Raising the head of the bed by even a few centimeters increases the shearing force over the sacral area. Therefore, the semireclining position is avoided in patients at risk. Proper positioning with adequate support is important when a patient is sitting in a chair. Polyester sheepskin pads are thought to reduce shear and friction and may be used with at-risk patients.

Nursing Alert *To avoid shearing forces when repositioning the patient, the nurse lifts and avoids dragging the patient across a surface.*

Minimizing Moisture

Continuous moisture on the skin must be prevented by meticulous hygienic measures. Perspiration, urine, stool, and drainage must be removed from the skin promptly. The soiled skin should be washed immediately with mild soap and water and blotted dry with a soft towel. The skin may be lubricated with a bland lotion to keep it soft and pliable. Drying agents and powders are avoided. Topical barrier ointments (eg, petroleum jelly) may be helpful in protecting the skin of patients who are incontinent.

Absorbent pads that wick moisture away from the body should be used to absorb drainage. Patients who are incontinent need to be checked and their wet incontinence pads and linens changed promptly. All efforts must be made to keep the skin clean and dry.

Promoting Pressure Ulcer Healing

Regardless of the stage of the pressure ulcer, the pressure on the area must be eliminated. The ulcer will not heal until all pressure is removed. The patient must not lie or sit on the pressure ulcer, even for a few minutes. Individualized positioning and turning schedules must be written in the plan of nursing care and followed meticulously.

In addition, inadequate nutritional status and fluid and electrolyte abnormalities must be corrected to promote healing. Wounds that drain body fluids and protein place the patient in a catabolic state and predispose to hypoproteinemia and serious secondary infections. Protein deficiency must be corrected to heal the pressure ulcer. Carbohydrates are necessary to "spare" the protein and to provide an energy source. Vitamin C and trace elements, especially zinc, are necessary for collagen formation and wound healing.

STAGE I PRESSURE ULCERS

To permit healing of stage I pressure ulcers, the pressure is removed to permit increased tissue perfusion, improved nutritional and fluid and electrolyte status, reduction of friction and shear, and avoidance of moisture to the skin.

STAGE II PRESSURE ULCERS

Stage II pressure ulcers have broken skin. In addition to measures listed for stage I pressure ulcers, a moist environment is desired to aid wound healing. A heat lamp is not used to dry the open wound. Migration of epidermal cells over the ulcer surface occurs more rapidly in a moist environment. The ulcer is gently cleansed with sterile saline solution. Use of antiseptic solutions that damage healthy tissues and delay wound healing is avoided. Semipermeable occlusive dressing, hydrocolloid wafers, or wet saline dressings are helpful in providing a moist environment for healing and in minimizing the loss of fluids and proteins from the body.

STAGE III AND IV PRESSURE ULCERS

Stage III and IV pressure ulcers are characterized by extensive tissue damage. In addition to measures listed for stage I, these advanced draining, necrotic pressure ulcers must be cleaned (débrided) to create an area that will heal. Necrotic, devitalized tissue favors bacterial growth, delays granulation, and inhibits healing. Wound cleaning and dressing are uncomfortable; therefore, the nurse must prepare the patient, explain the procedure, and administer prescribed analgesia when needed.

Débridement may be accomplished by wet-to-damp dressing changes, mechanical flushing of necrotic and infective exudate, application of prescribed enzyme preparations that dissolve necrotic tissue, or surgical dissection. If an eschar covers the ulcer, it is removed surgically to ensure a clean, vitalized wound. Exudate may be absorbed by dressings or special hydrophilic powders, beads, or gels. Cultures of infected pressure ulcers are obtained to guide selection of antibiotic therapy.

After the pressure ulcer is clean, a topical treatment is prescribed. The goal of therapy is to promote granulation. New granulation tissue must be protected from reinfection, drying, and damage. Care should be taken to prevent pressure and further trauma to the area. Dressings, solutions, and ointments applied to the ulcer should not disrupt the healing process. Multiple agents and protocols are used to treat pressure ulcers. Consistency is an important key to success. In addition, objective evaluation of the pressure ulcer (eg, measuring the pressure ulcer, inspecting for granulation tissue) for response to the treatment protocol must be made every 4 to 6 days. Taking photographs at weekly intervals is a reliable strategy for monitoring the healing process. Pressure ulcers can take a long time to heal.

Surgical intervention is necessary when the ulcer is extensive, when potential complications (such as fistula) exist, and when the ulcer does not respond to treatment. Surgical procedures include débridement, incision and drainage, bone resection, skin grafting, skin flaps, and myocutaneous flaps.

PREVENTING RECURRENCE

Recurrence of pressure ulcers should be anticipated; therefore, active, preventive intervention and frequent continuing assessment are essential. The patient's tolerance for sitting or lying on the healed pressure area is increased gradually; the time that pressure is allowed on the area is increased in 5- to 15-minute increments. The patient is taught to increase mobility and to follow a regimen of turning, weight shifting, and repositioning. The patient teaching plan includes instruction on strategies to reduce the risk for developing pressure ulcers and methods to detect, inspect, and minimize pressure areas. Early recognition and intervention are keys to long-term management of potential impaired skin integrity.

Evaluation

Expected Outcomes

Expected outcomes may include:

1. Maintains intact skin
   a. Exhibits no areas of nonblanchable erythema at bony prominences
   b. Avoids massage of bony prominences
   c. Exhibits no breaks in skin
2. Limits pressure on bony prominences
   a. Changes position every 1 to 2 hours
   b. Uses bridging techniques to remove pressure
   c. Uses special equipment as appropriate
   d. Raises self from seat or wheelchair every 15 minutes
3. Increases mobility
   a. Performs range-of-motion exercises
   b. Adheres to turning schedule
   c. Advances sitting time as tolerated
4. Sensory and cognitive ability improved
   a. Demonstrates improved level of consciousness
   b. Inspects potential pressure ulcer areas every morning and evening
5. Demonstrates improved tissue perfusion
   a. Exercises to increase circulation
   b. Elevates body parts susceptible to edema
6. Attains and maintains adequate nutritional status
   a. Verbalizes the importance of protein and vitamin C in diet
   b. Eats balanced diet high in protein and vitamin C
   c. Maintains hemoglobin, electrolyte, albumin, transferrin, and creatinine levels at acceptable levels
7. Avoids friction and shear
   a. Avoids semireclining position
   b. Uses sheepskin pad and heel protectors when appropriate
   c. Lifts body instead of sliding across surfaces
8. Maintains clean, dry skin
   a. Avoids prolonged contact with wet or soiled surfaces
   b. Keeps skin clean and dry
   c. Uses lotion to keep skin lubricated
9. Experiences healing of pressure ulcer
   a. Avoids pressure on area
   b. Improves nutritional status
   c. Participates in therapeutic regimen
   d. Demonstrates behaviors to prevent new pressure ulcers
   e. States early indicators of pressure ulcer development

NURSING PROCESS: THE PATIENT WITH ALTERED ELIMINATION PATTERNS

Urinary and bowel incontinence or constipation and impaction are problems that occur often in disabled patients. Incontinence curtails a person's independence, causing embarrassment and isolation. It occurs in up to 15% of the community-based elderly population, whereas almost half of nursing home residents are bowel or bladder incontinent or both. In addition, constipation may be a problem for the patients with disabilities. Complete and predictable evacuation of the bowel are goals. If a bowel routine is not established, the person may experience abdominal distention, small, frequent oozing of stool, or impaction.

Assessment

Urinary incontinence can be classified as urge, reflex, stress, functional, or total incontinence (AHCPR, 1996). **Urge incontinence** is involuntary elimination of urine associated with a strong perceived need to void. **Reflex (neurogenic) incontinence** is associated with a spinal cord lesion that interrupts cerebral control, resulting in no sensory awareness of the need to void. **Stress incontinence** is associated with weakened perineal muscles that permit leakage of urine when intra-abdominal pressure is increased (eg, with coughing or sneezing). **Functional incontinence** refers to incontinence in patients with intact urinary physiology who experience mobility impairment, environmental barriers, or cognitive problems. They are unable to reach and use the toilet before soiling themselves. **Total incontinence** occurs in patients who are unable to control excreta because of physiologic or psychological impairment; management of the excreta is the focus of nursing care. Urinary incontinence may result from multiple causes (eg, urinary tract infection, detrusor instability, bladder outlet obstruction or incompetence, neurologic impairment, bladder spasm or contracture, inability to reach the toilet in time).

The health history is used to explore bladder and bowel function, symptoms associated with dysfunction, physiologic risk factors for elimination problems, perception of micturition and defecation cues, and functional toileting abilities. Previous and current fluid intake and voiding patterns may be helpful in designing the plan of nursing care. A record of times of voiding and amounts voided is kept for at least 48 hours. In addition, episodes of incontinence and associated activity (eg, coughing, sneezing, lifting), fluid intake time and amount, and medications are recorded. This record is analyzed and used to determine patterns and relationships of incontinence to other activities and factors.

The ability to get to the bathroom, manipulate clothing, and use the toilet are important functional factors that may be related to incontinence. Also, related cognitive functioning (perception of need to void, verbalization of need to void, and ability to learn to control urination) must be assessed. In addition, the nurse reviews the results of the diagnostic studies (eg, urinalysis, urodynamic tests, postvoiding residual volumes).

Bowel incontinence and constipation may result from multiple causes (eg, diminished or absent sphincter control, cognitive or perceptual impairment, neurogenic factors, diet, immobility). The origin of the bowel problem must be determined.

The nurse assesses the patient's normal bowel patterns, nutritional patterns, use of laxatives, gastrointestinal problems (eg, colitis), bowel sounds, anal reflex and tone, and functional abilities. The character and frequency of bowel movements are recorded and analyzed.

Nursing Diagnosis

Based on the assessment data, major nursing diagnoses for the patient may include the following:

- Altered bowel elimination
- Altered urinary elimination

Planning and Goals

The major goals of the patient may include control of urinary incontinence or urinary retention, control of bowel incontinence, and regular elimination patterns.

Nursing Interventions

Promoting Urinary Continence

After the nature of the urinary incontinence has been identified, a nursing plan of care is developed based on analysis of the assessment data. Various approaches to promotion of urinary continence have been designed. Most approaches attempt to condition the body to control urination or to minimize the occurrence of unscheduled urination. Selection of the approach depends on the cause and type of the patient's incontinence. For the program to be successful, the patient's participation and desire to avoid incontinence episodes are crucial. An optimistic attitude with positive feedback for even slight gains is essential for success. Accurate recording of intake and output and response to selected strategies is essential for evaluation.

At no time should the fluid intake be restricted to decrease frequency of urination. Sufficient fluid intake (2,000 to 3,000 mL/day according to patient needs) must be ensured. To optimize the likelihood of voiding as scheduled, measured amounts of fluids may be administered about 30 minutes before voiding attempts. In addition, most of the fluids should be consumed before evening to minimize the need to void frequently during the night.

GERONTOLOGIC CONSIDERATIONS

Factors Altering Elimination Patterns in the Older Adult

- Decreased bladder capacity
- Decreased muscle tone
- Increased residual volumes
- Delayed perception of elimination cues
- Medications that alter elimination patterns, such as diuretics (increase volume of urine produced), sedatives (alter bladder sensitivity to cues), and adrenergics or anticholinergics (cause urinary retention)
- Functional immobility
- Activity intolerance

The goal of bladder training is to restore the bladder to normal function. It can be used with cognitively intact patients experiencing urge incontinence. A voiding and toileting schedule is formulated based on analysis of the assessment data. The schedule specifies times for the patient to try to empty the bladder using a bedpan, toilet, or commode. Privacy should be provided during voiding efforts. The interval between voiding times in the early phase of the bladder training period is short (1½ to 2 hours). The patient is encouraged not to void until the specified voiding time. Voiding success and episodes of incontinence are recorded. As the patient's bladder capacity and control increase, the interval is lengthened. Usually, there is a temporal relationship between drinking, eating, exercising, and voiding. The alert patient can participate in recording intake, activity, and voiding and can plan the schedule to achieve maximum continence.

Barrier-free access to the toilet and modification of clothing help the patient with functional incontinence to achieve self-care in toileting and continence.

Habit training is used to try to keep the patient dry by strictly adhering to a toileting schedule. It may be successful with stress, urge, or functional incontinence. With a confused person, the caregiver takes the person to the toilet according to the schedule before involuntary voiding occurs. Simple cuing and consistency promote success. Periods of continence and successful voidings are praised and rewarded.

Biofeedback is a system through which the patient learns consciously to contract excretory sphincters and control voiding cues. Cognitively intact patients who have stress or urge incontinence may gain bladder control through biofeedback.

Pelvic floor exercises (Kegel exercises) strengthen the pubococcygeus muscle. The patient is instructed to tighten pelvic floor muscles for 4 seconds 10 times, 4 to 6 times a day. Stopping and starting the stream during urination is recommended to increase control. Daily practice is essential. These exercises are helpful for cognitively intact women who experience stress incontinence.

Suprapubic tapping or stroking the inner thigh may produce voiding by stimulating the voiding reflex arc in patients with reflex incontinence. This method is not always effective, however, because of the presence of detrusor–sphincter dyssynergy. As the bladder reflexively contracts to expel urine, the bladder sphincter reflexively closes, producing a high residual urine volume and an increased incidence of urinary tract infection.

Intermittent self-catheterization is an appropriate alternative for managing reflex incontinence, urinary retention, and overflow incontinence due to an overdistended bladder. Emphasis of patient teaching is placed on the regular emptying of the bladder rather than sterility. Disabled patients reuse and clean catheters with bleach or hydrogen peroxide solutions or soap and water and may use a microwave oven to sterilize catheters. Aseptic intermittent catheterization technique is required in health care institutions because of the potential for bladder infection from resistant organisms. Intermittent self-catheterization may be difficult for patients with limited mobility, dexterity, or vision; however, family members can be taught the procedure.

Indwelling catheters are avoided if at all possible. The incidence of urinary tract infection with indwelling catheters is high. Short-term use may be needed during treatment of severe skin breakdown due to continued incontinence. Disabled patients who are unable to perform intermittent self-catheterization may elect to use a suprapubic catheter for long-term bladder management. Suprapubic catheters are easier to maintain than indwelling catheters. A fluid intake of 3000 mL/day must be encouraged.

External catheters (condom catheters) and leg bags to collect spontaneous voidings are useful for male patients with reflex or total incontinence. The appropriate design and size must be chosen for maximal success. The patient or caregiver must be taught how to apply the condom catheter and how to provide daily hygiene, including skin inspection. Instruction on emptying the leg bag must also be provided, and modifications can be made for patients with limited hand dexterity. External collection devices for women do exist, but difficulties with fit have precluded widespread use.

Incontinence pads (briefs) are used only as a last resort. They manage rather than solve the incontinence problem. Also, they have a negative psychological effect on the patient because many people think of them as diapers. Every effort should be made to reduce the incidence of incontinence episodes through other methods that have been described. Incontinence pads may be useful at times for patients with stress or total incontinence to protect clothing, but they should be avoided whenever possible. When incontinence pads are used, they should wick moisture away from the body to minimize contact of moisture and excreta with the skin. Wet incontinence pads must be changed promptly, the skin cleansed, and a moisture barrier applied to protect the skin.

Promoting Bowel Continence

The goals of a bowel training program are to develop regular bowel habits and to prevent uninhibited bowel elimination. Regular complete emptying of the lower bowel results in bowel continence. A bowel-training program takes advantage of the patient's natural reflexes. Regularity, timing, nutrition and fluids, exercise, and correct positioning promote predictable defecation.

The nurse records defecation time, character of stool, nutritional intake, cognitive abilities, and functional self-care toileting abilities for 5 to 7 days. Analysis of this record is helpful when designing a bowel program for the patient with fecal incontinence.

Consistency in implementing the plan is essential. A regular time for defecation is established. Attempts at evacuation should be within 15 minutes of the designated time daily. Natural gastrocolic and duodenocolic reflexes occur about 30 minutes after a meal. Therefore, after breakfast is one of the best times to plan for bowel evacuation. If the patient had a previously established habit pattern at a different time of day, it should be followed.

The anorectal reflex may be stimulated by rectal suppository (eg, glycerin) or mechanical stimulation (eg, digital stimulation with a lubricated gloved finger or anal dilator). Mechanical stimulation should only be used in disabled patients who have no voluntary motor function and no sensation as a result of injuries above the sacral segments of the spinal cord (ie, quadriplegic, high paraplegic, or severely brain-injured patients). The technique is not effective in patients who do not have an intact sacral reflex arc (ie, those with flaccid paralysis). Mechanical stimulation, suppository insertion, or both should be initiated about 30 minutes before the scheduled bowel elimination time. The interval between stimulation and defecation is noted for subsequent modification of the bowel program. Once the bowel routine is well established, stimulation with a suppository may not be necessary.

The patient should assume the normal squatting position (knees higher than the hips) and be in a private bathroom for defecation if at all possible. A padded commode chair or bedside toilet is an acceptable alternative. Seating time is limited in patients at risk for skin breakdown. Bedpans should be avoided. A disabled patient who is unable to sit on a toilet should be positioned on the left side with legs flexed and the head of the bed elevated 30 to 45 degrees to increase intra-abdominal pressure. Protective padding is placed behind the buttocks. When possible, the patient is instructed to bear down and to contract the abdominal muscles. Massaging the abdomen right to left facilitates movement of feces in the lower tract.

Preventing Constipation

The record of bowel elimination, character of stool, food and fluid intake, level of activity, bowel sounds, medications, and other assessment data are reviewed to develop the plan of care. Multiple approaches may be used to prevent constipation. The diet should be well balanced and include adequate intake of high-fiber foods (vegetables, fruits, bran) to prevent hard stools and stimulate peristalsis. Fluid intake should be between 2 and 3 L/day unless contraindicated. Prune juice or fig juice (120 mL) taken 30 minutes before a meal once daily is helpful to some when constipation is a problem. Physical activity and exercise are encouraged, as is self-care in toileting. The patient is encouraged to respond to the natural urge to defecate. Privacy during toileting is provided. Stool softeners, bulk-forming agents, mild stimulants, and suppositories may be prescribed to stimulate defecation and to prevent constipation.

Evaluation

Expected Outcomes

Expected outcomes may include:

1. Demonstrates control over excreta
   a. Experiences no episodes of incontinence
   b. Avoids constipation
   c. Achieves independence in toileting
   d. Expresses satisfaction in level of excreta control
2. Achieves urinary continence
   a. Uses therapeutic approach appropriate to type of incontinence
   b. Maintains adequate fluid intake
   c. Washes and dries skin after episodes of incontinence
3. Achieves bowel continence
   a. Participates in bowel program
   b. Verbalizes need for regular time for bowel evacuation
   c. Modifies diet to promote continence
   d. Uses bowel stimulants as prescribed and needed
4. Experiences relief of constipation
   a. Uses high-fiber diet, fluids, and exercise to promote defecation
   b. Responds to urge to defecate

SEXUALITY ISSUES

An issue confronting the disabled patient and an important component of self-concept is sexuality. Sexuality involves not only biologic sexual activity but also one's concept of masculinity or femininity. Sexuality affects the way a person reacts to others and is perceived by them, and is expressed not only by physical intimacy but also by caring and emotional intimacy.

Sexuality problems faced by disabled patients include limited access to information about sexuality, lack of opportunity to form friendships and loving relationships, impaired self-image, and low self-esteem. Frequently, rehabilitation programs focus only on helping the patient gain independence and forget that sexuality is part of the patient's identity. Recognizing and addressing sexual issues promotes feelings of self-worth, which are essential to total rehabilitation. The nurse should give the patient "permission" to discuss sexuality concerns and should show a willingness to listen and help the patient overcome these concerns. The disabled person may need sex education and communication, social, and assertiveness skills to develop relationships in general. The specialized services of a sex counselor or therapist are available to help those with specific sexual needs or conflicts. Classes, books, movies, and support groups also may be useful.

COPING WITH FATIGUE

People with disabilities frequently experience fatigue. Physical and emotional weariness may be caused by discomfort and pain associated with a chronic health problem, deconditioning associated with prolonged periods of bed rest and immobility, impaired motor function requiring excessive expenditure of energy to ambulate, and the frustrations of performing ADLs. Ineffective coping with the disability, unresolved grief, and depression can contribute to fatigue. The patient can use coping strategies to manage the psychological impact of the disability and pain management techniques to control the associated discomforts (see Chap. 12 for a discussion of pain management). In addition, the nurse can teach the patient to manage fatigue through priority setting and energy-conserving techniques.

The following may be useful in teaching patients how to reduce their energy output, thus conserving their strength to achieve a meaningful lifestyle:

Take Control of Your Life
- Face the reality of your disability.
- Emphasize areas of strength.
- Remain outward looking.
- Seek inventive ways to tackle problems.
- Share concerns and frustrations.
- Maintain and improve general health.
- Plan for recreation.

Have Well-Defined Goals and Priorities
- Keep priorities in order; eliminate nonessential activities.
- Plan and pace your activities.

Organize Your Life
- Plan each day.
- Organize work.
- Perform tasks in steps.
- Distribute heavy work throughout the day or week.

Conserve Energy
- Rest before undertaking difficult tasks.
- Stop the activity before fatigue occurs.
- Continue with an exercise conditioning program to strengthen muscles.

Control Your Environment
- Try to be well organized.
- Keep possessions in the same place, so that they can be found with a minimum of effort.
- Store equipment (personal care, crafts, work) in a box or basket.
- Use energy-conservation and work-simplification techniques.
- Keep work within easy reach and in front of you.
- Use adaptive equipment, self-help aids, and labor-saving devices.
- Recruit assistance of others; delegate when necessary.
- Take safety precautions.

PROMOTING HOME AND COMMUNITY-BASED CARE

An important goal of rehabilitation is to assist the person to return to the home environment after learning to manage the disability. A referral system maintains continuity of care when the patient is transferred to the home or to an extended care facility. The plan for discharge is formulated when the patient is first admitted to the hospital, and discharge plans are made with the patient's functional potential in mind.

The patient's support system (family, friends) is assessed. The attitudes of family and friends toward the patient, the disability, and the return home are important in successful transition to home. Not all families are able to carry on the arduous programs of exercise, physical training, and personal care that a patient may need. They may not have the resources or stability to care for a severely disabled family member. Even a stable family may be overwhelmed by the physical, emotional, economic, and energy strains of a disabling condition. Members of the rehabilitation team must not judge the family but rather should provide supportive interventions that help them attain their highest level of function.

The family needs to know as much as possible about the patient's condition and care so that they do not fear the patient's return home. The nurse develops with the patient and family methods for coping with problems that may arise. A skills checklist individualized for the patient and family can be developed to make certain that the family is proficient in assisting the patient with certain tasks.

Continuing Care

The home care nurse may visit the patient in the hospital, interview the patient and family, and review the ADL sheet to gain knowledge of the activities the patient can perform. This helps ensure continuity of care and that the patient does not "lose ground" but instead maintains the independence gained while in the hospital. The family may need to purchase, borrow, or improvise needed equipment, such as safety rails, raised toilet seat or commode, or tub bench. Ramps may have to be built or doorways widened to achieve full access.

Family members are taught how to use equipment and are given a copy of the equipment manufacturer's instruction booklet, the names of resource people, and lists of supplies and where these may be obtained. A written summary of the care plan is included in family teaching.

A network of support services and communication systems may be required to enhance opportunities for independent living. The nurse uses collaborative, administrative skills to coordinate these activities and to pull together the network of care. The nurse also provides skilled care, initiates additional referrals when indicated, and serves as the patient's advocate and counselor when obstacles are encountered. The nurse continues to reinforce the teaching that has been done and helps the patient to set and

HOME CARE TEACHING CHECKLIST: MANAGING THE THERAPEUTIC REGIMEN AT HOME

At the completion of the program, the patient or caregiver will be able to: **Patient** **Caregiver**

- State the impact of disability on physiologic functioning. ✔ ✔
- State changes in lifestyle necessary to maintain health. ✔ ✔
- State the name, dose, side effects, frequency, and schedule for all medications. ✔ ✔
- State how to obtain medical supplies after discharge. ✔ ✔
- Identify durable medical equipment needs, proper usage, and maintenance necessary for safe utilization: ✔ ✔
  - [ ] Wheelchair—manual/power
  - [ ] Cushion
  - [ ] Grab bars
  - [ ] Sliding board
  - [ ] Mechanical lift
  - [ ] Raised padded commode seat
  - [ ] Padded commode wheelchair
  - [ ] Bedside toilet
  - [ ] Crutches
  - [ ] Walker
  - [ ] Prosthesis
  - [ ] Orthosis
  - [ ] Specialty bed
- Demonstrate usage of adaptive equipment for activities of daily living: ✔ ✔
  - [ ] Long-handled sponge
  - [ ] Reacher
  - [ ] Universal cuff
  - [ ] Plate mat and guard
  - [ ] Rocker-knife, spork, weighted utensils
  - [ ] Special closures for clothing
  - [ ] Other
- Demonstrate mobility skills: ✔ ✔
  - [ ] Transfers: bed to chair; in and out of toilet and tub; in and out of car
  - [ ] Negotiate ramps, curbs, stairs
  - [ ] Assume sitting from supine position
  - [ ] Turn side to side in bed
  - [ ] Maneuver wheelchair; manage arm and leg rests; lock brakes
  - [ ] Ambulate safely using assistive devices
  - [ ] Range-of-motion exercises
  - [ ] Muscle-strengthening exercises
- Demonstrate skin care: ✔ ✔
  - [ ] Inspect bony prominences every morning and evening
  - [ ] Identify stage I pressure ulcer and actions to take if present
  - [ ] Change dressings for stage II to IV pressure ulcers
  - [ ] State dietary requirements to promote healing of pressure ulcers
  - [ ] Demonstrate pressure relief at prescribed intervals
  - [ ] State sitting schedule
  - [ ] Demonstrate adherence to bed turning schedule, bed positioning, and use of bridging techniques
  - [ ] Apply and wear protective boots at prescribed times
  - [ ] Demonstrate correct wheelchair sitting posture
  - [ ] Demonstrate techniques to avoid friction and shear in bed
  - [ ] Demonstrate proper hygiene to maintain skin integrity
- Demonstrate bladder care: ✔ ✔
  - [ ] State schedule for voiding, toileting, and catheterization
  - [ ] Identify relationship of fluid intake to voiding and catheterization schedule
  - [ ] State how to perform pelvic floor exercises
  - [ ] Demonstrate clean self-intermittent catheterization and care of catheterization equipment
  - [ ] Demonstrate indwelling catheter care
  - [ ] Demonstrate application of external condom catheter
  - [ ] Demonstrate application, emptying, and cleaning of urinary drainage bag
  - [ ] Demonstrate application of incontinence pads and performing perineal hygiene
  - [ ] State signs and symptoms of urinary tract infection
- Demonstrate bowel care ✔ ✔
  - [ ] State optimum dietary intake to promote evacuation
  - [ ] Identify schedule for optimum bowel evacuation
  - [ ] Demonstrate techniques to increase intra-abdominal pressure: Valsalva maneuver; abdominal massage; leaning forward
  - [ ] Demonstrate techniques to stimulate bowel movements: ingesting warm liquids, digital stimulation; insertion of suppositories
  - [ ] Demonstrate optimum position for bowel evacuation: up on toilet with knees higher than hips; left side in bed with knees flexed and head slightly elevated
  - [ ] Identify complications and corrective strategies for bowel retraining: constipation, impaction, diarrhea, hemorrhoids, rectal bleeding, anal tears
- Identify community resources for peer and family support ✔ ✔
  - [ ] Identify phone numbers for disabled support groups
  - [ ] State meeting locations and times

(*continued*)

Managing the Therapeutic Regimen at Home (Continued)

	Patient	Caregiver
• Demonstrate how to access transportation [ ] Identify locations of wheelchair accessibility for public buses or trains [ ] Identify phone numbers for private wheelchair van [ ] Contact Division of Motor Vehicles for handicapped parking permit [ ] Contact Division of Motor Vehicles for driving test when appropriate [ ] Identify resources for adapting private vehicle with hand controls or wheelchair lift	✔	✔
• Identify vocational rehabilitation resources [ ] State name and phone number of vocational rehabilitation counselor [ ] Identify educational opportunities that may lead to future employment	✔	✔
• Identify community resources for recreation [ ] State local recreation centers that offer programs for the disabled [ ] Identify leisure activities that can be pursued in the community	✔	✔

achieve attainable goals. The degree to which the patient adapts to the home and community environment depends on the confidence and self-esteem developed during the rehabilitation process and on the acceptance, support, and reactions of the family, employer, and community members.

There is a growing trend toward independent living by severely disabled people, either alone or in groups that share resources. Preparation for independent living should include training in managing a household and working with personal care attendants as well as training in mobility. The goal is integration into the community—living and working in the community with accessible housing, employment, public buildings, transportation, and recreation.

State rehabilitation administration agencies provide services to assist disabled people in obtaining the help they need to engage in gainful employment. These services include diagnostic, medical, and mental health services. There are counseling, training, placement, and follow-up services available to help people with disabilities select and attain jobs.

If the patient is transferred to an extended care facility, the transition is planned to promote continued progress. Independence gained continues to be supported, and progress is fostered. Adjustment to the extended care facility is facilitated through communication. The family is encouraged to visit, to be involved, and to take the patient home on weekends and holidays if possible.

Americans With Disabilities Act

For years, people with disabilities have been discriminated against in employment, public accommodations, and public and private services. In 1990, the U.S. Congress passed the Americans With Disabilities Act (ADA) (PL 101-336). This civil rights legislation is designed to permit those with disabilities access to the community and to job opportunities. It stipulates that communities must provide public transportation that is accessible to people with disabilities. Public facilities (eg, stores, restaurants, hotels) must be accessible and accommodate those with disabilities. Telecommunication providers must offer communication devices for the deaf. Employers must evaluate an applicant's ability to perform the job and not discriminate on the basis of a disability. Employers also must make "reasonable accommodations," such as equipment or access ramps, to facilitate employment of a person with a disability.

Although the regulations took effect in July 1992, compliance has been slow. Reasonable accommodation and "without undue hardship" provisions in the law permit businesses to continue with inaccessible conditions. All new construction and modifications of public facilities, however, must address access by people with disabilities. With increased awareness of the needs of people with disabilities, there will be changes to facilitate access and accommodate them. A higher quality of life for those with disabilities is an objective of the ADA.

People with disabilities are no longer an invisible minority; they are active members of society. Modification of the physical environment permits access to public and private facilities and services. Many employment opportunities require minimal modification for a qualified applicant with a disability to be successful. Nurses can serve as advocates for compliance with ADA legislation to eliminate discriminatory practices.

Critical Thinking Exercises

1. You are caring for a patient who is recovering from a stroke. You are discussing the patient's level of functioning with the physical rehabilitation team. Describe the kinds of self-care activities that you would assess to determine the rehabilitation plan for the patient.

2. An elderly patient who has limited mobility and ambulation abilities is to be discharged to his home and cared for by his family. The family members express particular concern about how to prevent pressure ulcers. Describe the instructions you would give them. How might your teaching strategies differ if family members converse primarily in their native tongue, which is not English?

3. You are caring for a young man who was injured in a motor vehicle crash. He is to return home to continue rehabilitation as an outpatient. You accompany the home health care nurse who is conducting an assessment of the patient's home environment in anticipation of his discharge. Compare the types of safety factors that might be considered if the patient lives in a single-story house, in a two-story house, in a two-room apartment in a high-rise building, or on a farm.

References and Selected Readings

BOOKS

Agency for Health Care Policy and Research, Public Health Service, U.S. Department of Health and Human Services. Panel for the Prediction and Prevention of Pressure Ulcers in Adults. (1992). *Pressure ulcers in adults: Prediction and prevention.* Clinical Practice Guideline, Number 3. AHCPR Publication No. 92-0047. Rockville, MD: Author, May.

Agency for Health Care Policy and Research, Public Health Service, U.S. Department of Health and Human Services. (1994). *Treatment of pressure ulcers.* Clinical Practice Guideline, Number 15. AHCPR Publication No. 95-0652. Rockville, MD: Author, December.

Agency for Health Care Policy and Research. Public Health Service, U.S. Department of Health and Human Services. Urinary Incontinence Guideline Panel. (1996). *Urinary incontinence in adults: Clinical practice guideline.* AHCPR Pub. No. 96-0682. Rockville, MD: Author.

Antorek, R., & Hanoch, L. (1997). *Psychosocial adaptation to chronic illness and disability.* Gaithersburg, MD: Aspen.

Association of Rehabilitation Nurses. (1993). *The specialty practice of rehabilitation nursing: A core curriculum* (3rd ed.). Skokie, IL: Author.

Association of Rehabilitation Nurses. (1994). *Standards and scope of rehabilitation nursing practice* (3rd ed.). Skokie, IL: Author.

Association of Rehabilitation Nurses. (1995). *Twenty-one rehabilitation nursing diagnoses: A guide to interventions and outcomes.* Glenview, IL: Author.

Association of Rehabilitation Nurses. (1996). *Scope and standards of advanced clinical practice in rehabilitation nursing.* Glenview, IL: Author.

Association of Rehabilitation Nurses. (1997). *Advanced practice in rehabilitation nursing: A core curriculum.* Glenview, IL: Author.

Dittmar, S., & Gresham, G. (1997). *Functional assessment and outcome measures for the rehabilitation health professional.* Gaithersburg, MD: Aspen.

Hoeman, S. (1996). *Rehabilitation nursing: Process and application* (2nd ed.). St. Louis: Mosby–Year Book.

Sipski, M. &, Alexander, C. (1997). *Sexual function in people with disability and chronic illness: A health professional's guide.* Gaithersburg, MD: Aspen.

Sussman, C., & Bates-Jenson, B. (1998). *Wound care: A collaborative practice manual for physical therapists and nurses.* Gaithersburg, MD: Aspen.

U.S. Department of Justice. (1996). *A guide to disability rights laws.* Washington, DC: U.S. Government Printing Office.

JOURNALS

Asterisks indicate nursing research articles.

*Ailinger, R., & Dear, M. (1997). An examination of self-care needs of clients with rheumatoid arthritis. *Rehabilitation Nursing, 22*(3), 135–140.

Baggerly, J. (1996). Pressure sore prevention in a rehabilitation setting: Implementing a programmatic approach. *Rehabilitation Nursing, 21*(5), 234–238.

Bohny, B. (1997). A time for self-care: Role of the home healthcare nurse. *Home Healthcare Nursing, 15*(4), 281–286.

Davidhizer, R. (1997). Disability does not have to be the grief that never ends: Helping patients adjust. *Rehabilitation Nursing, 22*(1), 32–35.

Davidhizer, R. (1997). Helping the client with chronic disability achieve high-level wellness. *Rehabilitation Nursing, 22*(3), 131–134.

Habel, M. (1997). Muscle tone abnormalities. *Rehabilitation Nursing, 22*(3), 118–123.

Hanna, B. (1996). Sexuality, body image, and self-esteem: The future after trauma. *Journal of Trauma Nursing, 3*(1), 13–16.

Hodges, C. (1997). Cushions are important to pressure sore prevention. *Nursing Times, 93*(26), 58, 60, 62.

Maklebust, J. (1996). Using wound care products to promote a healing environment. *Critical Care Nursing of North America, 8*(2), 141–158.

Mervine, J., & Temple, R. (1997). Using a microwave oven to disinfect intermittent-use catheters. *Rehabilitation Nursing, 22*(6), 318–320.

Palmer, M. (1997). Pelvic muscle rehabilitation: Where do we go from here? *Journal of Wound, Ostomy, and Continence Nursing, 24*(2), 98–105.

Patterson, J., & Bennett, R. (1995). Prevention and treatment of pressure sores. *Journal of American Geriatrics Society, 43*(8), 919–927.

Pinkowski, P. (1996). Prompted voiding in the long-term care facility. *Journal of Wound, Ostomy, and Continence Nursing, 23*(2), 110–114.

*Prieto-Fingerhut, T., Kresimer, B., & Lynne, C. (1997). A study comparing sterile and nonsterile urethral catheterization in patients with spinal cord injury. *Rehabilitation Nursing, 22*(6), 299–301.

*Resnick, B., & Daly, M. (1998). Predictors of functional ability in geriatric rehabilitation patients. *Rehabilitation Nursing, 23*(1), 23–29.

*Riley, P. (1996). Development of a COPD self-care action scale. *Rehabilitation Nursing Research, 5*(1), 3–8.

*Scherer, Y., Schmieder, L. E., & Schimmel, S. (1998). The effects of education alone and in combination with pulmonary rehabilitation on self-efficacy in patients with COPD. *Rehabilitation Nursing, 23*(2), 71–77.

*Sprung, P., Hou, Z., & Ladin, D. A. (1998). Hydrogels and hydrocolloids: An objective product comparison. *Ostomy/Wound Management, 44*(1), 36–52.

*Weeks, S. (1996). Taking on the family care giver role: Nurses' sensitivity to needs of prospective family care givers. *Rehabilitation Nursing Research, 5*(1), 16–22.

*Wells, J,. & Karr, D. (1998). Interface pressure, wound healing, and satisfaction in the evaluation of a non-powered fluid mattress. *Ostomy/Wound Management, 44*(2), 38–54.

Whittle, H., Fletcher, C., Hoskin, A., & Campbell, K. (1996). Nursing management of pressure ulcers using a hydrogel dressing protocol: Four case studies. *Rehabilitation Nursing, 21*(5), 238–242.

Resources

Accent on Living (AOL), P.O. Box 700, Bloomington, IL 61702; 1-309-378-2961

Access/Abilities, P.O. Box 458, Mill Valley, CA 94942; 1-415-388-3250

Association of Rehabilitation Nurses, 4700 W. Lake Avenue, Glenview, IL 60025-1485; 1-800-229-7530; fax 1-847-375-4710; http://www.rehabnurse.org

National Institute on Disability and Rehabilitation Research (NIDRR), Office of Special Education and Rehabilitation Research, U.S. Department of Education, Washington, DC 20202; 1-202-205-9151

National Rehabilitation Information Center (NARIC), 8455 Colesville Road, Silver Spring, MD 20910-3319; 1-800-346-2742; http://www.naric.com/naric

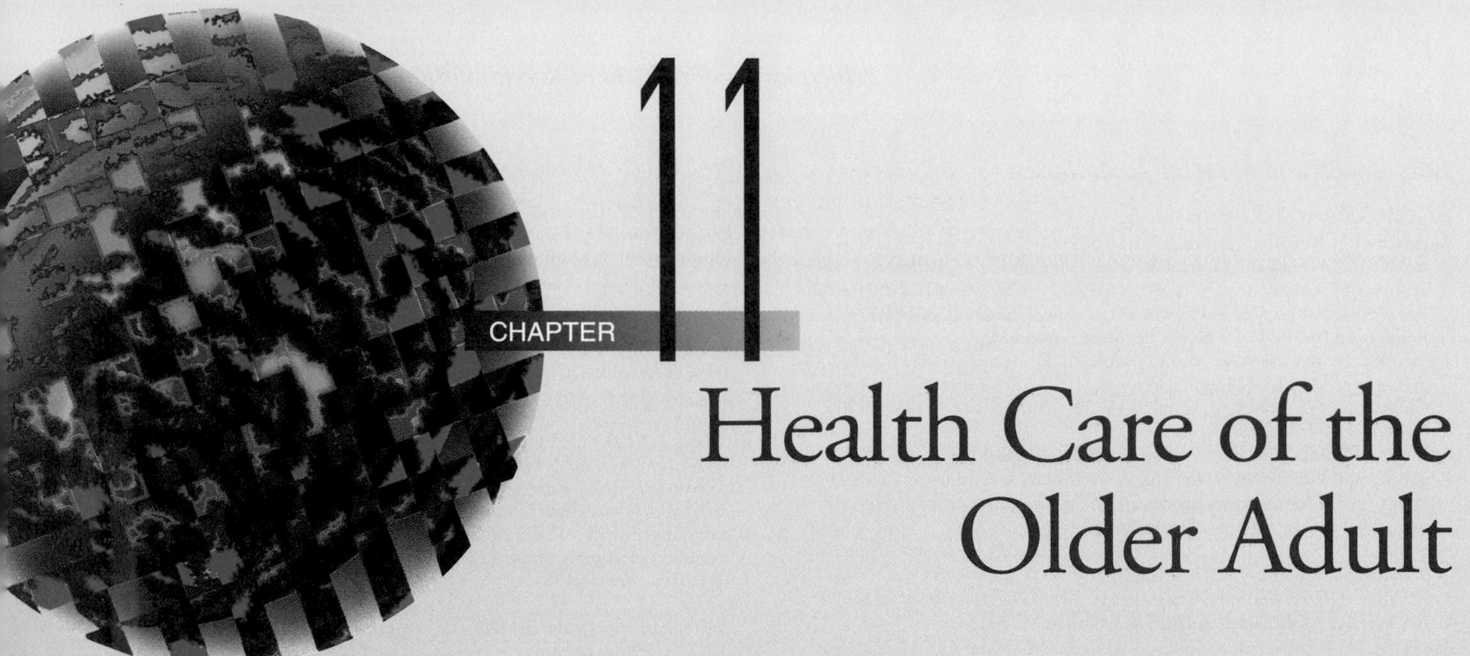

CHAPTER 11

Health Care of the Older Adult

Learning Objectives

On completion of this chapter, the learner will be able to:

1. Develop a definition of aging based on developmental and sociologic theories of aging.
2. Describe the aging American population based on demographic trends and statistical data.
3. Discuss the physiologic aspects of aging that occur as a result of both normal and pathologic changes.
4. Describe the significance of preventive health care and health promotion for the elderly.
5. Identify the important physical and mental health problems of aging and their effects on the functioning of older people and their families.
6. Identify the major geriatric syndromes and their effects on the individual patient.
7. Specify nursing implications relative to medication therapy in older people.
8. Examine the concerns of older people and their families in the home and community, in the acute care setting, and in a protected environment.
9. Identify major legal and ethical issues relevant to the care of older people.

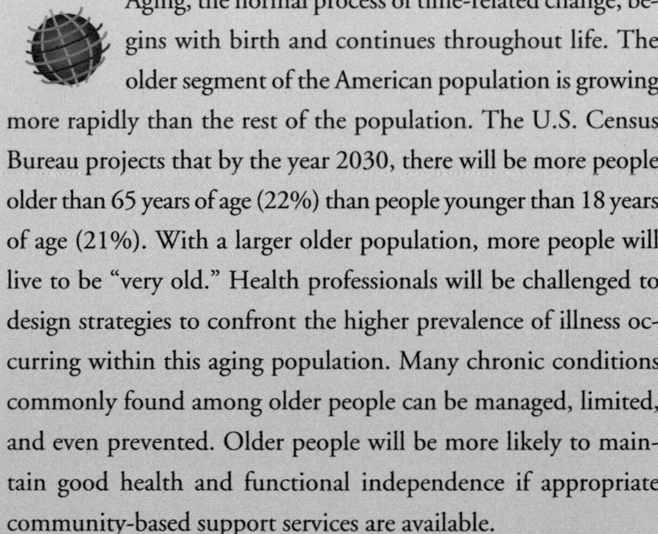

Aging, the normal process of time-related change, begins with birth and continues throughout life. The older segment of the American population is growing more rapidly than the rest of the population. The U.S. Census Bureau projects that by the year 2030, there will be more people older than 65 years of age (22%) than people younger than 18 years of age (21%). With a larger older population, more people will live to be "very old." Health professionals will be challenged to design strategies to confront the higher prevalence of illness occurring within this aging population. Many chronic conditions commonly found among older people can be managed, limited, and even prevented. Older people will be more likely to maintain good health and functional independence if appropriate community-based support services are available.

CARING FOR OLDER ADULTS

Life expectancy is the average number of years that a person can be expected to live. In the twentieth century, life expectancy from birth has risen dramatically from an average of 47.3 years (1900) to 75.4 years (1990), with women (79.0 years) living about 7 years longer than men (72.1 years). Early in this century, increased life expectancy was attributed to the decreased death rates of infants and young people. Since 1970, however, increases in life expectancy have resulted from decreased mortality among the middle-aged and elderly populations. Because more people are living longer, health professionals will be expected to help the geriatric patient make these added years healthy and productive.

Geriatrics, the study of old age, includes the physiology, pathology, diagnosis, and management of the diseases of older adults. The broader field of gerontology is the study of the aging process and includes the biologic, psychological, and sociologic sciences.

Gerontologic nursing is the field of nursing that specializes in care of the elderly. Standards and Scope of Gerontological Nursing Practice were originally developed in 1969 and revised in 1976 and 1987 by the American Nurses Association. The nurse gerontologist can be either a specialist or a generalist offering comprehensive nursing care to the older person. The basic nursing process of assessment, diagnosis, planning, implementation, and evaluation is used in combination with a specialized knowledge of aging. Gerontologic nursing can be provided in acute, chronic, or community settings. Emphasis of care is placed on promoting and maintaining functional status, thus promoting independence. Strengths of older adults are identified and used to help them achieve optimal independence. The nurse helps the older person to maintain dignity and maximum autonomy despite physical, social, and psychological losses.

Because old age is a normal occurrence that encompasses all experiences of life, care and concern for the elderly cannot be limited to one discipline. Optimal care of elderly people can best be provided through a cooperative effort. An interdisciplinary team, through comprehensive geriatric assessment, can combine expertise and resources to provide insight into all aspects of the aging process. Nurses collaborate with the interdisciplinary team to obtain non-nursing services and provide a holistic approach to care.

DEMOGRAPHICS OF AGING

Since 1900, the percentage of Americans 65 years of age and older has more than tripled (from 4.1% in 1900 to 12.8% in 1996), and the number has increased nearly 11 times (from 3.1 million to 33.9 million) (Fig. 11-1). The older population, 33.9 million in 1996, represents about one in every eight Americans. Since 1990, the number of older Americans has increased by 2.6 million, or 8%, compared with an increase of 6% for the population younger than 65 years of age. In 1996, there were 20.0 million older women and 13.9 million older men (a ratio of 145 women to every 100 men). The ratio of women to men increased with age, ranging from 120 for the 65 to 69 years of age group to a high of 257 for those aged 85 years and over.

The older population itself is getting older. In 1996, the 65 to 74-year-old age group (18.7 million) was eight times larger than in 1900, but the 75 to 84-year-old age group (11.4 million) was 16 times larger, and the 85 years of age and older group (3.8 million) was 31 times larger. In 1996, people reaching the age of 65 years had an average life expectancy of an additional 17.7 years (19.2 years for women and 15.5 years for men). A child born in 1996 could expect to live 76.1 years, about 29 years longer than a child born in 1900.

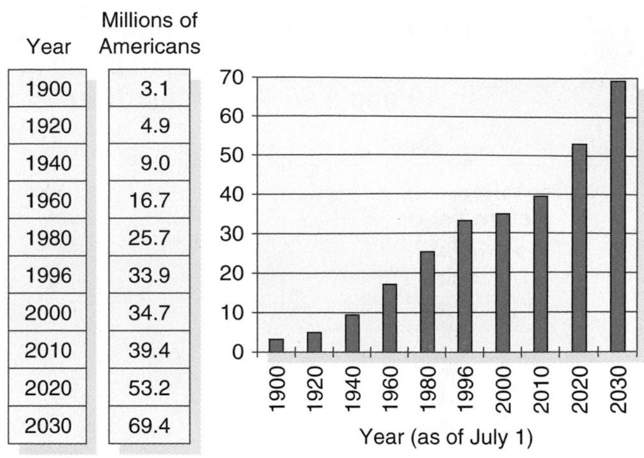

FIGURE 11•1 Profile of Americans aged 65 years and older (based on data from the U.S. Bureau of the Census; data from year 1900 to present used to predict millions of Americans aged 65 and older in the year 2030).

Although most older adults enjoy good health, physical disability is associated with aging. In national surveys, disability is reported by up to 40% of adults aged 65 years and older. Chronic disease is the major cause of disability. Heart disease, cancer, and stroke account for more than 75% of elderly deaths (Table 11-1). In clinical practice, however, "old age" is frequently described by older people as the cause of their decline in physical function (Williamson & Fried, 1996). Even though some older adults perceive no difficulty or decline, they modify the way they perform certain activities of daily living (ADLs) or instrumental activities of daily living (IADLs), thus demonstrating adaptation to a decline in physical performance (Fried, Bandeen-Roche, & Williamson, 1996). ADLs include bathing, dressing, eating, and getting around the house; IADLs include preparing meals, shopping, managing money, using the telephone, doing housework, and taking medication.

Despite the decrease in inpatient and outpatient hospital visits during the past 30 years by the population at large, an increase in utilization among older people has been observed. Hospitalization for diagnoses associated with end-stage cardiovascular disease, musculoskeletal disease, frailty, and iatrogenic and nosocomial conditions in the institutionalized elderly are clearly increasing substantially (Haan, Selby, Quesenberry, Schmittdiel, Fireman, & Rice, 1997). Older people accounted for 38% of all hospital stays and 48% of all days of care in hospitals in 1995. The average length of a hospital stay was 6.8 days for older people, compared with only 4.5 days for people younger than 65 years of age. Because hospitalized patients are being discharged to home "quicker and sicker" than ever before, there is a great need for nurses in all settings, including hospitals, home care rehabilitation, and outpatient settings, to be knowledgeable about geriatric nursing principles and skilled in meeting the needs of elderly patients.

PSYCHOSOCIAL ASPECTS OF AGING

Successful psychological aging is reflected in the older person's ability to adapt to physical, social, and emotional losses and to achieve contentment, serenity, and life satisfactions. Because changes in life patterns are inevitable over a lifetime, the older person needs resiliency and coping skills when confronting stresses and change.

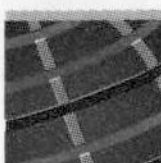

TABLE 11•1 **Deaths and Death Rates for the 10 Leading Causes of Death in People 65 Years and Older***

Rank	Cause of death	Number	Rate†
—	All causes	1,694,326	5,052.8
1	Heart diseases	615,426	1,835.3
2	Malignant neoplasms, including neoplasms of lymphatic and hematopoietic tissues	381,142	1,136.6
3	Cerebrovascular diseases	138,762	413.8
4	Chronic obstructive pulmonary diseases and allied conditions	88,478	263.9
5	Pneumonia and influenza	74,297	221.6
6	Diabetes mellitus	44,452	132.6
7	Accidents and adverse effects	29,099	86.8
	Motor vehicle crashes	7,626	22.7
	All other accidents and adverse effects	21,473	64.0
8	Alzheimer's disease	20,230	60.3
9	Nephritis, nephrotic syndrome, and nephrosis	20,182	60.2
10	Septicemia	16,899	50.4
	All other causes (residual)	265,359	791.4

* All races, both sexes, United States, 1995.
† Rates per 100,000 population.
Anderson, R. N., Kochanek, K. D., & Murphy, S. L. (1997). Report of final mortality statistics, 1995. *Monthly vital statistics report* (Vol. 45, No. 11, Supp. 2, Table 7). Hyattsville, MD: National Center for Health Statistics.

A positive self-image enhances risk taking and participation in new, untested roles.

Although attitudes toward old people differ in ethnic subcultures, a subtle theme of "ageism"—prejudice or discrimination against older people—predominates in our society. It is often based on stereotypes, simplified and often untrue beliefs, that reinforce society's negative image of the aged person. Elderly people make up an extremely heterogeneous group, yet negative stereotypes are attributed to all of them.

Fear of aging and the inability for many to confront their own aging process may trigger ageist beliefs. Retirement and perceived nonproductivity are also responsible for negative feelings. The younger working person may see the older person as one who is not contributing to society and is draining economic resources. This negative image is so common in American society that the elderly themselves often believe it. Only through an understanding of the aging process and respect for each person as an individual can the myths of aging be dispelled. If the elderly are treated with dignity and encouraged to maintain autonomy, the quality of their lives will improve.

Stress and Coping in the Older Adult

Coping patterns and the ability to adapt to stress are developed over the course of a lifetime and remain consistent with those of earlier life. Knowledge of successes in younger adulthood helps a person develop a positive self-image that remains solid even with adversities of old age. A person's abilities to adapt to changes, make decisions, and respond predictably are all determined by past experiences. A flexible, well-functioning person will probably continue as such. However, losses may accumulate within a short period of time and be overwhelming. The older person will have fewer choices and diminished resources to deal with stressful events. Common stressors of old age include normal aging changes that impair physical function, activities, and appearance; disabilities of chronic illness; social and environmental losses of income, roles, and activities; and the deaths of significant others. Many older adults rely strongly on their spiritual beliefs for comfort during stressful times.

Developmental Theories of Aging

Erikson (1963) developed the concept of eight stages of humans, each stage representing crucial turning points in the life-span stretching from birth to death. He delineated the major developmental task of old age as ego integrity versus despair. Ego integrity suggests an acceptance of one's lifestyle and a belief that choices made were the best that could be made at a particular time. One is still in control of one's life, a life of dignity. Despair, the opposite of ego integrity, implies that the older person feels dissatisfied and disappointed with his or her life. If given another chance, the person would live life differently.

Havighurst (1972) also suggests developmental tasks that occur during a lifetime. The tasks of the older person include adjusting to retirement from a lifetime of employment, possible reduction of income, a decrease in physical strength and health, and death of a spouse; establishing affiliation with one's age group; adapting to new social roles in a flexible way; and establishing satisfactory physical living arrangements.

Combining these concepts results in the following tasks: (1) maintenance of self-worth, (2) conflict resolution, (3) adjustment to the loss of dominant roles, (4) adjustment to the deaths of significant others, (5) environmental adaptation, and (6) maintenance of optimal levels of wellness.

Sociologic Theories of Aging

Sociologic theories of aging attempt to predict and explain the social interactions and roles that contribute to the older adult's successful adjustment to old age. The activity theory (Havighurst, 1972) proposes that life satisfaction in normal aging involves maintaining the active lifestyle of middle age. The continuity theory (Atchley, 1989; Neugarten, 1961) proposes that successful adjustment to old age rests with the ability of the person to continue life patterns across a lifetime. Continuity and a connection to the past are maintained through a continuation of well-established habits, values, and interests that are integral to the person's present lifestyle.

COGNITIVE ASPECTS OF AGING

Cognition can be affected by many variables, including sensory impairment, physiologic health, environment, and psychosocial influences. Older adults may experience temporary changes in cognitive function when hospitalized or admitted to skilled nursing facilities, rehabilitation centers, or long-term care facilities related to change in environment, medical therapy, or alteration in role performance. All of these factors contribute to cognitive functioning. Additionally, early research into intelligence and the elderly failed to consider these variables and others, possibly resulting in misconceptions about aging-induced decline in mental function (Eliopoulis, 1997).

Intelligence

When intelligence test scores from people of all ages are compared (cross-sectional testing), test scores for older adults show a progressive decline beginning in midlife; however, it has been demonstrated that environment and health have a considerable influence on scores and that certain types of intelligence (eg, spatial perceptions and retention of nonintellectual information) decline, whereas other types do not (problem-solving ability based on past experiences, verbal comprehension, mathematical ability). Cardiovascular health, a stimulating environment, high levels of education, occupational status, and income all appear to have a positive effect on intelligence scores in later life.

Learning and Memory

The ability to learn and acquire new skills and information decreases in the older adult, particularly, after the seventh decade of life. Despite this, many older people continue to learn and participate in varied educational experiences. Motivation, performance speed, and physical status all are important factors that influence learning.

Memory, an integral part of learning, has components that include short-term memory (5 to 30 seconds), recent memory (1 hour to several days), and long-term memory (lifetime). Acquisition of information, registration (recording), retention (storing), and recall (retrieval) are essential components of the memory process. Sensory losses, distractions, and disinterest interfere with acquiring and recording information. Age-related loss occurs more frequently with short-term and recent memory. In the absence of a pathologic process, it is called benign senescent forgetfulness. The process by which older adults learn is facilitated when the nurse undertakes the following:

- Supplies mnemonics to enhance recall of related data
- Encourages ongoing learning
- Links new information with familiar information
- Uses visual, auditory, and other sensory cues
- Encourages the learners to wear prescribed glasses and hearing aids
- Provides glare-free lighting
- Provides a quiet, nondistracting environment
- Sets short-term goals with input from the learner
- Keeps teaching periods short
- Paces learning tasks according to the endurance of the learner
- Encourages verbal participation by the learner
- Reinforces successful learning in a positive manner

NORMAL BIOLOGIC AGING

Intrinsic aging (from within the person) refers to those changes caused by the normal aging process that are genetically programmed and essentially universal within a species. Universality is the major criterion to use in distinguishing normal from abnormal aging. Extrinsic aging results from influences outside the person. Illness and disease, air pollution, and sunlight are examples of extrinsic factors that may hasten the aging process. These abnormal aging processes can be eliminated or reduced through effective health care interventions.

Cellular and extracellular changes of old age cause a change in physical appearance and decline in function. Measurable changes in the shape and body make-up occur. The body's ability to maintain homeostasis becomes increasingly diminished with cellular aging. Organ systems cannot function at full efficiency because of cellular and tissue deficits. Cells become less able to replace themselves and accumulate a pigment known as lipofuscin. A degradation of elastin and collagen causes connective tissue to become stiffer and less elastic.

BODY SYSTEM CHANGES AND HEALTH PROMOTION ACTIVITIES

The well-being of an aged person depends on physical, mental, social, and environmental factors. A total assessment includes evaluating all major body systems, social and mental status, and the ability of the person to function independently despite a chronic illness. See Table 11-2 for a summary of signs and symptoms of age-related changes in body systems functioning and suggested nursing interventions.

Cardiovascular System

Heart disease is a leading cause of death in the aged. The heart valves become thicker and stiffer, and the heart muscle and arteries lose their elasticity. Calcium and fat deposits accumulate within arterial walls, and veins become increasingly tortuous. Although function is maintained under normal circumstances, the cardiovascular system has less reserve and responds less efficiently to stress. The resting cardiac output (heart rate [HR] × stroke volume) decreases about 1% annually after 20 years of age. Under conditions of stress, both the maximum cardiac output and the maximum heart rate diminish gradually. The relationship between maximum heart rate and age is:

$$\text{maximum HR} = 220 - \text{age in years}$$

Hypertension has been shown to be a serious risk factor at all ages for cardiovascular disease and stroke. A diagnosis of hypertension is made only after it has been confirmed by at least two subsequent readings. In older people, the diagnosis of hypertension is classified as follows:

Isolated systolic hypertension: the systolic reading exceeds 140 mm Hg, and the diastolic measurement is normal or near normal (less than 90 mm Hg).

Primary hypertension: the diastolic pressure is greater than or equal to 90 mm Hg regardless of the systolic pressure.

Secondary hypertension: hypertension that can be attributed to an underlying cause.

Cardiovascular dysfunction may manifest as cardiac dysrhythmias, congestive heart failure, coronary artery disease, arteriosclerosis, hypertension, intermittent claudication (leg pain caused by walking), myocardial infarction, peripheral vascular disease, orthostatic hypotension, or cerebrovascular accidents (strokes).

Cardiovascular health can be promoted by regular exercise, proper diet, weight control, regular blood pressure measurements, stress management, and smoking cessation. To avoid lightheadedness, fainting, and possible falls caused by orthostatic hypotension, the older person should be counseled to rise slowly from a lying, to a sitting, to a standing position.

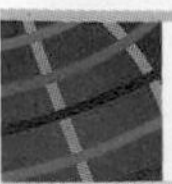

TABLE 11•2 Body Systems: Changes in Functional Status With Nursing Recommendations

Changes	Subjective and Objective Findings	Health Promotion Strategies
Cardiovascular System		
Decreased cardiac output; diminished ability to respond to stress; heart rate and stroke volume do not increase with maximum demand; slower heart recovery rate; increased blood pressure	Complaints of fatigue with increased activity Increased heart rate recovery time Normal BP ≤140/90 mm Hg	Exercise regularly; pace activities; avoid smoking; eat a low-fat, low-salt diet; participate in stress-reduction activities; check blood pressure regularly, medication compliance, weight control
Respiratory System		
Increase in residual lung volume; decrease in vital capacity; decreased gas exchange and diffusing capacity; decreased cough efficiency	Fatigue and breathlessness with sustained activity; impaired healing of tissues due to decreased oxygenation; difficulty coughing up secretions	Exercise regularly; avoid smoking; take adequate fluids to liquefy secretions; receive yearly influenza immunization; avoid exposure to upper respiratory tract infections
Integumentary System		
Decreased protection against trauma and sun exposure; decreased protection against temperature extremes; diminished secretion of natural oils and perspiration	Skin appears thin and wrinkled; complaints of injuries, bruises, and sunburn; complaints of intolerance to heat; bone structure is prominent; dry skin	Avoid solar exposure (clothing, sunscreen, stay indoors); dress appropriately for temperature; maintain a safe indoor temperature; shower preferable to tub bath; lubricate skin
Reproductive System		
Female: Vaginal narrowing and decreased elasticity; decreased vaginal secretions *Male:* Decreased size of penis and testes *Male and female:* Slower sexual response	*Female:* Painful intercourse; vaginal bleeding following intercourse; vaginal itching and irritation; delayed orgasm. *Male:* Delayed erection and achievement of orgasm	May require vaginal estrogen replacement; GYN/urology follow-up; use a lubricant with intercourse
Musculoskeletal System		
Loss of bone density; loss of muscle strength and size; degenerated joint cartilage	Height loss; prone to fractures; kyphosis; complaints of back pain; loss of strength, flexibility, and endurance; joint pain	Exercise regularly; eat a high-calcium diet; limit phosphorus intake; take hormones and calcium supplements as prescribed
Genitourinary System		
Male: Benign prostatic hyperplasia	Urinary retention; irritative voiding symptoms including frequency, feeling of incomplete bladder emptying, multiple nighttime voidings.	Seek referral to urological specialist; have ready access to toilet; wear easily manipulated clothing; drink adequate fluids; avoid bladder irritants (eg, caffeinated beverages, alcohol, artificial sweeteners); pelvic floor muscle exercises, preferably learned via biofeedback
Female: Relaxed perineal muscles, detrusor instability (urge incontinence), urethral dysfunction (stress urinary incontinence)	Urgency/frequency syndrome, decreased "warning time", bathroom mapping. Drops of urine lost with cough, laugh, position change.	Consider urologic workup
Gastrointestinal System		
Decreased salivation; difficulty swallowing food; delayed esophageal and gastric emptying; reduced gastrointestinal motility	Complaints of dry mouth; complaints of fullness, heartburn, and indigestion; constipation, flatulence, and abdominal discomfort	Use ice chips, mouthwash; brush, floss, and massage gums daily; receive regular dental care; eat small, frequent meals; sit up and avoid heavy activity after eating; limit antacids; eat a high-fiber, low-fat diet; limit laxatives; toilet regularly; drink adequate fluids
Nervous System		
Reduced speed in nerve conduction; increased confusion with physical illness and loss of environmental cues; reduced cerebral circulation (becomes faint, loses balance)	Slower to respond and react; learning takes longer; becomes confused with hospital admission; faintness; frequent falls	Pace teaching; with hospitalization, encourage visitors; enhance sensory stimulation; with sudden confusion, look for cause; encourage slow rising from a resting position
Special Senses		
Vision: Diminished ability to focus on close objects; inability to tolerate glare; difficulty adjusting to changes of light intensity; decreased ability to distinguish colors	Holds objects far away from face; complains of glare; poor night vision; confuses colors	Wear eyeglasses, use sunglasses outdoors; avoid abrupt changes from dark to light; use adequate indoor lighting with area lights and nightlights; use large printed books; use magnifier for reading; avoid night driving; use contrasting colors for color coding; avoid glare of shiny surfaces and direct sunlight
Hearing: Decreased ability to hear high-frequency sounds	Gives inappropriate responses; asks people to repeat words; strains forward to hear	Recommend a hearing examination; reduce background noise; face person; enunciate clearly; speak with a low-pitched voice; use nonverbal cues
Taste and smell: Decreased ability to taste and smell	Uses excessive sugar and salt	Encourage use of lemon, spices, herbs

Respiratory System

Age-related changes in the respiratory system affect lung capacity and function and include increased anteroposterior chest diameter, osteoporotic collapse of vertebrae resulting in kyphosis (increased convex curvature of the spine), calcification of the costal cartilages and reduced mobility of the ribs, diminished efficiency of the respiratory muscles, increased lung rigidity, and decreased alveolar surface area. Increased rigidity or loss of elastic recoil in the lung results in increased residual lung volume and decreased vital capacity. Gas exchange and diffusing capacity are diminished. Decreased cough efficiency, reduced ciliary activity, and increased respiratory dead space make the older person more vulnerable to respiratory infections.

Health promotion activities that help the elderly person maintain adequate respiratory function include regular exercise, appropriate fluid intake, regular pneumococcal vaccination, yearly influenza immunizations, and avoidance of smoking.

Integumentary System

The functions of the skin include protection, temperature regulation, sensation, and excretion. With aging, changes occur that affect the function and appearance of the skin. The epidermis and dermis become thinner. Elastic fibers are reduced in number; collagen becomes stiffer. Subcutaneous fat diminishes, particularly in the extremities. Decreased numbers of capillaries in the skin result in diminished blood supply. These changes result in a loss of resiliency and a wrinkling and sagging of the skin. Hair pigmentation decreases, resulting in gradual graying. The skin becomes drier and susceptible to irritations because of decreased activities of the sebaceous and sweat glands. These changes in the integument reduce tolerance to extremes of temperature and exposure to the sun.

Strategies to promote healthy skin function include avoiding exposure to the sun, using a lubricating skin cream, avoiding long soaks in the tub, and maintaining adequate (8 to 10 eight-ounce glasses per day) intake of water.

Reproductive System

Ovarian production of estrogen and progesterone ceases with menopause. Changes occurring in the female reproductive system include thinning of the vaginal wall with a narrowing in size and a loss of elasticity; decreased vaginal secretions, resulting in vaginal dryness, itching, and decreased acidity; involution (atrophy) of the uterus and ovaries; and decreased pubococcygeal muscle tone, resulting in a relaxed vagina and perineum. These changes contribute to vaginal bleeding and painful intercourse. In older men, the penis and testes decrease in size, and levels of androgens diminish. Erectile dysfunction may develop with concomitant cardiovascular disease, neurologic disorders, diabetes, or even respiratory disease, which limits exercise tolerance.

Sexual desire and activity decline but do not disappear. Due to a decrease in vaginal lubrication, local estrogen replacement enhances vaginal lubrication without the occasional side-effects of oral dosing. There are several treatment modalities for erectile dysfunction that is linked to either cardiovascular, neurologic, endocrine, or occasionally psychological dysfunction. The use of vacuum penile pumps, local injection or placement of vasostimulating medication into the urethral opening, or use of an oral medication, sildenafil citrate (Viagra), have all proved effective for some patients. Viagra is considered preferable to the other modalities for several reasons. A review of population subgroups demonstrated its efficacy regardless of baseline severity, etiology, race, or age. Viagra was effective in a broad range of patients with erectile dysfunction, including those with a history of coronary artery disease, hypertension, other cardiac disease, peripheral vascular disease, diabetes mellitus, depression, coronary artery bypass graft, radical prostatectomy, transurethral resection of the prostate, and spinal cord injury as well as in patients taking a wide variety of medications. There are special considerations that must be discussed with the patient who is currently taking other nitrate medications (Pfizer U.S. Pharmaceuticals, 1998). If significant dysfunction is present, referral to a gynecologist or urologist is warranted. For both men and women, maintaining a daily physical exercise routine promotes enhanced sexual performance.

Genitourinary System

The genitourinary system continues to function adequately in older people, although there is a decrease in kidney mass due primarily to loss of nephrons. Changes in kidney function include decreased filtration rate, diminished tubular function with less efficiency in resorbing and concentrating the urine, and a slower restoration of acid–base balance in response to stress. Older women often suffer from stress or urge incontinence, or both. Benign prostatic hyperplasia (enlarged prostate gland) is a common finding in older men. Enlargement of the prostate causes a gradual increase in urine retention and overflow incontinence. Prostate cancer, a slow-growing cancer, is most often seen in men older than 70 years of age. Kidney and bladder cancers are most frequently seen after the age of 50 years. Smoking is known to be a primary causative agent of these carcinomas.

Adequate consumption of fluids is necessary to reduce bladder infections and urinary incontinence. Other healthy habits include the following:

- Having ready access to toilet facilities
- Voiding every 3 to 4 hours while awake
- Practicing pelvic floor exercises

Pelvic floor exercises, first described by Kegel (1948), can be extremely useful in reducing the symptoms of stress and urge incontinence. Because achieving better muscle control takes at least several months to accomplish, the elderly person is encouraged to continue with the exercises. These daily exercises must continue indefinitely. The use of biofeedback to confirm the correct execution of these exercises has been documented to increase their effectiveness significantly. Teaching the patient how to do the exercises begins with identifying the pubococcygeus muscle. Point out that this muscle is the same one that is used to hold back flatus or to voluntarily stop the flow of urine, without contracting the abdomen, buttocks, or inner thigh muscles. The pelvic muscles are first tightened and then relaxed, with emphasis placed on maintaining a 5-second contraction, with 10-second rest intervals. This exercise should be routinely practiced for 30 to 80 repetitions each day. Additional repetitions are discouraged because of risk of fatigue of the muscle. These exercises are also recommended for men with dribbling incontinence related to post-prostatectomy surgery. The nurse instructs the patient to tighten the rectal sphincter until the penis retracts. Frequent repetition produces the desired muscle tone.

Constipation can be a major factor contributing to urinary incontinence. Encourage the patient to eat a high-fiber diet, drink adequate fluids, and increase mobility to promote regular bowel function. Additional health maintenance practices can be found in Table 11-2.

Gastrointestinal System

Sensory functions related to eating have nutritional consequences for the elderly (Yen, 1996). Periodontal disease leading to tooth decay and loss of teeth is common. Salivary flow diminishes, and the older person may experience a dry mouth. Major complaints often center on feelings of fullness, heartburn, and indigestion. Gastric motility may decrease, resulting in delayed emptying of stomach contents. Diminished secretion of acid and pepsin reduces the absorption of iron, calcium, and vitamin B_{12}. Absorption of nutrients in the small intestine also appears to diminish with age. The function of the liver, gallbladder, and pancreas is generally maintained, although some inefficiencies exist in absorption and tolerance to fat. The incidence of gallstones and common bile duct stones increases progressively with advanced years.

Constipation is common in aged people. When mild, the symptoms involve abdominal discomfort and flatulence. More serious consequences include fecal impaction that contributes to diarrhea around the impaction, fecal incontinence, and obstruction. Predisposing factors for constipation include lack of dietary bulk, prolonged use of laxatives, ignoring the urge to defecate, side effects of medications, inactivity, insufficient fluid intake, and excessive dietary fat.

Gastrointestinal health promotion practices include receiving regular dental care; eating small, frequent meals; avoiding heavy activity after eating; eating a high-fiber, low-fat diet; ingesting an adequate amount of fluids; establishing regular bowel habits; and avoiding the use of laxatives and antacids. Understanding the relationship between loss of smell and taste perception and food intake helps caregivers to intervene to maintain elderly patients' health (Yen, 1996).

NURSING RESEARCH

Bowel Hygiene and Laxative Use

Benton, J. M., O'Hara P. A., Chen H., et al. (1997). Changing bowel hygiene practice successfully: A program to reduce laxative use in a chronic care hospital. *Geriatric Nursing 18,* 12–17.

Purpose

This study describes the work of an interdisciplinary committee of a large long-term care facility to develop Bowel Hygiene Practice Guidelines that were designed to help patients restore and maintain patterns of normal bowel elimination without reliance on laxatives. The main elements of the guidelines were increased fluid and fiber intake, timely toileting habits, and regular exercise and activity as first-line interventions. Implementation of the guidelines resulted in successful change in clinical practice and positive clinical outcomes.

Study Sample and Design

A retrospective evaluation was conducted for 4 years of the medication records of patients on two comparable chronic care units; one of the units used the Bowel Hygiene Practice Guidelines, and the other unit served as a control group. Before the study, both units were similar in their proportion of patients who received regularly prescribed and PRN laxatives.

Findings

Use of PRN laxatives on the unit that implemented the Bowel Hygiene Practice Guidelines decreased from 91.2% of patients to less than 40% of patients. There was also a significant decrease in the use of regularly prescribed laxatives for the patients on this unit. There was no significant change in the use of PRN laxatives for the control group, and the use of regularly prescribed laxatives actually increased during the study period. Other clinical outcomes reported by the staff on the unit that implemented the Bowel Hygiene Practice Guidelines included less fecal incontinence, improved mental status functioning, decreased behavioral problems, decreased urinary tract infections, decreased skin problems, and improved physical functioning.

Nursing Implications

An interdisciplinary planning and implementation approach to establishing a bowel care program can be successful in improving the bowel patterns of long-term care patients. The clinical trends identified in this study need further validation but support the premise that a successful bowel care program can improve patients' quality of life.

Nutritional Health

The social, psychological, and physiologic functions of eating influence the dietary habits of the aged person. Decreased physical activity and a slower metabolic rate reduce the number of calories needed by the older adult to maintain an ideal weight. Apathy, immobility, depression, loneliness, poverty, inadequate knowledge, lack of oral health, and lack of taste discrimination contribute to suboptimal nutrient intake.

Health promotion teaching includes encouraging a diet low in sodium and saturated fats and high in vegetables, fruits, and fish. The older adult requires a variety of foods to maintain balanced nutrition. No more than 20% to 25% of dietary calories should be consumed as fat. Reducing salt intake is also advocated because sodium reduction has been shown to correct hypertension in some people. Protein intake should remain the same in later adulthood. Carbohydrates, a major source of energy, should supply the diet with 55% to 60% of the daily calories. Simple sugars should be avoided and complex carbohydrates encouraged. Potatoes, whole grains, brown rice, and fruit provide the person with minerals, vitamins, and fiber and should be encouraged. Drinking 8 to 10 eight-ounce glasses of water per day is recommended unless contraindicated by a medical condition.

Musculoskeletal System

A gradual, progressive decrease in bone mass begins before the age of 40 years. Excessive loss of bone density results in osteoporosis (see Chap. 62). Although it also affects men, this condition is most apparent in postmenopausal women and is associated with inactivity, inadequate calcium intake, and loss of estrogens (Fig. 11-2). Its incidence is higher in northern Europeans and other whites and in the Chinese and Japanese. The danger of fracture due to bone reabsorption is especially high for the dorsal vertebra, humerus, radius, femur, and tibia. A loss of height occurs in later life as a result of osteoporotic changes of the spine, kyphosis (excessive convex curvature of the spine), and flexion of the hips and knees. These changes negatively affect mobility, balance, and internal organ function.

The muscles diminish in size and lose strength, flexibility, and endurance with decreased activity and advanced age. Back pain is common. Beginning in middle age, the cartilage of joints progressively deteriorates. Degenerative joint disease is found in all older people past the age of 70 years.

Calcium supplements, vitamin D, fluoride, estrogens, and weight-bearing exercises are often prescribed for the person who is at high risk of or already has osteoporosis. Although osteoporosis cannot be reversed, the disease process can be prevented or arrested (Walsh, Scura, & Wipple, 1997). For skeletal health, the nurse can recommend the following:

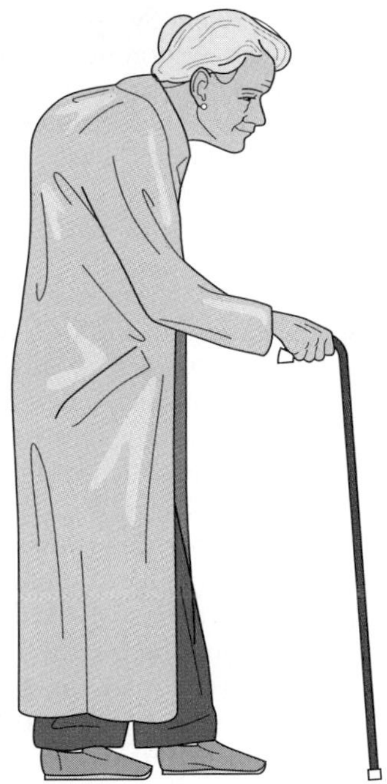

FIGURE 11•2 Age-related musculoskeletal changes affect posture, stance, and gait.

- A high calcium intake, 1500 mg/day, (dairy products and dark green vegetables are excellent sources, as are soups and broths made with a soup bone and cooked with added vinegar to leach calcium from the bone)
- A low-phosphorus diet (a calcium-to-phosphorus ratio of 1 : 1 is ideal; red meats, cola drinks, and processed foods that are low in calcium and high in phosphorus are avoided)
- Exercise (the pull of muscle insertions on the long bones strengthens them and retards calcium resorption)

Muscle strength and flexibility can be enhanced with a program of regular exercise. The axiom, "use it or lose it," is very relevant when considering the physical capacity of aged people. The nurse plays an important role by encouraging older adults to participate in a regular exercise program. Research shows that exercise enhances cardiovascular and respiratory efficiency. Regular exercise increases the strength and efficiency of heart contractions and improves oxygen uptake by cardiac and skeletal muscles, reduces fatigue, increases energy, and reduces cardiovascular risk factors. Muscle endurance, strength, and flexibility—all outcomes of regular exercise—help to promote independence and psychological well-being. Aerobic exercises are the foundation of programs of cardiovascular endurance conditioning. A physical examination by a physician or nurse practitioner is necessary before initiating an exercise program. The older person should perform exercises in moderation and use short rests to avoid undue fatigue. Swimming and brisk walking are often recommended because they are managed easily and usually enjoyed by the older person.

Nervous System

The structure and function of the nervous system change with advanced age. A progressive loss in brain mass is attributed to a loss of nerve cells. There is a reduction in the synthesis and metabolism of the major neurotransmitters. Because nerve impulses are conducted more slowly, older people take a longer time to respond and react. The autonomic nervous system performs less efficiently, and postural hypotension, which causes the person to feel lightheaded upon standing up quickly, may occur. Cerebral ischemia with related lightheadedness may interfere with mobility and safety. Homeostasis is more difficult to maintain, but in the absence of pathologic changes, the older person functions adequately and retains cognitive and intellectual abilities. Accompanying the nervous system changes is a reduction in cerebral blood flow.

A slowed reaction time places the older person at risk for falls and injuries. Loss of consciousness or a feeling of faintness may occur when the person rises too rapidly from a lying or sitting position. The nurse advises the person to allow a longer time to respond to a stimulus and to move more deliberately. Mental function is threatened by physical or emotional stresses. A sudden onset of confusion may be the first symptom of an infection or change in physical condition (pneumonia, urinary tract infection, medication interactions, dehydration, and others).

Sensory System

Sensory losses with old age affect all sensory organs. Sensory losses can be devastating to the person who cannot see to read or watch television, who cannot hear conversation well enough to communicate, or who cannot discriminate taste well enough to enjoy food.

Sensory Losses Versus Sensory Deprivation

Sensory losses can often be helped by assistive devices such as glasses or hearing aids. Sensory deprivation is the absence of stimuli in the environment, or the inability to interpret existing stimuli (perhaps as a result of a sensory loss). This deprivation can lead to boredom, confusion, irritability, disorientation, and anxiety. Meaningful sensory stimulation offered to the older person is often helpful in correcting this problem. One sense can substitute for another in observing and interpreting stimuli. The nurse can enhance sensory stimulation in the environment with colors, pictures, textures, tastes, smells, and sounds. The stimuli are most meaningful when they are interpreted to the older person and if they are changed often. The confused person responds well to touching and to familiar music.

Vision

As new cells form on the outside surface of the lens of the eye, the older central cells accumulate and become yellow, rigid, dense, and cloudy. Thus, only the outer portion of the lens is elastic enough to change shape (accommodate) and focus at near and far distances. As the lens becomes less flexible, the near point of focus gets farther away. This condition, presbyopia, usually begins in the fifth decade of life. Reading glasses to magnify objects are required. In addition, the yellowing, cloudy lens causes light to scatter and therefore makes the older person sensitive to glare. The ability to discern blue from green declines. The pupil dilates slowly and less completely because of increased stiffness of the muscles of the iris. The older person takes longer to adjust when going to and from light and dark environments or settings and needs brighter light for close vision. Although pathologic visual conditions are not a part of normal aging, there is an increased incidence of eye disease in older people, most commonly cataracts, glaucoma, senile macular degeneration, and diabetic retinopathy.

Hearing

Loss of the ability to hear high-frequency tones occurs in midlife. This age-related hearing loss, called presbycusis, is attributed to irreversible inner ear changes. Older people are often unable to follow conversation because tones of high-frequency consonants (letters *f, s, th, ch, sh, b, t, p*) all sound alike. Hearing loss may cause the older person to respond inappropriately, to misunderstand conversation, and to avoid social interaction. This behavior may be erroneously interpreted as confusion. Wax buildup or other correctable problems may be responsible for major hearing difficulties. A properly prescribed and fitted hearing aid may be useful in reducing hearing deficits.

Taste and Smell

The four basic tastes are sweet, sour, salty, and bitter. Of these, sweet tastes are particularly dulled in older people. Blunted taste may contribute to the preference for salty, highly seasoned foods. Herbs, onions, garlic, and lemon are encouraged as substitutes for salt to flavor food.

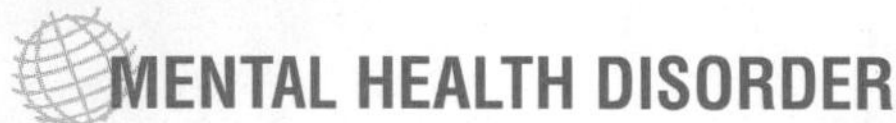

MENTAL HEALTH DISORDERS

Older adults are less likely than younger people to seek treatment for mental health symptoms. Health professionals are challenged to recognize, assess, refer, collaborate, treat, and support those older adults who exhibit noticeable changes in intellect or affect. In a community setting, the nurse may be the only health provider who has contact with the person. Symptoms should not be dismissed as age-related changes. A thorough assessment may reveal a treatable, reversible physical or mental condition. Related concerns include family involvement, access and quality of care, treatment costs and compliance, and ethical issues.

Depression

Depression is the most common affective or mood disorder of old age and is often responsive to treatment. Its classification and diagnosis vary according to the number, severity, and duration of symptoms. Depression disrupts quality of life, increases the risk of suicide, and becomes self-perpetuating. It can be an early sign of a chronic illness and a result of physical illness (Lesseig, 1996). Signs of depression include feelings of sadness, fatigue, diminished memory and concentration, feelings of guilt or worthlessness, sleep disturbances, appetite disturbances with excessive weight loss or gain, restlessness, impaired attention span, and suicidal ideation.

Although depression among the elderly is widespread, it is often undiagnosed and untreated. Attentive clinical evaluation is essential. Geriatric depression and symptoms of dementia often overlap, and cognitive impairment may be due to depression rather than the dementia. When depression and medical illnesses coexist, and they often do, neglect of the depression can retard physical recovery. Symptoms might be secondary to a medication interaction or an undiagnosed physical condition. Assessment of the patient's mental status, including assessment for depression, is vital and must not be overlooked (see Charts 11-1 and 11-2).

CHART 11•1 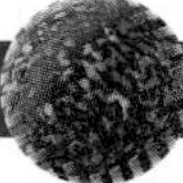 **Items of Mini-Mental State Examination**

Maximum Score	
	Orientation
5	What is the (year) (season) (date) (day) (month)?
5	Where are we (state) (county) (city) (hospital) (floor)?
	Registration
3	Name three objects: One second to say each. Then ask the patient all three after you have said them. Give one point for each correct answer. Repeat them until he learns all three. Count trials and record number: Number of trials
	Attention and calculation
5	Begin with 100 and count backwards by 7 (stop after five answers). Alternatively, spell "world" backwards.
	Recall
3	Ask for the three objects repeated above. Give one point for each correct answer.
	Language
2	Show a pencil and a watch, and ask subject to name them.
1	Repeat the following: "No 'if's,' 'and's,' or 'but's.'"
3	A three-stage command: "Take a paper in your right hand; fold it in half, and put it on the floor."
1	Read and obey the following: (show subject the written item). CLOSE YOUR EYES
1	Write a sentence.
1	Copy a design (complex polygon as in Bender-Gestalt).
30	Total score possible

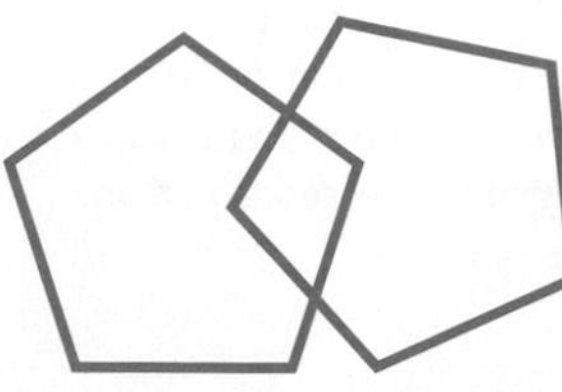

CHART 11•2 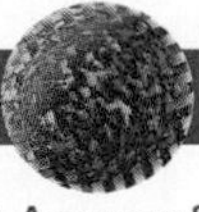 **Geriatric Depression Scale**

Choose the Best Answer for How You Felt This Past Week.

*1.	Are you basically satisfied with your life?	YES	NO
2.	Have you dropped many of your activities and interests?	YES	NO
3.	Do you feel that your life is empty?	YES	NO
4.	Do you often get bored?	YES	NO
*5.	Are you hopeful about the future?	YES	NO
6.	Are you bothered by thoughts you can't get out of your head?	YES	NO
*7.	Are you in good spirits most of the time?	YES	NO
8.	Are you afraid that something bad is going to happen to you?	YES	NO
*9.	Do you feel happy most of the time?	YES	NO
10.	Do you often feel helpless?	YES	NO
11.	Do you often get restless and fidgety?	YES	NO
12.	Do you prefer to stay at home, rather than going out and doing new things?	YES	NO
13.	Do you frequently worry about the future?	YES	NO
14.	Do you feel you have more problems with memory than most?	YES	NO
*15.	Do you think it is wonderful to be alive now?	YES	NO
16.	Do you often feel downhearted and blue?	YES	NO
17.	Do you feel pretty worthless the way you are now?	YES	NO
18.	Do you worry a lot about the past?	YES	NO
*19.	Do you find life very exciting?	YES	NO
20.	Is it hard for you to get started on new projects?	YES	NO
*21.	Do you feel full of energy?	YES	NO
22.	Do you feel that your situation is hopeless?	YES	NO
23.	Do you think that most people are better off than you are?	YES	NO
24.	Do you frequently get upset over little things?	YES	NO
25.	Do you frequently feel like crying?	YES	NO
26.	Do you have trouble concentrating?	YES	NO
*27.	Do you enjoy getting up in the morning?	YES	NO
28.	Do you prefer to avoid social gatherings?	YES	NO
*29.	Is it easy for you to make decisions?	YES	NO
*30.	Is your mind as clear as it used to be?	YES	NO

Score: ☐ (Number of "depressed" answers)

Norms	
Normal	5 ± 4
Mildly depressed	15 ± 6
Very depressed	23 ± 5

* Appropriate (nondepressed) answers = yes; all others = no.

Yesavage J. et al. (1983). Development and validation of a geriatric screening scale: A preliminary report. *Journal of Psychiatric Research 17*. Reprinted with permission from Pergamon Press Ltd., Headington Hill Hall, Oxford OX3 OBW, UK.

Depressive illness in late life should be vigorously treated with antidepressants. Psychosocial approaches have been found to be effective, and electroconvulsive treatment may be useful. The serotonin selective reuptake inhibitors, such as fluoxetine (Prozac) and paroxetine (Paxil), are clinically useful and exhibit rapid action with low occurrence of adverse effects. Central nervous system overstimulation, including such symptoms as anxiety and tremor, can occur. The tricyclic antidepressants, specifically nortriptyline, desipramine, and doxepine, are also clinically therapeutic for depression. Anticholinergic, cardiac, and orthostatic side effects, as well as interactions with other medications, require that these agents be used with care. Accordingly, the dosage must be managed carefully to relieve symptoms and at the same time avoid medication toxicity. It may take 4 to 6 weeks for symptoms to recede, so the nurse should offer explanations and encouragement during this period (Lebowitz, 1996).

Delirium

Delirium, often called acute confusional state, begins with confusion and progresses to disorientation. The patient may experience an altered level of consciousness ranging from stupor to excessive activity. Thinking is disorganized, and the attention span is characteristically short. Hallucinations, delusions, fear, anxiety, and paranoia may be evident. Because of the acute and unexpected onset of symptoms and the unknown underlying cause, this situation represents a medical emergency. Delirium occurs secondary to any number of causes, including physical illness, medication or alcohol toxicity, dehydration, fecal impaction, malnutrition, infection, head trauma, lack of environmental cues, and sensory deprivation or overload. Older adults are particularly vulnerable to acute confusion because of their marginal biologic reserve and the large number of medications they take. The nurse must recognize the grave implications of the acute symptoms and report them immediately. If the delirium goes unrecognized and the underlying cause is not treated, permanent, irreversible brain damage or death can follow. Delirium is sometimes mistaken for dementia (see Table 11-3 for a comparison of dementia and delirium).

Therapeutic interventions vary, depending on the reason for the symptoms. Because medication interactions and toxicity are often implicated, it is desirable that nonessential medications be withdrawn. Nutritional and fluid intake should be supervised and monitored. The environment should be quiet and calm. To increase orientation and provide familiar environmental cues, the nurse encourages family members or friends to touch and talk to the patient. With a newly admitted patient, it is important to question the family carefully about the patient's prior cognitive state. Ongoing mental status assessments using this baseline are helpful in evaluating responses to treatment and to the hospital or extended care facility admission.

ALZHEIMER'S DISEASE AND OTHER DEMENTIAS

Dementia is an acquired syndrome in which progressive deterioration in global intellectual abilities is of such severity that it interferes with the person's customary occupational and social performance. Alzheimer's disease and related dementias affect at least 2 million and possibly as many as 4 million U.S. residents. The National Institute on Aging estimates that $90 billion is spent annually for the treatment of Alzheimer's disease alone (Costa et al., 1996).

The dementias are characterized by a general decline in intellectual functioning that may include losses of memory, abstract reasoning ability, judgment, and language. Personality changes occur, and ability to perform ADLs deteriorates over time. Dementia is suspected when a person experiences a substantial decline in memory, other changes in cognition, or both. Symptoms are usually subtle in onset and often progress slowly until they are obvious and devastating. The changes characteristic of dementia fall into three

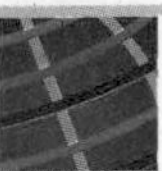

TABLE 11•3 Summary of Differences Between Dementia and Delirium

	Dementia		Delirium
	ALZHEIMER'S DISEASE (AD)	MULTI-INFARCT DEMENTIA	
Etiology	Familial (genetic [chromosomes 14, 19, 21]) Sporadic	Cardiovascular (CV) disease Cerebrovascular disease Hypertension	Drug toxicity and interactions; acute disease; trauma; chronic disease exacerbation Fluid and electrolyte disorder
Risk factors	Advanced age; genetic factor	Preexisting CV disease	Preexisting cognitive impairment
Occurrence	50%–60% of dementias	20% of dementias	20% of hospitalized older people
Onset	Slow	Often abrupt Follows a stroke or transient ischemic attack	Rapid, acute onset A harbinger of acute medical illness
Age of onset (yr)	Early onset AD: 30s–65 Late onset AD: 65+ Most commonly: 85+	Most commonly 50–70 yr	Any age, but predominantly in older persons
Gender	Males and females equally	Predominantly males	Males and females equally
Course	Chronic, irreversible; progressive, regular, downhill	Chronic, irreversible Fluctuating, stepwise progression	Acute
Duration	2–20 yr	Variable; years	Lasts 1 day to 1 month
Symptom progress	Onset insidious. *Early*—mild and subtle *Middle and late*—intensified Progression to death (infection or malnutrition)	Depends on location of infarct and success of treatment; death due to underlying CV disease	Symptoms are fully reversible with adequate treatment; can progress to chronicity or death if underlying condition is ignored
Mood	Early depression (30%)	Labile; mood swings	Variable
Speech/language	Speech remains intact until late in disease *Early*—mild anomia (cannot name objects); deficits progress until speech lacks meaning; echoes and repeats words and sounds; mutism.	May have speech deficit/aphasia depending on location of lesion	Fluctuating; often cannot concentrate long enough to speak
Physical signs	*Early*—no motor deficits *Middle*—apraxia [70%] (cannot perform purposeful movement) *Late*—Dysarthria (impaired articulation) *End stage*—loss of all voluntary activity; positive neurologic signs	According to location of lesion: focal neurologic signs, seizures Commonly exhibits motor deficits	Signs and symptoms of underlying disease
Orientation	Becomes lost in familiar places (topographic disorientation) Has difficulty drawing three-dimensional objects (visual and spatial disorientation) Disorientation to time, place, and person—with disease progression		May fluctuate between lucidity and complete disorientation to time, place, and person
Memory	Loss is an early sign of dementia; loss of recent memory is soon followed by progressive decline in recent and remote memory		Impaired recent and remote memory; may fluctuate between lucidity and confusion
Personality	Apathy, indifference, irritability *Early disease*—social behavior intact; hides cognitive deficits *Advanced disease*—disengages from activity and relationships; suspicious; paranoid delusions caused by memory loss; aggressive; catastrophic reactions		Fluctuating; cannot focus attention to converse; alarmed by symptoms (when lucid); hallucinations; paranoid
Functional status, activities of daily living	Poor judgment in everyday activities; has progressive decline in ability to handle money, use telephone, function in home and workplace		Impaired
Attention span	Distractable; short attention span		Highly impaired; cannot maintain or shift attention
Psychomotor activity	Wandering, hyperactivity, pacing, restlessness, agitation		Variable; alternates between high agitation, hyperactivity, restlessness, and lethargy
Sleep–wake cycle	Often impaired; wandering and agitation at nighttime		Takes brief naps throughout day and night

general categories: cognitive, functional, and behavioral. Reversible causes of dementia include alcohol abuse, medication use (polypharmacy), psychiatric disorders, and normal-pressure hydrocephalus. The three most common nonreversible dementias are Alzheimer's disease, multi-infarct dementia, and mixed Alzheimer's disease and multi-infarct dementia. Other non-Alzheimer's dementias include Parkinson's disease, acquired immunodeficiency disease (AIDS)–related dementia, and Pick's disease. The remaining dementias account for less than 5% of cases and are relatively uncommon (Costa et al., 1996).

The prevalence of dementia increases with age; however, the prevalence is affected not so much by the rate of new cases in the population as by the duration of the disorder, which equals the survival of affected individuals. In one study, almost 10% of nondemented people between the ages of 85 and 88 years became demented each year (Aevarsson & Skoog, 1996).

Multi-Infarct Dementia

Multi-infarct dementia is second only to Alzheimer's disease in incidence. About 15% of the cases of dementia are attributed to this disease. It is characterized by an uneven, downward decline in mental function. Multi-infarct dementia is sometimes confused with Alzheimer's disease, paranoia, or delirium because of its unpredictable clinical course. The diagnosis can be even more difficult if the patient is suffering from both Alzheimer's disease and multi-infarct dementia, the third type of dementia.

Cerebral damage occurs when blood supply to the brain is disrupted. Infarction, the death of brain tissue, occurs with striking rapidity. Multiple small cerebral infarctions, clinically manifested as small strokes, result in multi-infarct dementia. Instead of displaying the progressively downhill course of Alzheimer's disease, the progress of multi-infarct dementia is uneven. Every small infarct is followed by some recovery and a plateau until the next infarction occurs. Often, the patient has a history of cardiovascular and cerebrovascular disease. The age of onset is between 50 and 70 years; it occurs more frequently in men than in women.

Dizziness, headaches, and decreased mental and physical vigor are early signs of multi-infarct dementia. In more than half the cases, it appears acutely as sudden confusion. This is followed by gradual, spotty memory loss. The patient may hallucinate and display symptoms of delirium. Speech disturbances may be present. Early treatment of hypertension and vascular disease may prevent progression of the disease. In later stages, manifestations of the decline are similar to those of Alzheimer's disease, and often they cannot be distinguished.

Alzheimer's Disease

Alzheimer's disease is a progressive, irreversible, degenerative neurologic disease that begins insidiously and is characterized by gradual losses of cognitive function and disturbances in behavior and affect. Alzheimer's disease is not found exclusively in old people. In 1% to 10% of cases, its onset occurs in middle age. Family history of Alzheimer's disease and the presence of Down syndrome are two established risk factors for Alzheimer's disease. If family members have at least one other relative with Alzheimer's disease, then a familial component is said to exist. A familial component nonspecifically includes environmental triggers and genetic determinants. Genetic studies show that autosomal-dominant forms of Alzheimer's disease are associated with early onset and early death.

In 1987, chromosome 21 was first implicated in early-onset familial Alzheimer's disease (FAD). Soon after, the gene coding for amyloid precursor protein (APP) was also found to be on chromosome 21. Not until 1991 was an actual mutation in association with FAD found in the APP gene of chromosome 21. For these people, onset of Alzheimer's disease began in their 50s. Only a few of the cases of FAD have been found to have this genetic mutation. In 1992, chromosome 14 was found to contain an unidentified mutation also linked to FAD. In 1995, a new link, chromosome 1, was discovered. Newer studies suggest an association between alleles of the apolipoprotein E (apo E) gene locus on chromosome 19 and either increased risk for late-onset Alzheimer's disease (apo E-4) or protection against this risk (apo E-2 or E-3). Different studies have shown varying levels of association between the different apo E genotypes: 30% to 40% prevalence of Alzheimer's disease in people with the homozygous apo E genotype, and as low as 15% to 20% prevalence in older people who have either the apo E-2 or E-3 genotypes. For these reasons, it seems clear that other factors, such as other genes, life experiences, and environmental factors, must also play a role in late-onset Alzheimer's disease (Costa et al., 1996).

Pathophysiology

There are specific neuropathologic and biochemical changes found in patients with Alzheimer's disease. These include neurofibrillary tangles (a tangled mass of nonfunctioning neurons) and senile or neuritic plaques (deposits of β-amyloid protein, part of a larger protein, APP). This neuronal damage occurs primarily in the cerebral cortex and results in decreased brain size. Similar changes are found to a lesser extent in normal brain tissue of older adults. Cells principally affected by this disease are the ones that use the neurotransmitter acetylcholine. Biochemically, the enzyme active in producing acetylcholine is decreased. Acetylcholine is specifically involved in memory processing.

Clinical Manifestations

In the early stages of Alzheimer's disease, forgetfulness and subtle memory loss occur. There may be small difficulties in work or social activities, but the patient has adequate cognitive function to hide the loss and can function independently. Depression may occur at this time. With further progression of the disease, the deficits can no longer be concealed. Forgetfulness is manifested in many daily actions. These patients may lose their ability to recognize familiar faces, places, and objects and get lost in a familiar environment. They may repeat the same stories because they forget that they told them. Trying to reason with the person and use reality orientation only increase the patient's anxiety without increasing function because this is also forgotten. Conversation becomes difficult and there are word-finding difficulties. The ability to formulate concepts and think abstractly disappears. The patient can interpret a proverb only in concrete terms. The patient is often unable to appreciate the consequences of his or her actions and will therefore exhibit impulsive behavior. For example, on a hot day, the patient may decide to wade in the city fountain fully clothed. The patient has difficulty with everyday activities, such as operating simple appliances and handling money.

Personality changes are usually evident. The patient may become depressed, suspicious, paranoid, hostile, and even combative. Progression of the disease intensifies the symptoms. Speaking skills deteriorate to nonsense syllables; agitation and physical activity increase. The patient may wander at night. Eventually, assistance is needed for most ADLs, including eating and toileting; dysphagia (an inability or difficulty in swallowing) occurs, and incontinence develops. The terminal stage may last for months. The patient is usually immobile and requires total care. Occasionally, the patient may recognize family or caretakers. Death occurs as a result of complications such as pneumonia, malnutrition, or dehydration.

Assessment and Diagnostic Findings

Health history, including medical history; family history; social and cultural history; medication history; and physical examination, including functional and mental health status, are key in the diagnosis of probable Alzheimer's disease. Diagnostic tests, including complete blood count, VDRL, human immunodeficiency virus (HIV) testing, chemistry profile, and vitamin B_{12} and thyroid hormone levels, as well as screening with electroencephalography, computed tomography, magnetic resonance imaging and examination of the cerebrospinal fluid may all refute or support a diagnosis of probable Alzheimer's disease (Pruitt, 1995). Depression can closely mimic early-stage Alzheimer's disease and coexists in many patients. A depression scale and a cognitive function test, such as the Mini-Mental State Examination, should be used for screening. A clinical presentation of cognitive impairment may be due to depression and must be considered. The electroencephalographic changes are not always specific. The computed tomography and magnetic resonance imaging scans are useful for excluding hematoma, brain tumor, stroke, normal pressure hydrocephalus, and atrophy but are not reliable in making a definitive diagnosis of Alzheimer's disease. Infections, physiologic disturbances such as hypothyroidism, Parkinson's disease, and vitamin B_{12} deficiency can produce cognitive impairment that can be misdiagnosed as Alzheimer's disease. Biochemical abnormalities can be excluded by examination of the blood and cerebrospinal fluid, but findings are not specific enough to make the diagnosis. A diagnosis of "probable Alzheimer's disease" is made when the medical history, physical examination, and laboratory tests have excluded all known causes of other dementias. It can be confirmed only by cerebral biopsy on autopsy (Agency for Health Care Policy and Research, 1996; Mangino & Middlemiss, 1997). Chart 11-3 provides case studies relating to the differential diagnosis of Alzheimer's disease.

Medical Management

In the fall of 1993, the U.S. Food and Drug Administration approved the first Alzheimer's medication, tacrine hydrochloride, for the treatment of the symptoms of Alzheimer's disease. This agent enhances acetylcholine. Because this medication can cause liver toxicity, patients must be closely monitored. Since the introduction of this medication, other such medications have become available. All require ongoing monitoring and vary in their level of effectiveness from patient to patient. This is due in part to their window of effectiveness, which in general is limited to the early stages of dementia.

Nursing Management

Although Alzheimer's disease is the focus of this nursing management discussion, the interventions described apply to all patients with dementia, regardless of the cause. Nursing interventions are aimed at maintaining the patient's physical safety, reducing anxiety and agitation, improving communication, promoting independence in self-care activities, providing for the patient's needs for socialization and intimacy, maintaining adequate nutrition, managing sleep pattern disturbances, and supporting and educating family caregivers. Support for the caregivers of a community-dwelling patient with Alzheimer's disease is essential to prevent "caregiver burnout." This is particularly relevant for female caregivers, who often carry multiple roles. Early, continuous, and specific assessment of caregivers' social networks by nurses in all settings may help to identify those potentially at risk for inadequate support (Hibbard, Neufeld, & Harrison, 1996).

SUPPORTING COGNITIVE FUNCTION

As the patient's cognitive ability declines, the nurse provides a calm, predictable environment that helps the person interpret his or her surroundings and activities. Environmental stimuli are limited, and a regular routine is followed. A quiet, pleasant manner of speaking, clear and simple explanations, and use of memory aids and cues help to minimize confusion and disorientation and give the patient a sense of security. Prominently displayed clocks and calendars may enhance orientation to time. Color-coding the doorway may help the patient who has difficulty locating his or her room. Active participation may help the patient to maintain cognitive, functional, and social interaction abilities for a longer period of time (Kovach & Henschel, 1996).

PROMOTING PHYSICAL SAFETY

A safe environment allows the patient to move about as freely as possible and relieves the family of constant worry about safety. To prevent falls and other accidents, all obvious hazards are removed. Night lights are helpful. The patient's intake of medications and food is monitored. Smoking is allowed only with supervision. A hazard-free environment allows the patient maximum independence and a sense of autonomy. Because of a short attention span and forgetfulness, wandering behavior can often be reduced by gently persuading or distracting the patient. Restraints are avoided because they may increase agitation. Doors leading from the house must be secured. Outside the home, all activities must be supervised to protect the patient. The patient should wear an identification bracelet or neck chain in case he or she becomes separated from the caregiver.

REDUCING ANXIETY AND AGITATION

Despite profound cognitive losses, there will be times when the patient is aware of his or her rapidly diminishing abilities. The patient will need constant emotional support that will reinforce a positive self-image. When losses of skills occur, goals are adjusted to fit the patient's declining ability.

The environment should be kept simple, familiar, and noise free. Excitement and confusion can be upsetting and may precipitate a combative, agitated state known as a catastrophic reaction (overreaction to excessive stimulation). During such a reaction, the patient responds by screaming, crying, or becoming abusive (physical or verbal assault). This is his or her way of expressing an inability to deal with the environment. When this occurs, it is important to remain calm and unhurried. Measures such as listening to music, stroking, rocking, or distraction may quiet the patient. Frequently, the patient forgets what triggered the reaction. Structuring activities is also helpful. Being familiar with the person's predicted responses to certain stressors helps caregivers to avoid similar situations.

IMPROVING COMMUNICATION

To promote the patient's interpretation of messages, the nurse remains unhurried and reduces noises and distractions. Clear, easy-to-understand sentences are used to convey messages because the meaning of words is frequently forgotten or there is difficulty with organizing and expressing thoughts. Lists and simple written instructions can serve as reminders to the patient and are often helpful. Sometimes, the patient can point to an object or

CHART 11•3 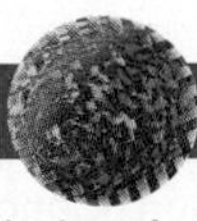 **Case Studies Relating to the Differential Diagnosis of Alzheimer's Disease**

Case Study: Alzheimer's Disease

Albert, age 87, had become increasingly forgetful over the past few years but had been able to hide it well. More recently, he failed to recognize his younger grandchildren, although his memory of events of long ago remained clear. Albert grew increasingly suspicious of those around him and often acted in ways that were socially inappropriate, such as exhibiting emotional outbursts. Such behavior was a departure from his former demeanor. He no longer slept through the night. Instead, his wife often found him wandering the house, seeming more confused at night than during the day. More recently, his hygiene and grooming had deteriorated noticeably. His appetite had diminished considerably and he began losing weight.

Case Study: Vascular Dementia

Mary had lived independently until the age of 93 with diagnoses of degenerative joint disease and osteoporosis with impaired mobility, HTN, and a history of a small stroke in the preceding year that left her with right-sided weakness. After that she went to live with her daughter and son-in-law. She was alert, oriented, and outgoing. Two months after her move, she had an episode of confused thinking and numbness in her left hand. Her blood pressure became elevated, and she required several drug trials to bring it under control over the next month. Four months later, she had an episode of lethargy that came on suddenly, in the dining room. The episode lasted for several minutes, then seemed to clear. Two other similar episodes occurred during the next few months.

At her annual physical, she was found to be somewhat forgetful and scored poorly on the mental status exam. Her daughter noted that this seemed to have come on rather suddenly in the past year. The physician listed the diagnosis of early Alzheimer's disease. Three weeks later, she was found unconscious in her bed and rushed to the hospital. A CT scan of the head revealed a new ischemic stroke as well as several small and apparently recent strokes throughout.

Case Study: Parkinson's Disease and B_{12} Deficiency

Norman was a 69-year-old nursing home resident with a diagnosis of SDAT [senile dementia, Alzheimer type]. He was nonverbal and transferred from bed to chair with a two-person assist; he required total care, including feeding. On physical exam, he presented with bilateral upper-extremity cogwheel rigidity, bradykinesia, and resting tremor. These findings, in combination with his lack of facial expression, known as *masked face*, and forward bent posture, were classic symptoms of Parkinson's disease, a diagnosis he did not carry. In addition, a routine CBC revealed a macrocytic anemia. Further testing revealed a B_{12} deficiency anemia. Norman was started on low-dose Sinemet [carbidopa/levodopa] and B_{12} injections. In about a week, he stood up and began to walk on his own, to everyone's amazement. After a loading dose of B_{12}, he began to talk in simple phrases and to answer questions appropriately. Unfortunately, the effects of the B_{12} anemia were not completely reversible.

Case Study: Hypothyroidism

Over a period of approximately 3 years, Adelaide, living with her unmarried son, became increasingly forgetful. In 1980, at the age of 87, she was diagnosed with SDAT. The family was advised of its progressive nature and the lack of treatment. Some time later, the son decided to change primary doctors. The new physician was unwilling to simply accept the diagnosis. He ordered several blood tests and found that she suffered from significant hypothyroidism. Once replacement hormones had restored her to a euthyroid state, she was again alert, fully oriented, and articulate. She resumed reading the paper and returned to her previous social routine. Adelaide lived to see her 100th birthday before she died from the effects of cardiovascular disease.

Case Study: Korsakoff's Dementia

Frances was a 72-year-old woman diagnosed with Alzheimer's disease by a geriatric assessment team in another state. Her son and daughter-in-law were informed of the diagnosis. They relocated her to their home in Philadelphia, where she was seen for a second opinion, at which time she was unable to express any clear thoughts independently. When interviewed on her initial visit, she had great difficulty with word finding and demonstrated short- and long-term memory impairment. She had a short attention span and confabulated repeatedly. In contrast to this, she was well groomed. Her clothing was coordinated and her hair and make-up were exact. Her daughter reported that she was able to do these things without any assistance. She had been driving in Florida until the time of her move without incident. In addition, Frances drank almost a gallon of wine a week. After a complete physical, including mental status exam and depression scale, neither of which she was able to focus on, a battery of lab tests was completed. They revealed combined B_{12} and folate deficiencies, elevated liver enzymes, and a blood alcohol level of 2.1. Over the next 2 months her family weaned her from the alcohol, and her mental status improved considerably. She was again able to participate in simple conversation with an improved attention span.

Case Study: Delirium—Medication Induced

Claire, age 91, was admitted to the hospital for open reduction-internal fixation of her fractured right hip. She had no history of dementia, confusion, or loss of memory. Three days post-op she was given medication for anxiety in the evening and later a sleeping pill. A few hours later she was found confused and on the floor. A stat CT scan of the head performed within the hour was normal, and a stat x-ray of the hip showed no damage to the repair from the fall. A neurologist saw her the next morning and diagnosed her as mildly demented on exam. No other tests were ordered. Claire's mental status cleared to baseline within 48 hours.

Reprinted with permission from Mangino, M., & Middlemiss, C. (1997). Alzheimer's disease: Preventing and recognizing a diagnosis. *Nurse Practitioner 22*(10), 73–74.

use nonverbal language to communicate. Tactile stimuli, such as a hug or a hand pat, are usually interpreted as signs of affection, concern, and security.

PROMOTING INDEPENDENCE IN SELF-CARE ACTIVITIES

Pathophysiologic changes in the brain make it difficult for a person with Alzheimer's disease to maintain physical independence. Efforts are directed toward helping the person remain functionally independent for as long as possible. One suggestion is to simplify daily activities by organizing them into short, achievable steps so that the patient experiences a sense of accomplishment. Frequently, an occupational therapist can suggest ways to simplify tasks or recommend adaptive equipment. Direct patient supervision is sometimes necessary. Maintaining personal dignity and autonomy is important for the person with Alzheimer's disease. He or she is encouraged to make choices when appropriate and to participate in self-care activities as much as possible.

PROVIDING FOR SOCIALIZATION AND INTIMACY NEEDS

Because socialization with old friends can be comforting, visits, letters, and phone calls are encouraged. Visits should be brief and nonstressful; limiting visitors to one or two at a time helps to reduce overstimulation. Because recreation is important, the person is encouraged to enjoy simple activities. Realistic goals that provide satisfaction are appropriate. Hobbies and activities (walking, exercise, socializing) can improve the quality of life. The confused, lonely person may find stimulation, comfort, and contentment in the nonjudgmental friendliness of a pet. Care of the pet by the patient can provide a satisfying activity and an outlet for energy.

Alzheimer's disease does not eliminate the need for intimacy. The patient and his or her spouse may or may not continue to enjoy sexual activity. The spouse should be encouraged to talk about any sexual concerns, and sexual counseling may be suggested if necessary. Simple expressions of love, such as touching and holding, are often meaningful.

PROMOTING ADEQUATE NUTRITION

Mealtime can be a pleasant, social occasion, or it can become a time of upset and distress. Mealtime should be kept simple and calm, without confrontations. The patient will prefer familiar foods that look appetizing and taste good. To avoid the patient's "playing" with the food, one dish is offered at a time. Food is cut into small pieces to prevent choking. Liquids may be easier to swallow if they are converted to gelatin. Hot food and beverages are served warm. The temperature of the foods should be checked to prevent burns.

When lack of coordination interferes with self-feeding, adaptive equipment is helpful. Some patients may do well eating with their fingers. If this is the case, an apron or a smock, rather than a bib, is used to protect clothing. As deficits progress, it may be necessary to feed the patient. Forgetfulness, disinterest, dental problems, incoordination, overstimulation, and choking can all serve as barriers to good nutrition.

PROMOTING BALANCED ACTIVITY AND REST

Many patients with Alzheimer's disease exhibit sleep disturbances, wandering, and other behaviors that may be deemed inappropriate. These behaviors are most likely to occur when there is an underlying physical or psychological need that is unmet. It is imperative that caregivers seek to learn the need of the patient who is exhibiting this type of behavior because further health decline could ensue if the source of the problem is not corrected. Adequate sleep and physical exercise is essential. If sleep is interrupted or the patient is unable to fall asleep, music, warm milk, or a back rub may help the person relax. During the day, the patient should be given sufficient opportunity to participate in exercise activities because a regular pattern of activity and rest will enhance nighttime sleep. Long periods of daytime sleeping are discouraged.

PROMOTING HOME AND COMMUNITY-BASED CARE

The emotional burden placed on the family of a patient with Alzheimer's disease is enormous. The physical health of the patient is often excellent, and the mental degeneration is gradual. Because the diagnosis is not specific, the family may cling to the hope that the diagnosis is incorrect and that the person will improve if he or she tries harder. Aggression and hostility exhibited by the patient are often misunderstood by the caregiver or family, who feel unappreciated, frustrated, and angry. Feelings of guilt, nervousness, and worry contribute to caregiver fatigue, depression, and family dysfunction.

The multiple needs of family caregivers have been addressed by the Alzheimer's Association. This national organization is a coalition of family members and professionals sharing the goals of family support and service, education, research, and advocacy. Family support groups, respite care, and adult day care are available through the Alzheimer's Association. Concerned volunteers are trained to provide structure to caregiver support groups. Through the use of respite care, a service commonly provided, the caregiver can get away from the home for short periods of time while someone else is tending to the patient's needs.

The nurse must be sensitive to the highly emotional issues that the family is confronting. Support and education of the caregivers are essential components of care. The family can contact the Alzheimer's Association or a comparable group that provides the opportunity to meet with others experiencing similar problems.

GERIATRIC SYNDROMES: MULTIPLE PROBLEMS WITH MULTIPLE ETIOLOGIC FACTORS

In the frail elderly, multiple problems, or syndromes, are frequently seen. Illness, whether acute or chronic, generally results from several factors rather than from a single cause. When combined with a decrease in host resistance, these factors lead to illness or injury. Because problems may have developed slowly, the onset of symptoms is often acute. Furthermore, the presenting symptoms may appear in other body systems before becoming apparent in the affected system. The term frailty is used to describe those elders at highest risk for adverse health outcomes or geriatric syndromes. There are no standard clinical criteria for frailty. The most widely agreed on definition of frailty applies to those elderly people who are most vulnerable to significant problems as a result of one or more of the following: extreme old age (85 years or older), inability to perform IADLs or ADLs independently, and the presence of multiple chronic diseases. As with specific illnesses, geriatric syndromes are never a normal consequence of aging. Early intervention can prevent further complications and help to maximize the quality of life for many older people (Hazzard, Bierman, Blass, Ettinger, & Halter, 1994).

Impaired Mobility

The causes of decreased mobility are multifactorial. More common causes include Parkinson's disease, diabetic neuropathy, cardiovascular compromise, osteoarthritis, osteoporosis, and sensory deficits. Environmental barriers and iatrogenic factors also weigh heavily. Elderly patients should be encouraged to stay as active as possible to avoid the downward spiral of immobility. During illness, periods of bed rest should be kept to a minimum. Even brief periods of bed rest quickly lead to deconditioning and, consequently, to a wide range of complications. When bed rest cannot be avoided, the patient should perform active range-of-motion and strengthening exercises with the unaffected extremities, and the affected extremities should receive passive range-of-motion exercises. Frequent position changes help offset the hazards of immobility. Staff and family can assist in maintaining the current level of mobility (Ham & Sloane, 1997).

Dizziness

Older people frequently seek help for dizziness. Dizziness presents a particular challenge because there are so many possible internal and external causes. For many, the problem is further complicated because of an inability to differentiate between the sensation of true dizziness (a sensation of disorientation in relation to position) and vertigo (a spinning sensation). Other simi-

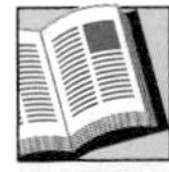

NURSING RESEARCH

What Is Frail?

Gealey, S. G. (1997). Quantification of the term frail as applied to the elderly client. *Journal of the American Academy of Nurse Practitioners 9*(11), 505–510.

Purpose

Although the term *frail* frequently appears in literature regarding the elderly, *frail* is infrequently defined. There is no consistent explanation of patient characteristics that prompts a clinician to use the label to describe some elderly patients and not others. The purpose of this quantitative study was to determine if there are objective measurements available to classify elderly people as frail or not frail.

Study Design

After an extensive literature review, a 10-item questionnaire about characteristics of frailty was developed. The questionnaire was verbally presented to five health care professionals: two geriatric physicians and three gerontologic nurse practitioners. Their responses suggested a relationship between frailty and inability to carry out activities of daily living (ADLs) and instrumental activities of daily living (IADLs), with frailty linked to functional decline.

A descriptive correlational study was subsequently completed to determine the relationship between ADLs and IADLs, and to validate the classification of frail versus not frail. A convenience sample of 34 subjects from two geriatric settings was used. Chart reviews were conducted to determine the subjects' ADL and IADL scores. Practitioners then rated the subjects as frail or not frail, and these ratings were compared with the ADL and IADL scores.

Findings

Findings revealed a consistent relationship between the classification of frail or not frail and the scores of the ADL and IADL scales.

Nursing Implications

Findings of the study indicated that assessment tools exist that provide for objective classification of the elderly as frail or not frail. Further studies are needed to provide information that can be used to refine these tools and enhance the ability of practitioners to plan care for the elderly, for example, to plan rehabilitation needs, home care needs, or long-term care needs.

lar sensations include near-syncope and dysequilibrium. The causes for these sensations range in severity from minor, as in buildup of ear wax, to significant, as in dysfunction of the cerebral cortex, cerebellum, brain stem, proprioceptive receptors, and the vestibular system. Even a minor culprit, such as an ear wax impaction, can result in the loss of balance and subsequent fall and injury (Hazzard et al., 1994).

Falls and Falling

Falling is a common and preventable source of mortality and mobility in older adults. A result of multiple possible physiologic and iatrogenic disorders, falls cause further negative sequelae. Overall, women appear to have more serious falls then men. The most common fracture occurring from a fall is hip fracture, resulting from the combined comorbidities of osteoporosis and the condition or situation that provoked the fall. Studies have shown that elderly people who fall experience greater decline in ability to perform ADLs and social activities, have a greater chance of being institutionalized than elderly people who do not fall, and utilize more health care services.

In institutionalized elderly people, restraints in the form of physical modalities (lap belts; geriatric chairs; vest, waist, and jacket restraints) and chemical modalities (medications) are known to precipitate many of the injuries they were meant to prevent. Documented injuries and deaths resulting from these restraints include strangulation, vascular and neurologic damage, pressure ulcers, skin tears, fractures, increased confusion, and significant emotional trauma. The time needed to supervise restrained patients adequately is better used addressing the unmet need that provoked the behavior that resulted in the use of restraint. Because of the overwhelming negative sequelae of restraint use, the accrediting agencies of nursing homes and acute care facilities now maintain stringent guidelines concerning their use (Strumpf, Evans, Wagner, & Patterson, 1992; Sullivan-Marx, 1996).

Urinary Incontinence

Urinary incontinence can be acute and develop during an illness, or it can develop chronically over a period of years. The older patient often does not report this very common problem unless specifically asked. Using the acronym DRIP, transient causes may be attributed to delirium, dehydration (D); restricted mobility, restraints (R); inflammation, infection, impaction (I); and pharmaceuticals, polyuria (P). Once identified, the causative factor can be eliminated. Established incontinence may be due to neurologic or structural abnormalities.

The pelvic floor serves as the supporting mechanism or "hammock" for the bladder, uterus, and rectum. It may have become

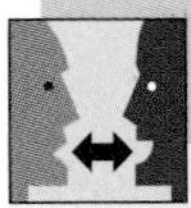

ETHICS AND RELATED ISSUES

Question

Should restraints be used without the patient's consent?

Situation

An elderly woman is admitted to the hospital with a diagnosis of pneumonia and dehydration. She is malnourished, underweight, and lethargic. IV fluids and antibiotics are prescribed. On the third day of hospitalization, her caloric intake is less than 500 calories per day. The physician orders tube feedings. The patient repeatedly removes her feeding tube, and the physician writes an order that her hands be restrained at all times so that the tube will not be pulled out. The patient, who is alert and oriented, says to the nurse, "Won't you please untie me? And take this thing out of my nose! I don't want it!"

Dilemma

The obligation to respect the patient's autonomy by releasing her from the restraints at her request conflicts with the obligation to protect her from harming herself by removing or dislodging the feeding tube (autonomy versus beneficence).

Discussion

What arguments would you offer *against* removing the restraints?

What arguments would you offer *in favor of* removing the restraints?

weakened as a result of pregnancy, labor and delivery, prior pelvic surgeries, or work that required prolonged standing or lifting. Dysfunction of the pelvic floor can be greatly improved with Kegel exercises. Other measures that help prevent accidents include having quick access to toilet facilities and wearing clothing that can be easily unfastened.

Incontinence can be as emotionally devastating as it is physically debilitating, especially to older women (Walsh Scura & Wipple, 1997). The patient with this problem should be urged to seek help from appropriate health personnel. Nurses who specialize in behavioral approaches to urinary incontinence management are particularly successful in assisting the individual either to regain continence or to significantly improve the level of continence. Although medications such as anticholinergics may decrease some of the symptoms of urge incontinence (detrusor instability), their side effects (dry mouth, slowed gastrointestinal motility, and confusion) may make them inappropriate choices for the elderly. Various surgical procedures are also used to manage urinary incontinence particularly in stress urinary incontinence.

Detrusor hyperactivity with impaired contractility is a type of urge incontinence that is predominantly seen in the elderly population. In this variation of urge incontinence, the patient has absolutely no warning that he or she is about to lose urine, and often when toileted has small volumes (if any) of urine, followed by a large incontinence episode after leaving the bathroom. It is essential that nursing staff be familiar with this form of incontinence and not show disapproval to the patient. Many patients with dementia suffer from this type of incontinence because both conditions are a result of dysfunction in similar areas of the brain. Prompted, timed voiding can be of assistance to these individuals, although clean intermittent catheterization is the preferred management.

AIDS IN OLDER ADULTS

AIDS is no longer only a disease of young people. It has been increasingly recognized that AIDS does not spare the older segment of society. According to a report of the Centers for Disease Control and Prevention, from 1981 to 1989, more than 10% of all AIDS patients nationwide were 50 years of age or older at the time of diagnosis, and about 3% were 60 years of age or older. In that database, male homosexual contact and blood transfusions were the predominant modes of transmission among older patients. A 1995 report of the San Francisco Department of Veteran Affairs Medical Center HIV Registry included 65 HIV-infected men who had at least one lymphocyte subset determination between 1987 and 1992. There has been a decline in recent years in transmission by contaminated blood products. The predominant mode of transmission in older people is through sexual contact. The most common AIDS-indicator disease in the older person is *Pneumocystis carinii* pneumonia. Wasting syndrome and HIV encephalopathy are also common in older HIV-infected people. Survival is significantly shorter in older patients than in younger patients with AIDS (Centers for Disease Control and Prevention, 1994; Chen, et al., 1998).

MEDICATIONS AND THE ELDERLY

Older people use more medications than any other age group. Representing 12.6% of the total population, they use 30% of the prescribed medications and 40% of all over-the-counter medications. Medications have improved the health and well-being of older people by alleviating symptoms of discomfort, treating chronic illnesses, and curing infectious processes. Problems commonly occur, however, because of medication interactions, multiple medication effects, multiple medication use (polypharmacy), and noncompliance. Combinations of prescription medications and some over-the-counter medications further complicate the problem.

Any medication is capable of altering nutritional status, which, in the elderly, may already be compromised by a marginal diet and chronic disease and its treatment. Medications can depress the appetite, cause nausea and vomiting, irritate the stomach, cause constipation or diarrhea, and decrease absorption of nutrients. In addition, they can alter electrolyte balance and carbohydrate and fat metabolism. A few examples of medications capable of altering the nutritional status are antacids (produce thiamine deficiency); cathartics (diminish absorption); antibiotics and phenytoin (reduce use of folic acid); and phenothiazines, estrogens, and steroid hormones (increase food intake and weight gain).

Altered Pharmacokinetics

Pharmacokinetics is the study of the actions of medications in the body, including the processes of absorption, distribution, metabolism, and excretion. Variability in these processes in older people (Table 11-4) is due, in part, to a reduced capacity of the liver and kidneys to metabolize and excrete the medications and to lowered levels of circulatory and nervous system efficiency in coping with the effect of certain medications. Many medications and their metabolites are excreted by the kidney. With advanced age, there are decreases in body weight, total body water, lean body mass, and plasma albumin (protein) and an increase in body fat. Consequently, highly protein-binding agents have fewer binding sites and higher pharmacologic activity. Fat-soluble agents have more binding sites, thus enhancing storage and delaying elimination.

Nursing Implications

The nurse administering medications to older people must be aware of the following:

- Medications removed from the body primarily by renal excretion remain in the body for a longer time in people with decreased renal function. Dosages often must be reduced. Overdosage and medication toxicity at usual therapeutic dosages are common.
- Medications with a narrow safety margin (eg, digitalis glycosides) must be administered cautiously.
- A decline in cardiac output may decrease the delivery rate to the target organ or storage tissue.
- The circulatory and central nervous systems of older people are less able to cope with the effect of certain medications, even when blood levels are normal.
- Paradoxical or unusual responses to medications may manifest as toxic reactions and complications.
- As a result of a slowing metabolism, medication levels may increase in the tissues and plasma, leading to prolonged medication action.
- Many elderly people have multiple medical problems that require treatment with one or more medications. The possibility of interactions between medications is further magnified if the older person is also taking one or more over-the-counter medications.

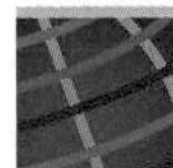

TABLE 11•4 Altered Drug Responses in Older People

Age-Related Changes	Impact of Age-Related Change	Applicable Drugs
Absorption		
Reduced gastric acid; increased pH (less acid)	Rate of drug absorption—possibly delayed	
Reduced GI motility; prolonged gastric emptying	Extent of drug absorption—not affected	
Distribution		
Decreased albumin sites	Serious alterations in drug binding to plasma proteins (the unbound drug gives the pharmacologic response); highly protein-bound drugs have fewer binding sites, leading to increased effects and accelerated metabolism and excretion	*Selected highly protein-binding drugs:* Oral anticoagulants (warfarin) Oral hypoglycemic agents (sulfonylureas) Barbiturates Calcium channel blockers furosemide (Lasix) Nonsteroidal anti-inflammatory drugs (NSAIDs) Sulfonamides quinidine phenytoin (Dilantin)
Reduced cardiac output	Decreased perfusion of many bodily organs	
Impaired peripheral blood flow	Decreased perfusion	
Increased percentage of body fat	Proportion of body fat increases with age and thus gives the body an increased ability to store fat-soluble drugs; this causes drug accumulation, prolonged storage, and delayed excretion	*Selected fat-soluble drugs:* Barbiturates diazepam (Valium) lidocaine Phenothiazines (antipsychotics)
Decreased lean body mass	Decreased body volume allows higher peak levels of drugs	Ethanol morphine
Metabolism		
Decreased cardiac output and decreased perfusion of the liver	Decreased metabolism and delay of breakdown of drugs, resulting in prolonged duration of action, accumulation, and drug toxicity	All drugs metabolized by the liver
Excretion		
Decreased renal blood flow; loss of functioning nephrons; decreased renal efficiency	Decreased rates of elimination and increased duration of action Danger of accumulation and drug toxicity	*Selected drugs with prolonged action:* Aminoglycoside antibiotics cimetidine (Tagamet) chlorpropamide (Diabinase) digoxin lithium procainamide

- A high-fiber diet and use of psyllium (Metamucil) or other laxatives may accelerate gastrointestinal transport and reduce absorption of medications taken concurrently.
- If for any reason the person is not dependable about taking medication, the nurse must be sure that the pill or capsule is actually swallowed and not retained between the cheeks and the gums or teeth.

Teaching self-administration of medication involves asking questions of the patient and requesting return demonstrations to ensure that learning has occurred. Sensory and memory losses, as well as decreased manual dexterity, can affect the patient's ability to carry out instructions properly, and the teaching plan will need to be adjusted to meet each patient's needs. The following steps taken by the nurse can help the patient to manage his or her medications and improve compliance:

- Explain the action, side effects, and dosage of each medication.
- Write out the medication schedule.
- Encourage the use of standard containers rather than safety lids (if there are no children in the household).
- Suggest using a multiple-day, multiple-dose medication dispenser to help patients adhere to the medication schedule (Fig. 11-3).
- Destroy old, unused medications.
- Review the medication schedule periodically.
- Discourage the use of over-the-counter medications without consulting a health professional.
- Encourage the patient to take all medications with him or her regularly, including over-the-counter medications, when visiting the primary health care provider.

THE OLDER PERSON IN THE COMMUNITY

Ninety-five percent of the elderly live in the community; 75% own their homes. In 1991, 31% were living alone (79% women). In the 65 years and older age group, half as many women as men

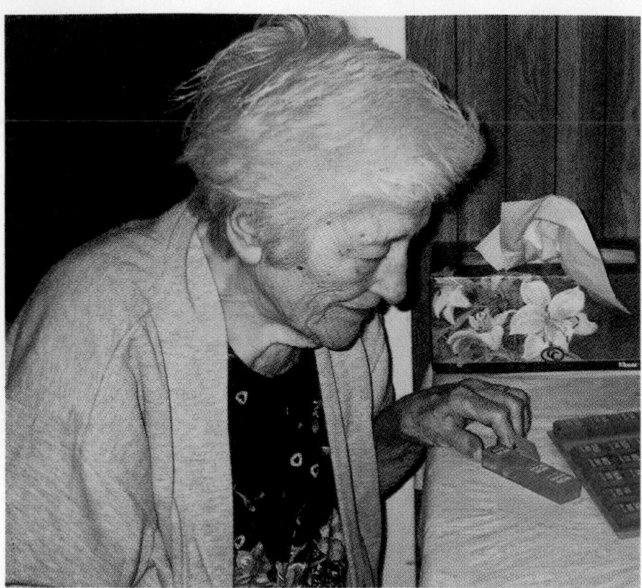

FIGURE 11•3 Commercially available, multiple-dose, multiple-day medication dispensers, such as this one, help older people to follow complex medication regimens safely at home.

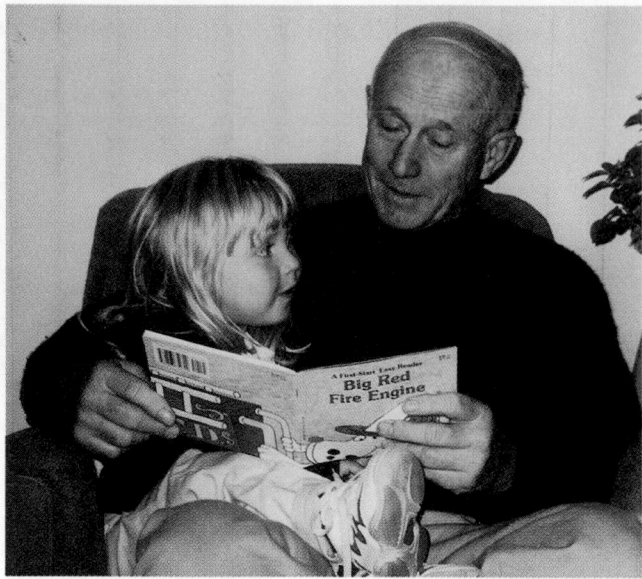

FIGURE 11•4 Families are an important source of psychosocial and physical support for elders and youngsters alike. Caring interaction among grandchildren, grandparents, and other family members typically contributes to the health of all.

were married and living with their spouses (40% of women, 74% of men). Half of the women older than 65 years of age (48%), but only 15% of the men, were widowed. This difference in marital status is due to several factors: women have a longer life expectancy than men, women tend to marry older men, and women remain widowed, whereas men often remarry.

Family

Planning for care and understanding the psychosocial issues confronting the older person must be accomplished within the context of the family. If dependency needs occur, the spouse assumes the role of primary caregiver. In the absence of the surviving spouse, an adult child usually assumes caregiver responsibilities and eventually may need help in providing care and support. A common myth within American society is that adult children and their aged parents are socially alienated. Furthermore, many believe that adult children abandon their parents when health and other dependency problems arise. Extensive research refutes these beliefs. The family is an important source of support for older people (Fig. 11-4). About 81% of the elderly have living children. Of those living alone, two thirds have at least one child living within 30 minutes of their home, and 62% see at least one adult child weekly.

Illness presents special problems for people who live alone. If community resources or adult children are unable to provide care, the elderly are at high risk for institutionalization. Social attitudes and cultural values often dictate that adult children should provide services and financial support and assume the burden of care if their aged parents are unable to care for themselves. Regardless of the amount of responsibility and love the adult child exhibits toward the dependent elderly parents, strains develop if care continues over a period of time. Research exploring the relationship between aged parents and their adult children shows that with poor health of the parent, the quality of the parent–child relationship declines. Under certain circumstances of high risk, strains in intergenerational relationships can result in elder abuse.

Elder abuse is an active or passive act or behavior that is harmful to the elderly person. Such behavior includes physical violence, personal neglect, financial exploitation, violation of rights, denial of health care, and self-inflicted abuse. Before elder abuse occurs, when strains are evident, preventive action should be taken. Interdisciplinary team members can be enlisted to help the caregiver develop self-awareness, increased insight, and understanding of the aging process. At the same time, community resources may be useful for both the aged person and the caregiver.

The Home Environment

Safety and Comfort

Injuries rank seventh as a cause of death for older people. Falls, the major cause of trauma in the elderly, are not often fatal but threaten health and the quality of life. Normal and pathologic consequences of aging that contribute to increased falls include visual changes, such as loss of depth perception, susceptibility to glare, loss of visual acuity, and difficulty in light accommodation. Neurologic changes include loss of balance, loss of position sense, and delayed reaction time. Cardiovascular changes may result in cerebral hypoxia and postural hypotension. Cognitive changes include confusion, loss of judgment, and impulsive behavior. Musculoskeletal changes include altered posture and decreased muscle strength. Many medications, medication interactions, and alcohol use precipitate falls by causing drowsiness, incoordination, and postural hypotension.

The nurse can encourage lifestyle and environmental changes that the older adult and his or her family can adopt. Adequate lighting with minimal glare and shadow can be achieved through the use of small area lamps, indirect lighting, sheer curtains to diffuse direct sunlight, dull rather than shiny surfaces, and night lights. Sharply contrasting colors can be used to mark the edges of stairs. Grab bars by the tub and toilet are useful. Loose clothing, improperly fitting shoes, scatter rugs, small objects, and pets create hazards and increase the risk of accidents. A person functions best in familiar settings if furniture and objects remain unchanged.

Personal Space

The older person needs a place of his or her own, a special location that can offer security, comfort, and privacy. This important "charted territory" can be a house, a room, or part of a room. It will contain treasures and mementos from a lifetime. The nurse can help the older person to maintain his or her own space. If moved, the patient will adjust more easily if he or she can establish a new area of privacy. These articles can be touched, thought about, and enjoyed regularly to enhance the quality of life. Personal items should *never* be removed without consent. Even if dementia is evident, it is preferable to clean up the area through a cooperative approach.

Community Programs and Health Services

Hospital and health services are used by the elderly more than by other age groups in the population. Disabilities resulting from chronic illnesses create the need in elders for help with basic activities of daily living. Twenty-two percent of the elderly are limited to a point at which they can no longer carry on regular daily activities. Community programs provide help beyond the capabilities of informal supports. Such valuable services as health care at home or in an adult day care center, opportunities for socialization, transportation, and home-delivered meals often keep the older person in the community and postpone or possibly eliminate the need for a nursing home.

Home Care

The older adult usually prefers to live independently, even if he or she has difficulty getting around the home. This may be against the wishes of the person's adult children. If the older person is capable of accepting responsibility for the personal risk involved, and other people are not endangered, the adult children should not interfere with this decision. There are many community supports that help the older person maintain independence. Informal sources of help, such as family, friends, the mail carrier, church members, and neighbors, can all keep an informal watch. Area Agencies on Aging perform many community services, including telephone reassurance, friendly visitors, home repair services, and home-delivered meals. Homemaker and chore services can be obtained at an hourly rate through these agencies or the local community nursing services. If the person is unable to pay, these services may be subsidized through local and state funds. Nursing care and rehabilitation services requiring the expertise of a registered nurse and other appropriate health professionals are usually paid for by Medicare (Schoen & Koenig, 1997).

Other community support services are available to help the older person outside of the home. Senior centers have social and health promotion activities; some provide a nutritious noontime meal. Adult day care facilities offer daily nursing care and social opportunities. Family members can carry on daily activities while the older person is at the day care center.

Hospice Services

Hospice services are a dignified alternative to the chaos of the acute care setting when a patient with an end-stage disease is expected to have 6 months to live or less. Hospice has been described as a program of supportive and palliative services for dying patients and their families that includes physical, psychological, social, and spiritual dimensions of care. Under Medicare and Medicaid, all needed medical and nursing services are provided to keep the patient as pain free and comfortable as possible. The family must agree to assist in the care of the patient, and services are brought into the home as needed. Hospice services may also be incorporated into the care of residents in long-term care facilities and include care for end-stage dementia (Cranmer, 1997; Keating, 1996; Wilson, Kovach, & Stearns, 1996).

ETHICAL AND LEGAL ISSUES AFFECTING THE OLDER ADULT

Loss of rights, victimization, and other grave problems face the person who has made no plans for personal and property management in the event of disability or death. The advice and services of a competent attorney regarding financial and personal issues can preserve future autonomy and self-determination. The nurse as an advocate can encourage the older person to prepare advance directives for future decision making in the event of incapacitation.

Power of attorney is a legal agreement that authorizes a person who is designated by the older person to act in specific, outlined purposes on behalf of the signer. This is a form of voluntary guardianship; permission is freely granted when the older person is competent. Unless stated otherwise, this power of attorney is invalidated on the incapacity of the signer. A durable power of attorney is a similar agreement that continues even if the older person is disabled or incapacitated. This power can include financial or personal decisions, depending on the desires of the person.

A trust is another option that the competent older person can consider. With a trust, the person designates someone to manage his or her property, stipulates how and under what circumstances the property will be managed, and designates a beneficiary. If incompetency or disability occurs, management of the property is undertaken according to the person's wishes.

If no advance arrangement has been made, and the older person appears unable to make decisions, anyone can petition the court for an incompetency hearing. If the court rules that the person is incompetent, the judge will appoint a guardian, a third party who is given powers by the court to assume responsibility for making financial or personal decisions for that person. There are two kinds of guardians—guardian of the person and guardian of the estate. Because such a court action strips the civil liberties and constitutional rights from the older person, there is potential for great harm. Safeguards include the following: (1) the older person must be given notice, (2) he or she must be given an opportunity to be legally represented, and (3) medical testimony can be cross-examined. A less restrictive form of guardianship, called the limited guardianship, transfers to the appointed guardian only those powers or duties that the older person cannot exercise. Although this alternative is not widely used, it remains an option.

Advance directives are formal, legally endorsed documents that provide instructions for care (living wills) or that name a proxy decision-maker (durable power of attorney) to be implemented in the event of future decision-making incapacity. This written document must be signed by the person and two witnesses. It should be given to the physician and incorporated into the medical record. The person must understand that this document is not meant to be used only when certain or all types of medical treatment are withheld, but rather allows for a detailed description of all health care preferences, including full use of all available medical interventions. The advance directive or a health care proxy has the authority to interpret the patient's wishes on the basis of the medical circumstances of the situation and is not restricted to deciding only if life-sustaining treatment can be withdrawn or withheld (Mezey, Bottrell, & Ramsey, 1996).

In 1990, the Patient Self-Determination Act (PSDA), a federally mandated law, was enacted to require patient education about advance directives at the time of hospital admission; documentation of this education is also required (PSDA, 1990; Markson et al., 1997). The PSDA is also mandated in nursing homes with the primary goal of enhancing resident autonomy by increasing involvement in health care decision making. There is a growing body of research that indicates that nursing homes implement the PSDA more vigorously than do hospitals. In both settings, there is considerable variation from facility to facility in the documentation and placement of advance directives in the medical record and in the education of patients about advance directives. Processes for fulfilling the requirements of the law are continuously being revised in many facilities to promote compliance. The PSDA has no guidelines regarding how often the advance directives of nursing home residents should be reviewed. In nursing homes in which ethics committees are present, there are more likely to be continuing quality improvement programs that establish guidelines for review (Mitty et al., 1996).

THE OLDER ADULT IN AN ACUTE CARE SETTING: ALTERED RESPONSES TO ILLNESS

The elderly person entering the acute care setting is at increased risk for complications, infections, and functional decline. The interdisciplinary team and the nursing staff can help avert negative outcomes by being knowledgeable about the physiologic and psychological responses of older adults to acute illnesses and by planning and implementing preventive measures. In addition to the interventions discussed later, general nursing measures that can be taken to avoid complications in the older adult include careful and frequent assessment of vital signs, mental status, fluid balance, and skin integrity; prompt identification and treatment of complications; promotion of independent self-care and mobility; assistance with frequent position changes and deep-breathing exercises; alertness to possible medication reactions; and assistance with ADLs and toileting.

Increased Susceptibility to Infection

Infectious diseases present a significant threat of morbidity and mortality to older people. In part, this is due to a blunted response of host defenses caused by a reduction in both cell-mediated and humoral immunity (see Chaps. 46 and 47). Also, age-related loss of physiologic reserve and chronic illnesses contribute to increased susceptibility. Pneumonia, urinary tract infections, tuberculosis (TB), gastrointestinal infections, and skin infections are some of the commonly occurring infections in older people.

The effects of influenza and pneumococcal infections on older people are also significant. Estimates place the number of deaths from influenza at 10,000 to 40,000 per year, whereas pneumococcal infections are responsible for 40,000 deaths annually. Of these deaths, at least 85% occur in older people. Safe and effective vaccines with few systemic reactions are available. Clinical studies show that the influenza vaccine is about 50% to 60% effective in preventing pneumonia and hospitalization and 60% to 70% effective in preventing death. It is estimated that the pneumococcal vaccine is about 60% to 70% effective in older people. The only contraindication is a history of anaphylactic hypersensitivity to eggs or a previous severe reaction (Centers for Disease Control and Prevention, 1998).

The influenza vaccine is prepared yearly to adjust for the specific immunologic characteristics that are present in the influenza viruses at that time. It is an inactivated preparation that should be taken annually in the fall, preferably in November. The pneumococcal vaccine has 23 type-specific capsular polysaccharides. Protection lasts 4 years or more. Revaccination is rarely recommended because of the higher incidence of local reaction on subsequent immunizations. Both of these injections can be received at the same time in separate injection sites. The nurse should urge older people to receive these vaccines. All health providers working with older people or high-risk chronically ill people should also be immunized.

TB also significantly affects older adults. The incidence of TB dropped from a peak of 84,000 cases in 1953 to a low of 22,000 cases in 1984. Between 1985 and 1993, there were about 60,000 more cases of TB than would have been predicted by previous trends (Griffith, 1998). Other than in HIV-infected people, case rates for TB are highest among the 65 years of age and older population. Nursing home residents account for the majority of the cases in the older population. Much of the infection rate is attributed to reactivation of old infection. Pulmonary and extrapulmonary TB often have subtle, nonspecific symptoms. This is of particular concern in the nursing home, because an active case of TB places patients and staff in jeopardy of infection.

The Centers for Disease Control and Prevention guidelines suggest that all new admissions to nursing homes receive a Mantoux test (PPD test) unless there is a history of TB or a previous positive response. All patients whose tests are not positive (positive = induration of more than 10 mm at 48 to 72 hours) should receive a second test in 1 week. The first PPD serves to boost the suppressed immune response that may occur with an older person. Chest x-rays and possibly sputum studies should be used to follow up on PPD-positive responders and converters. For positive converters, a course of preventive therapy for 6 to 12 months with isoniazid (INH) reduces the risk of active disease by 70%. All negative testers should be periodically retested. The nurse can facilitate this process within the care facility.

Altered Febrile and Pain Responses

Many altered physical, emotional, and systemic reactions to disease are attributed to age-related changes in older people. Useful and reliable physical indicators of illness in young and middle-aged people cannot be relied on for the diagnosis of potential life-threatening problems in older adults. The response to pain in older people may be lessened because of reduced acuity of touch, alterations in neural pathways, and diminished processing of sensory data. Research has demonstrated the absence of chest pain in many older adults experiencing a myocardial infarction. Hiatal hernia or upper gastrointestinal distress is often responsible for chest pain in elderly people. Acute abdominal conditions, such as mesenteric infarction and appendicitis, often go unrecognized in elderly people because of atypical signs and absence of pain.

The baseline body temperature in older people is about 1°F below that in younger people. Therefore, in the event of illness, the body temperature of an older person may not reach a sufficient elevation to qualify as the traditionally defined "fever." A temperature of 37.8°C (100°F), in combination with systemic symptoms, may signal infection. A temperature of 38.3°C (101°F) is almost certainly a serious infection that needs prompt attention. A blunted fever in the face of an infection often indicates a poor prognosis. Elevations in temperature rarely exceed 39.5°C (103°F). The nurse must be alert to other subtle signs of infection: mental confusion, increased respirations, tachycardia, and changed facial appearance and color.

Altered Emotional Impact

The emotional component of illness in older people may differ from that in younger people. Many elderly people equate good health with the absence of old age. "You are as old as you feel," is a belief of many. An illness that requires hospitalization or a change in lifestyle is an imminent threat to well-being. Admission to the hospital is often feared and actively avoided. Economic concerns and fear of becoming a burden to the family often lead to high anxiety in older people. The nurse must recognize the implications of fear, anxiety, and dependency in elderly patients. Autonomy and independent decision making are encouraged. A positive and confident demeanor in the nurse and the family promote a positive mental outlook in the elderly patient. In addition to anxiety and fear, older people are at high risk for disorientation, confusion, change in levels of consciousness, and other symptoms of delirium if they are admitted to the hospital.

Altered Systemic Response

The impact of illness on an aged person has far-reaching effects. The decline in organ function that occurs in every system of the aging body eventually forces one or more body systems to function at full capacity. Illness places new demands on body systems that have little or no reserve to meet this crisis. Homeostasis, the ability of the body to maintain an internal balance of function and chemical composition, is jeopardized. The older person may be unable to respond effectively to an acute illness or, if he or she has a chronic health condition, unable to sustain appropriate responses over a long period of time. Furthermore, the older person's ability to respond to definitive treatment is impaired. These responses reinforce the need for the nurse to monitor all of the older adult's body system functions closely, being alert to signs of impending systemic complication.

THE OLDER ADULT IN A PROTECTED ENVIRONMENT

Many housing communities for older people provide opportunities for socialization and recreation. Easier access to shopping and health care may convince the person that a new location will solve many residential problems. When preparation time is sufficient and money, energy, and health are adequate, a move to a new home can be a positive life experience. Retirement communities have living quarters of apartments, condominiums, and houses that are developed specifically for older people. An independent lifestyle is enhanced with social and recreational events. Health services are not provided. Life care (continuing care) communities offer all the features of retirement communities plus health care and skilled nursing care units. When entering such a community, the resident must be capable of independent living.

Until recently, about 5% of people between 65 and 84 years of age, and 22% of those 85 years of age or older, resided in nursing homes. With the onset of the "baby boomers" moving into retirement, residency ratio predictions for the year 2030 suggest that the percentages may decrease to 3.4% and 16.8%, respectively. These numbers are predicated on the effectiveness of preventative health maintenance.

Nursing homes offer a variety of health and personal services that include skilled nursing care and rehabilitation. They do not provide acute care, although an increasing number of facilities offer subacute care, which provides a step-down period of time from acute care in the skilled nursing environment (De La Cruz, 1997). Medicare will not pay for personal care and will only pay skilled nursing home costs for a limited number of days. The cost of nursing home care comes out of the patient's and family's funds. When money and assets are totally depleted, the costs may be paid by Medicaid.

Fundamental changes occur in the life patterns of a couple when one of them enters a nursing home. Changes that affect one member of the couple have significant effects on the spouse as well. With comprehensive preadmission planning and understanding of life patterns by the nurse, many of these issues can be explored and dealt with before placement to promote a more effective adjustment (Rosenkoetter, 1996). Research indicates that successful adjustment to the nursing home is enhanced if the older person participates in the decision-making process. The nurse and social worker can function as advocates, emphasizing this point and encouraging a family decision that includes the patient.

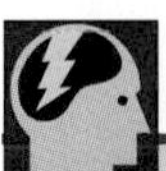

Critical Thinking Exercises

1. Your clinical assignment is in an adult day care center. Based on your knowledge of the aging process and theories about aging, describe the strategies and goals you would devise to enhance communication with the elderly patients.
2. A neighbor whose wife has recently been diagnosed with Alzheimer's disease approaches you expressing concern about his wife. He appears quite distraught and expresses anxiety about how he will be able to continue to care for her. Drawing on your knowledge about the course of this condition and the problems it presents to both the afflicted person and the caregiver, describe the guidance you would offer.
3. You are caring for an elderly patient in the home setting. Describe the focus of your assessment to determine if any changes need to be made in the patient's home environment and support systems to better meet his physical and psychosocial needs.

References and Selected Readings

BOOKS

Cohen, R. A., & Van Nostrand, J. F. (1995). *Trends in the health of older Americans: United States, 1994.* Washington, DC: U.S. Department of Health and Human Services.

Costa, P. T., Jr., Williams, T. F., Somerfield, M., et al. (1996). *Recognition and initial assessment of Alzheimer's disease and related dementias.* Clinical Practice Guideline No. 19. Rockville, MD: U.S. Department of Health and Human Services, Public Health Service, Agency for Health Care Policy and Research. AHCPR Publication No. 97-0702, November.

Cummings, E., & Henry, W. E. (1961). *Growing old: The process of disengagement.* New York: Basic Books.

Eliopoulis, C. (1997). *Gerontological nursing* (4th ed.). Philadelphia: Lippincott-Raven.

Erikson, E. H. (1963). *Childhood and society* (2nd ed.). New York: WW Norton.

Favus, M. J., & Christakos, S. (Eds.). (1997). *Osteoporosis: Fundamentals of clinical practice.* Philadelphia: Lippincott-Raven.

Gallo, J. J., Reichel, W., & Anderson, L. M. (1995). *Handbook of geriatric assessment* (2nd ed.). Gaithersburg, MD: Aspen.

Ham, R. J., & Sloane, P. D. (1997). *Primary care geriatrics: A case-based approach* (2nd ed.). St. Louis: Mosby–Year Book.

Havighurst, R. J. (1972). *Developmental tasks and education* (3rd ed.). New York: McKay.

Hazzard, W. R., Bierman, E. L, Blass, J. P., Ettinger, W. H., Jr., & Halter, J. B. (1994). *Principles of geriatric medicine and gerontology* (3rd ed.). New York: McGraw-Hill.

Neugarten, B. L. (1961). *Personality in middle and late life.* New York: Atherton Press.

Pfizer U.S. Pharmaceuticals. (1998). *Viagra: Full prescribing information.* Pamphlet No. HC041V98. Pfizer, Inc., April.

Pruitt, A. (1995). Evaluation of dementia. In Goroll, A. H., May, L. A., & Mulley, A. G. (Eds.), *Primary care medicine* (3rd ed.) (pp. 844–851). Philadelphia: J. B. Lippincott.

Schlenker, E. D. (1997). *Nutrition in aging* (2nd ed.). St. Louis: C. V. Mosby.

Siegel, J. (1996). *Aging into the 21st century.* Bethesda, MD: Administration on Aging, National Aging Information Center, May 31.

*Strumpf, N. E., Evans, L. K., Wagner, J., & Patterson, J. (1992). *Reducing restraints: Individualized approaches to behavior—a teaching guide.* Huntingdon Valley, PA: Geriatric Research & Training Center.

U.S. Department of Health and Human Services, Program Resources Department. (1997). *A profile of older persons.* Washington, DC: American Association of Retired Persons and U.S. Administration on Aging.

JOURNALS

Asterisks indicate nursing research articles.

Anderson, R. N., Kochanek, K. D, & Murphy, S. L. (1997). Report of final mortality statistics, 1995. *Monthly vital statistics report* (Vol. 45, No. 11, Suppl. 2, Table 7). Hyattsville, MD: National Center for Health Statistics.

Aevarsson, O., & Skoog, I. (1996). A population-based study on the incidence of dementia disorders between 85 and 88 years of age. *Journal of the American Geriatrics Society, 44,* 1455–1460.

Atchley, R. C. (1989). Continuity theory of normal aging. *Gerontologist, 29*(2), 183–190.

Branski, S. H. (1998). Delirium in hospitalized geriatric patients. *American Journal of Nursing, 98*(4), 16D–16L.

*Capezuti, E., Evans, L., Strumpf, N., & Maislin, G. (1996). Physical restraint use and falls in nursing home residents. *Journal of the American Geriatrics Society, 44,* 627–633.

Centers for Disease Control. (1991a). Purified protein derivative (PPD)—tuberculin anergy and HIV infection: Guidelines for anergy testing and management of anergic persons at risk of tuberculosis. *Morbidity and Mortality Weekly Report, 40*(RR-5), 27–32.

Centers for Disease Control. (1991b). Update on adult immunization: Recommendations of the Immunization Practices Advisory Committee (ACIP). *Morbidity and Mortality Weekly Report, 40*(RR-12), 33–36, 43, 44.

Centers for Disease Control and Prevention. (1994). Guidelines for preventing the transmission of *Mycobacterium tuberculosis* in health-care facilities, 1994. *Morbidity and Mortality Weekly Report, 43*(RR-13), 1–120.

Centers for Disease Control and Prevention. (1994). *HIV/AIDS surveillance report, 6,* 38–39.

Centers for Disease Control and Prevention. (1998). Prevention and control of influenza: Recommendations of the Advisory Committee on Immunization Practices. *Morbidity and Mortality Weekly Report, 47*(RR-6), 1–26.

Chen, H. X., Ryan, P. A., Ferguson, R. P., Yataco, A., Markowiz, J. A., & Raksis, K. (1998). Characteristics of acquired immunodeficiency syndrome in older adults. *Journal of the American Geriatrics Society, 46,* 153–156.

Cranmer, K. W. (1997). Hospice defined: Benefits, problems, and regulatory conflicts. *Nursing Home Medicine, 5*(7), 230–237.

*De La Cruz, P. (1997). Subacute nursing: Different stages of development. *MedSurg Nursing, 6*(4), 219–221.

*Evans, L. K., & Strumpf, N. E. (1989). Tying down the elderly: A review of the literature on physical restraints. *Journal of the American Geriatrics Society, 36*(1), 65–74.

Fantl, J. A., Newman, D. K., Colling, J., et al. (1996). *Managing acute and chronic urinary incontinence.* Clinical Practice Guideline. Quick Reference Guide for Clinicians, No. 2, 1996 Update. Rockville, MD: U.S. Department of Health and Human Services, Public Health Service, Agency for Health Care Policy and Research. AHCPR Pub. No. 96-0686, March.

Fried, L. P., Bandeen-Roche K., Williamson J. D., et al. (1996). Functional decline in older adults: Expanding methods of ascertainment. *Journal of Gerontology, 51,* M206–214.

*Grant, L. A., Kane, R. A., Potthoff, S. J. (1996). Staff training and turnover in Alzheimer special care units: Comparisons with non-special care units. *Geriatric Nursing, 17*(6), 278–282.

Griffith, D. E. (1998). Mycobacteria as pathogens of respiratory infection. *Infectious Disease Clinics of North America, 12*(3), 593–611.

Haan, M. N., Selby, J. V., Quesenberry, C. P., Jr., Schmittdiel, J. A., Fireman, B. H., & Rice D. P. (1997). The impact of aging and chronic disease on use of hospital and outpatient services in a large HMO: 1971–1991. *Journal of the American Geriatrics Society 45,* 667–674.

Havighurst, R. J. (1968). Personality and patterns of aging. *Gerontologist, 8*(3), 20–23.

*Hibbard, J., Neufeld, A., & Harrison, M. J. (1996). Gender differences in the support networks of caregivers. *Journal of Gerontological Nursing, 22*(9), 15–23.

*Hopkins, M. L., & Schoener, L. (1996). Tuberculosis and the elderly living in long-term care facilities. *Geriatric Nursing, 17*(1), 27–32.

*Keating, S. B. (1996). Hospice care and its relationship to home care services: A case study. *Geriatric Nursing, 17*(1), 41–43.

Kegel, A. H. (1948). Progressive resistance exercise in the functional restoration of the perineal muscles. *American Journal of Obstetrics and Gynecology, 56,* 238–248.

*Kovach, C. R., & Henschel, H. (1996). Planning activities for patients with dementia: A descriptive study of therapeutic activities on special care units. *Journal of Gerontological Nursing, 22*(9), 33–38.

Lebowitz, B. D. (1996). Diagnosis and treatment of depression in late life. *American Journal of Geriatric Psychiatry, 4*(Suppl. 1), S3–S6.

*Lesseig, D. Z. (1996). Primary care diagnosis and pharmacologic treatment of depression in adults. *Nurse Practitioner, 21*(10), 72–85.

*Mangino, M., & Middlemiss, C. (1997) Alzheimer's disease: Preventing and recognizing a misdiagnosis. *Nurse Practitioner, 22*(10), 58–78.

Markson L., et al. (1997). The doctor's role in discussing advance preferences for end-of-life care: Perception of physicians practicing in the VA. *Journal of the American Geriatrics Society, 45,* 399–406.

Mezey, M., Bottrell, M. M., & Ramsey, G. (1996). The Niche Faculty Advance Directives Protocol: Nurses helping to protect patient's rights. *Geriatric Nursing, 17*(5), 204–210.

Miller, C. A. (1996). Identify adverse medication effects when assessing function. *Geriatric Nursing, 17*(6), 295–296.

Mitty, E. L., et al. (1996). Ethics committees and implementation of the patient self-determination act in New York City nursing homes. *Nursing Home Medicine, 4*(1), 21–29.

National Center for Health Statistics. (1997). *Americans less likely to use nursing home care today.* U.S. Department of Health and Human Services, Press Release, January 23.

National Institute on Aging. (1994). *Discoveries in health for aging Americans: Progress report on Alzheimer's disease.* Washington, DC: U.S. Department of Health and Human Services, National Institutes of Health.

Patient Self-Determination Act (PSDA). (1990). *Omnibus Budget Reconciliation Act.* Title IV, Sec. 4206. Congress Record 12368, ct 26.

Pearlman, D. N., Branch, L. G., Ozminkowski, R. J., Experton, B., & Li, Z. (1997). Transitions in health care use and expenditures among older adults by payor/provider type. *Journal of the American Geriatrics Society, 45,* 550–557.

*Pontieri-Lewis, V. (1997). The role of nutrition in wound healing. *MedSurg Nursing, 6*(4), 187–221.

*Rosenkoetter, M. (1996). Changing life patterns of the resident in long-term care and the community-residing spouse. *Geriatric Nursing, 17*(6), 267–272.

*Schoen, M. A., & Koenig, R. J. (1997). Home health care nursing: Past and present—Part 1. *MedSurg Nursing, 6*(4), 231–232.

*Schwartz, D. (1996). Learning is a two-way street: Reciprocity and rewards. *Geriatric Nursing, 17*(1), 22–23.

*Stevenson, C., & Capezuti, E. (1991). Guardianship: Protection vs. peril. *Geriatric Nursing, 12*(1), 10–14.

*Sullivan-Marx, E. M. (1996). Restraint-free care: How does a nurse decide? *Journal of Gerontologic Nursing, 22*(9), 7–14.

U.S. Department of Health and Human Services, Public Health Service. (1992). *FDA safety alert: Potential hazards with restraint devices.* Rockville, MD: Food and Drug Administration, Center for Devices and Radiological Health, July 15.

*Walsh Scura, K., & Wipple, B. (1997). How to provide better care for the postmenopausal women. *American Journal of Nursing, 97*(4), 36–44.

Walton, J. C., & Miller, J. M. (1998). Evaluating physical and behavioral changes in older adults. *MEDSURG Nursing, 7*(2), 85–90.

Williamson, J. D., & Fried, L. P. (1996). Characterization of older adults who attribute functional decrements to "old age." *Journal of the American Geriatrics Society, 44,* 1429–1434.

Wilson, S. A., Kovach, C. R., & Stearns, S. A. (1996). Hospice concepts in the care for end-stage dementia. *Geriatric Nursing, 17*(1), 6–10.

Yen, P. K. (1996). When food doesn't taste good anymore. *Geriatric Nursing, 17*(1), 44–45.

Resources

AGENCIES

Administration on Aging, 330 Independence Avenue SW, Suite 4760, Washington, DC 20201; 1-202-619-0556 Statistical Information on Older Persons/ www.aoa.dhhs.gov/aoa/stats/statpage.html; Alzheimer's Disease/ www.aoa.dhhs.gov/factsheets/alz.html

Aging Network Services, Suite 907, 4400 East-West Highway, Bethesda, MD 20814; 1-301-657-4329

Alzheimer's Association, 919 Suite 1000, N. Michigan Avenue, Chicago, IL 60610; 1-312-335-8700

Alzheimer's Disease Education and Referral Center (ADEAR), P.O. Box 8250, Silver Spring, MD 20907-8250; 1-301-495-3311; 1-800-438-4380

American Association of Homes for the Aging, 901 E Street NW, Suite 500, Washington, DC 20004-2837; 1-202-783-2242

American Association for International Aging, 1133 20th Street W, Suite 330, Washington, DC 20036; 1-202-833-8893

American Association of Retired Persons, 601 E Street NW, Washington, DC 20049; 1-202-434-2277 www.aarp.org

American College of Health Care Administrators, 325 S. Patrick St., Alexandria, VA 22314; 1-703-549-5822

American Federation for Aging Research (AFAR), 1414 Avenue of the Americas, 18th Floor, New York, NY 10019; 1-212-572-2327

American Foundation for the Blind, 15 West 16th Street, New York, NY 10011; 1-212-620-2000

American Geriatrics Society, Inc., 770 Lexington Avenue, Suite 300, New York, NY 10021; 1-212-308-1414 www.aoa.dhhs.gov/aoa/dir/35.html

American Health Care Association, 1201 L Street NW, Washington, DC 20005; 1-202-842-8444

American Society for Geriatric Dentistry, 211 East Chicago Avenue, 17th Floor, Chicago, IL 60611; 1-312-440-2660

American Society on Aging, 833 Market Street, Suite 516, San Francisco, CA 94130; 1-415-974-9600

Association for Gerontology in Higher Education (AGHE), 1001 Connecticut Avenue NW, Suite 410, Washington, DC 20036; 1-202-429-9277

Children of Aging Parents (CAPS), Suite 302-A, 16098 Woodbourne Road, Levittown, PA 19057; 1-215-945-6900

Elderhostel, 75 Federal Street, Boston, MA 02110-1941; 1-617-426-7788

Gerontological Society of America, 1275 K Street NW, Suite 350, Washington, DC 20005-4006; 1-202-842-1275

Gray Panthers, 2025 Pennsylvania Avenue NW, Suite 821, Washington, DC 20006; 1-202-466-3132

Legal Services for the Elderly, 17th Floor, 130 West 42nd Street, New York, NY 10036; 1-212-391-0120

National Aging Resource Center on Elder Abuse (NARCEA), c/o American Public Welfare Association, Suite 500, 810 First Street NE, Washington, DC 20042-4205; 1-202-682-2470

National Association for Continence, P.O. Box 8306, Spartanburg, SC 29305-8306; 1-800-BLADDER (1-800-252-3337)

National Caucus and Center on Black Aged, Inc., Suite 500, 1424 K Street NW, Washington, DC 20005; 1-202-637-8400

National Council on the Aging, Inc., Suite 200, 409 Third Street SW, Washington, DC 20024; 1-202-479-1200

National Gerontological Nursing Association, 7250 Parkway Drive, Suite 510, Hanover, MD 21076; 1-800-723-0560

National Institute on Aging, P.O. Box 8057, Gaithersburg, MD 20898-8057; 1-800-222-2225

Simon Foundation for Continence, P.O. 835, Wilmette, IL 60091; 1-800-237-4666.

UNIT

3

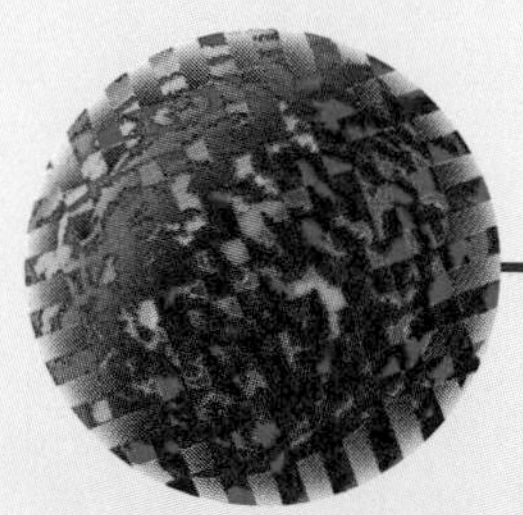

Concepts and Challenges in Patient Management

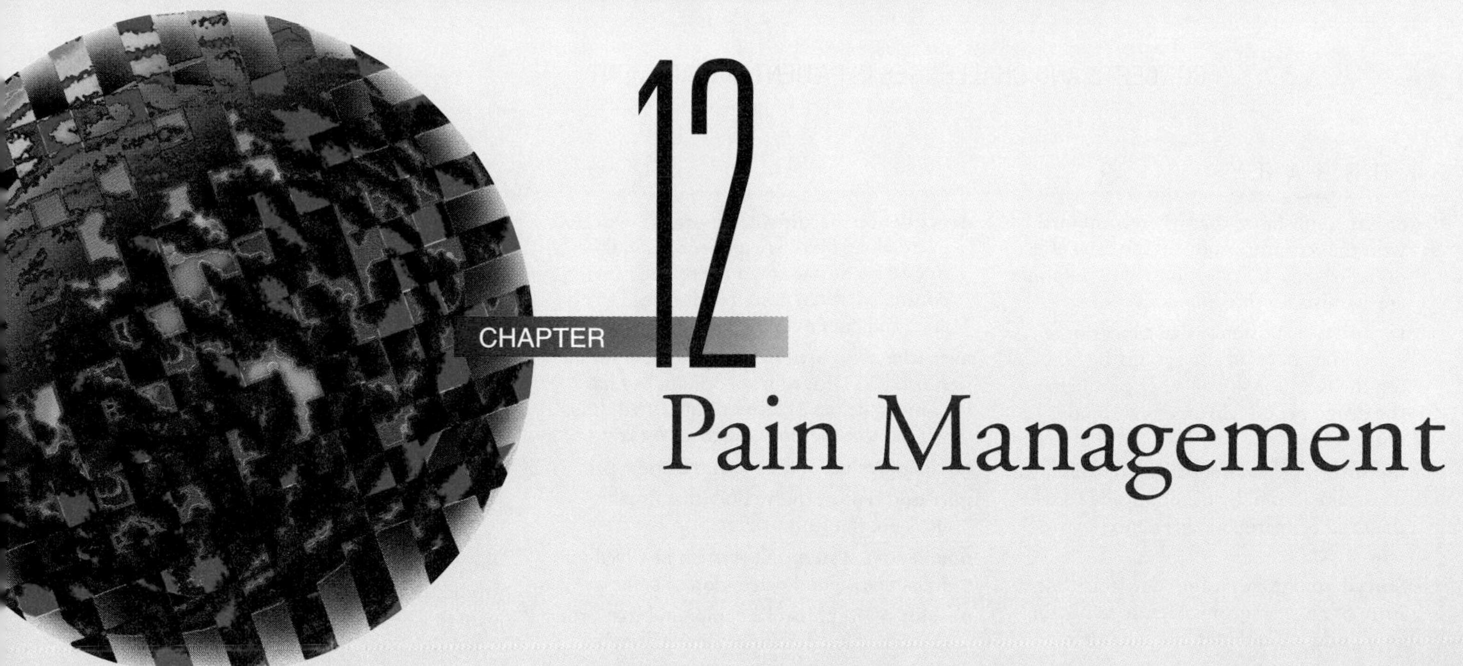

Pain Management

Learning Objectives

On completion of the chapter, the learner will be able to:

1. Differentiate between acute pain, chronic pain, and cancer pain.
2. Describe the negative consequences of pain.
3. Describe the neurophysiology of pain.
4. Explain the physiology of the pain relief interventions.
5. Explain the impact of aging on pain.
6. Demonstrate use of appropriate pain measurement instruments.
7. Describe physiologic and environmental factors that can alter the perception of pain.
8. Explain the differences between opioid dependency, tolerance, and addiction; discuss when opioid tolerance may be a problem.
9. Identify appropriate pain relief interventions for selected groups of patients.
10. Develop a plan to avoid adverse effects of opioid analgesics.
11. Use the nursing process as a framework for care of patients with pain.

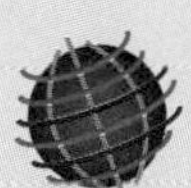

Pain is an unpleasant sensory and emotional experience resulting from actual or potential tissue damage. It is the most common reason for seeking health care. It occurs with many disorders and with some diagnostic tests and treatments. It disables and distresses more people than any single disease. Because nurses spend more time with the patient in pain than do other health care providers, nurses need to understand the physiologic basis of pain, the physiologic and psychological consequences of acute and chronic pain, and the methods used to treat pain. Nurses encounter patients in pain in a variety of settings, including acute care, outpatient, and long-term care settings, as well as the home. Thus, they must have the knowledge and skills to assess pain and its effects on the patient, to implement pain relief strategies, and to evaluate the effectiveness of these strategies, regardless of setting.

GLOSSARY

agonist: a substance that when combined with the receptor produces the drug effect or desired effect. Endorphins and morphine are agonists on the opioid receptors

antagonist: a substance that blocks or reverses the effects of the agonist by occupying the receptor site without producing the drug effect. Naloxone is an opioid antagonist

addiction: a behavioral pattern of substance use characterized by a compulsion to take the drug primarily to experience its psychic effects

balanced analgesia: using more than one form of analgesia concurrently to obtain more pain relief with fewer side effects

breakthrough pain: a sudden and temporary increase in pain occurring in a chronic pain patient (or cancer pain patient) being managed with opioid analgesia

endorphins and enkephalins: morphine-like substances produced by the body. Primarily found in the central nervous system, they have the potential to reduce pain.

dependence: occurs when a patient who has been taking opioids experiences a withdrawal syndrome when the opioids are discontinued; often occurs with opioid tolerance and does not indicate an addiction

narcotic: term used originally to describe all substances derived from opium, but has come to define a cluster of unrelated drugs whose distribution is regulated by law

nociceptor: nerve fiber that transmits pain

non-nociceptor: nerve fiber that usually does not transmit pain

nociceptive system: the system involved in transmission and perception of pain

opioid: a morphinelike compound that produces bodily effects including pain relief, sedation, constipation, and respiratory depression

pain: an unpleasant sensory and emotional experience resulting from actual or potential tissue damage

pain tolerance: the maximum intensity or duration of pain that a person is willing to endure

patient-controlled analgesia (PCA): self-administration of analgesics by a patient instructed about the procedure

placebo effect: analgesia that results from the expectation that a substance will work, not from the actual substance itself

prostaglandins: chemical substances that increase the sensitivity of pain receptors by enhancing the pain-provoking effect of bradykinin

referred pain: pain perceived as coming from an area different from that in which the pathology is occurring. An example would be the perception of left arm or jaw pain in a person having a myocardial infarction.

tolerance: occurs when a person who has been taking opioids becomes less sensitive to their analgesic (and usually side effect) properties. Characterized by the need for increasing dose requirements to maintain the same level of pain relief.

OVERVIEW

In health care, the primary care provider's role is to identify and treat the cause of the pain and prescribe medications and other treatments to relieve it. The nurse collaborates with the primary care provider but also with other health care professionals while administering most pain relief interventions, evaluating the effectiveness of the interventions, and serving as patient advocate when the intervention is ineffective. In addition, the nurse serves as an educator to the patient and family, teaching them to manage the pain relief (analgesic) regimen themselves when appropriate.

The nursing definition of pain is whatever bodily hurt the patient reports existing, whenever the patient says it does. The cardinal rule in the care of patients with pain is that all pain is real, even if its cause is unknown. Therefore, validation of the existence of pain is based simply on the patient's report that it exists. This definition is based on two important points.

First, the nurse believes patients when they indicate that they have pain. Pain is considered real even if no physical cause or origin can be identified. Although some painful sensations are associated with mental or psychological states, the patient actually feels a sensation of pain in such instances and does not merely imagine it. Most painful sensations are the result of physical stimuli and mental or emotional stimuli. Therefore, assessing a person's pain involves obtaining information about the physical causes of pain as well as the mental or emotional factors that influence the individual's perception of pain. Nursing interventions address both components.

The second point to keep in mind is that what the patient "says" about pain is not limited to verbal statements. Some patients cannot or will not verbally report that they have pain. Therefore, the nurse is also responsible for observing nonverbal behaviors that may occur with pain.

Although it is important to believe the patient who reports pain, it is equally important to be alert to patients who deny pain in situations where pain would be expected. A nurse who suspects pain in a patient who denies it should explore with the patient the reason for suspecting pain, such as the fact that the disorder or procedure is usually painful or that the patient grimaces when moving or avoids movement. Exploring the possible reasons why the patient is denying pain is also helpful. Some people deny pain because they fear the treatment that may result if they complain of pain. Others deny pain for fear of becoming addicted to opiates (substances derived from opium, also called narcotics) if these medications are prescribed.

TYPES OF PAIN

Three basic categories of pain are generally recognized: acute pain, chronic (nonmalignant) pain, and cancer-related pain.

Acute Pain

Usually of recent onset and commonly associated with a specific injury, acute pain indicates that damage or injury has occurred. Pain is significant in that it draws attention to its existence and teaches the person to avoid similar potentially painful situations. If no lasting damage occurs and no systemic disease exists, acute pain usually decreases along with healing, generally in less than 6 months and usually less than 1 month. For purposes of definition, acute pain can be described as lasting from seconds to 6 months.

Injuries or diseases that cause acute pain may heal spontaneously or may require treatment. For example, a prick of the finger heals rapidly, with the pain subsiding quickly. In a more severe condition, such as a fracture, treatment is required and the pain decreases in time as the bone heals.

Chronic (Nonmalignant) Pain

Chronic pain is constant or intermittent pain that persists over a period of time. It lasts beyond the expected healing time and often cannot be attributed to a specific cause or injury. It may not have a well-defined onset, and it is often difficult to treat because its cause or origin may be unclear. Although acute pain may be a useful signal that something is wrong, chronic pain usually becomes a problem in its own right.

Chronic pain may be defined as pain that lasts for 6 months or longer, although 6 months is an arbitrary period for differentiating between acute and chronic pain. An episode of pain may assume the characteristics of chronic pain before 6 months have elapsed, or some types of pain may remain primarily acute in nature for longer than 6 months. Nevertheless, after 6 months, most pain experiences are accompanied by problems related to the pain itself. Chronic pain serves no useful purpose. If it persists, it may become the major disorder.

Although the reason why some people develop chronic pain after an injury or disease is unknown, some experts suspect that nerve endings that normally do not transmit pain develop the ability to evoke painful sensations, or nerve endings that normally transmit only noxious (painful) stimuli transmit previously non-noxious (nonpainful) stimuli as painful stimuli.

The nurse may come in contact with patients with chronic pain when they are admitted to the hospital for treatment or when they are seen out of the hospital for home care. Frequently the nurse is called on in community-based settings to assist patients in managing pain. For more information on common pain syndromes, see Chart 12-1.

Cancer-Related Pain

Pain associated with cancer may be acute or chronic. Pain resulting from cancer is so ubiquitous that after fear of dying, it is the second most common fear of newly diagnosed cancer patients (Lema, 1997). Bonica (1985) estimated that more than 50% of patients with a diagnosis of cancer and 70% of patients with advanced cancer experience pain. Pain in the patient suffering from cancer can be directly associated with the cancer (eg, bony infiltration with tumor cells or nerve compression), a result of cancer treatment (eg, surgery or radiation), or not associated with the cancer (eg, trauma). Most pain associated with cancer, however, is a direct result of tumor involvement. An approach to cancer pain management is illustrated in Figure 12-1.

HARMFUL EFFECTS OF PAIN

Acute Pain

Regardless of its nature, pattern, or cause, pain that is inadequately treated has harmful effects beyond the discomfort it causes. Unrelieved pain impairs the postoperative patient's ability to sleep (Simpson, Lee, & Cameron, 1996). Zalon (1997) found that the most common response to severe pain in frail, elderly postoperative women was to lie absolutely still, a response very likely to result in postoperative complications. Unrelieved acute pain can affect the pulmonary, cardiovascular, gastrointestinal (GI), endocrine, and immunologic systems (Benedetti et al., 1984; Yeager et al., 1987). The stress response ("neuroendocrine response to stress") that occurs with trauma also occurs with other causes of severe pain. The widespread endocrine, immunologic, and inflammatory changes that occur with stress can have significant negative effects. This is particularly dangerous in patients compromised by age, illness, or injury.

The stress response generally consists of increased metabolic rate and cardiac output, impaired insulin response, increased production of cortisol, and increased retention of fluids (see Chap. 6 for details about the stress response). The stress response may increase the patient's risk for physiologic disorders (eg, myocardial infarction, pulmonary infection, thromboembolism, and prolonged paralytic ileus). The patient with severe pain and associated stress may be unable to take a deep breath and may experience increased fatigue and decreased mobility. Although these effects may be tolerated by a young healthy person, they may hamper recovery in an elderly, debilitated, or critically ill person. Effective pain relief may result in a speedier recovery and an earlier return to previous activities, including work.

Chronic Pain

Like acute pain, chronic pain also has adverse effects. Suppression of immune function associated with chronic pain may promote tumor growth. Also, chronic pain often results in depression and disability. Although health care providers express concern about the large quantities of opioid medications required to relieve chronic pain in some patients, it is safe to use large doses of these medications to control progressive chronic (eg, cancer-related) pain. In fact, failure to administer adequate pain relief may be unsafe because of the consequences of unrelieved pain (Liebeskind, 1991).

Regardless of how the patient copes with chronic pain, pain for an extended period often results in disability. Patients with a number of chronic pain syndromes report depression, anger, and fatigue. They also score lower on quality of life measures (Gatchel et al., 1994; Miaskowski & Dibble, 1995). The patient may be unable to continue the activities and interpersonal relationships he or she engaged in before pain began. Disabilities may range from curtailing participation in physical activities to being unable to take care of personal needs, such as dressing or eating. The nurse needs to understand the effects of chronic pain on the patient and family and to be knowledgeable about pain relief strategies and appropriate resources to assist effectively with pain management.

NEUROPHYSIOLOGIC MECHANISMS OF PAIN

Specific structures in the nervous system are involved in transforming a stimulus into a pain sensation. The system involved in the transmission and perception of pain is referred to as the **nociceptive system**. The sensitivity of the nociceptive system components can be affected by several factors and may differ among individuals. Not all people exposed to the same stimulus (appendicitis, for example) experience the same intensity of pain. A sensation that is painful to one person may be just noticeable to another. Further, a stimulus may result in pain at one time but not at another. For example, pain is often worse at night. Among those factors that can increase or decrease the sensitivity of the different components of the nociceptive system are the pain transmitter mechanisms, pain pathways, and control systems.

Pain Transmission

Among the nerve mechanisms and structures involved in the transmission of pain perceptions to and from the area of the brain that interprets pain are **nociceptors**, or pain receptors and chemical mediators.

Pain Receptors (Nociceptors)

Pain receptors are free nerve endings in the skin that respond only to intense, potentially damaging stimuli. Such stimuli may be mechanical, thermal, or chemical in nature. The joints, skeletal

CHART 12•1 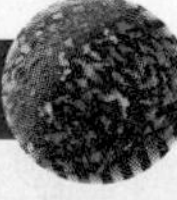 Pain Syndromes and Unusual Severe Pain Problems

Reflex Sympathetic Dystrophy (RSD)

Characterized by unexplained diffuse burning pain, usually in the periphery of an extremity, RSD is accompanied by weakness, skin color and temperature change relative to the other extremity, limited range of motion, hyperesthesia, hypoesthesia, edema, altered hair growth, and sweating. Pain, which worsens with movement, cutaneous stimulation, or stress, often occurs after surgery or trauma to the extremity, but is not limited to the area of surgery or trauma. RSD of the hand or wrist is often accompanied by shoulder pain (Veldman & Goris, 1995).

RSD is usually managed through a pain clinic. Currently, regional sympathetic blockade and regional IV bretylium offer promise. Tricyclic antidepressants may be tried as well.

Postmastectomy Pain Syndrome (PMP)

PMP occurs after mastectomy but is not necessarily related to the continuation of disease. Characterized by the sensation of constriction accompanied by a burning, prickling, or numbness in the posterior arm, axilla, or chest wall, PMP is often aggravated by movement of the shoulder, resulting in a frozen shoulder from immobilization (Miaskowski & Dibble, 1995).

Posttraumatic Headache

This disorder occurs after trauma to the head and is characterized by daily and persistent headache. It is more likely to follow mild head injury than moderate to severe injury (Uomoto & Esselman, 1993).

Fibromyalgia (Fibrositis)

Fibromyalgia, a chronic pain syndrome characterized by generalized musculoskeletal pain, trigger points, stiffness, fatigability, and sleep disturbances, is aggravated by stress and overexertion. Treatment consists of NSAIDs, trigger point injections with local anesthetics, tricyclic antidepressants, stress reduction, and regular exercise.

Hemiplegia-Associated Shoulder Pain

This pain syndrome occurs in as many as 80% of stroke patients. It may result from stretching of the shoulder joint due to the uncompensated pull of gravity on the impaired arm. It may be preventable with functional electrical stimulation of involved shoulder muscles.

Pain Associated With Sickle Cell Disease

Pain experienced by patients with sickle cell disease results from venous occlusion caused by the sickle shape of the blood cells, impaired circulation to a muscle or organ, ischemia, and infarction. Acute pain may be managed with IV opioid analgesics administered according to a schedule or by a patient-controlled analgesia (PCA) pump and NSAIDs. Warm soaks and elevating the affected body part may help as well. Meperidine (Demerol) therapy is not recommended in patients with compromised renal function, nor is cold therapy. Patients with sickle cell disease may have a long history of chronic pain. Some issues related to their history include tolerance, possible long-term dependence, racial prejudice, and inadequate pain treatment.

AIDS-Related Pain

As AIDS progresses, so do problems that produce increasing amounts of pain, such as neuropathy, esophagitis, headaches, postherpetic pain, and abdominal, back, bone, and joint pain. Pain relief interventions are individualized and may consist of NSAIDs, long-lasting opioids, such as fentanyl patches, and topical lidocaine. Tricyclic antidepressants may provide comfort in neuropathic and postherpetic pain.

Burn Pain

Possibly the most severe pain, burn pain tends to be underrated by health care professionals the longer they work with burn patients (Choiniere et al., 1990). Besides administration of IV opioid analgesics, current therapies to ameliorate pain in burn patients include débridement under general anesthesia; anxiety reduction; intervention with PCA devices, such as a hand-held nitrous oxide delivery system; and cognitive techniques, particularly hypnosis.

Guillain-Barré Syndrome and Pain

A progressive, inflammatory disorder of the peripheral nervous system, Guillain-Barré syndrome is characterized by flaccid paralysis accompanied by paresthesia and pain—muscle pain and severe, unrelenting, burning pain. Complaints of severe pain may be difficult to accept in the face of the characteristic flaccid facial response; therefore, the nurse must be sensitive and learn to disregard nonverbal cues that contradict the verbal complaint of pain. Treatment interventions include NSAIDs for muscle pain and opioids if NSAIDs are ineffective. Causalgia and neurogenic pain may be relieved by systemic or epidural opioids or, possibly, anticonvulsants or tricyclic antidepressants. To relieve the burning, some patients beg to have windows opened and clothing removed, even in cold weather. This suggests that gentle ice massage may help. Research is needed, however, to test this theory.

Opioid Tolerance

The opioid-tolerant patient is not uncommon among patients treated for chronic pain, especially in patients being treated by multiple health care providers. Opioid tolerance should be suspected when a patient (1) complains of significantly more pain than is usually associated with the condition, (2) requires unusually high doses of opioids to achieve pain relief, or (3) experiences an unusually low incidence and severity of side effects from opioids. Cancer patients also often develop a tolerance to opioids, requiring larger and larger doses of medication to obtain pain relief. In such cases, the nurse must first recognize what is happening, if necessary must seek additional information from the patient or family, and then must procure an additional medication prescription or an alternative intervention. In patients undergoing surgery, epidural local anesthetic agents provide excellent postoperative analgesia, but the problem of opioid tolerance must be elicited from the patient preoperatively.

Occasionally a recovering heroin addict is seen in an acute pain situation (surgery or trauma). This patient may be undergoing treatment with naltrexone (Trexan), a long-acting form of the opioid antagonist naloxone (Narcan). Both the short-acting naloxone and the long-acting naltrexone act by binding to the opioid receptors, so that opioids cannot be effective. If surgery is planned, the naltrexone should be discontinued a few days before the procedure. Should a patient receiving naltrexone be in immediate need of pain relief, very high doses of opioids are necessary. Alternative methods of pain relief (local or regional blockade and NSAIDs) should be incorporated in the pain management plan.

---

muscle, fascia, tendons, and cornea also have pain receptors that have the potential to transmit stimuli that produce pain. However, the large internal organs (viscera) do not contain nerve endings that respond only to painful stimuli. Pain originating in these organs results from intense stimulation of receptors that have other purposes. For example, inflammation, stretching, ischemia, dilation, and spasm of the internal organs all cause an intense response in these multipurpose fibers and can cause severe pain.

The pain receptors are part of complex multidirectional pathways. These nerve fibers branch very near their origin in the skin and send fibers to local blood vessels, mast cells, hair follicles, and sweat glands. When these fibers are stimulated, histamine is released from the mast cells and the blood vessels dilate (vasodilation).

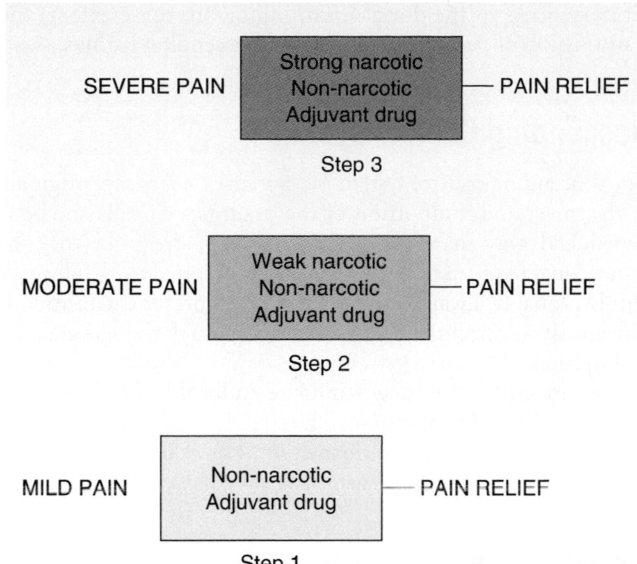

FIGURE 12•1 The World Health Organization three-step ladder approach to relieving cancer pain. Analgesic regimens are based on pain reported as ranging from mild to moderate to severe. Various opioid (narcotic) and nonopioid medications may be combined with other medications to control pain.

The cutaneous fibers located more centrally further branch and communicate with the paravertebral sympathetic chain of the nervous system and with large internal organs. As a result of the connections between these nerve fibers, pain is often accompanied by vasomotor, autonomic, and visceral effects. In a patient with severe acute pain, for example, GI peristalsis may decrease or stop.

Although intense activation of the pain receptor fibers in the skin causes a response in the visceral connection of that same fiber, the converse is also true. Intense stimulation of the visceral branch of a fiber may result in vasodilation and pain in the area of the body associated with that fiber. The result is called **referred pain.** The most widely recognized example of referred pain is pain in the left arm or jaw associated with cardiac ischemia or heart attack (myocardial infarction).

Chemical Mediators of Pain

A number of chemical substances that affect the sensitivity of the nerve endings or pain receptors are released into the extracellular tissue as a result of tissue damage. Histamine, bradykinin, acetylcholine, and substance P are chemicals that increase the transmission or perception of pain. **Prostaglandins** are chemical substances thought to increase the sensitivity of pain receptors by enhancing the pain-provoking effect of bradykinin. These chemical mediators also cause vasodilation and increased vascular permeability, resulting in redness, warmth, and swelling of the injured area.

Chemicals that reduce or inhibit the transmission or perception of pain include **endorphins** and **enkephalins**. These morphinelike neurotransmitters are endogenous—that is, they are produced by the body. They are examples of substances that reduce nociceptive transmission when applied to certain nerve fibers. The term "endorphin" is a combination of two words: endogenous and morphine. Endorphins and enkephalins are found in heavy concentrations in the central nervous system. Morphine and other **opioid** medications inhibit the transmission of noxious stimuli by mimicking enkephalin and endorphin.

Dorsal Horn and Ascending Pathways

The dorsal horn of the spinal cord has various functions, one of which is sensory processing. Peripheral fibers (eg, pain receptors) terminate here and the fibers of the ascending sensory tracts begin here (Fig. 12-2). Between the descending neuronal systems and the ascending sensory tracts are interconnections. The ascending tracts terminate on the lower and midportions of the brain and their impulses are relayed to the cortex of the brain.

The interconnections between the descending neuronal system and the ascending sensory tract are called inhibitory interneuronal fibers. These fibers contain enkephalin and are primarily activated through the activity of **non-nociceptor** peripheral fibers (fibers that normally do not transmit painful or noxious stimuli) in the same receptor field as the pain receptor, and descending fibers, grouped together in a system called descending control (discussed below). The enkephalins and endorphins are thought to inhibit pain impulses by stimulating the inhibitory interneuronal fibers, which in turn reduce the transmission of noxious impulses via the ascending system.

The existence of enkephalins and endorphins helps explain why different people feel different amounts of pain from similar stimuli. Endorphin levels vary among individuals, as do factors such as anxiety that influence endorphin levels. People with more endorphins feel less pain; those with fewer endorphins feel more pain.

For pain to be consciously perceived, neurons in the ascending system must be activated. Activation occurs as a result of input from the pain receptors located in the skin and internal organs. Once activated, the inhibitory interneuronal fibers in the dorsal horn inhibit or turn off the transmission of noxious or pain-stimulating information in the ascending pathway. Frequently this area is referred to as "the gate." The gate's natural tendency is to allow all noxious input from the periphery to activate the ascending pathways and result in pain.

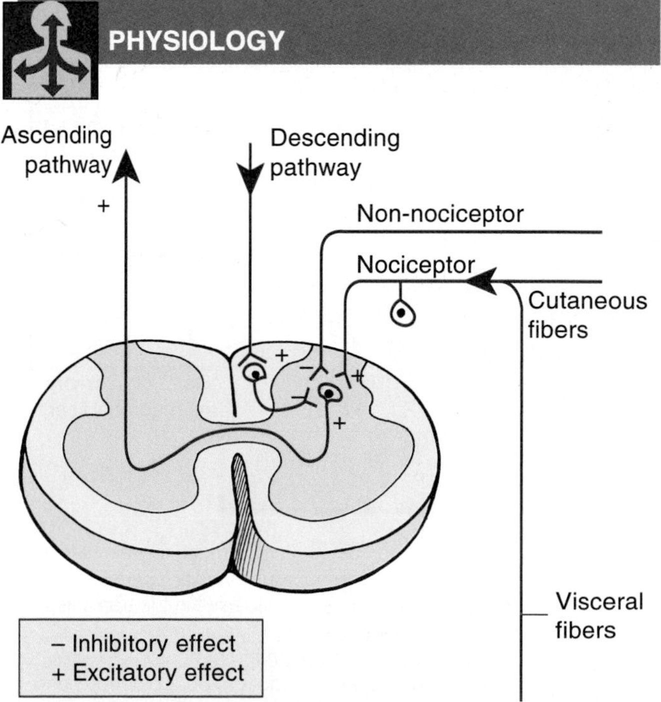

FIGURE 12•2 Representative nociception system, showing ascending and descending sensory pathways of the dorsal horn.

However, if this tendency went unopposed, many activities of daily living would be painful. Consequently, a system exists to "close the gate." Stimulation of inhibitory interneurons of the ascending system closes the gate to pain input and prevents the transmission of pain sensations (Fig. 12-3).

The classic gate control theory of pain (Wall, 1978) proposes that there is interaction between pain stimuli and other sensations and that stimulation of fibers that transmit nonpainful sensations blocks or decreases the transmission of pain impulses through an inhibitory gating. The inhibitory interneuronal fibers in the dorsal horn of the spinal cord are consistent with this theory.

This theory explains how certain activities decrease pain perception. The first response of a person who strikes a thumb with a hammer is to put the thumb in the mouth or in cold water. This action stimulates nonpain (non-nociceptive) fibers in the same receptor field as the pain-sensing fiber just activated. Stimulation of large numbers of non-nociceptive fibers, which synapse on inhibitory fibers in the dorsal horn, inhibit (to some extent) the transmission of painful sensation in the ascending pathways.

Descending Control System

The descending control system is a system of fibers that originate in the lower and midportion of the brain (specifically the periaqueductal gray matter) and terminate on the inhibitory interneuronal fibers in the dorsal horn of the spinal cord. This system is probably always somewhat active; it prevents continuous transmission of stimuli as painful, partly through the action of the endorphins.

Cognitive processes may stimulate endorphin production in the descending control system. The effectiveness of this system is illustrated by the effects of distraction. For example, people escaping a fire are often unaware that they have sustained burns

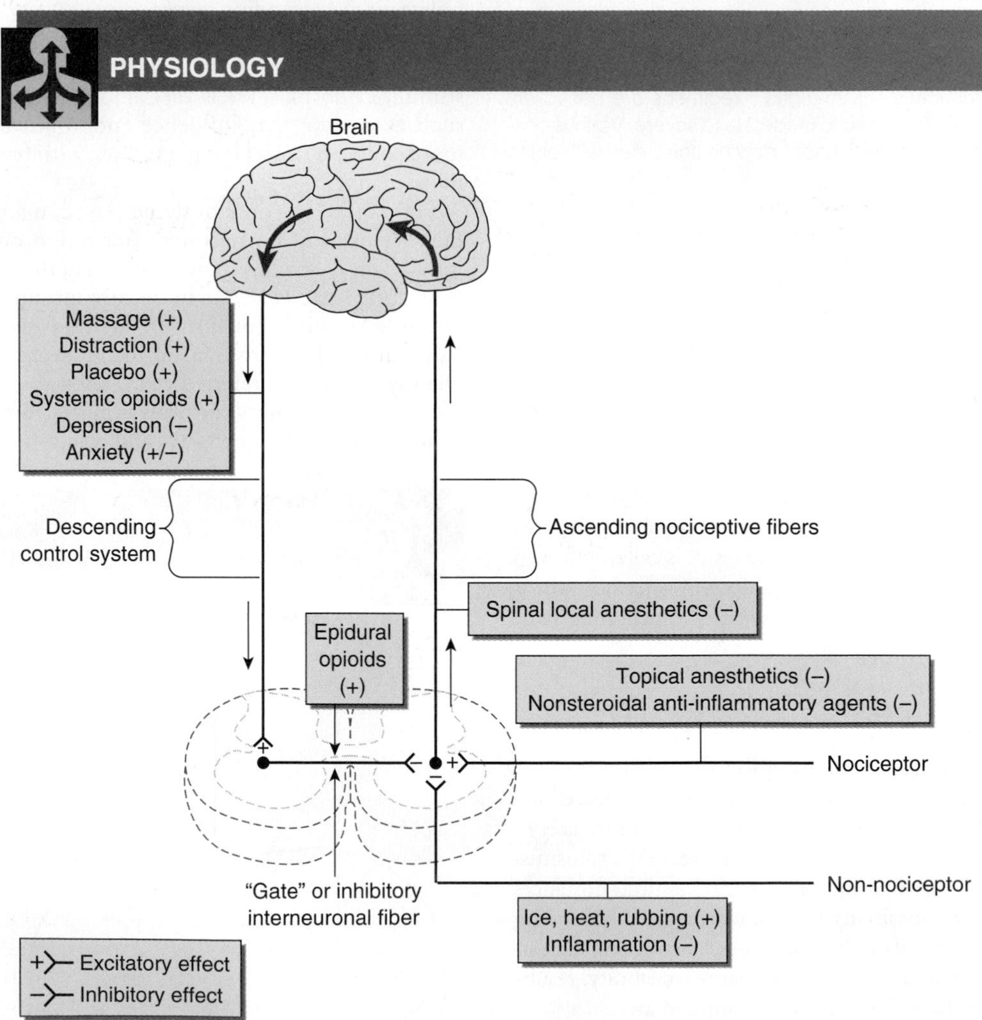

FIGURE 12•3 A schematic representation of the gate control system and aspects of the nociceptive system. The nervous system is made up of stimulatory and inhibitory fibers. For example, stimulation of the nociceptor will result in the transmission of an impulse that will be interpreted as pain. When it is stimulated it will stimulate transmission at the next fiber junction (represented as +≻). The interneuronal fiber is an inhibitory neuron (–≻). When it is stimulated it, in turn, inhibits or shuts off transmission at the next junction. So a placebo has a (+) stimulatory effect on the descending control system, which has a stimulatory effect (+) on the interneuronal fiber, which has an inhibitory effect (–) on the ascending control system. A topical anesthetic has an inhibitory effect (–) on nerve transmission at the nociceptor level and a spinal anesthetic has the same impact (–) on the ascending nociceptive fibers.

until reaching safety. For a person to reach safety, the brain shuts off the relatively less important pain perception by stimulating the descending control system. Similarly, intense physical activity is thought to increase endorphin production in the descending control system. In addition, the distractions of visitors or a favorite TV show may increase activity in the descending control system. Therefore, the person who has visitors may not report pain because activation of the descending control system results in less noxious or painful information being transmitted to consciousness. Once the distraction by the visitors ends, activity in the descending control system decreases, resulting in increased transmission of painful stimuli.

Depression can have the opposite effect of distraction. People who are depressed often report chronic pain. Unrelenting chronic pain can cause depression; depression in turn can lead to decreased activity in the descending control system and increased perception of pain. The difference in pain perception among individuals is probably a function of unconscious but persistent activity in the descending control system.

NURSING ASSESSMENT OF PAIN

In assessing a patient with pain, the nurse reviews the patient's description of the pain and other factors that may influence pain (ie, previous experience, anxiety, and age) as well as the person's response to pain relief strategies. Documentation of the pain level as rated on a pain scale becomes part of the patient's medical record, as does a record of the pain relief obtained from interventions.

Goals for Pain Relief

Pain assessment includes understanding what level of pain relief the acutely ill patient believes is needed to recover quickly or improve function, or what level of relief the chronically or terminally ill patient requires to maintain comfort. Patients with high levels of pain often report satisfaction with their pain management (Gordon & Ward, 1995). To understand this, it is necessary to understand patients' expectations and misconceptions about pain (Chart 12-2). A person who understands that pain relief not only contributes to comfort but also hastens recovery is more likely to request or self-administer medication appropriately.

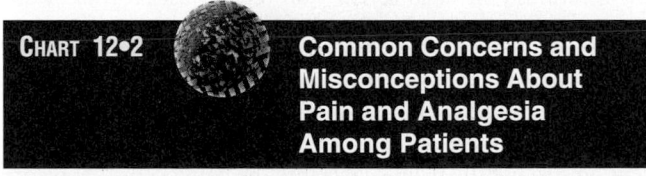

CHART 12•2 Common Concerns and Misconceptions About Pain and Analgesia Among Patients

- Complaining about pain will distract my doctor from his primary responsibility—curing my illness.
- I don't want to bother the nurse—he/she is busy with other patients.
- Pain medicine can't really control pain.
- People get addicted to pain medicine easily.
- It is easier to put up with pain than with the side effects that come from pain medicine.
- Good patients avoid talking about pain.
- Pain medicine should be saved in case the pain gets worse.
- Pain builds character. It's good for you.
- Patients should expect to have pain; it's part of almost every hospitalization.

Adapted with permission from Gordon, D. B., & Ward, S. E. (1995). Correcting patient misconceptions about pain. *American Journal of Nursing, 95*(7).

Tools for Assessing Perception of Pain

Only the patient can accurately describe and assess his or her pain. Nurses and physicians, on the other hand, consistently underestimate a patient's level of pain (Gujol, 1994; McCaffery & Ferrell, 1997; Puntillo et al., 1997; Thomas et al., 1998).

Therefore, various pain assessment tools may be needed to assess a patient's perception of pain (Fig. 12-4). Such tools may be used to document the need for intervention, to evaluate the effectiveness of the intervention, and to identify the need for alternative or additional interventions if the initial intervention is ineffective in relieving the person's pain. For a pain assessment tool to be useful, it must be easy to understand and use, require little effort on the part of the patient, be easily scored, and be sensitive to small changes in the intensity of pain.

Eliciting a Verbal Description of Pain

The patient is the best judge of his or her pain. Therefore, it is the patient who should be asked to describe the pain and rate its severity. The patient's pain is then described in the following ways:

- The intensity of the pain. The person may be asked to rate the pain on a verbal scale (eg, none, slight, moderate, severe, or very severe) or from 0 to 10, with 0 signifying no pain and 10 signifying the worst pain.
- Other characteristics of the pain. These may include location, duration (minutes, hours, days, months), rhythm (eg, continuous, intermittent, periods of waxing and waning of the intensity or existence of pain), and quality (eg, pricking, burning, aching, viselike).

Pain intensity scales

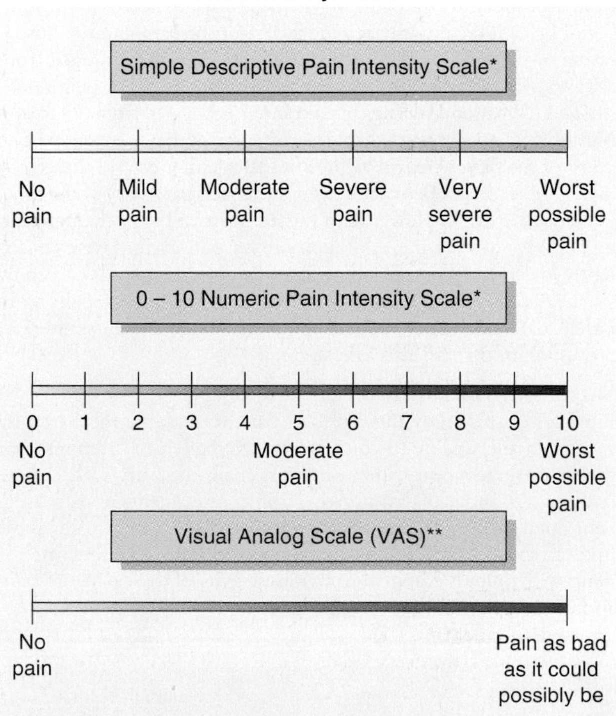

* If used as a graphic rating scale, a 10-cm baseline is recommended.

** A 10-cm baseline is recommended for VAS scales.

FIGURE 12•4 Examples of pain intensity scales.

NURSING RESEARCH

Pain Perception: By Patients and Nurses

Puntillo, K. A., Miaskowski, C., Kehrle, K., Stannard, D., Gleeson, S., & Nye, P. (1997). Relationship between behavioral and physiological indicators of pain, critical care patients' self-reports of pain, and opioid administration. *Critical Care Medicine, 25*(7), 1159–1166.

Purpose

The purpose of this study was to investigate nurses' assessment of a critical care patient's pain based on behavioral and physiologic indicators of pain. The authors note that the best indicator of a patient's pain is the patient's own report, but that critical care patients, often semiconscious or unable to communicate, may not be able to describe their pain.

Study Sample and Design

Subjects for this study were 14 registered nurses working in critical care or postanesthesia units. These nurses made 114 assessments on 31 patients who had undergone abdominal or thoracic surgical procedures and were mechanically ventilated or had been extubated within the previous 4 hours and had difficulty with communication.

Pain was assessed hourly over 5 hours by the nurses, using what the nurses believed to be a behavioral and physiologic indicator checklist that could be used when a patient was unable to communicate. In addition, patients completed a 0-to-10 horizontal numeric pain-intensity rating scale, the 0 extreme labeled "no pain" and the 10 extreme labeled "worst pain imaginable." The nurses rated the patients' pain using the behavioral and physiologic indicators and made an overall assessment of pain intensity using a scale similar to the patients'. Then the nurses asked the patients to rate their pain by pointing to the spot on the numeric rating scale that indicated their current pain. Finally, the nurses medicated the patients for pain using a sliding-scale opioid prescription.

Findings

Results of the study showed moderate correlations between the number of behavioral and physiologic indicators of pain and the nurses' rating of pain intensity. Correlations (reported as r^2) ranged from .001 to .77. Correlations between the nurses' ratings of pain intensity and the patients' ratings of pain intensity ranged from .09 to .45. Nurses' pain ratings were considered accurate if they were within one point of the patients' pain ratings (ie, 10% either way). Nurses' ratings were accurate 60% of the time, and inaccurate 40% of the time. Patients' scores were lower than nurses' scores 11% of the time and higher 29% of the time. Although nurses' pain ratings were consistently lower than the patients' ratings, the dose of opioids chosen by the nurses most frequently correlated with the nurses' pain score rather than the patients' pain score, even though the nurses were in possession of the patient's assessment.

Nursing Implications

Findings of this study indicate that patients who are mechanically ventilated and unable to communicate verbally can often indicate their pain perception using a numeric pain-intensity scale. These findings also indicate that nurses' indirect assessments of pain using behavioral and physiologic indicators are not accurate. Finally, these findings show that there continues to be a reluctance to medicate patients with opioids despite the obvious severity of these patients' pain and the short-term nature of the disorder.

- Factors that relieve pain (eg, movement, lack of movement, exertion, rest, over-the-counter medication) and what the person believes will help with the pain. Many people have definite ideas about what will relieve their pain, often based on experience or trial and error.
- Effects of pain on activities of daily living (eg, sleep, appetite, concentration, interactions with others, physical movement, work, and leisure activities). Acute pain is often associated with anxiety, chronic pain with depression.
- The person's concern about the pain. This may include a wide variety of concerns, such as financial burdens, prognosis, interference with roles, and body image changes.

Using Visual Analogue Scales

Visual analogue scales (VAS; see Fig. 12-4) are useful in assessing the intensity of pain. One version of the scale includes a horizontal 10-cm line, with anchors (ends) indicating the extremes of pain. The person is asked to place a mark indicating where the current pain lies on the line. The left anchor usually represents "none" or "no pain," whereas the right anchor usually represents "severe" or "worst possible pain." To score the results, a ruler is placed along the line and the distance the person marked the line from the bottom extreme is measured and reported in centimeters.

Some patients (eg, children, elderly patients, and visually or cognitively impaired patients) find it difficult to use an unmarked VAS. In those circumstances, ordinal scales (simple descriptive pain intensity scale, or 0 to 10 numeric pain intensity scale) may be used.

Using the FACES Pain Rating Scale

A FACES Pain Rating Scale (Wong et al., 1999) is a useful alternative, particularly for children and for patients with language problems or low literacy. This tool (Fig. 12-5) presents a series of cartoonlike faces ranging from a happy face to a crying face. The person experiencing pain is asked to point to the face that best represents how he or she feels. Patients' responses to this scale need to be evaluated carefully, and research that validates its use in adult patients is needed.

Guidelines for Using Pain Assessment Scales

Using a written scale to assess pain may not be possible if the person is seriously ill or in severe pain or has just returned from surgery. In these cases, the nurse can ask the patient, "On a scale of 0 to 10, 0 being no pain and 10 being pain as bad as it can be, how bad is your pain now?" For patients who have difficulty with a 0-to-10 scale, a 0-to-5 scale may be tried. Most patients usually can respond without difficulty. Ideally, the nurse instructs the patient how to use the pain scale before the pain occurs (ie, before surgery). The patient's numerical rating is documented and used to assess the effectiveness of the pain relief interventions.

If the person does not speak English or cannot communicate clearly information needed to manage pain, an interpreter, translator, or family member familiar with the person's method of communication should be consulted and a method established for pain assessment.

When a person with pain is cared for at home by family caregivers or the home care nurse, a pain scale may help in assessing the effectiveness of the interventions, if the scale is used before and after the interventions are administered. Scales that address the location and pattern of pain may be useful to the home care nurse in identifying new sources or sites of pain in the chronically or terminally ill patient and in monitoring changes in the patient's level of pain. The patient and family caregivers can be taught to use a pain as-

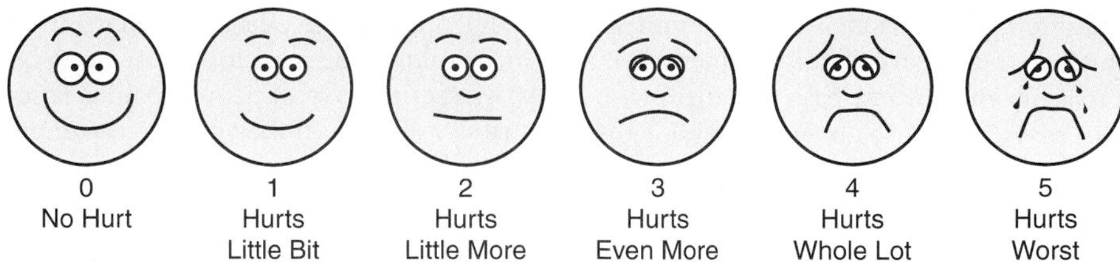

FIGURE 12•5 Wong-Baker FACES Pain Rating Scale. Instructions for using this scale: "Explain to the person that each face is for a person who feels happy because he has no pain (hurt) or sad because he has some or a lot of pain. Face 0 is very happy because he doesn't hurt at all. Face 1 hurts just a little bit. Face 2 hurts a little more. Face 3 hurts even more. Face 4 hurts a whole lot. Face 5 hurts as much as you can imagine, although you don't have to be crying to feel this bad. Ask the person to choose the face that best describes how he is feeling." Rating scale is recommended for persons age 3 and older. From Wong, D. L., Hockenberry-Eaton, M., Wilson, D., Winkelstein, M. L., Ahmann, E., & DiVito-Thomas, P. A. (1999). *Whaley and Wong's nursing care of infants and children* (6th ed.). St. Louis: Mosby, p. 1153. Copyrighted by Mosby–Year Book, Inc. Reprinted by permission.

sessment scale to assess and manage the patient's pain. The home care nurse who sees the patient only at intervals may thus benefit from the patient's or family's written record of the pain scores in evaluating how effective the pain management strategies have been over time.

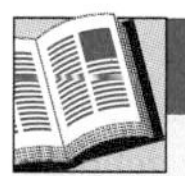

NURSING RESEARCH

Validity of Numeric Pain Rating

Paice, J. A., & Cohen, F. L. (1997). Validity of a verbally administered numeric rating scale to measure cancer pain intensity. *Cancer Nursing, 20*(2), 88–93.

Purpose

The purpose of this study was to test the validity of a verbally administered numeric pain rating scale (NRS).

Study Sample and Design

The verbal question "On a scale of 0–10, in which 0 is no pain and 10 is the most severe pain that you can possibly imagine, what number would you give your pain at this moment?" was administered to 50 subjects, all suffering from cancer and pain and able to understand English. The patients' scores on the NRS were compared with the patients' scores on a visual analogue scale (VAS) and a simple descriptor scale (SDS). (The VAS and SDS were very similar to those appearing in Figure 12-4, pain intensity scales.) All subjects were taking opioids.

Findings

Correlations between the patients' scores on the VAS and the NRS were high ($r = .847$) and support the validity of the NRS. When given a choice, most patients preferred the NRS, but the authors admit this may reflect a bias because the NRS is used widely and the patients may have been most familiar with this scale.

Eleven of the fifty subjects had difficulty with or were unable to complete the VAS. This difficulty was found most frequently in patients taking the higher doses of opioid.

Nursing Implications

This study lends support to the validity of the NRS when used clinically with ill patients. The difficulty some patients had with the VAS suggests that the VAS is difficult to use when the patient is suffering some cognitive impairment due to either opioids or a disease state. No subjects demonstrated difficulty with the NRS.

On occasion, a person will deny having pain when most people in similar circumstances would report significant pain. For example, it is not uncommon for a patient recovering from a total joint replacement to deny feeling "pain," but on further questioning will readily admit to having a "terrible ache, but I wouldn't call it pain." From then on, when evaluating this person's pain, the nurse would use the patient's words rather than the word "pain."

Assessment of Physiologic and Behavioral Responses to Pain

Assessing physiologic and behavioral indications of pain is sometimes difficult, if not impossible. Observable physiologic and behavioral indicators of pain may be minimal or absent; however, this does not mean that the patient does not have pain.

Many health care providers are more familiar with acute pain than chronic pain. Consequently, a health care provider unfamiliar with physiologic and behavioral pain responses may question the existence of pain in a patient who calmly reports severe pain or in someone who sleeps soundly immediately before or after reporting severe pain. However, not all patients with severe pain exhibit physiologic or behavioral signs of pain. The absence of these signs should not lead the nurse to conclude that pain is absent; conversely, the presence of these signs does not always mean that a patient has pain.

Identifying Physiologic Indicators of Pain

Involuntary physiologic changes were once considered more accurate indicators of pain than the patient's verbal report. However, these involuntary responses—increased pulse and respiratory rates, pallor, and perspiration—are indicators of autonomic nervous system arousal, not pain.

Some patients' heart rates may decrease in response to acute pain and increase only after the pain is relieved (Moltner et al., 1990). The heart rate may increase in anticipation of a painful procedure and decrease during the procedure itself (Porter et al., 1996). Patients experiencing severe acute pain may not demonstrate an increased respiratory rate, but may hold their breath. Any physiologic response to acute pain that a patient may demonstrate may only last a few minutes, even if the pain continues. Physiologic responses should be used as a substitute for verbal reports of pain only in the unconscious patient and should not be used to validate a person's verbal report of pain.

Because an intense physiologic reaction to pain cannot be maintained for weeks or years, or even several hours, patients usually respond differently to acute and chronic pain. A patient with very intense chronic pain may exhibit no apparent physiologic changes.

Recognizing Behavioral Responses to Pain

Behavioral responses to pain may include verbal statements, vocal behaviors, facial expressions, body movements, physical contact with others, or altered responses to the environment. A person in acute pain may cry, moan, frown, immobilize a body part, clench a fist, or withdraw. The person may become angry or irritable and apologize once the pain is relieved. Sounds from a radio or television may be very annoying to the person with pain. These behaviors vary greatly from one time to the next. Although a patient's behavioral responses may be the first indication that something is wrong, behavioral responses should not be used as a substitute for pain measurement except in unusual situations in which pain measurement is not possible (eg, the person is severely mentally retarded, cognitively impaired, or unconscious).

A person with pain of sudden onset may react very differently to pain that lasts more than a few minutes or becomes chronic. Pain may cause fatigue and leave the person too exhausted to moan or cry if such behavior is the normal response to pain. The patient may sleep, even with severe pain. The patient may appear relaxed and involved in activities by becoming a master at distraction from pain. The person who has succeeded in minimizing the effect of chronic pain on life should be encouraged rather than discouraged from coping in this way.

Understanding Factors Influencing the Pain Response

A person's pain experience is influenced by a number of factors, including past experiences with pain, anxiety, age, and expectations about pain relief (placebo effect). These factors may increase or decrease the person's perception of pain, increase or decrease tolerance for pain, and affect the manner of responses to pain. These factors are probably mediated through the gate previously described.

PAST EXPERIENCE

It is tempting to expect that a person who has had multiple or prolonged experiences with pain will be less anxious and more tolerant of pain than one who has had little pain. For most people, however, this is not true. Often, the more experience a person has had with pain, the more frightened he or she is about subsequent painful events. This person may be less able to tolerate pain; that is, he or she wants relief from pain sooner and before it becomes severe. This reaction is more likely to occur if the person has received inadequate pain relief in the past. A person with repeated pain experiences may have learned to fear the escalation of pain and its inadequate treatment. Once a person experiences severe pain, that person knows just how severe it can be. Conversely, someone who has never had severe pain may have no fear of such pain.

The way a person responds to pain is a result of many separate painful events during a lifetime. For some, past pain may have been constant and unrelenting, as in prolonged or chronic and persistent pain. The individual who has pain for months or years may become irritable, withdrawn, and depressed.

The undesirable effects that may result from previous experience point to the need for the nurse to be aware of the patient's past experiences with pain. If pain is relieved promptly and adequately, the person may be less fearful of future pain and better able to tolerate it.

ANXIETY AND DEPRESSION

Although it is commonly believed that anxiety will increase pain, this is not necessarily true. Research has demonstrated no consistent relationship between anxiety and pain, nor has it shown that preoperative stress reduction training reduces postoperative pain. Postoperative anxiety is most related to preoperative anxiety and postoperative complications. However, anxiety that is relevant or related to the pain may increase the patient's perception of pain. For example, a patient who was treated 2 years ago for breast cancer and now has hip pain may fear that the pain indicates metastasis. In this case, the anxiety may result in increased pain. Anxiety that is unrelated to the pain may distract the patient and may actually decrease the perception of pain. For example, a mother who is hospitalized with complications from a cholecystectomy and is anxious about her children may perceive less pain as her anxiety about her children increases.

The routine use of antianxiety medications to treat anxiety in someone with pain may prevent the person from reporting pain because of excessive sedation and may impair the patient's ability to take deep breaths, get out of bed, and cooperate with the treatment plan. Little evidence supports the old belief that antianxiety agents increase the effectiveness of analgesics. The most effective way to relieve pain is by directing the treatment at the pain rather than at the anxiety.

Just as anxiety is associated with pain because of underlying concerns and fears about the underlying disease, depression is associated with chronic pain and unrelieved cancer pain. In chronic pain situations, depression is associated with major life changes due to the limiting effects of the pain, specifically unemployment. Longer durations of pain are associated with an increased incidence of depression (Averill, Novy, Nelson, & Berry, 1996). Unrelieved cancer pain drastically interferes with the patient's quality of life. Relieving the pain may go a long way toward treating the depression.

CULTURE AND ETHNICITY

Culture and ethnicity have an influence on how a person responds to pain (how the pain is described or how the patient behaves in response to pain). However, culture and ethnicity do not affect pain perception (Calvillo & Flaskerud, 1993).

Old, often-cited research states that people from non–Anglo-Saxon origins have a lower **pain tolerance** (level or duration of pain that a person is willing to endure); however, this research is so seriously flawed that it is unacceptable by today's standards. Despite the widely held but erroneous belief that people of non–Anglo-Saxon ethnic groups have increased pain perception, and research findings that demonstrate that pain perception varies by individual rather than by ethnicity, people of nonwhite ethnic groups are prescribed and receive significantly less analgesia in emergency rooms (Todd et al., 1993), after surgery (McDonald, 1994; Ng et al., 1996a; 1996b), and for cancer-related pain (Cleeland et al., 1997).

Early in childhood, individuals learn from those around them what responses to pain are acceptable or unacceptable. For example, a child may learn that a sports injury is not expected to hurt as much as a comparable injury caused by a motor vehicle crash. The child also learns what stimuli are expected to be painful and what behavioral responses are acceptable. These beliefs vary from one culture to another; therefore, people from different cultures who experience the same intensity of pain may not report it or respond to it in the same ways. Rarely are the cultural expectations learned about pain altered by exposure to the opposing values of other cultures. Consequently, individuals believe that their perceptions of and reactions to pain are normal and acceptable.

The nurse's cultural values may differ from those of other cultures. The nurse's cultural expectations and values may include avoiding exaggerated expressions of pain, such as excessive crying and moaning, seeking immediate relief from pain, and giving complete descriptions of the pain. A patient's cultural expectations may be to moan and complain about pain, to refuse pain relief measures that do not cure the cause of the pain, and to use adjectives such as "unbearable" in describing the pain. A patient from another cultural background may behave in a quiet, stoic manner rather than expressing the pain loudly. The nurse must react to the person's pain perception and not to the pain behavior because the behavior is different from that of the nurse.

Recognizing the values of one's own culture and learning how these values differ from those of other cultures help to avoid evaluating the patient's behavior on the basis of one's own cultural expectations and values. It is equally important, however, to avoid stereotyping patients by culture. A nurse who recognizes cultural differences will have a greater understanding of the patient's pain and be more accurate in assessing pain and behavioral responses to pain, as well as more effective in relieving the patient's pain.

AGE

The influence of age on pain perception and pain tolerance is largely unstudied, but from what is known, pain perception does not change significantly with aging (Chakour et al., 1996; Heft et al., 1996). If pain perception is diminished in the elderly person, it is most likely secondary to a disease process (eg, diabetes), not aging (A.G.S. Panel on Chronic Pain in Older Persons, 1998). Although it does not appear that pain perception changes in the well elderly person, thermal perception may decline slightly.

Although many elderly people seek health care because of pain, others are reluctant to seek help even when in severe pain because they consider pain to be part of normal aging. Assessment of pain in older adults may be difficult because of the physiologic, psychosocial, and cognitive changes that often accompany aging. As many as 85% of nursing home residents are thought to be in pain, which contributes to the problems of depression, sleep disturbances, delayed rehabilitation, malnutrition, and cognitive dysfunction (Ferrell, 1995).

The way an older person responds to pain may differ from the way a younger person responds. Because elderly people have a slower metabolism and greater ratios of body fat to muscle mass than younger people, small doses of analgesics may be sufficient to relieve pain, and these doses may be effective longer. When given the opportunity to self-administer postoperative analgesia, elderly patients have been shown to obtain pain relief from smaller doses of opioids (Giuffre et al., 1991).

Elderly patients deal with pain according to their lifestyle, personality, and cultural background, as do younger adults. Many elderly people are very fearful of addiction and, as a result, will not report that they are in pain or ask for pain medication. Others fail to seek care because they fear that the pain may indicate serious illness or they fear loss of independence.

It is essential that the elderly patient receives adequate pain relief after surgery or trauma. When an elderly person becomes confused after surgery or trauma, the confusion is often attributed to medications, which are then discontinued. However, confusion in the elderly may be a result of untreated and unrelieved pain (Duggleby & Lander, 1994). In some cases postoperative confusion clears once the pain is relieved. Judgments about pain and the adequacy of treatment should be based on the patient's report of pain and pain relief rather than on age.

PLACEBO EFFECT

A **placebo effect** occurs when a person responds to the medication or other treatment because of an expectation that the treatment will work rather than because it actually does so. Simply receiving a medication or treatment may produce positive effects. The placebo effect results from the natural (endogenous) production of endorphins in the descending control system. It is a true physiologic response that can be reversed by naloxone, an opioid antagonist (Wall, 1993).

A patient's positive expectations about treatment may increase the effectiveness of a medication or other intervention. Often the more cues the patient receives about the intervention's effectiveness, the more effective it will be. A person who is informed that a medication is expected to relieve pain is more likely to experience pain relief than one who is told that a medication is unlikely to have any effect. A positive nurse–patient relationship may also serve an important role in enhancing the placebo effect.

Because of misperceptions about placebos and the placebo effect, the following principles and guidelines should be kept in mind:

- A placebo effect is not an indication that the person does not have pain; rather, it is a true physiologic response.
- Placebos should never be used to test the person's truthfulness about pain or as the first line of treatment.
- A positive response to a placebo (ie, reduction in pain) should never be interpreted as an indication that the person's pain is not real.
- A patient should never be given a placebo ("sugar pill" or saline injection) as a substitute for an analgesic medication. Although a placebo can produce analgesia, patients receiving a placebo may report that their pain is relieved or that they feel better simply to avoid disappointing the nurse.

NURSE'S ROLE IN PAIN MANAGEMENT

Before discussing what the nurse can do to intervene in the patient's pain, the nurse's role in pain management is reviewed. The nurse helps relieve pain by administering pain-relieving interventions (including both pharmacologic and nonpharmacologic approaches), assessing the effectiveness of those interventions, monitoring for adverse effects, and serving as an advocate for the patient when the prescribed intervention is ineffective in relieving pain. In addition, the nurse serves as an educator to the patient and family to enable them to manage the prescribed intervention themselves when appropriate.

Identifying Goals for Pain Management

The information the nurse obtains from the pain assessment is used to identify goals for managing the pain. The goals identified are shared or validated with the patient. For a few patients, the goal may be total elimination of the pain. For many, however, this expectation may be unrealistic. Other goals may include a decrease in the intensity, duration, or frequency of pain and a decrease in the negative effects the pain has on the patient. For example, pain may have a negative effect by interfering with sleep and thereby hampering recovery from an acute illness or decreasing appetite. In such instances, the goals might be to sleep soundly and to take adequate nutrition. Chronic pain may affect the person's quality of life by interfering with work or interpersonal relationships. Thus, a goal may be to decrease time lost from work or to increase the quality of interpersonal relationships.

To determine the goal, a number of factors are considered. The first is the severity of the pain, as judged by the patient. The second factor is the anticipated harmful effects of pain. A high-risk patient is at much greater risk for the harmful effects of pain than a young healthy patient. The third factor is the anticipated duration of the pain. In patients with pain from a disease such as cancer, the pain may be prolonged, possibly for the remainder of the patient's life. Therefore, interventions will be needed for some time and should not detract from the quality of life. A different set of interventions is required if the patient is likely to have pain for only a few days or weeks.

In a study of the dying experience, family members of 2,451 people who had died were interviewed (Lynn et al., 1997). Of these patients, 55% were conscious during their last 3 days of life. Four in 10 of the conscious patients were considered by their family members to be in severe pain most of the time. These findings strongly suggest that pain relief for dying patients should be a primary goal.

The goals for the patient may be accomplished by pharmacologic or nonpharmacologic means, but most success will be achieved with a combination of both. In the acute stages of illness, the patient may be unable to participate actively in relief measures, but when sufficient mental and physical energy is present, the patient may learn self-management techniques to relieve the pain. Thus, as the patient progresses through the stages of recovery, a goal may be to increase the patient's use of self-management pain relief measures.

Establishing the Nurse–Patient Relationship and Teaching

A positive nurse–patient relationship and teaching are key to managing analgesia in the patient with pain, because open communication and patient cooperation are essential to success.

A positive nurse–patient relationship characterized by trust is essential. By conveying to the patient the belief that the patient has pain, the nurse often helps reduce the patient's anxiety. Acknowledging to the patient, "I know that you have pain," often eases the patient's mind. Occasionally, patients who fear that no one believes the reported pain feel relieved when they know that the nurse can be trusted to believe the pain exists.

Teaching is equally important, because the patient or family may be responsible for managing the pain at home and preventing or managing side effects. Teaching patients about pain and strategies to relieve it may reduce pain in the absence of other pain relief measures and may enhance the effectiveness of the pain relief measures used.

The nurse also provides information by explaining how pain can be controlled. The patient is informed, for example, that pain should be reported in the early stages. When the patient waits too long to report pain, the pain may become so intense that it is difficult to relieve.

Providing Physical Care

The patient in pain may be unable to participate in the usual activities of daily living or to perform usual self-care and may need assistance to carry out these activities. The patient is usually more comfortable when physical and self-care needs have been met and efforts have been made to ensure as comfortable a position as possible. A fresh gown and change of bed linens, along with efforts to make the person feel refreshed (eg, brushing teeth, combing hair), often increase the level of comfort and improve the effectiveness of the pain relief measures.

Providing physical care to the patient also gives the nurse (in acute, long-term, and home settings) the opportunity to perform a complete assessment and to identify problems that may contribute to the patient's discomfort and pain. Appropriate and gentle physical touch during care may be reassuring and comforting. If fentanyl (a narcotic, or opioid, analgesic) patches are used, the skin under and around the patch should be assessed for integrity during physical care.

Managing Anxiety Related to Pain

Anxiety may affect a patient's response to pain. The patient who anticipates pain may become increasingly anxious. Teaching the patient about the nature of the impending painful experience and the ways to reduce pain often decreases anxiety; a person who is experiencing pain will use previously learned strategies to reduce anxiety and pain. Learning about measures to relieve pain may lessen the threat of pain and give the person a sense of control.

What the nurse explains about the available pain relief measures and their effectiveness may also affect anxiety. The patient's anxiety may be reduced by explanations that point out the degree of pain relief that can be expected from each measures. For example, the patient who is informed beforehand that an intervention may not eliminate pain completely is less likely to become anxious when a certain amount of pain persists. Anxiety resulting from anticipation of pain or the pain experience itself may often be managed effectively by establishing a relationship with the patient and by patient teaching.

A patient who is anxious about pain may be less tolerant of the pain, which in turn may increase the anxiety level. To prevent the pain and anxiety from escalating, the anxiety-producing cycle must be interrupted. Low levels of pain are easier to reduce or control than are more intense levels. Consequently, pain relief measures should be used before pain becomes severe. Many patients believe that they should not request pain relief measures until they cannot tolerate the pain, making it difficult for medications to provide relief. Therefore, it is important to explain to all patients that pain relief or control is more successful if such measures begin before the pain becomes unbearable.

PAIN MANAGEMENT STRATEGIES

Reducing pain to a "tolerable" level was once considered the goal of pain management. However, even patients who have described pain relief as adequate often report disturbed sleep and marked distress because of pain. In view of the harmful effects of pain and inadequate pain management, the goal of tolerable pain has been replaced by the goal of relieving the pain. Pain management strategies include both pharmacologic and nonpharmacologic approaches. These approaches are selected on the basis of the pa-

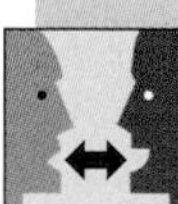

ETHICS AND RELATED ISSUES

Is It Acceptable to Ignore What You Believe to Be Inadequate Pain Management by a Colleague?

Situation

When taking over the care of ethnic minority patients at the change of shift from a particular colleague, you usually find these patients to be in a great deal of pain. Your nonsystematic observations have led you to conclude these patients receive only a small portion of the analgesia prescribed for them. You have heard a nurse colleague state a belief that people of certain ethnic groups have "no pain tolerance" and are "just looking for drugs."

Dilemma

Racial biases are difficult to change and deal with. To confront this nurse may not alter the behavior but will certainly disrupt the working relationships on the unit. It would be easier to look the other way. On the other hand, you believe that the nurse is giving inadequate and unethical care to selected patients and placing them at greater risk for postoperative complications.

Discussion

- What information would you need to collect before acting?
- From whom could you seek counsel?
- Are the two aspects of the dilemma equally important?

tient's requirements and goals. Appropriate analgesics are used as prescribed. They are not considered a last resort to be used only when other pain relief measures fail. Any intervention is most successful if initiated before the pain becomes severe, and the greatest success is usually achieved if several interventions are applied simultaneously.

Pharmacologic Interventions

Managing a patient's pain pharmacologically is accomplished in collaboration with the physician or other primary care provider, the patient, and often the family. The physician prescribes specific medications for pain or may establish an intravenous (IV) or epidural route for administering analgesic medications. However, it is the nurse who maintains the analgesia, assesses its effectiveness, and reports if the intervention is ineffective or produces side effects.

Pharmacologic management of pain requires close collaboration and effective communication among health care providers. In the home setting, it is often the family who manages the patient's pain and assesses the effectiveness of pharmacologic interventions, while it is the home care nurse who evaluates the adequacy of pain relief strategies and the family's ability to manage the pain. The home care nurse reinforces teaching and ensures communication among the patient, family care providers, physician, pharmacist, and other health care providers involved in the patient's care.

Premedication Assessment

Before administering any medication, the nurse asks the patient about allergies to medications and the nature of any previous allergic responses. True allergic or anaphylactic responses to opioids are rare, but it is not uncommon for a patient to report an allergy to one of the opioids. On further examination, the nurse often learns that the extent of the allergy was "itching" or "nausea and vomiting." These responses are not allergies; rather, they are side effects that, when necessary, can be managed while the patient receives pain relief. The patient's description of responses or reactions should be documented and reported before administering the medication.

The nurse obtains the patient's medication history (ie, current, usual, or recent use of prescription and over-the-counter medications), along with a history of health problems. Certain medications or conditions may affect the analgesic medication's effectiveness or the metabolism and excretion of analgesic agents.

Before administering analgesic agents, the nurse should assess the patient's status, including the intensity of current pain, changes in pain intensity after the previous dose of medication, and side effects of the medication.

Approaches for Using Analgesic Agents

Medications are most effective when the dose and interval between doses is individualized to meet the patient's needs. The only safe and effective way to administer analgesic medications is by asking the patient to rate the pain and by observing the response to medications.

BALANCED ANALGESIA

Pharmacologic interventions are most effective when a multimodal or **balanced analgesia** approach is used. Three general categories of analgesic agents are opioids, nonsteroidal anti-inflammatory drugs (NSAIDs), and local anesthetics. These agents work by different mechanisms. Using two or three types of agents simultaneously can maximize pain relief while minimizing the potentially toxic effects of any one agent. When one agent is used alone, it usually must be used in a higher dose to be effective. In other words, although it might require 15 mg of morphine to relieve a certain pain, it may take only 8 mg of morphine plus 30 mg of ketorolac (an NSAID) to relieve the same pain.

PRO RE NATA (PRN)

Until recently, the standard method used by most nurses and physicians in administering analgesia was to administer the analgesic on a *pro re nata* (PRN), or "as needed," basis. The standard was for the nurse to wait for the patient to complain of pain and then administer analgesia. As a result, many patients remained in pain because they did not know they needed to ask for medication.

By its very nature, the PRN approach to analgesia leaves the patient sedated or in severe pain a great deal of the time. To receive pain relief from an opioid analgesic, the serum level of that opioid must be maintained at a minimum therapeutic level (Fig. 12-6). By the time the patient complains of pain, the serum opioid level is below the therapeutic level. From the time the patient requests pain medication until the nurse administers the medication, the patient's serum level continues to fall. The lower the serum opioid level, the more difficult it is to achieve the therapeutic level with the next dose. The only way to ensure significant periods of analgesia, using this method, is to give doses large enough to produce periods of sedation.

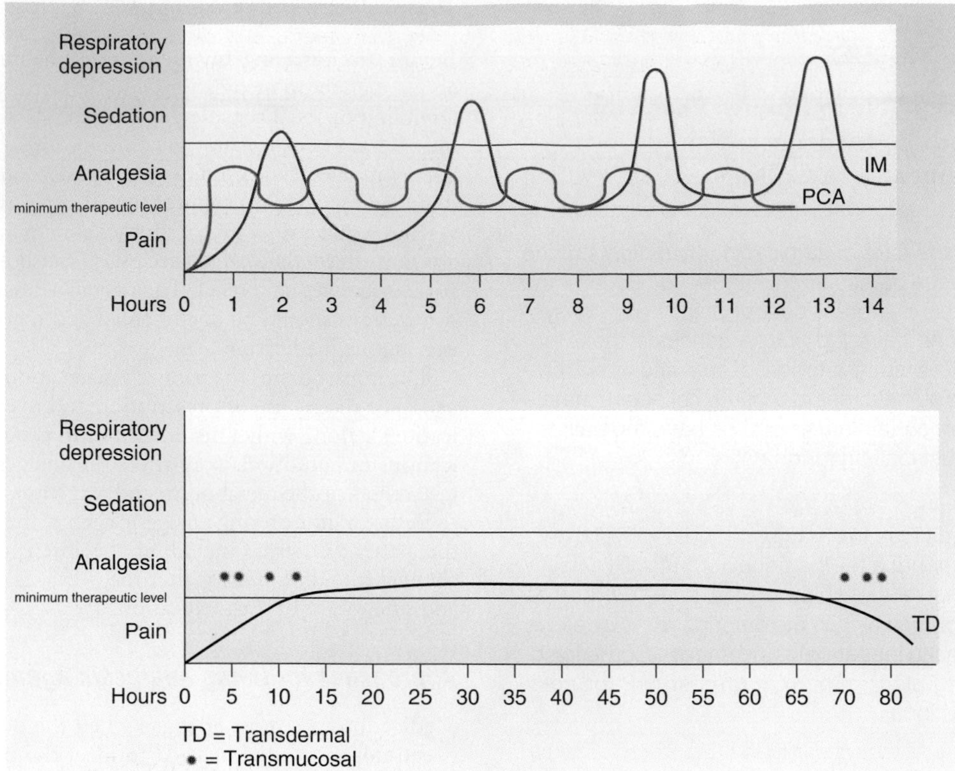

FIGURE 12•6 Relationship of mode of delivery of analgesia to serum analgesic level. *Top*: intramuscular (IM) and intravenous patient-controlled analgesia (PCA); *bottom*: transdermal (TD) and transmucosal (•).

PREVENTIVE APPROACH

Currently, a preventive approach to relieving pain by administering analgesics is considered the most effective strategy because a therapeutic serum level of medication is maintained. With the preventive approach, analgesics are administered at set intervals so that the medication acts before the pain becomes severe and the serum opioid level falls to a subtherapeutic level.

Administering analgesic medication on a time basis, rather than on the basis of the patient's complaint or report of pain, prevents the serum drug level from falling to subtherapeutic levels. An example of this would be giving the patient morphine or (as prescribed) the NSAID ibuprofen every 4 hours rather than waiting until the patient complains of pain. If the patient's pain is likely to occur around the clock or for a great portion of a 24-hour period, a regular around-the-clock schedule of administering analgesia may be indicated. Even if the analgesic is prescribed PRN, it can be administered on a preventive basis before the patient is in severe pain, as long as the prescribed interval between doses is observed. The preventive approach reduces the peaks and troughs in the serum level and provides more pain relief for the patient with fewer adverse effects.

Smaller doses of medication are needed with the preventive approach because the pain does not escalate to a level of severe intensity. Thus, a preventive approach may result in less medication over a 24-hour period, thereby helping prevent tolerance to analgesics and decreasing the severity of side effects (eg, sedation and constipation). Better pain control can be achieved with a preventive approach, reducing the amount of time the patient spends in pain.

In using the preventive approach, the nurse assesses for sedation before giving the next dose. The goal is to provide analgesia before the pain becomes severe. It would not be safe to medicate a patient (with an opioid) repeatedly if he or she was sedated or having absolutely no pain. It may be necessary to decrease the dosage of the opioid analgesic so that the patient receives pain relief with less sedation.

INDIVIDUALIZED DOSAGE

The dosage and the interval between doses should be based on the patient's requirements rather than on an inflexible standard or routine. People metabolize and absorb medications at different rates and experience different levels of pain. Therefore, one dose of an opioid medication given at specified intervals may be effective for one patient but ineffective for another.

Because of the fear of promoting addiction or causing respiratory depression, health care providers tend to prescribe and administer inadequate dosages of opioid agents to treat acute pain or chronic pain in the terminally ill patient. However, even prolonged administration of opioid agents is associated with an extremely low incidence (less than 1%) of addiction. Furthermore, small doses are not necessarily safe doses. For example, some patients receiving a relatively small dose (25 to 50 mg) of meperidine (Demerol) intramuscularly (IM) have experienced respiratory depression, whereas other patients have not exhibited any sedation or respiratory depression with very large doses of opioids.

Therefore, it is essential that the effects of opioid analgesics be monitored, especially when the first dose is given or when the dose is changed or given more frequently. The time, date, the patient's pain rating (scale of 0 to 10), the analgesic agent, other pain relief measures, side effects, and patient activity are recorded.

When the first dose of an analgesic is administered, the nurse needs to record a pain rating score, blood pressure, and respiratory and pulse rates. If the pain has not decreased in 30 minutes (sooner if an IV route is used) and the patient is reasonably alert and has a satisfactory respiratory status, blood pressure, and pulse rate, then some change in analgesia is indicated. Although the dose of analgesic medication is safe for this patient, it is ineffective in relieving the pain. Therefore, another dose of medication may be indicated. In such instances, the nurse consults with the physician to determine what further action is warranted.

PATIENT-CONTROLLED ANALGESIA

Used to manage postoperative pain as well as chronic pain, **patient-controlled analgesia** (PCA) allows patients to control the administration of their own medication within predetermined safety limits. This approach can be used with oral analgesics as well as with continuous infusions of opioid analgesics by IV, subcutaneous (SC), or epidural routes. PCA can be used in the hospital or home setting.

PCA pumps permit patients to self-administer continuous infusions of medication (basal rates) safely, thus enabling them to administer extra medication (bolus doses) with episodes of increased pain or painful activities. A PCA pump is electronically controlled by a timing device. Patients experiencing pain can administer small amounts of medication directly into their IV, SC, or epidural catheter by pressing a button. The pump then delivers a preset amount of medication.

The PCA pump also can be programmed to deliver a constant, background infusion of medication or basal rate and still allow the patient to administer additional bolus doses as needed. The timer can be programmed to prevent additional doses from being administered until a specified time period has elapsed and until the first dose has had time to exert its maximal effect. Even if the patient pushes the button multiple times in rapid succession, no additional doses are released. If another dose is required at the end of the delay period, the button must be pushed again to receive the dose. Patients who are controlling their own opioid administration usually become sedated and stop pushing the button before any significant respiratory depression occurs. Nevertheless, assessing respiratory status remains a major role for the nurse.

A continuous infusion plus bolus doses may be effective with cancer patients who require large doses of analgesia, or for postsurgical patients. Although this allows more uninterrupted sleep, the risk of sedation increases, especially when the patient has minimal or decreasing pain.

Patients who use PCA achieve better pain relief (Knapp-Spooner, Karlik, Pontieri-Lewis, & Yarcheski, 1995) and often require less pain medication than those who are treated in the standard PRN fashion. Because the patient can maintain a near-constant level of medication, periods of severe pain and sedation that occur with the traditional PRN regimen are avoided.

Initiating PCA. Whether PCA or any analgesia is used at home or in the hospital, it is important to avoid playing "catch-up." Pain should be brought under control before PCA starts, often by the use of an initial, larger bolus dose or loading dose. Then, after control is achieved, the pump is programmed to deliver small doses of medication at a time. If the patient with severe pain has a low serum level of opioid analgesic because of an inadequate basal rate, it is very difficult to regain control with the small doses available by pump. Before the PCA pump is used, repeated bolus doses of IV opioid may be administered as prescribed over a short time until the pain is relieved. Then PCA is initiated. If pain control is not achieved with the maximal dose of medication prescribed, further prescriptions are obtained. The goal is to achieve a minimum therapeutic level of analgesia and to allow the patient to maintain that level by using the PCA pump. The patient is instructed not to wait until the pain is severe before pushing the button to obtain a bolus dose. The patient is also reminded not to become so distracted by an activity or visitor that he or she forgets to self-administer a prescribed dose of medication. One potential drawback to distraction is that a patient who is using a PCA pump may not self-administer any analgesia during the time of effective distraction. When distraction ends suddenly (eg, the movie ends or the visitors leave), the patient may be left without a therapeutic opioid level in the serum. When intermittent distraction is used for pain relief, a continuous low-level background infusion of opioid through the PCA pump may be prescribed so that when the distraction ends, it will not be necessary to try to catch up.

PCA in Home Care. If PCA is to be used in the patient's home, the patient and family are taught about the operation of the pump and the side effects of the medication and strategies to manage them. Family members are cautioned not to push the button for the patient, especially if the patient is asleep, because this overrides some of the safety features of the system.

Local Anesthetic Agents

Local anesthetics work by blocking nerve conduction when applied directly to the nerve fibers. They can be applied directly to the site of injury (eg, a topical anesthetic spray for sunburn) or directly to nerve fibers by injection or at the time of surgery. They can also be administered through an epidural catheter.

TOPICAL APPLICATION

Local anesthetics have been successful in reducing pain associated with thoracic or upper abdominal surgery when injected by the surgeon intercostally. Local anesthetics are rapidly absorbed into the bloodstream, resulting in decreased availability at the surgical or injury site and an increased anesthetic level in the blood, increasing the risk of toxicity. Therefore, a vasoconstrictive agent (eg, epinephrine or phenylephrine) is added to the anesthetic agent to decrease its systemic absorption and to maintain its concentration at the surgical or injury site.

A topical anesthetic agent EMLA (eutectic mixture or emulsion of local anesthetics) cream has been effective for preventing pain associated with invasive procedures such as lumbar puncture or the insertion of IV lines. To be effective, EMLA must be applied to the site 60 to 90 minutes before the procedure.

INTRASPINAL ADMINISTRATION

Intermittent or continuous administration of local anesthetics through an epidural or spinal catheter has been used for years to produce anesthesia during surgery. Although the administration of local anesthetics in the spinal canal is still largely confined to acute pain, such as postoperative pain and pain associated with labor and delivery, the epidural administration of local anesthetics for pain management is increasing.

A local anesthetic administered through an epidural catheter is applied directly to the nerve root. The anesthetic can be administered continuously in low doses, intermittently on a schedule, or on demand as the patient requires it, and is often combined with the epidural administration of opioids. Surgical patients treated with this combination experience fewer complications after surgery, ambulate sooner, and have shorter hospital stays than patients receiving standard therapy (Yeager et al., 1987).

Opioid Analgesics

Opioids can be administered by various routes, including oral, IV, SC, intraspinal, rectal, and transdermal routes. The goal of administering opioids is to relieve pain and improve quality of life; therefore, the route of administration, dose, and frequency of administration are determined on an individual basis. Factors that are considered in determining the route, dose, and frequency of medication include characteristics of the pain (ie, its expected duration and severity), the overall status of the patient, the patient's response to analgesics, and his or her report of pain. Although the oral route is usually preferred for administering opioids, oral opioids must be given frequently enough and in large enough doses to be effective. Opioid analgesics given orally may provide a more consistent serum level than those given IM.

If the patient will need opioid analgesics at home, the patient's and the family's ability to administer opioids as prescribed is considered in planning. Steps are taken to ensure that the medication will be available to the patient. Many pharmacies, especially those in smaller rural areas or inner cities, may be reluctant to stock large amounts of opioids. Therefore, arrangements for obtaining these prescription medications must be made ahead of time.

With the administration of opioids by any route, side effects must be considered and anticipated. Anticipating and taking steps to minimize side effects increases the likelihood that the patient will receive adequate pain relief without interrupting therapy to treat these effects.

SIDE EFFECTS OF OPIOIDS

Respiratory Depression and Sedation. Respiratory depression is the most serious adverse effect of opioid analgesics administered by IV, SC, or epidural routes. However, it is relatively rare because doses administered through these routes are small, and tolerance increases if the dose is increased slowly. The risk of respiratory depression increases with age and the concomitant use of other opioids or other central nervous system depressants. The risk of respiratory depression also increases when the catheter is placed in the thoracic area and when the intra-abdominal or intrathoracic pressure is increased.

The patient receiving opioids by any route must be assessed frequently for changes in respiratory status. Specific notable changes are decreasing respiratory rate or shallow respirations. Despite the risks associated with their use, IV and epidural opioids are considered safe, with the risks related to epidural administration no greater than those related to IV or other systemic routes of administration. Sedation, which may occur with any method of administering opioids, is likely to occur when opioid doses are increased. However, the patient often develops tolerance quickly, so that in a short time the patient is no longer sedated by the dose that initially caused sedation. Increasing the time between doses or reducing the dose temporarily, as prescribed, usually prevents deep sedation from occurring. The patient at risk for sedation must be monitored closely for changes in respiratory status. The patient is also at risk for other problems associated with sedation and immobility. Therefore, the nurse must initiate strategies to prevent problems such as skin breakdown.

Nausea and Vomiting. Nausea and vomiting frequently occur with opioid use. Usually these effects occur some hours after the initial injection. Patients, especially postoperative patients, may not think to tell the nurse that they are nauseated, particularly if the nausea is mild. However, the patient receiving an opioid should be assessed for nausea and vomiting, which may be triggered by a position change and may be prevented by having the patient change positions very slowly. Adequate hydration and the administration of antiemetic agents may decrease the incidence. Opioid-induced nausea and vomiting often subside within a few days.

Constipation. Constipation, a common side effect of opioid use, may become so severe that the patient is forced to choose between relief of pain and relief of constipation. This situation can occur after surgery and in patients receiving large doses of opioids to treat cancer-related pain. Preventing constipation must be a high priority in all patients receiving opioids. Tolerance to this side effect does not occur; rather, it persists even with long-term use of opioids.

Several strategies may help prevent and treat opioid-related constipation. Mild laxatives and a high intake of fluid and fiber may be effective in managing mild constipation. Unless contraindicated, a mild laxative and a stool softener should be administered on a regular schedule. Continued severe constipation, however, often requires the use of a stimulating cathartic agent, such as senna derivatives (Senokot) or bisacodyl (Dulcolax). Oral laxatives and stool softeners may prevent constipation; rectal suppositories may be used if oral agents fail (Agency for Health Care Policy & Research, 1994).

Inadequate Pain Relief. One factor commonly associated with ineffective pain relief is an inadequate dose of opioid. This is most likely to occur when the caregiver underestimates the patient's pain, or the route of administration is changed without the differences in absorption and action being considered. Consequently, the patient receives doses too small to be effective and, possibly, too infrequently to relieve pain. For example, if opioid delivery is changed from the IV route to the oral route, the oral dose must be approximately three times greater than that given parenterally to provide relief. Because of differences in absorption of orally ingested opioids among individuals, the patient must be assessed carefully to ensure that the pain is relieved.

Table 12-1 lists opioids and dosages that are equivalent to morphine. In general, no recalculation needs to be done when switching from one brand of an agent to another brand of the same medication, with the exception of extended-release oral morphine. Currently, three brands of extended-release morphine (MSContin, Oramorph, and Kadian) are commonly used by cancer patients. Although these agents come in the same dosage form and contain the same drug, they are not considered therapeutically equivalent because they employ different release mechanisms. Patients who need to switch brands should be monitored carefully both for overdose and for inadequate pain relief.

Other Effects of Opioids. During the health history, when asked about drug allergies, patients with previous hospital experience (especially for surgery) may report that they are "allergic" to morphine. This report should be thoroughly investigated. Commonly, this "allergy" will be described as itching only. Pruritus (itching) is a frequent problem associated with opioids administered through any route, but it is not an allergic reaction. Itching can be relieved by administering antihistamines. Epidurally administered opioids may also cause urinary retention or pruritus. The patient should be monitored and may require urinary catheterization. Small doses of naloxone may be prescribed to relieve these problems in patients who are receiving epidural opioids for the relief of acute postoperative pain.

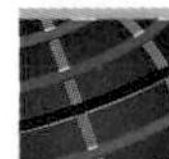

TABLE 12•1 Dosage Guidelines* for Equianalgesic Doses of Analgesics Equivalent to 10 mg of IM Morphine

Medication	Dose Equivalent to 10 mg of Morphine		Usual Starting Dose for Moderate to Severe Pain	
	PARENTERAL ROUTE	ORAL ROUTE	PARENTERAL ROUTE	ORAL ROUTE
Opioid Agonists				
morphine	10 mg	30 mg	10 mg q 3–4 h	30 mg q 3–4 h
codeine	75–130 mg	130–200 mg (NR)	60 mg q 2 h	60 mg q 3–4 h (IM or SC)
fentanyl	100 µg			
hydromorphone (Dilaudid)	1.5–2 mg	4–7.5 mg	1.5 mg q 3–4 h	6 mg q 3–4 h
meperidine (Demerol)	75–100 mg	300 mg (NR)	100 mg q 3 h	NR
hydrocodone (in Lorcet, Lortab, Vicodin, others)	NA	30 mg	NA	10 mg q 3–4 h
levorphanol (Levo-Dromoran)	2 mg	4 mg	2 mg q 6–8 h	4 mg q 6–8 h
methadone (Dolophine)	10 mg	20 mg	10 mg q 6–8 h	20 mg q 6–8 h
oxycodone (Percocet, Percodan, Tylox)	NA	30 mg	NA	10 mg q 3–4 h
oxymorphone (Numorphan)	1 mg	NA	1 mg q 3–4 h	NA
Opioid Agonist–Antagonist and Partial Agonist				
buprenorphine (Buprenex)	0.3–0.4 mg	NA	0.4 mg q 6–8 h	NA
butorphanol (Stadol)	2 mg	NA	2 mg q 3–4 h	NA
nalbuphine (Nubain)	10 mg	NA	10 mg q 3–4 h	NA
pentazocine (Talwin)	60 mg	150 mg	NR	50 mg q 4–6 h

* These are approximate and to be used only as a guideline. All doses must be based on individual patient's response.
NA = not available, NR = not recommended

Adapted from Agency for Health Care Policy and Research. (1994). *Acute pain management: Operative or medical procedures and trauma.* Clinical Practice Guideline, U.S. Department of Health and Human Services, and Agency for Health Care Policy and Research. (1992). *Management of Cancer Pain.* Clinical Practice Guideline, U.S. Department of Health and Human Services.

A number of factors may influence the safety and effectiveness of opioid administration. Opioid analgesics are primarily metabolized by the liver and excreted by the kidney. Therefore, metabolism and excretion of analgesic medications will be impaired in patients with liver or kidney disease, increasing the risk of cumulative or toxic effects. In addition, normeperidine, a metabolite of meperidine, may rapidly or unexpectedly accumulate to toxic levels. This is more likely to occur in patients with impaired kidney function. This accumulation may result in seizures in susceptible patients.

Patients with untreated hypothyroidism are more susceptible to the analgesic effects and side effects of opioids. In contrast, patients with hyperthyroidism may require larger doses for pain relief. Patients with a decreased respiratory reserve from disease or aging may be more susceptible to the depressant effects of opioids and must be carefully monitored for respiratory depression.

Dehydrated patients are at increased risk for the hypotensive effects of opioids. Patients who become hypotensive after the administration of an opioid should be kept recumbent and rehydrated unless fluids are contraindicated. Patients who are dehydrated are also more likely to experience nausea and vomiting with opioid use. Rehydration usually relieves these symptoms.

Patients receiving certain other medications, such as monoamine oxidase inhibitors, phenothiazines, or tricyclic antidepressants, may have an exaggerated response to the depressant effects of opioids. Patients taking these medications should receive small doses of opioids and must be monitored closely. Continued pain in these patients indicates that a therapeutic level of the analgesic has not been achieved. The patient must be monitored for sedation even if an analgesic effect has not been obtained.

Tolerance and Addiction. There is no maximal safe dosage of opioids, nor is there any easily identifiable therapeutic serum level. Both the maximal safe dosage and therapeutic serum level are relative and individual. **Tolerance** (the need for increasing doses of opioids to achieve the same therapeutic effect) will develop in almost all patients taking opioids over an extended period. Patients requiring opioids over a long term, especially cancer patients, will need increasing doses to relieve pain. After the first few weeks of therapy, the patient's dosing requirements usually level off. Patients who become tolerant to the analgesic effects of large doses of morphine may obtain pain relief by switching to a different opioid. Symptoms of physical **dependence** may occur when the opioids are discontinued; dependence often occurs with opioid tolerance and does not indicate an addiction.

Nursing Alert *Although patients may need increasing levels of opioids, they are not addicted. Physical tolerance usually occurs in the absence of addiction. Tolerance to opioids is common and becomes a problem primarily in terms of delivering or administering the medication (eg, how to administer thousands of milligrams of morphine a day to a patient). On the other hand, addiction is rare and should never be the primary concern of the nurse caring for a patient in pain.*

Addiction is a behavioral pattern of substance use characterized by a compulsion to take the drug primarily to experience its psychic effects. Fear of patients becoming addicted or dependent on opioids has contributed to inadequate treatment of pain. This fear is commonly expressed by health care providers as well as patients and results from lack of knowledge about the low risk of addiction.

In an often-cited classic study of more than 11,000 patients receiving opioids for a medical indication, only four patients without a history of substance abuse could be identified as becoming addicted (Porter & Jick, 1980). Addiction following therapeutic opioid administration is so negligible that it should not be a consideration when caring for the patient in pain. Thus, patients and health care providers should be dissuaded from withholding pain medication because of concerns about addiction.

Nonsteroidal Anti-Inflammatory Drugs

NSAIDs are thought to decrease pain by inhibiting the production of prostaglandin from traumatized or inflamed tissues, thereby preventing pain receptors from becoming sensitive to previously non-noxious stimuli. In addition to the anti-prostaglandin activity of NSAIDs, these agents may also have a central action.

Aspirin is the oldest NSAID. However, because it causes frequent and severe side effects, aspirin is infrequently used to treat significant acute or chronic pain. Ibuprofen (Advil, Motrin), another NSAID, is effective in relieving mild to moderate pain and has a low incidence of adverse effects.

NSAIDs are very helpful in the treatment of arthritic diseases and may be especially powerful in treating cancer-related bone pain. NSAIDs have been effectively combined with opioids to treat postoperative and other severe pain. The use of an NSAID with an opioid relieves pain more effectively than the opioid alone. In such cases, the patient may obtain pain relief with less opioid and fewer side effects. Repeated studies show that intraoperative administration of NSAIDs results in improved postoperative pain control and in some cases shorter hospital stays (McLaughlin, 1994).

A regimen of a fixed-dose, time-contingent NSAID (eg, every 4 hours) and a separately administered fluctuating dose of opioid may work very well in managing moderate to severe cancer pain. In more severe pain, the opioid dose will also be fixed, with an additional fluctuating dose as needed for **breakthrough pain** (a sudden pain increase despite administration of pain-relieving medications). These regimens result in better pain relief with fewer opioid-related side effects.

NSAIDs are well tolerated by most patients. However, those with impaired kidney function may require a smaller dose and must be monitored closely for side effects. Patients taking NSAIDs bruise easily because NSAIDs have some anticoagulant effect. Moreover, they may displace other medications, such as warfarin (Coumadin), from serum proteins and increase their effects. High doses or prolonged use can irritate the stomach and in some cases result in GI bleeding as well. Thus, monitoring the patient for GI bleeding is indicated.

Gerontologic Considerations

Physiologic changes in older adults require that analgesics be administered with caution. Drug interactions are more likely to occur in older adults because of the higher incidence of chronic illness and the increased use of prescription and over-the-counter medications. Although the elderly population is an extremely heterogeneous group, differences in response to pain or medications by a patient in this 40-year span (60 to 100 years) are more likely to be due to chronic illness or other individual factors than age. Before administering opioid and nonopioid analgesics to elderly patients, the nurse needs to obtain a careful medication history to identify potential drug interactions.

Absorption and metabolism of medications are altered in elderly patients because of decreased liver, renal, and GI function. In addition, changes in body weight, protein stores, and distribution of body fluid alter the distribution of medications in the body. As a result, medications are not metabolized as quickly and blood levels of the medication remain higher for a longer period. Elderly patients are more sensitive to medications and at an increased risk for drug toxicity (A.G.S. Panel on Chronic Pain in Older Persons, 1998).

Opioid and nonopioid analgesics can be given effectively to elderly patients but must be used cautiously because of increased susceptibility to depression of both the nervous and the respiratory systems. Although there is no reason to avoid opioids simply because a person is elderly, meperidine should be avoided because its active and neurotoxic metabolite, normeperidine, is more likely to accumulate in the elderly. In addition, because of decreased binding of meperidine by plasma proteins, blood concentrations of the medication twice those found in younger patients may result.

In many cases, the initial dose of analgesic medication prescribed for an elderly patient may be the same as that for a younger person or slightly smaller than the normal dose, but because of slowed metabolism and excretion related to aging, the safe interval for subsequent doses may be longer (or prolonged). As always, the best guide to pain management and administration of analgesics in all patients regardless of age is what the patient says. The elderly patient may obtain more pain relief for a longer time than a younger patient. As a result, smaller, less frequent doses may be required. The American Geriatrics Society (1998) has published clinical practice guidelines for managing chronic pain in elderly patients.

Tricyclic Antidepressants and Anticonvulsants

Pain of neurologic origin (eg, causalgia, tumor impingement on a nerve, postherpetic neuralgia) is difficult to treat and in general not responsive to opioid therapy. When these pain syndromes are accompanied by dysesthesia (burning or cutting pain), they may be responsive to a tricyclic antidepressant or an anticonvulsant agent. When indicated, tricyclic antidepressants, such as amitriptyline (Elavil) or imipramine (Tofranil), are prescribed in doses considerably smaller than those generally used for depression. The patient needs to know that a therapeutic effect may not occur before 3 weeks. Anticonvulsant medications, such as phenytoin (Dilantin) or carbamazepine (Tegretol), also are used in doses lower than those prescribed for seizure disorders. Because a variety of medications can be tried, the nurse should be familiar with the possible side effects and teach the patient and family how to recognize these effects.

Routes of Administration

The route selected for administering an analgesic (Table 12-2) depends on the patient's condition and the desired effect of the medication. Analgesics can be administered parenterally, transmucosally, gastrointestinally, transdermally, epidurally, or intraspinally. Each method of administration has advantages and disadvantages. The route selection should be based on the patient's needs.

PARENTERAL

Parenteral administration (IM, IV, or SC) of the analgesic produces effects more rapidly than oral administration, but these effects are of shorter duration. Parenteral administration may be indicated if the patient is not permitted oral intake or is vomiting.

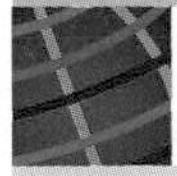

TABLE 12•2 Routes of Administration of Analgesics

Route	Site
parenteral	intramuscular (IM)
	intravenous (IV)
	subcutaneous (SC)
gastrointestinal	oral (PO)
	rectal (PR)
transdermal	skin
transmucosal	oral mucosa
	bronchial mucosa
epidural	epidural space
intraspinal	spinal canal

Medication administered IM enters the bloodstream more slowly than medication administered IV, and is metabolized slowly. The rate of absorption may be erratic and depends on the site selected and the amount of body fat.

The IV route is an alternative to IM injection for many but not all analgesics. The IV route is the preferred parenteral route in most acute care situations because it is much more comfortable for the patient. In addition, peak serum levels and pain relief occur more rapidly and reliably. Because it peaks rapidly (usually within minutes) and is metabolized quickly, an appropriate IV dose will be smaller and prescribed at shorter intervals than an IM dose.

IV opioids may be administered by IV push or slow push (eg, over a 5- to 10-minute period) or by continuous infusion with a pump. Continuous infusion provides a steady level of analgesia and is indicated when pain occurs over a 24-hour period (eg, after surgery for the first day or so, or in a patient with prolonged cancer pain who cannot take medication by other routes). The dose of analgesic is calculated carefully to relieve pain without producing respiratory depression and other side effects.

The SC route for infusion of opioid analgesics is used for patients with severe pain such as cancer pain; it is particularly useful for patients with limited IV access who cannot take oral medications, and patients who are managing their pain at home. The dose of opioid that can be infused through this route is limited because of the small volume that can be administered at one time into the subcutaneous tissue. However, this route is often an effective and convenient way to manage pain.

ORAL ROUTE

If the patient can take medication by mouth, oral administration is preferred over parenteral administration because it is easy, noninvasive, and not painful. Severe pain can be relieved with oral opioids if the doses are high enough (see Table 12-1).

In terminally ill patients with prolonged pain, doses may gradually be increased as the disease progresses and causes more pain or as the person builds up a tolerance to the medication. If these higher doses are increased gradually, they usually provide additional pain relief without producing respiratory depression or sedation. If the route of administration is changed from a parenteral route to the oral route at a dose that is not equivalent in strength (equianalgesic), the smaller oral dose may result in a withdrawal reaction and recurrence of pain.

RECTAL ROUTE

The rectal route of administration may be indicated in patients who cannot take medications by any other route. The rectal route may also be indicated for patients with bleeding problems, such as hemophilia. The onset of action of opioids administered rectally is unclear but is more delayed than with other routes of administration. Similarly, the duration of action is prolonged.

TRANSDERMAL ROUTE

The transdermal route has been used to achieve a consistent opioid serum level through absorption of the medication via the skin. This route is most often used for cancer patients who are at home or in hospice care and who have been receiving oral sustained-release morphine (SRM). Fentanyl is the only commercially available transdermal medication (Duragesic). The preparation is a patch consisting of a reservoir containing the medication and a membrane.

When the transdermal system is first applied to the skin, the fentanyl, which is fat-soluble, binds to the skin and fat layers. Then it is slowly and systemically absorbed. Therefore, there will be a delay in effect while the dermal layer is being saturated. A drug reservoir actually forms in the upper layer of skin. This results in a slowly rising serum level and a slow tapering of the serum level once the patch is removed (see Fig. 12-6). Because it takes 8 to 12 hours for the fentanyl levels to peak from the first patch, the last dose of SRM should be given at the same time the first patch is applied (Donner et al., 1996). Transdermal fentanyl is associated with slightly less constipation than oral opioids. Absorption is increased in the febrile patient. A heating pad should never be applied to the area where the patch is applied. Transdermal fentanyl is much more expensive than SRM but less costly than methods that deliver parenteral opioids.

Once it is determined that switching from other routes of morphine administration to the patch is appropriate, calculating the correct dosage for the patch is necessary. If the patient uses an opioid other than morphine, conversion to milligrams of oral morphine is the first step. After determining how many milligrams of morphine (or morphine equivalents) the patient has been using over 24 hours, an initial dose of transdermal fentanyl can be calculated.

Pasero (1997) suggests one method of calculating the initial dose of fentanyl: the patient's daily dose of morphine is divided by two. Thus, the equivalent of 400 mg of morphine used per day would be equivalent to 200 μg of fentanyl per hour. Patients switched from morphine from fentanyl need to be assessed not only for pain and potential side effects but also for dependence, reflected by withdrawal symptoms, which may consist of shivering, a feeling of coldness, sweating, headache, and paresthesia (Puntillo et al., 1997).

These conversions and the conversion-type table in the transdermal fentanyl (Duragesic) packet insert should be used only to establish the initial dose of fentanyl when the patient is switched from oral morphine to fentanyl (and not vice versa). These tables and equations are not meant to be used to determine the dosages of oral morphine for a patient who has been receiving transdermal fentanyl. Many patients will not achieve satisfactory analgesia from the initial dose of transdermal fentanyl and will require an increase in their fentanyl dose to treat breakthrough pain. If the table or equation is used incorrectly to calculate a morphine dose, there is a very real risk of overdose. If the patient requires a change from transdermal fentanyl back to oral or IV morphine (as in the case of surgery), the patch should be removed and IV morphine supplied on an assessed need basis.

Before applying a new patch, the patient should be carefully checked for any older, forgotten patches. These should be discarded. Patches should be replaced every 72 hours.

TRANSMUCOSAL ROUTE

The person with cancer pain who is being cared for at home may be receiving continuous opioids using SRM, hydromorphone, oxycodone, transdermal fentanyl, or other medications. These patients often experience short episodes of severe pain (eg, after coughing or moving), or they may experience sudden increases in their baseline pain resulting from a change in their condition. These periods, called breakthrough pain, can be well managed with a rapid onset but short-acting transmucosal opioid taken by mouth. Currently the only transmucosal opioid available is fentanyl, a lozenge on an applicator stick (often referred to as a lollipop by patients).

Currently the only approved and commercially available transmucosal opioid analgesic in a nasal spray form is butorphanol, a mixed opioid agonist–antagonist. This is a complex medication that simultaneously acts to induce or promote (**agonist**) and inhibit or reverse (**antagonist**) opioid effects. It works like an opioid agonist and an opioid antagonist at the same time. Butorphanol in any form cannot be combined with other opioids (eg, for cancer breakthrough pain) because the antagonist component will block the action of the opioids the patient is already receiving. The principal use of this agent is for brief, moderate to severe pain, such as migraine headaches.

INTRASPINAL AND EPIDURAL ROUTES

Infusion of opioids or local anesthetic agents into the subarachnoid space (intrathecal space or spinal canal) or epidural space has effectively controlled pain in postoperative patients and those with chronic pain unrelieved by other methods.

A catheter is inserted into the subarachnoid or the epidural space at the thoracic or lumbar level for administration of opioid or anesthetic agents (Fig. 12-7). With intrathecal administration, the medication infuses directly into the subarachnoid space and cerebrospinal fluid, which surrounds the spinal cord. With epidural administration, medication is deposited in the dura of the spinal canal and diffuses into the subarachnoid space. It is believed that pain relief from intraspinal administration of opioids is based on the existence of opioid receptors in the spinal cord.

Infusion of opioids and local anesthetics through an intrathecal or epidural catheter results in pain relief with fewer side effects—including sedation—than with systemic analgesia. Adverse effects associated with intraspinal administration include spinal headache resulting from loss of spinal fluid when the dura is punctured. This is more likely to occur in younger (less than 40 years of age) patients. The dura must be punctured with the intrathecal route, and dural puncture may occur inadvertently with the epidural route. When dural puncture inadvertently occurs, spinal fluid seeps out of the spinal canal. The resultant headache is likely to be more severe with an epidural needle because it is larger than a spinal needle, and therefore more spinal fluid escapes.

Although respiratory depression generally peaks 6 to 12 hours after epidural opioids are administered, it can occur earlier or up to 24 hours after the first injection. Therefore, the patient is monitored very closely for at least the first 24 hours after the first injection, longer if changes in respiratory status or level of consciousness occur. Opioid antagonists such as naloxone must be available to reverse respiratory depression if it occurs.

The patient is also observed for urinary retention, pruritus, nausea, vomiting, and dizziness. Precautions must be taken to minimize the risk of infection at the catheter site and catheter displacement. Only medications without preservatives should be administered into the subarachnoid or epidural space because of potential neurotoxic effects of preservatives.

During surgery, intrathecal opioids are used almost exclusively after a spinal anesthetic is administered. For patients undergoing large abdominal surgical procedures, especially those at risk for postoperative complications, a combination of a general inhaled anesthetic agent for the surgery and a local epidural anesthetic and epidural opioids administered after surgery results in excellent pain control with fewer postoperative complications.

Patients who have persistent, severe pain that fails to respond to other treatments, or those who obtain pain relief only with the risk of serious side effects, may benefit from medication administered by a long-term intrathecal or epidural catheter. After the physician tunnels the catheter through the subcutaneous tissue and places the inlet (or port) under the skin, the medication is injected through the skin into the inlet and catheter, which delivers the medication directly into the epidural space. The medication may need to be injected several times a day to maintain an adequate level of pain relief.

In patients who require more frequent doses or continuous infusions of opioid analgesics to relieve pain, an implantable infusion device or pump may be used to administer the medication continuously. The medication is administered at a small, con-

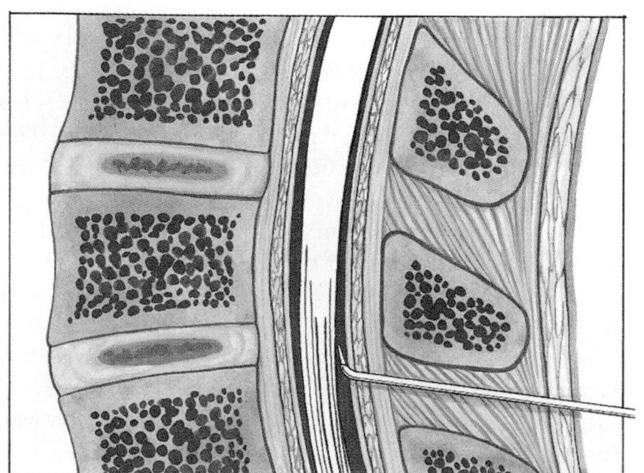

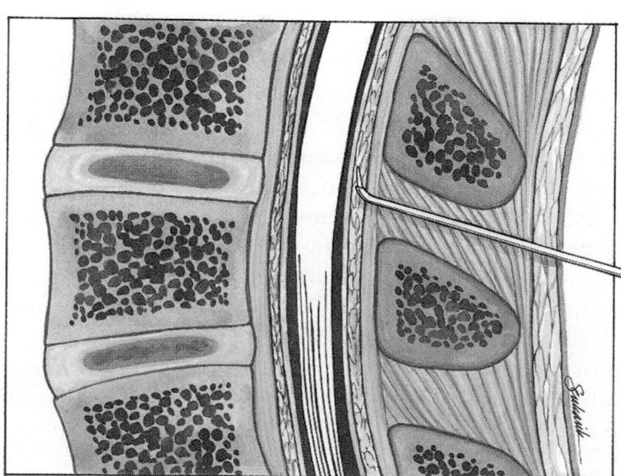

FIGURE 12•7 Placement of intraspinal catheters for administration of analgesic medications: (**A**) intrathecal route, (**B**) epidural route.

stant dose at a preset rate into the epidural or subarachnoid space. The reservoir of the infusion device stores the medication for slow release and needs to be refilled every 1 or 2 months, depending on the patient's needs. This eliminates the need for repeated injections through the skin.

Nursing Alert *An epidural catheter inserted for pain control is usually managed by the nurse. Baseline information necessary to provide safe and effective pain control includes the level or site of catheter insertion, the medications (eg, local anesthetics or opioids) that have been administered, and the medications anticipated in the future.*

Nursing Management of Side Effects. Headache resulting from spinal fluid loss may be delayed. Therefore, the nurse needs to assess for headache regularly after either type of catheter is placed. Should headache occur, the patient should remain flat in bed and should be given large amounts of fluids (provided the medical condition allows), and the physician should be notified.

Cardiovascular effects (hypotension and decreased heart rate) may result from relaxation of the vasculature in the lower extremities. Therefore, the nurse assesses frequently for decreases in blood pressure, pulse rate, and urine output.

For patients experiencing urinary retention and pruritus, the physician may prescribe small doses of naloxone. The nurse administers these doses in a continuous infusion that is small enough to reverse the side effects of the opioids without reversing the analgesic effects. Diphenhydramine (Benadryl) may also be used to relieve opioid-related pruritus.

Promoting Home and Community-Based Care. The patient who receives epidural analgesics at home and the family must be taught how to administer the prescribed medication using sterile technique and how to assess for infection. The patient and family also need to learn how to recognize side effects and what to do about them. Although respiratory depression is uncommon, urinary retention may be a problem, and patients and families must be prepared to deal with it if it occurs. Implanted analgesic delivery systems can be safely and confidently used at home only if health care personnel are available for consultation and, possibly, intervention on short notice.

Nonpharmacologic Interventions

Although pain medication is the most powerful pain relief tool available to nurses, it is not the only tool. Nonpharmacologic nursing activities can assist in relieving pain with usually low risk to the patient. Although such measures are not a substitute for medication, they may be all that is necessary or appropriate to relieve episodes of pain lasting only seconds or minutes. In instances of severe pain that lasts for hours or days, combining nonpharmacologic interventions with medications may be the most effective way to relieve pain.

Cutaneous Stimulation and Massage

The gate control theory of pain proposes that the stimulation of fibers that transmit nonpainful sensations can block or decrease the transmission of pain impulses. Several nonpharmacologic pain relief strategies, including rubbing the skin and using heat and cold, are based on this theory.

Massage, which is generalized cutaneous stimulation of the body, often concentrates on the back and shoulders. A massage does not specifically stimulate the nonpain receptors in the same receptor field as the pain receptors, but it may have an impact through the descending control system (see earlier discussion). Massage also promotes comfort because it produces muscle relaxation.

Ice and Heat Therapies

Ice and heat therapies may be effective pain relief strategies in some circumstances; however, their effectiveness and mechanism of action need further study. Proponents believe that ice and heat stimulate the nonpain receptors in the same receptor field as the injury.

For greatest effect, ice should be placed on the injury site immediately after injury or surgery. Ice therapy after joint surgery can significantly reduce the amount of analgesic medication required subsequently. Ice therapy may also relieve pain if applied later. Care must be taken to protect the skin from direct application of the ice. Ice should be applied to an area for no longer than 20 minutes at a time. Any longer may result in frostbite or nerve injury. Both ice and heat therapy must be applied carefully and monitored closely to avoid injuring the skin. Neither therapy should be applied to areas with impaired circulation.

Application of heat increases blood flow to an area and contributes to pain reduction by speeding healing. Both dry and moist heat may provide some analgesia, but their mechanisms of action are not well understood. Application of heat to inflamed joints, for example, may provide temporary comfort, but increasing the intra-articular temperature may impair healing (Oosterveld & Rasker, 1994a; 1994b).

Transcutaneous Electrical Nerve Stimulation

Transcutaneous electrical nerve stimulation (TENS) uses a battery-operated unit with electrodes applied to the skin to produce a tingling, vibrating, or buzzing sensation in the area of pain. It has been used in both acute and chronic pain relief. TENS is believed to decrease pain by stimulating the nonpain receptors in the same area as the fibers that transmit the pain. This mechanism is consistent with the gate control theory of pain and explains the effectiveness of cutaneous stimulation when applied in the same area as an injury. For example, when TENS is used in a postoperative patient, the electrodes are placed around the surgical wound.

Another possible explanation for the effectiveness of TENS is the placebo effect (the patient expects it to be effective). In a recent review of the literature, Carroll et al. (1996) found that in 15 of 17 studies with randomized control group designs, TENS was ineffective in relieving postoperative pain. In 17 of 19 studies that did not use this design, the authors of these studies concluded that TENS had a positive analgesic effect. The review of these studies suggests that a placebo effect may explain the effectiveness of TENS.

Distraction

Distraction helps relieve both acute and chronic pain (Johnson & Petrie, 1997). Distraction, which involves focusing the patient's attention on something other than the pain, may be the mechanism responsible for other effective cognitive techniques. Distraction is thought to reduce the perception of pain by stimulating the descending control system, resulting in fewer painful stimuli being transmitted to the brain. The effectiveness of distraction depends on the patient's ability to receive and create sensory input other than pain. Distraction techniques may range from simple activities, such as watching TV or listening to music, to highly complex physical and mental exercises. Pain relief generally increases in direct proportion to the person's active participation, the number of sensory modalities used, and the person's interest in the stimuli. Therefore, the stimulation of sight, sound, and touch is likely to be more effective in reducing pain than is the stimulation of a single sense.

Visits from family and friends are very effective in relieving pain. Watching an action-packed movie on a large screen with "SurroundSound" through headphones may be effective (provided the person finds it acceptable). Others may benefit from games and activities (eg, chess) that require concentration. Not all patients obtain pain relief with distraction, especially those in severe pain. With severe pain, the patient may be unable to concentrate well enough to participate in complex physical or mental activities.

Relaxation Techniques

Skeletal muscle relaxation is believed to reduce pain by relaxing tense muscles that contribute to the pain. Considerable evidence supports relaxation as effective in relieving chronic low back pain (NIH Technology Assessment Panel, 1996). Few studies, however, support its effectiveness in reducing postoperative pain. This may be due to the relatively small role skeletal muscles play in postoperative pain, or to the need for the patient to practice the relaxation technique for it to be effective. Practicing the technique may not be possible when it is taught only once, immediately before surgery. A patient who already knows a technique for relaxing may only need to be reminded to use it to reduce or prevent increased pain.

A simple relaxation technique consists of abdominal breathing at a slow, rhythmic rate. The patient may close the eyes and breathe slowly and comfortably. A constant rhythm can be maintained by counting silently and slowly with each inhalation ("in, two, three") and exhalation ("out, two, three"). When teaching this technique, the nurse may count out loud with the patient at first. Slow, rhythmic breathing may also be used as a distraction technique. Relaxation techniques, as well as other noninvasive pain relief measures, may require practice before the patient becomes skillful in using them.

Almost all people with chronic pain can benefit from some method of relaxation. Regular relaxation periods may help to combat the fatigue and muscle tension that occur with and increase chronic pain.

Guided Imagery

Guided imagery is using one's imagination in a special way to achieve a specific positive effect. Guided imagery for relaxation and pain relief may consist of combining slow, rhythmic breathing with a mental image of relaxation and comfort. The nurse instructs the patient to close the eyes and breathe slowly in and slowly out. With each slowly exhaled breath, the patient imagines muscle tension and discomfort being breathed out, carrying away pain and tension and leaving behind a relaxed and comfortable body. With each inhaled breath, the patient imagines healing energy flowing to the area of discomfort.

If guided imagery is to be effective, it requires a considerable amount of time to explain the technique and time for the patient to practice it. Usually, the patient is asked to practice guided imagery for about 5 minutes, three times a day. Several days of practice may be needed before the intensity of pain is reduced. Many patients begin to experience the relaxing effects of guided imagery the first time they try it. Pain relief can continue for hours after the imagery is used. The patient needs to be informed that guided imagery may work only for some people. Guided imagery should be used only in combination with all other forms of treatment that have demonstrated effectiveness.

Hypnosis

Hypnosis, which has been effective in relieving pain or decreasing the amount of analgesics required in patients with acute and chronic pain, may promote pain relief in particularly difficult situations (eg, burns). The mechanism by which hypnosis acts is unclear, but it does not appear to be mediated by the endorphin system (Moret et al., 1991). The effectiveness of hypnosis depends on the hypnotic susceptibility of the individual (Farthing et al., 1997). In some cases, hypnosis may be effective on the first session, with effectiveness increasing in additional sessions. In other cases it does not work at all. Usually, hypnosis must be induced by a specially skilled person (a psychologist or a nurse with specialized training in hypnosis). Sometimes patients learn to perform self-hypnosis.

Neurosurgical Methods

Several neurosurgical approaches have been used with qualified success in a few patients whose pain is debilitating and cannot be relieved or controlled with medications or other nonsurgical approaches. Neurolytic procedures—destructive nerve blocks—have limited usefulness because the loss of sensory components is usually accompanied by the loss of motor and sympathetic functions to the involved area as well. These procedures are discussed in Chapter 59.

Untested, Unproven Therapies

People suffering chronic, debilitating pain are often desperate. Often they will try anything, recommended by anyone, at any price. Information about an array of potential therapies can be found on the Internet and in the self-help section of the bookstore. Therapies specifically recommended for pain from these sources include but are not limited to chelation, therapeutic touch, music therapy, herbal therapy, reflexology, magnetic therapy, electrotherapy, polarity therapy, acupressure, emu oil, pectin therapy, aromatherapy, homeopathy, and macrobiotic dieting. Many of these "therapies" (with the exception of macrobiotic dieting) are probably not harmful. However, they have yet to be proven effective by the standards used to evaluate the effectiveness of medical and nursing interventions. The National Institutes of Health has established an office to examine the effectiveness of alternative therapies.

Despite this, a patient may find any one of these therapies helpful via the placebo response. It is important when caring for a patient who is using or considering using untested therapies (often referred to as alternative therapies) not to diminish the patient's hope and potential placebo response. This must be weighed against the professional nurse's responsibility to protect the patient from costly and potentially dangerous therapies that the patient is not in a position to evaluate scientifically.

Problems arise when patients do not find relief but are deprived of conventional therapy because the alternative therapy "should be helping," or when patients abandon conventional therapy for alternative therapy. In addition, few alternative therapies are free. Desperate patients may risk financial ruin seeking alternative therapies that do not work.

The nurse's role is to help the patient and family understand scientific research and how that differs from anecdotal evidence. Although not diminishing the placebo effects the patient may receive, the nurse encourages the patient to assess the effectiveness of the therapy continually using standard pain assessment techniques. In addition, the nurse encourages the patient using alternative therapies to combine them with conventional therapies and to discuss this use with the physician.

Promoting Home and Community-Based Care

Teaching Patients Self-Care

In preparing for pain management at home, the patient and family need to be taught and guided about what type of pain or discomfort to expect, how long the pain is expected to last, and when the pain indicates a problem that should be reported. The person who has experienced acute pain as a result of injury, illness, procedures, or surgery will probably receive one or more

PATIENT EDUCATION AND HOME CARE
Pain Management Plan

Pain control plan for

____

At home, I will take the following medicines for pain control:

Medicine	How to take	How many	How often	Comments

Medicines that you may take to help treat side effects:

Side effect	Medicine	How to take	How many	How often	Comments

Constipation is a very common problem when taking opioid medications. When this occurs, do the following:

- Increase fluid intake (8 to 10 glasses of fluid).
- Exercise regularly.
- Increase fiber in the diet (bran, fresh fruits, vegetables).
- Use a mild laxative, such as milk of magnesia, if no bowel movement in 3 days.
- Take ______________ every day at ______________ (time) with a full glass of water.
- Use a glycerin suppository every morning (this may help make a bowel movement less painful).

Nondrug pain control methods:

____

____

Additional instructions:

____

____

____

Important phone numbers:

Your doctor ______________________ Your nurse ______________________

Your pharmacy ______________________ Emergencies ______________________

Call your doctor or nurse immediately if your pain increases or if you have a new pain. Also call your doctor early for refill of pain medicines. Do not let your medicines get below 3 or 4 days' supply.

Agency for Health Care Policy and Research. (1994). *Management of Cancer Pain.* Clinical Practice Guidelines. Rockville, MD: Agency for Health Care Policy and Research, Public Health Service, U.S. Department of Health and Human Services.

prescriptions for analgesic medication. The patient and family need to understand the purpose of each medication, the appropriate time to use it, the side effects associated with each, and the strategies that can be used to prevent the problems associated with each. The patient and family often need reassurance that pain can be successfully managed at home.

Inadequate control of pain at home is a common reason people seek health care or are readmitted to the hospital. When chronic pain exists, anxiety and fear are multiplied at the time the patient is about to return home. The patient and family are instructed about the techniques for assessing pain, using pain assessment tools, and administering pain medications. These instructions are given verbally and in writing.

Opportunities are provided for the patient and family members to practice administering the medication until they are comfortable and confident with the procedure. They are instructed about the risks of respiratory and central nervous system depression associated with opioid drugs and ways to assess for these complications. If the medications cause other predictable effects, such as constipation, the instructions include measures for preventing and treating the problem, as described earlier. Steps are taken to ensure that required medications are available from the local pharmacy so that the patient receives the medication when required.

Education for patients and families must stress the need for keeping analgesic agents away from children, who might mistake them for candy. Elderly patients may become lax about this because no children live in the home, but visiting children can be placed at risk.

Continuing Care

If the patient is to receive parenteral or intraspinal analgesia at home, a referral to a home care nurse is indicated. The home care nurse makes a home visit to assess the patient and to determine if the pain management program is being implemented and if the technique for injecting or infusing the analgesia is being carried out safely and effectively. If the patient has an implanted infusion pump in place, the nurse examines the condition of the pump or

12•1

PLAN OF NURSING CARE

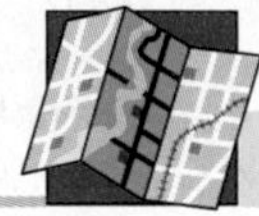

Care of the Patient With Pain

Nursing Interventions	Rationale	Expected Outcomes
Nursing Diagnosis: Pain **Goal:** Relief of pain or decrease in intensity of pain		
1. Reassure patient that you know pain is real and will assist him or her in dealing with it.	1. Fear that pain will not be accepted as real increases tension and anxiety and decreases pain tolerance.	• Reports relief that pain is accepted as real and that he or she will receive assistance in pain relief
2. Use pain assessment scale to identify intensity of pain.	2. Provides baseline for assessing changes in pain level and evaluating interventions	• Reports lower intensity of pain and discomfort after interventions implemented
3. Assess and record pain and its characteristics: location, quality, frequency, and duration.	3. Data assist in evaluating pain and pain relief and identifying multiple sources and types of pain.	• Reports less disruption from pain and discomfort after use of intervention • Uses pain medication as prescribed
4. Administer balanced analgesics as prescribed to promote optimal pain relief.	4. Analgesics are more effective if administered early in pain cycle. Simultaneous use of analgesics that work on different portions of the nociceptive system will provide greater pain relief with fewer side effects.	• Identifies effective pain relief strategies • Demonstrates use of new strategies to relieve pain and reports their effectiveness • Experiences minimal side effects of analgesia without interruption to treat side effects • Increases interactions with family and friends
5. Readminister pain assessment scale.	5. Permits assessment of effectiveness of analgesia and identifies need for further action if ineffective	
6. Document severity of patient's pain on chart.	6. Assists in demonstrating need for additional analgesic or alternative approach to pain management	
7. Seek additional prescriptions as needed.	7. Inadequate pain relief results in an increased stress response, suffering, and prolonged hospitalizations.	
8. Identify and encourage patient to use strategies that have been successful with previous pain.	8. Encourages use of pain relief strategies familiar to and accepted by patient	
9. Teach patient additional strategies to relieve pain and discomfort: distraction, relaxation, cutaneous stimulation.	9. Use of these strategies along with analgesia may produce more effective pain relief.	
10. Instruct patient and family about potential side effects of analgesics and their prevention and management.	10. Anticipating and preventing side effects enable the patient to continue analgesia without interruption because of side effects.	

injection site and may refill the reservoir with medication as prescribed or may supervise family members in the procedure. Any change in the patient's need for analgesic medications is assessed. In collaboration with the physician, the nurse then assists the patient and family in modifying the medication dose. These efforts enable the patient to obtain adequate pain relief while remaining at home and with family.

As tolerance develops, ever-increasing amounts of opioids are needed. It is important to assure the patient and family that slowly increasing doses will not cause an increased risk of respiratory depression and central nervous system depression, because the patient will become tolerant to these effects also. However, the patient will not become tolerant to the constipating effects of opioids and will require increased efforts to prevent constipation.

EVALUATING PAIN MANAGEMENT STRATEGIES

An important aspect of caring for the patient in pain is reassessing the pain after the intervention has been implemented. The measure's effectiveness is based on the patient's assessment of pain, as reflected in pain assessment tools. If the intervention was ineffective, the nurse needs to consider other measures. If these are ineffective, the pain relief goals need to be reassessed in collaboration with the physician. The nurse serves as a patient advocate in obtaining additional pain relief.

After interventions have had a chance to work, the patient is asked to rate the intensity of pain. This assessment is repeated at appropriate intervals after the intervention and compared with the previous rating. These assessments indicate the effectiveness of the pain relief measures and provide a basis for continuing or modifying the plan of care. See the accompanying Plan of Nursing Care for more information.

Expected Outcomes

Expected outcomes may include:

1. Achieves pain relief
   a. Rates pain at a lower intensity (on a scale of 0 to 10) after intervention
   b. Rates pain at a lower intensity for longer periods
2. Patient or family administers prescribed analgesic medications correctly
   a. States correct dose of medication
   b. Administers correct dose using correct procedure
   c. Identifies side effects of medication
   d. Describes actions taken to prevent or correct side effects
3. Uses nonpharmacologic pain strategies as recommended
   a. Reports practice of nonpharmacologic strategies
   b. Describes expected outcome of nonpharmacologic strategies
4. Reports minimal effects of pain and minimal side effects of interventions
   a. Participates in activities important to recovery (eg, drinking fluids, coughing, ambulating)
   b. Participates in activities important to self and to family (eg, family activities, interpersonal relationships, parenting, social interaction, recreation, work)
   c. Reports adequate sleep and absence of fatigue and constipation

Critical Thinking Exercises

1. Your patient has cancer and is nearing the end of his life. He is in severe discomfort, rating his pain as 9 on a visual analogue scale, but he is not receiving the maximum dose of opioids he could potentially receive. On discussing this with his sister, who is caring for him at home, it becomes apparent that she fears he is becoming addicted. She also knows that, in her words, "He is strong enough to take it." Describe the strategies you would use to ensure that your patient receives pain relief.

2. Earlier in your shift, you sent Ms. Jones to surgery for an exploratory laparotomy related to abdominal pain. She returns to the unit 4 hours later with a PCA pump for postoperative pain. The postanesthesia care unit nurse reports that while the patient was in the PACU, she received unusually large doses of an opioid analgesic but was never pain-free. Now she is screaming in pain. When asked the level of her pain, she indicates that it is off the pain scale. The patient's husband is yelling at you to do something. What assessment data would you collect, and what actions would you anticipate?

References and Selected Readings

BOOKS

Agency for Health Care Policy and Research, Public Health Service, Department of Health and Human Services. (1992). *Acute pain management: Operative or medical procedures and trauma. Clinical Practice Guidelines.* (AHCPR 92-0032). Washington, DC: U.S. Government Printing Office.

Agency for Health Care Policy and Research, Public Health Service, Department of Health and Human Services. (1994). *Management of cancer pain: Adults. Clinical Practice Guidelines* (AHCPR 94-0592). Washington, DC: U.S. Government Printing Office.

American Pain Society. (1999). *Principles of analgesic use in the treatment of acute pain and chronic cancer pain* (3rd ed.). Skokie, IL: Author.

Benedetti, C. (1984). Pathophysiology and therapy of postoperative pain. In: C. Benedetti, et al. (Eds.), *Recent advances in the management of pain.* New York: Raven Press.

Bonica, J. J. (1985). Treatment of cancer pain: Current status and future needs. In H. L. Fields, et al. (Eds.), *Advances in pain research and therapy: Vol. 9. Proceedings of the IVth World Congress on Pain* (pp. 589–616). New York: Raven Press.

*Levin, R., et al. (1989). Diagnostic content validity of the six most frequently cited nursing diagnostic categories: A construct replication. In R. M. Carroll-Johnson (Ed.), *Classification of nursing diagnoses: Proceedings of the eighth conference* (pp. 356–358). Philadelphia: J. B. Lippincott.

National Institutes of Health. *Integration of behavioral and relaxation approaches into the treatment of chronic pain and insomnia.* NIH Technology Assessment Statement, Oct. 16–18, 1995.

Patt, R. B. (1993). *Cancer pain.* Philadelphia: J. B. Lippincott.

Rowlingston, J. C. (Ed.). (1994). *Handbook of critical care pain management.* New York: McGraw-Hill.

Salerno, E., & Willens, J. S. (1996). *Pain management handbook: An interdisciplinary approach.* St. Louis: C. V. Mosby.

Sevarino, F. B., & Preble, L. M. (1992). *A manual for acute postoperative pain management.* New York: Raven Press.

Wall, P. D., et al. (Eds). (1994). *Textbook of pain.* New York: Churchill Livingstone.

JOURNALS

Asterisks indicate nursing research articles

Altmaier, E. M., Lehmann, T. R., Russell, D. W., Weinstein, J. N., & Kao, C. F. (1992). The effectiveness of psychological interventions for the rehabilitation of low back pain: A randomized controlled trial evaluation. *Pain, 49*(3), 329–335.

A.G.S. Panel on Chronic Pain in Older Persons. (1998). Clinical practice guidelines: The management of chronic pain in older patients. *Journal of the American Geriatric Society, 46*(5), 635–651.

Averill, P. M., et al. (1996). Correlates of depression in chronic pain patients: A comprehensive examination. *Pain, 65*(1), 93–100.

*Calvillo, E. R., & Flaskerud, J. H. (1993). Evaluation of the pain response by Mexican-American and Anglo-American women and their nurses. *Journal of Advanced Nursing, 18*(3), 451–459.

Cameron, J. C. (1992). Constipation related to narcotic therapy: A protocol for nurses and patients. *Cancer Nursing, 15*(5), 372–377.

Carroll, D., et al. (1996). Randomization is important in studies with pain outcomes: Systematic review of transcutaneous electrical nerve stimulation in acute postoperative pain. *British Journal of Anaesthesia, 77*(6), 798–803.

Chakour, M. C., Gibson, Bradbeer, & Helme, R. D. (1996). The effect of age on A delta- and C-fibre thermal pain perception. *Pain, 64*(1), 143–152.

Cleeland, C. S., et al. (1997). Pain and treatment of pain in minority patients with cancer. *Annals of Internal Medicine, 127*(9), 813–816.

*Conner, M., & Deane, D. (1995). Patterns of patient-controlled analgesia and intramuscular analgesia. *Applied Nursing Research, 8*(2), 67–92.

Donner, B., et al. (1996). Direct conversion from oral morphine to transdermal fentanyl: A multicenter study in patients with cancer pain. *Pain, 64*(3), 527–534.

*Donovan, M., et al. (1987). Incidence and characteristics of pain in a sample of medical-surgical inpatients. *Pain, 30*(1), 69–78.

Duggleby, W., & Lander, J. (1994). Cognitive status and post-operative pain. Older adults. *Journal of Pain Symptom Management, 9,* 19–27.

Ennis, J. H. (1991). Opioid analgesics and the burning pain of Guillain-Barré syndrome. *Anesthesiology, 75*(5), 913–914.

Farthing, G. W., et al. (1997). Internal and external distraction in the control of cold-pressor pain as a function of hypnotizability. *International Journal of Clinical & Experimental Hypnosis, 45*(4), 433–446.

Ferrell, B. A. (1995). Pain evaluation and management in the nursing home. *Annals of Internal Medicine, 123*(9), 681–687.

Foster, N. E., et al. (1996). Manipulation of transcutaneous electrical nerve stimulation variables has no effect on two models of experimental pain in humans. *Clinical Journal of Pain, 12*(4), 301–310.

Gatchel, R. D., et al. (1994). Psychopathology and the rehabilitation of patients with chronic low back pain disability. *Archives of Physical Medicine and Rehabilitation, 75*(6), 666–670.

Giuffre, M., et al. (1991). Postoperative joint replacement pain. Description and opioid requirement. *Journal of Post-Anesthesia Nursing, 6*(4), 239–245.

Gordon, D. B., & Ward, S. E. (1995). Correcting patient misconceptions about pain. *American Journal of Nursing, 95*(7), 43–45.

Gujol, M. C. (1994). A survey of pain assessment and management practices among critical care nurses. *American Journal of Critical Care, 3*(2), 123–128.

Gureje, O., Von Korff, M., Simon, G. E., & Gater, R. (1998). Persistent pain and well-being. *JAMA, 280*(2), 147–151.

Heft, M. W., Cooper, B. Y., O'Brien, K. K. K., Hemp, E., & O'Brien, R. (1996). Aging effects on the perception of noxious and non-noxious thermal stimuli applied to the face. *Aging (Milano), 8*(1), 35–41.

International Association for the Study of Pain, Subcommittee on Taxonomy. (1986). *Descriptions of chronic pain syndromes and definitions of pain terms. Pain* (Suppl), *3,* S1–226.

Johnson, M. H., & Petrie, S. M. (1997). The effects of distraction on exercise and cold presser tolerance for chronic low back pain sufferers. *Pain, 69*(1–2), 43–48.

Jurna, I., & Brine, K. (1990). Central effect of the common non-steroid anti-inflammatory agents, indomethacin, ibuprofen, and diclofenac, determined in C fibre-evoked activity in single neurones of the rat thalamus. *Pain, 41*(1), 71–80.

Keefe, F. J., & Williams, D. A. (1990). A comparison of coping strategies in chronic pain in patients in different age groups. *Journal of Gerontology, 45,* 161–165.

Kehlet, H. (1991). The surgical stress response: Should it be prevented? *Canadian Journal of Surgery, 34*(6), 565–567.

*Knapp-Spooner, C., Karlik, B. A., Pontieri-Lewis, V., & Yarcheski, A. (1995). Efficacy of patient-controlled analgesia in women cholecystectomy patients. *International Journal of Nursing Studies, 32*(5), 434–442.

Lema, M. J. (1997). Shooting flies with shotguns. *American Society of Anesthesiologists Newsletter, 61*(8), 4–5.

Liebeskind, J. C. (1991). Pain can kill. *Pain, 44*(1), 3–4.

Lynn, J., et al. (1997). Perceptions by family members of the dying experience of older and seriously ill patients. *Annals of Internal Medicine, 126*(2), 97–106.

*Malek, C. J. (1996). Pain management: Documenting the decision-making process. *Nursing Case Management, 1,* 64–74.

Marchiondo, K., & Thompson, A. (1996). Pain management in sickle cell disease. *MedSurg Nursing,* 5(1), 29–33.

Martic, B., & Meherg, D. (1994). Interpleural analgesia: A new technique. *Critical Care Nursing, 14*(5), 31–35.

McCaffery, M., & Ferrell, B. R. (1994). How to use the new AHCPR cancer pain guidelines. *American Journal of Nursing, 94*(7), 42–46.

McCaffery, M., & Ferrell, B. R. (1997). Nurses' knowledge of pain assessment and management: How much progress have we made? *Journal of Pain Symptom Management, 14*(3), 175–188.

*McDonald, D. D. (1994). Gender and ethnic stereotyping and narcotic analgesic administration. *Research in Nursing & Health, 17*(1), 45–49.

McLaughlin, M. E. (1994). The intraoperative administration of ketorolac tromethamine in evaluating length of stay in a same-day surgery unit. *AANA Journal, 62*(5), 433–436.

Melzack, R., et al. (1987). Pain on a surgical ward: A survey of the duration and intensity of pain and the effectiveness of medication. *Pain, 29*(1), 67–72.

*Miaskowski, C., & Dibble, S. L. (1995). The problem of pain in outpatients with breast cancer. *Oncology Nursing Forum, 22,* 791–797.

Moltner, A., et al. (1990). Heart rate changes as an autonomic component of the pain response. *Pain, 43*(1), 81–89.

Moret, V., et al. (1991). Mechanism of analgesia induced by hypnosis and acupuncture: Is there a difference? *Pain, 45*(2), 135–140.

Naber, L., et al. (1994). Epidural analgesia for effective pain control. *Critical Care Nurse, 14*(5), 69–83.

*Nam, H. K., & Park, Y. S. (1991). A study on comparisons of ice bag and heat lamp for the relief of perineal discomfort. *Kanho Hakhoe Chi: Journal of Nurses Academic Society, 21*(1), 27–40.

National Institutes of Health. (1997). Acupuncture. *NIH Consensus Statement, 15*(5): 1–34.

Ng, B., et al. (1996a). The effect of ethnicity on prescriptions for patient-controlled analgesia for post-operative pain. *Pain, 66*(1), 9–12.

Ng, B., et al. (1996b). Ethnic differences in analgesic consumption for post-operative pain. *Psychosomatic Medicine, 58*(2), 125–129.

NIH Technology Assessment Panel on Integration of Behavioral and Relaxation Approaches into the Treatment of Chronic Pain and Insomnia. (1996). Integration of behavioral and relaxation approaches into the treatment of chronic pain and insomnia. *Journal of the American Medical Association, 276*(4), 313–318.

Oosterveld, F. G., & Rasker, J. J. (1994a). Treating arthritis with locally applied heat or cold. *Seminars in Arthritis & Rheumatism, 24*(2), 82–90.

Oosterveld, F. G., & Rasker, J. J. (1994b). Effects of local heat and cold treatment on surface and articular temperature of arthritic knees. *Arthritis & Rheumatism, 37*(11), 1578–1582.

Parker, R. K., et al. (1994). Use of ketorolac after lower abdominal surgery. *Anesthesiology, 80*(1), 6–12.

Pasero, C. L. (1997). Using the FACES scale to assess pain. *American Journal of Nursing, 97*(7), 19–20.

Pasero, C. L., & McCaffery, M. (1994). Avoiding opioid-induced respiratory depression. *American Journal of Nursing, 94*(4), 25–30.

Pasero, C. L., & Vanderveer, B. L. (1994). Epidural infusions: Not just for labor anymore. *American Journal of Nursing, 94*(12), 51.

Porter, F. L., et al. (1996). Dementia and response to pain in the elderly. *Pain, 68*(2–3), 413–421.

Porter, J., and Jick, H. (1980). Addiction rare in patients treated with narcotics. *New England Journal of Medicine, 302*(2), 123.

*Puntillo, K., et al. (1997). Opioid and benzodiazepine tolerance and dependence: Application of theory to critical care practice. *Heart and Lung, 26*(4), 317–324.

*Puntillo, K. A., et al. (1997). Relationship between behavioral and physiological indicators of pain, critical care patients' self-reports of pain, and opioid administration. *Critical Care Medicine, 25*(7), 1159–1166.

*Puntillo, K., & Weiss, S. J. (1994). Pain: Its mediators and associated morbidity in critically ill cardiovascular surgical patients. *Nursing Research, 43*(1), 31–36.

*Simpson, T., et al. (1996). Relationships among sleep dimensions and factors that impair sleep after cardiac surgery. *Research in Nursing & Health, 19*(3), 213–223.

Sorkin, B. A., et al. (1990). Chronic pain in old and young patients: Differences appear less important than similarities. *Journal of Gerontology, 45,* 64–68.

Tanelian, D. L. (1996). Reflex sympathetic dystrophy. *Pain Forum, 5*(4), 247–256.

Thomas, T., et al. (1998). Prediction and assessment of the severity of post-operative pain and of satisfaction with management. *Pain, 75*(2–3), 177–185.

Todd, K. H., et al. (1993). Ethnicity as a risk factor for inadequate emergency department analgesia. *JAMA, 269*(12), 1537–1539.

Turner, J. A., & Jensen, M. P. (1993). Efficacy of cognitive therapy for chronic low back pain. *Pain, 52*(2), 169–177.

Uomoto, J. M., & Esselman, P. C. (1993). Traumatic brain injury and chronic pain: Differential types and rates by head injury severity. *Archives of Physical Medicine and Rehabilitation, 74*, 61–64.

Veldman, P. H. J. M., & Goris, J. A. (1995). Shoulder complaints in patients with reflex sympathetic dystrophy of the upper extremity. *Archives of Physical Medicine and Rehabilitation, 76*, 239–242.

Van der Does, A. J. (1989). Patients' and nurses' ratings of pain and anxiety during burn wound care. *Pain, 39*(1), 95–101.

Wall, P. D. (1978). The gate control theory of pain mechanisms: A re-examination and re-statement. *Brain, 101*, 1–18.

Wall, P. D. (1993). Pain and the placebo response. *Ciba Foundation Symposium, 174*, 187–211.

Wallace, M. (1994). Assessment and management of pain in the elderly. *MEDSURG Nursing, 3*(4), 293–298.

*Ward, S. E., Berry, P. E., & Misiewicz, H. (1996). Concerns about analgesia among patients and family caregivers in a hospice setting. *Research in Nursing & Health, 19*(3), 205–211.

Weisenberg, M., et al. (1984). Relevant and irrelevant anxiety in the reaction to pain. *Pain, 20*(4), 371–383.

Yeager, M. P., et al. (1987). Epidural anesthesia and analgesia in high-risk surgical patients. *Anesthesiology, 66*(6), 729–736.

*Zalon, M. L. (1997). Pain in frail, elderly women after surgery. *Image: Journal of Nursing Scholarship, 29*(1), 21–26.

Zatzick, D. F., & Dimsdale, J. E. (1990). Cultural variations in response to painful stimuli. *Psychosomatic Medicine, 52*(5), 544–557.

Resources

*American Pain Society, 4700 W. Lake Ave., Glenview, IL 60025; 1-847-375-4715; fax: 1-847-375-4777; http://www.ampainsoc.org/; e-mail: infor@ampainsoc.org

*International Pain Foundation, 909 NE 43rd St., Room 306, Seattle, WA 98105-6020; 1-206-547-6409; fax: 1-206-547-1703; http://dasnetO2.dokkyomed.ac.ip/IASPM/IASP.html; e-mail: IASP@locke.hs.washington.ed

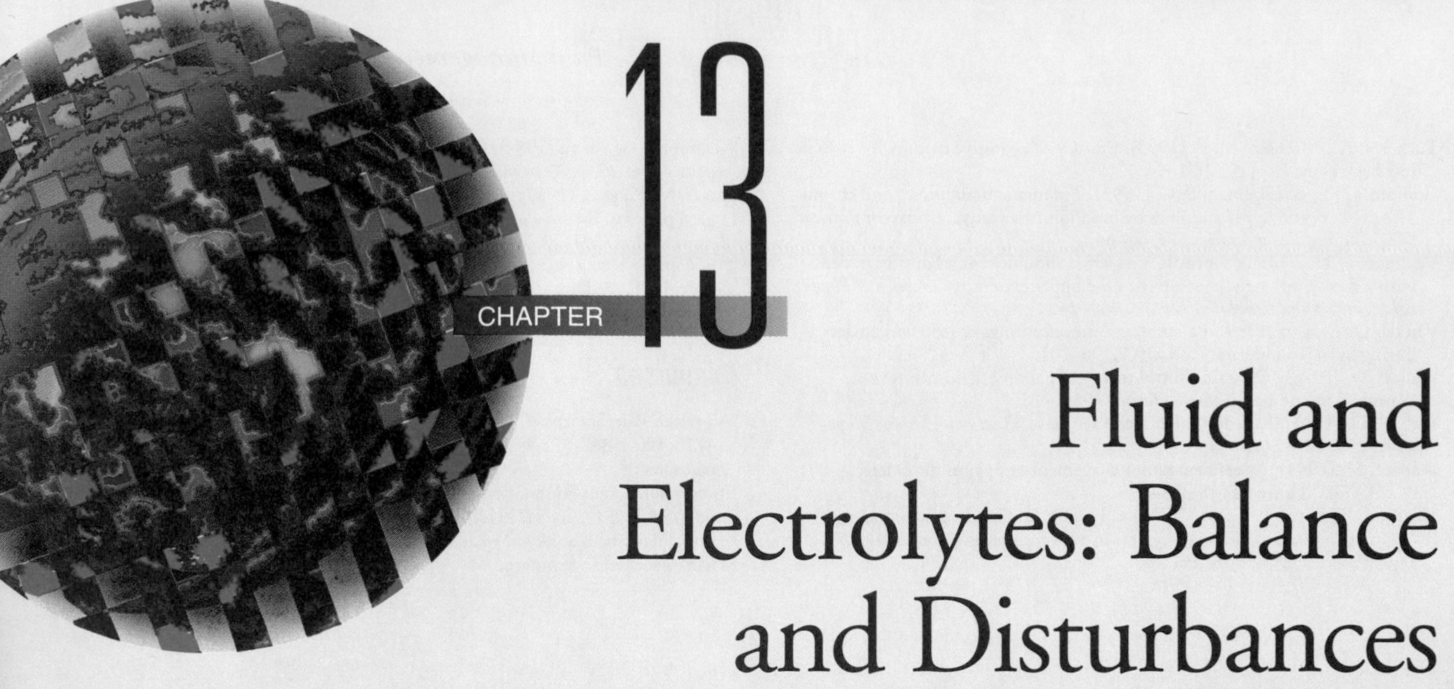

CHAPTER 13

Fluid and Electrolytes: Balance and Disturbances

Learning Objectives

On completion of this chapter, the learner will be able to:

1. Differentiate between osmosis, diffusion, filtration, and active transport.
2. Describe the role of the kidneys, lungs, and endocrine glands in regulation of the body's fluid composition and volume.
3. Identify the effects of aging on fluid and electrolyte regulation.
4. Plan effective care of patients with the following imbalances: fluid volume deficit and fluid volume excess; sodium deficit (hyponatremia) and sodium excess (hypernatremia); potassium deficit (hypokalemia) and potassium excess (hyperkalemia).
5. Describe the etiology, clinical manifestations, management, and nursing interventions for the following imbalances: calcium deficit (hypocalcemia) and calcium excess (hypercalcemia); magnesium deficit (hypomagnesemia) and magnesium excess (hypermagnesemia); phosphorus deficit (hypophosphatemia) and phosphorus excess (hyperphosphatemia); chloride deficit (hypochloremia) and chloride excess (hyperchloremia).
6. Explain the role of the lungs, kidneys, and chemical buffers in maintenance of acid–base balance.
7. Compare metabolic acidosis and alkalosis with regard to causes, clinical manifestations, diagnosis, and management.
8. Compare respiratory acidosis and alkalosis with regard to causes, clinical manifestations, diagnosis, and management.
9. Interpret arterial blood gas measurements.
10. Assess patients for evidence of acid–base imbalance.
11. Demonstrate a safe and effective procedure of venipuncture.
12. Describe measures used for preventing complications of intravenous therapy.

Fluid and electrolyte balance is a dynamic process that is crucial for life. Potential and actual disorders of fluid and electrolyte balance occur in every setting, with every disorder, and with a variety of changes that affect well people (eg, increased fluid and sodium loss with strenuous exercise and high environmental temperature; inadequate intake of fluid and electrolytes) as well as those who are ill.

GLOSSARY

acidosis: an acid–base imbalance characterized by an increase in H^+ concentration (decreased blood pH). A low arterial pH due to reduced bicarbonate concentration is called metabolic acidosis; a low arterial pH due to increased PCO_2 is respiratory acidosis

active transport: physiologic pump that moves fluid from an area of lower concentration to one of higher concentration; active transport requires adenosine triphosphate for energy

alkalosis: an acid–base imbalance characterized by a reduction in H^+ concentration (increased blood pH). A high arterial pH with increased bicarbonate concentration is called metabolic alkalosis; a high arterial pH due to reduced PCO_2 is respiratory alkalosis

diffusion: the process by which solutes move from an area of higher concentration to one of lower concentration; does not require expenditure of energy

hydrostatic pressure: the pressure created by the weight of fluid against the wall that contains it. In the body, hydrostatic pressure in blood vessels results from the weight of fluid itself and the force resulting from cardiac contraction

hypertonic solution: a solution with an osmolality higher than that of serum

hypotonic solution: a solution with an osmolality lower than that of serum

isotonic solution: a solution with the same osmolality as serum and other body fluids. Osmolality falls within normal range for serum (280–300 mOsm/L)

osmolality: the number of osmoles (the standard unit of osmotic pressure) per kilogram of solution. Expressed as mOsm/kg. Used more often in clinical practice than the term *osmolarity* to evaluate serum and urine. In addition to urea and glucose, sodium contributes the largest number of particles to osmolality

osmolarity: the number of osmoles, the standard unit of osmotic pressure per liter of solution. It is expressed as milliosmoles per liter (mOsm/L); describes the concentration of solutes or dissolved particles

osmosis: the process by which fluid moves across a semipermeable membrane from an area of low solute concentration to an area of high solute concentration; the process continues until the solute concentrations are equal on both sides of the membrane

tonicity: the measurement of the osmotic pressure of a solution

FUNDAMENTAL CONCEPTS

The nurse needs to understand the physiology of fluid and electrolyte balance and acid–base balance to anticipate, identify, and respond to possible imbalances in each. The nurse also must use effective teaching and communication skills to assist patients in preventing and treating various fluid and electrolyte disturbances.

Amount and Composition of Body Fluids

Approximately 60% of a typical adult's weight consists of fluid (water and electrolytes). Factors that influence the amount of body fluid are age, gender, and body fat. In general, younger people have a higher percentage of body fluid than older people, and men have proportionately more body fluid than women. Obese people have less fluid than thin people, because fat cells contain little water.

Body fluid is located in two fluid compartments: the intracellular space (fluid in the cells) and the extracellular space (fluid outside the cells). Approximately two thirds of body fluid is in the intracellular fluid compartment (ICF) and is located primarily in the skeletal muscle mass.

The extracellular fluid (ECF) compartment is further divided into the intravascular, interstitial, and transcellular fluid spaces. The intravascular space (the fluid within the blood vessels) contains plasma. Approximately 3 L of the average 6 L of blood volume is made up of plasma. The remaining 3 L is made up of erythrocytes, leukocytes, and thrombocytes. The interstitial space contains the fluid that surrounds the cell and totals about 8 L in an adult. Lymph is an example of interstitial fluid. The transcellular space is the smallest division of the ECF compartment and contains approximately 1 L of fluid at any given time. Examples of transcellular fluid are cerebrospinal, pericardial, synovial, intraocular, and pleural fluids; sweat; and digestive secretions.

Body fluid normally shifts between the two major compartments or spaces in an effort to maintain an equilibrium between the spaces. Loss of fluid from the body can disrupt this equilibrium. Sometimes fluid is not lost from the body but is unavailable for use by either the ICF or ECF. Loss of ECF into a space that does not contribute to equilibrium between the ICF and the ECF is referred to as a third-space fluid shift, or "third spacing" for short.

An early clue of a third-space fluid shift is a decrease in urine output despite adequate fluid intake. Urine output decreases because fluid shifts out of the intravascular space; the kidneys then receive less blood and attempt to compensate by decreasing urine output. Other signs and symptoms of third spacing that indicate an intravascular fluid volume deficit include increased heart rate, decreased blood pressure, decreased central venous pressure, edema, increased body weight, and imbalances in fluid intake and output (I&O). Third-space shifts occur in ascites, burns, peritonitis, bowel obstruction, and massive bleeding into a joint or body cavity.

Electrolytes

Electrolytes in body fluids are active chemicals (cations, which carry positive charges, and anions, which carry negative charges). The major cations in body fluid are sodium, potassium, calcium, magnesium, and hydrogen ions. The major anions are chloride, bicarbonate, phosphate, sulfate, and proteinate ions.

These chemicals unite in varying combinations. Therefore, electrolyte concentration in the body is expressed in terms of milliequivalents (mEq) per liter, a measure of chemical activity, rather than in terms of milligrams (mg), a unit of weight. More specifically, an milliequivalent is defined as being equivalent to the electrochemical activity of 1 mg of hydrogen. In a solution, cations and anions are equal in mEq/L.

Electrolyte concentrations in the ICF differ from those in the ECF, as reflected in Table 13-1. Because special techniques are required to measure electrolyte concentrations in the ICF, it is customary to measure the electrolytes in the most accessible portion of the ECF, namely the plasma.

Sodium ions, which are positively charged, far outnumber the other cations in the ECF. Because sodium concentration affects the overall concentration of the ECF, sodium is important in regulating the volume of body fluid. Retention of sodium is associated with fluid retention, and excessive loss of sodium is usually associated with decreased volume of body fluid.

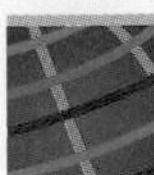

TABLE 13•1 Approximate Major Electrolyte Content in Body Fluid

Electrolytes	mEq/L
Extracellular Fluid (Plasma)	
Cations	
Sodium (Na^+)	142
Potassium (K^+)	5
Calcium (Ca^{++})	5
Magnesium (Mg^{++})	2
Total cations	154
Anions	
Chloride (Cl^-)	103
Bicarbonate (HCO_3^-)	26
Phosphate (HPO_4^{--})	2
Sulfate (SO_4^{--})	1
Organic acids	5
Proteinate	17
Total anions	154
Intracellular Fluid	
Cations	
Potassium (K^+)	150
Magnesium (Mg^{2+})	40
Sodium (Na^+)	10
Total cations	200
Anions	
Phosphates, Sulfates	150
Bicarbonate (HCO_3^-)	10
Proteinate	40
Total anions	200

Metheny, N. (1996). *Fluid and electrolyte balance: Nursing considerations* (3rd ed.). Philadelphia: Lippincott-Raven.

As shown in Table 13-1, the major electrolytes in the ICF are potassium and phosphate. The ECF has a low concentration of potassium and can tolerate only small changes in potassium concentrations. Therefore, release of large stores of intracellular potassium, typically caused by trauma to the cells and tissues, can be extremely dangerous.

The body expends a great deal of energy maintaining the high extracellular concentration of sodium and the high intracellular concentration of potassium. It does so by means of cell membrane pumps that exchange sodium and potassium ions. Normal movement of fluids through the capillary wall into the tissues depends on **hydrostatic pressure** (the pressure exerted by the fluid on the walls of the blood vessel) at both the arterial and the venous ends of the vessel and the osmotic pressure exerted by the protein of plasma. The direction of fluid movement depends on the differences in these two opposing forces (hydrostatic versus osmotic pressure).

In addition to electrolytes, the ECF transports other substances, such as enzymes and hormones. It also carries blood components, such as red and white blood cells, throughout the body.

Regulation of Body Fluid Compartments

Osmosis and Osmolality

When two different solutions are separated by a membrane impermeable to the dissolved substances, fluid shifts through the membrane from the region of low solute concentration to the region of high solute concentration until the solutions are of equal concentration; this diffusion of water caused by a fluid concentration gradient is known as **osmosis** (Fig. 13-1). The magnitude of this force depends on the number of particles dissolved in the solutions, not on their weights. The number of dissolved particles contained in a unit of fluid determines the **osmolality** of a solution, which influences the movement of fluid between the fluid compartments. **Tonicity** is the ability of all the solutes to cause an osmotic driving force that promotes water movement from one compartment to another. The control of tonicity determines the normal state of cellular hydration and cell size. Sodium, mannitol, glucose, and sorbitol are effective osmoles (capable of affecting water movement).

There are three other terms associated with osmosis: osmotic pressure, oncotic pressure, and osmotic diuresis.

- *Osmotic pressure* is the amount of pressure needed to stop the flow of water by osmosis. It is primarily determined by the concentration of solutes.
- *Oncotic pressure* is the osmotic pressure exerted by proteins (ie, albumin).
- *Osmotic diuresis* occurs when the urine output increases due to the excretion of substances such as glucose, mannitol, or contrast agents in the urine

Diffusion

Diffusion is the natural tendency of a substance to move from an area of higher concentration to one of lower concentration. It occurs through the random movement of ions and molecules. An example of diffusion is the exchange of oxygen and carbon dioxide between the pulmonary capillaries and alveoli.

Filtration

Hydrostatic pressure in the capillaries tends to filter fluid out of the vascular compartment into the interstitial fluid. An example of filtration is the passage of water and electrolytes from the arterial capillary bed to the interstitial fluid; in this instance, the hydrostatic pressure is furnished by the pumping action of the heart.

Sodium–Potassium Pump

As stated earlier, the sodium concentration is greater in the ECF than in the ICF; because of this, sodium tends to enter the cell by diffusion. This tendency is offset by the sodium–potassium

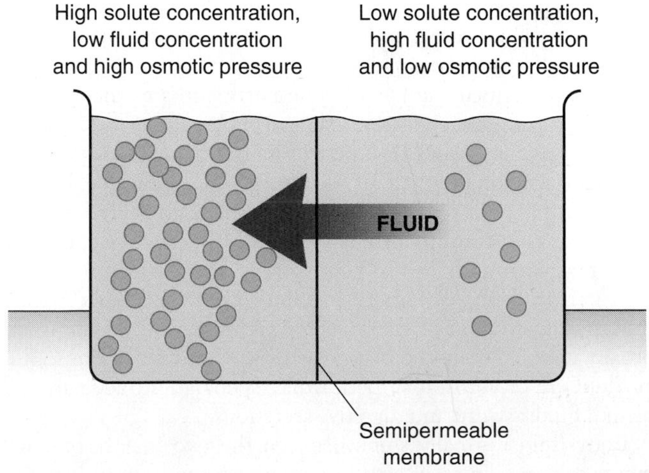

FIGURE 13•1 Osmosis. Adapted from Metheny, N. M. (1996). *Fluid and electrolyte balance: Nursing considerations* (3rd ed.). Philadelphia: Lippincott-Raven.

pump, which is located in the cell membrane and actively moves sodium from the cell into the ECF. Conversely, the high intracellular potassium concentration is maintained by pumping potassium into the cell. By definition, **active transport** implies that energy must be expended for the movement to occur against a concentration gradient.

Routes of Gains and Losses

Water and electrolytes are gained in various ways. A healthy person gains fluids by drinking and eating. In some disorders, fluids may be provided by the parenteral route (intravenously or subcutaneously) or by means of an enteral feeding tube in the stomach or intestine.

Nursing Alert *When fluid balance is critical, all routes of gain and all routes of loss must be recorded and the volumes compared. Organs of fluid loss include the kidneys, skin, lungs, and gastrointestinal (GI) tract.*

Kidneys

The usual daily urine volume in the adult is 1 to 2 L. A general rule is that the output is approximately 1 mL of urine per kilogram of body weight per hour (1 mL/kg/h) in all age groups.

Skin

Sensible perspiration refers to visible water and electrolyte loss through the skin (sweating). The chief solutes in sweat are sodium, chloride, and potassium. Actual sweat losses can vary from 0 to 1000 mL or more every hour, depending on the environmental temperature. Continuous water loss by evaporation (approximately 600 mL/day) occurs through the skin as insensible perspiration, a nonvisible form of water loss. Fever greatly increases insensible water loss through the lungs and the skin, as does loss of the natural skin barrier through major burns.

Lungs

The lungs normally eliminate water vapor (insensible loss) at a rate of 300 to 400 mL every day. The loss is much greater with increased respiratory rate or depth, or both.

GI Tract

The usual loss through the GI tract is only 100 to 200 mL daily, even though approximately 8 L of fluid circulates through the GI system every 24 hours (called the GI circulation). Because the bulk of fluid is reabsorbed in the small intestine, diarrhea and fistulas are associated with large losses.

In healthy people, the daily average intake and output of water are approximately equal (Table 13-2).

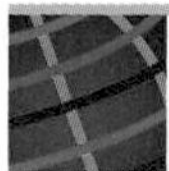

TABLE 13•2 Average Daily Intake and Output in an Adult

Intake		Output	
Oral liquids	1300 mL	Urine	1500 mL
Water in food	1000 mL	Stool	200 mL
Water produced by metabolism	300 mL	Insensible	
		Lungs	300 mL
		Skin	600 mL
Total	2600 mL	**Total**	2600 mL

Laboratory Tests for Evaluating Fluid Status

Osmolality reflects the concentration of fluid that affects the movement of water between fluid compartments by osmosis. Osmolality measures the solute concentration per kilogram in blood and urine. It is also a measure of a solution's ability to create osmotic pressure and affect the movement of water. Serum osmolality reflects the concentration of sodium and its anions. Urine osmolality is determined by urea, creatinine, and uric acid. When measured with serum osmolality, it is the most reliable indicator of urine concentration. Osmolality is reported as milliosmoles per kilogram of water (mOsm/kg).

Osmolarity, another term that describes the concentration of solutions, is measured in milliosmoles per liter (mOsm/L). The term osmolality, however, is used more often in clinical practice. Normal serum osmolality is 280 to 300 mOsm/kg, and normal urine osmolality is 50 to 1,400 mOsm/kg. Sodium predominates in ECF osmolality and holds water in this compartment.

Factors that increase and decrease serum and urine osmolality are identified in Table 13-3. Serum osmolality may be measured directly through laboratory tests or estimated at the bedside by doubling the serum sodium level or by using the following formula:

$$Na^{+} \times 2 + \frac{\text{Glucose}}{18} + \frac{\text{BUN}}{3} = \text{Approximate Value of Serum Osmolality}$$

The calculated value usually is within 10 mOsm of the measured osmolality.

Urine specific gravity measures the kidneys' ability to excrete or conserve water. The specific gravity of urine is compared to the weight of distilled water, which has a specific gravity of 1.000. The normal range of specific gravity is 1.010 to 1.025. Urine specific gravity can be measured at the bedside by placing a calibrated hydrometer or urinometer in a cylinder of approximately 20 mL of urine. Specific gravity can also be assessed with a refractometer or dipstick with a reagent for this purpose. Specific gravity varies inversely with urine volume; normally, the larger the volume of urine, the lower the specific gravity. Specific gravity is a less reliable indicator of concentration than urine osmolality; increased glucose or protein in urine can cause a falsely high specific gravity. Factors that increase or decrease urine osmolality are the same for urine specific gravity.

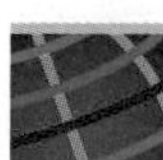

TABLE 13•3 Comparison of Serum and Urine Osmolality

Fluid	Factors Increasing Osmolality	Factors Decreasing Osmolality
Serum	Free water loss Diabetes insipidus Sodium overload Hyperglycemia Uremia	SIADH* Renal failure Diuretic use Adrenal insufficiency
Urine	Fluid volume deficit SIADH*	Fluid volume excess Diabetes insipidus

* Syndrome of inappropriate antidiuretic hormone

Blood urea nitrogen (BUN) is made up of urea, an end product of protein metabolism (from both muscle and dietary intake). Amino acid breakdown produces large amounts of ammonia molecules, which are absorbed into the bloodstream. Ammonia molecules are converted to urea and excreted in the urine. The normal BUN is 10 to 20 mg/dL (SI: 3.5–7 mmol/L). The BUN level varies with urine output. Factors that increase BUN include GI bleeding, dehydration, increased protein intake, fever, and sepsis. Those that decrease BUN include end-stage liver disease, a low-protein diet, starvation, and any condition that results in expanded fluid volume (eg, pregnancy).

Creatinine is the end product of muscle metabolism. It is a better indicator of renal function than BUN because it does not vary with protein intake and metabolic state. The normal serum creatinine is approximately 0.7 to 1.5 mg/dL (SI: 60–130 mmol/L); however, its concentration depends on lean body mass and varies from person to person.

Hematocrit measures the volume percentage of red blood cells (erythrocytes) in whole blood and normally ranges from 44% to 52% for males and 39% to 47% for females. Conditions that increase hematocrit are dehydration and polycythemia; those that decrease hematocrit are overhydration and anemia.

Urine sodium values change with sodium intake and the status of fluid volume (as sodium intake increases, excretion increases; as the circulating fluid volume decreases, sodium is conserved). Normal urine sodium levels range from 50 to 220 mEq/24 h (SI: 50–220 mmol/24 h). A random specimen usually contains more than 40 mEq/L of sodium.

Homeostatic Mechanisms

The body is equipped with remarkable homeostatic mechanisms to keep the composition and volume of body fluid within narrow limits of normal. Organs involved in homeostasis include the kidneys, lungs, heart, adrenal glands, parathyroid glands, and pituitary gland.

Kidney Functions

Vital to the regulation of fluid and electrolyte balance, the kidneys normally filter 170 L of plasma every day in the adult, while excreting only 1.5 L of urine. They act both autonomously and in response to blood-borne messengers, such as aldosterone and antidiuretic hormone (ADH). Major functions of the kidneys in maintaining normal fluid balance include the following:

- Regulation of ECF volume and osmolality by selective retention and excretion of body fluids
- Regulation of electrolyte levels in the ECF by selective retention of needed substances and excretion of unneeded substances
- Regulation of pH of the ECF by retention of hydrogen ions
- Excretion of metabolic wastes and toxic substances

Given these functions, it is readily apparent that renal failure will result in multiple fluid and electrolyte problems. Renal function declines with advanced age, as do muscle mass and daily exogenous creatinine production. Thus, high-normal and minimally elevated serum creatinine values may indicate substantially reduced renal function in the elderly.

Heart and Blood Vessel Functions

The pumping action of the heart circulates blood through the kidneys under sufficient pressure to allow for urine formation. Failure of this pumping action interferes with renal perfusion and thus with water and electrolyte regulation.

Lung Functions

The lungs are also vital in maintaining homeostasis. Through exhalation, the lungs remove approximately 300 mL of water daily in the normal adult. Abnormal conditions, such as hyperpnea (abnormally deep respiration) or continuous coughing, increase this loss; mechanical ventilation with excessive moisture decreases it. The lungs also have a major role in maintaining acid–base balance. Changes from normal aging result in decreased respiratory function, causing increased difficulty in pH regulation in older adults with major illness or trauma.

Pituitary Functions

The hypothalamus manufactures ADH, which is stored in the posterior pituitary gland and released as needed. ADH is sometimes called the water-conserving hormone because it causes the body to retain water. Functions of ADH include maintaining the osmotic pressure of the cells by controlling the retention or excretion of water by the kidneys and by regulating blood volume (Fig. 13-2).

Adrenal Functions

Aldosterone, a mineralocorticoid secreted by the zona glomerulosa (outer zone) of the adrenal cortex, has a profound effect on fluid balance. Increased secretion of aldosterone causes sodium retention (and thus water retention) and potassium loss. Conversely, decreased secretion of aldosterone causes sodium and water loss and potassium retention.

Cortisol, another adrenocortical hormone, has only a fraction of the mineralocorticoid potency of aldosterone. When secreted in large quantities, however, it can also produce sodium and fluid retention and potassium deficit.

Parathyroid Functions

The parathyroid glands, embedded in the thyroid gland, regulate calcium and phosphate balance by means of parathyroid hormone (PTH). PTH influences bone resorption, calcium absorption from the intestines, and calcium reabsorption from the renal tubules.

Other Mechanisms

Changes in the volume of the interstitial compartment within the ECF can occur without affecting body function. The vascular compartment, however, cannot tolerate change as readily and must be carefully maintained to ensure that tissues receive adequate nutrients.

BARORECEPTORS

The baroreceptors, which are small nerve receptors, detect changes in pressure within blood vessels and transmit this information to the central nervous system. They are responsible for monitoring the circulating volume, and they regulate sympathetic and parasympathetic neural activity as well as endocrine activities. They are categorized as low-pressure and high-pressure baroreceptor systems. Low-pressure baroreceptors are located in the cardiac atria, particularly the left atrium. The high-pressure baroreceptors are nerve endings in the aortic arch and in the cardiac sinus. Another high-pressure baroreceptor is located in the afferent arteriole of the juxtaglomerular apparatus of the nephron.

As arterial pressure decreases, baroreceptors transmit fewer impulses from the carotid sinuses and the aortic arch to the vasomotor center. A decrease in impulses stimulates the sympathetic

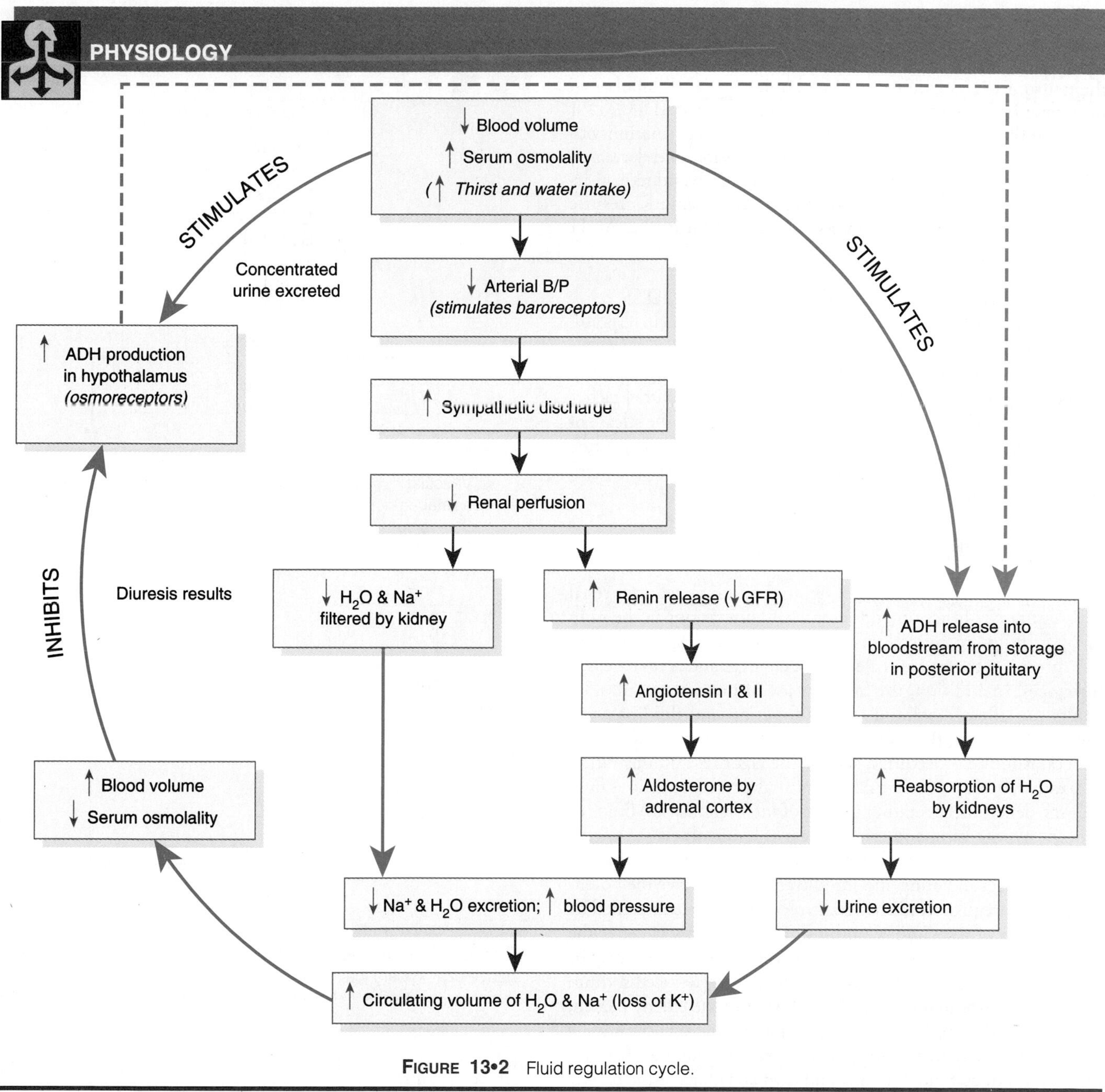

FIGURE 13•2 Fluid regulation cycle.

nervous system and inhibits the parasympathetic nervous system. The outcome is an increase in cardiac rate, conduction, and contractility and in circulating blood volume. Sympathetic stimulation constricts renal arterioles; this increases the release of aldosterone, decreases glomerular filtration, and increases sodium and water reabsorption.

RENIN–ANGIOTENSIN–ALDOSTERONE SYSTEM

Renin is an enzyme that converts angiotensinogen, an inactive substance formed by the liver, into angiotensin I and angiotensin II. Renin is released in response to decreased renal perfusion. An enzyme released within the lung capillaries converts angiotensin I to angiotensin II. Angiotensin II, with its vasoconstrictor properties, increases arterial perfusion pressure and stimulates thirst. As the sympathetic nervous system is stimulated, aldosterone is released in response to an increased release of renin. Aldosterone is a volume regulator and is also released as serum potassium increases, serum sodium decreases, or adrenocorticotropic hormone increases.

ADH AND THIRST

ADH and the thirst mechanism have important roles in maintaining sodium concentration and oral intake of fluids. Oral intake is controlled by the thirst center located in the hypothalamus. As serum concentration or osmolality increases or blood volume decreases, neurons in the hypothalamus are stimulated by intracellular dehydration; thirst then occurs, and the person increases oral intake of fluids. Water excretion is controlled by ADH, aldosterone, and baroreceptors, as mentioned previously. The presence or absence of ADH is the most significant factor in determining whether the urine that is excreted is concentrated or dilute.

OSMORECEPTORS

Located on the surface of the hypothalamus, osmoreceptors sense changes in sodium concentration. As osmotic pressure increases, the neurons become dehydrated and quickly release impulses to the posterior pituitary, which increases the release of ADH. ADH travels in the blood to the kidneys, where it alters permeability to water, causing an increased reabsorption of water and decreased urine output. The retained water dilutes the ECF and returns its concentration to normal. Restoration of normal osmotic pressure provides feedback to the osmoreceptors to inhibit further ADH release (see Fig. 13-2).

RELEASE OF ATRIAL NATRIURETIC PEPTIDE

Atrial natriuretic peptide is released by the cardiac atria in response to increased atrial pressure. Any disorder that results in volume expansion or increased cardiac filling pressures (eg, high sodium intake, congestive heart failure, chronic renal failure, atrial tachycardia, or use of vasoconstrictor agents) will increase the release of atrial natriuretic peptide. The action of atrial natriuretic peptide is the direct opposite of the renin–angiotensin–aldosterone system and decreases blood pressure and volume (Fig.13-3).

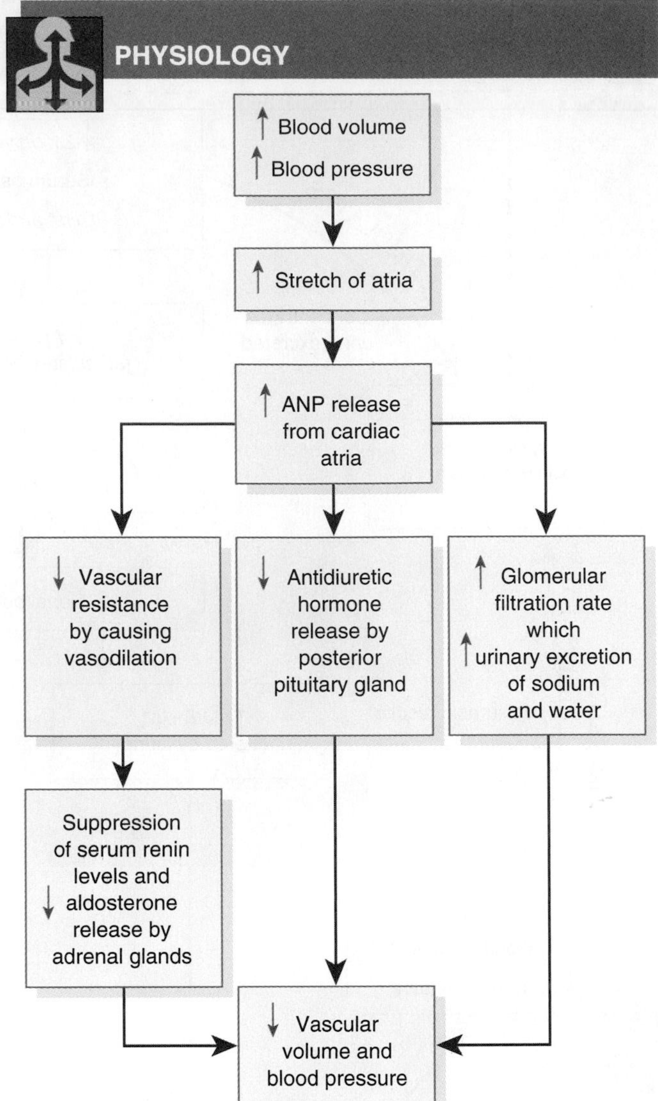

FIGURE 13•3 Role of atrial natriuretic peptide (ANP) in maintenance of fluid balance.

Gerontologic Considerations

Normal physiologic changes of aging, including reduced renal and respiratory function and reserve and alterations in the ratio of body fluids to muscle mass, may alter the responses of an elderly person to fluid and electrolyte changes and acid–base disturbances. In addition, the frequent use of medications in older adults can affect renal and cardiac function and fluid balance, thereby increasing the likelihood of fluid and electrolyte disturbances. Routine procedures, such as the vigorous administration of laxatives before colon x-ray studies, may produce a serious fluid volume deficit, necessitating the use of intravenous (IV) fluids to prevent hypotension and other effects of hypovolemia.

Alterations in fluid and electrolyte balance that may produce minor changes in young and middle-aged adults have the potential to produce profound changes in older adults, accompanied by a rapid onset of signs and symptoms. In other elderly patients, the clinical manifestations of fluid and electrolyte disturbances may be subtle or atypical. For example, fluid deficit or reduced sodium levels (hyponatremia) may cause confusion in the elderly person, whereas in young and middle-aged people the first sign commonly is increased thirst. Rapid infusion of an excessive volume of IV fluids may produce fluid overload and cardiac failure in the elderly patient. These reactions are likely to occur more quickly and with the administration of smaller volumes of fluid than in healthy young and middle-aged adults because of the decreased cardiac reserve and reduced renal function that accompany aging.

Increased sensitivity to fluid and electrolyte changes in the elderly patient requires careful assessment, with attention to intake and output of fluids from all sources and changes in daily weight, careful monitoring of side effects and interactions of medications, and prompt reporting and management of disturbances. Additional gerontologic considerations relating to specific fluid and electrolyte disturbances are discussed later in this chapter.

FLUID VOLUME DISTURBANCES

Fluid Volume Deficit (Hypovolemia)

Fluid volume deficit (FVD) results when water and electrolytes are lost in the same proportion as they exist in normal body fluids, so that the ratio of serum electrolytes to water remains the same. It should not be confused with the term *dehydration*, which refers to loss of water alone with increased serum sodium levels. FVD may occur alone or in combination with other imbalances. Unless other imbalances are present concurrently, serum electrolyte concentrations remain essentially unchanged.

Pathophysiology

FVD results from loss of body fluids and occurs more rapidly when coupled with decreased fluid intake. FVD can develop from inadequate intake alone if the decreased intake is prolonged. Causes of FVD include abnormal fluid losses, such as those resulting from vomiting, diarrhea, GI suction, and sweating, and decreased intake, as in the presence of nausea or inability to gain access to fluids.

Additional risk factors include diabetes insipidus, adrenal insufficiency, osmotic diuresis, hemorrhage, and coma. Third-space fluid shifts, or the movement of fluid from the vascular system to other body spaces (ie, with edema formation in burns or ascites with liver dysfunction), also produce FVD.

Clinical Manifestations

FVD can develop rapidly and can be mild, moderate, or severe, depending on the degree of fluid loss. Important characteristics of FVD include acute weight loss; decreased skin turgor; oliguria; concentrated urine; postural hypotension; a weak, rapid heart rate; flattened neck veins; increased temperature; decreased central venous pressure; cool, clammy skin related to peripheral vasoconstriction; thirst; anorexia; nausea; lassitude; muscle weakness; and cramps.

Assessment and Diagnostic Findings

Laboratory data useful in evaluating fluid volume status include BUN and its relation to the serum creatinine concentration. A volume-depleted patient has a BUN elevated out of proportion to the serum creatinine level (more than 10 : 1). The cause of hypovolemia may be determined through the health history and physical examination. The BUN can be elevated due to dehydration or decreased renal perfusion and function. Also, the hematocrit level is greater than normal because the red blood cells become suspended in a decreased plasma volume.

Serum electrolyte changes may also exist. Potassium and sodium levels can be reduced (hypokalemia, hyponatremia) or elevated (hyperkalemia, hypernatremia).

- Hypokalemia occurs with GI and renal losses.
- Hyperkalemia occurs with adrenal insufficiency.
- Hyponatremia occurs with increased thirst and ADH release.
- Hypernatremia results from increased insensible losses and diabetes insipidus

Urine specific gravity is increased related to the kidneys' attempt to conserve water and decreased with diabetes insipidus. Normal values for these tests are listed in Table 13-4.

Gerontologic Considerations

Elderly patients have special nursing care needs because of their propensity for developing fluid and electrolyte problems. Fluid balance in the elderly patient is often marginal at best because of certain physiologic changes associated with the aging process. Some of these changes include reduction in total body water (associated with increased body fat content and decreased muscle mass); reduction in renal function, resulting in decreased ability to concentrate urine; decreased cardiovascular and respiratory function; and disturbances in hormonal regulatory functions. Although these changes are viewed as normal in the aging process, they must be considered when the elderly person becomes ill, because age-related changes predispose the person to fluid and electrolyte imbalances. These physiologic changes must be considered during assessment of the elderly patient as well as before initiating treatment for fluid and electrolyte imbalances.

Assessment of the elderly patient should be modified somewhat from that of younger adults. For example, skin turgor is less valid in the assessment of elderly patients because their skin has lost some of its elasticity; therefore, other assessment measures (eg, slowness in filling of veins of the hands and feet) become more important in detecting FVD. In the elderly patient, skin turgor is best tested over the forehead or the sternum, because alterations in skin elasticity are less marked in these areas. As in any patient, skin turgor should be monitored serially to detect subtle changes.

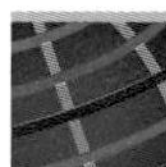

TABLE 13•4 Laboratory Values Used in Evaluating Fluid and Electrolyte Status

Test	Usual Reference Range	SI Units
Serum sodium	135–145 mEq/L	135–145 mmol/L
Serum potassium	3.5–5.5 mEq/L	3.5–5.5 mmol/L
Total serum calcium	8.5–10.5 mg/dL (approximately 50% in ionized form)	2.1–2.6 mmol/L
Serum magnesium	1.5–2.5 mEq/L	0.80–1.2 mmol/L
Serum phosphorus	2.5–4.5 mEq/L	0.80–1.5 mmol/L
Serum chloride	96–106 mEq/L	96–106 mmol/L
Carbon dioxide content	24–30 mEq/L	24–30 mmol/L
Serum osmolality	280–300 mOsm/kg	280–295 mmol/L
Blood urea nitrogen (BUN)	10–20 mg/dL	3.5–7 mmol/L of urea
Serum creatinine	0.7–1.5 mg/dL	62–133 μmol/L
BUN to creatinine ratio	10 : 1	
Hematocrit	Male: 44–52%	Volume fraction: 0.44–0.52
	Female: 39–47%	Volume fraction: 0.39–0.47
Serum glucose	70–110 mg/dL	3.9–6.1 mmol/L
Serum albumin	3.5–5.5 g/dL	3.5–5.5 g/L
Urinary sodium	50–220 mEq/day	50–220 mmol/day
Urinary potassium	40–80 mEq/day	40–80 mmol/day
Urinary chloride	110–250 mEq/day	110–250 mmol/day
Urinary specific gravity	1.025–1.035 = physiologic range after fluid restriction	1.025–1.035
	1.010–1.020 = random specimen with normal fluid intake	
Urine osmolality		
Extreme range	50–1400 mOsm/L	40–1400 mmol/kg
Typical urine	500–800 mOsm/L	500–800 mmol/kg
Urinary pH	4.5–8.0	4.5–8.0
Typical urine	<6.6	<6.6

The nurse should perform a functional assessment of the aged person's ability to determine fluid and food needs and to obtain adequate intake. For example, is the patient mentally clear? Is the patient able to ambulate and use both arms and hands to reach fluids and foods? Is the patient able to swallow? All of these questions have a direct bearing on how patients will be able to meet their own need for fluids and foods. During an elderly patient's hospital stay, the nurse must provide fluids for any patient who is unable to carry out self-care activities.

Another concern is that some elderly patients deliberately restrict their fluid intake to avoid embarrassing episodes of incontinence. In this situation, the nurse also identifies interventions to deal with the incontinence, such as encouraging the patient to wear protective clothing or devices, carry a urinal in the car, or pace fluid intake to allow access to toilet facilities during the day. Elderly people without cardiovascular or renal problems should be reminded to drink adequate fluids.

Medical Management

When planning the correction of fluid loss for the patient with FVD, the health care provider considers the usual maintenance requirements of the patient and other factors (such as fever) that can influence fluid needs. When the deficit is not severe, the oral route is preferred, provided the patient can drink. When fluid losses are acute or severe, however, the IV route is required. Isotonic electrolyte solutions (eg, lactated Ringer's or 0.9% sodium chloride) are frequently used to treat the hypotensive patient with FVD because they expand plasma volume. As soon as the patient becomes normotensive, a hypotonic electrolyte solution (eg, 0.45% sodium chloride) is often used to provide both electrolytes and water for renal excretion of metabolic wastes. These and additional fluids are listed in Table 13-5.

Accurate and frequent assessments of intake and output, weight, vital signs, central venous pressure, level of consciousness, breath sounds, and skin color should be performed to determine when therapy should be slowed to avoid volume overload. The rate of fluid administration is based on the severity of loss and the patient's hemodynamic response to volume replacement.

If the patient with severe FVD is not excreting enough urine and is therefore oliguric, the health care provider needs to determine whether the depressed renal function is the result of reduced renal blood flow secondary to FVD (prerenal azotemia) or, more seriously, to acute tubular necrosis from prolonged FVD. The test used in this situation is referred to as a fluid challenge test. During a fluid challenge test, volumes of fluid are administered at specific rates and intervals while the patient's hemodynamic response to this treatment is monitored (ie, vital signs, breath sounds, sensorium, central venous pressure, urine output).

A typical example of a fluid challenge involves administering 100 to 200 mL of normal saline solution over 15 minutes. The goal is to provide fluids rapidly enough to attain adequate tissue perfusion without compromising the cardiovascular system. The response by a patient with FVD but normal renal function will be increased urine output and an increase in blood pressure and central venous pressure. Shock can occur when the volume of fluid lost exceeds 25% of the intravascular volume, or when fluid loss is rapid. Shock and its causes and treatment are discussed in detail in Chapter 14.

Nursing Management

To assess for FVD, the nurse monitors and measures intake and output at least every 8 hours, and sometimes hourly. As FVD develops, body fluid losses exceed fluid intake. This loss may be in the form of excessive urination (polyuria), diarrhea, vomiting, and so on. Later, after FVD fully develops, the kidneys attempt to conserve needed body fluids, leading to a urine output of less than 30 mL/h in an adult. Urine in this instance is concentrated and represents a healthy renal response. Daily body weights are monitored; an acute loss of 0.5 kg (1 lb) represents a fluid loss of approximately 500 mL. (One liter of fluid weighs approximately 1 kg, or 2.2 lb.)

Vital signs are closely monitored. The nurse observes for a weak, rapid pulse and postural hypotension (ie, a drop in systolic pressure exceeding 15 mm Hg when the patient moves from a lying to a sitting position). A decrease in body temperature often accompanies FVD, unless there is a concurrent infection.

Skin and tongue turgor are monitored on a regular basis. In a healthy person, pinched skin immediately returns to its normal position when released. This elastic property, referred to as turgor, is partially dependent on interstitial fluid volume. In a person with FVD, the skin flattens more slowly after the pinch is released. When FVD is severe, the skin may remain elevated for many seconds. Tissue turgor is best measured by pinching the skin over the sternum, inner aspects of the thighs, or forehead.

Nursing Alert *The skin turgor test is not as valid in elderly people as in younger people because skin elasticity decreases with age.*

Evaluating tongue turgor, which is not affected by age, may be more valid than evaluating skin turgor. In a normal person, the tongue has one longitudinal furrow. In the person with FVD, there are additional longitudinal furrows and the tongue is smaller, because of fluid loss. The degree of oral mucous membrane moisture is also assessed; a dry mouth may indicate either FVD or mouth breathing.

Urinary concentration is monitored by measuring the urine specific gravity. In a volume-depleted patient, the urinary specific gravity should be above 1.020, indicating healthy renal conservation of fluid.

Mental function is eventually affected in severe FVD as a result of decreasing cerebral perfusion. Decreased peripheral perfusion can result in cold extremities. In patients with relatively normal cardiopulmonary function, a low central venous pressure is indicative of hypovolemia. Patients with acute cardiopulmonary decompensation require more extensive hemodynamic monitoring of pressures in both sides of the heart to determine if hypovolemia exists.

PREVENTING FVD

To prevent FVD, the nurse identifies patients at risk and takes measures to minimize fluid losses. For example, if the patient has diarrhea, diarrhea control measures should be implemented and replacement fluids administered. These measures may include administering antidiarrheal medications and small volumes of oral fluids at frequent intervals.

CORRECTING FVD

When possible, oral fluids are administered to help correct FVD, with consideration given to the patient's likes and dislikes. Also, the type of fluid the patient has lost is considered, and attempts are made to select fluids most likely to replace the lost electrolytes. If the patient is reluctant to drink because of oral discomfort, the nurse assists with frequent mouth care and provides nonirritating fluids. The patient may be offered small volumes of fluids at frequent intervals rather than a large volume all at once. If nausea is present, antiemetics may be needed before oral fluid replacement can be tolerated.

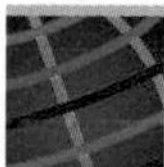

TABLE 13•5 **Selected Water and Electrolyte Solutions**

Solution	Comments
Isotonic Solutions	
0.9% NaCl (isotonic, also called normal saline) Na^+ 154 mEq/L Cl^- 154 mEq/L (308 mOsm/kg) Also available with varying concentrations of dextrose (the most frequently used is a 5% dextrose concentration)	• An isotonic solution that expands the extracellular fluid volume, used in hypovolemic states, resuscitative efforts, shock, diabetic ketoacidosis, metabolic alkalosis, hypercalcemia, mild Na^+ deficit • Supplies an excess of Na^+ and Cl^-; can cause fluid volume excess and hyperchloremic acidosis if used in excessive volumes, particularly in patients with compromised renal function, congestive heart failure, or edema • Not desirable as a routine maintenance solution, as it provides only Na^+ and Cl^- (and these are provided in excessive amounts) • When mixed with 5% dextrose, the resulting solution becomes hypertonic in relation to plasma and, in addition to the above described electrolytes, provides 170 calories/L • Only solution that may be administered with blood products
Lactated Ringer's solution (Hartmann's solution) Na^+ 130 mEq/L K^+ 4 mEq/L Ca^{2+} 3 mEq/L Cl^- 109 mEq/L Lactate (metabolized to bicarbonate) 28 mEq/L (274 mOsm/L) Also available with varying concentrations of dextrose (the most common is 5% dextrose)	• An isotonic solution that contains multiple electrolytes in roughly the same concentration as found in plasma (note that solution is lacking in Mg^{++}): provides 9 calories/L • Used in the treatment of hypovolemia, burns, fluid lost as bile or diarrhea, and for acute blood loss replacement • Lactate is rapidly metabolized into HCO_3^- in the body. Lactated Ringer's solution should not be used in lactic acidosis because the ability to convert lactate into HCO_3^- is impaired in this disorder. • Not to be given with a pH > 7.5, as bicarbonate is formed as lactate breaks down, causing alkalosis • Should not be used in renal failure because it contains potassium and can cause hyperkalemia
5% dextrose in water (D_5W) No electrolytes 50 g of dextrose	• An isotonic solution that supplies 170 calories/L and free water to aid in renal excretion of solutes • Used in treatment of hypernatremia, fluid loss, and dehydration • Should not be used in excessive volumes in the early postoperative period (when ADH secretion is increased due to stress reaction) • Should not be used solely in treatment of fluid volume deficit, because it dilutes plasma electrolyte concentrations • Contraindicated in head injury because it may cause increased intracranial pressure • Should not be used for fluid resuscitation as it can cause hyperglycemia • Should be used with caution in patients with renal or cardiac disease because of risk of fluid overload • Electrolyte-free solutions may cause peripheral circulatory collapse, anuria in patients with sodium deficiency, and increased body fluid loss.
Hypotonic Solutions	
0.45% NaCl (half-strength saline) Na^+ 77 mEq/L Cl^- 77 mEq/L (154 mOsm/L) Also available with varying concentrations of dextrose (the most common is a 5% concentration)	• Provides Na^+, Cl^-, and free water • Free water is desirable to aid the kidneys in elimination of solute. • Lacking in electrolytes other than Na^+ and Cl^- • When mixed with 5% dextrose, the solution becomes slightly hypertonic to plasma and in addition to the above-described electrolytes provides 170 calories. • Used to treat hypertonic dehydration, Na^+ and Cl^- depletion, and gastric fluid loss • Not indicated for third-space fluid shifts or increased intracranial pressure • Administer cautiously, as it can cause fluid shifts from vascular system into cells, resulting in cardiovascular collapse and increased intracranial pressure.
Hypertonic Solutions	
3% NaCl (hypertonic saline) Na^+ 513 mEq/L Cl^- 513 mEq/L (1026 mOsm/L)	• Highly hypertonic solution used only in critical situations to treat hyponatremia • Must be administered slowly and cautiously, as it can cause intravascular volume overload and pulmonary edema • Supplies no calories
5% NaCL (hypertonic solution) Na^+ 855 mEq/L Cl^- 855 mEq/L (1710 mOsm/L)	• Highly hypertonic solution used to treat symptomatic hyponatremia • Administered slowly and cautiously, as it can cause intravascular volume overload and pulmonary edema • Supplies no calories

If the patient cannot eat and drink, the nurse may need to administer fluid by an alternative route (enteral or parenteral) to prevent renal damage related to prolonged FVD.

Fluid Volume Excess (Hypervolemia)

Fluid volume excess (FVE) refers to an isotonic expansion of the ECF caused by the abnormal retention of water and sodium in approximately the same proportions in which they normally exist in the ECF. It is always secondary to an increase in the total body sodium content, which, in turn, leads to an increase in total body water. Because there is isotonic retention of body substances, the serum sodium concentration remains essentially normal.

Pathophysiology

FVE may be related to simple fluid overload or diminished function of the homeostatic mechanisms responsible for regulating fluid balance. Contributing factors can include congestive heart failure, renal failure, and cirrhosis of the liver. Another contributing factor is consumption of excessive amounts of table or other sodium salts. Excessive administration of sodium-containing fluids in a patient with impaired regulatory mechanisms may predispose him or her to a serious FVE as well.

Clinical Manifestations

Clinical manifestations of FVE stem from expansion of the ECF and include edema, distended neck veins, and crackles (abnormal lung sounds). Other manifestations include tachycardia; increased blood pressure, pulse pressure, and central venous pressure; increased weight; increased urine output; and shortness of breath and wheezing.

Assessment and Diagnostic Findings

Laboratory data useful in diagnosing FVE include BUN and hematocrit. In FVE, both of these values may be decreased because of plasma dilution. Other causes for abnormalities in these values include low protein intake and anemia. In chronic renal failure, both serum osmolality and sodium are decreased due to excessive retention of water. The urine sodium level is increased if the kidneys are attempting to excrete excess volume. Chest x-rays may disclose pulmonary congestion. Hypervolemia occurs when aldosterone is chronically stimulated (ie, cirrhosis, congestive heart failure, and nephrotic syndrome). Urine sodium levels, therefore, will not be increased in these conditions.

Medical Management

Management of FVE is directed at the causative factors. When the fluid excess is related to excessive administration of sodium-containing fluids, discontinuing the infusion may be all that is needed. Symptomatic treatment consists of administering diuretics and restricting fluids and sodium.

Diuretics are prescribed when dietary restriction of sodium alone is insufficient to reduce edema by inhibiting the reabsorption of sodium and water by the kidneys. The choice of diuretic is based on the severity of the hypervolemic state, the degree of impairment of renal function, and the potency of the diuretic. Thiazide diuretics block sodium reabsorption in the distal tubule, where only 5% to 10% of filtered sodium is reabsorbed. Loop diuretics (furosemide [Lasix], bumetanide [Bumex], torsemide [Demadex]) can cause a greater loss of both sodium and water because they block sodium reabsorption in the ascending limb of the loop of Henle, where 20% to 30% of filtered sodium is normally reabsorbed. Generally, thiazide diuretics (hydrochlorothiazide [HydroDiuril], trichlormethiazide [Diurese], methyclothiazide [Enduron]) are prescribed for mild to moderate hypervolemia and loop diuretics for severe hypervolemia.

Electrolyte imbalances may result from the effect of the diuretic. Hypokalemia can occur with all diuretics except those that work in the last distal tubule of the nephrons (eg, spironolactone). Potassium supplements can be prescribed to avoid this complication. Hyperkalemia can occur with diuretics that work in the last distal tubule, especially in patients with decreased renal function. Hyponatremia occurs with diuresis due to increased release of ADH secondary to reduction in circulating volume. Decreased magnesium levels occur with administration of loop and thiazide diuretics due to decreased reabsorption and increased excretion of magnesium by the kidney.

Azotemia (increased nitrogen levels in the blood) can occur with FVE when urea and creatinine are not excreted due to decreased perfusion by the kidneys and decreased excretion of wastes. High uric acid levels (hyperuricemia) can also occur from increased reabsorption and decreased excretion of uric acid by the kidneys.

HEMODIALYSIS

When renal function is severely impaired so that pharmacologic agents cannot act efficiently, other modalities are considered to remove sodium and fluid from the body. Hemodialysis or peritoneal dialysis may be used to remove nitrogenous wastes and control potassium and acid–base balance, and to remove sodium and fluid. Continuous arteriovenous hemofiltration may also be considered. See Chapter 40 for discussion of these treatment modalities.

NUTRITIONAL THERAPY

Treatment of FVE usually involves dietary restriction of sodium. An average daily diet not restricted in sodium contains 6 to 15 g of salt, whereas low-sodium diets can range from a mild restriction to as little as 250 mg of sodium per day, depending on the patient's needs. A mild sodium-restricted diet allows only light salting of food (about half the amount as usual) in cooking and at the table, and no addition of salt to commercially prepared foods that are already seasoned. Of course, foods high in sodium must be avoided. It is the sodium salt, sodium chloride, rather than sodium that contributes to edema formation. Therefore, patients need to read food labels carefully to determine salt content.

Because about half of ingested sodium is in the form of seasoning, the use of seasoning substitutes plays a major role in decreasing sodium intake. Lemon juice, onions, and garlic are excellent substitute flavoring agents; however, some patients prefer salt substitutes. Most salt substitutes contain potassium and must therefore be used cautiously by patients taking potassium-sparing diuretics (eg, spironolactone, triamterene, amiloride). They should not be used at all in conditions associated with potassium retention, such as advanced renal disease. Salt substitutes containing ammonium chloride can be harmful to patients with liver damage.

In some communities, the drinking water may contain too much sodium for a sodium-restricted diet. Depending on its source, water may contain as little as 1 mg or more than 1500 mg per quart. It may be necessary for patients to use distilled water when the local water supply is very high in sodium. Also, patients on sodium-restricted diets should be cautioned to avoid water softeners that add sodium to water in exchange for other ions, such as calcium.

Nursing Management

To assess for FVE, the nurse measures intake and output at regular intervals to identify excessive fluid retention. The patient is weighed daily and acute weight gain noted. An acute weight gain of 0.9 kg (about 2 lb) represents a gain of approximately 1 L of fluid.

The nurse needs to assess breath sounds at regular intervals in at-risk patients, particularly when parenteral fluids are being administered. The nurse monitors the degree of edema in the most dependent parts of the body, such as the feet and ankles in ambulatory patients and the sacral region in bedridden patients. The degree of pitting edema is assessed, and the extent of peripheral edema is monitored by measuring the circumference of the extremity with a tape marked in millimeters.

PREVENTING FVE

Specific interventions vary somewhat with the underlying condition and the degree of FVE. Most patients, however, require sodium-restricted diets in some form, and adherence to the prescribed diet is encouraged. The patient is instructed to avoid over-the-counter medications without first checking with a health care provider because these substances may contain sodium. When fluid retention persists despite adherence to a prescribed diet, hidden sources of sodium, such as the water supply or use of water softeners, should be considered.

DETECTING AND CONTROLLING FVE

Detecting FVE is of primary importance before the condition becomes critical. Interventions include providing rest, restricting sodium intake, monitoring parenteral fluid therapy, and administering appropriate medications.

Some patients benefit from regular rest periods, as bed rest favors diuresis of edema fluid. The mechanism is probably related to diminished venous pooling and the subsequent increase in effective circulating blood volume and renal perfusion. Sodium and fluid restriction should be instituted as indicated. Because most patients with FVE require diuretics, the patient's response to these agents is monitored. The rate of parenteral fluids and the patient's response to these fluids are also closely monitored. If dyspnea or orthopnea is present, the patient is placed in a semi-Fowler's position to promote lung expansion. The patient is turned and positioned at regular intervals because edematous tissue is more prone to skin breakdown than normal tissue.

Because conditions predisposing to FVE are likely to be chronic, the patient is taught to monitor his or her response to therapy by recording and evaluating fluid intake and output and body weight changes. The importance of adhering to the treatment regimen is emphasized.

TEACHING PATIENTS ABOUT EDEMA

Because edema is a common manifestation of FVE, patients need to recognize its symptoms and importance. The nurse gives special attention to edema when teaching patients with FVE. Edema can occur from increased capillary fluid pressure, decreased capillary oncotic pressure, or increased interstitial oncotic pressure, thus expanding the interstitial fluid compartment. Edema can be localized (eg, in the ankle, as in rheumatoid arthritis) or generalized (as in cardiac and renal failure). Severe generalized edema is called anasarca.

Edema occurs when there is a change in the capillary membrane, increasing the formation of interstitial fluid or decreasing the removal of interstitial fluid. Burns and infection are examples of conditions associated with increased interstitial fluid volume. Obstruction to lymphatic outflow or a decrease in plasma oncotic pressure contributes to increased interstitial fluid volume. The kidneys retain sodium and water when there is a decreased extracellular volume as a result of a decreased cardiac output from heart failure. A thorough medication history is necessary to identify any medications that may cause edema, such as nonsteroidal anti-inflammatory drugs, estrogens, corticosteroids, or antihypertensives.

Ascites is a form of edema in which fluid accumulates in the peritoneal cavity; it results from nephrotic syndrome or cirrhosis. Patients commonly report shortness of breath and a sense of pressure because of pressure on the diaphragm.

Edema usually affects dependent areas. It can be seen in the ankles, sacrum, scrotum, or the periorbital region of the face. Pitting edema is so named because a pit forms after a finger is pressed into edematous tissue. In pulmonary edema, the amount of fluid in the pulmonary interstitium and the alveoli increases. Manifestations include shortness of breath, increased respiratory rate, diaphoresis, and crackles and wheezing on auscultation of the lungs.

Decreased hematocrit resulting from hemodilution, arterial blood gas results indicative of respiratory alkalosis and hypoxemia, and decreased serum sodium and osmolality from retention of fluid may occur with edema. BUN and creatinine levels increase, urine specific gravity decreases as the kidneys attempt to excrete excess water, and the urine sodium level drops due to increased aldosterone production.

The goal of treatment is to preserve or restore the circulating intravascular fluid volume. In addition to treating the cause, other treatments may include diuretic therapy, restriction of fluids and sodium, elevation of the extremities, application of elastic pressure stockings, paracentesis, dialysis, or continuous arteriovenous hemofiltration in cases of renal failure or life-threatening fluid volume overload.

ELECTROLYTE IMBALANCES

Disturbances in electrolyte balances occur in clinical practice and must be corrected for the patient's health and safety. Table 13-6 summarizes the major fluid and electrolyte imbalances that follow in the text. An example of an electrolyte imbalance is an altered sodium balance.

Significance of Sodium

Sodium is the most abundant electrolyte in the ECF; its concentration ranges from 135 to 145 mEq/L (SI: 135–145 mmol/L). Consequently, sodium is the primary determinant of ECF osmolality. Decreased sodium is associated with parallel changes in osmolality. The fact that sodium does not easily cross the cell wall membrane, plus its abundance or high concentration, accounts for its primary role in controlling water distribution throughout the body. In addition, sodium is the primary regulator of ECF volume. A loss or gain of sodium is usually accompanied by a loss or gain of water. Sodium also functions in establishing the electrochemical state necessary for muscle contraction and the transmission of nerve impulses.

Sodium imbalance occurs frequently in clinical practice and can develop under simple and complex circumstances. Sodium deficit and excess are the two most common sodium imbalances.

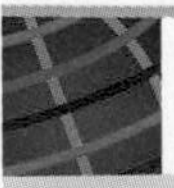

Table 13•6 Major Fluid and Electrolyte Imbalances

Imbalance	Contributing Factors	Signs/Symptoms and Laboratory Findings
Fluid volume deficit (hypovolemia)	Loss of water and electrolytes, as in vomiting, diarrhea, fistulas, fever, excess sweating, burns, blood loss, gastrointestinal suction, and third-space fluid shifts; and decreased intake, as in anorexia, nausea, and inability to gain access to fluid. Diabetes insipidus and uncontrolled diabetes mellitus also contribute to a depletion of extracellular fluid volume.	Acute weight loss, decreased skin turgor, oliguria, concentrated urine, weak rapid pulse, capillary filling time prolonged, low central venous pressure (CVP), ↓ blood pressure, flattened neck veins, dizziness, weakness, thirst and confusion, ↑ pulse, muscle cramps. *Labs indicate:* ↑ hemoglobin and hematocrit, ↑ serum and urine osmolality and specific gravity, ↓ urine sodium, ↑ BUN and creatinine
Fluid volume excess (hypervolemia)	Compromised regulatory mechanisms, such as renal failure, congestive heart failure, and cirrhosis; and overzealous administration of sodium-containing fluids. Prolonged corticosteroid therapy, severe stress, and hyperaldosteronism augment fluid volume excess.	Acute weight gain, edema, distended jugular veins, crackles, and elevated (CVP), shortness of breath, ↑ blood pressure, bounding pulse and cough. *Labs indicate:* ↓ hemoglobin and hematocrit, ↓ serum and urine osmolality, ↓ urine sodium and specific gravity
Sodium deficit (hyponatremia) Serum sodium <135 mEq/L	Loss of sodium, as in use of diuretics, loss of GI fluids, renal disease, and adrenal insufficiency. Gain of water, as in excessive administration of D_5W and water supplements for patients receiving hypotonic tube feedings; disease states associated with SIADH such as head trauma and oat-cell lung tumor; and drugs associated with water retention (oxytocin and certain tranquilizers). Hyperglycemia and congestive heart failure cause a loss of sodium.	Anorexia, nausea and vomiting, headache, lethargy, confusion, muscle cramps, muscular twitching, seizures, papilledema. *Labs indicate:* ↓ serum and urine sodium, ↓ urine specific gravity and osmolality
Sodium excess (hypernatremia) Serum sodium >145 mEq/L	Water deprivation in patients unable to drink at will, hypertonic tube feedings without adequate water supplements, diabetes insipidus, heatstroke, hyperventilation, and watery diarrhea. Excess corticosteroid, sodium bicarbonate, and sodium chloride administration, and salt water near-drowning victims.	Thirst, elevated body temperature, swollen dry tongue and sticky mucous membranes, hallucinations, lethargy, restless, irritability, focal or grand mal seizures, pulmonary edema. *Labs indicate.* ↑ serum sodium, ↓ urine sodium, ↑ urine specific gravity and osmolality
Potassium deficit (hypokalemia) Serum potassium <3.5 mEq/L	Diarrhea, vomiting, gastric suction, corticosteroid administration, hyperaldosteronism, carbenicillin, amphotericin B, bulimia, osmotic diuresis, alkalosis, starvation, and digoxin toxicity.	Fatigue, anorexia, nausea and vomiting, muscle weakness, decreased bowel motility, ventricular asystole or fibrillation, paresthesias, leg cramps, ↓ blood pressure, ileus, abdominal distention, hypoactive reflexes, *ECG:* flattened T waves, prominent U waves, ST depression, prolonged PR interval.
Potassium excess (hyperkalemia) Serum potassium >5.0 mEq/L	Pseudohyperkalemia oliguric renal failure, use of potassium-conserving diuretics in patients with renal insufficiency, acidosis, Addison's disease, crush injury, burns, stored bank blood transfusions, and rapid IV administration of potassium.	Vague muscular weakness, bradycardia, dysrhythmias, flaccid paralysis, paresthesias, intestinal colic, cramps, irritability, anxiety. *ECG:* tall tented T waves, prolonged PR interval and QRS duration, absent P waves, ST depression.
Calcium deficit (hypocalcemia) Serum calcium <8.5 mg/dL	Hypoparathyroidism (may follow thyroid surgery or radical neck dissection), malabsorption, pancreatitis, alkalosis, vitamin D deficiency, massive subcutaneous infection, generalized peritonitis, massive transfusion of citrated blood, and diuretic phase of renal failure.	Numbness, tingling of fingers, toes, and circumoral region; positive Trousseau's sign and Chvostek's sign; seizures, carpopedal spasms, hyperactive deep tendon reflexes, irritability, bronchospasm. *ECG:* prolonged QT interval.
Calcium excess (hypercalcemia) Serum calcium >10.5 mg/dL	Hyperparathyroidism, malignant neoplastic disease, prolonged immobilization, overuse of calcium supplements, vitamin D excess, oliguric phase of renal failure, acidosis, digoxin toxicity.	Muscular weakness, constipation, anorexia, nausea and vomiting, polyuria and polydipsia, hypoactive deep tendon reflexes, lethargy, deep bone pain, and pathologic features. *ECG:* shortened QT interval, bradycardia, heart blocks.
Magnesium deficit (hypomagnesemia) Serum magnesium <1.8 mg/dL	Chronic alcoholism, hyperparathyroidism, hyperaldosteronism, diuretic phase of renal failure, malabsorptive disorders, diabetic ketoacidosis, refeeding after starvation, and certain pharmacologic agents (such as gentamicin, cisplatin, and cyclosporine).	Neuromuscular irritability, positive Trousseau's and Chvostek's signs, insomnia, mood changes, anorexia and vomiting.
Magnesium excess (hypermagnesemia) Serum magnesium >2.7 mg/dL	Oliguric phase of renal failure (particularly when magnesium-containing medications are administered), adrenal insufficiency, excessive IV magnesium administration.	Flushing, hypotension, drowsiness, hypoactive reflexes, depressed respirations, cardiac arrest and coma, diaphoresis. *ECG:* tachycardia→bradycardia, prolonged PR interval and QRS.

(*continued*)

TABLE 13•6 Major Fluid and Electrolyte Imbalances *(Continued)*

Imbalance	Contributing Factors	Signs/Symptoms and Laboratory Findings
Phosphorus deficit (hypophosphatemia) Serum phosphorus < 2.5 mg/dL	Refeeding after starvation, alcohol withdrawal, diabetic ketoacidosis, respiratory alkalosis, ↓ magnesium, ↓ potassium, hyperparathyroidism, vomiting, diarrhea, hyperventilation, vitamin D deficiency associated with malabsorptive disorders.	Paresthesias, muscle weakness, bone pain and tenderness, chest pain, confusion, cardiomyopathy, respiratory failure, increased susceptibility to infection.
Phosphorus excess (hyperphosphatemia) Serum phosphorus > 4.5 mg/dL	Acute and chronic renal failure, excessive intake of phosphorus, vitamin D excess, respiratory acidosis, hypoparathyroidism, volume depletion, leukemia/lymphoma treated with cytotoxic agents, increased tissue breakdown, rhabdomyolysis.	Tetany, tachycardia, anorexia, nausea and vomiting, muscle weakness, signs and symptoms of hypocalcemia.
Chloride excess (hyperchloremia) Serum chloride > 108 mEq/L	Excessive sodium chloride infusions with water loss, head injury (sodium retention), hypernatremia, renal failure, corticosteroid use, dehydration, severe diarrhea (loss of bicarbonate), respiratory alkalosis, administration of diuretics, overdose of salicylates, Kayexalate, acetazolamide, phenylbutazone and ammonium chloride use, hyperparathyroidism, metabolic acidosis.	Tachypnea, lethargy, weakness, deep rapid respirations, decline in cognitive status, decreased cardiac output, dyspnea, tachycardia, pitting edema, dysrhythmias, coma. *Labs indicate:* increased serum chloride, increased serum sodium, decreased serum pH, decreased serum bicarbonate, normal anion gap, increased urinary chloride level.
Chloride deficit (hypochloremia) Serum chloride < 96 mEq/L	Addison's disease, reduced chloride intake or absorption, untreated diabetic ketoacidosis, chronic respiratory acidosis, excessive sweating, vomiting, gastric suction, diarrhea, sodium and potassium deficiency, metabolic alkalosis, loop, osmotic, or thiazide diuretic use, overuse of bicarbonate, rapid removal of sodium ascitic fluid, intravenous fluids that lack chloride (dextrose and water), draining fistulas and ileostomies, congestive heart failure, cystic fibrosis.	Agitation, irritability, tremors, muscle cramps, hyperactive deep tendon reflexes, hypertonicity, tetany, slow, shallow respirations, seizures, dysrhythmias, coma. *Labs indicate:* ↓ serum chloride, ↓ serum sodium, ↑ pH, ↑ serum bicarbonate, ↑ total carbon dioxide content, ↓ urine chloride level

Sodium Deficit (Hyponatremia)

Hyponatremia refers to a serum sodium level that is below normal (less than 135 mEq/L; SI: 135 mmol/L). Plasma sodium concentration represents the ratio of total body sodium to total body water. A decrease in this ratio can occur from a low quantity of total body sodium with a lesser reduction in total body water, normal total body sodium content with excess total body water, and an excess of total body sodium with an even greater excess of total body water. However, a hyponatremic state can be superimposed on an existing FVD or FVE.

Sodium may be lost by way of vomiting, diarrhea, fistulas, or sweating, or it may be associated with the use of diuretics, particularly in combination with a low-salt diet. A deficiency of aldosterone, as occurs in adrenal insufficiency, also predisposes the patient to sodium deficiency.

Dilutional Hyponatremia

In water intoxication (dilutional hyponatremia), the patient's serum sodium level is diluted by an increase in the ratio of water to sodium. This causes water to move into the cell, so that the patient develops an ECF volume excess. Predisposing conditions for this type of hyponatremia include syndrome of inappropriate ADH (SIADH), hyperglycemia, and increased water intake through the administration of electrolyte-poor parenteral fluids, the use of tap-water enemas, or the irrigation of gastric tubes with water instead of normal saline solution.

Water may be gained abnormally by the excessive parenteral administration of dextrose and water solutions, particularly during periods of stress. It may also be gained by compulsive water drinking (psychogenic polydipsia).

SIADH

The basic physiologic disturbances in SIADH are excessive ADH activity, with water retention and dilutional hyponatremia, and inappropriate urinary excretion of sodium in the presence of hyponatremia. SIADH can be the result of either sustained secretion of ADH by the hypothalamus or production of an ADH-like substance from a tumor (aberrant ADH production).

Conditions associated with SIADH include oat-cell lung tumors, head injuries, endocrine and pulmonary disorders, physiologic or psychological stress, and the use of medications such as oxytocin, cyclophosphamide, vincristine, thioridazine, and amitriptyline. SIADH is described in more detail in Chapter 38.

Clinical Manifestations

Clinical manifestations of hyponatremia depend on the cause, magnitude, and speed with which the deficit occurs. Poor skin turgor, dry mucosa, decreased saliva production, orthostatic fall in blood pressure, nausea, and abdominal cramping occur. Neurologic changes, including altered mental status, are probably related to the cellular swelling and cerebral edema associated with hyponatremia. As the extracellular sodium level decreases, the cellular fluid becomes relatively more concentrated and pulls water into the cells (Fig. 13-4). In general, patients with an acute decrease in serum sodium levels have more severe symptoms and higher mortality rates than do those with more slowly developing hyponatremia.

Features of hyponatremia associated with sodium loss and water gain include anorexia, muscle cramps, and a feeling of exhaustion. When the serum sodium level drops below 115 mEq/L (SI: 115 mmol/L), signs of increasing intracranial pressure, such as

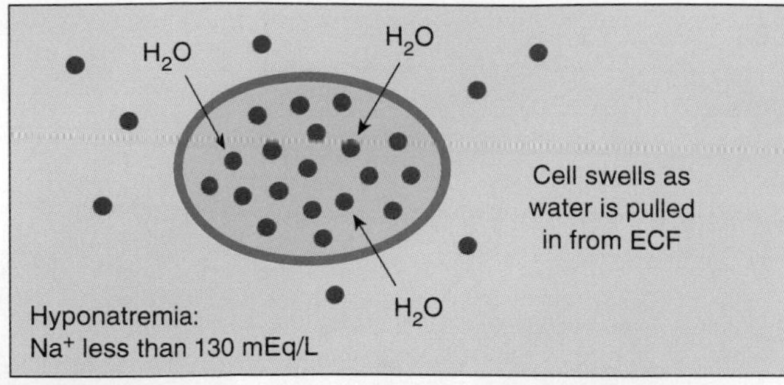

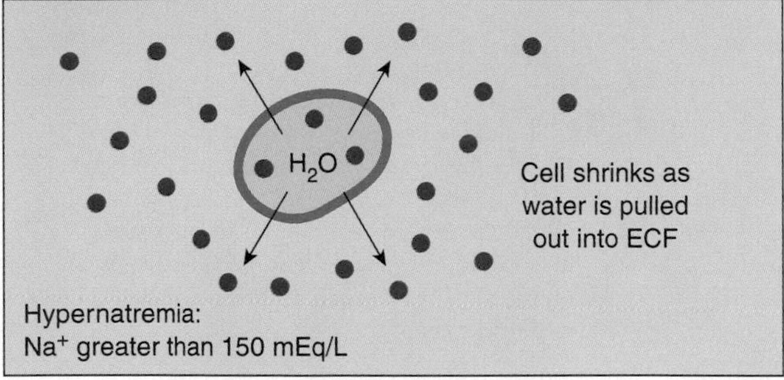

FIGURE 13•4 Effect of extracellular sodium level on cell size.

lethargy, confusion, muscle twitching, focal weakness, hemiparesis, papilledema, and seizures, may occur.

Assessment and Diagnostic Findings

Regardless of the cause of hyponatremia, the serum sodium level is less than 135 mEq/L; in SIADH it may be quite low, such as 100 mEq/L (SI: 100 mmol/L) or less. Serum osmolality is also decreased, except in azotemia or ingestion of toxins. When hyponatremia is due primarily to sodium loss, the urinary sodium content is less than 10 mEq/L (SI: 10 mmol/L), suggesting increased proximal reabsorption of sodium secondary to ECF volume depletion; the specific gravity is low, such as 1.002 to 1.004. When hyponatremia is due to SIADH, however, the urinary sodium content is greater than 20 mEq/L and the urine specific gravity is usually over 1.012. Although the patient with SIADH retains water abnormally and thus gains body weight, there is no peripheral edema; instead, fluid accumulates inside the cells. This phenomenon is sometimes manifested as "fingerprinting" when the finger is pressed over a bony prominence, such as the sternum.

Medical Management

The key to treating hyponatremia is knowing how rapidly it developed rather than knowing the actual serum sodium value.

SODIUM REPLACEMENT

The obvious treatment for hyponatremia is careful administration of sodium by mouth, nasogastric tube, or parenteral means. For patients who can eat and drink, sodium is easily replaced, because sodium is consumed abundantly in a normal diet. For those who cannot consume sodium, lactated Ringer's solution or isotonic saline (0.9% sodium chloride) solution may be prescribed. Table 13-5 describes the components of selected water and electrolyte solutions. The usual daily sodium requirement in adults is approximately 100 mEq, provided there are no abnormal losses.

In SIADH, the administration of hypertonic saline solution alone cannot change the plasma sodium concentration. Excess sodium would be excreted rapidly in a highly concentrated urine. With the addition of the diuretic furosemide, urine is not concentrated and isotonic urine is excreted to effect a change in water balance. In patients with SIADH, in whom water restriction is difficult, lithium or demeclocycline can antagonize the osmotic effect of ADH on the medullary collecting tubule.

WATER RESTRICTION

In a patient with normal or excess fluid volume, hyponatremia is treated by restricting fluid to a total of 800 mL in 24 hours. This is far safer than sodium administration and is usually effective. When neurologic symptoms are present, however, it may be necessary to administer small volumes of a hypertonic sodium solution, such as 3% or 5% sodium chloride. Incorrect use of these fluids is extremely dangerous because 1 L of 3% sodium chloride solution contains 513 mEq of sodium, and 1 L of 5% sodium chloride solution contains 855 mEq of sodium. If edema exists alone, sodium is restricted; if edema and hyponatremia occur together, both sodium and water are restricted.

Nursing Alert *Highly hypertonic sodium solutions (3% and 5% sodium chloride) should be administered only in intensive care settings under close observation, because only small volumes are needed to elevate the serum sodium level from a dangerously low value. These fluids are administered slowly and in small volumes, and the patient is monitored closely for fluid overload. The purpose is to relieve cerebral edema temporarily and to prevent neurologic complications rather than to correct the sodium concentration specifically. Along with the sodium solution, the patient may receive a loop diuretic to prevent ECF volume overload and to increase water excretion.*

Nursing Management

The nurse needs to identify patients at risk for hyponatremia so that they can be monitored. Early detection and treatment of this disorder are necessary to prevent serious consequences.

For patients at risk, the nurse monitors intake and output as well as daily body weight. Abnormal losses of sodium or gains of water are noted. GI manifestations, such as anorexia, nausea, vomiting, and abdominal cramping, are also noted. The nurse must be particularly alert for central nervous system changes, such as lethargy, confusion, muscle twitching, and seizures. In general, more severe neurologic signs are associated with very low sodium levels that have fallen rapidly because of fluid overloading. It is most important to monitor serum sodium levels closely in patients at risk for hyponatremia. When indicated, urinary sodium levels and specific gravity are also monitored.

Hyponatremia is a frequently overlooked cause of confusion in elderly patients. The elderly are at increased risk for hyponatremia because of changes in renal function and subsequent decreased ability to excrete excessive water loads. Administration of medications causing sodium loss or water retention is a predisposing factor.

DETECTING AND CONTROLLING HYPONATREMIA

For patients suffering abnormal losses of sodium who can consume a general diet, the nurse encourages foods and fluids with a high sodium content. For example, broth made with one beef cube contains approximately 900 mg of sodium; 8 oz of tomato juice contains approximately 700 mg of sodium. The nurse also needs to be familiar with the sodium content of parenteral fluids (see Table 13-5).

Nursing Alert *When administering fluids to patients with cardiovascular disease, the nurse assesses for signs of circulatory overload. The lungs are auscultated for crackles, and extreme care is taken when administering highly hypertonic sodium (eg, 3% or 5% sodium chloride) fluids, because these fluids can be lethal if infused carelessly.*

For patients taking lithium, the nurse observes for lithium toxicity, particularly when sodium is lost by an abnormal route. In such instances, supplemental salt and fluid are administered. Because diuretics promote sodium loss, patients taking lithium are instructed not to use diuretics without close medical supervision. For all patients on lithium therapy, adequate salt intake should be ensured.

Excess water supplements are avoided in patients receiving isotonic or hypotonic enteral feedings, particularly if abnormal sodium loss occurs or water is being abnormally retained (as in SIADH). Actual fluid needs are determined by evaluating fluid intake and output, urine specific gravity, and serum sodium levels.

RETURNING SODIUM LEVEL TO NORMAL

When the primary problem is water retention, it is safer to restrict fluid intake than to administer sodium. Administering sodium to a patient with normovolemia or hypervolemia predisposes the patient to fluid volume overload. As stated previously, the nurse must monitor patients with cardiovascular disease very closely.

In severe hyponatremia, the aim of therapy is to elevate the serum sodium level only enough to alleviate neurologic signs. It is generally recommended that the serum sodium concentration be raised no higher than 125 mEq/L (SI: 125 mmol/L) with a hypertonic saline solution.

Sodium Excess (Hypernatremia)

Hypernatremia is a higher-than-normal serum sodium level (exceeding 145 mEq/L [SI: 145 mmol/L]). It can be caused by a gain of sodium in excess of water or by a loss of water in excess of sodium. It can occur in patients with normal fluid volume or in those with FVD or FVE. With a water loss, the patient loses more water than sodium; as a result, the serum sodium concentration increases and the increased concentration pulls fluid out of the cell. This is both an extracellular and intracellular FVD. In sodium excess, the patient ingests or retains more sodium than water.

Pathophysiology

A common cause of hypernatremia is fluid deprivation in unconscious patients who cannot perceive, respond to, or communicate their thirst. Most often affected in this regard are very old, very young, and cognitively impaired patients. Administration of hypertonic enteral feedings without adequate water supplements leads to hypernatremia, as does watery diarrhea and greatly increased insensible water loss (eg, hyperventilation, denuding effects of burns).

Diabetes insipidus, a deficiency of ADH from the posterior pituitary gland, leads to hypernatremia if the patient does not experience, or cannot respond to, thirst or if fluids are excessively restricted. Less common causes are heat stroke, near-drowning in sea water (which contains a sodium concentration of approximately 500 mEq/L), and malfunction of either hemodialysis or peritoneal dialysis proportioning systems. Intravenous administration of hypertonic saline or excessive use of sodium bicarbonate also causes hypernatremia.

Clinical Manifestations

The clinical manifestations of hypernatremia are primarily neurologic and are presumably the consequence of cellular dehydration. Hypernatremia results in a relatively concentrated ECF, causing water to be pulled from the cells (see Fig. 13-4). Clinically, these changes may be manifested by restlessness and weakness in moderate hypernatremia and by disorientation, delusions, and hallucinations in severe hypernatremia. Dehydration (resulting in hypernatremia) is often overlooked as the primary reason for behavioral changes in the elderly patient. If hypernatremia is severe, permanent brain damage can occur (especially in children). Brain damage is apparently due to subarachnoid hemorrhages that result from brain contraction.

A primary characteristic of hypernatremia is thirst. Thirst is so strong a defender of serum sodium levels in healthy people that hypernatremia never occurs unless the person is unconscious or is denied access to water. Unfortunately, ill people may have an impaired thirst mechanism. Other signs include a dry, swollen tongue and sticky mucous membranes. Flushed skin, peripheral and pulmonary edema, postural hypotension, and increased muscle tone and deep tendon reflexes are additional signs and symptoms of hypernatremia. Body temperature may rise mildly but returns to normal when the hypernatremia is corrected.

Assessment and Diagnostic Findings

In hypernatremia, the serum sodium level exceeds 145 mEq/L (SI: 145 mmol/L) and the serum osmolality exceeds 295 mOsm/kg (SI: 295 mmol/L). The urine specific gravity and urine osmolality are increased as the kidneys attempt to conserve water (provided the water loss is from a route other than the kidneys).

Medical Management

Treatment of hypernatremia consists of a gradual lowering of the serum sodium level by the infusion of a hypotonic electrolyte solution (eg, 0.3% sodium chloride) or an isotonic nonsaline solution (eg, dextrose 5% in water [D_5W]). D_5W is indicated when water needs to be replaced without sodium. A hypotonic sodium solution is considered safer than D_5W by many clinicians because it allows a gradual reduction in the serum sodium level and thereby decreases the risk of cerebral edema. It is the solution of choice in severe hyperglycemia with hypernatremia. A rapid reduction in the serum sodium level temporarily decreases the plasma osmolality below that of the fluid in the brain tissue, causing dangerous cerebral edema. Diuretics also may be prescribed to treat the sodium gain.

There is no consensus about the exact rate at which serum sodium levels should be reduced. As a general rule, the serum sodium level is reduced at a rate no faster than 2 mEq/L/h to allow sufficient time for readjustment through diffusion across fluid compartments.

Desmopressin (DDAVP) may be prescribed to treat diabetes insipidus if it is the cause of hypernatremia.

Nursing Management

Fluid losses and gains are carefully monitored in patients at risk for hypernatremia. The nurse should assess for abnormal losses of water or low water intake and for large gains of sodium, as might occur with ingestion of over-the-counter medications with a high sodium content (such as Alka-Seltzer). Also, it is important to obtain a medication history because some prescription medications have a high sodium content.

The nurse notes the patient's thirst or elevated body temperature and evaluates it in relation to other clinical signs. The nurse monitors for changes in behavior, such as restlessness, disorientation, and lethargy.

PREVENTING HYPERNATREMIA

The nurse attempts to prevent hypernatremia by offering fluids at regular intervals, particularly in debilitated patients unable to perceive or respond to thirst. If fluid intake remains inadequate, the nurse consults with the physician to plan an alternate route for intake, either by enteral feedings or by the parenteral route. If enteral feedings are used, sufficient water should be administered to keep the serum sodium and BUN within normal limits. As a rule, the higher the osmolality of the enteral feeding, the greater the need for water supplementation.

For patients with diabetes insipidus, adequate water intake must be ensured. If the patient is alert and has an intact thirst mechanism, merely providing access to water may be sufficient. If the patient has a decreased level of consciousness or other disability interfering with adequate fluid intake, parenteral fluid replacement may be prescribed. This therapy in patients with neurologic disorders, particularly in the early postoperative period, can be anticipated.

CORRECTING HYPERNATREMIA

When parenteral fluids are necessary for managing hypernatremia, the nurse monitors the patient's response to the fluids by reviewing serial serum sodium levels and by observing for changes in neurologic signs. With a gradual decrease in the serum sodium level, the neurologic signs should improve. As stated in the discussion on management, too-rapid reduction in the serum sodium level renders the plasma temporarily hypo-osmotic to the fluid in the brain tissue, causing dangerous cerebral edema.

Significance of Potassium

Potassium is the major intracellular electrolyte; in fact, 98% of the body's potassium is inside the cells. The remaining 2% is in the ECF, and it is this 2% that is important in neuromuscular function. Potassium influences both skeletal and cardiac muscle activity. For example, alterations in its concentration change myocardial irritability and rhythm. Potassium is constantly moving in and out of cells according to the body's needs, under the influence of the sodium–potassium pump. The normal serum potassium concentration ranges from 3.5 to 5.5 mEq/L (SI: 3.5–5.5 mmol/L), and even minor variations are significant. Potassium imbalances are commonly associated with various diseases, injuries, medications (diuretics, laxatives, antibiotics), and special treatments, such as total parenteral nutrition (TPN) and chemotherapy.

To maintain potassium balance, the renal system must function because 80% of the potassium is excreted daily from the body by way of the kidneys; the other 20% is lost through the bowel and sweat glands. The kidneys are the primary regulators of potassium balance and accomplish this by adjusting the amount of potassium that is excreted in the urine. As serum potassium levels increase, so does the potassium level in the renal tubular cell. A concentration gradient occurs, favoring the movement of potassium into the renal tubule with the loss of potassium in the urine. Aldosterone also increases the excretion of potassium by the kidney. Because the kidneys do not conserve potassium as well as they conserve sodium, potassium may still be lost in urine in the presence of potassium depletion.

Potassium Deficit (Hypokalemia)

Hypokalemia, which is a below-normal serum potassium concentration, usually indicates an actual deficit in total potassium stores. Hypokalemia may occur in patients with normal potassium stores, however, when alkalosis is present a temporary shift of serum potassium into the cells occurs (see discussion of alkalosis later in this chapter).

As stated earlier, hypokalemia is a common imbalance. GI loss of potassium is probably the most common cause of potassium depletion. Vomiting and gastric suction frequently lead to hypokalemia, partly because potassium is actually lost when gastric fluid is lost, but more so because potassium is lost through the kidneys in association with metabolic alkalosis. Because relatively large amounts of potassium are contained in intestinal fluids, potassium deficit occurs frequently with diarrhea. Intestinal fluid may contain as much potassium as 30 mEq/L. Potassium deficit also occurs from prolonged intestinal suctioning, recent ileostomy, and villous adenoma (a tumor of the intestinal tract characterized by excretion of potassium-rich mucus).

Alterations in acid–base balance have a significant effect on potassium distribution. The mechanism involves shifts of hydrogen and potassium ions between the cells and the ECF. Hypokalemia can cause alkalosis, and in turn alkalosis can cause hypokalemia. For example, hydrogen ions move out of the cells in alkalotic states to help correct the high pH, and potassium ions move in to maintain an electrically neutral state. (This is discussed further in the section on acid–base balance.)

Hyperaldosteronism increases renal potassium wasting and can lead to severe potassium depletion. Primary hyperaldosteronism is seen in patients with adrenal adenomas. Secondary hyperaldosteronism occurs in patients with cirrhosis, nephrotic syndrome, congestive heart failure, and malignant hypertension.

Potassium-losing diuretics, such as the thiazides (eg, chlorothiazide [Diuril] and polythiazide [Renese]), can induce hypokalemia, particularly when administered in large doses to patients with poor potassium intake. Other medications that can lead to hypokalemia include corticosteroids, sodium penicillin, carbenicillin, and amphotericin B.

Entry of potassium into skeletal muscle and hepatic cells is promoted by insulin. Thus, patients with persistent insulin hypersecretion may experience hypokalemia, which is often the case in patients receiving high-carbohydrate parenteral fluids (as in TPN).

Patients unable or unwilling to eat a normal diet for a prolonged period are at risk for hypokalemia. This may occur in debilitated elderly people, alcoholics, and patients with anorexia nervosa. In addition to poor intake, people with bulimia frequently suffer increased potassium loss through self-induced vomiting and laxative and diuretic abuse.

Magnesium depletion causes renal potassium loss and must be corrected first; otherwise, urine loss of potassium will continue. Penicillins may produce renal potassium loss by acting as poorly reabsorbable anions and thus increasing distal sodium delivery and sodium-potassium loss.

Clinical Manifestations

Potassium deficiency can result in widespread derangements in physiologic function. Severe hypokalemia can cause death through cardiac or respiratory arrest. Clinical signs rarely develop before the serum potassium level has fallen below 3 mEq/L (SI: 3 mmol/L) unless the rate of fall has been rapid. Manifestations of hypokalemia include fatigue, anorexia, nausea, vomiting, muscle weakness, leg cramps, decreased bowel motility, paresthesias (numbness and tingling), dysrhythmias, and increased sensitivity to digitalis. If prolonged, hypokalemia can lead to an inability of the kidneys to concentrate urine, causing dilute urine (polyuria, nocturia) and excessive thirst. Potassium depletion depresses the release of insulin and results in glucose intolerance.

Assessment and Diagnostic Findings

In hypokalemia, the serum potassium concentration is less than the lower limit of normal. Electrocardiographic (ECG) changes can include flat T waves and/or inverted T waves, suggesting ischemia, and depressed ST segments (Fig. 13-5). An elevated U wave is specific to hypokalemia. Hypokalemia increases sensitivity to digitalis, predisposing the patient to digitalis toxicity at lower digitalis levels. Metabolic alkalosis is commonly associated with hypokalemia. This is discussed further in the section on acid–base disturbances.

The source of the potassium loss is usually evident from a careful history. When this is not the case, however, and the etiology of the loss is unclear, a 24-hour urinary potassium excretion test can be performed to distinguish between renal and extrarenal loss. Urinary potassium excretion exceeding 20 mEq/24 h with hypokalemia suggests that renal potassium loss is the cause.

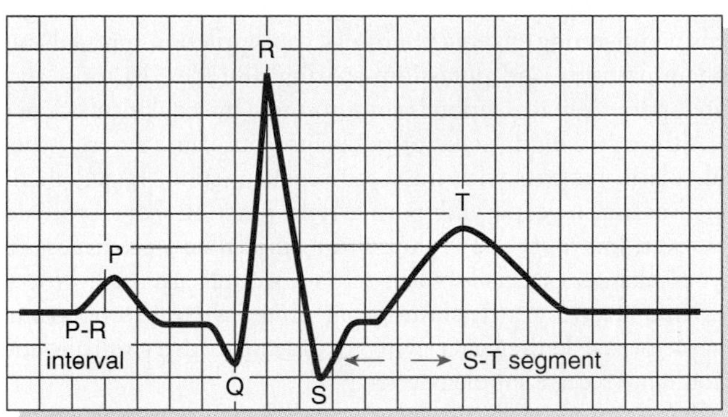

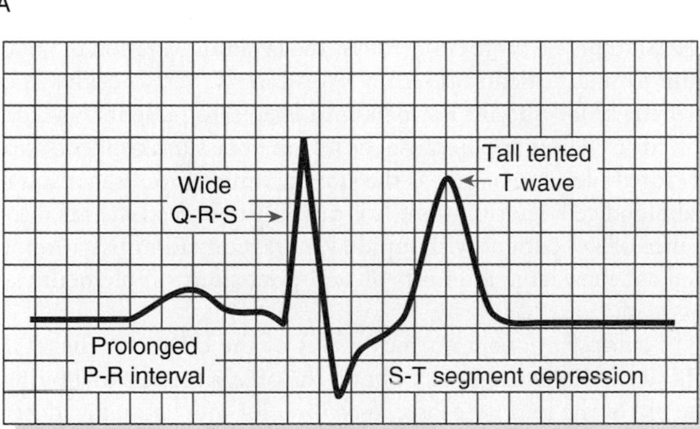

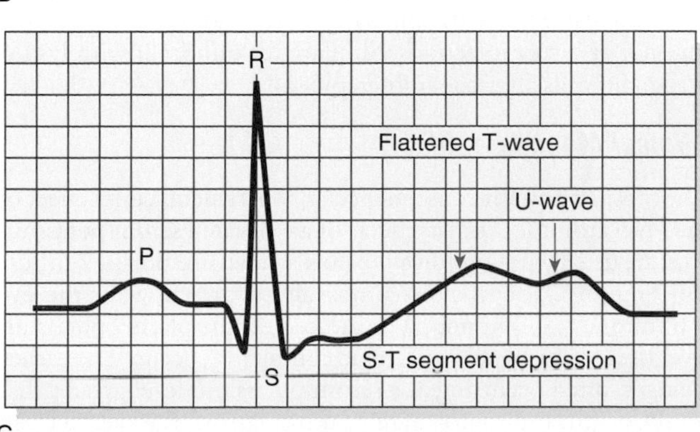

FIGURE 13•5 Effect of potassium on ECG. (**A**) Normal tracing; (**B**) serum potassium level above normal; (**C**) serum potassium level below normal.

Medical Management

If hypokalemia cannot be prevented by conventional measures such as increased intake in the daily diet, it is treated with oral or IV replacement therapy. Potassium loss must be corrected daily; administration of 40 to 80 mEq/day of potassium is adequate in the adult if there are no abnormal losses of potassium.

For patients at risk for hypokalemia, a diet containing sufficient potassium should be provided. Dietary intake of potassium in the average adult is 50 to 100 mEq/day. Foods high in potassium include fruit (especially raisins, bananas, apricots, and oranges), vegetables, legumes, whole grains, milk, and meat.

When dietary intake is inadequate for any reason, the physician may prescribe oral or IV potassium supplements. Many salt substitutes contain 50 to 60 mEq of potassium per teaspoon and may be all the patient needs.

Nursing Alert *Oral potassium supplements can produce small-bowel lesions; therefore, the patient must be assessed for and cautioned about abdominal distention, pain, or GI bleeding.*

When oral administration of potassium is not feasible, the IV route is indicated. The IV route is mandatory for patients with severe hypokalemia (eg, a serum level of 2 mEq/L). Although potassium chloride is usually used to correct potassium deficits, the physician may prescribe potassium acetate or potassium phosphate.

Nursing Management

Because hypokalemia can be life-threatening, the nurse needs to monitor for its early presence in patients at risk. Fatigue, anorexia, muscle weakness, decreased bowel motility, paresthesias, or dysrhythmias are signals that warrant assessing the serum potassium concentration. When available, the ECG may provide useful information. For example, patients receiving digitalis who are at risk for potassium deficiency should be monitored closely for signs of digitalis toxicity, because hypokalemia potentiates the action of digitalis. Physicians usually prefer to keep the serum potassium level above 3.5 mEq/L (SI: 3.5 mmol/L) in patients receiving digitalis medications such as digoxin.

PREVENTING HYPOKALEMIA

Measures are taken to prevent hypokalemia when possible. Prevention may involve encouraging intake of foods rich in potassium for the patient at risk (when the diet allows). Sources of potassium include fruit and fruit juices (bananas, melon, citrus fruit), fresh and frozen vegetables, fresh meats, and processed foods. When hypokalemia is due to abuse of laxatives or diuretics, patient education may help alleviate the problem. Part of the health history and assessment should be directed at identifying problems amenable to prevention through education. Careful monitoring of intake and output is necessary because 40 mEq of potassium is lost for every liter of urine output. The ECG is monitored for changes, and arterial blood gas values are checked for elevated bicarbonate and pH levels.

CORRECTING HYPOKALEMIA

Great care should be exercised when administering potassium, particularly in older adults, who have a lower lean body mass and total body potassium levels and therefore lower potassium requirements. Additionally, with the physiologic loss of renal function with advancing years, potassium may be retained more readily in older than in younger people.

ADMINISTERING IV POTASSIUM

Potassium should be administered only after adequate urine flow has been established. A decrease in urine volume to less than 20 mL/h for 2 consecutive hours is an indication to stop the potassium infusion until the situation is evaluated. Potassium is primarily excreted by the kidneys; therefore, when oliguria occurs, potassium administration can cause the serum potassium concentration to rise dangerously.

IV potassium must be administered using an infusion pump to avoid replacing potassium too quickly. When potassium is administered through a peripheral vein, the rate of administration must be decreased to avoid irritating the vein and causing a burning sensation during administration. Each health care facility has its own standard of care, which should be consulted; however, IV potassium should not be administered faster than 20 mEq/h or in concentrations greater than 30 to 40 mEq/L unless hypokalemia is severe, because this can cause life-threatening dysrhythmias.

Nursing Alert *Potassium is never administered IV push or intramuscularly. When prepared for IV infusions, it should be agitated well to prevent bolus doses that can result when the potassium concentrates at the bottom of the IV container. Stocking premixed 100-mL minibags of 20 mEq KCl is a safe alternative to adding a vial of KCl to an IV bag, because the KCl must be well distributed to prevent it from pooling at the insertion site at the bottom of the bag and causing a life-threatening elevation of the serum potassium level.*

In general, concentrations greater than 60 mEq/L are not administered in peripheral veins because venous pain and sclerosis may occur. For routine maintenance needs, potassium is suitably diluted and administered at a rate no faster than 10 mEq/h. In critical situations, more concentrated solutions (such as 40 mEq/h) may be administered through a central line. Even in extreme hypokalemia, however, potassium should be administered no faster than 20 to 40 mEq/h (suitably diluted). In such a situation, the patient must be monitored by electrocardiography and observed closely for other signs, such as changes in muscle strength.

Potassium Excess (Hyperkalemia)

Hyperkalemia, a greater-than-normal serum potassium concentration, seldom occurs in patients with normal renal function. Like hypokalemia, hyperkalemia is often due to iatrogenic (treatment-induced) causes. Although less common than hypokalemia, hyperkalemia is usually more dangerous because cardiac arrest is more frequently associated with high serum potassium levels.

There are a number of causes of "pseudo"-hyperkalemia. The most common are the use of a tight tourniquet around an exercising extremity while drawing a blood sample, and hemolysis of the sample before analysis. Other causes include marked leukocytosis (white blood cell count exceeding 200,000) or thrombocytosis (platelet count exceeding 1 million), drawing blood above a site where potassium is infusing, and familial pseudohyperkalemia, where potassium leaks out of the red blood cells while the blood is awaiting analysis. Failure to be aware of these causes of "pseudo"-hyperkalemia can result in aggressive treatment of nonexistent hyperkalemia, resulting in serious lowering of serum potassium levels. Thus, measurements of grossly elevated levels should be verified.

The major cause of hyperkalemia is decreased renal excretion of potassium. Thus, significant hyperkalemia is commonly seen in patients with untreated renal failure, particularly those in whom potassium levels rise as a result of infection or excessive intake of potassium in food or medications. In addition, patients with hypoaldosteronism and Addison's disease are at risk for hyperkalemia because these conditions are characterized by deficient adrenal hormones, leading to sodium loss and potassium retention.

Medications have been identified as a probable contributing factor in more than 60% of hyperkalemic episodes. Medications commonly implicated are potassium chloride, heparin, angiotensin-converting enzyme inhibitors, captopril, nonsteroidal anti-inflammatories, and potassium-sparing diuretics. In most such cases, potassium regulation is compromised by renal insufficiency.

Although a high intake of potassium can cause severe hyperkalemia in patients with impaired renal function, hyperkalemia rarely occurs in people with normal renal function. For all patients, however, improper use of potassium supplements predisposes to hyperkalemia, especially when salt substitutes are used. Not all patients receiving potassium-losing diuretics require potassium supplements. Patients receiving potassium-conserving diuretics should *not* receive supplements.

Potassium supplements are extremely dangerous when patients have impaired renal function and thus decreased ability to excrete potassium. Even more dangerous is the IV administration of potassium to such patients, as serum levels can rise very quickly. Aged (stored) blood should not be administered to patients with impaired renal function because the serum potassium concentration of stored blood increases as the storage time increases, a result of red blood cell deterioration. It is possible to exceed the renal tolerance of *any* patient with rapid IV potassium administration, as well as when large amounts of oral potassium supplements are ingested.

In acidosis, potassium moves out of the cells into the ECF. This occurs as hydrogen ions enter the cells, a process that buffers the pH of the ECF (see later in chapter for more about acidosis). An elevated extracellular potassium level should be anticipated when extensive tissue trauma has occurred, as in burns, crushing injuries, or severe infections. Similarly, it can occur with lysis of malignant cells after chemotherapy.

Clinical Manifestations

The most important consequence of hyperkalemia is its effect on the myocardium. Cardiac effects of an elevated serum potassium level are usually not significant below a concentration of 7 mEq/L (SI: 7 mmol/L), but they are almost always present when the level is 8 mEq/L (SI: 8 mmol/L) or greater. As the plasma potassium level rises, disturbances in cardiac conduction occur. The earliest changes, often occurring at a serum potassium level greater than 6 mEq/L (SI: 6 mmol/L), are peaked, narrow T waves; ST segment depression; and a shortened QT interval. If the serum potassium level continues to rise, the PR interval becomes prolonged and is followed by disappearance of the P waves. Finally, there is decomposition and prolongation of the QRS complex (see Fig. 13-5). Ventricular dysrhythmias and cardiac arrest may occur at any point in this progression.

Severe hyperkalemia causes skeletal muscle weakness and even paralysis, related to a depolarization block in muscle. Similarly, ventricular conduction is slowed. Although hyperkalemia has marked effects on the peripheral neuromuscular system, it has little effect on the central nervous system. Rapidly ascending muscular weakness leading to flaccid quadriplegia has been reported in patients with very high serum potassium levels. Paralysis of respiratory muscles and those required for speech can also occur.

GI manifestations, such as nausea, intermittent intestinal colic, and diarrhea, may occur in hyperkalemic patients.

Assessment and Diagnostic Findings

Serum potassium levels and ECG changes are crucial to the diagnosis of hyperkalemia, as discussed above. Arterial blood gas analysis may reveal metabolic acidosis, because hyperkalemia often occurs with acidosis.

Medical Management

An immediate ECG should be obtained to detect changes. Shortened repolarization and peaked T waves are seen initially. It is prudent as well to obtain a repeat serum potassium level from a vein without an IV infusion containing potassium to verify results.

In nonacute situations, restriction of dietary potassium and potassium-containing medications may suffice. For example, eliminating the use of potassium-containing salt substitutes in the patient taking a potassium-conserving diuretic may be all that is needed to deal with mild hyperkalemia.

Prevention of serious hyperkalemia by the administration, either orally or by retention enema, of cation exchange resins (eg, Kayexalate) may be necessary in patients with renal impairment. Cation exchange resins cannot be used if the patient has a paralytic ileus because intestinal perforation can occur.

EMERGENCY PHARMACOLOGIC MANAGEMENT

When serum potassium levels are dangerously elevated, it may be necessary to administer IV calcium gluconate. Within minutes after administration, calcium antagonizes the action of hyperkalemia on the heart. Infusion of calcium does not reduce the serum potassium concentration but immediately antagonizes the adverse cardiac conduction abnormalities. Calcium chloride and calcium gluconate are not interchangeable: calcium gluconate contains 4.5 mEq of calcium and calcium chloride contains 13.6 mEq of calcium. Monitoring the blood pressure is essential to detect hypotension, which may result from the rapid IV administration of calcium gluconate. The ECG should be continuously monitored during administration; the appearance of bradycardia is an indication to stop the infusion. The myocardial protective effects of calcium are transient, lasting about 30 minutes. Extra caution is required if the patient has been digitalized (received accelerated dosages of a digitalis-based cardiac glycoside to reach a desired serum digitalis level rapidly) because parenteral administration of calcium sensitizes the heart to digitalis and may precipitate digitalis toxicity.

IV administration of sodium bicarbonate may be necessary to alkalinize the plasma and cause a temporary shift of potassium into the cells. Also, sodium bicarbonate furnishes sodium to antagonize the cardiac effects of potassium. Effects of this therapy begin within 30 to 60 minutes and may persist for hours; however, they are temporary.

IV administration of regular insulin and a hypertonic dextrose solution causes a temporary shift of potassium into the cells. Glucose and insulin therapy has an onset of action within 30 minutes and lasts for several hours.

Beta-2 agonists also move potassium into the cells and may be used in the absence of ischemic cardiac disease.

The above stopgap measures only temporarily protect the patient from hyperkalemia. If the hyperkalemic condition is not transient, actual removal of potassium from the body is required; this may be accomplished by the use of cation exchange resins, peritoneal dialysis, or hemodialysis.

Nursing Management

Patients at risk for potassium excess, for example those with renal failure, should be identified so they can be monitored closely for signs of hyperkalemia. The nurse observes for signs of muscle weakness and dysrhythmias. The presence of paresthesias is noted, as are GI symptoms such as nausea and intestinal colic. For patients at risk, serum potassium levels are measured periodically.

Elevated serum potassium levels may be erroneous; thus, highly abnormal levels should always be verified. To avoid false reports of hyperkalemia, prolonged use of a tourniquet while drawing the blood sample is avoided, and the patient is cautioned not to exercise the extremity immediately before the blood sample is obtained. The blood sample is taken to the laboratory as soon as possible, because hemolysis of the sample results in a falsely elevated serum potassium level.

PREVENTING HYPERKALEMIA

Measures are taken to prevent hyperkalemia in patients at risk, when possible, by encouraging the patient to adhere to the prescribed potassium restriction. Potassium-rich foods to be avoided include coffee, cocoa, tea, dried fruits, dried beans, and whole-grain breads. Milk and eggs also contain substantial amounts of potassium. Conversely, foods with minimal potassium content include butter, margarine, cranberry juice or sauce, ginger ale, gumdrops or jellybeans, hard candy, root beer, sugar, and honey.

CORRECTING HYPERKALEMIA

As stated earlier, it is possible to exceed the tolerance for potassium in any person if the substance is administered rapidly by the IV route. Therefore, great care should be taken to monitor potassium solutions closely, paying careful attention to the solution's concentration and rate of administration. When potassium is added to parenteral solutions, the potassium is mixed with the fluid by inverting the bottle several times. Potassium chloride should *never* be added to a hanging bottle because the potassium might be administered as a bolus (potassium chloride is heavy and settles to the bottom of the container).

It is important to caution patients to use salt substitutes sparingly if they are taking other supplementary forms of potassium or potassium-conserving diuretics. Also, potassium-conserving diuretics (eg, spironolactone, triamterene, and amiloride), potassium supplements, and salt substitutes should not be administered to patients with renal dysfunction. Most salt substitutes contain approximately 60 mEq of potassium per teaspoon.

Significance of Calcium

Over 99% of the body's calcium is located in the skeletal system where it is a major component of bones and teeth. About 1% of skeletal calcium is rapidly exchangeable with blood calcium; the rest is more stable and only slowly exchanged. The small amount of calcium located outside the bone circulates in the serum, partly bound to protein and partly ionized. Calcium plays a major role in the transmission of nerve impulses and helps regulate muscle contraction and relaxation, including cardiac muscle. Calcium is instrumental in activating enzymes that stimulate many essential chemical reactions in the body, and it also plays a role in blood coagulation. Because many factors affect calcium regulation, both hypocalcemia and hypercalcemia are relatively common disturbances.

The normal total serum calcium level is 8.5 to 10.5 mg/dL (SI: 2.1–2.6 mmol/L). About 50% of the serum calcium exists in an ionized form that is physiologically active and important for neuromuscular activity and blood coagulation. The normal ionized serum calcium level is 4.5 to 5.1 mg/dL (SI: 1.1–1.3 mmol/L). The remainder of serum calcium is bound to serum proteins, primarily albumin. Calcium is absorbed from foods in the presence of normal gastric acidity and vitamin D. Calcium is excreted primarily in the feces, the remainder in urine. Serum calcium is controlled by PTH and calcitonin. As ionized serum calcium decreases, the parathyroid glands secrete PTH. This event then increases calcium absorption from the GI tract, increases calcium reabsorption from the renal tubule, and releases calcium from the bone. The increase in calcium ion concentration suppresses PTH secretion. When calcium increases excessively, the thyroid gland secretes calcitonin. It briefly inhibits calcium reabsorption from bone and decreases the serum calcium concentration.

Calcium Deficit (Hypocalcemia)

Hypocalcemia refers to a lower-than-normal serum concentration of calcium, which occurs in a variety of clinical situations. A patient, however, may have a total body calcium deficit (as in osteoporosis) and maintain a normal serum calcium level. Bed rest in the elderly person with osteoporosis is hazardous because impaired calcium metabolism with increased bone resorption is associated with immobilization.

Several factors can cause hypocalcemia. Primary hypoparathyroidism results in this disturbance, as does surgical hypoparathyroidism. The latter is far more common. Not only is hypocalcemia associated with thyroid and parathyroid surgery, but it can also occur after radical neck dissection and is most likely in the first 24 to 48 hours after surgery. Transient hypocalcemia can occur with massive administration of citrated blood (as in exchange transfusions in newborns), because citrate can combine with ionized calcium and temporarily remove it from the circulation.

Inflammation of the pancreas causes the breakdown of proteins and lipids. It is thought that calcium ions combine with the fatty acids released by lipolysis, forming soaps. As a result of this process, hypocalcemia occurs and is common in pancreatitis. It has also been suggested that hypocalcemia might be related to excessive secretion of glucagon from the inflamed pancreas, resulting in increased secretion of calcitonin (a hormone that lowers serum calcium).

Hypocalcemia is common in patients with renal failure because these patients frequently have elevated serum phosphate levels. Hyperphosphatemia usually causes a reciprocal drop in the serum calcium level. Other causes of hypocalcemia include inadequate vitamin D consumption, magnesium deficiency, medullary thyroid carcinoma, low serum albumin levels, alkalosis, and alcohol abuse. Medications predisposing to hypocalcemia include aluminum-containing antacids, aminoglycosides, caffeine, cisplatin, corticosteroids, mithramycin, phosphates, isoniazid, and loop diuretics.

Osteoporosis is associated with prolonged low intake of calcium and represents a total body calcium deficit, even though serum calcium levels are usually normal. This disorder occurs in millions of Americans, mostly postmenopausal women. It is characterized by loss of bone mass, causing bones to become porous and brittle and therefore susceptible to fracture (see Chap. 62).

Clinical Manifestations

Tetany is the most characteristic manifestation of hypocalcemia and hypomagnesemia. Tetany refers to the entire symptom complex induced by increased neural excitability. These symptoms are due to spontaneous discharges of both sensory and motor fibers in peripheral nerves. Sensations of tingling may occur in the tips of the fingers, around the mouth, and less commonly in the feet. Spasms of the muscles of the extremities and face may occur. Pain may develop as a result of these spasms.

Trousseau's sign (Fig. 13-6) can be elicited by inflating a blood-pressure cuff on the upper arm to about 20 mm Hg above systolic pressure; within 2 to 5 minutes, carpopedal spasm (an adducted thumb, flexed wrist and metacarpophalangeal joints, extended interphalangeal joints with fingers together) will occur as ischemia of the ulnar nerve develops. Chvostek's sign consists of twitching of muscles supplied by the facial nerve when the nerve is tapped about 2 cm anterior to the earlobe, just below the zygomatic arch.

Seizures may occur because hypocalcemia increases irritability of the central nervous system as well as of the peripheral nerves. Other changes associated with hypocalcemia include mental changes such as depression, impaired memory, confusion, delirium, and even hallucinations. Prolonged QT interval is seen on the ECG due to prolongation of the ST segment; a form of ventricular tachycardia called torsades de pointes may occur.

Assessment and Diagnostic Findings

When evaluating serum calcium levels, one must consider several other variables, such as the patient's serum albumin level and arterial pH. Because abnormalities in serum albumin levels may affect interpretation of the serum calcium level, it may be necessary to calculate the corrected serum calcium if the serum albumin level is abnormal. For every decrease in serum albumin of 1 g/dL below 4 g/dL, the total serum calcium level is underestimated by approximately 0.8 mg/dL. The following is a quick method to calculate the corrected serum calcium level:

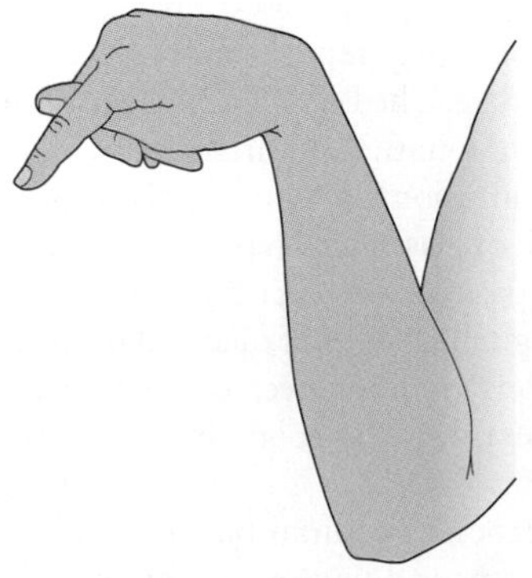

FIGURE 13•6 Trousseau's sign. Carpopedal spasm with hypocalcemia.

Measured total serum Ca^{2+} level (mg/dL) + 0.8 × (4.0 – measured albumin level [g/dL]) = corrected total calcium concentration (mg/dL)

An example to demonstrate the calculations needed to obtain the corrected total serum calcium level is as follows: A patient's reported serum albumin level is 2.5 g/dL; the reported serum calcium level is 10.5 mg/dL.

- The decrease in serum albumin level from normal level (difference from normal albumin of 4 g/dL) is calculated: 4 g/dL – 2.5 g/dL = 1.5 g/dL
- The following ratio is calculated:
  0.8 mg/dL : 1 g/dL = ? mg/dL : 1.5 mg/dL
  ? = 0.8 mg × 1.5
  ? = 1.2 mg/dL calcium
- Add 1.2 to 10.5 mg (reported serum calcium level) to obtain the corrected total serum calcium level of 11.7 mg/dL. 1.2 + 10.5 mg = 11.7 mg/dL

Clinicians often ignore a low serum calcium level in the presence of a similarly low serum albumin level. The ionized calcium level is usually normal in patients with reduced total serum calcium levels and concomitant hypoalbuminemia. When the arterial pH increases (**alkalosis**), more calcium becomes bound to protein. As a result, the ionized portion decreases. Symptoms of hypocalcemia may occur in the presence of alkalosis. **Acidosis** (low pH) has the opposite effect—that is, less calcium is bound to protein and thus more exists in the ionized form. However, relatively small changes in serum calcium levels occur during these acid–base abnormalities.

Ideally, the laboratory should measure the ionized level of calcium. In most laboratories, however, only the total calcium level is reported; thus, concentration of the ionized fraction must be estimated by simultaneous measurement of the serum albumin level. PTH levels are decreased in hypoparathyroidism. Magnesium and phosphorus levels need to be assessed to identify possible causes of decreased calcium.

Medical Management

Acute symptomatic hypocalcemia is life-threatening and requires prompt treatment with IV administration of calcium. Parenteral calcium salts include calcium gluconate, calcium chloride, and calcium gluceptate. Although calcium chloride produces a significantly higher ionized calcium level than calcium gluconate, it is not used as often because it is more irritating and can cause sloughing of tissue if it infiltrates. Too-rapid IV administration of calcium can cause cardiac arrest, preceded by bradycardia. IV calcium administration is particularly dangerous in patients receiving digitalis-derived medications because calcium ions exert an effect similar to that of digitalis and can cause digitalis toxicity, with adverse cardiac effects. IV calcium should be diluted in D_5W and given as a slow IV bolus or a slow IV infusion using a volumetric infusion pump. A 0.9% sodium chloride solution should not be used with calcium because it will increase renal calcium loss. Solutions containing phosphates or bicarbonate should not be used with calcium because they will cause precipitation when calcium is added. The nurse must clarify with the physician which calcium salt to administer, because calcium gluconate yields 4.5 mEq of calcium and calcium chloride provides 13.6 mEq of calcium. Calcium can cause postural hypotension; therefore, the patient is kept in bed for IV replacement and blood pressure is monitored.

Vitamin D therapy may be instituted to increase calcium absorption from the GI tract. Aluminum hydroxide antacids may be prescribed to decrease elevated phosphorus levels before treating hypocalcemia. Lastly, increasing the dietary intake of calcium to at least 1000 to 1500 mg/day in the adult is recommended (ie, milk products; green, leafy vegetables; canned salmon, sardines, and fresh oysters). Because hypomagnesemia can also cause tetany, if the tetany responds to IV calcium, then a low magnesium level is explored as a possible cause.

Nursing Management

It is important to observe for hypocalcemia in patients at risk. Seizure precautions are initiated when hypocalcemia is severe. The status of the airway is closely monitored because laryngeal stridor can occur. Safety precautions are taken, as indicated, if confusion is present.

People at high risk for osteoporosis are instructed about the need for adequate dietary calcium intake; if not consumed in the diet, calcium supplements should be considered. Also, the value of regular exercise in decreasing bone loss should be emphasized, as should the effect of medications on calcium balance. For example, alcohol and caffeine in high doses inhibit calcium absorption, and moderate cigarette smoking increases urinary calcium excretion. Additional teaching topics may involve discussion of hormone-replacement therapy and other medications such as alendronate (Fosamax) to prevent further bone loss.

Calcium Excess (Hypercalcemia)

Hypercalcemia refers to an excess of calcium in the plasma. It is a dangerous imbalance when severe; in fact, hypercalcemic crisis has a mortality rate as high as 50% if not treated promptly.

The most common causes of hypercalcemia are malignancies and hyperparathyroidism. Malignant tumors can produce hypercalcemia by a variety of mechanisms. The excessive PTH secretion associated with hyperparathyroidism causes increased release of calcium from the bones and increased intestinal and renal absorption of calcium.

Bone mineral is lost during immobilization, sometimes causing elevation of total (and especially ionized) calcium in the bloodstream. Symptomatic hypercalcemia from immobilization, however, is rare; when it does occur, it is virtually limited to people with high calcium turnover rates (eg, adolescents during a growth spurt). Most cases of hypercalcemia secondary to immobility occur after severe or multiple fractures or spinal cord injury.

Thiazide diuretics may cause a slight elevation in serum calcium levels because they potentiate the action of PTH on the kidneys, reducing urinary calcium excretion. The milk-alkali syndrome can occur in patients with peptic ulcer treated for a prolonged period with milk and alkaline antacids, particularly calcium carbonate. Vitamin A and D intoxication, as well as the use of lithium, can cause calcium excess.

Clinical Manifestations

As a rule, the symptoms of hypercalcemia are proportional to the degree of elevation of the serum calcium level. Hypercalcemia reduces neuromuscular excitability because it suppresses activity at the myoneural junction. Symptoms such as muscle weakness, incoordination, anorexia, and constipation may be due to decreased tone in smooth and striated muscle. Cardiac standstill can occur when the serum calcium is about 18 mg/dL (SI: 4.5 mmol/L). The inotropic effect of digitalis is enhanced by calcium; therefore, digitalis toxicity is aggravated by hypercalcemia.

Anorexia, nausea, vomiting, and constipation are common symptoms of hypercalcemia. Dehydration occurs with nausea, vomiting, anorexia, and calcium reabsorption at the proximal renal tubule. Abdominal and bone pain may also be present. Abdominal distention and paralytic ileus may complicate severe hypercalcemic crisis. Excessive urination due to disturbed renal tubular function produced by hypercalcemia may be present. Severe thirst may occur secondary to the polyuria caused by the high solute (calcium) load. Patients with chronic hypercalcemia may develop symptoms similar to those of peptic ulcer because hypercalcemia increases the secretion of acid and pepsin by the stomach.

Confusion, impaired memory, slurred speech, lethargy, acute psychotic behavior, or coma may occur. The more severe symptoms tend to appear when the serum calcium level is approximately 16 mg/dL (SI: 4 mmol/L) or above. However, some patients become profoundly disturbed with serum calcium levels of only 12 mg/dL (SI: 3 mmol/L). These symptoms resolve as serum calcium levels return to normal after treatment.

Hypercalcemic crisis refers to an acute rise in the serum calcium level to 17 mg/dL (SI: 4.3 mmol/L) or higher. Severe thirst and polyuria are characteristically present. Other findings may include muscle weakness, intractable nausea, abdominal cramps, obstipation (very severe constipation) or diarrhea, peptic ulcer symptoms, and bone pain. Lethargy, confusion, and coma may also occur. This condition is very dangerous and may result in cardiac arrest.

Assessment and Diagnostic Findings

The serum calcium level is greater than 10.5 mg/dL (SI: 2.6 mmol/L). Cardiovascular changes may include a variety of dysrhythmias and shortening of the QT interval and ST segment. The PR interval is sometimes prolonged. The double-antibody PTH test may be used to differentiate between primary hyperparathyroidism and malignancy as a cause of hypercalcemia: PTH levels are increased in primary or secondary hyperparathyroidism and suppressed in malignancy. X-rays may reveal the presence of osteoporosis, bone cavitation, or urinary calculi. The Sulkowitch urine test analyzes the amount of calcium in the urine; in hypercalcemia, dense precipitation is observed due to hypercalciuria.

Medical Management

Therapeutic aims in hypercalcemia include decreasing the serum calcium level and reversing the process causing hypercalcemia. Treating the underlying cause (eg, chemotherapy for a malignancy or partial parathyroidectomy for hyperparathyroidism) is essential.

General measures include administering fluids to dilute serum calcium and promote its excretion by the kidneys, mobilizing the patient, and restricting dietary calcium intake. IV administration of 0.9% sodium chloride solution temporarily dilutes the serum calcium level and increases urinary calcium excretion by inhibiting tubular reabsorption of calcium. Administering IV phosphate can cause a reciprocal drop in serum calcium. Furosemide is often used in conjunction with saline administration; in addition to causing diuresis, furosemide increases calcium excretion.

Calcitonin can be used to lower the serum calcium level and is particularly useful for patients with heart disease or renal failure who cannot tolerate large sodium loads. Calcitonin reduces bone resorption, increases the deposit of calcium and phosphorus in the bones, and increases urinary excretion of calcium and phosphorus. Although available in several forms, calcitonin derived from salmon is commonly used. Skin testing for allergy to salmon calcitonin is necessary before it is administered. Systemic allergic reactions are possible since this hormone is a protein; resistance to the medication may develop later because of antibody formation. Calcitonin is administered by intramuscular injection rather than subcutaneously because patients with hypercalcemia have poor perfusion of subcutaneous tissue.

For patients with malignant disease, treatment is directed at controlling the condition by surgery, chemotherapy, or radiation therapy. Corticosteroids may be used to decrease bone turnover and tubular reabsorption for patients with sarcoidosis, myelomas, lymphomas, and leukemias; patients with solid tumors are less responsive. The biphosphonates inhibit osteoclast activity. Pamidronate (Aredia) is the most potent of these agents and is given IV; it causes a transient, mild pyrexia, decreased white blood cell count, and myalgia. Etidronate (Didronel) is another biphosphonate that is given IV, but its action is slower. Mithramycin, a cytotoxic antibiotic, inhibits bone resorption and thus lowers the serum calcium level. This agent must be used cautiously because it has significant side effects, including thrombocytopenia, nephrotoxicity, rebound hypercalcemia when discontinued, and hepatotoxicity. Inorganic phosphate salts can be administered orally or by nasogastric tube (in the form of Phospho-Soda or Neutra-Phos), rectally (as retention enemas), or IV. IV phosphate therapy is used with extreme caution in the treatment of hypercalcemia because it can cause severe calcification in various tissues, hypotension, tetany, and acute renal failure.

Nursing Management

It is important to monitor for hypercalcemia in patients at risk. Interventions such as increasing patient mobility and encouraging fluids can help prevent hypercalcemia, or at least minimize its severity. Hospitalized patients at risk for hypercalcemia are encouraged to ambulate as soon as possible; outpatients and those cared for in their homes are informed of the importance of frequent ambulation.

When encouraging oral fluids, the nurse considers the patient's likes and dislikes. Fluids containing sodium should be administered unless contraindicated by other conditions, because sodium favors calcium excretion. Patients at home are encouraged to drink 3 to 4 quarts of fluid daily, if possible. Adequate bulk should be provided in the diet to offset the tendency for constipation. Safety precautions are taken, as necessary, when mental symptoms of hypercalcemia are present. The patient and family are informed that these mental changes are reversible with treatment. Increased calcium potentiates the effects of digitalis; therefore, the patient is assessed for signs and symptoms of digitalis toxicity. ECG changes (premature ventricular contractions, paroxysmal atrial tachycardia, and heart block) can occur; therefore, the patient's pulse is monitored for any abnormalities.

Significance of Magnesium

Next to potassium, magnesium is the most abundant intracellular cation. It acts as an activator for many intracellular enzyme systems and plays a role in both carbohydrate and protein metabolism. Magnesium balance is important in neuromuscular function. Because magnesium acts directly on the myoneural junction, variations in the serum concentration of magnesium affect neuromuscular irritability and contractility. For example, an excess of magnesium diminishes the excitability of the muscle cells, whereas a deficit increases neuromuscular irritability and contractility. Magnesium produces its sedative effect at the neuromuscular junction, probably by inhibiting the release of the neurotransmitter acetylcholine. It also increases the stimulus threshold in nerve fibers.

Magnesium exerts effects on the cardiovascular system, acting peripherally to produce vasodilation. Magnesium is thought to have a direct effect on peripheral arteries and arterioles, which results in a decreased total peripheral resistance. Magnesium disorders include hypomagnesemia and hypermagnesemia.

Magnesium Deficit (Hypomagnesemia)

Hypomagnesemia refers to a below-normal serum magnesium concentration. The normal serum magnesium level is 1.5 to 2.5 mEq/L (or 1.8–3.0 mg/dL; SI: 0.8–1.2 mmol/L). Approximately one third of serum magnesium is bound to protein; the remaining two thirds exist as free cations (Mg^{++}). Like calcium, it is the ionized fraction that is primarily involved in neuromuscular activity and other physiologic processes. As with calcium levels, magnesium levels should be evaluated in combination with albumin levels. Low serum albumin levels decrease total magnesium.

Hypomagnesemia is a common yet often overlooked imbalance in acutely and critically ill patients. It may occur with withdrawal from alcohol and administration of nourishment (tube feedings or TPN).

An important route for magnesium loss is the GI tract. Loss of magnesium from the GI tract may occur with nasogastric suction, diarrhea, or fistulas. Because fluid from the lower GI tract has a higher concentration of magnesium (10–14 mEq/L) than fluid from the upper tract (1–2 mEq/L), losses from diarrhea and intestinal fistulas are more likely to induce magnesium deficit than are those from gastric suction. Although magnesium losses are relatively small in nasogastric suction, hypomagnesemia will occur if losses are prolonged and magnesium is not replaced through IV infusion. Because the distal small bowel is the major site of magnesium absorption, any disruption in small bowel function, as in intestinal resection or inflammatory bowel disease, can lead to hypomagnesemia.

Alcoholism is currently the most common cause of symptomatic hypomagnesemia in the United States. It is particularly troublesome during treatment of alcohol withdrawal. Therefore, the serum magnesium level should be measured every 2 or 3 days in patients going through withdrawal from alcohol. The serum magnesium level may be normal on admission but fall as a result of metabolic changes, such as the intracellular shift of magnesium associated with IV glucose administration.

During nutritional repletion, the major cellular electrolytes move from the serum to newly synthesized cells. Thus, if the enteral or parenteral feeding formula is deficient in magnesium content, serious hypomagnesemia will occur. Because of this, serum magnesium levels should be measured at regular intervals during the administration of TPN and enteral feedings, especially to patients who have undergone a period of starvation. Other causes of hypomagnesemia include the administration of aminoglycosides, cyclosporine, cisplatin, diuretics, digitalis, and amphotericin and the rapid administration of citrated blood, especially to patients with renal or hepatic disease. Magnesium deficiency often occurs in diabetic ketoacidosis, secondary to increased renal excretion during osmotic diuresis and shifting of magnesium into the cells with insulin therapy. Other contributing causes are sepsis, burns, and hypothermia.

Clinical Manifestations

Clinical manifestations of hypomagnesemia are largely confined to the neuromuscular system. Some of the effects are due directly to the low serum magnesium level; others are due to secondary changes in potassium and calcium metabolism. Symptoms do not usually occur until the serum magnesium level is less than 1 mEq/L (SI: 0.5 mmol/L).

Among the neuromuscular changes are hyperexcitability with muscle weakness, tremors, and athetoid movements (slow, involuntary twisting and writhing). Others include tetany, generalized tonic-clonic or focal seizures, laryngeal stridor, and positive Chvostek's and Trousseau's signs (see earlier discussion on p. 222 of this chapter), which occur in part because of accompanying hypocalcemia.

Magnesium deficiency can disturb the ECG by prolonging the QRS, depressing the ST segment, and predisposing to cardiac dysrhythmias, such as premature ventricular contractions, supraventricular tachycardia, torsades de pointes (a form of ventricular tachycardia), and ventricular fibrillation. Increased susceptibility to digitalis toxicity is associated with low serum magnesium levels. This is important because patients receiving digoxin are also likely to be receiving diuretic therapy, predisposing them to renal loss of magnesium.

Hypomagnesemia may be accompanied by marked alterations in mood. Apathy, depression, apprehension, or extreme agitation have been noted, as well as ataxia, dizziness, insomnia, and confusion. At times, delirium, auditory or visual hallucinations, and frank psychoses may occur.

Assessment and Diagnostic Findings

On laboratory analysis, the serum magnesium level is less than 1.5 mEq/L or 1.8 mg/dL (SI: 0.75 mmol/L). Hypomagnesemia is frequently associated with hypokalemia and hypocalcemia. About 25% of magnesium is protein-bound, principally to albumin. A decreased serum albumin level can, therefore, reduce the measured total magnesium concentration; however, it does not reduce the ionized plasma magnesium concentration. ECG evaluations reflect magnesium, calcium, and potassium deficiencies, tachydysrhythmias, prolonged PR and QT intervals, widening QRS, ST segment depression, flattened T waves, and a prominent U wave. Torsades de pointes is associated with a low magnesium level. Premature ventricular contractions, paroxysmal atrial tachycardia, and heart block may also occur. Urinary magnesium levels may be helpful in identifying causes of magnesium depletion and are measured after a loading dose of magnesium sulfate. Two new diagnostic techniques (nuclear magnetic resonance spectroscopy and the ion selective electrode) are sensitive and direct means to measure ionized serum magnesium levels.

Medical Management

Mild magnesium deficiency can be corrected by diet alone. Principal dietary sources of magnesium are green leafy vegetables, nuts, legumes, whole grains, and seafood. Magnesium is also plentiful in peanut butter and chocolate. When necessary, magnesium salts can be administered orally to replace continuous excessive losses. Diarrhea is a common complication of excessive ingestion of magnesium. Patients receiving TPN require magnesium in the IV solution to prevent hypomagnesemia. IV administration of magnesium sulfate must be given by an infusion pump and at a rate not to exceed 150 mg/min. A bolus dose of magnesium sulfate given too rapidly can produce cardiac arrest. Vital signs must be assessed frequently during magnesium administration to detect changes in cardiac rate or rhythm, hypotension, and respiratory distress. Monitoring urine output is essential before, during, and after magnesium administration; the physician is notified if urine volume decreases to less than 100 mL over 4 hours. Calcium gluconate must be readily available to treat hypocalcemic tetany or hypermagnesemia.

Overt symptoms of hypomagnesemia are treated with parenteral administration of magnesium. Magnesium sulfate is the most commonly used magnesium salt. Serial magnesium concentrations can be used to regulate the dosage.

Nursing Management

The nurse should be aware of patients at risk for hypomagnesemia and observe for its presence. Patients receiving digitalis are monitored closely because a deficit of magnesium can predispose them to digitalis toxicity. When hypomagnesemia is severe, seizure precautions are implemented. Other safety precautions are instituted, as indicated, if confusion is present.

Because difficulty in swallowing (dysphagia) may occur in magnesium-depleted patients, the ability to swallow should be tested with water before oral medications or foods are offered. Dysphagia is probably related to the athetoid or choreiform (rapid, involuntary, and irregular jerking) movements associated with magnesium deficit.

Teaching plays a major role in the treatment of magnesium deficit, particularly that resulting from misuse of diuretic or laxative medications. In such cases, the nurse can instruct the patient about the need to consume magnesium-rich foods. For patients experiencing hypomagnesemia from misuse of alcohol, the nurse can provide teaching, counseling, support, and possible referral to alcohol abstinence programs or other professional help.

To determine neuromuscular irritability, the nurse needs to assess and grade deep tendon reflexes (see Chap. 56 for discussion of assessment and grading reflexes).

Magnesium Excess (Hypermagnesemia)

Hypermagnesemia refers to a greater-than-normal serum concentration of magnesium. A serum magnesium level can appear falsely elevated when blood specimens are allowed to hemolyze or are drawn from an extremity with an excessively tight tourniquet.

By far the most common cause of hypermagnesemia is renal failure. In fact, most patients with advanced renal failure have at least a slight elevation in serum magnesium levels. This condition is aggravated when such patients receive magnesium to control seizures or inadvertently take one of the many commercial antacids that contain magnesium salts.

Hypermagnesemia can occur in a patient with untreated diabetic ketoacidosis when catabolism causes the release of cellular magnesium that cannot be excreted because of profound fluid volume depletion and resulting oliguria. An excess of magnesium can also result from excessive magnesium administered to treat eclampsia and to lower serum magnesium levels. Increased serum magnesium levels can also occur in adrenocortical insufficiency, Addison's disease, or hypothermia. Excessive use of antacids (ie, Maalox, Riopan) and laxatives (Milk of Magnesia) also increases serum magnesium levels.

Clinical Manifestations

Acute elevation of the serum magnesium level depresses the central nervous system as well as the peripheral neuromuscular junction. At mildly elevated levels, there is a tendency for lowered blood pressure because of peripheral vasodilation. Nausea, vomiting, soft-tissue calcifications, facial flushing, and sensations of warmth may also occur. At higher magnesium concentrations, lethargy, difficulty speaking (dysarthria), and drowsiness can occur. Deep tendon reflexes are lost, and muscle weakness and paralysis may develop. The respiratory center is depressed when serum magnesium levels exceed 10 mEq/L (SI: 5 mmol/L). Coma, atrioventricular heart block, and cardiac arrest can occur when the serum magnesium level is greatly elevated and left untreated.

Assessment and Diagnostic Findings

On laboratory analysis, the serum magnesium level is greater than 2.5 mEq/L or 3.0 mg/dL (SI: 1.25 mmol/L). ECG findings may include a prolonged PR interval, tall T waves, and a widened QRS. ECG findings demonstrate a prolonged QT interval and atrioventricular blocks.

Medical Management

Hypermagnesemia can be prevented by avoiding administration of magnesium to patients with renal failure and by carefully monitoring seriously ill patients who are receiving magnesium salts. In patients with severe hypermagnesemia, all parenteral and oral magnesium salts are discontinued. In emergencies, such as respiratory depression or defective cardiac conduction, ventilatory support and IV calcium are indicated. In addition, hemodialysis with a magnesium-free dialysate can reduce the serum magnesium to a safe level within hours. Loop diuretics and 0.45% sodium chloride (half-strength saline) solution enhance magnesium excretion in patients with adequate renal function. IV calcium gluconate (10 mL of a 10% solution) antagonizes the neuromuscular effects of magnesium.

Nursing Management

Patients at risk for hypermagnesemia are identified and assessed. When hypermagnesemia is suspected, the nurse monitors the vital signs, noting hypotension and shallow respirations. The nurse also observes for decreased patellar reflexes and changes in the level of consciousness. Medications that contain magnesium are not given to patients with renal failure or compromised renal function, and patients with renal failure are cautioned to check with their health care providers before taking over-the-counter medications. Caution is essential when magnesium-containing fluids are prepared and administered parenterally because parenteral magnesium solutions are packaged in containers of various sizes (eg, 2-mL ampules or 50-mL vials).

Significance of Phosphorus

Phosphorus is a critical constituent of all the body's tissues. It is essential to the function of muscle and red blood cells, the formation of adenosine triphosphate (ATP) and 2,3-diphosphoglycerate, and the maintenance of acid–base balance, as well as to the nervous system and the intermediary metabolism of carbohydrate, protein, and fat. The normal serum phosphorus level is

2.5 to 4.5 mg/dL (SI: 0.8–1.5 mmol/L) and may be as high as 6 mg/dL (SI: 1.94 mmol/L) in infants and children. Serum phosphorus levels are presumably greater in children because of the high rate of skeletal growth. Phosphorus is the primary anion of the ICF. About 85% of phosphorus is located in bones and teeth, 14% in soft tissue, and less than 1% in the ECF. Phosphorus is critical to nerve and muscle function and provides structural support to bones and teeth. Phosphorus levels decrease with age.

Phosphorus Deficit (Hypophosphatemia)

Hypophosphatemia is a below-normal serum concentration of inorganic phosphorus. Although it often indicates phosphorus deficiency, hypophosphatemia may occur under a variety of circumstances in which total body phosphorus stores are normal. Conversely, phosphorus deficiency is an abnormally low content of phosphorus in lean tissues and may exist in the absence of hypophosphatemia.

Hypophosphatemia may occur during the administration of calories to patients with severe protein-calorie malnutrition. It is most likely to occur with overzealous intake or administration of simple carbohydrates. This syndrome can be induced in anyone with severe protein-calorie malnutrition (eg, patients with anorexia nervosa or alcoholism, or elderly debilitated patients unable to eat). As many as 50% of patients hospitalized because of chronic alcoholism have hypophosphatemia.

Marked hypophosphatemia may develop in malnourished patients who receive TPN if the phosphorus loss is not adequately corrected. Other causes of hypophosphatemia include prolonged intense hyperventilation, alcohol withdrawal, poor dietary intake, diabetic ketoacidosis, and major thermal burns. Low magnesium, low potassium, and hyperparathyroidism related to increased urinary losses of phosphorus contribute to hypophosphatemia. Respiratory alkalosis can cause a decrease in phosphorus because of an intracellular shift of phosphorus.

Excess phosphorus-binding by antacids containing magnesium, calcium, or albumin may decrease the phosphorus available from the diet to amounts below that required to maintain serum phosphorus balance. The degree of hypophosphatemia depends on the amount of phosphorus in the diet compared to the dose of antacid. Vitamin D regulates intestinal ion absorption; therefore, a deficiency of vitamin D may cause decreased calcium and phosphorus levels, which may lead to osteomalacia (softened, brittle bones).

Clinical Manifestations

Most of the signs and symptoms of phosphorus deficiency appear to result from a deficiency of ATP, 2,3-diphosphoglycerate, or both. ATP deficiency impairs cellular energy resources; diphosphoglycerate deficiency impairs oxygen delivery to tissues.

A wide range of neurologic symptoms may occur, such as irritability, fatigue, apprehension, weakness, numbness, paresthesias, confusion, seizures, and coma. Low levels of diphosphoglycerate may reduce the delivery of oxygen to peripheral tissues, resulting in tissue anoxia. Hypoxia then leads to an increase in respiratory rate and respiratory alkalosis, causing phosphorus to move into the cells and potentiating hypophosphatemia.

It is thought that hypophosphatemia predisposes a person to infection. In laboratory animals, hypophosphatemia is associated with depression of the chemotactic, phagocytic, and bacterial activity of granulocytes.

Muscle damage may develop as the ATP level in the muscle tissue declines. Clinical manifestations are muscle weakness, muscle pain, and at times acute rhabdomyolysis (disintegration of striated muscle). Weakness of respiratory muscles may greatly impair ventilation. Hypophosphatemia also may predispose a person to insulin resistance and thus hyperglycemia. Chronic loss of phosphorus can cause bruising and bleeding from platelet dysfunction.

Assessment and Diagnostic Findings

On laboratory analysis, the serum phosphorus level is less than 2.5 mg/dL (SI: 0.80 mmol/L) in adults. When reviewing laboratory results, the nurse should keep in mind that glucose or insulin administration causes a slight decrease in the serum phosphorus level. PTH levels are increased in hyperparathyroidism. Serum magnesium may decrease due to increased urinary excretion of magnesium. Alkaline phosphatase is increased with osteoblastic activity. X-rays may show skeletal changes of osteomalacia or rickets.

Medical Management

Prevention of hypophosphatemia is the goal. In patients at risk for hypophosphatemia, serum phosphate levels should be closely monitored and correction initiated before deficits become severe. Adequate amounts of phosphorus should be added to parenteral solutions, and attention should be paid to the phosphorus levels in enteral feeding solutions.

Severe hypophosphatemia is dangerous and requires prompt attention. Aggressive IV phosphorus correction is usually limited to patients whose serum phosphorus levels fall below 1 mg/dL (SI: 0.3 mmol/L) and whose GI tract is not functioning. Possible dangers of IV phosphorus administration include hypocalcemia and metastatic calcification from hyperphosphatemia. The rate of phosphorus administration should not exceed 10 mEq/h, and the site should be carefully monitored because tissue sloughing and necrosis can occur with infiltration. In less acute situations, oral phosphorus replacement is usually adequate.

Nursing Management

The nurse identifies patients at risk for hypophosphatemia and monitors for it. Because malnourished patients receiving TPN are at risk when calories are introduced too aggressively, preventive measures involve gradually introducing the feeding solution to avoid rapid shifts of phosphorus into the cells.

For patients with documented hypophosphatemia, careful attention is given to preventing infection because hypophosphatemia may alter the granulocytes. In patients requiring correction of phosphorus losses, the nurse frequently monitors serum phosphorus levels and documents and reports early signs of hypophosphatemia (apprehension, confusion, change in level of consciousness).

Phosphorus Excess (Hyperphosphatemia)

Hyperphosphatemia is a serum phosphorus level that exceeds normal. Various conditions can lead to this imbalance, but the most common is renal failure. Other causes include chemotherapy for neoplastic disease, hypoparathyroidism, respiratory acidosis or diabetic ketoacidosis, high phosphate intake, profound muscle necrosis, and increased phosphorus absorption. The primary complication of increased phosphorus is metastatic calcification (soft tissue, joints, and arteries), which results when the calcium–magnesium product (calcium × magnesium) exceeds 70 mg/dL.

Clinical Manifestations

An elevated serum phosphorus level causes few symptoms. Symptoms that do occur usually result from decreased calcium levels and soft-tissue calcifications. The most important short-term consequence is tetany. Because of the reciprocal relationship between phosphorus and calcium, a high serum phosphorus level tends to cause a low serum calcium concentration. Tetany can result, causing tingling sensations in the fingertips and around the mouth. Anorexia, nausea, vomiting, muscle weakness, hyperreflexia, and tachycardia may occur.

The major long-term consequence is soft-tissue calcification, which occurs mainly in patients with reduced glomerular filtration rates. High serum levels of inorganic phosphorus promote precipitation of calcium phosphate in nonosseous sites, decreasing urine output, impairing vision, and producing palpitations.

Assessment and Diagnostic Findings

On laboratory analysis, the serum phosphorus level exceeds 4.5 mg/dL (SI: 1.5 mmol/L) in adults. Serum phosphorus levels are normally higher in children, presumably because of the high rate of skeletal growth. The serum calcium level is useful also for diagnosing the primary problem and assessing the effects of treatments. X-ray studies may show skeletal changes with abnormal bone development. PTH levels are decreased in hypoparathyroidism. BUN and creatinine levels are used to assess renal function.

Medical Management

When possible, treatment is directed at the underlying disorder. For example, hyperphosphatemia related to tumor cell lysis might be lessened by prior administration of allopurinol to prevent urate nephropathy. For patients with renal failure, measures to decrease the serum phosphate level are indicated; these include administering phosphate-binding gels, restricting dietary phosphate, and dialysis.

Nursing Management

The nurse monitors patients at risk for hyperphosphatemia. When a low-phosphorus diet is prescribed, the patient is instructed to avoid phosphorus-rich foods, such as hard cheese, cream, nuts, whole-grain cereals, dried fruits, dried vegetables, kidneys, sardines, sweetbreads, and foods made with milk. When appropriate, the nurse instructs the patient to avoid phosphate-containing substances, such as laxatives and enemas that contain phosphate. The nurse also teaches the patient to recognize the signs of impending hypocalcemia and to monitor for changes in urine output.

Significance of Chloride

Chloride is the major anion of the ECF. It is found more in interstitial and lymph fluid compartments than in blood. Chloride is also contained in gastric and pancreatic juices as well as in sweat. Sodium and chloride in water make up the composition of the ECF and assist in determining osmotic pressure.

The serum level of chloride reflects a change in dilution or concentration of the ECF and does so in direct proportion to sodium. Aldosterone secretion increases sodium reabsorption, thereby increasing chloride reabsorption. The choroid plexus, where cerebrospinal fluid forms in the brain, depends on sodium and chloride to attract water to form the fluid portion of the cerebrospinal fluid. Bicarbonate has an inverse relationship with chloride. As chloride moves from plasma into the red blood cells (called the chloride shift), bicarbonate moves back into the plasma. Hydrogen ions are formed, which then help to release oxygen from hemoglobin. When the level of one of these three electrolytes (sodium, bicarbonate, or chloride) is disturbed, the other two will be affected as well.

Chloride Deficit (Hypochloremia)

Chloride control depends on the intake of chloride and the excretion and reabsorption of its ions in the kidneys. Chloride is produced in the stomach as hydrochloric acid; a small amount of chloride is lost in the feces. Chloride-deficient formulas, salt-restricted diets, GI tube drainage, and severe vomiting and diarrhea are risk factors for hypochloremia. As chloride decreases (usually because of volume depletion), sodium and bicarbonate ions are retained by the kidney to balance the loss. Bicarbonate accumulates in the ECF, which raises the pH and leads to hypochloremic metabolic alkalosis.

Clinical Manifestations

The signs and symptoms of hypochloremia are those of acid–base and electrolyte imbalances. The signs and symptoms of hyponatremia, hypokalemia, and metabolic alkalosis may also be noted. Metabolic alkalosis is a disorder that results in a high pH and a high serum bicarbonate level as a result of excess alkali intake or loss of hydrogen ions. With compensation, the $PaCO_2$ rises up to 50 mm Hg. Hyperexcitability of muscles, tetany, hyperactive deep tendon reflexes, weakness, twitching, and muscle cramps may result. Hypokalemia can cause hypochloremia, resulting in cardiac dysrhythmias. In addition, because low chloride levels parallel low sodium levels, a water excess may occur. Hyponatremia can cause seizures and coma.

Assessment and Diagnostic Findings

The normal serum chloride level is 96 to 106 mEq/L (SI: 96–106 mmol/L). Inside the cell, the chloride level is 4 mEq/L. In addition to the chloride level, sodium and potassium levels are also evaluated because these electrolytes are lost along with chloride. Arterial blood gas analysis identifies the acid–base imbalance, which is usually metabolic alkalosis. The urine chloride level, which is also measured, decreases in hypochloremia.

Medical Management

Treatment involves correcting the cause of hypochloremia and contributing electrolyte and acid–base imbalances. Normal saline (0.9% sodium chloride) or half-strength saline (0.45% sodium chloride) solution is administered IV to replace the chloride. The physician may reevaluate whether patients receiving diuretics (loop, osmotic, or thiazide) should discontinue these medications or change to another diuretic.

Foods high in chloride are provided; these include tomato juice, salty broth, canned vegetables, processed meats, and fruits. A patient who drinks free water (water without electrolytes) or bottled water will excrete large amounts of chloride; therefore, this kind of water should be avoided. Ammonium chloride, an acidifying agent, may be prescribed to treat metabolic alkalosis; the dosage depends on the patient's weight and serum chloride level. This agent is metabolized by the liver, and its effects last for about 3 days.

Nursing Management

The nurse monitors intake and output, arterial blood gas values, and serum electrolyte levels, as well as the patient's level of consciousness and muscle strength and movement. Changes are reported to the physician promptly. Vital signs are monitored and respiratory assessment carried out frequently. The nurse teaches the patient about foods with high chloride content.

Chloride Excess (Hyperchloremia)

Hyperchloremia exists when the serum level exceeds 106 mEq/L (SI: 106 mmol/L). Hypernatremia, bicarbonate loss, and metabolic acidosis can occur with high chloride levels. Hyperchloremic metabolic acidosis is also known as normal anion gap acidosis. It is usually caused by the loss of bicarbonate ions via the kidney or the GI tract with a corresponding increase in chloride ions. Chloride ions in the form of acidifying salts accumulate and acidosis occurs with a decrease in bicarbonate ions.

Clinical Manifestations

The signs and symptoms of hyperchloremia are the same as those of metabolic acidosis, hypervolemia, and hypernatremia. Tachypnea; weakness; lethargy; deep, rapid respirations; diminished cognitive ability; and hypertension occur. If untreated, hyperchloremia can lead to a decrease in cardiac output, dysrhythmias, and coma. A high chloride level is accompanied by a high sodium level and fluid retention.

Assessment and Diagnostic Findings

The serum chloride level is 108 mEq/L (SI: 108 mmol/L) or greater, the serum sodium level is greater than 145 mEq/L (SI: 145 mmol/L), the serum pH is less than 7.35, the serum bicarbonate level is less than 22 mEq/L (SI: 22 mmol/L), and there is a normal anion gap of 8 to 14 mEq/L (SI: 8–14 mmol/L). Urine chloride excretion increases.

Medical Management

Correcting the underlying cause of hyperchloremia and restoring electrolyte, fluid, and acid–base balance are essential. Lactated Ringer's solution may be prescribed to convert lactate to bicarbonate in the liver, which will increase the base bicarbonate level and correct the acidosis. Sodium bicarbonate may be given IV to increase bicarbonate levels, which leads to the renal excretion of chloride ions as bicarbonate and chloride compete for combination with sodium. Diuretics may be administered to eliminate chloride as well. Sodium, fluids, and chloride are restricted.

Nursing Management

Monitoring vital signs, arterial blood gas values, and intake and output is important to assess the patient's status and the effectiveness of treatment. Assessment findings related to respiratory, neurologic, and cardiac systems are documented and changes discussed with the physician. The nurse teaches the patient about the diet that should be followed to manage hyperchloremia.

ACID–BASE DISTURBANCES

Plasma pH is an indicator of hydrogen ion (H^+) concentration. Homeostatic mechanisms keep pH within a normal range (7.35–7.45). These mechanisms consist of buffer systems, the kidneys, and the lungs. The H^+ concentration is extremely important: the greater the concentration, the more acidic the solution and the lower the pH. The lower the H^+ concentration, the more alkaline the solution and the higher the pH. The pH range compatible with life (6.8–7.8) represents a tenfold difference in H^+ concentration in plasma.

Buffer Systems

Buffer systems prevent major changes in the pH of body fluids by removing or releasing H^+; they can act quickly to prevent excessive changes in H^+ concentration. Hydrogen ions are buffered by both intracellular and extracellular buffers. The body's major extracellular buffer system is the bicarbonate–carbonic acid buffer system. This is the system that is assessed when arterial blood gases are measured. Normally, there are 20 parts of bicarbonate (HCO_3^-) to one part of carbonic acid (H_2CO_3). If this ratio is altered, the pH will change. It is the ratio of HCO_3^- to H_2CO_3 that is important in maintaining pH, not absolute values. Carbon dioxide (CO_2) is a potential acid; when dissolved in water, it becomes carbonic acid ($CO_2 + H_2O = H_2CO_3$). Thus, when CO_2 is increased, the carbonic acid content is also increased, and vice versa. If either bicarbonate or carbonic acid is increased or decreased so that the 20 : 1 ratio is no longer maintained, acid–base imbalance results.

Less important buffer systems in the ECF include the inorganic phosphates and the plasma proteins. Intracellular buffers include proteins, organic and inorganic phosphates, and, in red blood cells, hemoglobin.

Kidneys

The kidneys regulate the bicarbonate level in the ECF; they can regenerate bicarbonate ions as well as reabsorb them from the renal tubular cells. In respiratory acidosis and most cases of metabolic acidosis, the kidneys excrete hydrogen ions and conserve bicarbonate ions to help restore balance. In respiratory and metabolic alkalosis, the kidneys retain hydrogen ions and excrete bicarbonate ions to help restore balance. The kidneys obviously cannot compensate for the metabolic acidosis created by renal failure. Renal compensation for imbalances is relatively slow (a matter of hours or days).

Lungs

The lungs, under the control of the medulla, control the CO_2 and thus the carbonic acid content of the ECF. They do so by adjusting ventilation in response to the amount of CO_2 in the blood. A rise in the partial pressure of CO_2 in arterial blood ($PaCO_2$) is a powerful stimulant to respiration. Of course, the partial pressure of oxygen in arterial blood (PaO_2) also influences respiration. Its effect, however, is not as marked as that produced by the $PaCO_2$.

In metabolic acidosis, the respiratory rate increases, causing greater elimination of CO_2 (to reduce the acid load). In metabolic alkalosis, the respiratory rate decreases, causing CO_2 to be retained (to increase the acid load).

Acute and Chronic Metabolic Acidosis (Base Bicarbonate Deficit)

Metabolic acidosis is a clinical disturbance characterized by a low pH (increased H^+ concentration) and a low plasma bicarbonate concentration. It can be produced by a gain of hydrogen ion or a loss of bicarbonate. It can be divided clinically into two forms, according to the values of the serum anion gap: high anion gap acidosis and normal anion gap acidosis. The anion gap reflects normally unmeasured anions (phosphates, sulfates, and proteins) in plasma. Measuring the anion gap is essential in analyzing acid–base disorders correctly. The anion gap can be calculated by subtracting the sum of the serum chloride and bicarbonate concentrations (anions, or negatively charged electrolytes) from the serum sodium level (a cation, or positively charged electrolyte) as follows:

$$\text{Anion gap} = Na^+ + K^+ - (Cl^- + HCO_3^-)$$

The normal value for an anion gap is 8 to 16 mEq/L (SI: 8–16 mmol/L). The unmeasured anions in the serum normally account for less than 16 mEq/L of the anion production. An anion gap greater than 16 mEq (SI: 16 mmol/L) suggests excessive accumulation of unmeasured anions.

Normal anion gap acidosis results from the direct loss of bicarbonate, as in diarrhea, lower intestinal fistulas, ureterostomies, and use of diuretics; early renal insufficiency; excessive administration of chloride; and the administration of parenteral nutrition without bicarbonate or bicarbonate-producing solutes (ie, lactate). Normal anion gap acidosis is also referred to as hyperchloremic acidosis.

High anion gap acidosis results from excessive accumulation of fixed acid. If it is increased to 30 mEq/L (SI: 30 mmol/L) or more, then a high anion gap metabolic acidosis is present regardless of what the pH and the HCO_3^- are. It occurs in ketoacidosis, lactic acidosis, the late phase of salicylate poisoning, uremia, methanol or ethylene glycol toxicity, and ketoacidosis with starvation. The hydrogen is buffered by HCO_3^-, causing the bicarbonate concentration to fall. In all of these instances, abnormally high levels of anions flood the system, increasing the anion gap above normal limits.

Clinical Manifestations

Signs and symptoms of metabolic acidosis vary with the severity of the acidosis. They may include headache, confusion, drowsiness, increased respiratory rate and depth, nausea, and vomiting. Peripheral vasodilation and decreased cardiac output occur when the pH falls below 7. Additional physical assessment findings include decreased blood pressure, cold and clammy skin, dysrhythmias, and shock.

Chronic metabolic acidosis is usually seen with chronic renal failure. The bicarbonate and pH decrease slowly; thus, the patient is asymptomatic until the bicarbonate is approximately 15 mEq/L or less.

Assessment and Diagnostic Findings

Arterial blood gas measurements are valuable in diagnosing metabolic acidosis. Expected blood gas changes include a low bicarbonate level (less than 22 mEq/L) and a low pH (less than 7.35). The cardinal feature of metabolic acidosis is a decrease in the serum bicarbonate level. Hyperkalemia may accompany metabolic acidosis as a result of the shift of potassium out of the cells. Later, as the acidosis is corrected, potassium moves back into the cells and hypokalemia may occur. Hyperventilation decreases the CO_2 level as a compensatory action. As stated previously, calculation of the anion gap is helpful in determining the cause of metabolic acidosis. An ECG will detect dysrhythmias caused by the increased potassium.

Medical Management

Treatment is directed at correcting the metabolic defect. If the problem results from excessive intake of chloride, treatment is aimed at eliminating the source of the chloride. When necessary, bicarbonate is administered if the pH is less than 7.1 and the bicarbonate level is less than 10. Although hyperkalemia occurs with acidosis, hypokalemia may occur with reversal of the acidosis and subsequent movement of potassium back into the cells. Therefore, the serum potassium level is monitored closely and hypokalemia is corrected as acidosis is reversed.

In chronic metabolic acidosis, low serum calcium levels are treated before treating chronic metabolic acidosis to avoid tetany resulting from an increase in pH and a decrease in ionized calcium. Treatment modalities may include alkalizing agents and hemodialysis or peritoneal dialysis.

Acute and Chronic Metabolic Alkalosis (Base Bicarbonate Excess)

Metabolic alkalosis is a clinical disturbance characterized by a high pH (decreased H^+ concentration) and a high plasma bicarbonate concentration. It can be produced by a gain of bicarbonate or a loss of H^+.

Probably the most common cause of metabolic alkalosis is vomiting or gastric suction with loss of hydrogen and chloride ions. The disorder also occurs in pyloric stenosis, in which only gastric fluid is lost. Gastric fluid has an acid pH (usually 1–3); therefore, loss of this highly acidic fluid increases the alkalinity of body fluids. Other situations predisposing to metabolic alkalosis include those associated with loss of potassium, such as diuretic therapy that promotes excretion of potassium (eg, thiazides, furosemide), and excessive adrenocorticoid hormones (as in hyperaldosteronism and Cushing's syndrome).

Hypokalemia produces alkalosis in two ways: (1) the kidneys conserve potassium, and thus H^+ excretion increases; and (2) cellular potassium moves out of the cells into the ECF in an attempt to maintain near-normal serum levels (as potassium ions leave the cells, hydrogen ions must enter to maintain electroneutrality). Excessive alkali ingestion from antacids containing bicarbonate or from using sodium bicarbonate during cardiopulmonary resuscitation can also cause metabolic alkalosis.

Chronic metabolic alkalosis can occur with long-term diuretic therapy (thiazides or furosemide), villous adenoma, external drainage of gastric fluids, significant potassium depletion, cystic fibrosis, and the chronic ingestion of milk and calcium carbonate.

Clinical Manifestations

Alkalosis is primarily manifested by symptoms related to decreased calcium ionization, such as tingling of the fingers and toes, dizziness, and hypertonic muscles. The ionized fraction of serum calcium decreases in alkalosis as more calcium combines with serum proteins. Because it is the ionized fraction of calcium that influences neuromuscular activity, symptoms of hypocalcemia are often the predominant symptoms of alkalosis. Respirations are depressed as a compensatory action by the lungs. Atrial tachycardias may occur. As the pH increases above 7.6 and hypokalemia develops, ventricular disturbances may occur. Decreased motility and paralytic ileus may also occur.

Symptoms of chronic metabolic alkalosis are the same as for acute metabolic alkalosis, and as potassium decreases, frequent premature ventricular contractions or U waves are seen on the ECG.

Assessment and Diagnostic Findings

Evaluation of arterial blood gases reveals a pH greater than 7.45 and a serum bicarbonate concentration greater than 26 mEq/L. The $PaCO_2$ increases as the lungs attempt to compensate for the excess bicarbonate by retaining CO_2. This hypoventilation is more pronounced in semiconscious, unconscious, or debilitated patients than in alert patients. The former may develop marked hypoxemia as a result of hypoventilation. Hypokalemia may accompany metabolic alkalosis.

Urinary chloride levels may help to identify the cause of metabolic alkalosis if the patient's history provides inadequate information. Metabolic alkalosis is the setting in which urine chloride concentration may be a more accurate estimate of volume than is the urine sodium concentration. Urine chloride concentrations help to differentiate between vomiting or diuretic ingestion or one of the causes of mineralocorticoid excess. Hypovolemia and hypochloremia in patients with vomiting or cystic fibrosis, those receiving nutritional repletion, or those taking diuretics produce urine chloride concentrations less than 25 mEq/L. Signs of hypovolemia are not present and the urine chloride concentration exceeds 40 mEq/L in patients with mineralocorticoid excess or alkali loading; these patients usually have expanded fluid volume. The urine chloride concentration should be less than 15 mEq/L when decreased chloride levels and hypovolemia occur.

Medical Management

Treatment aims at reversing the underlying disorder. Sufficient chloride must be supplied for the kidney to absorb sodium with chloride (allowing the excretion of excess bicarbonate). Treatment also includes restoring normal fluid volume by administering sodium chloride fluids (because continued volume depletion serves to maintain the alkalosis). In patients with hypokalemia, potassium is administered as KCl to replace both K^+ and Cl^- losses. Histamine-2 receptor antagonists, such as cimetidine (Tagamet), reduce the production of gastric HCl, thereby decreasing the metabolic alkalosis associated with gastric suction. Carbonic anhydrase inhibitors are useful in treating metabolic alkalosis in patients who cannot tolerate rapid volume expansion (eg, patients with congestive heart failure). Because of volume depletion from GI loss, intake and output must be monitored carefully. Management of chronic metabolic alkalosis is aimed at correcting the underlying acid–base disorder.

Acute and Chronic Respiratory Acidosis (Carbonic Acid Excess)

Respiratory acidosis is a clinical disorder in which the pH is less than 7.35 and the $PaCO_2$ is greater than 42 mm Hg. It may be either acute or chronic.

Respiratory acidosis is always due to inadequate excretion of CO_2 with inadequate ventilation, resulting in elevated plasma CO_2 levels and thus elevated carbonic acid (H_2CO_3) levels. In addition to an elevated $PaCO_2$, hypoventilation usually causes a decrease in PaO_2. Acute respiratory acidosis occurs in emergency situations, such as acute pulmonary edema, aspiration of a foreign object, atelectasis, pneumothorax, overdosage of sedatives, sleep apnea syndrome, administration of oxygen to a patient with chronic hypercapnia (excessive CO_2 in the blood), severe pneumonia, and acute respiratory distress syndrome. Respiratory acidosis can also occur in diseases that impair respiratory muscles, such as muscular dystrophy, myasthenia gravis, and Guillain-Barré syndrome.

Mechanical ventilation can be associated with hypercapnia if the rate of effective alveolar ventilation is inadequate. Ventilation is fixed in these patients, and CO_2 may be retained if the rate of CO_2 production is increased.

Clinical Manifestations

Clinical signs in acute and chronic respiratory acidosis vary. Sudden hypercapnia (elevated $PaCO_2$) can cause increased pulse and respiratory rate, increased blood pressure, mental cloudiness, and feeling of fullness in the head. An elevated $PaCO_2$ causes cerebrovascular vasodilation and increased cerebral blood flow, particularly when it is higher than 60 mm Hg. Ventricular fibrillation may be the first sign of respiratory acidosis in anesthetized patients.

If respiratory acidosis is severe, intracranial pressure may increase, resulting in papilledema and dilated conjunctival blood vessels. Hyperkalemia may result as hydrogen concentration overwhelms the compensatory mechanisms and moves into cells, causing a shift of potassium out of the cell.

Chronic respiratory acidosis occurs with pulmonary diseases such as chronic emphysema and bronchitis, obstructive sleep apnea, and obesity. As long as the $PaCO_2$ does not exceed the body's ability to compensate, the patient will be asymptomatic. However, if the $PaCO_2$ rises rapidly, cerebral vasodilation will increase intracranial pressure; cyanosis and tachypnea will develop. Patients with chronic obstructive pulmonary disease who gradually accumulate CO_2 over a prolonged period (days to months) may not develop symptoms of hypercapnia because compensatory renal changes have had time to occur.

Nursing Alert *When the $PaCO_2$ is chronically above 50 mm Hg, the respiratory center becomes relatively insensitive to CO_2 as a respiratory stimulant, leaving hypoxemia as the major drive for respiration. Oxygen administration may remove the stimulus of hypoxemia, and the patient develops "carbon dioxide narcosis" unless the situation is quickly reversed. Therefore, oxygen is only administered with extreme caution.*

Assessment and Diagnostic Findings

Arterial blood gas evaluation reveals a pH less than 7.35, a $PaCO_2$ greater than 42 mm Hg, and a variation in the bicarbonate level, depending on the duration of the acidosis in acute respiratory acidosis. When compensation (renal retention of bicarbonate) has fully occurred, the arterial pH may be within the lower limits of normal. Depending on the cause of respiratory acidosis, other diagnostic measures would include serum electrolyte evaluation, chest x-ray for determining any respiratory disease, and a drug screen if an overdose is suspected. An ECG to identify any cardiac involvement as a result of chronic obstructive pulmonary disease may be indicated as well.

Medical Management

Treatment is directed at improving ventilation; exact measures vary with the cause of inadequate ventilation. Pharmacologic agents are used as indicated. For example, bronchodilators help reduce bronchial spasm, antibiotics are used for respiratory infections, and thrombolytics or anticoagulants are used for pulmonary emboli.

Pulmonary hygiene measures are initiated, when necessary, to clear the respiratory tract of mucus and purulent drainage. Adequate hydration (2–3 L/day) is indicated to keep the mucous membranes moist and thereby facilitate the removal of secretions. Supplemental oxygen is used as necessary.

Mechanical ventilation, used appropriately, may improve pulmonary ventilation. Inappropriate mechanical ventilation (eg, increased dead space, insufficient rate or volume settings, high fraction of inspired oxygen [FiO_2] with excessive CO_2 production) may cause such rapid excretion of CO_2 that the kidneys will be unable to eliminate excess bicarbonate quickly enough to prevent alkalosis and seizures. For this reason, the elevated $PaCO_2$ must be decreased slowly. Placing the patient in a semi-Fowler's position facilitates expansion of the chest wall. Treatment of chronic respiratory acidosis is the same as for acute respiratory acidosis.

Acute and Chronic Respiratory Alkalosis (Carbonic Acid Deficit)

Respiratory alkalosis is a clinical condition in which the arterial pH is greater than 7.45 and the $PaCO_2$ is less than 38 mm Hg. As with respiratory acidosis, acute and chronic conditions can occur.

Respiratory alkalosis is always due to hyperventilation, which causes excessive "blowing off" of CO_2 and, hence, a decrease in the plasma carbonic acid concentration. Causes can include extreme anxiety, hypoxemia, the early phase of salicylate intoxication, gram-negative bacteremia, and inappropriate ventilator settings that do not match the patient's requirements.

Chronic respiratory alkalosis results from chronic hypocapnia, and decreased serum bicarbonate levels are the consequence. Chronic hepatic insufficiency and cerebral tumors are predisposing factors.

Clinical Manifestations

Clinical signs consist of lightheadedness due to vasoconstriction and decreased cerebral blood flow, inability to concentrate, numbness and tingling from decreased calcium ionization, tinnitus, and at times loss of consciousness.

Assessment and Diagnostic Findings

Analysis of arterial blood gases assists in the diagnosis of respiratory alkalosis. In the acute state, the pH is elevated above normal as a result of a low $PaCO_2$ and a normal bicarbonate level. (The kidneys cannot alter the bicarbonate level quickly.) In the compensated state, the kidneys have had sufficient time to lower the bicarbonate level to a near-normal level. Evaluation of serum electrolytes is indicated to identify any decrease in potassium as hydrogen is pulled out of the cells in exchange for potassium; decreased calcium, as severe alkalosis inhibits calcium ionization, resulting in carpopedal spasms and tetany; or decreased phosphate due to alkalosis, causing an increased uptake of phosphate by the cells. A toxicology screen should be performed to rule out salicylate intoxication.

Patients with chronic respiratory alkalosis are usually asymptomatic, and the diagnostic evaluation and plan of care are the same as for acute respiratory alkalosis.

Medical Management

Treatment depends on the underlying cause of respiratory alkalosis. If the cause is anxiety, the patient is instructed to breathe more slowly to allow CO_2 to accumulate or to breathe into a closed system (such as a paper bag). A sedative may be required to relieve hyperventilation in very anxious patients. Treatment for other causes of respiratory alkalosis is directed at correcting the underlying problem.

Mixed Acid–Base Disorders

At times patients can simultaneously experience two or more independent acid–base disorders. A normal pH in the presence of changes in the $PaCO_2$ and plasma HCO_3^- concentration immediately suggests a mixed disorder. The only mixed disorder that cannot occur is a mixed respiratory acidosis and alkalosis, because it is impossible to have alveolar hypoventilation and hyperventilation at the same time. An example of a mixed disorder is the simultaneous occurrence of metabolic acidosis and respiratory acidosis during respiratory and cardiac arrest.

Compensation

Generally, the pulmonary and renal systems compensate for each other to return the pH to normal. In a single acid–base disorder, the system not causing the problem will try to compensate by returning the ratio of bicarbonate to carbonic acid to the normal 20:1. The lungs compensate for metabolic disturbances by changing CO_2 excretion. The kidneys compensate for respiratory disturbances by altering bicarbonate retention and H^+ secretion.

In respiratory acidosis, excess hydrogen is excreted in the urine in exchange for bicarbonate ions. In respiratory alkalosis, the renal excretion of bicarbonate increases, and hydrogen ions are retained. In metabolic acidosis, the compensatory mechanisms increase the ventilation rate and the renal retention of bicarbonate.

In metabolic alkalosis, the respiratory system compensates by decreasing ventilation to conserve CO_2 and raise the $PaCO_2$. Because the lungs respond to acid–base disorders within minutes, compensation for metabolic imbalances occurs faster than compensation for respiratory imbalances.

Table 13-7 summarizes compensation effects.

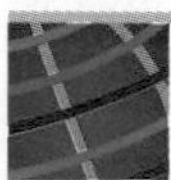

TABLE 13•7 Acid–Base Disturbances and Compensation

Disorder	Initial Event	Compensation
Respiratory acidosis	$\uparrow PaCO_2$, $\uparrow$ or normal HCO_3^-, $\downarrow$ pH	Kidneys eliminate H^+ and retain HCO_3^-
Respiratory alkalosis	$\downarrow PaCO_2$, $\downarrow$ or normal HCO_3^-, $\uparrow$ pH	Kidneys conserve H^+ and excrete HCO_3^-
Metabolic acidosis	$\downarrow$ or normal $PaCO_2$, $\downarrow HCO_3^-$, $\downarrow$ pH	Lungs eliminate CO_2, conserve HCO_3^-
Metabolic alkalosis	$\uparrow$ or normal $PaCO_2$, $\uparrow HCO_3^-$, $\uparrow$ pH	Lungs $\downarrow$ ventilation to $\uparrow PCO_2$, kidneys conserve H^+ to excrete HCO_3^-

Blood Gas Analysis

Blood gas analysis is often used to identify the specific acid–base disturbance and the degree of compensation that has occurred. The analysis is usually based on an arterial blood sample, but when an arterial sample cannot be obtained, a mixed venous sample may be used. Table 13-8 compares normal ranges of venous and arterial blood gas values. See also the accompanying display, Systematic Assessment of Arterial Blood Gases.

PARENTERAL FLUID THERAPY

IV fluid administration is performed both in the hospital and in the home to replace fluids, administer medications, and provide nutrients when no other route is available.

Purpose

The choice of an IV solution depends on the purpose for which it is intended. Generally, IV fluids are administered to achieve one or more of the following goals:

- To provide water, electrolytes, and nutrients to meet daily requirements
- To replace water and correct electrolyte deficits
- To administer medications

IV solutions contain dextrose or electrolytes mixed in various proportions with water. Pure, electrolyte-free water can never be administered IV because it rapidly enters red blood cells and causes them to rupture.

Types of IV Solutions

Solutions are often categorized as **isotonic, hypotonic,** or **hypertonic,** according to whether their total osmolality is the same as, less than, or greater than that of blood (see the section Laboratory Tests for Evaluating Fluid Status for a discussion of osmolality).

Electrolyte solutions are considered isotonic if the total electrolyte content (anions plus cations) is approximately 310 mEq/L. They are considered hypotonic if the total electrolyte content is less than 250 mEq/L and hypertonic if the total electrolyte content exceeds 375 mEq/L. The nurse must also consider a solution's osmolality, keeping in mind that the osmolality of plasma is approximately 300 mOsm/L (SI: 300 mmol/L). For example, a 10% dextrose solution has an osmolality of approximately 505 mOsm/L.

When administering parenteral fluids, then nurse monitors the patient's response to the fluids, considering the fluid volume, the content of the fluid, and the patient's clinical status.

TABLE 13•8 Normal Values: Arterial and Venous Blood

Parameter	Arterial Sample	Venous Sample
pH	7.35–7.45	7.32–7.38
$PaCO_2$	35–45 mm Hg	PCO_2 42–50 mm Hg
PaO_2	80–100 mm Hg	PO_2 40 mm Hg
Oxygen saturation	95%–100%	75%
Base excess or deficit	+ or −2	+ or −2
HCO_3^-	22–26 mEq/L	23–27 Eq/L

Isotonic Fluids

Fluids that are classified as isotonic have a total osmolality close to that of the ECF and do not cause red blood cells to shrink or swell. The composition of these fluids may or may not approximate that of the ECF. Isotonic fluids expand the ECF. One liter of isotonic fluid expands the ECF by 1 L; however, it expands the plasma by only 0.25 L because it is a crystalloid fluid and diffuses quickly into the ECF compartment.

For the same reason, 3 liters of isotonic fluid are needed to replace 1 L of blood loss. Because these fluids expand the intravascular space, patients with hypertension and congestive heart failure should be carefully monitored for signs of fluid overload.

D_5W

A solution of D_5W has a serum osmolality of 252 mOsm/L. Once administered, the glucose is rapidly metabolized, and this initially isotonic solution then disperses as a hypotonic fluid, one-third extracellular and two-thirds intracellular. It is essential to consider this action of D_5W, especially if the patient is at risk for increased intracranial pressure. During fluid resuscitation, this solution should not be used because it can cause hyperglycemia. Therefore, D_5W is used mainly to supply water and to correct an increased serum osmolality. About 1 L of D_5W provides fewer than 200 kcal and is a minor source of calories for the body's daily requirements.

NORMAL SALINE SOLUTION

Normal saline (0.9% sodium chloride) solution has a total osmolality of 308 mOsm/L. Because the osmolality is entirely contributed by electrolytes, the solution remains within the ECF. For this reason, normal saline solution is often used to treat an extracellular volume deficit. Although referred to as normal, it contains only sodium and chloride and does not actually simulate the ECF.

OTHER SOLUTIONS

Several other solutions contain ions in addition to sodium and chloride and are somewhat similar to the ECF in composition. Ringer's solution contains potassium and calcium in addition to sodium chloride. It is used to correct dehydration and sodium depletion and replace GI losses. Lactated Ringer's solution contains bicarbonate precursors as well. These solutions are marketed, with slight variations, under various trade names.

Hypotonic Fluids

One purpose of hypotonic solutions is to replace cellular fluid, because it is hypotonic as compared with plasma. Another is to provide free water for excretion of body wastes. At times, hypotonic sodium solutions are used to treat hypernatremia and other hyperosmolar conditions. Half-strength saline (0.45% sodium chloride) is frequently used. Multiple-electrolyte solutions are also available. Excessive infusions of hypotonic solutions can lead to intravascular fluid depletion, decreased blood pressure, cellular edema, and cell damage. These solutions exert less osmotic pressure than the ECF.

Hypertonic Fluids

When normal saline solution or Ringer's solution contains 5% dextrose, the total osmolality exceeds that of the ECF. The dextrose is quickly metabolized, however, and only the isotonic solution remains. Therefore, any effect on the intracellular compartment is temporary. Similarly, with hypotonic multiple-electrolyte solutions containing 5% dextrose, once the dextrose is metabolized, these solutions disperse as hypotonic fluids.

ASSESSMENT
ARTERIAL BLOOD GASES

The following steps are recommended to evaluate arterial blood gas values. They are based on the assumption that the average values are

$$pH = 7.4$$
$$PaCO_2 = 40 \text{ mm Hg}$$
$$HCO_3^- = 24 \text{ mEq/L}$$

1. *First, look at the pH.* It can be high, low, or normal, as follows:

   pH > 7.4 (alkalosis)
   pH < 7.4 (acidosis)
   pH = 7.4 (normal)

   A normal pH may indicate perfectly normal blood gases, *or* it may be an indication of a *compensated* imbalance. A compensated imbalance is one in which the body has been able to correct the pH by either respiratory or metabolic changes (depending on the primary problem). For example, a patient with primary metabolic acidosis starts out with a low bicarbonate level but a normal CO_2 level. Soon afterward, the lungs try to compensate for the imbalance by exhaling large amounts of CO_2 (hyperventilation). As another example, a patient with primary respiratory acidosis starts out with a high CO_2 level; soon afterward, the kidneys attempt to compensate by retaining bicarbonate. If the compensatory maneuver is able to restore the bicarbonate to carbonic acid ratio back to 20 : 1, full compensation (and thus normal pH) will be achieved.
2. *The next step is to determine the primary cause of the disturbance. This is done by evaluating the $PaCO_2$ and HCO_3^- in relation to the pH.*

   Example: pH > 7.4 (alkalosis)
   a. *If the $PaCO_2$ is <40 mm Hg,* the primary disturbance is respiratory alkalosis. (This situation occurs when a patient hyperventilates and "blows off" too much CO_2. Recall that CO_2 dissolved in water becomes carbonic acid, the acid side of the "carbonic acid–bicarbonate buffer system.")
   b. *If the HCO_3^- is >24 mEq/L,* the primary disturbance is metabolic alkalosis. (This situation occurs when the body gains too much bicarbonate, an alkaline substance. Bicarbonate is the basic or alkaline side of the "carbonic acid–bicarbonate buffer system.")

   Example: pH < 7.4 (acidosis)
   a. *If the $PaCO_2$ is >40 mm Hg,* the primary disturbance is respiratory acidosis. (This situation occurs when a patient hypoventilates and thus retains too much CO_2, an acidic substance.)
   b. *If the HCO_3^- is <24 mEq/L,* the primary disturbance is metabolic acidosis. (This situation occurs when the body's bicarbonate level drops, either because of direct bicarbonate loss or because of gains of acids such as lactic acid or ketones.)
3. *The next step involves determining if compensation has begun.* This is done by looking at the value other than the primary disorder. If it is moving in the same direction as the primary value, compensation is underway. Consider the following gases:

pH	$PaCO_2$	HCO_3^-
(1) 7.20	60 mm Hg	24 mEq/L
(2) 7.40	60 mm Hg	37 mEq/L

The first set (1) indicates acute respiratory acidosis without compensation (the $PaCO_2$ is high, the HCO_3^- is normal). The second set (2) indicates chronic respiratory acidosis. Note that compensation has taken place; that is, the HCO_3^- has elevated to an appropriate level to balance the high $PaCO_2$ and produce a normal pH.

Higher concentrations of dextrose, such as 50% dextrose in water, are administered to help meet calorie requirements. These solutions are strongly hypertonic and must be administered into central veins so that they can be diluted by rapid blood flow.

Saline solutions are also available in osmolar concentrations greater than that of the ECF. These solutions draw water from the ICF to the ECF and cause cells to shrink. If administered rapidly or in large quantity, they may cause an extracellular volume excess and precipitate circulatory overload and dehydration. As a result, these solutions must be administered cautiously and usually only when the serum osmolality has decreased to dangerously low levels. Hypertonic solutions exert an osmotic pressure greater than that of the ECF.

Other IV Substances

When the patient's GI tract cannot accept food, nutritional requirements are often met using the IV route. Parenteral solutions may include high concentrations of glucose, protein, or fat to meet nutritional requirements. The parenteral route may also be used to administer colloids, plasma expanders, and blood products. Examples of blood products include whole blood, packed red blood cells, albumin, and cryoprecipitate.

Many medications are also delivered by the IV route, either by infusion or directly into the vein. Because IV medications enter the circulation rapidly, administration by this route is potentially very hazardous. All medications can produce adverse reactions; however, medications given by the IV route can cause these reactions within 15 minutes after administration because the medications are delivered directly into the bloodstream. Administration rates and recommended dilutions for individual medications are available in specialized texts pertaining to IV medications and in manufacturers' package inserts; these should be consulted to ensure safe IV administration of medications. In addition, the nurse must assess the patient for a history of allergic reactions to medications; although this is important when any medication is to be administered, it is even more important with IV administration.

Nursing Management of the Patient Receiving IV Therapy

Venipuncture, or the ability to gain access to the venous system for administering fluids and medications, is an expected nursing skill in many settings. This responsibility includes selecting the appropriate venipuncture site and type of cannula and being proficient in the technique of vein entry.

Preparing to Administer IV Therapy

Before performing venipuncture, the nurse washes the hands, applies gloves, and informs the patient about the procedure. Next the nurse selects the most appropriate insertion site and type of cannula for a particular patient. Factors influencing these choices include the type of solution to be administered, the expected duration of IV therapy, the patient's general condition, and the availability of veins. The skill of the person initiating the infusion is also an important consideration.

Choosing an IV Site

Many sites can be used for IV therapy, but ease of access and potential hazards vary. Veins of the extremities are designated as peripheral locations and are ordinarily the only sites used by nurses. Because they are relatively safe and easy to enter, arm veins are most commonly used (Fig. 13-7). Leg veins should rarely, if ever, be used because of the high risk of thromboembolism. Additional sites to avoid include veins below a previous IV infiltration or phlebitic area, sclerosed or thrombosed veins, an arm with an arteriovenous shunt or fistula, or an arm affected by edema, infection, blood clot, or skin breakdown. The arm on the side of a mastectomy is avoided because of impaired lymphatic flow.

Central veins frequently used by physicians include the subclavian and internal jugular veins. It is possible to gain access to (or cannulate) these larger vessels even when peripheral sites have collapsed, and they allow for the administration of hyperosmolar solutions. Hazards are much greater, however, and may include inadvertent entry into an artery or the pleural space.

Ideally, both arms and hands are carefully inspected before choosing a specific venipuncture site that does not interfere with mobility. For this reason, the antecubital fossa is avoided, except as a last resort. The most distal site of the arm or hand is generally used first so that subsequent IV access sites can be moved progressively upward. The following are factors to consider when selecting a site for venipuncture:

- Condition of the vein
- Type of fluid or medication to be infused
- Duration of therapy
- Patient's age and size
- Whether the patient is right- or left-handed
- Patient's medical history and current health status
- Skill of the person performing the venipuncture

After applying a tourniquet, the nurse palpates and inspects the vein. The vein should feel firm, elastic, engorged, and round, not hard, flat, or bumpy. Because arteries lie close to veins in the antecubital fossa, the vessel should be palpated for arterial pulsation (even with a tourniquet on), and cannulation of pulsating vessels should be avoided. General guidelines for selecting a cannula include:

- Length: 3/4″ to 1.25″ long
- Diameter: narrow diameter of the cannula to occupy minimal space within the vein.
- Gauge: 20 to 22 gauge for most IV fluids; a larger gauge for caustic or viscous solutions; 18 gauge for blood administration.

Hand veins are easiest to cannulate. Cannula tips should not rest in a flexion area (eg, the antecubital fossa); this would inhibit the IV flow.

Selecting Venipuncture Devices

Equipment used to gain access to the vasculature includes cannulas, needleless IV delivery systems, and peripherally inserted central catheter or midline catheter access lines.

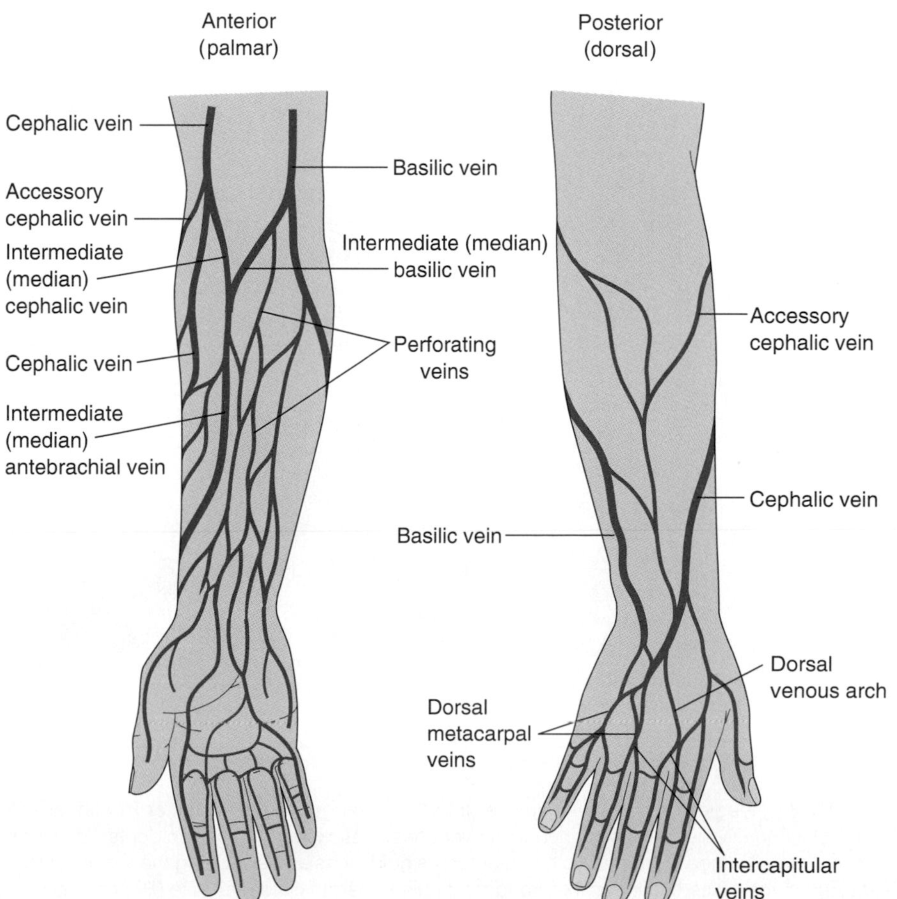

FIGURE 13•7 Sites of parenteral administration. Anterior (palmar) veins at left; posterior (dorsal) veins at right.

CANNULAS

The main types of cannula devices available are those with a steel scalp vein needle (also called a butterfly needle), indwelling plastic cannulas inserted over a steel needle, and indwelling plastic cannulas inserted through a steel needle. Scalp vein or butterfly needles are short steel needles with plastic wing handles. These are easy to insert, but because they are small and nonpliable, infiltration occurs easily. The use of these needles should be limited to bolus injections or infusions lasting only a few hours, as they increase the risk for vein injury and infiltration. Insertion of an over-the-needle catheter requires the additional step of advancing the catheter into the vein after venipuncture. Because these devices are less likely to cause infiltration, they are frequently preferred over scalp vein needles.

Plastic cannulas inserted through a hollow needle are usually called intracatheters. They are available in long lengths and are well suited for placement in central locations. Because insertion requires threading the cannula through the vein for a relatively long distance, these can be difficult to place.

Many types of cannulas are available for IV therapy. Some of the variations in these cannulas include thickness of the cannula wall (affects rate of flow), sharpness of insertion needles (determines needle insertion technique), softening properties of the cannula (influences the length of time the cannula can remain in place), safety features (minimizes risk of needlestick injuries and blood-borne exposure), and the number of lumens (determines the number of solutions that can be infused simultaneously). Cannula systems that help prevent needlesticks and transmission of blood-borne diseases are discussed below.

NEEDLELESS IV DELIVERY SYSTEMS

In an effort to decrease needlestick injuries and exposure to HIV, hepatitis, and other blood-borne pathogens, agencies have implemented needleless IV delivery systems. These systems have built-in protection against accidental needlesticks and provide a safe means of using and disposing of an IV administration set (which consists of tubing, an area for inserting the tubing into the container of IV fluid, and an adapter for connecting the tubing to the needle). Numerous companies produce needleless components. IV line connectors allow the simultaneous infusion of IV medications and other intermittent medications (known as a piggyback delivery) without the use of needles (Fig. 13-8).

PERIPHERALLY INSERTED CENTRAL CATHETER OR MIDLINE CATHETER ACCESS LINES

Patients who need moderate- to long-term parenteral therapy often receive a peripherally inserted central catheter or a midline catheter. These catheters are also used for patients with limited peripheral access (eg, obese people, IV drug users, emaciated patients) who require IV antibiotics, blood, and parenteral nutrition. For these devices to be used, the median cephalic, basilic, and cephalic veins must be pliable (not sclerosed or hardened) and not subject to repeated puncture. If these veins are damaged, then central venous access via the subclavian or internal jugular vein, or surgical placement of an implanted port or a vascular access device, must be considered as an alternative. Table 13-9 compares peripherally inserted central and midline catheter lines.

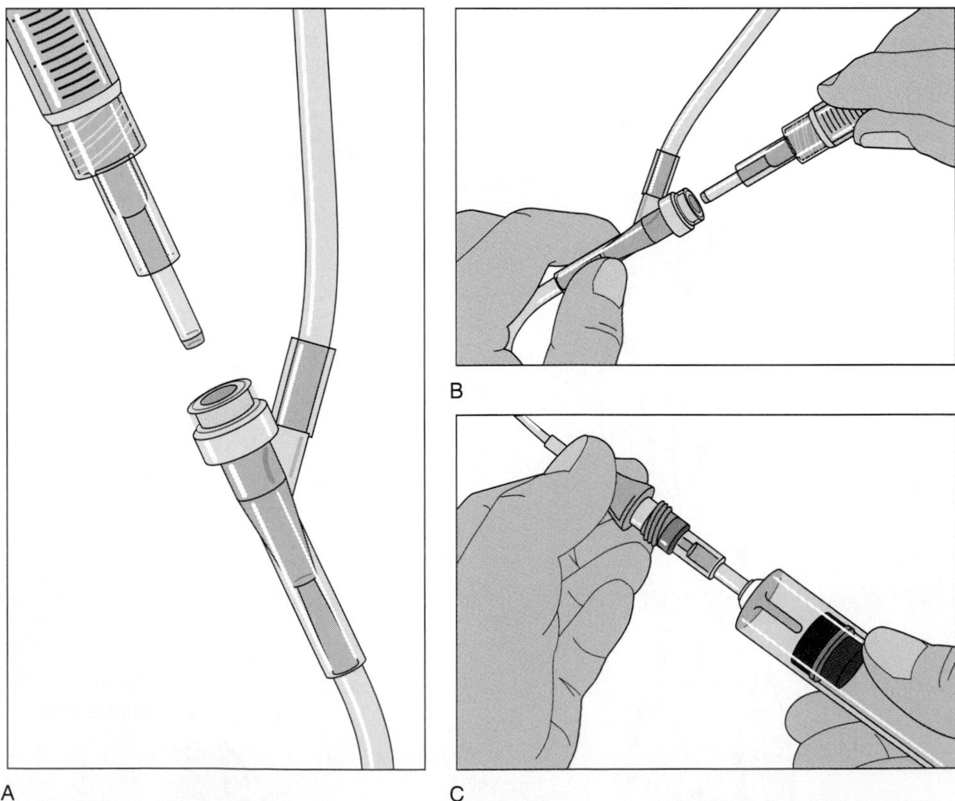

FIGURE 13•8 Needleless IV access device (InterLink Syringe Cannula, Baxter Healthcare Corp., Becton Dickinson Division) (**A**) designed to prevent needlesticks and other accidents. After drawing medication into a syringe according to manufacturer's guidelines and swabbing the Y-site intersection with antiseptic, the nurse can insert the syringe-cannula apparatus into the Y site (**B**) and deliver bolus dose medications. If a blood tube holder (**C**) is attached to the cannula, blood can be withdrawn safely without fear of contact or spills.

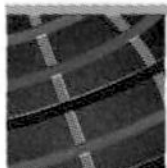

TABLE 13•9 **Comparison of Peripherally Inserted Central and Midline Catheters**

	Peripherally Inserted Central Catheter	Midline Catheter
Indications	Hyperalimentation, pain management, chemotherapeutic agents, antibiotics, intravenous hydration, blood drawing	Antibiotics, IV fluid hydration, removal of blood specimens, peripheral nutrition, pain management infusions
Features	Single- and double-lumen catheters available 40–60 cm long; gauge variable (16–24 g)	Single- and double-lumen catheters available 2 hours postinsertion, the catheter increases 2 gauges in size and 2.5 cm in length. Within 90 minutes of contact with body fluids, the catheter becomes 50× softer.
Material	Radiopaque, polymer (polyurethane), Silastic or aquavene materials	Elastomeric hydrogel
Insertion sites	Venipuncture performed in the antecubital fossa, above or below it into the basilic, cephalic, or axillary veins of the dominant arm. The median basilic is the ideal insertion site.	Venipuncture performed 2–3 fingerbreadths above the antecubital fossa or 1 fingerbreadth below the antecubital fossa into the cephalic, basilic, or median cubital vein
Catheter placement	The tip of the catheter lies in the superior vena cava or the brachiocephalic vein.	Between the antecubital area and the head of the clavicle (tip in axillary region). The tip terminates in the proximal portion of the extremity.
Insertion method	Through the needle technique, with or without a guidewire, breakaway needle with introducer or cannula with introducer (peelaway sheath). (A peripherally inserted central catheter can also be used as a midline catheter.)	No separate guidewire or introducer is needed. Stiff catheter is passed using the catheter advancement tab.
	Insertion can be accomplished at the bedside using sterile technique. Arm to be used should be positioned in abduction to 90 degree angle. Consent is required.	Insertion can be accomplished at the bedside using sterile technique. Arm to be used should be positioned in abduction to 90 degree angle. Consent is required.
	Catheter may stay in place for up to 6 months or as long as required without complications.	Catheter may stay in place for 2–4 weeks.
Potential complications	Malposition, pneumothorax, hemothorax, hydrothorax, dysrhythmias, nerve or tendon damage, respiratory distress, catheter embolism, thrombophlebitis, or catheter occlusion. Compared with centrally placed catheters, venipuncture in the antecubital space reduces risk of insertion complications.	Thrombosis, phlebitis, air embolism, infection, vascular perforation, bleeding, and catheter transection
Contraindications	Dermatitis, cellulitis, burns, high fluid volume infusions, rapid bolus injections, hemodialysis, and venous thrombosis. No clamping of this catheter or splinting of the arm permitted.	Dermatitis, cellulitis, burns, high fluid volume infusions, rapid bolus injection, hemodialysis, and venous thrombosis
Catheter maintenance	Dressing changes according to agency policy and procedure. Generally, dressing changes should be done 2–3 × /week or when wet, soiled, or nonocclusive. Line is flushed with 3 mL normal saline followed by heparin 3 mL (100 U/mL) per lumen every 12 hours.	Dressing changes according to policy and procedures. Generally the dressing should be changed 2–3 × /week, when wet, soiled, or nonocclusive. Line is flushed after each infusion or every 12 hours with 5–10 mL normal saline followed by 1 mL of heparin (100 U/mL). Catheter must be anchored securely, as the line may fall out.
Postplacement	Chest x-ray needed to confirm placement if inserted in superior vena cava.	Chest x-ray to assess placement may be obtained if unable to flush catheter, no free flow blood return, if difficulty with catheter advancement, or if guidewire difficult to remove or bent on removal.
Assessment	Daily measurement of arm circumference (4″ above insertion site) and length of exposed catheter	Daily measurement of arm circumference (4″ above insertion site) and length of exposed catheter
Removal	Catheter should be removed when no longer indicated for use, if contaminated, or if complications occur.	Catheter should be removed when no longer indicated for use, if contaminated, or if complications occur.
	Arm is abducted during removal.	Arm is abducted during removal.
	Pressure is applied on removal with a sterile dressing and antiseptic ointment to site. Dressing is changed every 24 hours until epithelialization occurs.	Pressure is applied on removal with a sterile dressing and antiseptic ointment to site. Dressing is changed every 24 hours until epithelialization occurs.
Advantages	Reduces cost and avoids repeated venipunctures as compared with centrally placed catheters	Reduces cost and avoids repeated venipunctures as compared with centrally placed catheters

The principles for inserting these lines are much the same as those for inserting peripheral catheters; however, their insertion should be undertaken only by those who are experienced and specially skilled in inserting IV lines. (See Resources at the end of the chapter for information about such training.)

The physician prescribes the line and the solution to be infused. Insertion of either line requires sterile technique. The size of the catheter lumen chosen is based on the type of solution, the size of the patient, and the vein to be used. The patient's consent is obtained before use of these catheters. Use of the dominant arm is recommended as the site for inserting the cannula into the superior vena cava to ensure adequate arm movement, which encourages blood flow and reduces the risk of dependent edema.

Teaching the Patient

Except in emergency situations, a patient should be prepared in advance for an IV infusion. The venipuncture, the expected length of infusion, and activity restrictions are explained. Then the patient should have an opportunity to ask questions and voice concerns. For example, some patients believe they will die if small bubbles in the tubing enter their veins. After acknowledging this fear, the nurse can explain that usually only relatively large volumes of air administered rapidly are dangerous.

Preparing the IV Site

Before preparing the skin, the nurse should ask the patient if he or she is allergic to latex and iodine, products commonly used in preparing for IV therapy. Excessive hair at the selected site may be removed by clipping to increase the visibility of the veins and to facilitate insertion of the cannula and adherence of dressings to the IV insertion site. Because infection can be a major complication of IV therapy, the IV device, the fluid, the container, and the tubing must be sterile. The insertion site is scrubbed with a sterile pad soaked in 10% povidone–iodine (Betadine) solution for 2 to 3 minutes, working from the center of the area to the periphery and allowing the area to air day. The site should not be wiped with 70% alcohol because the alcohol negates the effect of the povidone–iodine. (Alcohol pledgets are used for 30 seconds instead, only if the patient is allergic to iodine.) If agency policy dictates, an antibacterial ointment (eg, povidone–iodine) may be applied around the insertion site to serve as a barrier.The nurse must wear nonsterile disposable gloves during the venipuncture procedure because of the likelihood of coming into contact with the patient's blood.

Performing Venipuncture

Guidelines and a suggested sequence for venipuncture are presented in Guideline 13-1. For veins that are very small or particularly fragile, modifications in the technique may be necessary. Alternative methods can be found in journal articles or in specialized textbooks of IV therapy. Institutional policies and procedures determine whether all nurses must be certified to perform venipuncture. A nurse certified in IV therapy or an IV team can be consulted to assist with initiating IV therapy.

Maintaining Therapy

Maintaining an existing IV infusion is a nursing responsibility that demands knowledge of the solutions being administered and the principles of flow. In addition, patients must be assessed carefully for both local and systemic complications.

FACTORS AFFECTING FLOW

The flow of an IV infusion is governed by the same principles that govern fluid movement in general.

- *Flow is directly proportional to the height of the liquid column.* Raising the height of the infusion container may improve a sluggish flow.
- *Flow is directly proportional to the diameter of the tubing.* The clamp on IV tubing regulates the flow by changing the tubing diameter. In addition, the flow is faster through large-gauge rather than small-gauge cannulas.
- *Flow is inversely proportional to the length of the tubing.* Adding extension tubing to an IV line will decrease the flow.
- *Flow is inversely proportional to the viscosity of a fluid.* Viscous IV solutions, such as blood, require a larger cannula than do water or saline solutions.

Monitoring Flow

Because so many factors influence gravity flow, a solution does not necessarily continue to run at the speed originally set. Therefore, the nurse monitors IV infusions frequently to make sure that the fluid is flowing at the intended rate. The IV container should be marked with tape to indicate at a glance whether the correct amount has infused. The flow rate is calculated when the solution is originally started, then monitored at least hourly. To calculate the flow rate, the nurse determines the number of drops delivered per milliliter; this varies with equipment and is usually printed on the administration set packaging. A formula that can be used to calculate the drop rate is:

gtt/mL of given set/60 (min in hour) × total hourly vol. = gtt/min

A variety of infusion pumps are available to assist in IV fluid delivery. These devices allow more accurate administration of fluids and medications than is possible with routine gravity-flow setups. Some pumps have flow rates calibrated in mL/h and are referred to as volumetric pumps. Others are calibrated in drops/min and are referred to as infusion controllers. It is important to read the manufacturer's directions carefully before using any infusion pump or controller, because there are many variations in available models. Use of these devices does not eliminate the need for frequent monitoring of the infusion and the patient.

Discontinuing an Infusion

The removal of an IV catheter is associated with two possible dangers: bleeding and catheter embolism. To prevent excessive bleeding, a dry, sterile sponge should be held over the site as the catheter is removed. Firm pressure is applied until bleeding stops.

If a plastic IV catheter is severed, the loose fragment can travel to the right ventricle and block the blood flow. To detect this complication when the catheter is removed, the nurse compares the expected length of the catheter with its actual length. Plastic catheters should be withdrawn carefully and their length measured to make certain that no fragment has broken off.

Great care must be exercised when using scissors around the dressing site. If the catheter clearly has been severed, the nurse can attempt to occlude the vein above the site by applying a tourniquet to prevent the catheter from entering the central circulation (until surgical removal is possible). As always, however, it is better to prevent a potentially fatal problem than to deal with it after

13•1 GUIDELINES FOR STARTING AN INTRAVENOUS INFUSION

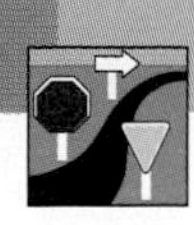

Nursing Action	Rationale
Preparation	
1. Verify order for IV therapy, check solution label, and identify patient.	1. Serious errors can be avoided by careful checking.
2. Explain procedure to patient.	2. Knowledge increases patient comfort and cooperation.
3. Wash hands and put on disposable nonlatex gloves.	3. Asepsis is essential to prevent infection. Prevents exposure of nurse to patient's blood.
4. Apply a tourniquet and identify a suitable vein.	4. This will distend the veins and allow them to be visualized.
5. Choose site.	5. Careful site selection will increase likelihood of successful venipuncture and preservation of vein.
6. Choose IV cannula.	6. Length and gauge of cannula should be appropriate for both site and purpose of infusion.
7. Connect infusion bag and tubing, and run solution through tubing to displace air; cover end of tubing.	7. Prevents delay; equipment must be attached immediately after successful venipuncture to prevent clotting.
8. Raise bed to comfortable working height and position for patient; adjust lighting. Position patient's arm below heart level to encourage capillary filling. Place protective pad on bed under patient's arm.	8. Proper positioning will increase likelihood of success and provide comfort for patient.
Procedure	
1. Depending on agency policy and procedure, lidocaine 1% (without epinephrine) 0.1–0.2 mL may be injected locally to the IV site or a transdermal analgesic cream may be applied to the site 30–60 minutes before IV placement or blood withdrawal.	1. Reduces pain locally from procedure and decreases anxiety about pain.
2. Ask the patient about sensitivity to latex, use blood-pressure cuff rather than latex tourniquet if there is possibility of sensitivity.	2. Prevents allergic reaction.
3. Apply a new tourniquet for each patient or a blood-pressure cuff 15 to 20 cm (6″–8″) above injection site. Palpate for a pulse distal to the tourniquet. Ask patient to open and close fist several times or position patient's arm in a dependent position to distend a vein.	3. The tourniquet distends the vein and makes it easier to enter; it should never be tight enough to occlude arterial flow. If a pulse cannot be palpated distal to the tourniquet, then it is too tight. A new and separate tourniquet should be used for each patient to prevent the transmission of organisms. A blood-pressure cuff may be used for elderly patients to avoid rupture of the veins. A clenched fist encourages the vein to become round and turgid.
4. Ascertain if the patient is allergic to iodine. Prepare site by scrubbing with three povidone–iodine swabs for 2–3 min. in circular motion, moving outward from injection site. Allow to dry. a. If the site elected is excessively hairy, clip hair. (Check agency's policy and procedure about this practice.) b. If the patient is allergic to povidone–iodine, then 70% alcohol is used in its place.	4. Strict asepsis and careful site preparation are essential to prevent infection.
5. With hand not holding the venous access device, steady patient's arm and use finger or thumb to pull skin taut over vessel.	5. Applying traction to the vein helps to stabilize it.
6. Holding needle bevel up and at 25–45 degree angle, depending on the depth of the vein, pierce skin to reach but not penetrate vein.	6. Bevel-up position usually produces less trauma to skin and vein.
7. Decrease angle of needle to 10–20 degrees or until nearly parallel with skin, then enter vein either directly above or from the side in one quick motion.	7. Two-stage procedure decreases chance of thrusting needle through posterior wall of vein as skin is entered.
8. If backflow of blood is visible, straighten angle and advance needle. Additional steps for catheter inserted over needle:	8. Backflow may not occur if vein is small; this position decreases chance of puncturing posterior wall of vein.
a. Advance needle 0.6 cm (¼″) after successful venipuncture.	a. Advancing the needle slightly makes certain the plastic catheter has entered the vein.
b. Hold needle hub, and slide catheter over the needle into the vein. Never reinsert needle into a plastic catheter or pull the catheter back into the needle.	b. Reinsertion of the needle or pulling the catheter back can sever the catheter, causing catheter embolism.
c. Remove needle, while pressing lightly on the skin over the catheter tip; hold catheter hub in place.	c. Slight pressure prevents bleeding before tubing is attached.

(continued)

13•1 Guidelines For Starting an Intravenous Infusion *(Continued)*

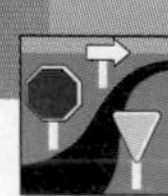

Nursing Action	Rationale
9. Release tourniquet and attach infusion tubing; open clamp enough to allow drip.	9. Infusion must be attached promptly to prevent clotting of blood in cannula. After two unsuccessful attempts at venipuncture, assistance by a more experienced health care provider is recommended.
10. Slip a sterile 2″ × 2″ gauze pad under the catheter hub.	10. The gauze acts as a sterile field.
11. Anchor needle firmly in place with tape.	11. A stable needle is less likely to become dislodged or to irritate the vein.
12. The insertion site is then covered with a bandage or sterile gauze; tape in place with nonallergenic tape but do not encircle extremity.	12. Tape encircling extremity can act as a tourniquet.
13. Tape a small loop of IV tubing onto dressing.	13. The loop decreases the chance of inadvertent cannula removal if the tubing is pulled.
14. Cover the insertion site with a dressing according to hospital policy and procedure. A gauze or transparent dressing may be used.	14. Transparent dressings allow assessment of the insertion site for phlebitis, infiltration, and infection without removing the dressing.
15. Label dressing with type and length of cannula, date, and initials.	15. Labeling facilitates assessment and safe discontinuation.
16. A padded, appropriate-length arm board may be applied to an area of flexion (neurovascular checks should be done frequently).	16. Secures cannula placement and allows correct flow rate (neurovascular checks assess nerve, muscle, and vascular function to be sure function is not affected by immobilization).
17. Calculate infusion rate and regulate flow of infusion.	17. Infusion must be regulated carefully to prevent overinfusion or underinfusion.
18. Document site, cannula size and type, time, solution, IV rate, and patient response to procedure.	18. Documentation is essential to facilitate care and for legal purposes.

it has occurred. Fortunately, catheter embolism can be prevented easily by following simple rules:

- Avoid using scissors near the catheter.
- Avoid withdrawing the catheter through the insertion needle.
- Follow the manufacturer's guidelines carefully (eg, cover the needle point with the bevel shield to prevent the catheter from being severed).

Managing Systemic Complications

IV therapy predisposes the patient to numerous hazards, including both local and systemic complications. Systemic complications occur less frequently but are usually more serious than local complications. They include circulatory overload, air embolism, febrile reaction, and infection.

FLUID OVERLOAD

Overloading the circulatory system with excessive IV fluids causes increased blood pressure and central venous pressure. Signs of fluid overload include moist crackles on auscultation, edema, weight gain, dyspnea, and respirations that are shallow and have an increased rate. Possible causes include rapid infusion of an IV solution or hepatic, cardiac, or renal disease. The risk for fluid overload and subsequent pulmonary edema is especially increased in elderly patients with cardiac disease; this is referred to as circulatory overload.

The treatment for circulatory overload is decreasing the IV rate, monitoring vital signs frequently, assessing breath sounds, and placing the patient in a high Fowler's position. The physician is contacted immediately. This complication can be avoided by using an infusion pump for infusions and by carefully monitoring all infusions. Complications of circulatory overload include congestive heart failure and pulmonary edema.

AIR EMBOLISM

The risk of air embolism is rare but ever-present. It is most often associated with cannulation of central veins. Manifestations of air embolism include dyspnea and cyanosis; hypotension; weak, rapid pulse; loss of consciousness; and chest, shoulder, and low back pain. Treatment calls for immediately clamping the cannula, placing the patient on the left side in the Trendelenburg position, assessing vital signs and breath sounds, and administering oxygen. Air embolism can be prevented by using a Luer-Lok adapter on all lines, filling all tubing completely with solution, and using an air detection alarm on an IV pump. Complications of air embolism include shock and death. The amount of air necessary to induce death in humans is not known; however, the rate of entry is probably as important as the actual volume of air.

SEPTICEMIA AND OTHER INFECTION

Pyrogenic substances in either the infusion solution or the IV administration set can induce a febrile reaction and septicemia. Signs and symptoms include an abrupt temperature elevation shortly after the infusion is started, backache, headache, increased pulse and respiratory rate, nausea and vomiting, diarrhea, chills and shaking, and general malaise. In severe septicemia, vascular collapse and septic shock may occur. Causes of septicemia include contamination of the IV product or a break in aseptic technique, especially in immunocompromised patients. Treatment is symptomatic and includes culturing of the IV cannula, tubing, or solution if suspect and establishing a new IV site for medication or fluid administration. See Chapter 14 for a discussion of septic shock.

Infection ranges in severity from local involvement of the insertion site to systemic dissemination of organisms through the bloodstream, as in septicemia. Measures to prevent infection are essential at the time the IV line is inserted and throughout the entire infusion. Prevention includes:

- Carefully washing one's hands before every contact with any part of the infusion system or patient
- Examining the IV containers for cracks, leaks, or cloudiness, which may indicate a contaminated solution
- Using strict aseptic technique
- Firmly anchoring the IV cannula to prevent to-and-fro motion
- Inspecting the IV site daily and replacing a soiled or wet dressing with a dry sterile dressing
- Removing the IV cannula at the first sign of local inflammation, contamination, or complication
- Replacing the peripheral IV cannula every 48 to 72 hours, or as indicated
- Replacing the IV cannula inserted during emergency conditions (with questionable asepsis) as soon as possible
- With all parenteral nutrition solutions, using a 0.2-micron air-eliminating filter as close to the cannula site as possible to decrease the possibility of an air embolism. The filter should be changed at the same time the entire administration set is changed.
- Replacing the solution bag and administration set in accordance with agency policy and procedure

Managing Local Complications

Local complications of IV therapy include infiltration and extravasation, phlebitis, thrombophlebitis, hematoma, and clotting of the needle.

INFILTRATION AND EXTRAVASATION

Infiltration is the administration of a nonvesicant solution or medication into surrounding tissue. This can occur when the IV cannula dislodges or perforates the wall of the vein. Infiltration is characterized by edema around the insertion site, leakage of IV fluid from the insertion site, discomfort and coolness in the area of infiltration, and a significant decrease in the flow rate. When the solution is particularly irritating, sloughing of tissue may result. Closely monitoring the insertion site is necessary to detect infiltration before it becomes severe.

Infiltration is usually easily recognized if the insertion area is larger than an identical region in the opposite extremity; however, it is not always so obvious. A common misconception is that a backflow of blood into the tubing proves that the catheter is properly placed within the vein. If the catheter tip has pierced the wall of the vessel, however, IV fluid will seep into tissues as well as flow into the vein. Although blood return occurs, infiltration has occurred as well. A more reliable means of confirming infiltration is to apply a tourniquet above or proximal to the infusion site and tighten it enough to restrict venous flow. If the infusion continues to drip despite the venous obstruction, infiltration is present.

As soon as the nurse notes infiltration, the infusion should be stopped, the IV discontinued, and a sterile dressing applied to the site after careful inspection to determine the severity of damage. The infiltration of any amount of blood product, irritant, or vesicant is considered the most severe.

The IV infusion should be started in a new site or proximal to the infiltration if the same extremity is used. A warm compress may be applied to the site if small volumes of noncaustic solutions have infiltrated over a long time, and the affected extremity should be elevated to promote the absorption of fluid. If the infiltration is recent, a cold compress may be applied to the area. Infiltration can be detected and treated early by inspecting the site every hour for redness, pain, edema, blood return, coolness at the site, and IV fluid draining from the IV site. Using the appropriate size and type of cannula for the vein prevents this complication.

Extravasation is similar to infiltration, with an inadvertent administration of vesicant solution or medication into the surrounding tissue. Medications such as dopamine, calcium preparations, and chemotherapeutic agents can cause pain, burning, and redness at the site. Blistering, inflammation, and necrosis of tissues can occur. The extent of tissue damage is determined by the concentration of the medication, the quantity that extravasated, the location of the infusion site, the tissue response, and the duration of the process of extravasation.

The infusion must be stopped and the physician notified promptly. The agency's extravasation protocol is initiated; the protocol may specify specific treatments, including antidotes specific to the medication that extravasated, and may indicate whether the IV line should remain in place or be removed before treatment. The protocol often specifies that the infusion site be infiltrated with an antidote prescribed after assessment by the physician and application of ice initially, followed by warm soaks and elevation of the extremity. This extremity should not be used for further cannula placement. Thorough neurovascular assessments of the affected extremity must be performed frequently.

Checking the institution's IV policy and procedures, incompatibility charts, and with the pharmacist before administering any IV medication, whether given peripherally or centrally, is a prudent way to determine incompatibilities and vesicant potential to prevent extravasation. Careful, frequent monitoring of the IV site, avoiding insertion of IV devices in areas of flexion, securing the IV line, and using the smallest catheter possible that accommodates the vein help minimize the incidence and severity of this complication. In addition, when vesicant medication is administered by IV push, it should be given through a side port of an infusing IV solution to dilute the medication and decrease the severity of tissue damage if extravasation occurs.

PHLEBITIS

Phlebitis is defined as inflammation of a vein related to a chemical or mechanical irritation, or both. It is characterized by a reddened, warm area around the insertion site or along the path of the vein, pain or tenderness at the site or along the vein, and swelling. The incidence of phlebitis increases with the length of time the IV line is in place, the composition of the fluid or medication infused (especially its pH and tonicity), the size and site of the cannula inserted, ineffective filtration, improper anchoring of the line, and the introduction of microorganisms at the time of insertion. The Intravenous Nursing Society assesses phlebitis according to specific standards, which appear in the accompanying chart, Assessment: Phlebitis.

Treatment consists of discontinuing the IV and restarting it in another site, and applying a warm, moist compress to the affected site. Phlebitis can be prevented by using aseptic technique during insertion, using the appropriate-size cannula and needle for the vein, considering the composition of fluids and medications when selecting a site, observing the site hourly for any complications, anchoring the cannula or needle well, and changing the IV site according to agency policy and procedures.

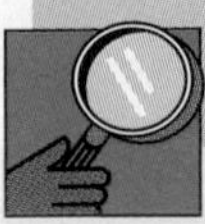

ASSESSMENT PHLEBITIS

According to the Intravenous Nursing Standards of Practice, the following phlebitis scale should be used to document the occurrence of phlebitis and to serve as a baseline for assessing further changes:

0 = No clinical symptoms
1 + = Erythema with or without pain
Edema may or may not be present
No streak formation
No palpable cord
2 + = Erythema with or without pain
Edema may or may not be present
Streak formation
No palpable cord
3 + = Erythema with or without pain
Edema may or may not be present
Streak formation
Palpable cord

Intravenous Nursing Society. (1998). *Revised intravenous nursing standards of practice.* Cambridge, MA: Author

THROMBOPHLEBITIS

Thrombophlebitis refers to the presence of a clot plus inflammation in the vein. It is evidenced by localized pain, redness, warmth, and swelling around the insertion site or along the path of the vein, immobility of the extremity because of discomfort and swelling, sluggish flow rate, fever, malaise, and leukocytosis.

Treatment includes discontinuing the IV infusion, applying a warm compress, elevating the extremity, and restarting the line in the opposite extremity. If the patient has signs and symptoms of thrombophlebitis, the IV line should not be flushed (although flushing may be indicated in the absence of phlebitis to ensure cannula patency and to prevent mixing incompatible medications and solutions). Thrombophlebitis can be prevented by avoiding trauma to the vein at the time the IV is inserted, observing the site every hour, and checking medication additives for compatibility.

HEMATOMA

Hematoma results when blood leaks into tissues surrounding the IV insertion site. Leakage can result from perforation of the opposite vein wall during venipuncture, the needle slipping out of the vein, and insufficient pressure applied to the site after removing the needle or cannula. The signs of a hematoma include ecchymosis, immediate swelling at the site, and the leakage of blood at the site.

Treatment includes removing the needle or cannula and applying pressure with a sterile dressing; applying an ice bag for 24 hours to the site and then a warm compress to increase absorption of blood; assessing the site; and restarting the line in the other extremity if indicated. A hematoma can be prevented by carefully inserting the needle and using diligent care when a patient has a bleeding disorder, takes anticoagulant medication, or has advanced liver disease.

CLOTTING AND OBSTRUCTION

Blood clots may form in the IV line as a result of kinked IV tubing, a very slow infusion rate, an empty IV bag, or failure to flush the IV line after intermittent medication or solution administrations. The signs are decreased flow rate and blood backflow into the IV tubing.

If blood clots in the IV line, the infusion must be discontinued and restarted in another site with a new cannula and administration set. The tubing should not be irrigated or milked. Neither the infusion rate nor the solution container should be raised, and the clot should not be aspirated from the tubing. Clotting of the needle or cannula may be prevented by not permitting the IV solution bag to run dry, taping the tubing to prevent kinking and maintain patency, maintaining an adequate flow rate, and flushing the line after intermittent medication or other solution administration. In some cases, a specially trained nurse or physician may inject a thrombolytic agent into the catheter to clear an occlusion resulting from fibrin or clotted blood.

Promoting Home and Community-Based Care

TEACHING PATIENTS SELF-CARE

At times, IV therapy must be administered in the home setting; consequently, much of the daily management rests with the patient and family. Teaching becomes essential to ensure that the patient and family can manage the IV fluid and infusion properly and prevent complications. Written instructions as well as demonstration and return demonstration help reinforce the key points for all these functions.

CONTINUING CARE

Home infusion therapies cover a wide range of treatments, including antibiotic, analgesic, and antineoplastic medications; blood or blood component therapy; and TPN. When direct nursing care is necessary, arrangements can be made to have an infusion nurse visit the home and administer the IV therapy as prescribed. In addition to implementing and monitoring the IV therapy, the nurse carries out a comprehensive assessment of the patient's condition and continues to teach the patient and family about the skills involved in overseeing the IV therapy setup. Any dietary changes that may be necessary because of fluid or electrolyte imbalances are explained or reinforced during such sessions.

Periodic laboratory testing may be necessary to assess the effects of IV therapy and the patient's progress. Blood specimens may be obtained by a laboratory near the patient's home, or a home visit may be arranged to obtain blood specimens for analysis.

Critical Thinking Exercises

1. Your patient is an 89-year-old man in a coma. His serum sodium level is 190 mEq/L; his serum glucose level is within normal range. What IV solution do you anticipate will be prescribed for him? Provide a rationale for its use, and discuss the nursing actions relevant to its administration.
2. A 29-year-old patient has been admitted to the emergency department with a history of laxative abuse in an effort to lose weight. Laboratory values in the emergency department are as follows: serum Na^+, 140 mEq/L; serum Cl^-, 90 mEq/L; serum bicarbonate, 34 mEq/L; serum K^+, 3.1 mEq/L; serum glucose, 120 mg/dL; BUN, 30 mg/dL; arterial blood gases: pH, 7.48; PCO_2, 47; HCO_3^-, 34. What is the acid–base disorder? What treatments and relevant nursing actions related to the underlying disorder and its treatment should the nurse anticipate?

3.
An elderly woman has been hospitalized with gastroenteritis and dehydration. While obtaining the patient's history, you learn that she intentionally avoids drinking liquids because of her fear of incontinence. Explain the potential fluid and electrolyte disorders that could occur as a result of her failure to consume an adequate fluid intake. What approaches would you use in teaching the patient about the potential risks and about strategies to prevent them?

The nurse collaborates with the case manager in assessing the patient, family, and home environment; developing a plan of care in accordance with the patient's treatment plan and level of ability; and arranging for appropriate referral and follow-up if necessary. Any necessary equipment may either be provided by the agency or purchased by the patient, depending on the terms of the home care arrangements. Appropriate documentation is necessary to assist in obtaining third-party payment for the service provided.

References and Selected Readings

BOOKS

American Heart Association. (1997). *Instructor's manual, advanced cardiac life support.* Atlanta, GA.

Booker, M. F., & Ignatavicius, D. D. (1996). *Infusion therapy. Techniques and medications.* Philadelphia: W. B. Saunders.

Brensilver, J. M., & Goldberger, E. (1996). *A primer of water, electrolyte and acid–base syndromes* (8th ed.). Philadelphia: F. A. Davis.

Fluid and electrolytes. Video and workbook. (1994). Springhouse, PA: Springhouse Corp.

Fluid and electrolyte disorders. Nursing Time Savers. (1994). Springhouse, PA: Springhouse Corp.

Fluids and electrolytes made incredibly easy! (1997). Springhouse, PA: Springhouse Corp.

Gahart, B. (1996). *Intravenous medications* (7th ed.). St. Louis: C. V. Mosby.

Guyton, A. C., & Hall, J. E. (1996). *Pocket companion to textbook of medical physiology.* Philadelphia: W. B. Saunders.

Halperin, M. L., & Goldstein, M. B. (1994). *Fluid, electrolyte and acid–base physiology: A problem-based approach.* Philadelphia: W. B. Saunders.

Horne, M. M., Hertz, U. E., & Swearingen, P. L. (1997). *Pocket guide: Fluid, electrolytes, and acid–base balance* (3rd ed.). St. Louis: Mosby–Year Book.

Intravenous Nursing Society. (1998). *Revised intravenous nursing standards of practice.* Cambridge, MA: Intravenous Nursing Society.

IV therapy. Clinical Skillbuilders. (1990). Springhouse, PA: Springhouse Corp.

Kee, J. L., & Paulanka, B. (1994). *Fluids and electrolytes with clinical applications* (5th ed.). Albany, NY: Delmar Publishers, Inc.

Kokko, J., & Tannen, R. (1996). *Fluids and electrolytes* (3rd ed.). Philadelphia, W. B. Saunders.

LaRocca, J. C., & Otto, S. E. (1997). *Pocket guide to intravenous therapy* (3rd ed.). St. Louis: C. V. Mosby.

Lee, C. A., Barrett, C. A., & Ignatavicius, D. (1996). *Fluids and electrolytes. A practical approach* (4th ed.). Philadelphia: F. A. Davis.

Lippincott Review Series. *Fluid and electrolytes.* (1995). Philadelphia: J. B. Lippincott.

McFarland, M. R., & Grant-Moeller, M. (1994). *Nursing implications of laboratory tests* (3rd ed.). Albany, NY: Delmar Publishers, Inc.

McMorrow, M., & Malarkey, L. (1998). *Laboratory and diagnostic tests. A pocket guide.* Philadelphia: W. B. Saunders.

Metheny, N. M. (1996). *Fluid and electrolyte balance: Nursing considerations* (3rd ed.). Philadelphia: Lippincott-Raven.

Preston, R. A. (1997). *Acid–base, fluids, and electrolytes made ridiculously simple.* Miami: MedMaster, Inc.

Price, S. A., & Wilson, L. M. (1997). *Pathophysiology. Clinical concepts of disease processes.* St. Louis: Mosby–Year Book.

Rose, B. (1994). *Clinical physiology of acid–base and electrolyte disorders* (4th ed.). New York: McGraw-Hill.

Steele, J. (1996). *Practical IV therapy* (2nd ed.). Springhouse, PA: Springhouse Corp.

Urden, L., Lough, M., & Stacy, K. (1996). *Priorities of critical care nursing.* St. Louis: Mosby–Year Book.

Weinstein, S. (1997). *Plumer's principles and practice of intravenous therapy* (6th ed.) Philadelphia: Lippincott-Raven.

Weldy, N. J. (1996). *Body fluids and electrolytes.* Programmed Presentation, 7th ed. St. Louis, C. V. Mosby.

JOURNALS

Asterisks indicate nursing research articles.

AARC Clinical Practice Guideline. (1992). Sampling for arterial blood gas analysis. *Respiratory Care, 37*(8), 913–917.

Beaumont, E. (1996). Technology scorecard–Are you up to date? Needlestick-prevention IV systems: Greater protection. *American Journal of Nursing, 96*(12), 23.

Brater, D. C. (1998). Diuretic therapy. *New England Journal of Medicine, 339*(6), 387–395.

Clayton, K. (1997). Cancer-related hypercalcemia: How to spot it, how to manage it. *American Journal of Nursing, 97*(5), 42–49.

Driscoll, M., et al. (1997). Inserting and maintaining peripherally inserted central catheters. *MedSurg Nursing, 6*(6), 350–358.

Faria, S. H., & Taylor, L. J. (1997). Interpretation of arterial blood gases by nurses. *Journal of Vascular Nursing, 15*(4), 128–130.

Fulop, M. (1998). Algorithms for diagnosing some electrolyte disorders. *American Journal of Emergency Medicine, 16*(1), 76–84.

Goldhill, D. R. (1997). Calcium and magnesium. *Care of the Critically Ill, 13*(3), 112–115.

Intravenous Nurses Society. (1997). Position paper: Midline and midclavicular catheters. *Journal of Intravenous Nursing, 20*(4), 175–178.

Intravenous Nurses Society. (1997). Position paper: Peripherally inserted central catheters. *Journal of Intravenous Nursing, 20*(4), 172–174.

Lilly, L. L., & Guanci, R. (1997). Persistent potassium problems. *American Journal of Nursing, 97*(6), 14.

Krzywda, E. A. (1998). Central venous access—Catheters, technology, and physiology. *MedSurg Nursing, 7*(3),132–139.

Renner, C., et al. (1996). Vascular access in home care: Current trends. *Infusion, 3*(1), 13–27.

Toffaletti, J. (1997). Blood gas testing in the laboratory and at the point of care: Finding the right mix. *Medical Lab Observer,* (Suppl. 14-7), 34–35.

Vonfrolio, L. (1995). Would you hang these IV solutions? *American Journal of Nursing,* June, 37–39.

Resources

Assessing Fluids and Electrolytes. Video Skill Series. (1989). Springhouse, PA, Springhouse Corp.

Detecting and Managing IV Problems. Video Skill Series. (1988). Springhouse, PA, Springhouse Corp.

Intravenous Nurses Society (National Chapter), Brighton St., Belmont, MA 02178. (617) 489-5205.

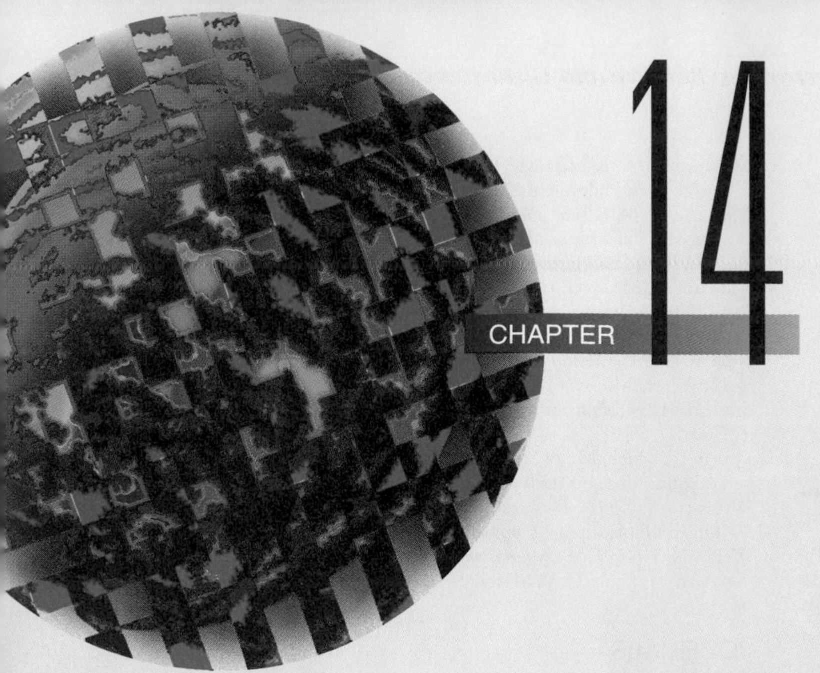

Shock and Multisystem Failure

Learning Objectives

On completion of this chapter, the learner will be able to:

1. Define shock and its underlying pathophysiology.
2. Compare clinical findings of the compensatory and progressive stages of shock.
3. Describe organ damage that may occur with shock.
4. Compare hypovolemic, cardiogenic, and distributive shock in terms of causes, pathophysiologic effects, and medical and nursing management.
5. Describe indications for varying types of fluid replacement.
6. Identify vasoactive medications used in treating shock, and describe nursing implications associated with their use.
7. Discuss the importance of nutritional support in all forms of shock.
8. Discuss the role of the nurse in psychosocial support of both the patient experiencing shock and the family.
9. Discuss the syndrome of multiple organ dysfunction.

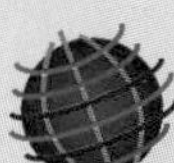

Shock is a life-threatening condition with a variety of underlying causes. It is characterized by inadequate tissue perfusion that, if untreated, results in cell death. The nurse caring for the patient with shock or at risk for shock must understand the underlying mechanisms of shock and recognize its subtle as well as more obvious signs. Rapid assessment and rapid response are essential to recovery.

Shock can best be defined as a condition in which systemic blood pressure is inadequate to deliver oxygen to vital organs (Jones, 1996). Adequate blood flow to the tissues and cells requires the following components: adequate cardiac pump, effective vasculature or circulatory system, and adequate blood volume.

When one component is impaired, blood flow to the tissues is threatened or compromised. Without treatment, inadequate blood flow to the tissues results in inadequate oxygen and nutrients to the cells, cellular starvation, cell death, organ dysfunction progressing to organ failure, and eventual death.

GLOSSARY

anaphylactic shock: shock state resulting from severe allergic reaction producing an overwhelming systemic vasodilation and relative hypovolemia

biochemical mediator: messenger substance that may be released by a cell to create an action at that site or be carried by the bloodstream to a distant site before being activated

cardiogenic shock: shock state resulting from impairment or failure of the myocardium

colloids: intravenous solutions that contain molecules that are too large to pass through capillary membranes

crystalloids: electrolyte solutions that move freely between the intravascular compartment and interstitial spaces

distributive shock: shock state resulting from displacement of blood volume creating a relative hypovolemia; also called vasogenic shock

hypovolemic shock: shock state resulting from decreased intravascular volume due to fluid loss

neurogenic shock: shock state resulting from loss of sympathetic tone causing relative hypovolemia

septic shock: distributive shock state resulting from overwhelming infection resulting in relative hypovolemia

shock: physiologic state in which there is inadequate blood flow to tissues and cells of the body

systemic inflammatory response syndrome (SIRS): overwhelming inflammatory response in the absence of infection causing relative hypovolemia and decreased tissue perfusion

SIGNIFICANCE OF SHOCK

Shock affects all body systems. It may develop rapidly or slowly depending on the underlying cause. During shock, the body struggles to survive, calling on all its homeostatic mechanisms to restore blood flow and tissue perfusion. Any insult to the body can create a cascade of events resulting in poor tissue perfusion. Therefore, almost any patient with any disease state may be at risk for developing shock.

Nursing care of the patient with shock requires ongoing systematic assessment. Many of the interventions required in caring for the patient with shock call for close collaboration with other members of the health care team and a physician's order. The nurse must anticipate such orders because they need to be executed with speed and accuracy.

CONDITIONS PRECIPITATING SHOCK

Classification of Shock

Shock can be classified by etiology and may be described as (1) **hypovolemic shock**, (2) **cardiogenic shock**, or (3) **distributive** or **vasogenic shock**. Some authors identify a fourth category, obstructive shock, which results from disorders that cause mechanical obstruction to blood flow through the central circulatory system despite normal myocardial function and intravascular volume. Examples include pulmonary embolism, cardiac tamponade, dissecting aortic aneurysm, and tension pneumothorax. In this discussion, obstructive disorders are discussed as examples of noncoronary cardiogenic shock. Hypovolemic shock occurs when there is a decrease in the intravascular volume. Cardiogenic shock occurs when the heart has an impaired pumping ability; it may be of coronary or noncoronary origin. Distributive shock results from a maldistribution or mismatch of blood flow to the cells.

Normal Cellular Function

Energy metabolism occurs within the cell where nutrients are chemically broken down and stored in the form of adenosine triphosphate (ATP). Cells use this stored energy to perform necessary functions, such as active transport, muscle contraction, and biochemical synthesis, as well as specialized cellular functions, such as the conduction of electrical impulses. ATP can be synthesized aerobically (in the presence of oxygen) or anaerobically (in the absence of oxygen). Aerobic metabolism yields far greater amounts of ATP per mole of glucose than does anaerobic metabolism and, therefore, is a more efficient and effective means of producing energy. Additionally, anaerobic metabolism results in the accumulation of the toxic end product, lactic acid, which must be removed from the cell and transported to the liver for conversion into glucose and glycogen.

Pathophysiology

In shock, the cells lack an adequate blood supply and are deprived of oxygen and nutrients; therefore, they must produce energy through anaerobic metabolism. This results in low energy yields from nutrients and an acidotic intracellular environment. Because of these changes, normal cell function ceases (Fig. 14-1). The cell swells, and its membrane becomes more permeable, allowing electrolytes and fluids to seep out of and into the cell. The sodium–potassium pump becomes impaired; cell structures, primarily the mitochondria, are damaged; and death of the cell results.

Vascular Responses

Oxygen attaches to the hemoglobin molecule in red blood cells, and the blood carries it to body cells. The amount of oxygen that is delivered to cells depends both on blood flow to a specific area and on blood oxygen concentration. Blood is continuously recycled through the lungs to be reoxygenated and to eliminate end products of cellular metabolism, such as carbon dioxide. The heart muscle is the pump that propels the freshly oxygenated blood out to the body tissues. This process of circulation is facilitated through an elaborate and dynamic vasculature consisting of arteries, arterioles, capillaries, veins, and venules. The vasculature can dilate or constrict based on central and local regulatory mechanisms. Central regulatory mechanisms stimulate dilation or constriction of the vasculature to maintain an adequate blood pressure. Local regulatory mechanisms, referred to as **autoregulation**, stimulate vasodilation or vasoconstriction in response to **biochemical mediators** released by the cell communicating its need for oxygen and nutrients (Robins, 1996). A biochemical mediator is a substance released by a cell; the substance triggers an action at a cell site or travels in the bloodstream to a distant site, where it triggers action.

PATHOPHYSIOLOGY

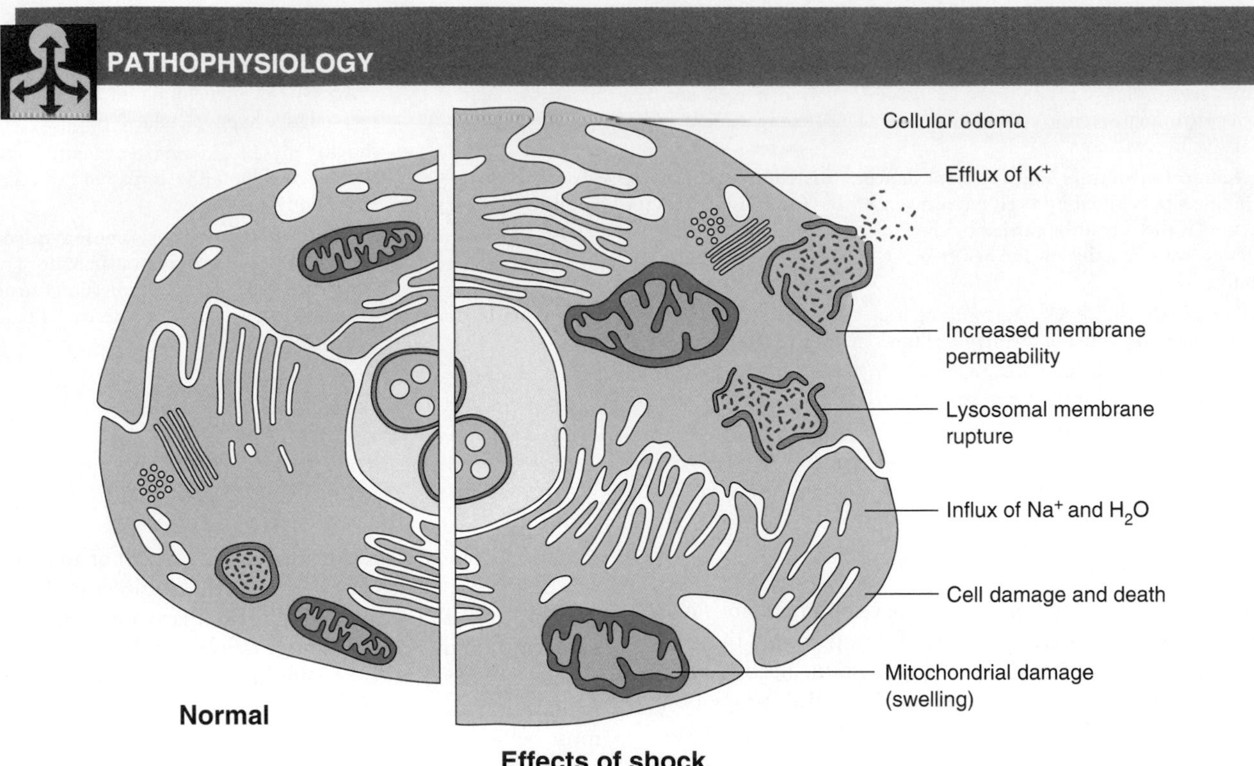

FIGURE 14•1 Cellular effects of shock. The cell swells and the cell membrane becomes more permeable, and fluids, and electrolytes seep from and into the cell. Mitochondria and lysosomes are damaged, and the cell dies.

Blood Pressure Regulation

Three major components of the circulatory system—blood volume, the cardiac pump, and the vasculature—must respond effectively to complex neural, chemical, and hormonal feedback systems to maintain an adequate blood pressure and ultimately perfuse body tissues.

Blood pressure is regulated through a complex interaction of neural, chemical, and hormonal feedback systems affecting both cardiac output and peripheral resistance. This relationship is expressed in the following equation:

$$\text{mean arterial blood pressure} = \text{cardiac output} \times \text{peripheral resistance}$$

Cardiac output is determined by stroke volume (the amount of blood ejected at systole) and heart rate. Peripheral resistance is determined by the diameter of the arterioles.

Tissue and organ perfusion depend on mean arterial pressure (MAP). The MAP is the average pressure at which blood moves through the vasculature. Although true MAP can only be calculated by complex methods, Chart 14-1 displays a convenient formula for clinical use in estimating MAP. MAP should exceed 80 mm Hg for cells to receive the oxygen and nutrients needed to metabolize energy in amounts sufficient to sustain life (Robins, 1996).

Blood pressure is regulated by the baroreceptors (pressure receptors) located in the carotid sinus and aortic arch. These pressure receptors convey impulses to the sympathetic nervous center in the medulla of the brain. When blood pressure drops, catecholamines (epinephrine and norepinephrine) are released from the adrenal medulla of the adrenal glands. This increases heart rate and vasoconstriction, thus restoring blood pressure. Chemoreceptors, also located in the aortic arch and carotid arteries, regulate blood pressure and respiratory rate using much the same mechanism in response to changes in oxygen and carbon dioxide concentrations in the blood. These primary regulatory mechanisms can respond to changes in blood pressure on a moment-to-moment basis.

The kidneys also play an important role in blood pressure regulation. They regulate blood pressure by releasing renin, an enzyme needed for the conversion of angiotensin I to angiotensin II, a potent vasoconstrictor. This effect indirectly leads to the release of aldosterone from the adrenal cortex, which promotes the retention of sodium and water. The increased concentration of sodium in the blood then stimulates the release of antidiuretic hormone (ADH) by the pituitary gland. ADH causes the kidneys to retain water further in an effort to raise blood volume and blood pressure. These secondary regulatory mechanisms may take hours or days to respond to changes in blood pressure.

To summarize, adequate blood volume, an effective cardiac pump, and an effective vasculature are necessary to maintain blood pressure and tissue perfusion. When one of the three components of this system begins to fail, the body is able to compen-

CHART 14•1 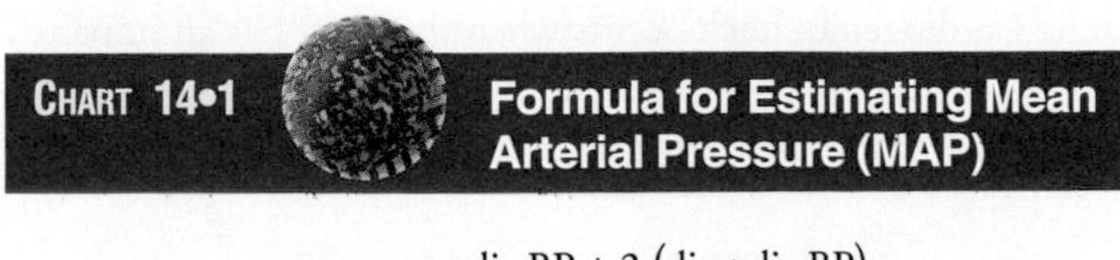 **Formula for Estimating Mean Arterial Pressure (MAP)**

$$\text{MAP} = \frac{\text{systolic BP} + 2\,(\text{diastolic BP})}{3}$$

Example: patient's BP = 125/75

$$\text{MAP} = \frac{125 + (2 \times 75)}{3}$$

$$\text{MAP} = 92\,(\text{rounded to nearest } 1/10)$$

sate through increased work by the other two (Fig. 14-2). When compensatory mechanisms can no longer compensate for the failed system, body tissues are inadequately perfused, and shock occurs. Without prompt intervention, shock progresses, resulting in organ dysfunction, organ failure, and death.

STAGES OF SHOCK

Some think of the shock syndrome as a continuum along which the patient struggles to survive. A convenient way to understand the physiologic responses and subsequent clinical signs and symptoms is to divide the continuum into separate stages: compensatory, progressive, and irreversible. (Although some authorities identify an initial stage of shock, changes attributed to this stage occur at the cellular level and are generally not detectable clinically.) The earlier that medical management and nursing interventions can be initiated along this continuum, the greater the patient's chance of survival.

Compensatory Stage

In the compensatory stage of shock, the patient's blood pressure remains within normal limits. Vasoconstriction, increased heart rate, and increased contractility of the heart contribute to maintaining adequate cardiac output. This results from stimulation of the sympathetic nervous system and subsequent release of catecholamines (epinephrine and norepinephrine). The patient is in the often-described "fight or flight" response. The body shunts blood from organs such as the skin, kidneys, and gastrointestinal (GI) tract to the brain and heart to ensure adequate blood supply to these vital organs. As a result, the patient's skin is cold and clammy, bowel sounds are hypoactive, and urine output decreases in response to the release of aldosterone and ADH.

Clinical Manifestations

Despite a normal blood pressure, the patient shows numerous clinical signs indicating inadequate organ perfusion. The result of

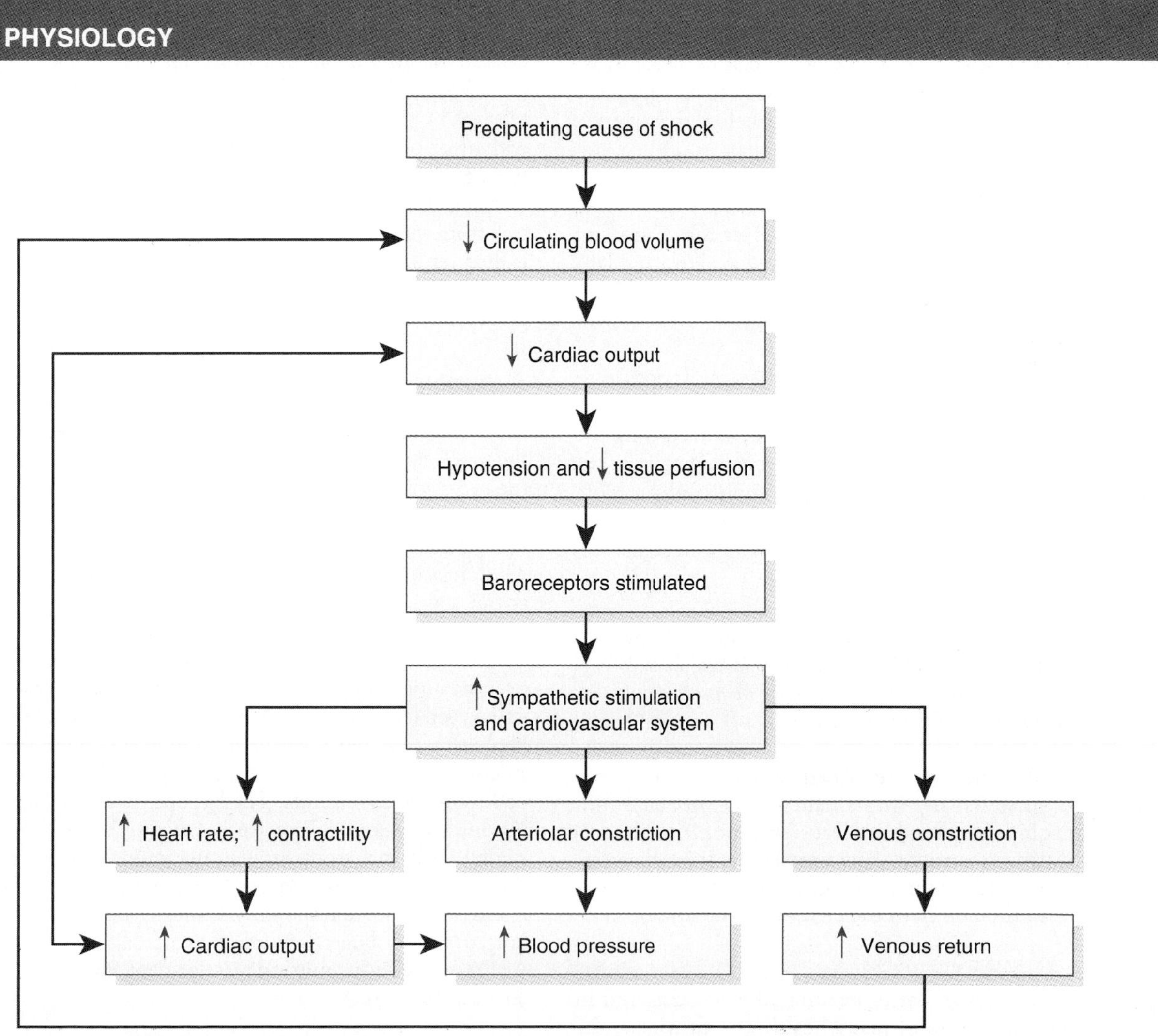

FIGURE 14•2 Compensatory mechanisms for the restoration of circulatory blood volume in shock. Adapted with permission from Jones, K. (1996). *Shock.* In J.M. Clochesy, & C. Breu, et al. (Eds.). *Critical care nursing* (2nd ed). Philadelphia, W. B. Saunders Company.

inadequate perfusion is anaerobic metabolism and buildup of lactic acid, producing metabolic acidosis. The respiratory rate increases in response to metabolic acidosis. This rapid respiratory rate facilitates removal of excess carbon dioxide (CO_2) but results in raising the blood pH and often causing a compensatory respiratory alkalosis. The alkalotic state causes mental status changes, such as confusion or combativeness, as well as arteriolar dilation. If treatment begins in this stage of shock, the prognosis for the patient is good.

Medical Management

Medical treatment is directed toward identifying the cause of the shock, correcting the underlying disorder so that shock does not progress, and supporting those physiologic processes that thus far have responded successfully to the threat. Because compensation cannot be effectively maintained indefinitely, measures such as fluid replacement and medication therapy must be initiated to maintain an adequate blood pressure and reestablish and maintain adequate tissue perfusion.

Nursing Management

Early intervention along the continuum of shock is the key to improving the patient's prognosis. Therefore, the nurse needs to assess systematically those patients at risk for shock to recognize the subtle clinical signs of the compensatory stage before the patient's blood pressure drops.

MONITORING TISSUE PERFUSION

In assessing tissue perfusion, the nurse observes for changes in level of consciousness, skin, urinary output, vital signs, and laboratory values. In the compensatory stage of shock, serum sodium and blood glucose levels are elevated in response to the release of aldosterone and catecholamines.

The role of the nurse at the compensatory stage of shock is to monitor the patient's hemodynamic status and promptly report deviations to the physician, assist in identifying and treating the underlying disorder by continuous in-depth assessment of the patient, administer prescribed fluids and medications, and promote patient safety. Vital signs are key indicators of the patient's hemodynamic status; however, blood pressure is an indirect method of monitoring tissue hypoxia.

Nursing Alert *By the time blood pressure drops, damage has already been occurring on the cellular and tissue levels. Therefore, it is imperative that the patient at risk for shock be assessed and monitored closely before the blood pressure falls.*

Although treatments are prescribed and initiated by the physician, the nurse usually implements them, operates and troubleshoots equipment used in treatment, monitors the patient's status during treatment, and assesses the immediate effects of treatment. Additionally, the nurse assesses the response of the patient and the family to the crisis and to treatment.

REDUCING ANXIETY

In experiencing a major threat to health and well-being and in being the focus of attention of many health care providers, the patient often becomes anxious and apprehensive. Providing brief explanations about the diagnostic and treatment procedures, supporting the patient during those procedures, and providing information about their outcomes are usually effective in reducing stress and anxiety and thus promoting the patient's physical and mental well-being.

PROMOTING SAFETY

Another nursing intervention is monitoring potential threats to the patient's safety because a high anxiety level and altered mental status typically impair a person's judgment. In this stage, patients who were previously cooperative and followed instructions may now disrupt intravenous lines and catheters and further complicate their condition. Therefore, close monitoring is essential.

Progressive Stage

In the progressive stage of shock, the mechanisms that regulate blood pressure can no longer compensate, and the MAP falls below normal limits, with an average systolic blood pressure of less than 90 mm Hg (Baxter, 1997).

Pathophysiology

Although all organ systems suffer from hypoperfusion at this stage, two events further perpetuate the shock syndrome. First, the overworked heart becomes ischemic. This leads to failure of the cardiac pump—even if the underlying cause of the shock is not of cardiac origin. Second, the autoregulatory function of the microcirculation fails in response to numerous biochemical mediators released by the cells, resulting in increased capillary permeability, with areas of arteriolar and venous constriction further compromising cellular perfusion. At this stage, the patient's prognosis worsens. The relaxation of precapillary sphincters causes fluid to leak from the capillaries, creating interstitial edema, and less fluid is then returned to the heart. Even if the underlying cause of the shock is reversed, the breakdown of the circulatory system itself perpetuates the shock state, and a vicious circle ensues.

Assessment and Diagnostic Findings

Chances of survival depend on the patient's general health before the shock state as well as the amount of time it takes to restore tissue perfusion. As shock progresses, organ systems decompensate.

RESPIRATORY PROBLEMS

The lungs, which become compromised early in shock, are affected at this stage. Subsequent decompensation of the lungs increases the likelihood that mechanical ventilation may be needed if shock progresses. Respirations are rapid and shallow. Crackles are heard over the lung fields. Decreased pulmonary blood flow causes arterial oxygen levels to decrease and carbon dioxide levels to increase. Hypoxemia and biochemical mediators cause pulmonary vasoconstriction, which further perpetuates the pulmonary capillary hypoperfusion and hypoxemia. The hypoperfused alveoli stop producing surfactant and subsequently collapse. Pulmonary capillaries begin to leak their contents, causing pulmonary edema and additional alveolar collapse (Baxter, 1997). This condition is sometimes referred to as acute respiratory distress syndrome (ARDS), shock lung, or noncardiogenic pulmonary edema. Further explanation of ARDS, as well as its nursing management, can be found in Chapter 21 of this text.

CARDIOVASCULAR PROBLEMS

A lack of adequate blood supply leads to dysrhythmias and ischemia (blood deficiency). The patient has a rapid heart rate, sometimes exceeding 150 bpm. The patient may complain of chest pain and even suffer a myocardial infarction. Cardiac enzyme levels (eg, lactate dehydrogenase, CPK-MB, and cTn-I) rise.

NEUROLOGIC PROBLEMS

As blood flow to the brain becomes impaired, the patient's mental status deteriorates. Changes in mental status occur as a result of decreased cerebral perfusion and hypoxia; the patient may initially exhibit confusion or a subtle change in behavior. Subsequently, lethargy increases, and the patient begins to lose consciousness. The patient's pupils dilate and are only sluggishly reactive to light.

RENAL PROBLEMS

When the MAP falls below 75 mm Hg, the glomerular filtration rate of the kidneys cannot be maintained, and drastic changes in renal function occur. Acute renal failure (ARF) can occur. ARF is characterized by an increase in blood urea nitrogen (BUN) and serum creatinine levels, fluid and electrolyte shifts, acid-base imbalances, and a loss of the renal-hormonal regulation of blood pressure. Urinary output usually decreases to below 30 mL/h but can be variable depending on the phase of ARF. For a further discussion of ARF, see Chapter 41.

HEPATIC PROBLEMS

Decreased blood flow to the liver impairs the liver cells' ability to perform metabolic and phagocytic functions. Consequently, the patient is less able to metabolize medications and metabolic waste products, such as ammonia and lactic acid. The patient becomes more susceptible to infection as the liver fails to filter bacteria out of the blood. Liver enzymes (aspartate aminotransferase [AST], formerly serum glutamic-oxaloacetic transaminase [SGOT]; alanine aminotransferase [ALT], formerly serum glutamate pyruvate transaminase [SGPT]; lactate dehydrogenase) and bilirubin levels are elevated, and the patient appears jaundiced.

GASTROINTESTINAL PROBLEMS

GI ischemia can cause stress ulceration in the stomach, placing the patient at risk for GI bleeding. In the small intestine, the mucosa can become necrotic and slough off, causing bloody diarrhea. Beyond the local effects of impaired perfusion, GI ischemia leads to the release of endotoxin, which enters the bloodstream through the lymph system. In addition to causing infection, endotoxin can cause cardiac depression and vasodilation and activate additional biochemical mediators that interfere with healthy cells, resulting in their inability to metabolize nutrients (Kellum & Decker, 1996; Swank & Deitch, 1996).

HEMATOLOGIC PROBLEMS

The combination of hypotension, sluggish blood flow, metabolic acidosis, and generalized hypoxemia can interfere with normal hemostatic mechanisms. Disseminated intravascular coagulation (DIC) can occur either as a cause or as a complication of shock. In this condition, widespread clotting and bleeding occur simultaneously. Bruises (ecchymoses) and bleeding (petechiae) may appear in the skin. Coagulation times (prothrombin time, partial thromboplastin time) are prolonged. Clotting factors and platelets are consumed and require replacement therapy to achieve hemostasis. Further discussion of disseminated intravascular coagulation appears in Chapter 30.

Medical Management

Specific medical management in the progressive stage of shock depends on the type of shock and its underlying cause. It is also based on the degree of decompensation in the organ systems. Medical management specific to each type of shock is discussed in later sections of this chapter. Although there are several differences in medical management by type of shock, some medical interventions are common to all types. These include use of appropriate intravenous fluids and medications to restore tissue perfusion by (1) optimizing intravascular volume, (2) supporting the pumping action of the heart, and (3) improving the competence of the vascular system. Other aspects of management may include early enteral nutritional support and use of antacids, histamine-2 (H_2)-blockers, or antipeptic agents to reduce risk of GI ulceration and bleeding.

Nursing Management

Nursing care of the patient in the progressive stage of shock requires expertise in assessing and understanding shock and the significance of changes in assessment data. The patient in the progressive stage of shock is often cared for in the intensive care setting to facilitate close monitoring (hemodynamic monitoring, electrocardiographic [ECG] monitoring, arterial blood gases, serum electrolyte levels, physical and mental status changes), rapid and frequent administration of various prescribed medications and fluids, and possibly, intervention with supportive technologies, such as mechanical ventilation, dialysis, and intra-aortic balloon pump.

Working closely with other members of the health care team, the nurse carefully documents treatments, medications, and fluids that are administered by all members of the team, recording the time, dosage or volume, and the patient's response. Additionally, the nurse coordinates both the scheduling of diagnostic procedures that may be carried out at the patient's bedside and the flow of health care personnel involved in the patient's care.

PREVENTING COMPLICATIONS

If supportive technologies are used, the nurse helps reduce the risk of related complications and monitors the patient for early signs of complications. Monitoring includes evaluating blood levels of medications, observing invasive vascular lines for signs of infection, and checking neurovascular status if arterial lines are inserted, especially in the lower extremities. Simultaneously, the nurse promotes the patient's safety and comfort by ensuring that all procedures, including invasive procedures, are carried out using correct aseptic techniques and that venous and arterial puncture and infusion sites are maintained with the goal of preventing infection. Positioning and repositioning the patient to promote comfort, prevent pulmonary complications, and maintain skin integrity are integral to caring for the patient in shock.

PROMOTING REST AND COMFORT

Efforts are made to minimize the cardiac workload by reducing the patient's physical activity and fear or anxiety. Promoting rest and comfort is a priority in the patient's care. To ensure that the patient gets as much uninterrupted rest as possible, the nurse performs only essential nursing activities. To conserve the patient's energy, the nurse protects the patient from temperature extremes (excessive warmth or shivering cold), which can increase the metabolic rate and subsequently the cardiac workload. The patient should not be warmed too quickly, and warming blankets should not be applied because they can cause vasodilation and a subsequent drop in blood pressure.

SUPPORTING FAMILY MEMBERS

Because the patient in shock is the object of intense attention by the health care team, the family members may feel neglected; but

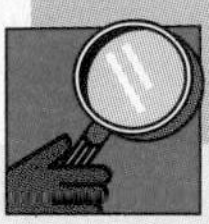

ASSESSMENT
CLINICAL FINDINGS IN STAGES OF SHOCK

Finding	Compensatory	Progressive	Irreversible
Blood pressure	Normal	Systolic < 80–90 mm Hg	Requires mechanical or pharmacologic support
Respiratory status	>20 breaths/min	Rapid, shallow respirations; crackles	Requires intubation
Heart rate	>100 bpm	>150 bpm	Erratic or asystole
Skin	Cold, clammy	Mottled, petechiae	Jaundice
Urinary output	Decreased	<30 mL/h	Anuric, requires dialysis
Mentation	Confusion	Lethargy	Unconscious
Acid–base balance	Respiratory alkalosis	Metabolic acidosis	Profound acidosis

they may be reluctant to ask questions or seek information for fear that they will be in the way or will interfere with the attention given to the patient. The nurse should make sure that the family is comfortably situated and kept informed about the patient's status. Often, family members need advice from the health care team to get some rest; they are more likely to take this advice if they feel that the patient is being well cared for and that they will be notified of any significant changes in the patient's status. A visit from the hospital chaplain may be comforting to the family and provides some attention to the family while the nurse concentrates on the patient.

Irreversible Stage

The irreversible (or refractory) stage of shock represents the point along the shock continuum at which organ damage is so severe that the patient does not respond to treatment and cannot survive. Despite treatment, blood pressure remains low. Complete renal and liver failure, compounded by the release of necrotic tissue toxins, creates an overwhelming metabolic acidosis. Anaerobic metabolism contributes to a worsening lactic acidosis. Reserves of ATP are almost totally depleted, and mechanisms for storing new supplies of energy have been destroyed. Multiple organ dysfunction progressing to complete organ failure has occurred, and death is imminent. Multiple organ dysfunction can occur as a progression along the shock continuum or as a syndrome unto itself and is further described later in this chapter.

Medical Management

Medical management during the irreversible stage of shock is usually the same as for the progressive stage. Although the patient's condition may have progressed from the progressive to the irreversible stage, the judgment that the shock is irreversible can be made only retrospectively on the basis of failure of the patient to respond to treatment. Strategies that may be experimental (ie, investigational medications, such as antibiotics and immunomodulation therapy) may be tried to reduce or reverse the severity of shock.

Nursing Management

As in the progressive stage of shock, the nurse focuses on carrying out prescribed treatments, monitoring the patient, preventing complications, protecting the patient from injury, and providing comfort. Offering brief explanations to the patient about what is happening is essential even if there is no certainty that the patient hears or understands what is being said.

As it becomes obvious that the patient is unlikely to survive, the patient's family needs to be informed about the prognosis and likely outcomes. Opportunities should be provided, throughout the patient's care, for the family to see, touch, and talk to the patient. A close family friend or clergy may be of comfort to the family in dealing with the inevitable death of the patient. Whenever possible and appropriate, the family should be approached regarding any living will or other written or verbal wishes the patient may have shared in the event that he or she cannot participate in end-of-life decisions. In some cases, ethics committees may assist the family and medical team in making difficult decisions.

During this stage of shock, families may misinterpret the actions of the health care team. They have been told that nothing has been effective in reversing the shock and that the patient's survival is very unlikely; yet, the health care team continues to work feverishly on the patient. A distraught, grieving family may interpret this as a chance for recovery when none exists. As a result, family members may become angry when the patient dies. If different members of the health care team confer with the family, family members will have an opportunity to understand the patient's prognosis and the purpose for the measures being taken. During these conferences, it is essential to explain that the equipment and treatments being provided are for the patient's comfort and do not suggest that the patient will recover. Families should be encouraged to express their wishes concerning the use of life-support measures.

OVERALL MANAGEMENT STRATEGIES IN SHOCK

As described previously and in the discussion of types of shock to follow, management in all types and all phases of shock includes the following:

- Fluid replacement to restore intravascular volume
- Vasoactive medications to restore vasomotor tone and improve cardiac function
- Nutritional support to address the metabolic requirements that are often dramatically increased in shock

Therapies described in this section require collaboration among all members of the health care team to ensure that the manifestations of shock are quickly identified and that adequate and timely treatment is instituted to achieve the best outcome possible.

Fluid Replacement

Fluid replacement is given in all types of shock. The selection of fluids and the speed of delivery vary, but fluids are given to enhance oxygenation, which in part depends on flow. The fluids administered may include **crystalloids** (electrolyte solutions that move freely between intravascular and interstitial spaces), **colloids** (large-molecule intravenous solutions), or blood components.

Crystalloid and Colloid Solutions

Selection of the best fluid to treat shock remains controversial. In emergency situations, the "best" fluid is often the fluid that is readily available. Both crystalloids and colloids, as described later, can be given to restore intravascular volume. Blood component therapy is used most frequently in hypovolemic shock.

Crystalloids are electrolyte solutions that move freely between the intravascular compartment and the interstitial spaces. Isotonic crystalloid solutions are often selected because they contain the same concentration of electrolytes as the extracellular fluid and therefore can be given without altering concentrations of electrolytes in the plasma.

Common intravenous fluids used for resuscitation in cases of hypovolemic shock include 0.9% sodium chloride solution (normal saline) and lactated Ringer's solution (Jones, 1996). Ringer's lactate is an electrolyte solution containing the lactate ion, which should not be confused with lactic acid. The lactate ion is converted to bicarbonate, which helps to buffer the overall acidosis that occurs in shock.

A disadvantage in using isotonic crystalloid solutions is that three parts of the volume are lost to the interstitial compartment for every one part that remains in the intravascular compartment. This occurs in response to mechanisms that store extracellular body fluid. Diffusion of crystalloids into the interstitial space necessitates that more fluid be administered than the amount lost (Robins, 1996).

Care is taken when rapidly administering isotonic crystalloids to avoid causing excessive edema, particularly pulmonary edema. For this reason, and depending on the cause of the hypovolemia, a hypertonic crystalloid solution, such as 3% sodium chloride, is sometimes administered in hypovolemic shock. Hypertonic solutions produce a large osmotic force that pulls fluid from the intracellular space to the extracellular space to achieve a fluid balance (Robins, 1996). The osmotic effect of hypertonic solutions results in fewer fluids being administered to restore intravascular volume. Complications associated with use of hypertonic saline solution include excessive serum osmolality, hypernatremia, hypokalemia, and altered thermoregulation (Robins, 1996).

Generally, intravenous colloidal solutions are considered to be plasma proteins, which are molecules that are too large to pass through capillary membranes. Colloids expand intravascular volume by exerting oncotic pressure, thereby pulling fluid into the intravascular space. Colloidal solutions have the same effect as hypertonic solutions in increasing intravascular volume, but less volume of fluid is required than is required with crystalloids. Additionally, colloids have a longer duration of action than crystalloids because the molecules remain within the intravascular compartment longer.

A 5% albumin solution is commonly used to treat hypovolemic shock. Albumin is a plasma protein; 5% albumin solution is prepared from human plasma and is heated to reduce its potential to transmit disease. The disadvantages in using albumin are its high cost and limited availability, which depends on blood donors. Synthetic colloid preparations, such as 6% hetastarch and 6% dextran solution, are now widely used. Dextran, however, may interfere with platelet aggregation and therefore is not indicated if hemorrhage is the cause of the hypovolemic shock or if the patient has a coagulation disorder (coagulopathy).

Nursing Alert *With all colloidal solutions, side effects include the rare occurrence of anaphylactic reactions, for which the nurse must monitor.*

Complications of Fluid Administration

Close monitoring of the patient during fluid replacement is necessary to identify side effects and complications. The most common and serious side effects of fluid replacement are cardiovascular overload and pulmonary edema.

Patients receiving fluid replacement must be monitored frequently for adequate urinary output, changes in mental status, skin perfusion, and changes in vital signs. The patient's lung sounds are auscultated frequently to detect signs of fluid accumulation. Adventitious lung sounds, such as crackles, may indicate pulmonary edema.

Often a right atrial pressure line (also known as a central venous pressure line) is inserted. In addition to physical assessment, the right atrial pressure value helps in monitoring the patient's progress with fluid replacement. A normal right atrial pressure value is 4 to 12 cm H_2O. Several readings are obtained to determine a range, and fluid replacement is continued to achieve a pressure within normal limits. Hemodynamic monitoring with arterial and pulmonary artery lines may be implemented to allow close monitoring of the patient's cardiac status and response to therapy.

Vasoactive Medication Therapy

Vasoactive medications are given in all forms of shock to improve the patient's hemodynamic stability when fluid therapy alone cannot maintain adequate MAP. Specific medications are selected to correct the particular hemodynamic alteration that is impeding cardiac output. Specific vasoactive medications are prescribed for the patient in shock because they can support the patient's hemodynamic status. These medications help to increase the strength of myocardial contractility, regulate the heart rate, reduce myocardial resistance, and initiate vasoconstriction.

Vasoactive medications are selected for their action on receptors of the sympathetic nervous system. These receptors are known as alpha-adrenergic and beta-adrenergic receptors. Beta-adrenergic receptors are further classified as $beta_1$- and $beta_2$-adrenergic receptors. When alpha-adrenergic receptors are stimulated, blood vessels constrict in the cardiorespiratory and GI systems, skin, and kidneys. When $beta_1$-adrenergic receptors are stimulated, heart rate and myocardial contraction increase. When $beta_2$-adrenergic receptors are stimulated, vasodilation occurs in the heart and skeletal muscles, and the bronchioles relax. The medications used in treating shock consist of various combinations of vasoactive medications to maximize tissue perfusion by stimulating or blocking the alpha- and beta-adrenergic receptors.

When vasoactive medications are administered, vital signs must be monitored frequently (at least every 15 minutes, or more often if indicated). Vasoactive medications should be administered through a central venous line because infiltration and extravasation of some vasoactive medications can cause tissue necrosis and sloughing. An intravenous pump or controller should be used to ensure that the medications are delivered safely and accurately.

Individual medication dosages are usually titrated by the nurse, who adjusts the intravenous drip rates based on the physician's prescription and the patient's response. Dosages are changed to maintain the patient's MAP (usually above 80 mm Hg) at a physiologic level that ensures adequate tissue perfusion.

Nursing Alert *When vasoactive medications are discontinued, they should never be stopped abruptly because this could cause severe hemodynamic instability, perpetuating the shock state.*

Dosages of vasoactive medications should be tapered and the patient weaned from the medication with frequent monitoring (every 15 minutes) of blood pressure. Table 14-1 presents some of the commonly prescribed vasoactive medications used in treating shock.

Nutritional Support

Nutritional support is an important aspect of care for the patient with shock. Increased metabolic rates during shock increase energy requirements and therefore caloric requirements. The patient in shock requires more than 3000 calories daily.

The release of catecholamines early in the shock continuum causes glycogen stores to be depleted in about 8 to 10 hours. Nutritional energy requirements are then met by breaking down lean body mass. In this catabolic process, skeletal muscle mass is broken down even when the patient has large stores of fat or adipose tissue. Loss of skeletal muscle can greatly prolong the recovery time for the patient in shock. Parenteral or enteral nutritional support should be initiated as soon as possible, with some form of enteral alimentation always being administered. The integrity of the GI system depends on direct exposure to nutrients. Additionally, glutamine (an essential amino acid during stress), is important in the immunologic structure of the GI tract, providing a fuel source for lymphocytes and macrophages. Glutamine is currently only available to be administered through enteral nutrition (Rauen & Munro, 1998).

Stress ulcers occur frequently in acutely ill patients because of the compromised blood supply to the GI tract. Therefore, antacids, H_2-blockers (eg, ranitidine), and antipeptic agents (eg, sucralfate) are prescribed to prevent ulcer formation by inhibiting gastric acid secretion or increasing gastric pH.

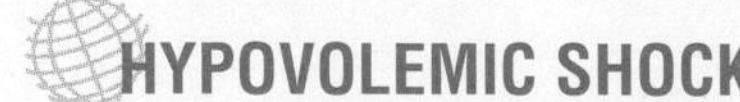

HYPOVOLEMIC SHOCK

In addition to caring for the patient through different stages of shock, the nurse needs to tailor interventions to the type of shock—whether it is hypovolemic, cardiogenic, or distributive shock.

Hypovolemic shock—the most common type of shock—is characterized by a decreased intravascular volume. Body fluid is contained in intracellular and extracellular compartments. Intracellular fluid accounts for about two thirds of the total body water. The extracellular body fluid is found in one of two compartments: intravascular (inside blood vessels) or interstitial (surrounding tissues). The volume of interstitial fluid is about three to four times that of intravascular fluid. Hypovolemic shock occurs when there is a reduction in intravascular volume of 15% to 25%. This would represent a loss of 750 to 1300 mL of blood in a 70-kg (154-lb) person.

Pathophysiology

Hypovolemic shock can be caused by external fluid losses, as in hemorrhage, or by internal fluid shifts, as in severe dehydration, severe edema, or ascites. Intravascular volume can be reduced both by fluid loss and fluid shifting between intravascular and interstitial compartments.

The sequence of events in hypovolemic shock begins with a decrease in the intravascular volume. This results in decreased venous return of blood to the heart and subsequent decreased ventricular filling. Decreased ventricular filling results in decreased stroke volume (amount of blood ejected from the heart) and decreased cardiac output. When cardiac output drops, blood pressure drops, and tissues cannot be adequately perfused (Fig. 14-3).

Medical Management

Major goals in treating hypovolemic shock are to (1) restore intravascular volume to reverse the sequence of events leading to inadequate tissue perfusion, (2) redistribute fluid volume, and (3) correct the underlying cause of the fluid loss as quickly as possible. Depending on the severity of shock and the patient's condition, it is likely that efforts will be made to address all three goals simultaneously.

TREATMENT OF THE UNDERLYING CAUSE

If the patient is hemorrhaging, efforts are made to stop the bleeding. This may involve applying pressure to the bleeding site or

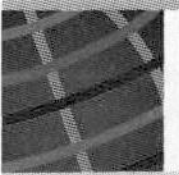

TABLE 14•1 Vasoactive Drugs Used in Treating Shock

Drug	Desired Action in Shock	Disadvantages
Sympathomimetics dopamine (Intropin) dobutamine (Dobutrex) epinephrine (Adrenaline) milrinone (Primacor)	Improve contractility, increase stroke volume, increase cardiac output	Increase oxygen demand of the heart
Vasodilators nitroprusside (Nipride) nitroglycerine (Tridil)	Reduce preload and afterload, reduce oxygen demand of heart	Cause hypotension
Vasoconstrictors phenylephrine (Neo-Synephrine) methoxamine (Vasoxyl)	Increase blood pressure by vasoconstriction	Increase afterload, thereby increasing cardiac work load; compromise perfusion to skin, kidneys, lungs, GI tract

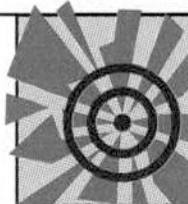

Risk Factors for HYPOVOLEMIC SHOCK

External: Fluid Losses
Trauma
Surgery
Vomiting
Diarrhea
Diuresis
Diabetes insipidus

Internal: Fluid Shifts
Hemorrhage
Burns
Ascites
Peritonitis

surgery to stop internal bleeding. If the cause of the hypovolemia is diarrhea or vomiting, medications to treat diarrhea and vomiting are administered.

FLUID AND BLOOD REPLACEMENT

Beyond reversing the primary cause for the decreased intravascular volume, fluid replacement (also referred to as fluid resuscitation) is of primary concern. At least two large-gauge intravenous lines are inserted to establish access for fluid administration. Two intravenous lines allow simultaneous administration of fluid and blood component therapy if required. Because the goal of the fluid replacement is to restore intravascular volume, it is necessary to administer fluids that will remain in the intravascular compartment and thus avoid creating fluid shifts from the intravascular compartment into the intracellular compartment. Table 14-2 summarizes fluids commonly used in treating shock.

Lactated Ringer's and 0.9% sodium chloride solutions are isotonic crystalloid fluids commonly used in treating hypovolemic shock (Robins, 1996). Large amounts of fluid must be administered to restore intravascular volume because isotonic crystalloid solutions move freely between the fluid compartments of the body and do not remain in the vascular system.

Colloids (eg, albumin, hetastarch, and 6% dextran) are now widely used. Dextran is not indicated if the cause of the hypovolemic shock is hemorrhage because it interferes with platelet aggregation.

Blood products, also colloids, may need to be administered, particularly when the cause of the hypovolemic shock is hemorrhage. Because of the risk of transmitting blood-borne viruses and the scarcity of blood products, however, these products are used only if other alternatives are unavailable or blood loss is extensive and rapid. Packed red blood cells are administered to replenish the patient's oxygen-carrying capacity in conjunction with other fluids that will expand volume. Current recommendations are to base the need for transfusions on the patient's oxygenation needs, which are determined by vital signs, blood gas values, and clinical appearance rather than using an arbitrary laboratory value. Synthetic forms of blood (ie, compounds capable of carrying oxygen in the same way that blood does) are potential alternatives.

Autotransfusion, the collection and retransfusion of the patient's own blood, may be initiated. This reduces the risk of transmitting a communicable disease or of a transfusion reaction and eliminates the prolonged time needed for typing and crossmatching blood. Autotransfusion may only be performed when the patient is bleeding within a closed cavity, such as the chest or abdominal cavity (Ley, 1995). A chest tube is inserted, and blood is collected through a filter in a specifically designed collection device often attached to routine chest tube drainage systems. The blood obtained must be transfused back to the patient within 4 hours of its collection. Potential complications of autotransfusion are rare but may include infection, hemolysis, coagulopathy, and the risk of microembolism (Ley, 1995).

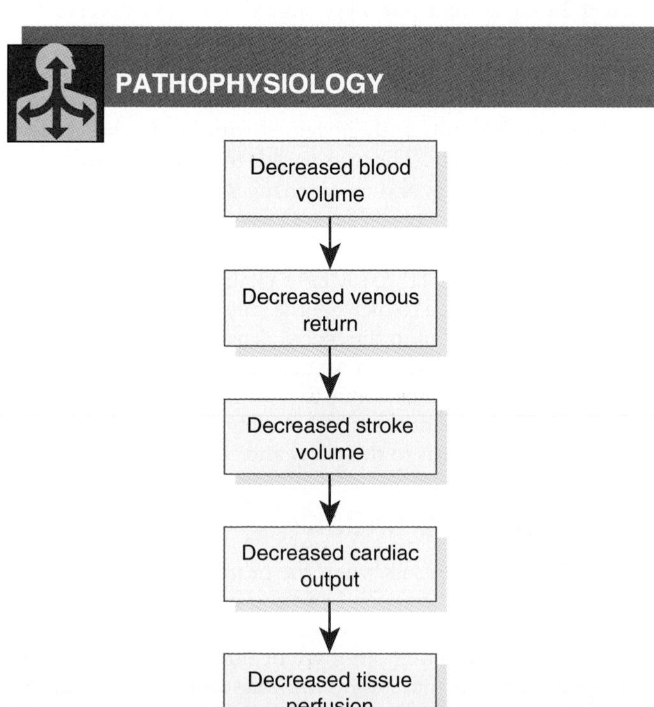

FIGURE 14•3 Pathophysiologic sequence of events in hypovolemic shock.

REDISTRIBUTION OF FLUID

In addition to administering fluids to restore intravascular volume, positioning the patient properly assists fluid redistribution. A modified Trendelenburg position (Fig. 14-4) is recommended in hypovolemic shock. Elevating the patient's legs promotes the return of venous blood. Positioning patients in a full Trendelenburg position, however, makes breathing difficult and therefore is not recommended.

Pharmacologic Therapy

If fluid administration fails to reverse hypovolemic shock, then the same medications given in cardiogenic shock are used because unreversed hypovolemic shock progresses to cardiogenic shock (the "vicious circle").

If the underlying cause of the hypovolemia is dehydration, medications are prescribed to reverse the cause of the dehydration. For example, insulin is administered if dehydration is secondary to hyperglycemia; desmopressin (DDVP) is administered for diabetes insipidus, antidiarrheal agents for diarrhea, and antiemetics for vomiting.

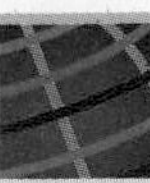

TABLE 14•2 **Fluid Replacement in Shock**

Fluids	Advantages	Disadvantages
Crystalloids		
0.9% sodium chloride (Normal saline solution)	Widely available, inexpensive	Requires large volume of infusion; can cause pulmonary edema
lactated Ringer's	Lactate ion helps buffer metabolic acidosis	Requires large volume of infusion; can cause pulmonary edema
hypertonic saline (3%, 5%, 7.5%)	Small volume needed to restore intravascular volume	Danger of hypernatremia
Colloids		
albumin (5%, 25%)	Rapidly expands plasma volume	Expensive; requires human donors; limited supply; can cause congestive heart failure
dextran (40, 70)	Synthetic plasma expander	Interferes with platelet aggregation; not recommended for hemorrhagic shock
hetastarch	Synthetic; less expensive than albumin; effect lasts up to 36 h	Prolongs bleeding and clotting times

Nursing Management

Primary prevention of shock is an essential focus of nursing intervention. Hypovolemic shock can be prevented in some instances by closely monitoring patients who are at risk for fluid deficits and assisting with fluid replacement before intravascular volume is depleted. In other circumstances, hypovolemic shock cannot be prevented, and nursing care focuses on assisting with treatment targeted at treating its cause and restoring intravascular volume.

General nursing measures include ensuring safe administration of prescribed fluids and medications and documenting their administration and effects. Another important nursing role is monitoring for signs of complications and side effects of treatment and reporting these signs early in treatment.

ADMINISTERING FLUIDS AND BLOOD SAFELY

Administering blood transfusions safely is a vital nursing role. In emergency situations, it is important to obtain blood specimens quickly for a baseline complete blood count and to type and cross-match the patient's blood in anticipation of blood transfusions. The patient who receives a transfusion of blood products must be monitored closely for adverse effects (see Chap. 30).

Fluid replacement complications can occur, often when large volumes are administered rapidly. Therefore, the nurse monitors the patient closely for cardiovascular overload and pulmonary edema. The risks of these complications increase in the elderly and in patients with pre-existing cardiac disease. Hemodynamic pressure, vital signs, arterial blood gases, hemoglobin and hematocrit levels, and fluid intake and output are among the parameters monitored. The patient's temperature should also be monitored closely to ensure that rapid fluid resuscitation does not precipitate hypothermia. Intravenous fluids may need to be warmed during administration of large volumes. Physical assessment focuses on observing the patient's jugular veins for distention and monitoring jugular venous pressure. Jugular venous pressure is low in hypovolemic shock; it increases with effective treatment and is significantly increased with fluid overload and congestive heart failure. The nurse needs to monitor cardiac and respiratory status closely and report changes in heart rate, rhythm, and lung sounds to the physician.

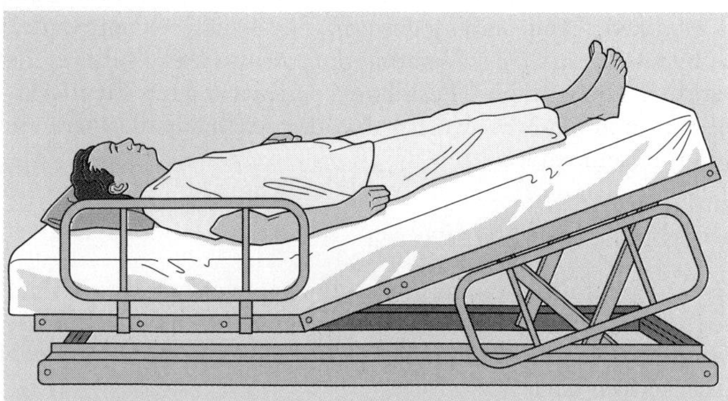

FIGURE 14•4 Proper positioning of the patient who shows signs of shock. The lower extremities are elevated to an angle of about 20 degrees; the knees are straight, the trunk is horizontal, and the head is slightly elevated.

IMPLEMENTING OTHER MEASURES

Oxygen is administered to increase the amount of oxygen carried by available hemoglobin in the blood. A patient who is confused may feel apprehensive with an oxygen mask or cannula in place, and frequent explanations about the need for the mask may reduce some of the patient's fear and anxiety. Simultaneously, the nurse must direct efforts to the safety and comfort of the patient.

CARDIOGENIC SHOCK

Cardiogenic shock occurs when the heart's ability to contract and to pump blood is impaired and the supply of oxygen is inadequate for the heart and tissues. The causes of cardiogenic shock are known as either coronary or noncoronary. Coronary cardiogenic shock is more common than noncoronary cardiogenic shock and is seen most often in patients with myocardial infarction. Coronary cardiogenic shock occurs when a significant amount of the left ventricular myocardium has been destroyed (Jones, 1996; Madding, 1996). Patients experiencing an anterior

Risk Factors for CARDIOGENIC SHOCK

Coronary Factors
Myocardial infarction

Noncoronary Factors
Cardiomyopathies
Valvular damage
Cardiac tamponade
Dysrhythmias

wall myocardial infarction are at the greatest risk of developing cardiogenic shock because of the potentially extensive damage to the left ventricle caused by occlusion of the left anterior descending coronary artery.

Pathophysiology

In cardiogenic shock, cardiac output, which is a function of both stroke volume and heart rate, is compromised. When stroke volume and heart rate decrease or become erratic, blood pressure drops, and tissue perfusion is compromised. Along with other tissues and organs being deprived of adequate blood supply, the heart muscle itself receives inadequate blood. The result is impaired tissue perfusion. Because impaired tissue perfusion weakens the heart and impairs its ability to pump blood forward, the ventricle does not fully eject its volume of blood at systole. As a result, fluid accumulates in the lungs. This sequence of events can occur rapidly or over a period of days (Fig. 14-5).

Clinical Manifestations

Patients in cardiogenic shock may experience angina pain and develop dysrhythmias.

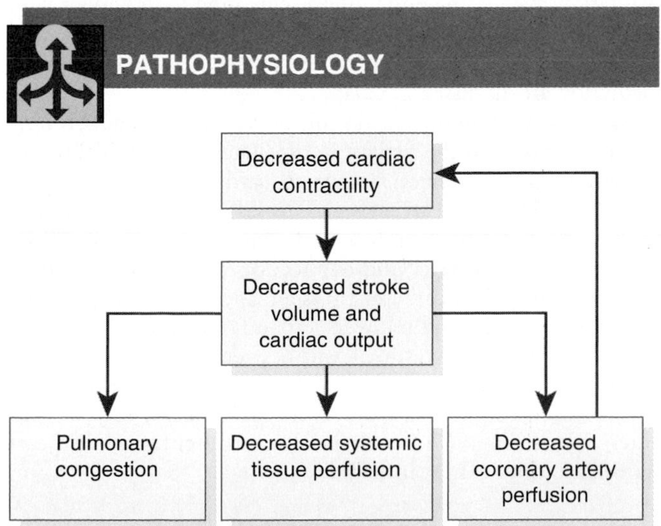

FIGURE 14•5 Pathophysiologic sequence of events in cardiogenic shock.

Medical Management

The goals of medical management are to (1) limit further myocardial damage and preserve the healthy myocardium, and (2) improve the cardiac function either by increasing cardiac contractility, decreasing ventricular afterload, or both (Magder, 1996). In general, these goals are achieved by increasing oxygen supply to the heart muscle, while reducing oxygen demands.

CORRECTION OF UNDERLYING CAUSES

As with all forms of shock, the underlying cause of cardiogenic shock must be corrected. It is necessary first to treat the oxygenation needs of the heart muscle to ensure its continued ability to pump blood to other organs. In the case of coronary cardiogenic shock, the patient may require thrombolytic therapy, angioplasty, or coronary artery bypass graft surgery. In the case of noncoronary cardiogenic shock, the patient may require a cardiac valve replacement or correction of a dysrhythmia. For further explanation of these procedures, refer to Chapters 24 and 25.

INITIATION OF FIRST-LINE TREATMENT

First-line treatment of cardiogenic shock involves the following actions:

- Supplying supplemental oxygen
- Controlling chest pain
- Administering vasoactive medications
- Controlling heart rate
- Providing selective fluid support
- Implementing mechanical cardiac support (transthoracic pacemaker)

Oxygenation. In the early stages of shock, supplemental oxygen is given by nasal cannula at a rate of 2 to 6 L/min to achieve an oxygen saturation exceeding 90%. Monitoring arterial blood gas values and pulse oximetry values helps to indicate whether the patient requires a more aggressive method of oxygen delivery.

Pain Control. If the patient experiences chest pain, morphine sulfate is given intravenously for pain relief. In addition to relieving pain, morphine dilates the blood vessels. This reduces the workload of the heart by both decreasing the cardiac filling pressure (preload) and reducing the pressure against which the heart muscle has to eject blood (afterload). Morphine also relieves the patient's anxiety. Cardiac enzyme levels are measured, and 12-lead ECG is performed daily to assess the degree of myocardial damage.

Hemodynamic Monitoring. Hemodynamic monitoring is initiated to assess the patient's response to treatment. In many institutions, this is performed in the intensive care unit where an arterial line can be inserted. The arterial line enables accurate and continuous monitoring of blood pressure and provides a port from which to obtain frequent arterial blood samples without having to perform repeated arterial punctures. A multilumen pulmonary artery catheter is inserted to allow measurement of the patient's pulmonary artery pressures and cardiac output. For more information, see Chapter 27.

Pharmacologic Therapy

Vasoactive medication therapy consists of multiple pharmacologic strategies to restore and maintain adequate cardiac output. In coronary cardiogenic shock, the aims of vasoactive medication therapy are improved cardiac contractility, decreased preload and afterload, or stable heart rate.

Because improving contractility and decreasing cardiac workload are opposing pharmacologic actions, two classifications of medications may be given in combination: sympathomimetics and vasodilators. Sympathomimetic medications increase cardiac output by mimicking the action of the sympathetic nervous system through vasoconstriction, increasing myocardial contractility, or increasing the heart rate. Vasodilators are used to decrease preload and afterload, thus reducing the workload of the heart and the oxygen demand. Two medications commonly combined to treat cardiogenic shock are dopamine and nitroglycerin.

DOPAMINE

Dopamine (Intropin) has varying vasoactive effects depending on the dose. Low-dose dopamine (0.5 to 3.0 μg/kg/min) increases renal and mesenteric blood flow, thereby preventing ischemia of these organs because shock causes blood to be shunted away from the kidneys and the mesentery. This dosage, however, does not improve cardiac output. Medium-dose dopamine (4 to 8 μg/kg/min) has the effect of improving contractility and slightly increasing the heart rate. At this dosage, dopamine increases cardiac output and therefore is desirable. High-dose dopamine (8 to 10 μg/kg/min) causes vasoconstriction. Vasoconstriction increases afterload and thus increases cardiac workload. This effect is not desired; therefore, dosages must be carefully titrated. Once the patient's blood pressure stabilizes, low-dose dopamine may be continued for its effect of promoting renal perfusion in particular. In severe metabolic acidosis, which occurs in the later stages of shock, dopamine's effectiveness is diminished. To maximize the effectiveness of any vasoactive agent, metabolic acidosis must first be corrected. The physician may prescribe intravenous sodium bicarbonate to treat the acidosis.

NITROGLYCERIN

Intravenous nitroglycerin (Tridil) in low doses acts as a venous vasodilator and therefore reduces preload. At higher doses, nitroglycerin causes arterial vasodilation and therefore reduces afterload as well. These actions, in combination with medium-dose dopamine, increase cardiac output while minimizing cardiac workload. Additionally, vasodilation enhances blood flow to the myocardium, improving oxygen delivery to the weakened heart muscle.

OTHER VASOACTIVE MEDICATIONS

Additional vasoactive agents that may be used in managing cardiogenic shock include dobutamine (Dobutrex), norepinephrine (Levophed), epinephrine (Adrenalin), isoproterenol (Isuprel), milrinone (Primacor), and amrinone (Inocor). Each of these medications stimulates different receptors of the sympathetic nervous system. A combination of these medications may be prescribed, depending on the patient's response to treatment. All vasoactive medications have adverse effects, making specific medications more useful than others at different stages phases of shock. Diuretics, such as furosemide (Lasix), may be administered to reduce the workload of the heart by reducing fluid accumulation.

ANTIARRHYTHMIC MEDICATIONS

Antiarrhythmic medication is also part of the medication regimen in cardiogenic shock. Multiple factors, such as hypoxemia, electrolyte imbalances, and acid–base imbalances, contribute to serious cardiac dysrhythmias in all patients with shock. Additionally, as a compensatory response to decreased cardiac output and blood pressure, the heart rate increases beyond normal limits. This impedes cardiac output further by shortening diastole and thereby decreasing time for ventricular filling. Consequently, antiarrhythmic medications are required to stabilize the heart rate. For a full discussion of cardiac dysrhythmias as well as commonly prescribed medications, see Chapter 24. General principles regarding the administration of vasoactive medications are discussed later in this chapter.

FLUID THERAPY

In addition to medications, appropriate fluid is necessary in treating cardiogenic shock. Administration of fluids must be monitored closely to detect signs of fluid overload. Incremental intravenous fluid boluses are cautiously administered to determine optimal filling pressures to improve cardiac output. A fluid bolus should never be given quickly because rapid fluid administration in patients with cardiac failure may result in acute pulmonary edema.

Mechanical Assistive Devices

In cases in which cardiac output does not improve despite supplemental oxygen, vasoactive medications, and fluid boluses, mechanical assistive devices are used temporarily to improve the heart's ability to pump. Intra-aortic balloon counterpulsation (IABC) is one means of providing temporary circulatory assistance (see Chap. 27). A polyurethane balloon catheter is inserted percutaneously through the common femoral artery and advanced into the descending thoracic aorta. The balloon catheter is connected to a console containing a gas-filled pump. The timing of the balloon inflation is synchronized electrocardiographically with the beginning of diastole, and the balloon deflation occurs just before systole. The goals of IABC include the following:

- Increased stroke volume
- Improved coronary artery perfusion
- Decreased preload
- Decreased cardiac workload
- Decreased myocardial oxygen demand (Jones, 1996)

Other means of mechanical assistance include left and right ventricular assist devices and total artificial hearts. These devices are electrical pumps or pumps driven by air. They assist or replace the ventricular pumping action of the heart. Human heart transplantation may be the only option remaining for a patient who has cardiogenic shock and who cannot be weaned from mechanical assistive devices. (Mechanical assistive devices and heart transplantation are discussed in Chap. 27.)

Another short-term means of providing cardiac or pulmonary support to the patient in cardiogenic shock is through an extracorporeal device similar to cardiopulmonary bypass (CPB) used in open heart surgery. The CPB system requires systemic anticoagulation, arterial and venous cannulation of the femoral artery and vein, and connection to a centrifugal, oxygenated pump. The catheter tip is advanced into the patient's right atrium. This system lowers left and right ventricular pressures, reducing the workload and oxygen needs of the heart. Complications of CPB include coagulopathies, myocardial ischemia, infection, and thromboembolism. CPB is used only in emergency situations until definitive treatment, such as heart transplantation, can be initiated.

Nursing Management

PREVENTING CARDIOGENIC SHOCK

In some circumstances, cardiogenic shock can be prevented by identifying patients at risk early and promoting adequate oxygenation of the heart muscle and decreasing cardiac workload. This can be accomplished by conserving the patient's energy, promptly relieving angina, and administering supplemental oxygen. Often, however, cardiogenic shock cannot be prevented. In such instances, nursing management includes working with other members of the health care team to prevent shock from progressing and to restore adequate cardiac function and tissue perfusion.

MONITORING HEMODYNAMIC STATUS

A major role of the nurse is monitoring the patient's hemodynamic and cardiac status. Arterial lines and ECG monitoring equipment must be maintained and functioning properly. The nurse anticipates the medications, intravenous fluids, and equipment that might be used and is ready to assist in implementing these measures. Changes in hemodynamic, cardiac, and pulmonary status are documented and reported promptly. Additionally, adventitious breath sounds, changes in cardiac rhythm, and other abnormal physical assessment findings are reported immediately.

ADMINISTERING MEDICATIONS AND INTRAVENOUS FLUIDS

The nurse has a critical role in safe and accurate administration of intravenous fluids and medications. Fluid overload and pulmonary edema are risks because of ineffective cardiac function and accumulation of blood and fluid in the pulmonary tissues. The nurse documents and records medications and treatments that are administered as well as the patient's response to treatment.

The nurse needs to be knowledgeable about the desired effects as well as side effects of medications. For example, it is important to monitor the patient for decreased blood pressure after administering morphine or nitroglycerin. The patient receiving thrombolytic therapy must be monitored for bleeding. Arterial and venous puncture sites must be observed for bleeding and pressure applied at the sites if bleeding occurs. Intravenous infusions must be observed closely because tissue necrosis and sloughing may occur if vasopressor medications infiltrate the tissues. Urine output, BUN, and serum creatinine levels are monitored to detect decreased renal function secondary to the effects of cardiogenic shock or its treatment.

MAINTAINING INTRA-AORTIC BALLOON COUNTERPULSATION

The nurse plays a critical role in caring for the patient receiving IABC. The nurse makes ongoing timing adjustments of the balloon pump to maximize its effectiveness by synchronizing it with the cardiac cycle. The patient is at great risk of circulatory compromise to the leg on the side where the catheter for the IABC has been placed. Therefore, the nurse must frequently check the neurovascular status of the lower extremities.

ENHANCING SAFETY AND COMFORT

Throughout the patient's care, the nurse must also take an active role in safeguarding the patient, enhancing his or her comfort, and reducing anxiety. This includes administering medication to relieve chest pain, preventing infection at the multiple arterial and venous line insertion sites, protecting the patient's skin, and monitoring respiratory function. Proper positioning of the patient promotes effective breathing without decreasing blood pressure and may also increase the patient's comfort while reducing anxiety.

Brief explanations about procedures that are being performed and the use of comforting touch often provide reassurance to the patient and family. Families are usually anxious and benefit from opportunities to see and talk to the patient. Explanations of treatments and the patient's response to them are often comforting to family members.

Risk Factors for DISTRIBUTIVE SHOCK

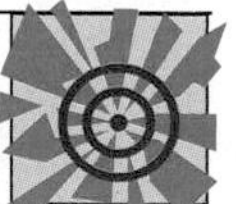

Neurogenic shock
Spinal cord injury
Spinal anesthesia

Anaphylactic shock
Penicillin sensitivity
Transfusion reaction
Bee sting allergy

Septic shock
Immunosuppression
Extremes of age (<1 yr and >65 yr)
Malnourishment
Chronic illness
Invasive procedures

DISTRIBUTIVE SHOCK

Distributive or vasogenic shock occurs when blood volume is abnormally displaced in the vasculature—for example, when blood volume pools in peripheral blood vessels. The displacement of blood volume causes a relative hypovolemia because not enough blood returns to the heart, which leads to subsequent inadequate tissue perfusion. The ability of the blood vessels to constrict helps return the blood to the heart. Thus, the vascular tone is determined both by central regulatory mechanisms, as in blood pressure regulation, and by local regulatory mechanisms, as in tissue demands for oxygen and nutrients. Therefore, distributive shock can be caused either by a loss of sympathetic tone or by release of biochemical mediators from cells.

The varied mechanisms leading to the initial vasodilation in distributive shock further subdivide this classification of shock into three types: (1) **septic shock**, (2) **neurogenic shock**, and (3) **anaphylactic shock**.

The different types of distributive shock cause variations in the pathophysiologic chain of events and are explained here separately. In all types of distributive shock, massive arterial and venous dilation allows blood to pool peripherally. Arterial dilation reduces systemic vascular resistance. Initially, cardiac output can be high in distributive shock, both from the reduction in afterload (systemic vascular resistance) and from the heart muscle's increased effort to maintain perfusion despite the incompetent vasculature secondary to arterial dilation. Pooling of blood in the periphery results in decreased venous return. Decreased venous return results in decreased stroke volume and decreased cardiac output. Decreased cardiac output, in turn, causes decreased blood pressure and ultimately decreased tissue perfusion. Figure 14-6 presents the pathophysiologic sequence of events in distributive shock.

Septic Shock

Septic shock is the most common type of distributive shock and is caused by widespread infection. Despite increased sophistica-

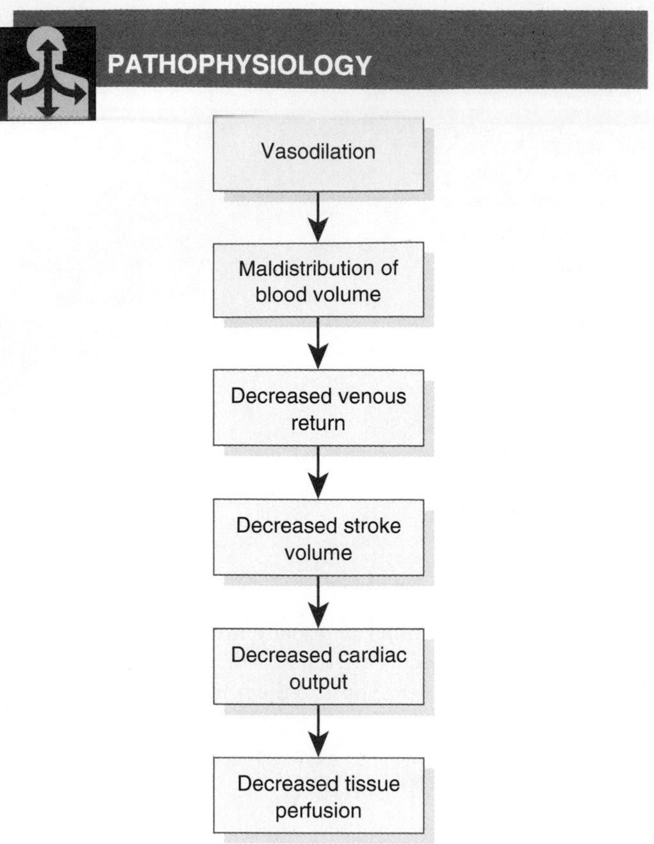

FIGURE 14•6 Pathophysiologic sequence of events in distributive shock.

tion of antibiotic therapy, the incidence of septic shock has continued to rise during the past 60 years. It is the most common cause of death in intensive care units in the United States, the 13th leading cause of death in the U.S. population (National Safety Council, 1996), and the 8th leading cause of death in elderly adults (Ackerman, 1994). Toxic shock syndrome, a specific form of septic shock, is described in Chapter 43.

The incidence of nosocomial infection (infections occurring in the hospital) in critically ill patients ranges from 20% to 25% (Osguthorpe & Ormond, 1995) The incidence of septic shock can be reduced by carrying out infection control practices and meticulous aseptic technique, débriding wounds to remove necrotic tissue, properly cleaning and maintaining equipment, and using thorough hand-washing techniques.

The most common causative microorganisms of septic shock are the gram-negative bacteria. Other infectious agents, however, such as gram-positive bacteria and viruses, also can cause septic shock. When a microorganism invades body tissues, the patient exhibits an immune response. This immune response provokes the activation of biochemical mediators that have a variety of effects leading to shock. Increased capillary permeability, which leads to fluid seeping from the capillaries, and vasodilation are two such effects.

Septic shock typically occurs in two phases. The first phase, referred to as the hyperdynamic, or warm, phase, is characterized by a high cardiac output with vasodilation. The patient becomes overheated or hyperthermic with warm, flushed skin. The respiratory rate is elevated. Urinary output may increase or may remain at normal levels. GI status may be compromised as evidenced by nausea, vomiting, or diarrhea. The patient may be febrile and may exhibit subtle changes in mental status, such as confusion or agitation. A decrease in blood pressure with concomitant tachycardia may occur.

The later phase, referred to as the hypodynamic, or cold, phase, is characterized by low cardiac output with vasoconstriction reflecting the body's effort to compensate for the hypovolemia caused by the loss of intravascular volume through the capillaries. In this phase, the patient's blood pressure drops, and the skin is cool and pale. Temperature may be normal or below normal. Heart and respiratory rates remain rapid. The patient no longer produces urine, and multiple organ failure may occur.

Systemic inflammatory response syndrome (SIRS) presents clinically like septic shock. The only difference between SIRS and sepsis is that there is no identifiable source of infection. SIRS stimulates an overwhelming inflammatory immunologic and hormonal response, similar to that seen in infected septic patients. Despite an absence of infection, antibiotics may still be administered because of the possibility of unrecognized infection. Additional therapies directed to the support of the patient with SIRS are similar to those for septic shock.

Medical Management

Current treatment of septic shock involves identifying and eliminating the cause of infection. Specimens of urine, blood, sputum, and wound drainage are collected for culture using aseptic technique.

Any potential routes of infection must be eliminated, including intravenous lines, which must be removed and reinserted elsewhere, and urinary catheters, which should be removed. Any abscesses should be drained and necrotic areas débrided. Fluid replacement must be instituted to correct the hypovolemia that results from the incompetent vasculature.

PHARMACOLOGIC THERAPY

If the infecting organism is unknown, broad-spectrum antibiotics are started until culture and sensitivity reports are received (Lynn & Cohen, 1995). A cephalosporin agent plus an aminoglycoside may be prescribed initially. This combination works against most gram-negative and some gram-positive organisms. When culture and sensitivity reports are available, the antibiotic may be changed to one that is more specific to the infecting organism and less toxic to the patient.

Research efforts show promise for improving the outcomes of septic shock. Although past treatments focused on destroying the infectious organism, emphasis is now on altering the immune response of the patient to the organism. The cell walls of gram-negative bacteria contain a lipopolysaccharide, an endotoxin released during phagocytosis (Kellum & Decker, 1996). Endotoxin is believed to trigger the release of the biochemical mediators whose effects lead to shock. Current research focuses on the development of medications that will inhibit the effects of biochemical mediators, such as endotoxin. The focus on immunotherapy in treating septic shock is expected to shed light on how the cellular response to infection leads to shock.

NUTRITIONAL THERAPY

Aggressive nutritional supplementation is critical in the management of septic shock because malnutrition further impairs the patient's resistance to infection. Nutritional supplementation should be initiated within the first 24 hours of the onset of shock (Wojnar, Hawkins, & Lang, 1995). Enteral feedings are preferred to the parenteral route because of the increased risk of iatrogenic infection associated with intravenous catheters; however, enteral feedings may not be possible if decreased perfusion to the GI tract limits peristalsis and absorption.

Nursing Management

The nurse caring for any patient in any setting must keep in mind the risks of sepsis and the high mortality rate associated with septic shock. All invasive procedures must be carried out with aseptic technique after careful hand washing. Additionally, intravenous lines, arterial and venous puncture sites, surgical incisions, trauma wounds, urinary catheters, and pressure ulcers are monitored for signs of infection in all patients. The nurse identifies patients at particular risk for sepsis and septic shock (ie, elderly and immunosuppressed patients or patients with extensive trauma or burns or diabetes), keeping in mind that these high-risk patients may not develop typical or classic signs of infection and sepsis. Confusion, for example, may be the first sign of infection and sepsis in elderly patients.

When caring for the patient with septic shock, the nurse collaborates with other members of the health care team to identify the site and source of sepsis and the specific organisms involved. Appropriate specimens for culture and sensitivity are often obtained by the nurse.

Elevated body temperature (hyperthermia) is common with sepsis and raises the patient's metabolic rate and oxygen consumption. Fever is one of the body's natural mechanisms for fighting infections. Thus, an elevated temperature may not be treated unless it reaches dangerous levels (more than 40°C [104°F]) or unless the patient is uncomfortable. Efforts may be made to reduce the patient's temperature by administering salicylates, hypothermia blankets, or ice packs. During these therapies, the nurse monitors the patient closely for shivering, which further increases oxygen consumption. Efforts to increase the patient's comfort are important if the patient experiences chills, fever, or shivering.

The nurse administers prescribed intravenous fluids and medications, including antibiotics and vasoactive medications to restore vascular volume. Because of decreased perfusion to the kidneys and liver, serum concentrations of antibiotics that are normally cleared by these organs may increase and produce toxic effects. Therefore, the nurse monitors blood levels (antibiotic levels, BUN, creatinine, white blood count) and reports increased levels to the physician.

As with other types of shock, the nurse monitors the patient's hemodynamic status, fluid intake and output, and nutritional status. Daily weighing and close monitoring of serum albumin levels help determine the patient's protein requirements.

Neurogenic Shock

In neurogenic shock, vasodilation occurs as a result of a loss of sympathetic tone. This can be caused by spinal cord injury, spinal anesthesia, or nervous system damage. It can also result from depressant action of medications or lack of glucose (eg, insulin reaction or shock).

Neurogenic shock may have a prolonged course (spinal cord injury) or a short one (syncope or fainting). It is characterized by dry, warm skin rather than the cool, moist skin seen in hypovolemic shock. Another characteristic is bradycardia, rather than the tachycardia that characterizes other forms of shock.

Medical Management

Treatment of neurogenic shock involves restoring sympathetic tone either through the stabilization of a spinal cord injury or, in the instance of spinal anesthesia, by positioning the patient properly. Specific treatment of neurogenic shock depends on its cause. Further discussion of managing the patient with a spinal cord injury is presented in Chapter 58. If hypoglycemia (insulin shock) is the cause, glucose is rapidly administered. Hypoglycemia and insulin reaction are described further in Chapter 37.

Nursing Management

It is important to elevate and maintain the head of the bed at least 30 degrees to prevent neurogenic shock when a patient is receiving spinal or epidural anesthesia. Elevation of the head of the bed helps to prevent the spread of the anesthetic up the spinal cord. In suspected spinal cord injury, neurogenic shock may be prevented by carefully immobilizing the patient to prevent further damage to the spinal cord.

Nursing interventions are directed toward supporting the patient's cardiovascular and neurologic functions until the usually transient episode of neurogenic shock resolves. Applying elastic pressure stockings and elevating the foot of the bed may minimize pooling of blood in the legs. Pooled blood increases the risk for thrombus formation. Therefore, the nurse needs to check the patient daily for a positive Homans' sign (calf pain on dorsiflexion of the foot) and any redness of the calves.

To elicit Homans' sign, the nurse lifts the patient's leg, flexing it at the knee and dorsiflexing the foot. If the patient complains of pain in the calf, the sign is positive and suggestive of deep vein thrombosis. Administering heparin as prescribed, applying elastic pressure stockings, and initiating pneumatic compression of the legs may prevent thrombus formation. Performing passive range of motion of the immobile extremities helps promote circulation.

Patients who have experienced a spinal cord injury may not report pain caused by internal injuries. Therefore, in the immediate postinjury period, the nurse must monitor the patient closely for signs of internal bleeding that could lead to hypovolemic shock.

Anaphylactic Shock

Anaphylactic shock is caused by a severe allergic reaction when a patient who has already produced antibodies to a foreign substance (antigen) develops a systemic antigen–antibody reaction. This process requires that the patient has previously been exposed to the substance. An antigen–antibody reaction provokes mast cells to release potent vasoactive substances, such as histamine or bradykinin, which cause widespread vasodilation and capillary permeability. Anaphylactic shock occurs rapidly and is life-threatening. Because anaphylactic shock occurs in patients already exposed to an antigen who have developed antibodies to it, it can often be prevented. Therefore, patients with known allergies need to understand the consequences of subsequent exposure to the antigen and wear medical identification of their sensitivities. This could prevent inadvertent administration of a medication that would lead to anaphylactic shock. Additionally, the patient and family need instruction about emergency use of medications to treat anaphylaxis.

Medical Management

Treatment of anaphylactic shock requires removing the causative antigen (eg, discontinuing an antibiotic), administering medications that restore vascular tone, and providing emergency support of basic life functions. Epinephrine is given for its vasoconstrictive action. Diphenhydramine (Benadryl) is administered to reverse the effects of histamine, thereby reducing capillary permeability. Aminophylline is given to reverse histamine-induced bronchospasm. These medications are given intravenously.

If cardiac arrest and respiratory arrest are imminent or have occurred, cardiopulmonary resuscitation is performed. Endotracheal intubation or tracheotomy may be necessary to establish an airway. Intravenous lines are inserted to provide access for administering fluids and medications. Further discussion of anaphylaxis and specific chemical mediators is presented in Chapter 49.

Nursing Management

The nurse has an important role in preventing anaphylactic shock: assessing all patients for allergies or previous reactions to antigens (eg, medications, blood products, foods, contrast agents, latex) and communicating the existence of these allergies or reactions to others. Additionally, the patient's understanding of previous reactions and steps taken by the patient and family to prevent further exposure to antigens are assessed. When new allergies are identified, the nurse advises wearing or carrying identification that names the specific allergen or antigen.

When administering any new medication, the nurse observes the patient for an allergic reaction. This is especially important with medications that are administered intravenously. Allergy to penicillin is one of the most common causes of anaphylactic shock.

In the hospital and outpatient testing settings, especially, the nurse needs to identify patients at risk for anaphylactic reactions to contrast agents (radiopaque, dyelike substances that may contain iodine) used for diagnostic studies: those with a well-known allergy to iodine or fish or those who have had previous allergic reactions to contrast agents. This information must be conveyed to the testing staff, and especially the radiography personnel.

The nurse must be knowledgeable about the clinical signs of anaphylaxis, take immediate action if signs and symptoms occur, and be prepared to begin cardiopulmonary resuscitation if cardiorespiratory arrest occurs. In addition to monitoring the patient's response to treatment, the nurse assists with intubation if needed, monitors the patient's hemodynamic status, ensures intravenous access for administration of medications, administers prescribed medications and fluids, and documents treatments and their effects.

Community health and home care nurses whose role includes administering medications, including antibiotics, in the patient's home or other setting must be prepared to administer epinephrine subcutaneously or intramuscularly in the event of an anaphylactic reaction.

After recovery from anaphylaxis, the patient and family require explanation of the event. Further, the nurse provides instruction about avoiding future exposure to antigens and administering emergency medications to treat anaphylaxis.

MULTIPLE ORGAN DYSFUNCTION SYNDROME

Multiple organ dysfunction syndrome (MODS) is altered organ function in an acutely ill patient that requires medical intervention to support the continued organ function. The disorder can be further categorized as primary and secondary MODS.

Pathophysiology

Primary MODS is the result of direct tissue insult, which then leads to impaired perfusion or ischemia. Secondary MODS is most often a complication of septic shock or SIRS. However, MODS may result as a complication of any form of shock because of inadequate tissue perfusion. As previously described, in shock, all organ systems singularly suffer damage from a lack of adequate perfusion that can result in organ failure. However, a syndrome of sequential organ failure has been further observed in patients. The exact mechanism that triggers this syndrome is unknown.

Although various causes of MODS have been identified, including dead or injured tissue, infection, and perfusion deficits, it is not yet possible to predict which patients will develop MODS. This is partly because much of the organ damage occurs at the cellular level and therefore cannot be directly observed or measured. The sequence of organ failure usually begins in the lungs and is followed by failure of the liver, GI system, and kidneys (McMahon, 1995). Advanced age, malnutrition, and coexisting diseases appear to increase the risk of MODS developing in an acutely ill patient.

Clinical Manifestations

The clinical course of MODS follows one of two patterns. In both patterns, there is an initial event that results in low blood pressure. The cause of the drop in blood pressure is treated, and the patient appears to respond. In the first pattern of MODS (primary MODS), which occurs most often when the initiating event is a pulmonary one, such as lung injury, the patient experiences respiratory compromise that necessitates intubation. This usually occurs within 72 hours of the initiating event. Respiratory failure leads rapidly to MODS, resulting in a mortality rate of 30% to 40% (McMahon, 1995).

In secondary MODS, the pattern is more insidious. It occurs most often in the patient with septic shock and progressively unfolds over about 1 month. The patient also experiences respiratory failure and requires intubation. The patient remains hemodynamically stable for about 7 to 14 days. Despite this apparent stability, the patient exhibits a hypermetabolic state characterized by hyperglycemia (elevated blood glucose level), hyperlactacidemia (excess of lactic acid in the blood), and polyuria (excessive urinary output). The patient's metabolic rate is 1.5 to 2 times basal metabolic rate. Infection is usually present, and skin breakdown begins to occur. During this stage, there is a severe loss of skeletal muscle mass, a process referred to as *autocatabolism.* In cases in which the hypermetabolic phase can be reversed, the mortality rate at this stage is 60% (McMahon, 1995).

In patients in whom the hypermetabolic phase cannot be reversed, MODS progresses and is characterized by jaundice, hyperbilirubinemia, and renal failure, often requiring dialysis. The patient becomes less hemodynamically stable and begins to require vasoactive medications and fluid support. This phase of MODS is prognostically significant in that the mortality rate increases from 40% to 60% in the early stage to 90% to 100% in the late stage.

Medical Management

Prevention remains the top priority in managing MODS. Elderly patients are at increased risk of MODS because of the lack of physiologic reserve associated with aging and the natural degenerative process, especially immune compromise (Rauen & Munro, 1998). Early detection and documentation of initial signs of infection are essential in managing elderly patients with MODS. Subtle changes in mentation or gradual rise in temperature are early warning signs. Other patients at risk of MODS are those with chronic illness, malnutrition, immunosuppression, and surgical or traumatic wounds.

If preventive measures fail, treatment measures to reverse MODS are aimed at (1) controlling the initiating event, (2) promoting adequate organ perfusion, and (3) providing nutritional support.

Nursing Management

The general plan of nursing care for the patient with MODS is the same as that for the patient in septic shock. Providing information and support to family members is a critical role of the nurse in caring for patients with MODS. Addressing end-of-life decisions is an important role of the health care team to ensure that supportive therapies are congruent with the wishes of the patient.

PROMOTING COMMUNICATION

The nurse encourages frequent and open communication about treatment modalities and options to ensure that the patient's wishes regarding medical management are met. For those patients who survive MODS, the massive loss of skeletal muscle mass makes rehabilitation a long, slow process.

PROMOTING HOME AND COMMUNITY-BASED CARE

Teaching Patients Self-Care. The patient who experiences and survives shock may have been unable to get out of bed for an extended period of time and is likely to have a slow, prolonged recovery. The patient and family are instructed about strategies to prevent further episodes of shock by identifying those factors implicated in the initial episode. In addition, the patient and family require instruction about assessments needed to identify complications that may occur after the patient is discharged from the hospital. Depending on the type of shock and its management, the patient or family may require instruction about treatment modalities (ie, emergency administration of medications, intravenous therapy, parenteral nutrition, skin care, exercise, ambulation). The patient and family are also instructed about the need for gradual increases in ambulation and other activity. The need for an adequate dietary intake is another crucial aspect of teaching.

Continuing Care. Because of the physical toll associated with recovery from shock, the patient may be cared for in an extended care facility or rehabilitation setting after hospital discharge. Alternatively, a referral may be made for home care. The home care nurse assesses the patient's physical status and monitors recovery. The nurse also assesses the adequacy of treatments that are continued at home and the ability of the patient and family to cope with these treatments. The patient is likely to require close medical supervision until complete recovery occurs. The home care nurse reinforces the importance of continuing medical care and assists the patient and family to identify and mobilize community resources.

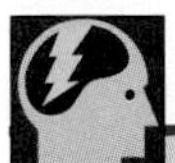

Critical Thinking Exercises

1. A patient in septic shock arrives in the emergency department. How would you explain septic shock to the patient's family? How might your approach differ if the family members are distraught and crying? If they do not speak English well?

2. You are on duty as the occupational health nurse for a large farm equipment manufacturer when an accident occurs in the plant. One worker is seriously injured and is bleeding profusely when you are notified. Describe the measures you would take at the scene to prevent or reduce the severity of shock, and discuss your reasons for these measures.

3. A patient has experienced second- and third-degree burns over 50% of his body. You know you must be alert for different types of shock that can occur during various phases of burn management. How would you assess for the various types of shock at different management stages, and how would the management of the different types of shock differ?

4. How would you distinguish anaphylactic shock from other forms of shock?

References and Selected Readings

BOOKS

Clochesy, J. M., Breu, C., et al. (Eds.). (1996). *Critical care nursing* (2nd ed.). Philadelphia: W. B. Saunders.

Cotran, R. S., et al. (Eds.). (1994). *Robbin's pathologic basis of disease* (5th ed.). Philadelphia: W. B. Saunders.

Dressler, D. K., et al. (Eds.). (1994). *Cardiovascular critical care nursing.* Albany, NY: Delmar Publishers.

Fein, A. M., et al. (Eds.). (1997). *Sepsis and multiorgan failure.* Baltimore: Williams & Wilkins.

Hudak, C. M., Gallo, M., & Morton, P. (Eds.). (1998). *Critical care nursing: A holistic approach* (7th ed.). Philadelphia: Lippincott-Raven.

Jones, K. (1996). Shock. In J. M. Clochesy, C. Breu, S. Cardin, A. A. Whittaker, & E. Rudy (Eds.), *Critical care nursing* (2nd ed.). Philadelphia: W. B. Saunders.

Madding, J. E. (1996). Cardiogenic shock in anterior wall myocardial infarction. In Melander, S. D., et al. (Eds.). *Review of critical care nursing.* Philadelphia: W. B. Saunders.

Magder, S. (1996). Shock physiology. In M. R. Pinsky & J. F. A. Dhainaut (Eds.), *Pathophysiologic foundations of critical care.* Baltimore, MD: Williams & Wilkins.

National Safety Council. (1996). *Accident facts 1996 edition.* Itasca, IL: Library of Congress.

Pinsky, M. R., et al. (Eds.). (1996). *Pathophysiologic foundations of critical care.* Baltimore: Williams & Wilkins.

Rauen, C. A. & Munro, N. (1998). Shock. In M. R. Kinney, S. B. Dunbar, J. A. Brooks-Brunn, N. Molter, & J. M. Vitello-Cicciu (Eds.), *AACN clinical reference for critical care nursing.* St. Louis: C. V. Mosby.

Reitschel, E. T., & Wagner, H. (1996). *Pathology of septic shock.* Berlin, NY: Springer.

Robins, E. V. (1996). Maldistribution of circulating volume. In V. H. Secor (Ed.), *Multiple organ dysfunction and failure: Pathophysiology and clinical implications.* St. Louis: C. V. Mosby.

Secor, V. H. (Ed.). (1996). *Multiple organ dysfunction and failure: Pathophysiology and clinical implications.* St. Louis: C. V. Mosby.

Thelan, L. A., et al. (Eds.). (1994). *Critical care nursing: Diagnosis and management* (2nd ed.). St. Louis: Mosby–Year Book.

JOURNALS

Ackerman, M. H. (1994). The systemic inflammatory response, sepsis, and multiple organ dysfunction: New definitions for an old problem. *Critical Care Clinics of North America, 6*(2), 243–250.

Barron, R. L. (1993). Pathophysiology of septic shock and implications for therapy. *Clinical Pharmacology and Therapy, 12*(11), 829–842.

Baxter, F. (1997). Septic shock. *Canadian Journal of Anaesthesia, 44*(1), 59–72.

Bone, R. C., et al. (1992). Definitions for sepsis and organ failure and guidelines for the use of innovative therapies in sepsis. *Chest, 101*(6), 1644–1655.

Bone, R. C., et al. (1996). Toward a theory regarding the pathogenesis of the systemic inflammatory response syndrome: What we do and do not know about cytokine regulation. *Critical Care Medicine, 24,* 163–172.

Bone, R. C., Grodzin, C. J., & Balk, R. A. (1997). Sepsis: A new hypothesis for pathogenesis of the disease process. *Chest, 112*(1), 253–243.

Carcillo, J. A., & Cunnion, R. E. (1997). Septic shock. *Critical Care Clinics, 13*(3), 553–574.

Effat, M. A. (1995). Pathophysiology of ischemic heart disease: An overview. *AACN Clinical Issues, 6*(3), 369–374.

Gullo, A., & Berlot, G. (1996). Ingredients of organ dysfunction or failure. *World Journal of Surgery, 20*(4), 430–436.

Heyland, D. K., et al. (1996). Maximizing oxygen delivery in critically ill patients: A methodologic appraisal of the evidence. *Critical Care Medicine, 24*(3), 517–523.

Jacobs, B. B. (1995). Emergent neurologic events. *Critical Care Clinics of North America, 7*(3), 427–444.

Kellum, J. A., & Decker, J. M. (1996). The immune system: Relation to sepsis and multiple organ failure. *AACN Clinical Issues, 7*(3), 339–350.

Ley, S. J. (1995). Intraoperative and postoperative blood salvage. *AACN Clinical Issues, 7*(2), 238–248.

Livingston, D. H., Mosenthal, A. C., & Deitch, E. A. (1995). Sepsis and multiple organ dysfunction syndrome. *New Horizons, 3*(2), 257–264.

Lynn, W. A., & Cohen, J. (1995). Adjunctive therapy for septic shock: A review of experimental approaches. *Clinical Infectious Diseases, 20*(1), 143–154.

Lynn, W. A., & Cohen, J. (1995). Management of septic shock. *Journal of Infection, 30*(3), 207–212.

McMahon, K. (1995). Multiple organ failure: The final compilation of critical illness. *Critical Care Nurse, 15*(6), 20–28.

O'Neal, P. V. (1994). How to spot early signs of cardiogenic shock. *American Journal of Nursing, 94*(5), 36–41.

Osguthorpe, S. G., & Ormond, L. (1995). Management constraints in infection control. *Critical Care Nursing Clinics of North America, 7*(4), 703–712.

Rangel-Frausto, M. S., et al. (1995). The natural history of the systemic inflammatory response syndrome. *Journal of the American Medical Association, 273*(2), 117–123.

Rauen, C. A., & Stamatos, C. A. (1997). Caring for geriatric patients with MODS. *American Journal of Nursing, 97*(5), 16BB–16II.

Sibbald, W. J., & Vincent, J. L. (1995). Round table conference on clinical trials for the treatment of sepsis. *Chest, 107*(2), 522–527.

Swank, G. M., & Deitch, E. A. (1996). Role of the gut in multiple organ failure. *World Journal of Surgery, 20*(4), 411–417.

Vincent, J. L. (1996). Prevention and therapy of multiple organ failure. *World Journal of Surgery, 20*(4), 465–470.

Wheeler, A. P., & Bernard, G. R. (1999). Treating patients with severe sepsis. *New England Journal of Medicine, 340*(3), 207–214.

Workman, M. L. (1995). Essential concepts of inflammation and immunity. *Critical Care Nursing Clinics of North America, 7*(4), 601–615.

Wojnar, M. M., Hawkins, W. G., & Lang, C. H. (1995). Nutritional support of the septic patient. *Critical Care Clinics, 11*(3), 717–733.

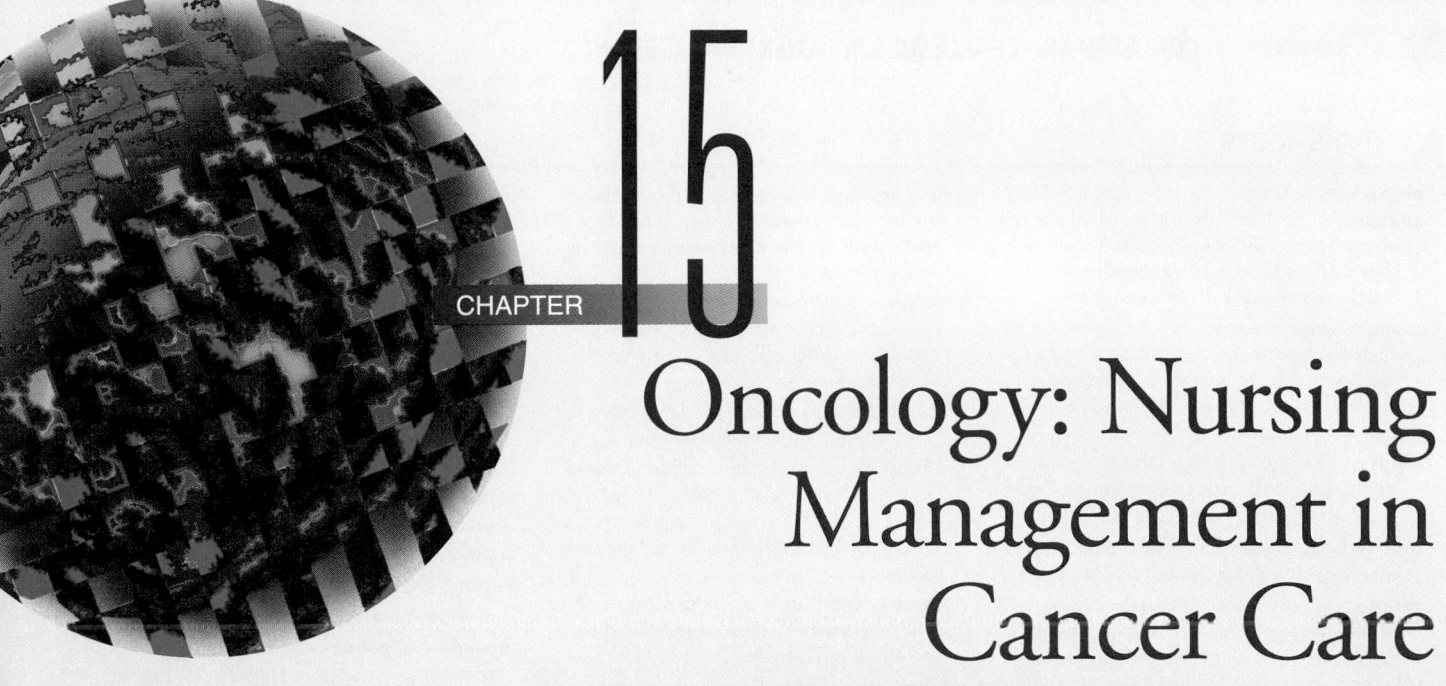

Oncology: Nursing Management in Cancer Care

Learning Objectives

On completion of this chapter, the learner will be able to:

1. Compare the structure and function of the normal cell and the cancer cell.
2. Differentiate between benign and malignant tumors.
3. Identify agents and factors that have been found to be carcinogenic.
4. Describe the significance of health education and preventive care in decreasing the incidence of cancer.
5. Differentiate among the purposes of surgical procedures used in cancer treatment, diagnosis, prophylaxis, palliation, and reconstruction.
6. Describe the roles of surgery, radiation therapy, chemotherapy, hyperthermia, biologic response modifiers, and gene therapy in treating cancer.
7. Describe the special nursing needs of patients receiving chemotherapy.
8. Describe common nursing diagnoses and collaborative problems of patients with cancer.
9. Use the nursing process as a framework for care of patients with cancer.
10. Describe the concept of hospice in providing care for patients with advanced cancer.
11. Discuss the role of the nurse in assessment and management of common oncologic emergencies.

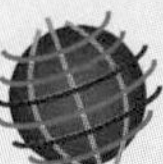

Cancer nursing practice covers all age groups and nursing specialties and is carried out in a variety of health care settings, including the home, community, acute care institutions, and rehabilitation centers. The scope, responsibilities, and goals of cancer nursing, also called **oncology** nursing, are as diverse and complex as those of any nursing specialty. Because many people associate cancer with pain and death, nurses need to identify their own reactions to cancer and set realistic goals to meet the challenges inherent in caring for patients with cancer.

In addition, the cancer nurse must be equipped to support the patient and family through a wide range of physical, emotional, social, cultural, and spiritual crises. Chart 15-1 identifies major areas of responsibility for nurses caring for patients with cancer.

GLOSSARY

alopecia: hair loss

anaplasia: cells that lack normal cellular characteristics and differ in shape and organization with respect to their cells of origin; usually, anaplastic cells are malignant

biologic response modifier therapy: use of agents or treatment methods that can alter the immunologic relationship between the tumor and the host to provide a therapeutic benefit

biopsy: a diagnostic procedure to remove a small sample of tissue to be examined microscopically to detect malignant cells

brachytherapy: the delivery of radiation therapy through internal implants

cancer: a disease process whereby cells proliferate abnormally, ignoring growth-regulating signals in the environment surrounding the cell

carcinogenesis: the process of transforming normal cells into malignant cells

chemotherapy: the use of drugs to kill tumor cells by interfering with cellular functions and reproduction

control: containment of the growth of cancer cells

cure: prolonged survival and disappearance of all evidence of disease so that the patient has the same life expectancy as anyone else in his or her age group

cytokines: substances produced by cells of the immune system to enhance production and functioning of components of the immune system

dysplasia: bizarre cell growth resulting in cells that differ in size, shape, or arrangement from other cells of the same type of tissue

extravasation: the leaking of drugs from the veins into the subcutaneous tissues

grading: identification of the type of tissue from which the tumor originated and the degree to which the tumor cells retain the functional and structural characteristics of the tissue of origin

hyperplasia: an increase in the number of cells of a tissue; most often associated with periods of rapid body growth

malignant: having cells or processes that are characteristic of cancer

metaplasia: the conversion of one type of mature cell into another type of cell

metastasis: the spread of cancer cells from the primary tumor to distant sites

myelosuppression: suppression of the blood cell–producing function of the bone marrow

nadir: the lowest point of white blood cell depression after therapy that has toxic effects on the bone marrow

neoplasia: uncontrolled cell growth that follows no physiologic demand

neutropenia: an abnormally low absolute neutrophil count

oncology: the field or study of cancer

palliation: the relief of symptoms associated with cancer

radiation therapy: the use of ionizing radiation to interrupt the growth of malignant cells

stomatitis: inflammation of the oral tissues, often associated with some chemotherapeutic agents

staging: the process of determining the size and spread, or metastasis, of a tumor

thrombocytopenia: a decrease in the number of circulating platelets; associated with the potential for bleeding

tumor-specific antigen (TSA): protein on the membrane of cancer cells that distinguishes the malignant cell from a benign cell of the same tissue type

vesicant: a substance that can cause tissue necrosis and damage, particularly when extravasated

xerostomia: dry oral cavity resulting from decreased function of salivary glands

CHART 15•1 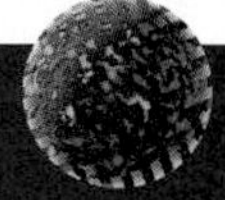 Responsibilities of the Nurse in Cancer Care

- Support the idea that cancer is a chronic illness that has acute exacerbations rather than one that is synonymous with death and suffering.
- Assess own level of knowledge relative to the pathophysiology of the disease process.
- Make use of current research findings and practices in the care of the patient with cancer and his or her family.
- Identify patients at high risk for cancer.
- Participate in primary and secondary prevention efforts.
- Assess the nursing care needs of the patient with cancer.
- Assess the learning needs, desires, and capabilities of the patient with cancer.
- Identify nursing problems of the patient and the family.
- Assess the social support networks available to the patient.
- Plan appropriate interventions with the patient and the family.
- Assist the patient to identify strengths and limitations.
- Assist the patient to design short-term and long-term goals for care.
- Implement a nursing care plan that interfaces with the medical care regimen and that is consistent with the established goals.
- Collaborate with members of a multidisciplinary team to foster continuity of care.
- Evaluate the goals and resultant outcomes of care with the patient, the family, and members of the multidisciplinary team.
- Reassess and redesign the direction of the care as determined by the evaluation.

EPIDEMIOLOGY

Although cancer affects every age group, most cancers occur in people older than 65 years of age. Overall, the incidence of cancer is higher in men than in women and higher in industrialized sectors and nations.

More than 1.2 million Americans are diagnosed each year with a cancer affecting one of various body sites (Fig. 15-1). Cancer is second only to cardiovascular disease as a leading cause of death in the United States. Each year, more than 560,000 Americans die of a **malignant** process. In order of frequency, the leading causes of cancer deaths in the United States are lung, prostate, and colorectal cancer in men and lung, breast, and colorectal cancer in women.

Relative 5-year survival rates in 1997 were 44% for African Americans and 60% for white Americans. In the United States, cancer mortality in African Americans is higher than in any other racial group. This finding is related to the higher incidence and later stage of diagnosis among African Americans. The increased cancer morbidity and mortality for this group are largely related to economic factors, education, and barriers to health care rather than to racial characteristics.

PATHOPHYSIOLOGY OF THE MALIGNANT PROCESS

Cancer is a disease process that begins when an abnormal cell is transformed by the genetic mutation of the cellular DNA. This abnormal cell forms a clone and begins to proliferate abnormally, ignoring growth-regulating signals in the environment surrounding the cell. The cells acquire invasive characteristics, and changes occur in surrounding tissues. The cells infiltrate these tissues and

Ten Leading Sites of Cancer in Men and Women

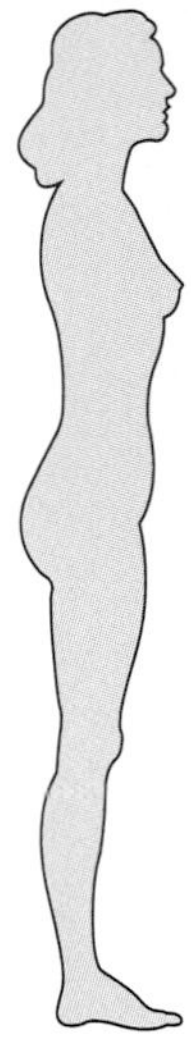

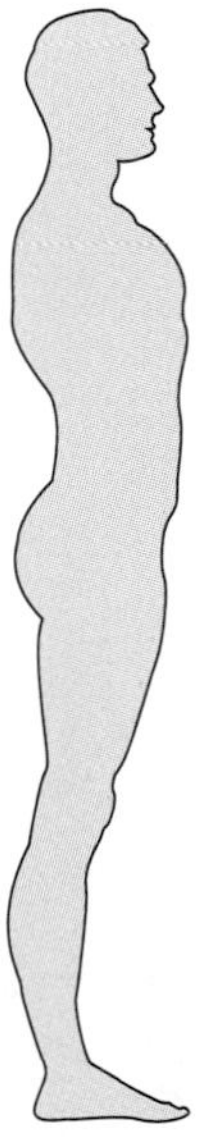

	New Cases*	Causes of Death*
Women	29% Breast	25% Lung and bronchus
	13% Lung and bronchus	16% Breast
	11% Colon and rectum	11% Colon and rectum
	6% Uterine corpus	5% Pancreas
	4% Non-Hodgkin's lymphoma	5% Ovary
	4% Ovary	5% Non-Hodgkin's lymphoma
	3% Melanoma of skin	4% Leukemia
	3% Urinary bladder	2% Uterine corpus
	2% Pancreas	2% Brain and other nervous system
	2% Thyroid	2% Stomach†
	23% All other sites	2% Multiple myeloma†
		21% All other sites
Men	29% Prostate	31% Lung and bronchus
	15% Lung and bronchus	13% Prostate
	10% Colon and rectum	10% Colon and rectum
	6% Urinary bladder	5% Pancreas
	5% Non-Hodgkin's lymphoma	5% Non-Hodgkin's lymphoma
	4% Melanoma of skin	4% Leukemia
	3% Kidney and renal pelvis	3% Esophagus
	3% Leukemia	3% Liver and intrahepatic bile duct
	3% Oral cavity and pharynx	3% Urinary bladder
	2% Stomach	3% Stomach
	20% All other sites	20% All other sites

*Excludes basal and squamous cell skin cancers and carcinoma in situ except bladder.
†These two cancers both received a ranking of 10; they have the same number of deaths and contribute the same percentage.

FIGURE 15•1 Estimated leading sites of cancer incidences and deaths—1999. *Cancer Facts and Figures, 1999.* American Cancer Society, Atlanta, Georgia.

gain access to lymph and blood vessels, which carry the cells to other areas of the body. This phenomenon is called **metastasis** (cancer spread to other parts of the body).

Although describable in general terms, cancer is not a single disease with a single cause; rather, it is a group of distinct diseases with different causes, manifestations, treatments, and prognoses.

Proliferative Patterns

During the life span, various body tissues normally experience periods of rapid or proliferative growth that must be distinguished from malignant growth activity. Several patterns of cell growth exist and are designated by the terms **hyperplasia, metaplasia, dysplasia, anaplasia,** and **neoplasia** (see Glossary).

Cancerous cells are described as malignant neoplasms. They demonstrate uncontrolled cell growth that follows no physiologic demand. Benign and malignant growths are classified and named by tissue of origin as described in Table 15-1.

Benign and malignant cells differ in many cellular growth characteristics, including method and rate of growth, ability to metastasize or spread, general effects, destruction of tissue, and ability to cause death. These differences are summarized in Table 15-2. The degree of anaplasia (lack of differentiation of cells) ultimately determines the malignant potential.

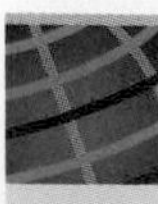

TABLE 15•1 **Tumors and Tissue Types**

Tissue Type	Benign Tumors	Malignant Tumors
Epithelial		
Surface	Papilloma	Squamous cell carcinoma
Glandular	Adenoma	Adenocarcinoma
Connective		
Fibrous	Fibroma	Fibrosarcoma
Adipose	Lipoma	Liposarcoma
Cartilage	Chondroma	Chondrosarcoma
Bone	Osteoma	Osteosarcoma
Blood vessels	Hemangioma	Hemangiosarcoma
Lymph vessels	Lymphangioma	Lymphangiosarcoma
Lymph tissue		Lymphosarcoma
Muscle		
Smooth	Leiomyoma	Leiomyosarcoma
Striated	Rhabdomyoma	Rhabdomyosarcoma
Neural Tissue		
Nerve cell	Neuroma	Neuroblastoma
Glial tissue	Glioma (benign)	Glioblastoma, astrocytoma, medulloblastoma, oligodendroglioma
Nerve sheaths	Neurilemmoma	Neurilemmal sarcoma
Meninges	Meningioma	Meningeal sarcoma
Hematologic		
Granulocytic		Myelocytic leukemia
Erythrocytic		Erythrocytic leukemia
Plasma cells		Multiple myeloma
Lymphocytic		Lymphocytic leukemia or lymphoma
Monocytic		Monocytic leukemia
Endothelial Tissue		
Blood vessels	Hemangioma	Hemangiosarcoma
Lymph vessels	Lymphangioma	Lymphangiosarcoma
Endothelial lining		Ewing's sarcoma

Reproduced with permission from Porth, C. M. (1998). *Pathophysiology: Concepts of altered health states* (5th ed.). Philadelphia: Lippincott Raven.

Characteristics of Malignant Cells

Despite their individual differences, all cancer cells share some common cellular characteristics in relation to the cell membrane, special proteins, the nuclei, chromosomal abnormalities, and the rate of mitosis and growth. The cell membranes are altered in cancer cells, which affects fluid movement in and out of the cell.

The cell membrane of malignant cells also contains proteins called **tumor-specific antigens**, for example, carcinoembryonic antigen and prostate-specific antigen, which develop as they become less differentiated (mature) over time. These proteins distinguish the malignant cell from a benign cell of the same tissue type. They may be useful in measuring the extent of disease in a person and in tracking the course of illness during treatment or relapse. Malignant cellular membranes also contain less fibronectin, a cellular cement. They are therefore less cohesive and do not adhere to adjacent cells as readily.

Typically, nuclei of cancer cells are large and irregularly shaped (pleomorphism). Nucleoli, structures within the nucleus that house ribonucleic acid (RNA), are larger and more numerous in malignant cells, perhaps because of increased RNA synthesis. Chromosomal abnormalities (translocations, deletions, additions) and fragility of chromosomes are commonly found when cancer cells are analyzed.

Mitosis (cell division) occurs more frequently in malignant cells than in normal cells. As the cells grow and divide, more glucose and oxygen are needed. If glucose and oxygen are unavailable, malignant cells use anaerobic metabolic channels to produce energy, which makes the cells less dependent on the availability of a constant oxygen supply.

Invasion and Metastasis

Malignant disease processes have the ability to spread or transfer cancerous cells from one organ or body part to another by invasion and metastasis. Patterns of metastasis can be partially explained by circulatory patterns and by specific affinity for certain malignant cells to bind to molecules in specific body tissue.

Invasion, which refers to the growth of the primary tumor into the surrounding host tissues, occurs in several ways. Mechanical pressure exerted by rapidly proliferating neoplasms may force fingerlike projections of tumor cells into surrounding tissue and interstitial spaces. Malignant cells are less adherent and may break off from the primary tumor and invade adjacent structures. Malignant cells are thought to possess or produce specific destructive enzymes (proteinases), such as collagenases (specific to collagen), plasminogen activators (specific to plasma), and lysosomal hydrolyses. These enzymes are thought to destroy surrounding tis-

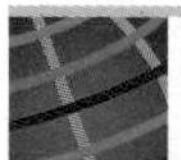

TABLE 15•2 **Characteristics of Benign and Malignant Neoplasms**

Characteristics	Benign	Malignant
Cell characteristics	Well-differentiated cells that resemble normal cells of the tissue from which the tumor originated	Cells are undifferentiated and often bear little resemblance to the normal cells of the tissue from which they arose
Mode of growth	Tumor grows by expansion and does not infiltrate the surrounding tissues; usually encapsulated	Grows at the periphery and sends out processes that infiltrate and destroy the surrounding tissues
Rate of growth	Rate of growth is usually slow	Rate of growth is variable and depends on level of differentiation; the more anaplastic the tumor, the faster its growth
Metastasis	Does not spread by metastasis	Gains access to the blood and lymphatic channels and metastasizes to other areas of the body
General effects	Is usually a localized phenomenon that does not cause generalized effects unless its location interferes with vital functions	Often causes generalized effects, such as anemia, weakness, and weight loss
Tissue destruction	Does not usually cause tissue damage unless its location interferes with blood flow	Often causes extensive tissue damage as the tumor outgrows its blood supply or encroaches on blood flow to the area; may also produce substances that cause cell damage
Ability to cause death	Does not usually cause death unless its location interferes with vital functions	Usually causes death unless growth can be controlled

Reproduced with permission from Porth, C. M. (1998). *Pathophysiology: Concepts of altered health states* (5th ed.). Philadelphia: Lippincott Raven.

sue, including the structural tissues of the vascular basement membrane, facilitating invasion of malignant cells. The mechanical pressure of a rapidly growing tumor may enhance this process.

Metastasis is the dissemination or spread of malignant cells from the primary tumor to distant sites by direct spread of tumor cells to body cavities or through lymphatic and blood circulation. Tumors growing in or penetrating body cavities may shed cells or emboli that travel within the body cavity and "seed" the surfaces of other organs. This can occur in ovarian cancer when malignant cells enter the peritoneal cavity and seed the peritoneal surfaces of such abdominal organs as the liver or pancreas.

Metastatic Mechanisms

The circulation of lymph and blood are key mechanisms by which cancer cells spread. Angiogenesis, a mechanism by which the tumor cells are ensured a blood supply, is another important process.

LYMPHATIC SPREAD

The most common mechanism of metastasis is lymphatic spread, which is transport of tumor cells through the lymphatic circulation. Tumor emboli enter the lymph channels by way of the interstitial fluid that communicates with lymphatic fluid. Malignant cells also may penetrate lymphatic vessels by invasion. After entering the lymphatic circulation, malignant cells either lodge in the lymph nodes or pass between lymphatic and venous circulation. Tumors arising in areas of the body with rapid and extensive lymphatic circulation are at high risk for metastasis through lymphatic channels. Breast tumors frequently metastasize in this manner through axillary, clavicular, and thoracic lymph channels.

HEMATOGENOUS SPREAD

Another metastatic mechanism is hematogenous spread, by which malignant cells are disseminated through the bloodstream. Hematogenous spread is directly related to the vascularity of the tumor. Few malignant cells can survive the turbulence of arterial circulation, insufficient oxygenation, or destruction by the body's immune system. In addition, the structure of most arteries and arterioles is far too secure to permit malignant invasion. Those malignant cells that do survive this hostile environment are able to attach to endothelium and attract fibrin, platelets, and clotting factors to seal themselves from immune system surveillance. The endothelium retracts, allowing the malignant cells to enter the basement membrane and secrete lysosomal enzymes. These enzymes then destroy surrounding body tissues and thereby allow implantation.

ANGIOGENESIS

Malignant cells also have the ability to induce the growth of new capillaries from the host tissue to meet their needs for nutrients and oxygen. This process is referred to as angiogenesis. It is through this vascular network that tumor emboli can enter the systemic circulation and travel to distant sites. Large tumor emboli that become trapped in the microcirculation of distant sites may further metastasize to other sites. Research into ways to prevent angiogenesis is ongoing.

Carcinogenesis

Malignant transformation, or **carcinogenesis**, is thought to be at least a three-step cellular process: initiation, promotion, and progression.

Initiation is the first step, in which initiators (carcinogens), such as chemicals, physical factors, and biologic agents, escape normal enzymatic mechanisms and alter the genetic structure of the cellular deoxyribonucleic acid (DNA). Normally, these alterations are reversed by DNA repair mechanisms, or the changes initiate programmed cellular suicide (apoptosis). Occasionally, cells escape these protective mechanisms, and permanent cellular mutations occur. These mutations usually are not significant to cells until the second step of carcinogenesis.

During *promotion*, repeated exposure to promoting agents (cocarcinogens) causes the expression of abnormal or mutant genetic information even after long latency periods. Latency periods for the promotion of cellular mutations vary with the type of agent and the dosage of the promoter as well as the innate characteristics of the target cell.

Cellular oncogenes, present in all mammalian systems, are responsible for the vital cellular functions of growth and differentiation. Cellular proto-oncogenes are present in cells and act as an "on switch" for cellular growth. Similarly, cancer suppressor genes "turn off" or regulate unneeded cellular proliferation. When the suppressor genes become mutated, rearranged, or amplified or lose their regulatory capabilities, malignant cells are allowed to reproduce. The p53 gene is a tumor suppressor gene that is frequently mutated in many human cancers. This gene regulates whether cells will repair or die after DNA damage. Mutant p53 gene is associated with a poor prognosis and may be associated with determining response to treatment. Once this genetic expression occurs in cells, the cells begin to produce mutant cell populations that are different from their original cellular ancestors.

Progression is the third step of cellular carcinogenesis. The cellular changes formed during initiation and promotion now exhibit increased malignant behavior. These cells now show a propensity to invade adjacent tissues and to metastasize. Agents that initiate or promote cellular transformation are referred to as carcinogens.

Etiology

Certain categories of agents or factors implicated in carcinogenesis include viruses and bacteria, physical agents, chemical agents, genetic or familial factors, dietary factors, and hormonal agents.

Viruses and Bacteria

Viruses as a cause of human cancers are hard to determine because viruses are difficult to isolate. Infectious causes are considered or suspected, however, when specific cancers appear in clusters. Viruses are thought to incorporate themselves in the genetic structure of cells, thus altering future generations of that cell population—perhaps leading to a cancer. For example, the Epstein-Barr virus is highly suspect as a cause in Burkitt's lymphoma, nasopharyngeal cancers, and some types of non-Hodgkin's lymphoma and Hodgkin's disease.

Herpes simplex virus type II, cytomegalovirus, and human papillomavirus types 16, 18, 31, and 33 are associated with dysplasia and cancer of the cervix. The hepatitis B virus is implicated in cancer of the liver; the human T-cell lymphotropic virus may be a cause of some lymphocytic leukemias and lymphomas; and the human immunodeficiency virus (HIV) is associated with Kaposi's sarcoma. The bacterium *Helicobacter pylori* has been associated with increased gastric malignancy, perhaps secondary to inflammation and injury of gastric cells.

Physical Agents

Physical factors associated with carcinogenesis include exposure to sunlight or radiation, chronic irritation or inflammation, and tobacco use.

Excessive exposure to the ultraviolet rays of the sun, especially in fair-skinned, blue- or green-eyed people, increases the risk for skin cancers. Factors such as clothing styles (sleeveless shirts or shorts), use of sunscreens, occupation, recreational habits, and environmental variables, including humidity, altitude, and latitude, all play a role in the amount of exposure to ultraviolet light.

Exposure to ionizing radiation can occur with repeated diagnostic x-ray procedures or with radiation therapy used to treat disease. Fortunately, improved x-ray equipment appropriately minimizes the risk for extensive radiation exposure. Radiation therapy used in disease treatment or exposure to radioactive materials at nuclear weapon manufacturing sites or nuclear power plants is associated with higher incidence of leukemias, multiple myeloma, and cancers of the lung, bone, breast, thyroid, and other tissues. Background radiation from the natural decay processes that produce radon has also been associated with lung cancer. Homes with high levels of trapped radon should be ventilated to allow the gas to disperse into the atmosphere.

Chemical Agents

About 85% of all cancers are thought to be related to the environment. Tobacco smoke, the single most lethal chemical carcinogen, accounts for at least 30% of cancer deaths. Smoking is strongly associated with cancers of the lung, head and neck, esophagus, pancreas, cervix, and bladder. Tobacco may also act synergistically with other substances, such as alcohol, asbestos, uranium, and viruses, to promote cancer development.

Chewing tobacco is associated with cancers of the oral cavity and primarily occurs in men younger than 40 years of age. Many chemical substances found in the workplace have proved to be carcinogens or co-carcinogens. The extensive list of suspected chemical substances continues to grow and includes aromatic amines and aniline dyes; pesticides and formaldehydes; arsenic, soot, and tars; asbestos; benzene; betel nut and lime; cadmium; chromium compounds; nickel and zinc ores; wood dust; beryllium compounds; and polyvinyl chloride.

Most hazardous chemicals produce their toxic effects by altering DNA structure in body sites distant from chemical exposure. The liver, lungs, and kidneys are the organ systems most often affected, presumably because of their roles in detoxifying chemicals.

Genetic and Familial Factors

Almost every cancer type has been shown to run in families. This may be due to genetics, shared environments, cultural or lifestyle factors, or chance alone. Genetic factors, however, do play a role in cancer cell development. Abnormal chromosomal patterns and cancer have been associated with extra chromosomes, too few chromosomes, or translocated chromosomes. Specific cancers with underlying genetic abnormalities include Burkitt's lymphoma, chronic myelogenous leukemia, meningiomas, acute leukemias, retinoblastomas, Wilms' tumor, and skin cancers, including malignant melanoma.

Some cancers of adulthood and childhood display familial predisposition. These cancers tend to occur at an early age and at multiple sites in one organ or pair of organs. In cancers with a hereditary predisposition, commonly two or more first-degree relatives share the same cancer type. Cancers associated with familial inheritance include retinoblastomas, nephroblastomas, pheochromocytomas, malignant neurofibromatosis, leukemias, and breast, endometrial, colorectal, stomach, prostate, and lung cancers.

Dietary Factors

Dietary factors are thought to be related to 40% to 60% of all environmental cancers. Dietary substances can be proactive (protective), carcinogenic, or co-carcinogenic. The risk for cancer increases with long-term ingestion of carcinogens or co-carcinogens or chronic absence of proactive substances in the diet.

Dietary substances associated with an increased cancer risk include fats, alcohol, salt-cured or smoked meats, food containing nitrates and nitrites, and a high caloric dietary intake. Food substances that appear to reduce cancer risk include high-fiber foods, cruciferous vegetables (cabbage, broccoli, cauliflower, Brussels sprouts, kohlrabi), carotenoids (carrots, tomatoes, spinach, apricots, peaches, dark-green and deep-yellow vegetables), and possibly vitamins E and C, zinc, and selenium.

Obesity is associated with endometrial cancer and possibly postmenopausal breast cancers. Obesity may also increase the risk for cancers of the colon, kidney, and gallbladder.

Hormonal Agents

Tumor growth may be promoted by disturbances in hormonal balance either by the body's own (endogenous) hormone production or by administration of exogenous hormones. Cancers of the breast, prostate, and uterus are thought to depend on endogenous hormonal levels for growth. Diethylstilbestrol has long been recognized as a cause of vaginal carcinomas. Oral contraceptives and prolonged estrogen replacement therapy are associated with slight increases in hepatocellular, endometrial, and breast cancers, whereas they appear to decrease the risk for ovarian and endometrial cancers. The combination of estrogen and progesterone appears safest in decreasing the risk for endometrial cancers. Hormonal changes with reproduction are also associated with cancer incidence. Increased numbers of pregnancies are associated with decreased incidence of breast, endometrial, and ovarian cancers.

Role of the Immune System

In humans, malignant cells are capable of developing on a regular basis. Some evidence indicates, however, that the immune system can detect the development of malignant cells and destroy them before cell growth becomes uncontrolled. When the immune system fails to identify and stop the growth of malignant cells, clinical cancer develops.

Patients who for various reasons are immunoincompetent have been shown to have an increased incidence of cancer. Organ transplant recipients who receive immunosuppressive therapy to prevent rejection of the transplanted organ have an increased incidence of lymphoma, Kaposi's sarcoma, squamous cell cancer of the skin, and cervical and anogenital cancers. Patients with immunodeficiency diseases, such as AIDS, have an increased incidence of Kaposi's sarcoma, lymphoma, and rectal and head and neck cancers. Some patients who have received alkylating chemotherapeutic agents to treat Hodgkin's disease have an increased incidence of secondary malignancies. Autoimmune diseases, such as rheumatoid arthritis and Sjögren's syndrome, are associated with increased cancer development. Finally, age-related changes, such as declining organ function, increased incidence of chronic diseases, and diminished immunocompetence, may contribute to an increased incidence of cancer in older people.

Normal Immune Responses

Normally, an intact immune system has the ability to combat cancer cells in several ways. Usually, the immune system recognizes as foreign certain antigens on the cell membranes of many cancer cells. These antigens are known as tumor-associated antigens (also called tumor cell antigens) and are capable of stimulating both cellular and humoral immune responses.

Along with the macrophages, T lymphocytes, the soldiers of the cellular immune response, are responsible for recognizing tumor-associated antigens. When T lymphocytes recognize tumor antigens, other T lymphocytes that are toxic to the tumor cells are stimulated. These lymphocytes proliferate and are released into the circulation. In addition to possessing cytotoxic (cell-killing) properties, T lymphocytes can stimulate other components of the immune system to rid the body of malignant cells.

Certain lymphokines, which are substances produced by lymphocytes, are capable of killing or damaging various types of malignant cells. Other lymphokines can mobilize other cells, such as macrophages, that disrupt cancer cells. Interferon (IFN), a substance produced by the body in response to viral infection, also possesses some antitumor properties. Antibodies produced by B lymphocytes, associated with the humoral immune response, also defend the body against malignant cells. These antibodies act either alone or in combination with the complement system or the cellular immune system.

Natural killer (NK) cells are a major component of the body's defense against cancer. NK cells are a subpopulation of lymphocytes that act by directly destroying cancer cells or by producing lymphokines and enzymes that assist in cell destruction.

Immune System Failure

How is it, then, that malignant cells can survive and proliferate despite the elaborate immune system defense mechanisms? Several theories suggest how tumor cells can evade an apparently intact immune system. If the body fails to recognize the malignant cell as different from "self," (non-self or foreign) the immune response may not be stimulated. When tumors do not possess tumor-associated antigens that label them as foreign, the immune response is not alerted. The failure of the immune system to respond promptly to the malignant cells allows the tumor to grow too large to be managed by normal immune mechanisms.

Tumor antigens may combine with the antibodies produced by the immune system and hide or disguise themselves from normal immune defense mechanisms. These tumor antigen–antibody complexes can suppress further production of antibodies. Tumors are also capable of changing their appearance or producing substances that impair usual immune responses. These substances not only promote tumor growth but also increase the patient's susceptibility to infection by various pathogenic organisms. As a result of prolonged contact with a tumor antigen, the patient's body may be depleted of the specific lymphocytes and no longer able to mount an appropriate immune response.

Abnormal concentrations of host suppressor T lymphocytes may play a role in developing cancers. Suppressor T lymphocytes normally assist in regulating antibody production and diminishing immune responses when they are no longer required. Low levels of serum antibodies and high levels of suppressor cells have been found in patients with multiple myeloma, a cancer associated with hypogammaglobulinemia (low amounts of serum antibodies). Carcinogens, such as viruses and certain chemicals, including chemotherapeutic agents, may weaken the immune system and ultimately enhance tumor growth.

DETECTION AND PREVENTION OF CANCER

Nurses and physicians have traditionally been involved with tertiary prevention, the care and rehabilitation of the patient after cancer diagnosis and treatment. In recent years, however, the American Cancer Society, the National Cancer Institute, clinicians, and researchers have placed greater emphasis on primary and secondary prevention of cancer. Primary prevention is concerned with reducing the risks of cancer in healthy people. Secondary prevention involves detection and screening to achieve early diagnosis and prompt intervention to halt the cancer process.

Primary Prevention

By acquiring the knowledge and skills necessary to educate the community about cancer risk, nurses in all settings play a key role in cancer prevention. Assisting patients to avoid known carcinogens is one way to reduce the risk for cancer. Another way involves adopting dietary and various lifestyle changes that epidemiologic and laboratory studies show influence the risk for cancer. Nurses can use their teaching and counseling skills to facilitate patient participation in cancer prevention programs and to promote healthful lifestyles.

Secondary Prevention

The evolving understanding of the role of genetics in cancer cell development has contributed to prevention and screening efforts. Individuals who have inherited specific genetic mutations have an increased susceptibility to cancer. For example, individuals who have familial adenomatosis polyposis have an increased risk for colon cancer. Women in whom the BRCA-1 and BRCA-2 genes have been identified have an increased risk for breast and ovarian cancer. To provide individualized education and recommendations for continued surveillance and care in high-risk populations, nurses need to be familiar with the ongoing developments in the field of genetics and cancer.

Numerous factors, such as race, cultural influences, access to care, physician–patient relationship, level of education, income, and age, influence the knowledge, attitudes, and beliefs people have about cancer. These factors also influence the type of health-promoting behaviors they practice. For example, Salazar (1996) examined Hispanic women's beliefs about breast cancer and mammography. The findings suggested that among other factors, cultural issues, social concerns, and belief in fate influenced the beliefs and health care practices among the women studied. Nurses can use this type of information in planning education, prevention, and screening programs.

Public awareness about health-promoting behaviors can be increased in a variety of ways. Health education and health maintenance programs are sponsored by community organizations such as churches, senior citizen groups, and parent–teacher associations. Although primary prevention programs may focus on the hazards of tobacco use or the importance of nutrition, secondary prevention programs may promote breast and testicular self-examination and Papanicolaou's tests. The American Cancer Society has developed a public education program, "Taking Control," that integrates diet, exercise, and general health habit tips that people can follow to reduce their risk for cancer (see Taking Steps to Minimize Cancer Risk Factors).

Similarly, nurses in acute care settings can develop programs that identify risks for patients and families and that incorporate teaching and counseling in discharge planning, particularly for patients and families with a high incidence of cancer.

Screening to detect early cancer usually focuses on cancers with the highest incidence or those that have improved survival rates if diagnosed early. Examples of these cancers include breast, colorectal, cervical, endometrial, testicular, skin, and oropharyngeal cancers. Nurses and physicians can encourage individuals to comply with detection efforts as suggested by the American Cancer Society (Table 15-3).

Risk Factors

TAKING STEPS TO MINIMIZE CANCER

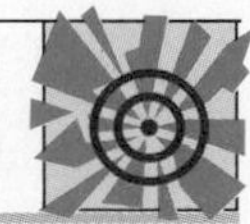

The following are cancer prevention strategies that nurses can recommend when teaching individual patients or groups:

1. Increase consumption of fresh vegetables (especially those of the cabbage family) because studies indicate that roughage and vitamin-rich food help to prevent cancer.
2. Increase fiber intake because high-fiber diets may reduce the risk for certain cancers (eg, breast, prostate, and colon).
3. Increase intake of vitamin A, which reduces the risk for esophageal, laryngeal, and lung cancers.
4. Increase intake of foods rich in vitamin C, such as citrus fruits and broccoli, which are thought to protect against stomach and esophageal cancers.
5. Practice weight control because obesity is linked to cancers of the uterus, gallbladder, breast, and colon.
6. Reduce intake of dietary fat because a high-fat diet increases the risk for breast, colon, and prostate cancers.
7. Practice moderation in consuming salt-cured, smoked, and nitrate-cured foods; these have been linked to esophageal and gastric cancers.
8. Stop smoking cigarettes and cigars, which are carcinogens.
9. Reduce alcohol intake because drinking large amounts of alcohol increases the risk of liver cancer. (*Note:* People who drink heavily and smoke are at greater risk for cancers of the mouth, throat, larynx, and esophagus.)
10. Avoid overexposure to the sun, wear protective clothing, and use a sunscreen to prevent skin damage from ultraviolet rays that increase the risk of skin cancer.

Adapted from the "Taking Control" program of the American Cancer Society.

DIAGNOSIS OF CANCER AND RELATED NURSING CONSIDERATIONS

A cancer diagnosis is based on the assessment for physiologic and functional changes and results of the diagnostic evaluation. Patients with suspected cancer undergo extensive testing to (1) determine the presence of tumor and its extent, (2) identify possible spread (metastasis) of disease or invasion of other body tissues, (3) evaluate the function of involved and uninvolved body systems and organs, and (4) obtain tissue and cells for analysis, including evaluation of tumor stage and grade. The diagnostic evaluation is guided by information obtained through a complete history and physical examination. Knowledge of suspicious symptoms and of the behavior of particular types of cancer assists in determining which diagnostic tests are most appropriate (Table 15-4).

A patient undergoing extensive testing is usually fearful of the procedures and anxious about the possible test results. The nurse can help relieve fear and anxiety by explaining the tests to be performed, the sensations likely to be experienced, and the patient's role in the test procedures. The nurse encourages the patient and family to voice their fears about the test results, supports the patient and family throughout the test period, and reinforces and clarifies information conveyed by the physician. The nurse also encourages the patient and family members to communicate and share their concerns and to discuss their questions and concerns with each other.

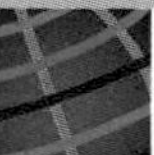

TABLE 15•3 American Cancer Society Recommendations for Early Detection of Cancer in Asymptomatic People

Test	Gender	Age	Frequency
Sigmoidoscopy, preferably flexible	Males and females	50 and older	Every 5 years
Fecal occult blood test	Males and females	50 and older	Every year
Digital rectal examination	Males and females	40 and older	Every year
Prostate examination*	Males	50 and older	Every year
Papanicolaou's (Pap) test	Females	All women who are, or who have been, sexually active, or who have reached 18 years of age, should have an annual Pap test and pelvic examination. After a woman has had three or more consecutive satisfactory normal annual examinations, the Pap test may be performed less frequently at the discretion of her physician.	
Breast self-examination	Females	20 and older	Every month
Breast clinical examination	Females	20 to 40	Every 3 years
		Older than 40	Every year
Mammography	Females	40 and older	Every year

* Men age 50 years and older should have an annual digital rectal examination and prostate-specific antigen (PSA) analysis. If the result of either test is abnormal, further evaluation should be considered.
Adapted from *Cancer Facts and Figures, 1999.* Atlanta, GA: American Cancer Society.

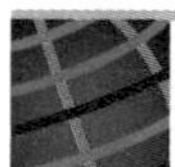

TABLE 15•4 Imaging Tests Used to Detect Cancer

Test	Description	Potential Uses
Tumor marker identification	Analysis of substances found in blood or other body fluids that are made by the tumor or by the body in response to the tumor	Breast, colon, lung, ovarian, testicular prostate cancers
Magnetic resonance imaging (MRI)	Use of magnetic fields and radiofrequency signals to create sectioned images of various body structures	Neurologic, pelvic, abdominal, thoracic cancers
Computed tomography (CT scan)	Use of narrow beam x-ray to scan successive layers of tissue for a cross-sectional view	Neurologic, pelvic, skeletal, abdominal, thoracic cancers
Fluoroscopy	Use of x-rays that identify contrasts in body tissue densities: may involve the use of contrast agents	Skeletal, lung, gastrointestinal cancers
Ultrasonography (ultrasound)	High-frequency sound waves echoing off body tissues are converted electronically into images; used to assess tissues deep within the body	Abdominal and pelvic cancers
Endoscopy	Direct visualization of a body cavity or passageway by insertion of an endoscope into a body cavity or opening; allows tissue biopsy, fluid aspiration and excision of small tumors; both diagnostic and therapeutic	Bronchial, gastrointestinal cancers
Nuclear medicine imaging	Uses intravenous injection or ingestion of radioisotope substances followed by imaging of tissues that have concentrated the radioisotopes	Bone, liver, kidney, spleen, brain, thyroid cancers
Positron emission tomography (PET scan)	Computed cross-sectional images of increased concentration of radioisotopes in malignant cells provides information about biologic activity of malignant cells; helps distinguish between benign and malignant processes and responses to treatment	Lung, colon, liver, and pancreatic cancers
Radioimmunoconjugates	Monoclonal antibodies are labeled with a radioisotope and injected intravenously into the patient; the antibodies that aggregate at the tumor site are visualized with scanners	Colorectal, breast, ovarian, head and neck cancers; lymphoma and melanoma

Tumor Staging and Grading

A complete diagnostic evaluation includes identifying the stage and grade of the tumor. This is accomplished before treatment begins to provide baseline data for evaluating outcomes of therapy and to maintain a systematic and consistent approach to ongoing diagnosis and treatment. Treatment options and prognosis are determined on the basis of staging and grading.

Staging determines the size of the tumor and the existence of metastasis. Several systems exist for classifying the anatomic extent of disease. The TNM system is frequently used. In this system, *T* refers to the extent of the primary tumor, *N* refers to lymph node involvement, and *M* refers to the extent of metastasis (Chart 15-2). A variety of other staging systems are used to describe the extent of cancers, such as central nervous system cancers, hematologic cancers, and malignant melanoma, that the TNM system does not describe appropriately.

Grading refers to the classification of the tumor cells. Grading systems seek to define the type of tissue from which the tumor originated and the degree to which the tumor cells retain the functional and histologic characteristics of the tissue of origin. Samples of cells to be used to establish the grade of a tumor may be obtained through cytology (examination of cells from tissue scrapings, body fluids, secretions, or washings), **biopsy**, or surgical excision.

This information assists the health care team to predict the behavior and prognosis of various tumors. The tumor is assigned a numeric value ranging from I to IV. Grade I tumors, also known as well-differentiated tumors, closely resemble the tissue of origin in structure and function. Tumors that do not clearly resemble the tissue of origin in structure or function are described as poorly differentiated or undifferentiated and are assigned grade IV. These tumors tend to be more aggressive and less responsive to treatment than well-differentiated tumors.

CHART 15•2 TNM Classification System

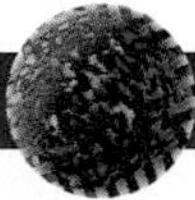

T subclasses

Tx—tumor cannot be adequately assessed
T0—no evidence of primary tumor
TIS—carcinoma in situ
T1, T2, T3, T4—progressive increase in tumor size and involvement

N subclasses

Nx—regional lymph nodes cannot be assessed clinically
N0—regional lymph nodes demonstrably normal
N1, N2, N3, N4—increasing degrees of demonstrable abnormalities of regional lymph nodes

M subclasses

Mx—not assessed
M0—no (known) distant metastasis
M1—distant metastasis present, specify site(s)

Histopathology

G1—well-differentiated grade
G2—moderately well-differentiated grade
G3, G4—poorly to very poorly differentiated grade

T, primary tumor; N, regional lymph nodes; M, distant metastasis. American Joint Committee on Cancer. *Manual for staging of cancer.* Chicago: Author.

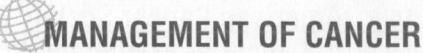

MANAGEMENT OF CANCER

Treatment options offered to cancer patients should be based on realistic and achievable goals for each specific type of cancer. The range of possible treatment goals may include complete eradication of malignant disease (**cure**), prolonged survival and containment of cancer cell growth (**control**), or relief of symptoms associated with the disease (**palliation**).

The health care team, the patient, and the patient's family must have a clear understanding of the treatment options and goals. Open communication and support are vital as the patient and family periodically reassess treatment plans and goals when complications of therapy develop or disease progresses.

Multiple modalities are commonly used in cancer treatment. A variety of therapies, including surgery, **radiation therapy**, **chemotherapy**, and **biologic response modifier** (BRM) **therapy** may be used at various times throughout treatment. Understanding the principles of each and how they interrelate is important in understanding the rationale and goals of treatment.

Surgery

Surgical removal of the entire cancer remains the ideal and most frequently used treatment method. The specific surgical approach, however, may vary for several reasons. Diagnostic surgery is the definitive method of identifying the cellular characteristics that inform all treatment decisions. Surgery may be the primary method of treatment, or it may be prophylactic, palliative, or reconstructive.

Diagnostic Surgery

Diagnostic surgery, such as a biopsy, is usually performed to obtain a tissue sample for analysis of cells suspected to be malignant. The three most common biopsy methods are the excisional, incisional, and needle methods.

Excisional biopsy is most frequently used for easily accessible tumors of the skin, breast, upper and lower gastrointestinal tract, and upper respiratory tract. In many cases, the surgeon can remove the entire tumor and surrounding marginal tissues as well. This removal of normal tissue beyond the tumor area decreases the possibility that residual microscopic disease cells may lead to a recurrence of the tumor. This approach not only provides the pathologist who stages and grades the cells with the entire tissue specimen but also decreases the chance of seeding the tumor (disseminating cancer cells through surrounding tissues).

Incisional biopsy is performed if the tumor mass is too large to be removed. In this case, a wedge of tissue from the tumor is removed for analysis. The cells of the tissue wedge must be representative of the tumor mass so that the pathologist can provide an accurate diagnosis. If the specimen does not contain representative tissue and cells, negative biopsy results do not guarantee the absence of cancer.

Excisional and incisional approaches are often performed through endoscopy. Surgical incision, however, may be required to determine the anatomic extent or stage of the tumor. For example, a diagnostic or staging laparotomy, the surgical opening of the abdomen to assess malignant abdominal disease, may be necessary to assess malignancies such as gastric cancer.

Needle biopsy is performed to sample suspicious masses that are easily accessible, such as some growths in the breasts, thyroid, lung, liver, and kidney. The procedure is fast, relatively inexpensive, and easy to perform and generally requires only local anesthesia. In general, the patient experiences minimal and temporary physical discomfort. In addition, the surrounding tissues are disturbed only minimally, thus decreasing the likelihood of seeding cancer cells. There is, however, a chance that even in the best of circumstances, a full description of the cellular types is not possible.

The choice of biopsy method is based on many factors. Of greatest importance is the type of treatment anticipated if the cancer diagnosis is confirmed. Definitive surgical approaches include the original biopsy site so that any cells disseminated during the biopsy are excised at the time of surgery. Nutrition and hematologic, respiratory, renal, and hepatic function are considered in determining the method of treatment as well. If the biopsy requires general anesthesia and if subsequent surgery is likely, the effects of prolonged anesthesia on the patient are considered.

The patient and family are given an opportunity to discuss the available options before definitive plans are made. The nurse, as the patient's advocate, serves as a liaison between the patient and the physician to facilitate this process. Time should be set aside to minimize interruptions. Time should be provided for questions and for thinking through all that has been discussed.

Surgery as Primary Treatment

When surgery is the primary approach in treating cancer, the goal is to remove the entire tumor or as much as is feasible (a procedure sometimes called debulking) and any involved surrounding tissue, including regional lymph nodes,

Two common surgical approaches used for treating primary tumors are local and wide excisions. Local excision is warranted when the mass is small. It includes removal of the mass and a small margin of normal tissue that is easily accessible. Wide or radical excisions (en bloc dissections) include removal of the primary tumor, lymph nodes, adjacent involved structures, and surrounding tissues that may be at high risk for tumor spread. This surgical method can result in disfigurement and altered functioning. Wide excisions are considered, however, if the tumor can be removed completely and the chances of cure or control are optimal.

In some situations, video-assisted endoscopic surgery is replacing surgeries associated with long incisions and extended recovery periods. In these procedures, an endoscope with intense lighting and an attached multichip minicamera is inserted through a small incision into the body. The surgical instruments are inserted into the surgical field through one or two additional small incisions, each about 3 cm long. The camera transmits the image of the involved area to a monitor so the surgeon can manipulate the instruments to perform the necessary procedure. This type of procedure is now being used for many thoracic and abdominal surgeries.

Salvage surgery is an additional treatment option that uses an extensive surgical approach to treat the local recurrence of the cancer after a less extensive primary approach is used. A mastectomy to treat recurrent breast cancer after primary lumpectomy and radiation is an example of salvage surgery.

In addition to the use of surgical blades or scalpels to excise the mass and surrounding tissues, several other types of surgical interventions are available. Electrosurgery makes use of electrical current to destroy the tumor cells. Cryosurgery uses liquid nitrogen to freeze tissue to cause cell destruction. Chemosurgery uses combined topical chemotherapy and layer-by-layer surgical removal of abnormal tissue. Laser surgery (*l*ight *a*mplification by *s*timulated *e*mission of *r*adiation) makes use of light and energy aimed at an exact tissue location and depth to vaporize cancer cells.

A multidisciplinary approach is essential during and after any type of surgery. The effects of surgery on body image, self-esteem, and functional abilities are addressed. If necessary, a plan for postoperative rehabilitation is made before the surgery is performed.

The growth and dissemination of cancer cells may have produced distant micrometastases by the time the patient seeks treatment. Therefore, attempting to remove wide margins of tissue in the hope of "getting all the cancer cells" may not be feasible. This reality substantiates the need for a coordinated multidisciplinary approach to cancer therapy. Once the surgery has been completed, one or more additional (or adjuvant) modalities may be chosen to increase the likelihood of destroying the cancer cells. However, some cancers that are treated surgically in the very early stages are considered to be curable (eg, skin cancers, testicular cancers).

Prophylactic Surgery

Prophylactic surgery involves removing nonvital tissues or organs that are likely to develop cancer. The following factors are considered when electing prophylactic surgery:

- Family history and genetic predisposition
- Presence or absence of symptoms
- Potential risks and benefits
- Ability to detect cancer at an early stage
- Patient's acceptance of the postoperative outcome

Colectomy and mastectomy are the two most common prophylactic operations. Some controversy, however, exists about adequate justification for prophylactic surgical procedures. For example, a strong family history of breast cancer, an abnormal physical finding on breast examination such as progressive nodularity and cystic disease, a proven history of breast cancer in the opposite breast, abnormal mammography findings, and abnormal biopsy results may be necessary to justify prophylactic mastectomy.

Because the long-term physiologic and psychological effects are unknown, prophylactic surgery is offered selectively to patients and discussed thoroughly with the patient and family. Preoperative teaching and counseling, as well as long-term follow-up, are provided.

Palliative Surgery

When cure is not possible, the goals of treatment are to make the patient as comfortable as possible and to promote a satisfying and productive life for as long as possible. Whether the period is extremely brief or lengthy, the major goal is a high quality of life—with quality defined by the patient and family. Honest and informative communication with the patient and family about the goal of surgery is essential to avoid false hope and disappointment.

Palliative surgery is performed in an attempt to relieve complications of cancer, such as ulcerations, obstructions, hemorrhage, pain, and malignant effusions (Table 15-5).

Reconstructive Surgery

Reconstructive surgery may follow curative or radical surgery and is carried out in an attempt to improve function or obtain a more desirable cosmetic effect. It may be performed in one operation or in stages. Patients are instructed about possible reconstructive

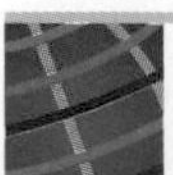

TABLE 15•5 Indications for Palliative Surgical Procedures

Procedure	Indications
Pleural drainage tube placement	Pleural effusion
Peritoneal drainage tube placement (Tenckoff catheter)	Ascites
Abdominal shunt placement (Levine shunt)	Ascites
Pericardial drainage tube placement	Pericardial effusion
Colostomy or ileostomy	Bowel obstruction
Gastrostomy, jejunostomy tube placement	Upper gastrointestinal tract obstruction
Biliary stent placement	Biliary obstruction
Ureteral stent placement	Ureteral obstruction
Nerve block	Pain
Cordotomy	Pain
Venous access device placement (for administering parenteral analgesics)	Pain
Epidural catheter placement (for administering epidural analgesics)	Pain
Hormone manipulation (removal of ovaries, testes, adrenals, pituitary)	Tumors that depend on hormones for growth

surgical options before the primary surgery by the surgeon who will perform the reconstruction. Reconstructive surgery may be indicated for breast, head and neck, and skin cancers.

The nurse must recognize the patient's needs and the impact that altered functioning and altered body image may have on quality of life. Providing the patient and family with opportunities to discuss these issues is imperative. The needs of the individual must be accurately assessed and validated in each situation for any type of reconstructive surgery.

Nursing Management in Cancer Surgery

The patient undergoing surgery for cancer requires general perioperative nursing care, as described in Unit 4, along with specific care related to the patient's age, organ impairment, nutritional deficits, disorders of coagulation, and altered immunity that may increase the risk for postoperative complications. Combining other treatment methods, such as radiation and chemotherapy, with surgery also contributes to postoperative complications, such as infection, impaired wound healing, altered pulmonary or renal function, and the development of deep vein thrombosis. In these situations, the nurse completes a thorough preoperative assessment for all factors that may affect patients undergoing surgical procedures.

The patient undergoing surgery for the diagnosis or treatment of cancer is often anxious about the surgical procedure, possible findings, postoperative limitations, changes in normal body functions, and prognosis. The patient and family require time and assistance to deal with the possible changes and outcomes resulting from the surgery.

The nurse provides education and emotional support by assessing patient and family needs and exploring with the patient and family their fears and coping mechanisms, encouraging them to take an active role in decision-making when possible. When the patient or family asks about the results of diagnostic testing and surgical procedures, the nurse's response is guided by the information the physician previously conveyed to them. The patient and family may also ask the nurse to explain and clarify information that the physician initially provided but that they did not grasp because they were anxious at the time. It is important for the nurse to communicate frequently with the physician and other health care team members to be certain that the information provided is consistent.

After surgery, the nurse assesses the patient's responses to the surgery and monitors for possible complications, such as infection, bleeding, thrombophlebitis, wound dehiscence, fluid and electrolyte imbalance, and organ dysfunction. The nurse also provides for patient comfort. Postoperative teaching addresses wound care, activity, nutrition, and medication information.

Plans for discharge, follow-up care, and treatment are initiated as early as possible to ensure continuity of care from hospital to home or from a cancer referral center to the patient's local hospital and health care provider. Patients and families are also encouraged to use community resources such as the American Cancer Society or Make Today Count for support and information.

Radiation Therapy

In radiation therapy, ionizing radiation is used to interrupt cellular growth. More than half of patients with cancer receive a form of radiation therapy at some point during treatment. Radiation may be used to cure the cancer, as in Hodgkin's disease, testicular seminomas, localized cancers of the head and neck, and cancers of the uterine cervix. Radiation therapy may also be used to control malignant disease when a tumor cannot be removed surgically or when local nodal metastasis is present, or it can be used prophylactically to prevent leukemic infiltration to the brain or spinal cord.

Palliative radiation therapy is used to relieve the symptoms of metastatic disease, especially when the cancer has spread to brain, bone, or soft tissue, or to treat oncologic emergencies, such as superior vena cava syndrome or spinal cord compression.

Two types of ionizing radiation—electromagnetic rays (x-rays and gamma rays) and particles (electrons [beta particles], protons, neutrons, and alpha particles)—can lead to tissue disruption. The most harmful tissue disruption is the alteration of the DNA molecule within the cells of the tissue. Ionizing radiation breaks the strands of the DNA helix, leading to cell death. Ionizing radiation can also ionize constituents of body fluids, especially water, leading to the formation of free radicals and irreversibly damaging

DNA. If the DNA is incapable of repair, the cell may die immediately, or it may initiate cellular suicide (apoptosis), a genetically programmed cell death.

Cells are most vulnerable to the disruptive effects of radiation during DNA synthesis and mitosis (early S, G_2, and M phases of the cell cycle). Therefore, those body tissues that undergo frequent cell division are most sensitive to radiation therapy. These tissues include bone marrow, lymphatic tissue, epithelium of the gastrointestinal tract, and gonads. Slower-growing tissues or tissues at rest are relatively radioresistant (less sensitive to the effects of radiation). Such tissues include muscle, cartilage, and connective tissues.

A radiosensitive tumor is one that can be destroyed by a dose of radiation that still allows for cell regeneration in the normal tissue. Tumors that are well oxygenated also appear to be more sensitive to radiation. In theory, therefore, radiation therapy may be enhanced if more oxygen can be delivered to tumors. In addition, if the radiation is delivered when most tumor cells are cycling through the cell cycle, the number of cancer cells destroyed (cell-killing) is maximal.

Certain chemicals, including chemotherapy agents, act as radiosensitizers and sensitize more hypoxic (oxygen-poor) tumors to the effects of radiation therapy. Radiation is delivered to tumor sites by external or internal means.

External Radiation

If external radiation therapy is used, one of several delivery methods may be chosen, depending on the depth of the tumor. Depending on the amount of energy they contain, x-rays can be used to destroy cancerous cells at the skin surface or deeper in the body. The higher the energy, the deeper the penetration into the body. Kilovoltage therapy devices deliver the maximal radiation dose to superficial lesions, such as lesions of the skin and breast, whereas linear accelerators and betatron machines produce higher-energy x-rays and deliver their dosage to deeper structures with less harm to the skin and less scattering of radiation within the body tissues. Gamma rays are another form of energy used in radiation therapy. This energy is produced from the spontaneous decay of naturally occurring radioactive elements such as cobalt 60. The gamma rays also deliver this radiation dose beneath the skin surface, sparing skin tissue from adverse effects.

A few centers nationwide treat more hypoxic, radiation-resistant tumors with particle-beam radiation therapy. This type of therapy accelerates subatomic particles (neutrons, pions, heavy ions) through body tissue. This therapy, which is also known as high linear energy transfer radiation, damages target cells as well as cells in its pathway.

Some centers are using intraoperative radiation therapy (IORT), which involves delivering a single dose of high-fraction radiation therapy to the exposed tumor bed while the body cavity is open during surgery. Cancers for which IORT is being used (and the effects tested) include gastric, pancreatic, colorectal, bladder, and cervical cancers and sarcomas. Toxicity with IORT is minimized because the radiation is precisely targeted to the diseased areas, and exposure to overlying skin and structures is avoided.

Internal Radiation

Internal radiation implantation, or **brachytherapy**, delivers a high dose of radiation to a localized area. The specific radioisotope for implantation is selected on the basis of its half-life, which is the time it takes for half of its radioactivity to decay. This internal radiation can be implanted by means of needles, seeds, beads, or catheters into body cavities (vagina, abdomen, pleura) or interstitial compartments (breast).

Intracavitary radioisotopes are frequently used to treat gynecologic cancers. In these malignancies, the radioisotopes are inserted into specially positioned applicators after the position is verified by radiography. These radioisotopes remain in place for a prescribed period and then are removed. Patients are maintained on bed rest and log-rolled to prevent displacement of the intracavitary delivery device. An indwelling urinary catheter is inserted to ensure that the bladder empties. Low-residue diets and antidiarrheal agents, such as diphenoxylate (Lomotil), are provided to prevent bowel movement during therapy, again to prevent the radioisotopes from being displaced.

Interstitial implants may be temporary or permanent, depending on the radioisotopes used. These implants usually consist of seeds, needles, wires, or small catheters positioned to provide a local radiation source and are less frequently dislodged. With internal radiation therapy, the farther the tissue is from the radiation source, the lower the dosage. This spares the noncancerous tissue from the radiation dose.

Because patients receiving internal radiation emit radiation while the implant is in place, contacts with the health care team are guided by principles of time, distance, and shielding to minimize exposure of personnel to radiation. Safety precautions used in caring for the patient receiving brachytherapy include assigning the person to a private room, posting appropriate notices about radiation safety precautions, having staff members wear dosimeter badges, making sure that pregnant staff members are not assigned to this patient's care, prohibiting visits by children or pregnant visitors, limiting visits from others to 30 minutes daily, and seeing that visitors maintain a 6-foot distance from the radiation source.

Radiation Dosage

The radiation dosage is dependent on the sensitivity of the target tissues to radiation and on the tumor size. The lethal tumor dose is defined as that dose that will eradicate 95% of the tumor yet preserve normal tissue. The total radiation dose is delivered over several weeks to allow healthy tissue to repair and to achieve greater cell kill by exposing more cells to the radiation as they begin active cell division. Repeated radiation treatments over time (fractionated doses) also allow for the periphery of the tumor to be reoxygenated repeatedly because tumors shrink from the outside inward. This increases the radiosensitivity of the tumor, thereby increasing tumor cell death.

Toxicity

Toxicity of radiation therapy is usually localized to the region being irradiated. Toxicity may be increased when concomitant chemotherapy is administered. Acute local reactions occur when normal cells in the treatment area are also destroyed and cellular death exceeds cellular regeneration. Body tissues most affected are those that normally proliferate rapidly, such as the skin, the epithelial lining of the gastrointestinal tract, including the oral cavity, and the bone marrow. Altered skin integrity is a common effect and can include **alopecia** (hair loss), erythema, and shedding of skin (desquamation). After treatments have been completed, reepithelialization occurs.

Alterations in oral mucosa secondary to radiation therapy include stomatitis, **xerostomia** (dryness of the mouth), change and loss of taste, and decreased salivation. The entire gastrointestinal mucosa may be involved, and esophageal irritation with chest pain and dysphagia may result. Anorexia, nausea, vomiting, and diarrhea may occur if the stomach or colon is in the irradiated field. Symptoms subside, and gastrointestinal reepithelialization occurs after treatments are complete.

Bone marrow cells proliferate rapidly, and if bone marrow–producing sites are included in the radiation field anemia, leukopenia (decreased white blood cells [WBCs]), and **thrombocytopenia** (a decrease in platelets) may result. Patients are then at increased risk for infection and bleeding until blood cell counts return to normal. Chronic anemia may occur. Research continues to develop radioprotective agents that can protect normal tissue from radiation damage.

Certain systemic side effects are also commonly experienced by patients receiving radiation therapy. These manifestations, which are generalized, include fatigue, malaise, headache, nausea, and vomiting. This syndrome may be secondary to substances released when tumor cells break down. The effects are temporary and subside with the cessation of treatment.

Late effects of radiation therapy may also occur in various body tissues. These effects are chronic, usually produce fibrotic changes secondary to a decreased vascular supply, and are irreversible. These late effects can be most severe when they involve vital organs such as the lungs, heart, central nervous system, and bladder. Toxicities may intensify when radiation is combined with other treatment modalities.

Nursing Management in Radiation Therapy

The patient receiving radiation therapy and the family often have questions and concerns about its safety. In a key position to answer questions and allay fears about the effects of radiation on others, on the tumor, and on the patient's normal tissues and organs, the nurse can explain the procedure for delivering radiation and describe the equipment, the duration of the procedure (often minutes only), the possible need for immobilizing the patient during the procedure, and the absence of new sensations, including pain, during the procedure. If a radioactive implant is used, the nurse informs the patient about the restrictions placed on visitors and health care personnel and other radiation precautions. Patients also need to understand their own role before, during, and after the procedure.

PROTECTING THE SKIN AND ORAL MUCOSA

The nurse assesses the patient's skin, nutritional status, and general feeling of well-being. The skin and oral mucosa are assessed frequently for changes (particularly if radiation therapy is directed to these areas). The skin is protected from irritation, and the patient is instructed to avoid using ointments, lotions, or powders on the area.

Gentle oral hygiene is essential to remove debris, prevent irritation, and promote healing. If systemic changes, such as weakness and fatigue, occur, the patient may need assistance with activities of daily living and personal hygiene. Additionally, the nurse offers reassurance by explaining that these symptoms are a result of the treatment and do not represent deterioration or progression of the disease.

PROTECTING THE CAREGIVERS

When a patient has a radioactive implant in place, nurses and other health care providers need to protect themselves as well as the patient from the effects of radiation. Specific instructions are usually provided by the radiation safety officer from the radiology department. The instructions identify the maximum time to spend safely in the patient's room, the shielding equipment to be used, and special precautions and actions to be taken if the implant is dislodged. The nurse should explain the rationale for these precautions to keep the patient from feeling unduly isolated.

Chemotherapy

In chemotherapy, antineoplastic agents are used in an attempt to kill tumor cells by interfering with cellular functions and reproduction. Chemotherapy is used primarily to treat systemic disease rather than lesions that are localized and amenable to surgery or radiation. Chemotherapy may be combined with surgery or radiation therapy, or both, to reduce tumor size preoperatively, to destroy any remaining tumor cells postoperatively, or to treat some forms of leukemia. The goals of chemotherapy (cure, control, palliation) must be realistic because they will define the medications to be used and the aggressiveness of the treatment plan.

Cell Kill and the Cell Cycle

Each time a tumor is exposed to a chemotherapeutic agent, a percentage of tumor cells (20% to 99%, depending on dosage) is destroyed. Repeated doses of chemotherapy are necessary over a prolonged period to achieve regression of the tumor. Eradication of 100% of the tumor is nearly impossible, but a goal of treatment is to eradicate enough of the tumor so that the remaining tumor cells can be destroyed by the body's immune system.

Actively proliferating cells within a tumor (growth fraction) are the most sensitive to chemotherapeutic agents. Nondividing cells capable of future proliferation are the least sensitive to antineoplastic medications and consequently are potentially dangerous. The nondividing cells must be destroyed, however, to eradicate a cancer completely. Repeated cycles of chemotherapy are used to kill more tumor cells by destroying these nondividing cells as they begin active cell division.

Reproduction of both healthy and malignant cells follows the cell cycle pattern (Fig. 15-2). The cell cycle time is the time required for one tissue cell to divide and reproduce two identical daughter cells. The cell cycle of any cell has four distinct phases, each with a vital underlying function:

1. G_1 phase—RNA and protein synthesis occur.
2. S phase—DNA synthesis occurs.
3. G_2 phase—premitotic phase; DNA synthesis is complete, mitotic spindle forms.
4. Mitosis—cell division occurs.

The G_0 phase, the resting or dormant phase of cells, can occur after mitosis and during the G_1 phase. In the G_0 phase are those dangerous cells that are not actively dividing but have the future potential for replicating. The administration of certain chemotherapeutic agents (as well as administration of some other forms of therapy) is coordinated with the cell cycle.

Classification of Chemotherapeutic Agents

Certain chemotherapeutic agents (cell cycle–specific drugs) destroy cells actively reproducing by means of the cell cycle. Many of these agents are phase specific to certain phases of the cell cycle. Most affect cells in the S phase by interfering with DNA and RNA synthesis. Others, such as the vinca or plant alkaloids, are specific to the M phase, where they halt mitotic spindle formation.

Chemotherapeutic agents that act independently of the cell cycle phases are termed cell cycle–nonspecific drugs. These agents usually have a prolonged effect on cells, leading to cellular damage or

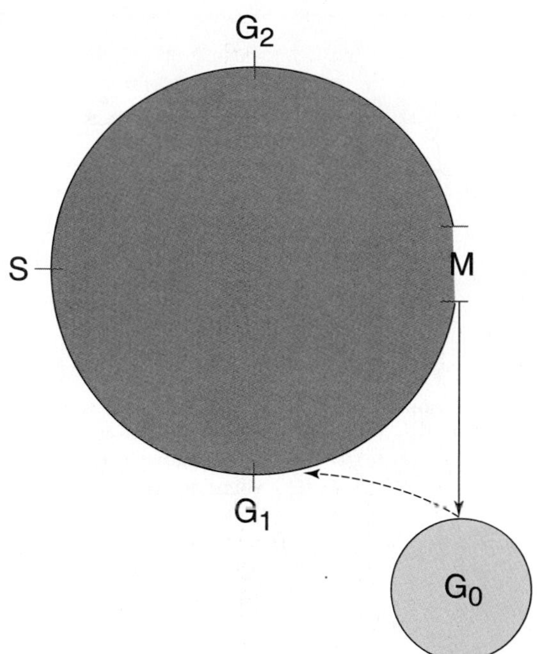

FIGURE 15•2 Phases of the cell cycle extend over the interval between the midpoint of mitosis to the subsequent end point in mitosis in a daughter cell. G_1 is the postmitotic phase during which ribonucleic acid (RNA) and protein synthesis are increased and cell growth occurs. G_0 is the resting, or dormant, phase of the cell cycle. In the S phase, nucleic acids are synthesized and chromosomes replicated in preparation for cell mitosis. During G_2, RNA and protein synthesis occurs as in G_1 from Porth, C. M. (1998). *Pathophysiology: Concepts of altered health states* (5th ed). Philadelphia: Lippincott-Raven.

death. Many treatment plans combine cell cycle–specific and cell cycle–nonspecific drugs to increase the number of vulnerable tumor cells killed during a treatment period.

Chemotherapeutic agents are also classified according to various chemical groups, each with a different mechanism of action. These include the alkylating agents, nitrosureas, antimetabolites, antitumor antibiotics, plant alkaloids, hormonal agents, and miscellaneous agents. The classification, mechanism of action, common drugs, cell cycle specificity, and common side effects of antineoplastic agents are listed in Table 15-6.

Chemotherapeutic agents from each category may be used to enhance the tumor cell kill during therapy by creating multiple cellular lesions. Combined drug therapy relies on medications of differing toxicities and with synergistic actions. Using combination drug therapy also prevents development of drug-resistant mechanisms.

Researchers continue to seek ways to combat the resistance of tumor cells to chemotherapeutic agents. Combining older drugs with other agents, such as levamisole, leukovorin, hormones, or IFN, has shown some benefit. Newer investigational agents are being studied for effectiveness in resistant tumor lines. For more information about investigative drugs, see the chart "Investigational Antineoplastic Therapies and Clinical Trials."

Administration of Chemotherapeutic Agents

Chemotherapeutic agents may be administered in the hospital, clinic, or home setting by topical, oral, intravenous, intramuscular, subcutaneous, arterial, intracavitary, and intrathecal routes. The administration route usually depends on the type of agent, the required dose, and the type, location, and extent of tumor being treated. Guidelines for the administration of chemotherapy are issued by the Oncology Nursing Society. Patient education is essential to maximize safety if chemotherapy is administered in the patient's home. See "Home Care Teaching Checklist: Home Chemotherapy Administration."

DOSAGE

Dosage of antineoplastic agents is based primarily on the patient's total body surface area, previous response to chemotherapy or radiation therapy, major organ function, and physical performance status.

SPECIAL PROBLEMS: EXTRAVASATION

Special care must be taken whenever intravenous vesicant agents are administered. **Vesicants** are those agents that, if deposited into the subcutaneous tissue (**extravasation**), cause tissue necrosis and damage to underlying tendons, nerves, and blood vessels. Although the complete mechanism of tissue destruction is unclear, it is known that the pH of many antineoplastic drugs is responsible for the severe inflammatory reaction as well as the ability of these drugs to bind to tissue DNA. Sloughing and ulceration of the tissue may be so severe that skin grafting may be necessary. The full extent of tissue damage may take several weeks to become apparent. Medications classified as vesicants include dactinomycin, daunorubicin, doxorubicin (Adriamycin), nitrogen mustard, mitomycin, vinblastine, vincristine, and vindesine.

Only specially trained physicians and nurses should administer vesicants. Careful selection of peripheral veins, skilled venipuncture, and careful drug administration are essential. Indications of extravasation during drug administration include the following:

- Absence of blood return from the intravenous catheter
- Resistance to flow of intravenous fluid
- Swelling, pain, or redness at the site

If extravasation is suspected, the drug administration is stopped immediately, and ice is applied to the site (unless the extravasated vesicant is a vinca alkaloid). The physician may aspirate any infiltrated drug from the tissues and inject a neutralizing solution into the area to reduce tissue damage. Selection of the neutralizing solution depends on the extravasated medication. Examples of neutralizing solutions include sodium thiosulfate, hyaluronidase, and sodium bicarbonate. Recommendations and guidelines for managing vesicant extravasation have been issued by individual drug manufacturers, pharmacies, and the Oncology Nursing Society, and they differ from one medication to the next.

When frequent, prolonged administration of antineoplastic vesicants is anticipated, right atrial Silastic catheters or venous access devices may be inserted to promote safety during drug administration and reduce problems with access to the circulatory system (Figs. 15-3 and 15-4). Complications associated with their use include infection and thrombosis.

TOXICITY

Toxicity associated with chemotherapy can be acute or chronic. Cells with rapid growth rates (eg, epithelium, bone marrow, hair follicles, sperm) are very susceptible to damage, and various body systems may be affected as well.

Gastrointestinal System. Nausea and vomiting are the most common side effects of chemotherapy and may persist for up to 24 hours after drug administration. The vomiting centers of the brain are stimulated by (1) activation of the receptors found in the chemoreceptor trigger zone (CTZ) of the medulla; (2) stimulation

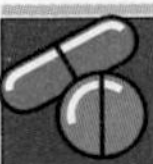

TABLE 15•6 Antineoplastic Agents

Drug Class and Examples	Mechanism of Action	Cell Cycle Specificity	Common Side Effects
Alkylating Agents			
busulfan, carboplatin, chlorambucil, cisplatin, cyclophosphamide, dacarbazine, hexamethyl melamine, ifosfamide, melphalan, nitrogen mustard, thiotepa	Alter DNA structure by misreading DNA code, initiating breaks in the DNA molecule, cross-linking DNA strands	Cell cycle–nonspecific	Bone marrow suppression, nausea, vomiting, cystitis (cyclophosphamide, ifosfamide), stomatitis, alopecia, gonadal suppression, renal toxicity (cisplatin)
Nitrosureas			
carmustine (BCNU), lomustine (CCNU), semustine (methyl CCNU), streptozocin	Similar to the alkylating agents; cross the blood–brain barrier	Cell cycle–nonspecific	Delayed and cumulative myelosuppression, especially thrombocytopenia; nausea, vomiting
Topoisomerase I Inhibitors			
irinotecan, topotecan	Induce breaks in the DNA strand by binding to enzyme topoisomerase I, preventing cells from dividing	Cell cycle–specific	Bone marrow suppression, diarrhea, nausea, vomiting, hepatotoxicity
Antimetabolites			
5-azacytadine, cytarabine, edatrexate fludarabine, 5-fluorouracil (5-FU), FUDR, gemcitabine, hydroxyurea, leustatin, 6-mercaptopurine, methotrexate, pentostatin, 6-thioguanine	Interfere with the biosynthesis of metabolites or nucleic acids necessary for RNA and DNA synthesis	Cell cycle–specific (S phase)	Nausea, vomiting, diarrhea, bone marrow suppression, proctitis, stomatitis, renal toxicity (methotrexate), hepatotoxicity
Antitumor Antibiotics			
bleomycin, dactinomycin, daunorubicin, doxorubicin (Adriamycin), idarubicin, mitomycin, mitoxantrone, plicamycin	Interfere with DNA synthesis by binding DNA; prevent RNA synthesis	Cell cycle–nonspecific	Bone marrow suppression, nausea, vomiting, alopecia, anorexia, cardiac toxicity (daunorubicin, doxorubicin)
Mitotic Spindle Poisons			
Plant alkaloids: etoposide, teniposide, vinblastine, vincristine (VCR), vindesine, vinorelbine	Arrest metaphase by inhibiting mitotic tubular formation (spindle); inhibit DNA and protein synthesis	Cell cycle–specific (M phase)	Bone marrow suppression (mild with VCR), neuropathies (VCR), stomatitis
Taxanes: puclitaxel, docetaxel	Arrest metaphase by inhibiting tubulin depolymerization	Cell cycle–specific (M phase)	Bradycardia, hypersensitivity reactions, bone marrow suppression, alopecia, neuropathies
Hormonal Agents			
androgens and antiandrogens, estrogens and antiestrogens, progestins and antiprogestins, aromatase inhibitors, luteinizing hormone–releasing hormone analogs, steroids	Bind to hormone receptor sites that alter cellular growth; block binding of estrogens to receptor sites (antiestrogens); inhibit RNA synthesis; suppress aromatase of P450 system, which decreases estrogen level	Cell cycle–nonspecific	Hypercalcemia, jaundice, increased appetite, masculinization, feminization, sodium and fluid retention, nausea, vomiting, hot flashes, vaginal dryness
Miscellaneous Agents			
asparaginase, procarbazine	Unknown or too complex to categorize	Varies	Anorexia, nausea, vomiting, bone marrow suppression, hepatotoxicity, anaphylaxis, hypotension, altered glucose metabolism

of peripheral autonomic pathways (gastrointestinal tract and pharynx); (3) stimulation of the vestibular pathways (inner ear imbalances, labyrinth input); (4) cognitive stimulation (central nervous system disease, anticipatory nausea and vomiting); and (5) a combination of factors.

Medications that can decrease nausea and vomiting include serotonin blockers, such as ondansetron and granisetron, which block serotonin receptors of the gastrointestinal tract and CTZ, and dopaminergic blockers, such as metoclopramide (Reglan), which block dopamine receptors of the CTZ. Phenothiazines,

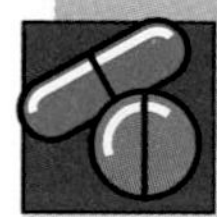

PHARMACOLOGY

Investigational Antineoplastic Therapies and Clinical Trials

Evaluation of the effectiveness and toxic potential of promising new modalities for preventing, diagnosing, and treating cancer is accomplished through clinical trials. Before new drug therapies are approved for clinical use, they are subjected to rigorous and lengthy evaluations to identify beneficial effects, adverse effects, and safety.

- *Phase I* clinical trials determine optimal dosing, scheduling, and toxicity.
- *Phase II* trials determine effectiveness with specific tumor types and further define toxicities. Participants in these early trials are most often those who have not responded to standard forms of treatment. Because phase I and II trials may be viewed as last-chance efforts, patients and families are fully informed about the experimental nature of the *trial* drugs. Although it is hoped that investigational therapy will effectively treat the disease, the purpose of early phase trials is to gather information concerning maximal tolerated doses, adverse effects, and effects of the drugs on tumor growth.
- *Phase III* clinical trials establish the effectiveness of new drugs or procedures as compared with conventional approaches. Nurses may assist in the recruitment, consent, and education processes for patients who participate. In many cases, nurses are instrumental in monitoring adherence, assisting patients to adhere to the parameters of the trial, and documenting data describing patients' responses. The physical and emotional needs of patients in clinical trials are addressed in much the same way as those of patients who receive standard forms of cancer treatment.
- *Phase IV* testing further investigates established drugs in terms of new uses, dosing schedule, and toxicities.

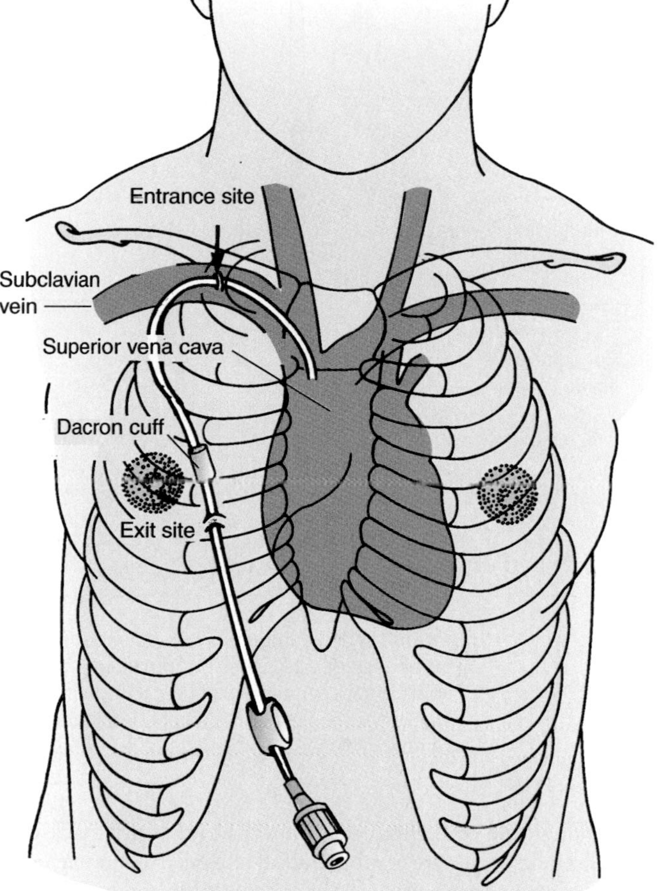

FIGURE 15•3 Right atrial catheter. The right atrial catheter is inserted into the subclavian vein and advanced until its tip lies in the superior vena cava just above the right atrium. The proximal end is then tunneled from the entry site through the subcutaneous tissue of the chest wall and brought out through an exit site on the chest. The Dacron cuff anchors the catheter in place and serves as a barrier to infection.

sedatives, steroids, and histamines, alone or in combination, are used with the more emetogenic chemotherapeutic regimens.

Delayed nausea and vomiting that occur later than 48 to 72 hours after chemotherapy are troublesome for some patients. To minimize discomfort, some antiemetic medications are necessary for the first week at home after chemotherapy. Relaxation techniques and imagery can also help to decrease stimuli contributing to symptoms. Altering the patient's diet to include small frequent meals, bland foods, and comfort foods may reduce the frequency or severity of these symptoms.

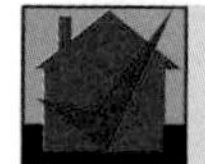

HOME CARE TEACHING CHECKLIST: CHEMOTHERAPY ADMINISTRATION

At the completion of the program, the patient or caregiver will be able to:	Patient	Caregiver
• Demonstrate how to administer the chemotherapy agent in the home.	✔	✔
• Demonstrate safe disposal of needles, syringes, IV supplies, or unused chemotherapy medications.	✔	✔
• List possible side effects of chemotherapeutic agents.	✔	✔
• List complications of medications necessitating a call to the nurse or physician.	✔	✔
• List complications of medications necessitating a visit to the emergency department.	✔	✔
• List names and telephone numbers of resource personnel involved in care (ie, home care nurse, infusion services, IV vendor, equipment company).	✔	✔
• Explain treatment plan (protocol) and upcoming visits to physician.	✔	✔

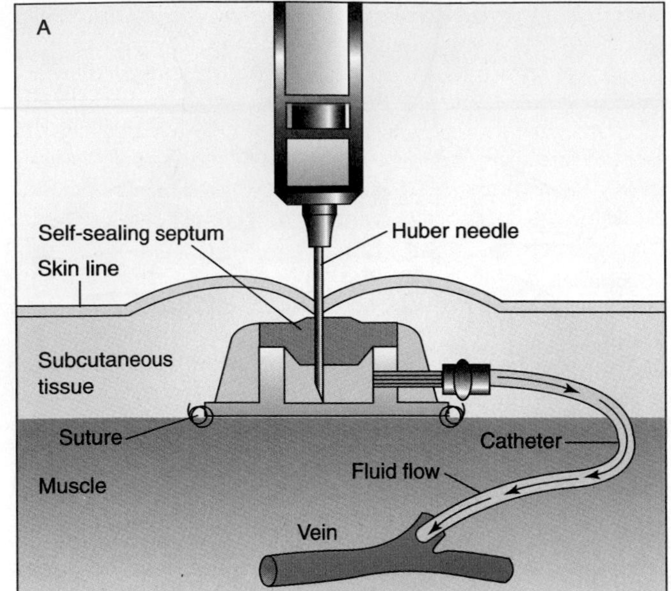

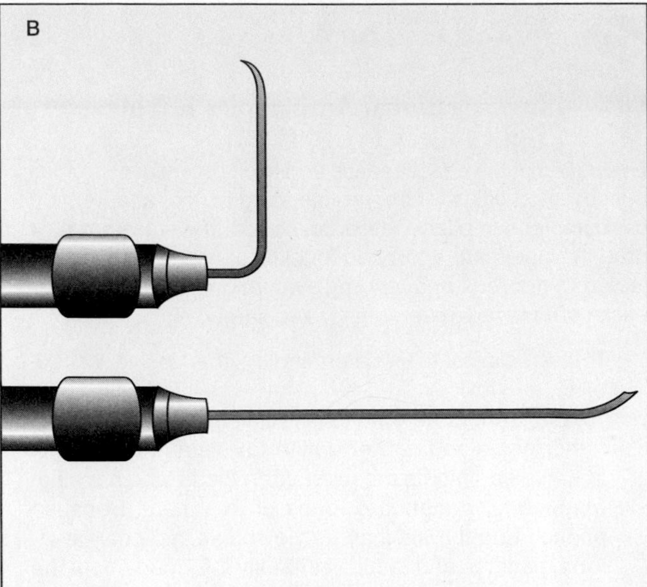

FIGURE 15•4 Implanted vascular access device.(**A**) A schematic diagram of an implanted vascular access device used for administering medication, fluids, blood products, and nutrition. The self-sealing septum permits repeated puncture by Huber needles without damage or leakage. (**B**) Two Huber needles used to enter the implanted vascular port. The 90-degree needle is used for top-entry ports for continuous infusions.

Although the epithelium that lines the oral cavity quickly renews itself, its rapid rate of proliferation makes it susceptible to the effects of chemotherapy. As a result, stomatitis and anorexia are common. The entire gastrointestinal tract is susceptible to mucositis (inflammation of the mucosal lining), and diarrhea is a common result. Antimetabolites and antitumor antibiotics are the major culprits in mucositis and other gastrointestinal symptoms.

Hematopoietic System. Most chemotherapeutic agents cause **myelosuppression** (depression of bone marrow function), resulting in decreased production of blood cells. Myelosuppression decreases the number of WBCs or leukocytes (leukopenia), red blood cells (anemia), and platelets or thrombocytes (thrombocytopenia) and increases the risk for infection and bleeding. Depression of these cells is the usual reason for limiting the dose of the chemotherapeutic agents. Monitoring blood cell counts frequently is essential, as is protecting the patient from infection and injury, particularly while the blood cell counts are depressed.

Other agents, called colony-stimulating factors (granulocyte colony-stimulating factor [G-CSF], granulocyte-macrophage colony-stimulating factor [GM-CSF], and erythropoietin [EPO]), are given after chemotherapy. G-CSF and GM-CSF stimulate the bone marrow to produce WBCs, especially neutrophils, at an accelerated rate, thus decreasing the duration of **neutropenia**. The colony-stimulating factors decrease the episodes of infection and the need for antibiotics and allow for more timely cycling of chemotherapy with less need to reduce the dosage. EPO stimulates red blood cell production, thus decreasing the symptoms of chronic anemia.

Renal System. Chemotherapeutic agents can damage the kidneys because of their direct effects during excretion and the accumulation of end products after cell lysis. Cisplatin, methotrexate, and mitomycin are particularly toxic to the kidneys. Rapid tumor cell lysis after chemotherapy results in increased urinary excretion of uric acid, which can cause renal damage. In addition, intracellular contents are released into the circulation, resulting in excessive levels of potassium and phosphates (hyperkalemia and hyperphosphatemia) and diminished levels of calcium (hypocalcemia). (See later discussion of tumor lysis syndrome.)

Monitoring blood urea nitrogen, serum creatinine, creatinine clearance, and serum electrolyte levels is essential. Adequate hydration, alkalinization of the urine to prevent formation of uric acid crystals, and the use of allopurinol are frequently indicated to prevent these side effects.

Cardiopulmonary System. Antitumor antibiotics (daunorubicin and doxorubicin) are known to cause irreversible cumulative cardiac toxicities, especially when total dosage reaches 550 mg/m^2. Cardiac ejection fraction (volume of blood ejected from the heart with each beat) and signs of congestive heart failure must be monitored closely. Bleomycin, carmustine (BCNU), and busulfan are known for their cumulative toxic effects on lung function. Pulmonary fibrosis can be a long-term effect of prolonged dosage with these agents. Therefore, the patient is monitored closely for changes in pulmonary function, including pulmonary function test results. Total cumulative doses of bleomycin are not to exceed 400 units.

Reproductive System. Testicular and ovarian function can be affected by chemotherapeutic agents, resulting in possible sterility. Normal ovulation, early menopause, or permanent sterility may result. In men, temporary or permanent azoospermia (absence of spermatozoa) may develop. Reproductive cells may be damaged during treatment and result in chromosomal abnormalities in offspring. Banking of sperm is recommended for men before treatments are initiated to protect against sterility or any mutagenic damage to sperm.

Patients and their partners need to be informed about potential changes in reproduction resulting from chemotherapy. They are advised to use reliable methods of birth control while receiving chemotherapy and not to assume that sterility has resulted.

Neurologic System. The taxanes and plant alkaloids, especially vincristine, can cause neurologic damage with repeated doses. Peripheral neuropathies, loss of deep tendon reflexes, and paralytic ileus may occur. These side effects are usually reversible and disappear after completion of chemotherapy. Cisplatin is also responsible for peripheral neuropathies and hearing loss due to damage to the acoustic nerve.

Miscellaneous. Fatigue is a distressing side effect for most patients that greatly affects quality of life. Fatigue can be debilitating and last for months after treatment.

Nursing Management in Chemotherapy

The nurse has an important role in assessing and managing many of the problems experienced by the patient undergoing chemotherapy. Because of the systemic effects on normal as well as malignant cells, these problems are often widespread, affecting many body systems.

ASSESSING FLUID AND ELECTROLYTE STATUS

Anorexia, nausea, vomiting, altered taste, and diarrhea put the patient at risk for nutritional and fluid and electrolyte disturbances. Changes in the mucosa of the gastrointestinal tract may lead to irritation of the oral cavity and intestinal tract, further threatening the patient's nutritional status. Therefore, it is important for the nurse to assess the patient's nutritional and fluid and electrolyte status frequently and to use creative ways to encourage an adequate fluid and dietary intake.

MODIFYING RISKS FOR INFECTION AND BLEEDING

Suppression of the bone marrow and immune system is an expected consequence of chemotherapy and frequently serves as a guide in determining appropriate chemotherapy dosage. However, this effect also increases the risk for anemia, infection, and bleeding disorders. Therefore, nursing assessment and care focus on identifying and modifying factors that further increase the patient's risk. Aseptic technique and gentle handling are indicated to prevent infection and trauma. Laboratory test results, particularly blood cell counts, are monitored closely. Untoward changes in blood test results and signs of infection and bleeding are reported promptly. The patient and family members are instructed about measures to prevent these problems at home (see Plan of Nursing Care 15-1 for more information).

ADMINISTERING CHEMOTHERAPY

The local effects of the chemotherapeutic agent are also of concern. The patient is observed closely during its administration because of the risk and consequences of extravasation (particularly of vesicant agents or those that may produce necrosis if deposited in the subcutaneous tissues). Local difficulties or problems with administration of chemotherapeutic agents are brought to the attention of the physician promptly so that corrective measures can be taken immediately to minimize local tissue damage.

IMPLEMENTING SAFEGUARDS

Nurses involved in handling chemotherapeutic agents may be exposed to low doses of the drugs by direct contact, inhalation, and ingestion. Urinalyses of personnel repeatedly exposed to cytotoxic drugs demonstrate mutagenic activity. Although not all mutagens are carcinogenic, they can produce permanent inheritable changes in the genetic material of cells.

Although long-term studies of nurses handling chemotherapeutic agents have not been conducted, it is known that chemotherapeutic agents are associated with secondary formation of cancers and chromosome abnormalities. Additionally, nausea, vomiting, dizziness, alopecia, and nasal mucosal ulcerations have been reported in health care personnel who have handled chemotherapeutic agents.

Because of known and potential hazards associated with handling chemotherapeutic agents, the Occupational Safety and Health Administration, Oncology Nursing Society, hospitals, and other health care agencies have developed specific precautions for those involved in the preparation and administration of chemotherapy (Guideline 15-1).

Bone Marrow Transplantation

Although surgery, radiation therapy, and chemotherapy have resulted in improved survival rates for cancer patients, many cancers that initially respond to therapy continue to recur. This is true of hematologic cancers that affect the bone marrow and solid tumor cancers treated with lower doses of antineoplastics to spare the bone marrow from larger, ablative doses of chemotherapy or radiation therapy.

The role of bone marrow transplantation (BMT) for malignant as well as some nonmalignant diseases continues to grow. Types of BMT based on the source of donor tissue include:

- Allogeneic (from an unrelated donor)
- Autologous (from self)
- Syngeneic (from an identical twin)
- Stem cell transplantation by apheresis

Allogeneic BMT, used primarily for disease of the bone marrow, depends on the availability of a human leukocyte antigen–matched donor. This greatly limits the number of transplants possible. The recipient must undergo ablative doses of chemotherapy and possibly total body irradiation to destroy all existing bone marrow and malignant disease. The harvested donor marrow is infused intravenously into the recipient and travels to sites in the body where it produces bone marrow and establishes itself. This establishment of the new bone marrow is known as engraftment. Once engraftment is complete (2 to 4 weeks, sometimes longer), the new bone marrow becomes functional and begins producing red blood cells, WBCs, and platelets.

Before engraftment, patients are at a high risk for infection, sepsis, and bleeding. Side effects of the high-dose chemotherapy and total-body irradiation (TBI) can be acute and chronic. Acute side effects include alopecia, hemorrhagic cystitis, nausea, vomiting, diarrhea, and severe stomatitis. Chronic side effects include sterility, pulmonary dysfunction, cardiac dysfunction, and liver disease. Patients receive immunosuppressant drugs, such as cyclosporine or azathioprine (Imuran), to prevent graft-versus-host disease (GVHD). In allogeneic transplant recipients, GVHD occurs when the T lymphocytes from the transplanted donor marrow mount an immune response against the recipient's tissues (skin, gastrointestinal tract, liver). T lymphocytes respond in this manner because they view the recipient's tissue as "foreign," immunologically differing from what they recognize as "self" in the donor. GVHD may occur acutely or chronically. The first 100 days after allogeneic transplantation are crucial days for BMT patients until the immune system and blood-making capacity (hematopoiesis)

(*text continues on page 290*)

15•1 **PLAN OF NURSING CARE** 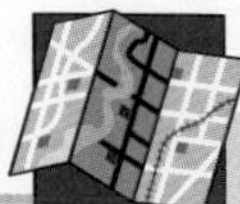

The Patient With Cancer

Nursing Interventions	Rationale	Expected Outcomes
Nursing Diagnosis: Risk for infection related to altered immunologic response		
Goal: Prevention of infection		
1. Assess patient for evidence of infection: a. Check vital signs every 4 hours. b. Monitor WBC count and differential each day. c. Inspect all sites that may serve as entry ports for pathogens (intravenous sites, wounds, skin folds, bony prominences, perineum, and oral cavity).	1. Signs and symptoms of infection may be diminished in the immunocompromised host. Prompt recognition of infection and subsequent initiation of therapy will reduce morbidity and mortality associated with infection.	• Demonstrates normal temperature and vital signs. • Exhibits absence of signs of inflammation: local edema, erythema, pain, and warmth. • Exhibits normal breath sounds on auscultation. • Takes deep breaths and coughs every 2 hours to prevent respiratory dysfunction and infection.
2. Report fever ≥38.3°C (101°F), chills, diaphoresis, swelling, heat, pain, erythema, exudate on any body surfaces. Also report change in respiratory or mental status, urinary frequency or burning, malaise, myalgias, arthralgias, rash, or diarrhea.	2. Early detection of infection facilitates early intervention.	
3. Obtain cultures and sensitivities as indicated before initiation of antimicrobial treatment (wound exudate, sputum, urine, stool, blood).	3. These tests identify the organism and indicate the most appropriate antimicrobial therapy. Use of inappropriate antibiotics enhances proliferation of additional flora and encourages growth of antibiotic-resistant organisms.	• Exhibits absence of pathologic bacteria on cultures.
4. Initiate measures to minimize infection. a. Discuss with patient and family (1) Placing patient in private room if absolute WBC count <1000/mm³ (2) Importance of patient avoiding contact with people who have known or recent infection or recent vaccination	4. Exposure to infection is reduced. a. Preventing contact with pathogens helps prevent infection.	• Avoids contact with others with infections. • Avoids crowds. • All personnel wash hands after each voiding and bowel movement. • Excoriation and trauma of skin are avoided. • Trauma to mucous membranes is avoided (avoidance of rectal temperatures, suppositories, vaginal tampons, perianal trauma). • Uses recommended procedures and techniques if participating in management of invasive lines or catheters. • Uses electric razor. • Is free of skin breakdown and stasis of secretions. • Adheres to dietary and environmental restrictions. • Exhibits no signs of septicemia or septic shock. • Exhibits normal vital signs, cardiac output, and arterial pressures when monitored. • Demonstrates ability to administer colony-stimulating factor.
b. Instruct all personnel in careful hand washing before and after entering room.	b. Hands are significant source of contamination.	
c. Avoid rectal or vaginal procedures (rectal temperatures, examinations, suppositories; vaginal tampons).	c. Incidence of rectal and perianal abscesses and subsequent systemic infection is high. Manipulation may cause disruption of membrane integrity and enhance progression of infection.	
d. Use stool softeners to prevent constipation and straining.	d. This minimizes trauma to tissues.	
e. Assist patient in practice of meticulous personal hygiene.	e. This prevents skin irritation.	
f. Instruct patient to use electric razor.	f. Minimizes skin trauma.	
g. Encourage patient to ambulate in room unless contraindicated.	g. Minimizes chance of skin breakdown and stasis of pulmonary secretions.	
h. Avoid fresh fruits, raw meat, fish, and vegetables if absolute WBC count <1000/mm³, also remove fresh flowers and potted plants.	h. Fresh fruits and vegetables harbor bacteria not removed by ordinary washing. Flowers and potted plants are also sources of organisms.	
i. Each day: change drinking water, denture cleaning fluids, and respiratory equipment containing water.	i. Stagnant water is a source of infection.	
5. Assess intravenous sites every day for evidence of infection:	5. Nosocomial staphylococcal septicemia is closely associated with intravenous catheters.	
a. Change intravenous sites every other day.	a. Incidence of infection is increased when catheter is in place >72 hr.	

(continued)

15•1

PLAN OF NURSING CARE

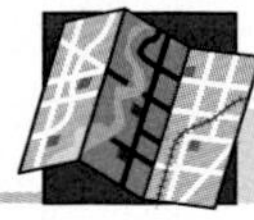

The Patient With Cancer (*continued*)

Nursing Interventions	Rationale	Expected Outcomes
b. Cleanse skin with povidone-iodine before arterial puncture or venipuncture.	b. Povidone-iodine is effective against many gram-positive and gram-negative pathogens.	
c. Change central venous catheter dressings every other day.	c. Allows observation of site and removes source of contamination.	
d. Change all solutions and infusion sets every 48 hours.	d. Once introduced into the system, microorganisms are capable of growing in infusion sets despite replacement of container and high flow rates.	
6. Avoid intramuscular injections.	6. Reduces risk for skin abscesses.	
7. Avoid insertion of urinary catheters; if catheters are necessary, use strict aseptic technique.	7. Rates of infection *greatly* increase after urinary catheterization.	
8. Teach patient or family member to administer granulocyte (or granulocyte-macrophage) colony-stimulating factor when prescribed.	8. Granulocyte colony-stimulating factor decreases the duration of neutropenia and the potential for infection.	

Nursing Diagnosis: Impaired skin integrity: erythematous and wet desquamation reactions to radiation therapy

Goal: Maintenance of skin integrity

Nursing Interventions	Rationale	Expected Outcomes
1. In erythematous areas: a. Avoid the use of soaps, cosmetics, perfumes, powders, lotions and ointments, deodorants. b. Use only lukewarm water to bathe the area. c. Avoid rubbing or scratching the area. d. Avoid shaving the area with a straight-edged razor. e. Avoid applying hot-water bottles, heating pads, ice, and adhesive tape to the area. f. Avoid exposing the area to sunlight or cold weather.	1. Care to the affected areas must focus on preventing further skin irritation, drying, and damage	• Avoids use of soaps, powders, and other cosmetics on site of radiation therapy. • States rationale for special care of skin. • Exhibits minimal change in skin. • Avoids trauma to affected skin region (avoids shaving, constricting, and irritating clothing, extremes of temperature, and use of adhesive tape). • Reports change in skin promptly. • Demonstrates proper care of blistered or open areas. • Exhibits absence of infection of blistered and opened areas.
g. Avoid tight clothing in the area. Use cotton clothing.	g. Allows air circulation to affected area.	
h. Apply vitamin A&D ointment to the area.	h. Aids healing.	
2. If wet desquamation occurs: a. Do not disrupt any blisters that have formed. b. Avoid frequent washing of the area. c. Report any blistering.	2. Open weeping areas are susceptible to bacterial infection. Care must be taken to prevent introduction of pathogens.	
d. Use *prescribed* creams or ointments.	d. Decreases irritation and inflammation of the area.	
e. If area weeps, apply a thin layer of gauze dressing.	e. Enhances drying.	

Nursing Diagnosis: Altered oral mucous membrane: stomatitis

Goal: Maintenance of intact oral mucous membranes

Nursing Interventions	Rationale	Expected Outcomes
1. Assess oral cavity daily.	1. Provides baseline for later evaluation.	• States rationale for frequent oral assessment and hygiene.
2. Instruct patient to report oral burning, pain, areas of redness, open lesions on the	2. Identification of initial stages of stomatitis will facilitate prompt interventions, includ-	

(*continued*)

15•1

PLAN OF NURSING CARE

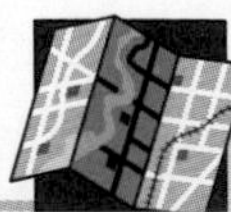

The Patient With Cancer (*continued*)

Nursing Interventions	Rationale	Expected Outcomes
lips, pain associated with swallowing, or decreased tolerance to temperature extremes of food.	ing modification of treatment as prescribed by physician.	• Identifies signs and symptoms of stomatitis to report to nurse or physician. • Participates in recommended oral hygiene regimen. • Avoids mouthwashes with alcohol. • Brushes teeth and mouth with soft toothbrush. • Uses lubricant to keep lips soft and non-irritated. • Avoids hard to chew, spicy, and hot foods. • Exhibits clean, intact oral mucosa. • Exhibits no ulcerations or infections of oral cavity. • Exhibits no evidence of bleeding. • Reports absent or decreased oral pain. • Reports no difficulty swallowing. • Exhibits healing (reepithelialization) of oral mucosa within 5 to 7 days (mild stomatitis). • Exhibits healing of oral tissues within 10 to 14 days (severe stomatitis). • Exhibits no bleeding or oral ulceration. • Consumes adequate fluid and food. • Exhibits absence of dehydration and weight loss.
3. Encourage and assist in oral hygiene.		
Preventive		
a. Avoid commercial mouthwashes.	a. Alcohol content of mouthwashes will dry oral tissues and potentiate breakdown.	
b. Brush with soft toothbrush; use non-abrasive toothpaste after meals and bedtime; floss every 24 h unless painful or platelet count falls below 40,000 cu/mm.	b. Limits trauma and removes debris.	
Mild stomatitis (generalized erythema, limited ulcerations, small white patches: *Candida*)		
c. Use normal saline mouth rinses every 2 h while awake; every 6 h at night.	c. Assists in removing debris, thick secretions, and bacteria.	
d. Use soft toothbrush or toothette.	d. Minimizes trauma.	
e. Remove dentures except for meals, be certain dentures fit well.	e. Minimizes friction and discomfort.	
f. Apply lip lubricant.	f. Promotes comfort.	
g. Avoid foods that are spicy or hard to chew and those with extremes of temperature.	g. Prevents local trauma.	
Severe Stomatitis (confluent ulcerations with bleeding and white patches covering more than 25% of oral mucosa)		
h. Obtain tissue samples for culture and sensitivity tests of areas of infection.	h. Assists in identifying need for antimicrobial therapy.	
i. Assess ability to chew and swallow; assess gag reflex.	i. Patient may be in danger of aspiration.	
j. Use oral rinses as prescribed or place patient on side and irrigate mouth; have suction available (may combine in solution saline, anti-*Candida* agent, such as Mycostatin, and topical anesthetic agent as described below).	j. Facilitates cleansing, provides for safety and comfort.	
k. Remove dentures.	k. Prevents trauma from ill-fitting dentures.	
l. Use toothette or gauze soaked with solution for cleansing.	l. Limits trauma, promotes comfort.	
m. Use lip lubricant.	m. Promotes comfort.	
n. Provide liquid or pureed diet.	n. Ensures intake of easily digestible foods.	
o. Monitor for dehydration.	o. Decreased oral intake and ulcerations potentiate fluid deficits.	
4. Minimize discomfort.		
a. Consult physician for use of topical anesthetic, such as dyclonine and diphenhydramine, or viscous lidocaine.	a. Alleviates pain and increases sense of well-being; promotes participation in oral hygiene and nutritional intake.	
b. Administer systemic analgesics as prescribed.		
c. Perform mouth care as described.	c. Promotes removal of debris, healing, and comfort.	

(*continued*)

15•1

PLAN OF NURSING CARE The Patient With Cancer (*continued*)

Nursing Interventions	Rationale	Expected Outcomes
Nursing Diagnosis: Impaired tissue integrity: alopecia		
Goal: Maintenance of tissue integrity; coping with hair loss		
1. Discuss potential hair loss and regrowth with patient and family.	1. Provides information so patient and family can begin to prepare cognitively and emotionally for loss.	• Identifies alopecia as potential side effect of treatment. • Identifies positive and negative feelings and threats to self-image. • Verbalizes meaning that hair and possible hair loss have for him or her. • States rationale for modifications in hair care and treatment. • Uses mild shampoo and conditioner and shampoos hair only when necessary. • Avoids hair dryer, curlers, sprays, and other stresses on hair and scalp. • Wears hat or scarf over hair when exposed to sun. • Takes steps to deal with possible hair loss before it occurs; purchases wig or hair piece. • Maintains hygiene and grooming. • Interacts and socializes with others. • States that hair loss and necessity of wig are temporary.
2. Explore potential impact of hair loss on self-image, interpersonal relationships, and sexuality.	2. Facilitates coping.	
3. Prevent or minimize hair loss through the following:	3. Retains hair as long as possible.	
a. Use scalp hypothermia and scalp tourniquets, if appropriate	a. Decreases hair follicle uptake of chemotherapy (not used for patients with leukemia or lymphoma because tumors cells may be present in blood vessels or scalp tissue).	
b. Cut long hair before treatment.	b–e. Minimizes hair loss due to the weight and manipulation of hair.	
c. Use mild shampoo and conditioner, gently pat dry, and avoid excessive shampooing.		
d. Avoid electric curlers, curling irons, dryers, clips, barrettes, hair sprays, hair dyes, and permanent waves.		
e. Avoid excessive combing or brushing; use wide-toothed comb.		
4. Prevent trauma to scalp.	4. Preserves tissue integrity.	
a. Lubricate scalp with vitamin A&D ointment to decrease itching.	a. Assists in maintaining skin integrity.	
b. Have patient use sunscreen or wear hat when in the sun.	b. Prevents ultraviolet light exposure.	
5. Suggest ways to assist in coping with hair loss:	5. Minimizes change in appearance.	
a. Purchase wig or hair piece before hair loss.	a. Wig that closely resembles hair color and style is more easily selected if hair loss has not begun.	
b. If hair loss has occurred, take photograph to wig shop to assist in selection.	b. Facilitates adjustment.	
c. Begin to wear wig before hair loss.		
d. Contact the American Cancer Society for donated wigs, or a store that specializes in this product.		
e. Wear hat, scarf, or turban.	e. Conceals loss.	
6. Encourage patient to wear own clothes and retain social contacts.	6. Assists in maintaining personal identity.	
7. Explain that hair growth usually begins again once therapy is completed.	7. Reassures patient that hair loss is usually temporary.	
Nursing Diagnosis: Altered nutrition, less than body requirements, related to nausea and vomiting		
Goal: Fewer episodes of nausea and vomiting before, during, and after chemotherapy		
1. Assess the patient's previous experiences and expectations of nausea and vomiting, including causes and interventions used.	1. Identifies patient concerns, misinformation, potential strategies for intervention. Also gives patient sense of empowerment and control.	• Identifies previous triggers of nausea and vomiting. • Exhibits decreased apprehension and anxiety.

(*continued*)

15•1 **PLAN OF NURSING CARE** 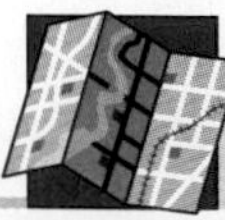 **The Patient With Cancer (*continued*)**

Nursing Interventions	Rationale	Expected Outcomes
2. Adjust diet before and after drug administration according to patient preference and tolerance.	2. Each patient responds differently to food after chemotherapy. A diet containing foods that relieve the patient's nausea or vomiting is most helpful.	• Identifies previously used successful interventions for nausea and vomiting. • Reports decrease in nausea. • Reports decrease in incidence of vomiting.
3. Prevent unpleasant sights, odors, and sounds in the environment.	3. Unpleasant sensations can stimulate the nausea and vomiting center.	• Consumes adequate fluid and food when nausea subsides.
4. Use distraction, music therapy, biofeedback, self-hypnosis, relaxation techniques, and guided imagery before, during, and after chemotherapy.	4. Decreases anxiety, which can contribute to nausea and vomiting. Psychological conditioning may also be decreased.	• Demonstrates use of distraction, relaxation, and imagery when indicated. • Exhibits normal skin turgor and moist mucous membranes.
5. Administer prescribed antiemetics, sedatives, and corticosteroids before chemotherapy and afterward as needed.	5. Administration of antiemetic regimen before onset of nausea and vomiting limits the adverse experience and facilitates control. Combination drug therapy reduces nausea and vomiting through various triggering mechanisms.	• Reports no additional weight loss.
6. Ensure adequate fluid hydration before, during, and after drug administration; assess intake and output.	6. Adequate fluid volume dilutes drug levels, decreasing stimulation of vomiting receptors.	
7. Encourage frequent oral hygiene.	7. Reduces unpleasant taste sensations.	
8. Provide pain relief measures, if necessary.	8. Increased comfort increases physical tolerance of symptoms.	
9. Assess other causes of nausea and vomiting, such as constipation, gastrointestinal irritation, electrolyte imbalance, radiation therapy, medications, and central nervous system metastasis.	9. Multiple factors may cause nausea and vomiting.	

Nursing Diagnosis: Altered nutrition: less than body requirements, related to anorexia, cachexia, or malabsorption

Goal: Maintenance of nutritional status and of weight within 10% of pretreatment weight

Nursing Interventions	Rationale	Expected Outcomes
1. Teach patient to avoid unpleasant sights, odors, sounds in the environment during mealtime.	1. Anorexia can be stimulated or increased with noxious stimuli.	• Exhibits weight loss no greater than 10% of pretreatment weight. • Reports decreasing anorexia and increased interest in eating.
2. Suggest foods that are preferred and well tolerated by the patient, preferably high-calorie and high protein foods. Respect ethnic and cultural food preferences.	2. Foods preferred, well tolerated, and high in calories and protein maintain nutritional status during periods of increased metabolic demand.	• Demonstrates normal skin turgor. • Identifies rationale for dietary modifications. • Participates in calorie counts and diet histories.
3. Encourage adequate fluid intake, but limit fluids at mealtime.	3. Fluids are necessary to eliminate wastes and prevent dehydration. Increased fluids with meals can lead to early satiety.	• Uses appropriate relaxation and imagery before meals.
4. Suggest smaller, more frequent meals.	4. Smaller, more frequent meals are better tolerated because early satiety does not occur.	• Exhibits laboratory and clinical findings indicative of adequate nutritional intake: normal serum protein and transferrin levels; normal serum iron levels; normal hemoglobin, hematocrit, and lymphocyte levels; normal urinary creatinine levels.
5. Promote relaxed, quiet environment during mealtime with increased social interaction as desired.	5. A quiet environment promotes relaxation. Social interaction at mealtime increases appetite.	
6. If possible, serve wine at mealtime with foods.	6. Wine often stimulates appetite and adds calories.	• Consumes diet high in required nutrients. • Carries out oral hygiene before meals.
7. Consider cold foods, if desired.	7. Cold, high-protein foods are often more tolerable and less odorous than hot foods.	• Reports that pain does not interfere with meals.
8. Advocate nutritional supplements and high-protein foods between meals.	8. Supplements and snacks add protein and calories to meet nutritional requirements.	• Reports decreasing episodes of nausea and vomiting.
9. Encourage frequent oral hygiene.	9. Oral hygiene stimulates appetite and increases saliva production.	• Participates in increasing levels of activity.

(*continued*)

15•1

PLAN OF NURSING CARE 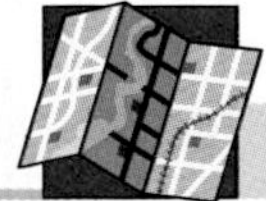 The Patient With Cancer (*continued*)

Nursing Interventions	Rationale	Expected Outcomes
10. Provide pain relief measures.	10. Pain impairs appetite.	• States rationale for use of tube feedings or hyperalimentation. • Participates in management of tube feedings or total parenteral nutrition.
11. Provide control of nausea and vomiting.	11. Nausea and vomiting increase anorexia.	
12. Increase activity level as tolerated.	12. Increased activity promotes appetite.	
13. Decrease anxiety by encouraging verbalization of fears, concerns; use of relaxation techniques; imagery at mealtime.	13. Relief of anxiety may increase appetite.	
14. Position patient properly at mealtime.	14. Proper body position and alignment are necessary to aid chewing and swallowing.	
15. For collaborative management, provide enteral tube feedings of commercial liquid diets, elemental diets, or blenderized foods as prescribed.	15. Tube feedings may be necessary in the severely debilitated patient who has a functioning gastrointestinal system.	
16. Provide total parenteral nutrition with lipid supplements as prescribed.	16. Total parenteral nutrition with supplemental fats supplies needed calories and proteins to meet nutritional demands, especially in the nonfunctional gastrointestinal system.	
17. Administer appetite stimulants as prescribed by physician.	17. Although the mechanism is unclear, medications such as Megace have been noted to improve appetite in patients with cancer and HIV infection.	

Nursing Diagnosis: Fatigue and activity intolerance

Goal: Increased activity tolerance and decreased fatigue level

Nursing Interventions	Rationale	Expected Outcomes
1. Encourage several rest periods during the day, especially before and after physical exertion.	1. During rest, energy is conserved and levels are replenished. Several shorter rest periods may be more beneficial than one longer rest period.	• Reports decreasing levels of fatigue. • Increases participation in activities gradually. • Rests when fatigued. • Reports restful sleep. • Requests assistance with activities appropriately. • Reports adequate energy to participate in activities important to him or her (eg, visiting with family, hobbies). • Consumes diet with recommended protein and caloric intake. • Uses relaxation exercises and imagery to decrease anxiety and promote rest. • Participates in planned exercise program gradually. • Reports no breathlessness during activities. • Exhibits acceptable hemoglobin and hematocrit levels. • Exhibits normal fluid and electrolyte balance. • Reports decreased discomfort. • Exhibits improved mobility.
2. Increase total hours of nighttime sleep.	2. Sleep helps to restore energy levels.	
3. Rearrange daily schedule and organize activities to conserve energy expenditure.	3. Reorganization of activities can reduce energy losses and stressors.	
4. Allow or ask for others' assistance with necessary chores, such as housework, child care, shopping, cooking.	4. Conserves energy.	
5. Encourage reduced job workload, if possible, by reducing number of hours worked per week.	5. Reducing workload decreases physical and psychological stress and increases periods of rest and relaxation.	
6. Encourage adequate protein and calorie intake.	6. Protein and calorie depletion decreases activity tolerance.	
7. Encourage use of relaxation techniques, mental imagery.	7. Promotion of relaxation and psychological rest decreases physical fatigue.	
8. Encourage participation in planned exercise programs.	8. Proper exercise programs increase endurance and stamina.	
9. For collaborative management, administer blood products as prescribed.	9. Lowered hemoglobin and hematocrit predispose patient to fatigue due to decreased oxygen availability.	
10. Assess for fluid and electrolyte disturbances.	10. May contribute to altered nerve transmission and muscle function.	
11. Assess for sources of discomfort.	11. Coping with discomfort requires energy expenditure.	
12. Provide strategies to facilitate mobility.	12. Impaired mobility requires increased energy expenditure.	

(*continued*)

15•1

PLAN OF NURSING CARE

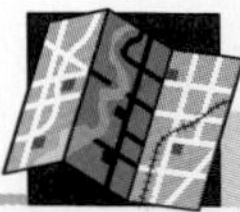

The Patient With Cancer (*continued*)

Nursing Interventions	Rationale	Expected Outcomes
Nursing Diagnosis: Pain and discomfort **Goal: Relief of pain and discomfort**		
1. Assess pain and discomfort characteristics: location, quality, frequency, duration, etc.	1. Provides baseline for assessing changes in pain level and evaluation of interventions.	• Reports decreased level of pain and discomfort.
2. Assure patient that you know that pain is real and will assist him or her in reducing it.	2. Fear that pain will not be considered real increases anxiety and reduces pain tolerance.	• Reports less disruption from pain and discomfort.
3. Assess other factors contributing to patient's pain: fear, fatigue, anger, etc.	3. Provides data about factors that decrease patient's ability to tolerate pain and increase pain level.	• Explains how fatigue, fear, etc., contribute to severity of pain and discomfort. • Accepts pain medication as prescribed.
4. Administer analgesics to promote optimum pain relief within limits of physician's prescription.	4. Analgesics tend to be more effective when administered early in pain cycle.	• Exhibits decreased physical and behavioral signs of pain and discomfort in acute pain (no grimacing, crying, moaning; displays interest in surroundings and activities around him).
5. Assess patient's behavioral responses to pain and pain experience.	5. Provides additional information about patient's pain.	• Takes an active role in administration of analgesia.
6. Collaborate with patient, physician, and other health care team members when changes in pain management are necessary.	6. New methods of administering analgesia must be acceptable to patient, physician, and health care team to be effective; patient's participation decreases the sense of powerlessness.	• Identifies additional effective pain relief strategies. • Uses alternative pain relief strategies appropriately. • Reports effective use of new pain relief strategies and decrease in pain intensity.
7. Encourage strategies of pain relief that patient has used successfully in previous pain experience.	7. Encourages success of pain relief strategies accepted by patient and family.	• Reports that decreased level of pain permits participation in other activities and events.
8. Teach patient new strategies to relieve pain and discomfort: distraction, imagery, relaxation, cutaneous stimulation, etc.	8. Increases number of options and strategies available to patient.	
Nursing Diagnosis: Anticipatory grieving related to loss; altered role functioning **Goal: Appropriate progression through grieving process**		
1. Encourage verbalization of fears, concerns, and questions regarding disease, treatment, and future implications.	1. An increased and accurate knowledge base decreases anxiety and dispels misconceptions.	• The patient and family progress through the phases of grief as evidenced by increased verbalization and expression of grief.
2. Encourage active participation of patient or family in care and treatment decisions.	2. Active participation maintains patient independence and control.	• The patient and family identify resources available to aid coping strategies during grieving.
3. Visit family frequently to establish and maintain relationships and physical closeness.	3. Frequent contacts promote trust and security and reduce feelings of fear and isolation.	• The patient and family use resources and supports appropriately.
4. Encourage ventilation of negative feelings, including projected anger and hostility, within acceptable limits.	4. This allows for emotional expression without loss of self-esteem.	• The patient and family discuss the future openly with each other. • The patient and family discuss concerns and feelings openly with each other.
5. Allow for periods of crying and expression of sadness.	5. These feelings are necessary for separation and detachment to occur.	• The patient and family use nonverbal expressions of concern for each other.
6. Involve clergy as desired by the patient and family.	6. This facilitates the grief process and spiritual care.	
7. Advise professional counseling as indicated for patient or family to alleviate pathologic grieving.	7. This facilitates the grief process.	
8. Allow for progression through the grieving process at the individual pace of the patient and family.	8. Grief work is variable. Not every person uses every phase of the grief process, and the time spent in dealing with each phase varies with every person. To complete grief work, this variability must be allowed.	

(*continued*)

15•1

PLAN OF NURSING CARE 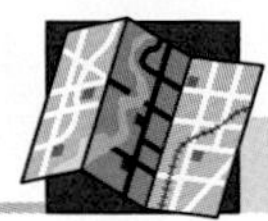 The Patient With Cancer (*continued*)

Nursing Interventions	Rationale	Expected Outcomes
Nursing Diagnosis: Body image disturbance and self-esteem disturbance related to changes in appearance, function, and roles		
Goal: Improved body image and self-esteem		
1. Assess patient's feelings about body image and level of self-esteem.	1. Provides baseline assessment for evaluating changes and assessing effectiveness of interventions.	• Identifies concerns of importance. • Takes active role in activities. • Maintains previous role in decision making. • Verbalizes feelings and reactions to losses or threatened losses. • Participates in self-care activities. • Permits others to assist in care when he or she is unable to be independent. • Exhibits interest in appearance and uses aids (cosmetics, scarves, etc.) appropriately. • Participates with others in conversations and social events and activities. • Verbalizes concern about sexual partner. • Explores alternative ways of expressing concern and affection.
2. Identify potential threats to patient's self-esteem (eg, altered appearance, decreased sexual function, hair loss, decreased energy, role changes). Validate concerns with patient.	2. Anticipates changes and permits patient to identify importance of these areas to him or her.	
3. Encourage continued participation in activities and decision making.	3. Encourages and permits continued control of events and self.	
4. Encourage patient to verbalize concerns.	4. Identifying concerns is an important step in coping with them.	
5. Individualize care for the patient.	5. Prevents or reduces depersonalization and emphasizes patient's self-worth.	
6. Assist patient in self-care when fatigue, lethargy, nausea, vomiting, and other symptoms prevent independence.	6. Physical well-being improves self-esteem.	
7. Assist patient in selecting and using cosmetics, scarves, hair pieces, and clothing that increase his or her sense of attractiveness.	7. Promotes positive body image.	
8. Encourage patient and partner to share concerns about altered sexuality and sexual function and to explore alternatives to their usual sexual expression.	8. Provides opportunity for expressing concern, affection, and acceptance.	
Collaborative Problem: Potential complication: risk for bleeding problems		
Goal: Prevention of bleeding		
1. Assess for potential for bleeding: monitor platelet count.	1. Mild risk: 50,000–100,000/mm^3 (SI: 0.05–0.1 × 10^{12}/L) Moderate risk: 20,000–50,000/mm^3 (SI: 0.02–0.05 × 10^{12}/L) Severe risk: less than 20,000/mm^3 (SI:0.02 × 10^{12}/L)	• Signs and symptoms of bleeding are identified. • Exhibits no blood in feces, urine, or emesis. • Exhibits no bleeding of gums or of injection or venipuncture sites. • Exhibits no ecchymosis (bruising). • Patient and family identify ways to prevent bleeding. • Uses recommended measures to reduce risk of bleeding (uses soft toothbrush, shaves with electric razor only). • Exhibits normal vital signs. • Reports that environmental hazards have been reduced or removed. • Consumes adequate fluid. • Reports absence of constipation. • Avoids substances interfering with clotting. • Absence of tissue destruction. • Exhibits normal mental status and absence of signs of intracranial bleeding.
2. Assess for bleeding:	2. Early detection promotes early intervention.	
a. Petechiae or ecchymosis	a. Indicates injury to microcirculation and larger vessels.	
b. Decrease in hemoglobin or hematocrit	b. Indicates blood loss.	
c. Prolonged bleeding from invasive procedures, venipunctures, minor cuts or scratches		
d. Frank or occult blood in any body excretion, emesis, sputum		
e. Bleeding from any body orifice		
f. Altered mental status	f. Indicates neurologic involvement.	
3. Instruct patient and family about ways to minimize bleeding:	3. Patient can participate in self-protection.	
a. Use soft toothbrush or toothette for mouth care.	a. Prevents trauma to oral tissues.	
b. Avoid commercial mouthwashes.	b. Contains high alcohol content that will dry oral tissues.	
c. Use electric razor for shaving.	c. Prevents trauma to skin.	

(*continued*)

15•1 PLAN OF NURSING CARE 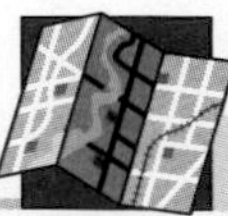 The Patient With Cancer (*continued*)

Nursing Interventions	Rationale	Expected Outcomes
d. Use emery board for nail care.		• Avoids medications that interfere with clotting (aspirin).
e. Avoid foods that are difficult to chew.	e. Prevents oral tissue trauma.	• Absence of epistaxis and cerebral bleeding.
4. Initiate measures to minimize bleeding.	4. Preserves circulating blood volume.	
a. Draw all blood for lab work with one daily venipuncture.	a. Minimizes trauma and blood loss.	
b. Avoid taking temperature rectally or administering suppositories and enemas.	b. Prevents trauma to rectal mucosa.	
c. Avoid intramuscular injections; use smallest needle possible.	c. Prevents intramuscular bleeding.	
d. Apply direct pressure to injection and venipuncture sites for at least 5 min.	d. Minimizes blood loss.	
e. Lubricate lips with petrolatum.	e. Prevents skin from drying.	
f. Avoid bladder catheterizations; use smallest catheter if catheterization is necessary.	f. Prevents trauma to urethra.	
g. Maintain fluid intake of at least 3 L/24 h unless contraindicated.	g. Hydration helps to prevent skin drying.	
h. Use stool softeners or increase bulk in diet.	h. Prevents constipation and straining that may injure rectal tissue.	
i. Avoid medications that will interfere with clotting (eg, aspirin).	i. Minimizes risk of bleeding.	
j. Recommend use of water-based lubricant before sexual intercourse.	j. Prevents friction and tissue trauma.	
5. When platelet count is less than 20,000/mm^3, institute the following:	5. Platelet count of less than 20,000/mm^3 is associated with increased risk of spontaneous bleeding.	
a. Bed rest with padded side rails.	a. Reduces risk of injury	
b. Avoidance of strenuous activity.	b. Increases intracranial pressure and risk of cerebral hemorrhage.	
c. Platelet transfusions as prescribed; administer prescribed diphenhydramine hydrochloride (Benadryl) or hydrocortisone sodium succinate (Solu-Cortef) to prevent reaction to platelet transfusion.	c. Allergic reactions to blood products are associated with antigen–antibody reaction that causes platelet destruction.	
d. Supervise activity when out of bed.		
e. Caution against forceful nose blowing.	e. Prevents trauma to nasal mucosa and increased intracranial pressure.	

have recovered sufficiently to prevent infection and hemorrhage. Most acute side effects, such as nausea, vomiting, and mucositis, also resolve in the initial 100 days after transplantation.

Autologous BMT is considered for patients with disease of the bone marrow who do not have a suitable donor for allogeneic BMT and for those patients who have healthy bone marrow but require bone marrow ablative doses of chemotherapy to cure their aggressive malignancy. Bone marrow is harvested from the patient and preserved for reinfusion and, if necessary, treated to kill any malignant cells within the marrow. The patient is treated with ablative chemotherapy and, possibly, TBI to eradicate any remaining tumor. Then, the harvested bone marrow is reinfused and engrafted. Until engraftment occurs in the bone marrow sites of the body, the patient is at high risk for infection, sepsis, and bleeding. Acute and chronic toxicities from chemotherapy and radiation therapy may be severe. No immunosuppressant medications are necessary after autologous BMT because the patient did not receive foreign tissue. A disadvantage of autologous transplantation is the risk for viable tumor cells remaining in the bone marrow despite conditioning regimens (high-dose chemotherapy).

Syngeneic BMT is the least common type of transplantation because it requires an identical sibling for harvest. Syngeneic transplantations result in fewer complications and no marrow rejection because the donor is an identical tissue match to the recipient. The transplantation and harvest process are the same with syngeneic BMT as with allogeneic BMT.

Peripheral blood stem cell BMT is the newest method. With this method, patients receive chemotherapy and hematopoietic growth factors to stimulate production of hematopoietic stem cells. These stem cells are then collected by apheresis for reinfusion at a later date. Stem cells are essentially bone marrow because they are responsible for engraftment and repopulation of hematopoietic tissue. Patients then receive the ablative therapy regimens, followed by reinfusion of the stem cells. Marrow recovery time after engraftment with stem cells is faster than with other types of transplantation.

15•1 GUIDELINES FOR SAFETY IN ADMINISTERING CHEMOTHERAPY

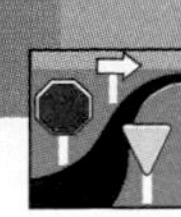

Safety recommendations from the Occupational Safety and Health Administration (OSHA), Oncology Nursing Society (ONS), hospitals, and other health care agencies for the preparation and handling of antineoplastic agents follow:

- Use a biologic safety cabinet for the preparation of all chemotherapy drugs.
- Wear surgical gloves when handling drugs and the excretions of patients who received chemotherapy.
- Wear disposable, long-sleeved gowns when preparing and administering chemotherapy drugs.
- Use Luer-Lok fittings on all intravenous tubing used to deliver chemotherapy.
- Dispose of all equipment used in chemotherapy preparation and administration in appropriate, leak-proof, puncture-proof containers.
- Dispose of all chemotherapy wastes as hazardous materials.

When followed, these precautions greatly minimize the risk of exposure.

Nursing Management in Bone Marrow Transplantation

Nursing care of patients undergoing BMT is complex and demands a high level of skill. Transplantation nursing can be extremely rewarding yet extremely stressful. The success of BMT is greatly influenced by nursing care throughout the transplantation process.

IMPLEMENTING PRETRANSPLANTATION CARE

All patients must undergo extensive pretransplantation evaluations to assess the current clinical status of the disease. Nutritional assessments, extensive physical examinations and organ function tests, and psychological evaluations are completed. Blood work includes assessing past antigen exposure, for example, to hepatitis virus, cytomegalovirus, herpes simplex virus, HIV, and syphilis. The patient's social support systems and financial and insurance resources are also evaluated. Informed consent and patient teaching about the procedure and pretransplantation and posttransplantation care are vital.

PROVIDING CARE DURING TREATMENT

Skilled nursing care is required during the treatment phase of BMT when high-dose chemotherapy (conditioning regimen) and total-body irradiation are administered. The acute toxicities of nausea, diarrhea, mucositis, and hemorrhagic cystitis require close monitoring and constant attention by the nurse.

Nursing management during the bone marrow or stem cell infusions consists of monitoring vital signs and blood oxygen saturation; assessing for adverse effects, such as fever, chills, shortness of breath, chest pain, cutaneous reactions, nausea, vomiting, hypotension or hypertension, tachycardia, anxiety, and taste changes; and providing ongoing support and patient teaching.

Through the period of bone marrow aplasia until engraftment of the new marrow occurs, patients are at high risk for dying from sepsis and bleeding. Patients require support with blood products and hemopoietic growth factors. Potential infection may be bacterial, viral, fungal, or protozoan in origin. Renal complications arise from nephrotoxic chemotherapy drugs used in the conditioning regimen or to treat infection (amphotericin B, aminoglycosides). Tumor lysis syndrome and acute tubular necrosis are also risks after BMT.

GVHD requires skillful nursing assessment to detect early effects on the skin, liver, and gastrointestinal tract. Veno-occlusive disease of the liver from conditioning regimens used in BMT can result in fluid retention, jaundice, abdominal pain, ascites, tender and enlarged liver, and encephalopathy. Pulmonary complications, such as pulmonary edema, interstitial pneumonia, and other pneumonias, often complicate the recovery after BMT.

PROVIDING POSTTRANSPLANTATION CARE

Ongoing nursing assessment in follow-up visits is essential to detect late effects of therapy in BMT patients. Late complications occur 100 days or later after BMT. Late effects include infections, such as varicella zoster infection, restrictive pulmonary abnormalities, and recurrent pneumonias. Sterility often results. Chronic GVHD involves the skin, liver, intestine, esophagus, eye, lungs, joints, and vaginal mucosa. Cataracts may develop as well after TBI.

Psychosocial assessments by nursing staff must be ongoing. In addition to the stressors affecting patients at each phase of the transplantation experience, marrow donors and family members also have psychosocial needs that must be addressed.

CARING FOR THE DONORS

Donors commonly experience mood alterations, decreased self-esteem, and guilt from feelings of failure if the transplantation fails. Family members must be educated and supported to reduce anxiety and promote coping during this difficult time. Family members must also be assisted to maintain realistic expectations of themselves as well as of the patient.

As BMT becomes more prevalent, many moral and ethical issues become apparent, including issues of informed consent, allocation of resources, and quality of life.

Hyperthermia

Hyperthermia (thermal therapy), the generation of temperatures greater than physiologic fever range (above 41.5°C [106.7°F]), has been used for many years to destroy tumors in human cancers. Research suggests that malignant cells are more sensitive than normal cells to the harmful effects of high temperatures for several reasons. Malignant cells lack repair mechanisms necessary to repair cell damage by elevated temperatures. Most tumor cells lack an adequate blood supply to provide needed oxygen during periods of increased cellular demand, such as during hyperthermia. Cancerous tumors lack blood vessels of adequate size for dissipation of heat. In addition, the body's immune system may be indirectly stimulated when hyperthermia is used.

Hyperthermia is most effective when combined with radiation therapy, chemotherapy, or biologic therapy. Hyperthermia and radiation therapy are thought to work well together because hypoxic tumor cells and cells in the S phase of the cell cycle are more sensitive to heat than radiation; the addition of heat damages tumor cells so that they cannot repair themselves after radiation therapy. Hyperthermia is thought to alter cellular membrane permeability when used with chemotherapy, allowing for an increased uptake of the chemotherapeutic agent. Hyperthermia may enhance function of immune system cells, such as macrophages and T cells, which are stimulated by many biologic agents.

Heat can be produced by using radiowaves, ultrasound, microwaves, magnetic waves, hot-water baths, or even hot-wax immersions. Hyperthermia may be local or regional, or it may include the whole body. Local or regional hyperthermia may be delivered to a cancerous extremity (for malignant melanoma) by regional perfusion, in which the affected extremity is isolated by a tourniquet and an extracorporeal circulator heats the blood flowing through the affected part. Hyperthermia probes may also be inserted around a tumor in a local area and attached to a heat source during treatment. Chemotherapeutic agents, such as melphalan, may also be heated and instilled into the region's circulating blood. Local or regional hyperthermia may also include infusion of heated solutions into cancerous body organs. Whole-body hyperthermia to treat disseminated disease may be achieved by extracorporeal circulation, immersion of patients in heated water or paraffin, or enclosure in heated suits.

Side effects of hyperthermic treatments include skin burns and tissue damage, fatigue, hypotension, peripheral neuropathies, thrombophlebitis, nausea, vomiting, diarrhea, and electrolyte imbalances. Resistance to hyperthermia may develop during the treatment because cells adapt to repeated thermal insult. Research into the effectiveness of hyperthermia, methods of delivery, and side effects is ongoing.

Nursing Management in Hyperthermia

Although hyperthermia has been used for many years, many patients and their families are unfamiliar with this cancer treatment. Consequently, they need explanations about the procedure, its goals, and its effects. The patient is assessed for adverse effects, and efforts are made to reduce their occurrence and severity. Local skin care at the site of the implanted hyperthermic probes is also required.

Biologic Response Modifiers

BRMs are naturally occurring or recombinant (reproduced through genetic engineering) agents or treatment methods that can alter the immunologic relationship between the tumor and the cancer patient (host) to provide a therapeutic benefit. Although the mechanisms of action vary with each type of BRM, the goal is to destroy or stop the malignant growth. The basis of BRM treatment lies in the restoration, modification, stimulation, or augmentation of the body's natural immune defenses against cancer.

Nonspecific Biologic Response Modifiers

Some of the early investigations of the stimulation of the immune system involved nonspecific agents such as bacille Calmette-Guérin (BCG) and *Corynebacterium parvum.* When injected into the patient, these agents serve as antigens that stimulate an immune response. The hope is that the stimulated immune system will then eradicate malignant cells. Extensive animal and human investigations with BCG have shown promising results, especially in treating localized malignant melanoma. Additionally, BCG is considered to be a standard form of treatment for localized bladder cancer. Use of nonspecific agents in advanced cancer remains limited, however, and research is continuing in an effort to identify other uses and other agents.

Monoclonal Antibodies

Monoclonal antibodies (MoAbs) are another type of BRM that became available through technologic advances, enabling investigators to grow and produce specific antibodies for specific malignant cells. The production of MoAbs involves injecting tumor cells that act as antigens into mice. Antibodies made in response to injected antigens can be found in the spleen of the mouse. Antibody-producing spleen cells are combined with a cancer cell that has the ability to grow indefinitely in culture medium and continue producing more antibodies. The combination of spleen cells and the cancer cells are referred to as hybridomas. From hybridomas that continue to grow in the culture medium, the desired antibodies are harvested, purified, and prepared for diagnostic or therapeutic use (Fig. 15-5). Alternative methods of producing MoAbs using human or genetically engineered sources are under investigation.

MoAbs are being used as aids in diagnostic evaluations. By attaching a radioactive substance to the MoAb, physicians can detect both primary and metastatic tumors through radiologic techniques. This process is referred to as radioimmunodetection. OncoScint (Cytogen Corporation, Princeton, NJ) is a U.S. Food and Drug Administration (FDA)-approved MoAb that is used to assist in diagnosing ovarian and colorectal cancers. The use of MoAbs in detecting breast, gastric, and prostate cancers and lymphoma is under investigation. MoAbs are also used in purging residual tumor cells from bone marrow or peripheral blood of patients who are undergoing BMT for peripheral stem cell rescue after high-dose cytotoxic therapy.

In cancer therapy, MoAbs may be used alone (unconjugated) to destroy cancer cells directly. Preliminary investigations of MoAbs in treating hematologic malignancies and solid tumors have demonstrated some effect, but further investigation is needed. Researchers are also exploring the feasibility of conjugating or combining MoAbs with other substances, such as radioactive materials, chemotherapeutic agents, toxins, hormones, or other BRMs. Immunoconjugate therapy, sometimes referred to as a "magic bullet," transports cancer killing substances to the cancer cells. Currently, no MoAbs have received FDA approval for treating cancer.

Cytokines

Cytokines, substances produced by cells of the immune system to enhance the production and functioning of components of the immune system, are also the focus of cancer treatment research. Cytokines are grouped into families, such as interferons, interleukins, colony-stimulating factors, and tumor necrosis factors (TNFs).

INTERFERONS

IFNs are examples of cytokines with both antiviral and antitumor properties. When stimulated, all nucleated cells are capable of producing these glycoproteins, which are classified according to their biologic and chemical properties: IFN-α is produced by leukocytes, IFN-β is produced by fibroblasts, and IFN-γ is produced by lymphocytes.

Although the exact antitumor effects of IFNs have not been thoroughly established, it is thought that they either stimulate the immune system or assist in preventing tumor growth. The antitumor effects are dependent on the type of IFN and the disease for

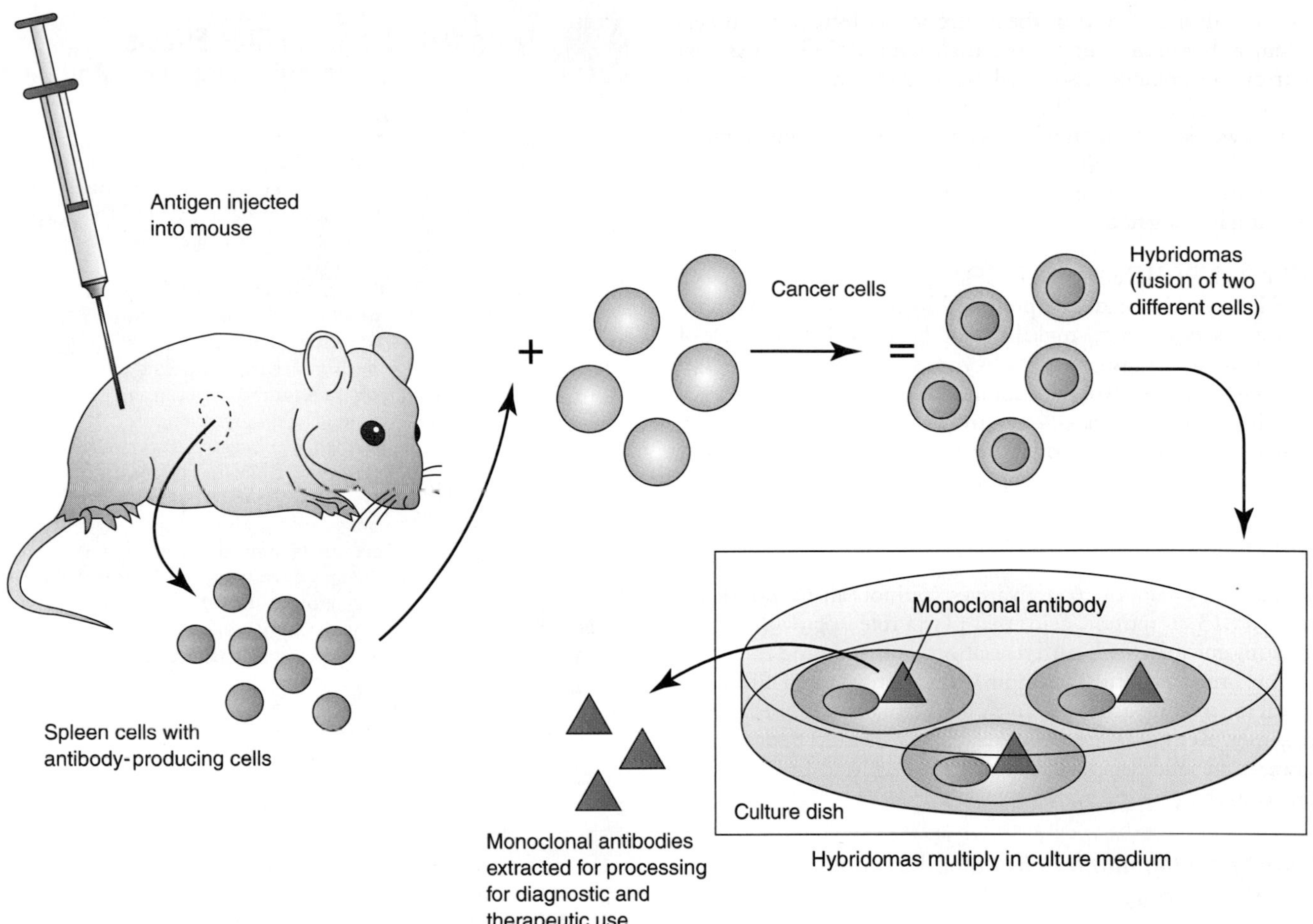

FIGURE 15•5 Antibody-producing spleen cells are fused with cancer cells. This process produces cells called hybridomas. These cells, which can grow indefinitely in a culture medium, produce antibodies that are harvested, purified, and prepared for diagnostic or treatment purposes.

which IFN is being used. IFNs enhance both lymphocyte and antibody production. They also facilitate the cytolytic or cell destruction role of macrophages and natural killer cells. Additionally, IFNs can inhibit cell multiplication by increasing the duration of various phases of the cell cycle.

The effects of IFN have been demonstrated in a variety of malignancies. IFN-α has been approved by the FDA for treating hairy-cell leukemia, Kaposi's sarcoma, chronic myelogenous leukemia, and melanoma. Other positive responses have been seen in hematologic malignancies and renal carcinomas. IFN-α, IFN-β, and IFN-γ have been approved by the FDA for the treatment of several nonmalignant diseases. IFN is administered through subcutaneous, intramuscular, intravenous, and intracavitary routes. Efforts are underway to establish the effectiveness of IFN for various malignancies in combination with other treatment regimens.

INTERLEUKINS

Interleukins are a subgroup of cytokines known as *lymphokines* and *monokines* because they are primarily produced by lymphocytes and monocytes. About 15 different interleukins have been identified. They act by signaling and coordinating other cells of the immune system. The FDA has approved interleukin-2 (IL-2) as a treatment option for renal cell cancer in adults. Originally referred to as T-cell growth factor, IL-2 is known to stimulate the production and activation of several different types of lymphocytes. In addition, IL-2 enhances the production of other types of cytokines and plays a role in influencing both humoral and cell-mediated immunity.

Clinical trials are beng conducted on IL-2 as well as other interleukins, such as IL-1, IL-4, and IL-6, for their roles in treating other cancers. Some clinical trials are assessing the effects of interleukins in combination with chemotherapy. In addition, interleukins are being investigated for their role as growth factors for treating myelosuppression after the use of some forms of chemotherapy.

HEMATOPOIETIC GROWTH FACTORS (COLONY-STIMULATING FACTORS)

Hematopoietic growth factors, also known as colony-stimulating factors, are hormonelike substances naturally produced by cells within the immune system. Hematopoietic growth factors of different types regulate the production of all cells in the blood, including neutrophils, macrophages, monocytes, red blood cells, and platelets. FDA approval of GM-CSF, G-CSF, and EPO has contributed significantly to the supportive care of patients with cancer.

Although these agents do not treat the underlying malignancy, they do target the effects of myelotoxic cancer therapies (adversely affecting the bone marrow), such as radiation and chemotherapy. Previously, the myelotoxic or bone marrow suppressive effects of chemotherapy had imposed limits on some chemotherapy agents and contributed to the development of life-threatening infections.

GM-CSF is used to treat the neutropenia (decreased numbers of neutrophils in the blood) associated with BMT. G-CSF is used to treat neutropenia associated with chemotherapy for solid tumor malignancies. EPO is used to treat anemia in cancer patients as well as in patients with chronic renal disease and in HIV-infected patients with zidovudine-induced anemia. Other growth factors, such as macrophage colony-stimulating factor and IL-3, are being investigated.

TUMOR NECROSIS FACTOR

TNF is a cytokine naturally produced by macrophages, lymphocytes, astrocytes, and microglial cells of the brain. The exact role of TNF is still under investigation. In vitro studies have shown TNF to stimulate other cells of the immune response and in animal studies to have direct tumor-killing activity. Clinical trials with TNF alone and in combination with other agents for treating melanoma, lung cancer, and renal cancer are underway.

Retinoids

Retinoids are vitamin A derivatives (retinol, all-*trans*-retinoic acid, and 13-*cis*-retinoic acid) that play a role in growth, reproduction, epithelial cell differentiation, and immune function. All-*trans*-retinoic acid (tretinoin) has been granted FDA approval for treating acute promyelocytic leukemia, a rare form of leukemia. Retinoids are being tested for treating hematologic cancers and solid tumors and for preventing head and neck and lung cancers.

Nursing Management in Biologic Response Modifier Therapy

Patients receiving BRM therapy have many of the same needs as cancer patients undergoing other treatment approaches. However, some BRM therapies are still investigational and considered a last chance effort by many patients who have not responded to standard treatments. Consequently, it is essential that the nurse assess the need for education, support, and guidance for both the patient and family and assist in planning and evaluating patient care.

MONITORING THERAPEUTIC AND ADVERSE EFFECTS

Nurses need to be familiar with each agent given and the potential effects (Table 15-7). Adverse effects, such as fever, myalgia, nausea, and vomiting, as seen with IFN therapy, may not be life-threatening. However, nurses must be aware of the impact of these side effects on the patient's quality of life. Other life-threatening adverse effects (eg, capillary leak syndrome, pulmonary edema, and hypotension) may occur with IL-2 therapy. Nurses work closely with physicians in assessing and managing potential toxicities of BRM therapy. Because of the investigational nature of many of these agents, the nurse will be administering them in a research setting. Accurate observations and careful documentation are essential components of patient assessment and data collection.

PROMOTING HOME AND COMMUNITY-BASED CARE

Teaching Patients Self-Care. Some BRMs, such as IFN, EPO, and G-CSF, can be administered by the patient or family in the home. Nurses teach patients and families, as needed, how to administer these agents through subcutaneous injections. Home care nurses monitor the patient's responses to treatment and provide teaching and continued care.

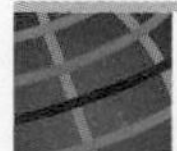

TABLE 15•7 Common Side Effects of Biologic Response Modifiers

Agent	Common Side Effects
Interferon	Influenza-like symptoms, fatigue, mental status changes, anorexia, alteration in lab values (hematology and LFTs [liver function tests]), weight loss because of anorexia
Interleukin-2	Influenza-like symptoms, fatigue, mental status changes, anorexia, nausea and vomiting, diarrhea, capillary leak syndrome, edema and fluid retention, hypotension, tachycardia and decreased systolic blood pressure, skin rash, erythema, and desquamation, inflammatory reactions/induration, at injection sites ("knots" may last 2–3 mo), weight gain during therapy, weight loss because of anorexia with long-term therapy, alterations in laboratory values (hematology, LFTs)
Monoclonal antibodies	Potential allergic reactions, including hives, pruritus, anaphylactic reactions, hypotension
Hematopoietic growth factors	Bone pain (sargramostim, filgrastim), mild constitutional symptoms (sargramostim)
Retinoids	Headache, fever, skin and mucous membrane dryness, bone pain, nausea and vomiting

Reproduced with permission from Sandstrom, S. K. (1996). Nursing management of patients receiving biologic therapy. *Seminars in Oncology Nursing 12* (2), 154.

Photodynamic Therapy

Photodynamic therapy, or phototherapy, is an investigational cancer treatment that uses photosensitizing agents, such as Photofrin. When administered intravenously, these agents are retained in higher concentrations in malignant tissue than in normal tissue. They are then activated by a light source, usually laser light, which penetrates body tissue. The light-activated agent then creates activated singlet oxygen molecules that are cytotoxic or harmful to body tissue cells. Because most of the photosensitizing agent has been retained in malignant tissue, a selective cytotoxicity can be achieved with minimal destruction to normal tissues.

Cancers treated with phototherapy include esophageal cancers, endobronchial tumors, skin cancers, breast cancers, intraperitoneal tumors, and malignant central nervous system disease. The major side effect of therapy is photosensitivity for 4 to 6 weeks after treatment. Patients must protect themselves from direct and indirect sunlight to prevent skin burns. In addition, local reactions are observed in the area treated. Liver and renal function should also be monitored for transient abnormalities. As with any investigational treatment, emotional support and education are vital to assist the patient and family.

Gene Therapy

As early as 1914, the somatic mutation theory of cancer suggested that cancer develops as a result of inherited or acquired genetic mutations that lead to a disturbance in the normal chromosomal balance regulating cell growth and reproduction. Technologic advances and information gained through intense study of genetics have assisted researchers in predicting, diagnosing, and treating cancer. Gene therapy includes approaches that correct genetic defects or manipulate genes to induce tumor cell destruction in the hope of preventing or combating disease. Somatic cell (any cell not contained in an embryo or destined to become an egg or sperm) gene therapy is the only approved form of gene therapy in the United States. This type of therapy involves the insertion of a desired gene into the targeted cells.

Although gene therapy is currently investigational, researchers predict it will have a profound impact on medical and health care in the 21st century. More than 100 clinical trials for gene therapy in treating cancer have been initiated. An example of one such trial involves inserting the gene associated with the production of TNF into lymphocytes. It is hypothesized that the lymphocytes migrate to the targeted tumors and produce TNF locally, resulting in tumor cell destruction. This approach has been used to treat melanoma. In another clinical trial, a "suicide gene" is inserted into tumor cells to facilitate cell death. When the gene for herpes simplex virus thymadine kinase is inserted into malignant cells, those cells become infected with the virus and susceptible to destruction by antiviral drugs, such as ganciclovir. This approach has been tried in treating brain, ovarian, and breast cancers. For more information about investigational therapies, see the earlier chart, "Investigational Antineoplastic Therapies and Clinical Trials."

Unproven and Unconventional Therapies

A diagnosis of cancer evokes many emotions in patients and families, including feelings of fear, frustration, and loss of control. Despite increasing 5-year survival rates with use of traditional methods of treatment, a significant number of patients use or seriously consider using some form of unconventional treatment. Hopelessness, desperation, unmet needs, ignorance, and family or social pressures are major factors that motivate patients to seek unconventional methods of treatment and allow them to fall prey to deceptive practices and quackery.

Caring for patients who choose unconventional methods may place members of the health care team in difficult situations professionally, legally, and ethically. Nurses must keep in mind those ethical principles that help guide professional practice, such as autonomy, beneficence, nonmaleficence, and justice.

Unconventional treatments have not demonstrated scientifically, in an objective, reproducible method, the ability to cure or control cancer. In addition to being ineffective, some unconventional treatments may also be harmful to patients and incur costs to patients and families in thousands of dollars. Most unproven cancer treatments can be categorized as machines and devices, drugs and biologicals, metabolic and dietary regimens, or mystical and spiritual approaches.

Machines and Devices

Electrical gadgets and devices are commonly reputed to cure cancers. Most are operated by people with questionable training who report incredulous success stories. Such machines are often decorated with elaborate lights and dials and produce vibrations or other sensations of currents or energy.

Drugs and Biologicals

Medicinal agents, herbs, proteins (such as shark cartilage), megavitamins, immune therapy, vaccines, enzymes, hydrogen peroxide, and sera have been frequent components of fraudulent cancer therapy. These agents have included oral, intravenous, and external medications derived from weeds, flowers, and herbs and the blood and urine of patients and animals. Many of these agents, especially in megadoses, can be toxic.

Metabolic and Dietary Regimens

Metabolic and dietary regimens emphasize the ingestion of only natural substances to purify the body and retard cancerous growth. These regimens include the grape diet, the carrot juice diet, garlic, onions, various teas, coffee enemas, and raw liver intake. Laetrile (vitamin B_{17}, amygdalin), one of the best-known forms of cancer quackery, was advocated as an agent to kill tumor cells by releasing cyanide, which is especially toxic to malignant cells. The National Cancer Institute, in response to public demand, investigated the effects of laetrile and reported no therapeutic benefits with its use. Many toxic effects (cyanide poisoning, fever, rash, headache, vomiting, diarrhea, and hypotension) were reported. Macrobiotic diets have also been advocated as a cancer treatment to reestablish balance between the major forces in the universe, yin and yang. People who adhere to macrobiotic diets tend to develop vitamin, mineral, and protein deficiencies; experience additional weight loss due to decreased calorie intake; and achieve no therapeutic benefits from the diet.

Mystical and Spiritual Approaches

Mystical or spiritual approaches to cancer therapy include such techniques as psychic surgery, faith healing, "laying on of hands," prayer groups, and invocation of mystical universal powers to kill cancerous growths. These techniques are difficult to disclaim because they are based on faith.

Nursing Management in Unconventional Therapies

A trusting relationship, supportive care, and promotion of hope in the patient and family are the most effective means of protecting them from fraudulent therapy and questionable claims of cancer cures. Truthful responses given in a nonjudgmental manner to questions and inquiries about unproven methods of cancer treatments may alleviate the fear and guilt on the part of the patient and family that they are not "doing everything" to obtain a cure. Characteristics common to fraudulent therapy may be shared with patients and their families so that they are informed and cautious in evaluating other forms of "therapy."

NURSING PROCESS: THE PATIENT WITH CANCER

The outlook for patients with cancer has greatly improved because of scientific and technologic advances. As a result of the underlying disease or various treatment modalities, however, the patient with cancer may experience a variety of secondary problems, such as infection, reduced WBC counts, bleeding, skin problems, nutritional problems, pain, fatigue, and psychological stress.

Assessment

Regardless of the type of cancer treatment or prognosis, many patients with cancer are susceptible to these problems and complications. An important role of the nurse on the oncology team is to assess the patient for these problems and complications.

Infection

In all stages of cancer, the nurse assesses factors that can promote infection. Infection is the leading cause of death in cancer patients. Factors predisposing patients to infection are summarized in Table 15-8. The nurse monitors laboratory studies to detect early changes in WBC counts. Common sites of infection, such as the pharynx, skin, perianal area, urinary tract, and respiratory tract, are assessed frequently. The typical signs of infection (fever, swelling, redness, drainage, and pain), however, may not occur in the immunosuppressed patient. The nurse also monitors the patient for sepsis, particularly if invasive catheters or infusion lines are in place.

The function of the WBCs is often impaired in cancer patients. A decrease in circulating WBCs is referred to as leukopenia or granulocytopenia. There are three types of WBCs: neutrophils, basophils, and eosinophils. The neutrophils, totaling 60% to 70% of all the body's WBCs, play a major role in combating infection by engulfing and destroying infective agents in a process called phagocytosis. Both the total WBC count and the concentration of neutrophils are important in determining the patient's ability to fight infection.

A differential WBC count identifies the relative numbers of WBCs and permits tabulation of polymorphonuclear neutrophils (mature neutrophils, reported as "polys," PMNs, or "segs") and immature forms of neutrophils (reported as bands, metamyelocytes, and "stabs"). These numbers are compiled and reported as the absolute neutrophil count (ANC). The ANC is calculated by the following formula:

$$\frac{\text{Total WBC count} \times (\text{\% segmented neutrophils} + \text{\% bands})}{100}$$

For example if the patient's total WBC count is 6000, with segmented neutrophils 25% and bands 25%, the ANC would be 3000.

Neutropenia, an abnormally low ANC, is associated with an increased risk for infection. The risk for infection rises as the ANC decreases and persists. An ANC of less than 1000 cells/mm^3 reflects a severe risk for infection. The term **nadir** is used to describe the lowest ANC after myelosuppressive chemotherapy or radiation therapy. Therapies that suppress bone marrow function are called myelosuppressive.

Bleeding

The nurse assesses cancer patients for factors that may contribute to bleeding. These include bone marrow suppression from radiation, chemotherapy, and other medications that interfere with

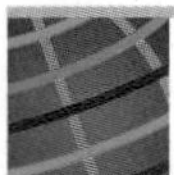

TABLE 15•8 **Factors Predisposing Cancer Patients to Infection**

Factors	Underlying Mechanisms
1. Impaired skin and mucous membrane integrity	• Loss of body's first line of defense against invading organisms.
2. Chemotherapy	• Many agents cause suppression of bone marrow, resulting in decreased production and function of white blood cells. Chemotherapy agents that cause mucositis impair skin and mucous membrane integrity. Organ damage associated with certain agents may also predispose patients to infection. Organ damage such as pulmonary fibrosis or cardiomyopathy that is associated with certain agents may also predispose patients to infection.
3. Radiation therapy	• Radiation involving sites of bone marrow production may result in bone marrow suppression. May also lead to impaired tissue integrity.
4. Biologic response modifiers	• Some biologic response modifiers may cause bone marrow suppression and organ dysfunction.
5. Malignancy	• Malignant cells may infiltrate the bone marrow and interfere with production of white blood cells and lymphocytes. Hematologic malignancies (leukemias and lymphomas) are associated with impaired function and production of blood cells.
6. Malnutrition	• Results in impaired function and production of cells of the immune response. May contribute to impaired skin integrity.
7. Medications	• Antibiotics disturb the balance of normal flora, allowing them to become pathogenic. This process occurs most commonly in the gastrointestinal tract. Corticosteroids and nonsteroidal anti-inflammatory drugs mask the inflammatory response.
8. Urinary catheter	• Creates port and mechanism of entry for organisms.
9. Intravenous catheter	• Results in impaired skin integrity and site of entry for organisms.
10. Other invasive procedures (surgery, paracentesis, thoracentesis, drainage tubes, endoscopies, mechanical ventilation)	• Creates port of entry and possible introduction of exogenous organisms into the system.
11. Contaminated equipment	• Environmental objects such as stagnant water in oxygen equipment are associated with growth of microorganisms.
12. Age	• Increasing age associated with declining organ function. Also associated with decreased production and functioning of the cells of the immune system.
13. Chronic illness	• Associated with impaired organ function and altered immune responses.
14. Prolonged hospitalization	• Allows increased exposure to nosocomial infection and colonization of new organisms.

coagulation and platelet functioning, such as aspirin, dipyridamole (Persantine), heparin, or warfarin (Coumadin). Common bleeding sites include skin and mucous membranes; the intestinal, urinary, and respiratory tracts; and the brain. Gross hemorrhage, as well as blood in the stools, urine, sputum, or vomitus (melena, hematuria, hemoptysis, hematemesis), oozing at injection sites, bruising (ecchymosis), petechiae, and changes in mental status, are monitored and reported.

Skin Problems

Skin and tissue integrity is at risk in cancer patients because of the effects of chemotherapy, radiation therapy, surgery, and invasive procedures carried out for diagnosis and therapy. As part of the assessment, the nurse identifies which of these predisposing factors are present and assesses the patient for other risk factors, including nutritional deficits, bowel and bladder incontinence, immobility, immunosuppression, and changes related to aging. Skin lesions or ulcerations secondary to the tumor are noted. Alterations in tissue integrity throughout the gastrointestinal tract are particularly bothersome to the patient. The oral mucous membranes and any lesions are noted, as are their effects on the patient's nutritional status and comfort level.

Hair Loss

Alopecia (hair loss) is another form of tissue disruption common to cancer patients who receive radiation therapy or chemotherapy. In addition to noting hair loss, the nurse also assesses the psychological impact of this side effect on the patient and the family.

Nutritional Concerns

Assessing the patient's nutritional status is an important nursing role. Impaired nutritional status may contribute to the progression of the disease, immune incompetence, increased incidence of infection, delayed tissue repair, diminished functional ability, and decreased capacity to continue antineoplastic therapy. Altered nutritional status and weight loss and cachexia (wasting, emaciation) may be secondary to decreased protein and caloric intake, the effect of a local tumor, systemic disease, side effects of the treatment, or the emotional status of the patient.

The patient's weight and caloric intake are monitored daily. Other information obtained through assessment includes diet history, any episodes of anorexia, changes in appetite, situations and foods that aggravate or relieve anorexia, and medication history. Difficulty in chewing or swallowing is determined and the occurrence of nausea, vomiting, or diarrhea is noted.

Clinical and laboratory data useful in assessing the patient's nutritional status include anthropometric measurements (triceps skin fold and middle-upper arm circumference), serum protein levels (albumin and transferrin), lymphocyte count, skin response to intradermal injection of antigens, hemoglobin levels, hematocrit, urinary creatinine levels, and serum iron levels.

Pain

Pain and discomfort in cancer may be related to the underlying disease, pressure exerted by the tumor, diagnostic procedures, or the cancer treatment itself. As in any other situation involving pain, cancer pain is affected by both physical and psychosocial influences.

In addition to assessing the source and site of pain, the nurse also assesses those factors that increase the patient's perception of pain, such as fear and apprehension, fatigue, anger, and social isolation. Pain assessment scales (see Chap. 12) are useful in assessing the patient's pain level before pain-relieving interventions are instituted and in evaluating their effectiveness in relieving pain.

Fatigue

Acute fatigue, which occurs after an energy-demanding experience, serves a protective function; chronic fatigue, however, does not. It is often overwhelming, excessive, and not responsive to rest, and it seriously affects quality of life. Fatigue is the most commonly reported side effect in patients who receive chemotherapy and radiation therapy. The nurse assesses for feelings of weariness, weakness, lack of energy, inability to carry out necessary and valued daily functions, lack of motivation, and inability to concentrate. Patients may become less verbal and appear pallid with relaxed facial musculature. The nurse assesses physiologic and psychological stressors that can contribute to fatigue, including pain, nausea, dyspnea, constipation, fear, and anxiety.

Psychosocial Status

Nursing assessment also focuses on the patient's psychological and mental status as the patient and the family face this life-threatening experience, unpleasant diagnostic tests and treatment modalities, and progression of disease. The patient's mood and emotional reaction to the results of diagnostic testing and prognosis are assessed along with evidence that the patient is progressing through the stages of grief and can talk about the diagnosis and prognosis with the family.

Body Image

Cancer patients are forced to cope with many assaults to body image throughout the course of disease and treatment. Entry into the health care system is often accompanied by depersonalization. Threats to self-concept are enormous as patients face the realization of illness, possible disability, and death. To accommodate treatments or because of the disease, many cancer patients are forced to alter their lifestyles. Priorities and values change when body image is threatened and physical characteristics become less important. Disfiguring surgery, hair loss, cachexia, skin changes, altered communication patterns, and sexual dysfunction are some of the devastating results of cancer and its treatment that threaten the patient's self-esteem and body image. The nurse identifies these potential threats and assesses the patient's ability to cope with these changes.

Diagnosis

Nursing Diagnoses

Based on the assessment data, nursing diagnoses of the patient with cancer may include the following:

- Impaired tissue integrity related to the effects of treatment and the disease
- Altered nutrition: less than body requirements related to anorexia and gastrointestinal changes
- Pain and discomfort related to disease and treatment effects
- Fatigue related to physical and psychological stressors
- Grieving related to anticipated loss and altered role function
- Body image disturbance related to changes in appearance and role functions

Collaborative Problems/Potential Complications

Based on the assessment data, potential complications that may develop include the following:

- Infection and sepsis
- Hemorrhage
- Superior vena cava syndrome
- Spinal cord compression
- Hypercalcemia
- Pericardial effusion
- Disseminated intravascular coagulation
- Syndrome of inappropriate secretion of antidiuretic hormone
- Tumor lysis syndrome

See the later section, Oncologic Emergencies, for more information.

Planning and Goals

The major goals for the patient may include maintenance of tissue integrity, maintenance of nutrition, relief of pain, relief of fatigue, effective progression through the grieving process, improved body image, and absence of complications.

Nursing Interventions

The patient with cancer is at risk for various adverse effects of therapy and complications. The nurse in all health care settings assists the patient and family in managing these problems.

Maintaining Tissue Integrity

Some of the most frequently encountered disturbances include skin and tissue reactions to radiation therapy, stomatitis, alopecia, and metastatic skin lesions.

The patient who is experiencing skin and tissue reactions to radiation therapy requires careful skin care to prevent further skin irritation, drying, and damage. The skin over the affected area is handled gently; rubbing and use of hot or cold water, soaps, powders, lotions, and cosmetics are avoided. Tissue injury is prevented by wearing loose-fitting clothes and avoiding clothes that constrict, irritate, or rub the affected area. If blistering occurs, care is taken not to disrupt the blisters, thus reducing the risk of introducing bacteria. Moisture and vapor-permeable dressings, such as hydrocolloids and hydrogels, are helpful in promoting healing and reducing pain. Aseptic wound care is indicated to minimize the risk for infection and sepsis. Topical antibiotics, such as 1% silver sulfadiazine cream (Silvadene) or bacitracin, are used on areas of moist desquamation (painful, red, moist skin).

Managing Stomatitis

Stomatitis, an inflammatory response of the oral tissues, commonly develops within 5 to 14 days after the patient receives certain chemotherapeutic agents, such as doxorubicin and 5-fluorouracil, and BRMs, such as IL-2 and IFN. It may also occur with radiation to the head and neck. Stomatitis is characterized by mild redness (erythema) and edema or, if severe, by painful ulcerations, bleeding, and secondary infection. In severe cases of stomatitis, cancer therapy may be temporarily halted until the inflammation decreases.

As a result of normal everyday wear and tear, the epithelial cells that line the oral cavity undergo rapid turnover and slough off routinely. Chemotherapy and radiation interfere with the body's ability to replace those cells. An inflammatory response develops as denuded areas appear in the oral cavity. Poor oral hygiene, existing dental disease, and impaired nutritional status contribute to morbidity associated with stomatitis. Radiation-induced xerostomia (dry mouth) associated with decreased salivary gland functioning may contribute to stomatitis in patients who have received radiation to the head and neck.

Myelosuppression (bone marrow depression) resulting from underlying disease or its treatment predisposes the patient to oral bleeding and infection. Pain associated with ulcerated oral tissues can significantly interfere with nutritional intake, communication, and a willingness to maintain oral hygiene.

Good oral hygiene that includes brushing, flossing, and rinsing is necessary to minimize the risk for oral complications associated with cancer therapies. Soft-bristled toothbrushes and nonabrasive toothpaste prevent or reduce trauma to the oral mucosa. Oral swabs with spongelike applicators may be used in place of a toothbrush for painful oral tissues. Flossing may be performed unless it causes pain or unless platelet levels are below 40,000 mm^3. Oral rinses with saline solution or tap water may be necessary for patients who cannot tolerate a toothbrush. Products that irritate oral tissues or impair healing, such as alcohol-based mouth rinses, are avoided. Foods that are difficult to chew or too hot or spicy are avoided to minimize further trauma. The patient's lips are lubricated to keep the tissues from becoming dry and cracked. Topical anti-inflammatory and anesthetic agents may be prescribed to promote healing and minimize discomfort. Products that coat or protect oral mucosa are used to facilitate comfort and prevent further trauma. The patient who experiences severe pain and discomfort with stomatitis requires systemic analgesics.

Adequate fluid and food intake is encouraged. In some instances, parenteral hydration and nutrition are needed. Topical or systemic antifungal and antibiotic drugs are prescribed to treat local or systemic infections.

Explaining Alopecia

The temporary or permanent thinning or complete loss of hair is a potential adverse effect of various radiation therapies and chemotherapeutic agents. The extent of alopecia depends on the dose and duration of therapy. These treatments cause alopecia by damaging stem cells and hair follicles. As a result, the hair is brittle and may fall out or break off at the surface of the scalp. Loss of other body hair is less frequent. Hair loss usually begins within 2 to 3 weeks after treatment; regrowth begins within 8 weeks after the last treatment. Some patients who undergo radiation to the head may sustain permanent hair loss. Many health professionals view hair loss as a minor problem when compared with the potentially life-threatening consequences of cancer. For many patients, however, hair loss is a major assault on body image, arousing feelings of anxiety, sadness, anger, rejection, and isolation. To patients and families, hair loss can serve as a constant reminder of the challenges cancer places on coping abilities, interpersonal relationships, and sexuality.

The nurse's role is to provide information about alopecia and to support the patient and family in coping with disturbing effects of therapy, such as hair loss and changes in body image. The nurse may encourage the patient to acquire a wig or hairpiece before hair loss occurs so that the replacement matches the patient's own hair. Use of attractive scarves and hats may make the patient feel less conspicuous. Nurses can refer patients to supportive programs, such as "Look Good, Feel Better," offered by the American Cancer Society. That hair usually begins to regrow after completing therapy may comfort some patients, although the color and texture of the new hair may change.

Managing Malignant Skin Lesions

Skin lesions may occur with local extension of the tumor or embolization of the tumor into the epithelium and its surrounding lymph and blood vessels. Secondary growth of cancer cells into the skin may result in redness (erythematous areas) or can progress to wounds involving tissue necrosis and infection. The most extensive lesions tend to disintegrate and are purulent and malodorous. In addition, these lesions are a source of considerable pain and discomfort. Although this type of wound is most often associated with breast cancer and head and neck cancers, it can also accompany lymphoma, leukemia, melanoma, and cancers of the lung, uterus, kidney, colon, and bladder. The development of severe skin lesions is usually associated with a poor prognosis for extended survival.

Ulcerating skin lesions usually indicate widely disseminated disease unlikely to be eradicated. Managing these lesions becomes a nursing priority. Nursing care includes carefully assessing and cleansing the skin, reducing superficial bacteria, controlling bleeding, reducing odor, and protecting the skin from pain and further trauma. The patient and family require assistance and guidance to care for these skin lesions at home. Referral for home care is indicated.

Promoting Nutrition

Most cancer patients experience some weight loss during their illness. Anorexia, malabsorption, and cachexia are examples of nutritional problems commonly seen in cancer patients.

ANOREXIA

Among the many causes of anorexia in the cancer patient are alterations in taste, manifested by increased salty, sour, and metallic taste sensations, and altered responses to sweet and bitter flavors, leading to decreased appetite, decreased nutritional intake, and protein-calorie malnutrition. Taste alterations may result from mineral (eg, zinc) deficiencies, increases in circulating amino acids and cellular metabolites, or the administration of chemotherapeutic agents. Patients undergoing radiation therapy to the head and neck may experience "mouth blindness," which is a severe impairment of taste.

Alterations in the sense of smell also alter taste, which is a common experience of patients with head and neck cancers. Anorexia may occur because the person feels full after eating only a small amount of food. This sense of fullness occurs secondary to a decrease in digestive enzymes, abnormalities in the metabolism of glucose and triglycerides, and prolonged stimulation of gastric volume receptors, which convey the feeling of being full. Psychological distress, such as fear, pain, depression, and isolation, throughout illness may also have a negative impact on appetite. The person may develop an aversion to food because of nausea and vomiting after treatment.

MALABSORPTION

Many cancer patients are unable to absorb nutrients from the gastrointestinal system as a result of tumor activity and cancer treatment. Tumors can affect the gastrointestinal activity in several ways. They may impair enzyme production or create fistulas. They secrete hormones and enzymes, such as gastrin, which leads to increased gastrointestinal irritation, peptic ulcer disease, and decreased fat digestion. They also interfere with protein digestion.

Chemotherapy and radiation can irritate and damage mucosal cells of the bowel, inhibiting absorption. Radiation therapy can cause sclerosis of the blood vessels in the bowel and fibrotic changes in the gastrointestinal tissue. Surgical intervention may change peristaltic patterns, alter gastrointestinal secretions, and reduce the absorptive surfaces of the gastrointestinal mucosa, all leading to malabsorption.

CACHEXIA

Cachexia is common in patients with cancer, especially in advanced disease. Cancer cachexia is related to inadequate nutritional intake along with increasing metabolic demand, increased energy expenditure due to anaerobic metabolism of the tumor, impaired glucose metabolism, competition of the tumor cells for nutrients, altered lipid metabolism, and a suppressed appetite. It is characterized by loss of body weight, adipose tissue, visceral protein, and skeletal muscle.

Food should be prepared in ways to make it look and taste appealing. Unpleasant smells and unappetizing looking food are avoided. Family members are included in the plan of care to encourage adequate food intake. The patient's preferences, as well as physiologic and metabolic requirements, are considered when selecting foods. Small, frequent meals are provided, with additional supplements between meals. Oral hygiene and pain relief measures are offered before mealtime to make meals more pleasant.

If malabsorption is a problem, enzyme and vitamin replacement may be instituted. Additional strategies include changing the feeding schedule, using simple diets, and relieving diarrhea. If malabsorption is severe, total parenteral nutrition (TPN) may be necessary. TPN can be administered in several ways: by a long-term venous access device device, such as a right atrial catheter, an implanted venous port, or a peripherally inserted central catheter (Fig. 15-6). The nurse teaches the patient and family how to care for venous access devices and how to administer TPN. Home care nurses may assist with or supervise TPN in the home.

Interventions to reduce cachexia usually do not prolong survival but may improve the patient's quality of life. Before invasive nutritional strategies are instituted, the nurse should assess the patient

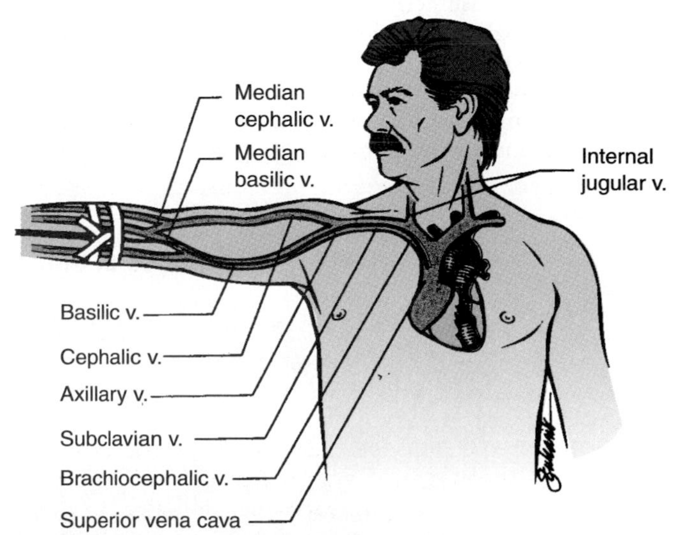

FIGURE 15•6 A peripherally inserted central catheter (PICC) is advanced through the cephalic or basilic vein to the axillary, subclavian, or brachiocephalic vein or the superior vena cava.

carefully and discuss the options with the patient and family. Creative dietary therapies, enteral (tube) feedings, or TPN may be chosen to deliver nourishment. Nursing care is also directed toward preventing trauma, infection, and other complications that increase metabolic demands.

Relieving Pain

Of all patients with progressive cancer, more than 60% experience pain. Although patients with cancer may have acute pain, their pain is more frequently characterized as chronic. (For more information on cancer-related pain, see Chap. 13.) As in other situations involving pain, the experience of cancer pain is influenced by both physical and psychosocial factors.

Cancer can cause pain in various ways (Table 15-9). Pain is also associated with various cancer treatments. Acute pain is linked with trauma from surgery. Occasionally, chronic pain syndromes, such as postsurgical neuropathies (pain related to nerve tissue injury), occur. Some chemotherapeutic agents cause tissue necrosis, peripheral neuropathies, and stomatitis—all potential sources of pain—whereas radiation therapy can cause skin or organ inflammation. Cancer patients may have other sources of pain, such as arthritis or migraine headaches, that are unrelated to the underlying cancer or its treatment.

In today's society, most people expect pain to disappear or resolve quickly, and in fact, it usually does. Although controllable, cancer pain is commonly irreversible and not quickly resolved. For many patients, pain is a signal that the tumor is growing and that death is approaching. As the patient anticipates the pain and anxiety increases, pain perception heightens, producing fear and additional pain. Chronic cancer pain, then, can be best described as a cycle progressing from pain to anxiety to fear and back to pain again.

Pain tolerance, the point past which pain can no longer be tolerated, varies among people. Pain tolerance is decreased by fatigue, anxiety, fear of death, anger, powerlessness, social isolation, changes in role identity, loss of independence, and past experiences. Adequate rest and sleep, diversion, mood elevation, empathy, and medications such as antidepressants, antianxiety agents, and analgesics enhance tolerance to pain.

Inadequate pain management is most often the result of misconceptions and insufficient knowledge about pain assessment and pharmacologic interventions on the part of patients, families, and health care providers. Successful management of cancer pain is based on a thorough and objective pain assessment that examines physical, psychosocial, environmental, and spiritual factors. A multidisciplinary team approach is essential to determine optimal management of the patient's pain. Unlike instances of chronic nonmalignant pain, systemic analgesics play a central role in managing cancer pain.

The World Health Organization advocates a three-step approach to treating cancer pain (see Chap. 13). Analgesics are administered based on the patient's level of pain. Nonopioid analgesics (eg, acetaminophen) are used for mild pain; weak opioid analgesics (eg, codeine) are used for moderate pain, and strong opioid analgesics (eg, morphine) are used for severe pain. If the patient's pain escalates, the strength of the analgesic medication is increased until the pain is controlled. Adjuvant medications are also administered to enhance the effectiveness of analgesics and to manage other symptoms that may contribute to the pain experience. Examples of adjuvant medications include antiemetics, antidepressants, anxiolytics, anticonvulsants, stimulants, local anesthetics, radiopharmaceuticals (radioactive agents that may be used to treat painful bone tumors), and corticosteroids.

Preventing and reducing pain help to decrease anxiety and break the pain cycle. This can be accomplished best by administering analgesics on a regularly scheduled basis as prescribed (the preventive approach to pain management), with additional analgesics administered for breakthrough pain as needed and as prescribed.

Various pharmacologic and nonpharmacologic approaches offer the best methods of managing cancer pain. No reasonable approaches, even those that may be somewhat invasive, should be overlooked because of a poor or terminal prognosis. Nurses help patients and families to play an active role in managing pain. Nurses provide education and support to correct fears and misconceptions about opioid use. Inadequate pain control leads to suffering, anxiety, fear, immobility, isolation, and depression. Improving a patient's quality of life is as important as preventing a painful death.

Decreasing Fatigue

Nurses help the patient and family to understand that fatigue is usually an expected and temporary side effect of the cancer process and the treatments employed. Fatigue also stems from the stress of coping with cancer. It does not always signify that the cancer is advancing or that the treatment is failing. Potential sources of fatigue are summarized in Chart 15-3.

Nursing strategies are implemented to minimize fatigue or assist the patient to cope with existing fatigue. Helping the patient to identify sources of fatigue aids in selecting appropriate and individualized interventions. Ways to conserve energy are developed to help the patient plan daily activities. Alternating periods of rest and activity are beneficial. Regular, light exercise may decrease fatigue

TABLE 15•9 Sources of Cancer Pain

Source	Descriptions	Underlying Cancer
Bone metastasis	Throbbing, aching	Breast, prostate, myeloma
Nerve compression, infiltration	Burning, sharp, tingling	Breast, prostate, lymphoma
Lymphatic or venous obstruction	Dull, aching, tightness	Lymphoma, breast, Kaposi's sarcoma
Ischemia	Sharp, throbbing	Kaposi's sarcoma
Organ obstruction	Dull, crampy, gnawing	Colon, gastric
Organ infiltration	Distention, crampy	Liver, pancreatic
Skin inflammation, ulceration, infection, necrosis	Burning, sharp	Breast, head and neck, Kaposi's sarcoma

NURSING RESEARCH

What Nurses Know and Do Not Know About Cancer Pain Management With Opioid Analgesics

Ferrell, B. R. & McCaffery, M. (1997). Nurses' knowledge about equianalgesia and opioid dosing. *Cancer Nursing 20*(3), 201–212.

Purpose

This study was conducted to identify the knowledge of nurses who regularly provide care to oncology patients and who are involved with patients receiving morphine and transdermal (TD) fentanyl. Nurses' knowledge about cancer pain management is crucial because nurses are the cornerstone of the interdisciplinary approach to care of patients with pain.

Study Sample and Design

Participants were nurse volunteers attending lectures on pain management throughout the United States during 1994. Of the 82 nurses who participated in this study, most (65.9%) practiced in a hospital setting. The others practiced in community home care or hospice settings. The most common clinical practice areas were oncology (50%), followed by medical-surgical areas (39.1%). Most nurses had experience with both extended-release morphine and TD fentanyl.

A descriptive study was conducted using a survey instrument designed to determine how much nurses who regularly care for cancer patients know about cancer pain management, particularly the use of morphine and TD fentanyl in relation to determining equianalgesic doses; calculation of breakthrough doses; calculation of the appropriate dose increases; and duration of action and indications for use. Content validity of the survey instrument was established by selecting content from established guidelines developed by the Agency for Health Care Policy and Research (1994) and the American Pain Society (1992). The investigators conducted pilot testing. Data were obtained before their attending an education program on pain management.

Findings

- About one third of the participants were unable to calculate equianalgesic doses despite having access to an equianalgesic chart. Errors of overdosing and underdosing were made.
- About one third of the participants did not understand the concept of extended- and immediate-release medications.
- Almost two thirds of the respondents selected breakthrough doses that would seriously undertreat pain.
- For almost half of the participants, selection of appropriate dose increases for ineffective opioid doses was problematic.
- There was some misunderstanding about indications for the use of TD fentanyl and opioid tolerance.

Nursing Implications

The results of the survey are troubling because the participants were probably among the more informed nurses caring for patients with cancer pain. Inadequate knowledge about pain management techniques would predictably result in grossly inadequate pain relief. In some instances, a lack of knowledge could result in overdosage. The authors present resources and an overview of guidelines for equianalgesic dosing, titration upward, breakthrough dosing, and the pharmacokinetics of fentanyl. They also discuss the importance of appropriate education for patients and nurses.

and facilitate coping, whereas lack of physical activity and "too much rest" can contribute to debilitation and associated fatigue.

Patients are encouraged to maintain as normal a lifestyle as possible by continuing with those activities they value and enjoy. Prioritizing necessary and valued activities can assist patients in planning for each day. Both patients and families are encouraged to plan to reallocate responsibilities, such as attending to child care, cleaning, and preparing meals. Patients who are employed full-time may need to reduce the number of hours worked each week. The nurse assists the patient and family in coping with these changing roles and responsibilities.

Nurses also address factors that contribute to fatigue and implement pharmacologic and nonpharmacologic strategies to manage pain. Nutrition counseling is provided to patients who are not eating enough calories or protein. Small, frequent meals require less energy for digestion. Serum hemoglobin and hematocrit levels are monitored for deficiencies, and blood products are administered as prescribed. Patients are monitored for alterations in oxygenation and electrolyte balances. Physical therapy and assistive devices are beneficial for patients with impaired mobility.

CHART 15•3 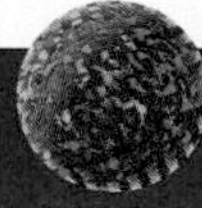 Sources of Fatigue in Cancer Patients

- Pain, pruritus
- Altered nutrition related to anorexia, nausea, vomiting, cachexia
- Electrolyte imbalance related to vomiting, diarrhea
- Altered protection related to neutropenia, thrombocytopenia, anemia
- Impaired tissue integrity related to stomatitis, mucositis
- Impaired physical mobility related to neurologic impairments, surgery, bone metastasis, pain, and analgesic use
- Knowledge deficit related to disease process, treatment
- Anxiety related to fear, diagnosis, role changes, uncertainty of future
- Ineffective breathing patterns related to cough, shortness of breath, and dyspnea
- Sleep pattern disturbance related to cancer therapies, anxiety, and pain

Improving Body Image and Self-Esteem

A positive approach is essential when caring for the patient with an altered body image. To help the patient retain control and a sense of self-worth, it is important to encourage independence and continued participation in self-care and decision making. The patient should be assisted to assume those tasks and participate in those activities that are personally of most value. Any negative feelings that the patient has or threats to body image should be expressed and discussed. The nurse serves as a listener and counselor to both the patient and the family. Referral to a support group provides additional assistance in coping with the changes resulting from cancer or its treatment. In many cases, a cosmetologist can provide ideas about hair or wig styling, makeup, and the use of scarves and turbans to help with body image concerns.

Patients who are experiencing alterations in sexuality and sexual function are encouraged to share and discuss concerns openly with their partner. Alternative forms of sexual expression are explored with the patient and partner to promote positive self-worth and acceptance. The nurse who identifies serious physiologic, psychological, or communication difficulties related to sexuality or sexual function is in a key position to assist the patient and partner to seek further counseling if necessary.

Assisting in the Grieving Process

A cancer diagnosis need not indicate a fatal outcome. Many forms of cancer are curable; others may be cured if treated early. Despite these facts, many patients and their families view cancer as a fatal disease that is inevitably accompanied by pain, suffering, debility, and emaciation. Grieving is a normal response to these fears and to the losses anticipated or experienced by the patient with cancer. These may include loss of health, normal sensations, body image, social interaction, sexuality, and intimacy. The patient, family, and friends may grieve the loss of quality time to spend with others, the loss of future and unfulfilled plans, and the loss of control over one's own body and emotional reactions.

The patient and family just informed of the cancer diagnosis frequently respond with shock, numbness, and disbelief. It is often during this stage that the patient and family are called on to make important initial decisions about treatment. They require the support of the physician, nurse, and other health care team members to make these decisions. An important role of the nurse is to answer any questions the patient and family may have and clarify information provided by the physician.

In addition to assessing the response of the patient and family to the diagnosis and planned treatment, the nurse assists them in framing their questions and concerns, identifying resources and support people (eg, clergy, counselor), and communicating and sharing their concerns with each other. Support groups for patients and families are available through hospitals and various community organizations. These groups provide direct assistance, advice, and emotional support.

As the patient and family progress through the grieving process, they may express feelings of anger, frustration, and depression. During this time, the nurse encourages the patient and family to verbalize their feelings in an atmosphere of trust and support. The nurse continues to assess their reactions and provides assistance and support as they confront and learn to deal with new problems.

If the patient enters the terminal phase of disease, the nurse may realize that the patient and family members are at different stages of grief. In such cases, the nurse assists the patient and family to come to grips with their reactions and feelings. Physical support, including holding the patient's hand or just being with the patient at home or at the bedside, frequently contributes to peace of mind. Maintaining contact with the surviving family members after death of the cancer patient may help them to work through their feelings of loss and grief.

Monitoring and Managing Potential Complications

Despite advances in cancer care, infection remains the leading cause of death. Defense against infection is compromised in many different ways. The integrity of the skin and mucous membrane, the body's first line of defense, is challenged by multiple invasive diagnostic and therapeutic procedures, by adverse effects of radiation and chemotherapy, and by the detrimental effects of immobility.

Impaired nutrition resulting from anorexia, nausea, vomiting, diarrhea, and the underlying disease alters the body's ability to combat invading organisms. Medications, such as antibiotics, disturb the balance of normal flora, allowing the overgrowth of pathogenic organisms. Other medications can also alter the immune response (see Chap. 46). Cancer itself may be immunosuppressive. Cancers such as leukemia and lymphoma are often associated with defects in cellular and humoral immunity. Advanced cancer can lead to tumors obstructing hollow viscera (such as the intestines), blood vessels, and lymphatic vessels, creating a favorable environment for proliferation of pathogenic organisms. In some patients, tumor cells infiltrate bone marrow and prevent normal production of WBCs. Most often, however, a decrease in WBCs is a result of bone marrow suppression after chemotherapy or radiation therapy.

The use of the hematopoietic growth factors, also called colony-stimulating factors (see the previous discussion of biologic response modifier therapy), has reduced the severity and duration of neutropenia associated with myelosuppressive chemotherapy or radiation therapy. The administration of these factors assists in reducing the risk for infection and, possibly, in maintaining treatment schedules, drug dosages, treatment effectiveness, and the quality of life.

INFECTION

Gram-positive organisms, such as *Streptococcus* and *Staphylococcus* species, are the most frequently isolated causes of infection. Gram-negative organisms, such as *Escherichia coli* and *Pseudomonas aeruginosa*, and fungal organisms, such as *Candida albicans*, also contribute to the incidence of serious infection.

Fever is probably the most important sign of infection in the immunocompromised patient. Although fever may be related to a variety of noninfectious conditions, including the underlying cancer, any temperature of 38.3°C (101°F) or higher is reported and dealt with promptly.

Antibiotics may be prescribed to treat infections after cultures of wound drainage, exudate, sputum, urine, stool, or blood are obtained. Patients with neutropenia are treated with broad-spectrum antibiotics before the infecting organism is identified because of the high incidence of mortality associated with untreated infection. Broad-spectrum antibiotic coverage or empiric therapy includes a combination of medications to defend the body against the major pathogenic organisms. An important component of the nurse's role is to administer these medications promptly according to the prescribed schedule to achieve adequate blood levels of the medications.

Strict asepsis is essential when handling intravenous lines, catheters, and other invasive equipment. Exposure of the patient to others with an active infection and to crowds is avoided. Patients with profound immunosuppression, such as recipients of bone marrow transplants, may need to be placed in a protective environment whereby the room and its contents are sterilized and the air filtered. These patients may also receive low-bacterial diets, avoiding fresh fruits and vegetables. Hand washing and appropriate hygiene are necessary to reduce exposure to potentially harmful bacteria and to eliminate environmental contaminants. Invasive procedures, such as injections, vaginal or rectal examinations, rectal temperatures, and surgery, are avoided. The patient is encouraged to do coughing and deep-breathing exercises frequently to prevent atelectasis and other potential respiratory problems. The nurse teaches the patient and family to recognize signs and symptoms of infection to report, perform effective hand washing, use antipyretics, maintain skin integrity, and self-administer hematopoietic growth factors when indicated.

SEPTIC SHOCK

The nurse assesses frequently for infection and inflammation throughout the course of the disease. Septicemia and septic shock are life-threatening complications that must be prevented or detected and treated early. Patients with signs and symptoms of impending sepsis and septic shock require immediate hospitalization and aggressive treatment.

Signs and symptoms of septic shock (see Chap. 14) include altered mental status, either subnormal or elevated temperature, cool and clammy skin, decreased urine output, hypotension, dysrhythmias, electrolyte imbalances, and abnormal arterial blood gas values. The patient and family members are instructed about signs of septicemia, methods for preventing infection, and actions to take if infection or septicemia occurs.

Septic shock is most often associated with overwhelming gram-negative bacterial infections. The nurse monitors the blood pressure, pulse rate, respirations, and temperature of the patient with shock every 15 to 30 minutes. Neurologic assessments are carried out to detect changes in orientation and responsiveness. Fluid and electrolyte status is monitored by measuring fluid intake and output and serum electrolytes. Arterial blood gas levels are obtained to determine tissue oxygenation. The nurse administers intravenous fluids, blood products, and vasopressor drugs as prescribed to maintain the patient's blood pressure and tissue perfusion. Supplemental oxygen is often necessary. Broad-spectrum antibiotics are administered as prescribed to combat the underlying infection (see Chap. 14).

BLEEDING AND HEMORRHAGE

Thrombocytopenia, a decrease in the circulating platelet count, is the most common cause of bleeding in cancer patients and is usually defined as a count of less than 100,000/mm^3 (SI: 0.1 $\times$ 10^{12}/L). When the count falls between 20,000 and 50,000/mm^3 (SI: 0.02 to 0.05 $\times$ 10^{12}/L), the risk for bleeding increases. Counts under 20,000/mm^3 (SI: 0.02 $\times$ 10^{12}/L) are associated with an increased risk for spontaneous bleeding, for which the patient requires a platelet transfusion. Platelets are essential for normal blood clotting and coagulation (hemostasis).

Thrombocytopenia often results from bone marrow depression after certain types of chemotherapy and radiation therapy. Tumor infiltration of the bone marrow can also impair the normal production of platelets. In some cases, platelet destruction is associated with an enlarged spleen (hypersplenism) and abnormal antibody function that occur with leukemia and lymphoma.

In addition to monitoring laboratory values, the nurse continues to assess the patient for bleeding. The nurse also takes steps to prevent trauma and minimize the risk for bleeding by encouraging the patient to use a soft, not stiff, toothbrush and an electric, not straight-edged, razor. Additionally, the nurse avoids unnecessary invasive procedures (eg, rectal temperatures, intramuscular injections, and catheterization) and assists the patient and family to identify and remove environmental hazards that may lead to falls or other trauma. Soft foods, increased fluid intake, and stool softeners, if prescribed, may be indicated to reduce trauma to the gastrointestinal tract. The joints and extremities are handled and moved gently to minimize the risk for spontaneous bleeding.

Hemorrhage may be related to various underlying abnormalities, such as thrombocytopenia and coagulation disorders. These clinical situations are often associated with the cancer itself or the adverse effects of cancer treatments. Sites of hemorrhage may include the gastrointestinal, respiratory, and genitourinary tracts and the brain. Blood pressure and pulse and respiratory rates are monitored every 15 to 30 minutes when hospitalized patients experience bleeding.

Serum hemoglobin and hematocrit are monitored carefully for changes indicating blood loss. The nurse tests all urine, stool, and emesis for occult blood. Neurologic assessments are performed to detect changes in orientation and behavior. The nurse administers fluids and blood products as prescribed to replace any losses. Vasopressor drugs are administered as prescribed to maintain blood pressure and ensure tissue oxygenation. Supplemental oxygen is used as necessary.

Promoting Home and Community-Based Care

TEACHING PATIENTS SELF-CARE

Patients with cancer usually return home from acute care facilities or receive treatment in the home or outpatient area rather than acute care facilities. The shift from the acute care setting also shifts the responsibility for care to the patient and family. As a result, families and friends must assume increased involvement in patient care, which requires teaching that enables them to provide care. Teaching initially focuses on providing information needed by the patient and family to address the most immediate care needs likely to be encountered at home.

Side effects of treatments and changes in the patient's status that should be reported are reviewed verbally and reinforced with written information. Strategies to deal with side effects of treatment are discussed with patients and their families. Other learning needs are identified based on the priorities conveyed by the patient and family as well as on the complexity of home-provided care.

Technologic advances allow home administration of chemotherapy, TPN, blood products, parenteral antibiotics, and parenteral analgesics; management of symptoms; and care of vascular access devices. Although home care nurses provide care and support for patients receiving this advanced technical care, the patient and family need instruction and ongoing support that allow them to feel comfortable and proficient in managing these treatments at home. Follow-up visits and telephone calls from the nurse are often reassuring to the patient and family and increase their comfort in dealing with complex and new aspects of care. Continued contact facilitates evaluation of patient progress and ongoing needs.

CONTINUING CARE

Referral for home care is often indicated for the patient with cancer. The responsibilities of the home care nurse include assessing the home environment, suggesting modifications to assist the patient and family in addressing the patient's physical needs, providing physical care, and assessing the psychological and emotional impact of the illness on the patient and the family.

Assessing changes in the patient's physical status and reporting relevant changes to the physician help to ensure that appropriate and timely modifications in therapy are made. The home care nurse also assesses the adequacy of pain management and the effectiveness of other strategies to prevent or manage the side effects of treatment modalities.

The patient's and family's understanding of the treatment plan and management strategies is assessed, and previous teaching is reinforced. The nurse often facilitates the coordination of patient care by maintaining close communication with all health care providers involved in each patient's care. The nurse may make referrals and coordinate available community resources (eg, local office of the American Cancer Society, home aides, church groups, and support groups) to assist patients and caregivers.

Evaluation

Expected Outcomes

For specific outcomes, see Plan of Nursing Care 15-1. Expected outcomes may include:

1. Maintains adequate tissue (skin and mucous membrane) integrity
2. Maintains adequate nutritional status
3. Achieves relief of pain and discomfort

4. Demonstrates increased activity tolerance and decreased fatigue
5. Progresses through the grieving process
6. Exhibits improved body image and self-esteem
7. Experiences no complications, such as inflammation, infection, or sepsis, and no episodes of bleeding or hemorrhage

CANCER REHABILITATION

Many cancer patients, including those who receive primary surgical treatment and adjuvant chemotherapy or radiation therapy, return to work and their usual activities of daily living. These patients may encounter a variety of problems, including changes in their functional abilities and in the attitudes of employers, coworkers, and families who still view cancer as a terminal, debilitating disease. Nurses play an important role in the rehabilitation of the cancer patient. Both the patient and family are included as part of any rehabilitation effort because cancer affects not only the patient but also the family members. In addition, with the shift away from inpatient care, family members are caring for many patients at home. To maximize beneficial outcomes, evaluation of patient needs related to cancer rehabilitation begins early in cancer treatment (Table 15-10).

Assessment for body image changes as a result of disfiguring treatments is necessary to facilitate the patient's adjustment to changes in appearance or functional abilities. The nurse can refer the patient and family to a variety of support groups sponsored by the American Cancer Society, such as those for people who have had laryngectomies or mastectomies. Nurses also collaborate with physical, occupational, and enterostomal therapists in improving the patient's abilities, in the use of prosthetic devices, and in altering the home environment as needed.

TABLE 15•10 Assessing Patient Needs for Cancer Rehabilitation

Area of Need	Factors to Assess
Functional	
Activities of daily living	Mobility Cognitive impairment Sensory impairments Communication barriers
Physiologic	
Nutrition	Need for enteral or parenteral nutrition
Elimination	Alterations in bowel and bladder function
Symptoms related to disease or treatment	Pain Nausea, vomiting, diarrhea Dyspnea, fatigue Skin impairment, alopecia
Psychosocial Resources	
Family	Availability of caregiver, home physical environment Availability of private transportation; affordability of transportation
Community	Availability of public transportation; affordability of transportation Availability and access to community organizations for assistance and support
Personal	Spiritual concerns Family relationships Body image Coping abilities Sexuality
Financial	Job security for patient and family member Need for vocational training

Patients often experience symptom distress (eg, pain, nausea) related to the underlying cancer or treatments. These symptoms may interfere with work and quality of life. Nurses assess for these problems and assist the patient in identifying strategies for coping with them. For patients with gastrointestinal disturbances after chemotherapy, altering work hours or receiving treatments in the evenings may prove helpful. Collaboration with physicians and pharmacists is helpful in identifying appropriate interventions.

Nurses collaborate with dietitians to help patients plan meals that will be acceptable and meet nutritional requirements. Nurses are also involved in the ongoing assessment of patients to detect any long-term consequences of cancer treatment.

Discrimination against recovering cancer patients has been demonstrated in several forms. Some employers do not understand that different kinds of cancers have different prognoses and different effects on functional ability. As a result, employers may hesitate to hire or continue to employ people with cancer, especially if ongoing treatment regimens require adjustments in work schedules. Employers, coworkers, and families may continue to view the person as being "sick" despite ongoing recovery or completion of treatment. Attitudes of coworkers can be a problem when the patient has a communication impairment, such as may occur in some head and neck cancers. The patient may benefit from vocational rehabilitation services of the American Cancer Society or other agencies.

Nurses can participate in efforts to educate employers and the public in general to ensure that the rights of patients with cancer are maintained. Whenever possible, nurses assist patients and families to resume preexisting roles. Psychologists and clergy are consulted to assist with psychosocial and spiritual concerns. Rehabilitation shifts the focus from what has been lost to what can be done with existing strengths and abilities. In that spirit, nurses encourage patients to regain the highest level of independence possible.

GERONTOLOGIC CONSIDERATIONS

As a result of an increased life expectancy and an increased risk for cancer with age, nurses are providing cancer-related care for growing numbers of elderly patients. More than 58% of all cancers occur in people older than 65 years of age, and about two thirds of all cancer deaths occur in people 65 years of age and older. Nursing care of this population addresses special needs, including physical, psychosocial, and financial concerns.

Age-Related Physiologic Changes

Oncology nurses working with the elderly population need to understand the normal physiologic changes that occur with aging. These changes include decreased skin elasticity; decreased skeletal mass, structure, and strength; decreased organ function and structure; impaired immune system mechanisms; alterations in neurologic and sensory functions; and altered drug absorption, distribution, metabolism, and elimination. These changes ultimately influence the elderly patient's ability to tolerate cancer treatment. In addition, many elderly patients have other chronic diseases and associated treatments that may limit tolerance to cancer treatments.

Potential chemotherapy-related toxicities, such as renal impairment, myelosuppression, fatigue, and cardiomyopathy, may increase as a result of declining organ function and diminished physiologic reserves. The recovery of normal tissues after radiation therapy may be delayed, and the patient may experience more severe adverse effects, such as mucositis, nausea and vomiting, and myelosuppression. Because of decreased tissue healing capacity and declining pulmonary and cardiovascular functioning, the older patient is slower to recover from surgery. Elderly patients are also at increased risk for developing complications such as atelectasis, pneumonia, and wound infections.

Other Age-Related Concerns

Access to cancer care for elderly patients may be limited by discriminatory or fatalistic attitudes of health care providers, caregivers, and patients. Issues such as the gradual loss of supportive resources, declining health or loss of a spouse, and unavailability of relatives or friends may result in limited access to care and unmet needs for assistance with activities of daily living. In addition, the economic impact of health care may be difficult for those living on fixed incomes.

The nurse must be aware of the special needs of the aging population. Cancer prevention, detection, and screening efforts are directed toward the elderly as well as the younger population. Nurses carefully monitor elderly patients receiving cancer treatments for signs and symptoms of adverse effects. In addition, the elderly patient is instructed to report all symptoms to the physician. It is not uncommon for the elderly patient to delay reporting symptoms, attributing them to "old age." Many elderly people do not want to report illness for fear of losing their independence or financial security. Information processing challenges, such as sensory losses and memory deficits, are considered when planning patient education. In such cases, the nurse needs to act as a patient advocate, encouraging independence and identifying resources for support when indicated.

CARE OF THE PATIENT WITH ADVANCED CANCER

The patient with advanced cancer is likely to experience many of the problems previously described, but all to a greater degree. Symptoms of gastrointestinal disturbances, nutritional problems, weight loss, and cachexia make the patient more susceptible to skin breakdown, fluid and electrolyte problems, and infection.

Although not all cancer patients experience pain, those who do commonly fear that it will not be adequately treated. Although treatment at this stage of illness is likely to be palliative rather than curative, prevention and appropriate management of problems can improve the quality of the patient's life considerably. For example, use of analgesia on a regular basis at set intervals rather than on an "as needed" basis usually breaks the cycle of tension and anxiety associated with waiting until pain becomes so severe that pain relief is inadequate once the analgesic is given. Working with the patient and family, as well as with other health care providers, on a pain-management program based on the patient's specific requirements frequently increases the patient's comfort and sense of control. In addition, the dose of opioid analgesic required is often reduced as pain becomes more manageable, and other medications (eg, sedatives, tranquilizers, muscle relaxants) are added to assist in relieving pain.

If the patient is a candidate for radiation therapy or surgical intervention to relieve severe pain, the consequences of these procedures (eg, percutaneous nerve block, cordotomy) are explained to the patient and family, and measures are taken to prevent complications resulting from altered sensation, immobility, and changes in bowel and bladder function.

With the appearance of each new symptom, patients may experience dread and fear that the disease is progressing. However, one cannot assume that all symptoms are related to the cancer. The new symptoms and problems are evaluated and treated aggressively if possible to increase the patient's comfort and improve quality of life.

Weakness, immobility, fatigue, and inactivity typically occur in the advanced stages of cancer as a result of the tumor, treatment, inadequate nutritional intake, or difficulty breathing (dyspnea). The nurse works with the patient to set realistic goals and to provide rest balanced with planned activities and exercise. Other measures include assisting the patient in identifying less energy-consuming methods for accomplishing tasks and promoting activities that the patient values the most.

Efforts are made throughout the course of the disease to provide the patient with as much control and independence as desired, but with assurance that support and assistance are available when needed. Additionally, the health care team works with the patient and family to ascertain and comply with the patient's wishes about treatment methods and care as the terminal phase of illness and death approach.

Hospice

For many years, society was unable to cope appropriately with patients in the most advanced stages of cancer, and patients died in acute care settings rather than at home or in facilities specifically designed to meet their needs. The needs of patients with terminal illnesses are well managed by a comprehensive multidisciplinary program that focuses on quality of life, palliation of symptoms, and provision of psychosocial and spiritual support for the patient and family when cure and control of disease progress are no longer possible. The concept of hospice, which originated in Great Britain, best addresses these needs. Most important, the focus of care is on the family, not just the patient. Hospice care can be provided in several settings: free-standing, hospital-based, and community or home-based settings.

Because of high costs associated with maintaining free-standing hospices, care is often delivered by coordinating services provided by both the hospital and community. Although physicians, social workers, clergy, dietitians, pharmacists, physical therapists, and volunteers are involved in patient care, nurses are most often the coordinators of all hospice activities. It is essential that home care and hospice nurses possess advanced skills in assessing and managing pain, nutrition, dyspnea, bowel dysfunction, and skin impairments.

In addition, hospice programs facilitate clear communication among family members and health care providers. Most patients and families are informed of the prognosis and are encouraged to participate in decisions regarding pursuing or terminating cancer treatment. Through collaboration with other support disciplines, nurses assist patients and families to cope with changes in role identity, family structure, grief, and loss. Hospice nurses are actively involved in bereavement counseling. In many instances, family support for survivors continues for about 1 year.

ONCOLOGIC EMERGENCIES

For information about these emergencies, see Table 15-11.

(*text continues on page 310*)

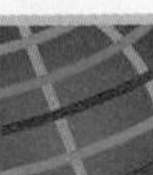

TABLE 15•11 Oncologic Emergencies: Manifestations and Management

Emergency	Clinical Manifestations and Diagnostic Findings	Management
Superior vena cava syndrome (SVCS) Compression or invasion of the superior vena cava by tumor, enlarged lymph nodes, intraluminal thrombus that obstructs venous circulation, or drainage of the head, neck, arms, and thorax. Typically associated with lung cancer, SVCS can also occur with lymphoma and metastases. If untreated, SVCS may lead to cerebral anoxia (because not enough oxygen reaches the brain), laryngeal edema, bronchial obstruction, and death.	*Clinical* Gradually or suddenly impaired venous drainage giving rise to • Progressive shortness of breath (dyspnea), cough, and facial swelling • Edema of the neck, arms, hands, and thorax and reported sensation of skin tightness and difficulty swallowing • Possibly engorged and distended jugular, temporal, and arm veins • Dilated thoracic vessels causing prominent venous patterns on the chest wall • Increased intracranial pressure, associated visual disturbances, headache, and altered mental status *Diagnostic* Diagnosis is confirmed by • Clinical findings • Chest x-ray • Thoracic CT scan • MRI Intraluminal thrombosis is identified by venogram.	*Medical* • Radiation therapy to shrink tumor size and relieve symptoms • Chemotherapy for radiation-resistant tumor (eg, lymphoma or small cell lung cancer) or when the mediastinum has been irradiated to maximum tolerance • Anticoagulant or thrombolytic therapy for intraluminal thrombosis • Surgery (less common), eg, vena cava bypass graft (synthetic or autologous) to redirect blood flow around the obstruction • Supportive measures such as oxygen therapy, corticosteroids, and diuretics *Nursing* • Identify patients at risk for SVCS. • Monitor and report clinical manifestations of SVCS. • Monitor cardiopulmonary and neurologic status. • Facilitate breathing by positioning the patient properly. This helps to promote comfort and reduce anxiety produced by difficulty breathing resulting from progressive edema. • Promote energy conservation to minimize shortness of breath. • Monitor the patient's fluid volume status and administer fluids cautiously to minimize edema. • Assess for thoracic radiation-related problems such as dysphagia (difficulty swallowing) and esophagitis. • Monitor for chemotherapy-related problems, such as myelosuppression. • Provide postoperative care as appropriate.
Spinal cord compression Potentially leading to permanent neurologic impairment and associated morbidity and mortality, compression of the cord and its nerve roots may result from tumor, lymphomas, or intervertebral collapse. The prognosis depends on the severity and rapidity of onset. About 70% of compressions occur at the thoracic level, 20% in the lumbosacral level and 10% in the cervical region. Metastatic cancers (breast, lung, kidney, prostate, myeloma, lymphoma) and related bone erosion are associated with spinal cord compression.	*Clinical* • Local inflammation, edema, venous stasis, and impaired blood supply to nervous tissues • Local or radicular pain along the dermatomal areas innervated by the affected nerve root (eg, thoracic radicular pain extends in a band around the chest or abdomen) • Pain exacerbated by movement, coughing, sneezing, or the Valsalva maneuver • Neurologic dysfunction, and related motor and sensory deficits (numbness, tingling, feelings of coldness in the affected area, inability to detect vibration, loss of positional sense) • Motor loss ranging from subtle weakness to flaccid paralysis • Bladder and/or bowel dysfunction depending on level of compression (above S2, overflow incontinence; from S3 to S5, flaccid sphincter tone and bowel incontinence)	*Medical* • Radiation therapy to reduce tumor size to halt progression and corticosteroid therapy to decrease inflammation and swelling at the compression site • Surgery only if symptoms progress despite radiation therapy • Chemotherapy as adjuvant to radiation therapy for patients with lymphoma or small cell lung cancer • *Note:* Despite treatment, patients with poor neurologic function before treatment are less likely to regain complete motor and sensory function; patients who develop complete paralysis usually do not regain all neurologic function. *Nursing* • Perform ongoing assessment of neurologic function to identify existing and progressing dysfunction. • Control pain with pharmacologic and nonpharmacologic measures.

(*continued*)

TABLE 15•11 **Oncologic Emergencies: Manifestations and Management** *(Continued)*

Emergency	Clinical Manifestations and Diagnostic Findings	Management
	Diagnostic • Percussion tenderness at the level of compression • Abnormal reflexes • Sensory and motor abnormalities • MRI, myelogram, spinal cord x-rays, bone scans, and CT scan	• Prevent complications of immobility resulting from pain and decreased function (ie, skin breakdown, urinary stasis, thrombophlebitis, and decreased clearance of pulmonary secretions). • Maintain muscle tone by assisting with range-of-motion exercises in collaboration with physical and occupational therapists. • Institute intermittent urinary catheterization and bowel training programs for patients with bladder or bowel dysfunction. • Provide encouragement and support to patient and family coping with pain and altered functioning, lifestyle, roles, and independence.
Hypercalcemia In cancer patients, hypercalcemia is a potentially life-threatening metabolic abnormality resulting when the calcium released from the bones is more than the kidneys can excrete or the bones can reabsorb. It may result from: • Bone destruction by tumor cells and subsequent release of calcium • Production of prostaglandins and osteoclast-activating factor, which stimulate bone breakdown and calcium release • Tumors that produce parathyroid-like substances that promote calcium release • Excessive use of vitamins and minerals and conditions unrelated to cancer, such as dehydration, renal impairment, primary hyperparathyroidism, thyrotoxicosis, thiazide diuretics, and hormone therapy	*Clinical* Fatigue, weakness, confusion, decreased level of responsiveness, hyporeflexia, nausea, vomiting, constipation, polyuria (excessive urination), polydipsia (excessive thirst), dehydration, and dysrhythmias *Diagnostic* Serum calcium level exceeding 11 mg/dL (SI: 2.74 mmol/L)	*Medical* See Chapter 13. *Nursing* • Identify patients at risk for hypercalcemia and assess for signs and symptoms of hypercalcemia. • Educate patient and family; prevention and early detection can prevent fatality. • Teach at-risk patients to recognize and report signs and symptoms of hypercalcemia. • Encourage patients to consume 2 to 3 L of fluid daily unless contraindicated by existing renal or cardiac disease. • Explain the use of dietary and pharmacologic interventions such as stool softeners and laxatives for constipation. • Advise patients to maintain nutritional intake without restricting normal calcium intake. • Discuss antiemetic therapy if nausea and vomiting occur. • Promote mobility by emphasizing its importance in preventing demineralization and breakdown of bones.
Pericardial Effusion and Cardiac Tamponade Cardiac tamponade is an accumulation of fluid in the pericardial space. The accumulation compresses the heart and thereby impedes expansion of the ventricles and cardiac filling during diastole. As ventricular volume and cardiac output fall, the heart pump fails, and circulatory collapse develops. With gradual onset, fluid accumulates gradually, and the outer layer of the pericardial space stretches to compensate for rising pressure. Large amounts of fluid accumulate before symptoms of heart failure occur. With rapid onset, pressures rise too quickly for the pericardial space to compensate. Cancerous tumors, particularly from adjacent thoracic tumors (lung, esophagus, breast cancers), and cancer treatment are the most common	*Clinical* • Neck vein distention during inspiration (Kussmaul's sign) • Pulsus paradoxus (systolic blood pressure decrease exceeding 10 mm Hg during inspiration; pulse gets stronger on expiration) • Distant heart sounds, rubs and gallops, cardiac dullness • Compensatory tachycardia (heart beats faster to compensate for decreased cardiac output) • Increased venous and vascular pressures *Diagnostic* • ECG helps diagnose pericardial effusion. • In small effusion, chest x-rays show small amounts of fluid in the pericardium; in large effusions, x-ray films disclose "water-bottle" heart (obliteration of vessel contour and cardiac chambers). • ECG and CT scans help diagnose pleural effusions and evaluate effect of treatment. • Narrow pulse pressure • Shortness of breath and tachypnea	*Medical* • Pericardiocentesis (the aspiration or withdrawal of the pericardial fluid by a large-bore needle inserted into the pericardial space). In malignant effusions, pericardiocentesis provides only temporary relief; fluid usually reaccumulates. Windows or openings in the pericardium can be created surgically as a palliative measure to drain fluid into the pleural space. Catheters may also be placed in the pericardial space and sclerosing agents (such as tetracycline, talc, bleomycin, 5-fluorouracil, or thiotepa) injected to prevent fluid from reaccumulating. • Radiation therapy or antineoplastic agents, depending on how sensitive the primary tumor is to these treatments. In mild effusions, prednisone and diuretic medications may be prescribed and the patient's status carefully monitored. *Nursing* • Monitor vital signs and oxygen saturation frequently. • Assess for pulsus paradoxus.

(continued)

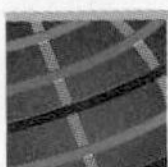

TABLE 15•11 Oncologic Emergencies: Manifestations and Management *(Continued)*

Emergency	Clinical Manifestations and Diagnostic Findings	Management
causes of cardiac tamponade. Radiation therapy of 4000 cGy or more to the mediastinal area has also been implicated in pericardial fibrosis, pericarditis, and resultant cardiac tamponade. Untreated pericardial effusion and cardiac tamponade lead to circulatory collapse and cardiac arrest.	• Weakness, chest pain, orthopnea, anxiety, diaphoresis, lethargy, and altered consciousness from decreased cerebral perfusion	• Monitor ECG tracings. • Assess heart and lung sounds, neck vein filling, level of consciousness, respiratory status, and skin color and temperature. • Monitor and record intake and output. • Review laboratory findings (eg, arterial blood gas and electrolyte levels). • Elevate the head of the patient's bed to ease breathing. • Minimize patient's physical activity to reduce oxygen requirements; administer supplemental oxygen as prescribed. • Provide frequent oral hygiene. • Reposition and encourage the patient to cough and take deep breaths every 2 hours. • As needed, maintain patent IV access, reorient the patient, and provide supportive measures and appropriate patient instruction.
Disseminated Intravascular Coagulation (DIC, also called consumption coagulopathy) Complex disorder of coagulation or fibrinolysis (destruction of clots), which results in thrombosis or bleeding. DIC is most commonly associated with blood cancers (leukemia); cancer of prostate, GI tract, and lungs; chemotherapy (methotrexate, prednisone, L-asparaginase, vincristine, and 6-mercaptopurine), and disease processes, such as sepsis, hepatic failure, and anaphylaxis. Blood clots form when normal coagulation mechanisms are triggered. Once activated, the clotting cascade continues to consume clotting factors and platelets faster than the body can replace them. Clots are deposited in the microvasculature, placing the patient at great risk for impaired circulation, tissue hypoxia, and necrosis. In addition, fibrinolysis occurs, breaking down clots and increasing the circulating levels of anticoagulant substances, thereby placing the patient at risk for hemorrhage.	*Clinical* *Chronic DIC:* Few or no observable symptoms or easy bruising, prolonged bleeding from venipuncture and injection sites, bleeding of the gums, and slow GI bleeding *Acute DIC:* life-threatening hemorrhage and infarction; clinical symptoms of this syndrome are varied and depend on the organ system involved in thrombus and infarction or bleeding episodes *Diagnostic* • Prolonged prothrombin time (PT or protime) • Prolonged partial thromboplastin time (PTT) • Prolonged thrombin time (TT) • Decreased fibrinogen level • Decreased platelet level • Decrease in clotting factors • Decreased hemoglobin • Decreased hematocrit • Elevated fibrin split products • Positive protamine sulfate precipitation test (thrombin activation test)	*Medical* • Chemotherapy, biologic response modifier therapy, radiation therapy, or surgery is used to treat the underlying cancer. • Antibiotic therapy is used for sepsis. • Anticoagulants, such as heparin or antithrombin III, decrease the stimulation of the coagulation pathways. • Transfusion of fresh frozen plasma or cryoprecipitates (which contain clotting factors and fibrinogen), packed red blood cells, and platelets may be used as replacement therapy to prevent or control bleeding. • Although controversial, antifibrinolytic agents such as aminocaproic acid (Amicar), which is associated with increased thrombus formation, may be used. *Nursing* • Monitor vital signs. • Measure and document intake and output. • Assess skin color and temperature; lung, heart, and bowel sounds; level of consciousness, headache, visual disturbances, chest pain, decreased urine output, and abdominal tenderness. • Inspect all body orifices, tube insertion sites, incisions, and bodily excretions for bleeding. • Review laboratory test results. • Minimize physical activity to decrease injury risks and oxygen requirements. • Prevent bleeding; apply pressure to all venipuncture sites, and avoid nonessential invasive procedures; provide electric rather than straight-edged razors; avoid tape on the skin and advise gentle but adequate oral hygiene. • Assist the patient to turn, cough, and take deep breaths every 2 hours. • Reorient the patient, if needed; maintain a safe environment; and provide appropriate patient education and supportive measures.

(continued)

TABLE 15•11 Oncologic Emergencies: Manifestations and Management *(Continued)*

Emergency	Clinical Manifestations and Diagnostic Findings	Management
Syndrome of Inappropriate Secretion of Antidiuretic Hormone (SIADH) The continuous, uncontrolled release of antidiuretic hormone (ADH), produced by tumor cells or by the abnormal stimulation of the hypothalmic–pituitary network, leads to increased extracellular fluid volume, water intoxication, hyponatremia, and increased excretion of urinary sodium. As fluid volume increases, stretch receptors in the right atrium respond by releasing a second hormone, atrial naturetic factor (ANF). The release of ANF causes increased renal excretion of sodium, which worsens hyponatremia. The most common cause of SIADH is cancer, especially small cell cancers of the lung. Antineoplastics—vincristine, vinblastine, cisplatin, and cyclophosphamide—and morphine also stimulate ADH secretion, which promotes conservation and reabsorption of water by the kidneys. As more fluid is absorbed, the circulatory volume increases, ANF is released, and sodium is actively excreted by the kidneys in compensation.	*Clinical* *Serum sodium levels below 120 mEq/L* (SI: 120 mmol/L): symptoms of hyponatremia including personality changes, irritability, nausea, anorexia, vomiting, weight gain, fatigue, muscular pain (myalgia), headache, lethargy, and confusion. *Serum sodium levels below 110 mEq/L* (SI: 110 mmol/L): seizure, abnormal reflexes, papilledema, coma, and death. Edema is rare. *Diagnostic* • Decreased serum sodium level • Increased urine osmolality • Increased urinary sodium level • Decreased BUN, creatinine, and serum albumin levels secondary to dilution • Abnormal water load test results	*Medical* Fluid intake range limited to 500 to 1000 mL/day to increase the serum sodium level and decrease fluid overload. If water restriction alone is not effective in correcting or controlling serum sodium levels, demeclocycline is often prescribed to interfere with the antidiuretic action of ADH and ANF. When neurologic symptoms are severe, parenteral sodium replacement and diuretic therapy are indicated. Electrolyte levels are monitored carefully to detect secondary magnesium, potassium, and calcium imbalances. After the symptoms of SIADH are controlled, the underlying cancer is treated. If water excess continues despite treatment, pharmacologic intervention (urea and furosemide) may be indicated. *Nursing* • Maintain intake and output measurements. • Assess level of consciousness, lung and heart sounds, vital signs, daily weight, and urine specific gravity; also assess for nausea, vomiting, anorexia, edema, fatigue, and lethargy. • Monitor laboratory test results, including serum electrolyte levels, osmolality, and blood urea nitrogen, creatinine, and urinary sodium levels. • Minimize the patient's activity; provide appropriate oral hygiene; maintain environmental safety; and restrict fluid intake if necessary. • Reorient the patient and provide instruction and encouragement as needed.
Tumor Lysis Syndrome Potentially fatal complication associated with radiation- or chemotherapy-induced cell destruction of large or rapidly growing cancers such as leukemia, lymphoma, and small cell lung cancer. The release of intracellular contents from the tumor cells, leads to electrolyte imbalances—hyperkalemia, hypocalcemia, hyperphosphatemia, and hyperuricemia—because the kidneys can no longer excrete large volumes of the released intracellular metabolites.	*Clinical* Clinical manifestations depend on the extent of metabolic abnormalities. • Neurologic: Fatigue, weakness, memory loss, altered mental status, muscle cramps, tetany, paresthesias (numbness and tingling), seizures • Cardiac: Elevated blood pressure, shortened QT complexes, widened QRS waves, dysrhythmias, cardiac arrest • GI: Anorexia, nausea, vomiting, abdominal cramps, diarrhea • Renal: Flank pain, oliguria, anuria, renal failure, acidic urine pH *Diagnostic* Electrolyte imbalances identified by laboratory test results.	*Medical* • To prevent renal failure and restore electrolyte balance, aggressive fluid hydration is initiated 48 hours before and after the initiation of cytotoxic therapy to increase urine volume and eliminate uric acid and electrolytes. Urine is alkalinized by adding sodium bicarbonate to IV fluid to maintain a urine pH of 7 or more; this prevents renal failure secondary to uric acid precipitation in the kidneys. • Diuretic therapy, with a carbonic anhydrase inhibitor or acetazolamide, to alkalinize the urine • Allopurinol therapy to inhibit the conversion of nucleic acids to uric acid • Administration of a cation-exchange resin, such as sodium polystyrene sulfonate (Kayexalate) to treat hyperkalemia by binding and eliminating potassium through the bowel • Administration of hypertonic dextrose and regular insulin temporarily shifts potassium into cells and lowers serum potassium levels. • Administration of phosphate-binding gels, such as aluminum hydroxide, to treat hyperphosphatemia by promoting phosphate excretion in the feces.

(continued)

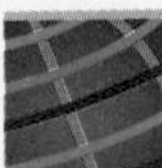

TABLE 15•11 **Oncologic Emergencies: Manifestations and Management** *(Continued)*

Emergency	Clinical Manifestations and Diagnostic Findings	Management
		• Hemodialysis when patients are unresponsive to the standard approaches for managing uric acid and electrolyte abnormalities *Nursing* • Identify at-risk patients, including those in whom tumor lysis syndrome may develop up to 1 week after therapy has been completed. • Institute essential preventive measures, (eg, fluid hydration and allopurinol). • Assess patient for signs and symptoms of electrolyte imbalances. • Assess urine pH to confirm alkalization. • Monitor serum electrolyte and uric acid levels for evidence of fluid volume overload secondary to aggressive hydration. • Instruct patients to report symptoms indicating electrolyte disturbances.

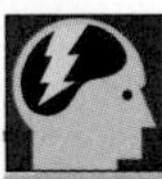

Critical Thinking Exercises

1.
A 45-year-old woman with a history of breast cancer developed irreversible lower extremity paralysis and urinary incontinence as a result of a spinal cord compression. She is otherwise in relatively good health and has no other areas of organ or tissue metastasis. On completion of radiation therapy, she would like to continue her job as a high school teacher. She is married and has two children ages 17 and 15 years. Identify this patient's learning needs in relation to radiation therapy, ongoing disease monitoring, and altered mobility. Describe the assessment, planning, and potential interventions needed to facilitate her continued roles as wife, mother, and teacher.

2.
One of your home care patients, a 64-year-old man with end-stage metastatic lung cancer, has been experiencing uncontrolled pain for which he has been taking a nonopioid analgesic. Both the patient and his spouse have refused to consider opioid analgesics because of a fear of addiction. The patient's wife confides that using "strong drugs for pain" signals a loss of hope and a desire to die. They both fear that hospitalization will be needed if other analgesics are used. What course of action would you take? What educational needs should be addressed?

3.
A female patient in the clinic has been given the choice of standard treatment for a malignant brain tumor or enrollment in a clinical trial of investigational therapy. She is concerned about the potential "unknowns" of the clinical trial, but is eager to support the physician's desire to participate in research activities. How would you assist her in the decision-making process?

References and Selected Readings

BOOKS

Agency for Health Care Policy and Research, Public Health Service, Department of Health and Human Services. (1992). *Acute pain management: Operative or medical procedures and trauma.* Clinical Practice Guideline (AHCPR 92-0032). Washington, DC: U.S. Government Printing Office.

Agency for Health Care Policy and Research, Public Health Service, Department of Health and Human Services. (1994). *Management of cancer pain: Adults.* Clinical Practice Guideline (AHCPR 94-0592). Washington, DC: U.S. Government Printing Office.

American Pain Society. (1999). *Principles of analgesic use in the treatment of acute pain and chronic cancer pain: A concise guide to medical practice* (4th ed.). Skokie, IL: American Pain Society.

Boik, J. (1995). *Cancer and natural medicine: A textbook of basic science and clinical research.* Princeton, MN: Oregon Medical Press.

Corwin. E. J. (1996). *Handbook of pathophysiology,* Philadelphia: Lippincott-Raven.

DeVita, V. T., Hellman, S., & Rosenberg, S. A. (Eds.). (1995). *Biologic therapy of cancer* (2nd ed.). Philadelphia: J. B. Lippincott.

Groenwald, S., Hansen-Frogge, M., Goodman, M., & Henke Yarbro, C. (Eds.). (1998). *Comprehensive cancer nursing review* (4th ed.). Boston: Jones and Bartlett.

Harvey, J. C., & Beattie, E. J. (Eds.). (1996). *Cancer surgery.* Philadelphia: W. B. Saunders.

McGuire, D. B., Yarbo, C. H., & Ferrell, B. R. (Eds.). (1995). *Cancer pain management* (2nd ed.). Boston: Jones & Bartlett.

Miaskowski, C. (1997). *Oncology nursing: An essential guide for patient care.* Philadelphia: W. B. Saunders.

Otto, S. E. (1997). *Oncology nursing* (3rd ed.). St. Louis: C. V. Mosby.

Parris, C. V. (1997). *Cancer pain management: Principles and practice.* Boston: Butterworth-Heinmann.

Perry, M. C. (Ed.). (1997). *The chemotherapy source book* (2nd ed.). Baltimore: Williams & Wilkins.

Varricchio, C., Pierce, M., Walker, C. L., & Ades, T. B. (Eds.). (1997). *A cancer source book for nurses* (7th ed.). Atlanta: American Cancer Society.

Wilkes, G. M., et al. (Eds.). (1997). *Oncology nursing drug handbook 1997–1998.* Boston: Jones & Bartlett.

JOURNALS

Asterisks indicate nursing research articles.

General

Ballinger, J. R. (1996). Radiologic imaging in cancer. *Medical Clinics of North America, 80*(1), 201–217.

Borton, D. (1996). WBC count and differential: Reviewing the defensive roster. *Nursing, 26*(9), 26–31.

*Cox, K., & Avis, M. (1996). Psychosocial aspects of participation in early anticancer drug trials: Report of a pilot study. *Cancer Nursing, 19*(3), 177–186.

Emmanoulides, C., & Glaspy, J. (1996). Opportunistic infections in oncologic patients. *Hematology/Oncology Clinics of North America, 10*(4), 841–860.

*Graydon, J. E., Bubela, N., Irvine, D., & Vincent, L. (1995). Fatigue-reducing strategies used by patients receiving treatment for cancer. *Cancer Nursing, 18*(1), 23–28.

Madeya, M. L. (1996). Oral complications from cancer therapy. I. Pathophysiology and secondary complications. *Oncology Nursing Forum, 23*(5), 801–807.

Madeya, M. L. (1996). Oral complications from cancer therapy. II. Nursing implications for assessment and treatment. *Oncology Nursing Forum, 23*(5), 808–819.

Markman, M. (1995). Surgery for support and palliation in patients with malignant disease. *Seminars in Oncology, 22*(Suppl. 2), 91–94.

Montbriand, M. J. (1994). An overview of alternative therapies chosen by patients with cancer. *Oncology Nursing Forum, 21*(9), 1547–1554.

Pamies, R. J., & Crawford, D. R. (1996). Tumor markers: An update. *Medical Clinics of North America, 80*(1), 185–199.

Salazar, M. K. (1996). Hispanic women's beliefs about breast cancer and mammography. *Cancer Nursing, 19*(6): 437–446.

Spanks, S., & Camp-Sorrell, D. (1997). Assessing the myelosuppressed patient. *American Journal of Nursing, 97*(Suppl. 5), 4–8.

Zaloznik, A. J. (1994). Unproven (unorthodox) cancer treatment. *Cancer Practitioner, 2*(1), 19–24.

Biologic Response Modifiers

DeLa Pena, L., et al. (1996). Programmed instruction: Biotherapy Module IV—Interleukins. *Cancer Nursing, 19*(1), 60–75.

DeLa Pena, L., et al. (1996). Programmed instruction: Biotherapy Module V—Hematopoietic growth factors. *Cancer Nursing, 19*(2), 135–150.

Gantz, S., et al. (1995). Programmed instruction: Biotherapy Module III—Interferons. *Cancer Nursing, 18*(6), 479–494.

Karius, D., & Marriott, M. A. (1997). Immunologic advances in monoclonal antibody therapy: Implications for oncology nursing. *Oncology Nursing Forum, 24*(3), 483–494.

Rieger, P. T. (Ed.). (1996). Biotherapy: Present accomplishments and future projections. *Seminars in Oncology Nursing, 12*(2), 1–175.

Tomaszewski, J. K., et al. (1995). Programmed instruction: Biotherapy—The Immune system and cancer. *Cancer Nursing, 18*(4), 313–331.

Tomaszewski, J. K., et al. (1995). Programmed instruction: Biotherapy Module II—Overview of biotherapy. *Cancer Nursing, 18*(5), 397–414.

Bone Marrow Transplantation

Applebaum, F. R. (1996) The use of bone marrow and peripheral blood cell transplantation in the treatment of cancer. *CA: A Cancer Journal for Clinicians, 46*(3), 142–164.

Buchsel, P. C., & Kapustay, P. M. (1995). Peripheral stem cell transplantation. *Oncology Nursing Update: Patient Treatment and Support, 2*(2), 1–14.

Buchsel, P. C., et al. (1996). Delayed complications of bone marrow transplantation: An update. *Oncology Nursing Forum, 23*(8), 1267–1291.

Hurley, C. (1997). Ambulatory care after bone marrow or peripheral blood stem cell transplantation. *Clinical Journal of Oncology Nursing, 1*(1), 19–21.

Larson, P. J. (1995). Perceptions of the needs of hospitalized patients undergoing bone marrow transplant. *Cancer Practitioner, 3*(3), 173–179.

Molassiotis, A., & van den Akker, O. (1995). Psychological stress in nursing and medical staff in bone marrow transplant units. *Bone Marrow Transplantation, 15*(3), 449–454.

Poliquin, C. M. (1997). Overview of bone marrow and peripheral blood stem cell transplantation. *Clinical Journal of Oncology Nursing, 1*(1), 11–17.

Carcinogenesis and Risk Factors

Cavenee, W. K., & White, R. L. (1995). The genetic basis of cancer. *Scientific American, 272*(3), 72–79.

Fraser, M. C., et al. (1997). Familial cancers: Evolving challenges for nursing practice. *Oncology Nursing Update: Patient Treatment and Support, 4*(3), 1–18.

Heath, C. W. (1996). Electromagnetic field exposure and cancer: A review of epidemiologic evidence. *CA: A Cancer Journal for Clinicians, 46*(1), 29–44.

Hines, J., et al. (1995). Human papillomaviruses: Their clinical significance in the management of cervical carcinoma. *Oncology, 9*(4), 279–285.

Lea, D. H., & Jenkins, J. (1997). Cancer genetics for nurses. I. The genetic basis of cancer. *Oncology Nursing Update: Patient Treatment and Support, 4*(5), 1–11.

Loescher, L. J. (1995). Genetics in cancer prediction, screening, and counseling. I. Genetics in cancer prediction and screening. *Oncology Nursing Forum, 22*(Suppl. 2), 10–15.

Stillman, J. M., & Stillman, S. D. (1996). Cancer and the workplace. *CA: A Cancer Journal for Clinicians, 46*(2), 70–92.

Woods, N. A. (1996). Cancer risk controversies: Women's exposure to exogenous ovarian hormones. *Oncology Nursing Update: Patient Treatment and Support, 3*(1), 1–16.

Chemotherapy

Boyle, D. M., & Engelking, C. (1995). Vesicant extravasation: Myths and realities. *Oncology Nursing Forum, 22*(1), 57–67.

Bociek, R. G., & Armitage, J. O. (1996). Hematopoietic growth factors. *CA: A Cancer Journal for Clinicians, 46*(3), 165–184.

Brogden, J. M., & Nevidjon, B. (1995). Vinorelbine tartrate (Navelbine): Drug profile and nursing implications of a new vinca alkaloid. *Oncology Nursing Forum, 22*(4), 635–646.

Crabbe, W. (1996). The tamoxifen controversy. *Oncology Nursing Forum, 23*(5), 761–766.

*Dodd, M. J., et al. (1996). Randomized clinical trials of chlorhexidine versus placebo for the prevention of oral mucositis in patients receiving chemotherapy. *Oncology Nursing Forum, 23*(6), 921–927.

Fessele, K. S. (1996). Managing the multiple causes of nausea and vomiting in the patient with cancer. *Oncology Nursing Forum, 23*(9), 1409–1415.

Giacome, G. (1995). New drugs in non-small cell lung cancer: An overview. *Lung Cancer, 12*(Suppl. 1), S155–S166.

Henry, D. H. (1996). Recombinant human erythropoietin treatment of anemic cancer patients. *Cancer Practitioner, 4*(4), 180–184.

Huizing, M., et al. (1995). Taxanec: A new class of antitumor agents. *Cancer Investigation, 13*(4), 381–404.

Johnson, M. H., et al. (1997). Relieving nausea and vomiting in patients with cancer: A treatment algorithm. *Oncology Nursing Forum, 24*(1), 51–57.

Krakoff, I. H. (1996). Systemic treatment of cancer. *CA: A Cancer Journal for Clinicians, 46*(3), 134–141.

*Messias, D. K. H., et al. (1997). Patients' perspectives of fatigue while undergoing chemotherapy. *Oncology Nursing Forum, 24*(1), 43–48.

Rieger, P. T., & Haeuber D. (1995). A new approach to managing chemotherapy-related anemia: Nursing implications of epoetin alpha. *Oncology Nursing Forum, 22*(1), 71–81.

Rhodes, V. A., et al. (1995). Expectations and occurrence of postchemotherapy side effects. *Cancer Practitioner, 3*(4), 247–253.

Toth, B., et al. (1995). Minimizing oral complications of cancer treatment. *Oncology, 9*(9), 851–857.

Wasaff, B. (1997). Current status of hormonal treatment for metastatic breast cancer in postmenopausal women. *Oncology Nursing Forum, 24*(9), 1515–1520.

Gene Therapy

Bowles Biesecker, B. (1997). Programmed instruction: Cancer genetics. Genetic testing for cancer predisposition. *Cancer Nursing, 20*(4), 285–300.

Dimond, E., Peters, J., & Jenkins, J. (1997). Programmed instruction: Human genetics. The genetic basis of cancer. *Cancer Nursing, 20*(3), 213–226.

Halsey, L. D. (1997). Gene therapy: Current and future implications for oncology nursing practice. *Seminars in Oncology Nursing, 13*(2), 115–122.

Peters, J. A. (1997). Applications of genetic technologies to cancer screening, prevention, diagnosis, prognosis and treatment. *Seminars in Oncology Nursing, 13*(2), 74–81.

Peters, J. A., Dimond, E., & Jenkins, J. (1997). Programmed instruction: Cancer genetics. Clinical applications of genetic technologies to cancer care. *Cancer Nursing, 20*(5), 359–377.

Williams, J. K. (1997). Principles of genetics and cancer. *Seminars in Oncology Nursing, 13*(2), 68–73.

Gerontology

Balducci, L., Lyman, G. H., & Fabri, P. J. (1996). Management of cancer in the aged. *Comprehensive Therapy, 22*(2), 88–93.

Lichtman, S. M. (1995). Physiologic aspects of aging: Implications for the treatment of cancer. *Drugs and Aging, 7*(3), 212–225.

Wells, N. L., & Balducci, L. (1997). Geriatric oncology: Medical and psychosocial perspectives. *Cancer Practitioner, 5*(2), 87–91.

Home Care and Hospice

Blesch, K. S. (1996). Rehabilitation of the cancer patient at home. *Seminars in Oncology Nursing, 12*(3), 219–225.

Cherny, N. I., Coyle, N., & Foley, K. M. (1996). Guidelines in the care of the dying cancer patient. *Hematology/Oncology Clinics of North America, 10*(1), 261–286.

Gorski, L. A., & Grothman, L. (1996). Home infusion therapy. *Seminars in Oncology Nursing, 12*(3), 193–201.
Magnum, L. C., Bentzen, C., & Landmark, S. (1996). Pain management in home care. *Seminars in Oncology Nursing, 12*(3), 202–218.
McEnroe, L. E. (1996). Role of the oncology nurse in home care: Family centered practice. *Seminars in Oncology Nursing, 12*(3), 188–192.
McNally, J. C., Bohnet, N. L., & Linquist, M. E. (1996). Hospice nursing. *Seminars in Oncology Nursing, 12*(3), 238–243.

Oncologic Emergencies

Barri, Y. M., & Knochel, J. P. (1996). Hypercalcemia and electrolyte disturbances in malignancy. *Hematology/Oncology Clinics of North America, 10*(4), 775–790.
Bick, R. L., Strauss, J. F., & Frenkel, E. P. (1996). Thrombosis and hemorrhage in oncology patients. *Hematology/Oncology Clinics of North America, 10*(4), 875–907.
Chisholm, M. A., Mulloy, A. L., & Taylor, A. T. (1996). Acute management of cancer-related hypercalcemia. *Annals of Pharmacotherapy, 30*(5), 507–513.
Clayton, K. (1997). Cancer-related hypercalcemia: How to spot it, how to manage it. *American Journal of Nursing, 97*(5), 42–49.
Goad, K. E., & Gralnick, H. R. (1996). Coagulation disorders in cancer. *Hematology/Oncology Clinics of North America, 10*(2), 457–484.
Rohaly-Davis, J., & Johnston, K. (1996) Hematologic emergencies in the intensive care unit. *Critical Care Nursing Quarterly, 18*(4), 35–43.
Shuey, K. M. (1994). Heart, lung, and endocrine complications of solid tumors. *Seminars in Oncology Nursing, 10*(3), 177–188.
Uage, C., Kahsen, K., & Parish, L. (1996). Oncology emergencies. *Critical Care Nursing Quarterly, 18*(4), 26–34.

Pain

Caraceni, A. (1996). Clinicopathologic correlates of common cancer pain syndromes. *Hematology/Oncology Clinics of North America, 10*(1), 57–78.
*Carpenter, J. S., & Brockopp, D. (1995). Comparison of patients' ratings and examination of nurses' responses to pain intensity rating scales. *Cancer Nursing, 18*(4), 292–298.
Cherny, N. I., & Foley, K. M. (1996). Nonopioid and opioid analgesic pharmacotherapy of cancer pain. *Hematology/Oncology Clinics of North America, 10*(1), 79–102.
*Ferrell, R. B., & McCaffery, M. (1997). Nurses' knowledge about equianalgesia and opioid dosing. *Cancer Nursing, 20*(3), 201–212.
Levy, M. H. (1996). Drug therapy: Pharmacologic treatment of cancer pain. *New England Journal of Medicine, 335*(15), 1124–1132.
Niles, R. (1995). Pharmacologic management of cancer pain. *Nursing Clinics of North America, 30*(4), 745–763.
Portenoy, R. K. (1995). Pharmacologic management of cancer pain. *Seminars in Oncology, 22*(Suppl 2), 112–120.
Portenoy, R. K. (1996). Adjuvant analgesic agents. *Hematology/Oncology Clinics of North America, 10*(1), 103–119.

Radiation Therapy

Blackman, A. (1997). Radiation-induced skin alterations. *Medsurg Nursing, 6*(3), 172–175.
Cash, J. C., & Dattoli, M. J. (1997). Management of patients receiving transperineal Palladium-103 prostate implants. *Oncology Nursing Forum, 24*(8), 1361–1367.
Dibble, S. L., et al. (1996). Mouth assessment: A new tool to evaluate mucositis in the radiation therapy patient. *Cancer Practitioner, 4*(3), 135–140.
Dunne-Daly, C. F. (1995). Programmed instruction: Radiation therapy. Skin and wound care in radiation oncology. *Cancer Nursing, 18*(2), 144–162.
Fieler, V. K. (1997). Side effects and quality of life in patients receiving high-dose brachytherapy. *Oncology Nursing Forum, 24*(3), 545–553.
Korinko, A., & Urick, A. (1997). Maintaining skin integrity during radiation therapy. *American Journal of Nursing, 97*(2), 40–44.
Porter, A. T., et al. (1995). Brachytherapy for prostate cancer. *CA: A Cancer Journal for Clinicians, 45*(3), 165–178.
Roach, M., et al. (1995). Radiation pneumonitis following combined modality therapy for lung cancer: Analysis of prognostic factors. *Journal of Clinical Oncology, 13*(10), 2606–2612.

Vascular Access Devices

Eastridge, B., & Lefor, A. (1995). Complications of indwelling venous devices in cancer patients. *Journal of Clinical Oncology, 13*(1), 233–238.
Howell, P., et al. (1995). Risk factors for infection of adult patients with cancer who have tunneled central catheters. *Cancer, 75*(6), 1367–1375.
Mayo, D. J., et al. (1997). Superior vena cava thrombosis associated with a central venous access device: A case report. *Clinical Journal of Oncology Nursing, 1*(1), 5–10.

Resources

PROFESSIONAL ORGANIZATIONS

American Association for Cancer Education (AACE), University of Texas, MD Anderson Cancer Center, Box 189, 1515 Holcombe Boulevard, Houston, Texas 77030; 1-713-792-3020.
American Society of Clinical Oncology, 225 Reinekers Lane, Suite 650, Alexandria, VA 22314'; 1-703-299-0150; e-mail: asco@asco.org.
Hospice Nurses Association (HNA), 5512 Northumberland Street, Pittsburgh, PA 15217-1131; 1-412-687-3231.
International Society of Nurses in Cancer Care, The Royal College of Nursing, 20 Cavendish Square, London WIM OAB, 1-071-495-6119.
Oncology Nursing Society (ONS), 510 Holiday Drive, Pittsburgh, PA 15220-2749; 1-412-921-7373; e-mail: member@nauticom.net.

ORGANIZATIONS FOR PATIENT/FAMILY SUPPORT AND EDUCATION

American Brain Tumor Association (ABTA), 2720 River Road, Suite 146, Des Plaines, IL 60018; 1-800-886-2282 (patient line); ABTA@aol.com (E-mail).
American Cancer Society (ACS), 1599 Clifton Road NE, Atlanta, GA; 1-800-ACS-2345 (check your local directory for the unit of division nearest you); www.cancer.org.
Bone Marrow Transplant Family Support Network, PO Box 845, Avon, CT 06001, 1-888-826-9376.
Cancer Care Inc. and the National Cancer Care Foundation, 1180 Avenue of the Americas, New York, NY 10036; 1-800-813-HOPE; e-mail: cancercare@aol.com.
Cancer Information Service (CIS), National Cancer Institute, Building 31, Room 10A16, Bethesda, MD 20892; 1-800-422-6237.
Cancernet: http://cancernet.nci.nih.gov.
Hospice Education Institute, 190 Westbrook Road, Essex, CT 06426; 1-800-331-1620.
Leukemia Society of America, Inc., 600 Third Avenue, New York, NY 10016; 1-212-573-8484; 1-800-955-4LSA (for chapter nearest you); www.leukemia.org.
Make Today Count, Mid Atlantic Cancer Center, 1235 East Cherokee, Springfield, MO 65804-2263; 1-800-432-2273.
National Alliance of Breast Cancer Organizations, 1180 Avenue of the Americas, 2nd Floor, New York, NY 10036; 1-212-719-0154; e-mail: NAB@aol.com.
National Coalition for Cancer Survivorship (NCCS), 1010 Wayne Ave, 5th Floor, Silver Spring, MD 20910; 1-301-650-8868.
National Hospice Organization (NHO), 1901 North Moore Street, Suite 901, Arlington, VA 22209; 1-800-658-8898; e-mail: drsnho@cais.com.
United Ostomy Association (UOA), 36 Executive Park, Suite 120, Irvine, CA 92714; 1-800-826-0826; e-mail: uoa@deltanet.com.
The Wellness Community, 2716 Ocean Park Blvd, Suite 1040, Santa Monica, CA 90405-5211; 1-310-314-5211.

UNIT

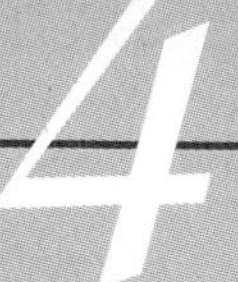

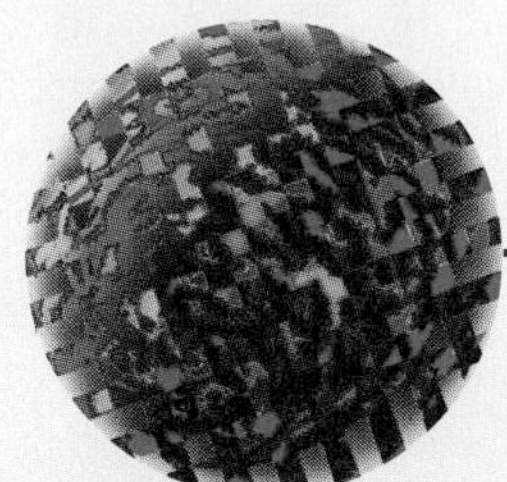

Perioperative Concepts and Nursing Management

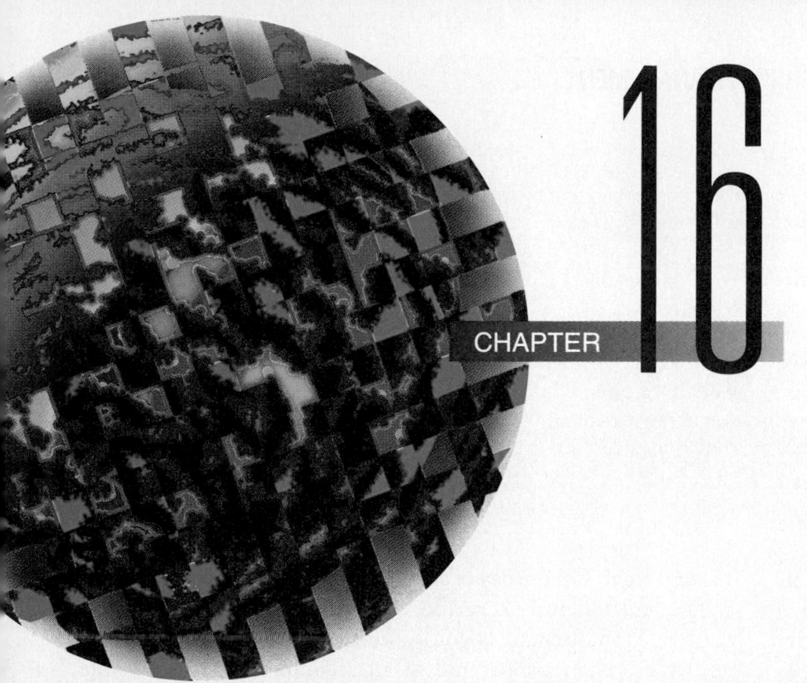

Preoperative Nursing Management

Learning Objectives

On completion of this chapter, the learner will be able to:

1. Identify the causes of preoperative anxiety and describe nursing measures to alleviate it.
2. Describe a comprehensive preoperative assessment to identify surgical risk factors.
3. Identify legal and ethical considerations related to informed consent.
4. Describe preoperative nursing measures that decrease the risk for infection and other postoperative complications.
5. Develop a preoperative teaching plan designed to promote the patient's recovery from anesthesia and surgery, thus preventing postoperative complications.
6. Describe the immediate preoperative preparation of the patient.

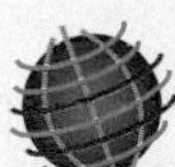

Surgery, whether elective or emergency, is a stressful, complex event. Today, as a result of advances in surgical techniques and instrumentation as well as in anesthesia, most surgical procedures are performed in an ambulatory or outpatient setting. The number of surgical patients admitted for overnight hospital stays is expected to continue to decrease. In the recent past, the patient scheduled for elective surgery would be admitted to the hospital at least one day before surgery for evaluation and preparation; these activities are now completed before the patient is admitted to the hospital. Today, many patients arrive at the hospital the morning of surgery and go home after recovering in the postanesthesia care unit (PACU) from the anesthesia. Surgical patients who require hospital stays are often trauma patients, acutely ill patients, patients undergoing major surgery, patients who require emergency surgery, and patients with a concurrent medical disorder.

Recent technologic advances have led to more complex procedures, more complicated microsurgical and laser technology, more sophisticated bypass equipment, increased use of laparoscopic surgery, and more sensitive monitoring devices. Surgery might now involve the transplantation of multiple human organs, the implantation of mechanical devices, or the reattachment of body parts. Advances in anesthesia have kept pace with the newer surgical technologies. More sophisticated monitoring and new pharmacologic agents, such as short-acting anesthetics and more effective antiemetics, have combined with improved postoperative pain management techniques to reduce procedure and recovery times.

GLOSSARY

ambulatory surgery (same-day surgery): surgery that does not require an overnight hospital stay

intraoperative phase: period of time from when the patient is transferred to the operating room table to when he or she is admitted to the postanesthesia care unit

informed consent: making autonomous decisions based on the nature of the condition, the treatment options, and the risks involved

perioperative period: period of time that constitutes the surgical experience; includes the preoperative, intraoperative, and postoperative phases

postoperative phase: period of time that begins with the admission of the patient to the postanesthesia care unit and ends after a follow-up evaluation in the clinical setting or home

preadmission testing (PAT): diagnostic testing done before admission to the hospital

preoperative phase: the period of time from when the decision for surgical intervention is made to when the patient is transferred to the operating room table

Concurrent with technologic advances have been changes in the delivery of and payment for health care. Pressure to reduce hospital lengths of stay and contain costs has resulted in patients undergoing diagnostic (**preadmission testing**, or PAT) and preoperative preparation before admission to the hospital. Patients also leave the hospital sooner, increasing the need for teaching, discharge planning, preparation for self-care, and referral for home care and rehabilitation services. It is now common for a patient to be admitted to the hospital, receive general anesthesia, undergo a surgical procedure, and be discharged home to the care of the family or friends all on the same day.

In the 1980s, seven of every eight surgeries required at least one overnight stay in the hospital. Today, it is estimated that more than 70% of all elective surgeries are performed on an ambulatory or outpatient basis. When combined with same-day admissions, this figure is closer to 80%. It is anticipated that in the 21st century, 85% of all elective surgical procedures will be performed in ambulatory or outpatient settings (White, 1997). Competent care of the ambulatory or same-day surgical patient requires a solid knowledge of all aspects of perioperative and perianesthesia nursing practice.

This unit focuses on the application of the nursing process for the patient receiving perioperative or perianesthesia care.

PERIOPERATIVE AND PERIANESTHESIA NURSING

Perioperative and perianesthesia nursing describes the wide variety of nursing functions associated with the patient's surgical experience. Perioperative and perianesthesia nursing addresses the nursing roles relevant to the three phases of the surgical experience—preoperative, intraoperative, and postoperative. As shown in Chart 16-1 each of these phases begins and ends at a particular point in the sequence of events that constitutes the surgical experience, and each includes a wide range of activities that the nurse performs using the nursing process and standards of practice.

The **preoperative phase** of perioperative and perianesthesia nursing begins when the decision for surgical intervention is made and ends with the transfer of the patient to the operating room table. The scope of nursing activities during this time can include establishing a baseline evaluation of the patient before the day of surgery by carrying out a preoperative interview (including physical and emotional assessment, previous anesthetic history, presence of known allergies), ensuring that necessary tests are performed (preadmission testing), arranging appropriate consultative services, and providing preparatory education about recovery from anesthesia and postoperative management. On the day of surgery, patient teaching is reviewed, the patient's identity is verified, and an intravenous infusion is started. If the patient is going home the same day, the availability of safe transport and of an accompanying responsible adult is verified. Depending on when the preadmission evaluation and testing were done, the nursing activities on the day of surgery may be limited to performing or updating the preoperative patient assessment and addressing questions the patient or family may have.

The **intraoperative phase** of perioperative and perianesthesia nursing begins when the patient is transferred to the operating room table and ends when he or she is admitted to the PACU. In this phase, the scope of nursing activity can include starting the intravenous infusion, administering intravenous medications, carrying out the full scope of physiologic monitoring throughout the surgical procedure, and providing for the patient's safety. In some instances, the nursing activities can be limited to providing emotional support by holding the patient's hand during general anesthesia induction, acting as scrub nurse or circulating nurse, or assisting in positioning the patient on the operating room table using basic principles of body alignment.

The **postoperative phase** begins with the admission of the patient to the postanesthesia care unit and ends with a follow-up evaluation in the clinical setting or at home. The scope of nursing covers a wide range of activities during this period. In the immediate postoperative phase, the focus includes assessing the effects of the anesthetic agents and the surgical procedure, monitoring vital functions, providing comfort and pain relief, and preventing complications. Nursing activities then focus on promoting the patient's recovery and initiating the teaching, follow-up care, and referrals essential for successful recovery and rehabilitation after discharge. Each phase is reviewed in more detail in this unit.

SURGICAL CLASSIFICATIONS

Surgery may be performed for a variety of reasons. It may be diagnostic, such as when a biopsy is obtained or an exploratory laparotomy is performed; it may be curative, such as when a tumor mass is excised or an inflamed appendix is removed; it may be reparative, such as when multiple wounds must be repaired; it may be reconstructive or cosmetic, such as when a mammoplasty or a face lift is performed; or it may be palliative, such as when pain must be relieved or a problem corrected—for example, when a gastrostomy tube is inserted to compensate for the inability to swallow food. Surgery may also be classified according to the degree of urgency involved, with use of the terms emergency, urgent, required, elective, and optional. These

CHART 16•1 Examples of Perioperative Nursing Activities

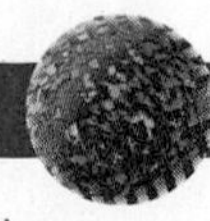

Preoperative Phase

Preadmission Testing

1. Initiates initial preoperative assessment
2. Initiates teaching appropriate to patient's needs
3. Involves family in interview
4. Verifies completion of preoperative testing
5. Assesses patient's need for postoperative transportation and care

Admission to Surgical Center or Unit

1. Completes preoperative assessment
2. Assesses for risks for postoperative complications
3. Reports unexpected findings or any deviations from normal
4. Verifies that operative consent has been signed
5. Coordinates patient teaching with other nursing staff
6. Reinforces previous teaching
7. Explains phases in perioperative period and expectations
8. Answers patient's and family's questions
9. Develops a plan of care

Holding Area

1. Assesses patient's status
2. Reviews chart
3. Identifies patient
4. Verifies surgical site
5. Establishes intravenous line
6. Administers medications if prescribed
7. Takes measures to ensure patient's comfort
8. Provides psychological support
9. Communicates patient's emotional status to other appropriate members of the health care team

Intraoperative Phase

Maintenance of Safety

1. Positions the patient
   a. Functional alignment
   b. Exposure of surgical site
   c. Maintenance of position throughout procedure
2. Applies grounding device to patient
3. Provides physical support
4. Ensures that the sponge, needle, and instrument counts are correct
5. Maintains aseptic, controlled environment
6. Effectively manages human resources

Physiologic Monitoring

1. Calculates effects on patient of excessive fluid loss or gain
2. Distinguishes normal from abnormal cardiopulmonary data
3. Reports changes in patient's pulse, respirations, temperature, and blood pressure

Psychological Support (Before Induction and if Patient Is Conscious)

1. Provides emotional support to patient
2. Stands near or touches patient during procedures and induction
3. Continues to assess patient's emotional status

Postoperative Phase

Transfer of Patient to Postanesthesia Care Unit

1. Communicates intraoperative information
   a. Identifies patient by name
   b. States type of surgery performed
   c. Identifies type of anesthetic used
   d. Reports patient's response to surgical procedure and anesthesia
   e. Describes intraoperative factors (ie, insertion of drains or catheters; administration of blood, analgesic agents or other medications during surgery; occurrence of unexpected events)
   f. Describes physical limitations
   g. Reports patient's preoperative level of consciousness
   h. Communicates necessary equipment needs

Postoperative Assessment Recovery Area

1. Determines patient's immediate response to surgical intervention
2. Monitors patient's physiologic status
3. Maintains patient's safety (airway, circulation, prevention of injury)
4. Administers medications, fluid, and blood component therapy, if prescribed
5. Provides oral fluids if prescribed for ambulatory surgery patient
6. Assesses patient's readiness for transfer to inhospital unit or for discharge home

Surgical Unit

1. Continues close monitoring of patient's physical and psychological response to surgical intervention
2. Provides teaching to patient during immediate recovery period
3. Assists patient in recovery and preparation for discharge home
4. Determines patient's psychological status
5. Assists with discharge planning

Home or Clinic

1. Provides follow-up care during office or clinic visit or by telephone contact
2. Reinforces previous teaching and answers patient's and family's questions about surgery and follow-up care
3. Assesses patient's response to surgery and anesthesia and their effects on body image and function
4. Determines family's perception of surgery and its outcome

terms are defined in Table 16-1, and examples of the types of surgery involved are given.

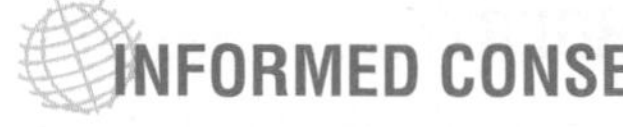

INFORMED CONSENT

Voluntary and informed written consent from the patient is necessary before surgery can be performed. Such written permission protects the patient from unsanctioned surgery and protects the surgeon from claims of an unauthorized operation. In the best interests of all parties concerned, sound medicolegal principles are followed. The nurse may ask the patient to sign the form and may witness the patient's signature; however, it is the physician's responsibility to provide appropriate information. Table 16-2 lists the criteria for a valid **informed consent**.

Before the patient signs the consent form, the surgeon should provide a clear and simple explanation of what the surgery will entail. The surgeon must also inform the patient of alternatives, possible risks, complications, disfigurement, disability, and removal of body parts as well as what to expect in the early and late postoperative periods. If the patient needs additional information to make his or her decision, the nurse notifies the physician about this. Also, the nurse ascertains that the consent form has been signed before administering psychoactive premedication; the consent form may not be valid if consent was obtained while the patient was under the influence of medications that can affect judgment and decision-

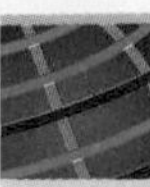

TABLE 16•1 Categories of Surgery Based on Urgency

Classification	Indications for Surgery	Examples
I. Emergency—Patient requires immediate attention; disorder may be life-threatening	Without delay	Severe bleeding Bladder or intestinal obstruction Fractured skull Gunshot or stab wounds Extensive burns
II. Urgent—Patient requires prompt attention	Within 24–30 h	Acute gallbladder infection Kidney or ureteral stones
III. Required—Patient needs to have surgery	Plan within a few weeks or months	Prostatic hyperplasia without bladder obstruction Thyroid disorders Cataracts
IV. Elective—Patient should be operated on	Failure to have surgery not catastrophic	Repair of scars Simple hernia Vaginal repair
V. Optional—Decision rests with patient	Personal preference	Cosmetic surgery

making capacity. Informed consent is necessary in the following circumstances:

- The procedure is invasive, such as a surgical incision, a biopsy, a cystoscopy, or paracentesis.
- Anesthesia is used.
- A nonsurgical procedure is performed in which there is more than slight risk to the patient, such as an arteriogram.
- A procedure is performed that involves radiation.

TABLE 16•2 Criteria for Valid Informed Consent

Component	Comments
Consent voluntarily given	Valid consent must be freely given, without coercion.
Incompetent subject	Legal definition: individuals who are *not* autonomous and cannot give or withhold consent (eg, individuals who are mentally retarded, mentally ill, or comatose)
Informed subject	Informed consent should be in writing It should contain the following: Explanation of procedure and its risks Description of benefits and alternatives An offer to answer questions about procedure Instructions that the patient may withdraw consent A statement informing the patient if the protocol differs from customary procedure
Subject able to comprehend	Information must be written and delivered in language understandable to the patient. Questions must be answered to facilitate comprehension if material is confusing.

The patient personally signs the consent if he or she is of legal age and is mentally capable. When the patient is a minor or is unconscious or incompetent, permission must be obtained from a responsible family member (preferably next of kin) or legal guardian. An emancipated minor (married or independently earning own living) may sign his or her own permit. State regulations and agency policy must be followed. In an emergency, it may be necessary for the surgeon to operate as a lifesaving measure without the patient's informed consent. Every effort, however, must be made to contact the patient's family. In such a situation, contact can be made by telephone, telegram, fax, or other electronic means.

When the patient has doubts and has not had the opportunity to investigate alternative treatments, a second opinion may be requested. No patient should be urged or coerced to sign an operative permit; refusing to undergo a surgical procedure is a person's legal right and privilege. However, such information must be documented and relayed to the surgeon so that other arrangements can be made; for instance, additional explanations may be provided to the patient and family, or the surgery may be rescheduled at a later time.

The consent process can be improved by providing audiovisual materials to supplement discussion, by ensuring that the wording of the consent form is understandable, and by using other strategies and resources as needed to help the patient understand its content.

Nursing Alert *The signed consent form is placed in a prominent place on the patient's chart and accompanies the patient to the operating room.*

NURSING PROCESS: PREPARING THE PATIENT FOR SURGERY

Assessment

Assessment of the surgical patient involves evaluating a wide range of physical and psychological factors. A variety of patient problems or nursing diagnoses can be anticipated or identified on the basis of the data. Detailed discussions of the psychosocial assessment and the physical examination of the surgical patient follow this section.

Nursing Diagnosis

Based on the assessment data, major preoperative nursing diagnoses of the surgical patient may include the following:

- Anxiety related to the surgical experience (anesthesia, pain) and the outcome of surgery
- Risk for ineffective management of therapeutic regimen related to knowledge deficit regarding preoperative procedures and protocols and postoperative expectations

Planning and Goals

The surgical patient's major goals may include relief of preoperative anxiety and increased knowledge of preoperative preparations and postoperative expectations.

Nursing Interventions

Reducing Preoperative Anxiety

Specific nursing interventions are discussed in detail under Psychosocial Nursing Assessment and Interventions.

Providing Patient Education

Specific nursing interventions are discussed in detail in other sections of this chapter under Preoperative Patient Education. See also Preoperative Nursing Interventions and Immediate Preoperative Nursing Interventions.

Evaluation

Expected Outcomes

Expected outcomes may include:

1. Anxiety is relieved
   a. Discusses concerns with anesthesiologist or anesthetist related to types of anesthesia and induction
   b. Verbalizes an understanding of the preanesthetic medication and general anesthesia
   c. Discusses last-minute concerns with nurse or physician
   d. Discusses financial concerns with social worker, when appropriate
   e. Requests visit with member of clergy when appropriate
   f. Relaxes quietly after being visited by health team members
2. Prepares for surgical intervention
   a. Participates in preoperative preparation
   b. Demonstrates and describes exercises he or she is expected to perform postoperatively
   c. Reviews information about postoperative care
   d. Accepts preanesthetic medication, if prescribed
   e. Remains in bed
   f. Relaxes during transportation to operating room or unit
   g. States rationale for use of side rails
3. Participates in discharge planning

PSYCHOSOCIAL NURSING ASSESSMENT AND INTERVENTIONS

Any surgical procedure is preceded by some type of emotional reaction by the patient, whether it is obvious or hidden, normal or abnormal. For example, preoperative anxiety may be an anticipatory response to an experience the patient views as a threat to his or her customary role in life, body integrity, or life itself. Psychological distress directly influences the functioning of the body. Therefore, it is imperative to identify the sources of the anxiety the patient is experiencing.

By taking a careful health history, the nurse elicits patient concerns that can have a bearing on the course of the surgical experience. Undoubtedly, a patient about to undergo surgery is faced with various fears, including fears of the unknown, of death, of anesthesia, of cancer. Concerns about loss of work time, the possible loss of job, the responsibility of family support, and the threat of permanent incapacity further contribute to the emotional strain created by the prospect of surgery. Less obvious concerns may occur because of previous experiences with the health care system and people the patient has known with the same condition. Consequently, the nurse must be a good listener, be empathetic, and provide information that helps alleviate concerns.

The extent of the patient's reaction is based on many factors, including the discomforts and changes anticipated—whether physical, financial, psychological, spiritual, or social—and the surgical outcome expected. Will the operation improve the condition? Will it result in disability? Is this just a temporary measure in a chronic condition?

An important outcome of the assessment is the determination of the role of the patient's family or friends. The value and reliability of all available support systems are also determined. Other information, such as usual level of functioning and typical daily activities, may assist in the patient's care and rehabilitation plans.

Alleviating Fear

Fear is expressed in different ways by different people. For example, fear may be expressed indirectly by the patient who repeatedly asks a lot of questions, even though answers were given previously. For another person, the reaction may be withdrawal—deliberately avoiding communication, perhaps by reading or watching television. Still others may talk about trivialities. When a patient expresses concern or worry about impending surgery, it is important to acknowledge these concerns by listening and communicating therapeutically. To respond to the patient's fears with unwarranted reassurance by saying, "Oh, there's nothing to be afraid of," immediately blocks communication and causes the patient to use less effective means of coping with his or her worries. A preoperative patient may experience a number of fears. Fear of anesthesia, fear of pain or death, fear of the unknown, or fear of deformity or other threats to body image may cause unease and anxiety. The nurse can do much to dispel false conceptions and misinformation and to provide reassurance when possible. In addition to the fears listed here, the patient often has other worries, such as financial problems, family responsibilities, and employment obligations, or fear of a poor prognosis or the probability of disability in the future. The nurse can explore these fears with the patient and arrange for the assistance of other health professionals if required.

Respecting Spiritual and Cultural Beliefs

Spiritual beliefs play an important role in how people cope with fears and anxiety. Regardless of the patient's religious affiliation, spiritual beliefs can be as therapeutic as medication. Every attempt must be made to help the patient obtain the spiritual help that he or she requests. Faith has great sustaining power; thus, the beliefs of each individual patient should be respected and supported.

Some nurses avoid the subject of a clergy visit on the premise that the suggestion may alarm the patient. However, asking if the patient's spiritual adviser knows about the impending surgery is a caring, nonthreatening approach.

Respect for a patient's cultural values and beliefs facilitates rapport and trust. Some areas of assessment include identifying the ethnic group to which the patient relates and the customs and beliefs the patient holds about illness and health care providers. For example, patients from some cultural groups are unaccustomed to expressing feelings openly. Nurses need to consider this pattern of self-control when assessing pain. As a sign of respect, people from other cultural groups may not make direct eye contact with others. It is important for the nurse to know that this lack of eye contact is not avoidance or a lack of interest.

Perhaps the most valuable skill at the disposal of the nurse is listening carefully to the patient, especially when obtaining the patient's history. By engaging in conversation and using communication and interviewing skills, the nurse can acquire invaluable information and insight. An unhurried, understanding, and caring nurse invites confidence on the part of the patient.

GENERAL PHYSICAL ASSESSMENT

Before treatment is initiated, a health history is obtained, a physical examination is performed during which vital signs are noted, and a database is established for future comparisons. During the physical examination, significant physical findings, such as pressure ulcers, edema, or abnormal breath sounds, that further describe the patient's overall condition are noted. Blood tests, x-rays, and other diagnostic testing should only be ordered when specifically indicated by information obtained from a thorough history and physical examination or according to anesthesiology standards of care.

These preliminary contacts with the health care team provide the patient with opportunities to ask questions and to become acquainted with those who might be providing care during and after surgery.

Nutritional Status

Nutritional needs may be determined by the patient's height and weight, body mass index (BMI), triceps skin fold, upper arm circumference, serum protein levels, or nitrogen balance. Any nutrient deficiency should be corrected before surgery to provide enough protein for tissue repair. Nutrients needed for wound healing are summarized in Table 16-3. Obesity greatly increases the risk and severity of complications associated with surgery. During surgery, fatty tissues are especially susceptible to infection. Additionally, obesity creates increased technical and mechanical problems. Therefore, dehiscence (wound separation) and wound infections are more common. The obese patient is often more difficult to care for because of the added weight; the patient tends to breathe poorly when supine, which increases the risk of hypoventilation and postoperative pulmonary complications. In addition, abdominal distention, phlebitis, and cardiovascular, endocrine, hepatic, and biliary diseases occur more readily in obese patients. It has been estimated that for each 30 pounds of excess weight, about 25 additional miles of blood vessels are needed. The increased demands on the heart are obvious.

Dehydration, hypovolemia, and electrolyte imbalances can be a significant problem in the elderly population or in patients with comorbid medical conditions. The degree of severity is often difficult to determine. Mild volume deficits may be treated during surgery; however, additional time may be needed to correct pronounced fluid and electrolyte deficits to promote the best possible preoperative condition.

Drug or Alcohol Use

People who use drugs or alcohol frequently deny or attempt to hide it. This calls for care and attention when obtaining the patient's history, patience, frank questions, and a nonjudgmental attitude on the part of the nurse.

The acutely intoxicated person is susceptible to injury. Therefore, surgery is postponed if possible. If emergency surgery is required, local or regional block anesthesia is used for minor surgery. Otherwise, to prevent vomiting and potential aspiration, a nasogastric tube is inserted before the administration of general anesthesia.

The person with a history of chronic alcoholism often suffers from malnutrition and other systemic problems that increase the surgical risk. Additionally, alcohol withdrawal delirium (delirium tremens) may be anticipated up to 72 hours after alcohol withdrawal, and it is associated with a significant mortality rate when it occurs postoperatively.

Respiratory Status

The goal for potential surgical patients is to have optimum respiratory function. All patients are urged to stop smoking 4 to 6 weeks before surgery and are taught breathing exercises and how to use an incentive spirometer if indicated. Because adequate ventilation is potentially compromised during all phases of surgical treatment, surgery is usually contraindicated when the patient has a respiratory infection. Patients with underlying respiratory disease (eg, asthma, chronic obstructive pulmonary disease) are assessed carefully for current threats to the pulmonary status; their use of medications that may affect their postoperative recovery is assessed.

Cardiovascular Status

The goal in preparing any patient for surgery is to have a well-functioning cardiovascular system to meet the oxygen, fluid, and nutritional needs throughout the perioperative period. If the patient has uncontrolled hypertension, surgery may be postponed until the blood pressure is under control.

Because cardiovascular disease increases risk, patients with these conditions demand greater than usual diligence during all phases of management and care. Depending on the severity of symptoms, surgery may be deferred until medical treatment can be instituted to improve the patient's condition. At times, surgical treatment can be modified to meet the cardiac tolerance of the patient. For example, in a patient with obstruction of the descending colon and coronary artery disease, a temporary simple colostomy may be performed rather than a more extensive colon resection.

Of particular importance in the patient with cardiovascular disease is the need to avoid sudden changes of position, prolonged immobilization, hypotension or hypoxia, and overloading of the circulatory system with fluids or blood.

Hepatic and Renal Function

The goal is to have maximum functioning of the liver and urinary systems so that medications, anesthetic agents, body wastes, and toxins are adequately removed from the body.

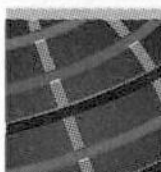

TABLE 16•3 **Nutrients Important for Wound Healing and Recovery**

Nutrient	Rationale for Increased Need	Possible Deficiency Outcome
Protein	To replace the lean body mass lost during the catabolic phase following stress To restore blood volume and plasma proteins lost from exudates, bleeding from the wound, and possible hemorrhage To replace losses resulting from immobility (increased excretion) To meet the increased needs for tissue repair and resistance to infection	Significant weight loss Impaired or delayed wound healing Shock related to decreased blood volume Edema related to decreased serum albumin Diarrhea related to decreased albumin Anemia Increased risk of infection related to decreased antibodies, impaired tissue integrity Decreased lipoprotein synthesis → fatty infiltration of the liver → liver damage Increased mortality
Calories	To replace losses related to NPO, hypermetabolism during catabolic phase following stress To spare protein To restore normal weight	Signs and symptoms of protein deficiency may develop when protein is used to meet energy requirements Extensive weight loss
Water	To replace losses through vomiting, hemorrhage, exudates, fever, drainage, diuresis To maintain homeostasis	Signs, symptoms, and complications of dehydration, such as poor skin turgor, dry mucous membranes, oliguria, anuria, weight loss, increased pulse rate, decreased central venous pressure
Vitamin C	Important for capillary formation, tissue synthesis, and wound healing through collagen formation Needed for antibody formation	Impaired or delayed wound healing related to impaired collagen formation and increased capillary fragility and permeability Increased risk of infection related to decreased antibodies
Thiamine, niacin, riboflavin	Requirements based on metabolic rate: increased metabolic rate → increased requirements	Decreased enzymes available for energy metabolism
Folic acid, vitamin B_{12}	Needed for cell proliferation and therefore tissue synthesis Important for maturation of red blood cells Impaired folic acid synthesis related to some antibiotics; impaired vitamin B_{12} absorption related to some antibiotics	Decreased or arrested cell division Megaloblastic anemia
Vitamin A	Important for tissue synthesis, wound healing, and immune function Enhances resistance to infection	Impaired or delayed wound healing related to decreased collagen synthesis; impaired immune function Increased risk of infection
Vitamin K	Important for normal blood clotting Impaired intestinal synthesis related to antibiotics	Prolonged prothrombin time
Iron	Needed to replace iron lost through blood loss	Signs, symptoms, and complications of iron deficiency anemia, such as fatigue, weakness, pallor, anorexia, dizziness, headaches, stomatitis, glossitis, cardiovascular and respiratory changes, possible cardiac failure
Zinc	Needed for protein synthesis and wound healing Needed for normal lymphocyte and phagocyte response	Impaired or delayed wound healing Impaired immune response

From Dudek, S. G. (1997). *Nutrition handbook for nursing practice* (3rd ed.). Philadelphia: Lippincott-Raven, with permission.

The liver is important in the biotransformation of anesthetic compounds. Therefore, any disorder of the liver has an effect on how an anesthetic is metabolized. Because acute liver disease is associated with a high surgical mortality, preoperative improvement in liver function is desired. Careful assessment is made with various liver function tests (see Chap. 36).

The kidneys are involved in the excretion of anesthetic drugs and their metabolites. Acid–base status and metabolism are also important considerations in anesthetic administration. Surgery is contraindicated when a patient has acute nephritis, acute renal insufficiency with oliguria or anuria, or other acute renal problems, unless the surgery is a lifesaving measure or is necessary to improve urinary function, as in the case of an obstructive uropathy.

Endocrine Function

The patient with diabetes who is undergoing surgery is at risk for hypoglycemia and hyperglycemia. Hypoglycemia may develop during anesthesia or from inadequate carbohydrates postoperatively or excessive administration of insulin. Hyperglycemia may occur with the stress of surgery and increased levels of stress hormones. Hyperglycemia may increase the risk for surgical wound infection. Other risks are acidosis and glucosuria. Although the surgical risk in the patient with controlled diabetes is not greater than that in the nondiabetic patient, the goal is to maintain the blood glucose level at less than 200 mg/dL. Frequent monitoring of blood glucose levels is important before, during, and after surgery (see Chap. 37 for discussion of the patient with diabetes undergoing surgery).

Patients receiving corticosteroids are at risk for adrenal insufficiency; therefore, the use of steroid medications for any purpose during the preceding year must be reported to the anesthesiologist and surgeon. Additionally, the patient is monitored for signs of adrenal insufficiency.

Patients with uncontrolled thyroid disorders are at risk for thyrotoxicosis (with hyperthyroid disorders) and respiratory failure (with hypothyroid disorders). Therefore, the patient is assessed for a history of these disorders.

Immunologic Function

An important function of preoperative assessment is to determine the existence of allergies, including the nature of previous allergic reactions. It is especially important to identify and document any sensitivities to medications and past adverse reactions to these agents. The patient is asked to identify any substances that precipitated previous allergic reactions, including medications, blood transfusions, contrast agents, latex, and food products, and to describe the signs and symptoms produced by these substances. A history of bronchial asthma is reported to the anesthesiologist.

Immunosuppression is common with corticosteroid therapy, renal transplantation, radiation therapy, chemotherapy, and disorders affecting the immune system (eg, acquired immunodeficiency syndrome [AIDS], leukemia). The mildest symptoms or slightest temperature elevation must be investigated. Because these patients are highly susceptible to infection, great care is taken to use strict asepsis.

Previous Medication Therapy

A medication history is obtained from each patient because of the possible effects of medications on the patient's perioperative and perianesthesia course and the possibility of drug interaction effects. Any medication the patient is using or has used in the past is documented, including over-the-counter (OTC) preparations and the frequency with which they are taken. Potent medications have an effect on physiologic functions; interactions of such medications with anesthetic agents can cause serious problems, such as arterial hypotension and circulatory collapse.

The potential effects of prior medication therapy are evaluated by the anesthesiologist or anesthetist, who considers the length of time the patient has used the medications, the physical condition of the patient, and the nature of the proposed surgery. Medications that cause particular concern include the following:

Adrenal corticosteroids—Corticosteroids are not to be discontinued abruptly before surgery. A person who has been taking steroids for some time may suffer cardiovascular collapse if the steroids are discontinued suddenly. Therefore, a bolus of steroid may be administered intravenously immediately before and after surgery.

Diuretics—Thiazide diuretics may cause excessive respiratory depression during anesthesia; this results from an associated electrolyte imbalance.

Phenothiazines—These medications may increase the hypotensive action of anesthetics.

Antidepressants—Monoamine oxidase (MAO) inhibitors increase the hypotensive effects of anesthetics.

Tranquilizers—Barbiturates, diazepam, and chlordiazepoxide may cause anxiety, tension, and even seizures if withdrawn suddenly.

Insulin—Interaction between anesthetics and insulin must be considered when a patient with diabetes is undergoing surgery.

Antibiotics—"Mycin" drugs, such as neomycin, kanamycin, and, less frequently, streptomycin, may present problems; when these medications are combined with a curariform muscle relaxant, nerve transmission is interrupted, and apnea due to respiratory paralysis may result.

For the reasons cited, it is imperative that the patient's medication history be assessed by the nurse and anesthesiologist or anesthetist.

Assessing the Ambulatory Surgical Patient

The health history of the ambulatory or same-day surgical patient is often obtained by telephone interview or at the time of preadmission testing. The interview includes questions relating to recent and past health history, allergies, medications, preoperative preparation, and psychosocial and demographic factors. The patient undergoing **ambulatory surgery** should be in stable medical condition and free of infection. It may be better for the person with a mild systemic disease to have a surgical procedure in the short-term facility than be exposed to the risks associated with hospitalization. Age is not usually a factor; however, it is desirable that the patient be psychologically willing to accept this mode of treatment. The physical assessment is completed the day of surgery.

Gerontologic Considerations

An older person undergoing surgery may have a combination of chronic illnesses and health problems in addition to the specific one for which surgery is indicated. Elderly people frequently do not report symptoms, perhaps because they fear that a serious illness may be diagnosed or because they accept such symptoms as part of the aging process. Subtle clues alert the nurse to underlying problems.

The hazards of surgery for the aged are proportional to the number and severity of coexisting health problems and the nature and duration of the operative procedure. The underlying principle that guides the preoperative assessment, surgery, and postoperative care is that the aged patient has less physiologic reserve (the ability of an organ to return to normal after a disturbance in its equilibrium) than the younger patient. Cardiac reserves are lower, renal and hepatic function are depressed, and gastrointestinal activity is likely to be reduced. Dehydration, constipation, and malnutrition may be evident.

Sensory limitations, such as impaired vision or hearing and reduced tactile sensitivity, are often the reasons for accidents, injuries, and burns. Therefore, the nurse must be alert to maintaining a safe environment. Arthritis is common in older people and may affect mobility, making it difficult for the patient to turn from one side to the other or ambulate without discomfort. Protective measures include adequate padding for tender areas, moving the patient slowly, protecting bony prominences from prolonged pressure, and providing gentle massage to promote adequate circulation.

The condition of the mouth is important to assess. Dental caries, dentures, and partial plates are particularly significant to the anesthesiologist or anesthetist because decayed teeth or dental prostheses may become dislodged during intubation and occlude the airway.

Decreased perspiration leads to dry, itchy skin. Such fragile skin is easily abraded, so added precautions are taken when moving an elderly person. Decreased subcutaneous fat makes older people more susceptible to temperature changes. A lightweight cotton blanket is an appropriate cover when an elderly patient is moved to and from the operating room.

The elderly person has undoubtedly experienced many personal illnesses and possibly life-threatening illnesses of friends and family. Such experiences may result in fears about the surgery and about the future. Providing an opportunity to express these fears enables the patient to gain some peace of mind and a sense of being understood.

Although important for every patient, the requirements for optimum results after surgery on an elderly patient are of even greater importance because of greater risks. These requirements include (1) skillful preoperative assessment and treatment, (2) skillful anesthesia and surgery, and (3) meticulous and competent postoperative and postanesthesia management.

In summary, the overall goal in the preoperative period is to have as many positive health factors as possible. Every attempt is made to stabilize those conditions that otherwise hinder a smooth recovery. When negative factors dominate, the risks of surgery and postoperative complications increase.

PREOPERATIVE PATIENT EDUCATION

The value of preoperative instruction has long been recognized. Each patient is taught as an individual, with consideration for any unique concerns or needs, so that a program of instruction based on the individual's learning needs can be planned and implemented. Teaching should begin as soon as possible. It may start in the physician's office and continue until the patient arrives in the operating room.

Ideally, instruction is spaced over a period of time to allow the patient to assimilate information and ask questions as they arise. Frequently, teaching sessions are combined with various preparation procedures to allow for an easy flow of information. In reality, the nurse must make a judgment about how much the patient wants and needs to know and can grasp in the limited time available. In some instances, too much detail raises the patient's anxiety level.

Teaching should go beyond descriptions of the procedure and should include explanations of the sensations the patient will experience. For example, telling the patient only that preoperative medication will relax him or her before the operation is not as effective as also noting that the medication may result in lightheadedness and drowsiness. Knowing what to expect will help the patient anticipate these reactions and thus attain a higher degree of relaxation than might otherwise be expected.

The ideal timing for preoperative teaching is not on the day of surgery but during the preadmission visit when diagnostic tests are being performed. At this time, the nurse or resource person answers questions and provides important patient teaching. During this visit, the patient can meet and ask questions of the perianesthesia nurse, view audiovisuals, receive written materials, and be given the telephone number to call as questions arise closer to the date of surgery.

Risk Factors for SURGICAL COMPLICATIONS

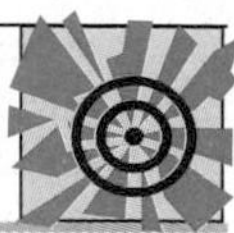

Systemic Factors

- Hypovolemia
- Dehydration or electrolyte imbalance
- Nutritional deficits
- Extremes of age
- Extremes of weight
- Infection and sepsis
- Toxic conditions
- Immunologic abnormalities
- Pulmonary disease
  - Obstructive disease
  - Restrictive disorder
  - Respiratory infection
- Renal or urinary tract disease
  - Decreased renal function
  - Urinary tract infection
  - Obstruction
- Pregnancy
  - Diminished maternal physiologic reserve
- Cardiovascular disease
  - Coronary artery disease or previous myocardial infarction
  - Cardiac failure
  - Dysrhythmias
  - Hypertension
  - Prosthetic heart valve
  - Thromboembolism
  - Hemorrhagic diathesis
  - Cerebrovascular disease
- Endocrine dysfunction
  - Diabetes mellitus
  - Adrenal disorders
  - Thyroid malfunction
- Hepatic disease
  - Cirrhosis
  - Hepatitis

Teaching Deep Breathing and Coughing Exercises

One goal of preoperative nursing care is to teach the patient how to promote optimal lung expansion and consequent blood oxygenation after anesthesia. The patient assumes a sitting position to enhance lung expansion. The nurse then demonstrates how to take a deep, slow breath (maximal sustained inspiration [MSI]) and how to exhale slowly. After practicing deep breathing several times, the patient is instructed to breathe deeply, exhale through the mouth, take a short breath, and cough from deep in the lungs (see illustrations in the patient education chart). In addition to enhancing respiration, these exercises may help the patient to relax.

If there will be a thoracic or abdominal incision, the nurse demonstrates how the incision line can be splinted so that pressure is minimized and pain is controlled. The patient should put the palms of both hands together, interlacing the fingers snugly. Placing the hands across the incisional site acts as an effective splint when coughing. In addition, the patient is informed that medications are available to relieve pain and that they should be taken regularly for pain relief to enable effective deep breathing and coughing exercises. The goal in promoting coughing is to mobilize secretions so they can be removed. When a deep breath is taken before coughing, the cough reflex is stimulated. If the patient does not cough effectively, hypostatic pneumonia and other lung complications may occur.

Encouraging Mobility and Active Body Movement

The goals of promoting mobility postoperatively are to improve circulation, prevent venous stasis, and promote optimal respiratory function.

The nurse explains the rationale for frequent position changes after surgery. The patient is then shown how to turn from side to side and how to assume the lateral position without causing pain or disrupting intravenous lines, drainage tubes, or other apparatus. Any special position the individual patient will need to maintain after surgery is discussed (eg, adduction or elevation of an extremity), as is the importance of maintaining as much mobility as possible despite restrictions. Reviewing the process before surgery is helpful to the patient who may be too uncomfortable after surgery to absorb new information.

Exercises of the extremities include extension and flexion of the knee and hip joints (similar to bicycle riding while lying on the side). The foot is rotated as though tracing the largest possible circle with the great toe (see illustrations in the patient education chart). The elbow and shoulder are also put through range of motion. At first, the patient is assisted and reminded to perform these exercises, but later, the patient is encouraged to do them independently. Muscle tone is maintained so that ambulation will be easier.

The nurse is reminded to use proper body mechanics and to instruct the patient to do the same. When the patient is placed in any position, his or her body is maintained in proper alignment.

Explaining Pain Management

Postoperatively, medications are administered to relieve pain and maintain comfort without increasing the risk for inadequate air exchange. The patient is instructed to take the medication as frequently as prescribed during the initial postoperative period for pain relief. Anticipated methods of administration of analgesic agents for inpatients are patient-controlled analgesia (PCA), epidural catheter bolus or infusion, or patient-controlled epidural analgesia (PCEA). A patient who is expected to go home would receive oral analgesic agents. These are discussed with the patient before surgery, and the inpatient's interest and willingness to participate in use of those methods are assessed. The patient is instructed in use of a pain intensity rating scale to promote effective postoperative pain management.

Teaching Cognitive Coping Strategies

Cognitive strategies may be useful for relieving tension, overcoming anxiety, and achieving relaxation. Examples of such strategies include the following:

Imagery—The patient is encouraged to concentrate on a pleasant experience or restful scene.

Distraction—The patient is encouraged to think of an enjoyable story or recite a favorite poem.

Optimistic self-recitation—The patient is encouraged to recite optimistic thoughts ("I know all will go well").

Providing Information

The patient benefits from knowing when family and friends will be able to visit after surgery and that a spiritual advisor will be available if desired. Knowing ahead of time about the possible need for a ventilator, the presence of drainage tubes, or other types of equipment will help the patient accept these devices in the postoperative period.

Teaching the Ambulatory Surgical Patient

Preoperative education for the same-day or ambulatory surgical patient comprises all the material presented earlier in this chapter as well as collaborative planning with the patient and family for discharge and follow-up home care. The major difference in outpatient preoperative education is the teaching environment.

Preoperative teaching content may be presented in a group meeting, on a videotape, during night classes, at preadmission testing, or by telephone in conjunction with the preoperative interview. In addition to answering questions and describing what to expect, the nurse tells the patient when and where to report, what to bring (insurance card, list of medications and allergies), what to leave at home (jewelry, watch, medications, contact lenses), and what to wear (loose-fitting, comfortable clothes; flat shoes). The nurse in the surgeon's office may initiate teaching before the perioperative telephone contact. The last preoperative phone call is designed to remind the patient not to eat or drink as directed.

PREOPERATIVE NURSING INTERVENTIONS

Managing Nutrition and Fluids

Until recently, fluid and food were restricted preoperatively overnight and often longer. However, recent review of this practice by the American Society of Anesthesiologists (ASA) has resulted in new recommendations for persons undergoing elective surgery who are otherwise healthy. The major purpose of withholding food and fluid before surgery is to prevent aspiration. However, studies have demonstrated that in the absence of coexisting diseases or disorders that affect gastric emptying or fluid volume (eg., pregnancy, obesity, diabetes, gastroesophageal reflux, enteral tube feeding, ileus or bowel obstruction) or of a compromised airway, lengthy restriction of fluid and food is unnecessary (American Society of Anesthesiologists, 1998).

The ASA recommends a fasting period for a light meal (eg., toast and a clear liquid) of 6 hours or more and clear liquids for 2 to 4 hours before surgical procedures requiring general anesthesia, regional anesthesia, or conscious sedation. Clear liquids include water, fruit juices without pulp, carbonated beverages, clear tea, and black coffee; they exclude alcohol. A fasting period of 8 hours or more is recommended for a meal that includes fried or fatty foods or meat. The anesthesiologist or anesthetist may restrict foods and fluids for longer periods of time depending on the patient's fluid status, age, pulmonary status, and the nature of the surgical procedure.

The purpose of withholding food before surgery is prevention of aspiration. Aspiration occurs when food or fluid is regurgitated from the stomach and enters the pulmonary system. Such inhaled material acts as a foreign substance, is irritating, and causes an inflammatory reaction that interferes with adequate air exchange. Aspiration is a serious problem and has a high mortality rate

(*text continues on page 326*)

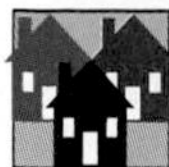

PATIENT EDUCATION AND HOME CARE

Preoperative Instructions to Prevent Complications

Preoperative teaching for patients undergoing surgery includes instruction in breathing and leg exercises used to prevent postoperative complications, such as pneumonia and deep vein thrombosis. These exercises may be performed in the hospital or at home.

Diaphragmatic Breathing

Diaphragmatic breathing refers to a flattening of the dome of the diaphragm during inspiration, with resultant enlargement of the upper abdomen as air rushes in. During expiration, the abdominal muscles contract.

1. Practice in the same position you would assume in bed after surgery: a semi-Fowler's position, propped in bed with the back and shoulders well supported with pillows.
2. With your hands in a loose-fist position, allow the hands to rest lightly on the front of the lower ribs, with your fingertips against lower chest to feel the movement.

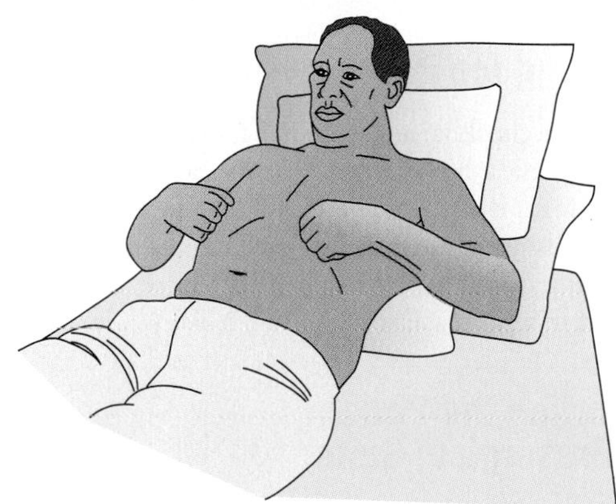

Diaphragmatic breathing

3. Breathe out gently and fully as the ribs sink down and inward toward midline.
4. Then take a deep breath through your nose and mouth, letting the abdomen rise as the lungs fill with air.
5. Hold this breath for a count of five.
6. Exhale and let out *all* the air through your nose and mouth.
7. Repeat this exercise 15 times with a short rest after each group of five.
8. Practice this twice a day preoperatively.

Coughing

1. Lean forward slightly from a sitting position in bed, interlace your fingers together, and place your hands across the incisional site to act as a splintlike support when coughing.

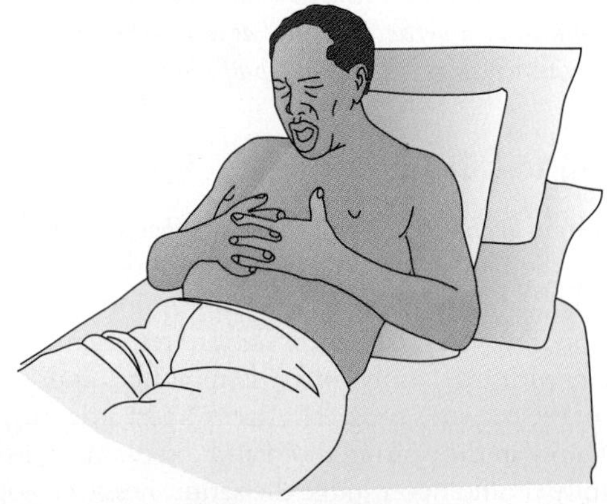

Splinting when coughing

2. Breathe with the diaphragm as described under "Diaphragmatic Breathing."
3. With your mouth slightly open, breathe in fully.
4. "Hack" out sharply for three short breaths.
5. Then, keeping your mouth open, take in a quick deep breath and immediately give a strong cough once or twice. This helps clear secretions from your chest. It may cause some discomfort but will not harm your incision.

Leg Exercises

1. Lie in a semi-Fowler's position and perform the following simple exercises to improve circulation.
2. Bend your knee and raise your foot—hold it a few seconds, then extend the leg and lower it to the bed.

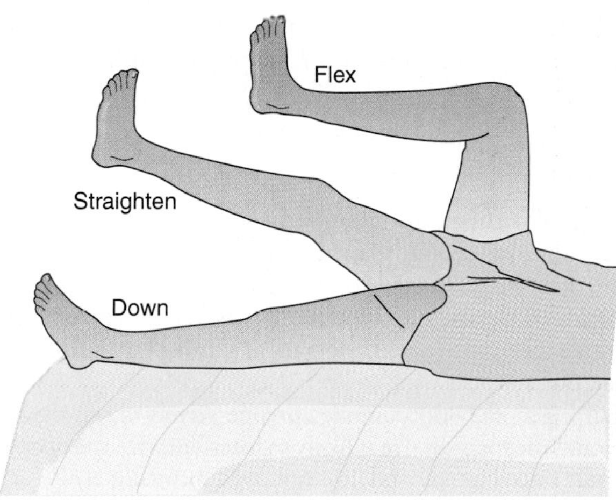

Leg exercises

3. Do this five times with one leg, then repeat with the other leg.
4. Then trace circles with the feet by bending them down, in toward each other, up, and then out.

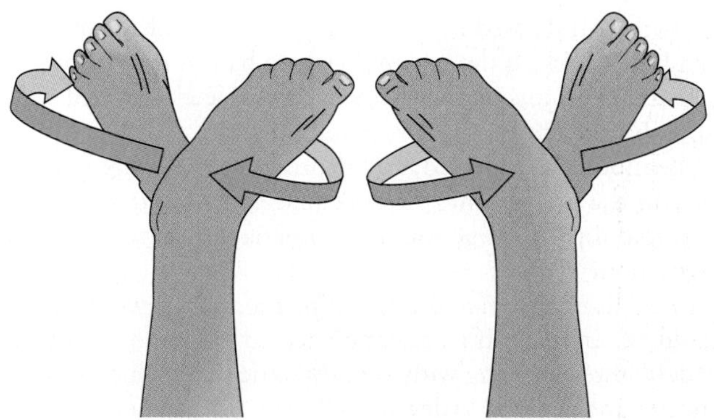

Foot exercises

5. Repeat these movements five times.

Turning to the Side

1. Turn on your side with the uppermost leg flexed most and supported on a pillow.
2. Grasp the side rail as an aid to maneuver to the side.
3. Practice diaphragmatic breathing and coughing while on your side.

Getting Out of Bed

1. Turn on your side.
2. Push yourself up with one hand as you swing your legs out of bed.

(60% to 70%) when it occurs. In those circumstances in which the patient is assessed as at high risk for aspiration, more stringent food and fluid restrictions are prescribed by the anesthesiologist or anesthetist. Fluids may be administered intravenously in some patients to ensure an adequate fluid volume when oral fluids are restricted.

Preparing the Bowel for Surgery

Enemas are not commonly ordered preoperatively unless the patient is undergoing abdominal or pelvic surgery. In this case, a cleansing enema or laxative may be prescribed the evening before surgery and may be repeated the morning of surgery. This is to allow satisfactory visualization of the surgical site and to prevent trauma to the intestine or accidental contamination of the peritoneum by feces. Unless the condition of the patient presents some contraindication, the toilet or bedside commode, rather than the bedpan, is used for evacuation of the enema if the patient is hospitalized during this time. Additionally, antibiotics may be prescribed to reduce intestinal flora.

Preparing the Skin

The goal of preoperative skin preparation is to decrease bacteria without injuring the skin. If the surgery is not an emergency, the patient may be instructed to use a soap containing a detergent-germicide to cleanse the skin area for several days before surgery to reduce the number of skin organisms; this preparation may be carried out at home.

Hair is generally not removed preoperatively unless the hair at or around the incision site is likely to interfere with the operation.

If hair must be removed, it is removed immediately before the operation using electric clippers.

IMMEDIATE PREOPERATIVE NURSING INTERVENTIONS

The patient is dressed in a hospital gown that is left untied and open in the back. If the patient has long hair, it may be braided; hairpins are removed, and the hair is completely covered with a disposable paper cap.

The mouth is inspected, and dentures or plates are removed. If left in the mouth, these items could easily fall to the back of the throat during induction of anesthesia and cause respiratory obstruction.

Jewelry is not worn to the operating room; even wedding rings should be removed. If a patient objects to the removal of a ring, securely fasten the ring with tape. All articles of value, including dentures and prosthetic devices, are given to family members or are labeled clearly with the patient's name and stored in a safe place according to agency policy.

All patients (except those with urologic disorders) should void immediately before going to the operating room to promote continence during low abdominal surgery and to make abdominal organs more accessible. Catheterization is performed in the operating room as necessary. The catheter is connected to a closed drainage system.

Administering Preanesthetic Medication

The use of preanesthetic medication (eg, sedatives, anxiolytics) is minimal with ambulatory or outpatient surgery and, if prescribed, is usually administered in the holding area. If a preanesthetic medication is administered, the patient is kept in bed with the side rails raised because the medication can cause lightheadedness or drowsiness. During this time, the nurse observes the patient for any untoward reaction to the medications. The immediate surroundings are kept quiet to promote relaxation.

Often, surgery is delayed or operating room schedules are changed, and it becomes impossible to request that a medication be given at a specific time. In these situations, the preoperative medication is prescribed "on call from operating room." The nurse can have the medication ready to give and administer it as soon as a call is received from the operating room staff. It usually takes 15 to 20 minutes to prepare the patient for the operating room. If the nurse gives the medication before attending to the other details of preoperative preparation, the patient will have at least partial benefit from the preoperative medication and will have a smoother anesthetic and operative course.

Maintaining the Preoperative Record

A preoperative checklist is shown in Figure 16-1. The completed chart accompanies the patient to the operating room. The surgical consent form is also attached, as are all laboratory reports and nurses' records. Any unusual last-minute observations that may have a bearing on the anesthesia or surgery are noted at the front of the chart in a prominent place.

Transporting the Patient to the Presurgical Suite

The patient is transferred to the holding area or presurgical suite in a bed or on a stretcher about 30 to 60 minutes before the anesthetic is to be given. The stretcher should be as comfortable as possible, with a sufficient number of blankets to ensure against chilling in air-conditioned rooms. A small pillow at the head is usually provided.

The patient is taken to the preoperative holding area and is greeted by name and made to feel in safe hands. The area must be quiet if the preoperative medication is to have maximal effect. Unpleasant sounds or conversation should be avoided because they might be misinterpreted by a sedated patient who overhears them.

Nursing Alert *It is important that someone be with the preoperative patient at all times. Someone must be present with the patient to provide reassurance as well as to ensure safety. Reassurance can be communicated verbally as well as nonverbally by facial expression, manner, or the warm grasp of a hand.*

Attending to Family Needs

Most hospitals and surgicenters have a special surgical waiting room where the family can wait while the patient is undergoing surgery. This room may be equipped with comfortable chairs, television, telephones, and facilities for light refreshment. Volunteers may remain with the family, offer them coffee, and keep them informed of the patient's progress. After surgery, the surgeon may meet the family in the waiting room and discuss the outcome.

The family should never judge the seriousness of an operation by the length of time the patient is in the operating room. A patient may be in surgery much longer than the actual operating time for several reasons:

1. Patient's name: ______ Date: ______ Height: ______ Weight: ______
   Identification band present: ______
2. Informed consent signed: ______ Special permits signed: ______ (Ex: Sterilization)
3. History & physical examination report present: ______ Date: ______
4. Laboratory records present: ______
   CBC: ______ Hgb: ______ Urinalysis: ______ Hct: ______

5. Item	Present	Removed
a. Natural teeth	______	______
Dentures; upper, lower, partial	______	______
Bridge, fixed; crown	______	______
b. Contact lenses	______	______
c. Other prostheses—type: ______	______	______
d. Jewelry:		
Wedding band (taped/tied)	______	______
Rings	______	______
Earrings: pierced, clip-on	______	______
Neck chains	______	______
e. Make-up	______	______
Nail polish	______	______
6. Clothing		
a. Clean patient gown	______	______
b. Cap	______	______
c. Sanitary pad, etc.	______	______

7. Family instructed where to wait? ______
8. Valuables secured? ______
9. Blood available? ______ Ordered? ______ Where? ______
10. Preanesthetic medication given: ______
    Signature Time
11. Voided: ______ Amount: ______ Time: ______ Catheter: ______
    Mouth care given: ______
12. Vital signs: Temperature: ______ Pulse: ______ Resp: ______ Blood Pressure: ______
13. Special problems/precautions: (Allergies, deafness, *etc.*): ______
14. Area of skin preparation: ______
15. ______ Date: ______ Time: ______
    Signature: Nurse releasing patient

FIGURE 16•1 Preoperative checklist.

- It is customary to send for the patient some time in advance of the actual operating time.
- Anesthesiologists and anesthetists often make additional preparations that may take from 30 to 60 minutes.
- Occasionally, the surgeon takes longer than expected with the preceding case, which delays the start of the next surgical procedure.
- After surgery, the patient is taken to the postanesthesia care unit (recovery room) to ensure satisfactory emergence from the anesthetic.

Those waiting to see the patient after surgery should be informed that the patient may have certain equipment or devices in place when returned to the room (ie, intravenous lines, indwelling urinary catheter, nasogastric tube, suction bottles, oxygen lines, monitoring equipment, and blood transfusion lines). When the patient returns to the room, the nurse provides explanations regarding the frequent postoperative observations. However, it is the responsibility of the surgeon—not the nurse—to relay the surgical findings and the prognosis, even when the findings are favorable.

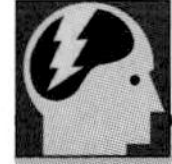

Critical Thinking Exercises

1. During the preoperative assessment of a patient scheduled for a major surgical procedure, the patient's responses suggest to you that he does not understand the procedure and the effect it will have on his ability to function postoperatively. What further assessment is indicated and what actions are warranted?

2. A patient with a long history of severe asthma is scheduled for major surgery. What effect would this information have on your preoperative care of this patient?

3. Two patients are admitted to the same-day surgery unit for a hip replacement. One patient is 40 years old and the other is 72 years old. How would your assessments and preoperative preparation differ for these two patients?

References and Selected Readings

BOOKS

Agency for Health Care Policy and Research. (1992). *Acute pain management: Operative or medical procedures and trauma.* Clinical Practice Guideline. Washington, DC: Public Health Service, U.S. Department of Health and Human Services.

American Society of Anesthesiology. (1995). *ASA standards for post anesthesia care.* Park Ridge, IL: American Society of Anesthesiology.

American Society of Anesthesiologists. (1998). *Practice guidelines for preoperative fasting and the use of pharmacologic agents to reduce the risk of pulmonary aspiration: Application to healthy patients undergoing elective procedures.* (http://www.asahq.org/practice/)

American Society of PeriAnesthesia Nurses. (1998). *Standards of perianesthesia nursing practice.* Thorofare, NJ: ASPAN.

Applegeet, C. J. (1993). *AORN patient classification instrument for perioperative nursing.* Denver: Association of Operating Room Nurses.

Benedetti, C., Chapman, R., & Giron, G. (Eds.). (1990). *Advances in pain research and therapy.* (Vol 14). New York: Raven Press.

DeFazio-Quinn, D. M. (Ed.). (1999). *Ambulatory surgical nursing core curriculum.* Philadelphia: W. B. Saunders.

Drain, C. B. (Ed.). (1996). *The postanesthesia care unit: A critical care approach to postanesthesia nursing.* Philadelphia: W. B. Saunders.

Economou, S. G., & Economou, T. S. (1999). *Instructions for surgery patients.* Philadelphia: W. B. Saunders.

Fairchild, S. (1996). *Perioperative nursing: Principles and practice.* Boston: Little, Brown.

Fitzpatrick, J. J. (1998). *Encyclopedia of nursing research.* New York: Springer Publishing Co.

Hanson, G. C. (Ed.). (1997). *Critical care of the surgical patient.* New York: Chapman and Hall Medical.

Kneedler, J. A., & Dodge, G. H. (1994). *Perioperative patient care: The nursing perspective* (3rd ed.). Boston: Jones & Bartlett.

Kost, M. (1998). Manual of conscious sedation. Philadelphia: W. B. Saunders.

Litwack, K. (Ed.). (1999). *Core curriculum for perianesthesia nursing practice.* Philadelphia: W. B. Saunders.

McGoldrick, K. E. (1995). *Ambulatory anesthesiology: A problem-oriented approach.* Baltimore: Williams & Wilkins.

Meeker, M. H., Rothrock, J. C., & Alexander, E. L. (Eds.). (1999). *Alexander's care of the patient in surgery.* St. Louis: Mosby–Year Book.

Merli, G., & Weitz, H. (Eds.). (1998). *Medical management of the surgical patient.* (2nd ed.). Philadelphia: W. B. Saunders.

Miller, T. A. (Ed.). (1998). *Modern surgical care: Physiologic foundations and clinical applications.* St. Louis: Quality Medical.

Schirmer, B. D., & Rattner, D. W. (1998). *Ambulatory surgery.* Philadelphia: W. B. Saunders.

Schwartz, S., & Shires, G. T. (1999). *Principles of surgery.* New York: McGraw-Hill.

JOURNALS

Asterisks indicate nursing research articles.

Ambulatory Surgery

Beatty A. M., Martin D. E., Couch, M., & Long N. (1997). Relevance of oral intake and necessity to void as ambulatory surgical discharge criteria. *Journal of Perianesthesia Nursing, 12*(6), 413–421.

Brockway, P. M. (1997). The ambulatory surgical nurse: Evolution, competency and vision. *Nursing Clinics of North America, 32*(2), 387–394.

*Coslow, B. I. F., & Eddy M. E. (1998). Effects of preoperative ambulatory gynecological education: Clinical outcomes and patient satisfaction. *Journal of Perianesthesia Nursing, 13*(1), 4–10.

DeFazio-Quinn, D. M. (1997). Ambulatory surgery: An evolution. *Nursing Clinics of North America, 32*(2), 377–386.

Dunn, D. (1998). Preoperative assessment criteria and patient teaching for ambulatory surgery patients. *Journal of Perianesthesia Nursing, 13*(5), 274–291.

*Hession, M. (1998). Factors influencing successful discharge after outpatient laparoscopic cholecystectomy. *Journal of Perianesthesia Nursing, 13*(1), 11–15.

Ireland, D. (1997). Legal issues in ambulatory surgery. *Nursing Clinics of North America, 32*(2), 469–476.

Lancaster, K. A. (1997). Patient teaching in ambulatory surgery. *Nursing Clinics of North America, 32*(2), 417–427.

Litwack, K. (1997). Care of the special needs patient. *Nursing Clinics of North America, 32*(2), 457–467.

New, S. W., & Gutierrez, L. (1997). Quality improvement in the ambulatory surgical setting. *Nursing Clinics of North America, 32*(2), 477–488.

Swan, B. A. (1996). Assessing symptom distress in ambulatory surgery patients. *MedSurg Nursing, 5*(5), 348–354.

Anesthesia and Surgery

Arsenault, C. (1998). Nurses' guide to general anesthesia. Part I. *Nursing, 28*(3), 32.

Booth, M. (1998). Clinical aspects of CRNA practice: Sedation and monitored anesthesia care. *Nursing Clinics of North America, 31*(3), 667–682.

Ferrara-Love, R. (1997). Laparoscopic surgery. *Nursing Clinics of North America, 32*(2), 429–440.

Goldstein, F. J. (1995). Preemptive analgesia: A research review. *MedSurg Nursing 4*, 305–308.

Oulette, S. M. (1998). Clinical aspects of CRNA practice: General anesthesia. *Nursing Clinics of North America, 31*(3), 623–642.

Perrin, L. S., Penta, B. A., & Patton, S. B. (1997). Designing a conscious sedation program: A collaborative approach. *Critical Care Nursing Clinics of North America, 9*(3), 251–272.

Spitzer, L E. (1998). Clinical aspects of CRNA practice: Regional anesthesia. *Nursing Clinics of North America, 31*(3), 643–665.

Wiklund, R. A., & Rosenbaum, S. H. (1997). Anesthesiology (the first of two parts). *New England Journal of Medicine, 337*(16), 1132–1141.

Wiklund, R. A., & Rosenbaum, S. H. (1997). Anesthesiology (the second of two parts). *New England Journal of Medicine, 337*(17), 1215–1219.

Perioperative Nursing

*Gatson-Grindel, C. (1996). Building nursing's minimum data set: The results of a pilot study. *MedSurg Nursing, 5*(6), 449–456.

Geier, K. (1998). Perioperative blood management. *Orthopaedic Nursing, 17*(Suppl.), 6–38.

McConnell, E. A. (1997). Reflections on the art and science of perianesthesia nursing. *Journal of Perianesthesia Nursing, 12*(4), 234–239.

Redmond, M. C. (1996). Latex allergy: Recognition and perioperative management. [Review] [14 refs] *Journal of Post Anesthesia Nursing, 11*(1): 6–12.

Salipante, D. M. (1998). Refusal of blood by a critically ill patient. *Critical Care Nurse, 18*(2), 68–76.

Warner, M. E. (1997). Risks and outcomes of perioperative pulmonary aspiration. *Journal of Perianesthesia Nursing, 12*(5), 352–357.

Preoperative Nursing

Posel, N. (1998). Preoperative teaching in the preadmission clinic. *Journal of Nursing Staff Development, 14*(1), 52–56.

Smetana, G. W. (1999). Preoperative pulmonary evaluation. *New England Journal of Medicine, 340*(12): 937–944.

Williams, G. D. (1997). Preoperative assessment and health history interview. *Nursing Clinics of North America, 32*(2), 395–416.

Zambricki, C. (1998). Clinical aspects of the preanesthetic evaluation. *Nursing Clinics of North America, 31*(3), 607–621.

Resources

American Society of PeriAnesthesia Nurses, 6900 Grove Road, Thorofare, NJ 08086; 1-609-845-5557; www.aspan.org.

Association of Operating Room Nurses, Inc., 2170 S. Parker Rd., Suite 300, Denver, CO 80231; 1-303-755-6304; www.aorn.org.

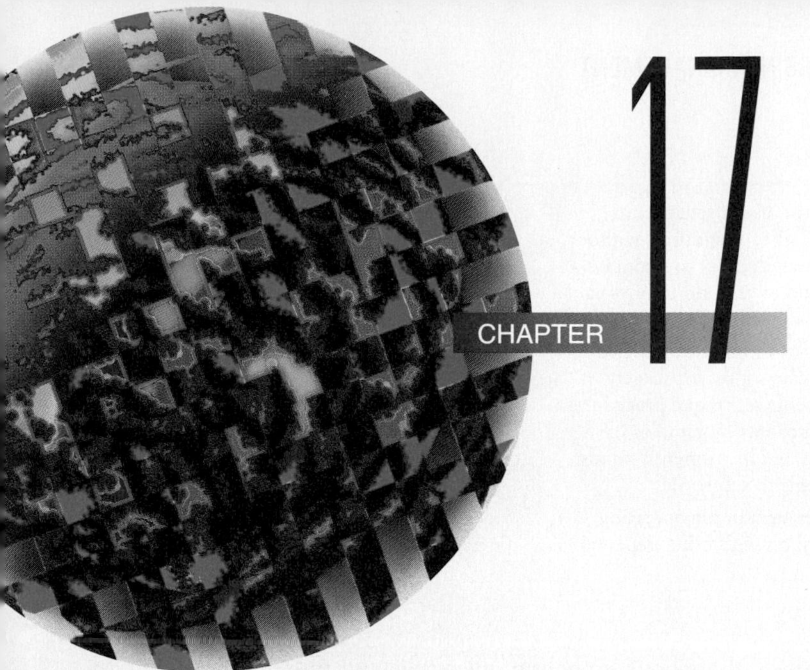

Intraoperative Nursing Management

Learning Objectives

On completion of this chapter, the learner will be able to:

1. Describe the interdisciplinary approach to the care of the patient during surgery.
2. Describe the principles and basic guidelines of surgical asepsis.
3. Describe the role of the anesthesiologist or anesthetist in the preoperative and intraoperative care of the patient.
4. Identify adverse effects of surgery and anesthesia.
5. Identify the risk factors related to surgery in elderly people and nursing interventions to reduce risks to the elderly surgical patient.
6. Compare the various types of anesthesia with regard to uses, advantages, disadvantages, and nursing responsibilities.

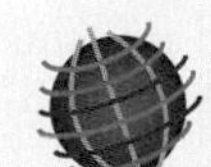

The patient in the intraoperative phase of the surgical experience is very vulnerable. Anesthesia and surgery place the patient at risk for multiple complications or adverse events. Consciousness or full awareness, mobility, protective biologic functions, and personal control are totally or partially relinquished by the patient on entering the operating room. The departments of anesthesia, nursing, and surgery and their staff work collaboratively to implement professional standards of care, to control iatrogenic and individual risks, and foster high-quality patient outcomes.

GLOSSARY

anesthesia: a state of narcosis, analgesia, relaxation and reflex loss

anesthesiologist: physician trained to deliver anesthesia and to monitor patient's condition during surgery

anesthetist: health care professional, such as a nurse anesthetist, who is trained to deliver anesthesia and to monitor patient's condition during surgery

circulating nurse: registered nurse in the operating room who coordinates and documents patient care in the operating room

conscious sedation: use of sedation to depress the level of consciousness without altering the patient's ability to maintain a patent airway and to respond to physical stimuli and verbal commands

scrub nurse: registered nurse or licensed practical nurse who scrubs for surgery and performs sterile technique procedures in the operating room (eg, handles sterile surgical supplies and instruments, hands sterile instruments to surgeon)

unrestricted zone: area in the operating room that interfaces with other departments; includes patient reception area and holding area

semirestricted zone: area in the operating room where scrub attire is required; may include areas where surgical instruments are processed

surgical asepsis: absence of microorganisms in the surgical environment to reduce the risk for infection

restricted zone: area in the operating room where scrub attire and surgical masks are required; includes operating room, substerile and sterile core areas

THE SURGICAL TEAM

The surgical team consists of the patient, the anesthesiologist or anesthetist, the surgeon, the intraoperative nurses, and the surgical technicians. The anesthesiologist or nurse anesthetist administers the anesthetic agent, places the patient in the proper position on the operating table, and monitors and manages the patient's physical status throughout the surgery; the surgeon and assistants scrub and perform the surgery; the intraoperative nurses and technicians manage the operating room.

The Patient Undergoing Anesthesia

As the patient enters the operating room, he or she may feel relaxed and prepared, or fearful and highly stressed. Fears about loss of control, the unknown, pain, death, alteration in body structure or function, and disruption of lifestyle all may contribute to a generalized anxiety. These fears can increase the anesthesia needed, the level of postoperative pain, and overall recovery time. The patient is also subject to multiple risks; infection, failure of the surgery to provide relief of symptoms, possible temporary or permanent complications related to the procedure or anesthesia, and death are all uncommon but potential outcomes of the surgical experience (Chart 17-1). In addition to these fears and risks, the patient undergoing sedation and anesthesia temporarily loses both cognitive function and biologic self-protective mechanisms. Loss of pain sense, reflexes, and ability to communicate subject the intraoperative patient to possible injury.

Gerontologic Considerations

Elderly patients face higher risks from anesthesia and surgery than do other adults. Statistically, perioperative risk increases with each decade over 60 years of age, often because of the increased incidence of coexisting disease. With modifications tailored to the biologic changes of later life (see Chap. 11) and the application of research findings for this population, the risks are reduced.

Biologic variations with particular impact include cardiovascular and pulmonary changes that occur with aging. The aging heart and blood vessels have a decreased ability to respond to stress. Reduced cardiac output and limited cardiac reserve make the elderly patient vulnerable to changes in circulating volume and blood oxygen levels. Excessive or rapid administration of intravenous solutions may cause pulmonary edema; a sudden or prolonged drop in blood pressure may lead to cerebral ischemia, thrombosis, embolism, infarction, and anoxemia. Reduced gas exchange can lead to cerebral hypoxia.

The older person needs less anesthetic to produce anesthesia and takes longer to eliminate anesthetic agents. One reason for reduction of anesthesia dosages is that, as people age, the percentage of fatty tissue steadily increases (from 20% to 30% at age 20 years to 35% to 45% at age 60 to 70 years); anesthetic agents that have an affinity for fatty tissue concentrate in body fat and the brain. Another reason is that the older patient, particularly when malnourished, may have low plasma protein levels. With decreased plasma proteins, more of the anesthetic agent remains free or unbound, resulting in a more potent action. In addition,

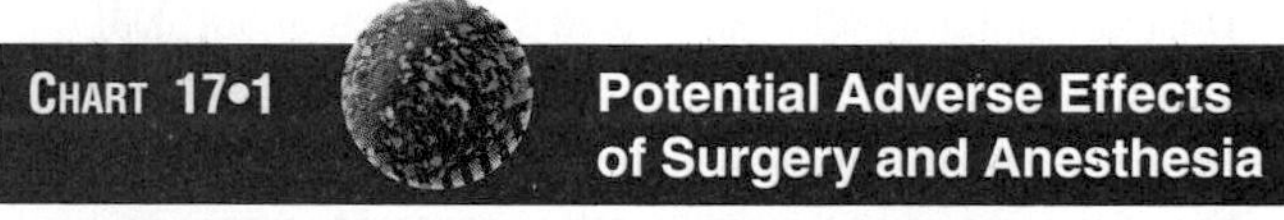

CHART 17•1
Potential Adverse Effects of Surgery and Anesthesia

All major body systems are disrupted by anesthesia and surgery. Although most patients can effectively compensate for surgical trauma and the effects of anesthesia, all patients are at risk during the operative procedure. These risks include the following:

- Cardiac dysrhythmia due to electrolyte imbalance or adverse effect of anesthetic agents
- Myocardial depression, bradycardia, and circulatory collapse due to toxic levels of local anesthetics
- Central nervous system agitation, seizures, and respiratory arrest due to toxic levels of local anesthetics
- Oversedation or undersedation during conscious sedation
- Agitation or disorientation, especially in the elderly
- Hypoxemia or hypercarbia due to hypoventilation and inadequate respiratory support during anesthesia
- Laryngeal trauma, oral trauma, and broken teeth due to difficult intubation
- Hypothermia due to cool operating room temperatures, exposure of body cavities, and impaired thermoregulation secondary to anesthetic agents
- Hypotension due to blood loss or adverse effect of anesthesia
- Infection
- Thrombosis due to compression of blood vessels or stasis
- Malignant hyperthermia secondary to adverse effect of anesthesia
- Nerve damage, skin breakdown due to prolonged or inappropriate positioning
- Electrical shock or burns
- Laser burns
- Drug toxicity, faulty equipment, and human error

body tissues made up predominantly of water and those with a rich blood supply, such as skeletal muscle, the liver, and kidneys, shrink. Reduction in liver size decreases the rate at which the liver can inactivate many anesthetics. The decreased functioning of the kidneys reduces elimination of waste products and anesthetics.

Other factors affecting the elderly surgical patient in the intraoperative period include the following:

- Bone loss (25% in women; 12% in men), which necessitates careful manipulation and positioning during surgery
- Reduced ability to adjust rapidly to emotional and physical stress, which influences surgical outcomes and requires meticulous observation of vital functions
- Impaired ability to increase metabolic rate and impaired thermoregulatory mechanisms, which increase susceptibility to hypothermia

As expected, the mortality rate is higher with emergency surgery than with elective surgery; continuous and careful monitoring and quick intervention are essential for older surgical patients.

The Intraoperative Nurses

Intraoperative nurses are responsible for the safety and well-being of the patient, the coordination of the operating room personnel, and the performance of scrub nurse and circulating nurse activities. Intraoperative nurses are also concerned about the patient's emotional state and continue the care begun by preoperative nurses by providing the patient with information and realistic reassurance, supporting coping strategies, and reinforcing the patient's ability to influence outcomes (ie, active participation in plan of care). As the patient's chief advocates, the intraoperative nurses monitor factors that can cause injury (such as patient position, equipment malfunction, and environmental hazards) and protect the patient's dignity and interests while he or she is anesthetized. In addition, the intraoperative nurses maintain surgical standards of care, identify existing patient risk factors, and assist in modifying complicating factors to help reduce operative risk.

The Circulating Nurse

The **circulating nurse** must be a registered nurse. He or she manages the operating room and protects the safety and health needs of the patient by monitoring the activities of members of the surgical team and checking the conditions in the operating room. The main responsibilities include verifying consent, coordinating the team, and ensuring cleanliness, proper temperature, humidity, and lighting; the safe functioning of equipment; and the availability of supplies and materials. The circulating nurse also monitors aseptic practices to avoid breaks in technique while coordinating the movement of related personnel (medical, radiography, and laboratory). The circulating nurse monitors the patient and documents specific activities throughout the operative procedure to ensure the patient's safety and well-being.

The Scrub Nurse

The activities of the **scrub nurse** and surgical technician include scrubbing for surgery; setting up the sterile tables; preparing sutures, ligatures, and special equipment; assisting the surgeon and the surgical assistants during the procedure by anticipating the required instruments, sponges, drains, and other equipment; and keeping track of the time the patient is under anesthesia and the time the wound is open. As the surgical incision is closed, the scrub nurse or surgical technician counts all needles, sponges, and instruments to be sure they are accounted for to ensure patient well-being. Specimens must also be labeled and sent to the laboratory. The scrub nurse may be a registered nurse or a licensed practical nurse. In some settings, surgical technicians may carry out these functions.

The Registered Nurse First Assistant

Another role of the nurse in the operating room is the registered nurse first assistant (RNFA). Although the scope of practice of the RNFA depends on each state's Nurse Practice Act, the RNFA practices under the direct supervision of the surgeon. RNFA responsibilities may include handling tissue, providing exposure at the operative field, using instruments, suturing, and providing hemostasis. The entire process requires a thorough understanding of anatomy, tissue care, and the principles of asepsis; an awareness of the objectives of the surgery; the knowledge and ability to anticipate needs and to work as a skilled member of a team; and the capacity to handle any emergency situation in the operating room.

The Anesthesiologist and Anesthetist

An **anesthesiologist** is a physician specifically trained in the art and science of anesthesiology. An **anesthetist** is a qualified nurse, dentist, or physician who administers anesthetics. Most anesthetists are nurses who have graduated from an accredited nurse anesthesia program and have passed certification by the American Association of Nurse Anesthetists to become a certified registered nurse anesthetist (CRNA). The anesthesiologist or anesthetist interviews and assesses the patient, selects the anesthesia, administers it, intubates the patient if necessary, manages any technical problems relating to the administration of the anesthetic agent, and supervises the patient's condition throughout the surgical procedure. Before the patient enters the operating room, the anesthesiologist or anesthetist visits the patient to provide information and answer questions. The type of anesthesia to be administered, previous reactions to anesthesia, and known anatomic abnormalities that would make intubation difficult are discussed. The anesthesiologist or anesthetist uses the American Society of Anesthesiology (ASA) Physical Status Classification System to classify the patient's status (Table 17-1).

When the patient arrives in the operating room, the anesthesiologist or anesthetist again assesses the patient's physical condition. The anesthetic is administered, and the patient is intubated and placed on a ventilator, if indicated. During surgery, the anesthesiologist or anesthetist monitors the patient's blood pressure, pulse, and respirations as well as the electrocardiogram (ECG), oxygen saturation, tidal volume, blood gas levels, blood pH, alveolar gas concentrations, and body temperature. Monitoring by electroencephalograph (EEG) may sometimes be required. Anesthetic levels in the body can also be determined; a mass spectrometer can provide instant readouts of critical concentration levels on display terminals. It also assesses the ability to breathe unassisted and indicates the need for mechanical assistance when the patient is not ventilating well independently.

THE SURGICAL ENVIRONMENT

Because the intraoperative patient's risk for serious infection is great, prophylactic antibiotics may be prescribed and given within 2 hours of the initial incision. External precautions include surgi-

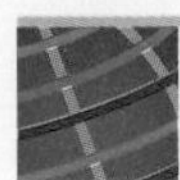

TABLE 17•1 American Society of Anesthesiology Physical Status Classification System

Classification	Description
I	A normally healthy patient *Examples:* No systemic abnormality, localized infection without fever, benign tumor, hernia
II	A patient with mild systemic disease *Examples:* well-controlled hypertension, well-controlled diabetes mellitus, chronic bronchitis, obesity, age over 80 yr
III	A patient with severe systemic disease that is not incapacitating *Examples:* severe disease, compensated heart failure, MI more than 6 mo ago, angina pectoris, severe dysrhythmia, cirrhosis, poorly controlled diabetes or hypertension, ileus
IV	A patient with an incapacitating systemic disease that is a constant threat to life *Examples:* Severe congestive heart failure, myocardial infarction less than 6 mo ago, severe respiratory failure, advanced liver or renal failure
V	A moribund patient who is not expected to survive for 24 hours with or without operation *Examples:* Unconscious patient with traumatic head injury and agonal cardiac rhythm

cal asepsis, which depends on strict control of the operating room environment. Policies governing this environment address such issues as the health of the staff; cleanliness of the rooms; sterility of equipment and surfaces; processes for scrubbing, gowning, and gloving; and operating room attire.

To provide the best possible conditions for surgery, the operating room is located in a section of the hospital free from contaminating particles, dust, other pollutants, radiation, and noise. Electrical hazards, emergency exit clearances, and storage of equipment and anesthetic gases are checked periodically by the state and the Joint Commission for the Accreditation of Healthcare Organizations (JCAHO). To help decrease microbes, the surgical area is divided into three zones: the **unrestricted zone**, where street clothes are allowed; the **semirestricted zone**, where attire consists of scrub clothes, shoe covers, and caps; and the **restricted zone**, where scrub clothes, shoe covers, caps, and masks are worn. The surgeons and other surgical team members wear additional sterile clothing and protective devices in the operating room.

The Association of Operating Room Nurses (AORN) has recommended practices for surgical attire to promote high-level cleanliness in a particular practice setting (Smith, 1995). Operating room attire includes close-fitting cotton dresses, pantsuits, jumpsuits, and gowns. Knitted cuffs on sleeves and pant legs prevent organisms shed from the perineum, legs, and arms from being released into the immediate surroundings. Shirts and waist drawstrings should be tucked inside the pants to prevent accidental contact with sterile areas and to contain skin sheddings. Wet or soiled garments should be changed.

Masks are worn at all times in the restricted zone of the operating room. High-filtration masks decrease the risk for postoperative wound infection by containing and filtering microorganisms from the oropharynx and nasopharynx. Masks must be tight-fitting, should cover the nose and mouth completely, and should not interfere with breathing, speech, or vision. Masks must be adjusted to prevent venting from the sides. Disposable masks have a filtration efficiency of greater than 95%. Masks are changed between patients and should not be worn outside the surgical department. Because the mask loses much of its effectiveness when it becomes moistened, it is also changed if it becomes damp. The mask must be either on or off; it must not be allowed to hang around the neck.

Headgear should completely cover the hair (head and neckline, including beard) so that single strands of hair, bobby pins, clips, particles of dandruff, and dust do not fall on the sterile field. The styles of headgear available are all disposable, lint-free, and clothlike.

Shoes should be comfortable and supportive; clogs, tennis shoes, sandals, and boots are not permitted because they are unsafe and difficult to clean. Shoes are covered with disposable shoe covers. Conductive covers establish an electrical ground for the wearer. The black strips provided with some conductive shoe covers should be placed inside the shoe in contact with the sole of the foot. Shoe covers are worn one time only and are removed upon leaving the restricted area.

Barriers such as scrub attire and masks do not entirely protect the patient from microorganisms. Colds, sore throats, and skin infections are sources of pathogenic organisms and must be reported. Good health is essential for any person in the operating room, and any perioperative team member with an infectious disease (eg, an upper respiratory tract infection, infected skin lesion) should not have direct patient care contact. Until the infectious process has resolved, the perioperative team members should not work in the operating room setting. Because artificial fingernails harbor microorganisms even after a 5-minute scrubbing (Edel et al., 1998), the wearing of artificial nails by operating room personnel is discouraged.

Principles of Perioperative Asepsis

Surgical asepsis prevents the contamination of surgical wounds. Although postoperative wound infection may be caused by natural skin flora or a previously existing infection, operating room personnel have the responsibility for using aseptic principles to minimize this risk.

All surgical material—any instruments, needles, sutures, dressings, gloves, covers, and solutions that may come in contact with the surgical wound and exposed tissues—must be sterilized before their use in surgery. In addition, the surgeon, surgical assistants, and nurses must prepare themselves by scrubbing their hands and arms with soap and water and donning long-sleeved, sterile gowns and gloves. Head and hair are covered with a cap, and a mask is worn over the nose and mouth to minimize the possibility of bacteria from the upper respiratory tract entering the wound. During surgery, the personnel who have scrubbed and gowned touch only sterilized objects. Nonscrubbed personnel refrain from touching or contaminating anything sterile.

An area of the patient's skin considerably larger than that requiring exposure during the surgery is meticulously cleansed, and an antiseptic agent is applied. The remainder of the patient's body is covered with sterile drapes.

Environmental Controls

In addition to the protocols described previously, surgical asepsis requires meticulous cleaning and maintenance of the operating room environment. Floors and horizontal surfaces are cleaned frequently with detergent, soap and water, or detergent germicide;

sterilizing equipment is inspected regularly to ensure optimal operation and performance.

All equipment that comes into direct contact with the patient must be sterile. Sterilized linens, drapes, and solutions are used; instruments are cleaned and sterilized in a unit near the operating room. Individually wrapped sterile items are used when additional individual items are needed.

As stated previously, airborne bacteria are a concern. To decrease the amount of bacteria in the air, standard operating room ventilation provides 16 to 20 air exchanges per hour. Staff members shed skin scales, which results in about 1000 bacteria-carrying particles (or colony-forming units [CFUs]) per cubic foot per minute. With the standard air exchanges, air counts of bacteria may be 50 CFUs/cubic foot/min to 150 CFUs/cubic foot/min. The number of personnel and unnecessary physical movements may be restricted to minimize bacteria in the air and achieve an operating room infection rate no greater than 3% to 5% in clean, infection-prone surgery.

Some operating rooms have laminar air-flow units. These units provide 400 to 500 air exchanges per hour. When used appropriately, laminar air-flow units result in fewer than 10 CFUs/cubic foot/min during surgery. The goal for a laminar flow-equipped operating room is an infection rate less than 1%. A room equipped with this unit is frequently used for total joint replacement surgery (Friberg, 1998).

Despite all these precautions, wound contamination may occasionally occur during surgery but only become apparent days or weeks later in the form of an incisional infection or abscess. Constant surveillance and conscientious technique in carrying out aseptic practices must be continuous to reduce the risk for contamination and infection.

Basic Guidelines for Maintaining Surgical Asepsis

GENERAL

- Sterile surfaces or articles may touch other sterile surfaces or articles and remain sterile; contact with unsterile objects at any point renders a sterile area contaminated.
- If there is any doubt about the sterility of an article or area, it is considered unsterile and contaminated.
- Whatever is sterile for one patient (an opened sterile tray or tables with sterile supplies) can be used for this patient only. Unused sterile supplies must be discarded or resterilized if they are to be used again.

PERSONNEL

- Scrubbed personnel remain in the area of the surgical procedure; if a scrubbed person leaves the room, that person's sterile status is lost. To return to surgery, this person is required to go through the procedure of scrubbing, gowning, and gloving.
- Only a small part of a scrubbed person's body is considered sterile: from front waist to the shoulder area; forearms and gloves. Therefore, the gloved hands must be kept in front between the shoulders and waistline.
- In some operating rooms, a special wrap-around gown is worn.
- The circulating nurse and any unscrubbed personnel remain at a safe distance to avoid contamination of any sterile area.

DRAPING

- During draping of a table or patient, the sterile drape is held well above the surface to be covered and is positioned from front to back.
- Only the top of the patient or table that is draped is considered sterile; drapes hanging over the edge are not regarded as sterile.
- Sterile drapes are kept in position by the use of clips or adherent material; drapes are not moved during the surgical procedure.
- A tear or puncture of the drape permitting access to an unsterile surface underneath renders the area unsterile. Such a drape must be replaced.

DELIVERY OF STERILE SUPPLIES

- Packages are wrapped or sealed in such a way that they can be opened easily without risk of contaminating contents.
- Sterile supplies, including solutions, are delivered to a sterile field or handed to a "scrubbed" person in such a way that sterility of the object or fluid remains intact.
- Edges of wrappers covering sterile supplies or outer lips of bottles or flasks containing sterile solutions are not considered sterile.
- The unsterile arm of the circulating nurse must not extend over a sterile area. Sterile articles are to be dropped onto the sterile field, a reasonable distance from the edge of the sterile area.

SOLUTIONS

- Sterile solutions are poured from a point high enough to prevent accidental touching of the sterile receiving cup or basin, but not so high as to produce splashing. (When a sterile surface becomes wet, it is contaminated.)

Health Hazards Associated With the Surgical Environment

Safety issues in the operating room include exposure to blood and body fluids, hazards associated with laser beams, and exposure to latex, radiation, and toxic agents. Internal monitoring of the operating room includes the analysis of swipe samples for infectious and toxic agents. In addition, policies and procedures for minimizing exposure to body fluids and reducing the dangers associated with lasers and radiation have been established.

Laser Risks

The AORN has recommended practices for laser safety. While lasers are in use, warning signs should be clearly posted to alert personnel. The safety requirements include but are not limited to the following issues: reducing the possibility of exposure to the eyes and skin, preventing inhalation of the laser plume (smoke and particulate matter), and protecting the patient and personnel from fire and electrical hazards. Because several types of lasers are available for clinical use, perioperative personnel should be familiar with the unique features, specific operation, and safety measures for each type of laser used in the practice setting.

Perioperative personnel working with lasers are required to have a thorough eye examination before participating in perioperative cases involving lasers. Special protective goggles, specific to the type of laser used in the procedure, are worn. There is controversy about the protection needed to avoid the laser plume and effects of its inhalation. Personnel equipped with a hooded air-pack system are provided with an individual breathing system that eliminates the risk for inhalation of room air. However, this equipment is relatively expensive. Smoke evacuators may be used in some procedures to remove the laser plume from the operative field.

NURSING RESEARCH

Pryor, F., & Messmer, P. R. (1998). The effect of traffic patterns in the OR on surgical site infections. *AORN Journal 68*(4), 649–659.

Purpose

Standards of care recommend that the numbers of people in the operating room (OR) and traffic through the OR be restricted; however, research on these issues is sparse. This study was conducted to explore the relationship between the number of people in the OR during surgery and the incidence of subsequent surgical site infections (SSIs). In addition, the study examined the effect of other variables (gender, age, American Society of Anesthesiologists [ASA] physical assessment score, length of preoperative stay, duration of surgery, and timely antibiotic prophylaxis) on SSIs.

Study Sample and Design

A retrospective chart review of patients undergoing clean surgical procedures in five surgical specialties in a large academic medical center was conducted to determine the contribution of selected variables on the incidence of surgical site infection. The researchers reviewed 2864 clean surgical procedures performed between January 1, 1995 and December 31, 1995. Infections were identified from monthly infection control reports.

Surgical procedure reports, anesthesia records, preoperative assessment records, discharge summaries, and medication administration records were reviewed using a standardized data collection form. A total of 69 reported SSI cases were identified and matched with noninfected cases for age, gender, type of procedure, and ASA score.

Findings

Significant differences were found by duration of surgery ($p = 0.022$), and infection rate tended to increase as duration of the surgical procedure increased. Further, as the number of people in the OR increased, infection rates tended to increase. On analysis by backward stepwise regression, both duration of surgical procedure and ASA score were statistically significant risk factors for SSIs.

Nursing Implications

An increased risk for SSI can be anticipated with lengthy surgical procedures. Because of the consequences of surgical site infections on patients' well-being and costs of care, more research on risk factors related to SSIs is warranted so that effective prevention programs can be developed and implemented.

Exposure to Blood and Body Fluids

Since the onset of the acquired immunodeficiency syndrome (AIDS) epidemic, operating room attire has changed drastically. Double gloving is routine, at least in trauma surgery where sharp bone fragments are present. In addition to the routine scrub suit and double gloves, some surgeons wear rubber boots, a waterproof apron, and sleeve protectors. Goggles or a wrap-around face shield are worn when the surgical wound is irrigated or bone drilling is performed and when splashing is expected to occur. In hospitals where numerous total joint procedures are performed, a full bubble mask is used. This mask provides full barrier protection from bone fragments and splashes and safe ventilation through an accompanying hood with a separate air-filtration system.

Latex Allergy

The American Society of Perianesthesia Nurses has published recommendations for the care of the patient with latex allergy in its 1995 Standards of PeriAnesthesia Nursing Practice. These recommendations include early identification of the latex allergy patient and maintenance of latex allergy precautions throughout the perianesthesia and perioperative period. Due to the increase in number of patients with latex allergies, more latex-free products are now available. It is the responsibility of all nurses, including perianesthesia and perioperative nurses, to be aware of latex allergies, the necessary precautions, and products that are latex free. Hospital staff are also at risk for developing a latex allergy secondary to repeated exposure to latex products.

THE SURGICAL EXPERIENCE

Anesthesia: An Overview

Anesthesia is a state of narcosis (severe central nervous system depression produced by pharmacologic agents), analgesia, relaxation, and reflex loss. Inhalation anesthesia is the most common method of administration because it can be controlled. The intake and elimination of the anesthetic agent are in large measure affected by pulmonary ventilation. Greater depth (or plane) of anesthesia requires a stronger concentration of the agent.

Anesthetics are divided into two classes: (1) those that suspend sensation in the whole body (general anesthesia, conscious sedation) and (2) those that suspend sensation in parts of the body (local, regional, epidural, or spinal anesthesia).

General Anesthesia

General anesthesia is most commonly achieved when the anesthetic is inhaled or administered intravenously. Inhaled anesthetic agents include volatile liquid agents and gas anesthetics. Volatile liquid anesthetics produce anesthesia when their vapors are inhaled. Included in this group are halothane (Fluothane), enflurane (Ethrane), isoflurane (Forane), sevoflurane (Ultrane), and desflurane (Suprane). All are administered with oxygen, and usually with nitrous oxide as well. Gas anesthetics are administered by inhalation and are always combined with oxygen. Nitrous oxide is the most common gas anesthetic agent used. When inhaled, the substances enter the blood through the pulmonary capillaries and act on cerebral centers to produce loss of consciousness and loss of sensation. When administration of the anesthetic is discontinued, the vapor or gas is eliminated through the lungs. Table 17-2 identifies the advantages, disadvantages, and implications of the different volatile liquid and gas anesthetics.

General anesthetics produce anesthesia because they are delivered to the brain at high partial pressure. Relatively large amounts of anesthetic must be administered during induction and the early maintenance phases because the anesthetic is recirculated and deposited in body tissues. As these sites become saturated, smaller amounts of the anesthetic agent are required to maintain anesthesia because equilibrium or near equilibrium has been achieved between brain, blood, and other tissues.

Anything that diminishes peripheral blood flow, such as vasoconstriction or shock, may result in only small amounts of anesthetic being required. Conversely, when peripheral blood flow is unusually high, as in the muscularly active or the apprehensive patient, induction is slower, and greater quantities of anesthetic are required because the brain receives a smaller quantity of anesthetic.

METHODS OF ADMINISTRATION

Liquid anesthetics may be administered by mixing the vapors with oxygen or nitrous oxide–oxygen and then having the patient inhale the mixture. The vapor is administered to the patient through a tube and a mask. The endotracheal technique for administering

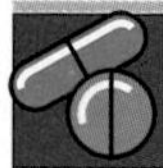

TABLE 17•2 **Inhalation Anesthetic Agents**

Agent	Administration	Advantages	Disadvantages	Implications
Volatile Liquids				
halothane (Fluothane)	Inhalation; special vaporizer	Not explosive or flammable Induction rapid and smooth Useful in almost every type of surgery Low incidence of postoperative nausea and vomiting	Requires skillful administration to prevent overdosage May cause liver damage May produce hypotension Requires special vaporizer for administration	In addition to observation of pulse and respiration postoperatively, it is important that blood pressure be monitored frequently.
methoxyflurane (Penthrane)	Inhalation; special vaporizer	Nonflammable Seldom causes postoperative nausea and vomiting Analgesic action continues several hours after surgery Excellent muscle relaxation	Requires skillful administration Renal damage may occur Unpleasant odor	Prolonged postoperative depressant action calls for careful observation by PACU/recovery room personnel.
enflurane (Ethrane)	Inhalation	Rapid induction and recovery Potent analgesic Not explosive or flammable	Respiratory depression may develop rapidly along with ECG abnormalities Not compatible with epinephrine	Observe for possible respiratory depression. Administration with epinephrine may cause ventricular fibrillation.
isoflurane (Forane)	Inhalation	Rapid induction and recovery Muscle relaxants are markedly potentiated	A profound respiratory depressant	Respirations must be monitored closely and supported when necessary.
sevoflurane (Ultrane)	Inhalation	Rapid induction and excretion; minimal side effects	Coughing and laryngospasm; trigger for malignant hyperthermia	Monitor for malignant hyperthermia.
desflurane (Suprane)	Inhalation	Rapid induction and emergence; rare organ toxicity	Respiratory irritation; trigger for malignant hyperthermia	Monitor for malignant hyperthermia, dysrhythmias.
Gases				
nitrous oxide (N_2O)	Inhalation (semiclosed method)	Induction and recovery rapid Nonflammable Useful with oxygen for short procedures Useful with other agents for all types of surgery	Poor relaxant Weak anesthetic May produce hypoxia	Most useful in conjunction with other agents with longer action. Monitor for chest pain, hypertension, and stroke

anesthetics consists of introducing a soft rubber or plastic endotracheal tube into the trachea usually by means of a laryngoscope. The endotracheal tube may be inserted through either the nose or mouth (Fig. 17-1). When in place, the tube seals off the lungs from the esophagus, so that if the patient vomits, none of the stomach contents enters the lungs.

STAGES OF GENERAL ANESTHESIA

Anesthesia consists of four stages, each associated with specific clinical manifestations. When opioids (narcotics) and neuromuscular blockers (relaxants) are administered, several of the stages are absent.

Stage I: Beginning Anesthesia. As the patient breathes in the anesthetic mixture, warmth, dizziness, and a feeling of detachment may be experienced. The patient may have a ringing, roaring, or buzzing in the ears and, though still conscious, may be aware of being unable to move the extremities easily. During this stage, noises are exaggerated; even low voices or minor sounds appear distressingly loud and unreal. For this reason, unnecessary noise or motion must be avoided when anesthesia is started.

Stage II: Excitement. The excitement stage—characterized variously by struggling, shouting, talking, singing, laughing, or crying—frequently may be avoided if the anesthetic is administered smoothly and quickly. The pupils become dilated but contract if exposed to light; the pulse rate is rapid and respirations irregular.

Because of the uncontrolled movements of the patient during this stage, the anesthesiologist or anesthetist must always be attended by someone ready to help restrain the patient. A strap may be in place across the patient's thighs, and the hands are secured to an armboard. The patient should not be touched except for purposes of restraint, but restraints should not be applied over the operative site. Manipulation increases circulation to the operative site, thereby increasing the potential for bleeding.

Stage III: Surgical Anesthesia. Surgical anesthesia is reached by continued administration of the vapor or gas. The patient is unconscious, lying quietly on the table. The pupils are small but contract when exposed to light. Respirations are regular, the pulse rate and volume are normal, and the skin is pink or slightly flushed. With proper administration of the anesthetic, this stage may be maintained for hours in one of several planes, ranging from light (1) to deep (4), depending on the depth of anesthesia needed.

Stage IV: Medullary Depression. This stage is reached when too much anesthesia has been administered. Respirations become shallow, the pulse is weak and thready, the pupils become widely dilated and no longer contract when exposed to light. Cyanosis

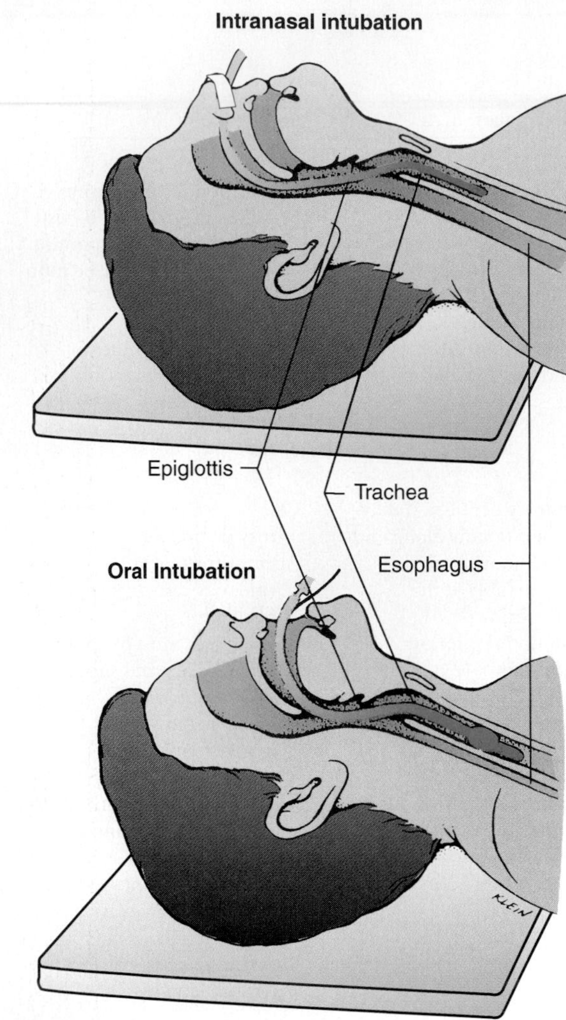

FIGURE 17•1 Endotracheal anesthesia. (*Top*) Nasal endotracheal catheter in proper position. (*Bottom*) Oral endotracheal intubation; tube in position with cuff inflated. For both methods, the head is tilted back to permit the airway to be open.

develops and, unless prompt action is taken, death rapidly follows. If this stage develops, the anesthetic is discontinued immediately, and respiratory and circulatory support is necessary to prevent death. Stimulants, although rarely used, may be administered if excessive anesthetic has been administered. Narcotic antagonists can be used if overdosage is due to opioids.

During smooth administration of an anesthetic, there is, of course, no sharp division between the first three stages, and there is no stage IV. The patient passes gradually from one stage to another, and it is only by close observation of the signs exhibited by the patient that an anesthesiologist or anesthetist can control the situation. The responses of the pupils, the blood pressure, and the respiratory and cardiac rates are probably the most reliable guides to the patient's condition.

INTRAVENOUS ANESTHESIA

General anesthesia can also be produced by the intravenous injection of various substances, such as barbiturates, benzodiazepines, nonbarbiturate hypnotics, dissociative agents, and opioids. These medications may be administered for induction (initiation) or maintenance of anesthesia. They are often used along with inhalation anesthetics but may be used alone. Additionally, they can be used to produce conscious sedation (see later discussion). Intravenous anesthetics are presented in Table 17-3.

One of the advantages of intravenous anesthesia is that the onset of anesthesia is pleasant; there is none of the buzzing, roaring, or dizziness known to follow administration of an inhalation anesthetic. For this reason, induction of anesthesia usually begins with an intravenous agent and is often preferred by patients who have experienced various methods. The duration of action is brief, and the patient awakens with little nausea or vomiting. Thiopental is often administered with other anesthetic agents in prolonged procedures.

Intravenous anesthetic agents have the advantages of being nonexplosive, requiring little equipment, and being easy to administer. The low incidence of postoperative nausea and vomiting makes the method useful in eye surgery because vomiting would increase intraocular pressure and endanger vision in the operated eye. Intravenous anesthesia is useful for short procedures but is used less often for the longer procedures of abdominal surgery. It is not indicated for children, who have small veins and require intubation because of their susceptibility to respiratory obstruction.

A disadvantage of intravenous anesthesia is the powerful respiratory depressant effect of thiopental. It must be administered by a skilled anesthesiologist or anesthetist and only when some method of oxygen administration is available immediately in case of difficulty. Sneezing, coughing, and laryngospasm are sometimes noted with its use.

CONSCIOUS SEDATION

Conscious sedation is a form of intravenous anesthesia. It is defined as a depressed level of consciousness without impairment of the patient's ability to maintain a patent airway and to respond appropriately to physical stimulation and verbal command. Its goal is a calm, tranquil amnesic patient who, when sedation is combined with analgesic agents, is relatively pain free during the procedure but able to maintain protective reflexes (Booth, 1996). Conscious sedation can be administered by an anesthesiologist, anesthetist, other physician, or nurse. When administered by an anesthesiologist or anesthetist, conscious sedation is referred to as *monitored anesthesia care.* The medications permitted for use in conscious sedation vary with the credentials of the person administering the conscious sedation. In addition, State Department of Health Regulations are very specific about who may administer the conscious sedation as well as specific training required for those individuals. These regulations vary greatly from state to state.

Intravenous conscious sedation may be used alone or in combination with local, regional, or spinal anesthesia. Its use is increasing as more surgical procedures and diagnostic studies are performed with the expectation that the patient will be discharged home within a few hours after the procedure is completed.

Midazolam (Versed) or diazepam (Valium) is used frequently for intravenous conscious sedation. In some states, the first dose must be administered by the physician; subsequent doses can then be administered by a nurse with special training. Other medications used include analgesic agents (eg, morphine, fentanyl) and reversal agonists (naloxone [Narcan]). The patient who receives conscious sedation must be continuously monitored by a nurse who is knowledgeable and skilled in detection of dysrhythmias, administration of oxygen, and resuscitation. The patient receiving this form of anesthesia is never left alone and is closely monitored for respiratory, cardiovascular, and central nervous system depression. Monitoring includes pulse oximetry, continuous electrocardiography, and frequent measurement of vital signs. The patient's level of sedation is monitored by his or her ability to maintain a patent airway and to respond to verbal commands.

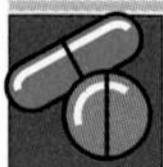

TABLE 17•3 **Intravenous Anesthetic Agents**

Agent	Administration	Advantages	Disadvantages	Implications/Considerations
Tranquilizers and Sedative Hypnotics				
Benzodiazepines				
midazolam (Versed)	Intravenously	Short acting; has antianxiety, sedative, amnesic, muscle relaxant effects.	Increased sensitivity to its effects in chronic obstructive pulmonary disease patients	Monitor respiratory status closely.
diazepam (Valium)	Intravenously Orally	Preoperative sedation Intraoperative tranquilization during regional anesthesia	Absorbed unpredictably when given intramuscularly	IV administration may produce thrombophlebitis (central vein is therefore preferred).
chlordiazepoxide (Librium)	Intramuscularly	Production of hypnosis during anesthetic induction		
droperidol (Inapsine)	Intravenously	Long duration of action	Weak antihistaminic action and α-adrenergic blocking action; inhibition of basic ganglionic dopaminergic pathways—may lead to extrapyramidal rigidity resembling parkinsonism	Major tranquilizer Keep IV fluids and vasopressors available to treat hypotension.
lorazepam (Ativan)	Intravenously	Long duration of action	Used with caution in patients with renal and liver impairment	Monitor laboratory values.
Opioids (Narcotics)				
morphine (high doses)	Intravenously	Not a myocardial depressant	Can depress arterial blood pressure by decreasing systemic vascular resistance Does not provide good amnesia Does not promote adequate muscular relaxation	Orthostatic hypotension may occur after morphine.
meperidine hydrochloride (Demerol)	Intravenously Subcutaneously Intramuscularly	Prompt onset Because of spasmolytic effect, it is drug of choice for surgery of bile duct, distal colon, and rectum; easily detoxified and excreted	May slow rate of respirations Adverse reactions: dizziness, nausea, and vomiting	In some patients, histamine may be released; treatment is diphenhydramine (Benadryl).
Neuroleptanalgesics				
The term *neuroleptanalgesic* refers to the combination of a short-acting synthetic opioid agent (fentanyl) and a butyrophenone (droperidol). Patient becomes very drowsy; responds to voice command, although analgesia is profound. Of significance, the combination produces peripheral vasodilation followed by a decrease in arterial blood pressure. If administered rapidly, it may cause skeletal muscular rigidity and possibly respiratory impairment. These agents are also called narcotic agonist analgesics.				
fentanyl (Sublimaze)	Intravenously Transdermally	75–100 times more potent than morphine and about 25% of duration of morphine (IV) Little effect on cardiovascular system	In very high dosage, an α-adrenergic blocking effect Respiratory depression	Short duration of action is due to its more rapid redistribution and more active metabolism by liver than other opioids.
sufentanil	Injection	Onset extremely rapid		Duration is only about one third that of fentanyl.
Dissociative Agents				
When under dissociative analgesia, the patient appears not to be asleep or anesthetized, but rather dissociated from the surroundings.				
ketamine (Ketalar; Ketaject)	Intravenously Intramuscularly	Rapid induction and short action; often used to supplement nitrous oxide Useful when hypotension may be hazardous; can be administered as analgesic or anesthetic	May cause elevated blood pressure and depressed respirations Patient may experience hallucinations Vomiting and aspiration may occur	Avoid verbal, visual, or tactile stimulation because this may trigger psychic aberration. Droperidol or diazepam (see below) may eliminate such psychic phenomena. Observe for signs of respiratory depression. Keep resuscitation equipment nearby.

(*continued*)

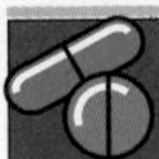

TABLE 17•3 **Intravenous Anesthetic Agents** *(Continued)*

Agent	Administration	Advantages	Disadvantages	Implications
Barbiturates				
thiopental sodium (Pentothal)	Intravenous injection (or rectal)	Rapid induction Nonexplosive Requires little equipment Low incidence of postoperative nausea and vomiting	Powerful depressant of breathing Poor relaxant May produce coughing, sneezing, and laryngospasm Not useful for children because of small veins	Requires intelligent and close observation because of potency and rapidity of drug action
methohexital sodium (Brevital)	Intravenous	Rapid onset	Respiratory depression, involuntary muscle movement, seizures; may cause necrosis if IV infiltrates	Monitor respiratory status closely, monitor for seizure activity, ensure IV in vein.
Nonbarbiturate Hypnotics				
etomidate (Amidate)	Intravenous	Few cardiovascular and respiratory effects; useful for fragile patients	Transient adrenal suppression; involuntary muscle movements	
propofol (Diprivan)	Intravenous	Rapid induction with minimal excitatory effects; may have antiemetic effect	Myocardial depression; hypotension; pain on injection	Monitor cardiac function and blood pressure closely; contraindicated in patients with allergy to eggs and soybean oil.

ADJUNCTIVE AGENTS: NEUROMUSCULAR BLOCKERS

Neuromuscular blockers (muscle relaxants) block transmission of nerve impulses at the neuromuscular junction of skeletal muscles. Muscle relaxants are used to relax muscles in abdominal and thoracic surgery, relax eye muscles in certain kinds of eye surgery, facilitate endotracheal intubation, treat laryngospasm, and assist in mechanical ventilation.

Purified curare was the first widely used muscle relaxant; tubocurarine was isolated as the active principle. Succinylcholine was later introduced because it acts more rapidly than curare. Several other agents are also used (Table 17-4). The ideal muscle relaxant has the following characteristics:

- Is nondepolarizing, with an onset time and duration of action similar to those of succinylcholine but without its problems of bradycardia and cardiac dysrhythmias
- Has a duration of action between those of succinylcholine and pancuronium
- Lacks cumulative and cardiovascular effects
- Is metabolizable and does not depend on the kidneys for its elimination

Regional Anesthesia

Regional anesthesia is a form of local anesthesia in which an anesthetic agent is injected around nerves so that the area supplied by these nerves is anesthetized. The effect depends on the type of nerve involved. Motor fibers are the largest fibers and have the thickest myelin sheath. Sympathetic fibers are the smallest and have a minimal covering. Sensory fibers are intermediate. Thus, a local anesthetic blocks motor nerves least readily and sympathetic nerves most readily. An anesthetic cannot be regarded as having "worn off" until all three systems (motor, sensory, and autonomic) are no longer affected by the anesthetic.

The patient under spinal or local anesthesia is awake and aware of his or her surroundings. Careless conversation, unnecessary noise, and unpleasant odors must be avoided—these may be noticed by the patient in the operating room and may contribute to a negative view of the surgical experience by the patient. A quiet environment is therapeutic. Even the diagnosis must not be stated aloud if the patient is not to know it at this time. Regional or spinal anesthetic agents may be supplemented with medications to produce mild sedation or to relieve the patient's anxiety.

SPINAL ANESTHESIA

Spinal anesthesia is a type of extensive conduction nerve block that occurs by introducing a local anesthetic into the subarachnoid space at the lumbar level, usually between L4 and L5 (Fig. 17-2). It produces anesthesia of the lower extremities, perineum, and lower abdomen. For the lumbar puncture procedure, the patient usually lies on his or her side in a knee–chest position. Sterile technique is used as a spinal puncture is made and the medication is injected through the needle. As soon as the injection has been made, the patient is placed on his or her back. If a relatively high level of block is sought, the head and shoulders are lowered.

The spread of the anesthetic agent and the level of anesthesia depend on the amount of fluid injected, the speed with which it is injected, the positioning of the patient after the injection, and the specific gravity of the agent. If the specific gravity of the agent is greater than that of cerebrospinal fluid (CSF), the agent moves to the dependent position of the subarachnoid space; if the specific gravity is less than that of CSF, the anesthetic moves away from the dependent portion. This is controlled by the anesthesiologist or anesthetist. Generally, the agents used are procaine, tetracaine (Pontocaine), lidocaine (Xylocaine), and bupivacaine (Marcaine) (Table 17-5).

In a few minutes, anesthesia and paralysis affect the toes and perineum and then gradually affect the legs and abdomen. If the anesthetic reaches the upper thoracic and cervical spinal cord in

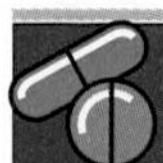

TABLE 17•4 Neuromuscular Blocking Agents

Muscle Relaxant	Action	Advantages	Disadvantages	Uses and Comments
Nondepolarizing Neuromuscular Blocking Agents				
tubocurarine chloride (Tubarine)	Peaks at 30–60 min	50%–70% excreted unchanged in 3–6 h	Histamine-like reaction Hypotension Increased airway resistance Skin erythema	Contraindicated with history of allergy, asthma
gallamine (Flaxedil)	⅕ as potent as curare Lasts 25% shorter time than curare Blocks vagal ganglia in heart	All excreted unchanged	Tachycardia	Used with cyclopropane or halothane
pancuronium bromide (Pavulon)	Similar to curare but 5 times more potent Duration, 60–85 min	Safe; stable Good muscle relaxant Reversible by neostigmine and atropine		Excellent for situations requiring complete relaxation Avoid with myasthenia gravis or renal disease Avoid with patients sensitive to bromide
vecuronium bromide (Norcuron)	Blocks depolarization	Facilitates endotracheal intubation; good muscle relaxant	Prolonged dose-related apnea	Related to Pavulon Well tolerated in patients with renal failure
Depolarizing Neuromuscular Blocking Agents				
These mimic the action of acetylcholine at the neuromuscular junction. Acetylcholine is discharged almost immediately on release, then repolarization of muscle takes place. When depolarizing neuromuscular blocking agents are used, skeletal muscle depolarizes.				
succinylcholine (Anectine; Sucostrin)	Onset is rapid: 1 min Duration: 4–8 min	Ideal for endotracheal intubation, fracture reduction; treatment of laryngospasm	Contraindicated in patients with low pseudocholinesterase On second IV injection, bradycardia and various dysrhythmias May cause fasciculations of the muscles and pain	Used to treat laryngospasm, status asthmaticus, and toxic reactions to local anesthetic drugs
decamethonium bromide (Syncurine)	Onset: 30–40 sec Duration: 15–20 min	Excreted unchanged by kidney	Some fasciculation of muscle: jaw masseter muscles; posterior calf muscles Difficult to reverse its action	Produces depolarization of end-plate region

high concentrations, a temporary partial or complete respiratory paralysis results. Paralysis of the respiratory muscles is managed by mechanical ventilation until the effects of the anesthetic on the respiratory nerves have worn off.

Nausea, vomiting, and pain may occur during surgery when spinal anesthesia is used. As a rule, these reactions result from manipulation of various structures, particularly those within the abdominal cavity. Such reactions may be avoided by the simultaneous intravenous administration of a weak solution of thiopental and inhalation of nitrous oxide.

Headache may occur after spinal anesthesia. Several factors are involved in the incidence of headache: the size of the spinal needle used, the leakage of fluid from the subarachnoid space through the puncture site, and the patient's hydration status. Measures that increase cerebrospinal pressure are helpful in relieving headache. These include keeping the patient lying flat, quiet, and well hydrated.

In continuous spinal anesthesia, the tip of a plastic catheter is left in the subarachnoid space during the surgical procedure so that more anesthetic may be injected as needed. This technique provides greater control of the dosage. However, there is greater potential for postanesthetic headache because of the large-gauge needle used.

CONDUCTION BLOCKS

There are many types of conduction blocks depending on the nerve groups injected.

Epidural anesthesia is achieved by injecting a local anesthetic into the spinal canal in the space surrounding the dura mater (see Fig. 17-2). Epidural anesthesia also blocks sensory, motor, and autonomic functions, but it is differentiated from spinal anesthesia by the injection site and the amount of anesthetic used. Epidural doses are much higher because the epidural anesthetic does not make direct contact with the cord or nerve roots.

An advantage of epidural anesthesia is the absence of headache that occasionally results from subarachnoid injection. A disadvantage is the greater technical challenge of introducing the anesthetic into the epidural rather than the subarachnoid space. If accidental subarachnoid injection occurs during epidural anesthesia and the anesthetic travels toward the head, "high" spinal anesthesia can result. High spinal anesthesia can produce severe hypotension and respiratory depression and arrest. Treatment of these complications includes airway support, intravenous fluids, and use of vasopressors.

The following are examples of other types of nerve blocks:

- Brachial plexus block, which produces anesthesia of the arm
- Paravertebral anesthesia, which produces anesthesia of the nerves supplying the chest, abdominal wall, and extremities

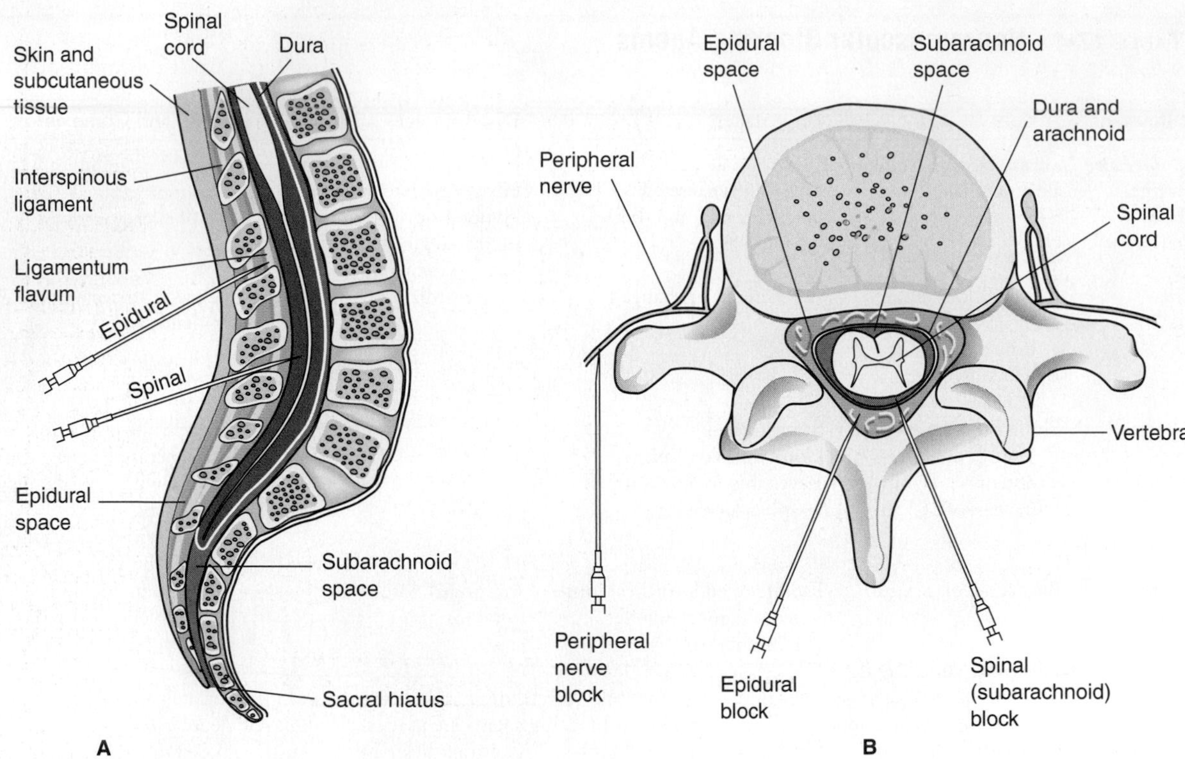

FIGURE 17•2 (**A**) Injection sites for spinal and epidural anesthesia. (**B**) Cross section showing injection sites for peripheral nerve, epidural, and spinal blocks.

- Transsacral (caudal) block, which produces anesthesia of the perineum and, occasionally, the lower abdomen

LOCAL INFILTRATION ANESTHESIA

Infiltration anesthesia is the injection of a solution containing the local anesthetic into the tissues at the planned incision site. Often, it is combined with a local regional block by injecting the nerves immediately supplying the area. The advantages of local anesthesia are as follows:

- It is simple, economical, and nonexplosive.
- Equipment is minimal.
- Postoperative recovery is shortened.
- Undesirable effects of general anesthesia are avoided.
- It is ideal for short and superficial surgical procedures.

Local anesthesia is often administered in combination with epinephrine. Epinephrine causes constriction of blood vessels, which prevents rapid absorption of the anesthetic agent and thus prolongs its local action; rapid absorption into the bloodstream, which could cause seizures, is also prevented.

Different types of local anesthetic agents are listed in Table 17-6.

Local anesthesia is the anesthesia of choice in any surgical procedure in which it can be used. However, it is contraindicated for surgery in highly nervous, apprehensive patients because surgery with local anesthesia may increase anxiety. A patient who begs to be put to sleep rarely does well under local anesthesia. For some surgical procedures, local anesthesia is impractical because of the number of injections and the amount of anesthetic that would be required—as in breast reconstruction, for example.

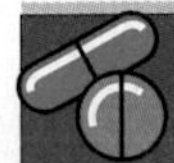

TABLE 17•5 Regional Anesthetic Agents

Agent	Advantages of Spinal Anesthesia (Includes All Agents)	Disadvantages of Spinal Anesthesia (Includes All Agents)
procaine (Novocaine)	Easily administered by a physician	Blood pressure may fall rapidly unless monitored carefully and treated with medications such as ephedrine.
tetracaine (Pontocaine)	Inexpensive	If the spinal anesthesia ascends to the chest, there may be respiratory distress.
lidocaine (Xylocaine)	Minimum of equipment required	Occasionally, postoperative complications occur, such as headache or, rarely, meningitis or paralysis.
bupivacaine (Marcaine)	Rapid onset	
	Excellent muscular relaxation	

The skin is prepared as for any surgical procedure, and a small-gauge needle is used to inject a modest amount of the anesthetic into the skin layers. This produces blanching or a wheal. Additional anesthetic is then injected in the skin until an area the length of the proposed incision is anesthetized. A larger, longer needle then is used to infiltrate deeper tissues with the anesthetic. The action of the agent is almost immediate, so surgery may begin as soon as the injection is complete. Anesthesia lasts anywhere from 45 minutes to 3 hours, depending on the anesthetic and the use of epinephrine.

Patient Position on the Operating Table

The position in which the patient is placed on the operating table depends on the surgical procedure to be performed as well as on the physical condition of the patient (Fig. 17-3). The potential for transient discomfort or even permanent injury is clear because many positions are awkward, hyperextending joints, compressing arteries, or pressing on nerves and bony prominences, or result in discomfort simply because the position is sustained for long periods. Factors to consider include the following:

- The patient should be in as comfortable a position as possible, whether asleep or awake.
- The operative area must be adequately exposed.
- The vascular supply should not be obstructed by an awkward position or undue pressure on a part.
- There should be no interference with the patient's respiration as a result of pressure of the arms on the chest or constriction of the neck or chest caused by a gown.
- Nerves must be protected from undue pressure. Improper positioning of the arms, hands, legs, or feet may cause serious injury or paralysis. Shoulder braces must be well padded to prevent irreparable nerve injury, especially when the Trendelenburg position is necessary.
- Precautions for patient safety must be observed, particularly with thin, elderly, or obese patients.
- The patient needs *gentle* restraint before induction, in case of excitement.

The usual position for surgery is flat on the back; one arm is at the side of the table, with the hand placed palm down; the other is carefully positioned on an armboard for intravenous infusion. This position, called the dorsal recumbent position, is used for most abdominal surgery, except for surgery of the gallbladder and the pelvis.

The Trendelenburg position usually is used for surgery on the lower abdomen and the pelvis to obtain good exposure by displacing the intestines into the upper abdomen. In this position, the head and body are lowered and the knees are flexed. The patient is held in position by padded shoulder braces (see Fig. 17-3*B*).

The lithotomy position is used for nearly all perineal, rectal, and vaginal surgical procedures (see Fig. 17-3*C*). The patient is laid on his or her back with the legs and thighs flexed at right angles. The position is maintained by placing the feet in stirrups.

The Sims or lateral position is used for renal surgery. The patient is placed on the nonoperative side with an air pillow 12.5 to 15 cm (5 or 6 inches) thick under the loin, or on a table with a kidney or back lift (see Fig. 17-3*D*).

Other procedures, such as brain surgery or abdomino-thoracic surgery, may require unique positioning and supplemental apparatus depending on the operative approach.

Induced Hypotension

There are times during surgery when it is desirable to lower blood pressure to reduce bleeding at the operative site because this

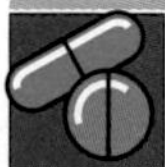

TABLE 17•6 Local Anesthetic Agents

Agent	Administration and Action	Advantages	Disadvantages	Implications and Use
lidocaine (Xylocaine) and mepivacaine (Carbocaine)	Topical or injection	Rapid Longer duration of action (compared with procaine) Free from local irritative effect	Occasional idiosyncrasy	Useful topically for cystoscopy Injected for use in dental work and surgery Observe for untoward reactions—drowsiness, depressed respiration.
bupivacaine (Marcaine)	Infiltration Peripheral nerve block Epidural	Duration is 2–3 times longer than lidocaine or mepivacaine	Use cautiously in patients with known drug allergies or sensitivities.	A period of analgesia persists after return of sensation; therefore, need for strong analgesics is reduced.
etidocaine (Duranest)	Infiltration Block			Greater potency and longer action than lidocaine
procaine (Novocaine)	Subcutaneously, intramuscularly, intravenously, or spinal	Low toxicity Inexpensive	Some idiosyncrasies Skin rash Poor stability	Observe for reaction: hypotension, bradycardia, weak pulse. Usually given with epinephrine, causing vasoconstriction, thereby slowing absorption and prolonging nerve-deadening effect
tetracaine (Pontocaine)	Topical Infiltration Nerve block	Same as procaine	Same as procaine	More than 10 times as potent as procaine Usually administered with epinephrine

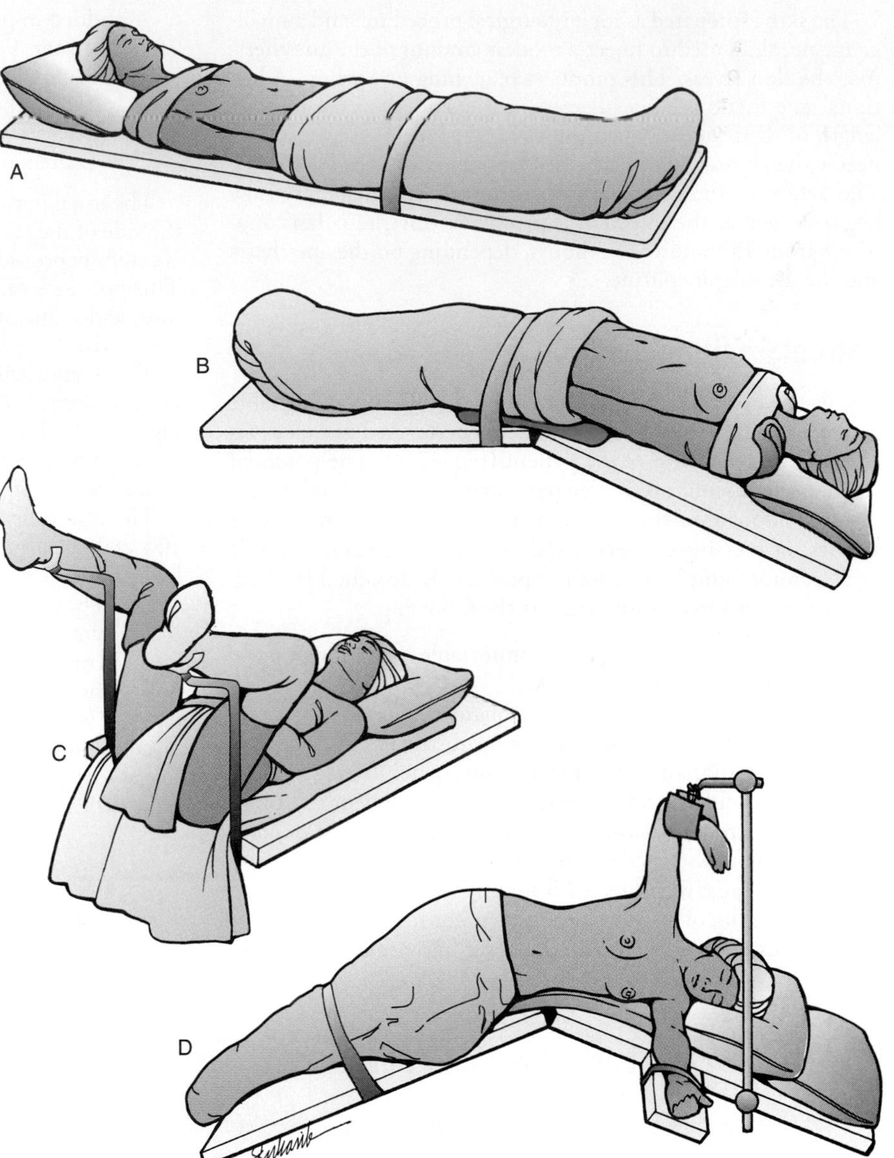

A Patient in position on the operating table for a laparotomy. Note the strap above the knees.
B Patient in Trendelenburg position on operating table. Note padded shoulder braces in place. Be sure that brace does not press on brachial plexus.
C Patient in lithotomy position. Note that the hips extend over the edge of the table.
D Patient lies on unaffected side for kidney surgery. Table is broken to spread apart space between the lower ribs and the pelvis. The upper leg is extended; the lower leg is flexed at the knee and the hip joints; a pillow is placed between the legs.
A
B
C
D

FIGURE 17•3 Positions on the operating table. Captions call attention to safety and comfort features. All surgical patients wear caps to cover the hair completely.

allows the surgery to be carried out more quickly with less blood loss. Artificially induced hypotension has been used for brain surgery, radical neck dissection, and radical pelvic surgery.

Deliberate hypotension is accomplished by inhalation or intravenous injection of medications that affect the sympathetic nervous system and peripheral smooth muscle. Halothane is the inhalation anesthetic agent commonly used. This anesthetic is supplemented with other measures to lower blood pressure, such as a head-up position, positive pressure applied to the airway, and administration of a ganglionic blocking agent, such as pentolinium (Ansolysen) or sodium nitroprusside.

POTENTIAL INTRAOPERATIVE COMPLICATIONS

As previously stated, the surgical patient is subject to many risks from anesthesia. These potential complications include nausea and vomiting, hypoxia, hypothermia, and malignant hyperthermia.

Nausea and Vomiting

Vomiting or regurgitation may occur, especially when the patient comes to the operating room with a full stomach. If gagging occurs, the patient is turned to the side, the head of the table is lowered, and a basin is provided to collect the vomitus. Suction is used to remove saliva and vomited gastric contents.

In some cases, the anesthesiologist administers oral antacids preoperatively to counteract a possible acid aspiration syndrome. If the patient aspirates vomitus, as an asthma-like attack with severe bronchial spasms and wheezing is triggered. The patient can subsequently develop pneumonitis and pulmonary edema, leading to extreme hypoxia. Increasing medical attention is being paid to silent regurgitation of gastric contents, which occurs more frequently than previously realized. The importance of pH in the etiology of acid aspiration is being studied, as is the value of perioperative administration of a histamine-2 receptor antagonist, such as cimetidine (Tagamet), and similar medications.

Hypoxia and Other Respiratory Complications

Inadequate ventilation, occlusion of the airway, inadvertent intubation of the esophagus, and hypoxia are significant potential problems of general anesthesia. Many factors can contribute to inadequate ventilation. Respiratory depression caused by anesthetic agents, aspiration of respiratory tract secretions or vomitus, and position on the operating room table can compromise the exchange of gases. Anatomic variation can make the trachea difficult to visualize and result in the artificial airway being inserted into the esophagus. In addition to these dangers, asphyxia caused by foreign bodies in the mouth, spasm of the vocal cords, relaxation of the tongue, or aspiration of vomitus, saliva, or blood can occur. Since brain damage from hypoxia occurs within minutes, vigilant assessment of the patient's oxygenation status is a primary function of the anesthesiologist or anesthetist and the circulating nurse. Peripheral perfusion is checked frequently, and pulse oximeter results are monitored continuously.

Hypothermia

During anesthesia, the patient's temperature may fall. Glucose metabolism is reduced, and as a result, metabolic acidosis may develop. This condition is called *hypothermia* and is indicated by a core body temperature below normal (36.6°C [98.0°F] or lower). Inadvertent hypothermia may occur as a result of a low temperature in the operating room, infusion of cold fluids, inhalation of cold gases, open body wounds or cavities, decreased muscle activity, advanced age, or the pharmaceutical agents used (vasodilators, phenothiazines, general anesthetics). Hypothermia may also be intentionally induced in selected surgical procedures to reduce the patient's metabolic rate.

Prevention of hypothermia is a major objective; if hypothermia occurs, the goal of intervention is to minimize or reverse the physiologic process. If hypothermia is intentional, the goal is safe return to normal body temperature. Environmental temperature in the operating room can temporarily be set at 25° to 26.6°C (78° to 80°F). Intravenous and irrigating fluids are warmed to 37°C (98.6°F). Wet gowns and drapes are removed promptly and replaced with dry materials because wet linens promote heat loss. Whatever methods are employed to rewarm the patient, warming must be accomplished gradually, not rapidly.

Conscientious monitoring of core temperature, urinary output, the electrocardiograph, blood pressure, arterial blood gases, and serum electrolytes is required. Attention to hypothermia management extends into the postoperative period to prevent significant nitrogen loss and catabolism. Treatment includes oxygen administration, adequate hydration, and proper nutrition.

Gerontologic Considerations

Heat loss in older patients in the operating room can be prevented by covering the patient's head with a heat-retaining cap during anesthesia. A disposable plastic cap can be effective and inexpensive. Also, the operating room temperature should be maintained at 26.6°C (80°F). Antiseptic solutions used in the initial preparation of the skin before the application of drapes should be comfortably warm, not cold.

Malignant Hyperthermia

Malignant hyperthermia is an inherited muscle disorder chemically induced by anesthetic agents. With the mortality rate exceeding 50%, identifying patients at risk for malignant hyperthermia is imperative. Susceptible people include those with bulky, strong muscles, a history of muscle cramps or muscle weakness and unexplained temperature elevation, and an unexplained death of a family member during surgery that was accompanied by a febrile response.

Pathophysiology

During anesthesia, potent agents such as inhalation anesthetics (halothane, enflurane) and muscle relaxants (succinylcholine) may trigger the symptoms of malignant hyperthermia. Such medications as sympathomimetics (epinephrine), theophylline, aminophylline, anticholinergics (atropine), and cardiac glycosides (digitalis) can also induce or intensify such a reaction. The process is also initiated by stress.

The pathophysiology is related to muscle cell activity. Muscle cells are composed of inner fluid (sarcoplasm) and an outer surrounding membrane. Calcium, an essential factor in the process of muscle contraction, is normally stored in sacs in the sarcoplasm. When nerve impulses stimulate the muscle, calcium is released, allowing contraction to occur. A pumping mechanism returns calcium to the sacs so that relaxation can take place. In malignant hyperthermia, this mechanism is disrupted. Calcium ions are not returned, and they accumulate, causing clinical symptoms of hypermetabolism, which in turn increases muscle contraction (rigidity), hyperthermia, and damage to the central nervous system.

Clinical Manifestations

The initial symptoms of malignant hyperthermia are related to cardiovascular and musculoskeletal activity. Tachycardia (heart rate above 150/min) is often the earliest sign. In addition to the tachycardia, sympathetic nervous stimulation leads to ventricular dysrhythmia, hypotension, decreased cardiac output, oliguria, and, later, cardiac arrest. With the abnormal transport of calcium, rigidity or tetany-like movements occur, often in the jaw. The rise in temperature is actually a late sign that develops rapidly, and it can increase 1° every 5 minutes.

Medical Management

Early recognition of symptoms and prompt discontinuation of anesthesia are imperative. Goals of treatment are to decrease metabolism, reverse metabolic and respiratory acidosis, correct dysrhythmias, decrease body temperature, provide oxygen and nutrition to tissues, and correct electrolyte imbalance. The Malignant Hyperthermia Association of North America (MHAUS) publishes a treatment protocol that should be posted in the operating room.

Although malignant hyperthermia usually presents about 10 to 20 minutes after induction of the anesthetic, it can also occur in the first 24-hour postoperative period. As soon as the diagnosis is made, anesthesia and surgery are halted, and the patient is hyperventilated with 100% oxygen. Dantrolene sodium, a skeletal muscle relaxant, and sodium bicarbonate are administered immediately. Continued monitoring of all parameters is necessary to evaluate the patient's status.

Nursing Management

Although malignant hyperthermia occurs infrequently, it is imperative that the nurse identify patients at risk, recognize the problem, have the appropriate medication and equipment available, and know the protocol to follow. This information may be lifesaving if malignant hyperthermia occurs.

THE NURSING PROCESS: CARING FOR THE PATIENT DURING SURGERY

Assessment

Nursing assessment of the intraoperative patient involves obtaining data from the patient and the patient record to identify variables that can affect care and serve as guidelines for developing an individualized plan of patient care. The nurse performs a focused preoperative nursing assessment. This includes assessing physiologic status (eg, health–illness level, level of consciousness), psychosocial status (eg, expressions of concern, anxiety level, verbal communication problems, coping mechanisms), and physical status (eg, operative site, skin condition and effectiveness of preparation; immobile joints).

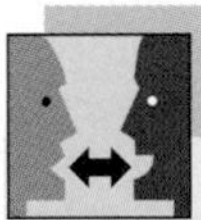

ETHICS AND RELATED ISSUES

The Do-Not-Resuscitate (DNR) Order in the Operating Room

Situation

Your hospital has developed a policy, authorized through the medical staff, that allows for patients to have a do not resuscitate order in place during a surgical procedure. This policy follows the American Society of Anesthesiologists guidelines for DNR in the Operating Room (OR). You are getting a patient ready for surgery and the anesthesiologist who will be administering the anesthetic writes an order for the DNR to be rescinded during surgery. The physician is refusing to talk to the patient concerning the DNR.

Problem

The patient believes his/her wishes will be followed with regard to resuscitation in the event of a cardiac arrest and the physician does not believe he can administer the anesthetic management if the DNR is in place.

Discussion

- What are the rights of the patient with regard to advance directives?
- What can you do to advocate for the patient?
- Should you call the ethics committee of the hospital?
- How do you access the ethics committee?

Diagnosis

Nursing Diagnoses

Based on the assessment data, the patient's major nursing diagnoses may include the following:

- Anxiety
- Risk for injury related to anesthesia and surgery
- Risk for perioperative positioning injury related to required position and loss of protective responses secondary to anesthesia
- Sensory/perceptual alteration (global) related to general anesthesia or conscious sedation

Collaborative Problems/Potential Complications

Based on the assessment data potential complications may include the following:

- Infection
- Hypothermia
- Hypoxia
- Malignant hyperthermia

Planning and Goals

Goals for care of the patient during surgery include reducing anxiety, maintaining safety, preventing positioning and other injuries, maintaining the patient's dignity, and absence of complications.

Nursing Interventions

Reducing Anxiety

The operating room environment can seem cold, clinical, and frightening to the patient, who may be experiencing feelings of isolation and apprehension. Introducing oneself, addressing the patient by name warmly and frequently, verifying details, providing explanations, and encouraging and answering questions provide a sense of professionalism and friendliness that can help the patient feel secure. When discussing what to expect, the nurse uses common, basic communication skills, such as touch and eye contact, to reduce anxiety. Attention to physical comfort (warm blankets, position changes) helps the patient feel more comfortable. Telling the patient who else will be present in the operating room, how long the procedure is expected to take, and other details helps the patient prepare for the experience and gain a sense of control over and participation in events.

Protecting the Patient's Safety

One way the nurse protects the patient from injury is by providing a safe environment. A variety of activities and functions address the diverse patient safety issues that arise in the operating room. Verifying information, checking the chart for completeness, and maintaining surgical asepsis and an optimal environment are critical nursing responsibilities. Verifying that all required documentation is completed is one of the first functions of the intraoperative nurse.

The patient is identified, and the planned surgical procedure and type of anesthesia are verified. It is important to review the patient's record for the following:

- Correct informed surgical consent with patient's signature
- Completed records for health history and physical examination
- Results of diagnostic studies
- Completed health history and assessment
- Preoperative checklist

In addition to checking that all necessary patient data are complete, the circulating nurse obtains the necessary equipment specific to the procedure. The need for nonroutine medications, blood components, instruments, and other equipment and supplies is assessed, and the readiness of the room, completeness of physical setup, and completeness of instrument, suture, and dressing setups are determined. Any aspects of the operating room environment that may negatively affect the patient are identified. These include physical features, such as room temperature and humidity; electrical hazards; potential contaminants (dust, blood, and discharge on floor or surfaces, uncovered hair, faulty attire of personnel, jewelry worn by personnel, dirty footwear); and unnecessary traffic. The nurse also sets up and maintains suction in working order, sets up invasive monitoring equipment, assists with line insertion (arterial, Swan-Ganz, central venous pressure, intravenous), and initiates appropriate physical comfort measures for patient.

Preventing physical injury includes using safety straps and bed rails and not leaving the sedated patient unattended. Transferring the patient from the stretcher to the operating room table requires safe transferring practices. Other safety measures include properly positioning the grounding pad under the patient to prevent electrical burns and shock, removing excess povidone-iodine (Betadine) or other surgical germicide from the patient's skin, and promptly and completely draping exposed areas after the sterile field has been created to decrease the risk for hypothermia.

Preventing Intraoperative Positioning Injury

Proper operating room positioning is determined by the type of surgery to be done; however, the nurse must be alert to what bodily areas are at risk as a result of positioning. Maintaining anatomic position, padding equipment that can constrict or compress body structures, and frequently assessing peripheral pulses are measures the nurse employs to prevent injury. Protecting the patient from electrical and laser hazards, such as fire, shock, and burns, involves maintaining properly functioning equipment, protecting surrounding tissue from burns, and properly positioning the patient grounding pad. The scrub nurse participates in the sponge and instrument count according to hospital protocols.

Serving as Patient Advocate

Because the patient undergoing general anesthesia or conscious sedation experiences temporary sensory/perceptual alteration or loss, he or she has an increased need for protection and advocacy. Patient advocacy in the operating room entails maintaining the patient's physical and emotional comfort, privacy, rights, and dignity. Patients, whether conscious or not, should not be subjected to excess noise, inappropriate conversation, and, most of all, ridicule. As surprising as this sounds, banter in the operating room occasionally includes jokes about the patient's physical appearance, job, personal history, and so forth. Cases have been reported in which seemingly deeply anesthetized patients were able to recall the entire surgical experience, including remembering disparaging personal remarks made by operating room personnel. As an advocate, the nurse never engages in this conversation and discourages others from doing so. Other advocacy activities include correcting for the clinical, dehumanizing aspects of being a surgical patient by making sure the patient is treated as a person, respecting cultural and spiritual values, providing physical privacy, and maintaining confidentiality.

Monitoring and Managing Potential Complications

It is the responsibility of the anesthetist or anesthesiologist to monitor and manage complications; however, intraoperative nurses also play an important role. Being alert to and reporting signs and symptoms of hypovolemia, hypotension, malignant hyperthermia, or hypothermia and assisting with their management are nursing functions. Maintaining asepsis is the responsibility of all members of the surgical team.

Evaluation

Expected Outcomes

Expected outcomes may include:

1. Exhibits low level of anxiety
2. Experiences no unexpected threats to safety
3. Remains free of surgical positioning injury
4. Maintains environmental safety
5. Has dignity preserved throughout operating room experience
6. Is free of complications or experiences successful management of adverse effects of surgery and anesthesia

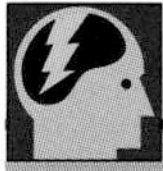

Critical Thinking Exercises

1. A patient in the holding area awaiting surgery indicates that he had not received instructions not to take his usual medications (ie, antihypertensive agent, diuretic, digoxin, potassium chloride, and insulin injection); as a result, he took them a few hours ago. What implications does this have for the patient's care and well-being while awaiting surgery, during surgery, and in the immediate postoperative period?

2. What are the differences in responsibility of the operating room nurse for care of patients who receive general anesthesia, conscious sedation, spinal anesthesia, and regional anesthesia?

3. While she is being assisted in transfer from the stretcher to the operating table, a patient indicates that she is very anxious about her surgery because of previous negative experiences. What assessment and interventions are indicated at this time?

References and Selected Readings

BOOKS

Agency for Health Care Policy and Research. (1992). *Acute pain management: Operative or medical procedures and trauma.* Clinical Practice Guideline. Washington, DC: Public Health Service, U.S. Department of Health and Human Services.

American Society of Anesthesiology. (1995). *ASA standards for post anesthesia care.* Park Ridge, IL: Author.

American Society of PeriAnesthesia Nurses. (1998). *Standards of periAnesthesia nursing practice.* Thorofare, NJ: ASPAN.

Drain, C. B. (Ed.). (1996). *The postanesthesia care unit: A critical care approach to postanesthesia nursing.* Philadelphia: W. B. Saunders.

DeFazio-Quinn, D. M. (Ed.). (1999). *Ambulatory surgical nursing core curriculum.* Philadelphia: W. B. Saunders.

Economou, S. G., & Economou, T. S. (1999). *Instructions for surgery patients.* Philadelphia: W. B. Saunders.

Fairchild, S. (1996). *Perioperative nursing: Principles and practice.* Boston: Little, Brown.

Fitzpatrick, J. J. (1998). *Encyclopedia of nursing research.* New York: Springer Publishing Co.

Groah, L. K. (1996). *Perioperative nursing.* Stamford, CT: Appleton & Lange.

Hanson, G. C. (1997). *Critical care of the surgical patient.* New York: Chapman & Hall Medical.

Kneedler, J. A., & Dodge, G. H. (1994). *Perioperative patient care: The nursing perspective* (3rd ed.). Boston: Jones & Bartlett.

Kost, M. (1998). *Manual of conscious sedation.* Philadelphia: W. B. Saunders.

Litwack, K. (Ed.). (1999). *Core curriculum for perianesthesia nursing practice.* Philadelphia: W. B. Saunders.

McGoldrick, K. E. (1995). *Ambulatory anesthesiology: A problem-oriented approach.* Baltimore: Williams & Wilkins.

Merli, G., & Weitz, H. (Eds.). (1998). *Medical management of the surgical patient* (2nd ed.). Philadelphia: W. B. Saunders.

Miller, T. A. (1998). *Modern surgical care: Physiologic foundations and clinical applications* (2nd ed.). St. Louis: Quality Medical.

Meeker, M. H., Rothrock, J. C., & Alexander, E. L. (Eds.). (1999). *Alexander's care of the patient in surgery.* (11th ed.). St. Louis: Mosby–Year Book.

Schirmer, B. D., & Rattner, D. W. (1998). *Ambulatory surgery.* Philadelphia: W. B. Saunders.

Schwartz, S., & Shires, G. T. (1999). *Principles of surgery.* New York: McGraw-Hill.

Summers, S., & Ebbert, D. W. (1992). *Ambulatory surgical nursing: A nursing diagnosis approach.* Philadelphia: J. B. Lippincott.

Watson, D. (1998). *Conscious sedation/analgesia.* St Louis: C. V. Mosby.

JOURNALS

Asterisks indicate nursing research articles.

Ambulatory Surgery

Brockway, P. M. (1997). The ambulatory surgical nurse: Evolution, competency and vision. *Nursing Clinics of North America, 32*(2), 387–394.

DeFazio-Quinn, D. M. (1997). Ambulatory surgery: An evolution. *Nursing Clinics of North America, 32*(2), 377–386.

Ireland, D. (1997). Legal issues in ambulatory surgery. *Nursing Clinics of North America, 32*(2), 469–476.

Lancaster, K. A. (1997). Patient teaching in ambulatory surgery. *Nursing Clinics of North America, 32*(2), 417–427.

Litwack, K. (1997). Care of the special needs patient. *Nursing Clinics of North America, 32*(2), 457–467.

New, S. W., & Gutierrez, L. (1997). Quality improvement in the ambulatory surgical setting. *Nursing Clinics of North America, 32*(2), 477–488.

Swan, B. A. (1996). Assessing symptom distress in ambulatory surgery patients. *MedSurg Nursing, 5*(5), 348–354.

Anesthesia and Surgery

(1998). Recommended practices for laser safety in practice settings. *AORN Journal, 67*(1), 263–264, 267–269.

Arsenault, C. (1998). Nurses' guide to general anesthesia. Part I. *Nursing, 28*(3), 32.

Booth, M. (1996). Clinical aspects of CRNA practice: Sedation and monitored anesthesia care. *Nursing Clinics of North America, 31*(3), 667–682.

Ferrara-Love, R. (1997). Laparoscopic surgery. *Nursing Clinics of North America, 32*(2), 429–440.

Friberg, B. (1998). Ultraclean laminar airflow ORs. *AORN Journal, 67*(4), 841–851.

Goldstein, F. J. (1995). Preemptive analgesia: A research review. *MedSurg Nursing, 4,* 305–308.

Gosden, P. E., McGowan A. P., & Bannister, G. C. (1998). Importance of air quality and related factors in the prevention of infection in orthopaedic implant surgery. *Journal of Hospital Infection, 39*(3), 173–180.

McLean, T. (1998). Air safety–not just for airplanes: Exposures and expectations in the health care environment. *Today's Surgical Nurse, 20*(2), 13–19, 35–36.

Oulette, S. M. (1996). Clinical aspects of CRNA practice: General anesthesia. *Nursing Clinics of North America, 31*(3), 623–642.

Perrin, L. S., Penta, B. A., & Patton, S. B. (1997). Designing a conscious sedation program: A collaborative approach. *Critical Care Nursing Clinics of North America, 9*(3), 251–272.

Romig, C. L., & Smalley P. J. (1997). Regulation of surgical smoke plume. *AORN Journal, 65*(4), 824–828.

Spitzer, L. E. (1996). Clinical aspects of CRNA practice: Regional anesthesia. *Nursing Clinics of North America, 31*(3), 643–665.

Sweet, C. (1997). Laser light: Waves of the future. *Today's Surgical Nurse, 19*(3), 11–17.

Walker, J. R. (1996). What is new with inhaled anesthetics: Part 2. *Journal of Perianesthesia Nursing, 11*(6): 404–9.

Wiklund, R. A., & Rosenbaum, S. H. (1997). Anesthesiology (the first of two parts). *New England Journal of Medicine, 337*(16), 1132–1141.

Wiklund, R. A., & Rosenbaum, S. H. (1997). Anesthesiology (the second of two parts). *New England Journal of Medicine, 337*(17), 1215–1219.

Williams, H., & Reeves, F. (1998). Anesthetic techniques and positioning: Implications for perioperative nurses. *Seminars in Perioperative Nursing, 7*(1): 14–20.

Wolford, E. T. (1997). Timing of perioperative antibiotic administration. *AORN Journal, 65*(1), 109–115.

Intraoperative Nursing

(1998). Revised AORN official statement on RN first assistants. *AORN Journal, 67*(1), 47–48, 51.

Copelin, C. (1998). Practical points in the use of albumin for hypovolemia. *Journal of Perianesthesia Nursing, 13*(2): 118–120.

Hlozek, C. C., Zacharias, W. M., & Mizener, K. A. (1998). RN first assistants expand their perioperative role. *AORN Journal, 67*(3), 560–563, 565–566.

Nathan, B. (1997). Use of scrubs and related apparel in health care facilities. *American Journal of Infection Control, 25*(5), 401–404.

Sessler, D. (1997). Mild perioperative hyperthermia. *New England Journal of Medicine, 336*(24), 1730–1737.

Smith, C. D. (1995). Covering gowns; surgical hand scrub; smoke evaculators; operative records abbreviations; open sterile setups. *AORN Journal, 61*(4): 753–754.

Vermette, E. (1998). Emergency! Malignant hyperthermia. *American Journal of Nursing, 98*(4), 45.

Perioperative Nursing

*Gatson-Grindel, C. (1996). Building nursing's minimum data set: The results of a pilot study. *MedSurg Nursing, 5*(6), 449–456.

Geier, K. (1998). Perioperative blood management. *Orthopaedic Nursing, 17*(Suppl.), 6–38.

McConnell, E. A. (1997). Reflections on the art and science of perianesthesia nursing. *Journal of Perianesthesia Nursing, 12*(4), 234–239.

Salipante, D. M. (1998). Refusal of blood by a critically ill patient. *Critical Care Nurse, 18*(2), 68–76.

Warner, M. E. (1997). Risks and outcomes of perioperative pulmonary aspiration. *Journal of Perianesthesia Nursing, 12*(5), 352–357.

Resources

American Society of PeriAnesthesia Nurses, 6900 Grove Road, Thorofare, NJ, 08086; 1-609-845-5557; www.aspan.org

Association of Operating Room Nurses, Inc., 2170 S. Parker Rd., Suite 300, Denver, CO 80231; 1-303-755-6304; www.aorn.org

Malignant Hyperthermia Association of the United States (MHAUS), 332 S. Main Street, Sherburne, NY 13460; www.medhelp.org/agsg/aqsg7059.htm

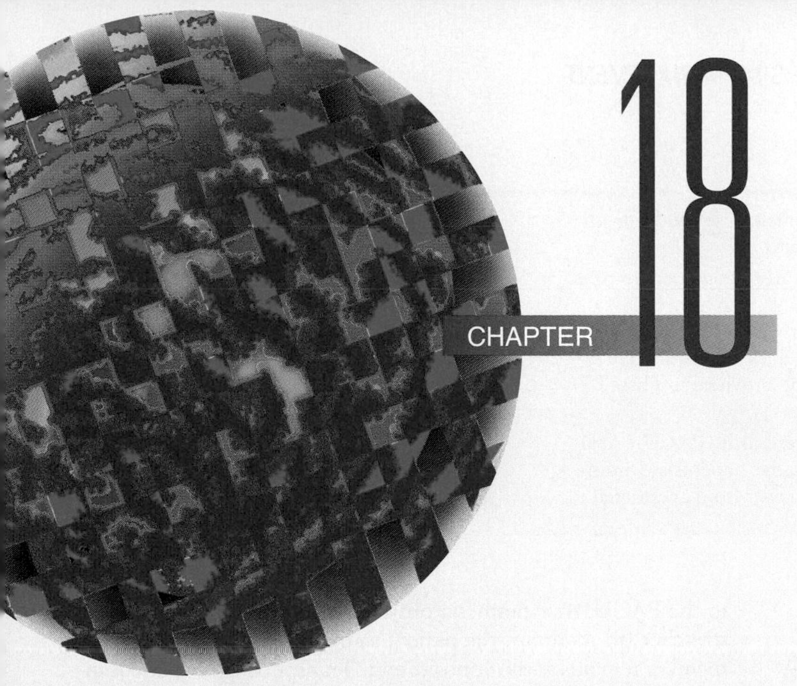

Postoperative Nursing Management

Learning Objectives

On completion of this chapter, the learner will be able to:

1. Describe the responsibilities of the post anesthesia care unit nurse in the prevention of immediate postoperative complications.
2. Compare postoperative care of the ambulatory surgery patient and the hospitalized surgery patient.
3. Identify common postoperative discomforts and their management.
4. Describe the gerontologic considerations related to postoperative management of patients.
5. Describe variables that affect wound healing.
6. Demonstrate sterile dressing technique.
7. Identify assessment parameters appropriate for the early detection of postoperative complications.

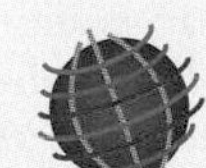

The postoperative period extends from the time the patient leaves the operating room until the last follow-up visit with the surgeon. This period may be as short as 1 week or as long as several months. During the postoperative period, nursing care is directed at reestablishing the patient's physiologic equilibrium, alleviating pain, preventing complications, and teaching the patient self-care. Careful assessment and immediate intervention assist the patient in returning to optimal function quickly, safely, and as comfortably as possible. Ongoing care in the community through home care, clinic visits, office visits or telephone follow-up facilitates an uncomplicated recovery.

GLOSSARY

dehiscence: partial or complete separation of wound edges

evisceration: protrusion of abdominal organs through the surgical incision

first intention healing: method of healing in which wound edges are surgically approximated and integumentary continuity is restored without granulating

Phase I PACU: area designated for care of surgical patients immediately after surgery and those patients whose condition warrants close monitoring

Phase II PACU: area designated for care of surgical patients who have been transferred from a Phase I PACU because their condition does not require the close monitoring provided in Phase I PACU

post anesthesia care unit (PACU): area where postoperative patients are monitored as they recover from anesthesia; formerly referred to as the recovery room or postanesthesia recovery room

second intention healing: method of healing in which wound edges are not surgically approximated and integumentary continuity is restored by granulations

third intention healing: method of healing in which surgical approximation of wound edges is delayed and integumentary continuity is restored by bringing apposing granulations together

THE POST ANESTHESIA CARE UNIT

The **post anesthesia care unit (PACU)**, also called the post anesthesia recovery room, is located adjacent to the operating rooms. Patients still under anesthesia or recovering from it are placed in this unit for easy access to experienced, highly skilled nurses, anesthesiologists or anesthetists, surgeons, advanced hemodynamic and pulmonary monitoring and support, special equipment, and medications.

The PACU is kept quiet, clean, and free of unnecessary equipment. It should be painted in soft, pleasing colors and have indirect lighting; a soundproof ceiling; equipment that controls or eliminates noise (eg, plastic emesis basins, rubber bumpers on beds and tables); and isolated but visible quarters for disruptive patients. The PACU should also be well ventilated. These features are of psychological value to the patient to decrease anxiety. The PACU bed provides easy access to the patient, is safe and easily movable, can be readily placed in shock position, and has features that facilitate care, such as intravenous poles, side rails, wheel brakes, and a chart storage rack.

Post anesthesia care in some hospitals and ambulatory surgical centers is divided into two phases. Phase I is the immediate recovery phase and requires intensive nursing care. Phase II post anesthesia care is reserved for patients who require less frequent observation and less nursing care. In the Phase II unit, the patient is prepared for discharge home. Recliners rather than stretchers or beds are standard in many Phase II units, which may also be referred to as Step Down, Sit Up, or Progressive Care units. Patients may remain in a Phase II PACU unit for as long as 4 to 6 hours or as short as 1 to 2 hours. In facilities without separate Phase I and Phase II units, the patient remains in the PACU and may be discharged home directly from this unit.

Both Phase I and Phase II PACU nurses have special skills. The **Phase I PACU** nurse must be vigilant in frequent (every 15 minutes) monitoring of the patient's pulse, electrocardiogram, respiratory rate, blood pressure, and pulse oximetry. In some cases, end-tidal carbon dioxide ($ETCO_2$) levels are monitored as well. The patient's airway may become obstructed because of the latent effects of recent anesthesia, and the PACU nurse must be prepared to assist in reintubation of the patient and in other emergencies that may occur. The nurse in the **Phase II PACU** must possess strong clinical assessment and patient teaching skills.

Admitting the Patient to the Post Anesthesia Care Unit

Transferring the postoperative patient from the operating room to the post anesthesia care unit is the responsibility of the anesthesiologist or anesthetist. During transport from the operating room to the PACU, the anesthesia provider remains at the head of the stretcher (to maintain the patient's airway), and a surgical team member remains at the opposite end. Transporting the patient involves special consideration of the patient's incision site, potential vascular changes, and exposure. The surgical incision is considered every time the postoperative patient is moved; many wounds are closed under considerable tension, and every effort is made to prevent further strain on the incision. The patient is positioned so that he or she is not lying on and obstructing drains or drainage tubes. Serious arterial hypotension may occur when a patient is moved from one position to another, such as from a lithotomy position to a horizontal position, or from a lateral to a supine position. Therefore, the patient must be moved slowly and carefully. As soon as the patient is placed on the stretcher or bed, the soiled gown is removed and replaced with a dry gown. The patient is covered with lightweight blankets and warmed. The side rails are raised to protect against falls.

The nurse who admits the patient to the PACU reviews the following information with the anesthesiologist or anesthetist:

1. Medical diagnosis and type of surgery performed
2. Patient's age and general condition, airway patency, vital signs
3. Anesthetic and other medications used (eg, opioids and other analgesics, muscle relaxant, antibiotics)
4. Any problems that occurred in the operating room that might influence postoperative care (eg, extensive hemorrhage, shock, cardiac arrest)
5. Pathology encountered (if malignancy, whether the patient or family has been informed)
6. Fluid administered, estimated blood loss and replacement
7. Any tubing, drains, catheters, or other supportive aids
8. Specific information about which the surgeon, anesthesiologist, or anesthetist wishes to be notified

Nursing Management in the Post Anesthesia Care Unit

The nursing management objectives for the patient in the PACU are to provide care until the patient has recovered from the effects of anesthesia (ie, until return of motor and sensory functions), is oriented, has stable vital signs, and shows no evidence of hemorrhage.

Assessing the Patient

Frequent skilled assessments of the patient's oxygen saturation, pulse volume and regularity, depth and nature of respirations, skin color, level of consciousness, and ability to respond to commands are the cornerstones of nursing care in the PACU. The nurse performs a baseline assessment followed by checking the surgical site for drainage or hemorrhage and connecting all drainage tubes and monitoring lines. After the initial assessment, vital signs are monitored, and the patient's general physical status is assessed at least every 15 minutes. Patency of the airway and respiratory function are always evaluated first, followed by assessment of cardiovascular function, the condition of the surgical site, and function of the central nervous system. It is also essential for the nurse to be aware of any pertinent information from the patient's history that may be significant (eg, patient is hard of hearing, has a history of seizures, has diabetes, is allergic to certain medications).

Maintaining a Patent Airway

The primary objective in the immediate postoperative period is to maintain pulmonary ventilation and thus prevent hypoxemia (reduced oxygen in blood) and hypercapnia (excess carbon dioxide in blood). Both can occur if the airway is obstructed and ventilation is reduced (hypoventilation). The nurse checks the orders for and applies supplemental oxygen and assesses respiratory rate and depth, ease of respirations, oxygen saturation, and breath sounds.

Patients who have experienced prolonged anesthesia usually are unconscious, with all muscles relaxed. This relaxation extends to the muscles of the pharynx; therefore, when the patient lies on his or her back, the lower jaw and the tongue fall backward, and the air passages become obstructed (Fig. 18-1*A*). Signs of occlusion include choking, noisy and irregular respirations, and, within minutes, a blue, dusky color (cyanosis) of the skin. Because movement of the thorax and the diaphragm do not necessarily indicate that the patient is breathing, this is ascertained by placing the palm of the hand at the patient's nose and mouth to feel the exhaled breath.

Nursing Alert *The treatment of hypopharyngeal obstruction involves tilting the head back and pushing forward on the angle of the lower jaw, as if to push the lower teeth in front of the upper teeth (Fig. 18-1B and C). This maneuver pulls the tongue forward and opens the air passages.*

The anesthesiologist or anesthetist may leave a hard rubber or plastic airway in the patient's mouth (Fig. 18-2) to maintain a patent airway. Such a device should not be removed until signs, such as gagging, indicate that reflex action is returning. Alterna-

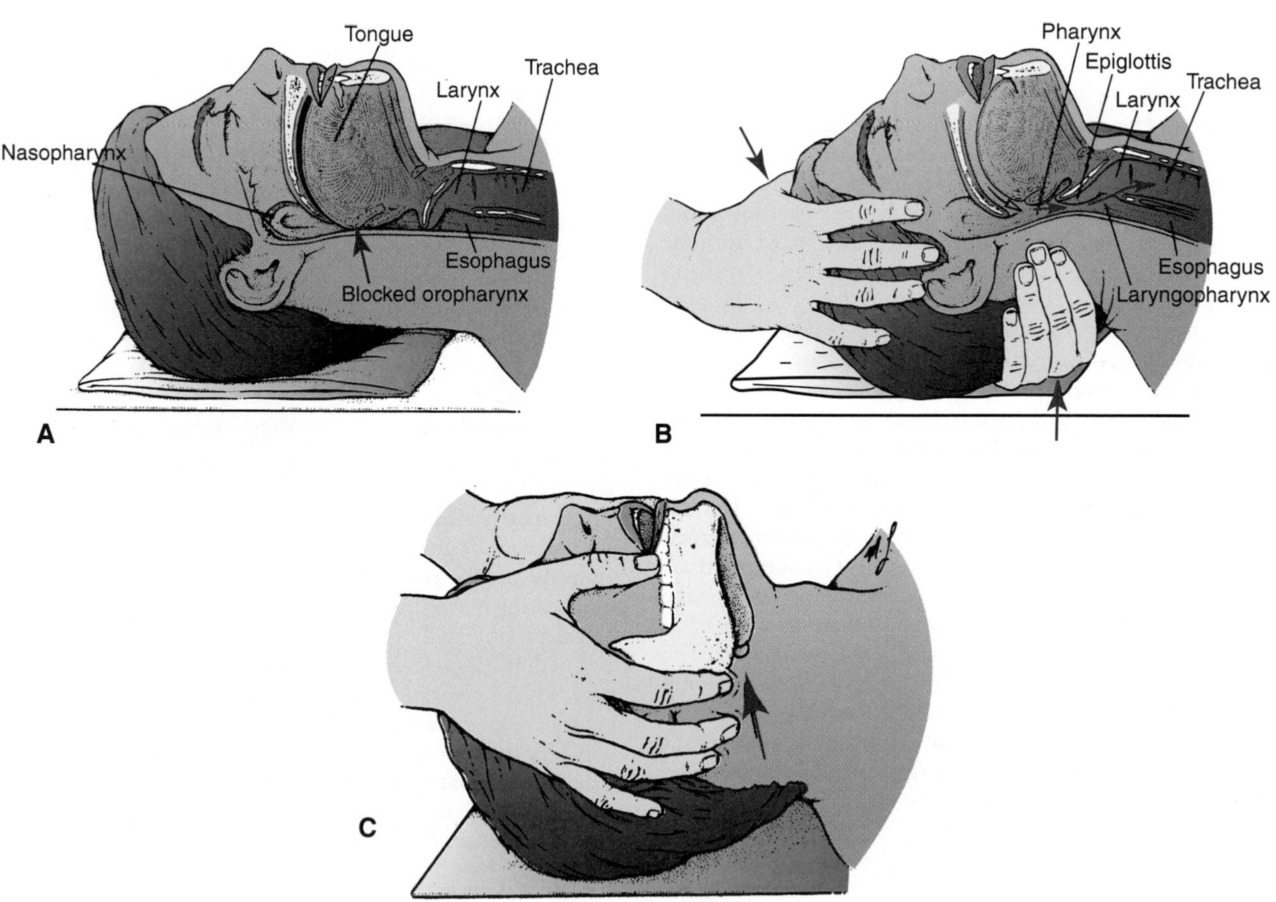

FIGURE 18•1 (**A**) A hypopharyngeal obstruction occurs when neck flexion permits the chin to drop toward the chest; obstruction almost always occurs when the head is in the midposition. (**B**) Tilting the head back to stretch the anterior neck structure lifts the base of the tongue off the posterior pharyngeal wall. The direction of the arrows indicates the pressure of the hands. (**C**) Opening the mouth is necessary to correct valvelike obstruction of the nasal passage during expiration, which occurs in about 30% of unconscious patients. Open the patient's mouth (separate lips and teeth) and move the lower jaw forward so that the lower teeth are in front of the upper teeth. To regain backward tilt of the neck, lift with both hands at the ascending rami of the mandible.

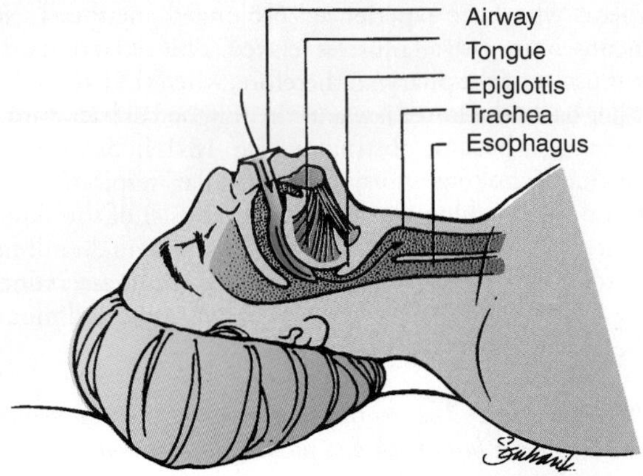

FIGURE 18•2 Use of an airway to prevent respiratory difficulty after anesthesia. The airway passes over the base of the tongue and permits air to pass into the pharynx in the region of the epiglottis. Patients often leave the operating room with an airway in place. The airway should remain in place until the patient recovers sufficiently to breathe normally. As the patient regains consciousness, the airway usually causes irritation and should be removed.

tively, the patient may be brought to the PACU with an endotracheal tube still in place and may require continued mechanical ventilation. The nurse then assists in initiating the use of the ventilator and in the weaning and extubation processes. Some patients, including those who have had extensive or lengthy surgical procedures, may be transferred from the operating room directly to the intensive care unit or may be transferred from the PACU to the intensive care unit while still intubated and on mechanical ventilation.

Respiratory difficulty can also result from excessive secretion of mucus or aspiration of vomitus. Turning the patient to one side allows the collected fluid to escape from the side of the mouth. If the patient's teeth are clenched, the mouth may be opened manually but cautiously with a padded tongue blade. The head of the bed is elevated 15 to 30 degrees unless contraindicated, and the patient is closely observed to maintain the airway as well as minimize the risk of aspiration. If vomiting occurs, the patient is turned to the side to prevent aspiration and the vomitus is collected in the emesis basin. Mucus or vomitus obstructing the pharynx or the trachea is suctioned with a pharyngeal suction tip or a nasal catheter introduced into the nasopharynx or the oropharynx. The catheter can be passed into the nasopharynx or the oropharynx safely to a distance of 15 to 20 cm (6 to 8 inches). Caution is necessary in suctioning the throat of a patient who has had a tonsillectomy or other oral or laryngeal surgery because of risk for bleeding and discomfort.

Maintaining Cardiovascular Stability

To monitor cardiovascular stability, the nurse assesses the patient's mental status; vital signs; cardiac rhythm; skin temperature, color, and moisture; and urine output. Central venous pressure, pulmonary artery pressure, and arterial lines are monitored if the patient's condition requires such assessment. The nurse also assesses the patency of all intravenous lines. The primary cardiovascular complications seen in the PACU include hypotension and shock, hemorrhage, hypertension, and dysrhythmias.

HYPOTENSION AND SHOCK

Hypotension can result from loss of blood, hypoventilation, position changes, pooling of blood in the extremities, or side effects of medications and anesthetics; the most common cause is loss of circulating volume through blood and plasma loss. If the amount of blood loss exceeds 500 mL (especially if the loss is rapid), replacement is usually indicated.

Shock, one of the most serious postoperative complications, can result from hypovolemia. Shock may be described as inadequate cellular oxygenation accompanied by the inability to excrete waste products of metabolism. Hypovolemic shock is characterized by a fall in venous pressure, a rise in peripheral resistance, and tachycardia. Neurogenic shock, a less common cause of shock in the surgical patient, occurs as a result of decreased arterial resistance caused by spinal anesthesia. It is characterized by a fall in blood pressure due to pooling of blood in dilated capacitance vessels (those with the ability to change volume capacity). Cardiogenic shock is unlikely in the surgical patient except in the presence of severe preexisting cardiac disease or if the patient experienced a myocardial infarction during surgery. See Chapter 14 for a detailed discussion of shock.

The classic signs of shock are as follows:

- Pallor
- Cool, moist skin
- Rapid breathing
- Cyanosis of the lips, gums, and tongue
- A rapid, weak, thready pulse
- Decreasing pulse pressure
- Usually, a low blood pressure and concentrated urine

Hypovolemic shock can be avoided largely by the timely administration of intravenous fluids, blood, and medications that elevate blood pressure. Other factors may contribute to hemodynamic instability, and the PACU nurse implements multiple measures to manage these factors. Pain is controlled by making the patient as comfortable as possible and by using opioids judiciously. Exposure is avoided, and normothermia is maintained to prevent vasodilation.

Volume replacement is the primary intervention. An infusion of lactated Ringer's solution or blood component therapy is initiated. Oxygen is administered by nasal cannula, face mask, or mechanical ventilation. Cardiotonics, vasodilators, and corticosteroids may be given to improve cardiac function and reduce peripheral vascular resistance. The patient is kept warm; however, overheating is avoided to prevent cutaneous vessels from dilating and depriving vital organs of blood. The patient is placed flat in bed with the legs elevated. Respiratory and pulse rate, blood pressure, O_2 concentration, urinary output, level of consciousness, central venous pressure, pulmonary artery pressure, pulmonary capillary wedge pressure, and cardiac output are monitored to provide information on the patient's respiratory and cardiovascular status. Vital signs are monitored continuously until the patient's condition has stabilized.

HEMORRHAGE

Hemorrhage is a serious complication of surgery that can result in death. It can present insidiously or emergently at any time in the immediate postoperative period or up to several days after surgery (Table 18-1). When blood loss is extreme, the patient is apprehensive, restless, and thirsty; the skin is cold, moist, and pale. The pulse rate increases, the temperature falls, and respirations are rapid and deep, often of the gasping type spoken of as "air hunger." If the hemorrhage progresses untreated, cardiac

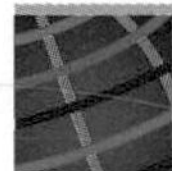

TABLE 18•1 **Classifications of Hemorrhage**

Classification	Defining Characteristic
Time Frame	
Primary	Hemorrhage occurs at the time of surgery.
Intermediary	Hemorrhage occurs during the first few hours after surgery when the rise of blood pressure to its normal level dislodges insecure clots from untied vessels.
Secondary	Hemorrhage may occur some time after surgery if a ligature slips because a blood vessel was insecurely tied, became infected, or was eroded by a drainage tube.
Type of Vessel	
Capillary	Hemorrhage is characterized by a slow, general ooze.
Venous	Darkly colored blood bubbles out quickly.
Arterial	Blood is bright red and appears in spurts with each heartbeat.
Visibility	
Evident	Hemorrhage is on the surface and can be seen.
Concealed	Hemorrhage is in a body cavity and cannot be seen.

output decreases, arterial and venous blood pressure and hemoglobin level fall rapidly, the lips and the conjunctivae become pallid, spots appear before the eyes, a ringing is heard in the ears, and the patient grows weaker but remains conscious until near death.

Giving a transfusion of blood or blood products and determining the cause of hemorrhage are the initial therapeutic measures. The surgical site and incision should always be inspected for bleeding. If bleeding is evident, a sterile gauze pad and a pressure dressing are applied, and the site of the bleeding is elevated to the level of the heart, if possible. The patient is placed in the shock position (lying flat on back with the legs elevated at a 20-degree angle while the knees are kept straight). If the source of bleeding is concealed, the patient may be taken back to the operating room for emergency exploration of the surgical site.

When intravenous fluids are given in cases of hemorrhage, it is important to remember that unless the hemorrhage has been well controlled, giving too large a quantity or administering the intravenous fluid too rapidly may raise the blood pressure enough to start the bleeding again. Additionally, special considerations must be given to patients who decline blood transfusions, such as Jehovah's Witnesses and those who identify specific requests on their advanced directives or living will.

HYPERTENSION AND DYSRHYTHMIAS

Hypertension is common in the immediate postoperative period secondary to sympathetic nervous system stimulation from pain, hypoxia, or bladder distention. Dysrhythmias are associated with electrolyte imbalance, altered respiratory function, pain, hypothermia, stress, and anesthetic medications. Both conditions are managed by treating the underlying causes.

Relieving Pain and Anxiety

Opioid analgesics are administered judiciously and often intravenously in the PACU. Intravenous administration provides immediate relief and is short acting, thus minimizing the potential for drug interactions or prolonged respiratory depression while anesthetics are still active in the patient's system. In addition to monitoring the patient's physiologic status and managing the patient's pain, the PACU nurse provides psychological support in an effort to relieve the patient's fears and concerns. The nurse checks the medical record for special needs and concerns of the patient. When the patient's condition permits, a close member of the family may visit in the PACU for a few moments. This often decreases the family's anxiety and makes the patient feel more secure.

Gerontologic Considerations

The elderly patient is transferred from the operating room table to the bed or stretcher *slowly* and *gently*. The effects of this action on blood pressure and ventilation are monitored. Special attention is given to keeping the patient warm because the elderly are more susceptible to hypothermia. Position is changed frequently to stimulate respirations and circulation and to promote comfort.

Immediate postoperative care for the elderly patient is the same as that for any surgical patient, but additional support is given if there is impaired function of the cardiovascular, pulmonary, or renal systems. With invasive monitoring, it is possible to detect cardiopulmonary deficits before obvious signs and symptoms are apparent. The elderly patient has less physiologic reserve, and physiologic responses to stress are diminished or slowed. These changes reinforce the need for close monitoring and prompt treatment of hypotension, shock, and hemorrhage. Because of monitoring and improved individualized preoperative preparation, many older adults tolerate surgery well and have an unremarkable and uneventful recovery.

Postoperative confusion is common in older patients. This is aggravated by social isolation, restraints, anesthetics and analgesics, and sensory deprivation. Reorienting the patient to the environment and using smaller amounts of sedatives, anesthetics, and analgesics may help prevent confusion. However, unrelieved pain—particularly pain at rest—may increase the risk for delirium and must be considered and addressed (Lynch, Lazor, Gellis, et al., 1998). It is also important to remember that hypoxia may present as confusion and restlessness, as can blood loss and electrolyte imbalance. Excluding all other causes of confusion must precede the assumption that confusion is related to age, circumstances, and medications.

Determining Readiness for Discharge From the Post Anesthesia Care Unit

A patient remains in the PACU until fully recovered from the anesthetic agent—that is, until the patient has a stable blood pressure, adequate respiratory function, an adequate O_2 saturation based on the patient's baseline or preoperative room air reading, and moves spontaneously or on command.

Usually the following measures are used to determine the patient's readiness for discharge from the PACU:

- Uncompromised pulmonary function
- Pulse oximetry readings of adequate O_2 saturation
- Stable vital signs
- Orientation to place, events, time
- Urine output not less than 30 mL/h
- Nausea and vomiting under control; pain minimal

Many hospitals use a scoring system to determine the patient's general condition and readiness to be transferred from the PACU. Throughout the recovery period, the patient's physical signs are observed and evaluated by means of a scoring system (ie, Aldrete score) based on a set of objective criteria. This evaluation guide, a modification of the Apgar scoring system used for evaluating newborns, makes possible a more objective assessment of the patient's physical condition in the PACU (Fig. 18-3). The patient's score is assessed at regular intervals, such as every 15 or 30 minutes, and totaled on the assessment record. Patients with a score of less than 7 must remain in the PACU until their condition improves or they are transferred to an intensive care area, depending on their preoperative baseline.

The patient is discharged from the Phase I PACU by the anesthesiologist or anesthetist to either the critical care unit, the medical-surgical unit, the Phase II PACU, or home with a responsible family member. Patients being discharged directly to home require teaching, written instructions, and information about follow-up care.

Post Anesthesia Care Unit:

MODIFIED ALDRETE SCORE

Patient: Final score:

Room: Surgeon:

Date: PACU nurse:

Area of Assessment	Point Score	Upon Admission	After		
			1 h	2 h	3 h
Muscle Activity:					
Moves spontaneously or on command:					
• Ability to move all extremities	2				
• Ability to move 2 extremities	1				
• Unable to control any extremity	0				
Respiration:					
• Ability to breathe deeply and cough	2				
• Limited respiratory effort (dyspnea or splinting)	1				
• No spontaneous effort	0				
Circulation:					
• BP ± 20% of preanesthetic level	2				
• BP ± 20%–49% of preanesthetic level	1				
• BP ± 50% of preanesthetic level	0				
Consciousness Level:					
• Fully awake	2				
• Arousable on calling	1				
• Not responding	0				
O_2 Saturation:					
• Able to maintain O_2 sat >92% on room air	2				
• Needs O_2 inhalation to maintain O_2 sat >90%	1				
• O_2 sat <90% even with O_2 supplement	0				
Totals:					

Required for discharge from Post Anesthesia Care Unit: 7–8 points

Time of release ______ Signature of nurse ______

FIGURE 18•3 Post anesthesia care unit record (O_2 sat: oxygen saturation).

Promoting Home and Community-Based Care

Expert patient teaching and discharge planning are necessary when a patient undergoes same-day or ambulatory surgery to ensure patient safety and recovery. Because anesthetics cloud memory for concurrent events, instructions should be given to both the patient and the adult who will be accompanying the patient home.

TEACHING PATIENTS SELF-CARE

The patient and caregiver (ie, family member or friend) are informed about expected outcomes and immediate postoperative changes anticipated in the patient's capacity for self-care. Written instructions about wound care, activity and dietary recommendations, medication, and follow-up visits to the same-day surgery unit or the surgeon are provided. The patient's caregiver at home is provided with verbal and written instructions about what to observe the patient for and about the actions to take if complications occur. Prescriptions are given to the patient. The nurse's or surgeon's telephone number is provided, and the patient and caregiver are encouraged to call if questions arise.

Although recovery time varies and is dependent on the type and extent of surgery and the patient's overall physical condition, instructions usually include limited activity for 24 to 48 hours. During this time, the patient is not to drive a vehicle, drink alcoholic beverages, or perform tasks that require energy or skill. Fluids may be consumed as desired, and smaller than normal amounts are eaten at mealtime. The patient is cautioned not to make important decisions at this time because the medications, anesthesia, and surgery may affect thinking ability.

CONTINUING CARE

Although most patients who undergo ambulatory surgery recover quickly and without complications, some patients require referral for home care. These may be elderly or frail patients, those who live alone, and patients with other health care problems that may interfere with self-care or resumption of usual activities. The home care nurse assesses the patient's physical status (ie, respiratory and cardiovascular status, adequacy of pain management, the surgical incision) and the patient's and family's ability to adhere to the recommendations given at the time of discharge. Previous teaching is reinforced as needed. The home care nurse may change surgical dressings, monitor patency of a drainage system, or administer medications. The patient is assessed for the occurrence of surgical complications. The patient and family are reminded about the importance of keeping follow-up appointments with the surgeon. Follow-up phone calls from the nurse or surgeon may also be used to assess the patient's progress and to answer any questions.

THE HOSPITALIZED POSTOPERATIVE PATIENT

The patient admitted to the clinical unit for postoperative care has multiple needs. Seriously ill patients or those who have undergone major cardiovascular, pulmonary, or neurologic surgery are admitted to specialized intensive care units for close monitoring and advanced interventions and support. The care required by these patients in the immediate postoperative period is discussed in specific chapters. Postoperative care for the surgical patient returning to the general medical-surgical floor is discussed below.

Receiving the Patient in the Clinical Unit

The patient's unit is readied by assembling the necessary equipment and supplies: intravenous pole, drainage receptacle holder, emesis basin, tissues, disposable pads (Chux), blankets, and postoperative charting forms. When the call comes to the unit about the patient's transfer from the PACU, the need for any additional items that might be needed is communicated. The PACU nurse reports the baseline data of the patient's condition to the receiving nurse. The report includes demographic data, medical diagnosis, procedure performed, comorbid conditions, unexpected intraoperative events, estimated blood loss, the type and amount of fluids received, medications administered for pain, whether the patient has voided, and information that the patient and family have received about the patient's condition. Usually, the surgeon speaks to the family after surgery and relates the general condition of the patient. The receiving nurse reviews the postoperative orders, admits the patient to the unit, performs an initial assessment, and attends to the patient's immediate needs (Chart 18-1).

Nursing Management During the First Hours After Surgery

Nursing care of the hospitalized patient on the general medical-surgical unit in the first hours up to the first 24 hours after surgery involves continuing to help the patient recover from the effects of anesthesia, frequently assessing the patient's physiologic status, monitoring for complications, managing pain, and implement-

HOME CARE TEACHING CHECKLIST: DISCHARGE FROM SAME-DAY SURGERY

At the completion of the program, the patient or caregiver will be able to:	Patient	Caregiver
• State procedure performed.	✔	✔
• Describe postoperative medication and treatments.	✔	✔
• Describe procedure for changing dressing and providing wound care.	✔	✔
• State activities to avoid (eg, driving, operating machinery).	✔	✔
• State allowed activities.	✔	✔
• State dietary restrictions.	✔	✔
• Describe signs and symptoms of complications.	✔	✔
• State time and date of follow-up appointment.	✔	✔
• State how to reach health provider with questions or complications.	✔	✔

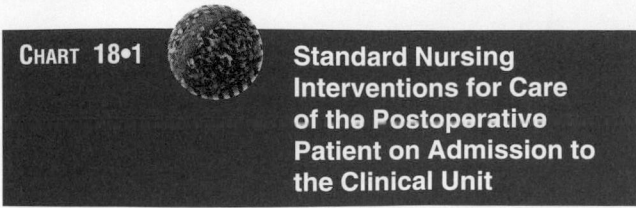

CHART 18•1 **Standard Nursing Interventions for Care of the Postoperative Patient on Admission to the Clinical Unit**

- Assess breathing and apply supplemental oxygen, if prescribed.
- Monitor vital signs and note skin warmth, moisture, and color.
- Assess the surgical site and wound drainage systems.
- Assess level of consciousness, orientation, and ability to move extremities.
- Connect all drainage tubes to gravity or suction as ordered and monitor closed drainage systems.
- Assess pain level, pain characteristics (location, quality) and timing, type, and route of administration of last pain medication.
- Position patient to enhance comfort, safety, and lung expansion.
- Assess intravenous sites for patency and infusions for correct rate and solution.
- Assess urine output in closed drainage system or the patient's urge to void and bladder distention.
- Reinforce need to begin deep-breathing and leg exercises.
- Place call light, emesis basin, ice chips (if allowed), and bedpan or urinal within reach.
- Provide information to patient and family.

ing measures designed to achieve the long-range goals of independence with self-care, successful management of the therapeutic regimen, discharge to home, and full recovery. In the initial hours after admission to the clinical unit, adequate ventilation, hemodynamic stability, incisional pain, surgical site integrity, nausea and vomiting, neurologic status, and spontaneous voiding are all primary concerns. Unless indicated more frequently, the pulse, blood pressure, and respirations are recorded every 15 minutes for the first hour and every 30 minutes for the next 2 hours. Thereafter, they are measured less frequently if they remain stable. The temperature is monitored every 4 hours for the first 24 hours.

Assessing and Managing Ventilation

Pulmonary complications are among the most frequent and serious problems encountered by the surgical patient. Monitoring and managing hypoventilation and preventing atelectasis and pneumonia are the goals of nursing care. The patient is observed for airway patency and the quality of respirations, including depth, rate, and sound, is noted. The chest is auscultated to verify that normal breath sounds are heard bilaterally; the findings are documented as a baseline for later comparisons. Often, because of the effects of pain medications, respirations are slow. Shallow and rapid respirations may be due to pain, constricting dressings, gastric dilation, or obesity. Noisy breathing may be due to obstruction by secretions or the tongue. Measures to maintain a patent airway are carried out as described earlier in this chapter.

The types of hypoxemia that can affect postoperative patients are subacute and episodic. Subacute hypoxemia is a constant low level of O_2 saturation, although the patient's breathing appears normal. Episodic hypoxemia develops suddenly, and the patient may be at risk for cerebral dysfunction, myocardial ischemia, and cardiac arrest. Patients at risk for hypoxemia include those who have undergone major surgery (particularly abdominal), are obese, or have preexisting pulmonary problems. Hypoxemia can be detected by pulse oximetry to determine O_2 saturation. The following factors may affect accuracy of pulse oximetry readings: cold extremities, tremors, atrial fibrillation, black or blue nail polish, and acrylic nails to name a few.

Crackles indicate static pulmonary secretions that need to be mobilized by coughing and deep-breathing exercises. When a mucus plug obstructs one of the bronchi entirely, the pulmonary tissue beyond the plug collapses, and a massive atelectasis—an incomplete expansion of the lung—results. To clear secretions and prevent pneumonia, the nurse encourages the patient to turn frequently and take deep breaths at least every 2 hours. Coughing is also encouraged to dislodge mucus plugs. These pulmonary exercises should begin as soon as the patient arrives on the clinical unit; they continue until the patient is discharged. Even if he or she is not fully awake from anesthesia, the patient can be asked to take several deep breaths. This helps to expel residual anesthetic agents, mobilize secretions, and prevent alveolar collapse (atelectasis). Careful splinting of abdominal or thoracic incision sites helps the patient overcome the fear that the exertion of coughing might open the incision. Pain medications are administered to permit more effective coughing, and oxygen is administered as prescribed to prevent or relieve hypoxemia or hypoxia. To encourage lung expansion, the patient can yawn or take sustained maximal inspirations to create a negative intrathoracic pressure of −40 mm Hg and expand lung volume to total capacity. Chest physical therapy may be prescribed if indicated. Coughing is contraindicated in patients who have head injuries or who have undergone intracranial surgery (because of risk of increasing intracranial pressure) as well as in patients who have undergone eye surgery (because of increasing intraocular pressure) or plastic surgery (because of increasing tension on delicate tissues).

Most postoperative patients, especially the elderly and those with an abdominal or thoracic incision, are given an incentive spirometer. Incentive spirometry is a method by which the patient performs sustained maximal inspirations and at the same time sees the results of these efforts as registered on the spirometer. Such feedback encourages the patient to continue to take deep breaths to maximize voluntary lung expansion. A target is established for each patient. The patient first exhales, then places the lips around the mouthpiece and slowly inhales, trying to drive

Risk Factors for
POSTOPERATIVE PULMONARY COMPLICATIONS

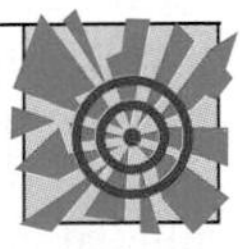

Type of surgery—greater incidence after all forms of abdominal surgery when compared with peripheral surgery
Location of incision—the closer the incision to the diaphragm, the higher the incidence of pulmonary complications
Preoperative respiratory problems
Age—greater risk after age 40 than before age 40
Sepsis
Obesity—weight greater than 110% of ideal body weight
Prolonged bed rest
Duration of surgical procedure—more than 3 hours
Aspiration
Dehydration
Malnutrition
Hypotension and shock
Immunosuppression

the piston on the device to a marked goal. Such a device offers several advantages: (1) the patient is encouraged to participate actively in the treatment; (2) it ensures that the maneuver is physiologically appropriate and is repeated; and (3) it is a cost-effective way of preventing complications. A common recommendation for use of the incentive spirometer is 10 deep breaths every hour while awake. Refer to Chapter 22 for additional discussion of incentive spirometry.

Assessing and Managing Hemodynamic Stability

The patient is still at risk for developing shock or hemorrhage. The patient's appearance, pulse, respirations, blood pressure, skin color (adequate or cyanotic), and skin (cold and clammy, warm and moist, or warm and dry) are used to determine cardiovascular function. If signs and symptoms of shock or hemorrhage occur, treatment and nursing care as described in the discussion of care in the PACU is implemented.

Nursing Alert *A systolic blood pressure of less than 90 mm Hg is usually considered reportable at once. However, the patient's preoperative or baseline blood pressure is used to make informed postoperative comparisons. A previously stable blood pressure that shows a downward trend of 5 mm Hg at each 15-minute reading should also be reported.*

Although most patients do not hemorrhage or go into shock, changes in circulating volume, the stress of surgery, and the effects of medications and preoperative preparations all affect cardiovascular function. Intravenous fluid replacement is standard for up to 24 hours after surgery or until the patient is stable and tolerating oral fluids. Close monitoring is indicated to detect and correct conditions such as fluid volume deficit, altered tissue perfusion, and decreased cardiac output—all of which can increase the patient's discomfort, place him or her at risk for complications, and prolong the hospital stay. Some patients are at risk for fluid volume excess secondary to existing cardiovascular or renal disease, advanced age, or the release of adrenocorticotropic hormone and antidiuretic hormone as a result of the stress of surgery. Consequently, fluid replacement must be carefully managed, and intake and output records must be accurate.

Nursing management includes assessing the patency of the intravenous lines and ensuring that the appropriate fluids are administered at the prescribed rate. Intake and output, including emesis and output from wound drainage systems, is recorded separately and totaled to determine fluid balance. If the patient has an indwelling urinary catheter, hourly outputs are monitored and rates of less than 30 mL/h are reported; if the patient is voiding, an output of less than 240 mL per shift is reported. Electrolyte levels and hemoglobin and hematocrit levels are monitored. Decreased hemoglobin and hematocrit levels can represent blood loss or dilution of circulating volume by intravenous fluids. If dilution is contributing to the decreased levels, the hemoglobin and hematocrit rise as the stress response abates and fluids are mobilized and excreted.

Venous stasis from dehydration, immobility, and pressure on leg veins during surgery put the patient at risk for deep vein thrombosis (DVT). Leg exercises and frequent position changes are initiated early in the postoperative period to stimulate circulation. Patients should avoid positions that compromise venous return, such as raising the bed's knee gatch or placing a pillow under the knees, sitting for long periods, and dangling the legs with pressure at the back of the knees. Venous return is promoted by antiembolism stockings and early ambulation. Early ambulation has a significant effect on recovery, and complication prevention and can begin, in many instances, the evening of surgery. Postoperative activity orders are checked before getting the patient out of bed. Sitting up at the edge of the bed for a few minutes may be all the patient can tolerate at first.

Assessing and Managing the Surgical Site

On the patient's arrival to the clinical unit, the surgical site is observed for bleeding, type and integrity of dressing, and drains. Wound drains are tubes exiting the peri-incisional area into either a portable wound suction device (closed) or into the dressings (open). The principle involved is to allow the escape of blood and serous fluids that can serve as a culture medium for bacteria. In portable wound suction, the use of gentle, constant suction enhances drainage of these fluids and collapses the skin flaps against the underlying tissue, thus removing "dead space." Types of wound drains include the Penrose, Hemovac, and Jackson-Pratt drains (Fig. 18-4). The PACU nurse empties the drains to tally the intake and output during the PACU stay, and all new drainage is recorded. Output from wound drainage systems and the amount of bloody drainage on the surgical dressing are assessed frequently. Spots of drainage on the dressings are marked and timed so that increased drainage can be easily seen. A certain amount of bloody drainage in a wound drainage system or on the dressing is expected; excessive amounts should be reported to the surgeon. Increasing amounts of fresh blood on the dressing should be reported immediately. Some wounds are irrigated heavily before closure in the operating room, and open drains exiting the wound may be embedded in the dressings. These wounds may drain large amounts of blood-tinged fluid that saturate the dressing. The dressing can be reinforced with sterile gauze bandages and the time recorded. If drainage continues, the surgeon should be notified so that he or she can change the dressing. Multiple similar drains are numbered or otherwise labeled (eg, left lower quadrant, left upper quadrant) so that outputs are reliable and consistently recorded.

Assessing and Managing Pain

Most patients experience some degree of pain after a surgical procedure. Many psychological factors (motivational, affective, cognitive, and emotional) influence the patient's total pain experience. Research findings have led to a better understanding of how perception, learning, personality, ethnic and cultural factors, and environment can affect anxiety, depression, and pain response. The degree and severity of postoperative pain and the patient's tolerance level for pain depend on the incision site, the nature of the surgical procedure, the extent of surgical trauma, the type of anesthetic agent, and how the agent was administered. The preoperative preparation received by the patient (including information about what to expect as well as reassurance and psychological support) is a significant factor in decreasing anxiety, apprehension, and even the pain experienced in the postoperative period.

The reasons for establishing effective pain control are compelling. There is a well-known correlation between frequency of complications and localization of pain (Benedetti, 1990). Intense pain stimulates the stress response, which adversely affects the cardiac and immune systems. When pain impulses are transmitted, muscle tension increases, as does local vasoconstriction. The ischemia in the affected area causes further stimulation of

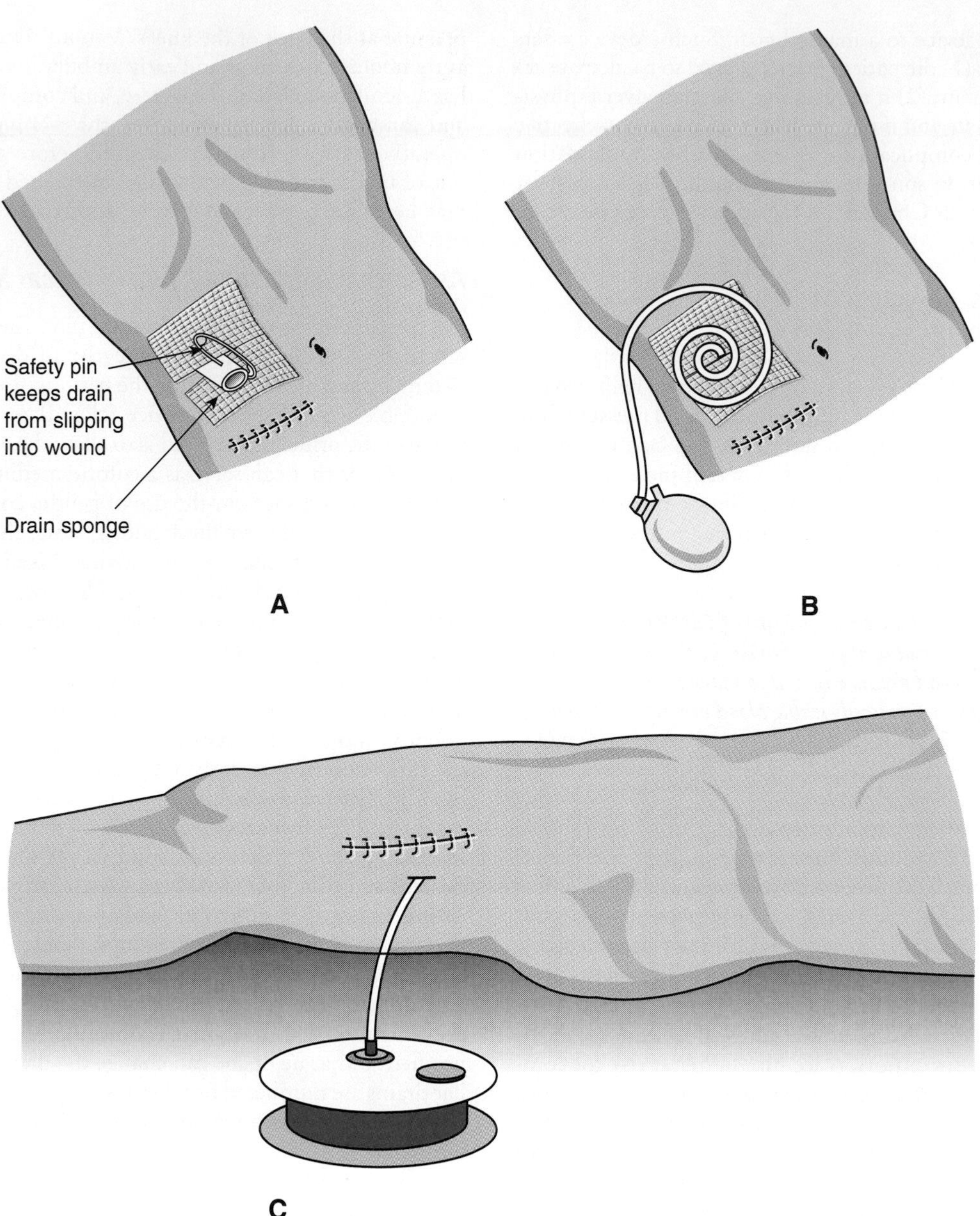

FIGURE 18•4 Types of surgical drains: (**A**) Penrose, (**B**) Jackson-Pratt, (**C**) Hemovac.

pain receptors. When these noxious impulses travel centrally, sympathetic activity is compounded, which increases myocardial demand and oxygen consumption. Research has shown that cardiovascular insufficiency occurs three times more frequently and the incidence of infection is five times greater in people with poor postoperative pain control (Benedetti, 1990). Hypothalamic stress response is also responsible for an increase in blood viscosity and platelet aggregation. This can lead to phlebothrombosis and pulmonary embolism.

The nurse assesses the patient's pain level using a verbal or visual analog scale and assesses the characteristics of the pain. Often, the physician has prescribed different medications or dosages to cover various levels of pain. The nurse should discuss the options with the patient to determine the best medication. The nurse should assess the effectiveness of the medication periodically beginning 30 minutes after administration or sooner if the medication is being delivered by patient-controlled analgesia (PCA).

OPIOIDS

With regard to the need for opioids (narcotics), about one third of patients complain of severe pain, one third of moderate pain, and one third of little or no pain. These statistics do not mean that the patients in the last group have no pain; rather, they appear to activate psychodynamic mechanisms that impair the registering of pain ("gate closing" theory and impaired nociceptive transmission). See Chapter 12 for a more detailed discussion of pain and factors influencing the experience of pain.

Opioid analgesics are often prescribed for pain and immediate postoperative restlessness. A preventive approach, rather than an "as needed" (PRN) approach, is more effective in relieving pain. With a preventive approach, the medication is administered at prescribed intervals rather than when the patient's pain becomes severe or unbearable. Many patients (and some health care providers) are overly concerned with the risk of drug addiction in the postoperative patient. This risk, however, is negligible with use of opioids for short-term pain control.

PATIENT-CONTROLLED ANALGESIA

In view of the negative impact of pain on recovery, nurses need to think "pain prevention" rather than sporadic pain control and encourage the use of PCA. Because patients recover more quickly when adequate pain measures are used, the clinical practice guidelines for postoperative analgesia issued by the Agency for Health Care Policy and Research (AHCPR, 1992) stress prevention rather than pain control and advocate PCA. PCA permits patients to self-administer pain medication when needed. The amount of medication delivered by the intravenous or epidural route and the time span during which the opioid is released are controlled by the PCA device. Self-administration promotes patient participation in care, eliminates delayed administration of pain medications, and maintains a therapeutic level of opioid.

Most patients are candidates for PCA. The two requirements for PCA are (1) an understanding of the need to self-dose and (2) the physical ability to self-dose. Upon sensing pain, the patient activates the pump with a hand-held button. PCA enables the patient to move, turn, cough, and take deep breaths with less pain, thus reducing postoperative pulmonary problems.

EPIDURAL INFUSIONS AND INTRAPLEURAL ANESTHESIA

For thoracic, orthopedic, obstetric, and major abdominal surgery, certain opioids may be administered by epidural or intrathecal infusion. Epidural infusions produce a more profound analgesia. Epidural infusions are used with caution in chest procedures because the effect of the analgesia may ascend along the spinal cord and affect respiration. Intrapleural anesthesia employs the administration of local anesthetic by a catheter between the parietal and visceral pleura. It provides sensory anesthesia without affecting motor function to the intercostal muscles. This anesthesia allows more effective coughing and deep breathing in conditions (eg, cholecystectomy, renal surgery, and rib fractures) in which pain in the thoracic region would interfere with these functions.

Local opioid or a combination anesthetic (use of opioid and local anesthetic agent) is used in the epidural infusion. Other local anesthetic methods may be used to provide analgesia and anesthesia. Intrapleural anesthesia has fewer adverse effects than systemic or spinal opioids and less urinary retention, vomiting, and pruritus when compared with a thoracic epidural.

OTHER PAIN RELIEF MEASURES

Complete absence of pain in the area of the surgical incision may not occur for a few weeks, depending on the site and nature of surgery. However, changing the patient's position, using distraction, applying cool washcloths to the face, and rubbing the back with a soothing lotion may be useful in relieving general discomfort temporarily and rendering the medication more effective when it is administered.

Maintaining Normal Body Temperature

In addition to monitoring respiration, hemodynamic status, the incisional site, and pain levels, the nurse monitors body system function and vital signs (Chart 18-2). The patient is still at risk for hypothermia or malignant hyperthermia; therefore, the temperature is monitored every 4 hours for the first 24 hours and every shift thereafter. Patients who have been anesthetized are susceptible to chills and drafts. Signs of hypothermia are reported to the physician. The room is maintained at a comfortable temperature, and blankets are provided to prevent chilling. The patient is also monitored for cardiac dysrhythmias. The risk for hypothermia is greater in the elderly and in those patients who have been in the cool operating room environment for a prolonged period of time. Efforts are made to identify malignant hyperthermia and to treat it early and promptly.

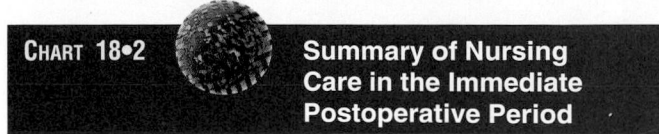

CHART 18•2 Summary of Nursing Care in the Immediate Postoperative Period

The nurse performs multiple tasks and functions in the immediate postoperative period. They include but are not limited to the following:

- Assessment and interpretation of respiratory rate, depth, and quality
- Initiation of supplemental oxygen, breathing exercises, or incentive spirometry use
- Assessment and interpretation of heart rate, blood pressure, color and moistness of the skin
- Assessment and interpretation of intake and output, electrolyte, and hemoglobin and hematocrit levels
- Assessment and care of surgical site
- Initiation of leg exercises and application of antiembolism hose or pneumatic compression stockings
- Assessment of urinary output and ability to void voluntarily
- Assessment of mental status
- Assessment and management of pain
- Positioning for comfort, lung expansion, and prevention of aspiration
- Assessment and treatment of nausea and vomiting
- Initiation of oral fluids (unless contraindicated by type of surgery)
- Assessment and management of patient's and family's psychosocial needs
- Maintaining the patient's safety

Assessing Mental Status

Upon the patient's return from the PACU, the nurse assesses the patient's mental status. The patient's level of consciousness, speech, and orientation should be determined and compared with preoperative baseline measures. Although a change in mental status or postoperative restlessness may be related to anxiety, pain, or medications, it may also be a symptom of oxygen deficit or hemorrhage. These serious causes must be investigated and excluded before other causes are pursued. General discomfort resulting from the patient lying in one position on the operating table, the surgeon's handling of tissues, and the body's reaction to recovery from anesthesia and anxiety are also common causes of restlessness. These discomforts may be relieved by administering the prescribed analgesics, changing the patient's position frequently, and assessing and alleviating the cause of anxiety. The nurse assesses for other possible causes of discomfort, such as tight, drainage-soaked bandages. Reinforcing or changing the dressing completely makes the patient more comfortable. The bladder is palpated for distention because urinary retention can cause restlessness.

Assessing Neurovascular Status

Any surgical procedure has the potential to disrupt neurovascular integrity, either by prolonged awkward positioning in the operating room, manipulation of tissues, inadvertent severing of nerves, or tight bandages. Any orthopedic surgery or surgery involving the extremities carries a risk of peripheral nerve damage. Vascular surgeries, such as replacing sections of diseased peripheral arteries or inserting an arteriovenous graft, put the patient at risk for thrombus formation at the surgical site and subsequent ischemia of tissues distal to the thrombus. Assessment includes having the patient move the hand or foot distal to the surgical site through a full range of motion, assessing that all surfaces have intact sensation, and assessing peripheral pulses.

Assessing and Managing Gastrointestinal Function

Gastrointestinal discomfort (nausea, vomiting, hiccups) and resumption of oral intake are issues for both the patient and the nurse. Nausea and vomiting are common after anesthesia. They are more common in women, people who are obese (fat cells act as reservoirs for the anesthesia), patients prone to motion sickness, and patients who have undergone lengthy surgical procedures. Other causes of postoperative vomiting include an accumulation of fluid in the stomach, inflation of the stomach, and the ingestion of food and fluid before peristalsis resumes.

Newer anesthetic agents and antiemetic medications have decreased the incidence of postoperative nausea, although inadequate ventilation during anesthesia can increase the incidence of vomiting. When vomiting is likely because of the nature of surgery, a nasogastric tube is inserted preoperatively and remains in place throughout the surgery and the immediate postoperative period. In addition, a nasogastric tube may be inserted when a patient who has food in the stomach requires emergency surgery.

After surgery, simple symptomatic therapy is usually all that is required. Many clinicians believe that most antiemetic medications (usually derivatives of phenothiazine) produce undesirable effects, such as hypotension and respiratory depression. If a medication is required, short-acting barbiturates are often prescribed. Intravenous or intramuscular administration of droperidol (Inapsine) may produce sedation and reduce the incidence of nausea and vomiting. The medication may be administered preoperatively and during surgery; its effects carry over into the postoperative period. Ondansetron (Zofran) is a frequently used, effective antiemetic, yet costly.

Nursing Alert *At the slightest indication of nausea, the patient is turned completely on one side to promote mouth drainage to prevent aspiration of vomitus, which can cause asphyxiation and death.*

Produced by intermittent spasms of the diaphragm secondary to irritation of the phrenic nerve, hiccups can occur after surgery. The irritation may be direct, such as from stimulation of the nerve by a distended stomach, subdiaphragmatic abscess, or abdominal distention; indirect, such as from toxemia or uremia that stimulates the center; or reflexive, such as irritation from a drainage tube or obstruction of the intestines. Usually, these occurrences are mild, transitory attacks that cease spontaneously. When hiccups persist, they may produce considerable distress and serious effects, such as vomiting, exhaustion, and possibly wound dehiscence. Phenothiazine medications may be prescribed for severe, persistent hiccups.

Once nausea and vomiting have subsided and the patient is fully awake and alert, the sooner he or she can tolerate a usual diet, the more quickly normal gastrointestinal function will resume. Taking food by mouth stimulates digestive juices and promotes gastric function and intestinal peristalsis. The return to normal dietary intake should proceed at the pace set by the patient. Of course, the nature of surgery and the type of anesthesia directly affect the rate of return. Liquids are the first substances desired and tolerated by the patient after surgery. Water, fruit juices, and tea may be given in increasing amounts. The fluids administered should be cool, not ice cold or tepid. Soft foods (gelatin, junket, custard, milk, and creamed soups) are added gradually after clear fluids have been tolerated. As soon as the patient tolerates soft foods well, solid food may be given.

Assessing and Managing Voluntary Voiding

Urinary retention after surgery can occur for a variety of reasons. Anesthesia, anticholinergic agents, and opioids interfere with the perception of bladder fullness and the urge to void and inhibit the ability to initiate voiding and completely empty the bladder. Abdominal, pelvic, and hip surgery may increase the likelihood of retention secondary to pain. Additionally, some patients find it difficult to use the bedpan or urinal in the recumbent position.

Bladder distention and urge to void should be assessed on the patient's arrival on the unit and frequently thereafter. The patient is expected to void within 8 hours of surgery (this includes time spent in the PACU). Also, if the patient has an urge to void and cannot, or if the bladder is distended and no urge is felt or the patient cannot void, catheterization is not delayed until after 8 hours. All methods to encourage the patient to void should be tried (eg, letting water run, applying heat to the perineum). A bedpan should be warm; a cold bedpan causes discomfort and automatic tightening of muscles (including the urethral sphincter). When a patient complains of not being able to use the bedpan, it may be permissible to use a commode rather than resort to catheterization. Male patients are often permitted to sit up or stand beside the bed to use the urinal, but safeguards should be taken to prevent the patient from falling or fainting due to loss of coordination from medications or orthostatic hypotension. If the patient is unable to void in the specified time frame, he or she is catheterized. The catheter is removed after the bladder has been emptied. Straight intermittent catheterization is preferred over indwelling catheterization because the risk for infection is increased with an indwelling catheter. If the patient does void, it does not necessarily mean the bladder has emptied. The nurse notes the amount of urine voided and palpates the suprapubic area for distention or tenderness or uses a portable ultrasound device to assess residual volume. Intermittent catheterization continues every 4 to 6 hours until the patient can void spontaneously and the postvoid residual is less than 100 mL.

Encouraging Activity

Most surgical patients are encouraged to be out of bed as soon as possible. Early ambulation reduces the incidence of postoperative complications, such as atelectasis, hypostatic pneumonia, gastrointestinal discomfort, and circulatory problems. Ambulation increases ventilation and reduces stasis of bronchial secretions in the lung. It also reduces postoperative abdominal distention by increasing gastrointestinal tract and abdominal wall tone and stimulating peristalsis. Thrombophlebitis or phlebothrombosis occurs less frequently because early ambulation prevents stasis of blood by increasing the rate of circulation in the extremities. Pain is often decreased when early ambulation is allowed. Finally, the hospital stay is shorter and less costly, a further advantage to the patient and the hospital.

Despite the advantages of early ambulation, patients may be reluctant to get up the evening of surgery. Reminding them of the importance of early mobility in preventing complications may help them overcome their fears. One concern when the patient is to get out of bed for the first time is orthostatic hypotension, also called postural hypotension. Orthostatic hypotension is an abnormal drop in blood pressure that occurs as the patient changes from a supine to a standing position. It is common after surgery because of changes in circulating volume and bed rest. Signs and symptoms include a 20 mm Hg decrease in systolic blood pressure or a 10 mm Hg decrease in diastolic blood pressure, weakness, dizziness, and fainting. Older adults are at increased risk for orthostatic hypotension secondary to age-related changes in vascular tone. To detect orthostatic hypotension, the nurse assesses the patient's feelings of dizziness and his or her blood pressure first in the supine position, after the patient sits up, again after the patient stands, and 2 to 3 minutes later. Gradual position change gives the circulatory system time to adjust. If the patient becomes dizzy, he or she should be returned to the supine position, and getting out of bed should be delayed for several hours.

To assist the postoperative patient in getting out of bed for the first time after surgery, the nurse performs the following actions:

- Helps the patient to move gradually from the lying position to the sitting position until dizziness passes, which can be achieved by raising the head of the bed
- Positions the patient completely upright (sitting) and turned so that both legs hang over the edge of the bed
- Assists the patient to stand beside the bed

When accustomed to the upright position, the patient may start to walk. The nurse should be at the patient's side to give physical support and encouragement. Care must be taken not to tire the patient; the extent of the first few periods of ambulation varies with the type of surgical procedure and the patient's physical condition and age.

Even when the patient ambulates early in the postoperative period, and especially if ambulation is not possible, bed exercises are encouraged to improve circulation.

Bed exercises consist of the following:

- Arm exercises (full range of motion, with specific attention to abduction and external rotation of the shoulder)
- Hand and finger exercises
- Foot exercises to prevent foot drop and toe deformities and to aid in maintaining good circulation
- Leg flexion and leg-lifting exercises to prepare the patient for ambulation
- Abdominal and gluteal contraction exercises

Maintaining a Safe Environment

The patient recovering from anesthesia should have all side rails up, and the bed should be in the low position. The nurse assesses the patient's level of consciousness and orientation and determines if the patient needs his or her glasses or hearing aid because problems with vision or inability to hear postoperative instructions places the patient at risk for injury. All objects the patient may need should be within reach, including, of course, the call bell. Any immediate postoperative orders concerning special positioning, equipment, or interventions should be implemented as soon as possible. The patient is asked to seek assistance with any activity. Although occasionally necessary for the disoriented patient, restraints should not be used if at all possible.

Providing Emotional Support to the Patient and Family

Although patients and families are undoubtedly relieved that the procedure is over, anxiety levels may remain high in the immediate postoperative period. Many factors contribute to this anxiety: pain, being in an unfamiliar environment, feeling unable to control one's circumstances, fear of the long-term effects of surgery, fear of complications, loss of ability to care for self, fatigue, spiritual distress, altered role responsibilities, ineffective coping, and altered body image are all potential reactions to the surgical experience. The nurse helps the patient and family work through their anxieties by providing reassurance and information and by spending time listening to and addressing their concerns. The nurse describes hospital routines and what to expect in the ensuing hours and days until discharge and explains the purpose of nursing assessments and interventions. Informing patients when they can take fluids or eat, when they will be getting out of bed, and when tubes and drains will be removed helps them gain a sense of control and participation in recovery and engages them in the plan of care. Acknowledging family members' concerns and accepting and encouraging their participation in the patient's care assists them to feel they are helping their loved one. The nurse can manipulate the environment to enhance rest and relaxation by providing privacy, reducing noise, adjusting the lighting, providing enough seating for family members, and performing any other measures that will produce a supportive atmosphere.

Gerontologic Considerations

Elderly patients continue to be at increased risk for postoperative complications. Age-related physiologic changes in respiratory, cardiovascular, and renal function and the increased incidence of comorbid conditions demand skilled assessment to detect early signs of deterioration. Anesthetics and opioids can cause confusion in the older adult, and altered pharmacokinetics results in delayed excretion and prolonged respiratory depressive effects. Careful monitoring of electrolyte, hemoglobin, and hematocrit levels and urine output are essential because older adults are less able to correct and compensate for fluid and electrolyte imbalances. Pneumonia, atelectasis, and venous stasis are greater threats to the older population. Initiating breathing and leg exercises helps reduce risk; however, the older adult's ability to perform these exercises may be diminished as a result of decreased activity tolerance. Age-related sensory deficits can interfere with postoperative instructions, and the elderly patient may need frequent reminders and demonstrations to participate in care effectively.

The First Postoperative Day to Day of Discharge

Patients usually begin to feel better several hours after surgery or after waking up the next morning. Although pain may still be intense, many patients feel more alert, less nauseous, and less anxious. They have begun their breathing and leg exercises, and many will have dangled over the edge of the bed, stood, and ambulated a few feet or been assisted out of bed to the chair at least once. Many will have tolerated a light meal and had intravenous fluids discontinued. The focus of care shifts from intense physiologic management and symptomatic relief of the adverse effects of anesthesia to regaining independence with self-care and preparing for discharge. Despite these gains, the postoperative patient is still at risk for complications. Atelectasis, pneumonia, DVT, pulmonary embolism, constipation, paralytic ileus, and wound infection are ongoing threats for the postoperative patient (Fig. 18-5).

NURSING PROCESS: THE PATIENT RECOVERING FROM SURGERY

Assessment

Ongoing assessment includes monitoring vital signs and completing a review of systems assessment each shift. Respiratory status, pain level, wound integrity, oral intake and nutritional status, bowel sounds, abdominal distention, passage of flatus or stool, fluid balance, blood chemistry levels, and hemoglobin and hematocrit levels are critical factors influencing recovery. Activity tolerance, functional status, and ability to participate in care are also assessed, as are the outcomes of specific patient teaching activities.

Diagnosis

Nursing Diagnoses

Based on the assessment data, major nursing diagnoses may include the following:

- Pain related to surgical incision
- Risk for ineffective airway clearance related to depressed respiratory function, pain, and bed rest
- Activity intolerance related to pain and weakness secondary to surgery
- Self-care deficit related to postoperative fatigue and pain
- Impaired skin integrity related to incision and drainage sites
- Risk for wound infection related to susceptibility to bacterial invasion
- Risk for altered nutrition: less than body requirements related to decreased intake and increased need for nutrients secondary to surgery
- Risk for colonic constipation related to effects of medications, surgery, dietary change, and immobility
- Risk for ineffective management of therapeutic regimen related to insufficient knowledge about wound care, dietary restrictions, activity recommendations, medications, follow-up care, or signs and symptoms of complications

Collaborative Problems/Potential Complications

Based on the assessment data, potential complications may include the following:

- Atelectasis or pneumonia
- Deep vein thrombosis (DVT)
- Wound infection, dehiscence, or evisceration
- Paralytic ileus

Planning and Goals

The major goals of the patient include relief of pain, optimal respiratory function, absence of complications, increased activity tolerance, unimpaired wound healing, maintenance of nutritional balance, resumption of usual pattern of bowel elimination, acquisition of sufficient knowledge to manage self-care after discharge, and absence of complications.

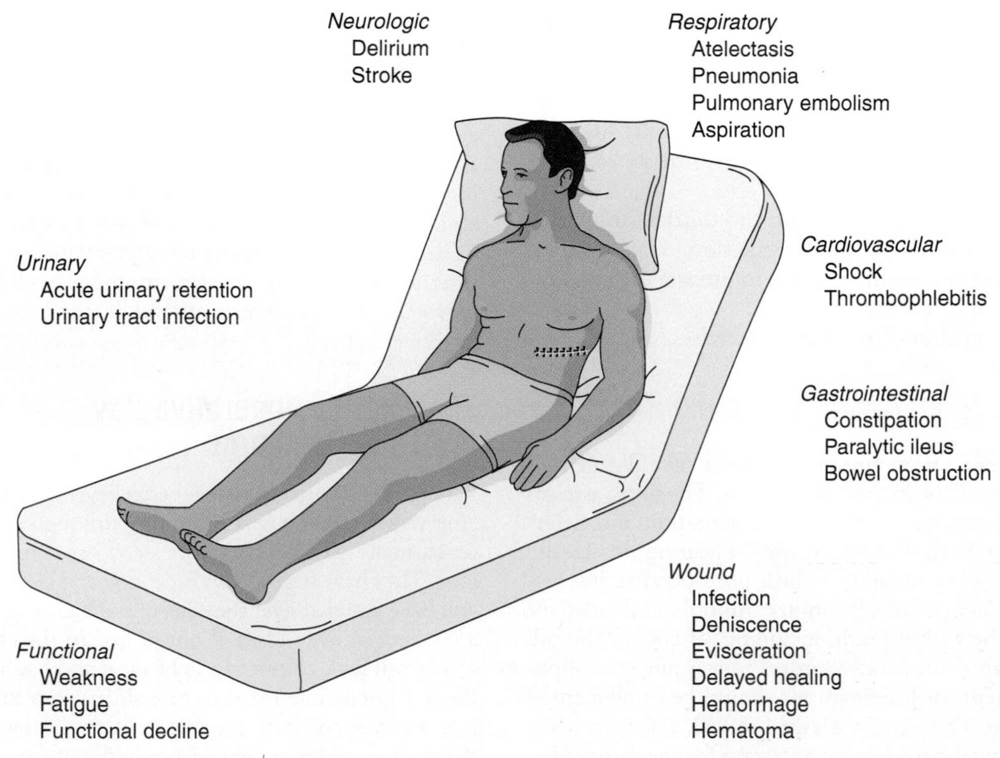

FIGURE 18•5 The postoperative patient is subject to a number of potential complications.

Nursing Interventions

Relieving Pain

The intensity of postoperative pain gradually subsides on subsequent days; however, pain control continues to be an important concern for the patient and the nurse. Effective pain management allows the patient to participate in care, perform deep-breathing and leg exercises, and tolerate activity. As stated previously, poor pain control contributes to postoperative complications and increased length of stay. The nurse continues to assess pain level, effectiveness of pain medication, and factors that influence pain tolerance (eg, energy level, stress level, cultural background, meaning of pain to the patient). The nurse explains that taking pain medication before the pain becomes intense is more effective and offers pain medication at intervals rather than waiting for the pain to request medication. Nonpharmacologic pain relief measures, such as imagery, relaxation, massage, application of heat or cold (if ordered), and distraction, can be used to supplement medications.

Preventing Respiratory Complications

Respiratory depressive effects of opioids, decreased lung expansion secondary to pain, and decreased mobility combine to keep the patient at risk for respiratory complications, particularly atelectasis and pneumonia (see Chap. 21). Atelectasis remains a risk for the patient who is not moving well or ambulating or is not performing deep-breathing and coughing exercises or using an incentive spirometer. Signs and symptoms include decreased breath sounds over the affected area, crackles, and cough. Pneumonia is characterized by chills and fever, tachycardia, and tachypnea. Cough may or may not be present and may or may not be productive. Hypostatic pulmonary congestion, caused by a weakened cardiovascular system that permits stagnation of secretions at lung bases, may develop in elderly or very weak patients. It occurs most frequently in elderly patients who are not mobilized effectively. The symptoms are often vague—perhaps a slight elevation of temperature, pulse, and respiratory rate and a cough. Physical examination reveals dullness and crackles at the base of the lungs. If the condition progresses, the outcome may be fatal.

Preventive measures and timely recognition of signs and symptoms help avert negative outcomes. Strategies to prevent respiratory complications include using an incentive spirometer and practicing deep-breathing and coughing exercises. If the patient has an abdominal or thoracic incision, he or she is taught to splint the incision while coughing. Early ambulation increases metabolism and pulmonary aeration and, in general, improves all body functions. The patient is encouraged to be out of bed as soon as possible (ie, on the day of surgery, or no later than the first postoperative day). This practice is especially valuable in preventing pulmonary complications in older patients.

Preventing Deep Vein Thrombosis

DVT and its possible consequence, pulmonary embolism, are serious potential complications of surgery. The stress response that is initiated as a result of surgery inhibits the fibrinolytic system, resulting in blood hypercoagulability. Dehydration, low cardiac output, blood pooling in the extremities, and bed rest add to the risk of thrombosis formation. Although all postoperative patients are at some risk, certain surgeries and patient populations carry a greater risk. The first symptom of DVT may be a pain or a cramp in the calf. Although not necessarily present in all cases, calf pain elicited on ankle dorsiflexion (Homans' sign) suggests thrombosis (Fig. 18-6). Initial pain and tenderness may be followed by a painful swelling of the entire leg, often accompanied by a slight fever and sometimes chills and diaphoresis.

Prophylactic treatment for postoperative patients at risk is common practice. Low-dose heparin may be prescribed and administered subcutaneously until the patient is ambulatory. Low-molecular-weight heparin and low-dose warfarin are other anticoagulants that may be used. External pneumatic compression and thigh-high elastic pressure stockings can be used alone or in combination with low-dose heparin.

Risk Factors for **POSTOPERATIVE DEEP VEIN THROMBOSIS**

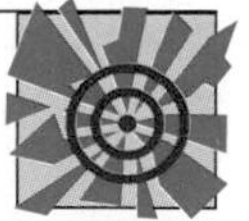

Patients at increased risk for postoperative deep vein thrombosis include the following:

Orthopedic patients having hip surgery, knee reconstruction, and other lower extremity surgery
Urologic patients having transurethral prostatectomy, and older patients having urologic surgery
General surgical patients over 40 years of age, those who are obese, those with a malignancy, those who have had prior deep vein thrombosis or pulmonary embolism, or those undergoing extensive, complicated surgical procedures
Gynecology (and obstetric) patients over 40 years of age with added risk factors (varicose veins, previous venous thrombosis, infection, malignancy, obesity)
Neurosurgical patients, similar to other surgical high-risk groups (in patients with stroke, eg, the risk of deep vein thrombosis in the paralyzed leg is as high as 75%)

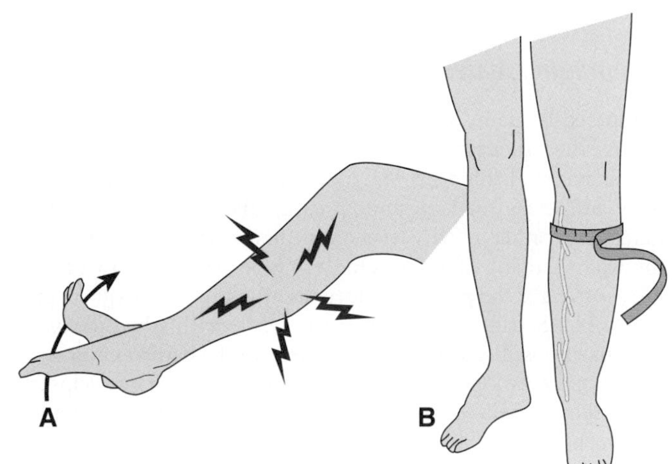

FIGURE 18•6 Assessment of signs and symptoms of phlebothrombosis. (**A**) With the knee flexed, the patient may complain of pain in the calf on dorsiflexion of the foot (Homans' sign). This is a sign of early and subclinical thrombosis, which may or may not be present. Gentle compression reveals tenderness of the calf muscles (note arrow). (**B**) The affected leg may swell; veins are more prominent and may be palpated easily.

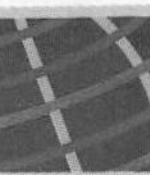

TABLE 18•2 Wound Classification and Associated Surgical Site Infection Risk

Surgical Category	Determinants of Category	Expected Risk of Postsurgical Infection (%)
Clean	Nontraumatic site Uninfected site No inflammation No break in aseptic technique No entry into respiratory, alimentary, genitourinary, or oropharyngeal tracts	1–3
Clean-contaminated	Entry into respiratory, alimentary, genitourinary, or oropharyngeal tracts without unusual contamination Appendectomy Minor break in aseptic technique Mechanical drainage	3–7
Contaminated	Open, newly experienced traumatic wounds Gross spillage from gastrointestinal tract Major break in aseptic technique Entry into genitourinary or biliary tract when urine or bile is infected	7–16
Dirty	Traumatic wound with delayed repair, devitalized tissue, foreign bodies, or fecal contamination Acute inflammation and purulent drainage encountered during procedure	16–29

The benefits of early ambulation and hourly leg exercises in the prevention of DVT cannot be overemphasized, and these activities are recommended for all patients, regardless of relative risk. It is important to avoid the use of blanket rolls, pillow rolls, or any form of elevation that can constrict vessels under the knees. Even prolonged "dangling" (having the patient sit on the edge of the bed with legs hanging over the side) can be dangerous and is not recommended in susceptible patients because pressure under the knees can impede circulation. Adequate hydration is also encouraged; the patient can be offered juices and water throughout the day to avoid dehydration. Refer to Chapter 28 for complete discussion of DVT and to Chapter 21 for discussion of pulmonary embolus.

Encouraging Activity and Promoting Self-Care

Hampered by pain, dressings, intravenous lines, or drainage apparatus, the patient is frequently unable to engage in activity without assistance. Prolonged inactivity may lead to pressure ulcers, DVT, atelectasis, or hypostatic pneumonia. Helping the patient increase his or her activity level on the first postoperative day is an important nursing function. One way to increase the patient's activity is to have the patient perform as much routine hygiene care as possible. Setting up the patient to bathe with a bedside wash basin or, if possible, assisting the patient to the bathroom to sit at a chair at the sink not only gets the patient moving but helps restore a sense of self-control and prepares the patient for discharge. Patients need to be able to ambulate a functional distance (length of the house or apartment), get in and out of bed unassisted, and be independent with toileting to be safely discharged to home. Patients can be asked to perform as much as they can and then to call for assistance. The patient and the nurse can collaborate on a schedule for progressive activity that includes ambulating in the room and hallway and sitting out of bed in the chair. Assessing the patient's vital signs before, during, and after a scheduled activity helps the nurse and patient determine the rate of progression. By providing physical support, the nurse maintains the patient's safety and by communicating a positive attitude about the patient's ability to perform the activity, the nurse promotes the patient's confidence. The nurse should make sure the patient continues to perform bed exercises, wears antiembolism stockings when in bed, and rests as needed.

Preventing Wound Infection and Providing Wound Care

The creation of a surgical wound disrupts the integrity of skin and its protective function. Exposure of deep body tissues to pathogens in the environment places the patient at risk for infection of the surgical site, a serious and potentially life-threatening complication. Surgical site infection increases hospital length of stay, costs of care, and risk for further complication. In postoperative patients, surgical site infection is the most common nosocomial infection, with 67% of these infections occurring within the incision and 33% occurring in an organ or space around the surgical site (CDC, 1999). Multiple factors place the patient at risk for wound infection.

One risk factor is the wound class. Surgical wounds are classified according to the degree of contamination. Table 18-2 defines the various terms used to describe surgical wounds and gives the expected rate of wound infection per category. Other risk factors include both patient-related factors and those associated with the surgical procedure. Patient-related factors include age, nutritional status, diabetes, smoking, obesity, remote infections, endogenous mucosal microorganisms, altered immune response, length of preoperative stay, and severity of illness. Risk factors related to the surgical procedure include method of preoperative skin preparation, the surgical attire of the team, method of sterile draping, duration of surgery, antimicrobial prophylaxis, aseptic technique, factors related to surgical technique, drains or foreign material, operating room ventilation, and exogenous microorganisms. Efforts to prevent wound infection are directed at re-

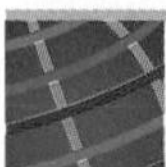

TABLE 18•3 Phases of Wound Healing

Phase	Duration	Events
Inflammatory (also called lag or exudative phase)	1–4 days	Blood clot forms Wound becomes edematous Debris of damaged tissue and blood clot are phagocytosed
Proliferative (also called fibroblastic or connective tissue phase)	5–20 days	Collagen produced Granulation tissue forms Wound tensile strength increases
Maturation (also called differentiation, resorptive, remodeling, or plateau phase)	21 days to months or even years	Fibroblasts leave wound Tensile strength increases Collagen fibers reorganize and tighten to reduce scar size

ducing these risks. Preoperative and intraoperative risks and interventions are discussed in Chapters 16 and 17. Although the conditions for surgical site infection and serious contamination of the wound occur in the preoperative and intraoperative time frames, postoperative care of the wound centers on assessing the wound, preventing contamination and infection before wound edges have sealed, and enhancing healing.

Assessment involves inspecting the wound for approximation of wound edges, integrity of sutures or staples, redness, discoloration, warmth, swelling, unusual tenderness, or drainage. The area around the wound should also be inspected for reactions to tape or trauma from tight bandages.

Healing occurs in three phases: the inflammatory, proliferative, and maturation phases (Table 18-3). Wounds also heal by different mechanisms, depending on the condition of the wound. These mechanisms include first, second, or third intention wound healing.

Wounds made aseptically, with a minimum of tissue destruction, and properly closed, heal with little tissue reaction by first intention (primary union) (Fig. 18-7). When wounds heal by **first intention healing**, granulation tissue is not visible, and scar formation is minimal. Postoperatively, these wounds are normally covered with dry sterile dressings.

Second intention healing (granulation) occurs in infected wounds (abscess) or in wounds in which the edges have not been approximated. When an abscess is incised, it collapses partly, but the dead and the dying cells forming its walls are still being released into the cavity. For this reason, drainage tubes or gauze packing are often inserted into the abscess pocket to allow drainage to escape easily. Gradually, the necrotic material disintegrates and escapes, and the abscess cavity fills with a red, soft, sensitive tissue that bleeds easily. This tissue is composed of minute, thin-walled capillaries and buds that later form connective tissue. These buds, called granulations, enlarge until they fill the area left by the destroyed tissue (see Fig. 18-7). The cells surrounding the capillaries change their round shape to become long, thin, and intertwined with each other to form a scar (cicatrix). Healing is complete when skin cells (epithelium) grow over these granulations. This method of repair is called healing by granulation, and it takes place whenever pus is formed or when loss of tissue has occurred for any reason. When the postoperative wound is allowed to heal by secondary intention, it is usually packed with saline-moistened sterile dressings and covered with a dry sterile dressing.

Third intention healing (secondary suture) is used for deep wounds that have either not been sutured early or break down and are resutured later, thus bringing together two apposing granulation surfaces. This results in a deeper and wider scar (see Fig. 18-7). These wounds are also packed postoperatively with moist gauze and covered with a dry sterile dressing.

As a wound heals, many elements, such as adequate nutrition, cleanliness, rest, and position, determine how quickly the process occurs. These factors are influenced by nursing interventions. Specific nursing assessments and interventions that address these factors and help to promote wound healing are presented in Table 18-4. Other nursing interventions include assessment and care of the wound.

Although postoperative dressings are initially changed by a member of the surgical team, subsequent dressing changes in the immediate postoperative period are usually done by the nurse. A dressing is applied to a wound for one or more of the following reasons: (1) to provide a proper environment for wound healing; (2) to absorb drainage; (3) to splint or immobilize the wound; (4) to protect the wound and new epithelial tissue from mechanical injury; (5) to protect the wound from bacterial contamination and from soiling by feces, vomitus, and urine; (6) to promote hemostasis, as in a pressure dressing; and (7) to provide mental and physical comfort for the patient.

The patient is told that the dressing is to be changed and that changing the dressing is a simple procedure associated with little discomfort. The dressing change is scheduled for a suitable time (ie, not at mealtimes or when visitors are present). Privacy is provided, and the patient is not unduly exposed. The incision should not be referred to as a "scar" because for some patients the term has negative connotations. Assurance is given that the incision will shrink as it heals and the redness will fade.

The nurse washes his or her hands before and after the dressing change. Disposable gloves are worn. The adhesive is removed by pulling it parallel with the skin surface and in the direction of hair growth, rather than at right angles. Alcohol wipes or nonirritating solvents aid in removing adhesive painlessly and quickly. The old dressing is removed and then deposited in a container designated for biomedical waste disposal. In accordance with standard precautions, dressings are never touched by ungloved hands because of the danger of transmitting pathogenic organisms.

The tray for a routine dressing change includes gloves, cotton balls, a packet of antiseptic solution, sterile saline, dressings, and forceps. When the sterile tray has been properly opened, the nurse places additional dressings on the field, if needed, and moistens the cotton balls with the antiseptic. Forceps are used in cleansing the wound and surrounding skin with the moistened cotton balls.

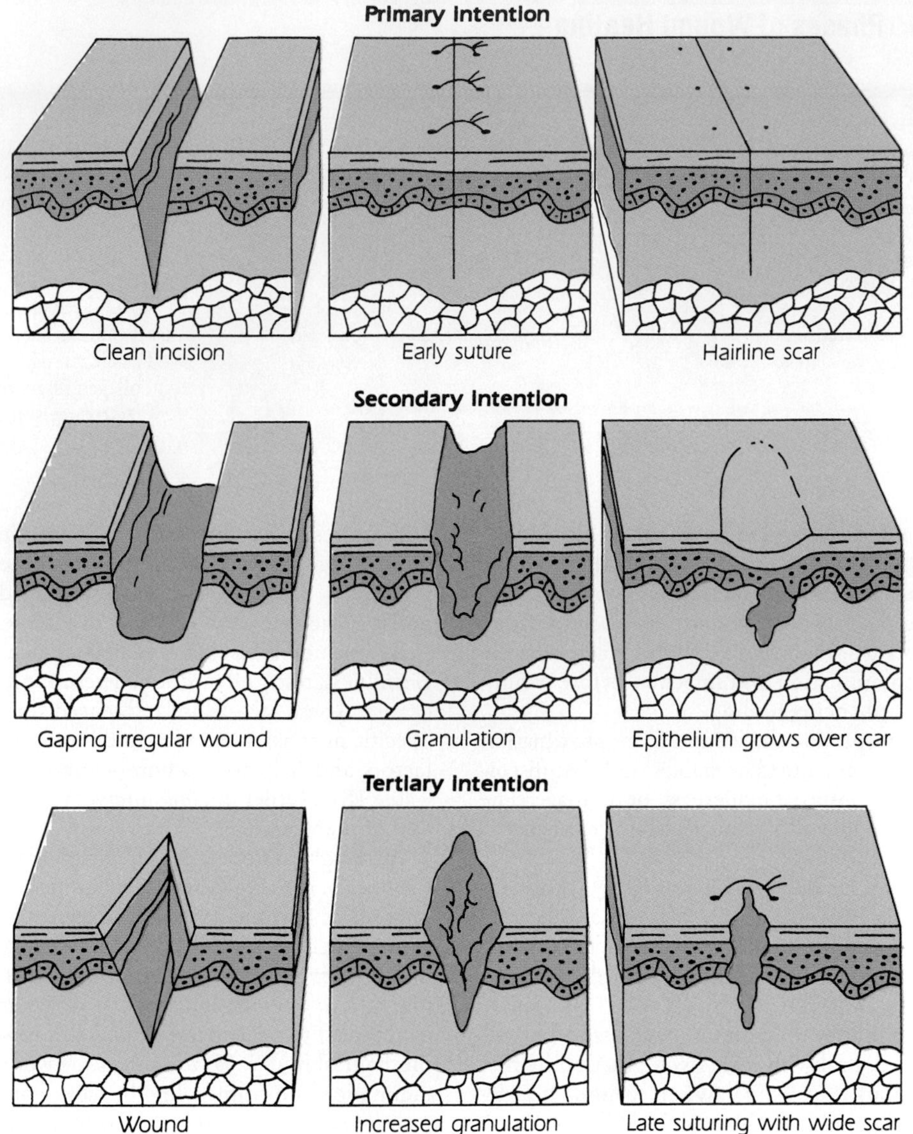

FIGURE 18•7 Types of wound healing: primary intention healing, secondary intention healing, and tertiary intention healing.

A separate cotton ball is used to clean around the drain tubing. The antiseptic solution is removed with sterile saline, and the new dressing (dry sterile dressing for a closed wound, saline-moistened gauze and a dry sterile dressing for an open wound) is then applied. A separate folded gauze pad or drain sponge is used to dress wound drains, and care is taken to avoid having drain tubing come in contact with the incision.

Dressings are held in place with tape. If the patient is sensitive to adhesive material, hypoallergenic tape is used. Many tapes are porous to permit ventilation and prevent maceration of the skin. The correct way to apply tape is to place the tape at the center of the dressing and then press the tape down on both sides, applying tension evenly away from the midline (Fig. 18-8). The wrong method of applying tape—fixing one end of the tape to the skin and pulling it tight over the dressing—often wrinkles and pulls the skin in the process. The resulting continuous and forceful traction produces a shearing effect, causing the epidermal layer to slip sideways and become separated from the deeper dermal layers. Some wounds become edematous after having been dressed, causing considerable tension on the tape. If the tape is not flexible, the stretching bandage will also cause a shear injury to the skin. This can result in denuded areas or large blisters. Elastic adhesive bandage (Elastoplast, Microfoam-3M) is preferable for holding dressings in place over mobile areas, such as the neck or the extremities, or where pressure is required.

A commercial silicone aerosol product is available that can be sprayed over the adhesive used to hold dressings in place; the silicone waterproofs the dressing so that the patient can bathe or swim, and it isolates the area from contamination. The spray is odorless, colorless, nonstaining, noninflammatory, heat stable, and hypoallergenic.

While changing the dressing, the nurse has an opportunity to teach the patient how to care for the incision and change the dressings at home. The nurse observes for indicators of the patient's readiness to learn, such as looking at the incision, expressing interest, or assisting in the dressing change. Information on self-care activities and possible signs of infection are summarized in the accompanying patient education box.

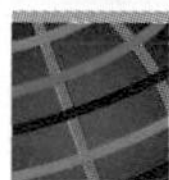

TABLE 18•4 Factors Affecting Wound Healing

Factors	Rationale	Nursing Interventions
Age of patient	The older the patient, the less resilient the tissues.	Handle all tissues gently.
Handling of tissues	Rough handling causes injury and delayed healing.	Handle tissues carefully and evenly.
Hemorrhage	Accumulation of blood creates dead spaces as well as dead cells that must be removed. The area becomes a growth medium for organisms.	Monitor vital signs. Observe incision site for evidence of bleeding and infection.
Hypovolemia	Insufficient blood volume leads to vasoconstriction and reduced oxygen and nutrients available for wound healing.	Monitor for volume deficit (circulatory impairment). Correct by fluid replacement as prescribed.
Local factors		
Edema	Reduces blood supply by exerting increased interstitial pressure on vessels	Elevate part; apply cool compresses.
Inadequate dressing technique		
Too small	Permits bacterial invasion and contamination	Follow guidelines for proper dressing technique.
Too tight	Reduces blood supply carrying nutrients and oxygen	
Nutritional deficits	Insulin secretion may be inhibited, causing blood glucose to rise.	Monitor blood glucose levels. Administer vitamin supplements as prescribed.
	Protein-calorie depletion may occur.	Correct deficits; this may require parenteral nutritional therapy.
Foreign bodies	Foreign bodies retard healing.	Keep wounds free of dressing threads, talcum, and powder from gloves.
Oxygen deficit (tissue oxygenation insufficient)	Insufficient oxygen may be due to inadequate lung and cardiovascular function as well as localized vasoconstriction.	Encourage deep breathing, turning, controlled coughing.
Drainage collection	Accumulated secretions hamper healing process.	Monitor closed drainage systems for proper functioning. Institute measures to remove accumulated secretions.
Medications		
Corticosteroids	May mask presence of infection by impairing normal inflammatory response	Be aware of action and effect of medications patient is receiving.
Anticoagulants	May cause hemorrhage	
Broad-spectrum and specific antibiotics	Effective if administered immediately before surgery for specific pathology or bacterial contamination. If administered after wound is closed, ineffective because of intravascular coagulation.	
Patient overactivity	Prevents approximation of wound edges. Resting favors healing.	Use measures to keep wound edges approximated: taping, bandaging, splints. Encourage rest.
Systemic disorders Hemorrhagic shock Acidosis Hypoxia Renal failure Hepatic disease Sepsis	These are depressants of cell function that directly affect wound healing.	Be familiar with the nature of the specific disorder. Administer prescribed treatment. Cultures may be indicated to determine appropriate antibiotic.
Immunosuppressed state	Patient is more vulnerable to bacterial and viral invasion; defense mechanisms are impaired.	Provide maximum protection to prevent infection. Restrict visitors with colds; institute mandatory hand washing by all staff.
Wound stressors Vomiting Valsalva maneuver Heavy coughing Straining	Produce tension on wounds, particularly of the torso.	Encourage frequent turning and ambulation and administer antiemetic medications as prescribed. Assist patient in splinting incision.

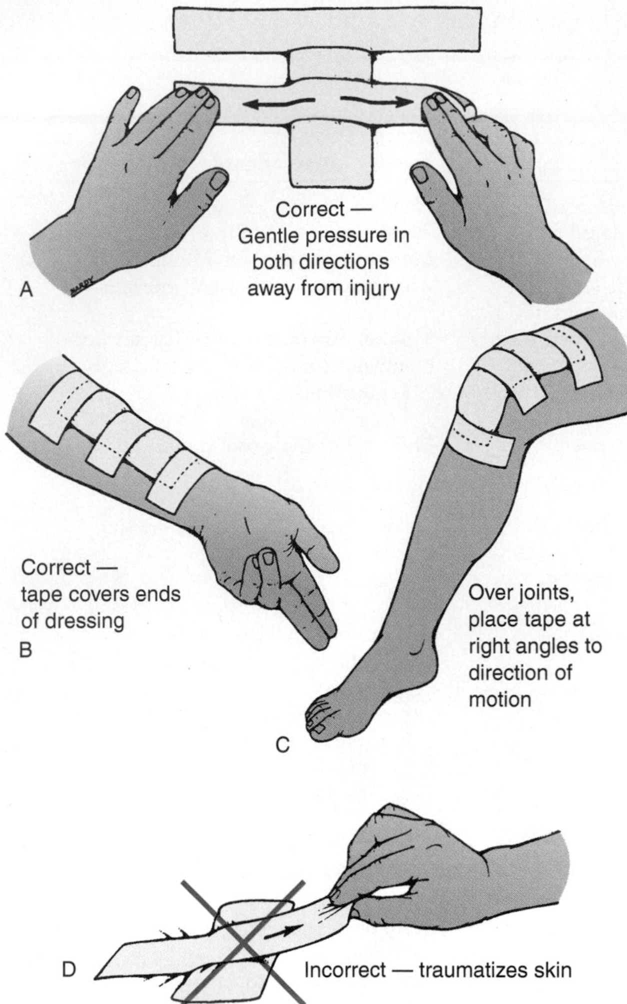

FIGURE 18•8 Application of tape. Views **A, B,** and **C** illustrate the correct ways to apply tape. The method shown in **D** is incorrect. (**A**) Pressure is applied evenly and directed away from the incision. (**B**) The proper way to cover the ends of a dressing for additional protection of the wound. (**C**) The correct way to position a dressing over a joint for maximum comfort and effectiveness. (**D**) In the incorrect method, the tape is pulling against the skin and exerting pressure over the wound.

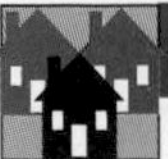

PATIENT EDUCATION AND HOME CARE
Wound Care Instructions

Until Sutures Are Removed

1. Keep the wound dry and clean.
   a. If there is no dressing, ask your nurse or physician if you can bathe or shower.
   b. If a dressing or splint is in place, do not remove it unless it is wet or soiled.
   c. If wet or soiled, change dressing yourself if you have been taught to do so; otherwise, call your nurse or physician for guidance.
   d. If you have been taught, instruction might be as follows:
      Cleanse area *gently* with sterile normal saline once or twice daily.
      Cover with a sterile Telfa pad or gauze square—large enough to cover wound
      Apply hypoallergenic tape (Dermacel or paper). Adhesive is not recommended because it is difficult to remove without possible injury to the incisional site.
2. Immediately report any of these signs of infection:
   a. Redness, marked swelling exceeding ½ inch (2.5 cm) from incision site; tenderness; or increased warmth around wound
   b. Red streaks in skin near wound
   c. Pus or discharge, foul odor
   d. Chills or temperature higher than 37.7°C (100°F)
3. If soreness or pain causes discomfort, apply a dry cool pack (containing ice or cold water) or take prescribed acetaminophen tablets (2) every 4–6 hours. Avoid aspirin without direction or instruction because bleeding can occur with its use.
4. Swelling after surgery is common. To help reduce swelling, elevate the affected part to the level of the heart.
   a. Hand or arm
      Sleep—elevate arm on pillow at side
      Sitting—place arm on pillow on adjacent table
      Standing—rest affected hand on opposite shoulder; support elbow with unaffected hand
   b. Leg or foot
      Sitting—place a pillow on a facing chair; provide support underneath the knee
      Lying—place a pillow under affected leg

After Sutures Are Removed

Although the wound appears to be healed when sutures are removed, it is still tender and will continue to heal and strengthen for several weeks.

1. Follow recommendations of physician or nurse regarding extent of activity.
2. Keep suture line clean; do not rub vigorously; pat dry. Wound edges may look red and may be slightly raised. This is normal.
3. Massage around wound gently using a bland baby oil, petrolatum, or moisturizing cream (twice a day).
4. If the site continues to be red, thick, and painful to pressure after 8 weeks, consult the health care provider. (This may be due to excessive collagen formation and should be checked.)

Managing Wound Complications

HEMATOMA

At times, concealed bleeding occurs beneath the skin at the surgical site. This hemorrhage usually stops spontaneously but results in clot formation (hematoma) within the wound. If the clot is small, it will be absorbed and need not be treated. When the clot is large, the wound usually bulges somewhat, and healing will be delayed unless the clot is removed. After several sutures are removed by the physician, the clot is evacuated, and the wound is packed lightly with gauze. Healing occurs usually by granulation, or a secondary closure may be performed.

INFECTION (WOUND SEPSIS)

Wound infection may not present until at least postoperative day 5. Most patients are discharged before that time, and more than half of wound infections are diagnosed after discharge, highlighting the importance of patient education regarding wound care. Risk factors for wound sepsis include wound contamination, foreign body, faulty suturing technique, devitalized tissue, hematoma, debilitation, dehydration, malnutrition, anemia, advanced age, extreme obesity, shock, length of preoperative hospitalization, duration of surgical procedure, and associated disorders (eg, diabetes mellitus, immunosuppression). Signs and symptoms of wound infection include pulse rate and temperature elevation; white blood cell count elevation; wound swelling, warmth, tenderness, or discharge; and incisional pain. Local signs may be absent if the infection is deep. *Staphylococcus aureus* accounts for many postoperative wound infections. Other infections may result from *Escherichia coli, Proteus vulgaris, Aerobacter aerogenes, Pseudomonas aeruginosa,* and other organisms. Although rare, beta-hemolytic streptococcal or clostridial infections can be rapid and deadly. If wound infection due to beta-hemolytic streptococcus or clostridium occurs, extreme care is needed to prevent spread of infection to others. The patient requires intensive medical and nursing care if the patient is to survive.

When a diagnosis of wound infection in a surgical incision is made, the surgeon may remove one or more sutures or staples and, under aseptic precautions, separate the wound edges with a pair of blunt scissors or a hemostat. Once the incision is opened, a drain is inserted. If the infection is deep, incision and drainage may be necessary. Antimicrobial therapy and a wound care regimen are also initiated.

WOUND DEHISCENCE AND EVISCERATION

Wound **dehiscence** (disruption of surgical incision or wound) and **evisceration** (protrusion of wound contents) are serious surgical complications (Fig. 18-9). Dehiscence and evisceration are especially serious when they involve abdominal incisions or wounds. These complications result from sutures giving way, from infection, and, more frequently, after marked distention or strenuous cough. They may also occur because of increasing age, poor nutritional status, and the presence of pulmonary or cardiovascular disease in patients who undergo abdominal surgery.

When the wound edges separate slowly, the intestines may protrude gradually or not at all, and the earliest sign may be a gush of bloody (serosanguineous) peritoneal fluid from the wound. When the rupture of a wound occurs suddenly, coils of intestine may push out of the abdomen. The patient may say that "something gave way." The evisceration causes pain and can be associated with vomiting.

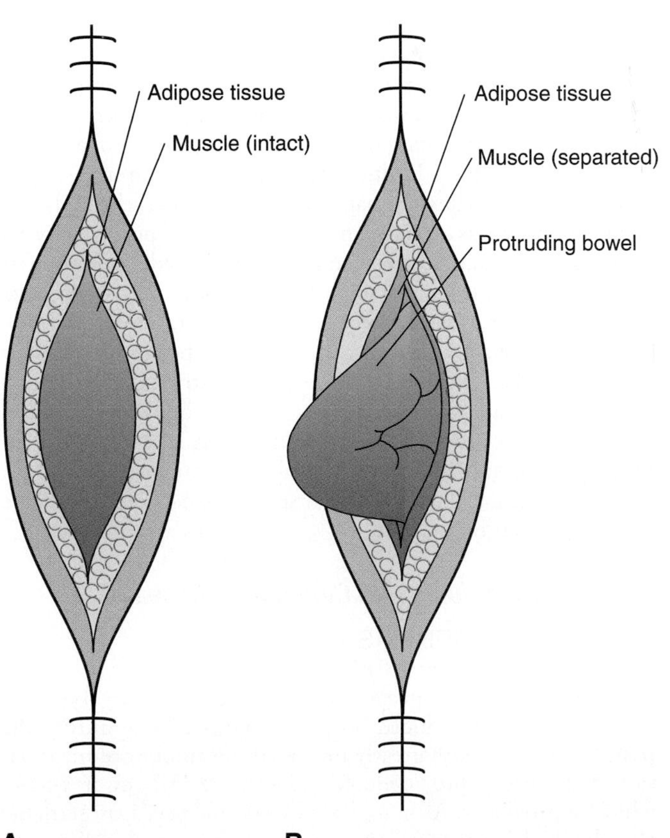

FIGURE 18•9 (**A**) Wound dehiscence; (**B**) wound evisceration.

Nursing Alert *When disruption of a wound occurs, the patient is placed in low Fowler's position and instructed to lie quietly. These actions minimize protrusion of body tissues. The protruding coils of intestine are covered with sterile dressings moistened with sterile saline solution, and the surgeon is notified at once.*

An abdominal binder, properly applied, is an excellent prophylactic measure against an evisceration of this kind and often is used along with the primary dressing, especially for surgery on patients with weak or pendulous abdominal walls or when rupture of a wound has occurred.

Resuming Oral Intake and Promoting Bowel Function

As previously discussed, oral intake resumes after the patient is awake and alert, nausea and vomiting have subsided, and peristalsis has returned. Patients who have not had gastrointestinal surgery may be started on soft foods or solids, depending on their desire; however, patients who have had surgery of the gastrointestinal tract may progress slowly to a full diet or have a modified diet. For example, oral surgery patients may have problems chewing and swallowing and require a liquid or puréed diet. Other surgical procedures, such as gastrectomy, small bowel resection, ileostomy, and colostomy, have a more drastic effect on the gastrointestinal system and require more extensive dietary considerations. These procedures are discussed in Chapters 34 and 35.

Constipation is common after surgery. The causes may be minor or serious. Decreased mobility, poor oral intake, and opioid analgesics contribute to difficulty having a bowel movement. In addition, irritation and trauma to the bowel during surgery may inhibit intestinal movement for several days. The combined effect of early ambulation, improved dietary intake, and a stool softener (if prescribed) promotes bowel elimination. Until the patient reports return of normal bowel function, the nurse should assess the abdomen for presence of distention and for presence and frequency of bowel sounds. If the abdomen is nondistended and bowel sounds are normal, and if the patient does not have a bowel movement by postoperative day 2 or 3, the physician should be notified so that a laxative can be given that evening.

Assessment and management of gastrointestinal function are important after surgery because the gastrointestinal tract is subject to uncomfortable or potentially life-threatening complications. Any postoperative patient may suffer from distention. Postoperative distention of the abdomen results from the accumulation of gas in the intestinal tract. Manipulation of the abdominal organs during the surgical procedure may produce a loss of normal peristalsis for 24 to 48 hours, depending on the type and extent of surgery. Even though nothing is given by mouth, swallowed air and gastrointestinal secretions enter the stomach and the intestines; if not propelled by peristaltic activity, they collect in the intestines, producing distention and causing the patient to complain of fullness or pain in the abdomen. Most often, the gas collects in the colon. Abdominal distention is further increased by immobility, anesthetic agents, and the use of opioid medications.

After major abdominal surgery, distention may be avoided by having the patient turn frequently, exercise, and ambulate as early as possible. This also alleviates distention produced by swallowing air, which is often done by anxious patients. When postoperative distention is anticipated, a nasogastric tube may be inserted before surgery. The nasogastric tube may remain in place until full peristaltic activity (indicated by passage of flatus) has resumed. The nurse can determine when peristaltic bowel sounds return by listening to the abdomen with a stethoscope. The presence of bowel sounds is reported so that the proper diet progression can be prescribed.

Paralytic ileus and intestinal obstruction are potential postoperative complications that occur more frequently in patients undergoing intestinal or abdominal surgery. Refer to Chapter 35 for discussion of treatment.

Gerontologic Considerations

Older adults recover more slowly and are at greater risk for developing postoperative complications. Delirium, pneumonia, decline in functional ability, exacerbation of comorbid conditions, pressure ulcers, decreased oral intake, gastrointestinal disturbance, and falls are all threats to the older adult's successful recovery. Expert nursing care can help the older adult avoid these complications or minimize their effects.

Postoperative delirium, characterized by confusion, perceptual and cognitive deficits, altered attention levels, disturbed sleep patterns, and impaired psychomotor skills, is a significant problem for postoperative older adults. Causes of delirium are multifactorial (Chart 18-3). Skilled and frequent assessment of mental status and of all physiologic factors influencing a change in mental status helps the nurse plan care because delirium may be the initial or only early indicator of infection, fluid and electrolyte imbalance, or deterioration of the elderly patient's respiratory or hemodynamic status. Factors that determine if the patient is at risk for delirium include age, history of alcohol abuse, preoperative cognitive function, physical function, serum chemistries, and type of surgery.

Recognizing postoperative delirium and identifying and treating its underlying cause are the goals of care. Postoperative delirium is sometimes mistaken for preexisting dementia or is attributed to age. In addition to monitoring and managing identifiable causes, nurses can implement supportive interventions. Keeping the patient in a well-lit room and close to the nurses' station can help with sensory deprivation. At the same time, distracting and unfamiliar noises should be kept to a minimum. Because unrelieved pain can contribute to postoperative delirium, the nurse can collaborate with the physician or geriatric nurse specialist and the patient to achieve pain relief without oversedation. The patient can be reoriented as often as necessary, and staff should introduce themselves each time they come in contact with the patient. Engaging the patient in conversation and care activities and placing a clock and calender nearby may help cognitive function. It is important that physical activity not be neglected while the patient is confused because physical deterioration can worsen delirium and place the patient at increased risk for other complications. Restraints should be avoided because they can also worsen confusion. If possible, a family member or staff member is asked to sit with the patient instead. Haloperidol (Haldol) or lorazepam (Ativan) may be given during episodes of acute confusion; however, these medications should be discontinued as soon as possible to avoid side effects.

Other problems confronting the older postoperative patient, such as pneumonia, altered bowel function, DVT, weakness, and functional decline, often can be prevented by early and progressive ambulation. Ambulation means walking, not sitting in a chair; sitting positions that promote venous stasis in the lower extremities are to be avoided. Adequate assistance is required to keep the patient from bumping into objects and falling. A physical therapy referral may be indicated to promote safe, regular exercise for the older adult.

Urinary incontinence can be prevented by providing easy access to the call bell and the commode and by prompting voiding. Early ambulation and familiarity with the room help the patient to become self-sufficient sooner.

Optimal nutritional status is important for wound healing, return of normal bowel function, and fluid and electrolyte balance. The nurse and patient can consult with the dietitian to plan appealing, high protein meals that provide sufficient fiber, calories, and vitamins. Nutritional supplements, such as Ensure or Sustacal, may be recommended. Multivitamins, iron, and vitamin C supplements aid tissue healing, formation of new red blood cells, and overall nutritional status and are commonly prescribed postoperatively.

In addition to monitoring and managing the older adult's physiologic recovery, the nurse identifies and addresses psychosocial needs. The older adult may require more encouragement and support to resume activities, and the pace may be slower. Sensory deficits may dictate the need for repeating instructions often, and decreased physiologic reserve may make frequent rest periods mandatory. The older adult may require extensive discharge planning to coordinate both professional and family care providers, and the nurse, social worker, or nurse case manager may institute the plan for continuing care.

CHART 18•3 Causes of Postoperative Delirium

- Electrolyte imbalance
- Dehydration
- Hypoxia
- Hypercarbia
- Acid–base balance disturbance
- Occult infection (urinary tract, wound, respiratory)
- Medications (anticholinergics, benzodiazepines, central nervous system depressants)
- Unrelieved pain
- Blood loss
- Decreased cardiac output
- Cerebral hypoxia
- Congestive heart failure
- Acute myocardial infarction
- Hypothermia or hyperthermia
- Unfamiliar surroundings and sensory deprivation
- Emergent surgery
- Alcohol withdrawal
- Urinary retention
- Fecal impaction

Promoting Home and Community-Based Care

TEACHING PATIENTS SELF-CARE

Patients have always required detailed discharge instructions to become proficient in special self-care needs after surgery; however, dramatically reduced hospital lengths of stay during the past decade have both greatly increased the amount of information that must be provided and reduced the amount of time in which to provide it. Although certain specific needs are germane to individual patients and the specific procedures they have undergone, the scope of patient education needs for postoperative care have been identified (Chart 18-4). Refer also to the Home

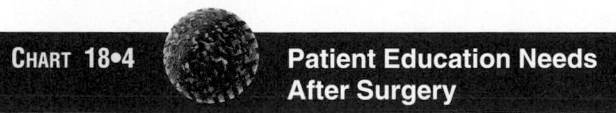

CHART 18•4 Patient Education Needs After Surgery

All postoperative patients need information and instruction in the following areas:

- The surgical procedure that was performed and any permanent changes in anatomic structure or function
- Interventions to adapt to any permanent changes in structure or function
- Potential complications, signs and symptoms of complications, and preventive measures
- Ongoing therapeutic regimen including
  - Medication
  - Diet
  - Progressive activity, including activities to avoid
  - Adjuvant therapies
  - Wound care
- Suggested health promotion activities (eg, smoking cessation, stress management)
- Community resources, home care referrals
- Follow-up appointments with surgeon and other practitioners

Care Teaching Checklist presented earlier in this chapter for the patient being discharged from the same-day surgery unit.

CONTINUING CARE

Continuing care by community-based services is frequently necessary after surgery. Older patients, patients who live alone, or patients without family support are often in greatest need. Planning for discharge involves arranging for necessary services early in the acute care hospitalization. Wound care, drain management, catheter care, infusion therapy, and physical or occupational therapy are some of the needs addressed by community health care providers. The home care nurse coordinates these activities and services. During home care visits, the nurse assesses the patient for postoperative complications; additionally, the nurse assesses the surgical incision, respiratory and cardiovascular status, adequacy of pain management, fluid and nutritional status, and the patient's progress in returning to preoperative status. The nurse assesses the patient's and family's ability to manage dressing changes, drainage systems, and other devices and to administer prescribed medications. The nurse may change dressings or catheters if needed. The nurse determines if any additional services are needed and assists the patient and family to arrange for them. Previous teaching is reinforced, and the patient is reminded to keep follow-up appointments. The patient and family are instructed about signs and symptoms to be reported to the surgeon. In addition, the nurse may provide information about how to obtain needed supplies and may suggest resources or support groups the patient may want to contact. In many settings, postoperative telephone calls are made to answer questions, assess recovery, and reassure patients and their families.

Evaluation

Expected Outcomes

Expected outcomes may include:

1. Indicates that pain is decreased in intensity
2. Maintains optimal respiratory function
   a. Performs deep-breathing exercises
   b. Displays clear breath sounds
   c. Uses incentive spirometer as prescribed
   d. Splints incisional site when coughing to reduce pain
3. Does not develop a DVT
4. Exercises and ambulates as prescribed
   a. Alternates periods of rest and activity
   b. Progressively increases ambulation
   c. Resumes normal activities within prescribed time frame
   d. Performs activities related to self-care
5. Wound heals without complication
6. Resumes oral intake and normal bowel function
   a. Reports absence of nausea; no vomiting
   b. Takes at least 75% of usual diet
   c. Is free of abdominal distress and gas pains
   d. Exhibits normal bowel sounds
   e. Resumes usual bowel elimination pattern
7. Acquires knowledge and skills necessary to manage therapeutic regimen
8. Experiences no complications and has normal vital signs

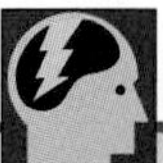

Critical Thinking Exercises

1. Your patient has a history of esophageal cancer. After undergoing ambulatory surgery to insert a gastric feeding tube, he is to be discharged from the PACU to home. Describe a teaching plan for the patient and his family. How would you modify the plan if the patient lives alone?

2. A patient who has undergone a lumbar fusion reports severe pain and as a result is unable to cough, deep breathe, or turn. When you check the patient's chart, you find that medication cannot be given for another hour. What assessment would you carry out at this time? How would you deal with this situation?

3. Your patient is a 72-year-old woman with poor nutritional status who has undergone emergency surgery. How would you modify your assessment, nursing care, and plans for home care management because of her poor nutritional status?

References and Selected Readings

BOOKS

Agency for Health Care Policy and Research. (1992). *Acute pain management: Operative or medical procedures and trauma.* Clinical Practice Guideline. Washington, DC: Public Health Service, U.S. Department of Health and Human Services.

American Pain Society. (1999). *Principles of analgesic use in the treatment of acute pain and cancer pain.* Glenview, IL: Author.

American Society of Anesthesiology. (1995). *ASA standards for post anesthesia care.* Park Ridge, IL: Author.

American Society of PeriAnesthesia Nurses. (1998). *Standards of perianesthesia nursing practice.* Thorofare, NJ: ASPAN.

Benedetti, C. (1990). The pathogenic effects of postoperative pain. In S. Lipton, E. Tunks, & M. Zoppi M (Eds.), *Advances in pain research and therapy: Vol. 13* (pp 279–285). New York: Raven Press.

DeFazio-Quinn, D. M. (Ed.). (1999). *Ambulatory surgical nursing core curriculum.* Philadelphia: W. B. Saunders.

Drain, C. B. (Ed.). (1996). *The postanesthesia care unit: A critical care approach to postanesthesia nursing.* Philadelphia: W. B. Saunders.

Economou, S. G. & Economou, T. S. (1999). *Instructions for surgery patients.* Philadelphia: W. B. Saunders.

Fairchild, S. (1996). *Perioperative nursing: Principles and practice.* Boston: Little, Brown.

Kost, M. (1998). *Manual of conscious sedation.* Philadelphia: W. B. Saunders.

Litwack, K. (1999). *Core curriculum for peri anesthesia nursing practice.* Philadelphia: W. B. Saunders.

Litwack, K. (1995). *Postanesthesia care nursing* (2nd ed.). St. Louis: Mosby–Year Book.

McGoldrick, K. E. (1995). *Ambulatory anesthesiology: A problem-oriented approach.* Baltimore: Williams & Wilkins.

Merli, G., & Weitz, H (Eds.). (1998). *Medical management of the surgical patient* (2nd ed.). Philadelphia: W. B. Saunders.

Meeker, M. H., & Rothrock, J. C. (1995). *Alexander's care of the patient in surgery.* St. Louis: Mosby–Year Book.

Schirmer, B. D., & Rattner D. W. (1998). *Ambulatory surgery.* Philadelphia: W. B. Saunders.

Schwartz, S., & Shires, G. T. (1999). *Principles of surgery.* New York: McGraw-Hill.

Summers, S., & Ebbert, D. W. (1992). *Ambulatory surgical nursing: A nursing diagnosis approach.* Philadelphia: J. B. Lippincott.

Vender, J., & Spiess, B. (Eds.). (1992). *Post anesthesia care.* Philadelphia: W. B. Saunders.

JOURNALS

Asterisks indicate nursing research articles.

Ambulatory Surgery

Aldreta, J. A. (1998). Modifications to the postanesthesia score for use in ambulatory surgery. *Journal of Perianesthesia Nursing, 12*(3), 148–155.

Beatty, A. M., Martin, D. E., Couch, M., & Long, N. (1997). Relevance of oral intake and necessity to void as ambulatory surgical discharge criteria. *Journal of Perianesthesia Nursing, 12*(6), 413–421.

Brockway, P. M. (1997). The ambulatory surgical nurse: Evolution, competency and vision. *Nursing Clinics of North America, 32*(2), 387–394.

Caslow, B. I. F., & Eddy, M. E. (1998). Effects of preoperative ambulatory gynecological education: Clinical outcomes and patient satisfaction. *Journal of Perianesthesia Nursing, 13*(1), 4–10.

DeFazio-Quinn, D. M. (1997). Ambulatory surgery: An evolution. *Nursing Clinics of North America, 32*(2), 377–386.

Hession, M. (1998). Factors influencing successful discharge after outpatient laparoscopic cholecystectomy. *Journal of Perianesthesia Nursing, 13*(1), 11–15.

Ireland, D. (1997). Legal issues in ambulatory surgery. *Nursing Clinics of North America, 32*(2), 469–476.

Lancaster, K. A. (1997). Patient teaching in ambulatory surgery. *Nursing Clinics of North America, 32*(2), 417–427.

Litwack, K. (1997). Care of the special needs patient. *Nursing Clinics of North America, 32*(2), 457–467.

Marley, R. A. (1996). Moline, B. M. Patient discharge from the ambulatory setting. *Journal of Post Anesthesia Nursing, 11*(1), 39–49.

New, S. W., & Gutierrez, L. (1997). Quality improvement in the ambulatory surgical setting. *Nursing Clinics of North America, 32*(2), 477–488.

Pain

American Society of Anesthesiologists. (1995). Practice guidelines for acute pain management in the perioperative setting—A report by the American Society of Anesthesiologists Task Force on Pain Management, Acute Pain Section. *Anesthesiology 82,* 1071–1081.

Association of Operating Room Nurses (1998). Recommended practices for managing the patient receiving local anesthesia. *AORN Journal, 67*(2), 454, 456–457.

*Auvil-Novak, S. E. (1997). A middle-range theory of chronotherapeutic intervention for post surgical pain. *Nursing Research, 46*(2), 66–71.

Goodwin, S. A. (1998). A review of preemptive analgesia. *Journal of Perianesthesia Nursing, 13*(2), 109–114.

Knowles, R. (1996). Standardization of pain management in the postanesthesia care unit. *Journal of Perianesthesia Nursing, 11*(6), 390–398.

Lynch, E. P., Lazor, M. A., Gellis, J. E., et al. (1998). The impact of postoperative pain in the development of postoperative delirium. *Anesthesia and Analgesia, 86,* 761–785.

Rittenmeyer, J., Dolezal, D., & Vogel, E. (1997). Pain management: A quality improvement project. *Journal of Perianesthesia Nursing, 12*(5), 329–333.

Seers, K., & Carroll, D. (1998). Relaxation techniques for acute pain management. *Journal of Advanced Nursing, 27*(3), 466–476.

*Taylor, L. K., Kuttler, K. L., Parks, T. A., & Milton, D. (1998). The effect of music in the perianesthesia care unit on pain levels in women who have had abdominal hysterectomies. *Journal of Perianesthesia Nursing, 13*(2), 88–94.

Postoperative and Postanesthesia Nursing

Brooks—Brunn, J. (1995). Minimizing pulmonary complications. *Heart and Lung, 24,* 94–115.

Dexter, F., & Rittenmeyer, H. (1997). Quantifying phase I postanesthesia nursing activities in the phase II post anesthesia care unit. *Nursing Outlook, 45*(2), 86–88.

Fox, V. J. (1998). Postoperative education that works. *AORN Journal, 67*(5), 1010, 1012–1017.

Ginsburg, W. H. (1996). Legal issues in the post anesthesia care unit. *Journal of Perianesthesia Nursing, 11*(4), 267–272.

Hayer, C. A., & Brncick, N. (1998). Fat embolism syndrome: A complication of orthopaedic trauma. *Orthopaedic Nursing, 17*(2), 41–43, 45, 58.

Hession, M. C. (1998). Factors influencing successful discharge after outpatient laparoscopic cholecystectomy. *Journal of Perianesthesia Nursing, 13*(1), 11–15.

*Hinojosa, R. J., & Hershey, J. (1997). Comparison of three rewarming methods in a post anesthesia care unit. *Plastic Surgery Nursing, 17*(4), 222–225.

Huffman, L. M. (1996). Regulations, standards, and guidelines protecting PACU healthcare workers. *Journal of Perianesthesia Nursing, 11*(4), 231–239.

Kerr, C. M., & Savage, G. T. (1996). Managing exposure to tuberculosis in the PACU: CDC guidelines and cost analysis. *Journal of Perianesthesia Nursing, 11*(3), 143–6.

Knowles, R. (1996). Standardization of pain management in the postanesthesia care unit. *Journal of Perianesthesia Nursing, 11*(6), 390–8.

Mamaril, M. (1997). The critical care setting: The post anesthesia care unit phase I. *Breathline, 17*(5), 16.

Mamaril, M., & Hooper, V. (1998). Fast tracking versus bypassing phase I. . . . rapid PACU progression. *Breathline, 17*(7), 12.

Marley, R. A. (1998). Postextubation laryngeal edema: A review with consideration for home discharge. *Journal of Perianesthesia Nursing, 13*(1), 39–53.

Redmond, M. C. (1996). Latex allergy: Recognition and perioperative management [Review]. *Journal of Post Anesthesia Nursing, 11*(1), 6–12.

Schwartz, L. B. (1998). Conventional and alternative therapies for acute deep vein thrombosis. *Journal of Care Management, 4,* 9–12, 32.

Tuller, S., McCabe, L., Cronenwett, L., et al. (1997). Patient, visitor, and nurse evaluations of visitation for adult post anesthesia care unit patients. *Journal of Perianesthesia Nursing, 12*(6), 402–412.

Vaughan, R. S. (1997). Airway management in the recovery room. *Anaesthesia 52* (7), 617–618.

Wounds and Infection

Centers for Disease Control and Prevention (1999). Guideline for prevention of surgical site infections. *Infection Control and Hospital Epidemiology, 20*(4), 247–280.

Csete, M. (1996). Special consideration for blood borne pathogens in the PACU. *Journal of Perianesthesia Nursing, 11*(4), 223–230.

Kerr, C. M., & Savage, G. T. (1996). Managing exposure to tuberculosis in the PACU: CDC guidelines and cost analysis. *Journal of Perianesthesia Nursing, 11*(3), 143–146.

Resources

AGENCIES

American Society of Anesthesiologists, 520 N. Northwest Highway, Park Ridge, IL, 60068; www.asahq.org/practice

American Society of PeriAnesthesia Nurses, 6900 Grove Road, Thorofare, NJ, 08086; 1-609-845-5557; www.aspan.org

Association of Operating Room Nurses, Inc., 2170 S. Parker Road, Suite 300, Denver, CO 80231; 1-303-755-6304; www.aorn.org

Malignant Hyperthermia Association of the United States (MHAUS), 332 S. Main Street, Sherburne, NY 13460; www.medhelp.org/agsg/aqsg7059.htm

UNIT

5

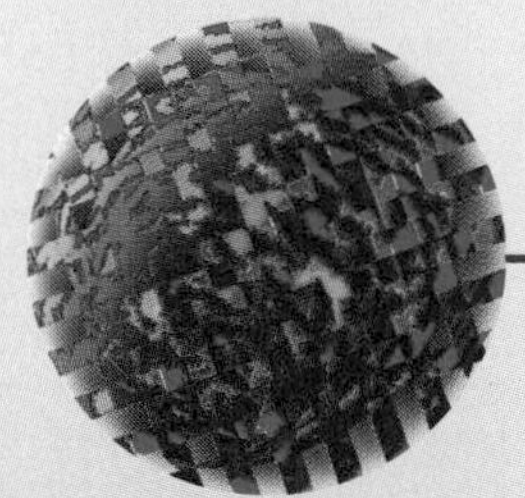

Gas Exchange and Respiratory Function

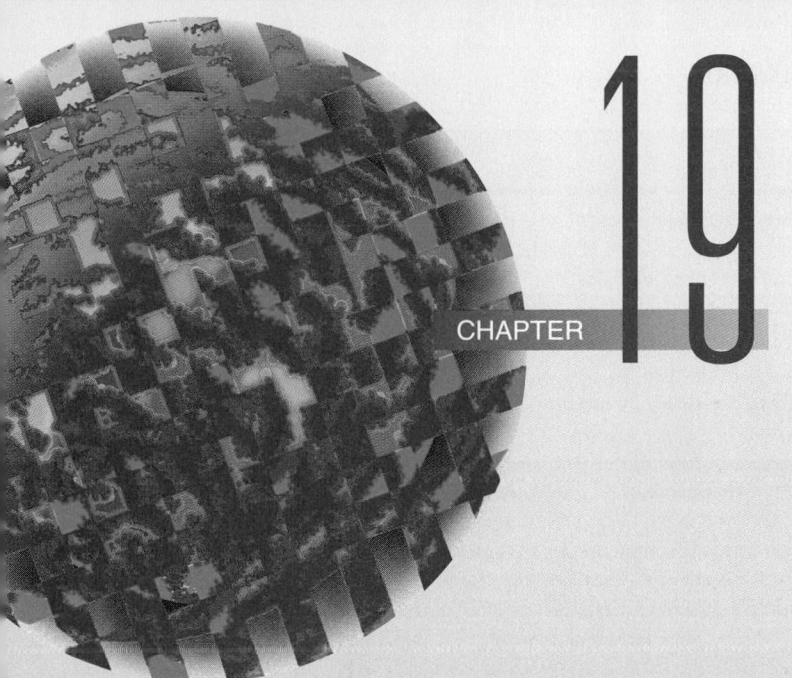

Assessment of Respiratory Function

Learning Objectives

On completion of this chapter, the learner will be able to:

1. Describe the structures and functions of the upper and lower respiratory tracts.
2. Describe ventilation, perfusion, diffusion, shunting, and the relationship of pulmonary circulation to these processes.
3. Discriminate between normal and abnormal breath sounds.
4. Use assessment parameters appropriate for determining the characteristics and severity of the major symptoms of respiratory dysfunction.
5. Identify the nursing implications of the various procedures used for diagnostic evaluation of respiratory function.

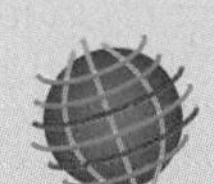

Disorders of the upper and lower respiratory tracts are common and are encountered by nurses in every setting from home and school settings to intensive care units. To assess upper and lower respiratory tract disorders, the nurse must be skilled at differentiating normal assessment findings from abnormal ones. Good assessment skills must be developed and used when caring for patients with acute and chronic respiratory problems. In addition, an understanding of respiratory function and the significance of abnormal pulmonary function and abnormal test results is essential.

GLOSSARY

apneustic center: area in lower pons that stimulates the inspiratory medullary center to promote deep, prolonged inspiration

bronchoscopy: direct examination of larynx, trachea, and bronchi using an endoscope

cilia: short hairs that provide a constant whipping motion that serves to propel mucus and foreign substances away from the lung toward the larynx

crackles: soft, high-pitched, discontinuous popping sounds during inspiration

diffusion: exchange of gas molecules from areas of high concentration to areas of low concentration

dyspnea: labored breathing or shortness of breath

hemoptysis: expectoration of blood from the respiratory tract

hypoxemia: low oxygen levels in the blood

hypoxia: low oxygen levels in the cells

orthopnea: inability to breathe easily except in an upright position

physiologic dead space: portion of the tracheobronchial tree that does not participate in gas exchange

pneumotaxic center: area in the upper pons that controls the pattern of respirations

pulmonary perfusion: blood flow through the pulmonary vasculature

respiration: gas exchange between atmospheric air and the blood and between the blood and cells of the body

sibilant wheezes: continuous, musical, high-pitched whistle-like sounds heard on inspiration and expiration

sonorous wheezes: deep, low-pitched, rumbling sounds heard primarily during expiration

ventilation: movement of air in and out of airways

ANATOMIC AND PHYSIOLOGIC OVERVIEW

The respiratory system is composed of the upper and lower respiratory tracts. Together, the two tracts are responsible for **ventilation** (movement of air in and out of the airways). The upper tract, known as the upper airway, warms and filters inspired air so that the lower respiratory tract (the lungs) can accomplish gas exchange. The gas exchange involves delivering oxygen to the tissues through the bloodstream and expelling waste gases, such as carbon dioxide, during expiration.

Anatomy of the Upper Respiratory Tract: Upper Airway

Upper airway structures consist of the nose, sinuses and nasal passages, pharynx, tonsils and adenoids, larynx, and trachea.

Nose

The nose is composed of an external and an internal portion. The external portion protrudes from the face and is supported by the nasal bones and cartilage. The anterior nares (nostrils) are the external openings of the nasal cavities.

The internal portion of the nose is a hollow cavity separated into the right and left nasal cavities by a narrow vertical divider, the septum. Each nasal cavity is divided into three passageways by the projection of the turbinates (also called conchae) from the lateral walls. The nasal cavities are lined with highly vascular ciliated mucous membranes called the nasal mucosa. Mucus secreted continuously by goblet cells covers the surface of the nasal mucosa and is moved back to the nasopharynx by the action of the **cilia** (fine hairs).

The nose serves as a passageway for air to pass to and from the lungs. It filters impurities and humidifies and warms the air as it is inhaled. It is responsible for olfaction (smell) because the olfactory receptors are located in the nasal mucosa. This function diminishes with age.

Paranasal Sinuses

The paranasal sinuses include four pairs of bony cavities that are lined with nasal mucosa and ciliated pseudostratified columnar epithelium. These air spaces are connected by a series of ducts that drain into the nasal cavity. The sinuses are named by their location—namely, frontal, ethmoidal, sphenoidal, and maxillary (Fig. 19-1). A prominent function of the sinuses is to serve as a resonating chamber in speech. The sinuses are a common site of infection.

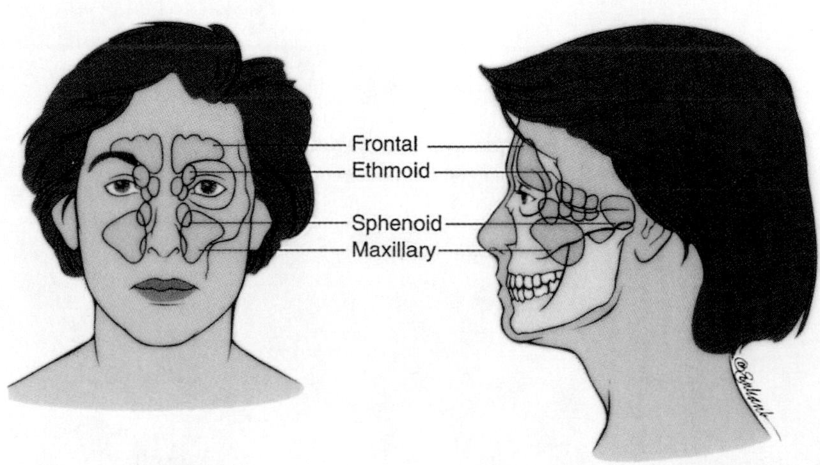

FIGURE 19•1 The paranasal sinuses.

Turbinate Bones (Conchae)

The turbinate bones, or conchae (the name suggested by their shell-like appearance), are adapted by shape and position to increase the mucous membrane surface of the nasal passages and to obstruct the air flowing through them slightly (Fig. 19-2).

Air entering the nostrils is deflected upward to the roof of the nose, and it follows a circuitous route before it reaches the nasopharynx. It comes into contact with a large surface of moist, warm mucous membrane that catches practically all the dust and organisms in the inhaled air. The air is moistened, warmed to body temperature, and brought into contact with sensitive nerves. Some of these nerves detect odors; others provoke sneezing to expel irritating dust.

Pharynx, Tonsils, and Adenoids

The pharynx, or throat, is a tubelike structure that connects the nasal and oral cavities to the larynx. It is divided into three regions: nasal, oral, and laryngeal. The nasopharynx is located posterior to the nose and above the soft palate. The oropharynx houses the faucial, or palatine, tonsils. The laryngopharynx extends from the hyoid bone to the cricoid cartilage. The entrance of the larynx is formed by the epiglottis.

The adenoids, or pharyngeal tonsils, are located in the roof of the nasopharynx. The throat is encircled by the tonsils, the adenoids, and other lymphoid tissue. These structures are important links in the chain of lymph nodes guarding the body from invasion by organisms entering the nose and the throat. The pharynx functions as a passageway for the respiratory and digestive tracts.

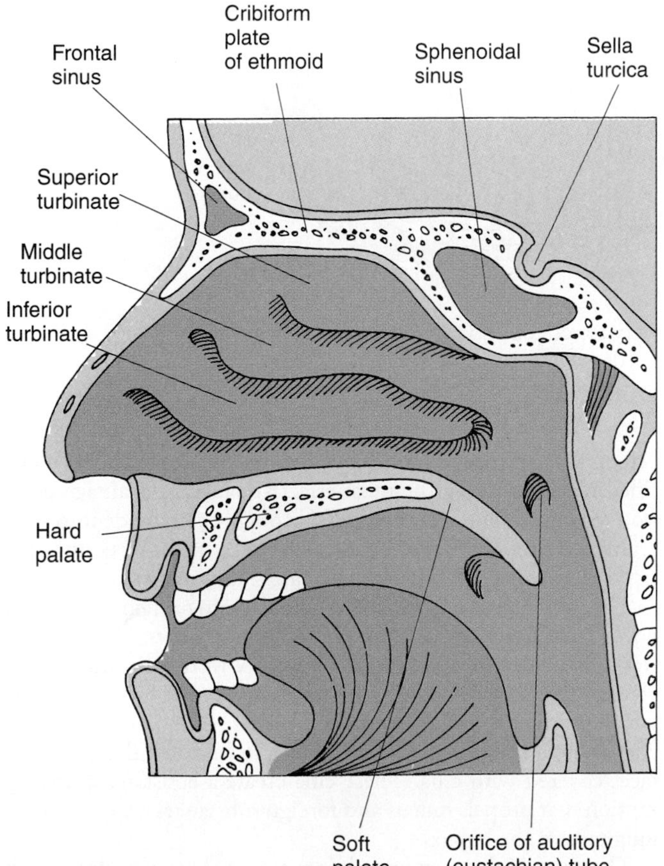

FIGURE 19•2 Cross-section of nasal cavity.

Larynx

The larynx, or voice organ, is a cartilaginous epithelium-lined structure that connects the pharynx and the trachea. The major function of the larynx is vocalization. It also protects the lower airway from foreign substances and facilitates coughing. It is frequently referred to as the voice box and consists of the following:

- Epiglottis—a valve flap of cartilage that covers the opening to the larynx during swallowing
- Glottis—the opening between the vocal cords in the larynx
- Thyroid cartilage—the largest of the cartilage structures; part of it forms the Adam's apple
- Cricoid cartilage—the only complete cartilaginous ring in the larynx (located below the thyroid cartilage)
- Arytenoid cartilages—used in vocal cord movement with the thyroid cartilage
- Vocal cords—ligaments controlled by muscular movements that produce sounds; located in the lumen of the larynx

Trachea

The trachea, or windpipe, is composed of smooth muscle with C-shaped rings of cartilage at regular intervals. The cartilaginous rings are incomplete on the posterior surface and give firmness to the wall of the trachea, preventing it from collapsing. The trachea serves as the passage between the larynx and the bronchi.

Anatomy of the Lower Respiratory Tract: Lungs

The lower respiratory tract consists of the lungs, which contain the bronchial and alveolar structures needed for gas exchange.

Lungs

The lungs are paired elastic structures enclosed in the thoracic cage, which is an airtight chamber with distensible walls (Fig. 19-3). Ventilation requires movement of the walls of the thoracic cage and of its floor, the diaphragm. The effect of these movements is alternately to increase and decrease the capacity of the chest. When the capacity of the chest is increased, air enters through the trachea (inspiration) because of the lowered pressure within and inflates the lungs. When the chest wall and diaphragm return to their previous positions (expiration), the lungs recoil and force the air out through the bronchi and trachea. The inspiratory phase of respiration normally requires energy; the expiratory phase is normally passive. Inspiration occupies the first third of the respiratory cycle, expiration the latter two thirds.

PLEURA

The lungs and wall of the thorax are lined with a serous membrane called the pleura. The visceral pleura covers the lungs; the parietal pleura lines the thorax. The visceral and parietal pleura and the small amount of pleural fluid between these two membranes serve to lubricate the thorax and lungs and permit smooth motion of the lungs within the thoracic cavity with each breath.

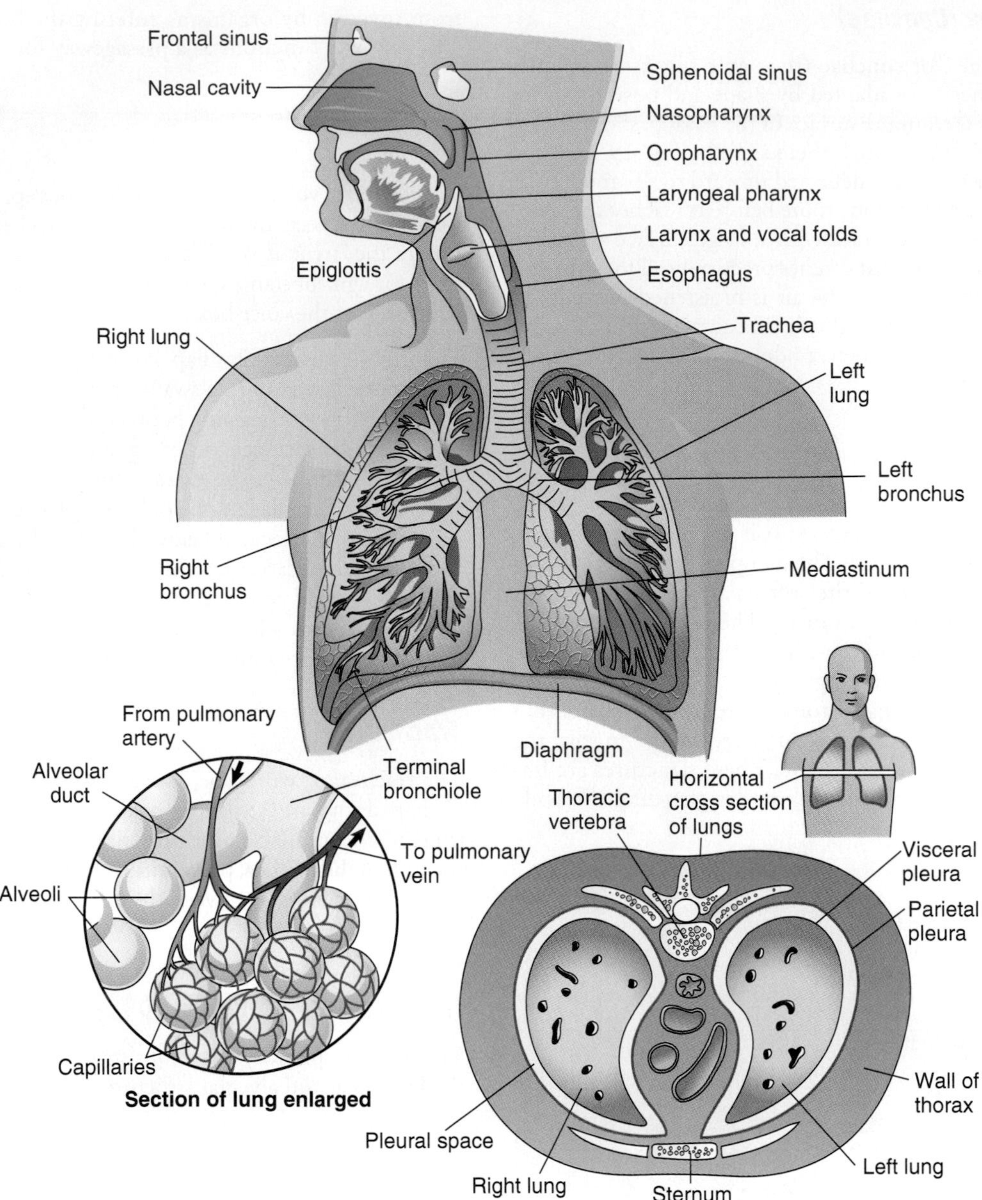

FIGURE 19•3 The respiratory system; upper respiratory structures and the structures of the thorax (*top*); alveoli and a horizontal cross section of the lungs (*bottom*).

MEDIASTINUM

The mediastinum is in the middle of the thorax, between the pleural sacs that contain the two lungs. It extends from the sternum to the vertebral column and contains all the thoracic tissue outside the lungs.

LOBES

Each lung is divided into lobes. The left lung consists of an upper and lower lobe, whereas the right lung has an upper, middle, and lower lobe (Fig. 19-4). Each lobe is further subdivided into two to five segments separated by fissures, which are extensions of the pleura.

BRONCHI AND BRONCHIOLES

There are several divisions of the bronchi within each lobe of the lung. First are the lobar bronchi (three in the right lung and two in the left lung). Lobar bronchi divide into segmental bronchi (10 on the right and 8 on the left), which are the structures identified when choosing the most effective postural drainage position for a given patient. Segmental bronchi then divide into subsegmental bronchi. These bronchi are surrounded by connective tissue that contains arteries, lymphatics, and nerves.

The subsegmental bronchi then branch into bronchioles, which have no cartilage in their walls. Their patency depends entirely on the elastic recoil of the surrounding smooth muscle and on the alveolar pressure. The bronchioles contain submucosal glands, which produce mucus that covers the inside lining of the airways. The bronchi and bronchioles are lined also with cells that have surfaces covered with cilia. These cilia create a constant whipping motion that propels mucus and foreign substances away from the lung toward the larynx.

The bronchioles then branch into terminal bronchioles, which do not have mucous glands or cilia. Terminal bronchioles then become respiratory bronchioles, which are considered to be the tran-

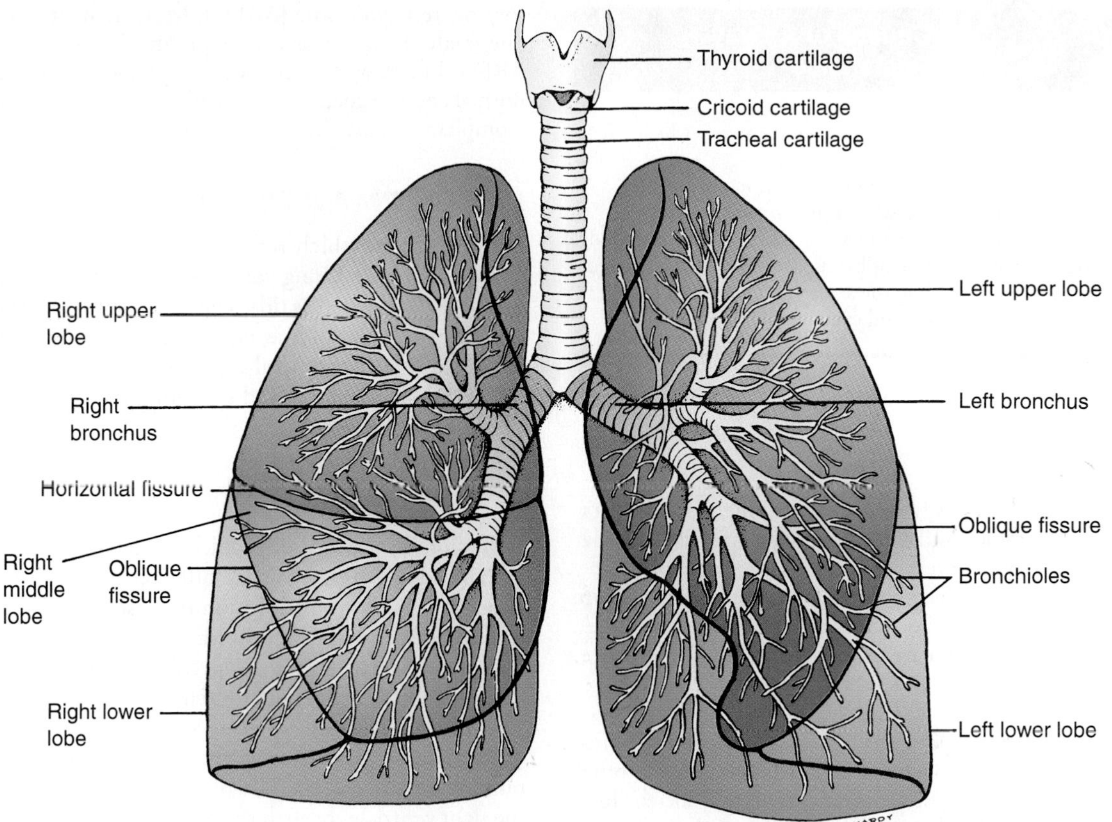

FIGURE 19•4 The lungs consist of five lobes. The right lung has three lobes (upper, middle, lower); the left has two (upper and lower). The lobes are further subdivided by fissures. The bronchial tree, another lung structure, inflates with air to fill the lobes.

sitional passageways between the conducting airways and the gas exchange airways. Up to this point, the conducting airways contain about 150 mL of air in the tracheobronchial tree that does not participate in gas exchange. This is known as **physiologic dead space**. The respiratory bronchioles then lead into alveolar ducts and alveolar sacs and then alveoli. Oxygen and carbon dioxide exchange takes place in the alveoli.

ALVEOLI

The lung is made up of about 300 million alveoli, which are arranged in clusters of 15 to 20. These alveoli are so numerous that if their surfaces were united to form one sheet, it would cover 70 square meters—the size of a tennis court.

There are three types of alveolar cells. Type I alveolar cells are epithelial cells that form the alveolar walls. Type II alveolar cells are metabolically active. These cells secrete surfactant, a phospholipid that lines the inner surface and prevents alveolar collapse. Type III alveolar cell macrophages are large phagocytic cells that ingest foreign matter (eg, mucus, bacteria) and act as an important defense mechanism.

Function of the Respiratory System

The cells of the body derive the energy they need from the oxidation of carbohydrates, fats, and proteins. As with any type of combustion, this process requires oxygen. Certain vital tissues, such as those of the brain and the heart, cannot survive for long without a continuing supply of oxygen. However, as a result of oxidation in the body tissues, carbon dioxide is produced and must be removed from the cells to prevent the buildup of acid waste products. The respiratory system performs this function by facilitating life-sustaining processes such as oxygen transport, respiration and ventilation, and gas exchange.

Oxygen Transport

Oxygen is supplied to, and carbon dioxide is removed from, cells by way of the circulating blood. Cells are in close contact with capillaries, whose thin walls permit easy passage or exchange of oxygen and carbon dioxide. Oxygen diffuses from the capillary through the capillary wall to the interstitial fluid. At this point, it diffuses through the membrane of tissue cells, where it is used by mitochondria for cellular respiration. The movement of carbon dioxide occurs by diffusion in the opposite direction—from cell to blood.

Respiration

After these tissue capillary exchanges, blood enters the systemic veins (where it is called venous blood) and travels to the pulmonary circulation. The oxygen concentration in blood within the capillaries of the lungs is lower than in the lungs' air sacs (alveoli). Because of this concentration gradient, oxygen diffuses from the alveoli to the blood. Carbon dioxide, which has a higher concentration in the blood than in the alveoli, diffuses from the blood into the alveoli. Movement of air in and out of the airways (ventilation) continually replenishes the oxygen and removes the carbon dioxide from the airways in the lung. This whole process of gas exchange between the atmospheric air and the blood and between the blood and cells of the body is called **respiration.**

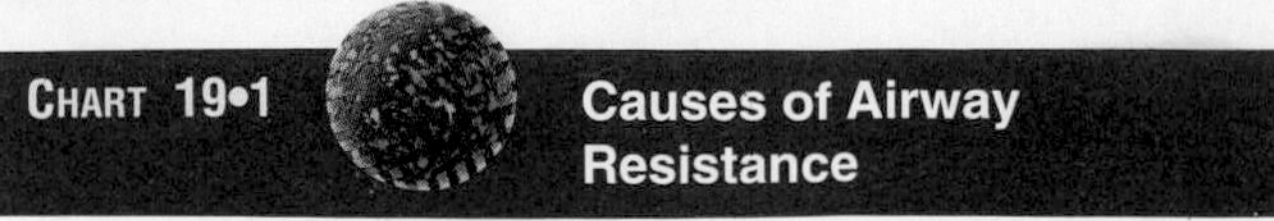

Common phenomena that may alter bronchial diameter, which affects airway resistance, include:

- Contraction of bronchial smooth muscle—as in asthma
- Thickening of bronchial mucosa—as in chronic bronchitis
- Obstruction of the airway—by mucus, a tumor, or a foreign body
- Loss of lung elasticity—as in emphysema, which is characterized by connective tissue encircling the airways, thereby keeping them open during both inspiration and expiration

Ventilation

During inspiration, air flows from the environment into the trachea, bronchi, bronchioles, and alveoli. During expiration, alveolar gas travels the same route in reverse.

Physical factors that govern air flow in and out of the lungs are collectively referred to as the mechanics of ventilation and include air pressure variances, resistance to air flow, and lung compliance.

AIR PRESSURE VARIANCES

Air flows from a region of higher pressure to a region of lower pressure. During inspiration, movement of the diaphragm and other muscles of respiration enlarges the thoracic cavity and thereby lowers the pressure inside the thorax to a level below that of atmospheric pressure. Therefore, air is drawn through the trachea and bronchi into the alveoli.

During normal expiration, the diaphragm relaxes and the lungs recoil, resulting in a decrease in the size of the thoracic cavity. The alveolar pressure then exceeds atmospheric pressure, and air flows from the lungs into the atmosphere.

AIRWAY RESISTANCE

Resistance is determined chiefly by the radius or size of the airway through which the air is flowing. Any process that changes the bronchial diameter or width affects airway resistance and alters the rate of air flow for a given pressure gradient during respiration (Chart 19-1). With increased resistance, greater-than-normal respiratory effort is required by the patient to achieve normal levels of ventilation.

COMPLIANCE

The pressure gradient between the thoracic cavity and the atmosphere causes air to flow in and out of the lungs. When pressure changes are applied in the normal lung, there is a proportional change in the lung volume. A measure of the elasticity, expandability, and distensibility of the lungs and thoracic structures is called compliance. Factors that determine lung compliance are the surface tension of the alveoli (normally low with the presence of surfactant) and the connective tissue (ie, collagen and elastin) of the lungs.

Compliance is determined by examining the volume–pressure relationship in the lungs and the thorax. In normal compliance (1.0 L/cm H_2O), the lungs and thorax easily stretch and distend when pressure is applied. High or increased compliance occurs when the lungs have lost their elasticity and the thorax is overdistended (ie, emphysema). When the lungs and thorax are "stiff," there is low or decreased compliance. Conditions associated with this include pneumothorax, hemothorax, pleural effusion, pulmonary edema, atelectasis, pulmonary fibrosis, and acute respiratory distress syndrome (ARDS). Measurement of compliance is one method used to assess the progression and improvement in ARDS. Lungs with decreased compliance require greater-than-normal energy expenditure to achieve normal levels of ventilation. Compliance is usually measured under static conditions.

Lung Volumes and Capacities

Lung function, which reflects the mechanics of ventilation, is viewed in terms of lung volumes and lung capacities. Lung volumes are categorized as tidal volume, inspiratory reserve volume, expiratory reserve volume, and residual volume. Lung capacity is evaluated in terms of vital capacity, inspiratory capacity, functional residual capacity, and total lung capacity. These terms are described in Table 19-1.

Diffusion and Perfusion

Diffusion is the process by which oxygen and carbon dioxide are exchanged at the air–blood interface. The alveolar–capillary membrane is ideal for diffusion because of its large surface area and thin membrane. In the normal healthy adult, oxygen and carbon dioxide travel across the alveolar–capillary membrane without difficulty as a result of differences in gas concentrations in the alveoli and capillaries.

Pulmonary perfusion is the actual blood flow through the pulmonary circulation. The blood is pumped into the lungs by the right ventricle through the pulmonary artery. The pulmonary artery divides into the right and left branches to supply both lungs. These two branches divide further to supply all parts of each lung. Normally about 2% of the blood pumped by the right ventricle does not perfuse the alveolar capillaries. This shunted blood drains into the left side of the heart without participating in alveolar gas exchange.

The pulmonary circulation is considered a low-pressure system because the systolic blood pressure in the pulmonary artery is 20 to 30 mm Hg and the diastolic pressure is 5 to 15 mm Hg. Because of these low pressures, the pulmonary vasculature normally can vary its capacity to accommodate the blood flow it receives. When a person is in an upright position, however, the pulmonary artery pressure is not great enough to supply blood to the apex of the lung against the force of gravity. Thus, when a person is upright, the lung may be considered to be divided into three sections: an upper part with poor blood supply, a lower part with maximal blood supply, and a section in between the two with an intermediate supply of blood. When a person lying down turns to one side, more blood passes to the dependent lung.

Perfusion also is influenced by alveolar pressure. The pulmonary capillaries are sandwiched between adjacent alveoli. If the alveolar pressure is sufficiently high, the capillaries will be squeezed. Depending on the pressure, some capillaries completely collapse, whereas others narrow.

Pulmonary artery pressure, gravity, and alveolar pressure determine the patterns of perfusion. In lung disease these factors vary, and the perfusion of the lung may become very abnormal.

Ventilation and Perfusion Balance and Imbalance

Ventilation is the flow of gas in and out of the lungs, and perfusion is the filling of the pulmonary capillaries with blood. Adequate gas exchange depends on an adequate ventilation–perfusion ratio. In different areas of the lung, the ratio may vary.

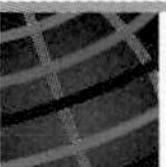

TABLE 19•1 **Lung Volumes and Lung Capacities**

Term	Symbol	Description	Normal Value*	Significance
Lung Volumes				
Tidal volume	V_T or TV	The volume of air inhaled and exhaled with each breath	500 mL or 5–10mL/kg	The tidal volume may not vary, even with severe disease.
Inspiratory reserve volume	IRV	The maximum volume of air that can be inhaled after a normal inhalation	3000 mL	
Expiratory reserve volume	ERV	The maximum volume of air that can be exhaled forcibly after a normal exhalation	1100 mL	Expiratory reserve volume is decreased with restrictive disorders, such as obesity, ascites, pregnancy.
Residual volume	RV	The volume of air remaining in the lungs after a maximum exhalation	1200 mL	Residual volume may be increased with obstructive disease.
Lung Capacities				
Vital capacity	VC	The maximum volume of air exhaled from the point of maximum inspiration VC = TV + IRV + ERV	4600 mL	A decrease in vital capacity may be found in neuromuscular disease, generalized fatigue, atelectasis, pulmonary edema, and COPD.
Inspiratory capacity	IC	The maximum volume of air inhaled after normal expiration IC = TV + IRV	3500 mL	A decrease in inspiratory capacity may indicate restrictive disease.
Functional residual capacity	FRC	The volume of air remaining in the lungs after a normal expiration FRV = ERV + RV	2300 mL	Functional residual capacity may be increased with COPD and decreased in ARDS.
Total lung capacity	TLC	The volume of air in the lungs after a maximum inspiration TLC = TV + IRV + ERV + RV	5800 mL	Total lung capacity may be decreased with restrictive disease (atelectasis, pneumonia) and increased in COPD.

*Values for healthy men; women are 20%–25% less.

Alterations in perfusion may occur with a change in the pulmonary artery pressure, alveolar pressure, and gravity. Airway blockages, local changes in compliance, and gravity may alter ventilation.

A ventilation–perfusion ($\dot{V}/\dot{Q}$) imbalance occurs from inadequate ventilation, inadequate perfusion, or both. There are four possible $\dot{V}/\dot{Q}$ states in the lung: normal $\dot{V}/\dot{Q}$ ratio, low $\dot{V}/\dot{Q}$ ratio (shunt), high $\dot{V}/\dot{Q}$ ratio (dead space), and absence of ventilation and perfusion (silent unit) (Chart 19-2).

Ventilation and perfusion imbalance causes shunting of blood, resulting in **hypoxia** (low cellular oxygen level). Shunting appears to be the main cause of hypoxia after thoracic or abdominal surgery and most types of respiratory failure. Severe hypoxia results when the amount of shunting exceeds 20%. Oxygen can eliminate hypoxia, depending on the type of $\dot{V}/\dot{Q}$ imbalance.

Gas Exchange

The air we breathe is a gaseous mixture consisting mainly of nitrogen (78.62%) and oxygen (20.84%), with traces of carbon dioxide (0.04%), water vapor (0.05%), helium, and argon. The atmospheric pressure at sea level is about 760 mm Hg. Partial pressure is the pressure exerted by each type of gas in a mixture of gases. The partial pressure of a gas is proportional to the concentration of that gas in the mixture. The total pressure exerted by the gaseous mixture is equal to the sum of the partial pressures.

PARTIAL PRESSURE OF GASES

Based on these facts, the partial pressures of nitrogen and oxygen can be calculated. The partial pressure of nitrogen is 79% of 760 (0.79×760), or 600 mm Hg; that of oxygen is 21% of 760 (0.21×760), or 160 mm Hg. Chart 19-3 spells out terms and abbreviations related to partial pressure of gases.

Once the air enters the trachea, it becomes fully saturated with water vapor, which displaces some of the gases so that the air pressure within the lung remains equal to the air pressure outside (760 mm Hg). Water vapor exerts a pressure of 47 mm Hg when it fully saturates a mixture of gases at the body temperature of 37°C (98.6°F). Nitrogen and oxygen are therefore now responsible for the remaining 713 mm Hg (760 − 47) pressure. Once this mixture enters the alveoli, it is further diluted by carbon dioxide. In the alveoli, the water vapor continues to exert a pressure of 47 mm Hg. The remaining 713 mm Hg pressure is now exerted as follows: nitrogen, 569 mm Hg (74.9%); oxygen, 104 mm Hg (13.6%), and carbon dioxide, 40 mm Hg (5.3%).

PARTIAL PRESSURE IN GAS EXCHANGE

When a gas is exposed to a liquid, the gas dissolves in the liquid until an equilibrium is reached. The dissolved gas also exerts a partial pressure. At equilibrium, the partial pressure of the gas in the liquid is the same as the partial pressure of the gas in the gaseous mixture. Oxygenation of venous blood in the lung illustrates this point. In the lung, venous blood and alveolar oxygen are separated by a very thin alveolar membrane. Oxygen diffuses across this membrane to dissolve in the blood until the partial pressure of oxygen in the blood is the same as that in the alveoli (104 mm Hg). Because carbon dioxide is a byproduct of oxidation in the cells, however, venous blood contains carbon dioxide at a higher partial pressure than that in the alveolar gas. In the lung, carbon dioxide diffuses out of venous blood into the alveolar gas. At

CHART 19•2 Ventilation–Perfusion Ratios

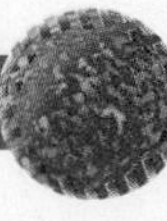

Normal Ratio

In the healthy lung, a given amount of blood passes an alveolus and is matched with an equal amount of gas (**A**). The ratio is 1 : 1 (ventilation matches perfusion).

Low Ventilation–Perfusion Ratio: Shunts

Low ventilation–perfusion states may be called shunt-producing disorders. When perfusion exceeds ventilation, a shunt exists (**B**). Blood bypasses the alveoli without gas exchange occurring. This is seen with obstruction of the distal airways, such as with pneumonia, atelectasis, tumor, or a mucus plug.

High Ventilation–Perfusion Ratio: Dead Space

When ventilation exceeds perfusion, dead space results (**C**). The alveoli do not have an adequate blood supply for gas exchange to occur. This is characteristic of a variety of disorders, including pulmonary emboli, pulmonary infarction, and cardiogenic shock.

Silent Unit

In the absence of ventilation and perfusion or with limited ventilation and perfusion, a condition known as a silent unit occurs (**D**). This is seen with pneumothorax and severe acute respiratory distress syndrome.

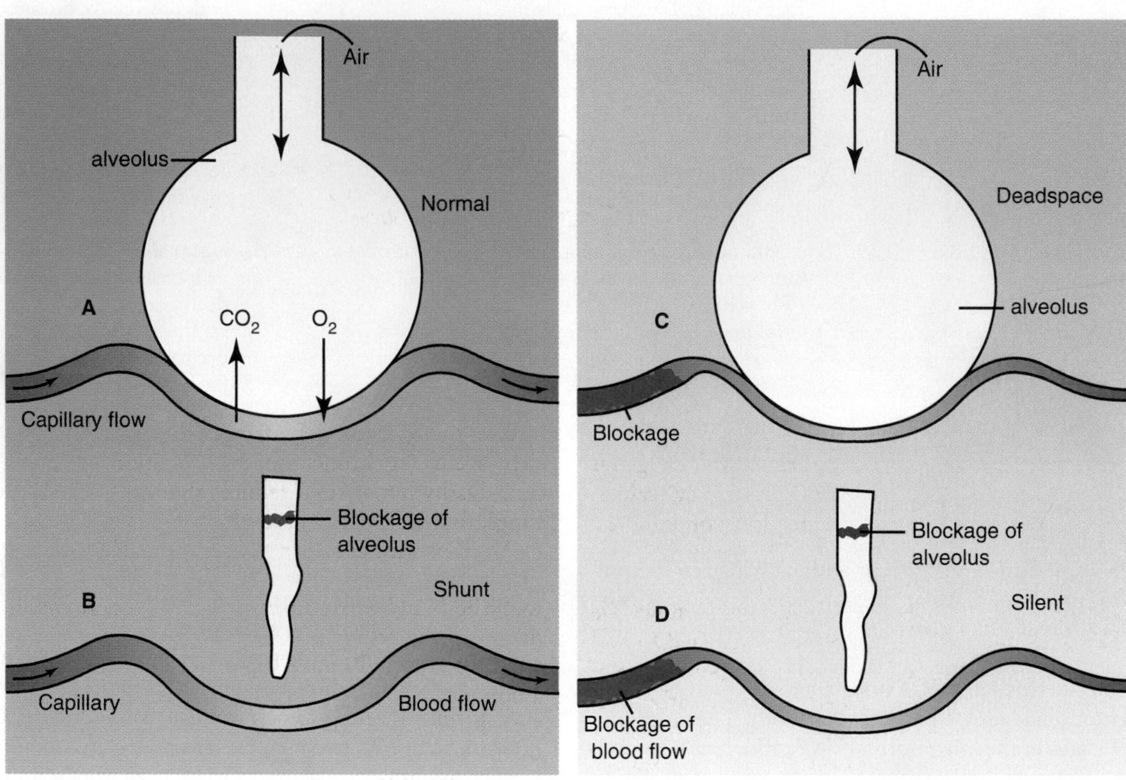

equilibrium, the partial pressure of carbon dioxide in the blood and in alveolar gas is the same (40 mm Hg). The changes in partial pressure are shown in Figure 19-5.

EFFECTS OF PRESSURE ON OXYGEN TRANSPORT

Oxygen and carbon dioxide are carried simultaneously by virtue of their abilities to dissolve in blood or to combine with some of the elements of blood. Oxygen is carried in the blood in two forms: first as physically dissolved oxygen in the plasma, and second in combination with the hemoglobin of the red blood cells. Each 100 mL of normal arterial blood carries 0.3 mL of oxygen physically dissolved in the plasma and 20 mL of oxygen in combination with hemoglobin. Large amounts of oxygen can be transported in the blood because it combines easily with hemoglobin to form oxyhemoglobin:

$$O_2 + Hgb \leftrightarrow HgbO_2$$

The volume of oxygen physically dissolved in the plasma varies directly with the partial pressure of oxygen in the arteries (PaO_2). The higher the PaO_2, the greater the amount of oxygen dissolved. For example, at a PaO_2 of 10 mm Hg, 0.03 mL of oxygen is dissolved in 100 mL of plasma. At 20 mm Hg, twice this amount is dissolved in plasma, and at 100 mm Hg, 10 times this amount is dissolved. Therefore, the amount of dissolved oxygen is directly proportional to the partial pressure, regardless of how high the oxygen pressure rises.

The amount of oxygen that combines with hemoglobin also depends on PaO_2, but only up to a PaO_2 of about 150 mm Hg. When the PaO_2 is 150 mm Hg, hemoglobin is 100% saturated and will not combine with any additional oxygen. When hemoglobin is 100% saturated, 1 g of hemoglobin will combine with 1.34 mL of oxygen. Therefore, in a person with 14 g/dL of hemoglobin, each 100 mL of blood will contain about 19 mL of

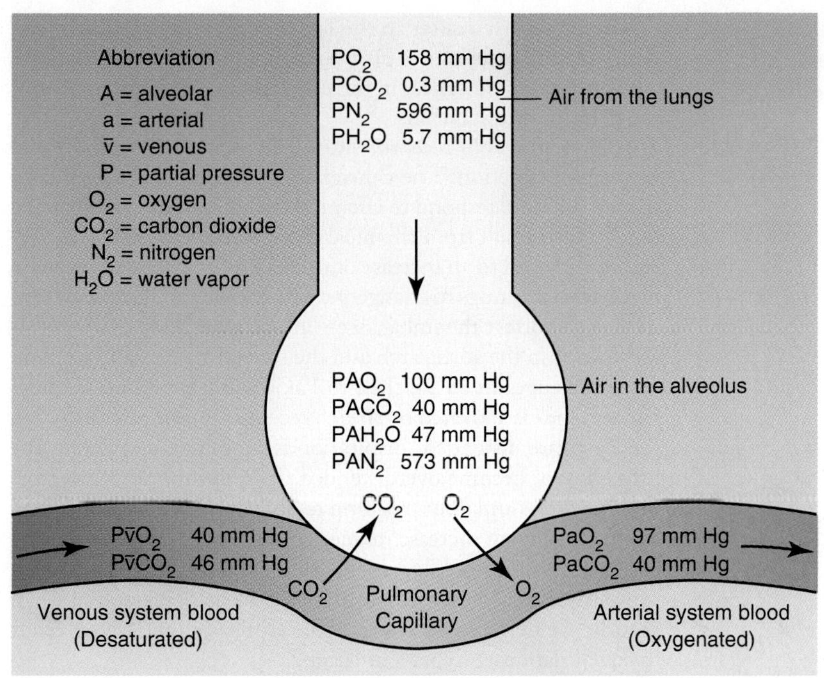

FIGURE 19•5 Changes occur in the partial pressure of gases during respiration. These values vary as a result of the exchange of oxygen and carbon dioxide and the changes that occur in their partial pressures as venous blood flows through the lungs. Adapted from Willis, M. C. (1996). *Medical terminology: The language of healthcare.* Baltimore: Williams & Wilkins.

oxygen associated with hemoglobin. If the PaO_2 is less than 150 mm Hg, the percentage of hemoglobin saturated with oxygen is lower. For example, at a PaO_2 of 100 mm Hg (normal value), saturation is 97%; at a PaO_2 of 40 mm Hg, saturation is 70%.

OXYHEMOGLOBIN DISSOCIATION CURVE

The oxyhemoglobin dissociation curve (Chart 19-4) shows the relationship between the partial pressure of oxygen (PaO_2) and the percentage of saturation of oxygen (SaO_2). The percentage of saturation can be affected by the following factors: carbon dioxide, pH, temperature, and 2,3-diphosphoglycerate. A rise in these factors shifts the curve to the right so that more oxygen is then released to the tissues at the same PaO_2. A reduction in these factors causes the curve to shift to the left, making the bond between oxygen and hemoglobin stronger, so that less oxygen is given up to the tissues at the same PaO_2. The unusual shape of the oxyhemoglobin dissociation curve is a distinct advantage to the patient for two reasons:

1. If the arterial PO_2 decreases from 100 to 80 mm Hg as a result of lung disease or heart disease, the hemoglobin of the arterial blood remains almost maximally saturated (94%) and the tissues will not suffer from hypoxia.
2. When the arterial blood passes into tissue capillaries and is exposed to the tissue tension of oxygen (about 40 mm Hg), hemoglobin gives up large quantities of oxygen for use by the tissues.

Clinical Significance. The normal value of PaO_2 is 80 to 100 mm Hg (95% to 98% saturation). With this level of oxygenation, there is a 15% margin of excess oxygen available to the tissues. With a normal hemoglobin level of 15 mg/dL and a PaO_2 level of 40 mm Hg (oxygen saturation 75%), there is adequate oxygen available for the tissues but no reserve for physiologic stresses that increase tissue oxygen demand. When a serious incident occurs (eg, bronchospasm, aspiration, hypotension, or cardiac dysrhythmias) that reduces the intake of oxygen from the lungs, tissue hypoxia will result.

An important consideration in the transport of oxygen is cardiac output, which determines the amount of oxygen delivered to the body and which affects lung and tissue perfusion. If the cardiac output is normal (5 L/min), the amount of oxygen delivered to the body per minute is normal. If cardiac output falls, the amount of oxygen delivered to the tissues also falls. Under normal conditions, most of the oxygen delivered to the body is not used. In fact, only 250 mL of oxygen is used per minute. Under normal conditions, this is approximately 25% of available oxygen. The rest of the oxygen returns to the right side of the heart, and the PO_2 of venous blood drops from 80 to 100 mm Hg to about 40 mm Hg.

CHART 19•3 Partial Pressure Abbreviations

P = pressure
PO_2 = partial pressure of oxygen
PCO_2 = partial pressure of carbon dioxide
PAO_2 = partial pressure of alveolar oxygen
$PACO_2$ = partial pressure of alveolar carbon dioxide
PaO_2 = partial pressure of arterial oxygen
$PaCO_2$ = partial pressure of arterial carbon dioxide
PVO_2 = partial pressure of venous oxygen
$PVCO_2$ = partial pressure of venous carbon dioxide
P_{50} = partial pressure of oxygen when the hemoglobin is 50% saturated

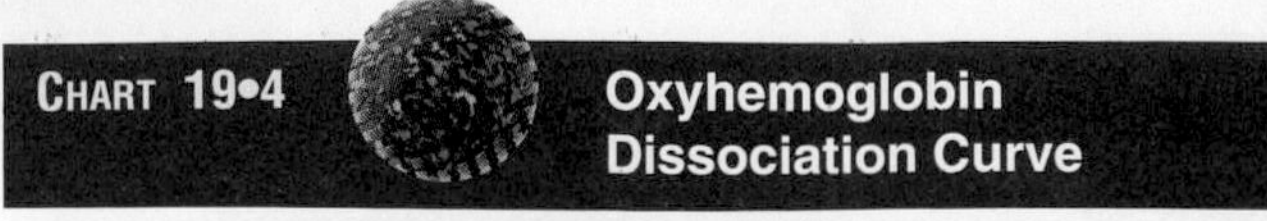

The oxyhemoglobin dissociation curve is marked to show three oxygen levels:

1. Normal levels—PaO_2 above 70 mm Hg
2. Relatively safe levels—PaO_2 45 to 70 mm Hg
3. Dangerous levels—PaO_2 below 40 mm Hg

The normal (middle) curve shows that 75% saturation occurs at a PaO_2 of 40 mm Hg. If the curve shifts to the right, the same saturation (75%) occurs at the higher PaO_2 of 57 mm Hg. If the curve shifts to the left, 75% saturation occurs at a PaO_2 of 25 mm Hg.

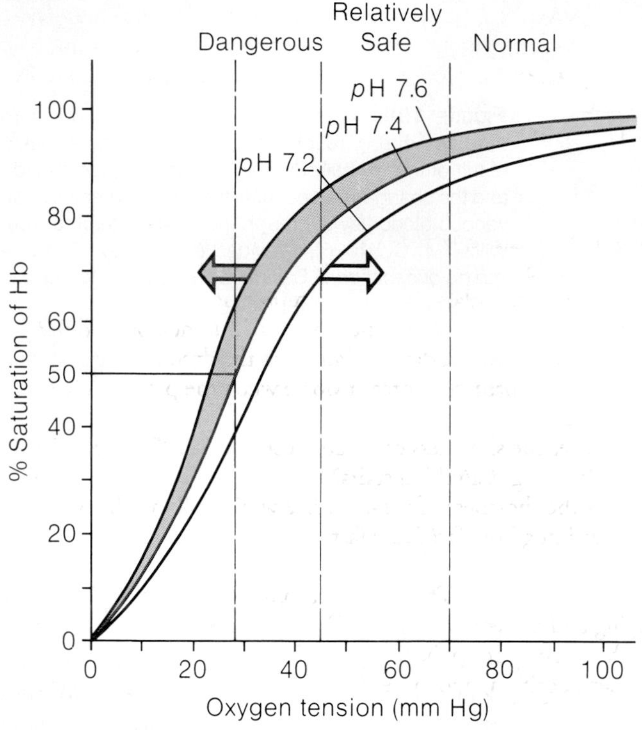

Carbon Dioxide Transport

At the same time that oxygen diffuses from the blood into the tissues, carbon dioxide diffuses in the opposite direction (ie, from tissue cells to blood) and is transported to the lungs for excretion. The amount of carbon dioxide in transit is one of the major determinants of the acid–base balance of the body. Normally, only 6% of the venous carbon dioxide is removed, and enough remains in the arterial blood to exert a pressure of 40 mm Hg. Most of the carbon dioxide (90%) enters the red blood cells; the small portion (5%) that remains dissolved in the plasma (PCO_2) is the critical factor that determines carbon dioxide movement in or out of the blood.

In summary, the many processes involved in respiratory gas transport do not occur in intermittent stages; rather, they are rapid, simultaneous, and continuous.

Neurologic Control of Ventilation

Resting respiration is the result of cyclical excitation of the respiratory muscles by the phrenic nerve. The rhythm of breathing is controlled by respiratory centers in the brain. The inspiratory and expiratory centers in the medulla oblongata and pons control the rate and depth of ventilation to meet the body's metabolic demands.

The **apneustic center** in the lower pons stimulates the inspiratory medullary center to promote deep, prolonged inspirations. The **pneumotaxic center** in the upper pons is thought to control the pattern of respirations.

Several groups of receptor sites assist in the brain's control of respiratory function. The central chemoreceptors are located in the medulla and respond to chemical changes in the cerebrospinal fluid, which result from chemical changes in the blood. These receptors respond to an increase or decrease in the pH and convey a message to the lungs to change the depth and then the rate of ventilation to correct the imbalance. The peripheral chemoreceptors are located in the aortic arch and the carotid arteries and respond first to changes in PaO_2, then to $PaCO_2$ and pH. The Hering–Breuer reflex is activated by stretch receptors in the alveoli. When the lungs are distended, inspiration is inhibited; as a result, the lungs do not become overdistended. In addition, proprioceptors in the muscles and joints respond to body movements, such as exercise, causing an increase in ventilation. Thus, range-of-motion exercises in an immobile patient stimulate breathing. Baroreceptors, also located in the aortic and carotid bodies, respond to an increase or decrease in arterial blood pressure and cause reflex hypoventilation or hyperventilation.

Gerontologic Considerations

A gradual decline in respiratory function begins in early to middle adulthood and affects the structure and function of the respiratory system. The vital capacity of the lungs and respiratory muscle strength peak between ages 20 and 25 and decrease thereafter. With aging (40 years and older), changes occur in the alveoli reducing the surface area available for the exchange of oxygen and carbon dioxide. At approximately age 50, alveoli begin to lose elasticity. A decrease in vital capacity occurs with loss of chest wall mobility, thus restricting tidal flow of air. The amount of respiratory dead space increases with age. These changes result in a decreased diffusion capacity for oxygen with age, producing lower oxygen levels in the arterial circulation. Elderly people have a decreased ability to move air rapidly in and out of the lungs. Despite these changes, in the absence of chronic pulmonary disease, elderly people are able to carry out activities of daily living, but they may have decreased tolerance for and require additional rest after prolonged or vigorous activity and excessive exertion.

ASSESSMENT

Health History

The health history focuses on the physical and functional problems of the patient and the effect of these problems on his or her life. The reason the patient is seeking health care often is related to one of the following: **dyspnea** (shortness of breath), pain, accumulation of mucus, wheezing, **hemoptysis** (blood spit up from the respiratory tract), edema of the ankles and feet, cough, and general fatigue and weakness.

In addition to identifying the chief reason why the patient is seeking health care, the nurse tries to determine when the health problem or symptom started, how long it lasted, if it was relieved at any time, and how relief was obtained. The nurse collects information about precipitating factors, duration, severity, and associated factors or symptoms. The nurse also assesses for risk factors that may contribute to the patient's lung condition.

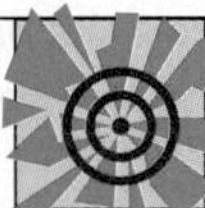

Risk Factors for RESPIRATORY DISEASE

Smoking (the single most important contributor to lung disease)
Personal or family history of lung disease
Occupation
Allergens and environmental pollutants
Recreational exposure

The nurse assesses the impact of signs and symptoms on the patient's ability to perform activities of daily living and to participate in usual work and family activities. In addition, psychosocial factors that may affect the patient are explored. These factors include anxiety, role changes, family relationships, financial problems, and employment status and the strategies the patient uses to cope with them.

Many respiratory diseases are chronic and progressively debilitating. Therefore, ongoing assessment of the patient's physical abilities, psychosocial supports, and quality of life is needed to plan appropriate interventions. It is important for the patient with a respiratory disorder to understand the condition and to be familiar with necessary self-care interventions. The nurse evaluates these factors over time and provides education as needed.

Signs and Symptoms

The major signs and symptoms of respiratory disease are dyspnea, cough, sputum production, chest pain, wheezing, clubbing of the fingers, hemoptysis, and cyanosis. These clinical manifestations are related to the duration and severity of the disease.

DYSPNEA

Dyspnea (difficult or labored breathing, shortness of breath) is a symptom common to many pulmonary and cardiac disorders, particularly when there is decreased lung compliance or increased airway resistance. The right ventricle of the heart will be affected ultimately by lung disease because it must pump blood through the lungs against greater resistance. It may also be associated with neurologic or neuromuscular disorders such as myasthenia gravis, Guillain-Barré syndrome, or muscular dystrophy.

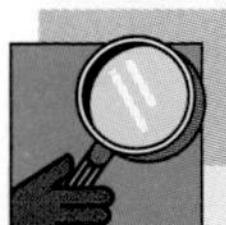

ASSESSMENT
PSYCHOSOCIAL FACTORS

Questions to consider when assessing psychosocial factors related to pulmonary disease and respiratory function include:

- What strategies does the patient use to cope with the signs and symptoms and challenges associated with pulmonary disease?
- Does the patient exhibit anxiety, anger, hostility, dependency, withdrawal, isolation, avoidance, noncompliance, acceptance, or denial?
- What support systems does the patient use to cope with the illness?
- Are resources (relatives, friends, or community groups) available? Do the patient and family use them effectively?

Significance. In general, acute diseases of the lungs produce a more severe grade of dyspnea than do chronic diseases. Sudden dyspnea in a healthy person may indicate pneumothorax (air in the pleural cavity), acute respiratory obstruction, or ARDS. In an ill patient or after surgery, sudden dyspnea may denote pulmonary embolism. **Orthopnea** (inability to breathe easily except in an upright position) may be found in patients with heart disease and occasionally in patients with chronic obstructive pulmonary disease (COPD); dyspnea with an expiratory wheeze occurs with COPD. Noisy breathing may result from a narrowing of the airway or localized obstruction of a major bronchus by a tumor or foreign body. The presence of both inspiratory and expiratory wheezing usually signifies asthma if the patient does not have congestive heart failure.

The circumstance that produces the patient's dyspnea must be determined. Therefore, it is important to ask the patient the following questions:

- How much exertion triggers shortness of breath?
- Is there an associated cough?
- Is dyspnea related to other symptoms?
- Was the onset of shortness of breath sudden or gradual?
- At what time of day or night does the dyspnea occur?
- Is the shortness of breath worse when the patient is flat in bed?
- Does the shortness of breath occur at rest? With exercise? Running? Climbing stairs?
- Is the shortness of breath worse while walking? If so, when walking how far? How fast?

Relief Measures. The management of dyspnea is aimed at identifying and correcting its cause. Relief of the symptom sometimes is achieved by placing the patient at rest with the head elevated (high Fowler's position) and, in severe cases, by administering oxygen.

COUGH

Cough results from irritation of the mucous membranes anywhere in the respiratory tract. The stimulus producing a cough may arise from an infectious process or from an airborne irritant, such as smoke, smog, dust, or a gas. The cough is the patient's chief protection against the accumulation of secretions in the bronchi and bronchioles.

Significance. Cough may indicate serious pulmonary disease. Of equal importance is the type of cough. A dry, irritative cough is characteristic of an upper respiratory tract infection of viral origin. Laryngotracheitis causes an irritative, high-pitched cough. Tracheal lesions produce a brassy cough. A severe or changing cough may indicate bronchogenic carcinoma. Pleuritic chest pain accompanying coughing may indicate pleural or chest wall (musculoskeletal) involvement.

The nurse also needs to evaluate the character of the cough—is it dry, hacking, brassy, wheezing, loose, or severe? The time of coughing is also noted. Coughing at night may herald the onset of left-sided heart failure or bronchial asthma. A cough in the morning with sputum production may indicate bronchitis. A cough that worsens when the patient is supine suggests postnasal drip (sinusitis). Coughing after food intake may indicate aspirated material in the tracheobronchial tree. A cough of recent onset is usually from an acute infection.

SPUTUM PRODUCTION

A patient who coughs long enough almost invariably produces sputum. Violent coughing causes bronchial spasm, obstruction, and further irritation of the bronchi and may result in syncope (fainting). A severe, repeated, or uncontrolled cough that is nonproductive is exhausting and potentially harmful. Sputum production is the reaction of the lungs to any constantly recurring irritant. It also may be associated with a nasal discharge.

Significance. A profuse amount of purulent sputum (thick and yellow, green, or rust-colored) or a change in color of the sputum probably indicates a bacterial infection. A thin, mucoid sputum frequently results from viral bronchitis. A gradual increase of sputum over time may indicate the presence of chronic bronchitis or bronchiectasis. Pink-tinged mucoid sputum suggests a lung tumor. Profuse, frothy, pink material, often welling up into the throat, may indicate pulmonary edema. Foul-smelling sputum and bad breath point to the presence of a lung abscess, bronchiectasis, or an infection caused by fusospirochetal or other anaerobic organisms.

Relief Measures. If the sputum is too thick for the patient to expectorate, it is necessary to decrease its viscosity by increasing its water content through adequate hydration (drinking water) and inhalation of aerosolized solutions, which may be delivered by any type of nebulizer. Methods for the nurse to use in assisting the patient to cough productively are discussed later in this chapter.

Smoking is contraindicated with excessive sputum production because it interferes with ciliary action, increases bronchial secretions, causes inflammation and hyperplasia of the mucous membranes, and reduces production of surfactant. Thus, smoking impairs bronchial drainage. When the person stops smoking, sputum volume decreases and resistance to bronchial infections increases.

The patient's appetite may decrease because of the odor of the sputum or the taste it leaves in the mouth. The nurse encourages adequate oral hygiene and wise selection of food, measures that will stimulate appetite. In addition, the nurse encourages the patient and family to remove sputum cups, emesis basins, and soiled tissues before mealtime. It is a good idea to encourage citrus juices at the beginning of the meal because they cleanse the palate of the sputum taste, thereby increasing the palatability of the rest of the meal.

CHEST PAIN

Chest pain or discomfort may be associated with pulmonary or cardiac disease. Chest pain associated with pulmonary conditions may be sharp, stabbing, and intermittent, or it may be dull, aching, and persistent. The pain usually is felt on the side where the pathologic process is located, but it may be referred elsewhere—for example, to the neck, back, or abdomen.

Significance. Chest pain may occur with pneumonia, pulmonary embolism with lung infarction, and pleurisy. It also may be a late symptom of bronchogenic carcinoma. In carcinoma the pain may be dull and persistent because the cancer has invaded the chest wall, mediastinum, or spine.

Lung disease does not always produce thoracic pain because the lungs and the visceral pleura lack sensory nerves and are insensitive to pain stimuli. However, the parietal pleura has a rich supply of sensory nerves that are stimulated by inflammation and stretching of the membrane. Pleuritic pain from irritation of the parietal pleura is sharp and seems to "catch" on inspiration; it is often described by patients as "like the stabbing of a knife." Patients are more comfortable when they lie on the affected side. This posture tends to splint the chest wall, limit expansion and contraction of the lung, and reduce the friction between the injured or diseased pleurae on that side. Pain associated with cough may be reduced manually by splinting the rib cage.

The nurse assesses the quality, intensity, and radiation of pain and identifies and explores precipitating factors, along with their relationship to the patient's position. Also, it is important to evaluate the relationship of pain to the inspiratory and expiratory phases of respiration.

Relief Measures. Analgesic medications may be effective in relieving chest pain, but care must be taken not to depress the respiratory center or a productive cough. Nonsteroidal anti-inflammatory drugs achieve this goal and thus are used for pleuritic pain. A regional anesthetic block may be performed to relieve extreme pain.

WHEEZING

Wheezing is often the major finding in a patient with bronchoconstriction or airway narrowing. It is heard with or without a stethoscope, depending on its location. Wheezing is a high-pitched, musical sound heard mainly on expiration.

Relief Measures. Oral or inhalant bronchodilator medications reverse wheezing in most instances.

CLUBBING OF THE FINGERS

Clubbing of the fingers as a sign of lung disease is found in patients with chronic hypoxic conditions, chronic lung infections, and malignancies of the lung. This finding may be manifested initially as sponginess of the nailbed and loss of the nailbed angle (Fig. 19-6).

HEMOPTYSIS

Hemoptysis (expectoration of blood from the respiratory tract) is a symptom of both pulmonary and cardiac disorders. The onset of hemoptysis is usually sudden, and it may be intermittent or continuous. Signs, which vary from blood-stained sputum to a large, sudden hemorrhage, always merit investigation. The most common causes are:

- Pulmonary infection
- Carcinoma of the lung

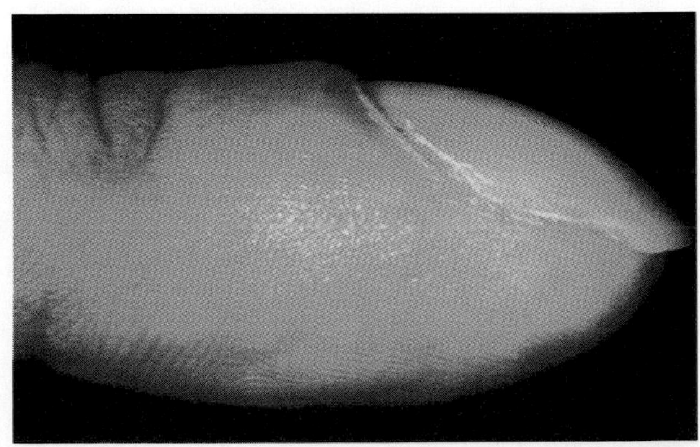

FIGURE 19•6 Clubbed finger. In clubbing, the distal phalanx of each finger is rounded and bulbous. The nail plate is more convex, and the angle between the plate and the proximal nail fold increases to 180 degrees or more. The proximal nail fold, when palpated, feels spongy or floating. Among the many causes are chronic hypoxia and lung cancer.

- Abnormalities of the heart or blood vessels
- Pulmonary artery or vein abnormalities
- Pulmonary emboli and infarction

Diagnostic evaluation to determine the cause includes several studies: chest x-ray, chest angiography, and bronchoscopy. A careful history and physical examination are necessary to establish a diagnosis of the underlying disease, irrespective of whether the bleeding involved a very small amount of blood in the sputum or a massive hemorrhage. The amount of blood produced is not always proportional to the seriousness of the cause.

First, it is important to determine the source of the bleeding—the gums, nasopharynx, lungs, or stomach. The nurse may be the only witness to the episode. When documenting the bleeding episode, the nurse considers the following points:

- Bloody sputum from the nose or the nasopharynx is usually preceded by considerable sniffing, with blood possibly appearing in the nose.
- Blood from the lung is usually bright red, frothy, and mixed with sputum. Initial symptoms include a tickling sensation in the throat, a salty taste, a burning or bubbling sensation in the chest, and perhaps chest pain, in which case the patient tends to splint the bleeding side. The term "hemoptysis" is reserved for the coughing up of blood arising from a pulmonary hemorrhage. This blood has an alkaline pH (greater than 7.0).
- If the hemorrhage is in the stomach, the blood is vomited (hematemesis) rather than coughed up. Blood that has been in contact with gastric juice is sometimes so dark that it is referred to as "coffee grounds." This blood has an acid pH (less than 7.0).

CYANOSIS

Cyanosis, a bluish coloring of the skin, is a very late indicator of hypoxia. The presence or absence of cyanosis is determined by the amount of unoxygenated hemoglobin in the blood. Cyanosis appears when there is 5 g/dL of unoxygenated hemoglobin. A patient with a hemoglobin level of 15 g/dL will not demonstrate cyanosis until 5 g/dL of that hemoglobin becomes unoxygenated, reducing the effective circulating hemoglobin to two thirds of the normal level. An anemic patient rarely manifests cyanosis, and a polycythemic patient may appear cyanotic even if adequately oxygenated. Therefore, cyanosis is *not* a reliable sign of hypoxia.

Assessment of cyanosis is affected by room lighting, the patient's skin color, and the distance of the blood vessels from the surface of the skin. In the presence of a pulmonary condition, central cyanosis is assessed by observing the color of the tongue and lips. This indicates a decrease in oxygen tension in the blood. Peripheral cyanosis results from decreased blood flow to a certain area of the body, as in vasoconstriction of the nailbeds or earlobes from exposure to cold, and does not necessarily indicate a central systemic problem.

Physical Assessment of the Upper Respiratory Structures

For a routine examination, only a simple light source, such as a penlight, is necessary. A more thorough examination requires the use of a nasal speculum.

Nose and Sinuses

The nurse inspects the external nose for lesions, asymmetry, or inflammation and then asks the patient to tilt the head backward. Gently pushing the tip of the nose upward, the nurse examines the internal structures of the nose, inspecting the mucosa for color, swelling, exudate, or bleeding. The nasal mucosa is normally redder than the oral mucosa, but it may appear swollen and hyperemic if the patient has a common cold. In allergic rhinitis, however, the mucosa appears pale and swollen.

Next the nurse inspects the septum for deviation, perforation, or bleeding. Most people have a slight degree of septal deviation, but actual displacement of the cartilage into either the right or left side of the nose may produce nasal obstruction. Such deviation usually causes no symptoms.

While the head is still tilted back, the nurse inspects the inferior and middle turbinates. In chronic rhinitis, nasal polyps may develop between the inferior and middle turbinates; they are distinguished by their gray appearance. Unlike the turbinates, they are gelatinous and freely movable.

Next the nurse may palpate the frontal and maxillary sinuses for tenderness (Fig. 19-7). Using the thumbs, the nurse applies gentle pressure in an upward fashion at the supraorbital ridges (frontal sinuses) and in the cheek area adjacent to the nose (maxillary sinuses). Tenderness in either area suggests inflammation. The frontal and maxillary sinuses can be inspected by transillumination (passing a strong light through a bony area, such as the sinuses, to inspect the cavity; Fig. 19-8). If the light fails to penetrate, the cavity is likely to contain fluid or pus.

Pharynx and Mouth

After the nasal inspection, the nurse may assess the mouth and pharynx, instructing the patient to open the mouth wide and take a deep breath. Usually this will flatten the posterior tongue and briefly allow a full view of the anterior and posterior pillars, tonsils, uvula, and posterior pharynx (Fig. 19-9). The nurse inspects these structures for color, symmetry, and evidence of exudate, ulceration, or enlargement. If a tongue blade is needed to depress the tongue to visualize the pharynx, it is pressed firmly beyond the midpoint of the tongue to avoid a gagging response.

Trachea

Next the position and mobility of the trachea are usually noted by direct palpation. This is performed by placing the thumb and index finger of one hand on either side of the trachea just above the ster-

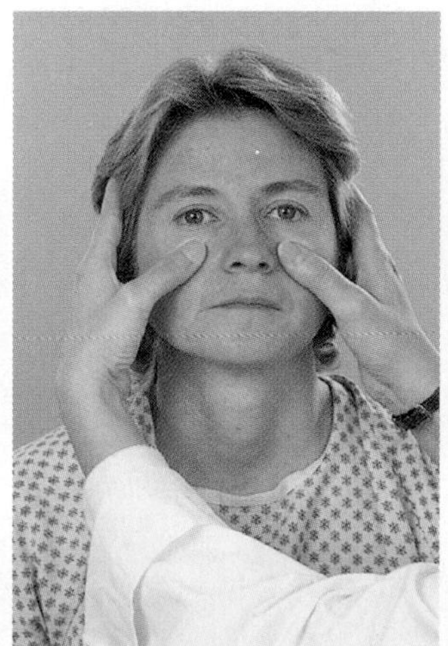

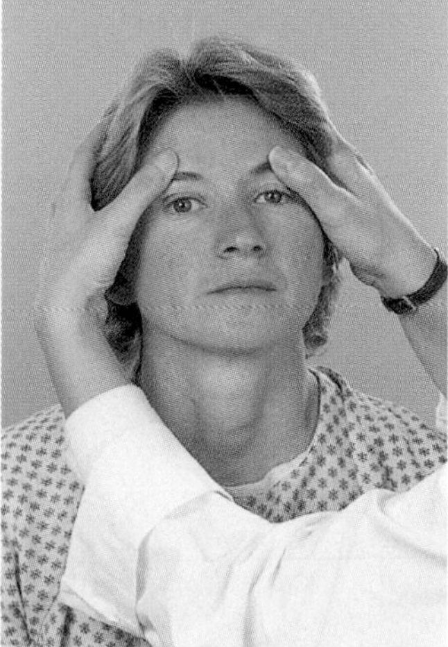

FIGURE 19•7 Technique for palpating the frontal sinuses at left and the maxillary sinuses at right. From Weber, J. & Kelley, J. (1998). *Health assessment in nursing*. Philadelphia: Lippincott-Raven.

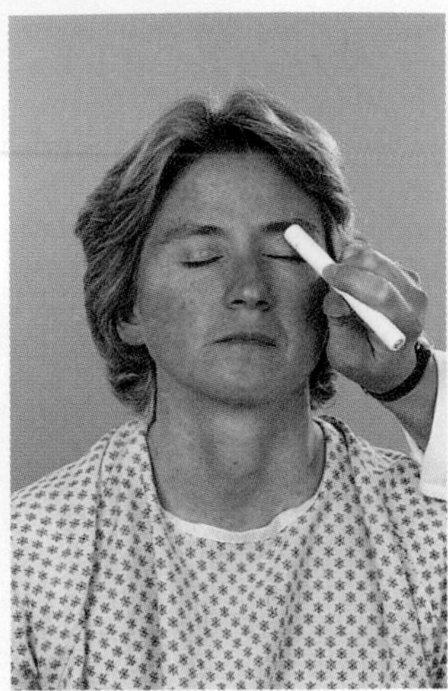

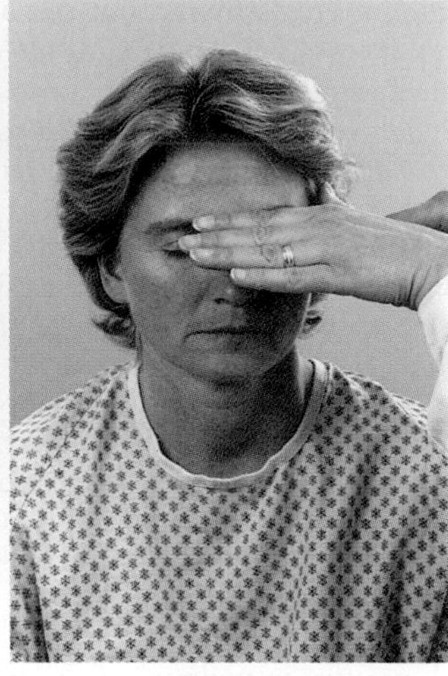

FIGURE 19•8 At left, the nurse positions the light source for transillumination of the frontal sinus. At right, the nurse shields the patient's brow and shines the light. In normal conditions (a darkened room), the light should shine through the tissues and appear as a reddish glow (above the nurse's hand) over the sinus. From Weber, J. & Kelley, J. (1998). *Health assessment in nursing.* Philadelphia: Lippincott-Raven.

nal notch. The trachea is highly sensitive, and palpating too firmly may trigger a coughing or gagging response. The trachea is normally in the midline as it enters the thoracic inlet behind the sternum, but it may be deviated by masses in the neck or mediastinum. Pleural or pulmonary disorders, such as a pneumothorax, may also displace the trachea.

Physical Assessment of the Lower Respiratory Structures and Breathing

Thorax

Inspection of the thorax provides information about the musculoskeletal structure, the patient's nutritional status, and the respiratory system. The nurse observes the skin over the thorax for color and turgor and for evidence of loss of subcutaneous tissue. It is important to note asymmetry, if present. When findings are recorded or reported, anatomic landmarks are used as points of reference (Chart 19-5).

CHEST CONFIGURATION

Normally, the ratio of the anteroposterior diameter to the lateral diameter is 1 : 2. However, there are four main deformities of the chest associated with respiratory disease that alter this relationship: barrel chest, funnel chest (pectus excavatum), pigeon chest (pectus carinatum), and kyphoscoliosis.

Barrel Chest. Barrel chest occurs as a result of overinflation of the lungs. There is an increase in the anteroposterior diameter of the thorax. In a patient with emphysema, the ribs are more widely spaced and the intercostal spaces tend to bulge on expiration. The appearance of the patient with advanced emphysema is thus quite characteristic and often allows the observer to detect its presence easily, even from a distance.

Funnel Chest (Pectus Excavatum). Funnel chest occurs when there is a depression in the lower portion of the sternum. This may compress the heart and great vessels, resulting in murmurs. Funnel chest may occur with rickets or Marfan's syndrome.

Pigeon Chest (Pectus Carinatum). A pigeon chest occurs as a result of displacement of the sternum. There is an increase in the anteroposterior diameter. This may occur with rickets, Marfan's syndrome, or severe kyphoscoliosis.

Kyphoscoliosis. A kyphoscoliosis is characterized by elevation of the scapula and a corresponding S-shaped spine. This deformity limits lung expansion within the thorax. It may occur with osteoporosis and other skeletal disorders that affect the thorax.

BREATHING PATTERNS AND RESPIRATORY RATES

Observing the rate and depth of respiration is a simple but important aspect of assessment. The normal adult who is resting comfortably breathes at 12 to 18 breaths per minute. Except for occasional sighs, respirations are regular in depth and rhythm.

Bradypnea, also called slow breathing, is associated with increased intracranial pressure, brain injury, and drug overdose.

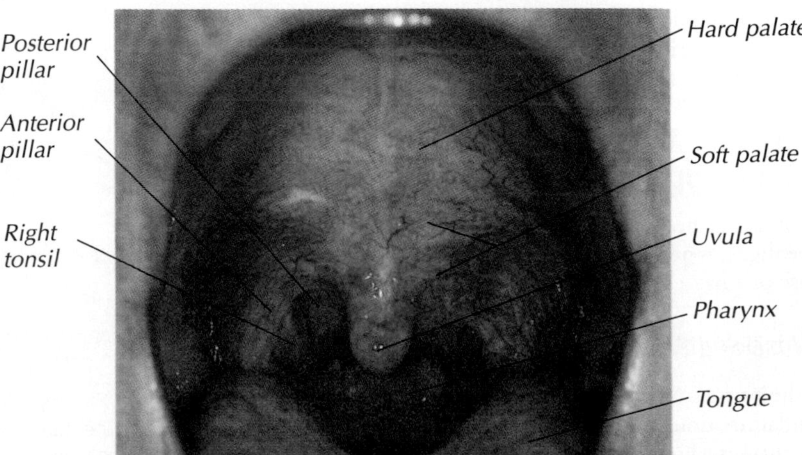

FIGURE 19•9 The pharynx and other oral structures—pillars, tonsils, uvula, hard and soft palates, posterior pharynx, and tongue—are easily seen when the mouth is open.

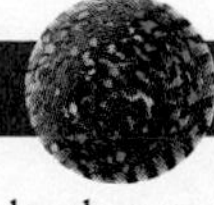

CHART 19•5 Locating Thoracic Landmarks

With respect to the thorax, location is defined both horizontally and vertically. With respect to the lungs, location is defined by lobe.

Horizontal Reference Points

Horizontally, thoracic locations are identified according to their proximity to the rib or the intercostal space under the examiner's fingers. On the anterior surface, identification of a specific rib is facilitated by first locating the angle of Louis. This is where the manubrium joins the body of the sternum in the midline. The second rib joins the sternum at this prominent landmark.

Other ribs may be identified by counting down from the second rib. The intercostal spaces are referred to in terms of the rib immediately above the intercostal space; for example, the fifth intercostal space is directly below the fifth rib.

Locating ribs on the posterior surface of the thorax is more difficult. The first step is to identify the spinous process. This is accomplished by finding the seventh cervical vertebra (*vertebra prominens*), which is the most prominent spinous process. When the neck is slightly flexed, the seventh cervical spinous process stands out. Other vertebrae are then identified by counting downward.

Vertical Reference Points

Several imaginary lines are used as vertical referents or landmarks to identify the location of thoracic findings. The *midsternal line* passes through the center of the sternum. The *midclavicular line* is an imaginary line that descends from the middle of the clavicle. The *point of maximal impulse* of the heart normally lies along this line on the left thorax.

When the arm is abducted from the body at 90°, imaginary vertical lines may be drawn from the anterior axillary fold, from the middle of the axilla, and from the posterior axillary fold. These lines are called, respectively, the *anterior axillary line,* the *midaxillary line,* and the *posterior axillary line.* A line drawn vertically through the superior and inferior poles of the scapula is called the *scapular line,* and a line drawn down the center of the vertebral column is called the *vertebral line.* Using these landmarks, for example, the examiner communicates findings by referring to an area of dullness extending from the vertebral to the scapular line between the seventh and tenth ribs on the right.

Lobes of the Lungs

The lobes of the lung may be mapped on the surface of the chest wall in the following manner. The line between the upper and lower lobes on the left begins at the fourth thoracic spinous process posteriorly, proceeds around to cross the fifth rib in the midaxillary line, and meets the sixth rib at the sternum. This line on the right divides the right middle lobe from the right lower lobe. The line dividing the right upper lobe from the middle lobe is an incomplete one that begins at the fifth rib in the midaxillary line, where it intersects the line between the upper and lower lobes and traverses horizontally to the sternum. Thus, the upper lobes are dominant on the anterior surface of the thorax and the lower lobes are dominant on the posterior surface. There is no presentation of the middle lobe on the posterior surface of the chest.

Anterior thorax
Clavicle
Suprasternal notch
First rib
First intercostal space
Angle of Louis
Manubrium
Xiphoid process
Costal angle
Costal margin
Midclavicular lines

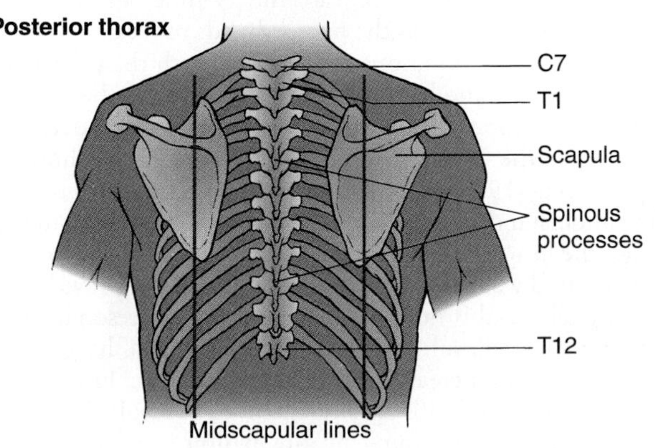

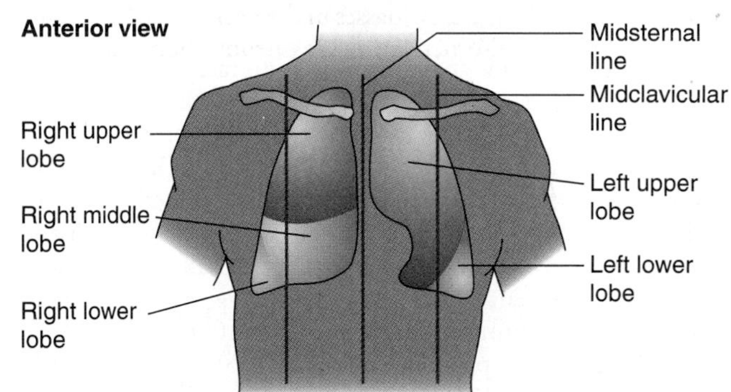

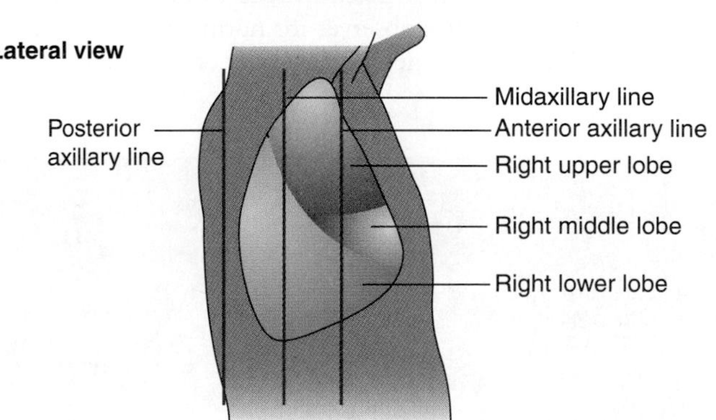

Tachypnea, or rapid breathing, is commonly seen in patients with pneumonia, pulmonary edema, metabolic acidosis, septicemia, severe pain, and rib fracture.

Accessory chest muscles are not normally used. An increase in depth is called hyperpnea. An increase in both rate and depth that results in a lowered arterial PCO_2 level is referred to as hyperventilation. With rapid breathing, inspiration and expiration are nearly equal in deviation. Hyperventilation that is marked by an increase in rate and depth, associated with severe acidosis of diabetic or renal origin, is called Kussmaul's respiration.

Cheyne-Stokes respiration is characterized by alternating episodes of apnea (cessation of breathing) and periods of deep breathing. It usually is associated with heart failure and damage to the respiratory center (drug-induced, tumor, trauma). The rate and depth of different patterns of respiration are presented in Figure 19-10.

In thin people, it is quite normal to note a slight retraction of the intercostal spaces during quiet breathing. Bulging during expiration implies obstruction of expiratory air flow, as in emphysema. Marked retraction on inspiration, particularly if asymmetric, implies blockage of a branch of the respiratory tree. Asymmetric bulging of the intercostal spaces, on one side or the other, is created by an increase in pressure within the hemithorax. This may be a result of air trapped under pressure within the pleural cavity where it does not normally appear (pneumothorax) or the pressure of fluid within the pleural space (pleural effusion).

Certain patterns of respiration are characteristic of specific disease states. Respiratory rhythms and their deviation from normal are important observations that the nurse reports and documents.

Thoracic Palpation

The nurse palpates the thorax for tenderness, masses, lesions, respiratory excursion, and vocal fremitus. If the patient has reported an area of pain or if lesions are apparent, the nurse performs direct palpation with the fingertips (for skin lesions and subcutaneous masses) or with the ball of the hand (for deeper masses or generalized flank or rib discomfort).

RESPIRATORY EXCURSION

Respiratory excursion is an estimation of thoracic expansion and may disclose significant information about thoracic movement during breathing. The nurse assesses the patient for range and symmetry of excursion. The patient is instructed to inhale deeply while the movement of the nurse's thumbs (placed along the costal margin on the anterior chest wall) during inspiration and expiration is observed. This movement is normally symmetric.

Posterior assessment is performed by placing the thumbs adjacent to the spinal column at the level of the tenth rib (Fig. 19-11). The hands lightly grasp the lateral rib cage. Sliding the thumbs medially about 2.5 cm (1 inch) raises a small skinfold between the thumbs. The patient is instructed to take a full inspiration and to exhale fully. The nurse observes for normal flattening of the skinfold and feels the symmetric movement of the thorax.

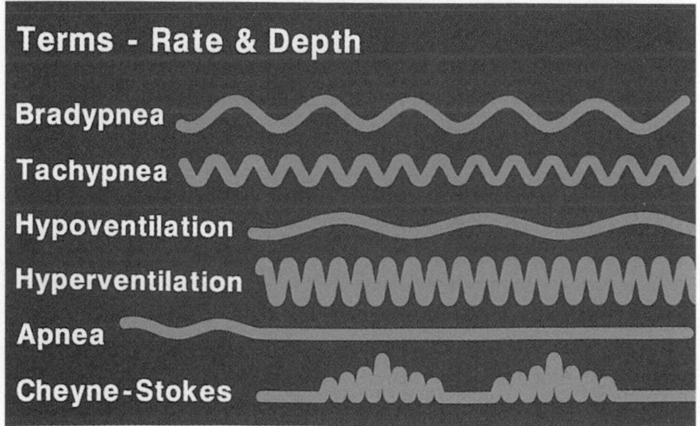

FIGURE 19•10 Graphic representation of different rates and depths of respiration.

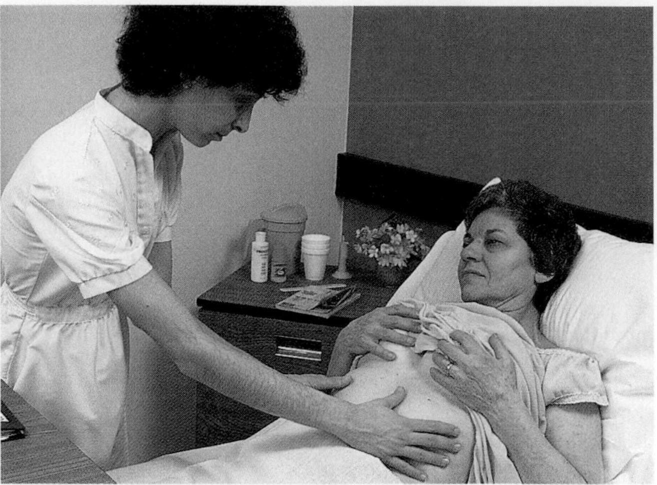

FIGURE 19•11 Method for assessing respiratory excursion. The nurse places both hands posteriorly along the rib cage at the tenth rib.

Decreased chest excursion may be due to chronic fibrotic disease. Asymmetric excursion may be due to splinting secondary to pleurisy, fractured ribs, trauma, or unilateral bronchial obstruction.

TACTILE FREMITUS

Sound generated by the larynx travels distally along the bronchial tree to set the chest wall in resonant motion. This is especially true of consonant sounds. The detection of the resulting vibration on the chest wall by touch is called tactile fremitus.

Normal fremitus is widely varied. It is influenced by the thickness of the chest wall, especially if that thickness is muscular. However, the increase in subcutaneous tissue associated with obesity may also affect fremitus. Lower-pitched sounds travel better through the normal lung and produce greater vibration of the chest wall. Thus, fremitus is more pronounced in men than in women because of the deeper male voice. Normally, fremitus is most pronounced where the large bronchi are closest to the chest wall and least palpable over the distant lung fields. Therefore, it is most palpable in the upper thorax, anteriorly and posteriorly.

The patient is asked to repeat "ninety-nine" or "one, two, three," or "eee, eee, eee" as the nurse's hands move down the patient's thorax. The vibrations are detected with the palmar surfaces of the fingers and hands, or the ulnar aspect of the extended hands, on the thorax. One hand is used as the nurse moves in sequence down the thorax. Corresponding areas of the thorax are compared (Fig. 19-12). Bony areas are not tested.

An understanding of the physics of sound transmission through the lungs aids in interpreting the findings. Air does not conduct sound well; a solid substance (tissue) does, provided that it has elasticity and is not compressed into a nonresonant mass. Thus, an increase in solid tissue per unit volume of lung will enhance fremitus; an increase in air per unit volume of lung will impede sound. Patients with emphysema, which results in the rupture of alveoli and trapping of air, exhibit almost no tactile fremitus. A patient with consolidation of a lobe of the lung from pneumonia will have increased tactile fremitus over that lobe. Air in the pleural space will not conduct sound.

Thoracic Percussion

Percussion sets the chest wall and underlying structures in motion, producing audible and tactile vibrations. The nurse uses percussion

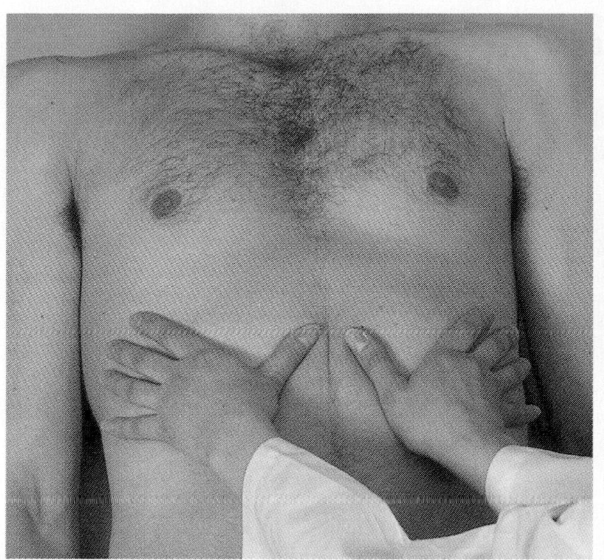

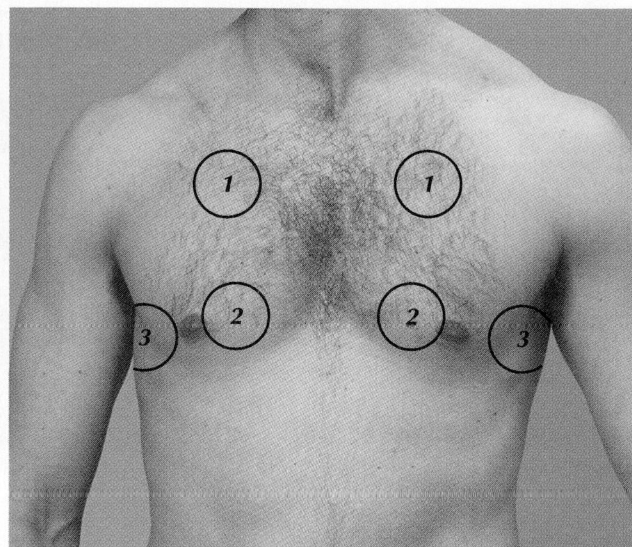

FIGURE 19•12 When palpating for tactile fremitus (*left*), the nurse places the ball or ulnar surface of the hands on the chest area being assessed. The palpation sequence is at right. From Bickley L. S. & Hoekelman, R. A. (1999). *Bates' guide to physical examination and history taking* (7th ed.). Philadelphia: Lippincott Williams & Wilkins.

to determine whether underlying tissues are filled with air, fluid, or solid material. Percussion also is used to estimate the size and location of certain structures within the thorax (eg, diaphragm, heart, liver).

Percussion usually begins with the posterior thorax. Ideally, the patient is in a sitting position with the head flexed forward and the arms crossed on the lap. This position separates the scapulae widely and exposes more lung area for assessment. The nurse percusses across each shoulder top, locating the 5-cm width of resonance overlying the lung apices (Fig. 19-13). Then the nurse proceeds down the posterior thorax, percussing symmetric areas at 5- to 6-cm (2- to 2.5-inch) intervals. The middle finger is positioned parallel to the ribs in the intercostal space; the finger is placed firmly against the chest wall before striking it with the middle finger of the opposite hand. Bony structures (scapulae or ribs) are not percussed.

Percussion over the anterior chest is performed with the patient in an upright position with shoulders arched backward and arms at the side. The nurse begins in the supraclavicular area and proceeds downward, from one intercostal space to the next. In the female patient, it may be necessary to displace the breasts for an adequate examination. Dullness noted to the left of the sternum between the third and fifth intercostal spaces is a normal finding because it is the location of the heart. Similarly, there is a normal span of liver dullness in the right thorax from the fifth intercostal space to the right costal margin at the midclavicular line.

The anterior and lateral thorax is examined with the patient in a supine position. If the patient cannot sit up, percussion of the posterior thorax is performed with the patient positioned on the side.

Dullness over the lung occurs when air-filled lung tissue is replaced by fluid or solid tissue. Examples include lobar pneumonia, in which consolidation results from accumulation of fluid, blood, fibrous tissue, and cells, or a tumor in the pleural space. Pneumothorax produces a tympanic or drumlike sound, whereas emphysema produces hyperresonance. Table 19-2 reviews percussion sounds and their characteristics.

DIAPHRAGMATIC EXCURSION

The normal resonance of the lung stops at the diaphragm. The position of the diaphragm is different during inspiration than during expiration.

To assess position and motion of the diaphragm, the nurse instructs the patient to take a deep breath and hold it while the

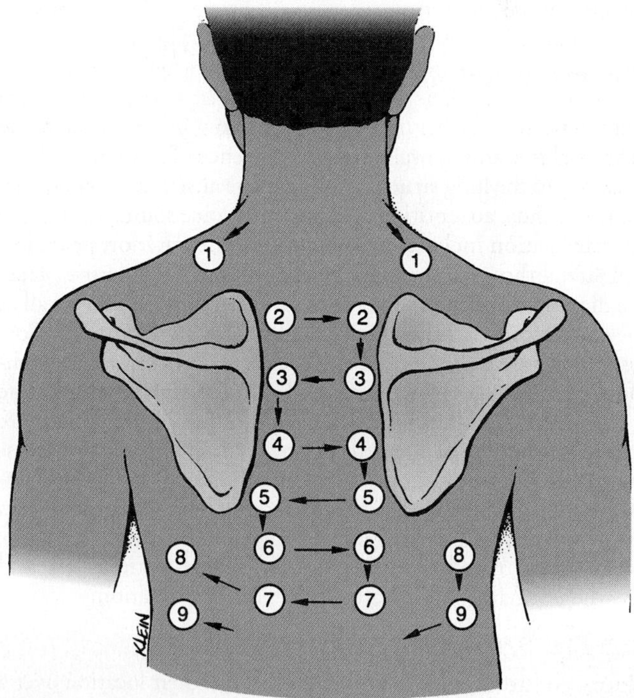

FIGURE 19•13 Percussion of the posterior thorax. With the patient in a sitting position, symmetric areas of the lungs are percussed at 5-cm intervals. This progression starts at the apex of each lung and concludes with percussion of each lateral chest wall.

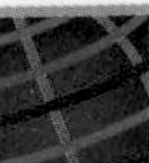

TABLE 19•2 **Characteristics of Percussion Sounds**

Sound	Relative Intensity	Relative Pitch	Relative Duration	Location Example	Examples
Flatness	Soft	High	Short	Thigh	Large pleural effusion
Dullness	Medium	Medium	Medium	Liver	Lobar pneumonia
Resonance	Loud	Low	Long	Normal lung	Simple chronic bronchitis
Hyperresonance	Very loud	Lower	Longer	None normally	Emphysema, pneumothorax
Tympany	Loud	High*	*	Gastric air bubble or puffed-out cheek	Large pneumothorax

*Distinguished mainly by its musical timbre

maximal descent of the diaphragm is percussed. The point at which the percussion note at the midscapular line changes from resonance to dullness is marked with a pen. The patient is then instructed to exhale fully and hold it while the nurse again percusses downward to the dullness of the diaphragm. This point is also marked. The distance between the two markings indicates the range of motion of the diaphragm.

Maximal excursion of the diaphragm may be as much as 8 to 10 cm (3 to 4 inches) in healthy, tall young men, but for most people it is usually 5 to 7 cm (2 to 2.75 inches). Normally, the diaphragm is 2 cm (0.75 inches) or so higher on the right because of the position of the heart and the liver above and below the left and right segments of the diaphragm, respectively. Decreased diaphragmatic excursion may occur with pleural effusion and emphysema. An increase in intra-abdominal pressure, as in pregnancy or ascites, may account for a diaphragm that is positioned high in the thorax.

Thoracic Auscultation

Auscultation is useful in assessing the flow of air through the bronchial tree and in evaluating the presence of fluid or solid obstruction in the lung structures. The nurse auscultates for normal breath sounds, adventitious sounds, and voice sounds.

Examination includes auscultation of the anterior, posterior, and lateral thorax and is performed as follows. The nurse places the diaphragm of the stethoscope firmly against the chest wall as the patient breathes slowly and deeply through the mouth. Corresponding areas of the chest are auscultated in a systematic fashion from the apices to the bases and along midaxillary lines. The sequence of auscultation and the positioning of the patient are similar to those used for percussion. It often is necessary to listen to two full inspirations and expirations at each anatomic location for valid interpretation of the sound heard. Repeated deep breaths may result in symptoms of hyperventilation (eg, lightheadedness); this is avoided by having the patient rest and breathe normally periodically during the examination.

BREATH SOUNDS

Normal breath sounds are distinguished by their location over a specific area of the lung and are identified as vesicular, bronchial (tubular), and bronchovesicular breath sounds (Table 19-3).

Vesicular sounds are quiet, low-pitched sounds with a long inspiratory phase and a short expiratory phase. They are heard normally throughout the entire lung field, except over the upper sternum and between the scapulae. Bronchial sounds are usually louder and higher-pitched than vesicular sounds. In comparison, the expiratory phase is longer than the inspiratory phase. Bronchial sounds are heard over the trachea. Bronchovesicular sounds are heard over the main bronchus; specifically, they can be heard between the scapulae and on either side of the sternum. Bronchovesicular breath sounds are medium in pitch; the inspiratory and expiratory phases are equal. Bronchial and bronchovesicular sounds that are audible elsewhere in the lungs signify pathology, usually indicating consolidation in the lung (eg, pneumonia, heart failure). They necessitate further evaluation.

The quality and intensity of breath sounds are determined during auscultation. When air flow is decreased by bronchial obstruction (atelectasis) or when fluid (pleural effusion) or tissue (obesity) separates the air passages from the stethoscope, breath sounds are diminished or absent. For example, the breath sounds of the patient with emphysema are faint or often completely inaudible. When heard, the expiratory phase is prolonged and may exhibit a high-pitched whistling tone called wheezing. This same sound is also heard in asthma and in any process associated with marked bronchoconstriction.

ADVENTITIOUS SOUNDS

An abnormal condition that affects the bronchial tree and alveoli may produce adventitious (additional) sounds. Adventitious sounds are divided into two categories: discrete, noncontinuous sounds (**crackles**) and continuous musical sounds (wheezes). The duration of the sound is the important distinction to make in identifying the sound as noncontinuous or continuous. Pleural friction rubs are specific examples of crackles (Table 19-4).

Crackles (formerly referred to as rales) are discrete, noncontinuous sounds that result from delayed reopening of deflated airways. Fine crackles, usually audible at the end of inspiration and originating from the alveoli, typically are heard in patients with interstitial pneumonia or fibrosis. Their sound can be recreated by rubbing several strands of hair together next to one's ear. Coarse crackles have a harsh, moist sound. They are produced in the large bronchi and are audible in early to mid-inspiration. Crackles may or may not be cleared by coughing. Crackles reflect underlying inflammation or congestion and are often present in such conditions as pneumonia, bronchitis, congestive heart failure, bronchiectasis, and pulmonary fibrosis.

Wheezes are associated with bronchial wall oscillation and changes in airway diameter. **Sibilant wheezes** (formerly called wheezes) are continuous musical sounds that are longer in dura-

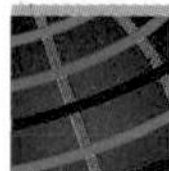

TABLE 19•3 **Breath Sounds**

	Duration of Sounds	Intensity of Expiratory Sound	Pitch of Expiratory Sound	Locations Where Heard Normally
Vesicular*	Inspiratory sounds last longer than expiratory ones.	Soft	Relatively low	Over most of both lungs
Broncho-vesicular	Inspiratory and expiratory sounds are about equal.	Intermediate	Intermediate	Often in the 1st and 2nd interspaces anteriorly and between the scapulae
Bronchial	Expiratory sounds last longer than inspiratory ones.	Loud	Relatively high	Over the manubrium, if heard at all
Tracheal	Inspiratory and expiratory sounds are about equal.	Very loud	Relatively high	Over the trachea in the neck

*The thickness of the bars indicates intensity; the steeper their incline, the higher the pitch.

tion than crackles. They may be audible during inspiration, expiration, or both. These sounds result from air passing through narrowed or partially obstructed passages. Obstruction is often due to the presence of secretions or edema, and wheezes may clear with coughing. Wheezes originate in the smaller bronchi and bronchioles; they are high-pitched and whistling. **Sonorous wheezes** (formally called rhonchi) originate in the larger bronchi or trachea and are lower-pitched and sonorous. They are heard in patients with increased secretions. Wheezes are commonly heard in patients with asthma, chronic bronchitis, and bronchiectasis.

Friction rubs result from inflammation of the pleural surfaces that induces a crackling, grating sound usually heard in inspiration and expiration. It sounds quite close to the ear and is enhanced by applying pressure to the chest wall with the head of the stethoscope. The sound is imitated by rubbing the thumb and index finger together near the ear. The grating sound of a friction rub is not altered by coughing. If audible only during inspiration, it may be difficult to distinguish from crackles, which may be multiple and so frequent that a continuous sound is perceived. A friction rub is best heard over the lower lateral anterior surface of the thorax.

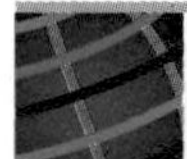

TABLE 19•4 **Abnormal (Adventitious) Breath Sounds**

Breath Sound	Description	Etiology
Crackles (rales)		
Crackles in general	Soft, high-pitched, discontinuous popping sounds that occur during inspiration	Secondary to fluid in the airways or alveoli or to opening of collapsed alveoli
Crackles in early inspiration	Same as above	Associated with obstructive pulmonary disease; fine crackles in early inspiration are associated with bronchitis or pneumonia.
Crackles in late inspiration	Same as above	Associated with restrictive pulmonary disease
Wheezes		
Sonorous wheezes (rhonchi)	Deep, low-pitched rumbling sounds heard primarily during expiration	Caused by air moving through narrowed tracheobronchial passages (narrowing may result from secretion or tumor)
Sibilant wheezes	Continuous, musical, high-pitched, whistle-like sounds heard during inspiration and expiration	Caused by narrow bronchioles and associated with bronchospasm, asthma, and buildup of secretions
Friction rubs		
Pleural friction rub	Harsh, crackling sound, like two pieces of leather being rubbed together Heard during inspiration alone or during both inspiration and expiration May subside when patient holds breath	Secondary to inflammation and loss of lubricating pleural fluid

TABLE 19•5 Assessment Findings in Common Respiratory Problems

Problem	Tactile Fremitus	Percussion	Auscultation
Consolidation (eg, pneumonia)	Increased	Dull	Bronchial breath sounds, crackles, bronchophony, egophony, whispered pectoriloquy
Bronchitis	Normal	Resonant	Normal to decreased breath sounds, wheezes
Emphysema	Decreased	Hyperresonant	Decreased intensity of breath sounds, usually with prolonged expiration
Asthma (severe attack)	Normal to decreased	Resonant to hyperresonant	Wheezes
Pulmonary edema	Normal	Resonant	Crackles at lung bases, possibly wheezes
Pleural effusion	Absent	Dull to flat	Decreased to absent breath sounds, bronchial breath sounds and bronchophony, egophony, and whispered pectoriloquy above the effusion over the area of compressed lung
Pneumothorax	Decreased	Hyperresonant	Absent breath sounds
Atelectasis	Absent	Flat	Decreased to absent breath sounds

VOICE SOUNDS

The sound heard through the stethoscope as the patient speaks is known as vocal resonance. The vibrations produced in the larynx are transmitted to the chest wall as they pass through the bronchi and alveolar tissue. During the process, the sounds are diminished in intensity and altered so that syllables are not distinguishable. Voice sounds are usually assessed by having the patient repeat "ninety-nine" or "eee" while the nurse listens with the stethoscope in corresponding areas of the chest from the apices to the bases.

Bronchophony describes vocal resonance that is more intense and clearer than normal. Egophony; describes voice sounds that are distorted. It is best appreciated by having the patient repeat the letter *E*. The distortion produced by consolidation transforms the sound into a clearly heard *A* rather than *E*. Bronchophony and egophony have precisely the same significance as bronchial breathing with an increase in tactile fremitus. When an abnormality is detected, it should be evident in more than one assessment method. A change in tactile fremitus is more subtle and can be missed, but bronchial breathing and bronchophony can be noted loudly and clearly.

Whispered pectoriloquy is a very subtle finding, heard only in the presence of rather dense consolidation of the lungs. Transmission of high-frequency components of sound is so enhanced by the consolidated tissue that even whispered words are heard, a circumstance not noted in normal physiology. The significance is the same as that of bronchophony.

The physical findings for the most common respiratory diseases are summarized in Table 19-5.

Physical Assessment of Breathing Ability

Tests of the patient's breathing ability are easily performed at the bedside by measuring the respiratory rate (see the section "Breathing Patterns and Respiratory Rates"), tidal volume, minute ventilation, vital capacity, inspiratory force, and compliance. These tests are particularly important for patients at risk for developing pulmonary complications, including those who have undergone chest or abdominal surgery, have had prolonged anesthesia, have preexisting pulmonary disease, or are elderly.

Patients whose chest expansion is limited by external restrictions such as obesity or abdominal distention and who cannot breathe deeply because of postoperative pain or sedation will inhale and exhale a low volume of air (referred to as low tidal volumes). Prolonged hypoventilation at low tidal volumes can produce alveolar collapse or atelectasis. The amount of air remaining in the lungs after a normal expiration (functional residual capacity) falls, the ability of the lungs to expand (compliance) is reduced, and the patient must breathe faster to maintain the same degree of tissue oxygenation. These events can be exaggerated in patients who have preexisting pulmonary diseases and in elderly patients whose airways are less compliant, because the small airways may collapse during expiration.

Nursing Alert *One should not rely only on visual inspection of the rate and depth of a patient's respiratory excursions to determine the adequacy of ventilation. Respiratory excursions may appear normal or exaggerated due to an increased work of breathing, but the patient may actually be moving only enough air to ventilate the dead space. If there is any question regarding adequacy of ventilation, auscultation and/or pulse oximetry should be used for additional assessment of respiratory status.*

Tidal Volume

The volume of each breath is referred to as the tidal volume (see Table 19-1 to review lung capacities and volumes). A spirometer is an instrument that can be used at the bedside to measure volumes. If the patient is breathing through an endotracheal tube or tracheostomy, the spirometer is directly attached to it and the exhaled volume is obtained from the reading on the gauge. In other patients, the spirometer is attached to a face mask or a mouthpiece positioned so that it is airtight, and the exhaled volume is measured.

The tidal volume may vary from breath to breath. To make the measurement reliable, it is important to measure the volumes of several breaths and to note the range of tidal volumes, together with the average tidal volume.

Minute Ventilation

Respiratory rates and tidal volume alone are unreliable indicators of adequate ventilation because both can vary widely from breath to breath. Together, however, the tidal volume and respiratory rate are important because the minute ventilation, which is useful in detecting respiratory failure, can be determined from them. Minute ventilation is the volume of air expired per minute. It is equal to the product of the tidal volume and the respiratory rate or frequency. In practice, the minute ventilation is not calculated but is measured directly using a spirometer.

Minute ventilation may be decreased by a variety of conditions that result in hypoventilation. When the minute ventilation falls, alveolar ventilation in the lungs also decreases, and the $PaCO_2$ increases. Risk factors for hypoventilation are listed in the risk factors chart.

Vital Capacity

Vital capacity is measured by having the patient take in a maximal breath and exhale fully through a spirometer. The normal value depends on the patient's age, sex, body build, and weight.

Nursing Alert *Most patients can generate a vital capacity twice the volume they normally breathe in and out (tidal volume). If the vital capacity is less than 10 mL/kg, the patient will be unable to sustain spontaneous ventilation and will require respiratory assistance.*

When the vital capacity is exhaled at a maximal flow rate, the forced vital capacity is measured. Most patients can exhale at least 80% of their vital capacity in 1 second (forced expiratory volume in 1 second, or FEV_1) and almost all of it in 3 seconds (FEV_3). A reduction in FEV_1 suggests abnormal pulmonary air flow. If the patient's FEV_1 and forced vital capacity are proportionately reduced, maximal lung expansion is restricted in some way. If the reduction in FEV_1 greatly exceeds the reduction in forced vital capacity, the patient may have some degree of airway obstruction.

Patients with respiratory disorders may be taught how to measure their peak flow rate (reflects maximal expiratory flow) at home using a spirometer. This allows them to monitor the progress of therapy, to alter medications and other interventions as needed based on caregiver guidelines, or to notify the health care provider if there is inadequate response to their own interventions. Home care teaching instructions are listed in the accompanying Home Care Teaching Checklist.

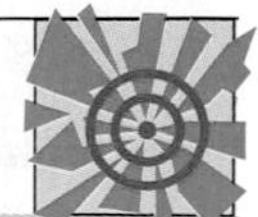

Risk Factors for HYPOVENTILATION

- Limited neurologic impulses transmitted from the brain to the respiratory muscles, as in spinal cord trauma, cerebrovascular accidents, tumors, myasthenia gravis, Guillain-Barré syndrome, polio, and drug overdose
- Depressed respiratory centers in the medulla, as with anesthesia and drug overdose
- Limited thoracic movement (kyphoscoliosis), limited lung movement (pleural effusion, pneumothorax), or reduced functional lung tissue (chronic pulmonary diseases, severe pulmonary edema)

Inspiratory Force

Inspiratory force evaluates the effort the patient is making during inspiration. It does not require patient cooperation and thus is useful in the unconscious patient. The equipment needed for this measurement includes a manometer that measures negative pressure and adapters that are connected to an anesthesia mask or a cuffed endotracheal tube. The manometer is attached and the airway is completely occluded for 10 to 20 seconds while the inspiratory efforts of the patient are registered on the manometer. The normal inspiratory pressure is about 100 cm H_2O. If the negative pressure registered after 15 seconds of occluding the airway is less than about 25 cm H_2O, mechanical ventilation is usually required because the patient lacks sufficient muscle strength for deep breathing or effective coughing.

DIAGNOSTIC EVALUATION

A wide range of diagnostic studies, described on the following pages, may be performed in patients with respiratory conditions. Some of these tests require a few seconds or minutes to complete; others are invasive procedures that require extensive patient preparation and the use of local anesthetics.

HOME CARE TEACHING CHECKLIST: PEAK FLOW MONITORING

At the completion of the program, the patient or caregiver will be able to:	Patient	Caregiver
• Define what peak flow measures and its importance: Peak flow measures how effectively air flows out of the lungs. It allows detection of early changes and monitors trends over time.	✔	✔
• Describe what values or trends require health care intervention: Large drop in value accompanied by other symptoms. Consistent decrease in number over several days.	✔	✔
• Demonstrate correct technique for obtaining measurement: Place the indicator at the base of the measured scale. Sit upright or stand. Take a deep breath. Place meter in mouth and close lips around the mouthpiece. Blow out as hard and fast as possible. Write down number that you get. Repeat measurement and recording at least two more times. Repeat if there is a large variation (>.75 mL/m) in values. Write the highest value in your diary. Clean your peak flow meter after each use.	✔	

Cultures

Throat cultures may be performed to identify organisms responsible for pharyngitis. Throat culture may also assist in identifying organisms responsible for infection of the lower respiratory tract. Nasal swabs also may be performed for the same purpose.

Sputum Studies

Sputum is obtained for study to identify pathogenic organisms and to determine whether malignant cells are present. It also may be used to assess for hypersensitivity states (in which there is an increase in eosinophils). Periodic sputum examinations may be necessary for patients receiving antibiotics, corticosteroids, and immunosuppressive medications for prolonged periods because these agents are associated with opportunistic infections. In general, sputum cultures are used in diagnosis, for drug sensitivity testing, and as a guide in treatment.

Expectoration is the usual method for collecting a sputum specimen. The patient is instructed to clear the nose and throat and rinse the mouth to decrease contamination of the sputum. After taking a few deep breaths, the patient coughs (rather than spits), using the diaphragm, and expectorates into a sterile container.

If the sputum cannot be raised spontaneously, the patient often can be induced to cough deeply by breathing an irritating aerosol of supersaturated saline, propylene glycol, or some other agent delivered with an ultrasonic nebulizer. Other methods of collecting sputum specimens include endotracheal aspiration, bronchoscopic removal, bronchial brushing, transtracheal aspiration, and gastric aspiration—usually for tuberculosis organisms (see Chap. 21). Generally, the deepest specimens (those from the base of the lungs) are obtained in the early morning after they have accumulated overnight.

The specimen is delivered to the laboratory within 2 hours by the patient or nurse. Allowing the specimen to stand for several hours in a warm room results in the overgrowth of contaminant organisms and may make it difficult to identify the organisms (especially *Mycobacterium tuberculosis*). The home care nurse may assist patients who need help obtaining the sample or who cannot deliver the specimen to the laboratory in a timely fashion.

Qualitative studies are often performed to determine if the secretions are saliva, mucus, or infectious material. A yellow-green color of the material expectorated usually implies infection (ie, pneumonia). This specimen may be cultured to identify organisms.

Nursing Interventions

For quantitative studies, the patient is given a special container in which to expectorate. The purpose of the study, the importance of collecting all sputum in the container, and safe handling of the container are explained. The container is weighed at the end of 24 hours and the amount and the character of the contents are recorded. Such a specimen is treated as biohazardous material and disposed of appropriately. To prevent odors, it is important to cover all sputum containers. The nurse reminds family members and caregivers to remove and discard soiled tissues promptly, to provide adequate room ventilation, and to practice frequent oral hygiene.

Pulmonary Function Tests

Pulmonary function tests are performed to assess respiratory function and to determine the extent of dysfunction. Such tests include measurements of lung volumes, ventilatory function, and the mechanics of breathing, diffusion, and gas exchange.

Pulmonary function tests are useful in following the course of a patient with an established respiratory disease and assessing the response to therapy. They are useful as screening tests in potentially hazardous industries, such as coal mining and those that involve exposure to asbestos and other noxious fumes, dusts, or gases. They are useful for patients scheduled for thoracic and upper abdominal surgery, patients with a history of smoking and cough, obese patients, older patients, and patients with pulmonary disease.

Pulmonary function tests generally are performed by a technician using a spirometer that has a volume collecting device attached to a recorder that demonstrates volume and time simultaneously. A number of tests are carried out because no single measurement provides a complete picture of pulmonary function. The most frequently used pulmonary function tests are described in Table 19-6.

Test results are interpreted on the basis of degree of deviation from normal, taking into consideration the patient's height, weight, age, and gender. For instance, vital capacity decreases about 25% in the elderly, while functional residual capacity increases. Because there is a wide range of normal values, pulmonary function tests may not detect early localized changes. The patient with respiratory symptoms (dyspnea, wheezing, cough, sputum production) usually undergoes a complete diagnostic evaluation, even though the results of pulmonary function tests are "normal." Trends of results provide feedback regarding disease progression as well as response to therapy.

Arterial Blood Gas Studies

Measurements of blood pH and of arterial oxygen and carbon dioxide tensions are obtained when managing patients with respiratory problems and in adjusting oxygen therapy as needed. The arterial oxygen tension (PaO_2) indicates the degree of oxygenation of the blood, and the arterial carbon dioxide tension ($PaCO_2$) indicates the adequacy of alveolar ventilation. Arterial blood gas studies aid in assessing the ability of the lungs to provide adequate oxygen and remove carbon dioxide and the ability of the kidneys to reabsorb or excrete bicarbonate ions to maintain normal body pH. Serial blood gas analysis also is a sensitive indicator of whether the lung has been damaged after chest trauma. Arterial blood gas levels are obtained through an arterial puncture at the radial, brachial, or femoral artery or through an indwelling arterial catheter. Arterial blood gas levels are discussed in detail in Chapter 13.

Pulse Oximetry

Pulse oximetry is a noninvasive method of continuously monitoring the oxygen saturation of hemoglobin (SaO_2). Although pulse oximetry does not replace arterial blood gas measurement, it is an effective tool to monitor for subtle or sudden changes in oxygen saturation. It is used in a variety of settings, including critical care units, the operating room, the postanesthesia care unit, general nursing units, and diagnostic and treatment areas when there is a need to monitor the patient's oxygen saturation during procedures; it is also used in the home care setting.

A disposable probe or sensor is attached to the fingertip (Fig. 19-14), forehead, earlobe, or bridge of the nose. A sensor detects changes in oxygen saturation levels by monitoring light signals generated by the oximeter and reflected by blood pulsing through the tissue at the probe. Normal SaO_2 values are 95% to 100%. Values less than 85% indicate that the tissues are not receiving enough oxygen, and the patient needs further evaluation. SaO_2 values obtained by pulse oximetry are unreliable in cardiac arrest and shock, when dyes (ie, methylene blue) or vasoconstrictor medications have been used, or when the patient has severe anemia or a high carbon monoxide level.

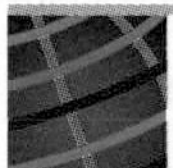

TABLE 19•6 Pulmonary Function Tests

Term Used	Symbol	Description	Remarks
Forced vital capacity	FVC	Vital capacity performed with a maximally forced expiratory effort	Forced vital capacity is often reduced in COPD because of air trapping.
Forced expiratory volume (qualified by subscript indicating the time intervals in seconds)	$FEVt_1$, usually FEV_1	Volume of air exhaled in the specified time during the performance of forced vital capacity	A valuable clue to the severity of the expiratory airway obstruction
Ratio of timed forced expiratory volume to forced vital capacity	FEVt/FVC%, usually FEV_1/FVC%	FEVt expressed as a percentage of the forced vital capacity	Another way of expressing the presence or absence of airway obstruction
Forced expiratory flow	$FEF_{200-1200}$	Mean forced expiratory flow between 200 and 1200 mL of the FVC	An indicator of large airway obstruction
Forced midexpiratory flow	$FEF_{25\%\ 75\%}$	Mean forced expiratory flow during the middle half of the FVC	Slowed in small airway obstruction
Forced end expiratory flow	$FEF_{75\%-85\%}$	Mean forced expiratory flow during the terminal portion of the FVC	Slowed in obstruction of smallest airways
Maximal voluntary ventilation	MVV	Volume of air expired in a specified period (12 seconds) during repetitive maximal effort	An important factor in exercise tolerance

Imaging Studies

Imaging studies, including x-rays, computed tomography scans, contrast studies, and magnetic resonance imaging, may be part of any diagnostic workup, ranging from a determination of the extent of infection in sinusitis to tumor growth in cancer.

Chest X-Ray Studies

Normal pulmonary tissue is radiolucent; therefore, densities produced by fluid, tumors, foreign bodies, and other pathologic conditions can be detected by x-ray examination. A chest x-ray may reveal an extensive pathologic process in the lungs in the absence of symptoms. The routine chest x-ray consists of two views—the posteroanterior projection and the lateral projection. Chest x-rays are usually taken after full inspiration (a deep breath) because the lungs are best visualized when they are well aerated. Also, the diaphragm is at its lowest level and the largest expanse of lung is visible. Taken on expiration, x-ray films may accentuate an otherwise unnoticed pneumothorax or obstruction of a major artery.

Computed Tomography

Computed tomography (CT) is an imaging method in which the lungs are scanned in successive layers by a narrow-beam x-ray. The images produced provide a cross-sectional view of the chest. Whereas a chest x-ray shows major contrast between body densities, such as bones, soft tissues, and air, CT scans can distinguish

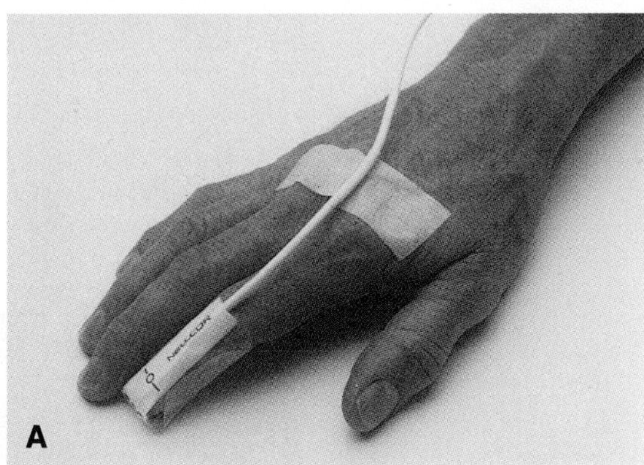

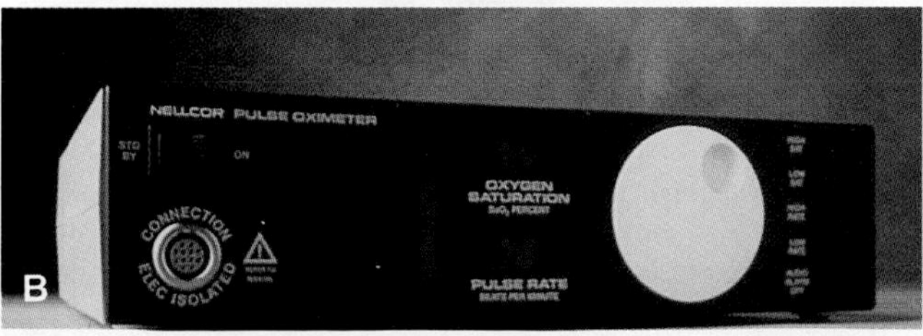

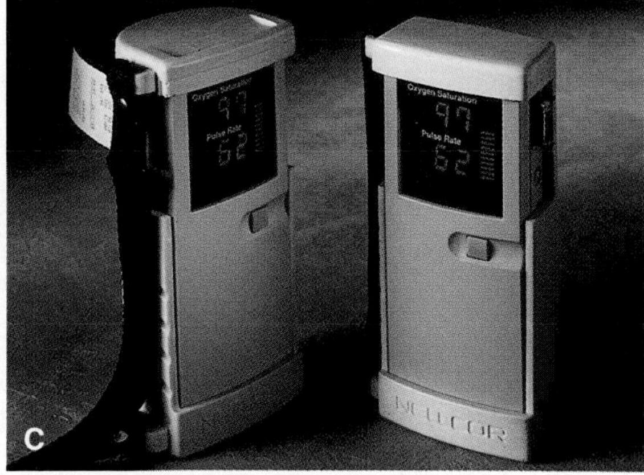

FIGURE 19•14 Measuring blood oxygenation with pulse oximetry eliminates the need for invasive procedures, such as drawing blood for analysis of oxygen levels. (**A**) The pulse oximeter sensor slips easily over a patient's finger. (**B**) The oxygen saturation level appears on the monitor. (**C**) Portable pulse oximeter is ideal for home use. Courtesy Nellcor Incorporated, Pleasanton, California.

fine tissue density. CT may be used to define pulmonary nodules and small tumors adjacent to pleural surfaces that are not visible on routine chest x-ray, and to demonstrate mediastinal abnormalities and hilar adenopathy, which are difficult to visualize with other techniques. Contrast agents are useful when evaluating the mediastinum and its contents.

Fluoroscopic Studies

Fluoroscopy is used to assist with invasive procedures, such as a chest needle biopsy or transbronchial biopsy, performed to identify lesions. It also may be used to study the movement of the chest wall, mediastinum, heart, and diaphragm, to detect diaphragm paralysis, and to locate lung masses.

BARIUM SWALLOW

A barium swallow outlines the esophagus and shows displacement of the esophagus and encroachment on its lumen by the heart, lungs, or mediastinal structures.

Angiographic Studies of the Pulmonary Vessels

Pulmonary angiography is most commonly used to investigate thromboembolic disease of the lungs, such as pulmonary emboli and congenital abnormalities of the pulmonary vascular tree. It involves the rapid injection of a radiopaque agent into the vasculature of the lungs for radiographic study of the pulmonary vessels. It can be performed by injecting the radiopaque agent into a vein in one or both arms (simultaneously) or into the femoral vein, with a needle or catheter. The agent also can be injected into a catheter that has been inserted in the main pulmonary artery or its branches or into the great veins proximal to the pulmonary artery.

Radioisotope Diagnostic Procedures (Lung Scans)

There are four types of lung scans: perfusion scan, ventilation scan, inhalation scan, and gallium scan. They are used to detect normal lung functioning, pulmonary vascular supply, and gas exchange.

A perfusion lung scan is performed by injecting a radioactive agent (technetium) into a peripheral vein and then obtaining a scan of the chest and body to detect radiation. The isotope particles pass through the right side of the heart and are distributed into the lungs in amounts proportional to the regional blood flow, making it possible to trace and measure blood perfusion through the lung. This procedure is used clinically to measure the integrity of the pulmonary vessels relative to blood flow and to evaluate blood flow abnormalities, as seen in pulmonary emboli. The nurse informs the patient that the imaging time is 20 to 40 minutes, during which the patient will lie under the camera with a mask fitted over the nose and mouth for the duration of the test.

A ventilation scan is performed after the perfusion scan. The patient takes a deep breath of a mixture of oxygen and radioactive gas (xenon, krypton), which diffuses throughout the lungs. A scan is performed to detect ventilation abnormalities, especially in patients who have regional differences in ventilation. It may be helpful in the diagnosis of bronchitis, asthma, inflammatory fibrosis, pneumonia, emphysema, and lung cancer.

An inhalation scan is performed by administering droplets of radioactive material by a positive-pressure ventilator. This scan is helpful, particularly in visualizing the trachea and major airways.

A gallium scan is a radioisotope lung scan used to detect inflammatory conditions, abscesses, adhesions, and the presence, location, and size of tumors. It is used to stage bronchogenic cancer and record tumor regression after chemotherapy or radiation. Gallium is injected intravenously, and scans are taken at 6, 24, and/or 48 hours to evaluate gallium uptake by the pulmonary tissues.

Endoscopic Procedures

Bronchoscopy

Bronchoscopy is the direct inspection and examination of the larynx, trachea, and bronchi through either a flexible fiberoptic bronchoscope or a rigid bronchoscope. The fiberoptic scope is used more frequently in current practice.

The purposes of diagnostic bronchoscopy are: (1) to examine tissues or collect secretions, (2) to determine the location and extent of the pathologic process and to obtain a tissue sample for diagnosis (by biting forceps, curettage, or brush biopsy), (3) to determine if a tumor can be resected surgically, and (4) to diagnose bleeding sites (source of hemoptysis).

Therapeutic bronchoscopy is used to: (1) remove foreign bodies from the tracheobronchial tree, (2) remove secretions obstructing the tracheobronchial tree when the patient cannot clear them, (3) treat postoperative atelectasis, and (4) destroy and excise lesions.

The fiberoptic bronchoscope is a thin, flexible bronchoscope that can be directed into the segmental bronchi (Fig. 19-15). Because of its small size, its flexibility, and its excellent optical system, it allows increased visualization of the peripheral airways and is ideal for diagnosing pulmonary lesions. Fiberoptic bronchoscopy allows biopsy of previously inaccessible tumors and can be performed at the bedside. It also can be performed through endotracheal or tracheostomy tubes of patients on ventilators. Cytologic examinations can be performed without surgical intervention.

The rigid bronchoscope is a hollow metal tube with a light at its end. It is used mainly for removing foreign substances, investigating the source of massive hemoptysis, or performing endobronchial surgical procedures. Rigid bronchoscopy is performed in the operating room, not at the bedside.

Possible complications of bronchoscopy include a reaction to the local anesthetic, infection, aspiration, bronchospasm,

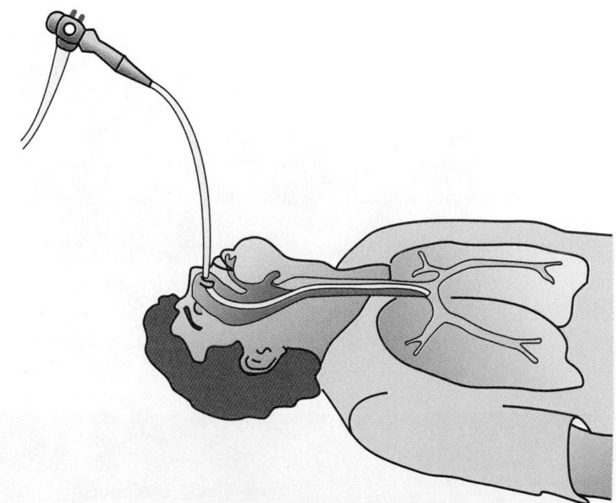

FIGURE 19•15 Endoscopic bronchoscopy permits visualization of bronchial structures. The bronchoscope is advanced into bronchial structures orally. Bronchoscopy permits the clinician not only to diagnose but also to treat various lung problems.

hypoxemia (low blood oxygen level), pneumothorax, bleeding, and perforation.

NURSING INTERVENTIONS

Before the procedure, the nurse obtains a signed consent form, and food and fluids are withheld for 6 hours before the test to reduce the risk of aspiration when the cough reflex is blocked by anesthesia. The nurse explains the procedure to the patient to reduce fear and decrease anxiety and administers preoperative medications (usually atropine and a sedative or opioid) as prescribed to inhibit vagal stimulation (thereby guarding against bradycardia, dysrhythmias, and hypotension), suppress the cough reflex, sedate the patient, and relieve anxiety.

Nursing Alert *Sedation given to patients with respiratory insufficiency may precipitate respiratory arrest.*

The patient must remove dentures and other oral prostheses. The examination is usually performed under local anesthesia, but general anesthesia may be needed for rigid bronchoscopy. A topical anesthetic such as lidocaine (Xylocaine) may be sprayed on the pharynx or dropped on the epiglottis and vocal cords and into the trachea to suppress the cough reflex and minimize discomfort. Sedatives or opioids are administered intravenously as prescribed to provide conscious sedation.

After the procedure, it is important that the patient takes nothing by mouth until the cough reflex returns, because the preoperative sedation and local anesthesia impair the protective laryngeal reflex and swallowing for several hours. Once the patient demonstrates a cough reflex, the nurse may offer ice chips and eventually fluids. The nurse assesses for confusion and lethargy in the elderly, which may be due to large doses of lidocaine given during the procedure. The nurse also monitors the patient's respiratory status and observes for hypoxia, hypotension, tachycardia, dysrhythmias, hemoptysis, and dyspnea. Any abnormality is reported promptly. The patient is not discharged from the recovery area to home or the nursing unit until adequate cough reflex and respiratory status are present. The nurse instructs the patient and family caregivers to report any shortness of breath or bleeding immediately.

Thoracoscopy

Thoracoscopy is a diagnostic procedure in which the pleural cavity is examined with an endoscope (Fig. 19-16). Small incisions are made into the pleural cavity in an intercostal space; the location of the incision depends on the clinical and diagnostic findings. After any fluid present in the pleural cavity is aspirated, the fiberoptic mediastinoscope is inserted into the pleural cavity, and its surface is inspected through the instrument. After the procedure, a chest tube may be inserted, and the pleural cavity is drained by negative-pressure water-seal drainage.

Thoracoscopy is primarily indicated in the diagnostic evaluation of pleural effusions, pleural disease, and tumor staging. Biopsies of the lesions can be performed under visualization for diagnosis.

Thoracoscopic procedures have expanded with the availability of video monitoring, which permits visualization of the lung. It has, in some cases, replaced thoracotomy as the standard for diagnosis of diffuse lung disorders, pulmonary infiltrates, and lung biopsy. It also has been used with the carbon dioxide laser in the removal of pulmonary blebs and bullae and in the treatment of spontaneous pneumothorax. Lasers have also been used in the excision of peripheral pulmonary nodules. Although the laser does not replace the need for thoracotomy in the treatment of some lung cancers, its use continues to expand because it is less invasive.

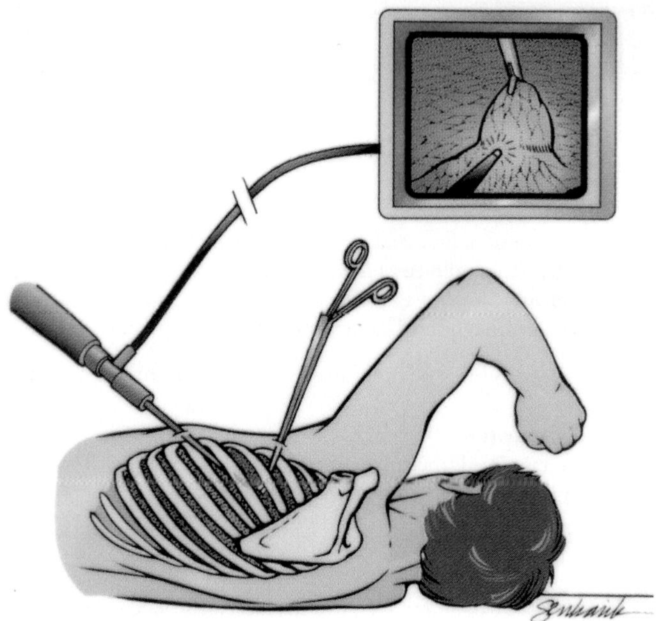

FIGURE 19•16 Endoscopic thoracoscopy. Like bronchoscopy, thoracoscopy uses fiberoptic instruments and video cameras for visualizing thoracic structures. Unlike bronchoscopy, thoracoscopy usually requires the surgeon to make a small incision before inserting the endoscope. A combined diagnostic–treatment procedure, thoracoscopy includes excising tissue for biopsy.

NURSING INTERVENTIONS

Home care involves monitoring the patient for shortness of breath (which might indicate a pneumothorax), and minor activity restrictions, which vary depending on the intensity of the procedure.

Thoracentesis

A thin layer of pleural fluid normally remains in the pleural space. An accumulation of pleural fluid may occur with some disorders. A sample of this fluid can be obtained by thoracentesis or by tube thoracotomy. Thoracentesis is the aspiration of pleural fluid for diagnostic or therapeutic purposes. It is important to position the patient as shown in Assisting the Patient Undergoing Thoracentesis.

A needle biopsy of the pleura may be performed at the same time. Studies of pleural fluid include Gram's stain culture and sensitivity, acid-fast staining and culture, differential cell count, cytology, pH, specific gravity, total protein, and lactic dehydrogenase.

Biopsy

Biopsy, the excision of a small amount of tissue, may be performed to permit examination of cells from the pharynx, larynx, and nasal passages. Local, topical, or general anesthesia may be administered, depending on the site and the procedure (see also Lung Biopsy Procedures below).

Pleural Biopsy

Pleural biopsy is accomplished by needle biopsy of the pleura or by pleuroscopy, a visual exploration through a fiberoptic bronchoscope inserted into the pleural space. Pleural biopsy is performed when there is pleural exudate of undetermined origin and when

19•1 Guidelines For 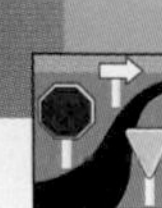 Assisting the Patient Undergoing Thoracentesis

A thoracentesis (aspiration of fluid or air from the pleural space) is performed on patients with various clinical problems. A diagnostic or therapeutic procedure, thoracentesis may be used for:

- Removal of fluid and air from the pleural cavity
- Aspiration of pleural fluid for analysis
- Pleural biopsy
- Instillation of medication into the pleural space

The responsibilities of the nurse and rationale for the nursing actions are summarized below.

Nursing Activities	**Rationale**
1. Ascertain in advance that a chest x-ray has been ordered and completed and the consent form has been signed.	1. Posteroanterior and lateral chest x-ray films are used to localize fluid and air in the pleural cavity and to aid in determining the puncture site. When fluid is loculated (isolated in a pocket of pleural fluid), ultrasound scans are performed to help select the best site for needle aspiration.
2. Assess the patient for allergy to the local anesthetic to be used. Also give sedation if prescribed.	2. If the patient is allergic to the initially prescribed anesthetic, assessment findings provide an opportunity to use a safer anesthetic.
3. Inform the patient about the nature of the procedure and: a. The importance of remaining immobile b. Pressure sensations to be experienced c. That no discomfort is anticipated after the procedure	3. An explanation helps to orient the patient to the procedure, assists the patient to mobilize resources, and provides an opportunity to ask questions and verbalize anxiety.
4. Position the patient comfortably with adequate supports. If possible, place the patient upright or in one of the following positions: a. Sitting on the edge of the bed with the feet supported and arms and head on a padded over-the-bed table	4. The upright position facilitates the removal of fluid that usually localizes at the base of the chest. A position of comfort helps the patient to relax.

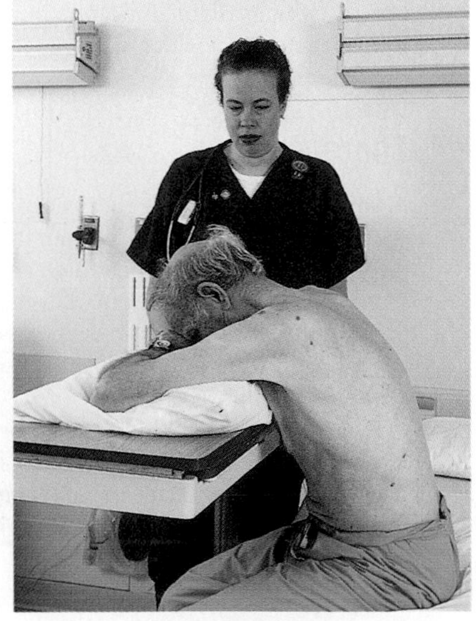

Patient positioned for thoracentesis.

b. Straddling a chair with arms and head resting on the back of the chair c. Lying on the unaffected side with the bed elevated 30 degrees to 45 degrees if unable to assume a sitting position	
5. Support and reassure the patient during the procedure. a. Prepare the patient for the cold sensation of skin germicide solution and for a pressure sensation from infiltration of local anesthetic agent. b. Encourage the patient to refrain from coughing.	5. Sudden and unexpected movement, such as coughing, by the patient can traumatize the visceral pleura and lung.

(*continued*)

19•1 GUIDELINES FOR ASSISTING THE PATIENT UNDERGOING THORACENTESIS (Continued)

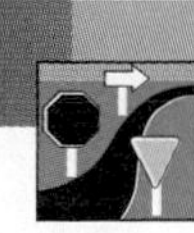

Nursing Activities	Rationale
6. Expose the entire chest. The site for aspiration is visualized by chest x-ray film and percussion. If fluid is in the pleural cavity, the thoracentesis site is determined by the chest x-ray, ultrasound scanning, and physical findings, with attention to the site of maximal dullness on percussion.	6. If air is in the pleural cavity, the thoracentesis site is usually in the second or third intercostal space in the midclavicular line because air rises in the thorax.
7. The procedure is performed under aseptic conditions. After the skin is cleansed, the physician uses a small-caliber needle to inject a local anesthetic slowly into the intercostal space.	7. An intradermal wheal is raised slowly; rapid injection causes pain. The parietal pleura is very sensitive and should be well infiltrated with anesthetic before the physician passes the thoracentesis needle through it.
8. The physician advances the thoracentesis needle with the syringe attached. When the pleural space is reached, suction may be applied with the syringe.	
a. A 20-mL syringe with a three-way stopcock is attached to the needle (one end of the adapter is attached to the needle and the other to the tubing leading to a receptacle that receives the fluid being aspirated).	a. When a large quantity of fluid is withdrawn, a three-way stopcock serves to keep air from entering the pleural cavity.
b. If a considerable quantity of fluid is removed, the needle is held in place on the chest wall with a small hemostat.	b. The hemostat steadies the needle on the chest wall. Sudden pleuritic chest pain or shoulder pain may indicate that the needle point is irritating the visceral or the diaphragmatic pleura.
9. After the needle is withdrawn, pressure is applied over the puncture site and a small, sterile dressing is fixed in place.	9. Pressure helps to stop bleeding and the dressing protects the site.
10. Advise the patient that he or she will be on bed rest and a chest x-ray will be obtained after thoracentesis.	10. A chest x-ray verifies that there is no pneumothorax.
11. Record the total amount of fluid withdrawn from the procedure and document the nature of the fluid, its color, and its viscosity. If indicated, prepare samples of fluid for laboratory evaluation. A specimen container with formalin may be needed for a pleural biopsy.	11. The fluid may be clear, serous, bloody, purulent, etc.
12. Monitor the patient at intervals for increasing respiratory rate; asymmetry in respiratory movement; faintness; vertigo; tightness in chest; uncontrollable cough; blood-tinged, frothy mucus; a rapid pulse; and signs of hypoxemia.	12. Pneumothorax, tension pneumothorax, subcutaneous emphysema, or pyrogenic infection are complications of a thoracentesis. Pulmonary edema or cardiac distress can occur after a sudden shift in mediastinal contents when large amounts of fluid are aspirated.

there is a need to culture or stain the tissue to identify tuberculosis or fungi.

Lung Biopsy Procedures

When the chest x-ray findings are inconclusive or show pulmonary density (indicating an infiltrate or lesion), biopsy may be performed to obtain lung tissue for examination to identify the nature of the lesion. There are several nonsurgical lung biopsy techniques that are used because they yield accurate information with low morbidity: (1) transcatheter bronchial brushing, (2) transbronchial lung biopsy, or (3) percutaneous (through-the-skin) needle biopsy.

In transcatheter bronchial brushing, a fiberoptic bronchoscope is introduced into the bronchus under fluoroscopy. A small brush attached to the end of a flexible wire is inserted through the bronchoscope. Under direct visualization, the area under suspicion is brushed back and forth, causing cells to slough off and adhere to the brush. The catheter port of the bronchoscope may be used to irrigate the lung tissue with saline solution to secure material for additional studies. The brush is removed from the bronchoscope and a microscopic slide is made. Sometimes the brush is cut off and sent to the pathology laboratory for testing.

This procedure is useful for cytologic evaluations of lung lesions and for the identification of pathogenic organisms (*Nocardia, Aspergillus, Pneumocystis carinii*, and other pathogens). It is especially useful in the immunologically compromised patient.

A transbronchial lung biopsy uses cutting forceps introduced by fiberoptic bronchoscope. A biopsy is indicated when a lung lesion is suspected and the results of routine sputum samples and bronchoscopic washings are negative.

Nursing care and complications for transcatheter bronchial brushing and transbronchial lung biopsy are the same as for fiberoptic bronchoscopy.

Another method of bronchial brushing involves the introduction of the catheter through the transcricothyroid membrane by needle puncture. After this procedure, the patient is instructed to hold a finger or thumb over the puncture site while coughing to prevent air from leaking into the surrounding tissues.

Percutaneous needle biopsy may be accomplished with a cutting needle or by aspiration with a spinal-type needle that provides a tissue specimen for histologic study. Analgesia may be administered before the procedure. The skin over the biopsy site is cleansed and anesthetized and a small incision is made. The biopsy needle is inserted through the incision into the pleura with the patient holding the breath in midexpiration. With fluoroscopic monitoring, the surgeon guides the needle into the periphery of the lesion and obtains a tissue sample from the mass. Possible complications include pneumothorax, pulmonary hemorrhage, and empyema.

NURSING INTERVENTIONS

After the procedure, recovery and home care are similar to those for bronchoscopy and thoracoscopy. Nursing care involves monitoring the patient for shortness of breath, bleeding, and infection.

Lymph Node Biopsy

The scalene lymph nodes are enmeshed in the deep cervical pad of fat overlying the scalenus anterior muscle. They drain the lungs and mediastinum and may show histologic changes from intrathoracic disease. When these nodes are palpable on physical examination, a scalene node biopsy may be performed. A biopsy of these nodes may be performed to detect lymph node spread of pulmonary disease and to establish a diagnosis or prognosis in such diseases as Hodgkin's disease, sarcoidosis, fungal disease, tuberculosis, and carcinoma.

Mediastinoscopy is the endoscopic examination of the mediastinum for exploration and biopsy of mediastinal lymph nodes that drain the lungs; this examination does not require a thoracotomy. Biopsy is usually performed through a suprasternal incision. Mediastinoscopy is carried out to detect mediastinal involvement of pulmonary malignancy and to obtain tissue for diagnostic studies of other conditions (eg, sarcoidosis).

An anterior mediastinotomy is thought to provide better exposure and diagnostic possibilities than a mediastinoscopy. An incision is made in the area of the second or third costal cartilage. The mediastinum is explored and biopsies are performed on any lymph nodes found. Chest tube drainage is required after the procedure. This diagnostic modality is particularly valuable to determine whether a pulmonary lesion is resectable.

Nursing Interventions

Postprocedure care focuses on providing adequate oxygenation, monitoring for bleeding, and providing pain relief. The patient may be discharged a few hours after the chest drainage system is removed. The nurse should instruct the patient and family about monitoring for changes in respiratory status.

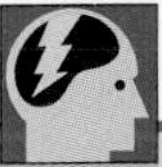

Critical Thinking Exercises

1. After a thoracentesis for diagnostic purposes, your patient reports shortness of breath and appears anxious. Based on your knowledge of the risks associated with thoracentesis, how would you focus your assessment because of those risks?

2. Your patient is scheduled for pulmonary function tests before heart surgery. You know that a patient who understands the purposes of the tests and what to expect during the procedures will be able to cooperate more during the tests. What teaching points would you emphasize when explaining the procedure to this patient? What types of details would you include?

3. Based on your understanding of clinical conditions, discuss at least one condition that would affect ventilation, diffusion, and perfusion.

References and Selected Readings

BOOKS

Ahrens, T. (1996). Respiratory monitoring. In J. Clochesy, C. Breu, S. Cardin, A. A. Whittaker, & E. B. Rudy (Eds.), *Critical care nursing* (2nd ed.). Philadelphia: W. B. Saunders.

Bickley, L. S., & Hoekelman, R. A. (1999). *Bates' guide to physical examination and history taking* (7th ed.). Philadelphia: Lippincott-Raven.

Burton, G. G., Hodgkin, J. E., & Ward, J. J. (Eds.). (1997). *Respiratory care: A guide to clinical practice* (4th ed.). Philadelphia: Lippincott-Raven.

Harrell, J. S. (1996). Age-related changes in the respiratory system. In M. Matteson, E. S. McConnell, & A. D. Linton (Eds.), *Gerontological nursing: Concepts and practice* (2nd ed.). Philadelphia: W. B. Saunders.

Hyatt, R. E., Scanlo, P. D., & Nakamura, M. (1997). *Interpretation of pulmonary function tests: A practical guide.* Philadelphia: Lippincott-Raven.

Levitzky, M. G. (1999). *Pulmonary physiology* (4th ed.). New York: McGraw Hill.

Madama, V. C., & Madama, V. (1997). *Pulmonary function testing and cardiopulmonary stress testing.* Albany, NY: Delmar.

Sole, M. L., & Byers, J. F. (1997). Ventilatory assistance. In J. C. Hartshorn, M. L. Sole, & M. L. Lamborn (Eds.), *Introduction to critical care nursing* (2nd ed.). Philadelphia: W. B. Saunders.

Stone, K. S. (1996). Respiratory physiology. In J. Clochesy, C. Breu, S. Cardin, A. A. Whittaker, & E. B. Rudy (Eds.), *Critical care nursing* (2nd ed.). Philadelphia: W. B. Saunders.

JOURNALS

Ferrin, M. S., & Tino, G. (1997). Acute dyspnea. *AACN Clinical Issues, 8*(3), 398–410.

Grap, M. J. (1998). Protocols for practice: Applying research at the bedside—pulse oximetry. *Critical Care Nurse, 18*(1), 94–99.

Haas, F., Salazar-Schicchi, J., Axen, K., & Fain, F. (1996). Pulmonary function testing. *Physical Medicine and Rehabilitation Clinics of North America, 7*(2), 223–239.

Misasi, R. S., & Keyes, J. L. (1996). Matching and mismatching ventilation and perfusion in the lung. *Critical Care Nurse, 16*(3), 23–38.

O'Hanlon-Nichols, T. (1998). The adult pulmonary system. *American Journal of Nursing, 98*(2), 39–45.

Tittle, M., & Flynn, M. B. (1997). Applied nursing research. Correlation of pulse oximetry and co-oximetry. *Dimensions of Critical Care Nursing, 16*(2), 88–95.

Weilitz, P. B., & Lueckenotte, A. (1995). Respiratory assessment of older adults: Part I. *Perspectives in Respiratory Nursing, 6*(1), 3–4.

Weilitz, P. B., & Lueckenotte, A. (1995). Respiratory assessment of older adults: Part II. *Perspectives in Respiratory Nursing, 6*(2), 3–4.

Resources

American Lung Association, 1740 Broadway, New York, NY 10019; 1-212-315-8700, 1-800-LUNG USA; http://www.lungusa.org

American Thoracic Society, 1740 Broadway, New York, NY 10019; 1-212-315-8700; http://www.lungusa.org

American Association for Respiratory Care, 11030 Ables Lane, Dallas, TX 75229; 1-972-243-2272

National Heart, Lung, and Blood Institute/National Institutes of Health, Rockville Pike, Bldg. 31, Bethesda, MD 20892; 1-301-496-5166; www.nhlbi.nih.gov/nhlbi/nhlbi.htm

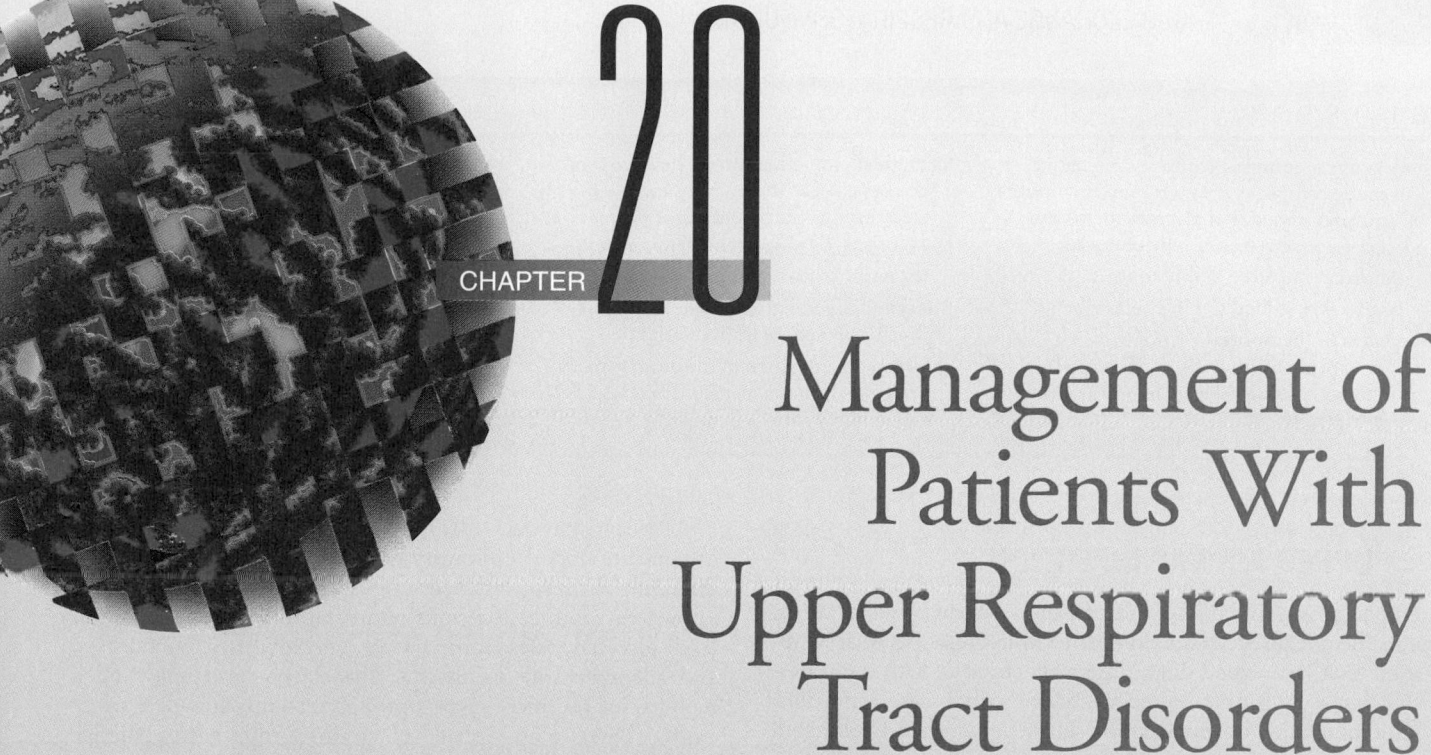

CHAPTER 20

Management of Patients With Upper Respiratory Tract Disorders

Learning Objectives

On completion of this chapter, the learner will be able to:

1. Describe nursing management of patients with upper airway disorders.
2. Compare and contrast the upper respiratory tract infections with regard to cause, incidence, clinical manifestations, management, and the significance of preventive health care.
3. Use the nursing process as a framework for care of patients with upper airway infection.
4. Describe nursing management of the patient with epistaxis.
5. Use the nursing process as a framework for care of patients undergoing laryngectomy.

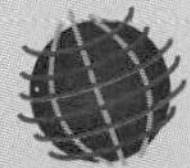

Many upper airway disorders are relatively minor and their effects are limited to mild and temporary discomfort and inconvenience for the patient. However, other upper airway disorders are acute, severe, and life-threatening and may require permanent alterations in breathing and speaking. Thus, the nurse must have good assessment skills, an understanding of the wide variety of disorders that may affect the upper airway, and an awareness of the impact of these alterations on patients.

Because many of the disorders are treated outside the hospital or at home by patients themselves, patient teaching is an important aspect of nursing care. When dealing with patients with acute, life-threatening disorders, the nurse needs highly developed assessment and clinical management skills, along with a focus on rehabilitation needs.

GLOSSARY

alaryngeal communication: alternative modes of speaking that do not involve the normal larynx; used by patients whose larynx has been surgically removed

aphonia: impaired ability to use one's voice

dysphagia: difficulties in swallowing

epistaxis: hemorrhage from the nose due to rupture of tiny, distended vessels in the mucous membrane of any area of the nose

laryngitis: inflammation of the larynx; may be due to voice abuse, exposure to irritants, or infectious organisms

laryngectomy: removal of all or part of the larynx and surrounding structures

pharyngitis: inflammation of the throat; usually viral or bacterial in origin

rhinitis: inflammation of the mucous membranes of the nose; may be infectious, allergic, or inflammatory in origin

rhinorrhea: drainage of a large amount of fluid from the nose

sinusitis: inflammation of the sinuses; may be acute or chronic; may be viral, bacterial, or fungal in origin

submucous resection: surgical procedure to correct nasal obstruction due to deviated septum; also called septoplasty

xerostomia: dryness of the mouth from a variety of causes

UPPER AIRWAY INFECTIONS

Upper airway infections are common conditions that affect most people on occasion. Some infections are acute, with symptoms that last several days; others are chronic, with symptoms that last a long time or recur. Patients with these conditions seldom require hospitalization. However, nurses working in community settings or long-term care facilities may encounter patients who have these infections. Thus, it is important for the nurse to recognize the signs and symptoms and to provide appropriate care.

Common Cold

The phrase "common cold" often is used when referring to symptoms of an upper respiratory tract infection characterized by nasal congestion, sore throat, and cough. The term *cold* refers to an afebrile, infectious, acute inflammation of the mucous membranes of the nasal cavity. More broadly, the term refers to an acute upper respiratory tract infection; terms such as *rhinitis, pharyngitis, laryngitis,* and *chest cold* distinguish the sites of the major symptoms. Colds are highly contagious because patients shed virus for about 2 days before the symptoms appear and during the first part of the symptomatic phase. Approximately 1 billion people in the United States acquire a common cold each year. Colds prevail among 15% of the working population at any time during the winter and account for almost half of all work absences and one fourth of the total time lost from work (Kirkpatrick, 1996).

Three waves of colds appear yearly in the United States:

- In September, just after school opens
- In late January
- Toward the end of April

Immunity after recovery is variable and depends on many factors, including a person's natural host resistance and the specific virus that caused the cold.

Clinical Manifestations

Signs and symptoms of a cold are nasal congestion, scratchy or sore throat, sneezing, tearing watery eyes, malaise, fever, chills, and often headache and muscle aches. As the cold progresses, cough usually appears. In some people a cold even exacerbates the herpes simplex, commonly called a cold sore (Chart 20-1)

Symptoms usually last 5 days to 2 weeks. If there is significant fever or more severe systemic respiratory symptoms, it is no longer considered a common cold but rather one of the other acute upper respiratory tract infections. More than 200 different viruses, classified into five major groupings, are known to produce the signs and symptoms of the common cold: picornaviruses, coronaviruses, myxoviruses, paraviruses, and adenoviruses. Rhinovirus, the classic head cold and a member of the picornavirus group, accounts for 40% of all colds. There are more than 100 strains of rhinovirus. Allergic conditions can also affect the nose and mimic the symptoms of a cold.

CHART 20•1 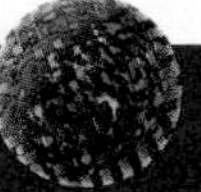 **Colds and Cold Sores (Herpes Simplex Virus)**

The herpes simplex virus (HSV-1) produces the familiar *herpes labialis,* commonly called a cold sore or fever blister. In the past, this painful blisterlike lip sore was thought to be caused by a cold or a fever. Even now that scientists recognize the origin of herpes labialis, the condition is still referred to as a cold sore. The herpes virus infection remains latent in cells of the lips or nose and is activated by stress, sunlight, and febrile illnesses from the common cold to streptococcal pneumonia, meningococcal meningitis, and even malaria.

The incubation period is 2 to 12 days. The virus is transmitted primarily by direct contact with infected secretions. The virus may also be transmitted from an asymptomatic person. Small vesicles, single or clustered, may erupt on the lips, inside the mouth, including the tongue, soft and hard palate, gums, buccal mucosa, and the pharynx. These soon rupture, forming sore shallow ulcers that increase in number. The gums may bleed and feel painful.

The herpes virus may subside spontaneously in 10 to 14 days. If it does not, acyclovir, an antiviral agent, may be administered orally or topically to minimize the symptoms and the duration or length of the flare-up. Analgesics, such as acetaminophen (Tylenol) with codeine or aspirin with codeine, are helpful in relieving pain and discomfort. Topical anesthetics, such as lidocaine (Xylocaine) or dyclonine (Dyclone), and over-the-counter preparations, such as Herpecin-L, may relieve oral pain. Applications of drying lotions or liquids may help to dry the lesions.

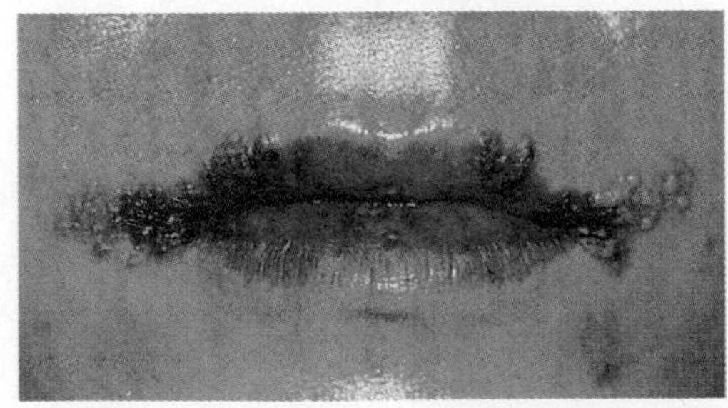

Medical Management

There is no cure for the common cold. Management consists of symptomatic therapy. Therapeutic measures include an adequate fluid intake, rest, prevention of chilling, aqueous nasal decongestants, antihistamines, vitamin C, and expectorants as needed. Warm salt water gargles soothe the sore throat, and aspirin, ibuprofen, or acetaminophen relieves the aches, pains, and fever. Antimicrobial agents do not affect the virus or reduce the incidence of bacterial complications; however, they may be used prophylactically for high-risk respiratory patients.

Nursing Management

Because most cold viruses are self-treated by patients at home and others are treated incidentally in long-term or acute care facilities, nursing management consists primarily of patient education.

TEACHING PATIENTS SELF-CARE

Most viruses are transmitted by hand-to-hand contact. It is important to teach the patient and the patient's family how to break the chain of infection. Hand washing remains the most effective preventive measure to reduce the transmission of organisms. The nurse teaches measures to prevent the common cold and methods to treat symptoms and prevent complications such as superinfection, bronchitis, and pneumonia. For more information, see the Home Care Teaching Checklist.

Acute Sinusitis

The sinuses are involved in a high proportion of upper respiratory tract infections. If their openings into the nasal passages are clear, the infections resolve promptly. However, if their drainage is obstructed by a deviated septum or by hypertrophied turbinates, spurs, nasal polyps, or tumors, sinus infection may persist as a

Home Care Teaching Checklist: Preventing and Managing Upper Respiratory Infections

At the completion of the program, the patient or caregiver will be able to:

	Patient	Caregiver
PREVENTION		
• **Identify strategies to prevent infection and, if infected, to prevent spread of infection to others by:**	✔	✔
• washing hands often		
• using disposable tissues		
• avoiding crowds during the flu season		
• avoiding individuals with known colds or respiratory infections		
• obtaining influenza vaccination, if recommended (especially if elderly or diagnosed with a chronic illness)		
• **Practice good health to prevent illness by:**	✔	✔
• eating a nutritious diet		
• getting plenty of rest and sleep		
• avoiding or reducing stress when possible		
• exercising appropriately		
• avoiding smoking and excessive intake of alcohol		
• increasing humidity in house, especially during winter		
• practicing adequate oral hygiene		
• **Avoid allergens, if allergies are associated with upper respiratory infections**	✔	
PREVENTION AND MANAGEMENT		
• **Identify strategies to control the environment by:**	✔	✔
• adequately humidifying (avoid overhumidifying) living quarters		
• placing a dehumidifier in the basement, if appropriate		
• providing central ventilation fans, air conditioning with microstatic air filters		
• reducing irritants (dust, chemical, tobacco smoke) when possible		
• limiting exposure to animals and house pets, particularly in the bedroom		
MANAGEMENT		
• **Describe strategies to relieve symptoms of upper respiratory infection, including:**	✔	✔
• gargling with salt water		
• increasing fluid intake, particularly of hot liquids		
• providing warm, moist air by shower or humidifier to relieve swollen mucous membranes		
• avoiding irritants (dust, chemicals, tobacco smoke) when possible		
• **Recognize signs and symptoms of infection and state when to contact a health care provider; for example, for**	✔	✔
• upper respiratory infection symptoms persisting longer than 7 to 10 days		
• extreme red throat or white patches on the back of the throat		
• discolored drainage or foul-smelling nasal discharge		
• prolonged fever of 100.5°F (38°C) >2 days		
• shortness of breath, wheezing		
• swollen glands		
• severe pain or tenderness around the eyes or persistent pain in sinus areas		
• severe headache		

smoldering secondary infection or progress to an acute suppurative process (causing purulent discharge). **Sinusitis** affects approximately 32 million people in the United States annually. The highest rates are seen in the Midwest and the South. Certain occupations, such as carpentry; leather tanning; and dye, paint, and solvent manufacturing, may expose workers to a greater occupational hazard because of chronic inflammation of the nasal passages (Kaliner et al., 1997).

Acute sinusitis is an inflammation of the sinuses for fewer than 8 weeks in an adult and 2 weeks in a child. It is frequently associated with the common cold.

Pathophysiology

Acute sinusitis frequently develops as a result of an upper respiratory infection (particularly a viral infection) or an exacerbation of allergic rhinitis. Nasal congestion, caused by inflammation, edema, and transudation of fluid, leads to obstruction of the sinus cavities. This provides an excellent medium for bacterial growth. Bacterial organisms account for more than 60% of the cases of acute sinusitis, namely *Streptococcus pneumoniae, Haemophilus influenzae,* and *Moraxella catarrhalis.* Tooth infections also have been associated with acute sinusitis.

Clinical Manifestations

Symptoms of acute sinus infections include pressure, pain over the sinus area, and purulent nasal secretions.

Assessment and Diagnostic Findings

A careful history and diagnostic assessment, including a computed tomography scan of the sinuses, is performed to rule out other local or systemic disorders, such as tumor, fistula, and allergy.

Complications

Acute sinusitis, if left untreated, may lead to severe and occasionally life-threatening complications, such as meningitis, brain abscess, ischemic infarction, and osteomyelitis. Other complications of sinusitis, although uncommon, include severe orbital cellulitis, subperiosteal abscess, and cavernous sinus thrombosis.

Medical Management

The goals of treatment of acute sinusitis are to treat the infection, shrink the nasal mucosa, and relieve pain. The antimicrobial agents of choice for bacterial infection are amoxicillin and amoxicillin/clavulanic acid (Augmentin). An alternative for patients allergic to penicillin is double-strength trimethoprim–sulfamethoxazole (Bactrim DS, Septra DS). The medication is administered for 7 to 10 days. Use of oral and topical decongestants is controversial, but these medications may decrease mucosal swelling of nasal polyps, thereby improving drainage of the sinuses. Heated mist and saline irrigation also may be effective for opening blocked passages. Decongestants have proven effective because of their vasoconstrictive properties. Common oral decongestants include pseudoephedrine (Sudafed) and phenylpropanolamine (Dimetapp). Topical decongestants such as oxymetazoline (Afrin) may be used for up to 72 hours. It is important to administer them with the patient's head tilted back to promote maximal dispersion of the medication. Guaifenesin, a mucolytic agent, also may be effective in reducing nasal congestion. If the patient continues to have symptoms after 7 to 10 days, the sinuses may need to be irrigated.

Nursing Management

TEACHING PATIENTS SELF-CARE

Patient teaching about self-care is an important aspect of nursing care for the patient with acute sinusitis. The nurse instructs the patient about methods to promote sinus drainage, such as inhaling steam (steam bath, hot shower, facial sauna), increasing fluid intake, and applying local heat (hot wet packs). The nurse also informs the patient about the side effects of nasal decongestant sprays and about rebound congestion. In the case of rebound congestion, the body's receptors, which have become dependent on the decongestant sprays to keep the nasal passages open, close and congestion results after the spray is discontinued.

The nurse stresses the importance of following the recommended medication regimen because a consistent level is critical to treat the infection. The nurse teaches the patient the early signs of a sinus infection and recommends preventive measures, such as following healthy practices and avoiding contact with people who have upper respiratory infections (see the checklist, Preventing and Managing Upper Respiratory Infections).

The nurse should explain to the patient that fever, severe headache, and nuchal rigidity are signs of potential complications. If fever persists despite antibiotic therapy, the patient should seek additional care.

Chronic Sinusitis

Chronic sinusitis is an inflammation of the sinuses that persists for more than 8 weeks in an adult or 2 weeks in a child.

Pathophysiology

Chronic sinusitis is usually caused by a narrowing or obstruction of the ostia of the frontal, maxillary, and anterior ethmoid sinuses, which drain into the middle meatus. This combined area is known as the osteomeatal complex. The blockage may occur because of infection, allergy, or structural abnormalities. This results in stagnant secretions, an ideal medium for infection. The organisms that cause chronic sinusitis are the same as those implicated in acute sinusitis. Immunocompromised patients, however, are more susceptible to fungal sinusitis. *Aspergillus fumigatus* is the most common organism associated with fungal sinusitis.

Clinical Manifestations

Clinical manifestations of chronic sinusitis include impaired mucociliary clearance and ventilation, cough (because of the constant dripping of the thick discharge backward into the nasopharynx), chronic hoarseness, chronic headaches in the periorbital area, and facial pain. These symptoms are generally most pronounced on awakening in the morning. Fatigue and nasal stuffiness are two additional common symptoms. In addition, some patients experience a decrease in smell and taste and a feeling of fullness in the ears.

Assessment and Diagnostic Findings

A careful history and diagnostic assessment, including a computed tomography scan of the sinuses or magnetic resonance imaging (if fungal sinusitis is suspected), is performed to rule out other local or systemic disorders, such as tumor, fistula, and allergy. Nasal endoscopy may be indicated to rule out underlying diseases, including tumors and sinus mycetomas (fungus balls). The fungus ball is usually a brown or greenish-black material with the consistency of peanut butter or cottage cheese.

Complications

Complications of chronic sinusitis, although uncommon, include severe orbital cellulitis, subperiosteal abscess, cavernous sinus thrombosis, meningitis, direct infection of the brain, and ischemic infarction.

Medical Management

The medical management of chronic sinusitis is almost the same as for acute sinusitis, except that the antimicrobial agents are administered for 21 days. Additional antimicrobial agents that may be used for chronic or recurrent sinusitis include cefuroxime axetil (Ceftin), cefixime (Suprax), clarithromycin (Biaxin), loracarbef (Lorabid), cefprozil (Cefzil), and azithromycin (Zithromax).

SURGICAL MANAGEMENT

When standard medical therapy fails, surgery, usually endoscopic, may be indicated to correct structural deformities that obstruct the ostia (openings) of the sinus. Excising and cauterizing nasal polyps, correcting a deviated septum, incising and draining the sinuses, aerating the sinuses, and removing tumors are some of the specific procedures performed. When sinusitis is caused by a fungal infection, surgery is required to excise the fungus ball and necrotic tissue and drain the sinuses. Oral and topical corticosteroids are usually prescribed.

Nursing Management

Because care measures for sinusitis are performed primarily by the patient at home, nursing management consists mainly of patient teaching.

TEACHING PATIENTS SELF-CARE

The nurse should teach the patient to promote sinus drainage by increasing the environmental humidity (steam bath, hot shower, facial sauna), increasing fluid intake, and applying local heat (hot wet packs). The nurse also instructs the patient about ways to prevent a sinus infection and how to recognize the early signs and symptoms.

Rhinitis

Rhinitis is an inflammation of the mucous membranes of the nose. It may be classified as infectious, allergic, or nonallergic. It is estimated that 10% to 20% of the U.S. population has allergic rhinitis (Ferguson, 1996). Rhinitis may be an acute or chronic condition.

Pathophysiology

Infectious rhinitis is most commonly caused by upper respiratory infections, from viruses (common cold), bacteria, and fungi. Rhinitis also occurs as a result of foreign bodies entering the nose, structural deformities, neoplasms and masses, chronic use of nasal decongestants, and use of oral contraceptives, cocaine, and antihypertensives. Rhinitis also may be a manifestation of an allergy (see Chap. 49), in which case it is referred to as allergic rhinitis. Figure 20-1 shows the pathologic processes involved in rhinitis and sinusitis.

Clinical Manifestations

The signs and symptoms of rhinitis include **rhinorrhea** (excessive nasal drainage, runny nose), nasal congestion, nasal discharge (purulent with bacterial rhinitis), nasal itchiness, and sneezing. Headache may occur, particularly if sinusitis is also present.

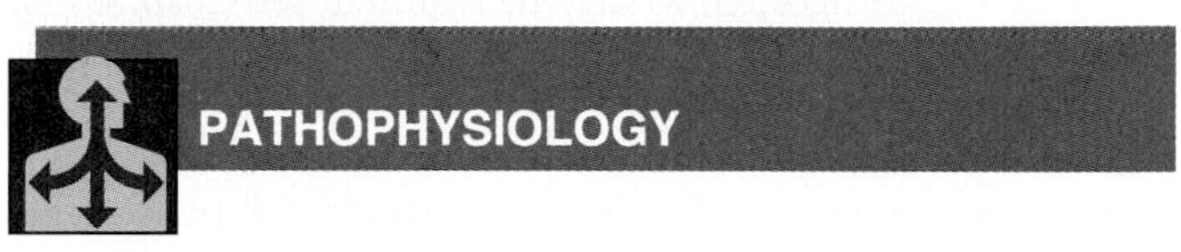

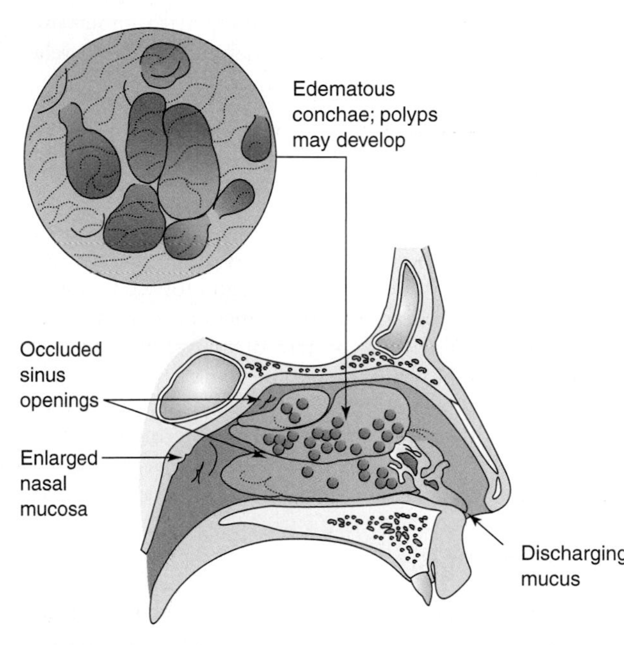

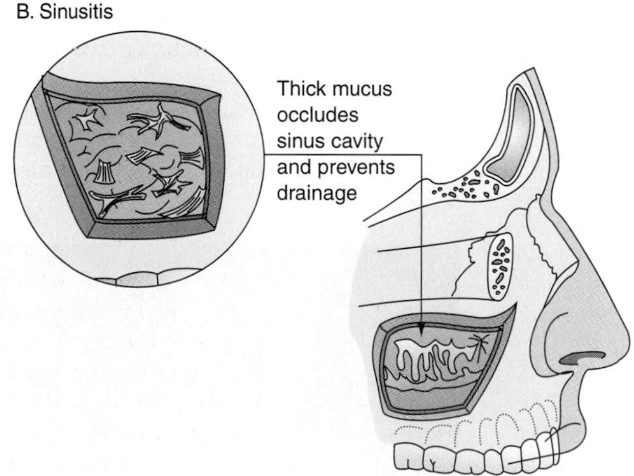

FIGURE 20•1 Pathophysiologic processes in rhinitis and sinusitis. Although pathophysiologic processes are similar in rhinitis and sinusitis, they affect different structures. In rhinitis (**A**), the mucous membranes lining the nasal passages become inflamed, congested, and edematous. The swollen nasal conchae block the sinus openings and mucus is discharged from the nostrils. Sinusitis (**B**) is also marked by inflammation and congestion, with thickened mucous secretions filling the sinus cavities and occluding the openings.

Medical Management

The management of rhinitis depends on the cause, which may be identified from the history and physical examination. If symptoms suggest a bacterial infection, an antimicrobial agent will be used (see the discussion of medical management of sinusitis). The examiner asks the patient about possible exposure to allergens in the home, environment, or workplace. In allergic rhinitis, tests may be performed to identify possible allergens. Depending on the severity of the allergy, desensitizing immunizations and corticosteroids may be required (see Chap. 49 for more details).

PHARMACOLOGIC THERAPY

Medication therapy for allergic and nonallergic rhinitis focuses on symptom relief. Antihistamines are administered for sneezing, itching, and rhinorrhea. Oral decongestants are administered for nasal obstruction. In addition, intranasal corticosteroids may be used for severe congestion and ophthalmic agents for relief of irritation, itching, and redness of the eyes.

Nursing Management

TEACHING PATIENTS SELF-CARE

The nurse instructs the patient with allergic rhinitis to avoid or reduce exposure to allergens and irritants, such as dusts, molds, animals, fumes, odors, powders, sprays, and tobacco smoke. The importance of controlling the environment at home and work is also explained. Saline nasal or aerosol sprays, or both, may be helpful in soothing mucous membranes, softening crusted secretions, and removing irritants. The nurse instructs the patient in the proper use of and technique for administering these types of medications. To achieve maximal relief, the patient must blow the nose before applying any medication into the nasal cavity.

Acute Pharyngitis

Acute **pharyngitis**, a febrile inflammation of the throat, is caused by a virus about 70% of the time. When group A streptococci cause the infection, the condition is referred to as strep throat. Group A streptococci are the most common bacterial organisms associated with acute pharyngitis (Fig. 20-2).

Uncomplicated viral infections usually subside promptly, within 3 to 10 days after the onset. However, pharyngitis caused by more virulent bacteria, such as group A streptococci, is a more severe illness during the acute stage and is more significant because of the increased incidence of dangerous complications, such as sinusitis, otitis media, peritonsillar abscess, mastoiditis, cervical adenitis, rheumatic fever, and nephritis.

Assessment and Diagnostic Findings

Rapid screening tests for streptococcal antigens, streptolysin titers, and throat cultures are used to determine the causative organism, after which appropriate therapy is prescribed. Nasal swabbings and blood cultures may also be necessary to identify the organism.

Clinical Manifestations

The signs of acute pharyngitis include a fiery-red pharyngeal membrane and tonsils, lymphoid follicles that are swollen and flecked with exudate, and enlarged and tender cervical lymph nodes. Fever, malaise, and sore throat also may be present. In addition, hoarseness, cough, and rhinitis are not uncommon.

Medical Management

Viral pharyngitis is treated with supportive measures since antibiotics will have no effect on a viral organism.

PHARMACOLOGIC THERAPY

If a bacterial cause is suggested or demonstrated, treatment may include the administration of antimicrobial agents. For group A streptococci, penicillin is the medication of choice. For patients who are allergic to penicillin or who have organisms resistant to erythromycin (one fifth of group A streptococci and most *Staphylococcus aureus* organisms are resistant to penicillin and erythromycin), cephalosporins and macrolides (clarithromycin and azithromycin) may be prescribed. Antibiotics are administered for at least 10 days to eradicate group A streptococci from the oropharynx.

Severe sore throats also can be relieved by analgesic medications taken as prescribed. For example, aspirin or acetaminophen (Tylenol) can be taken at 3- to 6-hour intervals; if required, acetaminophen with codeine may be taken three or four times daily. Antitussive medication, in the form of codeine, dextromethorphan (Robitussin DM), or hydrocodone bitartrate (Hycodan), may be required to control the persistent and painful cough that often accompanies acute pharyngitis.

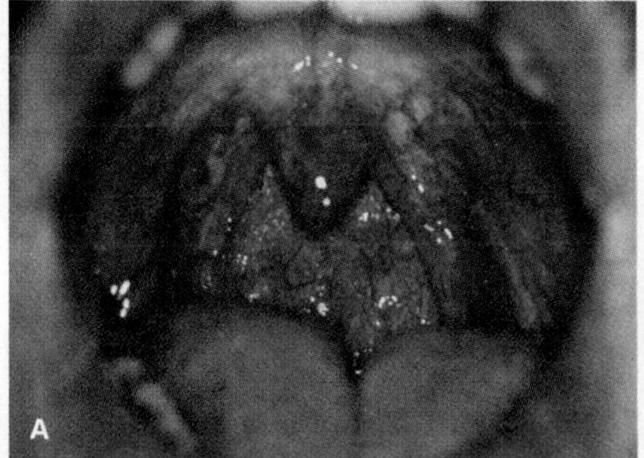

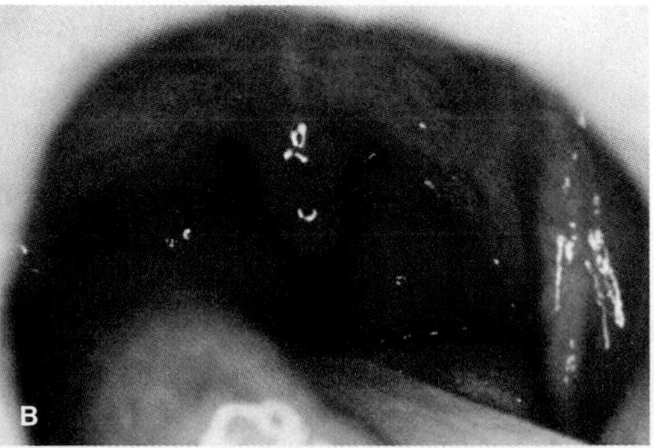

FIGURE 20•2 Pharyngitis—inflammation without exudate. (**A**) Redness and vascularity of the pillars and uvula are mild to moderate. (**B**) Redness is diffuse and intense. Each patient would probably complain of a sore throat. From Bickley, L. S., & Hoekelman, R. A. (1999). *Bates' guide to physical examination and history taking* (7th ed.). Philadelphia: Lippincott-Raven.

NUTRITIONAL THERAPY

A liquid or soft diet is provided during the acute stage of the disease, depending on the patient's appetite and the degree of discomfort with swallowing. Occasionally, the throat is so sore that liquids cannot be taken in adequate amounts by mouth. In severe situations, fluids are administered intravenously. Otherwise, the patient is encouraged to drink as much fluid as possible, at least 2 to 3 L per day.

Nursing Management

The nurse instructs the patient to stay in bed during the febrile stage of illness, to rest frequently once out of bed, and to dispose of tissues properly to prevent spreading the infection. It is important to examine the skin once or twice daily for possible rash because acute pharyngitis may precede some other communicable diseases.

Warm saline gargles or irrigations are used, depending on the severity of the lesion and the degree of pain. The benefits of this treatment depend on the degree of heat that is applied. The nurse teaches the patient about the recommended temperature of the solution—sufficiently high to be effective and as warm as the patient can tolerate, usually between 105°F and 110°F (40.6°C–43.3°C). Irrigating the throat properly is an effective means of reducing spasm in the pharyngeal muscles and relieving soreness of the throat. Unless the patient and family clearly understand the purpose of the procedure and its technique, however, the results may be less than satisfactory.

Severe sore throats also can be relieved by using an ice collar. The nurse encourages proper mouth care, which may increase the patient's comfort and prevent the development of lip fissures (cracking) and oral inflammation when bacterial infection is present. The nurse instructs the patient to resume activity gradually. A full course of antibiotic therapy is indicated in patients with hemolytic streptococcal infection in view of potential complications such as nephritis and rheumatic fever, which may occur 2 or 3 weeks after the pharyngitis subsides. The nurse instructs the patient or the family about the importance of taking the full course of therapy and about additional symptoms that indicate possible complications.

Chronic Pharyngitis

Chronic pharyngitis is common in adults who work or live in dusty surroundings, use the voice to excess, suffer from chronic cough, and habitually use alcohol and tobacco.

Three types of chronic pharyngitis are recognized:

- Hypertrophic: characterized by general thickening and congestion of the pharyngeal mucous membrane
- Atrophic: probably a late stage of the first type (the membrane is thin, whitish, glistening, and at times wrinkled)
- Chronic granular ("clergyman's sore throat"): characterized by numerous swollen lymph follicles on the pharyngeal wall

Clinical Manifestations

Patients with chronic pharyngitis complain of a constant sense of irritation or fullness in the throat; mucus, which collects in the throat and can be expelled by coughing; and difficulty swallowing.

Medical Management

The treatment of chronic pharyngitis is based on relieving symptoms, avoiding exposure to irritants, and correcting any upper respiratory, pulmonary, or cardiac condition that might be responsible for a chronic cough.

Nasal congestion may be relieved by short-term use of nasal sprays or medications containing ephedrine sulfate (Kondon's Nasal) or phenylephrine hydrochloride (Neo-Synephrine). If there is a history of allergy, one of the antihistamine decongestant medications, such as Drixoral or Dimetapp, is taken orally every 4 to 6 hours. Malaise is controlled by aspirin or acetaminophen.

Nursing Management

TEACHING PATIENTS SELF-CARE

To prevent the infection from spreading, the nurse instructs the patient to avoid contact with others until the fever subsides. Alcohol, tobacco, second-hand smoke, and exposure to cold are avoided, as are environmental or occupational pollutants if possible. The patient may minimize exposure to pollutants by wearing a disposable face mask.

The nurse encourages the patient to drink plenty of fluids. Gargling with warm saline solutions may relieve throat discomfort, and lozenges keep the throat moistened.

Tonsillitis and Adenoiditis

The tonsils are composed of lymphatic tissue and are situated on each side of the oropharynx. They frequently are the site of acute infection (tonsillitis). Chronic tonsillitis is less common and may be mistaken for other disorders, such as allergy, asthma, and sinusitis.

The adenoids consist of an abnormally large lymphoid tissue mass near the center of the posterior wall of the nasopharynx. Infection of the adenoids (adenoiditis) frequently accompanies acute tonsillitis. Group A streptococci are the most common organisms associated with tonsillitis and adenoiditis.

Clinical Manifestations

The symptoms of tonsillitis include sore throat, fever, snoring, and difficulty swallowing. Enlarged adenoids may cause mouth-breathing, earache, draining ears, frequent colds, bronchitis, foul-smelling breath, voice impairment, and noisy respiration. Unusually enlarged adenoids may cause nasal obstruction. Infection can extend to the middle ears by way of the auditory (eustachian) tubes and may result in acute otitis media, which can lead to spontaneous rupture of the eardrums and further extension of the infection into the mastoid cells, causing acute mastoiditis. The infection also may reside in the middle ear as a chronic, low-grade, smoldering process that eventually may cause permanent deafness.

Assessment and Diagnostic Findings

A thorough physical examination and a careful history are needed to rule out related or systemic conditions. The tonsillar site is cultured to determine the presence of bacterial infection. In adenoiditis, if recurrent episodes of suppurative otitis media result in hearing loss, a comprehensive audiometric examination is performed (see Chap. 55).

Medical Management

Tonsillectomy is usually performed for recurrent tonsillitis when conservative or symptomatic therapy is unsuccessful and when severe hypertrophy or peritonsillar abscess occludes the pharynx, making swallowing difficult and endangering the airway. Enlargement of the tonsils is rarely an indication for their removal; most children normally have large tonsils, which decrease in size with age. Despite the continuing debate over the effectiveness of tonsillectomy, it is still commonly performed in the United States.

Tonsillectomy or adenoidectomy is indicated for repeated bouts of tonsillitis, hypertrophy of the tonsils and adenoids that could cause obstruction and obstructive sleep apnea, repeated attacks of purulent otitis media, suspected hearing loss from serous otitis media associated with enlarged tonsils and adenoids, and other conditions such as rheumatic fever or exacerbation of asthma. Appropriate antibiotic therapy is initiated for patients undergoing tonsillectomy or adenoidectomy. The most common antimicrobial agent is oral penicillin, which is taken for 7 days; amoxicillin and erythromycin are alternatives.

Nursing Management

PROVIDING POSTOPERATIVE CARE

Continuous nursing observation is required in the immediate postoperative and recovery period because of the significant risk of hemorrhage. In the immediate postoperative period, the most comfortable position for the patient is prone with the head turned to the side to allow drainage from the mouth and pharynx. The nurse must not remove the oral airway until the patient demonstrates that the swallowing reflex has returned. The nurse applies an ice collar to the neck and provides a basin and tissues for the expectoration of blood and mucus.

Bleeding may be bright red if the patient expectorates blood without first swallowing it. Often, however, the patient swallows the blood, which immediately turns brown because of the action of the acidic gastric juice.

Hemorrhage is a potential complication after a tonsillectomy and adenoidectomy. If the patient vomits large amounts of altered blood or bright-red blood at frequent intervals, or if the pulse rate and temperature rise and the patient is restless, the nurse must notify the surgeon immediately. The nurse should have the following items ready for examination of the surgical site for bleeding: a light, a mirror, gauze, curved hemostats, and a waste basin.

Occasionally, suture or ligation of the bleeding vessel may be required. In such cases, the patient is taken to the operating room and given general anesthesia. After ligation, continuous nursing observation and postoperative care are required, as in the initial postoperative period.

If there is no bleeding, the nurse can give water and ice chips to the patient as soon as desired. It is important to instruct the patient to refrain from too much talking and coughing because they can produce throat pain.

TEACHING PATIENTS SELF-CARE

Tonsillectomy or adenoidectomy generally does not require hospitalization and is performed as outpatient surgery with a short length of stay. Because the patient will be sent home soon after surgery, it is critical that the patient and family understand the signs and symptoms of hemorrhage. If hemorrhage occurs, it usually does so in the first 12 to 24 hours. The nurse instructs the patient and family to report any bleeding to the physician.

Alkaline mouthwashes and warm saline solutions are useful in coping with the thick mucus and halitosis that may occur after tonsillectomy. It is important to explain to the patient that a sore throat, stiff neck, and vomiting may occur in the first 24 hours. A liquid or semiliquid diet is given for several days. Sherbet and gelatin are acceptable foods. The patient should avoid spicy, hot, cold, acidic, or rough foods. Milk and milk products (ice cream and yogurt) may be restricted because they tend to increase the amount of mucus in some people.

Peritonsillar Abscess

Peritonsillar abscess develops above the tonsil in the tissues of the anterior pillar and soft palate. As a rule, it occurs several days after an acute tonsillar infection and usually is caused by group A streptococci.

Clinical Manifestations

The usual symptoms of an infection are present, together with such local symptoms as **dysphagia** (difficulty in swallowing anything other than liquids), thickening of the voice, drooling, and local pain. An examination shows marked swelling of the soft palate, often partially obstructing the opening from the mouth into the pharynx.

Medical Management

Antibiotics (usually penicillin) are extremely effective in the control of the infection in peritonsillar abscess. If antibiotics are administered early in the course of the disease, the abscess may resolve without needing to be incised.

SURGICAL MANAGEMENT

If treatment is delayed, the abscess must be drained as soon as possible. The mucous membrane over the swelling is sprayed with a topical anesthetic and injected with a local anesthetic. Single or repeated needle aspirations are performed to decompress the abscess. The abscess may also be incised and drained. These procedures are performed best with the patient in the sitting position to make it easier to expectorate the pus and blood that accumulate in the pharynx. Almost immediate relief is experienced. Some laryngologists advocate tonsillectomy to prevent recurrence and to eliminate unsuspected asymptomatic pockets of infection.

Nursing Management

Considerable relief may be obtained by topical anesthetics and throat irrigations or the frequent use of mouthwashes or gargles, using saline or alkaline solutions at a temperature of 105°F to 110°F (40.6°C–43.3°C). The nurse instructs the patient to gargle every 1 or 2 hours for 24 to 36 hours. Liquids that are cool or at room temperature are usually well tolerated.

Laryngitis

Laryngitis, an inflammation of the larynx, often occurs as a result of voice abuse or exposure to dust, chemicals, smoke, and other pollutants, or as part of an upper respiratory tract infection. It also may be caused by isolated infection involving only the vocal cords.

The cause of this inflammation is almost always a virus. Bacterial invasion may be secondary. Laryngitis is usually associated with allergic rhinitis or nasopharyngitis. The onset of infection may be associated with exposure to sudden temperature changes, dietary deficiencies, malnutrition, and lack of immunity. Laryngitis is common in the winter and is easily transmitted.

Clinical Manifestations

Signs of acute laryngitis include hoarseness or **aphonia** (complete loss of voice) and severe cough. Chronic laryngitis is marked by persistent hoarseness. Laryngitis may be a complication of chronic sinusitis and chronic bronchitis.

Medical Management

Management of acute laryngitis includes resting the voice, avoiding smoking, resting, and inhaling cool steam or an aerosol. If the laryngitis is part of a more extensive respiratory infection due to a bacterial organism or if it is severe, appropriate antibacterial therapy is instituted. Most patients recover with conservative treatment; however, laryngitis tends to be more severe in elderly patients and may be complicated by pneumonia.

For chronic laryngitis, the treatment includes resting the voice, eliminating any primary respiratory tract infection, and eliminating smoking. The use of topical corticosteroids, such as beclomethasone dipropionate (Vanceril) inhalation, may also be used. These preparations have no systemic or long-lasting effects if used as recommended and may reduce local inflammatory reactions.

Nursing Management

The nurse instructs the patient to rest the voice and to maintain a well-humidified environment. If laryngeal secretions are present during acute episodes, expectorants and a daily fluid intake of 3 L are suggested to thin secretions.

NURSING PROCESS: THE PATIENT WITH UPPER AIRWAY INFECTION

Assessment

A health history reveals possible signs and symptoms of headache, sore throat, pain around the eyes and on either side of the nose, difficulty swallowing, cough, hoarseness, fever, stuffiness, and generalized discomfort and fatigue. Determining when the symptoms began, what precipitated them, what if anything relieves them, and what aggravates them is part of the assessment. It also is important to determine any history of allergy or the existence of a concomitant illness.

Inspection may reveal swelling, lesions, or asymmetry of the nose as well as bleeding or discharge. The nurse inspects the nasal mucosa for abnormal findings such as redness, swelling, or exudate and nasal polyps, which may develop in chronic rhinitis.

The nurse palpates the frontal and maxillary sinuses for tenderness, which suggests inflammation, and then inspects the throat by having the patient open the mouth wide and take a deep breath. The tonsils and pharynx are inspected for abnormal findings, such as redness, asymmetry, drainage, ulceration, or enlargement.

Next the nurse palpates the trachea to determine its midline position in the neck and to identify any masses or deformities. The neck lymph nodes are palpated to detect enlargement and tenderness.

Diagnosis

Nursing Diagnoses

Based on all the assessment data, the patient's major nursing diagnoses may include the following:

- Ineffective airway clearance related to excessive secretions secondary to inflammation
- Pain related to upper airway irritation secondary to an infection
- Impaired verbal communication related to upper airway irritation secondary to infection or swelling
- Fluid volume deficit related to increased fluid loss secondary to diaphoresis associated with a fever
- Knowledge deficit regarding prevention of upper respiratory infections, treatment regimen, surgical procedure, or postoperative care

Collaborative Problems/Potential Complications

Based on assessment data, potential complications may include:

- Sepsis
- Peritonsillar abscess
- Otitis media
- Sinusitis

Planning and Goals

The major goals for the patient may include maintenance of a patent airway, relief of pain, maintenance of effective means of communication, absence of fluid volume deficit, knowledge of how to prevent upper airway infections, and absence of complications.

Nursing Interventions

Maintaining a Patent Airway

An accumulation of secretions can block the airway in patients with an upper airway infection. As a result, changes in the respiratory pattern occur, and the work of breathing required to get beyond the blockage increases. The nurse can implement several measures to loosen thick secretions or to keep the secretions moist so that they can be easily expectorated. Increasing fluid intake helps thin the mucus. Humidifying the environment with room vaporizers or inhaling steam also loosens secretions and reduces inflammation of the mucous membranes. To enhance drainage from the sinuses, the nurse instructs the patient about the best position to assume; this depends on the location of the infection or inflammation. For example, drainage for sinusitis or rhinitis is achieved in the upright position. In some conditions, topical or systemic medications, when prescribed, help to relieve nasal or throat congestion.

Promoting Comfort

Upper respiratory tract infections usually produce localized discomfort. In sinusitis, pain may occur in the area of the sinuses or may produce a general headache. In pharyngitis, laryngitis, or tonsillitis, a sore throat occurs. The nurse encourages the patient to take analgesics, such as acetaminophen with codeine, as prescribed, which will help relieve this discomfort. Other helpful measures include topical anesthetics for symptomatic relief of herpes simplex blisters (see Chart 20-1) and sore throats, hot packs to relieve the congestion of sinusitis and promote drainage, and warm water gargles or irrigations to relieve the pain of a sore throat. The nurse encourages rest to relieve the generalized discomfort and fever that accompany many upper airway conditions (especially rhinitis, pharyngitis, and laryngitis). The nurse instructs the patient in general hygiene techniques to prevent the spread of infection. For postoperative care following tonsillectomy and adenoidectomy, an ice collar may reduce swelling and decrease bleeding.

Promoting Communication

Upper airway infections may result in hoarseness or loss of speech. The nurse instructs the patient to refrain from speaking as much as possible and to communicate in writing instead, if possible. Additional strain on the vocal cords may delay return of the full voice.

Encouraging Fluid Intake

In upper airway infections, the work of breathing and the respiratory rate increase as inflammation and secretions develop. This, in turn, may increase insensible fluid loss. Fever further increases the metabolic rate, diaphoresis, and increased fluid loss.

Sore throat, malaise, and fever may interfere with a patient's willingness to eat. The nurse encourages the patient to drink 2 to 3 L of fluid per day during the acute stage of airway infection, unless contraindicated, to thin secretions and promote drainage. Liquids (hot or cold) may be soothing, depending on the illness.

Promoting Home and Community-Based Care

TEACHING PATIENTS SELF-CARE

Prevention of most upper airway infections is difficult because of the many potential causes. However, most upper respiratory infections are transmitted by hand-to-hand contact. Therefore, it is important to teach the patient and family how to minimize spread of infection to others. Other preventive strategies are identified in the checklist Managing and Preventing Upper Respiratory Infections. The nurse advises the patient to avoid exposure to others at risk for serious illness if respiratory infection is transmitted. Those at risk include elderly adults, immunosuppressed people, and those with chronic health problems.

The nurse teaches patients and their families strategies to relieve symptoms of upper respiratory infections. These include increasing the humidity level, encouraging adequate fluid intake, getting adequate rest, using warm water gargles or irrigations and topical anesthetics to relieve sore throat, and applying hot packs to relieve congestion. The nurse reinforces the need to complete the treatment regimen, particularly when antibiotics are prescribed.

CONTINUING CARE

Referral for home care is rare. However, it may be indicated for the person whose health status was compromised before the onset of the respiratory infection and for those who cannot manage self-care without assistance. In such circumstances, the home care nurse assesses the patient's respiratory status and progress in recovery. The nurse may advise elderly patients and those who would be at increased risk from a respiratory infection to consider an annual influenza vaccine. A follow-up appointment with the primary care provider may be indicated for patients with compromised health status to ensure that the respiratory infection has resolved.

Evaluation

Expected Outcomes

Expected outcomes may include:

1. Maintains a patent airway by managing secretions
   a. Reports decreased congestion
   b. Assumes best position to facilitate drainage of secretions
2. Reports feeling more comfortable
   a. Follows comfort measures: analgesics, hot packs, gargles, rest
   b. Demonstrates adequate oral hygiene
3. Demonstrates ability to communicate needs, wants, level of comfort
4. Maintains adequate fluid intake
5. Identifies strategies to prevent upper airway infections and allergic reactions
6. Demonstrates an adequate level of knowledge and performs self-care adequately
7. Becomes free of signs and symptoms of infection
   a. Exhibits normal vital signs (temperature, pulse, respiratory rate)
   b. Absence of purulent drainage
   c. Free of pain in ears, sinuses, and throat

OBSTRUCTION AND TRAUMA OF THE UPPER RESPIRATORY AIRWAY

Obstruction During Sleep

A variety of respiratory disorders are associated with sleep, the most common being sleep apnea syndrome. Sleep apnea syndrome is defined as cessation of air flow (apnea) during sleep.

Pathophysiology

Sleep apnea is classified into three types:

- Obstructive—lack of air flow due to pharyngeal occlusion
- Central—simultaneous cessation of both air flow and respiratory movements
- Mixed—a combination of central and obstructive apnea within one apneic episode

The most common type of sleep apnea syndrome, obstructive sleep apnea, will be presented here.

Clinical Manifestations

Obstructive sleep apnea usually occurs in men, especially those who are older and overweight. Cigarette smoking is a risk factor. Obstructive sleep apnea is defined as frequent and loud snoring and breathing cessation for 10 seconds or more for five episodes per hour or more, followed by awakening abruptly with a loud snort as the blood oxygen level drops. From five apneic episodes per hour to several hundred per night can occur. Other symptoms include excessive daytime sleepiness, morning headache, sore throat, intellectual deterioration, personality changes, behavioral disorders, enuresis, impotence, obesity, and complaints by the partner that the patient snores loudly or is unusually restless during sleep.

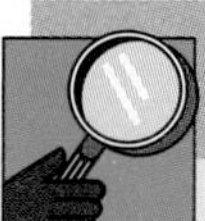

ASSESSMENT
OBSTRUCTIVE SLEEP APNEA

Clinical features of obstructive sleep apnea include:

Excessive daytime sleepiness
Frequent nocturnal awakening
Insomnia
Loud snoring
Morning headaches
Intellectual deterioration
Personality changes, irritability
Impotence
Systemic hypertension
Dysrhythmias
Pulmonary hypertension, cor pulmonale
Polycythemia

The obstruction may be caused by mechanical factors such as a reduced diameter of the upper airway or dynamic changes in the upper airway during sleep. The activity of the tonic dilator muscles of the upper airway is reduced during sleep. These sleep-related changes may predispose the patient to increased upper airway collapse with the small amounts of negative pressure generated during inspiration. Obstructive sleep apnea may be associated with obesity and with other conditions that reduce pharyngeal muscle tone (eg, neuromuscular disease, sedative/hypnotic medications, acute ingestion of alcohol). The diagnosis of sleep apnea is made based on clinical features plus polysomnographic findings (sleep test), in which the cardiopulmonary status of the patient is monitored during an episode of sleep.

The effects of obstructive sleep apnea can seriously tax the heart and lungs. Patients have a high prevalence of hypertension and an increased risk of myocardial infarction and stroke. In patients with underlying cardiovascular disease, the nocturnal hypoxemia may predispose to dysrhythmias.

Medical Management

Patients usually seek medical treatment because their partners express concern or because they experience excessive sleeplessness at inappropriate times or settings (eg, while driving a car). A variety of treatments are used. In mild cases, the patient is advised to avoid alcohol and medications that depress the upper airway and to lose weight. In more severe cases involving hypoxemia with severe CO_2 retention (hypercapnia), the treatment includes continuous positive airway pressure or bilevel positive airway pressure therapy with supplemental oxygen via nasal cannula. These treatment methods are described in Chapters 21 and 22.

Surgical procedures (eg, uvulopalatopharyngoplasty) may be performed to correct the obstruction. As a last resort, a tracheostomy is performed to bypass the obstruction if the potential for respiratory failure or life-threatening dysrhythmias exists. The tracheostomy is unplugged only during the patient's sleep. Although this is an effective treatment, it is used in a limited number of patients because of its associated physical disfigurement.

PHARMACOLOGIC THERAPY

The treatment of central sleep apnea also includes medication. Protriptyline given at bedtime is thought to increase the respiratory drive and improve upper airway muscle tone. Medroxyprogesterone acetate and acetazolamide have been recommended for sleep apnea associated with chronic alveolar hypoventilation, but their benefits have not been well established. Administration of low-flow nasal oxygen at night can help relieve hypoxemia in some patients but has little effect on the frequency or severity of apnea.

Nursing Management

The patient with obstructive sleep apnea may not recognize the potential consequences of the disorder. Therefore, the nurse explains the disorder in language that is understandable to the patient and relates symptoms (daytime sleepiness) to the underlying disorder. The nurse also instructs the patient about treatments, including the correct and safe use of oxygen, if prescribed.

Epistaxis (Nosebleed)

A hemorrhage from the nose, referred to as **epistaxis**, is caused by the rupture of tiny, distended vessels in the mucous membrane of any area of the nose. Rarely does epistaxis originate in the densely vascular tissue over the turbinates. Most commonly, the site is the anterior septum, where three major blood vessels enter the nasal cavity: (1) the anterior ethmoidal artery on the forward part of the roof (Kesselbach's plexus); (2) the sphenopalatine artery in the posterosuperior region; and (3) the internal maxillary branches (the plexus of veins located at the back of the lateral wall under the inferior turbinate).

There are a variety of causes associated with epistaxis, including trauma, infection, drugs, cardiovascular diseases, blood dyscrasias, nasal tumors, low humidity, a foreign body in the nose, and a deviated nasal septum. Vigorous nose-blowing and nose-picking have also been associated with epistaxis.

Medical Management

The management of epistaxis depends on the location of the bleeding site. A nasal speculum or headlight may be used to determine the site of bleeding in the nasal cavity. Most nosebleeds originate from the anterior portion of the nose. Initial treatment may include applying direct pressure. The patient sits upright with the head tilted forward to prevent swallowing and aspiration of blood and is directed to pinch the soft outer portion of the nose against the midline septum for 5 or 10 minutes continuously. If this measure is unsuccessful, additional treatment is indicated. In anterior nosebleeds, the area may be treated with a silver nitrate applicator and Gelfoam, or by electrocautery. Topical vasoconstrictors, such as adrenaline (1 : 1,000), cocaine (0.5%), and phenylephrine, may be prescribed.

If bleeding is from the posterior regions, cotton pledgets soaked in a vasoconstricting solution may be inserted into the nose to reduce the blood flow and improve the examiner's view of the bleeding site. Alternatively, a cotton tampon may be used to try to stop the bleeding. Suction can remove excess blood and clots from the field of inspection. The search for the bleeding site should shift from the anteroinferior quadrant to the anterosuperior, then to the posterosuperior, and finally to the posteroinferior area. The field is kept clear by suction and by shifting the

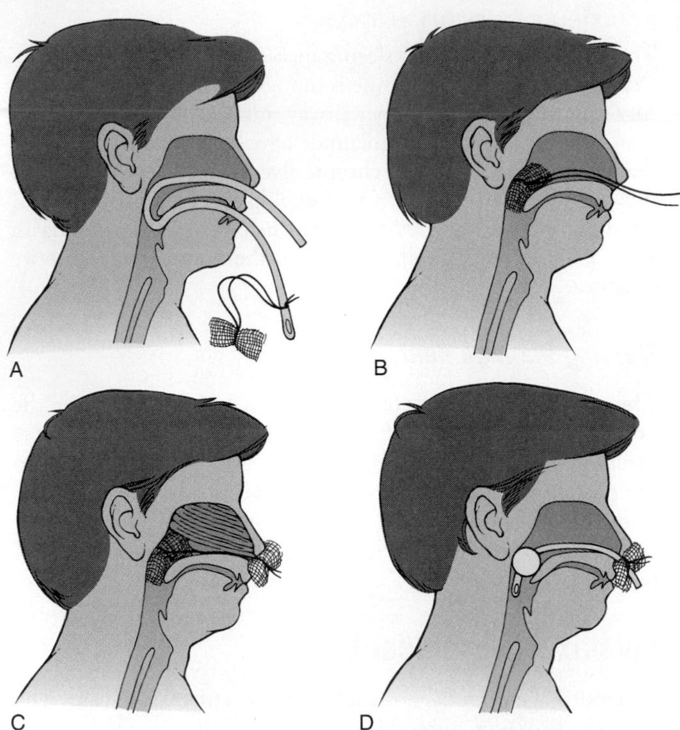

FIGURE 20•3 Packing to control bleeding from the posterior nose. (**A**) Catheter is inserted and packing is attached. (**B**) Packing is drawn into position as the catheter is removed. (**C**) Strip is tied over a bolster to hold the packing in place with an anterior pack installed "accordion pleat" style. (**D**) Alternative method, using a balloon catheter instead of gauze packing.

cotton tampons. Only about 60% of the total nasal cavity can actually be seen, however.

When the origin of the bleeding cannot be identified, the nose may be packed with gauze impregnated with petrolatum jelly or antibiotic ointment; a topical anesthetic spray and decongestant may be used before inserting the gauze packing, or a balloon-inflated catheter may be used (Fig. 20-3). The packing may remain in place for 48 hours or up to 5 or 6 days if necessary to control bleeding. Antibiotics may be given because of the risk of iatrogenic sinusitis and toxic shock syndrome.

Nursing Management

The nurse monitors the vital signs, assists in the control of bleeding, and provides tissues and an emesis basin to allow the patient to expectorate any excess blood. It is not uncommon for patients to be anxious in response to a nosebleed. Blood loss on clothing and handkerchiefs can be frightening, and the nasal examination and treatment are uncomfortable. Reassuring the patient in a calm, efficient manner that bleeding can be controlled can help reduce anxiety.

TEACHING PATIENTS SELF-CARE

Discharge teaching includes reviewing ways to prevent epistaxis: avoiding forceful nose-blowing, straining, high altitudes, and nasal trauma (including nose-picking). Adequate humidification may prevent drying of the nasal passages. In the case of a recurrent nosebleed, the nurse instructs the patient how to apply direct pressure to the nose with the thumb and the index finger for 15 minutes. If recurrent bleeding cannot be stopped, the nurse instructs the patient to seek medical attention.

Nasal Obstruction

The passage of air through the nostrils is frequently obstructed by a deviation of the nasal septum, hypertrophy of the turbinate bones, or the pressure of nasal polyps, which are grapelike swellings that arise from the mucous membrane of the sinuses, especially the ethmoids. This obstruction also may lead to a condition of chronic infection of the nose and result in frequent episodes of nasopharyngitis. Frequently, the infection extends to the sinuses of the nose (mucus-lined, air-filled cavities that drain normally into the nose). When sinusitis develops and the drainage from these cavities is obstructed by deformity or swelling within the nose, pain is experienced in the region of the affected sinus.

Medical Management

The treatment of nasal obstruction requires the removal of the obstruction, followed by measures to overcome whatever chronic infection exists. In many patients, an underlying allergy requires treatment. At times endoscopic surgery is necessary to drain the nasal sinuses. The specific procedure performed depends on the type of nasal obstruction found. Usually, surgery is performed under local anesthesia.

If a deviation of the septum is the cause of the obstruction, the surgeon makes an incision into the mucous membrane and, after raising the membrane from the bone, removes the deviated bone and cartilage with bone forceps. The mucosa then is allowed to fall back in place and is held there by tight packing. Generally, the packing is soaked in liquid petrolatum so that it can be removed easily in 24 to 36 hours. This operation is called a **submucous resection** or septoplasty.

Nasal polyps are removed by clipping them at their base with a wire snare. Hypertrophied turbinates may be treated by applying astringent to shrink them close to the side of the nose.

Nursing Management

Most of these procedures are conducted on an outpatient basis. If the patient is hospitalized, the nurse elevates the head of the bed to promote drainage and to help alleviate discomfort from edema. The nurse also encourages frequent oral hygiene to overcome dryness caused by breathing through the mouth.

Fractures of the Nose

The location of the nose makes it susceptible to injury by a wide variety of causes. In fact, the nose sustains fractures more often than any other bone in the body. Fractures of the nose usually result from direct trauma. As a rule, no serious consequences result, but the deformity that may follow often gives rise to obstruction of the nasal air passages and to facial disfigurement.

In some circumstances, more serious complications can occur. If a submucosal septal hematoma develops and is not drained, it eventually may become an abscess that destroys the septal cartilage. A saddle deformity of the nose results. Fracture of the cribriform plate may also occur with leakage of cerebrospinal fluid.

20•1 GUIDELINES FOR PERFORMING THE ABDOMINAL THRUST MANEUVER

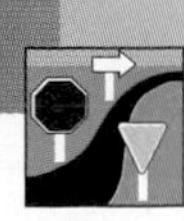

To assist a patient or other person who is choking on a foreign object, the nurse performs the abdominal thrust maneuver (sometimes called the Heimlich maneuver) according to guidelines set forth by the American Heart Association. (*Note:* Hands crossed at the neck is the universal sign for choking.)

1. Stand behind the person who is choking.
2. Place both arms around the person's waist.
3. Make a fist with one hand with the thumb outside the fist.
4. Place thumb side of fist against the person's abdomen above the navel and below the xiphoid process.
5. Grasp fist with other hand.
6. Quickly and forcefully exert pressure against the person's diaphragm, pressing upward with quick, firm thrusts.
7. Apply thrusts 6 to 10 times until the obstruction is cleared.
8. The pressure from the thrusts should lift the diaphragm, force air into the lungs, and create an artificial cough powerful enough to expel the aspirated object.

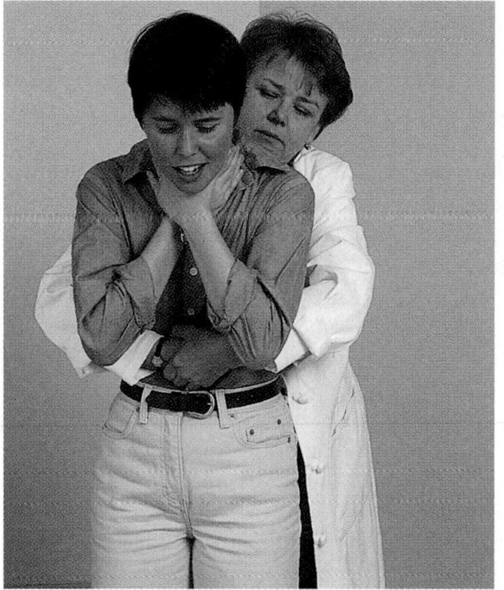

Clinical Manifestations

The signs of a nasal fracture are bleeding externally and internally into the pharynx, swelling of the soft tissues adjacent to the nose, and deformity.

Assessment and Diagnostic Findings

The nose is examined internally to rule out the possibility that the injury may be complicated by a fracture of the nasal septum and a submucosal septal hematoma. Because of the swelling and bleeding that occur with nasal fracture, an accurate diagnosis can be made only after the swelling subsides.

Clear fluid draining from either nostril suggests a fracture of the cribriform plate with leakage of cerebrospinal fluid. Because cerebrospinal fluid contains glucose, it can readily be differentiated from nasal mucus by means of a dipstick test (Dextrostix). Usually, careful inspection or palpation will disclose any deviations of the bone or disruptions of the nasal cartilages. An x-ray may reveal displacement of the fractured bones and may help rule out extension of the fracture into the skull.

Medical Management

As a rule, bleeding is controlled with the use of cold compresses. The nose is assessed for symmetry either before swelling has occurred or after it has subsided. The patient is referred to a specialist, usually 3 to 5 days after the injury, to evaluate the need to realign the bones. Nasal fractures are surgically reduced 7 to 10 days after the injury.

Nursing Management

The nurse instructs the patient to apply ice packs to the nose for 20 minutes four times a day to decrease swelling. The patient who experiences bleeding from the nose (epistaxis) because of injury or for unexplained reasons is usually frightened and anxious. The packing inserted to stop the bleeding may be uncomfortable and unpleasant, and obstruction of the nasal passages by the packing forces the patient to breathe through the mouth. This in turn causes the oral mucous membranes to become dry. Mouth rinses will help to moisten the mucous membranes and to reduce the smell and taste of dried blood in the oropharynx and nasopharynx.

Laryngeal Obstruction

Edema of the larynx is a serious, potentially fatal, condition. The larynx is a stiff box that will not stretch. It contains a narrow space between the vocal cords (glottis) through which air must pass. Therefore, swelling of the laryngeal mucous membranes may close off the opening tightly, leading to suffocation. Edema of the glottis occurs rarely in patients with acute laryngitis, occasionally in patients with urticaria, and more frequently in patients with severe inflammations of the throat, as in scarlet fever. It is an occasional cause of death in severe anaphylaxis (angioneurotic edema).

Foreign bodies (see Guideline 20-1) frequently are aspirated into the pharynx, the larynx, or the trachea and cause a twofold problem. First, they obstruct the air passages and cause difficulty in breathing, which may lead to asphyxia; later, they may be drawn farther down, entering the bronchi or a bronchial branch and causing symptoms of irritation, such as a croupy cough, expectoration of blood or mucus, or labored breathing. The physical signs and x-ray findings confirm the diagnosis.

Medical Management

When the obstruction is caused by edema resulting from an allergic reaction, treatment includes administering subcutaneous epinephrine or a corticosteroid (see Chap. 49) and applying an ice pack to the neck. In emergencies caused by obstruction by a foreign body, when the signs of asphyxia are evident, immediate treatment is necessary. Frequently, if the foreign body has lodged in the pharynx and can be visualized, it can be dislodged by the finger.

If the obstruction is in the larynx or the trachea, the nurse or other rescuer tries the subdiaphragmatic abdominal thrust maneuver. If these efforts are unsuccessful, an immediate tracheotomy is necessary.

CANCER OF THE LARYNX

Cancer of the larynx is potentially curable if detected early. It represents less than 1% of all cancers and occurs about eight times more frequently in men than in women and most commonly in people 50 to 70 years of age. The incidence of laryngeal cancer continues to decline. However, the incidence in women versus men continues to increase. Each year in the United States, approximately 10,600 new cases are discovered and 4,200 people with cancer of the larynx die (American Cancer Society, 1999).

A malignant growth may occur in three different areas of the larynx: the glottic area (vocal cords), the supraglottic area (area above the glottis, including the epiglottis and false cords), and the subglottis (area below the glottis to the cricoid). Two thirds of laryngeal cancers are in the glottic area. Supraglottic cancers account for approximately one third of the cases, subglottic tumors for less than 1%.

Clinical Manifestations

Hoarseness is noted early in the patient with cancer in the glottic area because the tumor impedes the action of the vocal cords during speech. The voice may sound harsh and lower in pitch. Affected voice sounds are not early signs of subglottic or supraglottic cancer; however, the patient may complain of pain and burning in the throat when drinking hot liquids and citrus juices. A lump may be felt in the neck. Later symptoms include difficulty swallowing or breathing (dyspnea), unilateral nasal obstruction or discharge, persistent hoarseness, persistent ulceration, and foul breath. Cervical lymphadenopathy, weight loss, a general debilitated state, and pain radiating to the ear may occur with metastasis.

Assessment and Diagnostic Findings

An initial assessment includes a complete history and physical examination of the head and neck. An indirect laryngoscopy initially is performed in the physician's office to evaluate the pharynx, larynx, and possible tumor. A direct laryngoscopic examination under local or general anesthesia is the primary method for evaluating all areas of the larynx. Samples of the suspicious tissue are obtained for histologic evaluation. The growth may involve any of the three areas of the larynx and may vary in appearance.

Risk Factors for
LARYNGEAL CANCER

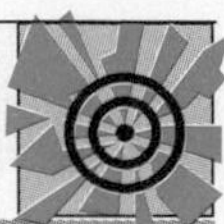

Carcinogens
Tobacco (smoke, smokeless)
Combined effects of alcohol and tobacco
Exposure to asbestos
Mustard gas
Wood dust
Cement dust
Tar products
Leather and metals

Other Factors
Straining the voice
Chronic laryngitis
Nutritional deficiencies (riboflavin)
Familial predisposition

Other diagnostic tests, including computed tomography and magnetic resonance imaging, may be used to assess regional adenopathy and soft tissue. Positron emission tomography scanning may be used to detect recurrence of a laryngeal tumor after treatment. Squamous cell carcinoma accounts for more than 90% of the cases of laryngeal carcinoma.

The TNM classification system developed by the American Joint Committee on Cancer is the accepted method used to classify tumors. The classification of the tumor determines the suggested treatment modalities. Because many of these lesions are submucosal, biopsy may require that an incision be made using microlaryngeal techniques or a CO_2 laser to transect the mucosa and reach the tumor.

It is important to assess the mobility of the vocal cords; if normal movement is limited, the growth may affect muscle, other tissue, and even the airway. The examiner palpates the lymph nodes of the neck and the thyroid gland for masses that may indicate spread of the malignancy.

Medical Management

Treatment of laryngeal cancer depends on the location, size, and histology of the tumor and cervical lymph node involvement. Treatment options include radiation therapy, chemotherapy, and surgery. Radiation therapy and surgery are both effective methods in the early stages. Chemotherapy may be used in conjunction with either radiation therapy or surgery. A complete dental examination is completed to rule out any oral disease. Any dental problems are resolved, if possible, before surgery. If surgery is to be

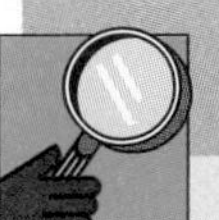

ASSESSING TUMOR STAGE: THE TNM CLASSIFICATION SYSTEM

In tumors that are staged and graded by the TNM system, the following factors are assessed:

T (tumor), or extent of the primary tumor
N (node), or location and extent of nodal involvement
M (metastasis), or spread of the tumor outside the site of origin

performed, a multidisciplinary team evaluates the needs of the patient and family to develop an effective plan of care.

RADIATION THERAPY

The goal of radiation therapy is to eradicate the cancer and preserve the function of the larynx. The decision to use radiation therapy is based on several factors: the stage of the tumor (usually for stage 1 and stage 2 tumors), the overall health status of the patient, the patient's lifestyle (including occupation), and the patient's preference. Excellent results have been achieved with radiation therapy in patients with early-stage glottic tumors when only one vocal cord is involved and there is normal mobility (ie, the cord moves with phonation). One advantage of radiation therapy is that patients retain a nearly normal voice. A few develop chondritis (inflammation of the cartilage) or stenosis; a few later require **laryngectomy** (surgical removal of some or all of the larynx).

Radiation therapy also may be used preoperatively to reduce the tumor size. Radiation therapy may be combined with surgery in advanced stages of laryngeal cancer, as adjunctive therapy to surgery or chemotherapy, and as a palliative measure. There are a variety of investigational protocols that combine chemotherapy and radiation therapy in the treatment of advanced laryngeal tumors. Early studies suggest that combined modality therapy may improve the tumor's response to radiation therapy. Radiation therapy combined with chemotherapy may be an alternative to a total laryngectomy.

The complications from radiation therapy may include acute mucositis, ulceration of the mucous membranes, pain, **xerostomia** (dry mouth), loss of taste, increased difficulty in swallowing and eating, fatigue, and skin reactions. Later complications may include laryngeal necrosis, edema and fibrosis.

SURGICAL MANAGEMENT

Recent advances in surgical techniques for the treatment of laryngeal cancer may minimize cosmetic and functional deficits. Depending on the location and staging of the tumor, four different types of surgery are considered:

- Partial laryngectomy
- Supraglottic laryngectomy
- Hemilaryngectomy
- Total laryngectomy

Some microlaryngeal surgery can be performed endoscopically. The CO_2 laser can be used to treat many laryngeal tumors, with the exception of large vascular tumors.

Partial Laryngectomy.

A partial laryngectomy (laryngofissure–thyrotomy) is recommended in the early stages of cancer in the glottic area when only one vocal cord is involved. The surgery is associated with a very high cure rate. A portion of the larynx is removed, along with one vocal cord or the tumor; all other structures remain. The airway remains intact and the patient should have no difficulty swallowing. The patient's voice quality may change, or the patient may be hoarse.

Supraglottic Laryngectomy.

A supraglottic laryngectomy is indicated in the management of early supraglottic tumors. The hyoid bone, glottis, and false cords are removed. The true vocal cords, cricoid cartilage, and trachea remain intact. During surgery, a radical neck dissection is performed on the involved side. A tracheostomy tube (see Chap. 22) is left in the trachea until the glottic airway is established. It is usually removed after a few days, and the stoma is allowed to close. Nutrition is provided through a nasogastric tube initially, followed by a semisolid diet. Postoperatively, the patient may have some difficulty swallowing for the first 2 weeks. Aspiration is a potential complication since the patient must learn a new method of swallowing (supraglottic swallowing). The chief advantage of this surgical approach is that it preserves the voice, even though the quality of the voice may change. Speech therapy is required before and after surgery. The major problem is recurrence of the cancer; therefore, patients are selected carefully.

Hemilaryngectomy.

A hemilaryngectomy is performed when the tumor extends beyond the vocal cord but is less than 1 cm and is limited to the subglottic area. In this procedure, the thyroid cartilage of the larynx is split in the midline of the neck and the portion of the vocal cord (one true cord and one false cord) is removed with the tumor. The arytenoid cartilage and half of the thyroid are also removed. The patient will have a tracheostomy tube and nasogastric tube in place after surgery for 10 to 14 days. The patient is at risk for aspiration after surgery. Some change may occur in the voice quality. The voice may be rough, raspy, and hoarse and have limited projection. The airway and the ability to swallow remain intact.

Total Laryngectomy.

A total laryngectomy is performed for cancer that extends beyond the vocal cords or for recurrent or persistent cancer following radiation therapy. In a total laryngectomy, the laryngeal structures are removed, including the hyoid bone, epiglottis, cricoid cartilage, and two or three rings of the trachea. The tongue, pharyngeal walls, and trachea are preserved. A total laryngectomy will result in the permanent loss of the voice and a change in the airway.

Many surgeons recommend that a radical neck dissection be performed on the same side as the lesion even if no lymph nodes are palpable, because metastases to the cervical lymph nodes are common. Surgery is more difficult when a lesion involves the midline structures or both vocal cords. With or without neck dissection, a total laryngectomy requires a permanent tracheal stoma because the larynx that provides the protective sphincter is no longer present. The tracheal stoma prevents the aspiration of food and fluid into the lower respiratory tract. The patient will have no voice, but will have normal swallowing. A total laryngectomy changes the manner in which airflow is used for breathing and speaking (Fig. 20-4). Complications that may occur include infection, wound breakdown, pharyngocutaneous fistula, stomal stenosis, and dysphagia secondary to pharyngeal and cervical esophageal stricture.

SPEECH THERAPY

The loss or alteration of speech is discussed before surgery with the patient and family, and the speech therapist conducts a preoperative evaluation. During this time, the nurse should inform the patient and family about methods of communication that will be available in the immediate postoperative period. These include writing, lip-speaking, and communication or word boards. A system of communication is established with the patient, family, nurse, and physician and implemented consistently after surgery.

A postoperative rehabilitation plan also is developed. The three most common techniques of **alaryngeal communication** are esophageal speech, artificial larynx (electrolarynx), and tracheoesophageal puncture. Training in these techniques begins once medical clearance is obtained from the physician.

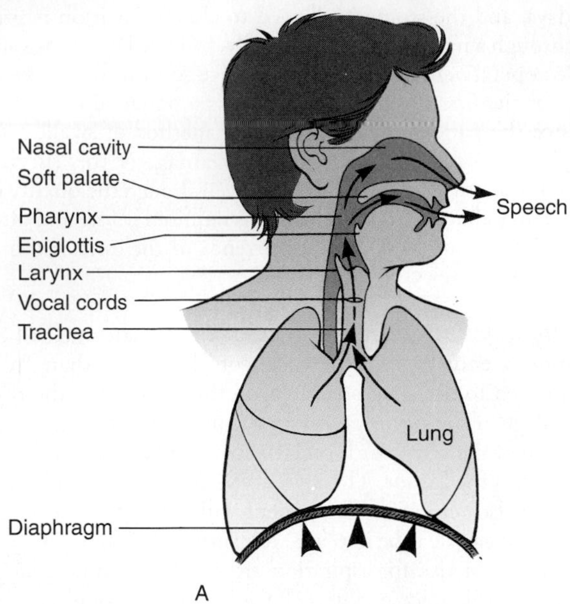

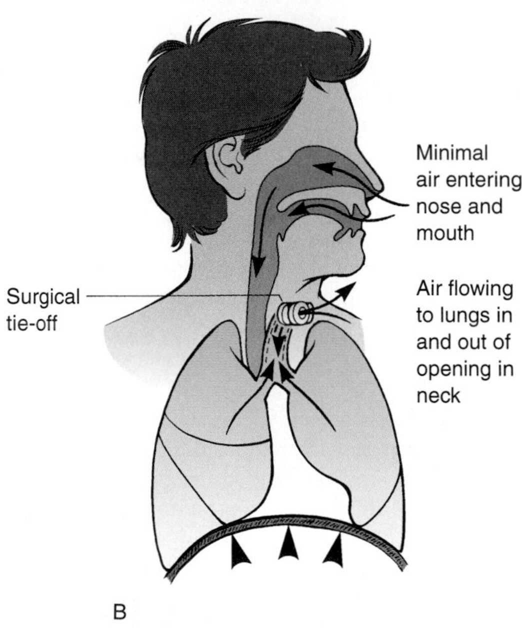

FIGURE 20•4 Laryngectomy requires a change in airflow for breathing and speaking. (**A**) Normal airflow. (**B**) Airflow after total laryngectomy.

Esophageal Speech. Esophageal speech was the primary method of alaryngeal speech taught to patients until the 1980s. The patient needs the ability to compress air into the esophagus and expel it, setting off a vibration of the pharyngeal esophageal segment. The technique can be taught once the patient begins oral feedings or 1 week after surgery. First, the patient learns to belch and is reminded to do so an hour after eating. Then the technique is practiced repeatedly. Later, this conscious belching action is transformed into simple explosions of air from the esophagus for speech purposes. Thereafter, the speech therapist works with the patient in an attempt to make speech intelligible and as close to normal as possible. Because it takes a long time to become proficient in esophageal speech, the success rate is low.

Electric Larynx. If esophageal speech is not successful, or until the technique is mastered, an electric larynx may be used for communication. This battery-powered apparatus projects sound into the oral cavity. When words are formed by the mouth (articulated), the sound from the electric larynx becomes audible words. The voice that is produced sounds mechanical, and some words may be difficult to distinguish. The advantage to patients is that they are able to communicate with relative ease while working to become proficient at either esophageal speech or tracheoesophageal puncture speech.

Tracheoesophageal Puncture. The third technique of alaryngeal speech is tracheoesophageal puncture (Fig. 20-5). This technique is the most widely used because speech associated with it most resembles normal speech and is easily learned. A valve is placed in the tracheal stoma to divert air into the esophagus and out the mouth. The sound produced is a combination of esophageal speech and voice. Once the puncture is surgically created and has healed, a voice prosthesis (Blom–Singer) is fitted through the puncture site between the anterior and posterior walls of the esophagus. The one-way valve allows air into the esophagus but prevents liquids from getting into the trachea. To prevent airway obstruction, the prosthesis is removed and cleaned when mucus builds up. A speech therapist teaches the patient how to produce sounds, but the speech is produced just as it was before surgery. Esophageal speech is created by moving the tongue and lips to form the sound into words, occluding the stoma, redirecting air from the trachea through the esophagus, and forcefully exhaling. Tracheoesophageal speech is successful in 80% to 90% of patients.

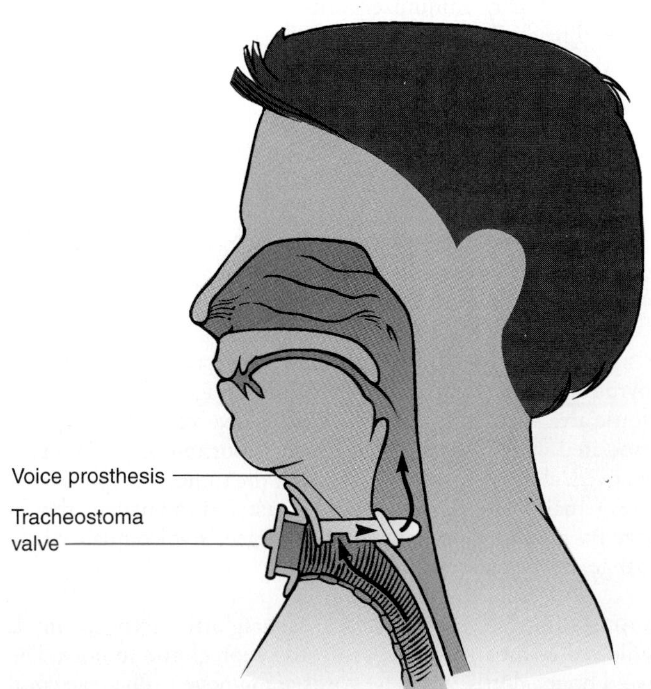

FIGURE 20•5 Schematic representation of tracheoesophageal puncture speech (TEP). Air travels from the lung through a puncture in the posterior wall of the trachea into the esophagus and out the mouth. A voice prosthesis is fitted over the puncture site.

NURSING PROCESS: THE PATIENT UNDERGOING LARYNGECTOMY

Assessment

The nurse assesses the patient for the following symptoms: hoarseness, sore throat, dyspnea, dysphagia, or pain and burning in the throat. The nurse palpates the patient's neck for swelling.

If treatment includes surgery, the nurse needs to know the nature of the surgery to plan appropriate care. If the patient is expected to have no voice, a preoperative evaluation by the speech therapist is indicated. The patient's ability to hear, see, read, and write is assessed because visual impairment and functional illiteracy may create additional problems with communication and require creative approaches to be sure that the patient can communicate after surgery. The nurse also assesses the psychological status and coping strategies of the patient and family before and after surgery.

Diagnosis

Nursing Diagnoses

Based on all the assessment data, major nursing diagnoses may include the following:

- Knowledge deficit about the surgical procedure and postoperative course
- Anxiety related to the diagnosis of cancer and impending surgery
- Ineffective airway clearance related to surgical alterations in the airway
- Impaired verbal communication related to removal of the larynx and to edema
- Altered nutrition: less than body requirements, related to swallowing difficulties
- Disturbance in body image, self-concept, and self-esteem related to major neck surgery
- Self-care deficit related to postoperative care
- Potential for noncompliance with rehabilitation program and home maintenance management

Collaborative Problems/Potential Complications

Based on assessment data, potential complications that may develop include:

- Respiratory distress (hypoxia, airway obstruction, tracheal edema)
- Hemorrhage
- Infection
- Wound breakdown

Planning and Goals

The major goals for the patient may include attainment of an adequate level of knowledge, reduction in anxiety, maintenance of a patent airway (patient is able to handle own secretions), effective use of alternative means of communication, attainment of optimal levels of nutrition and hydration, improvement in body image and self-esteem, adherence to rehabilitation program, home maintenance management, and absence of complications.

Nursing Interventions

Teaching the Patient Preoperatively

The diagnosis of laryngeal cancer is associated with misconceptions and fears. Many people assume that loss of speech and disfigurement are inevitable with this condition. Once the physician explains the diagnosis to the patient, the nurse clarifies any misconceptions by identifying the location of the larynx, its function, the nature of the surgical procedure, and its effect on the patient's speech. Informational materials (written and audiovisual) about the surgery are given to the patient and family for review and reinforcement.

If a complete laryngectomy is planned, the patient should know that the natural voice will be lost, but that special training can provide a means for communicating. However, the ability to sing, laugh, or whistle will be lost. Until this training is initiated, the patient needs to know that communication will be possible by using the call light or special communication board and by writing. The nurse answers questions about the nature of the surgery and reinforces the physician's explanation that the patient will lose the ability to vocalize, but that a rehabilitation program is available. The multidisciplinary team conducts an initial assessment of the patient and family. The team might include the nurse, physician, respiratory therapist, speech therapist, clinical nurse specialist, social worker, dietitian, and home care nurse.

Next, the nurse reviews equipment and treatments for postoperative care with the patient and family, teaches important coughing and deep-breathing exercises, and assists the patient to perform a return demonstration. The nurse clarifies the patient's role in the postoperative and rehabilitation periods.

Reducing Anxiety and Depression

Because surgery of the larynx is performed most commonly for a tumor that is malignant, the patient may have many questions: Will the surgeon be able to remove all of the tumor? Is it cancer? Will I die? Will I choke? Will I suffocate? Will I ever speak again? What will I look like? The psychological preparation of the patient is as important as the physical preparation.

Any patient undergoing surgery may have many fears. In laryngeal surgery, these fears may relate to the diagnosis of cancer and may be compounded by the possibility for permanent loss of one's voice and disfigurement. The nurse provides the patient and family with opportunities to ask questions, verbalize feelings, and share perceptions. It is important to address any questions and misconceptions the patient and family have. During the preoperative or postoperative period, a visit from someone who has had a laryngectomy may reassure the patient that people are available to help and that successful rehabilitation is possible.

Maintaining a Patent Airway

The nurse promotes a patent airway by positioning the patient in the semi-Fowler's or Fowler's position after recovery from anesthesia. Observing the patient for restlessness, labored breathing, apprehension, and increased pulse rate helps the nurse identify possible respiratory or circulatory problems. Medications that depress respiration, particularly opioids, should be used cautiously. As with other surgical patients, the nurse encourages the laryngectomy patient to turn, cough, and take deep breaths. If necessary, suctioning may be performed to remove secretions. The nurse also encourages and assists the patient with early ambulation to prevent atelectasis and pneumonia.

If a total laryngectomy was performed, a laryngectomy tube will most likely be in place. (In some instances a laryngectomy tube is not used; in others it is used temporarily, and in many it is used permanently.) The laryngectomy tube, which is shorter than a tracheostomy tube but has a larger diameter, is the patient's only airway. The care of this tube is the same as for a tracheostomy tube (see Chap. 22). The nurse cleans the stoma daily with saline solution or another prescribed solution. If a non–oil-based antibiotic ointment is prescribed, the nurse applies it around the stoma and suture line. If crusting appears around the stoma, the nurse removes the crusts with sterile tweezers and applies additional ointment.

Wound drains may be in place to assist in removal of fluid and air from the surgical site. Suction also may be used, but cautiously, to avoid trauma to the surgical site and incision. The nurse observes, measures, and records drainage. When drainage is less than 50 to 60 mL/day, the physician usually removes the drains.

Frequently, the patient coughs up rather large amounts of mucus through this opening. Because air passes directly into the trachea without being warmed and moistened by the upper respiratory mucosa, the tracheobronchial tree compensates by secreting excessive amounts of mucus. Therefore, the patient will have frequent coughing episodes and may develop a brassy-sounding, mucus-producing cough. The nurse should reassure the patient that these problems will diminish in time as the tracheobronchial mucosa adapts to the altered physiology.

After the patient coughs, the tracheostomy opening must be wiped clean and clear of mucus. A simple gauze dressing, washcloth, or even paper towel (because of its size and absorbency) worn below the tracheostomy may serve as a barrier to protect the clothing from the copious mucus that the patient may expel initially.

One of the most important factors in decreasing cough and mucus production, as well as crusting around the stoma, is adequate humidification of the environment. Mechanical humidifiers and aerosol generators (nebulizers) increase the humidity and are important for the patient's comfort.

The laryngectomy tube may be removed when the stoma is well healed, within 3 to 6 weeks after surgery. Until the tube is removed, the nurse can teach the patient how to clean and change the tube (see Chap. 22) and remove secretions.

Promoting Alternative Communication Methods

Understanding the patient's postoperative needs is critical. Alternative means of communication are established and used consistently by all personnel who come in contact with the patient—for example, a call bell or hand bell may be placed within easy reach of the patient. Because a Magic Slate often is used for communication, the nurse can document which hand the patient uses for writing so that the opposite arm can be used for intravenous infusions. (The nurse should be sure to discard any old notes used for communication to ensure the patient's privacy.) If the patient cannot write, a picture-word-phrase board or hand signals can be used. Preoperatively, the nurse reviews the system of communication to be used postoperatively with the patient.

Because it is very time-consuming to have to write everything or communicate through gestures, the inability to speak can be very frustrating. The patient may become impatient and angry when not understood. In such cases, other staff members need to be alert to the problem and also recognize that the patient will be unable to use the intercom system.

The return of communication is generally the ultimate goal in the rehabilitation of the laryngectomy patient. The nurse works with the patient, speech therapist, and family to encourage use of alternative communication methods.

Promoting Adequate Nutrition

Postoperatively, the patient may not be permitted to eat or drink for 10 to 14 days. Alternative sources of nutrition and hydration include intravenous fluids, enteral feedings through a nasogastric tube, and total parenteral nutrition.

Once the patient is ready to start oral feedings, the nurse explains to the patient that thick liquids will be used first because they are easy to swallow. The nurse instructs the patient to avoid sweet foods, which increase salivation and suppress the appetite. Solid foods are introduced as tolerated. The nurse instructs the patient to rinse the mouth with warm water or mouthwash and to brush the teeth frequently.

The patient can expect to have a diminished sense of taste and smell for a period of time after surgery. Inhaled air passes directly into the trachea, bypassing the nose and the olfactory end organs. Because taste and smell are so closely connected, taste sensations are altered. In time, however, the patient usually accommodates to this problem and olfactory sensation adapts, often with return of interest in eating. The nurse observes the patient for any difficulty swallowing, particularly when eating resumes, and reports its occurrence to the physician.

Promoting Self-Esteem

Disfiguring surgery and an altered communication pattern are a threat to a patient's self-concept, self-esteem, and body image. The reaction of family members and friends is a major concern for the patient. The nurse encourages the patient to express any feelings about the changes brought about by surgery, particularly those related to fear, anger, depression, and isolation.

A positive approach is important when caring for the patient. Promoting self-care activities is part of this approach. It is important for the patient and family to begin participating in self-care activities as soon as possible. The nurse needs to be a good listener and a support to the family, especially when explaining the tubes, dressings, and drains that are in place postoperatively. Referral to a support group, such as Lost Chord or New Voice clubs (through the International Association of Laryngectomees) and I Can Cope (through the American Cancer Society), may help the patient and family deal with the changes in their lives. Groups such as Lost Chord and New Voice promote and support the rehabilitation of people who have had a laryngectomy by providing an opportunity for exchanging ideas and sharing information.

Monitoring and Managing Potential Complications

The immediate potential complications after laryngectomy include respiratory distress and hypoxia, hemorrhage, infection, and wound breakdown.

RESPIRATORY DISTRESS AND HYPOXIA

The nurse monitors the patient for signs and symptoms of respiratory distress and hypoxia, particularly restlessness, irritation, agitation, confusion, tachypnea, use of accessory muscles, and decreased oxygen saturation. Any change in the patient's respiratory status requires immediate intervention. Obstruction needs to be ruled out immediately by suctioning and having the patient cough and breathe deeply. Hypoxia and airway obstruction, if not immediately treated, are life-threatening. The nurse contacts the physician immediately if nursing measures do not improve the patient's respiratory status.

HEMORRHAGE

Bleeding at the surgical site from the drains or with tracheal suctioning may signal the occurrence of hemorrhage. The nurse should notify the surgeon of any active bleeding immediately. Bleeding may occur at a variety of sites, including the surgical site, drains, or trachea. Rupture of the carotid artery is especially dangerous. Should this occur, the nurse should apply direct pressure over the artery, summon assistance, and provide emotional support to the patient until the vessel can be ligated. It is important to monitor vital signs for changes, particularly increased pulse rate, decreased blood pressure, and rapid deep respirations. Cold, clammy, pale skin may indicate active bleeding.

INFECTION

The nurse observes for postoperative infection. Early signs of infection include an increase in temperature and pulse, a change in the type of wound drainage, or increased areas of redness or tenderness at the surgical site. Other signs include purulent drainage, odor, and increased wound drainage. The nurse reports any significant change to the surgeon.

WOUND BREAKDOWN

Wound breakdown due to infection, poor wound healing, or development of a fistula, or as a result of radiation therapy or tumor growth, can create a serious, life-threatening emergency. The carotid artery, which is close to the stoma, may rupture from erosion if the wound does not heal properly. The nurse observes the stoma area for wound breakdown, hematoma, and bleeding and reports any significant changes to the surgeon. If wound breakdown occurs, the patient must be monitored carefully and identified as being at high risk for carotid hemorrhage.

Promoting Home and Community-Based Care

TEACHING PATIENTS SELF-CARE

The nurse has an important role in the recovery and rehabilitation of the laryngectomy patient. In an effort to facilitate the patient's ability to manage self-care, discharge instruction begins as soon as the patient is able to participate. Nursing care and patient teaching in the hospital, outpatient setting, and rehabilitation or long-term care facility must take into consideration the many emotions, physical changes, and lifestyle changes experienced by the patient. In preparing the patient to go home, the nurse assesses the patient's readiness to learn and the level of knowledge about self-care management. The nurse also reassures the patient and family that most self-care management strategies can be mastered. The patient will need to learn a variety of self-care behaviors, including tracheostomy and stoma care, wound care, and oral hygiene. In addition, the nurse instructs the patient about the need for safe hygiene and recreational activities.

Tracheostomy and Stoma Care. The nurse provides specific instructions to the patient and family about what to expect from the tracheostomy and its management. The nurse teaches the patient and family caregiver to perform suctioning and emergency measures and tracheostomy and stoma care. The nurse stresses the importance of humidification at home and instructs the family to set up a humidification system before the patient returns home. In addition, the nurse cautions the patient and family that air-conditioned air may be too cool or too dry, and thus too irritating, for the patient with a new laryngectomy. (See Chap. 22 for details about tracheostomy care.)

Hygiene and Safety Measures. The nurse instructs the patient and family about safety precautions needed because of the structural changes resulting from the surgery. Special precautions are needed in the shower to prevent water from entering the stoma. Wearing a loose-fitting plastic bib over the tracheostomy or simply holding the hand over the opening is effective. Swimming is not recommended, however, because people with a laryngectomy can drown without getting their face wet. Barbers and beauticians need to be alerted so that hair sprays, loose hair, and powder do not get near the stoma, because they can block or irritate the trachea and possibly cause infection. These self-care points are summarized in the Home Care Teaching Checklist, The Patient With a Laryngectomy.

Recreation and exercise are important, and all but very strenuous exercise can be enjoyed safely. Avoidance of strenuous exercise and fatigue is important because, when tired, the patient has more difficulty speaking, which can be discouraging. Additional safety points to address include the need for the patient to wear or carry medical identification, such as a card or bracelet, to alert first-aid personnel to the special requirements for resuscitation should this need arise. When resuscitation is needed, direct mouth-to-stoma ventilation should be performed. For home emergency situations, recorded emergency messages for police, the fire department, or other rescue services can be kept near the phone to be used quickly.

The nurse instructs and encourages the patient to perform oral care on a regular basis to prevent halitosis and infection. If the patient is receiving radiation therapy, there will be a decrease in saliva, and synthetic salivas may be required. The nurse instructs the patient to drink water or sugar-free liquids throughout the day and to use a humidifier at home. Brushing the teeth or dentures and rinsing the mouth several times a day will assist in maintaining proper oral hygiene.

CONTINUING CARE

Referral for home care is an important aspect of postoperative care for the patient who has had a laryngectomy and will assist the patient and family in the transition to the home. The home care nurse assesses the patient's general health status and the ability of the patient and family to care for the stoma and tracheostomy. The nurse assesses the patient's surgical incisions, nutritional and respiratory status, and the adequacy of pain management. The nurse assesses not only for signs and symptoms of complications but also for the patient's and family's knowledge of which signs and symptoms to report to the physician. During the home visit, the nurse identifies and addresses other learning needs of the patient and family, such as adaptation to physical, lifestyle, and functional changes. It is important to assess the patient's psychological status as well. The home care nurse reinforces previous teaching and provides reassurance and support to the patient and family as needed.

The nurse encourages the person who has had a laryngectomy to have regular physical examinations and to seek advice concerning any problems related to recovery and rehabilitation,

HOME CARE TEACHING CHECKLIST: THE PATIENT WITH A LARYNGECTOMY

At the completion of the program, the patient or caregiver will be able to:	Patient	Caregiver
• Demonstrate methods to clear the airway and handle secretions	✔	✔
• Explain the rationale for maintaining adequate humidification with a humidifier or nebulizer	✔	✔
• Demonstrate how to clean the skin around the stoma and how to use ointments and tweezers to remove encrustations	✔	✔
• State the rationale for wearing a loose-fitting protective cloth at the stoma	✔	✔
• Discuss the need to avoid cold air from air conditioning to prevent irritation of the airway	✔	✔
• Demonstrate safe technique in changing the laryngectomy tube	✔	✔
• Identify the signs and symptoms of wound infection and state what to do about them	✔	✔
• Describe safety or emergency measures to implement in case of breathing difficulty or bleeding	✔	✔
• State the rationale for wearing or carrying special medical identification and ways to obtain help in an emergency	✔	✔
• Explain the importance of covering the stoma when showering or bathing	✔	✔
• Identify fluid and caloric needs	✔	✔
• Describe mouth care and discuss its importance	✔	✔
• Demonstrate alternative communication methods	✔	✔
• Identify support groups and agency resources	✔	✔
• State the need for regular check-ups and reporting of any problems immediately	✔	✔

gently reminding the patient as appropriate about scheduled appointments with the physician, speech therapist, and other health care providers.

Evaluation

Expected Outcomes

Expected outcomes may include:

1. Acquires an adequate level of knowledge, verbalizing an understanding of the surgical procedure and performing self-care adequately
2. Demonstrates less anxiety and depression
   a. Expresses a sense of hope
   b. Meets with someone from the Lost Chord or New Voice club
   c. Participates in an I Can Cope support group
3. Maintains a clear airway and handles own secretions; also demonstrates practical and correct technique involved in cleaning and changing the laryngectomy tube
4. Acquires effective communication techniques
   a. Uses assistive devices for communication (Magic Slate, call bell, picture board, sign language, lip reading, computer aids)
   b. Practices the recommendations of the speech therapist
5. Maintains balanced nutrition and adequate fluid intake
6. Exhibits improved body image, self-esteem, and self-concept
   a. Expresses feelings and concerns
   b. Participates in self-care and decision making
   c. Accepts information about support group
7. Exhibits no complications
   a. Vital signs (blood pressure, temperature, pulse, respiratory rate) normal
   b. No redness, tenderness, or purulent drainage at surgical site
   c. Demonstrates a patent airway and appropriate respirations
   d. No bleeding from surgical site and minimal bleeding from drains
   e. No wound breakdown
8. Adheres to rehabilitation and home care program
   a. Practices recommended speech therapy
   b. Demonstrates proper methods for caring for stoma and laryngectomy tube (if present)
   c. Verbalizes understanding of symptoms that require medical attention
   d. States safety measures to take in emergencies
   e. Performs oral hygiene as prescribed

Critical Thinking Exercises

1. You are caring for a patient who is scheduled for a complete laryngectomy for cancer of the larynx. In anticipating the altered speech that will result from this surgery, describe the information you would share with the patient about methods of communicating in the early postoperative period, as well as in the long term.

2. You are making the first home visit to a patient who has just been discharged from the hospital following a laryngectomy. What will be the focus of your initial home visit? What aspects of assessment and nursing management are key at this point of your patient's rehabilitation?

3. A 20-year-old college student is diagnosed with acute viral pharyngitis and possible strep throat. What assessment and treatment should the nurse anticipate? What teaching and management strategies would you discuss with the patient? Why?

4. A 26-year-old man who has been hit in the face with a baseball comes to the urgent care center for treatment for a bleeding nose. What are the initial measures you would use to stop the bleeding? What other options are available if the bleeding does not stop within a reasonable period?

References and Selected Readings

BOOKS

American Cancer Society. (1999). *Cancer facts and figures.* Atlanta: Author.

Baum, G. L. et al. (1998). *Textbook of pulmonary diseases* (6th ed., Vols. 1 & 2). Philadelphia: Lippincott Williams & Wilkins.

DeVita, V. T., Hellman, S., & Rosenberg, S. A. (1997). *Cancer: Principles and practice of oncology* (5th ed., Vol. 1). Philadelphia: Lippincott-Raven.

Fishman, A. P. et al. (1997). *Fishman's pulmonary diseases and disorders* (3rd ed., Vol. 1). New York: McGraw-Hill.

Groenwald, S. et al., (Eds.).(1997). *Cancer nursing: Principles and practice* (4th ed.). Boston: Jones & Barlett Publishers.

Mandell, G. L. (1996). *Principles and practice of infectious diseases* (4th ed.). New York: Churchill Livingstone.

Meeker, M. H., Rothrock, J. C., & Alexander, E. L. (1999). *Alexander's care of the patient in surgery* (10th ed.). St. Louis: C. V. Mosby.

Otto, S. E. (Ed.). (1997). *Oncology nursing* (3rd ed.). St. Louis: Mosby–Year Book.

Roberts, J. R., & Hedges, J. R. (1998). *Clinical procedures in emergency medicine* (3rd ed.). Philadelphia: W. B. Saunders.

Schlossberg, D. (1996). *Current therapy of infectious disease.* St. Louis: C. V. Mosby.

Schwartz, S. I. et al. (1999). *Principles of surgery* (7th ed., Vol. 1). New York: McGraw-Hill.

JOURNALS

Al-Saden, P. (1994). Anticoagulation-induced epistaxis. *Nursing '94, 24*(12), 33.

Alvi, A., & Johnson, J. T. (1995). The neck mass, a challenging diagnosis. *Postgraduate Medicine, 97*(5), 87–97.

Aust, M. R., & McCaffrey, T. V. (1997). Early speech results with Provox Prosthesis after laryngectomy. *Archives of Otolaryngology—Head and Neck Surgery, 123*(9), 966–968.

Barbarito, C. (1998). Hypertension-induced epistaxis. *American Journal of Nursing, 98*(2), 48.

Blalock, D. (1997). Speech rehabilitation after treatment of laryngeal carcinoma. *Otolaryngologic Clinics of North America, 30*(2), 179–188.

Cherny, N. I., & Foley, K. M. (1997). Nonopioid and opioid analgesic pharmacotherapy of cancer pain. *Otolaryngologic Clinics of North America, 30*(2), 281–301.

Clements, K. S., et al. (1997). Communication after laryngectomy, an assessment of patient satisfaction. *Archives of Otolaryngology—Head and Neck Surgery, 123*(5), 493–496.

Courey, M. S., & Ossoff, R. H. (1997). Laser applications in adult laryngeal surgery. *Otolaryngologic Clinics of North America, 30*(2), 973–985.

Davis, R. K. (1997). Endoscopic surgical management of glottic laryngeal cancer. *Otolaryngologic Clinics of North America, 30*(1), 79–86.

DeShazo, R. D., Chapin, K., & Swain, R. E. (1997). Current concepts, fungal sinusitis. *New England Journal of Medicine, 337*(4), 254–259.

Deutsch, E. S. (1996). Tonsillectomy and adenoidectomy: Changing indications. *Pediatric Otolaryngology, 43*(6), 1319–1338.

Ferguson, B. J. (1996). Allergic rhinitis. *Postgraduate Medicine, 101*(5), 110–116.

Forth, R. (1998). Common questions about obstructive sleep apnea. *American Journal of Nursing, 98*(2), 60–64.

Galen, B. A. (1997). Chronic recurrent sinusitis. *Lippincott's Primary Care Practice, 1*(2), 183–198.

Galen, B. A. (1997). Rhinitis. *Lippincott's Primary Care Practice, 1*(2), 129–141.

Ganley, B. J. (1995). Effective mouth care for head and neck radiation therapy patients. *MedSurg Nursing, 4*(2), 133–141.

Graft, D. F. (1996). Allergic and nonallergic rhinitis. *Postgraduate Medicine, 100*(2), 64–74.

Kaliner, M. A., et al. (1997). Sinusitis: Bench to bedside current findings, future directions. *Journal of Allergy and Clinical Immunology, 99*(6), S829–847.

Katcher, M. L. (1996). Cold, cough and allergy medications: Uses and abuses. *Pediatrics in Review, 17*(1), 12–17.

Kirkpatrick, G. L. (1996). The common cold. *Primary Care, 23*(4), 657–675.

Koufman, J. A., & Burke, A. J. (1997). The etiology and pathogenesis of laryngeal carcinoma. *Otolaryngologic Clinics of North America, 30*(1), 1–19.

Kurz, J. M. (1997). A saline solution to allergic rhinitis symptoms? *American Journal of Nursing, 97*(6), 15.

Levine, P. A., Brasnu, D. F., Ruparelia, A., & Laccourreye, O. (1997). Management of advanced-stage laryngeal cancer. *Otolaryngologic Clinics of North America, 30*(1), 101–112.

Lockey, R. F. (1996). Management of chronic sinusitis. *Hospital Practice, 31*(3), 141–155.

McQuellan, R. P., & Hurt, G. J. (1997). The psychosocial impact of the diagnosis and treatment of laryngeal cancer. *Otolaryngologic Clinics of North America, 30*(2), 231–241.

Milgrom, H., & Bender, B. (1997). Adverse effects of medications for rhinitis. *Annuals of Allergy, Asthma & Immunology, 78*(5), 439–444.

Newland, J. A. (1998). Epistaxis. *American Journal of Nursing, 98*(3), 16.

Otto, R. A., et al. (1999). Impact of a laryngectomy on quality of life: perspective of the patient versus that of the health care provider. *Annals of Otlolaryngology, Rhinology, 106*(8), 693–699.

Ruppert, S. D. (1996). Differential diagnosis of common causes of pediatric pharyngitis. *Nurse Practitioner, 21*(4), 38–48.

Smith, L. J. (1995). Diagnosis and treatment of allergic rhinitis. *Nurse Practitioner, 20*(10), 58–66.

Watt-Watson, J., & Graydon, J. (1995). Impact of surgery on head and neck cancer patients and their caregivers. *Nursing Clinics of North America, 30*(4), 659–671.

Witt, M. E. (1998). Radiation and chemotherapy as combined treatment for advanced head and neck cancer. *MedSurg Nurs, 7*(3), 159–164.

Zeitels, S. M. (1997). Surgical management of early supraglottic cancer. *Otolaryngologic Clinics of North America, 30*(1), 59–78.

Resources

American Cancer Society, 1599 Clifton Rd., NE, Atlanta, GA 30329-4251; (404) 320-3333; (800) ACS-2345; www.cancer.org

American Lung Association, 1740 Broadway, New York, NY 10019-4374; (212) 315-8700; www.lungusa.org

International Association of Laryngectomees, 7400 N. Shadeland Ave., Suite 100, Indianapolis, IN 46250, (317) 570-4568; www.larynx.com

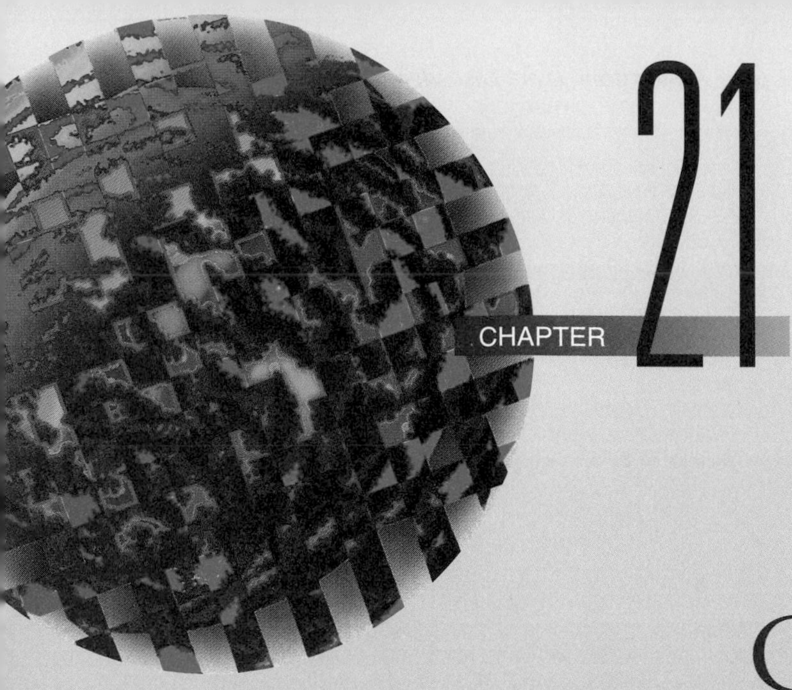

Management of Patients With Chest and Lower Respiratory Tract Disorders

Learning Objectives

On completion of this chapter, the learner will be able to:

1. Identify patients at risk for atelectasis and nursing interventions related to its prevention and management.
2. Compare the various pulmonary infections with regard to causes, clinical manifestations, nursing management, complications, and prevention.
3. Use the nursing process as a framework for care of the patient with pneumonia.
4. Relate pleurisy, pleural effusion, and empyema to pulmonary infection.
5. Describe smoking and air pollution as causes of pulmonary disease.
6. Compare and contrast chronic bronchitis, bronchiectasis, pulmonary emphysema, and asthma as chronic obstructive pulmonary diseases, and describe their relationship to pulmonary heart disease.
7. Use the nursing process as a framework for care of the patient with chronic obstructive pulmonary disease.
8. Develop a teaching plan for patients with chronic obstructive pulmonary disease.
9. Relate the therapeutic management techniques of acute respiratory distress syndrome to the underlying pathophysiology of the syndrome.
10. Describe risk factors for and measures appropriate for prevention and management of pulmonary embolism.
11. Describe preventive measures appropriate for controlling and eliminating the problem of occupational lung disease.
12. Discuss the modes of therapy and related nursing management for patients with lung cancer.
13. Describe the complications of chest trauma and their clinical manifestations and nursing management.
14. Describe nursing measures to prevent aspiration.

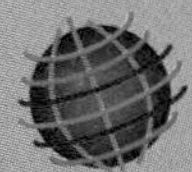

Conditions affecting the lower respiratory tract range from acute problems to long-term chronic disorders. Many of these disorders are serious and often life-threatening. The patient with a lower respiratory tract disorder requires care from nurses with astute assessment and clinical management skills as well as an understanding of the impact of the disorder on the patient's quality of life and ability to carry out usual activities of daily living. Patient and family teaching is an important nursing intervention in the management of all lower respiratory tract disorders.

GLOSSARY

acute respiratory distress syndrome (ARDS): nonspecific pulmonary response to a variety of pulmonary and nonpulmonary insults to the lung; characterized by interstitial infiltrates, alveolar hemorrhage, atelectasis, decreased compliance, and refractory hypoxemia

air trapping: incomplete emptying of alveoli during expiration due to loss of lung tissue elasticity (emphysema), bronchospasm (asthma), or airway obstruction

asbestosis: diffuse lung fibrosis resulting from exposure to asbestos fibers

atelectasis: collapse or airless condition of the alveoli caused by hypoventilation, obstruction to the airways, or compression

bronchiectasis: chronic dilation of a bronchus or bronchi; the dilated airways become saccular and are a medium for chronic infection

central cyanosis: bluish discoloration of the skin or mucous membranes due to hemoglobin carrying reduced amounts of oxygen

consolidation: lung tissue that has become more solid in nature due to collapse of alveoli or infectious process (pneumonia)

chronic obstructive pulmonary disease (COPD): disease state characterized by chronic airflow obstruction from chronic bronchitis, emphysema, or a combination of these two diseases; also known as chronic airway obstruction and chronic obstructive lung disease

cor pulmonale: "heart of the lungs"; enlargement of the right ventricle from hypertrophy or dilation or as a secondary response to disorders that affect the lungs

empyema: accumulation of purulent material in the pleural space

fine-needle aspiration: insertion of a needle through the chest wall to obtain cells of a mass or tumor; usually performed under fluoroscopy or chest CT guidance

hemoptysis: the coughing up of blood from the lower respiratory tract

induration: an abnormally hard lesion or reaction, as in a positive tuberculin skin test

nosocomial: pertaining to or originating from a hospital

open lung biopsy: biopsy of lung tissue through a limited thoracotomy

orthopnea: shortness of breath when reclining or in the supine position

pleural effusion: abnormal accumulation of fluid in the pleural space

pleural friction rub: localized grating or creaking sound caused by the rubbing together of inflamed parietal and visceral pleurae

pleural space: a potential space between the parietal and visceral pleurae

pneumothorax: partial or complete collapse of the lung due to positive pressure in the pleural space

pulmonary edema: increase in the amount of extravascular fluid in the lung

pulmonary embolism: obstruction of the pulmonary vasculature with an embolus; embolus may be due to blood clot, air bubbles, or fat droplets

purulent: consisting of, containing, or discharging pus

restrictive lung disease: disease of the lung that causes a decrease in lung volumes

spirometry: pulmonary function tests that measure specific lung volumes (eg, FEV_1, FVC) and rates ($FEF_{25-75\%}$); may be measured before and after bronchodilator administration

tension pneumothorax: pneumothorax characterized by increasing positive pressure in the pleural space with each breath; this is an emergency situation and the positive pressure needs to be decompressed or released immediately

transbronchial: through the bronchial wall, as in a transbronchial lung biopsy

ventilation–perfusion ratio: the ratio between ventilation and perfusion in the lung; matching of ventilation to perfusion optimizes gas exchange

ATELECTASIS

Atelectasis refers to closure or collapse of alveoli and often is described in relation to x-ray findings and clinical signs and symptoms. Atelectasis may be acute or chronic and may cover a broad range of pathophysiologic changes, from microatelectasis (which is not detectable on chest x-ray) to macroatelectasis with loss of segmental, lobar, or overall lung volume. The most commonly described atelectasis is acute atelectasis, which occurs frequently in the postoperative setting or in people who are immobilized and have a shallow, monotonous breathing pattern. Atelectasis also is observed in patients with a chronic airway obstruction that impedes or blocks air flow to an area of the lung (eg, obstructive atelectasis in the patient with lung cancer that is invading or compressing the airways). This type of atelectasis is more insidious and slower in onset.

Pathophysiology

Atelectasis may occur in the adult as a result of reduced alveolar ventilation or any type of blockage that impedes the passage of air to and from the alveoli that normally receive air through the bronchi and network of airways. The trapped alveolar air becomes absorbed into the bloodstream, but outside air cannot replace the absorbed air because of the blockage. As a result, the isolated portion of the lung becomes airless and shrinks. This may occur with altered breathing patterns, retained secretions, pain, alterations in small airway function, prolonged supine positioning, increased abdominal pressure, reduced lung volumes due to musculoskeletal or neurologic disorders, restrictive defects, and specific surgical procedures (eg, upper abdominal or open heart surgery). Persistent low lung volumes, secretions or a mass obstructing or impeding airflow, and compression of lung tissue may all cause collapse or obstruction of the airways, which leads to atelectasis.

The postoperative patient is at high risk for atelectasis because of the numerous respiratory changes that may occur. A monotonous low tidal breathing pattern may cause airway closure and alveolar collapse. This results from the effects of anesthesia or pain medications, supine positioning, splinting of the chest wall because of pain, and abdominal distention. The postoperative patient may also have secretion retention, airway obstruction, and an impaired cough reflex or may be reluctant to cough because of pain. Figure 21-1 shows the pathogenic mechanisms and consequences of acute atelectasis in the postoperative patient.

Atelectasis resulting from bronchial obstruction by secretions may occur in patients with impaired cough mechanisms (eg, musculoskeletal or neurologic disorders) or in debilitated, bedridden patients. Atelectasis may also result from excessive pressure on the lung tissue, which restricts normal lung expansion on inspiration. Such pressure may be produced by fluid accumulating within the pleural space (**pleural effusion**), air in the pleural space (**pneumothorax**), or blood in the pleural space (hemothorax). The **pleural space** is the area between the parietal and the visceral pleurae. Pressure may also be produced by a pericardium distended with fluid (pericardial effusion), tumor growth within the thorax, or an elevated diaphragm.

PATHOPHYSIOLOGY

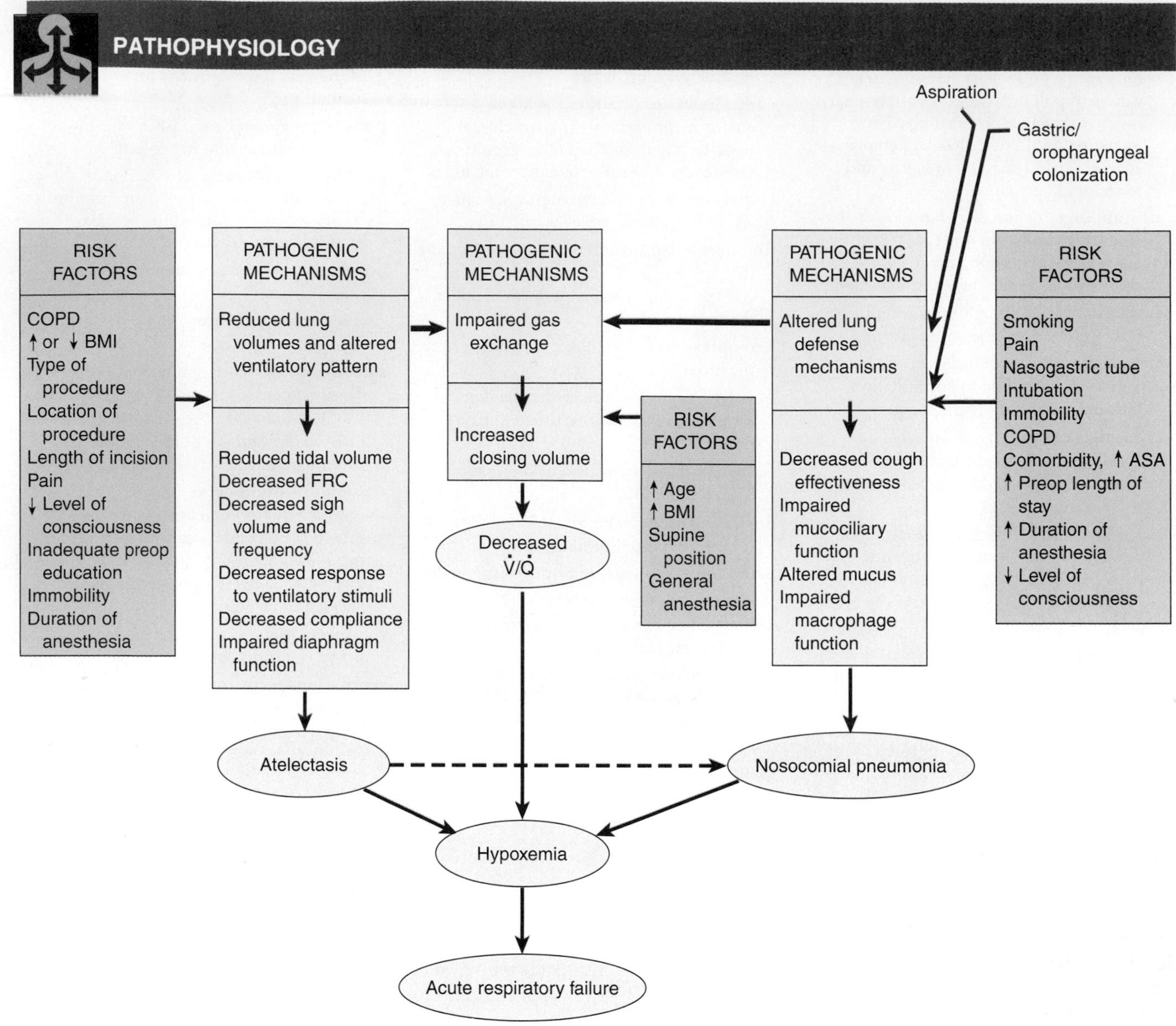

FIGURE 21•1 Relationship of risk factors, pathogenic mechanisms, and consequences of acute atelectasis in the postoperative patient. From the work of Jo Ann Brooks-Brunn, DNS, RN, FAAN, FCCP, Indiana University Medical Center, Indianapolis. COPD, chronic obstructive pulmonary disease; BMI, body mass index; FRC, functional residual capacity; diaphragm fx, diaphragm function; ASA, American Society of Anesthesiology Physical Status.

Clinical Manifestations

The development of atelectasis usually is insidious. Signs and symptoms include cough, sputum production, and low-grade fever. Fever is universally cited as a clinical sign of atelectasis, but there are few data to support this. Most likely the fever that accompanies atelectasis is due to infection/inflammation distal to the obstructed airway.

In acute atelectasis involving a large amount of lung tissue (lobar atelectasis), marked respiratory distress may be observed. In addition to the above signs and symptoms, dyspnea, tachycardia, tachypnea, pleural pain, and **central cyanosis** (a bluish skin hue that is a late sign of hypoxemia) may be anticipated. The patient characteristically has difficulty breathing in the supine position and is anxious. Signs and symptoms of chronic atelectasis are similar to those of acute atelectasis. Because the alveolar collapse is chronic, infection may occur distal to the obstruction. Thus, the signs and symptoms of a pulmonary infection also may be present.

Assessment and Diagnostic Findings

Decreased breath sounds and crackles are heard over the affected area. In addition, chest x-ray findings may reveal patchy or consolidated areas. Depending on the degree of hypoxemia, pulse oximetry (SpO_2) may demonstrate a low saturation of hemoglo-

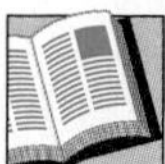

NURSING RESEARCH

Predicting Pulmonary Complications After Surgery

Brooks-Brunn, J. A. (1997). Predictors of postoperative pulmonary complications following abdominal surgery. *Chest, 111*(3), 564–571.

Purpose

Postoperative pulmonary complications are the leading cause of postoperative death and complications. Of the differing types of pulmonary complications, atelectasis and pneumonia occur frequently. The purpose of this study was to determine how risk factors could be combined to best predict the development of pulmonary complications after abdominal surgery.

Study Sample and Design

The population of interest was patients undergoing nonlaparoscopic, elective abdominal surgery. Inclusion criteria were age >18 years, anticipated hospital stay of ≤48 hours, first general anesthetic of the hospitalization, not previously a participant in the study, and able to understand the informed consent. Twenty-three risk factors were assessed, and a multicriteria outcome for postoperative pulmonary complication was used to collectively assess atelectasis and pneumonia.

The sample included 400 patients (65% female, mean age 52.5 years) who underwent abdominal surgery at four institutions. Informed consent was obtained, and patients were interviewed preoperatively and risk factors were assessed. After surgery, the patient's medical chart was reviewed for intraoperative risk factors and postoperative risk factors. Patients were visited daily after surgery. The research assistant asked a brief set of questions and performed a chest assessment.

Findings

Six risk factors were identified as independent by logistic regression techniques: age >60 years of age, impaired preoperative cognitive function, smoking history within the past 8 weeks, body mass index >27, a previous history of cancer, and an incision site that was either above the umbilicus (upper abdominal) or both above and below the umbilicus (upper and lower abdominal).

Nursing Implications

This study contributes to the increasing body of science regarding predicting outcomes, specifically postoperative pulmonary complications. Nursing plays a pivotal role in preventing or minimizing postoperative pulmonary complications. The six risk factors identified in this study are all accessible to the nurse in the preoperative or immediate postoperative setting. Although continued work is needed to develop a valid tool to be used clinically to predict postoperative pulmonary complications, the nurse should assess the patient for risk factors, develop an individualized plan of care, and intensify the postoperative respiratory interventions of "higher-risk" patients.

bin with oxygen (less than 90%) or a lower-than-normal partial pressure of arterial oxygen (PaO_2).

Prevention

Nursing measures to prevent atelectasis include frequent turning, early mobilization, and strategies to expand the lungs and to manage secretions. Deep-breathing maneuvers (at least every 2 hours) assist in preventing and treating atelectasis. The performance of these maneuvers requires a patient who is alert and cooperative. Patient education and reinforcement are key to the success of these interventions. The use of incentive spirometry or voluntary deep breathing enhances lung expansion, decreases the potential for airway closure, and may generate a cough. Secretion management techniques may include directed cough, suctioning, aerosol nebulizer treatments followed by chest physical therapy (postural drainage and chest percussion), or bronchoscopy. In some settings, a metered-dose inhaler (MDI) is used to dispense a bronchodilator rather than an aerosol nebulizer treatment. Guideline 21-1 summarizes measures to prevent atelectasis.

Management

The goal in treating the patient with atelectasis is to improve ventilation and remove secretions. The strategies to prevent atelectasis, which include frequent turning, early ambulation, lung volume expansion maneuvers (eg, deep-breathing exercises, incentive spirometry), and coughing, also serve as the first-line measures to minimize or treat atelectasis by improving ventilation. In patients who do not respond to first-line measures or who cannot perform deep-breathing exercises, other treatments such as positive expiratory pressure or PEP therapy (a simple mask and one-way valve system that provides varying amounts of expiratory resistance [usually 5 to 15 cm H_2O]; a manometer may be inserted between the valve and the resistance to measure PEP), continuous or intermittent positive pressure-breathing (IPPB), and bronchoscopy may be used. Although IPPB may be used in some settings, few data support its use in the postoperative setting (Duffy & Farley, 1993). Before initiating more complex, costly, and labor-intensive therapies, the nurse should ask several questions:

- Has the patient been given an adequate trial of deep-breathing exercises?
- Has the patient received adequate education, supervision, and coaching to carry out the deep-breathing exercises?
- Have other factors been evaluated that may impair ventilation (eg, lack of turning, mobilization; excessive pain; excessive sedation)?

If the cause of atelectasis is bronchial obstruction from secretions, the secretions must be removed by coughing or suctioning to permit air to reenter that portion of the lung. Chest physical therapy (chest percussion and postural drainage) may also be used to mobilize secretions. Nebulizer treatments with a bronchodilator medication may be used to assist in the expectoration of secretions. If respiratory care measures fail to remove the obstruction, a bronchoscopy is performed. Severe or massive atelectasis may lead to acute respiratory failure, especially in a patient with underlying lung disease. Endotracheal intubation and mechanical ventilation may be necessary. Prompt treatment reduces the risk for acute respiratory failure or pneumonia.

If atelectasis has resulted from compression of lung tissue, the goal is to decrease the compression. With a large pleural effusion that is compressing lung tissue and causing alveolar collapse, treatment may include thoracentesis, removal of the fluid by needle aspiration, or insertion of a chest tube. The measures to increase lung expansion described above also are used.

Management of chronic atelectasis focuses on removing the cause of the obstruction of the airways or the compression of the lung tissue. For example, bronchoscopy may be used to open an airway obstructed by lung cancer, and the procedure may involve cryotherapy or laser therapy. The goal is to reopen the airways and provide ventilation to the collapsed area. In some cases, surgical management may be indicated.

21•1
GUIDELINES FOR 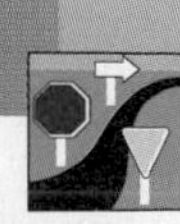 **PREVENTING ATELECTASIS**

1. Change patient's position frequently, especially from supine to upright position, to promote ventilation and prevent secretions from accumulating.
2. Encourage early mobilization from bed to chair followed by early ambulation.
3. Encourage appropriate deep breathing and coughing to mobilize secretions and prevent them from accumulating.
4. Teach/reinforce appropriate technique for incentive spirometry.
5. Administer prescribed opioids and sedatives judiciously to prevent respiratory depression.
6. Perform postural drainage and chest percussion, if indicated.
7. Institute suctioning to remove tracheobronchial secretions, if indicated.

RESPIRATORY INFECTIONS

Acute Tracheobronchitis

Acute tracheobronchitis, an acute inflammation of the mucous membranes of the trachea and the bronchial tree, often follows infection of the upper respiratory tract. A patient with a viral infection has decreased resistance and can readily develop a secondary bacterial infection. Thus, adequate treatment of upper respiratory tract infection is one of the major factors in the prevention of acute bronchitis. Aside from infection, inhalation of physical and chemical irritants, gases, and other air contaminants can also cause acute bronchial irritations.

Pathophysiology

In acute tracheobronchitis, the inflamed mucosa of the bronchi produces mucopurulent sputum, often in response to *Streptococcus pneumoniae, Haemophilus influenzae,* and *Mycoplasma pneumoniae.* In addition, a fungal infection (eg, *Aspergillus* tracheobronchitis) may also cause tracheobronchitis. A sputum culture is essential to identify the specific causative organism.

Clinical Manifestations

Initially, the patient has a dry, irritating cough and expectorates a scanty amount of mucoid sputum. The patient complains of sternal soreness from coughing and has fever or chills and night sweats, headache, and general malaise. As the infection progresses, the patient may be short of breath, inspiration and expiration may become noisy (inspiratory stridor and expiratory wheeze), and **purulent** (pus-filled) sputum may be present. With severe tracheobronchitis, blood-streaked secretions may be expectorated as a result of the irritation of the mucosa of the airways.

Medical Management

Antibiotic treatment may be indicated depending on the symptoms, sputum purulence, and results of the sputum culture. Antihistamines are usually not prescribed because they may cause excessive drying and make secretions more difficult to expectorate. Expectorants may be prescribed, although their efficacy is questionable. Fluid intake is increased to thin the viscous and tenacious secretions. Copious, purulent secretions that cannot be cleared by coughing place the patient at risk for increasing airway obstruction and the development of a more severe lower respiratory tract infection such as pneumonia. Suctioning and bronchoscopy may be needed to remove secretions. Rarely, endotracheal intubation may be required in cases of acute tracheobronchitis leading to acute respiratory failure. This may be necessary for patients who are severely debilitated or who have coexisting diseases that also impair the respiratory system.

In most cases, treatment of tracheobronchitis is largely symptomatic. The patient is advised to rest. Increasing the vapor pressure (moisture content) in the air will reduce irritation. Cool vapor therapy or steam inhalations may be beneficial in relieving the laryngeal and tracheal irritation. Moist heat to the chest may relieve the soreness and pain. Mild analgesics or antipyretics may be indicated.

Nursing Management

Acute tracheobronchitis is frequently treated in the home setting. Thus, patient teaching is a priority. A primary nursing function is to encourage bronchial hygiene, such as increasing fluid intake and directed coughing to remove secretions. The nurse should encourage and assist the patient to sit up frequently to cough effectively and to prevent retention of mucopurulent sputum. If the patient is treated with antibiotics for an underlying infection, it is important to emphasize the need to complete the full course of antibiotics prescribed. Fatigue is a consequence of tracheobronchitis; therefore, the nurse cautions the patient against overexertion, which can induce a relapse or extension of the infection.

Pneumonia

Pneumonia is an inflammation of the lung parenchyma that is caused by a microbial agent. Pneumonitis is a more general term that describes an inflammatory process in the lung tissue that may predispose a patient to or place a patient at risk for microbial invasion. Pneumonia is the most common cause of death from infectious diseases in the United States. It is the sixth leading cause of death in the United States for all ages (Ventura, Peters, Martin, & Maurer, 1997). It is treated extensively on both an inpatient and outpatient basis.

Pneumonia is caused by various microorganisms, including bacteria, mycobacteria, chlamydiae, mycoplasma, fungi, parasites, and viruses. Several systems are used to classify pneumonias. Classically, pneumonia has been categorized into one of four categories: bacterial or typical, atypical, anaerobic/cavitary, and opportunistic. However, there is overlap in the microorganisms thought to be responsible for typical and atypical pneumonias. A more widely used classification scheme categorizes the major pneumonias as community-acquired pneumonia, hospital-acquired pneumonia, pneumonia in the immunocompromised host, and aspiration pneumonia (Table 21-1). There is some overlap in how specific pneumonias are classified because they may occur in differing settings.

Community-acquired pneumonia (CAP) occurs either in the community setting or within the first 48 hours of hospitalization or institutionalization. Hospitalization for CAP depends on the severity of the pneumonia. The agents that most frequently cause CAP requiring hospitalization are *S. pneumoniae, Legionella, Pseudomonas aeruginosa,* and other gram-negative rods. The absence of a responsible caregiver in the home may be another indication for hospitalization. Of the approximately 4 million people who develop CAP each year, about 600,000 require hospitalization (Fine et al., 1996; Fine et al., 1997).

Hospital-acquired pneumonia (HAP), also known as **nosocomial** pneumonia, is defined as the onset of pneumonia symptoms more than 48 hours after admission to the hospital. HAP accounts for approximately 15% of hospital-acquired infections but is the most lethal nosocomial infection. It is estimated to occur in 0.5% to 1% of all hospitalized patients and in 15% to 20% of intensive care patients. Ventilator-associated pneumonia can be considered a type of nosocomial pneumonia that is associated with endotracheal intubation and mechanical ventilation.

The immunocompromised host is a growing component of the patient population. Examples of pneumonia in the immunocompromised host are *Pneumocystis carinii* pneumonia (PCP), fungal pneumonias, and mycobacterium tuberculosis. These types of pneumonia may also occur in the immunocompetent person and in different settings, but these are less common. Immunocompromised states occur with the use of corticosteroids or other immunosuppressive agents, chemotherapy, nutritional depletion, use of broad-spectrum antimicrobials, AIDS, genetic immune disorders, and long-term advanced life-support technology (mechanical ventilation). Patients with compromised immune systems commonly acquire pneumonia from organisms of low virulence. In addition, increasing numbers of patients with impaired defenses develop HAP pneumonia from gram-negative bacilli (*Klebsiella, Pseudomonas, Escherichia coli, Enterobacteriaceae, Proteus, Serratia*).

Aspiration pneumonia refers to the pulmonary consequences resulting from the entry of endogenous or exogenous substances into the lower airway. The most common form of aspiration pneumonia is bacterial infection from aspiration of bacteria that normally reside in the upper airways. Aspiration pneumonia may occur in the community or hospital setting; common pathogens are *S. pneumoniae, H. influenzae,* and *Staphylococcus aureus.* Other substances may be aspirated into the lung, such as gastric contents, exogenous chemical contents, or irritating gases. This type of aspiration or ingestion may impair the lung defenses, cause inflammatory changes, and lead to bacterial growth and a resulting pneumonia. (Aspiration is described in more detail at the end of this chapter.)

Pathophysiology

Upper airway characteristics normally prevent potentially infectious particles from reaching the normally sterile lower respiratory tract. Thus, patients with pneumonia caused by infectious agents often have acute or chronic underlying disease that impairs host defenses. Pneumonia arises from normally present flora in a patient whose resistance has been altered, or it results from aspiration of flora present in the oropharynx. It may also result from bloodborne organisms that enter the pulmonary circulation and are trapped in the pulmonary capillary bed, becoming a potential source of pneumonia.

Pneumonia often affects both ventilation and diffusion. An inflammatory reaction may occur in the alveoli and produces an exudate that interferes with the diffusion of oxygen and carbon dioxide. White blood cells, mostly neutrophils, also migrate into the alveoli and fill the normally air-containing spaces. Areas of the lung are not adequately ventilated because of secretions and mucosal edema that cause partial occlusion of the bronchi or alveoli, with a resultant decrease in alveolar oxygen tension. Bronchospasm may also occur in patients with reactive airway disease. Because of hypoventilation, a ventilation–perfusion mismatch occurs in the affected area of the lung. Venous blood entering the pulmonary circulation passes through the underventilated area and exits to the left side of the heart poorly oxygenated. The mixing of oxygenated and unoxygenated or poorly oxygenated blood eventually results in arterial hypoxemia.

If a substantial portion of one or more lobes is involved, the disease is referred to as lobar pneumonia. The term bronchopneumonia is used to describe pneumonia that is distributed in a patchy fashion, having originated in one or more localized areas within the bronchi and extending to the adjacent surrounding lung parenchyma. Bronchopneumonia is more common than lobar pneumonia (Fig. 21-2).

Risk Factors

Being knowledgeable about the factors and circumstances that commonly predispose a person to pneumonia will aid in identifying patients at high risk for pneumonia.

Increasing numbers of patients who have compromised defenses against infections are susceptible to pneumonia. Some types of pneumonia, such as those caused by viral infections, occur in previously healthy people and often follow a preceding viral illness.

Pneumonia is common with certain underlying disorders such as congestive heart failure, diabetes, alcoholism, chronic obstructive pulmonary disease (COPD), and AIDS. Certain diseases also have been associated with specific pathogens. For example, staphylococcal pneumonia has been noted after epidemics of influenza, and patients with COPD are at increased risk for developing pneumonia caused by pneumococci or *H. influenzae.* In addition, cystic fibrosis is associated with respiratory infection caused by pseudomonal and staphylococcal organisms, and PCP has been associated with AIDS. Pneumonias occurring in hospitalized patients often involve organisms not usually found in CAP, including enteric gram-negative bacilli and *S. aureus.*

The Centers for Disease Control and Prevention (CDC) has identified three specific strategies for preventing HAP: (1) staff education and infection surveillance, (2) interruption of transmission of microorganisms through person-to-person transmission and equipment transmission, and (3) modification of host risk of infection (CDC, 1997a). Providing anticipatory and preventive care is an important nursing measure.

To reduce or prevent serious complications of CAP in high-risk groups, vaccination against pneumococcal infection is advised for the following:

- People 65 years of age or older
- Immunocompetent people who are at increased risk for illness and death associated with pneumococcal disease because of chronic illness (eg, cardiovascular, pulmonary, diabetes mellitus, chronic liver disease)
- People with functional or anatomic asplenia
- People living in special environments or social settings in which the risk of disease is high
- Immunocompromised people at high risk for infection (CDC, 1997b)

(*text continues on page 430*)

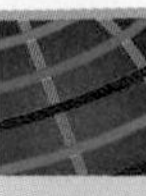

TABLE 21•1 Commonly Encountered Pneumonias

Type	Organism Responsible	Epidemiology
Community-Acquired Pneumonia		
Streptococcal pneumonia (pneumococcal)	*Streptococcus pneumoniae*	Highest occurrence in winter months. Incidence greatest in the elderly and in patients with COPD, congestive heart failure, alcoholism, splenectomy.
Haemophilus influenza	*Haemophilus influenzae*	Incidence greatest in alcoholics, the elderly, patients in chronic care facilities and nursing homes, patients with diabetes or COPD and children <5 years old. Accounts for 5% to 20% of community-acquired pneumonias. Mortality rate: 33%.
Legionnaires' disease	*Legionella pneumophila*	Highest occurrence in summer and fall. May cause disease sporadically or as part of an epidemic. Incidence greatest in middle-aged and older men, smokers, and patients with chronic diseases, those receiving immunosuppressive therapy, or those in close proximity to excavation site. Accounts for 15% of community-acquired pneumonias. Mortality rate: 15% to 50%.
Mycoplasma pneumonia	*Mycoplasma pneumoniae*	Highest occurrence in fall and early winter. Responsible for epidemics of respiratory illness that occur every 4 years. Most common type of atypical pneumonia. Accounts for 20% of community-acquired pneumonias. More common in children and young adults. Mortality rate: <0.1%.
Viral pneumonia	Influenza viruses types A, B adenovirus, parainfluenza, cytomegalovirus	Incidence greatest in winter months. Epidemics occur every 2 to 3 years. Most common organism in adults. Other organisms in children (eg, cytomegalovirus and respiratory syncytial virus). Accounts for 17% of community-acquired pneumonias.
Chlamydial pneumonia (TWAR pneumonia)	*Cipittaci*	Reported mainly in college students and military recruits. May be a common cause of community-acquired pneumonia. Mortality rate: 1% to 5%.
Hospital-Acquired Pneumonia		
Pseudomonas pneumonia	*Pseudomonas aeruginosa*	Incidence greatest in those with preexisting lung disease, cancer (particularly leukemia); those with homograft transplants, burns; debilitated persons; and patients receiving antimicrobial therapy and treatments such as tracheostomy, suctioning. It is almost always of nosocomial origin. Accounts for 5% to 15% of hospital-acquired pneumonias. Mortality rate: 40% to 60%.
Staphylococcal pneumonia	*Staphylococcus aureus*	Incidence greatest in immunocompromised patients, IV drug users, and as a complication of epidemic influenza. Commonly nosocomial in origin. Accounts for 10% to 30% of hospital-acquired pneumonias. Mortality rate: 25% to 60%.
Klebsiella pneumonia	*Klebsiella pneumoniae* (Friedlander's bacillus-encapsulated gram-negative aerobic bacillus)	Incidence greatest in the elderly, alcoholics; patients with chronic disease, such as diabetes, congestive heart failure, COPD; patients in chronic care facilities and nursing homes. Accounts for 2% to 5% of community-acquired and 10% to 30% of hospital-acquired pneumonias. Mortality rate: 40% to 50%.

Clinical Features	Treatment	Comments
Herpes simplex lesions often present on face. Usually involves one or more lobes. Bacteremia is common. Right lower lobe infiltrate common on chest x-ray, with occasional bronchopneumonia pattern.	penicillin G IV penicillin V PO amoxicillin Alternate antibiotic therapy, such as cefuroxime or a 3rd-generation cephalosporin (cefotaxime, ceftizoxime, ceftriaxone); erythromycin, clindamycin.	Complications include shock, pleural effusion, superinfections, pericarditis, and otitis media.
Frequently insidious onset associated with upper respiratory tract infection 2 to 6 weeks before onset of illness. Fever, chills, productive cough. Usually involves one or more lobes. Bacteremia is common. Infiltrate, occasional bronchopneumonia pattern in right lower lobe on chest x-ray.	Cephalosporin 2nd or 3rd generation TMP-SMZ	Complications include lung abscess, pleural effusion.
Flulike symptoms. High fevers with a pulse–temperature deficit (relative bradycardia), mental confusion, headache, pleuritic pain, myalgias, dyspnea, productive cough, hemoptysis. Patchy infiltrates, consolidation, possible pleural effusion on chest x-ray.	erythromycin +/– rifampin (in severely compromised patient) or TMP-SMZ, clarithromycin, or a fluoroquinolone (ofloxacin, levofloxacin, sparfloxacin)	Complications include hypotension, shock, and acute renal failure.
Onset is usually insidious. Patients not usually as ill as in other pneumonias. Sore throat, nasal congestion, ear pain, headache, low-grade fever, pleuritic pain, myalgias, diarrhea, erythema rash, pharyngitis.	erythromycin; tetracycline derivatives (doxycycline)	Complications include aseptic meningitis, meningoencephalitis, cerebral ataxia, Guillain-Barré syndrome, transverse myelitis, pericarditis, myocarditis.
Patchy infiltrate, small pleural effusion on chest x-ray. In majority of patients, influenza begins as an acute upper respiratory infection; others have bronchitis, pleurisy, etc., and still others develop gastrointestinal symptoms.	amantadine; rimantadine Treated symptomatically. Does not respond to treatment with currently available antimicrobials.	Complications include a superimposed bacterial infection, bronchopneumonia.
Hoarseness, fever, pharyngitis, rhinitis, nonproductive cough, myalgias, arthralgia. Single infiltrate on chest x-ray; pleural effusion possible.	doxycycline, erythromycin, clarithromycin, azithromycin	Complications include reinfection and ARDS.
Diffuse consolidation on chest x-ray.	Aminoglycoside and antipseudomonal beta-lactam (ticarcillin, piperacillin, mezlocillin, ceftazidine)	Complications include lung cavitation. Has capacity to invade blood vessels, causing hemorrhage and lung infarction. Usually requires hospitalization.
Severe hypoxemia, cyanosis, necrotizing infection. Bacteremia is common.	nafcillin/oxacillin +/– rifampin or gentamicin methicillin-resistant vancomycin +/– rifampin or gentamicin	Complications include pleural effusion/pneumothorax, lung abscess, empyema, meningitis, endocarditis. Frequently requires hospitalization. Treatment must be vigorous and prolonged because disease tends to destroy lungs.
Tissue necrosis occurs rapidly in lungs (mimics TB) with cavity formation in some patients.	gentamicin, tobramycin, third-generation cephalosporins (cefotaxime, ceftizoxime, ceftriaxone).	Complications include multiple lung abscesses with cyst formation, empyema, pericarditis, pleural effusion. May be fulminating, progressing to fatal outcome.

(*continued*)

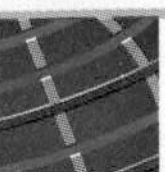

TABLE 21•1 **Commonly Encountered Pneumonias** *(Continued)*

Type	Organism Responsible	Epidemiology
Pneumonia in Immunocompromised Host		
Pneumocystis carinii pneumonia (PCP)	*Pneumocystis carinii*	Incidence greatest in patients with AIDS and patients receiving immunosuppressive therapy for cancer, organ transplants, and other disorders. Frequently seen with cytomegalovirus infection. Mortality rate 60% to 80%.
Fungal pneumonia	*Aspergillus fumigatus*	Incidence greatest in immunocompromised and neutropenic patients. Mortality rate: 15% to 20%.
Tuberculosis	*Mycobacterium tuberculosis*	Incidence increased in indigent, immigrant, and prison populations, people with AIDS, and the homeless. Mortality rate < 1% (depending on comorbidity)

+/− = may add depending upon situation

The vaccine provides specific prevention against pneumococcal pneumonia and other infections caused by this organism (otitis media, other upper respiratory tract infections). Vaccines should be avoided in the first trimester of pregnancy.

Community-Acquired Pneumonia

Pneumonia caused by *S. pneumoniae* (pneumococcus) is the most common CAP in people younger than 60 without comorbidity and in those older than 60 with comorbidity. It is most prevalent during the winter and spring, when upper respiratory tract infections are most frequent. *S. pneumoniae* is a gram-positive, capsulated, nonmotile coccus that resides naturally in the upper respiratory tract. The organism colonizes the upper respiratory tract and can cause the following types of illnesses: disseminated invasive infections, pneumonia and other lower respiratory tract infections, and upper respiratory tract infections, including otitis media and sinusitis (CDC, 1997b). It may occur as a lobar or bronchopneumonic form in patients of any age and may follow a recent respiratory illness.

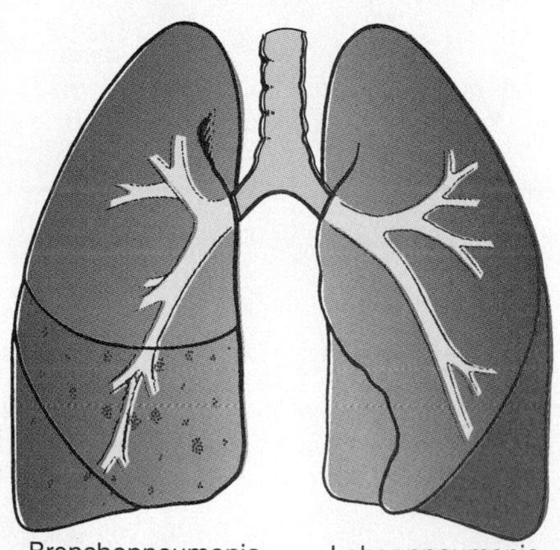

FIGURE 21•2 Distribution of lung involvement in bronchial and lobar pneumonia. In bronchopneumonia (*left*), patchy areas of consolidation occur. In lobar pneumonia, an entire lobe is consolidated.

Mycoplasma pneumonia, another type of CAP, occurs most often in older children and young adults, spread by infected respiratory droplets through person-to-person contact. Patients can be tested for mycoplasma antibodies. The inflammatory infiltrate is primarily interstitial rather than alveolar. It spreads throughout the entire respiratory tract, including the bronchioles, and has the characteristics of a bronchopneumonia. Earache and bullous myringitis are common. Impaired ventilation and diffusion may occur.

H. influenzae is another cause of CAP. It frequently affects elderly people or those with comorbid illnesses (eg, COPD, alcoholism, diabetes mellitus). The presentation of this pneumonia is indistinguishable from that of other forms of bacterial CAP. The presentation may be subacute, with cough or low-grade fever for weeks before diagnosis. Chest x-rays may reveal multilobar, patchy bronchopneumonia or areas of **consolidation** (tissue that solidifies as a result of collapsed alveoli or pneumonia).

Viruses are the most common cause of pneumonia in infants and children but are relatively uncommon causes of CAP in adults. The chief causes of viral pneumonia in the immunocompetent adult are influenza viruses types A and B, adenovirus, parainfluenza virus, and varicella-zoster virus. In immunocompromised adults, cytomegalovirus is the most common viral pathogen, followed by herpes simplex virus, adenovirus, and respiratory syncytial virus. The acute stage of a viral respiratory infection occurs within the ciliated cells of the airways. This is followed by infiltration of the tracheobronchial tree. With pneumonia, the inflammatory process extends into the alveolar area, resulting in edema and exudation. The clinical signs and symptoms of a viral pneumonia are often difficult to distinguish from those of a bacterial pneumonia.

Hospital-Acquired Pneumonia

The common organisms responsible for HAP include the pathogens *Enterobacter* species, *Escherichia coli, Klebsiella* species, *Proteus, Serratia marcescens, P. aeruginosa,* and methicillin-sensitive or methicillin-resistant *S. aureus.* These respiratory infections occur when at least one of three conditions exists: host defenses are impaired, an inoculum of organisms reaches the patient's

Clinical Features	Treatment	Comments
Pulmonary infiltrates on chest x-ray.	trimethoprim–sulfamethoxazole, dapsone, pentamidine.	Complications include respiratory failure.
Cough, hemoptysis, infiltrates, fungus ball on chest x-ray.	flucytosine with amphotericin B in non-neutropenic patients. ketoconazole Lobectomy of fungus ball	
Weight loss, fever, night sweats, cough, sputum production, hemoptysis, nonspecific infiltrate (lower lobe), hilar node enlargement, pleural effusion on chest x-ray	rifampin, streptomycin, ethambutol INH (isoniazid), pyrazinamide	Complications include reinfection and ARDS.

lower respiratory tract and overwhelms the host's defenses, or a highly virulent organism is present. Certain illnesses may predispose a patient to HAP because of impaired host defenses. Examples include severe acute or chronic illness, a variety of comorbid conditions, coma, malnutrition, prolonged hospitalization, hypotension, and metabolic disorders. The hospitalized patient is also exposed to potential bacteria from other sources (respiratory therapy devices and equipment, transmission of pathogens by the hands of health care personnel). Numerous intervention-related factors also may play a role in the development of HAP (eg, therapeutic agents leading to central nervous system depression with decreased ventilation, impaired removal of secretions, or poten-

Risk Factors for PNEUMONIA

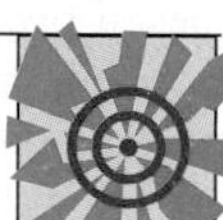

Risk Factor	Preventive Measure
Conditions that produce mucus or bronchial obstruction and interfere with normal lung drainage (eg, cancer, cigarette smoking, COPD)	Promote coughing and expectoration of secretions. Encourage smoking cessation.
Immunosuppressed patients and those with a low neutrophil count (neutropenic)	Initiate special precautions against infection.
Smoking, because cigarette smoke disrupts both mucociliary and macrophage activity	Encourage smoking cessation.
Prolonged immobility and shallow breathing pattern	Reposition frequently and promote lung expansion exercises and coughing. Initiate suctioning and chest physical therapy if indicated.
Depressed cough reflex (due to medications, a debilitated state, or weak respiratory muscles); aspiration of foreign material into the lungs during a period of unconsciousness (head injury, anesthesia, depressed level of consciousness), or abnormal swallowing mechanism	Reposition frequently to prevent aspiration and administer medications judiciously, particularly those that increase risk for aspiration. Perform suctioning and chest physical therapy if indicated.
Nothing-by-mouth (NPO) status; placement of nasogastric, orogastric, or endotracheal tube	Promote frequent oral hygiene. Minimize risk for aspiration by checking placement of tube and proper positioning.
Antibiotic therapy (in very ill people, the oropharynx is likely to be colonized by gram-negative bacteria)	
Alcohol intoxication (because alcohol suppresses the body's reflexes, may be associated with aspiration, and decreases white cell mobilization and tracheobronchial ciliary motion)	Encourage reduced or moderate alcohol intake (in case of alcohol stupor, position patient to prevent aspiration).
General anesthetic, sedative, or opioid preparations that promote respiratory depression, which causes a shallow breathing pattern and predisposes to the pooling of bronchial secretions and potential development of pneumonia	Observe the respiratory rate and depth during recovery from general anesthesia and before giving medications. If respiratory depression is apparent, withhold the medication and report the problem.
Advanced age, because of possible depressed cough and glottic reflexes and nutritional depletion	Promote frequent turning, early ambulation and mobilization, effective coughing, breathing exercises, and nutritious diet.
Respiratory therapy with improperly cleaned equipment	Make sure that respiratory equipment is cleaned properly; participate in continuous quality improvement monitoring with the respiratory care department.

tial aspiration; prolonged or complicated thoracoabdominal procedures, which may impair mucociliary function and cellular host defenses; endotracheal intubation; prolonged or inappropriate use of antibiotics; use of nasogastric tubes). In addition, immunocompromised patients are at particular risk. HAP is associated with a high mortality rate, in part because of the virulence of the organisms, their resistance to antibiotics, and the patient's underlying disorder.

Dominant pathogens for HAP are gram-negative bacilli (*P. aeruginosa* and *Enterobacteriaceae/Klebsiella* species, *Enterobacter, Proteus, Serratia*) and *S. aureus.* Pseudomonal pneumonia occurs in patients who are debilitated, those with altered mental status, and those with prolonged intubation or with tracheostomies. Staphylococcal pneumonia can occur through inhalation of the organism or spread through the hematogenous route. It is often accompanied by bacteremia and positive blood cultures. Although responsible for less than 10% of cases of CAP, staphylococcal pneumonia may be responsible for more than 30% of cases of HAP. Its mortality rate is high. Specific strains of staphylococci are resistant to all available antimicrobials except vancomycin. These strains of *S. aureus* are referred to as methicillin-resistant *S. aureus* (MRSA). Overuse and misuse of antimicrobial agents are major risk factors for the emergence of these resistant pathogens. Because MRSA is highly virulent, steps must be taken to prevent the spread of this organism. The patient with MRSA should be isolated in a private room and contact precautions (gown, mask, glove, and antibacterial soap) are used. The number of people in contact with the patient should be minimized, and appropriate precautions must be taken when transporting the patient within or between facilities.

The usual presentation of a HAP is a new pulmonary infiltrate on chest x-ray combined with evidence of infection such as fever, respiratory symptoms, purulent sputum, and/or leukocytosis. Pneumonias from *Klebsiella* or other gram-negative organisms (*E. coli, Proteus, Serratia*) are characterized by destruction of lung structure and alveolar walls, consolidation, and bacteremia. Elderly patients and those with alcoholism, chronic lung disease, or diabetes are at particular risk. A sudden onset of cough is a common presentation, and blood-tinged sputum may be present. In the debilitated or dehydrated patient, sputum production may be minimal or absent. Pleural effusions, high fevers, and tachycardia are often observed. Even with treatment, the mortality rate remains high.

Pneumonia in the Immunocompromised Host

Pneumonia in the compromised host may be caused by organisms also observed in CAP or HAP (*S. pneumoniae, S. aureus, H. influenzae, P. aeruginosa, M. tuberculosis*). PCP is rarely observed in the immunocompetent host and is often an initial AIDS-defining complication. Whether the patient is immunocompromised or immunocompetent, the clinical presentation of pneumonia is similar. PCP has a subtle onset with progressive dyspnea, fever, and a nonproductive cough.

Clinical Manifestations

Pneumonia varies in signs and symptoms depending on the organism and the patient's underlying disease. However, regardless of the type of pneumonia (CAP, HAP, immunocompromised host, aspiration), a specific type of pneumonia cannot be diagnosed by clinical manifestations alone. For example, the patient with streptococcal (pneumococcal) pneumonia usually has a sudden onset of shaking chills, rapidly rising fever (38.5° to 40.5°C [101° to 105°F]), and pleuritic chest pain that is aggravated by deep breathing and coughing. The patient is severely ill with marked tachypnea (25 to 45 breaths/min), accompanied by other signs of respiratory distress (eg, shortness of breath, use of accessory muscles in respiration). The pulse is rapid and bounding, and it usually increases about 10 beats/min for every degree of temperature (Celsius) elevation. A relative bradycardia for the amount of fever may suggest viral infection, mycoplasmic infection, or infection with a *Legionella* organism.

Some patients exhibit an upper respiratory tract infection (nasal congestion, sore throat), and the onset of symptoms of pneumonia is gradual and nonspecific. The predominant symptoms may be headache, low-grade fever, pleuritic pain, myalgia, rash, and pharyngitis. After a few days, mucoid or mucopurulent sputum is expectorated. In severe pneumonia, the cheeks are flushed and the lips and nailbeds demonstrate central cyanosis (a late sign of poor oxygenation [hypoxemia]).

Typically, the patient has **orthopnea** (shortness of breath when reclining); he or she prefers to be propped up in bed leaning forward (orthopneic position), trying to achieve adequate gas exchange without coughing or breathing deeply. Appetite is poor, and the patient is diaphoretic and tires easily. Sputum is often purulent; this is not a reliable indicator of the etiologic agent. Rusty, blood-tinged sputum may be expectorated with streptococcal (pneumococcal), staphylococcal, and *Klebsiella* pneumonia.

Signs and symptoms of pneumonia may also depend on underlying conditions. Differing signs occur in patients with other conditions, such as cancer, or in those who are undergoing treatment with immunosuppressants, which lower the resistance to infection. Such patients have fever, crackles, and physical findings that indicate consolidation of lung tissue, including increased tactile fremitus, percussion dullness, bronchial breath sounds, egophony (when auscultated, the spoken *E* becomes a loud, nasal-sounding *A*), and whispered pectoriloquy (whispered sounds are easily auscultated through the chest wall). These changes occur because sound is transmitted better through solid or dense tissue (consolidation) than through normal air-filled tissue; these sounds are described in Chapter 19.

Purulent sputum or slight changes in respiratory symptoms may be the only sign of pneumonia in patients with COPD. It may be difficult to determine whether an increase in symptoms is an exacerbation of the underlying disease process or an additional infectious process.

Assessment and Diagnostic Findings

The diagnosis of pneumonia is made by history (particularly of a recent respiratory tract infection), physical examination, chest x-ray studies, blood culture (bloodstream invasion, called bacteremia, occurs frequently), and sputum examination. The sputum sample is obtained by having the patient: (1) rinse the mouth with water to minimize contamination by normal oral flora, (2) breathe deeply several times, (3) cough deeply, and (4) expectorate the raised sputum into a sterile container.

More invasive procedures may be used to collect specimens. Sputum may be obtained by nasotracheal or orotracheal suctioning with a sputum trap or by fiberoptic bronchoscopy (see Chap. 19). Bronchoscopy is often used in patients with acute severe infection, those with chronic or refractory infection, or immunocompromised patients when a diagnosis cannot be made from an expectorated or induced specimen.

Medical Management

The treatment of pneumonia includes administration of the appropriate antibiotic as determined by the results of the Gram's stain. Penicillin G is clearly the antibiotic of choice for infection with *S. pneumoniae.* Other effective medications include erythromycin, clindamycin, the second- and third-generation cephalosporins, other penicillins, and trimethoprim–sulfamethoxazole (Bactrim, TMP-SMZ). Mycoplasma pneumonia responds to erythromycin, tetracycline, and tetracycline derivatives (doxycycline). PCP responds best to pentamidine and TMP-SMZ. Amantadine and rimantadine are effective with influenza A and have been shown to reduce the duration of fever and other systemic complications when administered within 24 to 48 hours of the onset of an uncomplicated influenza infection. These medications also reduce the duration and quantity of virus shedding in the respiratory secretions. They are most effective when used in combination with influenza vaccine. Ganciclovir is used to treat cytomegalovirus in the non-AIDS patient; cytomegalovirus immunoglobulin may also be used.

Treatment of viral pneumonia is primarily supportive. Antibiotics are ineffective in viral upper respiratory infections and pneumonia and may be associated with adverse effects. Treatment of viral infections with antibiotics is a major reason for the overuse of these medications in the United States. Antibiotics are indicated with a viral respiratory infection *only* when a secondary bacterial pneumonia, bronchitis, or sinusitis is present. Hydration is a necessary part of therapy because fever and tachypnea may result in insensible fluid losses. Antipyretics may be used to treat headache and fever; antitussive medications may be used for the associated cough. Warm, moist inhalations are helpful in relieving bronchial irritation. Antihistamines may provide benefit with reduced sneezing and rhinorrhea. Nasal decongestants may also be used to treat symptoms and improve sleep; however, excessive use may cause rebound nasal congestion. Treatment of viral pneumonia (with the exception of antimicrobial therapy) is the same as that for bacterial pneumonia. The patient is placed on bed rest until the infection shows signs of clearing. If hospitalized, the patient is observed carefully until the clinical condition improves.

If hypoxemia develops, oxygen is administered. Pulse oximetry or arterial blood gas analysis is performed to determine the need for oxygen and to evaluate the effectiveness of the therapy. A high concentration of oxygen is contraindicated in patients with COPD because it may worsen alveolar ventilation by decreasing the patient's ventilatory drive, leading to further respiratory decompensation. Respiratory support measures include high oxygen concentrations (fraction of inspired oxygen [FiO_2]), endotracheal intubation, and mechanical ventilation. Different modes of mechanical ventilation may be required; see Chapter 22.

Figure 21-3 provides an algorithm of pneumonia treatment.

Gerontologic Considerations

Pneumonia in the elderly patient may occur as a primary problem or as a complication of a chronic disease process. Pulmonary infections in the elderly frequently are difficult to treat and have a higher mortality rate than in younger patients. General deterioration, weakness, abdominal symptoms, anorexia, confusion, tachycardia, and tachypnea may signal the onset of pneumonia. The diagnosis of pneumonia may be missed because the classic symptoms of cough, chest pain, sputum production, and fever may be absent or masked in the elderly patient. Also, the presence of some signs may be misleading. Abnormal breath sounds, for example, may be due to microatelectasis that occurs in the aged as a result of decreased mobility, decreased lung volumes, and other respiratory function changes. Because chronic congestive heart failure is often seen in the elderly, chest x-rays may be obtained to assist in differentiating it from pneumonia as the cause of clinical signs and symptoms.

Supportive treatment includes hydration (with caution and frequent assessment because of the risk of fluid overload in the elderly), supplemental oxygen therapy, assistance with deep breathing, coughing, frequent position changes, and early ambulation. All of these are particularly important in the care of the elderly patient with pneumonia. To reduce or prevent serious complications of pneumonia in the elderly, vaccination against pneumococcal and influenza infections is recommended.

Complications

SHOCK AND RESPIRATORY FAILURE

Severe complications of pneumonia include hypotension and shock and respiratory failure (especially with gram-negative bacterial disease in elderly patients). These complications are encountered chiefly in patients who have received no specific treatment or inadequate or delayed treatment. These complications are also encountered when the infecting organism is resistant to therapy and when a comorbid disease complicates the pneumonia.

If the patient is seriously ill, aggressive therapy may include hemodynamic and ventilatory support to combat peripheral collapse, maintain arterial blood pressure, and provide adequate oxygenation. A vasopressor agent may be administered intravenously by continuous infusion and at a rate adjusted in accordance with the pressure response. Corticosteroids may be administered parenterally to combat shock and toxicity in patients who are extremely ill with pneumonia and in apparent danger of dying of the infection. Patients may require endotracheal intubation and mechanical ventilation. Congestive heart failure, cardiac dysrhythmias, pericarditis, and myocarditis also are complications of pneumonia that may lead to shock.

ATELECTASIS AND PLEURAL EFFUSION

Atelectasis (from obstruction of a bronchus by accumulated secretions) may occur at any stage of acute pneumonia. Pleural effusion, in which fluid collects in the pleural space, may signal the beginning of **empyema** (purulent fluid within the pleural space). After the pleural effusion is detected on a chest x-ray, a thoracentesis may be performed to remove the fluid. The fluid is sent to the laboratory for analysis. A chest tube may be inserted to treat pleural infection by establishing proper drainage of the empyema.

SUPERINFECTION

Superinfection may occur with the administration of very large doses of antibiotics, such as penicillin, or with combinations of antibiotics. Superinfection may also occur in the patient who has been receiving numerous courses and types of antibiotics. In such cases, bacteria may become resistant to the antibiotic therapy. If the patient improves and the fever diminishes after initial antibiotic therapy, but subsequently there is a rise in temperature with increasing cough and evidence that the pneumonia has spread, a superinfection is likely. Antibiotics are changed appropriately or discontinued entirely in some cases.

PHARMACOLOGY

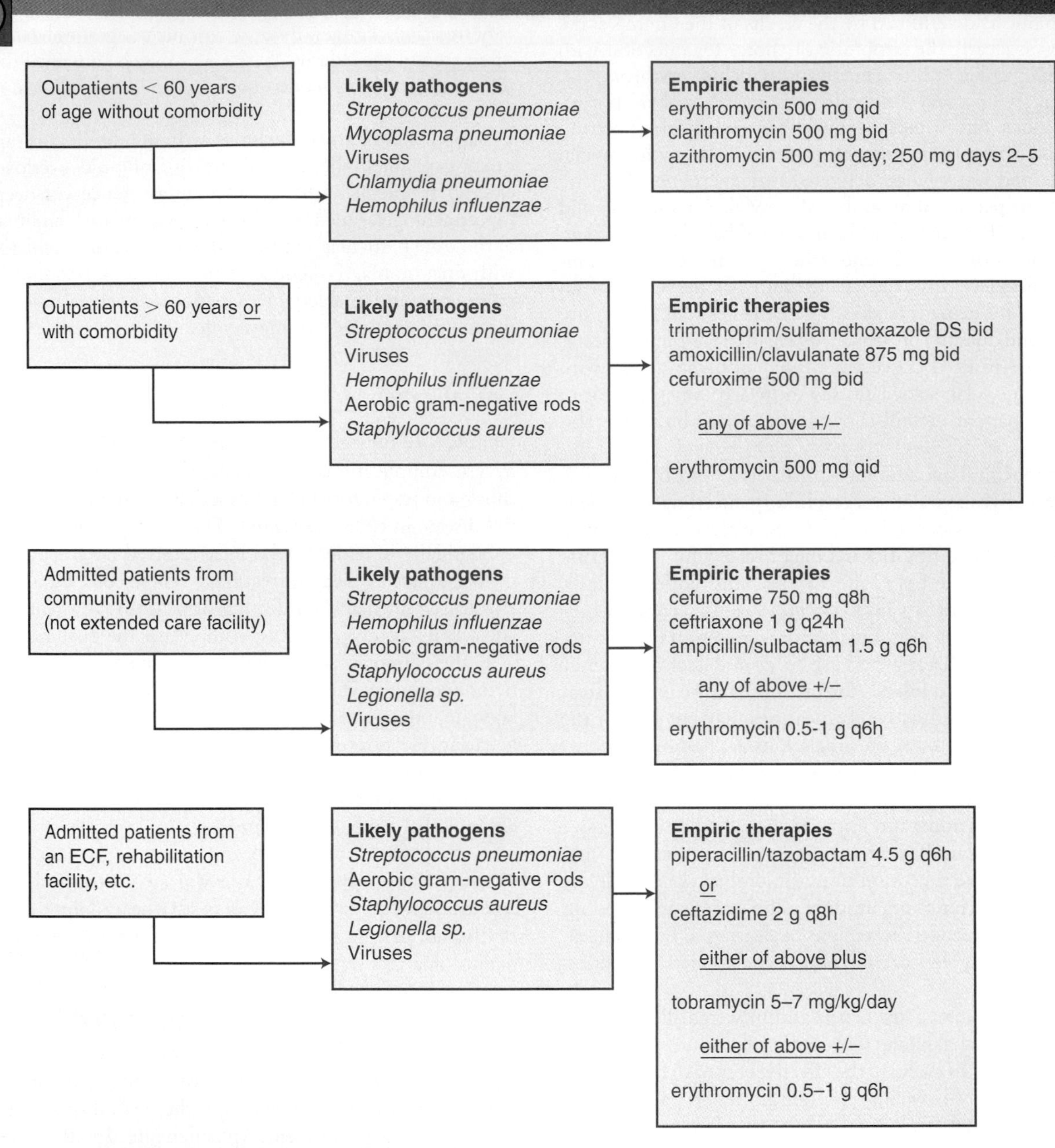

FIGURE 21•3 Guidelines for selecting antibiotic treatment in community-acquired pneumonia. Courtesy Clarian Health, Methodist * IU *Riley, Indianapolis, Indiana. (+/– = may add, depending on situation)

NURSING PROCESS: THE PATIENT WITH PNEUMONIA

Assessment

Nursing assessment is critical in detecting pneumonia. A fever, chills, or night sweats in any patient along with any respiratory symptoms should alert the nurse to the possibility of bacterial pneumonia. A respiratory assessment will further identify the clinical manifestations of pneumonia: pleuritic-type pain, fatigue, tachypnea, use of accessory muscles for breathing, bradycardia or relative bradycardia, coughing, and purulent sputum. It is important to identify the severity, location, and cause of the chest pain, along with any medications or procedures that provide relief. The nurse should monitor the following:

- Changes in temperature and pulse
- Amount, odor, and color of secretions
- Frequency and severity of cough
- Degree of tachypnea or shortness of breath
- Changes in physical assessment findings (primarily assessed by inspecting and auscultating the chest)

In addition, it is important to assess the elderly patient for unusual behavior, altered mental status, dehydration, prostration, and concomitant congestive heart failure.

Diagnosis

Nursing Diagnoses

Based on the assessment data, the patient's major nursing diagnoses may include:

- Ineffective airway clearance related to copious tracheobronchial secretions
- Activity intolerance related to altered respiratory function
- Risk for fluid volume deficit related to fever and dyspnea
- Altered nutrition: less than body requirements
- Knowledge deficit about the treatment regimen and preventive health measures

Collaborative Problems/Potential Complications

Based on the assessment data, collaborative problems or potential complications that may occur include:

- Continuing symptoms after initiation of therapy
- Hypotension and shock
- Respiratory failure
- Atelectasis
- Pleural effusion
- Delirium
- Superinfection

Planning and Goals

The major goals for the patient may include improved airway patency, enough rest to conserve energy, maintenance of proper fluid volume, maintenance of adequate nutrition, an understanding of the treatment protocol and preventive measures, and absence of complications.

Nursing Interventions

Improving Airway Patency

Removing secretions is important because retained secretions interfere with gas exchange and may slow recovery. The nurse encourages hydration (2 to 3 L/day) because adequate hydration thins and loosens pulmonary secretions. Humidification may be used to loosen secretions and improve ventilation. A high-humidity face mask (using either compressed air or oxygen) delivers warm, humidified air to the tracheobronchial tree, helps to liquefy secretions, and relieves tracheobronchial irritation. Coughing can be initiated either voluntarily or by reflex. Lung expansion maneuvers, such as deep breathing with an incentive spirometer, may induce a cough. A directed cough may be necessary to improve airway patency. The nurse encourages the patient to perform an effective, directed cough, which includes correct positioning, a deep inspiratory maneuver, glottic closure, contraction of the expiratory muscles against the closed glottis, sudden glottic opening, and an explosive expiration. In some cases, the nurse may assist the patient by placing his or her hands on the lower rib cage (anteriorly or posteriorly) to focus the patient on a slow deep breath, and then manually assisting the patient by applying external pressure during the expiratory phase.

Chest physiotherapy (percussion and postural drainage) is important in loosening and mobilizing secretions. Indications for chest physiotherapy include sputum retention not responsive to spontaneous or directed cough, a history of pulmonary problems previously treated with chest physiotherapy, continued evidence of retained secretions (decreased or abnormal breath sounds, change in vital signs), abnormal chest x-ray findings consistent with atelectasis or infiltrates, or deterioration in oxygenation. The patient is placed in the proper position to drain the involved lung segments, and then the chest is percussed and vibrated either manually or with a mechanical percussor.

After each position change, the nurse encourages the patient to breathe deeply and cough. If the patient is too weak to cough effectively, the nurse may need to remove the mucus by nasotracheal suctioning (see Chap. 22). It may take time for secretions to mobilize and move into the central airways for expectoration. Thus, it is important for the nurse to monitor the patient for cough and sputum production after the completion of chest physiotherapy.

The nurse administers oxygen as prescribed. The effectiveness of oxygen therapy is monitored by improvement in clinical signs and symptoms, and adequate oxygenation values measured by pulse oximetry or arterial blood gas analysis.

Promoting Rest and Conserving Energy

The nurse encourages the debilitated patient to rest and avoid overexertion and possible exacerbation of symptoms. The patient should assume a comfortable position to promote rest and breathing (eg, semi-Fowler's) and should change it frequently. It is important to instruct outpatients not to overexert themselves and to engage in only moderate activity during the initial phases of treatment.

Promoting Fluid Intake

The respiratory rate of a patient with pneumonia increases because of the increased workload imposed by labored breathing and fever. An increased respiratory rate leads to an increase in insensible fluid loss during exhalation, and the patient can dehydrate. Therefore, it is important to encourage increased fluid intake (at least 2 L/day).

Maintaining Nutrition

Patients with shortness of breath and fatigue often have a decreased appetite and will take only fluids. Fluids with electrolytes (commercially available drinks, such as Gatorade) may help provide fluid, calories, and electrolytes. In addition, fluids and nutrients may be administered intravenously if necessary.

Monitoring and Managing Potential Complications

CONTINUING SYMPTOMS AFTER INITIATION OF THERAPY

Patients usually begin to respond to treatment within 24 to 48 hours after antibiotic therapy is initiated. The patient is observed for response to antibiotic therapy. The patient is monitored for changes in physical status (deterioration of condition or resolution of symptoms) and also for persistent recurrent fever, which may be due to medication allergy (signaled possibly by a rash); medication resistance or slow response (greater than 48 hours) of the susceptible organism to therapy; superinfection (a subsequent infection with another bacteria during antibiotic therapy); pleural effusion; or pneumonia caused by an unusual organism, such as *Pneumocystis carinii* or *Aspergillus fumigatus.* Failure of the pneumonia to resolve or persistence of symptoms despite changes on the chest x-ray raises the suspicion of other underlying disorders, such as lung cancer. As described earlier, lung cancers may invade or compress airways, causing an obstructive atelectasis that may lead to pneumonia.

In addition to monitoring for continuing symptoms of pneumonia, the nurse also monitors for other complications, such as shock and multisystem failure, atelectasis, pleural effusion, and superinfection, which may develop during the first few days of antibiotic treatment.

SHOCK AND RESPIRATORY FAILURE

The nurse assesses for signs and symptoms of shock and respiratory failure by evaluating the patient's vital signs, pulse oximetry values, and hemodynamic monitoring parameters. The nurse reports signs of deteriorating patient status and assists in administering intravenous fluids and medications prescribed to combat shock. Intubation and mechanical ventilation may be required if respiratory failure occurs. Shock is described in detail in Chapter 14, and care of the patient receiving mechanical ventilation is described in Chapter 22.

ATELECTASIS AND PLEURAL EFFUSION

The patient is assessed for atelectasis, and preventive measures are initiated to prevent its development. If pleural effusion develops, the nurse assists in thoracentesis and explains the procedure to the patient. After thoracentesis, the nurse monitors the patient for pneumothorax. If a chest tube needs to be inserted, the nurse monitors the patient's respiratory status (see Chap. 22 for more information on care of the patient with a chest tube).

SUPERINFECTION

The patient is monitored for manifestations of superinfection (ie, rise in temperature with increasing cough, increasing fremitus and adventitious breath sounds on auscultation of the lungs). These signs are reported, and the nurse assists in implementing therapy to treat superinfection.

Promoting Home and Community-Based Care

TEACHING PATIENTS SELF-CARE

Depending on the severity of the pneumonia, treatment may occur in the hospital or in the outpatient setting. Patient education is crucial regardless of the setting. Proper administration of antibiotics is important. In some instances, the patient may be initially treated with intravenous antibiotics as an inpatient and then be discharged to continue the intravenous antibiotics in the home setting. It is important that a seamless system of care be maintained for the patient from hospital to home; this includes communication between the nurses caring for this patient. In addition, if oral antibiotics are prescribed, it is important to teach the patient about proper administration and potential side effects.

After the fever subsides, the patient may gradually increase activities. Fatigue and weakness may be prolonged after pneumonia. The nurse encourages breathing exercises to clear the lungs and promote full lung expansion. It is important to instruct the patient to return to the clinic or caregiver's office for a follow-up chest x-ray and physical examination. Often improvement in chest x-ray findings lags behind improvement in clinical signs and symptoms.

The nurse encourages the patient to stop smoking. Smoking inhibits tracheobronchial ciliary action, which is the first line of defense of the lower respiratory tract. Smoking also irritates the mucous cells of the bronchi and inhibits the function of alveolar macrophage (scavenger) cells. The patient is instructed to avoid fatigue, sudden changes in temperature, and excessive alcohol intake, all of which lower resistance to pneumonia. The nurse reviews with the patient the principles of adequate nutrition and rest, because one episode of pneumonia may make the patient susceptible to recurring respiratory tract infections.

CONTINUING CARE

Patients who are severely debilitated or who cannot care for themselves may require referral for home care. During home visits, the nurse assesses the patient's physical status, monitors for complications, assesses the home environment, and reinforces previous teaching. The nurse evaluates the patient's adherence to the therapeutic regimen (ie, taking medications as prescribed, performing breathing exercises, consuming an adequate fluid and dietary intake, and avoiding smoking, alcohol, and excessive activity). The nurse stresses to the patient and family the importance of monitoring for complications. The nurse encourages the patient to obtain an influenza vaccine at the prescribed times, because influenza increases susceptibility to secondary bacterial pneumonia, especially that caused by staphylococci, *H. influenzae,* and *S. pneumoniae.* The nurse also encourages the patient to seek medical advice about receiving the vaccine (Pneumovax) against *S. pneumoniae.*

Evaluation

Expected Outcomes

Expected outcomes may include:

1. Demonstrates improved airway patency, as evidenced by adequate oxygenation by pulse oximetry or arterial blood gas analysis, normal temperature, normal breath sounds, and effective coughing
2. Rests and conserves energy by remaining in bed while symptomatic and slowly increasing activities
3. Maintains adequate hydration, as evidenced by an adequate fluid intake and normal skin turgor
4. Exhibits no complications
   a. Has normal vital signs, pulse oximetry, and arterial blood gas measurements
   b. Reports productive cough that diminishes over time
   c. Has absence of signs or symptoms of shock, respiratory failure, or pleural effusion
   d. Remains oriented and aware of surroundings
   e. Maintains or increases weight
5. Complies with treatment protocol and prevention strategies

Pulmonary Tuberculosis

Tuberculosis (TB) is an infectious disease that primarily affects the lung parenchyma. It also may be transmitted to other parts of the body, including the meninges, kidneys, bones, and lymph nodes. The primary infectious agent, *Mycobacterium tuberculosis,* is an acid-fast aerobic rod that grows slowly and is sensitive to heat and ultraviolet light. *Mycobacterium bovis* and *Mycobacterium avium* have rarely been associated with the development of a TB infection.

TB is a worldwide public health problem, and the mortality and morbidity rates continue to rise. *M. tuberculosis* infects an estimated one third of the world's population and remains the leading cause of death from infectious disease in the world. It is the leading cause of death among HIV-positive people (World Health Organization, 1998). TB is closely associated with poverty, malnutrition, overcrowding, substandard housing, and inadequate health care.

In 1952, anti-TB medications were introduced, and the rate of reported cases of TB in the United States declined an average of 6% each year between 1953 and 1985. It was thought that by the early part of the 21st century, TB might be eliminated in the United States. However, since 1985 the trend has been reversed and the number of cases has increased. This change has been attributed to several factors, including increased immigration, the HIV epidemic, multidrug-resistant strains of TB, the increased homeless population, decreased interest and detection by health care providers, and inadequate funding of the U.S. public health system.

Transmission and Risk Factors

TB spreads from person to person by airborne transmission. An infected person releases droplet nuclei (generally particles 1 to 5 micrometers in diameter) through talking, coughing, sneezing, laughing, or singing. Larger droplets settle; smaller droplets remain suspended in the air and are inhaled by the susceptible person. Risk factors for TB are listed in the accompanying chart. Chart 21-1 summarizes the CDC's recommendations for prevention of TB transmission in health care settings.

Risk Factors for TUBERCULOSIS (TB)

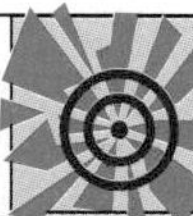

- Close contact with someone who has active TB. Inhalation of airborne nuclei from an infected person is proportional to the amount of time spent in the same air space, the proximity of the person, and the degree of ventilation.
- Immunocompromised status (eg, those with HIV, cancer, transplanted organs, and prolonged high-dose corticosteroid therapy)
- Substance abuse (IV or injection drug users and alcoholics)
- Any person without adequate health care (the homeless; impoverished; minorities, particularly children under age 15 years and young adults between ages 15 and 44 yrs)
- Preexisting medical conditions or special treatment (eg, diabetes, chronic renal failure, malnourishment, selected malignancies, hemodialysis, transplanted organ, gastrectomy, or jejunoileal bypass)
- Emigration from countries with a high prevalence of TB (southeastern Asia, Africa, Latin America, Caribbean)
- Institutionalization (eg, long-term care facilities, psychiatric institutions, prisons)
- Living in overcrowded, substandard housing
- Being a health care worker performing high-risk activities: administration of aerosolized pentamidine and other medications, sputum induction procedures, bronchoscopy, suctioning, coughing procedures, caring for the immunosuppressed patient, home care with the high-risk population, and administering anesthesia and related procedures (eg, intubation, suctioning)

Pathophysiology

A susceptible person inhales mycobacterium bacilli and becomes infected. The bacteria are transmitted through the airways to the alveoli, where they are deposited and begin to multiply. The bacilli also are transported via the lymph system and bloodstream to other parts of the body (kidneys, bones, cerebral cortex) and other areas of the lungs (upper lobes). The body's immune system responds by initiating an inflammatory reaction. Phagocytes (neutrophils and macrophages) engulf many of the bacteria, and TB-

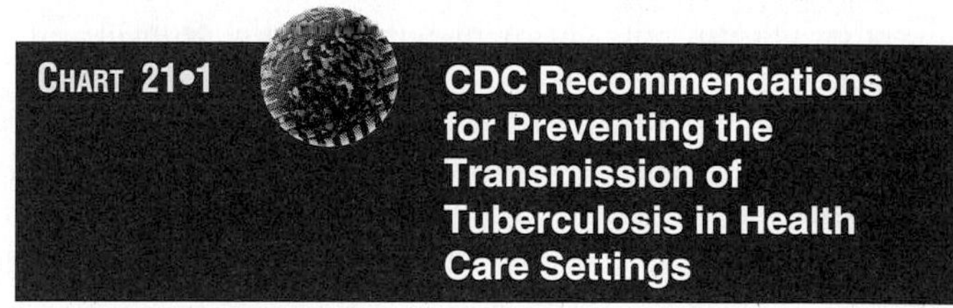

CHART 21•1 CDC Recommendations for Preventing the Transmission of Tuberculosis in Health Care Settings

1. Early identification and treatment of persons with active TB
   a. Maintain a high index of suspicion for TB to identify cases rapidly.
   b. Promptly initiate effective multidrug anti-TB therapy based on clinical and drug-resistance surveillance data.
2. Prevention of spread of infectious droplet nuclei by source control methods and by reduction of microbial contamination of indoor air
   a. Initiate acid-fast bacilli (AFB) isolation precautions immediately for all patients who are suspected or confirmed to have active TB and who may be infectious. AFB isolation precautions include use of a private room with negative pressure in relation to surrounding areas and a minimum of six air exchanges per hour. Air from the room should be exhausted directly to the outside. Use of ultraviolet lamps and/or high-efficiency particulate air filters to supplement ventilation may be considered.
   b. Persons entering the AFB isolation room should use disposable particulate respirators that fit snugly around the face.
   c. Continue AFB isolation precautions until there is clinical evidence of reduced infectiousness (ie, cough has substantially decreased, and the number of organisms on sequential sputum smears is decreasing). If drug resistance is suspected or confirmed, continue AFB precautions until the sputum smear is negative for AFB.
   d. Use special precautions during cough-inducing procedures.
3. Surveillance for TB transmission
   a. Maintain surveillance for TB infection among health care workers (HCWs) by routine, periodic tuberculin skin testing. Recommend appropriate preventive therapy for HCWs when indicated.
   b. Maintain surveillance for TB cases among patients and HCWs.
   c. Promptly initiate contact investigation procedures among HCWs, patients, and visitors exposed to an untreated, or ineffectively treated, infectious TB patient for whom appropriate AFB procedures are not in place. Recommend appropriate therapy or preventive therapy for contacts with disease or TB infection without current disease. Therapeutic regimens should be chosen based on the clinical history and local drug-resistance surveillance data.

specific lymphocytes lyse (destroy) the bacilli and normal tissue. This tissue reaction results in the accumulation of exudate in the alveoli, causing bronchopneumonia. The initial infection usually occurs 2 to 10 weeks after exposure.

Granulomas, new tissue masses of live and dead bacilli, are surrounded by macrophages, which form a protective wall around the granulomas. Granulomas are then transformed to a fibrous tissue mass, the central portion of which is called a Ghon tubercle. The material (bacteria and macrophages) becomes necrotic, forming a cheesy mass. This mass may become calcified and form a collagenous scar. At this point, the bacteria become dormant, and there is no further progression of active disease.

After initial exposure and infection, the person may develop active disease because of a compromised or inadequate immune system response. Active disease also may occur with reinfection and activation of dormant bacteria. In this case, the Ghon tubercle ulcerates, releasing the cheesy material into the bronchi. The bacteria then become airborne, resulting in further spread of the disease. Then the ulcerated tubercle heals and forms scar tissue. This causes the infected lung to become more inflamed, resulting in further development of bronchopneumonia and tubercle formation.

Unless the process is arrested, it spreads slowly downward to the hilum of the lungs and later extends to adjacent lobes. The process may be prolonged and characterized by long remissions when the disease is arrested, only to be followed by periods of renewed activity. Approximately 10% of people who are initially infected develop active disease. Some people develop reactivation TB (also called adult-type TB). This type of TB results from a breakdown of the host defenses. It most commonly occurs within the lungs, usually in the apical or posterior segments of the upper lobes, or the superior segments of the lower lobes (Gochuico & Bernardo, 1997).

Clinical Manifestations

The signs and symptoms of pulmonary TB are insidious. Most patients have a low-grade fever, cough, night sweats, fatigue, and weight loss. The cough may be nonproductive, or mucopurulent sputum may be expectorated. Hemoptysis also may occur.

Assessment and Diagnostic Findings

A complete history, physical examination, tuberculin skin test, chest x-ray, acid-fast bacillus smear, and sputum culture are used to diagnose TB. If the person is infected with TB, the chest x-ray usually reveals lesions in the upper lobes and the acid-fast bacillus smear contains mycobacterium.

TUBERCULIN SKIN TEST

The Mantoux test is used to determine if a person has been infected with the TB bacillus. The Mantoux test is a standardized procedure and should be performed only by those trained in its administration and reading. Tubercle bacillus extract (tuberculin), purified protein derivative (PPD), is injected into the intradermal layer of the inner aspect of the forearm, approximately 4 inches below the elbow (Fig. 21-4). Intermediate-strength (5 TU) PPD in a tuberculin syringe with a half-inch 26- or 27-gauge needle is used. The needle, with the bevel facing up, is inserted beneath the skin. Then 0.1 mL of PPD is injected, creating an elevation in the skin, a wheal or bleb. The site, antigen name, strength, lot number, date, and time of the test are recorded. The test result is read 48 to 72 hours after injection. A delayed localized reaction indicates that the person is sensitive to tuberculin.

A reaction occurs when both induration (hardening) and erythema (redness) are noted. After the area is inspected for induration, it is lightly palpated across the injection site, from the area of normal skin to the margins of the induration. The diameter of the

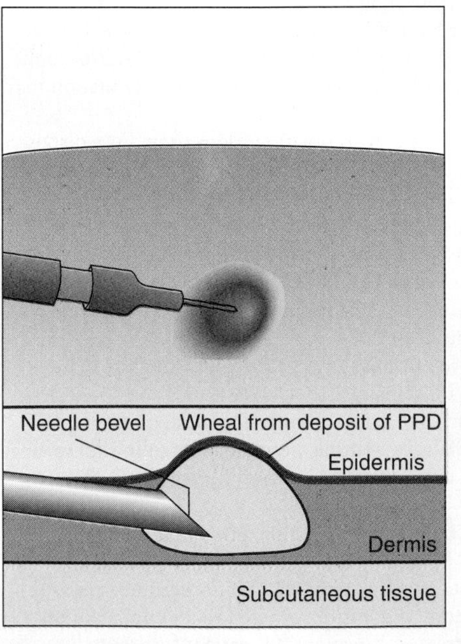

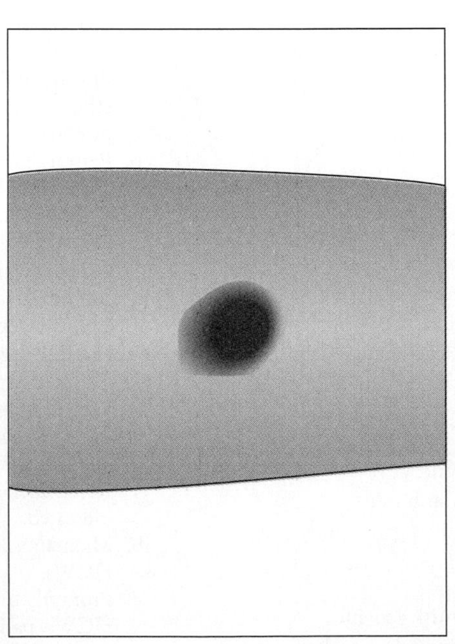

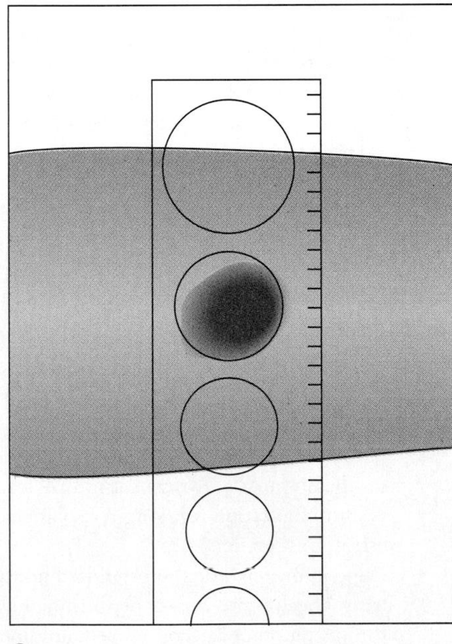

FIGURE 21•4 The Mantoux test for tuberculosis. (**A**) Correct technique for inserting the needle involves depositing the PPD subcutaneously with the needle bevel facing upward. (**B**) The reaction to the Mantoux test usually consists of a wheal, a hivelike, firm welt. (**C**) To determine the extent of the reaction, the wheal is measured using a commercially prepared gauge. A wheal measuring 5 mm or more is considered significant.

induration (not erythema) is measured in millimeters at its widest part (see Fig. 21-4), and the size of the induration is documented. Erythema without induration is not considered significant.

Interpretation of Results. The size of the induration determines the significance of reaction. A reaction of 0 to 4 mm is considered not significant; a reaction of 5 mm or greater may be significant. An induration of 10 mm or greater is usually considered significant. A significant reaction indicates that a patient has been exposed to *M. tuberculosis* recently or in the past or has been vaccinated with bacille Calmette-Guerin (BCG) vaccine. The BCG vaccine is given to produce a greater resistance to developing TB. It is effective in up to 76% of those who receive it. The vaccine is used in Europe and Latin America but not routinely in the United States.

A significant (positive) reaction does not necessarily mean that active disease is present in the body. Most (more than 90%) people who are tuberculin-significant reactors do not develop clinical TB. However, all significant reactors are candidates for active TB. In general, the more intense the reaction, the greater the likelihood of an active infection.

A nonsignificant (negative) skin test does not exclude TB infection or disease because patients who are immunosuppressed cannot mount an immune response adequate to produce a positive skin test (anergy).

The accuracy of the skin test depends on the skill of the person interpreting the test reaction. A recent study (Kendig, Kirkpatrick, Carter, Hill, Caldwell, & Entwistle, 1998) revealed that health care professionals tend to underestimate the size of induration: only 7% of a sample of 107 health care providers charted the correct size of induration.

OTHER SKIN TESTS

Multiple-puncture skin tests are used for surveying and screening large groups and are not intended to establish a positive diagnosis because there is no way to standardize the amount of tuberculin introduced. The test is conducted by introducing tuberculin into the skin either by puncturing the skin with a device with points coated with dried tuberculin or by puncturing the skin after a thin coat of liquid tuberculin has been spread on it. The test is read 48 to 72 hours after administration. If the reaction is in the form of papules, the diameter of the largest single papule or the largest diameter of coalescent induration is measured. If a blister is present, the person is sensitive to the tuberculin and is termed a reactor. However, not all reactors are infected with TB. All reactors should be retested with the Mantoux test and should obtain a chest x-ray.

CLASSIFICATION OF TUBERCULOSIS

Data from the history, physical examination, skin test, chest x-ray, and microbiologic studies are used to classify TB into one of five classes. A classification scheme provides public health officials with a systematic way to monitor epidemiology and treatment of the disease (CDC/American Thoracic Society, 1990):

- Class 0: no exposure; no infection
- Class 1: exposure; no infection
- Class 2: infection; no disease (eg, positive PPD reaction but no clinical evidence of active TB)
- Class 3: disease; clinically active
- Class 4: disease; not clinically active
- Class 5: suspected disease; diagnosis pending

Gerontologic Considerations

TB may have atypical manifestations in elderly patients, whose symptoms may include unusual behavior and altered mental status, fever, anorexia, and weight loss. Many elderly patients may have no reaction or delayed reactivity for up to a week (recall phenomenon). A second skin test is performed in 1 to 2 weeks.

Medical Management

Pulmonary TB is treated primarily with chemotherapeutic agents (antituberculosis agents) for 6 to 12 months. A prolonged treatment duration is necessary to ensure eradication of the organisms and to prevent relapse. A worldwide concern and challenge in TB therapy is the continuing (since the 1950s) and increasing resistance of *M. tuberculosis* to TB medications. Several types of drug resistance must be considered when planning effective therapy:

- Primary drug resistance: resistance to one of the first-line antituberculosis agents in a person who has not had previous treatment
- Secondary or acquired drug resistance: resistance to one or more antituberculosis agents in a patient undergoing therapy
- Multidrug resistance: resistance to two agents, isoniazid (INH) and rifampin. The populations at highest risk for multidrug resistance are those who are HIV-positive, institutionalized, or homeless.

The increasing prevalence of drug resistance points out the need to begin TB treatment with four or more medications, to ensure completion of therapy, and to develop and evaluate new anti-TB medications.

PHARMACOLOGIC THERAPY

In current TB therapy, five first-line medications are used (Table 21-2): INH, rifampin, pyrazinamide, and either streptomycin or ethambutol.

Combination medications, such as INH and rifampin (Rifamate) and medications administered twice a week (eg, rifapentine) are available to help improve patient adherence. Capreomycin, ethionamide, para-aminosalicylate sodium, and cycloserine are second-line medications. Additional potentially effective medications include other aminoglycosides, quinolones, ansamycin, clofazimine, and combinations of medications.

The CDC, the American Thoracic Society, and the American Academy of Pediatrics have recommended guidelines for treatment for newly diagnosed cases of pulmonary TB (American Thoracic Society and Centers for Disease Control, 1994), which consists of a multiple-medication regimen of INH, rifampin, pyrazinamide, and streptomycin or ethambutol. This initial intensive-treatment regimen is usually administered daily for at least 8 weeks. If cultures demonstrate that the organism is sensitive to the medications before the 8 weeks of therapy have been completed, either ethambutol or streptomycin can be discontinued. After 8 weeks of the three-medication therapy, pyrazinamide can be discontinued and INH and rifampin are administered for an additional 4 months. The medication regimen, however, may continue for 12 months. A person is considered noninfectious after 2 to 3 weeks of continuous medication therapy. Vitamin B_6 (pyridoxine) is usually administered with INH to prevent INH-associated peripheral neuropathy.

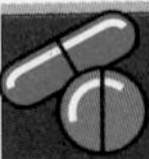

Table 21•2 First-Line Antituberculosis Medications

Commonly Used Agents	Adult Daily Dosage*	Most Common Side Effects	Drug Interactions†	Remarks*
isoniazid (INH)	5 to 20 mg/kg (300 mg maximum)	Peripheral neuritis, hepatitis, hypersensitivity	Phenytoin–synergistic Antabuse Alcohol	Bactericidal Pyridoxine as prophylaxis for neuritis. Monitor SGOT (AST) and SGPT (ALT).
rifampin	10 to 20 mg/kg (600 mg maximum)	Hepatitis, febrile reaction, purpura (rare), nausea, vomiting	Rifampin increases metabolism of oral contraceptives, quinidine, corticosteroids, coumarin derivatives and methadone, digoxin, oral hypoglycemics; PAS may interfere with absorption of rifampin.	Bactericidal. Orange urine and other body secretions. Discoloring of contact lenses. Monitor SGOT (AST) and SGPT (ALT).
streptomycin	15 to 20 mg/kg (1 g maximum)*	8th cranial nerve damage (may lead to deafness), nephrotoxicity	Neuromuscular blocking agents; may be potentiated to cause prolonged paralysis	Bactericidal in alkaline pH. Use with caution in elderly or in those with renal disease. Monitor vestibular function, audiograms, BUN/creatinine.
pyrazinamide	15 to 30 mg/kg (2.0 g maximum)*	Hyperuricemia, hepatotoxicity, skin rash, arthralgias, GI distress		Bactericidal. Monitor uric acid, SGOT (AST), SGPT (ALT).
ethambutol	15 to 25 mg/kg (2.5 g maximum)*	Optic neuritis (may lead to blindness; very rare at 15 mg/kg), skin rash		Bacteriostatic. Use with caution with renal disease or when eye testing is not feasible. Monitor visual acuity, color discrimination.‡
Combinations: INH + rifampin (eg, Rifamate)	150 mg INH 300 mg rifampin			

* Check product labeling for detailed information on dose, contraindications, drug interaction, adverse reactions, and monitoring.
† Reference should be made to current literature, particularly on rifampin, because it indicates hepatic microenzymes and therefore interacts with many drugs.
‡ Initial examination should be performed at start of treatment.
Modified from Lordi, G. M., & Reichman L. (1991). Treatment of tuberculosis. *American Family Physician, 44*(1):220; Treatment of tuberculosis and tuberculous infection in adults and children: Joint statement of the American Thoracic Society and the Centers for Disease Control. *Am J Respir Crit Care Med* 1994;149:1359–1374.

INH also may be used as a prophylactic (preventive) measure for those at risk for significant disease, including:

- Household family members of patients with active disease
- HIV-infected patients with a PPD test reaction of 5 mm of induration or more
- Patients with fibrotic lesions detected on a chest x-ray, suggestive of old TB, and a PPD reaction of 5 mm of induration or more
- Patients whose current PPD test results show a change from former test results, suggesting recent exposure to TB and possible infection (also called skin test converters)
- Drug (intravenous or injectable) users with PPD test results of 10 mm of induration or more
- Patients with high-risk comorbid conditions with a PPD result of 10 mm of induration or more

Other candidates for preventive INH therapy are those age 35 years or younger with PPD test results of 10 mm of induration or more and one of the following criteria:

- Foreign-born individuals from countries with a high prevalence of TB
- High-risk, medically underserved populations
- Institutionalized patients

Prophylactic INH treatment involves taking daily doses for 6 to 12 months. Liver enzyme, blood urea nitrogen, and creatinine levels are monitored monthly. Sputum culture results are monitored for acid-fast bacillus to evaluate the effectiveness of treatment and the patient's compliance with therapy.

Recently, the federal Advisory Council for the Elimination of Tuberculosis published recommendations for the development of TB vaccines. The recommendations include a focus on a "postinfection vaccine" to prevent people infected with TB from developing active disease (CDC, 1998a).

NURSING PROCESS: THE PATIENT WITH TUBERCULOSIS

Assessment

The nurse performs a complete history and physical examination. Clinical manifestations of fever, anorexia, weight loss, night sweats, fatigue, cough, and sputum production prompt a more thorough assessment of respiratory function—for example, assessing the lungs for consolidation by evaluating breath sounds (diminished, bronchial sounds, crackles), fremitus, egophony, and dullness on percussion. Enlarged, painful lymph nodes may be palpated as well. The nurse also assesses the patient's living arrangements, perceptions and understanding of TB and its treatment, and readiness to learn.

Diagnosis

Nursing Diagnoses

Based on the assessment data, the nursing diagnoses may include:

- Ineffective airway clearance related to copious tracheobronchial secretions
- Knowledge deficit about treatment regimen and preventive health measures and related ineffective individual management of the therapeutic regimen (noncompliance)
- Activity intolerance related to fatigue, altered nutritional status, and fever

Collaborative Problems/Potential Complications

Based on the assessment data, collaborative problems or potential complications that may occur include:

- Malnutrition
- Side effects of medication therapy: hepatitis, neurologic changes (deafness or neuritis), skin rash, gastrointestinal upset
- Multidrug resistance
- Spread of TB infection (miliary TB)

Planning and Goals

The major goals for the patient include maintenance of a patent airway, increased knowledge about the disease and treatment regimen and adherence to the medication regimen, increased activity tolerance, and absence of complications.

Nursing Interventions

Promoting Airway Clearance

Copious secretions obstruct the airways in many patients with TB and interfere with adequate gas exchange. Increasing fluid intake promotes systemic hydration and serves as an effective expectorant. The nurse instructs the patient about correct positioning to facilitate airway drainage (postural drainage); this is described in Chapter 22.

Advocating Adherence to Treatment Regimen

The multiple-medication regimen that a patient must follow can be quite complex. Understanding the medications, schedule, and side effects is important. The patient must understand that TB is a communicable disease and that taking medications is the most effective means of preventing transmission. The major reason treatment fails is that patients do not take their medications regularly and for the prescribed duration. The nurse carefully instructs the patient about important hygiene measures, including mouth care, covering the mouth and nose when coughing and sneezing, proper disposal of tissues, and hand washing.

Promoting Activity and Adequate Nutrition

Patients with TB are often debilitated from a prolonged chronic illness and impaired nutritional status. The nurse plans a progressive activity schedule that focuses on increasing activity tolerance and muscle strength. Anorexia, weight loss, and malnutrition are common in patients with TB. The patient's willingness to eat may be altered by fatigue from excessive coughing, sputum production, chest pain, or a generalized debilitated state. A nutritional plan that allows for small, frequent meals may be required. Liquid nutritional supplements may assist in meeting basic caloric requirements.

Monitoring and Managing Potential Complications

MALNUTRITION

This may be a consequence of the patient's lifestyle, lack of knowledge about adequate nutrition and its role in health maintenance, lack of resources, fatigue, or lack of appetite because of coughing and mucus production. To counter the effects of these factors, the nurse collaborates with the dietitian, physician, social worker, family, and patient to identify strategies to ensure an adequate nutritional intake and availability of nutritious food. Identifying facilities (eg, shelters, soup kitchens, Meals on Wheels, and other community resources) that provide meals in the patient's neighborhood may increase the likelihood that the patient with limited resources and energy will have access to a more nutritious intake. High-calorie nutritional supplements may be suggested as a strategy for increasing dietary intake using food products normally found in the home. Purchasing food supplements may be beyond the patient's budget, but a dietitian can help develop recipes to increase caloric intake despite minimal resources.

SIDE EFFECTS OF MEDICATION THERAPY

It is important to assess medication side effects because they are often a reason the patient fails to adhere to the prescribed medication plan. Efforts are made to reduce the side effects in an effort to increase the patient's willingness to take the medications as prescribed.

The nurse instructs the patient to take the medication either on an empty stomach or at least 1 hour before meals, because food interferes with medication absorption (although taking medications on an empty stomach frequently results in gastrointestinal upset). Patients taking INH should avoid foods containing tyramine and histamine (tuna, aged cheese, red wine, soy sauce, yeast extracts). Eating these types of foods while taking INH may result in headache, flushing, hypotension, light-headedness, palpitations, and diaphoresis.

In addition, rifampin can increase the metabolism of other medications, making them less effective. These medications include beta-blockers, oral anticoagulants such as warfarin (Coumadin), digoxin, quinidine, corticosteroids, oral hypoglycemic agents, oral contraceptives, theophylline, and verapamil. The nurse informs patients that rifampin may discolor contact lenses, so the patient may want to switch to wearing eyeglasses during treatment. The nurse monitors for other side effects of TB medications, including hepatitis, neurologic changes (hearing loss, neuritis), and rash. Liver enzyme, blood urea nitrogen, and serum creatinine levels are monitored to detect medication-related changes in liver and kidney function. Sputum culture results are monitored for acid-fast bacillus to evaluate the effectiveness of the treatment regimen and adherence to therapy.

MULTIDRUG RESISTANCE

The nurse carefully monitors vital signs and observes for spikes in temperature or changes in the clinical status. The nurse reports any change in the patient's respiratory status to the primary health care provider. The nurse instructs the patient about the risk of drug resistance if the medication regimen is not strictly and continuously followed.

SPREAD OF TB INFECTION

Spread of TB infection to nonpulmonary sites of the body is known as miliary TB. It is the result of invasion of the bloodstream by the tubercle bacillus (Ghon tubercle). Usually it results from late reactivation of a dormant infection in the lung or elsewhere. The origin of the bacilli that enter the bloodstream is either a chronic focus that has ulcerated into a blood vessel or multitudes of miliary tubercles lining the inner surface of the thoracic duct. The organisms migrate from these foci into the bloodstream, are carried throughout the body, and disseminate throughout all tissues, with tiny miliary tubercles developing in the lungs, spleen, liver, kidneys, meninges, and other organs.

The clinical course of miliary TB may vary from an acute, rapidly progressive infection with high fever to an indolent process with low-grade fever, anemia, and debilitation. At first, there may be no localizing signs except an enlarged spleen and a reduced number of leukocytes. Within a few weeks, however, the chest x-ray reveals small densities scattered diffusely throughout both lung fields; these are the miliary tubercles, which gradually grow.

The possibility of TB in nonpulmonary sites in the body requires careful monitoring for this very serious form of the infection. The nurse monitors vital signs and observes for spikes in temperature as well as changes in renal and cognitive function. Few physical signs may be elicited on physical examination of the chest, but at this stage the patient has a severe cough and dyspnea. Treatment of miliary TB is the same as for pulmonary TB.

Promoting Home and Community-Based Care

TEACHING PATIENTS SELF-CARE

The nurse plays a vital role in caring for the patient with TB and the family, which includes assessing the patient's ability to continue therapy at home. The nurse instructs the patient and family about infection control procedures, such as proper disposal of tissues, covering the mouth during coughing, and hand washing. Assessment of the patient's adherence to the medication regimen is imperative because of the risk of developing resistant strains of TB if the regimen is not followed faithfully. In some cases, when the ability of the patient to comply with the medication regimen is in question, referring the patient to an outpatient clinic for daily administration of medications may be required. This is referred to as directly observed therapy.

CONTINUING CARE

The nurse evaluates the patient's environment, including home, other residence, or social setting, to identify other people who may have been in contact with the patient during the infectious stage. It is important to arrange follow-up screening for any contacts of the infected person. Nurses who have contact with the patient in home, shelter, hospital, clinic, or work settings assess the patient's physical and psychological status and ability to adhere to the prescribed treatment. The nurse assesses the patient for adverse effects of medications and adherence to the therapeutic regimen (eg, taking medications as prescribed, practicing safe hygiene, consuming a nutritious and adequate diet, and participating in an appropriate level of activity). The nurse reinforces previous teaching and emphasizes the importance of keeping scheduled appointments with the primary health care provider.

Evaluation

Expected Outcomes

Expected outcomes may include:

1. Maintains a patent airway by managing secretions with hydration, humidification, coughing, and postural drainage
2. Demonstrates an adequate level of knowledge
    a. Lists medications by name, and the correct schedule for taking them
    b. Names expected side effects of medications
    c. Identifies how and when to contact health care provider
3. Adheres to treatment regimen by taking medications as prescribed and reporting for follow-up screening
4. Participates in preventive measures
    a. Disposes of used tissues properly
    b. Encourages people who are close contacts to report for testing
    c. Adheres to hand washing recommendations
5. Maintains activity schedule
6. Exhibits no complications
    a. Maintains adequate weight or gains weight if indicated
    b. Exhibits normal results of tests of liver and kidney function
7. Takes steps to minimize side effects of medications
    a. Takes supplemental vitamins (vitamin B_6), as prescribed, to minimize peripheral neuropathy
    b. Avoids use of alcohol
    c. Avoids foods containing tyramine and histamine
    d. Has regular physical examinations and blood tests to evaluate liver and kidney function, neuropathy, and visual acuity

Lung Abscess

A lung abscess is a localized necrotic lesion of the lung parenchyma containing purulent material that collapses and forms a cavity. Patients who have impaired cough reflexes and cannot close the glottis, or those with swallowing difficulties, are at risk for aspirating foreign material and developing a lung abscess. Other at-risk patients include those with central nervous system disorders (seizure, stroke), drug addiction, alcoholism, esophageal disease, or compromised immune function, as well as patients receiving nasogastric tube feedings and those with an altered state of consciousness from anesthesia.

Pathophysiology

Most lung abscesses are a complication of bacterial pneumonia or are caused by aspiration of oral anaerobes into the lung. Abscesses also may occur secondary to mechanical or functional obstruction of the bronchi by a tumor, foreign body, or bronchial stenosis, or from necrotizing pneumonias, TB, pulmonary embolism, or chest trauma.

Most abscesses are found in areas of the lung that may be affected by aspiration. The site of the lung abscess is related to gravity and is determined by the patient's position. For patients in a recumbent position, the posterior segment of an upper lobe and the superior segment of the lower lobe are the most common areas in which lung abscess occurs. However, atypical presentations may occur, depending on the position of the patient when the aspiration occurred.

Initially, the cavity in the lung may or may not extend directly into a bronchus, but eventually the abscess becomes surrounded, or encapsulated, by a wall of fibrous tissue. The necrotic process may extend at one or two points until it reaches the lumen of a bronchus or the pleural space and establishes communication with the respiratory tract, the pleural cavity, or both. If the bronchus is involved, the purulent contents are expectorated continuously in the form of sputum. If the pleura is involved, an empyema (collection of pus in the pleural cavity) results. A communication or connection between the bronchus and pleura is known as a bronchopleural fistula.

The organisms frequently associated with lung abscesses are *S. aureus*, *Klebsiella*, and other gram-negative species. Anaerobic organisms, however, may also be present. The organism varies depending on the underlying predisposing factors.

Clinical Manifestations

The clinical manifestations of a lung abscess may vary from a mild productive cough to acute illness. Most patients have a fever and a productive cough with moderate to copious amounts of foul-smelling, often bloody, sputum. Leukocytosis may be present. Pleurisy or dull chest pain, dyspnea, weakness, anorexia, and weight loss are common. Fever and cough may develop insidiously and may have been present for several weeks before diagnosis.

Assessment and Diagnostic Findings

Physical examination of the chest may reveal dullness on percussion and decreased or absent breath sounds with an intermittent **pleural friction rub** (grating or rubbing sound) on auscultation. Crackles may be present. Confirmation of the diagnosis is made by chest x-ray, sputum culture, and in some cases fiberoptic bronchoscopy. The chest x-ray reveals an infiltrate with an air–fluid level. A computed tomography (CT) scan of the chest may be required to provide more detailed pictures of different cross-sectional areas of the lung.

Prevention

The following measures will reduce the risk of lung abscess:

- Appropriate antibiotic therapy before any dental procedures in patients who must have teeth extracted while their gums and teeth are infected
- Adequate dental and oral hygiene, because anaerobic bacteria play a role in the pathogenesis of lung abscess
- Appropriate antimicrobial therapy for patients with pneumonia

Medical Management

The findings of the history, physical examination, chest x-ray, and sputum culture indicate the type of organism and the treatment required. Adequate drainage of the lung abscess may be achieved through postural drainage and chest physiotherapy. The patient should be assessed for an adequate cough. A few patients need a percutaneous catheter placed for drainage. The use of therapeutic bronchoscopy to drain an abscess is uncommon. A diet high in protein and calories is necessary because chronic infection is associated with a catabolic state, necessitating increased intake of calories and protein to facilitate healing. Surgical intervention is rare, but pulmonary resection (lobectomy) is performed when there is massive **hemoptysis** (coughing up of blood) or no response to medical management.

PHARMACOLOGIC THERAPY

Intravenous antimicrobial therapy depends on the results of the sputum culture and sensitivity and is administered for an extended period. Clindamycin is the medication of choice, followed by penicillin with metronidazole. Ceftazidime plus aminoglycoside or cefoperazone is used when the infecting organism is *P. aeruginosa. S. aureus* is treated with oxacillin, nafcillin, or a first-generation cephalosporin (cefuroxime). Large intravenous doses are generally required because the antibiotic must penetrate the necrotic tissue and the fluid in the abscess.

Long-term therapy with oral antibiotics replaces intravenous therapy after the patient shows signs of improvement (about 3 to 5 days). Improvement is demonstrated by normal temperature, decreased white blood cell count, and improvement on the chest x-ray (resolution of surrounding infiltrate, reduction in cavity size, absence of fluid). If treatment stops too soon, a relapse may occur. The duration of antibiotic therapy may be 6 to 16 weeks.

Nursing Management

The nurse administers antibiotics and intravenous therapies as prescribed and monitors for adverse effects. Chest physiotherapy is initiated as prescribed to facilitate drainage of the abscess. The nurse teaches the patient to perform deep-breathing and coughing exercises to help expand the lungs. To ensure proper nutritional intake, the nurse encourages a diet high in protein and calories. The nurse also offers emotional support because the abscess may take a long time to resolve.

PROMOTING HOME AND COMMUNITY-BASED CARE

Teaching Patients Self-Care. The patient who has had surgery may return home before the wound closes entirely or with a drain or tube in place. Thus, the patient or a caregiver needs instruction on how to change the dressings to prevent skin excoriation and odor, how to monitor for signs and symptoms of infection, and how to care for and maintain the drain or tube. The nurse instructs the patient to perform deep-breathing and coughing exercises every 2 hours during the day and shows a caregiver how to perform chest percussion and postural drainage to facilitate expectoration of lung secretions.

Continuing Care. Referral for home care may be required by some patients whose condition requires therapy at home. During visits to the patient at home, the nurse assesses the patient's physical condition, nutritional status, and home environment as well as the patient's and family's ability to carry out the therapeutic regimen. Patient teaching is reinforced during home visits, and nutrition counseling is provided for attaining and maintaining an optimal state of nutrition. To prevent a relapse, the nurse must emphasize the importance of completing the antibiotic regimen and of following the suggestions for rest and appropriate activity. If intravenous antibiotic therapy is to continue at home, the services of a home care nurse may be arranged to initiate intravenous therapy and to evaluate its administration by the patient or family. Although most outpatient intravenous therapy is administered in the home setting, a patient may visit a nearby clinic or physician's office for this treatment.

PLEURAL CONDITIONS

Pleural conditions are disorders that involve the membranes covering the lungs (visceral pleura) and the surface of the chest wall (parietal pleura) or disorders affecting the pleural space.

Pleurisy

Pathophysiology

Pleurisy (pleuritis) refers to inflammation of both layers of the pleurae (parietal and visceral). Pleurisy may develop in conjunction with pneumonia or an upper respiratory tract infection, TB, or collagen disease; after trauma to the chest, pulmonary infarction, or pulmonary embolism; in patients with primary and metastatic cancer; and after thoracotomy. The parietal pleura has nerve endings; the visceral pleura does not. When the inflamed pleural membranes rub together during respiration (intensified on inspiration), the result is severe, sharp, knifelike pain.

Clinical Manifestations

The key characteristic of pleuritic pain is its relationship to respiratory movement. Taking a deep breath, coughing, or sneezing worsens the pain. Pleuritic pain is restricted in distribution rather than diffuse and usually occurs only on one side. The pain may become minimal or absent when the breath is held, or it may be localized or may radiate to the shoulder or abdomen. Later, as pleural fluid develops, the pain lessens.

Assessment and Diagnostic Findings

In the early period, when little fluid has accumulated, a pleural friction rub can be heard with the stethoscope, only to disappear later as fluid accumulates and separates the inflamed pleural surfaces. Diagnostic tests may include chest x-rays, sputum examinations, thoracentesis to obtain a specimen of pleural fluid for examination, and less commonly a pleural biopsy.

Medical Management

The objectives of treatment are to discover the underlying condition causing the pleurisy and to relieve the pain. As the underlying disease (pneumonia, infection) is treated, the pleuritic inflammation usually resolves. At the same time, it is necessary to monitor for signs and symptoms of pleural effusion, such as shortness of breath, pain, assumption of a position that decreases pain, and decreased chest wall excursion.

Prescribed analgesics and topical applications of heat or cold provide symptomatic relief. Indomethacin, a nonsteroidal anti-inflammatory medication, may provide pain relief while allowing the patient to deep breathe and cough more effectively. If the pain is severe, an intercostal nerve block may be required.

Nursing Management

Because the patient has considerable pain on inspiration, the nurse can offer suggestions to enhance comfort, such as turning frequently onto the affected side to splint the chest wall and reduce the stretching of the pleurae. The nurse also can teach the patient to use the hands or a pillow to splint the rib cage while coughing.

Pleural Effusion

Pleural effusion, a collection of fluid in the pleural space, is rarely a primary disease process but is usually secondary to other diseases. Normally, the pleural space contains a small amount of fluid (5 to 15 mL), which acts as a lubricant that allows the pleural surfaces to move without friction (Fig. 21-5). Pleural effusion may be a complication of congestive heart failure, TB, pneumonia, pulmonary infections (particularly viral infections), nephrotic syndrome, connective tissue disease, pulmonary embolism, and neoplastic tumors. Bronchogenic carcinoma is the most common malignancy associated with a pleural effusion.

Pathophysiology

In certain disorders, fluid may accumulate in the pleural space to a point where it becomes clinically evident. This almost always has pathologic significance. The effusion can be composed of a relatively clear fluid, or it can be bloody or purulent. An effusion of clear fluid may be a transudate or an exudate. A transudate (filtrates of plasma that move across intact capillary walls) occurs when factors influencing the formation and reabsorption of pleural fluid are altered, usually by imbalances in hydrostatic or oncotic pressures. The finding of a transudative effusion generally implies that the pleural membranes are not diseased. The most common cause of a transudative effusion is congestive heart failure. An exudate (extravasation of fluid into tissues or a cavity) usually results from inflammation by bacterial products or tumors involving the pleural surfaces.

Clinical Manifestations

Usually the clinical manifestations are those caused by the underlying disease. Pneumonia causes fever, chills, and pleuritic chest pain, whereas a malignant effusion may result in dyspnea and coughing. The size of the effusion and the patient's underlying lung disease determine the severity of symptoms. A large pleural effusion causes shortness of breath. When a small to moderate pleural effusion is present, dyspnea may not be present. The severity of the symptoms assessed depends on the time course of the development of the pleural effusion.

Assessment and Diagnostic Findings

Assessment of the area of the pleural effusion reveals decreased or absent breath sounds, decreased fremitus, and a dull, flat sound when percussed. In an extremely large pleural effusion, the assessment reveals a patient in acute respiratory distress. Tracheal deviation away from the affected side may also be noted.

Physical examination, chest x-ray, chest CT scan, and thoracentesis confirm the presence of fluid. In some instances, a lateral decubitus x-ray is obtained. For this x-ray, the patient lies on the affected side in a side-lying position. A pleural effusion can be diagnosed because this position allows for the "layering out" of the fluid, and an air–fluid line is visible.

Pleural fluid is analyzed by bacterial culture, Gram's stain, acid-fast bacillus stain (for TB), red and white blood cell counts, chemistry studies (glucose, amylase, lactic dehydrogenase, protein), cytologic analysis for malignant cells, and pH. A pleural biopsy also may be performed.

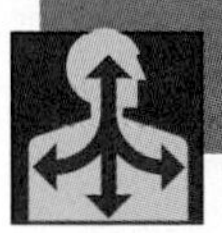

PATHOPHYSIOLOGY

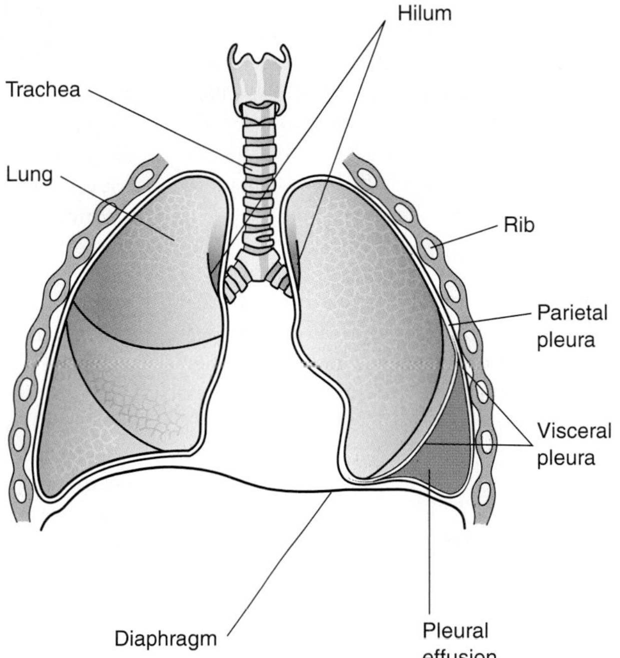

FIGURE 21•5 In pleural effusion, an abnormal volume of fluid collects in the pleural space causing pain and shortness of breath. Pleural effusion is usually secondary to other disease processes.

Medical Management

The objectives of treatment are to discover the underlying cause, to prevent reaccumulation of fluid, and to relieve discomfort and dyspnea. Specific treatment is directed at the underlying cause (eg, congestive heart failure, pneumonia, cirrhosis). If the pleural fluid is an exudate, more extensive diagnostic procedures are performed to determine the cause. Treatment for the primary cause is then instituted.

Thoracentesis is performed to remove fluid, to obtain a specimen for analysis, and to relieve dyspnea. Depending on the size of the pleural effusion, the patient may be treated with a chest tube connected to a water-seal drainage system or suction to evacuate the pleural space and reexpand the lung.

If the underlying cause is a malignancy, however, the effusion tends to recur within a few days or weeks. Repeated thoracenteses result in pain, depletion of protein and electrolytes, and sometimes pneumothorax. Once the pleural space is adequately drained, a chemical pleurodesis may be performed to obliterate the pleural space and prevent reaccumulation of fluid. Chemically irritating agents, such as doxycycline, minocycline, bleomycin, or talc, are instilled in the pleural space. After the agent is instilled, the chest tube is clamped and the patient is assisted to assume various positions to ensure uniform distribution of the agent and to maximize its contact with the pleural surfaces. The tube is unclamped as prescribed, and chest drainage may be continued several days longer to prevent reaccumulation of fluid and to promote the formation of adhesions between the visceral and parietal pleurae. Other treatments for malignant pleural effusions include surgical pleurectomy and diuretic therapy.

Nursing Management

The nurse's role in the care of the patient with a pleural effusion includes implementing the medical regimen. The nurse prepares and positions the patient for thoracentesis and offers support throughout the procedure. Pain management is a priority, and the nurse assists the patient to assume positions that are the least painful. However, frequent turning and ambulation are important to facilitate drainage. The nurse administers analgesics as prescribed and as needed.

If a chest tube drainage and water-seal system is used, the nurse is responsible for monitoring the system's function and recording the amount of drainage at prescribed intervals. Nursing care related to the underlying cause of the pleural effusion is specific to the underlying condition. Care of the patient with a chest tube is discussed in Chapter 22.

Empyema

An empyema is a collection of purulent liquid (pus) in the pleural cavity. Most empyemas occur as complications of bacterial pneumonia or lung abscess. Other causes include penetrating chest trauma, hematogenous infection of the pleural space, nonbacterial infections, or iatrogenic causes (after thoracic surgery or thoracentesis).

Pathophysiology

At first the pleural fluid is thin, with a low leukocyte count, but it frequently progresses to fibropurulent stage and, finally, to a stage where it encloses the lung within a thick exudative membrane (loculated empyema).

Clinical Manifestations

With an empyema, the patient is acutely ill and has signs and symptoms similar to those of an acute respiratory infection or pneumonia (fever, night sweats, pleural pain, cough, dyspnea, anorexia, weight loss). If the patient is immunocompromised, the symptoms may be more vague. If the patient has received antimicrobial therapy, the clinical manifestations may be less obvious.

Assessment and Diagnostic Findings

Chest auscultation demonstrates decreased or absent breath sounds over the affected area, and there is flatness on chest percussion as well as decreased fremitus (vocal vibration detected on palpation). The diagnosis is established by a chest x-ray or chest CT scan. Usually a diagnostic thoracentesis is performed.

Medical Management

The objectives of treatment are to drain the pleural cavity and to achieve full expansion of the lung. The fluid is drained and appropriate antibiotics are prescribed based on the causative organism. Large doses of the antibiotic are prescribed. Drainage of the pleural fluid depends on the stage of the disease and is accomplished by the following:

- Needle aspiration (thoracentesis) with a thin percutaneous catheter, if the volume is small and the fluid not too purulent or thick
- Tube thoracostomy (chest drainage using a large-diameter intercostal tube attached to water-seal drainage [see Chap. 22]) with fibrinolytic agents instilled through the chest tube in patients with loculated or complicated pleural effusions
- Open chest drainage via thoracotomy, including potential rib resection, to remove the thickened pleura, pus, and debris and to remove the underlying diseased pulmonary tissue

With longstanding inflammation, an exudate can form over the lung, trapping it and interfering with its normal expansion. This exudate must be removed surgically (decortication). The drainage tube is left in place until the pus-filled space is obliterated completely. The complete obliteration of the pleural space is monitored by serial chest x-rays, and the patient should be informed that treatment may be long term. Patients are frequently discharged from the hospital with a chest tube in place and with instructions to monitor fluid drainage at home.

Nursing Management

Resolution of empyema is a prolonged process. The nurse helps the patient cope with the condition and instructs the patient in lung expansion breathing exercises to restore normal respiratory function. The nurse also provides care specific to the method of drainage of the pleural fluid (eg, needle aspiration, closed chest drainage, or rib resection and drainage). When patients are discharged to home with a drainage tube or system in place, the nurse must instruct the patient and family on care of the drainage system and drain site, measurement and observation of drainage, signs and symptoms of infection, and how and when to contact the health care provider. (See Nursing Process: The Patient Undergoing Thoracic Surgery in Chap. 22.)

CHRONIC OBSTRUCTIVE PULMONARY DISEASE

Chronic obstructive pulmonary disease (COPD) is a disease state in which air flow is obstructed by emphysema, chronic bronchitis, or both. The air flow obstruction is usually progressive and irreversible, and it may be associated with airway hyperreactivity. Asthma used to be considered within the disease group of COPD, but it is now considered a separate disorder, classified as an abnormal airway condition characterized primarily by reversible inflammation. However, in some cases of asthma and in some cases of COPD, air flow obstruction may be uncharacteristically reversible or irreversible. Because of this overlap, asthma is included in this discussion of COPD.

COPD is the fourth leading cause of death in the United States. This represents a rise in the mortality rate at a time when death rates from other serious illnesses, such as heart disease and cerebral vascular disease, are declining (Ventura, Peters, Martin, & Maurer, 1997; Wilcox, 1998). Approximately 14 million people in the United States have COPD, an increase of 41.5% from 1982 to 1995. People with COPD commonly become symptomatic during the middle adult years, and the incidence of COPD increases with age. Although certain aspects of lung function normally decrease with age (eg, vital capacity [VC] and forced expiratory volume in one second [FEV_1]), COPD accentuates and accelerates these physiologic changes.

Pathophysiology

The airway obstruction that occurs to reduce air flow varies according to the underlying disease. In chronic bronchitis, excessive accumulation of mucus and secretions blocks the airways. In emphysema, impaired gas exchange (oxygen, carbon dioxide) results from destruction of the walls of overdistended alveoli. In asthma, inflamed and constricted airways obstruct airflow. Treatment regimens are related to the underlying pathophysiology and may overlap.

Smoking depresses the activity of scavenger cells and affects the ciliary cleansing mechanism of the respiratory tract, the function of which is to keep the breathing passages free of inhaled irritants, bacteria, and other foreign matter. When smoking damages this cleansing mechanism, air flow is obstructed and air becomes trapped behind the obstruction. The alveoli greatly distend, and the lung capacity is diminished. Smoking also irritates the goblet

Risk Factors for COPD

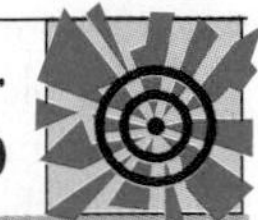

- Exposure to tobacco smoke accounts for an estimated 80% to 90% of COPD cases (Rennard, 1998)
- Passive smoking
- Occupational exposure
- Ambient air pollution
- Genetic abnormalities, including a deficiency of $alpha_1$-antitrypsin, an enzyme inhibitor that normally counteracts the destruction of lung tissue by certain other enzymes

cells and mucus glands, causing an increased accumulation of mucus. The accumulated mucus produces more irritation, infection, and damage to the lung. In addition, carbon monoxide (a byproduct of smoking) combines with hemoglobin to form carboxyhemoglobin. Hemoglobin that is bound by carboxyhemoglobin cannot carry oxygen efficiently.

Clinical Manifestations

COPD is characterized by dyspnea, cough, and increased work of breathing. Dyspnea may be severe and often interferes with the patient's activities. Weight loss is common because dyspnea interferes with eating. Often the patient cannot participate in even mild exercise because of dyspnea; as COPD progresses, dyspnea occurs even at rest. The work of breathing increases over time, and the accessory muscles are recruited in an effort to breathe. The patient with COPD is at risk for respiratory insufficiency and respiratory infections. Respiratory infections, in turn, increase the risk for acute and chronic respiratory failure. Clinical manifestations specific to the diseases that cause COPD (bronchitis and emphysema) are discussed in detail in later sections of this chapter.

Pulmonary function studies are used to determine disease severity and to follow the disease progression. Air flow obstruction is determined by the ratio of FEV_1 to forced vital capacity (FVC). With obstruction, the patient cannot forcibly exhale air from the lungs, reducing the FEV_1. Obstructive disease is defined as a FEV_1/FVC ratio of less than 70%. VC may also be reduced.

Complications

Because COPD is a broad classification of respiratory diseases, the potential complications may vary, depending on the underlying disorder. Respiratory insufficiency and failure are major life-threatening complications of COPD. Other complications of COPD (eg, pneumonia, atelectasis, pneumothorax) increase the risk for respiratory failure in this patient population.

The acuity of the onset and the severity of respiratory failure depend on the patient's baseline pulmonary function, pulse oximetry or arterial blood gas values, comorbid conditions, and the severity of other complications of COPD. Respiratory insufficiency and failure may be chronic (with longstanding emphysema) or acute (with severe bronchospasm or pneumonia in the patient with longstanding COPD). Acute respiratory insufficiency and failure may necessitate ventilatory support until other acute complications, such as infection, can be treated. Management of the patient requiring ventilatory support is discussed in Chapter 22. Other complications of COPD include atelectasis and pneumonia, pneumothorax, mediastinal or subcutaneous emphysema, and pulmonary hypertension (cor pulmonale).

Medical Management

Inhaled bronchodilators are often used to provide direct bronchodilator action to the airways, thereby improving air flow. These medications are delivered through an MDI or by nebulization. They are often given regularly throughout the day as well as on an as-needed basis. Bronchodilators may be used prophylactically to prevent dyspnea by taking the medication before an activity, such as eating or walking. Nebulized medications may be more effective in patients who cannot use an MDI properly; otherwise, the deposition of medication in the lungs is similar whether a nebulizer or an MDI is used.

OXYGEN THERAPY

Long-term oxygen therapy ultimately improves the quality of life and survival. Maintenance of a constant, adequate oxygen saturation (more than 90%) for those with an arterial oxygen pressure (PaO_2) of 55 mm Hg or less on room air is associated with a significant reduction in the mortality rate. Patients who are hypoxemic while awake are likely to be so during sleep. Therefore, nighttime oxygen therapy is recommended as well, and the prescription for oxygen therapy is for continuous, 24-hour use. Intermittent oxygen therapy is indicated for those who desaturate only during exercise or sleep.

Nursing Alert *Because hypoxemia is a stimulus for respiration in the patient with longstanding COPD, increasing the oxygen flow rate may raise the oxygen level in the patient's blood but lead to depression of the respiratory drive and retention of carbon dioxide. Monitoring the patient's respiratory response to oxygen administration is a priority.*

PULMONARY REHABILITATION

Pulmonary rehabilitation for patients with COPD is well established and widely accepted as a means to complement standard care to alleviate symptoms and optimize functional status. The primary goal of rehabilitation is to restore the patient to the highest level of independent function and to improve the patient's quality of life. A successful rehabilitation program is individualized for each patient, is multidisciplinary, and attends to both the physiologic and emotional needs of the patient. Most pulmonary rehabilitation programs consist of educational, psychosocial, behavioral, and physical components. Breathing exercises and retraining and exercise programs are used to improve functional status, and the patient is taught methods to alleviate symptoms.

Pulmonary rehabilitation may be used therapeutically in a variety of diseases in addition to COPD, including asthma, cystic fibrosis, lung cancer, interstitial lung disease, thoracic surgery, and lung transplantation. Pulmonary rehabilitation may be conducted in the inpatient or outpatient setting; the length of the program varies.

Nursing Management

The nurse plays a key role in identifying potential candidates for rehabilitation and also in facilitating and reinforcing the material learned in a rehabilitation program. Not all patients have access to a formal rehabilitation program. However, the nurse can be instrumental in teaching the patient and family as well as facilitating specific services for the patient (eg, respiratory therapy education, physical therapy for exercise and breathing retraining, and occupational therapy for conservation of energy techniques during activities of daily living). In addition, numerous educational materials are available to assist the nurse in teaching patients with COPD. Potential resources include the American Lung Association, the American Association of Cardiovascular and Pulmonary Rehabilitation, and the American Association of Respiratory Therapy.

TEACHING PATIENTS ABOUT COPD

Education of the COPD patient encompasses a broad variety of topics. Depending on the length and setting of the program, topics may include normal anatomy and physiology of the lung, pathophysiology and changes with COPD, medications and home oxygen therapy, nutrition, respiratory therapy treatments, symptom alleviation, smoking cessation, sexuality and COPD, coping with chronic disease, communicating with the health care team, and planning for the future (advance directives, living wills, informed decision making about health care alternatives).

Breathing Exercises. The respirations of most people with COPD are shallow, rapid, and inefficient. This type of upper chest breathing can be changed to diaphragmatic breathing with practice. Training in diaphragmatic breathing reduces the respiratory rate, increases alveolar ventilation, and sometimes helps expel as much air as possible during expiration (see Chap. 22 for technique). Pursed-lip breathing retraining helps to slow expiration, prevents collapse of small airways, and helps the patient to control the rate and depth of respiration. It also promotes relaxation. This enables the patient to gain control of dyspnea and feelings of panic.

Activity Pacing. A patient with COPD has decreased exercise tolerance during definite periods of the day. This is especially true on arising in the morning, because bronchial secretions collect in the lungs during the night while the person is lying down. The patient may have difficulty bathing or dressing. Activities requiring the arms to be supported above the level of the thorax may produce fatigue or respiratory distress. These activities may be tolerated better after the patient has been up and moving around for an hour or more. Because of these limitations, the patient must participate with the nurse in planning self-care activities and in determining the best time for bathing and dressing.

Inspiratory Muscle Training. Once the patient masters diaphragmatic breathing, a program of inspiratory muscle training may be prescribed to help strengthen the muscles used in breathing. This program requires that the patient breathe against resistance for 10 to 15 minutes every day. The resistance is gradually increased and the muscles become better conditioned. Conditioning of the respiratory muscles takes a long time, and the patient is instructed to continue practicing at home.

Self-Care Activities. As gas exchange, airway clearance, and the breathing pattern improve, the patient is encouraged to assume self-care activities. The patient is taught to try to coordinate diaphragmatic breathing with activities such as walking, bathing, bending, or climbing stairs. The patient should begin to bathe, dress, and take short walks, resting as needed to avoid fatigue and excessive dyspnea. Fluids should be readily available, and the patient should begin to drink fluids without having to be reminded. If postural drainage will be done at home, the nurse instructs and supervises the patient before discharge.

Physical Conditioning. Physical conditioning techniques include breathing exercises and general exercises intended to conserve energy and increase pulmonary ventilation. There is a close relationship between physical fitness and respiratory fitness. Graded exercises and physical conditioning programs employing treadmills, stationary bicycles, and measured level walks have been shown to improve symptoms and to increase work capacity and exercise tolerance. A physical activity that can be done on a regular sustained basis is helpful. A lightweight portable oxygen system is available for the ambulatory patient who requires oxygen therapy during physical activity to decrease hypoxemia.

Precautions for Oxygen Therapy. Oxygen supplied to the home comes in compressed gas, liquid, or concentrator systems. Portable oxygen systems allow the patient to exercise, work, and travel. To assist the patient in adhering to the oxygen prescription, the nurse explains the proper flow rate and required number of hours for oxygen use as well as the dangers of arbitrary changes in flow rates or duration of therapy. The nurse advises the patient that smoking with or near oxygen is extremely dangerous. Patient education also includes reassuring the patient that oxygen is not "addictive" and explaining the need for regular evaluations of blood oxygenation by pulse oximetry or arterial blood gas analysis.

Coping Measures. Any factor that interferes with normal breathing quite naturally induces anxiety, depression, and changes in behavior. Many patients find the slightest exertion exhausting. Constant shortness of breath and fatigue may make the patient irritable and apprehensive to the point of panic. Restricted activity (and reversal of family roles due to loss of employment), the frustration of having to work to breathe, and the realization that the disease is prolonged and unrelenting may cause the patient to react with anger, depression, and demanding behavior. Sexual function may be compromised, which also diminishes self-esteem.

It is important for the nurse and other health care personnel to encourage the patient to remain as active as possible without becoming overly fatigued. Emphasis should be on controlling symptoms and increasing self-esteem and a sense of mastery and well-being. Supportive medical and nursing care, ongoing patient teaching, exercise conditioning, and possibly group therapy sessions help somewhat to relieve an almost overwhelming burden.

The patient may also be directed to support groups conducted by the American Lung Association, to pulmonary rehabilitation programs, to smoking cessation programs (if still smoking), and to senior citizens groups for social interaction. These groups help improve the patient's knowledge and ability to cope with COPD and promote a sense of self-worth.

NURSING PROCESS: THE PATIENT WITH COPD

Assessment

Assessment involves obtaining information about current symptoms as well as previous disease manifestations. The accompanying chart, Assessment: COPD lists sample questions that may be used to obtain a clear history of the disease process.

Diagnosis

Nursing Diagnoses

Based on the assessment data, the patient's major nursing diagnoses may include the following:

- Impaired gas exchange related to ventilation–perfusion inequality
- Ineffective airway clearance related to bronchoconstriction, increased mucus production, ineffective cough, and bronchopulmonary infection
- Ineffective breathing pattern related to shortness of breath, mucus, bronchoconstriction, and airway irritants
- Self-care deficit related to fatigue secondary to increased work of breathing and insufficient ventilation and oxygenation
- Activity intolerance due to fatigue, hypoxemia, and ineffective breathing patterns

ASSESSMENT
COPD

Health History

- How long has the patient had respiratory difficulty?
- Does exertion increase the dyspnea? What type of exertion?
- What are limits of the patient's tolerance for exercise?
- At what times during the day does the patient complain most of fatigue and shortness of breath?
- Which eating and sleeping habits have been affected?
- What does the patient know about the disease and his or her condition?
- What is the patient's smoking history (primary and secondary)?
- Is there occupational exposure to smoke or other pollutants?
- What are the triggering events (exertion, strong odors, dust, exposure to animals, etc.)?

Inspection and Examination Findings

- What position does the patient assume during the interview?
- What are the pulse and the respiratory rates?
- What is the character of respirations? Even and without effort? Other?
- Can the patient complete a sentence without having to take a breath?
- Does the patient contract the abdominal muscles during inspiration?
- Does the patient use accessory muscles of the shoulders and neck when breathing?
- Does the patient take a long time to exhale (prolonged expiration)?
- Is central cyanosis evident?
- Are the patient's neck veins engorged?
- Does the patient have peripheral edema?
- Is the patient coughing?
- What is the color, amount, and consistency of the sputum?
- Is clubbing of the fingers present?
- What types of breath sounds (ie, clear, diminished or distant, crackles, wheezes) are heard? Describe and document findings and locations.
- What is the status of the patient's sensorium?
- Is there short-term or long-term memory impairment?
- Is there increasing stupor? Apprehension?

- Ineffective individual coping related to reduced socialization, anxiety, depression, lower activity level, and the inability to work
- Knowledge deficit of self-care to be performed at home

Collaborative Problems/Potential Complications

Based on the assessment data, potential complications that may develop include:

- Respiratory insufficiency or failure
- Atelectasis
- Pulmonary infection
- Pneumonia
- Pneumothorax
- Pulmonary hypertension

Planning and Goals

The major goals for the patient may include smoking cessation, improved gas exchange, airway clearance, improved breathing pattern, maximal self-management, improved activity tolerance, improved coping ability, adherence to the therapeutic program and home care, absence of complications, and improved health-related quality of life.

Nursing Interventions

Promoting Smoking Cessation

Once the COPD diagnosis is established, anyone who continues to smoke must be encouraged and assisted to quit. Unfortunately, sustained abstinence in pulmonary patients, even after counseling, is low. Factors associated with continued smoking vary among patients and may include the strength of nicotine addiction, continued exposure to smoking-associated stimuli (at work or in social settings), stress, depression, and habit. Continued smoking is also more prevalent among those with low incomes, a low level of education, and psychosocial problems.

Because there are multiple factors associated with continued smoking, successful cessation often requires multiple strategies. The health care provider should promote cessation by explaining the risks of smoking and personalizing the "at-risk" message to the patient. A strong warning regarding smoking should be given and a definite "quit date" established. Referral to a smoking cessation program may be helpful. Follow-up within 3 to 5 days after the quit date to review progress and to solve problems as needed is associated with increased success; this should be repeated as needed. Continued reinforcement with telephone calls or clinic visits is extremely beneficial. Relapses should be analyzed, and the patient and health care provider should jointly identify possible solutions to prevent future backsliding. It is important to emphasize successes rather than failures. Nicotine replacement therapy may be indicated, or other proven pharmacologic therapies (buproprion HCl) may be tried.

Smoking cessation can begin in a variety of health care settings—outpatient clinic, pulmonary rehabilitation, community, hospital, and the patient's home. Regardless of the setting, the nurse has the opportunity to begin teaching the patient about the risks of smoking and the benefits of smoking cessation. A variety of materials, resources, and programs are available to assist with this effort (eg, American Lung Association, American Cancer Society, hospital- or clinic-based smoking cessation programs).

Improving Gas Exchange

Bronchospasm, which occurs in many pulmonary diseases, reduces the caliber of the small bronchi and may cause dyspnea, static secretions, and infection. Bronchospasm can sometimes be detected when wheezing or diminished breath sounds are heard on auscultation with a stethoscope. Increased mucus production, along with decreased mucociliary action, contributes to further reduction in the caliber of the bronchi and results in decreased air flow and decreased gas exchange. This is further aggravated by the loss of lung elasticity observed with COPD.

These changes in the airway require that the nurse monitor the patient for dyspnea and hypoxemia. If bronchodilators or corticosteroids are prescribed, the nurse must administer the medications properly and be alert for potential side effects. The relief of bronchospasm is confirmed by measuring improvement in expiratory flow rates (how long it takes to exhale, and the amount of air exhaled) and assessing whether the patient has less dyspnea.

Achieving Airway Clearance

Diminishing the quantity and viscosity of sputum can clear the airway and improve pulmonary ventilation and gas exchange. All pulmonary irritants should be eliminated or reduced, particularly cigarette smoking, which is the most persistent source of pulmonary irritation. The nurse instructs the patient in directed or controlled coughing, which is more effective and reduces the fatigue associated with undirected forceful coughing. Directed coughing consists of a slow, maximal inspiration followed by breath-holding for several seconds and then two or three coughs. "Huff" coughing may also be effective. The technique consists of one or two forced exhalations ("huffs") from low to medium lung volumes with the glottis open. This reduces airway collapse and the triggering of bronchoconstriction.

Chest physiotherapy with postural drainage, intermittent positive-pressure breathing, increased fluid intake, and bland aerosol mists (with normal saline solution or water) may be useful for a few patients with COPD. The use of these measures must be based on the patient's response and tolerance.

Preventing Bronchopulmonary Infections

Bronchopulmonary infections must be controlled to diminish inflammatory edema and to permit recovery of normal ciliary action. Minor respiratory infections that are of no consequence to the person with normal lungs can be life-threatening to the person with COPD. The cough associated with bronchial infection introduces a vicious cycle with further trauma and damage to the lungs, progression of symptoms, increased bronchospasm, and increased susceptibility to bronchial infection. Infection compromises lung function and is a common cause of respiratory failure in patients with COPD.

In COPD, infection may be accompanied by subtle changes. The nurse instructs the patient to report any signs of infection, such as a fever or change in sputum color, character, consistency, or amount. Any worsening of symptoms (increased tightness of the chest, increased dyspnea and fatigue) also suggests infection and must be reported. Viral infections are hazardous to these patients because they are often followed by infections caused by bacterial organisms, such as *S. pneumoniae* and *H. influenzae.*

The nurse should encourage patients with COPD to be immunized against influenza and *S. pneumoniae* because these patients are prone to respiratory infection. It is important to caution patients to avoid going outdoors if the pollen count is high or if there is significant air pollution because of the risk of bronchospasm. The patient also should avoid exposure to high outdoor temperatures with high humidity.

Monitoring and Managing Potential Complications

The nurse caring for the patient with COPD must assess for various complications, such as life-threatening respiratory insufficiency and failure and respiratory infection and atelectasis, which may increase the patient's risk for respiratory failure. The nurse also monitors for cognitive changes (personality and behavioral changes, memory impairment), increasing dyspnea, tachypnea, and tachycardia, which may indicate increasing hypoxemia and impending respiratory failure.

The nurse monitors pulse oximetry values to assess the patient's need for oxygen and administers supplemental oxygen as prescribed. The nurse also instructs the patient about signs and symptoms of respiratory infection that may worsen hypoxemia and reports changes in the patient's physical and cognitive status to the physician. Other activities require assisting with the management of developing complications, with possible intubation and mechanical ventilation (see Chap. 22).

Promoting Home and Community-Based Care

TEACHING PATIENTS SELF-CARE

The nurse assists the patient to manage self-care by pointing out the importance of setting realistic goals, avoiding temperature extremes, and modifying lifestyle (particularly, stopping smoking) as applicable.

Setting Realistic Goals. A major area of teaching is the importance of setting and accepting realistic short-term and long-range goals. If the patient is severely disabled, the objectives of treatment are to preserve current pulmonary function and relieve symptoms as much as possible. If the disease is mild, the objectives are to increase exercise tolerance and prevent further loss of pulmonary function. It is important to plan and share the goals and expectations of treatment with the patient. The patient and those providing care need patience to achieve these goals.

Avoiding Temperature Extremes. The nurse instructs the patient to avoid extremes of heat and cold. Heat increases the body temperature, thereby raising oxygen requirements; cold tends to promote bronchospasm. Bronchospasm may be initiated also by air pollutants such as fumes, smoke, dust, and even talcum, lint, and aerosol sprays. High altitudes aggravate hypoxemia.

Altering Lifestyle. Patients with COPD should adopt a lifestyle of moderate activity, ideally in a climate with minimal shifts in temperature and humidity. As much as possible, the patient should avoid emotional disturbances and stressful situations that might trigger a coughing episode. The medication regimen for patients with COPD can be quite complex; patients receiving aerosol medications by an MDI may be particularly challenged. It is crucial to review this material and to have the patient perform a return demonstration before discharge, during follow-up visits to the caregiver's office or clinic, and during home visits.

Smoking cessation goes hand in hand with lifestyle changes, and reinforcement of the patient's efforts is a key activity of the nurse. Smoking cessation is the single most important therapeutic intervention for patients with COPD. There are many strategies, including prevention, cessation with or without oral or topical patch medications, and behavior modification techniques.

CONTINUING CARE

Referral for home care is important to enable the nurse to assess the patient's home environment and physical and psychological status, to evaluate the patient's adherence to the prescribed regimen, and to assess the patient's ability to cope with changes in lifestyle and physical status. The nurse assesses the patient's and family's understanding of the complications and side effects of medications. The home care visit provides an opportunity to reinforce information and activities learned in the inpatient or outpatient pulmonary rehabilitation program and to have the patient and family demonstrate correct administration of medications and oxygen, if indicated, and performance of exercises. If the patient does not have access to a formal pulmonary rehabilitation program, it is important for the nurse to provide the education and breathing retraining necessary to optimize the patient's functional status.

The nurse may direct patients to community resources such as pulmonary rehabilitation programs and smoking cessation programs to help improve their ability to cope with their chronic condition and the therapeutic regimen and to give them a sense of worth, hope, and well-being.

Evaluation

Expected Outcomes

Expected outcomes may include:

1. Demonstrates improved gas exchange
   a. Shows no signs of restlessness, confusion, or agitation
   b. Has stable pulse oximetry or arterial blood gas values (but not necessarily normal values due to chronic changes in the gas exchange ability of the lungs)
2. Achieves maximal airway clearance
   a. Stops smoking
   b. Avoids noxious substances and extremes of temperature
   c. Maintains adequate hydration
   d. If indicated, performs postural drainage correctly
   e. Knows signs of early infection and is aware of how and when to report them if they occur
   f. Performs controlled or "huff" coughing without experiencing excessive fatigue
3. Improves breathing pattern
   a. Practices and uses pursed-lip and diaphragmatic breathing
   b. Shows signs of decreased respiratory effort
4. Maintains maximum level of self-care and physical functioning
   a. Performs self-care activities within tolerance range
   b. Paces self to avoid fatigue and dyspnea
   c. Uses controlled breathing while performing activities
5. Achieves activity tolerance, and exercises and performs activities with less shortness of breath
6. Develops effective coping mechanisms and participates in a pulmonary rehabilitation program
7. Adheres to the therapeutic program
   a. Participates in determining the therapeutic program
   b. Understands the rationale for activities and medications
   c. Follows the medication plan
   d. Uses bronchodilators and oxygen therapy as prescribed
   e. Stops smoking
   f. Maintains acceptable activity level
8. Avoids or reduces complications
   a. Has no evidence of respiratory failure or insufficiency
   b. Maintains adequate pulse oximetry and arterial blood gas values
   c. Shows no signs of infection

Chronic Bronchitis

Chronic bronchitis is defined as a productive cough that lasts 3 months in each of 2 consecutive years in a patient in whom other causes for cough have been excluded. Cigarette smoking is by far the major risk factor for chronic bronchitis. Other risk factors include second-hand smoke inhalation, air pollution, and occupational exposure to hazardous airborne substances.

Patients with chronic bronchitis are more susceptible to recurring infections of the lower respiratory tract. A wide range of viral, bacterial, and mycoplasmal infections can produce acute episodes of bronchitis. Exacerbations of chronic bronchitis are most likely to occur during the winter.

Pathophysiology

Smoke or another environmental pollutant irritates the airways, resulting in hypersecretion of mucus and inflammation. Because of this constant irritation, the mucus-secreting glands and goblet cells increase in number, ciliary function is reduced, and more mucus is produced. The bronchial walls become thickened, the bronchial lumen is narrowed, and mucus may plug the airway. Alveoli adjacent to the bronchioles may become damaged and fibrosed, resulting in altered function of the alveolar macrophages. This is significant because the macrophages play an important role in destroying foreign particles, including bacteria. As a result, the patient becomes more susceptible to respiratory infection. Further bronchial narrowing follows as a result of the fibrotic changes that occur in the airways. Irreversible lung changes eventually may occur, possibly resulting in emphysema and **bronchiectasis** (chronic dilation of the bronchial structures). In chronic bronchitis, accumulated secretions in the bronchioles interfere with effective breathing.

Clinical Manifestations

A chronic, productive cough in the winter months is the earliest sign of chronic bronchitis. Cold weather, dampness, and pulmonary irritants may exacerbate the cough. Chronic bronchitis frequently presents in the fifth decade of life with a history of cigarette smoking and increasing frequency of respiratory infections.

Assessment and Diagnostic Findings

A complete history, including family, environmental exposure to irritating substances, occupation, and smoking habits (number of packs per day multiplied by number of years), is obtained. In addition, pulse oximetry, arterial blood gases, chest x-ray, and pulmonary function studies are performed and laboratory values (complete blood count, hemoglobin, hematocrit) are obtained.

In the patient with chronic bronchitis, pulmonary function studies will reveal a decrease in VC and FEV_1, an increased residual volume (the air remaining in the lungs after maximal exhalation), and a normal to slightly increased total lung capacity. The hematocrit and hemoglobin may be slightly increased. This may be caused by the body's response to chronic hypoxemia. Pulse oximetry may show desaturation, and the blood gas analysis may reveal hypoxemia with beginning hypercapnia. The typical chest x-ray of the patient with chronic bronchitis reveals an enlarged heart, with a normal or flattened diaphragm.

Prevention

Because of the disabling nature of chronic bronchitis, every effort is directed toward prevention. One essential measure is to avoid respiratory irritants (particularly tobacco smoke). People who are prone to respiratory tract infections should receive the vaccine against influenza and *S. pneumoniae.* All patients with acute upper respiratory tract infections should receive proper treatment, including antimicrobial therapy at the first sign of purulent sputum. For more information on nursing management and patient teaching, see Nursing Process: The Patient With COPD.

Medical Management

The objectives of treatment are to keep the bronchioles open and functioning, to facilitate removal of secretions to prevent infection, and to prevent disability. Changes in the sputum pattern (nature, color, amount, thickness) and in the cough pattern are important signs to note. Recurrent bacterial infections are treated with antibiotic therapy.

To help in removing bronchial secretions, bronchodilators are prescribed to relieve bronchospasm and reduce airway obstruction; thus, more oxygen is distributed throughout the lungs, and alveolar ventilation is improved. Postural drainage and chest percussion after treatments may be helpful, especially if bronchiectasis is present. Proper hydration helps to loosen secretions so they can be removed by coughing. Corticosteroid therapy may be used when the patient fails to respond to more conservative measures. The patient must stop smoking. Smoking increases bronchoconstriction; paralyzes the cilia, which are important in removing irritating particles; and inactivates surfactant, which plays an important role in enabling the alveoli to expand. Smokers also are more susceptible to bronchial infection.

Bronchiectasis

Bronchiectasis is a chronic, irreversible dilation of the bronchi and bronchioles that may be caused by a variety of conditions, including:

- Pulmonary infections and obstruction of the bronchus
- Aspiration of foreign bodies, vomitus, or material from the upper respiratory tract
- Pressure from tumors, dilated blood vessels, and enlarged lymph nodes

A person may be predisposed to bronchiectasis as a result of recurrent respiratory infections in early childhood, measles, influenza, TB, and immunodeficiency disorders.

Pathophysiology

The inflammatory process associated with pulmonary infections damages the bronchial wall, causing a loss of its supporting structure, and results in thick sputum that ultimately obstructs the bronchi. The walls become permanently distended and distorted, and mucociliary clearance is impaired. The inflammation and infection extend to the peribronchial tissues; in the case of saccular bronchiectasis, each dilated tube virtually amounts to a lung abscess, the exudate of which drains freely through the bronchus. Bronchiectasis is usually localized, affecting a lobe or segment of a lung. The lower lobes are most frequently involved.

The retention of secretions and subsequent obstruction ultimately cause the alveoli distal to the obstruction to collapse (atelectasis). Inflammatory scarring or fibrosis replaces functioning lung tissue. In time the patient develops respiratory insufficiency with reduced VC, decreased ventilation, and an increased ratio of residual volume to total lung capacity. There is impaired mixing of inspired gas (ventilation–perfusion imbalance) and hypoxemia.

Clinical Manifestations

Characteristic symptoms of bronchiectasis include chronic cough and the production of purulent sputum in copious amounts. A high percentage of patients with this disease have hemoptysis. Clubbing of the fingers also is very common because of respiratory insufficiency. The patient usually has repeated episodes of pulmonary infection.

Assessment and Diagnostic Findings

Bronchiectasis is not readily diagnosed because the symptoms can be mistaken for those of simple chronic bronchitis. A definite sign is offered by the prolonged history of productive cough, with sputum consistently negative for tubercle bacilli. The diagnosis is established on the basis of CT scan, which demonstrates either the presence or absence of bronchial dilation. Occasionally, a bronchogram is performed.

Medical Management

The objectives of treatment are to promote bronchial drainage to clear the affected portion of the lung or lungs of excessive secretions and to prevent or control infection. Postural drainage is part of all treatment plans because draining the bronchiectatic areas by gravity reduces the amount of secretions and the degree of infection. Sometimes mucopurulent sputum must be removed by bronchoscopy. Chest physiotherapy, including percussion and postural drainage, is important in secretion management.

Smoking cessation is important because smoking impairs bronchial drainage by paralyzing ciliary action, increasing bronchial secretions, and causing inflammation of the mucous membranes, resulting in hyperplasia of the mucous glands.

PHARMACOLOGIC THERAPY

Infection is controlled with antimicrobial therapy based on the results of sensitivity studies on organisms cultured from sputum. A year-round regimen of antibiotics may be prescribed, with different types of antibiotics at intervals. Some clinicians prescribe antibiotics throughout the winter or when acute upper respiratory tract infections occur. Patients should be vaccinated against influenza and pneumococcal pneumonia.

Bronchodilators may be given to patients who also have reactive airway disease. Patients with bronchiectasis almost always have associated bronchitis. Sympathomimetic medications, particularly beta-adrenergics, may be used to effect bronchodilation and to increase the mucociliary transport of secretions.

SURGICAL MANAGEMENT

Surgical intervention, although used infrequently, may be indicated for the patient who continues to expectorate large amounts of sputum and has repeated bouts of pneumonia and hemoptysis despite adhering to the treatment regimen. However, the disease must involve only one or two areas of the lung that can be removed without producing respiratory insufficiency. The goals of surgical treatment are to conserve normal pulmonary tissue and to avoid infectious complications. Diseased tissue is removed, provided that the postoperative lung function will be adequate. It may be necessary to remove a segment of a lobe (segmental resection), a lobe (lobectomy), or rarely an entire lung (pneumonectomy). Segmental resection is the removal of an anatomic subdivision of a pulmonary lobe. The chief advantage is that only diseased tissue is removed and healthy lung tissue is conserved. Chest CT scans aid in delineating the segment.

The surgery is preceded by a period of careful preoperative preparation. The objective is to obtain a dry (free of infection) tracheobronchial tree to prevent complications (atelectasis, pneumonia, bronchopleural fistula, and empyema). This is accomplished by postural drainage or, depending on the location, by direct suction through a bronchoscope. A course of antibacterial therapy may be prescribed. After the surgery, the care is the same as for any patient undergoing chest surgery, as discussed in Chapter 22. For nursing management and patient teaching, see Nursing Process: The Patient With COPD.

Emphysema

Emphysema is defined as an abnormal distention of the air spaces beyond the terminal bronchioles, with destruction of the walls of the alveoli. It is the end stage of a process that has progressed slowly for many years. In fact, by the time the patient develops symptoms, pulmonary function often is irreversibly impaired. Along with chronic obstructive bronchitis, it is a major cause of disability.

Smoking is the major cause of emphysema. In a small percentage of patients, however, there is a familial predisposition to emphysema associated with a plasma protein abnormality—a deficiency of alpha$_1$-antitrypsin, an enzyme inhibitor. Without it, certain enzymes destroy lung tissue. The genetically susceptible person is sensitive to environmental factors (smoking, air pollution, infectious agents, allergens) and in time develops chronic obstructive symptoms. Carriers of this genetic defect must be identified to permit modification of environmental factors to delay or prevent overt symptoms of disease. Genetic counseling should also be offered. Alpha$_1$-protease inhibitor replacement therapy is available for patients with this genetic defect to slow the progression of the disease, and for patients with severe disease. This therapy is required every 1 to 2 weeks because the half-life of the medication is approximately 7 days.

Pathophysiology

In emphysema, several factors cause airway obstruction—inflammation of bronchial mucosa, excessive mucus production, loss of elastic recoil of the airways, and collapse of bronchioles and redistribution of air to the functional alveoli. As the walls of the alveoli are destroyed (a process accelerated by recurrent infections), the alveolar surface area in direct contact with the pulmonary capillaries continually decreases, causing an increase in dead space (lung area where no gas exchange can occur) and impaired oxygen diffusion. Impaired oxygen diffusion causes hypoxemia. In the later stages of the disease, the elimination of carbon dioxide is impaired, resulting in increased carbon dioxide tension in arterial blood (hypercapnia). This causes respiratory acidosis.

As the alveolar walls continue to break down, the pulmonary capillary bed is reduced. Pulmonary blood flow is increased, and the right ventricle is forced to maintain a higher blood pressure in the pulmonary artery. Thus, right-sided heart failure (cor pulmonale) is one of the complications of emphysema. Congestion, dependent edema, distended neck veins, or pain in the region of the liver suggests the development of cardiac failure.

Secretions are also a problem in emphysema. This is especially true in the patient who has combined problems of chronic bronchitis and emphysema. Secretions are increased and retained because the person cannot generate a forceful cough to expel them. Chronic and acute infections thus persist in emphysematous lungs.

The person with emphysema has a chronic obstruction (marked increase in airway resistance) to the inflow and outflow of air from the lungs. The lungs are in a state of chronic hyperexpansion. To move air into and out of the lungs, negative pressure is required during inspiration and an adequate level of positive pressure must be attained and maintained during expiration. The resting position is one of inflation. Instead of being an involuntary passive act, expiration becomes active and requires muscular effort. The patient becomes increasingly short of breath, the chest becomes rigid, and the ribs are fixed at their joints. The chronic hyperinflation of the patient with emphysema leads to the "barrel chest" thorax configuration commonly seen in many of these patients. This results when the ribs become fixed in the inspiratory position due to hyperinflation, and also from the loss of lung elasticity (Fig. 21-6).

Retraction of the supraclavicular fossae occurs on inspiration, causing the shoulders to heave upward (Fig. 21-7). In advanced emphysema, the abdominal muscles also contract on inspiration. There is a progressive reduction of VC. Normal exhalation becomes increasingly difficult and finally impossible. The total VC may be normal, but the ratio of FEV_1 to FVC is low because the elasticity of the alveoli is greatly diminished. The effort required by the patient to move air from the damaged alveoli and narrowed airway increases the work of breathing. The ability to adapt to changing oxygenation needs is greatly compromised.

Classifications

There are two main types of emphysema, based on the changes taking place in the lung: panlobular (panacinar) and centrilobular (centroacinar) (Fig. 21-8).

In the panlobular (panacinar) type, there is destruction of the respiratory bronchiole, alveolar duct, and alveoli. All air spaces within the lobule are essentially enlarged, but there is little inflammatory disease. The patient with this type of emphysema typically has a hyperinflated chest (barrel chest on physical examination), marked dyspnea on exertion, and weight loss.

In the centrilobular (centroacinar) form, the pathologic changes take place mainly in the center of the secondary lobule, and the peripheral portions of the acinus are preserved. Frequently, there is a derangement of ventilation–perfusion ratios, producing chronic hypoxemia, hypercapnia (increased CO_2 in the arterial blood), polycythemia, and episodes of right-sided heart failure. This leads to central cyanosis, peripheral edema, and respiratory failure. In addition to the management outlined below, the patient may receive diuretic therapy for edema. Both types of emphysema may occur in the same patient.

Clinical Manifestations

Patients with emphysema usually have a long history of cigarette smoking and increasing dyspnea on exertion. They commonly are in their fifth decade (symptoms develop after about 20 years of smoking) and initially seek medical care for either an acute chest illness or increasing dyspnea. Dyspnea develops insidiously and becomes the major symptom in emphysema. This difficulty in breathing progresses and occurs with even the simplest activities of daily living, such as eating, bathing, walking, or bending over (exertional dyspnea). This contributes to the development of anorexia, weight loss, weakness, and inactivity. The patient develops a vicious downward spiral of shortness of breath leading to decreased activity and muscle deconditioning. Pursed-lip breathing and the use of accessory muscles (sternocleidomastoid) are common. Because of pooling of excessive secretions, the patient becomes prone to exacerbations in which inflammation and infection are present. There is an increased cough, purulent sputum, wheezing, dyspnea, and occasionally fever.

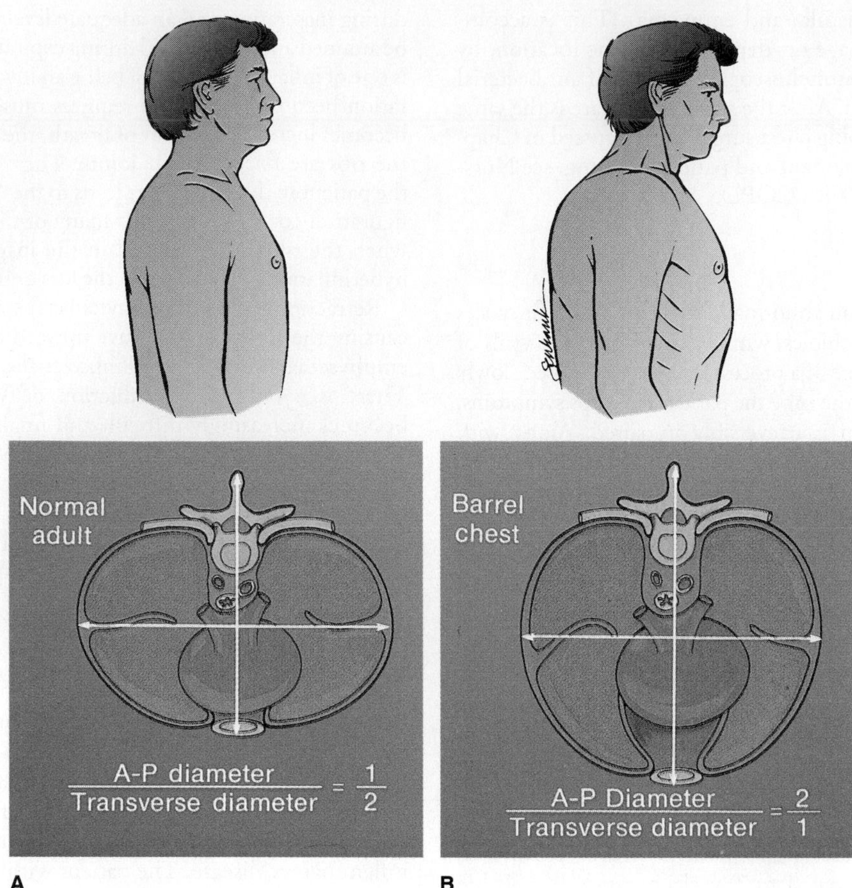

FIGURE 21•6 Characteristics of normal chest wall and chest wall in emphysema. The normal chest wall and its cross section are illustrated on the left (**A**). The barrel shaped chest of emphysema and its cross section are illustrated on the right (**B**).

Assessment and Diagnostic Findings

On inspection, the patient is tachypnic and usually has a barrel chest from **air trapping** in the lungs and generalized muscle wasting. Central cyanosis may be observed. When the chest is examined, hyperresonance and decreased fremitus are found throughout the lung fields. Auscultation reveals distant heart sounds and diminished breath sounds with prolonged expiration. Dry crackles may be heard at the bases, and wheezes are sometimes heard, especially with forced expiration. Evidence of pulmonary hypertension with an increased second heart sound, jugular venous distention, and a right ventricular heave may be present. In advanced stages of the disease, there are low oxygen levels (hypoxemia) and high carbon dioxide levels (hypercapnia). Morning headaches suggest hypercapnia. Cor pulmonale with right-sided heart failure and peripheral edema may develop in patients with chronic hypoxemia and hypercapnia.

The patient's symptoms and the clinical findings on physical examination provide the initial clues to the patient's problem. Other diagnostic tests include chest x-rays, chest CT scans, pulmonary function studies (particularly spirometry and diffusing capacity), pulse oximetry, arterial blood gas analysis (to assess ventilatory function and pulmonary gas exchange), and a complete blood count.

The chest x-ray reveals hyperinflation with a low, flat diaphragm, spreading of the ribs, and a long, narrow heart shadow. Pulmonary function studies are used to determine disease severity and to follow the disease progression. Air flow obstruction is determined by the FEV_1 to FVC ratio. With obstruction, the patient cannot forcibly exhale air from the lungs, reducing the FEV_1 measurement. Obstructive disease is defined as an FEV_1/FVC ratio of less than 70%. The VC may also be reduced. Lung volume measurements show an increase in total lung capacity, functional residual capacity, and residual volume because of air trapping. Diffusing capacity is decreased because of the loss of functional alveoli.

With advanced disease, the arterial blood gas analysis may reveal hypoxemia with hypercapnia. Hemoglobin and hematocrit levels are normal initially and then may increase as the disease progresses to compensate for the hypoxemia.

Medical Management

The major objectives of treatment are to improve the quality of life, to slow the progression of the disease process, and to treat the obstructed airways to relieve hypoxemia. Maximal medical management of patients includes bronchodilators, antimicrobial agents, oxygen therapy, pulmonary rehabilitation, smoking cessation, and

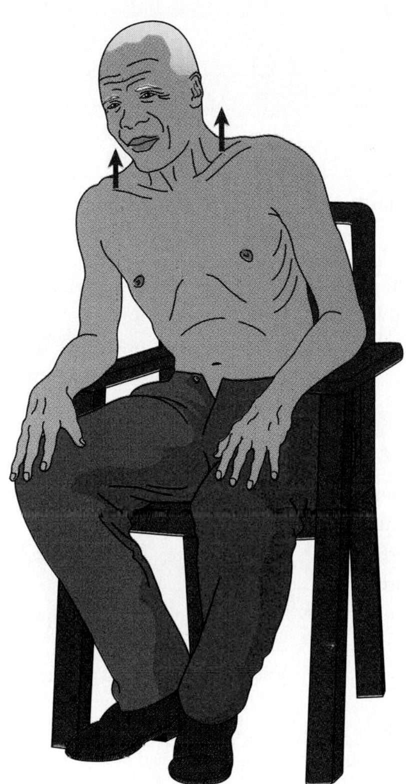

FIGURE 21•7 Typical posture of person with COPD—primarily emphysema. The person tends to lean forward and uses the accessory muscles of respiration to breathe, forcing the shoulder girdle upward and causing the supraclavicular fossae to retract on inspiration.

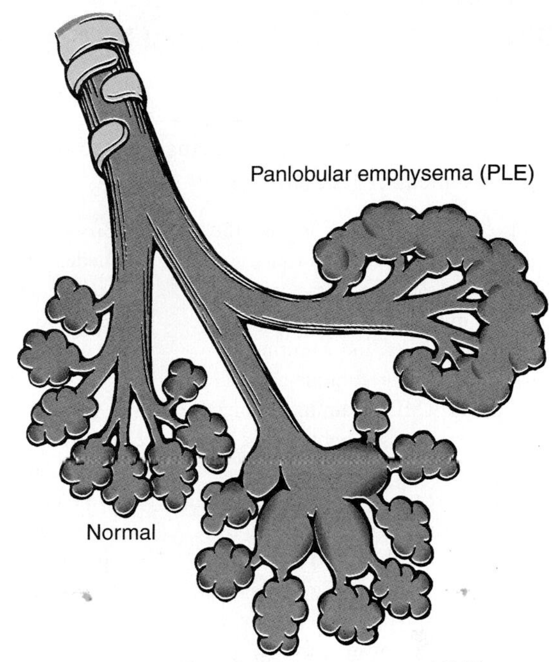

FIGURE 21•8 Changes in alveolar structure in centrilobular and panlobular emphysema. In panlobular emphysema, the bronchioles, alveolar ducts, and alveoli are destroyed and the air spaces within the lobule are enlarged. In centrilobular emphysema, the pathologic changes occur in the lobule, while the peripheral portions of the acinus are preserved.

corticosteroid boluses for episodic exacerbations. The therapeutic approach includes:

- Treatment measures designed to improve ventilation and decrease the work of breathing
- Prevention and prompt treatment of infection
- Physical therapy techniques to improve energy conservation techniques and increase pulmonary ventilation
- Maintenance of proper environmental conditions to facilitate breathing
- Psychological support
- Ongoing patient education and pulmonary rehabilitation

OXYGEN THERAPY

Oxygen therapy is the only therapy for COPD that has been demonstrated to be life-preserving. Severe hypoxemia is treated with low concentrations of oxygen to raise the PaO_2 to 65 to 80 mm Hg. In severe emphysema, oxygen is administered at least 16 hours per day, with 24 hours preferable. This modality may alleviate the patient's symptoms and improve the quality of life. Some patients require long-term home use of oxygen. General nursing care of the patient with COPD is discussed in the Plan of Nursing Care and in Nursing Process: The Patient With COPD.

PHARMACOLOGIC THERAPY

Bronchodilators. Bronchodilators are prescribed to reverse bronchospasm, thereby reducing obstruction and improving air flow. The preferred route is via an MDI. This allows for direct administration to the affected area, minimizing side effects and systemic action.

$Beta_2$-adrenergic agonists produce less bronchodilation in COPD than in asthma but are helpful in rapid reversal of bronchospasm on an as-needed basis. The $beta_2$-adrenergic agonists of choice include albuterol, pirbuterol, metaproterenol, terbutaline, and isoetherine. These medications are more selective than epinephrine, isoproterenol, and ephedrine and, when used appropriately, produce fewer side effects.

Anticholinergic agents may be more effective than $beta_2$-adrenergic agonists in COPD. The only currently available preparation is ipratropium bromide (Atrovent). Once the patient has daily symptoms, the regular use of ipratropium is recommended. Because it has a slower onset of action, ipratropium is not as helpful on an as-needed basis.

The methylxanthines (theophylline and aminophylline) have experienced a decline in popularity due to the potential for toxicity, incompatibility with many other medications, and multiple systemic side effects. Theophylline may be helpful, however, particularly for patients who cannot use an MDI effectively or who comply poorly.

Antimicrobials. Patients with emphysema are susceptible to lung infections and must be treated at the earliest signs of infection. *S. pneumoniae, H. influenzae,* and *Branhamella catarrhalis* are the most common organisms involved. Antimicrobial therapy is usually prescribed. An antimicrobial regimen is used at the first sign of respiratory infection, as evidenced by purulent sputum, increased cough, and fever. Patients should receive the pneumococcal vaccine every 5 to 10 years and a yearly influenza vaccine as preventive measures.

(*text continues on page 460*)

21•1

Plan of Nursing Care

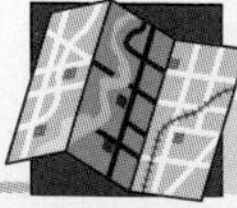

Care of the Patient With COPD

Nursing Interventions	Rationale	Expected Outcomes
Nursing Diagnosis: Impaired gas exchange related to ventilation–perfusion inequality **Goal:** Improvement in gas exchange		
1. Administer bronchodilators as prescribed: a. Inhalation is the preferred route. b. Observe for side effects: tachycardia, dysrhythmias, central nervous system excitation, nausea, and vomiting. c. Assess for correct technique of metered dose inhaler (MDI) administration.	1. Bronchodilators dilate the airways. The medication dosage is carefully adjusted for each patient, in accordance with clinical response.	• Verbalizes need for bronchodilators and for taking as prescribed • Evidences minimal side effects; heart rate near normal, absence of dysrhythmias, normal mentation • Reports a decrease in dyspnea • Shows an improved expiratory flow rate • Uses and cleans respiratory therapy equipment as applicable • Demonstrates diaphragmatic breathing and coughing • Uses oxygen equipment appropriately when indicated • Evidences improved arterial blood gases or pulse oximetry • Demonstrates correct technique for use of MDI
2. Evaluate effectiveness of nebulizer or MDI treatments. a. Assess for decreased shortness of breath, decreased wheezing or crackles, loosened secretions, decreased anxiety. b. Ensure that treatment is given before meals to avoid nausea and to reduce fatigue that accompanies eating.	2. Combining medication with aerosolized bronchodilators is typically used to control bronchoconstriction in an acute exacerbation. Generally, however, the MDI with spacer is the preferred route (less cost and time to treatment).	
3. Instruct and encourage patient in diaphragmatic breathing and effective coughing.	3. These techniques improve ventilation by opening airways to facilitate clearing the airways of sputum. Gas exchange is improved and fatigue is minimized.	
4. Administer oxygen by the method prescribed. a. Explain rationale and importance to patient. b. Evaluate effectiveness; observe for signs of hypoxemia. Notify physician if restlessness, anxiety, somnolence, cyanosis, or tachycardia is present. c. Analyze arterial blood gases and compare with baseline values. When arterial puncture is performed and a blood sample is obtained, hold puncture site for 5 minutes to prevent arterial bleeding and development of ecchymoses. d. Initiate pulse oximetry to monitor oxygen saturation. e. Explain that no smoking is permitted by patient or visitors while oxygen is in use.	4. Oxygen will correct the hypoxemia. Careful observation of the liter flow or the percentage administered and its effect on the patient is important. If the patient has chronic CO_2 retention, excessive oxygen could suppress the hypoxic drive and respirations. These patients generally need low-flow oxygen rates of 1 to 2 L/min. Periodic arterial blood gases and pulse oximetry help to evaluate adequacy of oxygenation. Smoking may render pulse oximetry inaccurate because the carbon monoxide from cigarette smoke also saturates hemoglobin.	
Nursing Diagnosis: Ineffective airway clearance related to bronchoconstriction, increased mucus production, ineffective cough, and bronchopulmonary infection **Goal:** Achievement of airway clearance		
1. Adequately hydrate the patient.	1. Systemic hydration keeps secretions moist and easier to expectorate. Fluids must be given with caution if right- or left-sided heart failure is present.	• Verbalizes need to drink fluids • Demonstrates diaphragmatic breathing and coughing • Performs postural drainage correctly • Coughing is minimized • Does not smoke • Verbalizes that pollens, fumes, gases, dusts, and extremes of temperature and humidity are irritants to be avoided
2. Teach and encourage the use of diaphragmatic breathing and coughing techniques.	2. These techniques help to improve ventilation and mobilize secretions without causing breathlessness and fatigue.	
3. Assist in administering nebulizer or MDI.	3. This ensures adequate delivery of medicine to the airways.	

(continued)

21•1

Plan of Nursing Care

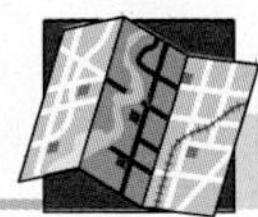

Care of the Patient With COPD (*continued*)

Nursing Interventions	Rationale	Expected Outcomes
4. If indicated, perform postural drainage with percussion and vibration in the morning and at night as prescribed. 5. Instruct patient to avoid bronchial irritants such as cigarette smoke, aerosols, extremes of temperature, and fumes. 6. Teach early signs of infection that are to be reported to the clinician immediately: a. Increased sputum production b. Change in color of sputum c. Increased thickness of sputum d. Increased shortness of breath, tightness in chest, or fatigue e. Increased coughing f. Fever or chills	4. Uses gravity to help raise secretions so they can be more easily expectorated or suctioned. 5. Bronchial irritants cause bronchoconstriction and increased mucus production, which then interferes with airway clearance. 6. Minor respiratory infections that are of no consequence to the person with normal lungs can produce fatal disturbances in the lungs of the person with emphysema. Early recognition is crucial.	• Identifies signs of early infection • Is free of infection (no fever, no change in sputum, lessening of dyspnea) • Verbalizes need to notify health care provider at the earliest sign of infection • Verbalizes need to stay away from crowds or people with colds in flu season • Discusses flu and pneumonia vaccines with clinician to help prevent infection
7. Administer antibiotics as prescribed.	7. Antibiotics may be prescribed to prevent or treat infection.	
8. Encourage patient to be immunized against influenza and *Streptococcus pneumoniae.*	8. People with respiratory conditions are prone to respiratory infections and are encouraged to be immunized.	

Nursing Diagnosis: Ineffective breathing pattern related to shortness of breath, mucus, bronchoconstriction, and airway irritants

Goal: Improvement in breathing pattern

Nursing Interventions	Rationale	Expected Outcomes
1. Teach patient diaphragmatic and pursed-lip breathing.	1. Helps patient prolong expiration time and decreases air trapping. With these techniques, patient will breathe more efficiently and effectively.	• Practices pursed-lip and diaphragmatic breathing and uses them when short of breath and with activity • Shows signs of decreased respiratory effort and paces activities • Uses inspiratory muscle trainer as prescribed
2. Encourage alternating activity with rest periods. Allow patient to make some decisions (bath, shaving) about care based on tolerance level.	2. Pacing activities permit patient to perform activities without excessive distress.	
3. Encourage use of an inspiratory muscle trainer if prescribed.	3. Strengthens and conditions the respiratory muscles.	

Nursing Diagnosis: Self-care deficits related to fatigue secondary to increased work of breathing and insufficient ventilation and oxygenation

Goal: Independence in self-care activities

Nursing Interventions	Rationale	Expected Outcomes
1. Teach patient to coordinate diaphragmatic breathing with activity (eg, walking, bending).	1. This will allow the patient to be more active and to avoid excessive fatigue or dyspnea during activity.	• Uses controlled breathing while bathing, bending, and walking • Paces activities of daily living to alternate with rest periods to reduce fatigue and dyspnea
2. Encourage patient to begin to bathe self, dress self, walk, and drink fluids. Discuss energy conservation measures.	2. As condition resolves, patient will be able to do more but needs to be encouraged to avoid increasing dependence.	• Describes energy conservation strategies
3. Teach postural drainage if appropriate.	3. Encourages patient to become involved in own care. Prepares patient to manage at home.	• Performs same self-care activities as before • Performs postural drainage correctly

Nursing Diagnosis: Activity intolerance due to fatigue, hypoxemia, and ineffective breathing patterns

Goal: Improvement in activity tolerance

Nursing Interventions	Rationale	Expected Outcomes
1. Support patient in establishing a regular regimen of exercise using treadmill and	1. Muscles that are deconditioned consume more oxygen and place an additional	• Performs activities with less shortness of breath

(*continued*)

21•1

Plan of Nursing Care

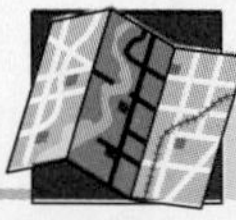

Care of the Patient With COPD (*continued*)

Nursing Interventions	Rationale	Expected Outcomes
exercycle, walking, or other appropriate exercises, such as mall walking. a. Assess the patient's current level of functioning and develop exercise plan based on baseline functional status. b. Suggest consultation with a physical therapist or pulmonary rehabilitation program to determine an exercise program specific to the patient's capability. Have portable oxygen unit available if oxygen is prescribed for exercise.	burden on the lungs. Through regular, graded exercise, these muscle groups become more conditioned, and the patient can do more without getting as short of breath. Graded exercise breaks the cycle of debilitation.	• Verbalizes need to exercise daily and demonstrates an exercise plan to be carried out at home • Walks and gradually increases walking time and distance to improve physical condition • Exercises both upper and lower body muscle groups

Nursing Diagnosis: Ineffective individual coping related to less socialization, anxiety, depression, lower activity level, and the inability to work

Goal: Attainment of an optimal level of coping

Nursing Interventions	Rationale	Expected Outcomes
1. Help the patient develop realistic goals.	1. Developing realistic goals will promote a sense of hope and accomplishment rather than defeat and hopelessness.	• Expresses interest in the future • Participates in the discharge plan • Discusses activities or methods that can be performed to ease shortness of breath • Uses relaxation techniques appropriately • Expresses interest in a pulmonary rehabilitation program
2. Encourage activity to level of symptom tolerance.	2. Activity reduces tension and decreases degree of dyspnea as patient becomes conditioned.	
3. Teach relaxation technique or provide a relaxation tape for patient.	3. Relaxation reduces stress, anxiety, and dyspnea and helps patient to cope with disability.	
4. Enroll patient in pulmonary rehabilitation program where available.	4. Pulmonary rehabilitation programs have been shown to promote a subjective improvement in a patient's status and self-esteem as well as increased exercise tolerance and decreased hospitalizations.	

Nursing Diagnosis: Knowledge deficit about self-management to be performed at home.

Goal: Adherence to therapeutic program and home care

Nursing Interventions	Rationale	Expected Outcomes
1. Help patient understand short- and long-term goals. a. Teach the patient about disease, medications, procedures, and how and when to seek help. b. Refer patient to pulmonary rehabilitation.	1. Patient needs to be a partner in developing the plan of care and needs to know what to expect. Teaching about the condition is one of the most important aspects of care; it will prepare the patient to live and cope with the condition and improve quality of life.	• Understands disease and what affects it • Verbalizes the need to preserve existing lung function by adhering to the prescribed program • Understands purposes and proper administration of medications • Stops smoking or enrolls in a smoking cessation program • Identifies when and whom to call for help
2. Give strong message to stop smoking. Discuss smoking cessation strategies. Provide information about resource groups (eg, SmokEnders, American Cancer Society, American Lung Association).	2. Smoking causes permanent damage to the lung and diminishes the lungs' protective mechanisms. Air flow is obstructed and lung capacity is reduced. Smoking increases morbidity and mortality and is also a risk factor for lung cancer.	

Collaborative Problems: Potential complications of COPD include atelectasis, pneumothorax, respiratory failure, pulmonary hypertension, and status asthmaticus.

Atelectasis

Nursing Interventions	Rationale	Expected Outcomes
1. Monitor respiratory status, including rate and pattern of respirations, breath sounds, signs and symptoms of respiratory distress, and pulse oximetry.	1. A change in respiratory status, including tachypnea, dyspnea, and diminished or absent breath sounds, may indicate atelectasis.	• Normal (baseline for patient) respiratory rate and pattern • Normal breath sounds for patient • Demonstrates diaphragmatic breathing and effective coughing

(*continued*)

21•1 **Plan of Nursing Care** 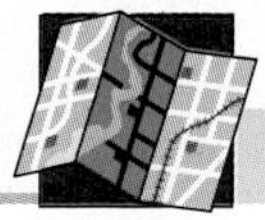 **Care of the Patient With COPD (*continued*)**

Nursing Interventions	Rationale	Expected Outcomes
2. Instruct in and encourage diaphragmatic breathing and effective coughing techniques.	2. These techniques improve ventilation and lung expansion and ideally improve gas exchange.	• Performs deep-breathing exercises, incentive spirometry as prescribed • Pulse oximetry is ≥ 90%
3. Promote use of lung expansion techniques (eg, deep-breathing exercises, incentive spirometry) as prescribed.	3. Deep-breathing exercises and incentive spirometry promote maximal lung expansion.	
Pneumothorax		
1. Monitor respiratory status, including rate and pattern of respirations, symmetry of chest wall movement, breath sounds, signs and symptoms of respiratory distress, and pulse oximetry.	1. Dyspnea, tachypnea, tachycardia, acute pleuritic chest pain, tracheal deviation away from the affected side, absence of breath sounds on the affected side, and decreased tactile fremitus may indicate pneumothorax.	• Normal respiratory rate and pattern for patient • Normal breath sounds bilaterally • Normal pulse for patient • Normal tactile fremitus • Absence of pain • Tracheal position is midline • Pulse oximetry ≥ 90% • Maintains normal oxygen saturation and arterial blood gas measurements for patient • Exhibits no hypoxemia and hypercapnia (or returns to baseline values) • Absence of pain • Symmetric chest wall movement • Lung is reexpanded on chest x-ray • Breath sounds are heard on the affected side
2. Assess pulse.	2. Tachycardia is associated with pneumothorax and anxiety.	
3. Assess for chest pain and precipitating factors.	3. Pain may accompany pneumothorax.	
4. Palpate for tracheal deviation/shift away from the affected side.	4. Early detection of pneumothorax and prompt intervention will prevent other serious complications.	
5. Monitor pulse oximetry and if indicated arterial blood gases (ABGs).	5. Recognition of a deterioration in respiratory function will prevent serious complications.	
6. Administer supplemental oxygen therapy, as indicated.	6. Oxygen will correct hypoxemia; administer it with caution.	
7. Administer analgesics, as indicated, for chest pain.	7. Pain interferes with deep breathing, resulting in a decrease in lung expansion.	
8. Assist with chest tube insertion and use pleural drainage system, as prescribed.	8. Removal of air from the pleural space will reexpand the lung.	
Respiratory Failure		
1. Monitor respiratory status, including rate and pattern of respirations, breath sounds, and signs and symptoms of acute respiratory distress.	1. Early recognition of a deterioration in respiratory function will avert further complications, such as respiratory failure, severe hypoxemia, and hypercapnia.	• Normal respiratory rate and pattern for patient with no acute distress • Recognizes hypoxemia and hypercapnia • Maintains normal ABGs/pulse oximetry or returns to baseline values
2. Monitor pulse oximetry and arterial blood gases.	2. Recognition of changes in oxygenation and acid–base balance will guide in correcting and preventing complications.	
3. Administer supplemental oxygen and initiate mechanisms for mechanical ventilation, as prescribed.	3. Acute respiratory failure is a medical emergency. Hypoxemia is a hallmark sign. Administration of oxygen therapy and mechanical ventilation (if indicated) are critical to survival.	
Pulmonary Hypertension		
1. Monitor respiratory status, including rate and pattern of respirations, breath sounds, pulse oximetry, and signs and symptoms of acute respiratory distress.	1. Dyspnea is the primary symptom of pulmonary hypertension. Other symptoms include fatigue, angina, near syncope, edema, and palpitations.	• Normal respiratory rate and pattern for patient • Exhibits no signs and symptoms of right-sided failure • Maintains baseline pulse oximetry values and ABGs
2. Assess for signs and symptoms of right-sided heart failure, including peripheral edema, ascites, distended neck veins, crackles, and heart murmur.	2. Right-sided heart failure is a common clinical manifestation of pulmonary hypertension due to increased right ventricular workload.	
3. Administer oxygen therapy, as prescribed.	3. Continuous oxygen therapy is a major component of management of pulmonary hypertension by preventing hypoxemia and thereby reducing pulmonary vascular constriction (resistance) secondary to hypoxemia.	

(*continued*)

21•1 **Plan of Nursing Care** 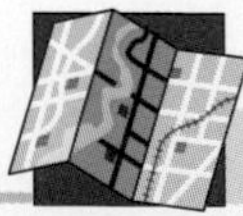 **Care of the Patient With COPD (*continued*)**

Nursing Interventions	Rationale	Expected Outcomes
Status Asthmaticus		
1. Monitor respiratory status, including rate and pattern of respirations, breath sounds, signs and symptoms of acute respiratory distress, and blood pressure.	1. Dyspnea, tachypnea, central cyanosis, labored, wheezy breathing, or diminished breath sounds are signs of respiratory distress due to status asthmaticus.	• Normal respiratory rate and pattern for patient • Normal or baseline breath sounds for patient • Maintains normal/baseline pulse oximetry values and ABGs • Improvement in respiratory function
2. Monitor pulse oximetry and arterial blood gases.	2. Hypoxemia and hypercapnia are signs of severe bronchospasm and impaired gas exchange.	
3. Administer supplemental oxygen therapy, as prescribed.	3. Oxygen will correct hypoxemia once the bronchospasm diminishes.	
4. Administer medications (beta-agonists and corticosteroids), as prescribed.	4. Beta-agonists are used initially to dilate bronchial smooth muscle. 5. Corticosteroids will decrease mucosal inflammation.	

Anti-Inflammatory Therapy. The place of regular use of corticosteroids remains unclear in the treatment of emphysema. Approximately one third of patients with COPD improve with chronic oral corticosteroid therapy. Because the dangers of corticosteroid therapy are so numerous, documentation of its efficacy for each patient is warranted before its institution, and the lowest effective dose should be determined. In some patients, inhaled corticosteroids may suffice; this route is preferable.

SURGICAL MANAGEMENT

Lung Volume Reduction Surgery. Treatment options for patients with end-stage emphysema are limited, although lung volume reduction surgery is an option for a specific subset of patients (ie, when optimal medical management is ineffective and when the patient is not a candidate for lung transplantation). Careful selection of patients for this procedure is essential to decrease the morbidity and mortality. Lung volume reduction surgery involves the removal of a portion of the diseased lung parenchyma that is not contributing to ventilation but occupies a space in the thorax. This allows the functional tissue to expand, resulting in improved elastic recoil of the lung and improved chest wall and diaphragmatic mechanics. This type of surgery does not cure the emphysema, but it may decrease dyspnea, improve lung function, and improve the patient's overall quality of life.

A large, multicenter randomized clinical trial is in progress in an attempt to answer the many questions regarding the risks and benefits of this procedure. The results of this large clinical trial will help to determine the role of lung volume reduction surgery for patients with severe emphysema (National Institutes of Health, 1996).

Lung Transplantation. Single lung transplantation is a viable alternative for definitive surgical treatment of end-stage emphysema. It is usually reserved for younger patients with alpha$_1$-antitrypsin deficiency. Generally, patients must be younger than 60 years of age and in relatively good health. Although lung transplantation is an alternative, organs are in short supply and many patients die while waiting for a transplant.

Asthma

Asthma is a chronic inflammatory disease of the airways, resulting in airway hyperresponsiveness, mucosal edema, and mucus production. This inflammation ultimately leads to recurrent episodes of asthma symptoms: cough, chest tightness, wheezing, and dyspnea. Asthma differs from the other obstructive lung diseases in that it is largely a reversible process, either spontaneously or with treatment. Acute exacerbations may occur, which last from minutes to hours or days, interspersed with symptom-free periods. Asthma can occur at any age and is the most common chronic disease of childhood. Despite increased knowledge regarding the pathology of asthma and the development of better medications and management plans, the death rate from asthma continues to increase. For most patients, however, it is a disruptive disease, affecting school and work attendance, occupational choices, physical activity, and quality of life in general.

Allergy is the strongest predisposing factor for the development of asthma. Chronic exposure to airway irritants or allergens also increases one's risk for developing asthma. Common allergens can be seasonal (eg, grass, tree, and weed pollens) or perennial (eg, mold, dust, roaches, or animals [especially cats]). Common triggers for asthma symptoms and exacerbations in patients with asthma include airway irritants (eg, air pollutants, cold, heat, weather changes, strong odors or perfumes, smoke), exertion, stress or emotional upsets, laughing, sinusitis with postnasal drip, and gastroesophageal reflux. Most people who have asthma are sensitive to a variety of triggers.

Pathophysiology

The underlying pathology in asthma is reversible, diffuse airway inflammation. The inflammation leads to obstruction from the following: swelling of the membranes that line the airways (mucosal edema), reducing the airway diameter; contraction of the bronchial smooth muscle that encircles the airways, causing further narrowing; and increased mucus production, which diminishes airway size and may entirely plug the bronchi.

The bronchial muscles and mucus glands enlarge; thick, tenacious sputum is produced; and the alveoli hyperinflate. Some patients may have airway sub-basement membrane fibrosis, which may cause irreversible air flow limitation.

Cells that play a key role in the inflammation of asthma are mast cells, neutrophils, eosinophils, and lymphocytes. Mast cells, when activated, release several chemicals called mediators. These chemicals, which include histamine, bradykinin, prostaglandins, and leukotrienes, perpetuate the inflammatory response, causing increased blood flow, vasoconstriction, fluid leak from the vasculature, attraction of white blood cells to the area, and bronchoconstriction. Regulation of these chemicals is the aim of much of the current research regarding pharmacologic therapy for asthma.

Further, alpha- and beta-adrenergic receptors of the sympathetic nervous system are located in the bronchi. When the alpha-adrenergic receptors are stimulated, bronchoconstriction occurs; bronchodilation occurs when the $beta_2$-adrenergic receptors are stimulated. The balance between alpha- and $beta_2$ receptors is controlled primarily by cyclic adenosine monophosphate (cAMP). Alpha-adrenergic receptor stimulation results in a decrease in cAMP, which leads to an increase of chemical mediators released by the mast cells and bronchoconstriction. $Beta_2$ receptor stimulation results in increased levels of cAMP, which inhibits the release of chemical mediators and causes bronchodilation.

Clinical Manifestations

The three most common symptoms of asthma are cough, dyspnea, and wheezing. In some instances, cough may be the only symptom. Asthma attacks often occur at night. The causes are not completely understood, but this may be related to circadian variations that influence airway receptor thresholds.

An asthma exacerbation may begin abruptly but most frequently is preceded by increasing symptoms over the previous few days. There is cough, with or without mucus production. At times the mucus is so tightly wedged in the narrowed airway that the patient cannot cough it up. There may be wheezing (the sound of air flow through narrowed airways), first on expiration and then possibly during inspiration as well. Generalized chest tightness and dyspnea occur. Expiration requires effort and becomes prolonged. As the exacerbation progresses, hypoxemia may occur, along with central cyanosis, diaphoresis, tachycardia, and a widened pulse pressure.

The occurrence of a severe, continuous reaction is referred to as status asthmaticus and is considered life-threatening. Other possible allergic reactions that may accompany asthma include eczema, rashes, and temporary edema. Asthma is categorized according to symptoms and objective measures of air flow obstruction (Table 21-3).

Assessment and Diagnostic Findings

A complete family, environmental, and occupational history is essential. To establish the diagnosis, the clinician must determine that periodic symptoms of air flow obstruction are present, air flow is at least partially reversible, and other etiologies have been excluded. A positive family history and environmental factors, including seasonal changes, high pollen counts, mold, climate changes (particularly cold air), and air pollution, are primarily associated with asthma. In addition, a variety of occupation-related chemicals and compounds have been associated with the development of asthma, including metal salts, wood and vegetable dust, medications (eg, aspirin, antibiotics, piperazine, cimetidine), industrial chemicals and plastics, biologic enzymes (eg, laundry detergents), animal and insect dusts, sera, and secretions.

During acute episodes, sputum and blood tests may disclose eosinophilia (elevated levels of eosinophils). There may be an elevation in serum levels of immunoglobulin E if allergy is present. Arterial blood gas analysis and pulse oximetry reveal hypoxemia during acute attacks. Initially, hypocapnia and respiratory alkalosis are present. As the condition worsens and the patient becomes more fatigued, the PCO_2 may rise. A normal PCO_2 value may be a signal of impending respiratory failure. Because PCO_2 is 20 times more diffusible than oxygen, it is rare for PCO_2 to be normal or elevated in a person who is breathing very rapidly. During an exacerbation, the FEV_1 and FVC are markedly decreased but improve with bronchodilators (demonstrating reversibility). Pulmonary function is usually normal between exacerbations.

Prevention

Patients with recurrent asthma should undergo tests to identify the substances that precipitate the symptoms. Possible causes could be dust, dust mites, roaches, certain types of cloth, pets, horses, detergents, soaps, certain foods, molds, and pollens. If the attacks are seasonal, pollens can be strongly suspected. The patient is instructed to avoid the causative agents whenever possible.

Complications

Complications of asthma may include status asthmaticus, rib fracture, pneumonia, and atelectasis. Airway obstruction, particularly during acute asthmatic episodes, often results in hypoxemia, requiring the administration of oxygen and the monitoring of pulse oximetry and arterial blood gases. Fluids are administered because people with asthma are frequently dehydrated from diaphoresis and insensible fluid loss with hyperventilation.

Medical Management

Immediate intervention is necessary because the continuing and progressive dyspnea leads to increased anxiety, aggravating the situation.

PHARMACOLOGIC THERAPY

Two general classes of asthma medications are: (1) long-term control medications to achieve and maintain control of persistent asthma and (2) quick relief medications for immediate treatment of asthma symptoms and exacerbations. Because the underlying pathology of asthma is inflammation, control of persistent asthma is accomplished primarily with regular use of anti-inflammatory medications. The route of choice is via MDI because these devices allow for topical administration of medications. These medications have systemic side effects when used in the long term. Critical to the success of inhaled therapy is the proper use of MDIs. If the patient has difficulty with this procedure, the addition of a spacer device is indicated. Table 21-3 presents a stepwise approach for managing asthma.

Long-Acting Control Medications. Corticosteroids are the most potent and effective anti-inflammatory medications currently available. Initially, the inhaled form is used. A spacer should be used with inhaled corticosteroids, and the patient should rinse the mouth after administration to prevent thrush, a common complication of inhaled corticosteroid use. A systemic preparation may be used to gain rapid control of the disease; to manage severe, persistent asthma; to treat moderate to severe exacerbations; to accelerate recovery; and to prevent recurrence.

(*text continues on page 464*)

TABLE 21•3 Stepwise Approach for Managing Asthma in Adults and Children Over 5 Years Old

Goals of Asthma Treatment

- Prevent chronic and troublesome symptoms (eg, coughing or breathlessness in the night, in the early morning, or after exertion)
- Maintain near-normal pulmonary function
- Maintain normal activity levels (including exercise and other physical activity)
- Prevent recurrent exacerbations of asthma and minimize the need for emergency department visits or hospitalizations
- Provide optimal pharmacotherapy with minimal or no adverse effects
- Meet patients' and families' expectation of and satisfaction with asthma care

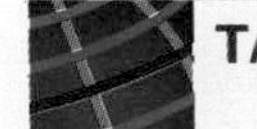	Symptoms**	Nighttime Symptoms	Lung Function	Long-Term Control	Quick Relief	Education
STEP 4 Severe Persistent	• Continual symptoms • Limited physical activity • Frequent exacerbations	Frequent	• FEV_1 or PEF ≤60% predicted • PEF variability >30%	Daily medications: • Anti-inflammatory: inhaled corticosteroid (high dose) and • Long-acting bronchodilator: either long-acting inhaled $beta_2$-agonist, sustained-release theophylline, or long-acting $beta_2$-agonist tablets AND • Corticosteroid tablets or syrup long term (2 mg/kg/day, generally do not exceed 60 mg per day).	• Short-acting bronchodilator: inhaled $beta_2$-agonists as needed for symptoms. • Intensity of treatment will depend on severity of exacerbation; see "Managing Exacerbations of Asthma." • Use of short-acting inhaled $beta_2$-agonists on a daily basis, or increasing use, indicates the need for additional long-term control therapy.	Steps 2 and 3 actions plus: • Refer to individual education/ counseling
STEP 3 Moderate Persistent	• Daily symptoms • Daily use of inhaled short-acting $beta_2$-agonist • Exacerbations affect activity • Exacerbations ≥2 times a week; may last days	>1 time a week	• FEV_1 or PEF >60% ≤80% predicted • PEF variability >30%	Daily medication: • Either - Anti-inflammatory: inhaled corticosteroid (medium dose) OR - Inhaled corticosteroid (low–medium dose) and add a long-acting bronchodilator, especially for nighttime symptoms; either long-acting inhaled $beta_2$-agonist, sustained-release theophylline, or long-acting $beta_2$-agonist tablets. • If needed - Anti-inflammatory: inhaled corticosteroids (medium–high dose) AND - Long-acting bronchodilator, especially for nighttime symptoms; either long-acting inhaled $beta_2$-agonist, sustained-release theophylline, or long-acting $beta_2$-agonist tablets.	• Short-acting bronchodilator: inhaled $beta_2$-agonists as needed for symptoms. • Intensity of treatment will depend on severity of exacerbation; see "Managing Exacerbations of Asthma." • Use of short-acting inhaled $beta_2$-agonists on a daily basis, or increasing use, indicates the need for additional long term control therapy.	Step 1 actions plus: • Teach self-monitoring • Refer to group education if available • Review and update self-management plan

STEP 2 **Mild Persistent**	• Symptoms > 2 times a week but < 1 time a day • Exacerbations may affect activity	> 2 times a month	• FEV_1 or PEF ≥ 80% predicted • PEF variability 20%–30%	Daily medication: • Anti-inflammatory: either inhaled corticosteroid (low doses) or cromolyn or nedocromil (children usually begin with a trial of cromolyn or nedocromil). • Sustained-release theophylline to serum concentration of 5–15 µg/mL is an alternative. Zafirlukast or zileuton may also be considered for patients ≥ 12 years of age, although their position in therapy is not fully established.	• Short-acting bronchodilator: inhaled $beta_2$-agonists as needed for symptoms. • Intensity of treatment will depend on severity of exacerbation; see "Managing Exacerbations of Asthma." • Use of short-acting inhaled $beta_2$-agonists on a daily basis, or increasing use, indicates the need for additional long-term-control therapy.	Step 1 actions plus: • Teach self-monitoring • Refer to group education if available • Review and update self-management plan
STEP 1 **Mild Intermittent**	• Symptoms ≤ 2 times a week • Asymptomatic and normal PEF between exacerbations • Exacerbations brief (from a few hours to a few days); intensity may vary	≤ 2 times a month	• FEV_1 or PEF ≥ 80% predicted • PEF variability < 20%	• No daily medication needed.	• Short-acting bronchodilator: inhaled $beta_2$-agonists as needed for symptoms. • Intensity of treatment will depend on severity of exacerbation; see "Managing Exacerbations of Asthma." • Use of short-acting inhaled $beta_2$-agonists more than 2 times a week may indicate the need to initiate long-term-control therapy.	• Teach basic facts about asthma • Teach inhaler/spacer/holding chamber technique • Discuss roles of medications • Develop self-management plan • Develop action plan for when and how to take rescue actions • Discuss appropriate environmental control measures to avoid exposure to known allergens and irritants

↓ STEP DOWN
Review treatment every 1 to 6 months; a gradual stepwise reduction in treatment may be possible.

↑ STEP UP
If control is not maintained, consider step up. First, review patient medication technique, adherence, and environmental control (avoidance of allergens or other factors that contribute to asthma severity).

Notes:

- The stepwise approach presents general guidelines to assist clinical decision making; it is not intended to be a specific prescription. Asthma is highly variable; clinicians should tailor specific medication plans to the needs and circumstances of individual patients.
- Gain control as quickly as possible; then decrease treatment to the least medication necessary to maintain control. Gaining control may be accomplished either by starting treatment at the step most appropriate to the initial severity of the condition or by starting at a higher level of therapy (eg, a course of systemic corticosteroids or higher dose of inhaled corticosteroids).
- A rescue course of systemic corticosteroid may be needed at any time and at any step.
- Some patients with intermittent asthma experience severe and life-threatening exacerbations separated by long periods of normal lung function and no symptoms. This may be especially common with exacerbations provoked by respiratory infections. A short course of systemic corticosteroids is recommended.
- At each step, patients should control their environment to avoid or control factors that make their asthma worse (eg, allergens irritants); this requires specific diagnosis and education.

PEF, peak expiratory flow
* The presence of one of the features of severity is sufficient to place a patient in that category. An individual should be assigned to the most severe grade in which any feature occurs. The characteristics noted in this figure are general and may overlap because asthma is highly variable. Furthermore, an individual's classification may change over time.

** Patients at any level of severity can have mild, moderate, or severe exacerbations. Some patients with intermittent asthma experience severe and life-threatening exacerbations separated by long periods of normal lung function and no symptoms.

Highlights of the Expert Panel Report 2. (1997). *Guidelines for the diagnosis and management of asthma.* National Institutes of Health, National Heart, Lung, and Blood Institute, NIH Publication No 97-4051A, p. 29.

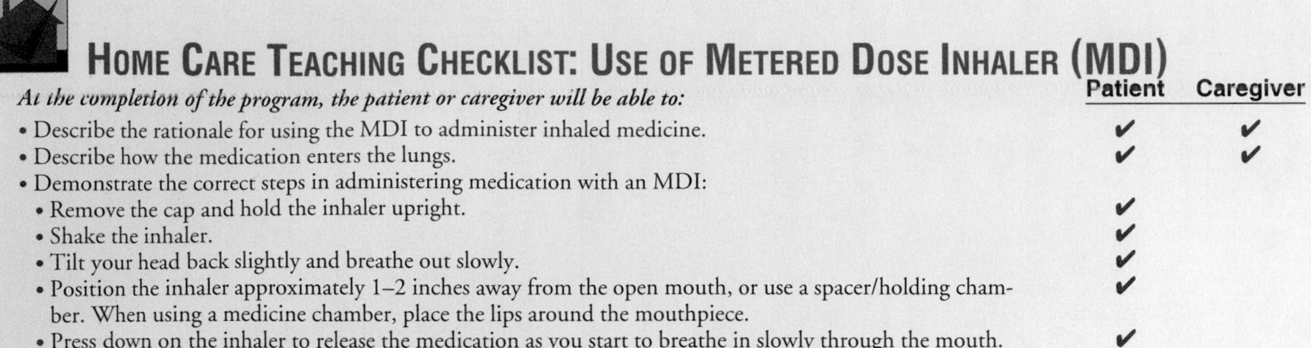

HOME CARE TEACHING CHECKLIST: USE OF METERED DOSE INHALER (MDI)

At the completion of the program, the patient or caregiver will be able to:	Patient	Caregiver
• Describe the rationale for using the MDI to administer inhaled medicine.	✔	✔
• Describe how the medication enters the lungs.	✔	✔
• Demonstrate the correct steps in administering medication with an MDI:		
• Remove the cap and hold the inhaler upright.	✔	
• Shake the inhaler.	✔	
• Tilt your head back slightly and breathe out slowly.	✔	
• Position the inhaler approximately 1–2 inches away from the open mouth, or use a spacer/holding chamber. When using a medicine chamber, place the lips around the mouthpiece.	✔	
• Press down on the inhaler to release the medication as you start to breathe in slowly through the mouth. Continue breathing in as the medication is released (press the cartridge down).	✔	

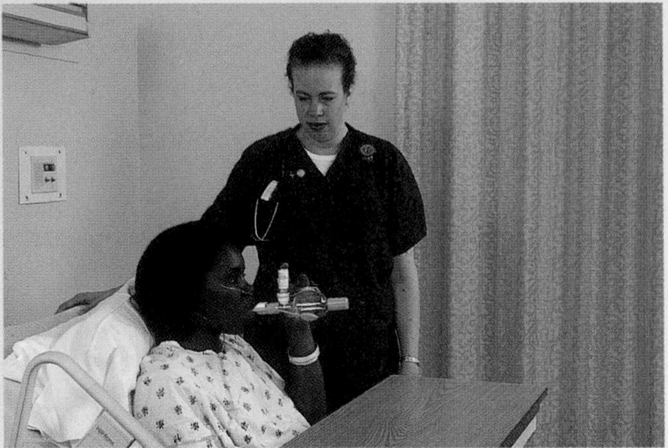

Nurse teaches patient to use a metered dose inhaler. © B. Proud.

	Patient	Caregiver
• Breathe in slowly and deeply for 3–5 seconds.	✔	
• Hold your breath for 8–10 seconds to allow the medication to reach down into your airways.	✔	
• Repeat puffs as directed, allowing 1–2 minutes between puffs.	✔	
• Apply the cap to the MDI for storage.	✔	
• After inhalation, rinse mouth with water when using a corticosteroid-containing MDI.	✔	
• Describe how to clean the MDI.	✔	✔
• Describe how to assess the amount of medication remaining in the MDI.	✔	✔
• Describe how and when to contact the health care provider for assessment, and how to obtain a refill of the MDI prescription.	✔	✔

Cromolyn sodium and nedocromil are mild to moderate anti-inflammatory agents that are used more commonly in children. They also are effective on a prophylactic basis to prevent exercise-induced asthma or in unavoidable exposure to known triggers.

Long-acting $beta_2$-adrenergic agonists are used with anti-inflammatory medications to control asthma symptoms, particularly those that occur during the night. These agents are also effective for preventing exercise-induced asthma. Long-acting $beta_2$-adrenergic agonists are not indicated for immediate relief of symptoms.

Methylxanthines (eg, theophylline) are mild to moderate bronchodilators usually used in addition to inhaled corticosteroids, mainly for relief of nighttime asthma symptoms. There is some evidence that theophylline may have a mild anti-inflammatory effect.

Leukotriene modifiers are a new class of medications. At this time, they may provide an alternative to inhaled corticosteroids for mild persistent asthma, or may be added to a regimen of inhaled corticosteroids in more severe asthma to attain further control.

Quick Relief Medications. Short-acting $beta_2$-adrenergic agonists are the medications of choice for relieving acute symptoms and preventing exercise-induced asthma. They have a rapid onset of action. Anticholinergics (eg, ipratropium bromide) may bring added benefit in severe exacerbations, but they are used more frequently in COPD patients.

PEAK FLOW MONITORING

Daily peak flow monitoring is recommended for all patients with moderate and severe asthma. It is a method of measuring asthma severity and, when added to symptom monitoring, is an indicator of the current degree of asthma control. The patient is instructed in the proper technique, particularly to give maximal effort. The

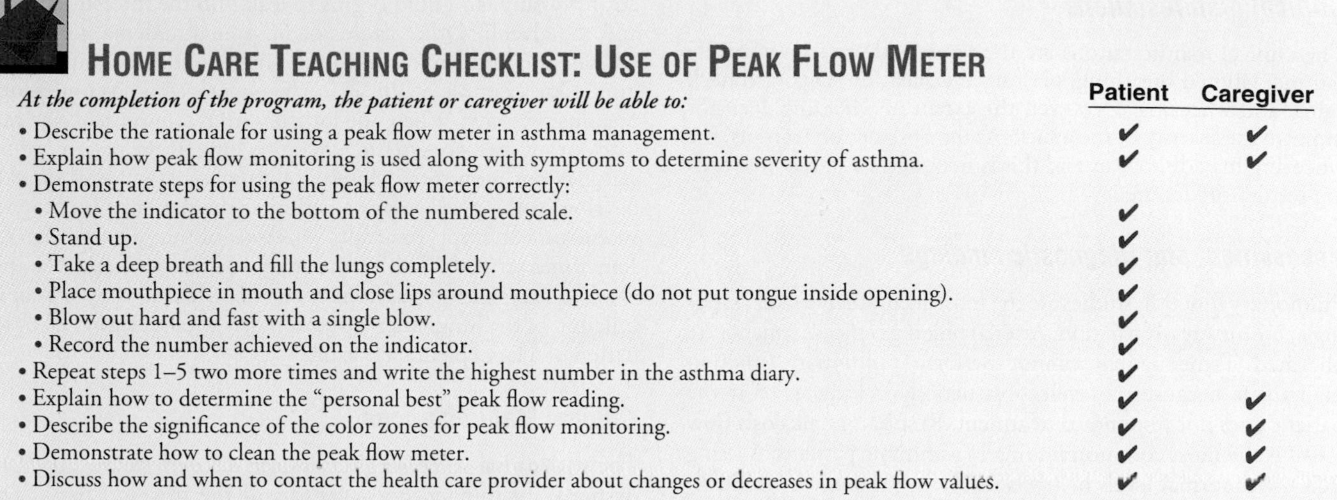

HOME CARE TEACHING CHECKLIST: USE OF PEAK FLOW METER

At the completion of the program, the patient or caregiver will be able to:	Patient	Caregiver
• Describe the rationale for using a peak flow meter in asthma management.	✔	✔
• Explain how peak flow monitoring is used along with symptoms to determine severity of asthma.	✔	✔
• Demonstrate steps for using the peak flow meter correctly:		
• Move the indicator to the bottom of the numbered scale.	✔	
• Stand up.	✔	
• Take a deep breath and fill the lungs completely.	✔	
• Place mouthpiece in mouth and close lips around mouthpiece (do not put tongue inside opening).	✔	
• Blow out hard and fast with a single blow.	✔	
• Record the number achieved on the indicator.	✔	
• Repeat steps 1–5 two more times and write the highest number in the asthma diary.	✔	
• Explain how to determine the "personal best" peak flow reading.	✔	✔
• Describe the significance of the color zones for peak flow monitoring.	✔	✔
• Demonstrate how to clean the peak flow meter.	✔	✔
• Discuss how and when to contact the health care provider about changes or decreases in peak flow values.	✔	✔

"personal best" is determined after monitoring peak flows for 2 or 3 weeks after receiving optimal asthma therapy. The green (80% to 100% of personal best), yellow (60% to 80%), and red (less than 60%) zones are determined, and specific actions are delineated for each zone, enabling the patient to monitor and manipulate his or her own therapy after careful instruction. This reinforces compliance, independence, and self-efficacy.

Nursing Management

The immediate nursing care of the patient with asthma depends on the severity of the asthma symptoms. The patient may be treated successfully as an outpatient if asthma symptoms are relatively mild, or he or she may require hospitalization and intensive care for acute and severe asthma.

The patient and family are often frightened and anxious because of the patient's dyspnea. Thus, an important aspect of care is a calm approach. The nurse assesses the patient's respiratory status by monitoring the severity of symptoms, breath sounds, peak flow, pulse oximetry, and vital signs. The nurse obtains a history of allergic reactions to medications before administering medications and identifies the patient's current use of medications. The nurse administers medications as prescribed and monitors the patient's responses to those medications. Fluids may be administered if the patient is dehydrated, and antibiotics may be prescribed if the patient has an underlying respiratory infection. If the patient requires intubation because of acute respiratory failure, the nurse assists with the intubation procedure, continues close monitoring of the patient, and keeps the patient and family informed about procedures.

PROMOTING HOME AND COMMUNITY-BASED CARE

Teaching Patients Self-Care. Patient teaching is a critical component of care for the patient with asthma. Multiple inhalers, different types of inhalers, antiallergy therapy, antireflux medications, and avoidance measures are all integral for long-term control. This complex therapy requires a patient–provider partnership to determine the desired outcomes and to formulate a plan to achieve those outcomes. The patient then carries out daily therapy as part of self-care management, with input and guidance by the health care provider. Before a partnership can be established, the patient needs to understand the following:

- The nature of asthma as a chronic inflammatory disease
- The definition of inflammation and bronchoconstriction
- The purpose and action of each medication
- Triggers to avoid, and how to do so
- Proper inhalation technique
- How to perform peak flow monitoring
- How to implement an action plan
- When to seek assistance, and how to do so

Continuing Care. The nurse who has contact with the patient in the hospital, clinic, school, or office uses the opportunity to assess the patient's respiratory status and ability to manage self-care to prevent serious exacerbations. The nurse emphasizes adherence to the prescribed therapy, preventive measures, and the need to keep follow-up appointments with the primary health care provider. A home visit to assess the home environment for allergens may be indicated for the patient with recurrent exacerbations. The nurse refers the patient to community support groups.

Status Asthmaticus

Status asthmaticus is severe and persistent asthma that does not respond to conventional therapy. The attacks can last longer than 24 hours. Infection, anxiety, nebulizer abuse, dehydration, increased adrenergic blockage, and nonspecific irritants may contribute to these episodes. An acute episode may be precipitated by hypersensitivity to aspirin.

Pathophysiology

The basic characteristics of asthma (constriction of the bronchiolar smooth muscle, swelling of the bronchial mucosa, and thickened secretions) decrease the diameter of the bronchi and are apparent in status asthmaticus. A ventilation–perfusion abnormality results in hypoxemia and respiratory alkalosis initially, followed by respiratory acidosis. There is a reduced PaO_2 and an initial respiratory alkalosis, with a decreased $PaCO_2$ and an increased pH. As status asthmaticus worsens, the $PaCO_2$ increases and the pH falls, reflecting respiratory acidosis.

Clinical Manifestations

The clinical manifestations are the same as those seen in severe asthma: labored breathing, prolonged exhalation, engorged neck veins, and wheezing. However, the extent of wheezing does not indicate the severity of the attack. As the obstruction worsens, the wheezing may disappear, and this is frequently a sign of impending respiratory failure.

Assessment and Diagnostic Findings

Pulmonary function studies are the most accurate means of assessing acute airway obstruction. Arterial blood gas measurements are obtained if the patient cannot perform pulmonary function maneuvers because of severe obstruction or fatigue, or if the patient does not respond to treatment. Respiratory alkalosis (low CO_2) is the most common finding in asthmatic patients. A rising PCO_2 (to normal levels or levels indicating respiratory acidosis) frequently is a danger sign of impending respiratory failure.

Medical Management

In the emergency setting, the patient is treated initially with beta-adrenergic agonists (eg, albuterol) and corticosteroids. The patient usually requires supplemental oxygen and intravenous fluids for hydration. Oxygen therapy is initiated to treat dyspnea, central cyanosis, and hypoxemia. Low-flow humidified oxygen by either Venturi mask or nasal catheter is administered. The flow is based on pulse oximetry or arterial blood gas values. The PaO_2 is maintained at 65 to 85 mm Hg. Sedatives are contraindicated. If there is no response to repeated treatments, hospitalization is required. Low pulmonary function test results and deteriorating blood gas levels (respiratory acidosis), which may indicate that the patient is tiring and will require mechanical ventilation, are other criteria calling for hospitalization. Although most patients do not need mechanical ventilation, it is used for patients in respiratory failure, for those who tire and are too fatigued by the attempt to breathe, or for those whose conditions do not respond to initial treatment.

Nursing Management

Constant monitoring of the patient by the nurse is important for the first 12 to 24 hours, or until status asthmaticus is halted. The nurse also assesses the patient's skin turgor to identify signs of dehydration. Fluid intake is essential to combat dehydration, to loosen secretions, and to facilitate expectoration. The nurse administers intravenous fluids as prescribed, up to 3 to 4 L/day, unless contraindicated. The patient's energy needs to be conserved, and the room should be quiet and free of respiratory irritants, including flowers, tobacco smoke, perfumes, or odors of cleaning agents. A nonallergenic pillow should be used.

PULMONARY EDEMA

Pulmonary edema is defined as abnormal accumulation of fluid in the lung tissue and/or alveolar space. It is a severe, life-threatening condition.

Pathophysiology

Pulmonary edema most commonly occurs as a result of increased microvascular pressure from abnormal cardiac function. The backup of blood into the pulmonary vasculature resulting from inadequate left ventricular function causes an increased microvascular pressure, and fluid begins to leak into the interstitial space and the alveoli. Other causes of pulmonary edema are hypervolemia or a sudden increase in the intravascular pressure in the lung. One example of this is in the patient who has undergone pneumonectomy. When one lung has been removed, all the cardiac output then goes to the remaining lung. If the patient's fluid status is not monitored closely, pulmonary edema can quickly develop in the postoperative period as the patient's pulmonary vasculature attempts to adapt. This type of pulmonary edema is sometimes termed "flash" pulmonary edema. A second example is called reexpansion pulmonary edema, which is due to a rapid inflation of the lungs after aspiration of a pneumothorax or evacuation of a large pleural effusion.

Clinical Manifestations

The patient has increasing respiratory distress, characterized by dyspnea, air hunger, and cyanosis of the lips and nails. The patient is usually very anxious. As the fluid leaks into the alveoli and mixes with air, a foam or froth is formed. The patient coughs up, or the nurse suctions out, these foamy or frothy and often blood-tinged secretions. The patient is in acute respiratory distress and may become confused or stuporous.

Assessment and Diagnostic Findings

Auscultation reveals crackles in the lung bases that rapidly progress toward the apices of the lungs. These crackles are due to the movement of air through the alveolar fluid. The chest x-ray reveals increased interstitial markings. The pulse oximetry values begin to fall, and arterial blood gas analysis demonstrates increasing hypoxemia.

Medical Management

Management focuses on correcting the underlying disorder. If the pulmonary edema is cardiac in origin, then improvement in left ventricular function is the goal. Vasodilators, inotropic medications, afterload or preload agents, or contractility medications may be given. Additional cardiac measures (eg, intra-aortic balloon pump) may be indicated if the patient does not respond. If the problem is fluid overload, diuretics are given and the patient is placed on fluid restrictions. Oxygen is administered to correct the hypoxemia; in some circumstances, intubation and mechanical ventilation are necessary. The patient is extremely anxious, and morphine is administered to reduce anxiety and control pain.

Nursing Management

Nursing management of the patient with pulmonary edema includes assisting with administration of oxygen and intubation and mechanical ventilation if respiratory failure occurs. The nurse also administers medications (ie, morphine, vasodilators, inotropic medications, preload and afterload agents) if prescribed and monitors the patient's response. Nursing management in pulmonary edema is described in more detail in Chapter 27.

ACUTE RESPIRATORY FAILURE

Respiratory failure is a sudden and life-threatening deterioration of the gas exchange function of the lung. It exists when the exchange of oxygen for carbon dioxide in the lungs cannot keep up with the rate of oxygen consumption and carbon dioxide production by the cells of the body.

Acute respiratory failure (ARF) is defined as a fall in arterial oxygen tension (PaO_2) to less than 50 mm Hg (hypoxemia) and a rise in arterial carbon dioxide tension ($PaCO_2$) to greater than 50 mm Hg (hypercapnia), with an arterial pH of less than 7.35. In ARF, the ventilation and/or perfusion mechanisms in the lung are impaired. Respiratory system mechanisms leading to ARF include:

- Alveolar hypoventilation
- Diffusion abnormalities
- Ventilation–perfusion mismatching
- Shunting

It is important to distinguish between ARF and chronic respiratory failure. Chronic respiratory failure is defined as a deterioration in the gas exchange function of the lung that has developed insidiously or has persisted for a long period after an episode of ARF. The absence of acute symptoms and the presence of a chronic respiratory acidosis suggest the chronicity of the respiratory failure. Two causes of chronic respiratory failure are COPD and neuromuscular diseases. These patients develop a tolerance to the gradually worsening hypoxemia and hypercapnia. However, a patient with chronic respiratory failure may develop ARF. This is seen in the COPD patient who develops an exacerbation or infection that causes additional deterioration of the gas exchange mechanism. The principles of management of acute versus chronic respiratory failure are different; the following discussion will be confined to ARF.

Pathophysiology

Common causes of ARF can be classified into four categories: decreased respiratory drive, dysfunction of the chest wall, dysfunction of the lung parenchyma, and other causes.

DECREASED RESPIRATORY DRIVE

Decreased respiratory drive may occur with severe brain injury, large lesions of the brain stem (multiple sclerosis), use of sedative medications, and metabolic disorders such as hypothyroidism. These disorders impair the normal response of chemoreceptors in the brain to normal respiratory stimulation.

DYSFUNCTION OF THE CHEST WALL

The impulses arising in the respiratory center travel through nerves that extend from the brain stem down the spinal cord to receptors in the muscles of respiration. Thus, any disease or disorder of the nerves, spinal cord, muscles, or neuromuscular junction involved in respiration seriously affects ventilation and may ultimately lead to ARF. These include musculoskeletal disorders (muscular dystrophy, polymyositis), neuromuscular junction disorders (myasthenia gravis, poliomyelitis), some peripheral nerve disorders, and spinal cord disorders (amyotrophic lateral sclerosis, Guillain-Barré syndrome, and cervical spinal cord injuries).

DYSFUNCTION OF LUNG PARENCHYMA

Pleural effusion, hemothorax, pneumothorax, and upper airway obstruction are conditions that interfere with ventilation by preventing expansion of the lung. These conditions, which may cause respiratory failure, usually are produced by an underlying lung disease, pleural disease, or trauma and injury. Other diseases and conditions of the lung that lead to ARF include pneumonia, status asthmaticus, lobar atelectasis, pulmonary embolism, and pulmonary edema.

OTHER FACTORS

In the postoperative period, especially after major thoracic or abdominal surgery, inadequate ventilation and respiratory failure may occur because of several factors. The causes of ARF during this period include the effects of anesthetic agents, analgesics, and sedatives; they may depress respiration as described earlier or enhance the effects of opioids and lead to hypoventilation. Pain may interfere with deep breathing and coughing. A mismatch of ventilation to perfusion is the usual cause of respiratory failure after major abdominal and thoracic surgery.

Clinical Manifestations

Early signs are those associated with impaired oxygenation and may include restlessness, fatigue, headache, dyspnea, air hunger, tachycardia, and increased blood pressure. As the hypoxemia progresses, more obvious signs may be present, including confusion, lethargy, tachycardia, tachypnea, central cyanosis, diaphoresis, and finally respiratory arrest. Physical findings are those of acute respiratory distress, including use of accessory muscles, decreased breath sounds if the patient cannot adequately ventilate, and other findings related specifically to the underlying disease process and cause of ARF.

Medical Management

The objectives of treatment are to correct the underlying cause and to restore adequate gas exchange in the lung. Intubation and mechanical ventilation may be required to maintain adequate ventilation and oxygenation while the underlying cause is corrected.

Nursing Management

Nursing management of the patient with ARF includes assisting with intubation and maintaining mechanical ventilation (described in Chap. 22). The nurse assesses the patient's respiratory status by monitoring the patient's level of response, arterial blood gases, pulse oximetry, and vital signs, and assessing the respiratory system. The nurse implements strategies (eg, turning schedule, mouth care, skin care, range of motion of extremities) to prevent complications. The nurse also assesses the patient's understanding of the management strategies that are used and initiates some form of communication to enable the patient to express his or her needs to the health care team. Nursing care also addresses the problems that led to ARF. As the patient's status improves, the nurse assesses the patient's knowledge of the underlying disorder and provides teaching as appropriate to address the underlying disorder.

ACUTE RESPIRATORY DISTRESS SYNDROME

Acute respiratory distress syndrome (ARDS; previously called adult respiratory distress syndrome) is a clinical syndrome characterized by a sudden and progressive pulmonary edema, increasing bilateral infiltrates on chest x-ray, hypoxemia refractory to oxygen supplementation, and reduced lung compliance. These signs occur in the absence of left-sided heart failure. Patients with ARDS usually require mechanical ventilation with a higher-than-normal airway pressure. A wide range of factors are associated with the development of ARDS (Chart 21-2), including direct injury to the lungs (eg, smoke inhalation) or indirect insult to the lungs (eg, shock). ARDS has been associated with a mortality rate as high as 50% to 60%. The major cause of death in ARDS is nonpulmonary multiple-system organ failure, often with sepsis.

CHART 21•2 Etiologic Factors Related to ARDS

- Aspiration (gastric secretions, drowning, hydrocarbons)
- Drug ingestion and overdose
- Hematologic disorders (disseminated intravascular coagulopathy, massive transfusions, cardiopulmonary bypass)
- Prolonged inhalation of high concentrations of oxygen, smoke, or corrosive substances
- Localized infection (bacterial, fungal, viral pneumonia)
- Metabolic disorders (pancreatitis, uremia)
- Shock (any cause)
- Trauma (pulmonary contusion, multiple fractures, head injury)
- Major surgery
- Fat or air embolism
- Systemic sepsis

Pathophysiology

ARDS occurs as a result of an inflammatory trigger that initiates the release of cellular and chemical mediators, causing injury to the alveolar capillary membrane. This results in leakage of fluid into the alveolar interstitial spaces and alterations in the capillary bed.

Severe ventilation–perfusion mismatching occurs in ARDS. Alveoli collapse because of the inflammatory infiltrate, blood, fluid, and surfactant dysfunction. Small airways are narrowed because of interstitial fluid and bronchial obstruction. The lung compliance becomes markedly decreased (stiff lungs), and the result is a characteristic decrease in functional residual capacity and severe hypoxemia. The blood returning to the lung for gas exchange is pumped through the nonventilated, nonfunctioning areas of the lung, causing a shunt to develop. This means that blood is interfacing with nonfunctioning alveoli and gas exchange is markedly impaired, resulting in severe, refractory hypoxemia. Figure 21-9 shows the sequence of pathophysiologic events leading to ARDS.

Clinical Manifestations

Clinically, ARDS is marked by a rapid onset of severe dyspnea that usually occurs 12 to 48 hours after an initiating event. The patient is anxious and has labored breathing and tachypnea.

Assessment and Diagnostic Findings

Intercostal retractions and crackles, as the fluid begins to leak into the alveolar interstitial space, are evident on physical examination. A diagnosis of ARDS may be made based on the following criteria: a history of systemic or pulmonary risk factors, acute onset of respiratory distress, bilateral pulmonary infiltrates, clinical absence of left-sided heart failure, and a ratio of partial pressure of oxygen of arterial blood to fraction of inspired oxygen (PaO_2/FiO_2) less than 200 mm Hg (severe refractory hypoxemia).

Medical Management

The primary focus in the management of ARDS includes identification and treatment of the underlying condition. Aggressive, supportive care must be provided to compensate for the severe respiratory dysfunction. This supportive therapy almost always includes intubation and mechanical ventilation. In addition, circulatory support, adequate fluid volume, and nutritional support are important. Supplemental oxygen is used as the patient begins the initial spiral of hypoxemia. As the hypoxemia progresses, intubation and mechanical ventilation are instituted. The concentration of oxygen and ventilator settings and modes are determined by the patient's status. This is monitored by arterial blood gas analysis, pulse oximetry, and bedside pulmonary function testing.

Positive end-expiratory pressure (PEEP) is a critical part of the treatment of ARDS. PEEP usually improves oxygenation, but it does not influence the natural history of the syndrome. Use of PEEP helps to increase functional residual capacity and reverse alveolar collapse by keeping the alveoli open, resulting in improved arterial oxygenation and a reduction in the severity of the ventilation–perfusion imbalance. By using PEEP, a lower FiO_2

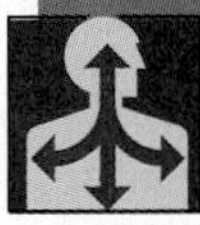

PATHOPHYSIOLOGY

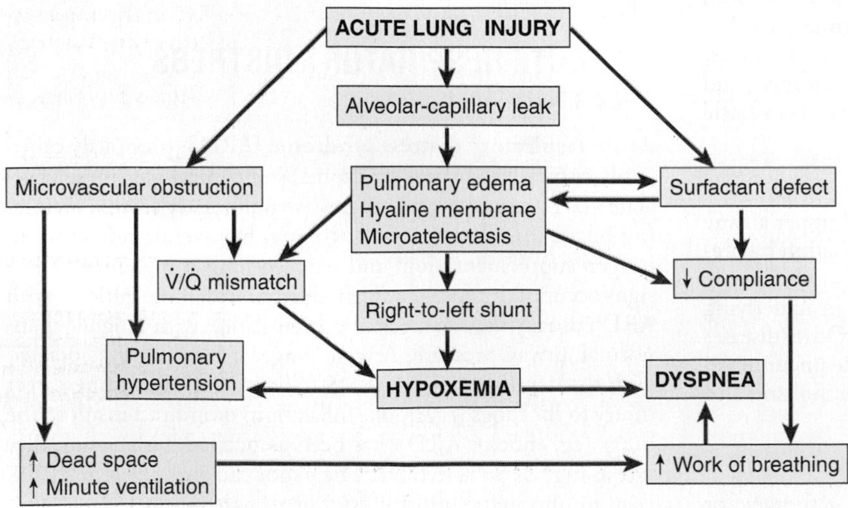

FIGURE 21•9 Pathogenesis and pathophysiology of acute respiratory distress syndrome. Adapted from Farzan, S. (1997). *A concise handbook of respiratory diseases* (4th ed.). Stamford, CT: Appleton & Lange.

may be required. The goal is a PaO_2 greater than 60 mm Hg or an oxygen saturation level of greater than 90% at the lowest possible FiO_2. PEEP is discussed in Chapter 22.

Systemic hypotension may occur in ARDS as a result of hypovolemia secondary to leakage of fluid into the interstitial spaces and depressed cardiac output from high levels of PEEP therapy. Hypovolemia must be carefully treated without causing further overload. Intravenous crystalloid solutions are administered, with careful monitoring of pulmonary status. Inotropic or vasopressor agents may be required. Pulmonary artery pressure catheters are used to monitor the patient's fluid status and the severe and progressive pulmonary hypertension sometimes observed in ARDS.

PHARMACOLOGIC THERAPY

Numerous pharmacologic treatments are under investigation to stop the cascade of events leading to ARDS. These include human recombinant interleukin-1 receptor antagonist, neutrophil inhibitors, pulmonary-specific vasodilators, surfactant replacement therapy, antioxidant therapy, and corticosteroids late in the course of ARDS. The use of corticosteroids early in the treatment of ARDS is controversial. Some believe that their use may contribute to deterioration in pulmonary function and the development of superinfections. A new pharmacologic therapy being investigated is the use of inhaled nitric oxide (a pulmonary vasodilator).

NUTRITIONAL THERAPY

Adequate nutritional support is vital in the treatment of ARDS. Patients with ARDS require 35 to 45 kcal/kg per day to meet normal requirements. Enteral feeding is the first consideration; however, total parenteral nutrition also may be required.

Nursing Management

GENERAL MEASURES

The patient with ARF and ARDS is critically ill and requires close monitoring because the condition could quickly change to a life-threatening situation. Most of the respiratory modalities discussed in Chapter 22 are used in this situation (oxygen administration, nebulizer therapy, chest physiotherapy, endotracheal intubation or tracheostomy, mechanical ventilation, suctioning, bronchoscopy). Frequent assessment of the patient's status is necessary to evaluate the effectiveness of treatment.

In addition to implementing the medical plan of care, the nurse considers other needs of the patient. Positioning is important. The nurse should turn the patient frequently to improve ventilation and perfusion in the lungs and enhance secretion drainage. However, the nurse must closely monitor the patient for rapid changes in oxygenation with changes in position. Oxygenation in the ARDS patient is sometimes improved in the prone position; studies to assess the benefits of such positioning are ongoing.

The patient is extremely anxious because of the increasing hypoxemia and dyspnea. The nurse should explain all procedures and deliver care in a calm, reassuring manner. It is important to reduce the patient's anxiety because anxiety prevents rest and increases oxygen expenditure. Rest is essential to reduce oxygen consumption, thereby reducing oxygen needs.

VENTILATOR CONSIDERATIONS

If the patient is intubated and receiving mechanical ventilation with PEEP, several considerations must be addressed. PEEP, which causes increased end-expiratory pressure, is an unnatural pattern of breathing and feels strange to the patient. The patient may be anxious and "fight" the ventilator. Nursing assessment is important to assess for problems with ventilation that may be causing the anxiety reaction: tube blockage by kinking or secretion retained; other acute respiratory problems (eg, pneumothorax, pain); a sudden drop in the oxygen level; the patient's level of dyspnea; or ventilator malfunction. In some cases, sedation may be required to decrease the patient's oxygen consumption, allow the ventilator to provide full support of ventilation, and decrease the patient's anxiety. Possible sedatives are diazepam, lorazepam, midazolam, haloperidol, propofol, and short-acting barbiturates.

If the PEEP level cannot be maintained despite the use of sedatives, neuromuscular blocking agents, such as pancuronium, vecuronium, atracurium, and rocuronium, may be given to paralyze the patient. This allows the patient to be ventilated more easily. With paralysis, the patient appears unconscious, loses motor function, and cannot breathe, talk, or blink independently. However, the patient retains sensation and is awake and able to hear. The nurse must reassure the patient that the paralysis is a result of the medication and is temporary. Paralysis should be used for the shortest possible time and never without adequate sedation.

Use of paralytic agents has many dangers and side effects. The nurse must be sure the patient does not become disconnected from the ventilator, because respiratory muscles are paralyzed and the patient will be apneic. Consequently, the nurse ensures that the patient is closely monitored at all times. All ventilator and patient alarms should be on at all times. Eye care is important as well because the patient cannot blink, increasing the risk of corneal abrasions. Neuromuscular blockers predispose patients to the development of deep venous thrombi, muscle atrophy, and skin breakdown. Nursing assessment is essential to minimize the complications related to neuromuscular blockade. The patient may have discomfort or pain but cannot communicate these sensations. Analgesia is usually administered concurrently with neuromuscular blocking agents. The nurse must anticipate the patient's needs regarding pain and comfort. The nurse checks the patient's position to ensure it is comfortable and talks to, and not about, the patient while in the patient's presence.

In addition, it is important for the nurse to describe the purpose and effects of the paralytic agents to the family. This experience can be very frightening to family members if they are unaware that these agents have been given.

PULMONARY HYPERTENSION

Pulmonary hypertension is a condition that is not clinically evident until late in its progression. Pulmonary hypertension exists when the systolic pulmonary artery pressure exceeds 30 mm Hg or the mean pulmonary artery pressure exceeds 25 mm Hg. These pressures cannot be measured indirectly as can systemic blood pressure; instead, they must be measured during right-sided heart catheterization. In the absence of these measurements, clinical recognition becomes the only indicator for the presence of pulmonary hypertension.

There are two forms of pulmonary hypertension: primary (or idiopathic) and secondary. Primary pulmonary hypertension is an uncommon disease in which the diagnosis is made by excluding all other possible causes. The exact cause is unknown, but there are several possible causes (Chart 21-3). The clinical presentation of primary pulmonary hypertension exists with no evidence of pulmonary and cardiac disease or pulmonary embolism. It occurs most often in women 20 to 40 years of age and is usually fatal within 5 years of diagnosis.

CHART 21•3 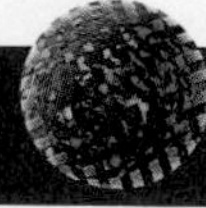 **Causes of Pulmonary Hypertension**

Primary or Idiopathic

- Altered immune mechanisms
- Silent pulmonary emboli
- Raynaud's phenomenon
- Oral contraceptives
- Sickle cell disease
- Collagen diseases

Secondary

- Pulmonary vasoconstriction due to hypoxemia
  - Chronic obstructive pulmonary disease
  - Kyphoscoliosis
  - Obesity
  - Smoke inhalation
  - High altitude
  - Neuromuscular disorders
  - Diffuse interstitial pneumonia
- Reduction of the pulmonary vascular bed (must impair 50% to 75% of the vascular bed)
  - Pulmonary emboli
  - Vasculitis
  - Widespread interstitial lung disease (sarcoidosis, systemic sclerosis)
  - Tumor emboli
- Primary Cardiac Disease
  - Congenital (patent ductus arteriosus, atrial septal defect, ventricular septal defect)
  - Acquired (rheumatic valvular disease, mitral stenosis, myxoma, left ventricular failure)

Secondary pulmonary hypertension is more common and results from existing cardiac or pulmonary disease. The prognosis depends on the severity of the underlying disorder and the changes in the pulmonary vascular bed. A common cause of secondary pulmonary hypertension is pulmonary artery constriction due to hypoxemia from COPD.

Pathophysiology

Normally, the pulmonary vascular bed can handle the blood volume delivered by the right ventricle. It has a low resistance to blood flow and compensates for increased blood volume by dilation of the vessels in the pulmonary circulation. However, if the pulmonary vascular bed is destroyed or obstructed, as in pulmonary hypertension, the ability to handle whatever flow or volume of blood it receives is impaired, and the increased blood flow then increases the pulmonary artery pressure. As the pulmonary arterial pressure increases, the pulmonary vascular resistance also increases. Both pulmonary artery constriction (as in hypoxemia or hypercapnia) and a reduction of the pulmonary vascular bed (which occurs with pulmonary emboli) result in an increase in pulmonary vascular resistance and pressure. This increased workload affects right ventricular function. The myocardium ultimately cannot meet the increasing demands imposed on it, leading to right ventricular hypertrophy (enlargement and dilation) and failure.

Clinical Manifestations

Dyspnea is the main symptom of pulmonary hypertension, occurring at first with exertion and eventually at rest. Substernal chest pain also is common, affecting 25% to 50% of patients. Other signs and symptoms include weakness, fatigue, syncope, and signs of right-sided heart failure (peripheral edema, ascites, distended neck veins, liver engorgement, crackles, heart murmur).

Assessment and Diagnostic Findings

A complete diagnostic evaluation includes a history, physical examination, chest x-ray, pulmonary function studies, electrocardiogram (ECG), echocardiogram, ventilation–perfusion scan, and cardiac catheterization. In some cases, an **open lung biopsy**, performed by thoracotomy, may be needed to make a definite diagnosis. Cardiac catheterization of the right side of the heart reveals elevated pulmonary arterial pressure. An echocardiogram can assess the progression of the disease and rule out other conditions with similar signs and symptoms. The ECG reveals right ventricular hypertrophy, right axis deviation, and tall peaked P waves in inferior leads, tall anterior R waves, and ST-segment depression and/or T-wave inversion anteriorly. The PaO_2 also is decreased (hypoxemia). A ventilation–perfusion scan or pulmonary angiography detects defects in pulmonary vasculature, such as pulmonary emboli. Pulmonary function studies may be normal or show a slight decrease in VC and lung compliance, with a mild decrease in the diffusing capacity.

Medical Management

The goal of treatment is to manage the underlying cardiac or pulmonary condition. Most patients with primary pulmonary hypertension do not have hypoxemia at rest but require supplemental oxygen with exercise. However, patients with severe right ventricular failure, decreased cardiac output, and progressive disease may have resting hypoxemia and require continuous oxygen supplementation. Appropriate oxygen therapy (see Chap. 22) reverses the vasoconstriction and reduces the pulmonary hypertension in a relatively short time.

In the presence of cor pulmonale, treatment should include fluid restriction, diuretics to decrease fluid accumulation, cardiac glycosides (eg, digitalis) in an attempt to improve cardiac function, calcium channel blockers for vasodilation, and rest. In primary pulmonary hypertension, vasodilators have been administered with variable success. Anticoagulants such as warfarin have been given to patients because of chronic pulmonary emboli. Heart–lung transplantation has been successful in select patients with primary hypertension who have not been responsive to other therapies.

Nursing Management

The major nursing goals are to identify patients at high risk for pulmonary hypertension. High-risk patients include those with COPD, pulmonary emboli, congenital heart disease, and mitral valve disease. The nurse also must be alert for signs and symptoms, administer oxygen therapy appropriately, and instruct patients and their families about the use of home oxygen supplementation.

PULMONARY HEART DISEASE (COR PULMONALE)

Cor pulmonale is a condition in which the right ventricle of the heart enlarges (with or without right-sided heart failure) as a result of diseases that affect the structure or function of the lung or its vasculature. Any disease affecting the lungs and accompanied by hypoxemia may result in cor pulmonale. The most frequent cause is severe COPD in which changes in the airway and retained secretions reduce alveolar ventilation. Other causes are conditions that restrict or compromise ventilatory function, leading to hypoxemia or acidosis (deformities of the thoracic cage, massive obesity), or conditions that reduce the pulmonary vascular bed (primary idiopathic pulmonary arterial hypertension, pulmonary embolus). Certain disorders of the nervous system, respiratory muscles, chest wall, and pulmonary arterial tree also may be responsible for cor pulmonale.

Pathophysiology

Pulmonary disease can produce physiologic changes that in time affect the heart and cause the right ventricle to enlarge and eventually fail. Any condition that deprives the lungs of oxygen can cause hypoxemia and hypercapnia, resulting in ventilatory insufficiency. Hypoxemia and hypercapnia cause pulmonary arterial vasoconstriction and possibly reduction of the pulmonary vascular bed, as in emphysema or pulmonary emboli. The result is increased resistance in the pulmonary circulatory system, with a subsequent rise in pulmonary blood pressure (pulmonary hypertension). A mean pulmonary arterial pressure of 45 mm Hg or more may occur in cor pulmonale. Right ventricular hypertrophy may result, followed by right ventricular failure. In short, cor pulmonale results from pulmonary hypertension, which causes the right side of the heart to enlarge because of the increased work required to pump blood against high resistance through the pulmonary vascular system.

Clinical Manifestations

Symptoms of cor pulmonale are usually related to the underlying lung disease, such as COPD. Shortness of breath and cough are key signs in COPD. As the right ventricle fails, the patient may develop increasing edema of the feet and legs, distended neck veins, an enlarged palpable liver, pleural effusion, ascites, and a heart murmur. Headache, confusion, and somnolence may occur as a result of increased levels of carbon dioxide (hypercapnia).

Medical Management

The objectives of treatment are to improve the patient's ventilation and to treat both the underlying lung disease and the manifestations of heart disease. Supplemental oxygen is administered to improve gas exchange and to reduce pulmonary arterial pressure and pulmonary vascular resistance. Improved oxygen transport relieves the pulmonary hypertension that is causing the cor pulmonale.

Better survival rates and greater reduction in pulmonary vascular resistance have been reported with continuous, 24-hour oxygen therapy for patients with severe hypoxemia. Substantial improvement may require 4 to 6 weeks of oxygen therapy, usually in the home. Periodic assessment of pulse oximetry and arterial blood gases is necessary to determine the adequacy of alveolar ventilation and to monitor the effectiveness of oxygen therapy.

Ventilation is further improved with chest physical therapy and bronchial hygiene maneuvers as indicated to remove accumulated secretions, and the administration of bronchodilators. Further measures depend on the patient's condition. If the patient is in respiratory failure, endotracheal intubation and mechanical ventilation may be necessary. If the patient is in heart failure, hypoxemia and hypercapnia must be relieved to improve cardiac function and output. Bed rest, sodium restriction, and diuretic therapy also are instituted judiciously to reduce peripheral edema (to lower pulmonary arterial pressure through a decrease in total blood volume) and the circulatory load on the right side of the heart. Digitalis may be given to relieve pulmonary hypertension if the patient also has left ventricular failure, a supraventricular dysrhythmia, or right ventricular failure that does not respond to other therapy.

ECG monitoring may be indicated because of the high incidence of dysrhythmias in patients with cor pulmonale. Any pulmonary infection must be treated promptly to avoid further impaired gas exchange and exacerbations of hypoxemia and pulmonary heart disease. The prognosis depends on whether the pulmonary hypertension is reversible. (Management of acute respiratory failure is discussed earlier in this chapter.)

Nursing Management

Nursing care of the patient with cor pulmonale addresses the underlying disorder leading to cor pulmonale as well as the problems related to pulmonary hyperventilation and right-sided cardiac failure. If intubation and mechanical ventilation are required to manage ARF, the nurse assists with the intubation procedure and maintains mechanical ventilation. The nurse assesses the patient's respiratory and cardiac status and administers medications as prescribed.

During the patient's hospital stay, the nurse instructs the patient about the importance of close monitoring and adherence to the therapeutic regimen, especially the 24-hour use of oxygen. Factors that affect the patient's adherence to the treatment regimen are explored and addressed.

PROMOTING HOME AND COMMUNITY-BASED CARE

Teaching Patients Self-Care. Most of the care and monitoring of the patient with cor pulmonale is performed by the patient and family in the home because it is a chronic disorder. If supplemental oxygen is administered, the nurse instructs the patient and the family in its use. Nutrition counseling is warranted if the patient is on a sodium-restricted diet or is taking diuretics. The nurse teaches the family to monitor for signs and symptoms of right ventricular failure and about emergency interventions and when to call for assistance. Most importantly, the nurse urges the patient to stop smoking.

CONTINUING CARE

A referral for home care may be warranted for the patient who cannot manage self-care or for the patient whose physical condition warrants close assessment. During the home visit, the home care nurse evaluates the patient's status and the patient's and family members' understanding of the therapeutic regimen and their adherence to it. If oxygen is used in the home, the nurse determines if it is being administered safely and as prescribed. It is important to assess the patient's progress in stopping smoking and to reinforce the importance of smoking cessation with the patient and family. The nurse identifies strategies to assist with smoking cessation and refers the patient and family to community support groups.

PULMONARY EMBOLISM

Pulmonary embolism (PE) refers to the obstruction of the pulmonary artery or one of its branches by a thrombus (or thrombi) that originates somewhere in the venous system or in the right side of the heart. Most commonly, PE is due to a blood clot or thrombus. However, there are other types of emboli: air, fat, amniotic fluid, and septic (from bacterial invasion of the thrombus). It is estimated that more than half a million people develop PE yearly, resulting in more than 50,000 deaths. PE is a common disorder and often is associated with trauma, surgery (orthopedic, major abdominal, pelvic, gynecologic), pregnancy, congestive heart failure, age older than 50 years, hypercoagulable states, and prolonged immobility. It also may occur in an apparently healthy person. Risk factors for developing PE are identified in the accompanying chart.

Although most thrombi originate in the deep veins of the legs, other sites include the pelvic veins and the right atrium of the heart. A venous thrombosis can result from slowing of blood flow (stasis), secondary to damage to the blood vessel wall (particularly the endothelial lining, or changes in the blood coagulation mechanism.

Pathophysiology

When a thrombus completely or partially obstructs a pulmonary artery or its branches, the alveolar dead space is increased. The area, although continuing to be ventilated, receives little or no blood flow. Thus, gas exchange is impaired or absent in this area.

Risk Factors for
PULMONARY EMBOLUS

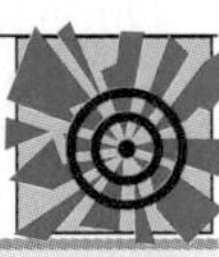

Venous Stasis (slowing of blood flow in veins)
Prolonged immobilization (especially postoperative)
Prolonged periods of sitting/traveling
Varicose veins
Spinal cord injury

Hypercoagulability (due to release of tissue thromboplastin after injury/surgery)
Injury
Tumor (pancreatic, GI, GU, breast, lung)
Increased platelet count (polycythemia, splenectomy)

Venous Endothelial Disease
Thrombophlebitis
Vascular disease
Foreign bodies (IV/central venous catheters)

Certain Disease States (combination of stasis, coagulation alterations, and venous injury)
Heart disease (especially congestive heart failure)
Trauma (especially fracture of hip, pelvis, vertebra, lower extremities)
Postoperative state/postpartum period
Diabetes mellitus
Chronic obstructive pulmonary disease

Other Predisposing Conditions
Advanced age
Obesity
Pregnancy
Oral contraceptive use
History of previous thrombophlebitis, pulmonary embolism
Constrictive clothing

In addition, various substances are released from the clot and surrounding area, causing regional blood vessels and bronchioles to constrict. This causes an increase in pulmonary vascular resistance. This reaction compounds the ventilation–perfusion imbalance.

The hemodynamic consequences are increased pulmonary vascular resistance from the regional vasoconstriction and reduced size of the pulmonary vascular bed. This results in an increase in pulmonary arterial pressure and, in turn, an increase in right ventricular work to maintain pulmonary blood flow. When the work requirements of the right ventricle exceed its capacity, right ventricular failure occurs, leading to a decrease in cardiac output followed by a decrease in systemic blood pressure and the development of shock.

Clinical Manifestations

The symptoms of PE depend on the size of the thrombus and the area of the pulmonary artery occluded by the thrombus; they may be nonspecific. Dyspnea is the most frequent symptom, tachypnea (very rapid respiratory rate) the most frequent sign (Goldhaber, 1998). The duration and intensity of the dyspnea depend on the extent of embolization. Chest pain is common and is usually sudden and pleuritic. It occasionally is substernal and may mimic angina pectoris or a myocardial infarction. Other symptoms include fever, tachycardia, apprehension, cough, diaphoresis, hemoptysis, and syncope.

A massive embolism occluding the outflow tract of the main pulmonary artery or the bifurcation of the pulmonary arteries can produce pronounced dyspnea, sudden substernal pain, rapid and weak pulse, shock, syncope, and sudden death. Multiple small emboli can lodge in the terminal pulmonary arterioles, producing multiple small infarctions of the lungs. A pulmonary infarction is ischemic necrosis of an area of the lung and occurs in 10% to 20% of cases of PE. The clinical picture may simulate that of bronchopneumonia or heart failure. In atypical instances, the disease causes few signs and symptoms, whereas in other instances it mimics various other cardiopulmonary disorders.

Assessment and Diagnostic Findings

Death from PE commonly occurs within 1 hour of symptoms; thus, early recognition and diagnosis are priorities. Because the symptoms of PE can vary from few to severe, a diagnostic workup is performed to rule out other diseases. Deep venous thrombosis is closely associated with the development of PE. Typically, patients report sudden onset of pain and/or swelling of the proximal or distal extremity. This pain is usually relieved with elevation. The diagnostic workup includes a ventilation–perfusion scan, pulmonary angiography, chest x-ray, ECG, peripheral vascular studies, impedance plethysmography, and arterial blood gas analysis.

The chest x-ray is usually normal but may show infiltrates, atelectasis, elevation of the diaphragm on the affected side, or a pleural effusion. The chest x-ray is most helpful in excluding other possible causes. The ECG usually shows sinus tachycardia, PR-interval depression, and nonspecific T-wave changes. Peripheral vascular studies may include impedance plethysmography, Doppler ultrasonography, or venography. Test results confirm or exclude the diagnosis of PE. Arterial blood gas analysis may show hypoxemia and hypocapnia (from tachypnea); however, arterial blood gas measurements are normal in up to 20% of patients with PE.

A ventilation–perfusion scan is the test of choice in patients with suspected PE. The perfusion portion of the scan may indicate areas of diminished or absent blood flow and is the most useful test to rule out clinically important PE (Goldhaber, 1998). A ventilation scan may show whether there is also a ventilation abnormality present. A normal perfusion scan rules out the diagnosis of PE. If there is a ventilation–perfusion mismatch, the probability of PE is high.

If lung scan results are not definitive, pulmonary angiography can be used to confirm the diagnosis of PE; pulmonary angiography is the gold standard for the diagnosis of PE. This test is performed in the interventional radiology department. A contrast agent is injected into the pulmonary arterial system, allowing visualization of obstructions to blood flow and abnormalities.

Prevention

For those at risk, the most effective approach in preventing PE is to prevent deep venous thrombosis. Active leg exercises to avoid venous stasis, early ambulation, and use of elastic pressure stockings are general preventive measures. Additional strategies for prevention are listed in the accompanying checklist.

Patients who are older than 40, whose hemostasis is adequate, and who are undergoing major elective abdominal or thoracic surgery may receive anticoagulant therapy. Low doses of heparin may be given before surgery to reduce the risk of postoperative deep venous thrombus and PE. Heparin should be administered subcutaneously 2 hours before surgery and continued every 8 to 12 hours until the patient is discharged. Low-dose heparin is thought to enhance the activity of antithrombin III, a major plasma inhibitor of clotting factor X. This regimen is not recommended for patients with an active thrombotic process or for those undergoing major orthopedic surgery, open prostatectomy, or surgery on the eye or brain. Low-molecular-weight heparin is an alternative therapy. It has a longer half-life but is expensive.

The intermittent pneumatic leg compression device is useful in preventing thromboembolism. The device inflates a bag that intermittently compresses the leg from the calf to the thigh, thereby improving venous return. It may be applied before surgery and continued until the patient is ambulatory. The device is particularly useful for patients who are not candidates for anticoagulant therapy.

Medical Management

Because PE is often a medical emergency, emergency management is of primary concern. After emergency measures have been taken and the patient's condition stabilizes, the treatment goal is to dissolve (lyse) the existing emboli and prevent new ones from forming. The treatment of PE may include a variety of modalities:

- General measures to improve respiratory and vascular status
- Anticoagulation therapy
- Thrombolytic therapy
- Surgical intervention

EMERGENCY MANAGEMENT

Massive PE is a life-threatening emergency. The immediate objective is to stabilize the cardiopulmonary system. Most patients who die of massive PE do so in the first 1 to 2 hours after the embolic event. Emergency management consists of the following:

- Nasal oxygen is administered immediately to relieve hypoxemia, respiratory distress, and central cyanosis.
- Intravenous infusion lines are started to establish routes for medications or fluids that will be needed.
- A perfusion scan, hemodynamic measurements, and arterial blood gas determinations are performed. In some circumstances, pulmonary angiography is performed. A sud-

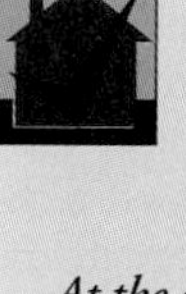

HOME CARE TEACHING CHECKLIST: PREVENTION OF RECURRENT PULMONARY EMBOLISM

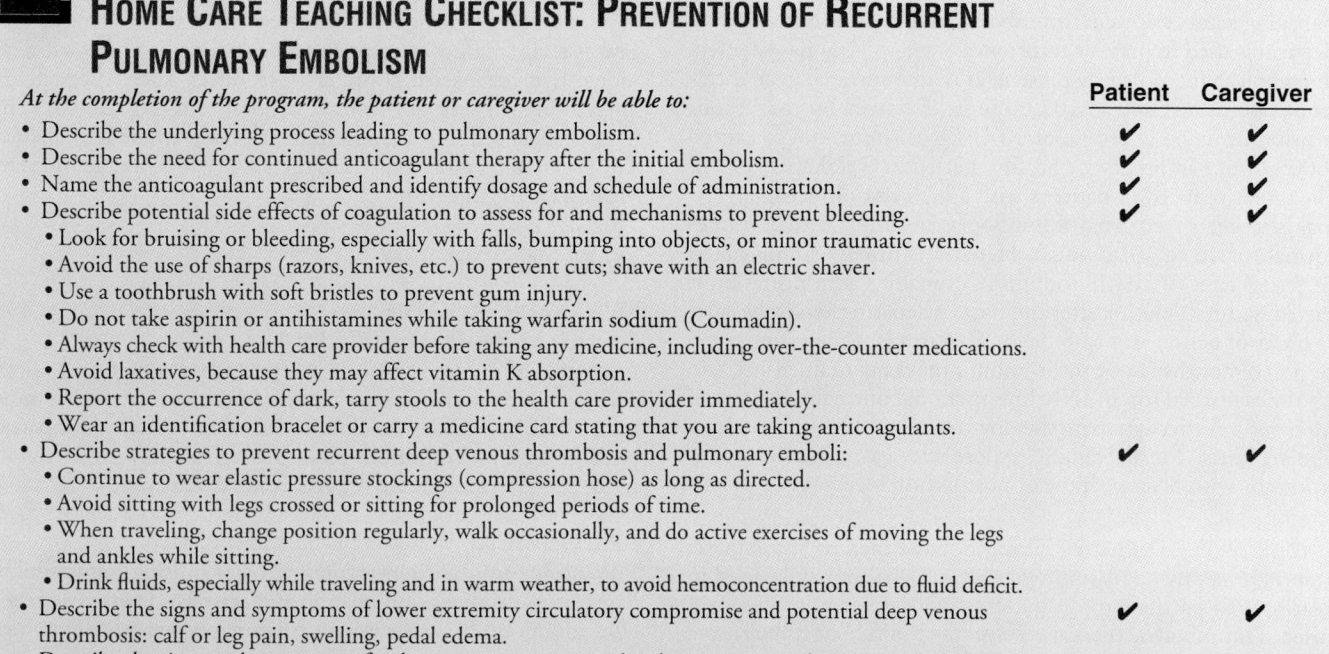

At the completion of the program, the patient or caregiver will be able to:

	Patient	Caregiver
• Describe the underlying process leading to pulmonary embolism.	✔	✔
• Describe the need for continued anticoagulant therapy after the initial embolism.	✔	✔
• Name the anticoagulant prescribed and identify dosage and schedule of administration.	✔	✔
• Describe potential side effects of coagulation to assess for and mechanisms to prevent bleeding.	✔	✔
• Look for bruising or bleeding, especially with falls, bumping into objects, or minor traumatic events.		
• Avoid the use of sharps (razors, knives, etc.) to prevent cuts; shave with an electric shaver.		
• Use a toothbrush with soft bristles to prevent gum injury.		
• Do not take aspirin or antihistamines while taking warfarin sodium (Coumadin).		
• Always check with health care provider before taking any medicine, including over-the-counter medications.		
• Avoid laxatives, because they may affect vitamin K absorption.		
• Report the occurrence of dark, tarry stools to the health care provider immediately.		
• Wear an identification bracelet or carry a medicine card stating that you are taking anticoagulants.		
• Describe strategies to prevent recurrent deep venous thrombosis and pulmonary emboli:	✔	✔
• Continue to wear elastic pressure stockings (compression hose) as long as directed.		
• Avoid sitting with legs crossed or sitting for prolonged periods of time.		
• When traveling, change position regularly, walk occasionally, and do active exercises of moving the legs and ankles while sitting.		
• Drink fluids, especially while traveling and in warm weather, to avoid hemoconcentration due to fluid deficit.		
• Describe the signs and symptoms of lower extremity circulatory compromise and potential deep venous thrombosis: calf or leg pain, swelling, pedal edema.	✔	✔
• Describe the signs and symptoms of pulmonary compromise related to recurrent pulmonary embolism.	✔	✔
• Describe how and when to contact the health care provider if symptoms of circulatory compromise or pulmonary compromise are identified.	✔	✔

den rise in pulmonary resistance increases the work of the right ventricle, which can cause acute right-sided heart failure with cardiogenic shock.

- If the patient has suffered massive embolism and is hypotensive, an indwelling urinary catheter is inserted to monitor urinary output.
- Hypotension is treated by a slow infusion of dobutamine (has a dilating effect on the pulmonary vessels and bronchi) or dopamine.
- The ECG is monitored continuously for dysrhythmias and right ventricular failure, which may occur suddenly.
- Digitalis glycosides, intravenous diuretics, and antiarrhythmic agents are administered when appropriate.
- Blood is drawn for serum electrolytes, complete blood count, and hematocrit.
- If clinical assessment and arterial blood gas analysis indicate the need, the patient is intubated and placed on a mechanical ventilator.
- Small doses of intravenous morphine are given to relieve the patient's anxiety, to alleviate chest discomfort, to improve tolerance of the endotracheal tube, and to ease adaptation to the mechanical ventilator.

GENERAL MANAGEMENT

Measures are initiated to improve the patient's respiratory and vascular status. Oxygen therapy is administered to correct the hypoxemia, relieve the pulmonary vascular vasoconstriction, and reduce the pulmonary hypertension. Using elastic stockings or intermittent pneumatic leg compression devices reduces venous stasis. These measures compress the superficial veins and increase the velocity of blood in the deep veins by redirecting the blood through the deep veins. Elevating the leg (above the level of the heart) also increases venous flow.

PHARMACOLOGIC THERAPY

Anticoagulation Therapy. Anticoagulant therapy (heparin, warfarin sodium) has traditionally been the primary method for managing acute deep vein thrombosis and PE (Goldhaber, 1998). Heparin is used to prevent recurrence of emboli but has no effect on emboli that are already present. It is administered as an intravenous bolus of 5000 to 10,000 units, followed by continuous infusion initiated at a dose of 18 U/kg per hour, not to exceed 1600 U/hour in otherwise healthy patients (Goldhaber, 1998). The rate is reduced in patients with a high risk of bleeding. The goal is to keep the partial thromboplastin time 1.5 to 2.5 times normal (or 46 to 70 seconds). Heparin is usually administered for 5 to 7 days. Warfarin sodium (Coumadin) administration is started within 24 hours after the start of heparin therapy because its onset of action is 4 to 5 days. Warfarin is usually continued for 3 to 6 months. The prothrombin time is maintained at 1.5 to 2.5 times normal (or an INR [international normalized ratio] of 2.0 to 3.0). Anticoagulation therapy is contraindicated in patients who are at risk for bleeding (eg, those with gastrointestinal conditions or with postoperative or postpartum bleeding).

Thrombolytic Therapy. Thrombolytic therapy (urokinase, streptokinase, tissue plasminogen activator) also may be used in treating PE, particularly in patients who are severely compromised. Thrombolytic therapy resolves the thrombi or emboli more quickly and restores more normal hemodynamic functioning of the pulmonary circulation, thereby reducing pulmonary hypertension and improving perfusion, oxygenation, and cardiac output. Bleeding, however, is a significant side effect. Contraindications to thrombolytic therapy include cerebrovascular accident within the past 2 months, other active intracranial processes, active bleeding, surgery within the past 10 days of the thrombotic event, recent labor and delivery, trauma, or severe hypertension. Consequently, thrombolytic agents are advocated only for PE affecting a significant area of blood flow to the lung and causing hemodynamic instability.

Before thrombolytic therapy is started, prothrombin time, partial thromboplastin time, hematocrit values, and platelet counts are obtained. During therapy, all but essential invasive procedures are avoided because of potential bleeding. If necessary, fresh whole blood, packed red cells, cryoprecipitate, or frozen plasma is given to replace blood loss and reverse the bleeding tendency. After the thrombolytic infusion is completed (which varies in duration according to the agent used and the condition being treated), the patient is given anticoagulants.

SURGICAL MANAGEMENT

A surgical embolectomy may be indicated if the patient has a massive PE or hemodynamic instability or if there are contraindications to thrombolytic therapy. Pulmonary embolectomy requires a thoracotomy with cardiopulmonary bypass technique. Transvenous catheter embolectomy is a technique in which a vacuum-cupped catheter is introduced transvenously into the affected pulmonary artery. Suction is applied to the end of the embolus and the embolus is aspirated into the cup. The surgeon maintains suction to hold the embolus within the cup, and the entire catheter is withdrawn through the right side of the heart and out the femoral vein. Newer catheters are available that pulverize the clot with high-velocity jets of normal saline solution (Goldhaber, 1998). An inferior caval filter is usually inserted at the time of surgery to protect against a recurrence.

Interrupting the inferior vena cava is another surgical technique used when PE recurs or when the patient is intolerant of anticoagulant therapy. This approach prevents dislodged thrombi from being swept into the lungs while allowing adequate blood flow. The preferred approach is the application of Teflon clips to the inferior vena cava to divide the lumen into small channels without occluding caval blood flow. Also, the use of transvenous devices that occlude or filter the blood through the inferior vena cava is a fairly safe way to prevent recurrent PE. One such technique involves inserting a filter (Greenfield filter) through the internal jugular vein or common femoral vein (Fig. 21-10). This filter is advanced into the inferior vena cava, where it is opened. The perforated umbrella permits the passage of blood but prevents the passage of large thrombi.

Nursing Management

MINIMIZING THE RISK OF PULMONARY EMBOLISM

A key role of the nurse is to identify patients at high risk for PE and to minimize the risk of PE in all patients. The nurse must have a high degree of suspicion for PE in any patient, but particularly those with conditions predisposing to a slowing of venous return (see the accompanying risk factors chart).

PREVENTING THROMBUS FORMATION

Preventing thrombus formation is a major nursing responsibility. The nurse encourages ambulation and active and passive leg exercises to prevent venous stasis in patients on bed rest. The nurse instructs the patient to move the legs in a "pumping" exercise so that the leg muscles can help increase venous flow. The nurse also advises the patient not to sit or lie in bed for prolonged periods, not to cross the legs, and not to wear constricting clothing. Legs should

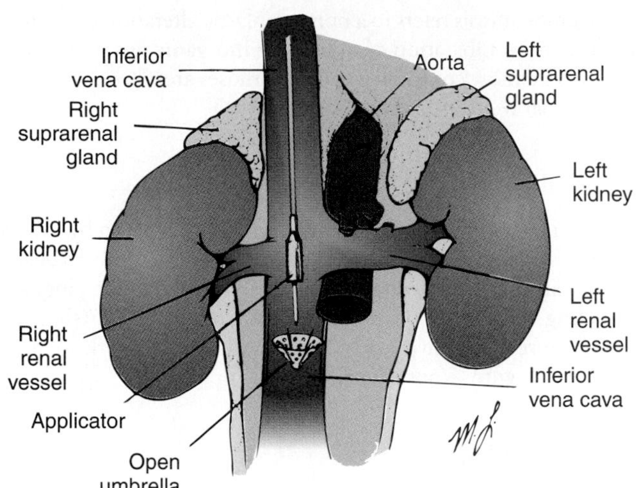

FIGURE 21•10 An umbrella filter is in place in the inferior vena cava to prevent pulmonary embolism. The filter (compressed within an applicator catheter) is inserted through an incision in the right internal jugular vein. The applicator is withdrawn when the filter fixes itself to the wall of the inferior vena cava after ejection from the applicator.

not be dangled or feet placed in a dependent position while the patient sits on the edge of the bed; instead, the patient's feet should rest on the floor or on a chair. In addition, intravenous catheters (for parenteral therapy or measurements of central venous pressure) should not be left in place for prolonged periods.

ASSESSING POTENTIAL FOR PULMONARY EMBOLISM

The nurse examines patients who are at risk for developing PE for a positive Homans' sign, which may or may not indicate impending thrombosis of the leg veins (see Chap. 28). To test for Homans' sign, the patient assumes a supine position, lifts the leg, and dorsiflexes the foot. The nurse asks the patient to report whether calf pain occurs during this maneuver. The occurrence of pain—a positive Homans' sign—may indicate deep venous thrombosis.

MONITORING THROMBOLYTIC THERAPY

The nurse is responsible for monitoring thrombolytic and anticoagulant therapy. Thrombolytic therapy (streptokinase, urokinase, tissue plasminogen activator) causes lysis of deep vein thrombi and pulmonary emboli, which helps dissolve the clots. During thrombolytic infusion, the patient remains on bed rest, vital signs are assessed every 2 hours, and invasive procedures are limited. Tests to determine prothrombin time or partial thromboplastin time are performed 3 to 4 hours after the thrombolytic infusion is started to confirm that the fibrinolytic systems have been activated. Because of the prolonged clotting time, only essential arterial punctures or venipunctures are performed, and manual pressure is applied to any puncture site for at least 30 minutes. Pulse oximetry is used to monitor changes in oxygenation. The nurse immediately discontinues the infusion if uncontrolled bleeding occurs. See Chapter 28 for nursing management for the patient receiving anticoagulant or thrombolytic therapy.

MANAGING PAIN

Chest pain, if present, is usually pleuritic rather than cardiac in origin. A semi-Fowler's position provides a more comfortable position for breathing. However, it is important to continue to turn the patient frequently and reposition the patient to improve the ventilation–perfusion ratio in the lung. The nurse administers opioid analgesics as prescribed for severe pain.

MANAGING OXYGEN THERAPY

Careful attention is given to the proper use of oxygen. It is important to ensure that the patient understands the need for continuous oxygen therapy. The nurse assesses the patient frequently for signs of hypoxemia and monitors the pulse oximetry values to evaluate the effectiveness of the oxygen therapy. Deep breathing and incentive spirometry are indicated for all patients to minimize or prevent atelectasis and improve ventilation. Nebulizer therapy or percussion and postural drainage may be used for management of secretions.

RELIEVING ANXIETY

The nurse encourages the stabilized patient to talk about any fears or concerns growing out of this frightening episode, answers the patient's questions concisely and accurately, explains the therapy, and describes how to recognize untoward effects early.

MONITORING FOR COMPLICATIONS

When caring for a patient who has had PE, the nurse must be alert for the potential complication of cardiogenic shock or right ventricular failure subsequent to the effect of PE on the cardiovascular system. Nursing activities for managing shock are found in Chapter 14.

PROVIDING POSTOPERATIVE NURSING CARE

After surgery, the nurse measures the patient's pulmonary arterial pressure and urinary output. The nurse assesses the insertion site of the arterial catheter for hematoma formation and infection. It is important to maintain the blood pressure at a level that can support perfusion of vital organs. To prevent peripheral venous stasis and edema of the lower extremities, the nurse elevates the foot of the bed and encourages isometric exercises, elastic pressure stockings, and walking when the patient is permitted out of bed. Sitting is discouraged because hip flexion compresses the large veins in the legs.

PROMOTING HOME AND COMMUNITY-BASED CARE

Teaching Patients Self-Care. Before hospital discharge and at follow-up visits to the clinic or during home visits, the nurse instructs the patient about how to prevent recurrence and what signs and symptoms to report immediately. Patient instructions, as presented in the accompanying checklist, are intended to help prevent recurrences and side effects of treatment.

SARCOIDOSIS

Sarcoidosis is a multisystem, granulomatous disease of unknown etiology. It may involve almost any organ or tissue but most commonly involves the lungs, lymph nodes, liver, spleen, central nervous system, skin, eyes, fingers, and parotid glands. The worldwide prevalence of sarcoidosis is 10 cases per 100,000 population; in the United States, the prevalence is 10 to 40 cases per 100,000 (National Institutes of Health, 1993). The disease is not gender-specific, but some manifestations are more common in women. In the United States, the disease is ten times more common in African Americans than in whites, and the disease usually begins in the third or fourth decade of life (Tanoue & Elias, 1998).

Pathophysiology

Sarcoidosis is thought to be a hypersensitivity response to one or more agents (bacteria, fungi, virus, chemicals) in people with an inherited or acquired predisposition to the disorder. The hypersensitivity response results in granuloma formation due to the release of cytokines and other substances that promote replication of fibroblasts. In the lung, granuloma infiltration and fibrosis may occur, resulting in low lung compliance, impaired diffusing capacity, and reduced lung volumes (Kelley, 1997).

Clinical Manifestations

A hallmark of this disease is its insidious onset and lack of prominent clinical signs or symptoms. The clinical picture depends on the systems involved. With pulmonary involvement, signs and symptoms may include dyspnea, cough, hemoptysis, and congestion. Generalized symptoms include anorexia, fatigue, and weight loss. Other signs include uveitis, joint pain, fever, and granulomatous lesions of the skin, liver, spleen, kidney, and central nervous system. The granulomas may disappear or gradually convert to fibrous tissue. With multisystem involvement, the patient has fatigue, fever, anorexia, weight loss, and joint pain.

Assessment and Diagnostic Findings

Chest x-rays and CT scans are used to assess pulmonary adenopathy. The chest x-ray may show hilar adenopathy and disseminated miliary and nodular lesions in the lungs. A mediastinoscopy or **transbronchial** biopsy (in which a tissue specimen is obtained through the bronchial wall) may be used to confirm the diagnosis. In rare cases, an open lung biopsy is performed. Diagnosis is confirmed by a biopsy that shows noncaseating granulomas. Pulmonary function test results are abnormal if there is restriction of lung function (reduction in total lung capacity). Arterial blood gas measurements may be normal or may show reduced oxygen levels (hypoxemia) and increased carbon dioxide levels (hypercapnia).

Medical Management

Many patients undergo remission without specific treatment. Corticosteroid therapy may benefit some patients because of its anti-inflammatory effect, which relieves symptoms and improves organ function. It is useful for patients with ocular and myocardial involvement, skin involvement, extensive pulmonary disease that compromises pulmonary function, hepatic involvement, and hypercalcemia. There is no single test that monitors the progression or recurrence of sarcoidosis. Multiple tests are used to monitor the involved systems.

OCCUPATIONAL LUNG DISEASES: PNEUMOCONIOSES

Diseases of the lungs occur in numerous occupations as a result of exposure to organic and inorganic (mineral) dusts and noxious gases (fumes and aerosols). The effects of inhaling these materials depend on the composition of the substance, its concentration, its ability to initiate an immune response, its irritating properties, the duration of exposure, and the individual's response or susceptibility to the irritant. Smoking may compound the problem and may increase the risk of lung cancers in people exposed to the mineral asbestos.

Pneumoconiosis refers to a non-neoplastic alteration of the lung resulting from inhalation of mineral or inorganic dust (eg, "dusty lung"). The most common pneumoconioses are silicosis, asbestosis, and coal workers' pneumoconiosis.

Silicosis

Silicosis is a chronic fibrotic pulmonary disease caused by inhalation of silica dust (crystalline silicon dioxide particles). Exposure to silica and silicates occurs in almost all mining, quarrying, and tunneling operations. Glass manufacturing, stone-cutting, the manufacture of abrasives and pottery, and foundry work are other occupations with exposure hazards.

Pathophysiology

When the silica particles, which have fibrogenic properties, are inhaled, nodular lesions are produced throughout the lungs. With the passage of time and further exposure, the nodules enlarge and coalesce. Dense masses form in the upper portion of the lungs, resulting in the loss of pulmonary volume. **Restrictive lung disease** (inability of the lungs to expand fully) and obstructive lung disease from secondary emphysema result. Cavities can form as a result of superimposed TB. Exposure of 15 to 20 years is usually required before the onset of the disease and shortness of breath are manifested. Fibrotic destruction of pulmonary tissue can lead to emphysema, pulmonary hypertension, and cor pulmonale.

Clinical Manifestations

The patient may have symptoms indicative of hypoxemia, severe air flow obstruction, and right-sided heart failure. Edema may occur because of the cardiac failure.

Medical Management

There is no specific treatment for silicosis, because the fibrotic process in the lung is irreversible. Supportive therapy is directed at managing complications and preventing infection. Testing is performed to rule out other lung diseases, such as TB, lung cancer, and sarcoidosis. If TB is present, it is aggressively treated. Additional therapy might include oxygen, diuretics, inhaled beta-adrenergic agonists, anticholinergics, and bronchodilator therapy.

Asbestosis

Asbestosis is a disease characterized by diffuse pulmonary fibrosis from the inhalation of asbestos dust. Current laws restrict the use of asbestos, but many industries used it in the past. Therefore, exposure occurred, and may still occur, in numerous occupations, including asbestos mining and manufacturing, shipbuilding, demolition work, and roofing. Materials such as shingles, cement, vinyl asbestos tile, fireproof paint and clothing, brake linings, and filters all contained asbestos at one time, and many of these materials are still in existence. Additional diseases related to asbestos exposure include lung cancer, mesothelioma, and asbestos pleural effusion.

Pathophysiology

Inhaled asbestos fibers enter the alveoli, where they are surrounded by fibrous tissue. The fibrous tissue eventually obliterates the alveoli. Fibrous changes also affect the pleura, which thickens and develops plaque. The result of these physiologic changes is a restrictive lung disease, with a decrease in lung volume, diminished exchange of oxygen and carbon dioxide, and hypoxemia.

Clinical Manifestations

The onset of the disease is insidious, and the patient has progressive dyspnea, persistent cough, sputum production, mild to moderate chest pain, anorexia, and weight loss. Early physical findings include bibasilar end-inspiratory crackles and in more advanced cases clubbing of the fingers. Cor pulmonale and respiratory failure occur as the disease progresses. A high proportion of workers who have been exposed to asbestos dust die of lung cancer, especially those who smoke or have a history of smoking. Cancer also can occur in other tissues.

Medical Management

There is no effective treatment for asbestosis: the lung damage is permanent and progressive. Management is directed at controlling infection and treating the lung disease. When oxygen–carbon dioxide exchange becomes severely impaired, continuous oxygen therapy may help improve activity tolerance. The patient must be instructed to avoid additional exposure to asbestos and to stop smoking.

Coal Workers' Pneumoconiosis

Coal workers' pneumoconiosis ("black lung disease") includes a variety of respiratory diseases found in coal workers who have inhaled coal dust over the years. Coal miners are exposed to dusts that are mixtures of coal, kaolin, mica, and silica.

Pathophysiology

When coal dust is deposited in the alveoli and respiratory bronchioles, macrophages engulf the particles (by phagocytosis) and transport them to the terminal bronchioles, where they are removed by mucociliary action. In time, the clearance mechanisms cannot handle the excessive dust load, and the macrophages aggregate in the respiratory bronchioles and alveoli. Fibroblasts appear and a network of reticulin is laid down surrounding the dust-laden macrophages. The bronchioles and the alveoli become clogged with coal dust, dying macrophages, and fibroblasts. This leads to the formation of the coal macule, the primary lesion of the disorder. Macules appear as blackish dots on the lungs. Fibrotic lesions develop and, as the macules enlarge, the weakening bronchioles dilate, with subsequent development of a localized emphysema. The disease begins in the upper lobes of the lungs but may progress to the lower lobes.

Clinical Manifestations

The first signs are a chronic cough and sputum production, similar to the signs encountered in chronic bronchitis. As the disease progresses, the patient develops dyspnea and coughs up large amounts of sputum with varying amounts of black fluid (melanoptysis), particularly if the individual is a smoker. Eventually, cor pulmonale and respiratory failure result. The diagnosis may first be made based on chest x-ray findings and a history of exposure.

Medical Management

Preventing this disease is key because there is no effective treatment. Instead, treatment focuses on early diagnosis and management of complications. (See also the section on emphysema above.)

Nursing Management

TEACHING ABOUT PREVENTION

The occupational health nurse serves as an employee advocate, making every effort to promote measures to reduce the exposure of workers to industrial products. Laws require that the work environment be ventilated properly to remove any noxious agent. Dust control can prevent many of the pneumoconioses. Dust control includes ventilation, spraying an area with water to control dust, and effective and frequent floor cleaning. Air samples need to be monitored. Toxic substances should be enclosed and placed in restricted areas. Workers must wear or use protective devices (face masks, hoods, industrial respirators) to provide a safe air supply when a toxic element is present. Employees who are at risk should be carefully screened and followed. There is a risk of developing serious smoking-related illness (cancer) in industries in which there are unsafe levels of certain gases, dusts, fumes, fluids, and other toxic substances. Ongoing educational programs should teach workers to take responsibility for their own health and to stop smoking and receive an influenza vaccination.

The Right to Know law stipulates that employees must be informed about all hazardous and toxic substances in the workplace. Specifically, they must be educated about any hazardous or toxic substances they work with, what effects these substances can have on their health, and the measures they can take to protect themselves. The responsibility for implementing these controls inevitably falls on the federal or state government.

CHEST TUMORS

Tumors of the lung may be benign or malignant. A malignant chest tumor can be primary, arising within the lung, chest wall, or mediastinum, or it can be a metastasis from a primary tumor site elsewhere in the body. Metastatic lung tumors occur frequently because the bloodstream transports cancer cells from primary cancers elsewhere in the body to the lungs.

Lung Cancer (Bronchogenic Carcinoma)

Lung cancer is the number-one cancer killer among men and women in the United States (American Cancer Society, 1999; Landis, Murray, Bolder, & Wingo, 1998). For men, the incidence of lung cancer has remained relatively constant, but in women it continues to rise. In approximately 70% of lung cancer patients, the disease has spread to regional lymphatics and other sites by the time of diagnosis (Reardon & Theodore, 1997). As a result, the long-term survival rate for lung cancer patients is low. Evidence indicates that carcinoma tends to arise at sites of previous scarring (TB, fibrosis) in the lung. More than 85% of lung cancers are caused by the inhalation of carcinogenic chemicals, most commonly cigarette smoke (Reardon & Theodore, 1997).

Pathophysiology

Lung cancers arise from a single transformed epithelial cell in the tracheobronchial airways. A carcinogen (cigarette smoke, radon gas, other occupational and environmental agents) binds to a cell's DNA and damages it. This damage results in cellular changes, abnormal cell growth, and eventually a malignant cell. As the damaged DNA is passed on to daughter cells, the DNA undergoes further changes and becomes unstable. With the accumulation of genetic changes, the pulmonary epithelium undergoes malignant transformation from normal epithelium to eventual invasive carcinoma (Kelley, 1997).

Squamous cell carcinoma arises from the bronchial epithelium and is more centrally located (Reardon & Theodore, 1997). Adenocarcinoma presents as peripheral masses or nodules and often metastasizes. Large cell carcinoma is a fast-growing tumor that tends to arise peripherally. Bronchioalveolar cell cancer arises from the terminal bronchus and alveoli and is usually slow-growing.

Classification and Staging

Non–small cell carcinoma represents 70% to 75% of tumors; small cell carcinoma represents 15% to 20% of tumors. For non-small cell carcinoma, the cell types include squamous cell or epidermoid carcinoma (25% to 40%), large cell carcinoma (10% to 15%), and adenocarcinoma, including bronchioalveolar carcinoma (25% to 45%). Most small cell carcinomas arise in the major bronchi and spread by infiltration along the bronchial wall. Early invasion of lymphatics and blood vessels is usual, and metastases have often occurred by the time of presentation (Reardon & Theodore, 1997).

In addition to cell type, lung cancers also are staged. The stage of the tumor refers to the size of the tumor, whether lymph nodes are involved, and whether the cancer has spread (Mountain, 1997). Tissue biopsy, lymph node biopsy, or mediastinoscopy determines initial staging. Staging helps determine whether the tumor should be removed. For further information on staging, see Chapter 15.

Risk Factors

Various factors have been associated with the development of lung cancer, including tobacco smoke, second-hand (passive) smoke, environmental and occupational exposures, genetics, and dietary deficits. Other factors that have been associated with lung cancer include genetic predisposition and other underlying respiratory diseases, such as COPD and TB.

TOBACCO SMOKE

Tobacco use is responsible for more than one of every six deaths in the United States from pulmonary and cardiovascular diseases. Smoking is the most important single preventable cause of death and disease in this country. More than 85% of lung cancers are attributable to inhalation of carcinogenic chemicals, such as cigarette smoke (Reardon & Theodore, 1997). Lung cancer is ten times more common in cigarette smokers than nonsmokers. Risk is determined by the pack-year history (number of packs of cigarettes used each day, multiplied by the number of years smoked). In addition, the younger a person is when he or she starts smoking, the greater the risk of developing lung cancer. Another factor is the type of cigarettes smoked (tar content, filtered versus nonfiltered). The risk of lung cancer decreases as the duration of smoking cessation increases.

SECOND-HAND SMOKE

Passive smoking has been identified as a possible cause of lung cancer in nonsmokers. In other words, people who are involuntarily exposed to tobacco smoke in a closed environment (home, car, building) are at increased risk for developing lung cancer as compared to unexposed nonsmokers. Local and federal agencies have passed numerous laws to restrict smoking in public places, such as restaurants, public buildings, and airplanes.

NURSING RESEARCH

Smoking After Lung Cancer Diagnosis

Sarna, L. (1995). Smoking behaviors of women after diagnosis with lung cancer. *Image: Journal of Nursing Scholarship, 27*(1), 35–41.

Purpose

As part of a larger study, this study described the smoking behavior of women who were recently diagnosed with lung cancer or recurrence of lung cancer. It also explored relationships among smoking behavior, physical function, and symptom distress. Lastly, the subjects described their perception of the effect of their diagnosis on the smoking behaviors of others.

Study Sample and Design

The sample was recruited from a university medical center, private physician's offices, and health maintenance organizations. Subjects must have had a recent diagnosis of lung cancer or a recurrence of lung cancer.

Data were collected over a 2-year period, and subjects participated in audiotaped interviews and completed self-report questionnaires on symptom distress and functional status. Content analysis was used to classify responses of women obtained during interviews. Convenience sampling was used, and 65 women agreed to participate in the study. The mean age was 62 ± 11 years. A total of 8% of the sample were current smokers and 78% were former smokers; 14% of the subjects had no smoking history.

Findings

Overall, the subjects had minimal compromise in functional ability, and there were no statistical differences in symptom distress or physical ability when analyzed by smoking history. The diagnosis of lung cancer had an impact on smoking behavior of family members. Twenty-six percent of subjects' family or friends changed or quit smoking. More than half of the subjects who were former smokers and quit at diagnosis had family members who continued to smoke. The subjects' responses to family members' smoking behavior were primarily described in terms of distress and resignation. Some described the positive effect their diagnosis of cancer had on the behavior of others.

Nursing Implications

Lung cancer in women is an area that has not received adequate attention. Although breast cancer is the most frequent type of cancer diagnosed in women, lung cancer is the leading cause of cancer-related death in women. This study has important implications for nursing. First, nurses must continue to focus on patient education and community education regarding the dangers of smoking. Second, this study provides insight into women diagnosed with lung cancer and some of the challenges they face. Although there were no statistical differences in symptom distress and functional status when analyzed by smoking status (current, ex-smoker, nonsmoker), this could be due to the small group sizes. Women with lung cancer have unique needs that must be further studied. This study highlights the importance of nursing in smoking cessation efforts. Nurses must always make smoking history an important part of the nursing assessment and initiate patient teaching.

ENVIRONMENTAL AND OCCUPATIONAL EXPOSURE

Various carcinogens have been identified in the atmosphere, including motor vehicle emissions and pollutants from refineries and manufacturing plants. Evidence suggests that the incidence of lung cancer is greater in urban areas as a result of the buildup of pollutants and motor vehicle emissions.

Radon is a colorless, odorless gas found in soil and rocks. For many years it has been associated with uranium mines, but it is now known to seep into homes through ground rock. High levels of radon have been associated with the development of lung cancer, especially when combined with cigarette smoking. Home owners are advised to have radon levels checked in their houses and to arrange for special venting if the levels are high.

Chronic exposure to industrial carcinogens, such as arsenic, asbestos, mustard gas, chromates, coke oven fumes, nickel, oil, and radiation, has been associated with the development of lung cancer. Laws have been passed to control exposure to such elements in the workplace.

GENETICS

Some familial predisposition to lung cancer seems apparent, because the incidence of lung cancer in close relatives of patients with lung cancer appears to be two to three times that of the general population regardless of smoking status (Bordow & Moser, 1996; Kelley, 1997).

DIETARY FACTORS

Research has demonstrated that smokers who eat a diet low in fruits and vegetables, which are high in vitamin A, have an increased risk of developing lung cancer. It is postulated that the increased risk is related to eating less beta-carotene or other compounds in fruits and vegetables rather than less vitamin A itself.

Clinical Manifestations

Often, lung cancer develops insidiously and is asymptomatic until late in its course. The signs and symptoms depend on the location and size of the tumor, the degree of obstruction, and the existence of metastases to regional or distant sites.

The most frequent symptom of lung cancer is cough or change in a chronic cough. People frequently ignore this symptom and attribute it to smoking or a respiratory infection. The cough starts as a dry, persistent cough, without sputum production. When obstruction of airways occurs, the cough may become productive due to infection.

Nursing Alert *A cough that changes in character should arouse suspicion of lung cancer.*

Wheezing is noted (occurs when a bronchus becomes partially obstructed by the tumor) in about 20% of patients with lung cancer. Patients also may report dyspnea. Hemoptysis or blood-tinged sputum may be expectorated. In some patients, a recurring fever occurs as an early symptom in response to a persisting infection in an area of pneumonitis distal to the tumor. In fact, cancer of the lung should be suspected in people with repeated unresolved upper respiratory tract infections. Chest or shoulder pain may indicate chest wall or pleural involvement by a tumor. Pain also is a late manifestation and may be related to bone metastasis.

If the tumor spreads to adjacent structures and regional lymph nodes, the patient may present with chest pain and tightness, hoarseness (involving the recurrent laryngeal nerve), dysphagia, head and neck edema, and symptoms of pleural or pericardial effusion. The most common sites of metastases are lymph nodes, bone, brain, contralateral lung, adrenal glands, and liver. Nonspecific symptoms of weakness, anorexia, and weight loss also may be diagnostic.

Assessment and Diagnostic Findings

If pulmonary symptoms occur in a heavy smoker, cancer of the lung is suspected. A chest x-ray is performed to search for pulmonary density, a solitary peripheral nodule (coin lesion), atelectasis, and infection. CT scans of the chest are used to identify small nodules not visualized on the chest x-ray and also to examine serially areas of the thoracic cage not clearly visible on the chest x-ray.

Sputum cytology may be used to make a diagnosis of lung cancer; however, fiberoptic bronchoscopy is more commonly used and provides a detailed study of the tracheobronchial tree and allows for brushings, washings, and biopsies of suspicious areas. For peripheral lesions not amenable to brochoscopic biopsy, a transthoracic **fine-needle aspiration** may be performed under CT or fluoroscopic guidance to aspirate cells from a suspicious area. In some circumstances, an endoscopy with an esophageal ultrasound may be used to obtain a transesophageal biopsy of subcarinal lymph nodes that are not easily accessible by other means.

A variety of scans may be used to assess for metastasis of the cancer. These may include bone scans, abdominal scans, and liver ultrasound or scans. CT of the brain, magnetic resonance imaging, and other neurologic diagnostic procedures are used to detect central nervous system metastases. Mediastinoscopy may be used to determine whether the tumor has spread to the hilar lymph nodes of the right lung, and a mediastinotomy gives some access to the hilar lymphatics of the left lung.

If surgery is a potential treatment, the patient is evaluated to determine whether the tumor is resectable and whether the physiologic impairment resulting from such surgery can be tolerated. Pulmonary function tests, arterial blood gas analysis, ventilation–perfusion scans, and exercise testing may all be used as part of the preoperative assessment.

Medical Management

The objective of management is to provide a cure, if possible. Treatment depends on the cell type, the stage of the disease, and the physiologic status (particularly cardiac and pulmonary status) of the patient. In general, treatment may involve surgery, radiation therapy, and chemotherapy—separately or in combination. Immunotherapy, which has met with minimal success in the past, is still investigational. Newer and more specific therapies to modulate the immune system (gene therapy, therapy with defined tumor antigens) are under study and show promise in treating lung cancer.

SURGICAL MANAGEMENT

Surgical resection is the preferred method of treating patients with localized tumors, no evidence of metastatic spread, and adequate cardiopulmonary function. If the patient's cardiovascular status, pulmonary function, and functional status are satisfactory, surgery is generally well tolerated. Coronary artery disease, pulmonary insufficiency, and other comorbidities, however, may contraindicate surgical intervention. The cure rate of surgical resection depends on the type and stage of the cancer. Surgery is primarily used for non–small cell carcinomas because small cell cancer of the lung grows rapidly and metastasizes early and extensively. Unfortunately, in many patients with bronchogenic cancer, the lesion is inoperable at the time of diagnosis.

Several different types of lung resections may be performed (Chart 21-4). The most common surgical procedure for a small, apparently curable tumor of the lung is lobectomy (removal of a lobe of the lung). In some cases, an entire lung may be removed (pneumonectomy).

RADIATION THERAPY

Radiation therapy may cure a small percentage of patients. It is useful in controlling neoplasms that cannot be surgically resected but are responsive to radiation (small cell and epidermoid tumors are usually radiation-sensitive). Radiation also may be used to reduce the size of a tumor to make an inoperable tumor operable or to relieve the pressure of the tumor on vital structures. It can control symptoms of spinal cord metastasis and superior vena caval compression. Also, prophylactic brain irradiation is used in certain patients to treat microscopic metastases to the brain. Radiation may help relieve cough, chest pain, dyspnea, hemoptysis, and bone and liver pain. Relief of symptoms may last from a few weeks to many months and is important in improving the quality of the remaining period of life.

Radiation therapy usually is toxic to normal tissue within the radiation field, and this may lead to complications such as esophagitis, pneumonitis, and radiation lung fibrosis. These may impair ventilatory and diffusion capacity and significantly reduce pulmonary reserve. The patient's nutritional status, psychological outlook, fatigue level, and signs of anemia and infection are monitored throughout the treatment. See Chapter 15 for management of the patient receiving radiation therapy.

CHEMOTHERAPY

Chemotherapy is used to alter tumor growth patterns, to treat patients with distant metastases or small cell cancer of the lung, and to supplement surgery or radiation therapy. Combinations of two or more medications may be more beneficial than single-dose regimens. A large number of medications act against lung cancer. A variety of chemotherapeutic agents are used, including alkylating agents (ifosfamide), platinum analogues (cisplatin and carboplatin), taxanes (paclitaxel, docetaxel), mitomycin C, vinca alkaloids (vinblastine and vindesine), doxorubicin, gemcitabine, navelbine, irinotecan (CPT-11), and etoposide (VP-16). The choice of agent depends on the growth of the tumor cell and the specific phase of the cell cycle that the medication affects. These agents are toxic and have a narrow margin of safety.

CHART 21•4 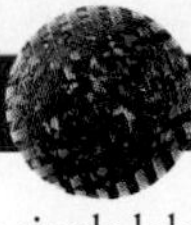 **Types of Lung Resections**

- Lobectomy: a single lobe of lung is removed
- Bilobectomy: two lobes of the lung are removed
- Sleeve resection: cancerous lobe(s) is removed and a segment of the main bronchus is resected
- Pneumonectomy: removal of entire lung
- Segmentectomy: a segment of the lung is removed
- Wedge resection: removal of a small, pie-shaped area of the segment
- Chest wall resection with removal of cancerous lung tissue: for cancers that have invaded the chest wall

Chemotherapy may provide relief, especially of pain, but it does not usually cure the disease, nor does it prolong life to any great degree. Chemotherapy is also accompanied by side effects. It is valuable in reducing pressure symptoms of lung cancer and in treating brain, spinal cord, and pericardial metastasis. See Chapter 15 for a discussion of chemotherapy for the patient with cancer.

PALLIATIVE THERAPY

Palliative therapy may include radiation therapy to shrink the tumor to provide pain relief, a variety of bronchoscopic interventions to open a narrowed bronchus or airway, and pain management and other comfort measures. Evaluation and referral for hospice care are important in planning for comfortable and dignified end-of-life care for the patient and family.

Treatment-Related Complications

A variety of complications may occur as a result of lung cancer treatments. Radiation therapy may result in diminished cardiopulmonary function and other complications, such as pulmonary fibrosis, pericarditis, myelitis, and cor pulmonale. Chemotherapy, particularly in combination with radiation therapy, can cause pneumonitis. Pulmonary toxicity is a potential side effect of chemotherapy. Surgical resection may result in respiratory failure, particularly when the cardiopulmonary system is compromised before surgery. Surgical complications and prolonged mechanical ventilation are potential outcomes.

Nursing Management

Nursing care of the patient with lung cancer is similar to that of other patients with cancer (see Chap. 15) and addresses the physiologic and psychological needs of the patient. The physiologic problems are primarily due to the respiratory manifestations of the disease. Nursing care includes strategies to ensure relief of pain and discomfort and to prevent complications.

MANAGING SYMPTOMS

The nurse instructs the patient and family about the potential side effects of the specific treatment and strategies to manage them. Strategies for managing such symptoms as dyspnea, fatigue, nausea and vomiting, and anorexia will assist the patient and family to cope with the therapeutic measures.

RELIEVING BREATHING PROBLEMS

Airway clearance techniques are key to maintaining airway patency through the removal of excess secretions. This may be accomplished through deep-breathing exercises, chest physiotherapy, directed cough, suctioning, and in some instances bronchoscopy. Bronchodilator medications may be prescribed to promote bronchial dilation. As the tumor enlarges or spreads, it may compress a bronchus or involve a large area of lung tissue, resulting in an impaired breathing pattern and poor gas exchange. At some stage of the disease, supplemental oxygen will probably be necessary.

Nursing measures focus on decreasing dyspnea by encouraging the patient to assume positions that promote lung expansion, breathing exercises for lung expansion and relaxation, and educating the patient on energy conservation and airway clearance techniques. Many of the techniques used in pulmonary rehabilitation can be applied to the lung cancer patient. Depending on the severity of disease and the patient's wishes, a referral to a pulmonary rehabilitation program may be helpful in managing respiratory symptoms.

REDUCING FATIGUE

Fatigue is a devastating symptom that affects quality of life in the cancer patient. It is commonly experienced by the lung cancer patient and may be related to the disease itself, the cancer treatment and complications (eg, anemia), sleep disturbances, pain and discomfort, hypoxemia, poor nutrition, or the psychological ramifications of the disease (eg, anxiety, depression) (Nail, 1998). The nurse is pivotal in thoroughly assessing the patient's level of fatigue, identifying potentially treatable causes, and validating with the patient that fatigue is indeed an important symptom. Educating the patient in energy conservation techniques or referring the patient to a physical therapy, occupational therapy, or pulmonary rehabilitation program may be helpful. In addition, guided exercise has been recently identified as a potential intervention for treating fatigue in cancer patients. This is an important area for research because few studies have been conducted, and only in select populations of cancer patients (Nail, 1998).

PROVIDING PSYCHOLOGICAL SUPPORT

Another important part of the nursing care of the lung cancer patient is psychological support and identification of potential resources for the patient and family. Often, the nurse must help the patient and family deal with the poor prognosis and relatively rapid progression of this disease. The nurse must help the patient and family with informed decision making regarding the possible treatment options, methods to maintain the patient's quality of life during the course of this disease, and end-of-life treatment options.

Tumors of the Mediastinum

Tumors of the mediastinum include neurogenic tumors, tumors of the thymus, lymphomas, germ cell, cysts, and mesenchymal tumors. These tumors may be malignant or benign.

Clinical Manifestations

Nearly all the symptoms of mediastinal tumors result from the pressure of the mass against important intrathoracic organs. Symptoms may include cough, wheezing, dyspnea, anterior chest or neck pain, bulging of the chest wall, heart palpitations, angina, other circulatory disturbances, central cyanosis, superior vena caval syndromes (ie, swelling of the face, neck, and upper extremities), marked distention of the veins of the neck and the chest wall (evidence of the obstruction of large veins of the mediastinum by extravascular compression or intravascular invasion), and dysphagia and weight loss from pressure or invasion into the esophagus.

Assessment and Diagnostic Findings

Chest x-rays are the major method used to diagnose mediastinal tumors and cysts. Lateral and oblique x-rays can localize the tumor. CT scans are the gold standard for assessment of the mediastinum and surrounding structures. Magnetic resonance imaging may be used in some circumstances. The biopsy of an enlarged lymph node removed from above the clavicle (supraclavicular) or one removed during mediastinoscopy may provide the diagnosis. Blood studies are of value in excluding other causes of lymph node enlargement, such as leukemia.

Medical Management

If the tumor is malignant and has infiltrated surrounding tissue, radiation therapy and chemotherapy are the therapeutic modalities used when complete surgical removal (discussed below) is not feasible.

SURGICAL MANAGEMENT

Many mediastinal tumors are benign and operable. The location of the tumor (anterior, visceral, or posterior compartments) in the mediastinum dictates the type of incision. The common incision used is a median sternotomy; however, a thoracotomy may be used depending on the location of the tumor. Additional approaches may include a bilateral anterior thoracotomy (clamshell incision) or video-assisted thoracoscopic surgery. The care is the same as for any patient undergoing thoracic surgery. The major complications include hemorrhage, injury to the phrenic or recurrent laryngeal nerve, and infection.

CHEST TRAUMA

Approximately 50% of all trauma victims have some type of chest or thoracic trauma. In fact, chest trauma accounts for 20% to 25% of all trauma-related deaths in the United States and may be a contributing factor in an additional 25% of deaths (Johnson, Kearney, & Smith, 1995).

Chest trauma is classified as either blunt or penetrating. Blunt chest trauma results from sudden compression or positive pressure inflicted to the chest wall. Automobile crashes, falls, and bicycle handlebars are the most common causes of blunt chest trauma. Penetrating trauma occurs when a foreign object penetrates the chest wall. The most common causes of penetrating chest trauma include gunshot wounds and stabbing.

Blunt Trauma

Although blunt chest trauma is more common, it is often difficult to identify the extent of the damage because the symptoms may be generalized and vague. In addition, patients may not seek immediate medical attention, which may complicate the problem.

Pathophysiology

Injuries to the chest are often life-threatening and result in one or more of the following pathologic mechanisms:

- Hypoxemia from disruption in the airway; injury to the lung parenchyma, rib cage, and respiratory musculature; massive hemorrhage; collapsed lung; and pneumothorax
- Hypovolemia from massive fluid loss from the great vessels, cardiac rupture, or hemothorax
- Cardiac failure from cardiac tamponade, cardiac contusion, or increased intrathoracic pressure

These mechanisms frequently result in impaired ventilation and perfusion leading to ARF, hypovolemic shock, and death.

Assessment and Diagnostic Findings

Time is critical in treating chest trauma. Therefore, it is essential to assess the patient immediately to determine the following:

- When the injury occurred
- Mechanism of injury
- Level of responsiveness
- Specific injuries
- Estimated blood loss
- Recent drug or alcohol use
- Prehospital treatment

The physical examination includes inspection of the airway, thorax, neck veins, and breathing difficulty. Specifics include assessing the rate and depth of breathing for abnormalities, such as stridor, cyanosis, nasal flaring, use of accessory muscles, drooling, and overt trauma to the face, mouth, or neck. The chest should be assessed for symmetric movement, symmetry of breath sounds, open chest wounds, entrance or exit wounds, impaled objects, tracheal shift, distended neck veins, subcutaneous emphysema, and paradoxical chest wall motion. In addition, the chest wall should be assessed for bruising, petechiae, lacerations, and burns. The vital signs and skin color are assessed for signs of shock. The thorax is palpated for tenderness and crepitus; the position of the trachea is also assessed.

The initial diagnostic workup includes a chest x-ray, complete blood count, clotting studies, type and cross-match, electrolytes, oxygen saturation, arterial blood gas analysis, and ECG. A CT scan may also be obtained. The patient is completely undressed to avoid missing additional injuries that can complicate care. Many patients with injuries involving the chest have associated head and abdominal injuries that require attention. Ongoing assessment is essential to monitor the patient's response to treatment and to detect early signs of a deteriorating condition.

Medical Management

The goals of treatment are to evaluate the patient's condition and to initiate aggressive resuscitation. An airway is immediately established with oxygen support and, in some cases, intubation and ventilatory support. Reestablishing fluid volume and negative intrapleural pressure and draining intrapleural fluid and blood are essential.

The potential for massive blood loss and exsanguination with blunt or penetrating chest injuries is high because of injury to the great blood vessels. Many patients die at the scene or are in shock by the time help arrives. Agitation and irrational and combative behavior are signs of decreased oxygen delivery to the cerebral cortex. Strategies to restore and maintain cardiopulmonary function include ensuring an adequate airway and ventilation, stabilizing and reestablishing chest wall integrity, occluding any opening into the chest (open pneumothorax), and draining or removing any air or fluid from the thorax to relieve pneumothorax or hemothorax or cardiac tamponade. Hypovolemia and low cardiac output must be corrected. Many of these treatment efforts, along with the control of hemorrhage, are usually carried out simultaneously at the scene of the injury or in the emergency department. Depending on the ability to control the hemorrhage in the emergency department, the patient may be taken immediately to the operating room. Principles of management are essentially those pertaining to care of the postoperative thoracic patient (see Chap. 22).

Rib Fractures

Rib fractures are the most common type of chest trauma, occurring in more than 60% of patients admitted with blunt chest injury. Most rib fractures are benign and are treated conservatively. Fractures of the first three ribs are rare but can result in a high mortality rate because they are associated with laceration of the subclavian artery or vein. The fifth through ninth ribs are the most common sites of fractures. Fractures of the lower ribs are associated with injury to the spleen and liver, which may be lacerated by fragmented sections of the rib.

CLINICAL MANIFESTATIONS

If conscious, the patient has severe pain, point tenderness, and muscle spasm over the area of the fracture, which is aggravated by coughing, deep breathing, and movement. The area around the fracture may be bruised. To reduce the pain, the patient splints the chest by breathing in a shallow manner and avoids sighs, deep breaths, coughing, and movement. This reluctance to move or breathe deeply results in diminished ventilation, collapse of unaerated alveoli (atelectasis), pneumonitis, and hypoxemia. Respiratory insufficiency and failure can be the outcomes of such a cycle.

ASSESSMENT AND DIAGNOSTIC FINDINGS

A crackling, grating sound in the thorax (subcutaneous crepitus) may be detected with auscultation. The diagnostic workup may include a chest x-ray, rib films, ECG, continuous pulse oximetry, and arterial blood gas analysis.

MEDICAL MANAGEMENT

The goals of treatment are to control pain and to detect and treat the injury. Sedation is used to relieve pain and to allow deep breathing and coughing. Care must be taken to avoid oversedation and suppression of the respiratory drive. Alternative strategies to relieve pain include an intercostal nerve block and ice over the fracture site; a chest binder may decrease pain on movement. Usually the pain abates in 5 to 7 days, and discomfort can be controlled with epidural analgesia, patient-controlled analgesia, or nonopioid analgesia. Most rib fractures heal in 3 to 6 weeks. The patient is monitored closely for signs and symptoms of associated injuries.

Flail Chest

Flail chest is frequently a complication of blunt chest trauma from a steering wheel injury. It occurs when two or more adjacent ribs (multiple contiguous ribs) are fractured at two or more sites, resulting in free-floating rib segments. As a result, the chest wall loses stability and there is subsequent respiratory impairment and usually severe respiratory distress.

PATHOPHYSIOLOGY

During inspiration, as the chest expands, the detached part of the rib segment (flail segment) moves in a paradoxical manner (pendalluft movement) in that it is pulled inward during inspiration, reducing the amount of air that can be drawn into the lungs. On expiration, because the intrathoracic pressure exceeds atmospheric pressure, the flail segment bulges outward, impairing the patient's ability to exhale. The mediastinum then shifts back to the affected side (Fig. 21-11). This paradoxical action results in increased dead space, a reduction in alveolar ventilation, and decreased compliance. Retained airway secretions and atelectasis frequently accompany flail chest. The patient has hypoxemia, and if gas exchange is greatly compromised, a respiratory acidosis develops as a result of CO_2 retention. Hypotension, inadequate tissue perfusion, and metabolic acidosis often follow as the paradoxical motion of the mediastinum decreases cardiac output.

MEDICAL MANAGEMENT

Management includes providing ventilatory support, clearing secretions from the lungs, and controlling pain. The specific management depends on the degree of respiratory dysfunction. If only a small segment of the chest is involved, the objectives are to clear the airway through positioning, coughing, deep breathing, and suctioning to aid in the expansion of the lung, and to relieve pain by intercostal nerve blocks, high thoracic epidural blocks, or cautious use of intravenous opioids.

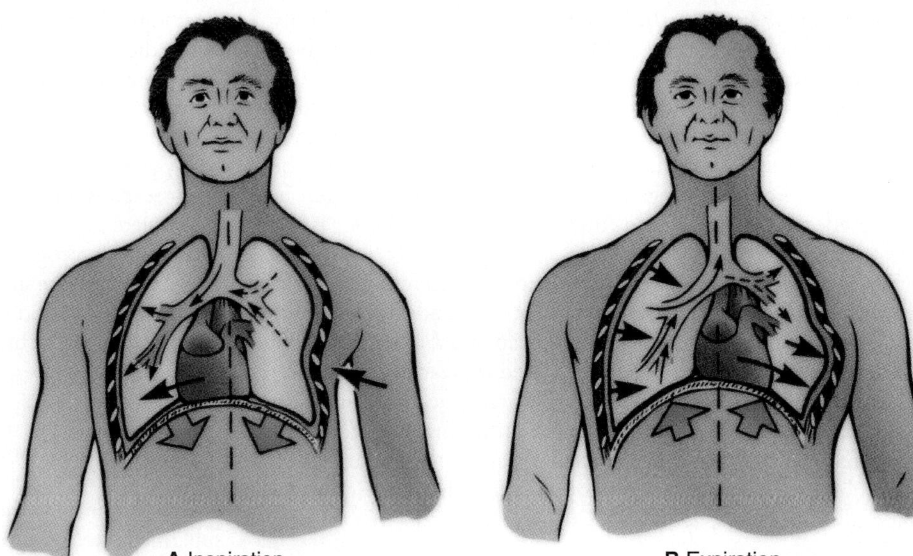

FIGURE 21•11 Flail chest is caused by a free-floating segment of rib cage resulting from multiple rib fractures. (**A**) Paradoxical movement on inspiration occurs when the flail rib segment is sucked inward and the mediastinal structures shift to the unaffected side. The amount of air drawn into the affected lung is reduced. (**B**) On expiration, the flail segment bulges outward and the mediastinal structures shift back to the affected side.

For mild to moderate flail chest injuries, the underlying pulmonary contusion is treated by monitoring fluid intake and appropriate fluid replacement, while relieving chest pain. Pulmonary physiotherapy focusing on lung volume expansion and secretion management techniques are performed. The patient is closely monitored for further respiratory compromise.

When a severe flail chest injury is encountered, endotracheal intubation and mechanical ventilation with a volume-cycled ventilator and PEEP are used to splint the chest wall (internal pneumatic stabilization) and to correct abnormalities in gas exchange. This helps to treat the underlying pulmonary contusion, serves to stabilize the thoracic cage to allow the fractures to heal, and improves alveolar ventilation and intrathoracic volume by decreasing the work of breathing. This treatment modality requires endotracheal intubation and ventilator support. Differing modes of ventilation are used depending on the patient's underlying disease and specific needs.

Regardless of the type of treatment, the patient is carefully monitored by serial chest x-rays, arterial blood gas analysis, pulse oximetry, and bedside pulmonary function monitoring. Pain management is key to successful treatment. Patient-controlled analgesia, intercostal nerve blocks, epidural analgesia, and intrapleural administration of opioids may be used to control thoracic pain.

Pulmonary Contusion

Pulmonary contusion is damage to the lung tissues resulting in hemorrhage and localized edema. It is associated with chest trauma when there is rapid compression and decompression to the chest wall (ie, blunt trauma). It may not be evident initially on examination but will develop in the post-traumatic period.

PATHOPHYSIOLOGY

The primary pathologic defect is an abnormal accumulation of fluid in the interstitial and intra-alveolar spaces. It is thought that injury to the lung parenchyma and its capillary network results in a leakage of serum protein and plasma. The leaking serum protein exerts an osmotic pressure that enhances loss of fluid from the capillaries. Blood, edema, and cellular debris (from cellular response to injury) enter the lung and accumulate in the bronchioles and alveolar surface, where they interfere with gas exchange. An increase in pulmonary vascular resistance and pulmonary artery pressure occurs. The patient has hypoxemia and carbon dioxide retention. Occasionally, a contused lung occurs on the other side of the point of body impact; this is called a contrecoup contusion.

CLINICAL MANIFESTATIONS

Pulmonary contusion may be mild, moderate, or severe. The clinical manifestations vary from tachypnea, tachycardia, pleuritic chest pain, hypoxemia, and blood-tinged secretions to more severe tachypnea, tachycardia, crackles, frank bleeding, severe hypoxemia, and respiratory acidosis. Changes in sensorium, including increased agitation or combative irrational behavior, may be signs of hypoxemia.

In addition, the patient with moderate pulmonary contusion has a large amount of mucus, serum, and frank blood in the tracheobronchial tree; the patient often has a constant cough but cannot clear the secretions. A patient with severe pulmonary contusion has the signs and symptoms of ARDS; signs and symptoms may include central cyanosis, agitation, combativeness, and productive cough with frothy, bloody secretions.

ASSESSMENT AND DIAGNOSTIC FINDINGS

The efficiency of gas exchange is determined by pulse oximetry and arterial blood gas measurements. Pulse oximetry is also used to measure oxygen saturation continuously. The chest x-ray may show pulmonary infiltration. The initial chest x-ray may show no changes; in fact, changes may not appear for 1 or 2 days after the injury.

MEDICAL MANAGEMENT

The goals of treatment include maintaining the airway, providing adequate oxygenation, and controlling pain. In mild pulmonary contusion, adequate hydration via intravenous fluids and oral intake is important to mobilize secretions. However, fluid intake must be closely monitored to avoid hypervolemia. Volume expansion techniques, postural drainage, physiotherapy including coughing, and endotracheal suctioning are used to remove the secretions. Pain is managed by intercostal nerve blocks or by opioids via patient-controlled analgesia or other methods. Usually, antimicrobial therapy is administered because the damaged lung is susceptible to infection. Supplemental oxygen is usually given by mask or cannula for 24 to 36 hours.

The patient with moderate pulmonary contusion may require bronchoscopy to remove secretions; intubation and mechanical ventilation with PEEP may also be necessary to maintain the pressure and keep the lungs inflated. Diuretics may be given to reduce edema. A nasogastric tube is inserted to relieve gastrointestinal distention.

The patient with severe contusion may develop respiratory failure and may require aggressive treatment with endotracheal intubation and ventilatory support, diuretics, and fluid restriction. Colloids and crystalloid solutions may be used to treat hypovolemia.

Antimicrobial medications may be prescribed for the treatment of pulmonary infection. This is a common complication of pulmonary contusion (especially pneumonia in the contused segment), because the extravasation of fluid and blood into the alveolar and interstitial spaces serves as an excellent culture medium.

Penetrating Trauma: Gunshot and Stab Wounds

Gunshot and stab wounds are the most common types of penetrating chest trauma. They are classified according to their velocity. Stab wounds are generally considered of low velocity because the weapon destroys a small area around the wound. Knives and switchblades cause most stab wounds. The appearance of the external wound may be very deceptive, because pneumothorax, hemothorax, lung contusion, and cardiac tamponade, along with severe and continuing hemorrhage, can occur from any small wound, even one caused by a small-diameter instrument such as an ice pick.

Gunshot wounds to the chest may be classified as of low, medium, or high velocity. The factors that determine the velocity and resulting extent of damage include the distance from which the gun was fired, the caliber of the gun, and construction and size of the bullet. A gunshot wound can produce a variety of pathophysiologic changes. A bullet can cause damage at the site of penetration and along its pathway. It also may ricochet off bony structures and damage the chest organs and great vessels. If the diaphragm is involved in either a gunshot wound or a stab wound, injury to the chest cavity must be considered.

Medical Management

The objective of immediate management is to restore and maintain cardiopulmonary function. After an adequate airway is ensured and ventilation is established, the patient is examined for shock and intrathoracic and intra-abdominal injuries. The patient is undressed completely so that additional injuries will not be missed. There is a high risk for associated intra-abdominal injuries with stab wounds below the level of the fifth anterior intercostal space. Death can result from exsanguinating hemorrhage or intra-abdominal sepsis.

After the status of the peripheral pulses is assessed, a large-bore intravenous line is inserted. The diagnostic workup includes a chest x-ray, chemistry profile, arterial blood gas analysis, pulse oximetry, and ECG. Blood typing and cross-matching are done in case blood transfusion is required. An indwelling catheter is inserted to monitor urinary output. A nasogastric tube is inserted to prevent aspiration, minimize leakage of abdominal contents, and decompress the gastrointestinal tract.

Shock is treated simultaneously with colloid solutions, crystalloids, or blood, as indicated by the patient's condition. Chest x-rays are obtained, and other diagnostic procedures are carried out as dictated by the needs of the patient (eg, CT scans of chest or abdomen, flat plate of the abdomen, abdominal tap to check for bleeding).

A chest tube is inserted into the pleural space in most patients with penetrating wounds of the chest to achieve rapid and continuing reexpansion of the lungs. The chest tube frequently results in a complete evacuation of the blood and air. The chest tube also allows early recognition of continuing intrathoracic bleeding, which would make surgical exploration necessary. If the patient has a penetrating wound of the heart and great vessels, the esophagus, or the tracheobronchial tree, surgical intervention is required.

Pneumothorax

Pneumothorax occurs when the parietal or visceral pleura is breached and the pleural space is exposed to positive atmospheric pressure. Normally the pressure in the pleural space is negative or subatmospheric compared to atmospheric pressure; this negative pressure is required to maintain lung inflation. When either pleura is breached, air enters the pleural space, and the lung or a portion of it collapses. Types of pneumothorax include simple, traumatic, and tension pneumothorax.

Simple Pneumothorax

A simple, or spontaneous, pneumothorax occurs when air enters the pleural space through either a breach of the parietal or visceral pleura. Most commonly this occurs as air enters the pleural space through the rupture of a bleb or a bronchopleural fistula. A spontaneous pneumothorax may occur in an apparently healthy person in the absence of trauma due to rupture of an air-filled bleb, or blister, on the surface of the lung, allowing air from the airways to enter the pleural cavity. It may be associated with diffuse interstitial lung disease and severe emphysema.

Traumatic Pneumothorax

Traumatic pneumothorax occurs when air escapes from a laceration in the lung itself and enters the pleural space or enters the pleural space through a wound in the chest wall. It can occur with blunt trauma (eg, rib fractures) or penetrating chest trauma. It may also occur from abdominal trauma (eg, stab wounds or gunshot wounds to the abdomen) and from diaphragmatic tears. Pneumothorax may occur with invasive thoracic procedures (ie, thoracentesis, transbronchial lung biopsy, insertion of a subclavian line) in which the pleura is inadvertently punctured, or with barotrauma from mechanical ventilation.

Traumatic pneumothorax resulting from major injury to the chest is often accompanied by hemothorax (collection of blood in the pleural space resulting from torn intercostal vessels, lacerations of the great vessels, and lacerations of the lungs). Often both blood and air are found in the chest cavity (hemopneumothorax) after major trauma. Chest surgery can cause what is classified as a traumatic pneumothorax as a result of the entry into the pleural space and the accumulation of air and fluid in the pleural space.

Open pneumothorax is one form of traumatic pneumothorax. It occurs when a wound in the chest wall is large enough to allow air to pass freely in and out of the thoracic cavity with each attempted respiration. Because the rush of air through the hole in the chest wall produces a sucking sound, such injuries are termed sucking chest wounds. In such patients, not only does the lung collapse, but the structures of the mediastinum (heart and great vessels) also shift toward the uninjured side with each inspiration and in the opposite direction with expiration. This is termed mediastinal flutter or swing, and it produces serious circulatory problems.

Clinical Manifestations

The signs and symptoms associated with pneumothorax depend on its size and cause. Pain is usually sudden and may be pleuritic. The patient may have only minimal respiratory distress with slight chest discomfort and tachypnea with a small simple or uncomplicated pneumothorax. If the pneumothorax is large and the lung collapses totally, acute respiratory distress occurs. The patient is anxious, has dyspnea and air hunger, has increased use of the accessory muscles, and may develop central cyanosis from severe hypoxemia. Severe chest pain may occur, accompanied by tachypnea, decreased movement of the affected side of the thorax, a tympanic sound on percussion of the chest wall, and decreased or absent breath sounds and tactile fremitus on the affected side.

Medical Management

Medical management of pneumothorax depends on its cause and severity. The goal of treatment is to evacuate the air or blood from the pleural space. A small chest tube (28 F) is inserted near the second intercostal space; this space is used because it is the thinnest part of the chest wall, minimizes the danger of contacting the thoracic nerve, and leaves a less visible scar. If the patient also has a hemothorax, a large-diameter chest tube (32 F or greater) is inserted usually in the fourth or fifth intercostal space at the midaxillary line. The tube is directed posteriorly to drain the fluid and air. Once the chest tube or tubes are inserted and suction is applied (usually to 20 mm Hg suction), effective decompression of the pleural cavity (drainage of blood or air) occurs.

If an excessive amount of blood enters the chest tube in a relatively short period, an autotransfusion may be needed. This technique involves taking the patient's own blood that has been drained from the chest, filtering it, and then transfusing it back into the patient's vascular system.

Nursing Alert *Traumatic open pneumothorax calls for emergency interventions. Stopping the flow of air through the opening in the chest wall is a life-saving measure.*

In such an emergency, anything may be used that is large enough to fill the chest wound—a towel, a handkerchief, or the heel of the hand. If conscious, the patient is instructed to inhale and strain against a closed glottis. This action assists in reexpanding the lung and ejecting the air from the thorax. In the hospital, the opening is plugged by sealing it with gauze impregnated with petrolatum. A pressure dressing is applied. Usually, a chest tube connected to water-seal drainage is inserted to permit air and fluid to drain. Antibiotics usually are prescribed to combat infection from contamination.

The severity of open pneumothorax depends on the amount and rate of thoracic bleeding and the amount of air in the pleural space. The pleural cavity can be decompressed by needle aspiration (thoracentesis) or chest tube drainage of the blood or air. The lung is then able to reexpand and resume the function of gas exchange. As a rule of thumb, the chest wall is opened surgically (thoracotomy) when more than 1500 mL of blood is aspirated initially by thoracentesis (or is the initial chest tube output) or when chest tube output continues at greater than 200 mL/hour. The urgency with which the blood must be removed is determined by the respiratory compromise. An emergency thoracotomy may also be performed in the emergency department if there is suggested cardiovascular injury secondary to chest or penetrating trauma.

Tension Pneumothorax

A **tension pneumothorax** occurs when air is drawn into the pleural space from a lacerated lung or through a small hole in the chest wall. It may be a complication of other types of pneumothorax. In contrast to open pneumothorax, the air that enters the chest cavity with each inspiration is trapped; it cannot be expelled during expiration through the air passages or the hole in the chest wall. In effect, a one-way valve or ball valve mechanism occurs where air enters the pleural space but cannot escape. With each breath, tension (positive pressure) is built up within the affected pleural space. This causes the lung to collapse and the heart, the great vessels, and trachea to shift toward the unaffected side of the chest (mediastinal shift). Both respiration and circulatory function are compromised because of the increased intrathoracic pressure. The increased intrathoracic pressure decreases venous return to the heart, causing decreased cardiac output and impairment of peripheral circulation. In extreme cases, the pulse may be undetectable—this is known as pulseless electrical activity.

CLINICAL MANIFESTATIONS

The clinical picture is one of air hunger, agitation, increasing hypoxemia, central cyanosis, hypotension, tachycardia, and profuse diaphoresis. A comparison of open and tension pneumothorax is shown in Figure 21-12.

Nursing Alert *Relief of tension pneumothorax is considered an emergency measure.*

MEDICAL MANAGEMENT

If a tension pneumothorax is suspected, the patient should immediately be given a high concentration of supplemental oxygen to treat the hypoxemia, and a pulse oximeter should be placed to monitor oxygen saturation.

In an emergency situation, a tension pneumothorax can be decompressed or quickly converted to a simple pneumothorax by inserting a large-bore needle (14 G) at the second intercostal space, midclavicular line on the affected side. This relieves the pressure and vents the positive pressure to the external environment. A chest tube is then inserted and connected to suction to remove the remaining air and fluid, reestablish the negative pressure, and reexpand the lung. If the lung reexpands and air leakage from the lung parenchyma stops, further drainage may be unnecessary. If a prolonged air leak continues despite chest tube drainage to underwater seal, surgery may be necessary to close the leak.

Cardiac Tamponade

Cardiac tamponade is the compression of the heart as a result of fluid within the pericardial sac. It usually is caused by blunt or penetrating trauma to the chest. A penetrating wound of the heart is associated with a high mortality rate. Cardiac tamponade also may follow diagnostic cardiac catheterization, angiographic procedures, and pacemaker insertion, which can produce perforations of the heart and great vessels. Pericardial effusion with fluid compressing the heart also may develop from metastases to the pericardium from malignant tumors of the breast, lung, and mediastinum and may occur with lymphomas and leukemias, renal failure, TB, and high-dose radiation to the chest. Cardiac tamponade is discussed in detail in Chapter 27.

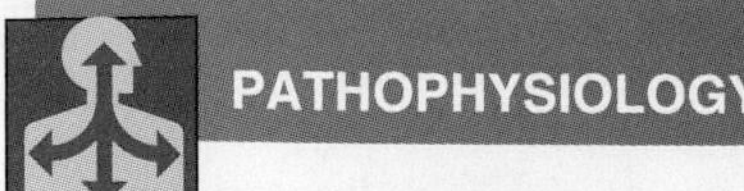

PATHOPHYSIOLOGY

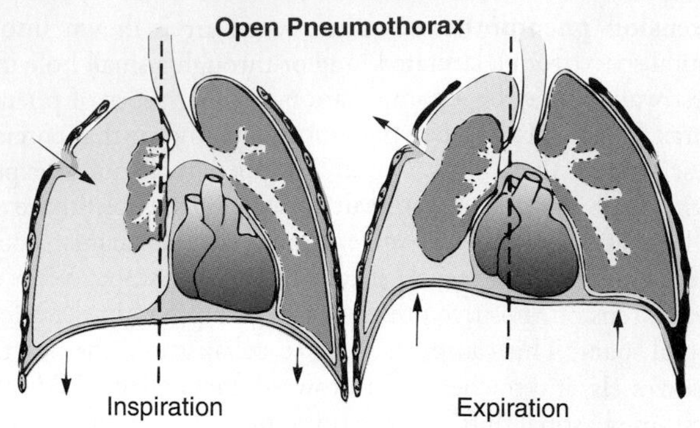

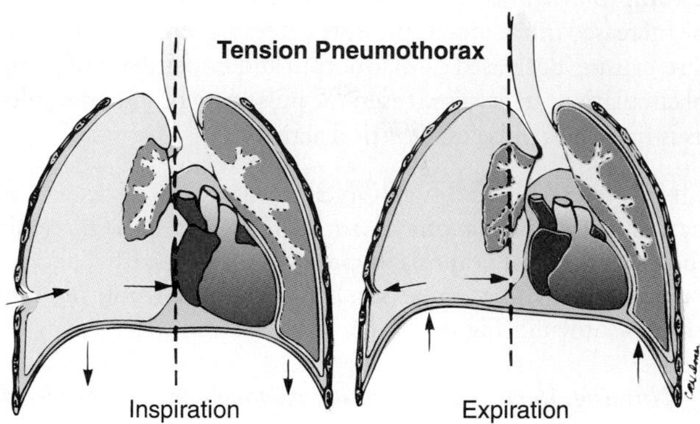

FIGURE 21•12 Open pneumothorax (*top*) and tension pneumothorax (*bottom*). In open pneumothorax, air enters the chest during inspiration and exits during expiration. A slight shift of the affected lung may occur because of a decrease in pressure as air moves out of the chest. In tension pneumothorax, air enters but cannot leave the chest. As the pressure increases, the heart and great vessels are compressed and the mediastinal structures are shifted toward the opposite side of the chest. The trachea is pushed from its normal midline position toward the opposite side of the chest, and the unaffected lung is compressed.

Subcutaneous Emphysema

No matter what kind of chest trauma the patient has, when the lung or the air passages are injured, air may enter the tissue planes and pass for some distance under the skin (eg, neck, chest). The tissues give a crackling sensation when palpated, and the subcutaneous air produces an alarming appearance as the face, neck, body, and scrotum become misshapen by subcutaneous air. Fortunately, subcutaneous emphysema is of itself not a serious complication. The subcutaneous air is spontaneously absorbed if the underlying air leak is treated or stops spontaneously. In severe cases in which there is widespread subcutaneous emphysema, a tracheostomy is indicated if airway patency is threatened.

ASPIRATION

Aspiration of stomach contents into the lungs is a serious complication that may cause pneumonia and the following clinical syndrome: tachycardia, dyspnea, central cyanosis, hypertension, hypotension, and finally death. It can occur when the protective airway reflexes are decreased or absent from a variety of factors.

Risk Factors for **ASPIRATION**

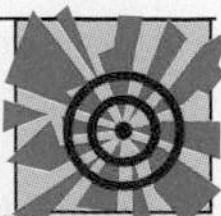

- Seizure activity
- Decreased level of consciousness from trauma, drug or alcohol intoxication, excessive sedation, or general anesthesia
- Nausea and vomiting in the patient with a decreased level of consciousness
- Stroke
- Swallowing disorders
- Cardiac arrest
- Silent aspiration

Nursing Alert *When a nonfunctioning nasogastric tube allows the gastric contents to drain around the tube, a condition known as silent aspiration may result. Silent regurgitation often occurs unobserved and may be more common than suspected. If untreated, massive inhalation of gastric contents develops in a period of several hours.*

Pathophysiology

The primary factors responsible for death and complications after aspiration of gastric contents are the volume and character of the aspirated gastric contents. For example, a small, localized aspiration from regurgitation can cause pneumonia and acute respiratory distress; a massive aspiration is usually fatal.

A full stomach contains solid particles of food. If these are aspirated, the problem then becomes one of mechanical blockage of the airways and secondary infection. During periods of fasting, the stomach contains acidic gastric juice, which, if aspirated, may be very destructive to the alveoli and capillaries. Fecal contamination (more likely seen in intestinal obstruction) increases the likelihood of death because the endotoxins produced by intestinal organisms may be absorbed systemically, or the thick proteinaceous material found in the intestinal contents may obstruct the airway, leading to atelectasis and secondary bacterial invasion.

Chemical pneumonitis may develop from aspiration of substances with a pH of less than 2.4. This results in the destruction of alveolar–capillary endothelial cells, with a consequent outpouring of protein-rich fluids into the interstitial and intra-alveolar spaces. As a result, surfactant is lost, which in turn causes the airways to close and the alveoli to collapse. Finally, the impaired exchange of oxygen and carbon dioxide causes respiratory failure.

Prevention

Prevention is the primary goal when dealing with patients at risk for aspiration.

LACK OF REFLEXES

Aspiration is likely to occur if the patient cannot adequately coordinate protective glottic, laryngeal, and cough reflexes. This hazard is increased if the patient has a distended abdomen, is in a supine position, has the upper extremities immobilized by intravenous infusions or hand restraints, receives local anesthetics to the oropharyngeal or laryngeal area for diagnostic procedures, has been sedated, or has had long-term intubation.

When vomiting, a person can normally protect the airway by sitting up or turning on the side and coordinating breathing, coughing, gag, and glottic reflexes. If these reflexes are active, an oral airway should not be inserted. If an airway is in place, it should be pulled out the moment the patient gags so as not to stimulate the pharyngeal gag reflex and promote vomiting and aspiration. Suctioning of oral secretions with a catheter should be performed with minimal pharyngeal stimulation.

DURING TUBE FEEDINGS

Even when the patient is intubated, aspiration may occur even with a nasogastric tube in place. This aspiration may result in nosocomial pneumonia. Blue dye may be added to the tube feeding to assess for aspiration by monitoring the pulmonary secretions. The patient who is receiving continuous or timed-interval tube feedings is positioned properly. The patient receiving a continuous infusion is given small volumes under low pressure in an upright position, which helps to prevent aspiration. Patients receiving tube feedings at timed intervals are maintained in an upright position during the feeding and for 30 minutes afterward to allow the stomach to empty partially. Tube feedings must be given only when it is certain that the feeding tube is positioned correctly in the stomach. Many patients today receive enteral feeding directly into the duodenum through a small-bore flexible feeding tube or surgically implanted tube. Feedings are given slowly and regulated by a feeding pump. Correct placement is confirmed by chest x-ray.

DELAYED STOMACH EMPTYING

A full stomach may cause aspiration because of increased intragastric or extragastric pressure. The following clinical situations cause a delayed emptying time of the stomach and may contribute to aspiration: intestinal obstruction; increased gastric secretions during anxiety, stress, or pain; or abdominal distention because of ileus, ascites, peritonitis, use of opioids and sedatives, severe illness, or vaginal delivery.

When a feeding tube is present, contents are aspirated, usually every 4 hours, to determine the amount of the last feeding left in the stomach (residual volume). If more than 50 mL is aspirated, there may be a problem with delayed emptying, and the next feeding should be delayed or the continuous feeding stopped for a period of time.

AFTER PROLONGED ENDOTRACHEAL INTUBATION

Prolonged endotracheal intubation or tracheostomy can depress the laryngeal and glottic reflexes because of disuse. Patients with prolonged tracheostomies are encouraged to phonate and exercise their laryngeal muscles. For patients who have had long-term intubation or tracheostomies, it may be helpful to have a rehabilitation therapist experienced in speech and swallowing disorders work with the patient to assess the swallowing reflex.

Critical Thinking Exercises

1.
Use of an MDI has been prescribed for the first time for your patient, a 35-year-old with asthma. Describe the teaching approach you would use to ensure correct use of the MDI. How would your approach differ if the patient had a learning disability or did not speak English?

2.
Your patient has a diagnosis of COPD and is short of breath. Oxygen is prescribed at 2 L/min. His family wants the oxygen flow increased to relieve his shortness of breath. How would you explain to the patient and family the need to keep the oxygen at the prescribed rate? What actions would you take to assist in decreasing the patient's breathlessness?

3.
During a home visit to a patient with advanced lung cancer, the patient says he cannot do anything except sit in a chair because of shortness of breath with any exertion. Describe the strategies you would plan with the patient to minimize his shortness of breath, improve his comfort level, and improve the quality of his life.

4.
Your patient, a 54-year-old employee at a homeless shelter, has just been diagnosed with active TB. She has been started on treatment at home, with specific instructions about her medication. She cannot take time off from work and has close contact with the adults and children in the shelter. What are the public health concerns, and what strategies will you provide to the patient and to those who live and work at the shelter?

5.
You are working on a surgical unit. Your patient is a 75-year-old man who had colon surgery 2 days ago for cancer. He is drowsy and reluctant to move in bed or mobilize to the chair, and he uses his patient-controlled analgesia pump on a regular basis. The family does not want him disturbed so that he can rest. What are the potential postoperative pulmonary complications? What information would you provide to the patient and family regarding care? What interventions would you implement to prevent pulmonary complications in this patient?

References and Selected Readings

BOOKS

American Association of Cardiovascular & Pulmonary Rehabilitation. (1998). *Guidelines for pulmonary rehabilitation programs* (2nd ed.). Champaign, IL: Human Kinetics.

Bartlett, J. G. (1997). *Management of respiratory tract infections.* Baltimore: Williams & Wilkins.

Berk, J. (1997). Pneumothorax. In R. H. Goldstein, J. J. O'Connell, & J. B. Karlinsky (Eds.), *A practical approach to pulmonary medicine* (pp. 206–223). Philadelphia: Lippincott-Raven.

Bordow, R. A., & Moser, K. M. (1996). *Manual of clinical problems in pulmonary medicine* (4th ed.). Boston: Little, Brown.

Cherniack, N. S., Homma, I., & Altose, M. (Eds.). (1999). *Rehabilitation of the patient with respiratory disease.* New York: McGraw-Hill.

Cordova, F., & Criner, G. (1997). Occupational lung disease. In R. H. Goldstein, J. J. O'Connell, & J. B. Karlinsky (Eds.), *A practical approach to pulmonary medicine* (pp. 472–494). Philadelphia: Lippincott-Raven.

Dantzker, D. R., MacIntyre, N. R., & Bakow, E. D. (1995). *Comprehensive respiratory care.* Philadelphia: W. B. Saunders.

*Duffy, S. Q., & Farley, D. E. (1993). *Intermittent positive pressure breathing: Old technologies rarely die* (AHCPR Publication No. 94-0001). Division of Provider Studies Research Note 18, Agency for Health Care Policy and Research, Rockville, MD: Public Health Service.

Expert Panel Report II. (1997). *Guidelines for the diagnosis and management of asthma.* National Asthma Education and Prevention Program, National Institutes of Health.

Farzan, S. (1997). *A concise handbook of respiratory diseases.* Stamford, CT: Appleton & Lange.

Gochuico, B. R., & Bernardo, J. (1997). Tuberculosis. In R. H. Goldstein, J. J. O'Connell, & J. B. Karlinsky (Eds.), *A practical approach to pulmonary medicine* (pp. 147–159). Philadelphia: Lippincott-Raven.

Goldstein, R. H., O'Connell, J. J., & Karlinsky, J. B. (Eds.). (1997). *A practical approach to pulmonary medicine*. Philadelphia: Lippincott-Raven.

Harber, P., Schenker, M., & Balmes, J. (1996). *Occupational and environmental respiratory disease*. St. Louis: Mosby.

Hudak, C. M., Gallo, B. M., & Morton, P. G. (1998). *Critical care nursing: A holistic approach* (7th ed.). Philadelphia: Lippincott-Raven.

Kelley, W. N. (1997). *Textbook of internal medicine* (3rd ed.). Philadelphia: Lippincott-Raven.

Nail, L. (1998). Interventions for cancer treatment-related fatigue. In *Anemia and fatigue in cancer patients: nursing care management* (pp. 18–25). Newton, PA: Associates in Medical Marketing Company, Inc.

National Institutes of Health, National Heart, Lung and Blood Institute. (1996). *Clinical study of effectiveness of lung reduction surgery*. National Emphysema Treatment Trial (NETT).

Reardon, C. C., & Theodore, A. C. (1997). Lung cancer. In R. H. Goldstein, J. J. O'Connell, & J. B. Karlinsky (Eds.), *A practical approach to pulmonary medicine* (pp. 129–146). Philadelphia: Lippincott-Raven.

*Respiratory Nursing Society and American Nurses Association. (1994). *Standards and scope of respiratory nursing practice/Joint Standards Task Force for Respiratory Nursing Practice.* Washington, DC: Author.

Stitik, T., & Beneveneto, B. T. (1997). Cardiac and pulmonary disease. In M. L. Sipski & C. J. Alexander (Eds.), *Sexual function in people with disability and chronic illness.* Gaithersburg, MD: Aspen.

Tanoue, L. T., & Elias, J. A. (1998). Systemic sarcoidosis. In G. L. Baum, J. D. Crapo, B. R. Celli, & J. B. Karlinsky (Eds.), *Textbook of pulmonary disease* (pp. 407–430). Philadelphia: Lippincott-Raven.

Wilcox, W. (1998). *Public health sourcebook* (vol. 34, p. 49). Detroit: Omnigraphics.

World Health Organization. (1998). *Tuberculosis fact sheet*. Geneva, Switzerland: Author.

Zimmerman, L. H. (1997). Pleural effusions. In R. H. Goldstein, J. J. O'Connell, & J. B. Karlinsky (eds.), *A practical approach to pulmonary medicine* (pp. 195–205). Philadelphia: Lippincott-Raven.

JOURNALS

Asterisks indicate nursing research articles.

General

Bryce, J. C. (1995). Aspiration: causes, consequences, and prevention. *ORL Head and Neck Nursing, 13*(2), 14–19.

Christie, F. (1998). Clinical snapshot: Pulmonary embolism. *American Journal of Nursing, 98*(11), 36–37.

Elpern, E. H. (1997). Pulmonary aspiration in hospitalized adults. *Nutrition in Clinical Practice, 12*(1), 5–13.

Goldhaber, S. Z. (1998). Medical progress: Pulmonary embolism. *New England Journal of Medicine, 339*(2), 93–104.

Handler, J. A., & Feied, C. F. (1995). Acute pulmonary embolism. Aggressive therapy with anticoagulants and thrombolytics. *Postgraduate Medicine, 97*(1), 61–72.

Lomotan, J. R., George, S. S., & Brandsetter, R. D. (1997). Aspiration pneumonia: Strategies for early recognition and prevention. *102*(2), 225–231.

Miniati, M., Pistolesi, M., Marini, C., et al. (1996). Value of perfusion lung scan in the diagnosis of pulmonary embolism: Results of the prospective investigative study of acute pulmonary embolism diagnosis (PISA-PED). *American Journal of Critical Care Medicine, 154*(5), 1387–1393.

National Institutes of Health. (1993). *Sarcoidosis.* Publication 91-3093.

Stein, P. D. (1996). Diagnosis and management of pulmonary embolism. *Current Opinion in Cardiology, 11*(5), 543–549.

van Beek, E. J., Kuijer, P. M., Buller, H.R., et al. (1997). The clinical course of patients with suspected pulmonary embolism. *Archives of Internal Medicine, 157*(22), 2593–2598.

Acute Respiratory Failure and ARDS

Bernard, G. R., Artigas, A., Brigham, K. L., et al. (1994). Report of the American-European consensus conference on acute respiratory distress syndrome: Definitions, mechanisms, relevant outcomes, and clinical trial coordination. *American Journal of Critical Care, 9*(1), 72–81.

Davidson, T. A., Caldwell, E. S., Curtis, J. R. et al. (1999). Reduced quality of life in survivors of acute respiratory distress syndrome compared with critically ill control patients. *Journal of American Medical Association, 281*(4), 354–360.

Gerber, B. G., Hebert, P., Yelle, J., Hodder, R., & McGown, J. (1996). Adult respiratory distress syndrome: A systemic overview of incidence and risk factors. *Critical Care Medicine, 24*(4), 687–695.

Hudson, L., Milberg, J., Anardi, D., & Maunder, R. (1995). Clinical risks for development of the acute respiratory distress syndrome. *American Journal of Critical Care Medicine, 151*(2 pt. 1), 293–301.

Kollef, M. H., & Schuster, D. P. (1995). The acute respiratory distress syndrome. *New England Journal of Medicine, 332*(1), 27–37.

Vollman, K. M. (1997). Prone positioning for the ARDS patient. *DCCN, 16*(4), 184–193.

COPD

ACCP/AACVPR Pulmonary Rehabilitation Guidelines Panel. (1997). Pulmonary rehabilitation: Joint ACCP/AACVPR evidence-based guidelines. *Chest, 112*(5), 1363–1396.

American Thoracic Society. (1995). Standards for the diagnosis and care of patients with chronic obstructive pulmonary disease. *American Journal of Respiratory Critical Care Medicine, 152*(5), S77–S121.

*Anderson, K. L. (1995). The effect of chronic obstructive pulmonary disease on quality of life. *Research in Nursing & Health, 18*(6), 547–556.

Borkgren, M. W., & Gronkiewicz, C. A. (1995). Update your asthma care from hospital to home. *American Journal of Nursing, 95*(1), 26–35.

*Devine, E. C. (1996). Meta-analysis of the effects of psychoeducational care in adults with asthma. *Research in Nursing & Health, 19*(5), 367–376.

Drazen, J. M., Israel, E., & O'Byrne, P. M. (1999). Treatment of asthma with drugs modifying the leukotriene pathway. *New England Journal of Medicine, 340*(3), 197–206.

Fein, A. (1998). Lung volume reduction surgery. *Chest, 113*(4), 277S–282S.

Garvey, C. (1998). COPD and exercise. *Lippincott's Primary Care Practice, 2*(6), 589–598.

Janson, S. (1998). National Asthma Education and Prevention Program, Expert Panel Report II: Overview and application for primary care. *Lippincott's Primary Care Practice, 2*(6), 578–588.

Kwiatkowski, M., & Jain, M. (1998). Current trends and treatments in chronic obstructive pulmonary disease. *Lippincott's Primary Care Practice, 2*(6), 545–558.

Lacasse, Y., Guyatt, G., & Goldstein, R. (1997). The components of a respiratory rehabilitation program: A systematic overview. *Chest, 111*(4), 1977–1088.

*Leidy, N. K., & Traver, G. A. (1995). Psychophysiologic factors contributing to functional performance in people with COPD: Are there gender differences? *Research in Nursing & Health, 18*(6), 535–546.

*Leidy, N. K., & Traver, G. A. (1996). Adjustment and social behavior in older adults with chronic obstructive pulmonary disease: The family's perspective. *Journal of Advanced Nursing, 23*(2), 252–259.

McGann, E. (1999). Medication compliance in adults with asthma. *American Journal of Nursing, 99*(3), 45–46.

Newsome, E. A., & Ott, B. B. (1997). Lung volume reduction: Surgical treatment for emphysema. *Journal of Critical Care, 6*(6), 423–427.

Owen, C. L. (1999). New directions in asthma management. *American Journal of Nursing, 99*(3), 26–33.

Petty, T. (1998). The national lung health education program (NLHEP). *Chest, 113*(2), 123S–163S.

Renkema, T. E. J., Schouten, J. P., Koeter, G. H., & Postma, D. S. (1996). Effects of long-term treatment with corticosteroids in COPD. *Chest, 109*(5), 1156–1162.

Rennard, S. I. (1998). COPD: Overview of definitions, epidemiology, and factors influencing its development. *Chest, 113*(4, suppl.), 235S–241S.

Robertson, R., Osman, L. M., & Douglas, J. G. (1997). Adult asthma review in general practice: Nurses' perception of their role. *Family Practice, 14*(3), 227–232.

*Scherer, Y. K., & Schmieder, L. E. (1997). The effect of a pulmonary rehabilitation program on self-efficacy, perception of dyspnea, and physical endurance. *Heart and Lung, 26*(1), 15–22.

*Scherer, Y. et al. (1998). The effects of education alone and in combination with pulmonary rehabilitation on self-efficacy in patients with COPD. *Rehabilitation Nursing, 23*(2), 71–77.

*Schott-Baer, D., & Christensen, M. (1999). A pilot program to increase self-care of adult asthma patients. *MedSurg Nursing, 8*(3), 178–183.

*Skilbeck, J., Mott, L., Smith, D., Page, H., & Clark, D. (1997). Research and development. Nursing care for people dying from chronic obstructive airway disease. *International Journal of Palliative Nursing, 3*(2), 100–106.

*Trudeau, M. E., & Solano-McGuire, S. M. (1999). Evaluating the quality of COPD care. *American Journal of Nursing, 99*(3), 47–50.

Van Ganse, E., Leufkens, H. G., Vincken, W., et al. Assessing asthma management from interviews of patients and family physicians. *Journal of Asthma, 34*(3), 203–209.

Zolty, P. (1998). Nutrition in COPD patients. *RT, 11*(3), 31–34.

Lung Cancer

American Cancer Society (1999). *Cancer Facts and Figures, 1999.* Atlanta, GA: Author.

Brown, J. K., & Radke, K. J. (1998). Nutritional assessment, intervention, and evaluation of weight loss in patients with non-small-cell lung cancer. *Oncology Nursing Forum, 25*(3), 547–554.

Landis, S. H., Murray, T., Bolden, S., & Wingo, P. A. (1998). Cancer statistics, 1998. *CA: A Cancer Journal for Clinicians, 48*(1), 6–29.

Mountain, C. F. (1997). Revisions in the international system for staging lung cancer. *Chest, 111*(6), 1710–1717.

*Sarna, L. (1995). Smoking behaviors of women after diagnosis with lung cancer. *Image: Journal of Nursing Scholarship, 27*(1), 35–41.

Shopland, D. R., Eyre, H. J., & Pechacek, T. F. (1992). Smoking-attributable cancer mortality in 1991: Is lung cancer now the leading cause of death among smokers in the United States? *Journal of the National Cancer Institute, 83*, 1142–1148.

Sugarbaker, D. J. (1997). Multimodality therapy of chest malignancies—update 1996. *Chest, 112*(4, suppl.), 181S–300S.

Vale, D. (1997). Lung cancer. *Journal of the American Academy of Nurse Practitioners, 9*(3), 143–150.

*Wewers, M. E., Jenkins, L., & Mignery, T. (1997). A nurse-managed smoking cessation intervention during diagnostic testing for lung cancer. *Oncology Nursing Forum, 24*(8), 1419–1422.

Pulmonary Infections

American College of Chest Physicians/American Thoracic Society Consensus Conference. (1995). Institutional control measures for tuberculosis in the era of multiple drug resistance. *Chest, 108*, 1690–1720.

American Thoracic Society. (1993). Guidelines for the initial management of adults with community-acquired pneumonia: Diagnosis, assessment of severity and initial antimicrobial therapy. *American Review of Respiratory Disease, 148*(5), 1418–1426.

American Thoracic Society. (1995). Hospital-acquired pneumonia in adults: Diagnosis, assessment of severity, initial antimicrobial therapy, and preventive strategies. A consensus statement. *American Journal of Critical Care Medicine, 153*(5), 1711–1725.

American Thoracic Society and Centers for Disease Control. (1994). Treatment of tuberculosis and tuberculosis infection in adults and children: Joint statement of the American Thoracic Society and Centers for Disease Control. *American Journal of Critical Care Medicine, 149*(5), 1359–1374.

Becker, K. L., & Appling, S. (1998). Acute bronchitis. *Lippincott's Primary Care Practice, 2*(6), 643–646.

*Brooks-Brunn, J. A. (1995). Postoperative atelectasis and pneumonia. *Heart and Lung, 24*(2), 94–115.

*Brooks-Brunn, J. A. (1997). Predictors of postoperative pulmonary complications following abdominal surgery. *Chest, 111*(3), 564–571.

Centers for Disease Control and Prevention. (1997a). Guidelines for prevention of nosocomial pneumonia. *Morbidity and Mortality Weekly Report, 46*: RR1, 3–79.

Centers for Disease Control and Prevention. (1997b). Prevention of pneumococcal disease: Recommendations of the advisory committee on immunization practices. *Morbidity and Mortality Weekly Report, 46*:RR-08, 1–24.

Centers for Disease Control and Prevention. (1998a). Development of new vaccines for tuberculosis. *Morbidity and Mortality Weekly Report, 47*: RR13, 1–6.

Centers for Disease Control and Prevention. (1998b). Tuberculosis morbidity, United States. *Morbidity and Mortality Weekly Report, 47*(13), 253–257.

Centers for Disease Control and Prevention/American Thoracic Society. (1990). Diagnostic standards and classification of tuberculosis: Joint statement of the American Thoracic Society and the Centers for Disease Control. *American Review of Respiratory Disease, 142*, 725–735.

Fine, M. J., Auble, T. E., Yealy, D. M., et al. (1997). A prediction rule to identify low-risk patients with community acquired pneumonia. *New England Journal of Medicine, 336*(4), 243–250.

Fine, M. J., Smith, M. A., Carson, C. A., et al. (1996). Prognosis and outcomes of patients with community acquired pneumonia: A meta analysis. *Journal of the American Medical Association, 75*(2), 134–141.

Goodwin, R. S. (1996). Prevention of aspiration pneumonia: A research-based protocol. *Dimensions of Critical Care Nursing, 15*(2), 58–74.

Grap, M. J., & Munro, C. (1997). Ventilator-associated pneumonia: Clinical significance and implications for nursing. *Heart and Lung, 26*(6), 419–429.

Harris, R. S. (1998). The integration of a tuberculosis control plan into a standard of care for tuberculosis. *MedSurg Nursing, 7*(1), 19–27.

Hecht, A., et al. (1995). Diagnosis and treatment of pneumonia in the nursing home. *Nurse Practitioner, 20*(5), 24–39.

Kendig, E. L., Kirkpatrick, B. V., Carter, W. H., Hill, F. A., Caldwell, K., & Entwistle, M. (1998). Underreading of the tuberculin skin test reaction. *Chest, 113*(5), 1175–1177.

Kollef, M. H. (1999). The prevention of ventilator-associated pneumonia. *New England Journal of Medicine, 340*(8), 627–634.

Lemasters, C. Z. (1999). Treatment of pulmonary tuberculosis. *Lippincott's Primary Care Practice, 3*(1), 55–58.

Long, C. O., Holmes, N. J., & Ismeurt, R. L. (1993). The tuberculin skin test. *Home Healthcare Nurse, 11*(3), 13–18.

Mackin, L. A. (1998). Screening for tuberculosis in the primary care setting. *Lippincott's Primary Care Practice, 2*(6), 599–610.

Mackin, L. A. (1998). Respiratory tract infection. *Lippincott's Primary Care Practice, 2*(6), 650–653.

Niederman, M. S. (1998). Disease management of pulmonary infections. *Chest, 113*(3), 165S–232S.

Tasota, F. J., Fisher, E. M., Coulson, C. F., & Hoffman, L. A. (1998). Protecting ICU patients from nosocomial infections: Practical measures for favorable outcomes. *Critical Care Nurse, 18*(1), 54–67.

Ventura, S. J., Peters, K. D., Martin, J. A., & Maurer, J. D. (1997). Births and deaths: United States, 1996. *Monthly Vital Statistics Report, 46*(1, suppl.), 32–33.

Williams, R. M. (1998). Pneumococcal vaccination. *Lippincott's Primary Care Practice, 2*(6), 625–633.

Zimmer, J. G., & Hall, W. J. (1997). Nursing home-acquired pneumonia: Avoiding the hospital. *Journal of the American Geriatrics Society, 45*(3), 380–381.

Trauma

Barmada, H., & Gibbons, J. R. (1994). Tracheobronchial injury in blunt and penetrating chest trauma. *Chest, 106*(1), 74–78.

Johnson, S. B., Kearney, P. A., & Smith, M. D. (1995). Echocardiography in the evaluation of thoracic trauma. *Surgical Clinics of North America, 75*(2), 193–205.

Karlet, M. C. (1997). Update for nurse anesthetists: Thoracic trauma. *AANA Journal, 65*(1), 73–80.

Stallard, T., & Smith, D. (1996). Chest injuries. *Emergency, 28*(5), 42–47.

Resources

GOVERNMENTAL AGENCIES

Centers for Disease Control and Prevention, 1600 Clifton Road, NE, Atlanta, GA 30333; www.cdc.gov

National Heart, Lung and Blood Institute, National Institutes of Health, 900 Rockville Pike, Bldg. 31, Bethesda, MD 20892; 1-301-496-5166; www.nhlbi.nih.gov

National Cancer Institute, National Institutes of Health, 31 Center Drive MSC 2580, Bldg. 31, Room 10A16, Bethesda, MD 20892; 1-800-4-CANCER (Cancer Information Services); www.nci.nih.gov

U.S. Department of Labor, Occupational Safety and Health Administration (OSHA), Directorate of Technical Support, 200 Constitution Avenue, NW, Washington, DC 20210; 1-202-219-7047; www.osha.gov

VOLUNTARY AGENCIES

American Association for Respiratory Care, 1720 Regal Row, Dallas, TX 75235; 1-214-630-3540; www.aarc.org

American Lung Association, 1740 Broadway, New York, NY 10019-4374; 1-212-315-8700; www.lungusa.org

American Thoracic Society, 1740 Broadway, New York, NY 10019; 1-212-315-8700; www.thoracic.org

Respiratory Nursing Society, 7794 Grow Drive, Pensacola, FL 32514; rns@puetzamc.com

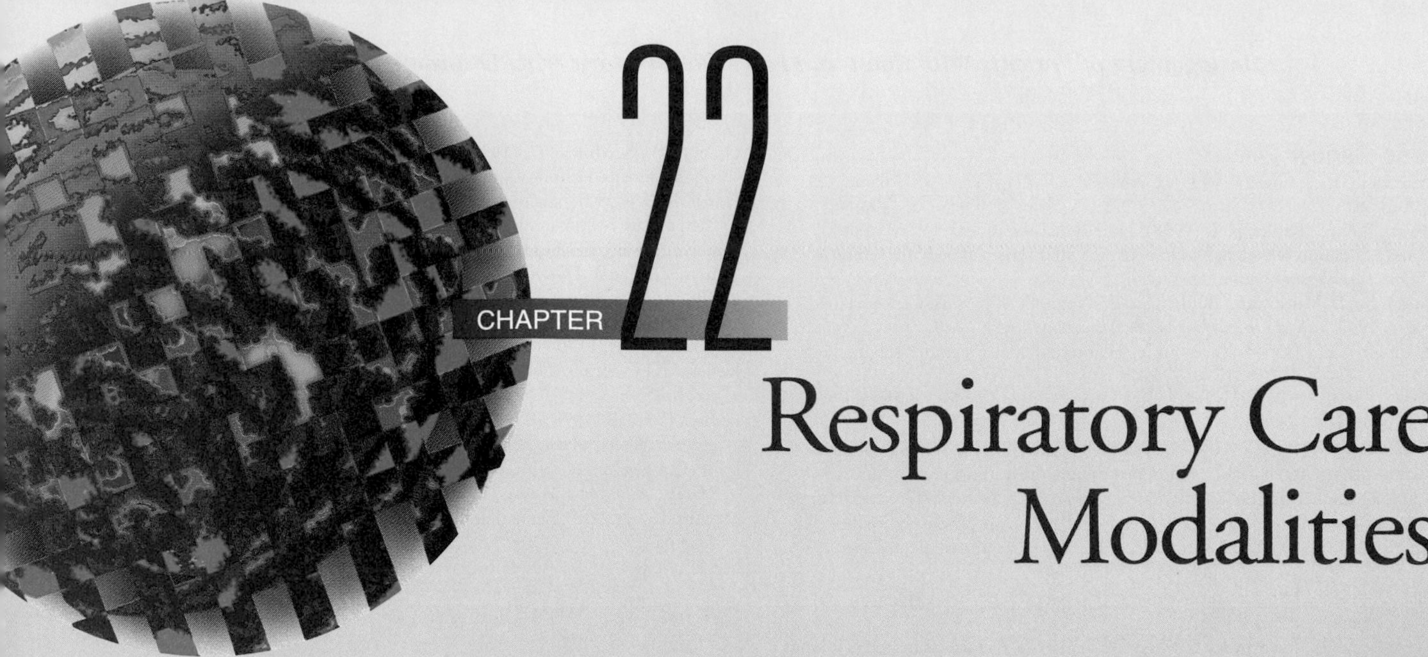

Respiratory Care Modalities

Learning Objectives

On completion of this chapter, the learner will be able to:

1. Describe the nursing management for patients receiving oxygen therapy, intermittent positive-pressure breathing, mini-nebulizer therapy, incentive spirometry, chest physiotherapy, and breathing retraining.
2. Describe the nursing care for a patient with an endotracheal tube and for a patient with a tracheostomy.
3. Demonstrate the procedure of tracheal suctioning.
4. Use the nursing process as a framework for care of patients who are mechanically ventilated.
5. Describe the significance of preoperative nursing assessment and patient teaching for the patient who is to have thoracic surgery.
6. Explain the principles of chest drainage and the nursing responsibilities related to the care of the patient with water-seal drainage.
7. Describe the patient education and home care considerations for patients who have had thoracic surgery.

Numerous treatment modalities are used when caring for patients with various respiratory conditions. The choice of modality is based on the oxygenation disorder and whether there is a problem with gas ventilation, diffusion, or both. Therapies range from simple and noninvasive modalities (oxygen and nebulizer therapy, chest physiotherapy, breathing retraining) to complex and highly invasive treatments (intubation, mechanical ventilation, surgery). Assessment and management of the respiratory patient are best accomplished when the approach is multidisciplinary and collaborative.

GLOSSARY

assist–control ventilation: mode of mechanical ventilation in which the patient's breathing pattern may trigger the ventilator and the patient will receive a preset tidal volume; in the absence of spontaneous breathing, the machine delivers a controlled breath at a minimum rate and preset tidal volume

chest drainage system: use of a chest tube and closed drainage system to reexpand the lung and to remove excess air, fluid, and blood

chest percussion and vibration: a technique to mobilize or dislodge mucus in the lungs

controlled ventilation: mode of mechanical ventilation in which the ventilator completely controls the patient's ventilation according to set tidal volumes and respiratory rate. Because of problems with synchrony, it is rarely used except in paralyzed or anesthetized patients

endotracheal intubation: insertion of a breathing tube into the trachea. The route of insertion can be nasal or oral

fraction of inspired oxygen (FiO_2): concentration of oxygen delivered (1.0 = 100% oxygen)

hypoxemia: decrease in arterial oxygen tension in the blood

hypoxia: decrease in oxygen supply to the tissues

mechanical ventilator: a positive- or negative-pressure breathing device that supports ventilation and oxygenation

positive end-expiratory pressure (PEEP): positive pressure maintained by the ventilator at the end of exhalation (instead of a normal zero pressure) to increase functional residual capacity and open collapsed alveoli; improves oxygenation with lower FiO_2

postural drainage: positioning the patient to allow drainage from all the lobes of the lungs and airways

pressure support ventilation: mode of mechanical ventilation in which preset positive pressure is delivered with spontaneous breaths to decrease work of breathing

respiratory weaning: process of gradual, systematic withdrawal and/or removal of ventilator, breathing tube, and oxygen

synchronized intermittent mandatory ventilation (SIMV): mode of mechanical ventilation in which the ventilator allows the patient to breathe spontaneously while providing a preset number of breaths to ensure adequate ventilation; ventilated breaths are synchronized with spontaneous breathing

thoracotomy: surgical opening into the chest cavity

tracheotomy: surgical opening into the trachea

tracheostomy tube: indwelling tube inserted directly into the trachea to assist with ventilation

NONINVASIVE RESPIRATORY THERAPIES

Oxygen Therapy

Oxygen therapy is the administration of oxygen at a concentration greater than that found in the environmental atmosphere. At sea level, the concentration of oxygen in room air is 21%. The goal of oxygen therapy is to provide adequate transport of oxygen in the blood while decreasing the work of breathing and reducing stress on the myocardium.

Oxygen transport to the tissues depends on factors such as cardiac output, arterial oxygen content, concentration of hemoglobin, and metabolic requirements. These factors must be kept in mind when oxygen therapy is considered. (Respiratory physiology and oxygen transport are discussed in Chap. 19.)

Indications

A change in the patient's respiratory rate or pattern may be one of the earliest indicators of the need for oxygen therapy. The change in respiratory rate or pattern may result from hypoxemia or hypoxia. **Hypoxemia** (a decrease in the arterial oxygen tension in the blood) is manifested by changes in mental status (progressing through impaired judgment, agitation, disorientation, confusion, lethargy, and coma), dyspnea, increase in blood pressure, changes in heart rate, dysrhythmias, central cyanosis (late sign), diaphoresis, and cool extremities. Hypoxemia usually leads to **hypoxia**, which is a decrease in oxygen supply to the tissues. Hypoxia, if severe enough, can be life-threatening.

The signs and symptoms signaling the need for oxygen may depend on how suddenly this need develops. With rapidly developing hypoxia, changes occur in the central nervous system because the higher neurologic centers are very sensitive to oxygen deprivation. The clinical picture may resemble that of alcohol intoxication, with the patient exhibiting incoordination and impaired judgment. Longstanding hypoxia (as seen in chronic obstructive pulmonary disease [COPD] and chronic congestive heart failure) may produce fatigue, drowsiness, apathy, inattentiveness, and delayed reaction time. The need for oxygen is assessed by arterial blood gas analysis and pulse oximetry as well as by clinical evaluation. For more information about hypoxia, see Chart 22-1.

Cautions in Oxygen Therapy

As with other medications, the nurse administers oxygen with caution and carefully assesses its effects on each patient. Oxygen is a medication and except in emergency situations is administered only when prescribed by a physician.

In general, patients with respiratory conditions are given oxygen therapy only to raise the arterial oxygen pressure (PaO_2) back to the patient's normal baseline, which may vary from 60 to 95 mm Hg. In terms of the oxyhemoglobin dissociation curve (see Chap. 19), the blood at these levels is 80% to 98% saturated with oxygen; higher inspired oxygen flow (FiO_2) values add no further significant amounts of oxygen to the red blood cells or plasma. Instead of helping, increased amounts of oxygen may produce toxic effects on the lungs and central nervous system or may depress ventilation (see discussion below).

It is important to observe for subtle indications of inadequate oxygenation when oxygen is administered by any method. Therefore, the nurse assesses the patient frequently for confusion, restlessness progressing to lethargy, diaphoresis, pallor, tachycardia, tachypnea, and hypertension. Intermittent or continuous pulse oximetry is used to monitor oxygen levels.

OXYGEN TOXICITY

Oxygen toxicity may occur when too high a concentration of oxygen (greater than 50%) is administered for an extended period (longer than 48 hours). The pathophysiology of oxygen toxicity is not fully understood, but it is related to the destruction and decrease of surfactant, the formation of a hyaline membrane lining

CHART 22•1 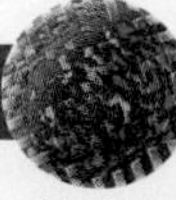 **Types of Hypoxia**

Hypoxia can occur from either severe pulmonary disease (inadequate oxygen supply) or from extrapulmonary disease (inadequate oxygen delivery) affecting gas exchange at the cellular level. The four general types of hypoxia are hypoxemic hypoxia, circulatory hypoxia, anemic hypoxia, and histotoxic hypoxia.

Hypoxemic Hypoxia

Hypoxemic hypoxia is a decreased oxygen level in the blood resulting in decreased oxygen diffusion into the tissues. It may be caused by hypoventilation, high altitudes, ventilation–perfusion mismatch (as in pulmonary embolism), shunts in which the alveoli are collapsed and cannot provide oxygen to the blood (commonly caused by atelectasis), and pulmonary diffusion defects. It is corrected by increasing alveolar ventilation or providing supplemental oxygen.

Circulatory Hypoxia

Circulatory hypoxia is hypoxia resulting from inadequate capillary circulation. It may be caused by decreased cardiac output, local vascular obstruction, low-flow states such as shock, or cardiac arrest. Although tissue partial pressure of oxygen (PO_2) is reduced, arterial oxygen (PaO_2) remains normal. Circulatory hypoxia is corrected by identifying and treating the underlying cause.

Anemic Hypoxia

Anemic hypoxia is a result of decreased effective hemoglobin concentration, which causes a decrease in the oxygen-carrying capacity of the blood. It is rarely accompanied by hypoxemia. Carbon monoxide poisoning, because it reduces the oxygen-carrying capacity of hemoglobin, produces similar effects but is not strictly anemic hypoxia because hemoglobin levels may be normal.

Histotoxic Hypoxia

Histotoxic hypoxia occurs when a toxic substance, such as cyanide, interferes with the ability of tissues to use available oxygen.

the lungs, and the development of pulmonary edema that is not cardiac in origin.

Signs and symptoms of oxygen toxicity include substernal distress, paresthesias, dyspnea, restlessness, fatigue, malaise, progressive respiratory difficulty, and alveolar infiltrates evident on chest x-rays.

Prevention of oxygen toxicity is achieved by using oxygen only as prescribed. If high concentrations of oxygen are necessary, it is important to minimize the duration of administration and reduce it as soon as possible. Often, **positive end-expiratory pressure** (PEEP) or continuous positive airway pressure (CPAP) is used with oxygen therapy to reverse or prevent microatelectasis, thus allowing a lower percentage of oxygen to be used. The level of PEEP that allows the best oxygenation without hemodynamic compromise is known as best PEEP.

SUPPRESSION OF VENTILATION

In patients with COPD, the stimulus for respiration is a decrease in blood oxygen rather than an elevation in carbon dioxide levels. Thus, administration of a high concentration of oxygen removes the respiratory drive that has been created largely by the patient's chronic low oxygen tension. The resulting decrease in alveolar ventilation can cause a progressive increase in arterial carbon dioxide pressure ($PaCO_2$), ultimately leading to the patient's death from carbon dioxide narcosis and acidosis. Oxygen-induced hypoventilation is prevented by administering oxygen at low flow rates (1 to 2 L/min).

OTHER COMPLICATIONS

Because oxygen supports combustion, there is always a danger of fire when it is used. It is important to post "no smoking" signs when oxygen is in use. Oxygen therapy equipment is also a potential source of bacterial cross-infection; thus, the nurse changes the tubing according to infection control policy and the type of oxygen delivery equipment.

Methods of Oxygen Administration

Oxygen is dispensed from a cylinder or a piped-in system. A reduction gauge is necessary to reduce the pressure to a working level, and a flow meter regulates the flow of oxygen in liters per minute. When oxygen is used at high-flow rates, it should be moistened by passing it through a humidification system to prevent the mucous membranes of the respiratory tract from becoming dry.

Many different oxygen devices are used, and all deliver oxygen if used as prescribed and maintained correctly (Table 22-1). The amount of oxygen delivered is expressed as a percentage concentration (eg, 70%). The appropriate form of oxygen therapy is best determined by arterial blood gas levels, which indicate the patient's oxygenation status.

The nasal cannula is used when the patient requires a low to medium concentration of oxygen for which precise accuracy is not essential. This method is relatively simple and allows the patient to move about in bed, talk, cough, and eat without interrupting oxygen flow. Flow rates in excess of 6 to 8 L/min may lead to swallowing of air; this may cause irritation and drying of the nasal and pharyngeal mucosa.

The oropharyngeal catheter is rarely used but may be prescribed for short-term therapy to administer low to moderate concentrations of oxygen. This method can lead to irritation of the nasal mucosa. Patients with chronic oxygen therapy need may use a transtracheal oxygen catheter, which is inserted directly into the trachea. These catheters are more comfortable, less dependent on breathing patterns, and less obvious than other oxygen delivery methods.

When oxygen is administered via cannula or catheter, the percentage of oxygen reaching the lungs varies with the depth and rate of respirations, particularly if the nasal mucosa is swollen or if the patient is a mouth breather.

Oxygen masks come in several forms. Each is used for different purposes (Fig. 22-1). Simple masks are used for low to moderate concentrations of oxygen, whereas partial rebreathing or nonrebreathing masks are used for moderate to high concentrations of oxygen. Although widely used, these masks cannot be used for controlled oxygen concentrations and must be adjusted for proper fit. They should not press too tightly against the skin, because this may cause a sense of claustrophobia and skin breakdown; adjustable elastic bands are provided to ensure comfort and security. Bags on partial rebreathing and nonrebreathing masks must remain inflated during both inspiration and expiration. This is accomplished by adjusting the flow so that the bag does not collapse on inspiration.

The Venturi mask is the most reliable and accurate method for delivering precise concentrations of oxygen through noninvasive means. The mask is constructed in a way that allows a constant flow of room air blended with a fixed flow of oxygen. It is used primarily for patients with COPD because it can provide low levels of supplemental oxygen, thus avoiding the risk of suppressing the hypoxic drive.

The Venturi mask employs the principle of air entrainment (trapping the air like a vacuum), which provides a high air flow with controlled oxygen enrichment. Excess gas leaves the mask

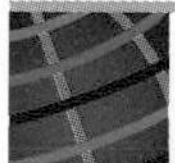

TABLE 22•1 Oxygen Administration Devices

Device	Suggested Flow Rate (L/min)	O_2 Percentage Setting	Advantages	Disadvantages
Cannula	1–2 3–5 6	23–30 30–40 42	Lightweight, comfortable, inexpensive, continuous use with meals and activity	Nasal mucosal drying, variable FiO_2
Catheter	1–6	23–42	Inexpensive	Variable FiO_2, requires frequent change (q8h), gastric distention can occur
Mask, simple	6–8	40–60	Simple to use, inexpensive	Poor fitting, variable FiO_2, must remove to eat
Mask, partial rebreather	8–11	50–75	Moderate O_2 concentration	Warm, poorly fitting, must remove to eat
Mask, non-rebreather	12	80–100	High O_2 concentration	Poorly fitting
Mask, Venturi	4–6 6–8	24, 26, 28 30, 35, 40	Provides low levels of supplemental O_2 Precise FiO_2, additional humidity available	Must remove to eat
Mask, aerosol	8–10	30–100	Good humidity, accurate FiO_2	Uncomfortable for some
Tracheostomy collar	8–10	30–100	Good humidity, comfortable, fairly accurate FiO_2	
T-piece, Briggs	8–10	30–100	Same as tracheostomy collar	Heavy with tubing
Face tent	8–10	30–100	Good humidity, fairly accurate FiO_2	Bulky and cumbersome

through the perforated cuff, carrying with it the exhaled carbon dioxide. This method allows a constant oxygen concentration to be inhaled regardless of the depth or rate of respiration.

The mask should fit snugly enough to prevent oxygen from flowing into the eyes. The nurse should check the patient's skin for irritation. It is necessary to remove the mask so that the patient can eat, drink, and take medications.

Other oxygen devices include aerosol masks, tracheostomy collars, and face tents, all of which are used with aerosol devices (nebulizers) that can be adjusted for oxygen concentrations from 27% to 100% (0.27 to 1.00). If the gas mixture flow falls below patient demand, room air is pulled in, diluting the concentration. The aerosol mist must be available for the patient during the entire inspiratory phase.

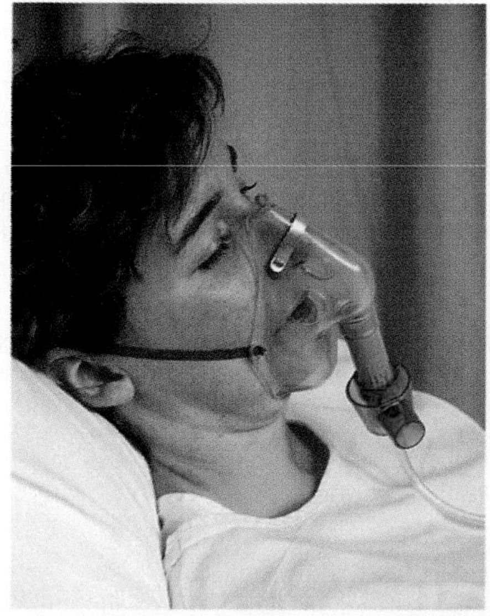

Venturi mask

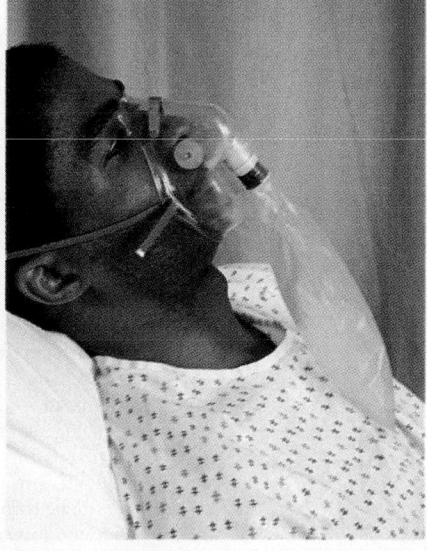

Nonrebreather mask

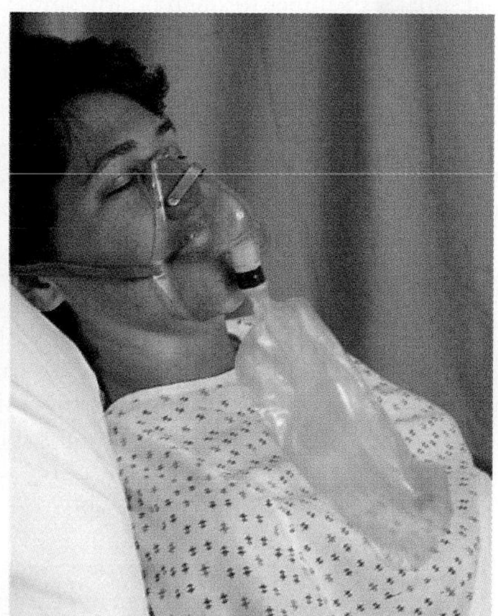

Partial rebreather mask

FIGURE 22•1 Types of oxygen masks used to deliver varying concentrations of oxygen. Photos © Ken Kaspar.

Oxygen concentrators are another means of providing varying amounts of oxygen, especially in the home setting. These devices are relatively portable, easy to operate, and cost-effective. However, they also require more maintenance than tank or liquid systems and probably cannot deliver flows in excess of 4 liters (which provides an FiO_2 of about 36%).

Promoting Home and Community-Based Care

TEACHING PATIENTS SELF-CARE

At times oxygen must be administered to the patient at home. The nurse instructs the patient or family in the methods for administering oxygen and informs the patient or family that oxygen is available in gas, liquid, and concentrated forms. The gas and liquid forms come in portable devices so that the patient can leave home while receiving oxygen therapy. Humidity must be provided while oxygen is used (except with portable devices) to counteract the dry, irritating effects of compressed oxygen on the airway.

CONTINUING CARE

Home visits by a home health nurse or respiratory therapist may be arranged based on the patient's status and needs. It is important to assess the patient's home environment, the patient's physical and psychological status, and the need for further teaching. The nurse reinforces the teaching points on how to use the oxygen safely and effectively, including fire safety tips because oxygen is flammable. To maintain a consistent quality of care and to maximize the patient's financial reimbursement for home oxygen therapy, the nurse ensures that the physician's order includes the disorder, the prescribed oxygen flow, and conditions for use (eg, continuous use, nighttime use only).

Intermittent Positive-Pressure Breathing

IPPB is the breathing of air or oxygen (or a combination) at a pressure higher than atmospheric pressure to produce air flow into the lungs during inhalation. IPPB is applied by a mechanical device that inflates the lungs through positive pressure, dispersing a prescribed medication. When the patient inhales, the negative inspiratory force triggers the machine to deliver a positive-pressure breath. After a preset pressure is reached on the machine, the machine cycles off and there is passive exhalation. The IPPB machine may be powered by electricity or gas and may be connected with a mouthpiece, mask, or tracheostomy adapter.

Indications

General indications for IPPB include difficulty in raising respiratory secretions, reduced vital capacity with ineffective deep breathing and coughing, or unsuccessful trials of simpler and less costly methods for loosening secretions, delivering aerosol, or expanding the lungs.

Complications

IPPB therapy is used infrequently because of its inherent hazards, which may include pneumothorax, mucosal drying, increased intracranial pressure, hemoptysis, gastric distention, vomiting with possible aspiration, psychological dependency (especially with long-term use, as in COPD patients), hyperventilation, excessive oxygen administration, and cardiovascular problems.

Mini-Nebulizer Therapy

The mini-nebulizer is a hand-held apparatus that disperses a moisturizing agent or medication, such as a bronchodilator or mucolytic agent, into microscopic particles and delivers it to the lungs as the patient inhales. The mini-nebulizer is usually air-driven by means of a compressor through connecting tubing. In some instances, the nebulizer is oxygen-driven rather than air-driven. To be effective, a visible mist must be available for the patient to inhale.

Indications

The indications for use of a mini-nebulizer are similar to the indications for IPPB, except that the patient must be able to generate a deep breath without the aid of the positive-pressure machine. Diaphragmatic breathing is a helpful technique to prepare for the proper use of the mini-nebulizer. Frequently, mini-nebulizers are

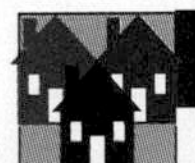

PATIENT EDUCATION AND HOME CARE
Breathing Exercises

General Instructions

- Breathe slowly and rhythmically to exhale completely and empty the lungs completely.
- Inhale through the nose to filter, humidify, and warm the air before it enters the lungs.
- If you feel out of breath, breathe more slowly by prolonging the exhalation time.
- Keep the air moist with a humidifier.

Diaphragmatic Breathing

Goal: To use and strengthen the diaphragm during breathing

- Place one hand on the abdomen (just below the ribs) and the other hand on the middle of the chest to increase the awareness of the position of the diaphragm and its function in breathing.
- Breathe in slowly and deeply through the nose, letting the abdomen protrude as far as possible.
- Breathe out through pursed lips while tightening (contracting) the abdominal muscles.
- Press firmly inward and upward on the abdomen while breathing out.
- Repeat for 1 minute; follow with a rest period of 2 minutes.
- Gradually increase duration up to 5 minutes, several times a day (before meals and at bedtime).

Pursed-Lip Breathing

Goal: To prolong exhalation and increase airway pressure during expiration, thus reducing the amount of trapped air and the amount of airway resistance

- Inhale through the nose while counting to 3—the amount of time needed to say "Smell a rose."
- Exhale slowly and evenly against pursed lips while tightening the abdominal muscles. (Pursing the lips increases intratracheal pressure; exhaling through the mouth offers less resistance to expired air.)
- Count to 7 while prolonging expiration through pursed lips—the length of time to say "Blow out the candle."
- While sitting in a chair:
  - Fold arms over the abdomen.
  - Inhale through the nose while counting to 3.
  - Bend forward and exhale slowly through pursed lips while counting to 7.
- While walking:
  - Inhale while walking two steps.
  - Exhale through pursed lips while walking four or five steps.

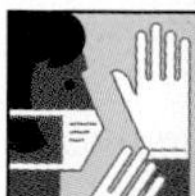

HEALTH PROMOTION AND ILLNESS PREVENTION

Assisting the Patient to Perform Incentive Spirometry

- Explain the reason and objective for the therapy: the inspired air helps to inflate the lungs. The ball or weight in the spirometer will rise in response to the intensity of the intake of air. The higher the ball rises, the deeper the breath.
- Assess the patient's level of pain and administer pain medication if prescribed.
- Position the patient in semi-Fowler's position or in an upright position (although any position is acceptable).
- Demonstrate how to use diaphragmatic breathing.
- Instruct the patient to place the mouthpiece of the spirometer firmly in the mouth, to breathe air in (inspire) and hold the breathe at the end of inspiration for about 3 seconds. The patient then exhales slowly.
- Encourage approximately 10 breaths per hour with the spirometer during waking hours.
- Set a reasonable volume and repetition goal (to provide encouragement and give the patient a sense of accomplishment).
- Encourage coughing during and after each session.
- Assist the patient to splint the incision when coughing postoperatively.
- Place the spirometer within easy reach of the patient.
- For the postoperative patient, begin the therapy immediately. (If the patient begins to hypoventilate, atelectasis can start to occur within an hour.)
- Record how effectively the patient performs the therapy and the number of breaths achieved with the spirometer every 2 hours.

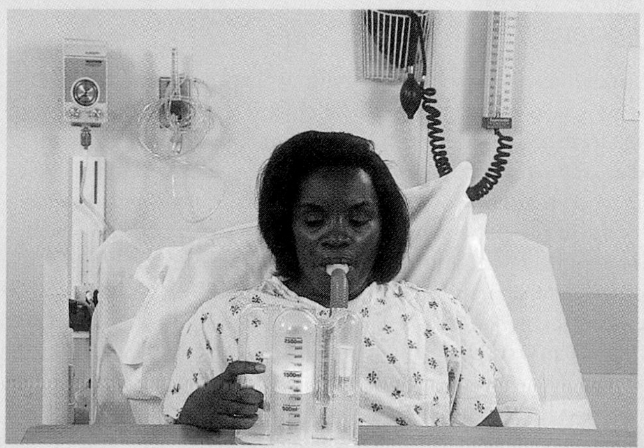

© B. Proud.

used for patients with COPD to dispense inhaled medications and are commonly used at home on a long-term basis.

Promoting Home and Community-Based Care

TEACHING PATIENTS SELF-CARE

The nurse instructs the patient to breathe through the mouth, taking slow, deep breaths, and then to hold the breath for a few seconds at the end of inspiration to increase intrapleural pressure and reopen collapsed alveoli, thereby increasing functional residual capacity. The nurse encourages the patient to cough and to monitor the effectiveness of the therapy. The nurse instructs the patient and family about the purpose of the treatment, equipment set-up, medication additive, and proper cleaning and storage of the equipment.

Incentive Spirometry (Sustained Maximal Inspiration)

The incentive spirometer gives visual feedback to help the patient inhale slowly and deeply to maximize lung inflation. Ideally, the patient assumes a sitting or semi-Fowler's position to enhance diaphragmatic excursion. However, this procedure may be performed with the patient in any position.

Incentive spirometers may be one of two types: volume or flow. In the volume type, the tidal volume of the spirometer is set according to the manufacturer's instructions. The purpose of the device is to ensure that the volume of air inhaled is increased gradually as the patient takes deeper and deeper breaths. The patient takes a deep breath through the mouthpiece, pauses at peak lung inflation, and then relaxes and exhales. Taking several normal breaths before attempting another with the incentive spirometer helps avoid fatigue. The volume is periodically increased as tolerated.

A flow spirometer has the same purpose as a volume spirometer, but the volume is not preset. The spirometer contains a number of movable balls that are pushed up by the force of the breath and held suspended in the air while the patient inhales. The amount of air inhaled and the flow of the air are estimated by how long and how high the balls are suspended.

Indications

Incentive spirometry is used after surgery, especially thoracic and abdominal surgery, to promote the expansion of the alveoli and to prevent or treat atelectasis. As a preventive measure, incentive spirometry may be more effective than IPPB because it maximizes the amount of air inhaled while maintaining relatively low airway pressures.

Nursing Management

Nursing management of the patient using incentive spirometry includes placing the patient in the proper position, teaching the technique for using the incentive spirometer, setting realistic goals for the patient, and recording the results of the therapy.

Chest Physiotherapy

Chest physiotherapy includes **postural drainage, chest percussion and vibration**, and breathing exercises/breathing retraining. In addition, teaching the patient effective coughing technique is an important part of chest physiotherapy. The goals of chest physiotherapy are to remove bronchial secretions, improve ventilation, and increase the efficiency of the respiratory muscles.

Postural Drainage (Segmented Bronchial Drainage)

Postural drainage uses specific positions that allow the force of gravity to assist in the removal of bronchial secretions. The secretions drain from the affected bronchioles into the bronchi and trachea and are removed by coughing or suctioning. It is used to prevent or relieve bronchial obstruction caused by accumulation of secretions.

Because the patient usually sits in an upright position, secretions are likely to accumulate in the lower parts of the lungs. With postural drainage, different positions (Fig. 22-2) are used so that the force of gravity helps to move secretions from the smaller bronchial airways to the main bronchi and trachea. The secretions then are removed by coughing. Instructing the patient to inhale prescribed bronchodilators and mucolytic agents before postural drainage assists in draining the bronchial tree.

Postural drainage exercises can be directed at any of the segments of the lungs. The lower and middle lobe bronchi drain more effectively when the head is down; the upper lobe bronchi drain more effectively when the head is up. Frequently, five positions are used, one for drainage of each lobe: head down, prone, right and left lateral, and sitting upright.

Nursing Management

The nurse should be aware of the patient's diagnosis as well as the lung lobes or segments involved, the cardiac status, and any structural deformities of the chest wall and spine. Auscultating the chest before and after the procedure helps to identify the areas needing drainage and to assess the effectiveness of treatment. The nurse teaches family members who will be assisting the patient at home to evaluate breath sounds before and after treatment. The nurse explores strategies that will enable the patient to assume indicated positions at home. This may require the creative use of objects readily available at home, such as pillows, cushions, or cardboard boxes.

Postural drainage is usually performed two to four times daily, before meals (to prevent nausea, vomiting, and aspiration) and at bedtime. Prescribed bronchodilators, water, or saline may be nebulized and inhaled before postural drainage to dilate the bronchioles, reduce bronchospasm, decrease the thickness of mucus and sputum, and combat edema of the bronchial walls.

The nurse makes the patient as comfortable as possible in each position and provides an emesis basin, sputum cup, and paper

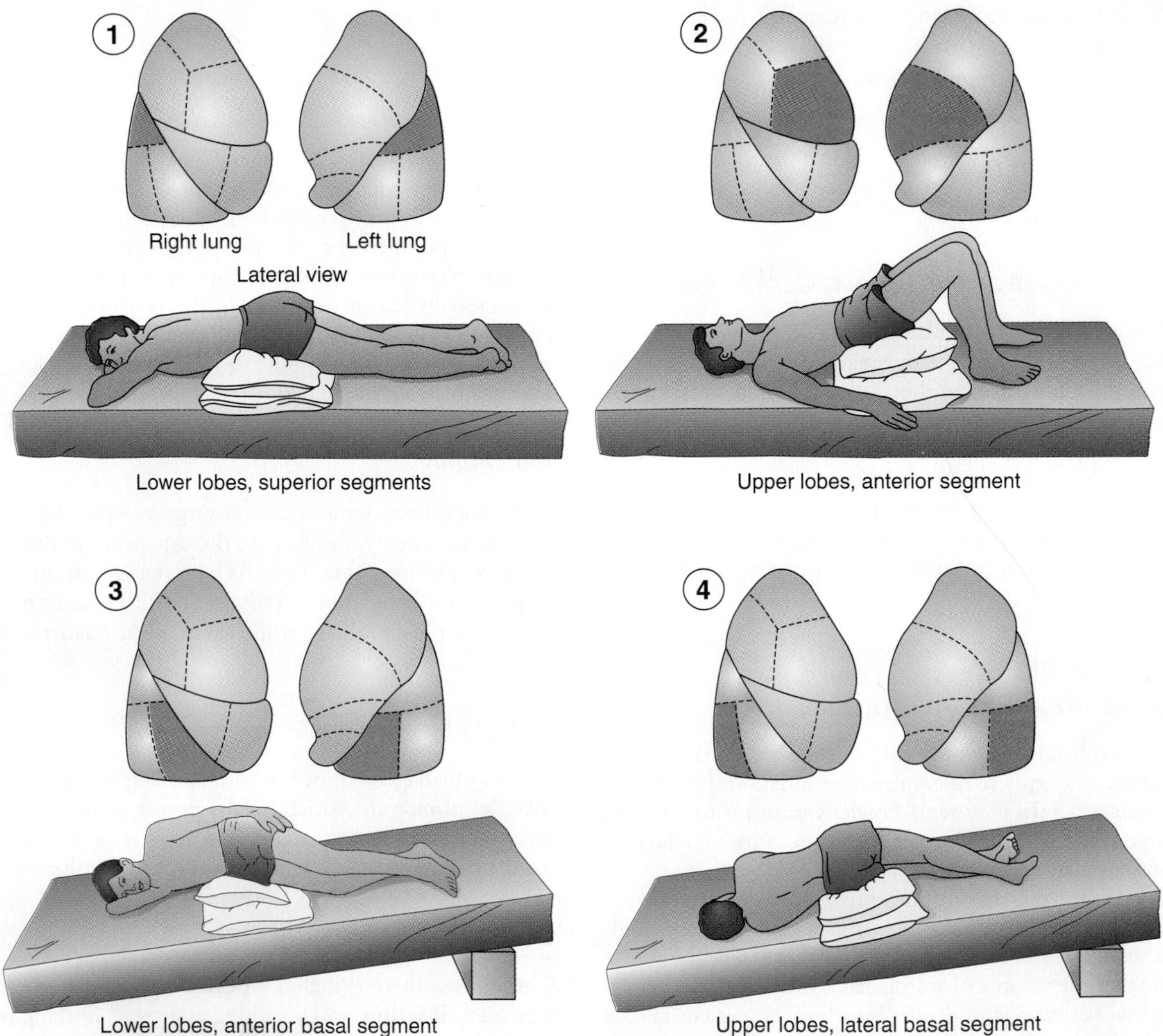

FIGURE 22•2 Postural drainage positions and the areas of lung drained by each position.

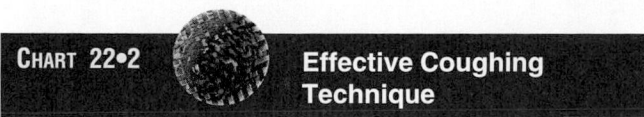

CHART 22•2 **Effective Coughing Technique**

1. The patient assumes a sitting position and bends slightly forward. This upright position permits a stronger cough.
2. The knees and hips are flexed to promote relaxation and reduce the strain on the abdominal muscles while coughing.
3. The patient inhales slowly through the nose and exhales through pursed lips several times.
4. The patient should cough twice during each exhalation while contracting (pulling in) the abdomen sharply with each cough.
5. The patient splints the incisional area, if any, with firm hand pressure or supports it with a pillow or rolled blanket while coughing. (The nurse can initially demonstrate this by using the patient's hands.)

tissues. The nurse instructs the patient to remain in each position for 10 to 15 minutes and to breathe in slowly through the nose and then breathe out slowly through pursed lips to help keep the airways open so that secretions can drain while in each position. If a position cannot be tolerated, the nurse helps the patient to assume a modified position. When the patient changes position, the nurse explains how to cough and remove secretions (Chart 22-2).

If the patient cannot cough, the nurse may need to suction the secretions mechanically. It also may be necessary to use chest percussion and vibration to loosen bronchial secretions and mucus plugs that adhere to the bronchioles and bronchi and to propel sputum in the direction of gravity drainage. If suctioning is required at home, the nurse instructs caregivers in safe suctioning technique.

After the procedure, the nurse notes the amount, color, viscosity, and character of the ejected sputum. It is important to evaluate the patient's skin color and pulse the first few times the procedure is performed. It may be necessary to administer oxygen during postural drainage.

If the sputum is foul-smelling, it is important to perform postural drainage in a room away from other patients and/or family members and to use deodorizers. After the procedure, the patient may find it refreshing to brush the teeth and use a mouthwash before resting.

Chest Percussion and Vibration

Thick secretions that are difficult to cough up may be loosened by tapping (percussing) and vibrating the chest. Chest percussion and vibration help to dislodge mucus adhering to the bronchioles and bronchi.

Percussion is carried out by cupping the hands and lightly striking the chest wall in a rhythmic fashion over the lung segment to be drained. The wrists are alternately flexed and extended so that the chest is cupped or clapped in a painless manner (Fig. 22-3). A soft cloth or towel may be placed over the segment of the chest that is being cupped to prevent skin irritation and redness from direct contact. Percussion, alternating with vibration, is performed for 3 to 5 minutes for each position. The patient uses diaphragmatic breathing during this procedure to promote relaxation (see the section on breathing retraining below). As a precaution, percussion over chest drainage tubes, the sternum, spine, liver, kidneys, spleen, or breasts (in women) is avoided. Percussion is performed cautiously in the elderly because of their increased incidence of osteoporosis and risk of rib fracture.

Vibration is the technique of applying manual compression and tremor to the chest wall during the exhalation phase of respiration (see Fig. 22-3). This helps to increase the velocity of the air expired from the small airways, thus freeing the mucus. After three or four vibrations, the patient is encouraged to cough, using the abdominal muscles. (Contracting the abdominal muscles increases the effectiveness of the cough.)

A scheduled program of coughing and clearing sputum, together with hydration, reduces sputum in most patients. The number of times the percussion and vibration cycle is repeated depends on the patient's tolerance and clinical response. It is important to evaluate breath sounds before and after the procedures.

Nursing Management

When performing chest physiotherapy, it is important to make sure the patient is comfortable, is not wearing restrictive clothing, and has not just eaten a meal. The uppermost areas of the lung are

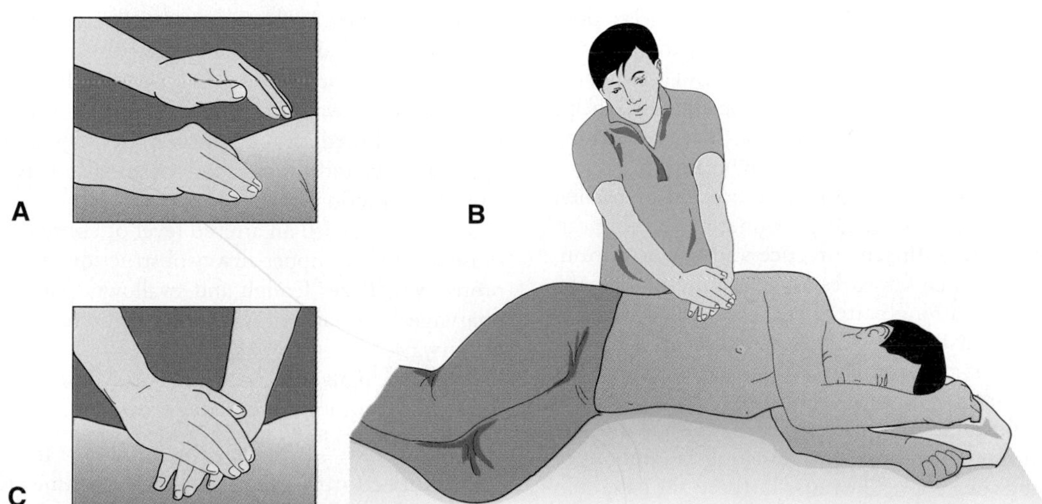

FIGURE 22•3 Percussion and vibration. (**A**) Proper hand position for percussion. (**B**) Proper technique for vibration. The wrists and elbows remain stiff and the vibrating motion is produced by the shoulder muscles. (**C**) Proper hand position for vibration.

treated first. The nurse gives medication for pain, as prescribed, before percussion and vibration and splints the incision and provides pillows for support as needed. The positions are varied, but focus is placed on the affected areas. On completion of the treatment, the nurse assists the patient to assume a comfortable position.

The nurse must stop treatment if any of the following symptoms occur: increased pain, increased shortness of breath, weakness, light-headedness, or hemoptysis. Therapy is indicated until the patient has normal respirations, can mobilize secretions, and has normal breath sounds, and when the chest x-ray is normal.

PROMOTING HOME AND COMMUNITY-BASED CARE

Teaching Patients Self-Care. Chest physiotherapy is frequently indicated at home for patients with COPD, bronchiectasis, and cystic fibrosis. The techniques are the same as described above, but gravity drainage is achieved by placing the hips over a box, a stack of magazines, or pillows (unless a hospital bed is available). The nurse instructs the patient and family in the positions and techniques of percussion and vibration so that therapy can be continued in the home. In addition, the nurse instructs the patient to maintain an adequate fluid intake and air humidity to prevent secretions from becoming thick and tenacious. It also is important to teach the patient to recognize early signs of infection, such as fever and a change in the color or character of sputum. Resting 5 to 10 minutes in each postural drainage position before chest physiotherapy maximizes the amount of secretions obtained.

Continuing Care. Chest physical therapy may be carried out during visits by a home care nurse. The nurse also assesses the patient's physical status, understanding of the treatment plan, and compliance with recommended therapy and the effectiveness of therapy. It is important to reinforce patient and family teaching during these visits. The nurse reports deterioration of the patient's physical status and inability to clear secretions to the patient's physician.

Breathing Retraining

Breathing retraining consists of exercises and breathing practices designed to achieve more efficient and controlled ventilation and to decrease the work of breathing. Breathing retraining is especially indicated in patients with COPD and dyspnea. These exercises enhance maximal alveolar inflation, promote muscle relaxation, relieve anxiety, eliminate ineffective, uncoordinated patterns of respiratory muscle activity, slow the respiratory rate, and decrease the work of breathing. Slow, relaxed, and rhythmic breathing also helps to control the anxiety that occurs with dyspnea. Specific breathing exercises include diaphragmatic and pursed-lip breathing.

The goal of diaphragmatic breathing is to use and strengthen the diaphragm during breathing. Diaphragmatic breathing can become automatic with sufficient practice and concentration. Pursed-lip breathing, which improves oxygen transport, helps to induce a slow, deep breathing pattern and assists the patient to control breathing, even during periods of stress. This type of breathing helps prevent airway collapse secondary to loss of lung elasticity in emphysema. The goal of pursed-lip breathing is to train the muscles of expiration to prolong exhalation and increase airway pressure during expiration, thus lessening the amount of airway trapping and resistance. The nurse instructs the patient in diaphragmatic breathing and pursed-lip breathing (see the chart on breathing exercises earlier in this chapter). Breathing exercises may be practiced in several positions because air distribution and pulmonary circulation vary with the position of the chest. Many patients require additional oxygen, using a low-flow method, while performing breathing exercises. Emphysema-like changes in the lung occur as part of the natural aging process of the lung; therefore, breathing exercises are appropriate for all elderly patients who are hospitalized and elderly patients in any setting who are sedentary, even without primary lung disease.

PROMOTING HOME AND COMMUNITY-BASED CARE

Teaching Patients Self-Care. The nurse instructs the patient to breathe slowly and rhythmically in a relaxed manner and to exhale completely to empty the lungs. The nurse instructs the patient always to inhale through the nose because this filters, humidifies, and warms the air. If short of breath, the patient should concentrate on breathing slowly and rhythmically. To avoid initiating a cycle of increasing shortness of breath and panic, it is often helpful to instruct the patient to concentrate on prolonging the length of exhalation rather than merely slowing down the rate of breathing. Minimizing the amount of dust or particles in the air and providing adequate humidification may also make it easier for the patient to breathe.

AIRWAY MANAGEMENT

Adequate ventilation is dependent on free movement of air through the upper and lower airways. In many conditions, the airway becomes narrowed or blocked as a result of disease, bronchoconstriction (narrowing of airway by contraction of muscle fibers), a foreign body, or secretions. Maintaining a patent (open) airway is achieved through meticulous airway management, whether in an emergency situation such as airway obstruction or in long-term management, as in caring for a patient with an endotracheal or a **tracheostomy tube**.

Emergency Management of Upper Airway Obstruction

Upper airway obstruction has a variety of causes. Acute upper airway obstruction may be caused by food particles, vomitus, blood clots, or any other particle that enters and obstructs the larynx or trachea. It also may occur from enlargement of tissue in the wall of the airway, as in epiglottitis, laryngeal edema, laryngeal carcinoma, or peritonsillar abscess, or from thick secretions. Pressure on the walls of the airway, as occurs in retrosternal goiter, enlarged mediastinal lymph nodes, hematoma around the upper airway, and thoracic aneurysm, also may result in upper airway obstruction.

The patient with an altered level of consciousness from any cause is at risk for upper airway obstruction because of loss of the protective reflexes (cough and swallowing) and the tone of the pharyngeal muscles, causing the tongue to fall back and block the airway.

The nurse makes the following rapid observations to assess for signs and symptoms of upper airway obstruction:

- Inspection—Is the patient conscious? Is there any inspiratory effort? Does the chest rise symmetrically? Is there use or retraction of accessory muscles? What is the skin color? Are there any obvious signs of deformity or obstruction (trauma, food, teeth, vomitus)? Is the trachea midline?

- Palpation—Do both sides of the chest rise equally with inspiration? Are there any specific areas of tenderness, fracture, or subcutaneous emphysema (crepitus)?
- Auscultation—Is there any audible air movement, stridor (inspiratory sound), or wheezing (expiratory sound)? Are breath sounds present bilaterally in all lobes?

As soon as an upper airway obstruction is identified, the nurse takes emergency measures (Guideline 22-1).

Endotracheal Intubation

Endotracheal intubation involves passing an endotracheal tube through the mouth or nose into the trachea (Fig. 22-4). Intubation provides a patent airway when the patient is having respiratory distress that cannot be treated by simpler methods. It is the method of choice in emergency care. Endotracheal intubation is a means of providing an airway for patients who cannot maintain an adequate airway on their own (eg, comatose patients or patients with upper airway obstruction), for mechanical ventilation, and for suctioning secretions from the pulmonary tree.

An endotracheal tube usually is passed with the aid of a laryngoscope by specifically trained medical, nursing, or respiratory therapy personnel. Once the tube is inserted, a cuff around the tube is inflated to prevent air from leaking around the outer part of the tube, to minimize the possibility of subsequent aspiration, and to prevent movement of the tube.

Suctioning of the tracheobronchial secretions is performed through the tube. Warmed, humidified oxygen should always be introduced through the tube, whether the patient is breathing spontaneously or is on ventilatory support. Endotracheal intubation may be used for no more than 3 weeks, by which time a tracheostomy must be considered to decrease irritation of and trauma to the tracheal lining, to reduce the incidence of vocal cord paralysis (secondary to laryngeal nerve damage), and to decrease the work of breathing. Guideline 22-2 discusses nursing care of the patient with an endotracheal tube.

There are several disadvantages of endotracheal and tracheostomy tubes. First, the tube causes discomfort. In addition, the cough reflex is depressed because closure of the glottis is hindered. Secretions tend to become thicker because the warming and

22•1 Guidelines For Clearing an Upper Airway Obstruction

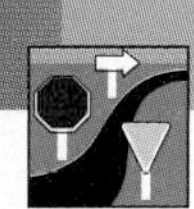

Clearing the Airway

- Hyperextend the patient's neck by placing one hand on the forehead and placing the fingers of the other hand underneath the jaw and lifting upward and forward. This action pulls the tongue away from the back of the pharynx.

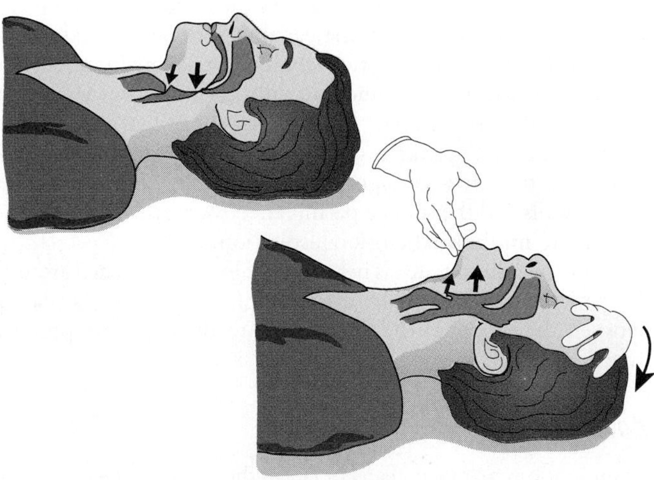

Opening the airway.

- Assess the patient by observing the chest and listening and feeling for the movement of air.
- Use a cross-finger technique to open the mouth and observe for obvious obstructions such as secretions, blood clots, or food particles.

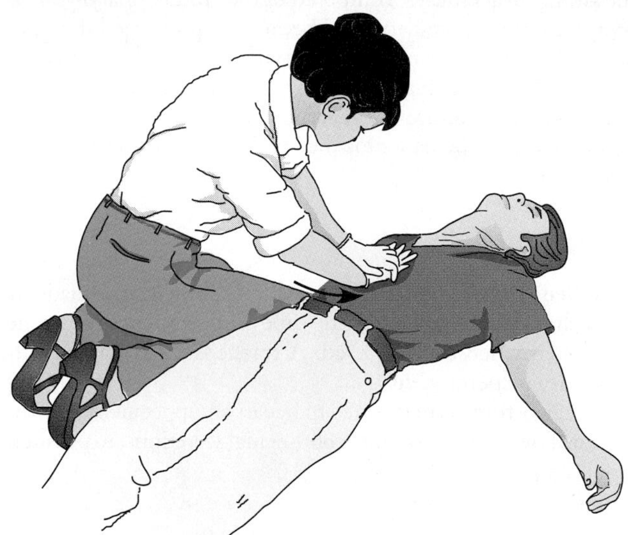

Abdominal thrust (Heimlich) maneuver administered to unconscious patient.

- If no passage of air is detected, apply five quick sharp abdominal thrusts just below the xiphoid process to expel the obstruction (Heimlich maneuver). Repeat this procedure until the obstruction is expelled.
- After the obstruction is expelled, roll the patient as a unit onto the side for recovery.
- When the obstruction is relieved and the patient can breathe spontaneously but not cough, swallow, or gag, insert an oral or nasopharyngeal airway.

(*continued*)

22•1 GUIDELINES FOR

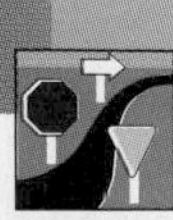

CLEARING AN UPPER AIRWAY OBSTRUCTION (*Continued*)

Bag and Mask Resuscitation

- Use a resuscitation bag and mask if assisted ventilation is required.
- Apply the mask to the patient's face and create a seal by pressing the thumb of the nondominant hand on the bridge of the nose and the index finger on the chin. Use the rest of the fingers on the hand and pull on the chin and the angle of the mandible to maintain the head in extension. Use the dominant hand to inflate the lungs by squeezing the bag to its full volume.

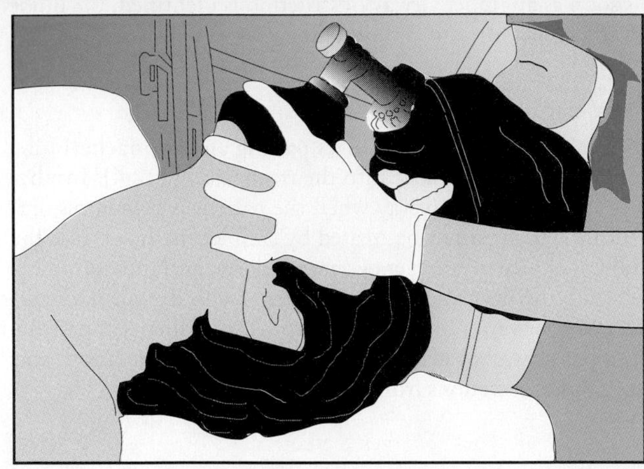

Resuscitation via bag and mask apparatus.

humidifying effect of the upper respiratory tract has been bypassed. The swallowing reflexes, composed of the glottic, pharyngeal, and laryngeal reflexes, are depressed because of prolonged disuse and the mechanical trauma of the endotracheal or tracheostomy tube, which puts the patient at increased risk for aspiration. In addition, ulceration and stricture of the larynx or trachea may develop. Of great concern to the patient is the inability to talk and to communicate needs.

Tracheostomy

A **tracheotomy** is a procedure in which an opening is made into the trachea. When an indwelling tube is inserted into the trachea, the term tracheostomy is used. A tracheostomy may be either temporary or permanent.

A tracheostomy is performed to bypass an upper airway obstruction, to allow removal of tracheobronchial secretions, to permit the long-term use of mechanical ventilation, to prevent aspiration of oral or gastric secretions in the unconscious or paralyzed patient (by closing off the trachea from the esophagus), and to replace an endotracheal tube. There are many disease processes and emergency conditions that make a tracheostomy necessary.

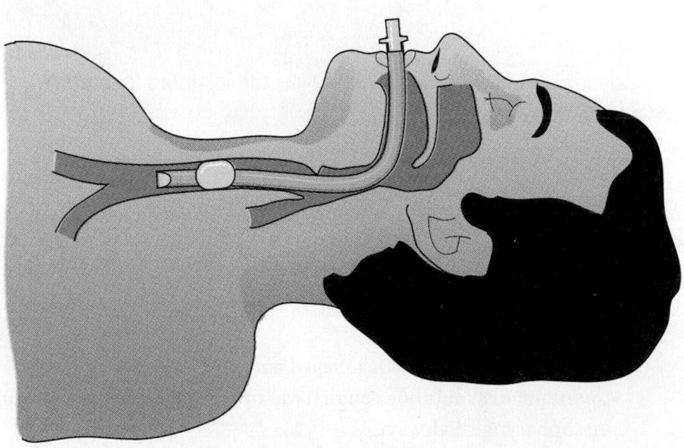

FIGURE 22•4 Endotracheal tube in place.

Procedure

The procedure is usually performed in the operating room or in an intensive care unit, where the patient's ventilation can be well controlled and optimal aseptic technique can be maintained. An opening is made in the second and third tracheal rings. After the trachea is exposed, a cuffed tracheostomy tube of an appropriate size is inserted. The cuff is an inflatable attachment to the tracheostomy tube that is designed to occlude the space between the trachea walls and the tube to permit effective mechanical ventilation and to minimize the risk of aspiration.

The tracheostomy tube is held in place by tapes fastened around the patient's neck. Usually, a square of sterile gauze is placed between the tube and the skin to absorb drainage and prevent infection.

Complications

Complications may occur early or late in the course of tracheostomy tube management. They may even occur years after the tube has been removed. Early complications include bleeding, pneumothorax, air embolism, aspiration, subcutaneous or mediastinal emphysema, recurrent laryngeal nerve damage, and posterior tracheal wall penetration. Long-term complications include airway obstruction from accumulation of secretions or protrusion of the cuff over the opening of the tube, infection, rupture of the innominate artery, dysphagia, tracheoesophageal fistula, tracheal dilation, and tracheal ischemia and necrosis. Tracheal stenosis may develop after the tube is removed.

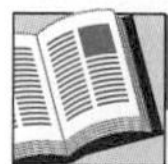

NURSING RESEARCH

Comparing Hyperoxygenation Methods

Grap, M. J., Glass, C., Corley, M., & Parks, M. (1996). Endotracheal suctioning: Ventilator vs. manual delivery of hyperoxygenation breaths. *American Journal of Critical Care, 5*(3), 192–197.

Purpose

Comparison of manually and mechanically delivered hyperoxygenation before and after endotracheal suctioning to determine each method's effectiveness.

Study Sample and Design

The investigators used a quasi-experimental, repeated-measures design to compare manual and mechanical delivery of hyperoxygenation before and after endotracheal suctioning with a convenience sample of 29 mechanically ventilated lung injury patients. When these patients needed to be suctioned, they randomly received either manual or ventilator hyperoxygenation. The next time they needed to be suctioned, the other hyperventilation method was used. Three breaths were given 5 seconds apart before and after each suctioning pass. Ventilator breaths were 100% oxygen breaths at the patient's ordered tidal volume. The manual method used a manual resuscitation bag with an FiO_2 of at least 0.85. A spirometer was used to ensure that manual breaths were ±10% of the patient's ventilator tidal volume. Two passes using normal suctioning technique with an in-line catheter were used. Outcomes studied were arterial blood pressure, arterial blood gas parameters, capillary oxygen saturation, heart rate, and cardiac rhythm.

Findings

Although both techniques prevented hypoxemia, arterial oxygen pressures were significantly higher ($p < 0.01$) and peak inspiratory pressures were lower ($p = 0.01$) using the ventilator method. Mean arterial blood pressure significantly increased with both methods.

Nursing Implications

This study was the first that evaluated the current clinical practice of delivering hyperoxygenation at normal tidal volumes. Although both methods prevented hypoxemia and were safe, ventilator hyperoxygenation was more effective. Based on the findings of this study, clinicians should use the ventilator rather than manual technique to hyperoxygenate patients during suctioning.

22•2 GUIDELINES FOR CARE OF THE PATIENT WITH AN ENDOTRACHEAL TUBE

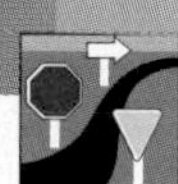

Immediately After Intubation

1. Check symmetry of chest expansion.
   - Auscultate breath sounds of anterior and lateral chest bilaterally.
   - Obtain order for chest x-ray to verify proper tube placement.
2. Ensure high humidity; a visible mist should appear in the T-piece or ventilator tubing.
3. Administer oxygen concentration as prescribed by physician.
4. Secure the tube to the patient's face with tape, and mark the proximal end for position maintenance.
   - Cut proximal end of tube if it is longer than 7.5 cm (3 inches) to prevent kinking.
   - An oral airway or mouth device may be inserted to prevent the patient from biting and obstructing the tube.
5. Use sterile suction technique and airway care to prevent iatrogenic contamination and infection.
6. Continue to reposition patient every 2 hours and as needed to prevent atelectasis and to optimize lung expansion.
7. Provide oral hygiene and suction the oropharynx whenever necessary.

Extubation (Removal of Endotracheal Tube)

1. Explain procedure.
2. Have self-inflating bag and mask ready in case ventilatory assistance is required immediately after extubation.
3. Suction the tracheobronchial tree and oropharynx, remove tape, and then deflate the cuff.
4. Give oxygen for a few breaths, then insert a new, sterile suction catheter inside tube.
5. Have the patient inhale. At peak inspiration remove the tube, suctioning the airway through the tube as it is pulled out.
   Note: In some hospitals this procedure can be performed by respiratory therapists; in others, by nurses. Check hospital policy.

Care of Patient Following Extubation

1. Give heated humidity and oxygen by face mask.
2. Monitor respiratory rate and quality of chest excursions. Note stridor, color change, and change in mental alertness or behavior.
3. Monitor the patient's oxygen level using a pulse oximeter, if available.
4. Keep NPO or give only ice chips for next few hours.
5. Provide mouth care.
6. Teach patient how to perform coughing and deep-breathing exercises.

22•3 GUIDELINES FOR CARE OF THE PATIENT WITH A TRACHEOSTOMY TUBE

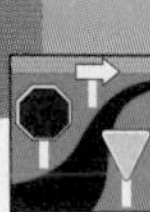

Nursing Intervention	Rationale
1. Gather the needed equipment; including sterile gloves, hydrogen peroxide, normal saline solution or sterile water, cotton-tipped applicators, dressing and twill tape (and the type of tube prescribed, if the tube is changed). A cuffed tube (air injected into cuff) is required during mechanical ventilation. A low-pressure cuff is most commonly used. Patients requiring long-term use of a tracheostomy tube and who can breathe spontaneously commonly use an uncuffed, metal tube.	Everything needed to care for a tracheostomy should be readily on hand for the most effective care. A cuffed tube prevents air from leaking during positive-pressure ventilation and also prevents tracheal aspiration of gastric contents. An adequate seal is indicated by the disappearance of any air leakage from the mouth or tracheostomy or by the disappearance of the harsh, gurgling sound of air coming from the throat. Low-pressure cuffs exert minimal pressure on the tracheal mucosa and thus reduce the danger of tracheal ulceration and stricture.
2. Provide patient and family instruction on the key points for tracheostomy care, beginning with how to inspect the tracheostomy dressing for moisture or drainage.	The tracheostomy dressing is changed as needed to keep the skin clean and dry. To prevent potential breakdown, moist or soiled dressings should not remain on the skin.
3. Wash hands.	Hand washing reduces bacteria on hands.
4. Explain procedure to patient and family as appropriate.	A patient with a tracheostomy is apprehensive and requires ongoing assurance and support.
5. Put on clean gloves; remove and discard the soiled dressing.	Observing body substance isolation reduces cross-contamination from soiled dressings.
6. Prepare sterile supplies, including hydrogen peroxide, normal saline solution or sterile water, cotton-tipped applicators, dressing, and tape.	Having necessary supplies and equipment readily available allows the procedure to be completed efficiently.
7. Put on sterile gloves. (Some physicians approve clean technique for long-term tracheostomy patients in the home.)	Sterile equipment minimizes transmission of surface flora to the sterile respiratory tract. Clean technique may be used in the home because of decreased exposure to potential pathogens.
8. Cleanse the wound and plate of the tracheostomy tube with sterile cotton-tipped applicators moistened with hydrogen peroxide. Rinse with sterile saline solution.	Hydrogen peroxide is effective in loosening crusted secretions. Rinsing prevents skin residue.
9. Soak inner cannula in peroxide and rinse with saline solution or replace with a new disposable inner cannula.	Soaking loosens and removes secretions from the inner lumen of the tracheostomy tube.
10. Remove soiled twill tape with clean tape, after the new tape is in place. Place clean twill tape in position to secure the tracheostomy tube by inserting one end of the tape through the side opening of the outer cannula. Take the tape around the back of the patient's neck and thread it through the opposite opening of the outer cannula. Bring both ends around so that they meet on one side of the neck. Tighten the tape until only two fingers can be comfortably inserted under it. Secure with a knot. For a new tracheostomy, two people should assist with tape changes.	This taping technique provides a double thickness of tape around the neck, which is needed because the tracheostomy tube can be dislodged by movement or by a forceful cough if left unsecured. A dislodged tracheostomy tube is difficult to reinsert, and respiratory distress may occur. Dislodgement of a new tracheostomy is a medical emergency.
11. Remove old tapes and discard in a biohazard container.	Tapes with old secretions may harbor bacteria.

(*continued*)

Postoperative Nursing Management

The patient requires continuous monitoring and assessment. The newly made opening must be kept patent by proper suctioning of secretions. After the vital signs are stable, the patient is placed in a semi-Fowler's position to facilitate ventilation, promote drainage, minimize edema, and prevent strain on the suture lines. Analgesia and sedatives must be administered with caution because of the risk of suppressing the cough reflex.

A major objective of nursing care is to alleviate the apprehension of the patient and provide an effective means of communication. Paper and pencil or a Magic Slate and the patient call light are kept within reach to ensure a means of communication. The care of the patient with a tracheostomy tube is summarized in Guideline 22-3.

SUCTIONING THE TRACHEAL TUBE (TRACHEOSTOMY OR ENDOTRACHEAL TUBE)

When a tracheostomy tube or an endotracheal tube is present, it is usually necessary to suction the patient's secretions because the effectiveness of the cough mechanism is decreased. Tracheal suctioning is performed when adventitious breath sounds are detected or whenever secretions are obviously present. Unnecessary suctioning can initiate bronchospasm and cause mechanical trauma to the tracheal mucosa.

22•3 GUIDELINES FOR

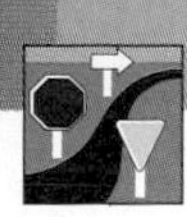

CARE OF THE PATIENT WITH A TRACHEOSTOMY TUBE (Continued)

Nursing Intervention	Rationale
12. Although some long-term tracheostomies with healed stomas may not require a dressing, other tracheostomies do. In such cases, use a sterile tracheostomy dressing, fitting it securely under the twill tapes and flange of tracheostomy tube so that the incision is covered, as shown below.	Healed tracheostomies with minimal secretions do not need a dressing. Dressings that will shred are not used around a tracheostomy because of the risk that pieces of material, lint, or thread may get into the tube, and eventually into the trachea, causing obstruction or abscess formation. Special dressings that do not have a tendency to shred are used.

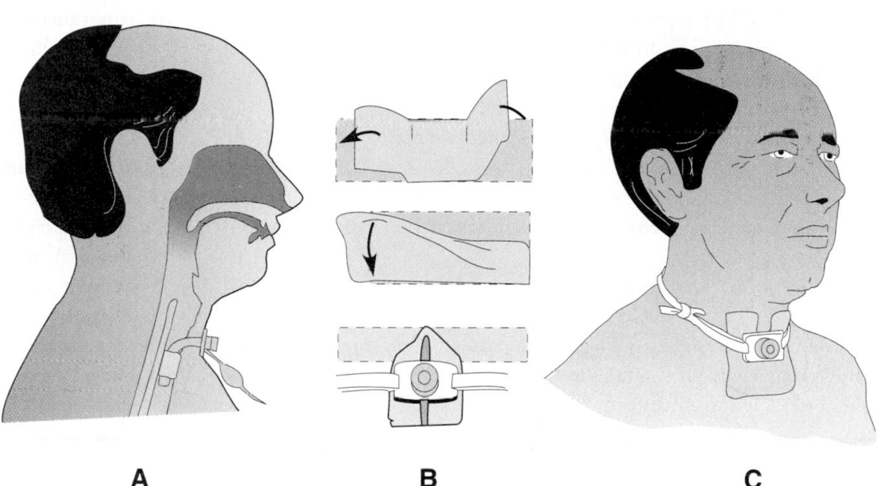

(**A**) The cuff of the tracheostomy tube fits smoothly and snugly in the trachea in a way that promotes circulation but seals off the escape of secretions and air surrounding the tube. (**B**) For a dressing change, a 4 × 4-inch gauze pad may be folded (cutting would promote shredding, placing the patient at risk for aspiration) around the tracheostomy tube and (**C**) stabilized by slipping the neck tape ties through the neck plate slots of the tracheostomy tube. The ties may be fastened to the side of the neck to eliminate the discomfort of lying on the knot.

All equipment that comes into direct contact with the patient's lower airway must be sterile to prevent overwhelming pulmonary and systemic infections. The procedure for suctioning a tracheostomy is presented in Guideline 22-4. In mechanically ventilated patients, an in-line suction catheter may be used to allow rapid suction when needed and to minimize cross-contamination of airborne pathogens. An in-line suction device allows the patient to be suctioned without being disconnected from the ventilator circuit.

MANAGING THE CUFF

As a general rule, the cuff on an endotracheal or tracheostomy tube should be inflated. The pressure within the cuff should be the lowest possible that allows delivery of adequate tidal volumes and prevents pulmonary aspiration. Usually the pressure is maintained at less than 25 cm H_2O to prevent injury and at more than 20 cm H_2O to prevent aspiration. Cuff pressure must be monitored at least every 8 hours by attaching a hand-held pressure gauge to the pilot balloon of the tube or by using minimal leak volume or minimal occlusion volume techniques. With long-term intubation, higher pressures may be needed to maintain an adequate seal.

PROMOTING HOME AND COMMUNITY-BASED CARE

Teaching Patients Self-Care. If the patient is at home with a tracheostomy, the nurse instructs the patient and family about daily care of the tracheostomy as well as measures to take in the event of an emergency. The nurse also makes sure the patient and family are aware of community contacts for education and support needs.

MECHANICAL VENTILATION

Mechanical ventilation may be required for a variety of reasons, including the need to control the patient's respirations during surgery and during treatment of severe head injury, to oxygenate the blood when the patient's ventilatory efforts are inadequate, and to rest the respiratory muscles. Many patients placed on a ventilator can breathe spontaneously but the effort needed to do so may be exhausting to the patient.

A **mechanical ventilator** is a positive- or negative-pressure breathing device that can maintain ventilation and oxygen delivery for a prolonged period. Caring for a patient on mechanical ventilation has become an integral part of nursing care in critical care units, on general medical-surgical units, in extended care facilities, and in the home. Nurses, physicians, and respiratory therapists must understand each patient's specific pulmonary needs and work together to set realistic goals. Essential for positive patient outcomes are understanding the principles of mechanical ventilation and the care needs of the patient, as well as open communication among members of the health care team about the goals of therapy, weaning plans, and the patient's tolerance of changes in ventilator settings.

Indications

If a patient has a continuous decrease in oxygenation (PaO_2), an increase in arterial carbon dioxide levels ($PaCO_2$), and a persistent acidosis (a decreased pH), mechanical ventilation may be necessary. Conditions such as thoracic or abdominal surgery, drug overdose, neuromuscular disorders, inhalation injury, COPD, multiple

22•4 GUIDELINES FOR TRACHEAL SUCTIONING

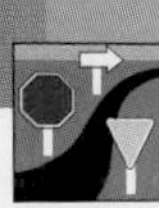

Equipment

- Suction catheters
- Gloves
- Goggles for eye protection
- Basin for sterile normal saline solution for irrigation
- Manual resuscitation bag with supplemental oxygen
- Suction source

Procedure

1. Explain the procedure to the patient before beginning and offer reassurance during suctioning; the patient may be apprehensive about choking and about an inability to communicate.
2. Begin by washing hands thoroughly.
3. Turn on suction source (pressure should not exceed 120 mm Hg).
4. Open suction catheter kit.
5. Fill basin with sterile normal saline solution.
6. Ventilate the patient with manual resuscitation bag and high-flow oxygen.
7. Put sterile glove on dominant hand.
8. Pick up suction catheter in gloved hand and connect to suction.
9. Hyperinflate or hyperoxygenate the patient's lungs for several deep breaths with the manual resuscitation bag. Instill normal saline solution into airway only if there are thick, tenacious secretions.
10. Insert suction catheter at least as far as the end of the tube without applying suction, just far enough to stimulate the cough reflex.
11. Apply suction while withdrawing and gently rotating the catheter 360° (no longer than 10 to 15 seconds, because hypoxia and dysrhythmias may develop, leading to cardiac arrest).
12. Reoxygenate and inflate the patient's lungs for several breaths.
13. Repeat previous three steps until the airway is clear.
14. Rinse catheter in basin with sterile normal saline solution between suction attempts if necessary.
15. Suction oropharyngeal cavity after completing tracheal suctioning.
16. Rinse suction tubing.
17. Discard catheter, gloves, and basin appropriately.

trauma, shock, multisystem failure, and coma all may lead to respiratory failure and the need for mechanical ventilation. The criteria for mechanical ventilation (Chart 22-3) guide the decision to place a patient on a ventilator. A patient with apnea that is not readily reversible also is a candidate for mechanical ventilation.

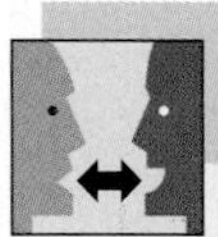

ETHICS AND RELATED ISSUES

What If a Patient Refuses Mechanical Ventilation?

Situation

Mechanical ventilation is a life-support treatment that can be used in a variety of clinical settings for acute and chronic conditions. Does a patient have the right to refuse a life-support treatment that is keeping him or her alive, even when the prognosis with continued treatment is favorable? If the withdrawal of mechanical ventilation results in the patient's death, is the health care provider who removed the ventilator guilty of killing the patient?

Dilemma

The patient's right to refuse treatment conflicts with the health care provider's obligation to help, not harm, the patient (autonomy versus beneficence).

Discussion

- What arguments would you pose in favor of withdrawing mechanical ventilation at the patient's request?
- What arguments would you pose against withdrawing mechanical ventilation at the patient's request?

Classification of Ventilators

Several types of mechanical ventilators exist; they are classified according to the manner in which they support ventilation. The two general categories are negative-pressure and positive-pressure ventilators. The most common category in use today is the positive-pressure ventilator.

Negative-Pressure Ventilators

Negative-pressure ventilators exert a negative pressure on the external chest. Decreasing the intrathoracic pressure during inspiration allows air to flow into the lung, filling its volume. Physiologically, this type of assisted ventilation is similar to spontaneous ventilation. It is used mainly in chronic respiratory failure associated with neuromuscular conditions, such as poliomyelitis, muscular dystrophy, amyotrophic lateral sclerosis, and myasthenia gravis. It is inappropriate for the unstable or complex patient or the patient whose condition requires frequent ventilatory changes. Negative-pressure ventilators are simple to use and do not require intubation of the patient's airway; consequently, they are especially adaptable for home use.

CHART 22•3 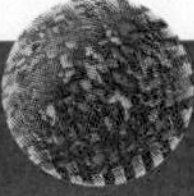 **Indications for Mechanical Ventilation**

$PaO_2 < 50$ mm Hg with $FiO_2 > 0.60$
$PaO_2 > 50$ mm Hg with pH < 7.25
Vital capacity < 2 times tidal volume
Negative inspiratory force < 25 cm H_2O
Respiratory rate > 35/min

There are several types of negative-pressure ventilators: iron lung, body wrap, and chest cuirass.

DRINKER RESPIRATOR TANK (IRON LUNG)

The iron lung is a negative-pressure chamber used for ventilation. It was used extensively during polio epidemics in the past and currently is used by polio survivors and patients with other neuromuscular disorders.

BODY WRAP (PNEUMOWRAP) AND CHEST CUIRASS (TORTOISE SHELL)

Both of these portable devices require a rigid cage or shell to create a negative-pressure chamber around the thorax and abdomen. Because of problems with proper fit and system leaks, these types of ventilators are used only with carefully selected patients.

Positive-Pressure Ventilators

Positive-pressure ventilators inflate the lungs by exerting positive pressure on the airway, similar to a bellows mechanism, forcing the alveoli to expand during inspiration. Expiration occurs passively. Endotracheal intubation or tracheostomy is necessary in most cases. These ventilators are widely used in the hospital setting and are increasingly used in the home for patients with primary lung disease. There are three types of positive-pressure ventilators, which are classified by the method of ending the inspiratory phase of respiration: pressure-cycled, time-cycled, and volume-cycled. Another type of positive-pressure ventilator used for selected patients is noninvasive positive-pressure ventilation.

PRESSURE-CYCLED VENTILATORS

The pressure-cycled ventilator is a positive-pressure ventilator that ends inspiration when a preset pressure has been reached. In other words, the ventilator cycles on, delivers a flow of air until a predetermined pressure is reached, and then cycles off. The major limitation of this type of ventilator is that the volume of air or oxygen can vary as the patient's airway resistance or compliance changes. The result is an inconsistency in the tidal volume delivered and possible compromised ventilation. Consequently, in adults, pressure-cycled ventilators are intended only for short-term use. The most common type is the IPPB machine.

TIME-CYCLED VENTILATORS

Time-cycled ventilators terminate or control inspiration after a preset time. The volume of air the patient receives is regulated by the length of inspiration and the flow rate of the air. Most ventilators have a rate control that determines the respiratory rate, but pure time-cycling is rarely used for adults. These ventilators are used in newborns and infants.

VOLUME-CYCLED VENTILATORS

Volume-cycled ventilators are by far the most commonly used positive-pressure ventilators today (Fig. 22-5). With this type of ventilator, the volume of air to be delivered with each inspiration is preset. Once this preset volume is delivered to the patient, the ventilator cycles off and exhalation occurs passively. From breath to breath, the volume of air delivered by the ventilator is relatively constant, ensuring consistent, adequate breaths despite varying airway pressures.

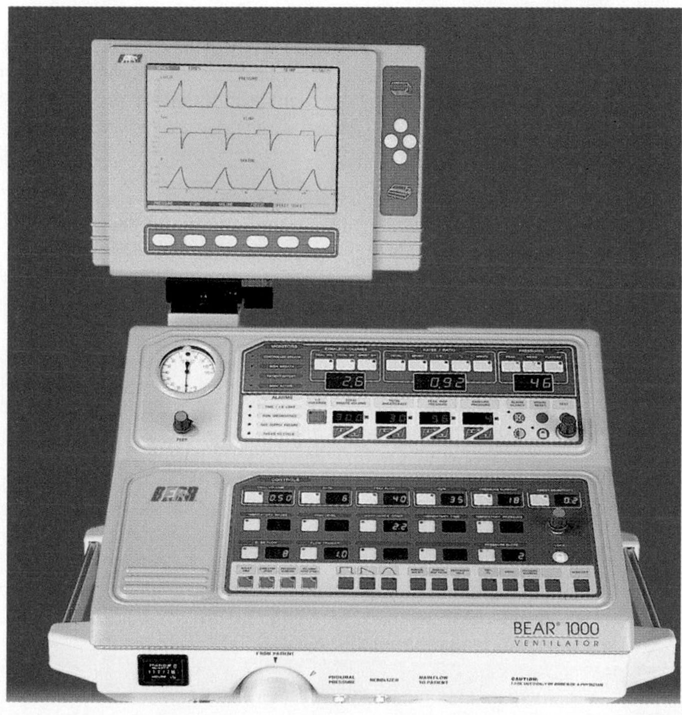

A

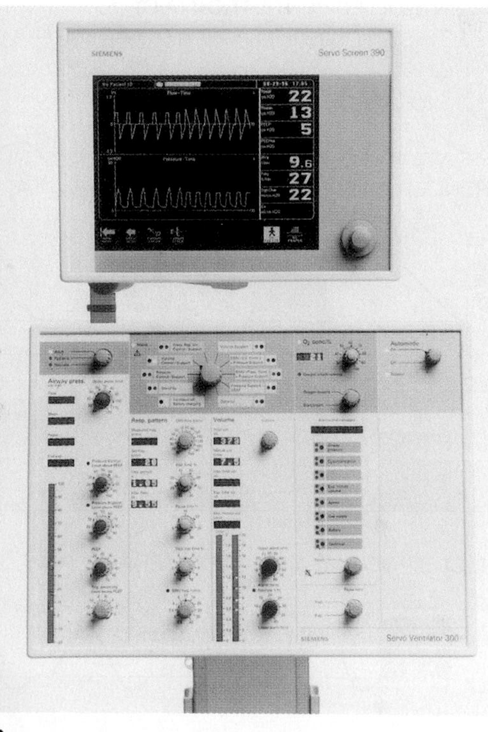

B

FIGURE 22•5 Control panels of ventilators in current use illustrate functions made possible by technologic advances. (**A**) Bear 1000 ventilator. Courtesy Bear Medical Systems. (**B**) Servo Ventilator 300 with Automode allows weaning to begin with the patient still intubated. Courtesy Siemens Medical Systems, Inc.

NONINVASIVE POSITIVE-PRESSURE VENTILATION

Positive-pressure ventilation can be given via face masks that cover the nose and mouth, nasal masks, or other nasal devices. This eliminates the need for endotracheal intubation or tracheostomy. Ventilation can be delivered by a volume ventilator, pressure-controlled ventilator, continuous positive airway device, or bilevel positive airway pressure (bi-PAP) ventilator. The most comfortable mode for the patient is pressure-controlled ventilation with pressure support. This eases the work of breathing and enhances gas exchange. The ventilator can be set with a minimum backup rate for patients with periods of apnea.

Patients are considered for noninvasive ventilation if they have acute or chronic respiratory failure, acute pulmonary edema, COPD, or chronic congestive heart failure with a sleep-related breathing disorder. The device also may be used at home to improve tissue oxygenation and to rest the respiratory muscles while the patient sleeps at night. Critically ill patients and cognitively impaired patients are not candidates for this therapy. Unique nursing considerations for patients with noninvasive positive-pressure ventilation include assessment for nasal mask intolerance, facial skin breakdown, and eye irritation (Hillberg & Johnson, 1997).

Bi-PAP ventilation offers independent control of inspiratory and expiratory pressures while providing pressure support ventilation. It is provided via a nasal or oral mask, nasal pillow, or mouthpiece with a tight seal and a portable ventilator. It is most often used for patients who require ventilatory assistance at night, such as patients with severe COPD or sleep apnea. Tolerance is variable; it is usually most successful with highly motivated patients.

Adjusting the Ventilator

The ventilator is adjusted so that the patient is comfortable and "in sync" with the machine. Minimal alteration of the normal cardiovascular and pulmonary dynamics is desired. Modes of mechanical ventilation are described in Figure 22-6. If the volume ventilator is adjusted appropriately, the patient's arterial blood gas values will

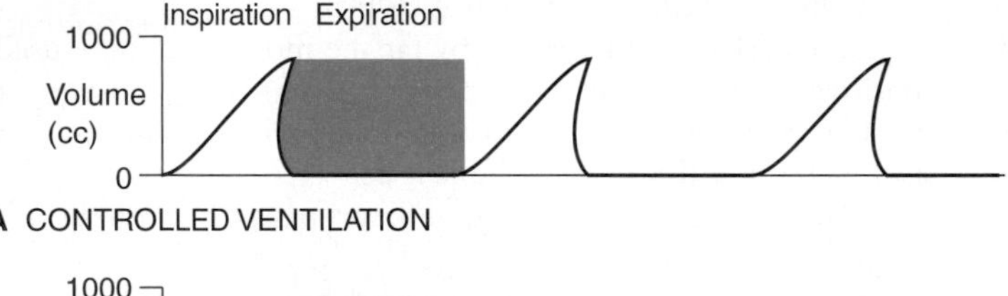

A Flow in the controlled ventilation mode. A preset volume of gas is delivered to the patient under positive pressure while spontaneous patient respiratory effort is "locked out."

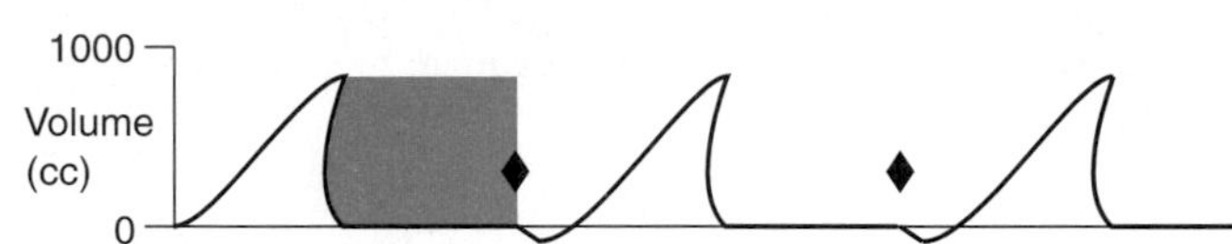

B Gas flow in the assist/control ventilation mode. In this mode, a preset volume of gas is delivered to the patient at a preset rate, but the patient may trigger a ventilator breath with negative inspiratory effort.

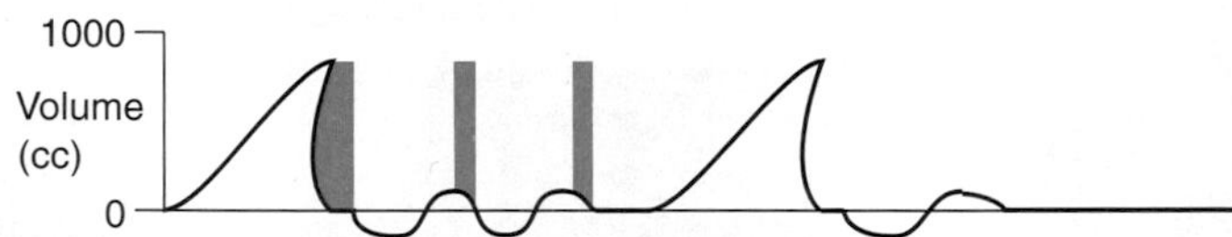

C Gas flow in the synchronized intermittent mandatory ventilation (SIMV) mode. A preset minimum number of breaths are synchronously delivered to the patient but the patient may also take spontaneous breaths of varying volumes. Note how inspiratory and expiratory pressures differ between spontaneous and ventilator breaths.

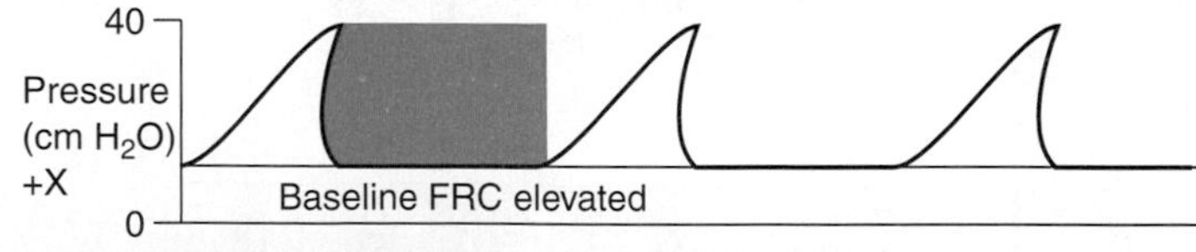

D Airway pressure with varying levels of positive end-expiratory pressure (PEEP). Note that at end expiration, the airway is not allowed to return to zero.

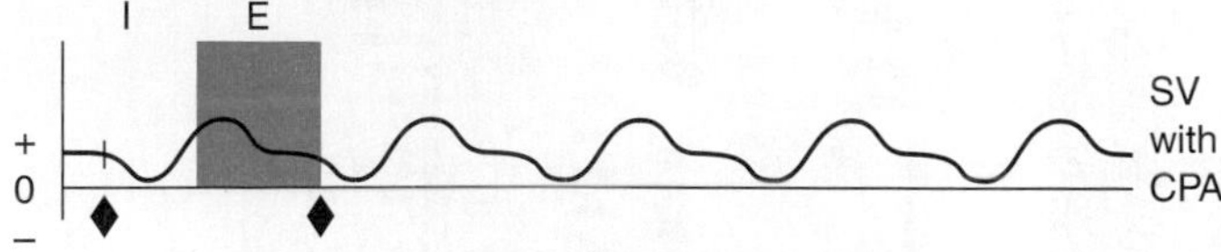

E Spontaneous ventilation with continous positive airway pressure (CPAP). This ventilatory adjunct is used only with spontaneous ventilation; the patient breathes spontaneously through the ventilator at an elevated baseline pressure throughout the breathing cycle.

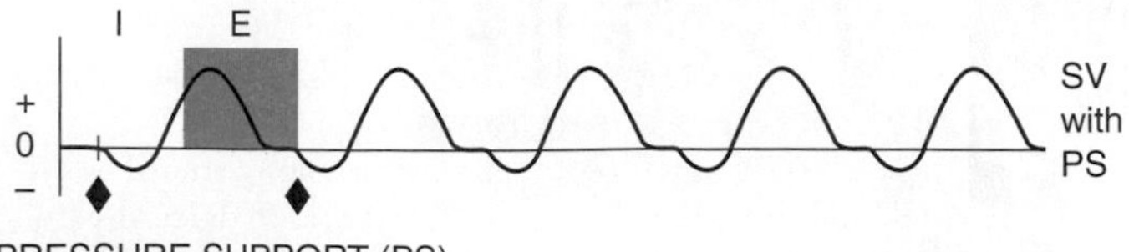

F Spontaneous ventilation with pressure support (PS). The patient breathes spontaneously with pressure assistance to each spontaneous inspiration.

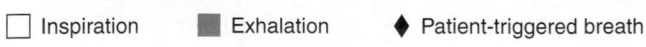

☐ Inspiration ■ Exhalation ♦ Patient-triggered breath

FIGURE 22•6 Modes of mechanical ventilation with air flow waveforms.

be satisfactory and there will be little or no cardiovascular compromise. Guideline 22-5 discusses how to achieve adequate mechanical ventilation for each patient.

Assessing the Equipment

The ventilator also needs to be assessed to make sure that it is functioning properly and that the settings are appropriate. Even though the nurse is not primarily responsible for adjusting the settings on the ventilator or measuring ventilator parameters (usually the responsibility of the respiratory therapist), the nurse is responsible for the patient and therefore needs to evaluate how the ventilator affects the patient's overall status.

In monitoring the ventilator, the nurse should note the following:

- Type of ventilator (volume-cycled, pressure-cycled, negative-pressure)
- Controlling mode (**controlled ventilation, assist–control ventilation, synchronized intermittent mandatory ventilation**)
- Tidal volume and rate settings (tidal volume is usually 10 to 15 mL/kg; rate is usually 12 to 16/min)
- FiO_2 (**fraction of inspired oxygen**) setting
- Inspiratory pressure reached and pressure limit (normal is 15 to 20 cm H_2O; this increases in conditions where there is increased airway resistance or decreased compliance)
- Sensitivity (a 2-cm H_2O inspiratory force should trigger the ventilator)
- Inspiratory-to-expiratory ratio (usually 1 : 3 [1 second of inspiration to 3 seconds of expiration] or 1 : 2)
- Minute volume (tidal volume × respiratory rate, usually 6 to 8 L/min)
- Sigh settings (usually 1.5 times the tidal volume and range from 1 to 3 per hour), if applicable
- Water in the tubing, disconnection or kinking of the tubing
- Humidification (humidifier filled with water) and temperature
- Alarms (functioning properly)
- PEEP and/or pressure support level, if applicable. PEEP is usually 5 to 15 cm H_2O.

Nursing Alert *If a malfunction of the ventilator system occurs and if the problem cannot be identified and corrected immediately, the nurse must be prepared to ventilate the patient with a manual resuscitation bag until the problem is resolved.*

Problems With Mechanical Ventilation

Because of the seriousness of the patient's condition and the highly complex and technical nature of mechanical ventilation, a number of problems or complications can occur. Such situations basically fall into two categories: ventilator problems or actual patient problems. In either case, the patient must be supported while the problem is being identified and corrected. Ventilator complications include cardiovascular compromise, pneumothorax, and pulmonary infection. These problems, their probable causes, and solutions are listed in Table 22-2.

BUCKING THE VENTILATOR

The patient is in synchrony with the ventilator when thoracic expansion coincides with the inspiratory phase of the machine and exhalation occurs passively. The patient is said to fight or buck the ventilator when out of phase with the machine. This is manifested when the patient attempts to breathe out during the ventilator's mechanical inspiratory phase or when there is jerky and increased abdominal muscle effort. The following factors contribute to this problem: anxiety, hypoxia, increased secretions, hypercarbia, inadequate minute volume, and pulmonary edema. These problems must be corrected before resorting to the use of paralyzing agents to reduce bucking; otherwise, the underlying problem is simply masked and the patient's condition will continue to deteriorate.

Muscle relaxants, tranquilizers, analgesics, and paralyzing agents are sometimes given to patients on mechanical ventilation. Their purpose is ultimately to increase the patient–machine synchrony by decreasing the patient's anxiety, hyperventilation, or excessive muscle activity. The selection and dose of the appropriate drug are determined carefully and are based on the patient's requirements and the cause of his or her restlessness. Paralyzing agents are always used as a last resort, and always in conjunction with a sedative.

22•5 GUIDELINES FOR INITIAL VENTILATOR SETTINGS

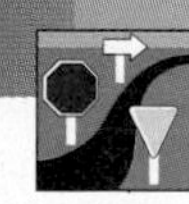

The following guide is an example of the steps involved in operating a mechanical ventilator. In practice, the nurse always reviews the manufacturer's instructions, which vary according to the equipment, before beginning mechanical ventilation.

1. Set the machine to deliver the tidal volume required (10 to 15 mL/kg).
2. Adjust the machine to deliver the lowest concentration of oxygen to maintain normal PaO_2 (80 to 100 mm Hg). This setting may be high initially but gradually reduced based on arterial blood gas results.
3. Record peak inspiratory pressure.
4. Set mode (assist–control or synchronized intermittent mandatory ventilation) and rate according to physician order. (See the glossary for definitions of modes of mechanical ventilation.) Set PEEP and pressure support if ordered.
5. Adjust sensitivity so that the patient can trigger the ventilator with a minimal effort (usually 2 mm Hg negative inspiratory force).
6. Record minute volume and measure carbon dioxide partial pressure (PCO_2), pH, and PO_2 after 20 minutes of continuous mechanical ventilation.
7. Adjust setting (FiO_2 and rate) according to results of arterial blood gas analysis to provide normal values or those set by the physician.
8. If the patient suddenly becomes confused or agitated or begins bucking the ventilator for some unexplained reason, assess for hypoxia and manually ventilate on 100% oxygen with a resuscitation bag.

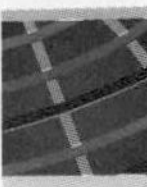

TABLE 22•2 Ventilator Problems

Problem	Cause	Solution
Ventilator		
Increase in peak airway pressure	Coughing or plugged airway tube	Suction airway for secretions, empty condensation fluid from circuit.
	Patient "bucking" ventilator	Adjust sensitivity.
	Decreasing lung compliance	Manually ventilate patient. Assess for hypoxia or bronchospasm. Check blood gases. Sedate only if necessary.
	Tubing kinked	Check tubing; reposition patient; insert oral airway if necessary.
	Pneumothorax	Manually ventilate patient; notify physician.
	Atelectasis or bronchospasm	Clear secretions.
Decrease in pressure or loss of volume	Increase in compliance	None
	Leak in ventilator or tubing; cuff on tube/humidifier not tight	Check entire ventilator circuit for patency. Correct leak.
Patient		
Cardiovascular compromise	Decrease in venous return due to application of positive pressure to lungs	Assess for adequate volume status by measuring heart rate, blood pressure, central venous pressure, pulmonary capillary wedge pressure, and urine output. Notify physician if values are abnormal.
Barotrauma/pneumothorax	Application of positive pressure to lungs; high mean airway pressures lead to alveolar rupture	Notify physician. Prepare patient for chest tube insertion. Avoid high pressure settings for patients with COPD, ARDS, or history of pneumothorax.
Pulmonary infection	Bypass of normal defense mechanisms; frequent breaks in ventilator circuit; decreased mobility; impaired cough reflex	Meticulous aseptic technique Frequent mouth care Optimize nutritional status.

Promoting Home and Community-Based Care

Increasingly, patients are being cared for in extended care facilities or their homes while on mechanical ventilators, with tracheostomy tubes, or on oxygen therapy. Patients on home ventilator care usually have chronic neuromuscular conditions or COPD.

TEACHING PATIENTS SELF-CARE

Caring for the patient with mechanical ventilator support at home can be accomplished quite successfully. The family must be emotionally, educationally, and physically able to assume the role of primary caregiver. A home care team consisting of nurse, physician, respiratory therapist, social service or home care agency, and equipment supplier needs to be available. The home itself is evaluated to determine if it is adequate for the safe operation of all electrical equipment. A summary of the basic assessment criteria needed for successful home care is presented in the accompanying chart.

Once the decision is made to initiate mechanical ventilation at home, the nurse prepares the patient and family for home care. It is important to teach the patient and family about the ventilator, suctioning, tracheostomy care, signs of pulmonary infection, cuff inflation and deflation, and assessment of vital signs. Teaching often begins in the hospital and continues in the home. Nursing responsibilities include evaluating the patient's and the family's understanding of the information presented.

The nurse teaches the family cardiopulmonary resuscitation, including mouth-to-tracheostomy tube (instead of mouth-to-mouth) breathing. It also is important to teach how to handle a power failure, which usually involves conversion of the ventilator from an electrical power source to a battery power source. Conversion is automatic in most types of home ventilators and lasts approximately 1 hour. The nurse teaches the family how to use a manual self-inflation bag should it be necessary. The patient and family responsibilities at home include those listed in the accompanying checklist.

CONTINUING CARE

A home care nurse is involved in monitoring and evaluating how well the patient and family are adapting to providing care in the home environment. The adequacy of ventilation and oxygenation is assessed, as is airway patency. The nurse addresses any unique adaptation problems the patient may have and listens to the patient's and the family's anxieties and frustrations, offering appropriate support and encouragement where possible. The home care nurse helps identify and contact appropriate community resources that may assist in home management of the patient with mechanical ventilation.

The technical aspects of the ventilator are managed by vendor follow-up. A respiratory therapist usually is assigned to the patient and makes frequent home visits to evaluate the patient and perform a maintenance check of the ventilator.

Transportation services are identified to determine the procedure for providing patient transportation in an emergency. These arrangements must be made before an emergency arises.

Providing the opportunity for ventilator-dependent patients and their families to return home to live in familiar surroundings can be a positive experience. The ultimate goal for the patient on home ventilator therapy is to enhance the quality of life, not simply to support or prolong it.

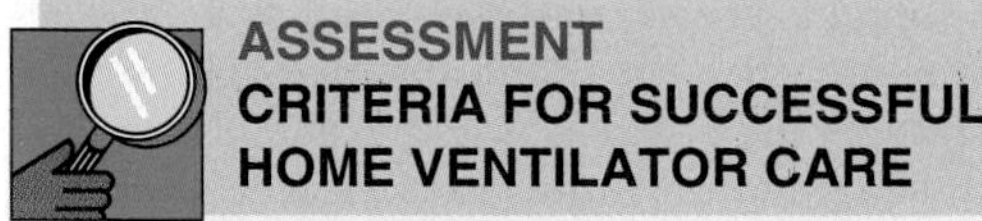

ASSESSMENT CRITERIA FOR SUCCESSFUL HOME VENTILATOR CARE

The decision to proceed with home ventilation therapy is usually based on the following parameters.

Patient Criteria

1. The patient has chronic underlying pulmonary abnormalities.
2. The patient's clinical pulmonary status is stable.
3. The patient is willing to go home on mechanical ventilation.

Home Criteria

1. The home environment is conducive to care of the patient.
2. The electrical facilities are adequate to operate all equipment safely.
3. The home environment is controlled, without drafts in cold weather and with proper ventilation in warm weather.
4. Space is available for cleaning and storing ventilator equipment.

Family Criteria

1. Family members are competent, dependable, and willing to spend the time required for proper training with available professional support.
2. Family members understand the diagnosis and prognosis.
3. Family has sufficient financial and supportive resources.

NURSING PROCESS: THE PATIENT ON A VENTILATOR

Assessment

The nurse has a vital role in assessing the patient's status and the functioning of the ventilator. In assessing the patient, the nurse evaluates the patient's physiologic status and psychosocial coping with mechanical ventilation.

Physical assessment includes systematic assessment of all body systems, with an in-depth focus on the respiratory system. Respiratory assessment includes vital signs, respiratory rate and pattern, breath sounds, evaluation of spontaneous ventilatory effort, and potential evidence of hypoxia. Increased adventitious breath sounds may indicate a need for suctioning. The nurse also evaluates the settings and functioning of the mechanical ventilator, as described previously.

Assessment also addresses the patient's neurologic status and effectiveness of coping with the need for assisted ventilation and the changes that accompany it. The nurse should assess the patient's comfort level and ability to communicate as well. Finally, successful weaning from mechanical ventilation requires adequate nutrition. Therefore, it is important to assess the function of the gastrointestinal system and nutritional status.

Diagnosis

Nursing Diagnoses

Based on the assessment data, the patient's major nursing diagnoses may include:

- Impaired gas exchange related to underlying illness, or ventilator setting adjustment during stabilization or weaning. (Note: The nursing diagnosis of impaired gas exchange is, by its complex nature, multidisciplinary and collaborative.)
- Ineffective airway clearance related to increased mucus production associated with continuous positive-pressure mechanical ventilation
- Risk for trauma and infection related to endotracheal intubation or tracheostomy
- Impaired physical mobility related to ventilator dependency
- Impaired verbal communication related to endotracheal tube and attachment to ventilator

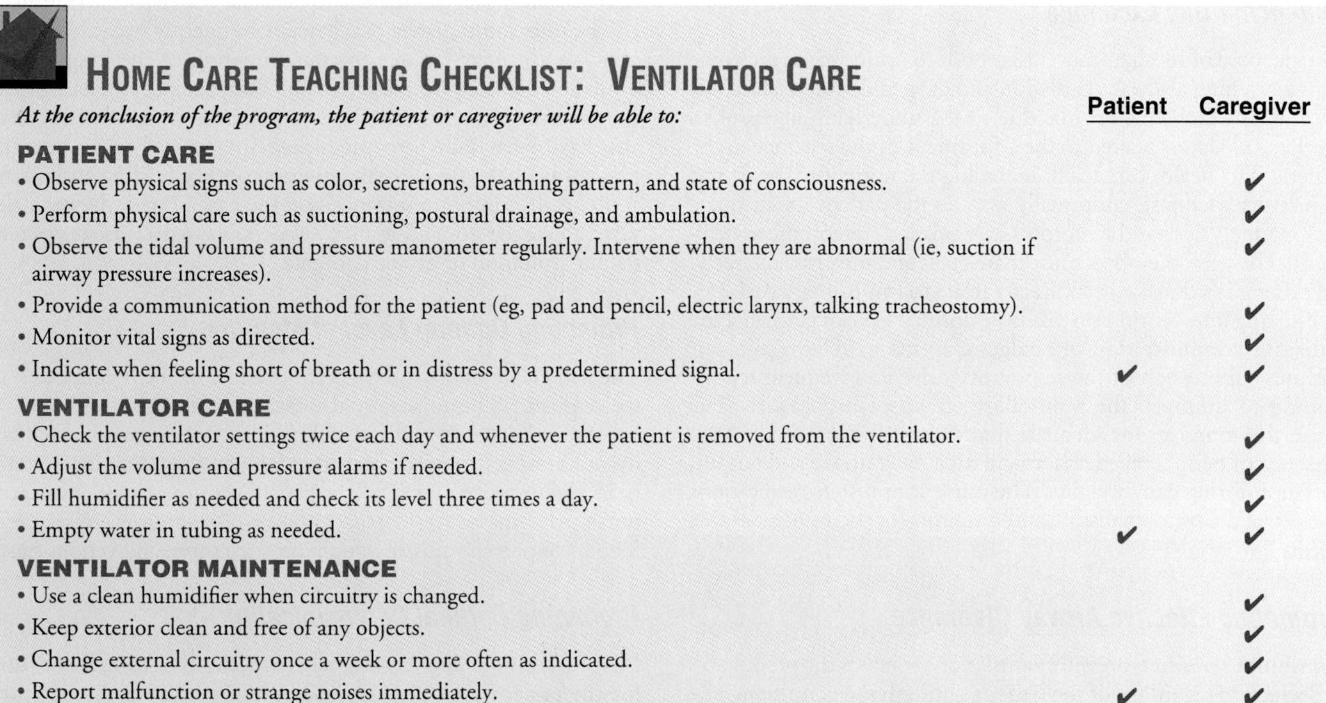

HOME CARE TEACHING CHECKLIST: VENTILATOR CARE

At the conclusion of the program, the patient or caregiver will be able to:	Patient	Caregiver
PATIENT CARE		
• Observe physical signs such as color, secretions, breathing pattern, and state of consciousness.		✔
• Perform physical care such as suctioning, postural drainage, and ambulation.		✔
• Observe the tidal volume and pressure manometer regularly. Intervene when they are abnormal (ie, suction if airway pressure increases).		✔
• Provide a communication method for the patient (eg, pad and pencil, electric larynx, talking tracheostomy).		✔
• Monitor vital signs as directed.		✔
• Indicate when feeling short of breath or in distress by a predetermined signal.	✔	✔
VENTILATOR CARE		
• Check the ventilator settings twice each day and whenever the patient is removed from the ventilator.		✔
• Adjust the volume and pressure alarms if needed.		✔
• Fill humidifier as needed and check its level three times a day.		✔
• Empty water in tubing as needed.	✔	✔
VENTILATOR MAINTENANCE		
• Use a clean humidifier when circuitry is changed.		✔
• Keep exterior clean and free of any objects.		✔
• Change external circuitry once a week or more often as indicated.		✔
• Report malfunction or strange noises immediately.	✔	✔

- Defensive coping and powerlessness related to ventilator dependency

Collaborative Problems/Potential Complications

Based on assessment data, potential complications may include:

- Alterations in cardiac function
- Barotrauma and pneumothorax
- Pulmonary infection

Planning and Goals

The major goals for the patient may include achievement of optimal gas exchange, maintenance of a patent airway, absence of trauma or infection, attainment of optimal mobility, adjustment to nonverbal methods of communication, acquisition of successful coping measures, and absence of complications.

Nursing Interventions

Nursing care of the mechanically ventilated patient requires unique technical and interpersonal skills. Nursing interventions are similar regardless of the setting; however, the frequency of interventions and the stability of the patient vary from setting to setting. Nursing interventions for the mechanically ventilated patient are not uniquely different from other pulmonary patients, but astute nursing observation and a therapeutic nurse–patient relationship are critical. The specific interventions used by the nurse are determined by the underlying disease process and the patient's response.

Two general nursing interventions important in the care of the mechanically ventilated patient are pulmonary auscultation and interpretation of arterial blood gas measurements. The nurse is often the first to note changes in physical assessment findings or significant trends in blood gases that signal the development of a significant problem (pneumothorax, tube displacement, pulmonary embolus).

Enhancing Gas Exchange

The purpose of mechanical ventilation is to optimize gas exchange by maintaining alveolar ventilation and oxygen delivery. The alteration in gas exchange may be due to the underlying illness or to mechanical factors related to the adjustment of the machine to the patient. The health care team, including the nurse, physician, and respiratory therapist, continually assesses the patient for adequate gas exchange, signs and symptoms of hypoxia, and response to treatment. The team members must share goals and information freely. All other goals directly or indirectly relate to this primary goal.

Nursing interventions to promote optimal gas exchange include judicious administration of analgesic agents to relieve pain but without suppression of the respiratory drive and frequent repositioning to diminish the pulmonary effects of immobility. The nurse also monitors for adequate fluid balance by assessing for the presence of peripheral edema, calculating daily intake and output, and monitoring daily weights. The nurse administers medications to control the primary disease and monitors for their potential side effects.

Promoting Effective Airway Clearance

Continuous positive-pressure ventilation increases the production of secretions regardless of the patient's underlying condition. The nurse must identify the presence of secretions by lung auscultation at least every 2 to 4 hours. Measures to clear the airway of secretions include suctioning, chest physiotherapy, frequent position changes, and increased mobility as soon as possible. Because of well-documented damage to the intima of the tracheobronchial tree, suctioning should be performed when clinically indicated rather than on a routine schedule.

The sigh mechanism on the ventilator may be adjusted to deliver at least one to three sighs per hour at 1.5 times the tidal volume if the patient is on assist–control. Because of the risk of hyperventilation and trauma to pulmonary tissue from excess ventilator pressure (barotrauma, pneumothorax), this feature is not being used as frequently in recent years. If the patient is on the synchronized intermittent mandatory ventilation (SIMV) mode, the mandatory ventilations act as sighs because they are of greater volume than the patient's spontaneous breaths. Periodic sighing prevents atelectasis and the further retention of secretions.

Humidification of the airway via the ventilator is maintained to help liquefy secretions so they are more easily removed. Bronchodilators and mucolytic agents, either intravenous or inhaled, are administered as prescribed to dilate the bronchioles and liquefy secretions so that they are more easily mobilized.

Preventing Trauma and Infection

Airway management must involve maintaining the endotracheal or tracheostomy tube. The nurse positions the ventilator tubing so that there is minimal pulling or distortion of the tube in the trachea, which reduces trauma to the trachea. It is important to monitor cuff pressure every 8 hours to maintain the pressure at less than 25 cm H_2O. The nurse evaluates for the presence of a cuff leak at the same time.

Patients with endotracheal intubation or a tracheostomy tube do not have the normal defenses of the upper airway. In addition, these patients frequently have multiple additional body system disturbances that lead to immunocompromise. It is important to perform tracheostomy care at least every 8 hours and more frequently if needed because of the increased risk of infection. The ventilator circuit and in-line suction tubing is replaced periodically, according to guidelines, to decrease the risk of infection.

The nurse administers oral hygiene frequently because the oral cavity is a primary source of contamination of the lungs in the intubated and compromised patient. The presence of a nasogastric tube and the use of antacids in the mechanically ventilated patient also have been shown to predispose the patient to nosocomial pneumonia from subclinical aspiration of tube feeding and gastric contents. It is important to position the patient with the head elevated above the stomach as much as possible to decrease the potential for aspiration of gastric contents.

Promoting Optimal Level of Mobility

The patient's mobility is limited because he or she is connected to the ventilator. The nurse should assist a patient whose condition has become stable out of bed and to a chair as soon as possible. Mobility and muscle activity are beneficial because they stimulate respirations and improve morale. If the patient cannot get out of bed, the nurse performs active or passive range-of-motion exercises every 8 hours to prevent muscle atrophy, contractures, and venous stasis.

Promoting Optimal Communication

It is important to develop alternative methods of communication for the patient on a ventilator. The nurse assesses the patient's communication abilities to evaluate for limitations. Questions to consider when assessing the ventilated patient's ability to communicate include the following:

- Is the patient conscious and able to communicate? Can the patient nod or shake the head?
- Is the patient's mouth unobstructed by the tube so that words can be mouthed?
- Is the patient's hand strong and available for writing? (If the patient is right-handed, the intravenous line is placed in the left arm if possible so that the right hand is free.)

Once the patient's limitations are known, the nurse offers several appropriate communication approaches: lip reading (use single key words), pad and pencil or Magic Slate, communication board, gesturing, or electric larynx. Use of a "talking" or fenestrated tracheostomy tube may be suggested to the physician to allow the patient to talk while on the ventilator. If indicated, the nurse should make sure that the patient's eyeglasses and hearing aid and a translator are available to enhance the patient's ability to communicate.

The patient must be assisted to find the most suitable communication method. Some methods may be frustrating to the patient, family, and nurse; these need to be identified and minimized. A speech therapist can assist in determining the most appropriate method for the patient.

Promoting Coping Ability

Dependence on a ventilator is frightening to both the patient and the family and disrupts even the most stable families. Encouraging the family to verbalize their feelings about the ventilator, the patient's condition, and the environment in general is beneficial. Explaining procedures every time they are performed helps to reduce anxiety and familiarizes the patient with ventilator procedures. To restore a sense of control, the nurse encourages the patient to participate in decisions about care, schedules, and treatment when possible. The patient may become withdrawn or depressed while on mechanical ventilation, especially if its use is prolonged. To promote effective coping, the nurse informs the patient about progress when appropriate. It is important to provide diversions such as watching television, playing music, or taking a walk (if appropriate and possible). Stress reduction techniques (eg, a backrub, relaxation measures) help release tension and help the patient to deal with any anxieties and fears about both the condition and the dependence on the ventilator.

Monitoring and Managing Potential Complications

ALTERATIONS IN CARDIAC FUNCTION

Alterations in cardiac output may occur as a result of positive-pressure ventilation. The positive intrathoracic pressure during inspiration compresses the heart and great vessels, thereby reducing venous return and cardiac output. This is usually corrected during exhalation when the positive pressure is off. Patients may have decreased cardiac output and resultant decreased tissue perfusion and oxygenation.

To evaluate cardiac function, the nurse first looks for signs and symptoms of hypoxia (restlessness, apprehension, confusion, tachycardia, tachypnea, labored breathing, pallor progressing to cyanosis, diaphoresis, transient hypertension, and decreased urine output). If a pulmonary artery catheter is in place, cardiac output, cardiac index, and other hemodynamic values can be used to assess the patient's status.

BAROTRAUMA AND PNEUMOTHORAX

Excessive positive pressure may cause barotrauma (trauma to the alveoli), which results in a spontaneous pneumothorax. This may quickly develop into a tension pneumothorax, further compromising venous return, cardiac output, and blood pressure. The nurse should consider any sudden onset of changes in oxygen saturation or respiratory distress a life-threatening emergency requiring immediate action.

PULMONARY INFECTION

The patient is at high risk for infection, as described above. The nurse should report fever or a change in color or odor of sputum to the physician for follow-up.

Evaluation

Expected Outcomes

Expected outcomes may include:

1. Exhibits adequate gas exchange, as evidenced by normal breath sounds, acceptable arterial blood gas levels, and vital signs
2. Demonstrates adequate ventilation with minimal mucus accumulation
3. Is free of injury or infection, as evidenced by normal temperature and white blood count
4. Is mobile within limits of ability
   a. Gets out of bed to chair, bears weight, or ambulates as soon as possible
   b. Performs range-of-motion exercises every 6 to 8 hours
5. Communicates effectively through written messages, gestures, or other communication devices
6. Copes effectively
   a. Verbalizes fears and concerns about condition and equipment
   b. Participates in decision making when possible
   c. Uses stress reduction techniques when necessary
7. Absence of complications
   a. Absence of cardiac compromise, as evidenced by stable vital signs and adequate urine output
   b. Absence of pneumothorax, as evidenced by bilateral chest excursion, normal chest x-ray, and adequate oxygenation
   c. Absence of pulmonary infection, as evidenced by normal temperature, clear pulmonary secretions, and negative sputum cultures

Weaning the Patient From the Ventilator

Respiratory weaning—weaning the patient from dependence on the ventilator—takes place in three stages: the patient is gradually weaned from the ventilator, the tube, and oxygen. Weaning from mechanical ventilation is performed at the earliest possible time consistent with patient safety. The decision must be made from a physiologic rather than from a mechanical viewpoint. A thorough understanding of the patient's clinical status is required in making this decision. Weaning is started when the patient is recovering from the acute stage of medical and surgical problems and when the cause of respiratory failure is sufficiently reversed.

Successful weaning involves collaboration among the physician, respiratory therapist, and nurse. Each health care provider must understand the scope and function of other team members in relation to patient weaning to conserve patient strength, use resources efficiently, and maximize successful outcomes.

Criteria for Weaning

The objective measurements of the patient's ventilatory capacities include:

- An ability to generate a minimal vital capacity of 10 to 15 mL/kg, or a vital capacity twice as large as the predicted normal resting tidal volume. The minimal required volume is usually in the range of 1000 mL in a normal adult.
- A spontaneous inspiratory force of at least −20 cm H_2O
- A PaO_2 of greater than 60 mm Hg with an FiO_2 of less than .40%
- Stable vital signs

When the decision has been made that the patient has adequate ventilatory capacity, it is important to note the following baseline measurements:

- Vital capacity
- Inspiratory force
- Respiratory rate
- Resting tidal volume
- Minute ventilation (frequency times total volume)
- Arterial blood gas levels
- FiO_2

It is important to follow the trend of these values as the weaning progresses rather than to rely on isolated measurements.

Patient Preparation

To maximize the success of weaning, the nurse must consider the patient as a whole. It is important to consider factors that impair the delivery of oxygen and elimination of carbon dioxide, as well as those that increase oxygen demand (sepsis, seizures, thyroid imbalances) or decrease the patient's overall strength (nutrition, neuromuscular disease). Adequate psychological preparation is necessary before and during the weaning process. Patients need to know what is expected of them during the procedure. They are often frightened by having responsibility for their own breathing again and need the reassurance that they are improving and are well enough to handle spontaneous breathing. The nurse explains what will happen during weaning and what role the patient will play in the procedure. The nurse emphasizes that someone will be with or near the patient at all times, and allows time to answer any questions simply and concisely. Proper preparation of the patient can reduce the weaning time.

Methods of Weaning

Considerable effort has been devoted to finding the best method of weaning from mechanical ventilation, but actually there is no best way appropriate for all patients: success depends on the combination of adequate patient preparation, available equipment, and a interdisciplinary approach to solving patient problems. The two most common weaning methods in use today are described below.

TRADITIONAL METHOD

The traditional method involves switching from the assist–control or SIMV mode to one or more T-piece trials. This method of weaning is usually used when there is short-term ventilatory assistance (less than 2 days) and when the patient is awake and alert, is breathing without difficulty, has good gag and cough reflexes, and is hemodynamically stable. The patient breathes spontaneously with the aid of humidified oxygen. During the weaning process, the patient is maintained on the same or a higher oxygen concentration than when on the ventilator.

While on the T-piece, the patient is observed for signs and symptoms of hypoxia or increasing fatigue, as manifested by the following:

- Tachycardia, premature ventricular contractions, ischemic electrocardiogram changes, or any other sign of increasing cardiac irritability
- Restlessness
- Respiratory rate greater than 35 breaths/min
- Use of accessory muscles for breathing
- Paradoxical chest movement

Fatigue or exhaustion is initially manifested by an increased respiratory rate associated with a gradual reduction in tidal volume. Later there is a slowing of the respiratory rate.

If the patient appears to be tolerating the T-tube trial, a second set of arterial blood gas measurements is drawn 20 minutes after the patient has been on spontaneous ventilation at a constant FiO_2. (Alveolar–arterial equilibration takes 15 to 20 minutes to occur.)

Signs of exhaustion and hypoxia correlated with a deterioration in the blood gas measurements indicate the need for ventilatory support. The patient is placed back on the ventilator each time signs of fatigue or deterioration develop.

If clinically stable, the patient usually can be extubated within 2 or 3 hours of weaning and allowed spontaneous ventilation by means of a mask with humidified oxygen. Patients who have had prolonged ventilatory assistance usually require more gradual weaning, which may take days or even weeks. They are weaned primarily during the day and placed back on the ventilator at night to rest.

SYNCHRONIZED INTERMITTENT MANDATORY VENTILATION METHOD

Some patients are difficult to wean from mechanical ventilation. SIMV is indicated if the patient satisfies all the criteria for weaning but cannot sustain adequate spontaneous ventilation for long periods. After initiation of SIMV, serial determinations of the following are made and recorded:

- Respiratory rate
- Minute volume
- Spontaneous and machine-generated tidal volume
- FiO_2
- Arterial blood gas levels

If no deterioration is apparent in these parameters, and if the patient maintains adequate tidal volumes, the rate of the ventilator is progressively decreased and the patient is allowed to rely more on spontaneous respiration until weaning is complete. **Pressure support**, frequently used as an adjunct to SIMV weaning, provides a set inspiratory pressure boost with spontaneous breaths. This decreases the patient's work of breathing. Pressure support is reduced gradually as the patient's strength increases.

Successful weaning from the ventilator is supplemented by intensive pulmonary care. The following are continued:

- Oxygen therapy
- Arterial blood gas evaluation
- Pulse oximetry
- Bronchodilator therapy
- Chest physiotherapy

- Adequate nutrition, hydration, and humidification
- Incentive spirometry

These patients still have borderline pulmonary function and need vigorous supportive therapy before their respiratory status returns to a level that supports activities of daily living.

Weaning From the Tube

The tracheostomy or endotracheal tube can be removed if the following criteria are met:

- Spontaneous ventilation is adequate.
- Pharyngeal and laryngeal gag reflexes are active.
- The patient is maintaining an adequate airway and can swallow, move the jaw, or clench the teeth, or voluntary cough is effective in bringing up secretions.

If these are ineffective, the tube is needed so that tracheobronchial secretions can be suctioned.

Before the patient is weaned from the tracheostomy tube, a trial period of mouth breathing or nose breathing is conducted. This is accomplished by:

- Changing to a smaller size tube to increase the resistance to air flow and plugging the tracheostomy tube (deflating the cuff) at the same time
- Switching to a cuffless tracheostomy tube
- Changing to a fenestrated tube (one with an opening or window in the bend of the tube), which permits air to flow around and through the tube to the upper airway and permits talking
- Changing to a tracheostomy button
- Removing the tracheostomy tube completely

Weaning From Oxygen

The patient who has been successfully weaned from the ventilator, cuff, and tube and has adequate respiratory function is then weaned from oxygen. The FiO_2 is gradually reduced until the PO_2 is in the range of 70 to 100 mm Hg while the patient is breathing room air. If the PO_2 is less than 70 mm Hg on room air, supplemental oxygen is recommended. The Health Care Financing Administration requires that the patient's PaO_2 on room air be less than 55 mm Hg for the patient to be eligible for financial reimbursement for in-home oxygen.

Success in weaning the long-term ventilator-dependent patient requires early and aggressive but judicious nutritional support. Respiratory musculature (diaphragm and especially intercostals) quickly become weak or atrophied after just a few days of mechanical ventilation, especially if nutrition is inadequate. High carbohydrate loads increase carbon dioxide production and thus may increase the work of breathing in patients with borderline pulmonary function. Consultation with a dietitian or nutrition support team soon after admission to plan the best form of nutritional replacement may decrease the duration of mechanical ventilation and prevent other complications, especially sepsis.

Research continues in a number of areas related to the mechanically ventilated patient and strategies for weaning. Areas of particular interest are the effectiveness of respiratory muscle training, nutritional support, modes and pressures of mechanical ventilation, suctioning frequency, and patient–nurse interactions.

THE PATIENT UNDERGOING THORACIC SURGERY

Assessment and management are particularly important in the patient undergoing thoracic surgery. Various types of thoracic surgical procedures are performed for a wide variety of reasons (Chart 22-4). Frequently these patients also have obstructive pulmonary disease with compromised breathing. Preoperative preparation and careful postoperative management are crucial for successful patient outcomes because these patients may have a very narrow range of what allows them to be functional and what causes distress.

Fortunately, the lungs have a large functional reserve. More advanced anesthesia techniques, respiratory therapy, surgical techniques, and intensive postoperative care have made possible more extensive and sometimes less invasive thoracic surgery.

The objectives of preoperative care are to ascertain the patient's functional reserve to determine if the patient can survive the surgery and to ensure the optimal condition of the patient for surgery.

Preoperative Management

Assessment and Diagnostic Findings

The nurse performs chest auscultation to assess breath sounds in the different regions of the lungs (see Chap. 19). It is important to note if breath sounds are normal, indicating a free flow of air in and out of the lungs. (In the patient with emphysema, the breath sounds may be markedly decreased or even absent on auscultation.) The nurse notes crackles and wheezes and assesses hyperresonance and decreased diaphragmatic motion. Unilateral diminished breath sounds and rhonchi can be the result of occlusion of the bronchi by mucous plugs. The nurse assesses for retained secretions during auscultation by asking the patient to cough. It is important to note any signs of rhonchi or wheezing. The patient history and assessment should include the following questions:

- What signs and symptoms are present: cough, sputum expectorated (amount and color), hemoptysis, chest pain, dyspnea?
- How long has the patient been smoking? Does the patient smoke currently? How many packs each day?
- What is the patient's cardiopulmonary tolerance while resting, eating, bathing, walking?
- What is the patient's breathing pattern? How much exertion is required to produce dyspnea?
- Does the patient need to sleep in an upright position?
- What is the physiologic status of the patient (eg, general appearance, mental alertness, behavior, nutritional status)?
- What other medical conditions exist (eg, allergies, cardiac disorders, diabetes)?

A number of tests are performed to determine the preoperative status of the patient and to assess physical assets and limitations. The decision to perform any pulmonary resection is based on the patient's cardiovascular status and pulmonary reserve. Pulmonary function studies (especially lung volume and vital capacity) are performed to determine whether the planned resection will leave sufficient functioning lung tissue. Arterial blood gas values are assessed to provide a more complete picture of the functional capacity of the lung. Exercise tolerance tests are useful to determine if the patient who is a candidate for pneumonectomy can tolerate removal of one of the lungs.

Preoperative studies are performed to provide a baseline for comparison during the postoperative period and to detect any unsuspected abnormalities. These studies include chest x-ray,

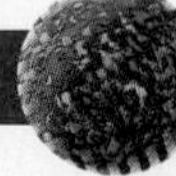

CHART 22•4 Types of Thoracic Surgeries and Procedures

Pneumonectomy

The removal of an entire lung (pneumonectomy) is performed chiefly for cancer when the lesion cannot be removed by a less extensive procedure. It also may be performed for lung abscesses, bronchiectasis, or extensive unilateral tuberculosis. The removal of the right lung is more dangerous than the removal of the left, because the right lung has a larger vascular bed and its removal imposes a greater physiologic burden.

A posterolateral or anterolateral thoracotomy incision is made, sometimes with resection of a rib. The pulmonary artery and the pulmonary veins are ligated and severed. The main bronchus is divided and the lung removed. The bronchial stump is stapled, and usually no drains are used because the accumulation of fluid in the empty hemithorax prevents mediastinal shift.

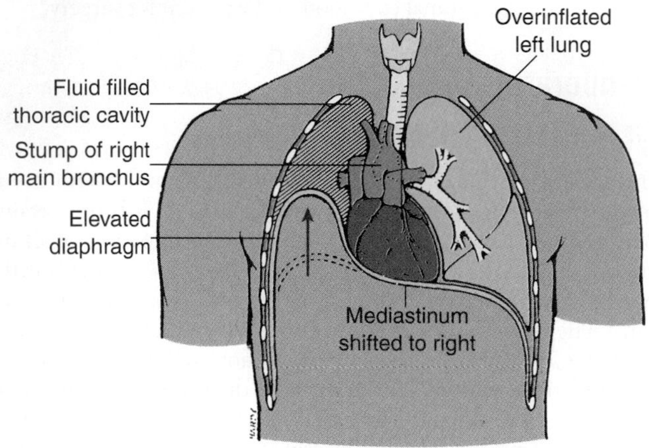

Pneumonectomy

Lobectomy

When the pathology is limited to one area of a lung, a lobectomy (removal of a lobe of a lung) is performed. Lobectomy, which is more common than pneumonectomy, may be carried out for bronchogenic carcinoma, giant emphysematous blebs or bullae, benign tumors, metastatic malignant tumors, bronchiectasis, and fungus infections.

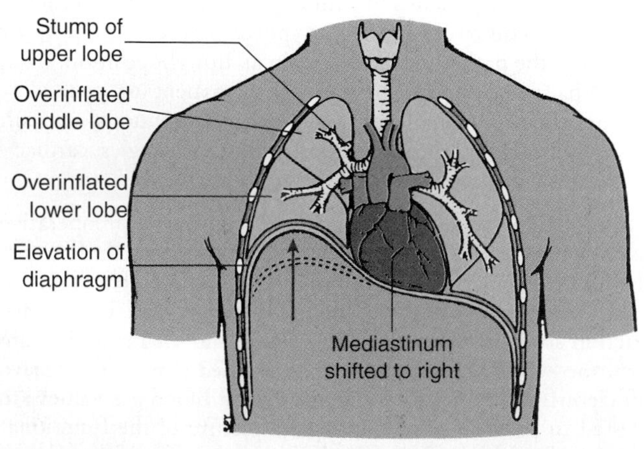

Lobectomy

The surgeon makes a thoracotomy incision; its exact location depends on the lobe to be resected. When the pleural space is entered, the involved lung collapses and the lobar vessels and the bronchus are ligated and divided. After the lobe is removed, the remaining lobes of the lung are reexpanded. Usually, two chest catheters are inserted for drainage. The upper tube is for the removal of air; the lower one is for drainage of fluid. Sometimes, only one catheter is needed. The chest tube is connected to a chest drainage apparatus for several days.

Segmentectomy (Segmental Resection)

Some lesions are located in only one segment of the lung. Bronchopulmonary segments are subdivisions of the lung that function as individual units. They are held together by delicate connective tissue. Disease processes may be limited to a single segment. Care is used to preserve as much healthy and functional lung tissue as possible, especially in patients who already have limited cardiopulmonary reserve. Single segments can be removed from any lobe; the right middle lobe, which has only two small segments, invariably is removed entirely. On the left side, corresponding to a middle lobe, is a "lingular" segment of the upper lobe. This can be removed as a single segment or by lingulectomy. This segment frequently is involved in bronchiectasis.

Wedge Resection

A wedge resection of a small, well-circumscribed lesion may be performed without regard for the location of the intersegmental planes. The pleural cavity usually is drained because of the possibility of an air or blood leak. This procedure is performed for diagnostic lung biopsy and for the excision of small peripheral nodules.

Bronchoplastic or Sleeve Resection

Bronchoplastic resection is a procedure in which only one lobar bronchus, together with a part of the right or left bronchus, is excised. The distal bronchus is reanastomosed to the proximal bronchus or trachea.

Lung Reduction

Surgeries are being evaluated for patients with severe emphysema (Newsome & Ott, 1997; Vaca, Osterloh, Daake, & Noedel, 1996). Giant bullae are excised to reduce lung volume and to allow for the reexpansion of compressed alveoli. A sternal or thoracoscopic approach is used.

Video Thoracoscopy

A video thoracoscopy is an endoscopic procedure that allows the surgeon to look into the thorax without making a large incision, to obtain specimens of tissue for biopsy, to treat recurrent spontaneous pneumothorax, and to diagnose either pleural effusions or pleural masses. Some advantages of video thoracoscopy include rapid diagnosis and treatment of some conditions, possibly less intense postoperative care, and a shortened hospital stay.

electrocardiogram (for arteriosclerotic heart disease, conduction defects), nutritional assessment, determination of blood urea nitrogen and serum creatinine (renal function), glucose tolerance or blood glucose (diabetes), assessment of serum electrolytes and protein levels, blood volume determinations, and complete blood cell count.

Preoperative Nursing Management

Improving Airway Clearance

The underlying lung condition often is associated with increased respiratory secretions. Before surgery, the airway is cleared of secretions to reduce the possibility of postoperative atelectasis or infection. This is accomplished through humidification, postural drainage, and chest percussion after bronchodilators are administered, if prescribed. The nurse estimates the volume of sputum in patients who expectorate large amounts of secretions. Such measurements are carried out to determine if and when the amount decreases. Antibiotics are administered as prescribed for infection, which may be causing the excessive secretions.

Teaching the Patient

Increasingly, patients are admitted on the day of surgery, which does not provide much time for the acute care nurse to talk with the patient. Nurses in all settings must take an active role in educating the patient and relieving anxiety. The nurse informs the patient what to expect, from administration of anesthesia to surgical opening of the chest (**thoracotomy**) and the likely use of chest tubes and a drainage system in the postoperative period. The patient is also informed about the usual postoperative administration of oxygen to facilitate breathing, and the possible use of a ventilator. It is important to explain the importance of frequent turning to promote drainage of lung secretions. Instruction in the use of incentive spirometry begins before surgery to familiarize the patient with its correct use. The nurse should teach diaphragmatic and pursed-lip breathing, and the patient should begin practicing these techniques.

Because a coughing schedule will be necessary in the postoperative period to promote the clearance or removal of secretions, the nurse instructs the patient in the technique of coughing and warns the patient that the coughing routine may be uncomfortable. The nurse teaches the patient to splint the incision with the hands, a pillow, or a folded towel (see Chart 22-2).

Another technique, "huffing," may be helpful for the patient with diminished expiratory flow rates or for the patient in severe pain who refuses to cough. Huffing is the expulsion of air through an open glottis. This type of forceful exhalation stimulates pulmonary expansion and assists in alveolar inflation. The nurse instructs the patient as follows:

- Take a deep diaphragmatic breath and exhale forcefully against your hand. Exhale forcefully in a quick, distinct pant, or huff.
- Practice doing small huffs and progress to one strong huff during exhalation.

Relieving Anxiety

The nurse listens to the patient to evaluate feelings about the illness and proposed treatment. The nurse also determines the patient's motivation to return to normal or baseline function. The patient may reveal significant reactions: fear of hemorrhage because of bloody sputum, fear of discomfort of a chronic cough and chest pain, fear of ventilator dependence, or fear of death because of dyspnea and the underlying disease (eg, tumor).

The nurse helps the patient to overcome many of these fears and to cope with the stress of surgery by correcting any false impressions, supporting the patient's decision to undergo surgery, reassuring the patient that the incision will "hold," and dealing honestly with questions about pain and discomfort and their treatment. The management and control of pain begin before surgery, when the nurse informs the patient that many postoperative problems can be overcome by following certain routines related to deep breathing, coughing, turning, and moving. If patient-controlled analgesia or epidural analgesia is to be used after surgery, the nurse instructs the patient in its use.

Postoperative Management

Mechanical Ventilation

Depending on the nature of the surgery, the patient's underlying condition, the intraoperative course, and the depth of anesthesia, the patient may require mechanical ventilation after surgery. The physician is responsible for determining the ventilator settings and modes, as well as determining the overall method and pace of weaning. However, the physician, nurse, and respiratory therapist work together closely to assess the patient's tolerance and weaning progress.

Chest Drainage

A crucial intervention for improving gas exchange and breathing in the postoperative period is the proper management of chest drainage and the **chest drainage system**. After thoracic surgery, chest tubes and a closed drainage system are used to reexpand the involved lung and to remove excess air, fluid, and blood. Chest drainage systems also are used in spontaneous pneumothorax and trauma resulting in pneumothorax.

BASIC PRINCIPLES

The normal breathing mechanism operates on the principle of negative pressure; that is, the pressure in the chest cavity normally is lower than the pressure of the atmosphere, causing air to move into the lungs during inspiration. Whenever the chest is opened, there is a loss of negative pressure, which can result in the collapse of the lung. The collection of air, fluid, or other substances in the chest can compromise cardiopulmonary function and can even cause the lung to collapse. Pathologic substances that collect in the pleural space include fibrin, or clotted blood; liquids (serous fluids, blood, pus, chyle); and gases (air from the lung, tracheobronchial tree, or esophagus).

Surgical incision of the chest wall almost always causes some degree of pneumothorax. Air and fluid collect in the intrapleural space, restricting lung expansion and reducing gas exchange. It is necessary to keep the pleural space evacuated after surgery and to maintain negative pressure within this potential space. Therefore, during or immediately after thoracic surgery, chest tubes or catheters are positioned strategically in the pleural space, sutured to the skin, and connected to a drainage apparatus to remove the residual air and drainage fluid from the pleural or mediastinal space. This results in the reexpansion of remaining lung tissue.

COMMERCIAL SYSTEMS

A chest drainage system must be capable of removing whatever collects in the pleural space so that a normal pleural space and normal cardiopulmonary function may be restored and maintained. Commercially available systems are the most common methods currently in use to provide chest drainage. These systems use the same principles as a three-bottle water-seal system. The chest tube or catheter is attached to the drainage system, using a one-way valve. Water in the second chamber acts as a seal and allows air and fluid to drain from the chest into the first chamber, but air cannot reenter the chest tube. Drainage accumulates in the first chamber and air exits through and from the second chamber. The water level fluctuates as the patient breathes, moving up when the patient inhales and down when the patient exhales. Suction may be added to the second chamber to create a negative pressure to promote drainage of fluid and removal of air. The addition of suction creates constant bubbling in the third chamber; if constant bubbling occurs in the absence of suction, there may be leakage of air from the lung or a leak in the system. Some commercial systems maintain the water-seal principle and/or suction without the use of water; in this instance, an air leak indicator is provided. Autotransfusion systems can also be attached for patients with large amounts of thoracic bleeding. Care of the patient with chest drainage systems is discussed in Guideline 22-6.

Traditional chest drainage systems are single-, two-, or three-bottle systems. Their principles are reviewed to assist in understanding the commercial systems.

Single-Bottle System. The end of the drainage tube from the patient's chest is submerged in water, which permits drainage of air and fluid from the pleural space but does not allow air to move back into the chest. Functionally, drainage depends on gravity and on the mechanics of respiration. As the fluid level in the bottle increases, it becomes progressively more difficult for air and fluid to exit the chest. Therefore, suction may be added.

Two-Bottle System. The two-bottle system consists of the same water-seal chamber plus a fluid collection bottle. Drainage is similar to that of a single unit, except that when pleural fluid accumulates, the underwater-seal system is not affected by the volume of drainage.

Effective drainage depends on gravity or on the amount of suction added to the system. When vacuum (suction) is added to the system from a vacuum source, such as wall suction, the connection is made at the vent stem of the underwater-seal bottle. The amount of suction applied to the system is regulated by the wall gauge.

Three-Bottle System. The three-bottle system is similar in all respects to the two-bottle system except for the addition of a third bottle to control the amount of suction applied. The amount of suction is determined by the depth to which the tip of the venting glass tube is submerged. (For example, submersion to 10 cm below the surface of the water equals 10 cm of water suction applied to the patient.) The amount of suction in this system is controlled by the manometer bottle. The mechanical suction motor or wall suction creates and maintains a negative pressure throughout the entire closed drainage system.

When the vacuum in the system becomes greater than the depth to which the tube is submerged, outside air is sucked into the system. This results in constant bubbling in the manometer (or pressure-regulator) bottle, which indicates that the system is functioning properly.

Nursing Alert *When the wall vacuum is turned off, the drainage system must be open to the atmosphere so that intrapleural air can escape from the system. This can be done by detaching the tubing from the suction port to provide a vent.*

The commercially available systems are safer because they are self-contained, unbreakable, and disposable and have no connections (except to the chest catheter) that can become loose. Nursing care is easier to provide, and the convenience of the systems encourages easier and earlier ambulation for the patient.

NURSING PROCESS: THE PATIENT UNDERGOING THORACIC SURGERY

Postoperative Assessment

The character and depth of respirations and the patient's color serve as important criteria in evaluating whether the lungs are being adequately expanded. Patients with thoracic surgery average a reduction in FEV_1 from baseline of 0.6 L/sec (Hallfeldt, Siebeck, Thetter, & Schweiberer, 1995). FEV_1 is the volume of air that a patient can forcibly expel in the first second. Decreased FEV_1 from baseline indicates decreased respiratory strength. This results in decreased tidal volumes, placing the patient at risk for respiratory failure. Additional risk factors for postoperative atelectasis and pneumonia are listed in the accompanying chart.

It is important to monitor the heart rate and rhythm by auscultation and electrocardiogram because major dysrhythmic episodes are common after thoracic and cardiac surgery. Dysrhythmias can occur at any time but frequently are seen between the second and sixth postoperative days. The incidence of dysrhythmias increases in patients older than 50 years of age and in those undergoing pneumonectomy or esophageal surgery.

In the immediate postoperative period, an arterial line may be maintained to allow frequent monitoring of blood gases, serum electrolytes, hemoglobin and hematocrit values, and arterial pressure. Central venous pressure may be monitored to detect early signs of fluid volume disturbances. These monitoring devices are being used less frequently and for shorter periods of time than in the past.

Diagnosis

Nursing Diagnoses

Based on the assessment data, the patient's major postoperative nursing diagnoses may include:

- Impaired gas exchange related to lung impairment and surgery
- Ineffective airway clearance related to lung impairment, anesthesia, and pain
- Pain related to incision, drainage tubes, and the surgical procedure
- Impaired physical mobility of the upper extremities related to thoracic surgery
- Risk for fluid volume deficit related to the surgical procedure
- Nutrition, less than body requirements related to dyspnea and anorexia
- Knowledge deficit about care procedures at home

Collaborative Problems/Potential Complications

Based on assessment data, potential complications may include:

- Respiratory distress
- Dysrhythmias
- Atelectasis, pneumothorax, and bronchopleural fistula
- Blood loss; hemorrhage
- Pulmonary edema

(*text continues on page 519*)

22•6 GUIDELINES FOR 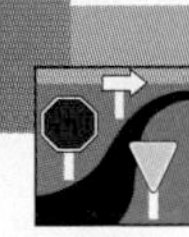 MANAGING CHEST DRAINAGE SYSTEMS

After most intrathoracic procedures, an intrapleural drainage system is needed. The system consists of one or more chest catheters held in the pleural space by suture to the chest wall. These tubes are then attached to a drainage system. The system removes liquids and gas from the pleural space or thoracic cavity and the mediastinal space, facilitates reexpansion of the lung, and restores normal cardiorespiratory function after surgery, trauma, or medical conditions by establishing negative pressure in the pleural cavity. Nursing actions and the reasons for them follow.

Nursing Action	Rationale
1. Fill the water-seal chamber with sterile water to the level specified by the manufacturer.	Water-seal drainage allows air and fluid to escape into a drainage bottle. The water acts as a seal and keeps the air from being drawn back into the pleural space.
2. When using suction, fill the suction-control chamber with sterile water to the 20-cm level or as prescribed. Alternatively, position the dial at the appropriate suction level.	The water level or dial setting determines the degree of suction applied.
3. Attach the drainage catheter exiting the patient's pleural space to the tubing coming from the collection chamber of the water seal system. Tape securely with adhesive tape.	In disposable drainage units, the system is closed. The only connection is the one to the patient's catheter.
4. If suction is used, connect the suction-control chamber tubing to the suction unit. Turn on the suction unit and increase pressure until slow but steady bubbling appears in the suction-control chamber.	The degree of suction is determined by the amount of water in the suction-control chamber and is not dependent on the rate of bubbling or the pressure gauge setting on the suction unit.

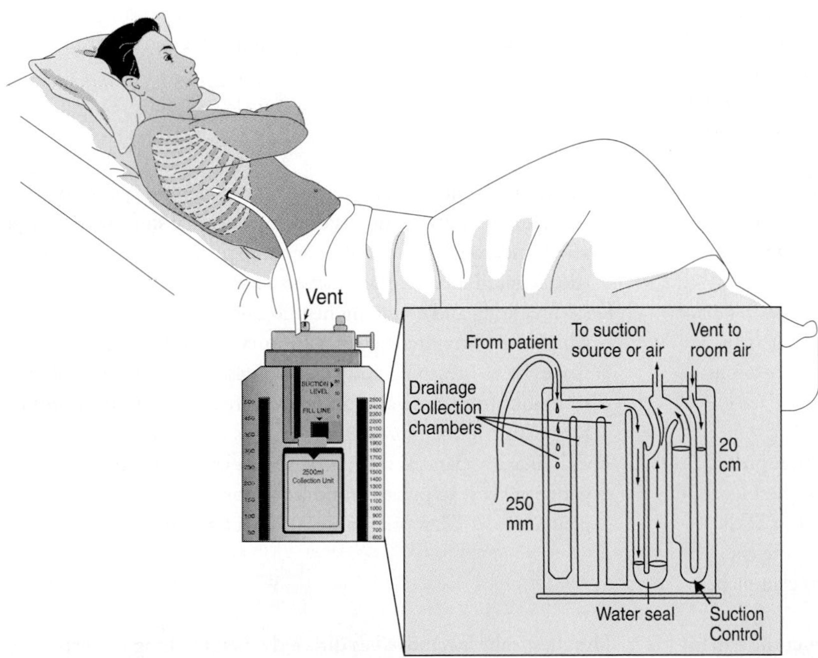

Example of a disposable chest drainage system.

Nursing Action	Rationale
5. Mark the original fluid level with tape on the outside of the drainage unit. Mark hourly/daily increments (date and time) at the drainage level.	This marking shows the amount of fluid loss and how fast fluid is collecting in the drainage bottle. It serves as a basis for determining the need for blood replacement, if the fluid is blood. Visibly bloody drainage will appear in the bottle in the immediate postoperative period. The drainage gradually becomes serous. Excessive drainage may indicate the need for reoperation or autotransfusion. Usually, however, drainage decreases progressively in the first 24 hours.
6. Ensure that the drainage tubing does not kink, loop, or interfere with the patient's movements.	Kinking, looping, or pressure on the drainage tubing can produce back-pressure, which may force drainage back into the pleural space or impede drainage from the pleural space.

(*continued*)

22•6 Guidelines For Managing Chest Drainage Systems *(Continued)*

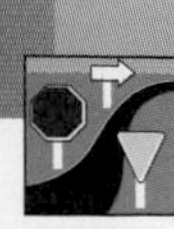

Nursing Action	Rationale
7. Encourage the patient to assume a position of comfort with good body alignment. When the patient is in the lateral position, make sure that the patient's body does not compress the tubing. Encourage the patient to change position frequently.	The patient's position should be changed frequently to promote drainage, and the body should be kept in good alignment to prevent postural deformities and contractures. Proper positioning helps breathing and promotes better air exchange. Analgesics may be needed to enhance comfort and deep breathing.
8. Put the arm and shoulder of the affected side through range-of-motion exercises several times daily. Analgesics may be necessary to relieve pain.	Exercise helps to prevent ankylosis of the shoulder and assists in reducing postoperative pain and discomfort.
9. Gently "milk" the tubing in the direction of the drainage chamber as needed.	"Milking" prevents the tubing from becoming obstructed by clots and fibrin. Constant attention to maintaining the patency of the tube facilitates prompt expansion of the lung and minimizes complications.
10. Make sure there is fluctuation ("tidaling") of the fluid level in the water-seal chamber or air leak indicator area. Note: Fluid fluctuations in the water-seal chamber or air leak indicator area will stop when • the lung has reexpanded • the tubing is obstructed by blood clots, fibrin, or kinks • a loop of tubing hangs below the rest of the tubing • suction motor or wall suction is not working properly.	Fluctuation of the water level shows effective communication between the pleural cavity and the drainage bottle and indicates that the drainage system remains patent. Fluctuation is also a gauge of intrapleural pressure.
11. Observe for air leaks in the drainage system; they are indicated by constant bubbling in the water-seal chamber or air leak detector. Also assess the chest tube system for correctable external leaks. Notify the physician immediately of excessive bubbling in the water-seal chamber not due to external leaks.	Leaking and trapping of air in the pleural space can result in tension pneumothorax.
12. Observe and immediately report rapid and shallow breathing, cyanosis, pressure in the chest, subcutaneous emphysema, symptoms of hemorrhage, or significant changes in vital signs.	Many clinical conditions may cause these signs and symptoms, including tension pneumothorax, mediastinal shift, hemorrhage, severe incisional pain, pulmonary embolus, and cardiac tamponade. Surgical intervention may be necessary.
13. Encourage the patient to breathe deeply and cough at frequent intervals. Provide adequate analgesia. If needed, request an order for patient-controlled analgesia. Also teach the patient how to perform incentive spirometry.	Deep breathing and coughing help to raise the intrapleural pressure, which promotes drainage of accumulated fluid in the pleural space. Deep breathing and coughing also promote removal of secretions from the tracheobronchial tree, which in turn promotes lung expansion and prevents atelectasis (alveolar collapse).
14. If the patient is lying on a stretcher and must be transported to another area, place the drainage system below the chest level. If the tubing disconnects, cut off the contaminated tips of the chest tube and tubing, insert a sterile connector in the cut ends, and reattach to the drainage system. Do *not* clamp chest tube during transport.	The drainage apparatus must be kept at a level lower than the patient's chest to prevent fluid from flowing backward into the pleural space. Clamping can result in a tension pneumothorax.
15. When assisting in the chest tube's removal, instruct the patient to perform a gentle Valsalva maneuver or to breathe quietly. Then the chest tube is clamped and quickly removed. Simultaneously, a small bandage is applied and made airtight with petrolatum gauze covered by a 4 × 4-inch gauze pad and thoroughly covered and sealed with nonporous tape.	The chest tube is removed as directed when the lung is reexpanded (usually 24 hours to several days), depending on the cause of the pneumothorax. During tube removal, the chief priorities are preventing air from entering the pleural cavity as the tube is withdrawn and preventing infection.

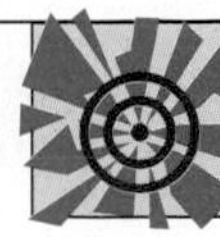

Risk Factors for
ATELECTASIS AND PNEUMONIA RELATED TO SURGERY

Preoperative Risk Factors
Increased age
Obesity
Poor nutritional status
Smoking history
Abnormal pulmonary function tests
Preexisting lung disease
Emergent surgery
History of aspiration
Comorbid states
Intraoperative Risk Factors
Thoracic incision
Prolonged anesthesia
Postoperative Risk Factors
Immobilization
Supine position
Decreased level of consciousness
Inadequate pain management
Prolonged intubation/mechanical ventilation
Presence of nasogastric tube
Inadequate preoperative education

Planning and Goals

The major goals for the patient may include improvement of gas exchange and breathing, improvement of airway clearance, relief of pain and discomfort, increased arm and shoulder mobility, maintenance of adequate fluid volume and nutritional status, understanding of self-care procedures, and absence of complications.

Nursing Interventions

Improving Gas Exchange and Breathing

Gas exchange is determined by evaluating oxygenation and ventilation. In the immediate postoperative period, this is achieved by measuring vital signs (blood pressure, pulse, and respirations) at least every 15 minutes for the first 1 to 2 hours, then less frequently as the patient's condition stabilizes.

Pulse oximetry is used for continuous monitoring of the adequacy of oxygenation. It is important to draw blood for arterial blood gas measurements early in the postoperative period to establish a baseline to assess the adequacy of oxygenation and ventilation and the possible retention of CO_2. The frequency with which postoperative arterial blood gases are measured depends on whether the patient is mechanically ventilated or exhibits signs of respiratory distress; the blood gas measurements can help determine appropriate therapy. It also is common practice for patients to have an arterial line in place to obtain blood for blood gas measurements and to monitor blood pressure closely. Hemodynamic monitoring may be used to assess hemodynamic stability.

Breathing techniques, such as diaphragmatic and pursed-lip breathing, that were taught before surgery should be practiced by the patient every 2 hours to expand the alveoli and prevent atelectasis. Another technique to improve ventilation is sustained maximal inspiration therapy or incentive spirometry. This technique optimizes lung inflation, improves the cough mechanism, and allows early assessment of acute pulmonary changes.

Positioning also improves breathing. When the patient is oriented and blood pressure is stabilized, the head of the bed is elevated 30 degrees to 40 degrees during the immediate postoperative period. This facilitates ventilation, promotes chest drainage from the lower chest tube, and helps residual air to rise in the upper portion of the pleural space, where it can be removed through the upper chest tube.

The nurse should consult with the surgeon about patient positioning. There is controversy regarding the best side-lying position. Most commonly, the patient is instructed to lie on the side of the surgery. However, the patient with unilateral lung pathology may not be able to turn well onto that side because of pain. In addition, positioning the patient with the "good lung" (the non-operative lung) down allows a better match of ventilation and perfusion, and therefore may actually improve oxygenation. The patient's position is changed from horizontal to semi-upright as soon as possible, because remaining in one position tends to promote the retention of secretions in the dependent portion of the lungs. After a pneumonectomy, the side that was operated on should be dependent so that fluid in the pleural space remains below the level of the bronchial stump, and the other lung can fully expand.

The procedure for turning the patient is as follows:

1. Instruct the patient to bend the knees and use the feet to push.
2. Have the patient shift hips and shoulders to the opposite side of the bed while pushing with the feet.
3. Bring the patient's arm over the chest, pointing it in the direction toward which the patient is being turned. Have the patient grasp the side rail with the hand.
4. Turn the patient in log-roll fashion to prevent twisting at the waist and pain from possible pulling on the incision.

Improving Airway Clearance

Retained secretions are a threat to the thoracotomy patient after surgery. Trauma to the tracheobronchial tree during surgery, diminished lung ventilation, and diminished cough reflex all result in the accumulation of excessive secretions. If the secretions are retained, airway obstruction occurs. This, in turn, causes air in the alveoli distal to the obstruction to become absorbed and the affected portion of the lung to collapse. Atelectasis, pneumonia, and respiratory failure may result.

Several techniques are used to maintain a patent airway. First, secretions are suctioned from the tracheobronchial tree before the endotracheal tube is discontinued. Secretions continue to be removed by suctioning until the patient can cough up secretions effectively. Nasotracheal suctioning may be needed to stimulate a deep cough and aspirate secretions that the patient cannot cough up. However, it should be used only after other methods to raise secretions have been unsuccessful (Guideline 22-7).

Coughing technique is another measure used in maintaining a patent airway. The patient is encouraged to cough effectively; ineffective coughing results in exhaustion and retention of secretions (see Chart 22-2). To be effective, the cough must be low-pitched, deep, and controlled. Because it is difficult to cough in a supine position, the patient is helped to a sitting position on the edge of the bed, with the feet resting on a chair. The patient should cough at least every hour during the first 24 hours and when necessary thereafter. If audible crackles are present, it may be necessary to use chest percussion with the cough routine until the lungs are clear.

22•7 GUIDELINES FOR NASOTRACHEAL SUCTIONING

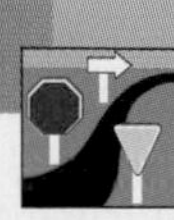

Sterile Technique to Be Used

1. Explain procedure to the patient.
2. Medicate patient for pain if necessary.
3. Place the patient in a sitting or semi-Fowler's position. Make sure the patient's head is not flexed forward. Remove excess pillows if necessary.
4. Oxygenate the patient several minutes before initiating the suctioning procedure. Have oxygen source ready nearby during procedure.
5. Put on sterile gloves.
6. Lubricate catheter with water-soluble gel.
7. Gently pass catheter through the patient's nose to the pharynx. If it is difficult to pass the catheter, and repeated suctioning is expected, a soft rubber nasal trumpet may be placed nasopharyngeally to provide easier catheter passage. Check the position of the tip of the catheter by asking the patient to open the mouth and inspecting it; the tip of the catheter should be in the lower pharynx.
8. Instruct the patient to take a deep breath or stick out the tongue. This action opens the epiglottis and promotes downward movement of the catheter.
9. Advance the catheter into the trachea only during inspiration. Listen for cough or for passage of air through the catheter.
10. Attach the catheter to suction apparatus. Apply intermittent suction while slowly withdrawing the catheter. Do not let suction exceed 120 mm Hg.
11. Do not suction for longer than 10 to 15 seconds, as dysrhythmias, bradycardia, or cardiac arrest may occur in patients with borderline oxygenation.
12. If additional suctioning is needed, withdraw the catheter to the back of the pharynx. Reassure patient and oxygenate for several minutes before resuming suctioning.

Aerosol therapy is helpful in humidifying and mobilizing secretions so that they can be readily cleared by coughing. To minimize incisional pain during coughing, the nurse supports the incision firmly over the operative side and against the opposite chest (Fig. 22-7).

After helping the patient to cough, the nurse should listen to both lungs, anteriorly and posteriorly, to determine whether there are any changes in breath sounds. Diminished breath sounds may indicate collapsed or hypoventilated alveoli.

Chest physiotherapy is the final technique for maintaining a patent airway. If a patient is identified as being at high risk for developing postoperative pulmonary complications, then chest physiotherapy is started immediately (perhaps even before surgery). The techniques of postural drainage, vibration, and percussion help to loosen and mobilize the secretions so that they can be coughed up or suctioned.

Relieving Pain and Discomfort

Pain after a thoracotomy may be severe, depending on the type of incision and the patient's reaction to and ability to cope with pain. Deep inspiration is very painful after thoracotomy. Pain can lead to postoperative complications if it reduces the patient's ability to breathe deeply and cough, and if it further limits chest excursions so that effective ventilation is decreased.

Immediately after the surgical procedure and before the incision is closed, the surgeon may perform a nerve block with a long-acting local anesthetic, which can reduce postoperative pain. The nurse administers small intravenous or epidural doses of a narcotic as prescribed. These medications are titrated to relieve pain while allowing the patient to cooperate in deep breathing, coughing, and mobilization. However, it is important to avoid depressing the respiratory system with excessive analgesia: the patient should not be so somnolent as to be unable to cough.

Because of the need to maximize patient comfort without depressing the respiratory drive, patient-controlled analgesia is often used. Patient-controlled analgesia, administered through an intravenous pump or epidural catheter, allows the patient to control the frequency and total dose of opioid analgesia. Preset limits on the pump avoid overdosage. With proper instruction, these methods are well tolerated and allow earlier mobilization and cooperation with the treatment regimen. (See Chap. 12 for a more extensive discussion of patient-controlled analgesia and pain management.)

Nursing Alert *It is important not to confuse the restlessness of hypoxia with the restlessness caused by pain. Dyspnea, restlessness, increasing respiratory rate, increasing blood pressure, and tachycardia are warning signs of impending respiratory insufficiency. The nurse uses pulse oximetry to monitor oxygenation and to differentiate causes of restlessness.*

Promoting Mobility and Shoulder Exercises

Because large shoulder girdle muscles are transected during a thoracotomy, the arm and shoulder must be mobilized by full range of motion of the shoulder. As soon as physiologically possible, usually within 8 to 12 hours, the patient is helped to get out of bed. Although this may be painful initially, the earlier the patient moves, the sooner the pain will subside. In addition to getting out of bed, the patient begins arm and shoulder exercises to restore movement and prevent painful stiffening of the affected arm and shoulder.

Maintaining Fluid Volume and Nutrition

INTRAVENOUS THERAPY

During the surgical procedure or immediately after, the patient may receive a blood transfusion, followed by a continuous intravenous infusion. The rate of administration must be titrated (as

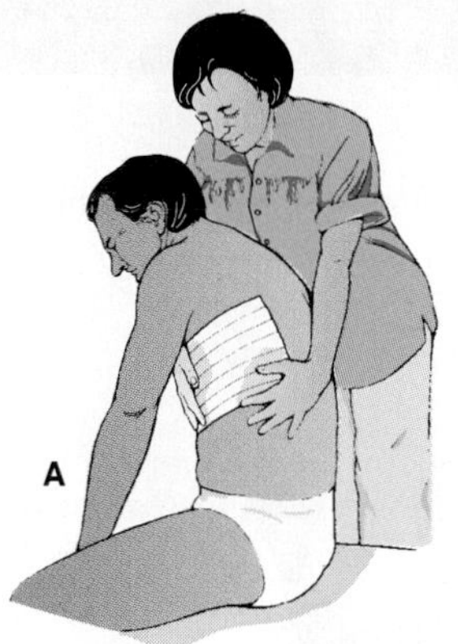

A The nurse's hands should support the chest incision anteriorly and posteriorly. The patient is instructed to take several deep breaths, inhale, and then cough forcibly.

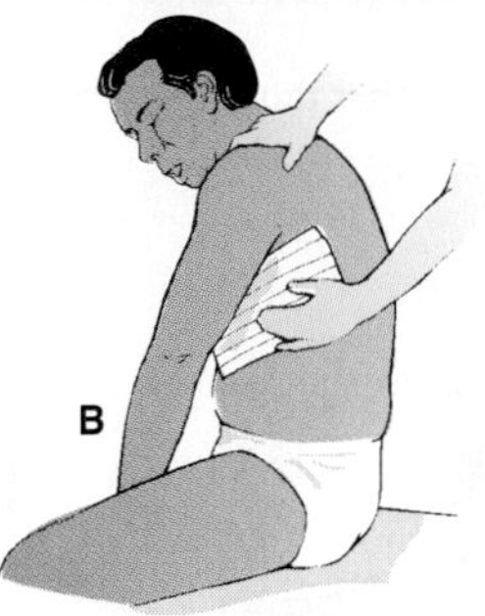

B With one hand, the nurse exerts downward pressure on the shoulder of the affected side while firmly supporting the area beneath the wound with the other hand. The patient is instructed to take several deep breaths, inhale, and then cough forcibly.

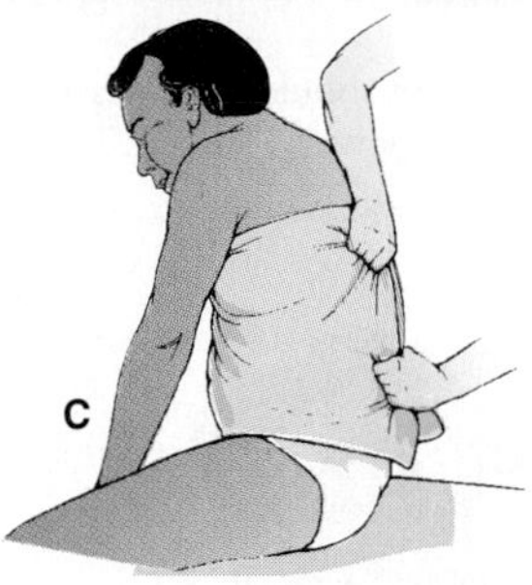

C The nurse can wrap a towel or sheet around the patient's chest and hold the ends together, pulling slightly as the patient coughs, and releasing during deep breaths.

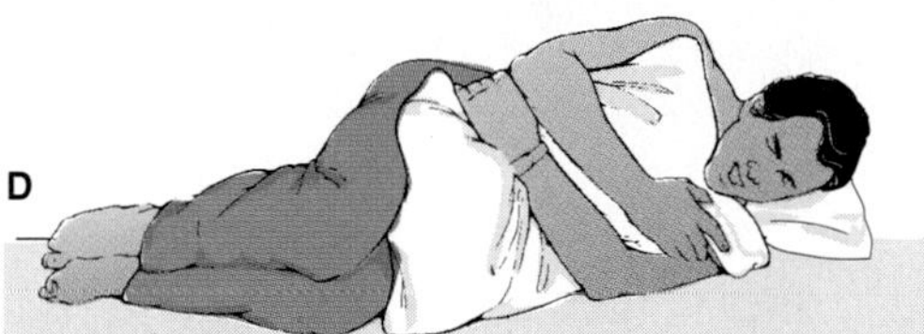

D The patient can be taught to hold a pillow firmly against the incision while coughing. This can be done while lying down or sitting in an upright position.

FIGURE 22•7 Techniques for supporting incision while a patient recovering from thoracic surgery coughs.

prescribed) based on the nurse's assessment of patient tolerance, especially when there is evidence of limited cardiopulmonary reserve and when the pulmonary vascular bed has been greatly reduced, as in pneumonectomy. Additional assessment includes monitoring of intake and output, vital signs, and jugular vein distention (see Plan of Nursing Care 22-1.).

DIET

It is not unusual for patients undergoing thoracotomy to have poor nutritional status before surgery because of dyspnea, sputum production, and poor appetite. Therefore, it is especially important that the patient's nutrition be supported as soon as feasible after surgery. A liquid diet is provided as soon as there is evidence of bowel sounds, and the patient is progressed to a full diet as soon as possible. Small, frequent, well-balanced meals are better tolerated and are crucial to the recovery and maintenance of lung function.

Monitoring and Managing Potential Complications

Complications after thoracic surgery are always a possibility and must be identified and managed early. In addition, the nurse monitors the patient at regular intervals for signs of respiratory distress or developing respiratory failure, dysrhythmias, bronchopleural fistula, hemorrhage and shock, atelectasis, and pulmonary infection.

Respiratory distress is treated by identifying and eliminating its cause while providing supplemental oxygen. If the patient progresses to respiratory failure, intubation and mechanical ventilation are necessary, eventually requiring weaning.

Dysrhythmias are often related to the effects of hypoxia or the surgical procedure. They are treated with antiarrhythmic medication and supportive therapy. Pulmonary infections or effusion, often preceded by atelectasis, may occur a few days into the postoperative course.

Bronchopleural fistula is a serious but rare complication preventing the return of negative intrathoracic pressure and lung reexpansion. Depending on its severity, it is treated with closed chest drainage, mechanical ventilation, and possibly talc pleurodesis (described in Chap. 21).

Hemorrhage and shock are managed by treating the underlying cause, whether by reoperation or by administration of blood products or fluids. Pulmonary edema from overinfusion of intravenous fluids is a significant danger. The early symptoms are dyspnea, crackles, bubbling sounds in the chest, tachycardia, and pink, frothy sputum. This constitutes an emergency and must be reported immediately.

Promoting Home and Community-Based Care

TEACHING PATIENTS SELF-CARE

The nurse instructs the patient and family about postoperative care that will be continued at home. The nurse explains signs and symptoms that should be reported to the physician. These include:

- Change in respiratory status: increasing shortness of breath, fever, increased restlessness or other changes in mental or cognitive status, increased respiratory rate, change in respiratory pattern, change in amount or color of sputum
- Bleeding or other drainage from the surgical incision or chest tube exit sites
- Increased chest pain

In addition, respiratory care modalities (oxygen, incentive spirometer, chest physiotherapy, and oral, inhaled, or intravenous

PATIENT EDUCATION AND HOME CARE

Performing Arm and Shoulder Exercises

Arm and shoulder exercises are performed after thoracic surgery to restore movement, prevent painful stiffening of the shoulder, and improve muscle power.

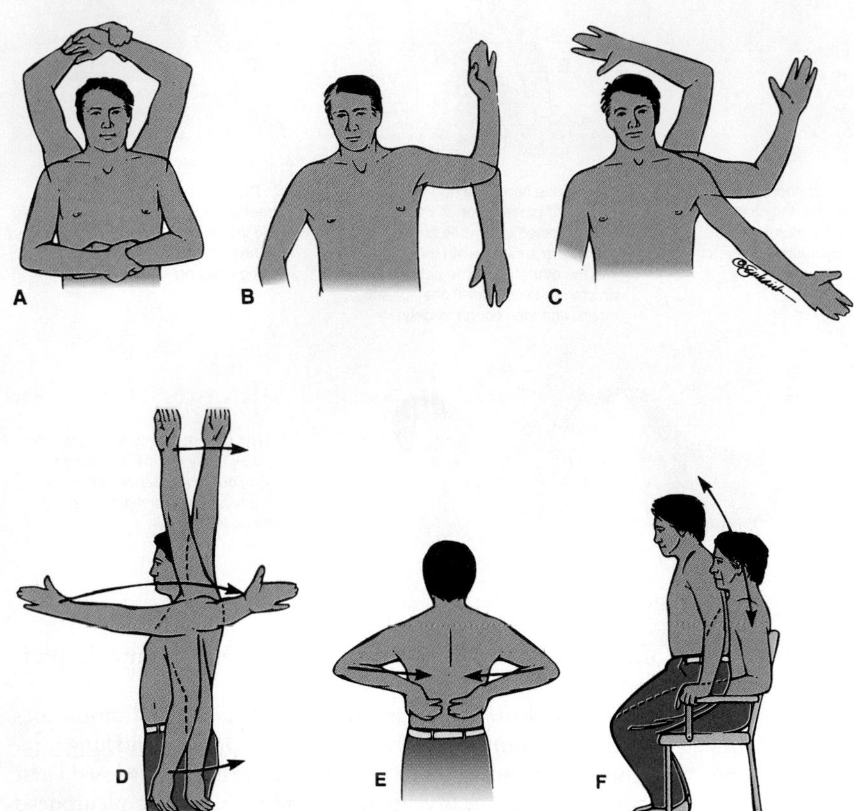

(**A**) Hold hand of the affected side with the other hand, palms facing in. Raise the arms forward, upward, and then overhead, while taking a deep breath. Exhale while lowering the arms. Repeat five times. (**B**) Raise arm sideward, upward, and downward in a waving motion. (**C**) Place arm at side. Raise arm sideward, upward, and over the head. Repeat five times. These exercises can also be done while lying in bed. (**D**) Extend the arm up and back, out to the side and back, down at the side and back. (**E**) Place hands in small of back. Push elbows as far back as possible. (**F**) Sit erect in an armchair; place the hands on the arms of the chair directly opposite either side of the body. Press down on hands, consciously pulling the abdomen in and stretching up from the waist. Inhale while raising the body until the elbows are extended completely. Hold this position a moment, and begin exhaling while lowering the body slowly to the original position.

medications) may be continued at home. Therefore, the nurse needs to instruct the patient and family in their correct and safe use.

The nurse emphasizes the importance of progressively increased activity. The nurse instructs the patient to ambulate within limits and explains that return of strength is likely to be very gradual. Another important aspect of patient teaching addresses shoulder exercises. It is important to instruct the patient to do these exercises five times daily. Additional patient teaching is described in the accompanying checklist.

CONTINUING CARE

Depending on the patient's physical status and the availability of family assistance, a home care referral may be indicated. The home care nurse assesses the patient's recovery from surgery, with special attention to respiratory status, the surgical incision, chest drainage, pain control, ambulation, and nutritional status. In addition, the nurse assesses the patient's compliance with the postoperative treatment plan. It is important to assess for acute complications and late complications. It also is important to assess the use of respiratory modalities to ensure they are being used correctly and safely.

Evaluation

Expected Outcomes

Expected outcomes may include:

1. Demonstrates improved gas exchange, as reflected in arterial blood gas measurements, breathing exercises, and use of incentive spirometry
2. Shows improved airway clearance, as evidenced by deep, controlled coughing and clear breath sounds or decreased presence of adventitious sounds
3. Has decreased pain and discomfort by splinting incision during coughing and increasing activity level
4. Shows improved mobility of shoulder and arm; demonstrates arm and shoulder exercises to relieve stiffening
5. Maintains adequate fluid intake and maintains nutrition for healing
6. Exhibits less anxiety by using appropriate coping skills, and demonstrates a basic understanding of technology used in care

(*text continues on page 526*)

22•1

PLAN OF NURSING CARE

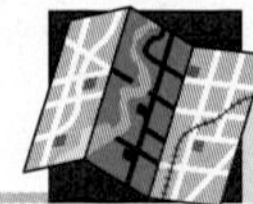

Care of the Patient After Thoracotomy

Nursing Interventions	Rationale	Expected Outcomes
Nursing Diagnosis: Impaired gas exchange related to lung impairment and surgery **Goal:** Improvement of gas exchange and breathing		
1. Monitor pulmonary status as directed and as needed: a. Auscultate breath sounds. b. Check rate, depth, and pattern of respirations. c. Assess blood gases for signs of hypoxemia or CO_2 retention. d. Evaluate patient's color for cyanosis.	1. Changes in pulmonary status indicate improvement or onset of complications.	• Lungs are clear on auscultation • Respiratory rate is within normal range with no episodes of dyspnea • Vital signs are stable • Dysrhythmias are not present or are under control • Demonstrates deep, controlled, effective breathing to allow maximal lung expansion • Uses incentive spirometer every 2 hours while awake • Demonstrates deep, effective coughing technique • Lungs are expanded to capacity (evidenced by chest x-ray)
2. Monitor and record blood pressure, apical pulse, and temperature every 2–4 hours, central venous pressure (if indicated) every 2 hours.	2. Aid in evaluating effect of surgery on cardiac status.	
3. Monitor continuous electrocardiogram for pattern and dysrhythmias.	3. Dysrhythmias (especially atrial fibrillation and atrial flutter) are more frequently seen after thoracic surgery. A patient with total pneumonectomy is especially prone to cardiac irregularity.	
4. Elevate head of bed 30 degrees–40 degrees when patient is oriented and hemodynamic status is stable.	4. Maximum lung excursion is achieved when patient is as close to upright as possible.	
5. Encourage deep-breathing exercises (see section on Breathing Retraining) and effective use of incentive spirometer (sustained maximal inspiration).	5. Helps to achieve maximal lung inflation and to open closed airways.	

(*continues on page 524*)

HOME CARE TEACHING CHECKLIST: THE PATIENT WITH A THORACOTOMY

At the conclusion of the program, the patient or caregiver will be able to:

	Patient	Caregiver
• Use local heat and oral analgesia to relieve intercostal pain.	✔	✔
• Alternate walking and other activities with frequent rest periods, expecting weakness and fatigue for the first 3 weeks.	✔	✔
• Practice breathing exercises several times daily for the first few weeks at home.	✔	
• Avoid lifting more than 20 pounds until complete healing has taken place; the chest muscles and incision may be weaker than normal for 3 to 6 months after surgery.	✔	
• Walk at a moderate pace, gradually and persistently extending walking time and distance.	✔	
• Immediately stop any activity that causes undue fatigue, increased shortness of breath, or chest pain.	✔	
• Avoid bronchial irritants (smoke, fumes, air pollution, aerosol sprays).	✔	✔
• Avoid others with known colds or lung infections.	✔	✔
• Obtain an annual influenza vaccine and discuss vaccination against pneumonia with the physician.	✔	
• Report for follow-up care by the surgeon or clinic as necessary.	✔	✔
• Stop smoking, if applicable.	✔	✔

22•1

PLAN OF NURSING CARE

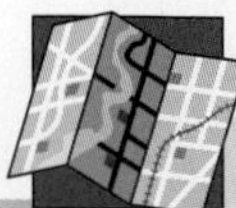

Care of the Patient After Thoracotomy (*continued*)

Nursing Interventions	Rationale	Expected Outcomes
6. Encourage and promote an effective cough routine to be performed every 1–2 hours during first 24 hours.	6. Coughing is necessary to remove retained secretions.	
7. Assess and monitor the chest drainage system:* a. Assess for leaks and patency as needed. b. Monitor amount and character of drainage and document every 2 hours. Notify physician if drainage is 150 mL/h or greater. c. See Guideline 25-6 for summary of nurse's role in management of chest drainage systems.	7. System is used to eliminate any residual air or fluid after thoracotomy.	

Nursing Diagnosis: Ineffective airway clearance related to lung impairment, anesthesia, and pain
Goal: Improvement of airway clearance and achievement of a patent airway

Nursing Interventions	Rationale	Expected Outcomes
1. Maintain an open airway.	1. Provides for adequate ventilation and gas exchange.	• Airway is patent • Coughs effectively • Splints incision while coughing • Sputum is clear or colorless • Lungs are clear on auscultation
2. Perform endotracheal suctioning until patient can raise secretions effectively.	2. Endotracheal secretions are present in excessive amounts in post-thoracotomy patients due to trauma to the tracheobronchial tree during surgery, diminished lung ventilation, and cough reflex.	
3. Assess and medicate for pain. Encourage deep-breathing and coughing exercises. Help splint incision during coughing.	3. Helps to achieve maximal lung inflation and to open closed airways. Coughing is painful; incision needs to be supported.	
4. Monitor amount, viscosity, color, and odor of sputum. Notify physician if sputum is excessive or contains bright-red blood.	4. Changes in sputum suggest presence of infection or change in pulmonary status. Colorless sputum is not unusual; opacification or coloring of sputum may indicate dehydration or infection.	
5. Administer humidification and mini-nebulizer therapy as prescribed.	5. Secretions must be moistened and thinned if they are to be raised from the chest with the least amount of effort.	
6. Perform postural drainage, percussion, and vibration as prescribed. Do not percuss or vibrate directly over operative site.	6. Chest physiotherapy uses gravity to help remove secretions from the lung.	
7. Auscultate both sides of chest to determine changes in breath sounds.	7. Indications for tracheal suctioning are determined by chest auscultation.	

Nursing Diagnosis: Pain related to incision and surgical procedure
Goal: Relief of pain and discomfort

Nursing Interventions	Rationale	Expected Outcomes
1. Evaluate location, character, quality, and severity of pain. Administer pain medication as prescribed and as needed. Observe for respiratory effect of opioid analgesic. Is patient too somnolent to cough? Are respirations depressed?	1. Pain limits chest excursions and thereby decreases ventilation.	• Asks for pain medication, but verbalizes that he or she expects some discomfort while deep breathing and coughing • Verbalizes that he or she is comfortable and not in acute distress • No signs of incisional infection evident

* A patient with a pneumonectomy usually does not have water-seal chest drainage because it is desirable that the pleural space fill with an effusion, which eventually obliterates this space. Some surgeons do use a modified water-seal system.

(*continued*)

22•1

PLAN OF NURSING CARE

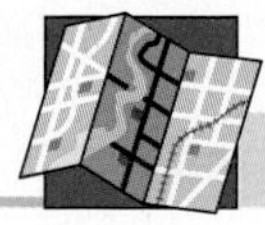

Care of the Patient After Thoracotomy (*continued*)

Nursing Interventions	Rationale	Expected Outcomes
2. Maintain care postoperatively in positioning the thoracotomy patient: a. Place patient in semi-Fowler's position. b. Patients with limited respiratory reserve may not be able to turn on unoperated side. c. Assist or turn patient every 2 hours.	2. The patient who is comfortable and free of pain will be less likely to splint the chest while breathing. A semi-Fowler's position permits residual air to rise to upper portion of pleural space and be removed via the upper chest catheter.	
3. Assess incision area every 8 hours for redness, heat, induration, swelling, separation, and drainage.	3. These signs indicate possible infection.	
4. Request order for patient-controlled analgesia pump if appropriate for patient.	4. Allowing patient control over frequency and dose improves comfort and compliance with treatment regimen.	

Nursing Diagnosis: Anxiety related to outcomes of surgery, pain, technology
Goal: Reduction of anxiety to a manageable level

Nursing Interventions	Rationale	Expected Outcomes
1. Explain all procedures in simple terms.	1. Explaining what can be expected in understandable terms decreases anxiety and increases cooperation.	• States that anxiety is at a manageable level • Participates with health care team in treatment regimen
2. Assess for pain and medicate, especially before potentially painful procedures.	2. Premedication before painful procedures or activities improves comfort and minimizes undue anxiety.	• Uses appropriate coping skills (verbalization, pain relief, use of support systems such as family, clergy)
3. Silence all *unnecessary* alarms on technology (monitors, ventilators).	3. Unnecessary alarms increase the risk of sensory overload and may increase anxiety.	• Demonstrates basic understanding of technology used in care
4. Encourage and support patient while increasing activity level.	4. Positive reinforcement improves patient motivation and independence.	
5. Mobilize resources (family, clergy, social worker) to help patient cope with outcomes of surgery (diagnosis, change in functional abilities).	5. A multidisciplinary approach promotes the patient's strengths and coping mechanisms.	

Nursing Diagnosis: Impaired physical mobility of the upper extremities related to thoracic surgery
Goal: Increased mobility of the affected shoulder and arm

Nursing Interventions	Rationale	Expected Outcomes
1. Assist patient with normal range of motion and function of shoulder and trunk: a. Teach breathing exercises to mobilize thorax. b. Encourage skeletal exercises to promote abduction and mobilization of shoulder (see chart). c. Assist out of bed to chair as soon as pulmonary and circulatory systems are stable (usually by evening of surgery).	1. Necessary to regain normal mobility of arm and shoulder and to speed recovery and minimize discomfort.	• Demonstrates arm and shoulder exercises and verbalizes intent to perform them on discharge • Regains previous range of motion in shoulder and arm
2. Encourage progressive activities according to development of fatigue.	2. Increases patient's use of affected shoulder and arm.	

Nursing Diagnosis: Fluid volume deficit related to the surgical procedure
Goal: Maintenance of adequate fluid volume

Nursing Interventions	Rationale	Expected Outcomes
1. Monitor and record hourly intake and output. Urine output should be at least 30 mL hourly after surgery.	1. Fluid management may be altered before, during, and after surgery, and patient's response to and need for fluid management must be assessed.	• Patient is adequately hydrated, as evidenced by: • Urine output greater than 30 mL/h

(*continued*)

22•1 PLAN OF NURSING CARE

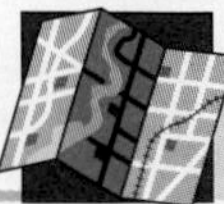

Care of the Patient After Thoracotomy (*continued*)

Nursing Interventions	Rationale	Expected Outcomes
2. Administer blood component therapy and parenteral fluids or diuretics as prescribed to restore and maintain fluid volume.	2. Pulmonary edema due to transfusion or fluid overload is an ever-present threat; after pneumonectomy, the pulmonary vascular system has been greatly reduced.	• Vital signs stable, heart rate, and central venous pressure approaching normal • No excessive peripheral edema
Nursing Diagnosis: Knowledge deficit of home care procedures **Goal:** Increased ability to carry out care procedures at home		
1. Encourage patient to practice arm and shoulder exercises five times daily at home.	1. Exercise accelerates recovery of muscle function and reduces long-term pain and discomfort.	• Demonstrates arm and shoulder exercises • Verbalizes need to try to assume an erect posture • Verbalizes the importance of relieving discomfort, alternating walking and rest, practicing breathing exercises, avoiding heavy lifting, avoiding undue fatigue, avoiding bronchial irritants, preventing colds or lung infections, getting flu vaccine, keeping follow-up visits, and stopping smoking
2. Instruct patient to practice assuming a functionally erect position in front of a full-length mirror.	2. Practice will help restore normal posture.	
3. Instruct patient in following aspects of home care:	3. Knowing what to expect speeds recovery.	
a. Relieve intercostal pain by local heat or oral analgesia.	a. Some soreness may persist for several weeks.	
b. Alternate activities with frequent rest periods.	b. Weakness and fatigability are common for the first 3 weeks.	
c. Practice breathing exercises at home.	c. Effective breathing is necessary to prevent splinting of affected side, which may lead to atelectasis.	
d. Avoid heavy lifting until complete healing has occurred.	d. Chest muscles and incision may be weaker than normal for 3–6 months.	
e. Avoid undue fatigue, increased shortness of breath, or chest pain.	e. Undue stress may prolong the healing process.	
f. Avoid bronchial irritants.	f. The lung is more susceptible to irritants.	
g. Prevent colds or lung infection.	g. The lung is more susceptible to infection during the recovery phase.	
h. Get annual influenza vaccine.	h. Vaccination helps prevent flu.	
i. Keep follow-up appointment with physician.	i. This allows timely follow-up assessment.	
j. Stop smoking.	j. Smoking will slow healing process by decreasing oxygen delivery to tissues and make lung susceptible to infection and other complications.	

7. Adheres to therapeutic program and home care
8. Is free of complications, as evidenced by normal vital signs and temperature, improved arterial blood gas measurements, clear lung sounds, and adequate respiratory function

For a detailed plan of nursing care for the patient who has had a thoracotomy, see the Plan of Nursing Care 22-1.

Critical Thinking Exercises

1.
Your 55-year-old patient is to be sent home on mechanical ventilation in the care of his wife. Develop a checklist to use in teaching the patient and his family about care in the home. Identify resources that would be helpful to this family in providing care for the patient in the home.

2.
A patient is returning to the nursing unit after chest surgery with an endotracheal tube, a chest tube, and two intravenous lines in place. Identify the priorities of assessment and interventions for this patient.

3.
A patient who has had a tracheostomy tube inserted 12 hours ago becomes confused and removes the tracheostomy tube. What are the immediate actions that are indicated in this situation? What nursing assessments and nursing interventions are needed once the immediate situation has been corrected?

References and Selected Readings

BOOKS

Burton, G. G., Hodgkin, J. E., & Ward, J. J. (Eds.). (1997). *Respiratory care: A guide to clinical practice.* Philadelphia: Lippincott-Raven.

Dumo, P. J., & McInturff, S. L. (1997). *Respiratory home care: The essentials.* Philadelphia: F. A. Davis.

Providing respiratory care (New Nursing Photobooks). (1995). Springhouse, PA: Springhouse.

Sole, M. L., & Byers, J. F. (1997). Ventilatory assistance. In J. C. Hartshorn, M. L. Sole, & M. L. Lamborn (Eds.), *Introduction to critical care nursing* (2nd ed.). Philadelphia: W. B. Saunders.

Wilson, D. J. (1996). Care of the chronic mechanically ventilated patient. In J. Clochesy, C. Breu, S. Cardin, A. A. Whittaker, & E. B. Rudy (Eds.), *Critical care nursing* (2nd ed.). Philadelphia: W. B. Saunders.

Wright, J., Doyle, P., & Yoshihara, G. (1996). Mechanical ventilation: current uses and advances. In J. Clochesy, C. Breu, S. Cardin, A. A. Whittaker, & E. B. Rudy (Eds.), *Critical care nursing* (2nd ed.). Philadelphia: W. B. Saunders.

Wyka, K. A. (1997). *Respiratory care in alternate sites.* Albany, NY: Delmar.

JOURNALS

Asterisks indicate nursing research articles.

*Berg, J. (1996). Quality of life in COPD patients using transtracheal oxygen. *MedSurg Nursing, 5*(1), 36–40.

Brenner, Z. R., & Addona, C. (1995). Caring for the pneumonectomy patient: Challenges and changes. *Critical Care Nurse, 15*(5), 65–72.

Brooks-Brunn, J. A. (1995). Postoperative atelectasis and pneumonia: Risk factors. *American Journal of Critical Care, 4*, 340–349.

Chang, V. M. (1995). Protocol for prevention of complications of endotracheal intubation. *Critical Care Nurse, 15*(5), 19–27.

Druding, M. C. (1997). Re-examining the practice of normal saline instillation prior to suctioning. *MedSurg Nursing, 6*(4), 209–212.

Gallagher, J. (1997). Taking the pressure off mechanically ventilated patients. *Nursing '97, 27*(5 Crit Care), CC1–7.

Glass, C. A., & Grap, M. J. (1995). Ten tips for safer suctioning. *American Journal of Nursing, 95*(5), 51–53.

Glass, C., Grap, M. J., & Battle, G. (1999). Preparing the patient and family for home mechanical ventilation. *MedSurg Nursing, 8*(2), 99–107.

*Gordon, P. A., Norton, J. M., Guerra, J. M., & Perdue, S. T. (1997). Position of chest tubes: Effects on pressure and drainage. *American Journal of Critical Care, 6*(1), 33–38.

Grap, M. J., Glass, C., & Lindamood, M. O. (1995). Factors related to unplanned extubation of endotracheal tubes. *Critical Care Nurse, 15*(4), 57–65.

*Grap, M. J., Glass, C., Corley, M., & Parks, T. (1996). Endotracheal suctioning: Ventilatory vs manual delivery of hyperoxygenation breaths. *American Journal of Critical Care, 5*(3), 192–197.

Hallfeldt, K. K. J., Siebeck, M., Thetter, O., & Schweiberer, L. (1995). The effect of thoracic surgery on pulmonary function. *American Journal of Critical Care, 4*, 352–354.

Hillberg, R. E., & Johnson, D. C. (1997). Noninvasive ventilation. *New England Journal of Medicine, 337*(24), 1746–1752.

Jacavone, J., & Young, J. (1998). Use of pulmonary rehabilitation strategies to wean a difficult-to-wean patient: A case study. *Critical Care Nurse, 18*(6), 29–37.

Kanacki, L. (1997). How to guide ventilator-dependent patients from hospital to home. *American Journal of Nursing, 97*(2 Cont Care), 37–39.

Knebel, A. R. (1996). Ventilator weaning protocols and techniques: Getting the job done. *AACN Clinical Issues: Advanced Practice in Acute and Critical Care, 7*(4), 550–559.

McGowan, C. M. (1998). Non-invasive ventilatory support: Use of bi-level positive airway pressure in respiratory failure. *Critical Care Nurse, 18*(6), 47–53.

Newsome, E. A., & Ott, B. B. (1997). Lung volume reduction: Surgical treatment for emphysema. *American Journal of Critical Care, 6*(6), 423–427.

O'Hanlon-Nichols, T. (1996). Commonly asked questions about chest tubes. *American Journal of Nursing, 96*(5), 60–64.

Rice, R. (1995). Procedures in home care. Home mechanical ventilator management. *Home Healthcare Nurse, 13*(1), 73–75.

Roman, M., et al. (1998). Breaking the boundaries: Collaborating to develop a model ventilator training program. *MedSurg Nursing, 7*(1), 9–17.

Ruggles, L. (1995). Auto-PEEP: Measurement issues and nursing interventions. *Critical Care Nurse, 15*(4), 30–38.

Schakenbach, L. (1997). Consult stat. Caring for patients with TTO transtracheal oxygen therapy. *RN, 60*(5), 69–73.

*Scherer, V. K., & Schmieder, L. E. (1997). The effect of a pulmonary rehabilitation program on self-efficacy, perception of dyspnea, and physical endurance. *Heart and Lung, 26*(1), 15–22.

Somerson, S. J., Husted, C. W., Somerson, S. W., & Sicilia, M. R. (1996). Mastering emergency airway management. *American Journal of Nursing, 96*(5), 24–30.

Turner, P., Glass, C., & Grap, M. J. (1997). Care of the patient requiring mechanical ventilation. *MedSurg Nursing, 6*(2), 68–76.

Vaca, K. J., Osterloh, J. F., Daake, C. J., & Noedel, N. R. (1996). Nursing care of the thoracoscopic lung volume reduction patient. *American Journal of Critical Care, 5*(6), 412–419.

Yaksic, J. R., DeWoody, S., & Campbell, S. (1996). Care management of chronic ventilator patients: Reduce average length of stay and cost by half. *Nursing Case Management, 1*(1), 2–10.

Zavotsky, K. E. (1995). Bedside percutaneous tracheostomy: Implications for critical care nurses. *Critical Care Nurse, 15*(5), 37–43.

RESEARCH-BASED PRACTICE PROTOCOLS

Burns, S. M. (1998). *Weaning from long-term mechanical ventilation.* Aliso Viejo, CA: American Association of Critical Care Nurses.

Glass, C. (1998). *Home care management of ventilator-assisted patients.* Aliso Viejo, CA: American Association of Critical Care Nurses.

Hanneman, S. K. (1998). *Weaning from short-term mechanical ventilation.* Aliso Viejo, CA: American Association of Critical Care Nurses.

Henneman, E. A., Ellstrom, K., & St. John, R. (1998). *Airway Management.* Aliso Viejo, CA: American Association of Critical Care Nurses.

Luer, J. M. (1998). *Sedation and neuromuscular blockade in patients with acute respiratory failure.* Aliso Viejo, CA: American Association of Critical Care Nurses.

Parrish, C. R., Krenitsky, J., & McCray, S. (1998). *Nutritional support for the mechanically ventilated patient.* Aliso Viejo, CA: American Association of Critical Care Nurses.

Pierce, L. (1998). *Mechanical ventilation: Traditional and non-traditional modes.* Aliso Viejo, CA: American Association of Critical Care Nurses.

Resources

American Association for Respiratory Care, 11030 Ables Lane, Dallas, TX 75229; 1-972-243-2272

American Lung Association, 1740 Broadway, New York, NY 10019; 1-212-315-8700, 1-800-LUNG-USA; http://www.lungusa.org

American Thoracic Society, 1740 Broadway, New York, NY 10019; 1-212-315-8700; http://www.lungusa.org

National Heart, Lung and Blood Institute, National Institutes of Health, 900 Rockville Pike, Bldg 31, Bethesda, MD 20892; 1-301-496-5166; http://www.nhlbi.gov

UNIT

6

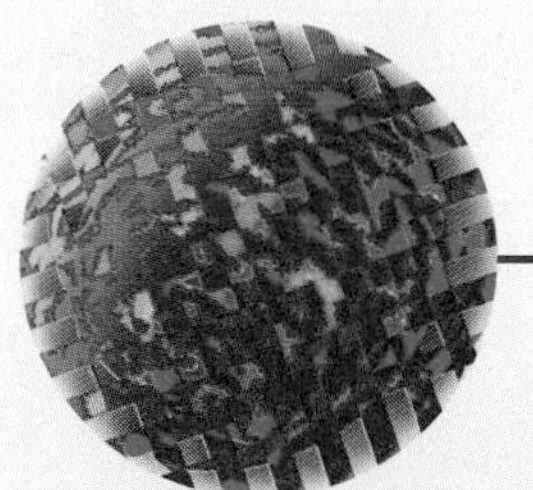

Cardiovascular, Circulatory, and Hematologic Function

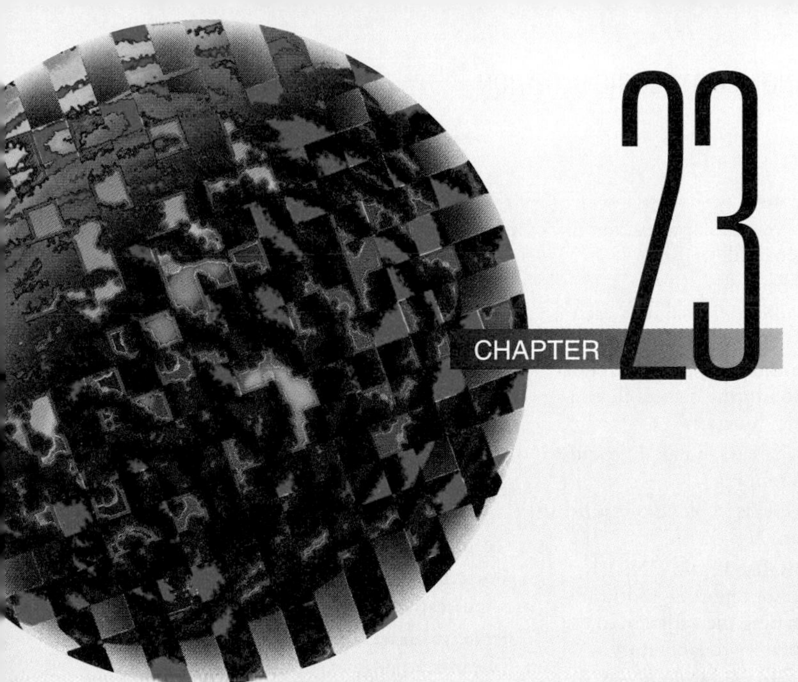

Assessment of Cardiovascular Function

Learning Objectives

On completion of this chapter, the learner will be able to:

1. Explain cardiac physiology in relation to cardiac anatomy and the conduction system of the heart.
2. Incorporate assessment of functional health patterns and cardiac risk factors into the health history and physical assessment of the patient with cardiac problems.
3. Use assessment parameters appropriate for determining the status of cardiovascular function.
4. Identify the clinical significance and related nursing implications of the various tests and procedures used for diagnostic assessment of cardiac function.
5. Compare central venous pressure monitoring, pulmonary artery pressure monitoring, and systemic intra-arterial monitoring with regard to clinical usefulness and significance, possible complications, and nursing responsibilities.

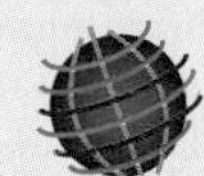

Patients with cardiovascular disease being cared for at any point in the continuum of care, whether in a home, hospital, or rehabilitation setting, all require similar assessment skills. Key components of the cardiovascular assessment include obtaining a health history, performing a physical assessment, and monitoring a variety of laboratory and diagnostic test results. An accurate and timely assessment of cardiovascular function provides the data necessary to identify nursing diagnoses, formulate a plan of care, and evaluate the response of the patient to the care provided. Essential to the development of these assessment skills is an understanding of the structure and function of the heart in health and in disease.

GLOSSARY

afterload: pressure the ventricular myocardium must overcome to eject blood during systole

apical impulse (also called **point of maximum impulse [PMI]**): impulse palpated at the fifth intercostal space, left midclavicular line caused by contraction of the left ventricle

baroreceptors: specialized nerve cells located in the aortic arch and carotid arteries that aid in regulating blood pressure

cardiac catheterization: an invasive procedure used to measure cardiac chamber pressure and patency of the coronary arteries

cardiac conduction system: specialized electrical cells strategically located throughout the heart responsible for methodically generating and coordinating the transmission of electrical impulses to the myocardial cells

cardiac output: amount of blood pumped by each ventricle in liters per minute; normal cardiac output is 5 L/min in the resting adult heart

cardiac stress test: a test used to evaluate the functioning of the heart during a period of increased oxygen demand

depolarization: electrical activation of the cell caused by the influx of sodium into the cell, while potassium exits the cell

diastole: period of ventricular relaxation resulting in ventricular filling

ejection fraction: percentage of the end-diastolic blood volume ejected with each heartbeat

hemodynamic monitoring: use of intravascular pressure monitoring devices to measure cardiovascular function

hypertension: an increase in blood pressure to above 140/90 mm Hg

hypotension: a decrease in blood pressure to below 100/60 mm Hg

international normalized ratio (INR): a standard method for reporting prothrombin levels, eliminating the variation in test results from laboratory to laboratory

murmurs: sounds created by abnormal, turbulent flow of blood in the heart

myocardial ischemia: decrease in oxygenation of the myocardium

myocardium: muscle layer of the heart responsible for the pumping action of the heart

normal heart sounds: sounds produced when the valves close; normal heart sounds are S_1 (semilunar valves) and S_2 (atrioventricular valves)

postural (orthostatic) hypotension: a significant drop in blood pressure after an upright posture is assumed

preload: degree of stretch of the cardiac muscle fibers at the end of diastole

pulmonary vascular resistance: resistance of the pulmonary pressure to right ventricle ejection

radioisotopes: unstable atoms that emit small amounts of energy in the form of gamma rays; used in cardiac nuclear medicine studies

repolarization: return of the cell to resting state caused by potassium reentering the cell, while sodium exits the cell

sinoatrial (SA) node: primary pacemaker of the heart, located in the right atrium

stroke volume: amount of blood ejected per heartbeat; normal stroke volume is 70 mL in the resting heart

systemic vascular resistance: resistance of the systemic pressure to left ventricle ejection

systole: period of ventricular contraction resulting in ejection of blood into the pulmonary artery and aorta

telemetry: the process of continuously monitoring the ECG by the transmission of radiowaves from a battery-operated transmitter worn by the patient

ANATOMIC AND PHYSIOLOGIC OVERVIEW

The heart is a hollow, muscular organ located in the center of the thorax, where it occupies the space between the lungs (mediastinum) and rests on the diaphragm. It weighs approximately 300 g (10.6 oz), although heart weight and size are influenced by age, gender, body weight, extent of physical exercise and conditioning, and heart disease. The heart pumps blood to the tissues, supplying them with oxygen and other nutrients.

The pumping action of the heart is accomplished by the rhythmic contraction and relaxation of its muscular wall. During **systole** (contraction of the muscle), the chambers of the heart become smaller as the blood is ejected. During **diastole** (relaxation of the muscle), the heart chambers fill with blood in preparation for the subsequent ejection. A normal resting adult heart beats approximately 60 to 80 times per minute. Each ventricle ejects approximately 70 mL of blood per beat and has an output of approximately 5 L per minute.

Anatomy of the Heart

The heart is composed of three layers (Fig. 23-1). The inner layer, or endocardium, consists of endothelial tissue, which lines the inside of the heart and valves. The middle layer, or **myocardium**, is made up of muscle fibers and is responsible for the pumping action. The exterior layer of the heart is called the epicardium.

The heart is encased in a thin, fibrous sac called the pericardium, which is composed of two layers. Adhering to the epicardium is the visceral pericardium. Enveloping the visceral pericardium is the parietal pericardium, a tough fibrous tissue that attaches to the great vessels, diaphragm, sternum, and vertebral column and supports the heart in the mediastinum. The space between these two layers (pericardial space) is filled with about 30 mL of fluid, which lubricates the surface of the heart and reduces friction during systole.

Heart Chambers

The four chambers of the heart constitute the right- and left-sided pumping systems. The right heart, made up of the right atrium and right ventricle, distributes venous blood (deoxygenated blood) to the lungs via the pulmonary artery (pulmonary circulation) for oxygenation. The right atrium receives blood returning from the superior vena cava (head, neck, and upper extremities), inferior vena cava (trunk and lower extremities), and coronary sinus (coronary circulation). The left side of the heart, composed of the left atrium and left ventricle, distributes oxygenated blood to the remainder of the body via the aorta (systemic circulation). The left atrium receives oxygenated blood from the pulmonary circulation via the pulmonary veins. The relationship of the four heart chambers is shown in Figure 23-1.

The varying thicknesses of the atrial and ventricular walls relate to the workload required by each chamber. The atria are thin-walled because blood returning to these chambers generates low pressures. In contrast, the ventricular walls are thicker because they generate greater pressures during systole. The right ventricle has thinner walls than the left ventricle. The right ventricle contracts against low pulmonary vascular pressure, whereas the left

PHYSIOLOGY

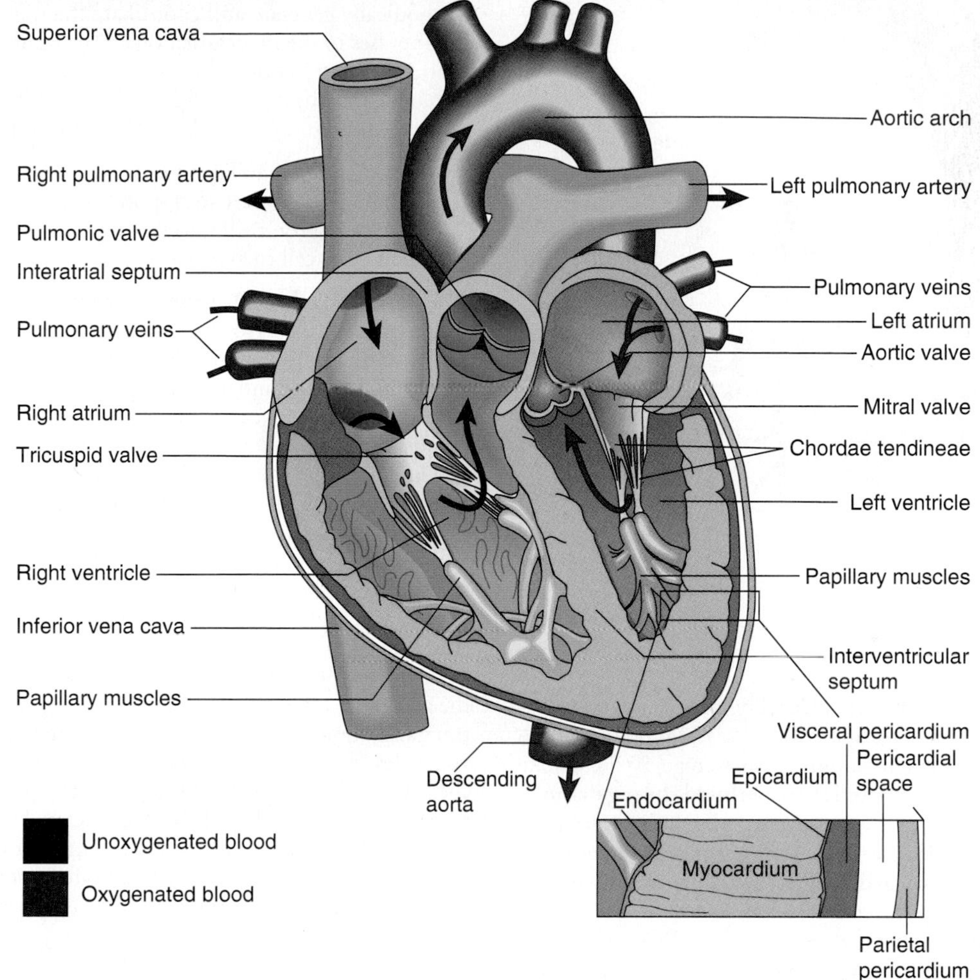

FIGURE 23•1 Structure of the heart. Arrows show course of blood flow through the heart chambers.

ventricle, with walls two-and-a-half times more muscular than the right, contracts against high systemic pressure.

Because the heart lies in a rotated position within the chest cavity, the right ventricle lies anteriorly (just beneath the sternum) and the left ventricle is situated posteriorly. The left ventricle is responsible for the apex beat or the point of maximum impulse (PMI), which is normally palpable in the left midclavicular line of the chest wall at the fifth intercostal space.

Heart Valves

The four valves in the heart permit blood to flow in only one direction. Valves, which are composed of thin leaflets of fibrous tissue, open and close in response to the movement of blood and pressure changes within the chambers. There are two types of valves: atrioventricular and semilunar.

ATRIOVENTRICULAR VALVES

The valves that separate the atria from the ventricles are termed atrioventricular valves. The tricuspid valve, so named because it is composed of three cusps or leaflets, separates the right atrium from the right ventricle. The mitral, or bicuspid, valve (two cusps) lies between the left atrium and the left ventricle (see Fig. 23-1).

Normally, when the ventricles contract, ventricular pressure rises, closing the atrioventricular valve leaflets. Two additional structures, the papillary muscle and the chordae tendineae, maintain valve closure. The papillary muscles, located on the sides of the ventricular walls, are connected to the valve leaflets by thin fibrous bands called chordae tendineae. During systole, contraction of the papillary muscles causes the chordae tendineae to become taut, keeping the valve leaflets approximated and closed.

SEMILUNAR VALVES

The two semilunar valves are composed of three half-moon–like leaflets. The valve between the right ventricle and the pulmonary artery is called the pulmonic valve; the valve between the left ventricle and the aorta is called the aortic valve.

Coronary Arteries

The left and right coronary arteries and their branches (Fig. 23-2) supply arterial blood to the heart. These arteries originate from the

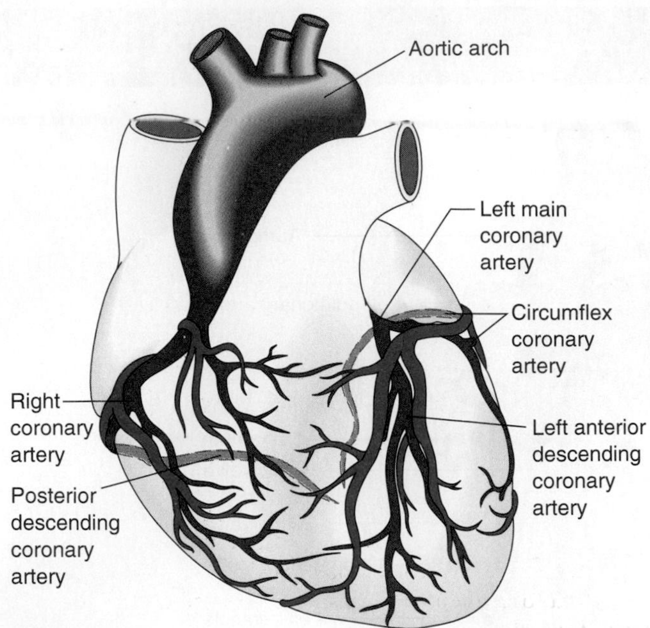

FIGURE 23•2 Coronary arteries (red vessels) arise from the aorta and encircle the heart. Coronary veins (*above*) are represented by blue.

aorta just above the aortic valve leaflets. The heart has large metabolic requirements, extracting approximately 70% to 80% of the oxygen delivered (other organs consume, on average, 25%). Unlike other arteries, the coronary arteries are perfused during diastole. An increase in heart rate shortens diastole and can decrease myocardial perfusion. Patients, particularly those with coronary artery disease, can develop **myocardial ischemia**, inadequate oxygen supply when the heart rate accelerates.

The left coronary artery has three branches. The artery from the point of origin to the first major branch is called the left main coronary artery. Two bifurcations arise off the left main coronary artery. These are the left anterior descending artery, which courses down the anterior wall of the heart, and the circumflex artery, which circles around to the lateral left wall of the heart.

The right side of the heart is supplied by the right coronary artery, which progresses around to the bottom or inferior wall of the heart. The posterior wall of the heart receives its blood supply by an additional branch called the posterior descending artery.

Superficial to the coronary arteries are the coronary veins. Venous blood through these veins returns to the heart primarily through the coronary sinus located posteriorly in the right atrium.

Cardiac Muscle

The myocardium is composed of specialized muscle tissue. Microscopically, myocardial muscle resembles striated (skeletal) muscle, which is under conscious control. Functionally, however, myocardial muscle resembles smooth muscle because it is involuntary. The myocardial muscle fibers are arranged in an interconnected manner (called a syncytium) that allows for coordinated myocardial contraction and relaxation. The sequential pattern of contraction and relaxation of individual muscle fibers ensures the rhythmic behavior of the myocardium as a whole and enables it to function as an effective pump.

Function of the Heart: Conduction System

The specialized electrical cells of the **cardiac conduction system** methodically generate and coordinate the transmission of electrical impulses to the myocardial cells. The result is sequential atrioventricular contraction, which provides for the most effective flow of blood, thereby optimizing cardiac output. Three physiologic characteristics of the electrical cells account for this synthesis:

- Automaticity: ability to initiate an electrical impulse
- Excitability: ability to respond to an electrical impulse
- Conductivity: ability to transmit an electrical impulse from one cell to another

The **sinoatrial (SA) node**, referred to as the primary pacemaker of the heart, is located at the junction of the superior vena cava and the right atrium (Fig. 23-3). The SA node in a normal resting heart has an inherent firing rate of 60 to 100 impulses per minute, but the rate can change in response to the metabolic demands of the body.

The electrical impulses initiated by the SA node are conducted along the myocardial cells of the atria via specialized tracts called internodal pathways. The impulses cause electrical stimulation and subsequent contraction of the atria. The impulses are then conducted to the atrioventricular (AV) node. The AV node (located in the right atrial wall near the tricuspid valve) consists of another group of specialized muscle cells similar to the SA node. The AV node coordinates the incoming electrical impulses from the atria and, after a slight delay (allowing the atria time to contract and complete ventricular filling), relays an impulse to the ventricles. This impulse is then conducted through a bundle of specialized electrical cells (bundle of His) that travel in the septum separating the left and right ventricles. The bundle of His divides into the right bundle branch (conducting impulses to the right ventricle) and the left bundle branch (conducting impulses to the left ventricle). To transmit impulses to the largest chamber

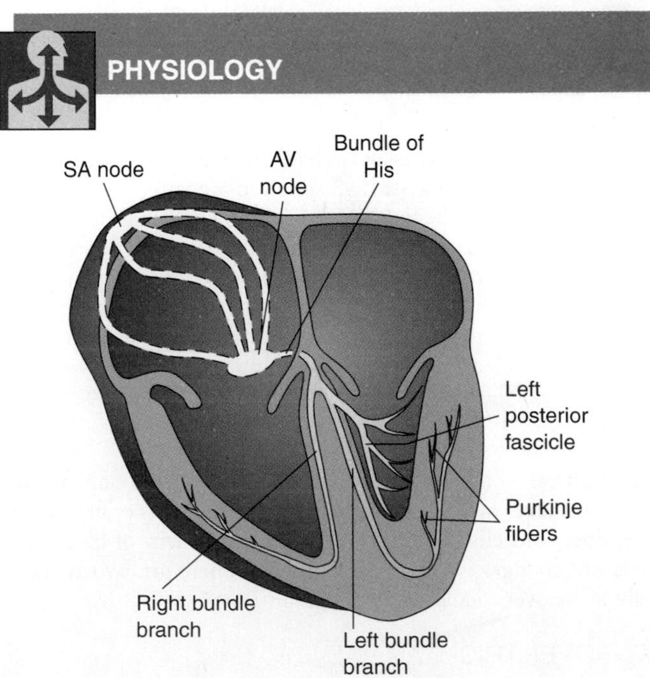

FIGURE 23•3 The cardiac conduction system.

of the heart, the left bundle branch bifurcates into the left anterior and left posterior bundle branches. Impulses travel through the bundle branches to reach the terminal point in the conduction system, called the Purkinje fibers. This is the point at which the myocardial cells are stimulated, causing ventricular contraction.

The heart rate is determined by the myocardial cells with the fastest inherent firing rate. Under normal circumstances, the SA node has the highest inherent rate, the AV node has the second-highest rate (40 to 60 impulses per minute), and the ventricular pacemaker sites have the lowest (30 to 40 impulses per minute). If the SA node malfunctions, the AV node generally takes over the pacemaker function of the heart at its lower rate. Should both the SA and AV nodes fail in their pacemaker function, a pacemaker site in the ventricle will fire at its inherent bradycardic rate of 30 to 40 impulses per minute.

Physiology of Cardiac Conduction

Cardiac electrical activity is the result of ions (charged particles such as sodium, potassium, and calcium) moving across the cell membrane. The electrical changes recorded within a single cell result in what is known as the cardiac action potential (Fig. 23-4).

In the resting state, cardiac muscle cells are polarized, which means an electrical difference exists between the negatively charged inside and the positively charged outside of the cell membrane. As soon as an electrical impulse is initiated, cellular permeability changes and sodium moves rapidly into the cell, while potassium exits the cell. This ionic exchange begins **depolarization** (electrical activation of the cell), converting the internal charge of the cell to a positive one (see Fig. 23-4). Contraction of the myocardium follows depolarization. The interaction between changes in membrane voltage and muscle contraction is called electromechanical coupling. As one cardiac muscle cell is depolarized, it acts as a stimulus to its neighboring cell, causing it to depolarize. Sufficient depolarization of a single specialized conduction system cell, therefore, results in depolarization and contraction of the entire myocardium. **Repolarization** (return of the cell to its resting state) occurs as the cell returns to its baseline or resting state; this corresponds to relaxation of myocardial muscle.

After the rapid influx of sodium into the cell during depolarization, the permeability of the cell membrane to calcium is changed, allowing for uptake of calcium into the cell. The influx of calcium, occurring during the plateau phase of repolarization, is much slower than that of sodium and continues for a longer period.

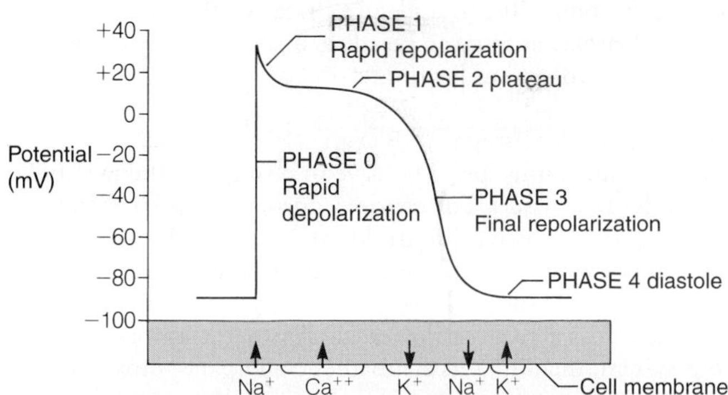

FIGURE 23•4 Cardiac action potential. The arrows below the diagram indicate the approximate time and direction of movement of each ion influencing membrane potential. The phase of Ca^{++} moving out of the cell is not well defined but is thought to occur during phase 4.

Cardiac muscle, unlike skeletal or smooth muscle, has a prolonged refractory period during which it cannot be restimulated to contract. There are two phases of the refractory period, referred to as absolute refractory period and relative refractory period. The absolute refractory period is the time when the heart cannot be restimulated to contract regardless of the strength of the electrical stimulus. This period corresponds with depolarization and the early part of repolarization. During the latter part of repolarization, however, if the electrical stimulus is stronger than normal, the myocardium can be stimulated to contract. This short period at the end of repolarization is called the relative refractory period.

Refractoriness protects the heart from sustained contraction (tetany), which would result in sudden cardiac death. Normal electromechanical coupling and contraction of the heart depend on the composition of the interstitial fluid surrounding the heart muscle cells. In turn, the composition of this fluid is influenced by the composition of the blood. A change in serum calcium concentration, therefore, may alter the contraction of the heart muscle fibers. A change in blood potassium concentration is also important, because potassium affects the normal electrical voltage of the cell.

Cardiac Hemodynamics

An important determinant of blood flow in the cardiovascular system is related to the principle that states that fluid flows from a region of higher pressure to one of lower pressure. The pressures responsible for blood flow in the normal circulation are generated during systole and diastole. Figure 23-5 depicts these pressure differences in the great vessels and the four chambers of the heart during systole and diastole.

CARDIAC CYCLE

Beginning with systole, the pressure inside the ventricles rapidly rises, forcing the atrioventricular valves to close. As a result, blood ceases to flow from the atria into the ventricles and regurgitation (backflow) of blood into the atria is prevented. The rapid rise of pressure inside the right and left ventricles forces the pulmonic and aortic valves to open, and blood is ejected into the pulmonary artery and aorta, respectively. The exit of blood is at first rapid; then, as the pressure in each ventricle and its corresponding artery equalizes, the flow of blood gradually decreases. At the end of systole, pressure within the right and left ventricles rapidly decreases. This lowers pulmonary artery and aortic pressure, causing closure of the semilunar valves. These events mark the onset of diastole.

During diastole, when the ventricles are relaxed and the atrioventricular valves are open, blood returning from the veins flows into the atria and then into the ventricles. Toward the end of this diastolic period, the atrial muscles contract in response to an electrical impulse initiated by the SA node (atrial systole). The resultant contraction raises the pressure inside the atria, ejecting blood into the ventricles. Atrial systole augments ventricular blood volume by 15% to 25% and is sometimes referred to as the "atrial kick." At this point, ventricular systole begins in response to propagation of the electrical impulse that began in the SA node some milliseconds previously. The following section reviews the chamber pressures generated during systole and diastole.

Chamber Pressures. In the right heart, the pressure generated during ventricular systole (15 to 25 mm Hg) exceeds the pulmonary artery diastolic pressure (8 to 15 mm Hg), and blood is

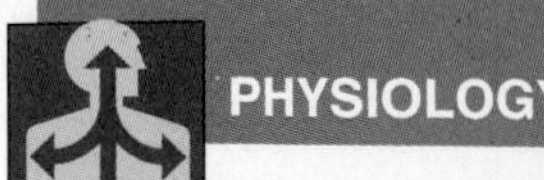

PHYSIOLOGY

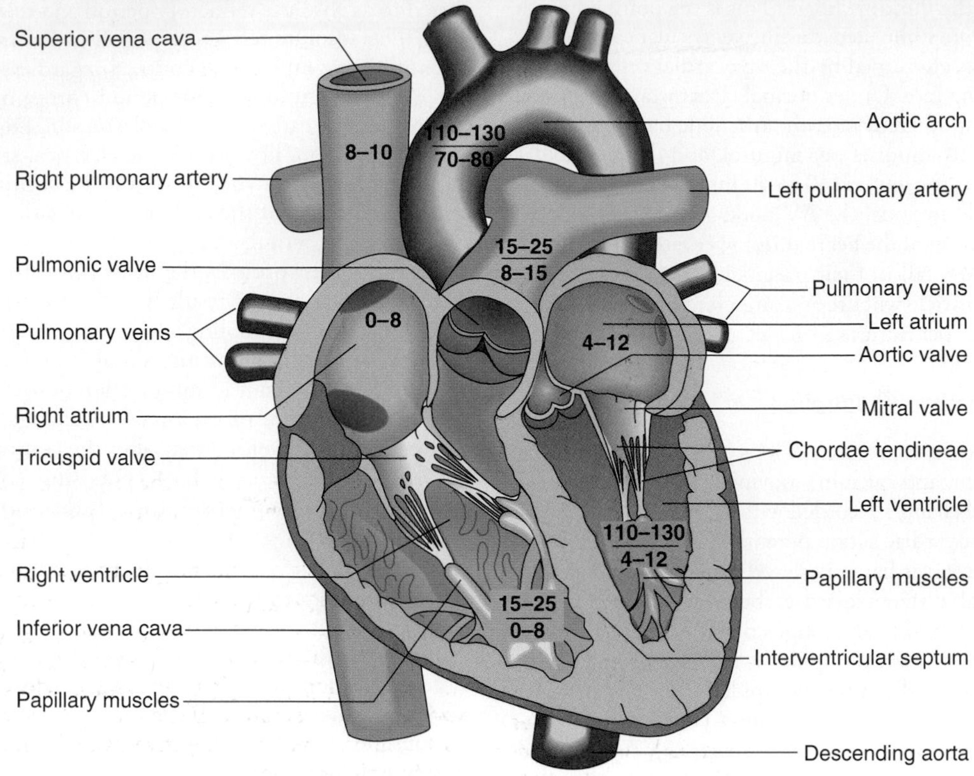

FIGURE 23•5 Great vessel and chamber pressures. Pressures are identified in mm Hg with systolic over diastolic pressure.

ejected into the pulmonary circulation. During diastole, venous blood flows into the atrium because pressure in the superior and inferior vena cava (8 to 10 mm Hg) is higher than that of the atrium. Blood flows through the open tricuspid valve and into the right ventricle until the two right chamber pressures equalize (0 to 8 mm Hg).

In the left heart, similar events are occurring, although higher pressures are generated. As pressure mounts in the left ventricle during systole (110 to 130 mm Hg), resting aortic pressure is exceeded (80 mm Hg) and blood is ejected into the aorta. During left ventricular ejection, the resultant aortic pressure (110 to 130 mm Hg) forces blood progressively through the arteries. Forward blood flow into the aorta ceases as the ventricle relaxes and pressure drops. During diastole, oxygenated blood returning from the pulmonary circulation via the four pulmonary veins flows into the atria, where pressure remains low. Blood readily flows into the left ventricle because ventricular pressure is also low. At the end of diastole, pressure in the atrium and ventricle equilibrates (4 to 12 mm Hg). Figure 23-5 depicts the systolic and diastolic pressures in the four chambers of the heart.

Pressure Measurement. Chamber pressures are measured using special monitoring catheters and equipment. This technique is called **hemodynamic monitoring**. Nurses caring for critically ill patients must have a sophisticated working knowledge of normal chamber pressures and the hemodynamic changes that occur during serious illnesses. The data obtained from hemodynamic monitoring assist with the diagnosis and management of pathophysiologic conditions affecting critically ill patients and are covered in more detail at the end of this chapter.

Cardiac Output

Cardiac output is the amount of blood pumped by each ventricle during a given period. The cardiac output in a resting adult is about 5 L per minute but varies greatly depending on the metabolic needs of the body. Cardiac output is computed by multiplying the stroke volume by the heart rate. **Stroke volume** is the amount of blood ejected per heartbeat. The average resting stroke volume is about 70 mL and heart rate is 60 to 80 beats per minute. Cardiac output can be affected, therefore, by changes in either stroke volume or heart rate.

CONTROL OF HEART RATE

Cardiac output must be responsive to changes in the metabolic demands of the tissues. For example, during exercise the total cardiac output may increase fourfold, to 20 L per minute. This increase is normally accomplished by approximately doubling both the heart rate and the stroke volume. Changes in heart rate are accomplished by reflex controls mediated by the autonomic nervous system, including its sympathetic and parasympathetic divisions. The parasympathetic impulses, which travel to the heart through the vagus nerve, can slow the cardiac rate, whereas sympathetic impulses increase it. These effects on heart rate result from action on the SA node, either to decrease or increase its inherent rate. The balance between these two reflex control systems normally determines the heart rate. The heart rate is stimulated also by an increased level of circulating catecholamines (secreted by the adrenal gland) and by excess thyroid hormone, which produces a catecholamine-like effect.

Heart rate is also affected by central nervous system and baroreceptor activity. **Baroreceptors** are specialized nerve cells located in the aortic arch and both right and left internal carotid arteries (at the point of bifurcation from the common carotid arteries). The baroreceptors are sensitive to blood pressure (BP) changes. During elevations in BP (**hypertension**), these cells increase their rate of discharge, transmitting impulses to the medulla. This initiates parasympathetic activity and inhibits sympathetic response, lowering heart rate and BP. The opposite is true during **hypotension** (low BP). Hypotension results in less baroreceptor stimulation. This prompts a decrease in parasympathetic inhibitory activity in the SA node, allowing for enhanced sympathetic activity. The resultant vasoconstriction and increased heart rate elevate BP.

CONTROL OF STROKE VOLUME

Stroke volume is primarily determined by three factors: preload, afterload, and contractility.

Preload is the term used to describe the degree of stretch of the cardiac muscle fibers at the end of diastole. The end of diastole is the period when filling volume in the ventricles is the highest and the degree of stretch on the muscle fibers is the greatest. Therefore, the volume of blood within the ventricle at the end of diastole determines preload. Preload has a direct effect on stroke volume. As the volume of blood returning to the heart increases, muscle fiber stretch also increases (increased preload), resulting in stronger contraction and a greater stroke volume. This relationship, called the Frank-Starling law of the heart (or sometimes the Starling law of the heart), is maintained until the physiologic limit of the muscle is reached. The Frank-Starling law is based on the fact that, within limits, the greater the initial length or stretch of the cardiac muscle, the greater the degree of shortening that will occur. This results from increased interaction between the thick and thin filaments of the sarcomeres (similar to the interaction discussed more fully in Chap. 60). Preload is decreased by a reduction in the volume of blood returning to the ventricles. Diuresis, venodilating agents such as nitrates, and loss of blood or body fluids from excessive diaphoresis, vomiting, or diarrhea reduce preload. Preload is increased by increasing the return of circulating blood volume to the ventricles. Controlling the loss of blood or body fluids and replacing fluids (ie, blood transfusions and intravenous fluid administration) are examples of ways to increase preload.

The second determinant of stroke volume is **afterload**, the pressure the ventricular myocardium must overcome to eject blood during systole. The resistance of the systemic pressure to left ventricle ejection is called **systemic vascular resistance**. The resistance of the pulmonary pressure to right ventricle ejection is called **pulmonary vascular resistance**. There is an inverse relationship between afterload and stroke volume. For example, afterload is increased from arterial vasoconstriction, which leads to decreased stroke volume. The opposite is true with arterial vasodilation. In this case, afterload is reduced because there is less resistance to ejection, and stroke volume increases.

Contractility is a term used to denote the force generated by the contracting myocardium under any given condition. Contractility is increased by circulating catecholamines, sympathetic neuronal activity, and certain medications (eg, digoxin and intravenous dopamine or dobutamine). Increased contractility results in increased stroke volume. Contractility is depressed by hypoxemia, acidosis, and certain medications (eg, beta-adrenergic blocking agents).

The heart can achieve a greatly increased stroke volume (eg, during exercise) by increasing preload (through increased venous return), by increasing contractility (through sympathetic nervous system discharge), and by decreasing afterload (through peripheral vasodilation with decreased aortic pressure).

The percentage of the end-diastolic volume that is ejected with each stroke is called the **ejection fraction**. With each stroke, about 42% (right ventricle) to 50% (left ventricle) or more of the end-diastolic volume is ejected by the normal heart. The ejection fraction can be used as an index of myocardial contractility; the ejection fraction decreases if contractility is depressed.

Gerontologic Considerations

Changes in cardiac structure and function are clearly observed in the older heart. To understand the changes specifically related to aging, it is helpful to isolate the normal aging process from cardiovascular disease–related changes. The anatomic and functional changes in the aging heart are listed in Table 23-1.

Studies show that the normal aging heart can produce adequate cardiac output under ordinary circumstances but may have a limited ability to respond to situations that cause physical or emotional stress. In an elderly person who is less active, the left ventricle may become smaller (atrophy) as a consequence of physical deconditioning. Aging also results in decreased elasticity and widening of the aorta, thickening and rigidity of the cardiac valves, and increased connective tissue in the SA and AV nodes and bundle branches.

These changes lead to decreased myocardial contractility, increased left ventricular ejection time (prolonged systole), and delayed conduction. Thus, stressful physical and emotional conditions, especially those that occur suddenly, may have adverse effects on the aged person. The heart cannot respond to such conditions with an adequate rate increase and needs more time to return to normal resting rates after even a minimal increase. In some patients, the added stress may precipitate heart failure.

Gender Differences in Cardiac Structure and Function

Compared to a man's heart, a woman's heart tends to be smaller. It weighs less and has smaller coronary arteries. These structural differences have significant implications. Because the coronary arteries of a woman are smaller, they occlude from atherosclerosis more easily, making procedures such as cardiac catheterization and angioplasty technically more difficult, with a higher incidence of postprocedure complications. In addition, the resting rate, stroke volume, and ejection fraction of a woman's heart are higher than those of a man's, and the conduction time of an electrical impulse coursing from the SA node through the AV node to the Purkinje fibers is also briefer.

Another significant difference between the genders is associated with female hormones. Women are thought to be protected from developing coronary artery disease by the beneficial effects of natural estrogen. Studies (PEPI Trial, 1995) have demonstrated that estrogen affects cholesterol levels, reducing low-density lipoprotein levels, raising high-density lipoprotein levels, and improving blood flow. However, these beneficial effects disappear after menopause, as the incidence of coronary artery disease in postmenopausal women not receiving estrogen replacement therapy equals that in their male counterparts.

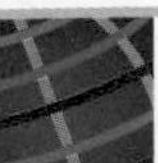

TABLE 23•1 **Age-Related Changes of the Cardiac System**

Cardiovascular System	Structural Changes	Functional Changes	History and Physical Findings
Atria	↑ size of left atrium Thickening of the endocardium	↑ atrial irritability	Irregular heart rhythm from atrial dysrhythmias
Left ventricle	Endocardial fibrosis Myocardial thickening (hypertrophy) Infiltration of fat into myocardium	Left ventricle stiff and less compliant Progressive decline in cardiac output ↑ risk for ventricular dysrhythmias Prolonged systole	Fatigue ↓ exercise tolerance Signs and symptoms of CHF or ventricular dysrhythmias Point of maximal impulse palpated lateral to the midclavicular line ↓ intensity S_1, S_2, split S_2 S_4 may be present
Valves	Thickening and rigidity of A-V valves Calcification of aortic valve	Abnormal blood flow across valves during cardiac cycle	Murmurs may be present Thrill palpated if significant murmur present
Conduction system	Connective tissue collects in SA node, AV node, and bundle branches ↓ number SA node cells ↓ number AV, bundle of His, right and left bundle branch cells	Slower SA node rate of impulse discharge Slowed conduction across AV node and ventricular conduction system	Bradycardia Heart block ECG changes consistent with slowed conduction (↑ PR interval, ↑ QRS complex)
Sympathetic nervous system	↓ response to beta-adrenergic stimulation	↓ adaptive response to exercise: contractility and heart rate slower to respond to exercise demands Heart rate takes more time to return to baseline	Fatigue Diminished exercise tolerance ↓ ability to respond to stress
Aorta and arteries	Stiffening of vasculature ↓ elasticity and widening of aorta Elongation of aorta, displacing the brachiocephalic artery upward	Left ventricular hypertrophy	Progressive increase in systolic BP; slight ↑ in diastolic BP Widening pulse pressure Pulsation visible above right clavicle
Baroreceptor response	↓ sensitivity of baroreceptors in the carotid artery and aorta to transient episodes of hypertension and hypotension	Baroreceptors unable to regulate heart rate and vascular tone, causing slow response to postural changes in body position	Postural blood pressure changes and reports feeling dizzy, fainting when moving from lying to sitting or standing position

ASSESSMENT

The severity of the patient's symptoms, the practice setting of the nurse, and the purpose of the assessment are variables to consider in determining the frequency and extent of nursing assessment required. The assessment of the acutely ill cardiac patient will be different from that of a patient with stable or chronic cardiac problems. For example, an assessment performed by an emergency department nurse caring for a patient experiencing an acute myocardial infarction (MI) must be very focused and must be performed rapidly. The nurse must assess the patient for complications associated with the MI, screen the patient for contraindications to thrombolytic therapy, and evaluate the patient's response to medical and nursing interventions. For this patient, the health history, physical assessment, and important nursing interventions, such as cardiac monitoring and administration of intravenous medications, are performed simultaneously.

Health History and Clinical Manifestations

For the patient experiencing an acute MI, the nurse obtains the health history using a few well-chosen questions about the onset and severity of chest discomfort, associated symptoms, current medications, and allergies. At the same time, the nurse observes the patient's general appearance and evaluates hemodynamic status (heart rate and rhythm, BP). Once the condition of the patient stabilizes, a more extensive history can be obtained.

With stable patients, a complete health history is obtained during the initial contact. Often, it is helpful to have the patient's spouse or partner available during the health history interview. Initially, demographic information regarding age, gender, and ethnic origin is obtained. Height, current weight, and usual weight (if there has been a recent weight loss or gain) are established. During the interview, the nurse conveys sensitivity to the cultural background and religious practices of the patient. This may remove barriers to communication that may result if the interview is based only on the nurse's personal frame of reference. Different cultural and ethnic groups may have different ways of describing symptoms such as pain and may engage in different health practices before seeking formal medical attention.

The baseline information derived from the history assists in identifying pertinent problems related to the patient's illness and educational and self-care needs. Once these problems are clearly identified, a plan of care can be instituted. During subsequent contacts or visits with the patient, a more focused health history is performed to determine if goals have been met, if the plan needs to be modified, or if new problems have developed. During the interview, the nurse asks questions to evaluate cardiac symptoms and health status.

Cardiac Symptoms

Patients with cardiovascular disorders commonly have one or more of the following signs and symptoms:

- Chest discomfort (angina pectoris or MI, valvular heart disease)
- Shortness of breath or dyspnea (left ventricular failure or congestive heart failure [CHF])
- Edema and weight gain (isolated right ventricular failure or CHF)
- Palpitations (dysrhythmias resulting from myocardial ischemia, valvular heart disease, ventricular aneurysm, stress, or electrolyte imbalance)
- Fatigue (earliest symptom associated with several cardiovascular disorders)
- Dizziness and syncope or loss of consciousness (postural hypotension, dysrhythmias, vasovagal effect, cerebrovascular disorders)

When a patient has chest discomfort, questions should focus on differentiating a serious, life-threatening condition such as MI from conditions that are less serious or that would be treated differently. Not all chest discomfort is related to myocardial ischemia. Table 23-2 summarizes the characteristics and patterns of the more common cardiac and noncardiac causes of chest pain.

Nursing Alert *Points to remember when evaluating chest discomfort include the following:*

- There is little correlation between the severity of the chest discomfort and the gravity of its cause. Some patients (eg, elderly or diabetic patients) may not have pain with angina or MI. Fatigue or shortness of breath may be the predominant symptom.
- There is poor correlation between the location of chest discomfort and its source.
- The patient may have more than one clinical problem occurring simultaneously.
- In a patient with a history of coronary artery disease, assume that the chest discomfort is secondary to ischemia until proven otherwise.

HEALTH PERCEPTION AND MANAGEMENT

The nurse may determine how patients perceive their current health status. To explore these concepts with patients, the nurse might ask some of the following questions:

- How has your health been recently? Have you noticed any changes from last year? or 5 years ago?
- Do you have a cardiologist or primary care provider? How often do you go for checkups?
- What do you do to stay healthy and to care for your heart?
- Can you identify any of your risk factors for heart disease?
- What do you think caused this illness?

Some patients may not be aware of their own medical diagnosis. For example, patients may not realize that their heart attack was caused by coronary artery disease. Patients who do not understand that their behaviors or diagnosis pose a threat to their health will be less motivated to make lifestyle changes or manage their illness effectively. On the other hand, patients who perceive that their modifiable cardiovascular risk factors have contributed to their health problems may be more likely to change these behaviors.

The patient's ability to recognize cardiac symptoms and to know what to do when they occur is essential for effective self-care management. However, numerous studies (eg, Dracup & Moser, 1997; Scherck, 1997) indicate that all too often, patients' new symptoms or symptoms of progressing cardiac illness go unrecognized. This results in delays in seeking life-saving treatment. Two major barriers to seeking prompt medical care include lack of knowledge about the relationship between symptoms and disease, and psychological factors—specifically, denial of symptoms when they occur.

An additional issue to consider is the patient's medication history, including prescription and over-the-counter medications, dosages, and schedule. Is the patient independent in taking medications? Are the medications taken as prescribed? Does the patient understand why the medication regimen is important? Are doses ever forgotten or skipped, or does the patient ever decide to stop taking a medication? An aspirin a day is a common nonprescription medication that improves patient outcomes after an MI. However, if patients are not aware of this benefit, they may be inclined to stop taking what they think is a trivial medication. A careful medication history will often uncover common medication errors and causes for nonadherence to the medication regimen.

Table 23-3 identifies typical questions nurses use to assess cardiac symptoms, as well as those used to determine the patient's ability to recognize and manage them. Other areas may need to be pursued for further clarification as necessary.

NUTRITION AND METABOLISM

Dietary modifications are important strategies for managing three major cardiovascular risk factors: hyperlipidemia, hypertension, and hyperglycemia (diabetes mellitus). Diets that are restricted in sodium, fat, cholesterol, and/or calories are commonly prescribed. The nurse should obtain the following dietary information:

- Food preferences (including cultural or ethnic)
- Typical diet
- Eating habits (canned or commercially prepared foods versus fresh foods, and restaurant cooking versus home cooking)
- Who shops for groceries
- Who prepares the meals

ELIMINATION

Typical bowel and bladder habits need to be identified. Nocturia (awakening at night to urinate) may be common for patients with CHF. Nocturia occurs when fluid that has collected in the tissues of the extremities is redistributed into the circulatory system once the patient lies down. Patients need to be aware of their response to diuretic therapy. Have there been any changes in urination?

To avoid straining, patients who become easily constipated need to establish a regular bowel regimen. When straining, the patient tends to bear down (the Valsalva maneuver), which momentarily increases pressure on the baroreceptors. This triggers a vagal response, causing the heart rate to slow down and causing syncope in some patients. For the same reason, straining during urination should be avoided. Because many cardiac medications can cause gastrointestinal side effects, the nurse asks about bloating, diarrhea, constipation, stomach upset, heartburn, loss of appetite, nausea and vomiting. Patients taking anticoagulants, such as low-molecular-weight heparin, heparin, or warfarin (Coumadin), are screened for bloody urine or stools.

TABLE 23•2 Assessment of Chest Pain

	Character, Location, and Radiation	Duration	Precipitating Events	Relieving Measures
Angina Pectoris	Substernal or retrosternal pain spreading across chest; may radiate to inside of arm, neck, or jaws	5–15 min	Usually related to exertion, emotion, eating, cold	Rest, nitroglycerin, oxygen
Myocardial Infarction	Substernal pain or pain over precordium; may spread widely throughout chest. Painful disability of shoulders and hands may be present.	>15 min	Occurs spontaneously but may be sequela to unstable angina	Morphine sulfate, successful reperfusion of blocked coronary artery
Pericarditis	Sharp, severe substernal pain or pain to the left of sternum; may be felt in epigastrium and may be referred to neck, arms, and back	Intermittent	Sudden onset. Pain increases with inspiration, swallowing, coughing, and rotation of trunk.	Sitting upright, analgesia, anti-inflammatory medications

(*continued*)

TABLE 23•2 **Assessment of Chest Pain** *(Continued)*

	Character, Location, and Radiation	Duration	Precipitating Events	Relieving Measures
Pleuritic Pain	Pain arises from inferior portion of pleura; may be referred to costal margins or upper abdomen. Patient may be able to localize the pain.	30+ min	Often occurs spontaneously. Pain occurs or increases with inspiration.	Rest, time. Treatment of underlying cause, bronchodilators.
Esophageal Pain (Hiatal hernia, reflux esophagitis or spasm)	Substernal pain; may be projected around chest to shoulders.	5–60 min	Recumbency, cold liquids, exercise. May occur spontaneously.	Food, antacid. Nitroglycerin relieves spasm.
Anxiety	Pain over chest; may be variable. Does not radiate. Patient may complain of numbness and tingling of hands and mouth.	2–3 min	Stress, emotional tachypnea	Removal of stimulus, relaxation

ACTIVITY AND EXERCISE

The effect of heart disease on the patient's functioning can be determined by assessing the patient's current activity level. Decreases in activity tolerance are typically gradual and may go unnoticed by the patient. In addition, the nurse needs to be certain that the patient describes symptoms, such as fatigue, angina pain, shortness of breath, or palpitations, that he or she has during exercise. Fatigue is an early indication of disease progression. Patients with fatigue may benefit from learning energy conservation techniques.

Additional areas to ask about include possible architectural barriers in the home, and what the patient does for exercise. If the patient exercises, the nurse asks additional questions: What is the intensity, and how long and how often is exercise performed? Has the patient ever participated in a cardiac rehabilitation program? Functional levels are known to improve for almost all patients who participate in a cardiac rehabilitation program (Wenger et al., 1995); therefore, attendance is highly recommended.

SLEEP AND REST

Clues to worsening cardiac disease, especially CHF, can be revealed by sleep-related events. Determining where the patient sleeps or rests is important. Recent changes, such as sleeping upright in a chair instead of in bed, increasing the number of pillows used, awakening short of breath at night (paroxysmal nocturnal dyspnea), or awakening with angina (nocturnal angina) are all indicative of worsening CHF.

COGNITION AND PERCEPTION

Evaluating cognitive ability helps to determine if the patient has the mental capacity to provide safe and effective self-care. Is the patient's short-term memory intact? Is there any history of

TABLE 23•3 Asking Questions to Evaluate Cardiac Problems

Symptoms	Assessing Signs and Symptoms	Assessing Patient's Capacity for Self-Care
Chest pain, chest discomfort, angina pain	• Where is your pain (ask patient to point to location on chest) • What does the pain feel like? (pressure, heaviness, burning) • How severe is it on a scale of 0 to 10? • What causes the pain? (exertion, stress) • Does anything relieve it? (rest, or nitroglycerin) • Does it spread to your arms, neck, jaw, shoulders, or back? • How long does the pain last? • Do you have any additional symptoms? (shortness of breath, palpitations, dizziness, sweating)	***Symptom Recognition*** • If you have angina, what does it usually feel like? • If you have angina, how do your angina symptoms differ from the discomfort caused by your other medical problems? (indigestion, other GI diseases) • How do you think you would tell the difference between the symptoms of angina and a heart attack? • What were you doing when the pain started? ***Symptom Management*** • What did you do when the pain started? • How long did you wait before seeking medical attention (calling the doctor, coming to the emergency department, or calling the ambulance) ***Use of Nitroglycerin*** • Do you have a prescription for nitroglycerin (NTG) tablets or spray? • At the time of your chest pain, did you use your NTG? • How many tablets or sprays did you use and how frequently? • If you have NTG and did not take it with this angina episode, why do you think you did not take it? • When did you first open your NTG container? Where is it stored?
Shortness of breath, edema, weight gain	• When did you first notice feeling short of breath? • Do you have a cough? If yes, what do you cough up? • What makes you short of breath? Does anything make your breathing better or worse? • What activities are you no longer able to do because you are short of breath? • Do you ever wake up at night feeling short of breath? • What is your normal weight? • Have you had a recent weight gain? • Do you get up at night to urinate? Have you noticed an increase or decrease in the amount you usually urinate? • Have you noticed any weight gain or swelling in your feet, ankles, legs, or abdomen (sacrum if bedridden)? Do your shoes feel tight or clothes feel tight around your waist? • How many pillows do you sleep on, and has this changed recently? • Do you sleep in your bed, or do you breathe easier sleeping in a chair?	• Has anyone ever told you that you have heart failure? What does this mean to you? • Do you ever forget to take your diuretic medication (water pill) or other heart medicines or decide not to take them? If so, why do you think this happens? • What do you typically eat or drink? Who does the food shopping and meal preparation? • Are you on a sodium- or fluid-restricted diet? Have you been able to follow your special diet? • Do you have a scale to weigh yourself? How often do you weigh yourself? • What are important signs or symptoms to report to your doctor?
Palpitations	• Do you ever feel your heart racing, skipping beats, or pounding? • Do you ever feel lightheaded or dizzy? • Are there any other symptoms that occur at the same time? • How much caffeine do you consume? • Do you use tobacco (cigarettes, cigars)? • Do you use any other stimulants? • Have there been any changes in the amount of stress you experience?	• What did you do when your symptoms first occurred? • Is your primary health care provider aware of these symptoms? • Are you on medication for this problem, and have you been taking it as directed?
Fatigue	• How would you describe your usual activity level? • What is your current activity level? • What were you able to do 1 month and 6 months ago? • What activities can you no longer do because of fatigue? • Do you feel rested when you wake up in the morning? • Can you rest during the day? • How often do you awaken at night, and for what reason?	• Have you spoken with your primary care provider about decreases in your activity level? • Has anyone ever taught you energy conservation techniques? If so, are you able to use them?

(*continued*)

TABLE 23•3 **Asking Questions to Evaluate Cardiac Problems** *(Continued)*

Symptoms	Assessing Signs and Symptoms	Assessing Patient's Capacity for Self-Care
Dizziness, syncope	• Do you ever feel dizzy or lightheaded? • Do you ever pass out or have fainting spells? • Does this happen when you move from a lying to a sitting or standing position? • Do you strain while having a bowel movement or when urinating? • Have you been urinating more than usual? • Have you decreased the amount of fluids you normally drink? • Do you have headaches?	• Have you ever been told you have high or low blood pressure? Has it been checked recently? • Are you on any medications that can lower your blood pressure? • Before standing from a lying position, do you sit for a few minutes? Does that help the dizziness? • What are you using to prevent constipation?

dementia? Is there evidence of depression or anxiety? Can the patient read? Can the patient read English? What is the patient's reading level or highest educational level? What is the patient's preferred learning style? What information does the patient perceive as important?

Providing the patient with written information can be a valuable adjunct to patient education, but only if the patient can read and comprehend information. Related assessments include possible hearing or visual impairments. If vision is impaired, patients with heart failure may not be able to weigh themselves independently and keep a daily record of variations in weight.

SELF-PERCEPTION AND SELF-CONCEPT

"Type A personality" has been considered a risk factor for coronary artery disease for more than two decades. A person with type A behavior may be characterized as aggressive, ambitious, competitive, impatient, easily angered, and hostile. Studies generated in the 1980s show that of all these characteristics, the strongest link to coronary artery disease is hostility.

During this portion of the health history, the nurse discovers how patients feel about themselves by asking questions such as: How would you describe yourself? Have you changed the way you feel about yourself since your heart attack or surgery? Do you find that you are easily angered or hostile? How do you feel right now? What helps to manage these feelings?

ROLES AND RELATIONSHIPS

Determining the patient's social support systems is vitally important in today's health care environment. Hospital stays for cardiac illnesses are getting shorter. Many invasive diagnostic cardiac procedures, such as cardiac catheterization and angioplasty, are now performed as outpatient procedures. Patients are being discharged back into the community with activity limitations, such as driving restrictions, and with greater nursing care and educational needs. These needs have significant implications for people who are, under normal circumstances, independent, as well as people, such as older adults, who are at higher risk for problems.

To assess support systems, the nurse needs to ask: Who is the primary caregiver? With whom does the patient live? Are there adequate services in place to provide a safe home environment? The nurse also assesses for any significant effects the cardiac illness has had on the patient's role in the family. Are there adequate finances and health insurance? The answers to these questions will assist the nurse in developing a plan to meet the patient's home care needs.

SEXUALITY AND REPRODUCTION

Research (Steinke & Patterson-Midgley, 1996) has shown that cardiac patients more than likely are not asked about concerns they have regarding sexual activity, nor are they given adequate information to help them resume their normal sex life. Patients recovering from MI and cardiac surgery have reported reduced frequency and satisfaction with sexual intercourse. The health history can be used to identify reasons for changes in sexuality.

The most commonly cited reasons for changes in sexual activity are fear of another heart attack or sudden death, untoward symptoms such as angina, dyspnea, or palpitations, or problems with impotence or depression. In men, impotence may develop as a side effect of cardiac medications (beta-adrenergic blocking agents), which may prompt the patient to stop taking them. Other medications can be substituted, and the patient should be encouraged to discuss this with his or her health care provider. Often, patients and their partners do not have adequate information about the physical demands related to sexual activity and ways these can be modified. Research indicates that the physiologic demands of intercourse are equivalent to walking up two flights of stairs. Having this information may make patients and their partners more comfortable with resuming sexual activity.

A reproductive history is necessary for women of childbearing age, particularly those with seriously compromised cardiac function. These women may be advised by their physicians not to become pregnant. The reproductive history includes information about previous pregnancies, plans for future pregnancies, oral contraceptive use (especially in women older than age 35 who are smokers), and hormone replacement therapy.

COPING AND STRESS TOLERANCE

The patient may experience four phases of emotional healing after an acute cardiac event such as MI. In the first 24 to 48 hours, patients and their spouses typically experience shock and disbelief. Patients exhibit anxiety or denial, while the partners may feel anxiety and guilt. The second phase (convalescent phase) occurs once the patient is hemodynamically stable and begins to internalize the significance of the cardiac event. Patients and spouses ask, "Why me?" or "Why my husband, wife, or companion?" Anxiety, depression, and, for the patient, aggressive sexual behavior may be demonstrated at this time. After hospital discharge, the third phase begins and may last up to 3 months. The patient is beginning to adapt to the diagnosis and starts to make decisions about lifestyle changes. The previously experienced responses continue. In addition, the partner may exhibit overprotective behavior to compensate for the patient's emotional distress. The last phase (up to 6 months

Risk Factors for HEART DISEASE

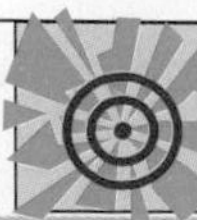

Nonmodifiable risk factors include the following:
Positive family history for premature coronary artery disease
Increasing age
Gender (men and postmenopausal women)
Race (higher incidence in African Americans than in whites)

Modifiable risk factors include the following:
Hyperlipidemia
Hypertension
Cigarette smoking
Elevated blood glucose level (ie, diabetes mellitus)
Obesity
Physical inactivity
Type A personality characteristics, particularly hostility
Use of oral contraceptives

from discharge) is a time for reorganization. A good predictor of long-term emotional adjustment is the patient's level of coping at 2 months (Oka, Burke, & Froelicher, 1995).

Being mindful of the emotional phases of healing after a cardiac event is necessary to identify how well the patient and spouse are coping with the illness. This is achieved by asking questions about recent stressors, previous coping styles and their effectiveness, and the patient's perception of his or her current coping ability.

Additional features of the health history include identification of risk factors and measures taken by the patient to prevent disease. The nurse's questions need to focus on the patient's health promotion practices. Epidemiologic studies show that certain conditions or behaviors, called risk factors, are associated with a greater incidence of coronary artery, peripheral vascular, and cerebrovascular diseases. Risk factors are classified by the extent to which they can be modified by changing one's lifestyle or modifying personal behavior.

Once the patient's risk factors are clear, the nurse assesses whether the patient has a plan for making necessary behavioral changes, or if assistance is needed to support these lifestyle changes. For example, research shows that about 10% of current smokers will quit with no other intervention but firm advice from their physician to quit, whereas others may need further encouragement. For patients with hyperlipidemia, hypertension, and diabetes, it is important to determine the frequency with which serum lipid levels, BP, and glucose levels are monitored and what the plan for management has been, such as diet, exercise, and/or medications. A detailed discussion of these risk factors appears later in this unit.

Recent studies (Smith et al., 1995; Wenger et al., 1995) in patients with coronary artery disease demonstrate that comprehensive secondary prevention strategies (early diagnosis and prompt intervention to halt or slow disease process and its sequelae) aimed at reducing cardiovascular risk factors improve overall survival, improve quality of life, reduce the need for revascularization procedures (angioplasty, coronary artery bypass surgery), and reduce the incidence of subsequent MIs. The overall benefits of secondary prevention also apply to other patient groups with atherosclerotic vascular disease, including patients with transient ischemic attacks, stroke, and peripheral vascular disease (the leading cause of disability and death in these patients being coronary artery disease).

Despite these findings, only one third of eligible patients, over the long term, adhere to risk factor interventions. Patient compliance increases significantly with a team approach that includes long-term follow-up with office or clinic visits and telephone contact (Smith et al., 1995).

Physical Assessment

A physical examination is performed to confirm the data obtained in the health history. In addition to observing the patient's general appearance, a cardiac physical assessment should include an evaluation of the following:

- Effectiveness of the heart as a pump
- Filling volumes and pressures
- Cardiac output
- Compensatory mechanisms

Indications that the heart is not contracting sufficiently or functioning effectively as a pump include reduced pulse pressure, cardiac enlargement, and murmurs and gallop rhythms (abnormal heart sounds).

The amount of blood filling the atria and ventricles and the resulting pressures (called filling volumes and pressures) are estimated by the degree of jugular vein distention and the presence or absence of congestion in the lungs, peripheral edema, and postural changes in BP that occur when the person sits up or stands.

Cardiac output is reflected by heart rate, pulse pressure, color and texture of the skin, urine output, and sensorium. Examples of compensatory mechanisms that help maintain cardiac output are increased filling volumes and elevated heart rate. Note that the findings on the physical examination are correlated with data obtained from diagnostic procedures, such as invasive hemodynamic monitoring (discussed later in this chapter).

The examination, which proceeds logically from head to toe, can be performed in about 10 minutes with practice: (1) general appearance, (2) skin, (3) BP, (4) arterial pulses, (5) jugular venous pulsations and pressures, (6) heart, (7) extremities, (8) lungs, and (9) abdomen.

General Appearance

The nurse observes the patient's level of distress, level of consciousness, and thought processes as an indication of the heart's ability to propel oxygen to the brain (cerebral perfusion). The nurse also observes for evidence of anxiety, along with any effects these emotional factors may have on cardiovascular status. The nurse attempts to put the anxious patient at ease throughout the examination.

Inspection of the Skin

Examination of the skin begins while evaluating the general appearance of the patient and continues throughout the assessment. It includes all body surfaces, starting with the head and finishing with the lower extremities. Skin color, temperature, and texture are assessed. The more common findings associated with cardiovascular diseases include:

- Pallor, or decrease in the color of the skin, is due to lack of oxyhemoglobin. It is caused by anemia or decreased arterial perfusion. Pallor is best observed around the fingernails, lips, and oral mucosa. In patients with dark skin, the nurse observes the palms of the hands and soles of the feet.

- Peripheral cyanosis, a bluish tinge, most often of the nails and skin of the nose, lips, earlobes, and extremities, suggests decreased flow rate of blood to a particular area, allowing more time for the hemoglobin molecule to become desaturated. This may occur normally with peripheral vasoconstriction associated with a cold environment, anxiety, or disease states such as CHF.
- Central cyanosis, a bluish tinge observed in the tongue and buccal mucosa, denotes serious cardiac conditions (pulmonary edema and congenital heart disease) in which venous blood passes through the pulmonary circulation without being oxygenated.
- Xanthelasma, yellowish, slightly raised plaques in the skin, may be observed along the nasal portion of one or both eyelids and may indicate elevated cholesterol levels (hypercholesterolemia).
- Reduced skin turgor occurs with dehydration and aging.
- Temperature and moistness are controlled by the autonomic nervous system. Normally the skin is warm and dry. Under stress, hands may become cool and moist. In cardiogenic shock, sympathetic nervous system stimulation causes vasoconstriction, and the skin becomes cold and clammy. During an acute MI, diaphoresis is common.
- Ecchymosis (bruise), a purplish-blue fading to green, yellow, or brown over time, is associated with blood outside of the blood vessels and is usually due to trauma. Patients receiving anticoagulant therapy should be carefully observed for unexplained ecchymosis. In these patients, excessive bruising indicates prolonged clotting times (prothrombin or partial thromboplastin times) caused by too high a dose of anticoagulant.
- Wounds, scars, and tissue surrounding implanted devices should also be examined. Wounds are assessed for adequate healing, and any scars from previous surgeries are noted. The skin surrounding pacemaker or implantable cardioverter defibrillator generators is examined for thinning, which could indicate erosion of the device through the skin.

Blood Pressure

Systemic arterial BP is the pressure exerted on the walls of the arteries during ventricular systole and diastole. It is affected by factors such as cardiac output, distention of the arteries, and the volume, velocity, and viscosity of the blood. BP usually is expressed as the ratio of the systolic pressure over the diastolic pressure, with normal adult values ranging from 100/60 to 140/90. The average normal BP usually cited is 120/80. An increase in BP above the upper normal range is called hypertension (see Chap. 29 for further definitions and management), whereas a decrease below the lower range is called hypotension.

BLOOD PRESSURE MEASUREMENT

BP can be measured using invasive arterial monitoring systems (discussed at the end of this chapter) or noninvasively by using a sphygmomanometer and stethoscope or with an automated BP monitoring device. A detailed description of the procedure for obtaining BP can be found in nursing skills textbooks, while specific manufacturer's instructions review the proper use of the automated monitoring devices. Several important details must be observed to ensure that BP measurements are accurate; these are highlighted in Chart 23-1.

CHART 23•1 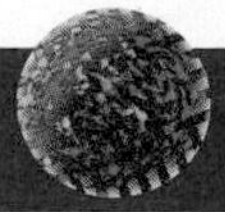 **Ensuring Accurate Blood Pressure Measurement**

- Cuff size must be appropriate for the patient. (The cuff size should have a bladder width 40% and length 80% of limb circumference.) The average adult cuff is 12 to 14 cm wide and 30 cm long. Using a cuff that is too small will give a high reading, whereas, too large a cuff results in a falsely low reading.
- Calibration of the sphygmomanometer should be performed routinely to ensure accuracy of blood pressure reading.
- Cuff is firmly wrapped around the arm, and cuff bladder is centered over the brachial artery.
- Patient's arm should be at heart level.
- Initial recordings are made on both arms, and subsequent measurements are taken on the arm with the higher pressure. Normally, in the absence of disease of the vasculature, there is a difference of no more than 5 mm Hg between arm pressures.
- Position of the patient and site of blood pressure measurement (eg, RA for right arm) are recorded.
- Palpation of the systolic pressure before auscultation helps to detect an auscultatory gap more readily.
- The patient is asked not to talk during blood pressure measurements. Researchers have found a significant increase in blood pressure and heart rate when subjects are talking.

PULSE PRESSURE

The difference between the systolic and the diastolic pressures is called the pulse pressure and is a reflection of stroke volume, ejection velocity, and systemic vascular resistance. Pulse pressure, which is normally 30 to 40 mm Hg, indicates how well the patient maintains cardiac output. The pulse pressure increases in conditions that elevate the stroke volume (anxiety, exercise, bradycardia), reduce systemic vascular resistance (fever), and reduce distensibility of the arteries (atherosclerosis, aging, hypertension). Decreased pulse pressure is an abnormal condition reflecting reduced stroke volume and ejection velocity (shock, heart failure, and hypovolemia) or obstruction to blood flow during systole (mitral or aortic stenosis). A pulse pressure of less than 30 mm Hg signifies a serious reduction in cardiac output and requires further cardiovascular assessment.

POSTURAL BLOOD PRESSURE CHANGES

Usually accompanied by dizziness, lightheadedness, or syncope, **postural (orthostatic) hypotension** occurs when the BP drops significantly after the patient assumes an upright posture.

Although there are many causes of postural hypotension, the three most common in patients with cardiac problems are a reduced volume of fluid or blood in the circulatory system (intravascular volume depletion), inadequate vasoconstrictor mechanisms, and insufficient autonomic effect on vascular constriction. Postural changes in BP and appropriate history help care providers differentiate among these causes. The following recommendations are important when assessing postural BP changes:

- Position the patient supine and flat as symptoms permit for 10 minutes before taking the initial BP and heart rate measurements.
- Check supine measurements before checking upright measurements.
- Record both heart rate and BP and indicate the corresponding position (eg, lying, sitting, standing).

- Do not remove the BP cuff between position changes, but check to see that it is still correctly placed.
- Assess postural BP changes with the patient sitting on the edge of the bed with feet dangling and, if appropriate, with the patient standing at the side of the bed.
- Wait 1 to 3 minutes after each postural change before measuring BP and heart rate.
- Be alert for any signs or symptoms of patient distress. If necessary, return the patient to bed before completing the test.
- Record any signs or symptoms that accompany the postural change.

Normal postural responses that occur when a person stands up or goes from a lying to a sitting position include: (1) a heart rate increase of 5 to 20 beats above the resting rate (to offset reduced stroke volume and maintain cardiac output), (2) an unchanged systolic pressure, or a slight decrease of up to 10 mm Hg, and (3) a slight increase of 5 mm Hg in diastolic pressure.

A decrease in the amount of blood or fluid in the circulatory system should be suspected after diuretic therapy or bleeding, when a postural change results in an increased heart rate and either a decrease in systolic pressure by 15 mm Hg or a drop in the diastolic pressure by 10 mm Hg. Vital signs alone will not help differentiate between a decrease in intravascular volume or inadequate constriction of the blood vessels as a cause of postural hypotension. With intravascular volume depletion, the reflexes that maintain cardiac output (increased heart rate and peripheral vasoconstriction) will function correctly; the heart rate will increase and the peripheral vessels will constrict. However, because of lost volume, the BP falls. With inadequate vasoconstrictor mechanisms, the heart rate again responds appropriately but, because of diminished peripheral vasoconstriction, the BP drops. The following is an example of a postural BP recording showing either intravascular volume depletion or inadequate vasoconstrictor mechanisms:

Lying down: BP 120/70, heart rate 70; sitting, BP 100/55, heart rate 90; standing, BP 98/52, heart rate 94

In autonomic insufficiency, the heart rate is unable to increase to compensate for the gravitational effects of an upright posture. Peripheral vasoconstriction may be absent or diminished. Autonomic insufficiency does not rule out a concurrent decrease in intravascular volume. The following is an example of autonomic insufficiency as demonstrated by postural BPs changes:

Lying down: BP 150/90, heart rate 60; sitting, BP 100/60, heart rate 60

Arterial Pulses

Factors to be evaluated in examining the pulse are rate, rhythm, quality, configuration of the pulse wave, and quality of the arterial vessel.

PULSE RATE

The normal pulse rate varies from a low of 50 in healthy, athletic young adults to rates well in excess of 100 after exercise or during times of excitement. Anxiety frequently raises the pulse rate during the physical examination. If the rate is higher than expected, it is appropriate to reassess it near the end of the physical examination, when the patient may be more relaxed.

PULSE RHYTHM

The rhythm of the pulse is as important to assess as the rate. Minor variations in the regularity of the pulse are normal. The pulse rate, particularly in young people, increases during inspiration and slows during expiration. This is called sinus arrhythmia.

For the initial cardiac examination, or if the pulse rhythm is irregular, the heart rate should be counted by auscultating the apical pulse for a full minute while simultaneously palpating the radial pulse.

Any discrepancy between contractions heard and pulses felt is noted. Disturbances of rhythm (dysrhythmias) often result in a pulse deficit, a difference between the apical rate (heart rate heard at the apex of the heart) and the peripheral rate. Pulse deficits commonly occur with atrial fibrillation, atrial flutter, premature ventricular contractions, and varying degrees of heart block. See Chapter 24 for a detailed discussion of these dysrhythmias.

To understand the complexity of dysrhythmias that may be encountered during the examination, the nurse needs to have a sophisticated knowledge of cardiac electrophysiology, obtained through advanced education and training.

PULSE QUALITY

The quality, or amplitude, of the pulse can be described as absent, diminished, or normal. It should be assessed bilaterally. Scales can be used to rate the strength of the pulse. The following is an example of a 0-to-4 scale:

0—not palpable or absent

+1—difficult to palpate; weak, thready pulse; obliterated with pressure

+2—diminished pulse, cannot be obliterated

+3—easy to palpate, full; cannot be obliterated

+4—strong bounding pulse; may be abnormal

Numerical classification is quite subjective; thus, when documenting the pulse quality, it helps to specify the scale range (eg, left radial +3/+4).

PULSE CONFIGURATION

The configuration, or contour, of the pulse conveys important information. In stenosis of the aortic valve, in which the valve opening is narrowed, reducing the amount of blood ejected into the aorta, the pulse pressure is narrow and the pulse feels feeble. With aortic insufficiency, in which the aortic valve does not close completely, allowing blood to flow back or leak from the aorta into the left ventricle, the rise of the pulse wave is abrupt and its fall is precipitous—a "collapsing" pulse. The true configuration of the pulse is best appreciated by palpating over the carotid artery rather than the distal radial artery, because the dramatic characteristics of the pulse wave may be distorted when the pulse is transmitted to smaller vessels.

EFFECT OF VESSEL QUALITY ON PULSE

The condition of the vessel wall also influences the pulse and is of concern, especially in older patients. Once rate and rhythm have been determined, the quality of the vessel is assessed by palpating along the radial artery and comparing it with normal vessels. Does it appear to be thickened? Is it tortuous?

To assess peripheral circulation, locate and evaluate all arterial pulses. Arterial pulses are palpated at points where the arteries are near the skin surface and are easily compressed against bones or firm musculature. Pulses are detected over the temporal, carotid, brachial, radial, femoral, popliteal, dorsalis pedis, and posterior tibial arteries. A reliable assessment of the pulses of the lower extremities depends on accurately identifying the location of the artery and carefully palpating the area. Light palpation is essential; firm finger pressure can easily obliterate the dorsalis pedis and posterior tibial pulses and confuse the examiner. In approximately 10% of patients, the dorsalis pedis pulses are not palpable. In such circumstances, both are usually absent together, and the posterior tibial arteries alone provide adequate blood supply to the feet.

Jugular Venous Pulsations

An estimate of right heart function can be made by observing the pulsations of the jugular veins of the neck. This provides a means of estimating central venous pressure, which reflects right atrial or right ventricular end-diastolic pressure (the pressure immediately preceding the contraction of the right ventricle).

Jugular vein distention is caused by increased filling volume and pressure on the right side of the heart. Jugular venous pressure is measured as follows:

- Begin with the patient supine, with the head of the examination table or bed elevated 15 degrees to 30 degrees.
- Turn the patient's head slightly away from the side of the neck that is being examined.
- Identify the external jugular vein.
- Locate the pulsations of the internal jugular vein. (Distinguish these pulsations from those of the adjacent carotid artery.)
- Identify the highest point at which the internal jugular vein pulsations can be seen.
- Find the sternal angle, which is the point where the manubrium joins the body of the sternum at the second rib. (The right atrium is 5 cm below the sternal angle.)
- Place a metric ruler at the sternal angle. Place a straightedge, such as a tongue blade, at the highest level of the internal jugular vein so that it intersects the ruler at a 90 degree angle. Measure the vertical distance above the sternal angle to the point where the straightedge intersects the ruler (Fig. 23-6).
- Record the distance in centimeters, and indicate the angle at which the patient was lying (eg, "The jugular venous pressure is 5 cm with the head elevated to 30 degrees.").

Measurements greater than 3 to 4 cm above the sternal angle are considered elevated.

When the internal jugular veins are difficult to see, the pulsations of the external jugular veins can be noted. These are more superficial and visible just above the clavicles, adjacent to the sternocleidomastoid muscles. They are frequently distended while the patient lies supine on the examining table or bed. As the patient's head is elevated, the distention of the veins will disappear. The veins are not normally apparent if the head of the bed or examining table is elevated more than 30 degrees.

Obvious distention of the veins with the patient's head elevated 45 degrees to 90 degrees indicates an abnormal increase in the volume of the venous system. This is associated with right-sided heart failure, less commonly with obstruction of blood flow in the superior vena cava, and rarely with acute massive pulmonary embolism.

Heart Inspection and Palpation

The heart is examined indirectly by inspection, palpation, percussion, and auscultation of the chest wall. A systematic approach is the cornerstone of a thorough assessment. Examination of the chest wall is performed in the following six areas (Fig. 23-7):

1. Aortic area—second intercostal space to the right of the sternum. To determine the correct intercostal space, start at the angle of Louis by locating the bony ridge near the top of the sternum at the junction of the body and the manubrium. From this angle, locate the second intercostal space by sliding one finger to the left or right of the sternum. Subsequent intercostal spaces are located from this reference point by palpating down the rib cage.
2. Pulmonic area—second intercostal space to the left of the sternum
3. Erb's point—third intercostal space to the left of the sternum
4. Right ventricular or tricuspid area—fourth and fifth intercostal spaces to the left of the sternum
5. Left ventricular or apical area—fifth intercostal space to the left of the sternum on the midclavicular line
6. Epigastric area—below the xiphoid process

For most of the examination, the patient lies supine, with the head slightly elevated. The right-handed examiner is positioned at the right side of the patient and the left-handed examiner at the left side.

In a systematic fashion, each area of the precordium is inspected and then palpated. Oblique lighting is used to assist the

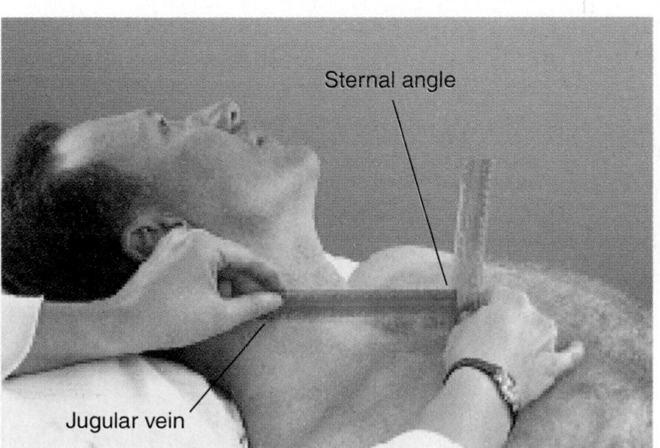

FIGURE 23•6 Assessing jugular venous pressure. Using a metric ruler, the nurse notes the highest point of visible jugular vein pulsations. The vertical distance between this point and the sternal angle is measured and recorded in centimeters. From Weber, J. W., & Kelley, J. (1998). *Health assessment in nursing.* Philadelphia: Lippincott-Raven.

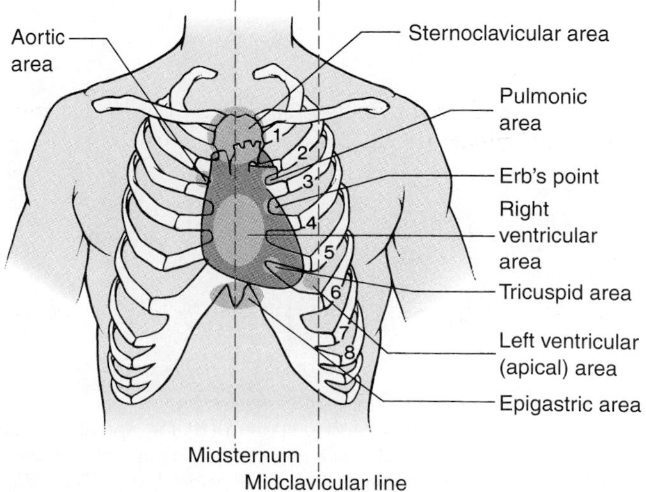

FIGURE 23•7 Areas of the precordium to be assessed when evaluating heart function. (Numerals identify ribs of adjacent intercostal spaces.)

examiner in identifying subtle pulsation. A normal impulse that is distinct and located over the apex of the heart is called the **apical impulse,** or **point of maximal impulse**. It may be observed in young people and in older people who are thin. The apical impulse is normally located and auscultated in the left fifth intercostal space in the midclavicular line (Fig. 23-8).

In many cases, the apical impulse is palpable and normally felt as a light pulsation, 1 to 2 cm in diameter. It is felt at the onset of the first heart sound and lasts only half of systole. (See the next section for a discussion of heart sounds.) The nurse uses the palm of the hand to locate the apical impulse initially and the fingerpads to assess its size and quality. A broad and forceful apical impulse is known as a left ventricular heave or lift. It is so named because it appears to lift the hand from the chest wall during palpation.

Nursing Alert *An apical impulse below the fifth intercostal space or lateral to the midclavicular line usually denotes left ventricular enlargement from left ventricular failure. Normally, the apical impulse is palpable in only one intercostal space; palpability in two or more adjacent intercostal spaces indicates left ventricular enlargement. If the apical impulse can be palpated in two distinctly separate areas and the pulsation movements are paradoxical (not simultaneous), a ventricular aneurysm should be suspected.*

Abnormal, turbulent blood flow within the heart may be palpated by the palm of the hand as a purring sensation. This phenomenon is called a thrill and is associated with a loud murmur. A thrill is always indicative of significant pathology within the heart. Thrills also may be palpated over vessels when blood flow is significantly and substantially obstructed and over the carotid arteries if aortic stenosis is present or if the aortic valve is narrowed.

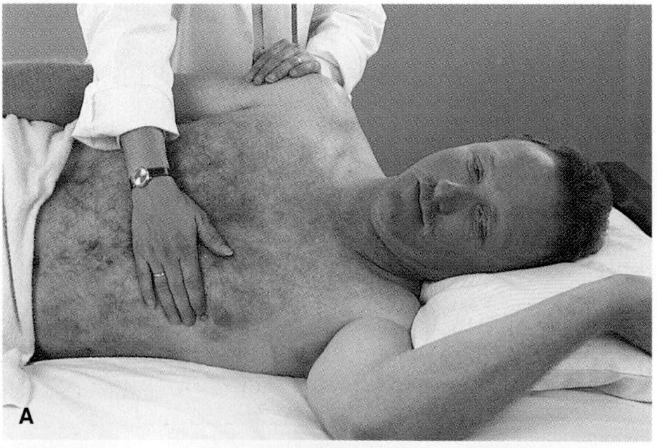

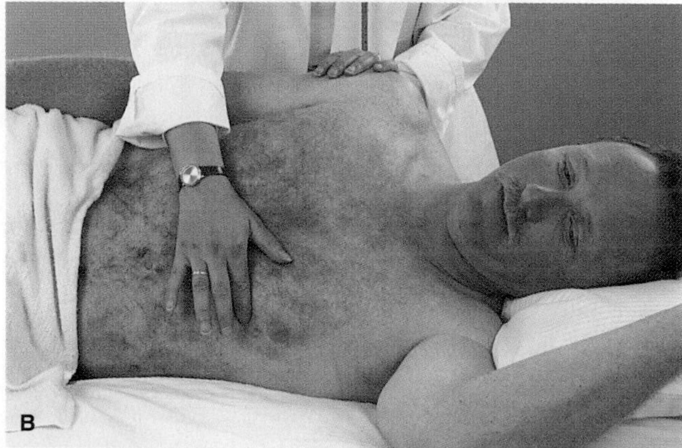

FIGURE 23•8 Locating (**A**) and palpating (**B**) the apical impulse (also called the point of maximal impulse, PMI). The apical impulse is located at the fifth intercostal space to the left of the sternum in the midclavicular line. The nurse locates the impulse with the palm of the hand and palpates with the fingerpads. From Weber, J. W., & Kelley, J. (1998). *Health assessment in nursing.* Philadelphia: Lippincott-Raven.

Chest Percussion

Normally, only the left border of the heart can be detected by percussion. It extends from the sternum to the midclavicular line in the third to fifth intercostal spaces. The right border lies under the right margin of the sternum and is not detectable. Enlargement of the heart to either the left or right usually can be noted. In people with thick chests, obesity, or emphysema, the heart may lie so deeply under the thoracic surface that not even its left border can be noted unless the heart is enlarged. Unless the nurse detects a displaced apical impulse and suspects cardiac enlargement, percussion is omitted.

Cardiac Auscultation

All areas identified in Figure 23-7, except the epigastric area, are auscultated. These include the aortic area, the pulmonary area, Erb's point, the tricuspid area, and the apical area. The actions of the four valves are uniquely reflected at specific locations on the chest wall. These locations do not correspond to the anatomic location of the valve within the chest; rather, they reflect the patterns by which heart sounds radiate toward the chest wall. Sound in vessels through which blood is flowing is always reflected downstream. For example, the actions of the mitral valve are usually heard best in the fifth intercostal space at the midclavicular line. This is called the mitral valve area.

HEART SOUNDS

The **normal heart sounds**, S_1 and S_2, are produced primarily by the closing of the heart valves. The time between S_1 and S_2 corresponds to systole (Fig. 23-9). This is normally shorter than the time between S_2 and S_1 (diastole). As the heart rate increases, diastole shortens.

In normal physiology, the periods of systole and diastole are silent. Ventricular disease, however, can give rise to transient sounds in systole and diastole that are called gallops, snaps, or clicks. Significant narrowing of the valve orifices at times when they should be open, or residual gapping of valves at times when they should be closed, gives rise to prolonged sounds called murmurs.

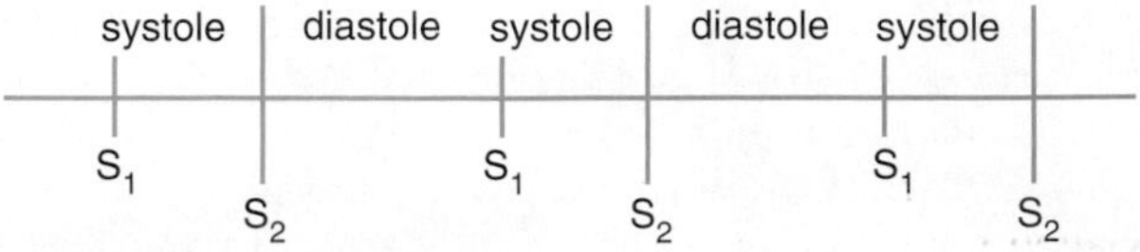

FIGURE 23•9 Normal heart sounds. The first heart sound (S_1) is produced by the simultaneous closing of the mitral and tricuspid valves and is best heard at the apex of the heart (*left ventricular or apical area*). The second heart sound (S_2) is produced by the closing of the aortic and pulmonic valves and is loudest at the base of the heart. The time between S_1 and S_2 corresponds to systole. The time between S_2 and S_1 is diastole.

S_1: First Heart Sound. Simultaneous closure of the mitral and tricuspid valves creates the first heart sound (S_1), although vibration of the myocardial wall also may contribute to this sound. Although heard over the entire precordium, S_1 is heard best at the apex of the heart (apical area). Its intensity increases when the valve leaflets are made rigid by calcium in rheumatic heart disease and in any circumstance in which ventricular contraction occurs at a time when the valve is caught wide open. The latter circumstance will occur, for example, when a premature ventricular contraction interrupts the normal cardiac cycle. The first heart sound varies in intensity from beat to beat when atrial contraction is not synchronous with ventricular contraction. This is because the valve may be fully or partially closed on one beat and open on the subsequent one as a function of irregular atrial activity. The first heart sound is easily identifiable and serves as the point of reference for the remainder of the cardiac cycle.

S_2: Second Heart Sound. Closing of the aortic and pulmonic valves produces the second heart sound (S_2). Although these two valves close almost simultaneously, the pulmonic valve usually lags slightly behind. Therefore, under certain circumstances, the two components of the second sound may be heard separately (split S_2). The splitting is more likely to be accentuated on inspiration and to disappear on expiration. (More blood is ejected from the right ventricle during inspiration; less blood is ejected during expiration.)

S_2 is heard loudest at the base of the heart. The aortic component of the second sound is heard clearly in both the aortic and pulmonic areas, and is heard less clearly at the apex. The pulmonic component of the second sound, if present, may be heard only over the pulmonic area. Thus, one may hear a "single" second heart sound in the aortic area and a split second heart sound in the pulmonic area.

Gallop Sounds. If the blood filling the ventricle is impeded during diastole, as occurs in certain disease states, then a temporary vibration may occur in diastole, similar to, although usually softer than, the first and second heart sounds. Heart sounds then come in triplets and have the acoustic effect of a galloping horse; they are therefore called gallops. This may occur early in diastole, during the rapid-filling phase of the cardiac cycle, or later at the time of atrial contraction.

A gallop sound occurring during rapid ventricular filling is called a third heart sound (S_3) and represents a normal finding in children and young adults (Fig. 23-10**A**). Such a sound is heard in patients who have myocardial disease or in those who have CHF and whose ventricles fail to eject all of their blood during systole. An S_3 gallop is heard best with the patient lying on the left side.

Gallop sounds heard during atrial contraction are called fourth heart sounds (S_4) (Fig. 23-10**B**). An S_4 is often heard when the ventricle is enlarged or hypertrophied and therefore resistant to filling. Such a circumstance may be associated with coronary artery disease, hypertension, or stenosis of the aortic valve. On rare occasions, all four heart sounds are heard within a single cardiac cycle, giving rise to what is called a quadruple rhythm.

Gallop sounds are very low-frequency sounds and may be heard only with the bell of the stethoscope placed very lightly against the chest. They are heard best at the apex, although occasionally, when emanating from the right ventricle, they may be heard to the left of the sternum.

Snaps and Clicks. Stenosis of the mitral valve resulting from rheumatic heart disease gives rise to an unusual sound very early in diastole that is high-pitched and best heard along the left sternal border. The sound is caused by high pressure in the left atrium with abrupt displacement of a rigid mitral valve. The sound is called an opening snap. It occurs too long after the second sound to be mistaken for a split second sound and too early in diastole to be mistaken for a gallop. It almost always is associated with the murmur of mitral stenosis and is specific for this disorder.

In a similar manner, stenosis of the aortic valve gives rise to a short, high-pitched sound immediately after the first heart sound that is called an ejection click. This is due to very high pressure within the ventricle, displacing a rigid and calcified aortic valve.

Murmurs. **Murmurs** are created by the turbulent flow of blood. The causes of the turbulence may be a critically narrowed valve, a malfunctioning valve that allows regurgitant blood flow, a congenital defect of the ventricular wall or a defect between the aorta and the pulmonary artery, or an increased flow of blood through a normal structure (eg, with fever, pregnancy, hyperthyroidism). Murmurs are characterized and consequently described by several characteristics, including timing in the cardiac cycle, location on the chest wall, intensity, pitch, quality, and pattern of radiation (Chart 23-2).

Friction Rub. In pericarditis, a harsh grating sound that can be heard in both systole and diastole is called a friction rub. It is caused by the abrasion of the pericardial surfaces during the cardiac cycle. Because friction rub may be confused with a murmur, care should be taken to identify the sound when appropriate and to distinguish it from murmurs that may be heard in both systole and diastole. A pericardial friction rub can be heard best using the diaphragm of the stethoscope, with the patient sitting up and leaning forward.

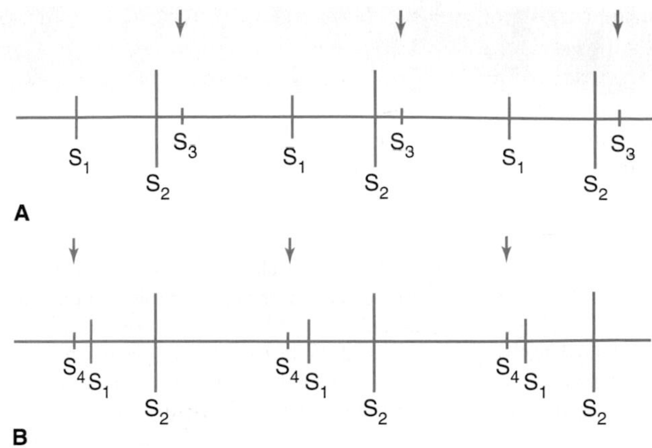

FIGURE 23•10 Gallops. (**A**) An S_3 gallop is heard immediately following the S_2 and occurs when the blood filling the ventricle is impeded during diastole, resulting in temporary vibrations. The heart sounds come in triplets and resemble the sound of a galloping horse. Myocardial disease and congestive heart failure are associated with this sound. (**B**) An S_4 gallop is heard immediately preceding the S_1. The S_4 sound occurs during atrial contraction and is often heard when the ventricle is enlarged or hypertrophied. Associated conditions include coronary artery disease (CAD), hypertension, and stenosis of the aortic valve.

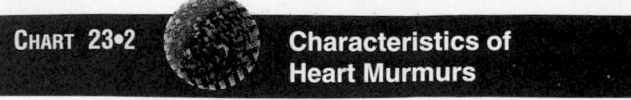

CHART 23•2 Characteristics of Heart Murmurs

Heart murmurs are described in terms of timing, location, intensity, pitch, and radiation. These characteristics provide data about the location and nature of the cardiac abnormality.

Timing

Timing of the murmur in the cardiac cycle is vital. The examiner first determines whether the murmur is occurring in systole or in diastole. Then, does it begin simultaneously with the first heart sound, or is there some delay between the sound and the beginning of a systolic murmur? Does the murmur continue to (or through) the second heart sound, or is there again a delay between the end of the murmur and the second heart sound? Are diastolic murmurs continuous, or do they subside in mid- or late diastole?

Location

The location of the murmur (where it is detected on the chest wall) is crucial. Depending on the type of valvular disorder, a murmur can be heard only at the apex or more widely over the chest wall, or along the left sternal border between the third and fourth interspaces.

Intensity

The intensity of murmurs is conventionally graded from I through VI. Sometimes, grade I murmurs are difficult to hear. However, a grade II cardiac murmur can be easily perceived by the experienced examiner. Murmurs of grades IV or louder are usually associated with thrills that may be palpated on the surface of the chest wall. A grade VI murmur often can be heard with the stethoscope off the chest. A murmur may vary in intensity from its beginning to its conclusion. This is very characteristic of certain valvular disorders.

Pitch

The next important quality of a murmur is its pitch, which may be a low, rumbling sound, often heard only with the bell placed lightly on the chest wall, or a very high-pitched murmur, occasionally "whistling," heard best with the stethoscope's diaphragm. Other murmurs contain the full spectrum of sound frequency and make the murmur sound harsh.

Radiation

The last feature of concern is radiation of the murmur. A murmur can radiate into the axilla, the carotid arteries in the neck, the left shoulder, or the back.

Auscultation Procedure

During auscultation, the patient remains supine and the examining room is as quiet as possible. A stethoscope with a diaphragm and a bell is necessary for accurate auscultation of the heart.

Using the diaphragm of the stethoscope, the examiner starts at the apical area and progresses upward along the left sternal border to the pulmonic and aortic areas. If desired, the examiner may choose to begin the examination at the aortic and pulmonic areas and progress downward to the apex of the heart. Initially, S_1 is identified and evaluated with respect to its intensity and splitting. Next, S_2 is identified and its intensity noted. After concentrating on S_1 and S_2, the examiner listens for extra sounds in systole and then in diastole.

Sometimes it helps to ask the following questions: Do I hear snapping or clicking sounds? Do I hear any high-pitched blowing sounds? Is this sound in systole, or diastole, or both? The examiner again proceeds to move the stethoscope to all of the designated areas of the precordium, listening carefully for these sounds. Finally, the patient is turned on the left side and the stethoscope is placed on the apical area, where an S_3 and a mitral murmur are more readily detected.

Once an abnormality is heard, the entire chest surface is reexamined to determine the exact location of the sound and its radiation. Also, the patient who may be concerned about the prolonged examination must be supported and reassured. Once the characteristics of each phase of the cycle have been determined, the relationship of one to another and the synthesis of events within the cardiac cycle may be summarized.

Interpretation of Cardiac Sounds

Interpreting cardiac sounds requires detailed knowledge of cardiac physiology and the pathophysiology of cardiac diseases. There are different levels of performance at which the nurse may be expected to function. The first level is simply recognizing that what one is hearing is not normal—for example, a third heart sound, a murmur in systole or diastole, a pericardial friction rub over the midsternum, or a second heart sound that is widely split. These findings are reported to the physician and acted on accordingly. This level of function is useful in screening. It is the kind of activity involved in performing physical examinations in schools on normal children or in performing routine physical examinations or screening examinations.

The second level involves recognizing patterns. The nurse correctly observes the findings and can recognize the constellation of sounds and the diagnostic significance of common ones.

At its most sophisticated level, cardiac diagnosis can be interpretive. Highly skilled nurses can differentiate among dysrhythmias and respond accordingly. They can determine the significance of the appearance and disappearance of gallops during the treatment of patients who have had MIs or who are in heart failure. This is the role that the coronary care nurse and the cardiovascular advanced practice RN assume. They function with a team of other health professionals who have highly tuned skills of cardiovascular assessment and diagnosis.

Inspection of the Extremities

The hands, arms, legs, and feet are observed for skin and vascular changes. The most noteworthy changes include:

- *Decreased capillary refill time* indicates a slower peripheral flow rate from sluggish reperfusion and is often observed in patients with hypotension or CHF. Capillary refill time provides the basis for estimating the rate of peripheral blood flow. To test capillary refill, briefly compress the nailbed so it blanches, then release the pressure. Normally, reperfusion occurs within 2 seconds, as evidenced by a return of skin color.
- *Vascular changes* from decreased arterial circulation include decrease in quality or loss of pulse, discomfort or pain, paresthesia, numbness, decrease in temperature, pallor, and loss of movement. During the first few hours after invasive cardiac procedures, such as cardiac catheterization, affected extremities should be assessed for vascular changes frequently.
- *Hematoma,* or a localized collection of clotted blood in the tissue, may be observed in patients who have undergone invasive cardiac procedures such as cardiac catheterization, angioplasty, or cardiac electrophysiology testing. Major blood vessels of the arms and legs are selected for catheter

insertion. During these procedures, systemic anticoagulation with heparin is necessary, and minor or small hematomas may occur at the catheter puncture site. However, large hematomas are a serious complication that can compromise circulating blood volume and cardiac output, requiring blood transfusions. All patients who have undergone these procedures must have their puncture sites frequently observed until hemostasis is adequately achieved.

- *Peripheral edema* is fluid accumulation in dependent areas of the body (feet and legs, sacrum in the bedridden patient). Assess for pitting edema (a depression over an area of pressure) by pressing firmly for 5 seconds with the thumb over the dorsum of each foot, behind each medial malleolus, and over the shins. Pitting edema is graded as absent, slight (1+) to very marked (4+). It is observed in patients with CHF and peripheral vascular diseases such as deep vein thrombosis or chronic venous insufficiency.
- *Clubbing* of the fingers and toes implies chronic hemoglobin desaturation, as in congenital heart disease.
- *Lower extremity ulcers* are observed in patients with arterial or venous insufficiency. Chapter 28 provides a complete description of differentiating characteristics.

Other Systems

LUNGS

The details of respiratory assessment are described in Chapter 19. Findings frequently exhibited by cardiac patients include the following:

- *Tachypnea:* Rapid, shallow breathing may be noted in patients who have heart failure or pain, or who are extremely anxious.
- *Cheyne-Stokes respirations:* Patients with severe left ventricular failure may exhibit Cheyne-Stokes breathing, a pattern of rapid respirations alternating with apnea. It is important to note the duration of the apnea.
- *Hemoptysis:* Pink, frothy sputum is indicative of acute pulmonary edema.
- *Cough:* A dry, hacking cough from irritation of small airways is common in patients with pulmonary congestion from heart failure.
- *Crackles:* Heart failure or atelectasis associated with bed rest, splinting from ischemic pain, or the effects of pain medication and sedatives often results in the development of crackles. Typically, crackles are first noted at the bases (because of gravity's effect on fluid accumulation and decreased ventilation of basilar tissue) but may progress to all portions of the lung fields.
- *Wheezes:* Compression of the small airways by interstitial pulmonary edema may cause wheezing. Beta-adrenergic blocking agents (beta-blockers), such as propranolol, may precipitate airway narrowing, especially in patients with underlying pulmonary disease.

ABDOMEN

For the cardiac patient, two components of the abdominal examination are frequently performed.

- *Hepatojugular reflux:* Liver engorgement occurs because of decreased venous return secondary to right ventricular failure. The liver will be enlarged, firm, nontender, and smooth. The hepatojugular reflux may be demonstrated by pressing firmly over the right upper quadrant of the abdomen for 30 to 60 seconds and noting a 1-cm rise in jugular venous pressure. This rise indicates an inability of the right side of the heart to accommodate increased volume.
- *Bladder distention:* Urine output is an important indicator of cardiac function, especially when urine output is reduced. This may indicate inadequate renal perfusion or a less serious problem such as one caused by urinary retention. When the urine output is decreased, the patient needs to be assessed for a distended bladder or difficulty voiding. The suprapubic area is palpated for an oval mass and is percussed for dullness, indicative of a full bladder.

Gerontologic Considerations

When performing a cardiovascular assessment examination on an elderly patient, the nurse may note such differences as more readily palpable peripheral pulses because of increased hardness of the arteries and a loss of adjacent connective tissue. Palpating the precordium in the elderly is affected by the changes in the shape of the chest. For example, a cardiac impulse may not be palpable in patients with chronic obstructive pulmonary disease because these patients usually have an increased anterior-posterior chest diameter. Kyphoscoliosis, a spinal deformity that occurs frequently in elderly patients, may dislocate the cardiac apex downward so that the diagnostic significance of palpating the apical impulse is obscured.

Systolic BP increases with age, but diastolic BP usually plateaus after 50 years. Medication therapy is usually initiated for high BP when consistent systolic readings of 160 mm Hg or diastolic readings of 95 mm Hg are observed. For the elderly patient, however, many factors are considered before initiating treatment. Orthostatic hypotension may reflect a decreasing sensitivity of postural reflexes, which must be considered when medication therapy is prescribed.

An S_4 is heard in about 90% of elderly patients; this is thought to be due to decreased compliance of the left ventricle. The S_2 is usually split. About 60% or more of elderly patients have murmurs, the most common being a soft systolic ejection murmur from sclerotic changes of the aortic leaflets (see Table 23-1).

DIAGNOSTIC EVALUATION

Diagnostic tests and procedures are used to confirm the data obtained by history and physical assessment. Some tests are easy to interpret, but others must be interpreted by expert clinicians. All tests should be explained to the patient. Some necessitate special preparation before they are performed and special monitoring by the nurse after the procedure.

Laboratory Tests

Laboratory tests may be requested for the following reasons:

- To assist in diagnosing an acute MI. (Angina pectoris, chest pain from an insufficient supply of blood to the heart, cannot be confirmed by either blood or urine studies.)
- To identify abnormalities in the blood that affect the prognosis of a patient with cardiac problems
- To assess the degree of inflammation
- To screen for risk factors associated with atherosclerotic coronary artery disease
- To determine baseline values before performing therapeutic interventions
- To identify serum levels of medications

- To assess the effects of medications (eg, the effects of diuretics on serum potassium levels)
- To screen generally for abnormalities

Because different laboratories use different equipment and different methods of measurements, normal test values may vary depending on the laboratory and the health care institution.

Cardiac Enzyme Analysis

Plasma cardiac enzyme analysis is part of a diagnostic profile, which also includes the health history, symptoms, and electrocardiogram (ECG), associated with acute MI. Enzymes are released from injured cells when the cell membranes rupture. Most enzymes are nonspecific in relation to the particular organ that has been damaged. Certain isoenzymes, however, come only from myocardial cells and are released when the cells are damaged by sustained hypoxia, resulting in infarction. The isoenzymes leak into the interstitial spaces of the myocardium and are carried into the general circulation by the lymphatic system and the coronary circulation, resulting in elevated enzyme levels.

Because different enzymes are released into the blood at varying periods after MI, enzyme levels should be tested in relation to the time of onset of chest discomfort or other symptoms. Creatine kinase (CK) and its isoenzyme CK-MB are the most specific enzymes analyzed in acute MI, and they are the first enzyme levels to rise. Lactic dehydrogenase and its isoenzymes also are analyzed in patients who have delayed seeking medical attention because these blood levels rise and peak in 2 to 3 days, much later than CK levels (see Table 25-3 in Chap. 25 for the time course of cardiac enzymes).

Troponin I is a relatively new laboratory test that has several advantages over traditional enzyme studies. Troponin I is a contractile protein found only in cardiac muscle. After myocardial injury, elevated serum troponin I levels can be detected within 3 to 4 hours; they peak in 4 to 24 hours and remain elevated for 1 to 3 weeks. These early and prolonged elevations make very early diagnosis of MI possible or allow for late diagnosis if the patient has delayed seeking treatment.

Blood Chemistry

LIPID PROFILE

Cholesterol, triglycerides, and lipoproteins are measured to evaluate a person's risk for developing atherosclerotic disease, especially if there is a family history of premature heart disease, or to diagnose a specific lipoprotein abnormality. Cholesterol and triglycerides are transported in the blood by combining with protein molecules to form lipoproteins. The lipoproteins are referred to as low-density lipoproteins (LDL) and high-density lipoproteins (HDL). The risk of coronary artery disease increases as the ratio of LDL to HDL or total cholesterol (LDL + HDL) to HDL increases. Although cholesterol levels remain relatively constant over 24 hours, the blood specimen for the lipid profile should be obtained after a 12-hour fast.

CHOLESTEROL LEVELS

Cholesterol (normal level less than 200 mg/dL) is a lipid required for hormone synthesis and cell membrane formation. It is found in large quantities in brain and nerve tissue. Two major sources of cholesterol are diet (animal products) and the liver, where cholesterol is synthesized. Elevated cholesterol levels are known to increase the risk for coronary artery disease. Factors that contribute to variations in cholesterol levels include age, gender, diet, exercise patterns, and stress levels.

LDLs (normal level less than 130 mg/dL) are the primary transporters of cholesterol and triglycerides into the cell. One harmful effect of LDL is the deposition of these substances in the walls of arterial vessels. Elevated LDL levels are associated with a greater incidence of coronary artery disease. In people with known coronary artery disease, the primary goal for lipid management is reduction of LDL levels to less than 100 mg/dL.

HDLs (normal range in males 35 to 65 mg/dL, normal range in females 35 to 85 mg/dL) have a protective action. They transport cholesterol away from the tissue and cells of the arterial wall to the liver for excretion. Therefore, there is an inverse relationship between HDL levels and risk for coronary artery disease. Factors that lower HDL levels include smoking, diabetes, obesity, and physical inactivity. In patients with coronary artery disease, a secondary goal of lipid management is the increase of HDL levels to more than 35 mg/dL.

Triglycerides (normal range 40 to 150 mg/dL), composed of free fatty acids and glycerol, are stored in the adipose tissue and are a source of energy. Triglyceride levels increase after meals and are affected by stress. Diabetes, alcohol use, and obesity can elevate triglyceride levels. These levels have a direct correlation with LDL and an inverse one with HDL.

SERUM ELECTROLYTE LEVELS

Sodium, potassium, and calcium are ions vital to cellular depolarization and repolarization. In addition, the serum sodium level reflects relative fluid balance. Generally, hyponatremia (low sodium level) indicates fluid excess and hypernatremia (high sodium level) indicates fluid deficit.

Serum potassium is affected by renal function and may be decreased by diuretic agents that are used to treat CHF. A decrease in potassium causes cardiac irritability and predisposes the patient receiving a digitalis preparation to digitalis toxicity and dysrhythmias. The effect of an elevated serum potassium level is myocardial depression and ventricular irritability. Both hypokalemia and hyperkalemia can lead to ventricular fibrillation or cardiac standstill. Calcium is necessary for blood coagulability and neuromuscular activity. Hypocalcemia and hypercalcemia can cause dysrhythmias.

Magnesium is integral to the absorption of calcium and the maintenance of potassium stores. It is required in the metabolism of adenosine triphosphate, playing a major role in protein synthesis, carbohydrate metabolism, and muscular contraction. Initial symptoms of hypermagnesemia are lethargy and decreased neuromuscular activity. On the ECG, hypomagnesemia lengthens the QT interval, predisposing the patient to life-threatening dysrhythmias.

BLOOD UREA NITROGEN LEVEL

Blood urea nitrogen is an end product of protein metabolism and is excreted by the kidneys. In the patient with cardiac disease, an elevated blood urea nitrogen level may reflect reduced renal perfusion (from decreased cardiac output) or intravascular fluid volume deficit (from diuretic therapy).

SERUM GLUCOSE LEVEL

The serum glucose level is important to monitor because many patients with cardiac disease also have diabetes mellitus. In addition, the serum glucose level may be mildly elevated in stressful situations, when mobilization of endogenous epinephrine results in conversion of liver glycogen to glucose.

COAGULATION STUDIES

The formation of a thrombus is initiated by injury to a vessel wall or to the tissue. These events activate the coagulation cascade, a complex series of interactions among phospholipids, calcium, and various clotting factors that convert prothrombin to thrombin. The coagulation cascade has two pathways, the intrinsic pathway and the extrinsic pathway.

Partial thromboplastin time (PTT) and activated partial thromboplastin time (aPTT) measure the activity of the intrinsic pathway. The values of PTT and aPTT are used to assess patients receiving heparin therapy. Patients receiving heparin have their PTT or aPTT levels maintained at 1.5 to 2.5 times their baseline values (reference range, 25 to 38 seconds). Prothrombin time (PT) measures the extrinsic pathway activity and is used to monitor patients receiving therapeutic anticoagulation with warfarin. Treatment goals for patients receiving warfarin include maintaining the PT at 1.5 to 2.5 times control (reference range, less than 13 seconds). Laboratory results of PT also include the **International Normalized Ratio** (INR). The INR provides a standard method for reporting PT levels, eliminating the variation from laboratory to laboratory. Patients receiving warfarin therapy should have their INR levels followed and maintained between 2.0 and 3.0 (2.5 to 3.5 for patients with mechanical heart valves).

Chest X-Ray and Fluoroscopy

A chest x-ray usually is obtained to determine the size, contour, and position of the heart. It reveals cardiac and pericardial calcifications and demonstrates physiologic alterations in the pulmonary circulation. It does not help diagnose acute MI but can help diagnose some complications (eg, CHF). Correct placement of cardiac catheters, such as pacemakers and pulmonary artery catheters, is also confirmed by chest x-ray.

Fluoroscopy allows visualization of the heart on a luminescent x-ray screen. It shows cardiac and vascular pulsations and unusual cardiac contours. Fluoroscopy is useful for positioning intravenously advanced pacing electrodes and for guiding catheter insertion during cardiac catheterization.

Electrocardiography

The ECG is a universal diagnostic tool used in assessing the cardiovascular system. It is a graphic recording of the electrical activity of the heart; a 12-lead ECG shows the activity from 12 different views. The ECG is obtained by placing disposable electrodes in standard positions on the skin of the chest wall and extremities. The heart's electrical impulses are recorded as a tracing on special graph paper.

The 12-lead ECG is particularly useful in diagnosing dysrhythmias, conduction abnormalities, enlarged heart chambers, myocardial ischemia or infarction, high or low calcium and potassium levels, and certain drug effects. To enhance interpretation of the ECG, the patient's age, gender, BP, height, weight, symptoms, and medications (especially digitalis and antiarrhythmic agents) should be noted on the ECG requisition. The details of electrocardiography are covered in Chapter 24.

Continuous ECG Monitoring

Continuous ECG monitoring is standard for patients at high risk for dysrhythmias. Two continuous ECG monitoring techniques are hardwire monitoring, found in critical care units and specialty stepdown units, and telemetry, found on general nursing care units. Patients who are receiving continuous ECG monitoring need to be informed of its purpose and cautioned that this monitoring method will not detect symptoms such as dyspnea or chest pain. Therefore, patients need to be advised to call the nurse whenever symptoms develop.

HARDWIRE CARDIAC MONITORING

The patient's ECG can be continuously observed on an oscilloscope at the bedside and at a central monitoring station by a hardwire monitoring system. This system is composed of three to five electrodes positioned on the patient's chest, a lead cable, and a bedside monitor. Hardwire monitoring systems vary in sophistication, but in general can do the following:

1. Monitor one or two leads simultaneously
2. Provide graded visual and audible alarms (based on priority, asystole would be highest)
3. Computerize rhythm monitoring (dysrhythmias are interpreted and stored in memory)
4. Print an ECG

Two leads commonly used for continuous monitoring are lead II and a modification of V_1 (MCL_1) (Fig. 23-11). Lead II provides the best visualization of atrial depolarization (represented by the P wave). MCL_1 is selected to identify the ventricle responsible for ectopic or abnormal beats.

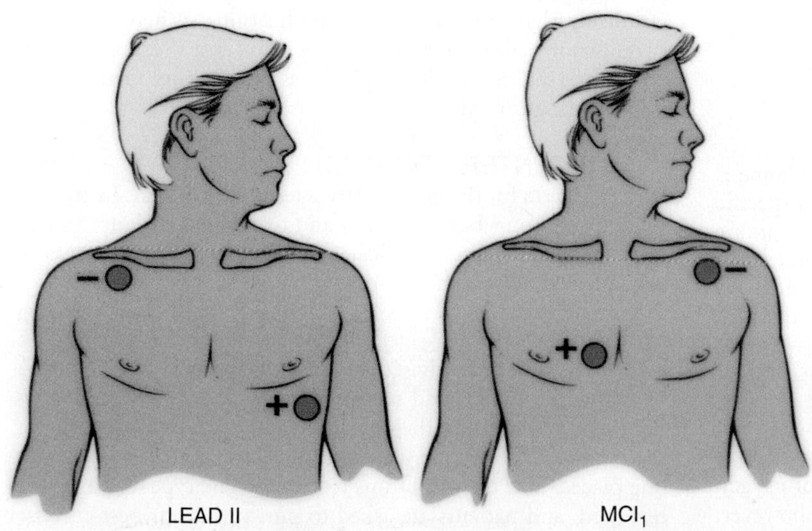

FIGURE 23•11 Two leads (*views of the heart*) commonly used for continuous monitoring. To monitor lead II, the negative electrode is placed on the right upper chest; the positive electrode is placed on the left lower chest. To monitor MCl_1, the negative electrode is placed on the left upper chest; the positive electrode is placed in the V_1 position. If three electrodes are used, the third electrode, which is the ground electrode, can be placed anywhere on the chest.

TELEMETRY

In addition to hardwire monitoring systems, the ECG can be continuously observed by **telemetry**, the transmission of radiowaves from a battery-operated transmitter, worn by the patient, to a central bank of monitors. Although telemetry systems have the same capabilities as hardwire systems, they are wireless, thereby allowing the patient to ambulate while being monitored. Following a few guidelines for electrode placement will ensure good conduction and a clear picture of the patient's rhythm on the monitor:

- Clean the skin surface with soap and water and dry well (or as recommended by the manufacturer) before applying the electrodes. If the patient has much hair where the electrodes need to be placed, shave or clip the hair.
- Apply a little benzoin to the skin if the patient is diaphoretic (sweaty) and the electrodes do not adhere well.
- Change the electrodes every 24 to 48 hours and examine the skin for irritation. Apply the electrodes to different locations each time they are changed.
- If the patient is sensitive to the electrodes, use hypoallergenic electrodes.

SIGNAL-AVERAGED ECG

For some patients considered at high risk for sudden cardiac death, a signal-averaged ECG is performed. This high-resolution ECG assists in identifying risk for life-threatening dysrhythmias and helps to determine the need for invasive diagnostic procedures. Signal averaging works by averaging about 150 to 300 QRS waveforms (QRS waveforms represent depolarization of the ventricle). The resulting averaged QRS complex is analyzed for certain characteristics that are likely to lead to lethal ventricular dysrhythmias. The recording is performed at the bedside and requires about 15 minutes.

CONTINUOUS AMBULATORY MONITORING

In ambulatory ECG monitoring, which may occur in the hospital but is more commonly prescribed for outpatients, one lead of the patient's ECG can be monitored by a Holter monitor. This monitor is a small tape recorder that continuously (from 10 to 24 hours) documents the heart's electrical activity on a magnetic tape. The tape recorder weighs approximately 2 pounds and can be carried over the shoulder or worn around the waist day or night to detect dysrhythmias or evidence of myocardial ischemia during activities of daily living. The patient keeps a diary of activity, noting the time of any symptoms, experiences, or unusual activities performed. The tape recording is then examined with a special scanner, analyzed, and interpreted. Evidence obtained in this way helps diagnose dysrhythmias and myocardial ischemia and evaluate therapy, such as antiarrhythmic and antianginal medications, or pacemaker function.

TRANSTELEPHONIC MONITORING

Another method of evaluating the ECG of a patient at home is by transtelephonic monitoring. The patient attaches a specific lead system for transmitting the signals and places a telephone mouthpiece over the transmitter box; the ECG is recorded and evaluated at another location. This method is often used for diagnosing dysrhythmias and in follow-up evaluation of permanent cardiac pacemakers.

Cardiac Stress Testing

Normally, the coronary arteries dilate four times their usual diameter in response to increased metabolic demands for oxygen and nutrients. Coronary arteries with atherosclerosis, however, dilate much less, compromising blood flow to the myocardium and cause ischemia. Therefore, abnormalities in cardiovascular function are more likely to be detected during times of increased demand, or "stress." The **cardiac stress test** procedures—the exercise stress test, the pharmacologic stress test, and more recently the mental or emotional stress test—are noninvasive ways to evaluate the response of the cardiovascular system to stress. The stress test helps determine the following: (1) coronary artery disease, (2) cause of chest pain, (3) functional capacity of the heart after an MI or heart surgery, (4) effectiveness of antianginal or antiarrhythmic medications, (5) dysrhythmias that occur during physical exercise, and (6) specific goals for a physical fitness program. Contraindications to stress testing include severe aortic stenosis, acute myocarditis or pericarditis, severe hypertension, suspected left main coronary artery disease, CHF, and unstable angina. Because complications associated with stress testing can be life-threatening (MI, cardiac arrest, CHF, and severe dysrhythmias), testing facilities have the staff and equipment necessary to provide advanced cardiac life support.

Mental stress testing for diagnostic purposes in patients with coronary artery disease is currently investigational. Preliminary results (McFetridge & Yarandi, 1997) indicate that mental stress induced, for example, when the patient performs a mental arithmetic test evokes a myocardial ischemia response similar to that evoked by conventional exercise testing.

Stress testing is often combined with echocardiography or radionuclide imaging. These techniques are performed during the resting state and immediately after stress.

Exercise Stress Testing

In an exercise stress test, the patient walks on a treadmill (most common) or pedals a stationary bicycle. Exercise intensity progresses according to established protocols. The Bruce protocol, for example, is a common treadmill protocol in which the speed and grade of the treadmill are increased every 3 minutes. The goal of the test is to increase the heart rate to the "target heart rate." This is 80% to 90% of the maximum predicted heart rate and is based on the age and gender of the patient. During the test, the following are monitored: two or more ECG leads for heart rate, rhythm, and ischemic changes, BP, skin temperature, physical appearance, perceived exertion, and symptoms including chest pain, dyspnea, dizziness, leg cramping, or fatigue. The test is terminated when the target heart rate is achieved or the patient experiences chest pain, extreme fatigue, a drop in BP or pulse rate, serious dysrhythmias, or other complications. When significant ECG abnormalities occur during the stress test (ST segment depressions), the test result is reported as positive and further diagnostic testing is required.

NURSING INTERVENTIONS

In preparation for the exercise stress test, the patient is instructed to fast for 4 hours before the test and to avoid stimulants such as tobacco and caffeine. Medications may be taken with sips of water. The physician may instruct patients not to take certain cardiac medications, such as beta-blockers, before the test. Clothes and sneakers or rubber-soled shoes suitable for exercising are to be worn. Women are advised to wear a bra that provides adequate support. Equipment and sensations or experiences that the patient may have during the test are reviewed. The nurse explains the monitoring equipment used, the need to have an intravenous line placed, and the symptoms to report. The type of exercise is reviewed, and patients are asked to put forth their best exercise effort. If the test is to be performed with echocardiography or radionuclide imaging, this information is reviewed as well. After the test, patients are monitored for 10 to 15 minutes. Once stable, they may resume their usual activities.

Pharmacologic Stress Testing

Physically handicapped or deconditioned patients will not be able to achieve their target heart rate by exercising on a treadmill or bicycle. Two vasodilating agents, dipyridamole (Persantin) and adenosine (Adenogard), administered intravenously, are used to mimic the effects of exercise by maximally dilating the coronary arteries. The effects of dipyridamole last about 15 to 30 minutes. The side effects are related to its vasodilating action and include chest discomfort, dizziness, headache, flushing, and nausea. Adenosine has similar side effects. although patients report these symptoms as more severe. A unique property of adenosine is that it has an extremely short half-life of less than 10 seconds, so any severe effects rapidly subside. Dipyridamole and adenosine are the agents of choice used in conjunction with radionuclide imaging techniques. Aminophylline, theophylline, and other xanthines, such as caffeine, block the effects of dipyridamole and adenosine and must be avoided before undergoing either of these pharmacologic stress tests.

Dobutamine is another medication that may be used for patients who cannot exercise. Dobutamine, a synthetic sympathomimetic agent, increases heart rate, myocardial contractility, and BP, thereby increasing the metabolic demands of the heart. It is the drug of choice when echocardiography is used because of its effects on altering myocardial wall motion (due to enhanced contractility). In addition, dobutamine is used for patients who have bronchospasm or pulmonary diseases and cannot tolerate having doses of theophylline withheld.

NURSING INTERVENTIONS

In preparation for the pharmacologic stress test, patients are instructed not to eat or drink anything for at least 4 hour before the test. This includes chocolate, caffeine, caffeine-free coffee, tea, carbonated beverages, or medications with caffeine (Anacin or Darvon). If caffeine is ingested before a dipyridamole or adenosine stress test, the test will have to be rescheduled. Patients taking aminophylline or theophylline are instructed to stop taking these medications for 24 to 48 hours before the test (if tolerated). Oral doses of dipyridamole are to be withheld as well. Patients are informed about the transient sensations they may experience during infusion of the vasodilating agent, such as flushing or nausea, which will pass quickly. The patient is instructed to report any other symptoms occurring during the test to the cardiologist or nurse. An explanation of echocardiography or radionuclide imaging is also provided as necessary. The stress test may take about 1 hour, or up to 3 hours if imaging is performed.

Echocardiography

Echocardiography is a noninvasive ultrasound test used to examine the size, shape, and motion of cardiac structures. It is a particularly useful tool for diagnosing pericardial effusions, determining the etiology of heart murmurs, evaluating the function of prosthetic heart valves, determining chamber size, and evaluating ventricular wall motion. It involves the transmission of high-frequency sound waves into the heart through the chest wall and the recording of the return signals. The ultrasound is generated by a hand-held transducer applied to the front of the chest. The transducer picks up the echoes, converts them to electrical impulses, and transmits them to the echocardiography machine for display on an oscilloscope and for recording on a videotape. An ECG is recorded simultaneously to time events within the cardiac cycle.

M-mode (motion), the unidimensional mode that was first introduced, provides information about the cardiac structures and their motion. Two-dimensional or cross-sectional echocardiography (Fig. 23-12), an enhancement of the technique, creates a sophisticated, spatially correct image of the heart. Other techniques, such as Doppler and color flow imaging echocardiography, show the direction and velocity of the blood flow through the heart.

As previously mentioned, echocardiography may be performed with an exercise or a dobutamine stress test, where resting and stress images are obtained. Myocardial ischemia from decreased perfusion during stress causes abnormalities in ventricular wall motion and is easily detected by echocardiography. A stress test using echocardiography is considered positive if abnormalities in ventricular wall motion are detected during stress but not during rest. These findings are highly suggestive of coronary artery disease and require further evaluation, such as a cardiac catheterization.

Transesophageal Echocardiography

A significant limitation of traditional echocardiography has been the poor quality of the images produced. Ultrasound loses its clarity as it passes through tissue, lung, and bone. A more recent echocardiographic technique involves threading a small transducer through the mouth and into the esophagus. This technique, called transesophageal echocardiography (TEE), provides clearer images because ultrasound waves are passing through less tissue. Pharmacologic stress testing using dobutamine and TEE can also be performed. The high-quality imaging obtained during TEE makes this technique an important adjunct to the technology available for detecting and evaluating the severity of coronary artery disease. Complications are uncommon during TEE,

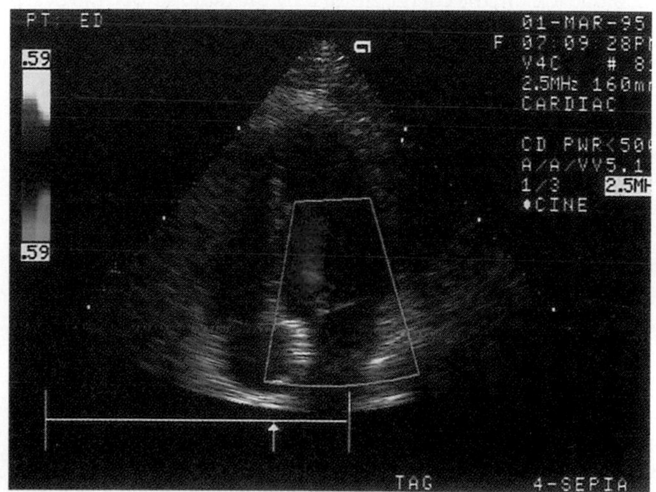

FIGURE 23•12 Two-dimensional echocardiogram, four-chamber view in a normal patient. The ventricles and atria are the dark areas outlined by the lighter coppery tones.

but if they do occur they are serious. These complications are due to sedation and impaired swallowing from topical anesthesia (respiratory depression and aspiration) and insertion and manipulation of the transducer into the esophagus and stomach (vasovagal response or esophageal perforation). The patient must be assessed before TEE for a history of dysphagia or radiation therapy to the chest that would increase the risk for complications.

NURSING INTERVENTIONS

Before traditional echocardiography, the nurse informs the patient about the test, explaining that it is painless. Echocardiographic monitoring is performed while a transducer that emits the sound waves is moved about the chest. Gel applied to the skin helps transmit the sound waves. Periodically, the patient will have to turn onto the left side or hold a breath. The test takes about 30 to 45 minutes. If the patient is to undergo an exercise or dobutamine stress test with echocardiography, information on stress testing is also reviewed.

In preparation for a TEE study, the following information is reviewed:

- The patient must fast for 6 hours before the study.
- An intravenous line is started for administering dobutamine and a sedative.
- The throat is anesthetized before the probe is inserted.
- BP and the ECG are monitored throughout the study.

The nurse may reassure the patient that he or she will be kept comfortable but not heavily sedated. The patient must be alert enough to follow instructions and report symptoms such as chest pain. After the study, monitoring continues for 30 to 60 minutes, after which the patient is to remain fasting for 4 hours. The patient may have a sore throat for the next 24 hours.

Radionuclide Imaging

These studies involve the use of radioisotopes to evaluate coronary artery perfusion noninvasively, to detect myocardial ischemia and infarction, and to assess left ventricular function. **Radioisotopes** are atoms in an unstable form. Thallium 201 and technetium 99m are two of the most common radioisotopes used in cardiac nuclear medicine studies. As they decay, they give off small amounts of energy in the form of gamma rays. When injected intravenously into the bloodstream, the energy emitted by the radioisotope can be detected outside as a scintillation or flash of light. Different imaging techniques can then be performed using a gamma scintillation camera positioned over the body. Planar imaging, used with thallium, is a technique that provides a one-dimensional view of the heart from three locations. A relatively new technique called single photon emission tomography (SPECT) provides three-dimensional images. With SPECT, the camera moves around the patient's chest in a 180 degree to 360 degree arc to identify the areas of decreased myocardial perfusion more precisely.

Myocardial Perfusion Imaging

Thallium 201, a radioisotope, is used to assess myocardial perfusion. It resembles potassium and readily crosses into the cells of healthy myocardium. It is taken up slowly and in smaller amounts by myocardial cells that are ischemic from decreased blood flow. Thallium, however, will not cross into the necrotic tissue resulting from an MI.

Often, thallium is used with stress testing to assess changes in myocardial perfusion immediately after exercise (or injection of one of the pharmacologic agents) and at rest. One or two minutes before the end of the stress test, a dose of thallium 201 is injected into the intravenous line, allowing the radioisotope to be distributed into the myocardium. Images are taken immediately. Areas that do not show thallium uptake are noted as defects and indicate either an area of infarction or stress-induced myocardial ischemia. The resting images taken 3 hours later help to differentiate infarction from ischemia. Infarcted tissue is unable to take up thallium regardless of when the scan is taken. The defect will remain the same size. This is called a fixed defect, indicating that there is no perfusion in that area of the myocardium. Ischemic myocardium, however, will take a few hours to recover. Once perfusion is restored, thallium crosses into the myocardial cells, and the area of defect on the resting images is either smaller or completely reversed. These are called reversible defects and constitute positive stress test findings. Usually, cardiac catheterization is recommended after a positive test result to determine whether angioplasty or coronary artery bypass graft surgery is needed.

Technetium (Tc-99m) is a newer and better radioisotope used for cardiac imaging. Technetium can be combined with various chemical compounds, giving it an affinity for different types of cells. For example, Tc-99m sestamibi (Cardiolite) is distributed to myocardial cells in proportion to their amount of perfusion, making this tracer excellent for assessing perfusion to the myocardium. The procedure for cardiac imaging using Tc-99m sestamibi with stress testing is similar to the one just described using thallium, with two differences. Patients receiving Tc-99m sestamibi can have their resting images recorded before or after the exercise images. Timing of the images is not important because the half-life of Tc-99m is short, and Tc-99m needs to be injected before each scan. Also, SPECT imaging with Tc-99m sestamibi provides high-quality images.

NURSING INTERVENTIONS

The patient undergoing nuclear imaging techniques with stress testing should be prepared for the type of stressor to be used (exercise or medications) and the type of imaging technique (planar or SPECT). The patient may be concerned about receiving a radioactive substance and needs to be assured that these tracers are safe, having radiation exposure similar to that of other diagnostic x-rays. No postprocedure radiation precautions are necessary.

Important teaching points for patients undergoing SPECT include instructing patients to keep their arms over their head for about 20 to 30 minutes. If they cannot do this, thallium with planar imaging will need to be used instead.

ERNA or MUGA: Test of Ventricular Function and Wall Motion

Equilibrium radionuclide angiocardiography (ERNA), also known as multiple-gated acquisition (MUGA) scanning, is a common noninvasive technique that uses a conventional scintillation camera interfaced with a computer to record images of the heart during several hundred heart beats. The computer processes the data and allows for sequential viewing of the functioning heart. The sequential images are analyzed to evaluate left ventricular function, wall motion, and ejection fraction. The ejection fraction is the percentage of the end-diastolic volume that is ejected with each stroke. Normal right ventricular ejection fraction exceeds 42%; normal left ventricular ejection fraction exceeds 50%. MUGA scanning can also be used to assess the differences in left ventricular function during rest and exercise.

The patient is assured that there is no known radiation danger and is instructed to remain motionless during the scan.

Positron Emission Tomography

Positron emission tomography (PET) is a noninvasive scan used in the past primarily to study neurologic dysfunction. More recently and with increasing frequency, PET has also been used to diagnose cardiac dysfunction. For cardiac patients, including those without symptoms, PET, which provides more specific information about myocardial perfusion and viability than do TEE or thallium scans, helps in planning treatment (eg, coronary artery bypass surgery or angioplasty). PET also helps evaluate the patency of native and previously grafted vessels and the collateral circulation.

In the patient undergoing a PET scan, radioisotopes are administered by injection; one compound is used to determine blood flow in the myocardium and another shows the metabolic function. The PET camera provides detailed three-dimensional images of the distributed compounds. The viability of the myocardium is determined by comparing the extent of glucose metabolism in the myocardium to the degree of blood flow. For example, ischemic but viable tissue would show decreased blood flow and elevated metabolism. For this patient, revascularization through surgery or angioplasty would be likely to improve heart function. Restrictions of food intake before the test vary among institutions, but because PET evaluates glucose metabolism, the patient's blood glucose level should be in the normal range. Although PET equipment is costly, it is increasingly valued and available.

NURSING INTERVENTIONS

Nurses involved in PET and other scanning procedures may instruct the patient to refrain from using tobacco and ingesting caffeine for 4 hours before the procedure. They should also reassure the patient that radiation exposure is at safe and acceptable levels, similar to those in thallium studies.

Cardiac Catheterization

Cardiac catheterization is an invasive diagnostic procedure in which radiopaque arterial and venous catheters are introduced into selected blood vessels of the right and left sides of the heart. Catheter advancement is guided by fluoroscopy. The catheters are inserted most commonly percutaneously through the blood vessels, or via a cutdown procedure if the patient has poor vascular access. Pressures and oxygen saturations in the four heart chambers are measured. Cardiac catheterization is used most commonly to assess coronary artery patency and to determine if revascularization procedures are necessary (percutaneous transluminal coronary angioplasty or coronary artery bypass surgery) if the patient has atherosclerosis (see Chap. 25). During cardiac catheterization, the patient will have an intravenous line in place, and BP and ECG tracings are continuously monitored. Resuscitation equipment must be readily available during the procedure because the introduction of catheters into the ventricles can induce potentially fatal dysrhythmias. Staff are prepared to provide advanced cardiac life support measures as necessary.

The patient is assessed before the procedure for previous reactions to contrast agents or allergies to shellfish (which contain iodine). Contrast agents are radiopaque agents used to visualize the coronary arteries; some contrast agents contain iodine. In addition, the following blood tests are performed to identify abnormalities that may complicate recovery: blood urea nitrogen and creatinine levels, PT, PTT, hematocrit and hemoglobin values, platelet count, and electrolyte levels.

Diagnostic cardiac catheterizations are commonly performed on an outpatient basis and require 8 hours or less of bed rest for recovery. Variations in recovery time are most often due to the method used for arterial and venous hemostasis once catheters are removed. Patients in whom manual pressure and mechanical hemostatic devices are used require longer bed rest. There are new hemostasis devices that allow for earlier ambulation and discharge. These devices (sutures [Perclose], a collagen plug [Vasoseal], or a combination of both [Angio-Seal]) are placed percutaneously at the arteriotomy site after the procedure has been completed. Patients hospitalized for angina or acute MI may also require cardiac catheterization. After the procedure, these patients usually return to their hospital rooms for recovery. In some cardiac catheterization laboratories, an angioplasty may be performed immediately after the catheterization if indicated.

Angiography

Cardiac catheterization is usually performed with angiography, a technique of injecting a contrast agent into the vascular system to outline the heart and blood vessels. When a particular heart chamber or blood vessel is singled out for study, the procedure is known as selective angiography. Angiography makes use of cineangiograms, a series of rapidly changing films or movies on an intensified fluoroscopic screen that records the passage of the contrast agent through the vascular site(s). The recorded information allows for comparison of information over time. Common sites for selective angiography are the aorta, the coronary arteries, and the right and left sides of the heart.

Aortography

An aortogram is a form of angiography that outlines the lumen of the aorta and the major arteries arising from it. In thoracic aortography, a contrast agent is used to study the aortic arch and its major branches. The catheter may be introduced into the aorta using the translumbar or retrograde brachial or femoral artery approach.

Coronary Arteriography

In coronary arteriography, the catheter is introduced into the right or left brachial or femoral artery and is passed into the ascending aorta and manipulated into the appropriate coronary artery. Coronary arteriography is used to evaluate the degree of atherosclerosis and to determine the mode of treatment. It is also used to study suspected congenital anomalies of the coronary arteries.

Right-Heart Catheterization

Right-heart catheterization usually precedes left-heart catheterization. It involves the passage of a catheter from an antecubital or femoral vein into the right atrium, right ventricle, pulmonary artery, and pulmonary capillary. Pressures and oxygen saturations from each of these areas are obtained and recorded.

Nursing Alert *Although right-heart catheterization is considered a relatively safe procedure, potential complications include cardiac dysrhythmias, venous spasm, infection of the insertion site, cardiac perforation, and, rarely, cardiac arrest.*

Left-Heart Catheterization

Left-heart catheterization is performed by retrograde catheterization of the left ventricle (most common technique) or by trans-septal catheterization of the left atrium. In the retrograde technique, the physician inserts the catheter into the right brachial artery or femoral artery and advances it into the aorta and left ventricle.

In the trans-septal approach, the physician advances the catheter from the right femoral vein into the right atrium, then a long needle is passed up through the catheter to puncture the septum separating the right and left atria. The needle is withdrawn and the catheter is advanced into the left ventricle.

Left-heart catheterization is performed to evaluate the patency of the coronary arteries and the function of the left ventricle and the mitral and aortic valves. Potential complications include dysrhythmias, MI, perforation of the heart or great vessels, and systemic embolization.

After the procedure, the catheter is carefully withdrawn and arterial hemostasis is achieved using manual pressure or other techniques previously described. If the physician opened the artery in a cutdown approach, the arteriotomy is sutured and a sterile dressing applied.

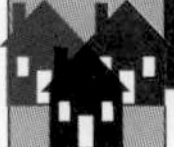

PATIENT EDUCATION AND HOME CARE

Guide to Self-Care After Cardiac Catheterization

After discharge from the hospital for cardiac catheterization, guidelines for self-care include the following:

- For the next 24 hours, do not bend, strain, or lift heavy objects.
- Avoid tub baths, but shower as desired.
- Talk with your physician about when you may return to work, drive, or resume strenuous activities.
- Call your physician if any of the following occur: bleeding, swelling, new bruising or pain from your procedure puncture site, temperature of 101.5°F (38.6°C) or more.
- If test results show that you have coronary artery disease, talk with your physican about options for treatment, including cardiac rehabilitation programs in your community. Also talk with your physician about lifestyle changes to reduce your risk for further or future heart problems, such as quitting smoking, lowering your cholesterol level, initiating dietary changes, beginning an exercise program, or losing weight.

NURSING INTERVENTIONS

Nursing responsibilities before cardiac catheterization include the following:

- Instruct the patient to fast, usually for 8 to 12 hours, before the procedure. If catheterization is to be performed as an outpatient procedure, explain that a friend, family member, or other responsible person must help transport the patient home.
- Prepare the patient for the expected duration of the procedure; indicate that it will involve lying on a hard table for less than 2 hours.
- Prepare the patient to experience certain sensations during the catheterization. Knowing what to expect can help the patient cope with the experience. Reassure the patient that mild sedatives will be given intravenously to relieve anxiety. The patient will feel sleepy but will awaken easily.
- Explain that an occasional pounding sensation (palpitation) may be felt in the chest because of extrasystoles that almost always occur, particularly when the catheter tip touches the myocardium. The patient may be asked to cough and breathe deeply, especially after the injection of contrast agent. Coughing may help to disrupt a dysrhythmia and help to clear the contrast agent from the arteries. Breathing deeply and holding the breath helps to lower the diaphragm for better visualization of heart structures. The injection of a contrast agent into either side of the heart may produce a flushed feeling throughout the body and a sensation similar to the need to void, which subsides in a minute or less.
- Encourage the patient to express fears and anxieties. Provide teaching and reassurance to reduce apprehension.

Nursing responsibilities after cardiac catheterization may include the following:

- Observe the catheter access site for bleeding or hematoma formation, and assess the peripheral pulses in the affected extremity (dorsalis pedis and posterior tibial pulses in the lower extremity, radial pulse in the upper extremity) every 15 minutes for 1 hour, and then every 1 to 2 hours until stable.
- Evaluate temperature and color of the affected extremity and any patient complaints of pain, numbness, or tingling sensations in the affected extremity to determine signs of arterial insufficiency. Report changes promptly.
- Observe for dysrhythmias by observing the cardiac monitor or by assessing the apical and peripheral pulses for changes in rate and rhythm. A vasovagal reaction, consisting of bradycardia, hypotension, and nausea, can be precipitated by a distended bladder or discomfort during the removal of the arterial catheter, especially if a femoral site has been used. Prompt intervention is critical; this includes raising the feet and legs above the head and administering intravenous fluids and intravenous atropine as prescribed, if necessary.
- Inform the patient that if the procedure was performed percutaneously through the femoral artery and without the use of a homeostasis device, bed rest must continue for 4 to 6 hours with the affected leg straight and the head elevated to 30 degrees or less until hemostasis is adequately achieved. The patient may be turned from side to side with the affected extremity straight as needed for comfort. Analgesic medication is administered as prescribed for discomfort.
- Instruct the patient to report chest pain and bleeding or sudden discomfort from the catheter insertion sites immediately.
- Encourage fluids to increase urinary output and flush out the dye.
- Ensure safety by instructing the patient to ask for help when getting out of bed the first time after the procedure, because orthostatic hypotension may occur and the patient may feel faint.

For patients being discharged from the hospital the same day as the procedure, additional instructions are provided. They appear in the accompanying chart, Guide to Self-Care After Cardiac Catheterization.

Electrophysiologic Testing

The electrophysiology study is an invasive procedure performed under laboratory conditions. Electrophysiologic testing plays a

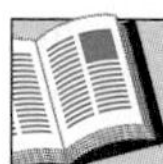

NURSING RESEARCH

Preferred Positions After Cardiac Catheterization

Rein A., et al. (1995). Positioning post-outpatient cardiac catheterization. *Progress in Cardiovascular Nursing, 10*(4), 4–10.

Vascular complications caused by trauma to the femoral artery during insertion or removal of catheters used during cardiac catheterization include bleeding, hematoma, pseudoaneurysm, distal embolization, and arterial thrombosis. The risk for these complications can be minimized by instructing the patient not to bend the affected extremity, to apply pressure at the site when coughing, and to refrain from raising the head off the pillow. Health care providers achieve hemostasis initially by using a variety of techniques, including manual pressure or mechanical devices. Five- to ten-pound sandbags over the catheter access site or sheet tucks over the affected extremity have also been used to immobilize the extremity.

Traditionally, patients have been positioned supine with the head of bed (HOB) flat or elevated no greater than 30 degrees after the procedure. Back discomfort or pain, however, from bed rest restrictions is a common complaint from patients recovering from this procedure.

Purpose

This study sought to explore the influence of three different post-procedural positions on the incidence of complications and patients' preferences for position.

Study Sample and Design

Sixty-nine patients who had undergone cardiac catheterization were randomly assigned to one of three positions after hemostasis was achieved at the puncture site. The three positions were (1) supine with HOB flat (control group), (2) side-lying with affected extremity straight, and (3) supine with HOB elevated to 15° to 30°. Before discharge, patients were asked which position they would have preferred.

Findings

No significant differences in rate of complications (bleeding or hematoma) were found among the three groups. However, the control group reported significantly more pain than the other two groups ($p = 0.028$). These findings are consistent with patient preferences: 85% of the control group preferred another position, compared with 24% of the patients in the other two groups ($p < 0.001$).

Nursing Implications

These findings are consistent with those of similar studies. Head of bed elevations to 30 degrees and side-lying with the affected extremity straight are safe and more comfortable alternatives to the traditional supine position. This study demonstrates the importance of examining current standards of practice and identifying opportunities for quality improvement.

major role in the diagnosis and management of serious dysrhythmias and is used (1) to distinguish atrial from ventricular tachycardias that cannot be determined by the 12-lead ECG, (2) to evaluate how readily a life-threatening rhythm, such as ventricular tachycardia or ventricular fibrillation, can be induced, (3) to evaluate AV node function, (4) to evaluate the effectiveness of antiarrhythmic medications in suppressing the dysrhythmia, and (5) to determine the need for other therapeutic interventions, such as a pacemaker, implantable cardioverter defibrillator, or radiofrequency ablation (discussed in Chap. 24). The electrophysiology study is indicated for patients with syncope and/or palpitations and for survivors of cardiac arrest from ventricular fibrillation (sudden cardiac death).

The initial study can take up to 4 hours. The patient is conscious but sedated. Catheters with recording and electrical stimulating capabilities (pacing) are inserted into the heart through the femoral and right subclavian veins to record electrical activity in the right and left atrium, bundle of His, and right ventricle. Fluoroscopy guides the positioning of these catheters. Baseline intracardiac recordings are obtained; programmed electrical stimulations of the atrium or ventricle are then administered in an attempt to induce the patient's dysrhythmia. If the dysrhythmia is induced, various antiarrhythmic medications are administered intravenously. The study is repeated after each medication to evaluate which medication or combination of medications is most effective in controlling the dysrhythmia.

After the study, the patient receives an equivalent oral antiarrhythmic agent, and subsequent studies may be necessary to evaluate the effectiveness of that medication before discharge. Results of the study may indicate the need for other therapeutic interventions, such as a pacemaker or implantable cardioverter defibrillator.

During an electrophysiologic study, lethal dysrhythmias may be induced; therefore, the procedure is performed in a controlled environment with resuscitation equipment (eg, defibrillator) readily available. Possible complications include bleeding and hematoma from the catheter insertion sites, pneumothorax (air in the pleural cavity), deep vein thrombosis, stroke, or sudden death.

Nursing Interventions

Patients receive nothing to eat or drink for 8 hours before the procedure, and antiarrhythmic medications are withheld for 24 hours before the study. This necessitates careful monitoring of the cardiac rate and rhythm for dysrhythmias. Other medications may be taken with sips of water.

Nurses help prepare patients for the study by explaining the reason for the study and describing the study and aftercare. Postprocedural interventions include carefully monitoring for complications. The nurse takes vital signs, reviews tracings of continuous ECG monitoring, assesses the apical pulse, auscultates for pericardial friction rub (indicates bleeding into the pericardial sac), and inspects the catheter insertion sites for bleeding or hematoma formation.

In addition, the nurse assists the patient to maintain bed rest with the affected extremity kept straight and the head of the bed elevated to 30 degrees for 4 to 6 hours. The frequency of assessments and the length of time on bed rest may vary based on institutional policy and physician preference.

Hemodynamic Monitoring

Critically ill patients require continuous assessment of their cardiovascular system to diagnose and manage their complex medical conditions. This is achieved by using direct pressure monitoring systems, often referred to as hemodynamic monitoring. Central venous pressure (CVP), pulmonary artery pressure, and intra-arterial BP monitoring are common forms of hemodynamic monitoring. Patients requiring hemodynamic monitoring are cared for in specialty critical care units. Some critical care step-down units also admit stable patients with central venous or intra-arterial BP monitoring.

To perform this type of monitoring, specialized equipment is necessary and includes the following:

- A central venous pressure, pulmonary artery, or arterial catheter, which is introduced into the appropriate artery or heart chamber
- A flush system composed of intravenous solution (often with heparin), tubing, stopcocks, and a flush device, which provides continuous and manual flushing of the system
- A pressure bag placed around the flush solution and maintained at 300 mm Hg of pressure; the pressurized flush system delivers 3 to 5 mL of solution per hour through the catheter to prevent clotting and backflow of blood into the pressure monitoring system
- A transducer to convert the pressure coming from the artery or heart chamber into an electrical signal
- An amplifier or monitor that increases the size of the electrical signal for display on an oscilloscope

Central Venous Pressure Monitoring

The CVP, the pressure in the vena cava or the right atrium, is used to assess right ventricular function and venous blood return to the right heart. The CVP can be continuously measured by connecting either a catheter positioned in the vena cava or the proximal port of a pulmonary artery catheter to a pressure monitoring system. The pulmonary artery catheter, described in greater detail below, is used for critically ill patients. Patients on general medical-surgical units requiring CVP monitoring may have a single-lumen or multilumen catheter placed into the superior vena cava. Intermittent measurement of the CVP can then be obtained by using a water manometer.

Because the pressures in the right atrium and right ventricle are equal at the end of diastole (0 to 8 mm Hg), the CVP is also an indirect method of determining right ventricular filling pressure (preload). This makes the CVP a useful hemodynamic parameter to observe when managing an unstable patient's fluid volume status. CVP monitoring is most valuable when pressures are followed over time and are correlated with the patient's clinical status. A rising pressure may be due to hypervolemia or a condition, such as CHF, that causes a decrease in myocardial contractility. (CVP monitoring is not clinically useful in a patient with CHF in which left ventricular failure precedes right ventricular failure, making an elevated CVP a very late sign of CHF.) Pulmonary artery monitoring is preferred for a patient with CHF. Decreased CVP indicates reduced right ventricular preload, most often caused by hypovolemia. This diagnosis can be substantiated when a rapid intravenous infusion causes the CVP to rise.

Before insertion of a CVP catheter, the site is prepared by shaving if necessary and cleansing with an antiseptic solution. A local anesthetic may be used. The physician threads a single-lumen or multilumen catheter through the external jugular, antecubital, or femoral vein into the vena cava just above or within the right atrium. Once the CVP catheter is inserted, it is secured and a dry sterile dressing is applied. Catheter placement is confirmed by a chest x-ray, and the site is inspected daily for signs of infection. The dressing, pressure monitoring system, or water manometer are changed according to hospital policy. CVP catheters can be used for infusing intravenous fluids, administering intravenous medications, and drawing blood specimens in addition to monitoring pressure.

When measuring the CVP, the transducer (when using a pressure monitoring system) or the zero mark on the manometer (when using the water manometer) must be placed at a standard reference point called the phlebostatic axis (Fig. 23-13). After locating this position, the nurse makes an ink mark on the patient's chest to indicate the location. If the phlebostatic axis is used, CVP can be measured correctly with the patient supine at any backrest position up to 45 degrees. The range for a normal CVP is 0 to 8 mm Hg (pressure monitoring system) or 3 to 8 cm H_2O (water manometer). The most common complications of CVP monitoring are infection and air embolism.

Pulmonary Artery Pressure Monitoring

Pulmonary artery pressure monitoring is an important tool used in critical care for assessing left ventricular function, diagnosing the etiology of shock, and evaluating the patient's response to medical interventions (eg, fluid administration or vasoactive medications). Pulmonary artery pressure monitoring is achieved by using one of many types of pulmonary artery catheters and the pressure monitoring system described previously. Catheters vary in the number of lumens and the types of measurement (eg, cardiac output and oxygen saturation) or pacing capabilities. All types require that a balloon-tipped, flow-directed catheter be inserted into a large vein (usually the subclavian, jugular, or femoral vein); it is then passed into the vena cava and right atrium. In the right atrium, the balloon tip is inflated, and the catheter is carried rapidly by the flow of blood through the tricuspid valve, into the right ventricle, through the pulmonic valve, and into a branch of the pulmonary artery. When the catheter reaches a small pulmonary artery, the balloon is deflated and the catheter is secured with sutures. Fluoroscopy may be used during insertion to visualize the progression of the catheter through the heart chambers to the pulmonary artery. This procedure can be performed in the operating room or cardiac catheterization laboratory or at the bedside in the critical care unit. During insertion of the pulmonary artery catheter, the bedside monitor is observed for waveform changes as the catheter is moved through the heart chambers on the right side to the pulmonary artery.

With the catheter correctly positioned, the following can be measured: CVP or right atrial pressure, pulmonary artery systolic and diastolic pressures, mean pulmonary artery pressure, and pulmonary capillary wedge pressure. When a thermodilution catheter is used, the cardiac output can be measured and systemic vascular resistance and pulmonary vascular resistance can be calculated.

Normal pulmonary artery pressure is 25/9, with a mean pressure of 15 mm Hg (see Fig. 23-5 for normal ranges). When the balloon tip is inflated, usually with 1 mL of air, the catheter floats farther out into the pulmonary artery until it becomes wedged. This is an occlusive maneuver impeding blood flow through that segment of the pulmonary artery. A pressure measurement, called pulmonary capillary wedge pressure, is taken within seconds of wedging the pulmonary artery catheter, then the balloon is immediately deflated and blood flow is restored. The nurse obtaining the wedge reading ensures that the balloon has returned to its normal position in the pulmonary artery by evaluating the pulmonary artery pressure waveform. The pulmonary artery diastolic reading and the wedge pressure reflect the pressure in the ventricle at end-diastole and are particularly important to monitor in critically ill patients, because they are used to evaluate left ventricular filling pressures (preload). At end-diastole, when the mitral valve is open, the wedge pressure is the same as the pressure in the left atrium and the left ventricle, unless the patient has mitral valve disease or pulmonary hypertension. Pulmonary capillary wedge pressure is a mean pressure and is normally 4.5 to 13 mm Hg. Critically ill patients usually require higher left ventricular filling pressures to optimize car-

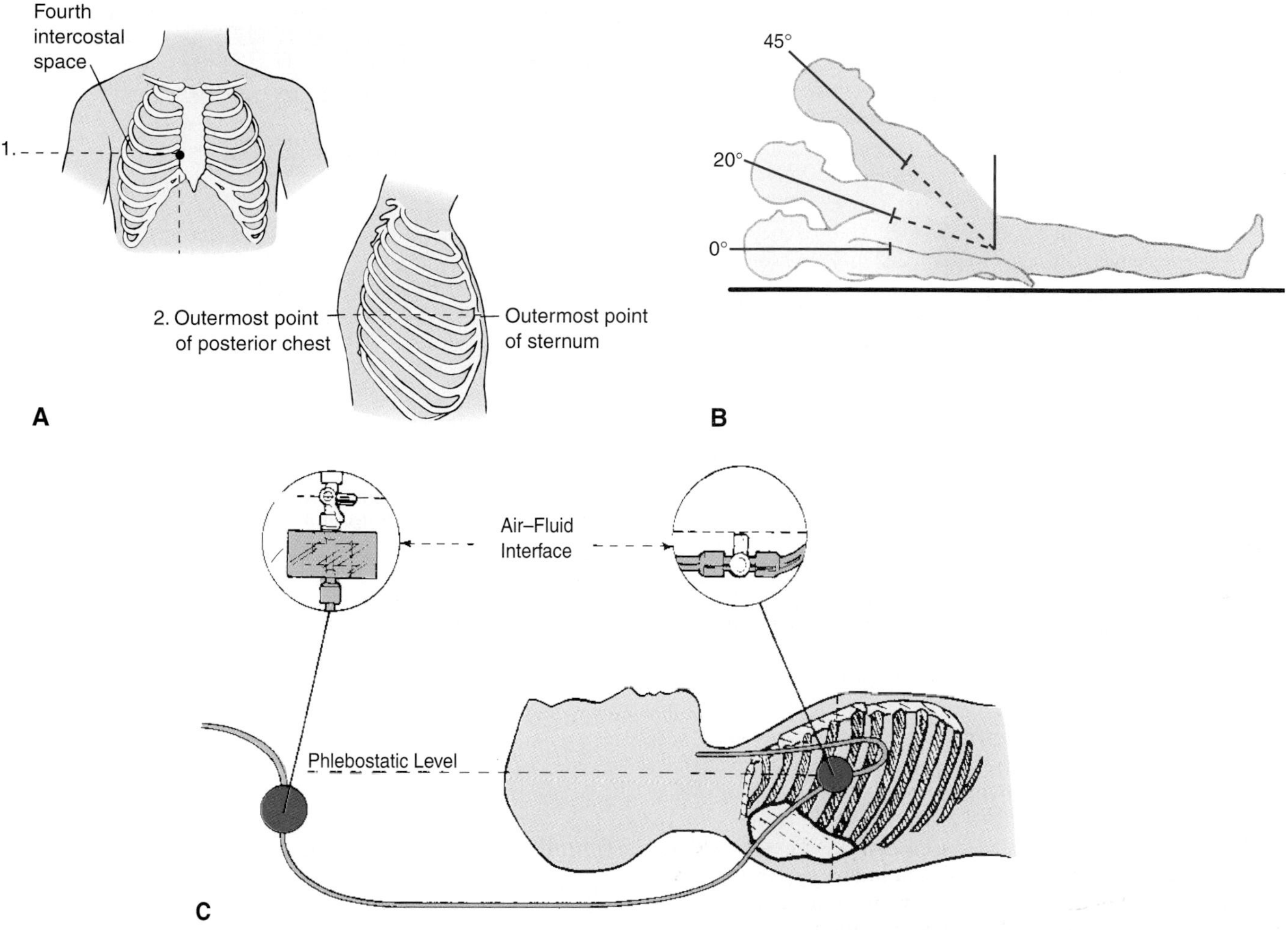

FIGURE 23•13 The phlebostatic axis and the phlebostatic level. (**A**) The phlebostatic axis is the crossing of two reference lines: (1) a line from the fourth intercostal space at the point where it joins the sternum, drawn out to the side of the body beneath the axilla; and (2) a line midway between the anterior and posterior surfaces of the chest. (**B**) The phlebostatic level is a horizontal line through the phlebostatic axis. The air–fluid interface of the stopcock of the transducer or the zero mark on the manometer must be level with this axis for accurate measurements. Moving from the flat to erect positions, the patient moves the chest and therefore the reference level: the phlebostatic level stays horizontal through the same reference point. Adapted from Shinn JA, Woods SL, Huseby JS: Effect of intermittent positive pressure ventilation upon pulmonary capillary wedge pressures in acutely ill patients. *Heart and Lung B*(2): 324, 1979. (**C**) Two methods for referencing the pressure system to the phlebostatic axis. The system can be referenced by placing the air–fluid interface of either the in-line stopcock or stopcock on top of the transducer at the phlebostatic level.

diac output. These patients may need to have their wedge pressure maintained as high as 18 mm Hg.

NURSING INTERVENTIONS

Catheter site care is essentially the same as for a CVP catheter. See Chapter 13 for more specific guidelines. As in measuring CVP, the transducer must be positioned at the phlebostatic axis to ensure accurate readings. Complications of pulmonary artery pressure monitoring include infection, pulmonary artery rupture, pulmonary thromboembolism, pulmonary infarction, catheter kinking, dysrhythmias, and air embolism.

Systemic Arterial Pressure Monitoring

Intra-arterial monitoring is used to obtain direct and continuous BP measurements in critically ill patients with severe high BP or hypotension. Arterial catheters are also useful when arterial blood gas measurements and blood samples need to be obtained frequently (Fig. 23-14).

Once an arterial site is selected (radial, brachial, femoral, or dorsalis pedis), collateral circulation to the area must be confirmed before the catheter is placed. If no collateral circulation exists, and the cannulated artery were to become occluded, ischemia and infarction of the area distal to the cannulated site could occur. Collateral circulation can be checked by the Allen test to evaluate the radial and ulnar arteries or by using an ultrasonic Doppler test for any of the arteries. With the Allen test, the nurse compresses the radial and ulnar arteries simultaneously and asks the patient to make a fist, causing the hand to blanch. After the patient opens the fist, the nurse releases the pressure on the ulnar artery while maintaining pressure on the radial artery. The patient's hand will turn pink if the ulnar artery is patent.

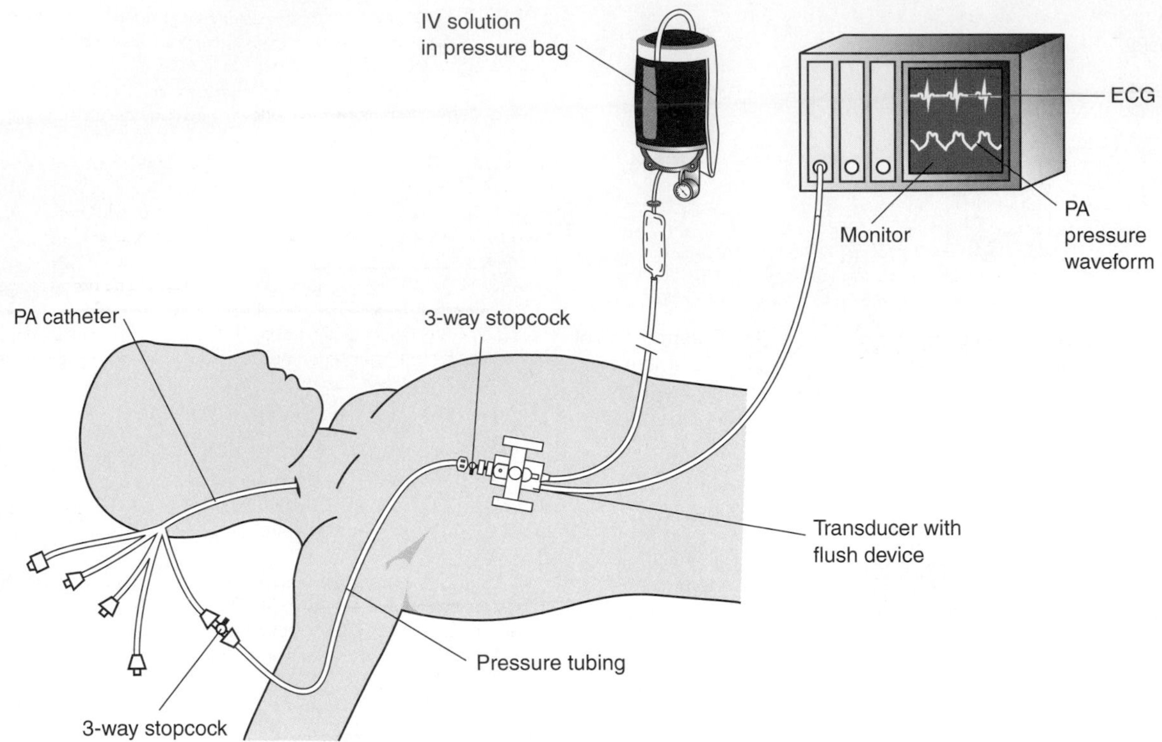

FIGURE 23•14 Example of a pulmonary artery (PA) pressure monitoring system, PA catheter is inserted into the internal jugular vein and advanced into the pulmonary artery. From Daily, E. (1994). *Techniques in bedside hemodynamic monitoring* (6th ed.). Mosby.

Site preparation and care are the same as for CVP catheters. The catheter flush solution is the same as for pulmonary artery catheters. A transducer is attached and pressures are measured in millimeters of mercury (mm Hg). Complications include local obstruction with distal ischemia, external hemorrhage, massive ecchymosis, dissection, air embolism, blood loss, pain, arteriospasm, and infection.

Critical Thinking Exercises

1.
Your patient is an elderly woman who has just been discharged from the cardiac telemetry unit of the local hospital. This is her second hospitalization within the last 6 weeks for CHF. As her home care nurse, you are in the process of identifying her home care needs. What questions will you include in this patient's health history to help you identify potential causes for her frequent hospitalizations?

2.
During rounds, the physician tells your patient that she will need a stress test. She has limited range of motion of both her upper and lower extremities. Based on these findings, what type of a stress test and radionuclide imaging technique do you anticipate the physician will order? What implications will this have for patient preparation?

3.
You are called into the room of a middle-aged man who had an MI 2 days ago. He tells you that he is experiencing chest pain. Keeping in mind the common causes of chest pain, what history and physical assessment information will you elicit from this patient to determine the source of his chest pain?

References and Selected Readings

BOOKS

American Nurses Association, Division on Medical-Surgical Nursing, and American Heart Association Council on Cardiovascular Nursing. (1994). *Standards of cardiovascular nursing practice.* Kansas City: American Nurses Association.

Bickley, L. S. & Hoekelman, R. A. (1999). *Bates' guide to physical examination* (7th ed.). Philadelphia: Lippincott Williams & Wilkins.

Braunwald, E. (1997). *Heart disease: A textbook of cardiovascular medicine* (Vols. I & II, 5th ed.). Philadelphia: W. B. Saunders.

Daily, E. (1994). *Techniques in bedside hemodynamic monitoring* (5th ed.). Mosby.

Darvic, G. (1995). *Hemodynamic monitoring: Invasive and noninvasive clinical application* (2nd ed.). Philadelphia: W. B. Saunders.

Ellestad, M. (1996). *Stress testing: Principles and practices* (4th ed.). Philadelphia: F. A. Davis.

Fuller, J., & Schaller-Ayers, J. (2000). *Health assessment: A nursing approach* (3rd ed.). Philadelphia: Lippincott Williams & Wilkins.

Huff, J. (1997). *ECG workout: Exercises in arrhythmia interpretation* (3rd ed.). Philadelphia: Lippincott-Raven.

Lipson, J. G., et al. (1996). *Culture & nursing care: A pocketbook guide.* San Francisco: UCSF Nursing Press.

Miller, C. (1995). *Nursing care of older adults: Theory and practice* (2nd ed.). Philadelphia: J. B. Lippincott.

Oka, R. K., Burke, L. E., & Froelicher, E. S. S. (1995). Emotional responses and inpatient education. In: S. Woods, et al. (Eds.), *Cardiac nursing* (3rd ed.). Philadelphia: J. B. Lippincott.

VanRiper, S., & VanRiper, J. (1997). *Cardiac diagnosis: A guide for nurses.* Philadelphia: W. B. Saunders.

Wenger, N. K., et al. (1995). *Cardiac Rehabilitation as Secondary Prevention.* Clinical Practice Guideline No. 17 (AHCPR Pub. 96-0673). Rockville, MD: US Department of Health and Human Services, Public Health Service, Agency for Health Care and Policy and Research and National Heart, Lung and Blood Institute.

Woods, S., et al. (1995). *Cardiac nursing* (3rd ed.). Philadelphia: J. B. Lippincott.

JOURNALS

Asterisks indicate nursing research articles.

Arnold, E. (1997). Cardiac stress testing. *Nursing '97, 27*(1), 58–61.

Bridges, E. J., & Woods, S. L. (1993). Pulmonary artery pressure measurement: State of the art. *Heart and Lung 22*(2), 101.

DeJong, M. A., & Morton, P. G. (1997). Control of vascular complications after cardiac catheterization: A research-based protocol. *Dimensions in Critical Care Nursing, 16*(4), 170–179.

*Dracup, K., & Bryan-Brown, C. (1997). Reducing patient delay in seeking treatment. *American Journal of Critical Care, 6*(6), 415–417.

*Dracup, K., & Moser, D. K. (1997). Beyond sociodemographics: Factors influencing the decision to seek treatment for symptoms of acute myocardial infarction. *Heart and Lung, 26*(4), 253–262.

Fleury, J., et al. (1997). Promoting wellness in individuals with coronary heart disease. *Journal of Cardiovascular Nursing, 11*(3), 26–42.

Gawlinski, A. (1997). Facts and fallacies of patient positioning and hemodynamic measurement. *Journal of Cardiovascular Nursing, 12*(1), 1–15.

Ide, B. (1995). Bedside electrocardiographic assessment. *Journal of Cardiovascular Nursing, 9*(4), 10–23.

Ishii, K. (1995). Physical capacity assessment of the acute cardiovascular patient. *Journal of Cardiovascular Nursing, 9*(4), 53–63.

Jenson, G. A., & Miller, D. S. (1995). The heart of aging: Special challenges of cardiac ischemic disease and failure in the elderly. *AACN Clinical Issues, 6*(3), 471–481.

Jenson, L., & King, K. (1997). Women and heart disease: The issues. *Critical Care Nursing, 17*(2), 45–52.

Kelly, C. S., & Stevens, K. R. (1997). Cultural considerations in promoting wellness. *Journal of Cardiovascular Nursing, 11*(3), 15–25.

Laurienzo, J. M. (1995). Transesophageal dobutamine stress echocardiography: The nurse's role. *Journal of Cardiovascular Nursing, 9*(4), 24–35.

Litin, S. C., & Gastineau, D. A. (1995). Concise review for primary care physicians: Current concepts in anticoagulant therapy. *Mayo Clinic Proceedings, 70*, 266–272.

McFetridge, J. A., & Yarandi, H. N. (1997). Cardiovascular function during cognitive stress in men before and after CABG. *Nursing Research, 46*(4), 188–194.

Minarik, P. (1995). Cognitive assessment of the cardiovascular patient in the acute care setting. *Journal of Cardiovascular Nursing, 9*(4), 36–52.

Montes, P. (1997). Managing outpatient cardiac catheterization. *American Journal of Nursing, 97*(8), 34–37.

Moser, D. (1997). Correcting misconceptions about women and heart disease. *American Journal of Nursing, 97*(4), 26–43.

PEPI Trial. (1995). Effects of estrogen or estrogen/progestin regimens on heart disease risk factors in postmenopausal women. *Journal of the American Medical Association, 273*(3), 199–208.

*Reiley, P., et al. (1996). Discharge planning: Comparison of patients' and nurses' perceptions of patients following hospital discharge. *Image: Journal of Nursing Scholarship, 28*(2), 143–147.

Romeo, K. C. (1995). The female heart: Physiologic aspects of cardiovascular disease in women. *Dimensions in Critical Care Nursing, 14*(4), 170–177.

Severson, A. L., et al. (1997). International Normalized Ratio in anticoagulant therapy: Understanding the issues. *American Journal of Critical Care, 6*(2), 88–92.

*Scherck, K. A. (1997). Recognizing a heart attack: The process of determining illness. *American Journal of Critical Care, 6*(4), 267–273.

Shinn, J. A., Woods, S. L., & Huseby, J. S. (1979). Effect of intermittent positive pressure ventilation upon pulmonary capillary wedge pressures in acutely ill patients. *Heart and Lung B*(2), 324.

Smith, S. C., et al. (1995). Preventing heart attack and death in patients with coronary artery disease. *Circulation, 92*(1), 2–4.

Steinke, E., & Patterson-Midgley, P. (1996). Sexual counseling of MI patients. *Dimensions in Critical Care Nursing, 15*(4), 216–223.

Stillman, F. A. (1997). Smoking cessation for the hospitalized cardiac patient: Rationale for and report of a model program. *Journal of Cardiovascular Nursing, 9*(2), 25–36.

Titler, M. G., & Pettit, D. M. (1995). Discharge readiness assessment. *Journal of Cardiovascular Nursing, 9*(4), 64–74.

Thompson, E. J., et al. (1996). Dobutamine stress echocardiography: A new, noninvasive method for detecting ischemic heart disease. *Heart and Lung, 25*(2), 87–97.

Warner, C. D. (1997). Triage and interpreting chest pain. *Journal of Cardiovascular Nursing, 12*(1), 84–92.

Weld, L. (1997). Developing a cardiac catheterization education program. *Journal of Cardiovascular Nursing, 11*(2), 47–57.

Zaret, B. L., & Wackers, F. J. (1993). Nuclear cardiology. Part I. *New England Journal of Medicine, 329*(11), 775–783.

Zaret, B. L., & Wackers, F. J. (1993). Nuclear cardiology. Part II. *New England Journal of Medicine, 329*(12), 855–863.

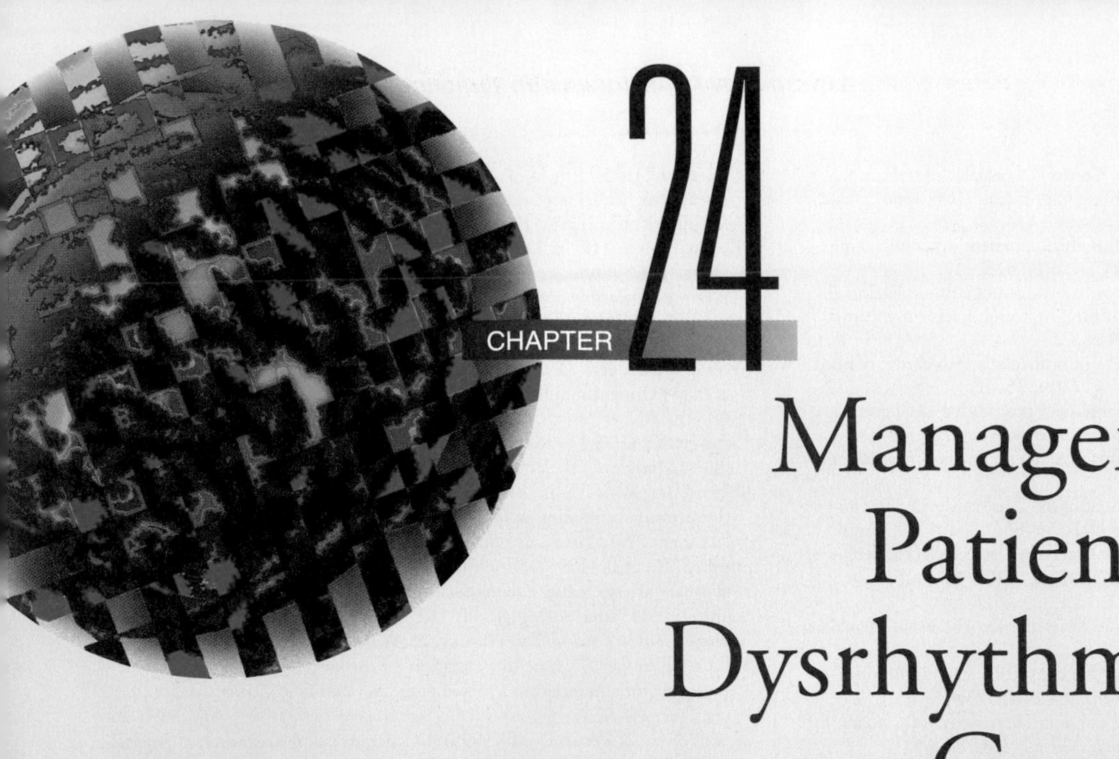

Management of Patients With Dysrhythmias and Conduction Problems

Learning Objectives

On completion of this chapter, the learner will be able to:

1. Correlate the components of the ECG with physiologic events of the heart.
2. Define the ECG as a waveform that represents the cardiac electrical event in relation to the lead depicted (placement of electrodes).
3. Analyze elements of an ECG rhythm strip: ventricular and atrial rate, ventricular and atrial rhythm, P wave and shape, QRS complex and shape, QRS duration, PR interval, and P:QRS ratio.
4. Identify the ECG criteria, etiologies, and management of several dysrhythmias, including conduction disturbances.
5. Describe the key points of using a defibrillator.
6. Describe the noninvasive and invasive methods used to diagnose and treat chronic dysrhythmias, and discuss the nursing implications.
7. Describe the purpose of an implantable cardioverter defibrillator (ICD), the types available, and their nursing implications.
8. Compare the different types of pacemakers, their uses, possible complications, and nursing implications.
9. Use the nursing process as a framework for care of patients with dysrhythmias.
10. Use the nursing process as a framework for care of patients with pacemakers.

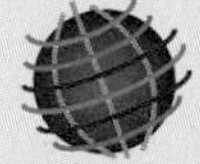

Without a regular rate and rhythm, the heart could not perform efficiently as a pump to circulate oxygenated blood and other life-sustaining nutrients to all the body organs (including itself) and tissues. With an irregular or erratic rhythm, the heart is considered to be dysrhythmic (sometimes called arrhythmic). This is a dangerous condition.

GLOSSARY

ablation: purposeful destruction of heart muscle cells, usually in an attempt to control a dysrhythmia

antidysrhythmic: a medication that suppresses or prevents a dysrhythmia

automaticity: ability of the cardiac muscle to initiate an electrical impulse

cardioversion: electrical current administered to a patient synchronized with his or her own QRS to stop a dysrhythmia.

conductivity: ability of the cardiac muscle to transmit electrical impulses

defibrillation: electrical current administered to a patient to stop a dysrhythmia, not synchronized with the patient's QRS complex

depolarization: process by which cardiac muscle cells change from a more negatively charged intracellular condition to a more positively charged state

dysrhythmia: abnormal conduction of electrical activity through the heart

inhibited: in reference to pacemakers, term used to describe the pacemaker withholding an impulse (not firing)

P wave: an ECG characteristic reflecting conduction of an electrical impulse through the atrium; atrial depolarization

PR interval: component of an ECG tracing reflecting conduction of an electrical impulse through the AV node

proarrhythmic: an agent (eg, a medication) that causes or exacerbates a dysrhythmia

QRS complex: an ECG characteristic reflecting conduction of an electrical impulse through the ventricles—ventricular depolarization

QT interval: an ECG characteristic reflecting the time from ventricular depolarization to repolarization

repolarization: process by which cardiac muscle cells return to a more negatively charged intracellular condition, their resting state

sinus rhythm: electrical activity of the heart initiated by the SA node

ST segment: an ECG characteristic reflecting the degree of synchrony of ventricular depolarization and repolarization

T wave: an ECG characteristic reflecting repolarization of the ventricles

triggered: in reference to pacemakers, term used to describe the release of an impulse in response to some stimulus

U wave: an ECG characteristic that may reflect Purkinje fiber repolarization; usually seen when a patient's serum potassium level is low

DYSRHYTHMIAS

Dysrhythmias are disorders of the formation and/or conduction of the electrical impulse within the heart. These can cause disturbances of the heart rate, the heart rhythm, or both. Dysrhythmias may initially be evidenced by the hemodynamic effect that they cause. They are diagnosed by analyzing the electrocardiographic waveform. Dysrhythmias are named according to the site of origin of the impulse and the mechanism of formation or conduction involved (Chart 24-1). For example, an impulse that originates in the sinoatrial (SA) node and that has a slow rate is called sinus bradycardia.

Normal Electrical Conduction

The electrical impulse that stimulates and paces the cardiac muscle normally originates in the sinus node, located near the vena cava in the right atrium. Normally, the impulse occurs at a rate ranging between 60 and 100 times a minute in the adult. The impulse quickly travels from the sinus node through the atria to the atrioventricular (AV) node (Fig. 24-1), causing the atria to contract. The structure of the AV node slows the impulse, which allows time for the atria to contract and the ventricles to fill with blood. From the AV node, the impulse travels very quickly along the right and left bundle branches and the Purkinje fibers, located in the ventricular muscle. The electrical stimulation of the ventricles, in turn, causes the ventricles to contract (systole). Then the electromechanical impulse completes the circuit and the cycle begins again. In this way, sinus rhythm promotes cardiovascular circulation. The electrical stimulus causes (and, therefore, is followed by) the mechanical event of the heart. The electrical stimulation is called **depolarization**; the mechanical contraction is called systole. Electrical relaxation is called **repolarization** and mechanical relaxation is called diastole. See Chapter 23 for a more complete explanation of cardiac function.

CHART 24•1 Identifying Dysrhythmias

Sites of Origin
- Sinus node
- Atria
- AV node or junction
- Ventricles

Mechanisms of Formation or Conduction
- Normal (idio) rhythm
- Bradycardia
- Tachycardia
- Dysrhythmia
- Flutter
- Fibrillation
- Premature complexes
- Blocks

Influences on Heart Rate and Contractility

The heart rate is influenced by the autonomic nervous system, which consists of sympathetic and parasympathetic fibers. Sympathetic (also referred to as adrenergic) nerve fibers are attached to the heart and arteries as well as several other areas in the body. Stimulation of the sympathetic system increases heart rate (positive chronotropy), conduction through the AV node (positive dromotropy), and the force of myocardial contraction (positive inotropy). Sympathetic stimulation also causes the constriction of peripheral blood vessels and, therefore, an increase in blood pressure. Parasympathetic nerve fibers are also attached to the heart and arteries. Conversely, parasympathetic stimulation slows the heart rate (negative chronotropy) and AV conduction (negative dromotropy) and reduces the force of contraction (negative inotropy), therefore lowering the blood pressure.

Manipulation of the autonomic nervous system may increase or decrease the incidence of dysrhythmias. Increased sympathetic stimulation, for example, with exercise, anxiety, fever, and administration of catecholamines (eg, dopamine, aminophylline, and

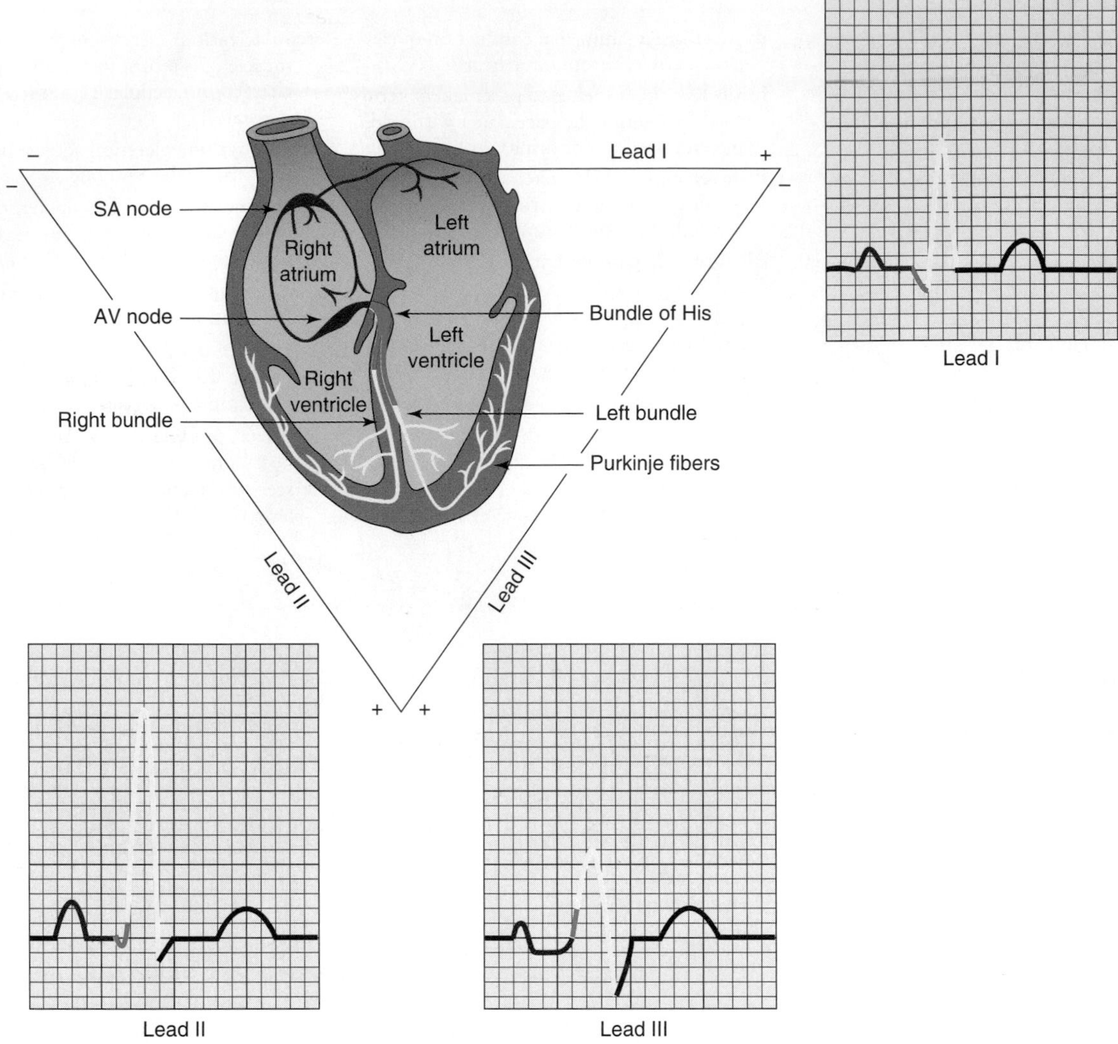

FIGURE 24•1 Relationship of electrocardiogram (ECG) complex, lead system, and electrical impulse. The heart conducts electrical activity, which the ECG measures and shows. The configurations of electrical activity displayed on the ECG vary depending on the lead (or view) of the ECG and on the rhythm of the heart. Therefore, the configuration of a normal rhythm tracing from lead I will differ from the configuration of a normal rhythm tracing from lead II, and lead II will differ from lead III and so on. The same is true for abnormal rhythms and cardiac disorders. To make an accurate assessment of the heart's electrical activity or to identify where, when, and what abnormalities occur, the ECG needs to be evaluated from every lead, not just from lead II. Here the different areas of electrical activity are identified by number and color.

dobutamine), may increase the incidence of dysrhythmias. Decreased sympathetic stimulation (eg, with rest, anxiety-reduction methods such as therapeutic communication or prayer, and administration of beta-adrenergic blocking agents) may decrease the incidence of dysrhythmias.

ECG INTERPRETATION

The electrical impulse that travels through the heart can be viewed by means of electrocardiography, the end product of which is an electrocardiogram (ECG). Each phase of the cardiac cycle is reflected by specific waveforms on the screen of a cardiac monitor or on a strip of ECG graph paper.

An ECG is obtained by slightly abrading or scraping the skin and placing electrodes on the body at specific areas. Electrodes come in various shapes and sizes, but all have two components: (1) an adhesive substance that attaches to the skin to secure the electrode in place and (2) a substance that reduces the skin's electrical impedance and promotes detection of the electrical current.

The number and placement of the electrodes depend on the type of ECG needed. Most continuous monitoring machines use two to five electrodes, usually placed on the limbs and the chest. These electrodes create an imaginary line, called a lead, that serves as a reference point from which the electrical activity is viewed. A lead is like an eye of a camera; it has a narrow peripheral field of vision, looking only at the electrical activity directly in front of it. Therefore, the ECG waveforms that appear on the paper or cardiac monitor represent the electrical current in relation to the lead (see Fig. 24-1). A change in the waveform can be caused by a change in the electrical current (where it originates or how it is conducted) or a change in the lead.

Obtaining an ECG

Electrodes are attached to cable wires, which are connected to one of the following:

- A cardiac monitor in the room for continuous reading. This kind of monitoring is usually called hardwire monitoring and is associated with intensive care units.
- An ECG machine placed at the patient's side for an immediate recording (standard 12-lead ECG)
- A small box that the patient carries and that continuously transmits the recording by radio waves to a central monitor located elsewhere (called telemetry)
- A small, lightweight tape recorder–like machine (called a Holter monitor) that the patient wears and that continuously records the ECG on a tape. The ECG on the Holter tape is later viewed and analyzed with a scanner

The placement of electrodes for continuous monitoring, telemetry, and Holter monitoring varies with the type of technology that is appropriate and available, the purpose of monitoring, and the standards of the institution. For a standard 12-lead ECG, 10 electrodes (six on the chest and four on the limbs) are placed on the body (Fig. 24-2). To prevent interference from the electrical activity of skeletal muscle, the limb electrodes are usually placed on areas that are not bony or have significant movement. These electrodes obtain the first six leads: lead I, II, and III, and aV_R, aV_L, and aV_F. The six chest electrodes are attached to the chest at very specific areas. The chest electrodes obtain the V or precordial leads, V_1 through V_6. To locate the fourth intercostal space and the placement of V_1, locate the sternal angle and then the sternal notch, which is about 1 or 2 inches below. When the fingers are moved to the patient's immediate right, the second rib can be palpated. The second intercostal space is the indentation felt just below the second rib.

Locating the specific intercostal space is critical for correct chest electrode placement. Errors in diagnosis can occur if they are incorrectly placed. Sometimes, when the patient is in the hospital and needs to be monitored closely for ECG changes, the chest electrodes are left in place to ensure the same placement for follow-up ECGs.

A standard 12-lead ECG reflects the electrical activity primarily in the left ventricle. Placement of additional electrodes for other leads may be needed to obtain more complete information. For example, in patients with suspected right-sided heart damage, right-sided precordial leads are required to evaluate the right ventricle (see Fig. 24-2).

ECG Analysis

The ECG waveform represents the function of the heart's conduction system, which normally initiates and conducts the electrical activity, in relation to the lead. When analyzed accurately, the ECG offers important information about the electrical activity of the myocardium. ECG waveforms are printed on graph paper that is divided by light and dark vertical and horizontal lines at standard intervals (Fig. 24-3). Time and rate are measured on the horizontal axis of the graph, and amplitude or voltage is measured on the vertical axis. When an ECG waveform moves toward the top of the paper, it is called a positive deflection. When it moves toward the bottom of the paper, it is called a negative deflection. When reviewing an ECG, each waveform should be examined and compared with the others.

Supplemental right precordial leads

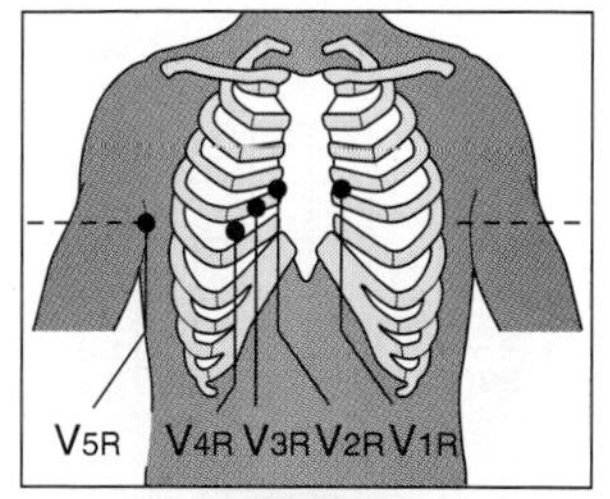

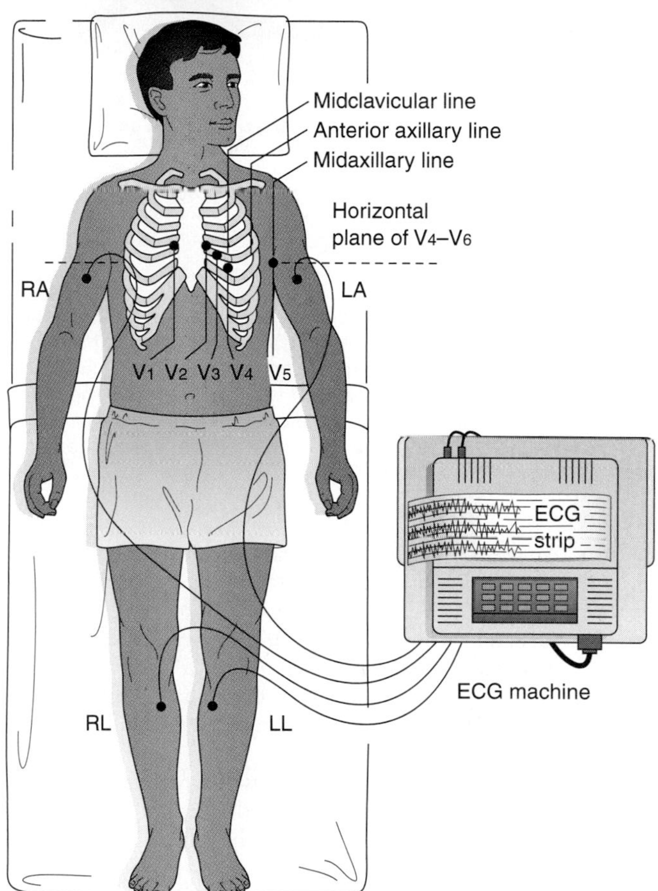

FIGURE 24•2 ECG electrode placement. The standard left precordial leads are V_1: 4th intercostal space, right sternal border; V_2: 4th intercostal space, left sternal border; V_3: diagonally between V_2 and V_4; V_4: 5th intercostal space, left midclavicular line, V_5: same level as V_4, anterior axillary line; V_6: same level as V_4 and V_5, midaxillary line. The right precordial leads, placed across the right side of the chest, are the mirror opposite of the left leads. From Hosley, J. B., & Molle-Matthews, E. (1999). *Lippincott's pocket guide to medical assisting.* Philadelphia: Lippincott Williams & Wilkins.

Waves, Complexes, and Intervals

The ECG is composed of waveforms (including the P wave, the QRS complex, the T wave, and possibly a U wave) and of segments or intervals (including the PR interval, the ST segment, and the QT interval) (see Fig. 24-3).

The **P wave** represents the electrical impulse starting in the SA node and spreading through the atria. Therefore, the P wave represents atrial muscle depolarization. It is normally 2.5 mm or less in height and 0.11 second or less in duration.

The **QRS complex** represents ventricular muscle depolarization. Not all QRS complexes have all three waveforms. The

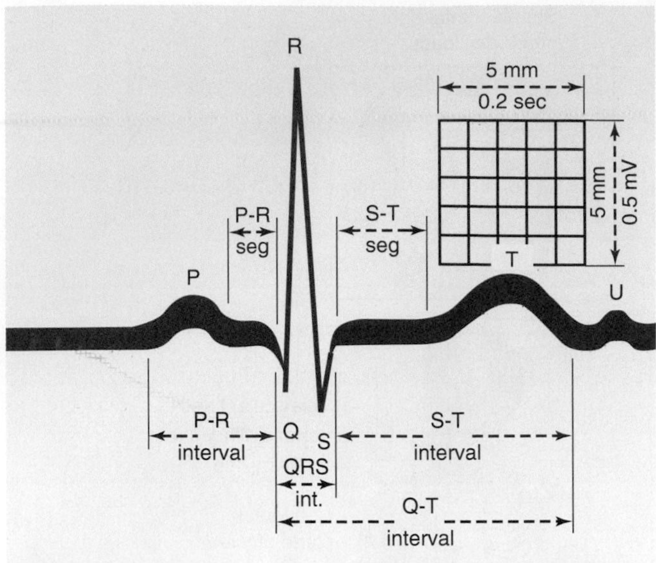

FIGURE 24•3 ECG graph and commonly measured complex components. Each small box represents 0.04 seconds on the horizontal axis and 1 mm or 0.1 millivolt on the vertical axis. The PR interval is measured from the beginning of the P wave to the beginning of the QRS complex; the QRS complex is measured from the beginning of the Q wave to the end of the S wave; the QT interval is measured from the beginning of the Q wave to the end of the T wave.

first negative deflection after the P wave is the Q wave, which is normally less than 0.04 second in duration and less than 25% of the R wave amplitude; the first positive deflection after the P wave is the R wave; and the S wave is the first negative deflection after the R wave. When a wave is less than 5 mm in height, small letters (q, r, s) are used; when a wave is taller than 5 mm, capital letters (Q, R, S) are used. The QRS complex is normally less than 0.12 seconds in duration.

The **T wave** represents ventricular muscle repolarization (when the cells regain a negative charge; also called the resting state). It follows the QRS complex and is usually of the same direction as the QRS complex.

The **U wave** is thought to represent repolarization of the Purkinje fibers, but it sometimes is seen in patients with hypokalemia (low potassium levels), hypertension, or heart disease. If present, the U wave follows the T wave and is usually smaller than the P wave. However, if tall, it may be mistaken for an extra P wave.

The **PR interval** is measured from the beginning of the P wave to the beginning of the QRS complex and represents the time needed for SA node stimulation, atrial depolarization, and conduction through the AV node before ventricular depolarization. In adults, the PR interval normally ranges from 0.12 to 0.20 seconds in duration.

The **ST segment**, which represents early ventricular repolarization, lasts from the end of the QRS complex to the beginning of the T wave. The beginning of the ST segment is usually identified by a change in the thickness or angle of the terminal portion of the QRS complex. It is normally isoelectric (see TP interval). It is analyzed to identify if it is above or below the isoelectric line, which may be, among other causes, a sign of cardiac ischemia (see Chap. 25).

The **QT interval**, which represents the total time for ventricular depolarization and repolarization, is measured from the beginning of the QRS complex to the end of the T wave. The QT interval varies with heart rate, sex, and age, and the measured QT interval needs to be corrected for these variables through a specific calculation. Several ECG interpretation books contain a chart of these calculations. It is usually 0.32 to 0.40 seconds in duration if the heart rate is 65 to 95 beats per minute. If the QT interval becomes prolonged, the patient may be at risk for a lethal ventricular dysrhythmia called torsades de pointes.

The PP interval is measured from the beginning of one P wave to the beginning of the next. The PP interval is used to determine atrial rhythm and atrial rate. The RR interval is measured from one QRS complex to the next QRS complex. The RR interval is used to determine ventricular rate and rhythm (Fig. 24-4).

When no electrical activity is detected, the line on the graph remains flat; this is called isoelectric. The TP interval, which represents the isoelectric period, is measured from the end of the T wave to the beginning of the next P wave. The ST segment is compared with this interval to detect changes.

Determining Ventricular Heart Rate From ECG

Heart rate can be obtained from the ECG strip by several methods. A 1-minute strip contains 300 large boxes and 1,500 small boxes. Therefore, an easy and accurate method of determining heart rate with a regular rhythm is to count the number of small boxes during an RR interval and divide the number into 1,500. If, for example, 10 small boxes are between two R waves, the heart rate is 150 (1500 ÷ 10); if there are 25 large boxes, the heart rate is 60 (1500 ÷ 25) (see Fig. 24-4**A**).

An alternative but less accurate method for estimating heart rate, which is usually used when the rhythm is irregular, is to count the number of RR intervals in 6 seconds and multiply that number by 10. The top of the ECG paper is usually marked at 3-second intervals, which is 15 large boxes horizontally (see Fig. 24-4**B**). The RR intervals are counted rather than QRS complexes because a computed heart rate based on the latter might be inaccurately high. The same methods may be used for determining atrial rate, using the PP interval instead of the RR interval.

Determining Heart Rhythm From ECG

The rhythm is often identified at the same time the rate is determined. The RR interval is used to determine ventricular rhythm, the PP interval to determine atrial rhythm. If the intervals are the same or nearly the same throughout the strip, the rhythm is called regular. If the intervals are different, the rhythm is called irregular.

Analyzing the ECG Rhythm Strip

The ECG must be analyzed in a systematic manner to determine the patient's cardiac rhythm and to detect dysrhythmias and conduction disorders, as well as evidence of myocardial ischemia, injury, and infarction. Chart 24-2 is an example of a method that can be used to analyze the patient's rhythm.

Once the rhythm has been analyzed, then the findings are compared with and matched to the ECG criteria for dysrhythmias to arrive at a diagnosis. It is important for the nurse to assess the patient to determine the physiologic effect of the dysrhythmia and to identify possible etiologies. Treatment of dysrhythmias is based on the etiology and effect of the dysrhythmia, not the dysrhythmia alone.

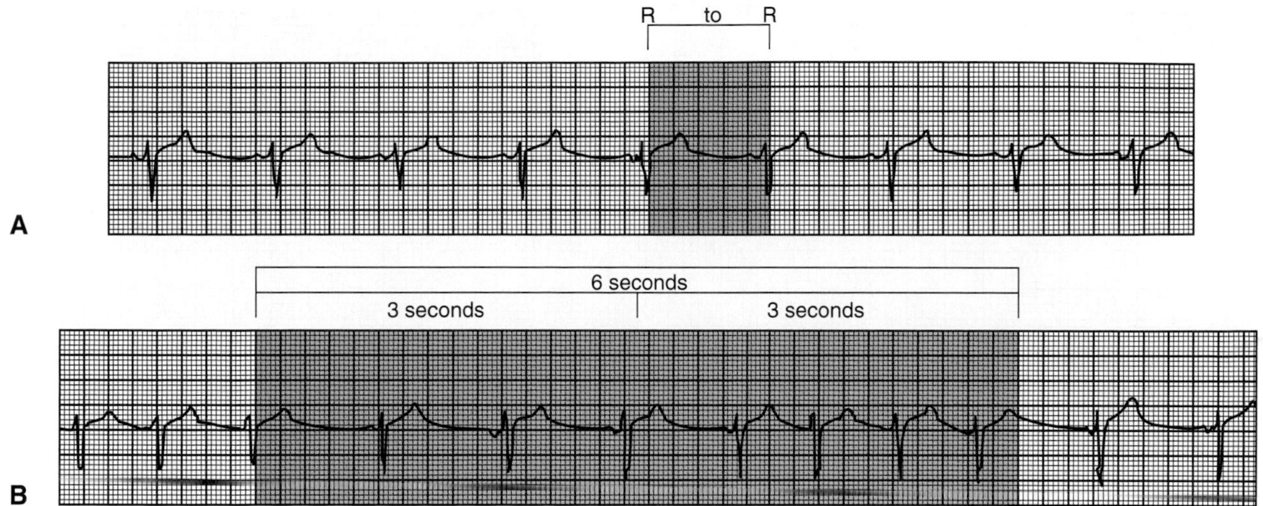

FIGURE 24•4 (**A**) Heart rate determination for a regular rhythm. 1500 divided by the number of small boxes between two R waves (there are 25 in this example) equals the ventricular heart rate. The heart rate in this example is 60. (**B**) Heart rate determination if the rhythm is irregular. There are approximately seven RR intervals in 6 seconds. Seven times 10 equals 70. The heart rate is 70. Woods, S. L., et al. (1995). *Cardiac nursing* (3rd ed.). Philadelphia: J. B. Lippincott, p. 294.

Normal Sinus Rhythm

Normal **sinus rhythm** occurs when the electrical impulse starts at a regular rate and rhythm in the SA node and travels through the normal conduction pathway. The following are the ECG criteria for normal sinus rhythm (Fig. 24-5):

Ventricular and atrial rate: 60 to 100 in the adult

Ventricular and atrial rhythm: Regular

QRS shape and duration: Usually normal, but may be regularly abnormal

P wave: Normal and consistent shape; always in front of the QRS

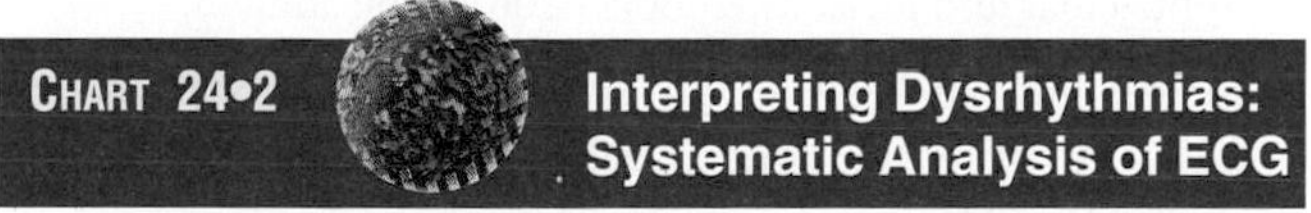

CHART 24•2 Interpreting Dysrhythmias: Systematic Analysis of ECG

When examining an ECG rhythm strip to learn more about a patient's dysrhythmia, the nurse takes the following criteria into consideration.

1. Determine the ventricular rate.
2. Determine the ventricular rhythm.
3. Determine QRS duration.
4. Is QRS duration consistent throughout the strip? If not, identify other duration.
5. Identify QRS shape; if not consistent, then identify other shapes.
6. Identify P waves; is there a P in front of every QRS?
7. Identify P-wave shape; identify whether it is consistent or not.
8. Determine the atrial rate.
9. Determine the atrial rhythm.
10. Determine each PR interval.
11. Determine if the PR intervals are consistent, irregular but with a pattern to the irregularity, or just irregular.
12. Determine how many P waves for each QRS (P:QRS ratio).

In many cases, the nurse may use a checklist and document the findings next to the appropriate ECG criterion.

PR interval: Consistent interval between 0.12 and 0.20 seconds

P:QRS ratio: 1:1

TYPES OF DYSRHYTHMIAS

Various kinds of dysrhythmias include sinus node, atrial, junctional, and ventricular and their various subcategories.

Sinus Node Dysrhythmias

Sinus Bradycardia

Sinus bradycardia occurs when the sinus node creates an impulse at a slower-than-normal rate. Etiologies include slower metabolic needs (eg, sleep, athletic training, hypothermia, hypothyroidism), vagal stimulation (eg, from vomiting, suctioning, severe pain, extreme emotions), medications (eg, calcium channel blockers, amiodarone, beta-blockers), increased intracranial pressure, and myocardial infarction (MI), especially of the inferior wall.

The following are characteristics of sinus bradycardia (Fig. 24-6):

Ventricular and atrial rate: Less than 60 in the adult

Ventricular and atrial rhythm: Regular

QRS shape and duration: Usually normal, but may be regularly abnormal

P wave: Normal and consistent shape; always in front of the QRS

PR interval: Consistent interval between 0.12 and 0.20 seconds

P:QRS ratio: P wave in front of every QRS, 1:1

All characteristics of sinus bradycardia are the same as those of normal sinus rhythm, except for the rate. The patient is assessed to determine the hemodynamic effect and the possible etiology of the dysrhythmia. If the decrease in heart rate results from vagal

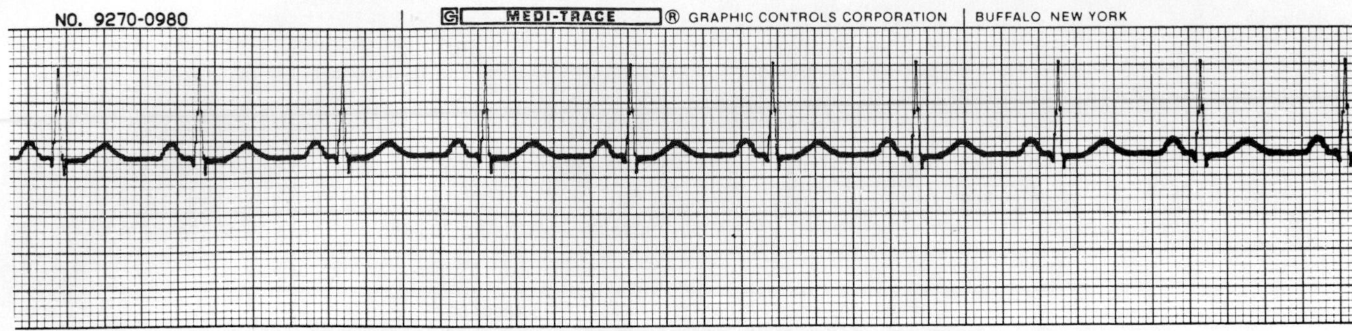

FIGURE 24•5 Normal sinus rhythm.

stimulation (stimulation of the vagus nerve), such as bearing down during defecation or vomiting, attempts are made to prevent further vagal stimulation. If the bradycardia is from a medication such as a beta-blocker, the medication is withheld. If the slow heart rate causes significant hemodynamic changes, resulting in shortness of breath, decreased level of consciousness, angina, hypotension, ST-segment changes, or premature ventricular complexes, treatment is directed toward increasing the heart rate.

Atropine, 0.5 to 1.0 mg given quickly and intravenously (IV) as a bolus, is the medication of choice in treating sinus bradycardia. It blocks vagal stimulation, thus allowing a normal rate to occur. Catecholamines and emergency transcutaneous pacing also may be implemented.

Sinus Tachycardia

Sinus tachycardia occurs when the sinus node creates an impulse at a faster-than-normal rate. It may be caused by acute blood loss, anemia, shock, hypervolemia, hypovolemia, congestive heart failure, pain, hypermetabolic states, fever, exercise, anxiety, or sympathomimetic medications. The ECG pattern for sinus tachycardia follows (Fig. 24-7):

Ventricular and atrial rate: Greater than 100 in the adult

Ventricular and atrial rhythm: Regular

QRS shape and duration: Usually normal, but may be regularly abnormal

P wave: Normal and consistent shape; always in front of the QRS, but may be buried in the preceding T wave.

PR interval: Consistent interval between 0.12 and 0.20 seconds

P:QRS ratio: P wave in front of every QRS, 1:1

All aspects of sinus tachycardia are the same as those of normal sinus rhythm, except for the rate. As the heart rate increases, the diastolic filling time decreases, possibly resulting in reduced cardiac output and subsequent symptoms of syncope and low blood pressure. If the rapid rate persists and the heart cannot compensate for the decreased ventricular filling, the patient may develop acute pulmonary edema.

Treatment of sinus tachycardia is usually directed at abolishing its cause. Calcium channel blockers (eg, diltiazem) and beta-blockers (eg, propranolol) may be used to reduce the heart rate quickly.

Sinus Arrhythmia

Sinus arrhythmia occurs when the sinus node creates an impulse at an irregular rhythm; the rate increases with inspiration and decreases with expiration. Nonrespiratory causes include heart disease and valvular disease, but these are rarely seen. The ECG criteria for sinus arrhythmia follow (Fig. 24-8):

Ventricular and atrial rate: 60 to 100 in the adult

Ventricular and atrial rhythm: Irregular

QRS shape and duration: Usually normal, but may be regularly abnormal

P wave: Normal and consistent shape; always in front of the QRS

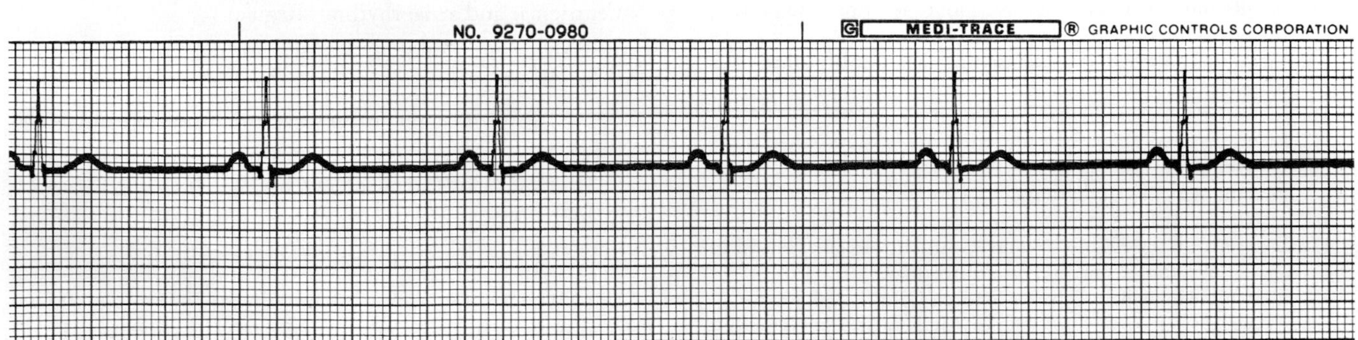

FIGURE 24•6 Sinus bradycardia.

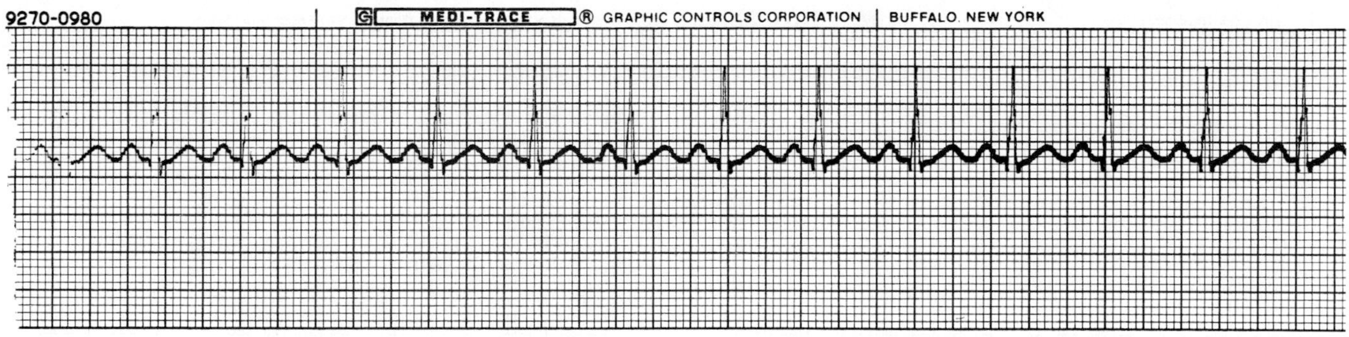

FIGURE 24•7 Sinus tachycardia.

PR interval: Consistent interval between 0.12 and 0.20 seconds

P: QRS ratio: 1:1

Sinus arrhythmia does not cause any significant hemodynamic effect and therefore is usually not treated.

Atrial Dysrhythmias

Premature Atrial Complex

A premature atrial complex (PAC) is a single ECG complex that occurs when an electrical impulse starts in the atrium before the next normal impulse of the SA node. The PAC may be caused by caffeine, alcohol, nicotine, stretched atrial myocardium as in hypervolemia, anxiety, hypokalemia (low potassium levels), atrial ischemia, injury, infarction, or hypermetabolic states. PACs are often seen with sinus tachycardia.

PACs have the following characteristics (Fig. 24-9):

Ventricular and atrial rate: Depends on the underlying rhythm (eg, sinus tachycardia)

Ventricular and atrial rhythm: Irregular due to early P waves, creating a PP interval that is shorter than the others

QRS shape and duration: The QRS that follows the early P wave is usually normal, but it may be abnormal (aberrantly conducted PAC). It may even be absent (blocked PAC).

P wave: An early and different P wave may be seen or may be hidden in the T wave; other P waves in the strip will be consistent.

PR interval: The early P wave will have a shorter than-normal PR interval, but still between 0.12 and 0.20 seconds.

P: QRS ratio: 1:1

PACs are not uncommon in normal hearts. The patient may say, "My heart skipped a beat." A pulse deficit (a difference between the apical and radial pulse rate) may exist.

If PACs are infrequent, no treatment is necessary. If they are frequent (more than six per minute), this may herald a worsening disease state or the onset of more serious dysrhythmias, such as atrial fibrillation. Treatment is directed toward the cause.

Paroxysmal Atrial Tachycardia

Paroxysmal atrial tachycardia is a term used to indicate a tachycardia characterized by abrupt onset and abrupt cessation and a QRS of normal duration. Because recent studies have indicated that this rhythm most often is caused by a conduction problem in the AV node, it is now called AV nodal reentry tachycardia, which is described later in the chapter.

Atrial Flutter

Atrial flutter occurs in the atrium and creates impulses at an atrial rate between 250 and 400 times per minute. Because the atrial rate is faster than the AV node can conduct, not all atrial impulses are conducted into the ventricle, causing a therapeutic block at the AV node. This is an important feature of this dysrhythmia. If all atrial impulses were conducted to the ventricle, the ventricular rate

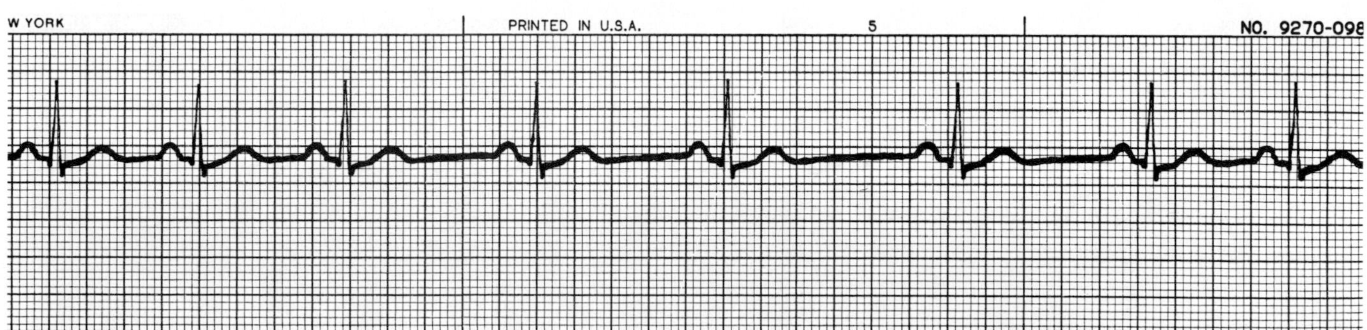

FIGURE 24•8 Sinus arrhythmia.

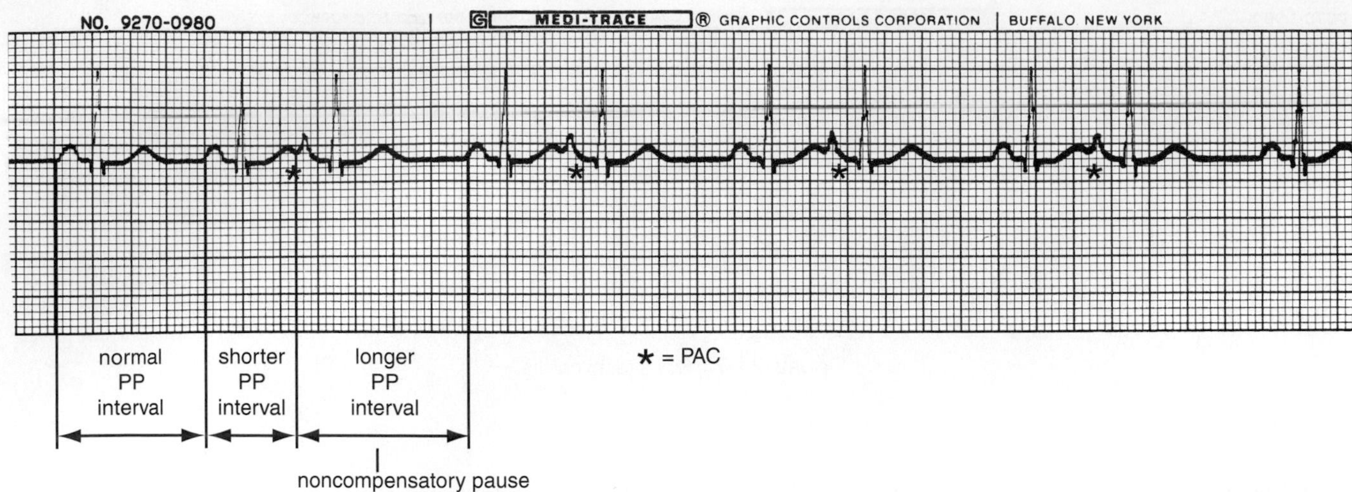

FIGURE 24•9 Premature atrial complexes (PACs).

would also be 250 to 400, which would result in ventricular fibrillation, a life-threatening dysrhythmia.

Atrial flutter is characterized by the following (Fig. 24-10):

Ventricular and atrial rate: Atrial rate ranges between 250 and 400; ventricular rate usually ranges between 75 and 150.

Ventricular and atrial rhythm: The atrial rhythm is regular; the ventricular rhythm is usually regular but may be irregular because of a change in the AV conduction.

QRS shape and duration: Usually normal, but may be abnormal or may be absent

P wave: Saw-toothed shape. These waves are referred to as F waves.

PR interval: Multiple F waves may make it difficult to determine the PR interval.

P:QRS ratio: 2:1, 3:1, or 4:1

Atrial flutter may cause serious signs and symptoms, such as chest pain, shortness of breath, and low blood pressure. If the patient is unstable, electrical cardioversion is usually indicated. If the patient is stable, diltiazem, verapamil, beta-blockers, or digitalis may be administered IV to slow the ventricular rate. These medications can slow conduction through the AV node. A Type 1A antidysrhythmic medication or amiodarone may be given to promote conversion to sinus rhythm. If medication therapy is unsuccessful, electrical cardioversion is often successful.

Atrial Fibrillation

Atrial fibrillation causes a rapid, disorganized, and uncoordinated twitching of atrial musculature. It is the most common dysrhythmia causing patients to seek medical attention. It may occur for a very short time, or it may be chronic. Causes are similar to those of atrial flutter. Atrial fibrillation is usually associated with advanced age, valvular heart disease, cardiomyopathy, hyperthyroidism, pulmonary disease, moderate to heavy ingestion of alcohol ("holiday heart" syndrome), and the aftermath of open heart surgery. Sometimes it may occur in people without any underlying pathophysiology (termed lone atrial fibrillation). Atrial fibrillation is characterized by the following (Fig. 24-11):

Ventricular and atrial rate: Atrial rate is 300 to 600. Ventricular rate is usually 120 to 200 in untreated atrial fibrillation.

Ventricular and atrial rhythm: Highly irregular

QRS shape and duration: Usually normal, but may be abnormal

P wave: No discernible P waves; irregular undulating waves are seen and are termed fibrillatory or f waves.

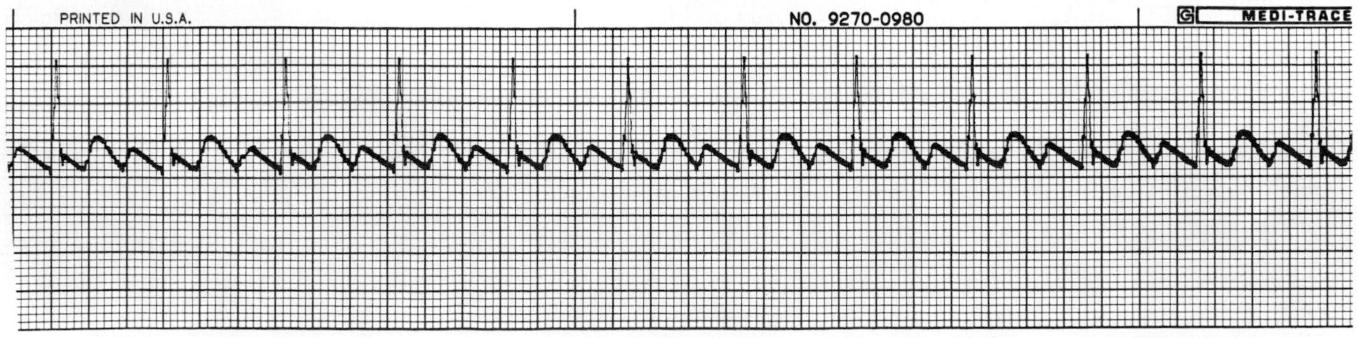

FIGURE 24•10 Atrial flutter.

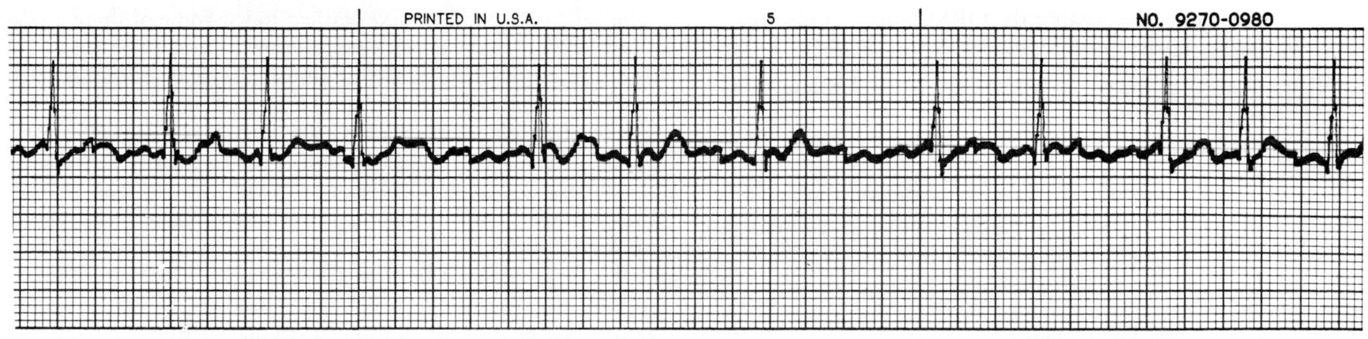

FIGURE 24•11 Atrial fibrillation.

PR interval: Cannot be measured

P : QRS ratio: many : 1

A rapid ventricular response reduces the time for ventricular filling and hence the stroke volume. Because this rhythm causes the atria and ventricles to contract at different times, the atrial kick (the last part of diastole and ventricular filling that accounts for 25% to 30% of the cardiac output) is also lost. There is usually a pulse deficit, a numerical difference between apical and radial pulse rates. The shorter time in diastole reduces the time available for coronary artery perfusion, thereby increasing the risk for myocardial ischemia. The erratic atrial contraction promotes the formation of a thrombus, increasing the risk for an embolic event, including stroke.

Treatment of atrial fibrillation depends on its cause and duration and the patient's symptoms and instability. In many patients, atrial fibrillation converts to sinus rhythm within 24 hours and without treatment. Both stable and unstable atrial fibrillation of short duration are treated the same as stable and unstable atrial flutter. For atrial fibrillation of acute onset, the medications used for atrial flutter and another medication, ibutilide (Corvert), may be given slowly IV to achieve conversion to sinus rhythm. IV adenosine has also been used for conversion as well as to assist in the diagnosis. To prevent recurrence and to promote heart rate control over a long period, quinidine, procainamide, flecainide, sotalol, or amiodarone may be prescribed. In addition, anticoagulation therapy is usually indicated if the patient is elderly or has hypertension, heart failure, or a history of stroke. Pacemaker implantation or surgery is sometimes indicated for patients who are unresponsive to medications.

Junctional Dysrhythmias

Premature Junctional Complex

A premature junctional complex is an impulse that starts in the AV nodal area before the next normal sinus impulse. Premature junctional complexes are less common than PACs. Causes of premature junctional complex include digitalis toxicity, congestive heart failure, and coronary artery disease. The ECG criteria for premature junctional complex are the same as for PACs except for the P wave and the PR interval. The P wave may be absent, may follow the QRS, or may occur before the QRS but with a PR interval of less than 0.12 seconds. Premature junctional complexes rarely produce any significant symptoms. For frequent premature junctional complexes, the treatment is the same as for frequent PACs.

Junctional Rhythm

Junctional or nodal rhythm occurs when the AV node, instead of the SA node, becomes the pacemaker of the heart. When the SA node slows (eg, from increased vagal tone) or when the impulse cannot be conducted through the AV node (eg, because of complete heart block), the AV node automatically discharges an impulse. The following are the ECG criteria when the junctional rhythm is not due to complete heart block (Fig. 24-12):

Ventricular and atrial rate: Ventricular rate 40 to 60; atrial rate also 40 to 60 if P waves are discernible

Ventricular and atrial rhythm: Regular

QRS shape and duration: Usually normal, but may be abnormal

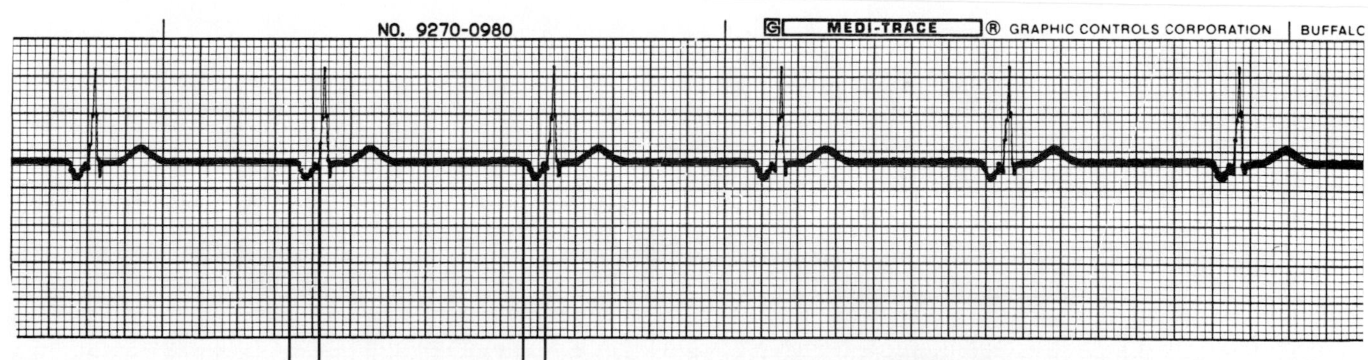

FIGURE 24•12 Junctional rhythm; note short PR intervals.

P wave: May be absent, after the QRS complex, or before the QRS; may be inverted, especially in lead II

PR interval: If P wave is in front of the QRS, PR interval is less than 0.12 second.

P:QRS ratio: 1:1

Junctional rhythm may produce signs and symptoms of reduced cardiac output. If so, the treatment is the same as for sinus bradycardia. Emergency pacing may be needed.

AV Nodal Reentry Tachycardia

AV nodal reentry tachycardia occurs when an impulse is conducted to an area in the AV node that causes the impulse to be rerouted back into the same area over and over again at a very fast rate. Each time the impulse is conducted through this area, it is also conducted down into the ventricles, causing a fast ventricular rate. Factors associated with the development of AV nodal reentry tachycardia include caffeine, nicotine, hypoxemia, and stress. Underlying pathophysiologies include coronary artery disease and cardiomyopathy. The ECG criteria are as follows (Fig. 24-13):

Ventricular and atrial rate: Atrial rate range usually 150 to 250; ventricular rate range usually 75 to 250

Ventricular and atrial rhythm: Regular; sudden onset and termination of the tachycardia

QRS shape and duration: Usually normal, but may be abnormal

P wave: Usually very difficult to discern

PR interval: If P wave is in front of the QRS, PR interval is less than 0.12 seconds.

P:QRS ratio: 1:1, 2:1

The clinical symptoms vary with the rate and duration of the tachycardia and the patient's underlying condition. It usually is of short duration, resulting only in palpitations. A fast rate may also reduce cardiac output, resulting in significant signs and symptoms such as restlessness, chest pain, shortness of breath, pallor, hypotension, and loss of consciousness.

Treatment is aimed at breaking the reentry of the impulse. Vagal maneuvers, such as carotid sinus massage (Fig. 24-14), gag reflex, breath holding, and immersing the face in ice water, increase parasympathetic stimulation, causing slower conduction through the AV node and blocking the reentry of the rerouted impulse. Some patients have learned to use some of these methods to terminate the episode on their own. Because of the risk of a cerebral embolic event, carotid sinus massage is contraindicated in patients with carotid bruits. If the vagal maneuvers are ineffective, the patient may then receive a bolus of adenosine, verapamil, or diltiazem. Cardioversion is the treatment of choice if the patient is unstable or does not respond to the medications. Intravenous adenosine may be prescribed to cause a conversion to sinus rhythm.

If P waves cannot be identified, the rhythm may be called supraventricular tachycardia, which indicates only that it is not ventricular tachycardia. Supraventricular tachycardia could be atrial fibrillation, atrial flutter, AV nodal reentry tachycardia, or other tachycardias. Vagal maneuvers and adenosine are used to slow conduction in the AV node to allow visualization of the P waves.

Ventricular Dysrhythmias

Premature Ventricular Complex

Premature ventricular complex (PVC) is an impulse that starts in a ventricle before the next normal sinus impulse. PVCs can occur in healthy people, especially with the use of caffeine, nicotine, and alcohol. They are also caused by cardiac ischemia or infarction, increased workload on the heart (eg, exercise, fever, hypervolemia, congestive heart failure, and tachycardia), digitalis toxicity, hypoxia, acidosis, and electrolyte imbalances, especially hypokalemia.

In the absence of disease, PVCs are not serious. The concern, however, lies in their ability to indicate the possibility of ensuing ventricular tachycardia. In the patient with acute MI, PVCs may indicate the need for more aggressive therapy. The following are often considered as warning or complex PVCs; in other words, precursors of ventricular tachycardia: (1) more than six per minute, (2) multifocal (having different shapes), (3) two in a row (pair), and (4) occurring on the T wave (the vulnerable period of ventricular depolarization). Although medical therapy has been used in the past for these types of PVCs to prevent ventricular tachycardia, recent studies do not always show these PVCs to be harbingers of more lethal dysrhythmias.

In a rhythm called bigeminy, every other complex is a PVC. Trigeminy is a rhythm in which every third complex is a PVC, and quadrageminy is a rhythm in which every fourth complex is a PVC.

PVCs have the following characteristics on the ECG (Fig. 24-15):

Ventricular and atrial rate: Depends on the underlying rhythm (eg, sinus tachycardia)

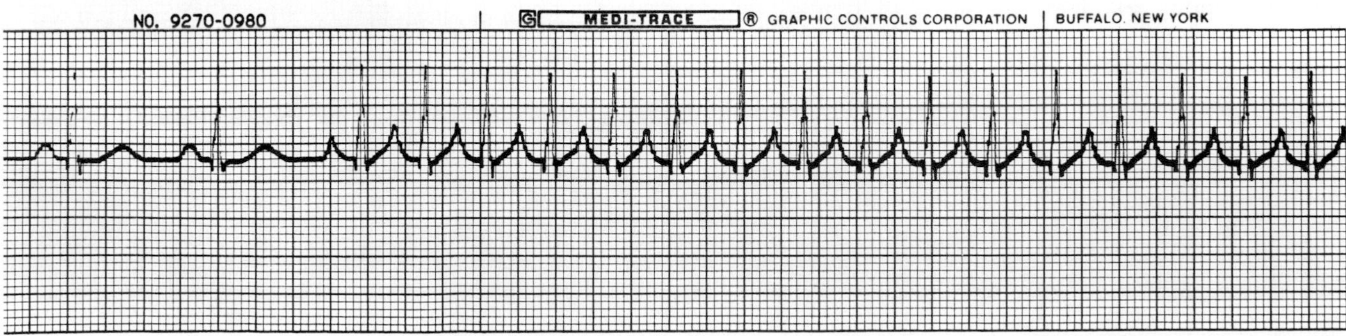

FIGURE 24•13 AV nodal reentry tachycardia.

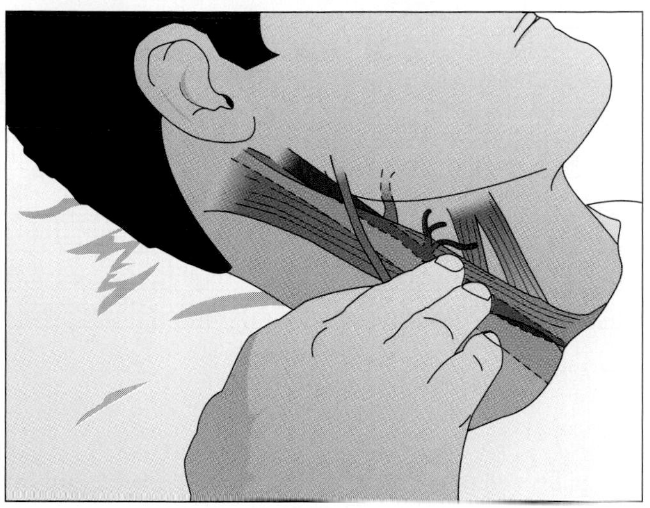

FIGURE 24•14 Carotid sinus massage.

Ventricular and atrial rhythm: Irregular due to early QRS, creating one RR interval that is shorter than the others. PP interval may be regular, indicating that the PVC did not depolarize the SA node.

QRS shape and duration: Duration is 0.12 seconds or more; bizarre, abnormal shape

P wave: Visibility of P wave depends on the timing of the PVC; may be absent (hidden in the QRS or T wave) or in front of the QRS. If the P wave follows the QRS, the shape of the P wave will be different.

PR interval: If P wave is in front of the QRS, PR is less than 0.12 seconds.

P:QRS ratio: 0:1; 1:1

The patient may feel nothing or say that the heart "skipped a beat." The effect of a PVC depends on its timing in the cardiac cycle and how much blood was in the ventricles when they contracted. Initial treatment is aimed at correcting the cause, if possible. Lidocaine is the medication most commonly used for immediate, short-term therapy. The need for long-term medication therapy for PVCs only is not indicated.

Ventricular Tachycardia

Ventricular tachycardia is defined as three or more PVCs in a row, occurring at a rate exceeding 100 beats per minute. The causes are similar to those for PVC. Ventricular tachycardia is usually associated with coronary artery disease and may precede ventricular fibrillation. Ventricular tachycardia is an emergency because the patient is usually unresponsive and pulseless. Ventricular tachycardia has the following characteristics (Fig. 24-16):

Ventricular and atrial rate: Ventricular rate is 100 to 200 beats per minute; atrial rate depends on the underlying rhythm (eg, sinus rhythm).

Ventricular and atrial rhythm: Usually regular; atrial rhythm may also be regular.

QRS shape and duration: Duration is 0.12 seconds or more; bizarre, abnormal shape

P wave: Very difficult to detect, so atrial rate and rhythm may be undeterminable

PR interval: Very irregular, if P waves seen.

P:QRS ratio: Difficult to determine, but if P waves are apparent, there are usually more QRS complexes than P waves.

The patient's tolerance or lack of tolerance for this rapid rhythm depends on the ventricular rate and underlying disease. If the patient is stable, simply continuing the assessment, especially obtaining a 12-lead ECG, may be the only action necessary. If medication is indicated, lidocaine is often the initial choice. Cardioversion (discussed later in this chapter) may be indicated if the medications are ineffective or if the patient becomes unstable. Ventricular tachycardia in a patient who is unconscious and without a pulse is treated in the same manner as ventricular fibrillation; immediate defibrillation is the action of choice.

Ventricular Fibrillation

Ventricular fibrillation is a rapid but disorganized ventricular rhythm that causes ineffective quivering of the ventricles. There is no atrial activity. Ventricular fibrillation has the following characteristics (Fig. 24-17):

Ventricular rate: Greater than 300 per minute

Ventricular rhythm: Extremely irregular, without specific pattern

QRS shape and duration: Irregular, undulating waves

This dysrhythmia is always characterized by the absence of an audible heartbeat, a palpable pulse, and respirations. Because there is no coordinated cardiac activity, cardiac arrest and death are imminent if ventricular fibrillation is uncorrected. Treatment includes immediate defibrillation and activation of emergency services. The importance of defibrillation is evident in one of the recent changes in basic life support: placing a call for emergency assistance takes precedence over initiating cardiopulmonary resuscitation in the adult victim. After successful defibrillation, eradicating causes and administering antidysrhythmic medication are treatments imposed to prevent the recurrence of ventricular fibrillation.

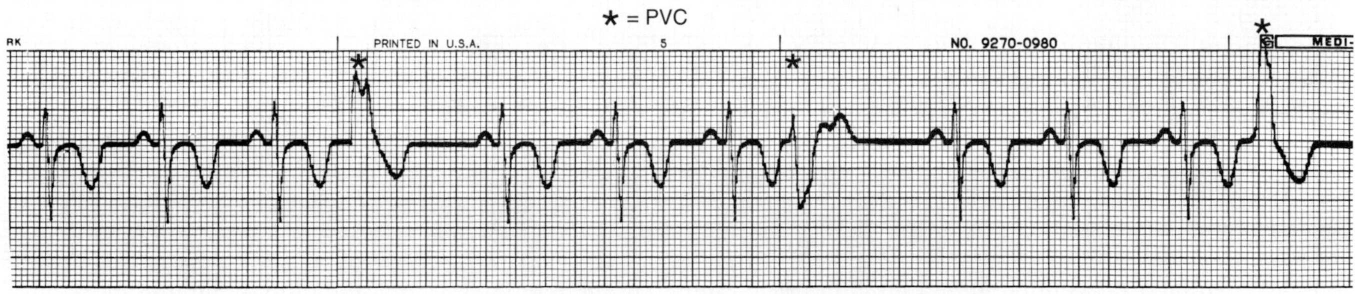

FIGURE 24•15 Multifocal PVCs in quadrageminy.

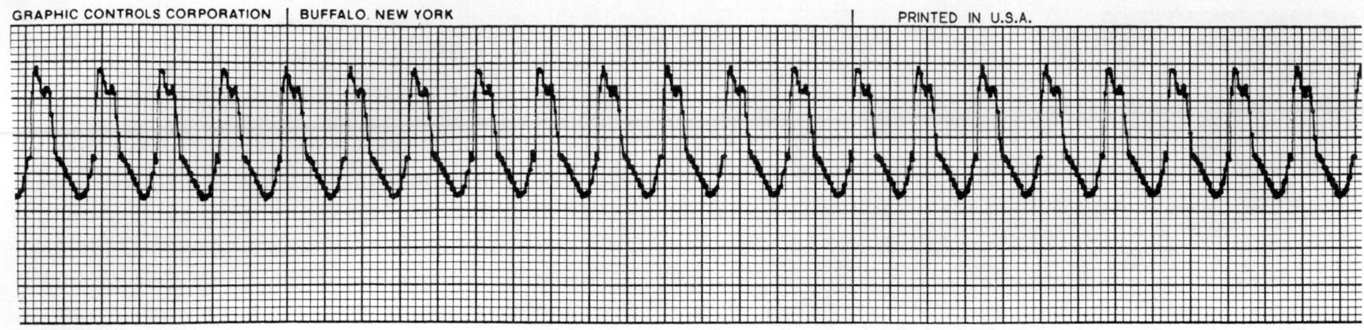

FIGURE 24•16 Ventricular tachycardia.

Idioventricular Rhythm

Idioventricular rhythm, also called ventricular escape rhythm, occurs when the impulse starts in the conduction system below the AV node. When the SA node fails to create an impulse (eg, from increased vagal tone) or when the impulse is created but cannot be conducted through the AV node (eg, due to complete AV block), the Purkinje fibers automatically discharge an impulse. The following are the ECG criteria when idioventricular rhythm is not due to AV block (Fig. 24-18):

Ventricular rate: Ranges between 20 and 40; if the rate exceeds 40, the rhythm is known as accelerated idioventricular rhythm.

Ventricular rhythm: Regular

QRS shape and duration: Bizarre, abnormal shape; duration is 0.12 seconds or more

Idioventricular rhythm commonly causes the patient to lose consciousness and experience other signs and symptoms of reduced cardiac output. In such cases, the treatment is the same as for any bradycardia, including identifying the underlying etiology, administering IV atropine, and initiating emergency transcutaneous pacing. Idioventricular rhythm may also cause no symptoms of reduced cardiac output. However, bed rest is prescribed so as not to increase the cardiac workload.

Ventricular Asystole

Commonly called flatline, ventricular asystole (Fig. 24-19) is characterized by absent QRS complexes, although P waves may be apparent for a short duration. There is no heartbeat, no palpable pulse, and no respiration. Without immediate treatment, ventricular asystole is fatal. Cardiopulmonary resuscitation and emergency services are necessary to keep the patient alive. The guidelines for advanced cardiac life support state that the key to successful treatment is rapid assessment to identify a possible cause, which may include hypoxia, acidosis, severe electrolyte imbalance, drug overdose, and hypothermia. Intubation and establishment of IV access are the first recommended actions. Transcutaneous pacing may be attempted. A bolus of IV epinephrine should be administered and repeated at 3- to 5-minute intervals. Sodium bicarbonate may be administered IV. Because of the poor prognosis associated with asystole, if the patient does not respond to these actions and others aimed at correcting underlying causes, resuscitation efforts are usually ended ("the code is called") unless special circumstances exist (eg, hypothermia).

Conduction Abnormalities

When assessing the rhythm strip, the nurse takes care first to identify the underlying rhythm (eg, sinus rhythm or sinus arrhythmia). Then the PR interval is assessed for the possibility of an AV block. AV blocks occur when the conduction of the impulse through the AV nodal area is decreased or stopped. These blocks can be caused by medications (eg, digitalis, calcium channel blockers, beta-blockers), myocardial ischemia and infarction, valvular disorders, and myocarditis. If the AV block is caused by increased vagal tone (eg, suctioning, pressure above the eyes or on large vessels, anal stimulation), it is commonly accompanied by sinus bradycardia.

The clinical signs and symptoms of a heart block vary with the resulting ventricular rate and the severity of any underlying disease processes. Whereas first-degree AV block rarely causes any

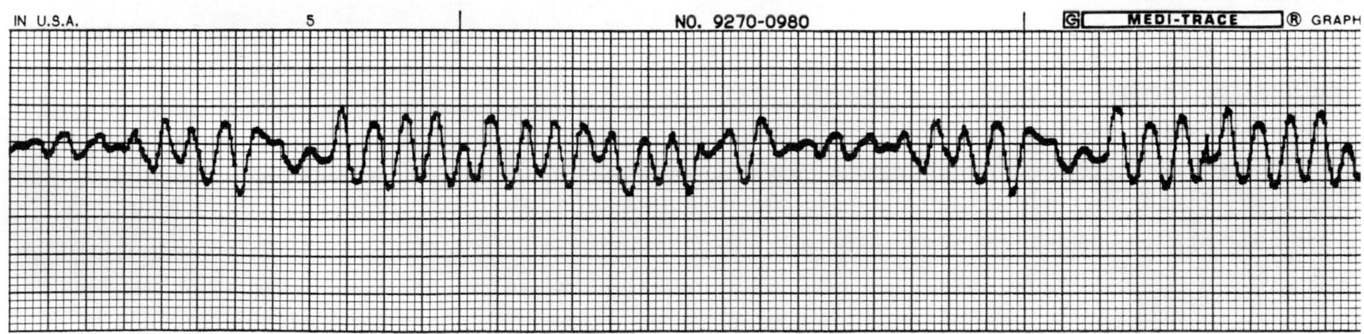

FIGURE 24•17 Ventricular fibrillation.

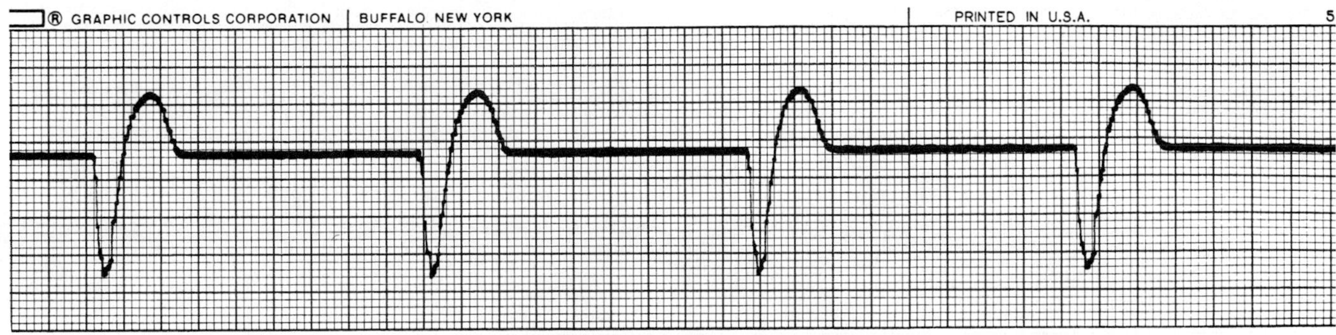

FIGURE 24•18 Idioventricular rhythm.

hemodynamic effect, the other blocks may result in a decrease in heart rate, causing a decrease in perfusion to vital organs, such as the brain, heart, kidneys, lungs, and skin. A patient with third-degree AV block caused by digitalis toxicity may be stable; another patient with the same rhythm caused by acute MI may be in cardiac arrest. Health care providers always keep in mind the need to treat the patient, not the rhythm.

First-Degree AV Block

First-degree heart block occurs when all the atrial impulses are conducted through the AV node into the ventricles at a rate slower than normal. This conduction disorder has the following characteristics (Fig. 24-20):

Ventricular and atrial rate: Depends on the underlying rhythm

Ventricular and atrial rhythm: Depends on the underlying rhythm

QRS shape and duration: Usually normal, but may be abnormal

P wave: In front of the QRS complex; shows sinus rhythm, regular shape

PR interval: 0.20 seconds or more; PR interval measurement is constant.

P:QRS ratio: 1:1

Second-Degree AV Block, Type I

Second-degree, type I heart block occurs when all but one of the atrial impulses are conducted through the AV node into the ventricles. Each atrial impulse takes a longer time for conduction until one impulse is fully blocked. Because the AV node is not depolarized by the blocked atrial impulse, the AV node has time to repolarize fully, so that the next atrial impulse can be conducted within the shortest amount of time. Second-degree AV block, type I has the following characteristics (Fig. 24-21):

Ventricular and atrial rate: Depends on the underlying rhythm

Ventricular and atrial rhythm: The PP interval is regular if the patient has an underlying normal sinus rhythm; the RR interval characteristically creates a pattern of change. Starting from the RR that is the longest, the RR interval gradually shortens until there is another long RR interval.

QRS shape and duration: Usually normal, but may be abnormal

P wave: In front of the QRS complex; shape depends on underlying rhythm

PR interval: PR interval becomes longer with each succeeding ECG complex until there is a P wave not followed by a QRS. The changes in the PR interval will be repeated between each "dropped" QRS, creating a pattern in the irregular PR interval measurements.

P:QRS ratio: 3:2, 4:3, 5:4, and so forth

Second-Degree AV Block, Type II

Second-degree, type II heart block occurs when only some of the atrial impulses are conducted through the AV node into the ven-

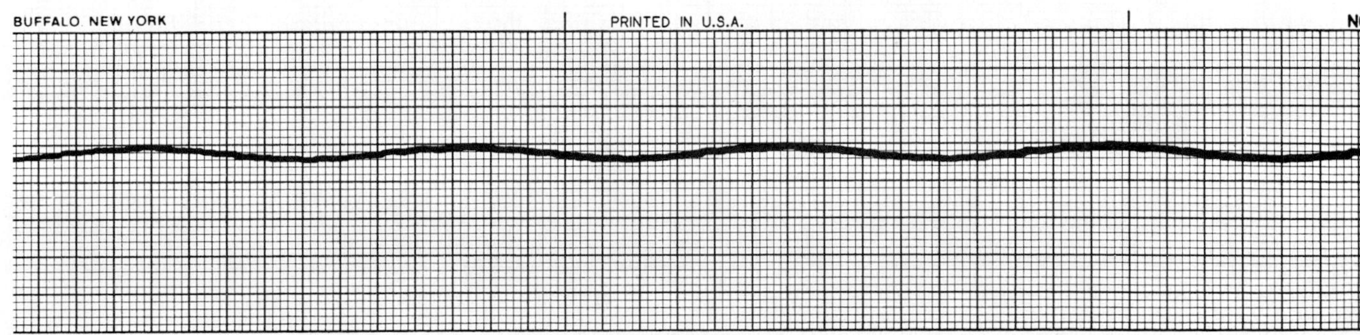

FIGURE 24•19 Asystole.

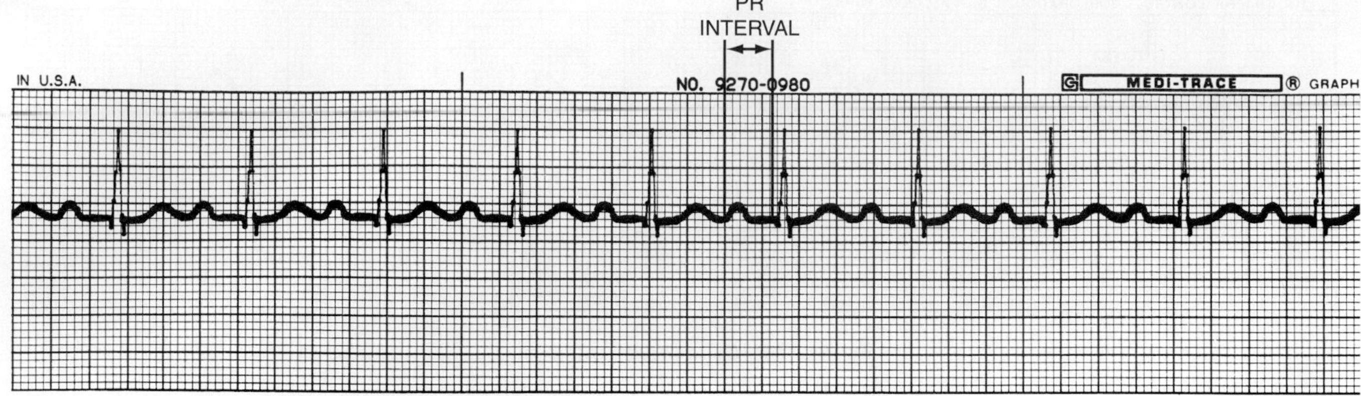

FIGURE 24•20 Sinus rhythm with first-degree AV block.

tricles. Second-degree AV block has the following characteristics (Fig. 24-22):

Ventricular and atrial rate: Depends on the underlying rhythm

Ventricular and atrial rhythm: The PP interval is regular if the patient has an underlying normal sinus rhythm. The RR interval is usually regular but may be irregular, depending on the P : QRS ratio.

QRS shape and duration: Usually abnormal, but may be normal

P wave: In front of the QRS complex; shape depends on underlying rhythm.

PR interval: PR interval is constant for those P waves just before QRS complex.

P : QRS ratio: 2 : 1, 3 : 1, 4 : 1, 5 : 1, and so forth

Third-Degree AV Block

Third-degree heart block occurs when no atrial impulse is conducted through the AV node into the ventricles. In third-degree heart block, two impulses stimulate the heart: one stimulates the ventricles (eg, junctional or ventricular escape rhythm), represented by the QRS complex, and one stimulates the atria (eg, sinus rhythm, atrial fibrillation), represented by the P wave. P waves may be seen, but the atrial electrical activity is not conducted down into the ventricles to cause the QRS complex, the ventricular electrical activity. This is called AV dissociation. Complete block (third-degree AV block) has the following characteristics (Fig. 24-23):

Ventricular and atrial rate: Depends on the escape and underlying atrial rhythm

Ventricular and atrial rhythm: The PP interval is regular and the RR interval is regular; however, the PP interval is not equal to the RR interval.

QRS shape and duration: Depends on the escape rhythm; in junctional escape, QRS shape and duration are usually normal, and in ventricular escape, QRS shape and duration are usually abnormal.

P wave: Depends on underlying rhythm

PR interval: Very irregular

P : QRS ratio: More P waves than QRS complexes

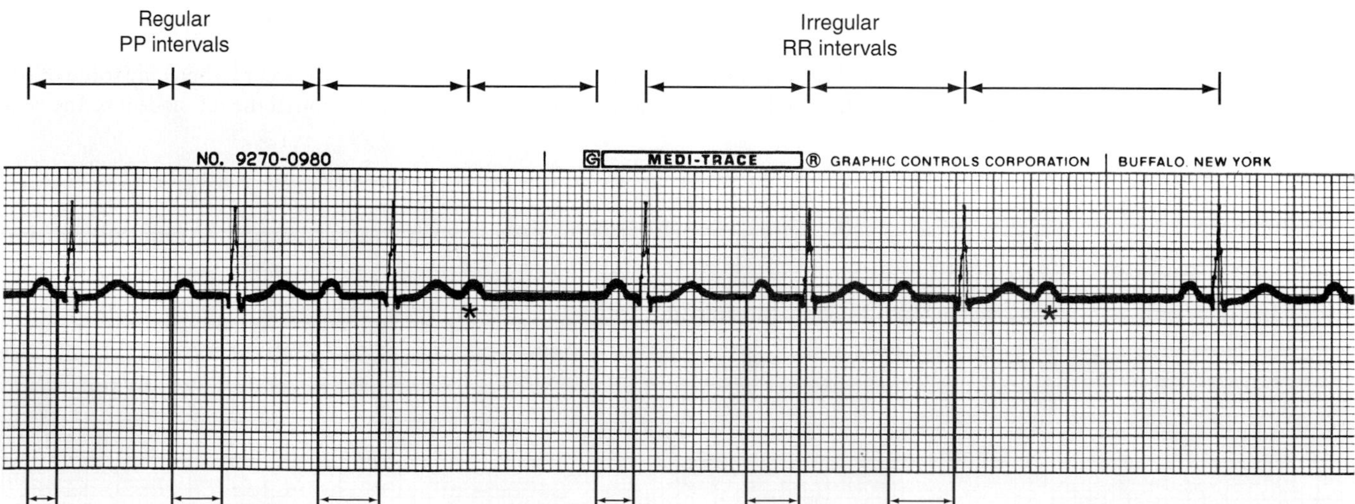

FIGURE 24•21 Sinus rhythm with second-degree AV block, type I, with progressively longer PR durations until there is a nonconducted P wave.

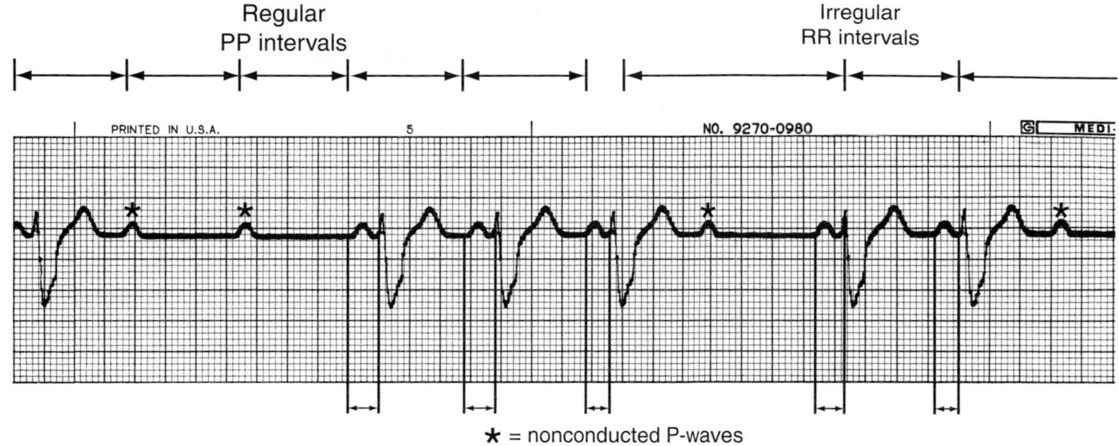

FIGURE 24•22 Sinus rhythm with second-degree AV block, Type II; note constant PR interval.

Based on the cause of the AV block and the stability of the patient, treatment is directed toward increasing the heart rate to maintain a normal cardiac output. If the patient is stable and has no symptoms, no treatment is indicated other than decreasing or eradicating the cause (eg, withholding the medication or treatment). If the patient is short of breath, complains of chest pain and lightheadedness, and has low blood pressure, an IV bolus of atropine is the initial treatment of choice. If the patient does not respond to atropine or has an acute MI, transcutaneous pacing should be started. A permanent pacemaker may be necessary if the block persists.

NURSING PROCESS: THE PATIENT WITH A DYSRHYTHMIA

Assessment

Major areas of assessment include possible causes of the dysrhythmia and the dysrhythmia's effect on the heart's ability to pump an adequate blood volume. When cardiac output is reduced, the amount of oxygen reaching the tissues and vital organs is diminished. This diminished oxygenation produces the signs and symptoms associated with dysrhythmias. If these signs and symptoms are severe or if they occur frequently, the patient may experience significant distress and disruption of daily life.

A health history is obtained to identify possible causes and past incidences of syncope (fainting), lightheadedness, dizziness, fatigue, chest discomfort, and palpitations. Any or all of these signs and symptoms can be present if the dysrhythmia causes decreased cardiac output. A thorough psychosocial assessment is also performed to identify the possible effects of the dysrhythmia.

The nurse conducts a physical assessment to confirm the data obtained from the history and to observe for signs of diminished cardiac output during the dysrhythmic event, especially changes in level of consciousness. The nurse then directs attention to the skin, which may be pale and cool. Signs of fluid retention, such as neck vein distention, and crackles and wheezes auscultated in the lungs may be detected. The rate and rhythm of apical and peripheral pulses are also assessed, and any pulse deficit is noted. The nurse auscultates the chest for extra heart sounds, especially S_3 and S_4, measures blood pressure, and determines pulse pressures. A declining pulse pressure indicates reduced cardiac output. Just one assessment may not disclose significant changes in cardiac output; therefore, the nurse compares the multiple assessment findings over time.

Diagnosis

Nursing Diagnoses

Based on assessment data, major nursing diagnoses of the patient may include:

- Potential/actual decrease in cardiac output
- Anxiety related to fear of the unknown
- Lack of knowledge about the dysrhythmia and its treatment

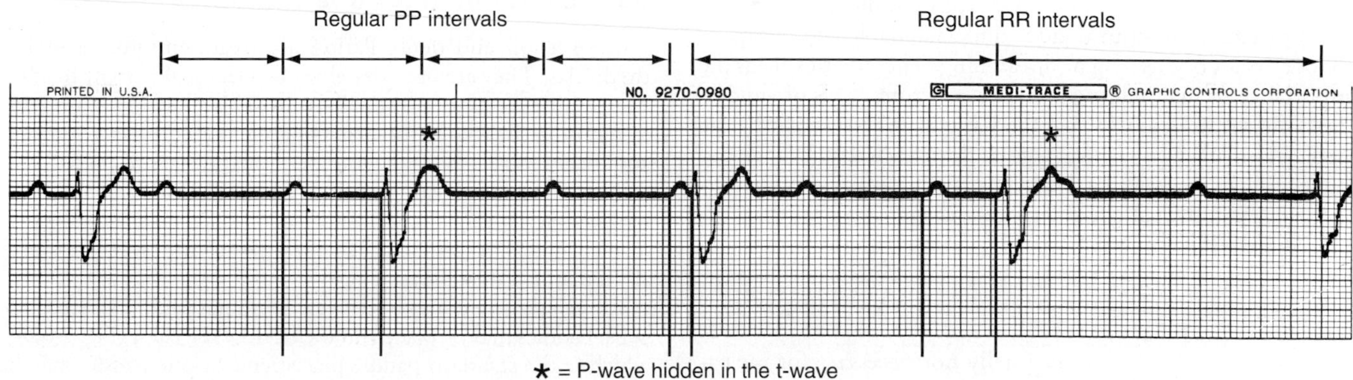

FIGURE 24•23 Sinus rhythm with third-degree AV block and idioventricular rhythm; note irregular PR intervals.

Collaborative Problems/Potential Complications

Based on the assessment data, a potential complication that may develop is ischemic heart disease.

Planning and Goals

The major goals of the patient may include eradicating or decreasing the incidence of the dysrhythmia (by decreasing contributory factors) to maintain cardiac output, minimizing anxiety, and acquiring knowledge about the dysrhythmia and its treatment.

Nursing Interventions

Monitoring and Managing the Dysrhythmia

Controlling the incidence and/or the effect of the dysrhythmia is most often achieved by the use of antidysrhythmic medications. The nurse manages medication administration carefully so that a constant serum blood level of the medication is maintained at all times. This maximizes beneficial effects and minimizes adverse effects. If the patient with a threatening dysrhythmia is hospitalized, an ECG is initiated and rhythm strips are analyzed to track the dysrhythmia. Blood pressure, rate and depth of respirations, and pulse rate and rhythm are evaluated regularly to determine the hemodynamic effect of the dysrhythmia.

Minimizing Anxiety

When the patient experiences episodes of dysrhythmia, the nurse maintains a calm and reassuring attitude. This demeanor fosters a trusting relationship with the patient and assists in reducing anxiety. Successes are emphasized with the patient to promote a sense of confidence in living with a dysrhythmia. For example, if a patient is experiencing episodes of dysrhythmia and a medication is administered that begins to reduce the incidence of the dysrhythmia, the nurse shares that information with the patient. The nursing goal is to maximize the patient's control and to make the unknown less threatening.

Promoting Home and Community-Based Care

TEACHING PATENTS SELF-CARE

When teaching patients about dysrhythmias, the nurse presents the information in terms that are understandable and in a manner that is not frightening or threatening. The nurse explains the importance of maintaining therapeutic serum levels of antidysrhythmic medications so that the patient understands why the medications are to be taken at regular times each day. In addition, the relationship between a dysrhythmia and cardiac output is explained so that the patient understands the rationale for the medical regimen. It is also important to establish with the patient and family a plan of action to take in case of an emergency. This allows the patient and family to feel in control and prepared for possible eventualities.

A referral for home care is usually not necessary for the patient with a dysrhythmia unless the patient is hemodynamically unstable and has significant symptoms of decreased cardiac output.

Evaluation

Expected Outcomes

Expected outcomes may include:

1. Cardiac output is maintained.
   a. Demonstrates heart rate, blood pressure, respiratory rate, and level of consciousness within normal ranges
   b. Demonstrates no or decreased episodes of dysrhythmia
2. Anxiety is minimized.
   a. Expresses a positive attitude about living with the dysrhythmia
   b. Expresses confidence in ability to take appropriate actions in an emergency
3. The patient knows about the dysrhythmia and its treatment.
   a. Explains the dysrhythmia and its effects
   b. Describes the medication regimen and its rationale
   c. Explains the need for therapeutic serum level of the medication
   d. States actions to take in the event of an emergency

ADJUNCTIVE MODALITIES AND MANAGEMENT

Dysrhythmia treatments depend on whether the disorder is acute or chronic as well as on the etiology of the dysrhythmia and the actual or potential hemodynamic effects.

Acute dysrhythmias may be treated with medications or external electrical therapy. Many antidysrhythmic medications (also called antiarrhythmics) are used to treat atrial and ventricular tachydysrhythmias. These medications are summarized in Table 24-1. The choice of medication depends on the specific dysrhythmia, the underlying cardiac failure and other diseases, and the patient's response to previous treatment. The nurse is responsible for monitoring and documenting the patient's responses to the medication and making sure that the patient has the knowledge and ability to manage the medication regimen.

When medications alone are ineffective in eradicating or decreasing the dysrhythmia, certain adjunctive mechanical therapies are available. The most common are elective cardioversion and defibrillation for acute tachydysrhythmia and implantable devices for chronic tachydysrhythmia. Surgical treatment, although less common, is also available.

Cardioversion and Defibrillation

Cardioversion and defibrillation are treatments for tachydysrhythmias. They are used to deliver an electrical current to stimulate a critical mass of myocardial cells. This allows the sinus node to recapture its role as the heart's pacemaker. One major difference between cardioversion and defibrillation has to do with the timing of the delivery of electrical current. Another major difference concerns the circumstance: defibrillation is usually performed as an emergency treatment, whereas cardioversion is usually a planned procedure.

Electrical current may be delivered through paddles or electrode pads. Paddles may be placed on the front of the chest (Fig. 24-24), which is the standard paddle placement, or one paddle may be placed on the chest and the other connected to an adapter with a long handle and placed under the patient's back, which is called an anteroposterior placement (Fig. 24-25).

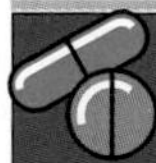

TABLE 24•1 Summary of Antiarrhythmic Medications*

Class	Action	Drugs: Generic (Trade) Names	Side Effects	Nursing Interventions
1 A	Moderate depression of depolarization; prolongs repolarization Treats and prevents atrial and ventricular dysrhythmias	quinidine (Quinaglute, Quinalan, Quinora, Quinidex, Cardioquin) procainamide (Pronestyl) disopyramide (Norpace)	Decreased cardiac contractility Prolonged QRS, QT Proarrhythmia Hypotension with IV administration Lupus-like syndrome with Pronestyl Anticholinergic effects: dry mouth, decreased urine output	Observe for cardiac failure Monitor QRS duration for > 50% baseline Monitor for prolonged QT Monitor blood pressure with administration Monitor NAPA lab values during procainamide therapy
1 B	Minimal depression of depolarization; shortened repolarization Treats ventricular dysrhythmias	lidocaine (Xylocaine) mexiletine (Mexitil) tocainide (Tonocard)	CNS side effects, eg, confusion, lethargy	Discuss decreasing the dose in elderly patients and/or patients with cardiac/liver dysfunction
1 C	Marked depression of depolarization; little effect on repolarization Treats atrial and ventricular dysrhythmias	flecainide (Tambocor)	Proarrhythmia CHF Bradycardia AV blocks	Discuss patient's left ventricular function with physician
II	Decreases automaticity and conduction Treats atrial and ventricular dysrhythmias	atenolol (Tenormin) esmolol (Brevibloc) metoprolol (Lopressor) nadolol (Corgard) propranolol (Inderal) sotalol (Betapace)	Bradycardia, AV block, Decreased contractility, Bronchospasm Hypotension with IV administration Masks hypoglycemia and thyrotoxicosis; CNS disturbances	Monitor heart rate, PR interval, signs and symptoms of heart failure Monitor blood glucose level in patients with type II diabetes mellitus
III	Prolongs repolarization	amiodarone (Cordarone)	Pulmonary toxicity Corneal microdeposits Photosensitivity Hypotension with IV administration	Make sure patient is sent for baseline pulmonary function tests Closely monitor patient
	Treats and prevents primarily ventricular dysrhythmias; amiodarone may also be used to treat atrial dysrhythmias	bretylium (Bretylol)	Hypotension Nausea and vomiting	Not recommended to be used undiluted in conscious patient
IV	Blocks calcium channel Treats atrial dysrhythmias Treats hypertension and vasospasm	verapamil (Calan, Isoptin, Verlan) diltiazem (Cardizem,Dilacor) nicardipine (Cardene) nifedipine (Procardia, Adalatz)	Bradycardia, AV blocks Hypotension with IV administration CHF, peripheral edema	Monitor heart rate, PR interval Monitor blood pressure closely with IV administration Monitor for signs and symptoms of CHF

* Based on Vaughn-Williams classification. *Note:* Medications in the antiarrhythmic drug class treat dysrhythmias.

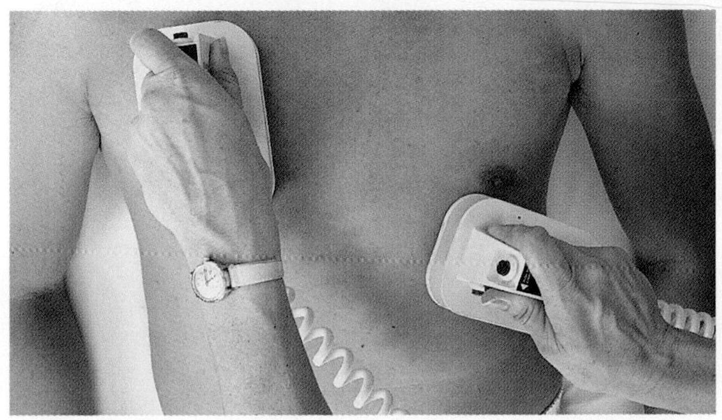

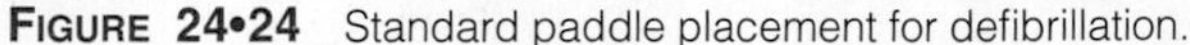

FIGURE 24•24 Standard paddle placement for defibrillation.

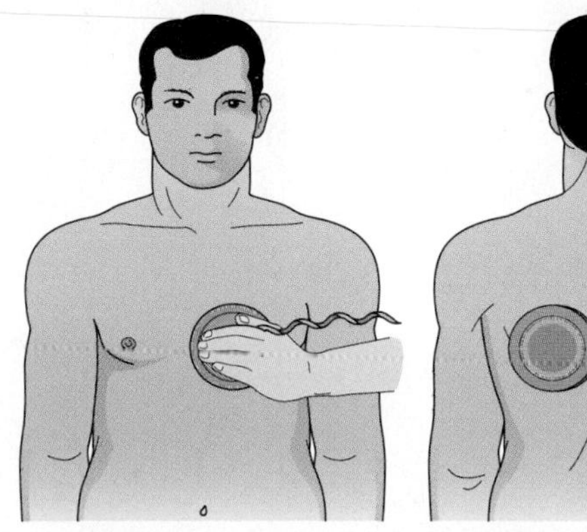

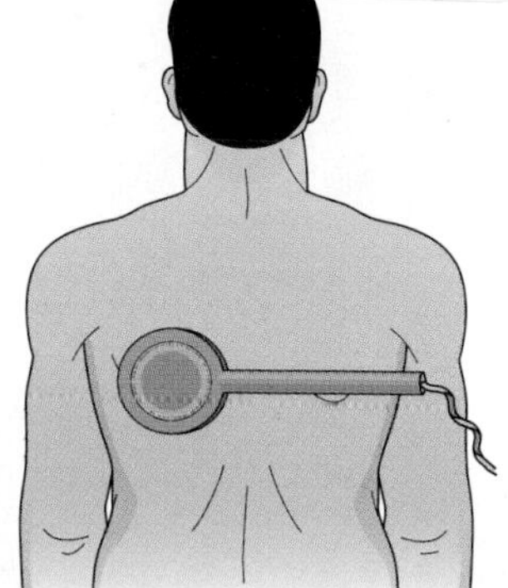

FIGURE 24•25 Anteroposterior paddle placement for defibrillation.

Nursing Alert *When using paddles, apply the appropriate conductant between the paddles and the patient's skin. Do not substitute any other type of conductive medium, such as ultrasound gel.*

Instead of paddles, defibrillator multifunction pads (Fig. 24-26) may be used. These pads, which are placed in the same position as the paddles and connected to the defibrillator, allow for hands-off defibrillation, thereby reducing the risk of touching the patient during the procedure and increasing electrical safety.

Whether using pads or paddles, two safety measures must be observed. First, maintain good contact between the paddles and the patient's skin; otherwise, the electrical current will leak into the air, "arcing" when the defibrillator is discharged. Second, avoid touching the patient or the bed when the defibrillator is discharged; if that were to happen, the electrical current may be conducted through the patient or bed into the person in contact with the patient.

The following are some key points to remember when performing defibrillation or cardioversion:

- Use a conducting agent between the skin and the paddles, such as defibrillation pads, gel, or paste.
- Place paddles or pads so that they do not touch the patient's clothing or bed linen and are not near medication patches or direct oxygen flow.
- Exert 20 to 25 pounds of pressure on each paddle to ensure good skin contact.
- Keep thumbs and fingers off the discharge buttons until paddles or pads are on the chest and ready to deliver electrical charge.
- Call "all clear" just before discharge; verify that no one is touching the bed or the patient when the electrical current is discharged.
- Record the delivered energy and the resulting cardiac rhythm.
- After the procedure is completed, inspect the skin under the pads or paddles for burns; if detected, discuss the method of treatment with the physician and a wound care nurse.

Cardioversion

Cardioversion involves the delivery of a "timed" electrical current to terminate a tachydysrhythmia. In cardioversion, the defibrillator is set to synchronize with a cardiac monitor so that the electrical impulse is timed to discharge during ventricular depolarization (QRS complex). Because there may be a short delay until the recognition of the QRS, the discharge buttons must be held down until the shock has been delivered. The synchronization prevents the discharge from occurring during the vulnerable period of repolarization (T wave), which could result in ventricular tachycardia or ventricular fibrillation. When the synchronizer is on, no electrical current will be delivered if the defibrillator does not discern a QRS complex. Sometimes the lead and the electrodes must be changed for the monitor to recognize the patient's QRS complex.

For an elective cardioversion, the patient usually prepares by avoiding food or fluid the night before or at least 8 hours before the procedure. Digoxin is usually withheld for 48 hours before cardioversion to ensure the resumption of sinus rhythm with normal conduction. Paddles or pads are positioned front and back (anteroposteriorly) for cardioversion. The patient is usually given conscious sedation before cardioversion. Respiration is then supported with supplemental oxygen delivered by a bag-mask-valve device; patients rarely require intubation. The amount of voltage used varies from 25 to 400 watt-seconds. If ventricular fibrillation occurs after cardioversion, the defibrillator must be recharged immediately. Then the synchronizer is turned off to defibrillate the patient.

Indications of a successful response are conversion to sinus rhythm, adequate peripheral pulses, and adequate blood pressure. Airway patency must be maintained and the patient's state of consciousness assessed. Vital signs, including oxygen saturation, should be monitored and recorded until the patient's condition stabilizes. ECG monitoring is required during and after cardioversion.

Defibrillation

Defibrillation is used in emergency situations as the treatment of choice for ventricular fibrillation and pulseless ventricular tachycardia. Defibrillation depolarizes a critical mass of myocardial cells at once, allowing the sinus node to recapture its role as the pace-

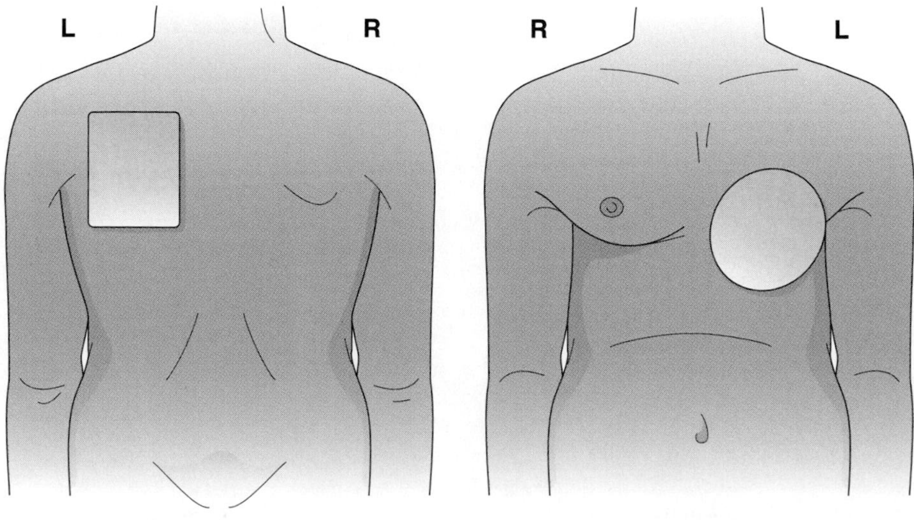

FIGURE 24•26 Multifunction pads for defibrillation.

maker. The electrical voltage required to defibrillate the heart is usually greater than that required for cardioversion. If three defibrillations of increasing voltage have been unsuccessful, cardiopulmonary resuscitation is resumed and advanced life support treatments are begun immediately.

The use of epinephrine may make the fibrillation easier to convert with defibrillation. It also increases cerebral and coronary artery blood flow. The patient may be intubated while the etiology of the arrest is investigated. Hypoxic lactic acidosis is no longer treated with sodium bicarbonate, but with increased ventilations. Sodium bicarbonate is prescribed only if the patient had a preexisting acidosis or is thought to have a drug overdose. Blood pressure is supported using vasopressors. After a medication is administered and 1 minute of cardiopulmonary resuscitation performed, defibrillation is again performed. This continues until a stable rhythm resumes or until it is determined that the patient cannot be revived.

Pacemaker Therapy

A pacemaker is an electronic device that provides electrical stimuli to the heart muscle. Pacemakers are usually used when a patient has a slower-than-normal impulse formation and/or a conduction disturbance that then causes symptoms. They may also be used to control tachydysrhythmias that do not respond to medication therapy.

Pacemakers can be permanent or temporary. Permanent pacemakers are used most commonly for irreversible complete heart block. Temporary pacemakers are used (eg, after MI or open heart surgery) to support patients until they improve or receive a permanent pacemaker.

Pacemaker Design and Types

Pacemakers consist of two components: an electronic pulse generator and pacemaker electrodes, which are located on leads or wires. The generator contains the circuitry and batteries that generate the rate (measured in beats per minute) and strength (measured in milliamps [mA]) of the electrical stimulus delivered to the heart. The pacemaker electrodes detect the intrinsic electrical activity in the heart and send this information through the lead to the generator; the generator's response to the received information is then transmitted to the heart.

Leads can be threaded through a major vein into the right ventricle (endocardial leads) or can be lightly sutured onto the outside of the heart and brought through the chest wall during open heart surgery (epicardial wires). The epicardial wires are always temporary and are removed by a gentle tug within a few days after surgery. The endocardial leads may be temporarily placed with catheters through the femoral, antecubital, brachial, or jugular vein (transvenous wires), usually guided by fluoroscopy. The transvenous wires are then connected to a temporary generator, which is about the size of a small paperback book (Fig. 24-27). The energy source for a temporary generator is a common household battery; monitoring for battery failure is a nursing responsibility.

The endocardial leads also may be placed permanently, usually through the external jugular vein, and connected to a permanent generator, which is usually implanted underneath the skin in a subcutaneous pocket in the pectoral region or below the clavicle. Sometimes an abdominal site is selected. This procedure is usually performed in a catheterization laboratory with the patient receiving a local anesthetic. Permanent generators are insulated to protect against body moisture and warmth. There are different energy sources for permanent generators: mercury–zinc batteries (lasting 3 to 4 years), lithium cell units (lasting up to 10 years), and nuclear-powered sources (eg, plutonium 238, which lasts up to 20 years). Some of the batteries are rechargeable. If the battery is not rechargeable and failure is impending, the old generator is removed and the new one is connected to the existing leads and reimplanted in the already existing subcutaneous pocket. This is usually performed with the patient receiving a local anesthetic.

When a patient suddenly develops a bradycardia, emergency pacing may be started with transcutaneous pacing, which most defibrillators are now equipped to perform. Large pacing ECG electrodes are placed on the patient's chest and back. The electrodes are connected to the defibrillator, which serves as the pacemaker generator (Fig. 24-28). Because the impulse must travel through the patient's skin and tissue before reaching the heart, transcutaneous pacing may cause significant discomfort and is intended to be used only in emergencies. If the patient is alert, the use of sedation and analgesia should be discussed with the physician.

Pacemaker Generator Functions

Because of the sophistication and wide use of pacemakers, a universal code has been adopted to provide a means of safe communication about their function. The coding is referred to as the ICHD code because it is sanctioned by the Inter-Society Commission for Heart Disease. The complete code consists of five letters, but usually only the first three are used in common practice.

The first letter of the code identifies the chamber(s) being paced, that is, the chamber containing a pacing electrode. The letter characters for this code are A (atrium), V (ventricle), or D (dual, meaning both A and V).

The second letter describes the chamber(s) being sensed by the pacemaker generator. Information from the electrode within the

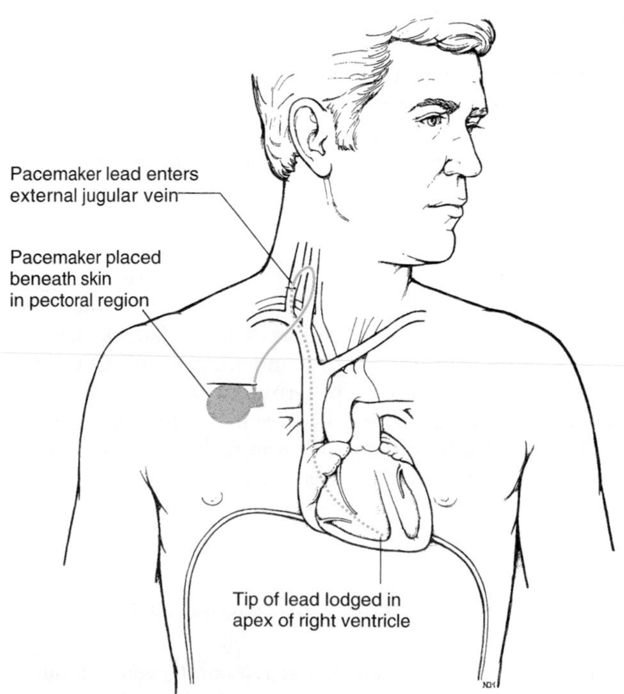

FIGURE 24•27 Implanted transvenous pacing electrode and pacemaker generator.

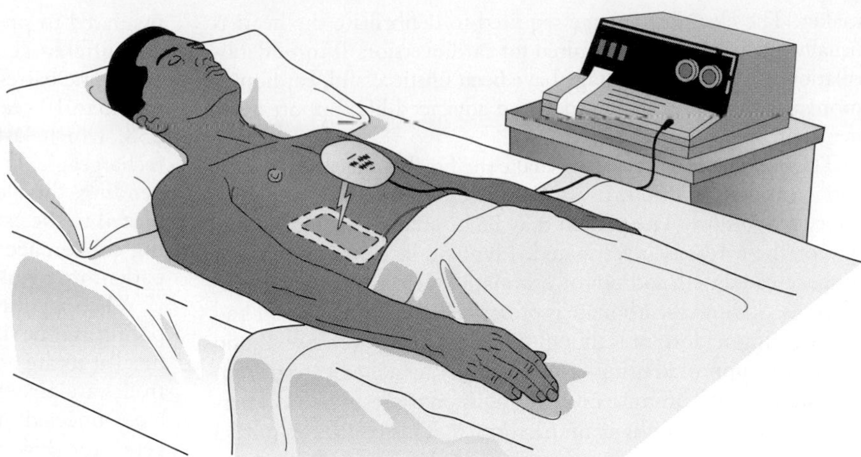

FIGURE 24•28 Transcutaneous pacemaker with electrode pads connected to the anterior and posterior chest walls.

chamber is sent to the generator for interpretation and action by the generator. The possible letter characters here are A (atrium), V (ventricle), D (dual), and O (indicating that the sensing function has been turned off).

The third letter of the code describes the type of response by the pacemaker to sensing. The possible letter characters used to describe this response are I for **inhibited**, T for **triggered**, D for inhibited and triggered, and O for none. Inhibitory response means that the response of the pacemaker is controlled by the activity of the patient's heart; that is, the pacemaker will not function when the patient's heart beats. In contrast, triggered response means that the pacemaker will trigger a response based on intrinsic heart activity.

The fourth and fifth letters are used only with permanent generators at this time. The fourth letter of the code is related to a permanent generator's ability to be programmed or reset. The possible letters are O (none), P (simple programmability), M (multiprogrammability; ability to change at least three factors, such as the rate pacing is initiated, the rate of pacing, and the amount of energy delivered), C (communicative or telemetry ability—information about the generator may be read or interrogated with a hand-held device held above the chest), and R (rate responsive capabilities; the ability of the rate to change from moment to moment based on parameters such as physical activity, acid–base changes, temperature, rate and depth of respirations, and oxygen saturation). A pacemaker with rate responsive ability will be capable of improving cardiac output during times of increased cardiac demand, such as with exercise.

The fifth letter of the code indicates that the permanent generator has antitachycardia and/or defibrillation capability. The possible letters are P (antitachycardia pacing), S (shock; defibrillation), D (antitachycardia pacing and shock), and O (none). Antitachycardia pacing is used to terminate tachycardias caused by a conduction disturbance called reentry, which is repetitive restimulation of tissue by the same impulse. An impulse or series of impulses are delivered to the heart at a fast rate to collide with and stop the impulses in the reentry conduction, and therefore to stop the tachycardia.

An example of an ICHD code is DVI:

D: Both the atrium and the ventricle have a pacing electrode in place.

V: The pacemaker is sensing the activity of the ventricle only.

I: The pacemaker's stimulating effect is inhibited by ventricular activity—in other words, it does not create an impulse when the patient's ventricle is active.

The type of generator and its selected settings depend on the patient's dysrhythmia, underlying cardiac function, and age. A straight vertical line usually can be seen on the ECG when pacing is initiated. The line that represents pacing is called a pacemaker spike. The appropriate ECG complex should immediately follow the pacing spike; therefore, a QRS complex should follow a ventricular pacing spike and a P wave should follow an atrial pacing spike. Because the impulse starts in a different place than the patient's normal rhythm, the QRS complex and/or P wave that responds to pacing looks very different from the patient's normal ECG complex. Capture is a term used to denote that the appropriate complex followed the pacing spike.

Pacemakers are generally set to sense and respond to intrinsic activity, which is called on-demand pacing (Fig. 24-29). If the pacemaker is set to pace but not to sense, it is called a fixed or asynchronous pacemaker (Fig. 24-30); this is written in code as AOO or VOO. The pacemaker will pace at a constant rate, independent of the patient's intrinsic rhythm. Because AOO pacing stimulates only the atrium, it may be used in a patient who has undergone open heart surgery and develops sinus bradycardia. AOO pacing ensures synchrony between the atrial and ventricular stimulation (and therefore contraction), as long as the patient has no conduction disturbances in the AV node. VOO is rare because of the risk of the pacemaker delivering an impulse during the vulnerable repolarization phase, leading to ventricular tachycardia.

Complications of Pacemakers

Complications associated with pacemakers relate to their presence within the body, and improper functioning. The following complications may arise from a pacemaker:

- Local infection at the entry site of the leads or at the subcutaneous site, for permanent generator placement
- Bleeding and hematoma at the lead-entry sites, or at the subcutaneous site for permanent generator placement
- Hemothorax from puncture of the subclavian vein or internal mammary artery
- Ventricular ectopy and tachycardia from irritation of the ventricular wall by the endocardial electrode
- Movement or dislocation of the lead placed transvenously (perforation of the myocardium)
- Phrenic nerve, diaphragmatic (hiccuping may be a sign of this), or skeletal muscle stimulation may occur if the lead is dislocated or if the delivered energy (mA) is set high.

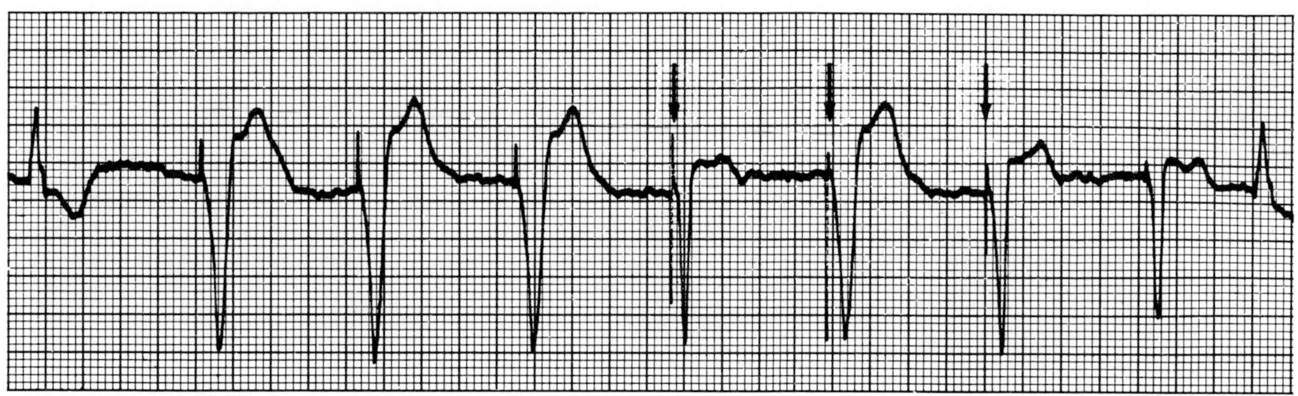

FIGURE 24•29 Pacing with appropriate sensing (on-demand pacing). Arrows denote pacing spike.

- Rarely, cardiac tamponade occurs after removal of epicardial wires

In the initial hours after a temporary or permanent pacemaker is inserted, the most common complication is dislodgement of the pacing electrode. Minimizing patient activities can help to prevent this complication. If a temporary electrode is in place, the extremity through which the catheter has been advanced is immobilized. With a permanent pacemaker, the patient is instructed initially to restrict activity on the side of the implantation.

Improper pacemaker function, which can arise from failure in one or more components of the pacing system, is outlined in Table 24-2. The following data should be noted on the patient's record: the model of pacemaker, type of generator, date and time of insertion, location of the pulse generator, stimulation threshold, pacer settings (eg, rate, energy output [mA], and duration between atrial and ventricular impulses [AV delay]). This information is important for identifying normal pacemaker function and diagnosing pacemaker malfunction. It is essential to monitor the ECG very carefully to detect pacemaker malfunction; the patient is usually placed in a cardiac-care unit.

In a patient experiencing pacemaker malfunction, signs and symptoms of decreased cardiac output may develop. The degree to which these symptoms become apparent depends on the severity of the malfunction, the patient's level of dependency on the pacemaker, and the patient's underlying condition. The diagnosis of pacemaker malfunction is made by analyzing the ECG. Manipulating the electrodes, changing the generator's settings, or replacing the pacemaker generator or leads or both may be necessary.

Inhibition of permanent pacemakers can occur with exposure to electromagnetic fields (electromagnetic interference), although most patients with a permanent pacemaker can safely use most household appliances and devices (eg, microwave ovens, electric tools, remote devices). The metal in some pacemakers may trigger some store and airport security alarms, but these alarm systems will not interfere with the pacemaker function. The patient should be instructed to carry the pacemaker identification card. Some electrical equipment, such as held-held metal detectors and old elevator switches, may inadvertently trigger or inhibit the pacemaker, but usually the interference is so brief that no clinical mishap occurs. However, large electromagnetic fields, such as those produced by magnetic resonance imaging, electrical substations, or direct or close contact of the generator with engines (eg, in a car or lawn mower), will cause electromagnetic interference. Therefore, the patient should be cautioned to avoid such situations and to wear or carry medical identification to alert emergency health care personnel to the presence of the pacemaker.

Pacemaker Surveillance

Pacemaker clinics have been established to monitor patients and to test pulse generators for impending pacemaker battery failure. Several other factors, such as lead fracture, muscle inhibition, and insulation disruption, are assessed, depending on the type of pacemaker and the equipment available. If indicated, the pacemaker is turned off, using a magnet or a programmer, for a few seconds while the ECG is recorded to assess the patient's underlying cardiac rhythm.

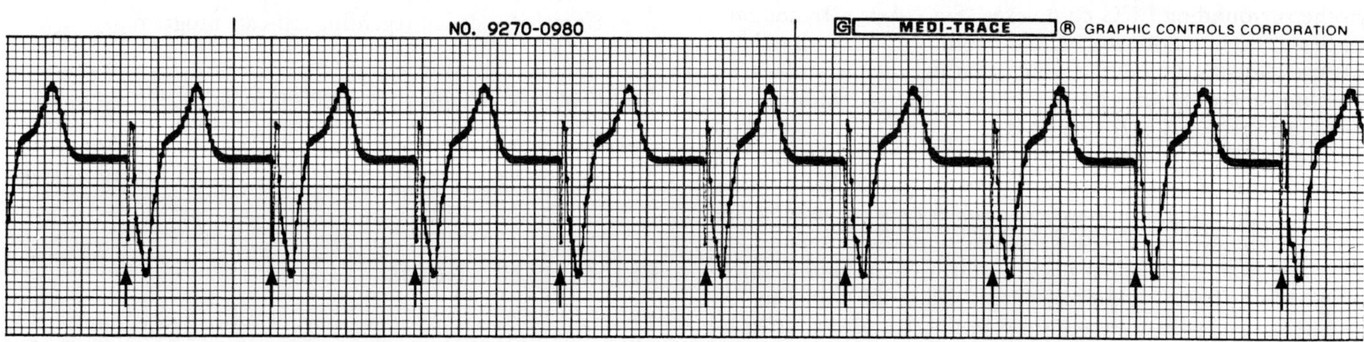

FIGURE 24•30 Fixed pacing or total loss of sensing pacing; arrows denote pacing spikes.

Table 24•2 Assessing Pacemaker Malfunction

Problem	Possible Cause	Intervention
Loss of capture—Complex does *not* follow pacing spike	Inadequate stimulus	Check security of all connections; increase milliamperage.
	Catheter malposition	Reposition limb; turn patient to left side.
	Battery depletion	Change battery.
	Electronic insulation break	Change generator.
Undersensing—Pacing spike occurs too soon (earlier than preset interval) after previous complex	Sensitivity setting too low	Increase sensitivity by turning dial clockwise to *lower* value.
	Electrical interference (eg, by a magnet)	Eliminate interference.
	Faulty generator	Replace generator.
Oversensing—Loss of pacing artifact; pacing does *not* occur at preset interval despite lack of intrinsic rhythm	Sensitivity at too high a setting	Decrease sensitivity by turning dial counterclockwise to *higher* value.
	Electrical interference	Eliminate interference.
	Battery depletion	Change battery.
Loss of pacing—Total absence of pacing spikes	Battery depletion	Change battery.
	Loose or disconnected wires	Check security of all connections.
	Perforation	Obtain 12-lead ECG and portable chest x-ray. Assess for murmur. Call physician.
Change in pacing QRS shape	Septal perforation	Obtain 12-lead ECG and portable chest x-ray. Assess for murmur. Call physician.
Rhythmic diaphragmatic or chest wall twitching or hiccuping	Output too high	Decrease milliamperage.
	Myocardial wall perforation	Turn pacer off. Call physician at once. Monitor closely for decreased cardiac output.

Another follow-up method is transtelephonic transmission of the generator's pulse rate. Special equipment is used to transmit information about the patient's pacemaker over the telephone to a receiving system at a pacemaker clinic. The information is converted into tones, which are then converted at the clinic into an electronic signal and permanently recorded on an ECG strip. The pacemaker rate and other data concerning pacemaker function are obtained and evaluated by a cardiologist. This simplifies the diagnosis of a failing generator, reassures the patient, and improves the management of the patient who is physically remote from pacemaker testing facilities.

NURSING PROCESS: THE PATIENT WITH A PACEMAKER

Assessment

After a temporary or a permanent pacemaker is inserted, the patient's heart rate and rhythm are monitored by ECG. The pacemaker's settings are noted and compared with the ECG recordings to assess pacemaker function. Pacemaker malfunction is detected by examining the pacemaker spike and its relationship to the surrounding ECG complexes (Fig. 24-31). In addition, cardiac output and hemodynamic stability are assessed to identify the patient's response to pacing and the adequacy of pacing. The appearance or increasing frequency of dysrhythmia is observed and reported to the physician.

The incision site where the pulse generator was implanted (or the entry site for the pacing electrode, if the pacemaker is temporary) is observed for bleeding, hematoma formation, or infection, evidenced by swelling, unusual tenderness, unusual drainage, and increased heat. The patient may complain of continuous throbbing or pain. These symptoms are reported to the physician.

The patient with a temporary pacemaker is also assessed for electrical interference and the development of microshock. The nurse observes for potential sources of electrical hazards. All electrical equipment used in the vicinity of the patient should be grounded. Improperly grounded equipment can generate leakage currents capable of producing ventricular fibrillation. Exposed wires must be carefully covered with nonconductive material to prevent accidental ventricular fibrillation from stray currents. The nurse, working with a biomedical engineer or electrician, should make certain that the patient is in an electrically safe environment.

Patients should be assessed for anxiety, especially those receiving a permanent pacemaker. In addition, for those receiving permanent pacemakers, the level of knowledge and learning needs of the patient and the family and the history of therapeutic adherence should be identified.

Diagnosis

Nursing Diagnoses

Based on assessment data, major nursing diagnoses of the patient may include the following:

- Risk for infection related to pacemaker lead or generator insertion
- Knowledge deficit regarding self-care program

Collaborative Problems/Potential Complications

Based on the assessment findings, potential complications that may develop include decreased cardiac output related to pacemaker malfunction.

Planning and Goals

The major goals of the patient may include absence of infection, adherence to a self-care program, and maintenance of pacemaker function.

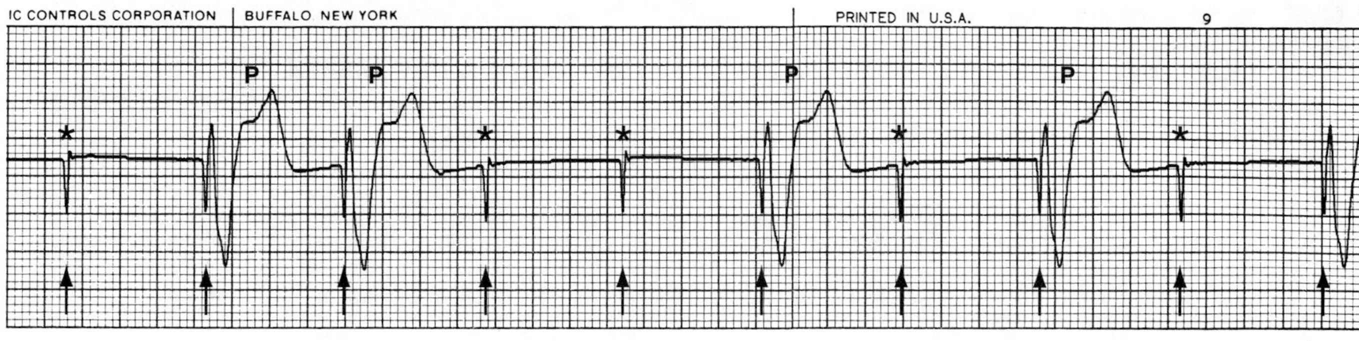

A

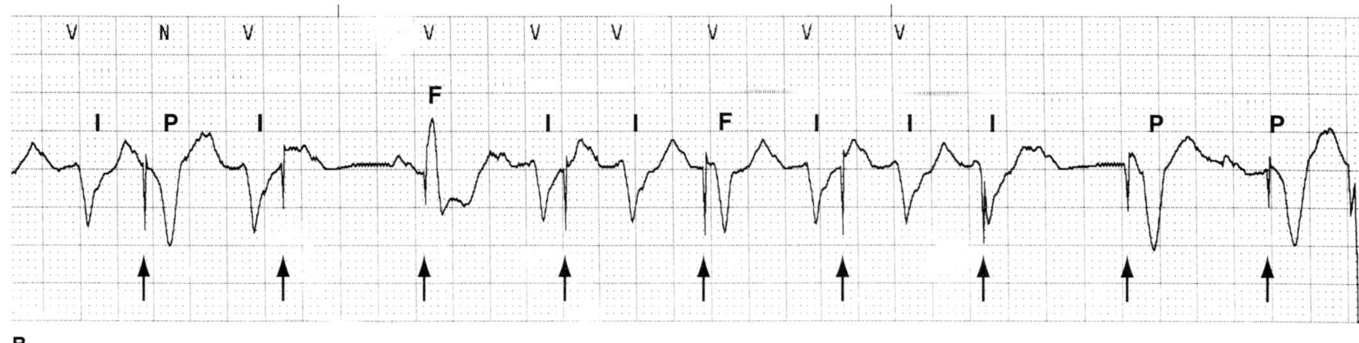

B

FIGURE 24•31 (**A**) Ventricular pacing with intermittent loss of capture (a pacing spike not followed by a QRS complex). (**B**) Ventricular pacing with loss of sensing (a pacing spike occurring at an inappropriate time). Key: ↑ = pacing spike; * = loss of capture; P = pacemaker-induced QRS complex; I = patient's intrinsic QRS complex; F = fusion (a QRS complex formed by a merging of the patient's intrinsic QRS complex and the pacemaker-induced QRS complex).

Nursing Interventions

Preventing Infection

The nurse changes the dressing regularly and inspects the wound site for redness, swelling, soreness, or any unusual drainage. An increase in temperature should be reported to the physician. Changes in the wound appearance are also reported to the physician.

Promoting Home and Community-Based Care

TEACHING PATIENTS SELF-CARE

The patient needs to understand the prescribed home care program and follow-up care. See the checklist The Patient With a Pacemaker for details.

Evaluation

Expected Outcomes

Expected outcomes may include:

1. The patient is free of infection.
   a. Has normal temperature
   b. Has white blood cell count within normal range (5000 to 10,000/mm^3)
   c. Exhibits no redness or swelling of pacemaker insertion site
2. The patient adheres to a self-care program.
   a. Responds appropriately when queried about the signs and symptoms of infection
   b. Identifies when to seek medical attention (as demonstrated in responses to signs and symptoms)
3. Pacemaker function is maintained (see the checklist The Patient With a Pacemaker).
   a. Measures and records pulse rate at regular intervals
   b. Experiences no abrupt changes in pulse rate or rhythm

Electrophysiologic Studies

An electrophysiology study is used to evaluate and treat various dysrhythmias that have caused cardiac arrest or significant symptoms. It also is indicated for patients with symptoms that suggest a dysrhythmia that has gone undetected and undiagnosed by other methods. An electrophysiology study is used to:

- Identify the impulse formation and propagation through the cardiac electrical conduction system
- Assess the function or dysfunction of the SA and AV nodal areas
- Identify the location and mechanism (called mapping) of dysrhythmogenic foci
- Assess the effectiveness of antiarrhythmic medications and devices for the patient with a dysrhythmia
- Treat certain dysrhythmias through the destruction of the causative cells (**ablation**)

An electrophysiology study is a type of cardiac catheterization that is performed in a specially equipped cardiac catheterization laboratory. Usually a catheter with multiple electrodes is inserted through the femoral vein, threaded through the vena cava, and ad-

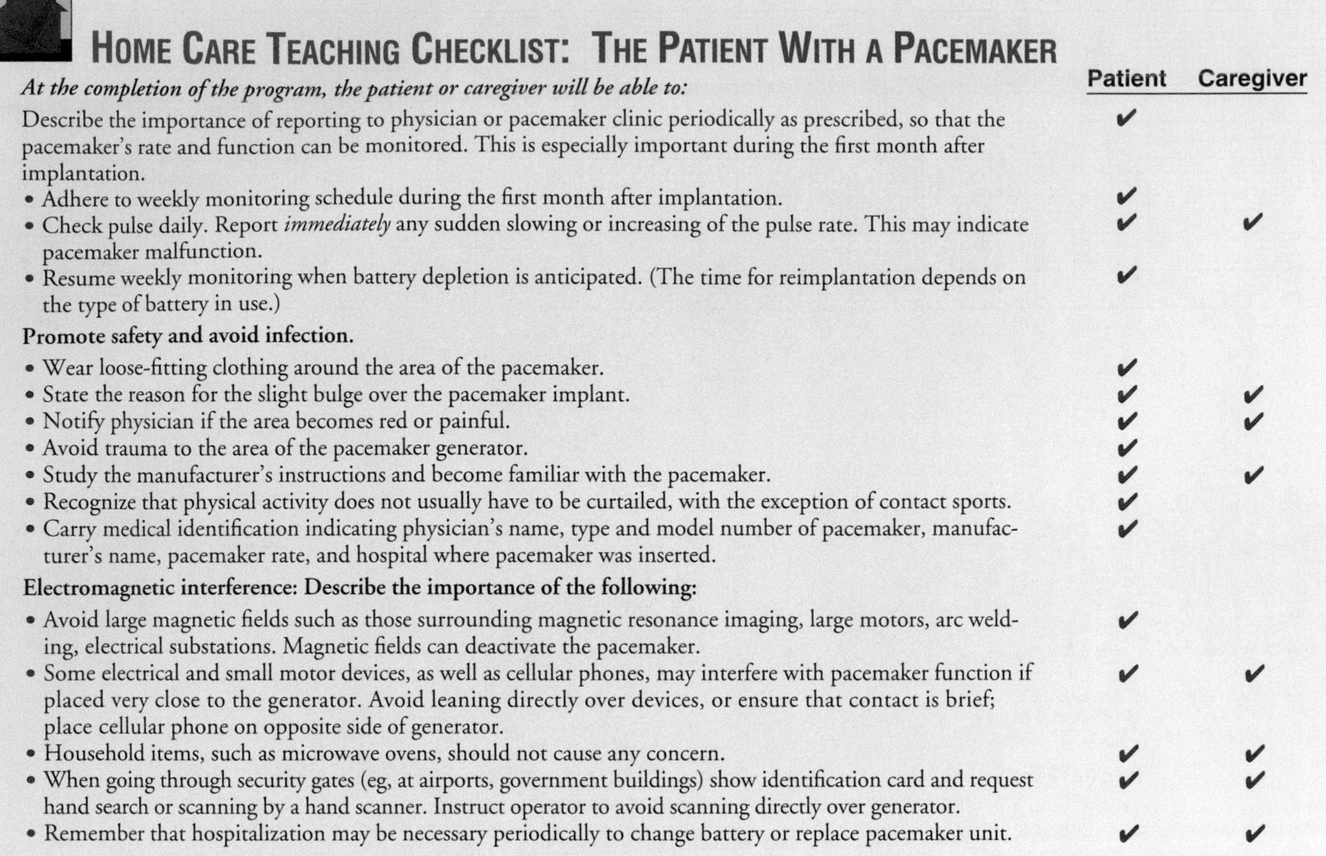

HOME CARE TEACHING CHECKLIST: THE PATIENT WITH A PACEMAKER

At the completion of the program, the patient or caregiver will be able to:	Patient	Caregiver
Describe the importance of reporting to physician or pacemaker clinic periodically as prescribed, so that the pacemaker's rate and function can be monitored. This is especially important during the first month after implantation.	✔	
• Adhere to weekly monitoring schedule during the first month after implantation.	✔	
• Check pulse daily. Report *immediately* any sudden slowing or increasing of the pulse rate. This may indicate pacemaker malfunction.	✔	✔
• Resume weekly monitoring when battery depletion is anticipated. (The time for reimplantation depends on the type of battery in use.)	✔	
Promote safety and avoid infection.		
• Wear loose-fitting clothing around the area of the pacemaker.	✔	
• State the reason for the slight bulge over the pacemaker implant.	✔	✔
• Notify physician if the area becomes red or painful.	✔	✔
• Avoid trauma to the area of the pacemaker generator.	✔	
• Study the manufacturer's instructions and become familiar with the pacemaker.	✔	✔
• Recognize that physical activity does not usually have to be curtailed, with the exception of contact sports.	✔	
• Carry medical identification indicating physician's name, type and model number of pacemaker, manufacturer's name, pacemaker rate, and hospital where pacemaker was inserted.	✔	
Electromagnetic interference: Describe the importance of the following:		
• Avoid large magnetic fields such as those surrounding magnetic resonance imaging, large motors, arc welding, electrical substations. Magnetic fields can deactivate the pacemaker.	✔	
• Some electrical and small motor devices, as well as cellular phones, may interfere with pacemaker function if placed very close to the generator. Avoid leaning directly over devices, or ensure that contact is brief; place cellular phone on opposite side of generator.	✔	✔
• Household items, such as microwave ovens, should not cause any concern.	✔	✔
• When going through security gates (eg, at airports, government buildings) show identification card and request hand search or scanning by a hand scanner. Instruct operator to avoid scanning directly over generator.	✔	✔
• Remember that hospitalization may be necessary periodically to change battery or replace pacemaker unit.	✔	✔

vanced into the heart. The electrodes are positioned within the heart at specific locations—for instance, the right atrium near the SA node, the coronary sinus, near the tricuspid valve, and the apex of the right ventricle. The number and placement of electrodes depend on the type of study being conducted. These electrodes allow the electrical signal to be recorded from within the heart (intracardiogram).

The electrodes also allow the clinician to introduce a pacing stimulus to the intracardiac area at a precisely timed interval and rate, thereby stimulating the area (programmed stimulation). An area of the heart may be paced at a rate much faster than the normal rate of **automaticity** (rate that impulses are spontaneously formed; eg, in the SA node), allowing the pacemaker to become an artificial focus of automaticity and to assume control (overdrive suppression). Then the pacemaker is stopped suddenly, and the time it takes for the SA node to resume control is assessed. A prolonged time indicates dysfunction of the area.

One of the main purposes of programmed stimulation is to assess the ability of the area surrounding the electrode to cause a reentry dysrhythmia. One or a series of premature impulses are delivered to an area in an attempt to cause the tachydysrhythmia. Because the precise location of the suspected area and the specific timing of the pacing needed are unknown, the electrophysiologist uses several different techniques to cause the dysrhythmia during the study. If the dysrhythmia can be reproduced by programmed stimulation, it is called inducible. Once a dysrhythmia is induced, a treatment plan is determined and implemented. If on the follow-up electrophysiology study, the tachydysrhythmia cannot be induced, then the treatment is determined to be effective. Different medications may be administered and combined with electrical devices (pacemakers, internal cardioverter defibrillators) to determine the most effective treatment to suppress the dysrhythmia. Tachydysrhythmias that are caused by abnormal impulse formation (automaticity) cannot be induced and are not evaluated by electrophysiology studies.

Complications of an electrophysiology study are the same as those that can occur with cardiac catheterization. Because the artery is usually not used, there is a lesser incidence of vascular complications than with other catheterization procedures. Cardiac arrest may occur, but the incidence is low (less than 1%).

Patients who are to undergo an electrophysiology study are usually very anxious about the procedure and about its outcome. A detailed discussion between patients and their families and the electrophysiologist usually occurs to ensure that patients are able to give informed consent and to reduce anxiety about the procedure. Before the procedure they should receive instructions about the procedure and its usual duration, the environment where the procedure is performed, and what to expect. Although an electrophysiology study is not painful, it does cause discomfort and can be tiring. It may also cause feelings that were experienced when the dysrhythmia occurred in the past. In addition, patients also learn what will be expected of them (eg, lying very still during the procedure, reporting symptoms or concerns).

Patients need to know that the dysrhythmia may occur during the procedure, but under very controlled circumstances. It often stops on its own; if it does not, treatment is given immediately to restore the patient's normal rhythm. During the procedure, patients benefit from a calm, reassuring approach.

Postprocedural care includes restriction of activity to promote hemostasis at the insertion site. To identify any complications and to ensure healing, the patient's vital signs and the appearance of the insertion site are assessed frequently.

Implantable Cardioverter Defibrillator

The implantable cardioverter defibrillator (ICD) is a device that detects and terminates life-threatening episodes of ventricular tachycardia or ventricular fibrillation in high-risk patients. Patients at high risk are those who have survived sudden cardiac death syndrome, survived ventricular fibrillation, experienced symptomatic ventricular tachycardia, or experienced syncope secondary to ventricular tachycardia. In addition, an ICD may be indicated for patients who have survived a heart attack but who are at high risk for cardiac arrest. Many of these patients are unresponsive to or cannot tolerate medications, surgery, or ablation procedures.

An ICD consists of a generator and at least one lead, which can sense intrinsic electrical activity and deliver an electrical impulse. The device is usually implanted much like a pacemaker (Fig. 24-32). Epicardial patches also may be used as leads to assist with defibrillation, but the implantation of patches necessitates open heart surgery.

The leads are designed to respond to two criteria: a rate that exceeds a predetermined level, or a change in the isoelectric line segments. When a dysrhythmia occurs, rate sensors take 5 to 10 seconds to sense the dysrhythmia. Then the device takes several seconds to charge and deliver the programmed amount of energy through the lead to the heart. Battery life usually is 3 to 5 years, depending on its use over time.

The battery is checked during follow-up visits. The ICD does not eliminate the patient's need for antidysrhythmic medication therapy. Antidysrhythmic medication is usually administered with this technology to prevent the occurrence of the tachydysrhythmia and to reduce the need for the ICD.

The first defibrillator, which was implanted in 1980 at Johns Hopkins University, just defibrillated the heart. Today, however, several devices are available, and many are programmed for multiple treatments. Each device offers different delivery sequences, but all of the devices deliver high-energy defibrillation to treat a tachycardia. The device may deliver up to six shocks if necessary. Some ICDs can respond with antitachycardia pacing, in which the device delivers an electrical impulse at a fast rate in an attempt to disrupt the tachycardia by low-energy cardioversion, and/or defibrillation. Some also have pacemaker capability (usually in a VVI mode) if the patient develops bradycardia, which sometimes occurs after treating the tachycardia. Some ICDs also deliver low-energy cardioversion. Which device is used and how it is programmed depend on the dysrhythmia.

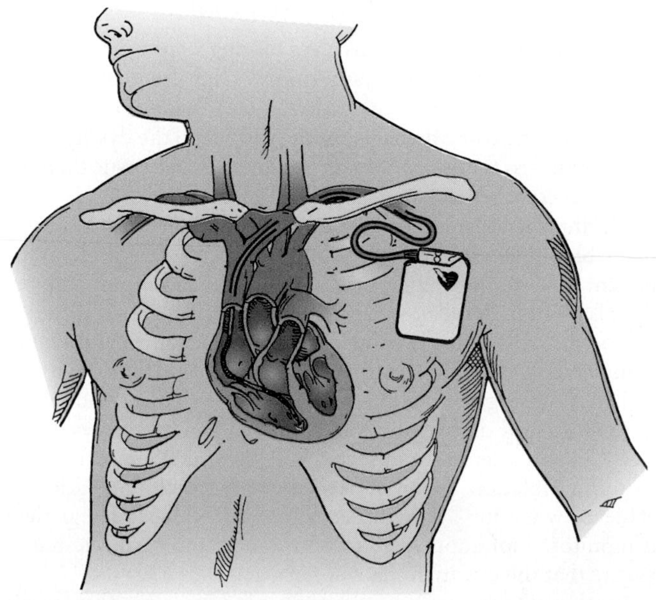

FIGURE 24•32 The implantable cardioverter defibrillator (ICD) mechanical system consists of a generator and a sensing/pacing/defibrillating electrode. Two epicardial patches may also be used.

The complications are similar to those associated with pacemaker insertion. The primary complication associated with the ICD is surgery-related infection. There are fewer complications associated with the technical aspects of the equipment, such as premature battery depletion and dislodged or fractured leads. Despite the possible complications, the consensus among clinicians is that the benefits of ICD therapy exceed the risks.

The nursing interventions for the patient with an ICD occur throughout the preoperative, perioperative, and postoperative phases. In addition to providing the patient and family with explanations regarding the implantation of the ICD in the preoperative phase, the nurse may need to manage acute episodes of life-threatening dysrhythmias. In the perioperative and postoperative phases, the nurse needs to observe the patient and his or her responses to the ICD carefully and to provide the patient and family with further teaching as needed (see The Patient With an ICD). The nurse can also assist them in making life-style changes necessitated by the dysrhythmia and resulting ICD implantation.

Cardiac Conduction Surgery

Atrial and ventricular tachycardias that do not respond to medications and are not suitable for antitachycardia pacing may be treated by methods other than medications and devices. Such methods include endocardial isolation, endocardial resection, and ablation. An ICD may be used with these surgical interventions.

Endocardial Isolation

Endocardial isolation involves making an incision into the endocardium, separating the area where the dysrhythmia originates from the surrounding endocardium. The edges of the incision are then sutured together. The incision and its resulting scar tissue prevent the dysrhythmia from affecting the whole heart.

Endocardial Resection

In endocardial resection, the origin of the dysrhythmia is identified, and that area of the endocardium is peeled away. No reconstruction or repair is necessary.

Catheter Ablation Therapy

Catheter ablation is a procedure that destroys specific cells that have been identified as the cause or central conduction method of a tachydysrhythmia. It is usually performed with or after an electrophysiologic study. Usually the indications for ablation are AV nodal reentry tachycardia, atrial fibrillation, or ventricular tachycardia that was unresponsive to previous therapy (or the therapy produced significant side effects).

Ablation is also indicated for accessory AV pathways or bypass tracts, also called preexcitation syndrome. During normal embryonic development, all connections between the atrium and ventri-

Home Care Teaching Checklist: The Patient With an ICD

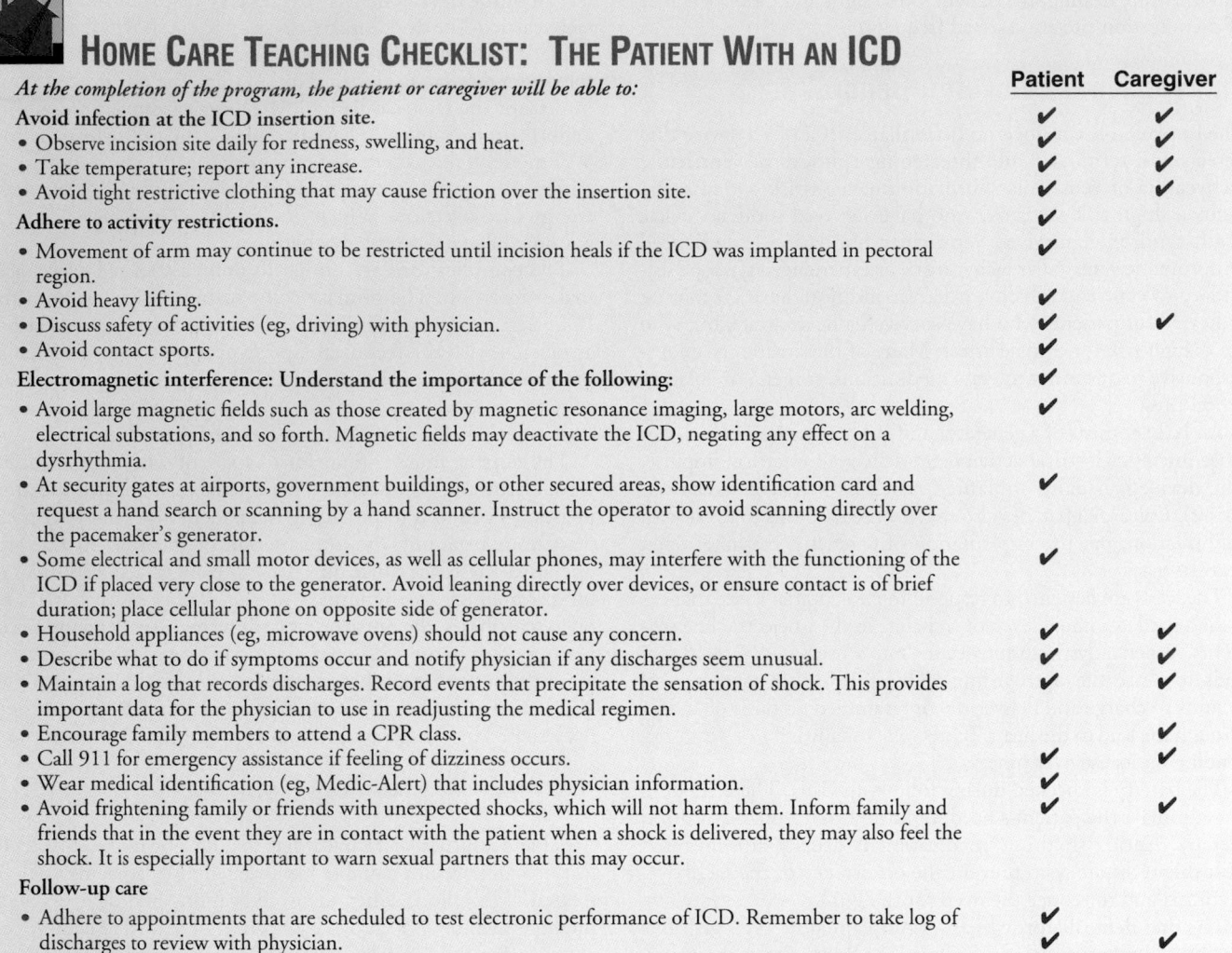

At the completion of the program, the patient or caregiver will be able to:	Patient	Caregiver
Avoid infection at the ICD insertion site.	✔	✔
• Observe incision site daily for redness, swelling, and heat.	✔	✔
• Take temperature; report any increase.	✔	✔
• Avoid tight restrictive clothing that may cause friction over the insertion site.	✔	✔
Adhere to activity restrictions.	✔	
• Movement of arm may continue to be restricted until incision heals if the ICD was implanted in pectoral region.	✔	
• Avoid heavy lifting.	✔	
• Discuss safety of activities (eg, driving) with physician.	✔	✔
• Avoid contact sports.	✔	
Electromagnetic interference: Understand the importance of the following:	✔	
• Avoid large magnetic fields such as those created by magnetic resonance imaging, large motors, arc welding, electrical substations, and so forth. Magnetic fields may deactivate the ICD, negating any effect on a dysrhythmia.	✔	
• At security gates at airports, government buildings, or other secured areas, show identification card and request a hand search or scanning by a hand scanner. Instruct the operator to avoid scanning directly over the pacemaker's generator.	✔	
• Some electrical and small motor devices, as well as cellular phones, may interfere with the functioning of the ICD if placed very close to the generator. Avoid leaning directly over devices, or ensure contact is of brief duration; place cellular phone on opposite side of generator.	✔	
• Household appliances (eg, microwave ovens) should not cause any concern.	✔	✔
• Describe what to do if symptoms occur and notify physician if any discharges seem unusual.	✔	✔
• Maintain a log that records discharges. Record events that precipitate the sensation of shock. This provides important data for the physician to use in readjusting the medical regimen.	✔	✔
• Encourage family members to attend a CPR class.		✔
• Call 911 for emergency assistance if feeling of dizziness occurs.	✔	✔
• Wear medical identification (eg, Medic-Alert) that includes physician information.	✔	
• Avoid frightening family or friends with unexpected shocks, which will not harm them. Inform family and friends that in the event they are in contact with the patient when a shock is delivered, they may also feel the shock. It is especially important to warn sexual partners that this may occur.	✔	✔
Follow-up care	✔	
• Adhere to appointments that are scheduled to test electronic performance of ICD. Remember to take log of discharges to review with physician.	✔	✔
• Attend an ICD support group within the area.	✔	

cles disappear, except for that between the AV node and the bundle of His. In some, however, these connections are not severed and normal heart muscle between the atrium and ventricles remains, providing an accessory electrical pathway or a tract through which the impulse can bypass the AV node. These pathways can be located in several different areas. If the patient develops atrial fibrillation, the impulse may be conducted into the ventricle at a rate of 300 times per minute or more, which can lead to ventricular fibrillation and sudden cardiac death. Tachycardia associated with specific ECG findings (shortened PR interval, prolonged QRS duration, and slurring [called a delta wave] of the initial QRS deflection) is called Wolff-Parkinson-White syndrome (Fig. 24-33).

Ablation may be accomplished by three different methods: cryoablation, electrical ablation, or radiofrequency ablation. Cryoablation involves placing a special probe, cooled to a temperature of −60°C (−76°F), on the endocardium at the site of the dysrhythmia's origin for 2 minutes. The frozen area becomes a small scar and the origin of the dysrhythmia is eliminated.

In electrical ablation, a catheter is placed at or near the origin of the dysrhythmia, and one to four shocks of 100 to 300 joules are administered through the catheter directly to the endocardium and surrounding tissue. The cardiac tissue burns and scars, thus eliminating the source of the dysrhythmia.

Radiofrequency ablation involves placing a special catheter at or near the origin of the dysrhythmia. High-frequency sound waves are passed through the catheter, destroying the dysrhythmic tissue. The tissue damage is more specific to the dysrhythmic tissue, with less trauma to the surrounding cardiac tissue than occurs with cryoablation or electrical ablation.

During the ablation procedure, defibrillation pads, an automatic blood pressure cuff, and a pulse oximeter are placed on the patient, and an indwelling urinary catheter is inserted. The patient is given light sedation, and the ablation catheter is placed at the origin of the dysrhythmia. With radiofrequency ablation, a high-frequency, low-energy current is passed through the catheter, causing thermal injury and cellular changes and resulting in localized destruction and scarring. An electrophysiologic study and an attempt to induce the dysrhythmia are performed. Multiple ablations may be necessary. Successful ablation is achieved when the dysrhythmia cannot be induced. The patient is monitored for another 30 to 60 minutes and then retested to ensure that the dysrhythmia will not recur.

Postprocedural care is similar to that for an electrophysiologic study, with the exception that the patient may be monitored more closely, depending on the time needed for recovery from sedation.

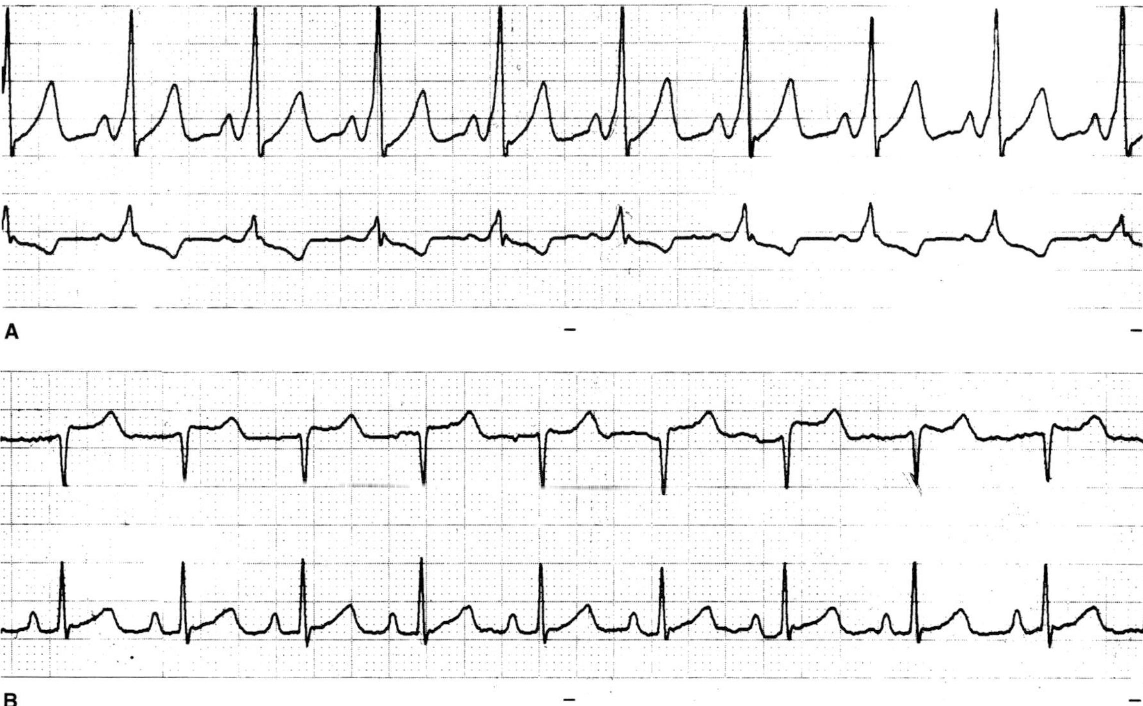

FIGURE 24•33 Wolfe-Parkinson-White syndrome. (**A**) Sinus rhythm. Note the short PR interval, slurred initial upstroke of the QRS complex (delta wave) and a prolonged QRS duration. (**B**) Rhythm strip of same patient following ablation. ECG strips courtesy of Linda Ardini and Catherine Berkmeyer, Inova Fairfax Hospital, Falls Church, VA.

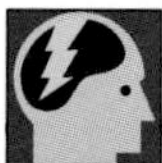

Critical Thinking Exercises

1. You are working in a clinic when a patient enters complaining of dizziness and fatigue. She tells you that she has been diagnosed as having an atrial dysrhythmia. How would you focus your assessment of this patient, and what key assessment factors would you highlight in reporting to the primary care provider?
2. You are caring for a patient who is being prepared for cardioversion. He indicates that he is very anxious about the procedure because it is the same as the "defibrillation" that his brother had when he died. In offering an explanation to the patient, how would you describe the differences in the two treatments?

References and Selected Readings

BOOKS AND PAMPHLETS

American Heart Association. (1997). *Advanced cardiac life support.* Dallas: Author.

Braunwald, E. (1997). *Heart disease: A textbook of cardiovascular medicine.* Philadelphia: W. B. Saunders.

Braunwald, E. (1996). *Atlas of heart diseases. Arrhythmias: Electrophysiologic principles* (Vol. IX). St. Louis: Mosby.

Conover, M. B. (1996). *Understanding electrocardiography* (7th ed.). St. Louis: Mosby.

Kinney, M., et al. (1998). *AACN Clinical reference for critical care nursing* (4th ed.). St. Louis: Mosby.

Marriott, H. J., & Conover, M. B. (1998). *Advanced concepts in arrhythmias.* St. Louis: Mosby.

Schlant, R. C., et al. (1994). *Hurst's The heart: Arteries and veins.* New York: McGraw-Hill.

Woods, S. L., et al. (1995). *Cardiac nursing* (3rd ed.). Philadelphia: J. B. Lippincott.

JOURNALS

Asterisks indicate nursing research articles.

Bernstein, J. E. (1997). Recognizing when long QT intervals mean trouble. *Nursing '97, 27*(4), 32aa–32ff.

Brannon, P. H., & Johnson, R. (1992). The internal cardioverter defibrillator: Patient–family teaching. *Focus on Critical Care, 19*(1), 41–46.

Burke, L. J. (1996). Securing life through technology acceptance: The first six months after transvenous internal cardioverter defibrillator implantation. *Heart and Lung, 25*(5), 352–366.

Collins, M. (1994). When your patient has an implantable cardioverter-defibrillator. *American Journal of Nursing, 94*(3), 34–38.

*Craney, J. M., et al. (1997). Implantable cardioverter defibrillators: Physical and psychosocial outcomes. *American Journal of Critical Care, 6*(6), 445–451.

Kellen, J. C., Ettinger, A., Todd, L., et al. (1996). The cardiac arrhythmia suppression trial: Implications for nursing practice. *American Journal of Critical Care, 5*(1), 19–25.

Knight, L., et al. (1997). Caring for patients with third-generation implantable cardioverter defibrillators: From decision to implant to patient's return home. *Critical Care Nursing, 17*(5), 46–63.

McCauley, K. M., Lloyd, C. T., & Doherty, J. U. (1997). Dysrhythmia update. Case study: Analysis of dual chamber rate responsive pacing in atrial fibrillation. *Journal of Cardiovascular Nursing, 11*(3), 93–96.

Petrosky-Pacini, A. J. (1996). The automatic implantable cardioverter defibrillator in home care. *Home Health Nursing, 14*(4), 238–243.

Scrima, D. (1993). Managing dobutamine infusions. *MedSurg Nursing, 2*(6), 459–465.
Smith, D. F., & Bumann, R. (1993). Assessing and treating decreased cardiac output. *MedSurg Nursing, 2*(5), 351–357.
Stahl, L. (1995). How to manage common arrhythmias in medical patients. *American Journal of Nursing, 95*(3), 36–41.
*Tyndall, A., Nystrom, K. V., & Funk, M. (1997). Nausea and vomiting in patients undergoing radiofrequency catheter ablation. *American Journal of Critical Care, 6*(6), 437–444.

Resources

National Heart, Lung, and Blood Institute, National Institutes of Health, Building 31, Room 5A52, Bethesda, MD 20892
American Heart Association, 7320 Greenville Ave., Dallas, TX 75231; 1-800-242-8721; http://www.americanheart.org/aha.html
Coronary Club, 9500 Euclid Ave., Cleveland, OH 44106; 1-800-478-4255; http://www.heartline-news.org/HL02/02.html
Heartlife, P.O. Box 54305, Atlanta, GA 30308; 1-800-241-6993

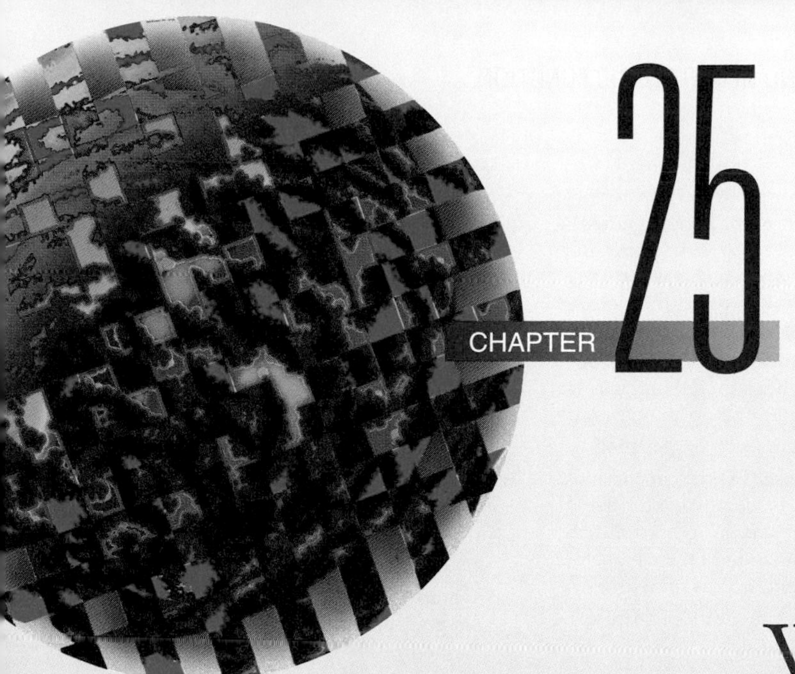

Management of Patients With Coronary Vascular Disorders

Learning Objectives

On completion of this chapter, the learner will be able to:

1. Describe the relationship between coronary atherosclerosis, angina pectoris, and myocardial infarction.
2. Develop teaching plans for patients with angina pectoris and myocardial infarction.
3. Use the nursing process as a framework for care of patients with angina pectoris.
4. Describe the essential elements of nursing assessment, patient teaching, and psychological support during preparation of the patient for cardiac surgery.
5. Use the nursing process as a framework for the care of patients before and after cardiac surgery.
6. Describe the postoperative management of the patient who has had cardiac surgery.
7. Identify the possible complications of cardiac surgery, the measures to prevent these complications, and assessment parameters appropriate for their identification.
8. Use the nursing process as a framework for care of patients with myocardial infarction.

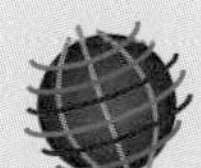

In the past, identification and treatment of heart disease focused on white, middle-aged men. More recently, however, studies have shown that other segments of the population are also seriously affected by cardiac problems. Cardiovascular disease is the leading cause of death in the United States for men and women of all racial and ethnic groups, and more women die of cardiovascular disease than of all the types of cancers combined.

GLOSSARY

angina pectoris: chest pain brought on by physical or emotional stress, relieved by rest or medication

atherosclerosis: abnormal accumulation of lipid deposits and fibrous tissue within arterial walls and lumens

atheromas: fibrous caps composed of smooth muscle cells that form over lipid deposits within arterial vessels and that protrude into the lumen of the vessel, narrowing it and obstructing blood flow; also called plaques

contractility: ability of the cardiac muscle to shorten in response to an electrical impulse

coronary artery bypass graft (CABG): a surgical procedure in which a blood vessel from another part of the body is grafted onto the occluded blood vessel above and below the occlusion in such a way that coronary blood flow bypasses the blockage.

creatine kinase (CK): an enzyme found in human tissues; one of the three types of CK is specific to heart muscle and may be used as an indicator of heart muscle injury

ischemia: insufficient tissue oxygenation

lactic dehydrogenase (LDH): an enzyme found in human tissues; two of the five types of LDH are specific to heart muscle. Comparing the amount of these two types of LDH may indicate heart muscle injury

myocardial infarction: death of heart tissue caused by ischemia

percutaneous transluminal coronary angioplasty (PTCA): an interventional procedure used to improve coronary artery blood flow by breaking the atheroma and opening the vessel lumen

sudden cardiac death: immediate cessation of heart activity

thrombolytic: an agent or process that breaks down blood clots

troponin: myocardial protein; measurement is used to indicate heart muscle injury

vasoconstrictor: an agent (usually a drug) that narrows the blood vessel lumen

vasodilator: an agent (usually a drug) that enlarges blood vessel lumens

CORONARY ARTERY DISEASE

The most prevalent type of cardiovascular disease is coronary artery disease (CAD). For this reason it is important for nurses to become familiar with the various types of cardiac problems and the methods for assessing, preventing, and treating these disorders, both medically and surgically.

Coronary Atherosclerosis

The most common heart disease in the United States is **atherosclerosis**, which is an abnormal accumulation of lipid, or fatty, substances and fibrous tissue in the vessel wall. These substances create blockages, or narrow the vessel, in a way that reduces blood flow to the myocardium. Recent studies (Crea et al., 1997; Kinlay & Ganz, 1997; Leibovitz et al., 1997; Mehta, Saldeen, & Rand, 1998) now indicate that atherosclerosis involves a repetitious inflammatory response to artery wall injury and an alteration in the biophysical and biochemical properties of the arterial walls. Although authorities disagree about how atherosclerosis begins, they agree that atherosclerosis is a progressive disease that can be curtailed and in some cases reversed.

Pathophysiology

Atherosclerosis begins as fatty streaks, lipids that are deposited on the intima of the arterial wall. Although they are thought to be the precursors of atherosclerosis, fatty streaks are not uncommon, even in childhood. Moreover, not all develop into more advanced lesions. It is not fully known why some fatty streaks continue to develop, but it is agreed that both genetic and environmental factors are involved. The continued development of atherosclerosis involves an inflammatory response. T lymphocytes and monocytes (that become macrophages) infiltrate the area to ingest the lipids and then die; this causes smooth muscle cells within the vessel to proliferate and form a fibrous cap to the dead fatty core. These deposits, called **atheromas** or plaques, protrude into the lumen of the vessel, narrowing it and obstructing blood flow (Fig. 25-1). If the fibrous cap of the plaque is thick and the lipid pool remains relatively stable, it is resistant to the stress from blood flow and vessel movement. If the cap is thin, the lipid core may grow, causing it to rupture and hemorrhage into the plaque, thereby allowing a thrombus to develop. The thrombus may obstruct blood flow, leading to **sudden cardiac death** or an acute **myocardial infarction** (MI), which is the death of heart tissue resulting from ischemia.

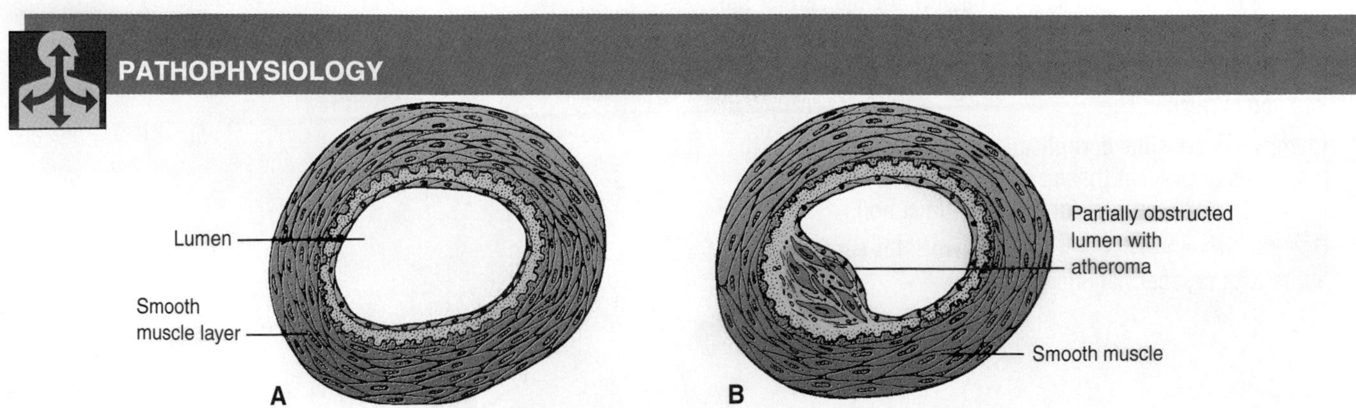

FIGURE 25•1 Cross-section of a normal and an atherosclerotic artery. (**A**) Cross-section of normal artery in which the lumen is fully patent, or open. (**B**) Cross-section of artery with diminished patency resulting from atheroma.

The anatomic structure of the coronary arteries makes them particularly susceptible to the mechanisms of atherosclerosis. As Figure 25-2 shows, they twist and turn as they supply blood to the heart, thereby creating sites susceptible to atheroma development. Although heart disease is most often due to atherosclerosis of the coronary arteries, other phenomena also decrease blood flow to the heart. Examples include vasospasm (a sudden constriction or narrowing) of a coronary artery, myocardial trauma from internal or external forces, structural disease, congenital anomalies, decreased oxygen supply (from acute blood loss, anemia, or low blood pressure), and increased demand for oxygen (from rapid heart rate, thyrotoxicosis, or ingestion of cocaine).

Clinical Manifestations

Coronary atherosclerosis produces symptoms and complications according to the degree of narrowing of the arterial lumen, thrombus formation, and obstruction of blood flow to the myocardium. This impediment to blood flow is usually progressive, and the inadequate blood supply that results deprives the muscle cells of oxygen needed for their survival. The condition is known as **ischemia**. **Angina pectoris** refers to recurrent chest pain that is brought about by physical exertion or emotional stress and relieved promptly by rest or medication. Most often, but not always, angina pectoris is caused by significant coronary atherosclerosis. If the decrease in blood supply is significant, of significant duration, or both, irreversible damage and death of myocardial cells, MI, may result. Over time, irreversibly damaged myocardium undergoes degeneration and is replaced by scar tissue, causing varying degrees of myocardial dysfunction. Significant myocardial damage may cause inadequate cardiac output—in other words, the heart cannot support the body's needs for blood. A decrease in blood supply from CAD may even cause the heart to stop immediately, an event that is called **sudden cardiac death**.

The most common manifestation of myocardial ischemia is acute onset of chest pain. However, an epidemiologic study of the people in Framingham, Massachusetts, showed that nearly 15% of men and women who had MI were totally asymptomatic (Kannel, 1986). Other clinical manifestations of CAD may be abnormalities signaled by changes on the electrocardiogram (ECG), dysrhythmias, and sudden death.

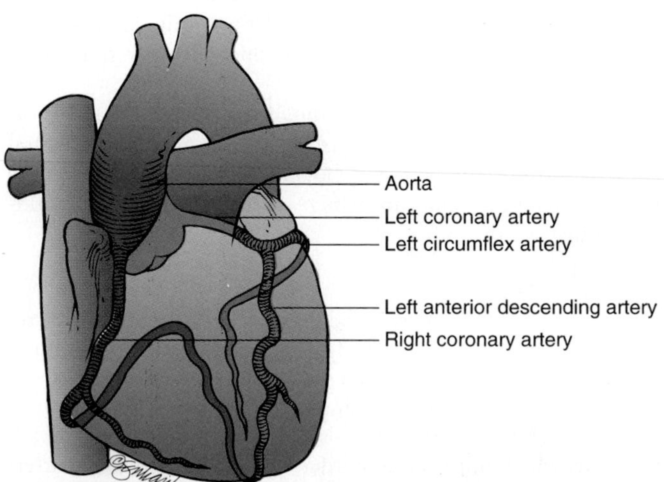

FIGURE 25•2 Angles of the coronary arteries. The many angles and curves of the coronary arteries contribute to the vessels' susceptibility to atheromatous plaques. Arteries shown in orange supply the posterior wall of the heart.

Risk Factors

Epidemiologic studies point to several factors that increase the probability that heart disease will develop. The incidence of CAD and MI increases with age. More than half of the people with CAD are at least 65 years old. A positive family history is also associated with a higher risk of heart disease.

Prevention

Four modifiable risk factors—cholesterol abnormalities, cigarette smoking, hypertension, and diabetes mellitus—have been cited as major causes of CAD and its consequent complications. They have received a great deal of attention in health promotion programs.

HIGH BLOOD CHOLESTEROL LEVEL

The association of a high blood cholesterol level with heart disease is well established and accepted. The metabolism of fats is highly complex and difficult to understand, but several key components are important in understanding the development of heart disease.

Fats, which are insoluble in water, are encased in water-soluble lipoproteins to allow them to be transported within a circulatory system that is water-based. Three elements of fat metabolism—

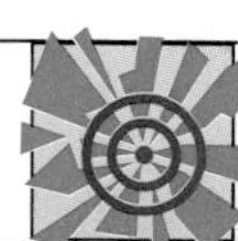

Risk Factors for CORONARY HEART DISEASE

A modifiable risk factor is one over which individuals may exercise control, such as by changing a lifestyle or personal habit or by using medication. A nonmodifiable risk factor is a circumstance over which individuals have no control, such as age or heredity. A risk factor may operate independently or in tandem with other risk factors. The more risk factors individuals have, the greater the likelihood of coronary artery disease. Those at risk are advised to seek regular medical examinations and, to engage in "heart-healthy" behavior, a deliberate effort to reduce the number and extent of risks.

Nonmodifiable Risk Factors

Family history of coronary heart disease
Increasing age
Gender (heart disease occurs three times more often in men than in premenopausal women)
Race (higher incidence of heart disease in African Americans than in whites)

Modifiable Risk Factors

High blood cholesterol level
Cigarette smoking
Hypertension
Diabetes mellitus
Lack of estrogen in women
Physical inactivity
Obesity
Stress

total cholesterol, low-density lipoprotein (LDL), and high-density lipoprotein (HDL)—are primary factors affecting the development of heart disease. Keeping the serum levels of total cholesterol and the balance of LDL with HDL within a therapeutic range is the goal of dietary management of heart disease. A cholesterol level of less than 200 mg/dL and a ratio of LDL to HDL of less than 3.5 to 1 is considered acceptable.

LDL exerts a harmful effect on the arterial wall and accelerates atherosclerosis. In contrast, HDL promotes the use of total cholesterol by transporting LDL to the liver, where it is biodegraded and then excreted. The desired goal is to have low LDL values and high HDL values. The desired level of LDL depends on the patient:

- Less than 160 mg/dL for primary prevention in patients with one or no risk factors
- Less than 130 mg/dL for primary prevention in patients with two or more risk factors
- Less than 100 mg/dL for secondary prevention

The level of HDL should exceed 35 mg/dL and should ideally be more than 60 mg/dL. A high HDL level is a strong negative risk factor for heart disease.

Serum cholesterol levels can usually be controlled by diet and exercise. Reducing the amount of fat eaten daily will reduce the fat available for metabolism and conversion to cholesterol. The HDL level can be increased by smoking cessation, weight loss, and exercise. The LDL level can be decreased by a low-fat diet, smoking cessation, and, if needed, medication therapy.

DIET

Dietary control has been made easier because food manufacturers are required to provide comprehensive nutritional data on product labels. The label information of interest to a person attempting to control cholesterol is as follows:

- Serving size, expressed in household measure
- Amount of fat per serving
- Amount of saturated fat per serving

The average American diet contains about 33% fat. The American Heart Association (AHA) recommends a diet that contains less than 30% fat (with less than 10% from saturated fat) and less than 300 mg of cholesterol for the general public. If the person has elevated LDL or low HDL levels or has been diagnosed with CAD, the AHA recommends a diet containing less than 30% fat (with less than 7% from saturated fat) and less than 200 mg of cholesterol. Many resources are available to assist people who are attempting to control their cholesterol levels. Registered dietitians, self-help groups, and literature from the AHA are a few examples.

Soluble dietary fiber may also help lower cholesterol levels. Soluble fibers such as pectin (found in fresh fruit) enhance the excretion of metabolized cholesterol. The ability of fiber to reduce serum cholesterol continues to be investigated. Intake of at least 25 to 30 grams of fiber each day is recommended.

MEDICATIONS

Medications are used in some instances to control cholesterol levels. If diet alone cannot normalize serum cholesterol levels, several medications have a synergistic effect with the prescribed diet. These agents, which help reduce an elevated LDH level, are usually grouped into four types:

- HMG-CoA reductase inhibitors or statins (eg, lovastatin, pravastatin, and simvastatin), which block cholesterol synthesis
- Niacins, which decrease lipoprotein synthesis
- Fibrates (eg, clofibrate and gemfibrozil), which decrease the synthesis of cholesterol
- Bile acid sequestrants or resins (eg, cholestyramine), which bind cholesterol in the intestine, increase its breakdown, and lower LDL levels

Significant side effects can occur from using these medications. Medication therapy is, therefore, reserved for at-risk patients and is not regarded as a substitute for dietary modification. The usefulness of medications in reversing heart disease remains under scrutiny, but it is broadly accepted that lowering LDL levels can have a significant impact on reducing the risk of heart disease.

Patients with elevated cholesterol levels need to be monitored for compliance with the medical plan, the effect on cholesterol levels, and the development of side effects from cholesterol-lowering medications. Home test kits are available for monitoring blood cholesterol levels between physician visits. The kits are available without a prescription, but patients should use them under the management of a physician.

CIGARETTE SMOKING

Cigarette smoking contributes to the development and severity of CAD in three ways. First, the inhalation of smoke increases the blood carbon monoxide level, causing hemoglobin, the oxygen-carrying component of blood, to combine more readily with carbon monoxide than with oxygen. A decreased amount of available oxygen may decrease the heart's ability to pump.

Second, the nicotinic acid in tobacco triggers the release of catecholamines, which raise both heart rate and blood pressure. Nicotinic acid can also cause the coronary arteries to constrict. Smokers have a tenfold increase in risk for sudden cardiac death. The increase in catecholamines may be a factor in the increased incidence of sudden cardiac death.

Third, cigarette smoking causes a detrimental vascular response and increases platelet adhesion, leading to a higher probability of thrombus formation. A person with increased risk for heart disease is encouraged to stop smoking through any means possible: counseling, consistent motivation and reinforcement messages, support groups, and medications. Some people have found complementary therapies (eg, acupuncture, guided imagery, hypnosis) to be helpful. People who stop smoking reduce their risk of heart disease by 30% to 50% within the first year, and the risk continues to decline as long as they refrain from smoking.

Exposure to other smokers' smoke (passive or second-hand smoke) is believed to cause heart disease in nonsmokers. Oral contraceptive use by women who smoke is inadvisable because these medications significantly increase the risk of CAD and sudden cardiac death.

HYPERTENSION

Hypertension is defined as blood pressure measurements that repeatedly exceed 140/90 mm Hg. Longstanding elevated blood pressure may result in increased stiffness of the vessel walls, leading to vessel injury and a resulting inflammatory response within the intima. Hypertension can also increase the work of the left ventricle, which must pump harder to eject blood into the arteries. Over time, the increased workload causes the heart to enlarge and thicken (hypertrophy), a condition that may eventually lead to cardiac failure.

Early detection of high blood pressure and compliance with a therapeutic regimen can prevent the serious consequences associated with untreated elevated blood pressure. Blood pressure is discussed in detail in Chapter 23.

DIABETES MELLITUS

The relationship between diabetes mellitus and heart disease has been substantiated. Hyperglycemia fosters increased platelet aggregation and altered red blood cell function, which can lead to thrombus formation. It has also been suggested that insulin injures the vessel wall, leading to the inflammatory response. Controlling hyperglycemia without modifying other risk factors does not reduce the risk of heart disease. If other risk factors such as high cholesterol levels are present, they must be brought under control.

GENDER AND ESTROGEN LEVEL

In women younger than age 60, the incidence of CAD is significantly lower than in men. However, after age 60, the incidence is approximately equal. The difference may be related to estrogen. Postmenopausal women who take estrogen have lower rates of CAD than women who do not, although estrogen use may increase the risk of breast cancer. Unopposed estrogen can also increase the risk of endometrial cancer in women with an intact uterus; estrogen is usually combined with progestin therapy for these women. The patient's risk of cancer should be assessed against the risk of CAD when making the decision for estrogen replacement therapy.

Because heart disease used to be considered to affect white men primarily, the disease was not as readily recognized and treated in women. Women tend to have a higher incidence of death and complications from CAD. Black women have a mortality rate twice that of white women. Women tend not to recognize the symptoms as early as men and to wait longer to report their symptoms and seek medical assistance. In the past, women were less likely than men to be referred for coronary artery diagnostic procedures, to receive medical therapy (eg, nitroglycerin and **thrombolytic** therapy to break down the blood clots that cause acute MI), and to be treated with invasive interventions (eg, angioplasty). It is hoped that with better education of the general public and health care professionals, gender and racial difference will have little influence on the diagnosis, treatment, and incidence of complications of heart disease.

BEHAVIOR PATTERNS

Most clinicians believe that stress and certain behaviors contribute to the pathogenesis of CAD and a cardiac event, especially in women. Psychological and epidemiologic studies describe behaviors that characterize people who are prone to heart disease: excessive competitiveness, a sense of time urgency (or impatience), aggressiveness, and hostility. A person with these behaviors is classified as type A coronary-prone. The type A coronary-prone classification may not be as significant as was once thought; evidence of its precise role remains inconclusive. To be on the safer side, however, such a person may be wise to alter behaviors and responses to triggering events and to reduce other risk factors. Nurses can assist these people by teaching them cognitive restructuring and relaxation techniques.

Angina Pectoris

Angina pectoris is a clinical syndrome usually characterized by episodes or paroxysms of pain or pressure in the anterior chest. The cause is usually insufficient coronary blood flow. The insufficient flow results in a decreased oxygen supply to meet an increased myocardial demand for oxygen in response to physical exertion or emotional stress. In other words, the need for oxygen exceeds the supply.

Pathophysiology

Angina is usually caused by atherosclerotic disease. Almost invariably, angina is associated with a significant obstruction of a major coronary artery. The characteristics of the various types of angina are listed in Chart 25-1. Several factors are associated with typical anginal pain:

- Physical exertion, which can precipitate an attack by increasing myocardial oxygen demands
- Exposure to cold, which can cause vasoconstriction and an elevated blood pressure, with increased oxygen demand
- Eating a heavy meal, which increases the blood flow to the mesenteric area for digestion, thereby reducing the blood supply available to the heart muscle. In a severely compromised heart, the shunting of blood for digestion can be sufficient to induce anginal pain.
- Stress or any emotion-provoking situation, causing the release of adrenaline and increasing blood pressure, which may accelerate the heart rate and thus increase myocardial workload

Identifying angina requires a careful history. Effective treatment begins with reducing the demands placed on the heart and teaching the patient about the condition.

Clinical Manifestations

Ischemia of the heart muscle may produce pain or other symptoms, varying in severity from a feeling of indigestion to a choking or heavy sensation in the upper chest that ranges from discomfort to agonizing pain accompanied by severe apprehension and a feeling of impending death. The pain is often felt deep in the chest behind the upper or middle third of the sternum (retrosternal). Typically, the pain or discomfort is poorly localized and may radiate to the neck, jaw, shoulders, and inner aspects of the upper arms, usually the left arm. The patient often feels a tightness or a heavy, choking, or strangling sensation that has a viselike, insistent quality.

The patient with diabetes mellitus may not have severe pain with angina because the neuropathy that accompanies diabetes can interfere with neuroreceptors, thus dulling the pain.

A feeling of weakness or numbness in the arms, wrists, and hands may accompany the pain, as may shortness of breath, pallor, diaphoresis, dizziness or light-headedness, and nausea and

CHART 25•1 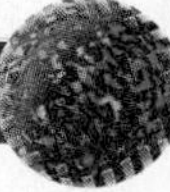 **Types of Angina**

- **Stable angina:** predictable and consistent pain that occurs on exertion and is relieved by rest
- **Unstable angina** (also called preinfarction angina or crescendo angina): symptoms occur when the patient is at rest; symptoms occur more frequently and last longer. The threshold for pain is lower as well.
- **Intractable or refractory angina:** severe incapacitating chest pain
- **Variant angina** (also called Prinzmetal's angina): pain at rest with reversible ST-segment elevation; thought to be due to coronary artery vasospasm
- **Silent ischemia:** objective evidence of ischemia (such as ECG changes with a stress test), but patient reports no symptoms

vomiting. Anxiety may accompany the pain. An important characteristic of anginal pain is that it promptly subsides with rest or nitroglycerin.

Gerontologic Considerations

The elderly person with angina may not exhibit the typical pain profile because of the diminished responses of neurotransmitters that occur in the aging process. Often the pain is atypical—for example, pain may be in the jaw rather than the chest, or fainting may occur. When exposed to cold temperatures, elderly people may experience anginal symptoms more quickly than younger people because they have less subcutaneous fat to provide insulation. They should be encouraged to wear extra clothing and to recognize feelings of weakness as an indication that they should rest or take prescribed medications.

Assessment and Diagnostic Findings

The diagnosis of angina is often made by evaluating the clinical manifestations of pain and the patient's history. ECG changes are also helpful in making the diagnosis, but obtaining an ECG when the patient is complaining of pain may be difficult. The patient may undergo an exercise or pharmacologic stress test in which the heart is monitored by ECG, echocardiogram, or both. The patient may also be referred for an echocardiogram, nuclear scan, or invasive procedures (eg, cardiac catheterization, coronary artery angiography).

Medical Management

The objectives of medical management of angina are to decrease the oxygen demands of the myocardium and to increase the oxygen supply. Medically, these objectives are met through pharmacologic therapy and control of risk factors.

Revascularization procedures that restore the blood supply to the myocardium include **coronary artery bypass graft** surgery (CABG) and invasive interventional procedures, such as **percutaneous transluminal coronary angioplasty** (PTCA), a procedure used to improve coronary artery blood flow by breaking the atheroma and opening the lumen of the vessel; intracoronary stents; and rotational atherectomy. All are discussed below.

A newer procedure, called minimally invasive direct coronary artery bypass (MIDCAB), involves special bypass surgery followed immediately or the next day with one of the invasive interventional techniques (eg, PTCA). Because this approach to treating CAD combines cardiac surgery and an invasive intervention, it has been termed "the hybrid."

Pharmacologic Therapy

Among medications used to control angina are nitroglycerin, beta-adrenergic blocking agents, calcium channel blockers, and antiplatelet agents, such as aspirin, ticlopidine, and heparin.

NITROGLYCERIN

The nitrates remain the mainstay for treating angina pectoris. A vasoactive agent, nitroglycerin (Nitrostat, Nitrol, Nitrobid IV) is administered to reduce myocardial oxygen consumption, which decreases ischemia and relieves pain. Nitroglycerin dilates primarily the veins and also the arteries. It also helps to increase coronary blood flow by preventing vasospasm and increasing perfusion through the collateral vessels.

Dilation of the veins causes venous pooling of blood throughout the body. As a result, less blood returns to the heart, and filling pressure (preload) is reduced. If the patient is hypovolemic (does not have adequate circulating fluid volume), the decrease in filling pressure can cause a significant decrease in cardiac output and blood pressure.

Nitrates also relax the systemic arteriolar bed and lower blood pressure (decreased afterload). Nitrates may increase blood flow to diseased coronary arteries and through collateral coronary arteries, arteries that have been underused until the body recognizes poorly perfused areas. These effects decrease myocardial oxygen requirements and increase oxygen supply, bringing about a more favorable balance between supply and demand.

Nitroglycerin may be administered by several routes: sublingual, topical, and intravenous. Sublingual nitroglycerin is generally placed under the tongue or in the cheek (buccal pouch) and alleviates the pain of ischemia within 3 minutes. Topical nitroglycerin is also fast-acting and is a convenient way to administer the medication. Both routes are suitable for patients who self-administer the medication. (For more information, see the accompanying chart.)

Intravenous nitroglycerin, however, is usually administered by the nurse. A continuous or intermittent intravenous infusion of nitroglycerin may be administered to the hospitalized patient with recurring signs and symptoms of ischemia or after a revascularization procedure. The amount of nitroglycerin administered is based on the patient's symptoms while avoiding side effects such as hypotension. Generally, once the patient is symptom-free, the patient may be switched to a topical preparation within 24 hours.

BETA-ADRENERGIC BLOCKING AGENTS

Beta blockers such as propranolol (Inderal) and atenolol (Tenormin) appear to reduce myocardial oxygen consumption by blocking the beta-adrenergic sympathetic stimulation to the heart. The result is a reduction in heart rate, blood pressure, and myocardial **contractility** (force of contraction) that establishes a more favorable balance between myocardial oxygen needs and the amount of oxygen available. This helps to control chest pain and allows the patient to work or exercise.

Cardiac side effects include hypotension, bradycardia, and worsening of congestive heart failure. If a beta blocker is given intravenously for an acute cardiac event, the ECG, blood pressure, and heart rate are monitored closely for up to 2 hours after the medication has been administered. Because some beta-blockers also affect the beta-adrenergic receptors in the bronchioles, causing bronchoconstriction, they are contraindicated in patients with significant pulmonary constrictive diseases, such as asthma. Other side effects include worsening of hyperlipidemia, depression, fatigue, decreased libido, and masking of symptoms of hypoglycemia.

Patients taking beta-blockers are cautioned not to stop taking them abruptly, because angina may worsen and MI may develop. Beta-blocker therapy needs to be decreased gradually over several days before discontinuing it. Diabetic patients on beta-blocker therapy are instructed to assess their blood glucose levels more often to identify their hypoglycemia that may result from the medication.

CALCIUM CHANNEL BLOCKING AGENTS

Calcium channel blockers (also called calcium ion antagonists) have different effects. Some decrease sinoatrial node automaticity and atrioventricular node conduction, resulting in a slower

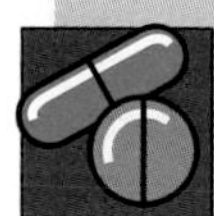

PHARMACOLOGY

Self-Administration of Nitroglycerin

Most patients with angina pectoris must self-administer nitroglycerin on a day-to-day basis. A key nursing role in such cases is educating patients about the medication and how to take it.

Teaching About Sublingual Nitroglycerin

- Instruct the patient to make sure the mouth is moist, the tongue is still, and saliva is not swallowed until the nitroglycerin tablet dissolves. If the pain is severe, the patient can crush the tablet between the teeth to hasten sublingual absorption.
- Advise the patient to carry the medication at all times as a precaution. However, because nitroglycerin is very unstable, it should be carried securely in its original container (a capped dark glass bottle); it should never be removed and stored in metal or plastic pillboxes.
- Explain that nitroglycerin is volatile and is inactivated by heat, moisture, air, light, and time. Instruct the patient to renew the nitroglycerin supply every 6 months.
- Inform the patient that the medication should be taken in anticipation of any activity that may produce pain. Because nitroglycerin increases tolerance for exercise and stress when taken prophylactically (ie, before angina-producing activity, such as exercise, stair-climbing, or sexual intercourse), it is best taken before pain develops.
- Recommend that the patient note how long it takes for the nitroglycerin to relieve the discomfort. If pain persists after taking three sublingual tablets at 5-minute intervals, advise the patient to go to the nearest emergency care facility.
- Discuss possible side effects of nitroglycerin, including flushing, throbbing headache, hypotension, and tachycardia. Explain also that the use of long-acting nitrate preparations is controversial. Isosorbide dinitrate (Isordil), for example, appears to be effective for up to 2 hours if taken sublingually but has an uncertain effect if taken orally.

Teaching About Topical Nitroglycerin

Nitroglycerin is also available in a lanolin-petrolatum base that is applied to the skin as a paste or a patch. Patients who use topical nitroglycerin need additional instruction.

- Advise the patient to read the instructions that accompany the product, because instructions vary according to the preparation. Also remind the patient to rotate the site of application to avoid skin irritation.
- Explain that the area of application needs to be an area that is well perfused for absorption to occur. Therefore, the medication should not be applied to areas with extensive body hair or scar tissue.
- Recommend that the patient protect clothing from the oil base in the paste.
- Explain that a long-term equally spaced dosing schedule of application of topical nitroglycerin is generally avoided to prevent tolerance (when the body does not respond as well to the same amount of medication). Most physicians prescribe application of topical nitroglycerin paste three or four times daily or every 6 hours (excluding the midnight dose), and the nitroglycerin patch to be applied every morning and removed at 10 PM. This dosing regimen allows for a 6- to 8-hour nitrate-free period to prevent the body's development of tolerance.

heart rate and a decrease in the strength of the heart muscle contraction (negative inotropic effect). These effects decrease the workload of the heart. Calcium channel blockers also relax the blood vessels, causing a decrease in blood pressure and an increase in coronary artery perfusion. Calcium channel blockers increase myocardial oxygen supply by dilating the smooth muscle wall of the coronary arterioles; they decrease myocardial oxygen demands by reducing systemic arterial pressure and thus the workload of the left ventricle.

The three calcium channel blockers most commonly used are nifedipine (Procardia), verapamil (Calan), and diltiazem (Cardizem). They may be used by patients who cannot take beta-blockers, who develop significant side effects from beta-blockers and/or nitrates, or who still have pain despite beta-blocker and nitroglycerin therapy. Calcium channel blockers are used to prevent and treat vasospasm, which commonly occurs after an invasive interventional procedure.

Calcium channel blockers should be avoided or used with great caution in people with heart failure because they decrease myocardial contractility. Hypotension may occur after the intravenous administration of any of the calcium channel blockers. Other side effects that may occur include atrioventricular blocks, bradycardia, constipation, and gastric distress.

ANTIPLATELET AND ANTICOAGULANT MEDICATIONS

Antiplatelet medications are administered to prevent platelet aggregation, which impedes blood flow.

Aspirin and Ticlopidine. Aspirin prevents platelet aggregation and has been shown to reduce the incidence of MI and death in patients with CAD. A daily dose of aspirin should be given to the patient with angina as soon as the diagnosis is made (eg, in the emergency room or physician's office). Although it may be one of the most important medications in the treatment of CAD, aspirin may be overlooked because of its low cost and common use.

Because aspirin may cause gastrointestinal upset and bleeding, some patients are given ticlopidine (Ticlid). Unlike aspirin, ticlopidine takes a few days to achieve its antiplatelet effect. It also causes gastrointestinal upset, including nausea, vomiting, and diarrhea, and decreases the neutrophil level.

Heparin. Heparin prevents the formation of new blood clots. If the patient's angina is considered to indicate a significant risk for a cardiac event (eg, MI), the patient is given an intravenous bolus of heparin and started on a continuous infusion or given an intravenous bolus every 4 to 6 hours. The amount of heparin administered is based on the results of the activated partial thromboplastin time (aPTT). Heparin therapy is usually considered therapeutic when the aPTT is 1.5 to 2 times the normal aPTT. Use of heparin alone in treating patients with unstable angina reduces the occurrence of MI. Because heparin increases the risk of bleeding, however, the patient is monitored for signs and symptoms of external and internal bleeding, such as low blood pressure, an increased heart rate, and a decrease in serum hemoglobin and hematocrit values. The patient receiving heparin is placed on bleeding precautions, including the following:

- Holding the site of any needle puncture for a longer time than usual
- Avoiding tissue injury and bruising from trauma or use of constrictive devices (eg, continuous use of an automatic blood pressure cuff)

OXYGEN ADMINISTRATION

Oxygen therapy is usually initiated at the onset of chest pain in an attempt to increase the amount of oxygen delivered to the myocardium and to decrease pain. Oxygen inhaled directly increases the amount of oxygen in the blood. The therapeutic effectiveness of oxygen is determined by observing the rate and rhythm of respiratory exchange. Blood oxygen saturation is monitored by pulse oximetry. Patients should have an oxygen saturation (SpO_2) level of more than 93%. Studies are being conducted to assess the use of oxygen in patients without respiratory distress and its effect on outcome.

NURSING PROCESS: THE PATIENT WITH ANGINA PECTORIS

Assessment

The nurse gathers information about the patient's symptoms and activities, especially those that precede and precipitate attacks of anginal pain. Appropriate questions may include:

- Where is the pain usually located? Does it occur anywhere else?
- How would you describe the pain (throbbing, crushing, knifelike, steady, intermittent)?
- How would you rate the pain on a scale of 0 (no pain) to 10 (worst pain)?
- What other symptoms occur with the pain?
- What usually brings on the pain? What usually relieves it? What makes it worse?
- How long does the pain usually last?
- How many minutes after taking nitroglycerin does the pain usually last?

The answers to these questions form a basis for designing a logical program of treatment and prevention. In addition to assessing anginal pain, the nurse also assesses the patient's risk factors for CAD, the patient's response to angina, the patient's and family's understanding of the diagnosis, and adherence to the current treatment plan.

Diagnosis

Nursing Diagnoses

Based on the assessment data, major nursing diagnoses for the patient may include the following:

- Altered myocardial tissue perfusion secondary to CAD, as evidenced by chest pain (or equivalent symptoms)
- Anxiety related to fear of death
- Knowledge deficit about the underlying disease and methods for avoiding complications
- Ineffective management of therapeutic regimen, noncompliance, related to failure to accept necessary lifestyle changes

Collaborative Problems/Potential Complications

Potential complications of angina include MI and its complications.

Planning and Goals

The major patient goals include immediate and appropriate treatment when pain occurs, prevention of pain, reduction of anxiety, awareness of the disease process and understanding of the prescribed care, adherence to the self-care program, and absence of complications.

Nursing Interventions

Treating Pain

If the patient complains of pain (or the individualized equivalent to pain), the nurse takes immediate action. When a patient senses chest pain, the nurse should direct the patient to stop all activities and sit or rest in bed in a semi-Fowler's position to reduce the oxygen requirements of the ischemic myocardium. The nurse assesses the patient's pain, asking the standard questions to determine whether the pain is the same as the patient typically describes. A difference may indicate a worsening of the disease or a different cause. The nurse then continues to assess the patient, measuring vital signs and observing for signs of respiratory distress. If the patient is in the hospital, a 12-lead ECG is usually obtained and scrutinized for ST-segment and T-wave changes. Nitroglycerin is administered sublingually and the patient's response is assessed (relief of chest pain and effect on blood pressure and heart rate). If the patient has been placed on cardiac telemetry with continuous ST-segment monitoring, the ST segment is also assessed for changes. If the chest pain is unchanged or is lessened but still present, nitroglycerin administration is repeated up to three doses. Each time, blood pressure, heart rate, and if indicated the ST segment are assessed. The nurse administers oxygen therapy as indicated if the patient's respiratory rate is increased or the oxygen saturation level is decreased. Although there is no documentation of its effect on outcome, oxygen is usually administered at 2 L/min by nasal cannula, even without evidence of respiratory distress. If the pain is significant and continues after these interventions, the patient is usually transferred to a higher acuity unit.

Preventing Pain

The nurse reviews the assessment findings, identifies the level of activity that causes the patient's pain, and plans the patient's activities accordingly. If the patient has pain frequently or with minimal activity, the nurse alternates the patient's activities with rest periods. The activity–rest balance is an important aspect of the educational plan for the patient and family.

Reducing Anxiety

Patients with angina often fear loss of their roles within society and the family. Exploring the implications that the diagnosis has for the patient and providing information about the illness, its treatment, and methods of preventing its progression are important nursing interventions.

HOME CARE TEACHING CHECKLIST: MANAGING ANGINA PECTORIS

At the completion of the program, the patient or caregiver will be able to:	Patient	Caregiver
• Reduce the probability of an episode of anginal pain by balancing rest with activity:	✔	
• Participate in a regular daily program of activities that do not produce chest discomfort, shortness of breath, or undue fatigue.		
• Avoid exercises requiring sudden bursts of activity; avoid isometric exercise.		
• Alternate activity with periods of rest.		
• Use appropriate resources for support during emotionally stressful times (eg, counselor, nurse, clergy, physician).	✔	✔
• Avoid using medications (eg, diet pills, nasal decongestants, or any over-the-counter medication that can increase the heart rate and blood pressure) without first discussing with health care provider.	✔	✔
• Stop smoking, because smoking increases the heart rate, blood pressure, and blood carbon monoxide levels. Also try to avoid second-hand smoke, which has the same effects.	✔	✔
• Understand that temperature extremes (particularly cold) may induce anginal pain; therefore, avoid exercise in temperature extremes.	✔	
• Carry nitroglycerin at all times, know when and how to use it, and know its side effects.	✔	✔

Promoting Home and Community-Based Care

TEACHING PATIENTS SELF-CARE

Learning to avoid, modify, or adapt the triggers for anginal pain is essential. The teaching program for the patient with angina is designed so that the patient and family can explain the illness, identify the symptoms of myocardial ischemia, state the actions to take when symptoms develop, and discuss methods to prevent chest pain and the advancement of CAD. The goals of the educational program are to reduce the frequency and severity of anginal attacks, to delay the progress of the underlying disease if possible, and to provide protection from other complications. The factors outlined in the accompanying checklist are important in educating the patient with angina pectoris.

The self-care program is prepared in collaboration with the patient and family or friends. Activities should be planned to minimize the occurrence of angina episodes. The patient needs to understand that any pain unrelieved within 30 minutes by the usual methods should be treated at the closest emergency center.

Evaluation

Expected Outcomes

Expected outcomes may include:

1. Reports that pain is relieved promptly
   a. Recognizes symptoms
   b. Takes immediate action
   c. Seeks medical assistance if pain persists or changes in quality
2. Understands ways to avoid complications and demonstrates freedom from complications
   a. Describes the process of angina
   b. Explains reasons for measures to prevent complications
   c. Exhibits normal ECG and cardiac enzyme level
   d. Experiences no signs and symptoms of acute MI
3. Reports anxiety decreased
   a. Expresses acceptance of diagnosis
   b. Expresses control over choices within medical regimen
   c. Does not exhibit specific signs and symptoms of anxiety
4. Adheres to self-care program
   a. Takes medications as prescribed
   b. Keeps health care appointments
   c. Implements plan for reducing risk factors

Invasive Interventions and Surgical Management

Angina pectoris may persist for many years in a stable form with brief attacks. However, unstable angina is a serious disease that can progress to MI or sudden cardiac death. Invasive interventional measures, such as PTCA, directional atherectomy, and stent implantation as well as surgical procedures, are treatments for unstable angina.

PERCUTANEOUS TRANSLUMINAL CORONARY ANGIOPLASTY

PTCA may be used to treat patients with recurrent chest pain that is unresponsive to medical therapy, those with atheromas that occlude at least 70% of the internal lumen of a major coronary artery, placing a large area of the myocardium at risk for ischemia, or those with conditions that do not respond to medical treatments. The procedure is attempted when the cardiologist believes that PTCA can improve blood flow to the myocardium. PTCA alone is seldom attempted in the patient with occlusions of the left main coronary artery that do not demonstrate collateral flow to the left anterior descending and circumflex arteries. The purpose of PTCA is to improve blood flow within a coronary artery by "cracking" the atheroma.

This invasive interventional procedure is carried out in the cardiac catheterization laboratory. The coronary arteries are examined by angiography, as they were during the diagnostic cardiac catheterization, and the location, extent, and calcification of the atheroma are verified. Hollow catheters, called sheaths, are inserted, usually in the femoral vein and/or artery, providing a conduit for other catheters. After the atheroma is verified, a balloon-tipped dilation catheter is passed through the guide catheter and positioned over the lesion. The physician guides the positioning by examining the markers on the balloon that can be seen with x-rays. When the catheter is properly positioned, the balloon is inflated with a radiopaque contrast agent (commonly called dye), not only to visualize the blood vessels but also to provide a steady or oscillating pressure. The balloon is inflated to a certain pressure for several seconds and then deflated. The pressure "cracks" and possibly compresses the atheroma (Fig. 25-3). The coronary artery's media and adventitia are also stretched.

Several inflations and several balloon sizes may be required to achieve the desired goal, usually defined as a residual stenosis of less than 20%. Other gauges of the success of a PTCA are an increase in the artery's lumen, a difference of less than 20 mm Hg in blood pressure from one side of the lesion to the other, and no clinically obvious arterial trauma.

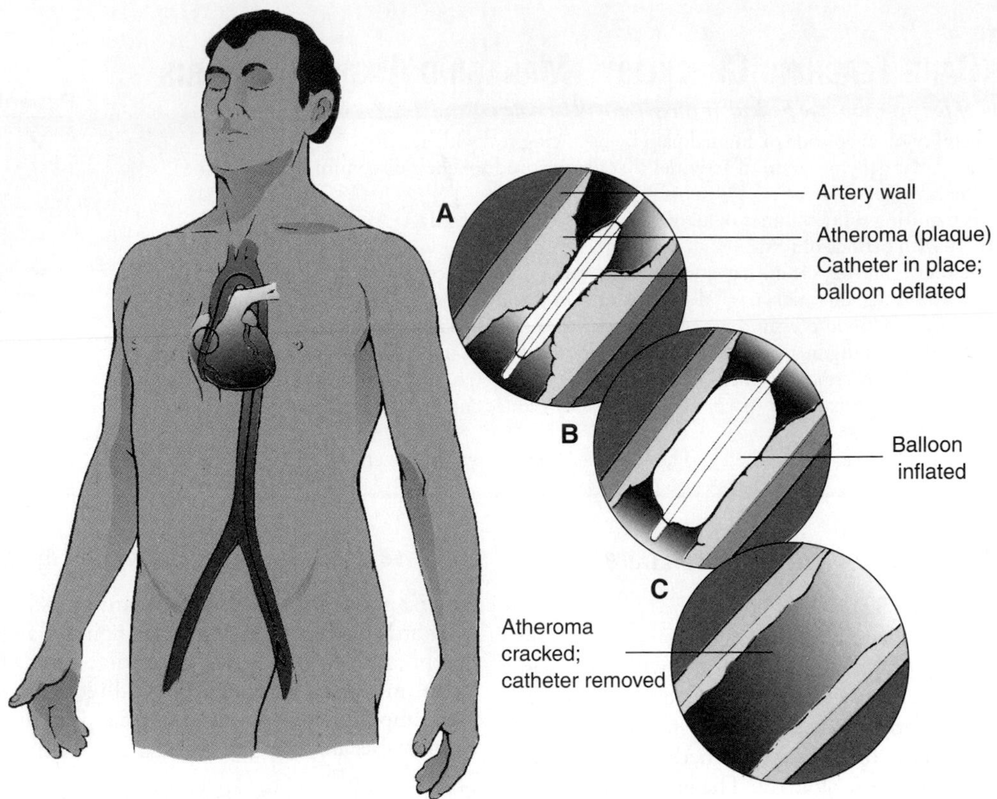

FIGURE 25•3 Percutaneous transluminal coronary angioplasty. (**A**) A balloon-tipped catheter is passed into the affected coronary artery and placed within the area of the atheroma (plaque). (**B**) The balloon is then rapidly inflated and deflated with controlled pressure. (**C**) After the atheroma is cracked, the catheter is removed, and blood flow improves.

Patient care is similar to that for a cardiac catheterization. Because the blood supply to the coronary artery decreases while the balloon is inflated, the patient may complain of chest pain (often called "stretch pain") and the ECG may display significant ST-segment changes.

Complications. Possible complications during the PTCA procedure include dissection, perforation, abrupt closure, or vasospasm of the coronary artery, acute MI, acute dysrhythmias (eg, ventricular tachycardia), and cardiac arrest. These may require emergency surgical treatment. Complications after the procedure may include abrupt closure and vascular complications, such as bleeding at the insertion site, retroperitoneal bleeding, hematoma, pseudoaneurysm, arteriovenous fistula, or arterial thrombosis and distal embolization (Table 25-1).

Postprocedure Care. Many patients are admitted to the hospital the day of the PTCA. Those with no complications go home the next day. During the PTCA, patients receive large amounts of heparin and are monitored closely for signs of bleeding. The patient often returns to the unit with the large peripheral vascular access sheaths in place. Most patients also receive intravenous nitroglycerin for a period after the procedure to prevent arterial spasm.

The sheaths are removed once blood studies (activated clotting time) indicate that the clotting time is within an acceptable range. This usually takes a few hours, depending on the amount of heparin given during the procedure. The patient must remain flat in bed and keep the affected leg straight until the sheaths are removed. The immobility usually causes the patient significant discomfort and is treated with analgesics and sedation.

Hemostasis after sheath removal is achieved by various methods: direct manual pressure, compression with a clamp, application of a collagen plug (eg, Vasoseal), or application of a surgical suture around the opening of the vessel. Removal of sheaths and the application of manual or mechanical pressure on the vessel insertion site may cause the heart rate to slow and the blood pressure to decrease (vasovagal response). An intravenous bolus of atropine is usually used to treat these side effects.

Some patients with unstable lesions and a high risk for abrupt vessel closure are restarted on heparin after sheath removal or receive an intravenous infusion of a GPIIb/IIIa inhibitor, a medication that prevents clot formation by inhibiting platelet aggregation. These patients are monitored more closely and progressed more slowly.

Patients usually can be weaned from the intravenous medications, resume self-care, and ambulate unassisted within 6 to 12 hours of the procedure. The duration of immobilization depends on the size of the sheath inserted, the amount of anticoagulant administered, the method of hemostasis, and the patient's underlying condition. Care for patients after PTCA is discussed later.

CORONARY ARTERY STENT

A stent is a woven stainless-steel mesh that provides structural support to a vessel at risk of acute closure. The stent is placed over the angioplasty balloon. When the balloon is inflated, the mesh expands and presses against the vessel wall, holding the artery open. The balloon is withdrawn, but the stent is left permanently

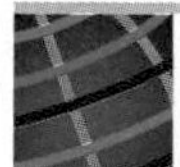

TABLE 25•1 **Complications After PTCA**

Complication	Signs and Symptoms	Possible Causes	Nursing Actions
Bleeding or hematoma	Hard lump or bluish tinge at sheath insertion site	Coughing, vomiting, bending leg or hip, obesity, bladder distention, high blood pressure	Keep the head of the bed flat. Insert indwelling urinary catheter if needed Apply manual pressure at site of sheath insertion. Outline extent of hematoma with a marking pen. If bleeding stops, apply ice bag to groin area insertion site. If bleeding does not stop, notify physician or nurse practitioner.
Lost or weakened pulse distal to sheath site	Extremity cool, cyanotic, pale, or painful	Arterial thrombus or embolus	Call physician or nurse practitioner. Anticipate surgery and anticoagulation or thrombolytic therapy.
Pseudoaneurysm and arteriovenous fistula	Pulsatile mass felt and bruit heard near insertion site	Vessel trauma during procedure	Call physician or nurse practitioner. Anticipate ultrasound-guided compression. Prepare patient for surgery to close fistula.
Retroperitoneal bleeding	Back or flank pain Low blood pressure Tachycardia Restlessness and agitation Decreased hemoglobin Decreased hematocrit	Arterial tear causing bleeding into flank area	Call physician or nurse practitioner immediately. Stop any anticoagulation medication. Anticipate need for intravenous fluids and/or administration of blood.

Courtesy of Washington Adventist Hospital. Care of the interventional cardiology patient nursing protocol, based on communication from Amy Dukovic, Cardiac Interventional Nurse Practitioner, 1998.

in place within the artery (Fig. 25-4). Eventually, endothelium covers the stent and it is incorporated into the vessel wall. Because of the risk of thrombus formation in the stent, the patient receives antiplatelet medications (eg, lifetime use of aspirin and ticlopidine therapy for 2 weeks).

ATHERECTOMY

Atherectomy is an invasive interventional procedure that involves the removal of the atheroma, or plaque, from a coronary artery. Directional and transluminal extraction atherectomy procedures involve the use of a catheter that shaves the lesion and removes the fragments. Rotational atherectomy uses a catheter with diamond chips impregnated on the tip (called a burr) that rotates like a dentist's drill at 130,000 to 180,000 rpm, pulverizing the lesion. Usually several passes of these catheters are needed to achieve satisfactory results. Postprocedural patient care is similar to that for PTCA.

TRANSMYOCARDIAL REVASCULARIZATION

Patients who have cardiac ischemia and who are not candidates for CABG may benefit from the experimental treatment of trans-

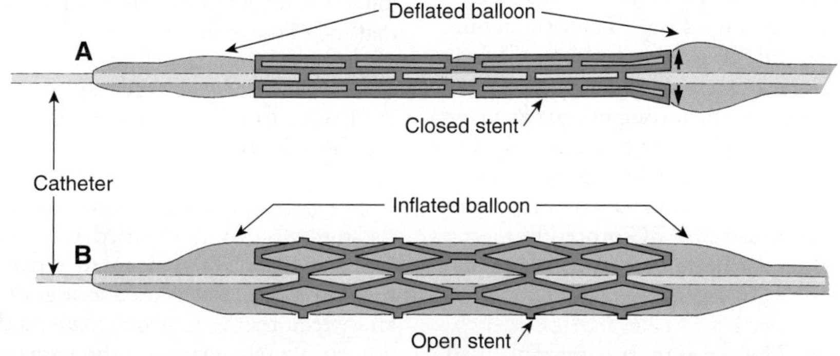

FIGURE 25•4 Intracoronary artery stent. (**A**) Stent closed, before balloon inflation. (**B**) Stent open, balloon inflated; stent will remain expanded after balloon is deflated and removed.

myocardial laser revascularization, also called percutaneous transmyocardial revascularization (PTMR). In the cardiac catheterization laboratory, a fiberoptic catheter is guided into the left ventricle, usually from the femoral artery. The tip of the catheter is held firmly against the ischemic area of the heart while a laser burns a channel into but not through the muscle. Each procedure usually involves making 20 to 40 channels. It is thought that some blood flows from the ventricle into the channels, decreasing the ischemia directly. Within the next few weeks to months, the channels close. The long-term result is the formation of new blood vessels in response to the inflammatory process that follows the laser burns. The new blood vessels provide enough blood to decrease the symptoms of cardiac ischemia. Nursing care before, during, and after the procedure is similar to that for PTCA.

CORONARY ARTERY REVASCULARIZATION: BYPASS

Advances in diagnostics, medical management, surgical and anesthesia techniques, and cardiopulmonary bypass, as well as the care provided in critical care and surgical units, home care, and rehabilitation programs, have helped make surgery a viable treatment option for patients with cardiac disease. CAD has been treated by some form of myocardial revascularization for approximately 40 years; current CABG techniques have been performed for approximately 30 years. CABG is a surgical procedure in which a blood vessel from another part of the body is grafted to the occluded blood vessel so that blood can flow around the occlusion.

Candidates for CABG are usually patients with the following conditions:

- Angina that cannot be controlled by medical therapies
- Unstable angina
- A positive exercise tolerance test and lesions or blockage that cannot be treated by PTCA
- A left main coronary artery lesion or blockage of more than 60%
- Complications from or unsuccessful PTCAs

In a patient considered for CABG, the coronary arteries to be bypassed have at least a 70% occlusion (50% if it is the left main coronary artery). If the blockage involves less than 70% of the artery, enough blood will still flow through the blocked artery to prevent adequate blood flow through the bypass graft. As a result, the graft would clot, effectively negating the surgery.

The CABG procedure is performed with the patient under a general anesthetic. Usually the surgeon makes a median sternotomy incision and connects the patient to the cardiopulmonary bypass machine (discussed below). Next, a blood vessel from another part of the patient's body (eg, saphenous vein, left internal mammary artery) is grafted distal to the coronary artery lesion, bypassing the obstruction (Fig. 25-5). Then cardiopulmonary bypass is discontinued and the incision is closed. The patient then is admitted to a critical care unit.

Alternatively, CABG can be performed using minimally invasive techniques such as thoroscopy (MIDCAB), with the patient under general anesthesia. The surgeon makes one or more 4-inch incisions in the chest wall. The internal mammary arteries are used to perform the minimally invasive CABG procedure. Some techniques are performed while the heart beats; others use cardiopulmonary bypass.

Graft Selection for CABG. The vessel most commonly used for CABG is the greater saphenous vein, followed by the lesser saphenous vein (Fig. 25-6). Cephalic and basilic veins are used also. The vein is removed from the leg (or arm) and grafted to the ascending aorta and to the coronary artery distal to the lesion. The saphenous veins are used in emergency CABG procedures because they can be obtained by one surgical team while another team performs the chest surgery. One side effect of using a large vein is edema, which may develop in the extremity from which it was taken. The degree of edema varies and may diminish over time. Approximately 5 to 10 years after CABG, symptomatic atherosclerotic changes develop in saphenous veins used for grafting. In arm veins, the same changes develop more quickly, approximately 3 to 6 years after the surgery.

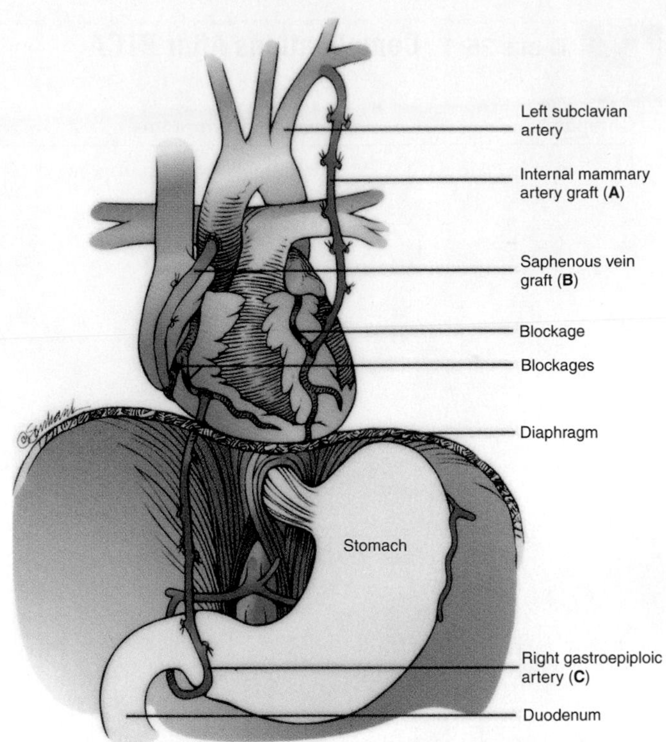

FIGURE 25•5 Three coronary artery bypass grafts. One or more procedures may be performed using various veins and arteries. (**A**) Left internal mammary artery, gaining in popularity because of its functional longevity. (**B**) Saphenous vein, the most frequently constructed bypass. (**C**) Right gastroepiploic artery, rarely used because this artery has a more extensive blood supply to its wall and because of the risk of gastrointestinal tract contamination of the abdominal and/or mediastinal wound.

The right and left internal mammary arteries, and occasionally radial arteries, are also used for CABG. Arterial grafts do not develop atherosclerotic changes as quickly and they remain patent longer than vein grafts. In general, the surgeon leaves the proximal end of the mammary artery intact and detaches the distal end of the artery from the chest wall. This distal end of the artery is then grafted to the coronary artery distal to the occlusion.

Disadvantages of using the internal mammary arteries are that they may not be long enough or wide enough for the bypass, and that ulnar nerve damage may result.

The gastroepiploic artery (located along the greater curvature of the stomach) may also be used. It has a much more extensive blood supply to its wall than the internal mammaries have, so it does not respond as well when used as a graft. Use of the gastroepiploic artery requires the surgeon to extend the chest incision to the abdomen, thereby exposing the patient to the additional risks of an abdominal incision and infection from contamination by the gastrointestinal tract at the surgical site.

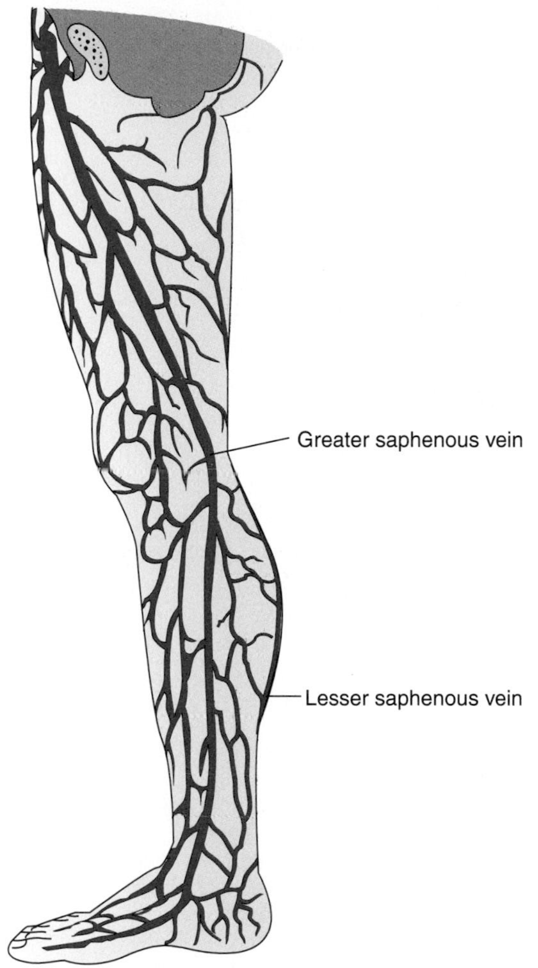

FIGURE 25•6 The greater and lesser saphenous veins are the vessels most commonly used in bypass graft procedures.

Implementing Cardiopulmonary Bypass. Many cardiac surgical procedures are possible because of cardiopulmonary bypass (also called extracorporeal circulation). The procedure mechanically circulates and oxygenates blood for the body while bypassing the heart and lungs. The heart–lung machine allows surgeons to work in a bloodless surgical field and maintains perfusion to other body organs and tissues.

Cardiopulmonary bypass, a common but complex technique, is accomplished by placing a cannula in the right atrium, vena cava, or femoral vein to withdraw blood from the body. The cannula is connected to tubing filled with an isotonic crystalloid solution (usually 5% dextrose in lactated Ringer's solution). Venous blood removed from the body by this cannula is filtered, oxygenated, cooled or warmed, and then returned to the body. The cannula used to return the oxygenated blood is usually inserted in the ascending aorta, but it may be inserted in the femoral artery (Fig. 25-7).

The patient receives heparin, an anticoagulant, to prevent thrombus formation and possible embolization that may occur when blood contacts the foreign surfaces of the cardiopulmonary bypass circuit and is pumped into the body by a mechanical pump (not the normal blood vessels and heart). After the patient is disconnected from the bypass machine, protamine sulfate is administered to reverse the effects of heparin.

During the procedure, hypothermia is maintained, usually 28°C to 32°C (82.4°F to 89.6°F). The blood is cooled during cardiopulmonary bypass and returned to the body. The cooled blood slows the body's basal metabolic rate, thereby decreasing its demand for oxygen. Cooled blood usually would have a higher viscosity, but the crystalloid solution used to prime the bypass tubing dilutes the blood. When the surgical procedure is completed, the blood is rewarmed as it passes through the cardiopulmonary bypass circuit. Urine output, blood pressure, arterial blood gas measurements, electrolytes, coagulation studies, and the ECG are monitored to assess the patient's status during cardiopulmonary bypass.

Postoperative Care. Initial postoperative care focuses on achieving or maintaining hemodynamic stability and recovery from general anesthesia. Care may be provided in the postanesthesia care unit or intensive care unit. Once hemodynamic stability and recovery from general anesthesia have been achieved, the patient is transferred to a surgical stepdown unit with telemetry. Care focuses on wound care, progressive activity, and diet. In addition, education about medications and risk factor modification is emphasized. Discharge from the hospital is usually 3 to 5 days after CABG. Patients can expect fewer symptoms from CAD and should enjoy an improved quality of life. However, CABG has not been shown to increase most patients' life spans (Davis et al., 1995).

Complications. CABG may result in complications such as MI, dysrhythmias, and hemorrhage. The patient's underlying heart disease remains; therefore, angina, exercise intolerance, or other symptoms experienced before CABG may develop again. Medications required before surgery may need to be continued. Lifestyle modifications recommended before surgery remain important, not just for the original pathology but for the continued viability of the newly implanted grafts.

An example of a clinical pathway for the postoperative management of the patient who has undergone a cardiac procedure can be found in Appendix A.

Preoperative Nursing Management

The cardiac surgery patient has many of the same needs and requires the same perioperative care as other surgical patients (see Chaps. 16 through 18). In addition, the patient and family are experiencing a major life crisis. The association of the heart with life and death intensifies their emotional and psychological needs. Patients frequently are admitted the same day as the procedure. For these patients, the nurse must prioritize needs carefully; in the time allowed, the nurse focuses on the needs that have the highest priority.

Before surgery, physical and psychological assessment establishes the baseline for future reference. The patient's understanding of the surgical procedure, informed consent, and adherence to treatment protocols are evaluated. Helping the patient to cope, understand the procedure, and maintain dignity are nursing responsibilities.

The preoperative phase of cardiac surgery begins before hospitalization. The nurse assesses other diseases, such as diabetes, hypertension, and respiratory, gastrointestinal, and hematologic diseases, and notes their treatment.

The nurse may clarify how the medication regimen is to be altered before surgery—for example, tapering corticosteroids and digoxin, decreasing or discontinuing anticoagulants, and maintaining medications for blood pressure, angina, diabetes, and dysrhythmias. The nurse also clarifies the need to maintain activity patterns, a balanced diet, healthful sleep habits, and cessation of smoking to minimize the risks of surgery.

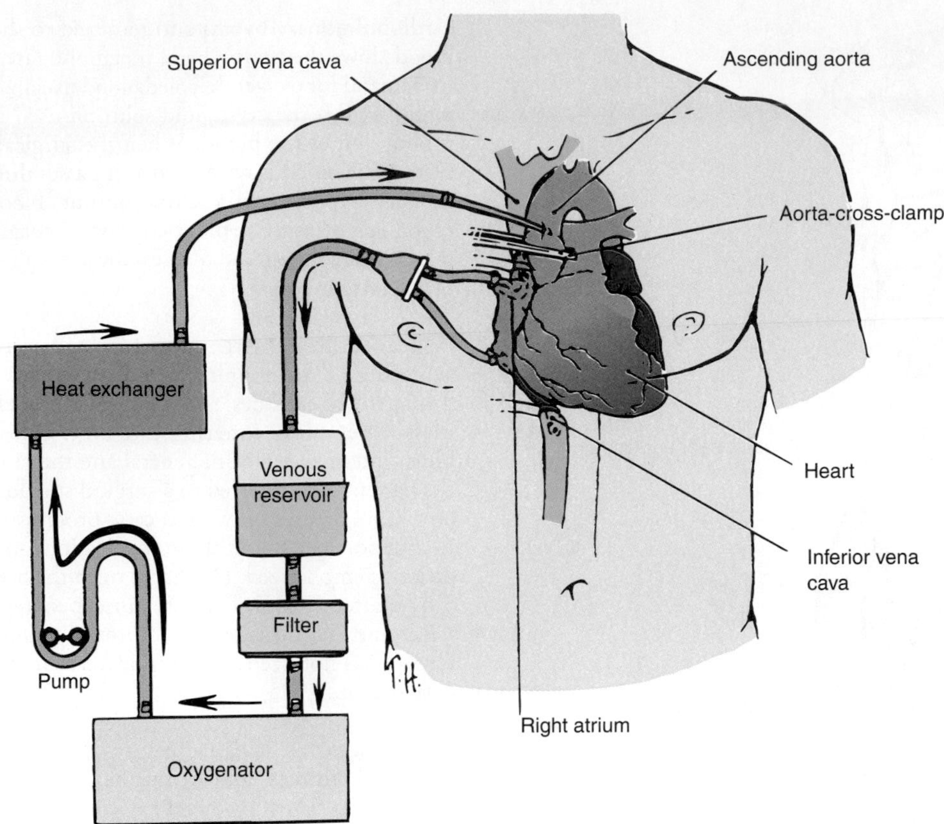

FIGURE 25•7 The cardiopulmonary bypass system, in which cannulae are placed through the right atrium into the superior and inferior vena cava to divert blood from the body and into the bypass system. The pump system creates a vacuum, pulling blood into the venous reservoir. The blood is cleared of air bubbles, clots, and particulates by the filter, and then it passes through the oxygenator, releasing carbon dioxide and obtaining oxygen. Next, the blood is pulled to the pump and pushed out to the heat exchanger, where its temperature is regulated. The blood is then returned to the body via the ascending aorta.

NURSING PROCESS: THE PATIENT AWAITING CARDIAC SURGERY

Assessment

Patients with nonacute heart disease may be admitted to the hospital the day of or the day before the surgery. Most of the preoperative evaluation is completed before the patient enters the hospital. Many surgeons' offices or hospitals mail an information packet to the patient's home.

A history and physical examination are performed by nursing and medical personnel. A chest x-ray, ECG, laboratory analyses, typing and cross-matching of blood, and autologous blood donation (the patient's own blood) may also be performed. The health assessment focuses on obtaining baseline physiologic, psychological, and social information. The patient's and family's learning needs are identified and addressed as necessary. Of particular importance is the patient's usual functional level, coping mechanisms, and support systems. These are important because the support of the family or significant others will affect the patient's postoperative course and rehabilitation. Discharge plans will be influenced by the lifestyle demands of the home situation and the physical environment of the home.

Health History

The preoperative history and health assessment should be thorough and well documented because they provide a basis for postoperative comparison. A systematic assessment of all systems is performed, with emphasis on cardiovascular functioning.

Functional status of the cardiovascular system is determined by reviewing the patient's symptoms, including past and present experiences with chest pain, hypertension, palpitations, cyanosis, breathing difficulty (dyspnea), leg pain that occurs with walking (intermittent claudication), orthopnea, paroxysmal nocturnal dyspnea, and peripheral edema. Because alterations in cardiac output can affect renal, respiratory, gastrointestinal, integumentary, hematologic, and neurologic functioning, these systems also are assessed thoroughly. History of major illnesses, previous surgeries, medication therapies, and use of drugs, alcohol, and tobacco are also explored.

Physical Assessment

A complete physical examination is performed, with special emphasis on the following:

- General appearance and behavior
- Vital signs

- Nutritional and fluid status, weight, and height
- Inspection and palpation of the heart, noting the point of maximal impulse, abnormal pulsations, and thrills
- Auscultation of the heart, noting pulse rate, rhythm, and quality, S_3, S_4, snaps, clicks, murmurs, and friction rub
- Jugular venous pressure
- Peripheral pulses
- Peripheral edema

Psychosocial Assessment

The psychosocial assessment and the assessment of the patient's and family's learning needs are as important as the physical examination. Anticipation of cardiac surgery is a source of great stress to the patient and family. They will be anxious and fearful and often have many unanswered questions. Their anxiety usually increases with the patient's admission to the hospital and the immediacy of surgery. An assessment of the level of anxiety is important. If it is low, this may indicate denial. If it is extremely high, it may interfere with the use of effective coping mechanisms and with preoperative teaching. Questions may be asked to obtain the following information:

- The meaning of the surgery to the patient and family
- Coping mechanisms that are being used
- Measures used in the past to deal with stress
- Anticipated changes in lifestyle
- Support systems in effect
- Fears regarding the present and the future
- Knowledge and understanding of the surgical procedure, postoperative course, and long-term rehabilitation

Adequate time should be allowed for the patient and family to express their fears. The fears most often expressed are fear of the unknown, fear of pain, fear of body image change, and fear of dying. During the assessment, the nurse determines how much the patient and family know about the impending surgery and the expected postoperative events. They are encouraged to ask questions and to indicate how much information they wish to have. Some patients prefer not to have detailed information, whereas others want to know as much as possible. Patients should be approached as unique individuals with their own specific learning needs, learning styles, and levels of understanding.

Patients requiring emergency heart surgery may have both cardiac catheterization and surgery within several hours of admission. The nurse will have little opportunity to assess and meet their emotional and learning needs before surgery. As a result, they will need extra help after surgery to adjust to the situation.

Diagnosis

Nursing Diagnoses

The nursing diagnoses for patients awaiting cardiac surgery vary from patient to patient according to each patient's cardiac disease and symptoms. Most patients have a nursing diagnosis of decreased cardiac output (see Cardiac Failure in Chap. 27). In addition, preoperative nursing diagnoses for most patients may include the following:

- Fear related to the surgical procedure, its uncertain outcome, and the threat to well-being
- Knowledge deficit regarding the surgical procedure and the postoperative course

Collaborative Problems/Potential Complications

The stress of impending cardiac surgery may precipitate complications that require collaborative management with the physician. Based on the assessment data, potential complications that may develop include:

- Angina (or anginal pain equivalent)
- Severe anxiety requiring an anxiolytic (anxiety-reducing) medication
- Cardiac arrest

Planning and Goals

The major goals of the patient may include reducing fear, learning about the surgical procedure and postoperative course, and avoiding complications.

Nursing Interventions

During the preoperative phase of cardiac surgery, the nurse develops a plan of care that includes emotional support and teaching for the patient and family. Establishing rapport, answering questions, listening to fears and concerns, clarifying misconceptions, and providing information about what to expect are all interventions the nurse uses to prepare the patient and family emotionally for the surgery and for the postoperative events.

Reducing Fear

The patient and family are allowed adequate time and repeated opportunities to express their fears. If there is fear of the unknown, other surgical experiences that the patient has had can be compared with the impending surgery. It is often helpful to describe to the patient the sensations that are expected. If the patient has already had a cardiac catheterization, the similarities and differences between that procedure and the surgery may be compared. Also, the patient is encouraged to talk about any concerns related to previous experiences.

A discussion of the patient's fears about pain is initiated. A comparison between the pain experienced with cardiac surgery and other pain experiences is made. The preoperative sedation, the anesthetic, and the postoperative pain medications are described. The nurse reassures the patient that the fear of pain is normal, that some pain will be experienced, and that the patient will be closely observed. Further, medication, positioning, and relaxation will make the pain more tolerable. Patients who have a fear of scarring from surgery are encouraged to discuss this concern; misconceptions are corrected. It may be helpful to indicate that the health care team members will keep the patient informed about the healing process.

The patient and family are encouraged to talk about their fear of dying. They should be reassured that this fear is normal. For those who only hint about this concern despite efforts to encourage them to talk about their fear, coaching may be helpful (eg, "Are you worrying about not making it through surgery? Most people who have heart surgery at least think about the possibility of dying."). Once the fear is expressed, the patient and family can be helped to explore their feelings.

By alleviating undue anxiety and fear, preparing the patient emotionally for surgery decreases the chance of preoperative problems, promotes smooth anesthesia induction, and enhances the patient's involvement in care and recovery after surgery. In addition, preparing the family for the events to come helps them to cope, be supportive to the patient, and participate in postoperative and rehabilitative care.

Monitoring and Managing Potential Complications

Angina may occur because of increased stress and anxiety related to the forthcoming surgery. The patient who develops angina usually responds to normal angina therapy, most commonly nitroglycerin placed under the tongue. Some patients require oxygen and intravenous nitroglycerin drips (see the angina pectoris section above).

For patients with extreme anxiety or fear and for whom emotional support and education are not successful, medication therapy may be helpful. The anxiolytic agents most commonly used before cardiac surgery are lorazepam and diazepam.

Should cardiac arrest occur in the preoperative period, advanced cardiac life support is provided.

Promoting Home and Community-Based Care

TEACHING PATIENTS SELF-CARE

Patient and family teaching is based on assessed learning needs. Teaching usually includes information about hospitalization, surgery (preoperative and postoperative care, length of surgery, pain and discomfort that can be expected, visiting hours, and procedures in the critical care unit), the recovery phase (length of hospitalization, what to expect from home care and rehabilitation, when normal activities such as housework, shopping, and work can be resumed), and ongoing lifestyle habits. Any changes made in medical therapy and preoperative preparations need to be explained and reinforced.

The patient is informed that physical preparation usually involves several showers or scrubs with an antiseptic solution. A sedative may be prescribed the night before and the morning of surgery. Most cardiac surgical teams use prophylactic antibiotic therapy, and the antibiotics are started before surgery.

If no preadmission teaching has been done and the preoperative hospitalization period is very short, teaching the patient and family together may be most effective. Anxiety often increases with the admission process and impending surgery. Unless the nurse has met the patient and family before the day of hospitalization, the time may be too short to establish a relationship that contributes to patient learning. Teaching the patient and family together capitalizes on their established support relationship. Teaching in this phase should be directed primarily by the patient's and family's questions. Too much detail may only increase anxiety.

The patient may be offered a tour of the critical care unit, the postanesthesia care unit, or both. (In some hospitals, the patient initially goes to the postanesthesia care unit.) The patient recovering from anesthesia may be reassured by having already seen the surroundings and having met someone from the unit. The patient and family are informed about the equipment, tubes, and lines that will be present after surgery and their purposes. They should know to expect monitors, several intravenous lines, chest tubes, and a urinary catheter. Explaining the purpose and the approximate time that these devices will be in place helps to reassure the patient. Most patients will remain intubated and on mechanical ventilation for 4 to 48 hours after surgery. They need to be aware that this prevents them from talking, and they should be reassured that the staff will be able to assist them with other means of communication.

The nurse takes care to answer the patient's questions about postoperative care and procedures. Deep breathing and coughing or huffing, use of the incentive spirometer, and foot exercises are explained and practiced by the patient before surgery. The family's questions at this time usually focus on the length of the surgery, who will discuss the results of the procedure with them after surgery and when this may occur, where to wait during the surgery, the visiting procedures for the critical care unit, and how they can support the patient before surgery and in the critical care unit.

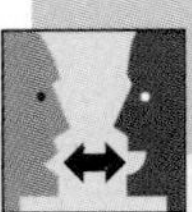

ETHICS AND RELATED ISSUES

When Is it Appropriate to Consider Withholding or Withdrawing Life Support?

Situation

Life-support devices include intra-aortic balloon pumps, ventilators, vasoactive infusions, CPR, and antibiotics. Patients who receive these treatments include the acutely, chronically, and terminally ill. When dependent on life support, a patient may be unable to make decisions about his or her own care, and the patient's family may be too confused and upset to make choices for the patient. At what point is it appropriate to raise the sensitive issue of withholding or withdrawing life support?

Dilemma

The patient's right to choose or refuse treatment conflicts with the obligation to do what is best for the patient (autonomy versus beneficence). The patient's right to choose or refuse treatment conflicts with the obligation not to harm the patient with threatening or inappropriate questions at the wrong time (autonomy versus nonmaleficence).

Discussion

- What arguments would you offer to support the view that discussions about the limitations of life-supporting treatment should be held when patients are admitted to the hospital?
- What arguments would you offer to support the view that discussions about the limitations of life-supporting treatment should be done only when certain circumstances arise?

Evaluation

Expected Outcomes

Expected outcomes may include:

1. Demonstrates reduced fear
   a. Identifies fears
   b. Discusses fears with family
   c. Uses past experiences as a focus for comparison
   d. Expresses positive attitude about outcome of surgery
   e. Expresses confidence in measures to be used to relieve pain
2. Learns about the surgical procedure and postoperative course
   a. Identifies the purposes of the preoperative preparation procedure

    b. Tours the critical care unit, if desired
    c. Identifies limitations expected after surgery
    d. Discusses expected immediate postoperative environment (eg, tubes, machines, nursing surveillance)
    e. Demonstrates expected activities after surgery (eg, deep breathing, coughing, foot exercises)
3. Shows no evidence of complications
    a. Reports anginal pain is relieved with medications and rest
    b. Takes medications as prescribed

Intraoperative Nursing Management

Most of the cardiac surgical procedures are performed through a median sternotomy incision, and the nurse needs to prepare the patient for continuous monitoring; electrodes, indwelling catheters, and probes are placed before the procedure. This facilitates assessment of the patient's status and the need for changes in therapy. Intravenous lines are inserted as needed to administer fluids, medications, and blood products. In addition, the patient will be intubated and placed on mechanical ventilation.

Before the chest incision is closed, chest tubes are positioned to evacuate air and drainage from the mediastinum and the thorax. Epicardial pacemaker electrodes are implanted on the surface of the right atrium and the right ventricle. These epicardial electrodes can be used to pace the heart and to monitor it for dysrhythmias via the atrial leads.

In addition to assisting with the surgical procedures, the surgical nurses are responsible for the comfort and safety of the patient. Some of the areas of intervention include positioning, skin care, wound care, and emotional support of the patient and family.

Possible intraoperative complications include dysrhythmias, hemorrhage, MI, cerebrovascular accident, embolization, and organ failure secondary to shock, embolus, or adverse drug reactions. Astute intraoperative patient assessment is critical in preventing these complications as well as detecting symptoms and initiating prompt therapy.

Postoperative Nursing Management

The immediate postoperative period for the patient who has undergone cardiac surgery presents many challenges to the health care team. All efforts are made to facilitate the transition from the operating room to the critical care unit or postanesthesia care unit with minimal risk. Specific information about the operation and important factors about postoperative management are communicated by the surgical team and anesthesia personnel to the critical care nurse, who then assumes responsibility for the patient's care. Figure 25-8 presents a graphic overview of the many aspects of postoperative care for the cardiac surgical patient.

NURSING PROCESS: THE PATIENT WHO HAS HAD CARDIAC SURGERY

Assessment

When the patient is admitted to the critical care unit, and at least every 12 hours thereafter, a complete assessment of all systems is performed to determine the postoperative status of the patient as compared with the preoperative baseline and to note anticipated changes since surgery. The following parameters are assessed:

- Neurologic status—level of responsiveness, pupil size and reaction to light, reflexes, movement of extremities, and hand grip strength
- Cardiac status—heart rate and rhythm, heart sounds, arterial blood pressure, central venous pressure (CVP), pulmonary artery pressure, pulmonary artery wedge pressure (PAWP), left atrial pressure, waveforms from the invasive blood pressure lines, cardiac output or index, systemic and pulmonary vascular resistance, pulmonary artery oxygen saturation ($S\bar{v}O_2$) if available, chest tube drainage, and pacemaker status and function
- Respiratory status—chest movement, breath sounds, ventilator settings (rate, tidal volume, oxygen concentration, mode [eg, synchronized intermittent mandatory ventilation], positive end-expiratory pressure, pressure support), respiratory rate, ventilatory pressure, arterial oxygen saturation (SaO_2), percutaneous oxygen saturation (SpO_2), end-tidal CO_2, chest tube drainage, arterial blood gases
- Peripheral vascular status—peripheral pulses; color of skin, nailbeds, mucosa, lips, and earlobes; skin temperature; edema; condition of dressings and invasive lines
- Renal function—urinary output, urine specific gravity, and osmolality
- Fluid and electrolyte status—intake, output from all drainage tubes, all cardiac output parameters, and the following indications of electrolyte imbalance:
    - Hypokalemia: digitalis toxicity, dysrhythmias (U wave, AV block, flat or inverted T waves)
    - Hyperkalemia: mental confusion, restlessness, nausea, weakness, paresthesias of extremities, dysrhythmias (tall, peaked T waves; increased amplitude, widening QRS complex; prolonged QT interval)
    - Hypomagnesemia: paresthesias, carpopedal spasm, muscle cramps, tetany, irritability, tremors, hyperexcitability, hyperreflexia, cardiac dysrhythmias (prolonged PR and QT intervals, broad flat T waves), disorientation, depression, hypotension, seizures
    - Hypermagnesemia: vasodilation, hypotension, hyporeflexia, slow gastrointestinal motility (hypoactive bowel sounds), lethargy, respiratory depression, coma, apnea, cardiac arrest
    - Hyponatremia: weakness, fatigue, confusion, seizures, coma
    - Hypocalcemia: paresthesias, carpopedal spasm, muscle cramps, tetany
    - Hypercalcemia: digitalis toxicity, asystole
- Pain—nature, type, location, duration (incisional pain must be differentiated from anginal pain); apprehension; response to analgesics.
- Some patients who have had CABG using an internal mammary artery experience ulnar nerve paresthesia on the same side of the body as the graft. The paresthesia may be temporary or permanent. Also, patients who have had CABG using the gastroepiploic artery may experience an ileus for a longer period after surgery and have abdominal pain at the site of the incision as well as pain at the site of the chest incision.

Assessment also includes observing all equipment and tubes to determine if they are functioning properly: endotracheal tube, ventilator, end-tidal CO_2 monitor, SaO_2 monitor, pulmonary artery catheter, $S\bar{v}O_2$ monitor, arterial and intravenous lines, intravenous infusion devices and tubing, cardiac monitor, pacemaker, chest tubes, and urinary drainage system.

As the patient regains consciousness and progresses through the postoperative period, the nurse expands the assessment to include parameters indicative of psychological and emotional status. The patient may exhibit behavior that reflects denial or depression or

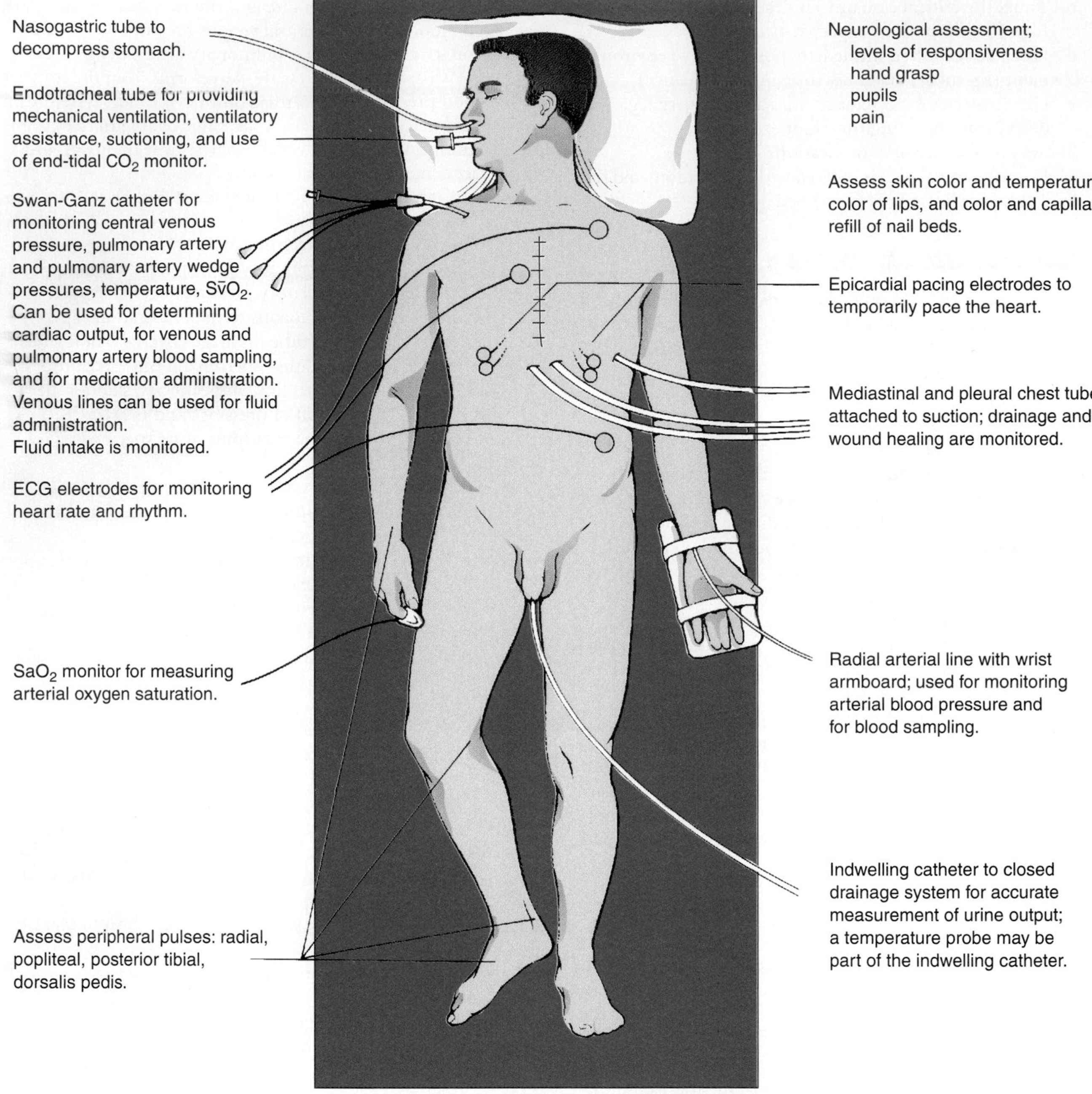

Nasogastric tube to decompress stomach.
Endotracheal tube for providing mechanical ventilation, ventilatory assistance, suctioning, and use of end-tidal CO_2 monitor.
Swan-Ganz catheter for monitoring central venous pressure, pulmonary artery and pulmonary artery wedge pressures, temperature, $S\bar{v}O_2$. Can be used for determining cardiac output, for venous and pulmonary artery blood sampling, and for medication administration. Venous lines can be used for fluid administration. Fluid intake is monitored.
ECG electrodes for monitoring heart rate and rhythm.
SaO_2 monitor for measuring arterial oxygen saturation.
Assess peripheral pulses: radial, popliteal, posterior tibial, dorsalis pedis.
Neurological assessment; levels of responsiveness hand grasp pupils pain
Assess skin color and temperature, color of lips, and color and capillary refill of nail beds.
Epicardial pacing electrodes to temporarily pace the heart.
Mediastinal and pleural chest tubes attached to suction; drainage and wound healing are monitored.
Radial arterial line with wrist armboard; used for monitoring arterial blood pressure and for blood sampling.
Indwelling catheter to closed drainage system for accurate measurement of urine output; a temperature probe may be part of the indwelling catheter.

FIGURE 25•8 Postoperative care of the cardiac surgical patient requires the nurse to be proficient in such skills as assessing pulse pressure, measuring urine output, maintaining various tubes and drains, and operating and interpreting various monitoring systems.

may experience postcardiotomy psychosis. Characteristic signs of psychosis include transient perceptual illusions, visual and auditory hallucinations, and disorientation and paranoid delusions.

The needs of the family also should be assessed. The nurse ascertains how they are coping with the situation; what their psychological, emotional, and spiritual needs are; and whether they are receiving adequate information about the patient's condition.

Assessing for Complications

The patient is continuously assessed for indications of impending complications (Table 25-2). The nurse and the surgeon function collaboratively to identify early signs and symptoms of complications and to institute measures to reverse their progression.

DECREASED CARDIAC OUTPUT

A decrease in cardiac output is always a threat to the patient who has had cardiac surgery. It can be due to a variety of causes:

- Preload alterations—too little or too much blood volume returning to the heart because of hypovolemia, persistent bleeding, cardiac tamponade, or fluid overload
- Afterload alterations—hypertension and arterioles that are too constricted or too dilated because of alterations in body temperature or use of vasoconstrictors and vasodilators
- Heart rate alterations—too fast, too slow, or dysrhythmias

(*text continues on page 615*)

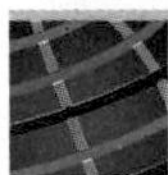

TABLE 25•2 Potential Complications of Cardiac Surgery

Complication	Description	Assessment and Management
Cardiac Complications (The patient may require interventions for more than one complication at a time. Collaboration between the nurses, physicians, pharmacists, and respiratory therapists is necessary to achieve the desired patient outcomes.)		
Preload Alterations (the amount of myocardial muscle fiber stretch at the end of diastole)		
Hypovolemia (most common cause of decreased cardiac output after cardiac surgery)	• Blood loss (although some blood may be replaced to provide sufficient hemoglobin to carry oxygen to the tissues) • Surgical hypothermia (As the reduced body temperature rises after surgery, blood vessels dilate. More volume is needed to fill the vessels.) • IV fluid loss to the interstitial spaces because cardiopulmonary bypass makes capillary beds more permeable • Arterial hypotension with low pulmonary artery wedge pressure (PAWP) and low central venous pressures (CVP) often are seen with an increased heart rate.	• Fluid replacement may be prescribed. Replacement fluids include: colloid (albumin or protein), starch (hetastarch), packed red blood cells, or crystalloid solution (normal saline, lactated Ringer's solution).
Persistent bleeding	• Cardiopulmonary bypass procedure, which may cause platelet malfunction (blood clots abnormally) and hypothermia, which alters clotting mechanisms • Surgical trauma causing tissues and blood vessels to ooze bloody drainage • Anticoagulant (heparin) therapy	• Accurate measurement of wound bleeding and drainage tube blood is essential. Bloody drainage should not exceed 200 mL/h for the first 4 to 6 hours. Drainage should decrease and stop within a few days, while progressing from sanguineous to serosanguineous and serous drainage. • Protamine sulfate may be administered to neutralize heparin; vitamin K and blood products may be used to treat hematologic deficiencies. • If bleeding persists, the patient may return to the operating room for corrective surgery.
Cardiac tamponade (may decrease preload to the heart by preventing available blood from entering the heart)	• Fluid accumulates in the pericardial sac, which compresses the heart, preventing blood from filling the ventricles. • Signs and symptoms include arterial hypotension, tachycardia, muffled heart sounds, decreasing urine output and equalizing of the PAWP, CVP, and pulmonary artery diastolic pressures. Additional signs and symptoms: arterial and pulmonary artery pressure waveforms demonstrating a pulsus paradoxus (decrease of more than 10 mm Hg during inspiration) and decreased chest tube drainage (suggesting that the drainage is trapped or clotted in the mediastinum).	• Equipment is checked to eliminate possible kinks or obstructions in the tubing. • Drainage system patency may be reestablished by milking the tubing (taking care not to strip the tubing, creating massive negative pressure within the chest, which may harm the surgical repair or trigger a dysrhythmia). • Chest film may show a widening mediastinum. • Emergency medical management is required; may include pericardiocentesis or return to surgery.
Fluid overload	• High PAWP, CVP, and pulmonary artery diastolic pressures as well as crackles indicate fluid overload.	• Diuretics are usually prescribed and the rate of IV fluid administration is reduced. • Fluid restriction may be prescribed. Alternative treatments are continuous arteriovenous hemofiltration, dialysis, and phlebotomy.
Afterload Alterations (The force that the ventricle must overcome to move blood forward. Vascular resistance may be calculated to assess afterload and the effects of any vasoactive treatments. Alteration in the patient's body temperature is the most common cause of alterations in afterload after cardiac surgery.)		
Hypothermia	• Blood vessel constriction, which increases afterload. (Blood vessel dilation from fever or other hyperthermic condition decreases afterload.)	• Patient is rewarmed gradually, although vasodilators may be required if the resistance is too great to wait for rewarming. The patient may require volume support or vasopressors during a fever or severe vasodilation.
Hypertension	• Various causes. Some patients have a history of this condition and the nurse can anticipate the need for treatment postoperatively. Other patients experience transient hypertension.	• Vasodilators (nitroglycerin, nitroprusside) may be used to treat hypertension. If patient had hypertension before surgery, the preoperative management regimen resumes as soon as possible.
Heart Rate Alterations		
Tachydysrhythmias	• May or may not result from preload or afterload alterations	• Rhythms are assessed to establish that they are not the result of preload or afterload alterations.

(*continued*)

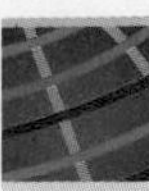

TABLE 25•2 **Potential Complications of Cardiac Surgery** *(Continued)*

Complication	Description	Assessment and Management
		• If a tachydysrhythmia is the primary symptom, the heart rhythm is assessed and medications (e.g., adenosine, digoxin, quinidine, verapamil, esmolol, propranolol, lidocaine, procainamide, bretylium) are prescribed. • Carotid massage may be performed by a physician to assist with diagnosing or treating the dysrhythmia. • Cardioversion and defibrillation are alternatives for symptomatic tachydysrhythmias.
Bradycardias	• Decreased heart rate	• Many postoperative patients will have temporary pacer wires that can be attached to a pulse generator (pacemaker) to stimulate the heart to beat faster. Less commonly, atropine, epinephrine or isoproterenol may be used to increase heart rate.
Dysrhythmias (may or may not affect cardiac output)	• Abnormal heart rates	• Dysrhythmias not affecting cardiac output are treated with medications, pacemakers, carotid massage, cardioversion, or defibrillation. Goal of treatment is to return the heart to a normal sinus rhythm. • In patients who cannot attain normal sinus rhythm, alternate goal may be to establish a stable rhythm that produces a cardiac output sufficient for the patient.
Contractility Alterations		
Cardiac failure	• Possible when the heart fails as a pump and the chambers cannot adequately empty	• The nurse observes for and reports falling mean arterial pressure; rising PAWP, pulmonary artery diastolic pressure, and CVP; increasing tachycardia; restlessness and agitation; peripheral cyanosis; venous distention; labored respirations; and edema. • Medical management includes diuretics and digitalization.
Myocardial infarction (may occur intraoperatively or postoperatively)	• Portion of the cardiac muscle dies, therefore contractility decreases. Until the infarcted area becomes edematous, the ventricular wall moves paradoxically during contractions, further decreasing cardiac output. Symptoms may be masked by the postoperative surgical discomfort or the anesthesia–analgesia regimen.	• Careful assessment to determine the type of pain the patient is experiencing; MI suspected if the mean blood pressure is low with normal preload. The systemic vascular resistance (afterload) and heart rate may be elevated to compensate for poor contractility. • Serial ECGs and cardiac enzymes assist in making the diagnosis. Analgesics are prescribed in small amounts while the patient's blood pressure and respiratory rate are monitored (because vasodilation secondary to analgesics or decreasing pain may occur and compound the hypotension). • Activity progression depends on the patient's activity tolerance.
Pulmonary Complications		
Impaired gas exchange	• Impaired gas exchange is a possible complication after cardiac surgery.	• Pulmonary complications are often detected during assessment of breath sounds, oxygen saturation levels, and end-tidal CO_2 levels, and when monitoring peak pressure and exhaled tidal volumes on the ventilator. Arterial blood gas results and mixed venous saturations also are monitored when available. • Extended periods of mechanical ventilation are often required while the complications are treated and until they are resolved.

(continued)

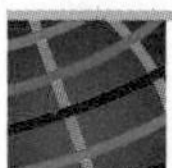

TABLE 25•2 **Potential Complications of Cardiac Surgery** *(Continued)*

Complication	Description	Assessment and Management
Pulmonary Complications (continued)		
		• In patients with hypoxia, ventricular stroke work index may be calculated to assist with assessment of contractility.
Fluid Volume Complications		
Hemorrhage	• Untoward and excessive bleeding may be life-threatening.	• Hemorrhage usually requires surgical intervention, and blood products are often administered in addition to autotransfusion if available. • Compression of a bleeding vessel is another treatment of hemorrhage. • Lungs may be used to compress bleeding mediastinal blood vessels, lung volume and pressure being increased by adding PEEP to the ventilator settings of an intubated patient. The lungs slow or stop the bleeding by pushing in on the mediastinum and create pressure on the bleeding vessels of the pericardium, coronary arteries, and bypass grafts.
Neurologic Complications		
Cerebrovascular accident (brain attack)	• Inability to follow simple command within 6 hours of recovery from anesthetic; different capabilities on right or left side of body	• Neurologically, most patients begin to recover from anesthesia in the operating room. • Patients who are elderly or who have renal or hepatic failure may take longer to recover. • Patient should be evaluated for brain attack or air embolism.
Pain (see Chapter 12)		
Renal Failure and Electrolyte Imbalance		
Renal failure	• Usually acute and resolves within 3 months, but may become chronic and require ongoing dialysis	• May respond to diuretics or may require dialysis
Acute tubular necrosis	• Often results from hypoperfusion of the kidneys or from injury to the renal tubules by medications in the filtrate or from exacerbation of a preexisting condition	• Fluids, electrolytes, and urine output are monitored continuously.
Hypokalemia (low potassium level; normal level is 3.5 to 5.0 mEq/L [3.5 to 5.0 mmol/L])	• May be caused by inadequate intake, diuretics, vomiting, diarrhea, excessive nasogastric drainage without potassium replacement, and stress due to surgery (increased aldosterone secretion produces decreased potassium and increased sodium retention). • Signs and symptoms: digitalis toxicity, dysrhythmias, metabolic alkalosis, a weakened myocardium, and cardiac arrest • One specific ECG change is a U wave (a positive deflection after the T wave) that is more than 1 mm high. Additional signs are AV block, flat or inverted T waves, and low voltage.	• Must be detected and treated immediately • Patient must be observed carefully when serum potassium rises or falls outside the normal level • Some cardiac surgeons strive to maintain potassium level at 4.0 mEq/L (4.0 mmol/L) or higher to avoid dysrhythmias in the postoperative period. • When necessary, the physician prescribes IV potassium replacement.
Hyperkalemia (high potassium level)	• Hyperkalemia may be caused by increased intake, red blood cell hemolysis caused by cardiopulmonary bypass or mechanical assist devices, acidosis, renal insufficiency, tissue necrosis, and adrenal cortical insufficiency. • Signs and symptoms: mental confusion, restlessness, nausea, weakness, and paresthesias of the extremities. • ECG changes specific for hyperkalemia are tall peaked T waves, increased amplitude and widening of the QRS complex, and a prolonged QT interval.	• The physician may prescribe an ion exchange resin, sodium polystyrene sulfonate (Kayexalate), which binds the potassium in the GI tract and results in decreased serum potassium. • Alternative treatments are IV sodium bicarbonate, IV insulin, and glucose to temporarily drive the potassium back into the cells from the extracellular fluid. • Hemodialysis or peritoneal dialysis may be used.

(continued)

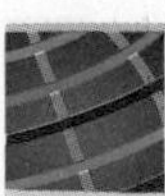

TABLE 25•2 Potential Complications of Cardiac Surgery *(Continued)*

Complication	Description	Assessment and Management
Hypomagnesemia (low magnesium level, <1.5 mEq/L (0.75 mmol/L), although symptoms usually develop with <1.0 mEq/L). Normal magnesium level ranges from 1.5–2.5 mEq/L (0.75–1.25 mmol/L)	• Can be caused by decreased intake, impaired absorption or increased excretion, and surgery, which causes the kidneys to excrete higher amounts of magnesium for 24 hours. Other causes may be decreased intake due to chronic alcoholism, malnutrition or starvation. Impaired absorption may be related to malabsorption syndromes (such as sprue, steatorrhea, or bowel resections) and excess intake of calcium. Increased excretion may result from diuretic use, loss of intestinal fluids (especially fistulas), diabetic ketoacidosis, primary aldosteronism, and primary hyperparathyroidism. Magnesium is important for the function of the neuromuscular system, so the signs and symptoms most often seen are neuromuscular. • Signs and symptoms: paresthesias, carpopedal spasm, muscle cramps, tetany, irritability, tremors, hyperexcitability, hyperreflexia, disorientation, depression, and seizures. Also, hypotension, dysrhythmias (atrial and ventricular), prolonged PR and QT intervals and broad flat T waves.	• Treatment is to correct the cause. If necessary, magnesium supplements may be given. The oral route is preferred to intramuscular injections, which are painful, and the IV route, which carries a significant risk for respiratory depression and hypotension. If the IV route is chosen for magnesium supplements, the nurse needs to assess the patient at least every 5 minutes for respiratory rate less than 16, hypotension, flushing, diaphoresis, and loss of the patellar reflex. If symptoms occur, the nurse slows or stops the infusion and notifies the physician.
Hypermagnesemia (high serum magnesium level, usually >3.0 Eq/L)	• Possibly caused by renal failure or intake of large amounts of medications with magnesium, such as some antacids and cathartics. • Signs and symptoms: vasodilation resulting in flushing, feeling warm, and hypotension. As the levels continue to rise, loss of reflexes, slowing bowel function, drowsiness, respiratory depression, coma, apnea and cardiac arrest may occur.	• Dialysis can be used to remove some magnesium but is not usually effective alone. Calcium gluconate is a temporary treatment until the cause can be identified and corrected.
Hypernatremia (high sodium level) and hyponatremia (low sodium level) Normal level is 135–145 mEq/L (135–145 mmol/L).	• Both may occur after cardiac surgery, but hyponatremia is more common. • Hyponatremia may result from reduced total body sodium or from increased water intake, which causes a dilution of body sodium. • Signs and symptoms of hyponatremia: weakness, fatigue, confusion, convulsions, and coma	• The patient must be observed for sodium values that vary from the normal ranges • When there is a true loss of sodium from the body, the physician prescribes sodium replacement. • Diuretics are prescribed when reduction in sodium is due to increased water intake.
Hypocalcemia (low calcium level) Normal level is 8.8–10.3 mg./100ml (2.20–2.58 mmol/L).	• May result from alkalosis, which reduces the amount of calcium in the extracellular fluid, or from transfusions of large amounts of citrated blood products—packed red blood cells or whole blood. Citrate binds with calcium, reducing the amount of circulating ionized calcium. Most blood banks now use less citrate to store blood as compared with the amounts used before 1985; however, after 5–6 units of packed cells or whole blood from the blood bank, calcium binding may become a concern. • Signs and symptoms: numbness and tingling in the fingertips, toes, ears, and nose; carpopedal spasm; and muscle cramps and tetany	• Calcium level is monitored to determine if it is within normal limits. • Any symptoms of hypocalcemia are reported promptly so that the physician can institute calcium replacement.
Hypercalcemia (high calcium level)	• Signs and symptoms: dysrhythmias that imitate those caused by digitalis toxicity (calcium can potentiate, or enhance, the action of digitalis)	• The nurse assesses the patient for signs of digitalis toxicity and reports these immediately so that the physician can institute treatment to prevent asystole and death.
Other Complications		
Hepatic failure	• Most common in patients with cirrhosis, hepatitis, or prolonged right-sided heart failure	• Use of medications metabolized by the liver must be minimized. If hepatic failure cannot be reversed, death is inevitable. • Bilirubin, albumin, and amylase levels are monitored, and nutritional support must be provided.

(continued)

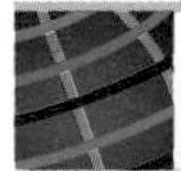

TABLE 25•2 **Potential Complications of Cardiac Surgery** *(Continued)*

Complication	Description	Assessment and Management
Coagulopathies	• Result of hypothermia, blood component depletion, anticoagulation, or liver dysfunction	• Each patient must be carefully evaluated to determine the cause. Appropriate therapy is then provided.
Infection	• Cardiopulmonary bypass and anesthesia alter the patient's immune system. Many invasive devices are used to monitor and support the patient's recovery and may serve as a source of infection.	• The following must be monitored to detect signs of possible infection: body temperature, white blood cell counts and differential counts, suture and puncture sites, cardiac output and systemic vascular resistance, urine (clarity, color, and odor), bilateral breath sounds, sputum (color, odor, amount), as well as nasogastric secretions. • Antibiotic therapy may be expanded or modified as necessary. • Invasive devices must be discontinued as soon as they are no longer required. Institutional protocols for maintaining and replacing invasive lines and devices must be followed to minimize the patient's risk for infection.

- Contractility alterations—cardiac failure, myocardial infarction, electrolyte imbalances, hypoxia

ALTERED FLUID AND ELECTROLYTE BALANCE

Alterations in fluid and electrolyte balance may occur after cardiac surgery. Nursing assessment for these complications includes monitoring of intake and output, weight, PAWP, left atrial pressure and CVP readings, hematocrit levels, distention of neck veins, edema, liver size, breath sounds (ie, fine crackles, wheezing), and electrolyte levels. Changes in serum electrolytes are reported promptly so that treatment can be instituted. Especially important are either dangerously high or dangerously low levels of potassium, magnesium, sodium, and calcium.

IMPAIRED GAS EXCHANGE

Impaired gas exchange is another possible complication after cardiac surgery. All body tissues require an adequate supply of oxygen and nutrients for survival. To achieve this after surgery, an endotracheal tube with ventilator assistance may be used for 48 or more hours. The assisted ventilation is continued until the patient's blood gas measurements are acceptable and the patient demonstrates the ability to breathe independently. Patients who are stable after surgery may be extubated as early as 2 to 4 hours after surgery, which reduces their anxiety regarding their limited ability to communicate.

The patient is continuously assessed for signs of impaired gas exchange: restlessness, anxiety, cyanosis of mucous membranes and peripheral tissues, tachycardia, and fighting the ventilator. Breath sounds are assessed often to detect fluid in the lungs and monitor lung expansion. Arterial blood gas values are monitored.

IMPAIRED CEREBRAL CIRCULATION

Brain function depends on a continuous supply of oxygenated blood. The brain does not have the capacity to store oxygen and must rely on adequate continuous perfusion by the heart. Thus, it is important to observe the patient for any symptoms of hypoxia: restlessness, headache, confusion, dyspnea, hypotension, and cyanosis. Arterial blood gases, SpO_2, $S\bar{v}O_2$, and end-tidal CO_2 are assessed for decreased oxygen and increased carbon dioxide. An assessment of the patient's neurologic status includes level of consciousness, response to verbal commands and painful stimuli, pupil size and reaction to light, movement of extremities, hand grip strength, presence of pedal and popliteal pulses, as well as temperature and color of extremities. Any indication of a changing status is documented, and any abnormal findings are reported to the surgeon because they may signal the beginning of a complication. Hypoperfusion or microemboli may produce central nervous system injury after cardiac surgery.

Diagnosis

Nursing Diagnoses

Based on the assessment data and the type of surgical procedure performed, major nursing diagnoses of the patient may include the following:

- Decreased cardiac output related to blood loss and compromised myocardial function
- Risk for impaired gas exchange related to trauma of extensive chest surgery
- Risk for fluid volume deficit (and electrolyte balance) related to alteration in circulating blood volume
- Risk for sensory–perceptual alterations related to sensory overload (critical care environment, surgical experience) and electrolyte imbalances
- Pain related to surgical trauma and pleural irritation caused by chest tubes
- Risk for altered tissue perfusion related to venous stasis, embolization, underlying atherosclerotic disease, effects of vasopressors, or coagulation problems
- Risk for alteration in renal tissue perfusion related to decreased cardiac output, hemolysis, or vasopressor drug therapy
- Risk for hyperthermia related to infection or postpericardiotomy syndrome
- Knowledge deficit about self-care activities

Collaborative Problems/Potential Complications

Based on the assessment data, potential complications that may develop include:

- Cardiac complications: congestive heart failure, MI, stunned myocardium, dysrhythmias, cardiac arrest
- Pulmonary complications: pulmonary edema, pulmonary emboli, pleural effusions, pneumothorax or hemothorax, respiratory failure, adult respiratory distress syndrome
- Hemorrhage
- Neurologic complications: cerebrovascular accident, air emboli
- Pain
- Renal failure, acute or chronic
- Electrolyte imbalances
- Hepatic failure
- Coagulopathies
- Infection, sepsis

Planning and Goals

The major goals for the patient include restoration of cardiac output, adequate gas exchange, maintenance of fluid and electrolyte balance, reduction of symptoms of sensory overload, relief of pain, promotion of rest, maintenance of adequate tissue perfusion, maintenance of adequate renal perfusion, maintenance of normal body temperature, learning self-care activities, and absence of complications.

Nursing Interventions

Restoring Cardiac Output

Nursing management of the patient involves continuously observing the patient's cardiac status and notifying the surgeon of any changes that indicate decreased cardiac output. The nurse and the surgeon then work collaboratively to correct the problem.

In evaluating the patient's cardiac status, the nurse primarily determines the effectiveness of cardiac output through clinical observations and routine measurements: serial readings of blood pressure, heart rate, CVP, arterial pressure, and left atrial or pulmonary artery pressure.

Renal function is related to cardiac function, as blood pressure and heart rate drive glomerular filtration; therefore, urinary output is measured and recorded. Urine output of less than 25 mL/h may indicate a decrease in cardiac output. Urine specific gravity also is assessed (normal: 1.010 to 1.025), as is urine osmolality. Inadequate fluid volume may be manifested by low urinary output and high specific gravity, whereas overhydration is exhibited by high urine output with low specific gravity.

The growth and function of body cells depend on adequate cardiac output to provide a continuous supply of oxygenated blood to meet the changing demands of the organs and body systems. Because the buccal mucosa, nailbeds, lips, and earlobes are sites with rich capillary beds, they should be observed for cyanosis or duskiness as possible signs of reduced heart action. Moist or dry skin may indicate vasodilation or vasoconstriction, respectively. Distention of the neck veins or of the dorsal surface of the hand raised to heart level may signal a changing demand or diminishing capacity of the heart. If cardiac output has fallen, the skin becomes cool, moist, and cyanotic or mottled.

Dysrhythmias, which may arise when poor perfusion of the heart exists, also serve as important indicators of cardiac function. The most common dysrhythmias encountered during the postoperative period are bradycardias, tachycardias, and ectopic beats. Continuous observation of the cardiac monitor for various dysrhythmias is an essential part of patient care and management.

Any indications of decreased cardiac output are reported promptly to the physician. These assessment data and results of diagnostic tests are used by the physician to determine the cause of the problem. Once a diagnosis has been made, the physician and the nurse work collaboratively to restore cardiac output and prevent further complications. When indicated, the physician prescribes blood components, fluids, digitalis or other antiarrhythmics, diuretics, vasodilators, or vasopressors. When further surgery is necessary, the patient and family are prepared for the procedure.

Promoting Adequate Gas Exchange

To ensure adequate gas exchange, the nurse assesses and maintains the patency of the endotracheal tube. The patient is suctioned when wheezes, coarse crackles, or rhonchi are present. Suctioning may be performed with an in-line suction catheter; the nurse and respiratory therapist determine if the ventilator's fractional inspired oxygen (FiO_2) should be increased for three or more breaths before the patient is suctioned. Alternatively, 100% oxygen is delivered to the patient by a manual resuscitation bag (Ambu-Bag) before and after suctioning to minimize the risk of hypoxia that can result from the suctioning procedure. Arterial blood gas determinations are compared with baseline data, and changes are reported to the physician promptly.

Because a patent airway is essential for oxygen and carbon dioxide exchange, the endotracheal tube must be secured to prevent it from slipping into the right mainstem bronchus and occluding the left bronchus. Frequent changes of position also provide for optimal pulmonary ventilation and perfusion by allowing the lungs to expand more fully. When the patient's condition stabilizes, body position is changed every 1 to 2 hours, and the nurse assesses breath sounds to detect crackles, wheezes, and fluid in the lungs.

The patient is usually weaned from the ventilator and extubated following a standard procedure. However, if the patient is gagging or fighting or bucking the ventilator, both physical assessment and arterial blood gas results may indicate the need for individualization of care. Before being extubated, the patient should have cough and gag reflexes and stable vital signs; be able to lift the head off the bed or give firm hand grasps; have adequate vital capacity, negative inspiratory force, and minute volume appropriate for body size; and have acceptable arterial blood gas levels while breathing warmed humidified oxygen without the assistance of the ventilator.

Extubation has been performed within these parameters without any adverse effects on the patient's condition or prognosis. During this time, the nurse assists with the weaning process and eventually the removal of the endotracheal tube. Deep breathing and huffing (or coughing) are encouraged at least every 1 to 2 hours after extubation to open the alveolar sacs and provide for increased perfusion. The patient should be taught and assisted to splint the chest incision before and during coughing to minimize discomfort.

Maintaining Fluid and Electrolyte Balance

To promote fluid and electrolyte balance, the nurse carefully assesses intake and output. Flow sheets are used to determine positive or negative fluid balance. All fluid intake is recorded, including intravenous fluids, flush solutions used in arterial and venous catheters and the nasogastric tube, and oral fluids. In addition, all output is recorded, including urine, nasogastric drainage, and chest drainage.

Hemodynamic parameters (blood pressure, pulmonary wedge and left atrial pressures, and CVP) are correlated with intake, output, and weight to determine the adequacy of hydration and cardiac output. Serum electrolytes are monitored, and the patient is observed for signs of potassium, magnesium, sodium, or calcium imbalance (hypokalemia, hyperkalemia, hypomagnesemia, hyponatremia, hypocalcemia).

Any indications of dehydration, fluid overload, or electrolyte imbalance are reported promptly, and the physician and nurse work collaboratively to restore fluid and electrolyte balance. The patient's response is monitored.

Reducing Symptoms of Sensory Overload

Sensory overload refers to a group of abnormal behaviors that occur in varying intensity and duration in a large number of patients. In the early years of cardiac surgery, this phenomenon occurred more frequently than it does today. At that time it was attributed to inadequate cerebral perfusion during surgery, microemboli, and the length of time that the patient remained on the cardiopulmonary bypass machine. Advances in surgical techniques have significantly decreased these factors. Today, when it occurs, it is thought to be caused by anxiety, sleep deprivation, increased sensory input, and disorientation to night and day when the patient loses track of time. An important finding is that patients who do not or cannot express anxiety before surgery are more prone to develop psychosis in the postoperative period. Psychosis may appear after a brief lucid interval.

The nurse monitors the patient for signs of denial and provides an opportunity for emotional expression during the preoperative period. Careful explanations of all procedures and of the need for cooperation help to keep the patient oriented throughout the postoperative course. Continuity of care is desirable; a familiar face and a nursing staff with a consistent approach promote the delivery of quality nursing care. A well-designed and individualized plan of nursing care will provide guidelines to assist the nursing team to coordinate their efforts for the emotional well-being of the patient.

Relieving Pain

Deep pain may not be reflected in the immediate area of injury but in a broader, more diffuse area. Patients who have had cardiac surgery experience pain caused by the interruption of intercostal nerves along the incision route and irritation of the pleura by the chest catheters.

It is essential to observe and listen to the patient for verbal and nonverbal clues about pain. The nurse accurately records the nature, type, location, and duration of the pain. (Incisional pain must be differentiated from anginal pain.) The patient is encouraged to use patient-controlled analgesia or accept medication as often as it is prescribed to reduce the amount of pain. Physical support of the incision during deep breathing and huffing (coughing) also helps to minimize pain. The patient should then be able to participate in respiratory exercises and to increase self-care progressively.

Pain produces tension, which may stimulate the central nervous system to release adrenalin, which in turn results in constriction of the arterioles. This can cause increased afterload and decreased cardiac output. Opioids alleviate anxiety and pain and induce sleep, which reduces the metabolic rate and oxygen demands. After the administration of opioids, any observations indicating relief of apprehension and pain are documented in the patient's record. The patient is observed for any respiratory depressant effects of the analgesic. If respiratory depression occurs, an opioid antagonist (eg, naloxone [Narcan]) is used to counteract the effect.

Promoting Rest

Basic comfort measures used in conjunction with prescribed analgesics potentiate the effects of the analgesics and promote rest. The patient is assisted in changing positions every 1 to 2 hours and is positioned in such a way to avoid strain on the incisional line and chest tubes. Nursing activities are scheduled as much as possible to provide undisturbed periods of rest. As the patient's condition stabilizes and the patient is disturbed less frequently for monitoring and therapeutic procedures, rest periods can be extended.

Maintaining Adequate Tissue Perfusion

Peripheral pulses (pedal, tibial, popliteal, femoral, radial, brachial) are routinely palpated to assess for arterial obstruction. If a pulse is absent in any extremity, the cause may be prior catheterization of that extremity. The newly identified absence of any pulse is immediately reported to the physician.

Thrombus formation and resulting embolization also can result from injury to the intima of the blood vessels, dislodging a clot from a damaged valve, loosening of mural thrombi, and coagulation problems. Air embolism may occur as a result of cardiopulmonary bypass. Symptoms of embolization vary according to site. The usual embolic sites are the lungs, coronary arteries, mesentery, spleen, extremities, kidneys, and brain. The patient is observed for the following:

- Chest pain and respiratory distress with pulmonary embolus or MI
- Midabdominal or mid-back pain
- Pain, cessation of pulses, blanching, numbness, or coldness in an extremity
- Decreased urine output
- One-sided weakness and pupillary changes, such as occur in cerebrovascular accident (CVA, brain attack)

All such symptoms are promptly reported to the physician.

After surgery, the following measures are taken to prevent venous stasis, which can cause thrombus formation and subsequent embolization:

- Applying elastic pressure stockings or elastic bandage wrap and pneumatic antiemboli stockings
- Discouraging crossing of legs
- Avoiding use of the knee gatch on the bed
- Omitting pillows in the popliteal space
- Instituting passive exercises followed by active exercises to promote circulation and prevent loss of muscle tone

Maintaining Adequate Renal Perfusion

Inadequate renal perfusion can occur as a complication of open-heart surgery. One possible cause is low cardiac output. In addition, trauma to blood cells during cardiopulmonary bypass can cause hemolysis of red blood cells. This leads to a buildup of toxic substances because the glomeruli are occluded by the debris of the damaged red blood cells. Use of vasopressor agents to increase blood pressure can also lead to reduction of the blood flow to the kidneys.

Nursing management includes accurate measurement of urine output. An output of less than 25 mL/h can indicate hypovolemia.

Specific gravity tests should be carried out to determine the kidneys' ability to concentrate urine in the renal tubules. Rapid-acting diuretics or inotropic medications (digitalis, isoproterenol) may be prescribed to increase cardiac output and renal blood flow. The nurse should be aware of the blood urea nitrogen and serum creatinine levels as well as urine and serum electrolyte levels. Abnormal levels are reported promptly because it may be necessary to adjust fluids and the dose or type of medication administered. If efforts to maintain renal perfusion are not effective, the patient may require dialysis or continuous renal replacement therapy (see Chap. 40).

Maintaining Normal Body Temperature

Patients are usually hypothermic when admitted to the critical care unit from the cardiac surgical procedure. The patient must be gradually warmed to a normal temperature. This is accomplished partially by the patient's own basal metabolic processes and often with the assistance of warmed ventilator air and warm blankets. Heat lamps may also be used. While the patient is hypothermic, the clotting process is less efficient, the heart is prone to dysrhythmias, and oxygen does not readily transfer from the hemoglobin to the tissues. Because anesthesia suppresses the basal metabolism, oxygen supply usually meets the cellular demand.

After cardiac surgery, the patient is at risk for developing elevated body temperature caused by infection or postpericardiotomy syndrome. The resultant increase in metabolic rate increases tissue oxygen demands and thus increases cardiac workload. Measures are taken to prevent this sequence of events or to halt it as soon as it is recognized.

Sites of infection include the lungs, urinary tract, incisions, and intravascular catheters. Meticulous care is used to prevent contamination at the sites of catheter and tube insertions. Aseptic technique is used when changing dressings and when providing endotracheal tube and catheter care. Clearance of pulmonary secretions is accomplished by frequent repositioning of the patient, suctioning, chest physical therapy, as well as deep breathing and huffing (or coughing). Closed systems are used to maintain all intravenous and arterial lines.

Postpericardiotomy syndrome occurs in approximately 10% to 40% of patients who undergo cardiac surgery. Its precise cause is unknown. A common factor appears to be trauma, with residual blood in the pericardial sac after surgery. The syndrome is characterized by fever, pericardial pain, pleural pain, dyspnea, pericardial effusion and pericardial friction rub, and arthralgia. There may be a combination of these signs and symptoms. Leukocytosis is present, along with elevation of the sedimentation rate. These symptoms frequently appear after the patient is discharged from the hospital.

The syndrome must be differentiated from other postoperative complications (incisional pain, MI, pulmonary embolus, bacterial endocarditis, pneumonia, atelectasis). The treatment depends on the severity of the symptoms. Bed rest and anti-inflammatory agents, such as salicylates and corticosteroids, produce a dramatic improvement in symptoms.

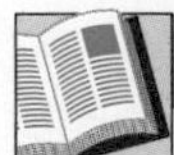

NURSING RESEARCH

Educational Needs of Patients After Cardiac Surgery

Goodman, H. (1997). Patients' perceptions of their education needs in the first six weeks following discharge after cardiac surgery. *Journal of Advanced Nursing, 25*(6), 1241–1251.

Purpose

The purpose of this study was to identify what information and support patients thought they needed in the first 6 weeks after hospital discharge following open heart surgery.

Study Sample and Design

A convenience sample of 10 patients who were within 2 days of discharge from the hospital was studied. The subjects were asked to keep a diary for the first 6 weeks after discharge. They were asked to record their thoughts, feelings, and questions regarding their recovery on the day that they occurred. On the day of their 6-week follow-up outpatient appointment, they participated in an audiotaped interview. The interview consisted of several open-ended questions that encouraged the subjects to talk about their perceptions of the recovery period.

Findings

Fourteen common themes emerged from the data. The themes of sleep and pain occurred primarily in the diaries and seemed to be limited to the early recovery period. Six themes focused on practical issues: dietary needs, lack of information, limitations to recovery, medical concerns, exercise, and medication. Four themes concerned the subjects' psychological state: negative, different, and positive psychological states and owning responsibility for care. The final two themes were concerned with emotional and physical support required in the community.

Nursing Implications

The results of this study are helpful to nurses in planning care after open heart surgery so that the health care team can meet the perceived needs of the patient. The patient's perceptions and needs for better pain management, information about sleep, rest, and relaxation techniques, information about hygiene and grooming while the sternotomy wound heals, and information about potential temporary psychological difficulties and expected progress toward recovery must be addressed. Further research is needed regarding patients' psychological preparation for discharge after open heart surgery.

Promoting Home and Community-Based Care

TEACHING PATIENTS SELF-CARE

Depending on the type of surgery and postoperative progress, the patient may be discharged from the hospital as early as 3 days after surgery. Although the patient may be anxious to return home, usually both patient and family have apprehensions about this transition. The family members often express the fear that they are not capable of caring for the patient at home. They often are concerned that complications will occur that they are unprepared to handle.

The nurse helps the patient and family to set realistic, achievable goals. A teaching plan that meets the patient's individual needs is developed with the patient and family. This is done before admission and reviewed each shift through the hospitalization or with each home care and rehabilitation contact. Specific instructions are provided about diet; activity progression and exercise; deep breathing, huffing (coughing), incentive spirometry, and smoking cessation; weight and temperature monitoring; the medication regimen; and follow-up visits with home care nurses, the rehabilitation program, the surgeon, and the cardiologist or internist.

Some patients may have difficulty learning and retaining information after cardiac surgery. Studies have documented that many patients have difficulties in cognitive function after cardiac surgery that do not occur after other types of major surgery. The patient may experience recent memory loss, short attention span, difficulty with simple math, poor handwriting, and visual disturbances. Patients with these difficulties often become frustrated when they try to resume normal activities and learn how to care for themselves at home. The patient and family are reassured that the difficulty is temporary and will subside, usually in 6 to 8 weeks. In the meantime, instructions are given to the patient at a much slower pace than normal, and a family member assumes responsibility for making sure that the prescribed regimen is followed.

CONTINUING CARE

Arrangements are made for a home care nurse to provide care. Since the length of time that the patient remains in the hospital is relatively short, it is particularly important for the nurse to assess the patient's and family's ability to manage care in the home. The education plan is continued by the home care nurse. Vital signs and incisions are monitored, the patient is assessed for signs and symptoms of complications, and support for the patient and family is provided. Additional interventions may include dressing changes, intravenous antibiotic administration, diet counseling, and smoking cessation strategies.

Patient teaching does not end at the time of discharge from home health. The patient is encouraged to maintain telephone contact with the surgeon, cardiologist, and nurses. This provides the patient and family with reassurance that questions can be answered and problems can be resolved if they arise. Many hospitals provide family support sessions that help family members to cope with their own stress related to the patient's home health care management. The patient is expected to have a follow-up visit with the surgeon.

Many patients and families benefit from supportive programs such as the postcardiac surgery rehabilitation programs offered by many medical centers. These programs provide exercise monitoring; instructions about diet and stress reduction; information about resuming exercise, work, driving, and sexual activity; and support groups for patients and families. The AHA sponsors the Mended Hearts Club, which provides information as well as an opportunity for families to share experiences.

Evaluation

Expected Outcomes

Expected outcomes may include:

1. Maintains adequate cardiac output
2. Maintains adequate gas exchange
3. Maintains fluid (and electrolyte) balance
4. Experiences decreased symptoms of sensory alterations; is oriented to person, place, and time
5. Experiences relief of pain
6. Maintains adequate tissue perfusion
7. Achieves adequate rest
8. Maintains adequate renal perfusion
9. Maintains normal body temperature
10. Performs self-care activities

A typical plan of postoperative nursing care for the cardiac surgery patient is presented in Plan of Nursing Care 25-1.

Myocardial Infarction (MI)

Pathophysiology

MI refers to the process by which areas of myocardial cells in the heart are permanently destroyed. Like unstable angina, MI is usually, but not always, caused by reduced blood flow in a coronary artery due to atherosclerosis and a complete occlusion of an artery by an embolus or thrombus. Other causes of an MI include vasospasm (a sudden constriction or narrowing) of a coronary artery, decreased oxygen supply (from acute blood loss, anemia, or low blood pressure), and increased demand for oxygen (from rapid heart rate, thyrotoxicosis, or ingestion of cocaine). In each case, a profound imbalance exists between myocardial oxygen supply and demand.

Coronary occlusion, heart attack, and MI are terms used synonymously, but the preferred term is MI. The area of infarction takes time to develop. Initially, as the cells are deprived of oxygen, ischemia develops, and over time the lack of oxygen results in infarction, or the death of cells. Thus, the expression "Time is muscle" may be used to indicate the urgency of appropriate treatment to improve patient outcomes. Each year in the United States, nearly 1 million people have an acute MI; one fourth of these people die from the MI. Half of those who die never even reach a hospital.

Various descriptions further define an MI: the location of the injury to the left ventricular wall (anterior, inferior posterior, or lateral wall) or to the right ventricle, or the point in time within the process of infarction (acute, evolving, or old). The location and timing are usually identified by an ECG. Regardless of the location, the goal of medical therapy in acute MI is to prevent or minimize myocardial tissue necrosis and to prevent complications.

The pathophysiology of heart disease and the risk factors involved were discussed earlier in this chapter.

Clinical Manifestations

Chest pain that occurs suddenly and continues despite rest and medication is the primary presenting symptom. Patients may be anxious and restless. They may have cool, pale, and moist skin. Their heart rate and respiratory rate may be faster than normal. These manifestations, which are due to stimulation of the sympathetic nervous system, may not be present; only some may be present; or they may be present for only a short while. In many cases, the signs and symptoms of MI cannot be distinguished from those of unstable angina.

Gerontologic Considerations

The gerontologic considerations for MI are the same as those for angina. However, age, other illnesses, and preexisting conditions may prevent the patient from receiving otherwise indicated treatment for acute MI (eg, thrombolytic therapy). The mortality rate is higher in patients older than age 65 with an acute MI.

Assessment and Diagnostic Findings

Diagnosis of MI is generally based on the history of the present illness, the ECG, and laboratory test results (eg, serial serum enzyme values). The prognosis depends on the severity of coronary artery obstruction and hence the extent of myocardial damage. Physical examination is always conducted, but the examination alone is insufficient to confirm the diagnosis.

PATIENT HISTORY

The patient history has two parts: the description of the current complaint of pain, and the history of previous illnesses and family health history, particularly of heart disease. Previous history should also include information about the patient's risk factors for heart disease.

(*text continues on page 625*)

25•1 **Plan of Nursing Care**

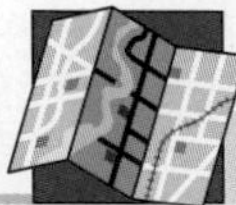

Care of the Patient After Cardiac Surgery

Nursing Interventions	Rationale	Expected Outcomes
Nursing Diagnosis: Decreased cardiac output related to blood loss and compromised myocardial function **Goal:** Restoration of cardiac output to maintain/attain desired lifestyle		
1. Monitor cardiovascular status. Serial readings of blood pressures (arterial, left atrial, pulmonary artery, pulmonary artery wedge pressure [PAWP], central venous pressure [CVP]), cardiac output/index, systemic and pulmonary vascular resistance, and cardiac rhythm and rate are obtained, recorded, and correlated with the patient's condition.	1. Effectiveness of cardiac output is determined by hemodynamic monitoring.	The following parameters are within the patient's normal ranges: • Arterial pressure • Left atrial pressures • PAWP • Pulmonary artery pressures • CVP • Heart sounds • Pulmonary and systemic vascular resistance • Cardiac output and cardiac index • Peripheral pulses • Cardiac rate and rhythm • Cardiac enzymes • Urine output • Skin and mucosal color • Skin temperature
a. Assess arterial pressure every 15 minutes until stable, and as directed thereafter.	a. Blood pressure is one of the most important physiologic parameters to follow; vasoconstriction after cardiopulmonary bypass may make auscultatory blood pressure unobtainable.	
b. Auscultate for heart sounds and rhythm.	b. Auscultation provides evidence of cardiac tamponade (muffled distant heart sounds), pericarditis (precordial rub), dysrhythmias.	
c. Assess peripheral pulses (pedal, tibial, popliteal, femoral, radial, brachial, carotid).	c. Presence or absence and quality of pulses provide data about cardiac output as well as obstructive lesions.	
d. Measure left atrial pressure, pulmonary artery diastolic (PAD) pressure, PAWP to determine left ventricular end-diastolic volume and to assess cardiac output.	d. Rising pressures may indicate congestive heart failure or pulmonary edema.	
e. Monitor PAWP, PAD, left atrial pressure, and CVP to assess blood volume, vascular tone, and pumping effectiveness of the heart. *Remember: Trends are more important than isolated readings;* mechanical ventilation may elevate CVP.	e. High PAWP, PAD, left atrial pressure, or CVP may result from hypervolemia, heart failure, cardiac tamponade. If blood pressure drop is due to low blood volume, PAWP, PAD, left atrial pressure, and CVP will show corresponding drop.	
f. Monitor ECG pattern for cardiac dysrhythmias (see Chap. 24 for discussion of dysrhythmias).	f. Dysrhythmias may occur with coronary ischemia, hypoxia, alterations in serum potassium, edema, bleeding, acid–base or electrolyte disturbances, digitalis toxicity, cardiac failure. ST-segment changes may indicate myocardial ischemia or coronary artery spasm. Pacemaker capture and antiarrhythmic medication effects are used to maintain a heart rate and rhythm to support stable blood pressures.	
g. Assess cardiac enzymes daily (if ordered).	g. Elevations may indicate myocardial infarction.	
h. Measure urine output every ½ to 1 hour at first, then with vital signs.	h. Urine output less than 25 mL/h indicates decreased cardiac output and decreased renal perfusion.	
i. Observe buccal mucosa, nailbeds, lips, earlobes, and extremities.	i. Duskiness and cyanosis may indicate decreased cardiac output.	
j. Assess skin; note temperature and color.	j. Cool moist skin indicates vasoconstriction and decreased cardiac output.	

(continued)

25•1 Plan of Nursing Care 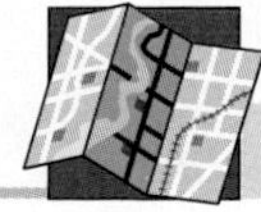

Care of the Patient After Cardiac Surgery (*continued*)

Nursing Interventions	Rationale	Expected Outcomes
2. Observe for persistent bleeding: steady, continuous drainage of blood; hypotension; low CVP; tachycardia. Prepare to administer blood products, IV solutions.	2. Bleeding can result from cardiac incision, tissue fragility, trauma to tissues, clotting defects.	• Less than 200 mL/h of drainage through chest tubes during first 4 to 6 hours • Vital signs stable
3. Observe for cardiac tamponade: hypotension; rising PAWP, PAD, left atrial pressure, or CVP; muffled heart sounds; weak, thready pulse; jugular vein distention; decreasing urinary output. Check for diminished amount of blood in chest drainage collection system. Prepare for pericardiocentesis. Assess for pulsus paradoxus.	3. Cardiac tamponade results from bleeding into the pericardial sac or accumulation of fluid in the sac, which compresses the heart and prevents adequate filling of the ventricles. Decrease in chest drainage may indicate fluid is accumulating in the pericardial sac.	• Vital signs stable • Chest tube drainage expected amount • CVP and left atrial pressures within normal limits • Urinary output within normal limits
4. Observe for cardiac failure: hypotension, rising PAWP, PAD, CVP, and left atrial pressure, tachycardia, restlessness, agitation, cyanosis, venous distention, dyspnea, moist crackles, ascites. Prepare to administer diuretics and digitalis.	4. Cardiac failure results from decreased pumping action of the heart; can cause deficient blood perfusion to vital organs.	• Vital signs stable • CVP and left atrial pressures within normal limits • Skin color normal • Respirations unlabored, clear breath sounds
5. Observe for myocardial infarction: ST-segment elevations, T-wave changes, decreased cardiac output in presence of normal circulating volume and filling pressures. Obtain serial ECGs and isoenzymes. Differentiate myocardial pain from incisional pain.	5. Symptoms may be masked by the patient's level of consciousness and pain medication.	• Vital signs stable • Pain limited to incision • ECG and isoenzymes negative for ischemic changes

Nursing Diagnosis: Risk for impaired gas exchange related to trauma of extensive chest surgery
Goal: Adequate gas exchange

Assess respiratory status and provide for adequate ventilation and tissue oxygenation.

Nursing Interventions	Rationale	Expected Outcomes
1. Maintain assist–control or intermittent (synchronous if possible) ventilation.	1. Ventilatory support may be used to decrease work of the heart, to maintain effective ventilation, and to provide an airway in the event of cardiac arrest.	• Airway patent • ABGs within normal range • Endotracheal tube correctly placed, as evidenced by x-ray • Breath sounds clear • Ventilator synchronous with respirations • Breath sounds clear after suctioning/huffing • Nailbeds and mucous membranes pink • Mental acuity consistent with amount of sedatives and analgesics received • Oriented to person; able to respond yes and no appropriately
2. Monitor arterial blood gases, tidal volumes, peak inspiratory pressures, and extubation parameters.	2. ABGs and tidal volume indicate effectiveness of ventilator and changes that need to be made to improve gas exchange.	
3. Auscultate chest for breath sounds.	3. Crackles indicate pulmonary congestion; decreased or absent breath sounds may indicate pneumothorax or hemothorax.	
4. Sedate patient adequately, as prescribed, and monitor respiratory rate and depth if ventilations are not "controlled."	4. Sedation helps the patient to tolerate the endotracheal tube and to cope with ventilatory sensations; sedatives can depress respiratory rate and depth.	
5. Provide chest physiotherapy as prescribed.	5. Aids in preventing retention of secretions and atelectasis.	
6. Promote deep breathing, coughing, and turning. Encourage use of incentive spirometer and compliance with breathing treatments. Teach incisional splinting with a "cough pillow" to decrease discomfort during deep breathing and huffing (coughing).	6. Aids in keeping airway patent, preventing atelectasis, and facilitating lung expansion.	

(*continued*)

25•1

Plan of Nursing Care 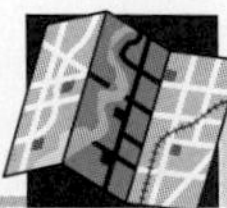 Care of the Patient After Cardiac Surgery (*continued*)

Nursing Interventions	Rationale	Expected Outcomes
7. Suction tracheobronchial secretions as needed, using strict aseptic technique.	7. Retention of secretions leads to hypoxia and possible cardiac arrest; retained secretions promote infection.	
8. Assist in weaning and endotracheal tube removal.		

Nursing Diagnosis: Risk for alteration in fluid volume and electrolyte balance related to alterations in blood volume
Goal: Fluid and electrolyte balance

Nursing Interventions	Rationale	Expected Outcomes
1. Maintain fluid and electrolyte balance.	1. Adequate circulating blood volume is necessary for optimal cellular activity; metabolic acidosis and electrolyte imbalance can occur after use of cardiopulmonary bypass.	• Fluid intake and output balanced • Hemodynamic assessment parameters negative for fluid overload and dehydration • Normal blood pressure with position changes • Absence of dysrhythmia
a. Keep intake and output flow sheets; record urine volume every ½ to 2 hours while in critical care unit; then every 4 to 8 hours.	a. Provides a method to determine positive or negative fluid balance and fluid requirements.	
b. Assess the following parameters: pulmonary artery pressures, left atrial pressures, blood pressure, CVP, PAWP, weight, electrolyte levels, hematocrit, jugular venous pressure, tissue turgor, liver size, breath sounds, urinary output, and nasogastric tube drainage.	b. Provides information about state of hydration.	
c. Measure postoperative chest drainage (should not exceed 200 mL/h for first 4 to 6 hours); cessation of drainage may indicate kinked or blocked chest tube. Ensure patency and integrity of the drainage system. Maintain autotransfusion system if in use.	c. Excessive blood loss from chest cavity can cause hypovolemia.	
2. Be alert to changes in serum electrolyte levels.	2. A specific concentration of electrolytes is necessary in both extracellular and intracellular body fluids to sustain life.	• Blood pH 7.35 to 7.45 • Serum potassium 3.5 to 5.0 mEq/L (3.5 to 5.0 mmol/L) • Serum magnesium 1.5 to 2.5 in mEq/L • Serum sodium 135 to 145 mEq/L (135 to 145 mmol/L) • Serum calcium 8.8 to 10.3 mg/100 mL (2.20 to 2.58 mmol/L)
a. Hypokalemia (low potassium) *Effects:* dysrhythmias, digitalis toxicity, metabolic alkalosis, weakened myocardium, cardiac arrest Observe for specific ECG changes. Administer IV potassium replacement as directed.	a. *Causes:* inadequate intake, diuretics, vomiting, excessive nasogastric drainage, stress from surgery	
b. Hyperkalemia (high potassium) *Effects:* mental confusion, restlessness, nausea, weakness, paresthesias of extremities Be prepared to administer an ion-exchange resin (sodium polystyrene sulfonate [Kayexalate]); IV sodium bicarbonate, or IV insulin and glucose.	b. *Causes:* Increased intake, hemolysis from cardiopulmonary bypass/mechanical assist devices, acidosis, renal insufficiency, tissue necrosis, adrenal cortical insufficiency. The resin binds potassium and promotes intestinal excretion of it. IV sodium bicarbonate drives potassium into the cells from extra-cellular fluid. Insulin assists the cells with glucose absorption. The glucose provides the energy to activate the sodium–potassium pumps, which pull potassium into the cell while pumping sodium out.	

(*continued*)

25•1

Plan of Nursing Care 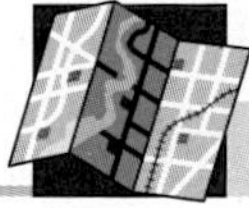 Care of the Patient After Cardiac Surgery (*continued*)

Nursing Interventions	Rationale	Expected Outcomes
c. Hypomagnesemia (low magnesium) *Effects:* paresthesias, carpopedal spasm, muscle cramps, tetany, irritability, tremors, hyperexcitability, hyperreflexia, disorientation, depression, seizures, hypotension, dysrhythmias, prolonged PR and QT intervals, broad flat T waves. Be prepared to treat the cause. Magnesium supplements may be given (po preferred, extreme caution if IV).	c. *Causes:* decreased intake (chronic alcoholism, malnutrition, starvation), impaired absorption (malabsorption syndromes, excess intake of calcium) and increased excretion normal for 24 hours after major surgery, diuretic loss of intestinal fluids, diabetic ketoacidosis, primary aldosteronism, primary hyperparathyroidism.	• See page 622 for expected outcomes
d. Hypermagnesemia (high magnesium) *Effects:* vasodilation, flushing, warm feeling, hypotension, loss of reflexes, slowing bowel function, drowsiness, respiratory depression, coma, apnea, cardiac arrest. Be prepared to treat cause; dialysis and calcium gluconate administration.	d. *Causes:* renal failure, excess intake of medications with magnesium (antacids, cathartics)	
e. Hyponatremia (low sodium) *Effects:* weakness, fatigue, confusion, seizures, coma. Administer sodium or diuretics as directed.	c. *Causes:* reduction of total body sodium, or increased water intake causing dilution of sodium	
f. Hypocalcemia (low calcium) *Effects:* numbness and tingling in fingertips, toes, ears, nose; carpopedal spasm; muscle cramps; tetany. Administer replacement therapy as directed.	f. *Causes:* alkalosis, multiple blood transfusions of citrated blood products	
g. Hypercalcemia (high calcium) *Effects:* dysrhythmias, digitalis toxicity, asystole. Institute treatment as directed.	g. *Cause:* prolonged immobility	

Nursing Diagnosis: Risk for sensory–perceptual alterations related to sensory overload
Goal: Reduction of symptoms of sensory overload; prevention of postcardiotomy psychosis

Nursing Interventions	Rationale	Expected Outcomes
1. Use measures to prevent postcardiotomy psychosis: a. Explain all procedures and the need for patient cooperation. b. Plan nursing care to provide for periods of uninterrupted sleep with day–night pattern. c. Decrease sleep-preventing environmental stimuli as much as possible. d. Promote continuity of care from nurse to nurse. e. Orient to time and place frequently. Encourage family to visit at regular times. f. Assess for medications that may contribute to delirium. g. Teach relaxation techniques and diversions.	1. Postcardiotomy psychosis may result from anxiety, sleep deprivation, increased sensory input, disorientation to night and day. Normally, sleep cycles are at least 50 minutes long. The first cycle may be as long as 90 to 120 minutes and then shorten during successive cycles. Sleep deprivation results when the sleep cycles are interrupted or there are not enough of them.	• Cooperates with procedures • Sleeps for long, uninterrupted intervals • Oriented to person, place, time • Experiences no perceptual distortions, hallucinations, disorientation, delusions

(*continued*)

25•1 Plan of Nursing Care

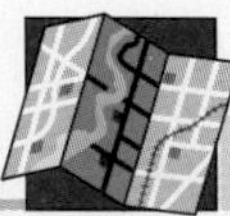

Care of the Patient After Cardiac Surgery (*continued*)

Nursing Interventions	Rationale	Expected Outcomes
h. Encourage self-care as much as tolerated to enhance self-control. Assess support systems and coping mechanisms		
2. Observe for symptoms: perceptual distortions, hallucinations, disorientation, paranoid delusions.		

Nursing Diagnosis: Pain related to operative trauma and pleural irritation caused by chest tubes and/or internal mammary artery dissection
Goal: Relief of pain

Nursing Interventions	Rationale	Expected Outcomes
1. Record nature, type, location, and duration of pain.	1. Pain and anxiety increase pulse rate, oxygen consumption, and cardiac workload.	• States pain is decreasing in severity • Reports absence of pain • Restlessness decreased • Vital signs stable • Participates in deep-breathing and coughing exercises • Verbalizes fewer complaints of pain each day • Positions self; participates in care activities • Gradually increases activity
2. Assist patient to differentiate between surgical pain and anginal pain.	2. Anginal pain requires immediate treatment.	
3. Encourage routine pain medication dosing for the first 24 to 72 hours and observe for side effects of lethargy, hypotension, tachycardia, respiratory depression.	3. Analgesia promotes rest, decreases oxygen consumption caused by pain, and aids patient in performing deep-breathing and coughing exercises.	

Nursing Diagnosis: Risk for alteration in renal perfusion related to decreased cardiac output, hemolysis, or vasopressor drug therapy
Goal: Maintenance of adequate renal perfusion

Nursing Interventions	Rationale	Expected Outcomes
1. Assess renal function:	1. Renal injury can be caused by deficient perfusion, hemolysis, low cardiac output, and use of vasopressor agents to increase blood pressure.	• Urine output consistent with fluid intake; greater than 25 mL/h • Urine specific gravity 1.015 to 1.025. • BUN, creatinine, electrolytes within normal limits
a. Measure urine output every ½ to 1 hour.	a. Less than 25 mL/h indicates decreased renal function.	
b. Measure urine specific gravity.	b. Indicates kidneys' ability to concentrate urine in renal tubules.	
c. Monitor and report lab results: BUN, serum creatinine, urine and serum electrolytes.	c. Indicate kidneys' ability to excrete waste products.	
2. Prepare to administer rapid-acting diuretics or inotropic drugs (dopamine, dobutamine).	2. Promote renal function and increase cardiac output and renal blood flow.	
3. Prepare patient for dialysis or continuous renal replacement therapy if indicated.		

Nursing Diagnosis: Risk for hyperthermia related to infection or postpericardiotomy syndrome
Goal: Maintenance of normal body temperature

Nursing Interventions	Rationale	Expected Outcomes
1. Assess temperature every hour.	1. Fever can indicate infectious process or postpericardiotomy syndrome.	• Normal body temperature • Incisions are free of infection and are healing • Absence of symptoms of postpericardiotomy syndrome
2. Use aseptic technique when changing dressings, suctioning endotracheal tube; maintain closed systems for all intravenous and arterial lines and for indwelling urinary catheter.	2. Decreases chance of infection.	
3. Observe for symptoms of postpericardiotomy syndrome: fever, malaise, pericardial effusion, pericardial friction rub, arthralgia.	3. Occurs in 10% to 40% of patients after cardiac surgery.	

(*continued*)

25•1

Plan of Nursing Care 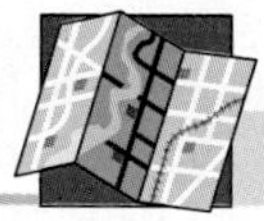 Care of the Patient After Cardiac Surgery (*continued*)

Nursing Interventions	Rationale	Expected Outcomes
4. Administer anti-inflammatory agents as directed.	4. Relieve symptoms of inflammation (eg, warmth or feverish sensation, swelling, fullness, stiffness or aching sensation, and fatigue).	
Nursing Diagnosis: Knowledge deficit about self-care activities **Goal:** Ability to perform self-care activities		
1. Develop teaching plan for patient and family. Provide specific instructions for the following: • Diet • Activity progression • Exercise • Deep breathing, huffing (coughing), lung expansion exercises • Temperature monitoring • Medication regimen • Pulse taking • CPR, if appropriate for the family to learn • Entry to the emergency medical system • Need for MedicAlert identification	1. Each patient will have unique learning needs.	• Patient and family members explain and comply with all therapeutic regimen • Patient and family members identify lifestyle changes necessitated by therapeutic regimen • Has copy of discharge instructions • Makes follow-up phone calls • Keeps follow-up appointments
2. Provide verbal and written instructions; provide several teaching sessions for reinforcement and answering questions.	2. Repetition promotes learning by allowing for clarification of misinformation. After cardiac surgery, patients have short-term memory difficulty; written information is helpful because it can be used as a resource after discharge. The less familiar or greater the amount of the content the patient and family need to learn, the more time it will take to learn.	
3. Involve family in all teaching sessions.	3. Family member responsible for home care is usually anxious and requires adequate time for learning.	
4. Provide information regarding follow-up phone call to surgeon, cardiologist, or liaison nurse; follow-up visit with surgeon.	4. Arrangements for phone contacts with health care personnel help to allay anxieties.	
5. Make appropriate referrals: home care agency, cardiac rehabilitation program, community support groups, Mended Hearts Club.	5. Learning and lifestyle changes continue after discharge from the hospital.	

ELECTROCARDIOGRAM

The ECG provides information that assists in diagnosing acute MI. It should be obtained within 10 minutes from the time a patient reports pain or arrives in the emergency department. By monitoring the ECG over time, the location, evolution, and resolution of an MI can be identified and followed.

The ECG changes that occur with an MI are seen in the leads that view the involved surface of the heart. Because infarction is time-mediated, the first ECG signs are those that represent myocardial ischemia and injury. Myocardial ischemia causes the T wave first to become enlarged and symmetric and later to be inverted because of altered late repolarization. Possibly, the ischemic region remains depolarized, whereas adjacent areas return to the resting state. Myocardial injury causes ST-segment changes. If there is epicardial myocardial injury, the injured cells depolarize normally but repolarize more rapidly than do normal cells; thus, the ST segment is above the isoelectric line (the area between the T wave and the next P wave is used as the reference for the isoelectric line). If the myocardial injury is on the endocardial surface, then the ST segment is depressed (1 mm or more) and is at least 0.08 seconds in duration. With injury, the ST-segment depression is usually horizontal or has a downward slope.

MI is classified either as Q-wave or non–Q-wave. With Q-wave infarction, abnormal Q waves develop within 1 to 3 days because there is no depolarization current conducted from necrotic tissue. The lead system then views the flow of current from other parts of the heart. An abnormal Q wave is 0.04 seconds or longer and is 25% of the R wave (provided the R wave itself exceeds 5 mm) in depth. Injury and ischemic changes are also present (Fig. 25-9). With non–Q-wave MI, the ST-segment and T-wave changes are not followed by a Q wave, but symptoms and cardiac enzyme analysis confirm the diagnosis.

During recovery from an MI, the ST segment often is the first to return to normal (1 to 6 weeks). The T wave becomes large and symmetric for 24 hours, and then inverts within 1 to 3 days for 1 to 2 weeks. Q-wave alterations are usually permanent. An old Q-wave MI is usually indicated by an abnormal Q wave without ST-segment and T-wave changes.

ECHOCARDIOGRAM

The echocardiogram is used to evaluate cardiac function, specifically ventricular function. It may be used to assist in diagnosing an MI, especially when the ECG is nondiagnostic. The ejection fraction can be determined by echocardiogram (see Chap. 23).

LABORATORY TESTS

Historically, laboratory tests included **creatine kinase** (CK) with isoenzymes and **lactic dehydrogenase** (LDH) evaluation. Other tests with a shorter run time, allowing for an earlier diagnosis, include myoglobin and **troponin** analysis. These tests are based on the release of cellular contents into the circulation when myocardial cells die. Table 25-3 shows the time courses of cardiac enzymes.

Creatine Kinase and Its Isoenzymes.

There are three CK isoenzymes: CK-MM (skeletal muscle), CK-MB (heart muscle), and CK-BB (brain tissue). CK-MB is the cardiac-specific isoenzyme—that is, CK-MB is found mainly in cardiac cells and therefore rises only when there has been damage to these cells. CK-MB is the most specific index for the diagnosis of acute MI. It starts to increase within 1 hour and peaks within 24 hours of an MI. If the area is reperfused (eg, from thrombolytic therapy or PTCA), it peaks earlier.

Lactic Dehydrogenase and Its Isoenzymes.

LDH is not as reliable an indicator of acute myocardial damage as CK. However, because it peaks later and is elevated longer than other cardiac enzymes, LDH is useful for diagnosing an MI in patients who may have delayed seeking treatment and admission to the hospital.

Of the five LDH isoenzymes, only two (LDH_1 and LDH_2) are important in diagnosing an acute MI. Both LDH_1 and LDH_2 predominate in the heart, kidney, and brain, but normally the percentage of LDH_2 compared with LDH_1 is greater. When the percentage of LDH_1 exceeds that of LDH_2, the pattern is said to have flipped, indicating an acute MI.

Myoglobin.

Myoglobin is a heme protein that helps to transport oxygen. Like CK-MB enzyme, myoglobin is found in cardiac and skeletal muscle. Myoglobin starts to increase within 1 or 2 hours and peaks within 6 hours after onset of symptoms. The test takes only a few minutes to run. An increase in myoglobin is not very specific in indicating an acute cardiac event; however, negative results are an excellent parameter for ruling out an acute MI. If the first myoglobin test results are negative, the test may be repeated 3 hours later. Another negative test result would confirm that the patient did not have an MI.

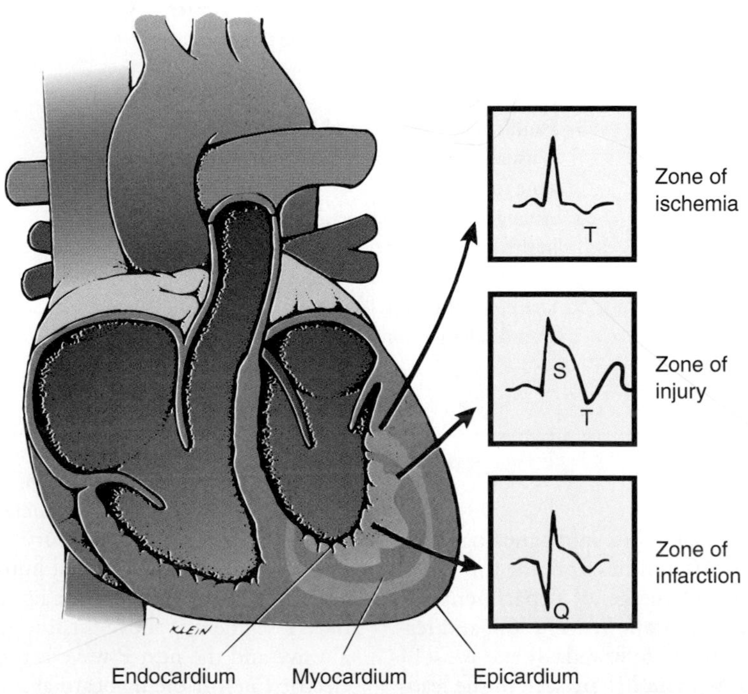

FIGURE 25•9 Effects of ischemia, injury, and infarction on ECG recording. Ischemia causes inversion of T wave because of altered repolarization. Cardiac muscle injury causes elevation of the ST segment and tall, symmetrical T waves. With Q-wave infarction, Q or QS waves develop because of the absence of depolarization current from the necrotic tissue and opposing currents from other parts of the heart.

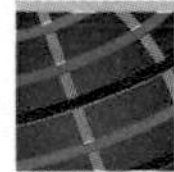

TABLE 25•3 **Serum Markers of Acute Myocardial Infarction**

Serum Lab Test	Earliest Increase	Test Running Time	Peak	Return to Normal
Total CK	3–6 hours	30–60 min	24–36 hours	3 days
CK-MB	2–8 hours	30–60 min	12–24 hours	3–4 days
	2–3 hours	10–40 min	10–18 hours	3–4 days
Myoglobin	1–3 hours	10–30 min	4–12 hours	12 hours
Troponin T or I	3–4 hours	30–60 min	4–24 hours	1–3 weeks

(Resource assistance by Kathy Senger, Laboratory Supervisor, Washington Adventist Hospital)

Troponin. Troponin, a protein found in the myocardium, regulates the myocardial contractile process. There are three isomers of troponin (C, I, and T). Because of its smaller size and the increased specificity for cardiac muscle, troponin I is the test more frequently used to identify a cardiac event. The increase in the amount of troponin in the serum starts and peaks approximately the same as CK-MB. However, it remains elevated for a longer period—up to 2 weeks. Unstable angina also causes an increase in troponin.

Medical Management

The goal of medical management is to minimize myocardial damage, preserve myocardial function, and prevent complications. These goals are now achieved by reperfusing the area by emergency use of PTCA or thrombolytic medications. Minimizing myocardial damage is also accomplished by reducing myocardial oxygen demand and increasing oxygen supply with medications, oxygen administration, and bed rest. The resolution of pain and ECG changes are the primary clinical indicators that demand and supply are in equilibrium; they may also indicate reperfusion. Visualization of blood flow through an open vessel in the catheterization laboratory is evidence of reperfusion.

EMERGENT PTCA

The patient in whom an acute MI is suspected may be referred for an immediate PTCA. PTCA may be used to open the occluded coronary artery in an acute MI and promote reperfusion to the area that has been deprived of oxygen. PTCA treats the underlying atherosclerotic lesion. Because the duration of the lack of oxygen is directly related to the number of cells that die, the time from the patient's arrival in the emergency room to the time of vessel access should be less than 60 minutes. Obviously, to perform an emergent PTCA within this short time, a cardiac catheterization laboratory and staff must be available.

PHARMACOLOGIC THERAPY

The patient with an acute MI receives the same medications as the patient with unstable angina, with the possible additions of thrombolytics, analgesics, and angiotensin-converting enzyme (ACE) inhibitors.

Thrombolytics. Thrombolytics are medications that are usually administered intravenously, although some may also be given directly into the coronary artery in the cardiac catheterization laboratory (Chart 25-2). The purpose of thrombolytics is to dissolve and lyse the thrombus in a coronary artery (thrombolysis), allowing blood to flow through the coronary artery again (reperfusion), minimizing the size of the infarction, and preserving ventricular function. Even though thrombolytics may dissolve the thrombus, they do not affect the underlying atherosclerotic lesion. Therefore, the patient is usually referred for a cardiac catheterization and other invasive interventions if needed at a later time.

Thrombolytics dissolve all clots, not just the one in the coronary artery. Therefore, thrombolytics are not to be used if the patient has formed a protective clot (eg, after major surgery or

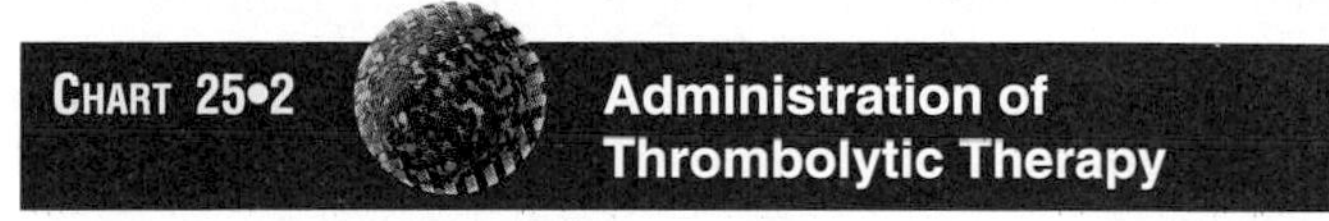

CHART 25•2 **Administration of Thrombolytic Therapy**

Indications

- Chest pain for longer than 20 minutes, unrelieved by nitroglycerin
- ST-segment elevation in at least two lead systems that face the same area of the heart
- Less than 24 hours from onset of pain

Absolute Contraindications

- Active bleeding
- Known bleeding disorder
- History of hemorrhagic stroke
- History of intracranial vessel malformation
- Recent major surgery or trauma
- Uncontrolled hypertension
- Pregnancy

Nursing Considerations

- Minimize the number of times the patient's skin is punctured.
- Avoid intramuscular injections.
- Draw blood for laboratory tests when starting the IV line.
- Start IV lines before thrombolytic therapy; designate one line to use for blood draws.
- Avoid continual use of noninvasive blood pressure cuff.
- Monitor for acute dysrhythmias, hypotension, and allergic reaction.
- Check for signs and symptoms of bleeding:
  decrease in hematocrit and hemoglobin values, decrease in blood pressure, increase in heart rate, oozing or bulging at invasive procedure sites, back pain, muscle weakness, changes in level of consciousness, complaints of headache
- Treat major bleeding by discontinuing thrombolytic therapy and any anticoagulants; apply direct pressure and notify the physician immediately.
- Treat minor bleeding by applying direct pressure if accessible and appropriate; continue to monitor.

hemorrhagic stroke). Moreover, thrombolytics reduce the patient's ability to form a stabilizing clot, so the patient is at risk for bleeding. Therefore, thrombolytics should not be used if the patient is bleeding or has a bleeding disorder. All patients who receive thrombolytic therapy are put on bleeding precautions to minimize the risk for bleeding. This means minimizing the number of punctures for inserting intravenous lines, avoiding intramuscular injections, preventing tissue trauma, and applying pressure for longer than usual after any puncture.

To be effective, thrombolytics must be administered as early as possible after the onset of symptoms that indicate an acute MI. They are not to be given to patients with unstable angina. Hospitals monitor their ability to administer these medications within 30 minutes from the time the patient arrives in the emergency room. This is called "door-to-needle" time.

The thrombolytic agents used most often are streptokinase and tissue-type plasminogen activator (t-PA). Others include reteplase, anistreplase, and urokinase.

Streptokinase. Streptokinase increases the amount of plasminogen activator, which then increases the amount of both circulating and clot-bound plasminogen. Because streptokinase is made from a bacteria, its use also entails a risk of an allergic reaction. Vasculitis has been noted up to 9 days after administration. Streptokinase is not used if the patient has been exposed to a recent *Streptococcus* infection or has received streptokinase in the past 6 to 12 months.

Tissue-Type Plasminogen Activator. t-PA, in contrast to streptokinase, activates the plasminogen on the clot more than the circulating plasminogen. Because it does not decrease the clotting factors as much as streptokinase does, heparin is used with t-PA to prevent another clot from forming at the same lesion site. The enzyme t-PA is a naturally occurring enzyme, so allergic reactions are minimized. t-PA costs considerably more than streptokinase.

Analgesics. The analgesic of choice for acute MI remains morphine sulfate administered in intravenous boluses. Not only does morphine reduce pain and anxiety, but it also reduces preload, which in turn decreases the workload of the heart, and relaxes bronchioles to enhance oxygenation. The cardiovascular response to morphine is monitored carefully, particularly the blood pressure, which can be lowered, and the respiratory rate, which can be depressed. Because morphine affects pain, careful assessment of ischemia by ST segment monitoring is needed.

Angiotensin-Converting Enzyme Inhibitor. A substance found in the lumen of all blood vessels, ACE converts angiotensin I to angiotensin II. Angiotensin I is formed when the kidneys release renin in response to decreased blood flow. Angiotensin I is converted to angiotensin II in the lungs. Angiotensin II causes the blood vessels to constrict and the kidneys to retain sodium and fluid while excreting potassium. These actions increase circulating fluid and raise the pressure against which the heart must pump, resulting in significantly increased cardiac workload. ACE inhibitors prevent the conversion of angiotensin from I to II. In the absence of angiotensin II, the blood pressure decreases and the kidneys excrete sodium and fluid (diuresis), so the oxygen demand of the heart is significantly decreased. Use of ACE inhibitors in patients after an MI has been shown to decrease the mortality rate and prevent the onset of congestive heart failure. Blood pressure, urine output, and serum sodium and potassium level need to be monitored closely because of the actions of ACE inhibitors.

NURSING PROCESS: THE PATIENT WITH MYOCARDIAL INFARCTION

Assessment

One of the most important aspects of care of the patient with an MI is the nursing assessment. This establishes a baseline on the patient's current status so that any deviations may be noted immediately. The nursing assessment systematically identifies the needs of the patient and determines the priority of these needs. Systematic assessment includes a careful history, particularly as it relates to symptoms: chest pain, difficulty breathing (dyspnea), palpitations, faintness (syncope), or sweating (diaphoresis). Each symptom must be evaluated with regard to time, duration, and the factors that precipitate the symptom and relieve it. A precise and complete physical assessment is critical to detect complications, and any change in patient status is reported immediately. The accompanying assessment chart identifies the aspects that need to be assessed and the possible assessment findings.

In addition, intravenous sites are examined frequently. The nurse inspects the lines for patency and the insertion site for signs of inflammation. At least one and possibly two intravenous lines are placed in any patient with chest pain to ensure that access is available for administering emergency medications. (Medications are administered intravenously to achieve rapid onset and to allow for timely adjustment. Intramuscular medications are avoided because of the risk of altering serum enzyme levels.) Once the patient's condition stabilizes, the intravenous line may be converted to a saline lock device to maintain access.

Diagnosis

Nursing Diagnoses

Based on the clinical manifestations, nursing history, and diagnostic assessment data, the patient's major nursing diagnoses may include the following:

- Decreased myocardial perfusion related to reduced coronary blood flow from coronary thrombus and atherosclerotic plaque
- Potential impaired gas exchange related to fluid overload from left ventricular dysfunction
- Potential altered peripheral tissue perfusion related to decreased cardiac output from left ventricular dysfunction
- Anxiety related to fear of death
- Knowledge deficit about post-MI self-care

Collaborative Problems/Potential Complications

Based on the assessment data, potential complications that may develop include:

- Acute pulmonary edema (see Chap. 27)
- Congestive heart failure (see Chap. 27)
- Cardiogenic shock (see Chap. 27)
- Pericardial effusion and cardiac tamponade (see Chap. 27)
- Myocardial rupture (see Chap. 27)
- Dysrhythmias and cardiac arrest (see Chaps. 24 and 27)

Planning and Goals

The major goals of the patient include relief of signs and symptoms of ischemia (eg, chest pain and ST-segment changes), prevention of further myocardial damage, absence of respiratory

ASSESSMENT
SIGNS AND SYMPTOMS OF AN ACUTE MI

Cardiovascular

Chest pain, palpitations. Heart sounds may include S_3, S_4, and new onset of a murmur. Increased jugular venous distention may be seen if the MI has caused heart failure. Blood pressure may be elevated because of sympathetic stimulation or decreased because of decreased contractility, impending cardiogenic shock, or medications. Pulse deficit may indicate atrial fibrillation. In addition to ST-segment and T-wave changes, ECG may show tachycardia, bradycardia, and dysrhythmias.

Respiratory

Shortness of breath, dyspnea, tachypnea, and crackles if MI has caused pulmonary congestion. Pulmonary edema may be present.

Gastrointestinal

Nausea and vomiting.

Genitourinary

Decreased urinary output may indicate cardiogenic shock.

Skin

Cool, clammy, diaphoretic, and pale appearance due to sympathetic stimulation from loss of contractility may indicate cardiogenic shock. Dependent edema may also be present due to poor contractility.

Neurologic

Anxiety, restlessness, light-headedness may indicate increased sympathetic stimulation or decrease in contractility and cerebral oxygenation. Same symptoms may also herald cardiogenic shock. Headache, visual disturbances, altered speech, altered motor function, and further changes in level of consciousness may indicate cerebral bleeding if patient is receiving thrombolytics.

Psychological

Fear with feeling of impending doom, or patient may deny that anything is wrong.

difficulties, maintenance or attainment of adequate tissue perfusion by decreasing the heart's workload, reduced anxiety, adherence to the self-care program, and absence or early recognition of complications.

Nursing Interventions

Relieving Chest Pain

Relieving chest pain is the top priority for the patient with an acute MI, and medication therapy is required to accomplish this goal. Thus, the management of chest pain is truly a collaborative effort between the physician and the nurse. However, because the chest pain is part of the patient's acute disease process and not a complication of the MI, management of the patient's chest pain is presented in this discussion of nursing interventions; collaboration between the patient, nurse, and physician is critical in assessing the patient's response to therapy and in altering the interventions accordingly.

The accepted method for relieving chest pain associated with MI is the intravenous administration of vasodilator and anticoagulant therapy. Nitroglycerin and heparin are the medications of choice, respectively. Thrombolytic therapy (eg, streptokinase, anistreplase) is highly desirable for patients who present to the health care facility immediately and who qualify clinically (ie, there is no major contraindication to the medication).

Vital signs are assessed frequently as long as the patient is experiencing pain.

Physical rest, in bed with the backrest elevated or in a cardiac chair, will help decrease chest discomfort and dyspnea. Elevation of the head is beneficial for the following reasons:

- Tidal volume improves because of reduced pressure from abdominal contents on the diaphragm and, thus, better lung expansion and gas exchange.
- Drainage of the upper lung lobes improves.
- Venous return to the heart decreases (preload), which reduces the work of the heart.

The nurse administers pain-relieving and related medications. The recommended medical treatment for an acute MI patient is thrombolytic therapy or emergent percutaneous angioplasty. These therapies are important because, in addition to relieving pain, they aid in minimizing or avoiding permanent injury to the myocardium. Other therapies include intravenous vasodilator, anticoagulant, and antiplatelet medications. Nitroglycerin, heparin, and aspirin are the medications of choice. Morphine is used for pain control.

Oxygen should be administered along with medication therapy to ensure relief of pain. Inhaling oxygen even in low doses raises the circulating level of oxygen and reduces pain associated with low levels of circulating oxygen. The route of administration, usually by nasal cannula, and the oxygen flow rate are documented. A flow rate of 2 to 4 L/min is usually adequate to maintain oxygen saturation levels of 96% to 100% if no other disease is present.

Improving Respiratory Function

Regular and careful assessment of respiratory function can help the nurse detect early signs of complications associated with the lungs. Scrupulous attention to fluid volume status prevents overloading the heart and hence the lungs. Encouraging the patient to breathe deeply and change position frequently helps keep fluid from pooling in the lung bases.

Promoting Adequate Tissue Perfusion

Keeping the patient on bed or chair rest is particularly helpful in reducing myocardial oxygen consumption ($M\dot{V}O_2$). Checking skin temperature and peripheral pulses frequently is important to ensure adequate tissue perfusion. Oxygen may be administered to enrich the supply of circulating oxygen.

Reducing Anxiety

Developing a trusting and caring relationship with the patient is critical in reducing anxiety. Frequent opportunities are provided for the patient to share concerns and fears privately. An atmosphere of acceptance helps the patient to know that these feelings are both realistic and normal.

NURSING RESEARCH

National Survey of Coronary Precautions in Nursing Care

Riegel, B., Thomason, T., Carlson, B., & Gocka, I. (1996). Are nurses still practicing coronary precautions? A national survey of nursing care of acute myocardial infarction patients. *American Journal of Critical Care, 5*(2), 91–98.

Purpose

Historically, many nurses have implemented measures (restriction of iced and hot fluids, caffeine, rectal temperature measurement, and vigorous backrubs; feeding patients; requiring bed rest; interventions to minimize the severity and frequency of the Valsalva maneuver) to prevent complications to patients with acute myocardial infarction (AMI). However, many of those practices are not based on research, and some of them have been shown by nursing research to be unnecessary. In the review of research literature, the researchers found that avoidance of the Valsalva maneuver is the only significant precaution supported by research.

The purpose of this study was to describe the nursing practices that are used nationwide related to coronary precautions for patients with AMI.

Study Sample and Design

A survey concerning precautionary nursing practices related to AMI patients was sent to two groups: (1) members of American Association of Critical Care Nurses (AACN) who worked in coronary care units, medical intensive care units, or progressive care units and (2) non-AACN nurses who responded to a request for volunteers in a letter sent to managers of intensive care units, telemetry units, and medical-surgical units in a random sample of proportionally geographic hospitals. The survey was developed by the researchers, reviewed by a panel of experts to establish face and content validity, and pilot tested with a convenience sample.

Of the 2549 surveys mailed, 882 were returned and acceptable. Almost 84% of those were from the AACN group. Nearly half of the respondents worked in units that admitted 10 to 30 AMI patients in a month, and about three quarters of the respondents personally cared for at least five AMI patients in a month. About 60% of the respondents were ages 31 to 45, and about 20% were 30 or younger. Years of nursing experience or years of experience with AMI patients were not reported.

Findings

Survey results revealed that 37.8% of the respondents restricted iced and hot fluids; 83.6% restricted stimulant beverages, such as coffee; 55.7% avoided rectal temperatures; and 33.8% offered complete bed baths and bedpans to stable, pain-free patients on the first day after admission. A total of 73% of the respondents taught patients to avoid the Valsalva maneuver. Although most (76.2%) stated that these practices were regulated by a written policy, 28.9% reported they used their own judgment to increase patient activity. Fewer (15.9%) reported that they were free to make an autonomous clinical decision about patient activity.

Nurses who were most apt to use the coronary precautions were licensed practical nurses (LVNs/LPNs) (versus RNs), nurses working on general medical-surgical units (versus those working on telemetry or intensive care units), nurses who were not members of AACN, and younger and older nurses, (20 to 35 years old and over 51 years old, versus 36 to 50 years old).

Nursing Implications

The study revealed that the data that support liberalization of coronary precautions have not been adequately disseminated. The study illustrates the difference between practice based on tradition and practice based on research. The use of coronary precautions (other than avoidance of the Valsalva maneuver) has little or no physiologic rationale. Basing hospital policies on current research results rather than "customary and usual standard" practice would facilitate the end of traditional but outdated practices. In addition, this study demonstrated that nurses are trading their independent decision-making role in progression of patient activity for safety by using unit standards or physician orders. AMI patient activity progression could be an independent nursing judgment.

Monitoring and Managing Potential Complications

Complications that can occur after acute MI are due to the damage that occurs to the myocardium and to the conduction system as a result of the reduced coronary blood flow. Because these complications can be lethal, early identification of the cardinal signs and symptoms of their onset is critical.

The nurse monitors the patient closely for changes in cardiac rate and rhythm, heart sounds, blood pressure, chest pain, respiratory status, urinary output, skin color and temperature, sensorium, and laboratory values. Any changes in the patient's condition are reported promptly to the physician, and emergency measures are instituted when necessary.

Promoting Home and Community-Based Care

TEACHING PATIENTS SELF-CARE

The most effective way to increase the probability that the patient will comply with a self-care regimen after discharge is to provide adequate education about the disease process and to facilitate the patient's involvement in a cardiac rehabilitation program. Working with patients in developing plans to meet their specific needs further enhances the potential for compliance. See the accompanying chart, Promoting Health After MI.

Evaluation

Expected Outcomes

Expected outcomes may include:

1. Experiences relief of pain
2. Shows no signs of respiratory difficulties
3. Maintains adequate tissue perfusion
4. Is less anxious
5. Complies with self-care program
6. Avoids complications

Care of the patient with an uncomplicated MI is summarized in Plan of Nursing Care 25-2.

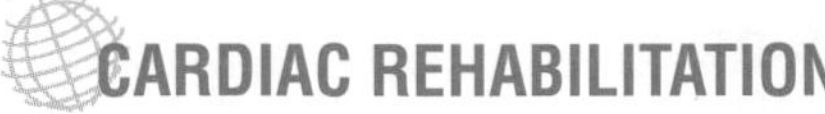

CARDIAC REHABILITATION

Once the MI patient is free of symptoms, an active rehabilitation program is initiated. Most insurance programs cover the cost of a cardiac rehabilitation program. However, some studies (Levknecht, Schriefer, & Maconis, 1997; Wenger et al., 1995) indicate that only 11% to 39% of patients who are candidates for cardiac rehabilitation services typically participate in these programs.

The goals of rehabilitation for the patient with an MI are to extend and improve the quality of life. The immediate objectives

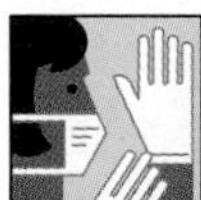

HEALTH PROMOTION AND ILLNESS PREVENTION

Promoting Health After MI

To extend and improve the quality of life, a patient who has had an MI must learn to regulate activity according to personal responses to each situation. With this in mind, the nurse and patient develop a program to help the patient achieve desired outcomes.

Changing Lifestyle During Convalescence and Healing

During this time, which starts early and lasts for varying periods, usually 6 to 8 weeks, patient goals include modification of activities so that complete recovery is achieved. Adaptation to a heart attack is an ongoing process and usually requires some modification of lifestyle. Some specific modifications include:

- Avoiding any activity that produces chest pain, dyspnea, or undue fatigue
- Avoiding extremes of heat and cold and walking against the wind
- Losing weight, if indicated
- Stopping smoking
- Alternating activity with rest periods. Some fatigue is normal and expected during convalescence.
- Using personal strengths to compensate for limitations
- Developing regular eating patterns (avoiding large meals and hurrying while eating; complying with prescribed diet, modifying calories, fat, and sodium as recommended)
- Adhering to medical regimen, especially in taking medications
- Pursuing activities that release tension

Adopting an Activity Program

Additionally, the patient needs to undertake an *orderly* program of increasing activity and exercise for long-term rehabilitation as follows:

- Engaging in a regimen of physical conditioning with a gradual increase in activity levels
- Walking daily, increasing distance and time as prescribed
- Monitoring pulse rate during physical activity until the maximum level of activity is attained
- Avoiding activities that tense the muscles: isometric exercise, weight-lifting, any activity that requires sudden bursts of energy
- Avoiding physical exercise immediately after a meal
- Shortening work hours when first returning to work
- Participating in a daily program of exercise that develops into a program of regular exercise for a lifetime

Managing Symptoms

The patient must learn to recognize and take appropriate action for possible recurrences of symptoms as follows:

- Reporting to the nearest emergency facility if chest pressure or pain is not relieved in 15 minutes by nitroglycerin
- Contacting the physician when the following occur: shortness of breath, fainting, slow or rapid heartbeat, swelling of feet and ankles

are to limit the effects and progression of atherosclerosis, return the patient to work and a pre-illness lifestyle, enhance the psychosocial and vocational status of the patient, and prevent another cardiac event. These objectives are accomplished by encouraging physical activity and physical conditioning, educating both patient and family, and providing counseling and behavioral interventions.

Throughout all phases of rehabilitation, the goals of activity and exercise tolerance are achieved through gradual physical conditioning, aimed at improving cardiac efficiency over time. Cardiac efficiency is achieved when work and activities of daily living can be performed at a lower heart rate and lower blood pressure, thereby reducing the heart's oxygen requirements and reducing cardiac workload.

Physical conditioning is performed under the care of a physician. The increase in activity should be gradual. It is not unusual for patients to "overdo it" in an attempt to achieve their goals too rapidly. Patients are observed for and instructed to stop exercise if chest pain, dyspnea, weakness, fatigue, or palpitations develop. In a monitored program, they are also monitored for an increase in heart rate above the target heart rate, an increase in systolic or diastolic blood pressure more than 20 mm Hg, a decrease in systolic blood pressure, onset or worsening of dysrhythmias, or ST-segment changes on the ECG.

The target heart rate in phase I is an increase of less than 10% from the resting heart rate, or 120 beats per minute. In phase II, the target heart rate is based on the results of the patient's stress test (usually 60% to 85% of the heart rate at which symptoms were noted), medications, and underlying condition. Oxygen saturation may also be assessed to ensure that it is greater than 93%. Should any signs or symptoms occur, the patient is instructed to slow down or stop exercising. If the patient is exercising in an unmonitored area, he or she is cautioned to cease activity immediately if signs or symptoms occur, and to seek appropriate medical attention.

Phases of Cardiac Rehabilitation

Cardiac rehabilitation occurs along the continuum of the disease and is typically categorized in three phases.

Phase I may begin with the diagnosis of atherosclerosis, which may occur when the patient is admitted to the hospital for unstable angina or acute MI. It consists of low-level activities and initial education for the patient and family. Because of the brief hospital stay, mobilization is earlier and patient teaching is now prioritized to the essentials of self-care, rather than instituting behavioral changes for risk reduction.

Priorities for in-hospital education include signs and symptoms that indicate the need to call 911, the medication regimen, activity restriction, and follow-up appointments with the physi-

(*text continues on page 634*)

25•2 **Plan of Nursing Care**

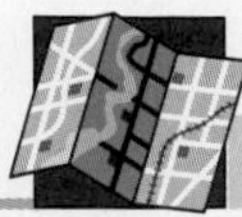

Care of the Patient With an Uncomplicated Myocardial Infarction

Nursing Interventions	Rationale	Expected Outcomes
Nursing Diagnosis: Chest pain related to reduced coronary blood flow **Goal:** Relief of chest pain		
1. Initially assess, document, and report to the physician the following:	1. These data assist in determining the cause and effect of the chest discomfort and provide a baseline with which post-therapy symptoms can be compared.	• Reports beginning relief of chest discomfort at once • Appears comfortable and pain free: Is rested Respiratory rate, cardiac rate, and blood pressure return to prediscomfort level Skin warm and dry • Adequate cardiac output as evidenced by: Heart rate and rhythm Blood pressure Mentation Urine output Serum BUN and creatinine Skin color, temperature, and moisture • Is pain free
a. The patient's description of chest discomfort, including location, radiation, duration of pain, and factors that affect it	a. There are many conditions associated with chest discomfort. There are characteristic clinical findings of ischemic pain.	
b. The effect of chest discomfort on cardiovascular hemodynamic perfusion—to the heart, to the brain, to the kidneys, and to the skin	b. MI decreases myocardial contractility and ventricular compliance and may produce dysrhythmias. Cardiac output is reduced, resulting in reduced blood pressure and decreased organ perfusion. The heart rate may increase as a compensatory mechanism to maintain cardiac output.	
2. Obtain a 12-lead ECG recording during pain, as prescribed, to determine extension of infarction.	2. An ECG during pain may be useful in the diagnosis of an extension of MI versus an anginal episode.	
3. Administer oxygen as prescribed.	3. Oxygen therapy may increase the oxygen supply to the myocardium if actual oxygen saturation is less than normal.	
4. Administer medication therapy as prescribed and evaluate the patient's response continuously.	4. Medication therapy is the first line of defense in preserving myocardial tissue. The side effects of these medications can be hazardous and the patient's status must be assessed.	
5. Ensure physical rest: use of the bedside commode with assistance; backrest elevated to promote comfort; full liquid diet as tolerated; arms supported during upper extremity activity; use of stool softener to prevent straining at stool. Provide a restful environment, and allay fears and anxiety by being supportive, calm, and competent. Visitor privileges are individualized, based on patient response.	5. Physical rest reduces myocardial oxygen consumption. Fear and anxiety precipitate the stress response; this results in increased levels of endogenous catecholamines, which increase myocardial oxygen consumption. Also, with increased epinephrine, the pain threshold is decreased, and pain increases myocardial oxygen consumption.	
Nursing Diagnosis: Potential ineffective air exchange related to fluid overload **Goal:** Absence of respiratory difficulties		
1. Initially and every 4 hours and with chest discomfort, assess, document, and report to the physician abnormal heart sounds (particularly S_3 and S_4 gallops and the holosystolic murmur of left ventricular papillary muscle dysfunction), abnormal breath sounds (particularly crackles), and patient intolerance to specific activities.	1. These data are useful in diagnosing left ventricular failure. Diastolic filling sounds (S_3 and S_4 gallop) result from decreased left ventricular compliance associated with MI. Papillary muscle dysfunction (from infarction of the papillary muscle) can result in mitral regurgitation and a reduction in stroke volume, leading to left ventricu-	• No shortness of breath, dyspnea on exertion, orthopnea, or paroxysmal nocturnal dyspnea • Respiratory rate less than 20 breaths/min with physical activity and 16 breaths/min with rest • Skin color normal • PaO_2 and $PaCO_2$ within normal range

(continued)

25•2 Plan of Nursing Care 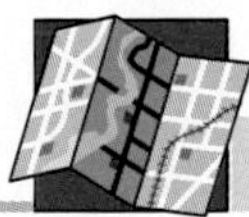

Patient With an Uncomplicated Myocardial Infarction (*continued*)

Nursing Interventions	Rationale	Expected Outcomes
	lar failure. The presence of crackles (usually at the lung bases) may indicate pulmonary congestion from increased left heart pressures. The association of symptoms and activity can be used as a guide for activity prescription and a basis for patient teaching.	• Heart rate less than 100 beats/min and greater than 60 beats/min, with blood pressure within patient's normal limits • Chest x-ray normal • Relief of chest discomfort • Appears comfortable: Appears rested Respiratory rate, cardiac rate, and blood pressure return to prediscomfort level Skin warm and dry
2. Teach patient: a. To adhere to the diet prescribed (for example, explain low-sodium, low-calorie diet)	2. a. Low-sodium diet may reduce extracellular volume, thus reducing preload and afterload, and thus myocardial oxygen consumption. In the obese patient, weight reduction may decrease cardiac work and improve tidal volume.	
b. To adhere to activity prescription	b. The activity prescription is determined individually to maintain the heart rate and blood pressure within safe limits.	

Nursing Diagnosis: Potential inadequate tissue perfusion related to decreased cardiac output
Goal: Maintenance/attainment of adequate tissue perfusion

Nursing Interventions	Rationale	Expected Outcomes
1. Initially and every 4 hours, and with chest discomfort, assess, document, and report to the physician the following: a. Hypotension b. Tachycardia and other dysrhythmia c. Fatigability d. Mentation changes (use family input) e. Reduced urine output (less than 250 mL per 8 hours) f. Cool, moist, cyanotic extremities	1. These data are useful in determining a low cardiac output state. An ECG with pain may be useful in the diagnosis of an extension of myocardial ischemia, injury, and infarction, and of variant angina.	• Blood pressure within the patient's normal range • Ideally, normal sinus rhythm without dysrhythmia is maintained, or patient's baseline rhythm is maintained between 60 and 100 beats/min without further dysrhythmia. • No complaints of fatigue with prescribed activity • Remains fully alert and oriented and without personality change • Appears comfortable Appears rested Respiratory rate, cardiac rate, and blood pressure return to prediscomfort level Skin warm and dry • Urine output greater than 40 mL/h • Extremities warm and dry with normal color

Nursing Diagnosis: Anxiety related to fear of death, change in health status
Goal: Reduction of anxiety

Nursing Interventions	Rationale	Expected Outcomes
1. Assess, document, and report to the physician the patient's and family's level of anxiety and coping mechanisms.	1. These data provide information about the psychological well-being and a baseline so that post-therapy symptoms can be compared. Causes of anxiety are variable and	• Reports less anxiety • Patient and family discuss their anxieties and fears about death • Patient and family appear less anxious

(*continued*)

25•2 **Plan of Nursing Care**

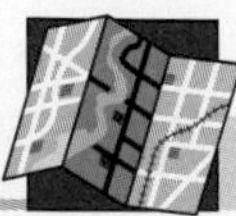

Patient With an Uncomplicated Myocardial Infarction (*continued*)

Nursing Interventions	Rationale	Expected Outcomes
	individual, and may include acute illness, hospitalization, pain, disruption of activities of daily living at home and at work, changes in role and self-image due to chronic illness, and lack of financial support. Because anxious family members can transmit anxiety to the patient, the nurse must also reduce the family's fear and anxiety.	• Appears restful, respiratory rate less than 16/min, heart rate less than 100/min without ectopic beats, blood pressure within patient's normal limits, skin warm and dry • Participates actively in a progressive rehabilitation program • Practices stress reduction techniques
2. Assess the need for spiritual counseling and refer as appropriate.	2. If a patient finds support in a religion, religious counseling may assist in reducing anxiety and fear.	
3. Allow patient (and family) to express anxiety and fear: a. By showing a genuine interest and concern b. By facilitating communication (listening, reflecting, guiding) c. By answering questions	3. Unresolved anxiety (the stress response) increases myocardial oxygen consumption.	
4. Use of flexible visiting hours allows the presence of a supportive family to assist in reducing the patient's level of anxiety.	4. The presence of supportive family members may reduce both patient's and family's anxiety.	
5. Encourage active participation in a cardiac rehabilitation program.	5. Prescribed cardiac rehabilitation may help to eliminate fear of death, may reduce anxiety, and may enhance feelings of well-being.	
6. Teach stress reduction techniques.	6. Stress reduction may help to reduce myocardial oxygen consumption and may enhance feelings of well-being.	

Nursing Diagnosis: Potential noncompliance with self-care program related to denial of diagnosis of MI
Goal: Complies with the home health care program

(See the earlier chart, Promoting Health After MI)

cian. The nurse needs to reassure the patient that although CAD is a life-long disease and must be treated life-long, most patients can resume a normal life after an MI. This positive approach helps to motivate and teach the patient while in the hospital to continue the education and lifestyle changes that are usually needed after discharge. The amount of activity allowed at discharge depends on the age of the patient, his or her condition before the cardiac event, the extent of the disease, the course of the hospital stay, and the development of any complications.

Phase II occurs after the patient has been discharged. It usually lasts for 4 to 6 weeks but may last up to 6 months. This outpatient program consists of supervised, if not ECG-monitored, exercise training that is individualized based on the results of an exercise stress test. In addition, support and guidance related to the treatment of the disease, and education and counseling related to lifestyle modification for risk-factor reduction are a significant part of this phase. Short-term and long-range goals are collaboratively determined based on the patient's needs. At each session, the patient is assessed for the effectiveness of and compliance with the current medical plan. To prevent complications and another hospitalization, the cardiac rehabilitation staff alert the referring physician to any problems.

These outpatient cardiac rehabilitation programs are designed to encourage patients and families to support each other. Many programs offer support sessions for spouses and significant others while the patients exercise. In addition, the programs involve group educational sessions for both patients and families that are given by cardiologists, exercise physiologists, dietitians, nurses, and other health care professionals. These sessions may take place outside a traditional classroom setting. For instance, a dietitian may take a group to a grocery store to examine labels and meat selections, or to a restaurant to discuss menu offerings for a "heart-healthy" diet.

Phase III focuses on maintaining cardiovascular stability and long-term conditioning. The patient is usually self-directed during this phase and does not require a supervised program, although it may be offered. The goals of each phase build on the accomplishments of the previous phase.

Critical Thinking Exercises

1. You are caring for a patient who was admitted to the hospital 6 hours earlier with angina pectoris. He complains of chest pain and states that he has received no relief from three nitroglycerin tablets. How would you determine what actions to take? How would your actions differ if this is a patient in a walk-in clinic?

2. You are caring for a patient who is scheduled to have CABG surgery. He appears quite anxious and states that he is afraid of the pain after surgery. His wife tends to minimize the significance of his concerns about pain. How would you respond to this patient and his wife? How might your response differ if the wife shares her husband's concerns?

3. You are caring for an elderly patient who underwent open-heart surgery 4 days ago and is progressing well. After ambulating in the corridor with his daughter, he returns to his room and bumps his nose, which begins to bleed profusely. His daughter is visibly upset. Explain what your first action will be and why. If your initial actions are not successful in decreasing the bleeding, how would you proceed? How would you explain the episode to the daughter to help her understand the bleeding?

4. The wife of a patient who is preparing for discharge after an MI approaches you and expresses concern about what to do if her husband suffers another heart attack. How might you instruct her in preparation for such an event? How would your instructions vary if the wife is in her 40s versus her late 60s, or lives in a rural community versus a suburban neighborhood?

References and Selected Readings

BOOKS AND PAMPHLETS

Agency for Health Care Policy and Research. (1994). *Unstable angina: Diagnosis and management.* Clinical Practice Guideline, Number 10, AHCPR Publication No. 94-0602. Rockville, MD: Public Health Service, U.S. Department of Health and Human Services.

American Heart Association. (1997). *Heart facts.* Dallas: Author.

Bates, B. (1999). *A guide to physical examination and history taking.* Philadelphia: Lippincott Williams & Wilkins.

Braunwald, E. (1997). *Heart disease: A textbook of cardiovascular medicine* (5th ed.). Philadelphia: W. B. Saunders.

Carpenito, L. J. (1997). *Nursing diagnosis: Application to clinical practice* (7th ed.). Philadelphia: Lippincott-Raven.

Chulay, M., Guzzetta, D., & Dossey, B. (1997). *AACN handbook of critical care nursing.* Stamford, CT: Appleton & Lange.

Diethrich, E. B., & Cohan, C. (1994). *Women and heart disease.* New York: Times Books.

Effron, D. M. (Ed.). (1998). *Cardiopulmonary resuscitation: CPR* (4th ed.). Tulsa, OK: CPR Publishers, Inc.

Hudak, C. M., Gallo, B. M., & Morton, P. G. (1998). *Critical care nursing: A holistic approach* (7th ed.). Philadelphia: Lippincott-Raven.

Schlant, R. C., et al. (1994). *Hurst's the heart: Arteries and veins* (8th ed.). New York: McGraw Hill.

Wenger, N. K. et al. (1995). *Cardiac rehabilitation.* Clinical Practice Guideline, Number 17, AHCPR Publication No. 96-0672. Rockville, MD: Public Health Service, Agency for Health Care Policy and Research and the National Heart, Lung, and Blood Institute.

Woods, S. L., et al. (1995). *Cardiac nursing.* Philadelphia: J. B. Lippincott.

JOURNALS

Asterisks indicate nursing research articles.

Anderson, J. J., & Gonzales, R.V. (1998). Transmyocardial laser revascularization: Old theory, new technology. *Critical Care Nursing Quarterly, 20*(4), 53–59.

Casey, K., Bedker, D. L., & Roussel-McElmeel, P. L. (1998). Myocardial infarction: Review of clinical trials and treatment strategies. *Critical Care Nursing, 18*(2), 39–54.

Crea, F., et al. (1997). Role of inflammation in the pathogenesis of unstable coronary artery disease. *American Journal of Cardiology, 80*(5A), 10E–16E.

Daniel, J., & Dattolo, J. (1998). Minimally invasive cardiac surgery: Surgical techniques and nursing considerations. *Critical Care Nursing Quarterly, 20*(4), 29–39.

Davis, D., VanRiper, S., Longstreet, J., et al. (1997). Vascular complications of coronary interventions. *Heart and Lung, 26,* 118–127.

Davis, K. B., et al. (1995). Comparison of 15-year survival for men and women after initial medical or surgical treatment for coronary artery disease: A CASS Registry study. *Journal of the American College of Cardiology, 25*(5), 1000–1009.

*Goodman, H. (1997). Patient's perceptions of their education needs in the first six weeks following discharge after cardiac surgery. *Journal of Advanced Nursing, 25*(6), 1241–1251.

Hammon, J. W. (1997). What's new in cardiac surgery. *Journal of the American College of Surgery, 184*(2), 105–108.

Harrison, H. (1999). Troponin I. *American Journal of Nursing, 99*(5), 24TT–26TT.

Howes, D. G. (1998). Cardiovascular disease and women. *Lippincott's Primary Care Practice, 2*(5), 514–524.

Hueta-Torres, V. (1998). Preparing patients for early discharge after CABG. *American Journal of Nursing, 98*(5), 49–51.

*Iezzoni, L. I., Ash, A. S., Shwartz, M., et al. (1997). Differences in procedure use, in-hospital mortality, and illness severity by gender for myocardial infarction patients. *Medical Care, 35*(2), 158–171.

Kannel, W. B. (1986). Silent myocardial ischemia and infarction: Insights from the Framingham study. *Cardiology Clinics, 4*(4), 583–591.

Kendler, B. S. (1997). Recent nutritional approaches to the prevention and therapy of cardiovascular disease. *Progress in Cardiovascular Nursing, 12*(3), 3–23.

*King, K. M., & Gortner, S. R. (1996). Women's short-term recovery from cardiac surgery. *Progress in Cardiovascular Nursing, 11*(2), 5–15.

Kinlay, S., & Ganz, P. (1997). Role of endothelial dysfunction in coronary artery disease and implications for therapy. *American Journal of Cardiology, 80*(9A), 11I–16I.

Kong, K., Kevorkian, C. G., & Rossi, C. D. (1996). Functional outcomes of patients on a rehabilitation unit after open heart surgery. *Journal of Cardiopulmonary Rehabilitation, 16*(6), 413–418.

Leibovitz, E., et al. (1997). Increased adhesiveness of white blood cells in patients with unstable angina: Additional evidence for an involvement of the immune-inflammatory system. *Clinical Cardiology, 20*(12), 1017–1020.

Levknecht, L., Schriefer, J., & Maconis, B. (1997). Combining case management pathways, and report cards for secondary cardiac prevention. *Jt Comm J Qual Improv, 23*(3), 162–174.

Lewandowski, D. M. (1995). Congestive heart failure. *American Journal of Nursing, 95*(3), 36.

Liu, B., et al. (1996). Factors influencing haemostasis and blood transfusion in cardiac surgery. *Perfusion, 11*(2), 131–143.

*Maxam-Moore, V. A., & Goedecke, R. S. (1996). The development of an early extubation algorithm for patients after cardiac surgery. *Heart and Lung, 25*(1), 61–68.

*McRae, M. E., et al. (1997). Development of a research-based standard for assessment, intervention, and evaluation of pain after neonatal and pediatric cardiac surgery. *Pediatric Nursing, 23*(3), 263–271.

*Meehan, D. A., et al. (1995). Analgesic administration, pain intensity, and patient satisfaction in cardiac surgical patients. *American Journal of Critical Care, 4*(6), 435–442.

Mehta, J. L., Saldeen, T. G., & Rand, K. (1998). Interactive role of infection, inflammation and traditional risk factors in atherosclerosis and coronary artery disease. *Journal of the American College of Cardiology, 31*(6), 1217–1225.

Miller, K. & Grindel, C. G. (1999). Coronary artery bypass surgery in women and men: Preoperative profile and postoperative outcomes. *MedSurg Nursing, 8*(3), 167–172.

Moser, D. K. (1997). Correcting misconceptions about women and heart disease. *American Journal of Nursing, 97*(4), 26–33.

*Nelson, S. (1996). Surgical nurse pre-admission education for patients undergoing cardiac surgery. *British Journal of Nursing, 5*(6), 335–340.

O'Meara, J. J., & Dehmer, G. J. (1997). Care of the patient and management of complications after percutaneous coronary artery interventions. *Annals of Internal Medicine, 127*(6), 458–471.

*Peterson, E. D., Shaw, L. K., DeLong, E. R., et al. (1997). Racial variation in the use of coronary revascularization procedures. *New England Journal of Medicine 1997, 336*(7), 480–486.

Reisz, W. G., & Robinson, D. J. (1998). Evaluating nontraumatic chest pain. *Primary Care Practice, 2*(5), 455–471.

*Riegel, B., et al. (1997). Effectiveness of a program of early hospital discharge of cardiac surgery patients. *Journal of Cardiovascular Nursing, 11*(3), 63–75.

Rose, E. A. (1996). What's new in cardiac surgery. *Journal of the American College of Surgery, 182*(2), 83–88.

*Schrott, H. G., Bittner, V., Bittinghoff, E., et al. (1997). Adherence to National Cholesterol Education Program treatment goals in post menopausal women with heart disease: The Heart and estrogen/progestin replacement study (HERS). *Journal of the American Medical Association, 277*(16), 1281–1286.

*Shih, F., et al. (1997). Turning points of recovery from cardiac surgery during the intensive care unit transition. *Heart and Lung, 26*(2), 99–108.

*Simpson, T., & Lee, E. R. (1996). Individual factors that influence sleep after cardiac surgery. *American Journal of Critical Care, 5*(3), 182–189.

Skillings, J. (1998). Atherosclerosis. *Primary Care Practice, 2*(5), 437–454

Skillings, J. (1998). Hyperlipidemia protocol. *Primary Care Practice, 2*(5), 525–528.

Skillings, J. (1998). Practical management of lipid disorders. *Primary Care Practice, 2*(5), 472–484.

Smith, S. C., Bliar, S. N., Criqui, M. H., et al. (1995). Preventing heart attack and death in patients with coronary disease. *Circulation, 92*, 2–4.

Strimike, C. L. (1995). Caring for a patient with an intracoronary stent. *American Journal of Nursing, 95*(1), 40–46.

Strong, J. P. (1999). Prevalence and extent of atherosclerosis in adolescents and young adults. *Journal of American Medical Association, 281*(8), 727–735.

*Valdix, S. W., & Puntillo, K. A. (1995). Pain, pain relief and accuracy of their recall after cardiac surgery. *Progress in Cardiovascular Nursing, 10*(3), 3–11.

Resources

American Heart Association 7320 Greenville Ave. Dallas, TX 75231; http://www.americanheart.org/aha.html

Coronary Club, 9500 Euclid Ave., Cleveland, OH 44106

Heartlife, P.O. Box 54305, Atlanta, GA 30308

Heartmates: http://www.heartmates.com/cardiac.html

National Heart, Lung, and Blood Institute, National Institutes of Health, Building 31, Room 5A52, Bethesda, MD 20892; http://www.nhlbi.nih.gov

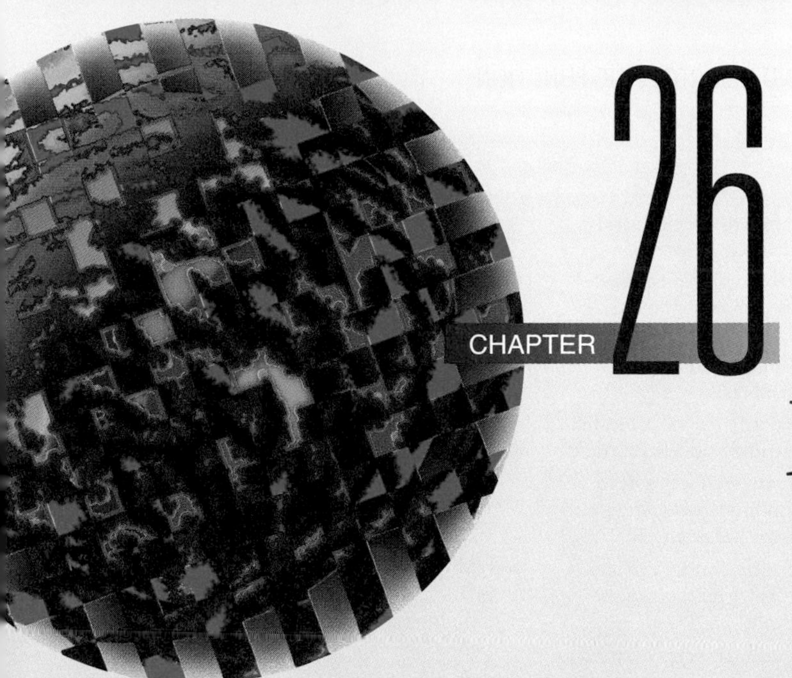

Management of Patients With Structural, Infectious, or Inflammatory Cardiac Disorders

Learning Objectives

On completion of this chapter, the learner will be able to:

1. Define valvular disorders of the heart and describe the pathophysiology, clinical manifestations, and management of patients with mitral and aortic disorders.
2. Describe types of cardiac valve repair and replacement procedures used to treat valvular problems and the care needed by patients who undergo these procedures.
3. Describe the pathophysiology, clinical manifestations, and management of patients with cardiomyopathies.
4. Describe the pathophysiology, clinical manifestations, and management of patients with infections of the heart.
5. Describe the significance of prophylactic antibiotic therapy for patients with mitral valve prolapse, valvular heart disease, rheumatic endocarditis, infective endocarditis, and myocarditis.

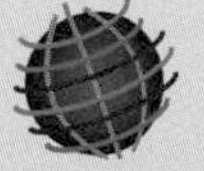

Structural disorders of the heart present many challenges for the patient, family, and health care team as do the conduction and vascular disorders discussed in Chapters 24 and 25. Problems with the heart valves, holes in the intracardiac septum, cardiomyopathies, and infectious diseases of the heart muscle result in altered cardiac output. Noninvasive treatments, such as medication therapy and activity and dietary modification, benefit patients with these diagnoses. Invasive treatments, such as valve repair or replacement, septal repair, ventricular assist devices, total artificial hearts, cardiac transplantation, and other procedures, may also be used. Nurses have an integral role in the care of patients with structural cardiac conditions as well as infectious and inflammatory disorders.

GLOSSARY

allograft: heart valve replacement made from a human heart valve (synonym: homograft)

annuloplasty: repair of a cardiac valve's outer ring

aortic valve: semilunar valve located between the left ventricle and the aorta

autograft: heart valve replacement made from the patient's own heart valve (ie, the pulmonic valve excised and used as an aortic valve)

cardiomyopathy: disease of the heart muscle

chordoplasty: repair of the stringy, tendinous fibers that connect the free edges of the atrioventricular valve leaflets to the papillary muscles

commissurotomy: splitting or separating fused cardiac valve leaflets

heterotopic transplant: procedure in which the recipient's heart remains in place and a donor heart is grafted to the right and anterior; patient has two hearts

homograft: heart valve replacement made from a human heart valve (synonym: allograft)

leaflet repair: repair of a cardiac valve's movable "flaps" (leaflets)

mitral valve: atrioventricular valve located between the left atrium and left ventricle

orthotopic transplant: recipient's heart is removed and a donor heart is grafted into the same site; patient has one heart

prolapse of a valve: stretching of an atrioventricular heart valve leaflet into the atrium during systole

pulmonic valve: semilunar valve located between the right ventricle and the pulmonary artery

regurgitation: backward flow of blood through a heart valve

stenosis: narrowing or obstruction of a cardiac valve's orifice

total artificial heart: mechanical device used to aid a failing heart, assisting both the right and left ventricles

tricuspid valve: atrioventricular valve located between the right atrium and right ventricle

valve replacement: insertion of a device at the site of a malfunctioning heart valve to restore blood flow in one direction through the heart

valvuloplasty: Repair of a stenosed or regurgitant cardiac valve by commissurotomy, annuloplasty, leaflet repair, and/or chordoplasty

ventricular assist device: mechanical device used to aid a failing ventricle, right or left

xenograft: heart valve replacement made of tissue from an animal heart valve

ACQUIRED VALVULAR DISORDERS

The valves of the heart control the flow of blood through the heart into the pulmonary artery and aorta by opening and closing in response to the blood pressure changes as the heart contracts and relaxes through the cardiac cycle.

The atrioventricular valves separate the atria from the ventricles and include the **tricuspid valve**, which separates the right atrium from the right ventricle, and the **mitral valve**, which separates the left atrium from the left ventricle. The tricuspid valve has three leaflets, the mitral valve two. Both valves have chordae tendineae that anchor the valve leaflets to the papillary muscles and ventricular wall.

The semilunar valves are located between the ventricles and their corresponding arteries. The **pulmonic valve** lies between the right ventricle and the pulmonary artery; the **aortic valve** lies between the left ventricle and the aorta. Figure 26-1 shows valves in the closed position.

When any of the heart valves do not open or close properly, blood flow is affected. When valves do not open completely, a condition called **stenosis**, the flow of blood through the valve is reduced. When valves do not close completely, blood flows backward through the valve in a process termed **regurgitation**.

Disorders of the mitral valve fall into the following categories: mitral valve prolapse (stretching of the valve leaflet into the atrium during systole), mitral stenosis, and mitral regurgitation. Disorders of the aortic valve are categorized as aortic stenosis and aortic regurgitation. These valvular disorders lead to various symptoms that, depending on their severity, may require surgical repair or replacement to correct the problem (Fig. 26-2). Tricuspid and pulmonic valve disorders also occur, usually with fewer symptoms and complications.

Mitral Valve Prolapse

Mitral valve prolapse, formerly known as mitral prolapse syndrome, is a deformity that usually produces no symptoms. Rarely, it progresses and can result in sudden death. Mitral valve prolapse occurs more frequently in women than in men. In recent years this disorder has been diagnosed more frequently, probably as a result of improved diagnostic methods.

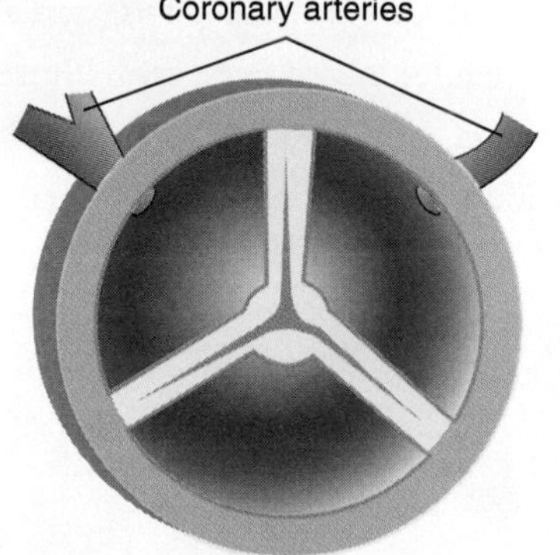

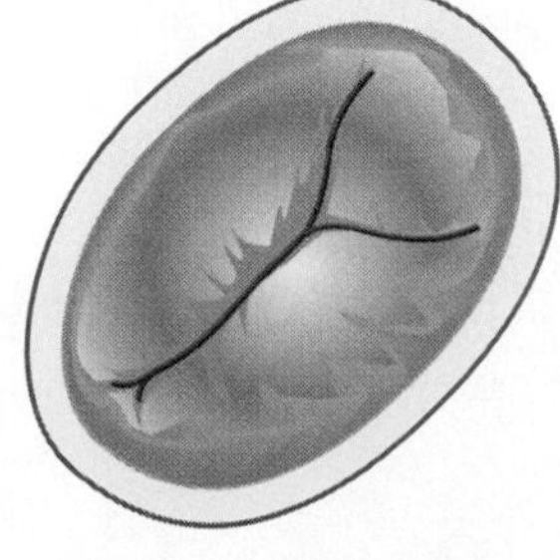

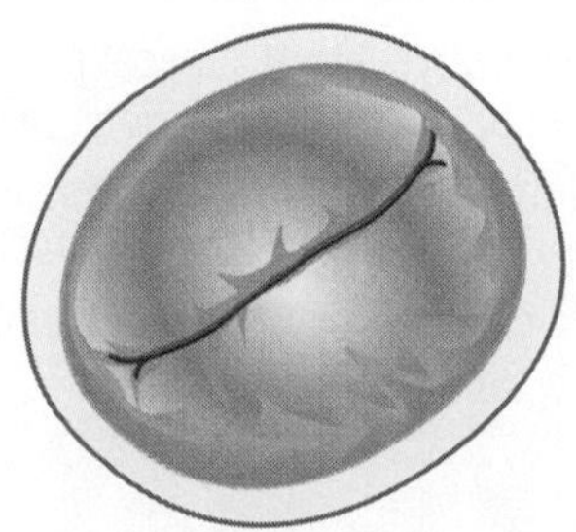

FIGURE 26•1 The valves of the heart (aortic or semilunar, tricuspid, and mitral) in closed position.

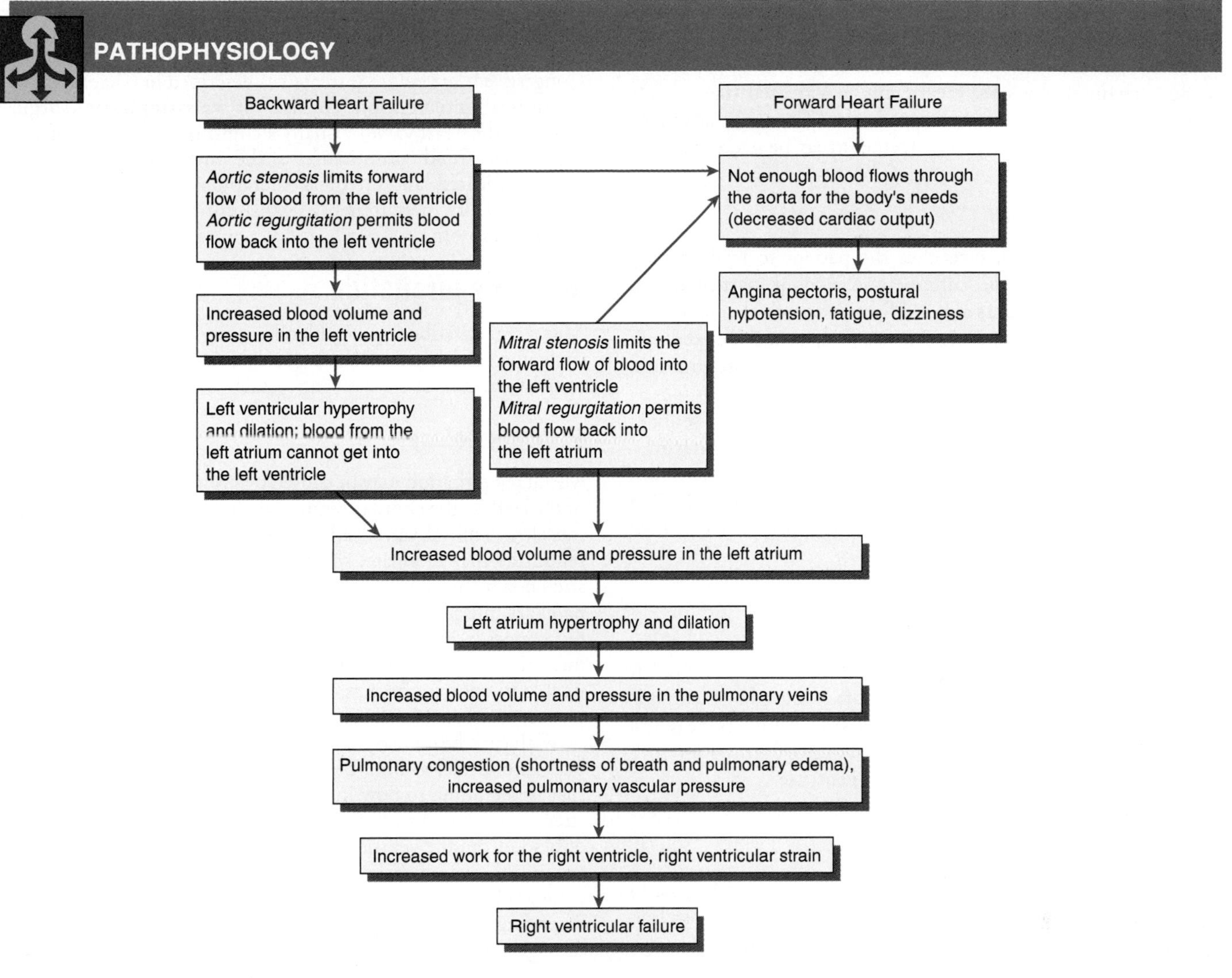

FIGURE 26•2 Valvular heart disease and the development of right ventricular failure.

Pathophysiology

In mitral valve prolapse, a portion of a mitral valve leaflet balloons back into the atrium during systole. The ballooning may stretch the leaflet to the point that the valve does not remain closed during systole (ventricular contraction). Blood then regurgitates from the left ventricle back into the left atrium.

Clinical Manifestations

Many people have a ballooned leaflet but no symptoms. Others have symptoms of fatigue, shortness of breath, light-headedness, dizziness, syncope, palpitations, chest pain, and anxiety.

Fatigue may be present regardless of the person's activity level and amount of rest or sleep. Shortness of breath is not correlated with activity levels or pulmonary function. Atrial or ventricular dysrhythmias may produce the sensation of palpitations, but palpitations have been reported while the heart has been beating normally. Another puzzling symptom is chest pain, which is often localized to the chest and may last for days.

Anxiety may be a response to the symptoms experienced by the patient; however, some patients report anxiety as the only symptom. Some clinicians speculate that the symptoms may be explained by dysautonomia, a dysfunction of the autonomic nervous system, although no consensus currently exists for the cause of the symptoms experienced by some patients with mitral valve prolapse.

Assessment and Diagnostic Findings

Often the first sign of mitral valve prolapse is identified when a physical examination of the heart discloses an extra heart sound, referred to as a mitral click. The systolic click is an early sign that a valve leaflet is ballooning into the left atrium. In addition to the mitral click, a murmur of mitral regurgitation may be heard. As the valve leaflet progressively stretches and regurgitation occurs, signs and symptoms of heart failure may occur.

Medical Management

Medical management is directed at controlling symptoms. If dysrhythmias are documented and cause symptoms, the patient is advised to eliminate caffeine and alcohol from the diet and stop smoking; antiarrhythmic medications may be prescribed.

Chest pain that does not respond to nitrates may respond to calcium channel blockers. Heart failure is treated traditionally (see Chap. 27 for a discussion of heart failure). In advanced stages, mitral valve repair or replacement may be necessary.

Nursing Management

As appropriate, the nurse teaches the patient to read product labels in a effort to avoid caffeine and alcohol, particularly in over-the-counter products and medications, such as cough medicine. The nurse also explains that alcohol, ephedrine, and epinephrine, which may be in some over-the-counter preparations, may produce dysrhythmias.

The nurse also educates patients with mitral valve prolapse about the need for prophylactic antibiotic therapy before undergoing invasive procedures (eg, dental work, genitourinary or gastrointestinal procedures) that may introduce infectious agents systemically. If in doubt about risk factors and the need for antibiotics, patients should consult their physician.

Mitral Stenosis

Mitral stenosis is an obstruction of blood flowing from the left atrium into the left ventricle. It is most often caused by rheumatic endocarditis, which progressively thickens and contracts the mitral valve leaflets. Eventually the mitral valve orifice narrows and progressively obstructs blood flow into the ventricle.

Pathophysiology

Normally, the mitral valve opening is as wide as three fingers. In cases of marked stenosis the opening narrows to the width of a lead pencil. The left atrium has great difficulty moving blood through the narrowed orifice into the ventricle; it dilates (stretches) and hypertrophies (thickens) because of the increased blood volume it now holds. Because no valve protects the pulmonary veins from a backward flow of blood from the atrium, the pulmonary circulation becomes congested. As a result, the right ventricle must contract against an abnormally high pulmonary arterial pressure and is thus subjected to excessive strain. Eventually the right ventricle fails.

Clinical Manifestations

Patients with mitral stenosis are likely to show progressive fatigue as a result of low cardiac output. They may expectorate blood (hemoptysis), have breathing difficulty (dyspnea) on exertion as a result of pulmonary venous hypertension, cough, and experience repeated respiratory infections.

Assessment and Diagnostic Findings

The pulse is weak and often irregular because of atrial fibrillation (caused by the strain on the atrium). A low-pitched, rumbling, diastolic murmur is heard at the apex. As a result of the increased blood volume and pressure, the atrium dilates and hypertrophies, becomes electrically unstable, and develops atrial dysrhythmias. Diagnostic aids include electrocardiography (ECG), echocardiography, and cardiac catheterization with angiography to determine the severity of the mitral stenosis.

Management

Antibiotic therapy is instituted to prevent recurrence of infections. Congestive heart failure is treated as described in Chapter 27.

Surgical intervention consists of **valvuloplasty** (surgical repair of the heart valve), usually a commissurotomy to open or rupture the fused commissures of the mitral valve. If surgery is contraindicated and medical therapy is not producing the desired results, percutaneous transluminal valvuloplasty may relieve symptoms.

Mitral Regurgitation

Mitral regurgitation involves blood flowing back from the left ventricle into the left atrium during systole. Often the margins of the mitral valve cannot close during systole.

Pathophysiology

Mitral regurgitation may be caused by problems with one or more of the leaflets, the chordae tendineae, the annulus, or the papillary muscles. A mitral valve leaflet may shorten or tear. The chordae tendineae may elongate, shorten, or tear. The annulus may be stretched by heart enlargement or deformed by calcification. The papillary muscle may rupture, stretch, or be pulled out of position by changes in the ventricular wall (eg, the scar from a myocardial infarction or ventricular dilation). The papillary muscle may be unable to contract because of ischemia. Regardless of the cause, blood regurgitates back into the atrium during systole.

With each beat of the left ventricle, some of the blood is forced back into the left atrium. Because this blood is added to the blood that is beginning to flow in from the lungs, the left atrium must stretch. It eventually hypertrophies and dilates. The backward flow of blood from the ventricle diminishes the volume of blood flowing into the atrium from the lungs. As a result, the lungs become congested, eventually adding extra strain on the right ventricle. Therefore, mitral regurgitation ultimately involves the lungs and the right ventricle.

Clinical Manifestations

Chronic mitral regurgitation is often asymptomatic, but acute mitral regurgitation (such as that resulting from a myocardial infarction) usually presents as severe congestive heart failure. Dyspnea, fatigue, and weakness are the most common symptoms. Palpitations, shortness of breath on exertion, and cough from pulmonary congestion also occur.

Assessment and Diagnostic Findings

A high-pitched, blowing systolic murmur is heard at the apex. The pulse may be regular and of good volume, or it may be irregular as a result of either extrasystolic or atrial fibrillation.

Medical Management

Management of mitral regurgitation is the same as that for congestive heart failure. Surgical intervention consists of mitral valve replacement or valvuloplasty.

Aortic Stenosis

Aortic valve stenosis is the narrowing of the orifice between the left ventricle and the aorta. In adults, the stenosis may involve congenital leaflet malformations or number of leaflets (one or two rather than three), or it may be a result of rheumatic endocarditis or cusp calcification of unknown cause. The leaflets of the aortic valve may fuse.

Pathophysiology

There is progressive narrowing of the valve orifice, usually over a period of several years to several decades. The left ventricle overcomes the obstruction to circulation by contracting more slowly but with greater energy than normal, forcibly squeezing the blood through the very small orifice. The obstruction to left ventricular outflow increases pressure on the left ventricle, which results in a thickening of the muscle wall. The heart muscle hypertrophies. When these compensatory mechanisms of the heart begin to fail, clinical signs develop.

Clinical Manifestations

Many patients with aortic stenosis are asymptomatic. Once symptoms develop, patients usually first have exertional dyspnea, caused by left ventricular failure. Other signs are dizziness and fainting because of reduced blood flow to the brain. Angina pectoris is a frequent symptom that results from the increased oxygen demands of the hypertrophied left ventricle, the decreased time in diastole for myocardial perfusion, and the decreased blood flow into the coronary arteries. Blood pressure can be low but is usually normal; there may be a low pulse pressure (30 mm Hg or less) because of diminished blood flow.

Assessment and Diagnostic Findings

On physical examination, a loud, rough systolic murmur may be heard over the aortic area. The sound to listen for is a systolic crescendo–decrescendo murmur, which may radiate into the carotid arteries and to the apex of the left ventricle. The murmur is low-pitched, rough, rasping, and vibrating. If one rests a hand over the base of the heart, a vibration may be felt. The vibration is caused by turbulent blood flow across the narrowed valve orifice. Evidence of left ventricular hypertrophy may be seen on a 12-lead ECG and echocardiogram.

Left-sided heart catheterization is necessary to measure the severity of this valvular abnormality. Pressure tracings are taken from the left ventricle and the base of the aorta. The systolic pressure in the left ventricle is considerably higher than that in the aorta during systole.

Medical Management

Antibiotic prophylaxis to prevent endocarditis is essential for anyone with aortic stenosis. Once left ventricular failure or dysrhythmias occur, medications are prescribed. Definitive treatment for aortic stenosis is surgical replacement of the aortic valve. Patients who are symptomatic and are not surgical candidates may benefit from one- or two-balloon percutaneous valvuloplasty procedures.

Aortic Regurgitation

Aortic regurgitation is the flow of blood back into the left ventricle from the aorta during diastole. It may be caused by inflammatory lesions that deform the leaflets of the aortic valve, preventing them from completely closing the aortic valve orifice. This valvular defect also may result from endocarditis, congenital abnormalities, diseases such as syphilis, and a dissecting aneurysm that cause dilation or tearing of the ascending aorta.

Pathophysiology

In aortic regurgitation, blood from the aorta returns to the left ventricle during diastole, in addition to the blood normally delivered by the left atrium. The left ventricle dilates, trying to accommodate the increased volume of blood. It also hypertrophies, trying to increase muscle strength to expel more blood with more-than-normal force—raising systolic blood pressure. The arteries attempt to compensate for the higher pressures by reflex vasodilation; the peripheral arterioles relax, reducing peripheral resistance and diastolic blood pressure.

Clinical Manifestations

Aortic insufficiency develops without symptoms in most patients. Some patients are aware of a forceful heartbeat, especially in the head or neck. There may be marked arterial pulsations that are visible or palpable at the carotid or temporal arteries. This is a result of the increased force and volume of the blood ejected from the hypertrophied left ventricle. Exertional dyspnea and fatigue follow. Progressive signs and symptoms of left ventricular failure include breathing difficulties, especially at night (orthopnea, paroxysmal nocturnal dyspnea).

Assessment and Diagnostic Findings

A high-pitched, blowing diastolic murmur is heard at the third or fourth intercostal space at the left sternal border. The pulse pressure (the difference between systolic and diastolic pressures) is considerably widened in patients with aortic regurgitation. One characteristic sign of the disease is the water-hammer pulse, in which the pulse strikes the palpating finger with a quick, sharp stroke and then suddenly collapses. Diagnosis is confirmed by ECG, echocardiogram, and cardiac catheterization.

Medical Management

Before the patient undergoes invasive and dental procedures, antibiotic prophylaxis is needed to prevent endocarditis. Heart failure and dysrhythmias are treated as described in Chapters 24 and 27. Aortic valve replacement is the treatment of choice, preferably performed before left ventricular failure. Surgery is recommended for any patient with left ventricular hypertrophy, regardless of the presence or absence of symptoms.

VALVE REPAIR AND REPLACEMENT PROCEDURES

Valvuloplasty

The repair, rather than replacement, of a cardiac valve is referred to as valvuloplasty. The type of valvuloplasty depends on the cause and type of valve dysfunction. Repair may be made to the commissures between the leaflets in a procedure known as commissurotomy, to the annulus of the valve by annuloplasty, or to the leaflets or the chordae by chordoplasty.

Most valvuloplasty procedures require general anesthesia and often cardiopulmonary bypass. Some procedures, however, can be performed in the cardiac catheterization laboratory; these procedures do not always require general anesthesia or cardiopulmonary bypass. Percutaneous partial cardiopulmonary bypass is now used in some cardiac catheterization laboratories.

The patient is managed in a critical care unit for the first 24 to 72 hours after surgery. Care focuses on hemodynamic stabilization and recovery from anesthesia. Most patients are then transferred to a telemetry or surgical unit for continued postsurgical care and teaching. Patients are discharged from the hospital in 1 to 7 days. In general, valves that have undergone valvuloplasty function longer than replacement valves, and the patients do not require continuous anticoagulation.

Commissurotomy

The most common valvuloplasty procedure is **commissurotomy**. Each valve has leaflets; the site where the leaflets meet is called the commissure. The leaflets may adhere to one another and close the commissure (stenosis). Less commonly, the leaflets fuse in such a way that in addition to stenosis, the leaflets are also prevented from closing completely, resulting in a backward flow of blood (regurgitation). A commissurotomy is the procedure performed to separate the fused leaflets.

Closed Commissurotomy

Closed commissurotomies do not require cardiopulmonary bypass. The patient receives a general anesthetic, a midsternal incision is made, a small hole is cut into the heart, and the surgeon's finger or a dilator is used to break open the commissure. The valve is not directly visualized. This type of commissurotomy has been performed for mitral, aortic, tricuspid, and pulmonary valve disease.

BALLOON VALVULOPLASTY

Balloon valvuloplasty (Fig. 26-3) is another type of closed commissurotomy that has been beneficial for mitral valve stenosis in younger patients, as well as aortic valve stenosis in elderly patients and patients with complex medical conditions that place them at high risk for the complications of more extensive surgical procedures. Most commonly used for mitral and aortic valve stenosis, balloon valvuloplasty also has been used for tricuspid and pulmonic valve stenosis. The procedure is performed in the cardiac catheterization laboratory, and the patient may receive a local anesthetic. Patients remain in the hospital 24 to 48 hours after the procedure.

Mitral valvuloplasty is contraindicated for patients with left atrial or ventricular thrombus, severe aortic root dilation, significant mitral valve regurgitation, thoracolumbar scoliosis, rotation of the great vessels, and other cardiac conditions that require open heart surgery. Mitral valvuloplasty involves advancing one or two catheters into the right atrium, through the atrial septum into the left atrium, across the mitral valve into the left ventricle, and out into the aorta. A guide wire is placed through each catheter, and the original catheter is removed. A large balloon catheter is then placed over the guide wire and positioned with the balloon across the mitral valve. The balloon is then inflated with a dilute liquid angiographic solution. When two balloons are used, they are inflated simultaneously. The advantage of two balloons is that they are each smaller than the one large balloon often used, making smaller atrial septal defects. Also, as the balloons are inflated they usually do not completely occlude the mitral valve, thus permitting some forward flow of blood during the inflation period.

All patients have some degree of mitral regurgitation after the procedure. Other possible complications include bleeding from the catheter insertion sites, emboli resulting in complications such as strokes, and rarely left-to-right atrial shunts through an atrial septal defect caused by the procedure.

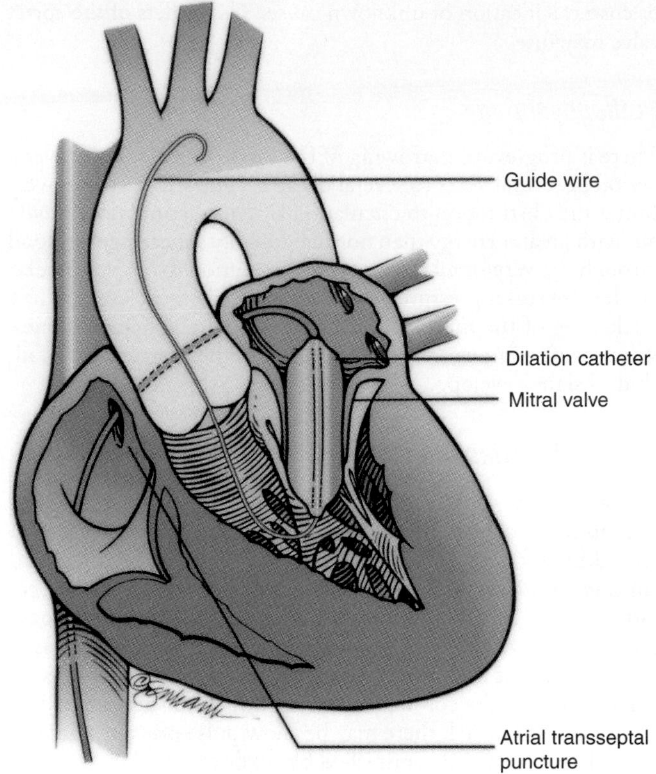

FIGURE 26•3 Balloon valvuloplasty: cross-section of heart illustrating guide wire and dilation catheter placed through an atrial transseptal puncture and across the mitral valve. The guide wire is extended out from the aortic valve into the aorta for catheter support.

Aortic valvuloplasty also may be performed by passing the balloon or balloons through the atrial septum, but it is performed more commonly by introducing a catheter through the aorta, across the aortic valve, and into the left ventricle. Either the one-balloon or the two-balloon technique can be used for aortic stenosis. Unfortunately, the aortic procedure is not as effective as the procedure for the mitral valve, and the rate of restenosis is nearly 50% in the first 12 to 15 months after the procedure. Possible complications include aortic regurgitation, emboli, ventricular perforation, rupture of the aortic valve annulus, ventricular dysrhythmias, mitral valve damage, and bleeding from the catheter insertion sites.

Open Commissurotomy

Open commissurotomies are performed with direct visualization of the valve. The patient is under general anesthesia, and a median sternotomy or left thoracic incision is made. Cardiopulmonary bypass is initiated, and an incision is made into the heart. A finger, scalpel, balloon, or dilator may be used to open the commissures. The added advantage of direct visualization of the valve is that thrombus may be noted and removed, calcifications can be seen, and if the valve has chordae or papillary muscles, they also may be surgically repaired (see the chordoplasty section of this chapter).

The patient is admitted to a critical care unit after surgery. Care focuses on recovery from anesthesia and hemodynamic stability. The patient is usually transferred to a telemetry or surgical unit in 24 to 48 hours and discharged from the hospital about 5 to 7 days after surgery. Wound care and patient teaching regarding diet, activity, medications, and self-care are the focus of nursing care throughout the continuum of care.

Annuloplasty

Annuloplasty is the repair of the valve annulus (the junction of the valve leaflets and the muscular heart wall). General anesthesia and cardiopulmonary bypass are required for all annuloplasties. The procedure narrows the diameter of the valve's orifice and is useful for the treatment of regurgitation.

There are two different annuloplasty techniques. One technique is to use an annuloplasty ring (Fig. 26-4). The leaflets of the valve are sutured to a ring, creating an annulus of the desired size. When the ring is in place, the tension created by the moving blood and the contracting heart is borne by the ring rather than by the valve or a suture line. Thus, progressive regurgitation is prevented by the repair. The other techniques involve tacking the valve leaflets to the atrium with sutures or taking tucks to tighten the annulus. The valve's leaflets and the suture lines are subjected to the direct forces of the blood and heart muscle movement, so the repair may degenerate more quickly than with the annuloplasty ring technique.

Leaflet Repair

Cardiac valve leaflets may be damaged by being stretched out of shape, being shortened, or developing holes. The repair for elongated, ballooning, or other excess tissue leaflets is removal of the extra tissue. The elongated tissue may be folded over onto itself (tucked) and sutured (leaflet plication). A wedge of tissue may be cut from the middle of the leaflet and the gap sutured closed (leaflet resection; Fig. 26-5). Short leaflets are most often repaired by chordoplasty (see next section). Once the short chordae are released, the leaflets often unfurl and can resume their normal function of closing the valve during systole. A piece of pericardium may also be sutured to the leaflet. Most commonly a pericardial patch is used when it is necessary to repair holes in the leaflets.

Chordoplasty

Chordoplasty is the repair of the chordae tendineae. The mitral valve is involved with chordoplasty (because it has the chordae tendineae); seldom is chordoplasty required for the tricuspid valve. Regurgitation may be caused by stretched, torn, or shortened chordae tendineae. Stretched chordae tendineae can be shortened, torn ones can be reattached to the leaflet, and shortened ones can be elongated. Regurgitation may also be caused by stretched papillary muscles, which can be shortened.

Valve Replacement

Prosthetic **valve replacement** began in the 1960s. When valvuloplasty or valve repair is not a viable alternative, such as when the annulus or leaflets of the valve are immobilized by calcifications, valve replacement is performed. General anesthesia and cardiopulmonary bypass are used for all valve replacements. Most procedures are performed through a median sternotomy (an incision through the sternum), although the mitral valve may be approached through a right thoracotomy incision.

Once the valve is visualized, the leaflets and other valve structures, such as the chordae and papillary muscles, are removed. Some surgeons leave the posterior mitral valve leaflet, its chordae, and papillary muscles in place to maintain the shape and function of the left ventricle. Sutures are placed around the annulus and then into the valve prosthesis. The replacement valve is slid down the suture into position and tied into place (Fig. 26-6). The incision is closed, and the surgeon evaluates the function of the heart and the quality of the prosthetic repair. The patient is weaned from cardiopulmonary bypass and surgery is completed.

Complications unique to valve replacement are related to the sudden changes in intracardiac blood pressures. Before surgery, the heart gradually adjusted to the pathology, but the surgery abruptly "corrects" the way blood flows through the heart.

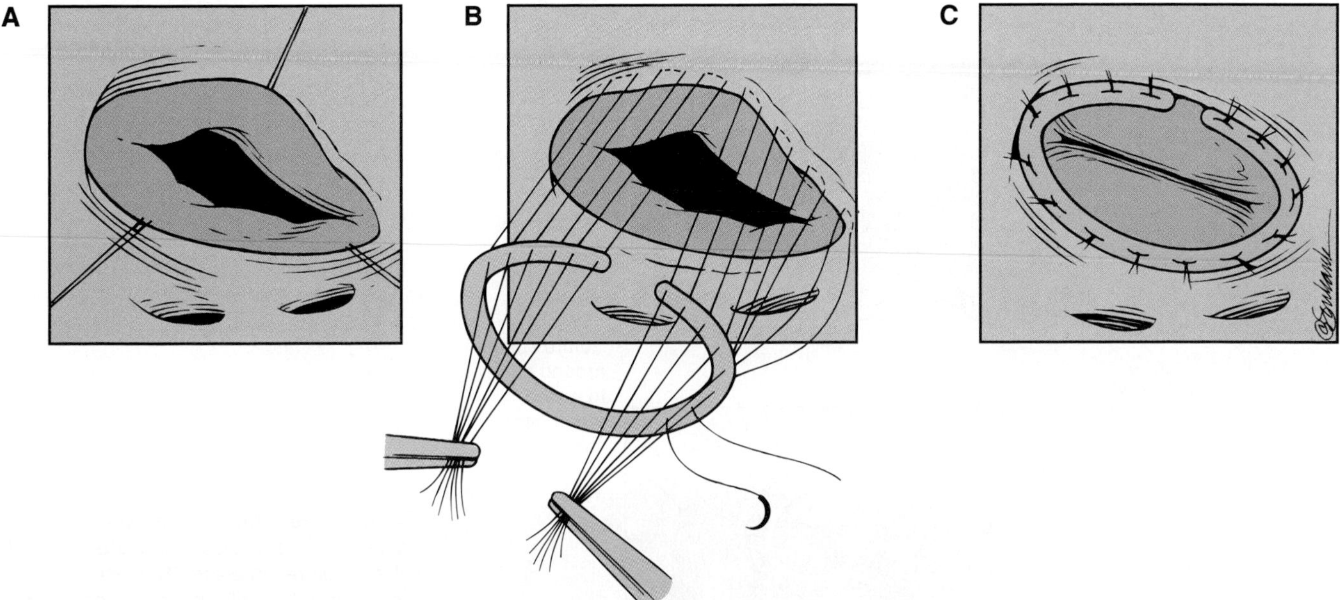

FIGURE 26•4 Annuloplasty ring insertion. (**A**) Mitral valve regurgitation; leaflets do not close. (**B**) Insertion of an annuloplasty ring. (**C**) Completed valvuloplasty; leaflets close.

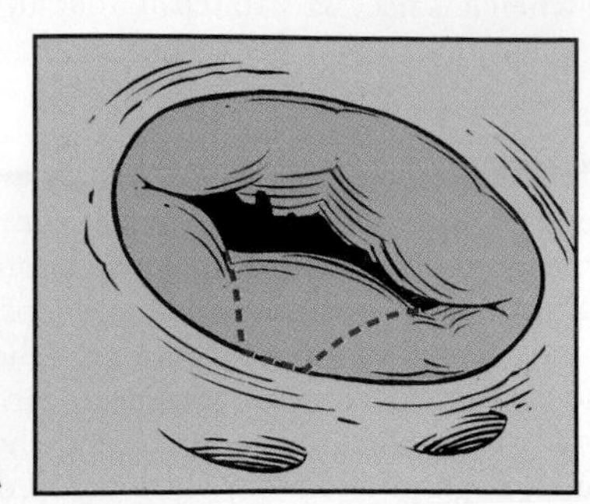

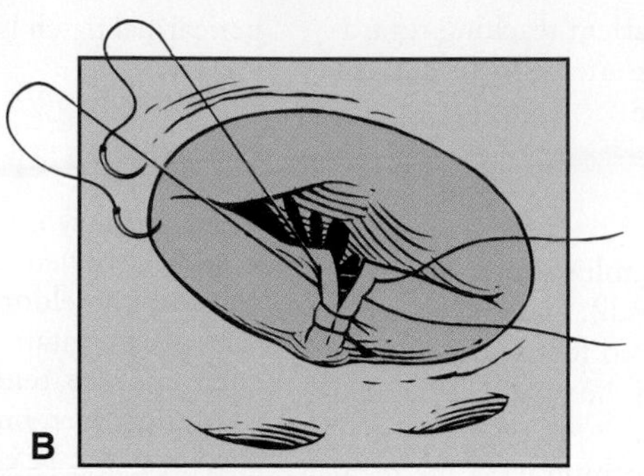

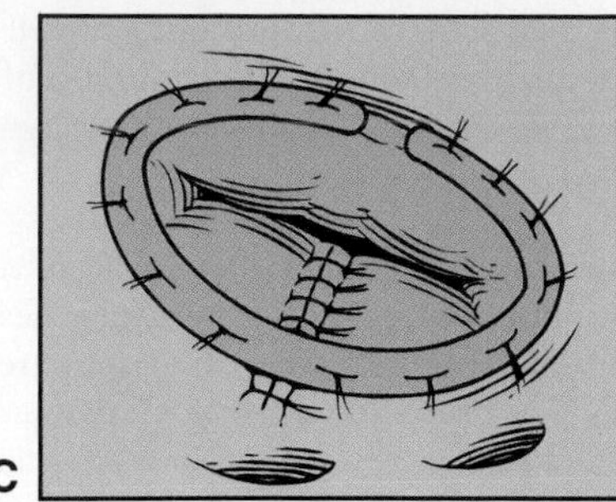

FIGURE 26•5 Valve leaflet resection and repair with a ring annuloplasty. (**A**) Mitral valve regurgitation; the section indicated by dashed lines will be excised. (**B**) Approximation of edges and suturing. (**C**) Completed valvuloplasty, leaflet repair, and annuloplasty ring.

Types of Valve Prostheses

Four types of valve prostheses may be used—mechanical valves, xenografts, homografts, and autografts. Figure 26-7 shows mechanical and xenograft valves.

The mechanical valves are of the ball-and-cage or disk design. Mechanical valves are thought to be more durable than the other types of prosthetic valves and often are used for younger patients. Thromboemboli are significant complications associated with mechanical valves, so long-term anticoagulation with warfarin is required.

Xenografts are tissue valves (bioprostheses, heterografts); most are from pigs (porcine), but valves from cows (bovine) may also be used. Their viability is 7 to 10 years. They do not generate thrombi, thus eliminating the need for long-term anticoagulation. They are used for women of childbearing age because the potential complications of long-term anticoagulation associated with menses, placental transfer to a fetus and those associated with delivery of a child do not exist. Xenografts also are used for patients older than age 70, patients with a history of peptic ulcer disease, and others who cannot tolerate long-term anticoagulation. Xenografts are used for all tricuspid valve replacements.

Homografts, or **allografts** (human valves), are obtained from cadaver tissue donations. The aortic valve and a portion of the aorta or the pulmonic valve and a portion of the pulmonary artery are harvested and stored cryogenically. Homografts are not always available and are very expensive. Homografts last for about 10 to 15 years, somewhat longer than xenografts. The homografts are not

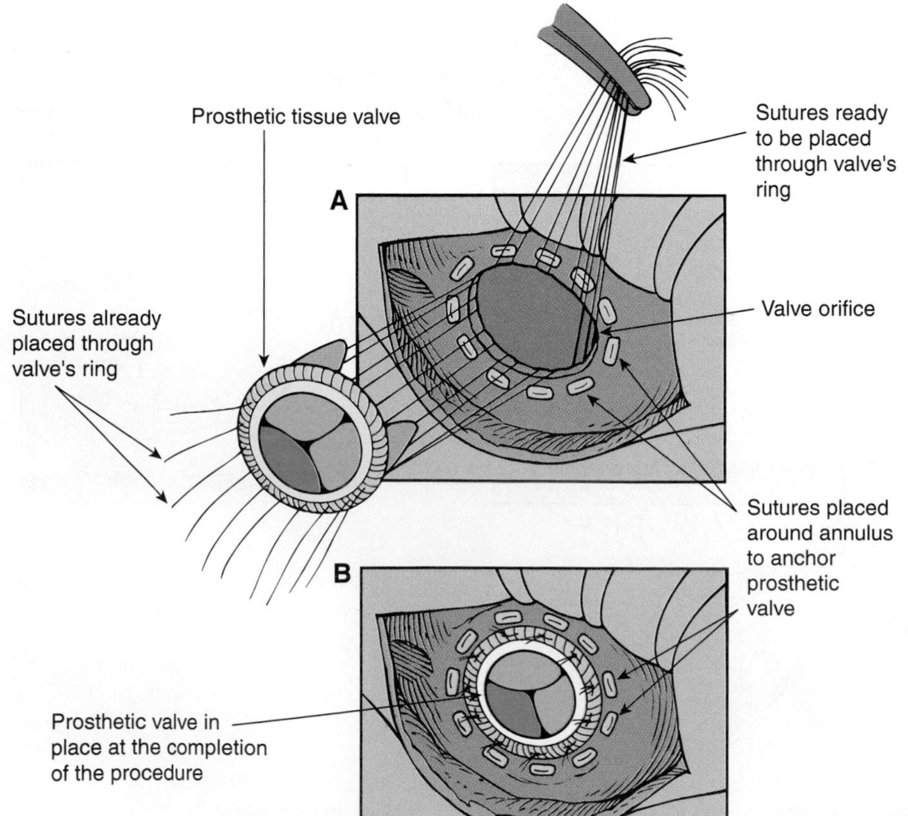

FIGURE 26•6 Valve replacement. (**A**) The native valve is excised and the prosthetic valve is sutured in place. (**B**) Once all sutures are placed through the ring, the surgeon slides the prosthetic valve down the sutures and into the natural orifice. The sutures are then tied off and trimmed.

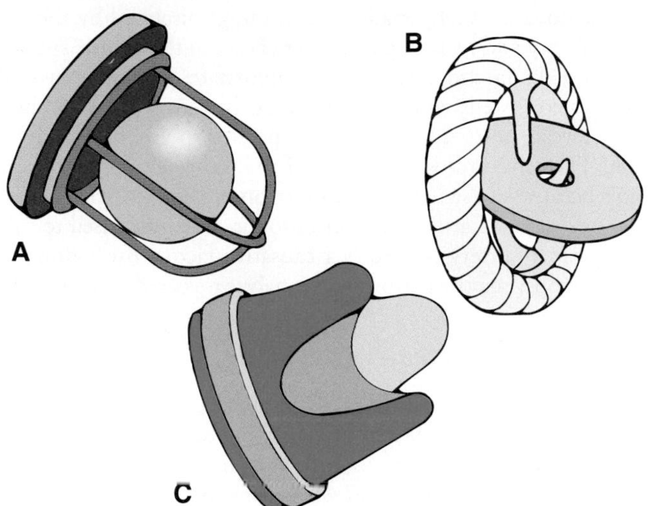

FIGURE 26•7 Common mechanical and biologic valve replacements. (**A**) Caged ball valve (Starr-Edwards, mechanical). (**B**) Tilting-disk valve (Medtronic-Hall, mechanical). (**C**) Porcine heterograft valve (Carpenter-Edwards, biologic).

thrombogenic and are resistant to subacute bacterial endocarditis. Homografts are used for aortic and pulmonic valve replacement.

Autografts (autologous valves) are obtained by excising the patient's own pulmonic valve and a portion of the pulmonary artery for use as the aortic valve. Anticoagulation is not necessary because the valve is the patient's own tissue and is not thrombogenic. The autograft is an alternative for children (it may grow as the child grows), women of childbearing age, young adults, patients with a history of peptic ulcer disease, and those who cannot tolerate anticoagulation. Aortic valve autografts have remained viable for more than 20 years.

Most aortic valve autograft procedures are double valve-replacement procedures: a homograft also is performed for pulmonic valve replacement. If pulmonary vascular pressures are normal, some surgeons elect not to replace the pulmonic valve. The patient can recover without a valve between the right ventricle and the pulmonary artery.

Complications

The sudden change in hemodynamics, as well as the surgical procedure, puts the patient at risk for many postoperative complications, such as bleeding, thromboembolism, infection, congestive heart failure, hypertension, dysrhythmias, hemolysis, and mechanical obstruction.

Nursing Management

Patients who have had valve replacements are admitted to the intensive care unit; care focuses on recovery from anesthesia and hemodynamic stability. The patient is usually transferred to a telemetry unit within 24 to 72 hours after surgery. Nursing care continues as for most postsurgical patients, including wound care and patient teaching regarding diet, activity, medication, and self-care.

In addition to needing education about long-term anticoagulant therapy, patients with a mechanical valve prosthesis require education regarding antibiotic prophylaxis to prevent bacterial endocarditis. Antibiotic therapy is prescribed for these patients before all dental and surgical interventions. Ideally, nurses should reinforce all new information and self-care instructions in 4 to 8 weeks after the procedure.

Septal Repair

The atrial or ventricular septum may have an abnormal opening between the right and left sides of the heart (septal defect). Although most septal defects are congenital and are repaired during infancy or childhood, adults may not have undergone early repair or may develop septal defects as a result of myocardial infarctions or diagnostic and treatment procedures.

Repair of septal defects requires general anesthesia and cardiopulmonary bypass. The heart is opened and a pericardial or synthetic (usually polyester or Dacron) patch is used to close the opening. Atrial septal defect repairs have low morbidity and mortality rates. When the mitral or tricuspid valve is involved, however, the procedure is more complicated. Generally, ventricular septal repairs are uncomplicated, but the proximity of the defect to the intraventricular conduction system and the valves may make this repair more complex.

CARDIOMYOPATHIES

Cardiomyopathy is a heart muscle disease of unknown cause, although some studies (Francis et al., 1998; Mestroni & Giacca, 1997) suggest that cardiomyopathy is an inherited genetic disorder. The three types of cardiomyopathy are classified according to the structural and functional abnormalities of the heart muscle: dilated cardiomyopathy (sometimes called congestive cardiomyopathy), hypertrophic cardiomyopathy, and restrictive or constrictive cardiomyopathy. Regardless of the category and the cause, these diseases may lead to severe heart failure, significant dysrhythmias, and death.

Pathophysiology

Dilated or congestive cardiomyopathy, the most common form of cardiomyopathy, is distinguished by significant dilation of the ventricles without significant concomitant hypertrophy (an increase in muscle wall thickness). The result is poor systolic functioning. A greater amount of blood remains within the ventricle after a contraction; this leads to stasis of the blood and the formation of atrial and ventricular thrombi. Microscopic examination of the muscle tissue shows a diminishing of the contractile elements of the muscle fibers and diffuse necrosis of myocardial cells. An infection, recent or remote, is often implicated as a source of this type of cardiomyopathy. Other causative factors include heavy alcohol intake and pregnancy.

In hypertrophic cardiomyopathy, which is less common, the heart muscle actually increases in size and mass, especially along the septum. The increase in the thickness of the heart muscle reduces the size of the ventricular cavities and causes the ventricles to take a longer time to relax, making it more difficult for the ventricles to fill with blood during the first part of diastole and more dependent on the atrial contraction for filling. Often the increase in septal size misaligns the papillary muscle so that during ventricular contraction, the mitral valve obstructs the flow of blood from the left ventricle into the aorta. Hence, hypertrophic cardiomyopathy is classified further as obstructive or nonobstructive.

Restrictive cardiomyopathy, the rarest category, is characterized by an impairment of ventricular stretch and therefore volume. Restrictive cardiomyopathy can be associated with amyloidosis (in which amyloid, a protein substance, is deposited within the cells) and other such infiltrative diseases.

Regardless of the distinguishing features, the pathophysiology of cardiomyopathy is a series of progressive events that culminate in an impaired pumping of the heart. The gradually decreasing stroke volume stimulates the sympathetic nervous system, resulting in increased systemic vascular resistance. As in heart failure from any cause, the left ventricle enlarges to accommodate the demands and eventually fails. Failure of the right ventricle usually accompanies this process (Fig. 26-8).

Clinical Manifestations

Cardiomyopathies may occur at any age; they affect both men and women. The patient may have the disease but remain stable and without symptoms for many years. The patient with hypertrophic cardiomyopathy is often active and may even be an athlete. As the disease progresses, so do symptoms; the patient may experience multiple hospitalizations, with a grim prognosis. Most patients with cardiomyopathy initially present with shortness of breath on exertion. Paroxysmal nocturnal dyspnea, cough, chest pain (may or may not be associated with exertion), palpitations, fatigue, dizziness, and syncope are other symptoms that occur early and as the disease progresses.

Assessment and Diagnostic Findings

Physical examination in the early stage reveals tachycardia and extra heart sounds. With progression of the disease, examination also reveals pulmonary auscultation of crackles, significant dysrhythmias and conduction abnormalities, jugular vein distention, pitting edema of dependent body parts, and an enlarged liver.

PATHOPHYSIOLOGY

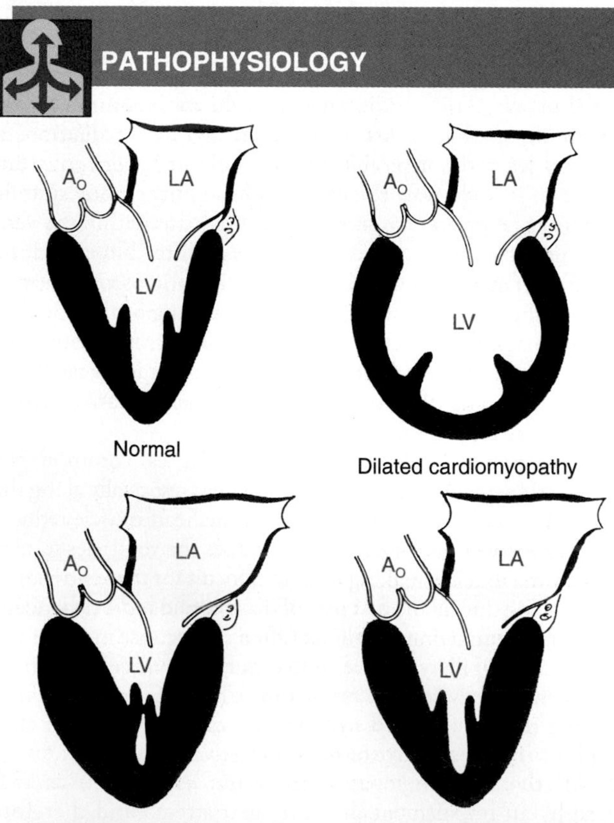

FIGURE 26•8 Cardiomyopathies that lead to congestive heart failure. With permission from Braunwald, E. (Ed.) (1997). *Heart disease: A textbook of cardiovascular medicine* (5th ed.). Philadelphia: W. B. Saunders.

Diagnosis is usually made from findings disclosed by the patient history and by ruling out other causes of the failure, such as myocardial infarction. The ECG demonstrates dysrhythmias and changes consistent with left ventricular hypertrophy. The chest x-ray reveals heart enlargement and possibly pulmonary congestion. The echocardiogram is one of the most helpful diagnostic tools because the structure and function of the ventricles can be observed easily. Cardiac catheterization is sometimes used to rule out coronary artery disease as a causative factor. An endomyocardial biopsy may be performed to analyze myocardial tissue cells.

Medical Management

Medical management is directed toward determining and managing possible underlying or precipitating causes; correcting the heart failure with medications, diet, and an exercise–rest regimen; and controlling dysrhythmias with antiarrhythmic medications and possibly an implanted electronic device, such as a pacemaker or an implantable cardioverter–defibrillator (see Chap. 24).

SURGICAL MANAGEMENT

When heart failure progresses to a point where medical treatment is ineffective, surgical intervention, including heart transplantation, is considered. In some cases ventricular assist devices are implanted to support the failing heart until a suitable donor heart becomes available.

When a patient with hypertrophic cardiomyopathy becomes symptomatic despite medical therapy and when a difference in pressure of 50 mm Hg or more exists between the left ventricle and the aorta, surgery is considered. The most common procedure is a myectomy (sometimes referred to as a myotomy–myectomy), in which some of the heart tissue is excised. Septal tissue approximately 1 cm wide and deep is cut from the enlarged septum below the aortic valve. The length of septum removed depends on the degree of obstruction caused by the hypertrophied muscle.

Instead of a septal myectomy, the surgeon may open the left ventricular outflow tract to the aortic valve by removing the mitral valve, chordae, and papillary muscles. The mitral valve then is replaced with a low-profile disk valve. The space taken up by the mitral valve is substantially reduced; then blood can move around the enlarged septum to the aortic valve in the area that the mitral valve once occupied. The primary complication of both procedures is dysrhythmias, in addition to surgical complications.

NURSING PROCESS: THE PATIENT WITH CARDIOMYOPATHY

Assessment

Nursing assessment for the patient with cardiomyopathy begins with a detailed history of the presenting signs and symptoms. The nurse identifies possible etiologic factors, such as heavy alcohol intake, recent illness or pregnancy, or history of the disease in immediate family members. If the patient complains of chest pain, a thorough review of the pain, including its precipitating factors, should be performed.

Because of the chronicity of cardiomyopathy, the nurse compiles a careful psychosocial history exploring the impact of the disease on the patient's role within the family and community. Identification of all perceived stressors helps the patient and the health care team to implement activities to relieve anxiety related to change in health status. Very early on, the patient's support systems should be identified and involved in the patient's care and therapeutic regimen.

The physical assessment should focus on signs and symptoms of congestive heart failure. The baseline assessment needs to include such key components as a careful evaluation of fluid volume status, documentation of vital signs (including calculation of pulse pressure), detection by palpation of a shift to the left of the point of maximal impulse, and auscultation for a systolic murmur and third and fourth heart sounds.

The physician may prescribe cardiac monitoring; however, once the diagnosis is made or once dysrhythmia is not a significant problem, the patient may not need to be monitored. The severity of the cardiac failure determines whether the patient needs to be in a critical care unit.

Diagnosis

Nursing Diagnoses

Based on the assessment data, major nursing diagnoses for the patient may include:

- Decreased cardiac output related to structural disorders secondary to cardiomyopathy or to dysrhythmia secondary to disease process and medical treatments
- Altered tissue perfusion related to decreased peripheral blood flow secondary to responses to decreased cardiac output
- Impaired gas exchange related to pulmonary congestion secondary to myocardial failure
- Activity intolerance related to decreased cardiac output and/or excessive fluid volume
- Anxiety related to the change in health status and change in role functioning
- Powerlessness related to disease process
- Noncompliance with medication and diet therapies

Collaborative Problems/Potential Complications

Based on the assessment data, potential complications include:

- Congestive heart failure
- Ventricular dysrhythmias
- Atrial dysrhythmias

These complications are discussed in Chapters 24 and 27.

Planning and Goals

The major goals for the patient include improved or maintained cardiac output, increased activity tolerance, reduction of anxiety, compliance with the self-care program, and absence of complications.

Nursing Interventions

Improving Cardiac Output

During a symptomatic episode, rest is indicated. Many patients find that leaning back in a chair is more comfortable than lying down in a bed. This position is helpful in pooling venous blood in the periphery and reducing preload. Oxygen, usually given through nasal prongs, may also be indicated.

Because the medical regimen is primarily palliative, careful monitoring is needed to correlate the intervention with the patient's response and then adjust the treatment plan accordingly. Documentation of the patient's response is critical in facilitating care across the health care continuum—from care in the emergency room and the intensive care unit to care provided at home. For example, determining the patient's weight every day and identifying a significant change is one way to monitor the patient's response to treatment. Identifying the activities that cause shortness of breath and then establishing whether more or less activity causes the same symptoms is another method. Assessing the patient's oxygen saturation at rest and during activity may also be indicated when determining a need for supplemental oxygen.

Attention to the timeliness of administering prescribed medications is vital. Ensuring that the patient receives or chooses food selections that are appropriate for the low-sodium diet is also important. In addition, helping the patient keep warm and change position frequently stimulates circulation and reduces the possibility of skin breakdown.

Increasing Activity Tolerance

The nurse plans the patient's activities so that they occur in cycles, alternating rest with activity periods. Not only will this benefit the patient's physiologic status, but it will also help teach the patient about the need for cycles of rest and activity. For example, working with the patient to determine which part of the bath can be completed without assistance, and then providing a period of rest before completing the bath, helps the patient conserve energy that is in short supply. The nurse can then make sure that the patient recognizes the symptoms that indicate the need for rest and the actions to take when the symptoms occur.

Reducing Anxiety

Spiritual, psychological, and emotional support may be indicated for the patient, family, and significant others. Interventions are directed toward eradicating or alleviating perceived stressors. The patient is provided with appropriate information about cardiomyopathy and encouraged to accomplish self-care activities. An atmosphere in which the patient feels free to verbalize any fears is provided, as is assurance that these concerns are legitimate. If the patient is facing death or awaiting transplant surgery, time must be provided to discuss these issues. Providing the patient with realistic hope helps to reduce anxiety while the patient awaits a donor heart. Nurses help the patient, family, and significant others with anticipating grieving. Accomplishing a goal, no matter how small, also promotes the patient's sense of well-being.

Promoting Home and Community-Based Care

TEACHING PATIENTS SELF-CARE

The patient with cardiomyopathy needs to learn to participate in and accomplish self-care activities within the boundaries of activity limitations. Teaching patients about the medication regimen and dietary restrictions is a key part of the plan of nursing care. The nurse is integral to this learning process as patients learn to balance their lifestyle and work and at the same time accomplish their therapeutic activities. Helping patients to cope and accept their disease status makes it easier for them to adjust their expectations and follow the self-care program at home.

CONTINUING CARE

Patients who have significant symptoms of congestive heart failure or other complications of cardiomyopathy may need a home care referral. The nurse reinforces previous teaching and performs ongoing assessment of the patient's symptoms and progress. The nurse also assists the patient and family to adjust to lifestyle changes imposed by activity limitations. Simple suggestions for organizing daily activities and for increasing tolerance to activity can be helpful. The patient's responses to diet and fluid restrictions and to the medication regimen are assessed, and explanations about symptoms that should be reported to the physician are emphasized. Establishing trust is vital to the relationship with these chronically ill patients and their families. This is particularly significant when the nurse is involved with the patient and family in discussions about end-of-life decisions.

Evaluation

Expected Outcomes

Expected outcomes may include:

1. Demonstrates improved cardiac function
   a. Exhibits heart and respiratory rates within normal limits
   b. Shows normal blood gas levels
   c. Reports decreased dyspnea and increased comfort
   d. Uses oxygen therapy as prescribed
   e. Reports no weight gain
2. Increases activity tolerance
   a. Carries out activities of daily living (eg, brushes teeth, feeds self)
   b. Transfers self from chair to bed
   c. Reports increased tolerance to activity
3. Is less anxious
   a. Discusses prognosis freely
   b. Verbalizes fears and concerns
   c. Participates in support groups if appropriate
4. Complies with the program of self-care
   a. Takes medications according to prescribed schedule
   b. Modifies diet to accommodate sodium/fluid restriction
   c. Modifies lifestyle to accommodate activity limitations
   d. Identifies signs and symptoms to be reported to the health care professional

HEART TRANSPLANTATION

The first human-to-human heart transplant was performed in 1967. Since then, transplant procedures, equipment, and medications continue to improve. Since 1983, when cyclosporine became available, heart transplantation has become a therapeutic option for patients with end-stage heart disease. Cyclosporine is an immunosuppressant that greatly decreases the body's rejection of foreign proteins, such as transplanted organs. Unfortunately, cyclosporine also decreases the body's ability to resist infections, so a fine balance must be achieved between suppressing rejection and avoiding infection.

Cardiomyopathy, ischemic heart disease, congenital heart disease, valvular disease, and rejection of previously transplanted hearts are the most common indications for transplantation. A typical candidate usually has severe symptoms uncontrolled by medical therapy, no other surgical options, and a prognosis of less than 12 months to live. A multidisciplinary team screens the candidate before recommending the transplantation procedure. The person's age, pulmonary status, other chronic health conditions, infections, history of other transplants, compliance, and current health status are considered in the screening.

When a donor heart becomes available, a computer generates a list of potential recipients on the basis of ABO blood group compatibility, the size of the donor and the candidate, and the distance between the donor and potential recipient (distance is a variable because the transplanted heart's function depends on its being implanted within 4 hours of harvest from the donor).

Transplantation Techniques

An **orthotopic transplant** is the most common surgical procedure for cardiac transplantation (Fig. 26-9). The recipient's heart is removed and the donor heart implanted at the vena cava and pulmonary veins. Some surgeons still prefer to remove the recipient's heart leaving a portion of the recipient's atria (with the vena cava and pulmonary veins) in place. The donor heart, which usually has been preserved in ice, is prepared for implant by cutting away a small section of the atria that corresponds with the sections of the recipient's heart that were left in place. The donor heart is implanted by suturing the donor atria to the residual atrial tissue of the recipient's native heart. Both techniques then connect the recipient's pulmonary artery and aorta to those of the donor heart.

The **heterotopic transplant** technique is less commonly performed (Fig. 26-10). The donor heart is placed to the right and slightly anterior to the recipient's heart; the recipient's heart is not removed. Initially it was thought that the original heart might provide some protection for the patient in the event that the transplanted heart was rejected. Although the protective effect has not necessarily been proved, other reasons for retaining the original heart have been identified: a small donor heart, a prolonged ischemic time for the donor heart, or a donor heart that may have been otherwise compromised but must be used in an emergency.

The transplanted heart has no nerve connections with the recipient's body (denervated heart); thus, the sympathetic and vagus

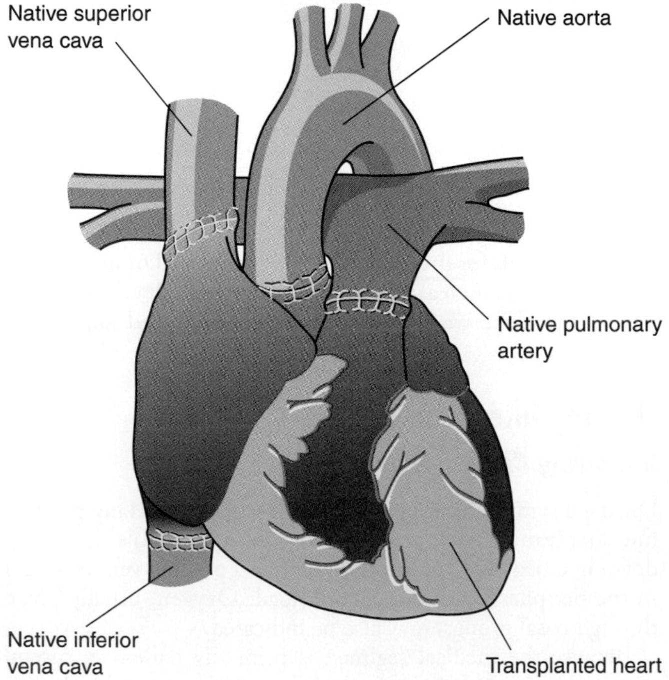

FIGURE 26•9 Orthotopic method of heart transplantation.

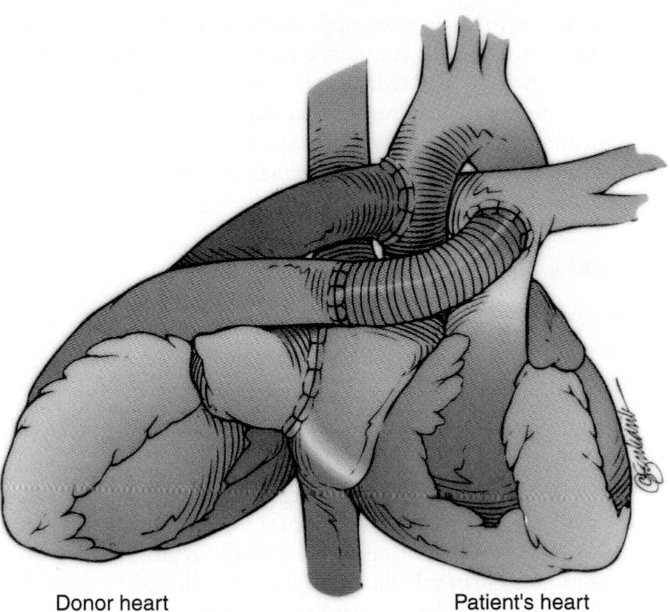

FIGURE 26•10 Heterotopic method of heart transplantation.

nerves do not affect the transplanted heart. The resting rate of the transplanted heart is approximately 70 to 90 beats per minute but increases gradually if catecholamines are in the circulation. Patients must gradually increase and decrease their exercise (extended warm-up and cool-down periods), because 20 to 30 minutes may be required to achieve the desired heart rate. Atropine does not increase the heart rate of these patients.

Postoperative Course

Heart transplant patients are constantly balancing the risk of rejection with the risk of infection. They must comply with a complex regimen of diet, medications, activity, follow-up laboratory studies, biopsies (to diagnose rejection), and clinic visits. Most commonly, patients receive cyclosporine and corticosteroids to minimize rejection.

In addition to rejection and infection, complications may include accelerated arteriosclerosis of the coronary arteries; hypertension and hypotension; central nervous system, respiratory, and gastrointestinal disturbances; renal failure; and responses to the psychosocial stresses imposed by organ transplantation.

The 1-year survival rate for heart transplant patients is approximately 80% to 90%; the 5-year survival rate is approximately 60% to 70%.

MECHANICAL ASSIST DEVICES AND TOTAL ARTIFICIAL HEARTS

The use of cardiopulmonary bypass for cardiovascular surgery and the possibility of performing heart transplantation for end-stage cardiac disease have increased the need for mechanical assist devices. Patients who cannot be weaned from cardiopulmonary bypass or patients with cardiogenic shock may benefit from a period of mechanical heart assistance. The most commonly used device is the intra-aortic balloon pump (see Chap. 27). This pump decreases the work of the heart during contraction but does not perform the actual work of the heart.

More complex devices that actually perform some or all of the pumping function for the heart also are being used. These more sophisticated **ventricular assist devices** (Fig. 26-11) can circulate as much blood per minute as the patient's heart, if not more. Each ventricular assist device is used to support one ventricle. Today, the most commonly used device is the centrifugal pump. Many pneumatically driven devices are being used, and the clinical results are very encouraging. Some ventricular assist devices can be combined with an oxygenator–extracorporeal membrane oxygenation. The oxygenator–ventricular assist device combination is used for the patient whose heart cannot pump adequate blood through their lungs or their body.

Total artificial hearts are designed to replace both ventricles. The patient's heart must be removed to implant the total artificial heart. All of these devices are experimental. The Jarvik-7 had some short-term success, but the long-term results have been disappointing. Researchers are hoping to develop a device that can be permanently implanted and that will eliminate the need for donated human heart transplantation for the treatment of end-stage cardiac disease.

Currently, ventricular assist devices and total artificial hearts are temporary treatments while the patient's own heart recovers or until a donor heart becomes available for transplantation. Bleed-

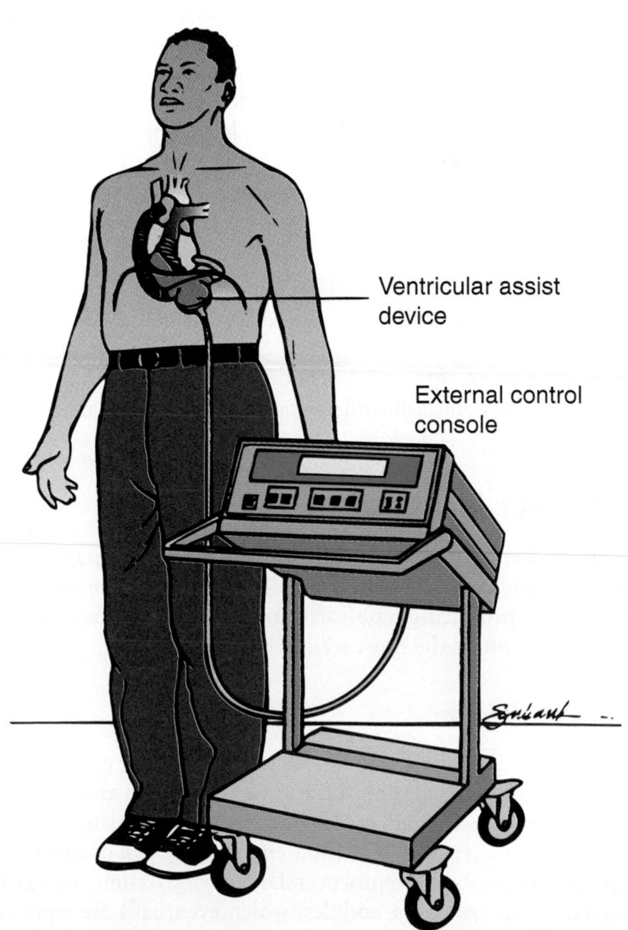

FIGURE 26•11 Left ventricular assist device.

ing disorders, hemorrhage, thrombus, emboli, hemolysis, infection, and mechanical failure are some of the possible complications of ventricular assist devices and total artificial hearts. The nursing care for these patients focuses on assessing for and minimizing these complications and also involves providing emotional support and education about the mechanical assist device.

CARDIAC TUMOR AND TRAUMA SURGERY

Tumor Excision

Tumors of the heart are quite rare. Most cardiac tumors are benign. Primary tumors occur in less than 1% of the population; metastatic tumors have been reported in 1.5% to 35% of oncology patients. Tumors may be a site for thrombus formation and therefore create a risk of embolism. Dysrhythmias may occur as the myocardium or conduction system is affected.

Surgical excision is performed to prevent obstruction of a chamber or valve. Cardiopulmonary bypass is used, except for epicardial tumors, which can be excised without entering the heart and without stopping the heart from beating. The tumor location may necessitate valve replacement, myocardial patching, or pacemaker implantation. The nursing care is the same as that for patients undergoing other forms of cardiac surgery.

Trauma Repair

Patients who require surgical treatment for cardiac trauma are those who have sustained a blunt force injury, a gunshot wound, or a stabbing. The repairs are typically to the valves or septum in blunt force injuries and to the ventricular and atrial walls in penetrating injuries. The wound is débrided and closed surgically when possible, but valve repair and replacement or patch grafts of the septum and atrial or ventricular walls may be required. The surgery is usually an emergency procedure, so the risk of complications from the injury and surgery is high.

INFECTIOUS DISEASES OF THE HEART

Among the most common infections of the heart are infective endocarditis, myocarditis, and pericarditis. The ideal management is prevention.

Rheumatic Endocarditis

Rheumatic endocarditis results directly from rheumatic fever caused by group A streptococcal infection. The disease affects all bony joints, producing a polyarthritis. The heart is also a target organ and is where the most serious damage occurs.

Pathophysiology

The heart damage and the joint lesions of rheumatic endocarditis are not infectious in origin, in the sense that these tissues are not invaded and directly damaged by destructive organisms; rather, they represent a sensitivity phenomenon or reaction occurring in response to hemolytic streptococci. Leukocytes accumulate in the affected tissues and form nodules, which eventually are replaced by scars. The myocardium is certain to be involved in this inflammatory process; that is, rheumatic myocarditis develops, which temporarily weakens the contractile power of the heart. The pericardium likewise is affected; that is, rheumatic pericarditis also occurs during the acute illness. These myocardial and pericardial complications usually are without serious sequelae. Rheumatic endocarditis, however, results in permanent and often crippling side effects.

Clinical Manifestations

Rheumatic endocarditis anatomically manifests itself first by tiny translucent vegetations or growths, which resemble pinhead-sized beads arranged in a row along the free margins of the valve flaps. These tiny beads look harmless enough and may disappear without injuring the valve leaflets. More often, however, they have serious effects. They are the starting point of a process that gradually thickens the leaflets, rendering them shorter and thicker than normal and preventing them from closing completely. The result is leakage, a condition called valvular regurgitation. The most common site of valvular regurgitation is the mitral valve. In other patients, the inflamed margins of the valve leaflets become adherent, resulting in valvular stenosis, a narrowed or stenotic valvular orifice.

A few patients with rheumatic fever become critically ill with intractable heart failure, serious dysrhythmias, and pneumonia. These patients are treated in an intensive care unit. Most patients recover quickly and usually completely. However, although the patient is free of symptoms, certain permanent residual effects remain that often lead to progressive valvular deformities. The extent of cardiac damage, or even its existence, may not have been apparent in clinical examinations during the acute phase of the disease. Eventually, however, the heart murmurs that are characteristic of valvular stenosis, regurgitation, or both become audible on auscultation and, in some patients, even detectable as thrills on palpation. Usually the myocardium can compensate for these valvular defects very well for a time. As long as the myocardium can compensate, the patient remains in apparently good health. Sooner or later, however, the myocardium fails to compensate. Decompensation, when it occurs, is signaled by the manifestations of congestive heart failure, as described in Chapter 27.

Assessment and Diagnostic Findings

During assessment, the symptoms that are disclosed depend on which side of the heart is involved. The mitral valve is most often affected, producing the symptoms of left-sided heart failure: shortness of breath with crackles and wheezes in the lungs. (See Chap. 27 for a discussion of left-sided versus right-sided failure.) The severity of the symptoms depends on the size and location of the lesion. The systemic symptoms that are present are proportionate to the virulence of the invading organism. When a new murmur is detected in a patient with a systemic infection, infectious endocarditis should be suspected. The patient is also at risk for embolic phenomena of the lung (recurrent pneumonia, pulmonary abscesses), kidney (hematuria, renal failure), spleen (left upper quadrant pain), heart (myocardial infarction), brain (stroke), or peripheral vessels.

Prevention

Rheumatic endocarditis is prevented through early and adequate treatment of streptococcal infections. A first-line approach in pre-

ASSESSMENT
RECOGNIZING AND PREVENTING RHEUMATIC FEVER

Rheumatic fever is a preventable disease. Eradicating rheumatic fever would eliminate rheumatic heart disease. Penicillin therapy in patients with streptococcal infections can prevent almost all primary attacks of rheumatic fever. A throat culture is the only method by which an accurate diagnosis can be determined.

The signs and symptoms of streptococcal pharyngitis are the following:

- Fever (38.9° to 40°C [101° to 104°F])
- Chills
- Sore throat (sudden in onset)
- Diffuse redness of throat with exudate on oropharynx (may not appear until after the first day)
- Enlarged and tender lymph nodes
- Abdominal pain (more common in children)
- Acute sinusitis and acute otitis media (may be due to streptococci)

venting initial attacks of rheumatic endocarditis is to recognize streptococcal infections, treat them adequately, and control epidemics in the community. Every nurse should be familiar with the signs and symptoms of streptococcal pharyngitis: high fever (38.9° to 40°C [101° to 104°F]), chills, sore throat, redness of the throat with exudate, enlarged lymph nodes, abdominal pain, and acute rhinitis.

Nursing Alert *A throat culture is the only method by which an accurate diagnosis can be made.*

Medical Management

The objectives of medical management are to eradicate the causative organism and prevent additional complications, such as a thromboembolic event. Long-term antibiotic therapy is the treatment of choice. Penicillin administered parenterally remains the medication of choice.

The patient who has rheumatic endocarditis, and whose valve function is faulty but whose disease is quiescent, does not require therapy as long as the heart pumps effectively. Nevertheless, the danger exists for recurrent attacks of acute rheumatic fever, bacterial endocarditis, embolism from vegetations or mural thrombi in the heart, and eventual cardiac failure.

Nursing Management

A key nursing role in infective endocarditis is teaching patients about the disease and its prevention and treatment. Susceptible patients need to know about long-term oral antibiotic therapy or, more commonly, about the need to take prophylactic antibiotics before procedures, such as dental work or examinations, that can introduce infection. These patients also must be reminded of less common procedures such as cystoscopy that may also require prophylactic antibiotic therapy.

Infective Endocarditis

Infective endocarditis (bacterial endocarditis) is an infection of the valves and endothelial surface of the heart. Infective endocarditis is more common in older people, probably because of decreased immunologic responses to infection, the metabolic alterations associated with aging, and the increased number of invasive diagnostic procedures, especially in genitourinary disease. There is a high incidence of staphylococcal endocarditis among intravenous drug users, the disease occurring for the most part on otherwise normal valves.

Pathophysiology

Infective endocarditis is caused by direct invasion by bacteria or other organisms and leads to deformity of the valve leaflets. Causative microorganisms include bacteria (streptococci, enterococci, pneumococci, and staphylococci), fungi, rickettsiae, and *Streptococcus viridans*. Infective endocarditis usually develops in patients who have a history of valvular heart disease. At great risk are patients with rheumatic heart disease or mitral valve prolapse and those who have had prosthetic valve surgery.

Hospital-acquired endocarditis occurs most often in patients with debilitating disease, those with indwelling catheters, and those receiving prolonged intravenous or antibiotic therapy. Patients receiving immunosuppressive medications or corticosteroids may develop fungal endocarditis.

Clinical Manifestations

Usually, the onset of infective endocarditis is insidious. The signs and symptoms develop from the toxic effect of the infection, from destruction of the heart valves, and from embolization of fragments of vegetative growths on the heart.

Assessment and Diagnostic Findings

The general manifestations, which may be mistaken for influenza, include vague complaints of malaise, anorexia, weight loss, cough, and back and joint pain. Fever is intermittent and may be absent in patients who are receiving antibiotics or corticosteroids or in those who are elderly or have congestive heart failure or renal failure. Splinter hemorrhages (hemorrhagic lines and streaks) may be noted under the fingernails and toenails, and petechiae may appear in the conjunctiva and mucous membranes. Hemorrhages with pale centers (Roth's spots) that may be seen in the fundi of the eyes are caused by emboli in the nerve fiber layer of the eye.

The cardiac manifestations include heart murmurs, which may be absent initially. Progressive changes in murmurs over time may be encountered and indicate valvular damage from vegetations or perforation of the valve or the chordae tendineae. Enlargement of the heart or evidence of congestive heart failure is also seen.

The central nervous system manifestations include headache, temporary or transient cerebral ischemia, and strokes, which may be caused by emboli involving the cerebral arteries. Embolization may be a presenting symptom; it may occur at any time and may involve other organ systems. Embolic phenomena may occur, as discussed in the section on rheumatic endocarditis.

Prevention

For those at risk, a key prevention strategy, antibiotic prophylaxis, is recommended immediately before and sometimes after the following procedures:

- Dental procedures that induce gingival or mucosal bleeding, including professional cleaning

Risk Factors for
INFECTIVE ENDOCARDITIS

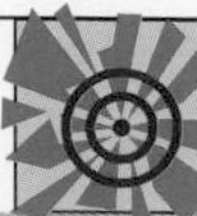

Structural abnormalities of the heart and great vessels, especially valvular heart disease
Patients with prosthetic cardiac valves
History of bacterial endocarditis (even without heart disease)
Congenital malformations or rheumatic and other acquired valvular dysfunction (even after valvular surgery), and mitral valve prolapse with valvular regurgitation
Hypertrophic cardiomyopathy
Any invasive procedure (eg, instrumentation) that introduces significant amounts of bacteria

- Tonsillectomy or adenoidectomy
- Surgical procedures that involve intestinal or respiratory mucosa
- Bronchoscopy with a rigid bronchoscope
- Sclerotherapy for esophageal varices
- Esophageal dilation
- Gallbladder surgery
- Cystoscopy
- Urethral dilation
- Urethral catheterization if urinary tract infection is present
- Urinary tract surgery if urinary tract infection is present
- Prostatic surgery
- Incision and drainage of infected tissue
- Vaginal hysterectomy
- Vaginal delivery in the presence of infection

Complications

Even if the patient responds to the therapy, endocarditis can be destructive to the heart and other organs. Congestive heart failure and cerebral vascular complications, such as stroke, may occur before, during, or after therapy. Valvular stenosis or regurgitation, myocardial damage, and mycotic (fungal) aneurysms are some potential heart complications. Many other organ complications can result from septic or nonseptic emboli, immunologic responses, or hemodynamic deterioration.

Medical Management

The objective of treatment is to eradicate the invading organism through adequate doses of an appropriate antimicrobial agent. The causative organism can be isolated by serial blood cultures. It is treated with a bactericidal agent or other appropriate medication that is known to be effective against the causative agent.

PHARMACOLOGIC THERAPY

Antibiotic therapy is usually administered parenterally in a continuous intravenous infusion for 4 to 6 weeks. Usually this therapy is delivered in the patient's home and is monitored by a home care nurse. Bactericidal serum levels of the selected antibiotic are monitored by titrating it against the causative organism. If the serum does not demonstrate bactericidal activity, increased dosages of the antibiotic are given, or a different antibiotic is used. There are numerous antimicrobial regimens in use, but penicillin is usually the medication of choice. Blood cultures are taken periodically to monitor the course of therapy.

In fungal endocarditis, an antifungal agent, such as amphotericin B, is the usual treatment. The patient's temperature is monitored at regular intervals because the course of the fever is one indication of the effectiveness of treatment. However, febrile reactions also may occur as a result of medication therapy. After adequate antimicrobial therapy is initiated, bacteria usually disappear. The patient should begin to feel better, regain an appetite, and have less fatigue. During this time, patients require a great deal of psychosocial support because, although they feel well, they may find themselves confined to the hospital or home with restrictive intravenous therapy.

SURGICAL MANAGEMENT

After the patient recovers from the infectious process, the valves may need to be replaced if they have been seriously damaged and cause severe symptoms. Surgical valve replacement greatly improves the prognosis for patients with severely damaged heart valves. Usually, valve excision and replacement are required for patients who develop congestive heart failure as a result of aortic or mitral valve involvement despite adequate medical treatment; patients who have more than one serious systemic embolic episode; and patients with uncontrolled infection, recurrent infection, or fungal endocarditis. Many patients who have prosthetic valve endocarditis (infected prostheses) require valve replacement.

Nursing Management

In addition to educating the patient and family about prevention and health promotion, the home care nurse may be called on to supervise and monitor intravenous antibiotic therapy delivered in the home setting. Additional nursing roles may involve postsurgical care and instruction.

Myocarditis

Myocarditis is an inflammatory process involving the myocardium. Myocarditis can cause heart dilatation, thrombi on the heart wall (mural thrombi), infiltration of circulating blood cells around the coronary vessels and between the muscle fibers, and degeneration of the muscle fibers themselves.

Pathophysiology

Myocarditis usually results from a viral, bacterial, mycotic, parasitic, protozoal, or spirochetal infection. It also may be seen in patients with acute systemic infections such as rheumatic fever, those receiving immunosuppressive therapy, or those with infective endocarditis. It is theorized that dilated cardiomyopathy is a latent manifestation of myocarditis.

Clinical Manifestations

The symptoms of acute myocarditis depend on the type of infection, the degree of myocardial damage, and the capacity of the myocardium to recover. The patient may be asymptomatic and the infection resolves on its own. The patient may develop mild to moderate symptoms and seek medical attention. The patient may also sustain sudden cardiac death or quickly develop severe congestive heart failure. The patient with mild to moderate symptoms often complains of fatigue and dyspnea, palpitations, and occasional discomfort in the chest and upper abdomen.

Assessment and Diagnostic Findings

Clinical assessment may disclose cardiac enlargement, faint heart sounds, gallop rhythm, and a systolic murmur. A pericardial friction rub may be heard if the patient has associated pericarditis. Pulsus alternans (a pulse in which there is a regular alternation of weak and strong beats) may be present. Fever and tachycardia are frequently seen, and symptoms of congestive heart failure may develop. The diagnosis can be confirmed by endomyocardial biopsy.

Prevention

Prevention of infectious diseases by means of appropriate immunizations and early treatment appears to be important in decreasing the incidence of myocarditis.

Medical Management

The patient receives specific treatment for the underlying cause, if it is known (eg, penicillin for hemolytic streptococci), and is placed on bed rest to decrease the cardiac workload. Bed rest also helps to decrease myocardial damage and the complications of myocarditis. The treatment is essentially the same as that used for congestive heart failure (see Chap. 27). After an episode of myocarditis, some residual heart enlargement may remain. Physical activity is increased slowly, and the patient is instructed to report any symptoms that occur with increasing activity, such as a rapidly beating heart. Competitive sports and alcohol must be avoided during recovery.

Nursing Management

Cardiac function and temperature are evaluated to determine whether the disease is subsiding and whether congestive heart failure has occurred. If a dysrhythmia occurs, the patient should be cared for in a unit with continuous cardiac monitoring so that personnel and equipment are readily available if a life-threatening dysrhythmia occurs.

Nursing Alert *Patients with myocarditis are sensitive to digitalis. Therefore, they must be closely monitored for digitalis toxicity (evidenced by dysrhythmia, anorexia, nausea, vomiting, headache, malaise; see Chap. 27).*

Elastic pressure stockings and passive and active exercises should be used, because embolization from venous thrombosis and mural thrombi can occur.

Pericarditis

Pericarditis refers to an inflammation of the pericardium, the membranous sac enveloping the heart. It may be a primary illness, or it may develop in the course of a variety of medical and surgical disorders.

Pathophysiology

The following are some of the causes underlying or associated with pericarditis:

- Idiopathic or nonspecific causes
- Infection: bacterial (eg, streptococci, staphylococci, meningococci, gonococci); viral (eg, coxsackie, influenza), and mycotic (fungal)
- Disorders of connective tissue: systemic lupus erythematosus, rheumatic fever, rheumatoid arthritis, polyarteritis
- Hypersensitivity states: immune reactions, drug reactions, serum sickness
- Diseases of adjacent structures: myocardial infarction, dissecting aneurysm, pleural and pulmonary disease (pneumonia)
- Neoplastic disease: secondary to metastasis from lung cancer or breast cancer, leukemia, and primary (mesothelioma)
- Radiation therapy
- Trauma: chest injury, cardiac surgery, during cardiac catheterization, pacemaker implantation
- Renal failure and uremia
- Tuberculosis

Clinical Manifestations

The characteristic symptom of pericarditis is pain; the characteristic sign is a friction rub. Pain is almost always present in acute pericarditis and is most common over the precordium. The pain may be felt beneath the clavicle and in the neck and left scapular region. Pericardial pain is aggravated by breathing, turning in bed, and twisting the body; it is relieved by sitting up. In fact, the patient prefers to adopt a forward-leaning or a sitting posture. Dyspnea may occur as the result of pericardial compression of the heart's movements, which leads to a decreased cardiac output. The patient may appear extremely ill. Pericarditis itself often gives rise to no signs other than fever, an increased white blood count, and a friction rub.

Assessment and Diagnostic Findings

Diagnosis is most often made on the basis of signs and symptoms. The ECG and echocardiogram help confirm the diagnosis.

Medical Management

The objectives of management are to determine the cause, administer therapy for the specific cause (when known), and be alert for cardiac tamponade (compression of the heart from fluid in the pericardial sac; see Chap. 27). The patient is placed on bed rest when cardiac output is impaired until the fever, chest pain, and friction rub have subsided.

Analgesics and nonsteroidal anti-inflammatory agents such as indomethacin (Indocin) may be prescribed for pain relief during the acute phase. They relieve pain and hasten the reabsorption of fluid in the patient with rheumatic pericarditis. Corticosteroids may be prescribed to control symptoms, hasten resolution of the inflammatory process in the pericardium, and prevent recurring pericardial effusion.

Nursing Management

The nurse, who has several primary concerns in caring for the patient with pericarditis, must be alert to the possibility of cardiac tamponade.

Nursing Alert *Nursing assessment skills are key to anticipating and identifying the triad of symptoms of cardiac tamponade: falling arterial pressure, rising venous pressure, and distant heart sounds.*

The nurse administers medications as prescribed to patients with infections of the pericardium once the organism causing the infection is identified. For example, patients with pericarditis associated with rheumatic fever may respond to penicillin. Patients with pericarditis resulting from tuberculosis may need administration of isoniazid, ethambutol hydrochloride, rifampin, and streptomycin, in various combinations. Amphotericin B is used in fungal pericarditis, and corticosteroids are administered in disseminated lupus erythematosus.

As the patient's condition improves, the nurse may encourage gradually increasing activity. If pain, fever, or friction rub reappear, however, bed rest must be resumed.

Chronic Constrictive Pericarditis

Chronic constrictive pericarditis is a condition in which chronic inflammatory thickening of the pericardium compresses the heart and prevents it from expanding to normal size. The ventricles cannot fill completely, and therefore less blood is pumped into the circulatory system. The adherent pericardium may become calcified, and heart action is greatly restricted by this tough, unyielding enclosure. Edema, ascites, and hepatic enlargement result. The fixation of the heart to the pericardium may produce a retraction of the chest wall with every beat.

Chronic restrictive pericarditis is caused by long-standing pyogenic infections, postviral infections, tuberculosis, or blood in the pericardial cavity (hemopericardium). The signs and symptoms are predominantly those of congestive heart failure (see Chap. 27), but dyspnea on exertion is the most prominent symptom. Chronic atrial fibrillation is common.

Surgical removal of the tough encasing pericardium (pericardiectomy) is the only treatment of any benefit. The objective of the surgery is to release both ventricles from the constrictive and restrictive inflammation.

NURSING PROCESS: THE PATIENT WITH PERICARDITIS

Assessment

Pain is the primary symptom of the patient with pericarditis. The pain of pericarditis is assessed by observing and evaluating the patient in various positions in bed. While observing the patient, the nurse tries to discover whether the pain is influenced by respiratory movements, with or without the actual passage of air; by flexion, extension, or rotation of the spine, including the neck; by movements of the shoulders and arms; by coughing; or by swallowing. Recognizing the events that precipitate or intensify pain may be very helpful in establishing a diagnosis and differentiating the pain of pericarditis from the pain of myocardial infarction.

A pericardial friction rub occurs when the pericardial surfaces lose their lubricating fluid because of inflammation. The rub is audible on auscultation and is synchronous with the heartbeat. However, it may be elusive and difficult to detect.

Nursing Alert *A pericardial friction rub is diagnostic of pericarditis and should be searched for diligently by placing the diaphragm of the stethoscope tightly against the thorax and auscultating the left sternal edge in the fourth intercostal space, the site where the pericardium comes into contact with the left chest wall. A pericardial friction rub has a scratching or leathery sound. The rub is louder at the end of exhalation and may be heard best with the patient sitting and leaning forward.*

If there is difficulty in distinguishing a pericardial friction rub from a pleural friction rub, patients are asked to hold their breath; a pericardial friction rub will continue.

The patient's temperature is monitored frequently. Pericarditis causes an abrupt onset of fever in a patient who has been afebrile.

Diagnosis

Nursing Diagnoses

Based on the assessment data, major nursing diagnoses of the patient may include the following:

- Pain related to inflammation of the pericardium

Collaborative Problems/Potential Complications

Based on the assessment data, potential complications that may develop include:

- Pericardial effusion
- Cardiac tamponade

Planning and Goals

The patient's major goals may include relief of pain and absence of complications.

Nursing Interventions

Relieving Pain

Relief of pain is achieved by having the patient remain on bed rest or chair rest, whichever is more comfortable. Because sitting upright and leaning forward is the posture that tends to relieve pain, chair rest may be more comfortable. As the chest pain and friction rub abate, activities of daily living may resume gradually. If the patient is receiving medications for the pericarditis, such as analgesics, antibiotics, or corticosteroids, his or her responses are monitored and recorded. If chest pain and friction rub recur, bed rest resumes.

Monitoring and Managing Potential Complications

PERICARDIAL EFFUSION

If the patient does not respond to medical management, fluid may accumulate between the pericardial linings or in the sac. This condition is called pericardial effusion (see Chap. 27). Fluid in the pericardial sac can constrict the myocardium and interrupt its ability to pump. Thus, cardiac output declines with each contraction. Failure to identify and treat this problem can lead to the development of cardiac tamponade and the possibility of sudden death.

The signs and symptoms of cardiac tamponade begin with falling arterial pressure. Usually the systolic pressure falls while the diastolic pressure remains stable; hence, the pulse pressure narrows. Heart sounds may progress from being distant to being imperceptible. Neck vein distention and other signs of rising central venous pressure are observed. These signs and symptoms occur because as the fluid-filled pericardial sac compresses the myocardium, blood continues to return to the heart from the periphery but cannot be pumped back into the circulation.

In such situations, the nurse notifies the physician immediately and prepares to assist with pericardiocentesis (see Chap. 27). The nurse stays with the patient and continues to assess and record signs and symptoms until the physician arrives to initiate more definitive therapy.

Evaluation

Expected Outcomes

Expected outcomes may include:

1. Patient is free of pain
   a. Performs activities of daily living comfortably
   b. Shows temperature returning to normal range
   c. Exhibits no pericardial friction rub
2. Avoids complications
   a. Sustains blood pressure in normal range
   b. Has heart sounds that are strong and can be auscultated
   c. Shows absence of neck vein distention

Critical Thinking Exercises

1.
One of your neighbors has just had a mitral valve replacement and says he does not understand why he has been instructed to take antibiotics before undergoing any dental work. How would you explain the rationale for these instructions?

2.
Discharge plans are being made for a middle-aged man with cardiomyopathy. His wife says she is prepared to care for him at home; she expects that he will be unable to participate extensively in his care. Based on your knowledge about developmental tasks of the middle years, how would you explain the husband's emotional and physical needs to the wife and the ways she can address these needs, as well as her own?

3.
A patient recovering from heart transplantation says he feels he has "a new lease on life" and is "looking forward to a normal life." What further information about the patient will be helpful in identifying his teaching and discharge planning needs? Another patient who has undergone the same surgical procedure seems depressed and apprehensive. How would you explain the different reactions, and how would your teaching strategies for these two patients differ?

4.
You are caring for a patient with pericarditis. His systolic blood pressure begins to fall and heart sounds cannot be heard. Describe the actions you would take and why.

References and Selected Readings

BOOKS AND PAMPHLETS

American Heart Association. (1997). *Heart facts.* Dallas: Author.
Bickley, L. S., & Hoekelman, R. A. (1999). *Bates's guide to physical examination and history taking* (7th ed.). Philadelphia: Lippincott Williams & Wilkins.
Braunwald, E. (1997). *Heart disease: A textbook of cardiovascular medicine* (5th ed.). Philadelphia: W. B. Saunders.
Hudak, C. M., Gallo, B. M., & Morton, P. G. (1998). *Critical care nursing: A holistic approach* (7th ed.). Philadelphia: Lippincott-Raven.
Kinny, M., et al. (1998). *AACN's clinical reference manual.* New York: McGraw-Hill.
Schlant, R. C., et al. (1998). *Hurst's the heart: Arteries and veins.* New York: McGraw-Hill.
Woods, S. L., et al. (1995). *Cardiac nursing* (3rd ed.). Philadelphia: J. B. Lippincott.

JOURNALS

Asterisks indicate nursing research articles.

Brown, K. K. (1998). Minimally invasive valve surgery. *Critical Care Nursing Quarterly, 20*(4), 40–52.
Canning, R. D., Dew, M. A., & Davidson, S. (1996). Psychological distress among caregivers to heart transplant recipients. *Social Science and Medicine, 42*(4), 599–608.
Chillcott, S. R., Atkins, P. J., & Adamson, R. M. (1998). Left ventricular assist as a viable alternative for cardiac transplantation. *Critical Care Nursing Quarterly, 20*(4), 64–79.
Constancia, P. E. (1991). The Ross procedure: Aortic valve replacement using autologous pulmonary valve. *Critical Care Clinics, 3*(4), 717–721.
*Corley, M. C., et al. (1995). Patient and nurse criteria for heart transplant candidacy. *MedSurg Nursing, 4*(3), 211–215.
Dajani, A. S., et al. (1997). Prevention of bacterial endocarditis: Recommendations by the American Heart Association. *Journal of the American Medical Association, 277*(22), 1794–1801.
Francis, S. E., et al. (1998). Interleukin-1 in myocardium and coronary arteries of patients with dilated cardiomyopathy. *Journal of Molecular Cell Cardiology, 30*(2), 215–223.
*Grady, K. L., & Jalowiec, A. (1995). Predictors of compliance with diet 6 months after heart transplantation. *Heart and Lung, 24*(5), 359–368.
Hammon, J. W. (1997). What's new in cardiac surgery. *Journal of the American College of Surgeons, 184*(2), 105–108.
Mestroni, L., & Giacca, M. (1997). Molecular genetics of dilated cardiomyopathy. *Current Opinion in Cardiology, 12*(3), 303–309.
Moroney, D.A., & Powers, K. (1997). Outpatient use of left ventricular assist devices: Nursing, technical, and educational consideration. *American Journal of Critical Care, 6*(5), 355–362.
Rafalowski, M. (1990). Cardiac valve replacement: The homograft. *Focus on Critical Care, 17*(2), 111–114.
Rose, E. A. (1996). What's new in cardiac surgery. *Journal of the American College of Surgeons, 182*(2), 83–88.
Scott, C., Schactman, M., & Graver, L. M. (1997). Aortic valve replacement with a pulmonary autograft: Case studies of the Ross procedure. *American Journal of Critical Care, 6*(6), 418–422.
Skillings, J. (1998). Endocarditis and endocarditis prophylaxis. *Primary Care Practice, 2*(5), 529–532.
Smith, A., & Fitzpatrick, E. (1993). Penetrating cardiac trauma: Surgical and nursing management. *Journal of Cardiovascular Nursing, 7*(2),52–70.
Usznski, H. J., et al. (1993). Hypertrophic cardiomyopathy: Medical, surgical, and nursing management. *Journal of Cardiovascular Nursing, 7*(2), 13–22.

Resources

American Heart Association: http://www.americanheart.org/aha.html
Heartmates: http://www.heartmates.com/cardiac.html
National Heart, Lung, & Blood Institute: http://www.nhlbi.nih.gov

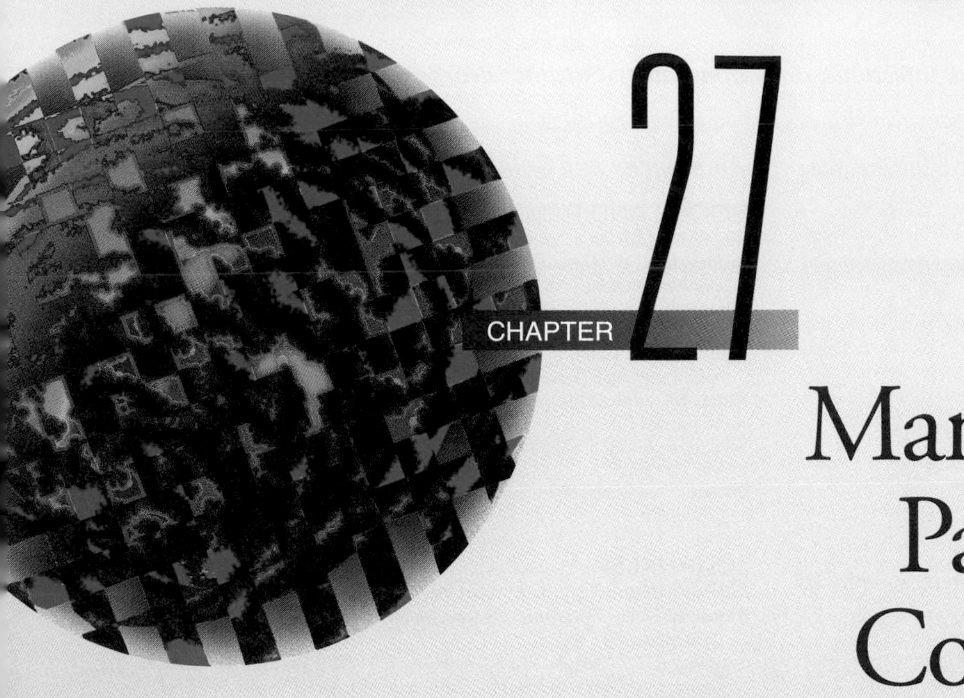

CHAPTER 27

Management of Patients With Complications From Heart Disease

Learning Objectives

On completion of this chapter, the learner will be able to:

1. Describe the management of patients with acute pulmonary edema.
2. Use the nursing process as a framework for care of patients with cardiac failure.
3. Develop teaching plans for patients with cardiac failure.
4. Describe the management of patients with cardiogenic shock.
5. Describe the management of patients with thromboembolic episodes, pericardial effusion and cardiac tamponade, and myocardial rupture.
6. Demonstrate the techniques of cardiopulmonary resuscitation.

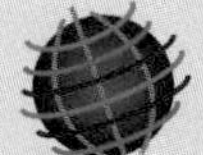

Today, the patient with heart disease can be assisted to achieve a quality of life far greater than anticipated even as recently as a decade ago. Through sophisticated diagnostic procedures that allow for earlier and more accurate diagnoses, treatment can begin well before significant debilitation occurs. New treatments, technologies, and pharmacotherapies are developing rapidly. However, heart disease remains a chronic condition and complications may develop. This chapter discusses the complications most often resulting from heart diseases and the treatments provided by the health care team for these complications.

GLOSSARY

afterload: the amount of resistance to ejection of blood from a ventricle

anuria: urine output of less than 50 mL per 24 hours

cardiac output: the amount of blood pumped out of the heart in 1 minute

congestive heart failure (CHF): the inability of the heart to pump sufficient blood to meet the needs of the tissues for oxygen and nutrients; a term commonly used when referring to left-sided or right-sided failure

contractility: the force of ventricular contraction; related to number and state of myocardial cells

dyspnea on exertion (DOE): shortness of breath that occurs with exertion

oliguria: diminished urine output; less than 400 mL per 24 hours

orthopnea: shortness of breath when lying flat

pericardiocentesis: procedure that involves surgically opening the pericardial sac

paroxysmal nocturnal dyspnea (PND): shortness of breath that occurs suddenly during sleep

preload: the amount of myocardial stretch just before systole caused by pressure created by a volume of blood within a ventricle before contraction

pulmonary edema: abnormal accumulation of fluid in the lungs, either in the interstitial spaces or in the alveoli

pulseless electrical activity (PEA): condition in which electrical activity is present but there is not an adequate pulse or blood pressure due to ineffective cardiac contraction or circulating blood volume

pulsus paradoxus: systolic blood pressure that is heard during expiration but not with inspiration; normally less than 10 mm Hg

stroke volume: amount of blood pumped out of the ventricle with each contraction

thermodilution: method of determining cardiac output, which involves injecting fluid into the pulmonary artery catheter. A thermistor measures the difference between the temperature of the fluid and the temperature of the blood ejected from the ventricle. Cardiac output is calculated from the change in temperature

ACUTE PULMONARY EDEMA

Pulmonary edema is the abnormal accumulation of fluid in the lungs. The fluid may accumulate either in the interstitial spaces or in the alveoli.

Pathophysiology

Although there are noncardiac causes, pulmonary edema usually is caused by a disorder, such as acute myocardial infarction, arterial hypertension, or valvular disease, that decreases the left ventricle's pumping ability. When the left ventricle cannot pump the blood out, the pressure in the ventricle increases. This phenomenon is known as elevated left ventricular end-diastolic pressure. Blood cannot then easily flow from the left atrium into the left ventricle. This causes the pressure to increase in the left atrium. The increase in atrial pressure may result in an increase in pulmonary venous pressure, which in turn produces an increase in hydrostatic pressure, which forces fluid out of the pulmonary capillaries into the interstitial spaces and alveoli.

Impaired lymphatic drainage also contributes to the accumulation of fluid in the lung tissues. The fluid mixes with air and is expelled from the mouth and nose, producing the classic symptom of pulmonary edema, frothy pink (blood-tinged) sputum. Because of the fluid within the alveoli, gas exchange is impaired and air cannot enter. The result is severe hypoxemia. Onset may be preceded by the premonitory symptoms of pulmonary congestion, but it also may develop quickly in the patient with a ventricle that has little reserve to meet increased oxygen needs.

CARDIAC HEMODYNAMICS

The basic function of the heart is pumping blood. The heart's ability to pump is measured by **cardiac output** (CO), the amount of blood pumped in 1 minute. CO is determined by measuring the heart rate (HR) and multiplying it by the **stroke volume** (SV). SV is the amount of blood pumped out with each contraction. The concept of CO is usually indicated by the equation $CO = HR \times SV$.

One of the factors controlling HR is the autonomic nervous system. When SV falls, the nervous system is stimulated to increase HR and thereby maintain adequate CO. SV depends on three factors: preload, contractility, and afterload.

Preload is the amount of myocardial stretch just before systole caused by the pressure created by the volume of blood within the ventricle before contraction. Like a rubber band, the ventricular muscle fibers need to be stretched (by the blood) to produce an optimal ejection of blood. Too little or too much muscle fiber stretching decreases the resulting volume of blood that is ejected. The major factor that determines preload is venous return, the volume of blood that enters the ventricle during diastole. Another factor that determines preload is ventricular compliance, the elasticity or amount of "give" when blood enters the ventricle. When cells die, they are replaced by fibrotic tissue that has little compliance, making the ventricle stiff, with little give. This causes an equal volume of blood to raise the pressure in a noncompliant ventricle.

Contractility, which refers to the force of contraction, is related to the number and status of myocardial cells. **Afterload** refers to the amount of resistance to the ejection of blood. To eject blood, the ventricle must overcome this resistance. Afterload is inversely related to SV. The major factors that determine afterload are the diameter and distensibility of the great vessels and the opening and competence of the semilunar valves (pulmonic and aortic). The more open the valves, the lower the resistance. If the patient has significant vasoconstriction from hypertension or a narrowed opening from a stenotic valve, then resistance (afterload) increases. Whenever afterload increases, the workload of the heart increases to overcome the resistance and eject blood.

In pulmonary edema, as well as in cardiac failure, preload, contractility, and afterload may be altered, thereby impairing CO. Technological advances in determining hemodynamic measurements with invasive monitoring procedures have made it easier to implement effective pharmacologic therapy in treating acute pulmonary edema.

Clinical Manifestations

The typical episode of pulmonary edema occurs after the patient has been lying down for a few hours. Recumbency increases the venous blood return to the heart. It also increases the reabsorption of extracellular fluid, especially that associated with peripheral edema in the legs, thereby expanding the circulating blood volume. The venous pressure rises and the right atrium fills with increasing rapidity. A corresponding increase in output from the right ventricle eventually surpasses the output from the left ventricle. The pulmonary vessels become engorged with blood and proceed to leak fluid. As a result of decreased cerebral oxygenation, the patient becomes increasingly restless and anxious. Along with a sudden onset of breathlessness and a sense of suffocation, the patient's hands become cold and moist, the nail beds become cyanotic (bluish), and the skin turns ashen (gray). In addition, the pulse is weak and rapid and the neck veins are distended. Incessant coughing may occur, producing increasing quantities of mucoid sputum. As pulmonary edema progresses, the patient's anxiety and restlessness increase; the patient becomes confused, and then stuporous. Breathing is rapid, noisy, and moist-sounding. Oxygen levels (saturation) are significantly decreased. The patient, nearly suffocated by the blood-tinged, frothy fluid now pouring into the bronchi and trachea, is literally drowning in secretions. The situation demands immediate action.

Assessment and Diagnostic Findings

The diagnosis is made by evaluating the clinical manifestations resulting from pulmonary congestion. An important method for evaluating the components of SV in a hemodynamically unstable patient is the use of the pulmonary artery (PA) catheter, used to obtain the hemodynamic data essential to diagnosis and treatment. Connected to a computerized transducer apparatus, the PA catheter serves as a fluid-filled conduit for detecting pressure changes within the heart. The pulsatile changes in pressure are converted into electrical signals, which are displayed as waveforms on a monitor (Fig. 27-1).

The PA catheter is inserted into the superior vena cava, usually via the subclavian, internal jugular, or femoral vein, and threaded into the right atrium. A balloon at the end of the catheter is then inflated, allowing the catheter to follow the blood flow through the tricuspid valve, the right ventricle, the pulmonic valve, into the main pulmonary artery, and then into the right (usually) or left PA, ultimately wedging into a branch of the pulmonary artery that is smaller than the inflated balloon. The balloon is deflated once the catheter is in the pulmonary artery. This causes the catheter to return from the wedged position to a larger area within the PA. It is then properly secured. The PA catheter may be inserted at the bedside.

Waveform and pressure readings are noted when the catheter enters each area during insertion. The methods for inserting the PA catheter, obtaining pressure readings, and providing follow-up care are described in Guideline 27-1.

The catheter contains several lumens with openings at various intervals. These lumens allow hemodynamic pressures to be measured at different points within the heart. Usually in the right atrium, the proximal port can measure central venous pressure, an indicator of right ventricular preload. The distal tip of the catheter rests in the PA and measures the PA systolic and diastolic pressures. When the balloon is inflated, the tip floats into smaller branches of the PA until it can no longer pass. The tip can then detect pressure only in front of it—that is, left atrial pressure and left ventricular end-diastolic pressure. The measurement is called PA capillary pressure, PA obstructive pressure, or PA wedge pressure. This pressure is an indicator of left ventricular preload. In most patients it equals the PA diastolic pressure.

CO is measured most often by the thermodilution method with the thermistor port of the catheter. The port is connected to a computer that calculates CO and other cardiac parameters. In **thermodilution**, a specific volume of fluid that is colder than the patient's blood is injected into the proximal port (right atrium). The fluid enters the right ventricle and is then ejected into the PA. The thermistor records the temperature before and after the ejection of fluid. The change in temperature is inversely related to CO: the greater the CO, the faster the blood and fluid moves, the less time the fluid has to mix with the blood to cause a change in temperature and the less change in temperature detected by the thermistor.

Cardiac parameters for afterload and contractility are calculated at the same time as CO (Table 27-1). Measurements of the various pressures are made at intervals. Therapy, especially intravenous medication, is adjusted based on the patient assessment and diagnostic findings.

Prevention

Like most complications, pulmonary edema is easier to prevent than to treat. To recognize it in its early stages, when the presenting signs and symptoms are solely those of pulmonary congestion, the nurse auscultates the lung fields. A dry, hacking cough, a complaint of fatigue, an increase in weight, and a decrease in activity tolerance may be early indicators of developing pulmonary edema.

In an early stage, the condition may be corrected by relatively simple measures. These include placing the patient in an upright position with the feet and legs dependent and eliminating overexertion and emotional stress to reduce the left ventricular load. A reexamination of the patient's treatment regimen and the patient's understanding of and compliance with it are also needed. The long-range approach to preventing pulmonary edema must be directed at its precursor, ventricular dysfunction and cardiac failure. Measures to control congestive heart failure are discussed later in the chapter.

Medical Management

Clinical management of a patient with acute pulmonary edema is directed toward improving the pumping ability of the left ventricle and improving respiratory exchange. These goals are accomplished through a combination of oxygen and medication therapies and nursing support.

PHARMACOLOGIC THERAPY

Various treatments and medications are prescribed for pulmonary edema, among them oxygen, morphine, diuretics, and various intravenous medications.

Oxygen Therapy. Oxygen is administered in concentrations adequate to relieve hypoxia and dyspnea. Usually a face mask or nonrebreathing mask is initially used. If respiratory failure is severe or persists despite optimal management, endotracheal intubation and mechanical ventilation are required. The use of positive end expiratory pressure (PEEP) is effective in reducing venous return, decreasing fluid movement out of the pulmonary capillaries, and improving oxygenation. Oxygenation is monitored with pulse oximetry and by measurement of arterial blood gases.

Morphine. Morphine is administered intravenously in small doses (2 to 5 mg) to reduce peripheral resistance and venous return so that blood can be redistributed from the pulmonary circulation to other parts of the body. This action decreases pressure in the pulmonary capillaries and decreases seepage of fluid into the lung tissue. The effect of morphine in decreasing anxiety is also beneficial.

Diuretic Therapy. Diuretics are medications used to increase the rate of urine production and the removal of excess extracel-

(text continues on page 661)

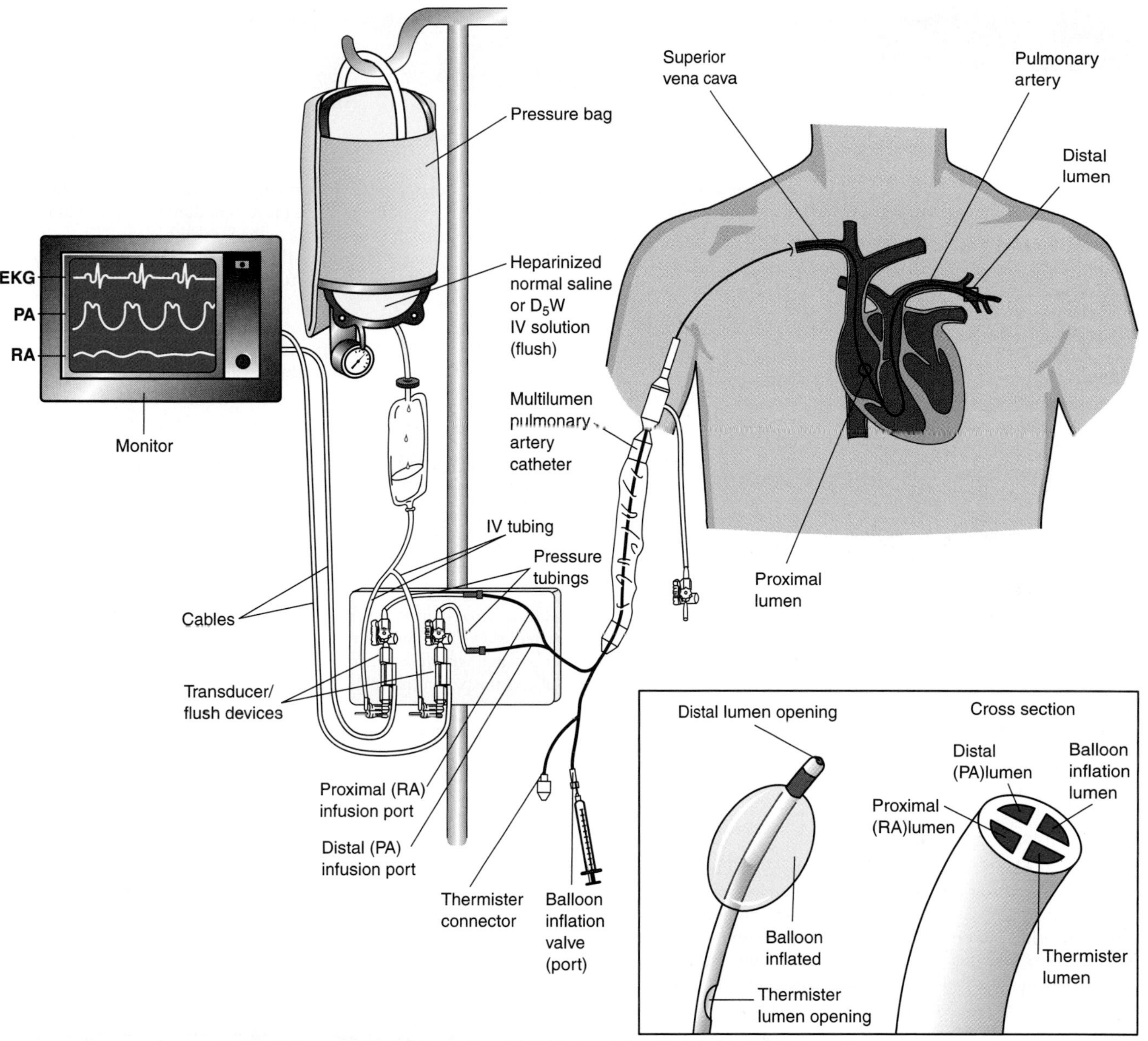

Figure 27•1 The pulmonary artery (PA) catheter system serves as a fluid-filled conduit for detecting pressure changes within the heart. The PA catheter is inserted through a sheath into the superior vena cava, usually via the internal jugular or subclavian vein. It is connected to pressure tubing which is then connected to a transducer. The transducer detects pulsatile changes in pressure and converts them into electrical signals. These signals are converted into waveforms, which are shown on a monitor. The transducer also contains a flush device that automatically infuses a small amount of IV fluid through the catheter to help maintain its patency. Because of the pressure that the heart generates, pressure is applied to the IV fluid to ensure that the IV fluid flows into the catheter and into the heart and that blood does not flow out of the heart and into the catheter. The PA catheter contains several lumens with openings located at various intervals. These lumens allow for the measurement of hemodynamic pressures at different points within the heart. The proximal port is usually in the right atrium and is used to measure central venous pressure (CVP). The distal tip of the catheter rests in the pulmonary artery and measures the pulmonary artery systolic and diastolic pressures. When the balloon is inflated, the tip floats into smaller branches of the pulmonary artery until it can no longer pass, that is, until it is "wedged" in the vessel. The distal tip then records the pressure in front of it, called pulmonary artery capillary pressure or wedge pressure (PAWP). Cardiac output is measured most often by the thermodilution method with the thermister port. The port is connected to a computer that calculates cardiac output and other cardiac parameters.

27•1 GUIDELINES FOR

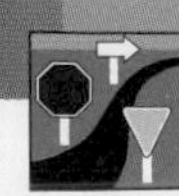

HEMODYNAMIC MONITORING: MULTILUMEN PULMONARY ARTERY CATHETER

Actions	Rationale/Amplification
Preparatory phase (nursing action)	
1. Explain the procedure to the patient, family, and significant others.	1. The information may assist in reducing the patient's anxiety, which may also help to limit the patient's movement during the procedure.
2. Check vital signs and apply ECG electrodes.	2. An initial assessment provides a baseline for comparison.
3. Position the patient to allow the physician access to the insertion site, decrease the risk of complications, and promote patient comfort. To ensure consistency, the angle of elevation should be documented if the patient cannot lie flat.	3. The patient is usually placed in a flat or Trendelenburg position to prevent complications and facilitate access.
4. Set up equipment according to manufacturer's directions.	4. Monitoring systems and setups vary according to manufacturer.
a. The pulmonary artery (PA) catheter requires pressure tubing, a transducer, a flush system, and a pressure amplifier connected to a monitoring–recording system. In addition, an IV pole and a transducer holder are usually needed.	a. The complexity of the setup requires an understanding of the equipment in use.
b. The pressure equipment is calibrated and flushed according to the manufacturer's directions.	b. Flushing the catheter system ensures patency and eliminates air bubbles.
c. The balloon is inflated with air or sterile water or saline solution to test for leakage evidenced by bubbles.	c. Testing for leakage ensures that the balloon is intact.
5. Prepare the skin over the insertion site.	5. Decreases risk of infection at insertion site
Performance phase (physician responsibility)	
1. The PA catheter that is inserted through an introducer sheath has been placed in the internal jugular, subclavian, or any easily accessible, large-diameter vein by percutaneous puncture or venotomy. The introducer sheath is surrounded by a protective sheath that maintains the sterility of the catheter.	1. The internal jugular vein insertion site has standard landmarks, establishes a straight route into the central venous system, and is associated with few complications. The subclavian insertion site allows the patient more mobility. It is also easier to secure the catheter from this site.
2. The catheter is advanced while monitoring the oscillations of the pressure waveforms, which indicate the placement of the tip of the catheter within the heart. Occasionally fluoroscopy is used to verify proper placement of the PA catheter.	2. Catheter placement is determined by characteristic waveforms and changes.
3. When the catheter is in the large vein, the balloon is inflated to its recommended volume.	3. The amount of air to be used is indicated on the catheter.
4. The patient's blood flow will gently pull the inflated balloon at the tip of the catheter through the right atrium and tricuspid valve into the right ventricle and into the main pulmonary artery. The monitoring equipment displays specific pressure waveforms as the catheter advances through the various chambers of the heart. These initial waveforms and pressures should be recorded.	4. Watching the ECG monitor for signs of ventricular irritability as the catheter enters the right ventricle allows signs of dysrhythmia to be reported to the physician in a timely manner. Subsequent pressure readings are taken from this baseline.
5. The flowing blood will continue to direct the catheter more distally into the pulmonary tree. When the catheter reaches a pulmonary vessel that is approximately the same size or slightly smaller in diameter than the inflated balloon, it will not advance any further. This is the wedge position from which pulmonary capillary wedge pressure (PCWP), pulmonary artery obstructive pressure (PAOP), or pulmonary artery wedge pressure (PAWP) is measured.	5. With the catheter in the wedge position, the balloon blocks the flow of blood from the right side of the heart toward the lungs. The resulting capillary wedge pressure correlates with the mean left ventricular end-diastolic pressure.
6. The pressure is recorded with the balloon wedged in the pulmonary vascular bed. A mean capillary wedge pressure between 8 and 12 mm Hg indicates optimal left ventricular function.	6. Wedge pressure is a valuable measure of cardiac function. Lower-than-normal pressure readings indicate hypovolemia. Higher-than-normal pressure readings indicate hypervolemia and/or left ventricular failure.
7. The balloon is then deflated, causing the catheter to retract spontaneously into a larger pulmonary artery. The change in the catheter tip position causes a reappearance of the pulmonary artery waveform. The pulmonary artery systolic, diastolic, and mean pressures are recorded.	7. The normal pulmonary artery systolic pressure is 15 to 30 mm Hg, and the diastolic pressure range is 10 to 15 mm Hg. The normal mean pulmonary artery pressure (average pressure in pulmonary artery throughout the entire cardiac cycle) ranges from 10 to 20 mm Hg. Elevated pulmonary pressures can indicate several clinical problems, such as pulmonary disease, mitral valve disease, and ventricular failure.
8. The protective sheath is attached to the introducer and secured to the catheter. The catheter is sutured in place and a dry dressing placed over the insertion site.	8. Maintaining catheter sterility in this manner allows for the advancement and repositioning of the catheter if needed. An antibiotic ointment may be placed around the site and covered with a sterile dressing.
9. A chest x-ray to confirm catheter position and to serve as a baseline for future reference is obtained after catheter insertion.	9. Accurate position will assure accurate readings and prevent complications.

27•1 GUIDELINES FOR HEMODYNAMIC MONITORING: MULTILUMEN PULMONARY ARTERY CATHETER *(Continued)*

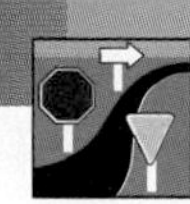

Actions	Rationale/Amplification
To obtain a wedge pressure reading	
1. Inflate the balloon slowly until the pulmonary artery pressure waveform changes (indicating a wedge pressure waveform) and an increase in resistance to injection is detected. Once these changes occur, no more air is introduced. (The amount of air to cause these changes should be less than 1.0–1.5 cc.) Most cardiac monitors allow for freezing the wedge pressure waveform and its immediate printing.	1. Do not allow the catheter to remain in the wedge position. The decrease in blood flow through the pulmonary artery that occurs when wedging the catheter may cause segmental pulmonary infarction.
2. Allow passive deflation of the balloon as soon as the wedge pressure is obtained by releasing pressure on the syringe. To make sure that the syringe cannot be inflated accidentally by removing it, push the plunger to the bottom of the barrel so that it is totally empty of air, and lock it closed.	2. These are standard safety measures.
Follow-up phase	
1. Inspect the insertion site daily. Observe for signs of infection, swelling, and bleeding.	1. Careful monitoring helps prevent complications. A foreign body (catheter) in the vascular system increases the risk of sepsis.
2. In accord with protocol, record date and time of dressing change and IV tubing change. If a peripheral vessel access site is used, assess the extremity for color, temperature, capillary filling, and sensation.	2. Ischemia may occur from inadequate arterial flow.
3. Evaluate pulse.	3. Absence of a pulse may indicate occlusion of the vessel.
4. Assess for complications: pneumothorax, pulmonary ischemia or infarction (due to persistent balloon wedging from inflation or catheter migration), pulmonary artery rupture (due to overinflation of the balloon), dysrhythmias, heart block, damage to tricuspid valve, knotting of catheter within the heart or blood vessels, thromboembolus, infection, balloon rupture.	4. These are standard nursing practices.
For removal of the catheter	
1. Explain the procedure to the patient, and make sure the balloon is not inflated.	1. An informed patient is less fearful; a deflated balloon is less likely to injure the patient during catheter removal.
2. Place the patient supine.	2. The supine position results in the least patient movement and is the best position for maintaining blood pressure and venous return.
3. Stop all IVs running through the PA catheter and turn stopcocks off.	3. This prevents fluid from infusing into tissues as the catheter is removed; it also prevents air from entering the catheter.
4. While the patient holds the breath or exhales, the catheter is removed gently and continuously, without excessive force or traction; a sterile dressing is applied over the site.	4. Positive intrathoracic pressure minimizes the chance of air entering the chest and vasculature through or around the catheter. Continuous gentle traction minimizes the risk of the catheter becoming kinked, knotted, or tangled. A sterile dressing minimizes the risk of infection from the skin wound.

lular fluid from the body. Of the types of diuretics prescribed for patients with edema from congestive heart failure, hepatic failure, renal failure or corticosteroid therapy, hypertension, and hyperaldosteronism, three types are most common: thiazide, loop, and potassium-sparing diuretics. These medications are classified according to their site of action in the kidney and their effects on renal electrolyte excretion and reabsorption. Thiazide diuretics, such as hydrochlorothiazide (HydroDIURIL), inhibit sodium and chloride reabsorption mainly in the early distal tubules. They also increase potassium and bicarbonate excretion. Loop diuretics, such as furosemide (Lasix), inhibit sodium and chloride reabsorption mainly in the ascending loop of Henle. Potassium-sparing diuretics, such as spironolactone (Aldactone), inhibit sodium reabsorption in the late distal tubule and collecting duct. They are used commonly as an adjunct to other diuretic therapy.

Dosages depend on the indications, patient age, clinical signs and symptoms, and renal function. Furosemide, for example, is administered intravenously to produce a rapid diuretic effect. Furosemide also causes vasodilation and pooling of blood in peripheral blood vessels, which in turn reduces the amount of blood returned to the heart, even before the diuretic effect. Some physicians may prescribe bumetanide (Bumex) and hydrochlorothiazide in place of furosemide. Table 27-2 lists commonly used diuretics, dosages, and pharmacokinetic parameters.

Other Intravenous Medications. Additional intravenous medications may also be used in patients with pulmonary edema. These include dobutamine, a catecholamine that increases myocardial contractility; amrinone, which dilates the arteries and increases CO; and digitalis, which increases contractility. These medications are discussed in more detail later in the chapter.

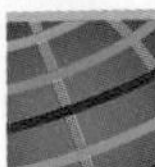

TABLE 27•1 **Hemodynamic Parameters**

Parameter	Right Ventricle	Left Ventricle
Preload		
Invasive normals	Central venous pressure (CVP): 0–8 mm Hg	Pulmonary artery wedge pressure (PAWP): 4–12 mm Hg
Afterload		
Invasive normals	Pulmonary vascular resistance (PVR): 20–120 dyne/sec/cm^{-5}	Systemic vascular resistance (SVR): 800–1500 dyne/sec/cm^{-5}
Calculation	$\frac{\text{mean PAP} - \text{PAWP}}{\text{CO}} \times 80$	$\frac{\text{Mean arterial pressure} - \text{CVP}}{\text{CO}} \times 80$
Contractility		
Invasive normals	Right ventricular stroke work index: 7–12 g/beat/m^2	Left ventricular stroke work index 35–85 g/beat/m^2
Calculation	$\frac{(\text{PA systolic pressure} - \text{CVP}) \times \text{SV} \times 0.0136}{\text{Body surface area (height and weight)}}$	$\frac{(\text{Systolic BP} - \text{PCWP}) \times 0.0136}{\text{Body surface area (height and weight)}}$

Nursing Management

Management of the patient in pulmonary edema with a hemodynamic catheter in place is highly specialized and is best provided in an intensive care environment (see Guideline 27-1).

POSITIONING THE PATIENT TO PROMOTE CIRCULATION

Proper positioning can help reduce venous return to the heart. The patient is positioned upright, preferably with the legs dangling over the side of the bed. This has the immediate effect of decreasing venous return, lowering the output of the right ventricle, and decreasing lung congestion. If the patient cannot sit with the lower extremities dependent, he or she may be placed in an upright position in bed.

PROVIDING PSYCHOLOGICAL SUPPORT

As the ability to breathe decreases, the patient's sense of fear and anxiety rises proportionately, which makes the condition more severe. Reassuring the patient and providing skillful anticipatory nursing care are integral parts of the therapy. Because this patient feels a sense of impending doom and has an unstable condition, the nurse must remain with the patient. The nurse should give the patient simple, concise information, in a reassuring voice, about what is being done to treat the condition and the expected results.

MONITORING MEDICATIONS

The patient receiving morphine is observed for excessive respiratory depression, hypotension, and vomiting; a morphine antagonist, such as naloxone hydrochloride (Narcan), is kept available and given to the patient who exhibits these side effects.

The patient receiving diuretic therapy will experience a large volume of urine formation within minutes after a potent diuretic is given. An indwelling catheter may be used to decrease the amount of energy required by the patient and to reduce the resultant increase in cardiac workload induced by getting on and off a bedpan.

Nursing Alert *Because of the resulting diuresis, the patient's electrolyte levels, especially potassium and sodium, need to be monitored closely. Fluid balance in some patients is very brittle—that is, they easily become hypovolemic or hypervolemic with small changes in the amount of circulating fluid. Falling blood pressure, increasing HR, and decreasing urine output indicate that the circulatory system is not tolerating diuresis and that measures must be taken to reverse the fluid imbalance that has occurred. In addition, men with prostatic hyperplasia must be observed for signs of urinary retention. Additional monitoring activities are discussed in Chart 27-1.*

CARDIAC FAILURE: CONGESTIVE HEART FAILURE

Congestive heart failure (CHF), often referred to as cardiac failure, is the inability of the heart to pump sufficient blood to meet the needs of the tissues for oxygen and nutrients. The term "congestive heart failure" is most commonly used when referring to left-sided and right-sided failure. Although the incidence and mortality rate of coronary artery disease are decreasing, just the opposite is true for CHF. As with coronary artery disease, the incidence of CHF increases with age. Nearly 5 million people in the United States have CHF. The condition is the most frequent reason for hospitalization in people older than age 65 and the second most frequent reason, after hypertension, for visits to a physician's office. The average length of hospital stay is 6.3 days, at an average cost of nearly $9,000. Many hospitalizations could be prevented by improved and appropriate outpatient care. Prevention and early intervention to arrest the progression of CHF are major health initiatives in the United States.

CHF is frequently classified according to the patient's symptoms. The New York Heart Association (NYHA) classification is described in Table 27-3. CHF may also be classified based on assessment of left ventricular functioning.

Pathophysiology

Cardiac failure most commonly occurs with disorders of cardiac muscle that result in decreased contractile properties of the heart. Common underlying conditions that lead to decreased myocardial contractility include myocardial dysfunction (especially from coronary atherosclerosis), arterial hypertension, and valvular dysfunction.

Myocardial dysfunction may be due to coronary artery disease, dilated cardiomyopathy, or inflammatory and degenerative diseases of the myocardium. Atherosclerosis of the coronary arteries is the primary cause of heart failure. Coronary artery disease is found in more than 60% of the patients with CHF. Ischemia

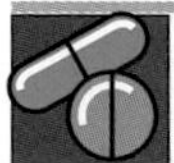

TABLE 27•2 **Diuretic Medications Used to Treat Cardiac Failure**

Diuretic	Usual Adult Dose	Onset (hours)	Peak (hours)	Duration (hours)
Thiazide diuretics				
bendroflumethiazide (Naturetin)	2.5–20 mg in single or divided dose, once a day, once every other day, or once a day for 3–5 days per week	2	4	12–16
benzthiazide (Exna)	12.5–200 mg in single or divided dose	2	4–6	16–18
chlorothiazide (Diuril)	Oral: 0.25–2 g as single or divided dose; may be given on alternate days	2	4	16–18
	IV: 0.5–1 g in single or divided dose (note: avoid extravasation)	15 min	30 min	
chlorthalidone (Hygroton)	12.5–200 mg once a day, once every other day, or once a day for 3 days per week	2	2–6	24–72
hydrochlorothiazide (HydroDIURIL, Esidrix, Oretic)	12.5–200 mg as single or divided dose once a day, once every other day, or once a day for 3–5 days per week	2	4–6	12–16
hydroflumethiazide (Diucardin, Saluron)	25–200 mg as single or divided dose once a day, once every other day, or once a day for 3–5 days per week	2	4	12–16
methyclothiazide (Enduron)	2.5–10 mg once a day	2	6	24
metolazone (Zaroxolyn, Mykrox)	Zaroxolyn: 2.5–20 mg once a day Mykrox: 0.5–1 mg once a day	1	2	12–24
polythiazide (Renese)	1–4 mg once a day, once every other day, or once a day for 3–5 days per week	2	6	24–28
quinethazone (Hydromox)	25–100 mg as single or divided dose; rarely, 200 mg once a day	2	6	18–24
trichlormethiazide (Metahydrin, Naqua)	1–4 mg once or twice a day	2	6	24
Loop diuretics				
bumetanide (Bumex)	0.5–2 mg once, twice or three times a day; may be given on alternate days or once every 3 days	30–60 min	1–2	4–6
	0.5–1 mg over 2 min; repeat every 2–3 h; a continuous infusion may be given at a rate of 1 mg/h.	5–10 min	15–30 min	½–1
ethacrynic acid (Edecrin)	50–400 mg as single or divided dose	<30 min	2	6–8
	0.5–1 mg/kg (max 100 mg) over several min; may be repeated within 2–6 h; repeat every hour in emergencies	<5 min	15–30 min	2
furosemide (Lasix)	20–600 mg as single daily dose, divided daily dose, as a dose given every other day or given once a day for 2–4 days per week	<1	1–2	6–8
	20–200 mg (max 6 mg/kg) given at a rate of 4 mg/min; after response obtained, given once or twice a day	<5 min	30 min	2
torsemide (Demadex)	5–200 mg as a daily single dose	<1	1–2	6–8
	IV and oral doses are equivalent. Give IV over 2 min.	<10 min	<1	6–8
Potassium-sparing diuretics				
amiloride (Midamor)	5–20 mg daily as single dose	2	6–10	24
spironolactone (Aldactone)	25–400 mg as single dose or divided up to 4 doses	24–48	48–72	48–72
triamterene (Dyrenium)	50–300 mg as single dose	2–4	6–8	12–16

causes myocardial dysfunction because of resulting hypoxia and acidosis (from accumulation of lactic acid). Myocardial infarction causes focal myocellular necrosis, the death of myocardial cells, and a loss of contractility; the extent of the infarction is prognostic of the severity of CHF.

Dilated cardiomyopathy causes diffuse cellular necrosis, leading to decreased contractility. Inflammatory and degenerative diseases of the myocardium, such as myocarditis, may also damage myocardial fibers, with a resultant decrease in contractility.

Systemic or pulmonary hypertension increases afterload (the resistance to ejection), which increases the workload of the heart and in turn leads to hypertrophy of myocardial muscle fibers; this can be considered a compensatory mechanism because it increases contractility. However, the hypertrophy may decrease the heart's ability to fill properly during diastole. In addition, the amount of resistance may be higher than the degree of hypertrophy. This too leads to CHF.

Valvular heart disease is also a cause of cardiac failure. The valves ensure that blood flows in one direction. With valvular dysfunction, blood has increasing difficulty moving forward. This decreases the amount of blood being ejected, increases pressure within the heart, and eventually leads to pulmonary and venous congestion. Chapter 26 discusses the effects of valvular heart disease.

ETIOLOGIC FACTORS

A number of systemic factors contribute to the development and severity of cardiac failure, including increased metabolic rate (eg, fever, thyrotoxicosis), hypoxia, and anemia (serum hematocrit less than 25). All conditions require increased CO to satisfy systemic

CHART 27•1 Administering and Monitoring Diuretic Therapy

When nursing care involves diuretic therapy for conditions such as pulmonary edema or cardiac failure, the nurse needs to administer the medication and monitor the patient's response carefully, as follows:

- Administer the diuretic at a time conducive to the patient's lifestyle; for example, early in the day to avoid nocturia.
- Give supplementary potassium with thiazide and loop diuretics as prescribed to replace potassium lost.
- Check laboratory results for electrolyte depletion, especially potassium, magnesium, and sodium; and for electrolyte elevation, especially potassium with potassium-sparing agents and calcium with thiazides.
- Monitor for adverse reactions, such as nausea and gastrointestinal distress, vomiting, diarrhea, weakness, headache, fatigue, anxiety or agitation, and cardiac dysrhythmias.
- Assess for signs of volume depletion, such as postural hypotension, dizziness, imbalance, and reduced jugular venous distention.
- Monitor for renal impairment.
- Monitor for glucose intolerance in patients with and without diabetes mellitus who are receiving thiazide diuretics.
- Anticipate potential ototoxicity in patients, especially those with renal failure, who are receiving a loop diuretic.
- Advise patients to avoid prolonged exposure to the sun because of the risk of photosensitivity.
- Monitor for elevated serum uric acid levels and the development of gout.
- Implement nursing actions to facilitate effect of medication, such as positioning patient upright with legs dangling.

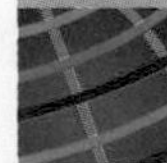

TABLE 27•3 NYHA Classification of Cardiac Failure

Classification	Symptoms	Prognosis
I	Ordinary physical activity does not cause undue fatigue, dyspnea, palpitations, or chest pain No pulmonary congestion or peripheral hypotension Patient is considered asymptomatic Usually no limitations on activities of daily living (ADLs)	Good
II	Slight limitation on ADLs Patient reports no symptoms at rest but increased physical activity will cause symptoms Basilar crackles and S_3 murmur may be detected	Good
III	Marked limitation on ADL Patient feels comfortable at rest but less than ordinary activity will cause symptoms	Fair
IV	Symptoms of cardiac insufficiency at rest	Poor

oxygen demand. Hypoxia or anemia also may decrease the supply of oxygen to the myocardium. Acidosis (respiratory or metabolic) and electrolyte abnormalities may decrease myocardial contractility. Cardiac dysrhythmias, which may be present independently or secondary to cardiac failure, decrease the overall efficiency of myocardial function.

A decrease in the amount of blood ejected from the ventricle stimulates the sympathetic nervous system. This stimulates the release of renin, which promotes the formation of angiotensin, causing fluid retention and vasoconstriction. The purpose of this compensatory response is to maintain or increase contractility to maintain CO. Because this response increases preload and afterload, the workload of the heart increases as well. This compensatory mechanism is the underlying feature of what is termed the "vicious cycle of CHF": the heart is not strong enough to pump, which causes a response that makes it work even harder.

VENTRICULAR FAILURE

The left and right ventricles can fail separately. Initially, the manifestations may differ according to whether left or right ventricular failure exists. However, because the outputs of the ventricles are coupled or synchronized, failure of either ventricle may lead to decreased output of the other. Dysrhythmias (especially tachycardias, ventricular ectopic beats, or atrioventricular [AV] and ventricular conduction defects) are common in CHF. They may be caused by the disease process as well as by the management of CHF (eg, a side effect of digitalis).

Left-Sided Cardiac Failure. Pulmonary congestion occurs when the left ventricle cannot pump the blood out of the chamber. This increases pressure in the left ventricle and decreases the blood flow from the left atrium. The pressure in the left atrium increases, which decreases the blood flow coming from the pulmonary vessels. The resultant increase in pressure in the pulmonary circulation forces fluid into the pulmonary tissues and alveoli, which impairs gas exchange. The clinical manifestations of pulmonary venous congestion that ensue include dyspnea, cough, pulmonary crackles (formerly called rales), and lower-than-normal oxygen saturation levels.

Dyspnea on exertion may be precipitated by minimal to moderate activity; dyspnea may even occur at rest. The patient may report **orthopnea**, difficulty in breathing when lying flat, as well. Patients with orthopnea usually prefer not to lie flat. They may need pillows to prop themselves up in bed, or they may sit in a chair and even sleep sitting up. Some patients have orthopnea only at night, a condition known as **paroxysmal nocturnal dyspnea.** This occurs when the patient, who has been sitting for a long period with the feet and legs in a dependent position, goes to bed. Fluid that has accumulated in the dependent extremities during the day begins to be reabsorbed into the circulating blood volume. When this happens, the impaired left ventricle cannot eject the increased fluid volume. As a result, the pressure in the pulmonary circulation increases and causes further shifting of fluid into the alveoli.

The cough associated with left ventricular failure may be dry and nonproductive, but usually it is moist. Large quantities of frothy sputum, which is sometimes pink (blood-tinged), may be produced, usually indicating severe pulmonary congestion—pulmonary edema.

Adventitious breath sounds may be heard in various lobes of the lungs. Usually, bi-basilar crackles are detected in the early phase of left ventricular failure. As the failure worsens and pulmonary congestion increases, crackles may be auscultated throughout all lung fields.

In addition to increased pulmonary pressures that cause decreased oxygenation, the amount of blood ejected from the left ventricle may decrease. A decrease in SV can decrease the amount of blood and oxygen delivered to all body organs, thereby stimulating the sympathetic nervous system. Because the brain is the organ most sensitive to a decrease in oxygenation and blood flow, the patient becomes restless and anxious. Restlessness and anxiety result from the decreased ability of the lungs to exchange gases, the decreased amount of blood being ejected from the ventricle into the body, the impaired tissue oxygenation, the stress associated with respiratory difficulty, and the knowledge that the heart is not functioning properly. As anxiety increases, so does dyspnea, in turn enhancing anxiety and creating a vicious cycle. The stimulation of the sympathetic system also causes the peripheral vessels to constrict, so the skin appears pale or ashen and feels cool and clammy.

The decrease in the ejected ventricular volume causes the HR to increase (tachycardia) and the patient to complain of palpitations. The pulses in turn become weak and thready. Without adequate output, the body cannot respond to increased energy demands, so the patient is easily fatigued and has decreased activity tolerance. Fatigue results from the increased energy expended in breathing and the insomnia that results from respiratory distress and coughing.

Right-Sided Cardiac Failure. When the right ventricle fails, congestion of the viscera and the peripheral tissues predominates. This occurs because the right side of the heart cannot eject blood and thus cannot accommodate all the blood that normally returns to it from the venous circulation.

The clinical manifestations that ensue include edema of the lower extremities (dependent edema), weight gain, hepatomegaly (enlargement of the liver), distended neck veins, ascites (accumulation of fluid in the peritoneal cavity), anorexia and nausea, nocturia, and weakness.

Edema usually affects the feet and ankles, worsening when the patient stands or dangles the legs. The swelling decreases when the patient elevates the legs. The edema can gradually progress up the legs and thighs and eventually into the external genitalia and lower trunk. Sacral edema is not uncommon for patients who are on bed rest, because the sacral area is dependent. Pitting edema, edema in which indentations in the skin remain after even slight compression with the fingertips (Fig. 27-2), is obvious only after retention of at least 4.5 kg (10 lb) of fluid.

Hepatomegaly and tenderness in the right upper quadrant of the abdomen result from venous engorgement of the liver. The increased pressure may interfere with the liver's ability to perform, termed secondary liver dysfunction. As hepatic dysfunction progresses, pressure within the portal vessels may rise enough to force fluid into the abdominal cavity, a condition known as ascites. This collection of fluid in the abdominal cavity may increase pressure on the stomach and intestines and cause gastrointestinal distress.

Anorexia (loss of appetite) and nausea or abdominal pain result from the venous engorgement and venous stasis within the abdominal organs. Hepatomegaly may also increase pressure on the diaphragm, causing respiratory distress. Nocturia, the need to urinate at night, occurs because renal perfusion is promoted by periods of recumbency. Diuresis results and is most common at night because CO is improved with rest. The weakness that accompanies right-sided failure is due to the reduced CO, impaired circulation, and inadequate removal of catabolic waste products from the tissues.

Clinical Manifestations

The dominant feature in cardiac failure is inadequate tissue perfusion. The diminished CO from cardiac failure has widespread manifestations because not enough blood reaches the tissues and organs (low perfusion) to provide the necessary oxygen. Some commonly encountered effects related to low perfusion are dizziness, confusion, fatigue, exercise or heat intolerance, cool extremities, and reduced urine output (oliguria). Renal perfusion pressure falls, which results in the release of renin from the kidney, which in turn leads to aldosterone secretion, sodium and fluid retention, and further increased intravascular volume.

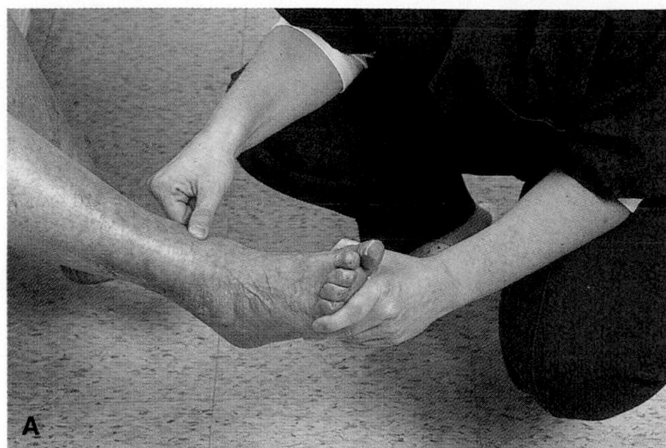

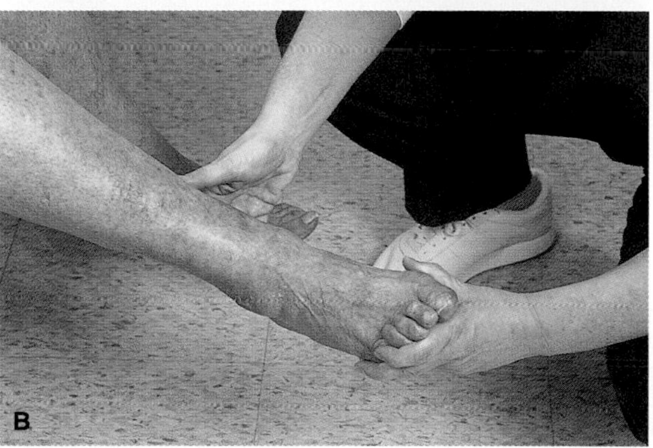

FIGURE 27•2 Example of pitting edema. (**A**) The nurse applies finger pressure to an area near the ankle. (**B**) When the pressure is released, an indentation remains in the edematous tissue. © B. Proud.

Congestion of tissues may occur from increased venous pressures due to decreased CO in the failing heart. Increased pulmonary venous pressure can cause fluid to pass from the pulmonary capillaries to the alveoli, resulting in pulmonary edema manifested by cough and shortness of breath. Increased systemic venous pressure can result in generalized peripheral edema and weight gain.

Assessment and Diagnostic Findings

The diagnosis of cardiac failure is made by evaluating the clinical manifestations of cardiac, pulmonary, and systemic congestion. An echocardiogram is usually performed to determine the patient's ejection fraction. Other tests may be performed to assist in determining the source of the congestion.

Medical Management

The basic objectives in treating patients with CHF are the following:

- Reducing the workload on the heart
- Increasing the force and efficiency of myocardial contraction

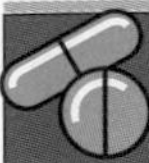

TABLE 27•4 ACE Inhibitors Used to Treat Cardiac Failure

ACE Inhibitor	Pharmacokinetics: Onset	Peak (hours)	Duration (hours)	Nursing Considerations
benazepril	within 1 h	2–4	24	Monitor blood pressure, urine output, and electrolyte levels.
captopril	15–60 min	60–90 min	6–12*	Monitor serum creatinine and urine creatinine clearance.
enalapril	1 h	4–6	24	Monitor for development of cough that is resistant to cough suppressants.
enalaprilat (IV)	15 min	1–4	6	Teach patient to change positions gradually and to report signs of dizziness or lethargy.
fosinopril	within 1 h	2–6	24	Instruct patient to weigh self daily and to report rapid weight gain and significant feet and hand swelling.
lisinopril	1 h	6	24	
quinapril	within 1 h	2–4	up to 24*	
ramipril	1–2 h	4–6	24	

*Duration of effect is related to the dose.

- Eliminating the excessive accumulation of body water by avoiding excess fluid intake, controlling the diet, and monitoring diuretic and angiotensin-converting enzyme (ACE) inhibitor therapy

Managing the patient with CHF includes general counseling and education concerning regular exercise, sodium restriction, and avoidance of excessive fluid intake, alcohol, and smoking. Medications are prescribed based on the patient's symptoms and compliance with the treatment plan. Oxygen therapy is based on the degree of pulmonary congestion and resulting hypoxia. Some patients may need supplemental oxygen therapy during activity. Others may require hospitalization and endotracheal intubation. If the patient has underlying coronary artery disease, coronary artery bypass surgery may be considered. If the patient's condition is unresponsive to advanced aggressive medical therapy, innovative therapies, including mechanical assist devices and transplantation, may be considered.

PHARMACOLOGIC THERAPY

If the patient is in mild failure, usually an ACE inhibitor is prescribed. A diuretic is added if there is no improvement or if there are signs of fluid overload. Next, digitalis is added if the symptoms continue. If symptoms are severe, all three medications are usually started immediately.

ACE Inhibitors. Of particular significance in managing cardiac failure are ACE inhibitors. Available as oral or intravenous medications, ACE inhibitors promote vasodilation and diuresis by decreasing afterload and preload. In so doing, they decrease the workload of the heart. Vasodilation reduces resistance to left ventricular ejection of blood and improves ventricular emptying. In promoting diuresis, ACE inhibitors decrease the secretion of aldosterone, a substance that causes the kidneys to retain sodium. Thus, ACE inhibitors stimulate the kidneys to excrete sodium and fluid (while retaining potassium), thereby reducing left ventricular filling pressure and decreasing pulmonary congestion. ACE inhibitors may be the first medication prescribed for patients in mild failure—that is, patients with fatigue or dyspnea on exertion but without symptoms of fluid overload and pulmonary congestion. Hydralazine and isosorbide dinitrate may be given to patients who cannot take ACE inhibitors.

Patients receiving ACE inhibitor therapy are monitored for hypotension, hypovolemia, and hyponatremia, especially if they are also receiving diuretics. When and for how long to observe for these effects depend on the onset, peak, and duration of the medication. Table 27-4 identifies several types of ACE inhibitors and their pharmacokinetics. Dosage depends on the patient's blood pressure, fluid status, renal status, and degree of cardiac failure. Hypotension is most likely to develop from ACE inhibitor therapy in patients older than age 75 and those with a systolic blood pressure of 100 mm Hg or less, a serum sodium level of less than 135 mEq/L, or severe cardiac failure.

Because ACE inhibitors cause the kidneys to retain potassium, the patient who is also receiving a diuretic may not need to take oral potassium supplements. However, patients receiving potassium-sparing diuretics (which do not cause potassium loss with diuresis) must be carefully monitored for hyperkalemia, an increased level of potassium in the blood. Other side effects include a dry persistent cough that may not respond to cough suppressants. However, the cough could also indicate a worsening of ventricular function and failure. Rarely, angioedema occurs. If angioedema affects the oropharyngeal area, the medication should be stopped immediately.

Diuretic Therapy. A diuretic is one of the first medications prescribed to a patient with CHF. Diuretics promote the excretion of sodium and water through the kidneys. These medications may not be necessary if the patient responds to activity recommendations, avoidance of excessive fluid intake, and a low-sodium diet (eg, 2 g/day).

Digitalis. The most commonly prescribed forms of digitalis for patients with CHF are digoxin (Lanoxin) and digitoxin. Although it is unknown whether digitalis decreases the mortality rate, it is known that it decreases symptoms of CHF and increases the ability to perform activities of daily living. The medication increases the force of myocardial contraction and slows conduction through the AV node. It improves contractility, thus increasing left ventricular output. The medication also enhances diuresis (which removes fluid and relieves edema). The effect of a given dose of medication depends on the state of the myocardium, electrolyte and fluid balance, and renal and hepatic function.

A key concern associated with digitalis therapy is digitalis toxicity. Chart 27-2 summarizes the actions and uses of digitalis, along with its actions and the nursing surveillance required when it is administered. During digitalis therapy, the patient is observed closely for relief of signs and symptoms of CHF: lessening dysp-

CHART 27•2 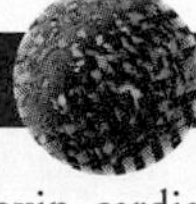 Digitalis Use and Toxicity in Cardiac Failure

Digoxin and digitoxin, cardiac glycosides derived from digitalis, are used for patients with CHF, atrial fibrillation, and atrial flutter. Digoxin improves cardiac function as follows:

- Increases the force of myocardial contraction
- Slows cardiac conduction through the AV node and therefore slows the ventricular rate in instances of supraventricular dysrhythmias
- Increases cardiac output by enhancing the force of ventricular contraction
- Promotes diuresis by increasing cardiac output.

Whether the patient receives digoxin or digitoxin depends on the desired speed of onset, the required duration of action, and individual patient response. The therapeutic level is usually 0.5 to 2.0 ng/mL. Blood is usually drawn to determine digitalis concentration at least 6 to 10 hours after the last dose. Toxicity may occur despite normal serum levels, and recommended dosages vary considerably.

Preparations

Digoxin

- Tablets: 0.125, 0.25, 0.5 mg (Lanoxin)
- Capsules: 0.05, 0.1, 0.2 mg (Lanoxicaps)
- Elixir: 0.05 mg/mL (Lanoxin Pediatric elixir)
- Injection: 0.25 mg/mL, 0.1 mg/mL (Lanoxin)

Digitoxin

- Tablets: 0.05, 0.1, 0.15, 0.2 mg (Crystodigin, Digitaline)

Digitalis Toxicity

A serious complication of digitalis therapy is toxicity. The incidence is high, and toxicity may occur even though the serum digitalis level remains within a normal range. Diagnosis of digitalis toxicity is based on the patient's clinical symptoms, which include the following:

- Fatigue, depression, malaise, anorexia, nausea, and vomiting (early effects of digitalis toxicity)
- Changes in heart rhythm: new onset of regular rhythm or new onset of irregular rhythm
- ECG changes indicating sinoatrial or AV block; new onset of irregular rhythm indicating ventricular dysrhythmias; and atrial tachycardia with block, junctional tachycardia, and ventricular tachycardia

Reversal of Toxicity

Digitalis toxicity is treated by holding the medication for at least a few days while monitoring the patient's symptoms and serum digitalis level. If the toxicity is severe, digoxin immune FAB (Digibind) may be prescribed. Digibind binds with digitalis and makes it unavailable for use. The Digibind dosage is based on the digitalis level and the patient's size. Serum digitalis values are not accurate for several days after administration of Digibind because they do not differentiate between bound and unbound digitalis. Because Digibind quickly decreases the amount of available digitalis, an increase in ventricular rate to atrial fibrillation and worsening of symptoms of CHF may ensue shortly after its administration.

Nursing Considerations and Actions

1. Assess the patient's clinical response to digitalis therapy by evaluating relief of symptoms, such as dyspnea, orthopnea, crackles, hepatomegaly, and peripheral edema.
2. Monitor serum potassium levels in patients receiving digitalis, especially those receiving both digitalis and diuretics. *An undetected, uncorrected potassium imbalance predisposes patients to dysrhythmias.*
3. Assess for symptoms of electrolyte depletion: lassitude, apathy, mental confusion, anorexia, decreasing urinary output, azotemia.
4. Monitor the patient for factors that increase the risk of toxicity:
   - Oral antibiotics, quinidine, amiodarone, calcium channel blocker therapy
   - Decreased potassium level (hypokalemia), which increases the action of digitalis and which may be caused by malnutrition, diarrhea, vomiting, or prolonged muscle wasting
   - Impaired renal function, particularly in patients age 65 and older with decreased renal clearance.
5. Take special precautions. Before administering digitalis, it is standard nursing practice to assess apical heart rate. When the patient's rhythm is atrial fibrillation and the heart rate is less than 60, or the rhythm becomes regular, the nurse may withhold the medication and notify the physician, because these signs indicate the development of AV conduction block. Although withholding digitalis is a common practice, the medication does not need to be withheld for a heart rate of less than 60 if the patient is in sinus rhythm because digitalis does not affect sinoatrial node automaticity.

   Note: If monitoring discloses that the patient is in sinus rhythm, the nurse then monitors the patient's PR interval instead of the patient's heart rate. If the patient is in atrial fibrillation, the nurse would monitor for the development of regular R-R intervals, indicating AV block.
6. Monitor for gastrointestinal side effects: anorexia, nausea, vomiting, abdominal pain and distention.
7. Monitor for neurologic side effects: headache, malaise, nightmares, forgetfulness, social withdrawal, depression, agitation, confusion, paranoia, hallucinations, decreased visual acuity, yellow or green halo around objects (especially lights), or "snowy" vision.
8. Observe for and anticipate potential drug interactions when other medications are added to the patient's regimen. This is an important step in preventing toxicity. For example, antidysrhythmic and antibiotic medications may increase the amount of digitalis available to the patient. Diuretics may decrease the amount of potassium and increase the availability of digitalis. In addition, because digitalis is eliminated by the kidneys, renal function (serum creatinine and urine creatinine clearance) should be monitored carefully.

---

nea and orthopnea, decrease in auscultation of pulmonary crackles, relief of peripheral edema, weight loss, and increase in activity tolerance. The serum potassium level is measured at intervals because diuresis may have produced hypokalemia. The effect of digitalis in the presence of hypokalemia is enhanced, so digitalis toxicity may occur.

Dobutamine. Dobutamine (Dobutrex) is an intravenous medication given to patients with significant left ventricular dysfunction. A catecholamine, it stimulates the $beta_1$-adrenergic receptors. Its major action is to increase cardiac contractility. However, with an increased dosage, it also increases the HR and incidence of ectopic beats and tachydysrhythmias. Because it also increases AV conduction, care must be taken in patients who have underlying atrial fibrillation. A medication that protects the AV node, such as digitalis, a beta blocker, or a calcium channel blocker, may be indicated before dobutamine therapy is initiated.

Milrinone. Milrinone (Primacor) is a phosphodiesterase inhibitor that prolongs the release and prevents the uptake of calcium. This, in turn, promotes vasodilation, causing a decrease in preload and afterload and decreasing the workload of the heart. Milrinone is given intravenously, usually to patients who have not responded to other therapies. It is not usually given to patients with renal failure. The major side effects are hypotension (usually asymptomatic), gastrointestinal dysfunction, an increase in ventricular dysrhythmias, and a decrease in platelets. The patient's blood pressure needs to be monitored closely.

Other Medications. Anticoagulants may be prescribed, especially if the patient has a history of an embolic event or atrial fibrillation or mural thrombus is present. Beta-adrenergic blockers, such as atenolol (Tenormin), metoprolol (Lopressor), and propranolol (Inderal), may be indicated in patients with mild or moderate failure. Other medications may be given to treat the underlying etiology of heart failure, such as antihypertensive or antianginal medications.

NUTRITIONAL THERAPY

A low-sodium diet and avoidance of excessive amounts of fluid are usually recommended. Although it has not been shown to affect the mortality rate, this recommendation reduces the symptoms of congestion. The purpose of sodium restriction is to decrease the amount of circulating volume, which would decrease the need for the heart to pump that volume. A balance needs to be achieved between the ability of patients to alter their diet and the amount of medications that are prescribed. Any change in diet needs to maintain good nutritional status and take into consideration the patient's likes, dislikes, and cultural food patterns.

Nursing Alert *The sources of sodium should be specified in describing the regimen, rather than simply saying "low-salt" or "salt-free," and the quantity should be indicated in milligrams. Keep in mind that salt is not 100% sodium: there are 393 mg of sodium in 1 g (1000 mg) of salt.*

Nursing Management

The nurse is responsible not only for administering the medication but also for assessing its effects, both beneficial and detrimental, on the patient. It is the balance of these effects that determines the type and dosage of pharmacologic therapy. Nursing actions to evaluate therapeutic effectiveness include the following:

- Keeping an intake and output record to identify a negative balance (more output than input)
- Weighing the patient daily at the same time, usually in the morning after urination
- Auscultating lung sounds at least daily to detect a decrease or an absence of pulmonary crackles
- Determining the degree of jugular vein distention
- Identifying and evaluating the severity of dependent edema
- Monitoring pulse rate and blood pressure, and making sure that the patient does not become hypotensive from dehydration
- Examining skin turgor and mucous membranes for signs of dehydration
- Assessing symptoms of fluid overload (orthopnea, paroxysmal nocturnal dyspnea, and dyspnea on exertion) and evaluating changes

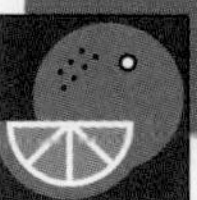

NUTRITION

Facts About Dietary Sodium

Although the major source of sodium in the average American diet is salt, many types of natural foods contain varying amounts of sodium. Even if no salt is added in cooking and if salty foods are avoided, the daily diet may still contain between 1,000 and 2,000 mg of sodium.

Additives in Food

Added food substances (additives), such as sodium alginate, which improves food texture; sodium benzoate, which acts as a preservative; and disodium phosphate, which improves cooking quality in certain foods, increase the sodium intake when included in the daily diet. Therefore, patients on low-sodium diets should be advised to check labels carefully for such words as "salt" or "sodium," especially on canned foods. Without looking at the labels, when given a choice between a serving of salt and vinegar potato chips and a cup of canned cream of mushroom soup, most would think that soup is lower in sodium. However, when the labels are examined, the lower sodium choice would be the chips.

Nonfood Sodium Sources

Sodium is also contained in toothpaste and municipal water. Patients on sodium-restricted diets should be cautioned against using nonprescription medications, such as antacids, cough syrups, laxatives, sedatives, or salt substitutes, because these products contain sodium or excessive amounts of potassium. Over-the-counter medications should not be used without first consulting the physician.

Promoting Dietary Adherence

If patients find food unpalatable because of the dietary sodium restrictions and/or the taste disturbances caused by the medications, they may refuse to eat or comply with the dietary regimen. For this reason, severe sodium restrictions should be avoided and the amount of medication should be balanced with the patient's ability to restrict dietary sodium. A variety of flavorings, such as lemon juice and herbs, may be used to improve the taste of the food and increase acceptance of the diet. The patient's food preferences should be taken into account—diet counseling and educational handouts can be geared to individual and ethnic preferences. It is very important to involve the family in the dietary teaching.

MONITORING AND MANAGING POTENTIAL COMPLICATIONS

Electrolyte Imbalances. Profuse and repeated diuresis can lead to hypokalemia (potassium depletion). Signs are weak pulse, faint heart sounds, hypotension, muscle flabbiness, diminished deep tendon reflexes, and generalized weakness. Hypokalemia poses new problems for the patient with CHF because hypokalemia markedly weakens cardiac contractions. In patients receiving digoxin, hypokalemia can lead to digitalis toxicity. Both digitalis toxicity and hypokalemia increase the likelihood of dangerous dysrhythmias (see Chart 27-2). Low levels of potassium may also indicate a low level of magnesium, which can add to the risk for dysrhythmias.

Nursing Alert *To reduce the risk for hypokalemia, the nurse advises patients to increase their dietary intake of potassium. Dried apricots, bananas, beets, figs, grapefruit (fresh and juice), orange or tomato juice, peaches and prunes, potatoes, raisins, spinach, squash, and watermelon are good dietary sources of potassium. An oral potassium supplement (potassium chloride) may also be prescribed for patients receiving diuretic medications.*

Prolonged diuretic therapy may also produce hyponatremia (deficiency of sodium in the blood), which results in apprehension, weakness, fatigue, malaise, muscle cramps and twitching, and a rapid, thready pulse.

Nursing Alert *Periodic assessment of the electrolyte levels will alert health team members to hypokalemia, hypomagnesemia, and hyponatremia. Serum levels are assessed frequently when the patient starts diuretic therapy and then usually every 3 to 12 months. It is important to remember that serum potassium levels do not always indicate the total amount of potassium within the body.*

Other problems associated with diuretic administration are hyperuricemia (excessive uric acid in the blood), volume depletion from excessive urination, and hyperglycemia.

GERONTOLOGIC CONSIDERATIONS

Elderly men require closer nursing surveillance because the incidence of urethral obstruction from an enlarged prostate gland is high in this age group. Signs of bladder distention should be observed for regularly by palpating over the bladder.

NURSING PROCESS: THE PATIENT WITH CARDIAC FAILURE

Assessment

The focus of the nursing assessment for the patient with cardiac failure is directed toward observing for signs and symptoms of pulmonary and systemic fluid overload. All signs and symptoms are recorded and reported.

Health History

The nurse explores sleep disturbances, particularly sleep suddenly interrupted by shortness of breath. The nurse also finds out about the number of pillows needed for sleep (an indication of dyspnea), activities of daily living, and the activities that cause shortness of breath.

Physical Examination

The lungs are auscultated at frequent intervals to detect crackles and wheezes or their absence. Crackles, which are produced by the sudden opening of small airways and alveoli that had been stuck together by edema and exudate, may be heard at the end of inspiration and are not cleared with coughing. They may also sound like gurgling that may clear with coughing or suctioning. The rate and depth of respirations are also noted.

The heart is auscultated for an S_3 heart sound, a sign that the heart pump is beginning to fail and that increased blood volume remains in the ventricle with each beat. HR and rhythm are also noted. Rapid rates indicate that SV has decreased and that the ventricle has less time to fill, with the result being some blood stagnation in the atria and eventually in the pulmonary bed.

Jugular vein distention is also assessed (see Chap. 23); distention greater than 3 cm above the sternal angle is considered abnormal. This is an estimate, not a precise measurement, of central venous pressure.

Sensorium and level of consciousness must be evaluated. As the volume of blood ejected by the heart decreases, so does the amount of oxygen transported to the brain.

The nurse makes sure that dependent parts of the patient's body are assessed for perfusion and edema. With significant decreases in SV, there is a decrease in perfusion to the periphery, causing the skin to appear pale or cyanotic, and cool. If the patient is sitting upright, the feet and lower legs are examined for edema; if the patient is supine in bed, the sacrum and back are assessed for edema. Fingers and hands may also become edematous. In extreme cases of cardiac failure, the patient may develop periorbital edema, in which the eyelids may be swollen shut.

The liver is examined for hepatojugular reflux. The patient is asked to breathe normally while manual pressure is applied over the upper right quadrant of the abdomen for 30 to 60 seconds. If neck vein distention increases more than 1 cm, the test finding is positive for increased venous pressure.

Because **oliguria** (diminished urine output; less than 400 mL per 24 hours) or **anuria** (urine output of less than 50 mL per 24 hours) may develop, the nurse measures output carefully to establish a baseline against which to measure the effectiveness of diuretic therapy. Intake and output records are rigorously maintained. It is important to know whether the patient has ingested more fluid than he or she has excreted (positive fluid balance).

Finally, the patient is weighed daily either in the hospital or at home, at the same time of day, with the same type of clothing, and on the same scales. If there is a significant change in weight, the patient is instructed to notify the physician and/or adjust the medications (eg, increase the diuretic dose).

Diagnosis

Nursing Diagnoses

Based on the assessment data, major nursing diagnoses for the patient may include the following:

- Activity intolerance related to imbalance between oxygen supply and demand secondary to decreased CO
- Fatigue secondary to cardiac failure
- Excess fluid volume related to excess fluid/sodium intake or retention secondary to CHF and its medical therapy
- Anxiety related to breathlessness and restlessness secondary to inadequate oxygenation
- Noncompliance related to lack of knowledge
- Powerlessness related to inability to perform role responsibilities secondary to chronic illness and hospitalizations

Collaborative Problems/Potential Complications

Based on the assessment data, potential complications that may develop include:

- Cardiogenic shock
- Dysrhythmias
- Thromboembolism
- Pericardial effusion and pericardial tamponade

Cardiogenic shock is described later in this chapter and in Chapter 14. The other complications are discussed in Chapters 25 and 26.

Planning and Goals

The major goals for the patient may include promoting activity while maintaining vital signs within identified range, reducing fatigue, relieving fluid overload symptoms, decreasing the incidence of anxiety or increasing the patient's ability to manage anxiety, teaching the patient about the self-care program, and encouraging the patient to verbalize his or her ability to make decisions and influence outcomes.

Nursing Interventions

Promoting Activity Tolerance

The patient's response to activities needs to be monitored. Although prolonged bed rest and even short periods of recumbency promote diuresis by improving renal perfusion, they also promote decreased activity tolerance. An acute event that causes hospitalization indicates the need for initial bed rest. Rest is also required in a patient with severe symptoms (NYHA class IV). Otherwise, regular activity should be encouraged. Prolonged bed rest and self-imposed bed rest should be avoided because of the deconditioning effects and hazards, such as pressure ulcers (especially in edematous patients), phlebothrombosis, and pulmonary embolism.

The patient is encouraged to perform an activity more slowly than usual, for a shorter duration, or with assistance initially. Barriers that could limit abilities to perform an activity are identified, and methods of adjusting an activity to ensure pacing but still accomplish the task are discussed. For example, objects that need to be taken upstairs can be put in a basket at the bottom of the stairs throughout the day. At the end of the day, the person can carry the objects up the stairs all at once. Likewise, cleaning supplies can be carried around in a basket or backpack rather than walking back and forth to obtain the items. Vegetables can be chopped or peeled while sitting at the kitchen table rather than standing at the kitchen counter. Pacing and prioritizing activities will maintain the patient's energy to allow participation in regular exercise.

Vital signs, especially pulse, should be taken before, during, and immediately after an activity to identify whether they are within the predetermined range. HR should return to baseline within 3 minutes. If the patient tolerates the activity, then short-term and long-term goals can be developed to increase gradually the intensity, duration, and/or frequency of activity. (For a discussion on physical conditioning and monitoring, see the section on cardiac rehabilitation in Chap. 10). Referral to a cardiac rehabilitation program may be needed, especially for CHF patients with a recent myocardial infarction, recent open heart surgery, or increased anxiety. A supervised program may also benefit those who need the structured environment, significant educational support, regular encouragement, and interpersonal contact.

Reducing Fatigue

The nurse and patient can collaborate to develop a schedule that promotes pacing and prioritization of activities. The schedule should alternate activities with periods of rest and avoid having two significant energy-consuming activities occur on the same day or in immediate succession. Family members can be encouraged to stagger their visits to allow for rest between visits or calls. Having a spokesperson relay messages from and to friends and family members may also help conserve the patient's energy. Identify the patient's peak and low periods of energy, and plan energy-consuming activities accordingly. For example, medical tests may need to be rearranged so that they occur in the morning. When home, the person may prepare the meals for the entire day in the morning. The nurse can explain that small, frequent meals tend to decrease the amount of energy needed for digestion while providing adequate nutrition. Finally, the nurse helps the patient develop a positive outlook focused on his or her strengths, abilities, and interests.

Managing Fluid Volume

Patients with severe CHF may receive intravenous diuretic therapy, but patients with less severe symptoms may receive oral diuretic medication. Oral diuretics should be administered early in the morning so that the resultant diuresis does not interfere with the patient's nighttime rest. Discussing the timing of medication administration is especially important for patients, such as elderly people, who may have urinary urgency or incontinence. (see Table 27-2 for a summary of diuretics in common use.) A single dose of a diuretic may cause the patient to lose a large volume of fluid shortly after administration.

The nurse monitors the patient's fluid status closely—auscultating the lungs, comparing daily body weights, monitoring intake and output, and assisting the patient to adhere to a low-sodium diet by reading food labels and avoiding commercially prepared convenience foods. If the diet includes fluid restriction, the nurse can assist the patient to plan the distribution throughout the day while respecting the patient's dietary preferences. If the patient is receiving intravenous fluids, the amount of fluid needs to be monitored closely and the physician or pharmacist needs to be consulted about the possibility of double-concentrating any medications.

The nurse needs to position the patient or teach the patient how to assume a position that shifts fluid away from the heart. The number of pillows may be increased, the head of the bed may be elevated, or the bed legs may be placed on 20- to 30-cm (8- to 10-in) blocks, or the patient may prefer to sit in a comfortable armchair. In this position the venous return to the heart (preload) is reduced, pulmonary congestion is alleviated, and impingement of the liver on the diaphragm is minimized. The lower arms should be supported with pillows to eliminate the fatigue caused by the constant pull of their weight on the shoulder muscles.

The patient who can breathe only in the upright position may sit on the side of the bed with the feet supported on a chair, the head and arms resting on an overbed table, and the lumbosacral spine supported by a pillow (Fig. 27-3). If pulmonary congestion is present, positioning the patient in an armchair is advantageous because this position favors the shift of fluid away from the lungs.

Because decreased circulation in edematous areas increases the risk of skin injury, the nurse needs to assess for skin breakdown and institute preventive measures. Frequent changes of position, positioning to avoid pressure, the use of elastic pressure stockings, and leg exercises may help to prevent skin injury.

Controlling Anxiety

Because patients in cardiac failure have difficulty maintaining adequate oxygenation, they are likely to be restless and anxious and feel overwhelmed by breathlessness. These symptoms tend to intensify at night. Emotional stress stimulates the sympathetic nervous system, which causes vasoconstriction, elevated arterial

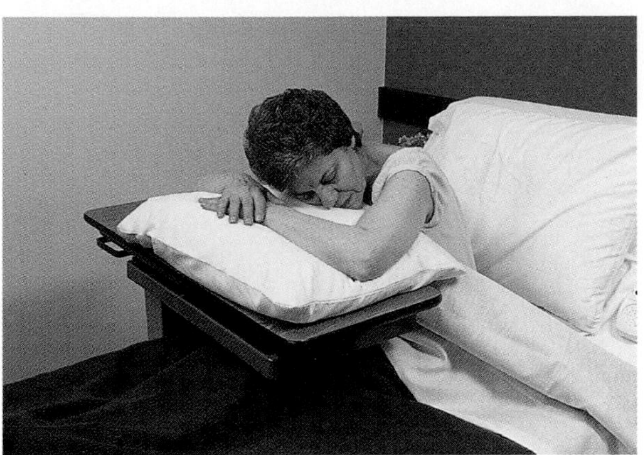

FIGURE 27•3 A patient with cardiac failure can be positioned as shown to reduce the amount of blood returning to the heart, which alleviates pulmonary congestion and breathing difficulties. The position may be maintained while the patient rests in bed or sits in a chair.

pressure, and increased HR. This sympathetic response increases the amount of work that the heart has to do. By decreasing anxiety, the patient's cardiac work also is decreased. Oxygen may be administered during the acute stage to diminish the work of breathing and to increase the comfort of the patient.

When the patient exhibits anxiety, the nurse takes steps to promote physical comfort and psychological support. In many cases, a family member's presence provides reassurance. Speaking in a slow, calm, and confident manner is helpful, and stating specific, brief directions for an activity, when necessary, is also helpful in decreasing the patient's anxiety.

Once the patient is comfortable, the nurse can begin teaching the patient ways to control anxiety and avoid anxiety-provoking situations. The patient is taught how to use relaxation techniques and is assisted in identifying factors that contribute to anxiety. Lack of sleep may increase anxiety, which in turn may prevent adequate rest. Other possible contributing factors include misinformation or lack of information, or poor nutritional status. Promoting physical comfort, providing accurate information, and teaching the patient to avoid situations that tend to promote anxiety and agitation may relax the patient.

Nursing Alert *Cerebral hypoxia with superimposed carbon dioxide retention may also be a problem in cardiac failure, causing the patient to react to sedative-hypnotic medications with confusion and increased anxiety. Hepatic congestion may result in a decrease of the liver's ability to metabolize the medication within a normal time frame to prevent toxicity. Therefore, many sedative-hypnotic medications must be administered with caution.*

In cases of confusion and anxiety reactions that affect the patient's safety, the use of restraints should be avoided. Restraints are likely to be resisted, and resistance inevitably increases the cardiac workload. The patient who insists on getting out of bed at night can be seated comfortably in an armchair. As cerebral and systemic circulation improves, the degree of anxiety decreases and the quality of sleep will improve.

Minimizing Powerlessness

Patients need to recognize that they are not helpless and that they can influence their direction, their lives, and their outcomes. The nurse needs to assess for factors contributing to a perception of powerlessness and intervene accordingly. Contributing factors may include lack of knowledge, hospital policies, and lack of opportunities to make decisions, particularly if health care providers and family members behave in maternalistic or paternalistic ways. Taking time to listen actively to patients often encourages them to express their concerns and questions. In some cases, the nurse may want to review hospital policies and standards that tend to promote powerlessness and advocate for their elimination or change.

Other strategies include providing the patient with decision-making opportunities, such as when activities are to occur or where objects are to be placed, and increasing the frequency and significance of those opportunities over time; providing encouragement and praise while identifying the patient's progress; and assisting the patient to differentiate between factors that can be controlled and those that cannot.

Promoting Home and Community-Based Care

TEACHING PATIENTS SELF-CARE

Providing patient education and involving the patient in implementing the therapeutic regimen promote understanding and compliance. Recurrences of cardiac failure, unnecessary hospitalizations, and a decreased life expectancy occur when the patient does not comply with the therapeutic recommendations, such as failing to follow the medication regimen properly, straying from dietary restrictions, failing to obtain adequate medical follow-up, engaging in excessive physical activity, and failing to recognize recurring symptoms. Although noncompliance is not well understood and the interventions that are needed to promote compliance are not clear, ensuring accurate understanding is an important part of the plan. A summary of teaching points for the patient with cardiac failure is presented in the accompanying home care teaching checklist.

The patient and family members need to be supported and encouraged to ask questions so that information can be clarified and understanding can be enhanced. The health care practitioner should be aware of cultural factors and adapt the teaching plan accordingly. Patients and their families should understand that the progression of the disease is influenced by compliance with the treatment plan. They need to understand that the health care providers are there to assist them in reaching their health care goals. Patients and family members need to make the decisions about the treatment plan, but they also need to understand the possible outcomes of those decisions. The treatment plan then will be based on what the patient wants, not just what the physician or other health care team members think is needed. Ultimately, the nurse needs to convey that monitoring symptoms and daily weights, restricting sodium intake, avoiding excess fluids, preventing infection, avoiding noxious agents (eg, alcohol and tobacco), and participating in regular exercise all aid in preventing the exacerbation of cardiac failure.

CONTINUING CARE

Depending on the patient's physical status and the availability of family assistance, a home care referral may be indicated. Assistance with transition to the home after hospitalization for an acute episode of CHF is often required by elderly patients and patients who have long-standing heart disease and whose physical stamina is compromised. It is important for the home care nurse to assess the physical environment of the home and the family or support system. Suggestions for adapting the home environment to meet the patient's activity limitations are important. If stairs are the concern, the patient can plan the day's activities so that stair climbing is minimized; for some patients, a temporary bedroom may be set up on the main level of the home.

Home Care Teaching Checklist: The Patient With Cardiac Failure

At the completion of the program, the patient or caregiver will be able to:	Patient	Caregiver
• Live within the limits of the cardiac reserve.	✔	
• Obtain adequate rest.	✔	
Have a regular daily rest period.	✔	
Shorten working hours if possible.	✔	
Avoid emotional upsets.	✔	
• Accept the fact that taking medications may be a permanent way of life.	✔	
Take medications daily, exactly as prescribed.	✔	
Check own pulse rate daily.		
Have a check-off system to ensure that medicine(s) has been taken.		
Know the signs and symptoms of potassium depletion; if taking oral potassium, keep a check-off system along with diuretic medication.		
• Monitor effects of medication.	✔	✔
Weigh at the same time daily to detect any tendency toward fluid accumulation.		
Report weight gain of more than 0.9 to 1.4 kg (2–3 pounds) in a few days.		
Learn to take own blood pressure at prescribed intervals.		
Know signs and symptoms of orthostatic hypotension and how to prevent it.		
• Accept that restricting sodium intake may be a permanent part of life.	✔	
Restrict sodium as directed: consulting the written diet plan and the list of permitted and restricted foods; examining labels to ascertain sodium content (antacids, laxatives, cough remedies, and the like); avoiding salt use; and avoiding excesses in eating and drinking.	✔	
• Review activity program.	✔	
Increase walking and other activities gradually, provided they do not cause fatigue and dyspnea.	✔	
In general, continue at whatever activity level can be maintained without the appearance of symptoms.	✔	
• Avoid extremes of heat and cold, which increase the work of the heart. Air conditioning may be essential in a hot, humid environment.	✔	
• Keep regular appointments with physician or clinic.	✔	
• Be alert for symptoms that may indicate recurring heart failure.		
Recall the symptoms experienced when illness began.	✔	✔
• Report immediately to the physician or clinic any of the following:	✔	✔
Gain in weight		
Loss of appetite		
Shortness of breath with activity		
Swelling of ankles, feet, or abdomen		
Persistent cough		

The home care nurse collaborates with the patient and family to maximize the benefits of these changes.

The home care nurse also reinforces and clarifies information about diet and fluid restrictions, monitoring symptoms and daily body weights, and reinforcing follow-up health care expectations. Assistance may be given in scheduling and keeping appointments as well. The patient is encouraged to gradually increase his or her self-care and responsibility for accomplishing the therapeutic regimen.

Evaluation

Expected Outcomes

Expected outcomes may include:

1. Demonstrates tolerance for increased activity
   a. Describes adaptive methods for usual activities
   b. Stops any activity that causes symptoms that indicate intolerance
   c. Maintains vital signs (pulse, blood pressure, respiratory rate, and pulse oximetry) within targeted range
   d. Identifies factors that contribute to activity intolerance and takes actions to avoid them
2. Has less fatigue and dyspnea
   a. Establishes priorities for activities
   b. Schedules activities to conserve energy and reduce fatigue and dyspnea
3. Maintains fluid balance
   a. Exhibits decreased peripheral and sacral edema
   b. Demonstrates methods for preventing edema
4. Is less anxious
   a. Avoids situations that produce stress
   b. Sleeps comfortably at night
   c. Reports decreased stress and anxiety
5. Adheres to self-care regimen
6. Makes decisions regarding care and treatment
   a. States ability to influence outcomes
7. Absence of complications

CARDIOGENIC SHOCK

Cardiogenic shock occurs when the heart cannot pump enough blood to supply the amount of oxygen needed by the tissues. This may occur because of one significant or multiple smaller infarctions in which more than 40% of the myocardium becomes necrotic, or because of a ruptured ventricle, significant valvular dysfunction, trauma to the heart resulting in myocardial contusion, or as the end stage of CHF. It also can occur with cardiac tamponade, pulmonary embolism, cardiomyopathy, and dysrhythmias.

Pathophysiology

The signs and symptoms of cardiogenic shock reflect the circular nature of the pathophysiology of cardiac failure. The degree of shock is proportional to the level of left ventricular dysfunction. The heart muscle loses its contractile power, resulting in a marked reduction in SV and CO, which is sometimes called "forward failure." The damage to the myocardium results in a decrease in CO, which in turn reduces arterial blood pressure and tissue perfusion in the vital organs (heart, brain, kidneys). Flow to the coronary arteries is reduced, resulting in decreased oxygen supply to the myocardium, which in turn increases ischemia and further reduces the heart's ability to pump. The inadequate emptying of the ventricle also leads to increased pulmonary pressures, pulmonary congestion, and pulmonary edema, exacerbating the hypoxia and resulting ischemia of vital organs. Thus, a vicious cycle is set in motion (Fig. 27-4).

Clinical Manifestations

The classic signs of cardiogenic shock are tissue hypoperfusion manifested as cerebral hypoxia (restlessness, confusion, agitation), low blood pressure, rapid and weak pulse, cold and clammy skin, increased respiratory crackles, hypoactive bowel sounds, and decreased urinary output. Initially, arterial blood gas analysis may show respiratory alkalosis. Dysrhythmias are common and result from a decrease in oxygen to the myocardium.

Assessment and Diagnostic Findings

As in pulmonary edema, the use of a PA catheter to measure left ventricular pressures and CO is important in assessing the severity of the problem and planning management. The PA wedge pressure is elevated and the CO is decreased as the left ventricle loses its ability to pump. The systemic vascular resistance is elevated due to the sympathetic nervous system stimulation that occurs as a compensatory response to the decrease in blood pressure. The decreased blood flow to the kidneys causes a hormonal response (increased catecholamines and activation of the renin-angiotensin-aldosterone system) that causes fluid retention and further vasoconstriction. The increases in HR, circulating volume, and vasoconstriction occur to maintain circulation to the brain, heart, and lungs, but at a cost: an increase in the workload of the heart.

Continued cellular hypoperfusion eventually results in organ failure. The patient becomes unresponsive, severe hypotension ensues, and the patient develops shallow respirations, cold, cyanotic or mottled skin, and absent bowel sounds. Arterial blood gas analysis shows metabolic acidosis, and all laboratory test results indicate organ dysfunction. Chapter 14 presents in more detail the pathophysiology and management of cardiogenic shock.

PATHOPHYSIOLOGY

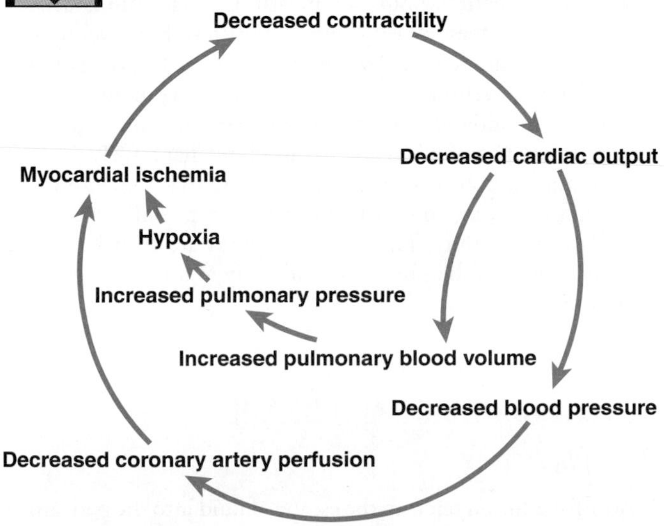

FIGURE 27•4 Pathophysiology of cardiogenic shock.

Medical Management

The major approach to treating cardiogenic shock is to correct the underlying problems, reduce any further demand on the heart, improve oxygenation, and restore tissue perfusion. Major dysrhythmias are corrected because they may have caused or contributed to the shock. If hypervolemia is present, diuresis is indicated. Diuretics, vasodilators, and mechanical devices (such as filtration and dialysis) have been used in cardiogenic shock. If hypovolemia or low intravascular volume is suspected or detected through pressure readings, the patient is given intravenous volume expanders (eg, normal saline solution, lactated Ringer's solution, or albumin) to increase the amount of circulating fluid. The patient is placed on strict bed rest to conserve energy. If the patient has hypoxemia, as detected by pulse oximetry or arterial blood gas analysis, oxygen administration is increased, often under positive pressure when regular flow is insufficient to meet tissue demands. Intubation and sedation may be necessary to maintain oxygenation balance. The settings for mechanical ventilation are adjusted according to the patient's oxygenation status and the need for conserving energy.

PHARMACOLOGIC THERAPY

Medication therapy is selected and guided according to CO, cardiac parameters, and mean arterial blood pressure. Because of the decreased perfusion to the gastrointestinal system and the need to adjust the dosage quickly, most medications are administered intravenously.

Pressor agents are medications used to raise blood pressure and increase CO. Many pressor medications are catecholamines (eg, norepinephrine and high-dose [more than 10 μg/kg/min] dopamine). Their purpose is to promote perfusion to the heart and brain. However, because they also tend to increase the workload of the heart by increasing oxygen demand, they are not administered early in the cardiogenic process.

Diuretics and vasodilators may be administered carefully to reduce the workload of the heart as long as they do not cause a worsening of the hypoperfusion to the tissues. Agents such as amrinone, milrinone, sodium nitroprusside, and nitroglycerin are effective vasoactive medications that lower the volume returning to the heart and decrease blood pressure and thus cardiac work. They cause the arteries and veins to dilate, thereby shunting much of the intravascular volume to the periphery and causing a reduction in preload and afterload.

Positive inotropic medications are given to increase myocardial contractility. Dopamine given at more than 2 μg/kg/min, dobutamine, and epinephrine are catecholamines that increase contractility. Each of these can cause tachydysrhythmias because they increase automaticity with increasing dosage. Therefore, monitoring baseline HR is important. As the baseline HR increases, so does the risk of developing tachydysrhythmias.

OTHER TREATMENTS

Other therapeutic modalities for cardiogenic shock include using circulatory assist devices. The most frequently used mechanical support system is the intra-aortic balloon pump (IABP). The IABP is a catheter with a inflatable balloon at the end. The catheter is usually inserted through the femoral artery and the balloon is positioned in the descending thoracic aorta (Fig. 27-5). IABP uses internal counterpulsation through the regular inflation and deflation of the balloon to augment the pumping action of the heart. The device inflates during diastole, increasing the pressure in the aorta during diastole and therefore increasing perfusion through the coronary and peripheral arteries. It deflates just before systole, lessening the pressure within the aorta before ventricular contraction, decreasing the amount of resistance the heart has to overcome to eject blood and therefore decreasing the amount of work the heart must complete to eject blood. The device is connected to a console that synchronizes its activities with systole and diastole, usually in synchrony with the electrocardiogram or the arterial pressure. Hemodynamic monitoring is essential to determine the patient's response to the IABP. Other ventricular assist devices are described in Chapter 26.

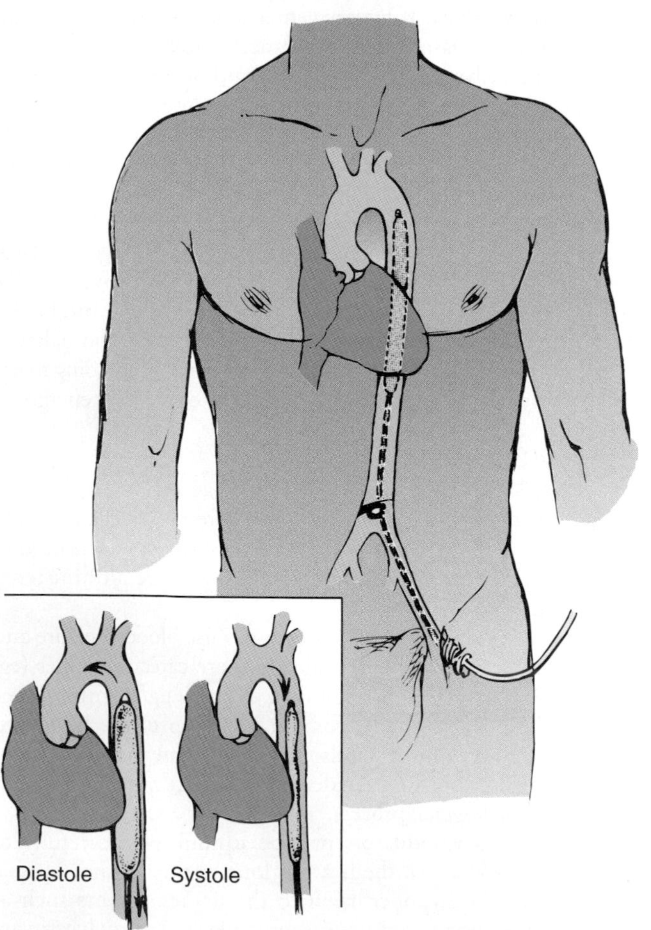

FIGURE 27•5 The intra-aortic balloon pump (IABP) inflates at the beginning of diastole, which results in increased perfusion of the coronary and peripheral arteries; it deflates just before systole, which results in a decrease in afterload (resistance to ejection) and in the left ventricular workload.

Nursing Management

The patient in cardiogenic shock requires constant monitoring and intensive care nursing. The nurse must carefully assess the patient, observe the cardiac rhythm, measure hemodynamic parameters, and record fluid intake and urinary output. The patient must be closely monitored for responses to the medical interventions and for the development of complications, which must be corrected immediately.

Because of the frequency of nursing interventions and the technology required for effective medical management in such cases, the patient is always treated in an intensive care environment. Intensive care unit nurses are responsible for the nursing management, which demands frequent assessments and timely adjustments to medications and therapies based on the assessment data. See Chapter 14 for more information about nursing management of the patient in cardiogenic shock.

THROMBOEMBOLISM

The decreased mobility of the patient with cardiac disease and the impaired circulation that accompany these disorders contribute to the development of intracardiac and intravascular thrombosis. Intracardiac thrombus is detected by an echocardiogram and treated with anticoagulants, such as warfarin (Coumadin). A part of the thrombus may become detached (the detached thrombus is called an embolus) and may be carried to the brain, kidneys, intestines, or lungs. The most common problem is pulmonary embolism. The symptoms of pulmonary embolism include chest pain, cyanosis, shortness of breath, rapid respirations, and hemoptysis (bloody sputum).

The pulmonary embolus may block the circulation to a part of the lung, producing an area of pulmonary infarction. Usually there is a significant decrease in oxygenation measured by arterial blood gas analysis or pulse oximetry. Pain experienced is usually pleuritic—that is, it increases with respiration and may subside when the patient holds the breath. Cardiac pain is usually continuous and does not vary with respirations. However, it may be difficult to differentiate by symptoms alone. The patient usually undergoes a ventilation—perfusion scan or a pulmonary arteriogram for definitive diagnosis. The treatment and care for patients with pulmonary embolism are discussed in Chapter 21.

Systemic embolism may present as cerebral, mesenteric, or renal infarction; an embolism can also compromise the blood supply to an extremity. The nurse must be aware of such possible complications and be prepared to identify and report signs and symptoms.

PERICARDIAL EFFUSION AND CARDIAC TAMPONADE

Pathophysiology

Pericardial effusion refers to the escape of fluid into the pericardial sac. This occurrence may accompany pericarditis (see Chap. 26), advanced CHF, metastatic carcinoma, cardiac surgery, trauma, or nontraumatic hemorrhage.

Normally, the pericardial sac contains less than 50 mL of fluid, which the heart needs to decrease friction for the beating heart. An increase in pericardial fluid raises the pressure within the pericardial sac and compresses the heart. This results in:

- Increased right and left ventricular end-diastolic pressures
- Decreased venous return
- Inability of the ventricles to distend adequately

Pericardial fluid may accumulate slowly without causing noticeable symptoms. A rapidly developing effusion, however, can stretch the pericardium to its maximum size and, because of increased pericardial pressure, and reduce venous return to the heart, and decrease cardiac output. The result is cardiac tamponade (compression of the heart).

Clinical Manifestations

The patient may complain of a feeling of fullness within the chest or may have substantial or ill-defined pain. The feeling of pressure in the chest may result from stretching of the pericardial sac. Because of increased pressure within the pericardium, venous pressure tends to rise, as evidenced by engorged neck veins. Other signs include shortness of breath and a drop and fluctuation in blood pressure. Systolic blood pressure that is detected during expiration but not heard with inspiration is called **pulsus paradoxus**. The difference in systolic pressure between the point that it is heard during expiration and the point that it is heard during inspiration is measured. Pulsus paradoxus exceeding 10 mm Hg is abnormal. The cardinal signs are falling systolic blood pressure, narrowing pulse pressure, rising venous pressure (increased jugular venous distention), and distant (muffled) heart sounds.

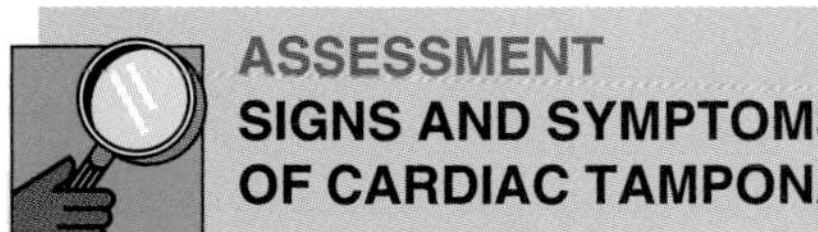

ASSESSMENT
SIGNS AND SYMPTOMS OF CARDIAC TAMPONADE

Assessment findings in cardiac tamponade resulting from pericardial effusion include feelings of faintness, shortness of breath, anxiety, and pain from decreased cardiac output, cough from pressure created in the trachea from swelling of the pericardial sac, distended neck veins from rising venous pressure, paradoxical pulse, and muffled or distant heart sounds.

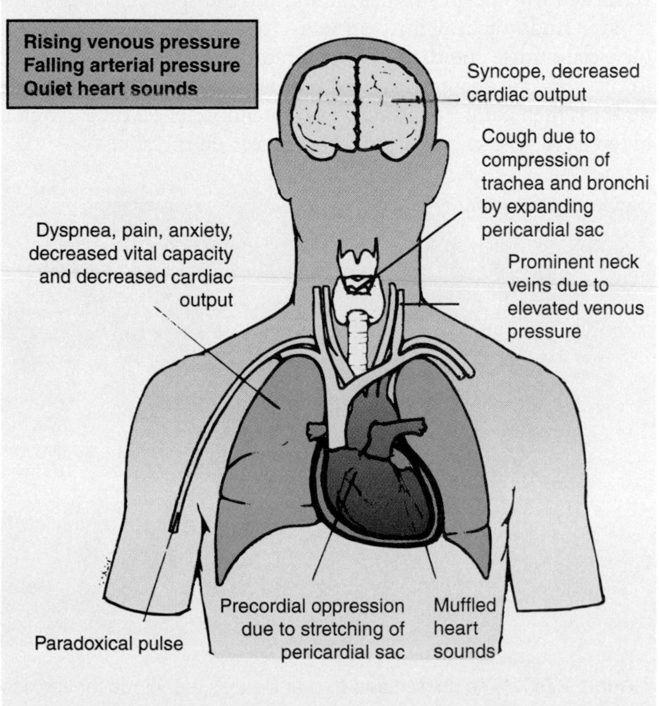

Nursing Alert *Pericardial tamponade is a life-threatening situation, demanding immediate intervention.*

Assessment and Diagnostic Findings

Pericardial effusion is detected by percussing the chest and noting an extension of flatness across the anterior aspect of the chest. The physician may order an echocardiogram to confirm the diagnosis. The clinical signs and symptoms and chest x-ray findings are usually sufficient to diagnose pericardial effusion.

Medical Management

PERICARDIAL FLUID ASPIRATION (PERICARDIOCENTESIS)

If cardiac function becomes seriously impaired, a **pericardiocentesis** (puncture of the pericardial sac) is performed to remove fluid from the pericardial sac. The major goal is to prevent cardiac tamponade, which restricts normal heart action.

During the procedure, the patient is monitored by electrocardiography and hemodynamic pressure measurements. Emergency resuscitative equipment should be readily available. The head of the bed is elevated to 45 degrees to 60 degrees, placing the heart in close proximity to the chest wall so that the needle can be inserted into the pericardial sac more easily. If a peripheral intravenous device is not already in place, one is inserted and a slow intravenous infusion is started in case it becomes necessary to administer emergency medications or blood products.

The pericardial aspiration needle is attached to a 50-mL syringe by a three-way stopcock. Several possible sites are used for pericardial aspiration. The needle may be inserted in the angle between the left costal margin and the xiphoid, near the cardiac apex; at the fifth or sixth intercostal space at the left sternal margin; or on the right sternal margin of the fourth intercostal space. The needle is advanced slowly until fluid is obtained. The V lead (precordial lead wire) of the electrocardiogram may be attached to the hub of the aspirating needle with alligator clips, because the electrocardiogram will help determine whether the needle has contacted the epicardium. Contact is evidenced by an elevated ST segment. The procedure may also be guided by echocardiographic monitoring. During the procedure, drainage fluid must be checked. Although not entirely accurate, the guideline is that pericardial blood does not clot readily, whereas blood obtained from inadvertent puncture of one of the heart chambers does clot.

A withdrawal of pericardial fluid with a resulting fall in central venous pressure and an associated rise in blood pressure indicates that the cardiac tamponade has been relieved. The patient almost always feels immediate relief. If there is a substantial amount of pericardial fluid, a small catheter may be left in place to drain recurrent bleeding or effusion. Pericardial fluid is sent to the laboratory for examination for tumor cells, bacterial culture, chemical and serologic analysis, and differential cell count.

Complications of pericardiocentesis include ventricular or coronary artery puncture, dysrhythmias, pleural laceration, gastric puncture, and myocardial trauma. After pericardiocentesis, the patient's heart rhythm, blood pressure, venous pressure, and heart sounds are monitored to detect any possible recurrence of cardiac tamponade. If it recurs, repeated aspiration is necessary. Cardiac tamponade may require treatment by open pericardial drainage. The patient is ideally in an intensive care unit.

PERICARDIOTOMY

Recurrent pericardial effusions, usually associated with neoplastic diseases, may be treated by a pericardiotomy (pericardial window). The patient receives a general anesthetic, but cardiopulmonary bypass is seldom necessary. A portion of the pericardium is excised to permit the pericardial fluid to drain into the lymphatic system. More rarely, catheters are placed between the pericardium and abdominal cavity to drain the pericardial fluid. The nursing care is the same as that described for other cardiac surgery (see Chap. 25).

MYOCARDIAL RUPTURE

Myocardial rupture is a rare event. However, it can occur when a myocardial infarction, infectious process, pericardial disease, or other myocardial dysfunction weakens the cardiac muscle (ventricular aneurysm) substantially. Persistent elevation of the ST segment is an indication of a ventricular aneurysm. In many cases the result of myocardial rupture is immediate death unless the patient undergoes immediate cardiac surgery. Other complications of a myocardial infarction include ventricular septal defect and mitral regurgitation due to papillary muscle dysfunction or rupture.

CARDIAC ARREST

Cardiac arrest occurs when the heart ceases to produce an effective pulse and blood circulation. It may be due to a cardiac electrical event, as when the HR is too fast (especially ventricular tachycardia or ventricular fibrillation) or too slow (bradycardia or AV block), or when there is no heart rate at all (asystole). Cardiac arrest may follow respiratory arrest; it may also occur when electrical activity is present but there is ineffective cardiac contraction or circulating volume, which is called **pulseless electrical activity** (PEA). Formerly called electrical–mechanical dissociation (EM), PEA can be caused by hypovolemia (eg, with excessive bleeding), cardiac tamponade, hypothermia, massive pulmonary embolism, drug overdoses (eg, tricyclics, digitalis, beta blockers, or calcium channel blockers), significant acidosis, and massive acute myocardial infarction.

Clinical Manifestations

Consciousness, pulse, and blood pressure are lost immediately. Ineffective respiratory gasping may occur. The pupils of the eyes begin dilating within 45 seconds. Seizures may or may not occur.

The risk of irreversible brain damage and death increases with every minute from the time that circulation ceases. The interval varies with the age and underlying condition of the patient. During this period, the diagnosis of cardiac arrest must be made and measures must be taken to restore circulation.

Nursing Alert *The most reliable sign of cardiac arrest is the absence of a pulse. In the adult and the child, the carotid pulse is assessed. In an infant, the brachial pulse is assessed. Valuable time should not be wasted taking the blood pressure, listening for the heartbeat, or checking proper contact of electrodes.*

Emergency Management: Cardiopulmonary Resuscitation

The ABCDs of basic cardiopulmonary resuscitation (CPR) are **A**irway, **B**reathing, **C**irculation, and **D**efibrillation. Once loss of consciousness has been established, the resuscitation priority for the adult victim is placing a phone call to activate the code team or the emergency medical system. However, because the underlying cause of arrest in an infant or child is usually respiratory, the priority becomes administering CPR; activating an emergency medical system after 1 minute of CPR. Because the care of the pediatric patient is individualized, the following discussion on the care of a cardiac arrest patient applies only to adults.

Resuscitation consists of:

1. Airway: maintaining an open airway
2. Breathing: providing artificial ventilation by rescue breathing
3. Circulation: promoting artificial circulation by external cardiac compression
4. Defibrillation: restoring the heartbeat

If the patient is monitored or is immediately placed on the monitor using the quick-look paddles that can be found on most defibrillators, and the electrocardiogram shows ventricular tachycardia or ventricular fibrillation, defibrillation, rather than CPR, is the treatment of choice. In this scenario, CPR is performed initially only if the availability of the defibrillator is delayed. The survival rate decreases by 10% for every minute that defibrillation is delayed. If the patient has not been defibrillated within 10 minutes, the chance of survival is close to zero. (See Chap. 24 for further discussion of defibrillation.)

MAINTAINING AIRWAY AND BREATHING

The first step in CPR is to obtain an open airway. Any obvious material in the mouth or throat should be removed. The chin is directed up and back or the jaw (mandible) is lifted forward. The rescuer "looks, listens, and feels" for air movement. An oropharyngeal airway is inserted if available. Two rescue ventilations over 3 to 4 seconds are provided using a bag or mouth-mask device (Fig. 27-6). An obstructed airway should be suspected when the rescuer cannot give the initial ventilations, and appropriate actions should be taken to relieve the obstruction.

If the first rescue ventilation entered easily, then the patient is ventilated with 12 breaths per minute and the open airway is maintained. Endotracheal intubation is frequently performed by a physician, nurse anesthetist, or respiratory therapist during a code to ensure an adequate airway and ventilation. The resuscitation bag device is then connected directly to the endotracheal tube. Arterial blood gas levels are measured to guide oxygen therapy.

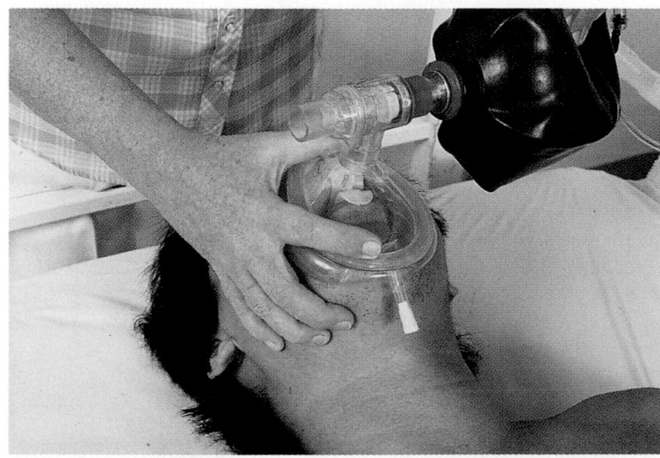

FIGURE 27•6 The chin lift and bag-and-mask technique for ventilating patients who need cardiopulmonary resuscitation.

RESTORING CIRCULATION

After performing ventilation, the carotid pulse is assessed and external cardiac compressions are provided when no pulse is detected. Compressions are performed with the patient on a firm surface, such as the floor, a cardiac board, or a meal tray. The rescuer (facing the patient's head) places the heel of one hand on the lower half of the sternum, two fingerwidths (3.8 cm [1.5 to 2 in]) from the tip of the xiphoid and positions the other hand on top of the first hand (Fig. 27-7). The fingers should not touch the chest wall.

Using the body weight while keeping the elbows straight, the rescuer presses quickly downward from the shoulder area to deliver a forceful compression to the victim's lower sternum—about 3.8 to 5 cm (1.5 to 2 in) toward the spine. The chest compression rate is 80 to 100 times per minute. If only one rescuer is available, the rate is two ventilations to every 15 cardiac compressions. When two rescuers are available, the first person performs the cardiac compressions, pausing after the fifth compression when the second rescuer ventilates the patient, with each ventilation taking 1.5 to 2 seconds.

When the code team or emergency medical personnel arrive, the patient is quickly assessed to determine cardiac rhythm and respiratory status, as well as possible causes for the arrest. The specific subsequent advanced life support interventions depend on the assessment results.

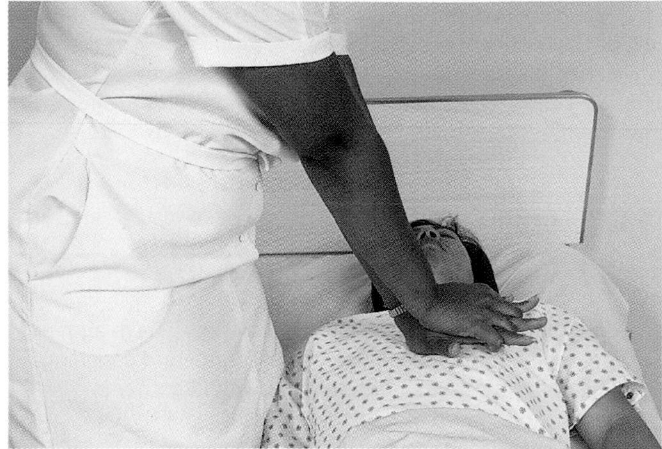

FIGURE 27•7 Chest compressions in cardiopulmonary resuscitation (CPR) are performed by placing the heel of one hand on the lower half of the sternum and the other hand on top of the first hand. Elbows are kept straight and body weight is used to apply quick, forceful compressions to the lower sternum.

FOLLOW-UP MONITORING

Once successfully resuscitated, the patient is transferred to an intensive care unit for close monitoring. Continuous electrocardiographic monitoring and frequent blood pressure assessment are essential until hemodynamic stability is reestablished. Etiologic factors that precipitated the arrest, such as metabolic and rhythm abnormalities, must be identified and treated. Possible contributing factors, such as electrolyte and acid–base imbalances, need to be identified and corrected. Selected medications, as described in Table 27-5, may be used during and after resuscitation.

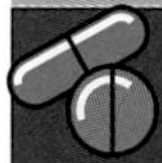

TABLE 27•5 Medications Used in Cardiopulmonary Resuscitation

Agent and Action	Indications	Nursing Considerations
Oxygen (improves tissue oxygenation and corrects hypoxemia)	Administered to all patients with acute cardiac ischemia or suspected hypoxemia, including those with COPD	• Use 100% FiO_2 during resuscitation. • Recognize that no lung damage occurs when used for less than 24 hours. • Monitor dose by end-tidal CO_2 or pulse oximeter.
Epinephrine (increases systemic vascular resistance and blood pressure; improves coronary and cerebral perfusion and myocardial contractility)	Given to patients in cardiac arrest caused by ventricular tachycardia, ventricular fibrillation, asystole, or pulseless electrical activity	• Administer by IV push (IVP) or through the endotracheal (ET) tube. • Avoid adding to IV lines that contain alkaline solution (eg, bicarbonate).
Atropine (blocks parasympathetic action; increases SA node automaticity and AV conduction)	Given to patients with symptomatic bradycardia (hemodynamically unstable, frequent premature ventricular contractions and symptoms of ischemia)	• Should be given rapidly as 2.0 to 2.5 mg IVP or through the ET tube. • Less than 0.5 mg in the adult can cause the heart rate to decrease to a worse bradycardia. • Monitor patient for reflexive tachycardia.
Sodium bicarbonate ($NaHCO_3$) (corrects metabolic acidosis)	Given to correct metabolic acidosis that is refractory to standard ACLS interventions (defibrillation, CPR, intubation, IVP epinephrine)	• Initial dose should be 1 mEq/kg IV; then the dose is based on the base deficit calculated from arterial blood gases. • To prevent rebound development of metabolic alkalosis, complete correction of acidosis is not indicated
Magnesium (promotes adequate functioning of the cellular sodium–potassium pump)	Given to patients with torsades de pointes	• May give diluted over 1–2 min or IVP. • Monitor for hypotension, asystole, bradycardia, respiratory paralysis.

If the patient does not respond to therapies given during the arrest, the resuscitation effort may be stopped or "called" by the physician. The decision to terminate resuscitation is based on medical considerations and will take into account the underlying condition of the patient and the chances for survival.

Critical Thinking Exercises

1. A patient who had a myocardial infarction 2 days ago begins to complain of shortness of breath and coughing. Describe the assessment data you would gather in preparing to report this development.
2. A patient is readmitted for cardiac failure for the third time in 2 months. Describe how you would assess for the factors that contribute to the patient's readmission.

References and Selected Readings

BOOKS

Agency for Health Care Policy and Research. (1994). *Heart failure: Evaluation and care of patients with left-ventricular systolic dysfunction.* Clinical Practice Guideline, Number 11, AHCPR Publication No. 94-0612. Public Health Service, U.S. Department of Health and Human Services, Rockville, MD: Author.

Alexander, R. W., Schlant, R. C., & Ruster, V. (1998). *Hurst's The heart.* New York: McGraw-Hill.

American Heart Association. (1997). *Heart facts.* Dallas: Author.

American Heart Association. (1997). *Textbook of advanced cardiac life support.* Dallas: Author.

Bickley, L. S. (1999). *Bates's guide to physical examination and history taking* (7th ed.). Philadelphia: Lippincott Williams & Wilkins.

Braunwald, E. (1997). *Heart disease: A textbook of cardiovascular medicine* (4th ed.). Philadelphia: W. B. Saunders.

CPR. (1998). Tulsa: CPR Publishers Inc.

Carpenito, L. J. (1997). *Nursing diagnosis: Application to clinical practice* (7th ed.). Philadelphia: Lippincott-Raven.

Chulay, M., Guzzetta, D., & Dossey, B. (1997). *AACN handbook of critical care nursing.* Stamford, CT: Appleton & Lange.

Darovic, G. I. (1995). *Hemodynamic monitoring: Invasive and noninvasive clinical application* (2nd ed.). Philadelphia: W. B. Saunders.

Fulmer, T. T., & Walker, M. K. (1992). *Critical care nursing of the elderly.* New York: Springer.

Guyton, A. C., & Hall, J. E. (1996). *Textbook of medical physiology* (9th ed.) Philadelphia: W. B. Saunders.

Hudak, C. M., & Gallo, B. M. (1998). *Critical care nursing: A holistic approach* (7th ed.). Philadelphia: Lippincott-Raven.

Woods, S. L., et al. (1995). *Cardiac nursing.* Philadelphia: J. B. Lippincott.

JOURNALS

Asterisks indicate nursing research articles.

Adams, K., & Zanna, F. (1998). Clinical definition and epidemiology of advanced heart failure. *American Heart Journal,* 135(6), S204–S215.

*Bennett, S. J., Huster, G. A., Baker, S. L., et al. (1998). Characteristics of the precipitants of hospitalization for heart failure decompensation. *American Journal of Critical Care,* 7, 168–174.

Cook, D. M. (1993). The use of central nervous manifestations in the early detection of digitalis toxicity. *Heart and Lung,* 22(6), 477–480.

Crumlish, C. M., & Hand, M. M. (1999). Reducing patient delay in seeking treatment for acute myocardial infarction. *MedSurg Nursing, 8*(2), 77–91.

Emergency Cardiac Care Committee and Subcommittees, American Heart Association. (1992). Guidelines for cardiopulmonary resuscitation and emergency cardiac care. *Journal of the American Medical Association,* 268, 172–183.

Halm, M., & Penque, S. (1999). Heart disease in women. *American Journal of Nursing, 99*(4), 26–32.

Happ, M. B., Naylor, M. D., & Roe-Prior, P. (1997). Factors contributing to rehospitalization of elderly patients with heart failure. *Journal of Cardiovascular Nursing,* 11(4), 75–84.

Kendler, B. S. (1997). Recent nutritional approaches to the prevention and therapy of cardiovascular disease. *Progress in Cardiovascular Nursing,* 12(3), 3–23.

Lewandowski, D. M. (1995). Congestive heart failure. *American Journal of Nursing,* 5(3), 36.

Mancini, M. E., & Kaye, W. (1999). AEDS. Changing the way you respond to cardiac arrest. *American Journal of Nursing, 99*(5), 26–30.

Rich, M. W., Beckham, V., Wittenberg, C., et al. (1995). A multidisciplinary intervention to prevent the readmission of elderly patients with congestive heart failure. *New England Journal of Medicine,* 333, 1190–1195.

Saver, C. L. (1994). Decoding the ACLS algorithms. *American Journal of Nursing,* 94(1), 27–36.

Schulman, K. A., Mark, D. B., & Califf, R. M. (1998). Outcomes and costs within a disease management program for advanced congestive heart failure. *American Heart Journal,* 135(6), S285–S292.

Resources

American Heart Association, 7320 Greenville Ave., Dallas, TX 75231; http://www.americanheart.org/aha.html

Coronary Club, 9500 Euclid Ave., Cleveland, OH 44106

Heartlife, PO Box 54305, Atlanta, GA 30308

Heartmates: http://www.heartmates.com/cardiac.html

National Heart, Lung, and Blood Institute, National Institutes of Health, Building 31, Room 5A52, Bethesda, MD 20892; http://www.nhlbi.nih.gov

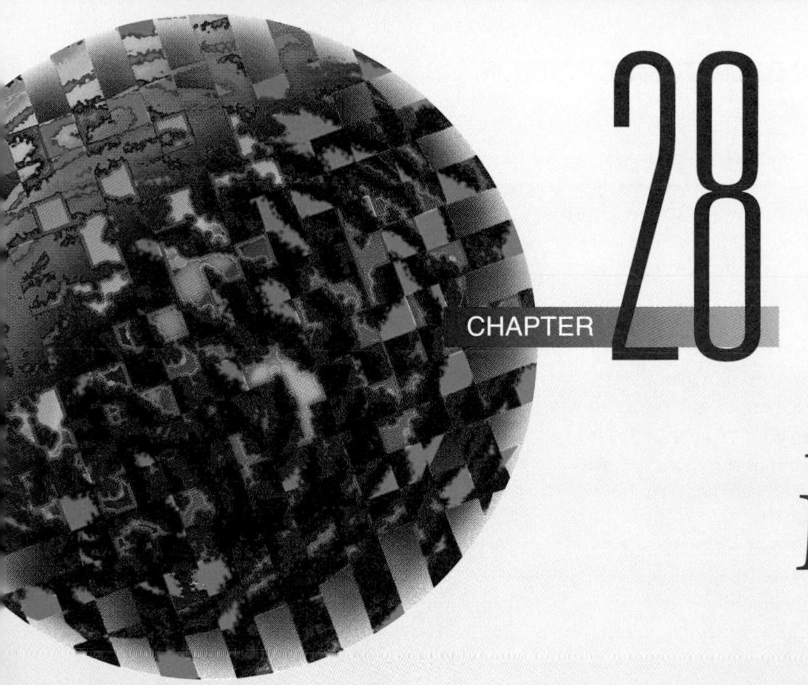

Assessment and Management of Patients With Vascular Disorders and Problems of Peripheral Circulation

Learning Objectives

On completion of this chapter, the learner will be able to:

1. Identify anatomic and physiologic factors that affect peripheral blood flow and tissue oxygenation.
2. Use appropriate parameters for assessment of peripheral circulation.
3. Use the nursing process as a framework of care for patients with circulatory insufficiency of the extremities.
4. Compare the various diseases of the arteries, their causes, pathologic and physiologic changes, clinical manifestations, management, and prevention.
5. Describe the prevention and management of venous thrombosis.
6. Compare the preventive management of venous insufficiency, leg ulcers, and varicose veins.
7. Use the nursing process as a framework of care for patients with leg ulcers.
8. Describe the relationship between lymphangitis and lymphedema.

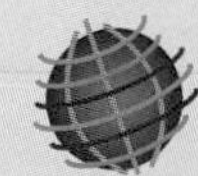

Adequate perfusion oxygenates and nourishes body tissues and depends in part on a properly functioning cardiovascular system. Adequate blood flow depends on the efficient pumping action of the heart, patent and responsive blood vessels, and adequate circulating blood volume. Nervous system activity, blood viscosity, and the metabolic needs of tissues influence the rate and hence the adequacy of blood flow.

GLOSSARY

anastomosis: a line of sutures joining two vessels

aneurysm: a localized sac or dilation of an artery formed at a weak point in the vessel wall

ankle–arm index (AAI) or ankle–brachial index (ABI): the ratio of the ankle systolic pressure to the arm systolic pressure; an objective measurement of arterial disease that allows quantification of the degree of stenosis

angioplasty: an invasive procedure that involves using a balloon-tipped catheter to dilate a stenotic area of a blood vessel

arteriosclerosis: diffuse process whereby the muscle fibers and the endothelial lining of the walls of small arteries and arterioles thicken

atherosclerosis: disease process that affects the intima of the large and medium-sized arteries; consists of the accumulation of lipids, calcium, blood components, carbohydrates, and fibrous tissue on the intimal layer of a large- or medium-sized artery

bruit: the sound produced by turbulent blood flow through an irregular, tortuous, stenotic, or dilated vessel

dissection: separation of the weakened elastic and fibromuscular elements in the medial layer of an artery

duplex ultrasound: combines B-mode–gray-scale imaging of tissue, organs, and blood vessels with capabilities of estimating velocity changes by use of a pulsed Doppler

intermittent claudication: a muscular, cramp-like pain in the extremities consistently reproduced with the same degree of exercise or activity and relieved by rest

international normalized ratio (INR): method of measuring anticoagulant levels, such as warfarin (Coumadin); devised to bring a universal application to the calibration of the system to monitor anticoagulation achieved by oral medications

ischemia: deficient blood supply

rest pain: persistent pain in the foot or digits when the patient is resting indicating a severe degree of arterial insufficiency

rubor: a reddish-blue discoloration of the extremities; indicative of severe peripheral arterial damage in vessels that remain dilated and unable to constrict

stenosis: a narrowing or constriction of a vessel

ANATOMIC AND PHYSIOLOGIC OVERVIEW

The vascular system consists of two interdependent systems: the right side of the heart pumps blood through the lungs to the pulmonary circulation, and the left side of the heart pumps blood to all other body tissues through the systemic circulation. The blood vessels in both systems channel the blood from the heart to the tissues and back to the heart. Contractions of the ventricles are the driving force that moves blood through the vascular systems.

Arteries distribute oxygenated blood from the left side of the heart to the tissues, whereas the veins carry deoxygenated blood from the tissues to the right side of the heart. Capillary vessels, located within the tissues, connect the arterial and venous systems and are the site of exchange of nutrients and metabolic wastes between the circulatory system and the tissues. Arterioles and venules immediately adjacent to the capillaries, together with the capillaries, make up the microcirculation (Fig. 28-1).

The lymphatic system complements the function of the circulatory system. Lymphatic vessels transport lymph (a fluid similar to plasma) and tissue fluids (containing smaller proteins, cells, and cellular debris) from the interstitial space to systemic veins.

Anatomy of the Vascular System

Arteries and Arterioles

Arteries are thick-walled structures that carry blood from the heart to the tissues. The aorta, which has a diameter of approximately 25 mm (1 in), gives rise to numerous branches, which in turn divide into smaller vessels, arteries, and arterioles, that measure about 4 mm (0.16 in) wide by the time they reach the tissues. Within the tissues, the vessels divide further, diminishing to approximately 30 μm in diameter; these vessels are called arterioles.

The walls of the arteries and arterioles are composed of three layers: the intima (an inner endothelial cell layer); the media (a middle layer of smooth elastic tissue); and the adventitia (an outer layer of connective tissue). The intima, a very thin layer, provides a smooth surface for contact with the flowing blood. The media makes up most of the vessel wall in the aorta and other large arteries of the body. This layer is composed chiefly of elastic and connective tissue fibers that give the vessels considerable strength and allow them to constrict and dilate to accommodate the blood ejected from the heart (stroke volume) and maintain an even, steady flow of blood. The adventitia is a layer of connective tissue that anchors the vessel to its surroundings. There is much less elastic tissue in the smaller arteries and arterioles, and the media in these vessels is composed primarily of smooth muscle.

Smooth muscle controls the diameter of the vessels by contracting and relaxing. Chemical, hormonal, and nervous system factors influence the activity of smooth muscle. Because arterioles can alter their diameter, thereby offering resistance to blood flow, they are often referred to as resistance vessels. Arterioles regulate the volume and pressure in the arterial system and the rate of blood flow to the capillaries. Because of the large amount of muscle, the walls of the arteries are relatively thick, accounting for approximately 25% of the total diameter of the artery. The walls of the arterioles account for approximately 67% of the total diameter of arterioles.

The intima and the inner third of the smooth muscle layer are in such close contact with the blood that the blood vessel receives its nourishment by direct diffusion. The adventitia and the outer media layers have a limited vascular system for nourishment and require their own blood supply to meet metabolic needs.

Capillaries

Capillary walls, which lack smooth muscle and adventitia, are composed of a single layer of endothelial cells. This thin-walled structure permits rapid and efficient transport of nutrients to the cells and removal of metabolic wastes. The diameter of capillaries ranges from 5 to 10 μm; this requires red blood cells to alter their shape to pass through these vessels. Changes in a capillary's diameter are passive and are influenced by contractile changes in the blood vessels that carry blood to and from a capillary. The

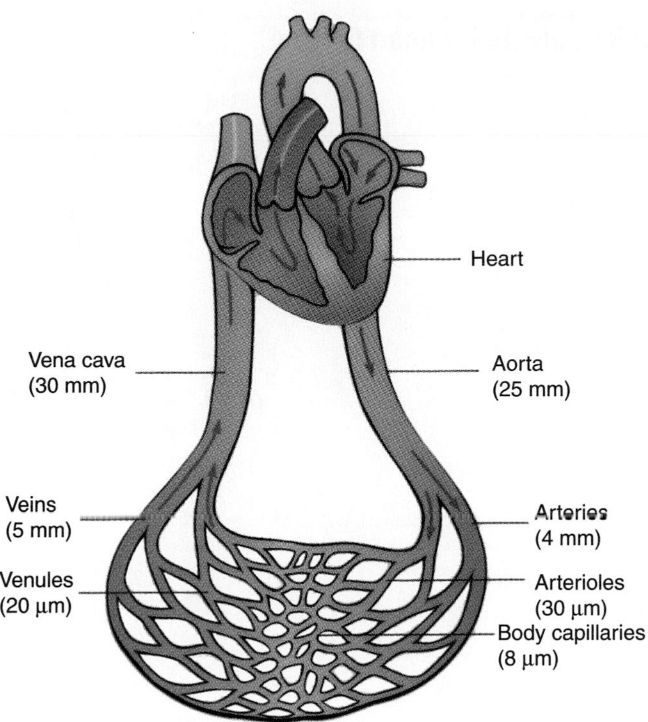

FIGURE 28•1 Systemic circulation. Oxygen-rich blood leaves the heart and goes through the aorta into the systemic arterial circulation until it reaches the capillaries, where the exchange of nutrients takes place. The deoxygenated blood returns to the heart by way of the venous system. Comparison of vessel size is demonstrated.

capillary's diameter also changes in response to chemical stimuli. In some tissues, a cuff of smooth muscle, called the precapillary sphincter, is located at the arteriolar end of the capillary and is responsible, along with the arteriole, for controlling capillary blood flow.

Some capillary beds, such as in the fingertips, contain arteriovenous anastomoses, through which blood passes directly from the arterial to the venous system. These vessels are believed to regulate heat exchange between the body and the external environment.

The distribution of capillaries throughout the tissues varies with the type of tissue. For example, skeletal tissue, which is metabolically active, has a denser capillary network than does cartilage, which is less active.

Veins and Venules

Capillaries join to form larger vessels called venules, which in turn join to form the veins. The venous system is therefore structurally analogous to the arterial system; venules correspond to arterioles, veins to arteries, and the vena cava to the aorta. Analogous types of vessels in the arterial and venous systems have approximately the same diameters (see Fig. 28-1).

The walls of the veins, in contrast to those of the arteries, are thinner and considerably less muscular. The wall of the average vein amounts to only 10% of the vein diameter, in contrast to 25% in the artery. The walls of a vein, like those of arteries, are composed of three layers; however, these layers are not as well defined.

The thin, less muscular structure of the vein wall allows these vessels to distend more than arteries. Greater distensibility and compliance permit large volumes of blood to be stored in the veins under low pressure. For this reason, veins are referred to as capacitance vessels. Approximately 75% of total blood volume is contained in the veins. The sympathetic nervous system, which innervates the vein musculature, can stimulate the veins to constrict (venoconstriction), thereby reducing venous volume and increasing the volume of blood in the general circulation.

Some veins, unlike arteries, are equipped with valves. In general, veins that transport blood against the force of gravity, as in the lower extremities, have one-way bicuspid valves that interrupt the column of blood to prevent blood from seeping backward as it is propelled toward the heart. Valves are composed of endothelial leaflets, the competency of which depends on the integrity of the vein wall.

Lymphatic Vessels

The lymphatic vessels are a complex network of thin-walled vessels similar to the blood capillaries. This network serves to collect lymphatic fluid from tissues and organs and to transport the fluid to the venous circulation. The lymphatic vessels converge into two main structures: the thoracic duct and the right lymphatic duct. These ducts empty into the junction of the subclavian and the internal jugular veins. The right lymphatic duct conveys lymph primarily from the right side of the head, neck, thorax, and upper arms. The thoracic duct conveys lymph from the remainder of the body. Peripheral lymphatic vessels join larger lymph vessels and pass through regional lymph nodes before entering the venous circulation. The lymph nodes play an important role in filtering foreign particles.

The lymphatic vessels are permeable to large molecules and provide the only means whereby interstitial proteins can return to the venous system. With muscular contraction, lymph vessels become distorted to create spaces between the endothelial cells, allowing protein and particles to enter. Muscular contraction of the lymphatic walls and surrounding tissues aids in propelling the lymph toward venous drainage points.

Function of the Vascular System

Circulatory Needs of Tissues

The amount of blood flow needed by body tissues constantly changes. The percentage of blood flow received by individual organs or tissues is determined by the rate of tissue metabolism, the availability of oxygen, and the function of the tissues (Table 28-1). When metabolic requirements increase, blood vessels dilate to increase the flow of oxygen and nutrients to the tissues. When metabolic needs decrease, vessels constrict and blood flow to the tissues decreases. Metabolic demands of tissues increase with physical activity or exercise, local heat application, fever, and infection. Reduced metabolic requirements of tissues accompany rest or decreased physical activity, local cold application, and cooling of the body. If the blood vessels fail to dilate in response to the need for increased blood flow, tissue **ischemia** (deficient blood supply to a body part) results. The mechanism by which blood vessels dilate and constrict to adjust for metabolic changes assumes that a normal arterial pressure is maintained.

As blood passes through tissue capillaries, oxygen is removed and carbon dioxide is added. The amount of oxygen extracted by each tissue is different. For example, the myocardium tends to extract about 50% of the oxygen from arterial blood in one pass through its capillary bed, whereas the kidneys extract only about 7% of the oxygen from the blood that passes through them. The

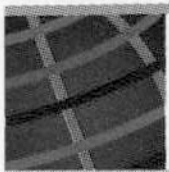

TABLE 28•1 **Blood Flow and Oxygen Consumption for Selected Human Organs**

		Blood Flow During Rest		Oxygen Usage During Rest	
Organ	Organ Weight (kg)	ORGAN BLOOD FLOW (ML/MIN)	% TOTAL CARDIAC OUTPUT	ORGAN O_2 USAGE (ML/MIN)	% TOTAL O_2 USAGE
Brain	1.4	750	14	45	18
Heart	0.3	250	5	25	10
Liver	1.5	1300	23	75	30
GI tract	2.5	1000			
Kidneys	0.3	1200	22	15	6
Muscle	35.0	1000	18	50	20
Skin	2.0	200	4	5	2
Remainder (eg, skeleton, bone marrow, fat, connective tissue)	27.0	800	14	35	14
TOTAL	70	6500	100	250	100

Folkow B. & Neil E. *Circulation.* New York: Oxford University Press.

average amount of oxygen removed collectively by all of the body tissues is about 25%. This means that the blood in the vena cavae contains about 25% less oxygen than aortic blood. This is known as the systemic arteriovenous oxygen difference. It increases when the amount of oxygen delivered to the tissues is decreased relative to their metabolic needs (see Table 28-1).

Blood Flow

Blood flow through the cardiovascular system always proceeds in the same direction: left side of the heart to the aorta, arteries, arterioles, capillaries, venules, veins, vena cavae, and finally to the right side of the heart. This unidirectional flow is caused by a pressure difference that exists between the arterial and venous systems. Because arterial pressure (approximately 100 mm Hg) is greater than venous pressure (approximately 4 mm Hg) and fluid always flows from an area of high pressure to an area of lower pressure, blood flows from the arterial to the venous system.

The pressure difference (ΔP) between the two ends of the vessel provides the impetus for the forward propulsion of blood. Impediments to blood flow offer the opposing force, which is known as resistance (R). Thus, the rate of blood flow is determined by dividing the pressure difference by the resistance:

$$\text{Flow rate} = \Delta P/R$$

This equation clearly shows that when resistance increases, a greater driving pressure is required to maintain the same degree of flow. In the body, an increase in driving pressure is accomplished by an increase in the force of contraction of the heart. If arterial resistance is chronically elevated, the myocardium hypertrophies (enlarges) to sustain the greater contractile force.

In most long smooth blood vessels, flow is laminar or streamlined, with blood in the center of the vessel moving slightly faster than the blood near the vessel walls. Laminar flow becomes turbulent when the blood flow rate increases, when blood viscosity increases, when the diameter of the vessel becomes greater than normal, or when segments of the vessel are narrowed or constricted. Turbulent blood flow creates a sound, called a **bruit**, that can be auscultated with a stethoscope.

Blood Pressure

See Chapters 23 and 29 for more information on physiology and measurement of blood pressure.

Capillary Filtration and Reabsorption

Fluid exchange across the capillary wall is continuous. This fluid, which has the same composition as plasma without the proteins, forms the interstitial fluid. The equilibrium between hydrostatic and osmotic forces of the blood and interstitium and capillary permeability govern the amount and direction of fluid movement across the capillary. Hydrostatic force is a driving pressure that is generated by the blood pressure. Osmotic pressure is the pulling force created by plasma proteins. Normally, the hydrostatic pressure at the arterial end of the capillary is relatively high compared with that at the venous end. This high pressure at the arterial end of the capillaries tends to drive fluid out of the capillary and into the tissue space. Osmotic pressure tends to pull fluid back into the capillary from the tissue space, but this osmotic force cannot overcome the high hydrostatic pressure at the arterial end of the capillary. At the venous end of the capillary, however, the osmotic force predominates over the low hydrostatic pressure, and there is a net reabsorption of fluid from the tissue space back into the capillary.

Except for a very small amount, the fluid that is filtered at the arterial end of the capillary bed is reabsorbed at the venous end. The excess filtered fluid enters the lymphatic circulation. These processes of filtration, reabsorption, and lymph formation aid in maintaining tissue fluid volume and removing tissue waste and debris. Under normal conditions, capillary permeability remains constant.

Under certain abnormal conditions, the fluid filtered out of the capillaries may greatly exceed the amounts reabsorbed and carried away by the lymphatic vessels. This imbalance can result from damage to capillary walls and subsequent increased permeability, obstruction of lymphatic drainage, elevation of venous pressure, or decrease in plasma protein osmotic force. The accumulation of fluid that results from these processes is known as edema.

Hemodynamic Resistance

The most important factor that determines resistance in the vascular system is the vessel radius. Small changes in vessel radius lead to large changes in resistance. The predominant sites of change in the caliber or width of blood vessels, and therefore in resistance, are the arterioles and the precapillary sphincter. Peripheral vascular resistance is the opposition to blood flow provided by the blood vessels. Poiseuille's law provides the method by which resistance can be calculated:

$$R = \frac{8\theta L}{\pi r^4}$$

where R = resistance, r = radius of the vessel, L = length of the vessel, θ = viscosity of the blood, and 8/π = a constant. This equation shows that the resistance is proportional to the viscosity or thickness of the blood and the length of the vessel, but inversely proportional to the fourth power of the vessel radius.

Under normal conditions, blood viscosity and vessel length do not change significantly. Therefore, these factors do not usually play an important role in blood flow. A large increase in hematocrit, however, may increase blood viscosity and reduce capillary blood flow.

Peripheral Vascular Regulating Mechanisms

Because the metabolic needs of body tissues, even at rest, are continuously changing, an integrated and coordinated regulatory system is necessary so that blood flow to individual areas is maintained in proportion to the needs of that area. As might be expected, this regulatory mechanism is complex and consists of central nervous system influences, circulating hormones and chemicals, and independent activity of the arterial wall itself.

Sympathetic (adrenergic) nervous system activity, mediated by the hypothalamus, is the most important factor in regulating the caliber, and thus the blood flow, of peripheral blood vessels. All vessels are innervated by the sympathetic nervous system except the capillary and precapillary sphincters. Stimulation of the sympathetic nervous system causes vasoconstriction. The neurotransmitter responsible for sympathetic vasoconstriction is norepinephrine. Sympathetic activation occurs in response to physiologic and psychological stressors. Removal of sympathetic activity by medications or sympathectomy results in vasodilation.

Other hormonal substances also affect peripheral vascular resistance. Epinephrine, released from the adrenal medulla, acts like norepinephrine in constricting peripheral blood vessels in most tissue beds. In low concentrations, however, epinephrine causes vasodilation in skeletal muscles, the heart, and the brain. Angiotensin, a potent substance formed from the interaction of renin (synthesized by the kidney) and a circulating serum protein, stimulates arterial constriction. Although the amount of angiotensin concentrated in the blood is usually small, its profound vasoconstrictor effects are important in certain abnormal states, such as congestive heart failure and hypovolemia.

Alterations in local blood flow are influenced by various circulating substances that have vasoactive properties. Potent vasodilators include histamine, bradykinin, prostaglandin, and certain muscle metabolites. A reduction in available oxygen and nutrients and changes in local pH also affect local blood flow. Serotonin, a substance liberated from platelets that aggregate at the site of vessel wall damage, constricts arterioles. The application of heat to parts of the body surface causes local vasodilation, whereas the application of cold causes vasoconstriction.

Pathophysiology of the Vascular System

Reduced blood flow through peripheral blood vessels characterizes all peripheral vascular diseases. The physiologic effects of altered blood flow depend on the extent to which tissue demands exceed the supply of oxygen and nutrients available. If tissue needs are high, even modestly reduced blood flow may be inadequate to maintain tissue integrity. Then, tissues fall prey to ischemia (deficient blood supply), become malnourished, and ultimately die if adequate blood flow is not restored.

Pump Failure

Inadequate peripheral blood flow occurs whenever the heart's pumping action becomes inefficient. Left-sided heart failure causes an accumulation of blood in the lungs and a reduction in forward flow or cardiac output, which results in inadequate arterial blood flow to the tissues. Right-sided heart failure causes systemic venous congestion and a reduction in forward flow (see Chap. 27).

Alterations in Blood and Lymphatic Vessels

Intact, patent, and responsive blood vessels are necessary to deliver adequate amounts of oxygen to tissues and to remove metabolic wastes. Arteries can become obstructed by atherosclerotic plaque, a thrombus, or an embolus. Arteries can become damaged or obstructed as a result of chemical or mechanical trauma, infections or inflammatory processes, vasospastic disorders, and congenital malformations. A sudden arterial occlusion causes profound and often irreversible tissue ischemia and tissue death. When arterial occlusions develop gradually, there is less risk for sudden tissue death because collateral circulation has an opportunity to develop.

Venous blood flow can be reduced by a thrombus obstructing the vein, by incompetent venous valves, or by a reduction in the effectiveness of the pumping action of surrounding muscles. A decrease in venous blood flow results in an increase in venous pressure, a subsequent rise in capillary hydrostatic pressure, a net filtration of fluid out of the capillaries into the interstitial space, and subsequent edema. Edematous tissues cannot receive adequate nutrition from the blood and consequently are more susceptible to breakdown or injury and to infection. Obstruction of lymphatic vessels also results in edema. Lymphatic vessels can become obstructed by tumor or by damage resulting from mechanical trauma or inflammatory processes.

GERONTOLOGIC CONSIDERATIONS

Aging produces changes in the walls of the blood vessels that affect the transport of oxygen and nutrients to the tissues. The intima thickens as a result of cellular proliferation and fibrosis. Elastin fibers of the media become calcified, thin, and fragmented, and collagen accumulates in both the intima and the media. These changes cause the vessels to stiffen, which results in increased peripheral resistance, impaired blood flow, and increased left ventricular workload.

Circulatory Insufficiency of the Extremities

Although many types of peripheral vascular diseases exist, most result in ischemia and produce some of the same symptoms: pain, skin changes, diminished pulse, and possible edema. The type and severity of symptoms depend in part on the type, stage, and extent of the disease process as well as the speed with which the disorder develops. Table 28-2 highlights the distinguishing features of arterial and venous insufficiency. For the purpose of the chapter, peripheral vascular disease will be categorized as arterial, venous, and lymphatic disorders.

ASSESSMENT

Health History and Clinical Manifestations

A muscular, cramp-type pain in the extremities consistently reproduced with the same degree of exercise or activity and relieved by rest is experienced by patients with peripheral arterial insufficiency.

Intermittent Claudication

Pain, referred to as **intermittent claudication**, is due to the inability of the arterial system to provide adequate blood flow to the tissues in the face of increased demands for nutrients during exercise. As the tissues are forced to complete the energy cycle without the nutrients, muscle metabolites and lactic acid are produced. Pain is experienced as the metabolites aggravate the nerve endings of the surrounding tissue. Usually about 50% of the arterial lumen or 75% of the cross-sectional area must be obstructed before intermittent claudication is experienced. When the patient rests, and thereby decreases the metabolic needs of the muscles, the pain subsides. The progression of the arterial disease can be monitored by documenting the amount of exercise or the distance a patient can walk before pain is produced. Persistent pain in the forefoot when the patient is resting indicates a severe degree of arterial insufficiency and a critical state of ischemia. Known as **rest pain**, this discomfort is often worse at night and may interfere with sleep. This pain frequently requires that the extremity be lowered to a dependent position to improve perfusion pressure to the distal tissues.

The site of arterial disease can be deduced from the location of claudication, because pain occurs in muscle groups below the disease. As a general rule, the pain of intermittent claudication occurs one joint level below the disease process. Calf pain may accompany reduced blood flow through the superficial femoral or popliteal artery, whereas pain in the hip or buttock may result from reduced blood flow in the abdominal aorta or common iliac or hypogastric arteries.

Changes in Skin Appearance and Temperature

Adequate blood flow warms the extremities and gives them a rosy coloring. Inadequate blood flow results in cool and pale extremities. Further reduction of blood flow to these tissues, which occurs when the extremity is elevated, for example, results in an even whiter or more blanched appearance (pallor). A reddish-blue discoloration of the extremities (**rubor**) may be observed within 20 seconds to 2 minutes after the extremity is dependent. Rubor suggests severe peripheral arterial damage in which vessels that cannot constrict remain dilated. Even with rubor present, the extremity begins to turn pale with elevation. Cyanosis, a bluish tint on the skin, is manifested when the amount of oxygenated hemoglobin contained in the blood is reduced.

Additional changes resulting from a chronically reduced nutrient supply include loss of hair, brittle nails, dry or scaling skin, atrophy, and ulcerations. Edema may be apparent either bilaterally or unilaterally and is related to the affected extremity's chronically dependent position because of severe rest pain. Gangrenous changes appear after prolonged severe ischemia and represent tissue necrosis. In elderly patients, gangrene may be the first sign of disease, because it is common for patients to adjust their lifestyle to accommodate the limitations imposed by the disease. Circulation is decreased, but this is not apparent to the patient until trauma occurs. At this point, gangrene develops when minimal arterial flow is impaired further by edema formation resulting from the traumatic event.

Pulses

Determining the presence or absence, as well as the quality, of peripheral pulses is important in assessing the status of peripheral arterial circulation (Fig. 28-2). Absence of a pulse may indicate

TABLE 28•2 Characteristics of Arterial and Venous Insufficiency

Characteristic	Arterial	Venous
Pain	Intermittent claudication to sharp, unrelenting, constant	Aching, cramping
Pulses	Diminished or absent	Present, but may be difficult to palpate through edema
Skin characteristics	Dependent rubor—elevational pallor of foot, dry, shiny skin, cool-to-cold temperature, loss of hair over toes and dorsum of foot, nails thickened and ridged	Pigmentation in gaitor area (area of medial and lateral malleolus), skin thickened and tough, may be reddish blue, associated dermatitis frequent
Ulcer characteristics		
Location	Tip of toes, toe webs, heel or other pressure areas if confined to bed	Medial malleolus; infrequently lateral malleolus or anterior tibial area
Pain	Very painful	Minimal pain if superficial
Depth of ulcer	Deep, often involving joint space	Superficial
Shape	Circular	Irregular border
Ulcer base	Pale to black and dry gangrene	Granulation tissue—beefy red to yellow fibrinous in chronic long-term ulcer
Edema	Minimal unless extremity kept in dependent position constantly to relieve pain	Moderate to severe

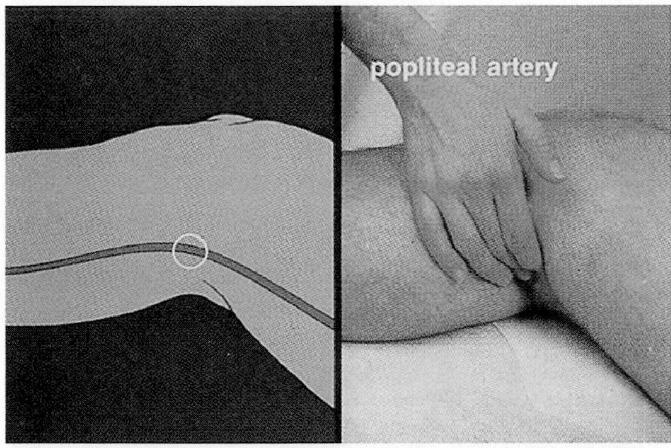

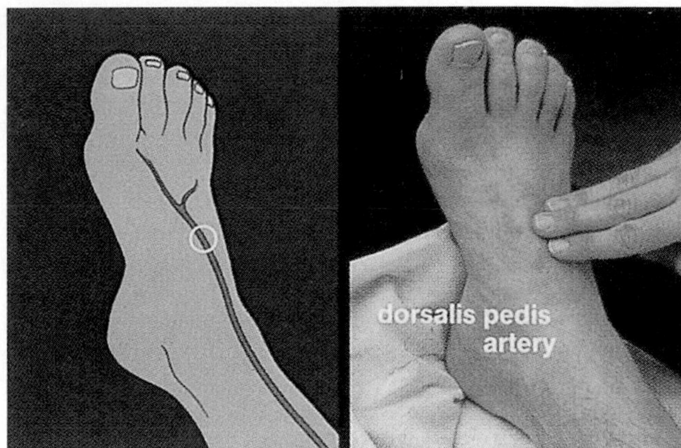

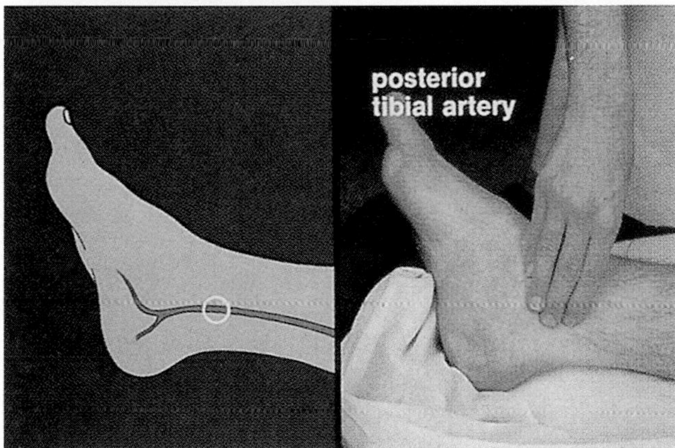

FIGURE 28•2 Assessing peripheral pulses. (*Left*) Popliteal pulse. (*Right*) Dorsalis pedis pulse. (*Bottom*) Posterior tibial pulse.

that the site of **stenosis** (narrowing or constriction) is proximal to that location. Occlusive arterial disease impairs blood flow and can reduce or obliterate palpable pulsations in the extremities. Pulses should be palpated bilaterally and simultaneously, comparing both sides for symmetry in rate, rhythm, and quality.

Gerontologic Considerations

In elderly people, symptoms of peripheral arterial disease may be more pronounced than in younger people because of the condition's duration and coexisting chronic disease. Intermittent claudication may occur after walking only a few short blocks or after walking up a slight incline. Any prolonged pressure on the foot can cause pressure areas that become ulcerated, infected, and gangrenous. The outcomes of arterial insufficiency in the elderly person include reduced mobility and activity, and loss of independence.

DIAGNOSTIC EVALUATION

In identifying and diagnosing the various abnormalities affecting the vascular structures (arteries, veins, and lymphatics), various tests may be performed.

Doppler Ultrasound Flow Studies

Palpating pulses is subjective, and the examiner may mistake his or her own pulse for that of the patient. To prevent this, the examiner should use light touch and avoid using only the index finger for palpation, because this finger has the strongest arterial pulsation of all the fingers. When pulses cannot be reliably palpated, use of a microphone-like hand-held Doppler ultrasound device (called a transducer or probe) may be helpful in detecting and assessing peripheral flow.

A continuous-wave (CW) Doppler ultrasound device may be used to hear (insonnate) the blood flow in vessels when pulses cannot be palpated. This hand-held device emits a continuous signal through the patient's tissues. These signals are reflected by (echo off) the moving blood cells and are received by the device. The filtered-output Doppler signal is then applied to a loudspeaker or headphones, where it can be heard for interpretation. Because a CW Doppler emits a continuous signal, all vascular structures in the path of the sound beam are insonnated. Therefore, differentiating arterial from venous flow and detecting the site of a stenosis may be difficult. The depth at which blood flow can be detected by Doppler is determined by the frequency (in megahertz [MHz]) it generates. The lower the frequency, the deeper the tissue penetration; a 5- to 10-MHz probe may be used to evaluate the peripheral arteries.

To evaluate the lower extremities, the patient is placed in a supine position with the head of bed elevated 20 degrees to 30 degrees; the legs are externally rotated, if possible, to permit adequate access to the medial malleolus. Acoustic gel is applied to the patient's skin to permit uniform transmission of the ultrasound wave (electrocardiogram gel is not used because it contains sodium, which may dissolve the epoxy that covers the transducer's tip). The tip of the Doppler transducer is positioned at a 45- to 60-degree angle over the expected location of the artery and angled slowly to identify arterial blood flow. Excessive pressure is avoided because severely diseased arteries will collapse with even minimal pressure.

The equipment can detect blood flow in advanced arterial disease states, especially if collateral circulation has developed, so identifying a signal only documents the presence of blood flow. However, it is clinically relevant to notify the primary care provider of the absence of a signal when one was detected during a previous examination.

The continuous wave (CW) Doppler device (Fig. 28-3) is more useful as a clinical tool when combined with ankle blood pressures, which are used to determine the **ankle–arm index** (AAI) or **ankle–brachial index** (ABI). The ABI is the ratio of the ankle systolic blood pressure to the arm systolic blood pressure. It is an objective indicator of arterial disease that allows one to quantify the degree of stenosis. With increasing degrees of arterial narrowing, there is a progressive decrease in systolic pressure distal to the involved sites.

The first step in determining the ABI is to have the patient rest in a supine position for at least 5 minutes (not seated). Then an appropriate-sized blood pressure cuff is applied to the patient's ankle above the malleolus (typically a 10-cm cuff). After identifying an arterial signal at the posterior tibial and dorsalis pedis arteries, the technician obtains systolic ankle pressures in both feet. Diastolic pressures cannot be measured with a Doppler device. If pressure in the arteries cannot be measured, pressure can be measured in the peroneal artery, which can also be assessed at the ankle (Fig. 28-4).

Next, the Doppler device may be used to measure brachial pressures in both arms. Both arms are evaluated because the patient may have an asymptomatic stenosis in the subclavian artery, causing brachial pressure on the affected side to be 20 mm Hg or more lower than systemic pressure. The abnormally low pressure should not be used for assessment.

To calculate ABI, the highest ankle pressure for each foot is divided by the higher of the two brachial pressures. To compute the ABI for a patient with right brachial, 160 mm Hg; left brachial, 120 mm Hg; right posterior tibial, 80 mm Hg; right dorsalis pedis, 60 mm Hg; left posterior tibial, 100 mm Hg; and left dorsalis pedis, 120 mm Hg, the highest tibial pressure for each ankle (80 for the right, 120 for the left) would be divided by the highest brachial pressure (160). The right ABI is 0.50, the left ABI 0.75. See Chart 28-1 for more information.

In general, systolic pressure in the ankle of a healthy person is the same or slightly higher than the brachial systolic pressure, resulting in an ABI of about 1.0 (no arterial insufficiency). Patients with claudication usually have an ABI of 0.50 to 0.95 (mild to

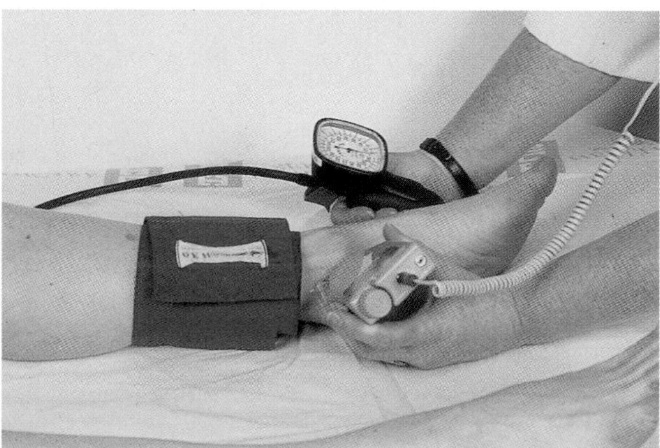

FIGURE 28•3 Continuous-wave (CW) Doppler ultrasound detects blood flow in peripheral vessels. Combined with computation of ankle or arm pressures, this diagnostic technique helps health care providers characterize the nature of peripheral vascular disease. Photo with permission from Cantwell-Gab, K. (1996). Identifying chronic PAD. *American Journal of Nursing, 96*(7), 40–46.

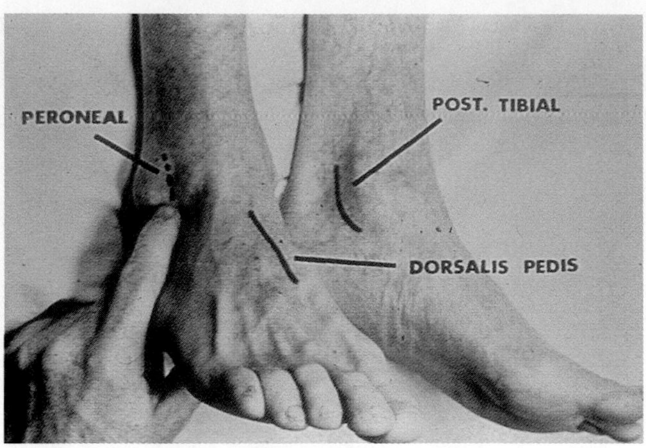

FIGURE 28•4 Location of peroneal artery; lateral malleolus. Photo with permission from Cantwell-Gab, K. (1996). Identifying chronic PAD. *American Journal of Nursing, 96*(7), 40–46.

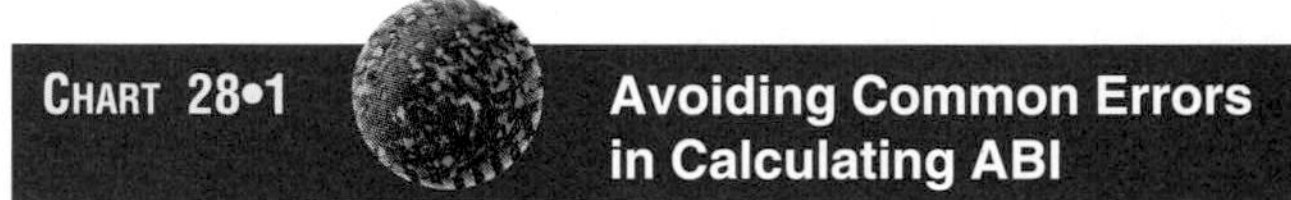

CHART 28•1 Avoiding Common Errors in Calculating ABI

Take the following precautions to ensure an accurate ABI calculation:

- *Use the correctly sized blood pressure cuffs.* To obtain accurate blood pressure measurements, use a cuff with a bladder that is 20% wider than the diameter of the patient's limb.
- *Document the blood pressure cuff sizes used on the nursing plan of care* (for example, "12-cm BP cuff used for brachial pressures; 10-cm BP cuff used for ankle pressures"). This minimizes the risk of shift-to-shift discrepancies in ABIs.
- *Use sufficient blood pressure cuff inflation.* To ensure complete closure of the artery and the most accurate measurements, inflate cuffs 20 to 30 mm Hg beyond the point at which the last arterial signal is detected.
- *Do not deflate blood pressure cuffs too rapidly.* Try to maintain a deflation rate of 2 to 4 mm Hg/second for patients without arrhythmias and 2 mm Hg/second or slower for patients with arrhythmias. Deflating the cuff more rapidly than that may cause you to miss the patient's highest pressure and record an erroneous (low) blood pressure measurement.
- *Be suspicious of arterial pressures recorded at less than 40 mm Hg.* This may mean the venous signal has been mistaken for the arterial signal. If you measure arterial pressure, which is normally 120 mm Hg at below 40 mm Hg, ask a colleague to double-check your findings before recording this as an arterial pressure.
- *Suspect medial calcific sclerosis anytime you calculate an ABI of 1.3 or greater or measure ankle pressure at more than 300 mm Hg.* This condition which is associated with diabetes mellitus, chronic renal failure, and hyperparathyroidism produces falsely elevated ankle pressures by making the vessels noncompressible.

From Cantwell-Gab, K. [1996]. Identifying chronic PAD. *American Journal of Nursing, 96*[7]; 40–46, with permission.)

moderate insufficiency); patients with ischemic rest pain have an ABI of less than 0.50, and patients with severe ischemia or tissue loss have an ABI of 0.25 or less.

Exercise Testing

Exercise testing is used to determine how long a patient can walk and to measure the ankle systolic blood pressure in response to walking. The patient walks on a treadmill at 1.5 mph with a 10% incline for a maximum of 5 minutes. Most patients can complete the test unless they have severe cardiac, pulmonary, or orthopedic problems. A normal response to the test is little or no drop in ankle systolic pressure after exercise. In a patient with true claudication, however, ankle pressure drops. Combining this hemodynamic information with the walking time helps the physician determine whether intervention is necessary.

Duplex Ultrasound

Duplex ultrasound scanning involves B-mode–gray-scale imaging of the tissue, organs, and blood vessels (both arterial and venous) and permits the estimation of velocity changes by use of a pulsed Doppler (Fig. 28-5). Color flow techniques, which can identify vessels, may be used as well to shorten the examination time. The procedure helps determine the level and extent of disease and is universally used to evaluate the venous system. The technique makes it possible to image and assess blood flow, evaluate the runoff status of the distal vessels, localize disease (stenosis versus occlusion), and determine anatomic morphology as well as the hemodynamic significance of plaque causing stenosis. Duplex ultrasound findings help in planning therapy and monitoring its outcomes. Moreover, the test is noninvasive and usually requires no patient preparation. The equipment is portable, making it useful anywhere for initial diagnosis or follow-up evaluations.

Computed Tomography (CT)

CT scanning provides cross-sectional images of soft tissue and can identify the area of volume changes to an extremity and the compartment where changes take places. CT of a lymphedematous arm or leg, for example, demonstrates a characteristic honeycomb pattern in the subcutaneous tissue.

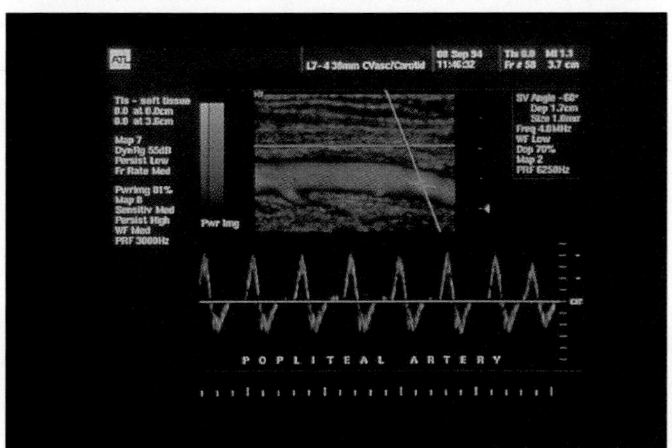

FIGURE 28•5 Color flow duplex image of popliteal artery with normal triphasic Doppler flow.

In spiral (also called volumetric) CT, the scan head moves circumferentially around the patient as the patient passes through the scanner, thus creating a series of overlapping images that are connected to one another in a continuous spiral (Verta & Verta, 1998). Using computer software, the slicelike images are reconstructed into three-dimensional images that can be rotated and viewed from multiple angles. Scan times are short; however, the patient is exposed to x-rays, and contrast agent usually must be injected to adequately visualize the blood vessels.

CT Angiography

In CT angiography, a spiral CT scanner and rapid intravenous infusion of contrast agent are used to image very thin (1-mm) sections of the target area; the results are configured in three dimensions so that the image closely resembles a regular angiogram (Verta & Verta, 1998). CT angiography shows the aorta and main visceral arteries better than it shows smaller branch vessels. Scan times are usually between 20 and 30 seconds. However, the large volume of contrast agent required limits the usefulness of this study in patients with sensitivity to contrast or with significantly impaired renal function.

Magnetic Resonance Angiography

Magnetic resonance angiography is performed with a standard magnetic resonance imaging scanner but with image-processing software specifically programmed to isolate the blood vessels. The images are reconstructed to resemble a standard angiogram, but because the images are reassembled in three dimensions, they can be rotated and viewed from multiple angles. Because no contrast agent is necessary, this study is useful in patients with poor renal function or contrast agent sensitivity. Scan time is long and motion artifacts are common; this restricts the use of the test to relatively short segments of the vascular system (Verta & Verta, 1998).

Angiography

An arteriogram produced by angiography may be used to confirm the diagnosis of occlusive arterial disease when considering surgery or other interventions. The procedure involves injecting a radiopaque contrast agent directly into the vascular system to visualize the vessels. The location of a vascular obstruction or an **aneurysm** (abnormal dilation of a blood vessel) and the collateral circulation can be demonstrated. Usually patients experience a temporary sensation of warmth as the contrast agent is injected. Local irritation may occur at the injection site as well. Infrequently, a patient may have an immediate or delayed allergic reaction to the iodine contained in the contrast agent. Manifestations include dyspnea, nausea and vomiting, sweating, tachycardia, and numbness of the extremities. Any such reaction must be reported at once; treatment may include the administration of epinephrine (adrenaline), antihistamines, or corticosteroids. Additional risks include vessel injury, bleeding, and stroke.

Lumbar Sympathetic Block

A lumbar sympathetic block is rarely used today but may be performed to evaluate peripheral circulation. An injection of a local anesthetic is made into the lumbar epidural space to block the sympathetic nerves to the legs. Because the sympathetic nerves control the tension in the muscles of the blood vessels, blocking these nerves should produce vasodilation and increased temperature in the legs. Because atherosclerotic vessels are incapable of vasodilation, there is either no increase in the temperature in the legs or only a slight increase. This test helps determine whether sympathectomy (interruption of afferent pathways in the sympathetic division of the autonomic nervous system) would benefit a patient with impaired circulation of the legs. Sympathectomy eliminates vasospasm and improves peripheral blood flow. Sympathectomy may be used if there are no other surgical options available and in cases of reflex sympathetic dystrophy. Reflex sympathetic dystrophy is a form of causalgic (intense burning) pain. This pain may be caused by ischemic damage to peripheral nerves after delayed revascularization, or it may follow inadvertent injury during surgery.

Air Plethysmography

Named for the standardized air chambers that fit around the lower leg and that are calibrated after being filled with a standard amount of air, air plethysmography quantifies venous reflux and calf muscle pump ejection. Changes in volume are measured with the patient's legs elevated, with the patient supine and standing, and after the patient performs toe-ups. Air plethysmography provides information about venous filling time, functional venous volume, ejected volume, and residual volume and is useful in evaluating patients with suspected valvular incompetence or chronic venous insufficiency.

Contrast Phlebography

Also known as venography, contrast phlebography involves injecting radiographic contrast media into the venous system through a dorsal foot vein. When a thrombus exists, an x-ray image will disclose an unfilled segment of vein in an otherwise completely filled vein. Injection of the contrast agent may cause a brief but painful inflammation of the vein. The test is generally performed if the patient is to undergo thrombolytic therapy, but duplex ultrasound is now accepted as the gold standard for diagnosing venous thrombosis.

Lymphangiography

Lymphangiography affords a means of detecting lymph node involvement by metastatic carcinoma, lymphoma, or infection in sites that are otherwise inaccessible to the examiner except by surgery. In this test, a lymphatic vessel in each foot (or hand) is injected with contrast agent. A series of x-rays are taken at the conclusion of the injection, 24 hours later, and periodically thereafter, as indicated. The failure to opacify subcutaneous collectors and the persistence of contrast agent in the tissue for days afterward contribute to a diagnosis of lymphedema.

Lymphoscintigraphy

Lymphoscintigraphy is a reliable alternative to lymphangiography. A radioactive-labeled colloid is injected subcutaneously in the second interdigital space. The extremity is then exercised to facilitate the uptake of the colloid by the lymphatic system. Serial images then are obtained at preset intervals. No adverse reactions have been reported.

MANAGEMENT OF ARTERIAL DISORDERS

Arteriosclerosis and Atherosclerosis

Arteriosclerosis is the most common disease of the arteries; it literally means "hardening of the arteries." It is a diffuse process whereby the muscle fibers and the endothelial lining of the walls of small arteries and arterioles become thickened. **Atherosclerosis** involves a different process, affecting the intima of the large and medium-sized arteries. These changes consist of the accumulation of lipids, calcium, blood components, carbohydrates, and fibrous tissue on the intimal layer of the artery. These accumulations are referred to as atheromas or plaques.

Although the pathologic processes of arteriosclerosis and atherosclerosis differ, rarely does one occur without the other, and thus the terms are often used interchangeably. Because atherosclerosis is a generalized disease of the arteries, when it is present in the extremities atherosclerosis is usually present elsewhere in the body.

Pathophysiology

The most common direct results of atherosclerosis in arteries include narrowing (stenosis) of the lumen, obstruction by thrombosis, aneurysm, ulceration, and rupture. Its indirect results are malnutrition and the subsequent fibrosis of the organs that the sclerotic arteries supply with blood. All actively functioning tissue cells require an abundant supply of nutrients and oxygen and are sensitive to any reduction in the supply of these nutrients. If such reductions are severe and permanent, these cells undergo ischemic necrosis (death of cells due to deficient blood flow) and are replaced by fibrous tissue, which requires much less nutrition.

Atherosclerosis can develop at any point in the body, but there are sites that are more vulnerable, typically bifurcation or branch areas. In the lower extremity, these include the distal abdominal aorta, the common iliac arteries, the orifice of the superficial femoral and profunda femoris arteries, and the superficial femoral artery in the adductor canal. The patterns distal to the knee are less distinct.

Although many theories exist about the development of atherosclerosis, no single theory fully explains the pathogenesis; however, parts of several theories have been combined into the reaction-to-injury theory. According to this theory, vascular endothelial cell injury results from prolonged hemodynamic forces, such as shearing stresses and turbulent flow, radiation, chemicals, or chronic hyperlipidemia in the arterial system. Injury to the endothelium increases the aggregation of platelets and monocytes at the site of the injury. Smooth muscle cells migrate and proliferate, allowing a matrix of collagen and elastic fibers to form. It may be that there is no single cause or mechanism for the development of atherosclerosis; rather, multiple processes may be involved.

Morphologically, atherosclerotic lesions are of two types: fatty streaks and fibrous plaque. Fatty streaks are yellow and smooth, protrude slightly into the lumen of the artery, and are composed of lipids and elongated smooth muscle cells. These lesions have been found in the arteries of people of all age groups, including infants. It is not clear whether fatty streaks predispose the person to the formation of fibrous plaques or whether they are reversible. They do not usually cause clinical symptoms.

The fibrous plaque characteristic of atherosclerosis is composed of smooth muscle cells, collagen fibers, plasma components, and lipids. It is white to whitish-yellow and protrudes in

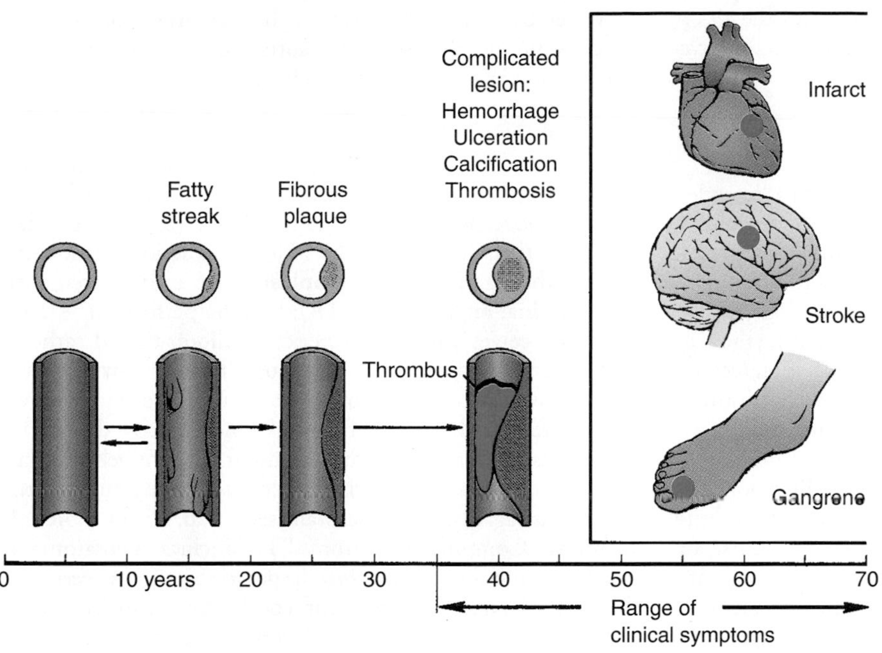

FIGURE 28•6 Schematic concept of the progression of atherosclerosis. Fatty streaks constitute one of the earliest lesions of atherosclerosis. Many fatty streaks regress, whereas others progress to fibrous plaques and eventually to atheroma, which may be complicated by hemorrhage, ulceration, calcification, or thrombosis and may produce myocardial infarction, stroke, or gangrene.

varying degrees into the arterial lumen, at times completely obstructing it. These plaques are found predominantly in the abdominal aorta and the coronary, popliteal, and internal carotid arteries. This plaque is believed to be an irreversible lesion (Fig. 28-6). Gradual narrowing of the arterial lumen as the disease process progresses stimulates the development of collateral circulation (Fig. 28-7). Collateral circulation consists of preexisting vessels that enlarge to reroute blood flow in the presence of a hemodynamically significant stenosis or occlusion. Collateral flow allows continued perfusion to the tissues beyond the arterial obstruction, but it is often inadequate to meet imposed metabolic demand, and ischemia results.

Lumbar
Inferior mesenteric
Superior hemorrhoidal
Middle hemorrhoidal
Inferior hemorrhoidal

FIGURE 28•7 Development of channels for collateral blood flow in response to occlusion of the right common iliac artery and the terminal aortic bifurcation.

Risk Factors

Many risk factors are associated with atherosclerosis. Although it is not completely clear whether modification of these risk factors prevents the development of cardiovascular disease, evidence indicates that it may slow the disease process. Some risk factors, such as age or gender, cannot be modified. However, some think that genetic factors can be modified indirectly by altering other risk factors.

Smoking may be one of the strongest risk factors in the development of atherosclerotic lesions. Nicotine decreases blood flow to the extremities and increases heart rate and blood pressure by stimulating the sympathetic nervous system, causing vasoconstriction. In addition, it increases the chances of clot formation by increasing the aggregation of platelets. By combining more readily with the hemoglobin, carbon monoxide deprives the tissues of oxygen. The number of cigarettes smoked is directly related to the

Risk Factors for **ATHEROSCLEROSIS**

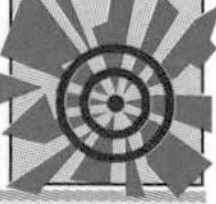

Controllable
Diet
High blood pressure
Diabetes (which speeds the atherosclerotic process by thickening the basement membranes of both the large and small vessels)
Stress
Sedentary lifestyle
Smoking

Not Controllable
Age
Gender

extent of the disease. Cessation of smoking reduces the risks. Many other factors such as obesity, stress, and lack of exercise have been identified as contributing to the disease process.

Prevention

Because a high-fat diet is suspected of contributing to atherosclerosis and because intermittent claudication is a sign of generalized atherosclerosis and may be a marker of occult coronary artery disease, it is reasonable to measure serum cholesterol to begin prevention efforts. Approximately 39% of the calories ingested by those living in the United States are from fats. To reduce the risk of cardiovascular disease, the American Heart Association recommends reducing the amount of fat ingested in the diet, substituting unsaturated fats for saturated fats, and decreasing cholesterol intake to no more than 300 mg daily.

Certain medications combined with dietary modification and exercise are being used to reduce blood lipid levels. There is limited evidence that these medications will alter the course of peripheral arterial disease, but they may reduce the mortality rate from cardiovascular disease. Several classes of medication are used to prevent atherosclerosis: bile acid sequestrants (cholestyramine or colestipol), nicotinic acid, statins (atorvastatin, lovastatin, pravastatin, and simvastatin), fibric acids (gemfibrozil), lipophilic substances (probucol), and estrogen replacement therapy. Patients receiving long-term therapy with these medications require close medical supervision.

Hypertension, which may accelerate the rate at which atherosclerotic lesions form in high-pressure vessels, can lead to stroke, ischemic renal disease, severe peripheral arterial disease, or coronary artery disease. The use of antihypertensive medication reduces the incidence of these diseases.

Although no single risk factor has been identified as the primary contributor to the development of atherosclerotic cardiovascular disease, it is clear that the greater the number of risk factors, the greater the likelihood of developing the disease. Therefore, the elimination of all controllable risk factors, particularly smoking, is strongly recommended.

Clinical Manifestations

The clinical signs and symptoms resulting from atherosclerosis depend on the organ or tissue affected. Coronary atherosclerosis (heart disease), angina, and acute myocardial infarction are discussed in Chapter 25. Cerebrovascular diseases, including transient cerebral ischemic attacks and stroke, are discussed in Chapter 59. Atherosclerosis of the aorta, including aneurysm, and atherosclerotic lesions of the extremities are discussed later in this chapter. Renovascular disease (renal artery stenosis and end-stage renal disease), including hypertension, is discussed in Chapter 41.

Medical Management

The traditional medical management of atherosclerosis involves modification of risk factors, a controlled exercise program to improve circulation and increase the functioning capacity of the circulation, medication, and interventional or surgical graft procedures.

SURGICAL MANAGEMENT

Vascular surgical procedures are divided into two groups: inflow procedures that provide blood supply from the aorta into the femoral artery, and outflow procedures that provide blood supply to vessels below the femoral artery. Inflow surgical procedures are discussed under diseases of the aorta, outflow procedures in the section on peripheral arterial occlusive disease.

RADIOLOGIC INTERVENTIONS

Several interventional radiologic techniques are important adjunctive therapies to surgical procedures. Rotational atherectomy removes lesions by abrading plaque that has completely occluded the artery. If an isolated lesion or lesions are identified during the arteriogram, **angioplasty**, also called percutaneous transluminal angioplasty (PTA), may be performed. After the patient receives a local anesthetic, a balloon-tipped catheter is maneuvered across the area of stenosis. Exactly how PTA works is controversial. Some theorize that it improves blood flow by overstretching the elastic fibers of (and thereby dilating) the nondiseased arterial segment. But most clinicians believe that the procedure widens the arterial lumen by cracking and flattening the plaque against the vessel wall (see Chap. 25 for more information). Complications from PTA include hematoma formation, embolus, **dissection** (separation) of the vessel, and bleeding. To decrease the risk of reocclusion, stents (small, stainless-steel mesh tubes) may be inserted to support the walls of blood vessels and prevent collapse immediately after balloon inflation (Fig. 28-8). Complications associated with stent use include distal embolization, intimal damage (dissection), and stent dislodgement. The advantage to angioplasty, stents, and atherectomy is the decreased length of hospital stay required for the treatment: many of the procedures are performed on an outpatient basis.

NURSING PROCESS: THE PATIENT WITH PERIPHERAL ARTERIAL INSUFFICIENCY OF THE EXTREMITIES

Assessment

The nursing assessment includes a complete health and medication history and identification of risk factors for peripheral artery disease. Signs and symptoms detected during the nursing assessment may include claudication pain; rest pain in the forefoot; pallor, rubor, or cyanosis; weak or absent peripheral pulses; and skin breakdown or ulcerations.

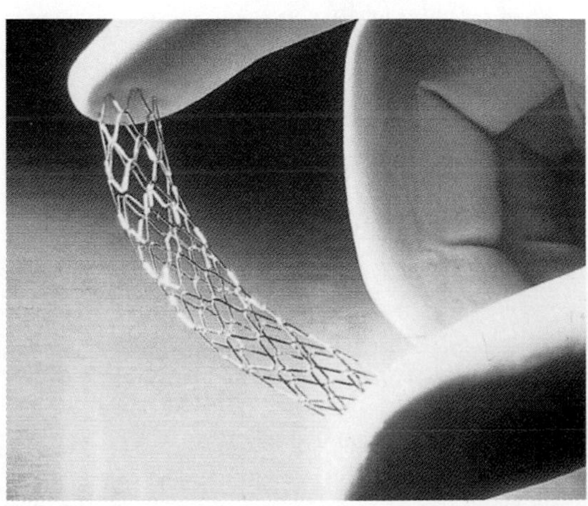

FIGURE 28•8 Flexible stent. Courtesy of Medtronics, Peripheral Division, Santa Rosa, California.

Nursing Diagnosis

Based on assessment data, major nursing diagnoses for the patient may include the following:

- Altered peripheral tissue perfusion related to compromised circulation
- Pain related to impaired ability of peripheral vessels to supply tissues with oxygen
- Risk for impaired skin integrity related to compromised circulation
- Knowledge deficit regarding self-care activities

Planning and Goals

The major goals for the patient may include increased arterial blood supply to the extremities, promotion of vasodilation, prevention of vascular compression, relief of pain, attainment or maintenance of tissue integrity, and adherence to the self-care program.

Measures used by the patient and members of the health care team to accomplish a single goal must be evaluated in terms of both the positive and the negative effects these measures may have on the simultaneous achievement of other goals. For an overview of the care of a patient with peripheral arterial problems, see the Plan of Nursing Care 28-1.

Nursing Interventions

Improving Peripheral Arterial Circulation

Arterial blood supply to a body part can be enhanced by positioning the part below the level of the heart. For the lower extremities, this is accomplished by elevating the head of the bed on 15-cm (6-in) blocks, using a reclining chair, or assuming a sitting position with the feet resting on the floor.

The nurse can assist the patient with walking or other moderate or graded isometric exercises that may be prescribed to promote blood flow and encourage the development of collateral circulation. Pain can serve as a guide in determining the amount of exercise appropriate for an individual. The onset of pain indicates that the tissues are not receiving adequate oxygen, signaling the patient to rest before continuing activity. However, a regular exercise program can result in an increased walking distance before the onset of claudication.

28•1

Plan of Nursing Care: The Patient With Peripheral Vascular Problems

Nursing Interventions	Rationale	Expected Outcomes
Nursing Diagnosis: Alteration in peripheral tissue perfusion related to compromised circulation **Goal:** Increased arterial blood supply to extremities		
1. Lower the extremities below the level of the heart. 2. Encourage moderate amount of walking or graded extremity exercises. 3. Encourage active postural exercise (Buerger-Allen exercises).	1. Dependency of lower extremities enhances arterial blood supply. 2. Muscular exercise promotes blood flow and the development of collateral circulation. 3. With postural exercises, gravity alternately fills and empties the blood vessels.	• Extremities warm to touch • Color of extremities improved • Experiences decreased muscle pain with exercise • Performs Buerger-Allen exercise series six times, four times per day as tolerated
Goal: Decrease in venous congestion		
1. Elevate extremities above heart level. 2. Discourage standing still or sitting for prolonged periods. 3. Encourage walking.	1. Elevation of extremities counteracts gravitational pull, promotes venous return, and prevents venous stasis. 2. Prolonged standing still or sitting promotes venous stasis. 3. Walking promotes venous return by activating the "muscle pump."	• Elevates lower extremities as prescribed • Decreased edema of extremities • Avoids prolonged standing still or sitting • Gradually increases walking time daily
Goal: Promotion of vasodilation and prevention of vascular compression		
1. Maintain warm temperature and avoid chilling. 2. Discourage nicotine use. 3. Counsel in ways to avoid emotional upsets; stress management.	1. Warmth promotes arterial flow by preventing the vasoconstriction effects of chilling. 2. Nicotine causes vasospasm, which impedes peripheral circulation. 3. Emotional stress causes peripheral vasoconstriction by stimulating the sympathetic nervous system.	• Protects extremities from exposure to cold • Avoids nicotine • Uses stress-management program to minimize emotional upset • Avoids constricting clothing and accessories • Avoids leg crossing • Takes medication as prescribed

(continued)

28•1 **Plan of Nursing Care**

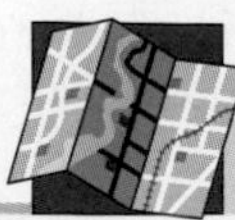

The Patient With Peripheral Vascular Problems (*continued*)

Nursing Interventions	Rationale	Expected Outcomes
4. Encourage avoidance of constrictive clothing and accessories.	4. Constrictive clothing and accessories impede circulation and promote venous stasis.	
5. Encourage avoidance of leg crossing.	5. Leg crossing causes compression of vessels with subsequent impediment of circulation, resulting in venous stasis.	
6. Administer vasodilator medications and adrenergic blocking agents as prescribed, with appropriate nursing considerations.	6. Vasodilators relax smooth muscle; adrenergic blocking agents block the response to sympathetic nerve impulses or circulating catecholamines.	

Nursing Diagnosis: Pain related to impaired ability of peripheral vessels to supply tissues with oxygen
Goal: Relief of pain

Nursing Interventions	Rationale	Expected Outcomes
1. Promote increased circulation.	1. Enhancement of peripheral circulation increases the oxygen supplied to the muscle and decreases the accumulation of metabolites that cause muscle spasms.	• Uses measures to increase arterial blood supply to extremities • Uses analgesics as prescribed
2. Administer analgesics as prescribed, with appropriate nursing considerations.	2. Analgesics help to reduce pain and allow the patient to participate in activities and exercises that promote circulation.	

Nursing Diagnosis: Risk for impaired skin integrity related to compromised circulation
Goal: Attainment/maintenance of tissue integrity

Nursing Interventions	Rationale	Expected Outcomes
1. Instruct in ways to avoid trauma to extremities.	1. Poorly nourished tissues are susceptible to trauma and bacterial invasion; healing of wounds is delayed or inhibited due to poor tissue perfusion.	• Inspects skin daily for evidence of injury or ulceration • Avoids trauma and irritation to skin • Wears protective shoes • Adheres to meticulous hygiene regimen • Eats well-balanced diet that contains adequate protein and vitamins B and C
2. Encourage wearing protective shoes and padding for pressure areas.	2. Protective shoes and padding prevent foot injuries and blisters.	
3. Encourage meticulous hygiene; bathing with neutral soaps, applying lotions, carefully trimming nails.	3. Neutral soaps and lotions prevent drying and cracking of skin.	
4. Caution to avoid scratching or vigorous rubbing.	4. Scratching and rubbing can cause skin abrasions and bacterial invasion.	
5. Promote good nutrition; adequate intake of vitamins B and C and protein; control of obesity.	5. Good nutrition promotes healing and prevents tissue breakdown.	

Nursing Diagnosis: Knowledge deficit regarding self-care activities
Goal: Adherence to the self-care program

Nursing Interventions	Rationale	Expected Outcomes
1. Include family/significant others in teaching program.	1. Adherence to the self-care program is enhanced when the patient receives support from family and from appropriate self-help groups and agencies.	• Practices frequent position changes as prescribed • Practices postural exercises as prescribed • Takes medications as prescribed • Avoids vasoconstrictors • Uses measures to prevent trauma • Uses stress-management program • Accepts condition as chronic but amenable to therapies that will decrease symptoms
2. Provide written instructions about foot care, leg care, and exercise program.	2. Written instructions serve as reminder and reinforcement of information.	
3. Assist to secure properly fitting clothing, shoes, stockings.		
4. Refer to self-help groups as indicated, such as smoking cessation clinics, stress management, weight management, and exercise program.		

The nurse can also assist the patient with postural exercises, such as the Buerger-Allen exercises. These may be prescribed for the patient with arterial insufficiency of the lower extremities. They involve placing the extremities in three positions: elevation, dependency, and horizontal. The patient lies flat in bed with both legs elevated above the heart for 2 to 3 minutes. Then, sitting on the edge of the bed with the legs relaxed and dependent, the patient exercises the feet and toes (upward and downward, inward and outward) for about 3 minutes. Finally, the patient lies flat with the legs at the same level as the heart for about 5 minutes. The times for each maneuver may vary, although the patient should attempt the series six times. Pain and dramatic color changes indicate the need to terminate the maneuver and to rest. This routine may be repeated (Fig. 28-9) four times daily or as tolerated.

Not all patients with peripheral vascular disease should exercise. Therefore, before recommending any exercise program, the primary care provider should be consulted. Conditions that worsen with activity include leg ulcers, cellulitis, gangrene, or acute thrombotic occlusions.

Promoting Vasodilation and Preventing Vascular Compression

Arterial dilation promotes increased blood flow to the extremities and is therefore a desirable goal for patients with peripheral arterial disease. However, if the arteries are severely sclerosed, inelastic, or damaged, dilation is not possible. For this reason, measures to promote vasodilation, such as medications or surgery, may be only minimally effective.

Nursing interventions may involve applications of warmth to promote arterial flow and instructions to avoid exposure to cold temperatures, which causes vasoconstriction. Adequate clothing and warm temperatures protect the patient from chilling. If chilling occurs, a warm bath or drink is helpful.

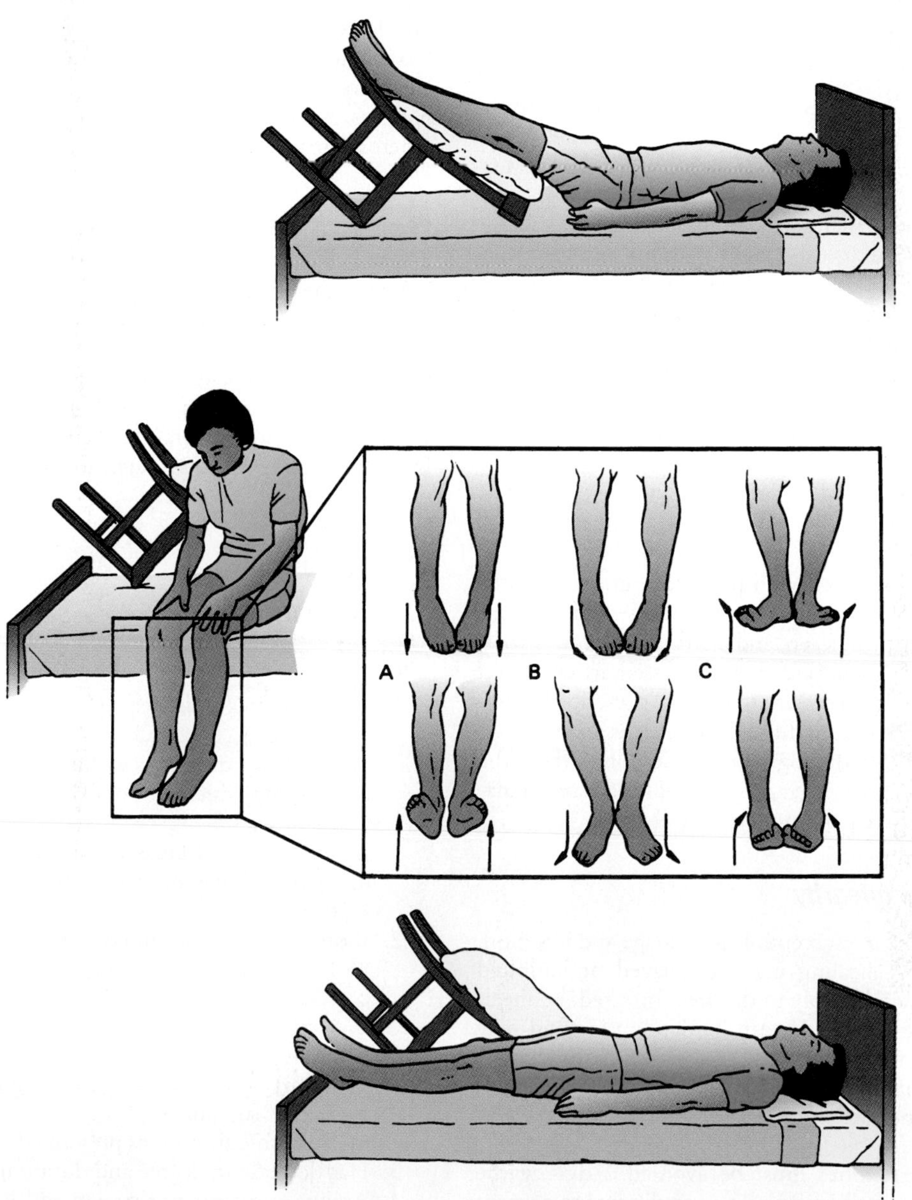

FIGURE 28•9 The Buerger-Allen exercise series is performed six times, four times a day to improve peripheral blood flow.

When heat is applied directly to ischemic extremities, the temperature of the heat source must not exceed body temperature. Even at lower temperatures, burn injuries can occur in ischemic extremities. In addition, excess heat may increase the metabolic rate of the extremities and thus increase the need for oxygen beyond that provided by the reduced arterial flow through the diseased artery.

Nursing Alert *Patients are instructed to test the temperature of bath water and to avoid using hot-water bottles and heating pads on the extremities. Applying a heating pad to the abdomen can cause reflex vasodilation in the extremities and is safer than direct application of heat to affected extremities.*

Nicotine causes vasospasm and can thereby dramatically reduce circulation to the extremities. Patients with arterial insufficiency who smoke must be fully informed of the effects of nicotine on circulation and encouraged to stop smoking.

Emotional upsets stimulate the sympathetic nervous system, resulting in peripheral vasoconstriction. Although emotional stress is unavoidable, it can be minimized to some degree by avoiding stressful situations when possible or by following a consistent stress-management program. Counseling services or relaxation training may be indicated for people who cannot cope effectively with situational stressors.

Constrictive clothing and accessories such as tight socks, panty girdles, and shoelaces impede circulation to the extremities and promote venous stasis and therefore should be avoided. Crossing the legs should be discouraged because it compresses vessels in the legs.

Vasodilator medications and adrenergic blocking agents may be administered as prescribed as adjunctive therapy. Vasodilators relax vascular smooth muscle, whereas adrenergic blocking agents block sympathetic response. Vasodilator therapy has not proved successful, however, and may worsen tissue perfusion if systemic blood pressure becomes too low.

Relieving Pain

Frequently, the pain associated with peripheral arterial insufficiency is chronic and continuous. It limits activities, affects work and responsibilities, disturbs sleep, and alters one's sense of well-being. Because of this, patients are often depressed, irritable, and unable to exert the energy necessary to execute prescribed therapies. As a result it can be more difficult to alleviate pain. Analgesics may be helpful in reducing pain to the point where the patient can participate in the therapies that will increase circulation and ultimately relieve pain more effectively.

Maintaining Tissue Integrity

Poorly nourished tissues are susceptible to damage and infection. When lesions develop, healing may be delayed or inhibited because of the poor blood supply to the area. Infected, nonhealing ulcerations of the extremities can be debilitating and may require prolonged and often expensive treatments. Amputation of an ischemic limb may eventually be necessary. Thus, measures to prevent these complications must be of high priority and vigorously implemented.

Trauma to the extremities must be avoided. Advising the patient to wear sturdy, well-fitting shoes, or slippers to prevent foot injury and blisters may be helpful, as may be recommending neutral soaps and body lotions to prevent drying and cracking of skin. Scratching and vigorous rubbing can abrade skin and create a site for bacterial invasion; therefore, feet should be patted dry. Stockings should be clean and dry. Fingernails and toenails should be carefully trimmed straight across and sharp corners filed to follow the contour of the nail. If nails are thick and brittle and cannot be trimmed safely, a podiatrist may be consulted. Corns and calluses need to be removed by a health care professional. Special shoe inserts may be needed to prevent calluses from recurring. All signs of blisters, ingrown toenails, infection, or other problems should be reported to health care professionals for treatment and follow-up. Patients with diminished vision may require assistance in periodically examining the lower extremities for trauma.

Good nutrition promotes healing and prevents tissue breakdown and is thus included in the overall therapeutic program for patients with peripheral vascular disease. Eating a well-balanced diet that contains adequate protein and vitamins is necessary for patients with arterial insufficiency. Key nutrients play specific roles in wound healing. Vitamin C is essential for collagen synthesis. Vitamin A enhances epithelialization. Zinc is necessary for cell mitosis and cell proliferation. Obesity strains the heart, increases venous congestion, and reduces circulation; therefore, a weight-reduction plan may be necessary for some patients. A diet low in lipids may be indicated for patients with atherosclerosis.

Promoting Home and Community-Based Care

The self-care program is planned with the patient so that activities that promote arterial and venous circulation, relieve pain, and promote tissue integrity will be acceptable. The patient and family should be helped to understand the reasons for each aspect of the program and the possible consequences of nonadherence. Long-term care of the feet and legs is of prime importance in the prevention of trauma, ulceration, and gangrene. Detailed patient instructions for foot and leg care are provided in the accompanying display.

Evaluation

Expected Outcomes

Expected outcomes may include:

1. Demonstrates an increase in arterial blood supply to extremities
   a. Exhibits extremities warm to touch
   b. Has improved color of extremities (is free of rubor or cyanosis)
   c. Experiences decreased muscle pain with exercise
   d. Demonstrates an increase in walking distance or duration
2. Promotes vasodilation; prevents vascular compression
   a. Protects extremities from exposure to cold
   b. Avoids nicotine use
   c. Uses a stress-management program to minimize emotional upset
   d. Wears nonconstricting clothing
   e. Avoids leg crossing
   f. Takes medication as prescribed
3. Has decrease in degree and duration of pain
4. Attains or maintains tissue integrity
   a. Avoids trauma and irritation to skin
   b. Wears protective shoes

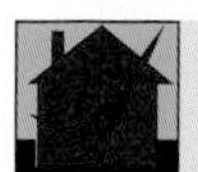

Home Care Teaching Checklist: Foot and Leg Care in Peripheral Vascular Disease

At the completion of the program, the patient or caregiver will be able to:	Patient	Caregiver
• Demonstrate daily foot bathing: Wash between toes with mild soap and lukewarm water, then rinse thoroughly and pat rather than rub dry.	✔	✔
• Recognize the dangers of thermal injury:	✔	
• Wear clean, loose, soft cotton socks (they are comfortable, allow air to circulate, and will absorb moisture)		
• In cold weather, wear extra socks in extra-large shoes.		
• Avoid heating pads, whirlpools, and hot tubs.		
• Avoid sunburn.		
• Identify safety concerns:	✔	✔
• Inspect feet daily with a mirror for redness, dryness, cuts, blisters, etc.		
• Always wear soft shoes or slippers when out of bed.		
• Trim nails straight across after showering.		
• Consult podiatrist to trim nails if vision is decreased; also for care of corns, blisters, ingrown nails.		
• Clear pathways in house to prevent injury.		
• Avoid wearing thong sandals.		
• Use lamb's wool between toes if they overlap or rub each other.		
• Demonstrate comfort measures:	✔	
• Wear leather shoes with an extra-depth toebox. Synthetic shoes do not allow air to circulate.		
• If feet become dry and scaly, use cream with lanolin. Never put cream between toes.		
• If feet perspire, especially between toes, use powder daily and/or lamb's wool between toes to promote drying.		
• Demonstrate ability to decrease risk of constricting blood vessels:	✔	
• Avoid promoting circular compression around feet or knees—for example, by applying knee-high stockings or tight socks.		
• Do not cross legs at knees.		
• Stop smoking (nicotine causes vasoconstriction and vasospasm).		
• Avoid applying tight, constricting bandages.		
• Participate in a regular walking exercise program to stimulate circulation.		
• Recognize when to seek medical attention:	✔	✔
• Contact health care provider at the onset of skin breakdown such as abrasions, blisters, athlete's foot, or pain.		
• Do not use any medication on feet or legs unless prescribed.		
• Avoid using iodine, alcohol, corn/wart-removing compound, or adhesive products before checking with health care provider.		

c. Adheres to meticulous hygienic regimen
d. Eats well-balanced diet that contains adequate protein, vitamins A and C, and zinc

5. Performs self-care activities

Peripheral Arterial Occlusive Disease

Arterial insufficiency of the extremities is usually found in individuals older than 50 years of age, most often in men. The legs are most frequently affected; however, the upper extremities may be involved. The age of onset and the severity are influenced by the type and number of atherosclerotic risk factors. In peripheral arterial disease, obstructive lesions are predominantly confined to segments of the arterial system extending from the aorta, below the renal arteries, to the popliteal artery (Fig. 28-10). However, distal occlusive disease is frequently seen in patients with diabetes mellitus and in elderly patients.

Clinical Manifestations

The hallmark is intermittent claudication. This pain may be described as aching, cramping, fatigue, or weakness that is consistently reproduced with the same degree of exercise or activity and relieved with rest. The pain commonly occurs in muscle groups one joint level below the stenosis or occlusion. As the disease progresses, the patient may relate a decreased ability to walk the same distance or may note increased pain with ambulation. When the arterial insufficiency becomes severe, the patient begins to have rest pain. This pain is associated with critical ischemia of the distal extremity and is persistent, aching, or boring; it may be so excruciating that it is unrelieved by opioids. Ischemic rest pain is usually worse at night and often wakes the patient. Elevating the extremity or placing it in a horizontal position increases the pain, whereas placing the extremity in a dependent position reduces the pain. In bed, some patients sleep with the affected leg hanging over the side of the bed. Some patients sleep in a reclining chair in an attempt to relieve the pain.

Assessment and Diagnostic Findings

A sensation of coldness or numbness in the extremities may accompany intermittent claudication and is a result of the reduced arterial flow. When the extremity is examined, it may feel cool to the touch and look pale when elevated or ruddy and cyanotic when placed in a dependent position. Skin and nail changes, ulcerations, gangrene, and muscle atrophy may be evi-

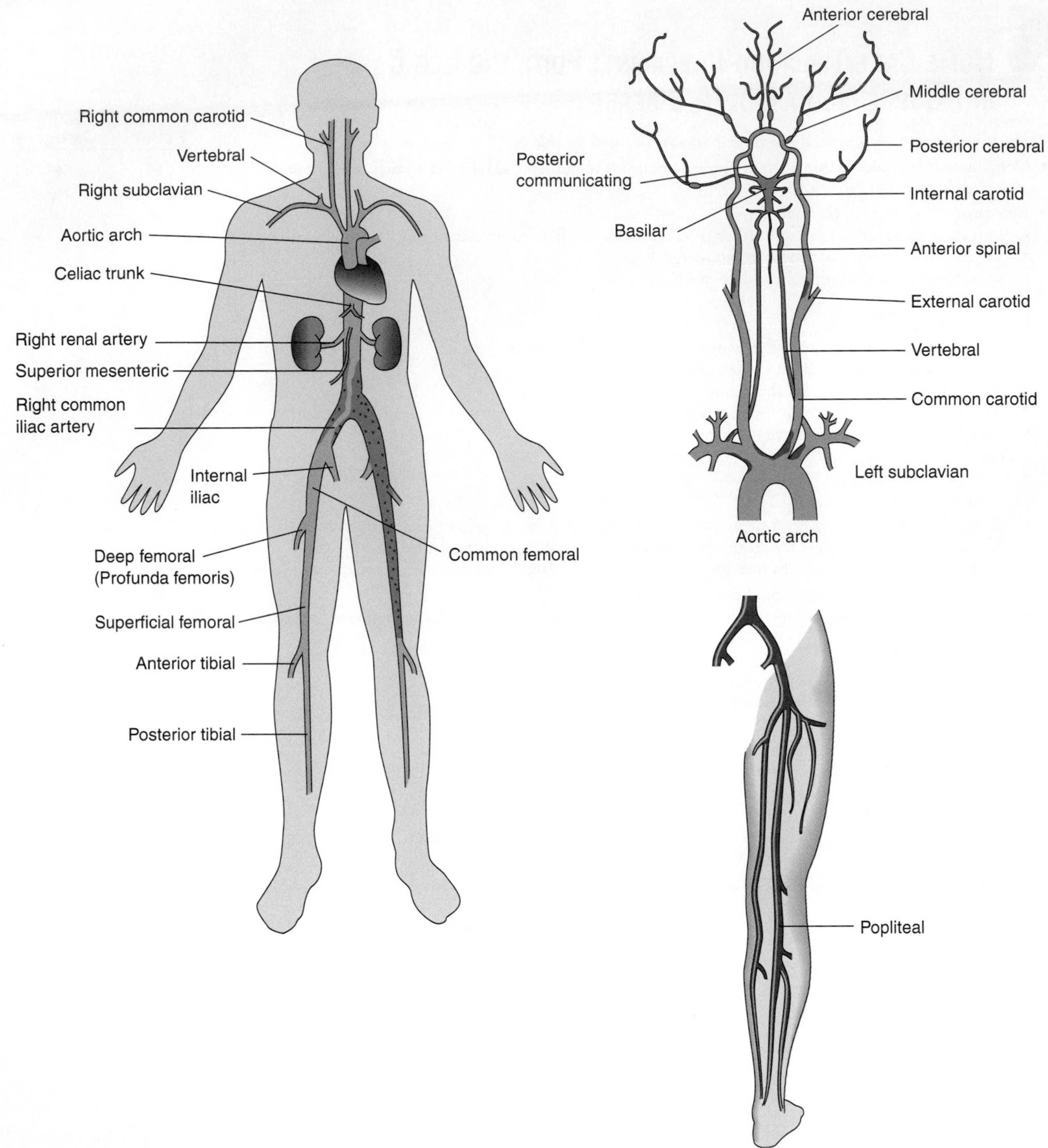

FIGURE 28•10 Common sites of atherosclerotic obstruction in major arteries.

dent. Bruits may be auscultated with a stethoscope (a bruit is the sound produced by turbulent blood flow through an irregular, tortuous, stenotic vessel or through a dilated segment of the vessel—an aneurysm). Peripheral pulses may be diminished or absent.

Examining the peripheral pulses is an important part of assessing for arterial occlusive disease. Unequal pulses between extremities or the absence of a normally palpable pulse is a sign of peripheral arterial disease. The femoral pulse in the groin and the posterior tibial pulse beside the medial malleolus are most easily palpated. The popliteal pulse is sometimes difficult to palpate; the location of the dorsalis pedis artery on the dorsum of the foot varies and is normally absent in about 7% of the population.

The presence, location, and extent of arterial occlusive disease are determined by a careful history of the symptoms and by physical examination. The color and temperature of the extremity are noted and the pulses palpated. The nails may be thickened and opaque, and the skin shiny, atrophic, and dry with sparse hair growth. A comparative assessment is made of the two extremities.

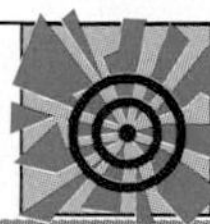

Risk Factors for PERIPHERAL ARTERIAL DISEASE

Controllable
Nicotine use
Hypertension
Diet (contributing to hyperlipidemia)
Obesity
Sedentary lifestyle
Stress
Diabetes mellitus

Not Controllable
Age
Gender
Familial predisposition

Medical Management

The diagnosis of peripheral arterial occlusive disease may be made using a CW Doppler and ankle-brachial indices, treadmill testing for claudication, duplex ultrasound, or other imaging studies previously described in this chapter.

Generally, patients feel better with some type of exercise program. If this program is combined with weight reduction and smoking cessation, patients often can improve their activity tolerance. Patients should not be promised that their symptoms will be relieved if they stop smoking, because claudication may persist, and they may lose their motivation to stop smoking.

SURGICAL MANAGEMENT

In most patients, when intermittent claudication becomes severe and disabling or when the limb is at risk for amputation because of tissue loss, vascular grafting or endarterectomy is the treatment of choice (Veith, 1994). The choice of the surgical procedure depends on the degree and location of the stenosis or occlusion. Another important consideration is the overall health of the patient, the length of the procedure that can be tolerated, and the patient's life expectancy. It is sometimes necessary to provide palliative therapy of primary amputation rather than an arterial bypass. If an endarterectomy is performed, an incision is made into the artery and the atheromatous obstruction is removed. The artery is then sutured closed to restore vascular integrity (Fig. 28-11).

Bypass grafts are performed to reroute the blood flow around the stenosis or occlusion. Before bypass grafting, the surgeon determines where the distal **anastomosis** (the site where the vessels are joined) will be placed. The distal outflow vessel must be at least 50% patent for the graft to remain patent. In addition, a higher primary patency rate is associated with keeping the length of the bypass as short as possible.

If the atherosclerotic occlusion is below the inguinal ligament in the superficial femoral artery, the surgical procedure of choice is the femoral-to-popliteal graft. This type of graft is further classified into above-knee and below-knee, referring to the location of the distal anastomosis. If the distal anastomosis is above the knee, prosthetic material may be used for the graft. If, however, the distal anastomosis is below the knee, an autologous vein (native; one of the patient's own veins) is preferred to ensure patency.

Lower leg or ankle vessels with occlusions may also require grafts. Occasionally the entire popliteal artery is occluded and only collateral circulation is identified. The distal anastomosis may be placed onto any of the tibial arteries (posterior tibial, anterior tibial, or peroneal arteries) or the dorsalis pedis or plantar artery. What determines the distal anastomosis site is the ease of exposure of the vessel in surgery as well as which vessel provides the best flow to the distal limb. These grafts require native vein to ensure patency. Native vein is autologous vein, usually the greater or lesser saphenous vein, or a combination of veins to meet the required length.

How long the graft remains patent is determined by several factors, including the size of the graft, graft location, and development of intimal hyperplasia at anastomosis sites. Bypass grafts may be either synthetic or autologous vein; however, native vein has a higher patency rate. Several synthetic materials are available

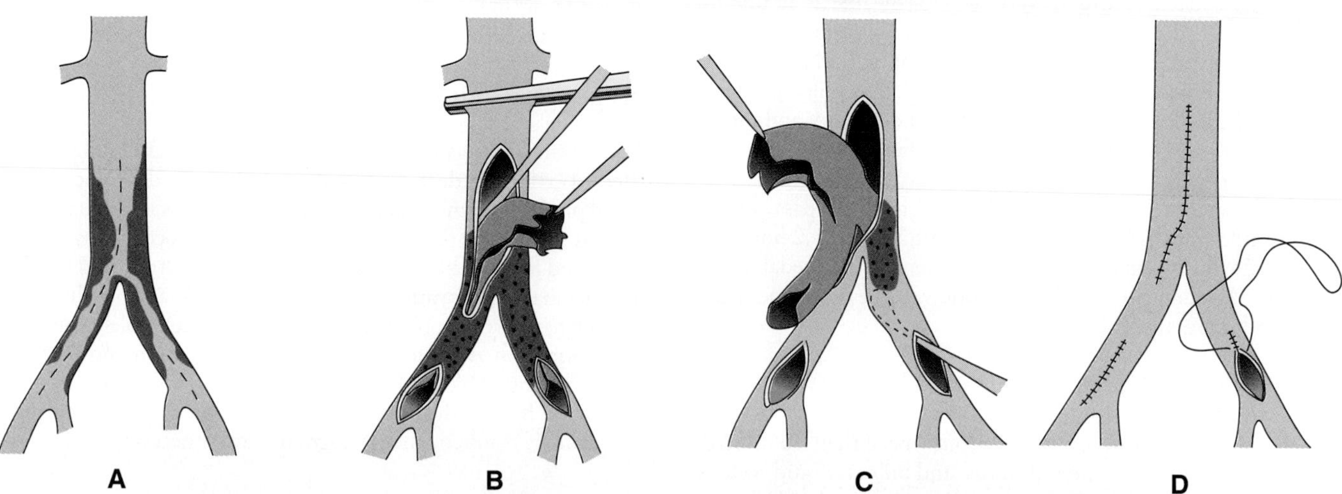

FIGURE 28•11 In an aortoiliac endarterectomy, the vascular surgeon (**A**) identifies the diseased area, (**B**) clamps off the blood supply to the vessel, (**C**) removes the plaque, and (**D**) sutures the vessel shut after which blood flow is restored. Adapted with permission from Rutherford, R. B. *Vascular surgery* (4th ed., Vol. I and II). Philadelphia: W. B. Saunders.

for use as a peripheral bypass graft: woven or knitted Dacron, expanded polytetrafluorethylene (ePTFE, such as Gore-Tex, Impra), and collagen-impregnated as well as umbilical vein may be used. Infection is a problem that threatens survival of the graft and almost always requires its removal.

Autologous vein has a higher patency rate, and because it is the patient's own tissue it is not antigenic. Anatomic and functional characteristics of the greater saphenous vein make it an excellent choice for a peripheral bypass. If the greater saphenous vein is not suitable for bypass, the cephalic or basilic veins from the arms or the lesser saphenous vein from the calf may be used. Sometimes synthetic materials are combined with autologous vein to form a composite bypass when a sufficient length of vein is not available. Vein grafts are further described based on the anatomic description of the vein used for the bypass graft:

In situ: The saphenous vein is used but is left in its anatomic location (in situ). A portion of the proximal and distal vein is dissected and brought over to the artery for anastomosis. Major branches from the saphenous vein are ligated, and the valves are rendered incompetent with an instrument called a valvulotome.

Reversed vein graft: The vein is harvested, removed from the extremity, reversed, and tunneled back into the extremity at the site of the stenosis to form a bypass graft. The venous valves remain intact; however, they no longer function and they collapse due to the high arterial pressure.

If a vein graft is the surgical choice, care must be taken in the operating room not to damage the vein after harvesting. The vein will be occluded at one end and inflated with a heparinized solution to check for leakage and competency. When this is done, the graft must be placed in a heparinized solution to keep it from becoming dry and brittle (Haimovici, 1996).

Nursing Management

MAINTAINING CIRCULATION

The primary objective in postoperative management of patients who have undergone vascular procedures is to maintain adequate circulation through the arterial repair. Pulses of the affected extremities are checked and recorded every hour for the first 24 hours and compared with those of the other extremity. Disappearance of a pulse that was present may indicate thrombotic occlusion of the graft, so the surgeon is immediately notified. The color and temperature of the extremity, capillary refill, and sensory and motor functions are also monitored every hour for 24 hours and any changes reported.

Doppler evaluation of the vessels distal to the bypass graft as well as ankle–arm indices should be monitored every 2 hours for the first 24 hours (may not be recommended for pedal artery bypasses). An adequate circulating blood volume should be established and maintained.

MONITORING AND MANAGING POTENTIAL COMPLICATIONS

Continuous monitoring of urine output (more than 30 mL/hr), central venous pressure, mental status, and pulse rate and volume permits the early recognition and treatment of fluid imbalances. Bleeding can result from the heparin administered during surgery or from an anastomotic leak. A hematoma may form as well.

Leg crossing and prolonged extremity dependency are avoided to prevent thrombosis. Edema is a normal postoperative finding; however, elevating the extremities and encouraging the patient to exercise the limbs while in bed reduces edema. Support hose may be used on some patients, but care must be taken to avoid compressing distal vessel bypass grafts. Severe limb edema, limb pain, and decreased sensation of fingers and toes can be an indication of compartment syndrome.

PROMOTING HOME AND COMMUNITY-BASED CARE

Discharge planning for the patient includes assessing his or her ability to manage independently. If the patient cannot do so, the nurse should assess whether the patient has a network of family and friends to assist with activities of daily living. Does the patient have the motivation to make the lifestyle changes necessary with a chronic disease? Does the patient have the knowledge and ability to assess for any postoperative complications such as infection, occlusion of the graft, and decreased blood flow? Has the patient stopped smoking?

Upper Extremity Arterial Occlusive Disease

Occlusions in the upper extremity occur less frequently and are not as symptomatic as those of the lower extremities because the collateral circulation is significantly better in the upper extremities (arms). Also, the arm has less muscle mass and is not subjected to the workload of the legs.

Clinical Manifestations

Stenosis and occlusions in the upper extremity result either from atherosclerosis or trauma. The stenosis usually occurs at the origin of the vessel proximal to the vertebral artery, setting up the vertebral artery as the major contributor of flow. The patient may develop a "subclavian steal" syndrome characterized by reverse flow in the vertebral and basilar artery to provide blood flow to the arm. This syndrome may cause vertebrobasilar (cerebral) symptoms. Most patients are asymptomatic; however, some report vertigo, ataxia, syncope, and bilateral visual changes.

The patient typically complains of arm fatigue and pain with exercise (forearm claudication) and inability to hold or grasp objects (painting, combing hair, placing objects on shelves above head). Some even note difficulties driving motor vehicles.

Assessment and Diagnostic Findings

Assessment findings include unilateral coolness and pallor of the affected extremity, decreased capillary refill, and a difference in arm blood pressures of more than 20 mm Hg. Noninvasive studies performed to evaluate for upper extremity arterial occlusions include upper and forearm blood pressures and duplex ultrasound to identify the anatomic location of the lesion as well as to evaluate the hemodynamics of the blood flow. Transcranial Doppler evaluation is performed to evaluate the intracranial circulation and to detect any siphoning of blood flow from the posterior circulation to provide blood flow to the affected arm. If a surgical or interventional procedure is planned, an arteriogram may be necessary.

Medical Management

If a short, focal lesion is identified in an upper extremity artery, a PTA may be performed. If the lesion involves the subclavian artery with documented siphoning of blood flow from the intracranial circulation, there are several surgical procedures available: carotid-to-subclavian-artery bypass, axillary-to-axillary-artery bypass, and autogenous reimplantation of the subclavian to the carotid artery.

Nursing Management

Nursing assessment involves a bilateral comparison of upper arm blood pressures; radial, ulnar, and brachial pulses; motor and sensory function; temperature; color changes; and capillary refill.

Nursing Alert *Before surgery, the arm is kept at heart level and protected from cold, venipunctures or arterial sticks, tape, and constrictive dressings. After surgery, the arm is kept at heart level or elevated, with the fingers at the highest level. Pulses are monitored with Doppler assessment of the arterial flow every hour for 24 hours. Motor and sensory function, warmth, color, and capillary refill are monitored every hour for 24 hours. Blood pressure is assessed every 2 hours for 24 hours.*

Thromboangiitis Obliterans (Buerger's Disease)

Buerger's disease is characterized by recurring inflammation of the intermediate and small arteries and veins of the lower and (in rare cases) upper extremities. It results in thrombus formation and occlusion of the vessels. It is differentiated from other vessel diseases by its microscopic appearance. In contrast to atherosclerosis, Buerger's disease is believed to be an autoimmune disease that results in occlusion of distal vessels.

The cause of Buerger's disease is unknown, but it is believed to be due to autoimmune vasculitis. It occurs most often in men between the ages of 20 and 35, and it has been reported in all races in many areas of the world. There is considerable evidence that heavy smoking or chewing of tobacco is either a causative or an aggravating factor. Generally, the lower extremities are affected, but arteries in the upper extremities or viscera can also be involved. Involvement is generally bilateral and symmetric with focal lesions. Superficial thrombophlebitis may be present.

Gerontologic Considerations

Although this condition is different from atherosclerosis, Buerger's disease in older patients may also be followed by atherosclerosis of the larger vessels after involvement of the smaller vessels.

Clinical Manifestations

Pain is the outstanding symptom of Buerger's disease. The patient complains of cramps in the feet, especially the arches (instep claudication), after exercise. The pain is relieved by rest; often there is a burning pain that is aggravated by emotional disturbances, nicotine, or chilling. Cold sensitivity of the Raynaud type is found in half the patients and is frequently confined to the hands. Digital rest pain is constantly present, and the characteristics of the pain do not change between activity and rest.

Physical signs include intense rubor (reddish-blue discoloration) of the feet, and absence of pedal pulses, with normal femoral and popliteal pulses. Radial and ulnar artery pulses are absent or diminished. Various types of paresthesia may develop.

As the disease progresses, definite redness or cyanosis of the part appears when the extremity is in a dependent position. Color changes may affect only one extremity or only certain digits. This may progress to ulceration. Ulceration with gangrene eventually occurs.

Assessment and Diagnostic Findings

Segmental limb blood pressures are taken to demonstrate the distal location of the lesions or occlusions. Duplex ultrasound is used to document patency of the proximal vessels and to visualize the extent of distal disease. Contrast angiography is performed to demonstrate the diseased portion of the anatomy.

Medical Management

The treatment of Buerger's disease is essentially the same as that for atherosclerotic peripheral arterial disease. The main objectives are to improve circulation to the extremities, prevent the progression of the disease, and protect the extremities from trauma and infection. Treatment of ulceration and gangrene is directed toward minimizing infection and conservative débridement of necrotic tissue. Tobacco use is highly detrimental, and patients are advised to stop using tobacco completely. Symptoms are often relieved by cessation of smoking.

Vasodilators are rarely prescribed because these medications cause dilation of only healthy vessels; therefore, vasodilators may even divert blood away from the partially occluded vessels, which makes the situation worse. A regional sympathetic block or ganglionectomy may be useful in some instances to produce vasodilation and thereby increase blood flow.

SURGICAL MANAGEMENT OF COMPLICATIONS

If gangrene of a toe develops as a result of arterial occlusive disease in the leg, it is unlikely that toe amputation or even transmetatarsal amputation will be sufficient: usually a below-knee amputation, or occasionally an above-knee amputation, is necessary. The indications for amputation are worsening gangrene, especially if the infected area is moist; severe rest pain; or fulminating sepsis.

Aortitis

The aorta, which is the main trunk of the arterial system, is divided into the ascending aorta (5 cm [2 in], contained in the pericardium), the aortic arch (extending upward, backward, and downward), and the descending aorta. The thoracic aorta is above the diaphragm; the abdominal aorta is below the diaphragm. The abdominal aorta is further designated as suprarenal (above renal artery level), perirenal level (at renal artery level), and infrarenal (below renal artery level).

Aortitis is inflammation of the aorta, particularly of the aortic arch. Two types are known to occur: Takayasu's disease and syphilitic aortitis. Takayasu's disease, or occlusive thromboaortopathy, is uncommon; today, syphilitic aortitis is rare.

Takayasu's disease, a chronic inflammatory disease of the aortic arch and its branches, primarily affects young or middle-aged women and is more common in those of Asian descent. It is nonatherosclerotic; the exact pathologic mechanism is unknown but thought to be immune complex-mediated. It progresses from a systemic inflammation with localized arteritis to end-organ ischemia because of large vessel stenosis or obstruction. Magnetic resonance angiography, CT, duplex ultrasound, or arteriography is used to diagnose and evaluate the lesions, which are typically

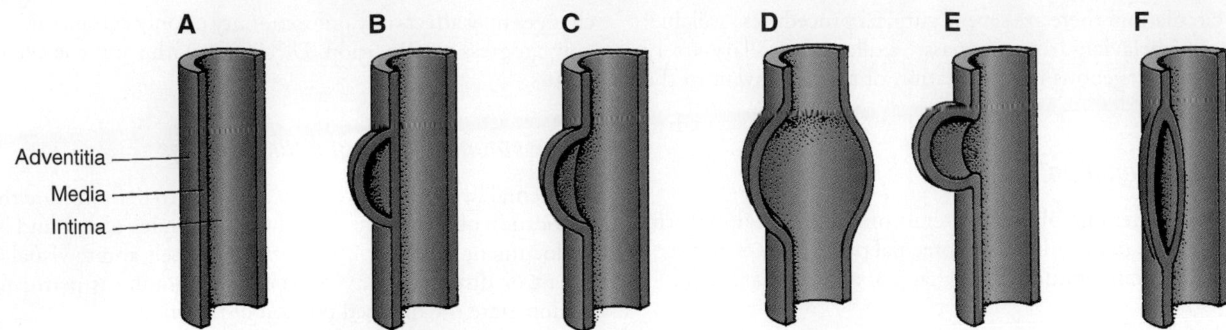

FIGURE 28•12 Characteristics of arterial aneurysm. (**A**) Normal artery. (**B**) False aneurysm—actually a pulsating hematoma. The clot and connective tissue are outside the arterial wall. (**C**) True aneurysm. One, two, or all three layers may be involved. (**D**) Fusiform aneurysm—symmetric, spindle-shaped expansion of entire circumference of involved vessel. (**E**) Saccular aneurysm—a bulbous protrusion of one side of the arterial wall. (**F**) Dissecting aneurysm—this usually is a hematoma that splits the layers of the arterial wall.

long, smooth areas of narrowing with or without aneurysms. In the early stages, the disease may respond to corticosteroids, and patients may benefit from the addition of cytotoxic immunosuppressive agents (Strider et al., 1996). Selective PTA and surgical revascularization may be performed after suppression of the systemic vascular inflammation.

Aortoiliac Disease

If collateral circulation has developed, patients with a stenosis or occlusion of the aortoiliac segment may be asymptomatic, or they may complain of buttock or low back discomfort associated with walking. Men may experience impotence. These patients may have decreased or absent femoral pulses.

Medical Management

The treatment of aortoiliac disease is essentially the same as that for atherosclerotic peripheral arterial occlusive disease. The surgical procedure of choice is the aorto–bi-iliac graft. If possible, the distal anastomosis is made to the iliac artery, and therefore the entire surgical procedure can be performed within the abdomen. If the iliac vessels are diseased, the distal anastomosis would be made to the femoral arteries (aorto–bifemoral). Bifurcated woven or knitted Dacron grafts are preferred for this surgical procedure.

Aortic Aneurysm

An aneurysm is a localized sac or dilation involving an artery formed at a weak point in the vessel wall (Fig. 28-12). It may be classified by either its shape or form. The most common forms of aneurysms are those that are saccular or fusiform. A saccular aneurysm projects from one side of the vessel only. If an entire arterial segment becomes dilated, a fusiform aneurysm develops. Very small aneurysms due to a localized infection are called mycotic aneurysms.

Historically, the cause of abdominal aortic aneurysm, the most common type of degenerative aneurysm, has been attributed to atherosclerotic changes in the aorta. Other causes of aneurysm formation are listed in Chart 28-2. Aneurysms are serious because they can rupture, leading to hemorrhage and death.

Thoracic Aortic Aneurysm

Approximately 85% of all cases of thoracic aortic aneurysm are caused by atherosclerosis. They occur most frequently in men between ages 40 and 70 years. The thoracic area is the most common site for a dissecting aneurysm. About one third of patients with thoracic aneurysms die from rupture of the aneurysm.

Clinical Manifestations

Symptoms are variable and depend on how rapidly the aneurysm dilates and how the pulsating mass affects surrounding intrathoracic structures. Some patients are asymptomatic. In most cases pain is the most prominent symptom. The pain is usually

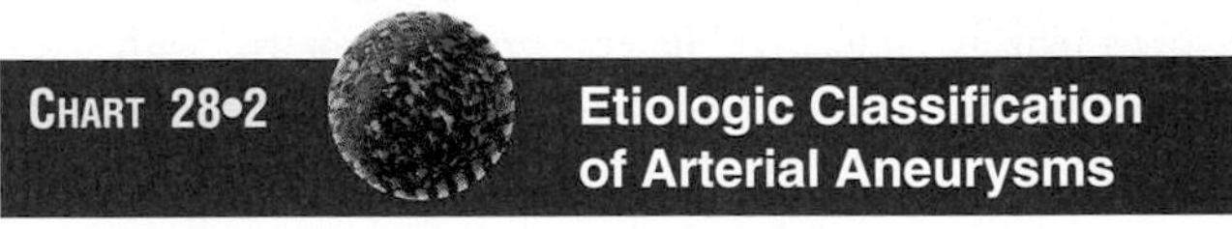

CHART 28•2 Etiologic Classification of Arterial Aneurysms

Congenital
Primary connective tissue disorders (Marfan's syndrome, Ehlers-Danlos syndrome) and other diseases (focal medial agenesis, tuberous sclerosis, Turner's syndrome, Menkes' syndrome)

Mechanical (Hemodynamic)
Poststenotic and arteriovenous fistula and amputation-related

Traumatic (Pseudoaneurysms)
Penetrating arterial injuries, blunt arterial injuries, pseudoaneurysms

Inflammatory (Noninfectious)
Associated with arteritis (Takayasu's disease, giant cell arteritis, systemic lupus erythematosus, Behçet's syndrome, Kawasaki's disease) and periarterial (ie, pancreatitis)

Infectious (Mycotic)
Bacterial, fungal, spirochetal

Pregnancy-Related Degenerative
Nonspecific, inflammatory variant

Anastomotic (Postarteriotomy) and Graft-Aneurysms
Infection, arterial wall failure, suture failure, graft failure

Adapted with permission from Rutherford, R. B. (1995). *Vascular surgery.* (4th ed., Vols. I and II.) Philadelphia: W. B. Saunders.

constant and boring but may occur only when the person is supine. Other conspicuous symptoms are dyspnea, the result of pressure of the sac against the trachea, a main bronchus, or the lung itself; cough, frequently paroxysmal and with a brassy quality; hoarseness, stridor, or weakness or complete loss of the voice (aphonia), resulting from pressure against the left recurrent laryngeal nerve; and dysphagia (difficulty in swallowing) due to impingement on the esophagus.

Assessment and Diagnostic Findings

When large veins in the chest are compressed by the aneurysm, the superficial veins of the chest, neck, or arms become dilated, and edematous areas on the chest wall and cyanosis are often evident. Pressure against the cervical sympathetic chain can result in unequal pupils. Diagnosis of a thoracic aortic aneurysm is principally made by chest x-ray, transesophageal echocardiography, and CT scan.

Medical Management

In most cases, an aneurysm is treated by surgical repair. General measures such as controlling blood pressure and correcting risk factors may be helpful. It is very important to control blood pressure in patients with dissecting aneurysms. Systolic pressure is maintained at about 100 to 120 mm Hg with antihypertensive medications (eg, nitroprusside, labetalol). Pulsatile flow is reduced by medications that reduce cardiac contractility (eg, propranolol). The goal of surgery is to remove the aneurysm and restore vascular continuity with a vascular graft (Fig. 28-13). Intensive monitoring is usually required after this type of surgery, and the patient is cared for in the critical care unit.

Abdominal Aortic Aneurysm

The most common cause of abdominal aortic aneurysm is atherosclerosis. The condition, which is more common among whites, affects men four times more often than women and is most prevalent in elderly patients. Most of these aneurysms occur below the renal arteries (infrarenal). Untreated, the eventual outcome may be rupture and death.

Pathophysiology

All aneurysms involve a damaged media layer of the vessel. This may be caused by congenital weakness, trauma, or disease. Once an aneurysm develops, it tends to grow. Risk factors include genetic predisposition, smoking, and hypertension; more than half of these patients have hypertension.

Clinical Manifestations

About two fifths of patients with abdominal aortic aneurysms have symptoms; the remainder do not. Some patients complain that they can feel their heart beating in their abdomen when lying down, or they may say they feel an abdominal mass or abdominal throbbing. If the abdominal aortic aneurysm is associated with thrombus, a major vessel may be occluded or smaller distal occlusions may result from emboli. An occlusion of a digital vessel causes "blue toe" syndrome.

Assessment and Diagnostic Findings

The most important diagnostic indication of an abdominal aortic aneurysm is a pulsatile mass in the middle and upper abdomen. About 80% of these aneurysms can be palpated. A systolic bruit

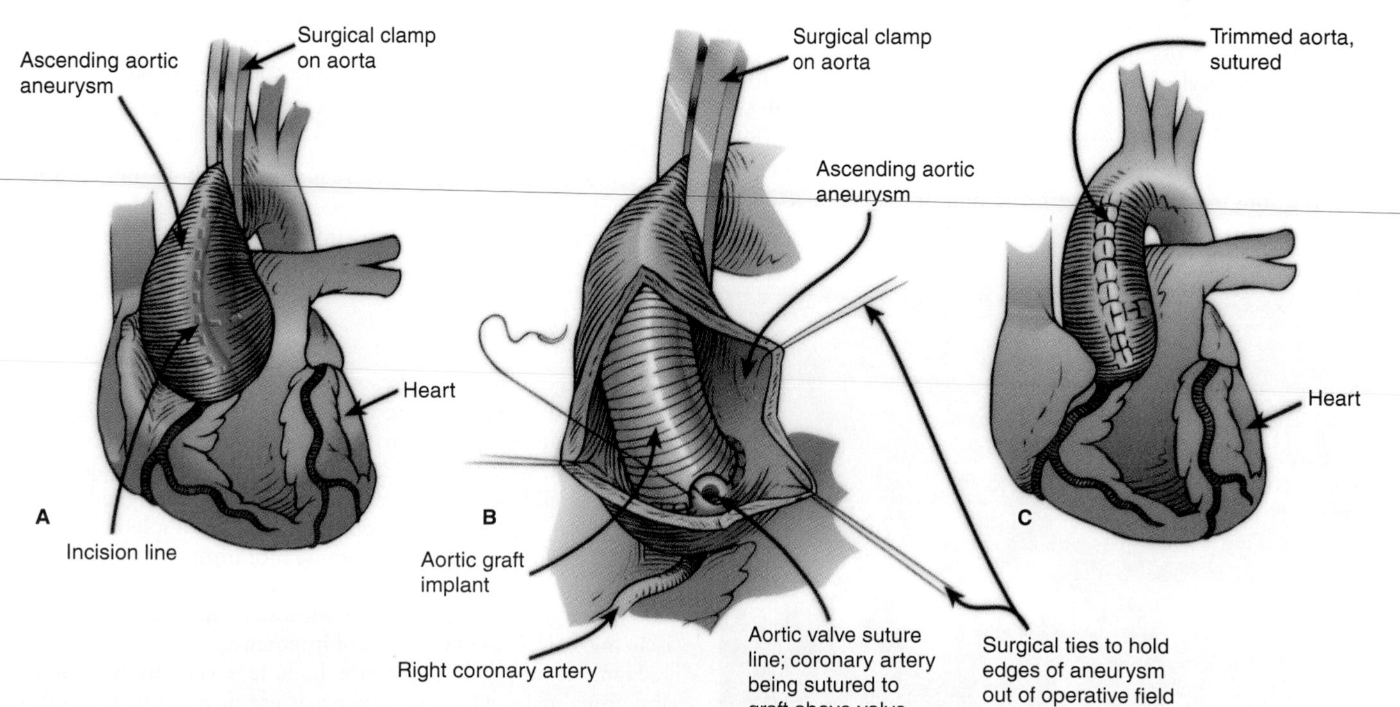

FIGURE 28•13 Repair of an ascending aortic aneurysm and aortic valve replacement: (**A**) incision into aortic aneurysm; (**B**) aortic valve replacement with aortic graft implant to repair ascending aortic aneurysm; (**C**) aortic aneurysm trimmed and closed over graft.

may be heard over the mass. Duplex ultrasound or CT scans are used to determine the size, length, and location of the aneurysm (Fig. 28-14). When the aneurysm is small, serial ultrasonography is conducted at 6-month intervals until the aneurysm reaches a size where an operation to prevent rupture is of more benefit than the possible complications of a surgical procedure. Some aneurysms remain stable over many years of observation.

Gerontologic Considerations

Most abdominal aneurysms occur in patients between ages 60 and 90 years. Rupture is likely with coexisting hypertension and with aneurysms larger than 6 cm. In most cases at this point, the chances of rupture are greater than the chance of death during surgical repair. If the elderly patient is considered at moderate risk for complications related to surgery or anesthesia, the aneurysm is not repaired until it reaches 5 cm (2 in). If the patient is a poor surgical risk, the aneurysm is not repaired until it reaches 6 cm. Some aneurysms remain the same size for many years.

Medical Management

An expanding or enlarging abdominal aneurysm is likely to rupture. Therefore, surgery is the treatment of choice for abdominal aneurysms larger than 5 cm (2 in) in diameter or those that are enlarging.

SURGICAL MANAGEMENT

The aneurysm is resected and a bypass graft is inserted (Fig. 28-15). The mortality rate associated with elective aneurysm repair, a major surgical procedure, is reported to be 1% to 4%. The prognosis for a patient with a ruptured aneurysm is poor, and surgery is performed immediately.

A new alternative for treating infrarenal abdominal aortic aneurysm is endovascular grafting. Endovascular grafting involves the transluminal placement and attachment of a sutureless aortic graft prosthesis across an aneurysm. This procedure can be performed under local or regional anesthesia. Endovascular grafting of abdominal aortic aneurysms may be performed if the patient's abdominal aorta is not extremely tortuous and if the aneurysm does not begin at the left renal artery level (perirenal). Potential complications include bleeding, hematoma or wound infection at the femoral insertion site, distal ischemia or embolization, dissection or perforation of the aorta, graft thrombosis, graft infection, attachment system break, graft migration break, proximal or distal graft leaks, delayed rupture, and bowel ischemia.

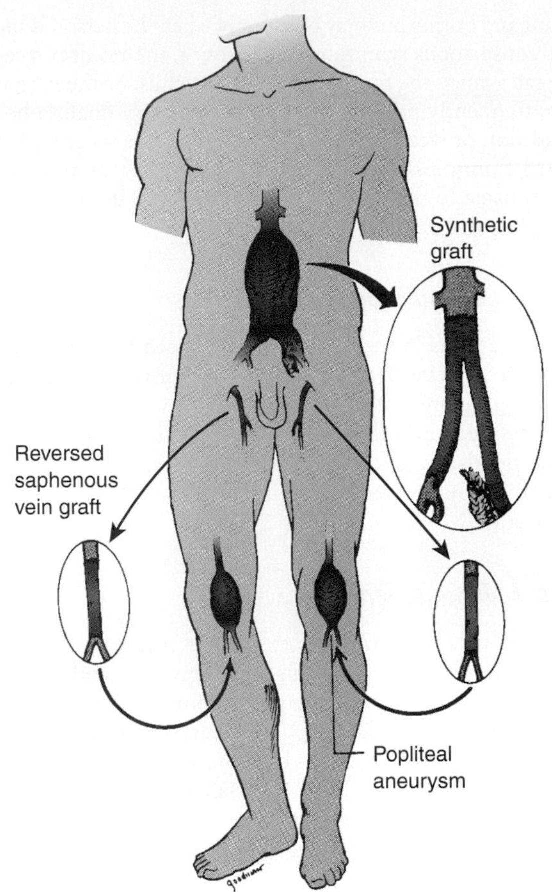

FIGURE 28•15 Surgical repair of an abdominal aneurysm and bilateral popliteal aneurysms. During the procedure, the surgeon replaces the abnormal section of the aorta with a synthetic graft and the popliteal aneurysms with reversed saphenous vein grafts, which are believed to function better than synthetic graft material. The saphenous vein graft is reversed so that the valves face in the same direction of the arterial flow and the valves collapse due to the arterial pressure.

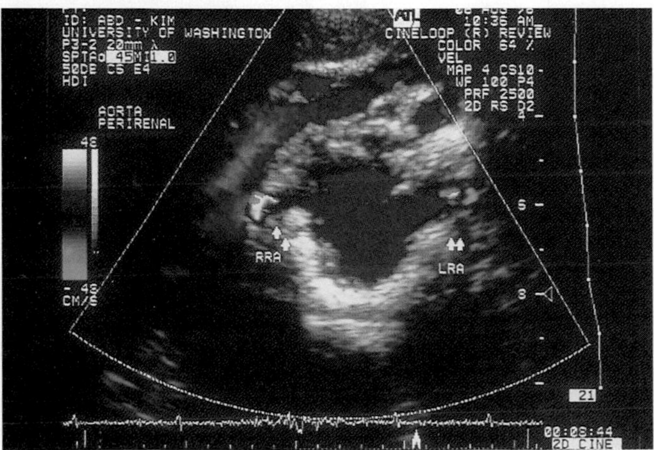

FIGURE 28•14 Duplex ultrasonic image of abdominal aortic aneurysm at the perirenal level. Cross-sectional image documents the location of right and left renal arteries.

Nursing Management

Before surgery, nursing assessment is guided by anticipating a rupture and by recognizing that the patient may have cardiovascular, cerebral, pulmonary, and renal impairment secondary to atherosclerosis. Therefore, the functional capacity of all organ systems should be established. Medical therapies designed to stabilize physiologic function should be promptly implemented.

Postoperative care requires intense monitoring of pulmonary, cardiovascular, renal, and neurologic status. Possible complications of surgery include arterial occlusion, hemorrhage, infection, ischemic colon, renal failure, and impotence.

Signs of impending rupture include severe back pain or abdominal pain, which may be persistent or intermittent and is often localized in the middle or lower abdomen to the left of the midline. Low back pain may also be present because of pressure of the aneurysm on the lumbar nerves. This is a serious symptom, usually indicating that the aneurysm is expanding rapidly and is about to rupture. Indications of a rupturing abdominal aortic aneurysm include a constant intense back pain, falling blood pressure, and decreasing hematocrit. A retroperitoneal rupture of an aneurysm may result in hematomas in the scrotum, perineum, flank, or penis. Signs of heart failure or a loud bruit may suggest a rupture into the vena cava. Rupture into the peritoneal cavity is rapidly fatal. The overall surgical mortality rate associated with a ruptured aneurysm is 50% to 75%.

Dissecting Aorta

Occasionally, in an aorta diseased by arteriosclerosis, a tear develops in the intima or the media degenerates, resulting in a dissection.

Pathophysiology

Arterial dissections (separations) are commonly associated with poorly controlled hypertension; they are three times more common in men than in women and occur in the 50- to 70-year-old age group. Dissection is caused by rupture in the intimal layer. A rupture may occur through adventitia or into the lumen through the intima, thereby allowing blood to reenter the main channel, resulting in chronic dissection or occlusion of branches of the aorta.

As the separation progresses, the arteries branching from the involved area of the aorta shear and occlude. The tear occurs most commonly in the region of the aortic arch, with the highest mortality rate associated with ascending aortic dissection. The dissection of the aorta may progress backward in the direction of the heart, obstructing the opening to the coronary arteries or producing hemopericardium (effusion of blood into the pericardial sac) or aortic insufficiency, or it may extend in the opposite direction, causing occlusion of the arteries supplying the gastrointestinal tract, the kidneys, the spinal cord, and even the legs.

Clinical Manifestations

Onset of symptoms is usually sudden. Severe and persistent pain, described as tearing or ripping, may be reported. The pain is in the anterior chest or back and extends to shoulders, epigastric area, or abdomen. Aortic dissection may be mistaken for an acute myocardial infarction, which could confuse the clinical picture and initial treatment. Cardiovascular, neurologic, and gastrointestinal symptoms are responsible for other clinical manifestations, depending on the location and extent of the dissection. The patient may appear pallid. Sweating and tachycardia may be detected. Blood pressure may be elevated or markedly different from one arm to the other if dissection involves the orifice of the subclavian artery on one side. Because of the variable clinical picture associated with this condition, early diagnosis is usually difficult.

Assessment and Diagnostic Findings

Arteriogram, CT scan, transesophageal echocardiography, duplex ultrasound, and magnetic resonance imaging aid in the diagnosis.

Medical Management

Medical or surgical treatment of a dissecting aneurysm depends on the type of dissection present and follows the general principles outlined for the treatment of thoracic aortic aneurysms.

Other Aneurysms

Aneurysms may also arise in the peripheral vessels, most often as a result of atherosclerosis. These may involve such vessels as the renal artery, the subclavian artery, the femoral artery, or (most frequently) the popliteal artery. Also, 50% to 60% of popliteal aneurysms are bilateral and may be associated with a higher incidence of abdominal aortic aneurysms.

The aneurysm produces a pulsating mass and disturbs peripheral circulation distal to it. Pain and swelling develop because of pressure on adjacent nerves and veins. Diagnosis is made by duplex ultrasonography and/or CT scans to determine the size, length, and extent of the aneurysm. Arteriography may be performed to evaluate the level of proximal and distal involvement.

Surgical repair is performed with replacement grafts.

Arterial Embolism and Arterial Thrombosis

Acute vascular occlusion may be due to an embolus or to acute thrombosis. Acute arterial occlusions may result from iatrogenic injury, which can occur during insertion of invasive catheters such as those used for arteriography, PTA/stent placement, or an intra-aortic balloon pump. Other causes include trauma from a fracture, crush injury, and penetrating wounds that disrupt the arterial intima. The accurate diagnosis of an arterial occlusion as embolic or thrombotic in origin is necessary to initiate appropriate treatment.

Pathophysiology

Arterial emboli arise most commonly from thrombi that develop in the chambers of the heart as a result of atrial fibrillation, myocardial infarction, infective endocarditis, or chronic congestive heart failure. These thrombi become detached and are carried from the left side of the heart into the arterial system, where they obstruct an artery that is smaller than the embolus. Emboli may also develop in advanced aortic atherosclerosis because the atheromatous plaques ulcerate or become rough. Acute thrombosis frequently occurs in patients with preexisting ischemic symptoms.

Clinical Manifestations

The symptoms of arterial emboli depend primarily on the size of the embolus, the organ involved, and the state of the collateral vessels. The immediate effect is cessation of distal blood flow. The blockage can progress above and below the obstruction. Secondary vasospasm can contribute to the ischemia. The embolus can fragment or break apart, resulting in occlusion of distal vessels. Emboli tend to lodge at arterial bifurcations and areas narrowed by atherosclerosis. Cerebral, mesenteric, renal, and coronary arteries are often involved in addition to the large arteries of the extremities.

The symptoms of acute arterial embolism in extremities with poor collateral flow are acute, severe pain and a gradual loss of sensory and motor function. The five P's associated with acute arterial embolism are pain, pallor, pulselessness, paresthesia, and paralysis. Eventually, superficial veins may collapse because of decreased blood flow to the extremity. The part of the extremity below the occlusion is markedly colder and paler (poikilothermia) than the part above the occlusion because of ischemia.

Arterial thrombosis can also acutely occlude an artery. A thrombosis is a slowly developing clot that usually occurs where the arterial wall has become damaged, generally as a result of atherosclerosis. Thrombi may also develop in an arterial aneurysm. The manifestations of an acute thrombotic arterial occlusion are similar to those described for embolic occlusion. However, treatment is more difficult with a thrombus because the arterial occlusion has occurred in a degenerated vessel and requires more extensive reconstructive surgery to restore flow than is required with an embolic event.

Assessment and Diagnostic Findings

An arterial embolus is usually diagnosed on the basis of the sudden or acute nature of the onset of symptoms and an apparent source for the embolus. Two-dimensional echocardiography or transesophageal echocardiography, chest x-ray, and electrocardiography may reveal underlying cardiac disease. Noninvasive duplex and Doppler ultrasonography can determine the presence and extent of underlying atherosclerosis. In addition, arteriography may be performed.

Medical Management

Management of arterial thrombosis depends on its cause. Management of acute embolic occlusion usually requires surgery because time is of the essence. Because the onset of the event is acute, collateral circulation has not developed and the patient quickly moves through the list of five Ps to paralysis, which is the most advanced stage. Heparin therapy is initiated immediately to prevent further development of emboli and to hamper the extension of existing thrombi. Typically an initial bolus of 5000 to 10,000 units is given, followed by a continuous infusion of 1000 U/hr.

SURGICAL MANAGEMENT

Emergency embolectomy is the procedure of choice only if the involved extremity is viable (Fig. 28-16). Arterial emboli are usually treated by insertion of an embolectomy catheter. The catheter is passed via a groin incision through the affected artery and distal to the occlusion. The balloon is inflated with sterile saline solution and the thrombus is extracted as the catheter is withdrawn. This involves incising the vessel and removing the clot.

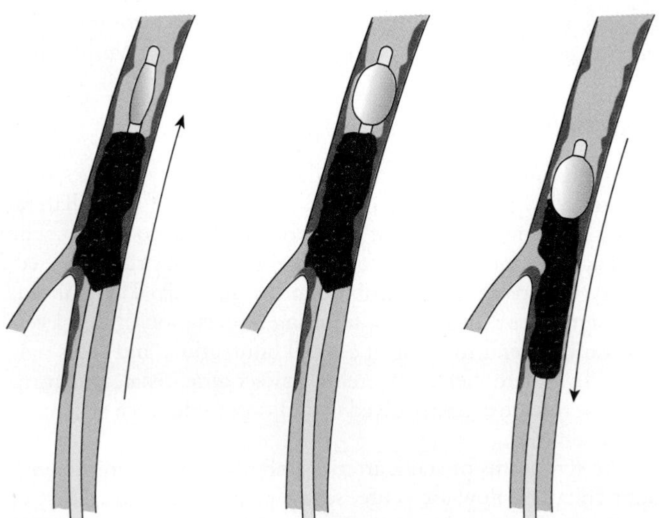

FIGURE 28•16 Extraction of an embolus by balloon-tipped embolectomy catheter. The deflated balloon-tipped catheter is advanced past the embolus, inflated and then gently withdrawn, carrying the embolic material with it. Adapted with permission from Rutherford, R. B. (1995). Vascular surgery (4th ed., Vols. I and II). Philadelphia: W. B. Saunders.

PHARMACOLOGIC THERAPY

When the patient has collateral circulation, treatment may include intravenous anticoagulation with heparin, which will prevent the clot from spreading and thus reduce muscle necrosis. The use of intra-arterial thrombolytic agents, such as streptokinase or urokinase, helps to dissolve the embolus.

Although these agents differ in their pharmacokinetics, they are administered in a similar manner. A catheter is advanced under x-ray visualization to the clot, and the thrombolytic agent is infused.

Thrombolytic therapy should not be used when there are known contraindications to therapy or when the extremity cannot tolerate the several additional hours of ischemia that it takes for the agent to lyse (disintegrate) the clot. Contraindications to thrombolytic therapy include active internal bleeding, stroke, recent major surgery, uncontrolled hypertension, and pregnancy.

Nursing Management

Before surgery, the patient remains on bed rest with the extremity level or slightly (15°) dependent. The affected part is kept at room temperature and protected from trauma. Heating and cooling pads are contraindicated because ischemic extremities are easily traumatized by alterations in temperature. Whenever possible, tape and electrocardiogram electrodes should not be used; sheepskin and foot cradles are used to protect the leg from mechanical trauma.

During the postoperative period, the nurse collaborates with the surgeon about the patient's appropriate activity level (based on the patient's condition). Generally every effort is made to encourage the patient to move the leg to stimulate circulation and prevent stasis. Anticoagulant therapy may be continued after surgery to prevent thrombosis of the affected artery and to diminish the development of subsequent thrombi at the initiating site. The nurse assesses for evidence of hemorrhage, both local and systemic, including mental status changes, which can occur when anticoagulants are administered. Pulses, Doppler signals, ABI, and motor and sensory function are assessed every hour because significant changes may indicate reocclusion. Metabolic abnormalities, renal failure, and compartment syndrome may be complications after an acute arterial occlusion.

Raynaud's Disease

Raynaud's disease is a form of intermittent arteriolar vasoconstriction that results in coldness, pain, and pallor of the fingertips or toes. The cause is unknown, although many patients with the disease seem to have immunologic disorders. Symptoms may result from a defect in basal heat production that eventually decreases the ability of cutaneous vessels to dilate. Episodes may be triggered by emotional factors or by unusual sensitivity to cold. The disease is most common in women ages 16 to 40 years and occurs more frequently in cold climates and during the winter.

The term "Raynaud's phenomenon" is currently used to refer to localized, intermittent episodes of vasoconstriction of small arteries of the feet and hands that cause color and temperature changes. Generally unilateral and affecting only one or two digits, the phenomenon is always associated with underlying systemic disease. It may occur with scleroderma, systemic lupus erythematosus, rheumatoid arthritis, obstructive arterial disease, or trauma.

The prognosis for Raynaud's disease varies; some patients slowly improve, some become progressively worse, and others show no change. Ulceration and gangrene are rare; however, chronic disease may cause atrophy of the skin and muscles. With appropriate patient teaching and lifestyle modifications, the disorder is generally benign and self-limiting.

Clinical Manifestations

The classic clinical picture reveals pallor brought on by sudden vasoconstriction. The skin then become bluish (cyanotic) due to pooling of deoxygenated blood during vasospasm. As a result of exaggerated reflow (hyperemia) due to vasodilation, a red color is produced (rubor). Thus, the characteristic sequence of color change of Raynaud's phenomenon is described as white, blue, and red. Numbness, tingling, and burning pain occur as the color changes. The involvement tends to be bilateral and symmetric.

Medical Management

Avoiding the particular stimuli (cold, smoking) that provoke vasoconstriction is a primary concern in controlling Raynaud's disease. In addition, calcium channel blockers may be effective in relieving symptoms. Studies indicate that nifedipine (Procardia, Adalat) is an effective calcium channel blocker for treating an acute episode of vasospasm (Kaufman & All, 1996). Sympathectomy (interrupting the sympathetic nerves by removing the sympathetic ganglia or dividing their branches) may help some patients.

Nursing Management

The nurse teaches patients to avoid situations that may be upsetting, stressful, or unsafe. Stress-management classes may be desirable. Exposure to cold must be minimized as well. In areas where the fall and winter months are cold, the patient should remain indoors as much as possible and wear layers of clothing when outdoors. Hats and mittens or gloves should be worn at all times when outside. Fabrics specially designed for cold climates (eg, Thinsulate) are recommended. Patients should warm up their vehicle before getting in so that they can avoid touching a cold steering wheel or door handle, which could elicit an attack. During summer, a sweater should be available when entering air-conditioned rooms.

Concerns about serious complications, such as gangrene and amputation, are common among patients. However, these consequences are uncommon. Patients should avoid nicotine; the nicotine gum or patches used to help people quit smoking may induce attacks.

Patients should be careful about safety. Sharp objects should be handled carefully to avoid injuring the fingers. Patients should be informed about the postural hypotension that may result from medications, such as calcium channel blockers, used to treat Raynaud's disease. The nurse also discusses safety precautions related to alcohol, exercise, and hot weather.

MANAGEMENT OF VENOUS DISORDERS

Venous Thrombosis, Deep Vein Thrombosis, Thrombophlebitis, and Phlebothrombosis

Although these four terms do not necessarily reflect identical disease processes, for clinical purposes they are often used interchangeably.

Pathophysiology

Although the exact cause of venous thrombosis remains unclear, three factors, known as Virchow's triad, are believed to play a significant role in its development: stasis of blood (venous stasis), vessel wall injury, and altered blood coagulation. At least two of the factors seem to be necessary for thrombosis to occur.

Venous stasis occurs when blood flow is reduced, as in heart failure or shock; when veins are dilated, as with some medication therapies; and when skeletal muscle contraction is reduced, as in immobility, paralysis of the extremities, or anesthesia. Moreover, bed rest reduces blood flow in the legs by at least 50%.

Damage to the intimal lining of blood vessels creates a site for clot formation. Direct trauma to the vessels, for example with fractures or dislocation, diseases of the veins, and chemical irritation of the vein from intravenous medications or solutions, can damage veins.

Increased blood coagulability occurs most commonly in patients who have been abruptly withdrawn from anticoagulant medications. Oral contraceptive use and several blood dyscrasias (abnormalities) also can lead to hypercoagulability.

Formation of a clot frequently accompanies thrombophlebitis, which is an inflammation of the vein walls. When a clot develops initially in the veins as a result of stasis or hypercoagulability, but without inflammation, the process is referred to as phlebothrombosis. Venous thrombosis can occur in any vein but occurs more in the veins of the lower extremities. Both the superficial and deep veins of the extremities may be affected.

Upper extremity venous thrombosis is not as common as lower extremity thrombosis. However, upper extremity venous thrombosis is more common in patients with intravenous catheters or in patients with an underlying disease that causes hypercoagulability. Internal trauma to the vessels may result from pacemaker leads, chemotherapy ports, dialysis catheters, or hyperalimentation lines. The lumen of the vein may be decreased as a result of the catheter or from external compression (eg, from neoplasms, an extra cervical rib). Effort thrombosis of the upper extremity is due to repetitive motion that irritates the vessel wall, causing inflammation and subsequent thrombosis.

Venous thrombi are aggregates of platelets attached to the vein wall, along with a tail-like appendage containing fibrin, white blood cells, and many red blood cells. The "tail" can grow or can propagate in the direction of blood flow as successive layers of the clot form. A propagating venous thrombosis is dangerous because parts of the clot can break off and produce an embolic occlusion of the pulmonary blood vessels. Fragmentation of the thrombus can occur spontaneously as the clot dissolves naturally, or it can occur in association with an elevation in venous pressure, as occurs when a person stands suddenly or engages in muscular activity after prolonged inactivity. After an episode of acute deep vein thrombosis, recanalization of the lumen typically occurs. The time required for complete recanalization is an important determinant of valvular incompetency, which is one complication of venous thrombosis (Meissner et al, 1995). Other complications of venous thrombosis are described in Chart 28-3.

Clinical Manifestations

A major problem associated with recognizing deep vein thrombosis is that the signs and symptoms are nonspecific. The exception to this is phlegmasia cerulea dolens (massive iliofemoral venous thrombosis), in which the entire extremity becomes massively swollen, tense, painful, and cool to the touch. Despite this variability, clinical signs should always be investigated.

Superficial veins, such as the greater saphenous, lesser saphenous, cephalic, basilic, and external jugular, are thick-walled muscular structures that lie just under the skin. Deep veins are thin-walled and have less muscle in the media. They run parallel to arteries and bear the same names as the arteries. Deep and superficial veins have valves that permit unidirectional flow back to the heart. The valves lie at the base of a segment of the vein that is expanded into a sinus. This arrangement permits the valves to open without coming into contact with the wall of the vein, thus permitting rapid closure when the blood starts to flow backward. Other kinds of veins are known as perforating veins. These vessels have valves that allow one-way blood flow from the superficial system to the deep system.

DEEP VEINS

With obstruction of the deep veins comes edema and swelling of the extremity because the outflow of venous blood is inhibited. The amount of swelling can be determined by measuring the circumference of the affected extremity at various levels with a tape measure and comparing one extremity with the other at the same level to determine size differences. If both extremities are swollen, a size difference may be difficult to detect. The affected extremity may feel warmer than the unaffected extremity, and the superficial veins may appear more prominent.

Tenderness, which usually occurs later, is produced by inflammation of the vein wall and can be detected by gently palpating the affected extremity. Homans' sign (pain in the calf after the foot is sharply dorsiflexed) is not specific for deep vein thrombosis because it can be elicited in any painful condition of the calf. In some cases, signs of a pulmonary embolus are the first indication of deep vein thrombosis.

CHART 28•3 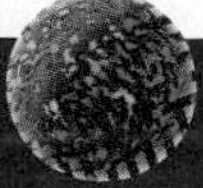 **Complications of Venous Thrombosis**

Chronic venous occlusion
Pulmonary emboli from dislodged thrombi
Valvular destruction
- Chronic venous insufficiency
- Increased venous pressure
- Varicosities
- Venous ulcers

Venous obstruction
- Increased distal pressure
- Fluid stasis
- Edema
- Venous gangrene

SUPERFICIAL VEINS

Thrombosis of superficial veins produces pain or tenderness, redness, and warmth in the involved area. The risk of the superficial venous thrombi becoming dislodged or fragmenting into emboli is very low because most of them dissolve spontaneously. Thus, this condition can be treated at home with bed rest, elevation of the leg, analgesics, and possibly anti-inflammatory medication.

Assessment and Diagnostic Findings

Careful assessment is invaluable in detecting early signs of venous disorders of the lower extremities. Patients with a history of varicose veins, hypercoagulation, neoplastic disease, cardiovascular disease, or recent major surgery or injury are at high risk. Also, the obese, the elderly, and women taking oral contraceptives are at risk.

Nursing Alert *When performing the nursing assessment, key concerns include limb pain, heaviness, functional impairment, ankle engorgement, and edema; differences in leg size (circumference) bilaterally from thigh to ankle; increase in the surface temperature of the leg, particularly the calf or ankle; and areas of tenderness or superficial thrombosis (cordlike venous segment).*

Prevention

Venous thrombosis, thrombophlebitis, and deep vein thrombosis can be prevented, especially if patients who are considered at high risk are identified and preventive measures are instituted without delay. Preventive measures include the application of elastic pressure stockings, the use of intermittent pneumatic compression devices, and special body positioning and exercise (all are

Risk Factors for **DEEP VEIN THROMBOSIS AND PULMONARY EMBOLISM** 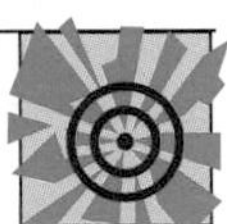

- Endothelial damage
  - Trauma
  - Surgery
  - Pacing wires
  - Central venous catheters
  - Dialysis access catheters
  - Local vein damage
  - Repetitive motion injury
- Venous stasis
  - Bed rest or immobilization
  - Obesity
  - History of varicosities
  - Spinal cord injury
  - Age (over 65)
- Coagulopathy
- Cancer
- Pregnancy
- Oral contraceptive use
- Congenital proteins C and S
- Anticardiolipin antibody
- Antithrombin III deficiency
- Polycythemia
- Septicemia

discussed below in the section on nursing management). A further method to prevent venous thrombosis in surgical patients is administration of subcutaneous heparin.

Medical Management

The objectives of treatment for deep vein thrombosis are to prevent the thrombus from growing and fragmenting (risking pulmonary embolism) and to prevent recurrent thromboemboli. Anticoagulant therapy (administration of a medication to delay the clotting time of blood, prevent the formation of a thrombus in postoperative patients, and forestall the extension of a thrombus once it has formed) can meet these objectives, although anticoagulants cannot dissolve a thrombus that has already formed.

ANTICOAGULATION THERAPY

Measures for preventing or reducing blood clotting within the vascular system are indicated in patients with thrombophlebitis, recurrent embolus formation, and persistent leg edema secondary to heart failure. They are also indicated in elderly patients with a hip fracture that may result in lengthy immobilization.

Heparin. Heparin, which is administered for 5 to 7 days by intermittent intravenous infusion or by continuous infusion, prevents the extension of a clot and the development of new clots. Oral anticoagulants, such as warfarin (Coumadin), are given with heparin therapy. Medication dosage is regulated by monitoring the partial thromboplastin time, the **international normalized ratio (INR)**, and the platelet count.

Low-Molecular-Weight Heparin. Subcutaneous low-molecular-weight heparin is an effective treatment for some cases of deep vein thrombosis. It has a longer half-life than unfractionated heparin, so doses can be given in one or two subcutaneous injections each day. Doses are adjusted according to weight. It is associated with fewer bleeding complications than unfractionated heparin. Because there are several preparations, the dosing schedule must be based on the product used and the protocol at each institution. The cost is higher than for unfractionated heparin; however, low-molecular-weight heparin may be used in pregnant women safely, and the patients are mobile and have an improved quality of life.

Thrombolytic Therapy. Unlike heparin, thrombolytic (fibrinolytic) therapy causes the clot to lyse and dissolve in 50% of patients. Thrombolytic therapy is given within the first 3 days after acute thrombosis, with either urokinase or streptokinase. The advantages of thrombolytic therapy include preservation of the venous valves and a reduced incidence of postthrombotic syndrome and chronic venous insufficiency. However, thrombolytic therapy results in approximately a threefold greater incidence of bleeding than does heparin. If bleeding occurs and cannot be stopped, the thrombolytic agent is discontinued.

SURGICAL MANAGEMENT

Surgery is necessary for deep vein thrombosis when (1) anticoagulant or thrombolytic therapy is contraindicated; (2) the danger of pulmonary embolism is extreme; and (3) the venous drainage is so severely compromised that permanent damage to the extremity will probably result. A thrombectomy (removal of the thrombosis) is the surgery of choice. A vena cava filter may be placed at the time of the thrombectomy; this filter will trap large emboli and prevent pulmonary emboli (for further details see Chap. 27).

Nursing Management

If the patient is receiving anticoagulant therapy, the nurse must frequently monitor the partial thromboplastin time, prothrombin time, hemoglobin and hematocrit values, platelet count, and fibrinogen level. Close nursing observation is also required to detect bleeding; if bleeding occurs, it must be reported immediately and therapy is discontinued.

ASSESSING AND MONITORING ANTICOAGULANT THERAPY

To prevent inadvertent infusion of large volumes of heparin, which could cause hemorrhage, continuous intravenous infusion by pump is the preferred method of administering sodium heparin. Dosage calculations are based on the patient's weight, and any possible bleeding tendencies are detected by a pretreatment clotting profile. If renal insufficiency exists, lower doses of heparin are required. Periodic coagulation tests and hematocrit evaluations are obtained. Heparin is in the effective range when the partial thromboplastin time is 1.5 times the control.

Intermittent intravenous injection is another means of administering heparin; a dilute aqueous solution of heparin is given every 4 hours. Administration may be facilitated by using a heparin lock, a small, butterfly-type scalp vein needle with an injection site at the end of the tubing.

Oral anticoagulants, such as warfarin, are monitored by the prothrombin time or INR. Because their effect is delayed for 3 to 5 days, they are usually administered with heparin until desired anticoagulation has been achieved (ie, when the prothrombin time is 1.5 to 2 times normal or the INR is 2.0 to 3.0).

MONITORING AND MANAGING POTENTIAL COMPLICATIONS

The principal complication of anticoagulant therapy is spontaneous bleeding anywhere in the body. Bleeding from the kidneys is detected by microscopic examination of the urine and is often the first sign of anticoagulant toxicity from excess dosage. Bruises, nosebleeds, and bleeding gums are also early signs. To reverse the effects of heparin promptly, intravenous injections of protamine sulfate may be prescribed. Reversing the effects of warfarin, a coumarin derivative, is more difficult, but effective measures that may be prescribed include vitamin K and possibly transfusion of fresh whole blood or plasma.

Thrombocytopenia. Another complication of therapy may be heparin-induced thrombocytopenia (a decrease in platelets), which may develop in patients who receive heparin for more than 5 days or on readministration after a brief interval of not receiving the medication. Beginning warfarin concomitantly with heparin will provide a stable INR or prothrombin time by day 5 of heparin treatment.

The use of low-molecular-weight heparin is less frequently associated with heparin-induced thrombocytopenia. The thrombocytopenia is thought to result from an immunologic mechanism that causes aggregation of platelets. This serious complication results in thromboembolic manifestations, and the prognosis is extremely guarded.

Prevention of thrombocytopenia depends on regular monitoring of platelet counts. Early signs are a falling platelet count to less than 100,000/mL or a decrease in platelet count exceeding 25% at one time, an increasing dose of heparin required to maintain a therapeutic level, thromboembolic or hemorrhagic complications, and a history of heparin sensitivity (Fahey, 1995). If thrombocytopenia does occur, platelet aggregation studies are conducted, the heparin is discontinued, and protamine sulfate is administered to reverse heparin's effects.

Drug Interactions. Because oral anticoagulants interact with many other medications, close monitoring of the patient's medication schedule is necessary. Medications that potentiate oral anticoagulants include salicylates, anabolic steroids, chloral hydrate, glucagon, chloramphenicol, neomycin, quinidine, and phenylbutazone (Butazolidin). Medications that decrease the anticoagulant effect include phenytoin, barbiturates, diuretics, and estrogen. It is advisable to identify medication interactions for patients taking specific oral anticoagulants.

Contraindications to anticoagulant therapy are summarized in the accompanying chart.

PROVIDING COMFORT

Bed rest, elevation of the affected extremity, elastic stockings, and analgesics for pain relief are adjuncts to therapy. They not only help to improve circulation, but they also increase comfort. Depending on the extent and location of a venous thrombosis, bed rest may be required for 5 to 7 days after diagnosis. This is approximately the time necessary for the thrombus to adhere to the vein wall, thus preventing embolization.

Warm, moist packs applied to the affected extremity reduce the discomfort associated with deep vein thrombosis, as do mild analgesics prescribed for pain control. When the patient begins to ambulate, elastic pressure stockings are used. Walking is better than standing or sitting for long periods. Bed exercises, such as dorsiflexion of the foot, are also recommended.

APPLYING ELASTIC PRESSURE STOCKINGS

Elastic pressure stockings are usually prescribed for patients with venous insufficiency. These stockings exert a sustained, evenly distributed pressure over the entire surface of the calves, thereby reducing the caliber of the superficial veins in the legs, resulting in increased flow in the deeper veins.

Nursing Alert *Any type of stocking, including the elastic type, can inadvertently become a tourniquet if applied incorrectly (ie, rolled tightly at the top). In such instances, the stockings will produce stasis rather than prevent it. Elastic pressure stockings are removed at night and reapplied before the legs are lowered from the bed to the floor in the morning.*

When the stockings are off, the skin is inspected for signs of irritation and the calves are examined for possible tenderness. Any skin changes or signs of tenderness are reported. Stockings are contraindicated in patients with severe pitting edema because they can produce severe pitting at the knee.

Gerontologic Considerations. Because of decreased strength and manual dexterity, elderly patients may be unable to apply elastic stockings properly. If such is the case, a family member or friend should be taught to assist the patient to apply the stockings so that they do not cause undue pressure on any part of the feet or legs.

USING INTERMITTENT PNEUMATIC COMPRESSION DEVICES

These devices can be used with elastic pressure stockings to prevent deep vein thrombosis. They consist of an electric controller that is attached by air hoses to plastic leg sleeves. The leg sleeves are divided into compartments, which sequentially fill to apply pressure to the ankle, calf, and thigh at 35 to 55 mm Hg pressure. These devices can increase blood velocity beyond that produced by the stockings. Nursing measures include ensuring that prescribed pressures are not exceeded, and assessing for patient comfort.

POSITIONING THE BODY AND ENCOURAGING EXERCISE

When the patient is on bed rest, the feet and lower legs should be elevated periodically above the level of the heart. This position allows the superficial and tibial veins to empty rapidly and to remain collapsed. Active and passive leg exercises, particularly those involving calf muscles, should be performed to increase venous flow. Early ambulation is most effective in preventing venous stasis. Deep-breathing exercises are beneficial because they produce increased negative pressure in the thorax, which assists in emptying the large veins.

PROMOTING HOME AND COMMUNITY-BASED CARE

In addition to teaching the patient how to apply elastic pressure stockings and advising him or her to elevate the legs and exercise adequately, the nurse teaches the patient about the medication, its purpose, and the need to take the correct amount at the specific times prescribed. The patient should also be aware that blood tests are scheduled periodically to determine whether a change in medication or dosage is required. If the patient fails to adhere to the therapeutic regimen, continuation of the medication therapy should be questioned. A person who refuses to discontinue the use of alcohol should not be receiving anticoagulants because chronic alcohol use decreases their effectiveness. In addition, in patients with liver problems, the potential for bleeding may be exacerbated by anticoagulant therapy.

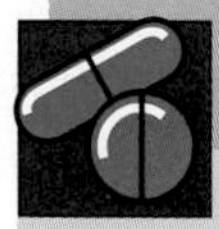

PHARMACOLOGY

Contraindications to Anticoagulation Therapy

- Lack of patient cooperation
- Bleeding from the following systems:
  - Gastrointestinal
  - Genitourinary
  - Respiratory
- Hemorrhagic blood dyscrasias
- Aneurysms
- Severe trauma
- Alcoholism
- Recent or impending surgery of:
  - Eye
  - Spinal cord
  - Brain
- Severe hepatic or renal disease
- Recent cerebrovascular hemorrhage
- Infections
- Open ulcerative wounds
- Occupations that involve a significant hazard for injury

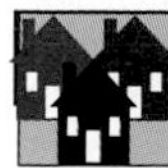

PATIENT EDUCATION AND HOME CARE

Taking Anticoagulant Medications

- Take the anticoagulant tablet at the same time each day, usually between 8:00 and 9:00 AM.
- Wear or carry identification indicating the anticoagulant being taken.
- Keep all appointments for blood tests.
- Because other medications affect the way the anticoagulant normally acts, do not take any of the following medications without consulting the physician: vitamins, cold medicines, antibiotics, aspirin, mineral oil, and anti-inflammatory agents, such as ibuprofen (Motrin) and similar medications. The physician should be contacted before taking any over-the-counter drugs.
- Avoid alcohol, because it may change the body's response to an anticoagulant.
- Avoid food fads, crash diets, or marked changes in eating habits.
- Do not take warfarin (Coumadin) unless directed by the physician.
- Do not stop taking Coumadin (when prescribed) unless directed to do so by the physician or nurse.
- When seeking treatment from another physician, a dentist, or a podiatrist, be sure to inform the caregiver that you are taking an anticoagulant.
- Contact your physician before having dental work or elective surgery.
- If any of the following signs appear, report them immediately to the physician:
  Faintness, dizziness, or increased weakness
  Severe headaches or abdominal pain
  Reddish or brownish urine
  Any bleeding—for example, cuts that do not stop bleeding
  Bruises that enlarge, nosebleeds, or unusual bleeding from any part of the body
  Red or black bowel movements
  Rash
- Avoid injury that can cause bleeding.
- For women: Notify the physician if you suspect pregnancy.

Chronic Venous Insufficiency

Venous insufficiency results from obstruction of the venous valves in the legs or a reflux of blood back through the valves. Both superficial and deep leg veins can be involved. Resultant venous hypertension can occur whenever there has been a prolonged increase in venous pressure, such as occurs with deep venous thrombosis. Because the walls of veins are thinner and more elastic than the walls of arteries, they distend readily when venous pressure is consistently elevated. In this state, leaflets of the venous valves are stretched and prevented from closing completely, thereby allowing a backflow or reflux of blood in the veins. Duplex ultrasound confirms the obstruction and identifies the level of valvular incompetence.

Clinical Manifestations

When the valves in the deep veins become incompetent after a thrombus has formed, postthrombotic syndrome may develop. This disorder is characterized by chronic venous stasis, resulting in edema, altered pigmentation, pain, and stasis dermatitis. The patient may notice the symptoms less in the morning and more in the evening. Obstruction or poor calf muscle pumping in addition to valvular reflux must be present for the development of severe postthrombotic syndrome, which includes stasis ulceration (Johnson & Strandness, 1997). Superficial veins may be dilated. The disorder is long-standing, difficult to treat, and often disabling.

Stasis ulcers develop as a result of the rupture of small skin veins and subsequent ulcerations. When these vessels rupture, red blood cells escape into surrounding tissues and then degenerate, leaving a brownish discoloration of the tissues. The pigmentation and ulcerations usually occur in the lower part of the extremity, in the area of the medial malleolus of the ankle. The skin becomes dry, cracks, and itches; subcutaneous tissues fibrose and atrophy. The risk of injury and infection of the extremities is increased.

Complications

Venous ulceration is the most serious complication of chronic venous insufficiency and can be associated with other conditions affecting the circulation of the lower extremities. The potential complications and the principles of care are the same.

Medical and Nursing Management

Management of the patient with venous insufficiency is directed at reducing venous stasis and preventing ulcerations. Measures that increase venous blood flow are antigravity activities, such as elevating the leg, and compression of superficial veins with elastic stockings.

Elevating the legs decreases edema, promotes venous return, and provides symptomatic relief. The legs should be elevated frequently throughout the day (at least 15 to 30 minutes every 2 hours). At night, the patient should sleep with the foot of the bed elevated about 15 cm (6 in). Prolonged sitting or standing still is detrimental; walking should be encouraged. When sitting, the patient should avoid placing pressure on the popliteal spaces, as occurs when crossing the legs or sitting with the legs dangling over the side of the bed. Constricting garments such as panty girdles or tight socks should be avoided.

Compression of the legs with elastic pressure stockings reduces the pooling of venous blood and enhances venous return to the heart. Thus, elastic pressure stockings are recommended for people with venous insufficiency. The stocking should fit so that pressure is greater at the foot and ankle and then gradually declines to a lesser pressure at the knee or groin. If the top of the stocking is too tight or becomes twisted, a tourniquet effect is created, which worsens venous pooling. Stockings should be applied after the legs have been elevated for a period of time, when the amount of blood in the leg veins is at its lowest.

Extremities with venous insufficiency must be carefully protected from trauma; the skin is kept clean, dry, and soft. Signs of ulceration are immediately reported to the health care provider for treatment and follow-up.

Leg Ulcers

A leg ulcer is an excavation of the skin surface that occurs when inflamed necrotic tissue sloughs off. About 75% of all leg ulcers result from chronic venous insufficiency. Lesions due to arterial insufficiency account for approximately 20%; the remaining 5% are due to burns, sickle cell anemia, and other factors.

Pathophysiology

Inadequate exchange of oxygen and other nutrients in the tissue is the metabolic abnormality that underlies the development of leg ulcers. When cellular metabolism cannot maintain energy balance, cell death (necrosis) results. Alterations in blood vessels at the arterial, capillary, and venous levels may affect cellular processes and lead to the formation of ulcers as well.

Clinical Manifestations

The clinical appearance and associated characteristics of leg ulcers are determined by the cause of the ulcer. Most ulcers, especially in an elderly patient, have more than one cause. The symptoms vary depending on whether the problem is arterial or venous in origin (see Table 28-2). The severity of the symptoms depends on the extent and duration of the vascular insufficiency. The ulcer itself appears as an open inflamed sore. Drainage may be present, or the area may be covered by eschar (dark, hard crust).

ARTERIAL ULCERS

Chronic arterial disease is characterized by intermittent claudication, which is pain caused by activity and relieved after a few minutes of rest. The patient may also complain of digital or forefoot pain at rest (previously discussed). If the onset of arterial occlusion is acute, ischemic pain is unrelenting and rarely relieved even with opioid analgesics. Typically, arterial ulcers are small, circular, deep ulcerations on the tips of toes or in the web spaces between toes. Ulcers often occur on the medial side of the hallux or lateral fifth toe and may be due to a combination of ischemia and pressure (Fig. 28-17).

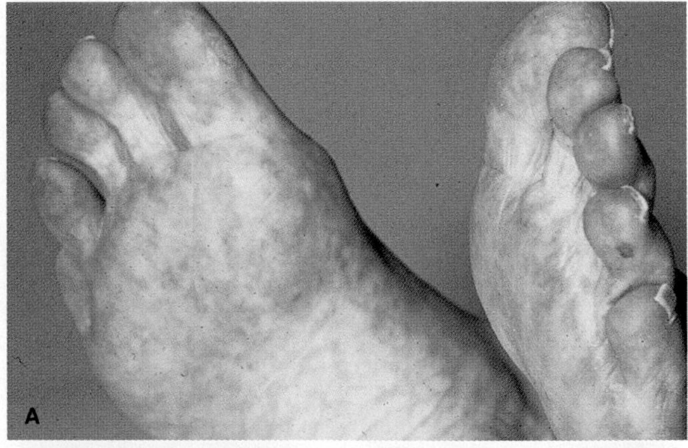

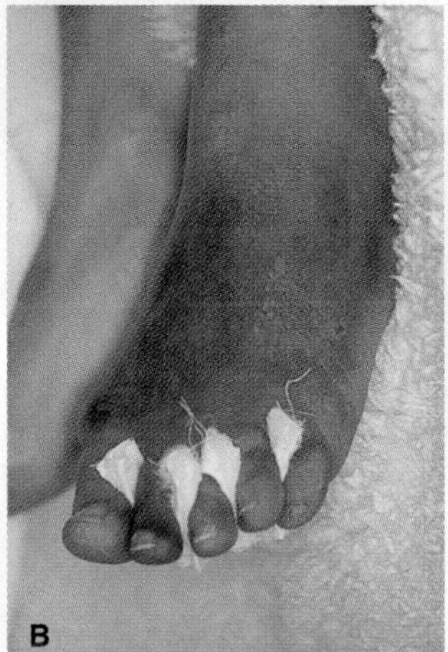

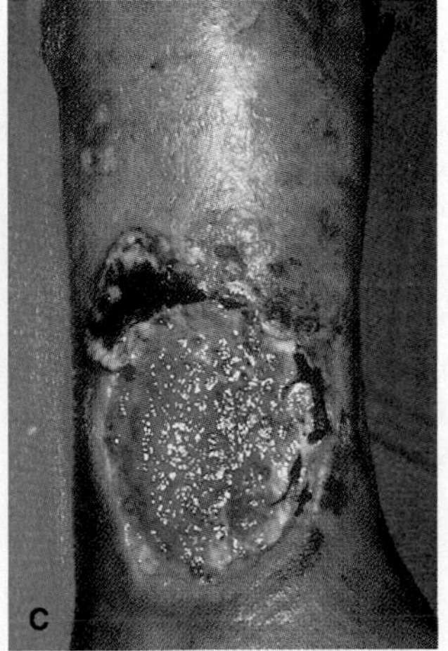

FIGURE 28•17 (**A**) Ulcers resulting from arterial emboli. (**B**) Gangrene of the toes resulting from severe arterial ischemia. (**C**) Ulcer from venous stasis.

Gangrene of the Toe. Arterial insufficiency may result in gangrene of the toe (digital gangrene), which is usually caused by trauma. The toe is stubbed and then turns black (see Fig. 28-17). Usually patients with this problem are elderly people without adequate circulation to provide revascularization. Débridement is contraindicated in these instances. Although the toe is gangrenous, it is dry. Managing dry gangrene is preferable to débriding the toe and causing an open wound that will not heal because of insufficient circulation. If the toe were to be amputated, the lack of adequate circulation would prevent healing and might make further amputation necessary—either a below-knee amputation or even an above-knee amputation. A higher level amputation in the elderly could result in a loss of independence and possible institutional care. Therefore, gangrene of the toe in an elderly person with poor circulation is usually left undisturbed.

VENOUS ULCERS

Chronic venous insufficiency is characterized by pain described as aching or heaviness. The foot and ankle may be edematous. Ulcerations are either in the area of the medial or lateral malleolus (gaiter area) and are typically large, superficial, and highly exudative. Venous hypertension causes extravasation of blood, which will discolor the pigment in the gaitor area (see Fig. 28-17). Patients with neuropathy frequently have ulcerations on the side of the foot over the metatarsal heads. These ulcers are painless and are described in further detail in Chapter 37.

Assessment and Diagnostic Findings

Because ulcers have many causes, their source needs to be identified so that appropriate therapy can be prescribed. The history of the condition is important in determining venous or arterial insufficiency. The pulses of the lower extremities (femoral, popliteal, posterior tibial, and dorsalis pedis) are carefully examined. More conclusive diagnostic aids are Doppler and duplex ultrasound studies, arteriography, and venography. Cultures of the ulcer drainage may be necessary to determine whether the infecting agent is the primary cause of the ulcer.

Medical Management

Patients with ulcers are effectively managed by advanced practice nurses in collaboration with physicians. All ulcers have the potential to become infected.

PHARMACOLOGIC THERAPY

Antibiotic therapy is prescribed when the ulcer is infected; the specific antibiotic is selected on the basis of culture and sensitivity test results. Oral antibiotics are usually prescribed because topical antibiotics have not proved to be effective for leg ulcers.

DÉBRIDEMENT

To promote healing, the wound is kept clean of drainage and necrotic tissue. The usual method is to flush the area with normal saline solution. If this is unsuccessful, débridement may be necessary. Débridement is the removal of nonviable tissue from wounds. Removing the dead tissue is important, particularly in instances of infection. Débridement can be accomplished by several different methods:

- Sharp surgical débridement is the fastest method and can be performed by the skilled advanced practice nurse in collaboration with the physician.

- Nonselective débridement can be accomplished by applying isotonic saline dressings of fine-mesh gauze to the ulcer. When the dressing dries, it is removed, along with the debris adhering to the gauze.
- Enzymatic débridement and the application of enzyme ointments may be prescribed to treat the ulcer. The ointment is applied to the lesion but not to normal surrounding skin. The lesion and ointment are then covered with a saline-soaked sponge that has been thoroughly wrung out. A gauze dressing and a loose bandage are then applied. The moist saline dressings are continued (without enzyme ointments) when pink granulating tissue develops.
- Débriding agents can be used. Dextranomer (Debrisan) beads are small, highly porous, spherical beads (0.1 to 0.3 mm in diameter) that can absorb wound secretions. Bacteria and the products of tissue necrosis and protein degradation are absorbed into the bead layer. When the beads are saturated, they take on a grayish-yellow color, at which point their cleansing action stops. They are then removed and a fresh layer is applied.
- Calcium alginate dressings can also be used for débridement and absorption of exudate. These dressings are changed daily or when the exudate seeps through the cover dressing. The dressing can also be used on areas that are bleeding, because the material helps stop the bleeding. As the dry fibers absorb exudate, they become a gel that is painlessly removed from the ulcer bed.

TOPICAL THERAPY

A variety of topical agents and soaps can be used in conjunction with washing and débridement therapies to promote healing of leg ulcers. The goals of treatment are to remove devitalized tissue and to keep the ulcer clean and moist while healing takes place. The treatment should not destroy developing tissue. For topical treatments to be successful, adequate nutritional therapy must be maintained.

WOUND DRESSING

Once the circulatory status has been assessed and determined to be adequate for healing (ABI of more than 0.5), surgical dressings can be used to promote a moist environment. The simplest method is to use a wound contact material (eg, Tegapore) next to the wound bed and cover it with gauze. Tegapore maintains a moist environment, can be left in place for several days, and does not disrupt the capillary bed when removed for evaluation. Hydrocolloids (DuoDerm CGF, Restore, Comfeel, Tegasorb) are also good choices to promote granulation tissue and reepithelialization. They also provide a barrier for protection because they adhere to the wound bed and surrounding tissue. However, a deep wound or an infected wound should never be covered with a hydrocolloid: the hydrocolloid dressing promotes an anaerobic environment and may increase the incidence of anaerobic infection.

Nursing Alert *Patient and family frustration, fear, and depression can lead to noncompliance; therefore, patient and family education is necessary before beginning wound dressing.*

STIMULATED HEALING

Tissue-engineered human skin equivalent along with therapeutic compression has been developed by Apligraf; it is a new skin product cultured from human dermal fibroblasts and keratinocytes. When applied, it seems to react to factors in the wound and may interact with the patient's cells to stimulate the production of growth factors. Application is not difficult, no suturing is involved, and the procedure is painless.

HYPERBARIC OXYGEN THERAPY

Hyperbaric oxygen therapy may be considered in addition to topical therapy. The increase in the level of oxygen tension to 30 mm Hg is thought to increase fibroblast and collagen proliferation.

NURSING PROCESS: THE PATIENT WITH LEG ULCERS

Assessment

A careful nursing history and assessment of symptoms are important. The extent and type of pain are carefully assessed, as are the appearance and temperature of the skin of both legs. The quality of all peripheral pulses is assessed, and comparisons are made of the pulses in both legs. The legs are checked for edema. If the extremity is edematous, the degree of edema is determined. Any limitation of mobility and activity that results from the vascular insufficiency is identified. In addition, the patient's nutritional status is assessed, and a history of diabetes, collagen disease, or varicose veins is obtained.

Diagnosis

Nursing Diagnoses

Based on the assessment data, major nursing diagnoses for the patient may include the following:

- Impairment of skin integrity related to vascular insufficiency
- Impaired physical mobility related to activity restrictions of the therapeutic regimen and pain
- Altered nutrition, less than body requirements, related to increased need for nutrients that promote wound healing

Collaborative Problems/Potential Complications

Based on the assessment data, potential complications that may develop include:

- Infection
- Gangrene

Planning and Goals

The major goals for the patient may include restoration of skin integrity, improved physical mobility, adequate nutrition, and avoidance of complications. The nursing challenge in caring for these patients is great, whether the patient is in the hospital, in a long-term care facility, or at home. The physical problem is often a long-term one that causes a substantial drain on the patient's physical, emotional, and economic resources.

Nursing Interventions

Restoring Skin Integrity

To promote wound healing, measures are used to keep the area clean. Cleansing requires very gentle handling, a mild soap, and lukewarm water. Positioning of the legs depends on whether the ulcer is of arterial or venous origin. If there is arterial insufficiency, the patient should be referred to be evaluated for vascular reconstruction. If there is venous insufficiency, dependent edema can be avoided by elevating the lower extremities. A decrease in edema will promote the exchange of cellular nutrients and waste products in the area of the ulcer; thus, healing is promoted.

Avoiding trauma to the lower extremities is imperative in promoting skin integrity. Protective boots may be used (eg, the Rooke Vascular boot, Lunax Boot, Bunny Boot); they are soft and provide warmth and protection from injury. If the patient is on bed rest, it is important to relieve pressure on the heels to prevent pressure ulcerations. When the patient is in bed, a bed cradle can be used to relieve pressure from bed linens and to prevent anything from touching the legs. When the patient is ambulatory, all obstacles are moved from the patient's path so that the patient's legs will not be bumped. Heating pads, hot-water bottles, or hot baths are avoided. Heat increases the oxygen demands and thus the blood flow demands of the tissue, which in this case are already compromised. The patient with diabetes mellitus suffers from neuropathy with decreased sensation; thus, heating pads may produce injury before the patient is aware of being burned.

Improving Physical Mobility

Generally, physical activity is initially restricted to promote healing. When infection resolves and healing begins, ambulation resumes gradually and progressively. Activity promotes arterial flow and venous return and is encouraged after the acute phase of the ulcer process. Until full activity resumes, the patient is encouraged to move about when in bed, to turn from side to side frequently, and to exercise the upper extremities to maintain muscle tone and strength. Meanwhile, diversional activities that interest the patient are encouraged. Consultation with an occupational therapist may be helpful if a prolonged period of limited mobility and activity is anticipated.

If pain limits the patient's activity, analgesics may be prescribed by the physician. The pain of peripheral vascular disease, whether it is arterial or venous, is typically chronic. Analgesics may be taken before scheduled activities to help the patient participate more comfortably.

Promoting Adequate Nutrition

Nutritional deficiencies are determined from the patient's report of usual dietary intake. Alterations in the diet are made to remedy these deficiencies. In addition, a diet that is high in protein, vitamins C and A, iron, and zinc is encouraged in an attempt to promote healing.

Many patients with peripheral vascular disease are elderly. Their caloric intake may need to be adjusted because of their decreased metabolic rate and level of activity. Particular consideration should also be given to their iron intake, because many elderly people are anemic.

Once a diet plan has been developed that meets the patient's nutritional needs and promotes healing, diet instruction is provided to the patient and family. The nurse and patient design the diet plan to be compatible with the patient's and family's lifestyle and preferences.

Evaluation

Expected Outcomes

Expected outcomes may include:

1. Demonstrates restored skin integrity
   a. Exhibits absence of inflammation
   b. Exhibits absence of drainage; negative wound culture
   c. Avoids trauma to the legs
2. Increases physical mobility
   a. Progresses gradually to optimal level of activity
   b. Reports that pain does not impede activity
3. Attains adequate nutrition
   a. Selects foods high in protein, vitamins, iron, and zinc
   b. Discusses with family members dietary modifications that need to be made at home
   c. Plans, with family, a diet that is nutritionally sound

Varicose Veins

Varicose veins (varicosities) are abnormally dilated, tortuous, superficial veins caused by incompetent venous valves (Fig. 28-18). Most commonly, this condition occurs in the lower extremities, the saphenous veins, or the lower trunk; however, it can occur elsewhere in the body (eg, esophageal varices; see Chap. 36).

It is estimated that varicose veins of the lower extremities affect one in five people in the world. The condition is most common in women and in people whose occupations require prolonged standing, such as salespeople, hair stylists, teachers, nurses, ancillary medical personnel, and construction workers. A hereditary weakness of the vein wall may contribute to the development of varicosities, and it is not uncommon to see this condition occur in several members of the same family.

Pathophysiology

Varicose veins may be considered primary (without involvement of deep veins) or secondary (resulting from obstruction of deep veins). A reflux of venous blood in the veins results in venous stasis. If only the superficial veins are affected, the person may have no symptoms but may be troubled by the appearance of the dilated veins.

Clinical Manifestations

Symptoms, if present, may take the form of dull aches, muscle cramps, and increased muscle fatigue in the lower legs. Ankle edema and a feeling of heaviness of the legs may occur. Nocturnal cramps are common. When deep venous obstruction results

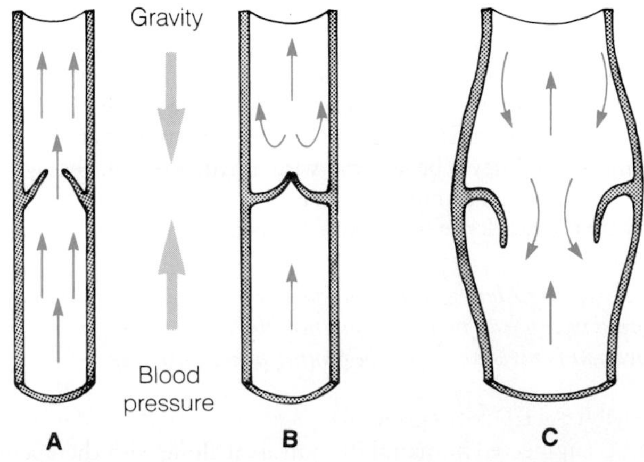

FIGURE 28•18 Competent valves showing blood flow patterns when the valve is open (**A**) and closed (**B**), allowing blood to flow against gravity. (**C**) With faulty or incompetent valves, the blood is unable to move toward the heart.

in varicose veins, patients may demonstrate the signs and symptoms of chronic venous insufficiency: edema, pain, pigmentation, and ulcerations. Susceptibility to injury and infection is increased.

Assessment and Diagnostic Findings

Diagnostic tests for varicose veins include the duplex scan, which documents the anatomic site of reflux and provides a quantitative measure of the severity of valvular reflux. Air plethysmography measures changes in venous blood volume. Venography is not routinely performed to evaluate for valvular reflux. When it is used, however, it involves injecting a radiographic contrast agent into the leg veins so that the vein anatomy can be visualized by x-ray studies during various leg movements.

Prevention

Activities that cause venous stasis should be avoided, such as wearing tight socks or a constricting panty girdle, crossing the legs at the thighs, and sitting or standing for long periods. Changing position frequently, elevating the legs when they are tired, and getting up to walk for several minutes of every hour promote circulation. The patient should be encouraged to walk 1 or 2 miles a day if there are no contraindications. Walking up the stairs rather than using the elevator or escalator is helpful in promoting circulation. Swimming is also good exercise for the legs.

Elastic stockings are useful, especially knee-high stockings. Patients are more likely to use knee-high stockings than thigh-high stockings. The overweight patient should be encouraged to begin a weight-reduction plan.

Medical Management

Surgery for varicose veins requires that the deep veins be patent and functional. The saphenous vein is ligated and divided. The vein is ligated high in the groin, where the saphenous vein meets the femoral vein. An incision is then made in the ankle, and a metal or plastic wire is passed the full length of the vein, "stripping" as it passes (Fig. 28-19). Pressure and elevation keep bleeding at a minimum during surgery.

SCLEROTHERAPY

In sclerotherapy, a chemical is injected into the vein, irritating the venous endothelium and producing localized phlebitis and fibrosis, thereby obliterating the lumen of the vein. This treatment may be performed alone for small varicosities or may follow vein ligation or stripping. Sclerosing is palliative rather than curative. After the sclerosing agent is injected, elastic compression bandages are applied to the leg. These are worn for approximately 5 days. The health care provider who performed sclerotherapy removes the first bandages. Compression stockings are then worn for an additional 5 weeks.

After sclerotherapy, patients are encouraged to perform walking activities as prescribed to maintain blood flow in the leg. Walking enhances dilution of the sclerosing agent.

Nursing Management

Surgery can be performed in an outpatient setting, or patients can be admitted to the hospital on the day of surgery and discharged the next day, but nursing measures are the same as if the patient were hospitalized. Bed rest is maintained for 24 hours, after which the patient begins walking every 2 hours for 5 to 10 minutes. Elastic pressure stockings are used to maintain compression of the leg. They are worn continuously for about 1 week after vein stripping. The nurse assists the patient to perform exercises and move the legs. The foot of the bed should be elevated. Standing still and sitting are discouraged.

PROMOTING COMFORT AND UNDERSTANDING

The nurse may administer analgesics to help patients move affected extremities more comfortably. Dressings are inspected for bleeding, particularly at the groin, where the risk of bleeding

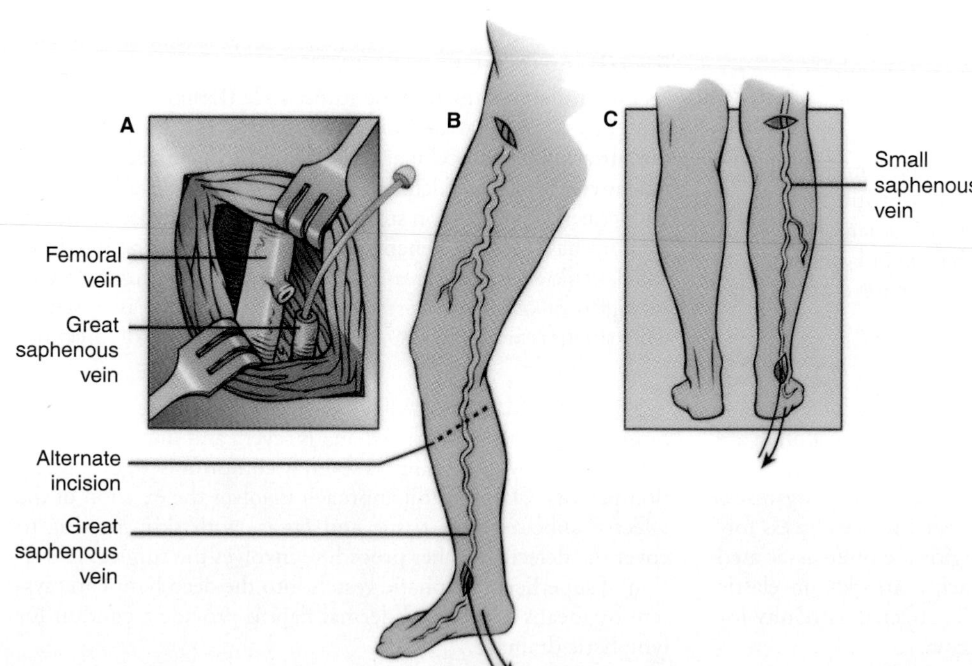

FIGURE 28•19 Ligation and stripping of the great and the small saphenous veins. (**A**) The tributaries of the saphenous vein have been ligated, and the saphenous vein has been ligated at the saphenofemoral junction. (**B**) The vein stripper has been inserted from the ankle superiorly to the groin. The vein is stripped from above downward. A number of alternate incisions may be needed to remove separate varicose masses. (**C**) The small saphenous vein is stripped from its junction with the popliteal vein to a point posterior to the lateral malleolus.

is greatest. In addition, the nurse is alert for reported sensations of "pins and needles." Hypersensitivity to touch in the involved extremity may indicate a temporary or permanent nerve injury resulting from surgery, because the saphenous vein and nerve are in close proximity in the leg.

If the patient underwent sclerotherapy and complains of a burning sensation in the injected leg for 1 or 2 days, the nurse may recommend a mild sedative and walking to provide relief. Because bathing may be a problem during this time, a plastic bag may be placed over the bandaged leg and secured above the bandage to allow the patient to shower.

PROMOTING HOME AND COMMUNITY-BASED CARE

Patients require long-term elastic support of the leg after discharge, and plans are made to obtain adequate supplies of elastic stockings or bandages as appropriate. Exercises of the legs also will be necessary; the development of an individualized plan requires consultation with the patient and the health care team.

MANAGEMENT OF LYMPHATIC DISORDERS

The lymphatic system consists of a set of vessels that spread throughout most of the body. These vessels start as lymph capillaries that drain unabsorbed plasma from tissue spaces. They unite to form the lymph vessels, which in turn pass through the lymph nodes and finally empty into the large thoracic duct that joins the jugular vein on the left side of the neck.

Lymph is the fluid found in lymph vessels. Tissue fluids are found outside of vessels in the cellular interspace. The lymphatic system of the abdominal cavity maintains a steady flow of digested fatty food (chyle) from the intestinal mucosa to the thoracic duct. In other parts of the body, the lymphatic system's function is regional; the lymphatic vessels of the head, for example, empty into clusters of lymph nodes located in the neck, and those of the extremities into nodes in the axillae and the groin. The flow of lymph depends on the intrinsic contractions of the lymph vessels, the contraction of muscles, respiratory movements, and gravity.

Lymphangitis and Lymphadenitis

Lymphangitis is an acute inflammation of the lymphatic channels. It arises most commonly from a focus of infection in an extremity. Usually, the infectious organism is a hemolytic streptococcus. The characteristic red streaks that extend up the arm or the leg from an infected wound outline the course of the lymphatic vessels as they drain.

The lymph nodes located along the course of the lymphatic channels also become enlarged, red, and tender (acute lymphadenitis). They can also become necrotic and form an abscess (suppurative lymphadenitis). The nodes involved most often are those in the groin, the axilla, or the cervical region.

Because these infections are nearly always caused by organisms that are sensitive to antibiotics, it is unusual to see abscess formation. Recurrent episodes of lymphangitis are often associated with progressive lymphedema. After acute attacks, an elastic stocking or sleeve should be worn on the affected extremity for several months to prevent long-term edema.

Lymphedema and Elephantiasis

Lymphedemas are classified as primary (congenital malformations) or secondary (acquired obstruction). A swelling of tissues in the extremities occurs because of an increased quantity of lymph that results from an obstruction of lymphatic vessels. It is especially marked when the extremity is in a dependent position. Initially the edema is soft, pitting, and relieved by treatment. As the condition progresses, the edema becomes firm, nonpitting, and unresponsive to treatment. The most common type is congenital lymphedema (lymphedema praecox), which is caused by hypoplasia of the lymphatic system of the lower extremity. This disorder is usually seen in women and first appears between ages 15 and 25.

The obstruction may be in both the lymph nodes and the lymphatic vessels. At times it is seen in the arm after a radical mastectomy for breast cancer, and in the leg in association with varicose veins or chronic thrombophlebitis. In the latter case, the lymphatic obstruction usually is due to a chronic lymphangitis. Lymphatic obstruction caused by a parasite (filaria) is seen frequently in the tropics. When chronic swelling is present, there may be frequent bouts of acute infection characterized by high fever and chills and increased residual edema after the inflammation has resolved. These lead to chronic fibrosis, thickening of the subcutaneous tissues, and hypertrophy of the skin. This condition, in which chronic swelling of the extremity recedes only slightly with elevation, is referred to as elephantiasis.

Medical Management

The goal of therapy is to reduce and control the edema and prevent infection. When the leg is affected, strict bed rest with the leg elevated may aid in mobilizing the fluids. Active and passive exercises assist in moving lymphatic fluid into the bloodstream. External compression devices milk the fluid proximally from the foot to the hip. When the patient is ambulatory, custom-fitted elastic stockings are worn; those with the highest compression strength (exceeding 40 mm Hg) are required.

PHARMACOLOGIC THERAPY

As initial therapy, the diuretic furosemide (Lasix) is taken intermittently to prevent the fluid overload that can result from the mobilization of extracellular fluid. Diuretics have also been used palliatively for lymphedema in conjunction with elevating the leg and wearing compression stockings. However, the use of diuretics alone has very little benefit because their main action is to limit capillary filtration by decreasing circulating blood volume. If lymphangitis or cellulitis is present, antibiotic therapy is initiated. The patient is taught to inspect the skin for evidence of infection.

SURGICAL MANAGEMENT

Surgery is performed if the edema is severe and uncontrolled by medical therapy, if mobility is severely compromised, or if infection persists. One surgical approach involves the excision of the affected subcutaneous tissue and fascia, with skin grafting to cover the defect. Another procedure involves the surgical relocation of superficial lymphatic vessels into the deep lymphatic system by means of a buried dermal flap to provide a conduit for lymphatic drainage.

After surgery, the management of skin grafts and flaps is the same as when these therapies are used for other conditions. Prophylactic antibiotics may be prescribed for 5 to 7 days. Constant elevation of the affected extremity and observations for complications are essential. Complications may include flap necrosis, hematoma or abscess under the flap, and cellulitis.

Critical Thinking Exercises

1. You are assigned to a medical clinic where many elderly patients receive care. Two patients, both with peripheral vascular disease, are overheard comparing their symptoms and their medical management. When they realize that many of their symptoms are similar but their medical management is distinctly different, they question you about this. What further information will be helpful in determining an accurate explanation to give to these two patients?
2. Your patient has been diagnosed with a calf vein deep vein thrombosis. The physician gives the patient two treatment options: hospitalization with intravenous sodium heparin therapy, or home treatment with low-molecular-weight heparin. How would you direct your assessment to identify the factors that might affect the patient's decision?
3. You are visiting a patient with a known venous ulceration of the right leg. During your home visit, she complains of right ankle swelling, constant pain in the right fourth and fifth digits of the foot, and pain that is worse when she tries to sleep at night. Physical examination reveals cyanotic digits and no palpable dorsalis pedis pulse. There is a 3-cm shallow, weeping ulcer in the medial malleolus region. Analyze these findings, indicate what you think the possible causes may be for these findings, and describe the actions you would take and explain why.

References and Selected Readings

BOOKS

Berne, R., & Levy, M. (1998). *Physiology.* St. Louis: Mosby–Year Book.

Bullock, B. (1996). *Pathophysiology: Adaptations and alterations in function* (4th ed.). Philadelphia: Lippincott-Raven.

Coleman, R. W., et al. (1994). *Hemostasis and thrombosis: Basic principles and clinical practice* (3rd ed.). Philadelphia: J. B. Lippincott.

Guyton, A., & Hall, J. (1996). *Textbook of medical physiology* (9th ed.). Philadelphia: W. B. Saunders.

Haimovici, H. (1996). *Vascular surgery principles and techniques* (4th ed.). Cambridge, MA: Blackwell Science.

Jarvis, C. (1998). *Physical examination and health assessment* (2nd ed.). Philadelphia: W. B. Saunders.

Moore, W. S. (1998). *Vascular surgery: A comprehensive review* (5th ed.). Philadelphia: W. B. Saunders.

Robbins, S., et al. (1995). *Pocket companion to pathologic basis of disease* (5th ed.). Philadelphia: W. B. Saunders.

Rodgers-Kinner, M. (1998). *AACN clinical reference for critical care nursing* (4th ed.). St. Louis: Mosby.

Rutherford, R. B. (1995). *Vascular surgery* (4th ed., Vols. I and II). Philadelphia: W. B. Saunders.

Tibbs, D. J., et al. (1997). *Varicose veins, venous disorders and lymphatic problems in the lower limbs.* New York: Oxford University Press.

Veith, F. J., et al. (1994). *Vascular surgery: Principles, and practice* (2nd ed.). New York: McGraw-Hill.

Zierler, B. (1998). *Integrated care pathway for venous thromboembolism.* RO3 HSO9348-02, Agency for Health Care Policy and Research.

Zierler, R. E., & Strandness, D. E., Jr. (1988). Diseases of the small arteries of the extremities. In: *Hardy's textbook of surgery* (2nd ed.). Philadelphia: J. B. Lippincott.

JOURNALS

Anticoagulant and Thrombolytic Therapy

Beckey, N. P. (1999). Outpatient management of patients on warfarin. *Lippincott's Primary Care Practice, 3*(3), 280–289.

Fahey, V. A. (1995). Heparin-induced thrombocytopenia. *Journal of Vascular Nursing, 13*(4), 112–116.

Nunnelee, J. D. (1997). Low-molecular-weight heparin. *Journal of Vascular Nursing, 15*(3), 94–96.

Arterial Conditions

Cantwell-Gab, K. (1996). Identifying chronic peripheral arterial disease. *American Journal of Nursing, 96*(7), 40–47.

Fellows, E. (1995). Abdominal aortic aneurysm: Warning flags to watch for. *American Journal of Nursing, 95*(5), 26–32.

Finkelmeier, B. A. (1997). Dissection of the aorta: A clinical update. *Journal of Vascular Nursing, 15*(3), 88–93.

Haji-Aghaii, M., & Fogarty, T. (1998). Balloon angioplasty, stenting and role of atherectomy. *Surgical Clinics of North America, 78*(4), 593–616.

Kaufman, M. W., & All, A. C. (1996). Raynaud's disease: Patient education as a primary nursing intervention. *Journal of Vascular Nursing, 14*(2), 34–39.

Lacey, K. O. (1996). Subclavian steal syndrome: A review. *Journal of Vascular Nursing, 14*(1), 1–7.

Lombardo, K. M. (1997). Endovascular grafting of abdominal aortic aneurysms. *Journal of Vascular Nursing, 15*(3), 83–87.

Sandler, R. L. (1995). Abdominal aortic aneurysm. *American Journal of Nursing, 95*(1), 38–39.

Strider, D., et al. (1996). Challenges with Takayasu's arteritis: A case study. *Journal of Vascular Nursing, 14*(1), 12–17.

Diagnosis and Assessment

Berdejo, G. L., et al. (1998). Color Duplex ultrasound evaluation of transluminally placed endovascular grafts for aneurysm repair. *Journal of Vascular Technology, 22*(4), 209–212.

Verta, K. F., & Verta, M. J. (1998). Alternative imaging techniques in vascular surgery. *Journal of Vascular Nursing, 16*(4), 78–83.

Zierler, R. E., &. Zierler, B. K. (1997). Duplex sonography of lower extremity arteries. *Seminars in Ultrasound, CT and MRI, 18*(1), 39–56.

Leg Ulcers

Kowallek, D. L., & DePalma, R. G. (1997). Venous ulceration: Active approaches to treatment. *Journal of Vascular Nursing, 15*(2), 50–57.

Venous Conditions

Johnson, B. F., & Strandness, D. E., Jr. (1997). Ultrasound and venous valvular reflux. *Journal of Vascular Investigation, 3*(2), 108–113.

Johnson, M. T. (1997). Treatment and prevention of varicose veins. *Journal of Vascular Nursing, 15*(3), 97–103.

Kurgan, A., & Nunnelee, J. D. (1995). Upper extremity venous thrombosis. *Journal of Vascular Nursing, 13*(1), 21–23.

Meissner, M. H., et al. (1995). Propagation, rethrombosis and new thrombus formation after acute deep vein thrombosis. *Journal of Vascular Surgery, 22*(5), 558–567.

Resources

National Heart, Lung and Blood Institute, Education Programs Information Center, 4733 Bethesda Ave, Suite 530, Bethesda MD 20814; E-mail: www.nhlbinih.gov/nhlbi/nhlbi.htm

Agency for Health Care Policy and Research, Public Health Service, U.S. Department of Health and Human Services, Center for Research Dissemination and Liaison AHCPR Publication Clearinghouse, P.O. Box 8547, Silver Spring, MD 20907; 1-800-358-9295; E-mail: www.ahcpr.gov

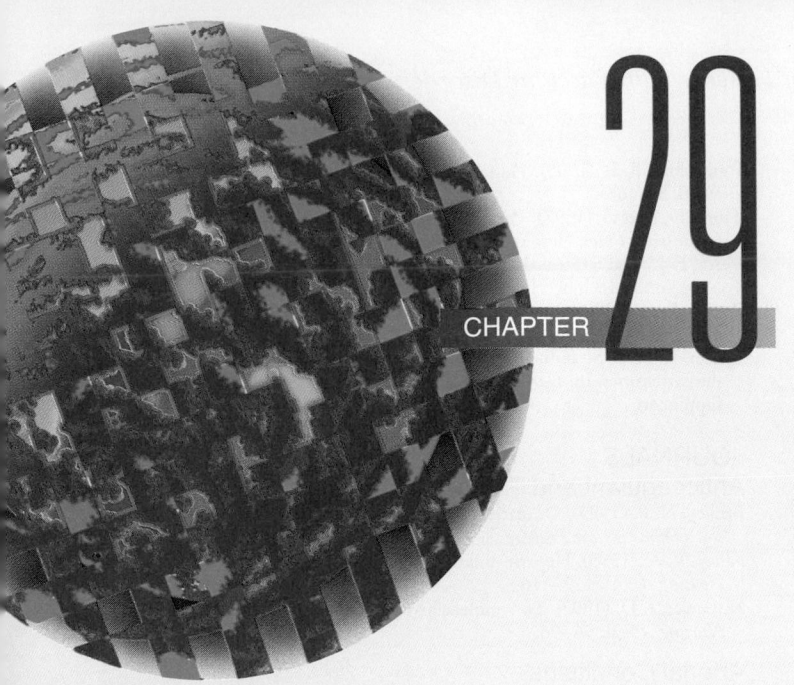

Assessment and Management of Patients With Hypertension

Learning Objectives

On completion of this chapter, the learner will be able to:

1. Define blood pressure and identify risk factors for hypertension.
2. Explain the difference between normal blood pressure and hypertension, and discuss the significance of hypertension.
3. Describe the treatment approach for hypertension, including lifestyle changes and medication therapy.
4. Use the nursing process as a framework for care of the patient with hypertension.
5. Describe the necessity for immediate treatment of hypertensive crisis.

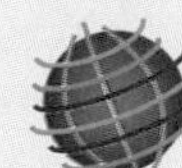

Blood pressure is the product of cardiac output multiplied by peripheral resistance. Cardiac output itself is the product of the heart rate multiplied by the stroke volume. In normal circulation, pressure is exerted by the flow of blood through the heart and blood vessels. High blood pressure, known as hypertension, can result from a change in cardiac output, a change in peripheral resistance, or both. The medications used in treatment of hypertension either decrease peripheral resistance, blood volume, or the strength and rate of myocardial contraction.

GLOSSARY

dyslipidemia: abnormally high or low blood lipid levels

hypertensive emergency: a situation in which blood pressure must be lowered immediately to prevent damage to target organs

hypertensive urgency: a situation in which blood pressure must be lowered within a few hours to prevent damage to target organs

JNC VI: Sixth Joint National Committee on the Prevention, Detection, Evaluation and Treatment of High Blood Pressure; body established to study and make recommendations about hypertension in the United States. Findings and recommendations of JNC VI are contained in an extensive report published in 1997.

monotherapy: medication therapy with a single medication

primary, hypertension: also called essential hypertension; denotes high blood pressure from an unidentified cause

rebound hypertension: blood pressure that is controlled with therapy and that becomes uncontrolled (abnormally high) with the discontinuation of therapy

secondary hypertension: high blood pressure from an identified cause, such as, renal disease

HYPERTENSION DEFINED

Officially, hypertension is defined as a systolic blood pressure greater than 140 mm Hg and a diastolic pressure greater than 90 mm Hg over a sustained period. Table 29-1 shows the categories of blood pressure levels established in 1997 by the Sixth Joint National Committee on the Prevention, Detection, Evaluation and Treatment of High Blood Pressure (**JNC VI**). The classification shows the direct relation between the risk of morbidity and mortality from hypertension and the level of systolic and diastolic blood pressures. The higher the pressure, either systolic or diastolic, the greater the risk.

Three stages (stages 1, 2, and 3) of hypertension are defined. The JNC used these terms, similar to those used to describe cancer progression, so that both the public and health care professionals would be aware that sustained elevations in blood pressure are associated with increased risks to health. Even within the normotensive range, three levels of blood pressure—optimal, normal, and high-normal—were specified to indicate that the lower the blood pressure, the lower the risk.

The JNC stated that the hypertension diagnosis must be based on the average of two or more blood pressure measurements taken in two or more contacts with the health care provider after an initial screening. The JNC also developed recommendations for follow-up monitoring according to initial blood pressure readings at the time of diagnosis (Table 29-2).

PRIMARY HYPERTENSION

Between 20% and 25% of the adult population in the United States has hypertension. Of this population, between 90% and 95% have **primary hypertension**, meaning the reason for the elevation in blood pressure cannot be identified. The remaining 5% to 10% of this group have high blood pressure related to specific causes, such as narrowing of the renal arteries, renal parenchymal disease, certain medications, pregnancy, and coarctation of the aorta. **Secondary hypertension** is the term used to signify high blood pressure from an identified cause.

Hypertension is sometimes called "the silent killer" because people who have it are often symptom free. In the most recent national survey (1991 to 1994), a total of 32% of people who had pressures exceeding 140/90 mm Hg were unaware of an elevation of blood pressure. Once identified, elevated blood pressure should be monitored at regular intervals because hypertension is a lifelong condition.

Hypertension often accompanies risk factors for atherosclerotic heart disease, such as **dyslipidemia** (abnormal blood fat levels) and diabetes mellitus. The incidence of hypertension is higher in the southeastern United States, particularly among African Americans. Cigarette smoking does not cause high blood

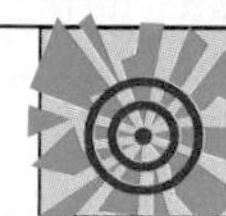

Risk Factors for HYPERTENSION

Age
Family history
Excess body weight
Sedentary lifestyle
Sodium intake (although current controversy continues over the role of salt in hypertension)

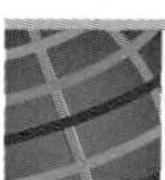

TABLE 29•1 Classification of Blood Pressure for Adults Age 18 and Older*

Category	Systolic (mm Hg)		Diastolic (mm Hg)
Optimal	<120	and	<80
Normal†	<130	and	<85
High-normal	130–139	or	85–89
Hypertension‡			
Stage 1	140–159	or	90–99
Stage 2	160–179	or	100–109
Stage 3	≥180	or	≥110

* Not taking antihypertensive drugs and not acutely ill. When systolic and diastolic blood pressures fall into different categories, the higher category should be selected to classify the individual's blood pressure status. For example, 160/92 mm Hg should be classified as stage 2 hypertension, and 174/120 mm Hg should be classified as stage 3 hypertension. Isolated systolic hypertension is defined as SBP of 140 mm Hg or greater and DBP below 90 mm Hg and staged appropriately (eg, 170/82 mm Hg is defined as stage 2 isolated systolic hypertension). In addition to classifying stages of hypertension on the basis of average blood pressure levels, clinicians should specify presence or absence of target organ disease and additional risk factors. This specificity is important for risk classification and treatment.

† Optimal blood pressure with respect to cardiovascular risk is below 120/80 mm Hg. However, unusually low readings should be evaluated for clinical significance.

‡ Based on the average of two or more readings taken at each of two or more visits after an initial screening.

From the Report of the Sixth Joint National Committee on Prevention, Detection, Evaluation, and Treatment of High Blood Pressure. (1997). *Archives of Internal Medicine, 157,* 2413–2446.

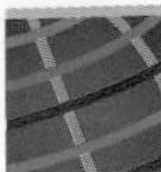

TABLE 29•2 **Recommendations for Follow-up Based on Initial Blood Pressure Measurements for Adults**

Initial Blood Pressure (mm Hg)*		
SYSTOLIC	DIASTOLIC	Follow-Up Recommended†
<130	<85	Recheck in 2 years
130–139	85–89	Recheck in 1 year‡
140–159	90–99	Confirm within 2 months
160–179	100–109	Evaluate or refer to source of care within 1 month
≥180	≥110	Evaluate or refer to source of care immediately or within 1 week depending on clinical situation

* If systolic and diastolic categories are different, follow recommendations for shorter time follow-up (eg, 160/86 mm Hg should be evaluated or referred to source of care within 1 month).

† Modify the scheduling of follow-up according to reliable information about past blood pressure measurements, other cardiovascular risk factors, or target organ disease.

‡ Provide advice about lifestyle modifications.

From the Report of the Sixth Joint National Committee on Prevention, Detection, Evaluation, and Treatment of High Blood Pressure. (1997). *Archives of Internal Medicine, 157,* 2413–2446.

pressure; however, if a person with hypertension smokes, his or her risk of dying from heart disease or related disorders increases significantly.

Hypertension can be viewed as three entities: a sign, a risk factor for atherosclerotic cardiovascular disease, and a disease. As a sign, nurses and other health professionals use blood pressure to monitor a patient's clinical status; an elevated pressure may indicate an excessive dose of vasoconstrictive medication or other problems. As a risk factor, hypertension contributes to the rate at which atherosclerotic plaque accumulates within arterial walls. When considered as a disease, hypertension is a major contributor to death from cardiac, renal, and peripheral vascular disease.

Prolonged blood pressure elevation eventually damages blood vessels throughout the body, particularly in target organs such as the heart, kidneys, brain, and eyes. Thus, the usual consequences of prolonged, uncontrolled hypertension are myocardial infarction, cardiac failure, renal failure, strokes, and impaired vision. In addition, the left ventricle of the heart becomes enlarged as it works to pump blood against the elevated pressure (left ventricular hypertrophy). An echocardiogram is the recommended method of identifying this hypertrophy.

Pathophysiology

Although the precise cause for most cases of hypertension cannot be identified, it is understood that hypertension is a multifactorial condition. Because hypertension is a sign, it is most likely to have many causes, just as fever has many causes. For hypertension to occur, there must a change in one of the factors in the blood pressure equation: peripheral resistance or cardiac output. Some of these factors are outlined in Figure 29-1. For hypertension to occur, there must be a problem with the control systems monitoring or regulating pressure, in addition to one or more alterations in the factors in the blood pressure equation. Single gene mutations have been identified for a few very rare types of hypertension, but most types of high blood pressure are thought to be polygenic (mutations in more than one gene).

Several hypotheses about the pathophysiologic bases of elevated blood pressure are associated with the concept of hypertension as a multifactorial condition. Given the overlap among these hypotheses, it is likely that aspects of all of them will eventually prove correct. Some of these hypotheses are listed below. Hypertension is a result of:

- Increased sympathetic nervous system activity related to dysfunction of the autonomic nervous system
- Increased renal reabsorption of sodium, chloride, and water related to a genetic variation in the pathways by which the kidneys handle sodium
- Increased activity of the renin-angiotensin-aldosterone system, resulting in expansion of extracellular fluid volume and increased systemic vascular resistance
- Decreased vasodilation of the arterioles related to dysfunction of the vascular endothelium
- Resistance to insulin action, which may be a common factor linking hypertension, type 2 diabetes mellitus, hypertriglyceridemia, obesity, and glucose intolerance

Gerontologic Considerations

Structural and functional changes in the heart and blood vessels contribute to increases in blood pressure that occur with age. These changes include accumulation of atherosclerotic plaque, fragmentation of arterial elastins, increased collagen deposits, and impaired vasodilation. The result of these changes is a decrease in the elasticity of the major blood vessels. Consequently, the aorta and large arteries are less able to accommodate the volume of blood pumped out by the heart (stroke volume); the energy that would have stretched the vessels instead elevates the systolic blood pressure. Isolated systolic hypertension is more common in older adults.

Clinical Manifestations

Physical examination may reveal no abnormalities other than high blood pressure. Occasionally retinal changes, such as hemorrhages, exudates (fluid accumulation), arteriolar narrowing, cotton wool spots (small infarctions), and in severe hypertension papilledema (swelling of the optic disc) may be seen. People with hypertension can be asymptomatic and remain so for many years. However, when specific signs and symptoms appear, they usually disclose vascular damage, with specific manifestations related to the organs served by the involved vessels. Coronary artery disease with angina and/or myocardial infarction is a common consequence of hypertension. Left ventricular hypertrophy occurs in response to the increased workload placed on the ventricle as it contracts against higher systemic pressure. When heart damage is extensive, heart failure ensues. Pathologic changes in the kidneys (increased blood urea nitrogen [BUN] and creatinine levels) may be manifested as nocturia. Cerebrovascular involvement may lead to a stroke or transient ischemic attack (TIA), manifested by alterations in vision or speech, dizziness, weakness, a sudden fall, or temporary paralysis on one side (hemiplegia). Cerebral infarctions account for about 80% of the strokes and TIAs in patients with hypertension.

Assessment and Diagnostic Evaluation

A thorough health history and physical examination are necessary. The retinas are examined, and laboratory studies are performed to assess possible target organ damage. Routine labora-

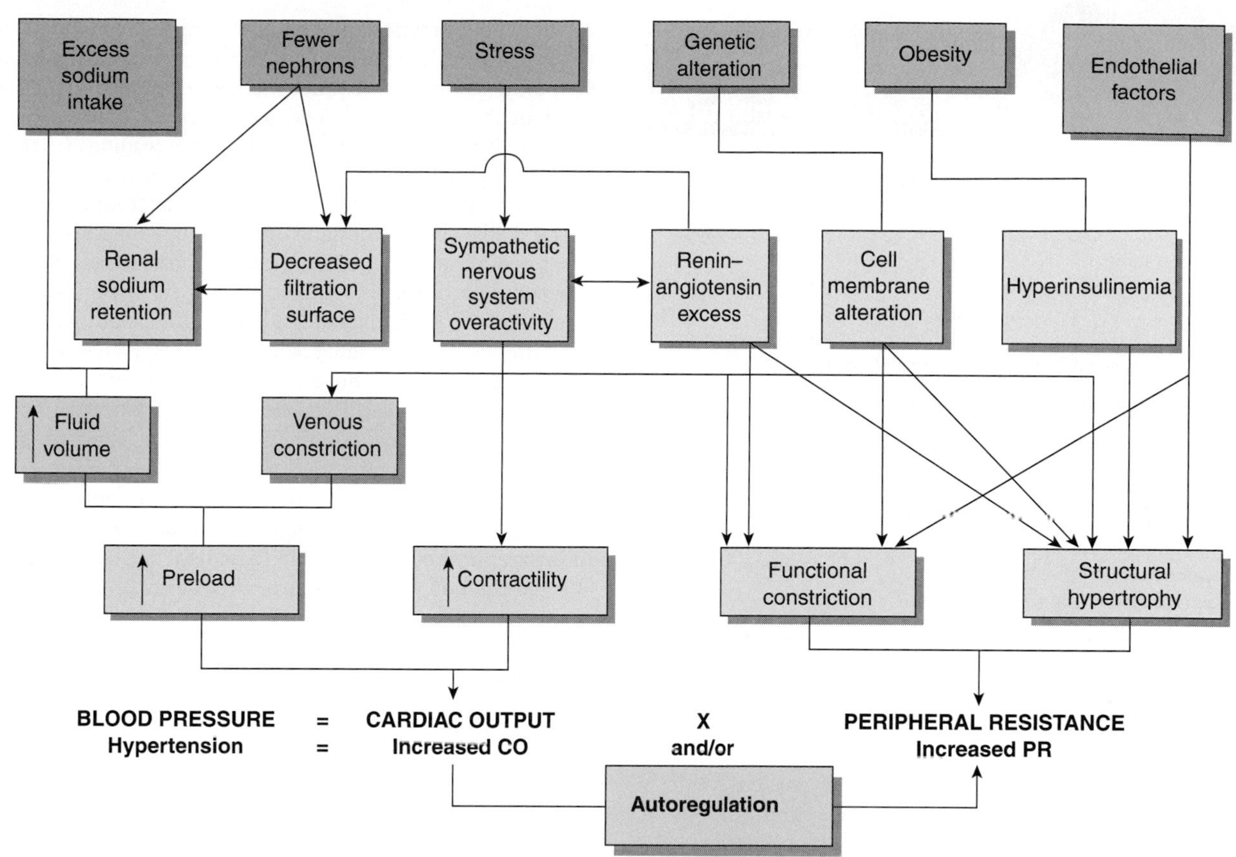

FIGURE 29•1 Factors involved in control of blood pressure, which is cardiac output multiplied by peripheral resistance. Adapted from Kaplan, N.M. (1997). *Clinical hypertension* (7th ed.). Philadelphia: Lippincott-Raven.

tory tests include urinalysis, blood chemistry (analysis of sodium, potassium, creatinine, fasting glucose, total and high-density lipoprotein [HDL] cholesterol levels), and a 12-lead electrocardiogram. Left ventricular hypertrophy can be assessed by echocardiography. Renal damage may be suggested by elevations in BUN and creatinine levels or by protein in the urine. Additional studies, such as creatinine clearance, renin level, urine tests, microalbuminuria, and 24-hour urine protein, may be performed.

A risk factor assessment, as advocated by the JNC, is needed to classify and guide treatment of hypertensive people at risk for cardiovascular damage. Risk factors and cardiovascular problems related to hypertension are presented in Chart 29-1 and Table 29-3.

Medical Management

The goal of hypertension treatment is to prevent death and complications by achieving and maintaining the arterial blood pressure at 140/90 mm Hg or even lower. The JNC has specified a lower goal pressure of 130/85 mm Hg for people with diabetes mellitus or with proteinuria greater than 1 g/24 hours. The optimal management plan is inexpensive and simple and causes the least possible disruption in the patient's life.

The management options for hypertension are summarized in the treatment algorithm issued in the JNC report (Fig. 29-2) and in Chart 29-2, which lists recommended lifestyle modifications. The clinician uses the algorithm in conjunction with the risk factor assessment data and the patient's blood pressure category (or stratum) to choose the initial and subsequent treatment plan for patients. Research findings demonstrate that weight loss, reduced alcohol and sodium intake, and regular physical activity are effective lifestyle adaptations to reduce blood pressure. Recent data show that a diet high in fruits and vegetables can prevent the development of hypertension and can lower elevated pressures.

PHARMACOLOGIC THERAPY

For patients with uncomplicated hypertension and no specific indications for another medication, the recommended initial medications include diuretics and/or beta blockers. Patients are first given low doses of medication. If blood pressure does not fall to less than 140/90 mm Hg, the dose is increased gradually and additional medications are included as necessary to achieve control. Table 29-4 describes the various pharmacologic agents used in treating hypertension. When the blood pressure has been less than 140/90 mm Hg for at least 1 year, gradual reduction of the types and doses of medication is recommended. To promote compliance, clinicians try to prescribe the simplest treatment schedule possible, ideally one pill once a day.

GERONTOLOGIC CONSIDERATIONS

Hypertension, particularly elevated systolic blood pressure, increases the risk of death and complications in elderly patients.

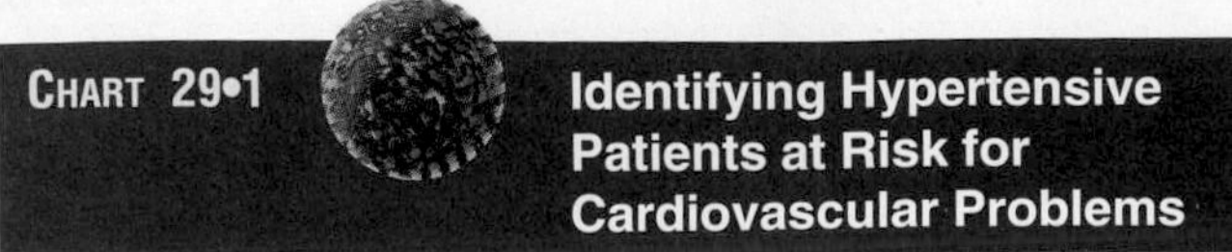

CHART 29•1
Identifying Hypertensive Patients at Risk for Cardiovascular Problems

Major Risk Factors (in Addition to Hypertension)

- Smoking
- Dyslipidemia
- Diabetes mellitus
- Age older than 60 years
- Gender (men and postmenopausal women)
- Family history of cardiovascular disease (in female relatives younger than age 65 or males younger than age 55)

Target Organ Damage/Clinical Cardiovascular Disease

- Heart diseases (left ventricular hypertrophy, angina or previous myocardial infarction, previous coronary revascularization, and heart failure)
- Stroke or TIA
- Nephropathy
- Peripheral arterial disease
- Retinopathy

Adapted from the Report of the Sixth Joint National Committee on the Prevention, Detection, Evaluation, and Treatment of High Blood Pressure. [1997]. *Archives of Internal Medicine, 157,* 2413–2446.

Treatment reduces this risk. Like younger patients, elderly patients should begin treatment with lifestyle modifications. If medications are needed to achieve the goal of blood pressure less than 140/90 mm Hg, the starting dose should be half that used in younger patients.

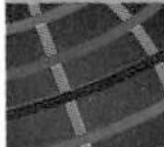

NURSING PROCESS: THE PATIENT WITH HYPERTENSION

Assessment

When hypertension is initially detected, nursing assessment involves carefully monitoring the blood pressure at frequent intervals and then, after diagnosis, at routinely scheduled intervals. The American Heart Association and the American Society of Hypertension have defined the standards for blood pressure measurement, including conditions required before measurements are made, equipment specifications, and techniques for measuring blood pressure to obtain an accurate and reliable reading (Chart 29-3). When the patient begins an antihypertensive treatment regimen, blood pressure assessments are needed to determine the effectiveness of medication therapy and to detect any changes in blood pressure that indicate the need for a change in the treatment plan.

A complete history is obtained to assess for symptoms that indicate target organ damage (ie, whether other body systems have been affected by the elevated blood pressure). Such symptoms may include anginal pain; shortness of breath; alterations in speech, vision, or balance; nosebleeds; headaches; dizziness; or nocturia.

During the physical examination, the nurse must also pay specific attention to the rate, rhythm, and character of the apical and peripheral pulses to detect effects of hypertension on the heart and blood vessels. A thorough assessment can yield valuable information about the extent to which the hypertension has affected the body as well as any other personal, social, or financial factors related to the problem.

Diagnosis

Nursing Diagnoses

Based on the assessment data, nursing diagnoses for the patient may include the following:

- Knowledge deficit regarding the relation between the treatment regimen and control of the disease process
- Noncompliance with therapeutic regimen related to side effects of prescribed therapy

Collaborative Problems/Potential Complications

Based on the assessment data, potential complications that may develop include:

- Left ventricular hypertrophy
- Myocardial infarction

TABLE 29•3 Risk Stratification and Treatment

Blood Pressure Stages (mm Hg)	Risk Group A (No Risk Factors No TOD/CCD)	Risk Group B (At Least 1 Risk Factor, Not Including Diabetes; No TOD/CCD)	Risk Group C (TOD/CCD and/or Diabetes, With or Without Other Risk Factors)
High-normal (130–139/85–89)	Lifestyle modification	Lifestyle modification	Medication therapy‡
Stage 1 (140–159/90–99)	Lifestyle modification (up to 12 months)	Lifestyle modification* (up to 6 months)	Medication therapy
Stages 2 and 3 (≥160/≥100)	Medication therapy	Medication therapy	Medication therapy

For example, a patient with diabetes and a blood pressure of 142/94 mm Hg plus left ventricular hypertrophy should be classified as having stage 1 hypertension with target organ disease (left ventricular hypertrophy) and with another major risk factor (diabetes). This patient would be categorized as Stage 1, Risk-Group C, and recommended for immediate initiation of pharmacologic treatment.

Lifestyle modification should be adjunctive therapy for all patients recommended for pharmacologic therapy.

TOD/CCD indicates target organ disease/clinical cardiovascular disease (see Chart 29-1).

*For patients with multiple risk factors, clinicians should consider medications as initial therapy plus lifestyle modifications.

‡For patients with heart failure, renal insufficiency, or diabetes.

From The Report of the Sixth Joint National Committee on the Prevention, Detection, Evaluation, and Treatment of High Blood Pressure. (1997). *Archives of Internal Medicine,* 157, 2413–2446.

Begin or continue lifestyle modifications

Not at goal blood pressure (<140/90 mm Hg)
Lower goals for patients with diabetes or renal disease

Initial drug choices*

Uncomplicated hypertension†
Diuretics
Beta-blockers

Specific indications for the following drugs
ACE inhibitors
Angiotensin II receptor blockers
Alpha-blockers
Beta-blockers
Calcium antagonists
Diuretics

Compelling indications†
Diabetes mellitus (type 1) with proteinuria
- ACE inhibitors

Heart failure
- ACE inhibitors
- Diuretics

Isolated systolic hypertension (older people)
- Diuretics preferred
- Long-acting dihydropyridine calcium antagonists

Myocardial infraction
- Beta-blockers (non-ISA)
- ACE inhibitors (with systolic dysfunction)

- Start with a low dose of a long-acting once-daily drug and titrate dose.
- Low-dose combinations may be appropriate.

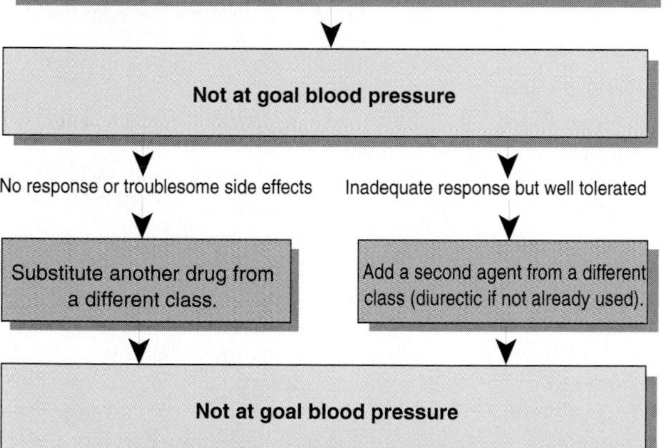
Not at goal blood pressure
No response or troublesome side effects
Inadequate response but well tolerated
Substitute another drug from a different class.
Add a second agent from a different class (diurectic if not already used).
Not at goal blood pressure

Continue adding agents from other classes.
Consider referral to a hypertension specialist.

* Unless contraindicated.
ACE = angiotensin-converting enzyme; ISA, intrinsic sympathomimetic activity.
†Based on randomized controlled trials

FIGURE 29•2 Algorithm of hypertension treatment. Treatment begins with lifestyle modifications and continues with various medication regimens. From the Report of the Sixth Joint National Committee on Prevention, Detection, Evaluation, and Treatment of High Blood Pressure, 1997.

- Heart failure
- TIAs
- Cerebrovascular accident (stroke)
- Renal insufficiency
- Retinal hemorrhage

Planning and Goals

The major goals for the patient include understanding of the disease process and its treatment, participation in a self-care program, and absence of complications.

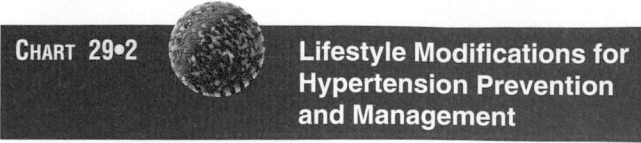

CHART 29•2 Lifestyle Modifications for Hypertension Prevention and Management

- Lose weight if overweight.
- Limit alcohol intake to no more than 1 oz (30 mL) ethanol (eg, 24 oz [720 mL] beer, 10 oz [300 mL] wine, or 2 oz [60 mL] 100-proof whiskey) per day or 0.5 oz (15 mL) ethanol per day for women and lighter-weight people.
- Increase aerobic physical activity (30 to 45 minutes most days of the week).
- Reduce sodium intake to no more than 100 mmol per day (2.4 g sodium or 6 g sodium chloride).
- Maintain adequate intake of dietary potassium (approximately 90 mmol per day).
- Maintain adequate intake of dietary calcium and magnesium for general health.
- Stop smoking and reduce intake of dietary saturated fat and cholesterol for overall cardiovascular health.

From the Report of the Sixth Joint National Committee on Prevention, Detection, Evaluation, and Treatment of High Blood Pressure. (1997). *Archives of Internal Medicine, 157,* 2413–2446.

Nursing Interventions

The objective of nursing care in hypertensive patients focuses on lowering and controlling the blood pressure without adverse effects and without undue cost. To achieve these goals, the nurse must support and teach the patient to adhere to the treatment regimen by implementing necessary lifestyle changes, taking medications as prescribed, and scheduling regular follow-up appointments with the health care provider to monitor progress or identify and treat any complications of disease or therapy.

Increasing Knowledge

It is important for the patient to understand the disease process as well as how lifestyle changes and medications can control hypertension. The nurse needs to emphasize the concept of controlling hypertension rather than curing it. The nurse can encourage the patient to consult a dietitian to help develop a plan for weight loss. The program usually consists of restricting sodium and fat intake, increasing intake of fruits and vegetables, and implementing regular physical activity. Explaining that it takes 2 to 3 months for the taste buds to adapt to changes in salt intake may help the patient adjust to reduced salt intake. The patient should be advised to drink no more than two alcoholic drinks per day, and tobacco should be avoided—not because smoking is related to hypertension, but because anyone with high blood pressure is already at increased risk for heart disease, and smoking makes this risk even higher. Support groups for weight control, smoking cessation, and stress reduction may be beneficial for some patients; others will benefit from the support of family and friends. The nurse assists the patient to develop and adhere to an appropriate exercise regimen because regular activity is a significant factor in weight reduction.

(*text continues on page 725*)

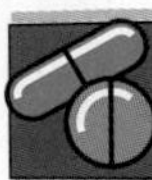

TABLE 29•4 Medication Therapy for Hypertension

Medications	Major Action	Advantages and Contraindications	Effects and Nursing Considerations
Purpose: To maintain blood pressure within normal ranges by the simplest and safest means possible with the fewest side effects for each individual patient			
Diuretics and Related Drugs			
Thiazide Diuretics			
chlorthalidone (Hygroton) quinethazone (Hydromox) chlorothiazide (Diuril) hydrochlorothiazide (Esidrix; Hydro-DIURIL)	Decrease of blood volume, renal blood flow, and cardiac output Depletion of extracellular fluid Negative sodium balance (from natriuresis), mild hypokalemia Directly affect vascular smooth muscle	Effective orally Effective during long-term administration Mild side effects Enhance other antihypertensive medications Counter sodium retention effect of other antihypertensive medications Contraindications: Gout, known sensitivity to sulfonamide-derived medications, and severely impaired kidney function	Side effects include dry mouth, thirst, weakness, drowsiness, lethargy, muscle aches, muscular fatigue, tachycardia, GI disturbance. Postural hypotension may be potentiated by alcohol, barbiturates, opioids, or hot weather. Because thiazides cause loss of sodium, potassium, and magnesium, monitor for signs of electrolyte imbalance. Encourage intake of potassium-rich foods (eg, fruits). *Gerontologic Considerations:* Risk of postural hypotension is significant because of volume depletion; measure blood pressure in three positions; caution patient to rise slowly.
Loop Diuretics			
furosemide (Lasix)	Volume depletion Blocks reabsorption of sodium chloride and water in kidney	Action rapid Potent Used when thiazides fail or patient needs rapid diuresis Contraindications: Same as for thiazides	Volume depletion is rapid—profound diuresis can occur. Electrolyte depletion— replacement is required. Thirst, nausea, vomiting, skin rash, postural hypotension. Sweet taste noted; oral and gastric burning. *Gerontologic Considerations:* Same as for thiazides.
Potassium-Sparing Diuretics			
spironolactone (Aldactone)	Competitive inhibitor of aldosterone	Spironolactone is effective in treating hypertension accompanying primary aldosteronism. Contraindications: Renal disease, Azotemia, Severe hepatic disease, Hyperkalemia	Drowsiness, lethargy, headache—decrease dosage. Monitor for hyperkalemia if given with angiotensin-converting enzyme inhibitor. Diarrhea and other GI symptoms—administer medication after meals. Skin eruptions, urticaria.
triamterene (Dyrenium)	Acts on distal tubule independently of aldosterone	Both spironolactone and triamterene cause retention of potassium.	Mental confusion, ataxia—dosage may need to be reduced. Gynecomastia (not for triamterene)
Adrenergic Inhibitors			
Peripheral Agents			
reserpine (Serpasil)	Impairs synthesis and reuptake of norepinephrine	Slows pulse, which counteracts tachycardia of hydralazine Contraindications: History of depression, psychosis, obesity, chronic sinusitis, peptic ulcer	May cause severe depression; report manifestations, as this may require that drug be omitted. Nasal stuffiness, which may require nasal vasoconstrictor. Increases appetite— therefore, weight control may be difficult. Recurrence of peptic ulcer Administer with meals or milk. *Gerontologic Considerations:* Depression and postural hypotension common in elderly

(*continued*)

TABLE 29•4 Medication Therapy for Hypertension *(Continued)*

Medications	Major Action	Advantages and Contraindications	Effects and Nursing Considerations
guanethidine (Ismelin)	Prevents release of sympathetic transmitter, norepinephrine. Is a depressant of adrenergic activity. Depletes tissue stores of norepinephrine Causes venous pooling, decreased venous return, and decreased cardiac output Decreases pulse rate, cardiac output, and renal blood flow	Potency Contraindications: Pheochromocytoma, because greatly enhances pressor effect of catecholamines	Severe postural hypotension accentuated by alcohol, exercise, hot weather Warn against standing suddenly or standing for a long time Diarrhea and nausea, nocturia Failure of ejaculation; counsel about possible sexual dysfunction Fatigue and giddiness; blackout
Central Alpha Agonists			
methyldopa (Aldomet)	Dopa-decarboxylase inhibitor; displaces norepinephrine from storage sites	Drug of choice for pregnant women with hypertension Useful in patients with renal failure Does not decrease cardiac output or renal blood flow Does not induce oliguria Contraindications: Liver disease	Drowsiness, dizziness Dry mouth; nasal stuffiness (troublesome at first but then tends to disappear). Hemolytic anemia (a hypersensitization reaction)—positive Coombs' test *Gerontologic Considerations:* May produce mental and behavioral changes in the elderly.
clonidine hydrochloride (Catapres)	Exact mode of action not understood, but acts through the central nervous system, apparently through centrally mediated alpha-adrenergic stimulation in the brain, producing blood pressure reduction	Little or no orthostatic effect. Moderately potent, and sometimes is effective when other medications fail to lower blood pressure. Contraindications: Severe coronary artery disease, pregnancy, children	Most common side effects are dry mouth, drowsiness, sedation, and occasional headaches and fatigue. Anorexia, malaise, and vomiting with mild disturbance of liver function have been reported. Rebound or withdrawal hypertension is relatively common; monitor blood pressure when going off medication.
Beta-Blockers			
propranolol (Inderal) metoprolol (Lopressor) nadolol (Corgard)	Block the sympathetic nervous system (beta-adrenergic receptors), especially the sympathetics to the heart, producing a slower heart rate and lowered blood pressure	Reduce pulse rate in patients with tachycardia and blood pressure elevation and are useful as an adjunct with medications that act at the neuroeffector site of the blood vessel Contraindications: Bronchial asthma, allergic rhinitis, right ventricular failure from pulmonary hypertension, congestive heart failure, depression, diabetes mellitus, dyslipidemia, heart block, peripheral vascular disease, heart rate under 60 pm	Mental depression manifested by insomnia, lassitude, weakness, and fatigue. Lightheadedness and occasional nausea, vomiting, and epigastric distress Check heart rate before giving. *Gerontologic Considerations:* Risk of toxicity is increased for elderly with decreased renal and liver function. Take blood pressure in three positions and observe for hypotension.
Alpha-Blocker			
prazosin hydrochloride (Minipress)	Peripheral vasodilator acting directly on the blood vessel; similar to hydralazine	Acts directly on the blood vessel and is an effective agent in patients with adverse reactions to hydralazine Contraindications: Angina pectoris and coronary artery disease. Induces tachycardia if not preceded by administration of propranolol and a diuretic.	Occasional vomiting and diarrhea, urinary frequency, and cardiovascular collapse, especially if given in addition to hydralazine without lowering the dose of the latter. Patients occasionally experience drowsiness, lack of energy, and weakness.

(continued)

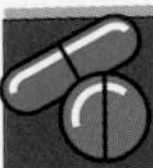

TABLE 29•4 Medication Therapy for Hypertension *(Continued)*

Medications	Major Action	Advantages and Contraindications	Effects and Nursing Considerations
Combined Alpha and Beta Blocker			
labetalol hydrochloride (Normodyne, Trandate)	Blocks alpha- and beta-adrenergic receptors; causes peripheral dilation and decreases peripheral vascular resistance	Fast-acting No decrease in renal blood flow Contraindications: Asthma, cardiogenic shock, severe tachycardia, heart block	Orthostatic hypotension, tachycardia
Vasodilators			
hydralazine hydrochloride (Apresoline)	Decreases peripheral resistance but concurrently elevates cardiac output Acts directly on smooth muscle of blood vessels	Not used as initial therapy; used in combination with other medications. Used also in eclampsia (pregnancy-induced hypertension) Contraindications: Angina or coronary disease, congestive heart failure, hypersensitivity	Headache, tachycardia, flushing, and dyspnea may occur—can be prevented by pretreating with reserpine. Peripheral edema may require diuretics. May produce lupus erythematosus-like syndrome
minoxidil	Direct vasodilating action on arteriolar vessels, causing decreased peripheral vascular resistance; reduces systolic and diastolic pressures	Hypotensive effect more pronounced than hydralazine No effect on vasomotor reflexes; thus does not cause postural hypotension Contraindications: Pheochromocytoma	Tachycardia, angina pectoris, ECG changes, edema; take blood pressure and apical pulse before administration; monitor intake and output and daily weights. Causes hirsutism
sodium nitroprusside (Nipride, Nitropress) nitroglycerin diazoxide (Hyperstat)	Peripheral vasodilation by relaxation of smooth muscle	Fast-acting Used only in hypertensive emergencies Contraindications: Sepsis, azotemia, high intracranial pressure.	Dizziness, headache, nausea, edema, tachycardia, palpitations. Can cause thiocyanate and cyanide intoxication.
Angiotensin-Converting Enzyme Inhibitors			
captopril (Capoten) enalapril (Vasotec) lisinopril (Prinivil, Zestril) ramipril (Altace) trandolapril (Mavik)	Inhibit conversion of angiotensin I to angiotensin II Lower total peripheral resistance	Fewer cardiovascular side effects Can be used with thiazide diuretic and digitalis Hypotension can be reversed by fluid replacement. Contraindications: Renal impairment, pregnancy	*Gerontologic Considerations:* Requires reduced dosages and loop diuretics with renal dysfunction
Angiotensin II Receptor Blockers			
losartan (Cozaar) valsartan (Diovan) irbesartan (Avapro)	Block the effects of angiotensin II at the receptor Reduce peripheral resistance	Minimal side effects Contraindications: Pregnancy Renovascular disease	Monitor for hypokalemia
Calcium Antagonists			
Nondihydropyridines			
diltiazem hydrochloride (Cardizem SR, Cardizem CD, Dilacor XR, Tiazac)	Inhibits calcium ion influx Reduces cardiac afterload	Inhibits coronary artery spasm not controlled by beta-blockers or nitrates Contraindications: Sick sinus syndrome; AV block; hypotension; heart failure	Do not discontinue suddenly. Observe for hypotension. Report irregular heartbeat, dizziness, edema. Instruct on regular dental care because of potential gingivitis.
verapamil, (Isoptin SR Calan SR, Verelan, Covera HS)	Inhibits calcium ion influx Slows velocity of conduction of cardiac impulse	Effective antidysrhythmic Rapid IV onset Blocks SA and AV node channels Contraindications: Sinus or AV node disease; severe heart failure; severe hypotension	Administer on empty stomach or before meal. Do not discontinue suddenly. Depression may subside when medication is discontinued. To relieve headaches, reduce noise, monitor electrolytes. Decrease dose for patients with liver or renal failure.

(continued)

TABLE 29•4 Medication Therapy for Hypertension *(Continued)*

Medications	Major Action	Advantages and Contraindications	Effects and Nursing Considerations
Dihydropyridines nifedipine (Procardia Adalat CC) amlodipine (Norvasc) felodipine (Plendil) nisoldipine (Sular)	Inhibit calcium ion influx across membranes Vasodilating effects on coronary and peripheral arteriole Decrease cardiac work and energy consumption, increase delivery of oxygen to myocardium	Rapid action Effective by oral or sublingual route No tendency to slow SA nodal activity or prolong AV node conduction Isolated systolic hypertension Contraindications: None (except heart failure for nifedipine)	Administer on empty stomach. Use with caution in diabetic patients. Small frequent meals if nausea. Muscle cramps, joint stiffness, sexual difficulties may disappear when dose decreased. Report irregular heartbeat, constipation, shortness of breath, edema. May cause dizziness.

Promoting Home and Community-Based Care

TEACHING PATIENTS SELF-CARE

Because the therapeutic regimen is the responsibility of the patient, in collaboration with the health care provider, education, goals, and social support can help the patient achieve blood pressure control. In addition, involving family members in education programs enables them to support the patient's efforts to control hypertension. The American Heart Association provides both printed and electronic (Web-based) patient education materials.

Written information about the expected effects and side effects of medications is very important. When side effects occur, patients need to understand the importance of reporting them and to whom they should be reported. Patients need to be informed that **rebound hypertension** can occur if antihypertensive medications are suddenly stopped. In addition, patients should know that some medications, such as beta blockers, may cause sexual dysfunction.

The nurse can encourage and teach patients to measure their blood pressure at home. This involves patients in their own care and emphasizes the fact that failing to take medications may result in an identifiable rise in blood pressure. Patients need to know that blood pressure varies continuously and that the range within which their pressure varies should be monitored.

CONTINUING CARE

Regular follow-up care is imperative so that the disease process can be assessed and treated, depending on whether control or progression is found. A history and physical examination should be completed at each clinic visit. The history should include all data that pertain to any potential problem, specifically medication-related problems such as postural (orthostatic) hypotension (dizziness or lightheadedness).

REINFORCING COMPLIANCE WITH SELF-CARE

Noncompliance with the therapeutic program is a significant problem in people with hypertension and other chronic conditions requiring lifetime management. It is estimated that 50% discontinue their medications within 1 year of beginning to take them. Blood pressure control is achieved by only 27%. However, when patients actively participate in self-care, including self-monitoring of blood pressure and diet, compliance increases—possibly because patients achieve immediate feedback, along with a greater sense of control.

Considerable effort is required by patients with hypertension to adhere to recommended lifestyle modifications and to take regularly prescribed medications. The effort needed may seem unreasonable to some, particularly when they have no symptoms without medications but do have side effects with medications. Continued education and encouragement are often needed to enable patients to formulate an acceptable plan that helps them live with their hypertension and adhere to the treatment plan. Compromises may have to be made on some aspects of therapy to achieve success in higher-priority goals.

GERONTOLOGIC CONSIDERATIONS

Compliance with the therapeutic program may be more difficult for elderly people. The medication regimen can be difficult to remember, and the expense can be a problem. **Monotherapy**

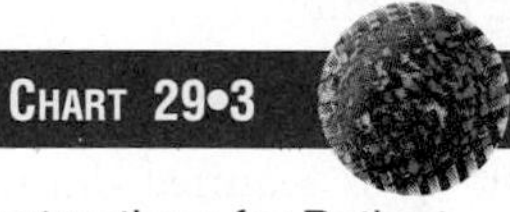

CHART 29•3 Measuring Blood Pressure

Instructions for Patient

- Avoid smoking cigarettes or drinking caffeine for 30 minutes before blood pressure is measured.
- Try to rest quietly for 5 minutes before the reading.
- Sit comfortably with forearm positioned at heart level.

Equipment

For Practitioner

- Mercury sphygmomanometer, recently calibrated aneroid manometer, or validated electronic device
- Several cuffs of different size chosen so that rubber bladder encircles at least two thirds of the adult arm

For Patient at Home

Automatic or semiautomatic device with digital display of readings.

Technique

Assessment is based on average of at least two readings. (If two readings differ by more than 5 mm Hg, additional readings are taken and an average reading is calculated from the results.)

Conclusion

Patient is informed of numeric blood pressure value and need for periodic reassessment. Patient who measures blood pressure at home is encouraged to keep a running, written record of readings.

(treatment with a single agent), if appropriate, may simplify the medication regimen and make it less expensive. Special care must be taken to ensure that the elderly patient understands the regimen and can see and read instructions, open the medication container, and get the prescription refilled. The elderly person's family or caregivers should be included in the teaching program so that they can understand the patient's needs, support adherence to the treatment plan, and know when and whom to call if problems arise or information is needed.

Nursing Alert *The patient and caregivers should be cautioned that antihypertensive medications can cause hypotension. Low blood pressure or postural hypotension should be reported immediately. Because elderly people have impaired cardiovascular reflexes, they are often more sensitive than younger people to the extracellular volume depletion caused by diuretic therapy and to the sympathetic inhibition caused by adrenergic antagonists. The nurse can teach patients to change positions slowly when moving from a lying or sitting position to a standing position. The nurse may also counsel elderly patients to use supportive devices such as handrails and walkers if necessary to prevent falls that could result from dizziness.*

Monitoring and Managing Potential Complications

Symptoms suggesting that hypertension is progressing and involving target organs must be detected early so that appropriate treatment can be initiated accordingly. When the patient returns for follow-up care, all body systems must be assessed to detect any evidence that vascular damage may be occurring. Examining the eyes is particularly important because retinal blood vessel damage is indicative of similar damage elsewhere in the vascular system. The patient is questioned about blurred vision, spots in front of the eyes, and diminished visual acuity. The heart, nervous system, and kidneys are also carefully assessed and examined. Any significant findings are promptly reported to determine whether additional diagnostic studies are required. Based on the findings, medications may be changed to improve blood pressure control.

Evaluation

Expected Outcomes

Expected outcomes may include:

1. Maintains adequate tissue perfusion
   a. Maintains blood pressure at less than 140/90 mm Hg with lifestyle modifications and/or medications
   b. Demonstrates no symptoms of angina, palpitations, or vision changes
   c. Has stable BUN and serum creatinine levels
   d. Has palpable peripheral pulses
2. Complies with the self-care program
   a. Adheres to the dietary regimen as prescribed: reduces calorie, sodium, and fat intake; increases fruit and vegetable intake
   b. Exercises regularly
   c. Takes medications as prescribed and reports any side effects
   d. Measures blood pressure routinely
   e. Abstains from tobacco and excessive alcohol intake
   f. Keeps follow-up appointments
3. Has no complications
   a. Reports no changes in vision
   b. Exhibits no retinal damage on vision testing
   c. Maintains pulse rate and rhythm and respiratory rate within normal ranges
   d. Reports no dyspnea or edema
   e. Maintains urine output consistent with intake
   f. Has renal function test results within normal range
   g. Demonstrates no motor, speech, or sensory deficits
   h. Reports no headaches, dizziness, weakness, changes in gait, or falls

HYPERTENSIVE CRISES

A **hypertensive emergency** is a situation in which blood pressure must be lowered immediately (not necessarily to less than 140/90 mm Hg) to halt or prevent damage to the target organs. Examples of conditions associated with a hypertensive emergency include acute myocardial infarction, a dissecting aortic aneurysm, and an intracranial hemorrhage. A **hypertensive urgency** is a situation in which blood pressure must be lowered within a few hours. Severe perioperative hypertension is considered a hypertensive urgency. Hypertensive emergencies are acute, life-threatening blood pressure elevations that require prompt treatment in an intensive care setting because of the serious target organ damage that may occur. Hypertensive urgencies and emergencies may occur in patients whose hypertension has been poorly controlled or in those who have abruptly discontinued their medications.

The medications of choice in hypertensive emergencies are those that have an immediate effect. Intravenous vasodilators, including sodium nitroprusside, nicardipine hydrochloride, fenoldopam mesylate, and nitroglycerin, have an immediate action that is short-lived (minutes to 4 hours); they are thus used as the initial treatment. Hypertensive urgencies are managed with oral doses of fast-acting agents such as loop diuretics, beta-blockers, angiotensin-converting enzyme inhibitors, calcium antagonists, or alpha$_2$-agonists.

Extremely close hemodynamic monitoring of the patient's blood pressure and cardiovascular status is required during treatment of hypertensive emergencies and urgencies. A precipitous drop in blood pressure can occur, which would require immediate action to restore blood pressure to an acceptable level.

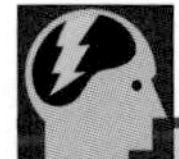

Critical Thinking Exercises

1.
You are a nursing student assigned to a hypertension clinic. One of the patients is a 58-year-old telemarketer. During the physical assessment, the patient, who is 5 feet 6 inches tall and weighs 180 lb, asks you why a complete physical examination is performed at every clinic visit. How would you answer this patient's question? Identify what additional data you needed to gather to support your answer.

2.
You are a home care nurse. One of your patients is an elderly man who lives alone and who has hypertension along with other health problems, including congestive

heart failure. In one of your visits with him, you learn that he has difficulty taking his medications as directed. What questions come to mind as you consider the situation? How will you direct your assessment to identify factors contributing to this problem? Using the factors identified, develop a sample follow-up home care teaching plan for this patient.

References and Selected Readings

BOOKS

Kaplan, N. (1998). *Clinical hypertension* (7th ed.). Baltimore: Williams & Wilkins.

Swales, J. D. (Ed.). (1994). *Textbook of hypertension.* Oxford: Blackwell.

JOURNALS

Alexander, L. M. (1998). Guidelines for hypertension treatment: Applications for primary care practice—A review of the JNC VI report. *Lippincott's Primary Care Practice, 2*(5), 485–497.

American Society of Hypertension. (1992). Recommendations for routine blood pressure measurement by indirect cuff sphygmomanometry. *American Journal of Hypertension, 5,* 207–209.

Appel, L. J., et al. (1997). A clinical trial of the effects of dietary patterns on blood pressure. *New England Journal of Medicine, 336,* 1117–1124.

Currey, R. (1998). Managing hypertensive urgencies in primary care. *Lippincott's Primary Care Practice, 2*(5), 498–504.

Miller, N. H., et al. (1997). The multilevel compliance challenge: Recommendations for a call to action. A statement for healthcare professionals. *Circulation, 95,* 1085–1090.

Pearce, K. A., et al. (1995). Does antihypertensive treatment of the elderly prevent cardiovascular events or prolong life? A meta-analysis of hypertension treatment trials. *Journal of Family Medicine, 4,* 943–949.

Perloff, D., et al. (1993). Human blood pressure determination by sphygmomanometry. *Circulation, 88,* 2460–2467.

Pickering, T. G. (1999). Contempo 1999: Advances in the treatment of hypertension. *Journal of the American Medical Association, 281*(2), 114–116.

Sixth Report of the Joint National Committee on Prevention, Detection, Evaluation, and Treatment of High Blood Pressure. (1997). *Archives of Internal Medicine, 157,* 2413–2446.

Wilkening, B. J. (1998). A patient with hypertension and hypokalemia. *Lippincott's Primary Care Practice, 2*(5), 539–544.

Resources

American Heart Association National Center, 7272 Greenville Ave., Dallas, TX 75231-4596; http://www.americanheart.org

National High Blood Pressure Education Program, NHLBI Information Center, P.O. Box 30105, Bethesda, MD 20824-1222; http://www.nhlbi.nih.gov/nhlbi/nhlbi.ntm

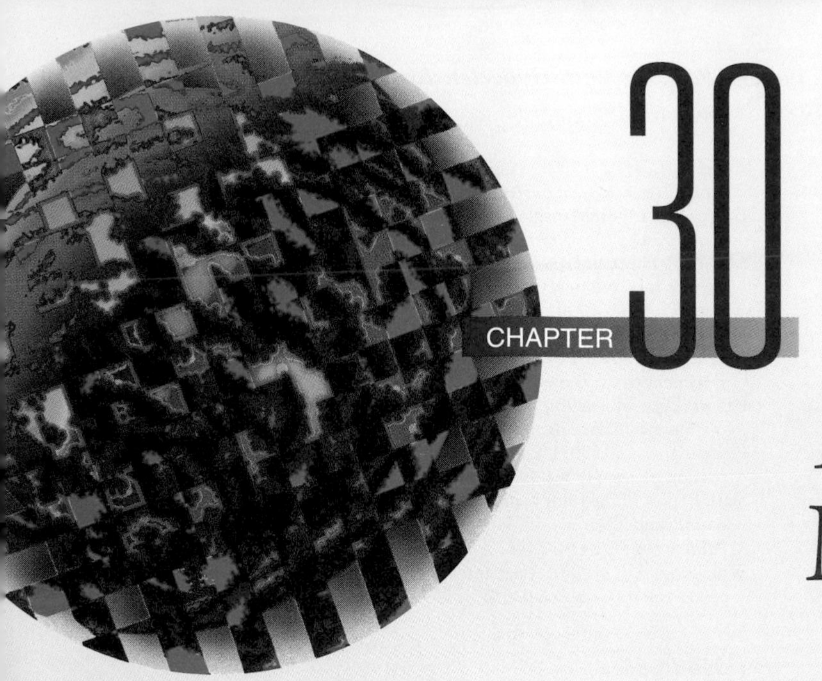

Assessment and Management of Patients With Hematologic Disorders

Learning Objectives

On completion of this chapter, the learner will be able to:

1. Describe the process of hematopoiesis.
2. Describe the processes involved in maintaining hemostasis.
3. Differentiate between the hypoproliferative and hemolytic anemias and compare and contrast the physiologic mechanisms, the clinical manifestations, medical management, and nursing interventions for each.
4. Use the nursing process as a framework for care of patients with anemia.
5. Compare the leukemias, their incidence, physiologic alterations, clinical manifestations, management, and prognosis.
6. Use the nursing process as a framework for care of patients with acute leukemia.
7. Use the nursing process as a framework for care of patients with disseminated intravascular coagulopathy.
8. Identify the common types of blood components, the implications for their use, and methods of administration.
9. Identify the appropriate nursing actions to take when a transfusion reaction is suspected.
10. Identify potential complications of blood component therapy.

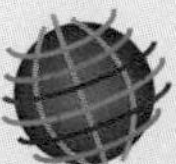

Unlike many other body systems, the hematologic system truly encompasses the entire human body. Patients with hematologic disorders can be quite challenging to nursing because they often have significant problems, but few or no symptoms. It is therefore imperative that nurses have a good understanding of the pathophysiology of the patient's condition and can make a thorough assessment that relies heavily on the interpretation of laboratory tests. It is equally important for the nurse to anticipate potential problems and target nursing interventions accordingly. Because it is so important to the understanding of most hematologic diseases, a basic understanding of blood cells and bone marrow function is necessary.

GLOSSARY

ANC: absolute neutrophil count

anemia: decreased red cell mass

anergy: reactivity to antigens (transient or complete)

angular cheilosis: cracking sore at corner of mouth

anisocytosis: variation in size of red cells

aplasia: arrested development (eg, of bone marrow)

apoptosis: complex process of programmed cell death

band cell: slightly immature neutrophil

blast cell: primitive white cell

D-dimer: test measuring fibrin breakdown; considered to be more specific than fibrin degradation products in relation to DIC

differentiation: development of functions and characteristics different from parent stem cell

Döhle bodies: inclusions of RNA fragments seen in cytoplasm of neutrophils

dysplasia: abnormal development (eg, of blood cells)

ecchymosis: bruising

erythrocyte sedimentation rate (ESR; "sed rate"): laboratory test measuring rate of settling of RBCs; indicative of inflammation

erythropoiesis: process of formation of red blood cells

erythropoietin: hormone produced by the kidney necessary for erythropoiesis

fibrin: filamentous protein; basis of blood clot

fibrinogen: protein converted into fibrin to form clot

glossitis: inflammation of tongue

granulocyte: granulated WBC (neutrophil, eosinophil, basophil); sometimes used synonymously with neutrophil

granulocytopenia: fewer than normal granulocytes

hematocrit: percent of total blood volume consisting of RBCs

hematopoiesis: formation and maturation of blood cells

hemoglobin: iron-containing protein of RBCs; delivers O_2 to tissues

hemolysis: destruction of RBCs

hemosiderin: iron-containing pigment derived from breakdown of hemoglobin

hemostasis: balance between clot formation and clot dissolution

histiocyte: cells present in all loose connective tissues capable of phagocytosis; part of RES

hyperplasia: increased proliferation of cells

hypochromia: pallor within the red cell due to decreased hemoglobin content

left shift: increased release of more immature forms of WBCs from the marrow in response to need

leukocyte: white blood cell

leukemia: uncontrolled proliferation of WBCs, often immature

leukopenia: less than normal amount of WBCs in circulation

lymphoid: pertaining to lymphocytes

lymphocyte: form of WBC involved in immune functions

lysis: destruction of cells

macrocytosis: larger than normal RBCs

macrophage: cells of the RES capable of phagocytosis

microcytosis: smaller than normal RBCs

monocyte: large WBC that becomes a macrophage when it leaves the circulation into body tissues

myeloid: pertaining to myeloid cells

myelopoiesis: formation and maturation of cells derived from myeloid stem cell

neutropenia: lower than normal neutrophils

neutrophil: fully mature form of WBC capable of phagocytosis; primary defense against bacterial infection

normochromic: normal RBC color, indicating normal amount of hemoglobin

normocytic: normal size of RBC

nucleated RBCs: immature form of RBC; portion of nucleus remains

oxyhemoglobin: combined form of O_2 and hemoglobin; found in arterial blood

pancytopenia: abnormal decrease in WBC, RBC, and platelets

petechiae: tiny capillary hemorrhages

phagocytosis: process of ingestion and digestion of bacteria

plasma: liquid portion of blood

plasminogen: protein used in dissolution of blood clot

poikilocytosis: variation in shape of red cells

polycythemia: excess of red cells

reticulocyte: slightly immature RBC, usually only 1% of total circulating RBCs

reticuloendothelial system (RES): system of cells throughout body capable of phagocytosis

rouleaux: stacking of RBCs onto one another due to coating with protein

serum: portion of blood remaining after coagulation occurs

spherocyte: RBC without central pallor; seen with hemolysis

stem cell: primitive cell, capable of self-replication and differentiating into myeloid or lymphoid stem cell

thrombin: enzyme necessary to convert fibrinogen into fibrin clot

thrombocyte: platelet

thrombocytopenia: lower than normal platelet count

thrombocytosis: higher than normal platelet count

ANATOMIC AND PHYSIOLOGIC OVERVIEW

The hematologic system consists of the blood and the sites where blood is produced, including the bone marrow and the **reticuloendothelial system** (RES). Blood is a specialized organ that differs from other organs in that it exists in a fluid state. Blood is composed of plasma and various types of cells. **Plasma** is the fluid portion of blood; it contains various proteins, such as albumin, globulin, **fibrinogen**, and other factors necessary for clotting as well as electrolytes, waste products, and nutrients. About 55% of blood volume is plasma.

The cellular component of blood consists of three primary cell types (Table 30-1): **leukocytes** (white blood cells [WBCs]), **erythrocytes** (red blood cells [RBCs]), and **thrombocytes** (platelets). These cellular components of blood normally make up 40% to 45% of the blood volume. Because most blood cells have a short life span, the need for the body to replenish its supply of cells is continual; this process is termed **hematopoiesis**. The primary site for hematopoiesis is the bone marrow. During embryonic development and in other conditions, the liver and spleen may also be involved.

Under normal conditions, the adult bone marrow produces about 175 billion RBCs, 70 billion **neutrophils** (mature form of white cell), and 175 billion platelets each day. When the body needs more blood cells, as in infection (when WBCs are needed to fight the invading pathogen) or in bleeding (requiring more RBCs), the marrow increases its production of the cells required. Thus, under normal conditions, the marrow responds to increased demand and releases adequate numbers of cells within the circulation.

The volume of blood in humans is approximately 7% to 10% of the normal body weight and amounts to 5 to 6 liters. Circulating through the vascular system and serving as a link between body organs, the blood carries oxygen absorbed from the lungs and nutrients absorbed from the gastrointestinal tract to the body cells for cellular metabolism. Blood also carries waste products

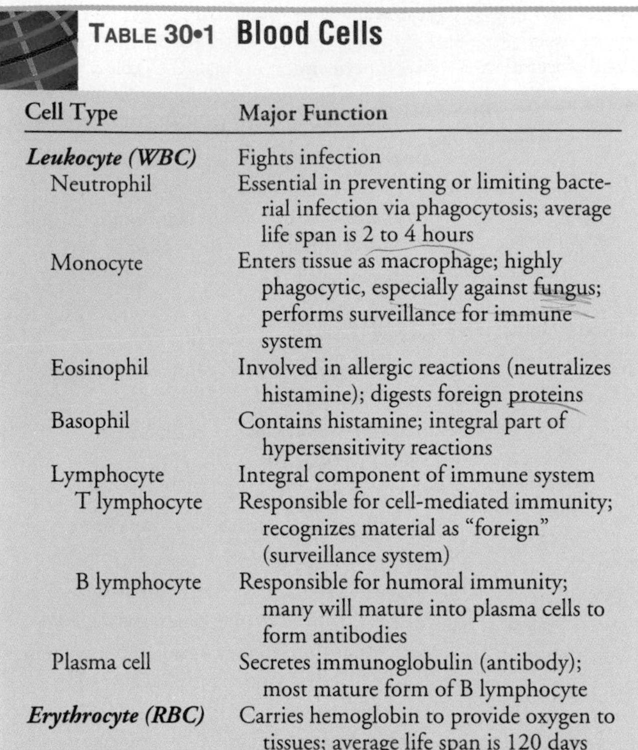

TABLE 30•1 Blood Cells

Cell Type	Major Function
Leukocyte (WBC)	Fights infection
Neutrophil	Essential in preventing or limiting bacterial infection via phagocytosis; average life span is 2 to 4 hours
Monocyte	Enters tissue as macrophage; highly phagocytic, especially against fungus; performs surveillance for immune system
Eosinophil	Involved in allergic reactions (neutralizes histamine); digests foreign proteins
Basophil	Contains histamine; integral part of hypersensitivity reactions
Lymphocyte	Integral component of immune system
T lymphocyte	Responsible for cell-mediated immunity; recognizes material as "foreign" (surveillance system)
B lymphocyte	Responsible for humoral immunity; many will mature into plasma cells to form antibodies
Plasma cell	Secretes immunoglobulin (antibody); most mature form of B lymphocyte
Erythrocyte (RBC)	Carries hemoglobin to provide oxygen to tissues; average life span is 120 days
Thrombocyte (platelet)	Fragment of megakaryocyte, not really a cell; provides basis for coagulation to occur; maintains hemostasis; average life span is 10 days

produced by cellular metabolism to the lungs, skin, liver, and kidneys, where they are transformed and eliminated from the body. Blood also carries hormones, antibodies, and other substances to their sites of action or use.

To function, blood must remain in its normally fluid state. Because blood is fluid, the danger always exists that trauma can lead to loss of blood from the vascular system. To prevent this, an intricate clotting mechanism is activated when necessary to seal any leak in the blood vessels. Excessive clotting is equally dangerous because it can obstruct blood flow to vital tissues. To prevent this complication, the body has a fibrinolytic mechanism that eventually dissolves clots formed within blood vessels. The balance between these two systems, clot formation and clot dissolution or fibrinolysis, is called **hemostasis.**

Bone Marrow

The bone marrow is the site of **hematopoiesis,** or blood cell formation (Fig. 30-1). In a child, all skeletal bones are involved, but as the person ages, marrow activity decreases. By adulthood, marrow activity is usually limited to the pelvis, ribs, vertebrae, and sternum.

Marrow is one of the largest organs of the body, making up 4% to 5% of total body weight. It consists of islands of cellular components (red marrow) separated by fat (yellow marrow). As the adult ages, the proportion of active marrow is gradually replaced by fat; however, in the healthy person, the fat can again be replaced by active marrow when more blood cell production is required. In adults with disease causing marrow destruction, fibrosis, or scarring, the liver and spleen can also resume production of blood cells by a process known as extramedullary hematopoiesis.

The marrow is highly vascular. Within it are primitive cells called **stem cells**. These stem cells have the ability to self-replicate, thereby ensuring a continuous supply of stem cells throughout the life cycle. When stimulated to do so, stem cells can begin a process of **differentiation** into either **myeloid** or **lymphoid** stem cells. These stem cells are committed to produce specific types of blood cells. Lymphoid stem cells produce either T or B **lymphocytes**. Myeloid stem cells differentiate into three broad cell types: erythrocytes, leukocytes, and platelets. Thus, with the exception of lymphocytes, all blood cells are derived from the myeloid stem cell, and thus it is easy to appreciate why a defect in the myeloid stem cell can cause problems not only with white cell production, but also with red cell and platelet production.

Blood Cells

Erythrocytes

The normal red cell is a biconcave disk resembling a soft ball compressed between two fingers (Fig. 30-2). It has a diameter of about 8 micrometers (μm) and is so flexible that it can pass easily through capillaries that may be as small as 2.8 μm in diameter. The RBC membrane is so thin that gases, such as oxygen and carbon dioxide, can easily diffuse across it; the disk shape provides a large surface area that facilitates the absorption and release of oxygen molecules.

Mature red cells consist primarily of **hemoglobin**, which contains iron and which makes up 95% of the cell mass. RBCs have no nuclei and have many fewer metabolic enzymes than do most other cells. The presence of a large amount of hemoglobin enables the erythrocyte to perform its principal function, the transport of oxygen between the lungs and tissues. Occasionally the marrow releases slightly immature forms of RBCs into the circulation, called **reticulocytes.** This occurs as a normal response to an increased demand for RBCs (as in bleeding) or in some disease states (described below).

The oxygen-carrying hemoglobin molecule is made up of four subunits, each containing a heme portion attached to a globin chain. Iron is present in the heme component of the molecule. An important property of heme is its ability to bind to oxygen loosely and reversibly. As a result, oxygen readily binds to hemoglobin in the lungs and is carried as **oxyhemoglobin** in arterial blood. Oxyhemoglobin is a brighter red than hemoglobin that does not contain oxygen (reduced hemoglobin), which is why arterial blood is a brighter red than venous blood. The oxygen readily dissociates from hemoglobin in the tissues, where the oxygen is needed for cellular metabolism. In venous blood, hemoglobin combines with hydrogen ions produced by cellular metabolism and thus buffers excessive acid. Whole blood normally contains about 15 g of hemoglobin per 100 mL of blood.

ERYTHROPOIESIS

Erythroblasts arise from the primitive myeloid stem cells in bone marrow. The erythroblast is a nucleated cell that, in the process of maturing within the bone marrow, accumulates hemoglobin and gradually loses its nucleus. At this stage, the cell is known as a reticulocyte. Further maturation into an erythrocyte entails the loss of dark-staining material and slight shrinkage. The mature erythrocyte is then released into the circulation. Under conditions of rapid **erythropoiesis** (erythrocyte production), reticulocytes and other immature cells (eg, nucleated RBCs) may be released prematurely into the circulation.

PHYSIOLOGY

Hematopoiesis

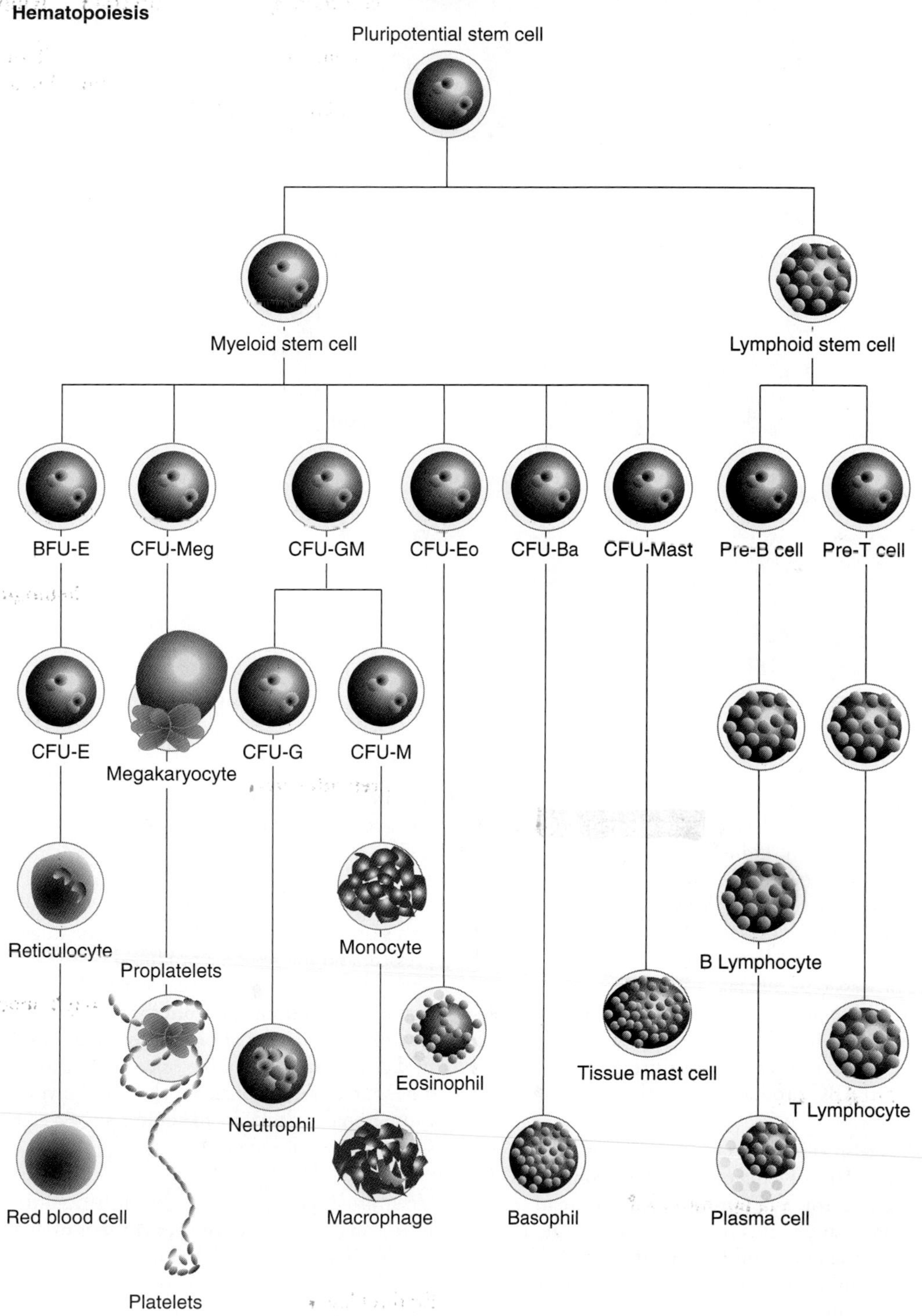

Pluripotential stem cell

Myeloid stem cell

Lymphoid stem cell

BFU-E

CFU-Meg

CFU-GM

CFU-Eo

CFU-Ba

CFU-Mast

Pre-B cell

Pre-T cell

CFU-E

Megakaryocyte

CFU-G

CFU-M

Reticulocyte

Proplatelets

Monocyte

B Lymphocyte

Eosinophil

Tissue mast cell

Neutrophil

T Lymphocyte

Red blood cell

Macrophage

Basophil

Plasma cell

Platelets

FIGURE 30•1 Hematopoiesis. Uncommitted (pluripotent) stem cells can differentiate into myeloid or lymphoid stem cells. These stem cells then undergo a complex process of differentiation and maturation into normal cells that are released into the circulation. The myeloid stem cell is responsible not only for all nonlymphoid white blood cells but also for the production of red blood cells and platelets. Each step of the differentiation process depends in part on the presence of specific growth factors for each cell type. When the stem cells are dysfunctional, they may respond inadequately to the need for more cells, or respond excessively, sometimes uncontrollably, as in leukemia. Adapted from Amgen, Inc., 1995, Thousand Oaks, CA.

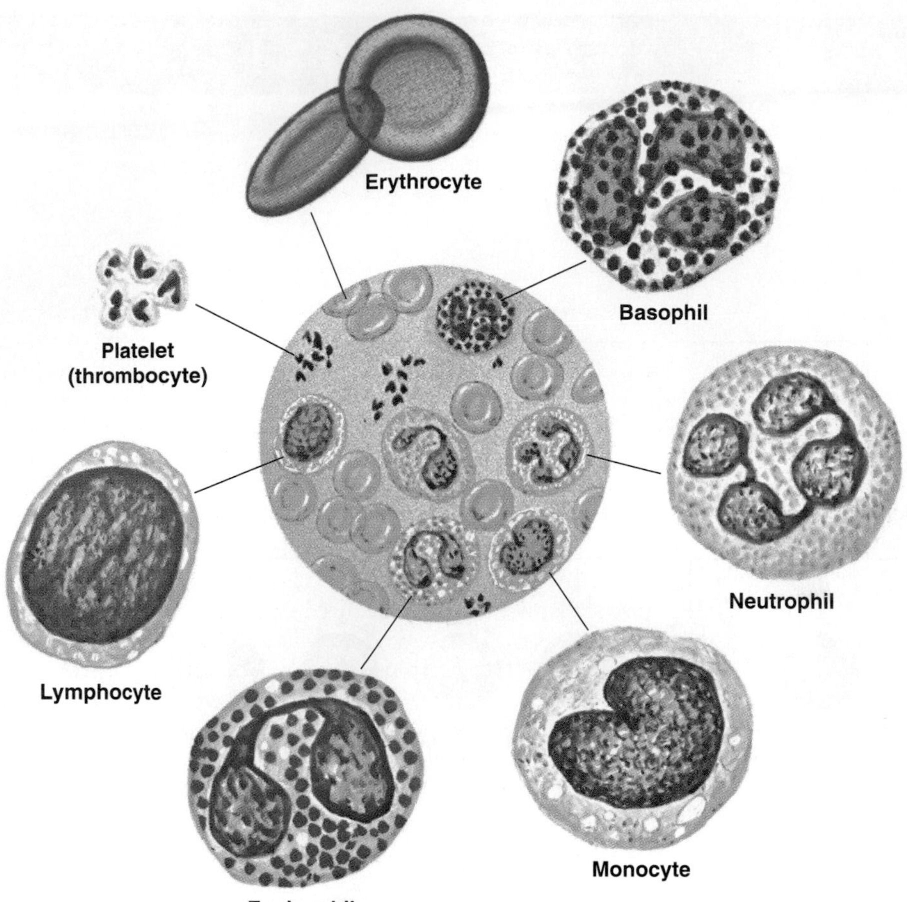

FIGURE 30•2 Normal types of blood cells.

Differentiation of the primitive myeloid stem cell of the marrow into an erythroblast is stimulated by **erythropoietin**, a hormone produced primarily by the kidney. If the kidney detects low levels of oxygen (as would occur in **anemia**, in which fewer RBCs are available to bind oxygen, or in people living at high altitudes), the release of erythropoietin is increased. The increased erythropoietin then stimulates the marrow to increase production of RBCs. The entire process typically takes 5 days.

For normal erythrocyte production, the bone marrow also requires iron, vitamin B_{12}, folic acid, pyridoxine (vitamin B_6), and other factors. A deficiency of these factors during erythropoiesis can result in decreased RBC production and thus anemia.

Iron Stores and Metabolism. The average daily diet in the United States contains 10 to 15 mg of elemental iron; normally 0.5 to 1 mg of ingested iron is absorbed from the small intestine. The rate of iron absorption is regulated by the amount of iron already stored in the body and by the rate of red cell production. Additional amounts of iron, up to 2 mg daily, must be absorbed by the adult female to replace blood lost during menstruation. Total body iron content in the average adult is approximately 3 g, most of which is present in hemoglobin or in one of its breakdown products. Iron is stored in the small intestine as ferritin and in reticuloendothelial cells. When required, the iron is released into the plasma, binds to transferrin, and is transported into the membranes of the normoblasts (erythrocyte precursor cells) within the marrow, where it is incorporated into hemoglobin. The entire process, from binding to the normoblast to incorporation into hemoglobin, takes only 6 to 8 minutes. Iron is lost in the feces, either in bile, blood, or mucosal cells from the intestine.

The concentration of iron in blood is normally about 75 to 175 μg/dL (13–31 μmol/L) for men and 65 to 165 μg/dL (11–29 μmol/L) for women. With iron deficiency, bone marrow iron stores are rapidly depleted; thus, hemoglobin synthesis is depressed, and the red cells produced by the marrow are small and low in hemoglobin. Iron deficiency in the adult generally indicates that blood has been lost from the body (eg, from bleeding in the gastrointestinal tract or heavy menstrual flow). In the adult, lack of dietary iron is rarely the sole cause of iron-deficiency anemia. The source of iron deficiency should be investigated promptly because iron deficiency in an adult may be a sign of bleeding in the GI tract or colon cancer.

Vitamin B_{12} and Folic Acid Metabolism. Vitamin B_{12} and folic acid are required for the synthesis of deoxyribonucleic acid (DNA) in many tissues, but deficiencies of either of these vitamins have the greatest effect on erythropoiesis. Both vitamin B_{12} and folic acid are derived from the diet. Folic acid is absorbed in the proximal small intestine, but only small amounts are stored within the body. If the diet is deficient in folic acid, stores within the body quickly become depleted. Because vitamin B_{12} is found only in foods of animal origin, strict vegetarians may ingest little B_{12}. B_{12} combines with intrinsic factor produced in the stomach. The vitamin B_{12}–intrinsic factor complex is absorbed in the distal ileum. People who have had a partial or total gastrectomy may have limited amounts of intrinsic factor, and thus the absorption of B_{12} may be diminished. The effects of either decreased absorption or decreased intake of B_{12} are not apparent for 2 to 4 years.

Vitamin B_{12} or folic acid deficiency is characterized by the production of abnormally large RBCs called megaloblasts. Because these cells are abnormal, many are sequestered while still in the bone marrow, and their rate of release is decreased. Some of these cells actually die in the marrow before they can be released into the circulation. This results in megaloblastic anemia.

RED BLOOD CELL DESTRUCTION

The average life span of a normal circulating RBC is 120 days. Aged RBCs lose their elasticity and become trapped in small blood vessels, particularly in the spleen. They are removed from the blood by the reticuloendothelial cells, particularly in the liver and the spleen. As the RBCs are destroyed, the hemoglobin is largely recycled. Some hemoglobin also breaks down to form bilirubin and is secreted in the bile. Most of the iron is recycled to form new hemoglobin molecules within the bone marrow; small amounts are lost daily in the feces and urine and monthly in menstrual flow.

Leukocytes

Leukocytes (WBCs) are divided into two general categories: **granulocytes** and lymphocytes. In normal blood, the total leukocyte count is 5000 to 10,000 cells per cubic millimeter. Of these, approximately 60% to 70% are granulocytes and 30% to 40% are lymphocytes. Primarily, leukocytes protect the body against infection and tissue injury.

Granulocytes

Granulocytes are defined by the presence of granules in the cytoplasm of the cell. Granulocytes are divided into three main subgroups, which are characterized by the staining properties of these granules (see Fig. 30-2). Eosinophils have bright-red granules in their cytoplasm, whereas the granules in basophils stain deep blue. The third, and by far the most numerous cell in this class, is the neutrophil, with granules that stain a pink to violet hue. Neutrophils are also called polymorphonuclear neutrophils (PMNs, or polys) or segmented neutrophils (segs).

The nucleus of the mature neutrophil generally has multiple lobes (usually two to five) connected by thin filaments of nuclear material and is usually twice the size of an RBC. The somewhat less mature granulocyte has a single-lobed nucleus and is called a **band cell**. Ordinarily, band cells account for only a small percentage of circulating granulocytes, although their percentage can increase greatly under conditions in which neutrophil production increases, such as infection.

MYELOPOIESIS (PRODUCTION OF NEUTROPHILS)

Granulocyte production from the myeloid stem cell pool results in the gradual differentiation of these cells from a myeloid **blast cell** into a fully mature neutrophil. The process is highly complex and depends on many factors. These factors, including specific cytokines such as growth factors, are normally present within the marrow itself. As the blast cell matures, the cytoplasm of the cell changes in color (from blue to violet) and granules begin to form with the cytoplasm. The shape of the nucleus also changes. The entire process of maturation and differentiation takes about 10 days (see Fig. 30-1). Once the neutrophil is released into the circulation from the marrow, it stays there for only about 6 hours before it migrates into the body tissues to perform its function of **phagocytosis** (ingestion and digestion of bacteria and particles) (Fig. 30-3). Here, neutrophils last no more than 1 to 2 days before they die. The number of circulating granulocytes found in the healthy person is relatively constant, but in infection, large numbers of these cells are rapidly released into the circulation.

Mononuclear Leukocytes (Agranulocytes)

Monocytes (also called mononuclear leukocytes) are white cells with a single-lobed nucleus and a granule-free cytoplasm—hence the term agranulocyte. In normal adult blood, monocytes account for approximately 5% of the total leukocytes. Monocytes are the largest of the leukocytes. Produced by the bone marrow, they remain in the circulation for a short time before entering the tissues and transforming into **macrophages**. Macrophages are particularly active in the spleen, liver, peritoneum, and the alveoli in the lung.

Mature lymphocytes are small cells with scanty cytoplasm. Immature lymphocytes are produced in the marrow from the lymphoid stem cells. A second major source of production is the cortex of the thymus. Cells derived from the thymus are known as T lymphocytes (or T cells); those derived from the marrow can also be T cells but are more commonly B lymphocytes (or B cells). Lymphocytes complete their differentiation and maturation primarily in the lymph nodes and in the lymphoid tissue of the intestine and spleen after exposure to a specific antigen. Thus, mature lymphocytes are antigen-specific cells.

FUNCTION OF LEUKOCYTES

Leukocytes protect the body from invasion by bacteria and other foreign entities. The major function of neutrophils is phagocytosis (see Fig. 30-3). Neutrophils arrive at the site within an hour of the onset of an inflammatory reaction and initiate phagocytosis, but they are short-lived. An influx of monocytes follows; these cells continue their phagocytic activities for long periods as macrophages. This process constitutes a second line of defense for the body against inflammation and infection. While neutrophils can often work adequately against bacteria without the need for excessive involvement with macrophages, macrophages are particularly effective against fungus and virus. Macrophages also digest senescent (aging or aged) blood cells, such as erythrocytes, primarily within the spleen.

The primary function of lymphocytes is to produce substances that aid in attacking foreign material. One group of lymphocytes (T lymphocytes) kills foreign cells directly or releases a variety of lymphokines, substances that enhance the activity of phagocytic cells. T lymphocytes are responsible for delayed allergic reactions, rejection of foreign tissue (eg, from transplants), or destruction of tumor cells. This process is known as cellular immunity. The other group of lymphocytes (B lymphocytes) is capable of differentiating into plasma cells. Plasma cells, in turn, produce immunoglobulin, or antibodies, which are protein molecules that destroy foreign material by several mechanisms. This process is known as humoral immunity.

Eosinophils and basophils function in hypersensitivity reactions. Eosinophils are important in the phagocytosis of parasites. The increase in eosinophil levels in allergic states indicates that these cells are involved in the hypersensitivity reaction; their function here is to neutralize histamine. Basophils produce and store histamine as well as other substances involved in hyper-

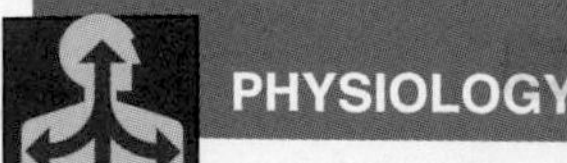

PHYSIOLOGY

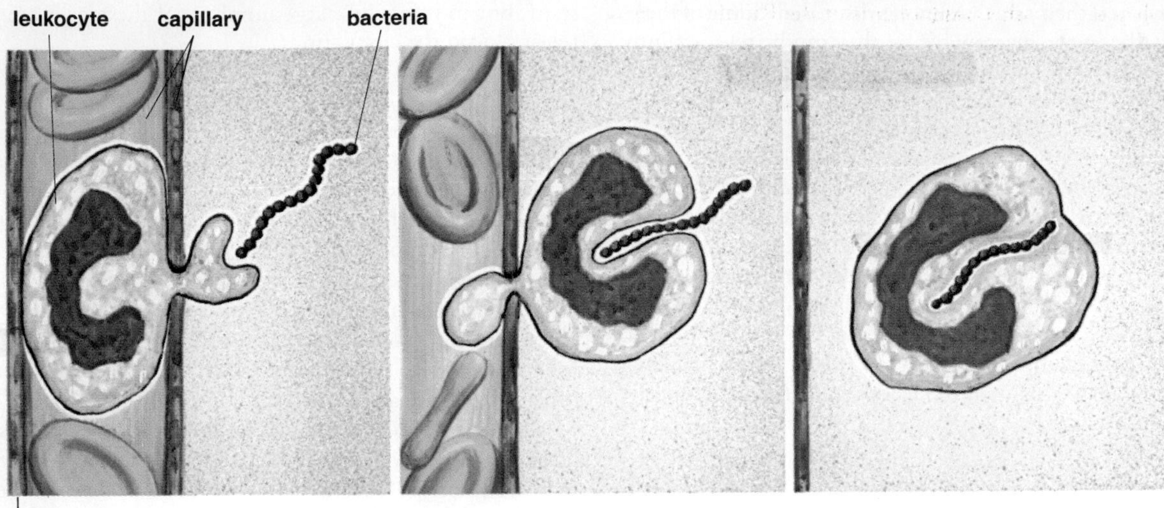

FIGURE 30•3 Phagocytosis. When foreign matter (such as bacteria or dead tissue) comes in contact with the cell membrane of the neutrophil, the membrane then surrounds and pinches off the area, leaving the membrane intact. Thus, the engulfed material is left in a vacuole within the neutrophil, where enzymes within the cell destroy the foreign material.

sensitivity reactions. The release of these substances provokes allergic reactions.

Thrombocytes (Platelets)

Platelets, or thrombocytes, are not actually cells. Rather, they are granular fragments of giant cells in the bone marrow called megakaryocytes. Platelet production in the marrow is regulated in part by the hormone thrombopoietin to stimulate the production and differentiation of megakaryocytes from the myeloid stem cell.

Platelets play an essential role in the control of bleeding. They circulate freely in the blood in an inactive state where they nurture the endothelium of the blood vessels, maintaining the integrity of the vessel. When vascular injury does occur, platelets collect at the site and are activated. They adhere to the site of injury and to each other, forming a platelet plug that temporarily stops bleeding. Substances are released from platelet granules that activate coagulation factors in the blood plasma and initiate the formation of a stable clot composed of **fibrin**, a filamentous protein. Platelets have a normal life span of 7 to 10 days.

Plasma

After cellular elements are removed from blood, the remaining liquid portion is called plasma. More than 90% of plasma is water. The remaining portion consists primarily of plasma proteins, clotting factors (particularly fibrinogen), and small amounts of other substances (eg, nutrients, enzymes, waste products, and gases). If plasma is allowed to clot, the remaining fluid is called **serum**. Serum has essentially the same composition as plasma, except that fibrinogen and several clotting factors have been removed in the clotting process.

Plasma Proteins

Plasma proteins consist primarily of albumin and globulins. The globulins can be separated into three main fractions, alpha, beta, and gamma, each of which consists of distinct proteins that have different functions. Important proteins in the alpha and beta fractions are the transport globulins and the clotting factors that are made in the liver. The transport globulins carry various substances in the bound form around the circulation. For example, thyroid-binding globulin carries thyroxin, and transferrin carries iron. The clotting factors, including fibrinogen, remain in an inactive form in the blood plasma until activated by the clotting cascade. The gamma globulins contain the immunoglobulins, or antibodies. These proteins are produced by the well-differentiated lymphocytes and plasma cells. The actual fractionation of the globulins can be seen on a specific laboratory test (serum protein electrophoresis).

Albumin is particularly important for the maintenance of fluid balance within the vascular system. Capillary walls are impermeable to albumin, so its presence in the plasma creates an osmotic force that keeps fluid within the vascular space. Albumin, which is produced by the liver, has the capacity to bind to several substances that are transported in plasma (eg, certain medications, bilirubin, and some hormones). People with poor hepatic function may have low concentrations of albumin, with a resultant decrease in osmotic pressure and the development of edema.

Reticuloendothelial System (RES)

The RES is composed of special tissue macrophages. Macrophages are derived from monocytes. When released from the marrow, monocytes spend a short time in the circulation (about 24 hours) and then enter the body tissues. Within the tissues, the monocytes continue to differentiate into cells called macrophages, which can survive for months. These macrophages, which have a variety of important functions (Chart 30-1), give rise to tissue **histiocytes**, including Kupffer cells of the liver, peritoneal macrophages, alveolar macrophages, and other components of the RES. Thus, the RES is a component of many other organs within the body, particularly the spleen, lymph nodes, lung, and liver.

The spleen is the site of activity for most macrophages. Most of the spleen is made of red pulp (75%); here the blood enters the venous sinuses through capillaries that are surrounded by macrophages. Within the red pulp are tiny aggregates of white pulp, consisting of B and T lymphocytes. The spleen sequesters newly released reticulocytes from the marrow, removing nuclear fragments and other materials (eg, denatured hemoglobin and iron) before the now fully mature erythrocyte returns to the circulation. Although a minority of red cells is pooled in the spleen (less than 5%), a significant proportion of platelets (20%–40%) is pooled here. If the spleen is enlarged, a greater proportion of RBCs and platelets can be sequestered here. The spleen is a major source of hematopoiesis in fetal life. It can resume hematopoiesis later in adulthood if necessary (eg, in bone marrow fibrosis). The spleen has important immunologic functions as well. It forms a substance that promotes the phagocytosis of neutrophils; it also forms the antibody IgM after exposure to antigen.

Hemostasis

Hemostasis is the process of preventing blood loss from intact vessels and of stopping bleeding from a severed vessel. The prevention of blood loss from intact vessels requires adequate numbers of functional platelets, because they nurture the endothelium and thereby maintain the structural integrity of the vessel wall. Two processes are involved in arresting bleeding: primary and secondary hemostasis.

In primary hemostasis, the severed blood vessel constricts. Circulating platelets aggregate at the site and adhere to the vessel and to one another. An unstable hemostatic plug is formed. The process of blood coagulation is highly complex. It can be activated by the intrinsic or the extrinsic pathway. Both pathways are needed for maintenance of normal hemostasis. For the coagulation process to be correctly activated, circulating coagulation factors are converted to active forms. This process occurs on the surface of the aggregated platelets at the site of vessel injury. The end result is the formation of fibrin, which reinforces the platelet plug and anchors it to the injury site. This process is termed secondary hemostasis (Fig. 30-4).

Many factors are involved in the reaction cascade that forms fibrin. When tissue is injured, the extrinsic pathway is activated by the release from the tissue of a substance called thromboplastin. As the result of a series of reactions, prothrombin is converted to **thrombin**, which in turn catalyzes the conversion of fibrinogen to fibrin. Clotting by the intrinsic pathway is activated when the collagen that lines blood vessels is exposed. Clotting factors are then activated sequentially until, as with the extrinsic pathway, fibrin is ultimately formed. Although slower, this sequence is probably most often responsible for clotting *in vivo*.

As the injured vessel is repaired and again covered with endothelial cells, the fibrin clot is no longer needed. The fibrin is digested via two systems: the plasma fibrinolytic system and the cellular fibrinolytic system. The substance **plasminogen** is required to lyse (break down) the fibrin. Plasminogen, which is present in all body fluids, circulates with fibrinogen and is therefore incorporated into the fibrin clot as it forms. When the clot is no longer needed, the plasminogen is activated to form plasmin. Plasmin

PHYSIOLOGY

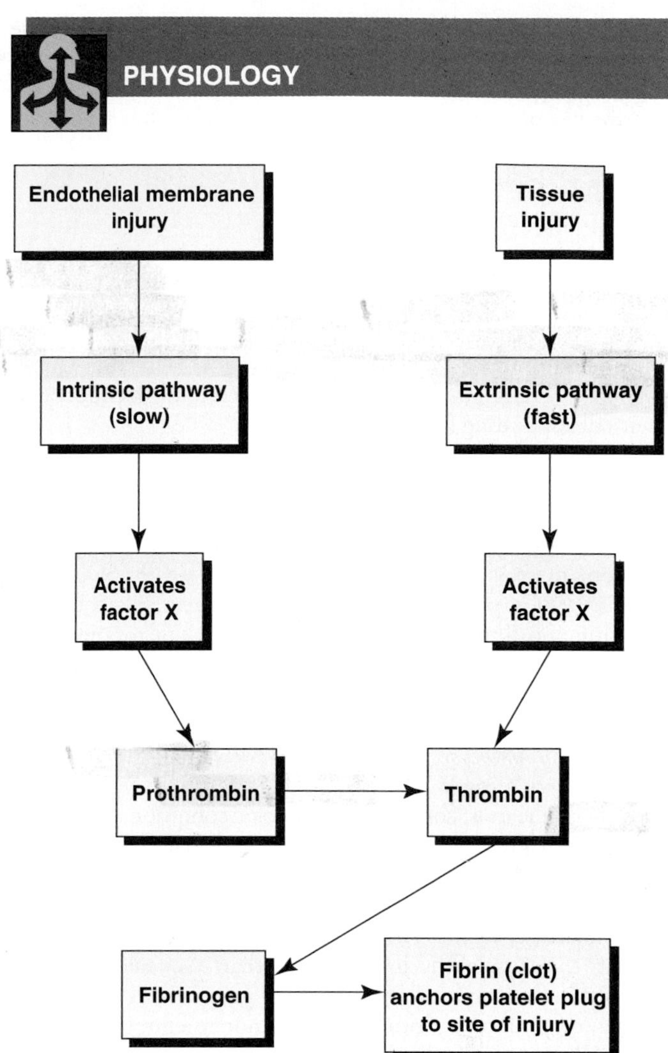

FIGURE 30•4 Secondary hemostasis. Based on the type of stimulus (injury to the endothelial membrane of a blood vessel or a tissue), one of two clotting pathways is initiated. The end result from either pathway is the conversion of prothrombin to thrombin. Thrombin is necessary for fibrinogen to be converted into fibrin, the stabilizing protein that anchors the fragile platelet plug to the site of injury to prevent further bleeding and permit the injured vessel or site to heal.

CHART 30•1 Functions of the Macrophages

- Defend body against foreign invaders (ie, bacteria and other pathogens) via phagocytosis
- Remove old or damaged cells from circulation
- Stimulate the inflammatory process
- Present antigen to the immune system (see Chap. 46)

actually digests the fibrinogen, and the breakdown particles of the clot (fibrin degradation products) are released into the circulation. Through this system, clots are dissolved as tissue is repaired, and the vascular system returns to its normal baseline state.

PATHOPHYSIOLOGY OF THE HEMATOLOGIC SYSTEM

Most hematologic diseases reflect a defect in the hematopoietic, hemostatic, or RES systems. The defect can be quantitative (eg, increased or decreased production of cells) or qualitative (eg, the cells that are produced are defective in their normal functional capacity). Chart 30-2 summarizes major blood disorders and their corresponding laboratory findings.

Gerontologic Considerations

In elderly patients, a common problem is the decreased ability of the bone marrow to respond to the body's need for blood cells (RBCs, WBCs, platelets). This inability is due to many factors, including the diminished production of growth factors necessary for hematopoiesis by the stromal cells within the marrow. Thus, when an elderly person needs more blood cells (eg, WBCs in infection, RBCs in anemia), the bone marrow may not be able to increase production of these cells adequately. **Leukopenia** (a decrease in circulating WBCs) or anemia can result.

Anemia, the most common hematologic condition affecting elderly patients, frequently results from iron deficiency (in the case of blood loss) or a nutritional deficiency, particularly folate deficiency or protein-calorie malnutrition. Management of the disorder varies depending on the etiology. Thus, it is important to identify the cause of the anemia rather than to consider it an inevitable consequence of aging. Elderly people with concurrent cardiac or pulmonary problems may not tolerate the anemia very well, and a prompt, thorough evaluation is warranted.

ASSESSMENT

Many hematologic conditions cause few symptoms. Therefore, the use of extensive laboratory tests is often required to diagnose a hematologic disorder. For most hematologic conditions, continued monitoring via specific blood tests is required because it is very important to assess for changes in test results over time.

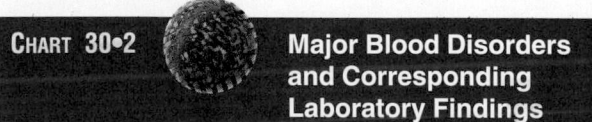

- Anemia: decreased hemoglobin and hematocrit values
- Polycythemia: increased hemoglobin and hematocrit values
- Leukopenia and neutropenia: decreased WBC and neutrophil counts
- Leukocytosis and hematologic cancers: increased WBC and neutrophil counts
- Thrombocytosis, thrombocythemia: increased platelet count
- Thrombocytopenia: decreased platelet count
- Other disorders (hemoglobinopathies, hemostatic disorders, thrombosis, bleeding): values vary

Hematologic Studies

The most common tests used are the complete blood count (CBC) and the peripheral blood smear (Table 30-2). The CBC identifies the total number of blood cells (WBCs, RBCs, and platelets) as well as the hemoglobin, hematocrit (percentage of blood consisting of RBCs), and RBC indices. Because cellular morphology (shape and appearance of the cells) is particularly important in most hematologic disorders, the diagnostician needs to examine the blood cells involved. This process is referred to as the examination of the peripheral smear, which may be part of the CBC. In this test, a drop of blood is spread on a glass slide, stained, and examined under a microscope. The shape and size of the RBCs and platelets as well as the actual appearance of the WBCs provides useful information in identifying hematologic conditions. Blood for the CBC is typically obtained by venipuncture.

Bone Marrow Aspiration and Biopsy

The bone marrow aspirate and biopsy are crucial when additional information is needed to assess how blood cells are formed within an individual and to assess the quantity and quality of each type of cell produced within the marrow. These tests are used also to document infection or tumor within the marrow.

Normal bone marrow is in a semifluid state and, therefore, can be aspirated through a special large needle. In adults, bone marrow is usually aspirated from the iliac crest and occasionally the sternum. The aspirate provides only a sample of cells. Aspirate alone may be adequate for evaluating certain conditions, such as anemia. However, when more information is required, a biopsy is also performed. Biopsy samples are taken from the posterior iliac crest; occasionally an anterior approach is required. A marrow biopsy shows the architecture of the bone marrow, as well as its degree of cellularity.

Most patients need no more preparation than a careful explanation of the procedure, but for some very anxious patients, an antianxiety agent may be useful. It is always important for the physician or nurse to describe and explain to the patient the procedure and the sensations that will be experienced. A signed informed consent is needed before the procedure is performed.

Using aseptic technique, the skin is cleansed as for any minor surgery. Then a small area is anesthetized with a local anesthetic through the skin and subcutaneous tissue to the periosteum of the bone. It is not possible to anesthetize the bone itself. The bone marrow needle is introduced with a stylet in place. When the needle is felt to go through the outer cortex of bone and enter the marrow cavity, the stylet is removed, a syringe is attached, and a small volume (0.5 mL) of blood and marrow is aspirated. Patients typically feel a pressure sensation as the needle is advanced into position. The actual aspiration always causes sharp but brief pain, resulting from the suction exerted as the marrow is aspirated into the syringe; the patient should be warned of this. Taking deep breaths or using relaxation techniques often helps ease the discomfort.

If a bone marrow biopsy is necessary, it is best performed after the aspiration and in a slightly different location, because the marrow structure may be altered after aspiration. A special biopsy needle is used. Because these needles are large, the skin is punctured first with a surgical blade to make a 3- or 4-mm incision. The biopsy needle is advanced well into the marrow cavity. When properly positioned, a portion of marrow is cored out, using a twisting or gentle rocking motion to free the sample and permit its removal within the biopsy needle. Patients feel a pressure sensation but should not feel actual pain. The nurse should instruct

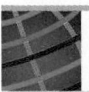

TABLE 30•2 Selected Blood Tests for Hematologic Disorders

Test	Normal Range	Description	Indications/Comments
Complete blood count (CBC)		General survey of bone marrow function; evaluates all three cell lines (WBCs, RBCs, platelets)	Important to note changes over time; many hematologic conditions show changes in CBC long before the patient has symptoms
Red blood cell (RBC) count	Male: $4.7–6.1 \times 10^6$ Female: $4.2–5.4 \times 10^6$	RBCs carry hemoglobin Survival time: 120 days	
Hemoglobin (Hgb)	Male: 13.5–17.5 g/dL Female: 11.5–15.5 g/dL	Delivers O_2 through circulation to body tissues and returns CO_2 from tissues to lungs	Decreased Hgb indicates anemia Increased Hgb indicates polycythemia
Hematocrit (Hct)	Male: 40%–52% Female: 36%–48%	Indicates relative proportions of plasma and RBCs (volume of RBCs/L whole blood)	Usually three times the hemoglobin level
Mean corpuscular volume (MCV)	81–96 μ^3	Indicates size of RBCs; very useful in differentiating types of anemia	Value of less than 80 indicates microcytic anemia Value exceeding 100 indicates macrocytic anemia
Mean corpuscular Hgb concentration (MCHC)	33–36 g/dL	Average concentration of Hgb in RBCs; independent of cell size	
RBC distribution width (RDW)	11%–14.5%	Measures degree of variation in RBC size	
Reticulocyte count	0.5%–1.5%	Measure of marrow production of erythrocytes; 1% of RBC mass is produced daily to replace the 1% of old cells that die	Indicates marrow's response to anemia (when anemia is present, reticulocyte level should rise)
Platelets	150,000–400,000/mm³	Total number of platelets in circulation; average life span: 7–10 days	Thrombocytopenia: <20,000 serious <10,000 may be life-threatening
Prothrombin time (PT)	Varies; compare with control; 11–12.5 seconds	Source of tissue factor added to plasma; measures time elapsed until clot forms Measures extrinsic and common depletion pathways	Increased prothrombin time seen in liver disease, disseminated intravascular coagulation, obstructive biliary disease, use of Coumarin, clotting factor depletion
Partial thromboplastin time (PTT)	Varies; compare with control; 25–35 seconds	Surface active agent added to plasma; measures time elapsed until clot forms Measures intrinsic and common pathway	Increased PTT seen in clotting factor depletion, disseminated intravascular coagulation, liver disease, biliary obstruction, circulating anticoagulants (heparin)
Thrombin time (TT)	Varies; compare with control; 8–11 seconds	Add diluted thrombin to patient's plasma; tests conversion of fibrinogen to fibrin	Time to clot is inversely proportional to fibrinogen level
Fibrinogen	170–340 mg/100 mL	Measurement of fibrinogen concentration within plasma available for conversion to fibrin clot	Decrease indicates bleeding disorder, pregnancy, malignancy, inflammatory disease
Fibrin degradation products (FDP)	<10 μg/mL	Byproduct of fibrinolysis	>40 μg/mL indicates disseminated intravascular coagulation
WBC	4500–11,000	Total WBC count	
Differential	% of various types of WBCs	% of cell type × total WBC = absolute number of that cell type	Shift to the left; bone marrow increased production of WBCs; more immature forms released into bloodstream
Neutrophils	40%–75% (2500–7500)	Essential in preventing or limiting bacterial infection (average life span: 2–4 hours)	Count exceeding 8000 occurs with infection, corticosteroids, other medications, myeloproliferative disease Decreased: neutropenia Absolute neutrophil count (ANC) <500: increased risk for infection Absolute neutrophil count (ANC) <100: infection certain (if neutropenia persists)
Lymphocytes	20%–50% (1500–5500)	Integral component of immune system	<1500 lymphopenia >4000 lymphocytosis; increase designates convalescent phase after bacterial infection, lymphoproliferative disease
Monocytes	1%–10% (100–800)	Enter tissue as macrophage; phagocytosis	Increase indicates acute and chronic infection
Eosinophils	0%–6% (0–440)	Involved in allergic reactions (neutralizes histamine); digest foreign proteins	Increase indicates allergic states; metastatic/necrotic tumors, chronic myeloid leukemia
Basophils	0%–2% (0–200)	Contain histamine; integral part of hypersensitivity reactions	Increase is very rare (chronic myeloid leukemia)

patients to inform the physician if they feel pain so that additional anesthetic can be administered.

The major hazard of either bone marrow aspiration or biopsy is a slight risk of bleeding and infection. The bleeding risk is somewhat increased if the patient's platelet count is low or if the patient has been taking a medication, such as aspirin, that alters platelet function. After the marrow sample is obtained, pressure is applied to the site for several minutes. The site is then covered with a sterile dressing. Most patients have no discomfort after a bone marrow aspiration, but the site of a biopsy may ache for 1 or 2 days. Warm tub baths or use of a mild analgesic (eg, acetaminophen) may be useful. Aspirin-containing analgesics should be avoided because they can aggravate or potentiate any bleeding that may occur.

MANAGEMENT OF HEMATOLOGIC DISORDERS

Commonly encountered blood disorders are anemia, polycythemia, leukopenia and neutropenia, leukocytosis, lymphoma, myeloma, leukemia, and various bleeding and coagulation disorders. Nursing management of patients with these disorders requires skillful assessment and monitoring as well as meticulous care and teaching to prevent deterioration and complications.

ANEMIA

Anemia, *per se*, is not a specific disease state but a sign of an underlying disorder. It is by far the most common hematologic condition. Anemia, a condition of a lower-than-normal level of hemoglobin, reflects fewer than normal RBCs within the circulation. As a result, the amount of oxygen delivered to body tissues is also diminished.

There are many different kinds of anemias (Table 30-3), but all can be classified into three broad etiologic categories:

- A loss of red cells: Loss of RBCs occurs with bleeding, potentially from any major source (gastrointestinal tract, uterus, nose, or wound).
- A decrease in production of red cells: Underproduction of red cells can be due to a deficiency in cofactors for erythropoiesis, including folic acid, vitamin B_{12}, and iron. RBC production may also be reduced if bone marrow is suppressed (by tumor, medications, or toxins) or is inadequately stimulated because of lack of erythropoietin, as occurs in chronic renal disease.
- An increase in destruction of red cells: Increased destruction of RBCs may occur because of an overactive RES (including hypersplenism) or because the bone marrow produces abnormal RBCs that are then destroyed by the RES (eg, sickle cell anemia).

A conclusion as to whether the anemia is caused by destruction of RBCs or inadequate production of RBCs usually can be reached on the basis of:

- The marrow's ability to respond to the decreased RBCs (as evidenced by an increased reticulocyte count in the circulating blood)
- The degree to which young RBCs proliferate in the bone marrow and the manner in which they mature (as observed on bone marrow biopsy)
- The presence or absence of end products of RBC destruction within the circulation (eg, elevated bilirubin level, decreased haptoglobin level)

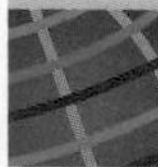

TABLE 30•3 Classification of Anemias

Kind of Anemia	Laboratory Findings
Classification: Hypoproliferative (Resulting From Defective RBC Production)	
Iron deficiency	Decreased reticulocytes, iron, ferritin, iron saturation, MCV Increased total iron binding capacity (TIBC)
Vitamin B_{12} deficiency (megaloblastic)	Decreased vitamin B_{12} level Increased MCV
Folate deficiency	Decreased folate level Increased MCV
Decreased erythropoietin production (eg, from renal dysfunction)	Decreased erythropoietin level Normal MCV and MCHC Increased creatinine level Decreased iron, TIBC
Cancer/inflammation	Normal MCV, MCHC Normal or decreased erythropoietin level Increased % of iron saturation, ferritin level
Classification: Bleeding (Resulting From RBC Loss)	
Bleeding from GI tract, menorrhagia (excessive menstrual flow), epistaxis (nosebleed), trauma	Increased reticulocyte level Normal Hgb and Hct if measured soon after bleeding starts, but levels decrease thereafter Normal MCV initially but decreased soon after bleeding starts Decreased ferritin and iron levels
Classification: Hemolytic (Resulting From RBC Destruction)	
Altered erythropoiesis (sickle cell anemia, thalassemia, other hemoglobinopathies)	Decreased MCV Fragmented RBCs Increased reticulocyte level
Hypersplenism (hemolysis)	Increased MCV
Drug-induced anemia	Vary depending on the drug
Autoimmune anemia	Increased spherocyte level
Mechanical heart-valve–related anemia	Fragmented red cells

Classification of Anemias

Anemia may be classified in several ways. The physiologic approach is to determine whether the deficiency in RBCs is due to a defect in production of RBCs (hypoproliferative anemia), destruction of RBCs (hemolytic anemia), or loss of RBCs (bleeding).

In the hypoproliferative anemias, RBCs usually survive normally, but the marrow cannot produce adequate numbers of these cells. The decreased production is reflected in a low reticulocyte count. Inadequate production of RBCs may be a result of marrow damage by medications or chemicals (eg, chloramphenicol, benzene) or may result from lack of factors necessary for RBC formation (eg, iron, vitamin B_{12}, folic acid, or erythropoietin).

Hemolytic anemias stem from a premature destruction of RBCs, resulting in a liberation of hemoglobin from the red cell into the plasma. The increased RBC destruction results in tissue hypoxia, which in turn stimulates erythropoietin production. This increased production is reflected in an increased reticulocyte count, as the bone marrow responds to the loss of RBCs. The released hemoglobin is converted in large part to bilirubin; thus, the bilirubin level rises. **Hemolysis** can result from an abnormality within the RBC itself (as in sickle cell anemia or glucose-6-phosphate dehydrogenase [G-6-PD] deficiency) or within the plasma (as in immune hemolytic anemias), or from direct injury to the RBC within the circulation (as in heart valve hemolysis). Chart 30-3 identifies the causes of hemolytic anemia.

Clinical Manifestations

Aside from the severity of the anemia itself, several factors influence the development of anemia-associated symptoms:

- Speed with which the anemia has developed
- Duration of the anemia (ie, its chronicity)
- Metabolic requirements of the individual
- Other disorders or disabilities (eg, cardiopulmonary disease)
- Special complications or concomitant features of the condition that produced the anemia

In general, the more rapidly an anemia develops, the more severe its symptoms. An otherwise healthy person can often tolerate as much as a 50% gradual reduction in hemoglobin without pronounced symptoms or significant incapacity, whereas the rapid loss of as little as 30% may precipitate profound vascular collapse in the same individual. A person who has been anemic for a very long time, with hemoglobin levels between 9 and 11 g/dL, usually has few or no symptoms other than slight tachycardia on exertion and fatigue.

Patients who customarily are very active or who have significant demands on their lives (eg, single mothers of small children working full-time) are more likely to have symptoms, and those symptoms are more likely to be pronounced than in a more sedentary person. A patient with hypothyroidism with decreased oxygen needs may be completely asymptomatic, without tachycardia or increased cardiac output, at a hemoglobin level of 10 g/dL. Similarly, patients with coexistent cardiac, vascular, or pulmonary disease may develop more pronounced symptoms of anemia (eg, dyspnea, chest pain, muscle pain or cramping) at a higher hemoglobin level than an individual without these concurrent health problems.

Finally, some anemic disorders are complicated by various other abnormalities that do not result from the anemia but are inherently associated with these particular diseases. These abnormalities may give rise to symptoms that completely overshadow those of the anemia, as in the painful crises of sickle cell anemia.

CHART 30•3 Causes of Hemolytic Anemia

Inherited Hemolytic Anemia

- Abnormal hemoglobin
  - Sickle cell anemia*
  - Thalassemia*
- Red blood cell membrane abnormality
  - Hereditary spherocytosis*
  - Hereditary elliptocytosis
  - Acathanthocytosis
  - Stomatocytosis
- Enzyme deficiencies
  - G-6-PD deficiency*

Acquired Hemolytic Anemia

- Antibody-related
  - Iso-antibody or transfusion reaction*
  - Autoimmune hemolytic anemia*
  - Cold agglutinin disease*
- Not antibody-related
  - Red blood cell membrane defects
    - Paroxysmal nocturnal hemoglobinuria
    - Liver disease
    - Uremia
    - Trauma
    - Mechanical heart valve
    - Microangiopathic hemolytic anemia
  - Infection
    - Bacterial
    - Parasitic
    - Disseminated intravascular coagulopathy (DIC)*
  - Toxins
  - Hypersplenism*

* Discussed in text

Assessment and Diagnostic Findings

A variety of hematologic studies are performed to determine the type and cause of the anemia. In an initial evaluation, the hemoglobin, hematocrit, reticulocyte count, and red cell indices, particularly the mean corpuscular volume (MCV), are particularly useful. Iron studies (serum iron level, total iron-binding capacity [TIBC], percent saturation, and ferritin), as well as serum vitamin B_{12} and folate levels, are also frequently obtained. Other tests include haptoglobin and erythropoietin levels. The remaining CBC values are useful in determining whether the anemia is an isolated problem or part of another hematologic condition, such as leukemia or myelodysplastic syndrome (MDS). Bone marrow aspiration may be performed. In addition, other diagnostic studies may be performed to determine the presence of underlying chronic illness such as malignancy and the source of any blood loss, such as polyps or ulcers within the gastrointestinal tract.

Complications

General complications of severe anemia include congestive heart failure (CHF), paresthesias, and confusion. At any given level of anemia, patients with underlying heart disease are far more likely to have angina or symptoms of congestive failure than someone without heart disease. Complications associated with specific types of anemia are included in the description of each type.

Medical Management

Management of anemia is directed toward correcting or controlling the cause of the anemia; if the anemia is severe, the RBCs that are lost or destroyed are replaced. The management of the various types of anemia is covered in the discussions below.

NURSING PROCESS: THE PATIENT WITH ANEMIA

Assessment

The health history and physical examination provide important data about the type of anemia involved, the extent and type of symptoms it produces, and the impact of those symptoms on the patient's life. Weakness, fatigue, and general malaise are common, as are pallor of the skin and mucous membranes (sclera, oral mucosa).

Jaundice may be present in patients with megaloblastic anemia or hemolytic anemia. The tongue may be smooth and red (in iron-deficiency anemia) or beefy red and sore (in megaloblastic anemia); the corners of the mouth may be ulcerated (**angular cheilosis**) in both types of anemia. Individuals with iron-deficiency anemia may crave ice, starch, or dirt (known as pica); their nails may be brittle, ridged, and concave.

The health history should include a medication history, because some medications can depress bone marrow activity or interfere with folate metabolism. An accurate history of alcohol intake, including the amount and duration of drinking, should be obtained. Family history is important because certain anemias are inherited. Athletic endeavors should be assessed because extreme exercise can decrease erythropoiesis and red cell survival in a few athletes.

A nutritional assessment is important because it may indicate deficiencies in essential nutrients such as iron, vitamin B_{12}, and folic acid. Children of indigent families may be at higher risk for developing anemia because of nutritional deficiencies. Strict vegetarians are also at risk for developing megaloblastic types of anemia if they do not supplement the diet with vitamin B_{12}.

Cardiac status should be carefully assessed. When the hemoglobin level is low, the heart attempts to compensate by pumping faster and harder in an effort to deliver more blood to hypoxic tissue. This increased cardiac workload can result in such symptoms as tachycardia, palpitations, dyspnea, dizziness, orthopnea, and exertional dyspnea. CHF may eventually develop, as evidenced by an enlarged heart (cardiomegaly) and liver (hepatomegaly) and by peripheral edema.

Assessment of the gastrointestinal system may disclose complaints of nausea, vomiting (with specific questions as to the appearance of any emesis [ie, "coffee grounds"]), melena or dark stools, diarrhea, anorexia, and **glossitis** (inflammation of the tongue). Stools should be tested for occult blood. Women should be questioned about their menstrual periods (eg, excessive menstrual flow or other vaginal bleeding) and the use of iron supplements during pregnancy.

Neurologic examination is also important because of the effect of pernicious anemia on the central and peripheral nervous systems. Assessment should include the presence and extent of peripheral numbness and paresthesias, ataxia, poor coordination, and confusion. Finally, it is important to monitor relevant laboratory test results and to note any changes over time.

Diagnosis

Nursing Diagnoses

Based on the assessment data, major nursing diagnoses for the anemic patient may include the following:

- Activity intolerance related to weakness, fatigue, and general malaise
- Altered nutrition, less than body requirements, related to inadequate intake of essential nutrients
- Altered tissue perfusion related to inadequate blood volume or hematocrit
- Noncompliance with prescribed therapy

Collaborative Problems/Potential Complications

Based on the assessment data, potential complications that may develop include:

- CHF
- Paresthesias
- Confusion

Planning and Goals

The major goals for the patient may include increased tolerance of normal activity, attainment or maintenance of adequate nutrition, maintenance of adequate tissue perfusion, compliance with prescribed therapy, and absence of complications.

Nursing Interventions

Managing Fatigue

The most frequent symptom and complication of anemia is fatigue. This distressing symptom is too often minimized by health care providers. Fatigue is often the symptom that has the most profoundly negative impact on the individual's level of functioning and subsequent quality of life. Patients describe the fatigue from anemia as oppressive; fatigue can be significant, yet the anemia may not be severe enough to warrant transfusion. Fatigue can interfere with an individual's ability to work, both inside and outside the home. It can harm relationships with family and friends. Patients often lose interest in hobbies and activities, including sexual activity. The distress from fatigue is often related to an individual's responsibilities and life demands as well as the amount of assistance and support received from others.

Nursing interventions can focus on assisting the patient to prioritize activities and to establish a balance between activity and rest that is realistic and feasible from the patient's perspective. Patients with chronic anemia need to maintain some physical activity and exercise to prevent deconditioning resulting from inactivity.

Maintaining Adequate Nutrition

Inadequate intake of essential nutrients, such as iron, vitamin B_{12}, and folic acid, can cause some anemias. The symptoms associated with anemias, such as fatigue and anorexia, can in turn interfere with maintaining adequate nutrition. A well-balanced diet should be encouraged. Because alcohol interferes with the utilization of essential nutrients, the nurse advises the patient to avoid alcoholic beverages or to limit their intake and provides a rationale for this recommendation. Dietary teaching sessions should be planned for the patient and the family because the diet plan should be acceptable to both the patient and family. Cultural aspects of nutrition must be considered. Dietary supplements (eg, vitamins, iron, folate) may be prescribed as well.

Equally important, the patient and family must understand the role of nutritional supplements in the proper context, because many forms of anemia are not the result of a nutritional deficiency. In such cases, excessive nutritional supplements will not improve the anemia. A potential problem in individuals with chronic transfusion requirements occurs with the indiscriminant use of iron. Unless an aggressive program of chelation therapy is implemented, these individuals are at risk for iron overload from their transfusions alone. Adding an iron supplement only exacerbates the problem.

Maintaining Adequate Perfusion

Patients with acute blood loss or severe hemolysis may have decreased tissue perfusion from decreased blood volume or reduced circulating RBCs (decreased hematocrit). Lost volume will be replaced with transfusions or intravenous fluids, based on the symptoms and the laboratory findings. Supplemental oxygen may be necessary, but it is rarely needed on a long-term basis unless there is underlying severe cardiac or pulmonary disease as well. Vital signs must be monitored closely; other medications, such as antihypertensive agents, may need to be adjusted or withheld.

Complying with Prescribed Therapy

For patients with anemia, medications and/or nutritional supplements are often prescribed to alleviate or correct the condition. These patients need to understand the purpose of the medication, how to take the medication and over what time period, and how to manage any side effects of therapy. To enhance compliance, the nurse can assist patients in developing ways to incorporate the therapeutic plan into their lives, rather than merely giving the patient a list of instructions. For example, many patients have difficulty taking iron supplements because of related gastrointestinal effects. Rather than seeking assistance from a health care provider in managing the problem, some of these patients simply stop taking the iron.

Abruptly stopping some medications may have serious consequences, as in the case of high-dose corticosteroids to manage hemolytic anemias. Some medications, such as growth factors, are extremely expensive. Patients receiving these medications may need assistance with obtaining needed insurance coverage or with exploring alternatives for obtaining these medications.

Monitoring and Managing Potential Complications

A significant complication of anemia is CHF from chronic diminished blood volume and the heart's compensatory effort to increase cardiac output. Patients with anemia should be assessed for signs and symptoms of CHF. A serial record of body weights can be more useful than recording dietary intake and output, because the intake and output measurements may not be accurate. In the case of fluid retention resulting from CHF, diuretics may be required.

In megaloblastic forms of anemia, the significant potential complications are neurologic. A neurologic assessment should be performed in patients known or suspected to have this form of anemia. Patients may initially complain of paresthesias in their lower extremities. These paresthesias are usually manifested as numbness and tingling on the bottom of the foot, and they gradually progress. As the anemia progresses and damage to the spinal cord occurs, other signs become apparent. Position and vibration sense may be diminished; difficulty maintaining balance is not uncommon, and some patients have gait disturbances as well. Initially mild but gradually progressive confusion may develop.

Evaluation

Expected Outcomes

Expected outcomes may include:

1. Tolerates activity at safe and acceptable level
   a. Follows a progressive plan of rest, activity, and exercise
   b. Prioritizes activities
   c. Paces activities according to energy level
2. Attains and maintains adequate nutrition
   a. Eats well-balanced diet
   b. Develops meal plan that promotes optimal nutrition
   c. Maintains adequate amounts of iron and vitamins from diet or supplements
   d. Adheres to nutritional supplement therapy when prescribed
   e. Verbalizes understanding of rationale for using or avoiding nutritional supplements
3. Maintains adequate perfusion
   a. Has vital signs within baseline for patient
   b. Has pulse oximetry (arterial oxygenation) value within normal limits
4. Experiences no or minimal complications
   a. Avoids or limits activities that cause dyspnea, palpitations, dizziness, or tachycardia
   b. Uses rest and comfort measures to alleviate dyspnea
   c. Has vital signs within baseline for patient
   d. Has no signs of increasing fluid retention (eg, peripheral edema, decreased urine output, neck vein distention)
   e. Answers to name and remains oriented to time, place, and situation
   f. Ambulates safely, using assistive devices as necessary
   g. Remains free of injury
   h. Verbalizes understanding of importance of serial CBC measurements
   i. Maintains safe home environment; obtains assistance as necessary.

HYPOPROLIFERATIVE ANEMIAS

Iron-Deficiency Anemia

Iron-deficiency anemia typically results when the intake of dietary iron is inadequate for hemoglobin synthesis. Because the body can store about one fourth to one third of its iron, it is not until those stores are depleted that iron-deficiency anemia actually begins to develop. Iron-deficiency anemia is the most common type of anemia in all age groups, and it is the most common anemia in the world. More than 500 million people are affected, more commonly in underdeveloped countries where inadequate iron stores can result from inadequate intake of iron (seen with vegetarian diets) and blood loss (as from intestinal hookworm). Iron deficiency is also common in the United States. A recent U.S. study (Looker et al., 1997) determined that 9% of toddlers and 10% of adolescent girls and women of childbearing age were iron-deficient; this deficiency resulted in anemia in 3% (ie, 700,000) of toddlers and 2% to 5% of adolescents and women (ie, 7.8 million women). In children, adolescents, and pregnant women, the cause is typically inadequate iron in the diet to keep up with increased growth. However, for most adults with iron-deficiency anemia, the cause is blood loss. In fact, in these people, the cause of iron-deficiency anemia should be considered to be bleeding until proven otherwise.

The common cause of iron deficiency in men and postmenopausal women is bleeding (eg, from ulcers, gastritis, inflammatory bowel disease, or gastrointestinal tumors). The most common cause of iron-deficiency anemia in premenopausal women is menorrhagia (excessive menstrual bleeding) and pregnancy with inadequate iron supplementation. Patients with chronic alcoholism often have chronic blood loss from the gastrointestinal tract, which causes iron loss and eventual anemia. Other causes include iron malabsorption, as seen after gastrectomy or with celiac disease.

Clinical Manifestations

Patients with iron deficiency primarily have the symptoms of anemia. If the deficiency is severe or prolonged, they may also have a smooth, sore tongue, brittle and ridged nails, and angular cheilosis (an ulceration of the corner of the mouth). These signs subside after iron-replacement therapy. The health history may be significant for multiple pregnancies, gastrointestinal bleeding, and pica (a craving for unusual substances, such as ice, clay, or laundry starch).

Assessment and Diagnostic Findings

The most definitive method of establishing the iron-deficiency anemia diagnosis is performing a bone marrow aspirate. The aspirate is stained to detect iron, which is at a low level or even absent. However, not all patients suspected of having iron-deficiency anemia undergo bone marrow aspiration. In many patients, the diagnosis can be established with other tests, particularly in patients with a history of conditions that predispose them to this type of anemia.

There is a strong correlation between laboratory values measuring iron stores and levels of hemoglobin. After the iron stores are depleted (reflected by low serum ferritin levels), the hemoglobin level falls. The diminished iron stores render the RBC small. Therefore, as the anemia progresses, the MCV, which measures the size of the RBC, also decreases. Hematocrit and RBC levels are also low in correlation with the hemoglobin level. Other laboratory tests that measure iron stores are useful but are not as consistent indicators as a low ferritin level, which reflects iron stores. Typically, patients with iron-deficiency anemia have a low serum iron level and an elevated TIBC, which measures the transport protein supplying the marrow with iron as needed (also referred to as transferrin). However, other disease states, such as infection and inflammatory conditions, can also cause a low serum iron level and TIBC and an increased ferritin level. Therefore, the most reliable laboratory findings in evaluating iron-deficiency anemia are the ferritin and hemoglobin values.

Medical Management

Except in the case of pregnancy, the cause of iron deficiency should be investigated. Anemia may be a sign of a curable gastrointestinal cancer or of uterine fibroid tumors. Stool specimens should be tested for occult blood. People 50 years or older should have a colonoscopy and/or endoscopy or other radiographic examination of the gastrointestinal tract to detect ulcerations, gastritis, polyps, or cancer.

IRON SUPPLEMENTATION

Several oral iron preparations—ferrous sulfate, ferrous gluconate, and ferrous fumarate—are available for treating iron-deficiency anemia. The least expensive and most effective preparation is ferrous sulfate. One tablet of iron sulfate provides 60 mg of elemental iron. Tablets with enteric coating may be poorly absorbed and thus should be avoided. An increase in the hemoglobin level may be seen in only a few weeks, and the anemia can be corrected in a few months, but iron store replenishment takes much longer. Thus, it is important to continue the iron for as long as 6 to 12 months.

In some cases, oral iron is poorly absorbed or poorly tolerated or needed in large amounts. In these situations, intramuscular or intravenous administration of iron dextran may be needed. The intramuscular injection causes some local pain and can stain the skin. Iron dextran should be injected deeply into each buttock using the Z-track technique. Before parenteral administration of a full dose, a small test dose should be administered to avoid the risk of anaphylaxis, which is greater with intramuscular injections than with intravenous injections. Because of these problems with intramuscular administration, the intravenous route is preferred for administering iron dextran.

Nursing Management

Preventive education is important because iron-deficiency anemia is common in menstruating and pregnant women. Food sources high in iron include organ meats (beef or calf's liver, chicken liver), other meats, beans (black, pinto, and garbanzo), leafy green vegetables, raisins, and molasses. Taking iron-rich foods with a source of vitamin C enhances the absorption of iron.

The nurse helps the patient select a well-balanced diet. Nutritional counseling can be provided for those whose normal diet is inadequate. Patients with a history of eating fad diets or strict vegetarian diets are counseled that such diets often contain inadequate amounts of absorbable iron. The nurse encourages patients to continue iron therapy as long as it is prescribed, even though they may no longer feel fatigued.

PROMOTING HOME AND COMMUNITY-BASED CARE

Because iron is best absorbed on an empty stomach, patients should be advised to take the supplement an hour before meals. Also, because many people have difficulty taking iron supplements because of gastrointestinal side effects (primarily constipation, but also cramping, nausea, and vomiting), compliance can be enhanced by specific patient teaching aids, such as the accompanying patient education guide.

If taking iron on an empty stomach causes gastric distress, the patient may need to take the iron supplement with meals. However, doing so diminishes iron absorption by as much as 50%. Thus, the time required to replenish the iron stores is prolonged. Antacids or dairy products should not be taken with iron because they greatly diminish the absorption of iron.

Liquid forms of iron that cause less gastrointestinal distress are available. However, they stain the teeth; patients should be instructed to take this medication through a straw, to rinse the mouth with water, and to practice good oral hygiene after taking this medication. Finally, patients should be informed that iron salts may color the stool dark green or black. However, iron replacement therapy does not cause a false-positive result on stool analyses for occult blood.

Anemias in Renal Disease

The degree of anemia in patients with end-stage renal disease varies greatly, but in general patients do not become anemic until the serum creatinine level exceeds 3 mg/100 mL. The symptoms

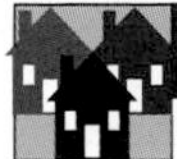

PATIENT EDUCATION AND HOME CARE

How to Take Iron Supplements

Iron supplements are usually given in oral form, typically as ferrous sulfate, or $FeSO_4$. Many people have difficulty tolerating iron supplements, primarily due to gastric problems (nausea, abdominal discomfort, and constipation). Here are guidelines for taking iron supplements:

- Take iron on an empty stomach (1 hour before meals, 2 hours after meals). Iron absorption is reduced with food, especially dairy products.
- If iron causes gastric upset, the following schedule may work better:
  - Start with only one tablet/day for a few days, then increase to two tablets/day, then three tablets/day. This method gradually permits the body to adjust to the iron.
- Increase the intake of vitamin C, (oranges, orange or grapefruit juice, broccoli, strawberries, tomatoes) as it enhances iron absorption.
- Eat foods high in fiber to diminish problems with constipation.
- Remember, stools will become quite dark from iron.
- If liquid forms of iron are taken, they may be better tolerated than solid forms. However, they can discolor teeth. Use a straw or place spoon at the back of the mouth to take the supplement; rinse mouth thoroughly afterward.

of anemia are often the most disturbing of the patient's symptoms. The hematocrit usually falls to between 20% and 30%, although in rare cases it may fall to less than 15%. The RBCs appear normal on the peripheral smear.

This anemia is due to both a mild shortening of RBC survival and a deficiency of erythropoietin necessary for erythropoiesis. As renal function decreases, erythropoietin, produced by the kidney, also decreases. Erythropoietin is also produced outside the kidney. Therefore, some erythropoiesis does continue, even in patients whose kidneys have been removed. However, the amount is small and the degree of erythropoiesis is inadequate.

Patients undergoing long-term hemodialysis lose blood into the dialyzer and thus may become iron-deficient. Folic acid deficiency develops because this vitamin passes into the dialysate. Therefore, dialysis patients who are anemic should be evaluated for iron and folate deficiency and treated as appropriate.

Medical Management

The availability of recombinant erythropoietin (epotin alpha) has dramatically altered the management of anemia in end-stage renal disease by decreasing the need for RBC transfusion, with its associated risks. Erythropoietin, in combination with oral iron supplements, can raise and maintain hematocrit levels to between 33% and 38%. This treatment has been successful with dialysis patients. Many patients report decreased fatigue, increased energy, increased feelings of well-being, improved exercise tolerance, better tolerance of dialysis treatments, and improved quality of life. Hypertension is the most serious side effect in this patient population when the hematocrit quickly rises to a high level. Therefore, the hematocrit should be checked frequently when a patient with renal disease begins erythropoietin therapy, and the amount of Epogen should be titrated to the hematocrit. In some patients, the elevated hematocrit and associated hypertension may require antihypertensive therapy.

Anemia of Chronic Disease

The term "anemia of chronic disease" is a misnomer in that only the chronic diseases of inflammation, infection, and/or malignancy cause this type of anemia. Many chronic inflammatory diseases are associated with a **normochromic**, **normocytic** (ie, the RBCs are normal in color and size) anemia. These disorders include rheumatoid arthritis; severe, chronic infections; and many cancers. It is therefore imperative that the "chronic disease" be identified when this form of anemia is seen.

The anemia is usually mild to moderate and nonprogressive. It develops gradually over 6 to 8 weeks and then stabilizes at a hematocrit seldom less than 25%. The hemoglobin level rarely falls below 9 g/dL, and the bone marrow has normal cellularity with increased stores of iron. Erythropoietin levels are low, perhaps because of decreased production, and iron use is blocked by erythroid cells. A moderate shortening of RBC survival also occurs.

Medical Management

Most of these patients have few symptoms and do not require treatment for the anemia. With successful treatment of the underlying disorder, the bone marrow iron is used to make RBCs and the hemoglobin level rises.

Aplastic Anemia

Aplastic anemia is a rather rare disease caused by a decrease in or damage to marrow stem cells, the microenvironment within the marrow, and replacement of the marrow with fat. It results in not only anemia but also neutropenia and **thrombocytopenia** (a deficiency of platelets).

Pathophysiology

Aplastic anemia can be congenital or acquired, or it may be idiopathic (ie, without apparent cause), which accounts for most cases. Certain infections and pregnancy can trigger it, or it may be caused by medications, chemicals, or radiation damage. Agents

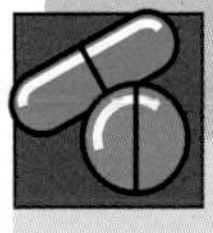

PHARMACOLOGY

Substances Associated with Aplastic Anemia

Analgesics
Anticonvulsants (mephenytoin, trimethadione*)
Antihistamines
Antimicrobials*
Antithyroid medications
Chloramphenicol*
Gold compounds*
Heavy metals
Hypoglycemic agents
Insecticides
Organic arsenicals*
Phenylbutazone*
Phenothiazines
Sulfonamides*
Sedatives

* Most common

that regularly produce marrow **aplasia** (arrested bone marrow development) include benzene and benzene derivatives (eg, airplane glue). Certain toxic materials, such as inorganic arsenic and several pesticides (eg, DDT [no longer used or available in the United States]), have also been implicated as potential causes. Various medications have been associated with aplastic anemia.

Clinical Manifestations

The manifestations of aplastic anemia are often insidious. Unless CBCs are obtained, complications resulting from the marrow failure may occur before the diagnosis is established. Typical complications are infection and symptoms of anemia (eg, fatigue, pallor, and dyspnea). Purpura (bruising) may develop later and should trigger a CBC and hematologic evaluation if these were not performed initially. If the patient has had repeated throat infections, cervical lymphadenopathy may be seen. Other lymphadenopathies and splenomegaly sometimes occur. Retinal hemorrhages are common.

Assessment and Diagnostic Findings

In many situations, aplastic anemia occurs when a medication or chemical is ingested in toxic amounts. However, in a few people, it develops after a medication has been taken at the recommended dosage. This may be considered an idiosyncratic reaction in those who are highly susceptible, possibly due to a genetic defect in the drug biotransformation or elimination process. A bone marrow aspirate shows an extremely hypoplastic or even aplastic (very few to no cells) marrow replaced with fat.

Medical Management

Despite its severity, aplastic anemia can be treated in most people. Potentially, those who are younger than age 60, who are otherwise healthy, and who have a compatible donor can be cured of the disease by a bone marrow or peripheral stem cell transplant. Others can be managed with immunosuppressive therapy. A combination of antithymocyte globulin and cyclosporine is used most frequently. If the patient relapses (becomes **pancytopenic** again), a reinstitution of the same immunologic agents may induce another remission.

Supportive therapy plays a major role in managing aplastic anemia. Any offending agent is discontinued. The patient is supported with transfusions of RBCs and platelets as necessary. Death is usually caused by hemorrhage or infection.

Nursing Management

Patients with aplastic anemia are vulnerable to problems related to leukocyte, erythrocyte, and platelet deficiencies. They should be assessed carefully for signs of infection and bleeding. Specific interventions are delineated in the sections on neutropenia and thrombocytopenia.

Megaloblastic Anemias

In the anemias caused by deficiencies of vitamin B_{12} and/or folic acid, identical bone marrow and peripheral blood changes occur because both vitamins are essential for normal DNA synthesis. In either anemia, the red cells that are produced are abnormally large and are called megaloblastic RBCs. Other cells derived from the myeloid stem cell (nonlymphoid white cells, platelets) are also abnormal. A bone marrow analysis reveals **hyperplasia** (abnormal increase in the number of cells), and the precursor erythroid and myeloid cells are large and bizarre in appearance. Many of these abnormal red and myeloid cells are destroyed within the marrow, however, so the mature cells that do leave the marrow are actually fewer in number. Thus, pancytopenia (a decrease in all myeloid-derived cells) can develop. In an advanced situation, the hemoglobin value may be as low as 4 to 5 g/dL, the WBC count 2000 to 3000/mm^3, and the platelet count less than 50,000/mm^3. Those cells that are released into the circulation are often abnormally shaped. The neutrophils are hypersegmented. The platelets may be abnormally large. The RBCs are abnormally shaped, and the shapes may vary widely (**poikilocytosis**). Because the RBCs are very large, the MCV is very high, usually exceeding 110 μ^3.

Pathophysiology

FOLIC ACID DEFICIENCY

Folic acid, a vitamin that is necessary for normal RBC production, is stored as different compounds, referred to as folates. The folate stores in the body are much smaller than those of vitamin B_{12}, so these stores are quickly depleted when the dietary intake of folate is deficient (about 4 months). Folate is found in green vegetables and liver. Thus, this deficiency occurs in people who rarely eat uncooked vegetables. Alcohol increases folic acid requirements; at the same time, patients with alcoholism usually have a diet that is deficient in the vitamin. Folic acid requirements are also increased in patients with chronic hemolytic anemias and women who are pregnant because the need for RBC production is increased in these conditions. Some patients with malabsorptive diseases of the small bowel, such as sprue, may not absorb folic acid normally.

VITAMIN B_{12} DEFICIENCY

A deficiency of vitamin B_{12} can occur in several ways. Inadequate dietary intake is rare but can develop in strict vegetarians who consume no meat or dairy products. Faulty absorption from the gastrointestinal tract is more common. This occurs in various conditions such as Crohn's disease, or after ileal resection or gastrectomy. Another cause is the absence of intrinsic factor, as in pernicious anemia. Intrinsic factor is normally secreted by cells within the gastric mucosa; normally it binds with the dietary vitamin B_{12} and travels with it to the ileum, where the vitamin is absorbed. Without intrinsic factor, orally consumed vitamin B_{12} cannot be absorbed, and RBC production is eventually diminished. Even if adequate vitamin B_{12} and intrinsic factor are present, a deficiency may occur if disease involving the ileum or pancreas impairs absorption. Pernicious anemia, which tends to run in families, is primarily a disorder of adults, particularly the elderly. The abnormality is in the gastric mucosa: the stomach wall atrophies and fails to secrete intrinsic factor. Thus, the absorption of vitamin B_{12} is significantly impaired.

Because the body normally has large stores of vitamin B_{12}, years may pass before the deficiency results in anemia. Because the body compensates so well, the anemia can be severe before the patient becomes very symptomatic. Patients with pernicious anemia have a higher incidence of gastric cancer than the general population.

Clinical Manifestations

Symptoms of folic acid and vitamin B_{12} deficiencies are similar, and the two anemias may coexist. However, the neurologic manifestations of vitamin B_{12} deficiency do not occur with folic acid deficiency, and they persist if B_{12} is not replaced. Therefore, careful distinction between the two anemias must be made. Serum levels of both vitamins can be measured. In the case of folic acid deficiency, even small amounts of folate will increase the serum folate level, sometimes to normal. Measuring the amount of folate within the RBC (red cell folate) is therefore a more sensitive test in determining true folate deficiency.

After the body stores of vitamin B_{12} are depleted, patients may begin to show signs of the anemia. However, because the onset and progression of the anemia are so gradual, the body can compensate very well until the anemia is severe, so that the typical manifestations of anemia (weakness, listlessness, fatigue) may not be apparent initially. The hematologic effects of deficiency are accompanied by effects on other organ systems, particularly the gastrointestinal tract and nervous system. Patients with pernicious anemia develop a smooth, sore, red tongue and mild diarrhea. They are extremely pale, particularly in the mucous membranes. They may become confused but more often have paresthesias in the extremities (particularly numbness and tingling in the feet and lower legs). They may have difficulty maintaining their balance because of damage to the spinal cord, and also lose position sense (proprioception). These symptoms are progressive, although the course of illness may be marked by spontaneous partial remissions and exacerbations. Without treatment, patients can die after several years, usually from CHF secondary to anemia.

Assessment and Diagnostic Findings

The method of determining the cause of vitamin B_{12} deficiency is the Schilling test, in which the patient receives a small oral dose of radioactive vitamin B_{12} followed in a few hours by a large, nonradioactive parenteral dose of vitamin B_{12} (this aids in renal excretion of the radioactive dose). If the oral vitamin is absorbed, more than 8% will be excreted in the urine within 24 hours; thus, if there is no radioactivity present in the urine (ie, the radioactive vitamin B_{12} stays within the gastrointestinal tract), the cause is gastrointestinal malabsorption of the vitamin B_{12}. Conversely, if the urine is radioactive, the cause of the deficiency is not ileal disease or pernicious anemia. Later, the same procedure is repeated, but this time intrinsic factor is added to the oral radioactive vitamin B_{12}. If radioactivity is now detected in the urine (ie, the B_{12} was absorbed from the gastrointestinal tract in the presence of intrinsic factor), the diagnosis of pernicious anemia can be made.

Medical Management

Folate deficiency is treated by increasing the amount of folic acid in the diet and administering 1 mg of folic acid daily. Folic acid is administered intramuscularly only in people with malabsorption problems. With the exception of the vitamins administered during pregnancy, most proprietary vitamin preparations do not contain folic acid, so it must be administered as a separate tablet. When the hemoglobin level returns to normal, the folic acid replacement can be stopped. However, patients with alcoholism should continue receiving folic acid as long as they continue alcohol consumption.

Vitamin B_{12} deficiency is treated by vitamin B_{12} replacement. Vegetarians can prevent or treat deficiency with oral supplements through vitamins or fortified soy milk. When, as is more common, the deficiency is due to defective absorption or absence of intrinsic factor, replacement is by monthly intramuscular injections of vitamin B_{12}, usually at a dose of 1000 µg. The reticulocyte count rises within a week, and in several weeks the blood counts are all normal. The tongue improves in several days. However, the neurologic manifestations require more time for recovery; if there is severe neuropathy, the patient may never recover fully. To prevent recurrence of pernicious anemia, vitamin B_{12} therapy must be continued life-long if the patient has had pernicious anemia or an inability to absorb B_{12}.

Nursing Alert *Even when the anemia is severe, RBC transfusions may not be used because the patient's body has compensated over time by expanding the total blood volume. Administering blood transfusions to such patients, particularly those who are elderly and/or who have cardiac dysfunction, can precipitate pulmonary edema. If transfusions are required, the RBCs should be transfused slowly, with careful attention to signs and symptoms of fluid overload.*

Nursing Management

Assessment of patients at risk for or with megaloblastic anemia includes inspecting the skin and mucous membranes. Mild jaundice may be apparent and is best seen in the sclera without using fluorescent lights. Vitiligo (patchy loss of skin pigmentation) and premature graying of the hair is often seen in pernicious anemia. The tongue is smooth, red, and sore. Because of the neurologic complications associated with these anemias, a careful neurologic assessment is important. The nurse pays particular attention to ambulation and assesses the patient's gait and stability. Position and vibration sense should also be tested.

PROMOTING HOME AND COMMUNITY-BASED CARE

The nurse needs to assess the need for assistive devices (eg, canes, walkers) and the patient's need for support and guidance in managing activities of daily living and the home environment. Of particular concern is ensuring safety when position sense, coordination, and gait are affected. Physical and/or occupational therapy referrals may be needed. When sensation is altered, patients need to be instructed to avoid excessive heat and cold.

Because mouth and tongue soreness may restrict nutritional intake, the nurse can advise patients to prepare bland, soft foods and to eat small amounts frequently. The nurse also may explain that other nutritional deficiencies, such as alcohol-induced anemia, can induce neurologic problems.

The Schilling test is useful only if the urine collections are complete; therefore, the nurse must promote the patient's understanding and ability to comply with this collection.

Patients must also be taught about the chronicity of their disorder and the necessity for monthly vitamin B_{12} injections even when the patient has no symptoms. Many patients can be instructed to self-administer their injections. The gastric atrophy associated with pernicious anemia increases the risk of gastric carcinoma, so these patients need to understand that ongoing medical follow-up and screening are important.

Myelodysplastic Syndromes (MDS)

MDS is a group of disorders of the myeloid stem cell causing **dysplasia** (abnormal development) in one or more types of cells. The most common feature of MDS—dysplasia of the RBCs—is manifested as a macrocytic anemia; however, the WBCs (myeloid cells, particularly neutrophils) and platelets can also be affected. Although the bone marrow is actually hypercellular, many of the cells within it die before being released into the circulation. Thus, the number of affected cells in the circulation is typically lower than normal. In addition to the quantitative defect (ie, fewer than normal cells), there is also a qualitative defect: the cells are not as functional as normal. Thus, the neutrophils have diminished ability to destroy bacteria by phagocytosis; platelets are less able to aggregate and are less adhesive than usual. The result of these qualitative defects is an increased risk for infection and bleeding, even when the actual number of circulating cells may not be excessively low. A significant proportion of MDS cases evolve into acute myeloid leukemia (AML); this type of leukemia tends to be very nonresponsive to standard therapy.

Primary MDS tends to be a disease of the elderly; more than 80% of patients with MDS are older than 60 years.

Secondary MDS may occur at any age and results from prior toxic exposure to chemicals, including chemotherapeutic medications (particularly alkylating agents). Secondary MDS tends to have a poorer prognosis than primary MDS.

Clinical Manifestations

The manifestations of MDS can vary widely. Many patients are asymptomatic, with the illness being discovered incidentally on a CBC performed for other purposes. Other patients have profound symptoms and complications from the illness. Fatigue is often present, at varying levels. Neutrophil dysfunction renders the person at risk for infection; recurrent pneumonias are not uncommon. Because platelet function can also be altered, bleeding can occur. These problems may persist at a fairly steady state for months, even years. They may also progress over time; as the dysplasia evolves into a leukemic state, the complications increase in severity.

Assessment and Diagnostic Findings

The CBC typically reveals a macrocytic anemia; WBC and platelet counts may be diminished as well. Serum erythropoietin levels may also be low, as is the reticulocyte count. As the disease evolves into AML, more immature blast cells are noted on the CBC.

Medical Management

With the exception of allogeneic bone marrow transplantation, there is no known cure for MDS. However, patients with mild cytopenias (low blood counts) actually require no therapy. For most patients with MDS, transfusions of RBCs are required to control the anemia and its symptoms. These patients can develop significant problems with iron overload from the repeated transfusions; this problem can be diminished with prompt initiation of chelation therapy to remove the excess iron (see below). Other patients may also require platelet transfusions on a chronic basis to prevent significant bleeding. Infections need to be managed aggressively and promptly. Growth factors, particularly granulocyte-colony-stimulating factor (G-CSF) and/or erythropoietin, have been successful in increasing neutrophils and diminishing anemia in certain patients; however, these agents are expensive and the effect is lost if the medications are stopped. Because MDS tends to occur in elderly people, the comorbid conditions that are present may have a significant role in selecting treatment options. Patients with secondary MDS or whose illness evolves into AML tend to be much more refractory to conventional therapy for leukemia.

Nursing Management

Caring for patients with MDS can be challenging because the illness can be unpredictable. As with other hematologic conditions, some patients (especially those with no symptoms) have difficulty perceiving that they have a serious illness that can place them at risk for life-threatening complications. At the other extreme, many patients have tremendous difficulty coping with the uncertain trajectory of the illness and fear that the illness will evolve into AML at a time when they are feeling very well physically.

Patients with MDS need extensive instruction about infection risk, measures to avoid it, signs and symptoms of developing infection, and appropriate actions to initiate should such symptoms occur. Instruction should also be initiated regarding the risk for bleeding. When hospitalized, patients with MDS may require neutropenic precautions.

Laboratory values need to be monitored closely to anticipate the need for transfusion and to determine response to growth factors. Patients with chronic transfusion requirements usually benefit from a vascular access device for this purpose. Chelation therapy is best administered as a subcutaneous infusion over 8 to 12 hours, often at night. Patients receiving growth factors or chelation must be educated about these medications, their side effects, and administration techniques.

Hemolytic Anemias

In hemolytic anemias, the erythrocytes have a shortened life span; thus, the number of RBCs in circulation is reduced. The reduction in RBCs and therefore the reduction in available oxygen cause renal hypoxia, which in turn stimulates an increase in erythropoietin release from the kidney. The erythropoietin stimulates the bone marrow to compensate by producing new RBCs and releasing the RBCs into the circulation somewhat prematurely as reticulocytes. When the RBC destruction persists, the hemoglobin is broken down excessively; about 80% of the heme is converted to bilirubin, conjugated in the liver, and excreted in the bile.

The mechanism of this RBC destruction varies, but all types of hemolytic anemia share certain laboratory features: the reticulocyte count is elevated; the fraction of indirect (unconjugated) bilirubin is increased; and the haptoglobin (a binding protein for free hemoglobin) supply is depleted as more hemoglobin is released, and therefore the plasma haptoglobin level is low. If the marrow cannot compensate to replace the RBCs (indicated by a decreased reticulocyte count), the anemia will progress.

Hemolytic anemia has various forms. Among the inherited forms are sickle cell anemia, thalassemia and thalassemia major, G-6-PD deficiency, and hereditary spherocytosis. Acquired forms include autoimmune hemolytic anemia and nonimmune-mediated paroxysmal nocturnal hemoglobinuria, microangiopathic hemolytic anemia, and heart valve hemolysis, as well as anemias associated with hypersplenism.

Sickle Cell Anemia

Sickle cell anemia is a severe hemolytic anemia resulting from the inheritance of the sickle hemoglobin gene (HbS). This gene causes the hemoglobin molecule to be defective. The sickle hemoglobin acquires a crystal-like formation when exposed to low oxygen tension. The oxygen level in venous blood can be low enough to cause this change; consequently, the cell containing S hemoglobin loses its round, very pliable concave disk shape and becomes deformed, rigid, and sickle-shaped (Fig. 30-5). These long, rigid cells can become lodged in small vessels; when they pile up against each other, blood flow to a region or an organ may be reduced. When ischemia or infarction results, the patient may have pain, swelling, and fever. The sickling process

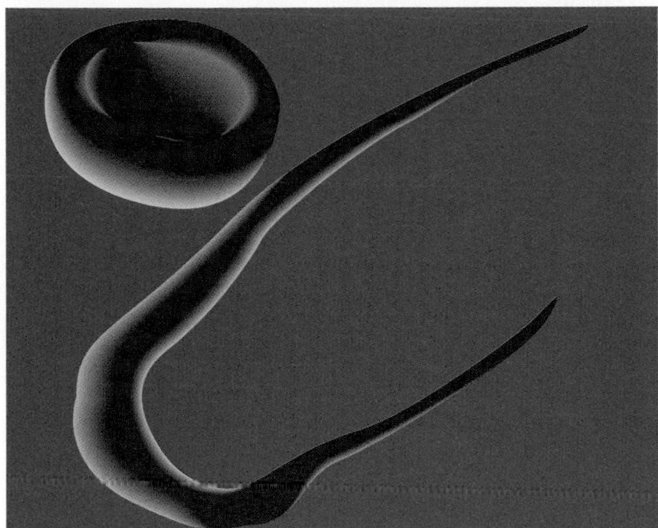

FIGURE 30•5 A normal red blood cell and a sickled cell.

takes time; if the RBC is again exposed to adequate amounts of oxygen (eg, when it travels through the pulmonary circulation) before the membrane becomes too rigid, it can revert to a normal shape. It is for this reason that the "sickling crises" are intermittent. Cold can aggravate the sickling process because vasoconstriction slows the blood flow.

The HbS gene is inherited in those of African descent and to a lesser extent in those of the Middle East, the Mediterranean, and aboriginal tribes in India. Sickle cell anemia is the most severe form of sickle cell disease. Less severe forms include sickle cell hemoglobin C (SC) disease, sickle cell hemoglobin D (SD) disease, and sickle cell beta thalassemia. The clinical manifestations and management are the same as for sickle cell anemia. Sickle cell trait refers to the carrier state for SC diseases; it is the most benign type of SC disease, in that less than 50% of the hemoglobin within an RBC is HbS. However, in terms of genetic counseling, it is still an important condition. If two people with sickle cell trait have children, the children may inherit two abnormal genes. These children will produce only hemoglobin S and therefore will have sickle cell anemia.

Assessment and Diagnostic Findings

The patient with sickle cell trait usually has normal hemoglobin levels, a normal hematocrit, and a normal blood smear. In contrast, the patient with sickle cell anemia has a low hematocrit and sickled cells on the smear. The diagnosis is confirmed by hemoglobin electrophoresis.

Clinical Manifestations

Symptoms of sickle cell anemia vary and are only somewhat based on the amount of hemoglobin S. Symptoms and complications result from chronic hemolysis or thrombosis. The sickled RBCs have a shortened life span. Patients are always anemic, usually with hemoglobin values of 7 to 10 g/dL. Jaundice is characteristic and is usually obvious in the sclerae. The bone marrow expands in childhood in a compensatory effort to offset the anemia, sometimes leading to enlargement of the bones of the face and skull. The chronic anemia is associated with tachycardia, cardiac murmurs, and often an enlarged heart (cardiomegaly). Dysrhythmias and heart failure may occur in adults.

Virtually any organ can be affected by thrombosis, but the primary sites involve those areas with slowed circulation, such as the spleen, lungs, and central nervous system. All the tissues and organs are constantly vulnerable to microcirculatory interruptions by the sickling process and therefore are susceptible to hypoxic damage or true ischemic necrosis. Patients with sickle cell anemia are unusually susceptible to infection, particularly pneumonia and osteomyelitis. Complications of sickle cell anemia include infection, stroke, renal failure, impotence, heart failure, and pulmonary hypertension. Table 30-4 summarizes the complications resulting from sickle cell anemia.

SICKLE CELL CRISIS

There are three types of sickle cell crisis in the adult population. The most common is the very painful sickle crisis, resulting from tissue hypoxia and necrosis due to inadequate blood flow to a specific region of tissue or organ. Aplastic crisis results from infection with the human parvovirus. The hemoglobin level falls rapidly, but the marrow cannot compensate, as evidenced by an absence of reticulocytes. Sequestration crisis results when other organs pool the sickled cells. Although the spleen is the most common organ responsible for sequestration in children, by age 10 most children with sickle cell anemia have had a splenic infarction and the spleen is then no longer functional (autosplenectomy). In adults, the common organs involved in sequestration are the liver and, more seriously, the lungs.

ACUTE CHEST SYNDROME

Acute chest syndrome is manifested by a rapidly falling hemoglobin level, tachycardia, fever, and bilateral infiltrates seen on the chest x-ray. These signs often mimic infection; in fact, recent studies have identified infection as a major cause of acute chest syndrome. Another common cause is pulmonary fat embolism. Measurement of secretory phospholipase A_2 levels has recently been identified as a predictor of impending acute chest syndrome; the increased amounts of free fatty acids can cause increased permeability of the pulmonary endothelium and leakage of the pulmonary capillaries.

Prognosis

Patients with sickle cell anemia are usually diagnosed in childhood because they become anemic in infancy and begin to have sickle cell crises at 1 or 2 years of age. Some children die in the first years of life, typically from infection, but the use of antibiotics and parent and patient teaching have greatly improved the outcomes for these children. However, with current management strategies, the average life expectancy is still suboptimal, at 42 years. These young adults are often forced to live with multiple, often severe complications from their disease. Interestingly, in some patients the symptoms and complications diminish by age 30; these patients live into the sixth decade or longer. At this time, there is no way to predict which patients will fall into this subgroup.

Medical Management

Treatment for sickle cell anemia is the focus of much research. Many trials of medications that have antisickling properties are being conducted. However, aside from the equally important aggressive symptom and complication management, currently there

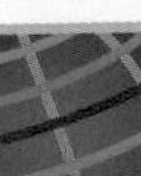

TABLE 30•4 Summary of Complications in Sickle Cell Anemia*

Organ Involved	Mechanisms*	Physical Findings	Symptom
Spleen	Primary site of sickling → infarctions → ↓ phagocytic function of macrophages	Autosplenectomy; ↑ infection (esp. pneumonia, osteomyelitis)	Abdominal pain; fever, signs of infection
Lungs	Infection Infarction → ↑ pulmonary pressure → pulmonary hypertension	Pulmonary infiltrate ↑ $sPLA_2$†	Chest pain; dyspnea
CNS	Infarction	Cerebral vascular accident	Weakness (if severe); learning difficulties (if mild)
Kidney	Sickling → damage to renal medulla	Hematuria; inability to concentrate urine; renal failure	Dehydration
Heart	Anemia	Tachycardia; cardiomegaly → heart failure	Weakness, fatigue, dyspnea
Bone	↑ erythroid production	Widening of medullary spaces and cortical thinning	Ache
	Infarction of bone	Osteosclerosis → avascular necrosis	Bone pain, especially hips
Liver	Hemolysis	Jaundice and gallstone formation; hepatomegaly	Abdominal pain
Skin and peripheral vasculature	↑ viscosity/stasis → infarction → skin ulcers	Skin ulcers; ↓ wound healing	Pain
Eye	Infarction	Scarring, hemorrhage, retinal detachment	↓ Vision; blindness
Penis	Sickling	Priapism → impotence	Pain, impotence

* Problems encountered in sickle cell anemia vary and are the result of a variety of mechanisms, as depicted in this table. Common physical findings and symptoms are also variable.
† $sPLA_2$: Secretory phospholipase A_2, a laboratory test that can predict impending acute chest syndrome (see text).

are only three primary treatment modalities for sickle cell diseases: bone marrow transplantation, hydroxyurea, and long-term RBC transfusion.

Bone marrow transplantation offers the potential of cure for this disease. However, this treatment modality is available to only a small subset of the patient population, either due to the lack of a compatible donor or to the severe organ (eg, renal, liver, lung) damage already present in the patient.

Hydroxyurea, a chemotherapy agent, has been shown to be effective in increasing hemoglobin F levels in patients with sickle cell anemia, thereby decreasing the permanent formation of sickled cells. Patients who receive hydroxyurea appear to have fewer painful episodes of sickle cell crisis, a lower incidence of acute chest syndrome, and less need for transfusions. Problems with hydroxyurea include its side effects (chronic suppression of WBC formation, teratogenesis, and potential for later development of a malignancy); patient response to the medication varies significantly. The incidence and severity of side effects are also highly variable within a dose range; some patients have toxicity when taking a very small dose (5 mg/kg/day), whereas others have little toxicity when taking a much higher dose (35 mg/kg/day). More research is needed to identify specific patient subgroups that are more likely to respond to this medication.

Chronic transfusions with RBCs have been shown to be highly effective in several situations: in an acute exacerbation of anemia (eg, aplastic crisis), in the prevention of severe complications from anesthesia and surgery, and in improving the response to infection (when it results in exacerbated anemia). Chronic transfusions have also been shown to be effective in diminishing episodes of sickle cell crisis in pregnant women; however, these transfusions have not been shown to improve fetal survival. Transfusion therapy may be effective in preventing complications from sickle cell disease. Although controversial, some data support the use of chronic transfusions in patients with cerebral ischemic injury (as seen on magnetic resonance imaging or Doppler studies) to prevent more severe injury (eg, stroke). More than 50% of asymptomatic patients have some cerebral ischemia documented by magnetic resonance imaging. A recent study (Adams et al., 1998) showed that chronic transfusion with RBCs resulted in a 90% reduction of stroke in children at risk for this complication. Transfusions may also be useful in the management of severe cases of acute chest syndrome.

The risk of complications from transfusion is important to consider. These risks include iron overload, necessitating chronic chelation therapy (see below); poor venous access, necessitating a vascular access device (and its risk for infection or thrombosis); infections (hepatitis, HIV); and alloimmunization from repeated transfusions. Another complication from transfusion is the increased viscosity of blood before actually reducing the concentration of hemoglobin S. Exchange transfusion may be performed to diminish the risk of excessively increasing viscosity.

Patients with sickle cell anemia require daily folic acid replacements to maintain the supply required for increased erythropoiesis from hemolysis. Infections must be treated promptly with appropriate antibiotics; infection remains a major cause of death in these patients.

Acute chest syndrome is managed by prompt initiation of antibiotics. Incentive spirometry has been shown to decrease the incidence of pulmonary complications significantly. In severe cases, bronchoscopy may be required to identify the source of pulmonary disease. Fluid restriction may be more beneficial than aggressive hydration, as was previously thought. Corticosteroids may also be useful. Transfusions reverse the hypoxia and decrease the secretory phospholipase A_2 levels. Pulmonary function should be monitored regularly, to detect pulmonary hypertension early, when therapy (hydroxyurea, transfusions, or transplantation) may have a positive impact.

Supportive care is equally important. A significant issue is pain management. The incidence of painful sickle crises is highly variable; many patients have pain on a daily basis. The severity of the pain may not be enough to cause the patient to seek assistance from health care providers but severe enough to interfere with the ability to work and function within the family. Acute pain episodes tend to be self-limited, lasting hours to days. If the patient cannot manage the pain at home, intervention is frequently sought in the acute care setting, usually urgent care or the emergency department. Adequate hydration is important during a painful sickling episode. Oral hydration is acceptable if the patient can maintain adequate amounts of fluids; intravenous hydration with dextrose 5% in water (D_5W) or dextrose 5% in 0.25 normal saline solution is usually required (3 L/m^2/24 hours) for sickle crisis. Supplemental oxygen may also be needed.

The use of pain medication is important (see Chap. 12 for discussion of pain management for sickle cell crisis). Aspirin is very useful in diminishing mild to moderate pain; it also diminishes inflammation and potential thrombosis (due to its ability to diminish platelet adhesion). Nonsteroidal anti-inflammatory drugs (NSAIDs) are useful for moderate pain or in combination with opioid analgesics. Although no tolerance develops with NSAIDs, a "ceiling effect" does develop whereby an increase in dosage does not increase analgesia. NSAID use must be carefully monitored because these medications can precipitate renal dysfunction. When opioid analgesics are used, morphine is the medication of choice for acute pain. Patient-controlled analgesia is frequently used.

Chronic pain increases in incidence as the patient ages. Here, the pain is due to complications from the sickling, such as avascular necrosis of the hip. With chronic pain management, the principal goal is to maximize functioning; pain may not be completely eliminated without sacrificing function. This concept may be difficult for patients to accept; they may need repeated explanations and support from nonjudgmental health care providers. Nonpharmacologic approaches to pain management are crucial in this setting. Examples include physical and occupational therapy, physiotherapy (including the use of heat, massage, and exercise), cognitive and behavioral intervention (including distraction, relaxation, motivational therapy), and support groups.

Working with patients who have multiple episodes of severe pain can be challenging. It is important for health care providers to realize that patients with sickle cell disease must face a life-long experience with severe and unpredictable pain. Such pain is disruptive to the person's level of functioning, including social functioning, and may result in a feeling of helplessness. Patients with inadequate social support systems may have more difficulty coping with chronic pain.

NURSING PROCESS: THE PATIENT WITH SICKLE CELL CRISIS

Assessment

Patients in sickle cell crisis should be assessed for factors that could have precipitated the crisis, such as symptoms of infection or dehydration, or situations that promote fatigue or emotional stress. In addition, patients are asked to recall factors that seemed to precipitate previous crises and measures they use to prevent and manage crises. Pain levels should always be monitored; this is best accomplished by a pain-rating scale, such as a 0 to 10 scale. The quality of the pain (eg, sharp, dull, burning), the frequency of the pain (constant versus intermittent), and factors that aggravate or alleviate the pain should be included in this assessment. When a patient is in sickle cell crisis, it is important to assess whether the pain currently experienced is the same as or different than the pain typically encountered in crisis.

Because the sickling process can interrupt circulation in any tissues or organs, with resultant hypoxia and ischemia, a careful assessment of all body systems is necessary. Particular emphasis is placed on assessing for pain, swelling, and fever. All joint areas are carefully examined for pain and swelling. The abdomen is assessed for pain and tenderness due to the possibility of splenic infarction.

The respiratory system must be assessed carefully, including auscultation of breath sounds, measurement of oxygen saturation levels, signs of cardiac failure, such as the presence and extent of dependent edema, an increased point of maximal impulse, and cardiomegaly (as seen on chest x-ray). The patient should be assessed for signs of dehydration by a history of fluid intake and careful examination of mucous membranes, skin turgor, urine output, and serum creatinine and blood urea nitrogen values.

A careful neurologic examination is important to elicit symptoms of cerebral hypoxia. However, ischemic findings on magnetic resonance imaging or Doppler studies may significantly precede the findings on the physical examination; therefore, they may be more beneficial to improve patient outcome.

Because patients with sickle cell anemia are so susceptible to infections, they are assessed for the presence of any infectious process. Particular attention is given to examination of the chest and long bones and femoral head, because pneumonia and osteomyelitis are especially common. Leg ulcers, which may be infected and are slow to heal, are not uncommon.

The extent of anemia (as measured by the hemoglobin level and hematocrit) and the ability of the marrow to replenish cells (as measured by the reticulocyte count) should be monitored and compared with the patient's baseline levels. The patient's current and past history of medical management should also be assessed, particularly chronic transfusion therapy, hydroxyurea use, and prior treatment for infection.

Diagnosis

Nursing Diagnoses

Based on the assessment data, major nursing diagnoses for the patient may include the following:

- Pain related to tissue hypoxia due to agglutination of sickled cells within blood vessels
- Risk for infection
- Powerlessness related to illness-induced helplessness
- Knowledge deficit regarding prevention of crisis

Collaborative Problems/Potential Complications

Based on the assessment data, potential complications may include:

- Hypoxia, ischemia, infection, and poor wound healing leading to skin breakdown and ulcers
- Dehydration
- Cerebrovascular accident (stroke)
- Anemia
- Renal dysfunction
- Heart failure, pulmonary hypertension, and acute chest syndrome
- Impotence
- Poor compliance
- Substance abuse related to chronic pain

Planning and Goals

The major goals for the patient are relief of pain, decreased incidence of crisis, enhanced sense of self-esteem and power, and absence of complications.

Nursing Interventions

Managing Pain

Acute pain during a sickle cell crisis can be severe and unpredictable. The patient's subjective description and rating of pain on a pain scale must guide the use of analgesics, which are valuable in controlling the acute pain of a sickle crisis. Any joint that is acutely swollen should be supported and elevated until the swelling diminishes. Relaxation techniques, breathing exercises, and distraction are helpful for some patients. When the acute painful episode has diminished, aggressive measures should be implemented to preserve function. Physical therapy, whirlpool baths, and transcutaneous nerve stimulation are examples of such modalities.

Preventing and Managing Infection

Nursing care focuses on monitoring the patient for signs and symptoms of infection. Prescribed antibiotics should be initiated promptly, and the patient should be assessed for signs of dehydration. If the patient is to take prescribed oral antibiotics at home, he or she must understand the need to complete the entire course of antibiotic therapy and must be able to identify a feasible administration schedule.

Promoting Coping Skills

This illness, because of its acute exacerbations that often result in chronic health problems, frequently leaves the patient feeling powerless and with a sense of decreased self-esteem. These feelings can be exacerbated in the setting of inadequate pain management. The patient's ability to use normal coping resources of physical strength, psychological stamina, and positive self-esteem is dramatically diminished. Enhancing pain management can be extremely useful in establishing a therapeutic relationship based on mutual trust. Nursing care that focuses on the patient's strengths rather than deficits can enhance effective coping skills. Providing the patient with opportunities to make decisions about daily care may increase his or her feelings of control.

Minimizing Knowledge Deficit

Patients with sickle cell anemia benefit from understanding what situations can precipitate a sickle cell crisis and the steps they can take to prevent or diminish such crises. Keeping warm and maintaining adequate hydration can be very effective in diminishing the occurrence and severity of attacks. Avoiding stressful situations is more challenging. Group education may be more effective if carried out by members of the community who are from the same ethnic group as those with the disease.

Monitoring and Managing Potential Complications

Management measures for many of the potential complications are delineated in the sections above. Other measures follow.

LEG ULCERS

When present, leg ulcers require careful management and protection from trauma and contamination. If they fail to heal, skin grafting may be necessary. Scrupulous aseptic technique is warranted to prevent nosocomial infections.

PRIAPISM LEADING TO IMPOTENCE

Male patients may develop sudden, painful episodes of priapism (persistent penile erection). The patient is taught to empty his bladder at the onset of the attack, exercise, and take a warm bath. If an episode persists more than 3 hours, medical attention is recommended. Repeated episodes may lead to extensive vascular thrombosis, resulting in impotence.

CHRONIC PAIN AND SUBSTANCE ABUSE

Many patients have considerable difficulty coping with chronic pain and repeated episodes of sickle crisis. Those who feel they have little control over their health and the physical complications that result from this illness may find it difficult to understand the importance of complying with a prescribed treatment plan. Being nonjudgmental and actively seeking involvement from the patient in establishing a treatment plan are useful strategies.

Unfortunately, some patients with sickle cell anemia develop problems with substance abuse. For many, this abuse results from inadequate management of acute pain during episodes of crisis. Some clinicians suggest that abuse may result from prescribing inadequate amounts of opioid analgesics for an inadequate time. Thus, the patient's pain may never be adequately relieved, promoting mistrust of the health care system and (from the patient's perspective) the need to seek care from a variety of sources or when the pain is not severe. This cycle is best managed by prevention. Receiving care from a single provider over time is much more beneficial than receiving care from rotating physicians and staff in an emergency department. When crises do arise, the staff in the emergency department should be in contact with the patient's primary health care provider so that optimal management can be achieved. Unfortunately, once the pattern of abuse is established, it is very difficult to manage, but continuity of care and establishing written contracts with the patient can be useful.

Evaluation

Expected Outcomes

Expected outcomes may include:

1. Reports control of pain
   a. Indicates that pain is relieved with analgesics
   b. Uses relaxation techniques, breathing exercises, distraction to help relieve pain
2. Is free of infection
   a. Has normal temperature
   b. Shows WBC count within normal range (5000 to 10,000/mm^3)
   c. Identifies importance of continuing antibiotics at home (if applicable)
3. Expresses improved sense of control
   a. Participates in goal setting and in planning and implementing daily activities
   b. Participates in decisions about care

4. Increases knowledge about disease process
    a. Identifies situations and factors that can precipitate sickle cell crisis
    b. Describes lifestyle changes needed to prevent crisis
    c. Describes the importance of warmth, adequate hydration, and prevention of infection in preventing crisis
5. Avoids complications

Thalassemia

Thalassemia is a group of hereditary disorders associated with defective hemoglobin-chain synthesis. These anemias occur worldwide, but the highest prevalence is found in people of Mediterranean, African, and Southeast Asian ancestry. Thalassemias are characterized by **hypochromia** (an abnormal decrease in the hemoglobin content of erythrocytes), extreme **microcytosis** (smaller-than-normal erythrocytes), destruction of blood elements (hemolysis), and variable degrees of anemia.

In thalassemia, the production of one or more globulin chains within the hemoglobin molecule is reduced. When this occurs, there is an imbalance in the configuration of the hemoglobin, and it precipitates in the erythroid precursors or the RBCs themselves. This increases the rigidity of the RBC and thus the premature destruction of these cells.

The thalassemias are classified into two major groups according to the globin chain diminished: alpha and beta. The alpha thalassemias occur mainly in people from Asia and the Middle East; the beta thalassemias are most prevalent in Mediterranean populations as well as those from the Middle and the Far East. The alpha thalassemias are milder than the beta forms and are often without symptoms. The RBCs are extremely microcytic, but the anemia, if present, is mild.

The severity of beta thalassemia varies depending on the extent to which the hemoglobin chains are affected. Patients with mild forms have a microcytosis and mild anemia. Untreated, severe beta thalassemia (thalassemia major, Cooley's anemia) can be fatal within the first few years of life. If treated with regular transfusion therapy, patients may survive into their 20s and 30s. Patient teaching during the reproductive years should include preconception counseling about the risk of congenital thalassemia major.

Thalassemia Major

Thalassemia major (Cooley's anemia) is characterized by severe anemia, marked hemolysis, and ineffective erythropoiesis (production of erythrocytes). With early regular transfusion therapy, growth and development through childhood is facilitated. Organ dysfunction due to iron overload results from the excessive amounts of iron obtained through the RBC transfusions. Regular chelation therapy (eg, via subcutaneous deferoxamine) has reduced the complications of iron overload and prolonged the life of these patients. This disease is potentially curable by bone marrow transplantation if the procedure can be performed before the liver sustains damage (ie, during childhood).

Glucose-6-Phosphate Dehydrogenase Deficiency

The abnormality in this disorder is in the G-6-PD gene; this gene produces an enzyme within the red cell that is essential for membrane stability. A few patients have inherited an enzyme so defective that they have a chronic hemolytic anemia, but the most common type of defect results in hemolysis only when the RBCs are stressed by certain situations, such as fever or the use of certain medications. The disorder came to the attention of researchers during World War II, when some soldiers developed hemolysis while taking primaquine, an antimalarial agent. African Americans and people of Greek or Italian origin are those primarily affected by this disorder. The type of deficiency found in the Mediterranean population is more severe than that in the African Caribbean population, resulting in greater hemolysis and sometimes in life-threatening anemias. All types of G-6-PD deficiency are inherited as X-linked defects; thus, many more men are at risk than women. In the United States, about 12% of African American males are affected. It is also common in those of Asian ancestry and certain Jewish populations.

Medications that have hemolytic effects for people with G-6-PD deficiency are oxidant drugs. These medications include antimalarial agents, sulfonamides, nitrofurantoin, common coal tar analgesics (including aspirin in high doses and phenacetin), thiazide diuretics, oral hypoglycemic agents, chloramphenicol, para-aminosalicylic acid, and vitamin K. In affected people, a severe hemolytic episode can result from ingesting fava beans.

Clinical Manifestations

Patients are asymptomatic and have normal hemoglobin levels and reticulocyte counts most of the time. However, several days after exposure to an offending medication, they may develop pallor, jaundice, and hemoglobinuria (hemoglobin in the urine). The reticulocyte count rises and symptoms of hemolysis develop. Special strains of the peripheral blood may then disclose Heinz bodies (degraded hemoglobin) within the RBCs. Hemolysis is often mild and self-limiting. However, in the more severe Mediterranean type of G-6-PD deficiency, this recovery may not occur and transfusions may be necessary.

Assessment and Diagnostic Findings

The diagnosis is made by a screening test or a quantitative assay of G-6-PD.

Medical Management

The treatment is to stop the offending medication. Transfusion is necessary only in the severe hemolytic states, more commonly seen with the Mediterranean variety of G-6-PD deficiency.

Nursing Management

The patient should be educated about the disease and given a list of medications to avoid. If hemolysis does develop, nursing interventions are the same as for hemolysis from other causes.

Hereditary Spherocytosis

Hereditary spherocytosis is a relatively common (1 : 5000) hemolytic anemia characterized by an abnormal permeability of the RBC membrane; this permits the cells to change into a spherical shape. These RBCs are destroyed prematurely in the spleen. The severity of this hemolytic anemia varies; jaundice can be intermittent, and splenomegaly (enlarged spleen) can also occur. Surgical removal of the spleen is the principal treatment for this disorder.

Immune Hemolytic Anemia

Hemolytic anemias can result from exposure of the RBC to antibodies. Alloantibodies result from the immunization of a person with foreign antigens. (An example is the immunization of an Rh-negative person with Rh-positive blood.) Alloantibodies tend to be large (IgM type) and cause immediate destruction of the sensitized RBCs, either within the blood vessel (intravascular hemolysis) or within the liver. The most common type of alloimmune hemolytic anemia in adults results from a hemolytic transfusion reaction.

Autoantibodies are developed by the person for varying reasons. In many instances, the person's immune system is dysfunctional, so that it falsely recognizes its own RBCs as foreign and produces antibodies against them; this mechanism is seen in people with chronic lymphocytic leukemia, for example. Another mechanism is a deficiency in suppressor lymphocytes that normally prevent antibody formation against the person's own antigens. Autoantibodies tend to be the IgG type. The RBCs are sequestered in the spleen and destroyed by the macrophages outside the blood vessel (extravascular hemolysis).

Autoimmune hemolytic anemias can be classified based on the body temperature involved when the antibodies react with the RBC antigen. Warm-body antibodies bind to RBCs most actively in warm conditions (37°C); cold-body antibodies react in cold (0°C). Most autoimmune hemolytic anemias are the warm-body type. Autoimmune hemolytic anemia is associated with other disorders in most cases (eg, medication exposure, lymphoma, chronic lymphocytic leukemia, other malignancy, collagen vascular disease, autoimmune disease, infection). In idiopathic autoimmune hemolytic states, the reason why the immune system produces the antibodies is not known. All ages and genders are equally vulnerable to this form, whereas the incidence of secondary forms is greater in people older than age 45 and in females.

Clinical Manifestations

Clinical manifestations can vary, and they usually reflect the degree of anemia. The hemolysis may be very mild, so that the patient's marrow compensates adequately, and the patient is asymptomatic. At the other extreme, the hemolysis can be so severe that the resultant anemia can be life-threatening. Most patients complain of fatigue and dizziness. Splenomegaly is the most common physical finding (in more than 80% of patients); hepatomegaly, lymphadenopathy, and jaundice are also common.

Assessment and Diagnostic Findings

The laboratory tests reveal a low hemoglobin level and hematocrit, most often with an accompanying increase in the reticulocyte count. RBCs appear abnormal; **spherocytes** are common. The serum bilirubin level is elevated, and if the hemolysis is severe, the haptoglobin level is low or absent. The Coombs' test shows a positive result.

Medical Management

Any possibly offending medication should be immediately discontinued. The treatment consists of high doses of corticosteroids (1 mg/kg/day) until hemolysis decreases. Corticosteroids decrease the macrophage's ability to clear the antibody-coated RBCs. If the hemoglobin level returns toward normal, usually after several weeks, the corticosteroid dose can be lowered or, in some cases, tapered and discontinued. However, corticosteroids rarely produce a lasting remission. In severe cases, blood transfusions may be required. Because the antibody may react with all possible donor cells, careful blood typing is necessary, and the transfusion should be administered slowly and cautiously.

Splenectomy (removal of the spleen) removes the major site of RBC destruction; therefore, it may be performed if corticosteroids do not produce a remission. If neither corticosteroid therapy nor splenectomy is successful, immunosuppressive agents may be administered. The two immunosuppressive agents most frequently used are cyclophosphamide (which has a more rapid effect but more toxicity) or azathioprine (less rapid effect but less toxicity). The synthetic androgen danazol can be useful in some patients, particularly in combination with corticosteroids. The mechanism for this success is unclear. When corticosteroids or immunosuppressive agents are used, the taper must be very gradual to prevent a rebound "hyperimmune" response and exacerbation of the hemolysis. Immunoglobulin administration is effective in about one third of patients, but the effect is transient and the medication expensive. Transfusions may be necessary if the anemia is severe; it may be extremely difficult to cross-match samples of available units of red cells with that of the patient.

For patients with cold-antibody hemolytic anemia, treatment may not be required, other than to advise the patient to keep warm; relocation to a warm climate may be necessary.

Nursing Management

Patients may have great difficulty understanding the pathologic mechanisms underlying the disease and need repeated explanations in terms they can understand. Patients who have had a splenectomy should be vaccinated against pneumococcal infections (Pneumovax) and informed that they are permanently at greater risk for infection. Patients receiving long-term corticosteroid therapy, particularly those with concurrent diabetes and/or hypertension, need careful monitoring. They must understand the need for this medication and the importance of never abruptly discontinuing it. A written explanation and a tapering schedule should be provided, and adjustments based on hemoglobin levels should be emphasized. Similar teaching should occur when immunosuppressive agents are used.

Nursing Alert *It can be difficult to cross-match blood when antibodies are present. When imperfectly cross-matched red cells need to be transfused, the nurse needs to begin the infusion very slowly (10 to 15 mL over 20 to 30 minutes) and monitor the patient very closely for signs and symptoms of a hemolytic transfusion reaction.*

HEREDITARY HEMOCHROMATOSIS

Hemochromatosis is a genetic condition in which iron is abnormally (excessively) absorbed from the gastrointestinal tract. The excessive iron is deposited in various organs, particularly the liver, myocardium, testes, thyroid, and pancreas; eventually the organs affected become dysfunctional. The actual incidence of hemochromatosis is not known; however, hereditary hemochromatosis is diagnosed in 0.5% of the population in the United States (ie, 1 million people). Recent data suggest that this defect may be a common cause of diabetes. Due to their natural loss of iron through menses, women are less affected than men.

Because the accumulation of iron in body organs occurs gradually, there often is no evidence of tissue injury until middle age. Symptoms of weakness, lethargy, arthralgia, weight loss, and loss of libido are common. The skin may be hyperpigmented with melanin deposits (occasionally **hemosiderin**, an iron-containing pigment). Cardiac dysrhythmias and cardiomyopathy can occur, with resulting dyspnea and edema. Endocrine dysfunction is manifested as hypothyroidism, diabetes mellitus, and hypogonadism (testicular atrophy, diminished libido, and impotence). A significant effect of hemochromatosis is the development of hepatocellular carcinoma in one third of those affected. CBC values are typically normal. The most useful laboratory findings are an elevated serum iron level and high transferrin saturation (more than 60%). The definitive diagnostic test is a liver biopsy.

Medical Management

Therapy involves the removal of excess iron via therapeutic phlebotomy (removing whole blood from a vein). To achieve this, a vigorous phlebotomy schedule is required over a 1- to 3-year period. Later the frequency of phlebotomy can be reduced to 1 unit of blood every several months to prevent reaccumulation of iron deposits. Removing excess iron appears to diminish the severity of diabetes and skin hyperpigmentation; cardiac function also tends to improve.

Nursing Management

Patients with hemochromatosis often believe it is important to limit their dietary intake of iron; however, this method has been shown to be very ineffective and should not be encouraged. However, it is important for these patients to avoid any additional insults to the liver, such as alcohol abuse. Serial screening tests for hepatoma are important; alpha-fetoprotein is used for this purpose. Other body systems should be monitored for signs of organ dysfunction, particularly the endocrine and cardiac systems. These systems should also be screened routinely for dysfunction so that appropriate management can be implemented quickly. Because patients with hemochromatosis require frequent phlebotomies (initially twice a week), problems with venous access are not uncommon.

POLYCYTHEMIA

Polycythemia refers to an increased volume of RBCs. It is a term used when the hematocrit is elevated (more than 55% in males and more than 50% in females). Dehydration (decreased volume of plasma) can cause an elevated hematocrit, but not typically to the level to be considered polycythemia. Polycythemia is classified as either primary or secondary.

Polycythemia Vera

Polycythemia vera, or primary polycythemia, is a proliferative disorder in which the myeloid stem cells seem to have escaped normal control mechanisms. The bone marrow is hypercellular, and the RBC, WBC, and platelet counts in the peripheral blood are elevated. However, the red cell elevation is predominant; the hematocrit can exceed 60%. This phase can last for an extended period of time (10 years or more). The spleen resumes its embryonic function of hematopoiesis and enlarges. Over time, the bone marrow may become fibrotic, with a resultant inability to produce as many cells ("burnt-out" or spent phase). The disease evolves into AML in a significant proportion of patients; this form of AML is usually refractory to standard forms of treatment.

Clinical Manifestations

Patients typically have a ruddy complexion and splenomegaly (enlarged spleen). The symptoms result from the increased blood volume (headache, dizziness, tinnitus, fatigue, paresthesias, and blurred vision) or increased blood viscosity (angina, claudication, dyspnea, and thrombophlebitis), particularly if the patient has atherosclerotic blood vessels. Another common and bothersome problem is generalized pruritus, which may be due to histamine release from the increased number of basophils. Erythromyalgia, a burning sensation in the fingers and toes, may be reported and is only partially relieved by cooling.

Assessment and Diagnostic Findings

Diagnosis is made by finding an elevated RBC mass (a nuclear medicine procedure), a normal oxygen saturation level, and an enlarged spleen. Other factors useful in establishing the diagnosis include an elevation in WBC and platelet counts, and elevated vitamin B_{12} and leukocyte alkaline phosphatase levels. The erythropoietin level is not as low as would be expected with an elevated hematocrit, but is normal or only slightly low.

Complications

Patients with polycythemia vera are at increased risk for thromboses resulting in a stroke or heart attack. Bleeding is also a complication, possibly due to the fact that the platelets (often very large) are somewhat dysfunctional. The bleeding can be significant and can occur in the form of nosebleeds, ulcers, and frank gastrointestinal bleeding.

Medical Management

The objective of management is to reduce the high blood cell mass. Phlebotomy (removing whole blood from a vein) is an important part of therapy and can be performed repeatedly to keep the hematocrit within normal range. This is achieved by removing enough blood (initially 500 mL once or twice weekly) to deplete the patient's iron stores, thereby rendering the patient iron-deficient and subsequently unable to continue to manufacture RBCs excessively. Patients need to be instructed to avoid iron supplements, including those within their multivitamin supplement. Radioactive phosphorus (^{32}P) or chemotherapeutic agents (eg, hydroxyurea) can be used to suppress marrow function, but they may increase the risk of leukemia. When the patient has an elevated uric acid level, allopurinol is used to prevent gouty attacks. Antihistamines are not particularly effective in controlling itching. If the patient develops ischemic symptoms, dipyridamole is sometimes used.

Nursing Management

The nurse's role is primarily that of teacher. Patients are usually advised to avoid aspirin and aspirin-containing medications because these medications alter platelet function. Minimizing alcohol intake should also be emphasized to further diminish any risk for bleeding. For patients with pruritus, the nurse may recommend bathing in tepid or cool water, along with applications of cocoa butter-based lotions and bath products.

Secondary Polycythemia

Secondary polycythemia is caused by excessive production of erythropoietin. This may occur in response to a reduced amount of oxygen, which acts as a hypoxic stimulus, as in cigarette smoking, chronic obstructive pulmonary disease, or cyanotic heart disease, or in nonpathologic conditions, such as high altitude. It can also result from certain hemoglobinopathies in which the hemoglobin has an abnormally high affinity for oxygen (eg, hemoglobin Chesapeake). It can also occur from neoplasms (ie, renal cell carcinoma) that stimulate erythropoietin production.

Medical Management

Management of secondary polycythemia may not be necessary; when it is, it involves treating the primary problem. If the cause cannot be corrected (by treating the renal cell carcinoma or improving pulmonary function), therapeutic phlebotomy may be necessary in symptomatic patients to reduce blood viscosity and volume.

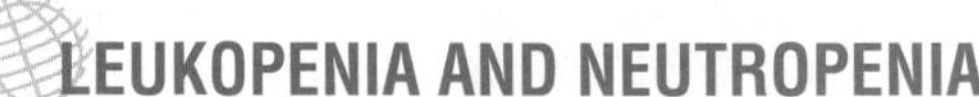

LEUKOPENIA AND NEUTROPENIA

Leukopenia, a condition in which there are fewer WBCs than normal, results from neutropenia (diminished neutrophils) or lymphopenia (diminished lymphocytes). Even when other WBC types are diminished (eg, monocytes, basophils), their numbers are too few to reduce the total WBC count significantly. Lymphopenia (lymphocytes less than 1500/mm^3) can result from ionizing radiation, long-term use of corticosteroids, uremia, some neoplasms (eg, breast, lung cancers, advanced Hodgkin's disease), and some protein-losing enteropathies (where the lymphocytes within the intestines are lost).

Neutropenia

Neutropenia (neutrophils less than 2000/mm^3) results from decreased production of neutrophils or increased destruction of these cells (Chart 30-4). Neutrophils are essential in preventing and limiting bacterial infection. A patient with neutropenia is at increased risk for infection, both exogenous and endogenous (the gastrointestinal tract and skin are common endogenous sources).

CHART 30•4 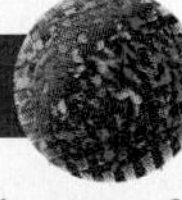 **Causes of Neutropenia**

Decreased production of neutrophils
- Aplastic anemia, secondary to medications or toxins
- Metastatic cancer, lymphoma, leukemia
- Myelodysplastic syndromes
- Chemotherapy
- Radiation therapy

Ineffective granulocytopoiesis
- Megaloblastic anemia

Increased destruction of neutrophils
- Hypersplenism
- Drug-induced*
- Immunologic disease (eg, systemic lupus erythematosus)
- Viral disease (eg, infectious hepatitis, mononucleosis)
- Bacterial infections

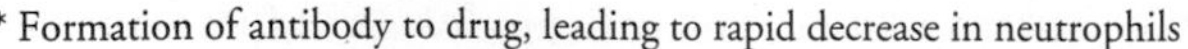

* Formation of antibody to drug, leading to rapid decrease in neutrophils

CHART 30•5 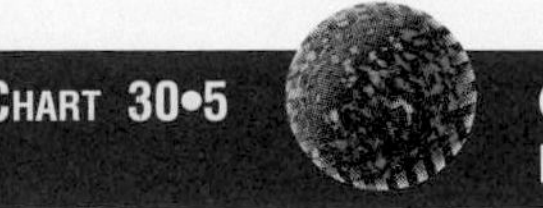 **Calculating the Absolute Neutrophil Count (ANC)**

$$\frac{\%\ \text{neutrophils} + \%\ \text{bands}}{100} \times \text{Total WBC count} = \text{ANC}$$

Normally, the neutrophil count is >2000/mm^3. The actual or absolute neutrophil count (ANC) is calculated using the above formula.

For example, if the total WBC is 3000 with 72% neutrophils and 3% bands, the ANC would be calculated as follows:

$$\frac{72 + 3}{100} \times 3000 = 2250$$

The finding (2250) does not identify neutropenia because the ANC exceeds 2000, although the total WBC count is low at 3000.

Conversely, in the following example, neutropenia is evident despite a normal WBC count: Total WBCs 5500, neutrophils 8%, bands 0%

$$\frac{8 + 0}{100} \times 5500 = 440$$

Here, the ANC is extremely low (440) despite the total WBC count being normal (5500).

When evaluating neutropenia, it is important to calculate the ANC and not to rely on the WBC count and percentage of neutrophils alone.

The risk for infection is based not only on the severity of the neutropenia (ie, how low the neutrophil count is), but also on the duration of the neutropenia. The longer the patient is neutropenic, the greater the chance for infection. The actual number of neutrophils, know as the absolute neutrophil count (ANC), is determined by a simple mathematical calculation using data obtained from the CBC and differential test (Chart 30-5). The risk of infection increases proportionately to the decrease in neutrophil count. Thus, the risk is significant when the ANC is less than 1000, is high when it is less than 500, and is almost certain when it is less than 100.

Clinical Manifestations

Unfortunately, there are no real symptoms of neutropenia until the patient becomes infected. Routine CBC with differential tests, such as those obtained after chemotherapy, can reveal neutropenia before the onset of infection.

Medical Management

Treatment of the neutropenia varies depending on the etiology. If the neutropenia is medication-induced, the offending agent needs to be stopped, if possible. Treating the underlying neoplasm can temporarily make the neutropenia worse, but with bone marrow recovery, treatment may improve it. Corticosteroids may be used if the cause is an immunologic disorder. The use of growth factors such as G-CSF or granulocyte/macrophage-colony-stimulating factor (GM-CSF) can be effective in increasing neutrophil production when the cause of the neutropenia is decreased production. Withholding or reducing the dose of chemotherapy or radiation therapy may be required when the neutropenia is due to these treatments. Should the neutropenia be accompanied by fever, the patient is automatically considered to be infected and usually is admitted to the hospital. Cultures of blood, urine, and sputum should be obtained, as well as a chest x-ray. To ensure adequate therapy against the invading infectious organisms, broad-spectrum antibiotics are initiated as soon as the cultures are obtained, although the medications may be changed when culture and sensitivity results are available.

Nursing Management

Nurses in all settings have a crucial role in assessing the severity of neutropenia and in preventing and managing infectious complications. Patient teaching is equally important, particularly in the outpatient setting, so that the patient can implement appropriate self-care measures and know when to seek medical care. Patients at risk for developing neutropenia should have CBCs drawn on an appropriate basis. Nurses need to be able to calculate the ANC and to assess the severity of neutropenia and the risk for infection. Chart 30-6 identifies nursing activities related to neutropenia.

LEUKOCYTOSIS AND MALIGNANCIES

Leukocytosis is an increased level of WBCs in the circulation. Typically, only one specific cell type is increased. Because the proportion of several types of WBCs is small (eg, eosinophils, basophils, monocytes), usually only an increase in neutrophils or lymphocytes can be great enough to elevate the total WBC count. Although leukocytosis can be a normal response to increased need (eg, in acute infection), the increase in WBCs should decrease as the need decreases. A prolonged or progressively increasing elevation in WBCs is abnormal and should be evaluated. A significant cause for leukocytosis is malignancy; Table 30-5 lists other causes of leukocytosis.

Hematopoiesis is characterized by a rapid, continuous turnover of cells. Normally, production of specific blood cells from their stem cell precursors is carefully regulated according to the body's needs. If the mechanisms that control the production of these cells are disrupted, the cells can proliferate to an excessive, potentially dangerous degree. Hematopoietic malignancies are often classified according to the cells involved. Leukemia, literally "white blood," is a neoplastic proliferation of one particular cell type (granulocytes, monocytes, lymphocytes, or megakaryocytes). The defect originates in the hematopoietic stem cell, the myeloid or the lymphoid stem cell. The lymphomas are neoplasms of lymphoid tissue, usually derived from B lymphocytes. Multiple myeloma is a malignancy of the most mature form of B lymphocyte, the plasma cell.

LEUKEMIAS

The common feature of the leukemias is an unregulated proliferation of WBCs in the bone marrow. In acute forms (or late stages of chronic forms), the proliferation of leukemic cells leaves little room for normal cell production. There can also be a proliferation of cells in the liver and spleen (extramedullary hematopoiesis), and with acute forms there can be infiltration of other organs, such as the meninges, lymph nodes, gums, and skin. The cause of leukemia is not fully known, but there is some evidence that genetic influence and viral pathogenesis may be involved. Bone marrow damage from radiation exposure or chemicals such as benzene and alkylating agents (eg, melphalan) can cause leukemia.

The leukemias are commonly classified according to the stem cell line involved, either lymphoid or myeloid. They are also classified as either acute or chronic, based on the time in which symptoms evolve and the phase of cell development that is halted, with few WBCs differentiating beyond that phase.

In acute leukemia, the onset of symptoms is abrupt, often occurring within a few weeks. WBC development is halted at the blast phase, so that most WBCs are undifferentiated or blasts. Acute leukemia progresses very rapidly; death occurs within weeks to months without aggressive treatment. In chronic leukemia, symptoms evolve over a period of months to years, and the majority of WBCs produced are mature. Chronic leukemia progresses more slowly; the disease trajectory can extend for years.

Acute Myeloid Leukemia

AML results from a defect in the hematopoietic stem cell that differentiates into all myeloid cells: monocytes, granulocytes (basophils, neutrophils, eosinophils), erythrocytes, and platelets. All age groups are affected; incidence rises with age, with a peak incidence at age 60. It is the most common nonlymphocytic leukemia.

Prognosis is highly variable and not consistently based on patient or disease variables. Patients with AML have a potentially curable disease. However, patients who are older or have a more undifferentiated form of AML tend to have a worse prognosis. Those who have preexisting MDS or who had previous alkylator therapy for cancer (secondary AML) have a much worse prognosis: the leukemia tends to be more resistant to treatment, resulting in a much shorter duration of remission. With treatment, these patients survive an average of less than 1 year, with death usually a result of infection or hemorrhage. Patients receiving supportive care also usually survive less than 1 year, again dying from infection or bleeding.

Clinical Manifestations

Most of the signs and symptoms evolve from insufficient production of normal blood cells. Fever and infection result from neutropenia, weakness and fatigue occur due to anemia, and bleeding tendencies arise as a result of thrombocytopenia. The proliferation of leukemic cells within organs leads to a variety of additional symptoms: pain from an enlarged liver or spleen, hyperplasia of the gums, and bone pain from expansion of marrow.

Assessment and Diagnostic Findings

The disorder develops without warning, with symptoms occurring over a period of weeks to months. CBC results show a decrease in both erythrocytes and platelets. Although the total leukocyte count can be low, normal, or high, the percentage of normal cells is usually vastly decreased. A bone marrow analysis reveals an excess of immature blast cells (more than 30%). AML can be further classified into seven different subgroups, based on cytogenetics, histology, and morphology (appearance) of the blasts. The actual prognosis varies somewhat between subgroups, but the clinical course and treatment differ substantially with only one subtype, acute promyelocytic leukemia (APL, or AML-M3). Patients with this leukemia often have significantly more problems with bleeding, in that they have underlying coagulopathy and a higher incidence of disseminated intravascular coagulation (DIC).

Complications

Complications of AML include bleeding and infection, the major causes of death. The risk of bleeding correlates with the level of platelet deficiency (thrombocytopenia). The low platelet count can result in **ecchymoses** (bruises) and **petechiae** (pinpoint red

CHART 30•6 Implementing Neutropenia Precautions

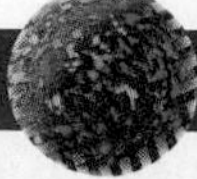

Nursing Diagnosis

Risk for infection secondary to impaired immunocompetence due to:

Diminished neutrophil count secondary to bone marrow invasion or hypocellularity secondary to medications

Dysfunctional neutrophils (eg, secondary to MDS)

Dysfunctional and/or diminished lymphocytes

Hypogammaglobulinemia

Diminished immune response and anergy

Malnutrition

Surgery or other invasive procedures

Antibiotic therapy (risk for superimposed infection).

- The risk of infection increases as the neutrophil count decreases: 500–1000 neutrophils, moderate risk; <500 neutrophils, severe risk.
- The duration of neutropenia can be more important than the degree of neutropenia in rendering a patient at risk for infection.
- When neutropenic, infected patients rarely exhibit the classic signs of infection (redness, purulent drainage, etc.). The only initial sign may be fever (and it usually occurs later in the infectious process with neutropenia).
- Skin and mucous membranes are the body's first line of defense against infection; loss of endothelial cell integrity allows organisms to enter the blood and lymphatic system.

Assessment

Patient

Assess the following areas thoroughly each shift/visit (with spot checks throughout shift if hospitalized) and notify physician of any signs of infection or worsening of status:

- Skin: Check for tenderness, edema, breaks in skin integrity, moisture, drainage, lesions (esp. under breasts, axillae, groin, skin folds, bony prominences, perineum). Check all puncture sites for signs and symptoms of inflammation/infection (eg, IV sites).
- Oral mucosa: Check for moisture, lesions, color (check palate, tongue, buccal mucosa, gums, lips, oropharynx).
- Respiratory: Check for cough, sore throat; auscultate breath sounds.
- GI: Check for abdominal discomfort/distention, nausea, change in bowel pattern; auscultate bowel sounds.
- GU: Check for dysuria, urgency, frequency. Check urine for color, clarity, odor.
- Neurologic: Check for complaints of headache, neck stiffness, visual disturbances.
  Assess level of consciousness, orientation, behavior.
- Temperature: Check q4h. Call physician if patient's temperature exceeds 101°F and patient is unresponsive to acetaminophen or shows decline in hemodynamic status.

Diagnostic Studies

- Monitor CBC and differential daily (especially ANC and lymphocyte count)
- Call physician for neutrophil count <1000, count has significantly changed from previous count, or whenever patient becomes symptomatic (eg, febrile).
- Monitor globulin, albumin, and total protein levels.
- Monitor all culture and sensitivity reports.
- Monitor x-ray reports.

Nursing Interventions to Prevent Complications

Environment and Staff

- Thorough hand washing *must* be done by *everyone* before entering patient's room *each* and *every time.*
- Allow no one with a cold/sore throat to care for patient, enter room, or come in contact with patient at home.
- Care for neutropenic patients before caring for other patients as much as possible.
- Use private room for patient when neutrophil count <1000.
- Allow no fresh flowers (stagnant water).
- Change water in containers every shift (including O_2 humidification systems q24h).
- Have room cleaned daily.

Dietary

- Provide low microbial diet.
- Restrict fresh salads, unpeeled fresh fruits or vegetables.

Patient

- Avoid suppositories, enemas, rectal temperatures.
- Encourage deep breathing (with incentive spirometer) q4h while patient is awake.
- Ambulate in hall; wear HEPA filter mask if neutropenia is severe.
- Prevent skin dryness with water-soluble lubricants (eg, lips, corners of mouth, elbows, feet, bony prominences).

Hygiene

- Provide meticulous total body hygiene daily (preferably with antimicrobial solution); perineal care after every bowel movement.
- Provide thorough oral hygiene after meals and q4h while patient is awake. Warm saline or salt and soda solution is effective; use quarter-strength hydrogen peroxide for very thick secretions. Avoid use of lemon-glycerine swabs and commercial mouthwashes.

IV Therapy

- Insert no plastic cannulas for peripheral IVs when neutrophil count <500 (if possible per agency) (vascular access device preferred for long-term/intensive IV therapy).
- Inspect IV sites each shift; monitor closely for any discomfort; erythema may not be present.
- Maintain meticulous IV site care.
- Cleanse skin with antimicrobial solution before venipuncture (unless allergic).
- Moisture-vapor-permeable dressings permissible with strict adherence to institutional protocol.
- Change IV tubing per institution policy, using aseptic technique.
- Administer antimicrobial agents on time.

Evaluation and Expected Outcome

1. Patient demonstrates absence of infection as evidenced by absence of fever, chills, inflammation, drainage, cough, dyspnea, sore throat, dysuria, or urinary frequency.
2. Patient demonstrates absence of infection as evidenced by vital signs within normal limits, including intact neurologic status and intact skin.

---

or purple hemorrhagic spots on the skin). Major hemorrhages also may develop when the platelet count drops to less than 10,000/mm^3. The most common sites of bleeding are gastrointestinal, pulmonary, and intracranial. For undetermined reasons, fever or infection also increases the likelihood of bleeding.

Due to the lack of mature and normal granulocytes, patients are always threatened by infection. The likelihood of infection increases with the degree and duration of neutropenia, so neutrophil counts that persist at less than 100/mm^3 make the chances of systemic infection extremely high.

HOME CARE TEACHING CHECKLIST: THE PATIENT AT RISK FOR INFECTION

At the completion of the program, the patient or caregiver will be able to:

	Patient	Caregiver
• Describe the function of the blood components called neutrophils, lymphocytes, and immunoglobulins.	✔	✔
• Verbalize the reason for being at risk for infection.	✔	✔
• Identify signs and symptoms of infection.	✔	✔
• Demonstrate how to monitor self for signs of infection.	✔	
• Describe to whom/how/when to report signs of infection.	✔	✔
• Identify appropriate ways to prevent infection: wash hands thoroughly and often; perform total body hygiene; maintain skin integrity; avoid fresh flowers, plants, garden work (soil); avoid bird cages and litter boxes; avoid fresh salads and unpeeled fruits or vegetables; maintain high-calorie, high-protein diet and fluid intake of 3000 mL (unless fluids are restricted); avoid people with infections and crowds; perform deep-breathing exercises use incentive spirometer q4h while awake; avoid anal intercourse; provide adequate lubrication with gentle vaginal manipulation in intercourse.	✔	✔
• Describe appropriate actions to take should infection occur.	✔	✔

Medical Management

The overall objective of treatment is to achieve complete remission, where there is no detectable evidence of residual leukemia remaining in the bone marrow. Attempts are made to reach remission by the aggressive administration of chemotherapy, called induction therapy, which usually requires hospitalization for several weeks. Induction therapy typically involves high doses of cytarabine (Cytosar, Ara-C) and daunorubicin (Daunomycin, Cerubidine) or mitoxantrone or idarubicin; sometimes etoposide (VP-16) is added to the regimen. The choice of agents is based on the patient's physical status and history of prior antineoplastic treatment.

The aim of induction therapy is to eradicate the leukemic cells, but this is often accompanied by the eradication of normal types of myeloid cells. Thus, the patient becomes severely neutropenic (an ANC of 0 is not uncommon), anemic, and thrombocytopenic (a platelet count of less than 10,000/mm^3 is common). During this time, the patient is typically very ill, with bacterial, fungal, and occasionally viral infections, bleeding, and severe mucositis, causing diarrhea and a marked decline in the ability to maintain adequate nutrition. Supportive care consists of administering blood products (RBCs and platelets) and promptly treating infections. The use of granulocytic growth factors, either G-CSF (filgrastim) or GM-CSF (sargramostim), can shorten the period of significant neutropenia by stimulating the bone marrow to produce leukocytes more quickly. Studies (eg, Rowe et al., 1995) indicate that the use of such growth factors does not increase the risk of producing more leukemic cells.

When the patient has recovered from the induction therapy (ie, the WBC and platelet counts have returned to normal and any infection has resolved), the patient typically receives consolidation therapy (postremission therapy). The goal of consolidation therapy is to eliminate any residual leukemia cells that are not clinically detectable, thereby diminishing the chance for recurrence. Multiple treatment cycles of various agents are used, usually containing some form of cytarabine. Frequently, the patient receives one cycle of treatment almost the same, if not identical, to the induction treatment but using lower dosages (and therefore resulting in less toxicity).

Unfortunately, despite the aggressive use of chemotherapy, the ability to remain in remission for a prolonged period of time is not great; about 70% of patients with AML suffer a relapse, and long-term survival (eg, 5 years) after initial relapse is less than 5%.

Another aggressive treatment option is bone marrow transplantation. When a suitable tissue match with a close relative can be obtained, the patient embarks on an even more aggressive regimen of chemotherapy (sometimes in combination with radiation therapy), with the treatment goal of virtually destroying the hematopoietic function of the patient's bone marrow. The patient is then "rescued" with the infusion of the donor bone marrow to provide blood cell production. Patients who undergo a

TABLE 30•5 Cell Types and Causes of Leukocytosis

Cell Type	Laboratory Values	Causes*
Neutrophils	>8000/mm^3 (normal range: 2500–7500/mm^3)	Inflammation, infection, malignancy, myeloproliferative disorders, adverse effects of medications, splenectomy, stress
Lymphocytes	>5000/mm^3 (normal range: 1500–5000/mm^3)	Lymphoid leukemias, viral infections, allergic reactions (some)
Monocytes	>800/mm^3 (normal range: 100–800/mm^3)	Inflammation, tuberculosis, infection, myeloproliferative disease, malignancy, myelodysplastic syndromes
Eosinophils	>600/mm^3 (normal range: 0–440/mm^3)	Allergic reactions, dermatitis, parasites, myeloproliferative disorders, adverse effects of medications, hypereosinophilic syndrome
Basophils	>100/mm^3 (normal range: 0–200/mm^3)	Hypersensitivity syndromes, myeloproliferative disorders, inflammation

* The clinical conditions associated with elevations of various types of WBCs vary, particularly in severity. Because the actual number of monocytes, eosinophils, and basophils is low, even a significant elevation in any of these cell types may not be adequate to raise the total WBC count above normal. Thus, it is important to evaluate the results in the differential as well as the WBC count.

marrow transplantation have a significant risk for problems with infection, potential graft-versus-host disease (where the donor's lymphocytes recognize the patient's body as "foreign" and set up reactions to attack the "foreign" host), and other complications.

Another important option for the patient to consider is supportive care alone. In this case, aggressive leukemia therapy is not used; occasionally, hydroxyurea is used briefly to control the rise in blast count. Patients are supported with antimicrobial therapy and transfusions as needed. Using this treatment approach provides the patient with some additional time at home, but death frequently occurs within months, typically from infection or bleeding.

COMPLICATIONS OF TREATMENT

The massive leukemic cell destruction resulting from chemotherapy increases uric acid levels and makes patients vulnerable to renal stone formation and renal colic. Therefore, patients require a high fluid intake, alkalinization of the urine, and prophylaxis with allopurinol to prevent crystallization of uric acid and subsequent stone formation. Gastrointestinal problems may result from the infiltration of abnormal leukocytes into the abdominal organs, as well as from the toxicity of the chemotherapeutic agents. Anorexia, nausea, vomiting, diarrhea, and severe mucositis are common.

Nursing Management

Nursing management of the patient with acute leukemia is discussed at the end of the leukemia section.

Chronic Myeloid Leukemia

Chronic myeloid leukemia (CML) also arises from a mutation in the myeloid stem cell. Normal myeloid cells continue to be produced, but there is a preference for immature (blast) forms as well. Therefore, a wide spectrum of cell types exists within the blood, from blast forms through mature neutrophils. Because there is an uncontrolled proliferation of cells, the marrow expands into the cavities of long bones (eg, the femur) and cells are also formed in the liver and spleen (extramedullary hematopoiesis), resulting in sometimes-painful enlargement of these organs. A cytogenetic abnormality termed the Philadelphia chromosome (Ph^1) is found in 90% to 95% of patients with CML. A more specific and sensitive marker, the BCR/ABL gene, is present in virtually all patients with this disease. CML is uncommon in people younger than age 20, but the incidence rises with age (median age, 40 to 50 years).

Patients diagnosed with CML in the chronic phase have an overall median life expectancy of 3 to 5 years. During that time, they have very few symptoms and complications from the disease itself. Problems with infections and bleeding are rare. However, once the disease transforms to the acute phase, overall survival rarely exceeds several months.

Clinical Manifestations

The clinical picture of CML varies. Many patients are without symptoms, with the diagnosis established when leukocytosis is detected by a CBC performed for some other reason. The WBC count commonly exceeds 100,000. Patients with extremely high WBC counts may be somewhat short of breath or slightly confused due to decreased capillary perfusion to the lungs and brain from leukostasis. Patients may complain of an enlarged, tender spleen. The liver may also be enlarged. Some patients have somewhat insidious symptoms, such as malaise, anorexia, and weight loss. Lymphadenopathy is rare. There are three stages in CML: chronic, transformation, and accelerated or blast crisis. Patients have more symptoms and complications as the disease progresses.

Medical Management

Therapies of choice depend on the stage of disease. In the chronic phase, the aim is to correct the chromosomal abnormality—in other words, to convert the malignant stem cell population back to normal. The agents typically used for this purpose are interferon and cytosine, often in combination. These agents are administered daily as subcutaneous injections. This therapy is not benign; many patients cannot tolerate the profound fatigue, depression, anorexia, mucositis, and inability to concentrate. A less aggressive therapeutic approach focuses on the reduction of the WBC count to a more normal level. This goal can be achieved by using oral chemotherapeutic agents, typically hydroxyurea or busulfan. In the case of an extreme leukocytosis at diagnosis (eg, WBC of more than 300,000), a more emergent treatment may be required. In this instance, leukopheresis (in which the patient's blood is removed and separated, with the leukocytes withdrawn and the remaining blood returned to the patient) can temporarily reduce the number of WBCs. An anthracycline chemotherapeutic agent (eg, daunomycin) may also be used to bring the WBC count quickly down to a safer level, when more conservative therapy can be instituted.

The transformation phase can be insidious but marks the process of evolving (or transforming) into the acute phase (blast crisis). In the transformation phase, the patient may complain of bone pain and may report fevers (without any obvious sign of infection) and weight loss. Even with chemotherapy, the spleen may continue to enlarge. The patient may become more anemic and thrombocytopenic; an increased basophil level is detected by the CBC. Despite being a myeloid stem cell disease, the disease will transform to resemble acute lymphoid leukemia (ALL), with lymphoid-appearing blasts, rather than AML in up to 30% of patients. Transformation into the acute phase can be gradual or rapid.

On transformation to a more acute form of leukemia, treatment may resemble induction therapy for acute leukemia, using the same medications as for AML or ALL. Patients whose disease evolves into a "lymphoid" blast crisis are more likely to be able to reenter a chronic phase after induction therapy. For those whose disease evolves into AML, therapy is largely ineffective in achieving a second chronic phase. Life-threatening infections and/or bleeding occur frequently in this phase.

CML is a disease that can potentially be cured with bone marrow transplantation. Patients who receive such transplants while still in the chronic phase of the illness tend to have a greater chance for cure than those who receive them in the acute phase. The transplantation procedure is now available for otherwise healthy patients younger than age 60.

Acute Lymphocytic Leukemia

ALL results from an uncontrolled proliferation of immature cells (lymphoblasts) derived from the lymphoid stem cell. It is most common in young children, with boys affected more often than girls; the peak incidence is 4 years of age. After age 15, ALL is uncommon. Because of improvements in therapy for ALL, more than 80% of children survive at least 5 years. Even when relapse occurs, resuming induction therapy can often achieve a second complete remission. Moreover, bone marrow transplants may be successful even after a second relapse.

Home Care Teaching Checklist: The Patient at Risk for Bleeding

At the completion of the program, the patient or caregiver will be able to:

	Patient	Caregiver
• Describe the source and function of platelets and clotting factors.	✔	✔
• Verbalize the reason for being at risk for bleeding.	✔	✔
• Identify medications and other substances to avoid (eg, aspirin-containing medications, and alcohol).	✔	✔
• Demonstrate how to monitor self for signs of bleeding.	✔	
• Describe to whom/how/when to report signs of bleeding.	✔	✔
• Express need to notify health care professional before having dental work.	✔	✔
• Describe appropriate ways to prevent bleeding (avoid use of suppositories, enemas, tampons; avoid constipation, vigorous sexual intercourse, anal sex; use only an electric razor for shaving and a soft-bristled brush for teeth).	✔	✔
• Demonstrate appropriate actions to take should bleeding occur.	✔	✔

Clinical Manifestations

Immature lymphocytes proliferate in the marrow and crowd the development of normal myeloid cells. As a result, normal hematopoiesis is inhibited, resulting in reduced numbers of leukocytes, RBCs, and platelets. Leukocyte counts may be either low or high but always include a high proportion of immature cells. Manifestations of leukemic cell infiltration into other organs are more common with ALL than with other forms of leukemia and include pain from an enlarged liver or spleen, bone pain, and headache and vomiting (because of meningeal involvement).

Medical Management

As in AML, the primary aim of treatment is complete remission. Lymphoid blast cells are typically sensitive to corticosteroids and vinca alkaloids; thus, these medications are an integral part of the initial induction therapy. Because ALL frequently invades the central nervous system, prophylaxis with cranial irradiation and/or intrathecal chemotherapy (eg, methotrexate) is another integral part of the treatment plan.

Treatment protocols for ALL tend to be complex, using a wide variety of chemotherapeutic agents. They often include a maintenance phase, when lower doses of medications are given for up to 3 years. Despite the complexity, treatment can be provided in the outpatient setting in some circumstances until severe complications develop.

Problems with infection are common, especially viral infections, and may result from the corticosteroids used in treating this illness. Patients with ALL tend to have a better response to treatment; however, bone marrow transplants offer patients a chance for prolonged remission or even cure if the illness recurs after therapy.

Nursing Management

The nursing management of the patient with acute leukemia follows the end of the leukemia section.

Chronic Lymphocytic Leukemia

Chronic lymphocytic leukemia (CLL) is a common malignancy of older adults; two thirds of all patients are older than 60 years at diagnosis. It is the most common form of leukemia in the United States and Europe but is rarely seen in Asia. The average survival for patients with CLL is 14 years (early stage) to 2.5 years (late stage).

Pathophysiology

CLL typically derives from a malignant clone of B lymphocytes (T-cell CLL is rare). Unlike the acute forms of leukemia, the preponderance of leukemia cells here are fully mature. It appears that these cells can escape **apoptosis** (programmed cell death), which results in an excessive accumulation of the cells in the marrow and circulation. The disease is classified into three or four stages (two classification systems are in use). In the early stage, an elevated lymphocyte count is seen (can exceed 300,000). Because the lymphocytes are small, they can easily travel through the small capillaries within the circulation, and the pulmonary and cerebral complications of leukocytosis (as seen with myeloid leukemias) are not found in CLL. Lymphadenopathy occurs, and nodes can become very large, sometimes painful. Hepatomegaly and splenomegaly then develop.

In later stages, anemia and thrombocytopenia may develop. Treatment is typically initiated in the later stages; earlier treatment does not appear to increase survival. Autoimmune complications can also occur at any stage, either as autoimmune hemolytic anemia or idiopathic thrombocytopenic purpura (ITP).

Clinical Manifestations

Many patients are asymptomatic and are diagnosed during physical examination or treatment for another disease. An increased lymphocyte count (lymphocytosis) is always present. The erythrocyte and platelet counts may be normal or, in later stages of the illness, decreased. Enlargement of lymph nodes (lymphadenopathy) is common; it can be severe and sometimes painful. The spleen can also be enlarged (splenomegaly).

Patients with CLL can develop "B symptoms," a constellation of symptoms including fevers, drenching sweats (especially at night), and unintentional weight loss. These patients have defects in their humoral and cell-mediated immune systems; therefore, infections are common. The defect in cellular immunity is evidenced by an absent or decreased reaction to skin sensitivity tests (eg, *Candida*, mumps); this inability is termed **anergy**. Problems with life-threatening infection are not infrequent. Viral infections, such as herpes zoster, can become widely disseminated.

Medical Management

In early stages, CLL may require no treatment. When symptoms are severe (drenching night sweats, painful lymphadenopathy, or advancement to later stages with resultant anemia and thrombocytopenia), chemotherapy with corticosteroids and chlorambucil (Leukeran) is often used. Other useful agents include cyclophosphamide, vincristine, and doxorubicin. A significant number of patients who do not respond to these medications have achieved remission with fludarabine. The major side effect of this medication is prolonged bone marrow suppression, manifested by prolonged periods of neutropenia, lymphopenia, and thrombocytopenia. Patients are then at risk for such infections as *Pneumocystis carinii* pneumonia, *Listeria*, mycobacteria, herpesviruses, and cytomegalovirus (CMV). Intravenous treatment with immunoglobulin may prevent recurrent bacterial infections in selected patients.

NURSING PROCESS: THE PATIENT WITH ACUTE LEUKEMIA

Assessment

Although the clinical picture varies with the type of leukemia involved as well as the treatment implemented, the health history may reveal a range of subtle symptoms reported by the patient that can be apparent before the problem is manifested by findings on physical examination. Weakness and fatigue are common manifestations, not only of the leukemia but also of the resulting complications of anemia and infection. While the patient is hospitalized, the assessments should be performed on a daily basis or more frequently as warranted. Because the physical findings may be subtle initially, a thorough, systematic assessment incorporating all body systems is essential. For example, a dry cough, mild dyspnea, and diminished breath sounds may indicate a pulmonary infection. However, the same infection may not be seen initially on the chest x-ray because of the lack of neutrophils within the body. The specific body system assessments are delineated in the neutropenic and bleeding precautions found in Charts 30-6 and 30-7, respectively. When performing serial assessments, current findings are compared with previous findings to evaluate new findings or improvement or worsening of previous findings.

The nurse also must closely monitor the results of laboratory studies. Flow sheets are particularly useful in tracking the WBC count, ANC, hematocrit, and platelet and creatinine levels. Hepatic function tests and electrolyte levels can also be tracked on flow sheets. Culture results need to be reported immediately so that appropriate antimicrobial therapy can begin or be modified.

Diagnosis

Nursing Diagnoses

Based on the assessment data, major nursing diagnoses for the acute leukemic patient may include the following:

- Risk for infection and bleeding
- Alterations in mucous membranes due to changes in epithelial lining of the gastrointestinal tract from chemotherapy or prolonged use of antimicrobial medications
- Pain and discomfort related to mucositis, leukocytic infiltration of systemic tissues, fever, and infection
- Altered nutrition, less than body requirements, related to hypermetabolic state, anorexia, mucositis, pain, and nausea
- Fatigue and activity intolerance related to anemia and infection
- Impaired physical mobility due to anemia and protective isolation
- Impaired skin integrity related to toxic effects of chemotherapy
- Diarrhea due to altered gastrointestinal flora, mucosal denudation
- Fluid imbalance due to potential for bleeding and renal dysfunction
- Self-care deficit due to fatigue and malaise
- Disturbance in body image related to change in appearance, function, and roles
- Anxiety due to knowledge deficit and uncertain future
- Potential for diminished spiritual well-being
- Grieving related to anticipatory loss and altered role functioning
- Knowledge deficit about disease process, treatment, complication management, self-care measures

Collaborative Problems/Potential Complications

Based on the assessment data, potential complications that may develop include:

- Infection
- Bleeding
- Renal dysfunction
- Tumor lysis syndrome
- Nutritional depletion
- Mucositis

Planning and Goals

The major goals for the patient may include attainment and maintenance of comfort, attainment and maintenance of adequate nutrition, self-care, activity tolerance, ability to cope with the diagnosis and prognosis, positive body image, understanding of the disease process and its treatment, and absence of complications.

Nursing Interventions

Preventing or Managing Infection and Bleeding

The nursing interventions for diminishing the risk for infection and for bleeding are delineated in Charts 30-6 and 30-7.

Managing Mucositis

Although emphasis is placed on the oral mucosa, it is important to realize that the entire gastrointestinal mucosa can be altered, not only by the effects of chemotherapy but also from prolonged administration of antibiotics. Assessment of the oral mucosa must be thorough; therefore, dentures must be removed. Areas to assess include the palate, buccal mucosa, tongue, gums, lips, oropharynx, and the area under the tongue. In addition to identifying and describing lesions, the color and moisture of the mucosa should be noted.

Oral hygiene is very important to diminish the bacteria within the mouth, maintain moisture, and provide comfort. Soft-bristled toothbrushes should be used until the neutrophil and platelet counts become very low; at that time, sponge-tipped applicators may be substituted. Lemon-glycerin swabs and commercial mouthwashes should never be used because the glycerin and alcohol within them are extremely drying to the tissues. Simple rinses with saline (or saline and baking soda) solutions are inexpensive but effective in cleaning and moistening the oral mucosa. Because the risk

CHART 30•7 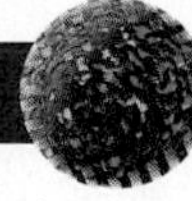 **Implementing Bleeding Precautions**

Nursing Diagnosis

Risk for bleeding and injury secondary to thrombocytopenia/altered coagulation due to:

Malignant invasion in bone marrow

Bone marrow suppression resulting from chemotherapy (particularly alkylators, antitumor antibiotics, antimetabolites) and radiation therapy

Hypersplenism

Disseminated intravascular coagulation

Altered coagulation

- Thrombocytopenia is usually defined as a platelet count < 100,000/mm^3 (normal: 150,000–350,000).
- Complications from thrombocytopenia (ie, serious spontaneous bleeding) are infrequent until the platelet count is < 20,000/mm^3.
- Prophylactic platelet transfusions are often administered if the platelet count drops to <10,000/mm^3 even if the patient remains asymptomatic.
- Other factors may increase risk for spontaneous hemorrhage, such as fever, sepsis, vomiting/cough → ↑ intravascular pressure.
- Serious hemorrhage is unusual in mildly thrombocytopenic patients in absence of local lesions (peptic ulcer, bleeding from hemorrhoids, cystitis).

Assessment

Patient

Assess the following areas thoroughly every shift or visit (with spot checks throughout the shift if inpatient) and notify physician if new onset of the following or worsening of status:

- Integument: Petechiae (usually located on trunk, legs), ecchymoses or hematomas, conjunctival hemorrhages, bleeding gums, bleeding at puncture sites (venipuncture, lumbar puncture, bone marrow)
- Cardiovascular: Hypotension, tachycardia, complaints of dizziness, epistaxis
- Respiratory: Respiratory distress, tachypnea
- GI: Hemoptysis, abdominal distention, rectal bleeding
- Genitourinary: Vaginal or urethral bleeding
- Neurologic: Headache, blurred vision, mental status

Laboratory Tests

- Monitor CBC, platelets at least daily, coagulation panel.
- Call physician if platelets < 10,000 count has significantly changed from previous count (including coagulation), or whenever patient becomes symptomatic.
- Ensure patient was HLA typed *before* transfusions or chemotherapy begins if admitted for induction therapy (eg, for acute leukemia).
- Obtain 1-hour posttransfusion platelet count if warranted.
- Test all urine, emesis, stools for occult blood.

Nursing Interventions to Prevent Complications

- Avoid aspirin or aspirin-containing medications or other medications known to inhibit platelet function if possible.
- Do not give IM injections.
- Insert no indwelling catheters.
- Take no rectal temps; use no suppositories, enemas.
- Use stool softeners, oral laxatives to prevent constipation.
- Induce amenorrhea in premenopausal women (eg, by birth control pills without placebos).
- Use smallest possible needles when performing venipuncture.
- Apply pressure to venipuncture sites for 5 minutes or until bleeding has stopped.
- Permit no flossing of teeth, and no commercial mouthwashes.
- Use only soft-bristled toothbrush for mouth care.
- Use only toothettes for mouth care if platelets <10,000, if gums bleed.
- Lubricate lips with water-soluble lubricant q2h while awake.
- Avoid suctioning if possible; if unavoidable, use only *gentle* suctioning.
- Discourage vigorous coughing or blowing nose.
- Use only electric razor for shaving.
- Pad side rails of bed as needed.
- Prevent falls by assisting patient to ambulate as necessary.

Control Bleeding

- Apply direct pressure (with sand bag as needed).
- For epistaxis, position patient in high Fowler's position; apply ice pack to back of neck and direct pressure to nose.
- Call physician for prolonged bleeding (eg, unable to stop within 10 minutes).
- Administer platelets, fresh-frozen plasma, packed red cells, as prescribed.

Evaluation and Expected Outcomes

1. Patient demonstrates absence of bleeding as evidenced by absence of: spontaneous petechiae, ecchymoses, epistaxis, hemoptysis, bleeding gums, conjunctival hemorrhage, vaginal bleeding, hematuria, guaiac positive stool, visual changes (ie, blurred vision), orthostatic hypotension, prolonged bleeding from puncture sites.
2. Patient demonstrates absence of bleeding as evidenced by the presence of: vital signs within normal limits, intact neurologic status.

of yeast or fungal infection in the mouth is great, other medications are often prescribed, such as chlorhexidine rinses or clotrimazole troches. The nurse may emphasize the importance of these medications to the patient to help enhance therapeutic compliance. Chlorhexidine rinses may discolor the teeth.

To diminish perirectal complications, it is important to cleanse the perirectal area thoroughly after each bowel movement. Women are instructed to cleanse the perineum from front to back. Sitz baths are a comfortable method of cleansing; the perianal region and buttocks must be carefully dried afterward to minimize the chance of excoriation. Stool softeners should be used to soften bowel movements; however, the stool frequency must be monitored so the softeners can be stopped if the stool becomes too loose.

Improving Nutritional Intake

The disease process can increase the patient's metabolic rate and therefore his or her nutritional requirements; sepsis adds to the problem. Nutritional intake is often reduced because of pain and discomfort associated with mucositis. Mouth care before and after meals and administration of analgesics before eating can help increase intake. If oral anesthetics are used, the patient must be warned to chew with extreme care to avoid inadvertently biting the tongue or buccal mucosa.

Nausea should not be a major contributing factor because recent advances in antiemetic therapy are highly effective. However, nausea can result from antimicrobial therapy; thus, some antiemetic therapy may still be required after the chemotherapy has been completed.

Small, frequent feedings of foods that are soft in texture and moderate in temperature may be better tolerated. Low-microbial diets are typically prescribed (avoiding uncooked fruits or vegetables or those without a peelable skin). Nutritional supplements are frequently used. Daily body weights (as well as intake and output measurements) are useful in monitoring fluid status. Calorie counts are useful as well as a formal nutritional assessment. Often total parenteral nutrition is required to maintain adequate nutrition.

Easing Pain and Discomfort

Recurrent fevers are common in acute leukemia; at times, they are accompanied by chills, even rigors. Myalgias and arthralgias can result. Acetaminophen is typically given to bring the fever down, but it does so by increasing diaphoresis. Sponging with cool water may be useful, but cold water or ice packs should be avoided because the heat cannot dissipate from constricted blood vessels. Bedclothes need frequent changing as well. Gentle back and shoulder massage may provide comfort.

Stomatitis can also cause significant discomfort. In addition to oral hygiene practices, patient-controlled analgesia can be effective in controlling the pain of mucositis.

Because patients with acute leukemia require extensive nursing care (either during induction or consolidation therapy or during resultant complications), sleep deprivation frequently results. Nurses need to implement creative strategies that permit uninterrupted sleep for at least a few hours while still administering necessary medications on time.

With the exception of severe mucositis, less pain is associated with acute leukemia than with many other forms of cancer. However, the amount of suffering that the patient must endure can be immense. Patients greatly benefit from active listening.

Decreasing Fatigue and Deconditioning

Fatigue is a common and oppressive problem. Nursing interventions should focus on assisting the patient to establish a balance between activity and rest that is realistic and feasible. Patients with acute leukemia need to maintain some physical activity and exercise to prevent deconditioning that results from inactivity. Using a HEPA filter mask can permit the patient to ambulate outside the room despite severe neutropenia. Although many patients lack the motivation to use them, stationary bicycles within the room can also be used. At a minimum, patients should be encouraged to sit up in a chair while awake rather than staying in bed; even this simple activity can improve the patient's tidal volume and enhance circulation. Physical therapy can also be beneficial.

Maintaining Fluid and Electrolyte Balance

Febrile episodes, bleeding, and inadequate or aggressive fluid replacement can alter the patient's fluid status. Similarly, repeated diarrhea, vomiting, and long-term use of certain antimicrobial agents can cause significant deficits in electrolytes. Intake and output need to be measured accurately; daily weights should also be obtained. The patient should be assessed for signs of dehydration as well as fluid overload. Laboratory test results, particularly electrolytes, blood urea nitrogen, creatinine, and hematocrit, should be monitored and compared with previous results. Replacement of electrolytes, particularly potassium and magnesium, is commonly required. Patients receiving amphotericin and some antibiotics are at increased risk for electrolyte depletion.

Improving Self-Care

Because hygiene measures are so important in this patient population, they must be performed by the nurse when the patient cannot do so. However, the patient should be encouraged to do as much as possible, to preserve mobility and function as well as self-esteem. Patients may often have feelings of self-depreciation, even disgust that they can no longer care for themselves. Empathetic listening is helpful, as is realistic assurance that these deficits are temporary. As the patient recovers from treatment, it is important to assist him or her to resume more self-care. Patients are usually discharged from the hospital with a vascular access device (eg, Hickman catheter), and most can care for the catheter with adequate instruction and practice under observation.

Managing Anxiety and Grief

Being diagnosed with acute leukemia can be extremely frightening. In many instances, the need to begin treatment is emergent; thus, patients have little time to process the fact that they have the illness before making decisions about therapy. Providing emotional support and discussing the uncertain future are crucial. The nurse also needs to assess how much information and understanding patients want to have regarding the illness, treatment, and potential complications. This desire should be reassessed at intervals as needs and interest in information change throughout the hospital stay. Priorities must be identified so that the procedures, assessments, and self-care expectations are adequately explained even to those who do not wish extensive information.

Many patients become depressed and begin to grieve for the losses they feel, such as normal family functioning, professional roles and responsibilities, and social roles as well as physical functioning. Nurses can assist patients to identify the source of the grief and encourage them to allow time to adjust to the major life changes produced by the illness. Role restructuring, both within family and professional lives, may be required. Again, when possible, permitting patients to identify options and to take time making significant decisions regarding such restructuring is helpful.

Discharge from the hospital can also provoke anxiety. Although most patients are extremely glad to be able to go home, they may lack confidence in their ability to manage potential complications. Close communication between nurses across care settings can reassure patients that they are not abandoned.

Encouraging Spiritual Well-Being

Because acute leukemia is a serious, potentially life-threatening illness, the nurse may offer support to enhance the patient's spiritual well-being. The patient's spiritual and religious practices should be assessed and pastoral services offered. Throughout the patient's illness, it is important that the nurse assist the patient to maintain hope. However, that hope should be realistic and will certainly change over the course of the illness. For example, the patient may initially hope to be cured, but with repeated relapses and a change to terminal care, the same patient may hope for a quiet, dignified death.

Monitoring and Managing Potential Complications

Nursing interventions for the potential complications have been described previously .

Promoting Home and Community-Based Care

TEACHING PATIENTS SELF-CARE

Most patients cope better when they have an understanding of what is happening to them. Based on their education, literacy level, and interest, teaching should focus on the disease (including some pathophysiology), its treatment, and certainly the significant risk for infection and bleeding that ensues.

Vascular access device management can be taught to most patients or adult family members. Follow-up and care for the devices may also need to be provided by nurses in an outpatient facility or from a home care agency.

CONTINUING CARE

Shortened hospital stays and outpatient care have significantly altered care for patients with acute leukemia. In many instances, when the patient is clinically stable but still requires parenteral antibiotics or blood products, these procedures can be performed outside the inpatient setting. Again, nurses in these different settings must communicate regularly. Patients need to learn which parameters are important for them to monitor, and how to monitor them. Specific instruction needs to be given as to when the patient should seek care from the physician.

Terminal Care. Patients and their families need to have a clear understanding of the disease and prognosis. The nurse acts as an advocate to ensure that this information is provided. When patients no longer respond to therapy, it is important to respect their choices about treatment, including measures to prolong life and other end-of-life measures. Advance directives and living wills provide patients with some measure of control during terminal illness.

Many patients in this stage still choose to be cared for at home, and families often need support when considering this option. Coordination of home care services and instruction can help to alleviate their anxiety about managing the patient's care in the home. As the patient becomes weaker, the caregivers must assume more care. In addition, caregivers often need to be encouraged to take care of themselves, allowing time for rest and accepting emotional support. Hospice staff can assist in providing respite for family members as well as care for the patient. Patients and families also need assistance to cope with changes in their roles and responsibilities. Anticipatory grieving is an essential task during this time.

In patients with acute leukemia, death typically occurs from infection or bleeding. Family members need to have information about these complications and the measures to take should either occur. Many family members cannot cope with the care required when a patient begins to bleed actively. It is important to delineate alternatives to keeping the patient at home. Should another option be sought, family members who may feel guilty that they could not keep the patient at home will require support from the nurse.

Evaluation

Expected Outcomes

Expected outcomes may include:

1. Demonstrates absence of infection
2. Demonstrates absence of bleeding
3. Exhibits intact oral mucous membranes
   a. Participates in oral hygiene regimen
   b. Reports no discomfort in mouth
4. Attains optimal level of nutrition
   a. Maintains weight with increased food and fluid intake
5. Reports less pain and discomfort
6. Has less fatigue and increases activity
7. Maintains fluid and electrolyte balance
8. Participates in self-care
9. Copes with anxiety and grief
   a. Discusses concerns and fears
   b. Uses stress management strategies appropriately
   c. Participates in decision regarding end-of-life care
10. Avoids complications

MALIGNANT LYMPHOMAS AND MULTIPLE MYELOMA

The lymphomas are neoplasms of cells of lymphoid origin. These tumors usually start in lymph nodes but can involve lymphoid tissue in the spleen, the gastrointestinal tract (eg, the wall of the stomach), the liver, or the bone marrow. They are often classified according to the degree of cell differentiation and the origin of the predominant malignant cell. Lymphomas can be broadly classified into two categories: Hodgkin's disease and non-Hodgkin's lymphoma.

Hodgkin's Disease

Hodgkin's disease is a relatively rare malignancy that has an impressive cure rate. It is somewhat more common in men than women and has two peaks of incidence: one in the early 20s and the other after age 50. Unlike other lymphomas, Hodgkin's disease is unicentric in origin; it spreads by contiguous extension along the lymphatic system. The cause of Hodgkin's disease is unknown. However, 20% of patients are also infected with the Epstein-Barr virus; this occurs more commonly in the younger patient population. There is a familial pattern associated with Hodgkin's disease: first-degree relatives have a higher-than-normal frequency of the disease. There is no increased incidence documented for nonblood relatives (eg, spouses).

The malignant cell of Hodgkin's disease is the Reed-Sternberg cell, a gigantic tumor cell that is morphologically unique and is thought to be of immature lymphoid origin. It is the pathologic hallmark and essential diagnostic criterion for Hodgkin's disease. However, the tumor is very heterogeneous and may actually contain few Reed-Sternberg cells. Repeated biopsies may be required to establish the diagnosis.

Hodgkin's disease is customarily classified into four subgroups based on pathologic analyses that reflect the grade of malignancy and suggest the prognosis. When lymphocytes predominate, for example, with few Reed-Sternberg cells and minimal involvement of the nodes, the prognosis is much more favorable than when the lymphocyte count is low and the lymph nodes are virtually replaced by tumor cells of the most primitive type. The majority of patients with Hodgkin's disease have the types currently designated "nodular sclerosis" or "mixed cellularity." The nodular sclerosis type tends to occur more often in young women, at an earlier stage but with a worse prognosis than the mixed cellularity subgroup, which occurs more commonly in men and causes more constitutional symptoms but has a better prognosis.

Clinical Manifestations

Hodgkin's disease usually begins as a painless enlargement of one or more lymph nodes on one side of the neck. The individual nodes are painless and firm but not hard. The most common sites for lymphadenopathy are the cervical, supraclavicular, and medi-

CHART 30•8 Staging Lymphomas and Hodgkin's Disease

Stage	I	Involvement of single lymph node region
	I_E	Involvement of single extralymphatic organ or site
Stage	II	Involvement of 2+ lymph node regions on same side of diaphragm
	II_E	Involvement of localized extralymphatic site on same side of diaphragm
Stage	III	Involvement of lymph node regions on both sides of diaphragm
	III_E	Localized involvement of extralymphatic organ or spleen
	III_S	Involvement of spleen
For Hodgkin's disease only:		
	III_1	Disease limited to upper abdomen
	III_2	Disease limited to lower abdomen
Stage	IV	Diffuse or disseminated involvement of 1+ extralymphatic organs, with or without lymph node involvement (liver, lung, marrow, skin)
B Symptoms:		Fever exceeding 38°C (100.4°F), night sweats, weight loss exceeding 10% body weight

astinal nodes; involvement of the iliac or inguinal nodes or spleen is much less common. A mediastinal mass may be seen on chest x-ray; occasionally, the mass is large enough to compress the trachea and induce dyspnea. Pruritus is common; it can be extremely distressing and is of unclear etiology. A fairly common finding (20%) is the development of brief but severe pain after drinking alcohol. The pain is usually at the site of the Hodgkin's disease, and the cause is unknown. All organs are vulnerable to invasion by Hodgkin's disease. Thus, symptoms result from the tumor compressing other organs, such as cough and pulmonary effusion (from pulmonary infiltrates); jaundice (from hepatic involvement or bile duct obstruction); abdominal pain (from splenomegaly or retroperitoneal adenopathy); or bone pain (from skeletal involvement). Herpes zoster infections are common. A cluster of constitutional symptoms has important prognostic implications. Referred to as "B symptoms", they include fever (without chills), drenching sweats (particularly at night), and unintentional weight loss of more than 10%. B symptoms are found in 40% of patients and are more common in advanced disease.

A mild anemia is the most common hematologic finding. The WBC count may be elevated or decreased. The platelet count is typically normal, unless the tumor has invaded the bone marrow, suppressing hematopoiesis. The **erythrocyte sedimentation rate** and serum copper levels are used by some clinicians to assess disease activity. Patients with Hodgkin's disease have a defect in their cellular immunity, as evidenced by an absent or decreased reaction to skin sensitivity tests (eg, *Candida*, mumps); this inability is termed anergy.

Assessment and Diagnostic Findings

Because many manifestations are similar to those occurring with infection, diagnostic studies are performed to rule out an infectious origin for the disease. The diagnosis is made by means of an excisional lymph node biopsy and the presence of the Reed-Sternberg cell. Once the diagnosis is confirmed and the histologic type established, it is necessary to assess the extent of the disease, a process referred to as staging (Chart 30-8).

The health history should assess for the presence of any B symptoms. Physical examination requires a careful, systematic evaluation of the lymph node chains, as well as the size of the spleen and liver. A chest x-ray and a computed tomography (CT) scan of the chest, abdomen, and pelvis are crucial to identify the extent of lymph-adenopathy within these regions. Laboratory tests include CBC, platelet count, sedimentation rate, and liver and renal function studies. A bone marrow biopsy is performed if there are signs of marrow involvement; in some settings, bilateral biopsies are routinely performed. Bone scans may be performed to identify any involvement in these areas. A staging laparotomy and lymphangiography are no longer considered mandatory, primarily because of the excellent visualization provided by computed tomography as well as changes in philosophy regarding treating early-stage disease.

Medical Management

The general intent of treating Hodgkin's disease, regardless of stage, is cure. Treatment is determined primarily by the stage of the disease, not the histologic type; however, extensive research is ongoing to target treatment regimens to histologic subtypes or prognostic features. Traditionally, early Hodgkin's disease was treated by staging laparotomy followed by radiation therapy. Recent data show improved results and decreased complications with a short course (2 to 4 months) of chemotherapy followed by radiation therapy in early-stage disease (IA and IIA). Combination chemotherapy (doxorubicin, bleomycin, vinblastine, and dacarbazine, referred to as ABVD) alone is now the standard treatment for more advanced disease (stages III and IV and all B stages).

Radiation therapy is still very useful for patients with extensive adenopathy (bulky disease). In this group, residual disease often persists when the chemotherapy treatment is finished; adding radiation therapy to the involved areas (remaining adenopathy) has been shown to improve survival.

Even when Hodgkin's disease does recur, the use of high doses of chemotherapeutic agents, followed by autologous bone marrow or stem cell transplantation, can be very effective in controlling the disease and extending survival.

LONG-TERM COMPLICATIONS OF THERAPY

Much is now known about the long-term effects of chemotherapy and radiation therapy, primarily from the large numbers of people who were cured of Hodgkin's disease by these treatments. The various complications of treatment are listed in Chart 30-9. Risk factors for other cancers should be assessed, and long-term surveillance is crucial. The potential development of a second malignancy is obviously of concern to patients, and this potential should be addressed with the patient when treatment decisions are made. However, it is important to consider that Hodgkin's disease is curable. Revised treatment approaches are aimed at diminishing the risk for complications without sacrificing the potential for cure.

Non-Hodgkin's Lymphomas

Non-Hodgkin's lymphomas are a heterogeneous group of cancers that originate from the neoplastic growth of lymphoid tissue. As in CLL, the neoplastic cells are thought to arise from a single clone of lymphocytes; however, in non-Hodgkin's lymphoma, the cells may vary morphologically. Most non-Hodgkin's lymphomas involve malignant B cells; only 5% involve T cells. Unlike Hodgkin's disease, the lymphoid tissues involved are largely

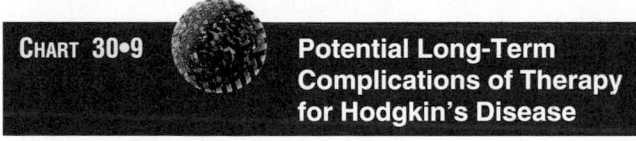

CHART 30•9 Potential Long-Term Complications of Therapy for Hodgkin's Disease

Immune dysfunction
Herpes infections (zoster and varicella)
Pneumococcal sepsis
Acute myeloid leukemia
Myelodysplastic syndromes
Non-Hodgkin's lymphoma
Solid tumors
Thyroid cancer
Thymic hyperplasia
Hypothyroidism
Pericarditis (acute or chronic)
Cardiomyopathy
Pneumonitis (acute or chronic)
Avascular necrosis
Growth retardation
Infertility
Impotence
Dental caries

infiltrated with malignant cells. The spread of these malignant lymphoid cells occurs unpredictably; true localized disease is uncommon. Lymph nodes from multiple sites may be infiltrated as well as tissue outside the lymphoid system (extranodal tissue). Although the cause is unknown, a viral etiology has been suggested, and there is an association with immunosuppressed states (eg, AIDS, immunosuppressive therapy for organ transplantation, and environmental toxins).

The prognosis varies greatly among the various types of non-Hodgkin's lymphoma. Long-term survival (more than 10 years) is commonly achieved in low-grade, localized lymphomas. Even with aggressive disease forms, cure is possible with aggressive treatment in at least one third of patients.

Clinical Manifestations

Symptoms are highly variable, reflecting the diverse nature of these diseases. With early-stage disease, or with the types that are considered more indolent, symptoms may be virtually absent or very minor. Thus, the illness is not typically diagnosed until it progresses to a later stage, when the patient is more symptomatic. At these stages (III or IV), lymphadenopathy is noticeable. One third of patients have the presence of B symptoms (recurrent fever, drenching night sweats, unintentional weight loss of 10% or more).

Assessment and Diagnostic Findings

The actual diagnosis of non-Hodgkin's lymphoma is categorized into a highly complex classification system based on histopathology and cytogenetic analyses of the malignant cells. The specific histopathologic type of the disease has important prognostic implications. Treatment also varies and is based on these features. Indolent types tend to have small cells and are distributed in a follicular pattern. Aggressive types tend to have large or immature cells distributed through the nodes in a diffuse pattern. For example, a low-grade lymphoma may not require treatment until the disease progresses to a later stage, whereas more aggressive types (eg, lymphoblastic lymphoma, Burkitt's lymphoma) require prompt initiation of chemotherapy. Staging, also an important factor, is typically based on data obtained from computed tomography (CT) scans, bone marrow biopsies, and occasionally cerebrospinal fluid analysis from lumbar puncture (see Chart 30-8). Stage is based on the site of disease and spread to other sites. For example, in stage I disease, only one area of involvement is detected; thus, stage I disease is highly localized and may respond well to localized therapy (eg, radiation therapy). In contrast, stage IV disease is detected in at least one extranodal site.

Medical Management

Treatment is based on the actual classification of disease, the stage of disease, prior treatment (if any), and the patient's ability to tolerate therapy. If the disease is not an aggressive form and is truly localized, radiation alone may be the treatment of choice. With aggressive types, aggressive combinations of chemotherapeutic agents are given even in early stages. More intermediate forms are commonly treated with combination chemotherapy and radiation therapy for stage I and II disease. The biologic agent interferon has recently been approved for treating follicular low-grade lymphomas, and an antibody to CD20 (rituximab) has been effective in achieving partial responses in patients with recurrent low-grade lymphoma. Studies of this agent in combination with conventional chemotherapy or as an adjuvant treatment are ongoing. Central nervous system involvement is also common with some forms of non-Hodgkin's lymphoma; in this situation, cranial radiation or intrathecal chemotherapy is used in addition to systemic chemotherapy. Treatment after relapse is controversial; bone marrow transplantation may be considered for patients younger than age 60.

Nursing Management

Most care for patients with Hodgkin's disease and non-Hodgkin's lymphoma is performed in the outpatient setting unless problems develop (eg, infection, respiratory compromise due to mediastinal mass). For patients who require treatment, chemotherapy and radiation therapy are most commonly used. Chemotherapy causes systemic side effects (eg, myelosuppression, nausea, hair loss, risk for infection), whereas the side effects from radiation therapy are specific to the area being irradiated. For example, patients receiving abdominal radiation therapy may experience nausea and diarrhea but not hair loss.

The risk of infection is significant for these patients, not only from treatment-related myelosuppression but also from the defective immune response that results from the disease itself. Thus, patients need to be taught to prevent infection, to recognize signs of possible infection, and to contact the health care professional should such signs develop (see Chart 30-6).

Many lymphomas can be cured with current treatments. However, as survival rates increase, the incidence of second malignancies, particularly AML (or MDS), also increases. Therefore, survivors should be regularly screened for second malignancies.

Lymphoma is a highly complex constellation of diseases. When caring for the patient with lymphoma, it is extremely important to know the specific disease type, stage of disease, treatment history, and current treatment plan.

Multiple Myeloma

Multiple myeloma is a malignant disease of the most mature form of B lymphocyte, the plasma cell. It is not classified as a lymphoma. Plasma cells secrete immunoglobulin, proteins necessary for antibody production to fight infection.

Pathophysiology

In myeloma, the malignant plasma cells produce an increased amount of a specific immunoglobulin that is not functional. Functional types of immunoglobulin are still produced (by nonmalignant plasma cells) but in lower-than-normal quantity. The specific immunoglobulin secreted by the myeloma cells is detectable in the blood and/or urine and is referred to as the monoclonal protein, or M-protein. This protein serves as a very useful marker to monitor the extent of disease and the patient's response to therapy. It is measured by serum or urine protein electrophoresis. Moreover, the patient's total protein level is typically elevated, again due to the production of monoclonal immunoglobulin protein. Occasionally the plasma cells infiltrate other tissue; this infiltration is referred to as plasmacytoma. Plasmacytomas can occur in the sinuses, spinal cord, and soft tissues. Median survival is 3 to 5 years. Death usually results from infection.

Clinical Manifestations

The classic presenting symptom of multiple myeloma is bone pain, usually in the back or ribs. Bone pain is reported by two thirds of all patients at diagnosis. Unlike arthritic pain, the bone pain associated with myeloma increases with movement and decreases with rest: patients may report that they have less pain on awakening but the pain intensity increases during the day. This pain is due to a substance secreted by the plasma cells, osteoclast activating factor, that stimulates bone breakdown. Thus, lytic lesions as well as osteoporosis may be seen on bone x-rays (they are not well visualized on bone scans). The bone destruction can be severe enough to cause fractures, including spinal fractures, which can impinge on the spinal cord and result in spinal cord compression.

Nursing Alert *Any elderly patient whose chief complaint is back pain, and who has an elevated total protein level, should be evaluated for possible myeloma.*

If the bone destruction is fairly extensive, excessive ionized calcium is lost from the bone and enters the serum; patients may therefore become hypercalcemic (frequently manifested by excessive thirst, dehydration, constipation, altered mental status, confusion, and potential coma). Renal failure may also be seen; the configuration of the immunoglobulin molecule (particularly the shape of lambda light chains) can damage the renal tubules.

As more and more malignant plasma cells are produced, the marrow has less space for red cell production, and the patient can become anemic. This anemia is also due to a great extent to a diminished production of erythropoietin by the kidney (a glycoprotein necessary for RBC production). Patients complain of fatigue and weakness, due to the anemia. In the late stage of the disease, a reduced number of leukocytes and platelets may also be seen because the bone marrow is infiltrated by malignant plasma cells.

Assessment and Diagnostic Findings

Finding an elevated monoclonal protein spike in the serum (via serum protein electrophoresis) or urine (via urine protein electrophoresis) or light chain in the urine (sometimes referred to as Bence Jones protein) is considered to be a major criterion in the diagnosis of multiple myeloma. The presence of lytic bone lesions on x-ray aids in the diagnosis, as does the presence of anemia or hypercalcemia. The diagnosis of myeloma can also be confirmed by bone marrow biopsy, where the presence of sheets of plasma cells is the hallmark diagnostic criterion. Because the infiltration of the marrow by these malignant plasma cells is not uniform, the extent of plasma cells may not be increased in a given sample (a false-negative result).

Gerontologic Considerations

The incidence of multiple myeloma increases with age; the disease rarely occurs in patients younger than 40. Because of the increasing older population, more patients are seeking treatment for this disease. Bone marrow transplantation is an option that can prolong remission and potentially cure some patients. However, it is unavailable to most because of age limitations. Back pain, which is often a presenting symptom in this disease, should be closely investigated in elderly patients.

Medical Management

There is no cure for multiple myeloma. Even bone marrow transplantation is considered by most authorities to extend remission rather than provide a cure. However, for many patients, it is possible to control the illness and maintain their level of functioning quite well for an extended period of time (several years or more). Chemotherapy is the primary mode of treatment; corticosteroids (particularly dexamethasone) are especially effective and are often combined with other agents (eg, melphalan, cyclophosphamide, doxorubicin, vincristine, and BCNU).

Radiation therapy is very useful in strengthening a specific bone lesion, particularly one at risk for bone fracture, or spinal cord compression; it is also useful in relieving bone pain and reducing the size of plasma cell tumors that occur outside the skeletal system. However, because it is a nonsystemic form of treatment, it will not diminish the source of the bone problems (ie, the production of malignant plasma cells). Thus, radiation therapy is typically used in conjunction with systemic treatment, such as chemotherapy.

The biologic agent alpha-interferon has been successful in maintaining remission in select types of myeloma. Newer forms of biphosphonates (eg, pamidronate) have been shown to strengthen bone (by diminishing the secretion of osteoclast activating factor) in this disease, controlling bone pain and potentially preventing bone fracture. They are also effective in managing and preventing hypercalcemia. Some evidence suggests that pamidronate may actually have activity against the myeloma cells themselves.

Nursing Management

Pain management is very important in this patient population. NSAIDs can be very useful for mild pain, or with opioid analgesics. However, care needs to be taken when using NSAIDs because they can cause renal dysfunction. Patients need to be educated about activity restrictions (eg, lifting no more than 10 pounds, proper body mechanics). Braces are occasionally needed to provide support to the spinal column.

Patients also need to be educated about the signs and symptoms of hypercalcemia. Maintaining mobility and hydration is important to diminish exacerbations of this complication; however, the primary cause is the disease itself. Renal function should also be monitored closely: renal failure can become severe, and dialysis may be needed.

Because antibody production is impaired, infections, particularly bacterial infections, are common and can be life-threatening. Patients need to be instructed in appropriate infection prevention measures (see Chart 30-6) and should be advised to contact their health care provider immediately if they have a fever or other signs and symptoms of infection.

BLEEDING DISORDERS

Normal hemostatic mechanisms can control bleeding from vessels and prevent spontaneous bleeding. When bleeding occurs, the severed vessel constricts and platelets aggregate at the site, forming an unstable hemostatic plug. Circulating coagulation factors are activated on the surface of these aggregated platelets, forming fibrin, which anchors the platelet plug to the site of injury.

The failure of normal hemostatic mechanisms can result in bleeding, which is severe at times. This bleeding is commonly provoked by trauma, but in certain circumstances it can occur spontaneously. When the source is platelet or coagulation factor abnormalities, the site of spontaneous bleeding can be anywhere in the body. When the defect is due to vascular abnormalities, the site of bleeding may be more localized. Some patients can have defects in more than one hemostatic mechanism simultaneously.

In a variety of situations, the bone marrow may be stimulated to increase platelet production (thrombopoiesis). The increased production may be a reactive response, as in a compensatory response to significant bleeding, or a more general response to increase hematopoiesis, as in iron-deficiency anemia. Sometimes, the increase in platelets does not result from increased production but from a loss in platelet pooling within the spleen. The spleen typically holds about one third of the circulating platelets at any time. When the spleen is lost (eg, splenectomy), the platelet reservoir is also lost, and an abnormally high amount of platelets enter the circulation. In time, the rate of thrombopoiesis slows to reestablish a more normal platelet level.

Clinical Manifestations

Signs and symptoms of bleeding disorders vary depending on the type of defect. A careful history and physical examination can be very useful in differentiating the source of the hemostatic defect. Abnormalities of the vascular system give rise to local bleeding, usually into the skin. Because platelets are primarily responsible for stopping bleeding from small vessels, patients with platelet defects develop petechiae, often in clusters; these are seen on the skin and mucous membranes but also occur throughout the body. Bleeding from platelet disorders can be highly significant. Unless the platelet disorder is severe, bleeding can often be stopped promptly when local pressure is applied; it does not typically recur when the pressure is released.

In contrast, coagulation factor defects do not tend to cause superficial bleeding because the primary hemostatic mechanisms are still intact. Instead, bleeding occurs deeper within the body, such as subcutaneous or intramuscular hematomas and hemorrhage into joint spaces. External bleeding diminishes very slowly when local pressure is applied; it often recurs several hours after pressure is removed. For example, severe bleeding may start several hours after a tooth extraction.

Medical Management

Management varies based on the underlying cause of the bleeding disorder. If bleeding is significant, transfusions of blood products are indicated. The specific blood product used is determined by the underlying defect. In specific situations where fibrinolysis is excessive, hemostatic agents such as aminocaproic acid (Amicar) can be used to inhibit this process. This agent must be used with caution because excessive inhibition of fibrinolysis can result in thrombosis.

Nursing Management

Patients who have bleeding disorders or who have the potential for developing such disorders as a result of disease or therapeutic agents must be taught to observe themselves carefully and frequently for bleeding. The skin is observed for petechiae and ecchymoses (bruises) and the nose and gums for bleeding. Hospitalized patients may be monitored for bleeding by testing all drainage and excreta (feces, urine, emesis, and gastric drainage) for occult as well as obvious blood. Outpatients are often given fecal occult blood screening cards to detect occult blood in stools.

Primary Thrombocythemia

Primary thrombocythemia (also called essential thrombocythemia) is a stem cell disorder within the bone marrow. Although the exact cause is unknown, it is similar to other myeloproliferative disorders, particularly polycythemia vera. The platelet count is consistently greater than 600,000/mm^3. Platelet size may be abnormal. Occasionally the platelet increase is accompanied by an increase in RBCs and/or WBCs; however, these cells are not increased to the extent that they are in polycythemia vera, CML, or myelofibrosis.

Clinical Manifestations

Many patients with primary thrombocythemia are asymptomatic; the illness is diagnosed as the result of finding an elevated platelet count on a CBC. Symptoms, when they do occur, result primarily from hemorrhage or vasoocclusion in the microvasculature. Symptoms may occur more when the platelet count exceeds 1 million/mm^3. However, symptoms do not always correlate with the extent to which the platelet count is elevated. Hemorrhage can be minor or major; it reflects platelet dysfunction. Bleeding from the mucous membranes of the nose and mouth is not uncommon, and significant gastrointestinal bleeding is also possible.

Vasoocclusive manifestations are most frequently seen in the form of erythromyalgia. Here, the toxic effects of platelet substances may induce painful burning, warmth, and redness in a localized distal area of the extremities. Neurologic manifestations may also be seen, such as numbness, tingling, and visual disturbance; these occlusive manifestations can progress to stroke and seizure and, less commonly, myocardial infarction. The spleen may be enlarged but usually not to a significant extent.

Assessment and Diagnostic Findings

As with other hematologic illnesses, the diagnosis of primary thrombocythemia is made by ruling out other potential causes. Iron deficiency should be excluded because a reactive increase in the platelet count often accompanies this deficiency. The myeloproliferative disorders identified above should also be excluded. Examining the CBC and other blood test results can frequently do this; analysis of the bone marrow (by aspiration and biopsy) is not usually necessary to establish the diagnosis. The disease, which affects men and women equally, tends to occur in late middle age. The median survival exceeds 10 years.

Medical Management

The management of primary thrombocythemia is highly controversial. Many studies (eg, Cortelazzo et al., 1995) show that the risk of significant thrombotic or hemorrhagic complications is not increased until the platelet count exceeds 1 million, and that earlier treatment is unnecessary. A careful assessment of other risk factors, such as history of peripheral vascular disease, smoking history, atherosclerosis, and prior thrombotic events, should be used in the decision of when to initiate therapy. In younger patients with no risk factors, low-dose aspirin therapy may be sufficient to prevent thrombotic complications; however, the use of aspirin can increase the risk for hemorrhagic complications.

More aggressive measures may be required in older patients or those with concurrent risk factors. Hydroxyurea is a chemotherapeutic agent that is very effective in lowering the platelet count. It is taken orally and causes minimal side effects, other than dose-related leukopenia. However, its potential for leukemogenesis is in question. The medication anagrelide is more specific in lowering the platelet count than hydroxyurea, but it has more side effects. Severe headaches cause many patients to stop taking the medication. Tachycardia and chest pain may also occur; anagrelide is contraindicated in patients with concurrent cardiac problems. Alpha-interferon has been shown to lower platelet counts by an unknown mechanism. The medication is administered subcutaneously at varying frequency; three times weekly is common. Interferon is very expensive. Significant side effects, such as fatigue, weakness, memory defects, dizziness, anemia, and liver dysfunction, limit its usefulness.

Rarely, the occlusive symptoms are so great that the platelet count must be reduced immediately. Platelet pheresis (see below) can reduce the amount of circulating platelets, but only transiently.

Nursing Management

Patients with primary thrombocythemia need to be educated about the accompanying risks of hemorrhage and thrombosis. Patients should be educated about signs and symptoms of thrombosis, particularly the neurologic manifestations, such as visual changes, numbness, tingling, and weakness. Risk factors for thrombosis should be assessed; measures to diminish any risk factors should be encouraged (eg, smoking cessation). Patients receiving aspirin therapy should be taught about the increased risk for bleeding. Patients at risk for bleeding should be taught about medications that can alter platelet function, such as aspirin, NSAIDs, and alcohol. Patients receiving interferon therapy should be taught how to self-administer the medication and manage side effects.

Secondary Thrombocytosis

Increased platelet production is the primary mechanism of secondary, or reactive, **thrombocytosis**. The platelet count is above normal, but unlike primary thrombocythemia an increase above 1 million/mm^3 is rare. Platelet function is normal; the platelet survival time is normal or decreased. Symptoms associated with hemorrhage or thrombosis are rare. Many disorders can cause a reactive increase in platelets. These include chronic inflammatory disorders, iron deficiency, malignant disease, acute hemorrhage, and splenectomy (see the section on primary thrombocythemia). Treatment is aimed at the underlying disorder. With successful management, the platelet count usually returns to normal.

Thrombocytopenia

Thrombocytopenia (low platelet level) can result from various factors: decreased production of platelets within the bone marrow, increased destruction of platelets, or increased consumption of platelets. Causes and treatments are summarized in Table 30-6.

Clinical Manifestations

Bleeding and petechiae usually do not occur with platelet counts above 50,000/mm^3, although excessive bleeding can follow surgery or other trauma. When the platelet count drops below 20,000, petechiae can appear, along with nose and gingival bleeding, excessive menstrual bleeding, and excessive bleeding after surgery or dental extractions. When the platelet count is less than 5000, spontaneous, potentially fatal central nervous system or gastrointestinal hemorrhage can occur. If the platelets are dysfunctional due to disease (eg, MDS) or medications (eg, aspirin), the risk of bleeding may be much greater even when the actual platelet count is not significantly reduced.

Assessment and Diagnostic Findings

A platelet deficiency that results from decreased production (eg, leukemia, MDS) can usually be diagnosed by examining the bone marrow (aspiration and biopsy). When platelet destruction is the

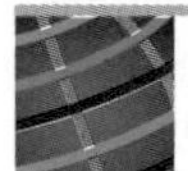

TABLE 30•6 Causes and Management of Thrombocytopenia

Cause	Management
Decreased Production	
Hematologic malignancy, especially acute leukemias	Treat leukemia; platelet transfusion
Myelodysplastic syndromes (MDS): metastatic involvement of bone marrow from solid tumors	Treat MDS; platelet transfusion Treat solid tumor
Aplastic anemia	Treat underlying condition
Megaloblastic anemia	Treat underlying anemia
Toxins	Remove toxin
Medications	Stop medication
Infection (esp. septicemia, viral infection, TB)	Treat infection
Alcohol	Refrain from alcohol consumption
Chemotherapy	Delay or decrease dose; platelet transfusion
Increased Destruction	
Due to Antibodies	Treat condition
ITP	
Lupus erythematosus	
Malignant lymphoma	
CLL	Treat CLL and/or treat as ITP
Medications	Stop medication
Due to Infection	Treat infection
Bacteremia	
Postviral infection	
Sequestration of platelets in enlarged spleen	If thrombocytopenia severe, may need splenectomy
Increased Consumption	
Disseminated intravascular coagulopathy (DIC)	Treat underlying condition triggering DIC; administer heparin, EACA, blood products

cause of thrombocytopenia, the marrow shows increased megakaryocytes (the cells from which the platelets originate) and normal or even increased platelet production as the body attempts to compensate for the decreased platelets in circulation.

Medical Management

The management for secondary thrombocytopenia is usually treatment of the underlying disease. If platelet production is impaired, platelet transfusions may raise platelet counts and stop bleeding or prevent spontaneous hemorrhage. If excessive platelet destruction occurs, transfused platelets will also be destroyed, and the platelet count will not rise. The most common cause of excessive platelet destruction is idiopathic thrombocytopenic purpura.

Nursing Management

The interventions to be taken in caring for a patient with thrombocytopenia are delineated in Chart 30-7.

Idiopathic Thrombocytopenic Purpura (ITP)

ITP is a disease that affects people of all ages, but it is more common among children and young women. There are two forms of ITP: acute and chronic. In the acute form, which occurs predominately in children, the disease is self-limiting, often 1 to 6 weeks after a viral illness. Remissions can occur spontaneously; occasionally corticosteroids may be needed for a brief time. Chronic ITP is often diagnosed by excluding other causes of thrombocytopenia.

Pathophysiology

Although the precise cause remains unknown, viral infections sometimes precede ITP in children. Occasionally medications such as sulfa drugs can induce ITP. Other conditions, such as systemic lupus erythematosus or pregnancy, can also induce ITP. ITP results from circulating antiplatelet autoantibodies that bind to a patient's platelets. When the platelets are bound to these antibodies, the body destroys them, using the RES or tissue macrophage system to ingest the platelets. The body attempts to compensate for this destruction by increasing platelet production within the marrow.

Clinical Manifestations

Many patients have no symptoms, and the low platelet count is an incidental finding. Common manifestations are easy bruising, heavy menses, and petechiae on the extremities or trunk. Patients with simple bruising or petechiae ("dry purpura") tend to have fewer complications from bleeding than those with bleeding from mucosal surfaces, such as the gastrointestinal tract (including the mouth) and pulmonary system (eg, hemoptysis). This phenomenon is termed "wet purpura." Patients with wet purpura have a greater risk for intracranial bleeding than those with dry purpura. Despite low platelet counts (eg, less than 20,000/mm^3; less than 5000 is not uncommon), the platelets are young and very functional in adhering to endothelial surfaces and one another; thus, spontaneous bleeding does not always occur.

Assessment and Diagnostic Findings

Patients may have an isolated decrease in platelets (less than 20,000) but may also have an increase in megakaryocytes (platelet precursors) within the marrow, as detected by bone marrow aspirate.

Medical Management

Treatment for ITP usually requires a combination of approaches. Obviously, if the patient is taking a medication that is known to cause ITP (eg, quinine, sulfa-containing medications), that medication must be stopped immediately. The mainstay of short-term therapy is the use of immunosuppressive agents that block the binding receptors on the macrophages so the platelets are not destroyed. Prednisone is the agent typically used (1 mg/kg) and is effective in about 75% of patients, but cyclophosphamide and azathioprine (Imuran) can also be used. Some studies (eg, Kühne et al., 1996) have found dexamethasone to be more effective in increasing the platelet count and in maintaining that increase longer. Platelet counts rise within a few days with corticosteroids; this effect takes longer with azathioprine. Because of the side effects associated with corticosteroids, patients cannot take high doses of corticosteroids indefinitely. Unfortunately, it is not unusual for the platelet count to drop once the corticosteroid dose is tapered.

Intravenous gamma globulin is also commonly used to treat ITP. It is very effective in binding the receptors on the macrophages, but it requires high doses (1 g/kg for 2 days), is very expensive, and can be difficult to obtain from the manufacturers. Splenectomy is an alternate treatment but results in a normal platelet count only 50% of the time; however, many patients can maintain a "safe" platelet count of more than 30,000 after removal of the spleen. Unfortunately, even for those who do respond to splenectomy, recurrences of severe thrombocytopenia may occur months or years later.

Other options for management include the use of the chemotherapy agent vincristine. Vincristine appears to work by blocking the receptors on the macrophages and therefore inhibiting platelet destruction; it may also stimulate thrombopoiesis as well.

A relatively new approach to the management of chronic ITP involves the use of anti-D in patients who are Rh(D)-positive. The actual mechanism of action is not known; one theory is that the anti-D binds to the patient's RBCs, which are in turn destroyed by the body's macrophages. (One can think of this as a sacrifice of some red cells to permit platelet survival, and in fact there is usually a drop in hematocrit after anti-D is infused.) Anti-D produces a transient increase in platelet counts in many but not all patients with ITP; it appears to be most effective in childhood ITP and least effective in patients who have undergone splenectomy.

Despite the extremely low platelet count, platelet transfusions are usually avoided. They tend to be ineffective because the transfused platelets bind to the antiplatelet antibodies and are subsequently destroyed. Platelet counts can actually drop after platelet transfusion. However, transfusion of platelets may help protect against catastrophic bleeding in patients with severe wet purpura.

Nursing Management

Nursing care for these patients should include obtaining a careful medication history, including over-the-counter medications. The nurse must be alert for sulfa-containing medications and medications that alter platelet function (medications that contain aspirin or other NSAIDs). The nurse should assess any history of recent viral illness and complaints of headache or visual disturbances that could be initial symptoms of intracranial bleeding. Patients admitted to the hospital with wet purpura and low platelet counts should have a neurologic assessment incorporated into their routine vital sign measurements. No intramuscular injections or rectal medications should be given, because the administration techniques can stimulate bleeding.

Patient teaching should address signs of exacerbation of disease (petechiae, ecchymoses); how to contact appropriate health care personnel; the name and type of medication inducing ITP (if appropriate); current medical treatment (medications, tapering schedule if relevant, side effects); and the frequency of platelet count monitoring. Patients should be instructed to avoid all medications that interfere with platelet function. The patient should avoid constipation, the Valsalva maneuver (eg, straining at stool), and flossing teeth. Electric razors should be used for shaving, and soft-bristled toothbrushes should replace stiff-bristled ones. Patients should also be counseled to refrain from vigorous sexual intercourse when the platelet count is less than 10,000/mm^3.

OTHER BLEEDING DISORDERS

Platelet Defects

Quantitative platelet defects are relatively common (thrombocytopenia), but qualitative defects can also occur. With qualitative defects, the number of platelets may be normal; however, the platelets cannot function normally. Platelet function is most commonly evaluated by the bleeding time; however, this test is a crude measurement at best.

An important functional platelet disorder is that induced by aspirin. Even small amounts of aspirin prevent normal platelet aggregation, and the bleeding time is prolonged for several days after aspirin ingestion. Although this defect does not cause bleeding in most people, patients with another coagulation disorder (eg, hemophilia) or thrombocytopenia can have significant bleeding after taking aspirin, particularly if invasive procedures or other trauma are involved.

NSAIDs can also inhibit platelet function, but the effect is not as prolonged as with aspirin (about 5 days versus 7 to 10 days). Other causes of platelet dysfunction include end-stage renal disease, possibly from metabolic products affecting platelet function; MDS; multiple myeloma (due to abnormal protein interfering with platelet function); cardiopulmonary bypass; and other medications.

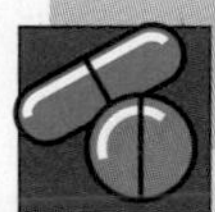

PHARMACOLOGY

Substances that Impair Platelet Function

- Anesthetic agents
  local
  halothane
- Antibiotics
  beta-lactams
    penicillins
    cephalosporins
  nitrofurantoin
  sulfonylureas
- Anticoagulation agents
  heparin
  fibrinolytic agents
- Nonsteroidal anti-inflammatory drugs (NSAIDs)
  aspirin
  ibuprofen
  naproxen
- Antineoplastic agents
  BCNU
  daunorubicin
  mithramycin
- Cardiovascular drugs
  beta blockers
  calcium channel blockers
  isosorbide
  nitroglycerine
  nitroprusside
  quinidine
- Medications that increase platelet cAMP
  caffeine
  dipyridamole
  prostacycline
  theophylline
- Food and food additives
  alcohol
  caffeine
  chinese black tree fungus
  clove
  cumin
  fish oils
  garlic
  onion extract
  turmeric
- Plasma expanders
  dextrans
  hydroxyethyl starch
- Psychotropic agents
  tricyclic antidepressants
  phenothiazines
- Miscellaneous
  antihistamines
  clofibrate
  furosemide
  heroin
  contrast agents
  ticlopidine
  vitamin E

Clinical Manifestations

Bleeding may be mild or severe. Its extent is not necessarily correlated with the platelet count or with tests that measure coagulation (prothrombin time, partial thromboplastin time). Ecchymoses are common, particularly on the extremities. Patients with platelet dysfunction are at risk for significant bleeding after trauma or invasive procedures (eg, biopsy, dental extraction).

Medical Management

Bleeding can often be prevented by transfusing normal platelets before invasive procedures. If the platelet dysfunction is due to medication, use of the offending medication needs to be stopped.

Nursing Management

Patients with significant platelet dysfunction need to be instructed to avoid medications that can diminish platelet function, such as over-the-counter medications and alcohol. They also need to be assisted to serve as their own advocates and to inform their health care providers (including dentists) of the underlying problem before any invasive procedure so that appropriate steps can be initiated to diminish the risk of bleeding. Bleeding precautions should be initiated as appropriate (see Chart 30-7).

Hemophilia

Two hereditary bleeding disorders are clinically indistinguishable but can be distinguished by laboratory tests: hemophilia A and hemophilia B. Hemophilia A is due to a genetic defect causing deficient or defective factor VIII; hemophilia B stems from a genetic defect resulting in deficient or defective factor IX. Hemophilia is a relatively rare disease; hemophilia A, which occurs in 1 : 10,000 births, is three times more common than hemophilia B. Both types of hemophilia are inherited as X-linked traits, so almost all affected people are males; females can be carriers but are almost always asymptomatic. The disease is recognized in early childhood, usually in the toddler age group. However, patients with mild hemophilia may not be diagnosed until the onset of severe trauma (eg, a high-school football injury) or surgery. Hemophilia occurs in all ethnic groups.

TABLE 30•7 Severity of Hemophilia*

Classification	Factor VIII Level (normal = 100%)	Clinical Problem
Severe	<1%	Spontaneous hemorrhages, particularly hemarthroses; hematomas; frequent factor replacement therapy required
Moderate	1%–5%	Hemorrhage secondary to trauma; spontaneous hemarthroses less common
Mild	6%–50%	Spontaneous hemorrhage rare; hemorrhage secondary to trauma

*Hemophilia is typically classified as mild, moderate, or severe, based on the degree of factor VIII deficiency. Related clinical problems vary with the severity of the deficiency.

Clinical Manifestations

The disease, which may be very severe, is manifested by hemorrhages into various parts of the body. Hemorrhage can occur even after minimal trauma. The frequency and severity of the bleeding depend on the degree of factor deficiency as well as the intensity of the precipitating trauma (Table 30-7).

About 75% of all bleeding occurs into joints. The most commonly affected joints are the knees, elbows, ankles, shoulders, wrists, and hips. Patients often note pain in a joint before they are aware of swelling and limitation of motion. Recurrent joint hemorrhages can result in damage so severe that chronic pain or ankylosis (fixation) of the joint occurs. Many patients with severe factor deficiency are crippled by the joint damage before they become adults. Hematomas (hemorrhages into muscle or subcutaneous tissue) can be superficial or deep. With severe factor deficiency, they can occur without known trauma and progressively extend in all directions. When the hematomas occur within muscle, particularly in the extremities, peripheral nerves can be compressed. Over time, this compression can result in decreased sensation, weakness, and atrophy of the area involved. Spontaneous hematuria and gastrointestinal bleeding can occur. Bleeding is also common in other mucous membranes, such as the nasal passages. The most dangerous site of hemorrhage is within the head (intracranial or extracranial). Any head trauma requires prompt evaluation and treatment. Surgical procedures typically result in excessive bleeding at the surgical site. Because clot formation is poor, wound healing is also poor. The most common type of such bleeding is that associated with dental extraction.

Medical Management

In the past, the only treatment for hemophilia was infusion of fresh-frozen plasma, which had to be administered in such large quantities that the patients experienced fluid volume overload. Now factor VIII and IX concentrates are available to all blood banks. Patients are given concentrates when they are actively bleeding or as a preventive measure before traumatic procedures, such as lumbar punctures, dental extractions, or surgery. The patient and family are taught how to administer the concentrate intravenously at home at the first sign of bleeding. It is crucial to initiate treatment as soon as possible so that bleeding complications can be avoided. A few patients eventually develop antibodies to the concentrates, so their factor levels cannot be increased. Treatment of this problem is extremely difficult and often unsuccessful.

Aminocaproic acid (Amicar) is a fibrinolytic enzyme inhibitor that can slow the dissolution of blood clots that do form; it is very effective as an adjunctive measure after oral surgery. It is also useful in treating mucosal bleeding in patients with hemophilia. Another agent, DDAVP (desmopressin), induces a transient rise in factor VIII levels; the mechanism for this response is not known. In patients with mild forms of hemophilia A, DDAVP is extremely useful, significantly reducing the amount of blood products required. However, DDAVP is not effective in patients with severe factor VIII deficiency.

Nursing Management

Most patients with hemophilia are diagnosed as children. These patients often require assistance in coping with the condition because it is chronic, places restrictions on their lives, and is an inherited disorder that can be passed to future generations. From childhood, patients are helped to accept themselves and the disease and to identify the positive aspects of their lives. They are encouraged to be self-sufficient and to maintain independence by preventing unnecessary trauma that can cause acute bleeding episodes and temporarily interfere with normal activities. As they work through their feelings about the condition and progress to accepting it, they can assume more and more responsibility for maintaining optimal health.

Patients with mild factor deficiency may not be diagnosed until adulthood if they do not experience significant trauma or surgery as children. These patients need extensive teaching about activity restrictions and self-care measures to diminish the chance of hemorrhage and complications of bleeding. The nurse should emphasize safety at home and in the workplace.

Patients with hemophilia must be instructed to avoid any medication that interferes with platelet aggregation, such as aspirin, NSAIDs, or alcohol. This restriction should be applied to over-the-counter medications such as cold remedies. Dental hygiene is very important as a preventive measure because dental extractions can be so hazardous. Applying pressure may be sufficient to control bleeding resulting from minor trauma if the factor deficiency is not severe. Nasal packing should be avoided because bleeding frequently resumes when the packing is removed. Splints and other orthopedic devices may be useful in patients with joint or muscle hemorrhages. All injections should be avoided; invasive procedures should be minimized or performed after administering appropriate factor replacement (eg, before endoscopy, lumbar puncture). Patients with hemophilia should be encouraged to carry or wear medical identification.

During hemorrhagic episodes, the extent of bleeding must be assessed carefully. Patients at risk for significant compromise (eg, bleeding into the respiratory tract or brain) warrant close observation and systematic assessment for emergent complications (eg, respiratory distress, altered level of consciousness). If the patient had recent surgery, the nurse frequently and carefully assesses the surgical site for bleeding. Frequent vital signs monitoring may be needed until the nurse is certain that there is no excessive postoperative bleeding. Analgesics are commonly required to alleviate the pain associated with hematomas and hemorrhage into joints. Many patients report that warm baths promote relaxation, improve mobility, and lessen pain. However, during bleeding episodes, heat, which can cause bleeding, is avoided; applications of cold are used instead.

Although recent technology (ie, the formulation of heat-treated or solvent- or detergent-treated factor concentrates) has rendered factor VIII and IX preparations free from viral infections (eg, HIV, hepatitis), many patients have already been exposed to these infections. These patients and their families may need assistance in coping with the diagnosis and the consequences of these infections.

In a significant portion (15% hemophilia A, 5% hemophilia B) of patients with severe hemophilia requiring frequent infusions of factor concentrate, antibodies to factor concentrates develop. This, of course, complicates factor replacement management. Patients with severe factor deficiency should be screened for antibodies (inhibitors), particularly before major surgery.

von Willebrand's Disease

von Willebrand's disease, a common bleeding disorder affecting males and females equally, is usually inherited as a dominant trait. The disease is due to a deficiency of von Willebrand factor (vWF), which is necessary for factor VIII activity. vWF is also necessary for platelet adhesion at the site of vascular injury. Although synthesis of factor VIII is normal, its half-life is shortened; hence, factor VIII levels are commonly mildly low (15% to 50% of normal).

Clinical Manifestations

Although they do not suffer from massive soft tissue or joint hemorrhages, patients commonly have nosebleeds, excessively heavy menses, bleeding from cuts, and postoperative bleeding. However, as the laboratory values fluctuate, so does the actual bleeding. For example, a careful history of prior bleeding may reveal little problem with postoperative bleeding but significant bleeding from a dental extraction.

Assessment and Diagnostic Findings

Laboratory test results show a normal platelet count but prolonged bleeding time and slightly prolonged partial thromboplastin time. These defects are not static; thus, laboratory test results can vary widely within the same patient over time.

Medical Management

Both the factor deficiency and the platelet impairment can be corrected by administering cryoprecipitate, which contains factor VIII, fibrinogen, and factor XIII (or fresh-frozen plasma, if cryoprecipitate is unavailable). Replacement continues for several days to ensure correction of the factor VIII deficiency; up to 7 to 10 days may be necessary after major surgery. Desmopressin (DDAVP), a synthetic vasopressin analogue, can be used to prevent bleeding associated with dental or surgical procedures or to manage mild bleeding after surgery. DDAVP provides a transient increase in factor VIII coagulant activity and may also correct the bleeding time. It can be administered as an intravenous infusion or intranasally. With major surgery or invasive procedures, both DDAVP and cryoprecipitate may be needed to prevent hemorrhage.

ACQUIRED COAGULATION DISORDERS

Liver Disease

With the exception of factor VIII, most blood coagulation factors are synthesized in the liver. Therefore, hepatic dysfunction (due to cirrhosis, tumor, or hepatitis) can result in diminished amounts of the factors needed for maintaining coagulation and hemostasis. Prolongation of the prothrombin time, unless it is due to vitamin K deficiency, may indicate severe hepatic dysfunction. Although minor bleeding is common (eg, ecchymoses), these patients are also at risk for significant bleeding, related especially to trauma or surgery. Transfusion of fresh-frozen plasma may be required to replace clotting factors and prevent or stop bleeding. They may also have life-threatening hemorrhage from peptic ulcers or esophageal varices. In these cases, replacement with fresh-frozen plasma, RBCs, and platelets is usually required.

Vitamin K Deficiency

The synthesis of many coagulation factors depends on vitamin K. Vitamin K deficiency is typical in malnourished patients, but some antibiotics are also known to deplete vitamin K stores by decreasing the intestinal flora that produces vitamin K. Administering vitamin K (typically as a subcutaneous injection) can correct the deficiency quickly; adequate synthesis of coagulation factors is reflected in a normalization of the prothrombin time.

Complications of Anticoagulant Therapy

Anticoagulants are used in the treatment or prevention of thrombosis. Excessive amounts of these agents, particularly warfarin or heparin, can result in bleeding. If excessive amounts of the agents are administered and bleeding has not occurred, the overdose can be managed by withholding additional medication. If severe, vitamin K is administered for warfarin toxicity; protamine sulfate is rarely needed for heparin toxicity, because the half-life of heparin is very short. With significant bleeding, fresh-frozen plasma is needed to replace the vitamin K-dependent coagulation factors. Other complications of anticoagulant therapy are discussed in Chapter 28.

Disseminated Intravascular Coagulopathy

Disseminated intravascular coagulopathy (DIC) is not a disease but rather a sign of a serious underlying disease mechanism. It is potentially life-threatening.

Pathophysiology

In DIC, the normal hemostatic mechanisms are altered so that an excessive formation of tiny clots exists within the microcirculation. When the intravascular thrombosis is extensive and uninhibited, initially the coagulation time is shortened. However, as the platelets and clotting factors are consumed to form the microthrombi, coagulation eventually fails. Thus, the paradoxical result of excessive clotting is bleeding. The clinical manifestations of DIC are reflected in the organs affected either by excessive clot formation (with resultant ischemia to that organ or part of organ) or bleeding. This bleeding is characterized by low platelet and fibrinogen levels; prolonged prothrombin time, partial thromboplastin time, and thrombin time; and elevated fibrin degradation products (D-dimers) (Table 30-8).

In DIC, the mortality rate can exceed 80%. Recognizing patients at risk for DIC and the early clinical manifestations of this syndrome may ensure earlier medical intervention, which can improve the prognosis. However, the primary prognostic factor is the ability to treat the underlying disease that precipitated DIC.

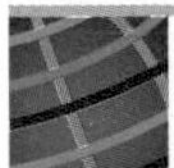

TABLE 30•8 Laboratory Values Commonly Found in DIC

Test	Function Evaluated	Normal Range	Ranges in DIC
Platelet count	Platelet number	150,000–450,000/mm^3	↓
Prothrombin time (PT)	Extrinsic pathway	11–12.5 sec	↑
Partial thromboplastin time (PTT)	Intrinsic pathway	23–35 sec	↑
Thrombin time (TT)	Clot formation	8–11 sec	↑
Fibrinogen	Amount available for coagulation	170–340 mg/dL	↓
D-dimer	Local fibrinolysis	0–250 ng/mL	Normal, if initially high; eventually >500 ng/mL
Fibrin degradation products (FDPs)	Fibrinolysis	0–5 μg/mL	↑
Euglobulin clot lysis	Fibrinolytic activity	≥2 hours	≤1 hour

* Because DIC is a dynamic disease state, the laboratory values measured here will change over time. Thus, a progressive increase or decrease in a given laboratory value is likely to be more important than the actual value of a test at a single point in time.

Clinical Manifestations

Patients with DIC may bleed from mucous membranes, venipuncture sites, and the gastrointestinal and urinary tracts. The bleeding can range from minimal occult internal bleeding to profuse hemorrhage from all orifices. Patients may also develop organ dysfunction, such as renal failure and pulmonary and multifocal central nervous system infarctions due to micro- and/or macrothromboses or hemorrhages.

Many serious illnesses may predispose a patient to DIC, including septicemia, premature separation of the placenta in pregnancy, metastatic malignancies, hemolytic transfusion reactions, massive tissue trauma, and shock. During the initial process of diffuse intravascular thrombosis, the patient has no new symptoms; the only manifestation is a progressive decrease in the platelet count. As the thrombosis becomes more extensive, the patient exhibits signs and symptoms of thrombosis in the organs involved. Then, as the clotting factors and platelets are consumed to form these thrombi, bleeding occurs. Initially the bleeding is subtle, but it can develop into frank hemorrhage. Signs and symptoms depend on the organs involved and are listed in Table 30-9.

Medical Management

The most important management issue is treating the underlying cause of DIC. Until the cause is controlled, the mechanism for DIC will persist. A second goal is to correct the secondary effects of tissue ischemia by improving oxygenation, replacing fluids, and administering vasopressor medications. If serious hemorrhage occurs, the depleted coagulation factors and platelets may be replaced to reestablish the potential for normal hemostasis and thus diminish bleeding. Cryoprecipitate is given to replace fibrinogen and factors V and VII; fresh-frozen plasma is administered to replace other coagulation factors.

A controversial method to interrupt the thrombosis process is the use of heparin infusion. Heparin may inhibit the formation of microthrombi and thus permit perfusion of the organs (skin, kidneys, or brain) to resume. When heparin is administered, bleeding may actually worsen initially until the thrombotic process is interrupted. Consumed platelets and clotting factors need to be replaced. The effectiveness of heparin can best be determined by observing for normalization of the plasma fibrinogen concentration and diminishing signs of bleeding.

An even more controversial management method involves administering fibrinolytic inhibitors, such as aminocaproic acid, which reduces the fibrin degradation products by decreasing the lysis of microthrombi. Aminocaproic acid should be used only with massive bleeding that does not respond to replacement therapy, because the medication keeps the vascular channels occluded with thrombus. Administering this agent is more dangerous if the patient has not been previously treated with heparin.

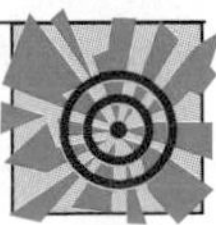

Risk Factors for DISSEMINATED INTRAVASCULAR COAGULATION

- Sepsis
- Viremia
- Cancer (especially acute promyelocytic leukemia and prostatic and pancreatic cancer)
- Trauma
- Acute hemolysis (eg, transfusion reaction)
- Obstetric complications
- Extensive burns or vasculitis

NURSING PROCESS: THE PATIENT WITH DIC

Assessment

Nurses need to be aware of patients at risk for DIC. Sepsis and acute promyelocytic leukemia are the most common causes of DIC. Patients need to be assessed thoroughly and frequently for signs and symptoms of thrombi and/or bleeding and monitored for any progression of these signs (see Table 30-9).

Diagnosis

Nursing Diagnoses

Based on the assessment data, major nursing diagnoses for the patient with DIC may include the following:

- Potential for fluid volume deficit related to bleeding
- Potential for impaired skin integrity related to ischemia or bleeding

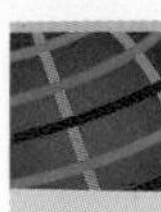

TABLE 30•9 Recognizing Thrombosis and Bleeding in DIC

System	Signs and Symptoms of Microvascular Thrombosis	Signs and Symptoms of Frank Bleeding
Integumentary system (skin)	↓ Temperature, sensation; ↑ pain; cyanosis in extremities, nose, earlobes; focal ischemia, superficial gangrene	Petechiae, including periorbital, oral mucosa; bleeding: gums, oozing from wounds, previous injection sites, around catheters (IVs, tracheostomies); epistaxis; diffuse ecchymoses; subcutaneous hemorrhage; joint pain
Circulatory system:	↓ Pulses; capillary filling time < 3 sec	Tachycardia
Respiratory system:	Hypoxia (secondary to clot in lung); dyspnea; chest pain with deep inspiration; ↓ breath sounds over areas of large embolism	High-pitched bronchial breath sounds; tachypnea; ↑ consolidation; signs and symptoms of acute respiratory distress syndrome
GI system:	Gastric pain; "heartburn"	Hemoptysis (heme⊕ NG output) melana (heme⊕ stools → tarry stools → bright-red blood from rectum) retroperitoneal bleeding (abdomen firm and tender to palpation; distended; ↑ abdominal girth)
Renal system:	↓ Urine output; ↑ creatinine, ↑ blood urea nitrogen	Hematuria
Neurologic system:	↓ Alertness and orientation; ↓ pupillary reaction; ↓ response to commands; ↓ strength and movement ability	Anxiety; restlessness; ↓ mentation, altered level of consciousness; headache; visual disturbances; conjunctival hemorrhage

Note: Signs of microvascular thrombosis are the result of an inappropriate activation of the coagulation system, causing thrombotic occlusion of small vessels within all body organs. As the clotting factors and platelets are consumed, signs of microvascular bleeding appear. This bleeding can quickly extend into frank hemorrhage. Treatment must be aimed at the disorder underlying the DIC; otherwise, the stimulus for the syndrome will persist.

- Potential for fluid volume excess
- Potential for diminished tissue perfusion related to microthrombi
- Fear of the unknown and possible death

Collaborative Problems/Potential Complications

Collaborative problems include the clinical conditions that precipitated the DIC. Based on the assessment data, potential complications can include:

- Renal failure
- Gangrene
- Pulmonary embolism or hemorrhage
- Altered level of consciousness
- Acute respiratory distress syndrome
- Stroke

Planning and Goals

Major patient goals include maintenance of hemodynamic status, intact skin and oral mucosa, maintenance of fluid balance, maintenance of tissue perfusion, enhanced coping, and prevention of complications.

Nursing Interventions

See Plan of Nursing Care 30-1 for nursing interventions, evaluation, and expected outcomes for the patient with DIC.

Monitoring and Managing Potential Complications

Despite aggressive measures, the lack of renal perfusion may result in acute renal failure, sometimes necessitating dialysis. Placement of a large-bore dialysis catheter is extremely hazardous in this patient population and should be accompanied by adequate platelet and plasma transfusions.

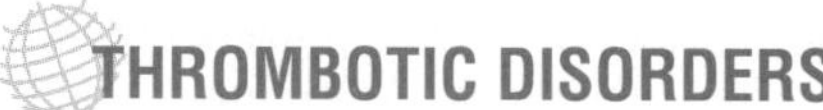

THROMBOTIC DISORDERS

As in many bleeding disorders, several conditions can alter the balance within the normal hemostasis process and cause excessive thrombosis. Abnormalities that predispose a person to thrombotic events involve decreased clotting inhibitors within the circulation (to inactivate coagulation factors), altered hepatic function (which serves to clear the activated coagulation factors), lack of fibrinolytic enzymes, and tortuous vessels (which promote platelet aggregation). Thrombosis can be caused by more than one predisposing factor. Several conditions can result from thrombosis, and many of them are discussed in Chapter 28.

In this chapter, however, several inherited or acquired deficiency conditions are discussed. Inherited conditions include homocystinemia, antithrombin III (ATIII) deficiency, protein C deficiency, activated protein C (APC) resistance and Factor V Leiden, and protein S deficiency. These conditions can predispose a patient to repeated episodes of thrombosis; they are referred to as hypercoaguable states or thrombophilia.

Thrombosis requires anticoagulation therapy. The duration of therapy varies with the location and extent of the thrombosis, precipitating events (eg, trauma, immobilization), and concurrent risk factors (eg, use of oral contraceptives, tortuous blood vessels, history of thrombotic events).

Homocystinemia

Increased plasma levels of homocystine are a significant risk factor for not only venous thrombosis (eg, deep venous thrombosis, pulmonary embolism) but also arterial thrombosis (eg, stroke, myocardial infarction). This disorder can be hereditary, or it can result from a nutritional deficiency of folic acid. In this condition, the endothelial lining of the vessel walls is denuded; this can precipitate unnecessary thrombus formation. Recent studies have identified this disorder as much more common than previously thought. In a long-term epidemiologic study (eg, Rimm et al., 1998) on nurses' health, women who used dietary supplements with folic acid

30•1

PLAN OF NURSING CARE

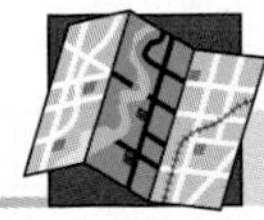

The Patient With DIC

Nursing Diagnosis: Potential for fluid volume deficit related to bleeding

Goals: Hemodynamic status maintained
Urine output ≥ 30 mL/hour

Nursing Interventions	Rationale	Expected Outcomes
1. Avoid procedures/activities that can increase intracranial pressure (eg, coughing, straining to have a bowel movement).	1. Prevents intracranial bleeding.	• Level of consciousness (LOC) stable. PERLA. • CVP 5–12 cm H_2O, systolic BP ≥ 70 mm Hg
2. Monitor vital signs closely, including neurologic checks: a. Monitor hemodynamics b. Monitor abdominal girth c. Monitor urine output	2. Ensures that signs of hemorrhage/shock are identified quickly.	• Urine output > 30 mL/hour • Decreased bleeding • Decreased oozing • Decreased ecchymoses • As above
3. Avoid medications that interfere with platelet function if possible (eg, ASA, NSAIDs, beta-lactam antibiotics).	3. Decreases problems with platelet aggregation and adhesion.	• Amenorrhea • Absence of oral, bronchial bleeding • Oral mucosa clean, moist, intact
4. Avoid rectal probes, rectal medications.	4. Decreases chance for rectal bleeding.	• Absence of bleeding
5. Avoid IM injections.	5. Decreases chance for intramuscular bleeding.	
6. Monitor amount of external bleeding carefully (number of dressings, % dressing is saturated; time to saturate a dressing is more objective than "dressing saturated a moderate amount"): a. Monitor suction output, all excreta b. Monitor pad counts in menstruating females.	6. Provides accurate, objective assessment of extent of bleeding.	
c. Females may receive progesterone to prevent menses.	c. Decreases chance for gynecologic source of hemorrhage.	
7. Use low pressure with any suctioning needed.	7. Prevents excessive trauma that could cause bleeding.	
8. Administer oral hygiene carefully. a. Avoid lemon-glycerine swabs, hydrogen peroxide, commercial mouthwashes. b. Use sponge-tipped swabs, salt/soda mouth rinses.	8. Glycerin and alcohol (in commercial mouthwashes) will dry mucosa, increasing risk for bleeding.	
9. Avoid dislodging any clots, including those around IV sites and injection sites.	9. Prevents excessive bleeding at sites.	

Nursing Diagnosis: Potential for impaired skin integrity secondary to ischemia or bleeding

Goals: Skin integrity remains intact
Oral mucosa remains intact

Nursing Interventions	Rationale	Expected Outcomes
1. Assess skin, with particular attention to bony prominences, skin folds.	1. Prompt identification of any area at risk for skin breakdown or showing early signs of breakdown can facilitate prompt intervention and thus prevent complications.	• Skin integrity remains intact; skin warm, of normal color • Oral mucosa intact, pink, moist, without bleeding
2. Reposition carefully; use pressure-reducing mattress. 3. Perform careful skin care q2h, emphasizing dependent areas, all bony prominences, perineum. 4. Use lamb's wool between digits, around ears, as needed.	2–4. Meticulous skin care and use of measures to prevent pressure on bony prominences decrease the risk of skin trauma.	
5. Use prolonged pressure after injection/procedure when such measures must be performed (at least 5 minutes)	5. Initial platelet plug is very unstable and easily dislodged, which can lead to increased bleeding.	
6. Administer oral hygiene carefully (see above).		

(continued)

30•1

PLAN OF NURSING CARE 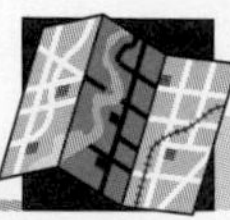 **The Patient With DIC (*continued*)**

Nursing Interventions	Rationale	Expected Outcomes
Nursing Diagnosis: Potential for fluid volume excess **Goals:** Absence of edema Absence of rales Intake not greater than output		
1. Auscultate breath sounds q2–4h.	1. Crackles can develop quickly.	• Breath sounds clear
2. Monitor extent of edema	2. Fluid may extend beyond intravascular system.	• Absence of edema • Intake does not exceed output
3. Monitor volume of IVs, blood products; decrease volume of IV medications if possible.	3. Helps prevent fluid overload.	• Weight stable
4. Administer diuretics as prescribed	4. Decreases fluid volume.	
Nursing Diagnosis: Potential for diminished tissue perfusion secondary to microthrombi **Goals:** Neurologic status remains intact Absence of hypoxemia Peripheral pulses remain intact Skin integrity remains intact Urine output remains ≥ 30 mL/hour		
1. Assess neurologic, pulmonary, integumentry systems.	1. Initial signs of thrombosis can be subtle.	• ABGs, O_2 saturation, pulse oximetry, level of consciousness, within normal limits. Above goals achieved
2. Monitor response to heparin therapy.	2. Response to heparin is most accurately reflected in fibrinogen level.	
3. Assess extent of bleeding.	3. Objective measurements of all sites of bleeding is crucial to accurately assess extent of blood loss.	
4. Monitor fibrinogen levels.	4. Response to heparin is most accurately reflected in fibrinogen level.	
5. Stop e-aminocaproic acid (EACA) if symptoms of thrombosis occur (see Table 30-9).	5. EACA should be used only in setting of extensive hemorrhage not responding to replacement therapy.	
Nursing Diagnosis: Potential for fear of unknown and possible death **Goal:** Fears verbalized/identified Maintain realistic hope		
1. Identify previous coping mechanisms, if possible: a. Encourage patient to use them as appropriate.	1. Identifying previous stressful situations can aid in recall of successful coping mechanisms.	• Previously used coping strategies identified and tried, to extent patient is able • Patient indicates comprehension of procedures, situation as condition permits
2. Explain all procedures and rationale for same in terms patient and family can understand.	2. Decreased knowledge and uncertainty can increase anxiety.	
3. Assist family in supporting patient.	3. Family can be useful in assisting patient to use coping strategies and to maintain hope.	
4. Use services from behavioral medicine, chaplain as needed.	4. Additional professional intervention may be necessary, particularly if previous coping mechanisms are maladaptive or ineffective. Spiritual dimension should not be ignored.	

and vitamin B_6 were found to have a lower incidence of thrombotic conditions such as deep vein thrombosis. Although the role of folic acid deficiency is fairly well known, B_6 and B_{12} deficiency can also be a factor. Patients who are found to have hyperhomocystinemia should receive folic acid, B_6, and/or B_{12} supplements and should be instructed in the rationale for their use to enhance compliance.

Antithrombin III Deficiency

Antithrombin is a protein that inhibits thrombin and certain coagulation factors. ATIII deficiency is a hereditary condition that can cause venous thrombosis, particularly when the level is less than 60% of normal. Patients with ATIII deficiency can develop venous thrombosis as young adults; by age 50, two thirds of these patients have developed a venous thrombosis. There is an increased resistance to heparin anticoagulation, so these patients may require greater amounts of heparin to achieve adequate anticoagulation. Patients with ATIII deficiency should be encouraged to have their family members tested for the deficiency.

Protein C Deficiency

Protein C is an enzyme that, when activated, inhibits coagulation. When levels of protein C are deficient, the risk of thrombosis increases. Protein C deficiency is more common than ATIII deficiency, and people who are protein C-deficient can develop thrombosis early in life, as early as age 15. An interesting and significant complication of anticoagulation management in patients with protein C deficiency is coumarin-induced skin necrosis. This complication appears to result from progressive thrombosis in the capillaries within the skin; the extent of the necrosis can be extreme.

Activated Protein C (APC) Resistance and Factor V Leiden

APC resistance is a common condition that can occur with other hypercoaguable states. APC is an anticoagulant; resistance to APC increases the risk for venous thrombosis. Recently, a molecular defect in the factor V gene has been identified in the majority (90%) of those with APC resistance; this defect is called Factor V Leiden. Factor V Leiden mutation has been identified as the most common cause of inherited hypercoaguability in whites; its incidence appears to be much lower in other ethnic groups. Factor V Leiden mutation synergistically increases the risk for thrombosis in patients with other risk factors (eg, use of oral contraceptives, hyperhomocystinemia, or increased age). It does not appear that the use of estrogen replacement therapy in postmenopausal women increases the risk for thrombotic events as does the use of oral contraceptives; the dose of estrogen in the former situation is much lower than in the latter.

Protein S Deficiency

Protein S is another natural anticoagulant normally produced in the liver. APC requires protein S to inactivate certain clotting factors. When the level of protein S is deficient, this inactivation process is diminished, and the risk for thrombosis can be increased. Like patients with protein C deficiency, those with protein S deficiency have a greater risk for recurrent venous thrombosis at a young age, as young as age 15.

Acquired Thrombophilia

Antibodies to phospholipids are common acquired causes for thrombophilia. The most common antibodies present against phospholipid are either lupus or anticardiolipin antibodies. Both of these antibodies can be transient, resulting from infection or certain medications. Most thrombotic events are venous, but arterial thrombosis can occur in one third of the cases. Patients who persistently test positive for either antibody and who have had a thrombotic event are at significant risk for recurrent thrombosis (more than 50%). Recurrent thromboses tend to be the same type—that is, venous thrombosis after an initial venous thrombosis, arterial thrombosis after an initial arterial thrombosis.

Another common acquired cause for thrombophilia is cancer. Specific types of stomach, pancreatic, lung, and ovarian cancers are most commonly associated with thrombophilia. Here, the type of thrombosis that results is unusual. Rather than deep vein thrombosis or pulmonary embolism, the thrombosis occurs in unusual sites, such as the portal, hepatic, or renal vein or the inferior vena cava. Migratory superficial thrombophlebitis or nonbacterial thrombotic endocarditis can also occur. In these patients, anticoagulation can be difficult to manage in that the thrombosis can progress despite standard amounts of anticoagulation.

Medical Management

The primary method of treating thrombotic disorders remains anticoagulation. However, in thrombophilic conditions, when to treat (prophylaxis or not) and how long to treat (life-long or not) can be controversial. Various agents can be used. The most common anticoagulant medications are identified below. Anticoagulation therapy is not without risks; the most significant is bleeding. Risks of anticoagulation therapy are identified in Chapter 28.

Concomitant with administering anticoagulant therapy is the importance of minimizing any risk factors that predispose a patient to thrombosis. When risk factors (eg, immobility after surgery, pregnancy) cannot be avoided, prophylactic anticoagulation may be necessary.

HEPARIN THERAPY

Heparin is a naturally occurring anticoagulant that enhances ATIII and inhibits platelet function. To prevent thrombosis, heparin is typically given as a subcutaneous injection, two or three times daily. To treat thrombosis, heparin is usually administered intravenously. The therapeutic effect of heparin is monitored by serial measurements of the activated partial prothrombin time; the dose is adjusted to maintain the range at 1.5 to 2.5 times the laboratory control.

LOW-MOLECULAR-WEIGHT HEPARIN THERAPY

Low molecular-weight heparin (LMWH) is a special form of heparin that has a more selective effect on coagulation. Based on its biochemical properties, LMWH has a longer half-life and a less variable anticoagulant response than standard heparin. These differences permit LMWH to be safely administered only once or twice daily, without the need for laboratory monitoring for dose adjustments. In certain conditions, the use of LMWH has allowed anticoagulation therapy to be moved entirely to the outpatient setting. Many patients with uncomplicated deep vein thrombosis are being managed outside the hospital setting. From the patient's perspective, a significant disadvantage to home therapy is that more than one injection may be required for the dose needed. Thus, the patient or family may have to administer multiple injections several times daily.

COUMARIN THERAPY

Coumarin anticoagulants are antagonists of vitamin K and, therefore, interfere with the synthesis of vitamin K-dependent clotting factors. They are bound to albumin, are metabolized in the liver, and have an extremely long half-life. Typically, a patient is treated initially with both heparin (either the standard form or LMWH) and a coumarin. When the International Normalized Ratio (INR) reaches the desired therapeutic range, the heparin is stopped. The dosage required to maintain the therapeutic range (typically using an INR of 2.0 to 3.0) varies widely between and even within patients. Frequent monitoring is extremely important. Coumarin is affected by many medications; consultation with a pharmacist is important to assess the extent to which concurrently administered medications may interact with coumarin.

Nursing Management

Patients with thrombotic disorders should avoid activities that promote circulatory stasis (eg, immobility, crossing the legs). Exercise, especially ambulation, should be performed frequently throughout the day, particularly during long trips by car or plane. Medications that alter platelet aggregation, such as low-strength aspirin, may be prescribed. Some patients require life-long therapy with anticoagulants, such as warfarin (Coumadin).

Patients with thrombotic disorders, particularly those with thrombophilia, should be assessed for concurrent risk factors for thrombosis and should avoid concomitant risk factors if possible. For example, smoking exacerbates the problem and should be avoided.

Just as for other diseases, patients with thrombotic disorders, particularly thrombophilia, should know the name of their specific condition and understand its significance. In many instances, younger patients with thrombophilia may not require prophylactic anticoagulation; however, with increasing age, concomitant risk factors (eg, pregnancy), or subsequent thrombotic events, prophylactic or life-long anticoagulation therapy may be required. Thus, being able to provide the health care provider with an accurate health history can be extremely useful and can help guide the selection of appropriate therapeutic interventions. Patients with hereditary disorders should be encouraged to have their siblings and children tested for the disorder.

When patients with thrombotic disorders are hospitalized, frequent assessments should be performed for signs and symptoms of beginning thrombus formation, particularly in the legs (deep vein thrombosis) and lungs (pulmonary embolism). Ambulation or range-of-motion exercises as well as the use of elastic pressure stockings should be initiated promptly to decrease stasis. Prophylactic anticoagulants are commonly prescribed.

THERAPIES IN BLOOD DISORDERS

Splenectomy

The surgical removal of the spleen (splenectomy) is sometimes necessary after trauma to the abdomen. Because the spleen is very vascular, severe hemorrhage can result if the spleen ruptures. Under such circumstances, splenectomy becomes an emergency procedure.

Splenectomy is also a possible treatment for other hematologic disorders. For example, an enlarged spleen may be the site of excessive destruction of blood cells. When this destruction is life-threatening, surgery may be lifesaving. This is the case in autoimmune hemolytic anemia or ITP when these disorders do not respond to more conservative measures, such as corticosteroid therapy. Some patients with severe anemia due to inherited RBC defects, such as thalassemia, may also benefit from splenectomy.

In general, the mortality rate after splenectomy is low. Laparoscopic splenectomy can be used in selected patients with a resultant decrease in the postoperative morbidity rate. Complications that may result from surgery are atelectasis, pneumonia, abdominal distention, and abscess formation. Although young children are at the highest risk after splenectomy, all age groups are vulnerable to overwhelming lethal infections and should receive pneumococcal vaccine before undergoing this surgical procedure if possible.

Patients are instructed to seek prompt medical attention when even relatively minor symptoms of infection occur. Often, patients with high platelet counts have even higher counts after splenectomy—more than 1 million/mm^3—which can predispose the patient to serious thrombotic or hemorrhagic problems. Fortunately, the increase is transient.

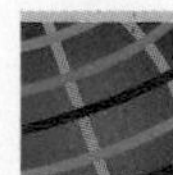

TABLE 30•10 Types of Apheresis

Procedure	Purpose	Examples of Clinical Use
Platelet pheresis	Remove platelets	Extreme thrombocytosis, essential thrombocythemia (temporary measure); single-donor platelets transfusion
Leukapheresis	Remove WBCs (can be specific to neutrophils or lymphocytes)	Extreme leukocytosis (eg, AML, CML) (very temporary measure); harvest WBCs for transfusion
Erythrocytapheresis (RBC exchange)	Remove RBCs	RBC dyscrasias (eg, sickle cell disease); RBCs replaced via transfusion
Plasmapheresis (plasma exchange)	Remove plasma proteins; treatment for some renal and neurologic diseases	Hyperviscosity syndromes (eg, Goodpasture's syndrome), Guillain-Barré

*Therapeutic apheresis can be used to treat a wide variety of conditions. When it is used to treat a disease that causes an increase in a specific cell type with a short life in circulation (ie, WBCs, platelets), the reduction in those cells is temporary. However, this temporary reduction permits a margin of safety while waiting for the effect of a longer-lasting treatment modality (eg, chemotherapy) to take effect.

Therapeutic Apheresis

Apheresis is a Greek word meaning separation. Therapeutic apheresis (or pheresis) simply means that only a specific component of blood is taken (Table 30-10) from the patient and passed through a centrifuge, where the specific component is separated from the blood and removed. The remaining blood is then returned to the patient. The entire system is closed, so the risk of bacterial contamination is extremely low. When platelets or WBCs are removed, the resultant decrease in these cells within the circulation is temporary. However, this temporary decrease permits a somewhat safer interval until therapeutic effects from suppressive medications occur (eg, chemotherapy).

Apheresis is also used to obtain larger amounts of platelets from a donor than can be provided from a single unit of whole blood. A unit of platelets obtained in such a way is equivalent to six to eight units of platelets from six to eight separate donors. WBCs can be obtained similarly, typically after the donor has received growth factors (G-CSF, GM-CSF) to stimulate the formation of additional WBCs and thus to increase the white cell count. Platelet donors can contribute blood cells as often as every 14 days.

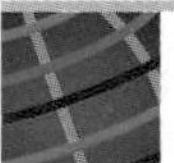

TABLE 30•11 **Blood and Blood Components Commonly Used in Transfusion Therapy**

Component	Composition	Indications and Considerations
Whole blood	Cells and plasma, hematocrit about 40%	Volume replacement and oxygen-carrying capacity; usually used only in significant bleeding (> 25% blood volume lost)
Red blood cells (RBCs)	RBCs with little plasma (hematocrit about 75%); some platelets and WBCs remain	Symptomatic anemia: platelets within the unit are not functional; WBCs within may cause reaction and are not functional ↑ RBC mass
Platelets–random	Platelets (5.5×10^{10} platelets/unit) Plasma; some RBCs, WBCs	Bleeding due to severe ↓ platelets Prevent bleeding when platelets <5000–10,000 Survival ↓ in presence of fever, chills, infection Repeated treatment → ↓ survival due to alloimmunization
Platelets–single donor	Platelets (3×10^{11} platelets/unit) 1 unit is equivalent to 6–8 units random platelets	Used for repeated treatment ↓ alloimmunization risk by limiting exposure to multiple donors
Plasma	Plasma; all coagulation factors Complement	Bleeding in patients with coagulation factor deficiencies; plasmapheresis
Granulocytes (pheresed)	Neutrophils (>1×10^{10}/unit); lymphocytes; some RBCs and platelets	Severe neutropenia in selected patients; stimulate graft-vs.-host disease; controversial
Cryoprecipitate	Fibrinogen ≥ 150 mg/bag, AHF (VIII:C) 80–110 units/bag, von Willebrand factor; fibronectin	von Willebrand's disease Hypofibrinoginemia Hemophilia A
Antihemophilic factor (AHF)	Factor VIII	Hemophilia A
Factor IX concentrate	Factor IX	Hemophilia B
Factor IX complex	Factor II, VII, IX, X	Hereditary factor VII, IX, X deficiency; Hemophilia A with factor VII inhibitors
Albumin	Albumin 5%, 25%	Hypoproteinemia; burns; volume expansion 5% leading to ↑ blood volume; 25% → ↓ hematocrit
Intravenous gamma globulin	IgG antibodies	Hypogammaglobulinemia (in CLL, recurrent infections); ITP; primary immunodeficiency states
Antithrombin III concentrate (ATIII)	ATIII (trace amounts of other plasma proteins)	ATIII deficiency with or at risk for thrombosis

Note: The composition of each type of blood component is described as well as the most common indications for using a given blood component. Red blood cells, platelets, and fresh-frozen plasma are the blood products most commonly used. When transfusing these blood products, the individual product is always "contaminated" with very small amounts of other blood products (eg, WBCs mixed in a unit of platelets). This contamination can cause some difficulties in certain patients.

Therapeutic Phlebotomy

Therapeutic phlebotomy is the removal of a certain amount of blood under controlled conditions. Patients with elevated hematocrits (eg, those with polycythemia vera) or excessive iron absorption (eg, hemochromatosis) can usually be managed by periodically removing 1 unit (about 500 mL) of whole blood. Eventually this process can produce iron deficiency, leaving the patient unable to produce as many RBCs. The actual procedure for therapeutic phlebotomy is similar to that for blood donation (see below).

Blood and Blood Component Therapy

A single unit of whole blood contains 450 mL blood and 50 mL anticoagulant. A unit of whole blood can be processed and dispensed for administration. However, it is more appropriate, economical, and practical to separate that unit of whole blood into its primary components: RBCs, platelets, and plasma. (WBCs are rarely used; see below.) Plasma can be further pooled and processed into blood derivatives, such as albumin, gamma globulin, factor VIII, and factor IX. Each component must be processed and stored differently to maximize the longevity of the viable cells and factors within it. It is for this reason that each individual blood component has a different storage life. RBCs are stored at 4°C. With special preservatives, they can be stored safely for up to 42 days before they must be discarded. In contrast, platelets must be stored at room temperature because they cannot withstand cold temperatures, and they can last for only 5 days before they must be discarded. To prevent clumping, platelets are gently agitated while stored. Plasma is immediately frozen to maintain the activity of the clotting factors within; it can last for 1 year if it remains frozen. Table 30-11 describes each blood component and how it is commonly used.

Special Preparations

Factor VIII concentrate (antihemophilic factor) is a lyophilized, freeze-dried concentrate of pooled fractionated human plasma. It is used in treating hemophilia A. Factor IX concentrate (prothrombin complex) is similarly prepared and contains factors II, VII, IX, and X. It is used primarily for treating patients with factor IX deficiency (hemophilia B, also called Christmas disease). Factor IX concentrate is also useful in treating patients with congenital factor VII and X deficiencies.

Plasma albumin is a large protein molecule that usually stays within vessels and is a major contributor to plasma oncotic pressure. This material is used to expand the blood volume of patients in hypovolemic shock and to elevate the level of circulating albumin in patients with hypoalbuminemia.

Immune globulin is a concentrated solution of the antibody IgG; it contains very little IgA or IgM. It is prepared from large pools of plasma. The intravenous form is used in various clinical situations to replace inadequate amounts in patients at risk for recurrent bacterial infection (eg, those with CLL and those receiving a bone marrow transplant). All of these preparations, in contrast to all other fractions of human blood, cells, or plasma, are subjected to heating at 60°C (140°F) for 10 hours to free them of viral contaminants.

Procuring Blood and Blood Products

BLOOD DONATION

To protect both the donor and the recipients, all prospective donors are examined and interviewed before they are allowed to donate their blood. The intent of the interview is to assess the general health status of the donor and to identify risk factors that might render the donor's blood to be considered contaminated—that is, potentially infected and therefore unable to be used. Donors should be in good health and should be free of any of the following disqualifying factors:

- A history of viral hepatitis, at any time in the past, or a history of close contact with a hepatitis or dialysis patient within 6 months
- A history of receiving a blood transfusion or an infusion of any blood derivative (other than serum albumin) within 6 months
- A history of untreated syphilis or malaria, because these diseases can be transmitted by transfusion even years later. A person who has been free of symptoms and off therapy for 3 years after malaria may be a donor.
- A history or evidence of drug abuse in which substances were self-injected, because many intravenous drug users are hepatitis carriers and because the AIDS risk is high in this group
- A history of possible exposure to the AIDS virus; the population at risk includes people who engage in anal sex, people with multiple sexual partners, intravenous/injection drug users, sexual partners of people at risk for AIDS, and people with hemophilia
- A skin infection, because of the possibility of contaminating the phlebotomy needle, and subsequently the blood itself
- A history of recent asthma, urticaria, or allergy to medications, because hypersensitivity can be transferred passively to the recipient
- Pregnancy within 6 months, because of the nutritional demands of pregnancy on the mother
- A history of tooth extraction or oral surgery within 72 hours, because such procedures are frequently associated with transient bacteremia
- A history of exposure to infectious disease within the past 3 weeks, because of the risk of transmission to the recipient
- Recent immunizations, because of the risk of transmitting live organisms (2-week waiting period for live, attenuated organisms; 1 month for rubella; 1 year for rabies)
- A history of recent tattoo, because of the risk of hepatitis
- Cancer, because of the uncertainty about transmission of the disease
- A history of whole blood donation within the past 56 days

Potential donors should be asked whether they have consumed any aspirin or aspirin-containing medications within the past 3 days. Although aspirin use does not render the donor ineligible, the platelets obtained would be dysfunctional and therefore not useful. The aspirin does not affect the RBCs and plasma obtained from the donor.

All donors are expected to meet the following minimal requirements:

- Body weight should exceed 50 kg (110 pounds) for a standard 450-mL donation. Donors weighing less than 50 kg donate proportionately less blood. People younger than age 17 and older than age 65 are usually disqualified from donation.
- The oral temperature should not exceed 37.5°C (99.6°F).
- The pulse rate should be regular and between 50 and 100 beats per minute.
- Systolic arterial pressure should be 90 to 180 mm Hg, and the diastolic pressure 50 to 100 mm Hg.
- The hemoglobin level should be at least 12.5 g/dL for women and 13.5 g/dL for men.

Directed Donation. At times friends and family of a patient will donate blood for that person. These blood donations are termed directed donations. Research has demonstrated that these donations are not any safer than those provided by random donors. Directed donors may not be as willing to identify themselves as having a history of any of the risk factors that disqualify a person from donating blood.

Standard Donation. Phlebotomy consists of venipuncture and blood withdrawal. Standard precautions are used. Donors are placed in a semirecumbent position. The skin over the antecubital fossa is carefully cleansed with an iodine preparation, a tourniquet applied, and venipuncture performed. Withdrawal of 450 mL of blood usually takes less than 15 minutes. After the needle is removed, donors are asked to hold the involved arm straight up, and firm pressure is applied with sterile gauze for 2 or 3 minutes or until bleeding stops. A firm bandage is then applied. Donors remain recumbent until they feel able to sit up, usually within a few minutes. Donors who experience weakness or faintness should rest for a longer period, after which they are given food and asked to remain another 15 minutes.

Donors should be instructed to leave the dressing on and to avoid heavy lifting for several hours, to avoid smoking for 1 hour, to avoid drinking alcoholic beverages for 3 hours, to increase fluid intake for 2 days, and to eat well-balanced meals for 2 weeks. Specimens from this donated blood are tested to detect infections and to identify the specific blood type (see below).

Autologous Donation. A patient's own blood may be collected for future transfusion; this method is useful for many elective surgeries where the potential need for transfusion is high (eg, orthopedic surgery). Preoperative donations are best collected 4 to 6 weeks before surgery. Iron supplements are prescribed during this period to prevent depletion of iron stores. Occasionally, erythropoietin is given to stimulate erythropoiesis to ensure that the donor's hematocrit remains high enough to be eligible for donation. Typically, 1 unit of blood is drawn each week; the number of units obtained varies with the type of surgical procedure to be performed (and thus the amount of blood anticipated to be transfused). Phlebotomies are not performed within 72 hours of surgery. Individual blood components can also be collected.

The primary advantage of autologous transfusions is the prevention of viral infections from another person's blood. Other advantages include safe transfusion for patients with a history of transfusion reactions, prevention of alloimmunization, and avoidance of complications in patients with alloantibodies. The policy of the American Red Cross requires autologous blood to be transfused only to the donor. If the blood is not required, it can be frozen until the donor needs it in the future (for up to 10 years). The blood is never returned to the general donor supply of blood products to be used by someone else.

The disadvantage of autologous donation is that it may be performed when the likelihood that the procedure will necessitate a transfusion is small. Needless autologous donation is expensive, takes time, and uses resources inappropriately. Moreover, in an emergent situation, the autologous units available may be inadequate, and the patient may still require additional units from the general donor supply.

Contraindications to autologous transfusion are acute infection, severely debilitating chronic disease, hemoglobin level less than 11 g/dL, hematocrit less than 33%, a history of active epilepsy, unstable angina, and acute cardiovascular or cerebrovascular disease. Patients with cancer may donate for themselves.

Intraoperative Blood Salvage. This transfusion method provides replacement for patients unable to donate before surgery and for patients undergoing vascular, orthopedic, or thoracic surgery. During a surgical procedure, blood lost into a sterile cavity (eg, hip joint) is suctioned into a cell-saver machine. The RBCs are washed, often with saline solution, and then returned to the patient as an intravenous infusion. Salvaged blood cannot be stored because bacteria cannot be completely removed from the blood.

Hemodilution. This transfusion method is initiated before or after induction of anesthesia. About 1 or 2 units of blood are removed from the patient through a venous or arterial line and simultaneously replaced with a colloid or crystalloid solution. The blood obtained is then reinfused after surgery. The advantage of this method is that the patient loses fewer RBCs during surgery, because the added intravenous solutions dilute the concentration of RBCs and lower the hematocrit. Patients who are at risk for myocardial injury, however, should not be further stressed by hemodilution.

COMPLICATIONS OF BLOOD DONATION

Excessive bleeding at the donor's venipuncture site is sometimes due to a bleeding disorder in the donor but more often results from a technique error: laceration of the vein, excessive tourniquet pressure, or failure to apply enough pressure after the needle is withdrawn.

Fainting is relatively common after blood donation and may be related to emotional factors, a vasovagal reaction, or prolonged fasting before donation. Because of the loss of blood volume, hypotension and syncope may occur when the donor assumes an erect position. A donor who appears pale or complains of faintness should immediately lie down or sit with head lowered below the knees; he or she should be observed for another 30 minutes.

Anginal chest pain may be precipitated in patients with unsuspected coronary artery disease. Seizures may occur in donors with epilepsy. Both angina and seizures require further medical evaluation.

Many people have the misconception that donating blood can cause AIDS and other infections. Potential donors need to be educated that the equipment used in donation is sterile, a closed system, and not reusable; they are at no risk for acquiring such infections from donating.

BLOOD PROCESSING

Samples of the unit of blood are always taken immediately after donation so that the blood can be typed and tested. Each donation is tested for antibodies to human immunodeficiency virus (HIV 1 and 2), hepatitis B core antibody (anti-HBc), hepatitis C virus (HCV), and human T-cell lymphotropic virus, type I (anti-HTLV-I/II). The blood is also tested for hepatitis B surface antigen (HbsAG) and syphilis. Negative reactions are required for the blood to be used, and each unit of blood is labeled certifying these results. Blood that tests positive for CMV can still be used, except in recipients who are negative for CMV and those who are immunocompromised, such as bone marrow transplant recipients.

Equally important to viral testing is accurately determining the blood type. More than 200 antigens have been identified on the surface of RBC membranes. Of these, the most important for safe transfusion are the ABO and Rh systems. The ABO system identifies which sugars are present on the membrane of an individual's RBCs: A, B, both A and B, and neither A nor B (O). Thus, to prevent a significant reaction, the same type of RBCs should be transfused. Previously, it was thought that in an emergent situation where the patient's blood type was not known, type O blood could be safely transfused. This practice is no longer advised by the American Red Cross.

The Rh antigen (also called D) is present on the surface of RBCs in 85% of the population (Rh-positive). Those who lack the D antigen are called Rh-negative. RBCs are routinely tested for the D antigen as well as ABO. Patients should receive RBCs with a compatible Rh type.

Transfusion

Administration of blood and blood components requires knowledge of correct administration techniques and possible complications. It is very important to be familiar with the agency's policies and procedures for transfusion therapy. Methods for transfusing blood components are presented in Guidelines 30-1 and 30-2. Potential complications of transfusion are presented below.

Setting

Although most blood transfusions are performed in the acute care setting, patients with chronic transfusion requirements often can receive transfusions in other settings. Freestanding infusion centers, ambulatory care clinics, a physician's office, and even the home may be appropriate settings for transfusion. Typically, patients who need chronic transfusions but are otherwise stable physically are appropriate candidates for outpatient therapy. Verification and administration of the blood product are performed much like in a hospital setting. Although most blood products can be transfused in the outpatient setting, the home is typically limited to transfusions of RBCs and factor components (eg, factor VIII for patients with hemophilia).

Pretransfusion Assessment

PATIENT HISTORY

Patient history is an important component of the pretransfusion assessment to determine the history of previous transfusions as well as previous reactions to transfusion. This should include the type of reaction, its manifestations, the interventions required, and whether any preventive interventions were used in subsequent

30•1 Guidelines For Transfusion of Whole Blood or Packed Cells

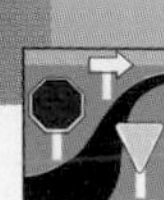

Preprocedure

1. Confirm that the transfusion has been prescribed.
2. Check that patient's blood has been typed and cross-matched.
3. Verify that patient has signed a written consent form per institution policy.
4. Explain the procedure to the patient. Instruct patient in signs and symptoms of transfusion reaction.
5. Take patient's temperature, pulse, respiration, and blood pressure to establish a baseline for comparing vital signs during transfusion.
6. Wash hands and wear gloves in accordance with standard precautions.
7. Use a 20-gauge or larger needle for placement in a large vein. Use special tubing that contains a blood filter to screen out fibrin clots and other particulate matter. Do not vent the blood container.

Procedure

1. Obtain the blood or blood components. (Institution policy may limit release of only one unit at a time.)
2. Double-check the labels with another nurse or physician to make sure that the ABO group and Rh type agree with the compatibility record.
   Check to see that the number and type on the donor blood label and on the patient's chart are correct.
   Check the patient's identification by asking the patient's name and checking the identification wristband.
3. Check the blood for gas bubbles and any unusual color or cloudiness. (Gas bubbles may indicate bacterial growth. Abnormal color or cloudiness may be a sign of hemolysis.)
4. Make sure blood is administered within 30 minutes of removing it from the blood bank refrigerator.
5. For first 15 minutes, run the transfusion slowly—no faster than 5 mL/min.
   Observe the patient carefully for adverse effects. If no adverse effects occur during the first 15 minutes, increase the flow rate unless the patient is at high risk for circulatory overload.
6. Observe the patient frequently throughout the transfusion. Monitor closely for 15–30 minutes to detect signs of reaction. Monitor vital signs at regular intervals per institution policy; compare results with baseline measurements. Increase frequency of measurements based on patient's condition.
7. Note that administration time does not exceed 4 hours because of the increased risk for bacterial proliferation.
8. Be alert for signs of adverse reactions: circulatory overload, sepsis, febrile reaction, allergic reaction, and acute hemolytic reaction.
9. Change blood tubing after every 2 units transfused to decrease chance of bacterial contamination.

Postprocedure

1. Obtain vital signs and compare with baseline measurements.
2. Dispose of used materials properly.
3. Document procedure in patient's medical record, including patient assessment findings and tolerance to procedure.
4. Monitor patient for response to and effectiveness of procedure.

Note: Never add medications to blood or blood products; if blood is too thick to run freely, normal saline solution may be added to the unit. If blood must be warmed, heat it by an in-line blood warmer with a monitoring system.

transfusions. It is useful to assess the number of pregnancies a woman has had, because an increased number can increase her risk for reaction due to antibodies developed from exposure to fetal circulation. Other concurrent health problems should also be noted, with careful attention to cardiac, pulmonary, and vascular disease.

PHYSICAL ASSESSMENT

A thorough, systematic physical assessment before transfusing any blood product is extremely important. In the event of a possible transfusion reaction, a comparison of physical findings can help differentiate between types of reactions.

Baseline vital signs are a crucial component. The respiratory system should be assessed, including careful auscultation of the lungs (crackles, wheezes) and use of accessory muscles. Cardiac system assessment should include a careful inspection for any edema as well as other signs of cardiac failure (eg, jugular venous distention). The skin should be observed for rashes, petechiae, or ecchymoses. The sclera should be examined for icterus.

PATIENT TEACHING

Reviewing the signs and symptoms of a potential transfusion reaction is crucial for patients who have not received a transfusion before. Signs and symptoms of a possible reaction include fever, chills, respiratory distress, low back pain, nausea, pain at the intravenous site, or anything "unusual." Although a thorough review is very important, it is also important to assure the patient that the blood is carefully tested with the patient's own blood (cross-matching) to diminish the likelihood of any untoward reaction. Such assurance can be extremely beneficial in allaying anxiety. Similarly, it can be useful to mention again the very low possibility of developing AIDS from the transfusion; this fear persists among many people.

Transfusion Complications

All patients who receive a blood transfusion may develop complications from that transfusion. When explaining the reasons for the transfusion, it is important to include the risks and benefits and what to expect during and after the transfusion. Patients must be informed that the supply of blood is not completely risk-free but that it has been tested carefully. Nursing management is directed toward preventing complications, promptly recognizing complications if they develop, and promptly initiating measures to control any complications that occur. The following are the most common or potentially severe transfusion-related complications.

30•2 GUIDELINES FOR TRANSFUSION OF PLATELETS OR FRESH-FROZEN PLASMA (FFP)

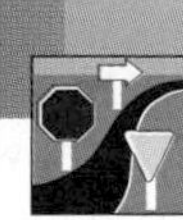

Preprocedure

1. Confirm that the transfusion has been prescribed.
2. Verify that patient has signed a written consent form per institution policy.
3. Explain the procedure to the patient. Instruct patient in signs and symptoms of transfusion reaction (itching, hives, swelling, shortness of breath, fever, chills).
4. Take patient's temperature, pulse, respiration, and blood pressure to establish a baseline for comparing vital signs during transfusion.
5. Wash hands and wear gloves in accordance with standard precautions.
6. Use a 22-gauge or larger needle for placement in a large vein, if possible. Use appropriate tubing per institution policy (platelets often require different tubing from that used for other blood products).

Procedure

1. Obtain the platelets/FFP from the blood bank (only *after* the IV is started).
2. Double-check the labels with another nurse or physician to make sure that the ABO group matches the compatibility record (not usually necessary for platelets; here only if compatible platelets are ordered).
   Check to see that the number and type on the donor blood label and on the patient's chart are correct.
   Check the patient's identification by asking the patient's name and checking the identification wristband.
3. Check the blood product for any unusual color or clumps. (Excessive redness indicates contamination with larger amounts of red cells.)
4. Make sure platelets/FFP are administered immediately when obtained.
5. Aseptically attach the blood infusion tubing to the blood component unit; prime the tubing (if not previously done) before connecting to patient's IV.
6. Infuse each unit as fast as patient can tolerate to diminish platelet clumping during administration. Observe the patient carefully for adverse effects, including circulatory overload. Decrease rate of infusion if necessary.
7. Observe the patient closely throughout the transfusion for any signs of adverse reaction, including restlessness, hives, nausea, vomiting, torso or back pain, shortness of breath, flushing, hematuria, fever, or chills. Should any adverse reaction occur, stop infusion immediately.
8. Monitor vital signs at end of transfusion per institution policy; compare results with baseline measurements.
9. Flush line with saline solution after transfusion to remove blood component from tubing.

Postprocedure

1. Obtain vital signs and compare with baseline measurements.
2. Dispose of used materials properly.
3. Document procedure in patient's medical record, including patient assessment findings and tolerance to procedure.
4. Monitor patient for response to and effectiveness of procedure. One hour after platelet transfusion platelet counts may be ordered to evaluate response.

Note: FFP requires ABO compatibility but not Rh. Platelets are *not* typically cross-matched for ABO compatibility. Never add medications to blood or blood products.

FEBRILE, NONHEMOLYTIC REACTION

Caused by antibodies to donor WBCs still present in the unit of blood or blood component, the nonhemolytic reaction is the most common type of transfusion reaction (accounting for more than 90% of reactions). It occurs more frequently in previously transfused patients (who have been exposed to multiple antigens from previous blood products) or Rh-negative women who have borne children (with subsequent exposures to Rh-positive fetuses, raising antibody levels in the mother). These reactions occur in 1% of RBC transfusions and 20% of platelet transfusions. More than 10% of patients with a chronic transfusion requirement develop this type of reaction.

The diagnosis of a febrile, nonhemolytic reaction is made by excluding other potential causes, such as a hemolytic reaction or bacterial contamination of the blood product. The signs and symptoms of a febrile, nonhemolytic transfusion reaction are chills (absent to severe) followed by fever (more than 1°C elevated). The fever typically begins within 2 hours after the beginning the transfusion. Although not life-threatening, the fever and particularly the rigors can be frightening to the patient.

These reactions can be diminished, even prevented, by further depleting the blood component of donor WBCs. This depletion can be accomplished by a leukocyte reduction filter. The blood product may be filtered during processing (better results, but more expensive) or during the actual transfusion by adding the filter to the blood administration tubing. Antipyretics can be given to prevent fever, but routine premedication is not advised because it can mask the beginning of a more serious transfusion reaction.

ACUTE HEMOLYTIC REACTION

The most dangerous—in fact, potentially life-threatening—type of transfusion reaction occurs when the donor blood is incompatible with that of the recipient. Antibodies already present in the recipient's plasma rapidly combine with antigens on donor erythrocytes, and these cells are hemolyzed (destroyed) in the circulation (intravascular hemolysis). The most rapid hemolysis occurs in ABO incompatibility. This reaction can occur after transfusion of as little as 10 mL of RBCs. Rh incompatibility is often less severe. The most common causes of acute hemolytic reactions result from errors in blood component labeling and/or patient identification.

Symptoms consist of fever, chills, low back pain, nausea, chest tightness, dyspnea, and anxiety. As the RBCs are destroyed, the hemoglobin within them is released and excreted by the kidneys,

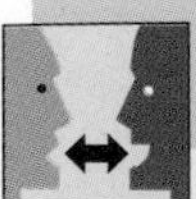

ETHICS AND RELATED ISSUES

Should a Lifesaving Blood Transfusion Be Withheld for Religious Reasons?

Situation

Blood transfusions are performed in the event of serious, often life-threatening health crises. They have the potential to save life in an otherwise hopeless situation. Jehovah's Witnesses are a sect of Christians who consent to aggressive medical treatment in case of illness or trauma but consistently refuse any blood or blood products because of their unique interpretation of the Bible. Should a Jehovah's Witness patient suffering from acute blood loss be allowed to die because of a religious belief if a relatively simple and accessible treatment (blood transfusion) could be performed that would most likely save his or her life?

Dilemma

The patient's right to refuse treatment conflicts with the professional obligation to help the patient (autonomy versus beneficence).

Discussion

- What arguments would you offer in support of the view that Jehovah's Witnesses *should* receive lifesaving transfusions against their will?
- What arguments would you offer to support the view that Jehovah's Witnesses *should not* receive blood transfusions if they refuse them?

and thus is present in the urine (hemoglobinuria). Hypotension, bronchospasm, and vascular collapse may result. Diminished renal perfusion results in acute renal failure, and DIC may also occur.

The reaction must be recognized promptly and the transfusion discontinued immediately. Appropriate blood and urine specimens must be analyzed for evidence of hemolysis. Treatment goals include maintaining blood volume and renal perfusion and preventing and managing DIC.

Acute hemolytic transfusion reactions are preventable. Meticulous attention to detail in labeling blood samples and blood components and identifying the recipient cannot be overemphasized.

ALLERGIC REACTION

Some patients may develop urticaria (hives) or generalized itching during a transfusion. The cause of these reactions is thought to be a sensitivity reaction to a plasma protein within the blood component being transfused. Symptoms of an allergic reaction are urticaria, itching, and flushing. The reactions are usually mild and respond to antihistamines. If the symptoms resolve after administering an antihistamine (eg, diphenhydramine), the transfusion may be resumed. Rarely, the allergic reaction is severe, with bronchospasm, laryngeal edema, and shock. These reactions are managed with epinephrine, corticosteroids, and pressor support, if necessary.

Giving the patient antihistamines before the transfusion may prevent future reactions. For severe reactions, future blood components are washed to remove any remaining plasma proteins. Leukocyte filters are not useful because the offending plasma proteins can pass through the filter.

CIRCULATORY OVERLOAD

If too much blood infuses too quickly, hypervolemia can occur. This condition can be aggravated in patients who already have increased circulatory volume (eg, those with CHF). Packed RBCs are safer to use than whole blood. If the administration rate is sufficiently slow, circulatory overload may be prevented. For patients at risk for or already in circulatory overload, diuretics are administered after the transfusion or between units of RBCs. Patients receiving fresh-frozen plasma or even platelets may also develop circulatory overload. Thus, the infusion rate of these blood components must also be titrated to the patient's tolerance.

Signs of circulatory overload include dyspnea, orthopnea, tachycardia, or sudden anxiety. Neck vein distention, crackles at the base of the lungs, and a rise in blood pressure can also occur. If the transfusion is continued, pulmonary edema can develop, as manifested by severe dyspnea and coughing of pink, frothy sputum.

The patient is placed in an upright position with the feet in a dependent position, the blood is discontinued, and the physician is notified. The intravenous line is kept patent with a very slow infusion of normal saline solution or a heparin lock device to retain access to the vein in case intravenous medications are necessary. Oxygen and morphine may be needed for severe dyspnea.

BACTERIAL CONTAMINATION

The incidence of bacterial contamination of blood components is low; however, receiving contaminated products puts the patient at great risk. Contamination can occur at any point in the procurement and processing process. Many bacteria cannot survive in the cold temperatures used to store RBCs (therefore, platelets are at greater risk for contamination because they are stored at room temperature), but some organisms can survive cold temperatures.

Preventive measures include meticulous care in the procurement and processing of blood components. When RBCs or whole blood are transfused, they should be administered within a 4-hour period, because warm room temperatures promote bacterial growth. A contaminated unit of blood product may not appear abnormal or have an abnormal odor.

The signs of bacterial contamination are fever, chills, and hypotension; these may not occur until the transfusion is complete, occasionally several hours after the transfusion. If not treated immediately with fluids and broad-spectrum antibiotics, shock can occur. Even with aggressive management, including vasopressor support, the mortality rate is high.

As soon as the reaction is recognized, any remaining transfusion is discontinued and the intravenous line is kept open with normal saline solution. The physician and blood bank are notified and the blood container is returned to the blood bank for testing and culture. Septicemia is treated with intravenous fluids, antibiotics, corticosteroids, and vasopressors.

TRANSFUSION-RELATED ACUTE LUNG INJURY

This is a potentially fatal, idiosyncratic reaction that occurs in fewer than 1 in 5000 transfusions. Plasma antibodies (usually in the donor's plasma) that are present in the blood component stimulate the recipient's WBCs; aggregates of these WBCs form and occlude the microvasculature within the lungs. This lung injury is manifested as pulmonary edema; it can occur within 4 hours after the transfusion.

Signs and symptoms include fever, chills, acute respiratory distress (in the absence of other signs of left ventricular failure, such as elevated central venous pressure), and bilateral pulmonary infiltrates. Aggressive supportive therapy (oxygen, intubation, diuretics) may prevent death.

DELAYED HEMOLYTIC REACTION

Delayed hemolytic reactions usually occur within 14 days after transfusion, when the level of antibody has been increased to the extent that a reaction can be mounted. The hemolysis of the RBCs is extravascular, via the RES, and occurs gradually.

Signs and symptoms of a delayed hemolytic reaction are fever, anemia, increased bilirubin level, decreased or absent haptoglobin, and possibly jaundice. Rarely is there hemoglobinuria. Generally, these reactions are not dangerous, but it is useful to recognize them because subsequent transfusions with blood products containing these antibodies may cause a more severe hemolytic reaction. However, recognition is also difficult, because the same patient may not be in a health care setting to be tested for this reaction; even if the patient is hospitalized, the reaction may be too mild to recognize clinically. Because the amount of antibody present can be too low to detect, it is difficult to prevent delayed hemolytic reactions. Fortunately, the reaction is usually mild and requires no intervention.

IRON OVERLOAD

One unit of RBCs contains 250 mg of iron. Patients with chronic transfusion requirements, therefore, can quickly acquire more iron than they can use. Over time, these excess iron deposits can cause organ damage, particularly in the liver, heart, testes, and pancreas. Promptly initiating a program of iron chelation therapy (eg, with deferoxamine) can prevent end-organ damage from iron toxicity.

DISEASES TRANSMITTED BY BLOOD TRANSFUSION

Despite the advances in donor screening and blood testing, certain diseases can still be transmitted by transfusion of blood components. The following diseases are examples of this phenomenon.

Hepatitis. Viral hepatitis is an important complication of transfusion therapy. Blood and blood products obtained from paid donors carry a higher risk than those from volunteer donors. Pooled blood products also carry a significantly higher risk. Tests are used to detect hepatitis B virus as well as hepatitis C, but the risk for acquiring hepatitis C is still estimated at 1 : 10,000. Hepatitis is discussed in Chapter 36.

AIDS. The human retroviruses (HIV and HTLV) have been associated with transfusion of blood products. For this reason, people who engage in high-risk behaviors (sex with multiple partners, anal sex, intravenous/injection drug use, sex with people at risk for AIDS) and people with signs and symptoms suggestive of the disease should not donate blood. All donated blood is now tested for antibodies to the AIDS virus. The risk of acquiring HIV from a transfusion is estimated to be 1 : 670,000.

Cytomegalovirus. CMV is hazardous when transmitted to premature newborns who have a CMV antibody-negative mother, and to other immunocompromised recipients who are CMV-negative (eg, those with acute leukemia or who have had bone marrow transplantation). Leukocyte-reduced blood transfusions have been effective in reducing the transmission of this virus.

Graft-Versus-Host Disease. Blood transfusion can be considered a type of tissue transplantation. In immunocompromised recipients, graft-versus-host disease can result when transfused lymphocytes engraft within the recipient and attack his or her lymphocytes or body tissues. This reaction occurs only in severely immunocompromised patients (eg, Hodgkin's disease, bone marrow transplant). Fever, skin rash that is diffuse and erythematous, nausea, vomiting, and diarrhea are symptoms. Irradiating blood products inactivates the donor lymphocytes, thus diminishing the risk for this complication. There are no known risks of radiation to the person receiving or administering this type of blood product. Leukocyte reduction filters also diminish the risk of developing this complication.

Creutzfeldt-Jakob Disease (CJD). CJD is a rare disease that results in irreversible brain damage. Although there is no evidence to support it, there has been concern that CJD could be transmitted by transfusion. In response to concerns from patients with hemophilia and others, the Food and Drug Administration has extended its requirement that all blood donors be screened for a positive family history of CJD. Any blood products (eg, factor VIII, immune globulin) developed from a donor who subsequently develops CJD are recalled. This policy has resulted in sporadic but severe shortages of these blood components.

Nursing Management for Transfusion Reactions

If a transfusion reaction is suspected, the transfusion must be immediately stopped and the physician notified. A thorough patient assessment is crucial because many complications have similar signs and symptoms. The following steps are taken to determine the type and severity of the reaction:

- Stop the transfusion. Maintain the intravenous line with normal saline solution, administered at a slow rate.
- Assess the patient carefully. Compare the vital signs with those from the baseline assessment. Assess the patient's respiratory status carefully. Note the presence of adventitious breath sounds, use of accessory muscles, extent of dyspnea (if any), and changes in mental status, including anxiety and confusion. Note any chills, diaphoresis, complaints of back pain, urticaria, and jugular vein distention.
- Notify the physician of the assessment findings, and implement any orders obtained. Continue to monitor the patient's vital signs and respiratory, cardiovascular, and renal status.
- Notify the blood bank that a suspected transfusion reaction has occurred.
- Send the blood container and tubing to the blood bank for repeat typing and culture. The identifying tags and numbers are verified.

If a hemolytic transfusion reaction or bacterial infection is suspected, the nurse should do the following:

- Obtain appropriate blood specimens from the patient.
- Collect a urine sample as soon as possible for a hemoglobin determination.
- Document the reaction, according to the institution's policy.

Pharmacologic Alternatives to Blood Transfusions

Researchers continue to seek a red cell substitute that is practical and safe. Products previously tried have not been successful. Thus, an effective but safe alternative to blood or blood components is still not available. However, recombinant technology has provided a means to produce hematopoietic growth factors necessary for the production of blood cells within the bone marrow. By increasing the body's production of blood cells, transfusions or complications resulting from diminished blood cells (eg, infection from neutropenia) may be avoided. However, the successful use of growth factors requires a functional marrow.

Erythropoietin

Erythropoietin (epoetin alpha) is an effective alternative treatment for patients with chronic anemia secondary to diminished levels of erythropoietin, as in chronic renal disease. This medication stimulates erythropoiesis. It also has been used for patients who are anemic from chemotherapy or AZT therapy, or who have diseases with bone marrow suppression, such as MDS. The use of erythropoietin can also enable a patient to donate several units of blood for future use (eg, preoperative autologous donation). The medication can be administered intravenously or subcutaneously. Plasma levels are more sustained with the subcutaneous route. Side effects are rare, but erythropoietin can cause or exacerbate hypertension. If the anemia is corrected too quickly or is overcorrected, the elevated hematocrit may cause headache and potentially seizures. This usually affects patients with renal failure, rarely others. Serial CBCs should be performed to evaluate the response to the medication. The dose and frequency of administration are titrated to the hematocrit.

Granulocyte-Colony Stimulating Factor

G-CSF is a cytokine that stimulates the proliferation and differentiation of myeloid stem cells; a rapid increase in neutrophils is seen within the circulation. G-CSF is effective in improving transient but severe neutropenia after chemotherapy or in some forms of MDS. It is particularly useful in preventing bacterial infections that would be likely to occur with neutropenia. G-CSF is administered subcutaneously on a daily basis. The primary side effect is bone pain; this probably reflects the increase in hematopoiesis within the marrow. Serial CBCs should be performed to evaluate the response to the medication and to ensure that the rise in WBCs is not excessive. Unfortunately, the effect of G-CSF on **myelopoiesis** is short; the neutrophil count drops once the medication is stopped.

Granulocyte-Macrophage Colony Stimulating Factor

GM-CSF is a cytokine that is naturally produced by a variety of cells, including monocytes and endothelial cells. It works either directly or synergistically with other growth factors to stimulate myelopoiesis. GM-CSF is not as specific to neutrophils as is G-CSF; thus, an increase in erythroid and megakaryocytic (platelet) production may also be seen. GM-CSF serves the same purpose as G-CSF. However, it may have a greater effect on macrophage function and thus be more useful against fungal infections, whereas G-CSF may be better used to fight bacterial infection. GM-CSF is also administered subcutaneously. Side effects include bone pain, fevers, and myalgias.

Bone Marrow Transplantation

Bone marrow transplantation is a therapeutic modality that offers the possibility of cure for some patients with hematologic disorders, such as severe aplastic anemia, some forms of leukemia, and thalassemia. Because most hematologic disease states arise from some form of bone marrow dysfunction, an autologous transplantation (receiving one's own stem cells back) is rarely an option. Instead, allogeneic transplantations are more common. Here, a patient receives intensive chemotherapy (sometimes with radiation therapy as well) with the goal of completely ablating the patient's bone marrow function. Stem cells from the donor (ideally a matched sibling) or actual marrow from the donor is then infused into the patient, using a process similar to an RBC transfusion. The stem cells travel to the marrow and slowly begin the process of resuming hematopoiesis.

Success of the treatment depends on tissue compatibility and the patient's tolerance of the immunosuppression that results from the ablative therapy. Patients require intensive nursing care that is directed toward preventing infection and assessing for early signs and symptoms of complications. One common complication involves the formation of lymphocytes that respond to their new host (ie, the patient) as foreign and mount a reaction against the body. This process is known as graft-versus-host-disease; it can involve the skin, gastrointestinal tract, and liver and can be life-threatening. In hematologic malignancies, some graft-versus-host-disease is actually desirable in that the donor lymphocytes can also mount a reaction against any lingering tumor cells; this process is referred to as graft-versus-leukemia. Late complications (after the initial 100 days after transplantation) are not infrequent; these patients, particularly those who receive an allogeneic transplant, require careful follow-up for a year or more after transplantation.

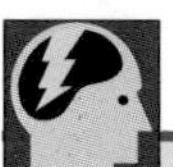

Critical Thinking Exercises

1. An elderly patient who is anemic says she believes that the anemia is due to her age, and she asks why she must have so many tests performed. What explanation would you give this patient about the rationale for the diagnostic tests?
2. You are caring for a young adult patient who has had repeated hospitalizations for sickle cell crisis. What factors should be assessed to determine the patient's educational, coping, and pain management needs?
3. You are caring for a patient diagnosed with leukemia. The family members are very concerned about the patient's risk for infection at home. What instructions should they be given about decreasing the risks for infection?
4. You are caring for a patient who is septic and is now receiving a transfusion of 2 units of packed RBCs. The patient spikes a temperature to 38.5°C after half of the second unit has been transfused. What are the possible causes of the fever? What are the appropriate nursing interventions?

References and Selected Readings

BOOKS

Chabner, B. A., & Longo, D. L. (1996). *Cancer chemotherapy and biotherapy: Principles and practice.* Philadelphia: Lippincott-Raven.

Committee on the Prevention, Detection, and Management of Iron. (1993). *Iron deficiency anemia: Recommended guidelines for the prevention, detection, and management among U.S. children and women of childbearing age.* Washington, DC: National Academy Press.

Engelking, C., & Hubbard, S. M. (1996). *Current issues and controversies in the management of non-Hodgkin's lymphoma.* New York: Triclinica Communications [Monograph].

Hirsh, J., & Brain, E. A. (1983). *Hemostasis and thrombosis: A conceptual approach* (2nd ed.). New York: Churchill Livingstone.

Hoffman, R., Benz, E. J., Shattil, S., Furie, B., Cohen, H., & Silberstein, L. E. (Eds.). (1995). *Hematology: Basic principles and practice* (2nd ed.). New York: Churchill Livingstone.

Kühne, T., Imbach, P., & Blanchette, V. S. (1996). Immune thrombocytopenic purpura: Intravenous immunoglobulin versus dexamethasone versus anti-D. In M. D. Kazatchkine & A. Morell (Eds.), *Intravenous immunoglobulin research and therapy.* Pearl River, NY: Parthenon Publishing Group.

Lee, G. R., Foerster, J., Lukens, J., Parastevas, F., et al. (1999). *Wintrobe's clinical hematology.* Baltimore: Williams & Wilkins.

Rieger, P. T. (1995). *Biotherapy: A comprehensive overview.* Boston: Jones and Bartlett.

Westphal, R. G. (1996). *Handbook of transfusion medicine* (3rd ed.). Washington, DC: American Red Cross Blood Services.

Wilkes, G. M., Ingwersen, K., & Burke, M. B. (1997). *1997–1998 oncology nursing drug handbook.* Boston: Jones and Bartlett.

Williams, W. J., et al. (Eds.). (1995). *Williams' hematology.* New York: McGraw-Hill, Inc., Health Professions Division.

JOURNALS

Asterisks indicate nursing research articles.

Anemia

Adams, R. J., McKie, V.C., Brambilla, D., et al. (1998). Stroke prevention in sickle cell anemia. *Controlled Clinical Trials, 19*(1), 110–129.

*Alleyne, J., & Thomas, V. J. (1994). The management of sickle cell crisis pain as experienced by patients and their caregivers. *Journal of Advanced Nursing, 19*(4), 725–732.

Cazzola, M., Mercuriali, F., & Brugnara, C. (1997). Use of recombinant human erythropoietin outside the setting of uremia. *Blood, 89*(12), 4248–4267.

Charache, S., Terrin, M. L., Moore, R., et al. Effect of Hydroxyurea on the Frequency of Painful Crises in Sickle Cell Anemia. (1995). *New England Journal of Medicine, 332*(20), 1317–1322.

Gorman, K. (1999). Sickle cell disease. *American Journal of Nursing, 99*(3), 38–43.

Hatton, C., & Mackie, P. H. (1996). Acquired haemolytic anaemia. *Medicine, 24*(1), 20–23.

Hatton, C., & Mackie, P. H. (1996). Haemolytic anaemias: Pathophysiology and classification. *Medicine, 24*(1), 11–13.

Hatton, C., & Mackie, P. H. (1996). Haemoglobinopathies and other congenital haemolytic anaemias. *Medicine, 24*(1), 14–19.

Looker, A. C., Dallman, P. R., Carroll, M. D., Gunter, E. W., & Johnson, C. L. (1997). Prevalence of iron deficiency in the United States. *Journal of the American Medical Association, 277*(12), 973–976.

Pippard, M. J., & Heppleston, A. D. (1996). Microcytic/macrocytic anaemias. *Medicine, 24*(1), 4–10.

Rosse, W., Bussel, J., & Ortel T. (1997). Challenges in managing autoimmune disease. *Hematology 1997: Education Program, American Society of Hematology*, pp. 92–102.

Serjeant, G. R. (1997). Chronic transfusion programmes in sickle cell disease: Problem or panacea? *British Journal of Haematology, 97*, 253–255.

Toh, B., van Driel, I. R., & Gleeson, P. A. (1997). Pernicious anemia. *New England Journal of Medicine, 337*(20), 1441–1448.

Vichinsky, E. P. (1997). Understanding the morbidity of sickle cell disease. *British Journal of Haematology, 99*, 974–982.

Coagulopathy and DIC

Bell, W. R. (1994). The pathophysiology of disseminated intravascular coagulation. *Seminars in Hematology, 31*(2), 19–24.

Giles, A. R., & Lillicrap, D. P. (1995). Haemophilia A and related disorders. *Medicine, 23*(12), 525–530.

Fatigue

*Dean, G. E., Spears, L., Ferrell, B. R., Quan, W. D. Y., Groshon, S., & Mitchell, M. S. (1995). Fatigue in patients with cancer receiving interferon alpha. *Cancer Practice, 3*(3), 164–172.

*Ferrell, B. R., Grant, M., Dean, G. E., Funk, B., & Ly, J. (1996). "Bone tired": The experience of fatigue and its impact on quality of life. *Oncology Nursing Forum, 23*(10), 1539–1547.

*Graydon, J. E., Bubela, N., Irvine, D., & Vincent, L. (1995). Fatigue-reducing strategies used by patients receiving treatment for cancer. *Cancer Nursing, 18*(1), 23–28.

Leukemia

*Bertero, C., Eriksson, B. E., & Ek, A. C. (1997). A substantive theory of quality of life of adults with chronic leukaemia. *International Journal of Nursing Studies, 34*(1), 9–16.

Bow, E., Sutherland, J. A., Kilpatrick, M. G., et al. (1996). Therapy of untreated acute myeloid leukemia in the elderly: Remission induction using a non-cytarabine-containing regimen plus etoposide. *Journal of Clinical Oncology, 14*, 1345–1352.

Caudell, K. A. (1996). Psychoneuroimmunology and innovative behavioral interventions in patients with leukemia. *Oncology Nursing Forum, 23*(3), 493–502.

Cohen, H. J., Rai, K. R., & Peterson, B. A. (1997). Lymphoproliferative disorders in the elderly. *Hematology 1997: Educational Program of the American Society of Hematology*, pp. 189–194.

Giralt, S., Kantarjian, H., & Talpaz, M. (1995). Treatment of chronic myelogenous leukemia. *Seminars in Oncology, 22*(4), 396–404.

Hagska, K., & McCartney, S. (1998). Nursing care of the patient with chronic lymphocytic leukemia. *Seminars in Oncology, 25*(1), 75–79.

Hern, B. (1996). Therapeutic leukapheresis in the patient with leukemia. *Journal of Intravenous Nursing, 19*(5), 269–272.

*Persson, L., Hallberg, I. R., & Ohlsson, O. (1997). Survivors of acute leukaemia and highly malignant lymphoma—retrospective views of daily life problems during treatment and when in remission. *Journal of Advanced Nursing, 25*(1), 68–78.

Rowe, J. M., Andersen, J. W., Mazza, J. J., et al. (1995). A randomized placebo-controlled phase III study of granulocyte-macrophage colony-stimulating factor in adult patients (>55 to 70 years of age) with acute myelogenous leukemia: A study of the Eastern Cooperative Oncology Group (E1490). *Blood, 86*(2), 457–462.

Lymphoma

Loeffler, M., Brostenanu, O., Hasenclever, D., et al. (1998). Meta-analysis of chemotherapy versus combined modality treatment trials in Hodgkin's disease. *Journal of Clinical Oncology, 16*(3), 818–829.

Mauch, P. (1998). What is the role for adjuvant radiation therapy in advanced Hodgkin's disease? *Journal of Clinical Oncology, 16*(3), 815–817.

*Persson, L., Hallberg, I. R., & Ohlsson, O. (1997). Survivors of acute leukaemia and highly malignant lymphoma—retrospective views of daily life problems during treatment and when in remission. *Journal of Advanced Nursing, 25*(1), 68–78.

*Sitzia, J., North, C., Stanley, J., & Winterberg, N. (1997). Side effects of CHOP in the treatment of non-Hodgkin's lymphoma. *Cancer Nursing, 20*(6), 430–439.

Multiple Myeloma

Barenson, J. R., Lichtenstein, A., Porter, L., et al. (1998). Long-term Pamidronate treatment of advanced multiple myeloma patients reduces skeletal events. *Journal of Clinical Oncology, 16*(2), 593–602.

Sheridan, C. A. (1996). Multiple myeloma. *Seminars in Oncology Nursing, 12*(1), 59–79.

Myelodysplastic Syndromes

Greenberg, P. (1996). Myeloproliferative and myelodysplastic syndromes. *Medicine, 24*(1), 34–37.

List, A. F., Brasfield, F., Heaton, R., et al. (1997). Stimulation of hematopoiesis by Amifostine in patients with myelodysplastic syndrome. *Blood, 90*(9), 3364–3369.

Utley, S. M. (1996). Myelodysplastic syndromes. *Seminars in Oncology Nursing, 12*(1), 51–58.

Neutropenia

Sparks, S., & Camp-Sorrell, D. (1997). Assessing the myelosuppressed patient. *American Journal of Nursing, 97*(Suppl.), 4–8.

Young, N. (1994). Agranulocytosis. *Journal of the American Medical Association, 271*(12), 935–938.

Platelet Disorders

Cortelazzo, S., Finazzi, G., Ruggeri, M., et al. (1995). Hydroxyurea for patients with essential thrombocytopenia and a high risk of thrombosis. *New England Journal of Medicine, 332*(17), 1132–1136.

Doyle, B., & Porter, D. L. (1997). Thrombocytopenia. *AACN Clinical Issues, 8*(3), 469–480.

George, J. N., Woolk, S. H., Raskob, G. E., et al. (1996). Idiopathic thrombocytopenic purpura: A practice guideline developed by explicit methods for the American Society of Hematology. *Blood, 88*, 3–40.

Shuey, K. M. (1996). Platelet-associated bleeding disorders. *Seminars in Oncology Nursing, 12*(1), 15–27.

Polycythemia Vera

Dickstein, J. I., & Vardiman, J. W. (1995). Hematopathologic findings in the myeloproliferative disorders. *Seminars in Oncology, 22*(4), 355–373.

Greenberg, P. (1996). Myeloproliferative and myelodysplastic syndromes. *Medicine, 24*(1), 34–37.

Knoop, T. (1996). Polycythemia vera. *Seminars in Oncology Nursing, 12*(1), 70–77.

Thrombosis

Barrowcliffe, T. W. (1995). Annotation: Low-molecular-weight heparin(s). *British Journal of Haematology, 90,* 1–7.

Griffin, J. H., Motulsky, A., & Hirsh, J. (1996). Diagnosis and treatment of hypercoaguable states. *Education Program, American Society of Hematology,* pp. 106–111.

Middeldorp, S., Henkens, C. M. A., Koopman, M. M. W., et al. (1998). The incidence of venous thromboembolism in family members of patients with factor V Leiden mutation and venous thrombosis. *Annals of Internal Medicine, 128*(1), 15–20.

Rimm, E. B., Willett, W. C., Hu, F. B., et al. (1998). Folate and vitamin B_6 from diet and supplements in relation to risk of coronary heart disease among women. *Journal of the American Medical Association, 279*(5), 359–364.

Welch, G. N., & Loscalzo, J. (1998). Homocystine and atherothrombosis. *New England Journal of Medicine, 338*(15), 1042–1050.

Transfusion

American College of Physicians. (1992). Practice strategies for elective red blood cell transfusion. *Annals of Internal Medicine, 116*(5), 403–406.

Buskard, N. A. (1996). Recent developments in blood transfusion. *Medicine, 24*(1), 26–33.

Ely, E. W., & Bernard, G. R. (1999). Transfusions in critically ill patients. *New England Journal of Medicine, 340*(6), 467–468.

Infectious disease testing for blood transfusions, NIH Consensus Statement (1995). 13(1), 1–27.

Roth, D. (1998). Adverse blood transfusion effects. *Journal of Vascular Access Devices, 3*(1), 10–15.

Schreiber, G. B., Busch, M. P., Kleinman, S. H., & Korelitz, J. J. (1996). The risk of transfusion-transmitted viral infections. *New England Journal of Medicine, 334*(26), 1685–1690.

Transplantation

Alcoser, P. W., and Burchetts, S. (1999). Bone marrow transplantation. *American Journal of Nursing, 99*(6), 26–30.

Buchsel, P. C., Leum, E. W., & Randolph, S. R. (1996). Delayed complications of bone marrow transplantation: An update. *Oncology Nursing Forum, 23*(8), 1267–1291.

Buchsel, P. C., Leum, E., & Randolph, S. R. (1997). Nursing care of the blood cell transplant recipient. *Seminars in Oncology Nursing, 13*(3), 172–183.

Yoder, L. H. (1997). Diseases treated with blood cell transplants. *Seminars in Oncology Nursing, 13*(3), 164–171.

Resources

American Cancer Society, 1599 Clifton Rd., N.E., Atlanta, GA 30329; www.cancer.org

American Hemochromatosis Society, 777 E. Atlantic Ave., Z-363, Delray Beach, FL 33483-5352; www.americanhs.org

American Red Cross, 1730 E Street NW, Washington, DC 20006; www.redcross.org

Aplastic Anemia Foundation of America, Inc., PO Box 613, Annapolis, MD 21404; www.aplastic.org

Blood and Marrow Transplant Newsletter, 1985 Spruce Ave., Highland Park, IL 60036

International Myeloma Foundation, 2129 Stanley Hills Dr., Los Angeles, CA 90046; www.myeloma.org

Leukemia Society of America, 600 Third Ave., New York, NY 10016; www.leukemia.org

Myelodysplastic Syndromes Foundation, PO Box 477, 464 Main St., Crosswicks, NJ 08515; www.mds-foundation.org

National Association for Sickle Cell Disease, Inc., 3345 Wilshire Boulevard, Suite 1106, Los Angeles, CA 90010-1880

National Association of Vascular Access Networks, 11417 S. 700 East, Suite 205, Draper, UT 84020

National Cancer Institute Cancer Information Service, 31 Center Drive MSC 2580, Building 31, Room 10A16, Bethesda, MD 20892-2580; 1-800-4-CANCER; www.nci.nih.gov

National Hemophilia Foundation, SoHo Building, 116 32nd St., 11th Floor, New York, NY 10011; www.hemophilia.org

National Marrow Donor Program, Suite 400, 3433 Broadway St. NE, Minneapolis, MN 55413; www.marrow.org

Oncology Nursing Society, 501 Holiday Dr., Pittsburgh, PA 15220-2749; www.ons.org

Sickle Cell Disease Association of America, Inc., 200 Corporate Pointe, Culver City, CA 90230-7633; www.stepstn.com/nord/org—sum/280.htm

UNIT

7

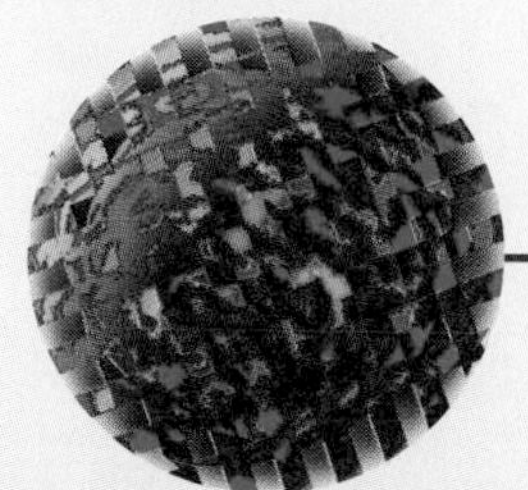

Digestive and Gastrointestinal Function

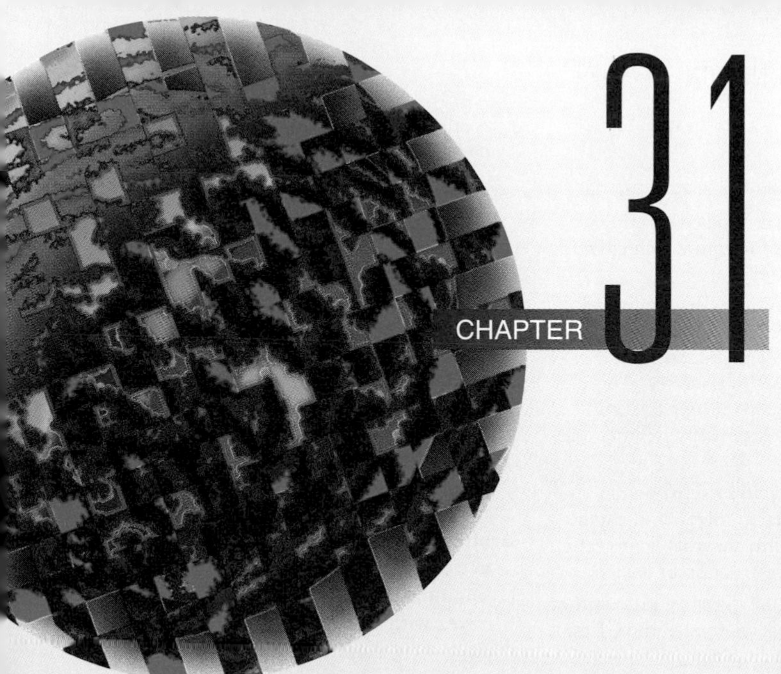

CHAPTER 31

Assessment of Digestive and Gastrointestinal Function

Learning Objectives

On completion of this chapter, the learner will be able to:

1. Describe the structure and function of the organs of the gastrointestinal tract.
2. Describe the mechanical and chemical processes involved in digesting and absorbing foods and eliminating waste products.
3. Use assessment parameters appropriate for determining the status of gastrointestinal function.
4. Describe the patient preparation, teaching, and follow-up care appropriate for patients having diagnostic testing of the gastrointestinal tract.

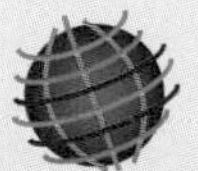

The gastrointestinal (GI) system is responsible for the ingestion, digestion, and absorption of nutrients and the elimination of the waste products of digestion. It consists of the digestive tract, the continuous tube beginning with the mouth and terminating at the anus, and the accessory organs. The accessory organs—the liver, gallbladder, and pancreas—aid in the digestive process but are not part of the alimentary canal.

GLOSSARY

absorption: phase of the digestive process that occurs when small molecules, vitamins, and minerals pass through the walls of the small and large intestine and into the bloodstream

amylase: an enzyme that aids in the digestion of starch

anus: last section of the GI tract; outlet for waste products from the system

chyme: mixture of food with saliva and ptyalin (salivary amylase) as it moves from the mouth through the esophagus to the stomach

digestion: phase of the digestive process that occurs when digestive enzymes and secretions mix with ingested food and when proteins, fats, and sugars are broken down into the component smaller molecules

elimination: phase of digestive process that occurs after digestion and absorption, when waste products are evacuated from the body

esophagus: collapsible tube connecting mouth to stomach through which chyme passes as it is ingested

fiberoscopy (gastrointestinal): intubation of a part of the GI system with a flexible, lighted tube to assist in diagnosis and treatment of diseases of that area. This can be an upper endoscopy (esophagus and stomach) or lower endoscopy (rectum and large intestine).

hydrochloric acid: acid secreted by the glands in the stomach; mixes with chyme to break it down into absorbable molecules and to aid in the destruction of bacteria

ingestion: phase of the digestive process that occurs when food is taken into the GI tract via the mouth and esophagus

intrinsic factor: a gastric secretion that combines with vitamin B_{12} so that it can be absorbed

large intestine: the portion of the GI tract into which waste material from the small intestine passes as absorption continues and elimination begins; consists of several parts—ascending segment, transverse segment, descending segment, sigmoid colon, and rectum

lipase: an enzyme that aids in the digestion of fats

mouth: first portion of the GI tract, through which ingestion of food takes place

pepsin: a gastric enzyme important in protein digestion

small intestine: longest portion of the GI tract, consisting of 3 parts—duodenum, jejunum, and ileum—through which food mixed with all secretions and enzymes passes as it continues to be digested and begins to be absorbed into bloodstream

stomach: distensible pouch into which chyme passes to be digested by gastric enzymes

trypsin: enzyme that aids in the digestion of protein

ANATOMIC AND PHYSIOLOGIC OVERVIEW

Anatomy of the Gastrointestinal Tract

The GI tract is a 23- to 26-foot-long pathway that extends from the **mouth** through the esophagus, stomach, and intestines to the anus (Fig. 31-1). The **esophagus** is located in the mediastinum in the thoracic cavity, anterior to the spine and posterior to the trachea and heart. This collapsible tube, which is about 25 cm (10 inches) in length, becomes distended when food passes through it.

The remaining portion of the GI tract is located within the peritoneal cavity. The **stomach** is situated in the upper portion of the abdomen to the left of the midline, just under the left diaphragm. It is a distensible pouch with a capacity of approximately 1500 mL. The inlet to the stomach is called the esophagogastric junction; it is surrounded by a ring of smooth muscle called the lower esophageal sphincter (or cardiac sphincter), which, on contraction, closes off the stomach from the esophagus. The stomach can be divided into four anatomic regions: the cardia (entrance), fundus, body, and pylorus (outlet). Circular smooth muscle in the wall of the pylorus forms the pyloric sphincter and controls the opening between the stomach and the small intestine.

The **small intestine** is the longest segment of the GI tract, accounting for about two thirds of the total length of the tract. It folds back and forth on itself, allowing for approximately 7000 cm of surface area for secretion and **absorption**, the process by which nutrients enter the bloodstream through the intestinal walls. The small intestine is divided into three anatomic parts: the upper part, called the duodenum; the middle part, called the jejunum; and the lower part, called the ileum. The common bile duct, which allows for the passage of both bile and pancreatic secretions, empties into the duodenum at the ampulla of Vater. The junction between the small and large intestine, the cecum, is located in the right lower portion of the abdomen. The ileocecal valve controls the passage of intestinal contents into the large intestine and prevents reflux of bacteria into the small intestine. The vermiform appendix is located near this junction.

The **large intestine** consists of an ascending segment on the right side of the abdomen, a transverse segment that extends from right to left in the upper abdomen, and a descending segment on the left side of the abdomen. The terminal portion of the large intestine consists of two parts: the sigmoid colon and the rectum. The rectum is continuous with the **anus**. The anal outlet is regulated by a network of striated muscle that forms both the internal and the external anal sphincters.

The GI tract receives blood from arteries that originate along the entire length of the thoracic and abdominal aorta. Of particular importance are the gastric artery and the superior and inferior mesenteric arteries. Oxygen and nutrients are supplied to the stomach by the gastric artery and to the intestine by the mesenteric arteries (Fig. 31-2). Blood is drained from these organs by veins that merge with others in the abdomen to form a large vessel called the portal vein. Nutrient-rich blood is then carried to the liver. The blood flow to the GI tract is about 20% of the total cardiac output and increases significantly after eating.

The GI tract is innervated by both the sympathetic and parasympathetic portions of the autonomic nervous system. In general, sympathetic nerves exert an inhibitory effect on the GI tract, decreasing gastric secretion and motility and causing the sphincters and blood vessels to constrict. Parasympathetic nerve stimulation causes peristalsis and increases secretory activities. The sphincters relax under the influence of parasympathetic stimulation. The only portions of the tract under voluntary control are the upper esophagus and the external anal sphincter.

Function of the Digestive System

All cells of the body require nutrients. These nutrients are derived from the intake of food that contains protein, fat, carbohydrates, vitamins and minerals, and cellulose fibers and other vegetable matter of no nutritional value.

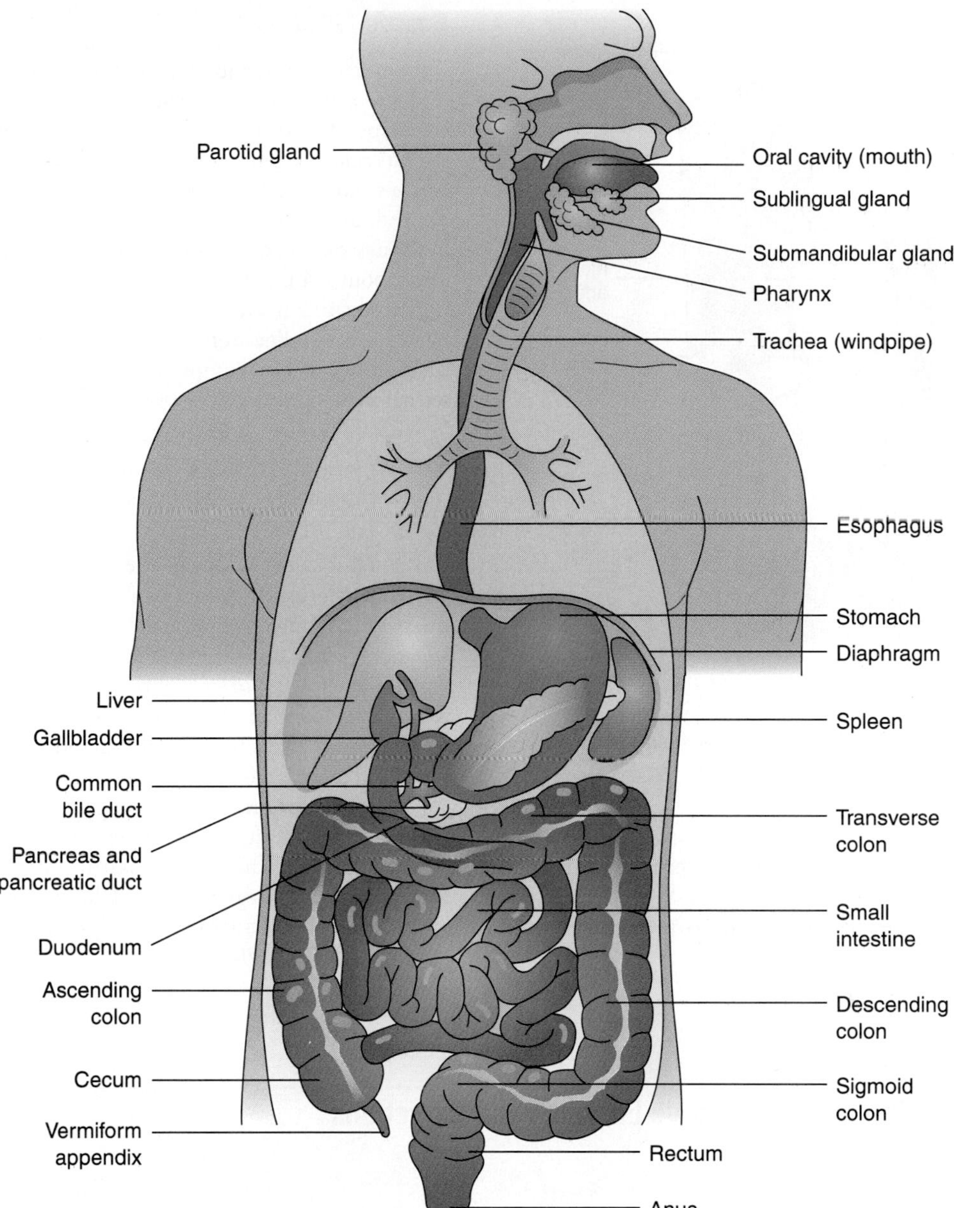

FIGURE 31•1 Organs of the digestive system and associated structures.

The primary digestive functions of the GI tract are to:

- Break down food particles into the molecular form for digestion
- Absorb into the bloodstream the small molecules produced by **digestion**
- Eliminate undigested and unabsorbed foodstuffs and other waste products from the body

After food is ingested, it is propelled through the GI tract, placing it in contact with a wide variety of secretions that aid in digestion, absorption, or **elimination** from the GI tract.

Chewing and Swallowing

The process of digestion begins with the act of chewing, in which food is broken down into small particles that can be swallowed and mixed with digestive enzymes. Eating, or even the sight, smell, or taste of food, can cause reflex salivation. Saliva is secreted from three pairs of glands: the parotid, the submaxillary, and the sublingual glands. Approximately 1.5 L of saliva are secreted daily. Saliva is the first secretion that comes in contact with food. Saliva contains the enzyme ptyalin, or salivary amylase, which begins the digestion of starches (Table 31-1). Saliva also contains mucus and water, which help to lubricate the food as it is chewed, thereby facilitating swallowing.

Swallowing begins as a voluntary act that is regulated by a swallowing center in the medulla oblongata of the central nervous system. As food is swallowed, the epiglottis moves to cover the tracheal opening and thus prevents aspiration of food into the lungs. Swallowing, which results in propelling the bolus of food into the upper esophagus, thus ends as a reflex action. The smooth muscle in the wall of the esophagus contracts in a rhythmic sequence from the upper esophagus toward the stomach to

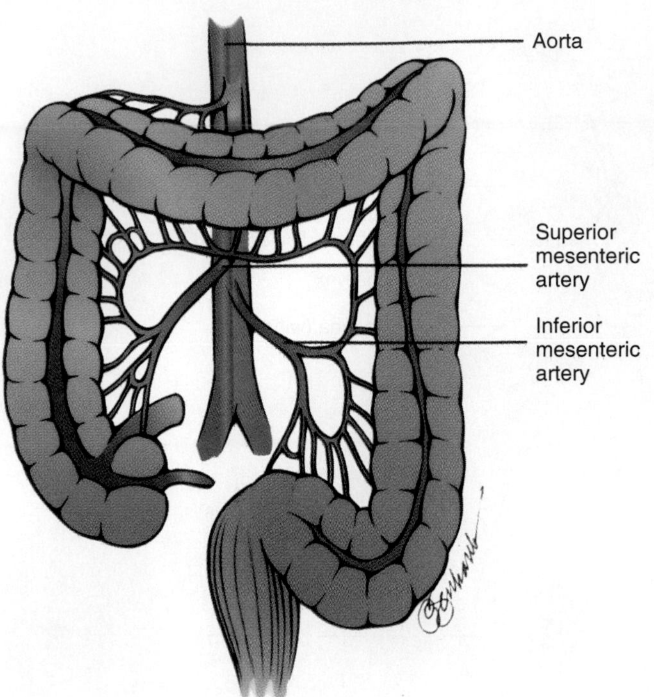

FIGURE 31•2 Anatomy and blood supply of the large intestine.

propel the bolus of food along the tract. During this process of esophageal peristalsis, the lower esophageal sphincter relaxes and permits the bolus of food to enter the stomach. Subsequently, the lower esophageal sphincter closes tightly to prevent reflux of stomach contents into the esophagus.

Gastric Function

The stomach stores and mixes the food with secretions. It secretes a highly acidic fluid in response to the presence or anticipated **ingestion** of food. This fluid, which may have a pH as low as 1, derives its acidity from the **hydrochloric acid** secreted by the glands of the stomach. The function of this gastric secretion is two-fold: to break down food into more absorbable components and to aid in the destruction of most ingested bacteria. The stomach can produce about 2.4 L per day of these gastric secretions. Gastric secretions also contain the enzyme **pepsin**, which is important for initiating protein digestion. **Intrinsic factor** is also secreted by the gastric mucosa. This compound combines with dietary vitamin B_{12} so that the vitamin can be absorbed in the ileum.

Nursing Alert *In the absence of intrinsic factor, vitamin B_{12} cannot be absorbed and pernicious anemia results (see Chap. 30).*

Peristaltic contractions in the stomach propel its contents toward the pylorus. Because large food particles cannot pass through the pyloric sphincter, they are churned back into the body of the stomach. In this way, food in the stomach is mechanically agitated and broken down into smaller particles. Food remains in the stomach for a variable length of time, from a half hour to several hours, depending on the size of food particles, the composition of the meal, and other factors. Peristalsis in the stomach and contractions of the pyloric sphincter allow the partially digested food to enter the small intestine at a rate that permits efficient absorption of nutrients. This food mixed with gastric secretions is called **chyme**. Hormones, neuroregulators, and local regulators found in the gastric secretions control the rate of gastric secretions and influence gastric motility (Table 31-2).

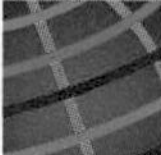

TABLE 31•1 The Major Digestive Enzymes and Secretions

Enzyme/Secretion	Enzyme Source	Digestive Action
Action of Enzymes That Digest Carbohydrates		
Ptyalin (salivary amylase)	Salivary glands	Starch→dextrin, maltose, glucose
Amylase	Pancreas and intestinal mucosa	Starch→dextrin, maltose, glucose Dextrin→maltose, glucose
Maltase	Intestinal mucosa	Maltose→glucose
Sucrase	Intestinal mucosa	Sucrose→glucose, fructose
Lactase	Intestinal mucosa	Lactose→glucose, galactose
Action of Enzymes/Secretions That Digest Protein		
Pepsin	Gastric mucosa	Protein→polypeptides
Trypsin	Pancreas	Proteins and polypeptides→polypeptides, dipeptides, amino acids
Aminopeptidase	Intestinal mucosa	Polypeptides→dipeptides, amino acids
Dipeptidase	Intestinal mucosa	Dipeptides→amino acids
Hydrochloric acid	Gastric mucosa	Protein→polypeptides, amino acids
Action of Enzymes That Digest Fat (Triglyceride)		
Pharyngeal lipase	Pharynx mucosa	Triglycerides→fatty acids, diglycerides, monoglycerides
Steapsin	Gastric mucosa	Triglycerides→fatty acids, diglycerides, monoglycerides
Pancreatic lipase	Pancreas	Triglycerides→fatty acids, diglycerides, monoglycerides
Bile	Liver and gallbladder	Fat emulsification

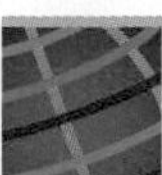

TABLE 31•2 **The Major Gastrointestinal Regulatory Substances**

Substance	Stimulus for Production	Target Tissue	Effect on Secretions	Effect on Motility
Neuroregulators				
Acetylcholine	Sight, smell, chewing food, stomach distention	Gastric glands, other secretory glands, gastrointestinal muscle	Increased gastric acid	Generally increased; decreased sphincter tone
Norepinephrine	Stress, other various stimuli	Secretory glands, gastrointestinal muscle	Generally inhibitory	Generally decreased; increased sphincter tone
Hormonal Regulators				
Gastrin	Stomach distention with food	Gastric glands	Increased secretion of gastric juice, which is rich in HCl	Increased motility of stomach, decreased time required for gastric emptying Relaxation of ileocecal sphincter Excitation of colon Constriction of gastroesophageal sphincter
Cholecystokinin	Fat in duodenum	Gallbladder	Release of bile into duodenum	
		Pancreas	Increased production of enzyme-rich pancreatic secretions	
		Stomach	Inhibits gastric secretion somewhat	Inhibits stomach contractions
Secretin	pH of chyme in duodenum below 4–5	Stomach	Inhibits gastric secretion somewhat	
		Pancreas	Increased production of bicarbonate-rich pancreatic juice	
Local Regulator				
Histamine	Unclear; substances in food	Gastric glands	Increased gastric acid production	

Small Intestine Function

The digestive process continues in the duodenum. Secretions in the duodenum come from the accessory digestive organs—the pancreas, liver, and gallbladder—and the glands in the wall of the intestine itself. These secretions contain digestive enzymes and bile. Pancreatic secretions have an alkaline pH because of high concentrations of bicarbonate. This neutralizes the acid entering the duodenum from the stomach. The pancreas also secretes digestive enzymes, including **trypsin**, which aids in digesting protein; **amylase**, which aids in digesting starch; and **lipase**, which aids in digesting fats. Bile (secreted by the liver and stored in the gallbladder) aids in emulsifying ingested fats, making them easier to digest and absorb.

The intestinal glands secrete mucus, hormones, electrolytes, and enzymes. The mucus coats the cells and protects the mucosa from injury by hydrochloric acid. Hormones, neuroregulators, and local regulators found in these intestinal secretions control the rate of intestinal secretion and also influence GI motility. Intestinal secretions total approximately 1 L/day of pancreatic juice, 0.5 L/day of bile, and 3 L/day from the glands of the small intestine. Tables 31-1 and 31-2 summarize the actions of digestive enzymes and GI regulatory substances.

Two types of contractions occur regularly in the small intestine. Segmentation contractions produce mixing waves that move the intestinal contents back and forth in a churning motion. Intestinal peristalsis propels the contents of the small intestine toward the colon. Both are stimulated by the presence of chyme.

Food, initially ingested in the form of fats, protein, and carbohydrates, is broken down into absorbable particles (constituent nutrients) by the process of digestion. Carbohydrates are broken down into disaccharides (eg, sucrose, maltose, and galactose) and monosaccharides (eg, glucose and fructose). Glucose is the major carbohydrate that the tissue cells use as fuel. Proteins are broken down into amino acids and peptides. Ingested fats are emulsified into monoglycerides and fatty acids. These smaller molecules are then ready to be absorbed.

Small, finger-like projections called villi are present throughout the entire intestine and function to produce digestive enzymes as well as to absorb nutrients. Vitamins and minerals are not digested but rather absorbed essentially unchanged. Absorption begins in the jejunum and is accomplished by both active transport and diffusion across the intestinal wall into the circulation.

Colonic Function

Within 4 hours after eating, residual waste material passes into the terminal ileum and slowly passes into the proximal portion of the colon through the ileocecal valve. This valve, which is normally closed, helps prevent colonic contents from refluxing into the small intestine. With each peristaltic wave of the small intestine, the valve opens briefly and permits some of the contents to pass into the colon.

The bacterial population is a major component of the contents of the large intestine. Bacteria assist in completing the breakdown of waste material, especially of undigested or unabsorbed proteins and bile salts. Two types of colonic secretions are added to the residual material—mucus and an electrolyte solution. The electrolyte solution is chiefly a bicarbonate solution that acts to neutralize the end products formed by the colonic bacterial action. The mucus protects the colonic mucosa from the interluminal contents and also provides adherence for the fecal mass.

Slow, weak peristaltic activity moves the colonic contents slowly along the tract. This slow transport allows efficient reabsorption of water and electrolytes. Intermittent strong peristaltic waves propel the contents for considerable distances. This generally occurs after another meal is eaten, when intestine-stimulating hormones are released. The waste materials from a meal eventually reach and distend the rectum, usually in about 12 hours. As much as one fourth of the waste materials from a meal may still be in the rectum 3 days after the meal was ingested.

Waste Products of Digestion

Feces consist of undigested foodstuffs, inorganic materials, water, and bacteria. Fecal matter is about 75% fluid and 25% solid material. The composition is relatively unaffected by alterations in diet, because a large portion of the fecal mass is of nondietary origin, derived from the secretions of the GI tract. The brown color of the feces results from the breakdown of bile by the intestinal bacteria. Chemicals formed by intestinal bacteria (especially indole and skatole) are responsible in large part for the fecal odor. Gases formed contain methane, hydrogen sulfide, and ammonia, among others. The GI tract normally contains approximately 150 mL of these gases. These gases are either absorbed into the portal circulation and detoxified by the liver or expelled from the rectum (flatus).

Elimination of stool begins with distention of the rectum, which reflexively initiates contractions of the rectal musculature and relaxes the normally closed internal anal sphincter. The internal sphincter is controlled by the autonomic nervous system; the external sphincter is under the conscious control of the cerebral cortex. During defecation, the external anal sphincter voluntarily relaxes to allow colonic contents to be expelled. Normally, the external anal sphincter is maintained in a state of tonic contraction. Thus, defecation is seen to be a spinal reflex (involving the parasympathetic nerve fibers) that can be voluntarily inhibited by keeping the external anal sphincter closed. Contracting the abdominal muscles (straining) facilitates emptying of the colon. The average frequency of defecation in humans is once daily, but the frequency varies among individuals.

ASSESSMENT

Health History and Clinical Manifestations

The nurse begins by taking a complete history, focusing on symptoms common to GI dysfunction. These symptoms include pain, indigestion, intestinal gas, nausea and vomiting, hematemesis, and changes in bowel habits and stool characteristics. Information about any previous GI disease is important. Past and current medication use and any previous treatment or surgery are noted. A dietary history is taken to assess nutritional status. Questioning about the use of tobacco and alcohol includes the details about type and amount. Changes in appetite and eating patterns are discussed. Patterns of unexplained weight gain or loss over the last year are elicited. Stool characteristics are assessed. The nurse records all abnormal findings and reports them to the physician.

Pain

Pain can be a major symptom of GI disease. The character, duration, pattern, frequency, location, and distribution of referred pain (Fig. 31-3) and time of the pain vary greatly depending on the underlying cause. Other factors, such as meals, rest, defecation, and vascular disorders, may directly affect this pain.

Indigestion

Upper abdominal discomfort or distress associated with eating is the most common complaint of patients with GI dysfunction. The basis for this abdominal distress may be the patient's own gastric peristaltic movements. Bowel movements may or may not relieve the pain. Indigestion can result from disturbed nervous control of the stomach or from a disorder in the GI tract or elsewhere in the body. Fatty foods tend to cause the most discomfort because they remain in the stomach longer than proteins or carbohydrates. Coarse vegetables and highly seasoned foods can also cause considerable distress.

Intestinal Gas

The accumulation of gas in the GI tract may result in belching (the expulsion of gas from the stomach through the mouth) or flatulence (the expulsion of gas from the rectum). It is through belching that swallowed air is quickly expelled when it reaches the stomach. Usually, gases in the small intestine pass into the colon and are released as flatus. Patients often complain of bloating, distention, or being "full of gas." Flatulence may be a symptom of gallbladder disease or food intolerance.

Nausea and Vomiting

Vomiting is another major symptom of GI disease. Vomiting is usually preceded by nausea, which can be triggered by odors, activity, or food intake. The emesis, or vomitus, may vary in color and content. It may contain undigested food particles or blood (hematemesis). When vomiting occurs soon after hemorrhage, the emesis is bright red. If blood has been retained in the stomach, it takes on a coffee-ground appearance because of the action of the digestive enzymes.

Change in Bowel Habits and Stool Characteristics

Changes in bowel habits may signal colon disease. Diarrhea (an abnormal increase in the frequency and liquidity of the stool or in daily stool weight or volume) commonly occurs when the contents move so rapidly through the intestine and colon that there is inadequate time for the GI secretions to be absorbed. Diarrhea is sometimes associated with abdominal pain or cramping and nausea or vomiting. Constipation (a decrease in the frequency of stool, or stools that are hard, dry, and of smaller volume than normal) may be associated with anal discomfort and rectal bleeding. See Chapter 35 for further discussion of diarrhea and constipation.

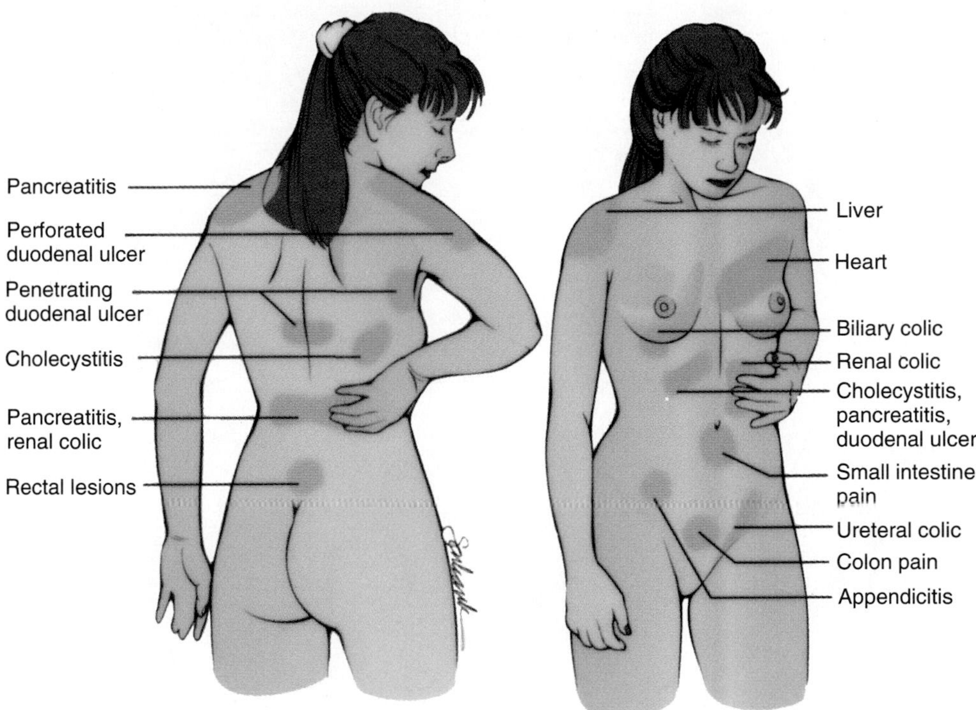

FIGURE 31•3 Common sites of referred abdominal pain.

The characteristics of the stool may vary greatly. Stool is normally light to dark brown. However, many circumstances, including the ingestion of certain foods and medications, can change the appearance of stool (Table 31-3). Blood in the stool must be investigated. It can present in various ways:

- If shed in sufficient quantities into the upper GI tract, blood produces a tarry-black color (melena).
- Blood entering the lower portion of the GI tract or passing rapidly through it will appear bright or dark red.
- Lower rectal or anal bleeding is suspected if there is streaking of blood on the surface of the stool or if blood is noted on toilet tissue.

Other common abnormalities in stool characteristics that the patient may describe during the health history include:

- Bulky, greasy, foamy stools that are foul in odor; stool color is gray, with a silvery sheen
- Light-gray or clay-colored stool because of the absence of urobilin
- Stool with mucus threads or pus that may be visible on gross inspection of the stool
- Small, dry, rock-hard masses called scybala are sometimes streaked with blood from rectal trauma as they pass through the rectum
- Loose, watery stool that may or may not be streaked with blood

TABLE 31•3 Foods and Medications That Alter Stool Color

Altering Substance	Color
meat protein	dark brown
spinach	green
carrots and beets	red
cocoa	dark red or brown
senna	yellow
bismuth, iron, licorice, and charcoal	black
barium	milky white

Physical Assessment

The physical examination includes assessment of the mouth, abdomen, and rectum. The mouth, tongue, buccal mucosa, teeth, and gums are inspected and ulcers, nodules, swelling, discoloration, or inflammation is noted. People with dentures should remove them during this part of the examination to allow good visualization.

The patient is placed in the supine position with knees flexed slightly for inspection, auscultation, palpation, and percussion of the abdomen (Fig. 31-4). Inspection is performed first, and skin changes and scars from previous operations are noted. Contour and symmetry of the abdomen are also noted, with the identification of localized bulging, distention, or peristaltic waves.

Auscultation is performed before percussion and palpation (which can increase intestinal motility and thereby change bowel sounds). The character, location, and frequency of bowel sounds are noted. Bowel sounds are assessed in all four quadrants using the diaphragm of the stethoscope; the high-pitched and gurgling sounds can be heard best in this manner. Findings are documented using the terms normal (sounds heard about every 5 to 20 seconds), hypoactive (one or two sounds in 2 minutes), hyperactive (5 to 6 sounds heard in less than 30 seconds), or absent (no sounds in 3 to 5 minutes).

Tympany or dullness is noted during percussion. Light palpation is used to identify areas of tenderness or swelling. Deep palpation is used to identify masses in any of the four quadrants. Rebound tenderness can be assessed in any area where the patient identifies discomfort. Pressure is exerted over the area and then released quickly. Pain experienced on withdrawal of the pressure

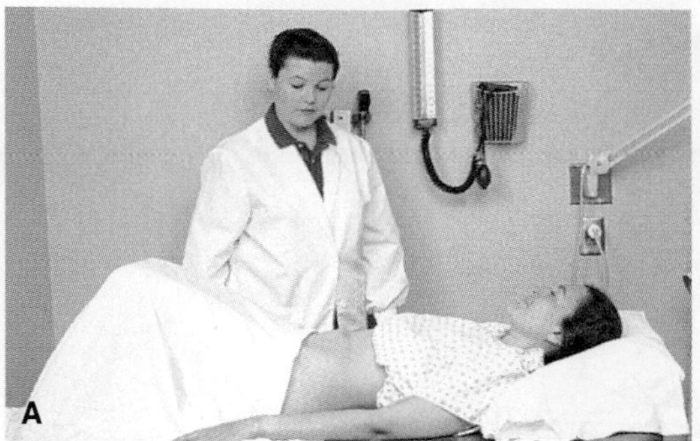

Inspecting the abdomen

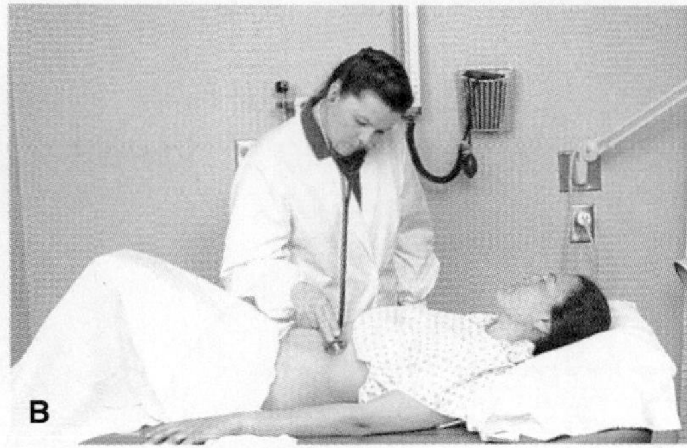

Auscultating the abdomen

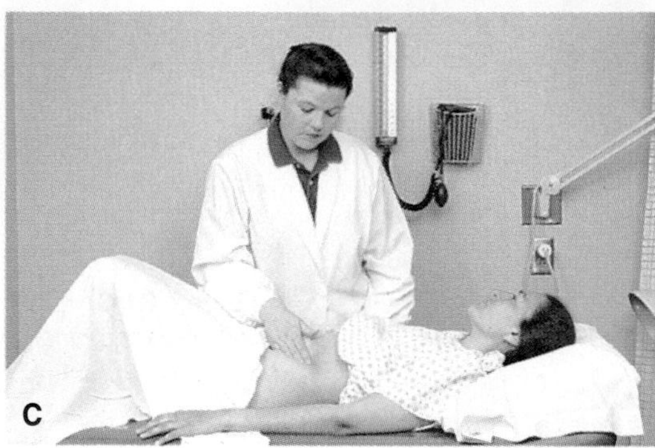

Palpating the abdomen

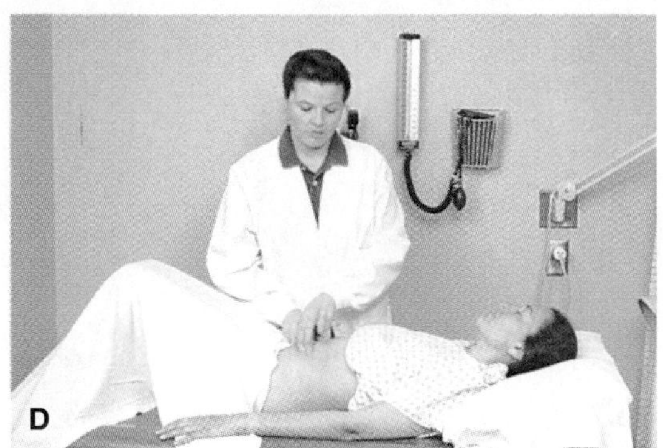

Percussing the abdomen

FIGURE 31•4 Examination of the abdomen includes inspection, auscultation, palpation, and percussion.

is noted. Any abnormal finding should be noted in relationship to the surface landmarks (xiphoid process, costal margins, anterior iliac spine, and symphysis pubis) or the four quadrants commonly used to describe the abdomen (RUQ, right upper quadrant; RLQ, right lower quadrant; LUQ, left upper quadrant; LLQ, left lower quadrant).

The examination is completed with inspection of the anal and perineal area. Areas of excoriation or rash, fissures or fistula openings, or external hemorrhoids should be inspected and palpated. A digital rectal examination can be performed to note any areas of tenderness or mass.

DIAGNOSTIC EVALUATION

Multiple modalities are available for the diagnostic assessment of the GI tract, including x-ray and ultrasound studies and direct visualization of portions of the GI tract through the passage of various gastric and intestinal tubes. The majority of these tests and procedures are performed on an outpatient basis in special units designed for this purpose (eg, endoscopy or GI laboratory). The nurse supports and educates patients undergoing diagnostic evaluation, whether in an inpatient or outpatient setting. Patients requiring such tests are frequently anxious, elderly, or debilitated. The preparation for many of these studies includes fasting and the use of laxatives or enemas, and ingestion or injection of contrast agent or a radiopaque dye. These measures are poorly tolerated by weak patients and have the potential to cause fluid and electrolyte imbalances. If further assessment or treatment is needed after any outpatient procedure, the patient may be admitted to the hospital.

Nursing interventions for the patient who is having GI diagnostic assessment include the following:

- Providing general information about a balanced diet and the nutritional factors that can cause GI disturbances. Information about specific nutrients that should be included in the diet is provided after a diagnosis has been confirmed.
- Providing needed information about the test and the activities required of the patient
- Providing instructions about postprocedure care, as well as activity restrictions
- Alleviating anxiety
- Helping the patient cope with discomfort
- Encouraging family members or others to offer emotional support to the patient during the diagnostic testing
- Assessing for adequate hydration before, during, and immediately after the procedure. Education should be provided about hydration concerns.

Upper Gastrointestinal Tract Study

The entire GI tract can be delineated by x-rays after the introduction of a contrast agent. A radiopaque liquid (such as barium sulfate) is one of the most commonly used agents. This tasteless, odorless, nongranular, and completely insoluble (hence, not absorbable) powder is ingested in the form of a thick or thin aqueous suspension for the purpose of studying the upper GI tract (upper GI series or barium swallow). The upper GI series enables the examiner to detect or exclude anatomic or functional derangement of the upper GI organs or sphincters. It also aids in the diagnosis of ulcers, varices, tumors, regional enteritis, and malabsorption syndromes. The procedure may be extended to examine the duodenum and small bowel (small bowel follow-through).

The patient swallows barium under direct fluoroscopic examination. As the barium descends into the stomach, the position, patency, and caliber of the esophagus are visualized, enabling the examiner to detect or exclude any anatomic or functional derangement of that organ. Fluoroscopic examination next extends to the stomach as its lumen fills with barium. The motility and the thickness of the gastric wall and the mucosal pattern are observed. The patency of the pyloric valve and the anatomy of the duodenum are also observed. Multiple x-rays are obtained during the procedure, and additional x-rays may be taken at intervals for up to 24 hours to evaluate the rate of gastric emptying. If small bowel follow-through is conducted, the motility of the small bowel is observed. Obstructions, ileitis, and diverticula can be detected if present.

Variations of the upper GI study include double-contrast studies and enteroclysis. The double-contrast method of examining the upper GI tract involves administering a thick barium suspension to outline the stomach and esophageal wall. Next, tablets that release carbon dioxide in the presence of water are given. This technique has the advantage of showing the esophagus and stomach in finer detail, thus permitting signs of early superficial neoplasms to be noted.

Enteroclysis is a very detailed, double-contrast study of the entire small intestine that involves the continuous infusion, through a duodenal tube, of 500 to 1000 mL of a thin barium sulfate suspension. Methylcellulose is then infused into the small intestine through the tube. The barium and methylcellulose fill the intestinal loops and are observed continuously by fluoroscope and filmed at frequent intervals as they progress through the jejunum and the ileum. This process (even with normal motility) can take up to 6 hours. The procedure aids in the diagnosis of partial small bowel obstructions or diverticula.

Nursing Interventions

The patient may be asked to maintain a low-residue diet for several days before the test. He or she should receive nothing by mouth after midnight before the test. A laxative may be prescribed to clean out the intestinal tract. Because smoking can stimulate gastric motility, the patient is discouraged from smoking the morning before the examination. All medications are withheld.

Follow-up care is needed after any of the above procedures to ensure that the ingested barium has been completely eliminated. Fluids must be increased to facilitate evacuation of stool. Stools must be monitored until they return to their normal color (the barium will look like clay). A laxative or enema may be needed.

Lower Gastrointestinal Tract Study

When barium is instilled rectally to visualize the lower GI tract, it is called a barium enema. The purpose of a barium enema is to detect the presence of polyps, tumors, and other lesions of the large intestine and to demonstrate any abnormal anatomy or malfunction of the bowel.

The radiopaque substance is instilled rectally in the radiology department during fluoroscopy. If the patient has been prepared adequately and the colon evacuated completely, the contour of the entire colon, including the cecum and appendix (if patent), is clearly visible and the motility of each portion readily observed. The procedure generally takes about 15 to 30 minutes. Radiographs (x-rays) are taken during the procedure.

Other means for visualizing the colon include double-contrast studies or a water-soluble contrast study. A double-contrast or air-contrast barium enema involves the instillation of a thicker barium solution, followed by the instillation of air. The patient may feel some cramping or discomfort with this process. This test provides a contrast between the air-filled lumen and the barium-coated mucosa. Smaller lesions can be more easily detected with this technique.

When the patient is suspected of having active inflammatory disease, fistulas, or perforation of the colon, a water-soluble iodinated contrast agent (eg, Gastrografin) can be used. The procedure is the same as for a barium enema; however, the patient must be assessed for iodine or contrast agent allergy. The contrast is readily eliminated after the procedure, so there is no need for postprocedure laxatives. A few patients complain of some diarrhea until the contrast agent is totally eliminated.

Nursing Interventions

Preparing the patient includes emptying and cleansing the lower bowel. This often includes a low-residue diet 1 to 2 days before the test (the preparation required by different radiology departments may vary); a clear liquid diet and a laxative the evening before; nothing by mouth after midnight; and cleansing enemas until returns are clear the following morning. Barium enemas should be scheduled before any upper GI studies. If the patient has active inflammatory disease of the colon, enemas are contraindicated. Active GI bleeding may prohibit the use of laxatives and enemas. Barium enema is contraindicated in patients with signs of perforation or obstruction; instead, a water-soluble contrast study may be performed in these situations.

An enema or laxative is administered after these tests to facilitate barium removal. Increasing fluid intake will assist in eliminating the barium. As with any barium study, the patient must be monitored for complete elimination of the barium.

Gastric Analysis, Gastric Acid Stimulation Test, and pH Monitoring

Analysis of the gastric juice yields information about the secretory activity of the gastric mucosa and the presence or degree of gastric retention in patients thought to have pyloric or duodenal obstruction. It is also useful in diagnosing diseases such as Zollinger-Ellison syndrome.

The patient receives nothing by mouth (NPO) for 8 to 12 hours before the procedure. Any medications affecting gastric secretions are withheld for 24 to 48 hours before the test. Smoking is not allowed the morning before the test because it increases gastric secretions. A small nasogastric tube with a catheter tip marked at various points is inserted through the nose. When the tube is at a point slightly less than 50 cm (21 inches) distant, it should be within the stomach, lying along the greater curvature. Once in place, the tube is secured to the patient's cheek and the patient is placed in a semireclining position. The entire stomach contents are aspirated by gentle suction into a syringe. Gastric samples are collected every 15 minutes for the next hour.

The gastric acid stimulation test is usually performed in conjunction with gastric analysis. Histamine or pentagastrin is given subcutaneously to stimulate gastric secretions. The patient is informed that this injection may produce a flushed feeling. Blood pressure and pulse are monitored frequently to detect hypotension. Gastric specimens are collected after the injection every 15 minutes for 1 hour and labeled to indicate the time after histamine injections. The volume and pH of the specimen are measured. In certain instances, cytologic study by the Papanicolaou technique may be used to determine the presence or absence of malignant cells. Enzyme analysis of the gastric juice may be indicated.

Important diagnostic information to be gained from gastric analysis is the ability of the mucosa to secrete hydrochloric acid, which is altered in various disease states:

- Patients with pernicious anemia secrete no acid under basal conditions or after stimulation.
- Patients with severe chronic atrophic gastritis or gastric cancer secrete little or no acid.
- Patients with peptic ulcer invariably secrete some acid.
- Patients with duodenal ulcers usually secrete an excess amount of acid.

Esophageal reflux of gastric acid may be diagnosed by ambulatory pH monitoring. Patients are maintained NPO for 6 hours. All medications affecting gastric secretions are withheld for 24 to 36 hours before the test. A probe that measures pH is placed through the nose and into position about 5 inches above the lower esophageal sphincter. It is connected to an external recording device and is worn for 24 hours while the patient continues his or her normal daily activities. The end result is a computer analysis and graphic display of the results.

Laparoscopy (Peritoneoscopy)

The use of laparoscopic techniques for the diagnosis of GI disease has been expanded. The procedure is performed with a special fiberoptic laparoscope that allows direct visualization of the organs and structures within the abdomen. It also allows biopsy samples to be taken from these structures and organs as necessary. This procedure is used to evaluate peritoneal disease, chronic abdominal pain, abdominal masses, and gallbladder and liver disease. The procedure is also being used to excise certain structures and masses.

Upper Gastrointestinal Fiberoscopy/ Esophagogastroduodenoscopy

Fiberscopes are flexible scopes equipped with fiberoptic lenses. **Fiberoscopy** of the upper GI tract allows direct visualization of the esophageal, gastric, and duodenal mucosa through a lighted endoscope (gastroscope) (Fig. 31-5). This procedure is called esophagogastroduodenoscopy (EGD). This procedure is especially valuable when esophageal, gastric, or duodenal abnormalities and inflammatory, neoplastic, or infectious processes are suspected. Esophageal and gastric motility can be evaluated. Secretions and tissue specimens can be collected for further analysis. Still or video photography taken through the scope allows for documentation of findings.

The gastroenterologist views the procedure through a viewing lens. Electronic video endoscopes are available that attach directly to a video processor, converting the electronic signals into pictures on a television screen. This allows larger and continuous viewing capabilities, as well as the simultaneous recording of the procedure. Side-viewing flexible scopes are used to visualize the common bile duct and the pancreatic and hepatic ducts through the ampulla of Vater in the duodenum. This procedure, called endoscopic retrograde cholangiopancreatography (ERCP), is helpful in evaluating jaundice, pancreatitis, tumors of the pancreas, common duct stones, and biliary tract disease.

Upper GI fiberoscopy also can be a therapeutic procedure when combined with other procedures. Therapeutic endoscopy can be used to remove common bile duct stones, dilate strictures, and treat gastric bleeding and esophageal varices. Laser-compatible scopes provide laser therapy for upper GI neoplasms. Sclerosing solutions can be injected through the scope in an attempt to control upper GI bleeding.

After the patient is sedated, the endoscope is lubricated with a water-soluble lubricant and passed smoothly and slowly along the back of the mouth and down into the esophagus. The gastroenterologist views the gastric wall and the sphincters. The endoscope is then advanced into the duodenum for further examination. Biopsy forceps to obtain tissue specimens or cytology brushes to obtain cells for microscopic study can be passed through the scope. The procedure generally takes about 30 minutes.

It is important to monitor and maintain the patient's oral airway during the procedure. Finger or ear oximeters are used to monitor oxygen saturation. Supplemental oxygen may be used if needed. Emergency equipment must be readily available. Precautions must be taken to protect the scope, because the fiberoptic bundles may be broken if the scope is bent at an acute angle. Mouth guards are essential to prevent the patient from biting the scope.

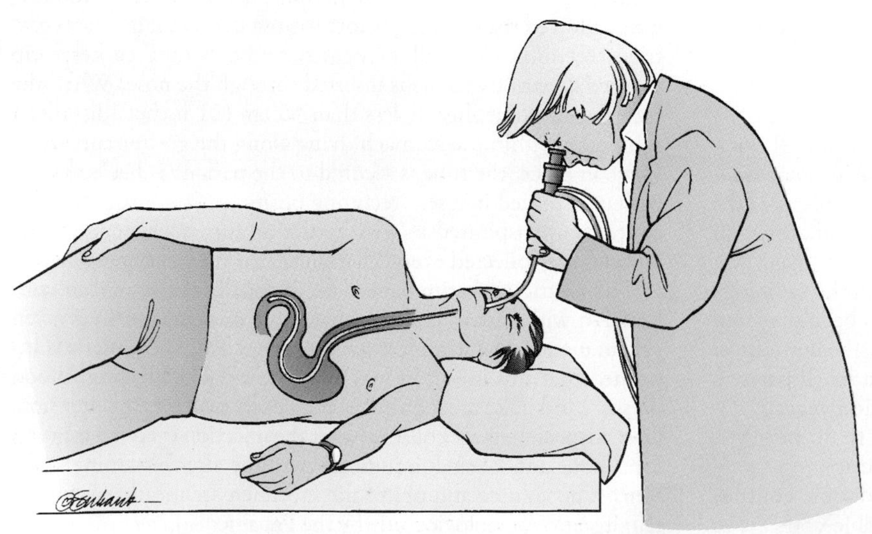

FIGURE 31•5 Patient undergoing gastroscopy.

Nursing Interventions

The patient is instructed not to eat or drink for 6 to 12 hours before the examination. Patient preparation includes spraying or gargling with a local anesthetic, along with administering midazolam (Versed) intravenously just before the scope is introduced. Midazolam is a sedative that provides conscious sedation and relieves anxiety during the procedure. Atropine may be administered to reduce secretions. Glucagon may be given, if needed, to relax smooth muscle. The patient is positioned on the left side to facilitate saliva drainage and to provide easy access for the endoscope.

After the procedure, the patient is instructed not to eat or drink until the gag reflex returns (in 1 to 2 hours) to prevent aspiration of food or fluids into the lungs. After gastroscopy, assessment by the nurse includes observing for signs of perforation, such as pain, bleeding, unusual difficulty swallowing, and an elevated temperature. Minor throat discomfort can be relieved with lozenges, saline gargle, and oral analgesics after the gag reflex has returned. Patients who were sedated for the procedure are maintained on bed rest until fully alert.

Anoscopy, Proctoscopy, and Sigmoidoscopy

The lower portion of the colon can also be viewed directly to evaluate rectal bleeding, acute or chronic diarrhea, or change in bowel habits and to observe for ulceration, tumors, polyps, or other pathologic processes. The scopes used can be rigid or flexible fiberoptic scopes. The anoscope is a rigid scope used to examine the anal canal. Proctoscopes and sigmoidoscopes are rigid scopes used to inspect the rectum and the sigmoid colon. The flexible fiberoptic sigmoidoscope (Fig. 31-6) permits the colon to be examined up to 40 to 50 cm (16 to 20 inches) from the anus. This is more than the 25 cm (10 inches) that can be seen with the rigid sigmoidoscope. The flexible scope has many of the same capabilities as the scopes used for the upper GI study. Still or video images can be used to document findings.

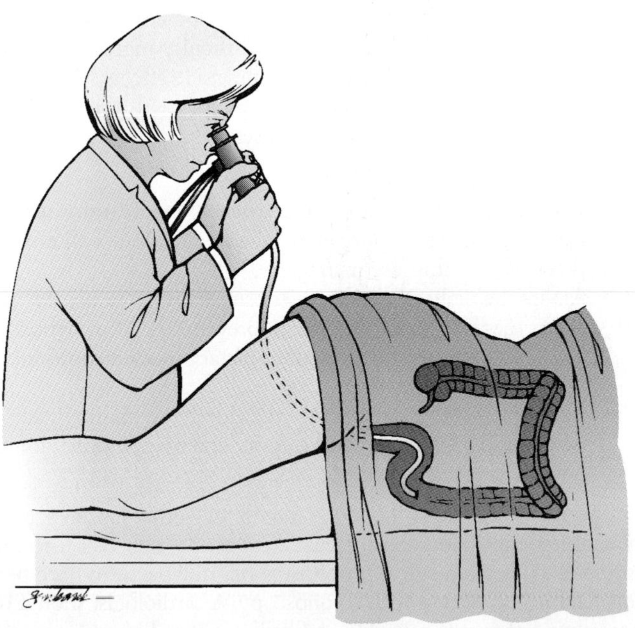

FIGURE 31•6 Flexible fiberoptic sigmoidoscopy. The instrument is advanced past the proximal sigmoid and then into the descending colon.

For rigid scope procedures, the patient assumes the knee–chest position at the edge of the bed or the examining table. With the back inclined at about a 45° angle, the patient is in proper position for the introduction of an anoscope, proctoscope, or sigmoidoscope. During the examination, the patient is kept informed about the progress of the examination. The patient is informed that the pressure exerted by the instrument will create the urge to have a bowel movement.

For flexible scope procedures, the patient is placed in a comfortable position on the left side with the right leg bent and placed anteriorly. Biopsies and polypectomies also can be performed during this procedure. The same nursing implications apply as for the rigid scope procedures.

One or more small pieces of tissue may be removed for biopsy. Biopsy is performed with small biting forceps introduced through the instrument. Rectal and sigmoid polyps, if present, may be removed with a wire snare, which is used to grasp the pedicle, or stalk. An electrocoagulating current is then used to sever the polyp and prevent bleeding. It is extremely important that all tissue that is excised by the endoscopist be placed immediately in moist gauze or in an appropriate receptacle, labeled correctly, and delivered without delay to the pathology laboratory for examination.

Nursing Interventions

These examinations require only limited bowel preparation. A warm tap-water enema or Fleet's enema is given until returns are clear. Dietary restrictions are not usually necessary. Sedation is not usually required.

After this procedure, the patient is monitored for rectal bleeding and signs of intestinal perforation (ie, fever, rectal drainage, abdominal distention, and pain). On completion of the examination, the patient can resume regular activities and dietary practices.

Fiberoptic Colonoscopy

Direct visual inspection of the colon to the cecum is possible by means of a flexible fiberoptic colonoscope (Fig. 31-7). The scopes have the same capabilities as those used for esophagogastroduodenoscopy; however, they are larger in diameter and longer. Still and video recordings can be used to document the procedure and findings. It is an effective procedure, with the distinct advantage of relatively low cost.

This procedure is commonly used as a diagnostic aid and screening device. It can be useful in the evaluation of patients with diarrhea of unknown etiology, occult bleeding, or anemia. It is used for further study of abnormalities detected on barium enema. It is most frequently used for screening for cancer (Table 31-4). Tissue biopsies can be obtained as needed, and polyps can be removed and evaluated. Inflammatory disease or other bowel disease can be diagnosed. Diagnoses can be clarified and the extent of the disease determined.

Therapeutically, the procedure can be used to remove polyps with a special snare and cautery through the colonoscope. Many colon cancers begin with adenomatous polyps of the colon; therefore, one goal of colonoscopic polypectomy is early detection and prevention of colorectal cancer. All visible polyps are removed. This procedure also can be used to treat areas of bleeding or stricture. Use of bipolar and unipolar coagulators, heater probes, and injections of sclerosing agents or vasoconstrictors are all possible during this procedure. Laser-compatible scopes provide laser therapy for bleeding lesions or colonic neoplasms. Bowel decompression can also be completed during the procedure.

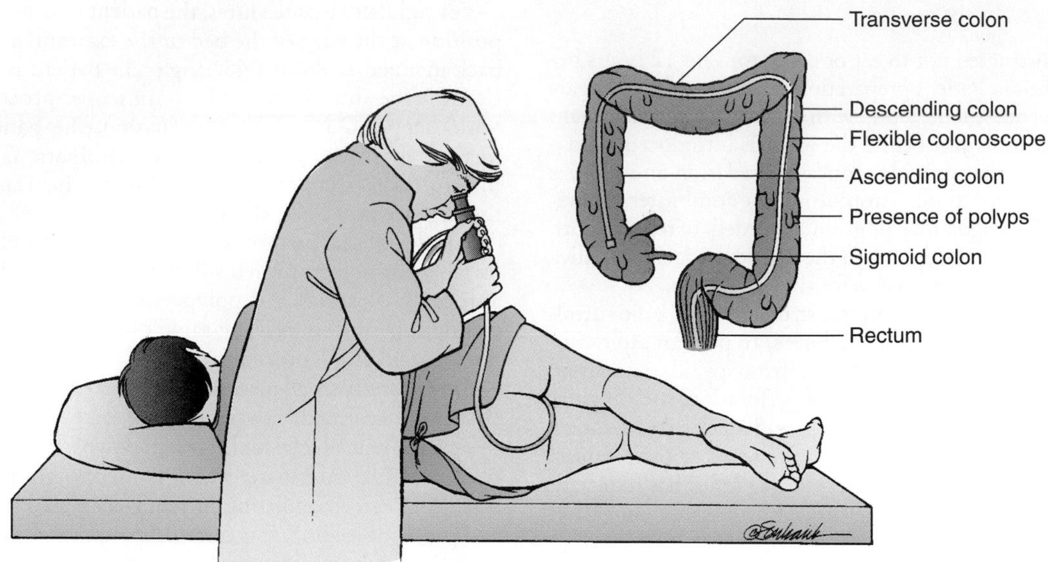

FIGURE 31•7. Colonoscopy. Flexible scope passes through rectum and sigmoid colon into the descending, transverse, and ascending colon.

Colonoscopy is performed with the patient lying on the left side with the legs drawn up toward the chest. The patient's position may be changed during the test to facilitate advancing the scope. The procedure generally takes about 1 hour. Discomfort may result from instilling air to expand the colon or from inserting and moving the scope. Biopsy forceps or a cytology brush may be passed through the scope to obtain specimens for histology and cytology examinations. Potential complications of colonoscopy include cardiac dysrhythmias and respiratory depression resulting from the medications administered, vasovagal reactions, and circulatory overload or hypotension resulting from overhydration or underhydration during bowel preparation. Therefore, it is important to monitor the patient's cardiac and respiratory function continuously. Oxygen saturation is monitored using a finger or ear oximeter. Supplemental oxygen should be used as necessary.

Nursing Interventions

The success of the procedure depends on how well the colon is prepared. Adequate colon cleansing will provide optimal visualization and decrease the time needed for the procedure. The intestinal tract is prepared by limiting the patient's intake of liquids for 24 to 72 hours before the examination. Cleansing of the colon can be accomplished in various ways. The physician may order a laxative for 2 nights before the examination and a Fleet's or saline enema until the return runs clear the morning of the test. More frequently, however, polyethylene glycol electrolyte lavage solutions (Golytely, Colyte, Nulytely) are used as effective intestinal lavages for cleansing of the bowel. The patient is placed on a clear liquid diet starting at noon the day before the procedure. The lavage solutions are then ingested orally at intervals over the next 3 to 4 hours. If necessary, this solution can be given through a feeding tube if the patient is unable to swallow. Patients with a colostomy can receive the same bowel preparation. Cleansing the bowel is fast (rectal effluent is clear in about 4 hours) and tolerated fairly well by most patients. Some side effects of the electrolyte solutions are nausea, bloating, cramps, or abdominal fullness, fluid and electrolyte imbalance, and hypothermia (patients are often told to drink the preparation as cold as possible to make it more palatable). The side effects are especially problematic for elderly patients. The elderly sometimes have difficulty ingesting the required volume of solution because of these side effects. The use of lavage solutions is contraindicated in patients with intestinal obstructions and inflammatory bowel disease.

Additional nursing actions include the following:

- Instruct the patient not to take routine medications when the lavage solution is ingested; the medications will not be digested and thus are ineffective.
- Advise the diabetic patient to consult with his or her doctor about medication adjustment to prevent hyper- or hypoglycemia because of the required dietary modifications in preparation for the test.
- Instruct all patients, especially the elderly, to maintain adequate fluid, electrolyte, and caloric intake while undergoing bowel cleansing (Raskin & Noed, 1995).

Special precautions must be taken in some patients. Implantable defibrillators and pacemakers are at high risk for malfunction if electrosurgical procedures (ie, polypectomy) are performed in conjunction with colonoscopy. A cardiologist should be consulted before the test. The defibrillator should be turned off. These patients require careful cardiac monitoring during the procedure. Colonoscopy cannot be performed if there is a suspected or documented colon perforation, acute severe diverticulitis, or

TABLE 31•4 Guidelines for Gastrointestinal Cancer Screening

Diagnostic Test	Guideline
Fecal occult blood testing	Annually after age 50
Sigmoidoscopy	Annually after age 50
Colonoscopy	Annually after age 50
Barium enema	Annually after age 50

fulminant colitis. Therapeutic colonoscopy may be contraindicated in patients with coagulopathies or those receiving anticoagulation therapy because of the high risk for excessive bleeding during and after the procedure. Nonsteroidal anti-inflammatory agents, aspirin, ticlopidine, and pentoxifylline must be discontinued before the test and for 2 weeks after the procedure. Patients taking coumarin or heparin must consult the physician for specific instructions. Those with prosthetic heart valves or a history of endocarditis require prophylactic antibiotics before the procedure (Raskin & Noed, 1995).

Informed consent is obtained before the test. The patient will be NPO after midnight before the test, but most medications can be taken with a small amount of water; the physician should be consulted about medication use. Before the examination, an opioid analgesic or a sedative (eg, midazolam) may be given intravenously to provide conscious sedation and relieve anxiety during the procedure. Glucagon may be used, if needed, to relax the colonic musculature and to reduce spasm during the test. Elderly or debilitated people may require a reduced dosage of medications to decrease the risks of oversedation and cardiopulmonary complications.

After the procedure, patients who were sedated are maintained on bed rest until fully alert. Some will have abdominal cramps caused by increased peristalsis stimulated by the air insufflated into the bowel during the procedure. The patient must be observed immediately after the test for signs and symptoms of bowel perforation (eg, rectal bleeding, abdominal pain or distention, fever, or focal peritoneal signs). If midazolam was used, its amnesic effects are explained. Written instructions are provided because the patient may be unable to recall verbal information. After a therapeutic procedure, the patient should be instructed to report any bleeding to the physician.

Small Bowel Enteroscopy

A small-caliber transnasal endoscope allows direct inspection of the small intestine wall. The endoscope used for this procedure is very long and flexible and has a balloon at its tip. When inflated, the balloon tip advances the scope by peristalsis through the small intestine. This procedure may take 10 or more hours to complete. The patient may be kept in the recovery area or sent home during this period of time.

Once the scope has entered the distal ileum, it is slowly retracted while the endoscopist examines the intestinal wall. This lengthy procedure is uncommon. Its use is limited to patients with continued bleeding even after extensive diagnostic testing has identified no other problem area.

Abdominal Ultrasonography

Ultrasonography is a noninvasive diagnostic technique in which high-frequency sound waves are passed into internal body structures and the ultrasonic echoes are recorded on an oscilloscope as they strike tissues of different densities. During abdominal ultrasonography, an image of the abdominal organs and structures is produced on the oscilloscope. This procedure is generally used to indicate the size and configuration of abdominal structures. It is particularly useful in the detection of cholelithiasis, cholecystitis, and appendicitis.

Advantages of abdominal ultrasonography are that it requires no ionizing radiation, there are no noticeable side effects, and it is relatively inexpensive. One disadvantage is that it cannot be used to examine structures that lie behind bony tissue, because bony tissue prevents sound waves from passing to deeper structures. Gas and fluid in the abdomen or air in the lungs also presents a problem because ultrasound is not well transmitted through gas, air, or fluid.

Endoscopic ultrasonography is a specialized enteroscopic procedure that aids in the diagnosis of GI disorders by providing direct imaging of a target area. It also helps to stage various GI cancers preoperatively. A high-frequency ultrasonic beam is added to the tip of the fiberoptic scope so that a transintestinal study can be completed. Intestinal gas, bone, and thick layers of adipose tissue—all of which hamper conventional ultrasonography—are not problems when this technique is used.

Nursing Interventions

Preparation includes fasting for 8 to 12 hours before the test to decrease the amount of gas in the bowel. If gallbladder studies are being done, a fat-free meal the evening before is ordered. If barium studies are to be performed, they must be scheduled after this test; otherwise, the barium will interfere with the transmission of the sound waves.

Computed Tomography

Computed tomography (CT) provides cross-sectional images of abdominal organs and structures. Multiple x-rays are taken from many different angles, computerized, reconstructed, and then viewed on a computer monitor. Indications for abdominal CT scanning are diseases of the liver, spleen, kidney, pancreas, and pelvic organs. Because the adequacy of detail in the test depends on the presence of fat, this diagnostic tool is not useful for very thin, cachectic patients. The procedure is completely painless, but radiation doses are considerable. Because a scanning time of 5 seconds is required, motion artifacts produced by heartbeat and respiration cannot be avoided, resulting in pictures that are less than clear.

Nursing Interventions

The patient has nothing to eat or drink for 6 to 8 hours before the test. An intravenous or oral contrast agent may be prescribed. If barium studies are to be performed, they must be scheduled after CT scanning so as not to interfere with imaging.

Magnetic Resonance Imaging

Magnetic resonance imaging (MRI) in gastroenterology is currently used to supplement ultrasonography and CT scanning. The use of oral contrast agents is increasing the application of this technique for the diagnosis of GI diseases. It is useful in evaluating abdominal soft tissue and blood vessels, abscesses, fistulas, neoplasms, and other sources of bleeding.

The physiologic artifacts of heartbeat, respiration, and peristalsis may create a less-than-clear image. Newer ultrafast MRI techniques may help to eliminate these physiologic motion artifacts.

MRI is contraindicated for patients with permanent pacemakers, artificial heart valves and defibrillators, implanted insulin pumps, and implanted transcutaneous electrical nerve stimulation devices because the magnetic field could cause malfunction. MRI is also contraindicated for patients with internal metal devices (eg, aneurysm clips).

Nursing Interventions

The patient has nothing to eat or drink for 6 to 8 hours before the test. All jewelry and other metals must be removed before the test. The patient lies in a machine that constructs an image based on the magnetic field created between the machine and the structures scanned. The entire procedure takes 30 to 90 minutes.

Patients should be warned that the close-fitting scanners used in many MRI facilities may induce feelings of claustrophobia and that the machine will make a knocking sound during the procedure. Open MRIs that are less close-fitting eliminate the claustrophobic concerns.

Gastrointestinal Motility Studies

Radionuclide testing is used to assess gastric emptying and colonic transit time. For gastric emptying studies, the liquid and solid components of a meal are tagged with radionuclide markers. After ingesting the meal, the patient is positioned under a scintiscanner, which measures the rate of passage of the radioactive substance out of the stomach. This is useful in diagnosing disorders of gastric motility.

Colonic transit studies are used to evaluate colonic motility in instances of chronic constipation and obstructive defecation syndromes. This is usually an outpatient study. The patient is given a capsule containing 20 radionuclide markers and instructed to follow a regular diet and normal daily activities. Abdominal x-rays are taken every 24 hours until all markers are passed. This process usually takes 4 to 5 days, but in the presence of severe constipation, it may take as long as 10 days. People with chronic diarrhea may be evaluated at 8-hour intervals. The amount of time it takes for the radioactive material to move through the colon indicates colonic motility.

Manometry and Electrophysiologic Studies

Manometry and electrophysiologic studies are other methods for evaluating patients with GI motility disorders. Disturbed motility can result in constipation, nausea, or both. Manometry is the measurement of pressures using a manometer. It is used to evaluate GI tract motility and intraluminal pressures. The pressures can be recorded manually or on a physiograph or a computer.

Esophageal manometry is used to detect motility disorders of the esophagus and the lower esophageal sphincter. Patients must refrain from eating or drinking for 8 to 12 hours before the test. Medications that could have a direct affect on motility are withheld for 24 to 48 hours (eg, calcium channel blockers, anticholinergics, and sedatives). A pressure-sensitive catheter is inserted through the nose and connected to a transducer and a video recorder. The patient then swallows small amounts of water while the resultant pressure changes are recorded.

Gastroduodenal, small intestine, and colonic manometry are used to evaluate delayed gastric emptying and gastric and intestinal motility disorders such as irritable bowel syndrome or atonic colon. This is often an ambulatory outpatient procedure lasting 24 to 72 hours. Anorectal manometry measures the resting tone of the internal anal sphincter and the contractibility of the external anal sphincter. It is helpful in evaluating patients with chronic constipation or fecal incontinence and is useful in biofeedback for the treatment of fecal incontinence. It can be done in conjunction with rectal sensory functioning tests. Phosphosoda or a saline cleansing enema is given 1 hour before the test. This test is performed with the patient in the prone or lateral position.

Electrogastrography, an electrophysiologic study, may also be performed to assess gastric motility disturbances. Electrodes are placed over the abdomen, and gastric electrical activity is recorded for up to 24 hours. Patients may exhibit rapid, slow, or irregular waveform activity. Electrogastrography can be useful in detecting motor or neurologic dysfunction in the stomach.

A rectal sensory function test is used to evaluate rectal sensory function and neuropathy. A catheter and balloon are passed into the rectum, and the balloon is inflated until the patient feels distention. The tone and pressure of the rectum and anal sphincter are measured. The results are especially helpful in the evaluation of patients with chronic constipation, diarrhea, or incontinence.

Defecography

Defecography measures anorectal function. Very thick barium paste is instilled into the rectum. Fluoroscopy is performed and the function of the rectum and anal sphincter is visualized while the patient attempts to expel the barium. The test requires no preparation. Newer features include digital subtraction methods that allow for more rapid imaging and mapping of rectal evacuation.

Electromyographic (EMG) techniques and other tests are being further developed to measure the integrity and function of the anal sphincters in an effort to treat functional bowel incontinence and constipation.

Stool Tests

Basic examination of the stool includes inspecting the specimen for consistency and color and testing for occult (not visible) blood. After the specimen is obtained it can be assessed for color and consistency. Occult blood testing can then be performed. Special tests, including tests for fecal urobilinogen, fat, nitrogen, parasites, pathogens, food residues, and other substances, require that the specimen be sent to the laboratory.

Stool samples are usually collected on a random basis unless a quantitative study such as fecal fat or urobilinogen is performed. Random specimens should be sent promptly to the laboratory for analysis. The quantitative 24- to 72-hour collections must be kept refrigerated until they are taken to the laboratory. Some stool collections require that a special diet be followed before the collection, or that certain medications be withheld. It is important to follow test guidelines closely for accurate results.

Fecal occult blood testing is probably one of the most commonly performed stool tests. It can be useful in initial screening for several disorders. It tests only for the presence of blood, thus requiring other follow-up testing. It is most frequently used in cancer screening programs and early cancer detection (see Table 31-3). The test can be performed at the bedside, in the laboratory, or at home. It tests for heme, the iron-containing portion of the hemoglobin molecule that is altered during transit through the intestines.

Probably the most widely used occult blood test is the Hemetest. It is inexpensive and noninvasive and carries no risk to the patient. It should not, however, be performed when there is hemorrhoidal bleeding. The stool specimen is smeared on a dry, guaiac-impregnated paper slide. The slide is mailed to the physician in an envelope provided for that purpose, and the stool specimen is examined. Serial 3- to 6-day testing is recommended. The test, however, is not perfect; certain factors interfere with the sensitivity and specificity of the test. False-positive results may occur if the patient has eaten rare meats, poultry, turnips, melons, salmon, sardines, or horseradish within 48 hours before or during the test. Medications such as iron, iodides, indomethacin, colchicine, salicylates, corticosteroids, and vitamin C may also cause false-positive results. Careful assessment of diet and the medication regimen reduces incorrect interpretation of results.

Other occult blood tests that may yield more specific and more sensitive readings include Hemetest II SENSA and HemoQuant. Immunologic tests are more specific to human hemoglobin and decrease the problem with dietary interference. Heme-porphyrin assays detect the broadest range of blood derivatives, but a strict dietary protocol is essential. Immunochemical tests using anti-human antibodies have now been developed that are extremely sensitive to human hemoglobin.

Hydrogen Breath Test

This breath test was developed to evaluate carbohydrate absorption. It can also be used to aid in the diagnosis of bacterial overgrowth in the intestine, and short bowel syndrome. This test determines the amount of hydrogen expelled in the breath after it is produced in the colon (on contact of galactose with fermenting bacteria) and absorbed into the blood.

Urea Breath Test

Urea breath tests detect the presence of *Helicobacter pylori*, the bacteria that can live in the mucosal lining of the stomach and cause peptic ulcer disease. The patient takes a capsule of carbon-labeled urea and then provides a breath sample 10 to 20 minutes later. Because *H. pylori* metabolizes urea rapidly, the labeled carbon is quickly absorbed; it can then be measured as CO_2 in the expired breath to determine if *H. pylori* is present. The patient should be advised to avoid antibiotics or loperamide (Pepto-Bismol) for 1 month before the test; sucralfate (Carafate) and omeprazole (Prilosec) for 1 week before the test; and cimetidine (Tagamet), famotidine (Pepcid), ranitidine (Zantac), or nizatidine (Axid) for 24 hours before urea breath testing. *H. pylori* can also be detected by assessing serum antibody levels.

Tagged Red Blood Cells and Leukocytes

Tagging red blood cells and leukocytes by injection of a radionuclide is performed to define areas of inflammation, abscess, blood loss, or neoplasm. A sample of blood is removed, mixed with a radioactive substance, and then reinjected into the patient. Abnormal concentrations of blood cells can then be detected by radiographic imaging, which is done at 24- and 48-hour intervals.

PATHOPHYSIOLOGIC AND PSYCHOLOGICAL CONSIDERATIONS

Abnormalities of the GI tract are numerous and exemplify every type of major pathology that can affect other organ systems: bleeding, perforation, obstruction, inflammation, and cancer. Congenital, inflammatory, infectious, traumatic, and neoplastic lesions have been encountered in every portion, and at every site, along the length of the GI tract. As with all other organ systems, the GI tract is subject to circulatory disturbances, faulty nervous system control, and aging.

Apart from the many organic diseases to which the GI tract is susceptible, there are many extrinsic factors that can interfere with its normal function and produce symptoms. Stress and anxiety, for example, often find their chief expression in indigestion, anorexia, or motor disturbances of the intestines, sometimes producing constipation or diarrhea. In addition to the state of mental health, physical factors such as fatigue and an unbalanced or abruptly changed dietary intake can markedly affect the GI tract. When assessing and instructing the patient, the nurse should realize that a combination of mental and physical factors affect the status of the GI tract.

GERONTOLOGIC CONSIDERATIONS

Normal physiologic changes occurring with aging can cause several problems in the GI system. Complaints and problems should be carefully assessed and monitored. They must be evaluated because some pathologic problems occur with increased frequency in older adults. A decrease in normal function can occur without much effect on the physiologic processes.

Age-related changes in the mouth include loss of teeth, diminished number of taste buds, decreased production of saliva, and atrophy of gingival tissue. These changes cause difficulty chewing and swallowing. Changes in the esophagus include decreased muscle tone and weakness in the lower esophageal sphincter, leading to reflux and heartburn.

Decreased gastric motility leads to delayed gastric emptying. Atrophy of the mucosa causes a decrease in hydrochloric acid production, and this can lead to food intolerances, malabsorption, or decrease in vitamin B_{12} absorption. Changes in the small and large intestine are largely evidenced by decreased motility and decreased transit time, which lead to complaints of indigestion and constipation. Other changes lead to decreased absorption of nutrients (dextrose, fats, calcium, and iron) in the large intestine. The nerve supply to the anal sphincter is sometimes impaired, causing fecal incontinence (Luekenotte, 1996).

Critical Thinking Exercises

1. You are caring for a patient who is to have a barium enema. The patient received a clear liquid diet and a laxative the evening before the test. On the morning of the test, she indicates that the laxative had caused her to have diarrhea during the night, and she refuses to have a cleansing enema. Based on your knowledge of intestinal physiology, how would you explain to this patient what has happened and why? Describe what the goals would be in this situation and the interventions that could be implemented to achieve them.

2. You accompany your patient to the endoscopy suite, where he is to have a colonoscopy. You notice that emergency equipment is readily available. After the procedure is completed, the nurse who assisted with the procedure must now assist with another procedure and asks you to monitor the patient's vital signs. You agree to carry out this function because you have a thorough understanding of the complications that can occur. Describe the changes in vital signs that you might detect as an indication that complications are developing, and the reasons these changes may occur.

References and Selected Readings

BOOKS

Achkar, E., et al. (1992). *Clinical gastroenterology.* Philadelphia: Lea & Febiger.

Bickley, L. S., & Hoekelman, R. A. (1999). *Bates' guide to physical examination and history taking* (7th ed.). Philadelphia: Lippincott Williams & Wilkins.

Beck, M., & Evans, N. (Eds.). (1993). *Gastroenterology nursing: A core curriculum.* St. Louis: Mosby–Year Book.

Gitnick, C. (Ed.). (1992). *Current gastroenterology.* (Vol. 12.) St. Louis: Mosby–Year Book.

Grendell, J., et al. (Eds.). (1996). *Current diagnosis and treatment in gastroenterology.* Stamford, CT: Appleton & Lange.

Jarvis, C. (1996). *Physical examination in health assessment* (2nd ed.). Philadelphia: W. B. Saunders.

Luekenotte, A. (1996). *Gerontologic nursing.* St. Louis: Mosby.

Raskin, J., & Noed, H. (1995). *Colonoscopy: Principles and techniques.* New York: Igakee-Shoin.

Yamada, T. (1992). *Atlas of gastroenterology.* Philadelphia: J. B. Lippincott.

JOURNALS

Butler, M. (1996). Preparing patients for endoscopic tests. *Practice Nurse, 11*(10), 707–712.

Cohen, L. (1996). Colorectal cancer: A primary care approach to screening. *Geriatrics, 51*(12), 45–50.

Dammel, T. (1997). Fecal occult blood testing. *Nursing '97, 27*(7), 44–45.

Kirton, C. (1997). Assessing bowel sounds. *Nursing '97, 27*(3), 64.

O'Hanlon-Nichols, T. (1998). Basic assessment series: Gastrointestinal system. *AJN, 98*(4), 48–53.

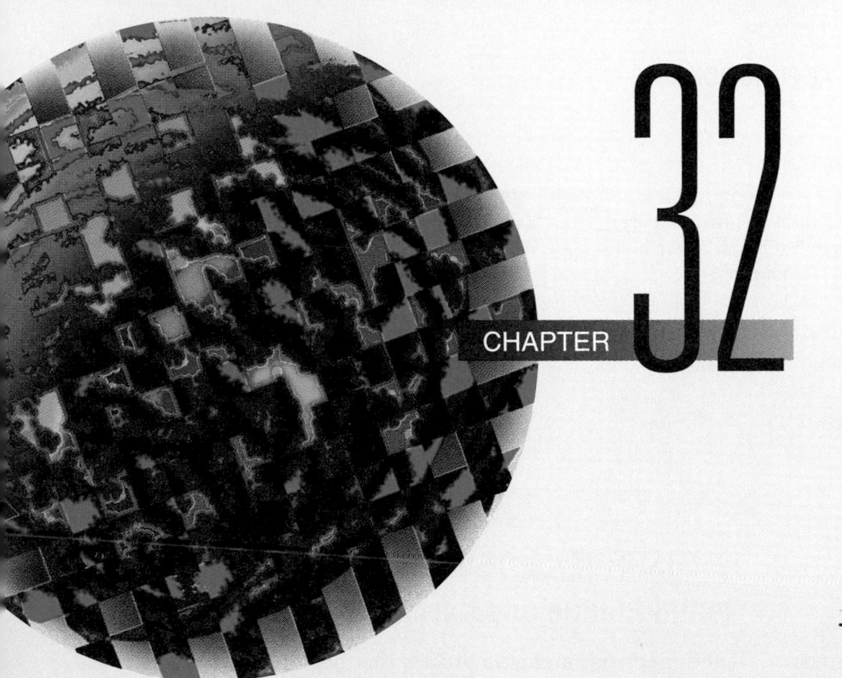

Management of Patients With Oral and Esophageal Disorders

Learning Objectives

On completion of this chapter, the learner will be able to:

1. Use the nursing process as a framework for care of patients with conditions of the oral cavity.
2. Describe the relationship of dental hygiene and dental problems to nutrition.
3. Describe the nursing management of patients with abnormalities of the lips, gums, teeth, mouth, and salivary glands.
4. Use the nursing process as a framework for care of patients with cancer of the oral cavity.
5. Identify the physical and psychosocial long-term needs of patients with oral cancer.
6. Use the nursing process as a framework for care of patients undergoing neck dissection.
7. Use the nursing process as a framework for care of patients with conditions of the esophagus.
8. Describe the various conditions of the esophagus and their clinical manifestations and management.

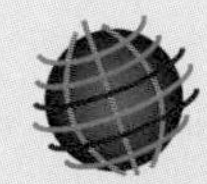

Because the process of ingestion normally begins in the mouth, adequate nutrition is related to good dental health and the general condition of the mouth. Any discomfort or adverse condition in the oral cavity can affect a person's nutritional status. Changes in the oral cavity may influence the type and amount of food ingested as well as the degree to which food particles are properly mixed with salivary enzymes. Esophageal problems related to swallowing can also adversely affect food and fluid intake, thereby jeopardizing general health and well-being. Given the close relationship between adequate nutritional intake and the structures of the upper gastrointestinal tract (lips, mouth, teeth, pharynx, esophagus), health teaching can help prevent disorders associated with these structures.

GLOSSARY

achalasia: absent or ineffective peristalsis (wavelike contraction) of the distal esophagus accompanied by failure of the esophageal sphincter to relax in response to swallowing

dysphagia: difficulty swallowing

gastroesophageal reflux: back-flow of gastric or duodenal contents into the esophagus

hernia: protrusion of an organ or part of an organ through the wall of the cavity that normally contains it

lithotripsy: use of shock waves to break up or disintegrate stones

parotitis: inflammation of the parotid gland

periapical abscess: abscessed tooth

sialadenitis: inflammation of the salivary glands

stomatitis: inflammation of the oral mucosa

temporomandibular disorders: a group of conditions that cause pain or dysfunction of the temporomandibular joint and surrounding structures

xerostomia: dry mouth

DISORDERS OF THE LIPS, MOUTH, AND GUMS

The oral cavity, which includes the lips, mouth, and gums, is subject to many disorders and diseases. Table 32-1 reviews common abnormalities, their possible causes, and nursing management.

DISORDERS OF THE TEETH

Dental Plaque and Caries

Tooth decay is an erosive process that begins with the action of bacteria on fermentable carbohydrates in the mouth, which produces acids that dissolve tooth enamel. The extent of damage to the teeth depends on:

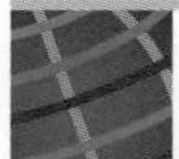

TABLE 32•1 Disorders of the Lips, Mouth, and Gums

Condition	Signs and Symptoms	Possible Causes	Nursing Considerations
Abnormalities of the Lips			
Actinic cheilitis	Irritation of lips associated with scaling, crusty, fissure. White overgrowth of horny layer of epidermis (hyperkeratosis).	Exposure to sun. More frequently occurring in fair-skinned people and in those whose occupations involve sun exposure, such as farmers. May lead to squamous cell cancer	Teach patient importance of protecting lips from the sun by using protective ointment such as sun block. Instruct patient to have a periodic checkup by physician.
Herpes simplex 1 (cold sore or fever blister)	Symptoms may be delayed up to 20 days after exposure. Singular or clustered painful vesicles that may rupture.	Herpes simplex virus—an opportunistic infection. Frequently seen in immunosuppressed patients. May recur with menstruation, fever, or sun exposure	Use acyclovir ointment or systemic medications as prescribed Administer analgesics as prescribed. Instruct patient to avoid irritating foods.
Chancre	Reddened circumscribed lesion that ulcerates and becomes crusted	Primary lesion of syphilis Very contagious	Comfort measures: cold soaks to lip, mouth care Administer antibiotics as prescribed. Instruct patient regarding contagion.
Contact dermatitis	Red area or rash. Itching.	Allergic reaction to lipstick, cosmetic ointments, or toothpaste	Instruct patient to avoid possible causes. Administer corticosteroids as prescribed.
Abnormalities of the Mouth			
Leukoplakia	White patches; may be hyperkeratotic. Usually in buccal mucosa. Usually painless.	Fewer than 2% are malignant.	Instruct patient to see a physician if it persists longer than 2 weeks.
Hairy leukoplakia	White patches with rough hair-like projections. Typically found on lateral border of the tongue.	Possibly viral Smoking and use of tobacco Often seen in people who are HIV positive	Instruct patient to see a physician if it persists longer than 2 weeks.
Lichen planus	White papules at the intersection of a network of interlacing lesions. Usually ulcerated and painful.	Recurrences are common. May lead to a malignant process	Administer viscous lidocaine for pain. Instruct the patient to hold this in the mouth for 2–3 minutes. Apply triamcinolone (Kenalog) or Orabase after meals or at bedtime to assist with healing.

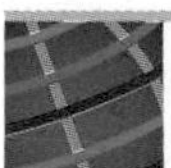

TABLE 32•1 Disorders of the Lips, Mouth, and Gums *(Continued)*

Condition	Signs and Symptoms	Possible Causes	Nursing Considerations
Abnormalities of the Mouth (continued)			
			Administer corticosteroids systemically or intralesionally as prescribed. Instruct the patient of need for follow-up if condition is chronic.
Candidiasis (moniliasis/thrush)	Cheesy white plaque that looks like milk curds. When rubbed off, it leaves erythematous and often bleeding base.	*Candida albicans* fungus. Predisposing factors include diabetes, antibiotic therapy, and immunosuppression.	Antifungal medications such as nystatin (Mycostatin), Amphotericin B, clotrimazole, or ketoconazole may be prescribed. These may be taken in pill form or as a suspension. When used as a suspension, instruct the patient to swish vigorously for at least 1 minute and then swallow.
Aphthous stomatitis (canker sore)	Shallow ulcer with a white or gray center and red border. Seen on the inner side of the lip and cheek or on the tongue. It begins with a burning or tingling sensation and slight swelling. Painful. Usually lasts 7–10 days and heals without a scar.	Associated with emotional or mental stress, fatigue, hormonal factors, minor trauma (such as biting), allergies, acidic foods, and juices Associated with HIV infection May recur	Instruct the patient in comfort measures, such as saline rinses, and a soft or bland diet. Antibiotics or corticosteroids may be prescribed.
Nicotine stomatitis (smoker's patch)	This has two stages. It begins as a red stomatitis. Over time the tongue and mouth become covered with a creamy, thick, white mucous membrane, which may slough, leaving a beefy red base.	Chronic irritation by tobacco.	Cessation of tobacco use. If condition exists for longer than 2 weeks a physician should be consulted and a biopsy may be needed.
Krythoplakia	Red patch on the oral mucous membrane	Nonspecific inflammation. More frequently seen in the elderly.	
Kaposi's sarcoma	Appears first on the oral mucosa as a red, purple, or blue lesion. May be a singular lesion or multiple lesions. May be flat or raised.	HIV infection	Instruct patient regarding side effects of planned treatment.
Abnormalities of the Gums			
Gingivitis	Painful, inflamed, swollen gums. Usually the gums bleed in response to light contact.	Poor oral hygiene: food debris, bacterial plaque, and calculus (tartar) accumulate. The gums may also swell in response to normal processes such as puberty and pregnancy.	Teach patient proper oral hygiene. See Preventive Oral Hygiene (page 810)
Necrotizing gingivitis (trench mouth)	Gray-white pseudomembranous ulcerations affecting the edges of the gums, mucosa of the mouth, tonsils, and pharynx. Foul breath. Painful, bleeding gums. Swallowing and talking are painful.	Poor oral hygiene. Bacterial infection, inadequate rest, overwork, emotional stress, and poor nutrition may contribute to development.	Teach patient proper oral hygiene. See Preventive Oral Hygiene (page 810) Irrigate with 2% to 3% hydrogen peroxide or normal saline.
Herpetic gingivostomatitis	Burning sensation with the appearance of small vesicles 24–48 hours later. Vesicles may rupture, forming sore, shallow ulcers covered with a gray membrane.	Herpes simplex virus. This occurs most frequently in people who are immunosuppressed. May occur in other infectious processes such as streptococcal pneumonia, meningococcal meningitis, and malaria.	Apply topical anesthetics as prescribed. May need opioids if pain is severe. Saline or 2% to 3% hydrogen peroxide irrigations Antiviral agents such as acyclovir may be prescribed.
Periodontitis	Little discomfort at onset. May have bleeding, infection, gum recession, and loosening of teeth. Later in the disease the teeth may fall out.	May result from untreated gingivitis Poor or inadequate dental hygiene and inadequate diet contribute to development.	Instruct patient in proper oral hygiene. Instruct patient to consult a dentist.

- The presence of dental plaque
- The strength of the acids and the ability of the saliva to neutralize them
- The length of time the acids are in contact with the teeth
- The susceptibility of the teeth to decay

Dental plaque is a gluey, gelatin-like substance that adheres to the teeth. The initial action that causes damage to a tooth occurs under dental plaque.

Dental decay begins with a small hole, usually in a fissure (a break in the tooth's enamel) or in an area that is hard to clean. Left unchecked, the affected area penetrates the enamel into the dentin. Because dentin is not as hard as enamel, decay progresses more rapidly and in time reaches the pulp. When the blood, lymph vessels, and nerves are exposed, they become infected, and an abscess may form, either within the tooth or at the tip of the root. Soreness and pain usually occur with an abscess. As the infection continues, the patient's face may become swollen, and there may be pulsating pain. The dentist can determine by x-ray the extent of damage and the type of treatment needed. Treatment for dental caries includes fillings, extraction, dental implants, and dentures. If treatment is not successful, it may be necessary to extract the tooth.

Prevention

Measures used to prevent and control dental caries include practicing effective mouth care, reducing the intake of sugars (refined carbohydrates), applying fluoride to the teeth or drinking fluoridated water, refraining from smoking, controlling diabetes, and using pit and fissure sealants.

MOUTH CARE

Healthy teeth must be conscientiously and effectively cleaned on a daily basis. Brushing and flossing are particularly effective in mechanically breaking up the bacterial plaque that collects around teeth.

The normal movement of the muscles of mastication and the normal flow of saliva also aid greatly in keeping the teeth clean. Because many ill patients do not eat adequate amounts of food, they produce less saliva, which in turn reduces the natural cleaning process of the teeth. The nurse may need to assume the responsibility for brushing the patient's teeth. In any case, merely wiping the patient's mouth and teeth with a swab is ineffective. The most effective method is mechanical cleansing (brushing). If it is not possible to brush, it is better to wipe the teeth with a gauze pad, then have the patient swish an antiseptic mouthwash several times before expectorating it into the emesis basin. A soft-bristled toothbrush is more effective than a sponge or foam stick. Lemon glycerin swabs, popular several years ago, are avoided because they are very drying to the oral mucosa. Instead, the lips may be coated with a water-soluble gel to prevent drying.

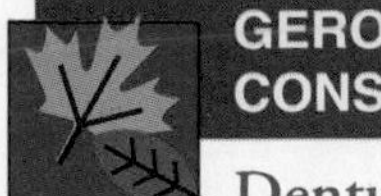

GERONTOLOGIC CONSIDERATIONS

Denture Care

Many older adults wear dentures. Mouth care and regular checkups remain part of the denture-wearing older adult's health promotion activities.

- Brush dentures daily.
- Remove dentures at night and soak them in water or a denture product.
- Rinse mouth with warm salt water in the morning, after meals, and at bedtime.
- Clean well under partial dentures, where food particles tend to get caught.
- Consume nonsticky foods that have been cut into small pieces; chew slowly.
- See dentist regularly to assess and readjust fit.

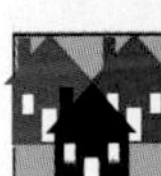

PATIENT EDUCATION AND HOME CARE

Preventive Oral Hygiene

- Brush teeth using a soft toothbrush at least two times daily. Hold toothbrush at a 45 degree angle between brush and the gums and teeth. Gums and tongue surface should be brushed.
- Floss at least once daily.
- Use an antiplaque mouth rinse.
- Visit a dentist at least every 6 months, or when you have a chipped tooth, an oral sore that persists longer than 2 weeks, or a toothache.
- Avoid alcohol and tobacco products, including smokeless tobacco.
- Maintain adequate nutrition and avoid sweets.
- Replace toothbrush at first signs of wear.

DIET

Dental caries may be prevented by decreasing the amount of sugar in the diet. Patients who snack should be encouraged to choose less cariogenic alternatives such as fruits, vegetables, nuts, and possibly cheeses.

FLUORIDATION

Fluoridation of public water supplies may decrease the amount of dental caries by 60%. Some areas of the country have natural fluoridation; other communities have mandated the addition of fluoride to public water supplies. Fluoridation may be attained by having a dentist apply a concentrated gel or solution to the teeth, adding fluoride to home water supplies, using fluoridated toothpaste, sodium fluoride tablets, drops, or lozenges.

PIT AND FISSURE SEALANTS

The occlusal surfaces of the teeth have pits and fissures, areas that are prone to caries. Some dentists apply a special coating to fill and seal these areas from potential exposure to cariogenic processes. These sealants may last up to 7 years.

Dentoalveolar Abscess or Periapical Abscess

Periapical abscess, more commonly referred to as an abscessed tooth, involves the collection of pus in the apical dental periosteum (fibrous membrane supporting the tooth structure) and the tissue surrounding the apex of the tooth (where it is suspended in the jaw bone). It may appear in two forms: acute and chronic. Acute periapical abscess is usually secondary to a suppurative pulpitis (a pus-producing inflammation of the dental pulp) that arises from an infection extending from dental caries. The infection of the dental pulp extends through the apical foramen of the tooth to form an abscess around the apex.

The abscess produces a dull, gnawing, continuous pain, often with a surrounding cellulitis and edema of the adjacent facial structures, and mobility of the involved tooth. The gum opposite the apex of the tooth is usually swollen on the cheek side. Swelling and cellulitis of the facial structures may make it difficult for the patient to open the mouth. In well-developed abscesses, there may be a systemic reaction, fever, and malaise.

Chronic dentoalveolar abscess is a slowly progressive infectious process. It differs from the acute form in that the process may progress to a fully formed abscess without the patient knowing it. The infection eventually leads to a "blind dental abscess," which is really a periapical granuloma. It may enlarge to as much as 1 cm in diameter. It is often discovered on x-ray and is treated by extraction or root canal therapy, often with apicectomy (excision of the apex of the tooth root).

In the early stages of an infection, a dentist or dental surgeon may perform a needle aspiration or drill an opening into the pulp chamber to relieve tension and pain and to provide drainage. Usually, the infection will have progressed to a periapical abscess. Drainage is provided by an incision through the gingivae down to the jaw bone. Pus (purulent material) escapes under pressure. This procedure is commonly performed in the dentist's office, but it may be performed in an outpatient surgery center or a same-day surgery department. After the inflammatory reaction has subsided, the tooth may be extracted or root canal therapy performed.

The nurse assesses the patient for bleeding after treatment and instructs the patient to use a warm saline or warm water mouth rinse to keep the area clean. The patient is also instructed to use antibiotics and analgesics and to advance from a liquid diet to a soft diet as tolerated.

Malocclusion

Malocclusion is a misalignment of the teeth of the upper and lower dental arcs when the jaws are closed. Malocclusion can be inherited or acquired (from thumb-sucking, accidents, or some medical conditions). Malocclusion makes the teeth difficult to clean and can lead to decay, gum disease, and excess wear on supporting bone and gum tissues. About 50% of the population has some form of malocclusion. Correction of malocclusion requires an orthodontist with special training, a patient who is motivated and cooperative, and adequate time. Most treatments begin when the patient has shed the last primary tooth and the last permanent successor has erupted, usually around 12 or 13 years of age, but treatment may occur in adulthood. Preventive orthodontics may be started at age 5 if malocclusion is diagnosed early. Studies have shown that the need for teeth straightening in adolescence is reduced if preventive orthodontics is started with the primary teeth.

People with malocclusion have an obviously misaligned bite, or crooked, crowded, widely spaced, or protruding teeth. To realign the teeth, the orthodontist gradually forces the teeth into a new location by using wires or plastic bands (braces). These devices may be unattractive, but this psychological burden must be overcome if good results are to be achieved. In the final phase of treatment, a retaining device is worn for several hours each day to support the tissues as they adjust to the new alignment of the teeth.

The patient must practice meticulous oral hygiene, and the nurse encourages the patient to persist in this important part of the treatment. An adolescent undergoing orthodontic correction admitted to the hospital for some other problem may have to be reminded to continue wearing the retainer (if it does not interfere with the problem requiring hospitalization).

DISORDERS OF THE JAW

Abnormal conditions affecting the mandible (jaw) and the temporomandibular joint include congenital malformation, fracture, chronic dislocation, cancer, and syndromes characterized by pain and limited motion. Temporomandibular disorders and jaw surgery (a treatment common in many structural abnormalities or cancer of the jaw) are discussed in this section.

Temporomandibular Disorders

Temporomandibular disorders (TMD) are a group of conditions that cause pain and/or dysfunction of the "temporomandibular joint and/or the muscles of mastication, as well as contiguous tissue components" (National Institutes of Health, 1996). Diagnosis and treatment of this condition remain somewhat ambiguous, but it is thought to affect about 10 million people in the United States. It is theorized that misalignment of the joints in the jaw and other problems associated with the ligaments and muscles of mastication result in tissue damage and muscle tenderness. Suggested causes include malocclusion, whiplash, arthritis of the jaw, head injury, sustained unnatural positions of the head and neck (eg, cradling the telephone, playing certain musical instruments), stress, habits of posture, and iatrogenic sequelae.

Clinical Manifestations

Patients have pain ranging from a dull ache to throbbing, debilitating pain that can radiate to the ears, teeth, neck muscles, and facial sinuses. They often have restricted jaw motion and may hear clicking and grating noises and have difficulty chewing and swallowing. Depression may accompany these symptoms.

Assessment and Diagnostic Findings

Diagnosis is based on the patient's subjective symptoms of pain, limitations in range of motion, dysphagia, difficulty chewing, difficulty with speech, and/or hearing difficulties. Magnetic resonance imaging, x-rays, and an arthrogram may be performed.

Management

Although some practitioners think the role of stress in temporomandibular joint disorders is overrated, patient education in stress management may be helpful (to reduce grinding and clenching of teeth). Patients may also be taught range of motion exercises. Pain management may include the use of nonsteroidal anti-inflammatory agents, with the possible addition of opioids, muscle relaxants, and/or mild antidepressants.

Correction of Mandibular Structural Abnormalities

The jaw may have to be repositioned or reconstructed for a variety of reasons. Simple fractures of the mandible without displacement, resulting from a blow on the chin, and planned surgical intervention, as in the correction of long or short jaw syndrome, may require treatment by these means. Jaw reconstruction may be necessary in the aftermath of trauma from a severe injury or cancer, both of which can cause loss of tissue and bone.

Mandibular fractures are usually closed fractures. In the past, immobilizing the lower jaw by wiring it to the upper jaw (internal maxillary fixation [IMF]) for approximately 6 weeks was the method used for treatment of mandibular fractures. This procedure

HOME CARE TEACHING CHECKLIST: RECOVERING FROM INTERNAL MAXILLARY FIXATION

At the completion of the program, the patient or caregiver will be able to:

	Patient	Caregiver
• State need to keep wire cutters immediately available.	✔	✔
• Demonstrate use of wire cutter.	✔	✔
• Demonstrate mouth care.	✔	✔
• State caloric/fluid needs.	✔	✔
• Demonstrate proper eating or feeding techniques.	✔	✔

is associated with several negative outcomes, however. Patients who have had this procedure cannot ingest adequate nutrition and have difficulties with oral hygiene, masticatory muscle atrophy, and temporomandibular joint dysfunction. They are also at high risk for aspiration, especially in the immediate postoperative period. Rigid plate fixation (insertion of metal plates and screws into the bone to approximate and stabilize the bone) is the current treatment of choice in many cases of mandibular fracture and in some mandibular reconstructive surgery procedures.

Nursing Management

Immediately after IMF surgery, the patient is placed on the side, with the head slightly elevated. The nasogastric suction tube inserted during surgery is connected to low intermittent pressure suction to remove stomach contents and reduce the danger of aspiration. Wire cutters are kept at the patient's bedside. If the patient vomits, the nurse must cut the wires to prevent aspiration. Surgery and rewiring will be performed later. Antiemetic medications are administered to prevent vomiting. Secretions of the nasopharyngeal area are cleared with a small catheter inserted through the nasal orifice. Mouth care and suctioning of oral secretions are performed with care.

The diet must necessarily be liquid, but of sufficient caloric and fluid intake to ensure adequate nutrition. A straw may be used without much difficulty, and soft foods are taken by spoon. Water is taken after each liquid feeding, followed by a mouthwash. The patient with rigid fixation should not chew food in the first 1 to 4 weeks after surgery.

PROMOTING HOME AND COMMUNITY-BASED CARE

The patient needs specific guidelines for mouth care and feeding. Any irritated areas in the mouth should be reported to the physician. For patients discharged after internal maxillary fixation, a wire cutter should be kept readily available, and the patient and family members are instructed about how to cut the wires in an emergency. The importance of keeping scheduled appointments with the physician for assessment of the stability of the fixation appliance is emphasized.

Consultation with a dietitian may be indicated. The patient and family are instructed about foods that are high in essential nutrients and ways that these foods can be prepared so that they can be consumed through a straw or spoon, while remaining tasty. The use of nutritional supplements may be recommended.

DISORDERS OF THE SALIVARY GLANDS

The salivary glands consist of the parotid glands, one on each side of the face below the ear; the submaxillary and sublingual glands, both in the floor of the mouth; and the buccal gland, beneath the lips. About 1200 mL of saliva is produced daily. The glands' primary functions are lubrication, antibacterial protection, and digestion.

Parotitis

Parotitis (inflammation of the parotid gland) is the most common inflammatory condition of the salivary glands; however, inflammation can occur in the other salivary glands as well. Mumps (epidemic parotitis), a communicable disease caused by viral infection and most commonly seen in children, is an inflammation of a salivary gland, usually the parotid.

Elderly, acutely ill, and debilitated people with decreased salivary flow from general dehydration or medications are at high risk for developing parotitis. The infecting organisms travel from the mouth through the salivary duct. The organism is usually *Staphylococcus aureus* (except in mumps). The onset of this complication is sudden, with an exacerbation of both the fever and the symptoms of the primary condition. The gland swells and becomes tense and tender. Pain is felt in the ear, and the swollen glands interfere with swallowing. The swelling increases rapidly, and the overlying skin soon becomes red and shiny.

Preventive measures are essential and include advising the preoperative patient to have necessary dental work performed before surgery. In addition, maintaining adequate nutritional and fluid intake, along with good oral hygiene, and discontinuing medications that may cause diminished salivation (eg, tranquilizers and diuretics) may help prevent the condition. If parotitis occurs, antibiotic therapy is necessary. Analgesics may also be prescribed to control pain. If antibiotic therapy is not effective, an incision and drainage of the gland is necessary. Parotidectomy may be necessary to treat chronic parotitis.

Sialadenitis

Sialadenitis (inflammation of the salivary glands) may be caused by dehydration, radiation therapy, stress, malnutrition, salivary gland calculi (stones), or improper oral hygiene and is associated with *S. aureus*, *Streptococcus viridans*, or pneumococcal infection. Symptoms include pain, swelling, and purulent discharge. Antibiotics are used to relieve acute symptoms; massage, hydration, and corticosteroids frequently cure the problem. Chronic sialadenitis with uncontrolled pain is treated by surgically draining the gland or excising the gland and its duct.

Salivary Calculus (Sialolithiasis)

Sialolithiasis, or salivary calculi (stones), occurs in the submandibular gland. Salivary gland ultrasound or sialograms (x-ray films taken after the injection of a radiopaque substance into the

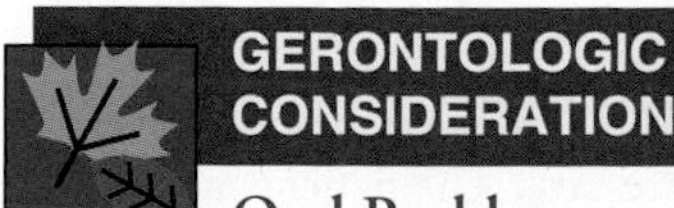

GERONTOLOGIC CONSIDERATIONS

Oral Problems

Many medications taken by the elderly cause dry mouth, which is uncomfortable, impairs communication, and increases the risk of oral infection. These medications include:

- Diuretics
- Antihypertensives
- Anti-inflammatories
- Antidepressants.

Poor dentition can exacerbate problems of aging, such as:

- Decreased food intake
- Loss of appetite
- Social isolation
- Increased susceptibility to systemic infection (from periodontal disease)
- Trauma to the oral cavity secondary to thinner, less vascular oral mucous membranes.

duct) may be required to demonstrate obstruction of the duct by stenosis. Salivary stones are formed mainly from calcium phosphate. If located within the gland, they are irregular and vary in diameter from 3 to 30 mm. Stones in the duct are small and oval.

Calculi within the salivary gland itself cause no symptoms unless infection arises; however, a calculus that obstructs the gland's duct causes sudden, local, and often colicky pain, which is abruptly relieved by a gush of saliva. This characteristic complaint is often elicited in the health history. On assessment, the gland is swollen and quite tender, the stone itself often is palpable, and its shadow may be seen on x-rays.

The calculus can be extracted fairly easily from the duct in the mouth; sometimes enlarging the ductal orifice permits the stone to pass spontaneously. **Lithotripsy**, a procedure used to disintegrate the stone with shock waves, may be used instead of surgical extraction. Lithotripsy requires no anesthesia, sedation, or analgesia. Side effects may include local hemorrhage and swelling. Surgery may be necessary to remove the gland if symptoms and calculi recur repeatedly.

Neoplasms

Although uncommon, neoplasms (tumors or growths) of almost any type may develop in the salivary gland. Tumors occur more frequently in the parotid gland. The incidence of salivary gland tumors is similar in men and women. Risk factors include exposure to radiation, employment in the rubber industry, smoking, and ingestion of alcohol. Diagnosis is based on the history and physical examination and biopsy results.

Management of salivary gland tumors is controversial, but the common procedure involves partial excision of the gland, along with all of the tumor and a wide margin. Dissection is carefully performed to preserve the seventh cranial nerve (facial nerve). For more involved tumors, it may not be possible to preserve the nerve. If the tumor is malignant, radiation therapy may follow surgery. Chemotherapy is usually used for palliative purposes. Local recurrences are common; the recurrent growth usually is more aggressive than the original. It has also been observed that these patients have an increased incidence of second primary cancers.

CANCER OF THE ORAL CAVITY

Cancers of the oral cavity, which can occur in any part of the mouth or throat, are curable if discovered early. These cancers are associated with the use of alcohol and tobacco. Many believe that the combination of alcohol and tobacco has a synergistic carcinogenic effect. About 75% of cases of oral cancer occur in people older than age 60, but the incidence is increasing in men younger than age 30 because of the use of smokeless tobacco, especially snuff.

Cancer of the oral cavity accounts for less than 2% of all cancer deaths in the United States. Men are afflicted more often than women; however, the incidence in women is increasing, possibly because they use tobacco and alcohol more frequently than they did in the past. The 5-year survival rate for cancer of the oral cavity and pharynx is 55% for whites and 33% for African Americans. Of the 8100 annual deaths from oral cancer (Landis et al., 1999), the distribution by site is estimated as follows:

Tongue 1800

Mouth 2300

Pharynx 2100

Other 1900

Chronic irritation by a warm pipe stem or prolonged exposure to the sun and wind may predispose to lip cancer. Predisposing factors for other oral cancers are exposure to tobacco (including smokeless tobacco), ingestion of alcohol, dietary deficiency, and ingestion of smoked meats.

Pathophysiology

Malignancies of the oral cavity are usually squamous cell cancers. Any area of the oropharynx can be a site for malignant growths, but the lips, the lateral aspects of the tongue, and the floor of the mouth are most commonly affected.

Clinical Manifestations

Many oral cancers produce few or no symptoms in the early stages. Later, the most frequent symptom is a painless sore or mass that will not heal. A typical lesion in oral cancer is a painless indurated (hardened) ulcer with raised edges. Any ulcer of the oral cavity that does not heal in 2 weeks should be examined through biopsy. As the cancer progresses, the patient may complain of tenderness; difficulty in chewing, swallowing, or speaking; coughing of blood-tinged sputum; or enlarged cervical lymph nodes.

Assessment and Diagnostic Findings

Diagnostic evaluation consists of an oral examination as well as an assessment of the cervical lymph nodes to evaluate for possible metastasis. Biopsies are performed on suspicious lesions (those that have not healed in 2 weeks). High-risk areas include the buccal mucosa and gingiva for people who use snuff or smoke cigars or pipes. For those who smoke cigarettes and drink alcohol, high-risk areas include the floor of the mouth, ventrolateral tongue, and soft palate complex (the soft palate, the anterior and posterior tonsillar area, the uvula, and the area behind the molar and tongue junction).

Medical Management

Management varies with the nature of the lesion, preference of the physician, and patient choice. Surgical resection, radiation therapy, chemotherapy, or a combination of these therapies may be effective.

In cancer of the lip, small lesions are usually excised liberally; larger lesions involving greater than one third of the lip may be more appropriately treated by radiation therapy because of superior cosmetic results. The choice depends on the extent of the lesion and what is necessary to cure the patient while preserving the best appearance. Tumors larger than 4 cm often recur.

Cancer of the tongue is treated aggressively because the recurrence rate is high. For cancer of the lateral margin of the tongue, the treatments of choice are radiation therapy and surgery. It is often necessary to perform a hemiglossectomy (surgical removal of half of the tongue). When cancer is present at the base of the tongue, surgical resection is more debilitating. Often radiation therapy is the primary treatment. A combination of radioactive interstitial implants and external beam radiation may be employed. For larger lesions, external beam therapy alone is used.

Often cancer of the oral cavity has metastasized through the extensive lymphatic channel in the neck region (Fig. 32-1), requiring a neck dissection and reconstructive surgery of the oral cavity. A common reconstructive technique involves use of a radial forearm free flap (use of a thin layer of skin from the forearm along with the radial artery).

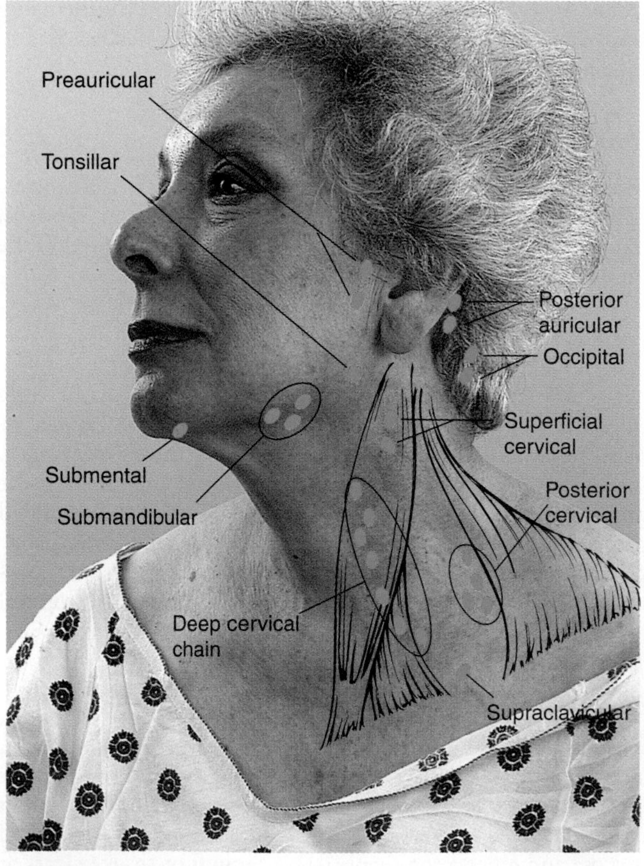

FIGURE 32•1 Lymphatic drainage of the head and neck. From Weber, J. W., & Kelley, J. (1998). *Health assessment in nursing.* Philadelphia: Lippincott-Raven.

Nursing Management

The patient's nutritional status is assessed preoperatively. A dietary consultation may be necessary. The patient may require enteral (through the intestine) or parenteral (intravenous) feedings before and after surgery to maintain adequate nutrition. If a radial graft is to be done, an Allen test on the donor arm must be performed to ensure that the ulnar artery is patent and can provide blood flow to the hand after removal of the radial artery. An Allen test is done by manually compressing the radial artery and asking the patient to make a fist. The patient's hand should turn pink, indicating ulnar artery patency.

Postoperatively, the patient is assessed for a patent airway. The patient may be unable to manage oral secretions, making suctioning necessary. If grafting was done, suctioning must be performed with care to prevent damage to the graft. The graft is assessed postoperatively for viability. Although color should be assessed (white may indicate arterial occlusion and blue mottling may indicate venous congestion), it may be difficult to assess the graft by looking into the mouth. A Doppler ultrasound may be used to locate the radial pulse at the graft site and to assess graft perfusion.

NURSING PROCESS: THE PATIENT WITH CONDITIONS OF THE ORAL CAVITY

Assessment

Obtaining a health history allows the nurse to determine the patient's learning needs concerning preventive oral hygiene, as well as to identify symptoms requiring medical evaluation. The history includes questions about the patient's normal brushing and flossing routine; frequency of dental visits; awareness of any lesions or irritated areas in the mouth, tongue, or throat; need to wear dentures or a partial plate; recent history of sore throat or bloody sputum; discomfort caused by certain foods; daily food intake; and use of alcohol and tobacco, including smokeless chewing tobacco.

A careful physical assessment follows the health history. Both the internal and external structures of the mouth and throat are inspected and palpated. Removal of dentures and partial plates is necessary to ensure a thorough inspection of the gums. In general, the examination can be accomplished with the use of a bright light source (penlight) and a tongue depressor. Gloves are worn to palpate the tongue and any abnormalities.

Lips

The examination begins with inspection of the lips for moisture, hydration, color, texture, symmetry, and the presence of ulcerations or fissures. The lips should be moist, pink, smooth, and symmetric. The patient is instructed to open the mouth wide; a tongue blade is then inserted to expose the buccal mucosa for an assessment of color and lesions. Stensen's duct of each parotid gland is visible as a small red dot in the buccal mucosa next to the upper molars.

Gums

The gums are inspected for inflammation, bleeding, retraction, and discoloration. The odor of the breath is also noted. The hard palate is examined for color and shape.

Tongue

The dorsum (back) of the tongue is inspected for texture, color, and lesions. A thin white coat and large, vallate papillae in a V formation on the distal portion of the dorsum of the tongue are normal findings. The patient is instructed to protrude the tongue and move it laterally. This provides the examiner with an opportunity to estimate the tongue's size as well as its symmetry and strength (to assess the integrity of the 12th cranial nerve [hypoglossal]).

Further inspection of the ventral surface of the tongue and the floor of the mouth is accomplished by asking the patient to touch the roof of the mouth with the tip of the tongue. Any lesions of the mucosa or any abnormalities involving the frenulum or superficial veins on the undersurface of the tongue are noted. This is a common area for oral cancer, which presents as a white or red plaque, an indurated ulcer, or a warty growth.

A tongue blade is used to depress the tongue for adequate visualization of the pharynx. It is pressed firmly beyond the midpoint of the tongue; proper placement avoids a gagging response. The patient is told to tip the head back, open the mouth wide, take a deep breath, and say "ah." Often this flattens the posterior tongue and briefly allows a full view of the anterior and posterior pillars, tonsils, uvula, and posterior pharynx (Fig. 32-2). These structures are inspected for color, symmetry, and evidence of exudate, ulceration, or enlargement. Normally, the uvula and soft palate rise symmetrically with a deep inspiration or "ah"; this indicates an intact vagus nerve (10th cranial nerve).

A complete assessment of the oral cavity is essential because many disorders such as cancer, diabetes, and immunosuppressive conditions from medication therapy or AIDS may be manifested by changes in the oral cavity. The neck is examined for enlarged lymph nodes (adenopathy).

Nursing Diagnosis

Based on all the assessment data, major nursing diagnoses may include the following:

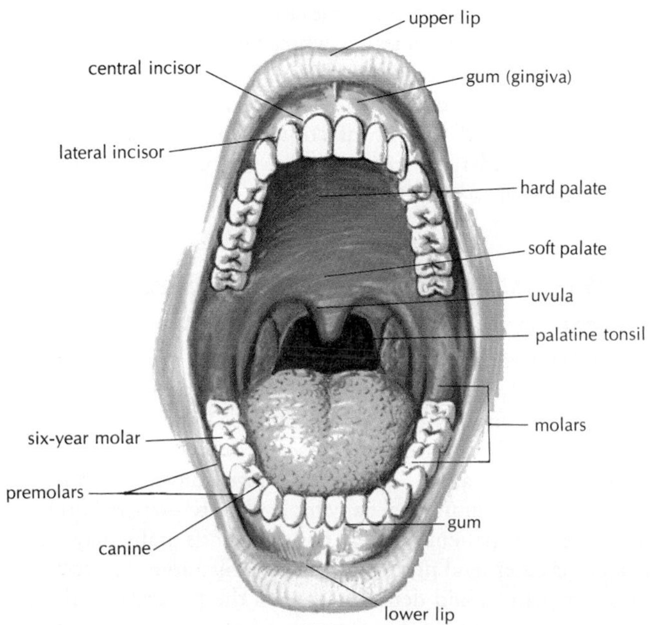

FIGURE 32•2 Structures of the mouth, including the tongue and palate.

- Altered oral mucous membrane related to a pathologic condition, infection, or chemical or mechanical trauma (eg, medications, ill-fitting dentures)
- Altered nutrition, less than body requirements, related to inability to ingest adequate nutrients secondary to oral or dental conditions
- Body image disturbance related to a physical change in appearance resulting from a disease condition or its treatment
- Fear of pain and social isolation related to disease or change in physical appearance
- Pain related to oral lesion or treatment
- Impaired verbal communication related to treatment
- Risk for infection related to disease or treatment
- Knowledge deficit about disease process and treatment plan

Planning and Goals

The major goals for the patient may include improving the condition of the oral mucous membrane, improving nutritional intake, attaining a positive self-image, relieving pain, identifying alternative communication methods, preventing infection, and understanding the disease and its treatment.

Nursing Interventions

Promoting Mouth Care

The nurse instructs the patient in the importance and techniques of preventive mouth care. If a patient cannot tolerate brushing or flossing, an irrigating solution of 1 teaspoon of baking soda to 8 ounces of warm water, half-strength hydrogen peroxide, or normal saline solution is recommended. The nurse reinforces the need to perform oral care, and provides such care to patients who are unable to do so themselves.

When a bacterial or fungal infection is present, the nurse administers the appropriate medication and instructs the patient in how to administer the medications at home. The nurse monitors the patient's physical and psychological response to treatment.

Xerostomia, dryness of the mouth, is a frequent sequela of oral cancer, particularly when the salivary glands have been exposed to radiation or major surgery. It is also seen in patients receiving psychopharmacologic agents, patients with HIV infection, or patients unable to close the mouth who therefore become mouth-breathers. To minimize this problem, the patient is advised to avoid dry, bulky, and irritating foods and fluids, as well as alcohol and tobacco. The patient is also encouraged to increase intake of fluids (when not contraindicated) and to use a humidifier during sleep. The use of synthetic saliva, a moisturizing antibacterial gel such as Oral Balance, or a saliva production stimulant such as Salagen may be helpful.

Stomatitis, or mucositis, which involves inflammation and breakdown of the oral mucosa, is often a side effect of chemotherapy or radiation therapy. Prophylactic mouth care is started when the patient begins receiving treatment; however, mucositis may become so severe that a break in treatment is necessary. If a patient receiving radiation therapy has poor dentition, extraction of the teeth is often recommended to prevent infection before treatment to the oral cavity is initiated. Many radiation therapy centers recommend the use of fluoride treatments for patients receiving radiation to the head and neck.

Home Care Teaching Checklist: The Patient With an Oral Condition

At the completion of the program, the patient or caregiver will be able to:	Patient	Caregiver
• Demonstrate use of suction equipment.	✔	✔
• State rationale for humidification.	✔	✔
• State foods necessary to meet caloric needs and dietary needs (ie, change in consistency, seasoning limitations, supplements).	✔	✔
• Demonstrate oral hygiene.	✔	✔
• Demonstrate care of incision.	✔	✔
• State when next medical/dental follow-up will be scheduled.	✔	✔

Ensuring Adequate Food and Fluid Intake

The patient's weight, age, and level of activity are recorded to determine if nutritional intake is adequate. A daily calorie count may be necessary to determine the exact quantity of food and fluid ingested. The frequency and pattern of eating are recorded to determine if any psychosocial or physiologic factors are affecting ingestion. The nurse recommends changes in the consistency of foods and the frequency of eating, based on the disease condition and the patient's preferences. Consultation with a dietitian can be helpful. The goal is to help the patient attain and maintain desirable body weight and level of energy, as well as to promote the healing of tissue.

Supporting a Positive Self-Image

A patient who has a disfiguring oral condition or has undergone disfiguring surgery may experience an alteration in self-image. The patient is encouraged to verbalize the perceived change in body appearance and realistically discuss actual changes or losses. The nurse offers support while the patient verbalizes fears and negative feelings (withdrawal, depression, anger). The nurse listens attentively and determines if the patient's needs are primarily psychosocial or cognitive-perceptual. This determination will help to individualize a plan of care. The patient's strengths, achievements, and positive attributes are reinforced.

The nurse should determine the patient's anxieties concerning relationships with others. Referral to support groups, a psychiatric liaison nurse, a social worker, or clergy may be useful in helping the patient to cope with anxieties and fears. Emphasizing that the patient's worth is not diminished by a physical change in a body part can be a helpful approach. The patient's progress toward developing positive self-esteem is documented. The nurse should be alert to signs of grieving and should record emotional changes. By providing acceptance and support, the nurse encourages the patient to verbalize feelings.

Minimizing Discomfort and Pain

Oral lesions may be painful. Strategies to reduce discomfort include avoiding foods that are spicy, hot, or hard (eg, pretzels, nuts). The patient is instructed about mouth care. It may be necessary to provide the patient with an analgesic such as viscous lidocaine (Xylocaine Viscous 2%) or opioids as prescribed. The nurse can reduce fear of pain by advising the patient regarding pain control methods.

Promoting Effective Communication

Verbal communication may be impaired by radical surgery for oral cancer. It is therefore vital to assess the patient's ability to communicate in writing before surgery. Pen and paper are provided postoperatively to patients who can use them to communicate. A communication board with commonly used words or pictures is obtained preoperatively and given to postoperative patients who cannot write so that they may point to needed items. A speech therapist is also consulted postoperatively.

Preventing Infection

Leukopenia (a decrease in white blood cells) may result from radiation, chemotherapy, AIDS, and some medications used to treat AIDS. This reduces defense mechanisms, increasing the risk for infections. Malnutrition, also common among these patients, may further decrease resistance to infection. If the patient is diabetic, the risk of infection increases further.

Laboratory results should be evaluated frequently and the patient's temperature checked every 4 to 8 hours for an elevation that may indicate infection. Visitors who might transmit microorganisms are prohibited because the patient's immunologic system is depressed. Sensitive skin tissues are protected from trauma to maintain skin integrity and prevent infection. Aseptic technique is necessary when changing dressings. Desquamation (shedding of the epidermis) is a reaction to radiation therapy that causes dryness and itching and can lead to a break in skin integrity and subsequent infection.

As discussed above, adequate nutrition is helpful in preventing infection. Signs of wound infection such as redness, swelling, drainage, or tenderness are reported to the physician. Antibiotics may be prescribed prophylactically.

Promoting Home and Community-Based Care

TEACHING PATIENTS SELF-CARE

The patient recovering from treatment of an oral condition is instructed about mouth care, nutrition, infection prevention, and signs and symptoms of complications. Methods of preparing nutritious foods that are properly seasoned and of the right temperature are explained. It may be more convenient for some patients to use commercial baby foods than to prepare liquid and soft diets. The patient who cannot take foods orally may receive enteral or parenteral nutrition; the administration of these feedings is explained and demonstrated to the patient and the care provider.

For patients with cancer, instructions are provided in the use and care of any prostheses. The importance of keeping dressings clean is emphasized, as is the need for conscientious oral hygiene.

CONTINUING CARE

The need for ongoing care in the home will depend on the patient's condition. The patient, family members or the person responsible for home care, the nurse, and other health care professionals (eg, speech therapist, nutritionist, psychologist) work together to prepare an individualized plan of care.

If suctioning the mouth or tracheostomy tube is required, the necessary equipment is obtained and the patient and care providers are taught how to use it. Humidification of the home, to keep secretions moist, and the control of odors may be considerations. The patient and the care providers are taught how to assess for obstruction, hemorrhage, and infection and what actions to take if they occur. The home care nurse may provide physical care, monitor for changes in the patient's physical status (eg, skin integrity, nutritional status, respiratory function), and assess the adequacy of pain control measures. The nurse also assesses the patient's and family's ability to manage incisions, drains, and feeding tubes and their use of recommended strategies for communication. The ability of the patient and family to accept physical, psychological, and role changes is assessed and addressed.

Follow-up visits to the physician are important to monitor the patient's condition and to determine the need for modifications in treatment and general care. The nurse reinforces instructions in an effort to promote the patient's self-care and comfort.

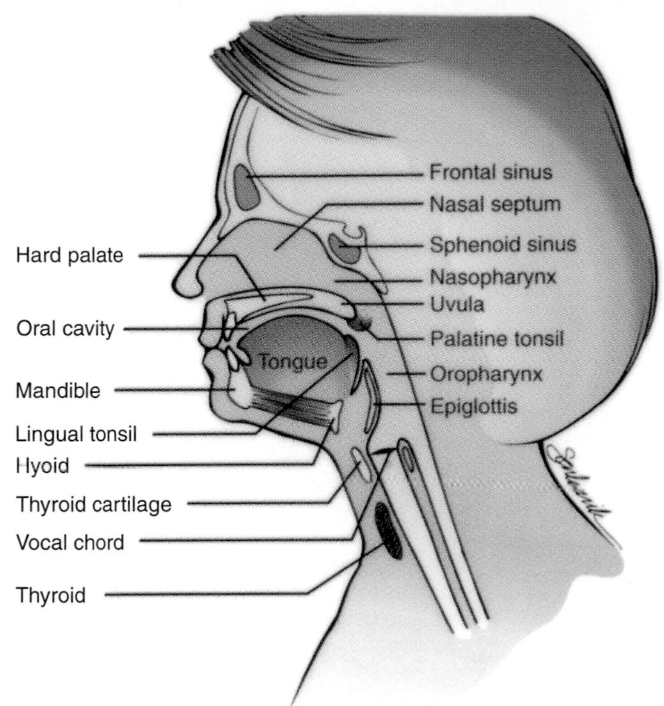

FIGURE 32•3 Anatomy of the head and neck.

Evaluation

Expected Outcomes

Expected outcomes may include:

1. Shows evidence of intact oral mucous membranes
   a. Is free of pain and discomfort in the oral cavity
   b. Has no visible alteration in membrane integrity
   c. Identifies and avoids foods that are irritating (nuts, pretzels, spicy foods)
   d. States measures necessary for preventive mouth care
   e. Complies with medication regimen
   f. Limits or avoids use of alcohol and tobacco (including smokeless tobacco)
2. Attains and maintains desirable body weight
3. Has a positive self-image
   a. Verbalizes anxieties
   b. Is able to accept change and modify self-concept accordingly
4. Attains an acceptable level of comfort
   a. Verbalizes that pain is absent or under control
   b. Avoids foods and liquids that cause discomfort
   c. Adheres to medication regimen
5. Has decreased fears related to pain, isolation, and the inability to cope
   a. Accepts that pain will be managed if not eliminated
   b. Freely expresses fears and concerns
6. Is free of infection
   a. Exhibits normal laboratory values
   b. Is afebrile
   c. Performs oral hygiene after every meal and at bedtime
7. Acquires information about disease process and course of treatment

NECK DISSECTION

Malignancies of the head and neck include those of the oral cavity, oropharynx, hypopharynx, nasopharynx, nasal cavity, paranasal sinus, and larynx (Fig. 32-3). (Laryngeal cancer is discussed in Chapter 20.) These cancers account for less than 5% of all cancers. Depending on the location and stage, treatment may consist of radiation therapy, chemotherapy, surgery, or a combination of these modalities. Deaths from malignancies of the head and neck are primarily attributable not to recurrence at the primary site but to local-regional metastasis to the cervical lymph nodes in the neck, which often takes place by way of the lymphatics before the primary lesion has been treated. This local-regional metastasis is not amenable to surgical resection and responds poorly to chemotherapy and/or radiation therapy.

A radical neck dissection involves removal of all cervical lymph nodes from the mandible to the clavicle and removal of the sternocleidomastoid muscle, internal jugular vein, and spinal accessory muscle. The associated morbidities include shoulder drop and poor cosmesis (visible neck depression). Modified radical neck dissection, which preserves one or more of the nonlymphatic structures, is used more often. This procedure preserves the internal jugular vein, the sternocleidomastoid muscle, and the spinal accessory nerve. A selective neck dissection (in comparison to a radical dissection) preserves one or more of the lymph node groups (Fig. 32-4).

Reconstructive techniques may be performed with a variety of grafts. A cutaneous flap (skin and subcutaneous tissue), such as the deltopectoral flap, may be used. A more frequently used graft for head and neck reconstruction is a myocutaneous flap (muscle and skin). The pectoralis major muscle is usually used. A microvascular free flap may be used for large defects. This involves the transfer of muscle, skin, or bone with an artery and vein to the area of reconstruction, using microinstrumentation. Areas used for a free flap include the scapula, the radial area of the forearm, or the fibula. The fibula provides a larger bone area if mandibular reconstruction is involved.

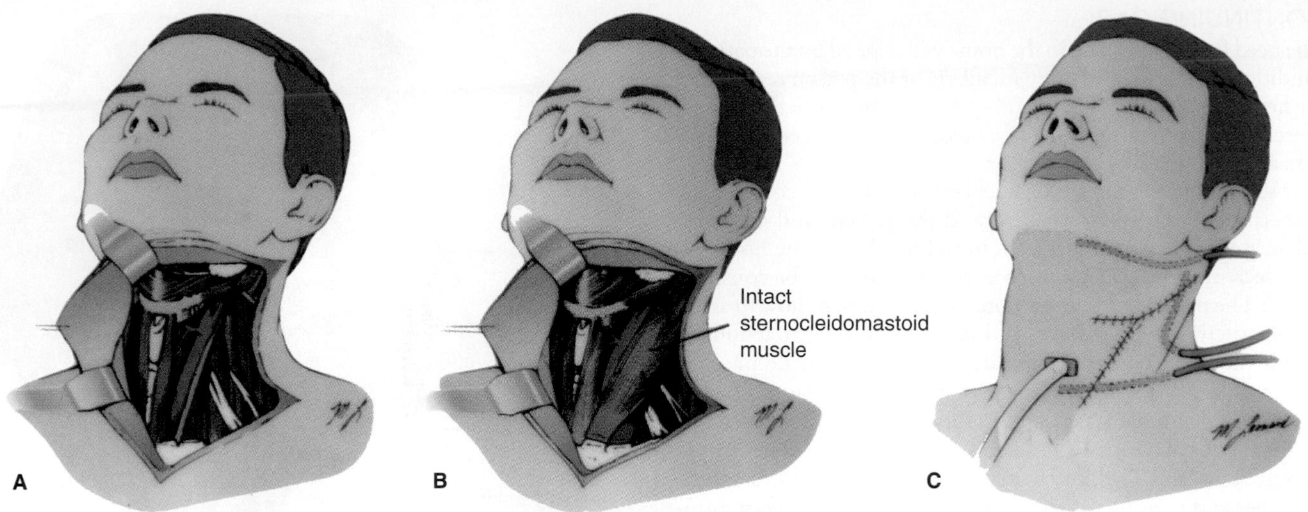

FIGURE 32•4 (**A**) A classic radical neck dissection in which the sternocleidomastoid and smaller muscles are removed. All tissue is removed, from the ramus of the jaw to the clavicle. The jugular vein has also been removed. The functional neck dissection (**B**) is similar but preserves the sternocleidomastoid muscle, internal jugular vein, and spinal accessory nerve. The wound is closed (**C**), and portable suction drainage tubes are in place.

NURSING PROCESS: THE PATIENT UNDERGOING A NECK DISSECTION

Assessment

Preoperatively, the patient's physical and psychological preparation for major surgery is assessed, along with his or her knowledge of the preoperative and postoperative procedures. Postoperatively, the patient is assessed for complications such as altered respiratory status, wound infection, and hemorrhage. As healing occurs, neck range of motion is assessed.

Diagnosis

Nursing Diagnoses

Based on all the assessment data, major nursing diagnoses may include the following:

- Knowledge deficit about preoperative and postoperative procedures
- Ineffective airway clearance related to obstruction by mucus, hemorrhage, or edema
- Risk for infection related to surgical intervention secondary to decreased nutritional status, or immunosuppression from chemotherapy or radiation therapy
- Impaired skin integrity secondary to surgery and graft
- Altered nutrition, less than body requirements, related to disease process or treatment
- Disturbance in self-esteem related to diagnosis or prognosis
- Pain related to surgical incision and the presence of abnormal epithelial cells
- Impaired communication secondary to surgical treatment
- Impaired physical mobility secondary to nerve injury

Collaborative Problems/Potential Complications

Potential postoperative complications that may develop include:

- Hemorrhage
- Nerve injury

Planning and Goals

The major goals for the patient include participation in the treatment plan, maintenance of respiratory status, absence of infection, viability of the graft, maintenance of adequate intake of food and fluids, effective coping strategies, attainment of comfort, effective communication, and absence of complications.

Nursing Interventions

Providing Preoperative Patient Education

Before surgery, the patient should be informed about the nature and extent of the surgery, and what the postoperative period will be like. The patient is encouraged to ask questions and to express concerns about the upcoming surgery. During this exchange, the nurse has an opportunity to assess the patient's coping abilities, answer questions, and develop a plan for offering assistance. A sense of mutual understanding and rapport will make the postoperative experience less traumatic for the patient. After the operation, the patient's expressions of concern, anxieties, and fears can guide the nurse in providing additional support.

Providing General Postoperative Care

The general postoperative nursing interventions are similar to those described in Chapter 18. For the patient who has had extensive neck surgery, specific postoperative interventions include maintenance of a patent airway and continuous assessment of respiratory

32•1

PLAN OF NURSING CARE

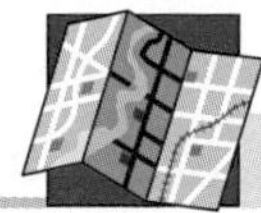

Care of the Patient Who Has Undergone Neck Dissection

Nursing Interventions	Rationale	Expected Outcomes
Nursing Diagnosis: Ineffective airway clearance related to obstruction secondary to edema, hemorrhage, or inadequate wound drainage **Goal:** Maintenance of normal respiratory function		
1. Place the patient in high Fowler's position.	1. High Fowler's position facilitates expansion of the lungs because the diaphragm is pulled downward and the abdominal viscera are pulled away from the lungs. Breathing is promoted. This position also increases lymphatic and venous drainage, decreases swallowing, and decreases venous pressure on the graft. Regurgitation and aspiration of stomach contents is prevented postoperatively.	• Achieves a normal respiratory rate • Breathes comfortably • Avoids use of accessory muscles of respiration • Maintains vital signs within normal range • Shows evidence of normal breath sounds
2. Monitor vital signs according to postoperative routine.	2. Edema, hemorrhage, or inadequate drainage will alter heart rate and respirations. Tachypnea and restlessness may indicate respiratory distress.	
3. Auscultate breath sounds as needed. In the immediate postoperative period, place the stethoscope over the trachea to assess for stridor.	3. Abnormal breath sounds may indicate ineffective ventilation, decreased perfusion, and fluid accumulation. Stridor, a harsh, high-pitched sound primarily heard on inspiration, indicates airway obstruction.	

(*continued*)

status, wound care and oral hygiene, maintenance of adequate nutrition, and observation for hemorrhage or nerve injury.

MAINTAINING THE AIRWAY

After the endotracheal tube or airway has been removed and the effects of the anesthesia have worn off, the patient may be placed in Fowler's position to facilitate breathing and promote comfort. This position also increases lymphatic and venous drainage, facilitates swallowing, and decreases venous pressure on the skin flaps.

In the immediate postoperative period, the nurse assesses for stridor (coarse, high-pitched sound on inspiration) by listening frequently over the trachea with a stethoscope. This finding must be reported immediately because it indicates obstruction of the airway. Signs of respiratory distress, such as dyspnea, cyanosis, changes in mental status, and changes in vital signs, are assessed because they may suggest edema, hemorrhage, inadequate oxygenation, and inadequate drainage.

Pneumonia may occur in the postoperative phase if pulmonary secretions are not removed. Coughing and deep breathing are encouraged to aid in the removal of secretions. The patient should assume a sitting position, with the nurse supporting the neck so that the patient may be able to bring up excessive secretions. If this is ineffective, the patient's respiratory tract may have to be suctioned. Care is taken to protect the suture lines during suctioning. If a tracheostomy tube is in place, suctioning is performed through this tube using sterile technique. The patient may also be instructed on use of the Yankauer suction (tonsil tip suction) to remove oral secretions. Temperature should not be taken orally.

PROVIDING WOUND CARE

Wound drainage tubes are usually inserted during surgery to prevent the collection of fluid subcutaneously. The drainage tubes are connected to portable suction (such as a Jackson-Pratt) and the container is emptied periodically. Between 80 and 120 mL of serosanguineous secretions may drain over the first 24 hours. If dressings are present, they may need to be reinforced from time to time. Dressings are observed for evidence of hemorrhage and constriction, which impairs respiration and graft perfusion. The graft is assessed for color and temperature, and the presence of a pulse if applicable, to determine viability. The graft should be pale pink and warm to the touch. The wound is also assessed for infection, which is reported immediately. The patient may be placed on prophylactic antibiotics.

MAINTAINING ADEQUATE NUTRITION

Nutritional status is assessed preoperatively; early intervention to correct nutritional imbalances may decrease the risk of postoperative complications. Frequently, nutrition is less than optimal because of inadequate intake, and the patient often requires enteral or parenteral supplements preoperatively to attain a positive nitrogen balance. This may need to be continued postoperatively if the patient cannot take enough calories by mouth. Supplements (eg, Ensure, Sustacal, or Carnation Instant Breakfast) provide a nutritionally dense adjunct and may help reestablish a positive nitrogen balance. They may be taken enterally by mouth, by nasogastric feeding tube, or by gastrostomy feeding tube. (See Plan of Nursing Care for further discussion.)

(*text continues on page 822*)

32•1 PLAN OF NURSING CARE 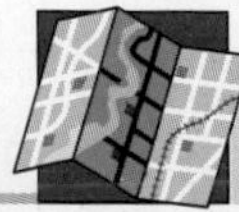

Care of the Patient Who Has Undergone Neck Dissection (*continued*)

Nursing Interventions	Rationale	Expected Outcomes
4. Encourage deep breathing and coughing. Place the patient in a sitting position and support the neck area with both hands.	4. Deep breathing before coughing promotes expansion of the airways and a more forceful cough. The coughing mechanism assists airway cilia with removal of secretions. Splinting the incision during coughing reduces strain and promotes the expulsion of secretions by allowing deeper inspirations.	• Coughs effectively • Maintains a patent airway • Does not develop a mucous plug
5. Suction the airway as needed using sterile technique and a soft catheter.	5. Suctioning assists in removal of secretions that the patient may be unable to cough up, thereby assisting with maintaining a patent airway.	
6. Provide humidified air or oxygen if the patient has a tracheostomy.	6. Keeps secretions thin.	

Nursing Diagnosis: Risk for infection
Goal: Absence of infection

Nursing Interventions	Rationale	Expected Outcomes
1. Instruct the patient in preoperative and postoperative oral hygiene using slightly alkaline solutions such as 8 oz of water mixed with 1 teaspoon of baking soda, or normal saline solution every 4 hours.	1. Oral care decreases oral bacteria, thereby decreasing the risk of bacterial infection postoperatively. Hydrogen peroxide should not be used as it may break down fresh granulation tissue.	• Patient performs oral hygiene preoperatively and postoperatively every 4 hours • Mouth remains clean • Wound drains less than 200 mL of serosanguineous drainage the first postoperative day • No hematoma at skin graft • Serosanguineous drainage is within normal limits • Dressing will remain intact with no constriction of airway or blood flow • Wound and surrounding skin remain clean and free of infection • Patient is afebrile with normal respirations and a normal heart rate • Patient is alert and aware of surroundings
2. Monitor wound suction drainage.	2. Suction drainage negates the need for pressure dressings because the skin flaps are pulled down tightly. Drainage should approximate 80–120 mL of serosanguineous secretions for the first 24 hours; then the secretions should decrease daily. Continuous bloody drainage indicates small vessel oozing.	
3. Note drainage quantity and odor.	3. Purulent, malodorous drainage indicates an infection. Drainage greater than 300 mL in the first 24 hours is considered abnormal.	
4. Assess condition of dressing and reinforce pressure dressings as needed. Assess for any possible constrictions that would affect respirations or decrease blood flow to graft.	4. If portable wound suction is not used, then pressure dressings may be applied to obliterate dead spaces and provide immobilization. These are reinforced, not changed, as needed.	
5. Use aseptic technique to cleanse skin around the drains; change the dressings as ordered by surgeon (usually the second through fifth postoperative days).	5. Aseptic technique prevents wound contamination. Sterile saline effectively cleans the skin around the drains.	
6. Monitor vital signs. Assess for symptoms of infection: chills, diaphoresis, altered level of consciousness.	6. An elevated temperature, tachypnea, and tachycardia may indicate an infection.	

(*continued*)

32•1 PLAN OF NURSING CARE 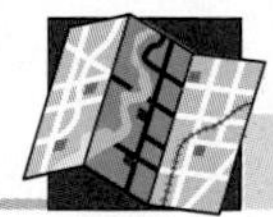

Care of the Patient Who Has Undergone Neck Dissection (*continued*)

Nursing Interventions	Rationale	Expected Outcomes
Nursing Diagnosis: Impaired skin integrity **Goal:** Maintenance of intact skin and viability of graft		
1. Assess condition of graft for viability.	1. Cyanotic, cool graft indicates possible necrosis. (Pale graft indicates arterial thrombosis; purple graft indicates venous congestion.)	• Graft will be pale pink in color and warm to touch • Tissue will blanch to gentle touch • Graft has pulse via Doppler ultrasound
2. Assess wound for signs and symptoms of infection.	2. Infected wound interferes with healing and threatens the viability of the graft.	• Patient will not have wound infection
Nursing Diagnosis: Altered nutrition, less than body requirements, related to anorexia and dysphagia **Goal:** Attainment/maintenance of adequate nutrition		
1. Assess nutritional status preoperatively, consult with dietitian.	1. Poor nutrition preoperatively decreases wound healing and increases potential for infection.	• Does not have weight loss greater than 10% of body weight. If patient does have weight loss greater than 10%, supplements are given to maintain/increase weight and obtain positive nitrogen balance
2. Administer tube feedings as prescribed. Keep head of bed elevated during feeding to prevent aspiration. Monitor for signs of tracheosophageal fistula (feeding in tracheal secretions).	2. A nasogastric tube may be in place for several days to administer enteral feedings.	• Tolerates tube feedings • No signs of aspiration • No sign of fistula • Expresses a desire for food • Swallows food easily
3. Provide oral hygiene before and after meals.	3. Oral hygiene enhances appetite.	• Is comfortable eating alone or with others
4. Assist with oral intake: a. Offer easily chewed foods; mash or blenderize if necessary. b. Suggest that the head be tilted to the unaffected side when swallowing. c. Inquire if privacy is desired when eating. d. Provide altered utensils as needed.	4. Soft-textured foods facilitate swallowing. Passage of food may be tolerated better when pressure occurs on the side opposite the surgery. Self-feeding difficulties may cause embarrassment and interfere with digestion.	
Nursing Diagnosis: Disturbance in self-esteem and body image related to changes in appearance and alterations in communication **Goal:** Attainment of positive self-image		
1. Assist the patient to communicate effectively: a. Provide materials for writing messages. b. Make certain that the call bell is readily accessible. c. Develop nonverbal ways to communicate (eg, finger-tapping, sign language, sign board). d. Consult speech/language therapist.	1. Temporary hoarseness is common after neck surgery. A tracheostomy may be performed and verbal communication may not be possible. Communication with head movement may be impossible because of incisional pain and need to maintain position of neck for graft. Speech/language therapist may assist with other forms of communication, such as esophageal speech or electrolarynx.	• Recognizes that hoarseness is temporary • Develops alternative forms of communication • Willingly conveys fears and concerns • Accepts prognosis with realistic limitations • Accepts support as offered • Absence of facial paralysis • Absence of drooling and dysphagia • Maintains normal shoulder function • Verbalizes methods to enhance physical appearance
2. Ecourage verbalization of fears: a. Provide time to listen. b. Project a positive, optimistic attitude. c. Reinforce reality.	2. Listening conveys acceptance and encourages further verbalization. An optimistic approach conveys interest and hope.	

(*continued*)

32•1

PLAN OF NURSING CARE

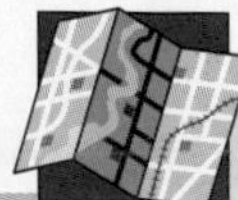

Care of the Patient Who Has Undergone Neck Dissection (*continued*)

Nursing Interventions	Rationale	Expected Outcomes
d. Collaborate with family members to elicit their support and encouragement. e. Consult support groups such as New Voice Club through the American Cancer Society.	Honesty will promote a trusting relationship. This includes confirming cosmetic and functional limitations. Family members or significant others can provide valuable support to the patient.	
3. Observe for facial paralysis.	3. Injury to facial nerve will cause lower facial paralysis.	
4. Observe for excessive drooling.	4. Damage to the hypoglossal nerve will result in excessive drooling and decreased ability to swallow.	
5. Check for normal shoulder position and function.	5. Damage to the spinal accessory nerve will result in drooping of the shoulder. Rehabilitation exercises are begun when the incision is healed.	
6. Provide information on clothing/cosmetics to deemphasize physical defects (offer information on "Look Good, Feel Better" program through American Cancer Society).	6. Physical appearance may be enhanced through use of cosmetics or clothing.	

The patient who is able to chew may take food by mouth, although the level of the patient's chewing ability will determine if some diet modification (eg, soft, puréed, or liquid foods) is necessary. Food preferences should also be discussed with the patient. Oral care before eating may enhance the patient's appetite, and oral care after eating is important to prevent infection. Most patients are able to maintain and gain weight.

SUPPORTING COPING MEASURES

Preoperatively, information about the planned surgery is given to the patient and family. The psychological postoperative nursing intervention is aimed at supporting the patient who has had a change in body image or who has major concerns regarding the prognosis. The patient may have difficulty communicating and may be concerned about his or her ability to breathe and swallow normally. The nurse enlists the support of family or friends in encouraging and reassuring the patient that adjusting to the results of this surgery will take time.

The person who has had extensive neck surgery often is sensitive about his or her appearance, either when the operative area is covered by bulky dressings or when the incision line is visible. If the nurse accepts the patient's appearance and expresses a positive, optimistic attitude, the patient is more likely to be encouraged. The patient also needs an opportunity to express concerns regarding the success of the surgery and the prognosis.

People with cancer of the head and neck frequently have used alcohol or tobacco before surgery; postoperatively, the patient is encouraged to abstain from these substances. Alternative methods of coping need to be explored and introduced slowly.

RELIEVING PAIN

Pain and the patient's fear of pain are assessed and managed. Patients with head and neck cancer often report less pain than patients with other types of cancer; however, the nurse needs to be aware that each person's pain experience is individual. The nurse administers analgesics as prescribed and assesses their effectiveness.

PROMOTING EFFECTIVE COMMUNICATION

If a laryngectomy was performed, the nurse explores other methods of communicating with the patient and obtains a consultation with a speech/language therapist.

MAINTAINING PHYSICAL MOBILITY

Excision of muscles and nerves results in weakness at the shoulder that can cause shoulder drop, a forward curvature of the shoulder. Many problems can be avoided with a conscientious exercise program. These exercises are usually begun when drains are removed and the neck incision is sufficiently healed. The purpose of the exercises depicted in Figure 32-5 is to promote maximal shoulder function and neck motion after surgery. Physical therapists and occupational therapists can assist patients in these exercises.

MONITORING AND MANAGING POTENTIAL COMPLICATIONS

Hemorrhage may occur from carotid artery rupture as a result of necrosis of the graft or damage to the artery itself from tumor or infection. The following measures are indicated to prevent or manage hemorrhage:

- Vital signs are assessed. Tachycardia, tachypnea, and hypotension may indicate impending hypovolemic shock subsequent to hemorrhage.
- The patient is instructed to avoid the Valsalva maneuver to prevent stress on the graft and carotid artery.
- Signs of impending rupture such as high epigastric pain or discomfort are reported.
- Dressings and wound drainage are observed for excessive bleeding.
- If hemorrhage occurs, assistance is summoned immediately.

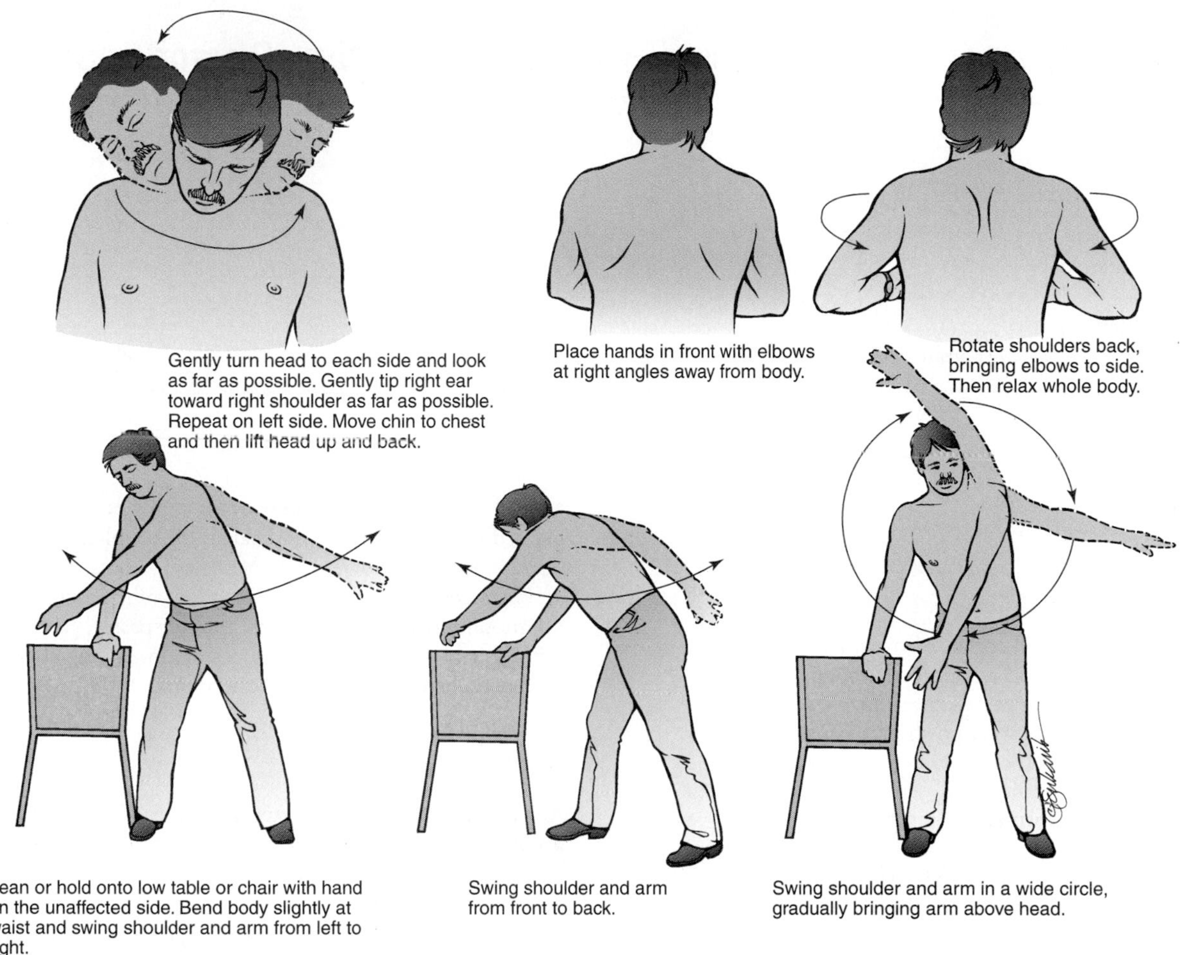

Gently turn head to each side and look as far as possible. Gently tip right ear toward right shoulder as far as possible. Repeat on left side. Move chin to chest and then lift head up and back.
Place hands in front with elbows at right angles away from body.
Rotate shoulders back, bringing elbows to side. Then relax whole body.
Lean or hold onto low table or chair with hand on the unaffected side. Bend body slightly at waist and swing shoulder and arm from left to right.
Swing shoulder and arm from front to back.
Swing shoulder and arm in a wide circle, gradually bringing arm above head.

FIGURE 32•5 Three rehabilitation exercises after head and neck surgery. The objective is to regain maximum shoulder function and neck motion after neck surgery. Exercise for Radical Neck Surgery Patients. Head and Neck Service, Department of Surgery, Memorial Hospital, New York, NY.

- Hemorrhage requires the continuous application of pressure to the bleeding site or major associated vessel.
- The head of the patient's bed is elevated to maintain airway patency and prevent aspiration.
- A controlled, calm manner will allay the patient's anxiety.
- The surgeon is notified immediately because a vascular or ligature tear requires surgical intervention.

Nerve injury can occur if the cervical plexus or spinal accessory nerves are severed during surgery. Because lower facial paralysis may occur as a result of injury to the facial nerve, this complication is observed for and reported. Likewise, if the superior laryngeal nerve is damaged, the patient may have difficulty swallowing liquids and food because of the partial lack of sensation of the glottis. Speech therapy may be indicated to assist with the problems related to nerve injury.

Promoting Home and Community-Based Care

TEACHING PATIENTS SELF-CARE

The patient and care provider will require instructions about management of the wound, dressing, and any drains that remain in place. Patients who require oral suctioning or who have a tracheostomy may be very anxious about their care at home; the transition to home can be eased if the care provider is given several opportunities to demonstrate the ability to meet the patient's needs.

If the patient cannot take food by mouth, detailed instructions and demonstration of enteral or parenteral feedings will be required. Techniques in effective oral hygiene are also important.

CONTINUING CARE

A referral for home care nursing may be necessary in the early period after discharge. The nurse will assess healing, ensure that feedings are being administered properly, and detect any complications. The home care nurse assesses the patient's adjustment to changes in physical appearance and status and ability to communicate and/or eat normally. Physical and speech therapy also may be continued at home.

The patient is given information regarding local support groups such as "I Can Cope" or "New Voice Club." The local chapter of the American Cancer Society may be contacted for information and equipment needed for the patient.

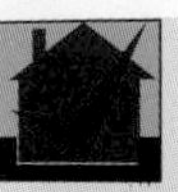

Home Care Teaching Checklist: Recovering From Neck Dissection Surgery

At the completion of the program, the patient or caregiver will be able to:	Patient	Caregiver
• Demonstrate use of suction equipment.	✔	✔
• State rationale for humidification.	✔	✔
• State dietary modifications needed to meet caloric needs.	✔	✔
• Demonstrate enteral or parenteral feeding techniques.	✔	✔
• Demonstrate care of incision and drains.	✔	✔
• State when next checkup is needed.	✔	✔
• Demonstrate exercises.	✔	✔
• Identify available support groups.	✔	✔

Evaluation

Expected Outcomes

Expected outcomes may include:

1. Discusses expected course of treatment
2. Demonstrates good respiratory exchange
   a. Lungs are clear to auscultation
   b. Breathes easily with no shortness of breath
   c. Demonstrates ability to use suction effectively
3. Remains free of infection
   a. Maintains normal laboratory values
   b. Is afebrile
4. Graft is pink and warm to touch
5. Maintains adequate intake of foods and fluids
   a. Accepts altered route of feeding
   b. Is well hydrated
   c. Maintains or gains weight
6. Demonstrates ability to cope
   a. Discusses emotional responses to the diagnosis
   b. Attends support groups
7. Verbalizes comfort
8. Attains maximal mobility
   a. Adheres to physical therapy exercises
   b. Attains maximal range of motion

The Plan of Nursing Care presents an overview of the care of a patient undergoing a neck dissection.

DISORDERS OF THE ESOPHAGUS

The esophagus is a mucus-lined, muscular tube that carries food from the mouth to the stomach. It begins at the base of the pharynx and ends about 4 cm below the diaphragm. Its ability to transport food and fluid is facilitated by two sphincters. The upper esophageal sphincter, also called the hypopharyngeal sphincter, is located at the junction of the pharynx and the esophagus. The lower esophageal sphincter, also called the gastroesophageal sphincter, is located at the junction of the esophagus and the stomach. An incompetent lower esophageal sphincter allows reflux (backward flow) of gastric contents.

Dysphagia (difficulty swallowing) is the most common symptom of esophageal disease. This symptom may vary from an uncomfortable feeling that a bolus of food is caught in the upper esophagus (before it eventually passes into the stomach) to acute pain on swallowing (odynophagia). Obstruction of food (solid and soft) and even liquids may occur anywhere along the esophagus. Often the patient can indicate if the problem is located in the upper, middle, or lower third of the esophagus.

There are many pathologic conditions of the esophagus, including motility disorders (achalasia, diffuse spasm), gastroesophageal reflux, hiatal hernias, diverticula, perforation, foreign bodies, chemical burns, benign tumors, and carcinoma.

Achalasia

Achalasia is absent or ineffective peristalsis of the distal esophagus, accompanied by failure of the esophageal sphincter to relax in response to swallowing. Narrowing of the esophagus just above the stomach results in a gradually increasing dilation of the esophagus in the upper chest. Achalasia may progress slowly and occurs most often in people aged 40 or older. There seems to be a familial incidence of achalasia.

Clinical Manifestations

The primary symptom of achalasia is difficulty in swallowing both liquids and solids. The patient has a sensation of food sticking in the lower portion of the esophagus. As the condition progresses, food is commonly regurgitated either spontaneously or intentionally by the patient to relieve the discomfort produced by prolonged distention of the esophagus by food that will not pass into the stomach. The patient may also complain of chest pain and heartburn (pyrosis). Pain may or may not be associated with eating. There may be secondary pulmonary complications from aspiration of gastric contents.

Assessment and Diagnostic Findings

Diagnostic x-ray studies show esophageal dilation above the narrowing at the gastroesophageal junction. Barium swallow and endoscopy may be used for diagnosis; however, the diagnosis is confirmed by manometry, a process in which the esophageal pressure is measured by a radiologist or gastroenterologist.

Management

The patient should be instructed to eat slowly and drink fluids with meals. Calcium channel blockers and nitrates have been used to decrease esophageal pressure and improve swallowing. Recently, injection of botulinum toxin to quadrants of the esophagus via endoscopy has been helpful because it inhibits the contraction of smooth muscle. If these methods are unsuccessful, pneumatic (forceful) dilation or surgical separation of the muscle fibers may be recommended.

Achalasia may be treated conservatively by stretching the narrowed area of the esophagus by pneumatic dilation (Fig. 32-6). Pneumatic dilation has a high success rate. Although perforation is a potential complication, its incidence is low. The procedure can be painful; therefore, an analgesic or tranquilizer is administered before the treatment. The patient is monitored for perforation. Complaints of abdominal tenderness and fever may be indications of perforation (see later discussion on perforation).

Achalasia may be treated surgically through an esophagomyotomy (Fig. 32-7). Either an abdominal or thoracic approach may be used to provide access to the lower esophagus. The esophageal muscle fibers are separated to relieve the lower esophageal stricture. Although patients with a history of achalasia have a slightly higher incidence of esophageal cancer, long-term follow-up with esophagoscopy has not proved beneficial.

Diffuse Spasm

Diffuse spasm is a motor disorder of the esophagus. The cause is unknown, but stressful situations can produce contractions of the esophagus. It is more common in women and generally presents in middle age.

Clinical Manifestations

Diffuse spasm is characterized by difficulty or pain on swallowing (dysphagia, odynophagia) and chest pain similar to that of coronary artery spasm.

Assessment and Diagnostic Findings

Esophageal manometry, which measures the motility of the esophagus and the pressure within the esophagus, indicates that simultaneous contractions of the esophagus occur irregularly. Diagnostic x-ray studies after ingestion of barium show separate areas of spasm.

Management

Conservative therapy includes administering sedatives and long-acting nitrates to relieve pain. Calcium channel blockers have also been used to manage diffuse spasm. Small, frequent feedings and a soft diet are usually recommended to decrease the esophageal pressure and irritation that lead to spasm. Dilation performed by bougienage (progressively sized, nonmercury- or mercury-filled flexible dilators), pneumatic dilation, or esophagomyotomy may be necessary if the pain becomes intolerable.

Gastroesophageal Reflux

Some degree of **gastroesophageal reflux** (back-flow of gastric or duodenal contents into the esophagus) is normal in both adults and children. Excessive reflux may occur because of an incompetent lower esophageal sphincter, pyloric stenosis, or a motility disorder. The occurrence of reflux seems to increase with age.

Clinical Manifestations

Symptoms may include pyrosis (burning sensation in the esophagus), dyspepsia (indigestion), regurgitation, dysphagia, or odynophagia (difficulty swallowing, pain on swallowing), hypersalivation, or esophagitis. The symptoms may mimic those of a heart attack. The patient's history aids in obtaining an accurate diagnosis.

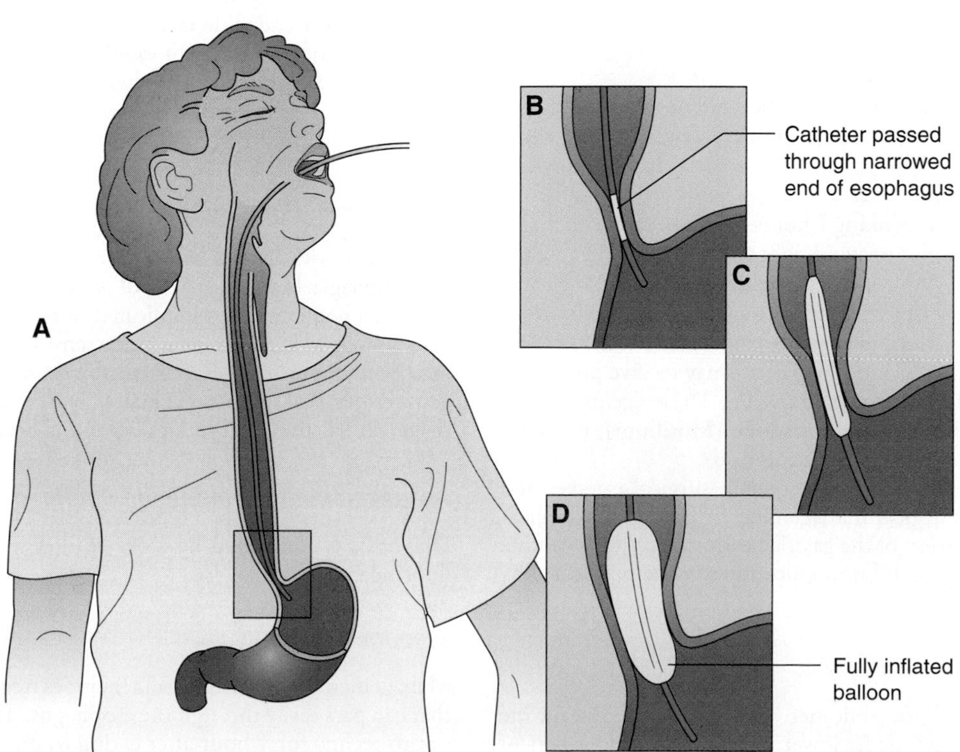

FIGURE 32•6 Treatment of achalasia by the conservative approach. (**A–C**) The dilator is passed, guided by a previously inserted guidewire. (**D**) When the balloon is in proper position, it is distended by pressure sufficient to dilate the narrowed area of the esophagus.

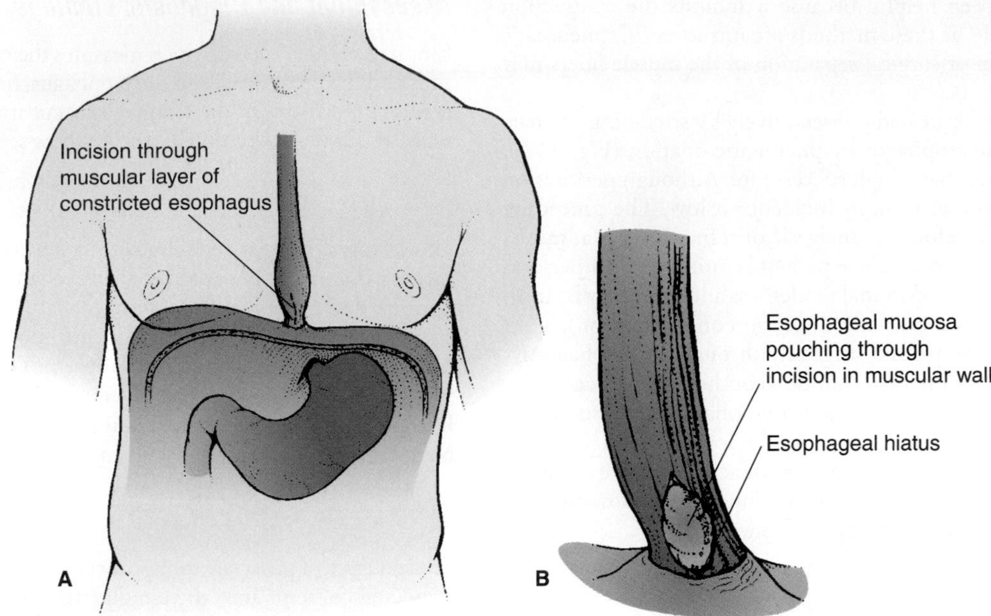

FIGURE 32•7 Treatment of achalasia: esophagomyotomy. (**A**) The esophagus is approached via thoracotomy from the front, on the left side. An incision is made through the muscularis of the esophagus extending about 1 cm into the gastric area. (**B**) The incision is large enough to allow a pouching of the esophageal mucosa. Separation of the muscular fibers relieves the narrowing at the lower end of the esophagus and permits the patient to swallow normally again.

Assessment and Diagnostic Findings

Diagnostic testing may include 12- to 36-hour esophageal pH monitoring to evaluate the degree of acid reflux; other tests include endoscopy or barium swallow.

Management

Management begins with teaching the patient to avoid factors that decrease lower esophageal sphincter pressure or cause esophageal irritation. The patient is instructed to eat a low-fat, high-fiber diet; to avoid caffeine, tobacco, and carbonated beverages; to avoid eating or drinking 2 hours before bedtime; to maintain normal body weight; to avoid tight clothes; and to elevate the head of the bed on 6- to 8-inch (15- to 20-cm) blocks. If gastroesophageal reflux persists, the patient may be given medications such as antacids, histamine receptor blockers, or gastric acid pump inhibitors. In addition, the patient may receive prokinetic agents, which accelerate gastric emptying. These agents include bethanechol (Urecholine), domperidone (Motilium), metoclopramide (Reglan), and cisapride (Propulsid).

If medical management is unsuccessful, surgical intervention may be necessary. Surgical management involves a fundoplication (wrapping a portion of the gastric fundus around the sphincter area of the esophagus). Fundoplication may be performed by laparoscopy.

Hiatal Hernia

The esophagus enters the abdomen through an opening in the diaphragm and empties at its lower end into the upper part of the stomach. Normally, the opening in the diaphragm encircles the esophagus tightly, and the stomach lies completely within the abdomen. In a condition known as hiatus (or hiatal) **hernia**, the opening in the diaphragm through which the esophagus passes becomes enlarged, and part of the upper stomach tends to move up into the lower portion of the thorax. Hiatal hernia occurs more often in women than men. There are two types of hiatal hernias: axial and paraesophageal. An axial, or sliding, hiatal hernia occurs when the upper stomach and the gastroesophageal junction are displaced upward and slide in and out of the thorax (Fig. 32-8**A**). About 90% of patients with esophageal hiatal hernias have sliding hernias. A paraesophageal hernia occurs when all or part of the stomach pushes through the diaphragm next to the gastroesophageal junction (Fig. 32-8**B**).

Clinical Manifestations

The patient with an axial hernia may have heartburn, regurgitation, and dysphagia, but at least 50% of patients are asymptomatic. Sliding hiatal hernia is often implicated in reflux. The patient with a paraesophageal hernia usually feels a sense of fullness after eating or may be asymptomatic. Reflux usually does not occur because the gastroesophageal sphincter is intact. The complications of hemorrhage, obstruction, and strangulation can occur.

Assessment and Diagnostic Findings

Diagnosis is confirmed by x-ray studies, barium swallow, and fluoroscopy.

Management

Management for an axial hernia includes frequent, small feedings that can pass easily through the esophagus. The patient is advised not to recline for 1 hour after eating to prevent reflux or movement of the hernia, and to elevate the head of the bed on 4- to 8-inch (10- to 20-cm) blocks to prevent the hernia from sliding upward. Surgery is indicated in about 15% of patients. Medical and surgical management of a paraesophageal hernia is similar to

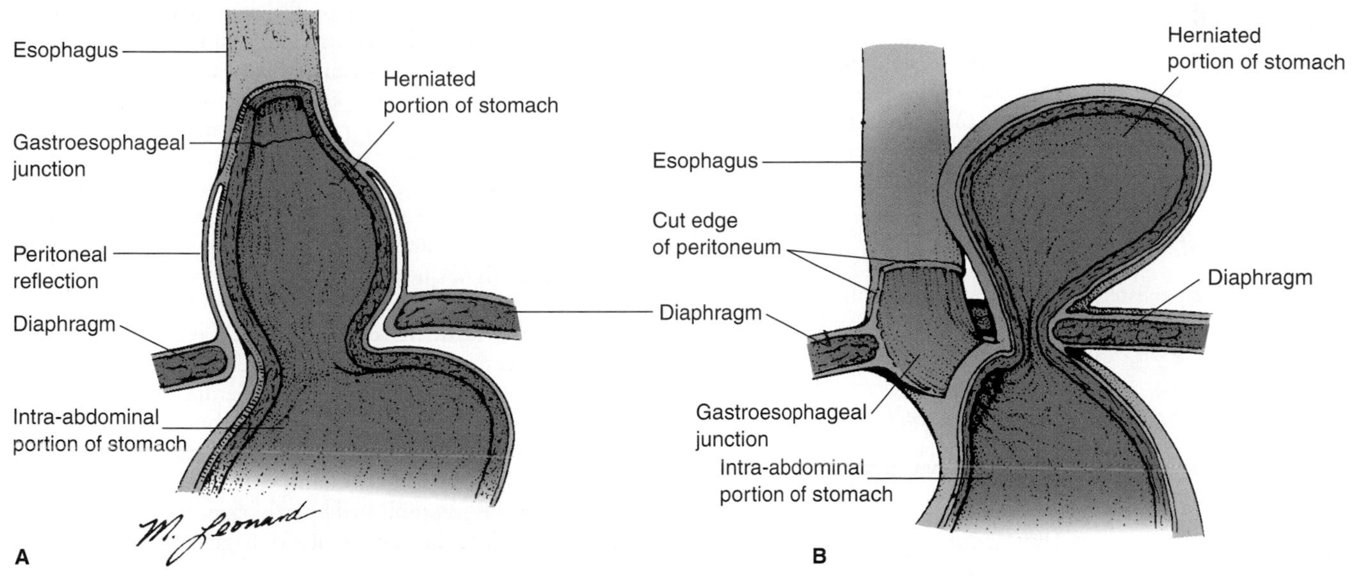

FIGURE 32•8 Sliding esophageal and paraesophageal hernias. (**A**) Sliding esophageal hernia. The upper stomach and cardioesophageal junction have moved upward and slide in and out of the thorax. (**B**) Paraesophageal hernia. All or part of the stomach pushes through the diaphragm next to the gastroesophageal junction.

that for gastroesophageal reflux; however, paraesophageal hernias may require emergency surgery.

Diverticulum

A diverticulum is an outpouching of mucosa and submucosa that protrudes through a weak portion of the musculature. Diverticula may occur in one of the three areas of the esophagus—the pharyngoesophageal or upper part of the esophagus, the midesophageal part, or the epiphrenic or lower part of the esophagus—or they may occur along the border of the esophagus intramurally.

The most common type of diverticulum, which is found three times more frequently in men than in women, is pharyngoesophageal pulsion diverticulum (Zenker's diverticulum). It occurs posteriorly through the cricopharyngeal muscle in the midline of the neck. It is usually seen in people older than 60 years of age. Other types of diverticula include midesophageal, epiphrenic, and intramural diverticula.

Midesophageal diverticula are uncommon. Symptoms are less acute, and usually the condition does not require surgery. Epiphrenic diverticula are usually larger diverticula in the lower esophagus just above the diaphragm. They are thought to be related to the improper functioning of the lower esophageal sphincter. Intramural diverticulosis is the occurrence of numerous small diverticula associated with a stricture in the upper esophagus.

Clinical Manifestations

Symptoms experienced by the patient with a pharyngoesophageal pulsion diverticulum include difficulty swallowing, fullness in the neck, belching, regurgitation of undigested food, and gurgling noises after eating. The diverticulum, or pouch, becomes filled with food or liquid. When the patient assumes a recumbent position, undigested food is regurgitated and may also cause coughing from irritation of the trachea. Halitosis and a sour taste in the mouth are also common because of the decomposition of food retained in the diverticulum.

Symptoms produced by midesophageal diverticula are less acute. One third of patients with epiphrenic diverticula are asymptomatic, with the remaining two thirds complaining of dysphagia and chest pain.

Assessment and Diagnostic Findings

A barium swallow may be performed to determine the exact nature and location of a diverticulum. Esophagoscopy usually is contraindicated because of the danger of perforating the diverticulum, with resulting mediastinitis. Blind insertion of a nasogastric tube should be avoided.

Management

Because pharyngoesophageal pulsion diverticulum is progressive, the only means of cure is surgical removal of the diverticulum. During surgery, care is taken to avoid trauma to the common carotid artery and internal jugular veins. The sac is dissected free and amputated flush with the esophageal wall. In addition to a diverticulectomy, a myotomy of the cricopharyngeal muscle is often performed to relieve spasticity of the musculature, which otherwise seems to contribute to a continuation of the previous symptoms. Postoperatively, the patient may have a nasogastric tube that usually is inserted at the time of surgery. The surgical incision must be observed for evidence of leakage from the esophagus and a developing fistula. Food and fluids are withheld until x-ray studies show no leakage at the surgical site. The diet is then begun with liquids and progressed as tolerated.

Surgery is indicated for epiphrenic and midesophageal diverticula only if the symptoms are troublesome and growing worse. Treatment consists of a diverticulectomy and long myotomy. Intramural diverticula usually regress when the esophageal stricture is dilated.

Perforation

The esophagus is not an uncommon site of injury. Perforation may result from stab or bullet wounds of the neck or chest, as well as from accidental puncture by a surgical instrument during examination or dilation. Spontaneous perforation of the esophagus has been known to occur during vomiting.

Clinical Manifestations

The patient has persistent pain followed by dysphagia. Infection, fever, leukocytosis, and severe hypotension may be noted. In some instances, signs of pneumothorax are observed.

Assessment and Diagnostic Findings

Diagnostic x-ray studies and fluoroscopy can localize the site of the injury.

Management

Because of the high risk of infection, broad-spectrum antibiotic therapy is initiated. A nasogastric tube is inserted to provide suction and to reduce the amount of gastric juice that can reflux into the esophagus and mediastinum. Nothing is given by mouth; nutritional needs are met by total parenteral nutrition. Total parenteral nutrition is preferred to gastrostomy because the latter might cause reflux into the esophagus.

Surgery may be necessary to close the wound, and postoperative nutritional support then becomes a primary concern. Depending on the incision site and nature of surgery, the postoperative nursing management is similar to that for patients who have had thoracic or abdominal surgery.

Foreign Bodies

Many swallowed foreign bodies pass through the gastrointestinal tract without the need for medical intervention. However, some swallowed foreign bodies (dentures, fish bones, pins, small batteries, items containing mercury or lead) may injure the esophagus or obstruct its lumen and must be removed. Pain and dysphagia may be present, and dyspnea may occur as a result of pressure on the trachea. The foreign body may be identified by x-ray.

If an impacted bolus of food is lodged in the esophagus, tartaric acid and sodium bicarbonate may be given to form a gas, thereby increasing the intraluminal pressure and possibly allowing the bolus to be dislodged. Glucagon, because of its relaxing effect on the esophageal muscle, may be injected intramuscularly. If these treatments are unsuccessful, an endoscope (with a covered hood or overtube) is used to remove the impacting food or object from the esophagus.

Chemical Burns

Chemical burns of the esophagus may be caused by undissolved medications in the esophagus. This occurs more frequently in the elderly than it does among the general adult population. Chemical burns of the esophagus occur most often when a patient, either accidentally or intentionally, swallows a strong acid or base (eg, lye). This patient is emotionally distraught as well as in acute physical pain. An acute chemical burn of the esophagus may be accompanied by severe burns of the lips, mouth, and pharynx, with pain on swallowing. There may be difficulty in breathing from either edema of the throat or a collection of mucus in the pharynx.

The patient, who may be profoundly toxic, febrile, and in shock, is treated immediately for shock, pain, and respiratory distress. Esophagoscopy and barium swallow are performed as soon as possible to determine the extent and severity of damage. The patient is given nothing by mouth, and intravenous fluids are administered. A nasogastric tube may be inserted by the physician. Emesis and gastric lavage are avoided to prevent further exposure of the esophagus to the caustic agent. The use of corticosteroids to reduce inflammation and minimize subsequent scarring and stricture formation is of questionable value. The value of the prophylactic use of antibiotics for these patients has also been questioned; however, these treatments continue to be prescribed.

After the acute phase has subsided, the patient may require further treatment to prevent or manage strictures of the esophagus. Dilation using bougies may be sufficient, but dilation treatment may need to be repeated periodically. For strictures that do not respond to dilation, surgical management is necessary. Reconstruction may be accomplished by esophagectomy or colon interposition to replace the portion of esophagus removed.

Benign Tumors

Benign tumors may arise anywhere along the esophagus. The most common lesion is a leiomyoma (tumor of the smooth muscle), which can occlude the lumen of the esophagus. Most benign tumors are asymptomatic and are distinguished from cancerous lesions by a biopsy. Small lesions are excised during esophagoscopy; lesions that occur within the wall of the esophagus may require a thoracotomy.

Cancer of the Esophagus

In the United States, carcinoma of the esophagus occurs more than three times as often in men as in women. It is seen more frequently in African Americans than in whites and usually occurs in the fifth decade of life. Cancer of the esophagus has a much higher incidence in other parts of the world, including China and northern Iran.

Chronic irritation is a risk factor for esophageal cancer. In the United States, cancer of the esophagus has been associated with the ingestion of alcohol and the use of tobacco. In other parts of the world, esophageal cancer has been associated with the use of opium pipes, ingestion of excessively hot beverages, and nutritional deficiencies, especially lack of fruits and vegetables (fruits and vegetables are thought to promote repair of irritated tissue).

Pathophysiology

Esophageal cancer is usually of the squamous cell epidermoid type; however, the incidence of adenocarcinoma of the esophagus is increasing in the United States. Tumor cells may spread beneath the esophageal mucosa or directly into, through, and beyond the muscle layers into the lymphatics. In the latter stages, obstruction of the esophagus is noted, with possible perforation into the mediastinum and erosion into the great vessels.

Clinical Manifestations

Unfortunately, the patient may have an advanced ulcerated lesion of the esophagus before symptoms are manifested. Symptoms include dysphagia, initially with solid foods and eventually with liquids; a feeling of a mass in the throat; painful swallowing; substernal pain or fullness; and, later, regurgitation of undigested food with foul breath and hiccups. The patient is first aware of intermittent and increasing difficulty in swallowing. As the tumor progresses and the obstruction becomes more complete, even liquids cannot pass into the stomach. Regurgitation of food and saliva occurs, hemorrhage may take place, and progressive loss of weight and strength occurs from starvation. Later symptoms include substernal pain, persistent hiccup, respiratory difficulty, and foul breath. The delay between the onset of early symptoms and the time when the patient seeks medical advice is often 12 to 18 months. Anyone with swallowing difficulties should be encouraged to consult a physician immediately.

Assessment and Diagnostic Findings

Diagnosis is confirmed in 95% of the cases by esophagogastroduodenoscopy (EGD) with biopsy and brushings. Bronchoscopy usually is performed, especially in tumors of the middle and the upper third of the esophagus, to determine whether the trachea has been affected and to help determine whether the lesion can be removed. Mediastinoscopy is used to determine if the cancer has spread to the nodes and other mediastinal structures. Cancer of the lower end of the esophagus may be due to adenocarcinoma of the stomach extending upward into the esophagus.

Medical Management

If esophageal cancer is found at an early stage, treatment goals may be directed toward cure; however, it is often found in late stages, making relief of symptoms the only reasonable goal of therapy. Treatment may include surgery, radiation, chemotherapy, or a combination of these modalities, depending on the extent of the disease.

Standard surgical management includes a total resection of the esophagus (esophagectomy) with removal of the tumor plus a wide tumor-free margin of the esophagus and the lymph nodes in the area. The surgical approach may be through the thorax or the abdomen, depending on the location of the tumor. When tumors occur in the cervical or upper thoracic area, esophageal continuity may be maintained by free jejunal graft transfer, in which the tumor is removed and the area replaced with a portion of the jejunum (Fig. 32-9). A segment of the colon may be used, or the stomach can be elevated into the chest and the proximal section of the esophagus implanted into the stomach.

Tumors of the lower thoracic esophagus are more amenable to surgery than are tumors located higher in the esophagus, and gastrointestinal tract integrity is maintained by implanting the lower esophagus into the stomach.

Surgical resection of the esophagus has a relatively high mortality rate because of infection, pulmonary complications, or leakage through the anastomosis. Postoperatively, the patient will have a nasogastric tube in place that should not be manipulated. The patient is given nothing by mouth until x-ray studies confirm that the anastomosis is secure and not leaking.

The use of preoperative radiation therapy and chemotherapy may be the treatment of choice, although only one treatment modality may be the treatment of choice based on type of cell, tumor spread, and patient condition.

Palliative treatment may be necessary to keep the esophagus open, to assist with nutrition, and to control saliva. Palliation may be accomplished with dilation of the esophagus, laser therapy, placement of an endoprosthesis (stent), radiation, and chemotherapy. Because the ideal method of treating esophageal cancer has not yet been found, treatment is individually determined.

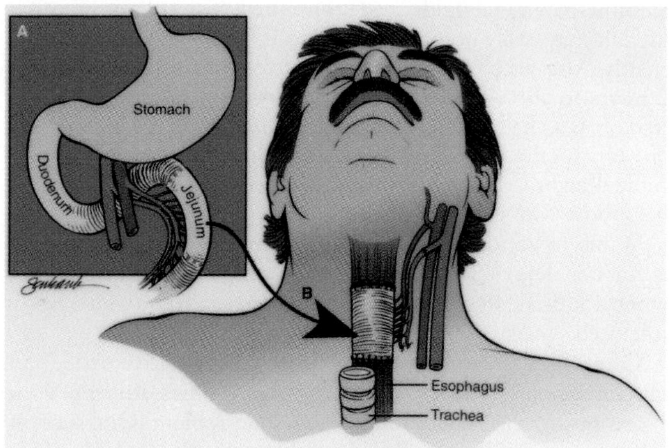

FIGURE 32•9 Esophageal reconstruction with free jejunal transfer. A portion of the jejunum is grafted between the esophagus and pharynx to replace the abnormal portion of the esophagus. The vascular structures are also anastomosed. A portion of the graft may be externalized through the neck wound to evaluate graft viability.

Nursing Management

Intervention is directed toward improving the patient's nutritional and physical condition in preparation for surgery, radiation therapy, or chemotherapy. A program to promote weight gain based on a high-caloric and high-protein diet, in liquid or soft form, is provided if adequate food can be taken by mouth. If not, total parenteral nutrition is initiated. Nutritional status is monitored throughout treatment. The patient is informed about the nature of the postoperative equipment that will be used, including that required for closed chest drainage, nasogastric suction, parenteral fluid therapy, and gastric intubation. Immediate postoperative care is similar to that provided for patients undergoing thoracic surgery. After recovering from the effects of anesthesia, the patient is placed in a semi-Fowler's position, and later in a Fowler's position, to assist in preventing reflux of gastric secretions. The patient is observed carefully for regurgitation and dyspnea. A common postoperative complication is aspiration pneumonia. Temperature is monitored to detect any elevation that may indicate seepage of fluid through the operative site into the mediastinum.

If grafting has been performed, the nurse checks for graft viability hourly for at least the first 12 hours. To make the graft visible, the surgeon usually brings a portion of the jejunum to the exterior neck by way of a small incision. A moist gauze covers the external portion of the graft. The gauze is removed briefly to assess the graft for color and to assess for the presence of a pulse by means of Doppler ultrasonography.

If an endoprosthesis has been placed or an anastomosis has been performed, a functioning continuum will exist between the throat and the stomach. Immediately after surgery, the nasogastric tube should be marked for position and the physician notified if displacement occurs. The nurse does not attempt to reinsert a displaced nasogastric tube, because damage to the anastomosis may occur. The nasogastric tube is removed 5 to 7 days after surgery, and a barium swallow is performed to evaluate for any anastomotic leak before the patient is fed.

Once feeding begins, the nurse encourages the patient to swallow small sips of water and, later, small amounts of puréed food. When the patient is able to increase food intake to an adequate amount, parenteral fluids are discontinued. If an endoprosthesis is used, it may easily become obstructed if food is not chewed sufficiently. After each meal, the patient is to remain upright for at least 2 hours to allow the food to move through the gastrointestinal tract. It is a challenge to encourage the patient to eat, because his or her appetite is usually poor. Family involvement and home-cooked favorite foods may help the patient to eat. Antacids may help those with gastric distress.

When radiation is part of the therapy, the patient's appetite is further depressed and esophagitis may occur, causing pain when food is eaten. Liquid supplements may be more easily tolerated.

Often, in either the preoperative or postoperative period, an obstructed or nearly obstructed esophagus causes difficulty with excess saliva, so that drooling becomes a problem. Oral suction may be provided if the patient is unable to handle oral secretions, or a wick-type gauze may be placed at the corner of the mouth to direct secretions to a dressing or emesis basin. The possibility that the patient may aspirate saliva into the tracheobronchial tree and develop pneumonia is of great concern.

When the patient is ready to go home, the family is instructed in the following: how to promote nutrition, what observations to make, what measures to take if complications occur, how to keep the patient comfortable, and how to obtain needed physical and emotional support.

NURSING PROCESS: THE PATIENT WITH A CONDITION OF THE ESOPHAGUS

Assessment

Emergency conditions of the esophagus (perforation, chemical burns) usually occur in the home or away from medical help and require emergency medical care. The patient is treated for shock and respiratory distress and transported as quickly as possible to a medical facility. Foreign bodies in the esophagus do not pose an immediate threat to life unless pressure is exerted on the trachea, resulting in dyspnea or interfering with respiration. Educating the public to prevent accidental swallowing of foreign bodies or corrosive agents is a major health issue.

For nonemergent symptoms, a complete health history may reveal the nature of the esophageal disorder. The nurse asks about the patient's appetite. Has it remained the same, increased, or decreased? Is there any discomfort with swallowing? If so, does it occur only with certain foods? Is it associated with pain? Does a change in position affect the discomfort? The patient is asked to describe the pain. Does anything aggravate it? Are there any other symptoms that occur regularly, such as regurgitation, nocturnal regurgitation, eructation (belching), heartburn, substernal pressure, a sensation that food is sticking in the throat, a feeling of becoming full after eating a small amount of food, nausea, vomiting, or weight loss? Are the symptoms aggravated by emotional upset? If the patient reports any of these complaints, the nurse asks about the time of their occurrence, their relationship to eating, and factors that relieve or aggravate them (eg, position change, belching, antacids, or vomiting).

This history also includes questions about past or present causative factors (eg, infections and chemical, mechanical, or physical irritants), the degree to which alcohol and tobacco are used, and the amount of daily food intake. The nurse determines if the patient appears emaciated and auscultates the patient's chest to determine whether pulmonary complications exist.

Nursing Diagnosis

Based on the assessment data, the nursing diagnoses may include the following:

- Altered nutrition, less than body requirements, related to difficulty swallowing
- Risk for aspiration due to difficulty swallowing and/or tube feeding
- Pain related to difficulty swallowing, ingestion of an abrasive agent, a tumor, or frequent episodes of gastric reflux
- Knowledge deficit about the esophageal disorder, diagnostic studies, medical management, surgical intervention, and rehabilitation

Planning and Goals

The major goals for the patient may include attainment of adequate nutritional intake, avoidance of respiratory compromise from aspiration, relief of pain, and increased knowledge level.

Nursing Interventions

Encouraging Adequate Nutritional Intake

The patient is encouraged to eat slowly and to chew all food thoroughly so that it can pass easily into the stomach. Small, frequent feedings of nonirritating foods are recommended to promote digestion and to prevent tissue irritation. Sometimes liquid swallowed with food will help the food pass through the esophagus. Food should be prepared in an appealing manner to help stimulate the appetite. Irritants such as tobacco and alcohol should be avoided. A baseline weight is obtained, and daily weights are recorded. The patient's intake of nutrients is assessed.

Decreasing Risk of Aspiration

The patient with difficulty swallowing or difficulty handling secretions should be kept in at least a semi-Fowler's position to decrease the risk of aspiration. The patient can be instructed in the use of oral suction to decrease the risk of aspiration further.

Relieving Pain

Small, frequent feedings are recommended because large quantities of food overload the stomach and promote gastric reflux. Very hot and cold beverages and spicy foods are avoided because they stimulate esophageal spasm and the secretion of hydrochloric acid. The patient is advised to avoid any activities that put strain on the thoracic area and increase pain, and to remain upright for 1 to 4 hours after each meal to prevent reflux. The head of the bed should be placed on 4- to 8-inch (10- to 20-cm) blocks. Eating before bedtime is discouraged.

The patient is advised that excessive use of over-the-counter antacids can cause rebound acidity. Antacid use should be directed by the primary care provider, who can recommend the daily, safe quantity needed to neutralize gastric juices and prevent esophageal irritation. Histamine antagonists are administered as prescribed to decrease gastric acid irritation.

Providing Patient Education

The patient is prepared physically and psychologically for diagnostic tests, treatments, and possible surgical intervention. The principal nursing interventions include reassuring the patient and dis-

HOME CARE TEACHING CHECKLIST: THE PATIENT WITH AN ESOPHAGEAL CONDITION

At the completion of the program, the patient or caregiver will be able to:

	Patient	Caregiver
• Demonstrate use of suction equipment.	✔	✔
• State dietary modifications needed to meet caloric needs.	✔	✔
• Demonstrate enteral or parenteral feeding techniques.	✔	✔
• Demonstrate care of incision.	✔	✔
• State when next checkup is needed.	✔	✔
• Identify available support groups.	✔	✔

cussing the procedures and their purposes. Some disorders of the esophagus evolve over time, whereas others are the result of trauma (eg, chemical burns or perforation). In instances of trauma, the emotional and physical preparation for treatment is more difficult because of the short time available and the circumstances of the injury. Treatment interventions must be evaluated continually; the patient is given sufficient information to participate in care and diagnostic efforts. If surgery is involved, immediate and long-term evaluation is similar to that of a patient undergoing thoracic surgery.

Promoting Home and Community-Based Care

TEACHING PATIENTS SELF-CARE

The self-care required of the patient will depend on the nature of the disorder and on the surgery or treatment measures used (eg, diet, positioning, or medications). If an ongoing condition exists, the nurse helps the patient plan for needed physical and psychological adjustment and for follow-up care.

The use of special equipment such as suction or enteral or parenteral feeding devices may be required. The patient may need help in planning meals, using medications as prescribed, and resuming activity. Education about nutritional requirements and how to measure the adequacy of nutrition is important. Elderly and debilitated patients in particular often need assistance and education in ways to adjust to their limitations and to resume activities that are important to them.

CONTINUING CARE

Patients with chronic esophageal conditions often require an individualized approach to their management at home. Food may need to be prepared in a special way (blenderized foods, soft foods), and the patient may need to eat more frequently (eg, four to six small servings per day). The medication schedule is adjusted to the patient's daily activities as much as possible. Analgesics and antacids can usually be taken as needed every 3 to 4 hours.

Postoperative home health care focuses on nutritional support, management of pain, and respiratory function. Some patients are discharged from the hospital with enteral feeding by means of a gastrostomy or jejunostomy tube or total parenteral nutrition. The patient and care provider need specific instructions about the management of the equipment and treatments. Home care visits by a nurse may be necessary to assess the patient's care and the care provider's ability to provide the necessary care. (See Chap. 33 for more information on parenteral nutrition and management of the patient with a gastrostomy.) For some patients, a multidisciplinary team comprising a nutritionist, social worker, and family members is helpful. Hospice care is appropriate for some patients.

Evaluation

Expected Outcomes

Expected outcomes may include:

1. Achieves an adequate nutritional intake
   a. Eats small, frequent meals
   b. Drinks water with small servings of food
   c. Avoids irritants (alcohol, tobacco, very hot beverages)
   d. Maintains desired weight
2. Does not aspirate or develop pneumonia
   a. Maintains upright position during feeding
   b. Uses oral suction equipment effectively
3. Is free of pain or able to control pain within a tolerable level
   a. Avoids large meals and irritating foods
   b. Takes medications as prescribed
   c. Maintains an upright position after meals for 1 to 4 hours
   d. States that there is less eructation and chest pain
4. Increases knowledge level of esophageal condition, treatment, and prognosis
   a. States cause of condition
   b. Discusses rationale for medical or surgical management and diet or medication regimen
   c. Describes treatment program
   d. Practices preventive measures so injuries are avoided

Critical Thinking Exercises

1. You are interviewing a patient in the medical clinic who has been treated in the clinic previously for gastroesophageal reflux. He complains that his symptoms are worse but that he has been taking his medications as prescribed. He states that he has tried many different kinds of antacids but none of them are helping him. Describe how you would continue to assess this patient to obtain the additional information that is needed. Speculate as to the different causes that may underlie this patient's inability to obtain relief.

2. You are caring for two postoperative patients. One patient is being treated for cancer of the mouth, the other for cancer of the esophagus. How will the nutritional care of these two patients differ?

References and Selected Readings

BOOKS

Ballenger, J., & Snow, J. (1996). *Otorhinolaryngology head and neck surgery* (15th ed.). Baltimore: Williams & Wilkins.

Bickley, L. S., & Hoekelman, R. A. (1999). *Bates' guide to physical examination and history taking* (7th ed.). Philadelphia: Lippincott Williams & Wilkins.

Bell, R., Rikkers, L., Mulholland, M. (1996). *Digestive tract surgery. A text and atlas* (4th ed.). Philadelphia: Lippincott-Raven.

DeVita, V. T., Hellman, S., & Rosenberg, S. A. (Eds.). (1997). *Cancer. Principles and practice of oncology* (5th ed.). Philadelphia: Lippincott-Raven.

Harris, N. O., & Garcia-Godoy (1999). *Primary preventive dentistry* (5th ed.). Norwalk, CT: Appleton & Lange.

Itano, J. K., & Taoka, K. N. (Eds.). (1998). *Core curriculum for oncology nursing* (3rd ed.). Philadelphia: W. B. Saunders.

McEvoy, G. R. (Ed.). (1999). *American Hospital Formulary Service.* Bethesda, MD: American Society of Health-System Pharmacists.

Myers, E. N. (Ed.). (1997). *Operative otolaryngology head & neck surgery.* Philadelphia: W. B. Saunders.

National Institutes of Health. (1996). *Management of temporomandibular disorders.* Technology Assessment Conference Statement.

Shankland, W. (1997). *TMJ: Its many faces* (2nd ed.). Columbus, OH: Anadem Publishers.

Woods, N. K., & Goaz, P. W. (1997). *Differential diagnosis of oral and maxillofacial lesions.* St. Louis: Mosby.

Yamada, T. (Ed.). (1995). *Textbook of Gastroenterology* (2nd ed.). Philadelphia: J. B. Lippincott.

Zuidema, G. D. (Ed.). (1996). *Shakelford's Surgery of the alimentary tract* (4th ed.). Philadelphia: W. B. Saunders.

JOURNALS

Conditions and Cancer of the Oral Cavity

American Academy of Periodontology. (1996). Position paper: Epidemiology of periodontal diseases. *Journal of Periodontology, 67*(9), 935–945.

Consensus report. Periodontal diseases: Prevention. (1996). *Annals of Periodontology, 1*(1), 250–255.

Genco, R. J. (1996). Current risk factors for periodontal diseases. *Journal of Periodontology, 67*(10 Suppl), 1041–1049.

Horn-Ross, P. L., et al. (1997). Environmental factors and the risk of salivary gland cancer. *Epidemiology, 8*(4), 414–419.

Jeffcoat, M. K., et al. (1997). Evidence-based periodontal treatment. Highlights from the 1996 world workshop in periodontics. *Journal of the American Dental Association, 128*(6), 713–724.

Kretzschmar, J. L., & Kretzschmar, D. P. (1996). Common oral conditions. *American Family Physician, 54*(1), 225–234.

Landis, S. H., et al. (1999). Cancer Statistics, 1999. *CA, 49*(1), 8–31.

Mandel, I. D. (1996). Caries prevention: Current strategies, new directions. *Journal of the American Dental Association, 127*(10), 1477–1488.

McEwen, D. R., & Sanchez, M. M. (1997). A guide to salivary gland disorders. *AORN Journal, 65*(3), 554–556.

Navalainen, M. J., et al. (1997). Oral mucosal lesions and oral hygiene habits on the home-living elderly. *Journal of Oral Rehabilitation, 24*(5), 332–337.

Nguyen, M. T., et al. (1996). Orally administered amphotericin B in the treatment of oral candidiases in HIV-infected patients caused by azole-resistant *Candida albicans. AIDS, 10*(14), 1745–1747.

Parker, S. L., et al. (1997). Cancer statistics, 1997. *CA, 47*(1), 5–27.

Patterson, M., & Baughman, R. (1996). Recurrent aphthous stomatitis: Primary care management. *Nurse Practitioner, 21*(5), 36–42.

Shugars, D., & Patton, L. (1997). Detecting, diagnosing, and preventing oral cancer. *Nurse Practitioner, 22*(6), 105–129.

Conditions and Treatment of the Esophagus

Bhutani, M. S. (1997). Gastrointestinal uses of botulinum toxin. *American Journal of Gastroenterology, 92*(6), 929–933.

Bosset, J. F., et al. (1997). Chemoradiotherapy followed by surgery compared with surgery alone in squamous cell cancer of the esophagus. *New England Journal of Medicine, 337*(3), 161–167.

Eckardt, V. F., et al. (1997). Complications and their impact after pneumatic dilation for achalasias: Perspective long-term follow-up study. *Gastrointestinal Endoscopy, 45*(5), 349–353.

Eypasch, E., et al. (1997). Laparoscopic antireflux surgery for gastroesophageal reflux disease (GERD). Results of a consensus development conference held at the fourth international congress of the European Association of Endoscopic Surgery, Trondheim, Norway, June 21–24, 1996. *Surgery and Endoscopy, 11*(5), 413–426.

Ilson, D. H., & Kelsen, D. P. (1996). Management of esophageal cancer. *Oncology, 10*(9), 1385–1396.

Larsen, R. R. (1997). Gastroesophageal reflux disease: Gaining control over heartburn. *Postgraduate Medicine, 101*(2), 181–182.

Paricha, P. J., & Kaltoo, A. N. (1997). Recent advances in the treatment of achalasia. *Gastrointestinal Endoscopy Clinics of North America, 7*(2), 191–206.

Stack, L. B., & Numter, D. W. (1996). Foreign bodies in the gastrointestinal tract. *Emergency Medicine Clinics of North America, 14*(3), 493–521.

Weant, C. (1995). Easing the pain of esophageal surgery. *RN,* August, 26–31.

Willekes, C. L., et al. (1997). Laparoscopic repair of paraesophageal hernia. *Annals of Surgery, 225*(1), 31–38.

Conditions and Treatment of the Head and Neck

Cordeiro, P. G., & Santamaria, E. (1997). The extended, pedicled rectus abdominis free tissue transfer for head and neck reconstruction. *Annals of Plastic Surgery, 39*(1), 53–59.

Forbes, K. (1997). Palliative care in patients with cancer of the head and neck. *Clinical Otolaryngology, 13*(3), 177–184.

Logemann, J. A., et al. (1997). Speech and swallowing rehabilitation for head and neck cancer patients. *Oncology, 11*(5), 651–656.

Miyata, K., & Kitamura, H. (1997). Accessory nerve damage and impaired shoulder movement after neck dissections. *American Journal of Otolaryngology, 18*(3), 197–201.

Zhenn, M. R., et al. (1997). Current role of the radial forearm free flap in mandibular reconstruction. *Plastic and Reconstructive Surgery, 99*(4), 1012–1017.

Resources

American Association of Public Health Dentists, New York University Dental Center, 325 East 24th St., New York, NY 10010

American Cancer Society, 1599 Clifton Rd. NE, Atlanta, GA 30329

American Dental Association, 211 E. Chicago Ave., Chicago, IL 60611

American Society of Geriatric Dentistry, 1121 W. Michigan St., Indianapolis, IN 46202

National Institute of Dental Research, National Institutes of Health, 900 Rockville Pike, Bethesda, MD 20892

National Oral Health Information Clearinghouse, 1 NOHIC Way, Bethesda, MD 20892-3500; 1-301-402-7364

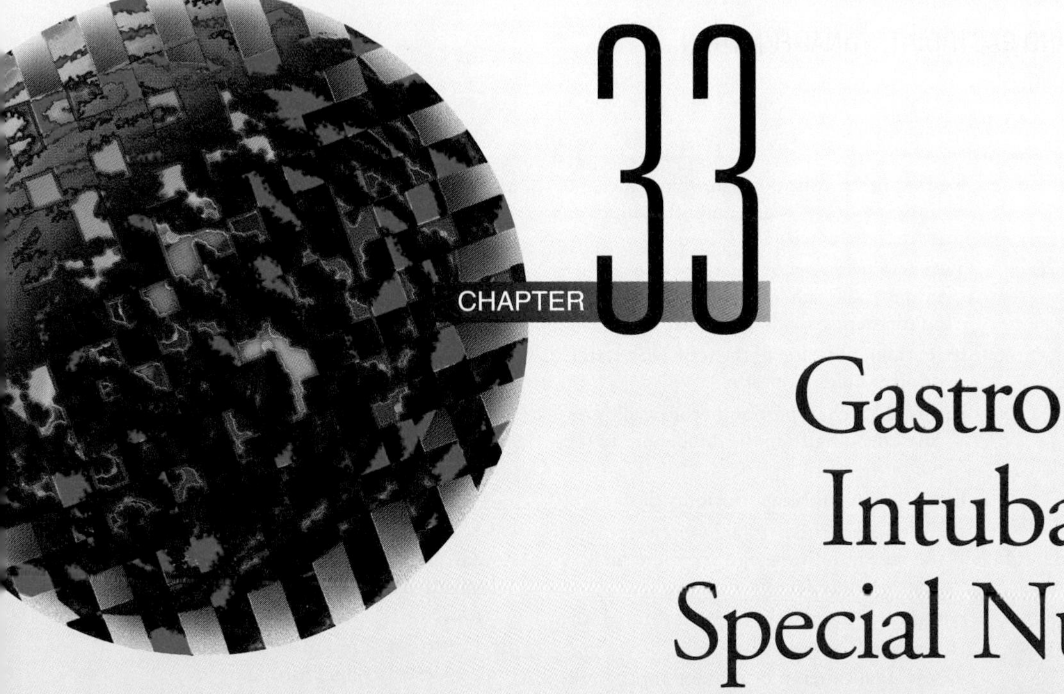

Gastrointestinal Intubation and Special Nutritional Modalities

Learning Objectives

On completion of this chapter, the learner will be able to:

1. Describe the purposes of gastrointestinal intubation and the care of patients with these therapies.
2. Use the nursing process as a framework for care of the patient receiving a tube feeding.
3. Explain the preoperative and postoperative care of the patient with a gastrostomy.
4. Use the nursing process as a framework for care of the patient with a gastrostomy.
5. Identify the purposes and uses of total parenteral nutrition.
6. Use the nursing process as a framework for care of the patient receiving total parenteral nutrition.
7. Describe the nursing measures used to prevent complications from total parenteral nutrition.

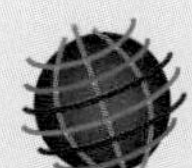

Nasogastric (NG) and nasoenteric tubes are commonly used for hospitalized patients as well as for those in skilled nursing facilities and the home setting. This chapter presents several topics related to NG and gastrointestinal (GI) intubation, including managing patients with NG and nasoenteric tubes, the various uses of these tubes, teaching points related to home health care, managing patients with gastrostomies, general indications for total parenteral nutrition, and nursing care of patients receiving these support measures.

GLOSSARY

antireflux valve: valve that prevents return or backward flow of fluid

aspiration: accidently breathing fluids or foods into the trachea and lungs; removal of substance by suction

bolus: a feeding administered into the stomach in large amounts and at designated intervals

CVAD: Central venous access device

cyclic feeding: periodic feeding/infusion given over a shorter period of time (8–12 hours)

decompression (intestinal): removal of intestinal contents to prevent gas and fluid from distending the coils of the intestine

dumping syndrome: rapid emptying of the stomach contents into the small intestine; characterized by sweating and weakness

duodenum: the first part of the small intestine, connecting with the pylorus of the stomach and extending to the jejunum

feeding tube: tube through which nutritional products, water, and other fluids can be introduced into the GI tract

gastrostomy: surgical creation of an opening into the stomach for the purpose of administering foods and fluids

irrigation: Flushing of the tube with water or other fluids to clear it

jejunum: Second portion of the small intestine extending from the duodenum to the ileum

LPGD: Low profile gastrostomy device

nasoduodenal tube: tube inserted through the nose into the beginning of the small intestine (duodenum)

nasogastric tube: tube inserted through the nose into the stomach

nasojejunal tube: tube inserted through the nose into the second portion of the small intestine (jejunum)

osmosis: passage of solvent through a semipermeable membrane. The solvent, usually water, passes through the membrane from a region of low concentration of solute to that of a higher concentration of solute

percutaneous endoscopic gastrostomy: an endoscopic procedure for placing a permanent feeding tube into the stomach

peristalsis: wavelike movement that occurs involuntarily in the alimentary canal

pH: the degrees of acidity or alkalinity of a substance or solution

PICC: peripherally inserted central catheter

stoma: artificially created opening between a body cavity (eg, stomach) and the body surface

total nutrient admixture: an amino acid–dextrose–lipid formula

total parenteral nutrition: an amino acid–dextrose-formula

GASTROINTESTINAL INTUBATION

GI intubation is the insertion of a rubber or plastic tube into the stomach, duodenum, or intestine. The tubes may be inserted through the mouth, the nose, or the abdominal wall (gastrostomy, jejunostomy). The tubes are either short, medium, or long, depending on their intended use; NG tubes are short, nasoduodenal tubes are of medium length, and nasoenteric tubes are long. GI intubation may be performed to:

- Decompress the stomach and remove gas and fluid
- Lavage the stomach and remove toxic ingested substances
- Diagnose GI motility and other disorders
- Administer medications and feedings
- Treat an obstruction
- Compress a bleeding site
- Aspirate gastric contents for analysis

A variety of tubes are used for decompression, aspiration, and lavage. The Sengstaken-Blakemore tube is a type of NG tube used to treat bleeding esophageal varices (refer to Chap. 36). Orogastric tubes are large-bore tubes with wide proximal outlets for removing particles of ingested substances (eg, pills); they are primarily used in emergency departments. Various other tubes are used to administer feedings and medications. The tubes are made of different materials (rubber, polyurethane, silicone) and vary in length (90 cm to 3 m [36 in to 10 ft]), size (6 to 18 Fr), purpose, and placement in the GI tract (stomach, duodenum, jejunum) (Table 33-1). Any solution administered through a tube is either poured through a syringe or delivered

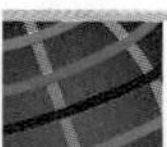

TABLE 33•1 Nasogastric, Nasoenteric, and Feeding Tubes

Tube Type	Length	Size (French)	Lumen	Other Characteristics
Nasogastric Tubes				
Levin (plastic or rubber)	125 cm	14–18	Single	Circular markings serve as guidelines for insertion
Gastric sump Salem (plastic)	120 cm	12–18	Double	Smaller lumen acts as a vent
Moss	90 cm	12–16	Triple	Contains both a gastric decompression lumen and a duodenal lumen for postoperative feedings
Sengstaken-Blakemore (rubber)			Triple	Two lumens are used to inflate the gastric and esophageal balloons
Nasoenteric Decompression Tubes				
Miller-Abbott (rubber)	300 cm	12–18	Double	One lumen uses mercury or air for balloon inflation
Harris	180 cm	14, 16	Single	Mercury-weighted tip
Cantor (rubber)	300 cm	16	Single	Mercury-weighted bag
Baker (plastic)	270 cm	16	Double	One lumen is used for balloon inflation
Nasoenteric Feeding Tubes				
Dobhoff or Keofeed II (polyurethane or silicone rubber)	160–175 cm	8–12	Single	Tungsten-weighted tip, radiopaque

by drip regulated by gravity or by an electric pump. **Aspiration** (suctioning) to remove gas and fluids is accomplished by using a syringe, an electric suction machine, or a built-in wall suction outlet.

Short Tubes

A **nasogastric tube** or short tube is introduced through the nose into the stomach. Commonly used short tubes include the Levin tube and the gastric sump tube. Short tubes are used in adults primarily to remove fluid and gas from the upper GI tract, and to obtain a specimen of gastric contents for laboratory studies. They are occasionally used for the short-term administration of medications or feedings (gavage). However, tubes that extend beyond the pylorus (nasoduodenal) or enter the GI tract percutaneously (gastrostomy tube, jejunostomy tube) are preferred for the administration of medications or feedings because the risk of aspiration is much less.

Levin Tube

The Levin tube has a single lumen (14 to 18 Fr) and is made of plastic or rubber with openings near its tip. It is 125 cm long (50 in). Circular markings at specific points on the tube serve as guides for insertion. A marking is made on the tube to indicate the midpoint (Fig. 33-1). The tube is advanced cautiously until this marking reaches the patient's nostril, thus suggesting the tube is in the stomach. Placement is checked by aspirating gastric contents with a syringe and testing the pH of the aspirated material. (The pH will vary according to the source of the aspirate.) An x-ray is the only sure way to verify the tube's location.

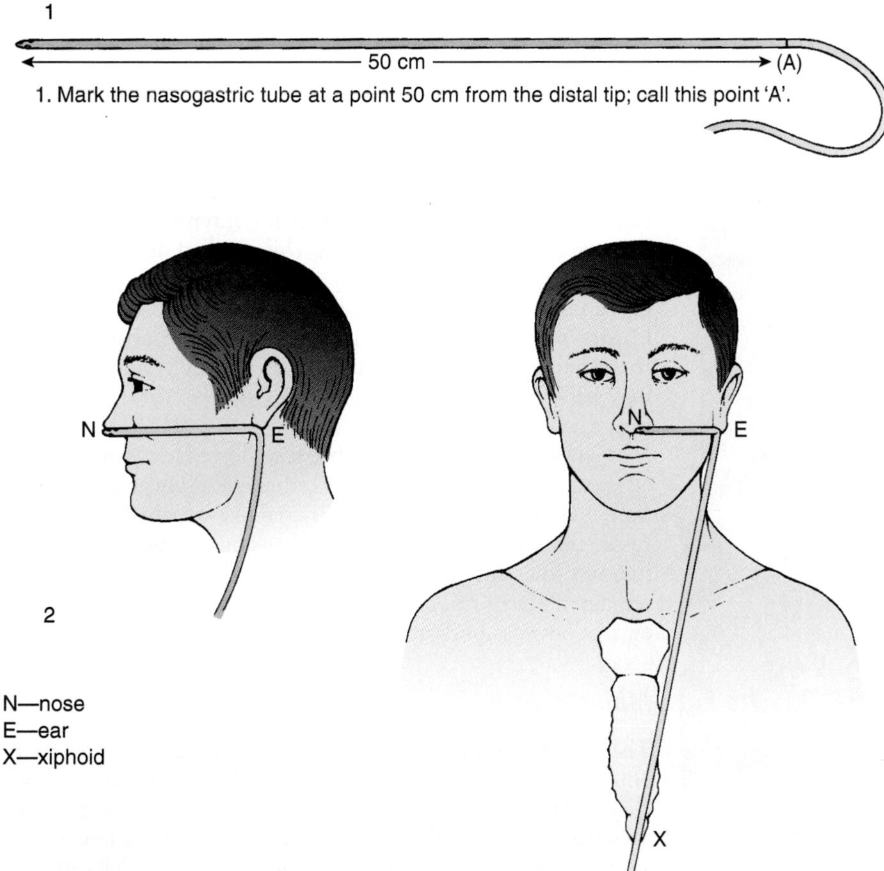
1
50 cm
(A)
1. Mark the nasogastric tube at a point 50 cm from the distal tip; call this point 'A'.
N
E
N
E
2
N—nose
E—ear
X—xiphoid
X
2. Have the patient sit in a neutral position with head facing forward. Place the distal tip of the tubing at the tip of the patient's nose (N); extend tube to the tragus (tip) of his ear (E), and then extend the tube straight down to the tip of his xiphoid (X). Mark this point 'B' on the tubing.
3

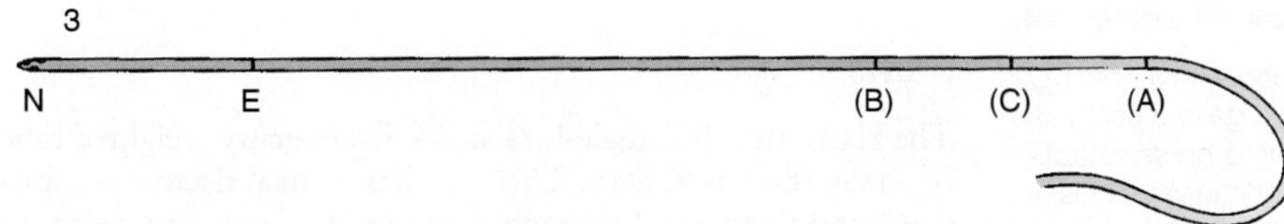
N
E
(B)
(C)
(A)
3. To locate point C on the tube, find the midpoint between points A and B. The nasogastric tube is passed to point C to ensure optimum placement in the stomach.

FIGURE 33•1 Measuring length of nasogastric tube for placement into stomach.

Gastric Sump

The gastric sump tube (Salem, Ventrol) is a radiopaque, clear plastic, double-lumen NG tube used to decompress the stomach and keep it empty. It is 120 cm long (48 in) and is passed into the stomach in the same way as the Levin tube. The inner, smaller tube vents the larger suction-drainage tube to the atmosphere by means of an opening at the distal end of the tube. This tube can protect gastric suture lines because, when used properly, the sump tube never allows the force of suction at the drainage openings, or outlets, to exceed 25 mm Hg, the level of capillary fragility. This action is controlled by the small vent tube (blue pigtail). If suction equipment is portable, continuous suction is set at a low pressure of 30 mm Hg and intermittent suction is set at 80 to 120 mm Hg. (Because of the cyclic setting, the suction will be reduced to about 25 mm Hg by the time it reaches the gastric mucosa.) When suction is available from a central source (ie, wall suction), both intermittent and continuous suction should be set low (30 to 40 mm Hg). The suction lumen is irrigated as ordered to maintain patency.

To prevent reflux of gastric contents through the vent lumen (blue pigtail), the vent lumen is kept above the patient's waist; otherwise it will act as a siphon. A one-way antireflux valve seated in the blue pigtail prevents the reflux of gastric contents out the vent lumen (Fig. 33-2). The valve should be removed after irrigating the suction lumen and 20 mL of air injected to reestablish a buffer of air between the gastric contents and the valve.

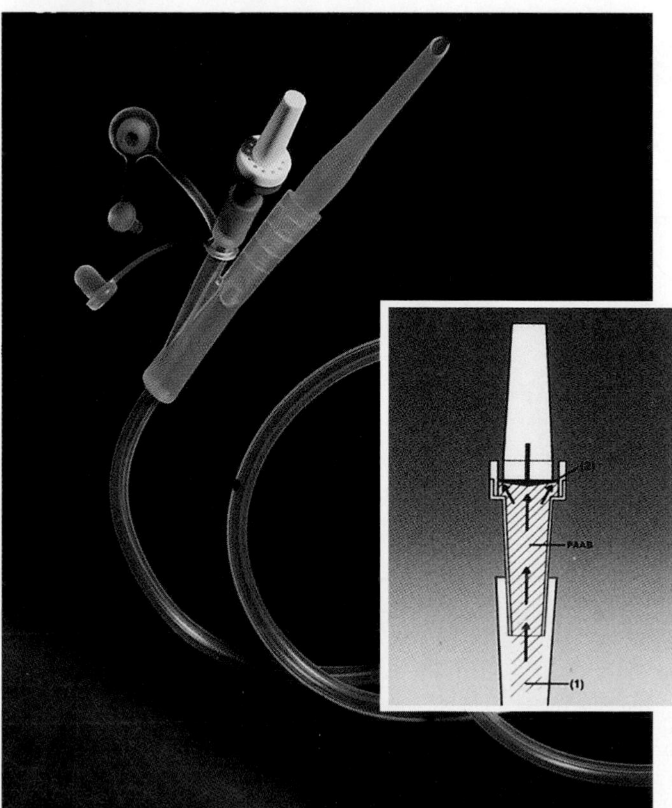

FIGURE 33•2 Gastric sump tube (Salem) equipped with a one-way antireflux valve that allows air to enter and prevents gastric contents from escaping. The antireflux valve is designed with a pressure activated air buffer (PAAB). The buffer is activated (**1**) and the valve closes (**2**) when pressure from gastric contents enters the tubing. Argyle Silicone Salem Sump Tube with preattached Argyle Salem Sump Anti-Reflux Valve courtesy of Sherwood Medical, St. Louis, Missouri.

Medium Tubes

Medium-length nasoenteric tubes are used for feeding and include the Dobbhoff and the Keofeed II tubes (Fig. 33-3). Feeding tubes placed in the duodenum are 160 cm (60 in) long; feeding tubes placed in the jejunum are 175 cm (66 in) long. They may be inserted under fluoroscopy or at the bedside. If inserted at the bedside, placement is verified by x-ray study. After insertion, the tip of the tube will initially be in the stomach; it usually takes 24 hours for the Dobbhoff or Keofeed II tube to pass through the stomach and into the intestines. Passage is facilitated by having the patient lie on the right side so that gravity and peristaltic motion can move the weighted tube into the duodenum.

Polyurethane or silicone rubber feeding tubes have small diameters (6 to 12 Fr) and tungsten tips (rather than weighted mercury-filled bags); some have a water-activated lubricant that makes it easier to insert the tube and insert and remove the stylet. The tubing may kink when a stylet is not used, particularly if the patient is uncooperative or unable to swallow. The stylet is used with caution in patients who are predisposed to esophageal punctures (elderly and frail with thin tissue). These tubes are passed in the same way as NG tubes—that is, with the patient in high Fowler's position. If this is not feasible, the patient is placed on the right side.

Nasoenteric Tubes

A long nasoenteric tube is introduced through the nose and passed through the esophagus and stomach into the intestinal tract. It is used to aspirate intestinal contents so that gas and fluid do not distend the intestine; this is called **decompression**. Three major nasoenteric tubes used for aspiration and decompression are the Miller-Abbott tube, the Harris tube, and the Cantor tube. These tubes are used to relieve obstruction of the small intestine. They are also used prophylactically; they may be inserted the night before GI surgery to prevent postoperative obstruction.

Because peristalsis is either absent or slowed for 24 to 48 hours after surgery as a result of the anesthesia and visceral manipulation, NG or nasoenteric suction is used to evacuate fluids and flatus so that vomiting is prevented, tension is reduced along the incision line, and obstruction is prevented. Usually, the tubes remain in place until peristalsis returns, as evidenced by the presence of bowel sounds and the passage of flatus.

Miller-Abbott

The Miller-Abbott tube is a double-lumen (12, 14, 16, 18 Fr), 300 cm (10-foot) rubber tube. One lumen is used to introduce mercury or air into the balloon at the end of the tube; the other lumen is used for aspiration. Before the tube is inserted, the balloon should be tested and its capacity measured, then it should be deflated completely. The tube should be lubricated sparingly and chilled well before the tip is inserted through the patient's nose. Markings on the tube indicate the distance it has been passed. Before removal, the balloon at the end of the lumen must be completely deflated.

Harris

The Harris tube is a single-lumen (14 Fr), mercury-weighted tube of about 180 cm (6 feet). This tube has a metal tip that is lubricated and introduced through the nose. The mercury-weighted bag follows. The weight of the mercury carries the bag by gravity. This tube is used solely for suction and irrigation. Usually, a

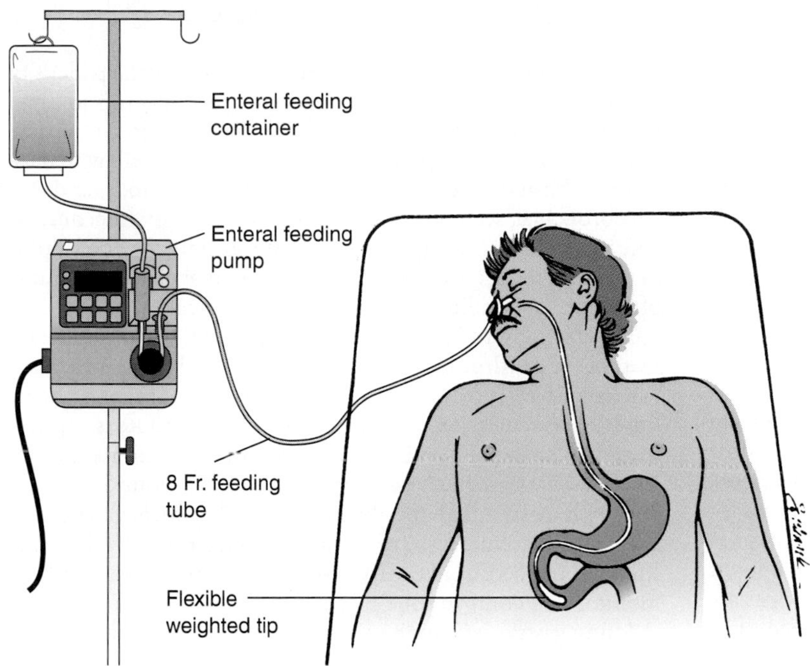

FIGURE 33•3 The enteral feeding tube (8 Fr) with a flexible weighted tip is readily passed into the stomach and through the pylorus into the duodenum or proximal jejunum. A pump is used for continuous tube feedings.

Y-tube is attached to the end of the Harris tube so that the suction apparatus is attached to one side and an outlet with a clamp is available on the other side for irrigating purposes.

Cantor

The Cantor tube is 300 cm (10 feet) long, with a 16 Fr lumen. Its distinguishing feature is that it is larger than the other long tubes and has 4 or 5 mL of mercury in the bag at the extreme end of the rubber tubing. Before the tube is inserted, the bag is wrapped around the tube. After the tube is lubricated, it is passed through the nose and advanced to the esophagus (Fig. 33-4). The patient is in a sitting position and is offered sips of water to facilitate passage of the tube. Fluoroscopy is helpful in verifying that the tube has passed into the duodenum.

Nursing Management of Nasogastric and Nasoenteric Intubation

Nursing interventions include:

- Instructing the patient about the purpose of the tube and the procedure required for inserting and advancing it
- Identifying the sensations to be expected during tube insertion
- Inserting the NG tube and assisting with the insertion of the nasoenteric tube
- Confirming the placement of the NG tube
- Advancing the nasoenteric tube
- Monitoring the patient and maintaining tube function
- Providing oral and nasal hygiene and care
- Monitoring for potential complications
- Removing the tube

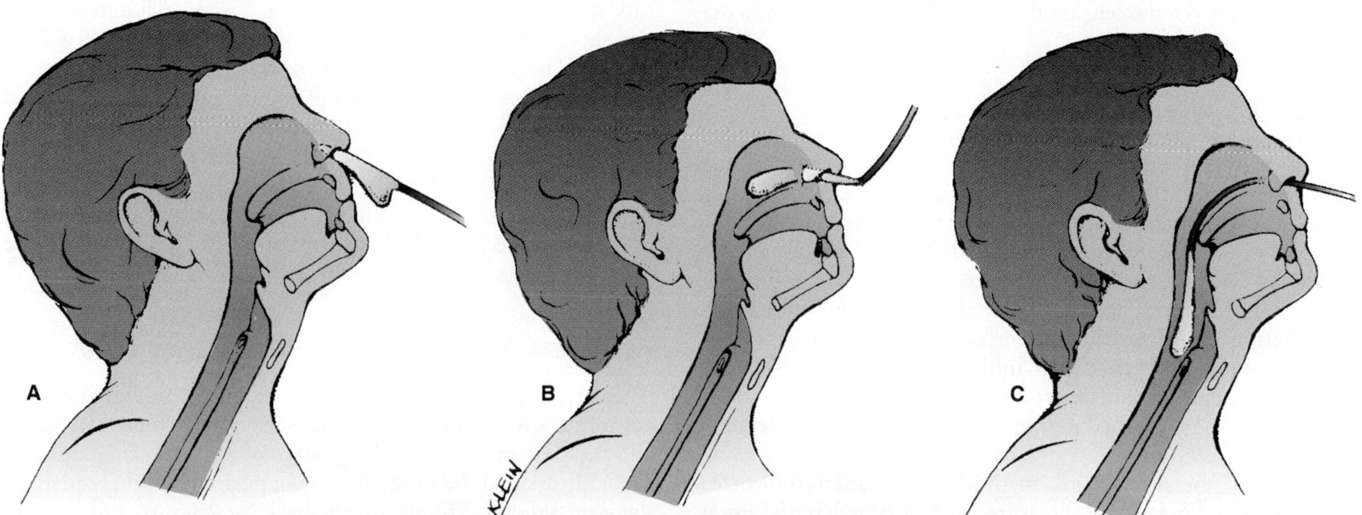

FIGURE 33•4 Passage of Cantor tube. (**A**) Tube with weighted mercury bag is introduced through the nose. Note the natural lift of the tubing. (**B**) After the mercury bag has entered the nostril, the catheter is tilted upward (head can also be tilted slightly upward) to facilitate gravity pull on the weighted bag. (**C**) The weight of the mercury pulls the bag downward.

Providing Instruction

Before the patient is intubated, the nurse explains the purpose of the tube; this information may make the patient more cooperative and tolerant of what can be an unpleasant procedure. The general activities related to inserting the tube are then reviewed, including the fact that the patient may have to breathe through the mouth and that the procedure may cause gagging until the tube has passed the gag reflex.

Inserting the Tube

Before inserting the tube, the clinician determines how much tubing will be needed to reach the stomach or the small intestine. A mark is made on the tube to indicate the desired length. Eisenberg (1994) recommends measuring the distance from the tip of the nose to the earlobe, and from the earlobe to the xiphoid process, and then adding 6 inches for NG placement or 8 to 10 inches for intestinal placement.

While the tube is being inserted, the patient usually sits upright with a towel spread bib-fashion over the chest. Tissue wipes are made available. Privacy and adequate light are provided. The physician may swab the nostril and spray the oropharynx with tetracaine (Pontocaine) to numb the nasal passage and suppress the gag reflex. This makes the entire procedure more tolerable. Having the patient gargle with a liquid anesthetic or hold ice chips in the mouth for a few minutes can have the same effect. Encouraging the patient to breathe through the mouth or pant often helps, as does swallowing water, if permitted.

A polyurethane tube may need to be warmed to make it more pliable. To make the tube easier to insert, it should be lubricated with a water-soluble substance (K-Y jelly) unless it has a dry coating called hydromer, which, when moistened, provides its own lubrication. The patient is placed in high Fowler's position. The nurse wears gloves during the procedure. The nostrils are inspected for any obstruction, and the more patent nostril is selected for use. The tip of the patient's nose is tilted and the tube is aligned to enter the nostril. When the tube reaches the nasopharynx, the patient is instructed to lower the head slightly and begin to swallow as the tube is advanced. The patient may also sip water through a straw to facilitate advancement of the tube. The oropharynx is inspected to ensure that the tube has not coiled in the pharynx or mouth.

Confirming Placement

To ensure patient safety, it is important to confirm that the tube has been placed correctly. Initially, an x-ray may be taken for this purpose. However, each time liquids or medications are administered, and once a shift for continuous feedings, the tube must be checked to ensure that it is properly placed. The traditional recommendation has been to inject air through the tube while auscultating the epigastric area with a stethoscope to detect air insufflation. However, studies indicate that this auscultatory method is not accurate in determining whether the tube has been inserted into the stomach, intestines, or respiratory tract (Metheny et al., 1990a, 1990b).

Instead of the auscultation method, a combination of three methods is recommended: measurement of tube length, visual assessment of aspirate, and pH measurement of aspirate. After the tube is inserted, the exposed tube is measured and the length is documented. The exposed tube length is then measured every shift and compared with the original measurement. An increase in the length of exposed tube may indicate dislodgement, or a leaking or a ruptured balloon.

Visual assessment of the color of the aspirate may help identify tube placement. Metheny et al. (1994) found that gastric aspirate is most frequently cloudy and green, tan or off-white, or bloody or brown. Intestinal aspirate is primarily clear and yellow to bile-colored. Pleural fluid is usually pale yellow and serous, and tracheobronchial secretions are usually tan or off-white mucus. They suggest that the appearance of the aspirate may be helpful in distinguishing between gastric and intestinal placement but is of little value in ruling out respiratory placement.

Determining the pH of the tube aspirate is a more accurate method of confirming tube placement. The pH of gastric aspirate is acidic (0 to 4, 0 to 6 if the patient is receiving acid-inhibiting medications), the pH of intestinal aspirate is approximately 6 or greater, and the pH of respiratory aspirate is more alkaline (7 or greater). Metheny et al. (1993) found that pH testing is best suited for distinguishing between gastric and intestinal placement. A pH sensor enteral tube (by Zinetics Medical Inc., Salt Lake City, Utah) may also be used to help monitor and confirm tube placement.

Using gastric aspiration as a means of verifying that the NG tube has been placed correctly may be a problem because of the characteristic properties and diameter of the tubes. Studies suggest that aspiration may be performed more easily with polyurethane tubes and tubes with a size 10 Fr diameter. Metheny et al. (1993) recommend the following steps if problems occur with aspirating fluid from small-bore feeding tubes:

1. Insufflate 20 mL of air through the tube with a large syringe (30 to 60 mL).
2. Pull back on the plunger.
3. If ineffective, insufflate another 20 mL of air and replace the large syringe with a smaller one (12 mL) and attempt to aspirate.
4. If still ineffective, repeat step 3.
5. Change the patient's position.

Securing the Tube

When the correct position of the tip has been confirmed, the NG tube is secured to the nose or cheek (Fig. 33-5**A**). A liquid skin barrier should be applied to the skin where the NG tube will be secured. The prepared area is covered with a strip of hypoallergenic tape or Op-site; the tube is then placed over the tape and secured with a second piece of tape. The nasoenteric tube can be secured by taping it to the cheek (use a slight U-shaped loop) or to the forehead (Fig. 33-5**B**). This secures the tube so that it does not become dislodged when the patient moves. Nasoenteric tubes are not taped immediately because it takes approximately 24 hours for these tubes to progress into the intestine.

Advancing the Nasoenteric Decompression Tube

After the tube has passed through the pyloric sphincter, it may be advanced 5 to 7.5 cm (2 to 3 in) every hour. To enable gravity and peristalsis to assist in the passage of the tube, the patient is generally asked to lie in the following positions in this order: on the right side for 2 hours, on the back for 2 hours, and then on the left side for 2 hours. Ambulation, if possible, also helps advance the tube. If the tube is advanced too rapidly, it will curl and kink in the stomach. The tube is irrigated with normal saline every 6 to 8 hours to prevent blockage.

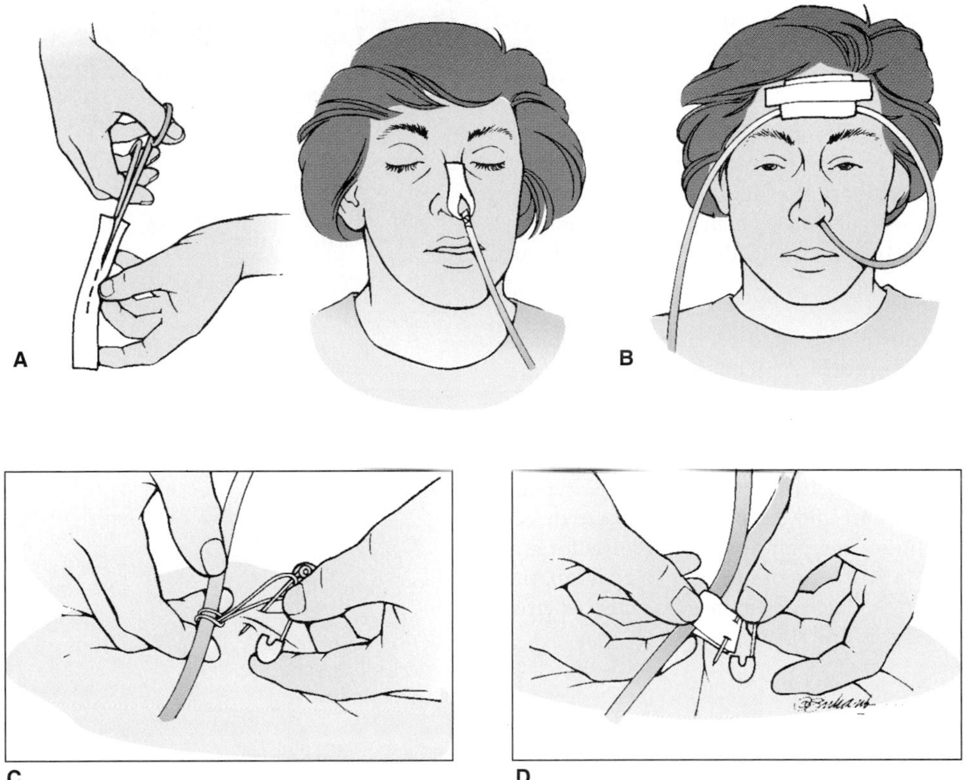

FIGURE 33•5 Securing nasogastric and nasoenteric tubes. (**A**) The nasogastric tube is secured to the nose with tape to prevent injury to the nasopharyngeal passages; the cheek may also be used. (**B**) Tape is placed on the forehead and the nasoenteric tube is taped to it, thereby allowing the tube to be advanced until desired placement is achieved. (**C, D**) Secure tubing to the patient's gown with either an elastic band or tape attached to a safety pin to prevent tension on the line during movement.

Monitoring the Patient and Maintaining Tube Function

If the NG tube is used for decompression, it is attached to intermittent low suction. If it is used for enteral nutrition, the end of the tube is plugged between feedings. Tube placement is confirmed before any fluids or medications are instilled and once a shift for continuous feedings. Displacement of the tube may be caused by tension on the tube (when the patient moves around in the bed or room), coughing, tracheal or nasotracheal suctioning, and airway intubation.

An accurate record is kept of all fluid intake, feedings, and irrigation. Irrigation with normal saline is recommended to avoid electrolyte loss through gastric drainage. The amount, color, and type of all drainage are recorded every 8 hours.

When double- or triple-lumen tubes are used, each lumen is labeled according to its intended use: aspiration, feeding, or balloon inflation. To avoid tension on the tube, the portion of the tube from the nose to the drainage unit is fixed in position, either with a safety pin or with adhesive tape loops that are pinned to the patient's pajamas or gown. The tube must be looped loosely to prevent tension and dislodgement (Figs. 33-5**C,D**).

Providing Oral and Nasal Hygiene

Regular and conscientious oral and nasal hygiene is a vital part of patient care, because the tube causes discomfort and pressure and may be in place for several days. Moistened cotton-tipped swabs can be used to clean the nose, followed by cleansing with a water-soluble lubricant. Frequent mouth care is comforting for the patient. The nasal tape is changed every other day and the nose is inspected for skin irritation. If the nasal and pharyngeal mucosa are excessively dry, steam or cool vapor inhalations may be beneficial. Throat lozenges, an ice collar, chewing gum or sucking on hard candies (if permitted), and frequent movement also assist in relieving patient discomfort. These activities keep the mucous membranes moist and help prevent infection of the parotid glands.

Monitoring and Managing Potential Complications

Patients with NG or nasoenteric intubation are susceptible to a variety of problems, including fluid volume deficit, pulmonary complications, and tube-related irritations. These potential complications require careful ongoing assessment.

Symptoms of fluid volume deficit include dry skin and mucous membranes, decreased urinary output, lethargy, and decreased body temperature. Assessment of fluid volume deficit involves maintaining an accurate record of intake and output. This includes measuring NG drainage, fluid instilled by irrigation of the NG tube, water taken by mouth, vomitus, water administered with tube feedings, and intravenous (IV) fluid. Laboratory values, particularly blood urea nitrogen and creatinine, are monitored. The 24-hour fluid balance is assessed, and negative fluid balance, increased NG output, interruption of IV therapy, or any other disturbance in fluid intake or output is reported.

Pulmonary complications from NG intubation occur because coughing and clearing the pharynx is impaired, and because tubes may become dislodged, retracting the distal end above the esophagogastric sphincter. Signs and symptoms of complications include coughing during the administration of foods or medications, difficulty clearing the airway, tachypnea, and fever. Assessment includes regular auscultation of lung sounds and routine assessment of vital signs. The patient is encouraged to cough and take deep breaths regularly. The nurse also carefully confirms the proper placement of the tube before instilling any fluids or medications.

Irritation of the mucous membranes is a common complication of NG intubation. The nostrils, oral mucosa, esophagus, and trachea are susceptible to irritation and necrosis. Visible areas are inspected frequently and the adequacy of hydration is assessed. When providing oral hygiene, the nurse carefully inspects the mucous membranes for signs of irritation or excessive dryness. The nurse palpates the area around the parotid glands to detect any soreness or lumps, indicating parotitis, and observes for any skin or mucous membrane irritation or necrosis. In addition, the patient is assessed for the presence of esophagitis and tracheitis; symptoms include sore throat and hoarseness.

Removing the Tube

Before removing a tube, the nurse may intermittently clamp and unclamp the NG tube for a trial period of 24 hours to ensure that the patient does not experience nausea, vomiting, or distention. Before it is removed, the tube is flushed with 10 mL of normal saline to ensure that it is free of debris and away from the gastric lining; then the balloon (if present) is deflated. Gloves are used when removing the tube. The tube is withdrawn gently and slowly for 15 to 20 cm (6 to 8 in) until the tip reaches the esophagus; the remainder is withdrawn rapidly from the nostril. If removing a nasointestinal tube, the tube is withdrawn at intervals of 10 minutes until the end reaches the esophagus. If the tube does not come out easily, force should not be used, and the problem is reported to the physician. As the tube is withdrawn, it is concealed in a towel, because the sight of it may be unpleasant to the patient. After the tube is removed, oral hygiene is provided.

NASOGASTRIC AND NASOENTERIC TUBE FEEDINGS

Tube feedings are given to meet nutritional requirements when oral intake is inadequate or not possible, as long as the GI tract is functioning normally. Tube feedings have several advantages over total parenteral nutrition: they are low in cost, safe, well tolerated by the patient, and easy to use both in extended care facilities and in the home setting. Tube feedings have other advantages:

- GI integrity is preserved by intraluminal delivery of nutrients.
- The normal sequence of intestinal and hepatic metabolism is preserved.
- Fat metabolism and lipoprotein synthesis are maintained.
- Normal insulin/glucagon ratios are maintained.

Tube feedings are delivered to the stomach (NG or gastrostomy) or to the distal duodenum or proximal jejunum (nasoduodenal or nasojejunal). Nasoduodenal or nasojejunal feeding is indicated when the esophagus and stomach need to be bypassed and when the patient is at risk for aspiration. The numerous conditions requiring enteral nutrition are summarized in Table 33-2.

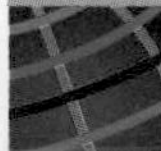

TABLE 33•2 Conditions Requiring Enteral Therapy

Condition or Need	Examples
Preoperative preparation with elemental diet	
Gastrointestinal problems with elemental diet	Fistulas, short bowel syndrome, Crohn's disease, ulcerative colitis, nonspecific maldigestion or malabsorption
Cancer therapy	Radiation, chemotherapy
Convalescent care	Surgery, injury, severe illness
Coma, semiconsciousness*	Stroke, head injury, neurologic disorders
Hypermetabolic conditions	Burns, trauma, multiple fractures, sepsis, AIDS, organ transplantation
Alcoholism, chronic depression, anorexia nervosa*	Chronic illness, psychiatric or neurologic disorder
Debilitation*	Disease or injury
Maxillofacial or cervical surgery	Disease or injury
Oropharyngeal or esophageal paralysis*	Disease or injury
Mental retardation*	

* Because some of these patients are at risk for regurgitating or vomiting and aspirating administered formula, each condition must be considered individually.

Osmosis and Osmolality

Fluid balance is maintained by **osmosis**, the process of water moving through membranes from a dilute solution of lower osmolality (ionic concentration) to a more concentrated solution of higher osmolality until both solutions are of nearly equal osmolality. The osmolality of normal body fluids is approximately 300 mOsm/kg. The body attempts to keep the osmolality of the contents of the stomach and intestines at approximately this level.

Highly concentrated solutions and certain foods can upset the normal fluid balance within the body. Individual amino acids and carbohydrates are small particles and have great osmotic effect. Proteins are extremely large particles and therefore have less osmotic effect. Fats are not water-soluble and do not form a solution in water; thus, they have no osmotic effect. Electrolytes such as sodium and potassium are comparatively small particles; they have a great effect on osmolality and consequently on the patient's ability to tolerate a given solution.

Therefore, osmolality is an important consideration for patients receiving tube feedings through the duodenum or jejunum. When a concentrated solution of high osmolality is taken in large amounts, water will move to the stomach and intestines from fluid surrounding the organs and the vascular compartment. The patient has a feeling of fullness, nausea, and diarrhea; this causes dehydration, hypotension, and tachycardia, collectively termed the **dumping syndrome**. This problem can generally be alleviated by starting with a more dilute solution and then increasing the concentration over several days.

Patients vary in the degree to which they tolerate the effects of osmolality. Usually, debilitated patients are more sensitive to such disorders. Therefore, the nurse should be knowledgeable about the osmolality of formulas and should observe for and actively prevent such disorders.

Tube Feeding Formulas

The choice of tube feeding formula is influenced by the status of the GI tract and the nutrient needs of the patient. The formula characteristics evaluated include the chemical composition of nutrient source (protein, carbohydrates, fat), caloric density, osmolality, residue, bacteriologic safety, vitamins, minerals, and cost.

Five major tube feeding types are available for use. Blenderized formulas can be made by the nurse or by the patient's family or can be obtained in a ready-to-use form that is carefully prepared according to directions. Commercially prepared polymeric formulas are composed of protein, carbohydrates, and fats in a high-molecular-weight form (Ensure Plus, Two Cal HN). Chemically defined formulas contain predigested and easy-to-absorb nutrients (Isocal, Osmolite). Modular products contain only one major nutrient, such as protein or carbohydrate (Promod). Disease-specific formulas are available for various conditions, such as renal failure (Nepro) or severe chronic obstructive pulmonary disease (Pulmocare). Nepro is high in calories and low in electrolytes. It is ideal for patients who require electrolyte and fluid restriction. Pulmocare is high in fat and low in carbohydrates. Its high density (1.5 calories/mL) is ideal for patients who require fluid restriction, and it is also designed to reduce carbon dioxide production. Fiber has also been added to formulas (Jevity, Ultracal) in an attempt to decrease the occurrence of diarrhea. Some feedings are given as supplements, and others are designed to meet the patient's total nutritional needs. Dietitians collaborate with physicians and nurses in determining the best formula for the individual patient.

Commercial formulas frequently present problems because the composition is fixed, and some patients may not be able to tolerate certain ingredients, such as sodium, protein, or potassium. Modular products may be substituted, and the critical constituents of sodium, potassium, and fat can be added. Attention is given to including all essential minerals and vitamins. Total intake of calories, nutrients, and fluids is assessed when there is a reduction in total intake or excessive dilution of feedings.

Tube Feeding Administration Methods

Many patients do not tolerate NG and nasoenteric tube feedings well. Often a medium- or fine-bore Silastic nasoenteric tube is tolerated better than a plastic or rubber tube. The finer-bore tube, however, requires a finely dispersed formula to ensure that the patency of the tube is maintained. For long-term tube feeding therapy, a gastrostomy or jejunostomy is used (see below).

The tube feeding method chosen depends on the location of the tube, patient tolerance, convenience, and cost. Intermittent bolus feedings are administered into the stomach (usually by gastrostomy) in large amounts at designated intervals. The intermittent gravity drip is another method for administering tube feedings into the stomach and is commonly used when the patient is at home. In this instance, the tube feeding is administered over 30 minutes at designated intervals. Both of these tube feeding methods are practical and inexpensive. However, the feedings delivered at variable rates may be poorly tolerated and time-consuming.

The continuous infusion method is used when feedings are administered into the small intestine. This method is preferred when patients are at risk for aspiration or tolerate the tube feedings poorly. The feedings are given continuously at a constant rate by means of a pump. The continuous tube feeding method decreases abdominal distention, gastric residuals, and the risk of aspiration. These methods (pumps) are expensive and permit the patient less flexibility than intermittent feedings.

An alternative to the continuous infusion method is **cyclic feeding**. The infusion is given at a more rapid rate over a shorter period of time (usually 8 to 12 hours at night) to avoid interrupting the patient's lifestyle. Cyclic continuous infusions may be appropriate for patients who are being weaned from tube feedings to an oral diet, as a supplement for a patient who cannot eat enough, and for patients at home who need day hours free from the pump (Forloines-Lynn, 1996a).

Tube feeding solutions vary in terms of required preparation, consistency, and the number of calories and supplemental vitamins they contain. The choice of solution depends on the size and location of the tube, the patient's nutrient needs, the type of nutritional supplement, the method of delivery, and convenience for the patient at home. A wide variety of containers, feeding tubes and catheters, delivery systems, and pumps (Corflo 300, Flexiflo III, Patrol, Kangaroo 324) are available for use with tube feedings.

NURSING PROCESS: THE PATIENT RECEIVING A TUBE FEEDING

Assessment

A preliminary assessment of the patient requiring a tube feeding includes several considerations, as well as the family's need for information:

- What is the patient's nutritional status, as judged by current physical appearance, dietary history, and recent weight loss?
- Are there any existing chronic illnesses or factors that will increase metabolic demands on the body (eg, surgical stress, fever)?
- What is the patient's hydration status? What are the electrolyte levels?
- Is the patient's digestive tract functioning?
- Are the kidneys functioning normally?
- Are fluid requirements (ie, 30 to 40 mL/kg body weight) being met?
- What medications and other therapies is the patient receiving that may affect digestive intake and function of the digestive system?
- Does the dietary prescription fulfill the patient's needs?

In addition, a more elaborate assessment is performed on patients who may require extensive nutritional therapy. This is conducted by a team that includes the nurse, physician, and dietitian. In addition to the history and physical examination (which includes anthropometric measurements), nutritional assessment consists of recording any weight change, determining serum albumin and transferrin levels and total lymphocyte count, testing for the delayed hypersensitivity reaction, and evaluating muscle function. (See Chap. 5 for a detailed description of nutritional assessment.)

Diagnosis

Nursing Diagnoses

Based on the assessment data, the major nursing diagnoses may include the following:

- Altered nutrition, less than body requirements, related to inadequate intake of nutrients

- Risk for diarrhea related to the dumping syndrome or tube feeding intolerance
- Risk for ineffective airway clearance related to aspiration of tube feeding
- Risk for fluid volume deficit related to hypertonic dehydration
- Risk for ineffective individual coping related to the discomfort imposed by the presence of the NG or nasoenteric tube
- Risk for ineffective management of therapeutic regimen related to knowledge deficit about home tube feeding regimen

Collaborative Problems/Potential Complications

Complications of NG and nasoenteric tube feeding therapy are classified as one of three types: GI, mechanical, and metabolic. Table 33-3 lists complications, possible causes, and appropriate interventions.

Planning and Goals

The major goals of the patient may include nutritional balance, normal bowel elimination pattern, adequate hydration, individual coping, knowledge of and skill in self-care, reduced risk of aspiration, and prevention of complications.

Nursing Interventions

Maintaining Nutritional Balance

The temperature and volume of the feeding, the flow rate, and the total fluid intake are important factors to be considered when tube feedings are administered. The schedule of tube feedings, including the correct quantity and frequency, is maintained. The nurse must carefully monitor the drip rate and avoid administering

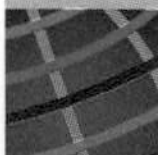

TABLE 33•3 Complications of Enteral Therapy

Complications	Causes	Selected Nursing Interventions
Gastrointestinal		
Diarrhea (most common)	Hyperosmolar feedings Rapid infusion/bolus feedings Bacteria-contaminated feedings Lactase deficiency Medications/antibiotic therapy Decreased serum osmolality level Food allergies Cold formula	Assess fluid balance and electrolyte levels; report findings. Assess rate of infusion and temperature of formula. Implement changes in tube feeding formula or rate. Replace formula every 4 hours; change tube feeding bag and tubing daily.
Nausea/vomiting	Change in rate Offensive smell Hyperosmolar formula Inadequate gastric emptying	Check residuals; if ≥100 mL, hold feeding for 1 hour and recheck, report if residual is still ≥100 mL.
Gas/bloating/cramping	Air in tube	Check rate and temperature of formula.
Dumping syndrome	Bolus feedings/rapid rate Cold formula	Check fiber and water content; report findings.
Constipation	High milk content Lack of fiber Inadequate fluid intake/dehydration	
Mechanical		
Aspiration pneumonia (atelectasis)	Improper tube placement Vomiting and aspirated tube feeding Flat in bed Tube too large	Implement reliable method for checking small-bore enteral tube placement (ie, measuring length of exposed tube). Keep head of bed elevated 30 degrees.
Tube displacement	Excessive coughing/vomitus Tension on the tube/unsecured tube Tracheal suctioning Airway intubation	Check tube placement before administering feeding.
Tube obstruction	Inadequate flushing/formula rate	Follow policy for crushing medications.
Residue	Inadequate crushing of medications and flushing after administration	Obtain liquid medications when possible. Flush feeding tube before and after medication administration.
Nasopharyngeal irritation	Tube position/improper taping Large tubes	Tape tube to prevent pressure on nares. Assess nasopharyngeal mucous membranes every 4 hours.
Metabolic		
Hyperglycemia	Glucose intolerance High carbohydrate feeding content	Check blood glucose levels periodically
Dehydration and azotemia (excessive urea in the blood)	Hyperosmolar feedings with insufficient fluid intake	Report signs and symptoms of dehydration. Implement changes in tube feeding formula, rate, or ratio to water.
Tube feeding syndrome	Excessive urea from high-protein mixture and formulas lacking fat Dehydration	

fluids too rapidly. Feedings are lactose-free, with an osmolality of only 300 mOsm/kg; a feeding may be given undiluted and provides 1 calorie/mL.

Feedings are administered by gravity (drip), bolus, or continuous controlled pump (either a volumetric cassette [mL/hour] or peristaltic pump [drops/hour]). Gravity feedings are placed above the level of the stomach and the speed of administration is determined by gravity. Bolus feedings are given in large volumes (300 to 400 mL every 4 to 6 hours). Continuous feeding is the preferred method; allowing the feeding to be given in small amounts over long periods reduces the incidence of aspiration, distention, nausea, vomiting, and diarrhea. Continuous administration rates of about 100 to 150 mL/hour (2400 to 3600 calories/day) are effective in inducing positive nitrogen balance and progressive weight gain without producing abdominal cramps and diarrhea. If the feeding is intermittent, 200 to 350 mL is given in 10 to 15 minutes.

Residual gastric content is measured before each intermittent feeding and every 4 to 8 hours during continuous feedings. (This aspirated fluid is readministered to the patient.) If the amount of aspirated gastric content exceeds 100 mL (or more than 10% to 20% above the hourly continuous feeding rate), the feeding is delayed and the patient's condition is reassessed in 1 hour. If this occurs twice, the problem is reported.

Enteral pumps use either a rotary peristaltic mechanism or a cassette mechanism. Rotary peristaltic mechanism pumps (Corflo 300, Clintec 2200, Flexiflo III, Patrol, Kangaroo 324) operate by wrapping a flexible section of the tubing around the pump rotor. As the rotor turns, the fluid is pushed through the tube. A drip sensor monitors the tube feeding's flow; therefore, the pump must remain upright for the drip sensor to operate properly. Cassette pumps (Quantum, Flexiflo Companion) operate by filling a small cassette with formula and pumping that volume. These pumps offer a more controlled infusion by preventing inadvertent free flow of tube feeding (Goff, 1997).

Electrical pumps commonly used to control the rate and pressure of the delivery of viscous fluids are relatively heavy and must be attached to an IV pole. There are several pumps specifically designed for enteral tube feedings that are lightweight and easy to handle at home. Two examples are the Kangaroo PET (Sherwood Davis & Geck, Columbus, Ohio), a rotary peristaltic pump that must remain upright to operate properly, and the Flexiflo Companion (Ross Products, Columbus, Ohio), a cassette pump that can operate in any position. Both pumps weigh about 4 pounds (including the rechargeable battery) and can be placed in a portable carrying case or backpack.

Maintaining tube function is an ongoing responsibility of the nurse, patient, or primary caregiver. To ensure patency and to decrease the chance of bacterial growth or crusting or occlusion of the tube, 15 to 30 mL of water is administered in each of the following instances:

- Before and after each dose of medication and each tube feeding
- After checking for gastric residuals and gastric pH
- Every 4 to 6 hours with continuous feedings
- If the tube feeding is discontinued for any reason

Some studies have demonstrated that water is superior to other liquids in preventing tube occlusion. When different types of medications are administered, each type is given separately using a bolus method that is compatible with its preparation (Table 33-4). The tube is flushed with 15 to 30 mL of water after each dose (Miller & Miller, 1995). Medications are not mixed with each other or with the tube feeding formula. When small-bore feeding tubes for continuous infusion are irrigated, a 30-mL or larger syringe is used because the pressure generated by smaller syringes can cause the tube to rupture. The bag and tubing are changed according to the agency's policy, usually every 24 to 72 hours (Hay et al., 1996). To avoid bacterial contamination, the amount of feeding formula hung is never more than what is expected to be infused in 4 hours.

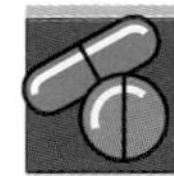

TABLE 33•4 Medication Administration by Way of Feeding Tube

Type	Preparation
Liquid	None
Simple compressed tablets	Crushed and dissolved in water
Buccal or sublingual tablets	Give as intended
Enteric-coated tablets	Cannot be crushed; change in form required
Time-release tablets	Some can be opened; cannot be crushed because doing so may release too much drug too quickly (overdose); check with pharmacist

The tube feeding regimen must be assessed frequently to evaluate its effectiveness and prevent complications. The following nursing measures are implemented:

- Assess tubing placement, patient's position (head of bed elevated 30 degrees), and flow rate.
- Determine the patient's ability to tolerate the formula (assess for feelings of fullness, bloating, urticaria, nausea, vomiting, diarrhea, and constipation).
- Check clinical responses, as noted in laboratory findings (blood urea nitrogen, serum protein, hemoglobin, hematocrit).
- Observe for signs of dehydration (dry mucous membranes, thirst, decreased urine output).
- Record the actual formula intake by the patient.
- Record incidents of vomiting and diarrhea or distention.
- Report a urine glucose concentration of +3 or +4, decreased urinary output, sudden weight gain, and periorbital or dependent edema.
- Replace formula every 4 hours with fresh formula. Formula should be room temperature or cool (not cold).
- Change tube feeding container and tubing every 24 to 48 hours.
- Assess residual volumes before each feeding, or in the case of continuous feedings every 4 hours. Stop feedings if residual exceeds 100 mL, and return the aspirate to the stomach.
- Monitor intake and output.
- Weigh the patient two or three times a week.
- Consult the dietitian.

Maintaining Normal Bowel Elimination Pattern

Patients receiving NG or nasoenteric tube feedings frequently have diarrhea (watery stools occurring three times in 24 hours). Pasty, unformed stool is expected with enteral therapy because many formulas have little or no residue. The dumping syndrome also leads to diarrhea. To confirm dumping syndrome as the cause of diarrhea, other possible causes must be ruled out:

NURSING RESEARCH

Improving Medication Administration Through an Enteral Feeding Catheter

Seifert, C. F., et al. (1995). A nursing survey to determine the characteristics of medication administration through enteral feeding catheters. *Clinical Nursing Research, 4*(3), 290–305.

Purpose

Patients receiving nutrition through an enteral feeding catheter also receive oral medications through the catheter. The researchers designed a survey to identify the current practices and problems encountered with medication administration through enteral feeding catheters.

Study Sample and Design

A random sample of nurses from the Oklahoma State Board of Nursing listing of registered and licensed practical nurses was invited to participate in the survey. A 55-question survey, developed by the investigators, was mailed to 399 nurses who had volunteered to be included in the study; 231 (57.9%) surveys were returned. Seventy-three percent of the nurses practiced in hospitals, 16% in long-term care, and 8% in home care.

The following information was obtained from the participants: estimated number of patients encountered in a typical day with feeding catheters and the number of oral medications and doses given through feeding catheters in a typical day, and estimated number of feeding catheters and obstructions encountered weekly. In addition, the participants were asked to respond to open-ended and multiple-choice questions regarding their current practices and learning experiences related to medication administration through enteral feeding catheters.

Findings

Participants estimated that a median of 10% of the patients they cared for on a daily basis had feeding catheters in place and that a median of 10% received medications through a feeding catheter. The estimated median occurrence for obstruction of feeding catheters was 1.5 times per week. The participants estimated that 50% of the cases of obstruction were caused by medications administered through the feeding catheter.

Responses to survey items related to medication administration techniques indicated that 97% of the participants believed that the use of liquid dosage forms decreased feeding catheter obstruction; however, they administered the liquid dosage form (when available) only 55% of the time. Only 45% of the participants indicated that medications for patients with feeding catheters were dispensed to the nursing unit in liquid forms; however, availability of pharmacy department assistance did influence administration practices. Participants who reported available pharmacy assistance were more likely to administer liquid dosage forms ($p < 0.001$), were less likely to administer medications that required crushing ($p < 0.001$), and encountered less feeding catheter obstruction ($p < 0.025$) than did participants who reported no available pharmacy assistance.

Nursing Implications

Although the results of the study are limited because of the reliance on the participants' recall of events that occurred in the past, there is evidence that nurses' techniques in administering medications via feeding catheters can be improved. Collaboration between nurses and pharmacists to ensure that patients with feeding catheters are receiving the most appropriate forms of their prescribed medications is important. In addition, nurses should consult with pharmacists to obtain current written information about drug compatibilities and medication absorption related to liquid formulations.

- Zinc deficiency (adding 15 mg of zinc to the tube feeding every 24 hours is recommended to maintain a normal serum level of 50 to 150 μg/dL [7.65 to 22.95 μmol/L])
- Contaminated formula
- Malnutrition (a decrease in the intestinal absorptive area resulting from malnutrition can cause diarrhea)
- Medication therapy. Antibiotics such as clindamycin (Cleocin) and lincomycin (Lincocin), antidysrhythmic medications (quinidine, propranolol [Inderal]), aminophylline (theophylline), and digitalis have been found to increase the frequency of the dumping syndrome in certain patients.

The dumping syndrome results from the rapid distention of the jejunum when hypertonic solutions are administered quickly (over 10 to 20 minutes). Foods high in carbohydrates and electrolytes draw extracellular fluid from the vascular system into the jejunum so that dilution and absorption can occur. The GI symptoms (diarrhea, nausea) associated with the dumping syndrome can be managed in the following manner:

- Decrease the instillation rate to provide time for carbohydrates and electrolytes to be diluted.
- Administer the feedings at room temperature, because temperature extremes stimulate peristalsis.
- Administer the feeding by continuous drip (if tolerated) rather than by bolus to prevent sudden distention of the intestine.
- Advise the patient to remain in semi-Fowler's position for 1 hour after the feeding (this position prolongs transit time by decreasing the influence of gravity).
- Instill the minimal amount of water needed to flush the tubing before and after a feeding, because fluid given with a feeding increases transit time.

Reducing the Risk of Aspiration

Aspiration pneumonia occurs when stomach contents or enteral feedings are regurgitated and aspirated, or when an NG tube is improperly placed and feedings are instilled into the pharynx or the trachea. Nasoenteric tubes, especially those that provide for gastric and esophageal or duodenal decompression (Moss), have helped decrease the frequency of regurgitation and aspiration.

To prevent aspiration, the nurse must check tube placement before giving every feeding, each time medications are administered, and every shift if the tube feeding is continuous. Feedings and medications should always be given with the patient in the proper position to prevent regurgitation. To reduce the risk of reflux and pulmonary aspiration, the semi-Fowler's position is necessary for an NG feeding, with the patient's head elevated at least 30 degrees. This position is maintained at least 1 hour after completion of intermittent tube feeding and is maintained at all times for patients receiving continuous tube feedings.

If aspiration is suspected, the feeding is stopped, the pharynx and trachea are suctioned, and the patient is placed on the right side with the head of the bed down. The physician is notified immediately.

Maintaining Adequate Hydration

Hydration is monitored carefully because the patient often cannot communicate the need for water. Water (at least 2 L/day) is given every 4 to 6 hours and after feedings to prevent hypertonic dehydration. At the beginning of administration, the feeding is diluted to at least half-strength and not more than 50 to 100 mL is given at a time, or 40 to 60 mL/hour is given in continuous drip administration. This gradual administration helps the patient to develop tolerance, especially for hyperosmolar solutions. The following nursing measures are important:

- Observe for signs of dehydration (dry mucous membranes, thirst, decreased urine output).
- Administer water routinely and as needed.
- Monitor intake, output, and fluid balance (24-hour intake versus output).

Promoting Coping Ability

The psychosocial goal of nursing care is to support and encourage the patient to accept the physical changes and convey hope that daily progressive improvement is possible. If the patient is having difficulty adjusting to the treatment, the nurse intervenes by:

- Encouraging self-care (eg, recording daily weight and intake and output), within the parameters of the patient's activity level
- Reinforcing an optimistic approach by identifying signs and symptoms that indicate progress (daily weight gain, electrolyte balance, absence of nausea and diarrhea)

Promoting Home and Community-Based Care

TEACHING PATIENTS SELF-CARE

Patients who require long-term tube feedings in the home care setting have conditions such as obstruction of the upper GI tract, malabsorption syndrome, surgery of the GI tract or head or neck region, or decreased level of consciousness. The following criteria must be met for a patient to be considered for tube feeding at home:

- The patient must be medically stable.
- The patient must have successfully completed a tube feeding trial (tolerated 70% of feeding).
- The patient must be capable of self-care or have a caregiver willing to assume the responsibility.
- The patient and/or caregiver must have access to and interest in education.

Preparing the patient for the home administration of enteral feedings begins while the patient is still hospitalized. Ideally, the nurse teaches while administering the feedings so that the patient can observe the mechanics of the procedure, participate in the procedure, ask questions, and express any concerns. Before discharge, information is provided about the equipment needed, formula purchase and storage, and administration of the feedings (frequency, quantity, rate of instillation).

Family members who will be active in the patient's home care are encouraged to participate in all teaching sessions. Available printed information about the equipment, formula, and procedure is reviewed. The patient and caregiver are encouraged to learn to use the equipment with the supervision of the nurse. Arrangements are made for the caregiver to obtain the equipment and formula and have it ready for use before the patient's discharge.

CONTINUING CARE

Referral to a home care agency is important so that a nurse can arrange to be present to supervise and provide support during the first feeding at home. Further visits will depend on the skill and comfort of the patient or caregiver in administering the feedings. During all visits, the nurse monitors progress (weight, vital signs, activity level, participation in the administration of the tube feedings) and assesses for any complications (dumping syndrome, nausea or vomiting, weight loss, lethargy, confusion, excessive thirst). The patient or caregiver is encouraged to keep a diary to record times and amounts of feedings and any symptoms that occur. The nurse reviews the diary with the patient and caregiver during home visits.

Evaluation

Expected Outcomes

Expected outcomes may include:

1. Attains or maintains nutritional balance
   a. Has positive nitrogen balance
   b. Maintains laboratory values within normal limits (ie, blood urea nitrogen, hemoglobin, hematocrit, serum protein)
   c. Attains or maintains hydration of body tissue
   d. Attains or maintains desired body weight
2. Is free of episodes of diarrhea
   a. Has fewer than three watery stools a day
   b. Does not have a bowel movement after a bolus feeding
   c. States that there is no intestinal cramping
   d. Has normal bowel sounds
3. Aspiration is prevented
   a. Lungs are clear to auscultation
   b. Exhibits normal heart rate and respirations
4. Attains or maintains hydration of body tissue
   a. Has a balanced intake and output every 24 hours
   b. Does not have dry skin or mucous membranes
5. Copes effectively with tube feeding regimen
6. Demonstrates skill in managing tube feeding regimen
7. Complications are prevented
   a. Has no GI disturbances
   b. Tube remains intact and patent for duration of therapy
   c. Maintains metabolic balance within normal limits

GASTROSTOMY

A **gastrostomy** is a surgical procedure to create an opening into the stomach for the purpose of administering food and fluids. In some instances, a gastrostomy is used for prolonged nutrition, as in the elderly or debilitated patient. Gastrostomy is preferred to NG feedings in the comatose patient because the gastroesophageal sphincter remains intact. Also, regurgitation is less likely to occur with a gastrostomy than with NG feedings.

Different types of feeding gastrostomies may be used: the Stamm (temporary and permanent), Janeway (permanent), and percutaneous endoscopic gastrostomy (temporary). The Stamm and Janeway gastrostomies (Fig. 33-6) require either an upper abdominal midline incision or a left upper quadrant transverse incision. The Stamm procedure requires the use of concentric pursestring sutures to secure a tube to the anterior gastric wall. To create the gastrostomy, an exit wound is created in the left upper abdomen to provide for the gastrostomy. The Janeway procedure necessitates the creation of a tunnel (called a gastric tube) that is brought out through the abdomen to form a permanent stoma.

A **percutaneous endoscopic gastrostomy** (PEG) is a procedure that requires the services of two physicians (or a physician and a specially trained nurse). One physician inserts a cannula into the stomach through an abdominal incision using local anesthesia

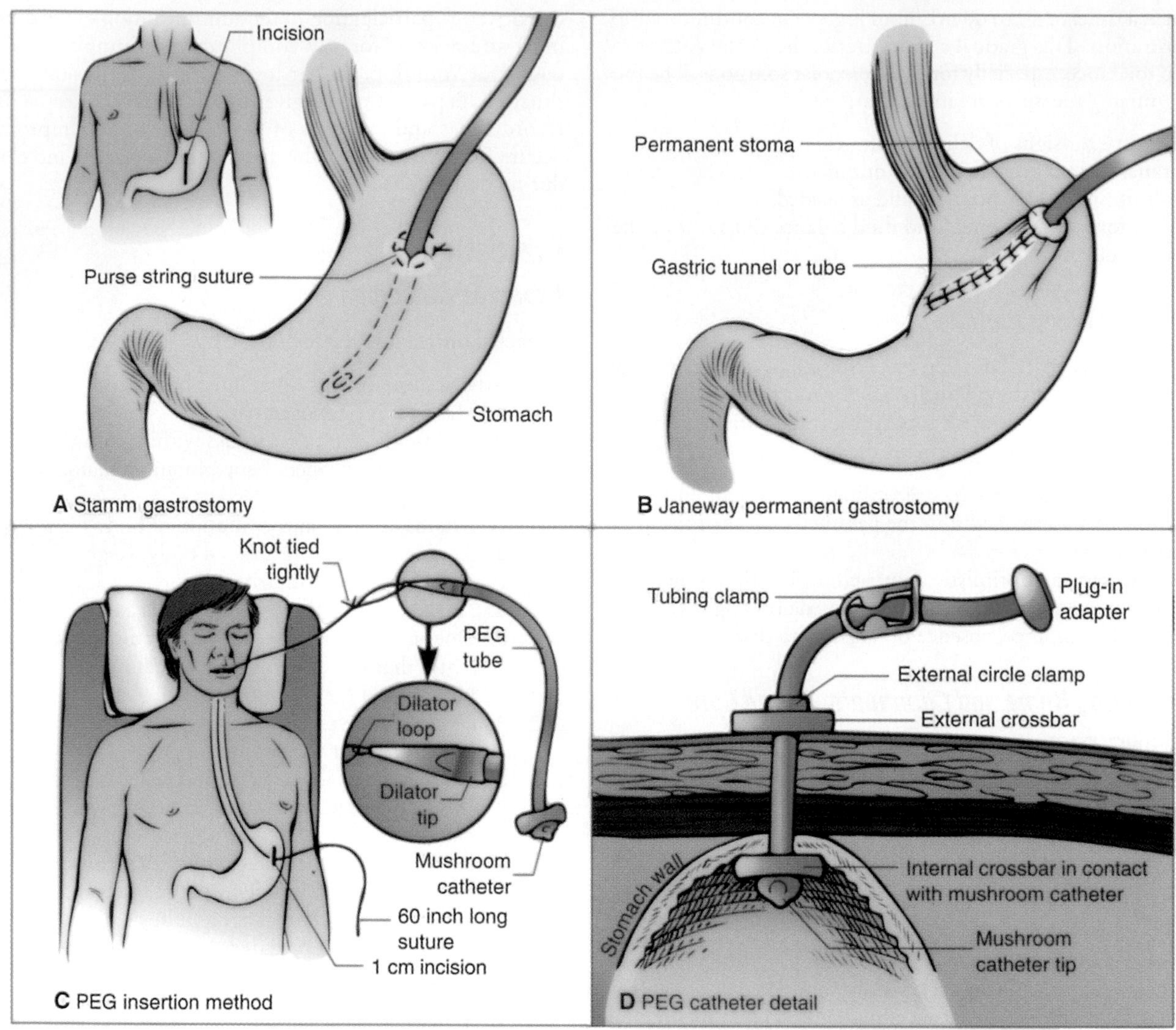

FIGURE 33•6 (**A**) Stamm gastrostomy, showing incision line and purse-string suture. (**B**) Janeway permanent gastrostomy. (**C**) Percutaneous endoscopic gastrostomy (PEG). (**D**) A detail of the abdomen and the PEG tube, showing catheter fixation.

and then threads a nonabsorbable suture through the cannula; a second physician, looking through an endoscope that has been passed into the upper GI tract, uses the endoscopic snare to grasp the end of the suture and guide it up through the patient's mouth. The suture is knotted to the dilator tip at the end of the PEG tube. The endoscopist then advances the dilator tip through the patient's mouth while the other physician pulls the suture through the cannula site. The attached PEG tube is guided down the esophagus, into the stomach, and out through the abdominal incision. The mushroom catheter tip and internal crossbar secure the tube against the stomach wall. An external crossbar or bumper keeps the catheter in place. A tubing adaptor is in place between feedings, and a clamp or plug is used to close or open the tubing.

The initial PEG device can be removed and replaced once the tract is well established (10 to 14 days after insertion). Replacing the PEG device is indicated if it is used for long-term nutritional support or to replace a clotted or migrated tube or to enhance patient comfort. The PEG replacement device should be fitted securely to the stoma to prevent leakage of gastric acid and is maintained in place through traction between the internal and anchoring devices.

An alternative to the PEG device is a low-profile gastrostomy device (LPGD). The low-profile gastrostomy device may be inserted 3 to 6 months after initial gastrostomy tube placement. These devices are inserted flush with the skin; they eliminate the possibility of tube migration and obstruction and have **antireflux valves** to prevent gastric reflux. Two types of devices may be used: obturated or nonobturated. The obturated devices (PEG Button or Gastro-Port II) have a dome tip that acts as an internal stabilizer. A major drawback is the need for a physician to obturate (insert a tube that is larger than the actual stoma). The nonobturated device (MIC-KEY) has an external skin disk and is inserted into the stoma without force; a balloon is inflated to secure placement. These devices can easily be inserted by a nurse in home settings. The drawbacks for both of the low-profile gastrostomy devices are the inability to check residual volumes (one-way valve) and the need for a special adaptor to connect the device to the feeding container.

Patients with severe gastroesophageal reflux are at risk for aspiration pneumonia and therefore are not candidates for a gastrostomy. A jejunostomy is preferred, or jejunal feeding through a nasojejunal tube may be recommended.

NURSING PROCESS: THE PATIENT WITH A GASTROSTOMY

Assessment

The focus of the preoperative assessment is to determine the patient's ability both to understand and to cope with the impending surgical experience. The ability to adjust to a change in body image and to participate in self-care is evaluated, along with the patient's and the family's psychological status.

The purpose of the operative procedure is explained so that the patient will have a better understanding of the expected postoperative course. The patient needs to know that the result of this surgery is to bypass the mouth and esophagus so that liquid feedings can be administered directly into the stomach by means of a rubber or plastic tube or a prosthesis. If the prosthesis is to be permanent, the patient should be made aware of this. Psychologically, this is often difficult for the patient to accept. When the procedure is being performed to relieve discomfort, prolonged vomiting, debilitation, and an inability to eat, the patient finds it more acceptable.

The nurse evaluates the patient's skin condition and determines whether a delay in wound healing may be anticipated because of a systemic disorder (eg, diabetes mellitus, cancer).

In the postoperative period, the patient's fluid and nutritional needs are assessed to ensure proper food and fluid intake. The nurse inspects the tube for proper maintenance and the wound for signs of infection. At the same time, the patient's response to the change in body image is evaluated, as is the understanding of the methods for carrying out the feeding procedure. Interventions are identified to help the patient cope with the tube and learn self-care measures.

Diagnosis

Nursing Diagnoses

Based on the assessment data, the major nursing diagnoses in the postoperative period may include the following:

- Altered nutrition, less than body requirements, related to enteral feeding problems
- Risk for infection related to presence of wound and tube
- Risk for impaired skin integrity at tube site
- Ineffective coping related to inability to eat normally
- Body image disturbance related to presence of tube
- Risk for ineffective management of therapeutic regimen related to knowledge deficit about home care and the feeding procedure

Collaborative Problems/Potential Complications

Potential complications that may develop include:

- Wound infection, cellulitis, and abdominal wall abscess
- GI bleeding
- Premature removal of the tube

Planning and Goals

The major goals of the patient may include attaining an optimal level of nutrition, preventing infection, maintaining skin integrity, enhancing coping, adjusting to changes in body image, acquiring knowledge of and skill in self-care, and preventing complications.

Nursing Interventions

Meeting Nutritional Needs

The first fluid nourishment is administered soon after surgery and usually consists of tap water and 10% glucose. At first, only 30 to 60 mL (1 to 2 oz) is given at one time, but the amount is gradually increased. By the second day, 180 to 240 mL (6 to 8 oz) may be given at one time, provided it is tolerated and no leakage of fluid occurs around the tube. Water and milk can be instilled after 24 hours for a permanent gastrostomy. High-calorie liquids are added gradually. In some settings, during the early postoperative period the nurse aspirates gastric secretions and reinstills them after adding enough feeding to bring the volume to the desired total. By this method, gastric dilation is avoided.

Blenderized foods are gradually added to clear liquids until a full diet is reached. Powdered feedings that are easily liquefied are commercially available. The patient who receives blenderized tube feedings typically is not forced to give up usual dietary patterns, which may prove to be psychologically more acceptable. In addition, near-normal bowel function is promoted because the fiber and residue are similar to that of a normal diet. Intake of milk is avoided in patients with lactase deficiency.

Providing Tube Care and Preventing Infection

A small dressing can be applied over the tube outlet and the gastrostomy tube can be held in place by a thin strip of adhesive tape that is first twisted about the tube and then firmly attached to the abdomen. The dressing protects the skin around the incision from the seepage of gastric acid and the spillage of feedings.

The tube's placement is verified, residuals are assessed, and the tube/stabilizing disk is rotated once daily to prevent skin breakdown. Some gastrostomy tubes have balloons that are inflated with water to anchor the tube in the stomach. The adequacy of balloon inflation is checked weekly by deflating the balloon using a Luer-tip syringe.

Providing Skin Care

The skin surrounding a gastrostomy requires special care because it may become irritated from the enzymatic action of gastric juices that leak around the tube. If untreated, the skin becomes macerated, red, raw, and painful. The area around the tube is washed with soap and water daily, rinsed well, and patted dry. Any encrustation is removed with saline and rinsed with water. Once the stoma is healed and there is no drainage, a dressing is not required. A long-term gastrostomy may require a special dressing to protect the skin around the tube from gastric secretions and to help stabilize the entry site (Fig. 33-7).

Skin at the tube site is evaluated daily for signs of breakdown, irritation, excoriation, and the presence of drainage or gastric leakage. The patient and family members should be encouraged to participate in this inspection and in hygiene activities. If skin problems do occur, an enterostomal therapist or wound care specialist can be of assistance.

Enhancing Body Image

The patient with a gastrostomy has experienced a major assault to body image. Eating, a physiologic and social function, can no longer be taken for granted. The patient is also aware that gastrostomy as a therapeutic intervention is performed only in the presence of a major, chronic, or perhaps terminal illness.

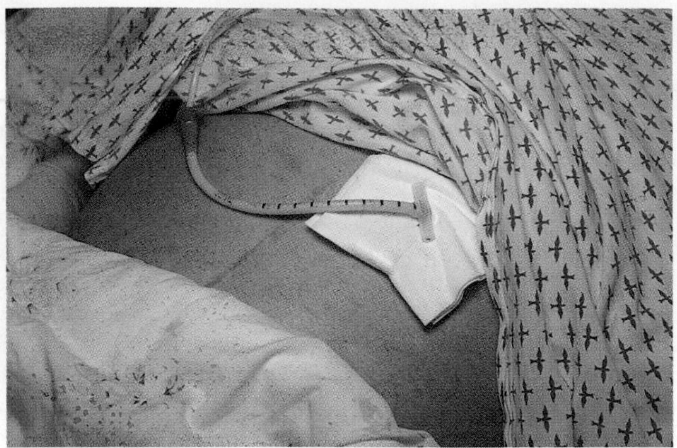

FIGURE 33•7 Protection at the gastrostomy site. A PEG tube may be protected by a dressing that allows access to the tube but covers the exit site. Typically the tube is stabilized with tape over the dressing. From Craven, R., & Hirnle, C. (1999). *Fundamentals of nursing: Human health and function* (3rd ed.). Philadelphia: Lippincott Williams & Wilkins.

Calm discussion of the purposes and routines of gastrostomy feeding can help keep the patient from feeling overwhelmed. Talking with a person who has had a gastrostomy can also help the patient to accept the expected changes. Adjusting to a change in body image takes time and requires family support and acceptance. Evaluating the existing family support system is necessary. One family member may emerge as the primary support person.

Monitoring and Managing Potential Complications

During the postoperative course, the nurse monitors the patient for potential complications. The most common complications are wound infection and other wound problems, including cellulitis at the wound site and abscesses in the abdominal wall. Because many patients who receive tube feedings are debilitated and have compromised nutritional status, any signs of infections are promptly reported to the physician so that appropriate antibiotic therapy can be instituted.

Bleeding from the insertion site in the stomach may also occur. The patient's vital signs are monitored closely, and all drainage from the operative site, vomitus, and stool are observed for evidence of bleeding. Any signs of bleeding are reported promptly.

Premature removal of the tube, whether it is done inadvertently by the patient or the caregiver, is another complication. If the tube is removed prematurely, the skin is cleansed and a sterile dressing is applied; the physician is notified immediately. The tract will close within 4 to 6 hours if the tube is not replaced.

Promoting Home and Community-Based Care

TEACHING PATIENTS SELF-CARE

The patient who is to receive gastrostomy tube feedings in the home setting must be capable of and responsible for administering the tube feedings or have a caregiver who is able to provide them. There must also be the physical, financial, and social resources to maintain care.

The patient's level of knowledge, interest in learning about the tube feeding, and ability to understand and apply the information are assessed. Detailed instructions about how to prepare the formula and manage the tube feeding are provided. Written materials for patients and caregivers are designed to outline the care instructions. To facilitate self-care, the patient is encouraged to participate in the tube feedings during hospitalization and to establish as normal a routine as possible.

Demonstration of the tube feeding begins by showing the patient how to check for residual gastric contents before the feeding. The patient then learns how to check and maintain the patency of the tube by administering room-temperature water before and after the feeding. This will establish patency before the feeding and then clear the tube of food particles, which could decompose if allowed to remain in the tube. All feedings are given at room temperature or near body temperature.

For a bolus feeding, the patient is shown how to introduce the liquid into the catheter by using a funnel or the barrel of a syringe. The receptacle is tilted to allow air to escape while the liquid is initially being instilled. As the funnel or syringe fills with liquid, the feeding is allowed to flow into the stomach by gravity by holding the barrel or syringe perpendicular to the abdomen (Fig. 33-8). The rate of flow is regulated by raising or lowering the receptacle to no higher than 45 cm (18 in) above the abdominal wall.

A bolus feeding of 300 to 500 mL usually is given for each meal and requires 10 to 15 minutes to complete. The amount is often determined by the patient's reaction. If the patient feels full, it may be desirable to give smaller amounts more frequently.

The patient and caregiver must understand that keeping the head of the bed elevated for at least 1 hour after feeding facilitates digestion and decreases the risk for aspiration. Any obstruction requires that the feeding be stopped and the physician notified.

The patient or caregiver is instructed to flush the tube with 30 mL of water after each bolus or medication administration, and otherwise to flush the tube daily to keep it patent. The equipment is cleaned with warm, soapy water and rinsed after each use.

The patient and caregiver are made aware that the tube is marked at skin level to provide the patient a baseline for later comparison. They are advised to monitor the tube's length and notify the physician or home care nurse if the segment of the tube outside the body becomes shorter or longer.

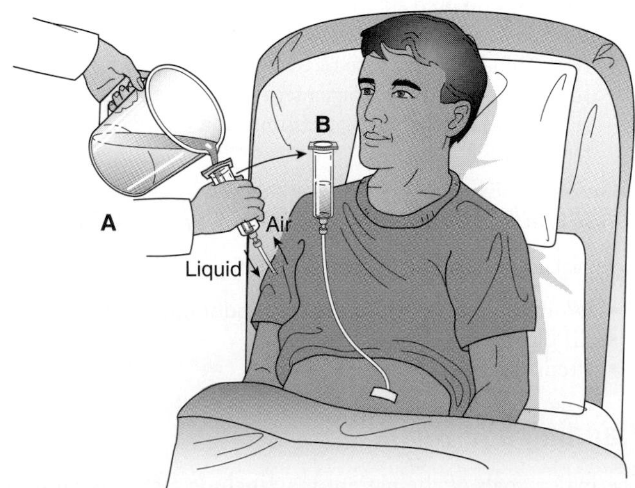

FIGURE 33•8 Gastrostomy feeding by gravity. (**A**) Feeding is instilled at an angle so that air does not enter the stomach. (**B**) Syringe is raised perpendicular to the abdomen so that feeding can enter by gravity.

If the patient is to use an intermittent or continuous pressure feeding pump at home, instruction in the use of the particular type of pump is essential. Most feeding pumps have built-in alarms that signal when the bag is empty, when the battery is low, or when an occlusion is present. The patient and caregiver will need to be aware of these alarms and how to trouble-shoot the pump.

CONTINUING CARE
Referral to a home care agency is important to provide initial supervision and support to the patient and caregiver. The home care nurse assesses the patient's status and progress and evaluates the techniques that are used in administering the tube feeding. Further instruction and supervision in the home setting may be required to help the patient and caregiver adapt to a physical environment and equipment that are different from the hospital setting. The nurse also reviews with the patient and caregiver information about complications to report (eg, dumping syndrome, nausea and vomiting, infection of the skin at the site of the tube).

The home care nurse assists the patient and family in establishing as normal a routine as possible. Some patients will want to experience a sensation of normal eating and are advised that they can try smelling, tasting, and chewing small amounts of food before taking their tube feedings. This stimulates the flow of salivary and gastric secretions and may give some sensation of a normal meal. The chewed food can then be deposited by the patient into a funnel or syringe attached to the gastrostomy tube for administration into the stomach.

The patient or caregiver is encouraged to keep a diary to record the times and amounts of feedings and any symptoms that occur. The diary is reviewed by the nurse during home visits.

When the tube is to be replaced, the patient or caregiver must be taught how to do this.

Evaluation

Expected Outcomes

Expected outcomes may include:

1. Achieves a balanced intake of nutrients
   a. Tolerates quantity and frequency of tube feedings
   b. Has 50 mL or less of residual gastric content before each feeding
   c. Has no diarrhea
   d. Maintains or gains weight
   e. Has normal electrolyte values
2. Is free from infection and skin breakdown
   a. Is afebrile
   b. Has no drainage from the incision
   c. Demonstrates intact skin surrounding the incision
   d. Inspects incision twice a day
3. Adjusts to change in body image
   a. Is able to discuss expected changes
   b. Verbalizes concerns
   c. Asks to speak with someone who has experienced this procedure
4. Avoids complications
   a. Exhibits adequate wound healing
   b. Has no abnormal bleeding from puncture site
   c. Tube remains intact for the duration of therapy
5. Demonstrates skill in managing feeding regimen
   a. Helps prepare prescribed formula or blenderized food
   b. Handles equipment competently
   c. Helps administer the feeding or does so independently
   d. Demonstrates how to maintain tube patency
   e. Cleans tubing as needed
   f. Keeps an accurate record of intake
   g. Can remove and reinsert the tube as appropriate and needed for feedings

TOTAL PARENTERAL NUTRITION (IV HYPERALIMENTATION)

Total parenteral nutrition (TPN) is a method of supplying nutrients to the body by an IV route. The goals of TPN are to improve nutritional status, establish a positive nitrogen balance, maintain muscle mass, promote weight gain, and enhance the healing process.

Preventing Negative Nitrogen Balance

When a patient's intake of protein and nutrients is significantly less than that required by the body to meet energy expenditures, a state of negative nitrogen balance results. In response, the body begins to convert the protein found in muscles into carbohydrates to be used to meet energy needs. The result is muscle wasting, weight loss, fatigue, and, if uncorrected, death.

The average postoperative adult patient requires approximately 1500 calories a day to keep the body from using its own store of protein. Traditional IV fluids do not provide sufficient calories or nitrogen to meet the body's daily requirements. TPN solutions, which supply nutrients such as dextrose, amino acids, electrolytes, vitamins, minerals, and fat emulsions, provide enough calories and nitrogen to meet the patient's daily nutritional needs. In general, TPN provides 30 to 35 kcal/kg and 1.0 to 1.5 g/kg protein.

The patient with fever, trauma, burns, major surgery, or hypermetabolic disease may require up to 10,000 additional calories daily. The volume of fluid necessary to provide these calories would surpass fluid tolerance and lead to pulmonary edema or congestive heart failure. To provide the required calories in small volume, it is necessary to increase the concentration of nutrients and use a route of administration (a large, high-flow vein [subclavian vein]) that will rapidly dilute incoming nutrients to the proper levels of body tolerance.

When highly concentrated glucose is administered, caloric requirements are satisfied and the body uses amino acids for protein synthesis rather than using them for energy. Additional potassium is added to the solution to maintain proper electrolyte balance and to transport glucose and amino acids across cell membranes. To prevent deficiencies and fulfill requirements for tissue synthesis, other elements, such as calcium, phosphorus, magnesium, and sodium chloride, are added.

Clinical Indications for TPN

The indications for TPN include a 10% deficit in pre-illness body weight, an inability to take oral food or fluids within 7 days after surgery, and hypercatabolic situations such as major infection with fever. In both the home and hospital setting, TPN is indicated in the following situations:

- The patient's intake is insufficient to maintain an anabolic state (eg, in cases of severe burns, malnutrition, short bowel syndrome, AIDS, sepsis, cancer).
- The patient's ability to ingest food orally or by tube is impaired (eg, paralytic ileus, Crohn's disease with

obstruction, postradiation enteritis, severe hyperemesis gravidarum in pregnancy).

- The patient is not interested in ingesting or is unwilling to ingest adequate nutrients (eg, anorexia nervosa, postoperative elderly patients).
- The underlying medical condition precludes being fed orally or by tube (eg, acute pancreatitis, high enterocutaneous fistula).
- Preoperative and postoperative nutritional needs are prolonged (eg, extensive bowel surgery).

Types of Nutritional Solutions

Two types of nutritional IV solutions are currently used in clinical practice: TPN and total nutrient admixture.

TPN refers to amino acid–dextrose formulas. A total of 2 to 3 L of solution is administered over a 24-hour period using a filter (1.2 micron particulate filter). Before administration, the TPN infusion must be inspected for clarity and any precipitate. The label is compared with the physician's order, noting the expiration date. Fat emulsions (Intralipid) are infused simultaneously with TPN through a Y-connector close to the infusion site. Fat emulsions should not be filtered. Before administration, the fat emulsion solution is inspected for frothiness, separation, or oily appearance. Usually 500 mL of a 10% emulsion is administered over 4 to 6 hours, one to three times a week. Fat emulsions can provide up to 30% of the total daily calorie intake.

The second type of parenteral nutrition solution is total nutrient admixture. Total nutrient admixture refers to amino acid–dextrose–lipid and is commonly called a "three-in-one" formulation. One liter is administered to the patient over a 24-hour period. A special final filter (1.5 microfilter) is used with this solution. Before administration, the solution is observed for oil droplets that have separated from the solution, forming a noticeable layer (cracking of lipid emulsion); such a solution should be discarded. Advantages of the three-in-one formula over TPN are cost savings in preparation and equipment, decreased chance of contamination with minimal IV line interruptions, less nursing time, and increased patient convenience and satisfaction.

Ideally, the nutritional support nurse, pharmacist, nutritionist, and physician collaborate to determine the specific formula needed.

Preparing the Solution and Initiating Therapy

The prescribed nutritional IV solution is prepared by a pharmacist under a filtered-air laminar flow hood using strict aseptic technique. The basic solution consists of 25% glucose and synthetic amino acids (FreAmine), which provides the patient with 1000 calories and 6 g of nitrogen per liter. Electrolytes are added as determined by the serum electrolyte needs of the patient. Solutions delivered to the nursing unit are refrigerated until needed and then allowed to warm to room temperature. Commercial preparations (eg, Aminosyn, Aminosyn II, Trophamine, FreAmine) are available and can be modified to meet individual needs.

TPN solutions are initiated slowly and gradually advanced each day to the desired rate and as the patient's fluid and glucose tolerance permits. The patient's laboratory values and response to TPN therapy are monitored on an ongoing basis by the nutritional support team. Standing orders are initiated for weighing the patient and obtaining a complete blood count, platelet count, prothrombin time, and electrolyte, magnesium, and blood glucose levels. In most hospitals, TPN solutions are prescribed by the physician on a daily parenteral nutrition order form. The formulation of the TPN solutions must be carefully calculated each day to meet the complete nutritional needs of each patient.

Methods of Administration

Various vascular access methods and devices are used to administer TPN solution in clinical practice. The method depends on the patient's condition and the anticipated length of therapy.

Peripheral Partial Method

To supplement oral intake when complete bowel rest is not indicated and NG or nasoenteric suction is not required, partial peripheral nutrition may be prescribed. Partial peripheral nutrition is administered by peripheral vein; this is possible because the solution is less hypertonic than TPN solution. Dextrose concentrations of more than 10% should not be administered through peripheral veins because they irritate the intima (innermost walls) of small veins, causing clinical phlebitis. The usual length of therapy using the partial peripheral method is 5 to 10 days.

Central Line Method

Because TPN solutions have five or six times the solute concentration of blood (and exert an osmotic pressure of about 2000 mOsm/L), they are injurious to the intima of peripheral veins. Therefore, to prevent phlebitis and other venous complications, these solutions are administered into the circulatory system through a catheter inserted into a high-flow, large blood vessel (the subclavian vein). Concentrated solutions are then very rapidly diluted to isotonic levels by the blood in this vessel.

Four groups of central venous access devices (CVAD) are available: nontunneled (or percutaneous) central catheters, peripherally inserted central catheters, tunneled catheters, and implanted ports. Whenever one of these catheters is inserted, the catheter tip's placement should be confirmed by x-ray before initiating TPN therapy. The optimal position is the midproximal third of the superior vena cava. The tip of the catheter should not be located in the right atrium.

NONTUNNELED (PERCUTANEOUS) CENTRAL CATHETERS

Percutaneously placed central venous catheters are used for short-term (less than 30 days) IV therapy in the acute care, long-term care, and home care settings. These catheters are inserted by the physician. The subclavian vein is the most common vessel used because the area provides a stable insertion site to which the catheter can be anchored, allows the patient freedom of movement, and provides easy access to the dressing site. Single-, double-, and triple-lumen central venous catheters are available for central lines. To ensure accessibility, a triple-lumen subclavian catheter should be used because it offers three ports for various uses (Fig. 33-9). The 16-gauge distal lumen can be used to infuse blood or other viscous fluids. The 18-gauge middle lumen is reserved for TPN infusion. The 18-gauge proximal port can be used for administering blood or medications. A port not being used for fluid administration can be used for drawing blood.

If a single-lumen percutaneous central catheter is used for administering TPN, various restrictions apply. Blood cannot be drawn from the catheter and medications cannot be administered through the catheter because the medication may be incompatible with the

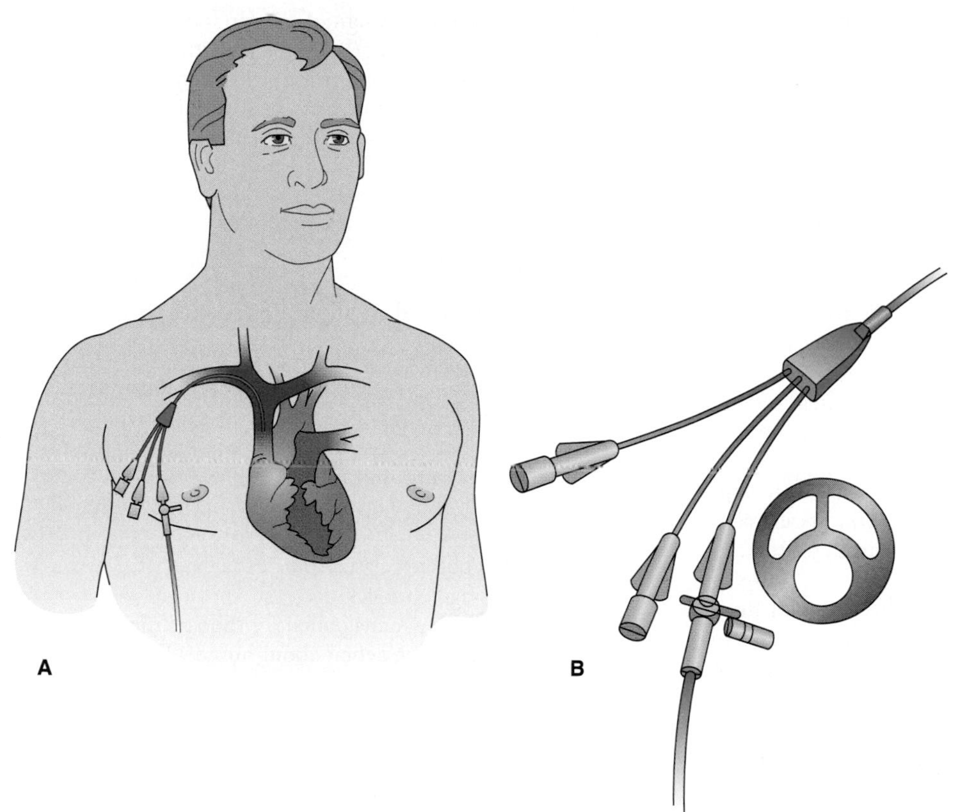

FIGURE 33•9 Subclavian triple-lumen catheter used for total parenteral nutrition and other adjunctive therapy. (**A**) The catheter is threaded through the subclavian vein and placed in the vena cava. (**B**) Each lumen is an avenue for solution administration; these are secured with Luer-Lok caps when not in use.

components of the nutritional solution (insulin is an exception). If medications must be given, they must be infused through a separate peripheral IV line, not by piggyback into the TPN line. Transfusions of blood products also cannot be given through the main line because red cells may possibly coat the lumen of the catheter, thereby reducing the flow of the nutritional solution.

PERIPHERALLY INSERTED CENTRAL CATHETERS

Peripherally inserted central catheters (PICC) are used for intermediate-length (3 to 12 months) IV therapy in the hospital, long-term care, or home setting. These catheters may be inserted at the bedside or in the outpatient setting by a specially trained nurse. The basilic or cephalic vein is accessed through the antecubital space and the catheter is threaded to a designated location, depending on the type of solution to be infused (superior vena cava for TPN).

TUNNELED CENTRAL CATHETERS

Tunneled central catheters may remain in place for many years. These catheters are cuffed and can have single or double lumens; two examples are the Hickman/Broviac catheter and the Groshong catheter. These catheters are inserted surgically. They are threaded under the skin (reduces risk of ascending infection) to the subclavian vein, and the distal end of the catheter is advanced into the superior vena cava 2 to 3 cm above the junction with the right atrium (see Chap. 15, Fig. 15-3).

IMPLANTED PORTS

Implanted ports are another device used for long-term home IV therapy (eg, Port-A-Cath, Mediport, Hickman Port, Infuse-A-Port, P.A.S. Port). Instead of exiting from the skin (as do the Hickman/Broviac and Groshong catheters), the end of the catheter is attached to a small chamber that is placed in a subcutaneous pocket, either on the anterior chest wall or on the forearm. The subcutaneous port requires minimal care and allows the patient complete freedom of activity. Implanted ports are more expensive than the external catheters, and access requires passing a special needle (Huber-tipped) through the skin into the chamber to initiate IV therapy (see Chap. 15, Fig. 15-4).

NONTUNNELED CENTRAL VENOUS CATHETER INSERTION

Patient Preparation. The procedure is explained so that the patient understands the importance of not touching the catheter insertion site and is aware of what to expect during the insertion procedure. To insert the catheter, the patient is placed supine, in head-low position (to produce dilation of neck and shoulder vessels, which makes entry easier and prevents air embolus). The area is shaved if necessary and the skin prepared with acetone and alcohol to remove surface oils. Final skin preparation includes cleaning with tincture of 2% iodine or povidone–iodine solution. If 2% iodine is used, it is removed with alcohol after 1 minute. To afford maximal accuracy in the placement of the tube, the patient is instructed to turn the head away from the site of venipuncture and to remain motionless while the catheter is inserted and the wound is dressed.

Inserting the Catheter. The preferred route is by way of the subclavian vein, which leads into the superior vena cava. The external jugular route can be used but is usually used only in emergency situations. Because a central venous catheter is always a potential source of serious infection, the site should be changed every 4 weeks or as recommended by the Centers for Disease Control and Prevention.

Sterile drapes are applied to the upper chest. The patient may be asked to wear a face mask to prevent the spread of microorganisms. Procaine or lidocaine is injected to anesthetize the skin and underlying tissues. The target area is the inferior border at the midpoint of the clavicle. A large-bore needle on a syringe is inserted and moved parallel to and beneath the clavicle until it enters the vein. The syringe is then detached and a radiopaque catheter is inserted through the needle into the vein.

When the catheter is positioned, the needle is withdrawn and the hub of the catheter is attached to the IV tubing. Until the syringe is detached from the needle and the catheter inserted, the patient may be asked to perform the Valsalva maneuver. (To do this, the patient is instructed to take a deep breath, hold it, and bear down with mouth closed. Compression of the abdomen may also accomplish the maneuver.) The Valsalva maneuver is performed to produce a positive phase in central venous pressure to lessen the possibility of air being drawn into the circulatory system (air embolism). The physician sutures the catheter to the skin to avoid accidental dislodgement.

The catheter insertion site is swabbed with an iodine solution. A gauze or transparent dressing is applied using strict sterile technique. An isotonic IV solution (eg, D_5W) is administered to keep the vein patent.

The position of the tip of the catheter is checked with fluoroscopy to confirm its location in the superior vena cava and to rule out a pneumothorax resulting from accidental puncture of the pleura. Once the catheter position is confirmed, the prescribed TPN solution is started. The initial rate of infusion is usually 50 mL/hour, and the rate is gradually increased to the maintenance rate or predetermined dose (100 to 125 mL/hour). An infusion pump is always used for administration of TPN and peripheral partial nutrition.

Each lumen of the catheter is secured with Luer-Lok caps and labeled according to location (proximal, middle, distal). To ensure patency, all lumens are flushed with a diluted heparin flush initially and two or three times a day when not in use, after each intermittent infusion, after blood drawing, and whenever an infusion is disconnected. Force is never used to flush the catheter. If resistance is met, aspiration may be effective in cleansing the lumen; if this is not effective, the physician is notified. A clot or fibrin sheath may need to be dissolved with low-dose urokinase. If attempts to clear the lumen are ineffective, the lumen is labeled as "clotted off."

Discontinuing TPN

The TPN solution is discontinued gradually to allow the patient to adjust to decreased levels of glucose. After terminating the TPN solution, isotonic glucose is administered for several hours to protect against rebound hypoglycemia. Oral carbohydrates will shorten the tapering time. Specific symptoms of rebound hypoglycemia include weakness, faintness, sweating, shakiness, feeling cold, confusion, and increased heart rate. Once all IV therapy is completed, the nurse (with a physician's order) may remove either the nontunneled central venous catheter or the peripherally inserted central catheter and apply an occlusive dressing to the exit site. Tunneled catheters and implanted ports are removed by a physician.

NURSING PROCESS: THE PATIENT RECEIVING TPN

Assessment

The nurse assists in identifying patients who may be candidates for TPN. Indicators include any significant weight loss (10% or more of usual weight), a decrease in oral food intake for more than 1 week, any significant sign of protein loss (serum albumin levels less than 3.2 g/dL [32 g/L], muscle wasting, decreased tissue healing, or abnormal urea nitrogen excretion), and persistent vomiting and diarrhea. The nurse carefully monitors the patient's hydration, electrolyte levels, and calorie intake.

Diagnosis

Nursing Diagnoses

Based on the assessment data, the major nursing diagnoses may include the following:

- Altered nutrition, less than body requirements, related to inadequate oral intake of nutrients
- Risk for infection related to contamination of the central catheter site or infusion line
- Risk for fluid volume excess or deficit related to altered infusion rate
- Risk for immobility related to fear that the catheter will become dislodged or occluded
- Risk for ineffective management of therapeutic regimen related to knowledge deficit about home TPN therapy

Collaborative Problems/Potential Complications

The most common complications include pneumothorax, air embolism, a clotted or displaced catheter, sepsis, hyperglycemia, rebound hypoglycemia, and fluid overload. These problems and the associated collaborative interventions are described in Table 33-5.

Planning and Goals

The major goals for the patient may include optimal level of nutrition, absence of infection, adequate fluid volume, optimal level of activity (within individual limitations), knowledge of and skill in self-care, and prevention of complications.

Nursing Interventions

Maintaining Optimal Nutrition

A continuous, uniform infusion of TPN solution over a 24-hour period is desired. In some cases, however (eg, home care patients), cyclic parenteral nutrition may be appropriate. With cyclic TPN, there is a set time during a 24-hour period when TPN is infused and a set time when it is not. The time periods for infusion are sufficient to meet the patient's nutritional and pharmacologic needs. Ideally, cyclic TPN is infused over an 8- to 10-hour period during the night.

The patient is weighed daily (this may be decreased to two or three times per week) at the same time of the day under the same conditions for accurate comparison. Under the TPN regimen (without additional energy expenditure), a satisfactory weight gain is usually achieved. Accurate intake and output records and calculations of fluid balance are kept. A calorie count is kept of any oral nutrients. Trace elements (copper, zinc, chromium, manganese, and selenium) are included in TPN solutions and are individualized for each patient. The TPN solutions are prescribed daily by the physician on a parenteral nutrition order form based on laboratory values and patient tolerance.

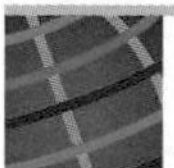

TABLE 33•5 **Complications of Total Parenteral Nutrition**

Complication	Cause	Nursing Actions and Collaborative Interventions
Pneumothorax	Improper catheter placement and inadvertent puncture of the pleura	Place in Fowler's position. Offer reassurance. Monitor vital signs. Prepare for thoracentesis or chest tube insertion.
Air embolism	Disconnected tubing	Tape all tubing connection sites securely. Replace tubing immediately and notify physician.
	Cap missing from port	Replace cap and notify physician.
	Blocked segment of vascular system	Turn patient on left side and place in the head-low position. Notify physician.
Clotted catheter line	Inadequate/infrequent heparin flushes	Administer heparin flush in unused lines twice a day.
	Disruption of infusion	Monitor infusion rate hourly and inspect the integrity of the line. On *rare* occasions, flush with urokinase as prescribed.
Catheter displacement	Excessive movement, possibly with a non-secured catheter	Stop the infusion and notify the physician.
	Separation of tubing and contamination	Tape all tubing connection sites. Avoid interrupting the main line or piggybacking other lines.
Sepsis	Separation of dressings	Reinforce or change dressing quickly using aseptic technique.
	Contaminated solution	Discard. Notify pharmacist.
	Infection at insertion site of catheter	Notify physician. Monitor vital signs every 4 hours. Change catheter site every 4 weeks.
Hyperglycemia	Glucose intolerance	Monitor glucose levels (blood and urine). Monitor urine output. Observe for stupor, confusion, lethargy. Notify physician; the addition of insulin to the TPN solution may be prescribed.
Fluid overload	Fluid infusing rapidly	Decrease infusion rate, use infusion pump. Monitor vital signs. Notify physician. Treat respiratory distress by sitting patient upright and administering oxygen as needed, if prescribed.
Rebound hypoglycemia	Feedings stopped too abruptly	Monitor for symptoms (weakness, tremors, diaphoresis, headache, hunger, and apprehension); notify physician. Gradually wean patient from TPN.

Preventing Infection

The high glucose content of TPN solutions makes these solutions ideal culture media for bacterial and fungal growth, and central venous catheters provide a port of entry. *Candida albicans* is the most common infectious organism. Other infectious organisms include *Staphylococcus aureus*, *Staphylococcus epidermidis*, and *Klebsiella pneumoniae*. Therefore, meticulous technique is essential to reduce the risk of infection.

Dressings are changed using sterile technique usually once or twice a week and as needed. The Centers for Disease Control and Prevention recommends changing dressings for central venous access devices only if they are damp, bloody, loose, or soiled. The nurse and patient wear masks during dressing changes to reduce the possibility of airborne contamination. Dressings are removed carefully to prevent the catheter from becoming dislodged. The area is checked for leakage, bloody drainage, a kinked catheter, and skin reactions such as inflammation, redness, swelling, tenderness, or purulent drainage. The nurse puts on sterile gloves and cleanses the area with acetone and alcohol swabs, followed by tincture of 2% iodine swabs; after 1 minute, the iodine is removed with alcohol. 1% povidone–iodine solution can be used instead of 2% iodine and left on the skin. Cleaning begins in a circular manner from the center moving outward. Alcohol may be used in the same manner to remove iodine. The insertion site is covered with a small dressing, slit to fit around the catheter. A gauze pad or transparent dressing is centered over the area.

The advantages of using a transparent dressing over the gauze pad are that it allows frequent examination of the catheter site without changing the dressing, it adheres well, and it is more comfortable for the patient. When the IV tubing extension is changed, it is replaced quickly to prevent contamination of the tubing. The connection (hub) of the catheter and tubing is then covered and secured with adhesive tape to prevent separation and exposure to air. Main-line IV tubing and filters are changed every 72 hours, and all connections are taped securely to avoid breaks in the integrity of the system. The dressing and tubing are labeled with the date, time of insertion, time of dressing change, and the initials of the person who carried out the procedure.

If the patient has a draining wound, such as a tracheostomy, in the nearby area, additional precautions are taken to keep the venous access device dressing dry by applying an occlusive dressing to ensure waterproofing. Hypoallergenic adhesive tape can be used if the patient complains of itching from conventional tape. The dressing change is documented, and the condition of the area and the patient's reaction are reported.

Maintaining Fluid Balance

An infusion pump is recommended for TPN to maintain an accurate rate. A designated rate in milliliters per hour is set. The rate is checked every 30 minutes to 1 hour; an alarm signals a problem. The infusion rate should not be increased or decreased to compensate for fluids that have infused too quickly or too slowly. If the IV runs out, 10% dextrose and water is infused until the next TPN solution is available from the pharmacy.

If the rate is too rapid, hyperosmolar diuresis occurs (excess sugar will be excreted), which if severe enough may cause intractable seizures, coma, and death. Symptoms of rapid hypertonic fluid intake include headache, nausea, fever, chills, and increasing lethargy.

If the flow rate is too slow, the patient does not get the maximal benefit of calories and nitrogen. Intake and output are recorded every 8 hours so that fluid imbalance can be readily detected. The patient is weighed two or three times a week; in ideal situations, the patient will show neither weight loss nor significant weight gain. The nurse assesses for signs of dehydration (eg, thirst, decreased skin turgor, decreased central venous pressure) and reports these findings to the physician immediately. It is essential to monitor blood glucose levels because hyperglycemia can cause diuresis and excessive fluid loss.

Encouraging Activity

Activities and ambulation are encouraged when the patient is physically capable. With a catheter in the subclavian vein, the patient is free to move the extremities and should be encouraged to maintain good muscle tone. If applicable, the teaching and exercise program initiated in the occupational and physical therapy departments should be reinforced.

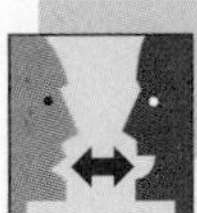

ETHICS AND RELATED ISSUES

Is It Ethical to Withhold or Withdraw Nutrition and Hydration?

Situation

It is generally agreed that patients (or their designated decision-makers) can refuse life-saving treatment, particularly if the means of treatment are extraordinary (eg, ventilators, dialysis machines, extracorporeal oxygenators). Extraordinary means are all medications, treatments, and procedures that can be obtained only at excessive cost, pain, or inconvenience and offer no reasonable hope of benefit. Nutrition and hydration therapy, however, are perceived as ordinary means.

Ordinary means are those medications, treatments, and procedures that offer a reasonable hope of benefit and can be obtained without excessive expense, pain, or inconvenience. Additionally, withdrawing or withholding nutrition and hydration can in and of itself cause death. Thus, some have argued that nutrition and hydration should always be provided to every patient, regardless of the patient's preference or condition.

Dilemma

The patient's desire to have nutrition or hydration withdrawn or withheld conflicts with the reluctance of others to harm the patient by withdrawing the food and water needed for survival (autonomy versus nonmaleficence).

Discussion

- What arguments would you offer against the withholding and withdrawing of nutrition and hydration?
- What arguments would you offer in favor of withholding and withdrawing nutrition and hydration?
- Are foods and fluids always "ordinary means," or are there instances in which they might be considered "extraordinary"? Support your answer.
- Answer the above questions using as an example a patient in a persistent vegetative state (ie, unable to express his or her wishes).

Promoting Home and Community-Based Care

TEACHING PATIENTS SELF-CARE

Successful home TPN requires teaching the patient and family specialized skills using an intensive training program and follow-up supervision in the home. This is accomplished through a team effort. The financial costs of such programs, although high, are less than those incurred in a hospital. Initiation of a home program may be the only way the patient can be discharged from the hospital.

Ideal candidates for home TPN are those who have a reasonable life expectancy after return home, have only a limited number of medical illnesses other than the one that has resulted in the need for TPN, and are highly motivated and fairly self-sufficient. In addition, ability to learn, availability of family interest and support, adequate finances, and the physical plan of the home are factors that must be assessed when the decision for home TPN is made.

Home health care agencies sponsoring home TPN programs have developed teaching brochures for every aspect of the treatment, including catheter and dressing care, use of an infusion pump, administration of fat emulsions, and instillation of heparin flushes. Teaching is begun in the hospital and is continued in the home setting or ambulatory infusion center.

CONTINUING CARE

The home care nurse should be aware that the average patient needs about 2 weeks of instruction and reinforcement.

Managing TPN. A home care teaching program prepares the patient to manage the appropriate form of TPN. The patient is taught how to store solutions, set up the infusion, flush the line with heparin, change the dressings, and trouble-shoot for problems. The most common complication is sepsis. The nurse emphasizes hand washing and strict asepsis in handling equipment, changing the dressing, and preparing the solution.

Managing Mechanical Difficulties. Mechanical problems usually arise from technical complications in the infusion pump or catheter site. The length of the external portion of the catheter is recorded. This measurement is used as a comparison if the line is pulled or dislodgement is suspected. The patient is taught how

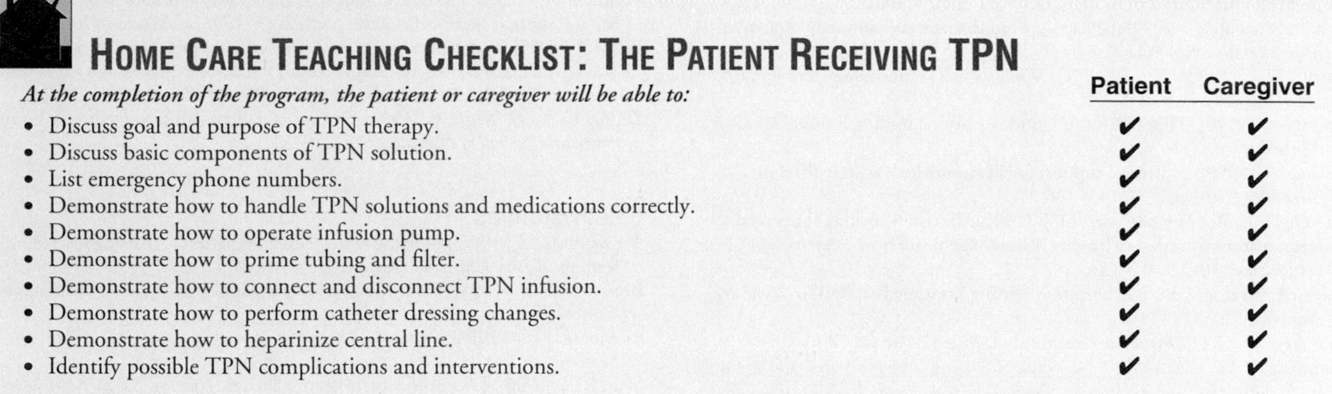

Home Care Teaching Checklist: The Patient Receiving TPN

At the completion of the program, the patient or caregiver will be able to:	Patient	Caregiver
• Discuss goal and purpose of TPN therapy.	✔	✔
• Discuss basic components of TPN solution.	✔	✔
• List emergency phone numbers.	✔	✔
• Demonstrate how to handle TPN solutions and medications correctly.	✔	✔
• Demonstrate how to operate infusion pump.	✔	✔
• Demonstrate how to prime tubing and filter.	✔	✔
• Demonstrate how to connect and disconnect TPN infusion.	✔	✔
• Demonstrate how to perform catheter dressing changes.	✔	✔
• Demonstrate how to heparinize central line.	✔	✔
• Identify possible TPN complications and interventions.	✔	✔

to trouble-shoot for catheter problems (eg, leakage, loose cap, blood clot, dislodgement) and is given a list of instructions explaining what to do for each problem.

Recognizing Metabolic Complications. The patient is given a list of symptoms that indicate metabolic complications (neuropathies, mentation changes, diarrhea, nausea, skin changes, decreased urine output) and directed to contact the home health care nurse or physician if any of these complications occurs. The patient is instructed to have weekly serum chemistry and hematology testing and to check the urine glucose level every day.

Obtaining Psychosocial Support. The psychosocial aspects of home parenteral nutrition are as important as the physiologic and technical concerns. These patients must cope with the loss of eating and the changes in lifestyle brought on by sleep disturbances (frequent urination during infusions, usually two or three times during the night). Major psychosocial reactions include depression, anger, withdrawal, anxiety, and altered self-image. A successful home parenteral nutrition program depends on motivation, emotional stability, and technical competence. Support groups are also available in the community to help patients and families cope with the transition and to minimize disruption of the patient's lifestyle.

Critical Thinking Exercises

1. You are caring for a patient with an NG feeding tube. Before administering the medications, you must confirm that the tube is placed correctly. Based on research findings, how will you check to make sure that the tube is properly placed?

2. A patient receiving NG tube feedings begins to have diarrhea. Explain what you think might be causing the diarrhea, describe the assessment data important in determining its possible causes, and discuss ways to control it.

3. When conducting a home visit with a patient receiving nightly 10-hour parenteral nutrition feedings, you find that the patient has chills, diarrhea, and a fever of 100°F (37.8°C). The patient's sister states that the previous evening's feeding solution looked "funny" and that she sped up the rate of the feeding so it would finish early. Analyze this situation and determine the actions you would take, explaining the reasoning behind your decision.

Evaluation

Expected Outcomes

Expected outcomes may include:

1. Attains or maintains nutritional balance
2. Is free of infection
   a. Is afebrile
   b. Has no purulent drainage from the catheter insertion site
   c. Has intact IV line
3. Is hydrated, as evidenced by good skin turgor
4. Achieves an optimal level of activity, within limitations
5. Demonstrates skill in managing TPN regimen
6. Prevents complications
   a. Maintains proper catheter and equipment function
   b. Has no symptoms of sepsis
   c. Maintains metabolic balance within normal limits
   d. Shows improved and stabilized nutritional status

References and Selected Readings

BOOKS

Centers for Disease Control and Prevention. (1995). Intravascular device-related infections prevention: Guideline availability. Department of Health and Human Services, Federal Register, 27; 60(187), 49978–50006.

Fischer, F. E. (Ed.). (1991). *Total parenteral nutrition* (2nd ed.). Boston: Little, Brown and Co.

Grant, J. P. (1992). *Handbook of total parenteral nutrition* (2nd ed.). Philadelphia: W. B. Saunders.

Rombeau, J. L., & Rolandelli, R. (1997). *Clinical nutrition: Enteral and tube feeding* (3rd ed.). Philadelphia: W. B. Saunders.

Schaik, T. V. (1993). *Gastroenterology nursing: A core curriculum.* St. Louis: Mosby–Year Book.

Spiro, H. M. (1993). *Clinical gastroenterology* (4th ed.). New York: McGraw-Hill.

Terry, J. (Ed.). (1995). *Intravenous therapy: Clinical principles and practice.* Philadelphia: W. B. Saunders.

Zeman, F. J. (1991). *Clinical nutrition and dietetics* (2nd ed.). New York: Macmillan.

JOURNALS

Asterisks indicate nursing research articles.

NG and Nasoenteric Intubation and Feeding

Bak, L. B., et al. (1996). Tube feeding your diabetic patient safely. *American Journal of Nursing, 96*(12), 47–49.

Barnie, D. C., & Currier, J. (1995). What's that GI tube being used for? *RN, 58*(8), 45–49.

Bowers, S. (1996). Tubes: A nurse's guide to enteral feeding devices. *MedSurg Nursing, 5*(5), 313–325.

Bowers, S. (1999). Nutrition support for malnourished, acutely ill adults. *MedSurg Nursing, 8*(3), 145–166.

Clevenger, F. W., & Rodriguez, D. J. (1995). Decision-making for enteral feeding administration: The why behind where and how. *Nutrition in Clinical Practice, 10*(3), 104–113.

Davis, A. E., et al. (1995). Preventing feeding-associated aspiration. *MedSurg Nursing, 4*(2), 111–119.

Eisenberg, P. G. (1994). Nasoenteral tubes. *RN, 57*(10), 62–70.

Eisenberg, P. G., et al. (1989). Nasoenteral feeding-tube properties and the ability to withdraw fluid via syringe. *Applied Nursing Research, 2*(4), 168–172.

Fater, K. H. (1995). Determining nasoenteral feeding tube placement. *MedSurg Nursing, 4*(1), 27–33.

Forloines-Lynn, S. (1996a). How to smooth the way for cyclic tube feedings. *Nursing '96, 26*(3), 57–60.

Forloines-Lynn, S. (1996b). Knowing how to manage complications of tube feeding. *Nursing '96, 26*(3), 32m–32p.

Gharib, A. M., et al. (1996). NG and feeding tubes. *Postgraduate Medicine, 99*(5), 165–176.

Goff, K. (1998). Enteral and parenteral nutrition: Transitioning from hospital to home. *Nursing Care Management, 3*(2), 67–74.

Goff, K. L. (1997). The nuts and bolts of enteral infusion pumps. *MedSurg Nursing, 6*(1), 9–15.

Hay, J., et al. (1996). Reducing the cost of enteral feeding. *Gastroenterology Nursing, 19*(1), 29–30.

Lord, L. M. (1997). Enteral access devices. *Nursing Clinics of North America, 32*(4), 685–704.

Lord, L. M., et al. (1996). Adult tube feeding formulas. *MedSurg Nursing, 5*(6), 407–420.

*Metheny, N., et al. (1986). Aspiration pneumonia in patients fed through nasoenteral tubes. *Heart and Lung, 15*(3), 256–261.

*Metheny, N. (1988). Measures to test placement of NG and nasointestinal feeding tubes: A review. *Nursing Research, 37*(6), 324–329.

*Metheny, N., et al. (1989). Effectiveness of pH measurements in predicting feeding tube placement. *Nursing Research, 38*(5), 280–285.

*Metheny, N., et al. (1990a). Detection of inadvertent respiratory placement of small-bore feeding tubes: A report of 10 cases. *Heart & Lung, 19*(6), 631–638.

*Metheny, N., et al. (1990b). Effectiveness of the auscultatory method in predicting feeding tube location. *Nursing Research, 39*(5), 262–267.

*Metheny, N., et al. (1993). How to aspirate fluid from small-bore feeding tubes. *American Journal of Nursing, 93*(5), 86–88.

*Metheny, N., et al. (1994). Visual characteristics of aspirates from feeding tubes as a method for predicting tube location. *Nursing Research, 43*(5), 282–287.

*Metheny, N., et al. (1998). Testing feeding tube placement: Auscultation vs. pH method. *American Journal of Nursing, 98*(5), 37–43.

Miller, D., & Miller, H. W. (1995). Giving meds through the tube. *RN, 58*(1), 44–48.

*Schmieding, N. J., & Waldman, R. C. (1997a). Gastric decompression in adult patients. *Clinical Nursing Research, 6*(2), 142–155.

*Schmieding, N. J., & Waldman, R. C. (1997b). NG tube feeding and medication administration: A survey of nursing practices. *Gastroenterology Nursing, 20*(4), 118–124.

*Schmieding, N. J., et al. (1997). NG tubes: Insertion, placement, and removal in adult patients. *Gastroenterology Nursing, 20*(1), 15–19.

*Seifert, C. F., et al. (1995). A nursing survey to determine the characteristics of medication administration through enteral feeding catheters. *Clinical Nursing Research, 4*(3), 290–305.

Towner, L. C., & Brown, A. J. B. (1996). Standardizing enteral feeding practice: An approach to achieve consistent practice with reduced documentation for long-term care nurses. *Geriatric Nursing, 17*(5), 211–216.

Viall, C. D. (1996). Location, location, location. *Nursing '96, 26*(9), 43–45.

Weinstein, D. S., & Furman, J. (1997). Enteral formulas. *Nursing Clinics of North America, 32*(4), 669–683.

Welch, S. K. (1996). Certification of staff nurses to insert enteral feeding tubes using a research-based procedure. *Nutrition in Clinical Practice, 11*(1), 21–27.

Willis, J. (1995). Enteral feeding pumps. *Professional Nurse, 10*(10), 635–640.

*Wilson, M. F., & Haynes-Johnson, V. (1987). Cranberry juice or water? A comparison of feeding tube irrigants. *Nutritional Support Services, 7*(7), 23–24.

Young, C. K., & White, S. (1992). Preparing patients for tube feeding at home. *American Journal of Nursing, 92*(4), 46–53.

Gastrostomies

Arrowsmith, H. (1996). Nursing management of patients receiving gastrostomy feeding. *British Journal of Nursing, 5*(5), 268–273.

Broscious, S. K. (1995). Preventing complications of PEG tubes. *Dimensions of Critical Care Nursing, 14*(1), 37–41.

Eisenberg, P. G. (1994). Gastrostomy and jejunostomy tubes. *RN, 57*(11), 54–60.

Hall, J. C. (1996). Low-profile gastrostomy devices. *Nursing '97, 27*(6), 62–64.

Hall, J. C., et al. (1996). Troubleshooting G-tubes. Balloon deflation problems. *RN, 59*(7), 25–28.

Heximer, B. (1996). Spontaneous balloon rupture. *RN, 59*(7), 22–28.

Kaufman, M. W., et al. (1995). Low-profile gastrostomy devices. *Gastroenterology Nursing, 18*(5), 171–176.

Moak, E. (1995). Laparoscopic gastrostomy/jejunostomy. *Today's OR Nurse, 17*(1), 23–27.

Thompson, L. (1995). Percutaneous endoscopic gastrostomy. *Nursing '95, 25*(4), 62–63.

TPN

Andris, D. A., & Krzywda, E. A. (1997). Central venous access. *Nursing Clinics of North America, 32*(4), 719–740.

ASPEN Board of Directors. (1993). Guidelines for the use of parenteral and enteral nutrition in adult and pediatric patients. *Journal of Parenteral and Enteral Nutrition, 17*(4, Suppl.).

Driscoll, M., et al. (1997). Inserting and maintaining peripherally inserted central catheters. *MedSurg Nursing, 6*(6), 350–358.

Galica, L. A. (1997). Parenteral nutrition. *Nursing Clinics of North America, 32*(4), 705–717.

Gianino, S., et al. (1996). The ABCs of TPN. *RN, 59*(2), 42–48.

Harrison, M. (1997). Central venous catheters: A review of the literature. *Nursing Standard, 11*(27), 43–45.

Kazywda, E. A. (1998). Central venous access—catheters, technology, and physiology. *MedSurg Nursing, 7*(3), 132–139.

Labow, C. A. (1995). Venous access device options. *Surgical Oncology Clinics of North America, 4*(3), 473–478.

Macklin, D. (1997). How to manage PICCs. *American Journal of Nursing, 97*(9), 26–33.

Masoorli, S. (1997). Managing complications of central venous access devices. *Nursing '97, 27*(8), 59–63.

Miller, K. D., & Dietrick, C. L. (1997). Experience with PICC at a university medical center. *Journal of Intravenous Nursing, 20*(3), 141–147.

Sweed, M. R., et al. (1995). Nursing implications for the adult patient receiving nutritional support. *MedSurg Nursing, 4*(2), 99–107.

Viall, C. (1995a). Taking the mystery out of TPN, part one. *Nursing '95, 25*(4), 35–43.

Viall, C. (1995b). Taking the mystery out of TPN, part two. *Nursing '95, 25*(5), 57–59.

Resources

Oley Foundation, 214 Hun Memorial, Albany, NY 12208

Society of Gastroenterology Nurses & Associates, Inc., 1070 Sibley Towers, Rochester, NY 14604

American Cancer Society, 1599 Clifton Rd. N.E., Atlanta, GA 30329; 1-404-320-3333; www.cancer.org

American Institute of Nutrition, 9650 Rockville Pike, Bethesda, MD 20014-3990

American Society for GI Endoscopy, 13 Elm St., Manchester, MA 01944

American Society of Parenteral and Enteral Nutrition (ASPEN), 8630 Fenton St., #412, Silver Spring, MD 20910-3805.

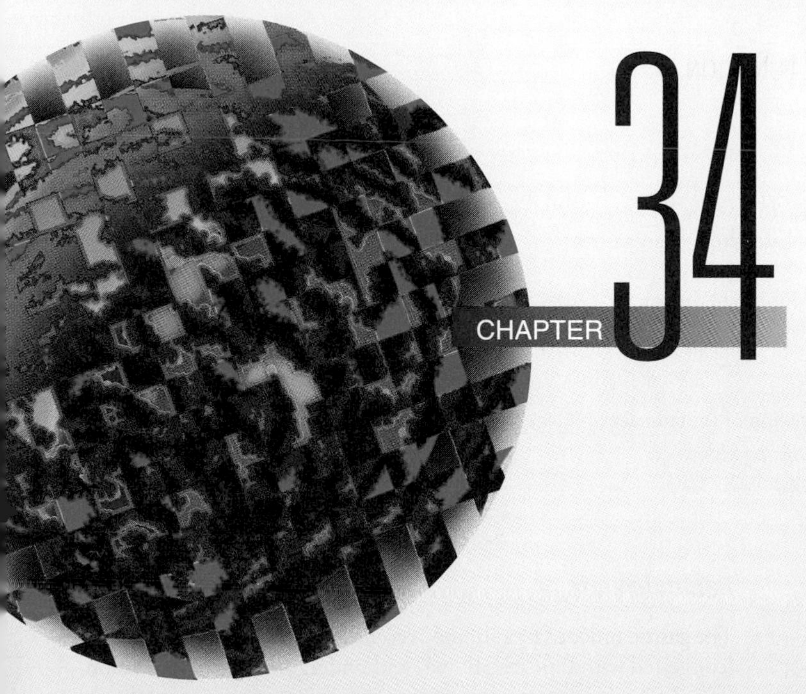

Management of Patients With Gastric and Duodenal Disorders

Learning Objectives

On completion of this chapter, the learner will be able to:

1. Compare the etiology, clinical manifestations, and management of acute gastritis, chronic gastritis, and peptic ulcer.
2. Use the nursing process as a framework for care of patients with gastritis.
3. Use the nursing process as a framework for care of patients with peptic ulcer.
4. Describe the dietary, pharmacologic, and surgical treatment of peptic ulcer.
5. Describe the nursing management of patients who undergo surgical procedures to treat obesity.
6. Use the nursing process as a framework for care of patients with gastric cancer.
7. Use the nursing process as a framework for care of patients undergoing gastric surgery.
8. Identify the complications of gastric surgery and their prevention and management.
9. Describe the home health care needs of the patient who has had gastric surgery.

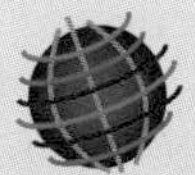

Nutritional status depends not only on the type and amount of intake but also on the functioning of the gastric and intestinal portions of the gastrointestinal (GI) system. This chapter describes disorders of the stomach and duodenum and their treatment.

GLOSSARY

antrectomy: removal of the pyloric (antrum) portion of the stomach with anastomosis (surgical connection) to the duodenum (gastroduodenostomy or Billroth I) or anastomosis to the jejunum (gastrojejunostomy or Billroth II)

dumping syndrome: physiologic response to rapid emptying of gastric contents into the jejunum, manifested by nausea, weakness, sweating, palpitations, syncope, and possibly diarrhea. Occurs in patients who have had partial gastrectomy and gastrojejunostomy.

duodenum: first portion of the small intestine, between the stomach and the jejunum

gastric: stomach

gastritis: inflammation of the stomach

hematemesis: vomiting blood

melena: tarry or black stools indicative of blood in stools

morbid obesity: 100 pounds or more over ideal body weight

pyloric orifice: opening between the stomach and the duodenum

pyloroplasty: surgical procedure to increase the opening of the pyloric orifice

pyrosis: heartburn

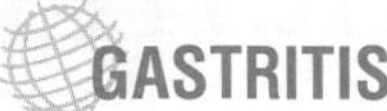

GASTRITIS

Gastritis (inflammation of the gastric or stomach mucosa) is a common GI problem. Gastritis may be acute, lasting several hours to a few days, or chronic, resulting from repeated exposure to irritating agents or recurring episodes of acute gastritis.

Acute gastritis is often due to dietary indiscretion—the person eats food that is contaminated with disease-causing microorganisms or that is irritating or too highly seasoned. Other causes of acute gastritis include overuse of aspirin and other nonsteroidal anti-inflammatory agents (NSAIDs), excessive alcohol intake, bile reflux, or radiation therapy. A more severe form of acute gastritis is caused by the ingestion of strong acid or alkali, which may cause the mucosa to become gangrenous or to perforate. Scarring can occur, resulting in pyloric obstruction. Gastritis also may be the first sign of an acute systemic infection.

Chronic gastritis and prolonged inflammation of the stomach may be caused by either benign or malignant ulcers of the stomach, or by the bacteria *Helicobacter pylori* (*H. pylori*) . Chronic gastritis is sometimes associated with autoimmune diseases such as pernicious anemia; dietary factors such as hot drinks or spices; the use of drugs, especially NSAIDs; alcohol; smoking; or reflux of intestinal contents into the stomach.

Pathophysiology

The gastric mucous membrane becomes edematous and hyperemic (congested with fluid and blood) and undergoes superficial erosion (Fig. 34-1). It secretes a scanty amount of gastric juice, containing very little acid but much mucus. Superficial ulceration may occur and can lead to hemorrhage.

Clinical Manifestations

The patient with acute gastritis may have abdominal discomfort, headache, lassitude, nausea, anorexia, vomiting, and hiccuping. Some patients, however, are asymptomatic. The patient with chronic gastritis may have symptoms of vitamin B_{12} deficiency or may complain of anorexia, heartburn after eating, belching, a sour taste in the mouth, or nausea and vomiting.

Assessment and Diagnostic Findings

Gastritis is sometimes associated with achlorhydria or hypochlorhydria (absence or low levels of hydrochloric acid) or with hyperchlorhydria (high levels of hydrochloric acid). Diagnosis

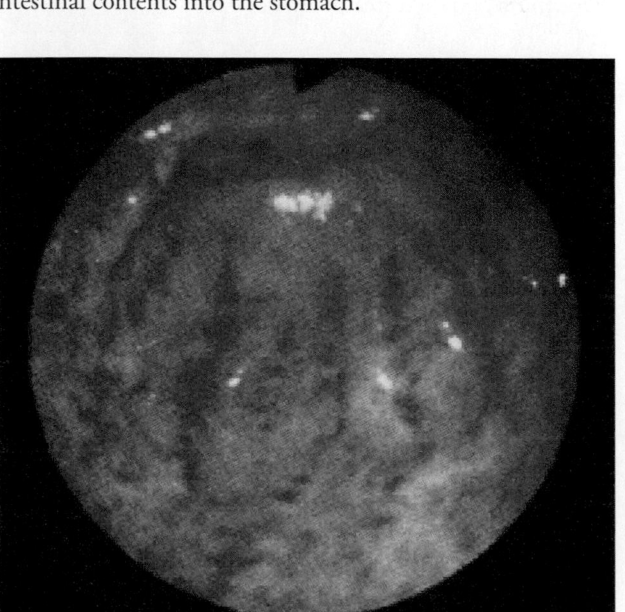

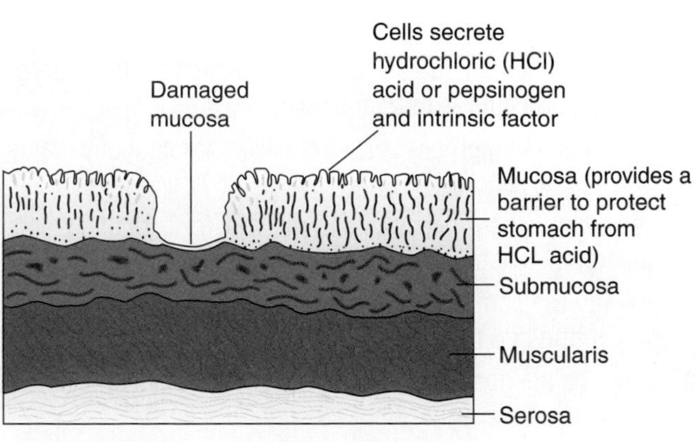

FIGURE 34•1 Endoscopic view of erosive gastritis (*left*). Damage from irritants (*right*) results in increased intracellular pH, impaired enzyme function, disrupted cellular structures, ischemia, vascular stasis, and tissue death. From Porth, C. (1998). *Pathophysiology: Concepts of altered health states* (5th ed.). Philadelphia: Lippincott Raven.

can be determined by endoscopy, an upper GI x-ray series, and histologic examination of a biopsy specimen. In addition to biopsy, other diagnostic measures for detecting *H. pylori* include serologic testing for antibodies for the *H. pylori* antigen, and a breath test.

Medical Management

The gastric mucosa is capable of repairing itself after a bout of gastritis. As a rule, the patient recovers in about a day, although the appetite may be diminished for an additional 2 or 3 days. Acute gastritis is also managed by instructing the patient to refrain from alcohol and food until symptoms subside. When the patient is able to take nourishment by mouth, a nonirritating diet is recommended. If the symptoms persist, fluids may need to be administered parenterally. If bleeding is present, management is similar to the procedures used for upper GI tract hemorrhage discussed later in this chapter.

If gastritis is due to ingestion of strong acids or alkalis, treatment consists of diluting and neutralizing the offending agent. To neutralize acids, common antacids (eg, aluminum hydroxide) are used; to neutralize an alkali, diluted lemon juice or diluted vinegar is used. If corrosion is extensive or severe, emetics and lavage are avoided because of the danger of perforation and damage to the esophagus.

Therapy is supportive and may include nasogastric intubation, analgesics and sedatives, antacids, and intravenous (IV) fluids. Fiberoptic endoscopy may be necessary. In extreme cases, emergency surgery may be required to remove gangrenous or perforated tissue. Gastrojejunostomy or gastric resection may be necessary to treat pyloric obstruction, a narrowing of the pyloric orifice.

Chronic gastritis is managed by modifying the patient's diet, promoting rest, reducing stress, and initiating pharmacotherapy. *H. pylori* may be treated with antibiotics (eg, tetracycline or amoxicillin) and bismuth salts (Pepto-Bismol). Patients with gastritis from vitamin deficiency usually have evidence of malabsorption of vitamin B_{12} caused by the presence of antibodies against intrinsic factor.

NURSING PROCESS: THE PATIENT WITH GASTRITIS

Assessment

When obtaining the history, the nurse asks about the patient's presenting signs and symptoms. Does the patient have heartburn, indigestion, nausea, or vomiting? Do the symptoms occur at any specific time of the day, before or after meals, after ingesting spicy or irritating foods, or after the ingestion of certain drugs or alcohol? Has there been recent weight gain or loss? Are the symptoms related to anxiety, stress, allergies, eating or drinking too much, or eating too quickly? How are the symptoms relieved? Is there a history of previous gastric disease or surgery? A diet history plus a 72-hour diet recall may be helpful. A thorough history is important in that it helps the nurse to identify whether known dietary excesses or other indiscretions are associated with the current symptoms, whether others in the patient's environment have similar symptoms, whether the patient is vomiting blood, and whether any known caustic element has been swallowed. The length of time that the current symptoms last and any methods used by the patient to treat these symptoms, and their effects, are also identified.

Signs to note during the physical examination include abdominal tenderness, dehydration, and evidence of any systemic disorder that might be responsible for the symptoms of gastritis.

Nursing Diagnosis

Based on the assessment data, the patient's major nursing diagnoses may include the following:

- Anxiety related to treatment
- Altered nutrition, less than body requirements, related to inadequate intake of nutrients
- Risk for fluid volume deficit related to insufficient fluid intake and excessive fluid loss subsequent to vomiting
- Knowledge deficit about dietary management and disease process
- Pain related to irritated stomach mucosa

Planning and Goals

The major goals of the patient may be reducing anxiety, avoiding irritating foods, ensuring adequate intake of nutrients, maintaining fluid balance, increasing awareness of dietary management, and relieving pain.

Nursing Interventions

Reducing Anxiety

If the patient has ingested acids or alkalis, emergency measures may be needed. Supportive therapy is offered to the patient and family during treatment and after the ingested acid or alkali has been neutralized or diluted. The patient may need to be prepared for additional diagnostic studies (endoscopy) or surgery. Anxiety about the pain and treatment modalities is usually present, as well as fear of permanent damage to the esophagus. The nurse uses a calm approach to assess the patient and to answer all questions as completely as possible. All procedures and treatments are explained according to the patient's interest and level of understanding.

Promoting Optimal Nutrition

For acute gastritis, physical and emotional support is provided and the patient is helped to manage the symptoms, which may include nausea, vomiting, heartburn, and fatigue. Foods and fluids by mouth will be withheld for hours or days until the acute symptoms subside, thus allowing the gastric mucosa to heal. If IV therapy is necessary, it is monitored regularly, as are serum electrolyte values. When the symptoms subside, the patient is offered ice chips followed by clear liquids. Solid food is introduced as soon as possible to provide oral nutrition, decrease the need for IV therapy, and minimize irritation to the gastric mucosa. As food is introduced, any symptoms suggesting a repeat episode of gastritis are evaluated and reported.

The intake of caffeinated beverages is discouraged because caffeine is a central nervous system stimulant that increases gastric activity and pepsin secretion. The use of alcohol is also discouraged, as is cigarette smoking because nicotine reduces the secretion of pancreatic bicarbonate and thus inhibits the neutralization of gastric acid in the duodenum. Nicotine also increases parasympathetic stimulation, which increases muscular activity in the bowel and can lead to nausea and vomiting. When appropriate, the patient is referred for alcohol counseling and smoking cessation programs.

Promoting Fluid Balance

Daily fluid intake and output are monitored to detect early signs of dehydration (minimal urine output of 30 mL/hour, minimal intake of 1.5 L/day). If food and fluids are withheld, IV fluids (3 L/day) are usually prescribed. Fluid intake plus caloric value

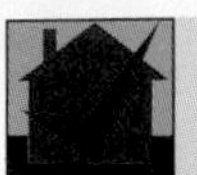

Home Care Teaching Checklist: The Patient With Gastritis

At the completion of the program, the patient or caregiver will be able to:

	Patient	Caregiver
• State foods and other substances that may cause gastritis.	✔	✔
• State medication regimen to follow.	✔	✔
• State need for vitamin B_{12} injections if patient has pernicious anemia.	✔	✔

is measured (1 L 5% dextrose in water = 170 calories of carbohydrate). Electrolyte values (sodium, potassium, chloride) may be assessed every 24 hours to detect imbalance.

The nurse must always be alert for any indicators of hemorrhagic gastritis: **hematemesis** (vomiting of blood), tachycardia, and hypotension. If these occur, the physician is alerted, vital signs are monitored as the patient's condition warrants, and the guidelines for managing upper GI tract bleeding, discussed later in the chapter, are followed.

Relieving Pain

The patient is instructed to avoid foods and beverages that may be irritating to the gastric mucosa (see above). The patient is also instructed in the use of medications to relieve chronic gastritis. The nurse assesses the patient's level of pain and the extent of comfort attained from the use of medications and avoidance of irritating substances.

Promoting Home and Community-Based Care

TEACHING PATIENTS SELF-CARE

The patient's knowledge about gastritis is evaluated and an individualized teaching plan is developed that includes information about stress management, diet, and medications. Dietary instructions take into account the patient's daily caloric needs, food preferences, and pattern of eating. Foods and other substances to be avoided (eg, spicy, irritating, or highly seasoned foods; caffeine; nicotine; alcohol) are reviewed. Consultation with a nutritionist may be indicated.

Providing information about prescribed antibiotics, bismuth salts, medications to decrease gastric secretion, and medications to protect mucosal cells from gastric secretions can help the patient recover and prevent recurrence. Patients with pernicious anemia need information about long-term vitamin B_{12} injections; a family member may be instructed in the administration of these injections, or arrangements can be made for the patient to receive the injections from a health care provider.

Evaluation

Expected Outcomes

Expected outcomes may include:

1. Exhibits less anxiety
2. Avoids eating irritating foods or drinking caffeinated beverages or alcohol
3. Maintains fluid balance
   a. Tolerates intravenous therapy of at least 1.5 L daily
   b. Drinks six to eight glasses of water daily
   c. Has a urinary output of about 1 L daily
   d. Displays adequate skin turgor
4. Adheres to medical regimen
   a. Selects nonirritating foods and beverages
   b. Takes medications as prescribed
5. Maintains appropriate weight
6. Reports less pain

PEPTIC ULCER

A peptic ulcer is an excavation (hollowed-out area) formed in the mucosal wall of the stomach, the pylorus (opening between stomach and duodenum), the duodenum (first part of small intestine), or the esophagus. A peptic ulcer is frequently referred to as a gastric, duodenal, or esophageal ulcer, depending on its location, or as peptic ulcer disease. It is caused by the erosion of a circumscribed area of mucous membrane (Fig. 34-2). This erosion may extend as deeply as the muscle layers or through the muscle to the peritoneum. Peptic ulcers are more likely to be in the duodenum than in the stomach. As a rule they occur alone, but they may occur in multiples. Chronic gastric ulcers tend to occur in the lesser curvature of the stomach, near the pylorus. Table 34-1 compares the features of gastric and duodenal ulcers.

Zollinger-Ellison syndrome (ZES), which consists of severe peptic ulcers, extreme gastric hyperacidity, and gastrin-secreting benign or malignant tumors of the pancreas, is a type of peptic ulceration. Stress ulcers, which are clinically different from peptic ulcers, are ulcerations in the mucosa that can occur in the gastroduodenal area. Both of these conditions are discussed with peptic ulcers.

The gram-negative bacteria *H. pylori* is present in 70% of patients with gastric ulcers and 95% of patients with duodenal ulcers. It is not associated with esophageal ulcers. Peptic ulcers treated with antibiotics to eradicate *H. pylori* have a 10% recurrence rate; those not treated for *H. pylori* have a 95% recurrence rate. The disease occurs with the greatest frequency in people between the ages of 40 and 60 years. It is relatively uncommon in women of childbearing age, but it has been observed in children and even in infants. After menopause, the incidence of peptic ulcers in women is almost equal to that in men. Peptic ulcers in the body of the stomach can occur without excessive acid secretion.

In the past, stress and anxiety were thought to be causative factors in ulcer occurrence. Ulcers do seem to develop more commonly in people who are tense, but whether this is a contributing factor to the condition is uncertain. The presence of excessive secretion of hydrochloric acid in the stomach may contribute to the formation of gastric ulcers, and stress may be associated with an increase in hydrochloric acid secretion. The ingestion of milk and caffeinated beverages, smoking, and alcohol may also increase hydrochloric acid secretion.

Familial tendency may be a significant predisposing factor. A further genetic link is noted in the finding that people with blood type O are more susceptible to peptic ulcers than those with blood type A, B, or AB.

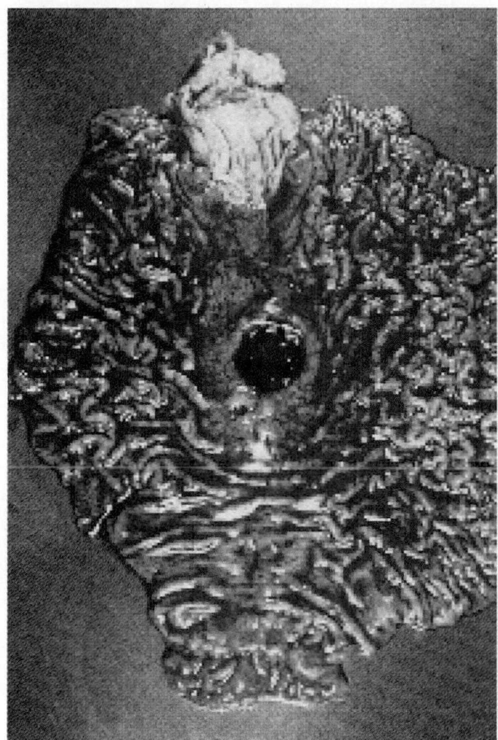

FIGURE 34•2 Deep peptic ulcer. From Porth, C. (1998). *Pathophysiology: Concepts of altered health states* (5th ed). Philadelphia: Lippincott Raven.

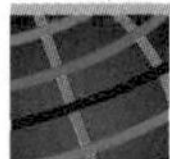

TABLE 34•1 Comparing Duodenal and Gastric Ulcers

Duodenal Ulcer	Gastric Ulcer
Incidence	
Age 30–60	Usually 50 and over
Male : female 2–3 : 1	Male : female 1 : 1
80% of peptic ulcers are duodenal	15% of peptic ulcers are gastric
Signs, Symptoms, and Clinical Findings	
Hypersecretion of stomach acid	Normal–hyposecretion of stomach acid
May have weight gain	Weight loss may occur
Pain occurs 2–3 hours after a meal; often awakened between 1–2 AM; ingestion of food relieves pain	Pain occurs ½ to 1 hour after a meal; rarely occurs at night; may be relieved by vomiting; ingestion of food does not help, sometimes increases pain
Vomiting uncommon	Vomiting common
Hemorrhage less likely than with gastric ulcer, but if present melena more common than hematemesis	Hemorrhage more likely to occur than with duodenal ulcer; hematemesis more common than melena
More likely to perforate than gastric ulcers	
Malignancy Possibility	
Rare	Occasionally
Risk Factors	
H. pylori, blood group O, chronic obstructive lung disease, chronic renal failure, alcohol, smoking, cirrhosis, stress	*H. pylori,* gastritis, alcohol, smoking, NSAIDs, stress

Predisposing factors associated with peptic ulcer include chronic use of NSAIDs, alcohol ingestion, and excessive smoking. Rarely, ulcers are due to excessive amounts of the hormone gastrin, produced by tumors (gastrinomas—ZES). Stress ulcers may also occur in patients exposed to stressful conditions. Esophageal ulcers occur as a result of the backward flow of hydrochloric acid from the stomach into the esophagus (gastroesophageal reflux disease).

Pathophysiology

In response to the ingestion of food, acetylcholine, gastrin, and histamine bind to specific receptors and stimulate the parietal cells in the fundus of the stomach to secrete hydrochloric acid (gastric acid). The parietal cells, with the assistance of the hydrogen–potassium adenosine triphosphatase (H^+, K^+-ATPase) pump, then transport the hydrochloric acid to the stomach lumen. Chief cells in the stomach secrete pepsinogen, which converts to pepsin in the presence of hydrochloric acid. The pepsin assists in the breakdown of food. Duodenal cells in the gastric epithelium secrete a mucous barrier to protect the lining of the gastroduodenal area.

Peptic ulcers occur mainly in the gastroduodenal mucosa because this tissue cannot withstand the digestive action of gastric acid (hydrochloric acid) and pepsin. The erosion is due to the increased concentration or activity of acid-pepsin, or to decreased resistance of the mucosa. A damaged mucosa cannot secrete enough mucus to act as a barrier against hydrochloric acid. The use of NSAIDs inhibits the secretion of mucus that protects the mucosa.

ZES is suspected when a patient has several peptic ulcers or an ulcer that is resistant to standard medical therapy. It is identified by the following findings: hypersecretion of gastric juice, duodenal ulcers, and gastrinomas (islet cell tumors) in the pancreas. Ninety percent of tumors are found in the "gastric triangle," which encompasses the cystic and common bile ducts, the second and third portions of the duodenum, and the neck and body of the pancreas. Approximately one third of gastrinomas are malignant. Diarrhea and steatorrhea (unabsorbed fat in the stool) may be evident. The patient may have coexistent parathyroid adenomas or hyperplasia and may therefore exhibit signs of hypercalcemia. The most common complaint is epigastric pain. *H. pylori* is not a risk factor for ZES.

Stress ulcer is the term given to the acute mucosal ulceration of the duodenal or gastric area that occurs after physiologically stressful events. Stressful conditions such as burns, shock, severe sepsis, and multiple organ trauma can initiate the development of stress ulcers. These ulcers seem to be most common in ventilator-dependent posttraumatic and postsurgical patients. Fiberoptic endoscopy within 24 hours of injury reveals shallow erosions of the stomach wall; by 72 hours, multiple gastric erosions are observed. As the stressful condition continues, the ulcers spread. When the patient recovers, the lesions are reversed. This pattern is typical of stress ulceration.

Differences of opinion exist as to the actual cause of mucosal ulceration in stress ulcers. Usually, it is preceded by shock; this leads to decreased gastric mucosal blood flow and to reflux of duodenal contents into the stomach. In addition, large quantities of pepsin are released. The combination of ischemia, acid, and pepsin creates an ideal climate for ulceration.

Stress ulcers should be distinguished from Cushing's ulcers and Curling's ulcers, two other types of gastric ulcers. Cushing's ulcers are common in patients with trauma to the brain. They may occur in the esophagus, stomach, or duodenum and are usually deeper and more penetrating than stress ulcers. Curling's ulcer is frequently observed about 72 hours after extensive burns and involves the antrum of the stomach or the duodenum.

Clinical Manifestations

Symptoms of an ulcer may last for a few days, weeks, or months and may disappear only to reappear, often without an identifiable cause. Many people have symptomless ulcers, and in 20% to 30% perforation or hemorrhage may occur without any preceding manifestations.

As a rule, the patient with an ulcer complains of dull, gnawing pain or a burning sensation in the midepigastrium or in the back. It is believed that the pain occurs when the increased acid content of the stomach and duodenum erodes the lesion and stimulates the exposed nerve endings. Another theory suggests that contact of the lesion with acid stimulates a local reflex mechanism that initiates contraction of the adjacent smooth muscle. Pain is usually relieved by eating, because food neutralizes the acid, or by taking alkali; however, once the stomach has emptied or the alkali's effect decreases, the pain returns. Sharply localized tenderness can be elicited by applying gentle pressure to the epigastrium at or slightly to the right of the midline. Some relief is obtained by applying local pressure on the epigastrium.

Other symptoms include **pyrosis** (heartburn), vomiting, constipation or diarrhea, or bleeding. Pyrosis is a burning sensation in the esophagus and stomach that moves up to the mouth, occasionally with sour eructation. Heartburn is often accompanied by eructation, or burping, which is common when the patient's stomach is empty.

Although rare in uncomplicated duodenal ulcer, vomiting may be a symptom of a complication of peptic ulcer. It results from obstruction of the pyloric orifice, caused by either muscular spasm of the pylorus or mechanical obstruction from scarring or acute swelling of the inflamed mucous membrane adjacent to the ulcer. Vomiting may or may not be preceded by nausea; usually it follows a bout of severe pain and bloating, which is relieved by ejection of the gastric contents. Emesis often contains undigested food eaten many hours earlier. Constipation or diarrhea can occur, probably as a result of diet and medications.

Twenty-five percent of patients with gastric ulcers experience bleeding. Patients may present with GI bleeding as evidenced by the passage of tarry stools. A small portion of patients who bleed from an acute ulcer have had no previous digestive complaints, but they develop symptoms thereafter.

Assessment and Diagnostic Findings

A physical examination may reveal pain, epigastric tenderness, or abdominal distention. A barium study of the upper GI tract may show an ulcer; however, endoscopy is the preferred diagnostic procedure because it allows direct visualization of inflammatory changes, ulcers, and lesions. Through endoscopy, a biopsy of the gastric mucosa and any suspicious lesions can be obtained. Endoscopy may reveal lesions not evident on x-ray studies because of their size or location.

Stools may be tested periodically until they are negative for occult blood. Gastric secretory studies are of value in diagnosing achlorhydria and ZES. *H. pylori* infection may be determined by biopsy and histology with culture. There is also a breath test that detects *H. pylori*, as well as a serologic test for antibodies to the *H. pylori* antigen. Pain that is relieved by ingesting food or antacids and the absence of pain on arising are also highly suggestive of an ulcer.

Medical Management

Once the diagnosis is established, the patient is informed that the problem can be kept under control, although remissions and recurrences are possible. The goal is to eradicate *H. pylori* and/or manage gastric acidity. Methods used for this include medications, lifestyle changes, and surgical intervention.

PHARMACOLOGIC THERAPY

Currently, the most commonly used therapy in the treatment of ulcers is a combination of antibiotics and bismuth salts that suppresses or eradicates *H. pylori*. Treatment may also include the following:

- Histamine receptor antagonists (H_2 receptor antagonists), which decrease the acid secretion in the stomach
- Proton pump inhibitors, which also decrease acid secretion
- Cytoprotective agents, which protect the mucosal cells from acid or NSAIDs
- Antacids

Table 34-2 lists some of the medications used in the treatment of peptic ulcers.

The patient is advised to adhere to the medication regimen to ensure complete healing of the ulcer. Because most patients become symptom-free in a week, it becomes a nursing goal to stress the importance of following the prescribed regimen so that the healing process can continue uninterrupted and the return of chronic ulcer symptoms can be prevented. Rest, sedatives, and tranquilizers may add to the patient's comfort and are used as needed. Maintenance dosages of H_2 receptor antagonists are usually recommended for 1 year.

For patients with ZES, hypersecretion of acid may be controlled with high doses of H_2 receptor antagonists. These patients may require twice the normal dose, and dosages usually need to be increased with prolonged use. Patients may also be prescribed octreotide (Sandostatin), a medication that suppresses gastrin levels.

Patients at risk for stress ulcers may be treated prophylactically with intravenous H_2 receptor antagonists, and cytoprotective agents because of the risk for upper GI tract hemorrhage. Frequent gastric aspiration is performed to monitor pH.

STRESS REDUCTION AND REST

Reducing environmental stress is a difficult task requiring physical and psychological interventions on the patient's part and the aid and cooperation of family members and significant others. The patient may need help in identifying situations that are stressful or exhausting. A rushed lifestyle and an irregular schedule may aggravate symptoms and interfere with regular meals taken in relaxed settings and with the regular administration of medications. The patient also may benefit from regular rest periods during the day, at least during the acute phase of the disease. Biofeedback, hypnosis, or behavior modification may be helpful.

SMOKING CESSATION

Studies have shown that smoking decreases the secretion of bicarbonate from the pancreas into the duodenum, resulting in increased acidity of the duodenum. Research indicates that

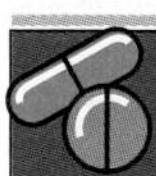

TABLE 34•2 **Drug Therapy for Peptic Ulcer Disease**

Medication	Major Action	Effects and Selected Nursing Considerations
Antibiotics and Bismuth Salts		
tetracycline (plus metronidazole and bismuth salts)	Exerts bacteriostatic effects to eradicate *H. pylori* bacteria in the gastric mucosa	May cause photosensitivity reaction; warn patient to use sunscreen. Use with caution in patients with renal or hepatic impairment. When taken with milk or dairy products, medication effectiveness may be reduced.
amoxicillin (plus metronidazole and bismuth salts or with high dose of proton pump inhibitor)	A bactericidal antibiotic that assists with eradicating *H. pylori* bacteria in the gastric mucosa	May cause diarrhea Do not use in patients allergic to penicillin.
metronidazole (Flagyl)	An amebicide that assists with eradicating *H. pylori* bacteria in the gastric mucosa	Give with meals to decrease GI distress. Given with other antibiotics and proton pump inhibitors
clarithromycin (Biaxin) (use with proton pump inhibitor or H_2 receptor antagonist)	Exerts bactericidal effects to eradicate *H. pylori* bacteria in the gastric mucosa	May cause GI upset
bismuth subsalicylate (Pepto-Bismol) (use with antibiotics)	Suppresses *H. pylori* bacteria in the gastric mucosa and helps mucosal lesions heal.	Given concurrently with antibiotics to cure *H. pylori* infection Should be taken on an empty stomach.
Histamine (H_2) Receptor Antagonists		
cimetidine (Tagamet)	Inhibits acid secretion by blocking the action of histamine on the histamine receptors of the parietal cell in the stomach	Least expensive of the H_2 receptor antagonists May cause confusion, agitation, or coma in the elderly or those with renal or hepatic insufficiency Long-term use may cause gynecomastia, impotence, and diarrhea.
ranitidine (Zantac)	Inhibits acid secretion by blocking the action of the histamine on the histamine receptors of the parietal cells in the stomach	Prolonged drug half-life in patients with renal and hepatic insufficiency Causes fewer side effects than cimetidine Rarely causes constipation, diarrhea, dizziness, and depression
famotidine (Pepcid)	Inhibits acid secretion by blocking the action of histamine on the histamine receptors on the parietal cells in the stomach.	Best choice for critically ill patients because it is known to have least risk of interaction with drugs other than cimetidine. (Unclear if other H_2 receptor antagonists are as safe as famotidine.) Does not alter drug metabolism in the liver. Prolonged half-life in patients with renal insufficiency Short-term relief for gastroesophageal reflux Dilute before IV injection. Rarely, causes constipation or diarrhea
nizantidine (Axid)	Inhibits acid secretion by blocking the action of histamine on the histamine receptors on the parietal cells in the stomach	Used for duodenal ulcers Prolonged half-life in patients with renal insufficiency Rarely, causes sweating, increased liver enzymes, nausea, urticaria
Proton (Gastric Acid) Pump Inhibitor		
omeprazole (Prilosec)	Decreases gastric acid secretion by slowing the hydrogen-potassium-adenosine triphosphatase (H^+, K^+-ATPase) pump on the surface of the parietal cells	Long-term use may cause gastric tumors and bacterial invasion.
Cytoprotective Medications		
misoprostol (Cytotec)	A synthetic prostaglandin. Protects the gastric mucosa from ulcerogenic agents. Increases mucus production and bicarbonate levels.	Used as a preventive method in patients using NSAIDs Administer with food. May cause diarrhea and cramping (including uterine cramping)
sucralfate (Carafate)	In the presence of gastric acid, sucralfate creates a viscous protective substance, forming a protective layer at the site of the ulcer, and prevents digestion by pepsin.	May cause constipation or nausea. Approved for duodenal ulcers, not gastric.

continuing to smoke cigarettes may significantly inhibit ulcer repair. Therefore, the patient is strongly encouraged to stop smoking. Smoking cessation support groups are helpful for many patients.

DIETARY MODIFICATION

The goal of the diet for patients with peptic ulcers is to avoid oversecretion of acid and hypermotility in the GI tract. These can be minimized by avoiding extremes of temperature and overstimulation by meat extracts, alcohol, caffeinated beverages, coffee (including decaffeinated coffee, which also stimulates acid secretion), and diets rich in milk and cream (which stimulate acid secretion). In addition, an effort is made to neutralize acid by eating three regular meals a day. Small, frequent feedings are not necessary as long as an antacid or a histamine blocker is taken. Diet compatibility becomes an individual matter: the patient eats foods that can be tolerated and avoids those that produce pain.

SURGICAL MANAGEMENT

The introduction of antibiotics to eradicate *H. pylori* and H_2 receptor antagonists as treatment for ulcers has greatly reduced the need for surgical interventions. However, surgery is usually recommended for patients with intractable ulcers (those that fail to heal after 12 to 16 weeks of medical treatment), life-threatening hemorrhage, perforation, or obstruction, or those with ZES not responding to medications. Surgical procedures include vagotomy, with or without pyloroplasty, or Billroth I or II (Fig. 34-3 and Table 34-3); see also the section on gastric surgery later in this chapter. Patients who need ulcer surgery may have had a long illness. They may be discouraged and have had interruptions in their work role and pressures in their family life.

FOLLOW-UP CARE

Recurrence within 1 year may be prevented with the prophylactic use of H_2 receptor antagonists given at a reduced dose. Not all patients require maintenance therapy; it may be prescribed only for those with two or three recurrences per year, those who have had a complication such as bleeding or outlet obstruction, or those who are candidates for gastric surgery but are at too high a risk for surgery. The likelihood of recurrence is reduced if the person avoids smoking, coffee (including decaffeinated coffee) and other caffeinated beverages, alcohol, and ulcerogenic medications (eg, NSAIDs).

NURSING PROCESS: THE PATIENT WITH A PEPTIC ULCER

Assessment

The patient is asked to describe the pain and the methods used to relieve it (food, antacids). Peptic ulcer pain is usually described as burning or gnawing; it occurs about 2 hours after a meal and frequently awakens the patient between midnight and 3 AM. The pain

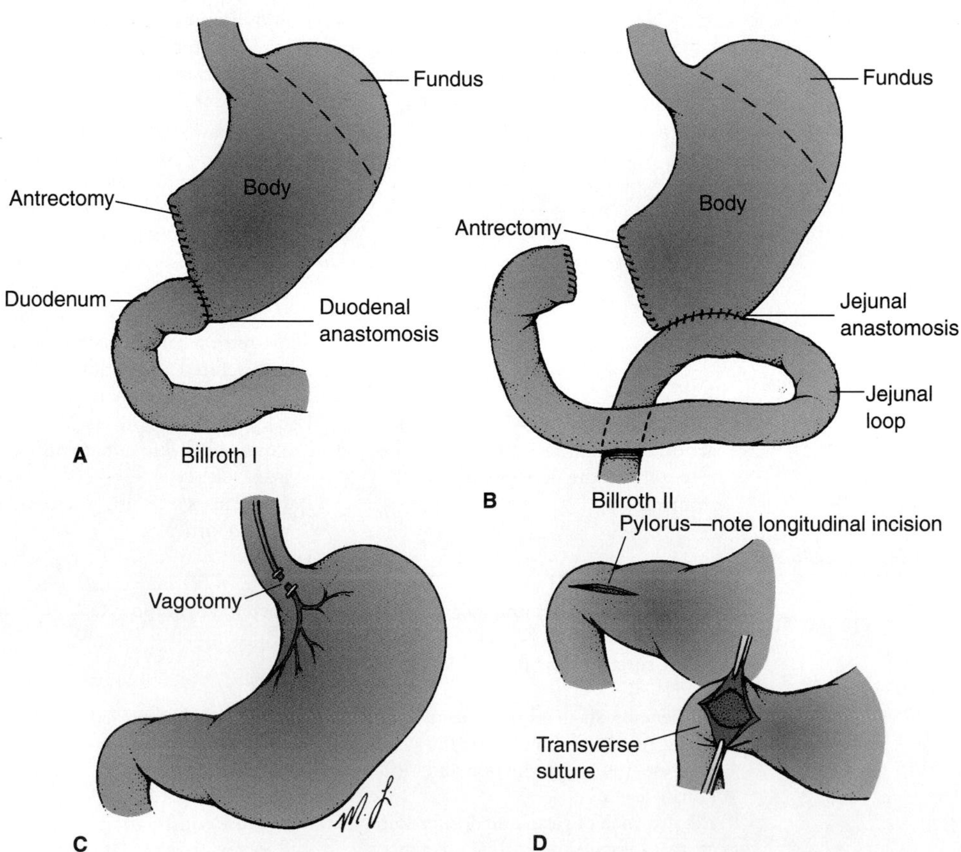

FIGURE 34•3 Surgical procedures for ulcer disease. (**A**) Antrectomy with anastomosis to the duodenum (gastroduodenostomy or Billroth I). (**B**) Antrectomy with anastomosis to the jejunum (gastrojejunostomy or Billroth II). (**C**) Severing of the vagus nerves (vagotomy). (**D**) Pyloroplasty—a longitudinal incision into the pylorus followed by a transverse suture to enlarge the opening.

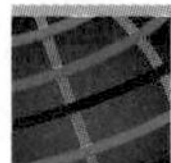

TABLE 34•3 **Surgical Procedures for Peptic Ulcer Disease**

Operation	Description	Comments
Vagotomy	Severing of the vagus nerve, which decreases gastric acid by diminishing cholinergic stimulation to the parietal cells, making them less responsive to gastrin	May be performed to reduce gastric acid secretion A drainage type of procedure (see pyloroplasty) is usually performed to assist with gastric emptying (as there is total denervation of the stomach). Some patients have problems with feelings of fullness, dumping syndrome, diarrhea, and gastritis.
Truncal vagotomy	Severing of the right and left vagus nerves as they enter the stomach at the distal part of the esophagus	This type of vagotomy is most commonly used to decrease acid secretions and reduce gastric and intestinal motility. Recurrence rate is 10%–15%.
Selective vagotomy	Severing of vagal innervation to the stomach but maintains innervation to the rest of the abdomen	
Proximal (parietal cell) gastric vagotomy without drainage	Denervates acid-secreting parietal cells but preserves vagal innervation to the gastric antrum and pylorus	No dumping syndrome. No need for drainage procedure Recurrence rate is 10–15%.
Pyloroplasty	A surgical procedure in which a longitudinal incision is made into the pylorus and transversely sutured closed to enlarge the outlet and relax the muscle	Usually accompanies truncal and selective vagotomies, which produce delayed gastric emptying due to decreased innervation
Antrectomy Billroth I (gastroduodenostomy) Billroth II (gastrojejunostomy)	Removal of the lower portion of the antral portion of the stomach (which contains the cells that secrete gastrin) as well as a small portion of the duodenum and pylorus. The remaining segment is anastomosed to the duodenum (Billroth I) or the jejunum (Billroth II).	May be performed in conjunction with a truncal vagotomy. The patient may have problems with feeling of fullness, dumping syndrome, and diarrhea. Recurrence rate is <1%.
Subtotal gastrectomy with Billroth I or II anastomosis	Removal of distal third of stomach; anastomosis with duodenum or jejunum. Removes gastrin-producing cells in the antrum and part of the parietal cells.	Dumping syndrome, anemia, malabsorption, weight loss; recurrence rate is 10%–15%.

is often relieved by taking antacids, eating, or vomiting. If the patient reports a recent history of vomiting, the nurse determines how often emesis has occurred and notes important characteristics of the vomitus—is it bright red, does it resemble coffee grounds, or is there undigested food from previous meals? Has the patient noted any bloody or tarry stools? The nurse also asks the patient to list the usual food intake for a 72-hour period and to describe food habits (speed of eating, regularity of meals, preference for spicy foods, use of seasonings, use of caffeinated beverages and coffee [both caffeinated and decaffeinated]). The patient's use of irritating substances is assessed. Does he or she smoke cigarettes? If yes, how many? Does the patient ingest alcohol? If yes, how much and how often? Are NSAIDs used? The nurse inquires about the patient's level of anxiety and his or her perception of current stressors. How does the patient express anger or cope with stressful situations? Is there occupational stress or problems within the family? Is there a family history of ulcer disease?

Vital signs are assessed and tachycardia and hypotension, which may indicate anemia from GI bleeding, are reported. The stool is examined for occult blood. A physical examination is performed, during which the abdomen is palpated for localized tenderness.

Diagnosis

Nursing Diagnoses

Based on the assessment data, the patient's nursing diagnoses may include the following:

- Pain related to the effect of gastric acid secretion on damaged tissue
- Anxiety related to coping with an acute disease
- Altered nutrition related to changes in diet
- Knowledge deficit about prevention of symptoms and management of the condition

Collaborative Problems/Potential Complications

Peptic ulcers may lead to the following complications:

- Hemorrhage
- Perforation
- Penetration
- Pyloric obstruction (gastric outlet obstruction)

Planning and Goals

The major goals of the patient may include relieving pain, reducing anxiety, maintaining nutrition requirements, learning about the management and prevention of ulcer recurrence, and avoiding complications.

Nursing Interventions

Relieving Pain

Pain relief can be attained with prescribed medications. Aspirin, foods and beverages that contain caffeine, and decaffeinated coffee are avoided. The patient is encouraged to eat regularly spaced meals in a relaxed atmosphere. The patient is further encouraged to learn relaxation techniques to help manage stress and pain and to enhance smoking cessation efforts.

Reducing Anxiety

The nurse assesses the patient's level of anxiety. Patients with peptic ulcers are usually anxious, but their anxiety is not always obvious. Information is provided at the patient's level of learning, and all questions are answered. The patient is encouraged to express fears openly. Diagnostic tests are explained, and medications are administered on schedule. The patient is assured that nurses are available to help with a problem. The nurse interacts with the patient in a relaxing manner and helps identify stressors and explains effective coping techniques and relaxation methods, such as biofeedback, hypnosis, or behavior modification. The nurse encourages the patient's family to participate in care and to provide emotional support.

Maintaining Optimal Nutritional Status

The patient is assessed for malnutrition and weight loss. Once recovered from an acute phase of peptic ulcer disease, the patient is instructed about the need to comply with the medication regimen and dietary restrictions.

Monitoring and Managing Potential Hemorrhage

Gastritis and hemorrhage from peptic ulcer are the two most common causes of upper GI tract bleeding. (Upper GI bleeding may also occur with esophageal varices, as discussed in Chap. 36.) Hemorrhage, the most common complication, occurs in about 20% of patients with peptic ulcers. The site of bleeding is usually the distal portion of the duodenum. Bleeding may be manifested by hematemesis or **melena** (tarry stools). The vomited blood can be bright red or have a "coffee grounds" appearance (which is dark) from the oxidation of hemoglobin to methemoglobin. When the hemorrhage is large (2000 to 3000 mL), most of the blood is vomited. Because large quantities of blood may be lost quickly, immediate correction of blood loss may be required to save the patient's life. When the hemorrhage is small, much or all of the blood is passed in the stools, which will appear tarry black because of the digested hemoglobin. Management depends on the amount of blood lost and the rate of bleeding.

The nurse assesses the patient for faintness or dizziness and nausea, which may precede or accompany bleeding. Vital signs are monitored frequently and the patient is evaluated for tachycardia, hypotension, and tachypnea. The hemoglobin and hematocrit are monitored. The stool is tested for gross or occult blood, and hourly urinary output is recorded to detect anuria or oliguria (absence or reduction of urine production).

Many times the bleeding from a peptic ulcer stops spontaneously; however, the incidence of recurrent bleeding is high. Because bleeding can be fatal, the cause and severity of the hemorrhage must be identified quickly and the blood loss treated to prevent hypovolemic shock. Management of upper GI tract bleeding consists of quickly determining the amount of blood lost and the rate of bleeding, rapidly replacing the blood that has been lost, stopping the bleeding, stabilizing the patient, and diagnosing and treating the cause. Related nursing and collaborative interventions include the following:

- Inserting a peripheral IV line for the infusion of saline or lactated Ringer's solution and blood. The nurse may need to assist with the placement of a pulmonary artery catheter for hemodynamic monitoring. Blood component therapy is initiated if there are signs of shock such as tachycardia, sweating, and coldness of the extremities.
- Monitoring the hemoglobin and hematocrit to assist in evaluating bleeding
- Inserting an indwelling urinary catheter and monitoring urinary output
- Inserting a nasogastric tube to distinguish fresh blood from "coffee grounds" material, to aid in the removal of clots and acid, to prevent nausea and vomiting, and to provide a means of monitoring further bleeding
- Monitoring the pH of gastric secretions hourly through the nasogastric tube, and administering antacids, if prescribed, for a pH less than 4
- Administering a room-temperature saline or water lavage
- Monitoring vital signs and oxygen saturation, and administering oxygen therapy
- Placing the patient in the recumbent position to prevent hypotension—or, to prevent aspiration from vomiting, placing the patient on the left side
- Treating hypovolemic shock (described in Chap. 14)

If bleeding cannot be managed by the measures just described, other treatment modalities may be used. Transendoscopic coagulation by laser, heat probe, medication, a sclerosing agent, or a combination of these therapies can halt bleeding and make surgical intervention unnecessary. There is much debate regarding how soon endoscopy should be performed. Some believe endoscopy should be performed in the first 24 hours after hemorrhage has been stabilized. Others believe endoscopy can be performed during acute bleeding, as long as the esophageal or gastric area can be visualized (visibility may be decreased because of the presence of blood).

Other methods to control bleeding include intra-arterial infusion of vasoconstricting medications and selective embolization. Intra-arterial infusion involves administering vasopressin by pump directly into the bleeding artery for 24 to 36 hours; a repeat arteriogram is needed to evaluate the efficacy of treatment. Selective embolization involves forcing emboli of autologous blood clots with or without Gelfoam (absorbable gelatin sponge) through a catheter to a point above the bleeding lesion. This procedure is performed by a radiologist.

Rebleeding may occur and often warrants surgical intervention. The patient is carefully monitored so that bleeding can be quickly detected. Signs of bleeding include tachycardia, tachypnea, hypotension, mental confusion, thirst, and oliguria. If bleeding recurs in 48 hours after medical therapy has begun, or if more than 6 to 10 units of blood are required in 24 hours to maintain blood volume, the patient is likely to require surgery. Some physicians rec-

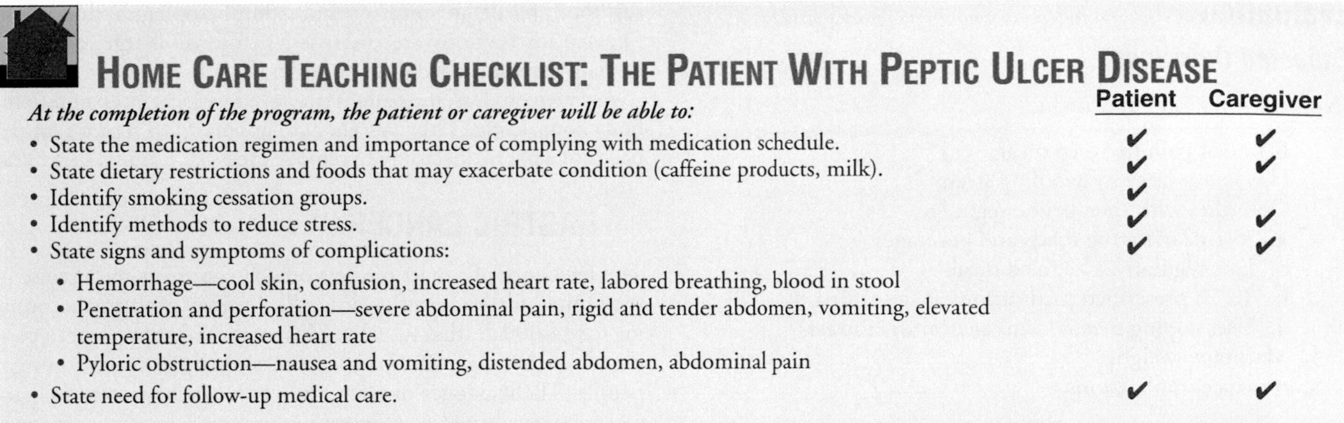

HOME CARE TEACHING CHECKLIST: THE PATIENT WITH PEPTIC ULCER DISEASE

At the completion of the program, the patient or caregiver will be able to:	Patient	Caregiver
• State the medication regimen and importance of complying with medication schedule.	✔	✔
• State dietary restrictions and foods that may exacerbate condition (caffeine products, milk).	✔	✔
• Identify smoking cessation groups.	✔	
• Identify methods to reduce stress.	✔	✔
• State signs and symptoms of complications:	✔	✔
• Hemorrhage—cool skin, confusion, increased heart rate, labored breathing, blood in stool		
• Penetration and perforation—severe abdominal pain, rigid and tender abdomen, vomiting, elevated temperature, increased heart rate		
• Pyloric obstruction—nausea and vomiting, distended abdomen, abdominal pain		
• State need for follow-up medical care.	✔	✔

ommend surgical intervention if a patient hemorrhages three times. Other criteria for surgery are the patient's age (in those older than age 60, massive hemorrhaging is three times more likely to be fatal), a history of chronic duodenal ulcer, and a coincidental gastric ulcer. The area of the ulcer is removed or the bleeding vessels are ligated. Many patients also undergo procedures aimed at controlling the underlying cause of the ulcers (eg, vagotomy and pyloroplasty, or gastrectomy).

Monitoring for Perforation and Penetration

Perforation is the erosion of the ulcer through the gastric serosa into the peritoneal cavity without warning. Perforation is an abdominal catastrophe and requires immediate surgery.

Penetration is erosion of the ulcer through the gastric serosa into adjacent structures such as the pancreas, biliary tract, or gastrohepatic omentum. Symptoms of penetration include back and epigastric pain not relieved by medications that were effective in the past. Like perforation, penetration usually requires surgical intervention.

Signs and symptoms of perforation include the following:

- Sudden, severe upper abdominal pain (persisting and increasing in intensity). Pain may be referred to the shoulders, especially the right shoulder, because of irritation of the phrenic nerve in the diaphragm.
- Vomiting and collapse (fainting)
- Extremely tender and rigid (boardlike) abdomen
- Hypotension and tachycardia, indicating shock

Immediate surgical intervention is indicated. Because chemical peritonitis develops within a few hours after perforation and is followed by bacterial peritonitis, the perforation must be closed as quickly as possible. In a few patients, it may be deemed safe and advisable to perform surgery for the ulcer disease in addition to suturing the perforation.

Postoperatively, the stomach contents are drained by means of a nasogastric tube. The nurse monitors fluid and electrolyte balance and assesses the patient for peritonitis or localized infection (increased temperature, abdominal pain, paralytic ileus, increased or absent bowel sounds, abdominal distention). Antibiotic therapy is given parenterally as prescribed.

Monitoring for Pyloric Obstruction

Pyloric obstruction occurs when the area distal to the pyloric sphincter becomes scarred and stenosed from spasm or edema or from scar tissue that forms when the ulcer alternately heals and breaks down. The patient has nausea and vomiting, constipation, epigastric fullness, anorexia, and (later) weight loss.

In treating the patient with pyloric obstruction, the first consideration is to insert a nasogastric tube to decompress the stomach. Confirming that obstruction is the cause of discomfort is accomplished by assessing the amount of fluid aspirated from the nasogastric tube. A residual of more than 200 mL is strongly suggestive of obstruction. Usually an upper GI study or endoscopy is performed to confirm gastric outlet obstruction. Decompressing the stomach and managing extracellular fluid volume and electrolyte balance may improve the patient's condition and avert the need for surgical intervention. If the obstruction is unrelieved by medical management, surgery (in the form of a vagotomy and antrectomy) may be required.

Promoting Home and Community-Based Care

TEACHING PATIENTS SELF-CARE

To manage ulcer disease successfully, the patient must understand the factors that will help or aggravate the condition. The nurse reviews information about medications to be taken at home, including name, dosage, frequency, and possible side effects, stressing the importance of continuing to take medications even after signs and symptoms have decreased or subsided. The patient is also instructed about medications to avoid. The patient is advised to avoid foods that exacerbate symptoms and to avoid substances that have acid-producing potential (eg, caffeinated beverages such as coffee, tea, and colas; alcohol). The patient is counseled regarding the importance of eating meals at regular times and in a relaxed setting, and avoiding overeating. If relevant, the patient is also informed about the irritant effects of smoking on the ulcer and is given information about smoking cessation programs.

The nurse reviews with the patient and family the signs and symptoms of complications to be reported:

- Hemorrhage: Cool skin, confusion, increased heart rate, labored breathing, blood in the stool
- Penetration and perforation: Severe abdominal pain, rigid and tender abdomen, vomiting, elevated temperature, increased heart rate
- Pyloric obstruction: Nausea, vomiting, distended abdomen, abdominal pain

The nurse reinforces the importance of follow-up care for approximately 1 year, the need to report recurrence of symptoms, and the need for treatment of possible postoperative sequelae such as intolerance to dairy products and sweet foods.

Evaluation

Expected Outcomes

Expected outcomes may include:

1. Is free of pain between meals
2. Has less anxiety by avoiding stress
3. Complies with therapeutic regimen
   a. Avoids irritating foods and beverages
   b. Eats regularly scheduled meals
   c. Takes prescribed medications as scheduled
   d. Uses coping mechanisms to deal with stress
4. Maintains weight
5. Avoids complications

MORBID OBESITY

One in three Americans is 20% or more over his or her ideal body weight. **Morbid obesity** is the term applied to people who are more than 100 pounds over their ideal body weight. Patients with morbid obesity are at higher risk for health complications such as cardiovascular disease, arthritis, asthmatic bronchitis, and diabetes. Conservative management consists of placing the person on a very-low-calorie diet in conjunction with behavioral modification; however, diet therapy is usually unsuccessful. If these conservative measures fail, surgery may be performed. (Some physicians recommend acupuncture and hypnosis before recommending surgery.)

The first surgical procedure to treat morbid obesity was the jejunoileal bypass. This procedure, which caused significant complications, has been largely replaced by gastric restriction procedures. Gastric bypass and vertical banded gastroplasty are the current reduction operations of choice. In gastric bypass surgery, the proximal segment of the stomach is transected to form a small pouch with a small gastroenterostomy stoma. The Roux-en-Y gastric bypass is the recommended procedure for long-term weight loss. In this procedure, a horizontal row of staples creates a stomach pouch with a 1-cm stoma that is anastomosed with a portion of distal jejunum, creating a gastroenterostomy. The transected proximal portion of the jejunum is anastomosed to the distal jejunum (Fig. 34-4**A**).

In vertical banded gastroplasty, a double row of staples is applied vertically along the lesser curvature of the stomach, beginning at the angle of His. A small stoma is created at the end of the staples by adding a circle of staples or a band of polypropylene mesh or silicone tubing (Fig. 34-4**B**).

General postoperative nursing care is similar to that for a patient recovering from a gastric resection, but with attention given to the risks of complications associated with morbid obesity. Postoperative complications that may occur in the immediate postoperative period include peritonitis, stomal obstruction, stomal ulcers, atelectasis and pneumonia, thromboembolism, and metabolic imbalances resulting from prolonged vomiting and diarrhea. After bowel sounds have returned and oral intake is resumed, six small feedings consisting of a total of 600 to 800 calories per day are provided and fluid intake is encouraged to prevent dehydration.

Patients are usually discharged in 1 week with detailed dietary instructions. They are instructed to report excessive thirst or concentrated urine, both of which are indications of dehydration. Psychosocial interventions are also essential for these patients. Efforts are directed toward helping them modify their eating behaviors and cope with changes in body image. Noncompliance by eating too much or too fast or eating high-calorie liquid and soft foods results in vomiting and painful esophageal distention. Dietary instructions are discussed before discharge, and outpatient visits are scheduled monthly.

After weight loss, the patient may need surgical intervention for body contouring. This may include lipoplasty to remove fat deposits or a panniculectomy to remove excess abdominal skin folds.

GASTRIC CANCER

The incidence of cancer of the stomach continues to decrease in the United States; however, it is still a serious problem, accounting for 14,000 deaths annually. Most of these deaths occur in people older than age 40, but they occasionally occur in younger people. The incidence of gastric cancer is much greater in Japan, which has instituted mass screening programs for earlier diagnosis. Diet appears to be a significant factor. A diet high in smoked foods and low in fruits and vegetables may increase the risk of gastric cancer. Other factors related to the incidence of gastric cancer include chronic inflammation of the stomach, pernicious anemia, achlorhydria, gastric ulcers, the presence of *H. pylori*, and heredity. The prognosis is poor because most patients have metastases at the time of diagnosis.

Pathophysiology

Most gastric cancers are adenocarcinomas and can occur in any portion of the stomach. The tumor infiltrates the surrounding mucosa, penetrating the wall of the stomach and adjacent organs and structures. The liver, pancreas, esophagus, and duodenum are often affected at the time of diagnosis. Metastasis through lymph to the peritoneal cavity occurs later in the disease.

Clinical Manifestations

The early symptoms of gastric cancer are often not definite because most of these tumors begin on the lesser curvature, where they cause little disturbance of gastric functions. In the early stages of gastric cancer, symptoms may be absent. Some studies have shown that early symptoms, such as pain relieved with antacids, resemble those of benign ulcers. Symptoms of progressive disease may include indigestion, anorexia, dyspepsia, weight loss, abdominal pain, constipation, anemia, and nausea and vomiting.

Assessment and Diagnostic Findings

Physical examination is usually not helpful because most gastric tumors are not palpable. Ascites may be present if there is metastasis to the liver. Endoscopy for biopsy and cytologic washings is the usual diagnostic study. X-ray examination of the upper GI tract with barium may also be done. Because metastasis often occurs before warning signs develop, a computed tomography (CT) scan, a bone scan, and a liver scan are valuable in determining the extent of the metastasis. Indigestion (dyspepsia) of more than 4 weeks' duration in any person older than age 40 calls for a complete x-ray examination of the GI tract.

Medical Management

There is no successful treatment for gastric carcinoma except removal of the tumor. If the tumor can be removed while it is still localized to the stomach, the patient can be cured. If the tumor has spread beyond the area that can be excised, cure is impossi-

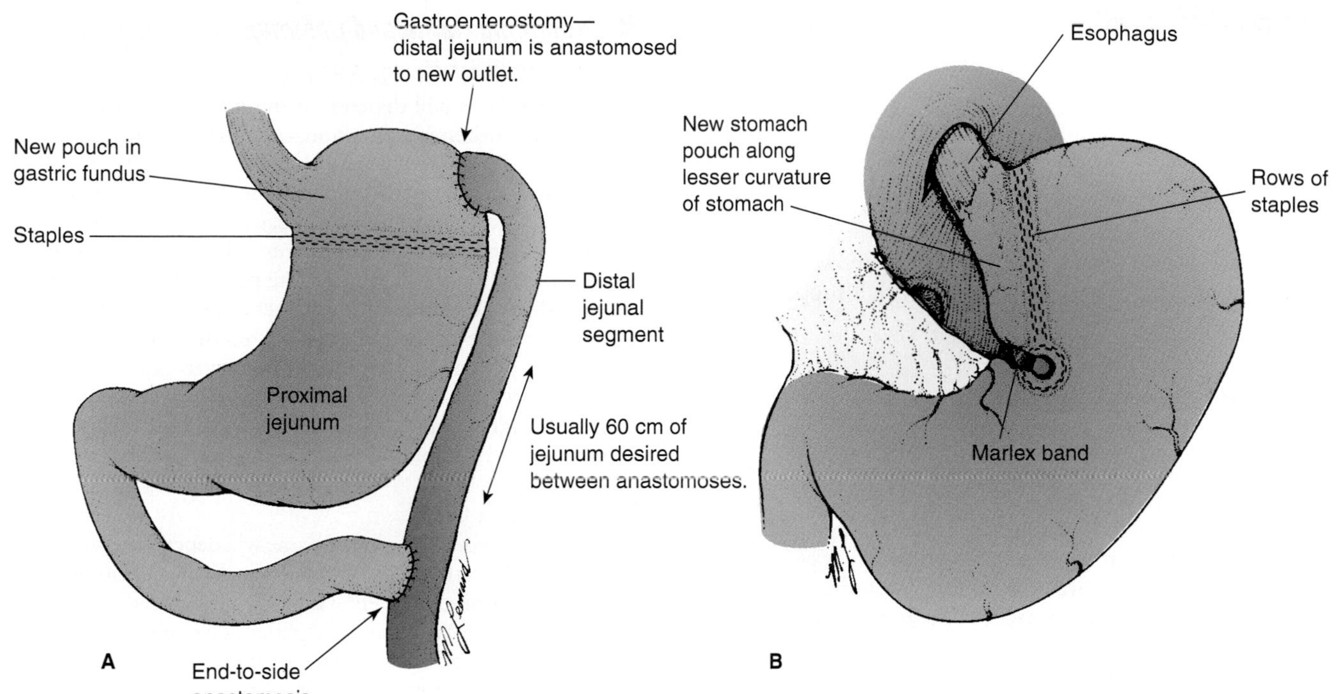

FIGURE 34•4 Surgical procedures for morbid obesity. (**A**) Gastric bypass with Roux-en-Y. A horizontal row of staples creates a pouch with a capacity of 50 mL or less. The proximal jejunum is transected and the distal end anastomosed to the new pouch. The proximal segment is anastomosed to the jejunum. (**B**) Vertical banded gastroplasty. A vertical row of staples along the lesser curvature of the stomach creates a new, smaller stomach pouch of 10–15 mL.

ble. In many of these patients, however, effective palliation to prevent symptoms such as obstruction may be obtained by resection of the tumor (see the section on gastric surgery below).

If a radical subtotal gastrectomy is performed, the stump of the stomach is anastomosed to the jejunum, as in the gastrectomy for ulcer. When a total gastrectomy is performed, GI continuity is restored by means of an anastomosis between the ends of the esophagus and jejunum. Palliative rather than radical surgery is performed if there is metastasis to other vital organs, such as the liver. Palliative surgery is performed to relieve symptoms of obstruction or dysphagia.

If surgical treatment does not offer cure, treatment with chemotherapy may offer further control of the disease or palliation. Commonly used chemotherapeutic drugs include a combination of 5-fluorouracil, doxorubicin (Adriamycin), and mitomycin-C. Radiation therapy may also be used for palliation. Assessment of tumor markers (blood analysis for antigens indicative of colon cancer) such as carcinoembryonic antigen, CA 19-9, and CA-50 may help determine the effectiveness of treatment. If these levels were elevated before treatment, they should decrease if the tumor is responding to the treatment.

NURSING PROCESS: THE PATIENT WITH GASTRIC CANCER

Assessment

The nurse elicits a dietary history from the patient, focusing on recent nutritional intake and status. Has the patient lost weight? If so, how much and over what period of time? Can the patient tolerate a full diet? If not, what foods can he or she eat? What other changes in eating habits have occurred? Does the patient have an appetite? Is the patient in pain? Do foods, antacids, or medications relieve the pain, make no difference, or worsen the pain? Is there a history of infection with *H. pylori* bacteria? Other health information to obtain includes the patient's smoking and alcohol history, as well as the family history: have any first- or second-degree relatives had gastric or other cancer? A psychosocial assessment including questions about social support, individual and family coping skills, and financial resources will help the nurse plan for care in acute and community settings.

After the interview, the nurse performs a complete physical examination and carefully assesses the abdomen for tenderness or masses. The nurse also observes for the presence of ascites.

Nursing Diagnosis

Based on the assessment data, the patient's major nursing diagnoses may include the following:

- Anxiety related to the disease and anticipated treatment
- Altered nutrition, less than body requirements, related to anorexia
- Pain related to the presence of abnormal epithelial cells
- Anticipatory grieving related to the diagnosis of cancer
- Knowledge deficit regarding self-care activities

Planning and Goals

The major goals for the patient may include reducing anxiety, attaining optimal nutrition, relieving pain, and adjusting to the diagnosis and to anticipated lifestyle changes.

Nursing Interventions

Reducing Anxiety

A relaxed, nonthreatening atmosphere is provided so that the patient can express fears, concerns, and possibly anger about the diagnosis and prognosis. The nurse encourages the family in their efforts to support the patient, offering assurance and supporting positive coping measures. The nurse advises the patient about any procedures and treatments so that the patient knows what to expect. The nurse also may suggest talking with a support person (eg, clergy), if desired.

Promoting Optimal Nutrition

The patient is encouraged to eat small, frequent portions of nonirritating foods to decrease gastric irritation. Food supplements should be high in calories as well as vitamins A and C and iron to enhance tissue repair. If the patient cannot eat enough to meet nutritional requirements, total parenteral nutrition may be necessary. Because the patient may develop dumping syndrome when enteral feeding resumes after gastric resection, the nurse explains ways to prevent and manage it (six small feedings daily that are low in carbohydrates and sugar; fluids between meals) and informs the patient that symptoms often resolve after several months. If a total gastrectomy is performed, parenteral vitamin B_{12} will be required indefinitely. The nurse monitors the IV therapy and nutritional status and records intake, output, and daily weights to ensure the patient is maintaining or gaining weight. Signs of dehydration (thirst, dry mucous membranes, poor skin turgor, tachycardia, decreased urine output) are assessed and the results of daily laboratory studies are reviewed to note any metabolic abnormalities (sodium, potassium, glucose, blood urea nitrogen). Antiemetics are administered as prescribed.

Relieving Pain

Analgesics are administered as prescribed. A continuous infusion of an opioid may be necessary for severe pain. The frequency, intensity, and duration of the pain are assessed to determine the effectiveness of the analgesic being administered. The nurse works with the patient to manage pain (eg, position changes). Nonpharmacologic methods for pain relief such as imagery, distraction, relaxation tapes, backrubs, and massage are suggested, and periods of rest and relaxation are encouraged.

Providing Psychosocial Support

The nurse helps the patient express fears, concerns, and grief about the diagnosis. The patient's questions are answered honestly, and the patient is encouraged to participate in treatment decisions. Some patients mourn the loss of a body part and perceive their surgery as a type of mutilation. Some express disbelief and need time and support to accept the diagnosis.

The nurse offers emotional support and involves family members and significant others whenever possible. This includes recognizing mood swings and defense mechanisms (denial, rationalization, displacement, regression) and reassuring the patient and family members that emotional responses are normal and expected. The services of clergy, psychiatric clinical nurse specialists, psychologists, social workers, and psychiatrists are made available, if needed. The nurse projects an empathetic attitude and spends time with the patient. Most patients will begin to participate in self-care activities when they have acknowledged their loss.

Promoting Home and Community-Based Care

TEACHING PATIENTS SELF-CARE

Self-care activities will depend on the mode of treatment used: surgery, chemotherapy, radiation, or palliative care. Patient and family teaching will include information about diet and nutrition, treatment regimens, activity and lifestyle changes, pain management, and possible complications. Consultation with a dietitian is essential to determine how the patient's nutritional needs can best be met at home. The patient or care provider is instructed about administration of enteral or parenteral nutrition. If chemotherapy or radiation is prescribed, explanations are given to the patient and family about what to expect: the length of treatments, the expected side effects (eg, nausea, vomiting, anorexia, fatigue, neutropenia), and the need for transportation to treatments. Psychological counseling may also be helpful.

CONTINUING CARE

The need for ongoing care in the home will depend on the patient's condition and treatment. Nutritional counseling is reinforced and the administration of any enteral or parenteral feedings is supervised by the home care nurse; the patient or family member must become skillful in administering the feeding and in detecting and preventing untoward effects or complications related to the feeding (see Chap. 33 to review management of enteral and parenteral feedings). The patient or family member is taught to record daily intake, output, and weight and is instructed how to manage pain, nausea, vomiting, or other symptoms. The patient or caregiver is also taught to recognize and report signs and symptoms of complications that require medical attention, such as bleeding, obstruction, perforation, or any symptoms that become progressively worse. The chemotherapy or radiation therapy regimen is explained. The patient and family need to know about the care that will be needed during and after treatments (see Chap. 15).

Evaluation

Expected Outcomes

Expected outcomes may include:

1. Is less anxious
   a. Expresses fears and concerns about surgery
   b. Seeks emotional support
2. Attains optimal nutrition
   a. Eats small, frequent meals high in calories, iron, and vitamins A and C
   b. Complies with enteral or parenteral nutrition as needed
3. Has less pain
4. Performs self-care activities and adjusts to lifestyle changes
   a. Resumes normal activities within 3 months
   b. Alternates periods of rest and activity
   c. Manages tube feedings

GASTRIC SURGERY

Gastric surgery may be performed on patients with peptic ulcers who have life-threatening hemorrhage, obstruction, perforation, or penetration or whose condition does not respond to medication. It also may be indicated for patients with gastric cancer or trauma. Surgical procedures include a partial gastrectomy (removal of the stomach) or total gastrectomy with either an end-to-end or end-to-side esophagojejunal anastomosis.

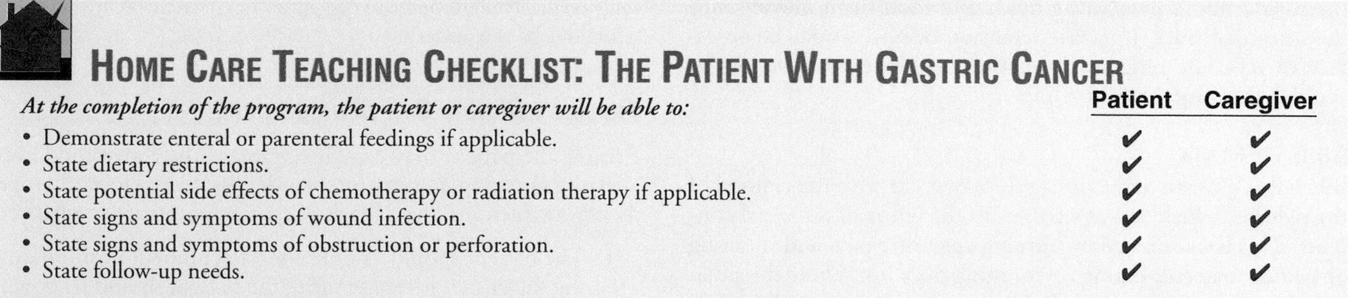

Home Care Teaching Checklist: The Patient With Gastric Cancer

At the completion of the program, the patient or caregiver will be able to:

	Patient	Caregiver
• Demonstrate enteral or parenteral feedings if applicable.	✔	✔
• State dietary restrictions.	✔	✔
• State potential side effects of chemotherapy or radiation therapy if applicable.	✔	✔
• State signs and symptoms of wound infection.	✔	✔
• State signs and symptoms of obstruction or perforation.	✔	✔
• State follow-up needs.	✔	✔

NURSING PROCESS: THE PATIENT UNDERGOING GASTRIC SURGERY

Assessment

Before surgery, the patient is assessed for knowledge of preoperative and postoperative surgical routines. The patient's and family's knowledge of the rationale for surgery is assessed. The patient's nutritional status is also assessed: Has the patient lost weight? How much? Over how much time? Does the patient have nausea and vomiting? Has the patient had hematemesis? The patient is assessed for the presence of bowel sounds. Palpation of the abdomen is performed to determine if masses can be felt or if there is tenderness.

After surgery, the patient is assessed for complications secondary to the surgical intervention such as hemorrhage, infection, abdominal distention, or decreased nutritional status. (See Nursing Process: Caring for The Postoperative Patient in Chap. 18, and The Patient Undergoing Thoracic Surgery in Chap. 22 for the patient who has had a total gastrectomy, because the chest cavity may be entered.)

Diagnosis

Nursing Diagnoses

Based on the assessment data, the patient's major nursing diagnoses may include the following:

- Anxiety related to surgical intervention
- Knowledge deficit about surgical procedures and postoperative course
- Altered nutrition, less than body requirements related to poor nutrition before surgery and altered GI system after surgery
- Pain related to surgical incision

Collaborative Problems/Potential Complications

In addition to the complications to which all postoperative patients are subject, the patient undergoing gastric surgery is at increased risk for hemorrhage.

Planning and Goals

The major goals for this patient may include reducing anxiety, increasing knowledge and understanding about the surgical procedure and postoperative course, attaining optimal nutrition and managing the complications that can interfere with nutrition, relieving pain, avoiding hemorrhage and steatorrhea, and enhancing the patient's self-care skills at home. General postoperative care for the patient who received general anesthesia, as discussed in Chapter 18, should be followed.

Nursing Interventions

Reducing Anxiety

An important part of the preoperative nursing care involves allaying the patient's fears and anxieties about the impending surgery and its implications. The nurse encourages the patient to express feelings and answers all questions. If the patient has an acute obstruction, a perforated bowel, or an active GI hemorrhage, adequate psychological preparation may not be possible. In this event, the nurse caring for the patient after surgery should anticipate the concerns, fears, and questions that are likely to surface and should be available for support and further explanations.

Increasing Knowledge

Routine preoperative and postoperative activities are explained to the patient: preoperative medications, nasogastric intubation, IV fluids, abdominal dressings, and pulmonary care. These explanations need to be reinforced after surgery, especially if the patient had emergency surgery.

Resuming Enteral Intake

The patient's nutritional status should be evaluated before surgery. Many patients with gastric cancer are malnourished and may require preoperative enteral or, more often, total parenteral nutrition (see Chap. 33). After surgery, parenteral nutrition may be continued to satisfy caloric needs, to replace fluids lost through drainage and vomitus, and to support the patient metabolically until oral intake is adequate.

After the return of bowel sounds and removal of the nasogastric tube, fluids may be given, followed by food in small portions. Foods are gradually added until the patient is able to eat six small meals a day and drink 120 mL of fluid between meals. The key to increasing the dietary content is to offer food and fluids gradually as tolerated and to recognize that each person's tolerance is different.

Recognizing Obstacles to Adequate Nutrition

DYSPHAGIA AND GASTRIC RETENTION

Dysphagia may occur in patients who have had truncal vagotomy, which can cause trauma to the lower esophagus. Gastric retention may be evidenced by abdominal distention, nausea, and vomiting. Regurgitation may also occur if the patient has eaten too much or too quickly. It also may indicate that edema along the suture line is preventing fluids and food from moving into the intestinal tract. If gastric retention occurs, it may be necessary to reinstate nasogastric suction; pressure must be low to avoid disrupting the suture line.

BILE REFLUX

Bile reflux gastritis and esophagitis may occur with the removal of the pylorus, which acts as a barrier to the reflux of duodenal contents. This is manifested by burning epigastric pain and vomiting of bilious material. Eating or vomiting does not relieve the situation. Binding agents such as cholestyramine (Questran), aluminum hydroxide gel, or metoclopramide hydrochloride (Reglan) have been used with some success.

DUMPING SYNDROME

The term **dumping syndrome** refers to an unpleasant set of vasomotor and GI symptoms that occur after meals in 10% to 50% of patients who have had GI surgery or a form of vagotomy. It may be the mechanical result of surgery in which a small gastric remnant connects into the jejunum through a large opening. Foods high in carbohydrates and electrolytes must be diluted in the jejunum before absorption can take place, but the passage of food from the stomach remnant into the jejunum is too rapid. The ingestion of fluid at mealtime is another factor that causes the stomach contents to empty rapidly into the jejunum. The symptoms that occur are probably a result of rapid distention of the jejunal loop anastomosed to the stomach. The hypertonic intestinal contents draw extracellular fluid from the circulating blood volume into the jejunum to dilute the high concentration of electrolytes and sugars.

Early symptoms include a sensation of fullness, weakness, faintness, dizziness, palpitations, diaphoresis, cramping pains, and diarrhea. Later, there is a rapid elevation of blood glucose, followed by increased insulin secretion. This results in a reactive hypoglycemia, which also is unpleasant for the patient. Vasomotor symptoms that occur 10 to 90 minutes after eating are pallor, perspiration, palpitations, headache, and feelings of warmth, dizziness, and even drowsiness. Anorexia may also be due to the dumping syndrome.

Steatorrhea may also occur in the patient with gastric surgery. It is partially the result of rapid gastric emptying, which prevents adequate mixing with pancreatic and biliary secretions. In mild cases, steatorrhea can be controlled by reducing the intake of fat and administering an antimotility medication.

VITAMIN AND MINERAL DEFICIENCIES

Other dietary deficiencies the nurse should be aware of include malabsorption of organic iron, which may require supplementation with oral or parenteral iron, and a low serum level of vitamin B_{12}, which may require supplementation by the intramuscular route. Total gastrectomy results in lack of intrinsic factor, a gastric secretion required for the absorption of vitamin B_{12} from the GI tract. Unless this vitamin is supplied by parenteral injection after gastrectomy, the patient inevitably suffers vitamin B_{12} deficiency, which eventually leads to a condition identical to pernicious anemia. All manifestations of pernicious anemia, including macrocytic anemia and combined system disease, may be expected to develop within a period of 5 years or less; they progress in severity thereafter and in the absence of therapy are fatal. This complication is avoided by the regular monthly intramuscular injection of 100 to 200 μg of vitamin B_{12}. This regimen should be started without delay after gastrectomy. Weight loss is a common long-term problem because the patient experiences early fullness, which curbs the appetite.

Teaching Dietary Self-Management

Because the patient may experience any of the above conditions affecting nutrition, nursing intervention is directed toward proper dietary instruction. The following teaching points are emphasized:

- The patient should assume a semirecumbent position during mealtime. After the meal, the patient should lie down for 20 to 30 minutes to delay stomach emptying.
- Fluids are discouraged with meals but may be given up to 1 hour before or 1 hour after mealtime.
- Fat may be given to tolerance, but carbohydrate intake should be kept low. Sucrose and glucose are avoided.
- Antispasmodics, as prescribed, also may aid in delaying the emptying of the stomach.
- Smaller but more frequent meals should be eaten.
- Meals should contain more dry than liquid items.
- Dietary supplements of vitamins and medium-chain triglycerides or injections of vitamin B_{12} and iron may be prescribed.

Instructions are also given regarding enteral or parenteral supplementation if it is needed.

Relieving Pain

Analgesics are administered after surgery as prescribed to maintain an acceptable level of comfort. Care must be taken to maintain the patient's ability to perform pulmonary care activities (deep breathing and coughing) and to ambulate. The nurse assesses the effectiveness of analgesic intervention. Positioning the patient in a modified Fowler's position promotes comfort and allows easy drainage of the stomach after a partial gastrectomy.

The functioning of the nasogastric tube is maintained to prevent distention and resultant pain. The amount of nasogastric drainage after a total gastrectomy is normally small.

Monitoring and Managing Potential Complications

Hemorrhage is occasionally a complication after gastric surgery. The patient has the usual signs of rapid blood loss and shock (see Chap. 14) and may vomit considerable amounts of bright-red blood. Nasogastric drainage should be assessed for type and amount; some bloody drainage is expected for the first 12 hours, but excessive bleeding should be reported. The abdominal dressing should also be assessed for bleeding. Because this situation is upsetting to the patient and family, the nurse should remain calm. Emergency measures are performed, such as nasogastric lavage and administration of blood and blood products.

Promoting Home and Community-Based Care

TEACHING PATIENTS SELF-CARE

Teaching is based on the assessment of the patient's physical and psychological readiness to participate in his or her care. Information is provided about nutrition, enteral or parenteral nutrition if required, nutritional supplements, pain management, and the symptoms of dumping syndrome and measures to use to prevent or minimize these symptoms.

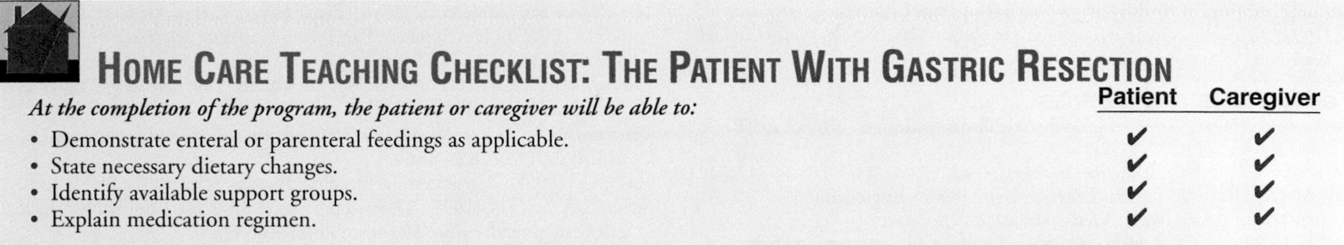

HOME CARE TEACHING CHECKLIST: THE PATIENT WITH GASTRIC RESECTION

At the completion of the program, the patient or caregiver will be able to:	Patient	Caregiver
• Demonstrate enteral or parenteral feedings as applicable.	✔	✔
• State necessary dietary changes.	✔	✔
• Identify available support groups.	✔	✔
• Explain medication regimen.	✔	✔

CONTINUING CARE

The patient and family benefit from a team approach to discharge planning. The team members include the home care nurse, physician, dietitian, and social worker. Written instructions about meals, activities, medications, and follow-up care are often helpful for the patient and family. The administration of any enteral or parenteral feedings is supervised by the home care nurse; information about detecting and preventing untoward effects or complications related to the feeding is emphasized. Information about community support groups is provided to the patient and family.

Evaluation

Expected Outcomes

Expected outcomes may include:

1. Is less anxious; expresses fears and concerns about surgery
2. Demonstrates knowledge regarding postoperative course by discussing the surgical procedure and postoperative course
3. Attains optimal nutrition
   a. Maintains a reasonable weight
   b. Does not have excessive diarrhea
   c. Tolerates 6 small meals a day
   d. Does not experience dysphagia, gastric retention, bile reflux, dumping syndrome, or vitamin and mineral deficiencies
4. Attains optimal level of comfort
5. Has no evidence of hemorrhage

Critical Thinking Exercises

1. You are visiting a resident of a retirement community. She tells you that she has begun to have symptoms of a peptic ulcer just like she had many years ago and that she is treating the ulcer as she did before, with a bland diet and antacids. Based on your knowledge of current theories about peptic ulcers, how would you advise her? If she is skeptical of your explanations, how might you convince her?

2. You are caring for a patient who has had a gastrectomy to treat gastric cancer. The patient's wife says she is eager for him to return home so that she can give him all of his favorite foods and help him regain the weight he has lost. Describe the conclusions you would draw from these statements, and explain how you would devise an instructional program that you believe would be helpful for this couple.

References and Selected Readings

BOOKS

Bell, R., et al. (1996). *Digestive tract surgery: A text and atlas* (4th ed.). Philadelphia: Lippincott-Raven.

DeVita, V. T., Hellman, S., Rosenberg, S. A. (Eds.). (1997). *Cancer: Principles and practice of oncology* (5th ed.). Philadelphia: Lippincott-Raven.

Haubrich, W. S., et al. (Eds.). (1995). *Bockus' Gastroenterology* (5th ed.). Philadelphia: W. B. Saunders.

Yamada, T., Alpers, D. H., Owyang, C., Powell, D. W., & Silverstein, F. E. (Eds.). (1995). *Textbook of gastroenterology* (2nd ed.). Philadelphia: J. B. Lippincott.

Zuidema, G. D. (Ed.). (1996). *Shakelford's Surgery of the alimentary tract* (4th ed.). Philadelphia: W. B. Saunders.

JOURNALS

Asterisks indicate nursing research articles.

Gastric Cancer

Burke, E. C., et al. (1997). Laparoscopy in the management of gastric adenocarcinoma. *Annals of Surgery, 225*(3), 262–267.

Evans, D. B., et al. (1997). Gastric cancer surgical practice guidelines. *Oncology, 11*(7), 1067–1072.

Jentschura, D., et al. (1997). Quality of life after curative surgery for gastric cancer: A comparison between total gastrectomy and subtotal gastric resection. *Hepatogastroenterology, 44*(16), 1137–1142.

Kirkwood, K. S. (1997). Prognostic indicators for cancer. Gastric cancer. *Surgical Oncology Clinics of North America, 6*(3), 495–514.

Lardis, S. H. et al. (1999). Cancer statistics, 1999. *Cancer, 49*(1): 8–31.

La Vecchia, C., et al. (1997). Diet diversity and gastric cancer. *International Journal of Cancer, 72*(2), 255–257.

Molloy, R. M., & Sonnenberg. A. (1997). Relation between gastric cancer and previous peptic ulcer disease. *Gut, 40*(2), 247–252.

McColl, K. E. (1997). The role of *Helicobacter pylori* in the pathophysiology of duodenal ulcer disease and gastric cancer. *Seminars in Gastrointestinal Disease, 8*(3), 142–155.

Nakajima, T., et al. (1997). Combined intensive chemotherapy and radical surgery for incurable gastric cancer. *Annals of Surgical Oncology, 4*(3), 203–208.

Noda, M. (1997). Possibilities and limitation of endoscopic resection for early gastric cancer. *Endoscopy, 29*(5), 361–364.

Pectasides, D., et al. (1997). CEA, CA 19-9, and CA-50 in monitoring gastric carcinoma. *American Journal of Clinical Oncology, 20*(4), 348–353.

Watanabe, Y., et al. (1997). *Helicobacter pylori* infection and gastric cancer. A nested case-control study in a rural area of Japan. *Digestive Disease Science, 42*(7), 1383–1387.

Morbid Obesity

Balsiger, B. M. (1997). Concise review for primary-care physicians. Surgical treatment of obesity: Who is an appropriate candidate? *Mayo Clinic Proceedings, 72*, 551–558.

Brolin, R. E. (1996). Update: NIH consensus conference. Gastrointestinal surgery for severe obesity. *Nutrition, 12*(6), 403–404.

Fried, M., & Peskova, M. (1997). Gastric binding in the treatment of morbid obesity. *Hepatogastroenterology, 44*(14), 582–587.

National Institutes of Health Consensus Development Conference Statement. (1992). Gastrointestinal surgery for severe obesity. *American Journal of Clinical Nutrition, 55*(Suppl 2), 615S–619S.

Peptic Ulcers and Gastritis

Belcaster, A. (1996). Reviewing Zollinger-Ellison syndrome—from A to ZES. *Nursing '96, 26*(3), 32C–32D.
Brozenec, S. A. (1996). Ulcer therapy update. *RN, 59*(9), 48–50.
Fay, M., & Jaffe, P. E. (1996). Diagnostic and treatment guidelines for *Helicobacter pylori. Nurse Practitioner, 21*(7), 28–35.
Forbes, G. M. (1997). Review: *Helicobacter pylori.* Current issues and new directions. *Journal of Gastroenterology and Hepatology, 12*(6), 419–424.
Garnett, W. R. (1996). Lanisoprazole: A proton pump inhibitor. *Annals of Pharmacotherapy, 30*(12), 1425–1436.
Heslin, J. M. (1997). Peptic ulcer disease: Making a case against the prime suspect. *Nursing '97, 27*(1), 34–39.
Hirshowitz, B. I. (1997). Zollinger-Ellison syndrome: Pathogenesis, diagnosis and management. *American Journal of Gastroenterology, 92*(4 Suppl), 44S–48S.
Lazzaroni, M. (1997). Triple therapy with ranitidine or lanisoprazole in the treatment of *Helicobacter pylori* associated with duodenal ulcer. *American Journal of Gastroenterology, 92*(4), 649–651.
Miehlke, S. (1997). An increasing dose of omeprazole combined with amoxicillin cures *Helicobacter pylori* infection more effectively. *Alimentary Pharmacology Therapy, 11*, 323–329.
NIH Consensus Conference. (1994). *Helicobacter pylori* peptic ulcer disease. NIH Consensus Development Panel on *Helicobacter pylori* in peptic ulcer disease. *JAMA, 272*(1), 65–69.
Owen, D. A. (1997). The morphology of gastritis. *Yale Journal of Biology and Medicine, 69*(1), 51–60.
Peterson, W. L., & Lee, W. M. (1997). Gastroenterology and hepatology. *JAMA, 277*(23), 1858–1860.
Rush, C. (1995). Gastrointestinal bleeding. *Nursing '95, 25*(8), 33.
Schurict, A. L., et al. (1997). Thorascopic vagotomy as a safe adjunct to remedial gastric surgery. *American Surgeon, 63*(6), 540–542.
Sontag, S. J. (1997). Guilty as charged: Bugs and drugs in gastric ulcer. *Massachusetts Journal of Gastroenterology, 92*(8), 1255–1261.
U.S. Dept. of Health and Human Services. (1994). Peptic ulcer disease. Feb. 7–9, 12(1).

Resources

American Cancer Society, 1599 Clifton Rd., N.E., Atlanta, GA 30329
American Digestive Disease Society, 420 Lexington Ave., New York, NY 10017
American Gastroenterological Association, 6900 Grove Rd., Thorofare, NJ 08086

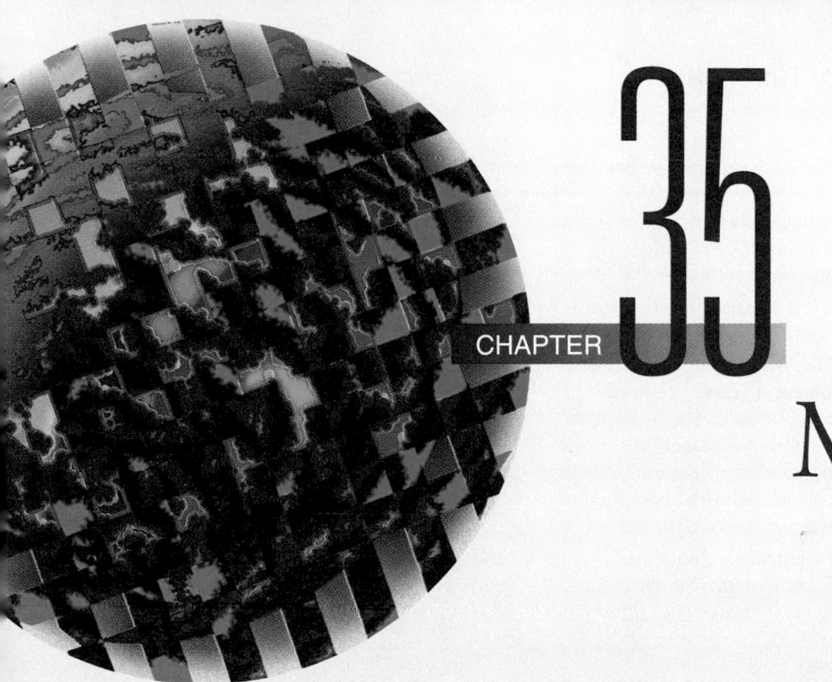

Management of Patients With Intestinal and Rectal Disorders

Learning Objectives

On completion of this chapter, the learner will be able to:

1. Identify the health care teaching needs of patients with constipation or diarrhea.
2. Compare the conditions of malabsorption with regard to their pathophysiology, clinical manifestations, and management.
3. Use the nursing process as a framework for care of patients with diverticulitis.
4. Compare regional enteritis and ulcerative colitis with regard to their pathophysiology, clinical manifestations, diagnostic evaluation, and medical, surgical, and nursing management.
5. Use the nursing process as a framework for care of the patient with an inflammatory bowel disease.
6. Describe the responsibilities of the nurse in meeting the needs of the patient with a fecal diversion.
7. Use the nursing process as a framework for care of the patient with cancer of the colon or rectum.
8. Describe the various types of intestinal obstructions and their management.
9. Use the nursing process as a framework for care of the patient with an anorectal condition.

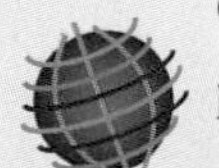

Gastrointestinal (GI) diseases constitute a major health problem, afflicting more than 34 million Americans. About 20 million of them have a chronic disorder and about 2 million are permanently disabled. The number of lives lost annually due to GI disease is 200,000. GI diseases are significant because a large part of the digestive process occurs on the intestinal surface and in the intestinal cells, where absorption occurs. The types of diseases and disorders that affect the lower GI tract are many and varied.

In all age groups, a fast-paced lifestyle, high levels of stress, irregular eating habits, insufficient intake of fiber and water, and lack of daily exercise contribute to these problems. Nurses can have an impact on these chronic problems by identifying behavior patterns that put patients at risk, by educating the public about prevention and management, and by helping those afflicted to improve their condition and prevent complications.

GLOSSARY

appendicitis: infectious and inflammatory process of the appendix creating acute abdominal pain and nausea

azotorrhea: excess of nitrogenous matter in the feces or urine

colostomy: surgical opening into the colon by means of a stoma to allow drainage of bowel contents; one type of fecal diversion

diverticulitis: inflammation of a diverticulum from obstruction (by fecal matter) resulting in abscess formation

diverticulum: sac-like outpouching of the lining of the bowel protruding through the muscle of the intestinal wall; usually caused by high intraluminal pressure

hemorrhoids: dilated portions of the anal veins; can occur inside or outside of the anal sphincter

ileostomy: surgical opening into the ileum by means of a stoma to allow drainage of bowel contents; one type of fecal diversion

inflammatory bowel disease: group of chronic disorders (most common are ulcerative colitis and Crohn's disease) that result in inflammation and/or ulceration of the bowel lining, associated with abdominal pain, diarrhea, fever, and weight loss

irritable bowel syndrome: functional disorder that affects frequency of defecation and/or consistency of stool; associated with crampy abdominal pain and bloating

lactose intolerance: occurs when there is a deficiency of the digestive enzyme lactase that breaks down milk sugar. It is associated with symptoms of cramping, bloating, and diarrhea

malabsorption: impaired transport across the mucosa

peritonitis: inflammation of the lining of the abdominal cavity, usually as a result of a bacterial infection of an area in the GI system with leakage of contents into the abdominal cavity

ABNORMALITIES OF FECAL ELIMINATION

Changes in patterns of fecal elimination are symptoms of functional disorders or disease states in the GI tract. The most common changes seen are constipation, diarrhea, and fecal incontinence. The nurse should be aware of the possible causes and therapeutic management of these problems, as well as the nursing management techniques. Education is important for patients with these abnormalities.

Constipation

Constipation is a term used to describe an abnormal infrequency or irregularity of defecation, abnormal hardening of stools that makes their passage difficult and sometimes painful, a decrease in stool volume, or retention of stool in the rectum for a prolonged period of time. Any variation from normal habits may be seen as a problem.

Constipation can be caused by certain medications (tranquilizers, anticholinergics, antidepressants, antihypertensives, opioids, antacids with aluminum, and iron); rectal or anal disorders (hemorrhoids, fissures); obstruction (cancer of the bowel); metabolic, neurologic, and neuromuscular conditions (diabetes mellitus, Hirschsprung's disease, Parkinson's disease, multiple sclerosis); endocrine disorders (hypothyroidism, pheochromocytoma); lead poisoning; and connective tissue disorders (scleroderma, lupus erythematosus). Constipation is a major problem for patients taking opioids for chronic pain. Diseases of the colon commonly associated with constipation are irritable bowel syndrome and diverticular disease. Constipation can also occur with an acute process in the abdomen (ie, appendicitis).

Other causes include weakness, immobility, debility, fatigue, and inability to increase intra-abdominal pressure to facilitate the passage of stools, such as occurs with emphysema. Many people develop constipation because they do not take the time to defecate or they ignore the urge to defecate. In the United States, constipation is also a result of dietary habits (low consumption of fiber and inadequate fluid intake), lack of regular exercise, and a stress-filled life.

Perceived constipation can also be a problem. This is a subjective problem that occurs when an individual's bowel elimination pattern is not consistent with what he or she perceives as normal. Chronic laxative use is attributed to this problem and is a major health concern in the United States, especially among the elderly population.

Pathophysiology

The pathophysiology of constipation is poorly understood. It is believed, however, to be related to interference with one of three major functions of the colon: (1) mucosal transport (mucosal secretions facilitate the movement of colon contents), (2) myoelectric activity (mixing of the rectal mass and propulsive actions), or (3) the processes of defecation. Any of the causative factors previously identified can interfere with any of these three processes. The urge to defecate is normally stimulated by rectal distention, which initiates a series of four actions: stimulation of the inhibitory rectoanal reflex, relaxation of the internal sphincter muscle, relaxation of the external sphincter muscle and muscles in the pelvic region, and increased intra-abdominal pressure. Interference with any of these four processes can thus lead to constipation.

If all organic causes are eliminated, idiopathic constipation is diagnosed. If the urge to defecate is ignored, the rectal mucous membrane and musculature become insensitive to the presence of fecal masses, and consequently a stronger stimulus is required to produce the necessary peristaltic rush for defecation. The initial effect of this fecal retention is to produce irritability of the colon, which at this stage frequently goes into spasm, especially after meals, giving rise to colicky midabdominal or low abdominal pains. After several years of this process, the colon loses muscular tone and becomes essentially unresponsive to normal stimuli. Atony or decreased muscle tone occurs with aging. This also leads to constipation because the stool is retained for longer periods of time.

Clinical Manifestations

Clinical manifestations include abdominal distention, borborygmus (intestinal rumbling), pain and pressure, decreased appetite, headache, fatigue, indigestion, a sensation of incomplete emptying, straining at stool, and the elimination of small-volume, hard, dry stool.

Assessment and Diagnostic Findings

The diagnosis of constipation is based on a patient history, physical examination, possibly a barium enema or a sigmoidoscopy, and stool testing for occult blood. These tests are completed to determine whether this symptom is due to spasm or narrowing of the bowel. Anorectal manometry (pressure studies) may be performed to determine malfunction of the muscle and sphincter. Defecography and bowel transit studies can also be completed (see Chap. 31 for discussion of these diagnostic studies).

Complications

Complications of constipation include hypertension, fecal impaction, hemorrhoids and fissures, and megacolon.

Increased arterial pressure can occur with defecation. Straining at stool, which results in the Valsalva maneuver (forcibly exhaling with the glottis closed), has a striking effect on arterial blood pressure. During active straining, the flow of venous blood in the chest is temporarily impeded because of increased intrathoracic pressure. This pressure tends to collapse the large veins in the chest. The atria and the ventricles receive less blood, and consequently less is delivered by the systolic contractions of the left ventricle; the cardiac output is decreased, and there is a transient drop in arterial pressure. Almost immediately after this period of hypotension, a rise in arterial pressure occurs; the pressure is elevated momentarily to a point far exceeding the original level (the rebound phenomenon). In patients with hypertension, this compensatory reaction may be exaggerated greatly, and the peaks of pressure attained may be dangerously high—sufficient to rupture a major artery in the brain or elsewhere.

Fecal impaction occurs when an accumulated mass of dry feces cannot be expelled. The mass may be palpable on digital examination, may produce pressure on the colon mucosa that results in ulcer formation, and may cause frequent seepage of liquid stools.

Hemorrhoids and anal fissures can develop as a result of constipation. Anal fissures may result from the passage of the hard stool through the anus, tearing the lining of the anal canal. Hemorrhoids develop as a result of perianal vascular congestion caused by straining.

Megacolon is a dilated and atonic colon caused by a fecal mass that obstructs the passage of colon contents. Symptoms include constipation, liquid fecal incontinence, and abdominal distention. Megacolon can lead to perforation of the bowel.

Gerontologic Considerations

Elderly people report problems with constipation five times more frequently than younger people. A number of factors contribute to this increased frequency. People who have loose-fitting dentures or have lost their teeth have difficulty chewing and frequently choose soft, processed foods that are low in fiber. Convenience foods, also low in fiber, are widely used by those who have lost interest in eating. Some older people reduce their fluid intake if they are not eating regular meals. Lack of exercise and prolonged bed rest also contribute to constipation by decreasing abdominal muscle tone and motility as well as intestinal and anal sphincter tone. Nerve impulses are dulled, and there is decreased sensation to defecate. In addition, many older people who overuse laxatives in an attempt to have a daily bowel movement become dependent on them.

Medical Management

Treatment is aimed at the underlying cause of constipation. Management includes discontinuing laxative abuse, inclusion of fiber in the diet with an increase in fluid intake, and performing an exercise routine to strengthen abdominal muscles. Biofeedback is a technique that can be used to help patients learn to relax the sphincter mechanism to expel stool. The daily addition to the diet of 6 to 12 teaspoonfuls of unprocessed bran is recommended, especially for the treatment of constipation in the elderly. If laxative use is necessary, one of the following may be prescribed: bulk-forming agents, saline and osmotic agents, lubricants, stimulants, or fecal softeners. The physiologic action and patient education information related to these laxatives are identified in Table 35-1. Enemas and rectal suppositories are generally not recommended for constipation and should be reserved for the treatment of impaction or for preparing the bowel for surgery or diagnostic procedures. If long-term laxative use is necessary, a bulk-forming agent may be prescribed in combination with an osmotic laxative.

Specific medication therapy can be used to increase the intrinsic motor function of the intestine. Studies indicate that the use of prokinetic agents such as cisapride can increase stool frequency.

Nursing Management

Information about the onset and duration of constipation, current and past elimination patterns, the patient's expectation of normal bowel elimination, and lifestyle information (eg, exercise and activity level, occupation, food and fluid intake, and stress level) should be elicited during the health history interview. Past medical and surgical history, current medications, and laxative and enema use are important, as is information about the sensation of rectal pressure or fullness, abdominal pain, excessive straining at defecation, and flatulence.

Patient teaching is an important function of the nurse. See the health promotion box for topics related to constipation. Once the health history is obtained, specific goals for teaching can be set. Goals for the patient would include restoring or maintaining a regular pattern of elimination, ensuring adequate intake of fluids and high-fiber foods, learning about methods to avoid constipation, relieving anxiety about bowel elimination patterns, and avoiding complications.

Diarrhea

Diarrhea is increased frequency of bowel movements (more than three per day), increased amount of stool (more than 200 g/day), and altered consistency (looseness) of stool. It is usually associated with urgency, perianal discomfort, incontinence, or a combination of these factors. Any condition that causes increased intestinal secretions, decreased mucosal absorption, or altered motility can produce diarrhea. Diarrhea can be acute or chronic. Acute diarrhea is most often associated with infection and is usually self-limiting; chronic diarrhea persists for a longer period of time and may return sporadically. Diarrhea can be caused by certain medications (thyroid hormone replacement, stool softeners and laxatives, antibiotics, chemotherapy, and antacids), certain tube feeding formulas, metabolic and endocrine disorders (diabetes, Addison's disease, thyrotoxicosis), and viral or bacterial infectious processes (dysentery, shigellosis, food poisoning). Other disease processes associated with diarrhea are nutritional and malabsorptive disorders (irritable bowel syndrome, ulcerative colitis, regional enteritis, and celiac disease), anal sphincter defect, Zollinger-Ellison syndrome, paralytic ileus, intestinal obstruction, and AIDS.

Pathophysiology

Types of diarrhea include secretory, osmotic, or mixed. Secretory diarrhea is usually high-volume diarrhea and is caused by increased production and secretion of water and electrolytes by the intestinal mucosa into the intestinal lumen. Osmotic diarrhea occurs when water is pulled into the intestines by the osmotic pressure of nonabsorbed particles, slowing the reabsorption of water. Mixed diarrhea is caused by increased peristalsis (usually from inflammatory bowel disease) and a combination of increased secre-

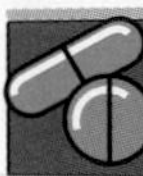

TABLE 35•1 Laxatives: Classification, Agent, Action, and Patient Education

Classification	Sample Agent	Action	Patient Education
Bulk forming	Psyllium hydrophilic muciloid (Metamucil)	Polysaccharides and cellulose derivatives mix with intestinal fluids, swell, and stimulate peristalsis.	Take with 8 ounces of water and follow with 8 ounces of water. Do not take dry. Report abdominal distention or unusual amount of flatulence
Saline agent	Magnesium hydroxide (Milk of Magnesia)	Nonabsorbable magnesium ions alter stool consistency by drawing water into the intestines by osmosis; peristalsis is stimulated. Action occurs within 2 hours.	The liquid preparation is more effective than the table form. Only short-term use is recommended because of toxicity (CNS or neuromuscular depression, electrolyte imbalance). Magnesium laxatives should not be taken by patients with renal insufficiency
Lubricant	Mineral oil	Nonabsorbable hydrocarbons soften fecal matter by lubricating the intestinal mucosa. The passage of stool is facilitated. Action occurs within 6–8 hours.	Do not take with meals because mineral oils may impair the absorption of fat-soluble vitamins and delay gastric emptying. Swallow carefully because drops of oil that gain access to the pharynx may produce a lipid pneumonia
Stimulant	Bisacodyl (Dulcolax)	Irritates the colon epithelium by stimulating sensory nerve endings and increasing mucosal secretions. Action occurs within 6–8 hours.	Catharsis may cause fluid and electrolyte imbalance, especially in the elderly. Tablets should be swallowed, not crushed or chewed. Avoid milk or antacids within 1 hour of taking the medication because the enteric coating may dissolve prematurely
Fecal softener	Dioctyl sodium sulfosuccinate (Colace)	Hydrates the stool by its surfactant action on the colonic epithelium (increases the wetting efficiency of intestinal water). Aqueous and fatty substances are mixed. The medication does not exert a laxative action.	Can be used safely by patients who should avoid straining (cardiac patients, patients with anorectal disorders)
Osmotic agent	Polyethyleneglycol and electrolytes (Colyte)	Cleanses colon rapidly and induces diarrhea.	This is a large volume product. It takes time to consume it safely. It may cause considerable nausea and bloating

tion or decreased absorption in the bowel. The physiology of diarrhea related to infection is discussed in Chapter 64.

Clinical Manifestations

In addition to the increased frequency and fluid content of stool, the patient usually has abdominal cramps, distention, intestinal rumbling (borborygmus), anorexia, and thirst. Painful spasmodic contractions of the anus and ineffectual straining (tenesmus) may occur with each defecation. Other symptoms depend on the cause and severity of the diarrhea but are related to dehydration and fluid and electrolyte imbalances.

Watery stools are characteristic of small bowel disease, whereas loose, semisolid stools are associated more often with disorders of the colon. Voluminous, greasy stools suggest intestinal malabsorption, and the presence of mucus and pus in the stools suggests inflammatory enteritis or colitis. Oil droplets on the toilet water are almost always diagnostic of pancreatic insufficiency. Nocturnal diarrhea may be a manifestation of diabetic neuropathy.

Assessment and Diagnostic Findings

When the cause of the diarrhea is not obvious, the following diagnostic tests may be performed: complete blood count, chemical profile, urinalysis, and a routine stool examination as well as stool examinations for infectious or parasitic organisms, bacterial toxins, blood, fat, and electrolytes. Endoscopy or barium enema may assist in identifying the cause.

Complications

Complications of diarrhea include the potential for cardiac dysrhythmias because of significant fluid and electrolyte loss (especially loss of potassium). Urinary output of less than 30 mL/hour

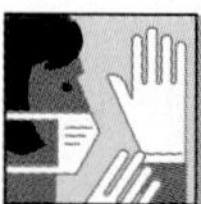

HEALTH PROMOTION AND ILLNESS PREVENTION
Preventing Constipation

- Describe the physiology of defecation.
- Emphasize heeding the urge to defecate.
- Discuss normal variations in patterns of defecation.
- Teach how to establish a bowel routine, and explain that having a regular time for defecation (eg, best time is after breakfast) may aid in initiating the reflex.
- Provide dietary information; suggest eating high-residue, high-fiber foods, adding bran daily (must be introduced gradually), and increasing fluid intake (unless contraindicated).
- Explain how an exercise regimen, increased ambulation, and abdominal muscle toning will increase muscle strength and help propel colon contents.
- Describe abdominal toning exercises (contracting abdominal muscles 4 times daily and leg to chest lifts 10 to 20 times a day).
- Explain that the normal position (semisquatting) maximizes use of abdominal muscles and force of gravity.

for 2 to 3 consecutive hours as well as muscle weakness, paresthesia, hypotension, anorexia, and drowsiness with a potassium level of less than 3.0 mEq/L (SI: 3 mmol/L) must be reported. Decreased potassium levels cause cardiac dysrhythmias (atrial and ventricular tachycardia, ventricular fibrillation, and premature ventricular contractions) that can lead to death.

Medical Management

Primary management is directed at controlling symptoms, preventing complications, and eliminating or treating the underlying disease. Certain medications (eg, antibiotics, anti-inflammatory agents) may reduce the severity of the diarrhea and the disease.

Nursing Management

The nurse's role includes assessing and monitoring the characteristics and pattern of diarrhea. A health history addresses medication therapy, past medical and surgical history, and dietary patterns and intake. Reports of recent exposure to an acute illness or recent travel to another geographic area are important. Assessment includes abdominal auscultation and palpation for abdominal tenderness. Inspection of the abdomen and mucous membranes and skin is important to determine hydration status. Stool samples are obtained for testing.

During an episode of acute diarrhea, bed rest and intake of liquids and foods low in bulk are encouraged until the acute attack subsides. When food intake is tolerated, a bland diet of semisolids and solids is recommended. Caffeine, carbonated beverages, and very hot and very cold foods are avoided because these stimulate intestinal motility. Milk products, fat, whole-grain products, fresh fruits, and vegetables may be restricted for several days. Antidiarrheal medications such as diphenoxylate (Lomotil) and loperamide (Imodium) are administered as prescribed. Intravenous (IV) fluid therapy may be necessary for rapid rehydration, especially for the elderly and those with preexisting GI conditions (eg, ulcerative colitis). Serum electrolyte levels must be monitored closely. Evidence of dysrhythmias or a change in the level of consciousness must be reported immediately.

Nursing Alert *Older people can quickly become dehydrated and suffer from low potassium levels (hypokalemia) as a result of diarrhea. The older person taking digitalis must be aware of how quickly dehydration and hypokalemia can occur with diarrhea. This person is also instructed to recognize the signs of hypokalemia, because low levels of potassium intensify the action of digitalis, which can lead to digitalis toxicity.*

The perianal area may become excoriated because diarrheal stool contains digestive enzymes that can irritate the skin. A perianal care routine should be followed to decrease irritation and excoriation. Skin sealants and moisture barriers are used as needed. The older person's skin is very sensitive because of decreased turgor and reduced subcutaneous fat layers.

Fecal Incontinence

The term fecal incontinence describes the involuntary passage of stool from the rectum. Several factors influence fecal continence: the ability of the rectum to sense and accommodate stool, the amount and consistency of stool, the integrity of the anal sphincters and musculature, and rectal motility.

Pathophysiology

Fecal incontinence can result from trauma (after surgical procedures involving the rectum), a neurologic disorder (eg, stroke, multiple sclerosis, diabetic neuropathy, dementia), inflammation, infection, radiation treatment, fecal impaction, pelvic floor relaxation, laxative abuse, medications, or advancing age (ie, weakness or loss of anal or rectal muscle tone). It is an embarrassing and socially incapacitating problem that requires a many-tiered approach to treatment and much adaptation on the patient's part.

Clinical Manifestations

Patients may have minor soiling, occasional urgency and loss of control, or complete incontinence. Poor control of flatus, diarrhea, or constipation may also be present.

Assessment and Diagnostic Findings

Because the treatment of fecal incontinence depends on the cause, diagnostic studies are necessary to define the cause. A rectal examination and other endoscopic examinations such as a flexible sigmoidoscopy are performed to rule out tumors, inflammation, or fissures. X-ray studies such as barium enema, computed tomography scans, anorectal manometry, and transit studies may be helpful in identifying alterations in intestinal mucosa and muscle tone, or other structural or functional problems.

Medical Management

If fecal incontinence is related to diarrhea, the incontinence may disappear when that process is successfully treated. Fecal incontinence is frequently a symptom of a fecal impaction. Once the impaction is removed and the rectum is cleansed, normal functioning of the anorectal area can resume. If the fecal incontinence is related to a more permanent condition, other treatments are initiated. Biofeedback therapy can be of assistance if the problem is decreased sensory awareness or sphincter control. Bowel training programs can also be effective. Surgical procedures include surgical reconstruction, sphincter repair, or fecal diversion.

Nursing Management

The nurse should take a thorough health history and complete an examination of the rectal area. Information about previous surgical procedures, chronic illnesses, bowel habits and problems, and current medication regimen should be obtained.

A bowel training program that involves setting a schedule to establish bowel regularity is initiated. Sometimes it is necessary to use suppositories to stimulate the anal reflex. Once a regular schedule is achieved, the suppository can be discontinued. Biofeedback can be used in conjunction with these therapies to help the patient improve sphincter contractility and rectal sensitivity.

Fecal incontinence is an embarrassing problem. It can also cause problems with perineal skin integrity. Maintaining skin integrity is a priority, especially in the debilitated or elderly patient. Incontinence briefs, although helpful in containing the fecal material, allow for increased skin contact with the feces and may cause excoriation of the skin. Meticulous skin hygiene must be encouraged and taught.

Sometimes continence cannot be achieved, and the nurse must assist the patient and family to accept and cope with this chronic situation. Special pouches can be used to contain fecal matter. Their use affords more freedom and assists in maintenance of skin integrity.

IRRITABLE BOWEL SYNDROME

Irritable bowel syndrome is one of the most common GI problems, affecting 8% to 14% of the population. It occurs more commonly in women than in men. The cause is still unknown. Although no anatomic or biochemical abnormalities have been found that explain the common symptoms, various factors are associated with the syndrome: heredity, psychological stress or illness, diet high in rich and stimulating or irritating foods, alcohol consumption, and smoking.

Pathophysiology

Irritable bowel syndrome results from a functional disorder of intestinal motility. The change in motility may be related to the neurologic regulatory system, infection or irritation, or a vascular or metabolic disturbance. The peristaltic waves are affected at specific segments of the intestine and in the intensity with which they propel the fecal matter forward. There is no evidence of inflammation or tissue changes in the intestinal mucosa.

Clinical Manifestations

The primary symptom is an alteration in bowel patterns—constipation, diarrhea, or a combination of both. This is often accompanied by pain, bloating, and abdominal distention. These symptoms vary in intensity and duration. The abdominal pain is sometimes precipitated by eating and is frequently relieved by defecation.

Assessment and Diagnostic Findings

Stool studies, contrast x-ray studies, and proctoscopy may be performed to rule out other colon diseases. Barium enema and colonoscopy may reveal spasm, distention, and/or mucus accumulation in the intestine (Fig. 35-1). Manometry and electromyography are used to study interluminal pressure changes generated by spasticity.

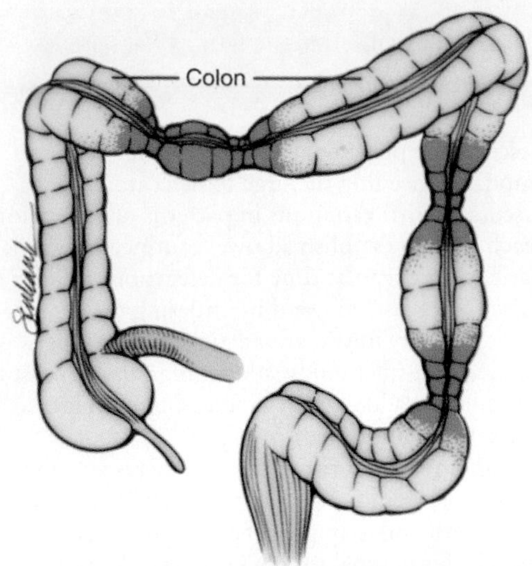

FIGURE 35•1 In irritable bowel syndrome the spastic contractions of the bowel can be seen in x-ray contrast studies.

Medical Management

The goals of treatment include relieving the abdominal pain, controlling the diarrhea and/or constipation, and reducing stress. A special diet may help determine what types of food are acting as irritants (eg, beans, caffeinated products, fried foods, alcohol, spicy foods). A well-balanced, high-fiber diet is prescribed to help control the diarrhea and constipation. Exercise can assist in reducing anxiety and increasing intestinal motility. Patients often find it helpful to participate in a stress reduction or behavior modification program. Hydrophilic colloids (bulk) and antidiarrheal agents may be given to control the diarrhea and fecal urgency. Antidepressants can assist in treating underlying anxiety and depression. Anticholinergics and calcium channel blockers decrease smooth muscle spasm, decreasing cramping and constipation.

Nursing Management

The nurse's role is to provide patient and family education. Emphasis is placed on teaching and reinforcing good dietary habits. The patient is encouraged to eat at regular times and to chew food slowly and thoroughly. The patient should understand that although adequate fluid intake is necessary, fluid should not be taken with meals because this results in abdominal distention. Alcohol use and cigarette smoking are discouraged.

CONDITIONS OF MALABSORPTION

Malabsorption is the inability of the digestive system to absorb one or more of the major nutrients—carbohydrates, fats, and proteins. Interruptions in the complex digestive process may occur anywhere in the digestive system and cause malabsorption.

Pathophysiology

The conditions that cause malabsorption can be grouped into five categories:

1. Mucosal disorders causing generalized malabsorption (celiac sprue, Crohn's disease, radiation enteritis)

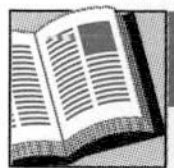

NURSING RESEARCH

Need for Increased Knowledge and Empathy for Patients With Irritable Bowel Syndrome

Leston, S., & Dancey, C. (1996). Nurses' perceptions of irritable bowel syndrome (IBS) and sufferers of IBS. *Journal of Advanced Nursing, 23;* 969–974.

Purpose

Irritable bowel syndrome (IBS) is a functional digestive disorder that affects many of our population. Patients have varied symptoms, and physicians have been unable to identify the cause of the problem or an effective treatment. Those living with this problem may have psychological consequences because of the way they perceive they are treated by health professionals. Studies have been conducted identifying physician response to the problem, but no studies before this one had been conducted with nurses. This study was designed to identify nurses' beliefs and attitudes toward IBS and its sufferers.

Study Sample and Study Design

Three hundred thirty-three randomly selected London nurses were surveyed. A 54-item questionnaire that had been previously piloted and revised was used. Two hundred fifty-three completed questionnaires were returned. The nurses were asked to respond to statements about IBS on a scale of 1 (agree) to 5 (disagree). There were four categories of statements: attitudes toward sufferers of IBS, beliefs about their knowledge of IBS, general awareness of IBS, and beliefs about knowledge and understanding displayed by health professionals toward those with IBS.

Findings

The nurses' perception of IBS sufferers was that they are demanding and difficult patients who are unable to cope with life and who crave attention, have a low pain tolerance, and tend to waste doctors' time. However, the nurses indicated that their knowledge of the syndrome was limited and that they could neither explain IBS to a patient nor recognize the symptoms.

They identified that IBS was a common disorder, but they were not very interested in it. They also indicated that health professionals have a poor understanding of IBS and that IBS is not taken seriously by health professionals.

Nursing Implications

The findings of this study indicate that nurses need a greater awareness and knowledge about IBS and the effects of this chronic illness on quality of life. Such an understanding could lead to improved communication with patients with IBS and reduce patients' fears and mistrust of others. Increased knowledge about IBS and its treatment could be shared with patients who seek knowledge and support.

2. Infectious diseases causing generalized malabsorption (small bowel bacterial overgrowth, tropical sprue, Whipple's disease)
3. Luminal problems causing malabsorption (bile acid deficiency, Zollinger-Ellison syndrome)
4. Postoperative malabsorption (after gastric or intestinal resection)
5. Disorders that cause malabsorption of specific nutrients (disaccharidase deficiency leading to lactose intolerance) (Grendell et al., 1996)

Table 35-2 lists the clinical and pathologic aspects of malabsorptive diseases.

Clinical Manifestations

The hallmarks of malabsorption syndrome, from whatever cause, are diarrhea or frequent, loose, bulky, foul-smelling stools that have increased fat content and are often grayish. Associated abdominal distention, increased flatus, weakness, weight loss, and a decreased sense of well-being are often present. The chief result of malabsorption is malnutrition, manifested by weight loss and other signs of vitamin and mineral deficiency (easy bruising, osteoporosis, anemia). Patients with a malabsorption syndrome, if untreated, become weak and emaciated because of starvation and dehydration. Failure to absorb the fat-soluble vitamins A, D, and K causes a corresponding avitaminosis.

Assessment and Diagnostic Findings

Several diagnostic tests may be ordered. Lactose tolerance tests, xylose absorption tests, and Schilling tests can be diagnostic of certain malabsorption diseases. Breath hydrogen testing is performed after ingestion of a measured amount of carbohydrate. Biopsy of the mucosa of the small intestine may be performed to assay for enzyme activity or to identify infection or destruction of mucosa. Ultrasound and radiologic testing can reveal pancreatic or intestinal tumors that may be the cause. A complete blood count is used to monitor for anemia. Fecal fat analysis may indicate a disorder in the digestion or absorption of fat.

Medical Management

Intervention is aimed at avoiding dietary substances that aggravate malabsorption as well as supplementing nutrients that have been lost. Common supplements are water-soluble vitamins (B_{12}, folic acid), fat-soluble vitamins (A, D, K), and minerals (calcium, iron). Primary disease states may be managed surgically or nonsurgically. Antibiotics are used to treat diseases of bacterial overgrowth. Antidiarrheal agents may be used to decrease intestinal spasms. Parenteral fluids may be necessary to treat dehydration.

Nursing Management

The nurse provides patient and family education regarding diet and the use of nutritional supplements. Patients with diarrhea must be monitored for fluid and electrolyte imbalances. Ongoing assessment needs to be conducted to determine if the clinical manifestations related to the nutritional deficits have abated.

ACUTE INFLAMMATORY INTESTINAL DISORDERS

Any part of the lower GI tract is susceptible to acute inflammation caused by bacterial, viral, or fungal infection. Two such situations are appendicitis and diverticulitis. These two conditions can lead to **peritonitis**, an inflammatory process within the abdomen.

Appendicitis

The appendix is a small, finger-like appendage about 10 cm (4 in) long, attached to the cecum just below the ileocecal valve. The appendix fills with food and empties regularly into the cecum. Because it empties inefficiently and its lumen is small, the appendix is prone to obstruction and is particularly vulnerable to infection (**appendicitis**).

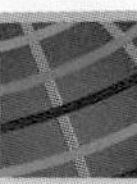

TABLE 35•2 Characteristics of Diseases of Malabsorption

Diseases/Disorders	Physiologic Pathology	Clinical Features
Gastric resection with gastrojejunostomy	Decreased pancreatic stimulation because of duodenal bypass; poor mixing of food, bile, pancreatic enzymes; decreased intrinsic factor, bacterial stasis in afferent loop	Weight loss, moderate steatorrhea, anemia (combination of iron deficiency, vitamin B_{12} malabsorption, folate deficiency)
Pancreatic insufficiency (chronic pancreatitis, pancreatic carcinoma, pancreatic resection, cystic fibrosis)	Reduced intraluminal pancreatic enzyme activity, with maldigestion of lipids and proteins	History of abdominal pain followed by weight loss; marked steatorrhea, azotorrhea; also frequent glucose intolerance (70% in pancreatic insufficiency)
Ileal dysfunction (resection or disease)	Loss of ileal absorbing surface leads to reduced bile-salt pool size and reduced vitamin B_{12} absorption; bile in colon inhibits fluid absorption	Diarrhea, weight loss with steatorrhea, especially when greater than 100 cm resection, decreased vitamin B_{12} absorption
Stasis syndromes (surgical strictures, blind loops, enteric fistulas, multiple jejunal diverticula, scleroderma)	Overgrowth of intraluminal intestinal bacteria, especially anaerobic organisms, to greater than 10^6/mL, results in deconjugation of bile salts, leading to decreased effective bile-salt pool size, also bacterial utilization of vitamin B_{12}	Weight loss, steatorrhea; low vitamin B_{12} absorption; may have low D-xylose absorption
Zollinger-Ellison syndrome	Hyperacidity in duodenum inactivates pancreatic enzymes	Ulcer diathesis, steatorrhea
Lactose intolerance	Deficiency of intestinal lactase results in high concentration of intraluminal lactose with osmotic diarrhea	Varied degrees of diarrhea and cramps after ingestion of lactose-containing foods; positive lactose intolerance test, decreased intestinal lactase
Celiac disease (gluten enteropathy)	Toxic response to a gluten fraction by surface epithelium results in destruction of absorbing surface	Weight loss, diarrhea, bloating, anemia (low iron, folate), osteomalacia, steatorrhea, azotorrhea, low D-xylose absorption; folate and iron malabsorption; diagnostic biopsy change
Tropical sprue	Unknown toxic factor results in mucosal inflammation, partial villous atrophy	Weight loss, diarrhea, anemia (low folate, vitamin B_{12}); steatorrhea; low D-xylose absorption, low vitamin B_{12} absorption; typical but nonspecific biopsy change
Whipple's disease	Bacterial invasion of intestinal mucosa	Arthritis, hyperpigmentation, lymphadenopathy, serous effusions, fever, weight loss; steatorrhea, azotorrhea, diagnostic biopsy change
Certain parasitic diseases (giardiasis, strongyloidiasis, coccidiosis, capillariasis)	Damage to or invasion of surface mucosa	Diarrhea, weight loss; steatorrhea; organism may be seen on jejunal biopsy or recovered in stool
Immunoglobulinopathy	Decreased local gut defenses, lymphoid hyperplasia, lymphopenia	Frequent association with *Giardia:* hypogammaglobulinemia or isolated IgA deficiency; diagnostic or typical biopsy changes

Appendicitis, the most common cause of acute inflammation in the right lower quadrant of the abdomen, is the most common reason for emergency abdominal surgery. About 7% of the population will have appendicitis at some time in their lives; males are affected more than females, and teenagers more than adults. Although it can occur at any age, it occurs most frequently between the ages of 10 and 30 years.

Pathophysiology

The appendix becomes inflamed and edematous as a result of either becoming kinked or occluded, possibly by a fecalith (hardened mass of stool), tumor, or foreign body. The inflammatory process increases intraluminal pressure, initiating a progressively severe generalized or upper abdominal pain that, within a few hours, becomes localized in the right lower quadrant of the abdomen. Eventually, the inflamed appendix fills with pus.

Clinical Manifestations

Right lower quadrant pain is present and is usually accompanied by a low-grade fever, nausea, and sometimes vomiting. Loss of appetite is common. Local tenderness is noted at McBurney's point (Fig. 35-2) when pressure is applied. Rebound tenderness (production or intensification of pain when pressure is released) may be present. Just how much tenderness and muscle spasm is present, and whether constipation or diarrhea occurs, depend not so much on the severity of the appendiceal infection as on the location of the appendix. If the appendix curls around behind the cecum, pain and tenderness may be felt in the lumbar region; if

PATIENT EDUCATION AND HOME CARE

Managing Lactose Intolerance

- Deficiency of lactase, a digestive enzyme essential for the absorption of lactose from the intestines, results in an intolerance to milk.
- Elimination of milk and milk substances can abolish symptoms.
- Many processed foods have fillers, such as dried milk, added to them.
- Pretreatment of foods with lactase preparations (ie, Lactaid drops) before ingestion can reduce symptoms.
- Most people can tolerate 1 to 2 cups of milk or milk products daily without major problems; best tolerated if ingested in small amounts during the day.
- Lactase activity of yogurt with "active cultures" helps digestion of lactose in intestine better than lactase preparations.
- Milk and milk products are rich sources of calcium and vitamin D. Elimination of milk from the diet may result in calcium and vitamin D deficiencies.
- Decreased intake without supplements can lead to osteoporosis.

its tip is in the pelvis, these signs may be elicited only on rectal examination. Pain on defecation suggests that the tip of the appendix is resting against the rectum; pain on urination suggests that the tip is near the bladder or impinges on the ureter. Some rigidity of the lower portion of the right rectus muscle may occur. Rovsing's sign may be elicited by palpating the left lower quadrant; this paradoxically causes pain to be felt in the right lower quadrant (see Fig. 35-2). If the appendix has ruptured, the pain becomes more diffuse; abdominal distention develops as a result of paralytic ileus, and the patient's condition worsens. Constipation can also occur with an acute process such as appendicitis. Laxatives administered in this instance may produce perforation of the inflamed appendix. In general, a cathartic should never be given while the person has fever, nausea, or pain.

Assessment and Diagnostic Findings

Diagnosis is based on a complete physical examination and laboratory and x-ray findings. A complete blood count is performed and will demonstrate an elevated white blood cell count. The leukocyte count may exceed $10,000/mm^3$ and the neutrophil count may exceed 75%. Abdominal x-rays and ultrasound studies may reveal a right lower quadrant density or localized distention of the bowel.

Complications

The major complication of appendicitis is perforation of the appendix, which can lead to peritonitis or an abscess. The incidence of perforation is 10% to 32%. The incidence is higher in young children and the elderly. Perforation generally occurs 24 hours after the onset of pain. Symptoms include a fever of 37.7°C (100°F) or greater, a toxic appearance, and continued abdominal pain or tenderness.

Gerontologic Considerations

In the elderly patient, the signs and symptoms of appendicitis may vary greatly. They may be very vague, suggesting bowel obstruction or another process. The patient may have no symptoms until the appendix ruptures. The incidence of perforated appendix is higher in the elderly population because many of these patients do not seek health care as quickly as younger patients.

Medical Management

Surgery is indicated if appendicitis is diagnosed. Antibiotics and IV fluids (to correct or prevent fluid and electrolyte imbalance and dehydration) are administered until surgery is performed.

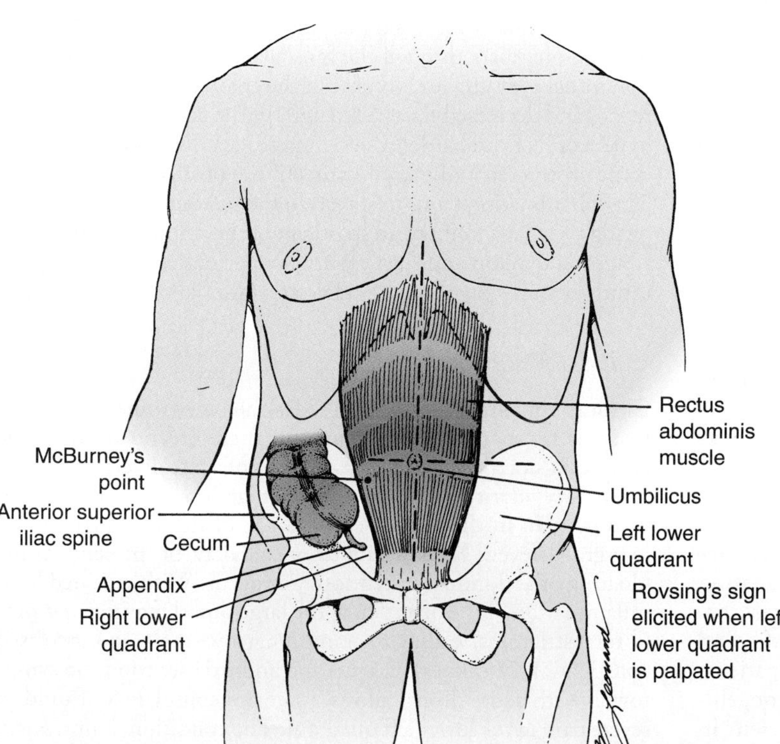

FIGURE 35•2 When the appendix is inflamed, tenderness can be noted in the right lower quadrant at McBurney's point, which is between the umbilicus and the anterior superior iliac spine. Rovsing's sign refers to pain felt in the right lower quadrant after the left lower quadrant has been palpated.

Analgesics can be administered after the diagnosis is made. The appendectomy (surgical removal of the appendix) is performed as soon as possible to decrease the risk of perforation. It may be performed under a general or spinal anesthetic with a low abdominal incision, or by laparoscopy.

Nursing Management

Goals include relieving pain, preventing fluid volume deficit, reducing anxiety, eliminating infection from the potential or actual disruption of the GI tract, maintaining skin integrity, and attaining optimal nutrition.

The nurse prepares the patient for surgery. An IV infusion is used to promote adequate renal function and replace fluid loss. Antibiotic therapy may be administered to prevent infection. If there is evidence or likelihood of paralytic ileus, a nasogastric tube may be inserted. An enema is not administered because it can lead to perforation.

After surgery, the patient is placed in a semi-Fowler's position. This position reduces the tension on the incision and abdominal organs, helping to reduce pain. An opioid, usually morphine sulfate, is given to relieve pain. Oral fluids are usually administered when they can be tolerated. Any patient who was dehydrated before surgery is given IV fluids. Food may be given as desired on the day of surgery if tolerated.

The patient may be discharged on the day of surgery, provided the temperature is within normal limits, there is no undue discomfort in the operative area, and the appendectomy was uncomplicated. Discharge teaching for the patient and family is imperative. The patient is instructed to make an appointment to have the surgeon remove the sutures between the fifth and seventh days after surgery. Incision care and activity guidelines are discussed. Normal activity can usually be resumed within 2 to 4 weeks.

If there is a possibility of peritonitis, a drain is left in place at the area of the incision. Patients at risk for this complication may be kept in the hospital for several days and are monitored carefully for signs of intestinal obstruction or secondary hemorrhage. Secondary abscesses may form in the pelvis, under the diaphragm, or in the liver, causing an elevation of temperature and pulse rate and an increased leukocyte count.

When the patient is ready for discharge, the patient and family must be taught to care for the wound and perform dressing changes and irrigations as prescribed. A home care nurse may be needed to assist with this care and to monitor the patient for complications and wound healing. Other potential complications of appendectomy are listed in Table 35-3.

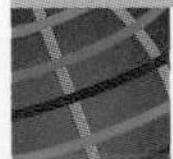

TABLE 35•3 Potential Complications and Nursing Interventions After Appendectomy

Complication	Nursing Interventions
Peritonitis	Observe for abdominal tenderness, fever, vomiting, abdominal rigidity, and tachycardia. Employ constant nasogastric suction. Correct dehydration as prescribed. Administer antibiotic agents as prescribed.
Pelvic or lumbar abscess	Evaluate for anorexia, chills, fever, and diaphoresis. Observe for diarrhea, which may indicate pelvic abscess. Prepare patient for rectal examination. Prepare patient for surgical drainage procedure.
Subphrenic abscess (abscess under the diaphragm)	Assess patient for chills, fever, and diaphoresis. Prepare for x-ray examination. Prepare for surgical drainage of abscess.
Ileus (paralytic and mechanical)	Assess for bowel sounds. Employ nasogastric intubation and suction. Replace fluids and electrolytes by intravenous route as prescribed. Prepare for surgery, if diagnosis of mechanical ileus is established.

Diverticular Disease

A **diverticulum** is a sac-like outpouching of the lining of the bowel that extends through a defect in the muscle layer. Diverticula may occur anywhere along the GI tract. Diverticulosis exists when multiple diverticula are present without inflammation or symptoms. More than 50% of Americans older than 60 have diverticulosis. The incidence increases to nearly 70% in those older than 80. **Diverticulitis** results when food and bacteria retained in a diverticulum produce infection and inflammation that can impede drainage and lead to perforation or abscess formation. Diverticulitis is most common in the sigmoid colon (95%). It has been estimated that approximately 20% of patients with diverticulosis have diverticulitis at some point. A congenital predisposition is suspected when the disorder is present in those younger than 40. A low intake of dietary fiber is considered a predisposing factor, but no exact cause is known. Diverticulitis may occur in acute attacks or may persist as a continuing, smoldering infection.

Pathophysiology

A diverticulum forms when the mucosa and submucosal layers of the colon herniate through the muscular wall because of high intraluminal pressure, low volume in the colon (fiber-deficient contents), and decreased muscle strength in the colon wall (muscular hypertrophy from hardened fecal masses). A diverticulum can become obstructed and then inflamed if the obstruction continues. The inflammation tends to spread to the surrounding bowel wall, giving rise to irritability and spasticity of the colon (diverticulitis). Abscesses develop and may eventually perforate, leading to peritonitis and erosion of the blood vessels (arterial) with bleeding.

Clinical Manifestations

Chronic constipation often precedes the development of diverticulosis by many years. Frequently there are no problematic symptoms noted in diverticulosis. Signs of acute diverticulosis are bowel irregularity and intervals of diarrhea, abrupt onset of crampy pain in the left lower quadrant of the abdomen, and a low-grade fever. Nausea and anorexia may be present. Some bloating or abdominal distention may occur. With repeated local inflammation of the diverticula, the large bowel may narrow with fibrotic strictures, leading to cramps, narrow stools, and increased constipation. Weakness, fatigue, and anorexia are common symptoms. With acute diverticulosis, there are complaints of mild to severe pain in the lower left quadrant. The condition, if untreated, can lead to septicemia.

Assessment and Diagnostic Findings

Diverticulosis may be diagnosed from x-ray studies such as barium enema that show narrowing of the colon and thickened muscle layers. If there are symptoms of peritoneal irritation and when the diagnosis is diverticulitis, barium enema is contraindicated because of the potential for perforation.

An abdominal x-ray may demonstrate free air under the diaphragm if a perforation has occurred from the diverticulitis. A computed tomography scan is the procedure of choice and can reveal abscesses. A colonoscopy may be performed if there is no acute diverticulitis or after resolution of an acute episode to visualize the colon, determine the extent of the disease, and rule out other conditions. Laboratory tests that will help in diagnosis are a complete blood count (the white cell count will be elevated) and sedimentation rate (will be elevated).

Complications

Complications of diverticulitis include peritonitis, abscess formation, and bleeding. If an abscess develops, there is tenderness, a palpable mass, fever, and leukocytosis. An inflamed diverticulum that perforates results in abdominal pain localized over the involved segment, usually the sigmoid; local abscess or peritonitis follows. Abdominal pain, a rigid board-like abdomen, loss of bowel sounds, and signs and symptoms of shock occur with peritonitis. Noninflamed or slightly inflamed diverticula may erode areas adjacent to arterial branches, thus causing massive rectal bleeding.

Gerontologic Considerations

The incidence of diverticular disease increases with age because of degeneration and structural changes in the circular muscle layers of the colon, as well as cellular hypertrophy. The symptoms are less pronounced in the elderly than in other adults. The elderly may not have abdominal pain until infection occurs. They may delay reporting symptoms because they fear surgery or are afraid that they may have cancer. Blood in the stool is frequently overlooked, especially in the elderly, because of a failure to examine the stool or the inability to see changes because of diminished vision.

Medical Management

Diverticulitis can be treated on an outpatient basis with dietary and medication therapy. Initially the diet is clear liquid until the inflammation subsides; then, a high-fiber, low-fat diet is recommended. This type of diet helps to increase stool volume, decrease colonic transit time, and reduce intraluminal pressure. Antibiotics are prescribed for 7 to 10 days. A bulk-forming laxative is also prescribed.

In acute cases of diverticulitis with significant symptoms, hospitalization is required. Hospitalization is often indicated for those who are elderly, immunocompromised, or taking corticosteroids. The bowel is rested by withholding oral intake, administering IV fluids, and instituting nasogastric suctioning if vomiting or distention is present. Broad-spectrum antibiotics are prescribed for 7 to 10 days. Meperidine (Demerol) is prescribed for pain relief (morphine is not used because it increases segmentation and intraluminal pressures). Oral intake is increased as symptoms subside. A low-fiber diet may be necessary until signs of infection decrease.

Antispasmodics such as propantheline bromide (Pro-Banthine) and oxyphencyclimine (Daricon) may be prescribed. Normal stools can be achieved by using bulk preparations (Metamucil) or stool softeners (Colace), by instilling warm oil into the rectum, or by inserting an evacuant suppository (Dulcolax). Such a prophylactic plan will reduce the bacterial flora of the bowel, diminish the bulk of the stool, and soften the fecal mass so that it moves more easily through the area of inflammatory obstruction.

SURGICAL MANAGEMENT

Although acute diverticulitis usually subsides with medical management, about 25% of the cases require immediate surgical intervention for complications (perforation, peritonitis, abscess formation, hemorrhage, or obstruction). Alternatively, when the acute episode of diverticulitis resolves, surgery may be recommended to prevent repeated episodes. Two types of surgery are considered:

1. A one-stage resection in which the inflamed area is removed and a primary end-to-end anastomosis is completed
2. Multiple-staged procedures for complications such as obstruction or perforation (Fig. 35-3)

The type of surgery performed depends on the extent of complications found during surgery. When possible, the area of diverticulitis is resected and the remaining bowel is joined end to end (primary resection and end-to-end anastomosis). A two-stage resection may be performed in which the diseased colon is resected (as in a one-stage procedure) but no anastomosis is performed; both ends of the bowel are brought out onto the abdomen as stomas. This "double-barrel" colostomy is then reanastomosed in a later procedure. Fecal diversion procedures are discussed later in this chapter.

NURSING PROCESS: THE PATIENT WITH DIVERTICULITIS

Assessment

During the health history, the patient is asked about the onset and duration of pain as well as past and present elimination patterns. Dietary habits are reviewed to determine fiber intake. The

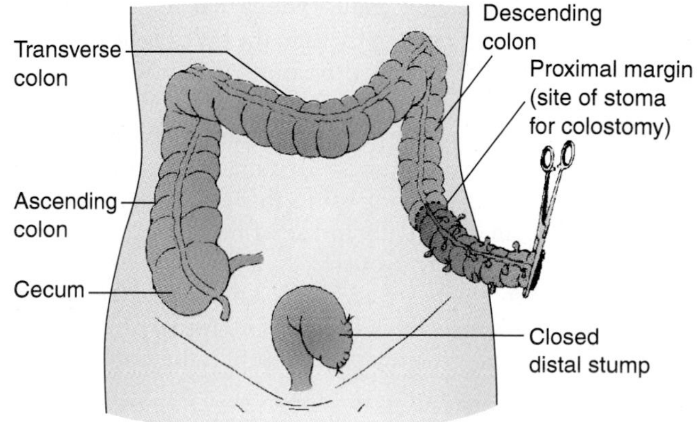

FIGURE 35•3 The Hartmann procedure for diverticulitis: primary resection for diverticulitis of the colon. The affected segment (clamp attached) has been divided at its distal end. In a primary anastomosis, the proximal margin (dotted line) is transected and the bowel attached end-to-end. In a two-stage procedure, a colostomy is constructed at the proximal margin with the distal stump oversewn (Hartmann procedure, as shown) or brought to the outer surface as a mucous fistula. The second stage consists of colostomy takedown and anastomosis.

patient is asked about straining at stool, history of constipation with periods of diarrhea, tenesmus (spasms of the anal sphincter with pain and persistent urge to defecate), abdominal bloating, and distention.

Assessment includes auscultating for the presence and character of bowel sounds and palpating for lower left quadrant pain, tenderness, or firm mass. The stool is inspected for pus, mucus, or blood. Temperature, pulse, and blood pressure are monitored for abnormal variations.

Diagnosis

Nursing Diagnoses

Based on the assessment data, the nursing diagnoses may include the following:

- Constipation related to narrowing of the colon secondary to thickened muscular segments and strictures
- Pain related to inflammation and infection

Collaborative Problems/Potential Complications

Potential complications that may develop include:

- Peritonitis
- Abscess formation
- Bleeding

Planning and Goals

The major goals for the patient may include attainment and maintenance of normal elimination patterns, pain reduction, and avoidance of complications.

Nursing Interventions

Maintaining Normal Elimination Patterns

A fluid intake of 2 L/day (within limits of the patient's cardiac and renal reserve) is recommended. Foods that are soft but have increased fiber are suggested to increase the bulk of the stool and to facilitate peristalsis, thereby promoting defecation. An individualized exercise program is encouraged to improve abdominal muscle tone. The patient's daily routine is reviewed to establish a schedule for meals and a set time for defecation. The patient is assisted in identifying habits that may have suppressed the urge to defecate. The daily intake of bulk laxatives such as Metamucil, which helps to propel feces through the colon, is encouraged. Stool softeners are administered as prescribed to decrease straining at stool, which decreases intestinal pressure. Oil retention enemas may be prescribed to soften the stool, making it easier to pass.

Relieving Pain

Analgesics (eg, meperidine) are administered to relieve the pain of diverticulitis. Antispasmodic agents are administered as prescribed to decrease intestinal spasm. The intensity, duration, and location of pain are recorded to determine if the inflammatory process worsens or subsides.

Monitoring and Managing Potential Complications

The major nursing focus is to prevent complications by identifying patients at risk and managing their symptoms as needed. The nurse assesses for the following signs of perforation:

- Increased abdominal pain and tenderness accompanied by abdominal rigidity
- Elevated white cell count
- Elevated sedimentation rate
- Increased temperature
- Tachycardia
- Hypotension

Perforation is a surgical emergency. The clinical manifestations of perforation and peritonitis and the care of the patient with peritonitis are presented in the next section.

Vital signs and urine output are monitored and IV fluids are administered to replace volume loss as needed.

Evaluation

Expected Outcomes

Expected outcomes may include:

1. Attains a normal pattern of elimination
   a. Reports less abdominal cramping and pain
   b. Reports the passage of soft, formed stool, without pain
   c. Adds unprocessed bran to foods
   d. Drinks at least 10 glasses of fluid a day (if fluid intake is tolerated)
   e. Exercises daily
2. Has less pain
   a. Requests analgesics as needed
   b. Adheres to a low-fiber diet during acute episodes
3. Recovers without complications
   a. Is afebrile
   b. Blood pressure remains normal
   c. Has a soft, nontender abdomen with normal bowel sounds
   d. Maintains adequate urine output
   e. Has no blood in the stool

Peritonitis

Peritonitis is inflammation of the peritoneum, the serous membrane lining the abdominal cavity and covering the viscera. Usually, it is a result of bacterial infection; the organisms come from diseases of the GI tract or, in women, from the internal reproductive organs. Peritonitis can also result from external sources such as injury or trauma (eg, gunshot or stab wound) or an inflammation that extends from an organ outside the peritoneal area, such as the kidney. The most common bacteria implicated are *Escherichia coli, Klebsiella, Proteus,* and *Pseudomonas.* Inflammation and paralytic ileus are the direct effects of the infection. Other common causes of peritonitis are appendicitis, perforated ulcer, diverticulitis, and bowel perforation (Fig. 35-4). Peritonitis may also be associated with abdominal surgical procedures and peritoneal dialysis.

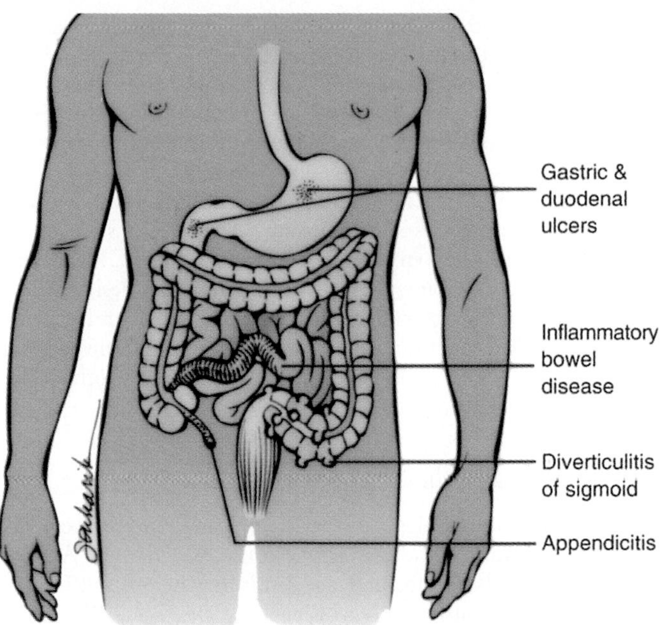

FIGURE 35•4 Common gastrointestinal causes of peritonitis.

Pathophysiology

Peritonitis is caused by leakage of contents from abdominal organs into the abdominal cavity, usually as a result of inflammation, infection, ischemia, trauma, or tumor perforation. Bacterial proliferation occurs. Edema of the tissues results, and in a short time exudation of fluid develops. Fluid in the peritoneal cavity becomes turbid with increasing amounts of protein, white cells, cellular debris, and blood. The immediate response of the intestinal tract is hypermotility, soon followed by paralytic ileus, with an accumulation of air and fluid in the bowel.

Clinical Manifestations

Symptoms depend on the location and extent of the inflammation. The early clinical manifestations of peritonitis frequently are the symptoms of the disorder causing the condition. At first a diffuse type of pain is felt. The pain tends to become constant, localized, and more intense near the site of the inflammation. It is usually aggravated by movement. The affected area of the abdomen becomes extremely tender and distended, and the muscles become rigid. Rebound tenderness and paralytic ileus may be present. Usually, nausea and vomiting occur and peristalsis is diminished. The temperature and pulse rate increase, and there is almost always an elevation of the leukocyte count.

Assessment and Diagnostic Findings

The leukocyte count will be elevated. The hemoglobin and hematocrit may be low if blood loss has occurred. Serum electrolytes may demonstrate altered levels of potassium, sodium, and chloride.

An abdominal x-ray is obtained and may show air and fluid levels as well as distended bowel loops. A CT scan of the abdomen may show abscess formation. Peritoneal aspiration and culture and sensitivity studies of the aspirated fluid may reveal infection and identify the causative organisms.

Complications

Frequently, the inflammation is not localized and the whole abdominal cavity becomes involved in a generalized sepsis. Sepsis is the major cause of death from peritonitis. Shock may result from septicemia or hypovolemia. The inflammatory process may cause intestinal obstruction, primarily from the development of bowel adhesions.

The two most common postoperative complications are wound evisceration and abscess formation. Any suggestion from the patient that an area of the abdomen is tender or painful or "feels as if something just gave way" must be reported. The sudden occurrence of serosanguineous wound drainage strongly suggests wound dehiscence (see Chap. 18).

Medical Management

Fluid, colloid, and electrolyte replacement is the major focus of medical management. The administration of several liters of an isotonic solution is prescribed. Hypovolemia occurs because massive amounts of fluid and electrolytes move from the intestinal lumen into the peritoneal cavity and deplete the fluid in the vascular space.

Analgesics are prescribed for pain. Antiemetics can be administered as prescribed for nausea and vomiting. Intestinal intubation and suction assist in relieving abdominal distention and in promoting intestinal function. Fluid in the abdominal cavity can cause pressure that restricts expansion of the lungs and causes respiratory distress. Oxygen therapy by nasal cannula or mask will promote adequate oxygenation, but occasionally airway intubation and ventilatory assistance are required.

Massive antibiotic therapy is usually initiated early in the treatment of peritonitis. Large doses of a broad-spectrum antibiotic are administered IV until the organism causing the infection is identified and the specific appropriate antibiotic therapy can be initiated.

Surgical objectives include removing the infected material and correcting the cause. Surgical treatment is directed toward excision (appendix), resection with or without anastomosis (intestine), repair (perforation), and drainage (abscess). With extensive sepsis, a fecal diversion may need to be created.

Nursing Management

Ongoing assessment of pain, vital signs, GI function, and fluid and electrolyte balance is important. The nature of the pain, its location in the abdomen, and any shifts in location are reported. Administering analgesic medication and positioning the patient for comfort are helpful in decreasing pain. The patient should be placed on the side with knees flexed; this decreases tension on the abdominal organs. Accurate recording of all intake and output and central venous pressure assists in calculating fluid replacement. IV fluids must be administered and monitored closely.

Signs that indicate that peritonitis is subsiding include a decrease in temperature and pulse rate, softening of the abdomen, return of peristaltic sounds, passing of flatus, and bowel movements. Fluid and food intake are gradually increased and parenteral fluids reduced. A worsening clinical condition may indicate a complication, and the nurse will need to prepare the patient for emergency surgery.

Drains are frequently inserted during the surgical procedure, and postoperatively the nurse must observe and record the character of the drainage. Care must be taken when moving and turning the patient to prevent the drains from being dislodged accidentally. It is also important for the nurse to prepare the patient and family for discharge. They must be taught to care for the incision and drains if the patient will be sent home with the drains still in place.

INFLAMMATORY BOWEL DISEASE

The term **inflammatory bowel disease** is used to designate two chronic inflammatory GI disorders: regional enteritis (Crohn's disease or granulomatous colitis) and ulcerative colitis.

The incidence of inflammatory bowel disease in the United States has increased in the last century: 10,000 to 15,000 new cases occur annually. In the past, a higher rate was noted among whites in general and the Jewish population in particular. Recent data now indicate a higher risk for African Americans and a lower risk for Jewish people, and women appear to be at higher risk than before. People ages 10 to 30 years are at greatest risk (Kirsner & Shorter, 1995).

Inflammatory bowel disease is thought to be triggered by environmental agents such as pesticides, food additives, tobacco, and radiation. An immunologic influence has also been suggested. Some research in the early 1990s linked *Mycobacterium* to inflammatory bowel disease, but the evidence remains inconclusive. The search for enteric pathogens as etiologic factors has gained popularity because of the use of antibiotics in treating the disease process (Kirsner & Shorter, 1995).

Regional Enteritis (Crohn's Disease)

Regional enteritis commonly occurs in adolescents or young adults but can appear at any time of life. It is seen frequently in the older population (50 to 80 years). It can occur anywhere along the GI tract, but the most common areas are the distal ileum and colon.

Pathophysiology

Regional enteritis is a subacute and chronic inflammation that extends through all layers (transmural) of the bowel wall from the intestinal mucosa. Fistulas, fissures, and abscesses form as the inflammation extends into the peritoneum. The lesions (ulcers) are not in continuous contact with one another and are separated by normal tissue. Granulomas occur in half of the cases. In advanced cases, the intestinal mucosa has a cobblestone appearance. As the disease advances, the bowel wall thickens and becomes fibrotic, and the intestinal lumen narrows.

Clinical Manifestations

With regional enteritis, the onset of symptoms is usually insidious, with prominent abdominal pain and diarrhea unrelieved by defecation. Diarrhea is present in 90% of patients. Scar tissue and the formation of granulomas interfere with the ability of the intestine to transport products of the upper intestinal digestion through the constricted lumen, resulting in crampy abdominal pains. Because intestinal peristalsis is stimulated by eating, the crampy pains occur after meals. To avoid these bouts of crampy pain, the patient tends to limit food intake, reducing the amounts and types of food to such a degree that normal nutritional requirements are not met. The result is weight loss, malnutrition, and secondary anemia. In addition, the ulcers in the membranous lining of the intestine and other inflammatory changes result in a weeping, swollen intestine that continually empties an irritating discharge into the colon. This causes chronic diarrhea and nutritional deficits because absorption is disrupted. The end result is a person who is thin and emaciated from inadequate food intake and constant fluid loss. In some patients, the inflamed intestine may perforate, leading to intra-abdominal and anal abscesses. Fever and leukocytosis occur. Abscesses, fistulas, and fissures are common. Symptoms extend beyond the GI tract and commonly include joint problems (arthritis), skin lesions (erythema nodosum), ocular disorders (conjunctivitis), and oral ulcers. The clinical course and symptoms can vary; in some patients periods of remission and exacerbation occur, but in others the disease follows a fulminating course.

Assessment and Diagnostic Findings

A proctosigmoidoscopic examination is usually performed initially to determine if the rectosigmoid area is inflamed. A stool examination is also performed; the result may be positive for occult blood and steatorrhea (excessive fat in the feces). The most conclusive diagnostic aid for regional enteritis is a barium study of the upper GI tract that shows the classic "string sign" on x-ray of the terminal ileum, indicating the constriction of a segment of intestine. A barium enema may also show ulcerations, the cobblestone appearance described earlier, fissures, and fistulas. A computed tomography scan may show bowel wall thickening and fistula tracts.

A complete blood count is performed to assess hematocrit and hemoglobin levels (usually decreased) as well as the white cell count (may be elevated). The sedimentation rate is usually elevated. Albumin and protein levels may be decreased, indicating malnutrition.

Complications

Complications of regional enteritis include intestinal obstruction or stricture formation, perianal disease, fluid and electrolyte imbalances, malnutrition from malabsorption, and fistula and abscess formation. A fistula is an abnormal communication between two body structures, either internal (between two structures) or external (between an internal structure and the outside surface of the body). The most common type of small bowel fistula that results from regional enteritis is the enterocutaneous fistula (between the small bowel and the skin). Abscesses can be the result of an internal fistula tract into an area that results in fluid accumulation and infection. Patients with regional enteritis are also at increased risk for colon cancer.

Ulcerative Colitis

Ulcerative colitis is a recurrent ulcerative and inflammatory disease of the mucosal layer of the colon and rectum. It most commonly affects whites, including people of Jewish heritage. The peak incidence is 30 to 50 years of age. It is a serious disease, accompanied by systemic complications and a high mortality rate. Eventually, 10% to 15% of the patients develop carcinoma of the colon.

Pathophysiology

Ulcerative colitis affects the superficial mucosa of the colon and is characterized by multiple ulcerations, diffuse inflammations, and desquamation or shedding of the colonic epithelium. Bleeding occurs as a result of the ulcerations. The lesions are continuous, occurring one after the other. The disease process begins in the rectum and may involve the entire colon. Eventually the bowel narrows, shortens, and thickens because of muscular hypertrophy and fat deposits.

Clinical Manifestations

The clinical course is usually one of exacerbations and remissions. The predominant symptoms of ulcerative colitis are diarrhea, abdominal pain, intermittent tenesmus, and rectal bleeding. The bleeding may be mild or severe. In addition, the patient may have anorexia, weight loss, fever, vomiting, and dehydration, as well as cramping, the feeling of an urgent need to defecate, and the passage of 10 to 20 liquid stools a day. Hypocalcemia and anemia frequently develop. Rebound tenderness may occur in the right lower quadrant. Other symptoms include skin lesions (erythema nodosum), eye lesions (uveitis), joint abnormalities (arthritis), and liver disease.

Assessment and Diagnostic Findings

The stool is positive for blood and laboratory tests reveal a low hematocrit and hemoglobin in addition to an elevated white cell count, low albumin levels, and an electrolyte imbalance. Sigmoidoscopy and barium enema are valuable in distinguishing this condition from other diseases of the colon with similar symptoms. A barium enema will show mucosal irregularities, shortening of the colon, and dilation of bowel loops. Endoscopy may reveal friable, inflamed mucosa with exudate and ulcerations.

Nursing Alert *In acute ulcerative colitis, cathartics are contraindicated when the patient is being prepared for barium enema or endoscopy because they may exacerbate the condition, which can lead to megacolon (excessive dilation of the colon), perforation, and death. If the patient needs to have these diagnostic tests, a liquid diet for a few days before the x-ray and a gentle tap-water enema on the day of the examination may be prescribed. Colonoscopy is contraindicated in severe disease because of the risk of perforation.*

Careful stool examination for parasites and other microbes is also performed to rule out dysentery caused by common intestinal organisms, especially *Entamoeba histolytica.*

Complications

Complications of ulcerative colitis include toxic megacolon, perforation, and bleeding as a result of ulceration, vascular engorgement, and highly vascular granulation tissue. In toxic megacolon, the inflammatory process extends into the muscularis, inhibiting its ability to contract and resulting in colonic distention. If the patient with toxic megacolon does not respond within 24 to 48 hours to medical management with IV fluids, corticosteroids, and antibiotics, surgical resection is indicated. Colonic perforation from toxic megacolon is associated with a high mortality rate (greater than 40%).

For many patients, surgery becomes necessary to relieve the effects of the disease and to treat these serious complications. Usually an ileostomy is performed. The surgical procedures involved and the care of patients with this type of fecal diversion are discussed below.

Management of Chronic Inflammatory Bowel Disorders

Medical treatment for both regional enteritis and ulcerative colitis is aimed at reducing inflammation, suppressing inappropriate immune responses, and providing rest for a diseased bowel so that healing may take place. Table 35-4 compares regional enteritis and ulcerative colitis.

Nutritional Therapy

Oral fluids and a low-residue, high-protein, high-calorie diet with supplemental vitamin therapy and iron replacement are prescribed to meet nutritional needs. Fluid and electrolyte imbalances from dehydration caused by diarrhea are corrected by IV therapy as necessary if the patient is hospitalized or by oral supplementation if the patient can be managed at home. Any foods that exacerbate diarrhea are avoided. Milk may contribute to diarrhea in those with lactose intolerance. In addition, cold foods and smoking are avoided because both increase intestinal motility. Total parenteral nutrition may be indicated.

Pharmacologic Therapy

Sedatives and antidiarrheal and antiperistaltic medications are used to reduce peristalsis to a minimum to rest the inflamed bowel. They are continued until the patient's stools approach normal frequency and consistency. Sulfonamides such as sulfasalazine (Azulfidine) or sulfisoxazole (Gantrisin) are often effective for mild or moderate inflammation. Antibiotics are used for secondary infections, particularly for purulent complications such as abscesses, perforation, and peritonitis. Sulfasalazine is helpful in preventing recurrences.

Parenteral adrenocorticotropic hormone (ACTH) and corticosteroids are effective in the treatment of acute inflammatory bowel disease. When the dosage of corticosteroids is reduced or stopped, however, the symptoms of disease may return. If corticosteroids are continued, adverse sequelae such as hypertension, fluid retention, cataracts, hirsutism (abnormal hair growth), and adrenal suppression may develop. New topical and oral aminosalicylates (eg, mesalamine [Asacol], olsalazine [Dipentum]) have been shown to be very effective in treatment. Immunosuppressive agents are also used to prevent relapses, and they allow the patient to receive lower doses of corticosteroids for shorter periods of time.

Surgical Management

When nonsurgical measures fail to relieve the severe symptoms of inflammatory bowel disease, surgery may be recommended. A technique that can be helpful is strictureplasty, in which the blocked or narrowed section of the bowel is widened, leaving the bowel intact.

If a lesion can be delineated in regional enteritis, or if a complication has occurred, the lesion is resected and the remaining portions of the bowel are anastomosed. Surgical removal of up to 50% of the small bowel can usually be tolerated. One of several surgical procedures is possible:

- Total colectomy (excision of the entire colon) with ileostomy
- Segmental colectomy (removal of a segment of the colon) with anastomosis (joining of the remaining portions of the colon)

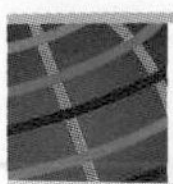

TABLE 35•4 **Comparison of Regional Enteritis and Ulcerative Colitis**

	Regional Enteritis	Ulcerative Colitis
Course	Prolonged, variable	Exacerbations, remissions
Pathology		
Early	Transmural thickening	Mucosal ulceration
Late	Deep, penetrating granulomas	Mucosal minute ulceration
Clinical Manifestations		
Location	Ileum, right colon (usually)	Rectum, left colon
Bleeding	Usually not, but may occur	Common—severe
Perianal involvement	Common	Rare—mild
Fistulas	Common	Rare
Rectal involvement	About 20%	Almost 100%
Diarrhea	Less severe	Severe
Diagnostic Study Findings		
X-ray	Regional, discontinuous lesions Narrowing of colon Thickening of bowel wall Mucosal edema Stenosis, fistulas	Diffuse involvement No narrowing of colon No mucosal edema Stenosis rare Shortening of colon
Sigmoidoscopy	May be unremarkable unless accompanied by perianal fistulas	Abnormal inflamed mucosa
Colonoscopy	Distinct ulcerations separated by relatively normal mucosa in right colon	Friable mucosa with pseudopolyps or ulcers in left colon
Therapeutic Management		
	Corticosteroids, sulfonamides (sulfasalazine [Azulfidine]) Antibiotics Total parenteral nutrition Partial or complete colectomy, with ileostomy or anastomosis Rectum can be preserved in some patients Recurrence common	Corticosteroids, sulfonamides; sulfasalazine useful in preventing recurrence Bulk hydrophilic agents Antibiotics Proctocolectomy, with ileostomy Rectum can be preserved in only a few patients "cured" by colectomy
Systemic Complications		
	Small bowel obstruction Right-sided hydronephrosis Nephrolithiasis Cholelithiasis Arthritis Retinitis, iritis Erythema nodosum	Toxic megacolon Perforation Hemorrhage Malignant neoplasms Pyelonephritis Nephrolithiasis Cholangiocarcinoma Arthritis Retinitis, iritis Erythema nodosum

- Subtotal colectomy (removal of nearly all of the colon) with ileorectal anastomosis (joining of the ileum and rectum)
- Total colectomy with continent ileostomy (formation of internal pouch)
- Total colectomy with ileoanal anastomosis (formation of a pouch with the anal sphincter intact)

The rate of recurrence after surgery is 20% to 40% in the first 5 years. Patients younger than 25 years of age have the highest recurrence rate.

Approximately 15% to 20% of patients with ulcerative colitis require surgical intervention. Indications for surgery include lack of improvement and continued deterioration, profuse bleeding, perforation, stricture formation, and cancer. The procedure of choice is a total colectomy and ileostomy; any procedure more limited will prove to be of only temporary benefit in most patients. A proctocolectomy (complete excision of colon, rectum, and anus) is recommended when the rectum is severely involved.

TYPES OF FECAL DIVERSIONS

An **ileostomy** is the surgical creation of an opening into the ileum or small intestine, usually by means of an ileal stoma on the abdominal wall. It allows for drainage of fecal matter (effluent) from the ileum to the outside of the body. The drainage is very mushy and occurs at frequent intervals. The ileostomy may be temporary or permanent. A permanent ileostomy is created after a total colectomy.

Another procedure is the continent ileal reservoir (Kock pouch). This procedure eliminates the need for an external fecal collection bag. Approximately 30 cm of the distal ileum is reconstructed to form a reservoir with a nipple valve that is created by pulling a portion of the terminal ileal loop back into the ileum. GI effluent (fecal matter) can accumulate in the pouch for several hours and then be removed by means of a catheter inserted through the nipple valve. The major problem with the Kock pouch is malfunction of the nipple valve, which occurs in 20% to 40% of the patients.

An ileoanal anastomosis is another surgical procedure that eliminates the need for a permanent ileostomy. It establishes an ileal reservoir, and anal sphincter control of elimination is retained. The procedure involves connecting a portion of the ileum to the anus (ileoanal anastomosis) in conjunction with removal of the colon and the rectal mucosa (a total abdominal colectomy and a mucosal proctectomy) (Fig. 35-5). A temporary diverting loop ileostomy is constructed at the time of surgery and closed about 3 months later.

With ileoanal anastomosis, the diseased colon and rectum are removed, voluntary defecation is maintained, and anal continence is preserved. The ileal reservoir decreases the number of bowel movements by 50%, from approximately 14 to 20 per day to 7 to 10 per day. Nighttime elimination is gradually reduced to one bowel movement. Complications of ileoanal anastomosis include irritation of the perianal skin from leakage of fecal contents, stricture formation at the anastomosis site, and small bowel obstruction.

Nursing Management

Nursing management of patients with inflammatory bowel disease may be medical, surgical, or both. Patients in the community setting or those recently diagnosed may primarily require education about diet and medications and referral to support groups. Hospitalized patients with long-standing or severe disease also require careful monitoring, parenteral nutrition and fluid replacement, and possibly emergent surgery. The surgical procedures may involve a fecal diversion, with attendant needs for physical care, emotional support, and extensive teaching in management of the ostomy.

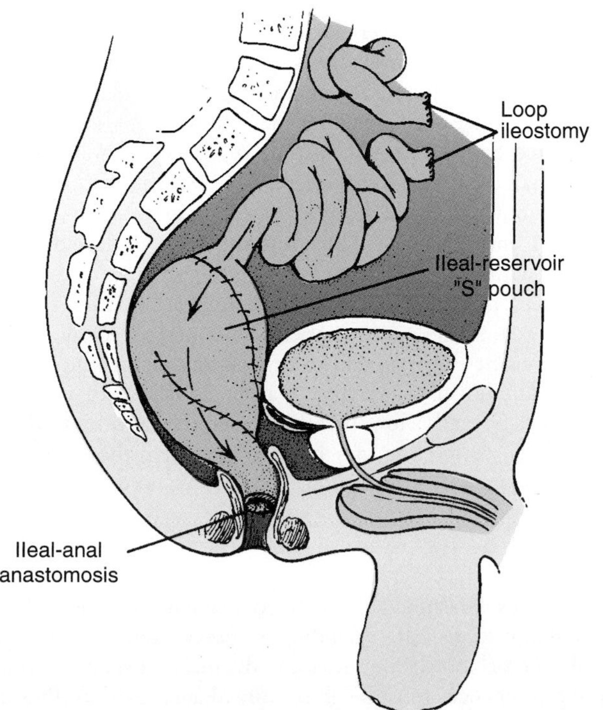

FIGURE 35•5 A mucosal proctectomy precedes anastomosis of the ileal reservoir. A temporary loop ileostomy diverts effluent for several months.

NURSING PROCESS: MANAGEMENT OF THE PATIENT WITH INFLAMMATORY BOWEL DISEASE

Assessment

A health history is taken to identify the onset, duration, and characteristics of abdominal pain; the presence of diarrhea or fecal urgency, straining at stool (tenesmus), nausea, anorexia, or weight loss; and family history of inflammatory bowel disease. Dietary patterns are discussed, including the amounts of alcohol, caffeine, and nicotine used daily and weekly. Patterns of bowel elimination are assessed, including character and frequency and presence of blood, pus, fat, or mucus. Allergies and food intolerances are important to document, especially milk (lactose) intolerance. The patient may identify sleep pattern disturbances if diarrhea or pain occurs at night.

Assessment includes auscultating the abdomen for bowel sounds and their characteristics; palpating the abdomen for distention, tenderness, or pain; and inspecting the skin for evidence of fistula tracts or symptoms of dehydration. The stool is inspected for blood and mucus.

With regional enteritis, pain is usually localized in the right lower quadrant, where hyperactive bowel sounds can be heard because of borborygmus (a gurgling bowel sound caused by passage of gas through the intestine) and increased peristalsis. Abdominal tenderness is noted on palpation. The most prominent symptom is intermittent pain that occurs with diarrhea but does not decrease after defecation. Pain in the periumbilical region usually indicates involvement of the terminal ileum. With ulcerative colitis, the abdomen may be distended and rebound tenderness may be present. Rectal bleeding is a significant sign.

Diagnosis

Nursing Diagnoses

Based on the assessment data, the nursing diagnoses may include the following:

- Diarrhea related to the inflammatory process
- Pain related to increased peristalsis and GI inflammation
- Fluid volume deficit related to anorexia, nausea, and diarrhea
- Altered nutrition, less than body requirements, related to dietary restrictions, nausea, and malabsorption
- Activity intolerance related to fatigue
- Anxiety related to impending surgery
- Ineffective individual coping related to repeated episodes of diarrhea
- Risk for impaired skin integrity related to malnutrition and diarrhea
- Risk for ineffective management of therapeutic regimen related to insufficient knowledge concerning the process and management of the disease

Collaborative Problems/Potential Complications

Potential complications that may develop include:

- Electrolyte imbalance
- Cardiac dysrhythmia related to electrolyte depletion
- GI bleeding with fluid volume loss
- Perforation of the bowel

Planning and Goals

The major goals for the patient include attainment of normal bowel elimination patterns, relief of abdominal pain and cramping, prevention of fluid volume deficit, maintenance of optimal nutrition and weight, avoidance of fatigue, reducing anxiety, promoting effective coping, absence of skin breakdown, learning about the disease process and therapeutic regimen, and avoidance of complications.

Nursing Interventions

Maintaining Normal Elimination Patterns

The nurse determines if there is a relationship between diarrhea and certain foods, activity, or emotional stress. Any precipitating factors are identified, as well as the frequency of bowel movements and the character, consistency, and amount of stool passed. Ready access to a bathroom or bedpan is provided, and the environment is kept clean and odor-free. Antidiarrheal medications are administered as prescribed, and the frequency and consistency of stools are recorded after therapy is initiated. Bed rest is encouraged to decrease peristalsis.

Relieving Pain

The character of the pain is described as dull, burning, or crampy. Its onset is relevant: Does it occur before or after meals, during the night, or before elimination? Is the pattern constant or intermittent? Is it relieved with medications? Anticholinergic medications are administered as prescribed 30 minutes before a meal to decrease intestinal motility, and analgesics are administered as prescribed for pain. Pain can also be reduced by position changes, the local application of heat (as prescribed), diversional activities, and the prevention of fatigue.

Maintaining Fluid Intake

To detect fluid volume deficit, an accurate record of oral and IV fluids is kept as well as a record of output (urine, liquid stool, vomitus, wound or fistula drainage). Daily weights are monitored for fluid gains or losses. The patient is assessed for signs of fluid volume deficit (dry skin and mucous membranes, decreased skin turgor, oliguria, exhaustion, decreased temperature, increased hematocrit, elevated urine specific gravity, and hypotension). Oral intake of fluids is encouraged, and the IV flow rate is monitored. Measures to decrease diarrhea are initiated (dietary restrictions, stress reduction, antidiarrheal agents).

Maintaining Optimal Nutrition

Total parenteral nutrition (TPN) is used when the symptoms of inflammatory bowel disease are severe. With TPN, the nurse maintains an accurate record of fluid intake and output as well as the patient's daily weight. The patient should gain 0.5 kg daily during therapy. Because TPN is very high in glucose and can cause hyperglycemia, the blood glucose is monitored every 6 hours. Elemental feedings high in protein and low in fat and residue are instituted after TPN therapy because they are digested primarily in the jejunum, do not stimulate intestinal secretions, and allow the bowel to rest. Intolerance is noted if the patient exhibits nausea, vomiting, diarrhea, or abdominal distention.

If oral foods are tolerated, small, frequent, low-residue feedings are given to avoid overdistending the stomach and stimulating peristalsis. Activities are restricted to conserve energy, reduce peristalsis, and reduce calorie requirements.

Promoting Rest

Intermittent rest periods during the day are recommended and activities are scheduled and/or restricted to conserve energy and reduce the metabolic rate. Activity within the limits of the patient's capacity is encouraged. Bed rest is suggested for a patient who is febrile, has frequent diarrheal stools, or is bleeding. The patient on bed rest is encouraged to perform active exercises to maintain muscle tone and prevent thromboembolic complications. If the patient is unable to do so, the nurse performs passive exercises and joint range of motion. Activity restrictions are modified as needed on a day-to-day basis.

Reducing Anxiety

Rapport can be established by being attentive and displaying a calm, confident manner. Time is provided for the patient to ask questions and express feelings. Careful listening and sensitivity to nonverbal indicators of anxiety (restlessness, tense facial expressions) are helpful. The patient may be emotionally labile because of the consequences of the disease; information about impending surgery should be tailored to the patient's level of understanding and desire for detail. Pictures and illustrations help to explain the surgical procedure and help the patient to visualize what a stoma looks like.

Enhancing Coping Measures

Because the patient may feel isolated, helpless, and out of control, understanding and emotional support are essential. The patient may respond to stress in a variety of ways that may alienate others, including anger, denial, and social self-isolation.

The nurse needs to recognize that the patient's behavior may be affected by a number of factors unrelated to inherent emotional characteristics. Any patient suffering the discomforts of frequent bowel movements and rectal soreness is anxious, discouraged, and depressed. Thus, it is important to develop a relationship with the patient that supports all attempts to cope with these stresses. It is important to communicate that the patient's feelings are understood: the patient is encouraged to talk and express his or her feelings and to discuss any disturbing matters. Stress reduction measures that may be used include relaxation techniques, visualization, breathing exercises, and biofeedback. Professional counseling may be needed to help the patient and family manage issues associated with chronic illness.

Preventing Skin Breakdown

The patient's skin should be examined frequently, especially the perianal skin. Perianal care, including the use of a skin barrier, is provided after each bowel movement. Reddened or irritated areas over bony prominences must be given immediate attention. Pressure-relieving devices should be used to avoid skin breakdown. Consultation with a wound care specialist or enterostomal therapist is often helpful.

HOME CARE TEACHING CHECKLIST: MANAGING INFLAMMATORY BOWEL DISEASE

At the completion of the program, the patient or caregiver will be able to:	Patient	Caregiver
• Verbalize an understanding of the disease process.	✔	✔
• Discuss nutritional management: bland, low-residue, high-protein, high-vitamin diet; identify foods to include and foods to be avoided.	✔	✔
• Describe medication regimen; identify medications by name, use, route, and frequency.	✔	✔
• Identify measures to be used to treat exacerbation of symptoms, to include rest, dietary modifications, medications.	✔	✔

Monitoring and Managing Potential Complications

Serum electrolyte levels are monitored daily. Evidence of dysrhythmias or change in level of consciousness is reported immediately. Electrolyte replacements are administered as prescribed.

Rectal bleeding is monitored closely. Blood component therapy and volume expanders are administered as prescribed to prevent hypovolemia. The blood pressure is monitored for hypotension. Coagulation and hematocrit and hemoglobin profiles are obtained frequently. Vitamin K may be prescribed to increase clotting factors.

The patient must be monitored closely for indications of perforation (acute increase in abdominal pain, rigid abdomen, vomiting, or hypotension) and obstruction and toxic megacolon (abdominal distention, decreased or absent bowel sounds, change in mental status, fever, tachycardia, hypotension, dehydration, and electrolyte imbalances).

Promoting Home and Community-Based Care

TEACHING PATIENTS SELF-CARE

The patient's understanding of the disease process and his or her need for additional information about medical management (medications, diet) and surgical interventions are assessed. Information about nutritional management is provided. A bland, low-residue, high-protein, high-calorie, and high-vitamin diet relieves symptoms and decreases diarrhea. The rationale for the use of corticosteroids and anti-inflammatory, antibacterial, antidiarrheal, and antispasmodic medications is provided. The importance of taking medications as prescribed and not abruptly discontinuing them (especially corticosteroids) is emphasized because serious medical problems may result. Ileostomy care is reviewed as necessary. Patient education information can be obtained from the National Foundation for Ileitis and Colitis.

CONTINUING CARE

Patients with chronic inflammatory disease are managed at home with follow-up care with their physician or through an outpatient clinic. Those whose nutritional status is compromised and who are receiving TPN will need home care nursing to ensure that their nutritional requirements are being met and that they or their caregivers can follow through with the instructions for TPN. Patients who are medically managed need to understand that their disease can be controlled and that they can lead a healthy life between exacerbations. Control implies management based on an understanding of the disease and its treatment. Patients in the home setting need information about their medications (name, dose, side effects, frequency of administration) and need to take medications on schedule. Medication reminders are helpful (containers that separate pills according to day and time, daily checklists).

During a flare-up, patients are encouraged to rest as needed and to modify activities according to their energy levels. They are advised to limit tasks that impose strain on the lower abdominal muscles. Patients should sleep in a room close to the bathroom because of the frequent diarrhea (10 to 20 times a day). Quick access to a toilet helps alleviate the worry of embarrassment if an accident occurs. Room deodorizers help control odors.

Dietary modifications can control but not cure the disease. A low-residue, high-protein, high-calorie diet is recommended, especially during an acute phase. Patients are encouraged to keep a record of the foods that irritate the bowel and to eliminate them from the diet. Fluid intake of at least eight glasses of water per day is encouraged.

The prolonged nature of the disease has an impact on the patient and often strains his or her family life and financial resources as well. Family support is vital; however, some family members may be resentful, guilty, and tired and feel unable to continue coping with the emotional demands of the illness as well as with the physical demands of caring for another. Some patients with inflammatory bowel disease do not socialize for fear of being embarrassed. Many prefer to eat alone. Because they have lost control over elimination, they may fear losing control over other aspects of their lives. They need time to express their fears and frustrations. Individual and family counseling may be helpful.

Evaluation

Expected Outcomes

Expected outcomes may include:

1. Reports a decrease in the frequency of diarrheal stools
   a. Complies with dietary restrictions; maintains bed rest
   b. Takes medications as prescribed
2. Has reduced pain
3. Maintains fluid volume balance
   a. Drinks 1 to 2 L of oral fluids daily
   b. Has a normal body temperature
   c. Displays adequate skin turgor and moist mucous membranes
4. Attains optimal nutrition—tolerates small, frequent feedings without diarrhea
5. Avoids fatigue
   a. Rests periodically during the day
   b. Adheres to activity restrictions

6. Is less anxious
7. Copes successfully with diagnosis
   a. Expresses feelings freely
   b. Uses appropriate stress reduction behaviors
8. Maintains skin integrity
   a. Cleans perianal skin after defecation
   b. Uses lotion or ointment as skin barrier
9. Acquires an understanding of the disease process
   a. Modifies diet appropriately to decrease diarrhea
   b. Adheres to medication regimen
10. Recovers without complications
    a. Maintains electrolytes within normal range
    b. Maintains normal sinus or baseline cardiac rhythm
    c. Maintains fluid balance
    d. Does not have perforation or rectal bleeding

Nursing Management of the Patient Requiring an Ileostomy

As previously discussed, some patients with inflammatory bowel disease eventually require permanent fecal diversion to manage symptoms and to treat or prevent complications.

Providing Preoperative Care

A period of preparation with intensive fluid, blood, and protein replacement is necessary before surgery is performed. Antibiotics may be prescribed. If the patient has been taking corticosteroids, they will be continued during the surgical phase. Usually, the patient is given a low-residue diet, offered in frequent, small feedings. All other preoperative measures are similar to those for general abdominal surgery. The abdomen is marked for the proper placement of the stoma by the surgeon or the enterostomal therapist. Care is taken to ensure that the ostomy stoma is conveniently placed—usually in the right lower quadrant about 2 inches below the waist crease, in an area away from previous scars, bony prominences, skin folds, or fistulas.

Information about an ileostomy is presented to the patient by means of written materials, models, and discussion. The patient must have a thorough understanding of the surgery to be performed and what to expect after surgery. Preoperative teaching will relate to managing the drainage from the stoma, the nature of drainage, and the need for nasogastric intubation, parenteral fluids, and possibly perineal packing and care.

Providing Postoperative Care

General abdominal surgery wound care is required. The stoma is observed for color and size. It should be pink to bright red and shiny. For the traditional ileostomy, a temporary plastic bag with an adhesive facing is placed over the ileostomy and firmly pressed onto surrounding skin. The ileostomy is monitored for fecal drainage, which should begin about 72 hours after surgery. The drainage is a continuous liquid from the small intestine because the stoma does not have a controlling sphincter. The contents drain into the plastic bag and are thus kept from coming into contact with the skin. They are collected and measured as the bag becomes full. If a continent ileal reservoir was created, as described for the Kock pouch, it will require continuous drainage by an indwelling reservoir catheter for 2 to 3 weeks after surgery. This allows the suture lines to heal.

Because these patients lose much fluid in the early postoperative period, an accurate record of fluid intake, urinary output, and fecal discharge is necessary to help gauge the fluid needs of the patient. There may be 1000 to 2000 mL of fluid lost each day, in addition to expected fluid loss through urine, perspiration, respiration, and other sources. With this loss, sodium and potassium are depleted. Laboratory values are monitored and electrolyte replacements administered as prescribed. IV fluids are given to replace fluid losses for 4 to 5 days.

Nasogastric suction is also a part of immediate postoperative care, with the tube requiring frequent irrigation, as prescribed. The purpose of nasogastric suction is to prevent a buildup of gastric contents. After the tube is removed, sips of clear liquids are offered and the diet is progressed gradually. Nausea and abdominal distention may indicate obstruction and are reported immediately. As with other patients undergoing abdominal surgery, those with ileostomies are encouraged to engage in early ambulation. Prescribed pain medications are administered as required.

By the end of the first week, rectal packing is removed. Because this procedure may be uncomfortable, an analgesic may be administered an hour before it is performed. After the packing is removed, the perineum is irrigated two or three times daily until full healing takes place.

Providing Emotional Support

The patient understandably may think that everyone is aware of the ileostomy, and may view the stoma as a mutilation in comparison with other abdominal incisions that heal and are hidden. Because there is loss of a body part and a major change in anatomy, the patient often goes through the various phases of grieving: shock, disbelief, denial, rejection, anger, and restitution. Nursing support through these phases is important, and understanding of the patient's emotional outlook in each instance should determine the approach taken. For example, teaching may be ineffective until the patient is ready to learn. Concern over body image may lead to questions related to family relationships, sexual function, and for women the ability to become pregnant and to deliver a baby normally. Patients need to know that someone understands and cares about them. A calm, nonjudgmental attitude exhibited by the nurse will aid in gaining the patient's confidence. It is important to recognize the dependency needs of these patients. Their prolonged illness can make them irritable, anxious, and depressed. The nurse can coordinate patient care through meetings attended by consultants such as the physician, psychologist, psychiatrist, social worker, enterostomal therapist, and dietitian. The team approach is important in facilitating the often complex care of this patient.

Conversely, a surgical procedure to create an ileostomy can produce dramatic positive changes in patients who have suffered from inflammatory bowel disease for several years. Once the continuous discomfort of the disease has decreased and patients learn how to take care of the ileostomy, they often develop a more positive outlook. Until they progress to this phase, an empathic and tolerant approach by the nurse will play an important part in recovery. The sooner the patient masters the physical care of the ileostomy, the sooner he or she will psychologically accept it.

The support of other ostomates is also helpful. The United Ostomy Association is dedicated to the rehabilitation of ostomates. This organization gives patients useful information about living with an ostomy through an educational program of literature, lectures, and exhibits. Local associations offer visiting services by qualified members who provide hope, and rehabilitation services to new ostomy patients. Hospitals and other health care agencies may have an enterostomal therapy nurse on staff who can serve as a valuable resource person for the ileostomy patient.

Managing Skin and Stoma Care

The patient with a traditional ileostomy cannot establish regular bowel habits because the contents of the ileum are fluid and are discharged continuously. Therefore, the patient must wear a pouch at all times. Stomal size and pouch size will vary initially; the stoma should be rechecked 3 weeks after surgery, when the edema has subsided. The final size and type of appliance is selected in 3 months, after the patient's weight has stabilized and the stoma shrinks to a stable shape.

The location and length of the stoma are significant in the management of the ileostomy by the patient. The surgeon positions the stoma as close to the midline as possible and at a location where even an obese patient with a protruding abdomen can care for it easily. Usually, the ileostomy stoma is about 2.5 cm (1 in) long, which makes it convenient for the attachment of an appliance.

Skin excoriation around the stoma can be a persistent problem. Peristomal skin integrity may be compromised by several factors, such as an allergic reaction to the ostomy appliance or skin barrier or paste, chemical irritation from the effluent, mechanical injury from the removal of the appliance, and possible infection. If irritation and yeast growth are present, nystatin powder (Mycostatin) is dusted lightly on the peristomal skin.

Changing an Ileostomy Appliance

A regular schedule for changing the pouch before leakage occurs must be established for those with a traditional ileostomy. The patient can be taught to change the pouch in a manner similar to that described in Guideline 35-1.

The amount of time a person can keep the appliance sealed to the body surface depends on the location of the stoma and on body structure. Usually, the normal wearing time is 5 to 7 days. The appliance is emptied every 4 to 6 hours, or at the same time the patient empties the bladder. An emptying spout at the bottom of the appliance is closed with a special clip made for this purpose.

Most pouches are disposable and odor-proof. Foods such as spinach and parsley act as deodorizers in the intestinal tract; foods that cause odors include cabbage, onions, and fish. Bismuth subcarbonate tablets, which may be prescribed and taken by mouth three or four times a day, are effective in reducing odor. A stool thickener, such as diphenoxylate (Lomotil), may also be prescribed to be taken by mouth to assist in odor control.

Irrigating a Continent Ileostomy

For a continent ileostomy (Kock pouch), the patient must be taught to drain the pouch, as described in Guideline 35-2. A catheter is inserted into the reservoir to drain the fluid. The length of time between drainage periods is gradually increased until the reservoir need only be drained every 4 to 6 hours and irrigated once a day. A pouch is not necessary; instead, most patients wear a small dressing over the opening.

When the fecal discharge is thick, water can be injected through the catheter to loosen and soften it. The consistency of the effluent is affected by food intake. At first, drainage is only 60 to 80 mL, but as time goes on it will increase significantly. The internal Kock pouch will stretch, eventually accommodating 500 to 1000 mL. The patient uses the sensation of pressure in the pouch as a gauge to determine how often the pouch should be drained.

Managing Dietary and Fluid Needs

A low-residue diet is followed for the first 6 to 8 weeks. Strained fruits and vegetables are given. These foods are important sources of vitamins A and C. Later there are few dietary restrictions, except for avoiding foods that are high in fiber or hard-to-digest kernels, such as celery, popcorn, corn, poppy seeds, caraway seeds, and coconut. Foods are reintroduced one at a time. The patient's tolerance for these foods is assessed, and he or she is reminded to chew food thoroughly.

Fluids may be a problem during the summer, when fluid lost through perspiration adds to the fluid loss through the ileostomy. Fluids such as Gatorade are helpful in maintaining electrolyte balance. If the effluent (fecal discharge) is too watery, fibrous foods (eg, whole-grain cereals, fresh fruit skins, beans, corn, and nuts) are restricted. If the effluent is excessively dry, salt intake is increased. An increased intake of water or fluid will not increase the effluent because excess water is excreted in the urine. See the Plan of Nursing Care 35-1 for a summary of caring for the patient with a fecal diversion.

Preventing Complications

Monitoring for complications is an ongoing activity for the patient with an ileostomy. Minor complications occur in about 40% of patients who have an ileostomy; less than 20% of the complications require surgical intervention.

Common complications include skin irritation, diarrhea, stomal stenosis, urinary calculi, and cholelithiasis. Peristomal skin irritation, the most common complication of an ileostomy, results from leakage of effluent. An ill-fitting pouch is often the cause. The pouch is adjusted by the nurse or an enterostomal therapist and skin barriers are applied. Diarrhea, manifested by very irritating effluent that rapidly fills the pouch (every hour or sooner), can quickly lead to dehydration and electrolyte losses. Supplemental water, sodium, and potassium are administered to prevent hypovolemia and hypokalemia. Antidiarrheal agents are administered. Stenosis is caused by circular scar tissue that forms at the stoma site. The scar tissue must be surgically released. Urinary calculi occur in about 10% of ileostomy patients because of dehydration secondary to decreased fluid intake. Intense lower abdominal pain that radiates to the legs, hematuria, and signs of dehydration indicate that the urine should be strained. Fluid intake is encouraged. Sometimes small stones are passed during urination; otherwise, treatment is necessary to crush or remove the calculi.

Cholelithiasis (gallstones) from cholesterol occurs three times more commonly in patients with an ileostomy than in the general population because of changes in the absorption of bile acids that occur postoperatively. Spasm of the gallbladder causes severe upper right abdominal pain that can radiate to the back and right shoulder.

Promoting Home and Community-Based Care

TEACHING PATIENTS SELF-CARE

The spouse and family should be familiar with the adjustment that will be necessary when the patient returns home. They need to know why it is necessary for the patient to occupy the bathroom for 10 minutes or more at certain times of the day, and why certain equipment is needed. Their understanding is necessary to reduce tension; a relaxed patient tends to have fewer problems. Visits from an enterostomal therapy nurse may be arranged to

35•1
GUIDELINES FOR CHANGING AN ILEOSTOMY APPLIANCE

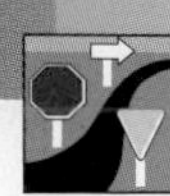

Changing an ileostomy appliance is necessary to prevent leakage (the bag is usually changed every 2 to 4 days), to allow for examination of the skin around the stoma, and to assist in controlling odor if this becomes a problem. The appliance should be changed at any time that the patient complains of burning or itching under the disk or pain in the area of the stoma; routine changes should be performed early in the morning before breakfast or 2 to 4 hours after a meal, when the bowel is least active.

Nursing Action	Rationale
1. Promote patient comfort and involvement in the procedure. • Have the patient assume a relaxed position. • Provide privacy. • Explain details of the procedure. • Expose the ileostomy area; remove the ileostomy belt (if worn).	Providing a relaxed atmosphere and adequate explanations help the patient to become an active participant in the procedure.
2. Remove the appliance. • Have the patient sit on the toilet or on a chair facing the toilet. A patient who prefers to stand should face the toilet. • The appliance (pouch) can be removed by gently pushing the skin away from the adhesive.	These positions facilitate disposal or drainage.

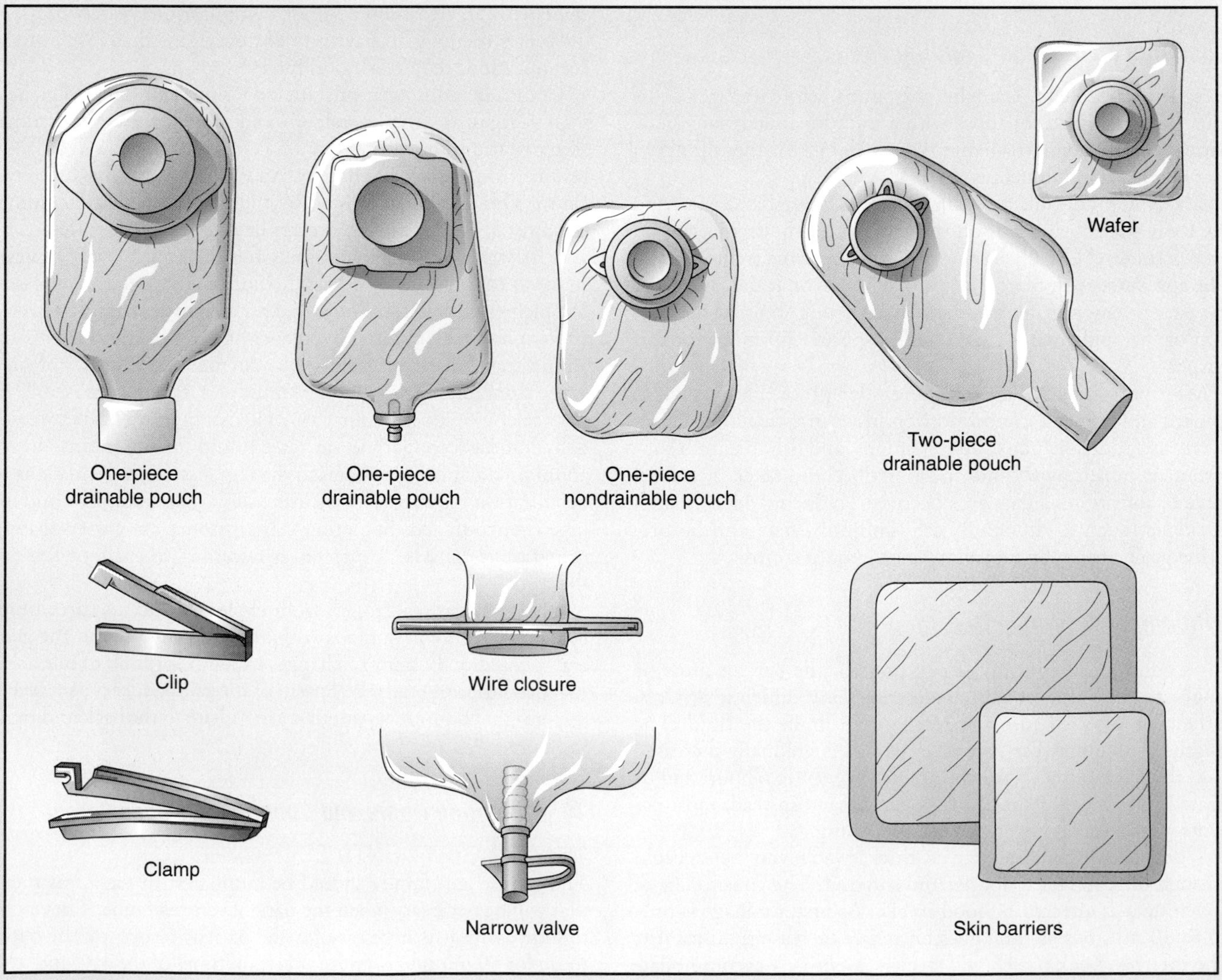

Selected ostomy pouches and accessories.

(continued)

35•1 GUIDELINES FOR 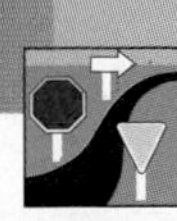 CHANGING AN ILEOSTOMY APPLIANCE (Continued)

Nursing Action	Rationale
3. Cleanse the skin:	
• Wash the skin gently with a soft cloth moistened with tepid water and mild soap; the patient may prefer to bathe before putting on a clean appliance.	The patient may shower with or without the pouch. Micropore or waterproof tape applied to the sides of the faceplate will keep it secure during bathing.
• Rinse and dry the skin thoroughly after cleansing.	Moisture or soap residue will interfere with appliance adhesion.
4. Apply appliance (when there is *no* skin irritation):	
• An appropriate skin barrier is applied to the peristomal skin before the pouch is applied.	Many pouches have a built-in skin barrier.
• Remove cover from adherent surface of disk of disposable plastic pouch and apply directly to the skin.	The skin should be thoroughly dried before applying the pouch.
• Press firmly in place for 30 seconds to ensure adherence.	
5. Apply appliance (when there is skin irritation):	
• Cleanse the skin thoroughly but gently; pat dry.	To remove debris.
• Apply Kenalog spray; blot excess moisture with a cotton pledget and dust lightly with nystatin (Mycostatin) powder.	The corticosteroid preparation (Kenalog) helps to decrease inflammation. The antifungal agent (nystatin) treats those types of infections that are common around stomas. A prescription is required for both medications.
Or apply as an alternative a wafer of Stomahesive (Squibb), which is commercially available. The stomal opening should be cut the same size as the stoma; use a cutting guide (supplied with Stomahesive). The wafer is applied directly to the skin.	Stomahesive is a substance that facilitates healing of excoriated skin. It adheres well even to moist, irritated skin.
• Another alternative is to moisten a karaya gum washer and apply when it is tacky. If the skin is moist, karaya powder may be applied first and any excess dusted off gently.	Karaya also facilitates skin healing. Tackiness promotes adherence.
• The pouch is then applied to the treated skin.	This will allow skin to heal while the appliance is in place.
6. Check the pouch bottom for closure; use the rubber band or clip provided.	Proper closure controls leakage.

ensure that the patient is progressing as expected and to provide additional guidance and teaching as needed.

The patient needs to know the commercial name of the pouch to be used so that he or she can obtain a ready supply, and information about obtaining other supplies. The names of the local enterostomal therapy nurse and local self-help groups are often helpful. Any special restrictions on driving or working also need to be reviewed. The patient should be taught about common postoperative complications and how to recognize and report them.

INTESTINAL OBSTRUCTION

Intestinal obstruction exists when blockage prevents the normal flow of intestinal contents through the intestinal tract. This flow can be impeded by two types of processes:

- Mechanical—an intraluminal obstruction or a mural obstruction from pressure on the intestinal walls occurs. Examples of conditions that can cause mechanical obstruction are intussusception, polypoid tumors and neoplasms, stenosis, strictures, adhesions, hernias, and abscesses.
- Functional—the intestinal musculature cannot propel the contents along the bowel. Examples are amyloidosis, muscular dystrophy, endocrine disorders such as diabetes mellitus, or neurologic disorders such as Parkinson's disease. It also can be temporary and the result of the manipulation of the bowel during surgery.

The obstruction can be partial or complete. Its severity depends on the region of bowel affected, the degree to which the lumen is occluded, and, especially, the degree to which the blood circulation in the bowel wall is disturbed.

Most bowel obstructions (85%) occur in the small intestine. Adhesions are the most common cause of small bowel obstruction (60% incidence), followed by hernias and neoplasms. Other causes include intussusception, volvulus (twisting of the bowel), and paralytic ileus. About 15% of intestinal obstructions occur in the large bowel; most of these are found in the sigmoid colon. The most common causes are carcinoma, diverticulitis, inflammatory bowel disorders, and benign tumors. Table 35-5 and Figure 35-6 list mechanical causes of obstruction and describe how they occur.

Small Bowel Obstruction

Pathophysiology

An accumulation of intestinal contents, fluid, and gas develops above the intestinal obstruction. The abdominal distention and retention of fluid reduce the absorption of fluids and stimulate

35•2 Guidelines For Draining a Continent Ileostomy (Kock Pouch)

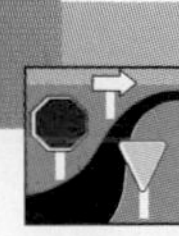

A continent ileostomy is the surgical creation of a pouch of small intestine that can serve as an internal receptacle for fecal discharge; a nipple valve is constructed at the outlet. Postoperatively, a catheter extends from the stoma and is attached to a closed drainage suction system. To ensure patency of the catheter, usually every 3 hours 10 to 20 mL of normal saline is instilled gently into the pouch; return flow is not aspirated but is allowed to drain by gravity.

After approximately 2 weeks, when the healing process has progressed to the point at which the catheter is removed from the stoma, the patient is taught to drain the pouch. The equipment required includes a catheter, tissues, water-soluble lubricant, gauze squares, a syringe, irrigating solution in a bowl, and an emesis or receiving basin.

The following procedure is used to drain the pouch; the patient is helped to participate in this procedure to learn to perform it unassisted.

Nursing Action	Rationale
1. Lubricate the catheter and gently insert it about 5 cm (2 in), at which some resistance may be felt at the valve or nipple.	When gentle pressure is used, the catheter usually will enter the pouch.
2. If there is much resistance, fill a syringe with 20 mL of air or water and inject it through the catheter, while still exerting some pressure on the catheter.	This will permit the catheter to enter the pouch.
3. Place the other end of the catheter in a drainage basin held below the level of the stoma. Later this process can be carried out at the toilet with drainage delivered into the toilet bowl.	Gravity facilitates drainage. Drainage may include flatus as well as effluent.
4. After drainage, the catheter is removed and the area around the stoma is gently washed with warm water. Pat dry and apply an absorbent pad over the stoma. Fasten the pad with hypoallergenic tape.	The entire procedure requires about 5 to 10 minutes; at first it is performed every 3 hours. The time between procedures is gradually lengthened to three times daily.

more gastric secretion. With increasing distention, pressure within the intestinal lumen increases, causing a decrease in venous and arteriolar capillary pressure. This, in turn, causes edema, congestion, necrosis, and eventual rupture or perforation of the intestinal wall, with resultant peritonitis.

Reflux vomiting may occur from the abdominal distention. Vomiting results in a loss of hydrogen ions and potassium from the stomach, leading to a reduction of chlorides and potassium in the blood and to metabolic alkalosis. Dehydration and acidosis develop from loss of water and sodium. With acute fluid losses, hypovolemic shock may occur.

Clinical Manifestations

The initial symptom is usually crampy pain that is wavelike and colicky. The patient may pass blood and mucus, but no fecal matter and no flatus. Vomiting occurs. If the obstruction is complete, the peristaltic waves initially become extremely vigorous and will eventually assume a reverse direction, the intestinal contents being propelled toward the mouth instead of toward the rectum. If the obstruction is in the ileum, fecal vomiting takes place. First, the patient vomits the stomach contents, then the bile-stained contents of the duodenum and the jejunum, and finally, with each paroxysm of pain, the darker, fecal-like contents of the ileum. The unmistakable signs of dehydration become evident: the patient has intense thirst, drowsiness, generalized malaise, and aching, and the tongue and mucous membranes become parched. The abdomen becomes distended. The lower the obstruction is in the GI tract, the more marked the abdominal distention. If the obstruction continues uncorrected, shock occurs from dehydration and loss of plasma volume.

Assessment and Diagnostic Findings

Diagnosis is based on the symptoms described above as well as on x-ray findings. Abdominal x-rays show abnormal quantities of gas and/or fluid in the bowel. Laboratory studies (electrolyte studies and a complete blood count) reveal a picture of dehydration and loss of plasma volume, and possibly infection.

Medical Management

Decompression of the bowel through a nasogastric or small bowel tube (see Chap. 33) is successful in the majority of cases. When the bowel is completely obstructed, the possibility of strangulation warrants surgical intervention. Before surgery, intravenous therapy is necessary to replace the depleted water, sodium, chloride, and potassium.

The surgical treatment of intestinal obstruction depends largely on the cause of the obstruction. In the most common causes of obstruction, such as hernia and adhesions, the surgical procedure involves repairing the hernia or dividing the adhesion to which the intestine is attached. In some instances, the portion of affected bowel may be removed and an anastomosis performed. The complexity of the surgical procedure for intestinal obstruction depends on the duration of the obstruction and the condition of the intestine found during surgery.

(text continues on page 901)

35•1

PLAN OF NURSING CARE 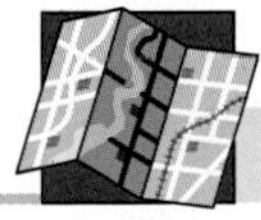 The Patient With a Fecal Diversion

Preoperative

Nursing Diagnosis: Knowledge deficit about the surgical procedure and preoperative preparation
Goal: Understands the surgical process and the necessary preoperative preparations

Nursing Interventions	Rationale	Expected Outcomes
1. Ascertain if the patient has had a previous surgical experience and ask for recollections of positive and negative impressions.	1. Fear of a repeated negative experience increases anxiety. Talking about the experience with a nurse helps clarify misconceptions and helps the patient ventilate any repressed emotions. Positive experiences are reinforced.	• Expresses anxieties and fears about the surgical process • Projects a positive attitude toward the surgical procedure • Repeats in own words information given by the surgeon • Identifies normal anatomy and physiology of gastrointestinal tract and how it will be altered. Can point to expected location of abdominal wound and stoma. Describes stoma appearance and size • Adheres to "bowel prep" regimen of antimicrobials or mechanical cleansing • Tolerates the presence of nasogastric/nasoenteric tube
2. Determine what information the surgeon gave the patient and family and whether it was understood. Clarify and elaborate as necessary. Determine whether the stoma is permanent or temporary. Be aware of the patient's prognosis if carcinoma exists.	2. Clarification prevents misunderstandings and alleviates anxiety. A positive affect may be more difficult to project if the ostomy is permanent or the prognosis poor.	
3. Use pictures or drawings to illustrate the location and appearance of the surgical wounds (abdominal, perineal) and the stoma if the patient is interested and receptive.	3. Knowledge, for some, alleviates anxiety because fear of the unknown is decreased. Others choose not to know because it makes them more anxious.	
4. Explain that oral/parenteral antimicrobials will be administered to cleanse the bowel preoperatively. Mechanical cleansing may also be required.	4. Antimicrobials and mechanical cleansing will reduce intestinal bacterial flora.	
5. Assist the patient during nasogastric/nasoenteric intubation. Measure drainage from the tube.	5. Nasoenteral intubation is used for decompression and drainage of gastrointestinal contents before surgery.	

Nursing Diagnosis: Body image disturbance
Goal: Attainment of a positive self-concept

Nursing Interventions	Rationale	Expected Outcomes
1. Encourage the patient to verbalize feelings about the stoma.	1. Free expression of feelings allows the patient the opportunity to verbalize and identify concerns. Expressed concerns can be therapeutically addressed by health care team members.	• Freely expresses concerns • Accepts support • Seeks help as needed • States is willing to talk with an ostomate
2. Offer to be present when the stoma is first viewed and touched.	2. Anxiety can be reduced if questions are immediately answered.	
3. Suggest that the spouse or significant other view the stoma.	3. Helps patient to overcome fears about partner's response.	
4. Offer counseling, if desired.	4. Provides opportunity for additional support.	
5. Arrange for a visit with an ostomate.	5. Ostomates can offer support and share mutual feelings.	

Postoperative

Nursing Diagnosis: Anxiety related to the loss of bowel control
Goal: Reduction of anxiety

Nursing Interventions	Rationale	Expected Outcomes
1. Provide information about expected bowel function: a. Characteristics of effluent b. Frequency of discharge	1. Emotional adjustment is facilitated if adequate information is provided at the level of the learner.	• Expresses interest in learning about altered bowel function • Handles equipment correctly • Changes the pouch unassisted

(continued)

35•1 **PLAN OF NURSING CARE**

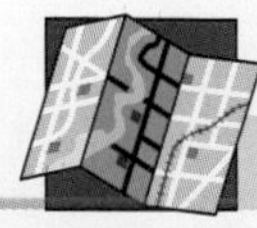

The Patient With a Fecal Diversion (*continued*)

Nursing Interventions	Rationale	Expected Outcomes
2. Teach the patient how to prepare the pouch for an adequate fit.		• Irrigates colostomy successfully • Progresses toward a regular schedule of elimination
a. Choose the drainage pouch that will provide a secure fit around the stoma. Measure the stoma size with a measuring guide provided by the ostomy manufacturer and compare with the opening on the pouch. About 3-mm (⅛-in) clearance should be provided around the stoma.	2. a. The pouch opening should be larger than the stoma for an adequate fit. Available brands come in different sizes to fit the stoma. Adjustments are made as necessary.	
b. Remove any plastic covering that protects the pouch adhesive. *Note:* The pouch is applied by pressing the adhesive for 30 seconds to the skin or skin barrier.	b. The pouch is ready to apply directly to the skin or skin protector.	
3. Demonstrate how to change the pouch before leakage occurs. Be aware that the elderly person may have diminished vision and difficulty handling equipment.	3. Manipulation of the appliance is a learned motor skill that requires practice and positive reinforcement.	
4. Demonstrate how to irrigate the colostomy (usually on the 4th–5th day). Recommend that irrigating be done at a consistent time, depending on the type of colostomy.		

Nursing Diagnosis: Risk for impaired skin integrity related to irritation of the peristomal skin by the effluent
Goal: Attainment of skin integrity

Nursing Interventions	Rationale	Expected Outcomes
1. Provide information about signs/symptoms of irritated or inflamed skin. Use pictures if possible.	1. Peristomal skin should be slightly pink without abrasions and similar to that of the entire abdomen.	• Describes appearance of healthy skin • Correctly cleanses the skin • Successfully applies a skin barrier • Gently removes the drainage pouch without skin damage • Demonstrates intact skin around the colostomy stoma
2. Teach patient how to cleanse the peristomal skin gently.	2. Mild friction with warm water and a gentle soap cleanses the skin and minimizes irritation and possible abrasions. Patting the skin dry prevents tissue trauma.	
3. Demonstrate how to apply a skin barrier (powder, gel, paste, wafer).	3. Skin barriers protect the peristomal skin from enzymes and bacteria.	
4. Demonstrate how to remove the pouch.	4. Gently separate adhesive from the skin to avoid irritation. Never pull!	

Nursing Diagnosis: Potential alteration in nutrition, less than body requirements, related to avoidance of foods that may cause GI discomfort
Goal: Achievement of an optimal nutritional intake

Nursing Interventions	Rationale	Expected Outcomes
1. Conduct a complete nutritional assessment to identify any foods that may increase peristalsis by irritating the bowel.	1. Patients react differently to certain foods because of individual sensitivity.	• Modifies diet to avoid offensive foods yet maintains a balanced nutritional intake • Avoids foods such as peanuts • Modifies intake of certain fruits
2. Advise the patient to avoid food products with a cellulose or hemicellulose base (nuts, seeds).	2. Cellulose food products are the nondigestible residue of plant foods. They hold water, provide bulk, and stimulate elimination.	
3. Recommend moderation in intake of certain irritating fruits such as prunes, grapes, and bananas.	3. These fruits tend to increase the quantity of effluent.	

(*continued*)

35•1 PLAN OF NURSING CARE 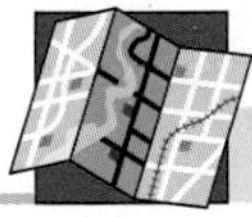 **The Patient With a Fecal Diversion (*continued*)**

Nursing Interventions	Rationale	Expected Outcomes
Nursing Diagnosis: Sexual dysfunction related to altered body image **Goal:** Attainment of satisfactory sexual performance		
1. Encourage the patient to verbalize fears. The sexual partner is welcomed to participate in the discussion.	1. Expressed needs help the therapist develop a plan of care.	• Expresses fears and concerns • Discusses alternative sexual positions • Accepts services of a professional counselor
2. Recommend alternative sexual positions.	2. Avoid patient embarrassment with the visual appearance of the stoma. Avoid peristomal skin irritation secondary to friction.	
3. Seek assistance from a sexual therapist, enterostomal therapist, or advanced practice nurse.	3. Some patients need professional sexual counseling.	
Nursing Diagnosis: Risk for fluid volume deficit related to anorexia and vomiting and increased loss of fluids and electrolytes from GI tract **Goal:** Attainment of fluid balance		
1. Estimate fluid intake and output: a. Strict intake and output	1. Provides indication of fluid balance. a. An early indicator of fluid imbalance is a daily, significant difference between intake and output. The average person ingests (food, fluids) and loses (urine, feces, lungs) about 3 L of fluid every 24 hours.	• Maintains fluid balance • Maintains normal serum and urinary values for sodium and potassium • Normal skin turgor • Surface of tongue is pink, with a moist mucous membrane
b. Daily weights	b. A gain/loss of 1 L of fluid is reflected in a body weight change of 2.2 pounds.	
2. Assess serum and urinary values of sodium and potassium.	2. Sodium is the major electrolyte regulating water balance. Vomiting results in decreased urinary and serum sodium levels. Urinary sodium values, in contrast to serum values, reflect early, sensitive changes in sodium balance. Sodium works in conjunction with potassium, which is also decreased with vomiting. A significant deficiency in potassium is associated with a decrease in intracellular potassium bicarbonate, which leads to acidosis and compensatory hyperventilation.	
3. Observe and record skin turgor and the appearance of the tongue.	3. Adequate hydration is reflected by the skin's ability to return to its normal shape after being grasped between the fingers. *Note:* In the older person, it is normal for the return to be delayed. Changes in the mucous membrane covering of the tongue are accurate and early indicators of hydration status.	

Nursing Management

Nursing management of the nonsurgical patient with a small bowel obstruction includes maintaining the function of the nasogastric tube, assessing and measuring the nasogastric output, assessing for fluid and electrolyte imbalance, monitoring nutritional status, and assessing for improvement (return of normal bowel sounds, decreased abdominal distention, subjective improvement in abdominal pain and tenderness, and passage of flatus or stool). The nurse reports discrepancies in intake and output, worsening of pain or abdominal distention, and increased nasogastric output. If the patient's condition does not improve,

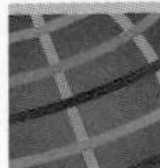

TABLE 35•5 Mechanical Causes of Intestinal Obstruction

Cause	Course of Events	Result
Adhesions	Loops of intestine become adherent to areas that heal slowly or scar after abdominal surgery.	3 or 4 days after surgery, adhesions produce a kinking of an intestinal loop.
Intussusception	One part of the intestine slips into another part located below it (like a telescope shortening).	Narrowing of the intestinal lumen
Volvulus	Bowel twists and turns on itself.	Intestinal lumen becomes obstructed. Gas and fluid accumulate in the trapped bowel.
Hernia	Protrusion of intestine through a weakened area in the abdominal muscle or wall.	Intestinal flow may be completely obstructed. Blood flow to the area may be obstructed as well.
Tumor	A tumor that exists within the wall of the intestine extends into the intestinal lumen, or a tumor outside the intestine causes pressure on the wall of the intestine.	Intestinal lumen becomes partially obstructed; if the tumor is not removed, complete obstruction results.

the nurse prepares him or her for surgery. The exact nature of the surgery will depend on the cause of the obstruction.

Nursing care of the patient after surgical repair of a small bowel obstruction is similar to that for other abdominal surgeries (see Chap. 18).

Large Bowel Obstruction

Pathophysiology

As in small bowel obstruction, large bowel obstruction results in an accumulation of intestinal contents, fluid, and gas proximal to the obstruction. Obstruction in the colon can lead to severe distention and perforation unless some gas and fluid can flow back through the ileal valve. Large bowel obstruction, even if complete, may be undramatic if the blood supply to the colon is not disturbed. If the blood supply is cut off, however, intestinal strangulation and necrosis (tissue death) occur; this condition is life-threatening. In the large intestine, dehydration occurs more slowly than in the small intestine because the colon can absorb its fluid contents and can distend to a size considerably beyond its normal full capacity.

Clinical Manifestations

Large bowel obstruction differs clinically from small bowel obstruction in that the symptoms develop and progress relatively slowly. In patients with obstruction in the sigmoid or the rectum, constipation may be the only symptom for days. Eventually, the abdomen becomes markedly distended, loops of large bowel become visibly outlined through the abdominal wall, and the patient has crampy lower abdominal pain. Finally, fecal vomiting develops. Symptoms of shock may occur.

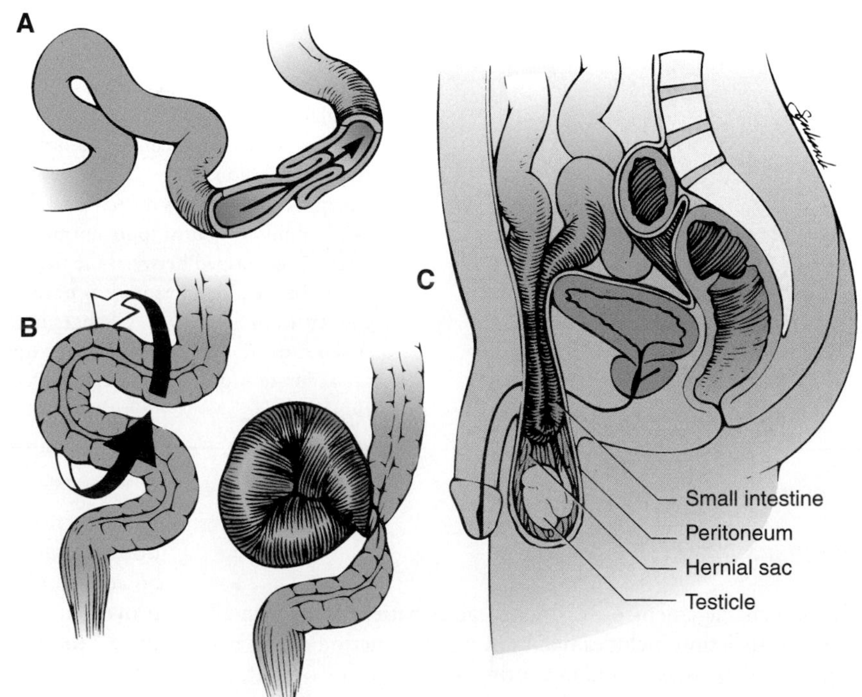

FIGURE 35•6 Three causes of intestinal obstruction. (**A**) Intussusception. Note invagination or shortening of colon by the movement of one segment of bowel into another. (**B**) Volvulus of the sigmoid colon. The twist is counterclockwise in most cases of sigmoid volvulus. Note the edematous bowel. (**C**) Hernia (inguinal). Note that the sac of the hernia is a continuation of the peritoneum of the abdomen and that the hernial contents are intestine, omentum, or other abdominal contents that pass through the hernial opening into the hernial sac.

Assessment and Diagnostic Findings

Diagnosis is based on symptoms and on x-ray studies. Abdominal x-rays (flat and upright) show a distended colon. Barium studies are contraindicated.

Medical Management

A colonoscopy may be performed to untwist and decompress the bowel. A cecostomy, in which a surgical opening is made into the cecum, may be performed in patients who are poor surgical risks and urgently need relief from the obstruction. The procedure provides an outlet for releasing gas and a small amount of drainage. A rectal tube may be used to decompress an area that is lower in the bowel. The usual treatment, however, is surgical resection to remove the obstructing lesion. A temporary or permanent colostomy may be necessary. An ileoanal anastomosis may be performed if it is necessary to remove the entire large colon.

Nursing Management

The nurse's role is to monitor the patient for symptoms indicating that the intestinal obstruction is worsening, as well as to provide emotional support and comfort. IV fluids and electrolytes are administered as prescribed. If the patient's condition does not respond to nonsurgical treatment, the nurse must prepare the patient for surgery. This preparation includes preoperative teaching as the patient's condition indicates. After surgery, general abdominal wound care is given and routine postoperative nursing care is required.

COLORECTAL CANCER

Tumors of the colon and rectum are relatively common—in fact, cancer of the colon and rectum is now the second most common type of internal cancer in the United States. It is a disease of Western cultures; 133,500 new cases of colorectal cancer are diagnosed in the United States each year (94,500 for colon, 39,000 for rectum). Colon cancer affects more than twice as many people as does rectal cancer.

The incidence increases with age (the incidence is highest in people older than 85) and is higher in people with a family history of colon cancer and in those with inflammatory bowel disease or polyps.

The distribution of cancer sites throughout the colon is shown in Figure 35-7. Changes in this distribution have occurred in recent years. The incidence of cancer in the sigmoid and rectal areas has decreased, whereas the incidence in the ascending and descending colon has increased.

Of the more than 133,000 people diagnosed each year, now less than half that number die annually, 46,400 from colon cancer and 8500 from rectal cancer. Almost three out of four people could be saved by early diagnosis and prompt treatment. Improved screening strategies have helped to reduce the number of deaths in recent years. The low 5-year survival rate of 40% to 50% is due primarily to late diagnosis and metastasis. Most people are asymptomatic for long periods and seek health care only when they notice a change in bowel habits or rectal bleeding.

The exact cause of colon and rectal cancer is unknown, but risk factors have been identified, including a family history of colon cancer or polyps, a history of inflammatory bowel disease, and a diet high in fat, protein, and low in fiber.

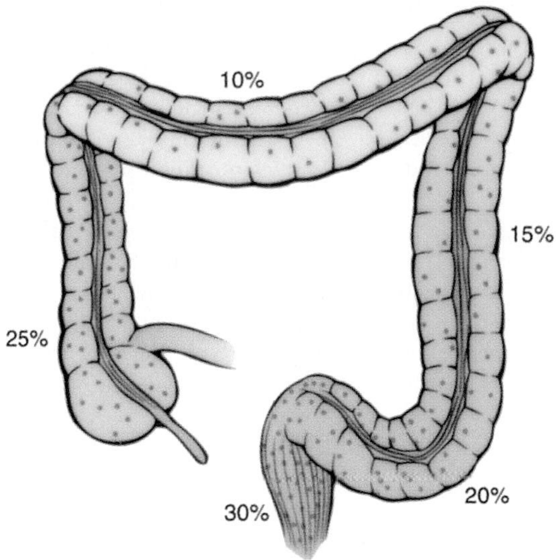

FIGURE 35•7 Percentage distribution of cancer sites in the colon and rectum.

Risk Factors for
COLORECTAL CANCER

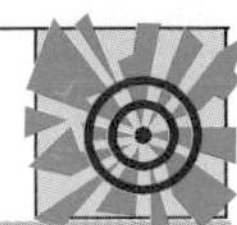

- Older than age 40
- History of rectal polyps or colon polyps
- Presence of adenomatous polyps or villous adenomas
- Family history of colon cancer or familial polyposis
- History of inflammatory bowel disease
- High-fat, high-protein (with high intake of beef), low-fiber diet

Pathophysiology

Cancer of the colon and rectum is predominantly (95%) adenocarcinoma (arising from the epithelial lining of the intestine). It may start as a benign polyp but may become malignant and invade and destroy normal tissues and extend into surrounding structures. Cancer cells may break away from the primary tumor and spread to other parts of the body (most often to the liver).

Clinical Manifestations

The symptoms are greatly determined by the location of the cancer, the stage of the disease, and the function of the intestinal segment in which it is located. The most common presenting symptom is a change in bowel habits. The passage of blood in the stools is the second most common symptom. Symptoms may also include unexplained anemia, anorexia, weight loss, and fatigue.

The symptoms most commonly associated with right-sided lesions are dull abdominal pain and melena (black, tarry stools). The symptoms most commonly associated with left-sided lesions are those associated with obstruction (abdominal pain and cramping, narrowing stools, constipation, and distention), as well as bright-red blood in the stool. Symptoms associated with rectal lesions are tenesmus (ineffective, painful straining at stool), rectal pain, the feeling of incomplete evacuation after a bowel movement, alternating constipation and diarrhea, and bloody stool.

Assessment and Diagnostic Findings

Along with the abdominal and rectal examination, the most important diagnostic procedures for cancer of the colon are fecal occult blood testing, barium enema, proctosigmoidoscopy, and colonoscopy (see Chap. 31). As many as 60% of colorectal cancer cases can be identified by sigmoidoscopy with biopsy or cytology smears.

Carcinoembryonic antigen (CEA) studies may also be performed. Although CEA may not be a highly reliable indicator in diagnosing colon cancer because not all lesions secrete CEA, studies show that CEA levels are reliable in predicting prognosis. With complete excision of the tumor, the elevated levels of CEA should return to normal within 48 hours. Elevations of CEA at a later date suggest recurrence.

Complications

Tumor growth may cause partial or complete bowel obstruction. Extension of the tumor and ulceration into the surrounding blood vessels results in hemorrhage. Perforation, abscess formation, peritonitis, sepsis, and shock may occur.

Gerontologic Considerations

The incidence of carcinoma of the colon and rectum increases with age. These cancers are considered the most common malignancies in old age, except for prostate cancer in men. Symptoms are often insidious. Fatigue is almost always present, primarily from iron-deficiency anemia. The symptoms most commonly reported by the elderly are abdominal pain, obstruction, tenesmus, and rectal bleeding.

Colon cancer in the elderly has been closely associated with dietary carcinogens. Lack of fiber is a major causative factor because the passage of feces through the intestinal tract is prolonged, which in turn prolongs exposure to possible carcinogens. Excess fat is believed to alter bacterial flora and convert steroids into compounds that have carcinogenic properties.

The elderly are also at increased risk for complications after surgery and may have difficulty managing colostomy care. They may have decreased vision and impaired hearing, as well as difficulty with fine motor coordination. It may be helpful for the patient to handle ostomy equipment and simulate cleaning the peristomal skin and irrigating the stoma before surgery. Skin care is a major concern in the elderly ostomate because of the skin changes that occur with aging: the epithelial and subcutaneous fatty layers become thin, and the skin is easily irritated. To prevent breakdown, special attention is paid to skin cleansing and the proper fit of an appliance. Arteriosclerosis causes decreased blood flow to the wound and stoma site. As a result, transport of nutrients is delayed, and healing time may be prolonged. Some patients have delayed elimination after irrigation because of decreased peristalsis and mucus production. Most patients require 6 months before they feel comfortable with their ostomy care.

Medical Management

The patient with symptoms of intestinal obstruction is treated with IV fluids and nasogastric suction. If there has been significant bleeding, blood component therapy may be required.

Treatment for colorectal cancer depends on the stage of the disease (Chart 35-1) and consists of surgery to remove the tumor, supportive therapy, and adjuvant therapy. Recent data demonstrate delays in tumor recurrence and increases in survival time for patients who receive some form of adjuvant therapy—chemotherapy, radiation therapy, and/or immunotherapy.

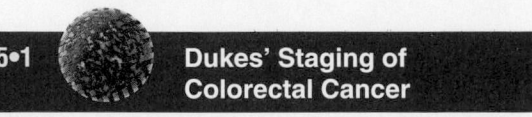

CHART 35•1 Dukes' Staging of Colorectal Cancer

Class A–Negative nodes, tumor limited to mucosa and submucosa

Class B_1–Negative nodes, tumor extends through mucosa but is still within bowel wall

Class B_2–Negative nodes, tumor extends through entire bowel wall

Class C_1–Positive nodes, tumor is limited to bowel wall

Class C_2–Positive nodes, tumor extends through entire bowel wall

Class D–Advanced and widespread regional metastasis

The standard adjuvant therapy administered to patients with Dukes' class C colon cancer is the 5-fluorouracil/levamisole regimen. Patients with Dukes' class B or C rectal cancer are given 5-fluorouracil and high doses of pelvic radiation. Mitomycin is also used. Radiation therapy is now being used before, during, and after surgery to shrink the tumor, to achieve better results from surgery, and to reduce the risk of recurrence. For inoperative or nonresectable tumors, radiation is used to provide significant relief from symptoms. Intracavity and implantable devices are used to deliver radiation to the site. The response to adjuvant therapy varies.

SURGICAL MANAGEMENT

Surgery is the primary treatment for most colon and rectal cancers. It may be curative or palliative. The type of surgery depends on the location and size of the tumor. Cancers limited to one site can be removed through the colonoscope. Laparoscopic colotomy with polypectomy minimizes the extent of surgery needed in some cases. A laparoscope is used as a guide in making an incision into the colon; the tumor mass is then excised. The Nd:YAG laser has proved effective with some lesions as well. Bowel resection is indicated for most class A lesions and all class B and C lesions. Surgery is sometimes recommended for class D colon cancer, but the goal of surgery in this instance is palliative. If the tumor has spread and involves surrounding vital structures, it is considered inoperable.

Surgical procedures include:

- Segmental resection with anastomosis (removal of the tumor and portions of the bowel on either side of the growth, as well as the blood vessels and lymphatic nodes) (Fig. 35-8)
- Abdominoperineal resection with permanent sigmoid colostomy (removal of the tumor and a portion of the sigmoid and all of the rectum and anal sphincter) (Fig. 35-9)
- Temporary colostomy followed by segmental resection and anastomosis and subsequent reanastomosis of the colostomy (allowing initial bowel decompression and bowel preparation before resection)
- Permanent colostomy or ileostomy (for palliation of unresectable obstructing lesions)

A **colostomy** is the surgical creation of an opening (stoma) into the colon. It can be created as a temporary or permanent diversion. It allows the drainage or evacuation of colon contents to the outside of the body. The consistency of the drainage is related to the placement of the colostomy, which in turn is dictated by the location of the tumor and the extent of invasion into sur-

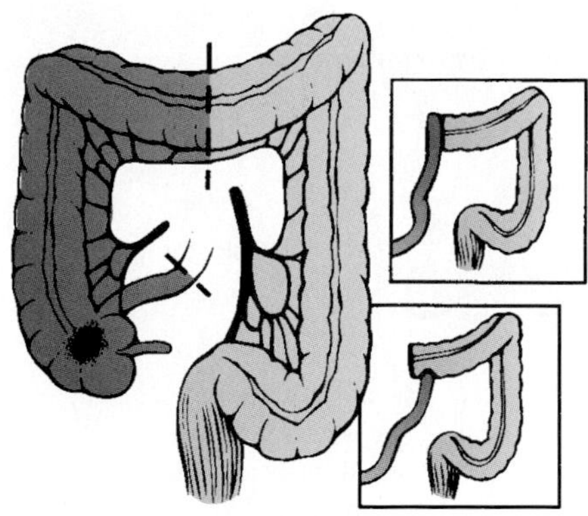

Cecum and lower ascending colon

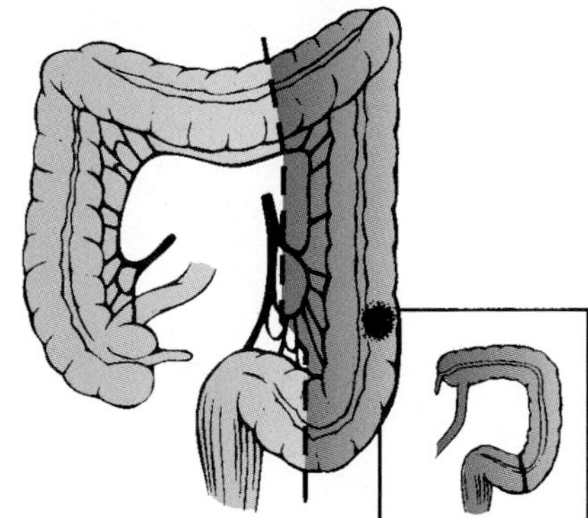

Descending colon and upper sigmoid

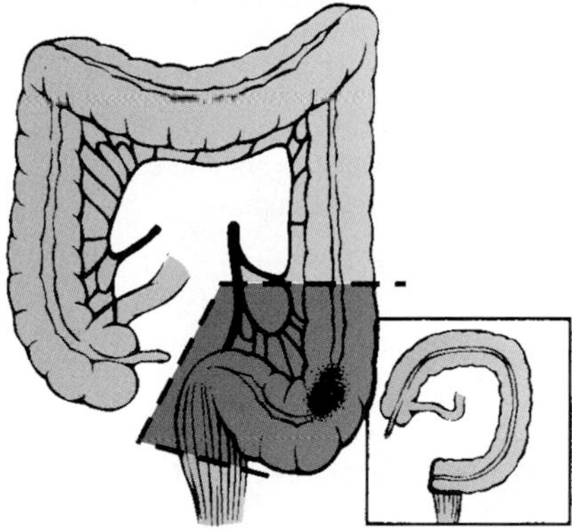

Low sigmoid and upper rectum

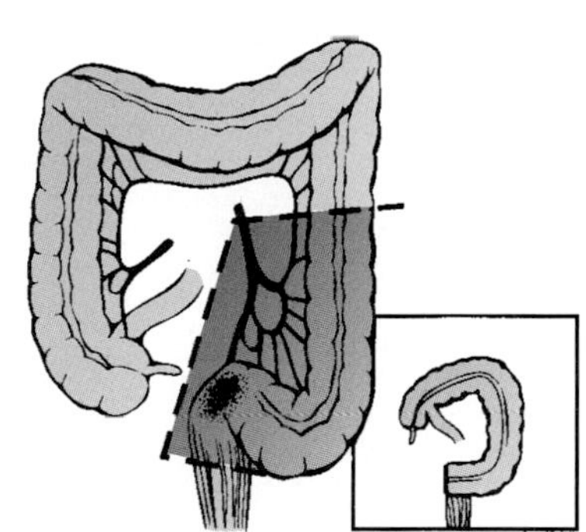

Rectal sigmoid resection

FIGURE 35•8 Examples of areas where cancer can occur, the area that is removed, and (in the very small diagrams) how the anastomosis is performed. Adapted from American Cancer Society.

rounding tissues (Fig. 35-10). With improved surgical techniques, colostomies are now performed on less than one third of patients with colorectal cancer.

NURSING PROCESS: THE PATIENT WITH COLORECTAL CANCER

Assessment

A health history is taken to obtain information about fatigue, abdominal or rectal pain (location, frequency, duration, association with eating or defecation), past and present elimination patterns, and characteristics of stool (color, odor, consistency, presence of blood or mucus). Additional information includes a past history of inflammatory bowel disease or colorectal polyps, a family history of colorectal disease, and current medication therapy. Dietary habits are identified, including fat and fiber intake as well as amounts of alcohol consumed. A history of weight loss is described and documented.

Assessment includes auscultating the abdomen for bowel sounds and palpating the abdomen for areas of tenderness, distention, and solid masses. Stool specimens are inspected for character and presence of blood.

Diagnosis

Nursing Diagnoses

Based on the assessment data, the major nursing diagnoses may include the following:

- Altered nutrition, less than body requirements, related to nausea and anorexia
- Risk for fluid volume deficit related to vomiting and dehydration
- Anxiety related to impending surgery and the diagnosis of cancer
- Risk for ineffective management of therapeutic regimen related to knowledge deficit concerning the diagnosis, the surgical procedure, and self-care after discharge
- Impaired skin integrity related to the surgical incisions (abdominal and perianal), the formation of a stoma, and frequent fecal contamination of peristomal skin
- Body image disturbance related to colostomy

Collaborative Problems/Potential Complications

Potential complications that may develop include:

- Intraperitoneal infection
- Complete large bowel obstruction
- GI bleeding
- Bowel perforation
- Peritonitis, abscess, and sepsis

Planning and Goals

The major goals for the patient may include attainment of optimal level of nutrition, maintenance of fluid and electrolyte balance, reduction of anxiety, learning about the diagnosis, surgical procedure, and self-care after discharge, maintenance of optimal tissue healing, protection of peristomal skin, learning how to irrigate the colostomy and change the appliance, expressing feelings and concerns about the colostomy and the impact on himself or herself, and avoidance of complications.

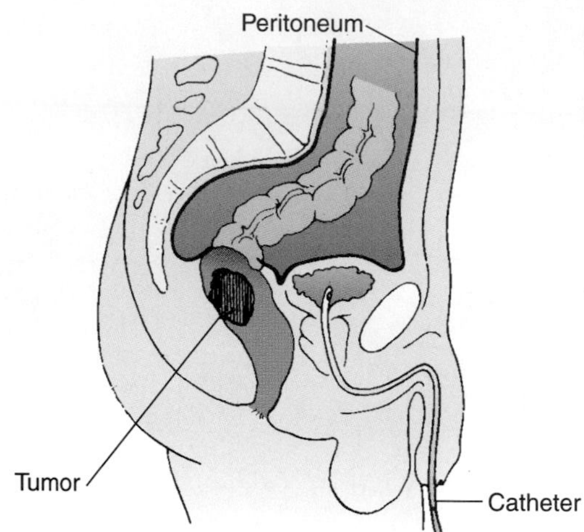

1. Prior to surgery. Note tumor in rectum.

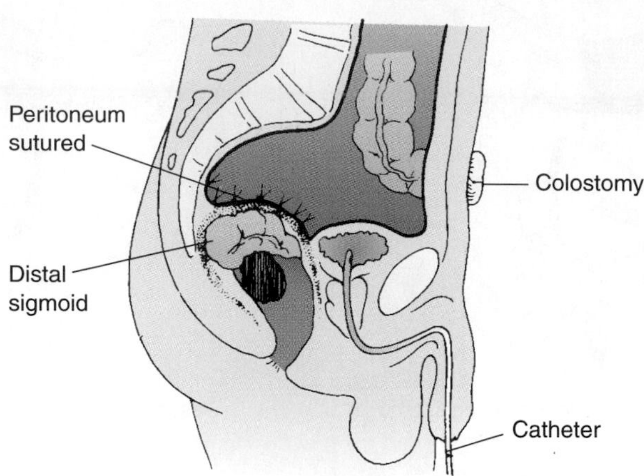

2. During surgery, the sigmoid is removed and colostomy established. The distal bowel has been dissected free to a point below the pelvic peritoneum, which is sutured over the closed end of the distal sigmoid and rectum.

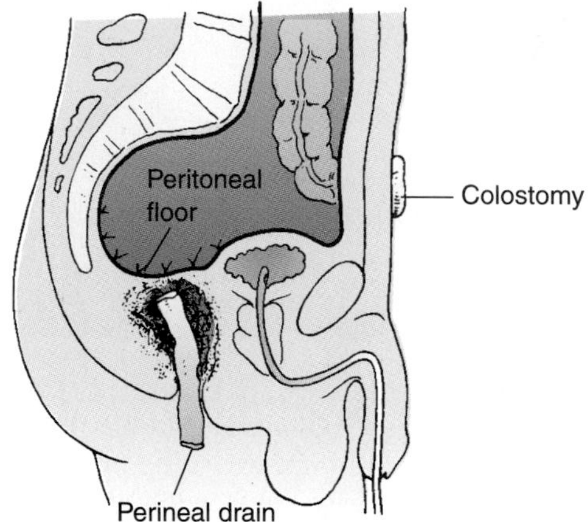

3. Perineal resection includes removal of the rectum and free portion of the sigmoid from below. A perineal drain is inserted.

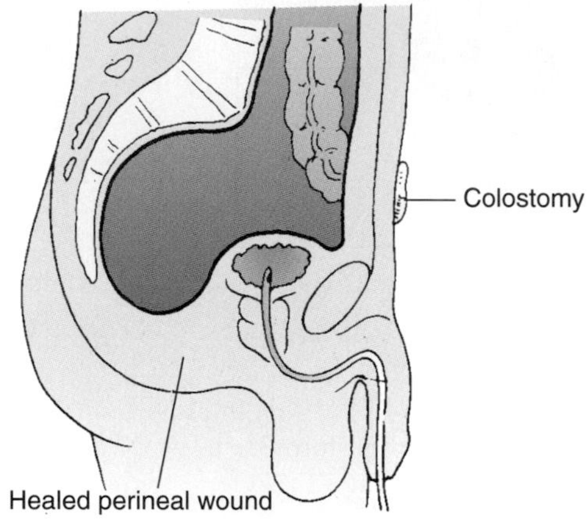

4. The final result after healing. Note healed perineal wound and the permanent colostomy.

FIGURE 35•9 Abdominoperineal resection for carcinoma of the rectum.

Preparing the Patient for Surgery

The patient anticipating surgery for colorectal cancer has many concerns, needs, and fears. He or she may be physically debilitated and emotionally distraught with concerns about finances, lifestyle changes after surgery, prognosis, and ability to perform in established roles. Priorities for nursing care include preparing the patient physically for surgery, providing information about postoperative care, including stoma care if a colostomy is to be created, and supporting the patient and family emotionally.

Physical preparation for surgery involves building the patient's stamina in the days preceding surgery and cleansing and sterilizing the bowel the day before surgery. If the patient's condition permits, a diet high in calories, protein, and carbohydrates and low in residue is recommended for several days before surgery to provide adequate nutrition and minimize cramping by decreasing excessive peristalsis. A full liquid diet may be prescribed 24 to 48 hours before surgery to decrease bulk. If the patient is hospitalized in the days preceding surgery, TPN may be required to replace depleted nutrients, vitamins, and minerals. In some instances, TPN may be given at home before surgery. Antibiotics such as kanamycin sulfate (Kantrex), erythromycin (Erythrocin), and neomycin sulfate are administered the day before surgery to reduce intestinal bacteria. In addition, the bowel is cleansed with laxatives, enemas, or colonic irrigations the evening before and the morning of surgery.

For the patient who is very ill and hospitalized, intake and output, including vomitus, are measured and recorded to provide an accurate record of fluid balance. The patient's intake of oral food and fluids may be restricted to prevent vomiting. Antiemetics are administered as prescribed. Full or clear liquids may be tolerated, or the patient may be allowed nothing by mouth. A nasogastric tube may be inserted to drain accumulated fluids and prevent abdominal distention. The abdomen is monitored for increasing distention, loss of bowel sounds, and pain or rigidity, which may indicate obstruction or perforation. IV fluids and electrolytes are monitored. Serum electrolyte levels are monitored to detect the hypokalemia and hyponatremia that occur with GI fluid loss. The nurse observes for signs of hypovolemia (tachycardia, hypotension, decreased pulse volume). Hydration status is assessed, and decreased skin turgor, dry mucous membranes, and concentrated urine are reported.

The patient's knowledge about the diagnosis, prognosis, surgical procedure, and expected level of functioning after surgery is assessed. Information about the physical preparation for surgery,

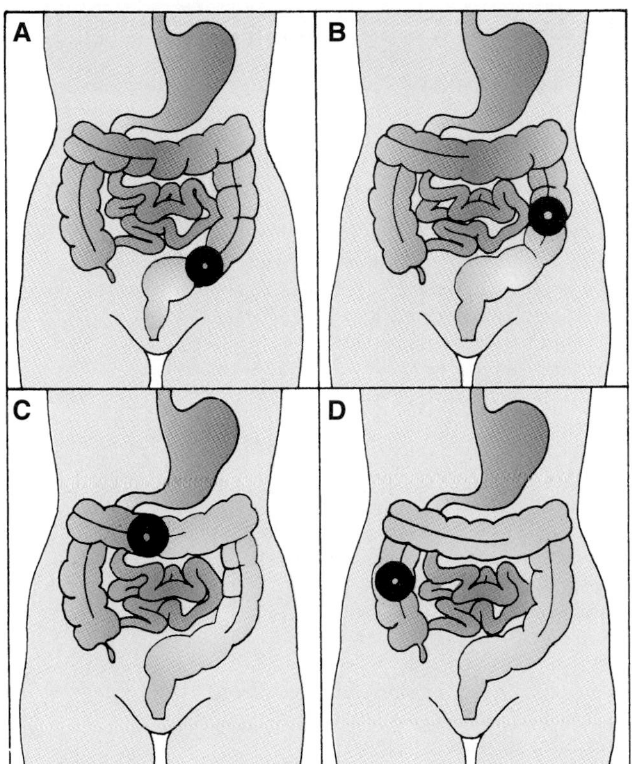

FIGURE 35•10 A diagrammatic representation of the placement of permanent colostomies. The nature of the discharge varies with the site. Shaded areas show sections of bowel removed. With a sigmoid colostomy (**A**) the feces are solid. With a descending colostomy (**B**) the feces are semimushy. With a transverse colostomy (**C**) the feces are mushy. With an ascending colostomy (**D**) the feces are fluid.

the expected appearance and care of the wound, the technique of ostomy care, dietary restrictions, pain control, and medication management are included in the teaching plan (see Plan of Nursing Care 35-1). If the patient will be admitted the day of surgery, the physician's office may arrange for the patient to be seen by an enterostomal therapist in the days preceding surgery. The therapist will help determine the optimal site for the stoma and provide teaching about care. If the patient is hospitalized before the day of surgery, the staff enterostomal therapist will be involved in the preoperative teaching. All procedures are explained in language the patient understands.

Providing Emotional Support

Patients anticipating bowel surgery for colorectal cancer may have very high levels of anxiety. They may grieve about the diagnosis, the impending surgery, and possible permanent colostomy. Patients undergoing surgery for a temporary colostomy may express fears and concerns similar to those of a person with a permanent stoma. All members of the health care team, including the enterostomal therapy nurse, should be available for assistance and support. The nurse's role is to assess the patient's anxiety level and coping mechanisms and suggest methods for reducing anxiety such as deep breathing exercises and visualizing a successful recovery from surgery and cancer. Other supportive measures include providing privacy if desired and teaching relaxation techniques to the patient. Time is set aside to listen to the patient who wishes to talk, cry, or ask questions. The nurse will arrange a meeting with a member of the clergy if the patient desires, or with the physicians if the patient wishes to discuss the treatment or prognosis. To promote patient comfort, the nurse projects a relaxed, professional, and empathetic attitude.

The patient undergoing a colostomy may find the anticipated changes in body image and lifestyle profoundly disturbing. Because the stoma is located on the abdomen, the patient may think that everyone will be aware of the ostomy. The nurse can help reduce this fear by presenting facts about the surgical procedure and the creation and management of the ostomy. If the patient is receptive, diagrams, photographs, and appliances may be used to explain and clarify. Because the patient is experiencing emotional stress, the nurse may need to repeat some of the information. Time should be provided for the patient and family to ask questions. The nurse's acceptance and understanding of the patient's concerns and feelings convey a caring, competent attitude that promotes confidence and cooperation. Consultation with an enterostomal therapist during the preoperative period can be extremely helpful, as can speaking with a person who is successfully managing a colostomy. The United Ostomy Association provides useful information about living with an ostomy, through literature, lectures, and exhibits. Visiting services by qualified members and rehabilitation services for new ostomy patients are provided.

Providing Postoperative Care

Postoperative nursing care for patients undergoing a colon resection and/or colostomy is similar to nursing care for any abdominal surgery patient (see Chap. 18). In addition, the patient is monitored for complications such as leakage from the site of the anastomosis, prolapse of the stoma, perforation, stoma retraction, fecal impaction, and skin irritation, as well as pulmonary complications associated with abdominal surgery. The abdomen is monitored for returning peristalsis, and the initial stool characteristics are assessed. Patients undergoing a colostomy are helped out of bed on the first postoperative day and encouraged to begin participating in managing the colostomy.

Providing Wound Care

The abdominal dressing is examined frequently during the first 24 hours after surgery to detect signs of hemorrhage. The patient is helped to splint the abdominal incision during coughing and deep breathing to lessen tension on the edges of the incision. Temperature, pulse, and respiratory rate are monitored for elevations, which may indicate an infectious process. If the patient has a colostomy, the stoma is examined for swelling (slight edema from surgical manipulation is normal), color (a healthy stoma is pink or red), discharge (a small amount of oozing is normal), and bleeding (an abnormal sign).

If the malignancy has been removed by the perineal route, the wound is observed carefully for signs of hemorrhage. This wound may contain a drain or packing, which is removed gradually. There may be sloughing of bits of tissue for a week. This process is hastened by mechanical irrigation of the wound or with sitz baths performed two or three times a day initially. The condition of the perineal wound and any bleeding, infection, or necrosis are documented.

Monitoring and Managing Complications

The patient is observed for signs and symptoms of complications. Frequent assessment of the abdomen, including decreasing or changing bowel sounds and increasing abdominal girth, is performed to detect bowel obstruction. Vital signs are monitored

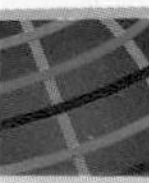

TABLE 35•6 **Potential Complications and Nursing Interventions After Intestinal Surgery**

Complication	Nursing Interventions
Paralytic ileus	Initiate or continue nasogastric intubation as prescribed. Prepare patient for x-ray study. Ensure adequate fluid and electrolyte replacement. Administer prescribed antibiotics if patient has symptoms of peritonitis.
Mechanical obstruction	Assess patient for intermittent colicky pain, nausea, and vomiting.
Intraperitoneal infection and abdominal wound infection	Monitor for evidence of constant or generalized abdominal pain, rapid pulse, and elevation of temperature. Prepare for tube decompression of bowel. Administer fluids and electrolytes by IV route as prescribed. Administer antibiotics as prescribed.
Intra-abdominal septic conditions	
Peritonitis	Evaluate patient for nausea, hiccups, chills, spiking fever, tachycardia. Administer antibiotics as prescribed. Prepare patient for drainage procedure. Institute parenteral fluid and electrolyte therapy as prescribed. Prepare patient for surgery if condition deteriorates.
Abscess formation	Administer antibiotics as prescribed. Apply warm compresses as prescribed. Prepare for surgical drainage.
Surgical wound complications	
Infection	Monitor temperature; report temperature elevation. Observe for redness, tenderness, and pain around wound. Assist in establishing local drainage. Obtain specimen of drainage material for culture and sensitivity studies.
Wound disruption	Observe for sudden appearance of profuse serous drainage from wound. Cover wound area with sterile towels held in place with binder. Prepare patient immediately for surgery.
Anastomotic complications	
Dehiscence of anastomosis	Prepare patient for surgery.
Fistulas	Assist in bowel decompression. Administer parenteral fluids as prescribed to correct fluid and electrolyte deficits.

for increased temperature, pulse, respirations, and decreased blood pressure, which could indicate an intra-abdominal infectious process. Rectal bleeding, indicative of hemorrhage, is reported immediately. Hematocrit and hemoglobin are monitored. Blood component therapy is administered as prescribed. Any abrupt change in abdominal pain is reported. Elevated white cell counts and temperature and/or symptoms of shock are reported; they may indicate sepsis. Antibiotics are administered as prescribed.

Pulmonary complications are always a concern with abdominal surgery. Patients older than 50 are at risk, especially if they are or have been receiving sedatives or are being maintained on bed rest for a prolonged period. Two primary pulmonary complications are pneumonia and atelectasis. These complications can be prevented by frequent activity (turning the patient from side to side every 2 hours), deep breathing, coughing, and early ambulation. Table 35-6 lists possible postoperative complications.

The incidence of complications related to the colostomy is about half that seen with an ileostomy. Some common complications are prolapse of the stoma (usually from obesity), perforation (from improper stoma irrigation), stoma retraction, fecal impaction, and skin irritation. Leakage from an anastomotic site can occur if the remaining bowel segments are diseased or weakened. Leakage from an intestinal anastomosis causes abdominal distention and rigidity, temperature elevation, and signs of shock. Surgical repair is necessary.

Removing and Applying the Colostomy Appliance

The colostomy will begin to function 3 to 6 days after surgery. The nurse manages the colostomy and teaches the patient about its care until the patient can take over. Skin care must be taught, along with how to apply and remove the drainage pouch. Care of the peristomal skin is an ongoing concern because excoriation or ulceration can develop quickly. The presence of such irritation makes adhering the ostomy bag difficult, and adhering the ostomy bag to irritated skin can worsen the skin condition. The effluent discharge and the degree to which it is irritating vary with the type of ostomy. With a transverse colostomy, the stool is soft and mushy and irritating to the skin. With a descending or sigmoid colostomy, the stool is fairly solid and only slightly irritating to the skin. Other skin problems include yeast infections and allergic dermatitis.

If the patient wants to bathe or shower before putting on the clean appliance, micropore tape applied to the sides of the pouch will keep it secure during bathing. To remove the appliance, the patient assumes a comfortable sitting or standing position and gently pushes the skin down from the faceplate while pulling the pouch up and away from the stoma. Gentle pressure prevents the skin from being traumatized and any liquid fecal contents from spilling out. The patient is advised to protect the peristomal skin by then washing the area gently with a moist, soft cloth and a mild soap. Soap acts as a mild abrasive agent to remove enzyme residue from fecal spillage. Any excess skin barrier is removed. While the skin is being cleansed, a gauze dressing can cover the stoma, or a vaginal tampon can be inserted gently to absorb excess drainage. After cleansing, the skin is patted completely dry with a gauze pad; rubbing the area is avoided. Nystatin powder (Mycostatin) can be lightly dusted on the peristomal skin if irritation or yeast growth is present.

Smoothly applying the drainage pouch for a secure fit requires practice and a well-fitting appliance. Patients can choose from a wide variety of pouches, depending on their individual needs. The stoma is measured to determine the correct size for the pouch; the pouch opening should be about 0.3 cm (1/8 in) larger than the stoma. After the skin is cleansed according to the above procedure, the peristomal skin barrier (wafer, paste, or powder) is applied. Mild skin irritation may require dusting the skin with karaya or stomahesive powder before attaching the pouch. The backing from the adherent surface of the pouch is removed and the bag is pressed down over the stoma for 30 seconds (Fig. 35-11). The drainage appliance is emptied or changed when it is one-third to one-fourth full so that the weight of its contents does not cause the pouch to separate from the adhesive disk and spill the contents. Most pouches are disposable and odor-resistant; commercially prepared deodorizers are available.

For some patients, colostomy bags are not always necessary. As soon as the patient has learned a routine for evacuation, bags may be dispensed with and a closed ostomy pouch or a simple dressing of disposable tissue (often covered with plastic wrap) is used, held in place by an elastic belt. Except for gas and a slight amount of mucus, nothing will escape from the colostomy opening between irrigations. Colostomy plugs (which expand on insertion to prevent passage of flatus and feces) are available.

Irrigating the Colostomy

The purpose of irrigating a colostomy is to empty the colon of gas, mucus, and feces so that the patient can go about social and business activities without fear of fecal drainage. A stoma on the abdomen does not have voluntary muscular control and may empty at irregular intervals. Regulating the passage of fecal material is achieved either by irrigating the colostomy or allowing the bowel to evacuate naturally without irrigations. The choice often depends on the individual and the nature of the colostomy. By irrigating the stoma at a regular time, there is less gas and retention of irrigants. The time for irrigating the colostomy should be consistent with the schedule the person will follow after leaving the hospital. Refer to Guideline 35-3 for the irrigating procedure and Figure 35-12 for the equipment.

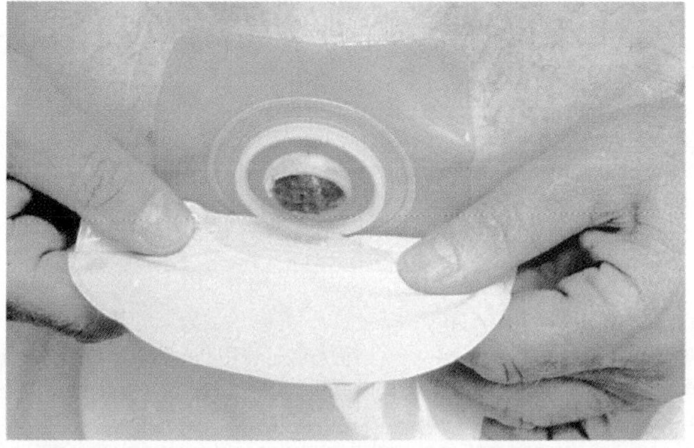

FIGURE 35•11 The colostomy appliance is pressed into place. Courtesy of Convatec, a Squibb Company.

Maintaining Optimal Nutrition

All patients undergoing surgery for colorectal cancer are taught about the health benefits to be derived from consuming a healthy diet. The diet is individualized as long as it is well balanced and does not cause diarrhea or constipation. The return to normal diet is rapid.

For patients with a colostomy, a complete nutritional assessment is performed. Foods that cause excessive odor and gas are avoided. These include foods in the cabbage family, eggs, fish, beans, and cellulose products such as peanuts. It is important to determine whether the elimination of specific foods is causing any nutritional deficiency. Nonirritating foods are substituted for those that are restricted so that deficiencies are corrected. The patient is advised to experiment with an irritating food several times before restricting it, because an initial sensitivity may decrease with time. The patient is helped to identify any foods or fluids that may be causing diarrhea, such as fruits, high-fiber foods, soda, coffee, tea, or carbonated beverages. Paregoric, bismuth subgallate, bismuth subcarbonate, or diphenoxylate with atropine (Lomotil) will help control the diarrhea. For constipation, prune or apple juice or a mild laxative is effective. At least 2 L of fluid per day is suggested.

Supporting a Positive Body Image

The patient is encouraged to verbalize feelings and concerns about altered body image and to discuss the surgery and the stoma (if one was created). A supportive environment and a supportive attitude on the nurse's part are crucial in promoting the patient's adaptation to the changes brought about by the surgery. Colostomy care must be learned and the patient must begin to plan for incorporating stoma care into daily life. Helping the patient overcome aversion to the stoma or fear of self-injury can be accomplished by providing care and teaching in an open, accepting manner, and encouraging the patient to talk about his or her feelings about the stoma.

Discussing Sexuality Issues

The patient is encouraged to discuss feelings about sexuality and sexual function. Some patients may initiate questions about sexual activity directly or give indirect clues about their fears. Some may view the surgery as mutilating and a threat to their sexuality; some fear impotence. Others may express worry about odor or leakage from the pouch during sexual activity. Although the pouch presents no deterrent to sexual activity, some patients wear silk or cotton covers and smaller pouches during sex. Alternative sexual positions are recommended, as well as alternative methods of stimulation to satisfy sexual drives. The nurse assesses the patient's needs and attempts to identify specific concerns. If the nurse is uncomfortable with this or if the patient's concerns seem complex, it may be appropriate for the nurse to seek assistance from an enterostomal therapy nurse, sex counselor or therapist, or advanced practice nurse.

Promoting Home and Community-Based Care

TEACHING PATIENTS SELF-CARE

Patient education and discharge planning require the combined efforts of the physician, nurse, enterostomal therapist, social worker, and dietitian. Patients are given specific information,

35•3
GUIDELINES FOR

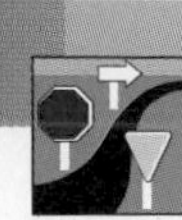

IRRIGATING A COLOSTOMY

A colostomy is irrigated to empty the colon of feces, gas, or mucus, cleanse the lower intestinal tract, and establish a regular pattern of evacuation so that normal life activities may be pursued. A suitable time for the irrigation is selected, preferably after a meal, so that this time is compatible with the patient's posthospital pattern of activity. Irrigation should be performed at the same time each day.

Before the procedure, the patient sits on a chair in front of the toilet or on the toilet itself. An irrigating reservoir with 500 to 1500 mL lukewarm tap water is hung 45 to 50 cm (18 to 20 in) above the stoma (shoulder height when the patient is seated). Dressings or pouch are removed. The following procedure is used; the patient is helped to participate in the procedure to learn to perform it unassisted.

Nursing Action	Rationale
1. Apply an irrigating sleeve or sheath to the stoma. Place the end in the commode (see Fig. 35-12).	This helps to control odor and splashing and allows feces and water to flow directly into the commode.
2. Allow some of the solution to flow through the tubing and catheter/cone.	Air bubbles in the setup are released so that air is not introduced into the colon, which would cause crampy pain.
3. Lubricate the catheter/cone and gently insert it into the stoma. Insert the catheter no more than 8 cm (3 in). Hold the shield/cone gently, but firmly, against the stoma to prevent backflow of water.	
4. If the catheter does not advance easily, allow water to flow slowly while advancing catheter. *Never force the catheter!*	A slow rate of flow helps to relax the bowel and facilitates passage of the catheter.
5. Allow tepid fluid to enter the colon slowly. If cramping occurs, clamp off the tubing and allow the patient to rest before progressing. Water should flow in over a 5- to 10-minute period.	Painful cramps are usually caused by too rapid a flow or by too much solution. 300 mL of fluid may be all that is needed to stimulate evacuation. Volume may be increased with subsequent irrigations to 500, 1000, or 1500 mL as needed by the patient for effective results.
6. Hold the shield/cone in place 10 seconds after the water has been instilled; then gently remove it.	
7. Allow 10 to 15 minutes for most of the return; then dry the bottom of the sleeve/sheath and attach it to the top, or apply the appropriate clamp to the bottom of the sleeve.	Most of the water, feces, and flatus will be expelled in 10 to 15 minutes.
8. Leave the sleeve/sheath in place about 30–45 minutes while the patient gets up and moves around.	Ambulation stimulates peristalsis and completion of the irrigation return.
9. Cleanse the area with a mild soap and water; pat the area dry.	Cleanliness and dryness will provide the patient with hours of comfort.
10. Replace the colostomy dressing or pouch.	The patient should use a pouch until the colostomy is sufficiently controlled. A dressing may be all that is needed.

individualized to their needs, about ostomy care and complications for which to observe. Dietary instructions are essential to help patients identify and eliminate irritating foods that can cause diarrhea or constipation. Patients are taught about their prescribed medications (action, purpose, and possible side effects).

Treatments (irrigations, wound cleansing) and dressing changes are reviewed, and the family is encouraged to participate. Because the hospital stay is so limited, the patient may not be able to become proficient in stoma care techniques before discharge. Many patients will need referral to a home care agency and the telephone number of the local chapter of the American Cancer Society. The home care nurse will come to the home to provide further care and teaching and to assess how well the patient and family are adjusting to the colostomy. In addition, the home environment is assessed for adequacy of resources that allow the patient to accomplish self-care. Someone in the family should assume responsibility for purchasing the equipment and supplies that will be needed at home.

Patients need very specific directions about when to call the physician. They need to know which complications require prompt attention (bleeding, abdominal distention and rigidity, diarrhea, fever, wound drainage, disruption of suture line). If radiation therapy is necessary, the possible side effects (anorexia, vomiting, diarrhea, and exhaustion) are reviewed.

CONTINUING CARE

Ongoing care of the patient with cancer and/or a colostomy often extends well beyond the initial hospital stay. Home care nurses manage ostomy follow-up care, manage the assessment and care of the debilitated patient, and coordinate adjuvant therapy. The home care visits also provide the nurse with opportunities to assess the patient's physical and emotional status and the patient's

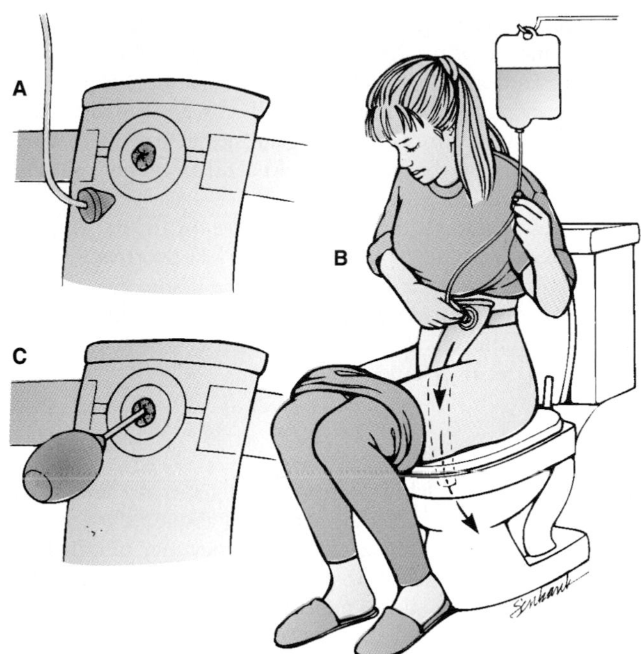

FIGURE 35•12 Colostomy irrigation. (**A**) Irrigating catheter has a cone attachment to prevent injury to stomal tissue. (**B**) Irrigating fluid is instilled with sleeve in place. Drainage contents empty into toilet. (**C**) The bulb syringe method can be used to stimulate fecal drainage. Note that a portion of the hard nozzle is removed and a catheter attached to minimize stomal irritation.

and family's ability to carry out recommended management strategies. Visits from an enterostomal therapy nurse are available to the patient and family as they learn to care for the ostomy and work through their feelings about it, the diagnosis of cancer, and the future. Some patients will be interested in and benefit from involvement in an ostomy support group.

Evaluation

Expected Outcomes

Expected outcomes may include:

1. Feels less anxious
   a. Expresses concerns and fears freely
   b. Uses coping measures to manage stress
2. Acquires information about diagnosis, surgical procedure, preoperative preparation, and self-care after discharge
   a. Discusses the diagnosis, surgical procedure, and postoperative self-care
   b. Demonstrates techniques of ostomy care
3. Maintains clean incision, stoma, and perineal wound
4. Expresses feelings and concerns about self
   a. Gradually increases participation in stoma and peristomal skin care
   b. Discusses feelings related to changed appearance
5. Recovers without complications
   a. Is afebrile
   b. Regains normal bowel activity
   c. Avoids perforation or bleeding

POLYPS OF THE COLON AND RECTUM

A polyp is a mass of tissue that protrudes into the lumen of the bowel. Polyps can occur anywhere in the intestinal tract and rectum. They can be classified as neoplastic (adenomas and carcinomas) or non-neoplastic (mucosal and hyperplastic). Adenomatous polyps (benign epithelial growths) are common in the Western world. They occur more commonly in the large intestine than in the small intestine. Although the vast majority of them do not develop into invasive neoplasms, their presence must be identified and closely followed. Polyps occur in 10% to 60% of the population; they occur most commonly in the fifth decade of life.

Clinical manifestations depend on the size of the polyp and the amount of pressure it exerts on intestinal tissue. The most common symptom is rectal bleeding. Lower abdominal pain may also occur. If the polyp is large enough, symptoms of obstruction occur. The diagnosis is based on history and digital rectal examination, barium enema studies, sigmoidoscopy, or colonoscopy.

Once a polyp is identified, it is removed through a colonoscope by the use of special equipment (biopsy forceps and snares). Microscopic examination of the polyp then identifies the type of polyp and indicates whether surgery is required. The principal reason for performing a colonic polypectomy is the possibility that malignancy is already present or may develop.

DISEASES OF THE ANORECTUM

Patients with anorectal disorders seek medical care primarily because of pain and rectal bleeding. Other common complaints are protrusion of hemorrhoids, anal discharge, perianal itching, swelling, anal tenderness, stenosis, and ulceration. Constipation results from delaying defecation because of pain.

Anorectal Abscess

An anorectal abscess is an infection in the pararectal spaces. People with regional enteritis or immunosuppressive conditions such as AIDS are particularly susceptible to these infections. Many of these abscesses result in fistulas.

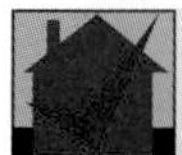

HOME CARE TEACHING CHECKLIST: MANAGING OSTOMY CARE

At the completion of the program, the patient or caregiver will be able to:	Patient	Caregiver
• Demonstrate ostomy care, including wound cleansing, irrigation, and appliance changing.	✔	✔
• Identify dietary restrictions (foods that can cause diarrhea and constipation).	✔	✔
• Describe medication regimen: identify medications by name, use, route, and frequency.	✔	✔
• Describe potential complications and necessary actions to be taken if complications occur.	✔	✔

An abscess may occur in a variety of spaces in and around the rectum. Often it contains a quantity of foul-smelling pus and is painful. If the abscess is superficial, swelling, redness, and tenderness are observed. A deeper abscess may result in toxic symptoms, lower abdominal pain, and fever.

Palliative therapy consists of sitz baths and analgesics. However, prompt surgical treatment to incise and drain the abscess is the treatment of choice. When a deeper infection exists, with the possibility of a fistula, the fistulous tract must be removed. If possible, the fistula is removed when the abscess is incised and drained, or a second procedure to do so may be necessary. The wound may be packed with gauze and allowed to heal by granulation.

Anal Fistula

An anal fistula is a tiny, tubular, fibrous tract that extends into the anal canal from an opening located beside the anus (Fig. 35-13**A**). Fistulas usually result from an infection. They may also develop from trauma, fissures, or regional enteritis. Pus or stool may leak constantly from the cutaneous opening. Other symptoms may be the passage of flatus or feces from the vagina or bladder, depending on the fistula tract. Untreated fistulas may cause systemic infection, with related symptoms.

Surgery is always recommended because few fistulas heal spontaneously. A fistulectomy (excision of the fistulous tract) is the recommended surgical procedure. The lower bowel is evacuated thoroughly with several prescribed enemas. During surgery, the sinus tract is identified by inserting a probe into it or by injecting the tract with methylene blue solution. The fistula is dissected out or laid open by an incision from its rectal opening to its outlet. The wound is packed with gauze.

Anal Fissure

An anal fissure is a longitudinal tear or ulceration in the lining of the anal canal (Fig. 35-13**B**). Fissures are usually caused by the trauma of passing a large, firm stool or from persistent tightening of the anal canal secondary to stress and anxiety (leading to constipation). Other causes include childbirth, trauma, and overuse of laxatives.

Fissures are characterized by extremely painful defecation, burning, and bleeding. Most of these fissures heal if treated by conservative measures, which include stool softeners and bulk agents, an increase in water intake, sitz baths, and emollient suppositories. A suppository combining an anesthetic with a corticosteroid helps relieve the discomfort. Anal dilation under anesthesia may be required.

If fissures do not respond to conservative treatment, surgery is indicated. Several types of procedures may be performed: in some cases, the anal sphincter is dilated and the fissure is excised; in others, a part of the external sphincter is divided. This produces a paralysis of the external sphincter, with consequent relief of spasm, and permits the ulcer to heal.

Hemorrhoids

Hemorrhoids are dilated portions of veins in the anal canal. They are very common. By the age of 50, about 50% of people have hemorrhoids to some extent. Pregnancy may initiate hemorrhoids or aggravate existing ones. Hemorrhoids are classified into two types: those above the internal sphincter are called internal hemorrhoids, and those appearing outside the external sphincter are called external hemorrhoids (Fig. 35-13**C**).

Hemorrhoids cause itching and pain and are the most common cause of bright-red bleeding with defecation. External hemorrhoids are associated with severe pain from the inflammation and edema caused by thrombosis (the clotting of blood within the hemorrhoid). This may lead to ischemia of the area and eventual necrosis. Internal hemorrhoids are not usually painful until they bleed or prolapse when they become enlarged.

Hemorrhoid symptoms and discomfort can be relieved by good personal hygiene and by avoiding excessive straining during defecation. A high-residue diet that contains fruit and bran may be all the treatment that is necessary; failing this, a laxative that absorbs water as it passes through the intestines may help. Sitz baths, ointments, and suppositories containing anesthetics, astringents (witch hazel), and bed rest allow the engorgement to subside.

There are several types of nonsurgical treatments for hemorrhoids. Infrared photocoagulation, bipolar diathermy, and laser therapy are newer techniques that are used to affix the mucosa to the underlying muscle. Injecting sclerosing solutions is also ef-

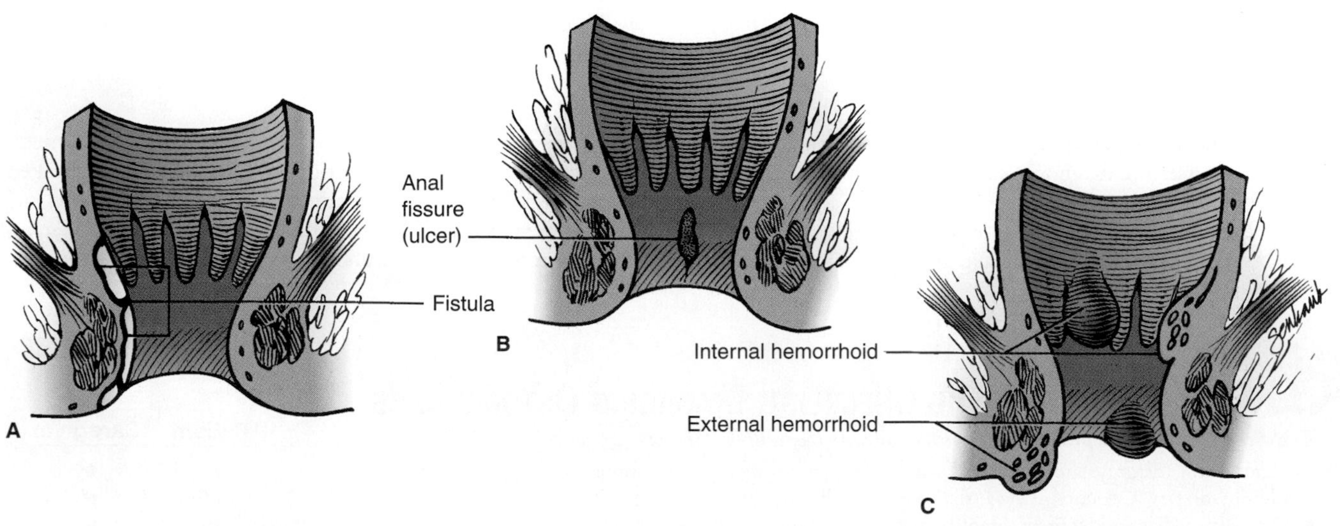

FIGURE 35•13 Various types of anal lesions. (**A**) Fistula. (**B**) Fissure. (**C**) External and internal hemorrhoids.

fective for small, bleeding hemorrhoids. These procedures help prevent prolapse.

A conservative surgical treatment of internal hemorrhoids is the rubber-band ligation procedure. The hemorrhoid is visualized through the anoscope, and its proximal portion above the mucocutaneous lines is grasped with an instrument. A small rubber band is then slipped over the hemorrhoid. Tissue distal to the rubber band becomes necrotic after several days and sloughs off. Fibrosis occurs; the result is that the lower anal mucosa is drawn up and adheres to the underlying muscle. Although this treatment has been satisfactory for some patients, it has proven painful for others and may cause some secondary hemorrhage. It has been known to cause perianal infection.

Cryosurgical hemorrhoidectomy, another method for removing hemorrhoids, involves freezing the hemorrhoid for a sufficient time to cause necrosis. Although it is relatively painless, this procedure is not widely used because the discharge is very foul-smelling and wound healing is prolonged. The Nd:YAG laser has been useful recently in excising hemorrhoids, particularly external hemorrhoidal tags. The treatment is quick and relatively painless. Hemorrhage and abscess are rare postoperative complications.

The methods of treating hemorrhoids just described are not effective for advanced thrombosed veins, which must be treated by more extensive surgery. Hemorrhoidectomy, or surgical excision, can be performed to remove all the redundant tissue involved in the process. During surgery, the rectal sphincter is usually dilated digitally and the hemorrhoids are removed with a clamp and cautery or by being ligated and then excised. After the operative procedures are completed, a small tube may be inserted through the sphincter to permit the escape of flatus and blood; pieces of Gelfoam or Oxycel gauze may be placed over the anal wounds.

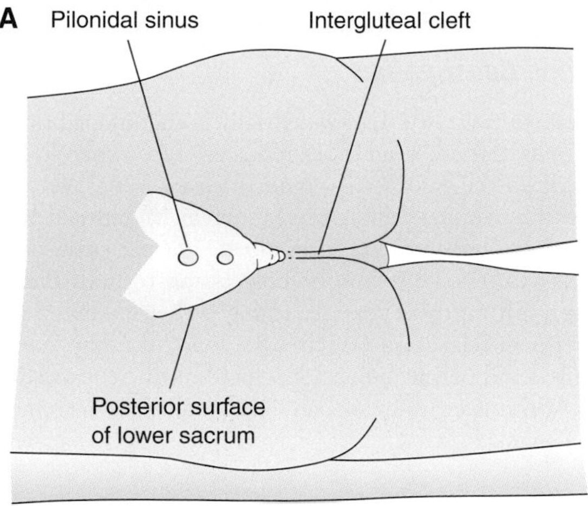

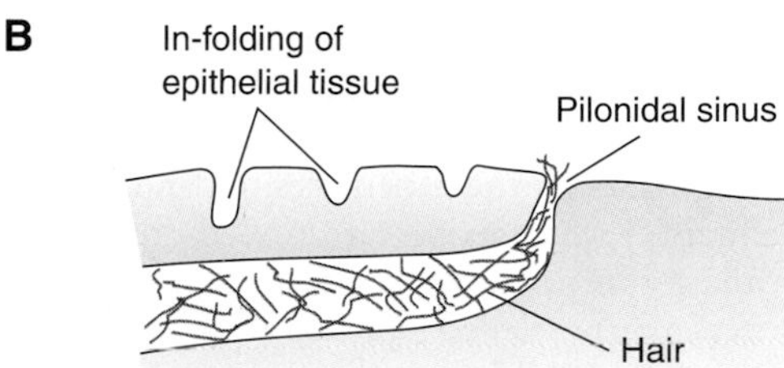

FIGURE 35•14 (**A**) Pilonidal sinus on lower sacrum about 5 cm (2 in) above the anus in the intergluteal cleft. (**B**) Note: Hair particles emerge from the sinus tract and localized indentations (pits) can appear on the skin near the sinus openings.

Pilonidal Sinus/Cyst

A pilonidal sinus or cyst is found in the intergluteal cleft on the posterior surface of the lower sacrum (Fig. 35-14). Current theories postulate that it results from the penetration of hairs into the epithelium and subcutaneous tissue. It may also be formed congenitally by an infolding of epithelial tissue beneath the skin, which may communicate with the skin surface through one or several small sinus openings. Hair frequently is seen protruding from these openings, and this gives the cyst its name—pilonidal (a nest of hair). The cysts rarely cause symptoms until adolescence or early adult life, when infection produces an irritating drainage or an abscess. This area is easily irritated by perspiration and friction.

In the early stages of the inflammation, the infection may be controlled by antibiotic therapy, but once an abscess has formed, surgery is indicated. The abscess is incised and drained under local anesthesia. After the acute process resolves, further surgery is performed to excise the cyst and the secondary sinus tracts. The wound is allowed to heal by granulation. Gauze dressings are placed in the wound to keep its edges separated while healing occurs.

NURSING PROCESS: THE PATIENT WITH AN ANORECTAL CONDITION

Assessment

A health history is taken to determine the presence and characteristics of itching, burning, or pain. Does it occur during bowel movements? How long does it last? Is any abdominal pain associated with it? Does any bleeding occur from the rectum? How much? How frequently? Is it bright red? Is there any other discharge, such as mucus or pus? Other questions relate to elimination patterns and laxative use, diet history (including fiber intake), the amount of exercise, activity levels, and occupation (especially one that involves prolonged sitting or standing). Assessment also includes inspection of the stool for blood or mucus, and the perianal area for hemorrhoids, fissures, irritation, or pus.

Diagnosis

Nursing Diagnoses

Based on the assessment data, the major nursing diagnoses may include the following:

- Constipation related to ignoring the urge to defecate because of pain during elimination
- Anxiety related to impending surgery and embarrassment
- Pain related to irritation, pressure, and sensitivity in the anorectal area secondary to anorectal disease and sphincter spasms after surgery
- Urinary retention related to postoperative reflex spasm and fear of pain
- Risk for ineffective management of the therapeutic regimen

Collaborative Problems/Potential Complications

Hemorrhage is a potential complication.

Planning and Goals

The major goals for the patient may include adequate elimination patterns, reduction of anxiety, pain relief, promotion of urinary elimination, managing the therapeutic regimen, and avoidance of complications.

Nursing Interventions

Relieving Constipation

The intake of at least 2 L of water daily is encouraged to provide adequate hydration. High-fiber foods are recommended to promote bulk in the stool and to make it easier to pass fecal matter through the rectum. Bulk laxatives such as Metamucil and stool softeners are administered as prescribed. The patient is advised to set aside a time for moving the bowels and to heed the urge to defecate as promptly as possible. It may be helpful to have the patient perform relaxation exercises before defecating to relax the abdominal and perineal muscles, which may be constricted or in spasm. Administering an analgesic before a bowel movement will be beneficial.

Reducing Anxiety

Patients facing rectal surgery may be upset and irritable because of discomfort, pain, and embarrassment. Specific psychosocial needs are identified and the plan of care is individualized. Privacy is provided by limiting visitors if the patient desires, and the patient's privacy is maintained when giving care. Soiled dressings are removed from the room promptly to prevent unpleasant odors; room deodorizers may be needed if dressings are foul-smelling.

Relieving Pain

During the first 24 hours after rectal surgery, painful spasms of the sphincter and perineal muscles may occur. Control of pain is a prime consideration. The patient is encouraged to assume a comfortable position. Flotation pads under the buttocks when sitting will help decrease the pain, as may ice and analgesic ointments. Warm compresses may promote circulation and soothe irritated tissues. Sitz baths, three or four times a day, will relieve soreness and pain by relaxing sphincter spasm. Twenty-four hours after surgery, topical anesthetic agents may be beneficial in relieving local irritation and soreness. Medications may include topical anesthetics (suppositories), astringents, antiseptics, tranquilizers, and antiemetics. Patients will be more compliant and less apprehensive if they are free of pain.

Wet dressings saturated with equal parts of cold water and witch hazel help relieve edema. When wet compresses are being used continuously, petrolatum should be applied around the anal area to prevent skin maceration. The patient is instructed to assume a prone position at intervals because this position promotes dependent drainage of edematous fluid.

Promoting Urinary Elimination

Voiding may be a problem after surgery because of a reflex spasm of the sphincter at the outlet of the bladder and a certain amount of muscle guarding from apprehension and pain. All methods to encourage voluntary voiding (increasing fluid intake, listening to running water, dripping water over the urinary meatus) should be tried before resorting to catheterization. After rectal surgery, urinary output should be monitored closely.

Monitoring and Managing Complications

The operative site must be examined frequently for rectal bleeding. The patient is assessed for systemic indicators of excessive bleeding (tachycardia, hypotension, restlessness, thirst). After hemorrhoidectomy, hemorrhage may occur from the veins that were cut. If a tube has been inserted through the sphincter after surgery, evidence of bleeding should be apparent on the dressings. If bleeding is obvious, direct pressure is applied to the area and the physician is notified. Moist heat is avoided because it will encourage vessel dilation and bleeding.

Promoting Home and Community-Based Care

TEACHING PATIENTS SELF-CARE

Most patients with anorectal conditions are not hospitalized. Those who have surgical procedures to correct the condition often are discharged directly from the outpatient surgical center. If they are hospitalized, it is for a short time, usually only 24 hours. Therefore, patient teaching is essential to facilitate recovery at home.

The patient is instructed to keep the perianal area as clean as possible by gently cleansing with warm water and then drying with absorbent cotton wipes. Rubbing the area with toilet tissue is avoided. Instructions about how to take a sitz bath and how to test the temperature of the water are provided. Sitz baths may be given in the bathtub or a plastic sitz bath unit three or four times a day. Sitz baths should follow each bowel movement for 1 to 2 weeks after surgery. The patient is encouraged to respond quickly to the urge to defecate so as to prevent constipation. Diet is modified to increase fluids and fiber. The patient is taught about the prescribed diet, the significance of proper eating habits and exercise, and the laxatives that can be taken safely. Moderate exercise is encouraged.

Evaluation

Expected Outcomes

Expected outcomes may include:

1. Attains a normal pattern of elimination
   a. Sets aside a time for defecation, usually after a meal or at bedtime
   b. Responds to the urge to defecate and takes the time to sit on the toilet and try to defecate
   c. Uses relaxation exercises as needed
   d. Increases fluid intake to 2 L per day
   e. Adds high-fiber foods to diet
   f. Reports passage of soft, formed stools
   g. Reports decreased abdominal discomfort
2. Is less anxious
3. Has less pain
   a. Modifies body position and activities to minimize pain and discomfort
   b. Applies warmth or cold to anorectal area
   c. Takes sitz baths four times a day
4. Voids without difficulty
5. Adheres to the therapeutic regimen
   a. Keeps perianal area dry
   b. Eats bulk-forming foods
   c. Has soft, formed stools on a regular basis
6. Avoids bleeding problems
   a. Has a clean incision
   b. Has normal vital signs
   c. Shows no signs of hemorrhage

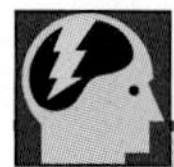

Critical Thinking Exercises

1. You are visiting a resident in an extended care facility. She complains that she has had pain throughout her abdomen for the past day. She has not had a bowel movement in 4 days, and she complains of loss of appetite. Physical examination reveals that her abdomen is distended and rigid and that bowel sounds are absent. Analyze these findings, indicate what you think the possible causes may be, and explain the actions you would take and why.

2. During a conversation with an elderly gentleman at a community center for senior citizens, he tells you he cannot have a bowel movement without taking a laxative each day. He asks if this is acceptable, given that he also takes "blood pressure medicine, a heart pill, and aspirin" each day. Explain how you would advise this patient, and give the rationale behind your advice.

3. You are caring for a patient who has been treated medically for ulcerative colitis for 5 years. The patient underwent a total colectomy and ileostomy yesterday. What are the similarities and differences between the care of this patient and that of a patient who has had a colon resection and colostomy? Explain how you would meet the emotional and health education needs of the patient with an ileostomy and the patient with a colostomy.

References and Selected Readings

BOOKS

American Cancer Society. (1998). *Cancer facts and figures.* Atlanta: Author.

Bryant, R., & Hampton, B. (1992). *Ostomies and continent diversions: Nursing management.* Baltimore: Mosby–Year Book.

Grendell, J.H., et al. (Eds.). (1996). *Current diagnosis and treatment in gastroenterology.* Stamford, CT: Appleton & Lange.

Hoebler, L., et al. (1997). *Cancer nursing: Principles and practice: Colon and rectal cancer.* Boston: Jones and Bartlett.

Kirsner, J., & Shorter, R. (1995). *Inflammatory bowel disease.* Philadelphia: Williams & Wilkins.

Lueckenotte, A. (1995). *Gerontologic nursing.* St. Louis: Mosby.

Raskin, J., & Noed, H. (1995). *Colonoscopy: Principles and techniques.* New York: Igaker-Shoin.

Richter, J., et al. (1994). *The functional GI disorders.* Boston: Little, Brown and Co.

Society of Gastroenterology Nurses and Associates. (1993). *Gastroenterology nursing: A core curriculum.* Baltimore: Mosby–Year Book.

Willian, N. (Ed.). (1996). *Colorectal cancer.* New York: Churchill Livingstone.

Yamada, T., Alpers, D. H., Owyang, C., Powell, D. W., & Silverstein, F. E. (Ed.). (1995). *Textbook of gastroenterology* (2nd ed.). Philadelphia: J. B. Lippincott.

JOURNALS

Abi-Hanna, P. (1997). Acute abdominal pain: A medical emergency in older patients. *Geriatrics, 52*(7), 72.

Black, P. (1996). Stoma appliances: What's new. *Community Nurse, 2*(3), 48–49.

Bond, J. (1997). Screening for colorectal cancer. *Hospital Practice, 32*(1), 59–78.

Borwell, B. (1996). Colostomies and their management. *Nursing Standard, 8*(11), 49–53.

Byade, A., & Mourad, F. (1996). Constipation: Common-sense care of the older patient. *Geriatrics, 51*(12) 28–36.

Cerda, J,, et al. (1996). Effective, compassionate management of IBS. *Patient Care, 30*(1), 131–144.

Cerda, J., et al. (1997). Diverticulitis: Cure and management strategies. *Patient Care, 33*, 170–186.

Clayton, H. A., et al. (1997). Development of an ostomy competency. *MedSurg Nursing, 6*(5), 256–269.

Cohen, L. (1996). Colorectal cancer: A primary care approach to screening. *Geriatrics, 51*(12), 45–49.

Collins, L. (1996). Laparoscopic extraperitoneal herniorrhaphy. *AORN Journal, 63*(6), 1089–1097.

Cox, J. (1995). Inflammatory bowel disease: Implications for the medical surgical nurse. *MedSurg Nursing, 4*(6), 427–434.

Cumbie, B., et al. (1996). Action stat, bowel obstruction. *Nursing '96, 26*(1), 33.

Epps, C. (1996). The delicate business of colostomy care. *RN, 22*(11), 32–36.

Gibson, P. (Ed.). (1997). Ulcerative colitis. *Clinical Gastroenterology, 11*(1).

Heitkemper, M., et al. (1995). Interventions for irritable bowel syndrome: A nursing model. *Gastroenterology Nursing, 18*(6), 224–230.

Hyman, N. (1997). Anorectal diseases: How to relieve pain and improve other symptoms. *Geriatrics, 52*, 75–91.

Kirkton, C. (1997). Assessing bowel sounds. *Nursing '97, 27*(3), 64–68.

Levitt, M., & Suarez, F. (1997). Lactose intolerance. *Patient Care, 28*, 185–188.

Mead, M. (1996a). Dealing with hemorrhoids. *Practice Nurse, 11*(2), 120–121.

Mead, M. (1996b). Detecting appendicitis. *Practice Nurse, 11*(7), 486–487.

Mead, M. (1997). Diverticular disease. *Practice Nurse, 13*(2), 104–105.

Meisner, J. (1996). Caring for patients with colorectal cancer. *Nursing '96, 26*(11), 60–61.

Mishkin, S. (1997). Dairy sensitivity, lactose malabsorption, and elimination diets in inflammatory bowel disease. *American Journal of Clinical Nutrition, 65*(2), 564–567.

Noe, C. A., & Barry, P. P. (1996). Healthy aging: Guidelines for cancer screening and immunizations. *Geriatrics, 51*(1), 75–83.

Self-Test: Understanding the GI system. *Nursing '96, 26*(3), 28–29.

Salter, M. (1996). Advances in ileostomy care. *Nursing Standard, 11*(9), 49–55.

Seaman, S. (1996). Basic ostomy management: Assessment and pouching. *Home Healthcare Nurse, 14*(5), 334–345.

Shaw, B. (1996). Primary care for women: Management and treatment of GI disorders. *Journal of Nurse Midwifery, 41*(2), 155–172.

Wald, A. (1997). Fecal incontinence: 3 steps to successful management. *Geriatrics, 52*, 44–52.

Willis, J. (1996). Stoma: Treatment and appliances. *Nursing Times 92*, (4), 48–50.

Resources

American Cancer Society, 1599 Clifton Rd. N.E., Atlanta, GA 30329; 1-404-320-3333; www.cancer.org

Crohn's & Colitis Foundation of America, 386 Park Avenue South, New York, NY 10016-8804

International Association for Enterostomal Therapy, 2081 Business Circle Dr., Suite 290, Irvine, CA 92715

International Foundation for Bowel Dysfunction, Box 17864, Milwaukee, WI 53217

National Foundation for Ileitis and Colitis, 295 Madison Ave., New York, NY 10017

United Ostomy Association, 2001 West Beverly Blvd., Los Angeles, CA 90057

UNIT

8

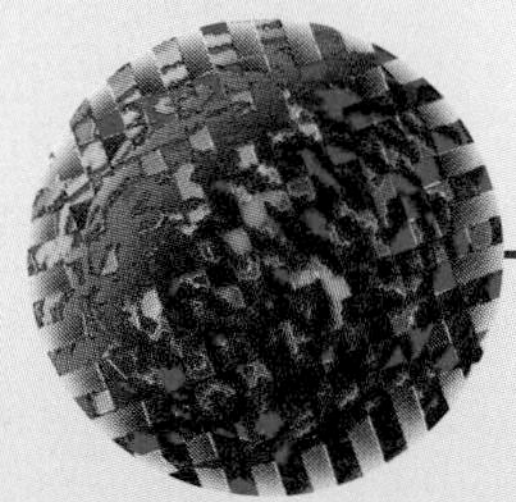

Metabolic and Endocrine Function

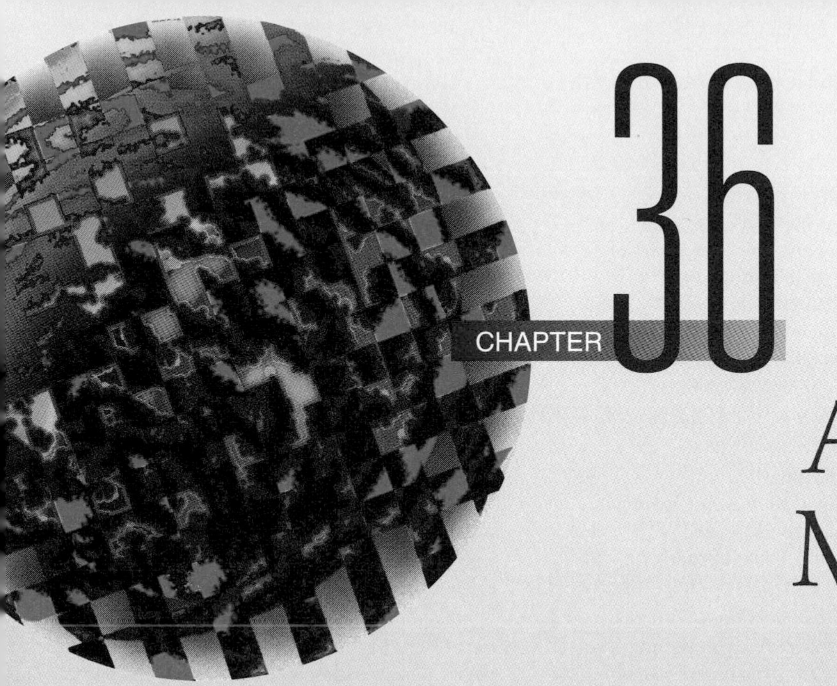

Assessment and Management of Patients With Hepatic and Biliary Disorders

Learning Objectives

On completion of this chapter, the learner will be able to:

1. Identify the metabolic functions of the liver and the alterations in these functions that occur with liver disease.
2. Explain liver function tests and clinical manifestations of liver dysfunction in relation to pathophysiologic alterations of the liver.
3. Relate jaundice, portal hypertension, ascites, nutritional deficiencies, and hepatic coma to pathophysiologic alterations of the liver.
4. Compare the various types of hepatitis and their causes, prevention, clinical manifestations, management, prognosis, and home health care needs.
5. Use the nursing process as a framework for care of the patient with cirrhosis of the liver.
6. Describe the medical, surgical, and nursing management of patients with esophageal varices.
7. Compare the nonsurgical and surgical management of patients with cancer of the liver.
8. Describe the postoperative nursing care of the patient undergoing liver transplantation.
9. Compare approaches to management of cholelithiasis.
10. Use the nursing process as a framework for care of patients with cholelithiasis and those undergoing cholecystectomy.

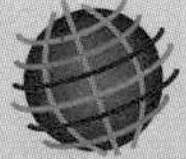

Disorders of the liver and biliary tract are common. Liver disorders may be viral in origin or a result of exposure to toxic substances, such as alcohol. It is not unusual for cancer to originate in the liver or to spread to the liver from other sites. Because of its complex functions, liver dysfunction affects all systems of the body. Biliary tract disorders, including gallbladder stones, are common. An understanding of the complex functions of the liver and biliary tract is essential. The nurse must have expert assessment and clinical management skills to care for patients undergoing complex diagnostic procedures and treatment that may involve recent technological advances in the management of liver and biliary tract disorders.

GLOSSARY

asterixis: involuntary flapping movements of the hands associated with metabolic liver dysfunction

balloon tamponade: use of balloons placed within the esophagus and proximal portion of the stomach and inflated to compress bleeding vessels (esophageal and gastric varices)

cholestatic diseases: hepatic dysfunction characterized by the body's inability to excrete bile

cirrhosis: a chronic liver disease characterized by fibrotic changes and the formation of dense connective tissue within the liver, subsequent degenerative changes and loss of functioning cells

constructional apraxia: inability to construct (draw) figures of two or three dimensions

cryoablation: a method of treatment of malignant hepatic lesions. A series of exposures of liver tissue (tumor) to extremely cold temperatures (below −20°C) and subsequent thawing. This surgical intervention is performed via a probe through which liquid nitrogen flows

dissolution therapy: use of medications to break up/dissolve gallstones

hepatic encephalopathy: central nervous system dysfunction resulting from liver disease; frequently associated with elevated ammonia levels producing changes in mental status, altered level of consciousness, and coma

endoscopic retrograde cholangiopancreatography (ERCP): an endoscopic procedure utilizing fiberoptic technology to visualize the biliary system

fulminant hepatic failure: sudden, severe onset of acute liver failure which occurs within 8 weeks of the first symptoms of jaundice

orthotopic liver transplantation (OLT): grafting of a donor liver into the normal anatomic location (with removal of diseased native liver)

portal hypertension: elevated pressure in the portal circulation resulting from obstruction of venous flow into and through the liver

sclerotherapy: use of substances injected into or around esophagogastric varices to cause constriction, thickening, and hardening of the vessel to stop bleeding

variceal banding: use of rubber bandlike device placed endoscopically over esophageal varices to ligate the area and stop bleeding

ANATOMIC AND PHYSIOLOGIC OVERVIEW

The liver, the largest gland of the body, can be considered a chemical factory that manufactures, stores, alters, and excretes a large number of substances involved in metabolism. The location of the liver is essential in this function, because it receives nutrient-rich blood directly from the gastrointestinal (GI) tract and then either stores or transforms these nutrients into chemicals that are used elsewhere in the body for metabolic needs. The liver is especially important in the regulation of glucose and protein metabolism. The liver manufactures and secretes bile, which has a major role in the digestion and absorption of fats in the GI tract. It removes waste products from the bloodstream and secretes them into the bile. The bile produced by the liver is stored temporarily in the gallbladder until it is needed for the process of digestion, at which time the gallbladder empties and bile enters the intestine. Figure 36-1 shows the liver and biliary system and their relation to the pancreas and spleen.

Anatomy of the Liver and Gallbladder

The liver is located behind the ribs in the upper right portion of the abdominal cavity. It weighs about 1500 g and is divided into four lobes. Each lobe is surrounded by a thin layer of connective tissue, which extends into the lobe itself and divides the liver mass into small units, called lobules.

The circulation of the blood into and out of the liver is of major importance in its function. The blood that perfuses the liver comes from two sources. Approximately 75% of the blood supply comes from the portal vein, which drains the GI tract and is rich in nutrients. The remainder of the blood supply enters by way of the hepatic artery and is rich in oxygen. Terminal branches of these two blood supplies join to form common capillary beds, which constitute the sinusoids of the liver (Fig. 36-2). Liver cells (hepatocytes) are thus bathed by a mixture of venous and arterial blood. The sinusoids empty into a venule that occupies the center of each liver lobule and is called the central vein. The central veins join to form the hepatic vein, which constitutes the venous drainage from the liver and empties into the inferior vena cava, close to the diaphragm. Thus, there are two sources of blood flowing into the liver and only one exit pathway.

In addition to hepatocytes, phagocytic cells belonging to the reticuloendothelial system are present in the liver. Other organs that contain reticuloendothelial cells are the spleen, bone marrow, lymph nodes, and lungs. In the liver, these cells are called Kupffer cells. Their main function is to engulf particulate matter (such as bacteria) that enters the liver through the portal blood.

The smallest bile ducts, called canaliculi, are located between the lobules of the liver. The canaliculi receive secretions from the hepatocytes and carry them to larger bile ducts, which eventually form the hepatic duct. The hepatic duct from the liver and the cystic duct from the gallbladder join to form the common bile duct, which empties into the small intestine. The flow of bile into the intestine is controlled by the sphincter of Oddi, located at the junction where the common bile duct enters the duodenum. The gallbladder, a pear-shaped, hollow, saclike organ, 7.5 to 10 cm (3 to 4 in) long, lies in a shallow depression on the inferior surface of the liver, to which it is attached by loose connective tissue. The capacity of the gallbladder is 30 to 50 mL of bile. Its wall is composed largely of smooth muscle. The gallbladder is connected to the common bile duct by the cystic duct (see Fig. 36-1).

Functions of the Liver

Glucose Metabolism

The liver plays a major role in the metabolism of glucose and the regulation of blood glucose concentration. After a meal, glucose is taken up from the portal venous blood by the liver and converted into glycogen, which is stored in the hepatocytes. Subsequently, the glycogen is converted back to glucose and released as needed into the bloodstream to maintain normal levels of blood glucose. Additional glucose can be synthesized by the liver through a process

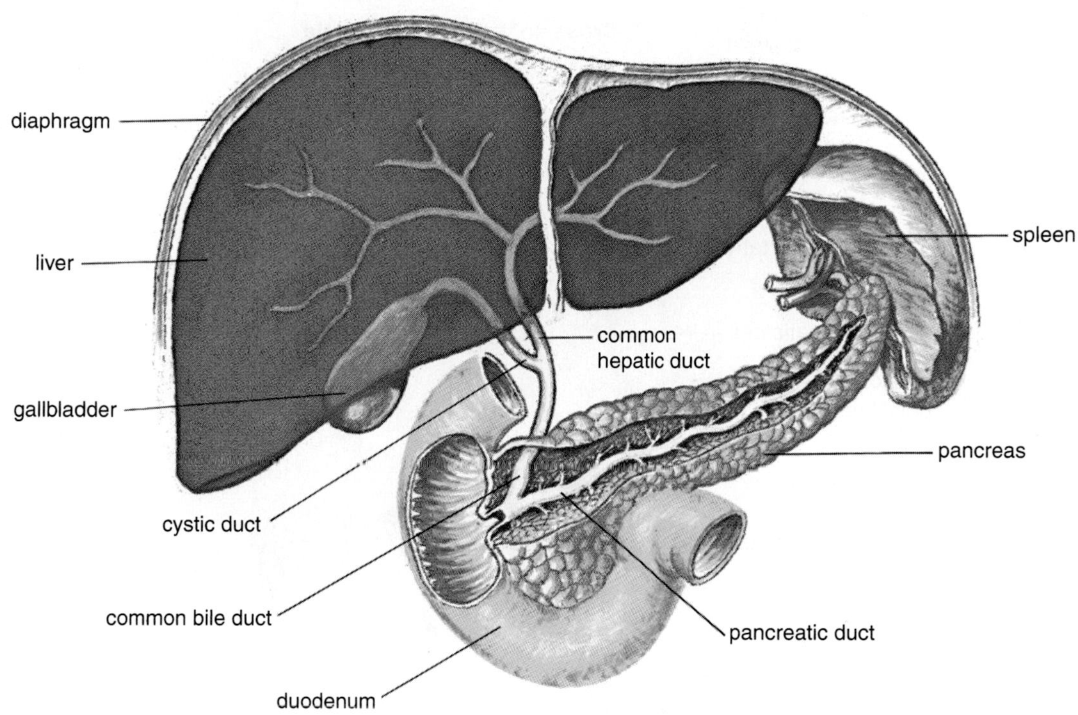

FIGURE 36•1 The liver and biliary system.

called gluconeogenesis. For this process, the liver uses amino acids from protein breakdown or lactate produced by exercising muscles.

Ammonia Conversion

Use of amino acids from protein for gluconeogenesis results in the formation of ammonia as a byproduct. The liver converts this metabolically generated ammonia into urea. Ammonia produced by bacteria in the intestines is also removed from portal blood for urea synthesis. In this way, the liver converts ammonia, a potential toxin, into urea, a compound that can be excreted in the urine.

Protein Metabolism

The liver also plays an important role in protein metabolism. It synthesizes almost all of the plasma proteins (except gamma globulin), including albumin, alpha and beta globulins, blood clotting factors, specific transport proteins, and most of the plasma lipoproteins. Vitamin K is required by the liver for synthesis of prothrombin and some of the other clotting factors. Amino acids serve as the building blocks for protein synthesis.

Fat Metabolism

The liver is also active in fat metabolism. Fatty acids can be broken down for the production of energy and the production of ketone bodies (acetoacetic acid, beta-hydroxybutyric acid, and acetone). Ketone bodies are small compounds that can enter the bloodstream and provide a source of energy for muscles and other tissues. Breakdown of fatty acids into ketone bodies occurs primarily when the availability of glucose for metabolism is limited, as during starvation or in uncontrolled diabetes. Fatty acids and their metabolic products are also used for the synthesis of cholesterol, lecithin, lipoproteins, and other complex lipids. Under some conditions, lipids may accumulate in the hepatocytes and result in the abnormal condition called fatty liver. – ETOH

Vitamin and Iron Storage

Vitamins A, B_{12}, and D and several of the B-complex vitamins are stored in large amounts in the liver. Certain substances, such as iron and copper, are also stored in the liver. Because the liver is rich in these substances, liver extracts have been used for therapy of a wide range of nutritional disorders.

Drug Metabolism

Many medications, such as barbiturates, opioids, sedatives, and amphetamines, are metabolized by the liver. Metabolism generally results in loss of activity of the medication, although in some cases activation of the medication may occur. One of the important pathways for medication metabolism involves conjugation (binding) of the medication with a variety of compounds, such as glucuronic or acetic acid, to form more soluble substances. The conjugated products may be excreted in the feces or urine, similar to bilirubin excretion. If an oral medication that is absorbed from the GI tract is metabolized by the liver to a great extent before it reaches the systemic circulation (first-pass effect), the amount of drug actually reaching the systemic circulation (oral bioavailability) will be decreased. Bioavailability is the percentage or fraction of the administered drug that reaches the systemic circulation. Some medications have such a large first-pass effect that their use is essentially limited to the parenteral route or oral doses are substantially larger than parenteral doses.

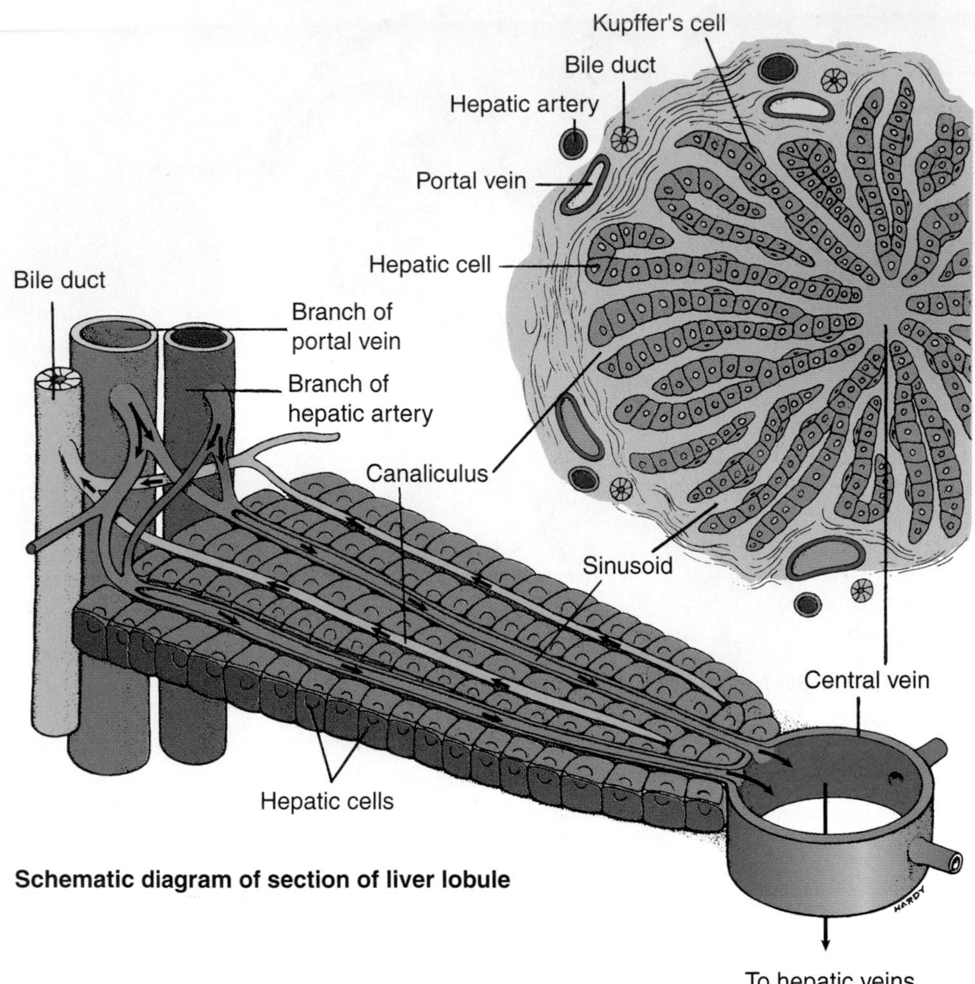

FIGURE 36•2 A section of liver lobule showing the location of hepatic veins, hepatic cells, liver sinusoids, and branches of the portal vein and hepatic artery.

Bile Formation

Bile is continuously formed by the hepatocytes and collected in the canaliculi and bile ducts. It is composed mainly of water and electrolytes, such as sodium, potassium, calcium, chloride, and bicarbonate, and it also contains significant amounts of lecithin, fatty acids, cholesterol, bilirubin, and bile salts. Bile is collected and stored in the gallbladder and is emptied into the intestine when needed for digestion. The functions of bile are excretory, as in the excretion of bilirubin; bile also serves as an aid to digestion through the emulsification of fats by bile salts.

Bile salts are synthesized by the hepatocytes from cholesterol. After conjugation or binding with amino acids (taurine and glycine), they are excreted into the bile. The bile salts, together with cholesterol and lecithin, are required for emulsification of fats in the intestine, which is necessary for efficient digestion and absorption. Bile salts are then reabsorbed, primarily in the distal ileum, into portal blood for return to the liver and are again excreted into the bile. This pathway from hepatocytes to bile to intestine and back to the hepatocytes is called the enterohepatic circulation. Because of the enterohepatic circulation, only a small fraction of the bile salts that enter the intestine are excreted in the feces. This decreases the need for active synthesis of bile salts by the liver cells.

Bilirubin Excretion

Bilirubin is a pigment derived from the breakdown of hemoglobin by cells of the reticuloendothelial system, including the Kupffer cells of the liver. Hepatocytes remove bilirubin from the blood and chemically modify it through conjugation to glucuronic acid, which makes the bilirubin more soluble in aqueous solutions. The conjugated bilirubin is secreted by the hepatocytes into the adjacent bile canaliculi and is eventually carried in the bile into the duodenum.

In the small intestine, bilirubin is converted into urobilinogen, which is in part excreted in the feces and in part absorbed through the intestinal mucosa into the portal blood. Much of this reabsorbed urobilinogen is removed by the hepatocytes and is secreted into the bile once again (enterohepatic circulation). Some of the urobilinogen enters the systemic circulation and is excreted by the kidneys in the urine. Elimination of bilirubin in the bile represents the major route of excretion for this compound.

The bilirubin concentration in the blood may be increased in the presence of liver disease, when the flow of bile is impeded (ie, with gallstones in the bile ducts), or with excessive destruction of red blood cells. With bile duct obstruction, bilirubin does not enter the intestine; as a consequence, urobilinogen is absent from the urine and decreased in the stool.

Function of the Gallbladder

The gallbladder functions as a storage depot for bile. Between meals, when the sphincter of Oddi is closed, bile produced by the hepatocytes enters the gallbladder. During storage, a large portion of the water in bile is absorbed through the walls of the gallbladder, so that gallbladder bile is five to ten times more concentrated than that originally secreted by the liver. When food enters the duodenum, the gallbladder contracts and the sphincter of Oddi relaxes, allowing the bile to enter the intestine. This response is mediated by secretion of the hormone cholecystokinin–pancreozymin from the intestinal wall.

Gerontologic Considerations

The most common change in the liver in the elderly is a decrease in size and weight accompanied by a decrease in total hepatic blood flow. In general, however, these decreases are in proportion to the decreases in body size and weight seen in normal aging. Results of liver function tests do not normally change in the elderly; abnormal results in an elderly patient indicate abnormal liver function and are not the result of the aging process itself.

The immune system is altered in the aged, and a less responsive immune system may be responsible for the increased incidence and severity of hepatitis B in the elderly and the increased incidence of liver abscesses secondary to decreased phagocytosis by the Kupffer cells. With the advent of hepatitis B vaccine as the standard for prevention, the incidence of hepatic diseases may decrease in the future.

Metabolism of medications by the liver appears to be decreased in the elderly, but such changes are usually accompanied by changes in intestinal absorption, renal excretion, and altered body distribution of some medications secondary to changes in fat deposition. These alterations necessitate careful administration and monitoring of all medications, with reduction of dosage to prevent medication toxicity.

ASSESSMENT

Physical Assessment

The liver may be palpable in the right upper quadrant. A palpable liver presents as a firm, sharp ridge with a smooth surface (Fig. 36-3). The size of the liver is estimated by percussion of the liver's upper and lower borders. When the liver is not palpable but tenderness is suspected, tapping the lower right thorax briskly may elicit tenderness. The patient's response is then compared by performing a similar maneuver on the left lower thorax.

If the liver is palpable, the examiner notes and records its size and consistency, whether it is tender, and whether its outline is regular or irregular. If the liver is enlarged, the degree to which it descends below the right costal margin is recorded to provide some indication of its size. The examiner determines whether the liver's edge is sharp and smooth or blunt and whether the enlarged liver is nodular or smooth. The liver of a patient with cirrhosis is small and hard, whereas the liver of a patient with acute hepatitis is quite soft and the edge is easily moved by the hand.

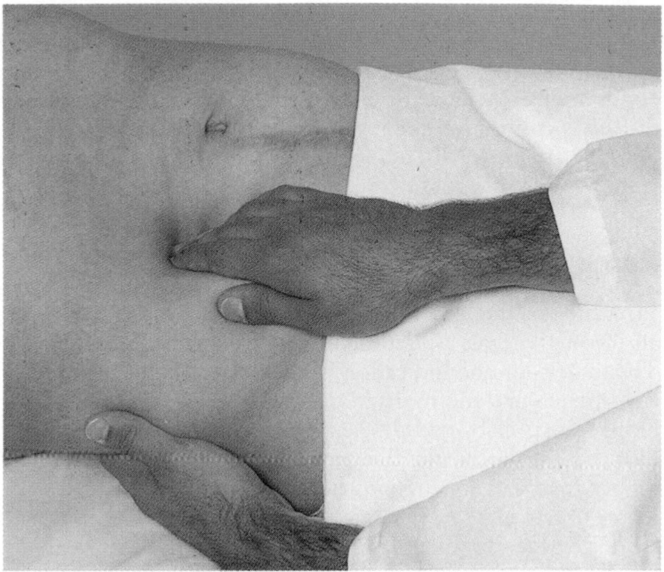

FIGURE 36•3 Technique for palpating the liver. The examiner places one hand under the right lower rib cage and presses downward with light pressure with the other hand. From Bickley, L. S. & Hoekelman, L. R., (1999). *Bates' guide to physical examination and history taking* (7th ed.). Philadelphia: Lippincott Williams & Wilkins.

Tenderness of the liver implies recent acute enlargement with consequent stretching of the liver capsule. The absence of tenderness may imply that the enlargement is of long-standing duration. The liver of a patient with viral hepatitis is tender, whereas that of a patient with alcoholic hepatitis is not. Enlargement of the liver is an abnormal finding requiring further evaluation.

DIAGNOSTIC EVALUATION

Liver Function Tests

More than 70% of the parenchyma of the liver may be damaged before liver function tests become abnormal. Function is generally measured in terms of serum enzyme activity (ie, alkaline phosphatase, lactic dehydrogenase, serum aminotransferases [transaminases]), and serum concentrations of proteins (albumin and globulins), bilirubin, ammonia, clotting factors, and lipids. Several of these tests may be helpful for assessing patients with liver disease; however, the nature and extent of hepatic dysfunction cannot be determined by these tests alone, as many other disorders can affect their results.

Serum aminotransferases (also called transaminases) are sensitive indicators of injury to the liver cells and are useful in detecting acute liver disease such as hepatitis. Alanine aminotransferase (ALT) (formerly called serum glutamic-pyruvic transaminase [SGPT]), aspartate aminotransferase (AST) (formerly called serum glutamic-oxalocetic transaminase [SGOT]), and gamma glutamyl transferase (GGT) (also called G-glutamyl transpeptidase) are the most frequently used tests of liver damage. ALT (SGPT) levels increase primarily in liver disorders and may be used to monitor the course of hepatitis or cirrhosis or the effects of treatments that may be toxic to the liver. AST (SGOT) is present in tissues that have high metabolic activity; thus, it may be increased in damage or death of tissues of organs such as the heart, liver, skeletal muscle, and kidney. Although not specific to liver disease, AST (SGOT) may be increased in cirrhosis, hepatitis, and liver cancer. Increased GGT is associated with cholestasis but can also be due to alcoholic liver disease. Despite the fact that the kidney has the highest level of the enzyme, the liver is considered the source of normal serum activity. The test determines liver cell dysfunction and is a sensitive indicator of cholestasis. Its main value in liver disease is confirming the hepatic origin of an elevated alkaline phosphatase level. A list of the commonly used liver function tests is shown in Table 36-1.

Percutaneous Needle Biopsy

Liver biopsy, the removal of a small amount of liver tissue usually through needle aspiration, permits examination of liver cells. The most common indication is to evaluate diffuse disorders of the parenchyma and to diagnose space-occupying lesions. Liver biopsy is especially useful when clinical findings and laboratory tests are not diagnostic. Bleeding and bile peritonitis after liver biopsy are the major complications; therefore, coagulation studies are obtained, their values are noted, and abnormal results are treated before liver biopsy is performed. Nursing responsibilities related to liver biopsy are summarized in Guideline 36-1.

Other Diagnostic Tests

Ultrasonography, computed tomography (CT) scanning, and magnetic resonance imaging (MRI) are used to identify normal structures and abnormalities of the liver and biliary tree. A radioisotope liver scan may be performed to assess liver size and hepatic blood flow and obstruction.

Laparoscopy (insertion of a fiber-optic endoscope through a small abdominal incision) is used to examine the liver and other pelvic structures. It is also used to perform guided liver biopsy, to determine the etiology of ascites, and to diagnose and stage tumors of the liver and other abdominal tumors.

HEPATIC DYSFUNCTION

Hepatic dysfunction results from damage to the liver parenchymal cells, either directly, from primary liver diseases, or indirectly, from obstruction of bile flow or derangements of hepatic circulation. Liver dysfunction may be acute or chronic; however, chronic dysfunction is far more common than acute.

Chronic liver disease, including cirrhosis, is the 11th most frequent cause of death in the United States. More than 40% of those deaths are associated with alcohol. The rates of chronic liver disease for men are two times higher than for women; it is more common among African Americans than whites (National Institutes of Health, 1997).

Pathophysiology

Disease processes that lead to hepatocellular dysfunction may be caused by infectious agents, such as bacteria and viruses, and by anoxia, metabolic disorders, toxins and medications, nutritional deficiencies, and states of hypersensitivity. The most common cause of parenchymal damage is malnutrition, especially in alcoholism.

The parenchymal cells respond to most noxious agents by replacing glycogen with lipids, producing fatty infiltration, with or without cell death or necrosis. This is commonly associated with inflammatory cell infiltration and growth of fibrous tissue. Cell regeneration can occur if the disease process is not too toxic to the cells. The end result of chronic parenchymal disease is the shrunken, fibrotic liver seen in cirrhosis.

Clinical Manifestations

The consequences of liver disease are numerous and varied. Their ultimate effects are often incapacitating or life-threatening; their presence is ominous, and their treatment is often difficult. Among the most frequent and important of consequences of liver disease are the following:

- Jaundice, resulting from increased bilirubin concentration in the blood
- Portal hypertension and ascites, resulting from circulatory changes within the diseased liver and producing severe GI hemorrhages and marked sodium and fluid retention
- Nutritional deficiencies, which result from the inability of the damaged liver cells to metabolize certain vitamins; responsible for impaired functioning of the central and peripheral nervous systems and for abnormal bleeding tendencies
- Hepatic encephalopathy or coma, reflecting accumulation of ammonia in the serum due to impaired protein metabolism by the diseased liver

Nursing care of the patient with impaired liver function is summarized in Plan of Nursing Care 36-1.

Jaundice

When the bilirubin concentration in the blood is abnormally elevated, all the body tissues, including the sclerae and the skin, become yellow-tinged or greenish yellow. This condition is called jaundice. Jaundice becomes clinically evident when the serum bilirubin level exceeds 2.5 mg/dL (SI: 43 μmol/L). Increased serum bilirubin levels and jaundice may result from impairment of hepatic uptake, conjugation of bilirubin, or excretion of bilirubin into the biliary system. There are several types of jaundice: (1) hemolytic, (2) hepatocellular, (3) obstructive, and (4) jaundice due to hereditary hyperbilirubinemia. Hepatocellular and obstructive jaundice are the two types commonly associated with liver disease.

HEMOLYTIC JAUNDICE

Hemolytic jaundice is the result of an increased destruction of the red blood cells, the effect of which is to flood the plasma with bilirubin so rapidly that the liver, although functioning normally, cannot excrete the bilirubin as quickly as it is formed. This type of jaundice is encountered in patients with hemolytic transfusion reactions and other hemolytic disorders. The bilirubin in the blood of these patients is predominantly of the unconjugated, or free, type. Fecal and urine urobilinogen levels are increased; conversely, the urine is free of bilirubin. Patients with this type of jaundice, unless their hyperbilirubinemia is extreme, do not experience symptoms or complications as a result of the jaundice per se. Very prolonged jaundice, however, even if mild, predisposes to the formation of pigment stones in the gallbladder, and extremely severe jaundice (levels of free bilirubin exceeding 20 to 25 mg/dL) poses a definite risk of brain stem damage.

HEPATOCELLULAR JAUNDICE

Hepatocellular jaundice is caused by the inability of damaged liver cells to clear normal amounts of bilirubin from the blood. The cellular damage may be from infection, such as in viral hepatitis (eg, hepatitis A, B, C, D, or E) or other viruses that affect the

(text continues on page 933)

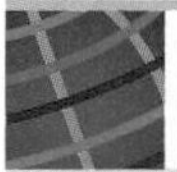

TABLE 36•1 **Liver Function Studies**

Test	Normal	Clinical Functions
Pigment Studies		
Serum bilirubin, direct	0–0.3 mg/dL (0–5.1 μmol/L)	These studies measure the ability of the liver to conjugate and excrete bilirubin. Results are abnormal in liver and biliary tract disease and are associated with jaundice clinically.
Serum bilirubin, total	0–0.9 mg/dL (1.7–20.5 μmol/L)	
Urine bilirubin	0(0)	
Urine urobilinogen	0.05–2.5 mg/24 h (0.09–4.23 μmol/24 h)	
Fecal urobilinogen (infrequently used)	40–200 mg/24 h (0.068–0.34 mmol/24 h)	
Protein Studies		
Total serum protein	7.0–7.5 g/dL (70–75 g/L)	Proteins are manufactured by the liver. Their levels may be affected in a variety of liver impairments.
Serum albumin	3.5–5.5 g/dL (35–55 g/L)	Albumin: Cirrhosis Chronic hepatitis Edema, ascites
Serum globulin	1.5–3.0 g/dL (15–30 g/L)	Globulin: Cirrhosis Liver disease Chronic obstructive jaundice Viral hepatitis
Serum protein electrophoresis	3.2–5.6 g/dL (32–56 g/L)	
Albumin		
α_1-Globulin	0.1–0.4 g/dL (1–4 g/L)	
α_2-Globulin	0.4–1.2 g/dL (4–12 g/L)	
β-Globulin	0.5–1.1 g/dL (5–11 g/L)	
γ-Globulin	0.5–1.6 g/dL (5–16 g/L)	
Albumin/globulin (A/G) ratio	A > G or 1.5:1–2.5:1	A/G ratio is reversed in chronic liver disease (decreased albumin and increased globulin).
Prothrombin Time	100% or 12–16 seconds	Prothrombin time may be prolonged in liver disease. It will not return to normal with vitamin K in severe liver cell damage.
Serum alkaline phosphatase	Varies with method: 2–5 Bodansky units 30–50 IU/L at 34°C (17–142 U/L at 30°C) (20–90 U/L at 30°C)	Serum alkaline phosphatase is manufactured in bones, liver, kidneys, and intestine and excreted through biliary tract. In absence of bone disease, it is a sensitive measure of biliary tract obstruction.
Serum Aminotransferase or Transaminase Studies		
AST, SGOT	10–40 units (4.8–19 U/L)	The studies are based on release of enzymes from damaged liver cells. These enzymes are elevated in liver cell damage.
ALT, SGPT	5–35 units (2.4–17 U/L)	
GGT, GGTP	10–48 IU/L	Elevated in alcohol abuse. Marker for biliary cholestasis.
LDH	100–200 units (100–225 U/L)	
Serum ammonia	20–120 μg/dL (11.1–67.0 μmol/L) 150–250 mg/dL (3.90–6.50 mmol/L)	Liver converts ammonia to urea. Ammonia level rises in liver failure.
Cholesterol		
Ester	60% of total (fraction of total cholesterol: 0.60)	Cholesterol levels are elevated in biliary obstruction and decreased in parenchymal liver disease.
HDL (high-density lipoprotein)	HDL Male: 35–70 mg/dL, Female: 35–85 mg/dL	
LDL (low-density lipoprotein)	LDL < 130 μg/dL	

Additional Studies	Clinical Functions
Barium study of esophagus	For varices, which indicate increased portal pressure
Abdominal x-ray	To determine gross liver size
Liver scan with radiotagged iodinated rose bengal, gold, technetium, or gallium	To show size and shape of liver; to show replacement of liver tissue with scars, cysts, or tumor
Cholecystogram and cholangiogram	For gallbladder and bile duct visualization
Celiac axis arteriography	For liver and pancreas visualization
Splenoportogram (splenic portal venography)	To determine adequacy of portal blood flow
Laparoscopy	Direct visualization of anterior surface of liver, gallbladder, and mesentery through a trocar
Liver biopsy (percutaneous or transjugular)	To determine anatomic changes in liver tissue
Measurement of portal pressure	Elevated in cirrhosis of the liver
Esophagoscopy/endoscopy	To search for esophageal varices and abnormalities
Electroencephalogram	Abnormal in hepatic coma and impending hepatic coma
Ultrasonography	To show size of abdominal organs and presence of masses
Computed tomography (CT scan)	To detect hepatic neoplasms; diagnose cysts, abscesses, and hematomas; and distinguish between obstructive and nonobstructive jaundice. Detects cerebral atrophy in hepatic encephalopathy.
Angiography	Visualizes hepatic circulation and detects presence and nature of hepatic masses
Magnetic resonance imaging (MRI)	To detect hepatic neoplasms; diagnose cysts, abscesses, and hematomas. Detects cerebral atrophy in encephalopathy.
Endoscopic retrograde cholangiopancreatography (ERCP)	Visualizes biliary structures via endoscopy

36•1 GUIDELINES FOR ASSISTING WITH LIVER BIOPSY

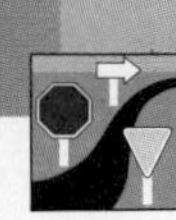

Nursing Activities	Rationale
Preprocedure	
1. Ascertain that results of coagulation tests (prothrombin time, PTT, and platelet count) are available and that compatible donor blood is available.	Many patients with liver disease have clotting defects and are at risk for bleeding.
2. Check for signed consent.	
3. Measure and record the patient's pulse, respirations, and blood pressure immediately before biopsy.	Prebiopsy values provide a basis on which to compare the patient's vital signs and evaluate status after the procedure.
4. Describe to the patient in advance: steps of the procedure; sensations expected; after-effects anticipated; restrictions of activity and monitoring procedures to follow.	Explanations serve to allay fears and ensure cooperation.
During Procedure	
5. Support the patient during the procedure.	Encouragement and support of the nurse enhance comfort and promote a sense of security.
6. Expose the right side of the patient's upper abdomen (right hypochondriac).	The skin at the site of penetration will be cleansed and a local anesthetic will be infiltrated.
7. Instruct the patient to inhale and exhale deeply several times, finally to exhale, and to hold breath at the end of expiration. The physician promptly introduces the biopsy needle by way of the transthoracic (intercostal) or transabdominal (subcostal) route, penetrates the liver, aspirates, and withdraws.	Holding the breath immobilizes the chest wall and the diaphragm; penetration of the diaphragm thereby is avoided, and the risk of lacerating the liver is minimized.
8. Instruct the patient to resume breathing.	

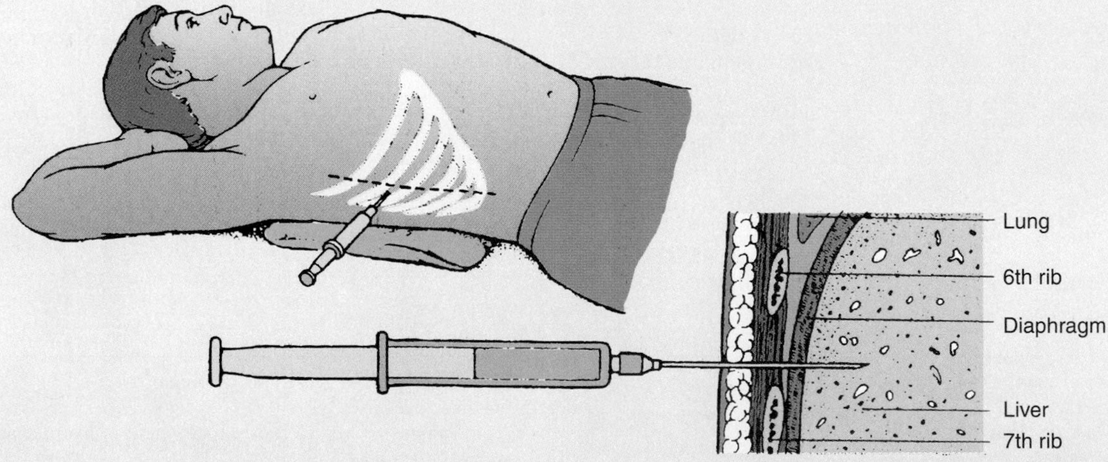

Nursing Activities	Rationale
Postprocedure	
9. Immediately after the biopsy, assist the patient to turn onto the right side; place a pillow under the costal margin, and caution the patient to remain in this position, recumbent and immobile, for several hours. Instruct the patient to avoid coughing or straining.	In this position, the liver capsule at the site of penetration is compressed against the chest wall, and the escape of blood or bile through the perforation is impeded.
10. Measure and record the patient's pulse, respiratory rate, and blood pressure at 10- to 15-minute intervals for the first hour, then every 30 minutes for the next 1 to 2 hours or until the patient's condition stabilizes.	Changes in vital signs may indicate bleeding, severe hemorrhage, or bile peritonitis, the most frequent complications of liver biopsy.
11. If the patient is discharged after the procedure, instruct the patient to avoid heavy lifting and strenuous activity for 1 week.	Cautious activity reduces the risk of bleeding at the biopsy puncture site.

36•1

PLAN OF NURSING CARE — The Patient With Impaired Liver Function

Nursing Interventions	Rationale	Expected Outcomes
Nursing Diagnosis: Activity intolerance related to fatigue, lethargy, and malaise **Goal:** Patient reports decrease in fatigue and reports increased ability to participate in activities		
1. Assess level of activity tolerance and degree of fatigue, lethargy, and malaise when performing routine ADLs.	1. Provides baseline for further assessment and criteria for assessment of effectiveness of interventions.	• Expresses anxieties and fears about condition • Exhibits increased interest in activities and events
2. Assist with activities and hygiene when fatigued.	2. Promotes exercise and hygiene within patient's level of tolerance.	• Participates in activities and gradually increases exercise within physical limits
3. Encourage rest when fatigued or when abdominal pain or discomfort occurs.	3. Conserves energy and protects the liver.	• Reports increased strength and well-being
4. Assist with selection and pacing of desired activities and exercise.	4. Stimulates patient's interest in selected activities.	• Reports absence of abdominal pain and discomfort
5. Offer high-protein, high-calorie diet.	5. Provides calories for energy and protein for healing.	• Reports increased strength and well-being • Plans activities to allow ample periods of rest
6. Give supplemental vitamins (A, B complex, C, and K).	6. Provides additional nutrients.	• Takes vitamins as prescribed
Nursing Diagnosis: Altered nutrition less than body requirements, related to abdominal distention and discomfort and anorexia **Goal:** Positive nitrogen balance, no further loss of muscle mass; achieves nutritional requirements		
1. Assess dietary intake and nutritional status through diet history and diary, daily weight measurements, laboratory data, and anthropometric assessment.	1. Identifies deficits in nutritional intake and adequacy of nutritional state.	• Exhibits improved nutritional status by increased weight (without fluid retention), improved laboratory data and anthropometric measurements
2. Provide diet high in carbohydrates with protein intake consistent with liver function.	2. Provides calories for energy, sparing protein for healing.	• States rationale for dietary modifications • Identifies foods high in carbohydrates and within protein requirements (high in cirrhosis and hepatitis, low in hepatic failure)
3. Assist patient in identifying low-sodium foods.	3. Reduces edema and ascites formation.	
4. Elevate the head of the bed during meals.	4. Reduces discomfort from abdominal distention and decreases sense of fullness produced by pressure of abdominal contents and ascites on the stomach.	• Reports improved appetite • Participates in oral hygiene measures • Reports increased appetite; identifies rationale for smaller, frequent meals
5. Provide oral hygiene before meals and pleasant environment for meals at meal time.	5. Promotes positive environment and increased appetite; reduces unpleasant taste	• Demonstrates intake of sufficient high-protein, high-calorie meals • Identifies foods and fluids that are nutritious and permitted on diet
6. Offer smaller, more frequent meals (6 per day).	6. Decreases feeling of fullness, bloating.	• Gains weight without increased edema or ascites formation
7. Encourage patient to eat meals and supplementary feedings.	7. Encouragement is essential for the patient with anorexia and gastrointestinal discomfort.	• Reports increased appetite and well-being • Excludes alcohol from diet
8. Provide attractive meals and an aesthetically pleasing setting at meal time.	8. Promotes appetite and sense of well-being.	• Takes medications for gastrointestinal disorders as prescribed
9. Eliminate alcohol.	9. Eliminates "empty calories" and avoids the gastric irritation produced by alcohol.	• Reports normal gastrointestinal function with regular bowel function
10. Apply an ice collar for nausea.	10. May reduce incidence of nausea.	
11. Administer medications prescribed for nausea, vomiting, diarrhea, or constipation.	11. Reduces gastrointestinal symptoms and discomforts that decrease the appetite and interest in food.	
12. Encourage increased fluid intake and exercise if the patient reports constipation.	12. Promotes normal bowel pattern and reduces abdominal discomfort and distention.	

(*continued*)

36•1

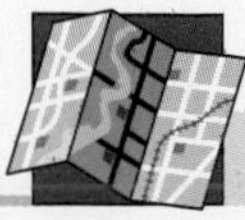

PLAN OF NURSING CARE The Patient With Impaired Liver Function (*continued*)

Nursing Diagnosis: Impaired skin integrity related to pruritus from jaundice and edema
Goal: Decrease potential for pressure sore development; breaks in skin integrity

Nursing Interventions	Rationale	Expected Outcomes
1. Assess degree of discomfort related to pruritus and edema.	1. Assists in determining appropriate strategies.	• Exhibits intact skin without redness, excoriation, or breakdown • Reports relief from pruritus • Exhibits no skin excoriation from scratching • Uses nondrying soaps and lotions. States rationale for use of nondrying soaps and lotions • Turns self periodically. Exhibits reduced edema of dependent parts of the body • Exhibits no areas of skin breakdown • Exhibits decreased edema; normal skin turgor
2. Note and record degree of jaundice and extent of edema.	2. Provides baseline for detecting changes and evaluating effectiveness of interventions.	
3. Keep patient's fingernails short and smooth.	3. Prevents skin excoriation and infection from scratching.	
4. Provide frequent skin care; avoid use of soaps and alcohol-based lotions.	4. Removes waste products deposited in skin while preventing dryness of skin.	
5. Massage every 2 h with emollients; turn every 2 hours	5. Promotes mobilization of edema.	
6. Initiate use of alternating-pressure mattress or low air loss bed.	6. Minimizes prolonged pressure on bony prominences susceptible to breakdown.	
7. Use nonallergenic linen; if at home avoid harsh detergents.	7. May decrease skin irritation and need for scratching.	
8. Assess skin integrity every 4–8 hours. Instruct patient and family in this activity.	8. Edematous skin and tissue has compromised nutrient supply and is vulnerable to pressure and trauma.	
9. Restrict sodium as prescribed.	9. Minimizes edema formation.	
10. Carry out range of motion exercises every 4 hours; elevate edematous extremities whenever possible.	10. Promotes mobilization of edema.	

Nursing Diagnosis: High risk for injury related to altered clotting mechanisms and altered level of consciousness
Goal: Reduced risk of injury

Nursing Interventions	Rationale	Expected Outcomes
1. Assess level of consciousness and cognitive level.	1. Assists in predicting patient's ability to protect self and comply with required self-protective actions; may detect deterioration of hepatic function.	• Is oriented to time, place, and person • Exhibits no ecchymoses (bruises), cuts, or hematoma • Exhibits no hallucinations, and demonstrates no efforts to get up unassisted or to leave hospital • Uses electric razor rather than sharp-edged razor • Exhibits absence of frank bleeding from gastrointestinal tract • Exhibits absence of restlessness, epigastric fullness, and other indicators of hemorrhage and shock • Exhibits negative results of test for occult gastrointestinal bleeding • Is free of ecchymotic areas or hematoma formation • Exhibits normal vital signs • Maintains rest and remains quiet if active bleeding occurs • Identifies rationale for blood transfusions and measures to treat bleeding • Uses measures to prevent trauma (eg, uses soft toothbrush, blows nose gently, avoids bumps and falls, avoids straining during defecation) • Experiences no side effects of medications
2. Provide safe environment (pad side rails, remove obstacles in room, prevent falls).	2. Minimizes falls and accidents and injury if falls occur.	
3. Provide frequent surveillance to orient patient and avoid use of restraints.	3. Protects patient from harm while stimulating and orienting patient; avoids use of restraints, which may disturb patient further.	
4. Replace sharp objects (razors) with safer items.	4. Avoids accidental cuts.	
5. Observe each stool for color, consistency, and amount.	5. Permits detection of bleeding in gastrointestinal tract.	
6. Be alert for symptoms of anxiety, epigastric fullness, weakness, and restlessness.	6. May indicate early signs of bleeding and shock.	
7. Test each stool and emesis for occult blood.	7. Detects early evidence of bleeding.	
8. Observe for hemorrhagic manifestations: ecchymosis, epistaxis, petechiae, and bleeding gums.	8. Indicates altered clotting mechanisms.	
9. Record vital signs at frequent intervals, depending on patient acuity (every 1–4 hours).	9. Provides baseline and evidence of hypovolemia, shock.	
10. Keep patient quiet and limit activity.	10. Minimizes risk of bleeding and straining.	
11. Assist physician in passage of tube for esophageal balloon tamponade.	11. Promote nontraumatic insertion of tube in anxious and combative patient for immediate treatment of bleeding.	

36•1 PLAN OF NURSING CARE

The Patient With Impaired Liver Function (*continued*)

Nursing Interventions	Rationale	Expected Outcomes
12. Observe during blood transfusions.	12. Permits detection of transfusion reactions (risk is increased with multiple blood transfusions needed for active bleeding from esophageal varices).	• Takes all medications as prescribed • Identifies rationale for precautions with use of all medications
13. Measure and record nature, time, and amount of vomitus.	13. Assists in evaluating extent of bleeding and blood loss.	
14. Maintain patient in fasting state, if indicated.	14. Reduces risk of aspiration of gastric contents and minimizes risk of further trauma to esophagus and stomach by preventing vomiting.	
15. Administer vitamin K as prescribed.	15. Promotes clotting by providing fat-soluble vitamin necessary for clotting mechanism.	
16. Stay in constant attendance during episodes of bleeding.	16. Reassures anxious patient and permits monitoring and detection of further needs of the patient.	
17. Offer cold liquids by mouth when bleeding stops (if prescribed).	17. Minimizes risk of further bleeding by promoting vasoconstriction of esophageal and gastric blood vessels.	
18. Institute measures to prevent trauma:	18. Promotes safety of patient.	
a. Maintain safe environment.	a. Minimizes risk of trauma and bleeding by avoiding falls and cuts, etc.	
b. Encourage *gentle* blowing of nose.	b. Reduces risk of nosebleed (epistaxis) secondary to trauma and decreased clotting.	
c. Provide soft toothbrush and avoid use of toothpicks.	c. Prevents trauma to oral mucosa while promoting good oral hygiene.	
d. Encourage intake of foods with high content of vitamin C.	d. Promotes healing.	
e. Apply cold compresses where indicated.	e. Minimizes bleeding into tissues by promoting local vasoconstriction.	
f. Record location of bleeding sites.	f. Permits detection of new bleeding sites and monitoring of previous sites of bleeding.	
g. Use small-gauge needles for injections.	g. Minimizes oozing and blood loss from repeated injections.	
19. Administer medications carefully; monitor for side effects.	19. Reduces risk of side effects secondary to damaged liver's inability to detoxify (metabolize) medications normally.	

Nursing Diagnosis: Body image disturbance related to changes in appearance, sexual dysfunction, and role function
Goal: Patient verbalizes feelings consistent with improvement of body image and self-esteem

Nursing Interventions	Rationale	Expected Outcomes
1. Assess changes in appearance and the meaning these changes have for patient and family.	1. Provides information for assessing impact of changes in appearance, sexual function, and role on the patient and family.	• Verbalizes concerns related to changes in appearance, life, and lifestyle • Shares concerns with significant others • Identifies past coping strategies that have been effective • Uses past effective coping strategies to deal with changes in appearance, life, and lifestyle • Maintains good grooming and hygiene • Identifies short-term goals and strategies to achieve them • Exercises an active role in decision making about self and care
2. Encourage patient to verbalize reactions and feelings about these changes.	2. Enables patient to identify and express concerns; encourages patient and significant others to share these concerns.	
3. Assess patient's and family's previous coping strategies.	3. Permits encouragement of those coping strategies that are familiar to patient and have been effective in the past.	
4. Assist and encourage patient to maximize appearance and explore alternatives to previous sexual and role functions.	4. Encourages patient to continue safe roles and functions while encouraging exploration of alternatives.	

(*continued*)

36•1

PLAN OF NURSING CARE 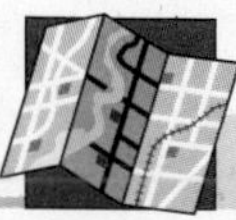 The Patient With Impaired Liver Function (*continued*)

Nursing Interventions	Rationale	Expected Outcomes
5. Assist patient in identifying short-term goals.	5. Accomplishing these goals serves as positive reinforcement and increases self-esteem.	• Identifies resources that are not harmful • Verbalizes that some of previous lifestyle practices have been harmful • Uses healthy expressions of frustration, anger, and so forth
6. Encourage and assist patient in decision making about care.	6. Promotes patient's control of life and improves sense of well-being and self-esteem.	
7. Identify with patient resources to provide additional support (counselor, clergy).	7. Assists patient in identifying resources and accepting assistance from others when indicated.	
8. Assist patient in identifying previous practices that may have been harmful to self (alcohol and drug abuse).	8. Recognition and acknowledgment of the harmful effects of these practices are necessary for identifying a healthier lifestyle.	

Nursing Diagnosis: Pain and discomfort related to enlarged tender liver and ascites
Goal: Increased level of comfort

Nursing Interventions	Rationale	Expected Outcomes
1. Maintain bed rest when patient experiences abdominal discomfort.	1. Reduces metabolic demands and protects the liver.	• Maintains bed rest and decreases activity in presence of pain • Takes antispasmodics and sedatives as indicated and as prescribed • Reports decreased pain and abdominal discomfort • Reports pain and discomfort if present • Reduces sodium and fluid intake to prescribed levels if indicated to treat ascites • Obtains pain relief • Exhibits decreased abdominal girth and appropriate weight changes • Reports decreased discomfort after paracentesis
2. Administer antispasmodics and sedatives as prescribed.	2. Reduces irritability of the gastrointestinal tract and decreases abdominal pain and discomfort.	
3. Observe, record, and report presence and character of pain and discomfort.	3. Provides baseline to detect further deterioration of status and to evaluate interventions.	
4. Reduce sodium and fluid intake if prescribed.	4. Minimizes further formation of ascites.	
5. Prepare patient and assist with paracentesis.	5. Removal of ascites fluid may decrease abdominal discomfort.	

Nursing Diagnosis: Fluid volume excess related to ascites and edema formation
Goal: Restoration of normal fluid volume

Nursing Interventions	Rationale	Expected Outcomes
1. Restrict sodium and fluid intake if prescribed.	1. Minimizes formation of ascites and edema.	• Consumes diet low in sodium and within prescribed fluid restriction • Takes diuretics, potassium, and protein supplements as indicated without experiencing side effects • Exhibits increased urine output • Exhibits decreasing abdominal girth • Identifies rationale for sodium and fluid restriction • Shows a decrease in ascites with decreased weight
2. Administer diuretics, potassium, and protein supplements as prescribed.	2. Promotes excretion of fluid through the kidneys and maintenance of normal fluid and electrolyte balance.	
3. Record intake and output every 1 to 8 hours depending on response to interventions and on patient acuity.	3. Assesses effectiveness of treatment and adequacy of fluid intake.	
4. Measure and record abdominal girth daily.	4. Monitors changes in ascites formation and fluid accumulation.	
5. Explain rationale for sodium and fluid restriction.	5. Promotes patient's understanding of restriction and cooperation with it.	
6. Prepare patient and assist with paracentesis.	6. Paracentesis will temporarily decrease amount of ascites present	

Nursing Diagnosis: Altered thought processes related to deterioration of liver function and increased serum ammonia level
Goal: Improved mental status; safety maintained

Nursing Interventions	Rationale	Expected Outcomes
1. Restrict dietary protein as prescribed.	1. Reduces source of ammonia (protein foods).	• Demonstrates improved mental status • Exhibits serum ammonia level within normal limits • Is oriented to time, place, and person • Reports normal sleep patterns
2. Give frequent, small feedings of carbohydrates.	2. Promotes adequate carbohydrate for energy requirements and spares protein from breakdown for energy.	
3. Protect from infection.	3. Minimizes risk of further increase in metabolic requirements.	

36•1

PLAN OF NURSING CARE — The Patient With Impaired Liver Function (*continued*)

Nursing Interventions	Rationale	Expected Outcomes
4. Keep environment warm and draft-free.	4. Minimizes shivering, which would increase metabolic requirements.	• Demonstrates an interest in events and activities in environment • Demonstrates normal attention span • Follows and participates in conversations appropriately • Reports no urinary or fecal incontinence • Experiences no seizures
5. Pad the side rails of the bed.	5. Provides protection for the patient in the event that hepatic coma and seizure activity occur.	
6. Limit visitors.	6. Minimizes patient's activity and metabolic requirements.	
7. Provide careful nursing surveillance to ensure patient's safety.	7. Provides close monitoring of new symptoms and minimizes trauma to the confused patient.	
8. Avoid opioids and barbiturates.	8. Prevents masking of symptoms of hepatic coma and prevents drug overdose secondary to reduced ability of the damaged liver to metabolize opioids and barbiturates.	
9. Rouse at intervals (every 2–4 hours).	9. Provides stimulation to the patient and opportunity for observing the patient's level of consciousness.	

Nursing Diagnosis: Altered body temperature: hyperthermia related to inflammatory process of cirrhosis or hepatitis
Goal: Maintenance of normal body temperature, free from infections complications

Nursing Interventions	Rationale	Expected Outcomes
1. Record temperature regularly (every 4 hours).	1. Provides baseline to detect fever and to evaluate interventions.	• Reports normal temperature and absence of chills or sweating • Demonstrates adequate intake of fluids • Exhibits no evidence of local or systemic infection
2. Encourage fluid intake.	2. Corrects fluid loss from perspiration and fever and increases patient's level of comfort.	
3. Apply cool sponges or icebag for elevated temperature.	3. Promotes reduction of fever by conduction and evaporation and increases patient's comfort.	
4. Administer antibiotics as prescribed.	4. Assures appropriate serum concentration of antibiotics to treat infection.	
5. Avoid exposure to infections.	5. Minimizes risk of further infection and further increases in body temperature and metabolic rate.	
6. Keep patient at rest while temperature is elevated.	6. Reduces metabolic rate.	
7. Assess for abdominal pain, tenderness.	7. May be present with spontaneous bacterial peritonitis	

Nursing Diagnosis: Ineffective breathing pattern related to ascites and restriction of thoracic excursion secondary to ascites, abdominal distention, and fluid in the thoracic cavity
Goal: Improved respiratory status

Nursing Interventions	Rationale	Expected Outcomes
1. Elevate head of bed to at least 30 degrees.	1. Reduces abdominal pressure on the diaphragm and permits fuller thoracic excursion and lung expansion.	• Experiences improved respiratory status • Reports decreased shortness of breath • Reports increased strength and sense of well-being • Exhibits normal respiratory rate (12–18/min) with no adventitious sounds • Exhibits full thoracic excursion without shallow respirations • Exhibits normal blood gases • Experiences absence of confusion or cyanosis
2. Conserve patient's strength by providing rest periods and assisting with activities.	2. Reduces patient metabolic and oxygen requirements.	
3. Change position every 2 hours.	3. Promotes expansion and oxygenation of all areas of the lungs.	
4. Assist patient during paracentesis or thoracentesis.	4. Paracentesis and thoracentesis (performed to remove fluid from the abdominal and thoracic cavities, respectively) may be frightening to the patient. Helps obtain patient's cooperation with procedures, minimizing discomfort and risks.	

(*continued*)

36•1 PLAN OF NURSING CARE 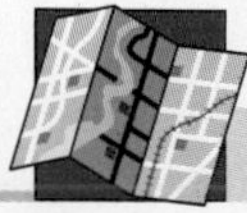

The Patient With Impaired Liver Function (*continued*)

Nursing Interventions	Rationale	Expected Outcomes
a. Have patient void before paracentesis.	a. Prevents inadvertent bladder injury.	
b. Support and maintain position during procedure.	b. Prevents inadvertent organ or tissue injury.	
c. Record both the amount and the character of fluid aspirated.	c. Provides record of fluid removed and indication of severity of limitation of lung expansion by fluid.	
d. Observe for evidence of coughing, increasing dyspnea, or pulse rate.	d. Indicates irritation of the pleural space and evidence of ventilatory function compromised by pneumothorax or hemothorax (air or blood accumulating in pleural space).	

Collaborative Problem: Gastrointestinal bleeding and hemorrhage
Goal: The patient will develop no episodes of gastrointestinal bleeding and hemorrhage

Nursing Interventions	Rationale	Expected Outcomes
1. Assess patient for evidence of gastrointestinal bleeding or hemorrhage. If bleeding does occur: a. Monitor vital signs (blood pressure, pulse, respiratory rate) every 4 hours or more frequently, depending on acuity. b. Assess skin temperature, level of consciousness every 4 hours or more frequently, depending on acuity. c. Monitor gastrointestinal secretions and output (emesis, stool for occult or obvious bleeding). Test emesis for blood once per shift and with any change. Hematest each stool. d. Monitor hematocrit and hemoglobin for trends and changes.	1. Allows early detection of signs and symptoms of bleeding and hemorrhage.	• Experiences no episodes of bleeding and hemorrhage • Vital signs are within acceptable range for patient • No evidence of bleeding from gastrointestinal tract • Hematocrit and hemoglobin levels within acceptable limits • Patient turns and moves without straining and increasing intra-abdominal pressure • No straining with bowel movements • No further bleeding episodes if aggressive treatment of bleeding and hemorrhage was needed • Patient and family state rationale for treatments
2. Avoid activities that increase intra-abdominal pressure (straining, turning). a. Avoid coughing/sneezing. b. Assist patient to turn. c. Keep all needed items within easy reach. d. Use measures to prevent constipation such as adequate fluid intake; stool softeners. e. Ensure small meals.	2. Minimizes increases in intra-abdominal pressure that could lead to rupture and bleeding of esophageal or gastric varices.	• Patient and family identify supports available to them • Patient and family describe signs and symptoms of a recurrent bleeding episode; know how to proceed
3. Have equipment (Blakemore tube, medications, intravenous fluids) available if indicated.	3. Equipment, medications, and supplies will be readily available if patient experiences bleeding from ruptured esophageal or gastric varices.	
4. Assist with procedures and therapy needed to treat gastrointestinal bleeding and hemorrhage.	4. Gastrointestinal bleeding and hemorrhage require emergency measures by entire health care team (ie, insertion of Blakemore tube).	
5. Monitor respiratory status every hour and minimize risk of respiratory complications if esophageal tamponade is needed.	5. The patient is at high risk for respiratory complications, including asphyxiation if gastric balloon of Blakemore tube ruptures or migrates upward.	
6. Prepare patient physically and psychologically for other treatment modalities if needed.	6. The patient who experiences hemorrhage is very anxious and fearful; minimizing anxiety assists in control of hemorrhage.	

36•1 PLAN OF NURSING CARE

The Patient With Impaired Liver Function (*continued*)

Nursing Interventions	Rationale	Expected Outcomes
7. Monitor patient for recurrence of bleeding and hemorrhage.	7. Risk of rebleeding is high with all treatment modalities used to halt gastrointestinal bleeding.	
8. Keep family informed of patient's status.	8. Family members are likely to be anxious about the patient's status; providing information will reduce their anxiety level and promote more effective coping.	
9. Once recovered from bleeding episode, provide patient and family with information regarding signs and symptoms of gastrointestinal bleeding.	9. Risk of rebleeding is high. Subtle signs may be more quickly identified.	

Collaborative Problem: Hepatic encephalopathy
Goal: Patient will be maintained safely and without injury

Nursing Interventions	Rationale	Expected Outcomes
1. Assess cognitive status every 4–8 hours: a. Assess patient's orientation to person, place, and time. b. Monitor patient's level of activity, restlessness, and agitation. Assess for presence of flapping hand tremors (asterixis). c. Obtain and record daily sample of patient's handwriting or ability to construct a simple figure (eg, star). d. Assess neurologic signs (deep tendon reflexes, ability to follow instructions).	1. Data will provide baseline of patient's cognitive status and enable detection of changes.	• Remains awake, alert, and aware of surroundings • Is oriented to time, place, and person • Exhibits no restlessness or agitation • Record of handwriting demonstrates no deterioration in cognitive function • States rationale for treatment used to prevent or treat hepatic encephalopathy • Demonstrates stable serum ammonia level within acceptable limits • Consumes adequate caloric intake and adheres to protein restriction • Takes medications as prescribed • Breath sounds are normal without adventitious sounds • Skin and tissue intact without evidence of pressure or breaks in integrity
2. Monitor medications to prevent administration of those that may precipitate hepatic encephalopathy (sedatives, hypnotics, analgesics).	2. Medications are a common precipitating factor in development of hepatic encephalopathy in patients at risk.	
3. Monitor laboratory data, especially serum ammonia level.	3. Increases in serum ammonia level are associated with hepatic encephalopathy and coma.	
4. Notify physician of even subtle changes in patient's neurologic status and cognitive function.	4. Allows early initiation of treatment of hepatic encephalopathy and prevention of hepatic coma.	
5. Limit sources of protein from diet if indicated.	5. Reduces breakdown and conversion of protein to ammonia.	
6. Administer medications prescribed to reduce serum ammonia level (eg, lactulose, antibiotics, glucose, flumazanil if indicated).	6. Reduces serum ammonia level.	
7. Assess respiratory status and initiate measures to prevent complications.	7. The patient who develops hepatic coma is at risk for respiratory complications (ie, pneumonia, atelectasis, infection).	
8. Protect patient's skin and tissue from pressure and breakdown.	8. The patient in coma is at risk for skin breakdown and pressure ulcer formation.	

liver (eg, yellow fever virus, Epstein–Barr virus), from medication or chemical toxicity (eg, carbon tetrachloride, chloroform, phosphorus, arsenicals, certain medications), or from alcohol. Cirrhosis of the liver is a form of hepatocellular disease that may produce jaundice. It is usually associated with excessive alcohol intake; however, it may also be a late result of liver cell necrosis caused by viral infection. In prolonged obstructive jaundice, cell damage eventually develops, so that both types appear together.

Patients with hepatocellular jaundice may be mildly or severely ill, with lack of appetite, nausea, malaise, fatigue, weakness, and possible weight loss. In some instances of hepatocellular disease, jaundice may not be obvious. The serum bilirubin concentration and urine urobilinogen level may be elevated. In addition, AST (SGOT) and ALT (SGPT) levels may be increased, indicating cellular necrosis. The patient may report headache, chills, and fever if the cause is infectious. Depending on the cause and extent of the liver cell damage, hepatocellular jaundice may or may not be completely reversible.

OBSTRUCTIVE JAUNDICE

Obstructive jaundice of the extrahepatic type may be caused by occlusion of the bile duct by a gallstone, an inflammatory process, a tumor, or pressure from an enlarged organ. The obstruction may also involve the small bile ducts within the liver (ie, intrahepatic obstruction), caused, for example, by pressure on these channels from inflammatory swelling of the liver or by an inflammatory exudate within the ducts themselves. Intrahepatic obstruction resulting from stasis and inspissation (thickening) of bile within the canaliculi may occur after the ingestion of certain medications, which are referred to as cholestatic agents. These include phenothiazines, antithyroid medications, sulfonylureas, tricyclic antidepressants, nitrofurantoin, androgens, and estrogens.

Whether the obstruction is intrahepatic or extrahepatic and whatever its cause may be, if bile cannot flow normally into the intestine but is backed up into the liver substance, it is reabsorbed into the blood and carried throughout the entire body, staining the skin, the mucous membranes, and the sclerae. It is excreted in the urine, which becomes deep orange and foamy. Because of the decreased amount of bile in the intestinal tract, the stools become light or clay-colored. The skin may itch intensely, requiring repeated soothing baths. Dyspepsia and an intolerance to fatty foods may develop because of impaired fat digestion in the absence of intestinal bile. AST (SGOT), ALT (SGPT), and GGT levels generally rise only moderately, but bilirubin and alkaline phosphatase levels are elevated.

HEREDITARY HYPERBILIRUBINEMIA

Increased serum bilirubin levels (hyperbilirubinemia) resulting from several inherited disorders can also produce jaundice. Gilbert's syndrome is a familial disorder characterized by an increased unconjugated bilirubin level that causes jaundice. Although serum bilirubin levels are increased, liver histology and liver function test results are normal, and there is no hemolysis. This syndrome affects 2% to 5% of the population.

Other conditions that are probably caused by inborn errors of biliary metabolism include Dubin–Johnson syndrome (chronic idiopathic jaundice, with pigment in the liver) and Rotor's syndrome (chronic familial conjugated hyperbilirubinemia without pigment in the liver); "benign" cholestatic jaundice of pregnancy, with retention of conjugated bilirubin, probably secondary to unusual sensitivity to the hormones of pregnancy; and probably also benign recurrent intrahepatic cholestasis.

Portal Hypertension and Ascites

PATHOPHYSIOLOGY

Obstruction to blood flow through the damaged liver results in increased blood pressure (**portal hypertension**) throughout the portal venous system. Although portal hypertension is commonly associated with hepatic cirrhosis, it can also occur with noncirrhotic liver disease.

Two major sequelae result from portal hypertension:

1. The formation of esophageal, gastric, and hemorrhoidal varicosities (varices). These varices develop because of the elevated pressures transmitted to all of the veins that drain into the portal system. These varicosities are prone to rupture and often are the source of massive hemorrhages from the upper GI tract and the rectum. The likelihood of bleeding is increased by the blood clotting abnormalities often seen in patients with cirrhosis.
2. The accumulation of fluid (ascites) in the abdominal cavity. As ascites develops, intravascular volume tends to fall and renin is released by the kidneys. The renin causes increased secretion of the hormone aldosterone by the adrenal glands, which in turn causes the kidneys to retain sodium and water in an attempt to return intravascular volume to normal. As portal hypertension continues, fluid retention contributes to the formation of even more ascites as the albumin in the ascitic fluid creates an osmotic gradient and pulls more fluid into the peritoneal cavity. (Although ascites is often a result of liver damage, it may also occur with other disorders including cancer, kidney disease, and heart failure.)

CLINICAL MANIFESTATIONS

Increased abdominal girth and rapid weight gain are common presenting symptoms of ascites. The patient may be short of breath and uncomfortable from the enlarged abdomen, and striae and distended veins may be visible over the abdominal wall. Fluid and electrolyte imbalances are common.

ASSESSMENT AND DIAGNOSTIC EVALUATION

The presence and extent of ascites are assessed by percussion of the abdomen. When fluid has accumulated in the peritoneal cavity, the flanks bulge when the patient assumes a supine position. The presence of fluid can be confirmed either by percussing for shifting dullness or by detecting a fluid wave (Fig. 36-4). A fluid wave is likely to be found only when there is a large amount of fluid present. Daily measurement and recording of abdominal girth and body weight are essential to assess the progression of ascites and its response to treatment.

MANAGEMENT

Dietary Modification. The goal of treatment for the patient with ascites is a negative sodium balance to reduce fluid retention. Table salt, salty foods, salted butter and margarine, and all ordinary canned and frozen foods (foods that are not specifically pre-

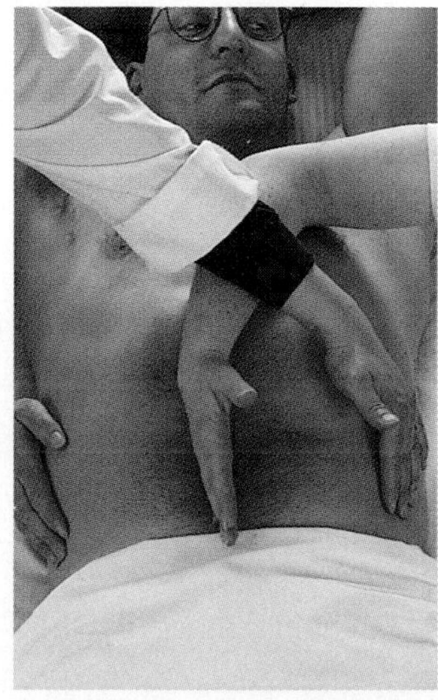

FIGURE 36•4 Assessing for abdominal fluid wave. The examiner places the hands along the side of the patient's flank, then strikes one flank sharply, detecting any fluid wave with the other hand. An assistant's hand is placed (ulnar side down) along the patient's midline to prevent the fluid wave from being transmitted through the tissues of the abdominal wall. From Weber, J. W., & Kelley, J. (1998). *Health assessment in nursing.* Philadelphia: Lippincott-Raven.

pared for low-sodium diets) should be avoided. The taste of unsalted foods can be improved by using salt substitutes, such as lemon juice, oregano, and thyme. Commercial salt substitutes need to be cleared with the physician because those containing ammonia could precipitate hepatic coma. Liberal use should be made of powdered, low-sodium milk and milk products. If fluid accumulation is not controlled with this regimen, the daily sodium allowance may be reduced further to 500 mg and diuretics may be administered.

Dietary control of ascites via strict sodium restriction is difficult to achieve at home. The likelihood that the patient will follow even a 2-g sodium diet is increased if the patient and the person preparing meals understand the rationale for the diet and receive periodic guidance about selecting and preparing appropriate foods. Approximately 10% of patients with ascites respond to these measures alone. Nonresponders and those who find sodium restriction difficult require diuretic therapy.

Diuretics. Use of diuretics along with sodium restriction is successful in 90% of patients with ascites. Spironolactone (Aldactone), an aldosterone-blocking agent, is often considered the first-line therapy in patients with ascites from cirrhosis. When used with other diuretics, it helps prevent potassium loss. Oral diuretics such as furosemide (Lasix) may be added but should be used cautiously, because with long-term use they may also induce severe sodium depletion (hyponatremia). Ammonium chloride and acetazolamide (Diamox) are contraindicated because of the possibility of precipitating hepatic coma. Daily weight loss should not exceed 1 to 2 kg (2.2 to 4.4 lb) in those with ascites and peripheral edema or 0.5 to 0.75 kg (1.1 to 1.65 lb) in those without edema. Fluid restriction is not attempted unless the serum sodium concentration is very low.

Possible complications of diuretic therapy include fluid and electrolyte disturbances and encephalopathy. Possible fluid and electrolyte problems include hypovolemia, hypokalemia, hyponatremia, and hypochloremic alkalosis. Encephalopathy may be precipitated by dehydration and hypovolemia. Also, when potassium stores are depleted, the amount of ammonia in the systemic circulation increases, which may cause impaired cerebral functioning and encephalopathy.

If a patient with ascites from liver disease is hospitalized, nursing measures include assessment and documentation of intake and output, abdominal girth, and daily weight to assess fluid status. Serum ammonia and electrolyte levels are monitored to assess electrolyte balance, response to therapy, and risk of encephalopathy.

PARACENTESIS

Paracentesis is the removal of fluid (ascites) from the peritoneal cavity through a small surgical incision or puncture made through the abdominal wall under sterile conditions. Paracentesis was once considered a routine form of treatment for ascites but is now performed primarily for diagnostic examination of ascitic fluid, for treatment of massive ascites that is resistant to nutritional and diuretic therapy and causing severe problems to the patient, and as a prelude to diagnostic imaging studies, peritoneal dialysis, or surgery. A sample of the ascitic fluid may be sent to the laboratory for analysis. Cell count, albumin and total protein levels, culture, and occasionally other tests are performed.

Use of large-volume (4 to 6 liters) paracentesis has been shown to be a cost-saving and safe method for treating hospitalized patients with severe ascites. This technique in combination with (in some cases) the intravenous (IV) infusion of salt-poor albumin has become the standard treatment for massive ascites, especially in patients with severe respiratory compromise, imminent umbilical hernia rupture, or refractory ascites (Sherlock & Dooley, 1997). The salt-poor albumin helps reduce edema by causing the ascitic fluid to be drawn back into the bloodstream and ultimately eliminated by the kidneys. The procedure provides only temporary removal of fluid; it rapidly recurs, necessitating repeated removal. Nursing care of the patient undergoing paracentesis is presented in Guideline 36-2.

OTHER METHODS OF TREATMENT

Insertion of a peritoneovenous shunt to redirect ascitic fluid from the peritoneal cavity into the systemic circulation is a treatment modality for ascites, but this procedure has largely been abandoned because of the high complication rate and high incidence of shunt failure.

PROMOTING HOME AND COMMUNITY-BASED CARE

Teaching Patients Self-Care. The patient treated for ascites is likely to be discharged home with some ascites still present. Before hospital discharge, the patient and family receive teaching about the treatment plan, including the need to adhere to a low-sodium diet and to take medications as prescribed. Patient and family teaching addresses skin care and the need to avoid all alcohol intake. They are also instructed about the need to weigh the patient daily and to watch for and report signs and symptoms of complications. The importance of checking with the physician before taking any new medications is emphasized.

Continuing Care. A referral for home care may be warranted, especially if the patient lives alone or cannot provide self-care. The home visit enables the nurse to assess changes in the patient's condition and weight, abdominal girth, skin, and cognitive and emotional status. The home care nurse can also assess the patient's home environment and the availability of resources needed to adhere to the treatment plan (eg, a scale to obtain daily weights, facilities to prepare and store appropriate foods, resources to purchase needed medications). The patient's adherence to the treatment plan and the ability to buy, prepare, and eat appropriate foods are also assessed. The nurse reinforces previous teaching and emphasizes the need for regular follow-up and the importance of keeping scheduled health care appointments.

Nutritional Deficiencies

Another group of problems common to patients with severe chronic liver disease of all types results from inadequate intake of sufficient vitamins. Among the specific deficiency states that occur on this basis are:

- Vitamin A deficiency, resulting in night blindness and eye and skin changes
- Thiamine deficiency, leading to beriberi, polyneuritis, and Wernicke–Korsakoff psychosis
- Riboflavin deficiency, resulting in characteristic skin and mucous membrane lesions
- Pyridoxine deficiency, resulting in skin and mucous membrane lesions and neurologic changes
- Vitamin K deficiency, resulting in hypoprothrombinemia, characterized by spontaneous bleeding and ecchymoses
- Vitamin C deficiency, resulting in the hemorrhagic lesions of scurvy
- Folic acid deficiency, resulting in macrocytic anemia

The threat of these avitaminoses provides the rationale for supplementing the diet of every patient with chronic liver disease

36•2 GUIDELINES FOR 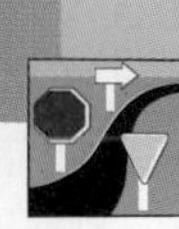

ASSISTING WITH A PARACENTESIS

Preprocedure

1. Prepare the patient by providing the necessary information and instructions about the procedure and by offering reassurance.
2. Instruct the patient to void.
3. Gather appropriate sterile equipment and collection receptacles.
4. Place patient in upright position on edge of bed with feet supported on stool, or place in chair. Fowler's position should be used for the patient confined to bed.
5. Place sphygmomanometer cuff around patient's arm to allow monitoring of blood pressure during the procedure.

Procedure

1. The physician, using aseptic technique, inserts the trocar through a puncture wound in the midline below the umbilicus. The fluid drains from the abdomen through a drainage tube into a container.
2. Help the patient maintain position throughout procedure.
3. Take and record blood pressure at frequent intervals from the beginning of the procedure.
4. Monitor the patient closely for signs of vascular collapse: pallor, increased pulse rate, or decreased blood pressure.

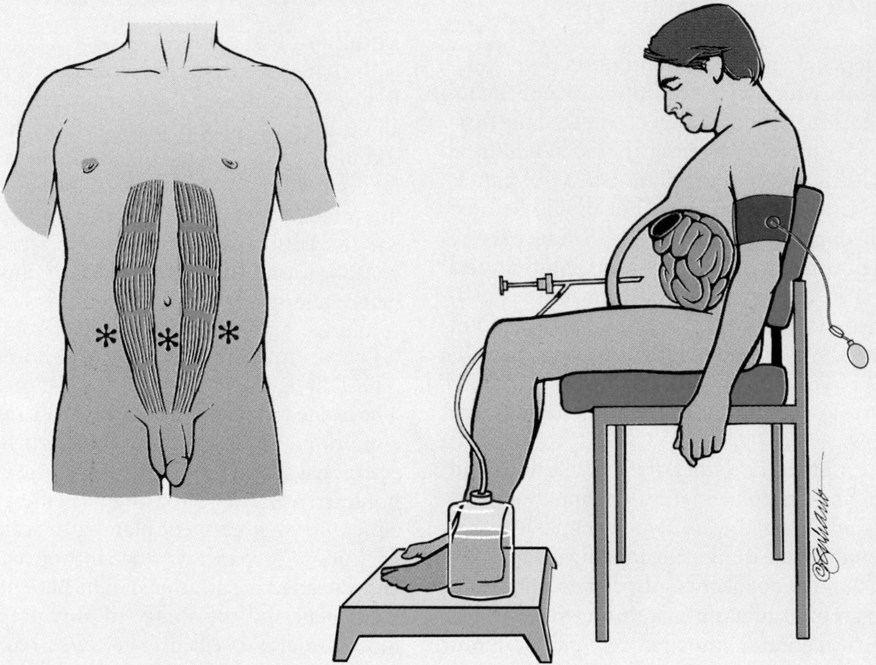

Postprocedure

1. Return patient to bed or to a comfortable sitting position.
2. Measure the fluid collected, describe, and record.
3. Label samples of fluid and send to laboratory.
4. Continue to monitor vital signs every 15 minutes for 1 hour, every 30 minutes over 2 hours, then every hour over 2 hours and then every 4 hours. Monitor temperature after procedure and every 4 hours.
5. Assess for hypovolemia, electrolyte loss, changes in mental status, and encephalopathy.
6. Check puncture sites when taking vital signs.

(especially if alcohol-related) with ample quantities of vitamins A, B complex, C, and K and folic acid.

Hepatic Encephalopathy and Coma

Hepatic encephalopathy, one of the dreaded complications of liver disease, occurs with profound liver failure and may result from the accumulation of ammonia and other toxic metabolites in the blood. Hepatic coma represents the most advanced stage of hepatic encephalopathy. Some researchers describe a false neurotransmitter as a cause, but the exact mechanism is not fully understood (Fabbri et al., 1996; Morgan, 1995).

PATHOPHYSIOLOGY

Ammonia accumulates because damaged liver cells fail to detoxify and convert to urea the ammonia that is constantly entering the bloodstream. Ammonia enters the bloodstream as a result of its absorption from the GI tract and its liberation from kidney

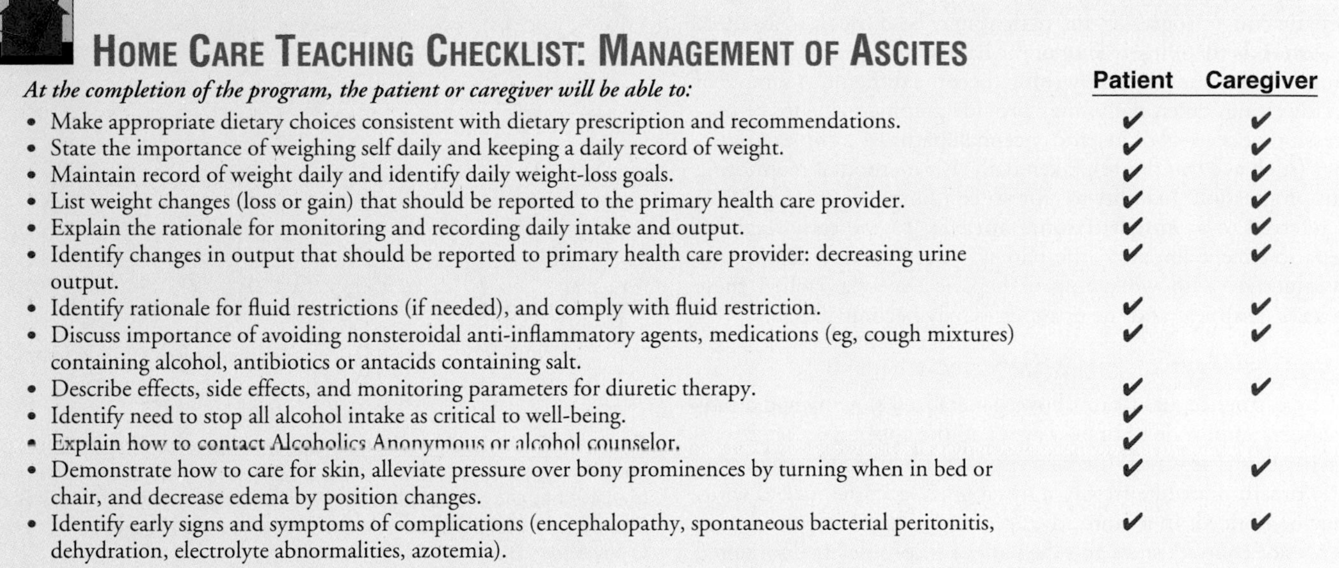

HOME CARE TEACHING CHECKLIST: MANAGEMENT OF ASCITES

At the completion of the program, the patient or caregiver will be able to:	Patient	Caregiver
• Make appropriate dietary choices consistent with dietary prescription and recommendations.	✔	✔
• State the importance of weighing self daily and keeping a daily record of weight.	✔	✔
• Maintain record of weight daily and identify daily weight-loss goals.	✔	✔
• List weight changes (loss or gain) that should be reported to the primary health care provider.	✔	✔
• Explain the rationale for monitoring and recording daily intake and output.	✔	✔
• Identify changes in output that should be reported to primary health care provider: decreasing urine output.	✔	✔
• Identify rationale for fluid restrictions (if needed), and comply with fluid restriction.	✔	✔
• Discuss importance of avoiding nonsteroidal anti-inflammatory agents, medications (eg, cough mixtures) containing alcohol, antibiotics or antacids containing salt.	✔	✔
• Describe effects, side effects, and monitoring parameters for diuretic therapy.	✔	✔
• Identify need to stop all alcohol intake as critical to well-being.	✔	
• Explain how to contact Alcoholics Anonymous or alcohol counselor.	✔	
• Demonstrate how to care for skin, alleviate pressure over bony prominences by turning when in bed or chair, and decrease edema by position changes.	✔	✔
• Identify early signs and symptoms of complications (encephalopathy, spontaneous bacterial peritonitis, dehydration, electrolyte abnormalities, azotemia).	✔	✔

and muscle cells. The increased ammonia concentration in the blood causes brain dysfunction and damage, resulting in hepatic encephalopathy.

Circumstances that increase serum ammonia levels tend to aggravate or precipitate hepatic encephalopathy. The largest source of ammonia is the enzymatic and bacterial digestion of dietary and blood proteins in the GI tract. Ammonia from these sources is increased as a result of GI bleeding (ie, bleeding esophageal varices or chronic GI bleeding), a high-protein diet, bacterial infections, and uremia. The ingestion of ammonium salts also increases the blood ammonia level. In the presence of alkalosis or hypokalemia, increased amounts of ammonia are absorbed from the GI tract and from the renal tubular fluid. Conversely, serum ammonia is decreased by elimination of protein from the diet and by the administration of antibiotics, such as neomycin sulfate, that reduce the number of intestinal bacteria capable of converting urea to ammonia.

Other factors unrelated to increased serum ammonia levels that may cause hepatic encephalopathy in susceptible patients include excessive diuresis, dehydration, infections, surgery, fever, and some medications (sedatives, tranquilizers, analgesics, and diuretics that cause potassium loss). Table 36-2 presents the stages of hepatic encephalopathy, common signs and symptoms, and potential nursing diagnoses for each stage.

Portal-systemic encephalopathy, the most common type of hepatic encephalopathy, occurs primarily in patients with cirrhosis with portal hypertension and portal-systemic shunting.

CLINICAL MANIFESTATIONS

The earliest symptoms of hepatic encephalopathy include minor mental changes and motor disturbances. The patient appears slightly confused, has alterations in mood, becomes unkempt, and has altered sleep patterns. The patient tends to sleep during

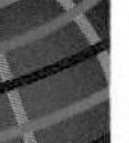

TABLE 36•2 Stages of Hepatic Encephalopathy and Possible Nursing Diagnoses*

Stage	Clinical Symptoms	Clinical Signs and EEG Changes	Selected Potential Nursing Diagnoses
1	Normal level of consciousness with periods of lethargy and euphoria; reversal of day–night sleep patterns	Asterixis; impaired writing and ability to draw line figures. Normal EEG.	Activity intolerance Self-care deficit Sleep pattern disturbances
2	Increased drowsiness; disorientation; inappropriate behavior; mood swings; agitation	Asterixis; fetor hepaticus. Abnormal EEG with generalized slowing.	Impaired social interaction Altered role performance Risk for injury
3	Stuporous; difficult to rouse; sleeps most of time; marked confusion; incoherent speech	Asterixis; increased deep tendon reflexes; rigidity of extremities. EEG markedly abnormal.	Altered nutrition Impaired mobility Impaired verbal communication
4	Comatose; may not respond to painful stimuli	Absence of asterixis; absence of deep tendon reflexes; flaccidity of extremities. EEG markedly abnormal.	Risk for aspiration Impaired gas exchange Impaired tissue integrity Sensory/perceptual alterations

*Nursing diagnoses are likely to progress so that most nursing diagnoses present at earlier stages will occur during later stages as well.

the day and to be restless and to have insomnia at night. As hepatic coma progresses, the patient may be difficult to awaken.

Asterixis (flapping tremor of the hands) may occur (Fig. 36-5). Simple tasks, such as handwriting, become difficult. A sample of handwriting, taken daily, may provide graphic evidence of progression or reversal of hepatic encephalopathy. A sample of drawings (such as a star figure), taken daily, is a method of monitoring this progression. Inability to reproduce a simple figure (Fig. 36-6) is referred to as **constructional apraxia**. In the early stages of hepatic encephalopathy, the patient's deep tendon reflexes are hyperactive; with worsening of hepatic encephalopathy, these reflexes disappear and the extremities may become flaccid.

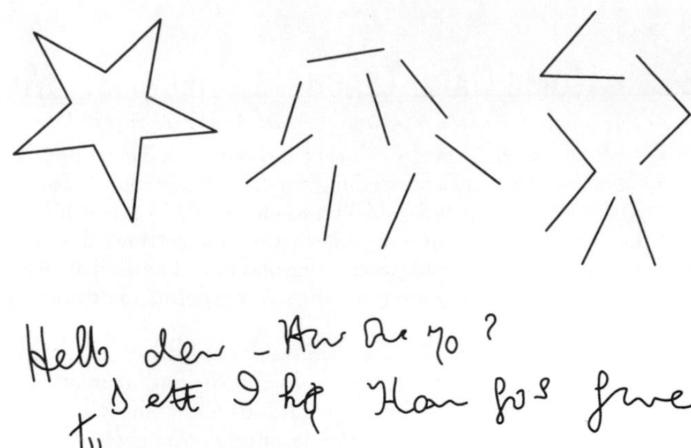

FIGURE 36•6 Effects of constructional apraxia. Deterioration of handwriting and inability to draw a simple star figure occurs with progressive hepatic encephalopathy. With permission from Sherlock S. & Dooley, J. (1997). *Diseases of the liver and biliary system* (10th ed). Olney Mead, Blackwell Scientific Ltd.

ASSESSMENT AND DIAGNOSTIC FINDINGS

The electroencephalogram shows generalized slowing and an increase in amplitude of brain waves and the appearance of characteristic triphasic waves. Occasionally, fetor hepaticus, a characteristic breath odor like freshly mowed grass, acetone, or old wine, may be noticed. In a more advanced stage, there are gross disturbances of consciousness and the patient is completely disoriented with respect to time and place. With further progression of the disorder, the patient lapses into frank coma and may have seizures. Approximately 35% of all patients with cirrhosis of the liver die in hepatic coma.

MANAGEMENT

Lactulose (Cephulac) is administered to reduce serum ammonia levels. It acts by several mechanisms that promote the excretion of ammonia in the stool: (1) ammonia is kept in the ionized state, resulting in a fall in colon pH, reversing the normal passage of ammonia from the colon to the blood; (2) evacuation of the bowel takes place, which decreases the ammonia absorbed from the colon; and (3) the fecal flora are changed to organisms that do not produce ammonia from urea. Two or three soft stools per day are desirable; this indicates that lactulose is performing as intended. Watery diarrheal stools, however, indicate medication overdose.

Possible side effects include intestinal bloating and cramps, which usually disappear in a week. To mask the sweet taste to which some patients object, lactulose can be diluted with fruit juice. The patient is closely monitored for hypokalemia and dehydration. Other laxatives are not prescribed during lactulose administration because their effects would disturb dosage regulation. Lactulose enemas have also been used effectively in acute hepatic encephalopathy for patients who are comatose or in whom oral administration is contraindicated or impossible.

Other aspects of management include IV administration of glucose to minimize protein breakdown, administration of vitamins to correct deficiencies, and correction of electrolyte imbalances (especially potassium). Additional principles of management of hepatic encephalopathy include the following:

- Therapy is directed toward treating or removing the cause.
- Neurologic status is assessed frequently. A daily record is kept of handwriting and performance in arithmetic to monitor mental status.
- Fluid intake and output and body weight are recorded each day.
- Vital signs are measured and recorded every 4 hours.
- Potential sites of infection (peritoneum, lungs) are assessed frequently, and abnormal findings are reported promptly.
- Serum ammonia level is monitored daily.
- Protein intake is restricted if signs of impending hepatic encephalopathy and coma occur.
- Reduction in the absorption of ammonia from the GI tract is accomplished by the use of enemas or oral antibiotics.
- Electrolyte status is carefully monitored and corrected if abnormal.
- Sedatives, tranquilizers, and analgesics are discontinued.
- Benzodiazepine antagonists may be given to improve encephalopathy whether or not the patient has previously taken benzodiazepines.

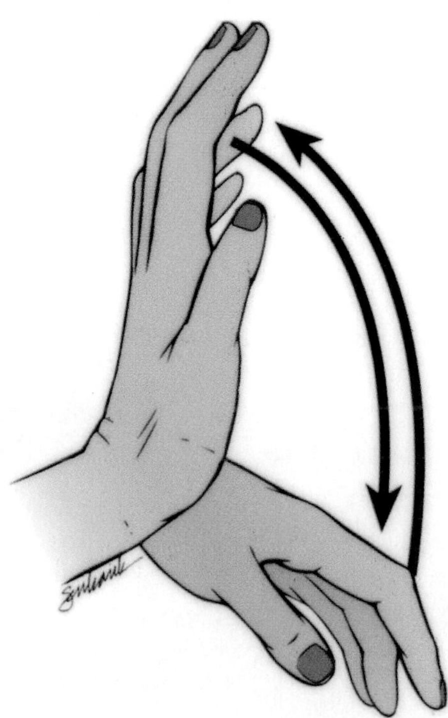

FIGURE 36•5 Asterixis or "liver flap" may occur in hepatic encephalopathy. The patient is asked to hold the arm out with the hand held upward (dorsiflexed). Within a few seconds, the hand falls forward involuntarily and then quickly returns to the dorsiflexed position.

PROMOTING HOME AND COMMUNITY-BASED CARE

Teaching Patients Self-Care. If the patient has recovered from hepatic encephalopathy and is to be discharged home, the family must be instructed to observe the patient for subtle signs of recurrent encephalopathy. In the acute phase of hepatic encephalopathy, dietary protein may be reduced to 20 g/day. During recovery, and in the home situation, the patient is instructed in maintenance of a low-protein, high-calorie diet. Protein may then be added in 10-g increments on alternate days. Any relapse is treated by a return to the previous level. The limits of tolerance are usually 40 to 60 g/day. Continued use of lactulose in the home environment is not uncommon, and its efficacy and side effects should be monitored closely by the patient and family after instruction. Use of vegetable rather than animal protein may be indicated in patients whose total daily protein tolerance is less than 1 g/kg per day. Vegetable protein intake may result in improved nitrogen balance without precipitating or advancing hepatic encephalopathy.

Continuing Care. Referral for home care is warranted in the patient who returns home after recovery from hepatic encephalopathy. The home care nurse assesses the patient's physical and mental status and collaborates closely with the patient's physician. The home visit also provides an opportunity for the nurse to assess the patient's home environment and the ability of the patient and family to monitor signs and symptoms and to follow the treatment regimen. Home care visits are particularly important if the patient lives alone, because encephalopathy may affect the patient's ability to remember or follow the treatment regimen. Previous teaching is reinforced, and the patient and family are reminded about the importance of dietary restrictions, close monitoring, and follow-up.

Other Manifestations of Liver Dysfunction

EDEMA AND BLEEDING

Many patients with liver dysfunction develop generalized edema from hypoalbuminemia that results from decreased hepatic production of albumin. The production of blood clotting factors by the liver is also reduced, leading to an increased incidence of bruising, nosebleeds, bleeding from wounds, and, as described above, GI bleeding.

VITAMIN DEFICIENCY

Decreased production of several clotting factors may be due, in part, to deficient absorption of vitamin K from the GI tract. This probably is caused by the inability of liver cells to use vitamin K to make prothrombin. Absorption of the other fat-soluble vitamins (vitamins A, D, and E) as well as dietary fats may also be impaired because of decreased secretion of bile salts into the intestine.

METABOLIC ABNORMALITIES

Abnormalities of glucose metabolism also occur; the blood glucose level may be abnormally high shortly after a meal (a diabetic-type glucose tolerance test result), but hypoglycemia may occur during fasting because of decreased hepatic glycogen reserves and decreased gluconeogenesis. Because the ability to metabolize medications is decreased, medications must be used cautiously and usual medication dosages must be reduced for the patient with liver failure.

Decreased metabolism of estrogens by the damaged liver can lead to gynecomastia, testicular atrophy, loss of pubic hair in the male, and menstrual irregularities in the female.

SPLENOMEGALY

Splenomegaly (enlarged spleen) with possible hypersplenism occurs commonly as a manifestation of portal hypertension.

ENDOCRINE IMBALANCES

Many endocrine abnormalities also occur with liver dysfunction because the liver cannot metabolize hormones normally, including androgens or sex hormones. Gynecomastia, amenorrhea, testicular atrophy, and other disturbances of sexual function and sex characteristics are thought to result from failure of the damaged liver to inactivate estrogens normally.

PRURITUS AND OTHER SKIN CHANGES

Patients with liver dysfunction resulting from biliary obstruction commonly develop severe itching (pruritus) due to retention of bile salts. Patients may develop vascular (or arterial) spider angiomas (Fig. 36-7) on the skin, generally above the waistline. These are numerous small vessels resembling a spider's legs. These are most frequently associated with cirrhosis, especially in alcoholic liver disease. Patients may also develop reddened palms ("liver palms" or palmar erythema).

HEPATIC DISORDERS

Viral hepatitis is a systemic, viral infection in which necrosis and inflammation of liver cells produce a characteristic cluster of clinical, biochemical, and cellular changes. To date, five definitive types of viral hepatitis have been identified: hepatitis A, B, C, D, and E. Hepatitis A and E are similar in mode of transmission (fecal–oral route), whereas hepatitis B, C, and D share many characteristics. A guide to the terminology associated with viral hepatitis is provided in Chart 36-1.

The increasing incidence of viral hepatitis is a growing public health concern. The disease is important because it is easy to transmit, has high morbidity, and causes prolonged loss of time from school or employment.

It is estimated that 60% to 90% of cases of viral hepatitis go unreported. The occurrence of subclinical cases, failure to recognize mild cases, and misdiagnosis are thought to contribute to the underreporting. Although approximately 50% of adults in the

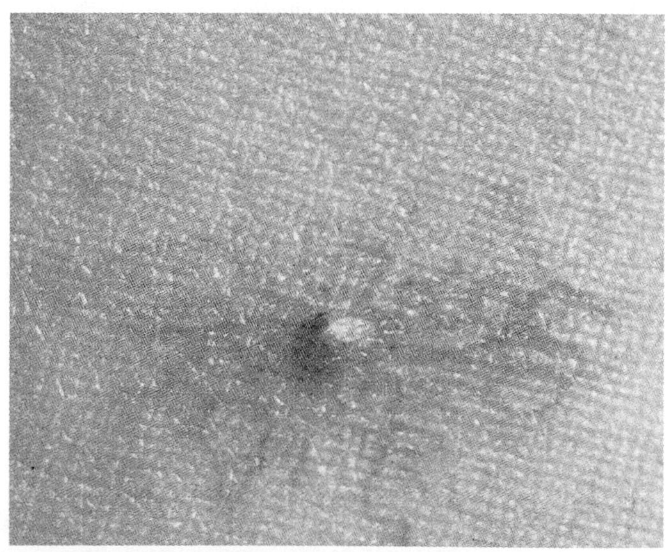

FIGURE 36•7 Spider angioma. This vascular (arterial) spider appears on the skin. Beneath the elevated center and radiating branches, the blood vessels are looped and tortuous.

CHART 36•1 Definition of Terms: Hepatitis

Hepatitis A	
HAV	Hepatitis A virus; etiologic agent of hepatitis A (formerly infectious hepatitis)
Anti-HAV	Antibody to hepatitis A virus; appears in serum soon after onset of symptoms; disappears after 3–12 months
IgM anti-HAV	IgM antibody to HAV; indicates recent infection with HAV; positive up to 6 months after infection
Hepatitis B	
HBV	Hepatitis B virus; etiologic agent of hepatitis B (formerly serum hepatitis)
HBsAG	Hepatitis B surface antigen (Australian antigen); indicates acute or chronic hepatitis B or carrier state; indicates infectious state
Anti-HBs	Antibody to hepatitis B surface antigen; indicates prior exposure and immunity to hepatitis; may indicate passive antibody from HBIG or immune response from hepatitis B vaccine
HBeAg	Hepatitis B e-antigen; present in serum early in course; indicates highly infectious stage of hepatitis B; persistence in serum indicates progression to chronic hepatitis
Anti-HBe	Antibody to hepatitis B e-antigen; suggests low titer of HBV
HBcAg	Hepatitis B core antigen; found in liver cells; not easily detected in serum
Anti-HBc	Antibody to hepatitis B core antigen; most sensitive indicator of hepatitis B; appears late in the acute phase of the disease; indicates infection of HBV at some time in the past
IgM anti-HBc	IgM antibody to HBcAg; present for up to 6 months after HBV infection
Hepatitis C	
HCV	Hepatitis C virus (formerly non-A, non-B virus); may be more than one virus
Hepatitis D	
HDV	Hepatitis D virus (delta agent); etiologic agent to hepatitis D; HBV required for replication
HDAg	Hepatitis delta antigen; detectable in early acute HDV infection
Anti-HDV	Antibody to HDV; indicates past or present infection with HDV
Hepatitis E	
HEV	Hepatitis E virus; etiologic agent of hepatitis E
Hepatitis G	
HGV	Hepatitis G virus; also known as GB virus C

United States have antibodies against hepatitis A virus, many cannot recall an earlier episode or the occurrence of the symptoms of hepatitis.

For a comparison of the many aspects of the major forms of viral hepatitis, see Table 36-3.

Hepatitis A Virus (HAV)

HAV accounts for 20% to 25% of cases of clinical hepatitis in the developed world. Hepatitis A, formerly designated infectious hepatitis, is caused by an RNA virus of the Enterovirus family. The mode of transmission of this disease is the fecal–oral route, primarily through the ingestion of food or liquids infected by the virus. The virus has been found in the stool of infected patients before the onset of symptoms and during the first few days of illness. Typically, a child or a young adult acquires the infection at school by poor hygiene, hand-to-mouth contact, or close contact at play. The virus is carried home, where haphazard sanitary habits spread it through the family. It is more prevalent in underdeveloped countries or in instances of overcrowding and poor sanitation. An infected food handler can spread the disease, and people can contract it by consuming water or shellfish from sewage-contaminated waters. Outbreaks have occurred in day care centers and institutions for the developmentally delayed because of lapses in hygiene. It is rarely, if ever, transmitted by blood transfusions.

The incubation period is estimated to be 15 to 50 days, with an average of 30 days. The course of the illness may be prolonged, lasting 4 to 8 weeks. It generally lasts longer and is more severe in those older than age 40. Recovery is the rule; hepatitis A rarely progresses to acute liver necrosis or fulminant hepatitis, terminating in cirrhosis of the liver or death. Hepatitis A confers immunity against itself; however, the person may contract other forms of hepatitis. The mortality rate of hepatitis A is approximately 0.5%. No carrier state exists, and no chronic hepatitis is associated with hepatitis A. The virus is present only briefly in the serum; by the time jaundice occurs, the patient is likely to be noninfectious.

Clinical Manifestations

Many patients are anicteric (without jaundice) and symptomless. When symptoms appear, they are of a mild, flulike upper respiratory tract infection, with low-grade fever. Anorexia is an early symptom and is often severe. It is thought to result from release of a toxin by the damaged liver or by failure of the damaged liver cells to detoxify an abnormal product. Later, jaundice and dark urine may become apparent. Indigestion is present, in varying degrees, marked by vague epigastric distress, nausea, heartburn, and flatulence. The patient may also develop a strong aversion to the taste of cigarettes or the presence of cigarette smoke and other strong odors. These symptoms tend to clear as soon as the jaundice reaches its peak—perhaps 10 days after its initial appearance. Although symptoms may be very mild in children, adults are more likely to be symptomatic, with the symptoms more severe and the course of the disease prolonged.

Assessment and Diagnostic Findings

The liver and the spleen are often moderately enlarged for a few days after onset; otherwise, apart from jaundice, there are few physical signs to be elicited. Hepatitis A antigen may be found in the stool a week to 10 days before illness and for 2 to 3 weeks after symptoms appear. HAV antibodies are detectable in the serum, but usually not until symptoms appear. Analysis of subclasses of immunoglobulins can help determine whether the antibody represents acute or past infection.

Prevention

A number of strategies exist to prevent transmission of HAV. Patients and their families need to be made aware of these and encouraged to consider them if recommended by their primary health care provider.

In February 1995, the first vaccine against hepatitis A was approved by the Food and Drug Administration for use in the

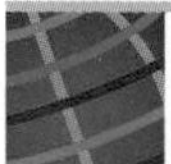

TABLE 36•3 **Comparison of Major Forms of Viral Hepatitis**

	Hepatitis A	Hepatitis B	Hepatitis C	Hepatitis D	Hepatitis E
Previous names	Infectious hepatitis	Serum hepatitis	Non-A, non-B hepatitis		
Epidemiology					
Cause	Hepatitis A virus (HAV)	Hepatitis B virus (HBV)	Hepatitis C virus (HCV)	Hepatitis D virus (HDV)	Hepatitis E virus (HEV)
Mode of transmission	Fecal–oral route; poor sanitation. Person-to-person contact. Water-borne; foodborne	Parenterally; or by intimate contact with carriers or those with acute disease; sexual and oral–oral contact. Perinatal transmission from mothers to infants. An important occupational hazard for health care personnel	Transfusion of blood and blood products; exposure to contaminated blood through equipment or drug paraphernalia	Same as HBV. HBV surface antigen necessary for replication; pattern similar to that of hepatitis B	Fecal–oral route; person to person contact may be possible, although risk appears low
Incubation (days)	15–50 days Average: 30 days	28–160 days Average: 70–80 days	15–160 days Average: 50 days	21–140 days Average: 35 days	15–65 days Average: 42 days
Immunity	Homologous	Homologous	Second attack may indicate weak immunity or infection with another agent	Homologous	Unknown
Nature of Illness					
Signs and symptoms	May occur with or without symptoms; flulike illness *Preicteric phase:* Headache, malaise, fatigue, anorexia, fever *Icteric phase:* Dark urine, jaundice of sclera and skin, tender liver	May occur without symptoms May develop arthralgias, rash	Similar to HBV; less severe and anicteric	Similar to HBV	Similar to HAV. Very severe in pregnant women
Outcome	Usually mild with recovery. Fatality rate: <1%. No carrier state or increased risk of chronic hepatitis, cirrhosis, or hepatic cancer	May be severe. Fatality rate: 1%–10%. Carrier state possible. Increased risk of chronic hepatitis, cirrhosis, and hepatic cancer	Frequent occurrence of chronic carrier state and chronic liver disease. Increased risk of hepatic cancer	Similar to HBV but greater likelihood of carrier state, chronic active hepatitis, and cirrhosis	Similar to HAV except very severe in pregnant women

United States. It is recommended that the two-dose vaccine be given to adults 18 years of age or older, with the second dose 6 to 12 months after the first. Protection against hepatitis A develops within several weeks after the first dose of the vaccine. Children and adolescents 2 to 18 years of age receive three doses, with the second dose 1 month after the first and the third dose 6 to 12 months later. It is estimated that protection against hepatitis A may last for at least 20 years (Marwick, 1995).

Hepatitis A vaccine is recommended for travelers to locations where sanitation and hygiene are unsatisfactory. Vaccination is also recommended for those from other high-risk groups (homosexual men, IV drug users, staff of day care centers, and health care personnel). As with other vaccinations, precautions must be taken to ensure prevention, detection, and treatment of hypersensitivity reactions to the vaccine.

Type A hepatitis can be prevented in those not previously vaccinated by the administration of globulin intramuscularly during the period of incubation, if given within 2 weeks of exposure. This bolsters the person's own antibody production and provides 6 to 8 weeks of passive immunity. Immune globulin may suppress overt symptoms of the disease; the resulting subclinical case of hepatitis A would produce active immunity to subsequent episodes of the virus.

Immune globulin is also recommended for household members and sexual contacts of people with hepatitis A. (Susceptible people in the same household as the patient with hepatitis A are usually also infected by the time the diagnosis is made and should receive immune globulin.)

Although rare, systemic reactions to immune globulin may occur. Caution is required when anyone who has previously had angioedema, hives, or other allergic reactions is treated with any human immune globulin. Epinephrine should be available in case a systemic, anaphylactic reaction occurs.

Preexposure prophylaxis is recommended for those traveling to developing countries and settings with poor or uncertain sanitation conditions but who do not have sufficient time to acquire protection by administration of hepatitis A vaccine.

Community interventions for preventing hepatitis A are outlined in Chart 36-2.

Medical Management

Bed rest during the acute stage and a diet that is both acceptable and nutritious are part of the treatment and nursing care. During the period of anorexia, the patient should receive frequent small feedings, supplemented, if necessary, by IV infusions of glucose. Because this patient often has an aversion to food, gentle persistence and creativity may be required to stimulate the appetite. Optimal food and fluid levels are necessary to counteract weight loss and slow recovery. Even before the icteric phase, however, many patients recover their appetites.

The patient's sense of well-being as well as laboratory test results are generally appropriate guides to bed rest and restriction of physical activity. Gradual but progressive ambulation seems to hasten recovery, provided the patient rests after activity and does not participate in activities to the point of fatigue.

Nursing Management

The patient is usually managed at home unless symptoms are particularly severe. Therefore, the patient and family need to be assisted to cope with the temporary disability and fatigue that are common problems in hepatitis and to be aware of the indications to seek additional health care if the symptoms persist or worsen. The patient and family also need specific guidelines about diet, rest, follow-up blood work, and the importance of avoiding alcohol, as well as sanitation and hygiene measures, particularly hand washing, to prevent spread of the disease to other family members.

Specific teaching to patients and families about reducing the risk of contracting hepatitis A include:

- Good personal hygiene, stressing careful hand washing (after bowel movements and before eating)
- Environmental sanitation—safe food and water supply, as well as effective sewage disposal

CHART 36•2 Community Prevention of Hepatitis A

- Proper community and home sanitation
- Conscientious individual hygiene
- Safe practices for preparing and dispensing food
- Effective health supervision of schools, dormitories, extended care facilities, barracks, and camps
- Community health education programs
- Mandatory reporting of viral hepatitis to local health departments

Hepatitis B Virus (HBV)

Unlike hepatitis A, which is transmitted primarily by the fecal–oral route, hepatitis B is transmitted primarily through blood (percutaneous and permucosal routes). HBV has been found in blood, saliva, semen, and vaginal secretions and can be transmitted through mucous membranes and breaks in the skin. HBV is also transferred from carrier mothers to their babies, especially in areas with a high incidence (ie, Southeast Asia). The infection is usually not via the umbilical vein, but from the mother at the time of birth and during close contact afterward.

HBV has a long incubation period. It replicates in the liver and remains in the serum for relatively long periods, allowing transmission of the virus. Those at risk for developing hepatitis B include surgeons, clinical laboratory workers, dentists, nurses, and respiratory therapists. Staff and patients in hemodialysis and oncology units and sexually active homosexual and bisexual men and injection drug users are also at increased risk.

Screening of blood donors has greatly reduced the occurrence of hepatitis B after blood transfusion. Most adults who do develop acute HBV infection recover fully within 6 months. The mortality rate from hepatitis B has been reported to be as high as 10%. Another 10% of patients who have hepatitis B progress to a carrier state or develop chronic hepatitis. It remains the chief cause of cirrhosis and hepatocellular carcinoma worldwide.

Clinical Manifestations

Clinically, the disease closely resembles hepatitis A. The incubation period, however, is much longer (between 1 and 6 months). Signs and symptoms of hepatitis B may be insidious and variable. Fever and respiratory symptoms are rare; some patients have arthralgias and rashes. The patient may have loss of appetite, dyspepsia, abdominal pain, generalized aching, malaise, and weakness. Jaundice may or may not be evident. If jaundice occurs, it is accompanied by light-colored stools and dark urine. The patient's liver may be tender and enlarged to 12 to 14 cm vertically. The spleen is enlarged and palpable in a few patients; the posterior cervical lymph nodes may also be enlarged. Subclinical episodes also occur frequently.

Assessment and Diagnostic Findings

HBV is a DNA virus composed of the following antigenic particles:

HBcAg—hepatitis B core antigen (antigenic material in an inner core)

HBsAg—hepatitis B surface antigen (antigenic material on surface of HBV)

HBeAg—an independent protein circulating in the blood

HBxAg—gene product of X gene of HBV/DNA

Each antigen elicits its specific antibody and is a marker for different stages of the disease process:

anti-HBc—antibody to core antigen or HBV; persists during the acute phase of illness; may indicate continuing HBV in the liver

anti-HBs—antibody to surface determinants on HBV; detected during late convalescence; usually indicates recovery and development of immunity anti-HBe—antibody to hepatitis B e-antigen; usually signifies reduced infectivity

anti-HBxAg—antibody to the hepatitis B x-antigen; may indicate ongoing replication of HBV

HBsAg appears in the circulation in 80% to 90% of infected patients 1 to 10 weeks after exposure to HBV and 2 to 8 weeks before the onset of symptoms or an increase in transferase (transaminase) levels. Patients with HBsAg that persists for 6 or more months after acute infection are referred to as HBsAg carriers.

HBeAg is the next antigen of HBV to appear in the serum. It usually appears within a week of the appearance of HBsAg and before changes in aminotransferase levels, disappearing from the serum within 2 weeks. HBV DNA, detected by polymerase chain reaction testing, appears in the serum at about the same time as HBeAg. HBcAg is not always detected in the serum in HBV infection.

About 15% of American adults are positive for anti-HBs, which indicates that they have had hepatitis B. Anti-HBs may be positive in as many as two thirds of injection drug users.

Risk Factors for HEPATITIS B

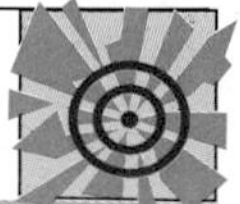

Frequent exposure to blood, blood products, or other body fluids:
- Health care workers: hemodialysis staff, oncology and chemotherapy nurses, personnel at risk for needlesticks, operating room staff, respiratory therapists, surgeons, dentists

Hemodialysis
Male homosexual and bisexual activity
IV/injection drug use
Close contact with carrier of HBV
Travel to or residence in area of uncertain sanitary conditions
Multiple sexual partners
Receipt of blood or blood products (eg, clotting factor concentrate)

Prevention

The goals of prevention are to interrupt the chain of transmission, to protect people at high risk with active immunization through the use of hepatitis B vaccine, and to use passive immunization for unprotected people exposed to HBV.

PREVENTING TRANSMISSION

Continued screening of potential blood donors for the presence of hepatitis B antigens will further decrease the risk of transmission by blood transfusion. The use of disposable syringes, needles, and lancets and the introduction of needleless IV delivery systems reduce the risk of spreading this infection from one patient to another or to health care personnel during the collection of blood samples or the administration of parenteral therapy. Good personal hygiene is fundamental to infection control. In the clinical laboratory, work areas should be disinfected daily. Gloves are worn when handling all blood and body fluids as well as HBAg-positive specimens, or when there is potential exposure to blood (blood drawing) or to patients' secretions. Eating and smoking are prohibited in the laboratory and in other areas exposed to patients' secretions, blood, or blood products.

ACTIVE IMMUNIZATION: HEPATITIS B VACCINE

Active immunization is recommended for individuals at high risk for hepatitis B (eg, health care personnel, hemodialysis patients). A yeast-recombinant hepatitis B vaccine (Recombivax HB) is used to provide active immunity. Long-term studies of healthy adults and children indicate that immunologic memory remains intact for at least 5 to 10 years, although antibody levels may become low or undetectable. Measurable levels of antibodies may not be essential for protection. In those with normal immune systems, booster doses are not generally required. The U.S. Public Health Service does not recommend booster doses at this time except for hemodialysis patients (Immunization Practices Advisory Committee, 1991).

A hepatitis B vaccine prepared from plasma of humans chronically infected with HBV is used only rarely and in patients who are immunodeficient or allergic to recombinant yeast-derived vaccines.

Both forms of the hepatitis B vaccine are administered in three doses, the second and third doses 1 and 6 months after the first dose. The third dose is very important in producing prolonged immunity. Hepatitis B vaccination should be administered to adults in the deltoid muscle: administration in the gluteal region may result in suboptimal response. Antibody response may be measured by anti-HBs levels 1 to 3 months after completing the basic course of vaccine, but this testing is not routine and not currently recommended (Katkov, 1996).

People at high risk, including nurses and other health care personnel exposed to blood or blood products, should receive active immunization. Health care workers who have had frequent contact with blood are screened for anti-HBs to determine whether immunity is already present from previous exposure. The vaccine produces active immunity to HBV in 90% of healthy people. It does not provide protection to those already exposed to HBV and provides no protection against other types of viral hepatitis. Side effects of immunization are infrequent. Soreness and redness at the injection site are the most common postinjection complaints.

Universal childhood vaccination for hepatitis B prevention has been recommended and instituted in the United States. The reason for this is that despite the advent of the safe and effective hepatitis B vaccine, the incidence of hepatitis B infection in the United States has not declined. Vaccination was initially targeted for select high-risk populations, but the U.S. Public Health Service and the Centers for Disease Control and Prevention have endorsed universal vaccination of all infants. In addition, nonvaccinated adolescents are also being targeted for vaccination against hepatitis B by the age of 11 to 12 years (Katkov, 1996; Recommended Childhood Immunization Schedule, U.S., 1996).

PASSIVE IMMUNITY: HEPATITIS B IMMUNE GLOBULIN

Hepatitis B immune globulin (HBIG) provides passive immunity to hepatitis B and is indicated for people exposed to HBV who have never had hepatitis B and have never received hepatitis B vaccine. Specific indications for postexposure vaccine with HBIG include: (1) accidental exposure to HBAg-positive blood through percutaneous (needlestick) or transmucosal (splashes in contact with mucous membrane) routes, (2) sexual contact with people positive for HBAg, and (3) perinatal exposure. HBIG, which provides passive immunity, is prepared from plasma selected for high titers of anti-HBs. There has been no evidence that HIV infection can be transmitted by HBIG. Prompt immunization with HBIG—that is, within hours to a few days after exposure to hepatitis B—increases the likelihood of protection. Both active and passive immunization are recommended for people exposed to hepatitis B through sexual contact or through percutaneous or transmucosal routes. If HBIG and hepatitis B vaccine are administered at the same time, separate sites and separate syringes should be used.

Gerontologic Considerations

The elderly patient who contracts hepatitis B has a serious risk of severe liver cell necrosis or fulminant hepatic failure, particularly if other illnesses are present. The patient is seriously ill and the prognosis is poor.

Medical Management

The goals of treatment are to minimize infectivity, normalize liver inflammation, and decrease symptoms. Of all the agents that have been used to treat chronic type B viral hepatitis, alpha interferon as the single modality of therapy offers the most promise. Approximately 30% to 40% of patients seroconvert from HBeAg-positive to HBeAg-negative and anti-HBe-positive after treatment, compared with a spontaneous seroconversion rate of approximately 10% per year (Fried, 1996; Sherlock & Dooley, 1997). The long-term benefits of this treatment are still being assessed. Interferon must be administered by daily injection and has significant side effects, including fever, chills, anorexia, nausea, myalgias, and fatigue. Late side effects are more serious and may necessitate dose reduction or discontinuation. These include bone marrow suppression, thyroid dysfunction, alopecia, and bacterial infections.

Bed rest may be recommended, regardless of other treatment, until the symptoms of hepatitis have subsided. The patient's activities are restricted until the hepatic enlargement and elevation of the levels of serum bilirubin and liver enzymes have disappeared. Patients may then participate in graduated activities.

Adequate nutrition should be maintained; proteins are restricted when the ability of the liver to metabolize protein byproducts is impaired, as demonstrated by symptoms. Therapeutic measures to control the dyspeptic symptoms and general malaise include the use of antacids and antiemetics. However, all medications should be avoided if vomiting is a problem. If vomiting persists, the patient may require hospitalization and fluid therapy. Because of the mode of transmission, the patient is evaluated for other bloodborne diseases (eg, HIV infection).

Nursing Management

Convalescence may be prolonged, with complete symptomatic recovery sometimes requiring 3 to 4 months or longer. During this stage, gradual resumption of physical activity is permitted and encouraged, after the jaundice has resolved.

Psychosocial considerations are identified by the nurse, particularly the effects of isolation and separation from family and friends during the acute and infective stages. Special planning is required to minimize alterations in sensory perception. The family is included in planning to decrease the fears and anxieties of the patient and family about the spread of the disease.

PROMOTING HOME AND COMMUNITY-BASED CARE

Teaching Patients Self-Care. Because of the prolonged period of convalescence, the patient and family must be prepared for home care. Provision for adequate rest and nutrition must be ensured before the patient's discharge. Family members and friends who have had intimate contact with the patient should be informed about the risks of contracting hepatitis B, and arrangements should be made for them to receive hepatitis B vaccine or hepatitis B immune globulin. Those at risk must be aware of early signs of hepatitis B and of ways to reduce risk to themselves by avoiding all modes of transmission. Patients with all forms of hepatitis are cautioned to avoid the use of alcohol.

Continuing Care. Follow-up visits by a home care nurse may be needed to assess the patient's progress and answer family members' questions about transmission of the disease. A home visit also permits assessment of the patient's physical and psychological status, evaluation of the understanding of the patient and family about the importance of adequate rest and nutrition, and reinforcement of previous instructions. Because of the risk of transmission through sexual intercourse, use of strategies to prevent exchange of body fluids is advised; these include abstinence or the use of condoms. The importance of keeping follow-up appointments is emphasized to the patient and family.

Hepatitis C Virus

A significant proportion of cases of viral hepatitis are neither hepatitis A, hepatitis B, nor hepatitis D; as a result, they are classified as hepatitis C (formerly referred to as non-A, non-B hepatitis or NANB hepatitis). Whereas blood transfusions and sexual contact used to account for most transmissions of hepatitis C in the United States, other parenteral means, such as sharing contaminated needles by IV/injection drug users and accidental needlesticks and other injuries in health care workers, now account for a significant number of cases.

Individuals at special risk for hepatitis C include IV/injection drug users, sexually active people with multiple partners, patients receiving frequent transfusions or those who require large volumes of blood, and health care personnel. The incubation period is variable and may range from 15 to 160 days. The clinical course of acute hepatitis C is similar to that of hepatitis B; symptoms are usually mild. A chronic carrier state occurs frequently, however, and there is an increased risk of chronic liver disease, including cirrhosis or liver cancer, after hepatitis C.

There is no benefit from rest, diet, or vitamin supplements. Recent studies have demonstrated that a combination of interferon and ribavirin, two antiviral agents, is effective in producing improvement in patients with hepatitis C and in treating relapses (Davis et al., 1998; McHutchison et al., 1998). Some patients experience complete remission with combination therapy. Hemolytic anemia is the most frequent side effect and may be severe enough to require that the treatment be discontinued. Ribavirin must be used with caution in women of childbearing age.

Screening of blood has reduced the incidence of hepatitis associated with blood transfusions, and public health programs are helping to reduce the number of cases associated with shared needles in illicit drug use. Chronic hepatitis C accounts for approximately 30% of liver transplantations in the United States.

Hepatitis D Virus

Hepatitis D (delta agent) occurs in some cases of hepatitis B. Because the virus requires hepatitis B surface antigen for its replication, only individuals with hepatitis B are at risk for hepatitis D. Anti-delta antibodies in the presence of HBAg on testing confirm the diagnosis. It is also common among IV/injection drug users, hemodialysis patients, and recipients of multiple blood transfusions. Sexual contact with those with hepatitis B is considered to be an important mode of transmission of hepatitis B and D. The incubation period varies between 21 and 140 days.

The symptoms of hepatitis D are similar to those of hepatitis B, except that patients are more likely to have fulminant hepatitis and to progress to chronic active hepatitis and cirrhosis. Treatment is similar to that of other forms of hepatitis; interferon as a specific treatment for hepatitis D is under investigation.

Hepatitis E Virus

Hepatitis E is believed to be transmitted by the fecal–oral route, principally through contaminated water in poor sanitation areas. The incubation period is variable, estimated to range between 15 and 65 days. In general, hepatitis E resembles hepatitis A. It has a self-limiting course with an abrupt onset. Jaundice is nearly always present. Chronic forms do not develop.

Avoiding contact with the virus through good hygiene, including hand washing, is the major method of prevention of hepatitis E. The effectiveness of immune globulin in protecting against hepatitis E virus is uncertain.

Hepatitis G Virus

It has long been believed that there is another non-A, non-B, non-C agent causing hepatitis in humans. The incubation periods for posttransfusion hepatitis is 14 to 145 days, too long for hepatitis B or C. In the United States, about 5% of chronic liver disease remains cryptogenic (non-A, non-B, non-C), and half the patients have been transfused. Thus, a new form of hepatitis (hepatitis G) has been described. Autoantibodies are absent.

The clinical significance of this virus remains uncertain. Risk factors are similar to those for hepatitis C. It is expected that this will not be the last type of hepatitis to be identified (Scheig, 1998; Sjogren, 1996).

Nonviral Hepatitis

Certain chemicals have toxic effects on the liver and when taken by mouth or injected parenterally produce acute liver cell necrosis, or toxic hepatitis. The chemicals most commonly implicated in this disease are carbon tetrachloride, phosphorus, chloroform, and gold compounds. These substances are true hepatotoxins. Many medications may induce hepatitis but are sensitizing rather than toxic. The result, drug-induced hepatitis, is similar to acute viral hepatitis; however, parenchymal destruction tends to be more extensive. Some examples of medications that can lead to hepatitis are isoniazid, halothane, acetaminophen, and certain antibiotics, antimetabolites, and anesthetic agents.

Toxic Hepatitis

Toxic hepatitis resembles viral hepatitis in onset. Obtaining a history of exposure to hepatotoxic chemicals, medications, or other agents assists in early initiation of treatment and removal of the offending agent. Anorexia, nausea, and vomiting are the usual symptoms; jaundice and hepatomegaly are noted on physical assessment. Symptoms are more intense for the more severely toxic patient.

Recovery from acute toxic hepatitis is rapid if the hepatotoxin is identified early and removed or if exposure to the agent has been limited. Recovery, however, is unlikely if there is a prolonged period between exposure and onset of symptoms. There are no effective antidotes. The fever rises; the patient becomes very toxic and prostrated. Vomiting may be persistent, with the emesis containing blood. Clotting abnormalities may be severe, and hemorrhages may appear under the skin. The severe GI symptoms may lead to vascular collapse. Delirium, coma, and seizures develop, and within a few days the patient may die of fulminant hepatic failure (discussed below) unless he or she receives a liver transplant.

Short of liver transplantation, few treatment options are available. Therapy is directed toward restoring and maintaining fluid and electrolyte balance, blood replacement, and provision of comfort and supportive measures. A few patients recover from acute toxic hepatitis only to develop chronic liver disease. In the event that the liver heals, there may be scarring, followed by postnecrotic cirrhosis.

Drug-Induced Hepatitis

Drug-induced hepatitis is responsible for up to 25% of cases of fulminant hepatic failure in the United States. Manifestations of sensitivity to a medication may occur on the first day of its use or not until several months later, depending on the medication. Usually, the onset is abrupt, with chills, fever, rash, pruritus, arthralgia, anorexia, and nausea. Later, there may be jaundice and dark urine and an enlarged and tender liver. When the offending medication is withdrawn, symptoms may gradually subside. Reactions may be severe, however, and even fatal, even though the medication is stopped. If fever, rash, or pruritus occurs from any medication, its use should be stopped immediately.

Although any medication can affect liver function, those most commonly associated with liver injury include but are not limited to anesthetic agents, medications used to treat rheumatic and musculoskeletal disease, antidepressants, psychotropic medications, anticonvulsants, and antituberculosis agents.

Halothane (Fluothane), a commonly used nonexplosive inhalation anesthetic, may cause serious, and sometimes fatal, liver damage; therefore, its use is contraindicated in (1) patients with known liver disease, (2) repeated instances, particularly in patients who have had a fever of unknown cause after the first administration of halothane, and (3) patients with evidence of prior sensitization. Such sensitization would have been evident during the second postoperative week, with such manifestations as fever, rash, eosinophilia, arthralgia, or jaundice.

Although its efficacy is uncertain, a short course of high-dose corticosteroids may be used in patients with very severe hypersensitivity. Liver transplantation is an option for drug-induced hepatitis, but outcomes may not be as successful as with other causes of liver failure.

Fulminant Hepatic Failure

Fulminant hepatic failure is the clinical syndrome of sudden and severely impaired liver function in a previously healthy person. The original and generally accepted definition of fulminant hepatic failure includes a time frame of development within 8 weeks of the first symptoms or jaundice.

Patterns of the progression from jaundice to encephalopathy have been identified and have led to proposals of time-based classifications, but agreement as to these classifications has not been reached. However, three categories are frequently cited: hyperacute, acute, and subacute liver failure. In hyperacute liver failure, the duration of jaundice before the onset of encephalopathy is 0 to 7 days; in acute liver failure, it is 8 to 28 days; and in subacute liver failure, it is 28 to 72 days. The prognosis for fulminant hepatic failure is much worse than for chronic liver failure, but in fulminant failure, the hepatic lesion is potentially reversible, with survival rates of approximately 50% to 85% (survival rates depend greatly on the etiology of liver failure). Those who do not survive die of massive hepatocellular injury and necrosis.

Viral hepatitis is the most common cause of fulminant hepatic failure; other causes include toxic medications (eg, acetaminophen) and chemicals (eg, carbon tetrachloride), metabolic disturbances (Wilson's disease, a hereditary syndrome with deposition of copper in the liver), and structural changes (Budd-Chiari syndrome, an obstruction to outflow in major hepatic veins).

Jaundice and profound anorexia may be the initial reasons the patient seeks health care. Fulminant hepatic failure is often accompanied by coagulation defects, renal failure and electrolyte disturbances, infection, hypoglycemia, encephalopathy, and cerebral edema.

Medical Management

The key to optimizing treatment is rapid recognition of acute liver failure and intensive interventions. Treatment modalities may include plasma exchanges or charcoal hemoperfusion for the removal (theoretically) of potentially harmful metabolites; however, more clinical trials are needed to determine their effects or outcomes. Hepatocytes within synthetic fiber columns have been tested as liver support systems (liver assist devices) and a bridge to transplantation.

Research into interventions for acute liver failure has begun to focus on techniques that combine the efficacy of a whole liver with the convenience and biocompatibility of hemodialysis. The acronyms ELAD (extracorporeal liver assist devices) and BAL (bioartificial liver) have been used to describe these hybrid devices. These are temporary devices that have enabled patients to survive until transplantation was possible. Definitive studies of these techniques are not yet available (Sherlock & Dooley, 1997). Although this approach is promising, more controlled study and evaluation are required.

Cerebral edema is a life-threatening complication, and intracranial pressure monitoring is indicated for effective management. Measures to promote adequate cerebral perfusion include careful fluid balance and hemodynamic assessments, a quiet environment, and diuresis with mannitol, an osmotic diuretic.

To prevent surges in intracranial pressure related to agitation, barbiturate anesthesia or pharmacologic paralysis and sedation are indicated. Other support measures include monitoring for and treating hypoglycemia, coagulopathies, and infection. Despite these treatment modalities, however, the mortality rate remains high. Consequently, liver transplantation has become the treatment of choice for fulminant hepatic failure. Liver transplantation is discussed later in this chapter.

Hepatic Cirrhosis

Cirrhosis is a chronic disease characterized by replacement of normal liver tissue with diffuse fibrosis that disrupts the structure and function of the liver. There are three types of cirrhosis or scarring of the liver:

- Alcoholic cirrhosis, in which the scar tissue characteristically surrounds the portal areas. This is most frequently due to chronic alcoholism and is the most common type of cirrhosis.
- Postnecrotic cirrhosis, in which there are broad bands of scar tissue, as a late result of a previous acute viral hepatitis.
- Biliary cirrhosis, in which scarring occurs in the liver around the bile ducts. This type usually is the result of chronic biliary obstruction and infection (cholangitis); its incidence is considerably lower than that of the other two types.

The portion of the liver chiefly involved in cirrhosis consists of the portal and the periportal spaces, where the bile canaliculi of each lobule communicate to form the liver bile ducts. These areas become the sites of inflammation, and the bile ducts become occluded with inspissated (thickened) bile and pus. An attempt is made by the liver to form new bile channels; hence, there is an overgrowth of tissue made up largely of disconnected, newly formed bile ducts and surrounded by scar tissue.

NURSING RESEARCH

The Lived Experience of Liver Failure and Liver Transplantation

Johnson, C. D., & Hathaway, D. K. (1996). The lived experience of end-stage liver failure and liver transplantation. *Journal of Transplant Coordination, 6*(3), 130–133.

Purpose

Because of the severity of their illnesses and the uncertainty associated with the possibility of receiving a liver transplant in time, patients' experiences associated with end-stage liver failure and liver transplantation are often extremely stressful. This phenomenologic study examined the lived experience of an individual who experienced end-stage liver failure and underwent liver transplantation.

Study Sample and Design

The patient, a 62-year-old African American woman, was interviewed and asked to describe what it was like for her to have experienced end-stage liver failure and liver transplantation. The interview was tape-recorded and data were analyzed.

Findings

Analysis revealed four categories and associated themes:

- Uncertainty (surprise and ambivalence), loss of control (dependence, confusion/disorientation, anger/frustration, and fear)
- Regaining control (returning independence, acts of prevention, concern for self-image, and preparedness)
- Social support (concern of family and health care providers)
- Spirituality (thankfulness to God and to the donor family).

The experience was described as uncertain throughout the course. Spirituality, faith in God, and support from family, friends, and health care workers were important throughout the experience.

Nursing Implications

Although the case study format limits the ability to generalize the findings, it is clear that the experience of developing end-stage liver failure and subsequently undergoing transplantation is a very difficult, uncertain one. The findings emphasize the importance of the nurse supporting the patient's faith in God and providing social support before, during, and after the stress, uncertainty, and loss of control that characterize the experience of liver transplantation. The findings of this study support the need for further research on the topic.

Clinical manifestations of this disease include intermittent jaundice and fever. Initially the liver is enlarged, hard, and irregular; eventually it atrophies. The treatment is the same as that for any form of chronic liver insufficiency.

Pathophysiology

Although several factors have been implicated in the etiology of cirrhosis, alcohol consumption is considered the major causative factor. Cirrhosis occurs with greatest frequency among alcoholics. Although nutritional deficiency with reduced protein intake contributes to liver destruction in cirrhosis, excessive alcohol intake is the major causative factor in fatty liver and its consequences. Cirrhosis, however, has also occurred in people who do not consume alcohol and in those who consume a normal diet and have a high alcohol intake.

Some people appear to be more susceptible than others to this disease, whether or not they are alcoholics or malnourished. Other factors may play a role, including exposure to certain chemicals (carbon tetrachloride, chlorinated naphthalene, arsenic, or phosphorus) or infectious schistosomiasis. Twice as many men as women are affected, and the majority of patients are 40 to 60 years of age. Each year more than 27,000 die of chronic liver diseases and cirrhosis in the United States (National Institutes of Health, 1997).

Alcoholic cirrhosis is a disease characterized by episodes of necrosis involving the liver cells, sometimes occurring repeatedly throughout the course of the disease. The destroyed liver cells are gradually replaced by scar tissue; eventually the amount of scar tissue exceeds that of the functioning liver tissue. Islands of residual normal tissue and regenerating liver tissue may project from the constricted areas, giving the cirrhotic liver its characteristic hobnail appearance. The disease usually has a particularly insidious onset and a very protracted course, occasionally proceeding over a period of 30 or more years.

The prognosis of different forms of cirrhosis caused by various liver diseases has been investigated in several studies. Of the many prognostic indicators, the Child's classification seems most useful in predicting the outcome of patients with liver disease (Table 36-4). It is also used in choosing management approaches.

Clinical Manifestations

Signs and symptoms of cirrhosis increase in severity as the disease progresses and worsens. The severity of the manifestations of cirrhosis helps to categorize the disorder into two main presentations.

Compensated cirrhosis, with its less severe, often vague symptoms, may be discovered secondarily at a routine physical examination. The hallmarks of decompensated cirrhosis result from failure of the liver to synthesize proteins, clotting factors, and other substances and manifestations of portal hypertension.

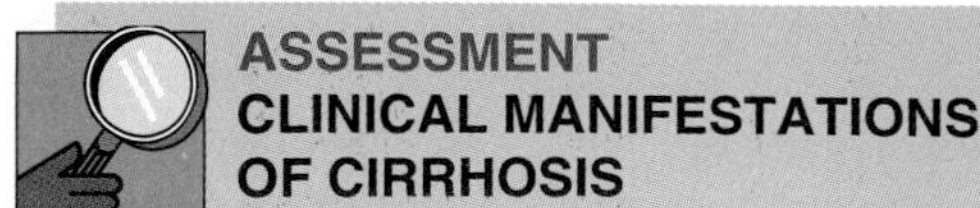

ASSESSMENT CLINICAL MANIFESTATIONS OF CIRRHOSIS

Compensated

Intermittent mild fever
Vascular spiders
Palmar erythema (reddened palms)
Unexplained epistaxis
Ankle edema
Vague morning indigestion
Flatulent dyspepsia
Abdominal pain
Firm, enlarged liver
Splenomegaly

Decompensated

Ascites
Jaundice
Weakness
Muscle wasting
Weight loss
Continuous mild fever
Clubbing of fingers
Purpura (due to decreased platelet count)
Spontaneous bruising
Epistaxis
Hypotension
Sparse body hair
White nails
Gonadal atrophy

LIVER ENLARGEMENT

Early in the course of cirrhosis, the liver tends to be large and its cells loaded with fat. The liver is firm and has a sharp edge noticeable on palpation. Abdominal pain may be present because of recent, rapid enlargement of the liver, producing tension on the fibrous covering of the liver (Glisson's capsule). Later in the course of the disease, the liver decreases in size as scar tissue contracts the liver tissue. The liver edge, if palpable, is nodular.

PORTAL OBSTRUCTION AND ASCITES

The late manifestations are due partly to chronic failure of liver function and partly to obstruction of the portal circulation. Practically all the blood from the digestive organs is collected in the

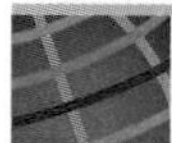

TABLE 36•4 Child's Classification of Hepatocellular Function in Cirrhosis

Group Designation	A (Least Severe)	B	C (Most Severe)
Serum bilirubin (mg/dL)	Below 2.0	2.0–3.0	Over 3.0
Serum albumin (g/dL)	Over 3.5	3.0–3.5	Under 3.0
Ascites	None	Easily controlled	Poorly controlled
Neurologic disorder (degree of encephalopathy)	None	Minimal	Advanced coma
Nutrition	Excellent	Good	Poor with "wasting"

From Sherlock, S., & Dooley, J. (1997). *Diseases of the liver and biliary system* (10th ed.). Oxford: Blackwell, p. 162.

portal veins and carried to the liver. Because a cirrhotic liver does not allow the blood free passage, it is backed up into the spleen and the GI tract, with the result that these organs become the seat of chronic passive congestion; that is, they are stagnant with blood and thus cannot function properly. Indigestion and altered bowel function ensue.

Fluid rich in protein may accumulate in the peritoneal cavity, producing ascites. This can be demonstrated through percussion for shifting dullness or a fluid wave (see Fig. 36-4).

INFECTION AND PERITONITIS

Bacterial peritonitis may develop in cirrhotic patients with ascites in the absence of an intra-abdominal source of infection or an abscess. This condition is referred to as spontaneous bacterial peritonitis. Bacteremia is generally believed to be the most likely route of infection. Clinical signs may be absent; paracentesis may be necessary for diagnosis. Antibiotic therapy is effective in the treatment and prevention of recurrent episodes of spontaneous bacterial peritonitis.

GI VARICES

The obstruction to blood flow through the liver resulting from the fibrotic changes also results in the formation of collateral blood vessels in the GI system and shunting of blood from the portal vessels into blood vessels with lower pressures. As a result, the patient with cirrhosis often has prominent, distended abdominal blood vessels, which are visible on abdominal inspection (caput medusae), and distended blood vessels throughout the GI tract. The esophagus, stomach, and lower rectum are common sites of collateral blood vessels. These distended blood vessels form varices or hemorrhoids, depending on their location (Fig. 36-8).

Because these vessels were not intended to carry the high pressure and volume of blood imposed by cirrhosis, they may rupture and bleed. Therefore, assessment must include observation for occult and frank bleeding from the GI tract. Approximately 25% of patients develop small hematemesis; others have profuse hemorrhage from gastric and esophageal varices.

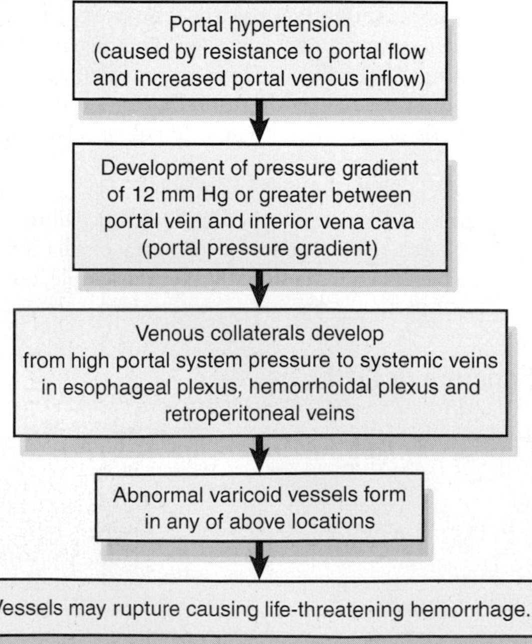

FIGURE 36•8 Pathogenesis of bleeding esophageal varices.

EDEMA

Other late symptoms of cirrhosis are attributable to chronic liver failure. The concentration of plasma albumin is reduced, predisposing to the formation of edema. Overproduction of aldosterone occurs, causing sodium and water retention and potassium excretion.

VITAMIN DEFICIENCY AND ANEMIA

Because of inadequate formation, use, and storage of certain vitamins (notably vitamins A, C, and K), signs of their deficiency are common, particularly hemorrhagic phenomena associated with vitamin K deficiency. Chronic gastritis and impaired GI function, together with inadequate dietary intake and impaired liver function, account for the anemia often associated with this disease. The anemia and the patient's poor nutritional status and poor state of health result in severe fatigue, which interferes with the ability to carry out routine daily activities.

MENTAL DETERIORATION

Additional clinical manifestations include deterioration of mental function with impending hepatic encephalopathy and hepatic coma. Therefore, neurologic assessment is indicated and includes the patient's general behavior, cognitive abilities, orientation to time and place, and speech patterns.

Assessment and Diagnostic Findings

The extent of liver disease and the type of treatment are determined after studying the laboratory findings. Because the functions of the liver are complex, there are many diagnostic tests that may provide information about liver function (see Table 36-1). The patient needs to know the reason these tests are being performed and ways to cooperate.

In severe parenchymal liver dysfunction, the serum albumin level tends to decrease, and the serum globulin level rises. Enzyme tests indicate liver cell damage: serum alkaline phosphatase, AST (SGOT), ALT (SGPT), and GGT levels increase, and the serum cholinesterase level may decrease. Bilirubin tests are performed to measure bile excretion or bile retention. Prothrombin time is prolonged.

Ultrasound scanning is used to measure the difference in density of parenchymal cells and scar tissue. CT scanning, MRI, and radioisotope liver scans give information about liver size and hepatic blood flow and obstruction. Diagnosis is confirmed by liver biopsy. Arterial blood gas analysis may reveal a ventilation–perfusion imbalance and hypoxia.

Medical Management

The management of the patient with cirrhosis is usually based on the presenting symptoms. For example, antacids are prescribed to decrease gastric distress and minimize the possibility of GI bleeding. Vitamins and nutritional supplements promote healing of damaged liver cells and improve the patient's general nutritional status. Potassium-sparing diuretics (spironolactone) may be indicated to decrease ascites, if present, and minimize the fluid and electrolyte changes common with other diuretic agents. An adequate balanced diet and avoidance of alcohol are essential. Although the fibrosis of the cirrhotic liver cannot be reversed, its progression may be halted or slowed by such measures.

Preliminary studies indicate that colchicine, an anti-inflammatory agent used to treat the symptoms of gout, may increase the length of survival in patients with mild to moderate cirrhosis.

NURSING PROCESS: THE PATIENT WITH HEPATIC CIRRHOSIS

Assessment

Nursing assessment focuses on the onset of symptoms and the history of precipitating factors, particularly long-term alcohol abuse, as well as dietary intake and changes in the patient's physical and mental status. The patient's past and current patterns of alcohol use (duration and amount) are assessed and documented. It is also important to document any exposure to toxic agents encountered in the workplace or during recreational activities. Exposure to potentially hepatotoxic medications or general anesthetic agents is documented and reported.

Mental status is assessed through the interview and other interactions with the patient; orientation to person, place, and time is noted. The patient's ability to carry on a job or household activities provides some information about physical and mental status. The patient's relationships with family, friends, and coworkers may give some indication about incapacitation secondary to alcohol abuse and cirrhosis. Abdominal distention and bloating, GI bleeding, bruising, and weight changes are noted.

Nutritional status, of major importance in cirrhosis, is assessed by daily weights, anthropometric measurements (see Chap. 5), and monitoring of plasma proteins, transferrin, and creatinine levels.

Diagnosis

Nursing Diagnoses

Based on all the assessment data, the patient's major nursing diagnoses may include the following:

- Activity intolerance related to fatigue, general debility, muscle wasting, and discomfort
- Altered nutrition, less than body requirements, related to chronic gastritis, decreased GI motility, and anorexia
- Impaired skin integrity related to compromised immunologic status, edema, and poor nutrition
- Risk for injury and bleeding related to altered clotting mechanisms

Collaborative Problems/Potential Complications

Based on assessment data, potential complications may include:

- Bleeding and hemorrhage
- Hepatic encephalopathy
- Fluid volume excess

Planning and Goals

The goals for the patient may include independence in activities, improvement of nutritional status, improvement of skin integrity, decreased potential for injury, improvement of mental status, and absence of complications.

Nursing Interventions

Providing Rest

The patient with active liver disease requires rest and other supportive measures to permit the liver to reestablish its functional ability. If the patient is hospitalized, weight and fluid intake and output are measured and recorded daily. The patient's position in bed is adjusted for maximal respiratory efficiency, which is especially important if ascites is marked, as it interferes with adequate thoracic excursion. Oxygen therapy may be required in liver failure to oxygenate the damaged cells and prevent further cell destruction.

Rest reduces the demands on the liver and increases the liver's blood supply. Because the patient is susceptible to the hazards of immobility, efforts to prevent respiratory, circulatory, and vascular disturbances are initiated. These measures may help prevent such problems as pneumonia, thrombophlebitis, and pressure ulcers. When nutritional status improves and strength increases, the patient is encouraged to increase activity gradually. Activity and mild exercise, as well as rest, are planned.

Improving Nutritional Status

The patient with cirrhosis who has no ascites or edema and exhibits no signs of impending coma should receive a nutritious, high-protein diet supplemented by vitamins of the B complex and others as indicated (including vitamins A, C, and K and folic acid). Because proper nutrition is so important, every effort is made to encourage the patient to eat. This is as important as any medication. Often small, frequent meals are tolerated better than three large meals because of the abdominal pressure exerted by ascites. Protein supplements may also be indicated.

Patient preferences are considered. Patients with prolonged or severe anorexia, or those who are vomiting or eating poorly for any reason, may receive nutrients enterally or total parenteral nutrition.

Patients with fatty stools (steatorrhea) should receive water-soluble forms of fat-soluble vitamins—A, D, and E (Aquasol A, D, and E). Folic acid and iron are prescribed to prevent anemia. If the patient shows signs of impending or advancing coma, the amount of protein in the diet is decreased temporarily. In the absence of hepatic encephalopathy, a moderate-protein, high-calorie intake is provided, with protein foods of high biologic value. A diet containing 1 to 1.5 g of protein per kilogram of body weight per day is required unless the patient is malnourished. Less protein is permitted if encephalopathy develops. The risk of encephalopathy may be decreased by incorporating vegetable protein to meet protein needs. Sodium restriction is also indicated to prevent ascites.

A high-calorie intake should be maintained, and supplemental vitamins and minerals should be provided (eg, oral potassium, if the serum potassium level is normal or low and if renal function is normal).

Providing Skin Care

Careful skin care is provided because of the presence of subcutaneous edema, the immobility of the patient, jaundice, and increased susceptibility to skin breakdown and infection. Frequent position changes are necessary to prevent pressure ulcers. Irritating soaps and the use of adhesive tape are avoided to prevent trauma to the skin. Lotion may be soothing to irritated skin; measures are taken to minimize the patient's scratching of the skin.

Reducing Risk of Injury

The patient with cirrhosis is protected from falls and other injuries. The side rails are in place and padded with soft blankets to minimize risks if the patient becomes agitated or restless. The patient is oriented to time and place and all procedures are explained to minimize the patient's agitation. The patient is instructed to ask for assistance to get out of bed. Any injury is evaluated carefully because of the possibility of internal bleeding.

Because of risk of bleeding from abnormal clotting, the patient is instructed and assisted to use an electric rather than a safety razor. Bleeding of the gums is minimized by use of a soft-bristled toothbrush. Pressure is applied to all venipuncture sites to minimize bleeding.

Monitoring and Managing Potential Complications

Bleeding and hemorrhage may occur because of the decreased production of prothrombin and the decreased ability of the diseased liver to synthesize the substances necessary for blood coagulation. Precautionary measures include protecting the patient with padded side rails, applying pressure to any injection site, and avoiding injury from sharp objects. The nurse should observe for melena and assess stools for blood as signs of possible internal bleeding. Vital signs also are monitored regularly. Precautions are taken to minimize rupture of esophageal varices by avoiding further increases in portal pressure. Dietary modification and appropriate use of stool softeners may help prevent straining during defecation. The patient is monitored closely for GI bleeding; equipment (Sengstaken-Blakemore tube), IV fluids, and medications needed to treat hemorrhage from esophageal varices are kept readily available.

If hemorrhage occurs, the nurse assists the physician in initiating measures to halt the bleeding, administering fluid and blood component therapy and medications. The patient with massive hemorrhage from bleeding esophageal or gastric varices may be transferred to the intensive care unit and may require emergency surgery or other treatment modalities. The patient and family require explanations about the event and the necessary treatment.

Hepatic encephalopathy, a possible complication of cirrhosis, includes deteriorating mental status and dementia as well as physical signs such as abnormal voluntary and involuntary movements. Hepatic encephalopathy is mainly caused by the accumulation of ammonia in the blood and its effect on cerebral metabolism. Many factors predispose the patient with cirrhosis to hepatic encephalopathy; therefore, the patient may require extensive diagnostic testing to identify hidden sources of bleeding and ammonia.

Treatment may include the use of lactulose and nonabsorbable intestinal tract antibiotics to decrease ammonia levels, modification in medications to eliminate those that may precipitate or worsen hepatic encephalopathy, and bed rest to minimize energy expenditure.

Monitoring is an essential nursing function to identify early deterioration in mental status. The nurse monitors the patient's mental status closely and reports changes so that treatment of encephalopathy can be initiated promptly. Because electrolyte disturbances can contribute to encephalopathy, serum electrolyte levels are carefully monitored and corrected if abnormal. Oxygen is administered if oxygen desaturation occurs. The nurse monitors for the presence of fever and/or abdominal pain, which may signal the onset of spontaneous bacterial peritonitis or other infection. (See the discussion of hepatic encephalopathy above.)

Promoting Home and Community-Based Care

TEACHING PATIENTS SELF-CARE

During hospitalization, the patient with cirrhosis is prepared for discharge by the nurse and other health care providers through dietary instruction. Of greatest importance is the exclusion of alcohol from the diet. The patient may need referral to Alcoholics Anonymous, psychiatric care, or counseling, or may benefit from support from clergy.

Sodium restriction will continue for a considerable time, if not permanently. If this restriction is to be followed correctly, the patient will require written instructions, teaching, reinforcement, and support from the staff as well as the family members.

The success of treatment depends on convincing the patient of the need to adhere completely to the therapeutic plan. This includes rest; probably a change in lifestyle; an adequate, well-balanced diet; and the elimination of alcohol. The patient and family are also instructed about the symptoms of impending encephalopathy and the possibility of bleeding tendencies and easy susceptibility to infection.

Recovery is neither rapid nor easy; there are frequent setbacks and apparent lack of improvement. Many patients find it difficult to refrain from using alcohol for comfort or escape. The nurse has a significant role in offering support and encouragement to this patient.

CONTINUING CARE

Referral of the patient to a home care nurse may assist the patient in dealing with the transition from hospital to home, where the use of alcohol may have been an important part of the patient's normal home and social life. The home care nurse assesses the patient's progress at home and the manner in which the patient and family cope with the elimination of alcohol and the dietary restrictions. The nurse also reinforces previous teaching and answers questions that may not have occurred to the patient or family until the patient is back home and trying to establish new patterns of eating, drinking, and lifestyle.

For an overall view of the nursing management of the patient with impaired liver function, refer to Plan of Nursing Care 36-1.

Evaluation

Expected Outcomes

Expected outcomes may include:

1. Participates in activities
   a. Plans activities and exercises to allow alternating periods of rest and activity
   b. Reports increased strength and well-being
   c. Participates in hygiene care
2. Increases nutritional intake
   a. Demonstrates intake of appropriate nutrients and avoidance of alcohol as reflected by diet log
   b. Gains weight without increased edema and ascites formation
   c. Reports decrease in GI disturbances and anorexia
   d. Identifies foods and fluids that are nutritious and allowed on diet or restricted from diet
   e. Adheres to vitamin therapy regimen
   f. Describes the rationale for small, frequent meals
3. Exhibits improved skin integrity
   a. Shows intact skin without evidence of breakdown, infection, or trauma
   b. Demonstrates normal turgor of skin of extremities and trunk, without edema
   c. Changes position frequently and inspects bony prominences daily
   d. Uses lotions to decrease pruritus

4. Avoids injury
   a. Is free of ecchymotic areas or hematoma formation
   b. States rationale for side rails and asks for assistance to get out of bed
   c. Uses measures to prevent trauma (eg, uses soft toothbrush, blows nose gently, arranges furniture to prevent bumps and falls, avoids straining during defecation)
5. Is free of complications
   a. Reports absence of frank bleeding from GI tract (ie, absence of melena and hematemesis)
   b. Is oriented to time, place, and person and demonstrates normal attention span
   c. Has serum ammonia level within normal limits
   d. Identifies early, reportable signs of impaired thought processes

Bleeding Esophageal Varices

Bleeding or hemorrhage from esophageal varices occurs in approximately one third of patients with cirrhosis and varices. The mortality rate resulting from the first bleeding episode is 45% to 50%; it is one of the major causes of death in patients with cirrhosis. The mortality rate increases with each subsequent bleeding episode.

Pathophysiology

Esophageal varices are dilated, tortuous veins usually found in the submucosa of the lower esophagus; however, they may develop higher in the esophagus or extend into the stomach. This condition nearly always is caused by portal hypertension, which, in turn, is due to obstruction of the portal venous circulation within the cirrhotic liver.

Because of increased obstruction of the portal vein, venous blood from the intestinal tract and spleen seeks an outlet through collateral circulation (new pathways of return to the right atrium). The effect is increased pressure, particularly in the vessels in the submucosal layer of the lower esophagus and upper part of the stomach. These collateral vessels are not very elastic but rather are tortuous and fragile and bleed easily. Other less common causes of varices are abnormalities of the circulation in the splenic vein or superior vena cava and hepatic venothrombosis.

Bleeding esophageal varices are life-threatening and can result in hemorrhagic shock, producing decreased cerebral, hepatic, and renal perfusion. In turn, there is an increased nitrogen load from bleeding into the GI tract and an increased serum ammonia level, which increase the risk of encephalopathy. Usually, the dilated veins cause no symptoms unless the portal pressure increases sharply and the mucosa or supporting structures become thin. Then massive hemorrhage takes place.

Factors that contribute to hemorrhage are muscular exertion from lifting heavy objects; straining at stool; sneezing, coughing, or vomiting; esophagitis; irritation of vessels by poorly chewed foods or irritating fluids; or reflux of stomach contents (especially alcohol). Salicylates and any medication that erodes the esophageal mucosa or interferes with cell replication also may contribute to bleeding.

Clinical Manifestations

The patient with bleeding esophageal varices may present with hematemesis, melena, or general deterioration in mental or physical status, and often has a history of alcohol abuse. Signs and symptoms of shock (cool clammy skin, hypotension, tachycardia) may be present.

Assessment and Diagnostic Findings

Endoscopy is used to identify the bleeding site, along with barium swallow, ultrasound, CT scan, and angiography.

ENDOSCOPY

Immediate endoscopy is indicated to identify the cause and the site of bleeding; at least 30% of patients suspected of bleeding from esophageal varices bleed from other sources (gastritis, ulcers). Nursing support can be effective in relieving anxiety during this often stressful experience. Careful monitoring can detect early signs of cardiac dysrhythmias, perforation, and hemorrhage.

After the examination, fluids are not given until the patient's gag reflex returns. Lozenges and gargles may be used to relieve throat discomfort if the patient's physical condition and mental status permit. If the patient is actively bleeding, oral intake will not be permitted and the patient will be prepared for further diagnostic and therapeutic procedures.

PORTAL HYPERTENSION MEASUREMENTS

Portal hypertension may be suspected if dilated abdominal veins and rectal hemorrhoids are detected. A palpable enlarged spleen (splenomegaly) and ascites may also be present.

Portal venous pressure can be measured directly or indirectly. Indirect measurement of the hepatic vein pressure gradient is the most commonly used procedure; it requires insertion of a fluid-filled balloon catheter into the antecubital or femoral vein. The catheter is advanced under fluoroscopy to a hepatic vein. A "wedged" pressure (similar to pulmonary artery wedge pressure) is obtained by occluding the blood flow in the blood vessel; pressure in the unoccluded vessel is also measured. Although the values obtained may underestimate portal pressure, this measurement may be obtained several times to evaluate the results of therapy.

Direct measurement of portal vein pressure can be obtained by several methods. One method is used when the patient is undergoing laparotomy by introducing a needle into the spleen; a manometer reading of more than 20 mL saline is abnormal. Another direct measurement requires insertion of a catheter into the portal vein or one of its branches. Endoscopic measurement of pressure within varices is used only in conjunction with endoscopic sclerotherapy.

LABORATORY TESTS

Laboratory tests that may be required include various liver function tests, such as serum aminotransferase (transaminase), bilirubin, alkaline phosphatase, and serum proteins. Blood flow and clearance studies also may be performed to assess cardiac output and hepatic blood flow.

Splenoportography involves serial or segmental x-rays to detect extensive collateral circulation in esophageal vessels, which would be indicative of varices. Other tests are hepatoportography and celiac angiography. These are usually performed in the operating room or radiology department.

Medical Management

Bleeding from esophageal varices can quickly lead to hemorrhagic shock and is an emergency. This patient is critically ill, requiring aggressive medical care and expert nursing care, and is usually transferred to the intensive care unit for close monitoring and management. See Chapter 14 for a discussion of care of the patient in shock.

The extent of bleeding is evaluated and vital signs are monitored continuously when hematemesis and melena are present.

Signs of potential hypovolemia are noted, such as cold clammy skin, tachycardia, a drop in blood pressure, decreased urine output, restlessness, and increased or shallow peripheral pulses. Blood volume is monitored by means of a central venous pressure or arterial catheter. Oxygen is administered to prevent hypoxia and to maintain adequate blood oxygenation.

Because patients with bleeding esophageal varices have intravascular volume depletion and are subject to electrolyte imbalance, IV fluids with electrolytes and volume expanders are provided to restore fluid volume and replace electrolytes. Transfusion of blood components also may be required. An indwelling urinary catheter is usually inserted to permit frequent monitoring of urine output.

A variety of pharmacologic, endoscopic, and surgical approaches are used to treat bleeding esophageal varices; however, none of them is ideal, and most are associated with considerable risk to the patient. Child's classification is used to identify appropriate treatment approaches (see Table 36-4).

NONSURGICAL MANAGEMENT

Nonsurgical treatment of bleeding esophageal varices is preferable because of the high mortality rate of emergency surgery for control of bleeding esophageal varices and because of the poor physical condition of the patient with severe liver dysfunction.

Pharmacologic Therapy. Vasopressin (Pitressin) may be the initial mode of therapy because it produces constriction of the splanchnic arterial bed and a resulting decrease in portal pressure. It may be administered intravenously or by intra-arterial infusion. Either method requires close monitoring by the nurse. The presence or absence of blood in the gastric aspirate and monitoring of vital signs provide indices of the effectiveness of vasopressin. Monitoring of fluid intake and output and electrolyte levels is necessary because hyponatremia may occur and vasopressin may have an antidiuretic effect.

Coronary artery disease in this patient is a contraindication to the use of vasopressin, because coronary vasoconstriction is a side effect that may precipitate myocardial infarction.

The combination of vasopressin and nitroglycerin (administered by the IV, sublingual, or transdermal route) has been effective in reducing or preventing the side effects (constriction of coronary vessels and angina) caused by vasopressin alone.

Somatostatin has been reported to be more effective than vasopressin in decreasing bleeding from esophageal varices without the vasoconstrictive effects of vasopressin. Propranolol, a beta-blocking agent that decreases portal pressure, has been shown to prevent bleeding from esophageal varices in some patients; however, it is recommended that it be used only in combination with other treatment modalities such as **sclerotherapy**, **variceal banding**, or **balloon tamponade**. Further studies of these and other medications are necessary to evaluate their use in the treatment and prevention of bleeding episodes.

Balloon Tamponade. To control the hemorrhage in certain patients, pressure is exerted on the cardia (upper orifice of the stomach) and against the bleeding varices by a double-balloon tamponade (Sengstaken–Blakemore tube) (Fig. 36-9). The tube has four openings, each with a specific purpose: gastric aspiration, esophageal aspiration, inflation of the gastric balloon, and inflation of the esophageal balloon.

The balloon in the stomach is inflated with 100 to 200 mL of air. An x-ray confirms proper positioning of the gastric balloon. Then the tube is pulled gently to exert a force against the cardia. Traction may be applied with weights or by attachment to a football helmet. Irrigation of the tubing is performed to detect bleeding; if returns are clear, the esophageal balloon is not inflated. If bleeding continues, the esophageal balloon is inflated. The desired pressure in the esophageal and gastric balloons is 25 to 40 mm Hg, as measured by the manometer. After the esophageal balloon is inflated, there is a possibility of injury or rupture of the esophagus. Constant nursing surveillance is necessary at this time.

Gastric suction is provided by connecting the proper catheter outlet to suction. The tubing is irrigated hourly, and drainage will indicate whether bleeding has been controlled. Room-temperature lavage or irrigation may be used in the gastric balloon. The pressure within the esophageal balloon is measured and recorded every 2 to 4 hours via the manometer to detect underinflation or overinflation with potential for esophageal injury. The balloons are carefully sequentially deflated. The esophageal balloon is deflated first and the patient is monitored for recurrent bleeding. After several hours without bleeding, the gastric balloon may be deflated safely. If there is still no bleeding, the tamponade tube is removed. The therapy is used for as short a time as possible (ie, several hours to 2 days) to stop the bleeding while avoiding complications.

Although balloon tamponade has been fairly successful, it is important to note some inherent dangers. Ulceration and necrosis of the nose, the mucosa of the stomach, or the esophagus may occur if the tube is left in place or inflated too long or at too high a pressure. Sudden rupture of the balloon is disastrous—airway obstruction and aspiration of gastric contents into the lungs can occur. Using a new tube that is tested before insertion may minimize this risk. Asphyxiation is another problem, caused by accidental pulling of the tube and inflated balloon into the oropharynx. Aspiration of blood and secretions into the lungs is frequently associated with the use of balloon tamponade, especially in the stuporous or comatose patient. Endotracheal intubation before insertion of the tube protects the airway and minimizes the risk of aspiration.

These potential complications necessitate intensive and expert care. A confused or restless patient with this tube in place and balloons inflated should not be left alone because of these risks. Nursing measures include frequent mouth and nasal care. For secretions that accumulate in the mouth, tissues should be within easy reach of the patient. Oral suction may be necessary to remove oral secretions.

The patient with esophageal hemorrhage is usually extremely anxious and frightened. Knowing that the nurse is nearby and will respond immediately can help alleviate some of this anxiety. Tube insertion is uncomfortable and never pleasant. Explanations during the procedure and while the tube is in place may be reassuring to the patient.

Although the use of balloon tamponade effectively stops the bleeding in most patients (90%), bleeding recurs in the majority of patients (60% to 70%), necessitating other treatment modalities (ie, sclerotherapy or banding). Once the balloons are deflated or the tube is removed, the patient must be assessed frequently because of the high risk of recurrent bleeding.

Endoscopic Sclerotherapy. In endoscopic sclerotherapy (Fig. 36-10) (also referred to as injection sclerotherapy), a sclerosing agent is injected through a fiber-optic endoscope into the bleeding esophageal varices to promote thrombosis and eventual sclerosis. Although the superiority of endoscopic sclerotherapy over other treatments continues to be the subject of study, the procedure has been used successfully to treat acute GI hemorrhage. In

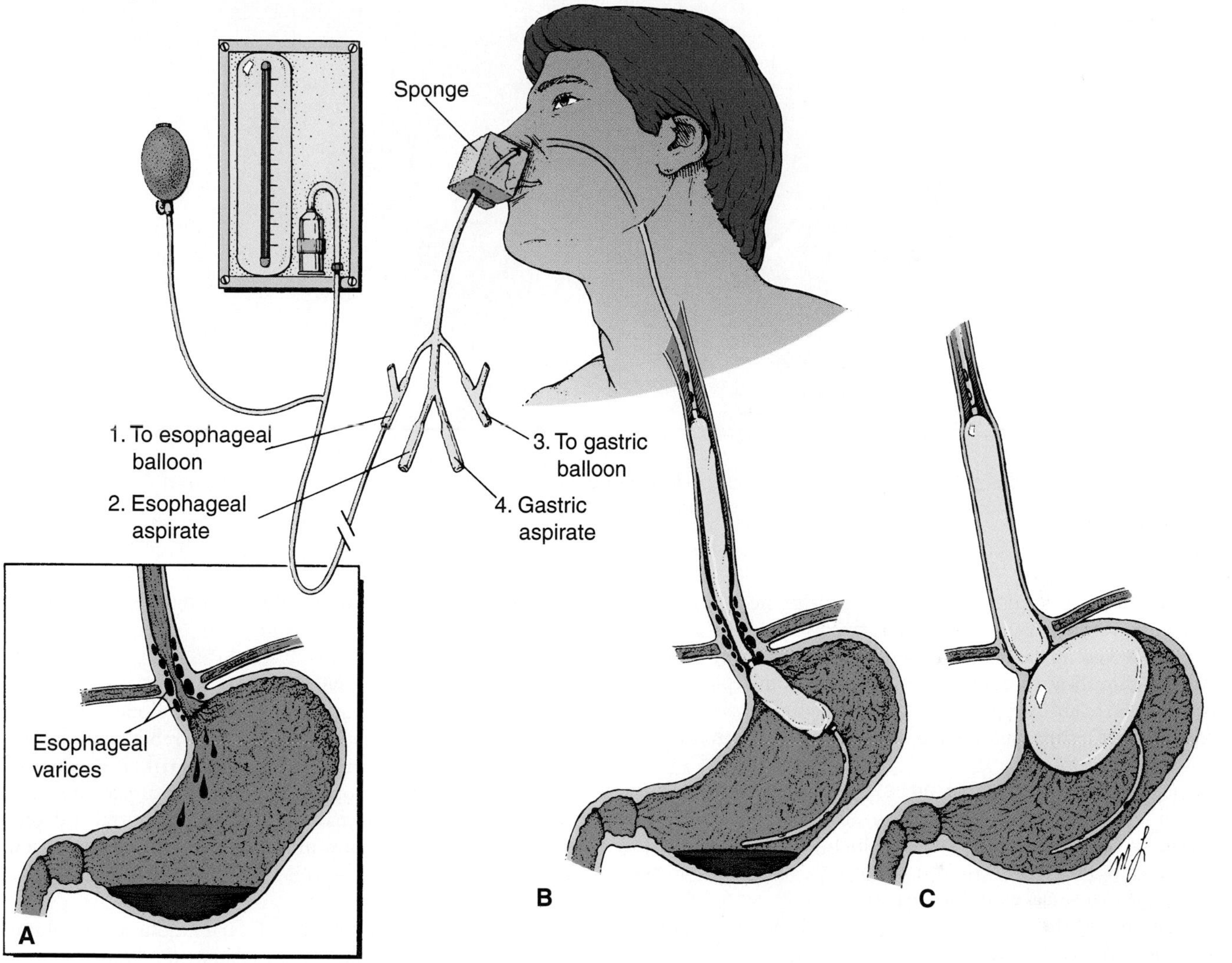

FIGURE 36•9 Esophageal balloon tamponade to treat esophageal varices. (**A**) Dilated, bleeding esophageal veins (varices) of the lower esophagus. (**B**) A four-lumen esophageal tamponade tube with balloons (uninflated) in place. (**C**) Compression of bleeding esophageal varices by inflated esophageal and gastric balloons. The gastric and esophageal outlets permit the nurse to aspirate secretions.

addition, it has been used to treat esophageal varices before bleeding has occurred; however, its use as a preventive measure is also controversial because of the inability to predict which patients with esophageal varices will bleed and which will not.

After treatment, the patient must be observed for bleeding, perforation of the esophagus, aspiration pneumonia, and esophageal stricture. Antacids may be administered after the procedure to counteract the effects of peptic reflux.

Repeated courses of sclerotherapy may be needed to obliterate all the varices. The patient and family need to be aware of the importance of these additional treatments and continued long-term follow-up, even though the patient may not be actively bleeding.

Esophageal Banding Therapy (Variceal Band Ligation). In esophageal banding therapy (Fig. 36-11), a modified endoscope loaded with an elastic rubber band is passed through an overtube directly onto the varix (or varices) to be banded. After suctioning the bleeding varix into the tip of the endoscope, the

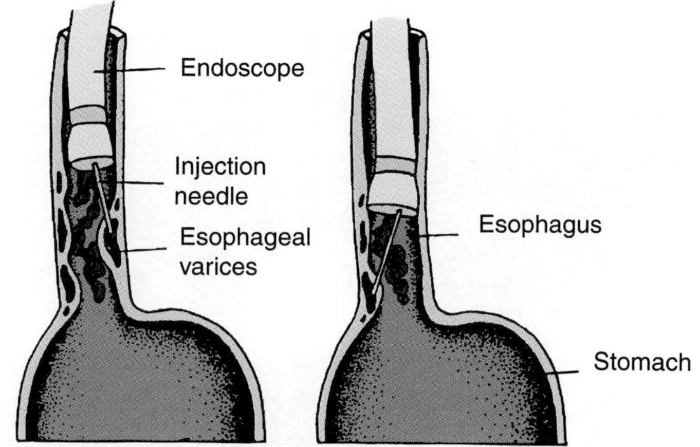

FIGURE 36•10 Injection sclerotherapy. Injection of sclerosing agent into esophageal varices through an endoscope promotes thrombosis and eventual sclerosis, thereby obliterating the varices.

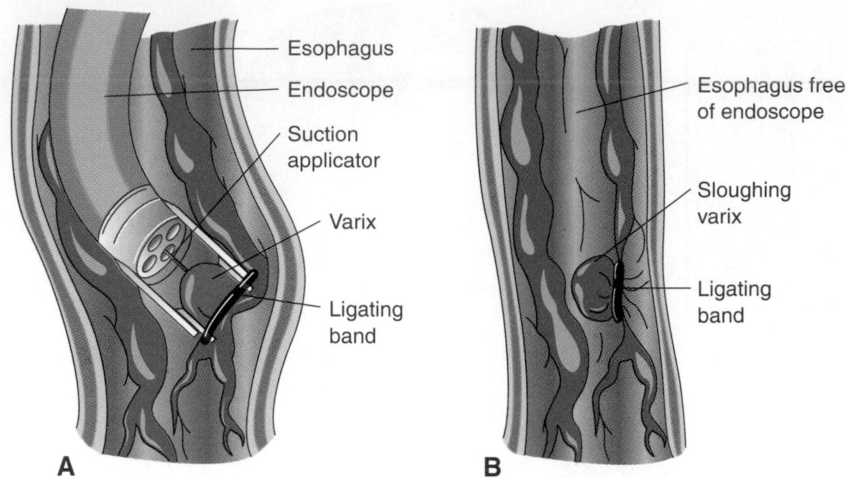

FIGURE 36•11 Esophageal banding. (**A**) A rubberband-like ligature is slipped over an esophageal varix via an endoscope. (**B**) Necrosis results and the varix eventually sloughs off.

rubber band is slipped over the tissue, causing necrosis, ulceration, and eventual sloughing of the varix.

There are completed and ongoing studies comparing the effectiveness, complications, and incidence of rebleeding episodes with banding and sclerotherapy. Although both techniques have advantages, further testing is needed to compare their effectiveness.

Transjugular Intrahepatic Portosystemic Shunting. Transjugular intrahepatic portosystemic shunting (TIPS) is a method of treatment for esophageal varices in which a cannula is threaded into the portal vein by the transjugular route. An expandable stent is inserted that serves as an intrahepatic shunt between the portal circulation and the hepatic vein (Fig. 36-12), thereby reducing portal hypertension.

Because results of studies of the effectiveness of TIPS are inconclusive, this approach is generally reserved for situations in which other approaches are unavailable or unsuccessful. Whereas sclerotherapy and esophageal banding are done to eradicate active bleeding sites, TIPS is usually performed afterward in an attempt to address the cause of the bleeding by decreasing portal hypertension.

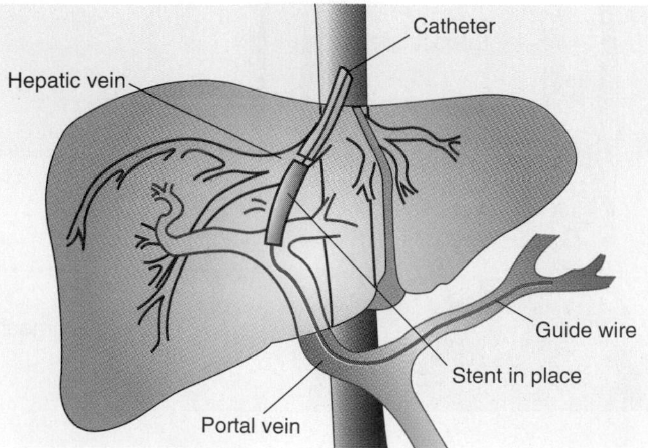

FIGURE 36•12 Transjugular intrahepatic portosystemic shunt (TIPS). A stent is inserted via catheter to the portal vein to divert blood flow and reduce portal hypertension.

SURGICAL MANAGEMENT

Several surgical procedures have been developed and used to treat esophageal varices and to minimize rebleeding; however, they are often accompanied by significant risk. Procedures that may be employed for esophageal varices are direct surgical ligation of varices; splenorenal, mesocaval, and portacaval venous shunts to relieve portal pressure; and esophageal transection with devascularization.

Surgical Bypass Procedures. Of the various surgical shunting procedures (Fig. 36-13), the distal splenorenal shunt described by Warren is the most widely used. This is a shunt made between the splenic vein and the left renal vein after splenectomy. A mesocaval shunt is created surgically by anastomosis of the superior mesenteric vein to the proximal end of the vena cava or to the side of the vena cava with grafting material. The goal of distal splenorenal and mesocaval shunts is to drain only a portion of venous blood from the portal bed to decrease portal pressure; thus, they are considered selective shunts. The liver continues to receive some portal flow, and the incidence of encephalopathy in the postoperative period may thus be reduced. Numerous controlled trials have demonstrated that the Warren distal splenorenal shunt carries the least risk of encephalopathy (Jaffe et al., 1996; Rosemurgy et al., 1996).

Portacaval shunts divert all portal flow to the vena cava via end-to-side or side-to-side approaches; therefore, they are considered nonselective shunts. Although still performed, this procedure is no longer standard surgical therapy because of the high risk of encephalopathy and other complications.

All of these procedures are extensive and are not always successful because of secondary thrombosis in the veins used for the shunt as well as resultant complications (encephalopathy, accelerated liver failure). There has been no difference shown in outcomes or mortality rates between the various surgical shunting procedures except for a decreased risk of encephalopathy with the selective shunts. Severity of the disease (by Child's classification) as well as the potential for future liver transplantation also guides the choice of intervention. If the cause of portal hypertension is the rare Budd-Chiari syndrome or other venous obstructive disease, a portacaval

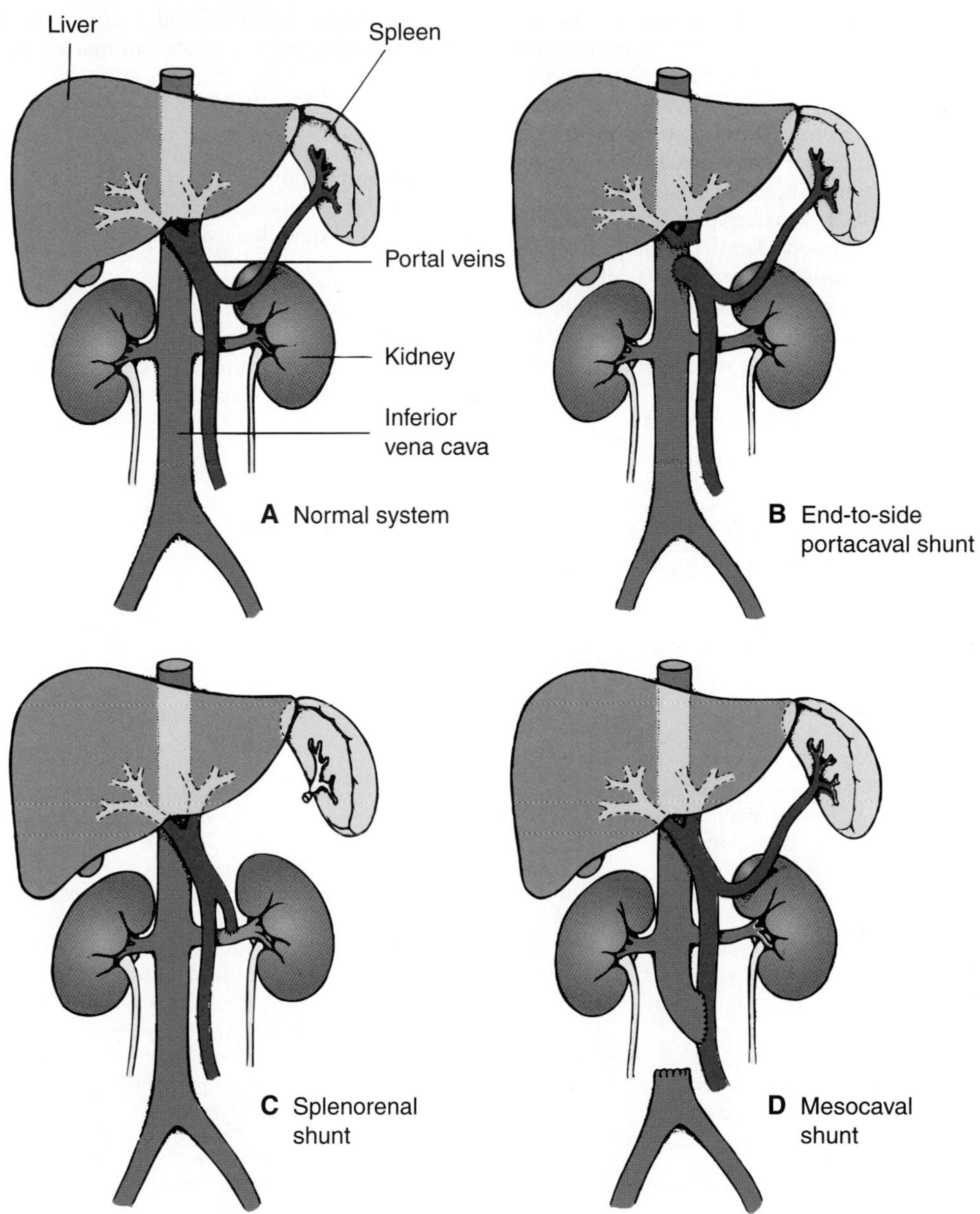

FIGURE 36•13 Portal systemic shunts. Normal portal system is shown in **A**; examples of portal shunts to reduce portal pressure are shown in **B** to **D**.

or a mesoatrial shunt may be performed (see Fig. 36-13). The mesoatrial shunt is required when the infrahepatic vena cava is thrombosed and must be bypassed.

Devascularization and Transection. Devascularization and staple-gun transection procedures to separate the bleeding site from the high-pressure portal system have been used in the emergency management of variceal bleeding. The lower end of the esophagus is reached through a small gastrostomy incision; a staple gun permits anastomosis of the transected ends of the esophagus. Rebleeding is a risk, and the outcomes of these procedures vary among patient populations.

Nursing Alert *Postoperative care is similar to that for any abdominal surgery, but the risk for complications (hypovolemic or hemorrhagic shock, hepatic encephalopathy, electrolyte imbalance, metabolic and respiratory alkalosis, alcohol withdrawal syndrome, and seizures) is high. The surgical procedures do not alter the course of the progressive liver disease, and bleeding may recur as new collateral vessels develop.*

Nursing Management

Overall nursing assessment includes monitoring the patient's physical condition and evaluating emotional responses and cognitive status. Vital signs are monitored and recorded, and the patient's nutritional status is assessed. Neurologic assessment will assist in identifying possible hepatic encephalopathy resulting from the breakdown of blood in the GI tract and a rising serum ammonia level. Manifestations range from drowsiness to encephalopathy and coma.

Bleeding may be treated by complete rest of the esophagus; therefore, total parenteral nutrition is initiated. Straining and vomiting must be prevented. Gastric suction usually is initiated to keep the stomach as empty as possible. The patient often complains of severe thirst, which may be relieved by frequent oral hygiene and moist sponges to the lips. The nurse closely monitors the patient's blood pressure. Vitamin K therapy and multiple blood transfusions often are indicated because of blood loss. A quiet environment and calm reassurance will help to relieve the patient's anxiety and reduce agitation.

Bleeding anywhere in the body is anxiety-provoking, resulting in a crisis situation for the patient and family. If the patient has been a heavy user of alcohol, delirium secondary to alcohol withdrawal can complicate the situation. The nurse provides support and pertinent explanations regarding medical and nursing interventions. Monitoring the patient closely will help in detecting and managing complications.

Management modalities and nursing care of the patient with bleeding esophageal varices are summarized in Table 36-5.

Cancer of the Liver

Hepatic tumors may be malignant or benign. Benign liver tumors were uncommon until the widespread use of oral contraceptives. With the use of oral contraceptives, benign tumors of the liver occur most frequently in women in their reproductive years.

Primary Liver Tumors

Few cancers originate in the liver. Primary liver tumors usually are associated with chronic liver disease, hepatitis B and C infections, and cirrhosis. Hepatocellular carcinoma (HCC) is by far

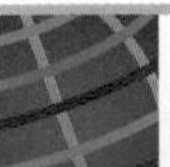

TABLE 36•5 Management Modalities and Nursing Care for the Patient With Bleeding Esophageal Varices

Treatment Modality*	Action	Nursing Priorities
Nonsurgical Modalities		
Pharmacologic agents		
vasopressin (Pitressin)	Reduces portal pressure by constricting splanchnic arteries	Observe response to therapy. Monitor for side effects. (*Vasopressin:* angina. Nitroglycerin may be prescribed to prevent or treat angina.
propranolol (Inderal)	Reduces portal pressure by β-adrenergic blocking action	*Propranolol:* decreased pulse and blood pressure, impaired cardiovascular response to hemorrhage.)
somatostatin	Reduces portal pressure by selective vasodilation of portal system	Administer medication as prescribed. Support patient during treatment.
Balloon tamponade	Exerts pressure directly to bleeding sites in esophagus and stomach	Monitor closely to prevent accidental removal or displacement of tube, subsequent airway obstruction, and aspiration. Explain procedure to patient briefly to obtain cooperation with insertion and maintenance of esophageal tamponade tube and reduce patient's fear of the procedure. Provide frequent oral hygiene. Report onset of chest pain.
Room-temperature saline lavage	Clears blood and secretions before endoscopy and other procedures	Ensure patency of the nasogastric tube to prevent aspiration. Observe gastric aspirate for blood and cessation of bleeding.
Injection sclerotherapy	Promotes thrombosis and sclerosing of bleeding sites by injection of sclerosing agent into the esophageal varices	Observe for aspiration, perforation of the esophagus, and recurrence of bleeding after treatment.
Variceal banding	Provides thrombosis and mucosal necrosis of bleeding sites by band ligation	Observe for recurrence of bleeding, esophageal perforation.
Transjugular intrahepatic portosystemic shunting (TIPS)	Reduces portal pressure by creating a shunt within the liver between the portal and systemic venous system.	Observe for rebleeding and signs of infection.
Surgical Modalities		
Portal-systemic shunting	Reduces portal hypertension by diverting blood flow away from obstructed portal system	Observe for development of portal-systemic encephalopathy (altered mental status, neurologic dysfunction), hepatic failure, and rebleeding. Requires intensive, expert nursing care for prolonged period.
Surgical ligation of varices	Ties off blood vessels at the site of bleeding	Observe for rebleeding.
Esophageal transection and devascularization	Separates bleeding site from portal system	Observe for rebleeding. Provide postthoracotomy care.

*Several modalities may be used concurrently or in sequence.

the most common type of primary liver cancer. HCC is usually nonresectable because of rapid growth and metastasis. Other types of primary liver cancer include cholangiocellular carcinoma and combined hepatocellular and cholangiocellular carcinoma. If found early, resection may be possible, but the likelihood of early detection is small.

Cirrhosis, chronic infection with hepatitis B and C, and exposure to certain chemical toxins (eg, vinyl chloride, arsenic) have been implicated as causes of HCC. Cigarette smoking has also been identified as a risk factor, especially when combined with alcohol use. Some evidence suggests that aflatoxin, a metabolite of the fungus *Aspergillus flavus,* may be a risk factor for HCC. This is especially true for areas where HCC is endemic (ie, Asia and Africa). Aflatoxin and other similar toxic molds can contaminate food such as ground nuts and grains and may act as a cocarcinogen with hepatitis B. The risk of contamination is greatest when storage conditions are tropical or subtropical.

Liver Metastases

Metastases from other primary sites are found in the liver in about half of all advanced cancer cases. Malignant tumors are likely to reach the liver eventually, by way of the portal system or lymphatic channels, or by direct extension from an abdominal tumor. Moreover, the liver apparently is an ideal place for these malignant cells to thrive. Often the first evidence of cancer in an abdominal organ is the appearance of liver metastases; unless exploratory surgery or an autopsy is performed, the primary tumor may never be identified.

Clinical Manifestations

The early manifestations of malignancy of the liver include pain, a continuous dull ache in the right upper quadrant, epigastrium, or back. Weight loss, loss of strength, anorexia, and anemia may also occur. The liver may be enlarged and irregular on palpation. Jaundice is present only if the larger bile ducts are occluded by the pressure of malignant nodules in the hilum of the liver. Ascites occurs if such nodules obstruct the portal veins or if tumor tissue is seeded in the peritoneal cavity.

Assessment and Diagnostic Findings

The diagnosis of cancer of the liver is made on the basis of clinical signs and symptoms, the history and physical examination, and the results of laboratory and x-ray studies. Increased serum levels of bilirubin, alkaline phosphatase, AST (SGOT), GGT, and lactic dehydrogenase may occur. Leukocytosis (increased white blood cells), erythrocytosis (increased red blood cells), hypercalcemia, hypoglycemia, and hypocholesterolemia may also be seen on laboratory assessment.

The serum level of alpha fetoprotein, which serves as a tumor marker, is abnormally elevated in 30% to 40% of patients with liver cancer. Carcinoembryonic antigen, which serves as a marker of advanced cancer of the digestive tract, may be elevated. These two markers together are useful to distinguish between metastatic liver disease and primary liver cancer.

Many patients have metastases from the primary liver tumor to other sites by the time diagnosis is made; metastases occur primarily to the lung but may also occur to regional lymph nodes, adrenals, bone, kidneys, heart, pancreas, and stomach.

X-rays, liver scans, CT scans, ultrasound studies, MRI, arteriography, and laparoscopy may be part of the diagnostic workup and may be performed to determine the extent of the cancer.

Confirmation of a tumor's histology can be made by biopsy under imaging guidance (CT scan or ultrasound) or laparoscopically. Local or systemic dissemination of the tumor by needle biopsy or fine-needle biopsy can occur but is rare. Some clinicians believe that these procedures should not be performed if the tumor is thought to be resectable; rather, diagnosis should be confirmed by frozen section at the time of laparotomy for primary HCC.

Nonsurgical Management

Although surgical resection of the liver tumor is possible in some patients, the underlying cirrhosis, so prevalent in cancer of the liver, increases the risks associated with surgery. Radiation therapy and chemotherapy have been used in the treatment of malignant disease of the liver with varying degrees of success. Although these therapies may prolong survival and improve the patient's quality of life by reducing pain and discomfort, their major effect is palliative.

RADIATION THERAPY

Pain and discomfort have been effectively reduced in 70% to 90% of patients with radiation therapy; anorexia, weakness, and fever also have been reduced. Liver function tests may improve temporarily. Methods of delivering radiation include: (1) IV injection of antibodies that are tagged with radioactive isotopes and specifically attack tumor-associated antigens and (2) percutaneous placement of a high-intensity source for interstitial radiation therapy. Their purpose is to deliver radiation directly to the tumor cells. External radiation therapy combined with chemotherapy has also been attempted, with no additional benefit demonstrated.

CHEMOTHERAPY

Chemotherapy has been used to improve the patient's quality of life and prolong survival; it also may be used as adjuvant therapy after surgical resection of hepatic tumors. Systemic chemotherapy and regional infusion chemotherapy are two methods used to administer antineoplastic agents to patients with primary and metastatic hepatic tumors.

An implantable pump has been used to deliver a high concentration of chemotherapy to the liver through the hepatic artery. This method provides a reliable, controlled, and continuous infusion of medication that can be carried out in the patient's home.

PERCUTANEOUS BILIARY DRAINAGE

Percutaneous biliary or transhepatic drainage is used to bypass biliary ducts obstructed by liver, pancreatic, or bile duct tumors in patients with inoperable tumors or in those considered poor surgical risks. Under fluoroscopy, a catheter is inserted through the abdominal wall, past the obstruction into the duodenum. Such procedures are used to reestablish biliary drainage, relieve pressure and pain from the buildup of bile behind the obstruction, and decrease pruritus and jaundice. As a result, the patient is made more comfortable and quality of life and survival are improved.

For several days after its insertion, the catheter is opened to external drainage. The bile is observed closely for the amount, color, and the presence of blood and debris. Complications of percutaneous biliary drainage include sepsis, leakage of bile, hemorrhage, and reobstruction of the biliary system by debris in the catheter or from encroaching tumor. Therefore, the patient is observed for fever and chills, bile drainage around the catheter, changes in vital signs, and evidence of biliary obstruction, including increased pain or pressure, pruritus, and recurrence of jaundice.

OTHER NONSURGICAL TREATMENTS

Laser hyperthermia has been used to treat hepatic metastases. Heat has been directed to tumors through several methods to cause necrosis of the tumors while sparing normal tissue. Immunotherapy is another treatment modality under investigation. In this therapy, lymphocytes with antitumor reactivity are administered to the patient with hepatic cancer. Regression of the tumor, the desired outcome, has been demonstrated in patients with metastatic cancer in whom standard treatment has failed. Transcatheter arterial embolization interrupts the arterial blood flow to small tumors by the injection of small particulate embolic and/or chemotherapeutic agents into the artery supplying the tumor. Ischemia and necrosis of the tumor result. For multiple small lesions, ultrasound-guided injection of alcohol causes dehydration of tumor cells and tumor necrosis.

Nursing Management

The patient with cancer of the liver may receive chemotherapy or radiation therapy in an effort to relieve symptoms and may go home while still receiving one or both of these therapies. The patient may also be discharged home with a biliary drainage system in place. Because of the need for the patient to participate in care and the family's role in care at home, the need for teaching is great.

PROMOTING HOME AND COMMUNITY-BASED CARE

Teaching Patients Self-Care. Patients are instructed to assess and report complications and side effects of the chemotherapy that may occur and are informed about the actions and desired and undesirable effects of the specific chemotherapy agent used. They are instructed about the importance of follow-up visits to permit frequent assessments of the response of the patient and the tumor to chemotherapy and radiation therapy. If the patient is receiving chemotherapy at home, the patient and family are instructed about their role in management of the chemotherapy infusion and in assessment of the chemotherapy infusion/insertion site. The patient is encouraged to resume routine activities as soon as possible but cautioned to avoid activities that may damage the pump.

The family and the patient at home with a biliary drainage system in place typically fear that the catheter will be dislodged. They need reassurance and instruction to reduce their fear that the catheter will fall out easily. The patient and family also require instruction on catheter care. They are instructed in techniques to keep the catheter site clean and dry and to assess the catheter and its insertion site. Irrigation of the catheter with sterile normal saline or water may be prescribed to keep the catheter patent and free of debris. The patient and caregivers are taught proper technique to avoid introducing bacteria into the biliary system or catheter during irrigation. They are instructed not to aspirate or draw back on the syringe during irrigation to prevent entry of irritating duodenal contents into the biliary tree or catheter. The patient and caregivers are also instructed about the signs of complications and are encouraged to notify the nurse or physician if problems or questions occur.

Continuing Care. Referral for home care may be important in allowing the patient with liver cancer to be at home in a familiar environment with family and friends available. Because of the poor prognosis associated with liver cancer, the home care nurse serves a vital role in assisting the patient and family to cope with the symptoms that may occur and the prognosis. The home care nurse assesses the patient's physical and psychological status, the adequacy of pain relief, nutritional status, and the presence of symptoms indicating complications of treatment or progression of disease. During home visits, the nurse assesses the function of the chemotherapy pump and the biliary drainage system, if indicated. The nurse collaborates with the other members of the health care team, the patient, and the family to ensure effective pain management and to manage other problems that may occur: weakness, pruritus, inadequate dietary intake, jaundice, and symptoms associated with metastasis to other sites. The home care nurse also assists the patient and family in making decisions about hospice care and assists with initiation of referrals. The patient is encouraged to discuss preferences for end-of-life care with family members and health care providers.

Surgical Management

Surgical resection is the treatment of choice when HCC is confined to one lobe of the liver and the function of the remaining liver is considered adequate for postoperative recovery. In the case of metastasis, hepatic resection can be performed when the primary site can be completely excised and the metastasis is limited. Metastases to the liver, however, are rarely limited or solitary. Capitalizing on the regenerative capacity of the liver cells, some surgeons have successfully removed 90% of the liver. However, the presence of cirrhosis limits the ability of the liver to regenerate. Staging of liver tumors aids in predicting the likelihood of surgical cure. A staging system for liver tumors is summarized in Table 36-6.

In preparation for surgery, the patient's nutritional, fluid, and general physical status is assessed and efforts are undertaken to ensure as optimal a physical condition as possible. Support, explanation, and encouragement are provided to help the patient prepare psychologically for the surgery.

Meanwhile, extensive and exhausting diagnostic studies may be performed. It may be necessary to prepare the intestinal tract by way of cathartics, colonic irrigation, and intestinal antibiotics to minimize the possibility of ammonium accumulation and to anticipate the possibility of incision into the intestines at surgery. Specific studies may include liver scan, liver biopsy, cholangiography, selective hepatic angiography, percutaneous needle biopsy, peritoneoscopy, laparoscopy, ultrasound, CT scans, MRI, and blood tests, particularly determinations of serum alkaline phosphatase, AST (SGOT), and GGT and its isoenzymes.

LOBECTOMY

Removal of a lobe of the liver is the most common surgical procedure used to remove a tumor of the liver. If it is necessary to restrict blood flow from the hepatic artery and portal vein beyond 15 minutes, it is likely that hypothermia will be used. Most surgeons prefer the anatomic (surgical) division of the lobes. Here the liver is divided into a right and a left lobe by a lobar fissure that is almost in line with the gallbladder bed and the inferior vena cava on the visceral surface. According to this division, the branching of hepatic vessels and the portal vein lends itself to a more even segmentation.

For a right-liver lobectomy or an extended right lobectomy (including the medial left lobe), a thoracoabdominal incision is used. An extensive abdominal incision is made for a left lobectomy.

CRYOSURGERY

Cryosurgery (**cryoablation**) is a technique in which tumors are destroyed using liquid nitrogen at −196°C. Two or three freeze-and-thaw cycles are administered via probes to cause tissue destruction during open laparotomy. This technique has been used alone or as an adjunct to hepatic resection in HCC and colorectal metas-

TABLE 36•6 **TNM* Staging for Hepatoma**

Stage I	T1	N0	M0
Stage II	T2	N0	M0
Stage III	T1	N1	M0
	T2	N1	M0
	T3	N0	M0
	T3	N1	M0
Stage IVA	T4	Any N	M0
Stage IVB	Any T	Any N	M1

Tumor (T)

T1 Solitary tumor 2 cm or less in greatest dimension without vascular invasion

T2 Solitary tumor 2 cm or less in greatest dimension with vascular invasion, *or*
Multiple tumors limited to one lobe none more than 2 cm in greatest dimension without vascular invasion, *or*
A solitary tumor more than 2 cm in greatest dimension without vascular invasion

T3 Solitary tumor more than 2 cm in greatest dimension with vascular invasion, *or*
Multiple tumors limited to one lobe, none more than 2 cm in greatest dimension, with vascular invasion, *or*
Multiple tumors limited to one lobe, any more than 2 cm in greatest dimension, with or without vascular invasion

T4 Multiple tumors in more than one lobe *or*
Tumor(s) involve(s) a major branch of portal or hepatic vein(s)

Lymph Node (N)

N0 No regional lymph node metastasis
N1 Regional lymph node metastasis

Distant Metastasis (M)

M0 No distant metastasis
M1 Distant metastasis

* T, tumor; N, node; M, metastasis
From Fleming, I. D., et al. (Eds.). (1997). *Manual for staging of cancer* (5th ed.). Philadelphia: Lippincott-Raven.

tases not amenable to radical surgical excision. The efficacy of cryosurgery is still being evaluated, with indications and outcomes requiring further investigation.

LIVER TRANSPLANTATION

Removal of the liver and its replacement by a healthy donor organ has been performed to treat liver cancer. Recurrence of the primary liver malignancy after transplantation, however, has been reported to be 70% to 85%, and there is often a short survival time after recurrence. Metastasis and recurrence may be enhanced by the immunosuppression necessary to prevent rejection. Transplantation tends to be reserved for patients unsuitable for resection because of severe hepatocellular disease, bilateral large lesions, or centrally located tumors. This procedure is effective when few, small (5 cm or less) lesions are present (Sherlock & Dooley, 1997). See the discussion of liver transplantation that follows.

Postoperative Nursing Management

Potential problems related to cardiopulmonary involvement include vascular complications and respiratory and liver dysfunction. Metabolic abnormalities require careful attention. A constant infusion of 10% glucose may be required in the first 48 hours to prevent a precipitous fall in blood glucose resulting from decreased gluconeogenesis. Protein synthesis and lipid metabolism are also altered, necessitating infusions of albumin. Extensive blood loss may occur; as a result, the patient will receive infusions of blood and IV fluids.

The patient requires constant, close monitoring and care for the first 2 or 3 days, as described for abdominal and thoracic postsurgical nursing care. The patient undergoing cryosurgery is monitored closely for hypothermia, hemorrhage, or bile leak; myoglobinuria can occur as a result of tissue necrosis and is minimized by hydration, diuresis, and at times medications (allopurinol) to bind to and aid in the excretion of toxic products.

Liver Transplantation

Liver transplantation involves total removal of the diseased liver and its replacement with a healthy liver in the same anatomic location (orthotopic). Removal of the patient's liver leaves a space for the new liver and permits anatomic reconstruction of the hepatic vasculature and biliary tract as close to normal as possible.

Liver transplantation is used to treat life-threatening, end-stage liver disease for which no other form of treatment is available. The success of liver transplantation depends on successful immunosuppression. Immunosuppressants currently in use include cyclosporine, corticosteroids, azathioprine, mycophenolate mofetil, OKT3 (a monoclonal antibody), tacrolimus, sirolimus, and antithymocyte globulin. Studies are underway to find the most effective combination of immunosuppressive agents and to identify new agents with fewer side effects.

Despite the success of immunosuppression in reducing the incidence of rejection of transplanted organs, liver transplantation is not a routine procedure and may be accompanied by complications related to the lengthy surgical procedure, immunosuppressive therapy, infection, and the technical difficulties encountered in the reconstruction of blood vessels and the biliary tract. Longstanding systemic problems resulting from the primary liver disease may complicate the preoperative and postoperative course. Previous surgery of the abdomen, including procedures to treat complications of advanced liver disease (ie, shunt procedures used to treat portal hypertension and esophageal varices), increase the complexity of the transplantation procedure.

The indications for liver transplantation are not as limited today as a result of advances in immunosuppressive therapy, improvements in biliary tract reconstruction, and in some cases the use of venovenous bypass. General indications for liver transplantation include irreversible advanced chronic liver disease, fulminant hepatic failure, metabolic liver diseases, and some hepatic malignancies. Examples of disorders that are indications for liver transplantation include hepatocellular liver disease (eg, viral hepatitis, drug- and alcohol-induced liver disease, and Wilson's disease) and **cholestatic diseases** (primary biliary cirrhosis, sclerosing cholangitis, and biliary atresia).

The patient being considered for liver transplantation frequently has many systemic problems that influence preoperative and postoperative care. Because transplantation is more difficult when the patient has developed severe GI bleeding and hepatic coma, efforts are made to perform the procedure before this stage.

Liver transplantation is now recognized as an established therapeutic modality rather than as an experimental procedure to treat these disorders. As a result, centers where liver transplantation is performed are increasing in number. Patients requiring transplantation are often referred from distant hospitals to these sites. To prepare the potential patient and family for liver transplantation, nurses in all settings must understand the process and procedure of liver transplantation.

Surgical Procedure

The donor liver is freed from other structures, the bile is flushed from the gallbladder to prevent damage to the walls of the biliary tract, and the liver is perfused with a preservative and cooled. Before the donor liver is placed in the recipient, it is flushed with cold lactated Ringer's solution to remove potassium and air bubbles.

Anastomoses of the blood vessels and bile duct between the donor liver and the recipient's liver are performed. Biliary reconstruction is performed with an end-to-end anastomosis of the donor and recipient common bile ducts; a stented T-tube is inserted for external drainage of bile. If an end-to-end anastomosis is not possible because of diseased or absent bile ducts, an end-to-side anastomosis is made between the common bile duct of the graft and a loop (Roux-en-Y portion) of jejunum; in this case, bile drainage will be internal and a T-tube will not be inserted.

Liver transplantation is a long surgical procedure, partly because the patient with liver failure often has portal hypertension and subsequently many venous collateral vessels that must be ligated. Blood loss during the surgical procedure may be extensive. If the patient has adhesions from previous abdominal surgery, lysis of adhesions is often necessary. If a shunt procedure was performed previously, it must be surgically reversed to permit adequate portal venous blood supply to the new liver.

During the lengthy surgery, the family is often very anxious about the patient's well-being. Updating the family about the progress of the surgery and the patient's status is often helpful during the procedure.

Postoperative Complications

The postoperative complication rate is high, related primarily to technical complications or infection. Immediate postoperative complications may include bleeding, infection, rejection, and impaired biliary drainage. Disruption, infection, or obstruction of the biliary anastomosis may occur. Vascular thrombosis and stenosis are other potential complications.

Bleeding is common in the postoperative period and may result from coagulopathy, portal hypertension, and fibrinolysis caused by ischemic injury to the donor liver. Hypotension may occur in this phase secondary to blood loss. Administration of platelets, fresh-frozen plasma, and other blood products may be necessary. Hypertension is more common; however, its cause is uncertain. This is treated if blood pressure elevation is significant or sustained.

Infection is the leading cause of death after liver transplantation. Pulmonary and fungal infections are common; susceptibility to infection is increased by the immunosuppression needed to prevent rejection. Therefore, precautions must be taken to prevent nosocomial infections by strict asepsis when manipulating arterial lines and urine, bile, and other drainage systems; obtaining specimens; and changing dressings. Meticulous hand washing is also crucial.

Rejection is a key concern. A transplanted liver is perceived by the immune system as a foreign antigen. It triggers an immune response, leading to the activation of T lymphocytes that attack and destroy the transplanted liver. Immunosuppressive agents are used to prevent this response and rejection of the transplanted liver. These agents inhibit the activation of immunocompetent T lymphocytes to prevent the production of effector T cells.

Although the 1- and 5-year survival rates have increased dramatically since the advent of new immunosuppressive therapy, these advances are not without major side effects. A major side effect of cyclosporine, widely used in transplantation, is nephrotoxicity; this problem seems to be dose-related, and renal dysfunction can be reversed if the dose of cyclosporine is appropriately decreased or if its use is not initiated immediately.

Corticosteroids, azathioprine, mycophenolate mofetil, antithymocyte globulin, OKT3, and tacrolimus are also elements of the various regimens of immunosuppression and may be used as the initial therapy to prevent or later to treat rejection. Liver biopsy and ultrasound may be required to investigate suspected episodes of rejection.

Retransplantation is usually attempted if failure of the transplanted liver occurs. The success rate of retransplantation does not approach that of the initial transplantation, however.

Nursing Management

The patient considering transplantation and the family have difficult decisions to make about treatment, use of financial resources, and relocating to another area to be closer to the medical center. They also must cope with long-standing health problems and perhaps social and family problems associated with behaviors that may be responsible for the patient's liver failure. Therefore, the time during which the patient and family are considering liver transplantation and awaiting the news that a liver is available is often very stressful. The nurse must be aware of these issues and attuned to the emotional and psychological status of the patient and family. Referral of the patient and family to a psychiatric liaison nurse, psychologist, psychiatrist, or clergy may be in order to help them deal with the stressors associated with chronic liver disease and liver transplantation.

PREOPERATIVE NURSING INTERVENTIONS

If irreversible, severe liver dysfunction has been diagnosed, the patient may be considered a potential candidate for transplantation. An extensive diagnostic evaluation will be carried out to determine whether the patient is a candidate. The patient and family are given full explanations about the procedure and about the chances of success of transplantation and its risks, including the side effects of long-term immunosuppression. The need for close follow-up and lifelong compliance with the therapeutic regimen, including immunosuppression, is explained to the patient and family.

Once the patient is accepted as a candidate, his or her name is placed on a waiting list at the transplant center; patient information is entered into the United Network Organ Sharing (UNOS) computer system so that candidates may be identified and matched when appropriate organs become available.

Because a liver becomes available for transplantation only with the death of another individual, usually healthy except for severe brain injury and brain death, the patient and family undergo a stressful waiting period. The nurse is often the major source of support for the patient and family during this period. The patient must be accessible at all times in case an appropriate liver becomes available. During this time, liver function may deteriorate further and the patient may experience other complications from the primary liver disease. Because of the current shortage of donor organs, many patients die awaiting transplantation.

Malnutrition, massive ascites, and fluid and electrolyte disturbances are treated before surgery to increase the patient's chances of a successful outcome. If the patient's liver dysfunction has a very rapid onset, as in fulminant hepatic failure, there is little time or opportunity for the patient to consider and weigh options and their consequences; often this patient is in a coma, and the decision to proceed with transplantation is made by the patient's family.

The nurse coordinator is an integral member of the transplant team and plays an important role in preparing the patient for liver transplantation. The nurse serves as a patient and family advocate and assumes the important role of link between the patient and the other members of the transplant team. The nurse also serves as a resource to other nurses and health care team members involved in evaluating and caring for the patient undergoing this procedure.

POSTOPERATIVE NURSING INTERVENTIONS

The patient is maintained in an environment as free from bacteria, viruses, and fungi as possible, because immunosuppressive medications reduce the body's natural defenses.

In the immediate postoperative period, the patient's cardiovascular, pulmonary, renal, neurologic, and metabolic functions are monitored continuously. Mean arterial and pulmonary artery pressures are monitored continuously. Cardiac output, central venous pressure, pulmonary capillary wedge pressure, arterial and mixed venous blood gases, oxygen saturation, urine output, heart rate, and blood pressure are used to evaluate the patient's hemodynamic status and intravascular fluid volume. Liver function tests, electrolyte levels, the coagulation profile, chest x-ray, electrocardiogram, and fluid output including urine, bile, and drainage from Jackson-Pratt tubes are monitored closely. Because the liver is responsible for the storage of glycogen and the synthesis of protein and clotting factors, monitoring and replacement of these substances in the immediate postoperative period are essential.

Because of the likelihood of atelectasis and an altered ventilation–perfusion ratio as a result of the insult to the diaphragm during the surgical procedure, prolonged anesthesia, immobility, and postoperative pain, the patient will have an endotracheal tube in place and will require mechanical ventilation during the initial postoperative period. Suctioning is performed as required and sterile humidification is provided.

As the patient's vital signs and condition stabilize, efforts are made to assist the patient to recover from the trauma of this complex surgery. After removal of the endotracheal tube, the patient is encouraged to use an incentive spirometer to decrease the risk for atelectasis. Once the arterial lines and the urinary catheter are removed, the patient is assisted to get out of bed and to ambulate as tolerated and to participate in self-care to prevent the complications associated with immobility. Close monitoring for signs and symptoms of liver dysfunction and rejection will continue throughout the patient's hospital stay. Plans will be made for close follow-up after discharge as well. Teaching, initiated during the preoperative period, continues after surgery. Although care of the patient undergoing liver transplantation is not routine, there have been efforts to minimize the length of hospital stay of patients undergoing this complex surgery (Cabello & Tahan, 1998).

PROMOTING HOME AND COMMUNITY-BASED CARE

Teaching Patients Self-Care. Teaching the patient and family about long-term measures to promote health is crucial for success of the transplant and represents an important role of the nurse. The patient and family must understand the reasons for the need to adhere continuously to the therapeutic regimen, with special emphasis on the methods of administration, rationale, and side effects of the prescribed immunosuppressive agents. The patient is given written as well as verbal instructions about how and when to take the medications and is instructed to take steps to be sure that an adequate supply of medication is available so that there is no chance of running out of the medication or skipping a dose. Instructions are also provided about the signs and symptoms that are indications of problems requiring consultation with the transplant team. The patient with a T-tube in place must be instructed in management of the tube.

Continuing Care. The importance of follow-up blood work and visits to the transplant team is emphasized. Tacrolimus and cyclosporine trough levels are obtained, along with other blood tests that indicate the function of the liver and kidneys. During the first months, the patient is likely to require blood work two or three times a week. As the patient's condition stabilizes, blood work and visits to the transplant team will be scheduled less frequently. The importance of routine ophthalmologic examinations is emphasized because of the increased incidence of cataracts and glaucoma with long-term corticosteroid therapy. Regular oral hygiene and follow-up dental care, with administration of prophylactic antibiotics before dental treatments, are recommended because of the immunosuppression.

The patient is advised that although a successful transplantation will not return him or her to normal, it does increase the chances for survival and a more normal life than before transplantation, if rejection and infection can be prevented. Many patients have lived successful and productive lives after liver transplantation. Several women have had normal pregnancies and delivered normal infants after liver transplantation.

Liver Abscesses

Two categories of liver abscess have been identified: amebic and pyogenic. Amebic liver abscesses are most commonly caused by *Entamoeba histolytica*. Most amebic liver abscesses occur in the developing countries of the tropics and subtropics because of poor sanitation and hygiene. Pyogenic liver abscesses are much less common but are more common in more developed countries than the amebic type.

Pathophysiology

Whenever an infection develops anywhere along the biliary or GI tract, infecting organisms may reach the liver through the biliary system, portal venous system, or hepatic arterial or lymphatic system. Most bacteria are promptly destroyed, but occasionally some gain a foothold. The bacterial toxins destroy the neighboring liver cells, and the resulting necrotic tissue serves as a protective wall for the organisms.

Meanwhile, leukocytes migrate into the infected area. The result is an abscess cavity full of a liquid containing living and dead leukocytes, liquefied liver cells, and bacteria. Pyogenic abscesses of this type may be either single or multiple and small. Examples of causes of pyogenic liver abscess include cholangitis and abdominal trauma.

Clinical Manifestations

The clinical picture is one of sepsis with few or no localizing signs. Fever with chills and diaphoresis, malaise, anorexia, nausea, vomiting, and weight loss may occur. The patient may complain of dull abdominal pain and tenderness in the right upper quadrant of the abdomen. Hepatomegaly, jaundice, anemia, and pleural effusion may develop. Sepsis and shock may be severe and life-threatening. In the past, the mortality rate was 100% because of the vague clinical symptoms, inadequate diagnostic tools, and

CHART 36•3 Definition of Terms: Biliary

Cholecystitis: inflammation of the gallbladder
Cholelithiasis: the presence of calculi in the gallbladder
Cholecystectomy: removal of the gallbladder
Cholecystostomy: opening and drainage of the gallbladder
Choledochotomy: opening into the common duct
Choledocholithiasis: stones in the common duct
Choledocholithotomy: incision of common bile duct for removal of stones
Choledochoduodenostomy: anastomosis of common duct to duodenum
Choledochojejunostomy: anastomosis of common duct to jejunum
Lithotripsy: disintegration of gallstones by shock waves
Laparoscopic cholecystectomy: removal of gallbladder through endoscopic procedure
Laser cholecystectomy: removal of gallbladder using laser rather than scalpel and traditional surgical instruments

inadequate surgical drainage of the abscess. With the aid of ultrasound, CT scanning, and liver scans, early diagnosis and surgical drainage of the abscess have greatly reduced the mortality rate.

Assessment and Diagnostic Findings

Blood cultures are obtained but may not identify the organism. Aspiration of the liver abscess, guided by ultrasound or CT scan, may be performed to assist in diagnosis and to obtain cultures of the organism. Percutaneous drainage of pyogenic abscesses is carried out to evacuate the abscess material and promote healing. A catheter may be left in place for continuous drainage; the patient is instructed about its management.

Medical Management

Treatment includes IV antibiotic therapy; the specific antibiotic used in treatment depends on the organism identified. Continuous supportive care is indicated because of the serious condition of the patient. Open surgical drainage may be required if antibiotic therapy and percutaneous drainage are ineffective.

BILIARY CONDITIONS

Several disorders affect the biliary system and interfere with normal drainage of bile into the duodenum. These disorders include carcinoma that obstructs the biliary tree and infection of the biliary system. Gallbladder disease with gallstones, however, is the most common disorder of the biliary system. Although not all occurrences of gallbladder infection (cholecystitis) are related to gallstones (cholelithiasis), more than 90% of patients with acute cholecystitis have gallstones. Most of the 15 million Americans with gallstones have no pain, however, and are unaware of the presence of stones. For a guide to the terminology associated with biliary disorders and procedures, see Chart 36-3.

Cholecystitis

Acute infection of the gallbladder causes pain, tenderness, and rigidity of the upper right abdomen and is associated with nausea, vomiting, and the usual signs of an acute inflammation. This condition is referred to as acute cholecystitis. If the gallbladder is found to be filled with purulent fluid, there is an empyema of the gallbladder.

Calculous cholecystitis occurs in more than 90% of patients with acute cholecystitis. In calculous cholecystitis, a gallbladder stone obstructs bile outflow. Bile remaining in the gallbladder initiates a chemical reaction; autolysis and edema occur; and the blood vessels in the gallbladder are compressed, compromising its vascular supply. Consequently, gangrene of the gallbladder with perforation may result. Bacteria play a minor role in acute cholecystitis; however, secondary infection with *Escherichia coli* and other enteric organisms occurs in about 40% of patients.

Acalculous cholecystitis describes acute gallbladder inflammation in the absence of obstruction by gallstones. Acalculous cholecystitis occurs after major surgical procedures, severe trauma, or burns. Other factors associated with this type of cholecystitis include torsion cystic duct obstruction, primary bacterial infections of the gallbladder, and multiple blood transfusions. It is speculated that acalculous cholecystitis results from alterations in fluids and electrolytes and in regional blood flow in the visceral circulation. Bile stasis (lack of gallbladder contraction) and increased viscosity of the bile are also thought to play a role. The occurrence of acalculous cholecystitis with major procedures or trauma makes its diagnosis difficult.

Cholelithiasis

Calculi, or gallstones, usually form in the gallbladder from the solid constituents of bile and vary greatly in size, shape, and composition (Fig. 36-14). Gallstones are uncommon in children and young adults but become increasingly prevalent after age 40. The incidence of cholelithiasis increases thereafter to such an extent that it has been estimated that by age 75, one of every three people will have gallstones.

Pathophysiology

There are two major types of gallstones: those composed predominantly of pigment and those composed primarily of cholesterol. Pigment stones probably form when unconjugated pigments in the bile precipitate to form stones; these stones account for about one third of cases in the United States. The risk of developing such stones is increased in patients with cirrhosis, hemolysis, and infections of the biliary tree. Pigment stones cannot be dissolved and must be removed surgically.

Cholesterol stones account for most remaining cases of gallbladder disease in the United States. Cholesterol, a normal constituent of bile, is insoluble in water. Its solubility depends on bile acids and lecithin (phospholipids) in bile. In gallstone-prone patients, there is decreased bile acid synthesis and increased cholesterol synthesis in the liver, resulting in a bile supersaturated with cholesterol, which precipitates out of the bile to form stones. The cholesterol-saturated bile predisposes to the formation of gallstones and acts as an irritant, producing inflammatory changes in the gallbladder.

Four times more women than men develop cholesterol stones and gallbladder disease; they are usually older than 40, multiparous, and obese. The incidence of stone formation is increased in users of oral contraceptives, estrogens, and clofibrate, which are known to increase biliary cholesterol saturation. The incidence of stone formation increases with age as a result of increased hepatic

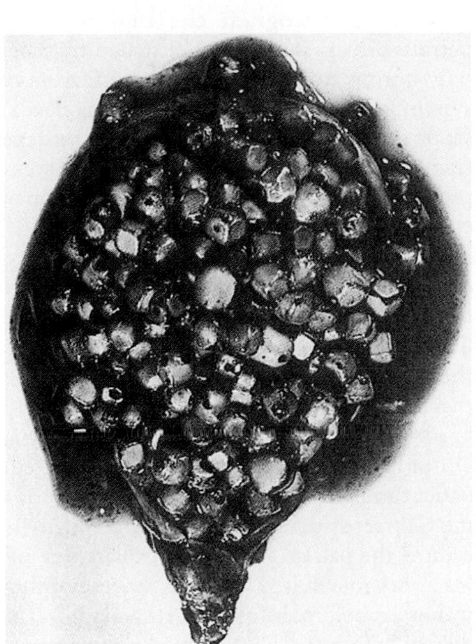

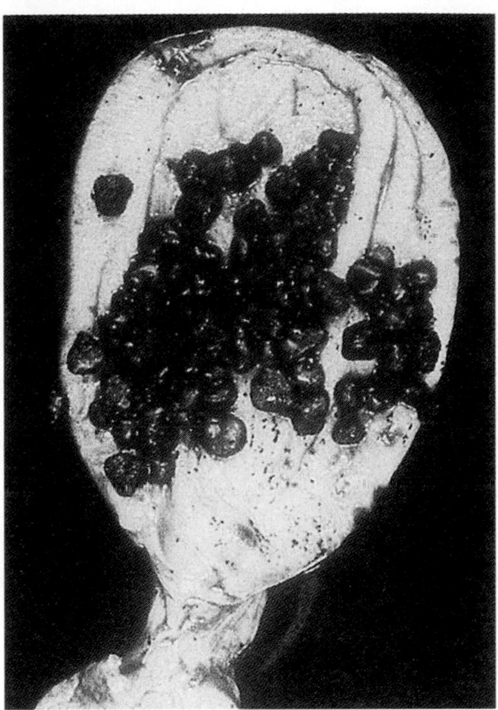

FIGURE 36•14 Examples of cholesterol gallstones (left) made up of a coalescence of multiple small stones (left) and pigment gallstones (right) composed of calcium bilirubinate. Rubin E., & Farber J. L. (1999). *Pathology* (3rd ed.) Philadelphia: Lippincott Williams & Wilkins.

secretion of cholesterol and decreased bile acid synthesis. In addition, there is increased risk because of malabsorption of bile salts in patients with GI disease or T-tube fistula or in those who have had ileal resection or bypass. There is also an increased incidence in people with diabetes.

Clinical Manifestations

Gallstones may be silent, producing no pain and only mild GI symptoms. Such stones may be detected incidentally during surgery or evaluation for unrelated problems.

The patient with gallbladder disease from gallstones may develop two types of symptoms: those due to disease of the gallbladder itself and those due to obstruction of the bile passages by a gallstone. The symptoms may be acute or chronic. Epigastric distress, such as fullness, abdominal distention, and vague pain in the right upper quadrant of the abdomen, may occur. This distress may follow a meal high in fried or fatty foods.

PAIN AND BILIARY COLIC

If a gallstone obstructs the cystic duct, the gallbladder becomes distended and eventually infected. The patient develops a fever and may have a palpable abdominal mass. The patient may have biliary colic with excruciating upper right abdominal pain that radiates to the back or right shoulder, is usually associated with nausea and vomiting, and is noticeable several hours after a heavy meal. The patient moves about restlessly, unable to find a comfortable position. In some patients the pain is constant rather than colicky in nature.

Such a bout of biliary colic is caused by contraction of the gallbladder, which cannot release bile because of obstruction by the stone. When distended, the fundus of the gallbladder comes in contact with the abdominal wall in the region of the right ninth and tenth costal cartilages. This produces marked tenderness in the right upper quadrant on deep inspiration and prevents full inspiratory excursion.

The pain of acute cholecystitis may be so severe that analgesics such as meperidine are required. Morphine is thought to increase spasm of the sphincter of Oddi and is therefore avoided.

JAUNDICE

Jaundice occurs in a few patients with gallbladder disease and usually occurs with obstruction of the common bile duct. The bile, no longer carried to the duodenum, is absorbed by the blood, giving the skin and mucous membrane a yellow color. This is frequently accompanied by marked itching of the skin.

CHANGES IN URINE AND STOOL COLOR

The excretion of the bile pigments by the kidneys gives the urine a very dark color. The feces, no longer colored with bile pigments, are grayish, like putty, and usually described as clay-colored.

VITAMIN DEFICIENCY

Obstruction of bile flow also interferes with absorption of the fat-soluble vitamins A, D, E, and K. Therefore, the patient may exhibit deficiencies (eg, bleeding caused by vitamin K deficiency) of these vitamins if biliary obstruction has been prolonged. Vitamin K deficiency interferes with normal blood clotting.

If the gallstone is dislodged and no longer obstructs the cystic duct, the gallbladder drains and the inflammatory process subsides after a relatively short time. If the gallstone continues to obstruct the duct, abscess, necrosis, and perforation with generalized peritonitis may result.

Diagnostic Evaluation

ABDOMINAL X-RAY

An abdominal x-ray may be obtained if gallbladder disease is suggested, to exclude other causes of symptoms. However, only 15% to 20% of gallstones are sufficiently calcified to be visible on such x-ray studies.

ULTRASONOGRAPHY

Ultrasonography has replaced oral cholecystography as the diagnostic procedure of choice because it is rapid and accurate and can be used in patients with liver dysfunction and jaundice. It does not expose patients to ionizing radiation. The procedure is most accurate if the patient fasts overnight so that the gallbladder is distended. The use of ultrasound is based on reflected sound waves. Ultrasonography can detect calculi in the gallbladder or a dilated common bile duct. It is reported to detect gallstones with 95% accuracy.

RADIONUCLIDE IMAGING OR CHOLESCINTIGRAPHY

Cholescintigraphy is used successfully in the diagnosis of acute cholecystitis. In this procedure, a radioactive agent is administered intravenously. It is taken up by the hepatocytes and rapidly excreted through the biliary system. The biliary tract is then scanned, and images of the gallbladder and biliary tree are obtained. This test is more expensive than ultrasonography, takes longer to perform, exposes the patient to radiation, and cannot detect gallstones. Its use may be limited to cases in which ultrasonography is not conclusive.

CHOLECYSTOGRAPHY

Although it has been replaced by ultrasonography as the test of choice, cholecystography is still used if ultrasound equipment is not available or if the ultrasound results are inconclusive. Oral cholangiography may be performed to detect gallstones and to assess the ability of the gallbladder to fill, concentrate its contents, contract, and empty. An iodide-containing contrast agent excreted by the liver and concentrated in the gallbladder is administered to the patient. The normal gallbladder fills with this radiopaque substance. If gallstones are present, they appear as shadows on the x-ray.

Contrast agents include iopanoic acid (Telepaque), iodipamide meglumine (Cholografin), and sodium ipodate (Oragrafin). These agents are administered orally 10 to 12 hours before the x-ray study. To prevent contraction and emptying of the gallbladder, the patient is permitted nothing by mouth after the contrast agent is administered.

The patient is asked about allergies to iodine or seafood. If no allergy is identified, the patient receives the oral form of the contrast agent the evening before the x-rays are obtained. An x-ray of the right upper abdomen is obtained. If the gallbladder is found to fill and empty normally and to contain no stones, it is concluded that no gallbladder disease is present. If gallbladder disease is present, the gallbladder may not be visualized because of obstruction by gallstones. A repeat of the oral cholecystogram with a second dose of the contrast agent may be necessary if the gallbladder is not visualized on the first attempt.

Cholecystography in the obviously jaundiced patient is not useful because the liver cannot excrete the radiopaque dye into the gallbladder in the presence of jaundice. Oral cholecystography is likely to continue to be used as part of the evaluation of the few patients who have been treated with gallstone **dissolution therapy** or lithotripsy.

ENDOSCOPIC RETROGRADE CHOLANGIOPANCREATOGRAPHY

Endoscopic retrograde cholangiopancreatography (ERCP) permits direct visualization of structures that could once be seen only during laparotomy. The examination of the hepatobiliary system is carried out via a side-viewing flexible fiber-optic endoscope inserted into the esophagus to the descending duodenum (Fig. 36-15). Multiple position changes are required during the procedure, beginning in the left semiprone position, to pass the endoscope.

Fluoroscopy and multiple x-rays are used during ERCP to evaluate the presence and location of ductal stones. Careful insertion of a catheter through the endoscope into the common bile duct is the most important step in sphincterotomy (division of the muscles of the biliary sphincter) for gallstone extraction via this technique.

Nursing Implications. The procedure requires a cooperative patient to permit insertion of the endoscope without damage to the GI tract structures, including the biliary tree. Before the procedure, the patient is given an explanation of the procedure and his or her role in it. The patient takes nothing by mouth for several hours before the procedure. Sedation is administered immediately before the procedure. Most endoscopists use a combination of an opioid and a benzodiazepine. Medications such as glucagon or anticholinergics may also be necessary to eliminate duodenal peristalsis to make cannulation of the papilla easier. The nurse observes closely for signs of respiratory and central nervous system depression, hypotension, oversedation, and vomiting (if glucagon is given). During ERCP, the nurse monitors IV fluids, administers medications, and positions the patient.

After the procedure, the nurse monitors the patient's condition, observing vital signs and monitoring for signs of perforation or infection. The nurse also monitors the patient for side effects of any medications received during the procedure and for return of the gag reflex after the use of local anesthetics.

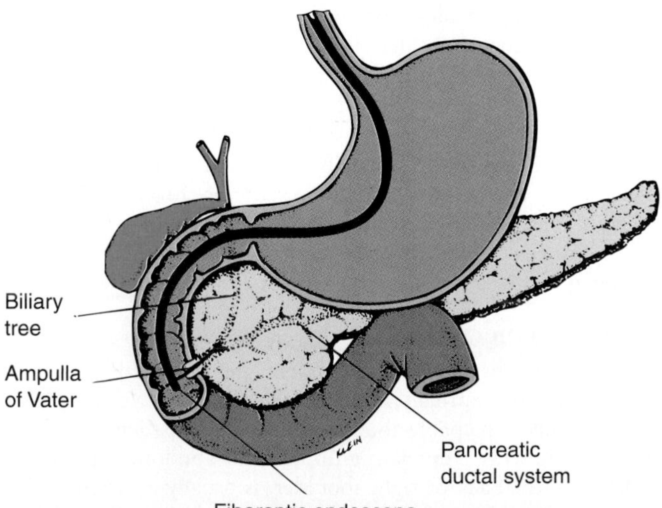

FIGURE 36•15 Endoscopic retrograde cholangiopancreatography (ERCP). A fiberoptic duodenoscope, with side-viewing apparatus, is inserted into the duodenum. The ampulla of Vater is catheterized and the biliary tree injected with contrast agent. The pancreatic ductal system is also assessed, if indicated. This procedure is of special value in visualizing neoplasms of the ampulla area and extracting a biopsy specimen.

PERCUTANEOUS TRANSHEPATIC CHOLANGIOGRAPHY

Percutaneous transhepatic cholangiography involves the injection of dye directly into the biliary tree. Because of the relatively large concentration of dye that is introduced into the biliary system, all components of the system, including the hepatic ducts within the liver, the entire length of the common bile duct, the cystic duct, and the gallbladder, are clearly outlined.

This procedure can be carried out even in the presence of liver dysfunction and jaundice. It is useful for distinguishing jaundice caused by liver disease (hepatocellular jaundice) from that caused by biliary obstruction, for investigating the GI symptoms of a patient whose gallbladder has been removed, for locating stones within the bile ducts, and for diagnosing cancer involving the biliary system.

Procedure. The patient, who is fasting and well sedated, lies supine on the x-ray table. The injection site, which is usually in the midclavicular line immediately beneath the right costal margin, is disinfected and anesthetized with lidocaine (Xylocaine). A small incision is made at this point and a thin, flexible needle with stylet is inserted posteriorly at a 45 degree angle and parallel to the midline. When the needle has penetrated to a depth of approximately 10 cm (4 in), the stylet is removed and replaced by a plastic connector tube with a 50-mL syringe attached. Gentle suction is applied while the needle is slowly withdrawn, until bile appears in the syringe. As much bile as possible is withdrawn, a radiopaque dye is injected, and an x-ray is obtained. Before the needle is removed, as much dye and bile as possible are aspirated to forestall subsequent leakage into the needle tract and eventually into the peritoneal cavity, to minimize the risk of bile peritonitis.

Nursing Alert *Although the complication rate after this procedure is low, the patient must be observed closely for symptoms of bleeding, peritonitis, and septicemia. Pain and indicators of these complications should be reported immediately. Antibiotics are administered if prescribed to minimize the risk of sepsis and septic shock.*

Medical Management

Removal of the gallbladder through traditional surgical approaches was considered the standard approach to management for more than 100 years. However, dramatic changes have occurred in the surgical management of gallbladder disease. Although nonsurgical approaches have the advantage of eliminating surgical risk, they are associated with persistent symptoms or recurrent stone formation. Most of the nonsurgical approaches, including lithotripsy and dissolution of gallstones, provide only temporary solutions to the problems associated with gallstones. They are, therefore, rarely employed in the United States. With the widespread use of laparoscopic cholecystectomy, whereby the gallbladder is removed through a small incision through the umbilicus, surgical risks have decreased, along with the length of hospital stay and the long recovery period associated with the standard surgical cholecystectomy. In some instances, other treatment approaches may be indicated; these are described below.

The major objectives of medical therapy are to reduce the incidence of acute episodes of gallbladder pain and cholecystitis by supportive and dietary management and, if possible, to remove the cause of cholecystitis by pharmacologic therapy, endoscopic procedures, or surgical intervention.

NUTRITIONAL AND SUPPORTIVE THERAPY

Approximately 80% of the patients with acute gallbladder inflammation achieve a remission with rest, IV fluids, nasogastric suction, analgesia, and antibiotics. Unless the patient's condition deteriorates, surgical intervention is delayed until the patient's acute symptoms subside and complete evaluation can be carried out.

The diet immediately after an episode is usually limited to low-fat liquids. Powdered supplements high in protein and carbohydrate can be stirred into skim milk. The following may then be added as tolerated: cooked fruits, rice or tapioca, lean meats, mashed potatoes, non–gas-forming vegetables, bread, coffee, or tea. Eggs, cream, pork, fried foods, cheese and rich dressings, gas-forming vegetables, and alcohol are avoided. The patient may need to be reminded that fatty foods may bring on an episode. Dietary management may be the major mode of therapy in patients who have had only dietary intolerance to fatty foods and vague GI symptoms.

PHARMACOLOGIC THERAPY

Ursodeoxycholic acid (UDCA) and chenodeoxycholic acid (chenodiol or CDCA) have been used to dissolve small, radiolucent gallstones composed primarily of cholesterol. UDCA has fewer side effects than chenodiol and can be administered in smaller doses to achieve the same effect. It acts by inhibiting the synthesis and secretion of cholesterol, thereby desaturating bile. Existing stones can be decreased in size, small ones dissolved, and new stones prevented from forming. Six to 12 months of therapy are required in many patients to dissolve stones, and monitoring of the patient is required during this time. The effective dose of medication depends on body weight; this method of treatment is generally indicated for patients who refuse surgery or for whom it is considered too risky.

Patients with significant, frequent symptoms, cystic duct occlusion, or pigment stones are not candidates for this therapy. Symptomatic patients with acceptable operative risk are better served with laparoscopic or open cholecystectomy.

NONSURGICAL REMOVAL OF GALLSTONES

Dissolving Gallstones. Several methods have been used to dissolve gallstones by infusion of a solvent (mono-octanoin or methyl tertiary butyl ether [MTBE]) into the gallbladder. The solvent can be infused through the following routes: through a tube or catheter inserted percutaneously directly into the gallbladder, through a tube or drain inserted through a T-tube tract to dissolve stones not removed at the time of surgery, through an ERCP endoscope, or through a transnasal biliary catheter.

In this last procedure, the catheter is introduced through the mouth and inserted into the common bile duct. The upper end of the tube is then rerouted from the mouth to the nose and left in place. This enables the patient to eat and drink normally while passage of stones is monitored or chemical solvents are infused to dissolve the stones. This method of dissolution of stones is not widely used in patients with gallstone disease.

Stone Removal by Instrumentation. Several nonsurgical methods are used to remove stones that were not removed at the time of cholecystectomy or have become lodged in the common bile duct (Fig. 36-16). A catheter and instrument with a basket attached are threaded through the T-tube tract or fistula formed at the time of T-tube insertion; the basket is used to retrieve and remove the stones lodged in the common bile duct.

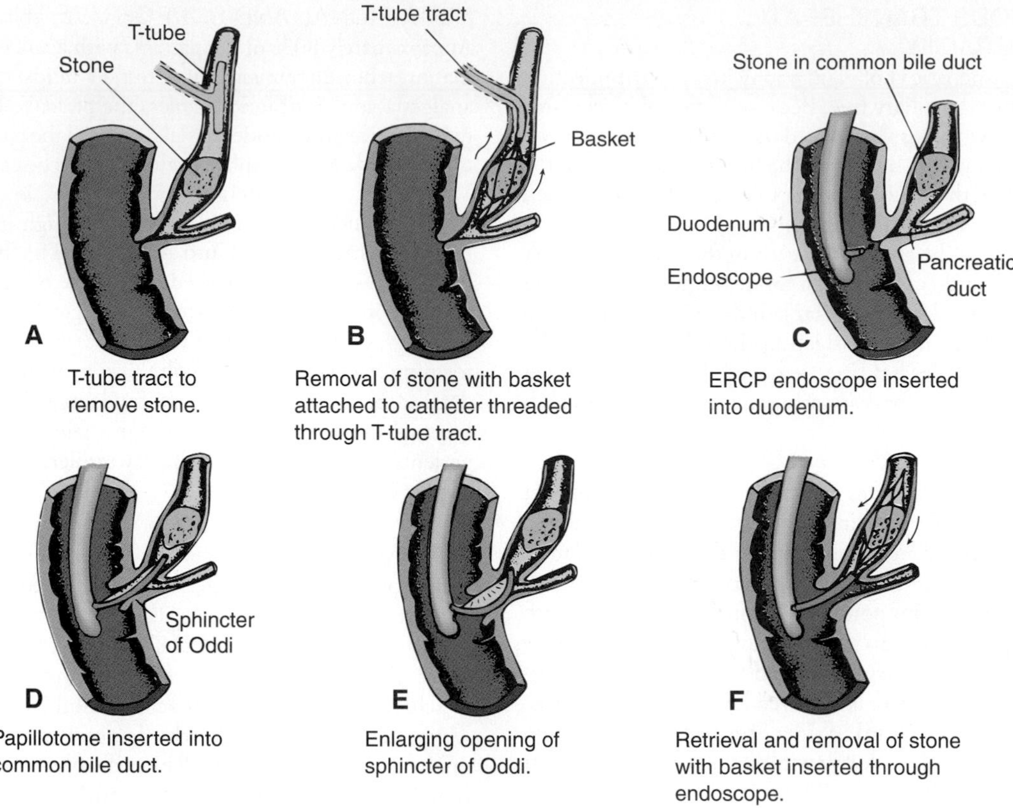
T-tube
Stone
T-tube tract
Basket
Stone in common bile duct
Duodenum
Endoscope
Pancreatic duct
A
T-tube tract to remove stone.
B
Removal of stone with basket attached to catheter threaded through T-tube tract.
C
ERCP endoscope inserted into duodenum.
Sphincter of Oddi
D
Papillotome inserted into common bile duct.
E
Enlarging opening of sphincter of Oddi.
F
Retrieval and removal of stone with basket inserted through endoscope.

FIGURE 36•16 Nonsurgical techniques for removing gallstones.

A second procedure involves the use of the ERCP endoscope. After the endoscope is inserted, a cutting instrument is passed through the endoscope into the ampulla of Vater of the common bile duct. It may be used to cut the submucosal fibers, or papilla, of the sphincter of Oddi, enlarging the opening, which may allow the lodged stones to pass spontaneously into the duodenum. Another instrument with a small basket or balloon at its tip may be inserted through the endoscope to retrieve the stones (see Fig. 36-16). Although complications after this procedure are rare, the patient must be observed closely for bleeding, perforation, and the development of pancreatitis or sepsis.

The ERCP procedure is particularly useful in the diagnosis and treatment of patients who have symptoms after biliary tract surgery, for patients with intact gallbladders, and for patients in whom surgery is particularly hazardous.

Extracorporeal Shock-Wave Lithotripsy. Extracorporeal shock-wave therapy (lithotripsy or ESWL) has been used for nonsurgical fragmentation of gallstones. The word "lithotripsy" is derived from *lithos*, meaning stone, and *tripsis*, meaning rubbing or friction.

This noninvasive procedure uses repeated shock waves directed at the gallstones in the gallbladder or common bile duct to fragment the stones. The energy is transmitted to the body through a water bath or fluid-filled bag. The converging shock waves are directed to the stones to be fragmented.

After the stones are gradually broken up, the stone fragments pass from the gallbladder or common bile duct spontaneously, are removed by endoscopy, or are dissolved with oral bile acid or solvents. Because the procedure requires no incision and no hospitalization, patients are usually treated as outpatients, but several sessions are generally necessary.

The advent of laparoscopic cholecystectomy has reduced the use of this method to treat gallbladder stones. It is used in some centers for a small percentage of suitable patients (those with common bile duct stones who may not be surgical candidates), sometimes in combination with dissolution therapy.

Intracorporeal Lithotripsy. With intracorporeal lithotripsy, stones in the gallbladder or common bile duct may be fragmented by ultrasound, pulsed laser, or hydraulic lithotripsy applied through an endoscope directly to the stones. The stone fragments or debris are then removed by irrigation and aspiration. The procedure may be followed by removal of the gallbladder through an incision or by laparoscopy. If the gallbladder is not removed, a drain may be inserted for 7 days.

Surgical Management

Surgical treatment of gallbladder disease and gallstones is carried out to relieve persistent symptoms, to remove the cause of biliary colic, and to treat acute cholecystitis. Surgery may be elective when the patient's symptoms have subsided or may be performed as an emergency procedure if the patient's condition necessitates it.

PREOPERATIVE MEASURES

A chest x-ray, electrocardiogram, and liver function tests (see Table 36-1) may be performed in addition to x-ray studies of the gallbladder. Vitamin K may be administered if the patient's prothrombin level is low. Blood component therapy may be administered before surgery.

Nutritional requirements are considered; if the patient's nutritional status is suboptimal, it may be necessary to provide IV glucose with protein hydrolysate supplements to aid wound healing and help prevent liver damage.

Preparation for gallbladder surgery is similar to that for any upper abdominal laparotomy or laparoscopy. Instructions and explanations are given before surgery with regard to turning and deep breathing. Pneumonia and atelectasis are possible postoperative complications that can be avoided by deep-breathing exercises and frequent turning. The patient should be informed that drainage tubes and a nasogastric tube and suction may be required during the immediate postoperative period if an open cholecystectomy is performed.

LAPAROSCOPIC CHOLECYSTECTOMY

Laparoscopic cholecystectomy (Fig. 36-17) has dramatically changed the approach to management of cholecystitis. Approximately 600,000 patients require surgery each year for removal of the gallbladder, and more than 85% of them are candidates for laparoscopic cholecystectomy (Evans & Ascher, 1998).

This procedure is performed through a small incision or puncture made through the abdominal wall in the umbilicus. The abdominal cavity is insufflated with carbon dioxide (pneumoperitoneum) to assist in inserting the laparoscope and to aid the surgeon in visualizing the abdominal structures. The fiber-optic scope is inserted through the small umbilical incision. Several additional punctures or small incisions are made in the abdominal wall to introduce other surgical instruments into the operative field. The surgeon can visualize the biliary system through the laparoscope; a camera attached to the scope permits a view of the intra-abdominal field to be transmitted to a television monitor.

Conversion to a traditional abdominal surgical procedure may be necessary if problems are encountered during the laparoscopic procedure; this occurs in about 5% of laparoscopic cases. The patient is informed that an open abdominal procedure may be necessary, and general anesthesia is administered. The advantage of the laparoscopic procedure is that the patient does not experience the paralytic ileus that occurs with open abdominal surgery and has less postoperative abdominal pain. The patient is often discharged from the hospital on the day of surgery or within a day or two and can resume full activity and employment within a week of the surgery.

Because of careful screening of patients and identification of those at low risk for problems, conversion to an open abdominal procedure is necessary only occasionally. With wider use of laparoscopic procedures, however, there may be an increase in the number of such conversions.

Nursing Alert *Because of the short hospital stay, written as well as verbal instructions must be provided about managing postoperative pain and reporting signs and symptoms of intra-abdominal complications, including loss of appetite, vomiting, pain, distention of the abdomen, and temperature elevation. Although recovery from laparoscopic cholecystectomy is rapid, patients are drowsy afterward. The nurse must ensure that the patient has assistance at home during the first 24 to 48 hours. If pain occurs in the right shoulder or scapular area (from migration of the* CO_2 *used to insufflate the abdominal cavity during the procedure), the nurse may recommend applying a heating pad for 15 to 20 minutes hourly, walking, and raising the upper torso when in bed.*

CHOLECYSTECTOMY

In this procedure, the gallbladder is removed through an abdominal incision after the cystic duct and artery are ligated. The procedure is performed for acute and chronic cholecystitis. A drain (Penrose) is placed in the gallbladder and brought out through a puncture wound to drain blood, serosanguineous fluids, and bile into absorbent dressings. Once one of the most common surgical procedures in the United States, this procedure has largely been replaced by laparoscopic cholecystectomy.

MINICHOLECYSTECTOMY

Minicholecystectomy is a surgical procedure in which the gallbladder is removed through a 3- to 4-cm incision. If needed, the surgi-

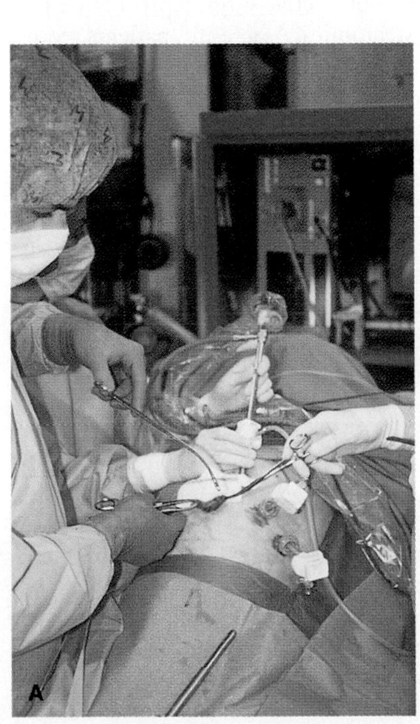

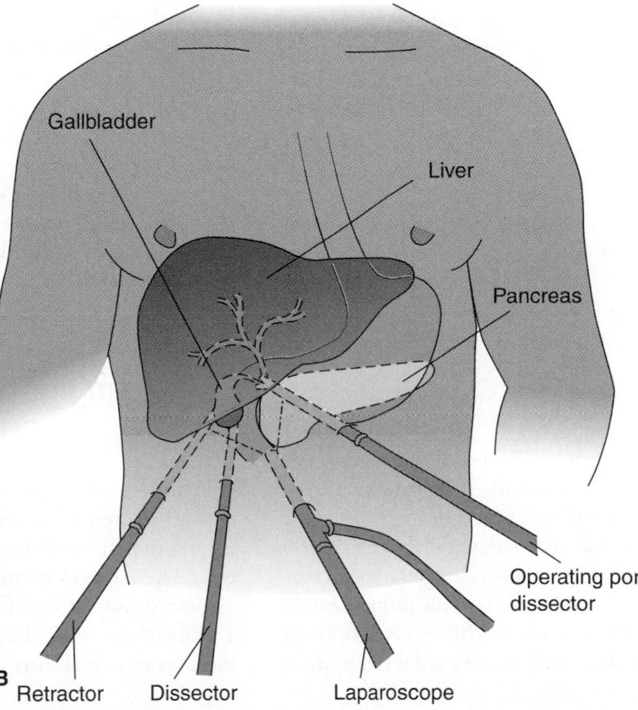

FIGURE 36•17 In (**A**) laparoscopic cholecystectomy, (**B**) the surgeon makes four small incisions (less than 1/2 inch each) in the abdomen and inserts a laparoscope with a miniature camera into the opening. The camera apparatus displays the gallbladder and adjacent tissues on a screen allowing the surgeon to visualize the sections of the organ for removal.

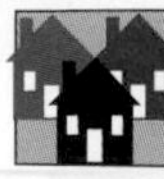

PATIENT EDUCATION AND HOME CARE

Managing Self-Care After Laparoscopic Cholecystectomy

Resuming Activity

- Begin light exercise (walking) immediately.
- Drive a car after 3 or 4 days.
- Take a shower or bath after 1 or 2 days.
- Resume sexual activity when desired.
- Avoid lifting objects exceeding 5 pounds after surgery, usually for 1 week.

Caring for the Wound

- Check puncture site daily for signs of infection.
- Wash puncture site with mild soap and water.
- Allow special adhesive strips on the puncture site to fall off. Do not pull them off.

Resuming Eating

- You may resume your normal diet.
- If you had fat intolerance before surgery, gradually add fat back into your diet in small increments.

Managing Pain

- You may experience pain or discomfort in your right shoulder from the gas used to inflate your abdominal area during surgery. Sometimes sitting upright in bed or a chair or walking may ease the discomfort.

Managing Follow-Up Care

- Make an appointment with your surgeon for 7 to 10 days from now.
- Call your surgeon if you see any signs of infection at or around the puncture site: redness, tenderness, swelling, heat, drainage.
- Call your surgeon if you experience a fever of 37.7°C (100°F) or more for 2 consecutive days.
- Call your surgeon if you develop nausea, vomiting, or abdominal pain.

cal incision is extended to remove large gallbladder stones. Drains may or may not be used. The cost savings resulting from patients' shorter hospital stays have been identified as major reasons for pursuing this type of procedure. Debate exists about this procedure because it limits exposure to all the involved biliary structures.

CHOLEDOCHOSTOMY

Choledochostomy involves an incision into the common duct for removal of stones. After the stones have been evacuated, a tube usually is inserted into the duct for drainage of bile until edema subsides. This tube is connected to gravity drainage tubing. The gallbladder also contains stones, and as a rule a cholecystectomy is performed at the same time.

SURGICAL CHOLECYSTOSTOMY

Cholecystostomy is performed when the patient's condition prevents more extensive surgery or when an acute inflammatory reaction is severe. The gallbladder is surgically opened, the stones and the bile or the purulent drainage are removed, and a drainage tube is secured with a purse-string suture. The drainage tube is connected to a drainage system to prevent bile from leaking around the tube or escaping into the peritoneal cavity. After recovery from the acute episode, the patient may return for cholecystectomy. Despite its lower risk, surgical cholecystostomy has a high mortality rate (reported as high as 20% to 30%) because of the patient's underlying disease process.

PERCUTANEOUS CHOLECYSTOSTOMY

Percutaneous cholecystostomy has been used in the treatment and diagnosis of acute cholecystitis in patients who are poor risks for any surgical procedure or for general anesthesia. These may include patients with sepsis or severe cardiac, renal, pulmonary, or liver failure. Under local anesthesia, a fine needle is inserted through the abdominal wall and liver edge into the gallbladder under the guidance of ultrasound or CT scan. Bile is aspirated to ensure adequate placement of the needle, and a catheter is inserted into the gallbladder to decompress the biliary tract. Almost immediate relief of pain and resolution of signs and symptoms of sepsis and cholecystitis have been reported with this procedure. Antibiotics are administered before, during, and after the procedure.

Gerontologic Considerations

Surgical intervention for disease of the biliary tract is the most common operative procedure performed in the elderly. Cholesterol saturation of bile increases with age due to increased hepatic secretion of cholesterol and decreased bile acid synthesis.

Although the incidence of gallstones increases with age, the elderly patient may not have the typical picture of fever, pain, chills, and jaundice. Symptoms of biliary tract disease in the elderly may be accompanied or preceded by those of septic shock: oliguria, hypotension, mental changes, tachycardia, and tachypnea.

Although surgery in the elderly presents a risk because of preexisting associated diseases, the mortality rate from serious complications from biliary tract disease itself is also high. The risk of death and complications is increased in the elderly patient who undergoes emergency surgery for life-threatening disease of the biliary tract. Despite the presence of chronic illness in many elderly patients, elective cholecystectomy is usually well tolerated and can be carried out with low risk if expert assessment and care are provided before, during, and after the surgical procedure.

Because of recent changes in the health care system, there has been a decrease in the number of elective surgical procedures performed, including cholecystectomies. As a result, patients requiring the procedure are seen in the later stages of disease. Simultaneously, patients undergoing surgery are increasingly older than 60 years of age and have complicated acute cholecystitis. The higher risk of complications and shorter hospital stays make it essential that older patients and their family members receive specific information about signs and symptoms of complications and measures to prevent them.

NURSING PROCESS: THE PATIENT UNDERGOING SURGERY FOR GALLBLADDER DISEASE

Assessment

The patient who is to undergo surgical treatment of gallbladder disease is often admitted to the hospital or same-day surgery unit on the morning of surgery. Preadmission testing has often been completed a week or more before admission.

Assessment should focus on the patient's respiratory status. If a traditional surgical approach is planned, the high abdominal incision required during surgery may interfere with full respiratory excursion. A history of smoking or previous respiratory problems is noted. Shallow respirations, a persistent or ineffective cough, and the presence of adventitious breath sounds are noted. Nutritional status is evaluated through dietary history, general examination, and the previously obtained laboratory results.

Diagnosis

Nursing Diagnoses

Based on all the assessment data, the major nursing diagnoses for the patient undergoing surgery for gallbladder disease may include the following:

- Pain and discomfort related to surgical incision
- Impaired gas exchange related to the high abdominal surgical incision (if traditional surgical cholecystectomy is performed)
- Impaired skin integrity related to altered biliary drainage after surgical intervention (if a T-tube is inserted because of stones in the common bile duct)
- Altered nutrition, less than body requirements, related to inadequate bile secretion
- Knowledge deficit about self-care activities related to incisional care, dietary modifications (if needed), medications, reportable signs or symptoms (fever, bleeding, vomiting)

Collaborative Problems/Potential Complications

Based on assessment data, potential complications may include:

- Bleeding
- GI symptoms

Planning and Goals

The goals for the patient include relief of pain, adequate ventilation, intact skin and improved biliary drainage, optimal nutritional intake, understanding of self-care routines, and absence of complications.

Postoperative Nursing Interventions

After recovery from anesthesia, the patient is placed in the low Fowler's position. IV fluids may be given, and nasogastric suction (a nasogastric tube was probably inserted immediately before surgery for a non-laparoscopic procedure) may be instituted to relieve abdominal distention. Water and other fluids may be given in about 24 hours, and a soft diet started later, after bowel sounds return.

Relieving Pain

The location of the subcostal incision in nonlaparoscopic gallbladder surgery is likely to cause the patient to avoid turning and moving and to splint the operative site by taking shallow breaths to prevent pain. Because full aeration of the lungs and gradually increased activity are necessary to prevent postoperative complications, analgesics should be administered as prescribed and the patient assisted to turn, cough, breathe deeply, and ambulate as indicated. Use of a pillow or binder over the incision may reduce pain during these maneuvers.

Improving Respiratory Status

Patients undergoing biliary tract surgery are especially prone to pulmonary complications, as are all patients with upper abdominal incisions. Thus, they should be reminded to take deep breaths every hour to expand the lungs fully and prevent atelectasis. Early ambulation prevents pulmonary complications as well as other complications, such as thrombophlebitis. Pulmonary complications are more likely to occur in the elderly and in obese patients.

Promoting Skin Care and Biliary Drainage

In patients who have undergone a cholecystostomy or choledochostomy, the drainage tubes must be connected immediately to a drainage receptacle. Tubing should be fastened to the dressings or to the bottom sheet, with enough leeway for the patient to move without dislodging or kinking it. Because a drainage system remains attached when the patient is ambulating, the drainage bag may be placed in a bathrobe pocket or fastened so that it is below the waist or common duct level. If a Penrose drain is used, as in standard abdominal surgical cholecystectomy, the dressings are changed as required.

After these surgical procedures, the patient is observed for indications of infection, leakage of bile into the peritoneal cavity, and obstruction of bile drainage. If bile is not draining properly, an obstruction is probably causing bile to be forced back into the liver and bloodstream. Because jaundice may result, the nurse should be particularly observant of the color of the patient's sclerae. The nurse should also note and report right upper quadrant abdominal pain, nausea and vomiting, bile drainage around the T-tube, clay-colored stools, and a change in vital signs.

Bile may continue to drain from the drainage tract in considerable quantities for a time, necessitating frequent changes of the outer dressings and protection of the skin from irritation. Skin pastes of zinc oxide, aluminum, or petrolatum prevent the bile from digesting the skin.

To prevent total loss of bile, the physician may want the drainage tube or collection receptacle elevated above the level of the abdomen, so that the bile drains externally only if pressure develops in the duct system. The bile collected is measured every 24 hours; the amount, color, and character of the drainage are documented. After several days of drainage, the tube may be clamped for an hour before and after each meal to deliver bile to the duodenum to aid in digestion. Within 7 to 14 days, the drainage tube is removed. The patient who goes home with a drainage tube in place requires instruction and reassurance about its function and care of the tube.

In all patients with biliary drainage, the stools should be observed daily and their color noted. Specimens of both urine and stool may be sent to the laboratory for examination for bile pigments. In this way, it is possible to determine that the bile pigment is disappearing from the blood and is draining again into the duodenum. A careful record of fluid intake and output is maintained.

Improving Nutritional Status

The patient's diet may be low in fats and high in carbohydrates and proteins immediately after surgery. At the time of hospital discharge, there are usually no special dietary instructions, other than to maintain a nutritious diet and avoid excessive fats. Fat restriction usually is lifted in 4 to 6 weeks when the biliary ducts dilate to accommodate the volume of bile once held by the gallbladder and when the ampulla of Vater again functions effectively. After this, when the patient eats fat, adequate bile will be released into the digestive tract to emulsify the fats and allow their digestion. Before surgery, fats may not be digested completely or adequately, and flatulence may occur. However, one purpose of gallbladder surgery is to allow a normal diet.

Monitoring and Managing Potential Complications

Bleeding may occur as a result of inadvertent puncture or nicking of a major blood vessel. Postoperatively, the patient's vital signs are monitored closely. Drainage (if a T-tube is present) and the surgical incisions are inspected for bleeding. The patient is also assessed periodically for increased tenderness and rigidity of the abdomen. If these signs and symptoms occur, they are reported to the surgeon The patient and family are instructed to report to the surgeon any change in the color of stools because this may indicate complications. GI symptoms, although unexpected, may occur with manipulation of the intestines during surgery.

After laparoscopic cholecystectomy, the patient is assessed for loss of appetite, vomiting, pain, distention of the abdomen, and temperature elevation. These may indicate infection or disruption of the GI tract and should be reported to the surgeon promptly. Because the patient is discharged soon after laparoscopic surgery, the patient and family are instructed verbally and in writing about the importance of reporting these symptoms promptly.

Promoting Home and Community-Based Care

TEACHING PATIENTS SELF-CARE

Because the patient may be discharged from the hospital while the drainage system is still in place, the patient and family may need instructions about its management. They must be instructed in proper care of the drainage tube and should know to report to the physician promptly any changes in the amount or characteristics of drainage. Assistance in securing the appropriate dressings will reduce the patient's anxiety about going home with the drain or tube still in place.

The patient should be instructed about which medications are required (vitamins, anticholinergics, and antispasmodics) and their actions. The patient and family also should be informed about symptoms that should be reported to the physician: jaundice, dark urine, pale-colored stools, pruritus, or signs of inflammation and infection, such as pain or fever.

Some patients report one to three bowel movements a day. This is the result of a continual trickle of bile through the choledochoduodenal junction after cholecystectomy. Usually, such frequency diminishes over a period of a few weeks to several months.

CONTINUING CARE

With sufficient support at home, most patients recover quickly from cholecystectomy. However, elderly or frail patients and those who live alone may require a referral for home care. During home visits, the nurse assesses the patient's physical status and progress toward recovery. The patient is assessed for adequacy of pain relief and pulmonary exercises. If the patient has a drainage system in place, it is assessed for patency and appropriate management by the patient and family. The patient is also assessed for signs of infection and is instructed about the signs and symptoms of infection. The patient's understanding of the therapeutic regimen (medications, gradual return to normal activities) is assessed, and previous teaching is reinforced. The importance of keeping follow-up appointments is emphasized to the patient and family.

Evaluation

Expected Outcomes

Expected outcomes may include:

1. Reports decrease in pain
   a. Splints abdominal incision to decrease pain
   b. Avoids foods that cause pain
   c. Uses postoperative analgesia as prescribed
2. Demonstrates appropriate respiratory function
   a. Can achieve full respiratory excursion, with deep inspiration and expiration
   b. Coughs effectively, using pillow to splint abdominal incision
   c. Uses postoperative analgesia as prescribed
   d. Exercises as prescribed (eg, turns, ambulates)
3. Exhibits normal skin integrity around biliary drainage site
   a. Is free of fever, abdominal pain, change in vital signs, or bile around drainage tube
   b. Exhibits or reports gradual decrease in bile drainage (if a T-tube is present) and normal color in urine and stool
   c. Demonstrates proper management of catheter (if applicable)
   d. Identifies signs and symptoms of biliary obstruction to be noted and reported
   e. Has serum bilirubin level within normal range
4. Obtains relief of dietary intolerance
   a. Maintains adequate dietary intake and avoids foods that cause GI symptoms
   b. Reports decreased or absent nausea, vomiting, diarrhea, flatulence, and abdominal discomfort
5. Is free of complications
   a. Has normal vital signs (blood pressure, pulse, respiratory rate and pattern, and temperature)
   b. Reports absence of bleeding from GI tract or T-tube (if present) and no evidence of bleeding in stool
   c. Reports return of appetite and no evidence of vomiting, abdominal distention, and pain
   d. Lists symptoms that should be reported to surgeon promptly

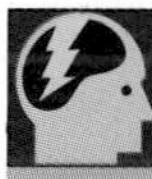

Critical Thinking Exercises

1.
A 50-year-old patient is admitted to the hospital with a diagnosis of cirrhosis and impending liver failure. What diagnostic workup and treatment would you anticipate, and what are the implications for nursing care of this patient?

2.
A 78-year-old patient is scheduled for a laparoscopic cholecystectomy. What postoperative care is indicated for this patient? What factors would you consider in preparing her for discharge? How would your care differ if she lived alone?

3.
A 20-year-old college student has been diagnosed with hepatitis B. What teaching is warranted for this patient to prevent transmission to others and to reduce the risk of complications?
4.
A 64-year-old man with a long history of alcohol abuse is admitted to the hospital with possible bleeding esophageal varices. Describe the possible treatments strategies for this patient and the nursing implications for each of the strategies.

References and Selected Readings

BOOKS

Berci, G., & Cuschieri, A. (Eds). (1997). *Bile duct and bile duct stones.* Philadelphia: W. B. Saunders.
Busuttil, R. W., & Klintmalm, G. B. (Eds). (1996). *Transplantation of the liver.* Philadelphia: W. B. Saunders.
Curley, S. A. (ed.) (1998). *Liver cancer.* New York: Springer.
Dagleish, A., & Weiss, R. F. (eds.) (1999). *HIV and the new viruses.* San Diego, CA: Academic Press.
Darzi, A., Grace, P. A., Pitt, H. A., & Bouchier-Hayes, D. (Eds). (1995). *Techniques in the management of gallstone disease.* Oxford: Blackwell.
Evans, S. R. T., & Ascher, S. M. (Eds.) (1998). *Hepatobiliary and pancreatic surgery.* New York: Wiley-Liss.
Fischbach, F. (1996). *A manual of laboratory and diagnostic tests* (5th ed.). Philadelphia: Lippincott-Raven.
Fleming, I. D., et al. (Eds.). (1997). *American joint committee on cancer* (5th ed.). Philadelphia: Lippincott-Raven.
Friedman, L. S., & Keefe, E. B. (eds.) (1998). *Handbook of liver disease.* Edinburgh: Churchill Livingstone.
Gitnick, G. (ed.) (1998). *Critical issues in gastroenterology.* Baltimore: Williams & Wilkins.
Holstege, A., Schölmerich, J., & Hahn, E. G. (Eds.). (1995). *Portal hypertension.* Dordrecht: Kluwer.
Hoogenraad, T. (1996). *Wilson's disease.* London: Saunders.
Kirsch, R., Robson, S., & Trey, C. (Eds.). (1995). *Diagnosis and management of liver disease.* London: Chapman and Hall.
Lee, W., & Williams, R. (Eds.). (1997). *Acute liver failure.* Cambridge: Cambridge University Press.
National Institutes of Health. National Institute on Alcohol Abuse and Alcoholism. (1997). *Ninth special report to the U.S. congress on alcohol and health.* Alexandria: U.S. Department of Health and Human Services.
Pitt, H.A., Carr-Locke, D.L., & Ferrucci, J.T. (Eds.). (1995). *Hepatobiliary and pancreatic disease: The team approach to management.* Boston: Little, Brown.
Schiff, E. R., Sorrell, M. F., & Maddrey, W. C. (Eds.). (1998). *Schiff's diseases of the liver* (8th ed.). Philadelphia: Lippincott-Raven.
Sherlock, S., & Dooley, J. (Eds.). (1997). *Diseases of the liver and biliary system* (10th ed.). Oxford: Blackwell.
Williams, R., Portmann, B., & Kai-Chah, T. (Eds.). (1995). *The practice of liver transplantation.* Edinburgh: Churchill Livingstone.
Zakim, D., & Boyer, T. D. (Eds.). (1996). *Hepatology: A textbook of liver disease* (3rd ed.). Philadelphia: W. B. Saunders.

JOURNALS

Asterisks indicate nursing research articles.

General

Fabbri, A., Magrini, N., Bianchi, G., et al. (1996). Overview of randomized clinical trials of oral branched chain amino acid treatment in chronic hepatic encephalopathy. *Journal of Parenteral and Enteral Nutrition, 20*(2), 159–165.
Goodman, Z. D., McNally, P. R., Davis, D. R., et al. (1995). Autoimmune cholangitis: A variant of primary biliary cirrhosis. *Digestive Disease Science, 40*(6), 1232–1242.
Jalan, R., Gooday, R., O'Carroll, R. E., et al. (1995). A prospective evaluation of changes in neuropsychological and liver function tests following transjugular intrahepatic portosystemic stent-shunt. *Journal of Hepatology, 23*(6), 697–702.
Letizia, M., & Noonan, M. A. (1997). Drug-induced hepatic injury. *MedSurg Nursing, 6*(3), 148–152.
Mahl, T. C. (1998). Approach to the patient with abnormal liver tests. *Lippincott's Primary Care Practice, 2*(4), 379–389.
Morgan, M. Y. (1995). The treatment of chronic hepatic encephalopathy. *Hepatogastroenterology, 38*(3), 377–382.
Moseley, R. H. (1996). Evaluation of abnormal liver function tests. *Medical Clinics of North America, 80*(5), 887–904.
Nunes, F. A., & Raper, S. E. (1996). Liver-directed gene therapy. *Medical Clinics of North America, 80*(5), 1201–1212.
Pasha, T. M., & Lindor, K. D. (1996). Diagnosis and therapy of cholestatic liver disease. *Medical Clinics of North America, 80*(5), 995–1016.
Riordan, S. M., & Williams, R. (1997). Treatment of hepatic encephalopathy. *New England Journal of Medicine, 337*(7), 473–478.
Rolla, G., Brussino, L., & Bucca, C. (1998). The hepatopulmonary syndrome. *Forum, 8*(1), 84–92.
Schenker, A., & Halff, G. A. (1995). Nutritional therapy in alcoholic liver disease. *Seminars in Liver Disease, 13*(2), 196–209.
Somberg, K. A., Riegler, J. L., LaBerge, J. M., et al. (1995). Hepatic encephalopathy after transjugular intrahepatic portosystemic shunts: Incidence and risk factors. *American Journal of Gastroenterology, 90*, 549–555.
Stone, R. (1998). Differential diagnosis. Acute abdominal pain. *Lippincott's Primary Care Practice, 2*(4), 341–57.
Tibbs, C., & Williams, R. (1995). Viral causes and management of acute liver failure. *Journal of Hepatology, 22*(suppl 1), 68–73.
Wright, J. A. (1997). Seven abdominal assessment signs every emergency nurse should know. *Journal of Emergency Nursing, 23*(5), 446–50.
Zimmerman, H. J., & Maddrey, W. C. (1995). Acetaminophen hepatotoxicity with regular intake of alcohol: Analysis of instances of therapeutic misadventure. *Hepatology, 22*(3), 767–770.

Cirrhosis

Gentilini, P., Casini-Raggi, V., DiFiore, G. et al. (1999). Albumin improves the response to diuretics in patients with cirrhosis and ascites: Results of a randomized, controlled trial. *Journal of Hepatology, 30*(4), 639–645.
Huonker, M., Schumacher, Y. O. Ochs, A, et al. (1999). Cardiac function and haemodynamics in alcoholic cirrhosis and effects of transjugular intrahepatic portosystemic stent shunt. *Gut., 44*(5), 743–748.
Klassen, L. W., Tuma, D., & Sorrell, M. F. (1995). Immune mechanisms of alcohol-induced liver disease. *Hepatology, 22*(2), 355–358.
Lieber, C. S. (1995). Medical disorders of alcoholism. *New England Journal of Medicine, 333*(16), 1058–1060.
Patel, N. H., Chalasani, N. & Jindal, R. M. (1998). Current status of transjugular intrahepatic portosystemic shunts. *Postgraduate Medical Journal, 74*(878), 716–720.
Sherlock, S. (1995). Alcoholic liver disease. *Lancet, 345*(8944), 227–231.

Esophageal Varices

Baroncini, D., Milandri, G. L., Piemontese, A., et al. (1997). A prospective randomized trial of sclerotherapy versus ligation in the elective treatment of bleeding esophageal varices. *Endoscopy, 29*, 235-240.
de la Pena, J., Rivero, M., Sanchez, E. et al. (1999). Variceal ligation compared with endoscopic schlerotherapy for variceal hemorrhage: Prospective randomized trial. *Gastrointestinal Endoscopy, 49*(4 pt 1), 417–423.
Hartigan, P. M., Gebhard, R. L., & Gregory, P. B. (1997). Sclerotherapy for actively bleeding esophageal varices in male alcoholics with cirrhosis. *Gastrointestinal Endoscopy, 46*(1), 1–7.
Huston, C. J. (1996). Ruptured esophageal varices. *American Journal of Nursing, 96*(4), 43.
Jaffe, D. L., Chung, R. T., & Friedman, L. S. (1996). Management of portal hypertension and its complications. *Medical Clinics of North America, 80*(5), 1021–1032.
Laine, L., & Cook, D. (1995). Endoscopic ligation compared with sclerotherapy for the treatment of esophageal variceal bleeding. *Annals of Internal Medicine, 123*(4), 280–287.
Navarro, V. J., & Garcia-Tsao, G. (1995). Variceal hemorrhage. *Critical Care Clinics, 11*(2), 391–414.
Teran, J. C., Imperiale, T. F., Mullen, K. D., et al. (1997). Primary prophylaxis of variceal bleeding in cirrhosis: A cost-effective analysis. *Gastroenterology, 112*(2), 473–482.

Gallbladder Disease

Attili, A., DeSantis, A., Capri, R., et al. (1995). The natural history of gallstones: The GREPCO experience. *Hepatology, 21*(3), 655.
Barie, P., & Fischer, E. (1995). Acute acalculous cholecystitis. *Journal of the American College of Surgery, 180*(2), 232.
Maxwell, J. G., Tyler, B. A., Rutledge, R. et al. (1998). Cholecystectomy in patients aged 80 and older. *American Journal of Surgery, 176*(6), 627–631.

Ponsky, J. L. (1996). Endoscopic approaches to common bile duct injuries. *Surgical Clinics of North America, 76*(3), 505–513.

Schwesinger, W. H., & Diehl, A. K. (1996). Changing indications for laparoscopic cholecystectomy. *Surgical Clinics of North America, 76*(3), 493–502.

Shea, J. A., Healey, M. J., Berlin, J. A., et al. (1996). Mortality and complications associated with laparoscopic cholecystectomy: A meta-analysis. *Annals of Surgery, 224*(5), 609–620.

Strasberg, S. M. (1999). Laparoscopic biliary surgery. *Gastroenterology Clinics of North America, 28*(1), 117–132.

Hepatitis

Advisory Committee on Immunization Practices, American Academy of Pediatrics, American Academy of Family Physicians and the National Immunization Program, Centers for Disease Control and Prevention. (1995). Recommended childhood immunization schedule—United States. *Morbidity and Mortality Weekly Report, 43*(51 & 52), 959–960.

Bizollon, T., Ducenf, C., Trepo, C., & Mutimer, D. (1999). Hepatitis C virus recurrence after liver transplantation. *Gut, 44*(4), 575–578.

Czaja, A. J. (1996). Diagnosis and therapy of autoimmune liver disease. *Medical Clinics of North America, 80*(5), 973–991.

Davis, G. L., et al. (1998). Interferon alfa-2b alone or in combination with ribavirin for the treatment of relapse of chronic hepatitis C. *New England Journal of Medicine, Nov 19,* 1493–1499.

DeMedina, M., & Schiff, E. R. (1995). Hepatitis C: Diagnosis assays. *Seminars in Liver Disease, 15*(1), 33–40.

Feng, X. (1999). Hepatitis C infection: A review. *Lippincott's Primary Care Practice, 3*(3), 345–353.

Fried, M. W. (1996). Therapy of chronic viral hepatitis. *Medical Clinics of North America, 80*(5), 957–972.

Herreid, J. A. (1995). Hepatitis C: Past, present, and future. *MedSurg Nursing, 4*(3), 179–186.

Hunt, C. M., & Sharara, A. I. (1999). Liver disease in pregnancy. *American Family Physician, 59*(4), 826–836.

Immunization Practices Advisory Committee. (1991). Hepatitis B virus: A comprehensive strategy for eliminating transmission in the United States. *Morbidity and Mortality Weekly Report, 40*(RR-13), 1–25.

Katkov, W. N. (1996). Hepatitis vaccines. *Medical Clinics of North America, 80*(5), 1189–1998.

Kowdley, K. (1996). Update on therapy for hepatobiliary diseases. *Nurse Practitioner, 21*(7), 78–88.

Marwick, C. (1995). Hepatitis A vaccine for 2-year-olds to adults. *Journal of American Medical Association, 273*(12): 906–907.

Mast, E. E., Alter, M. J., & Margolis, H. S. (1999). Strategies to prevent and control hepatitis B and C virus infections: A global perspective. *Vaccine, 17*(13-14), 1730–1733.

McHutchison, J. C., et al. (1998). Interferon alfa-2b alone or in combination with ribavirin as initial treatment for chronic hepatitis C. *New England Journal of Medicine, Nov 19,* 1485–1492.

Recommended childhood immunization schedule, United States—January to June (Special Medical Reports). (1996). *American Family Physician, 53,* 392–396.

Scheig, R. (1998). Acute and chronic viral hepatitis. *Lippincott's Primary Care Practice, 2*(4), 390–397.

Schvarcz, R., Yun, Z. B., Sonnerborg, A., et al. (1995). Combination treatment with Interferon alfa-2b and ribavirin for chronic hepatitis C in patients who have failed to achieve sustained response to interferon alone: Swedish experience. *Journal of Medical Virology, 46*(1), 43–47.

Sjogren, M. (1996). Serologic diagnosis of viral hepatitis. *Medical Clinics of North America, 80*(5), 929–953.

Strader, D. B., & Seeff, L. B. (1996). New hepatitis A vaccines and their role in prevention. *Drugs, 51*(3), 359–366.

Liver Cancer

Adam, R., Akpinar, E., Johann, M., et al. (1997). Place of cryosurgery in the treatment of malignant liver tumors. *Annals of Surgery, 225*(1), 39–50.

Brandt, B., DeAntonio, P., Dezort, M., & Eyman, L. (1996). Hepatic cryosurgery for metastatic colorectal carcinoma. *Oncology Nursing Forum, 23*(1), 29–38.

Di Carlo, V., Ferrari, G., Castoldi, R. et al. (1998). Preoperative chemoembolization of hepatocellular carcinoma in cirrhotic patients. *Hepato-Gastroenterology, 45*(24), 1950–1954.

Korpan, N. N. (1997). Hepatic cryosurgery for liver metastases. *Annals of Surgery, 225*(2), 193–201.

Leininger, S. M. (1997). Managing patients with cryosurgical ablation of the prostate and liver. *MedSurg Nursing, 6*(6), 359–386.

Saini, S. (1997). Imaging of the hepatobiliary tract. *New England Journal Medicine, 336*(26), 1889–1894.

Van Thiel, D. H., Colantoni, A. & De Maria, N. (1998). Liver transplant for hepatocellular carcinoma. *Hepato-Gastroenterology, 45*(24), 1944–2949.

Vauthey, J. N., et al. (1995). Factors affecting long-term outcome after hepatic resection for hepatocellular carcinoma. *American Journal of Surgery, 169*(1), 28–34.

Zuro, L. M., & Staren, E. D. (1996). Cryosurgical ablation of unresectable hepatic tumors. *AORN Journal, 64*(2), 231–248.

Liver Transplantation

Cabello, C. C., & Tahan, H. A. (1998). Implementation of an interdisciplinary clinical pathway for patients after a liver transplant. *Nursing Care Management, 3*(6), 255–265.

Chappell, S. M., & Case, P. (1997). Anxiety in liver transplant patients. *MedSurg Nursing, 6*(2), 98–103.

DeJong, W., Franz, H. G., Wolfe, S. M., et al. (1998). Requesting organ donation: An interview study of donor and nondonor families. *American Journal of Critical Care, 7*(1), 13–23.

Devlin, J., Wendon, J., Heaton, N., Tan, K., & Williams, R. (1995). Pretransplantation clinical status and outcome of emergency transplantation for acute liver failure. *Hepatology, 21*(4), 1018–1024.

Evanisko, M. J., Beasley, C. L., Brigham, L. E., et al. (1998). Readiness of critical care physicians and nurses to handle requests for organ donation. *American Journal of Critical Care, 7*(1), 4–12.

Evans, R. W. (1997). Liver transplants and the decline in deaths from liver disease. *American Journal of Public Health, 87*(5), 868–869.

Hasse, J. M. (1997). Diet therapy for organ transplantation. *Nursing Clinics of North America, 32*(4), 863–879.

*Johnson, C. D., & Hathaway, D. K. (1996). The lived experience of end-stage liver failure and liver transplantation. *Journal of Transplant Coordination, 6*(3), 130–133.

O'Connor, T. P., Lewis, W. D., & Jenkins, R. L. (1995). Biliary tract complications after liver transplantation. *Archives of Surgery, 130*(3), 312–317.

Rosen, H. R., Shackleton, C. R., & Martin, P. (1996). Indications for and timing of liver transplantation. *Medical Clinics North America, 80*(5), 1069–1093.

Siminoff, L. A. (1997). Withdrawal of treatment and organ donation. *Critical Care Nursing Clinics of North America, 9*(1), 85–95.

Thomas, D. J. (1996). Returning to work after liver transplant: Experiencing the roadblocks. *Journal of Transplant Coordination, 6*(3), 134–138.

van Hoek, B., de Boer, J., Boudjema, K., Williams, R. et al. (1999). Auxiliary versus orthotopic liver transplantation for acute liver failure. *Journal of Hepatology, 30*(4), 699–705.

Resources

Alcoholics Anonymous (AA) World Services, 475 Riverside Drive, 11th Floor, New York, NY 10115; (212) 870-3400; http://www.alcoholics-anonymous.org

Al-Anon Family Group Headquarters, 1600 Corporate Landing Parkway, Virginia Beach, VA 23454-5617; for meetings, 1-800-344-2666 (8 a.m. to 6 p.m., Monday through Friday); for information, 1-800-356-9996 (7 days a week, 24 hours); http://www.al-anon.alateen.org

Hepatitis Foundation International, 30 Sunrise Terrace, Cedar Grove, NJ 07009; 1-800-891-0707; http.//www.hepfi.org

American Liver Foundation, 1425 Pompton Ave., Cedar Grove, NJ 07009; 1-800-465-4837; http://www.gi.edu/alf/pubs.html

National Council on Alcoholism and Drug Dependence, 12 W. 21st St., New York, NY 10010; 1-800-NCA-CALL; http://www.ncadd.org

National Digestive Diseases Information Clearing House, 2 Information Way, Bethesda, MD 20892-3570; 1-301-654-3810; http://www.acg.gi.org/digest/gitract/

National Institute on Alcohol Abuse and Alcoholism, Scientific Communications Branch, 6000 Executive Boulevard, Suite 409, Bethesda, MD 20892-7003; 1-301-443-3860; http://www.niaaa.nih.gov

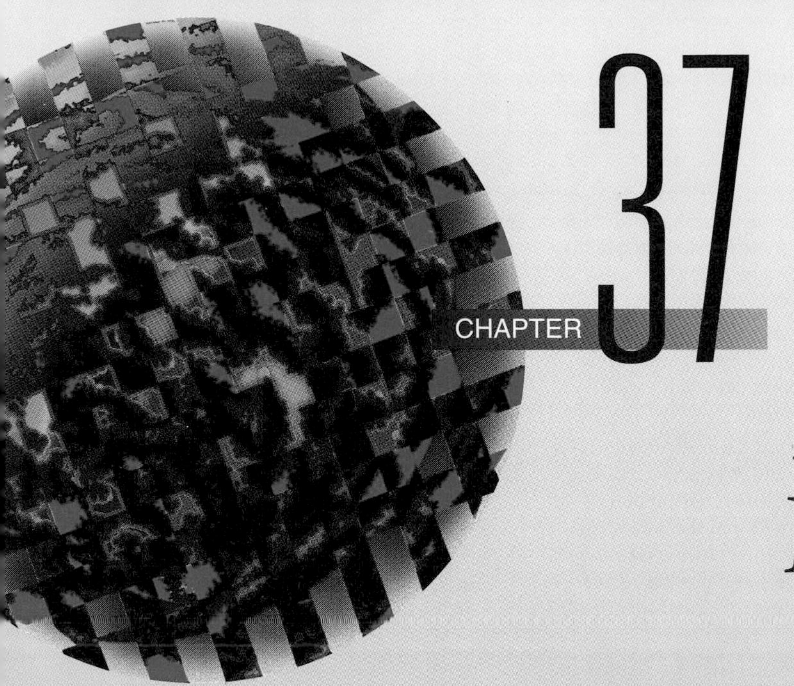

Assessment and Management of Patients With Diabetes Mellitus

Learning Objectives

On completion of this chapter, the learner will be able to:

1. Differentiate between type 1 and type 2 diabetes.
2. Describe etiologic factors associated with diabetes.
3. Relate the clinical manifestations of diabetes to the associated pathophysiologic alterations.
4. Identify the diagnostic and clinical significance of blood glucose tests.
5. Explain the dietary modifications used for management of people with diabetes.
6. Describe the relationship between diet, exercise, and medication (ie, insulin or oral hypoglycemic agents) for people with diabetes.
7. Develop a plan for teaching insulin self-administration.
8. Identify the role of oral antidiabetic agents in diabetic therapy.
9. Differentiate between hypoglycemia and diabetic ketoacidosis, and hyperosmolar nonketotic syndrome.
10. Describe management strategies for a person with diabetes to use during "sick days."
11. Describe the major macrovascular, microvascular, and neuropathic complications of diabetes and the self-care behaviors important in their prevention.
12. Identify the teaching aids and community support groups available for people with diabetes.
13. Use the nursing process as a framework for care of the patient with diabetes.

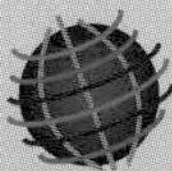

Diabetes mellitus is a group of metabolic diseases characterized by elevated levels of glucose in the blood (**hyperglycemia**) resulting from defects in insulin secretion, insulin action, or both (Expert Committee on the Diagnosis and Classification of Diabetes Mellitus, 1998).

Normally a certain amount of glucose circulates in the blood. The major source of this glucose is absorption of ingested food in the gastrointestinal tract and formation of glucose by the liver from food substances.

Insulin, a hormone produced by the pancreas, controls the level of glucose in the blood by regulating the production and storage of glucose. In the diabetic state, the cells may stop responding to insulin or the pancreas may stop producing insulin entirely. This leads to hyperglycemia, which may result in acute metabolic complications such as **diabetic ketoacidosis** and **hyperglycemic hyperosmolar nonketotic syndrome**. Long-term effects of hyperglycemia contribute to macrovascular complications (coronary artery disease, cerebrovascular disease, and peripheral vascular disease), chronic microvascular complications (kidney and eye disease), and neuropathic complications (diseases of the nerves).

GLOSSARY

American Association of Diabetes Educators: an organization of diabetes education specialists founded to promote diabetes self-management training and standards in diabetes education

alpha glucosidase inhibitor: a category of oral agents used to treat type 2 diabetes that delay the absorption of carbohydrate, resulting in lower postprandial blood glucose levels

self-monitoring of blood glucose (SMBG): a method of capillary blood glucose testing in which the patient pricks his/her finger and applies a drop of blood to a test strip that is read by a meter. The result is used to determine the effectiveness of treatment and to assist the patient and the health care professional to make decisions regarding diet, exercise, and medication

Certified Diabetes Educator: a health care professional who has pursued a career in diabetes education and has passed a certification examination

continuous subcutaneous insulin infusion: a small device that delivers insulin on a 24-hour basis as basal insulin; it is also programmed by the patient to deliver a bolus dose before eating a meal in an attempt to mimic normal pancreatic function

diabetes mellitus: a group of metabolic diseases characterized by hyperglycemia resulting from defects in insulin secretion, insulin action, or both

Diabetes Control and Complications Trial (DCCT): a 10-year prospective study of more than 1400 patients with type 1 diabetes that showed that the consistent normalization of blood glucose resulted in reduction of risk for and progression of retinopathy, nephropathy, and neuropathy

diabetic ketoacidosis (DKA): a metabolic derangement in type 1 diabetes that results from a deficiency of insulin. Highly acidic ketone bodies are formed, resulting in acidosis; usually requires hospitalization for treatment and is usually caused by nonadherence to insulin regimen, concurrent illness, or infection

fasting plasma glucose (FPG): blood glucose determination obtained in the laboratory after fasting for more than 8 hours

glycosylated hemoglobin (hemoglobin A_{1C}): a long-term measure of glucose control that is a result of glucose attaching to hemoglobin for the life of the red blood cell (120 days). The goal of diabetes therapy is a normal to near-normal level of glycosylated hemoglobin (Hgb A_{1C}), the same as in the nondiabetic population

hyperglycemia: elevated blood glucose level—fasting level greater than 126 mg/dL (6.9 mmol/L); 2-hour postprandial level greater than 200 mg/dL (11 mmol/L)

hyperglycemic hyperosmolar nonketotic coma: a metabolic disorder of type 2 diabetes resulting from a relative insulin deficiency initiated by an intercurrent illness that raises the demand for insulin; associated with polyuria and severe dehydration

hypoglycemia: low blood glucose (less than 50 mg/dL; less than 2.7 mmol/L) in a person with diabetes as a result of too much insulin, medication, too little food, and/or too much exercise that has not been compensated for with food; treated with fast-acting carbohydrate followed by a substantial meal or snack

Diabetes mellitus affects about 15 million people, 5 million of whom are undiagnosed. In the United States, approximately 650,000 new cases of diabetes are diagnosed yearly (Centers for Disease Control and Prevention, 1997). Diabetes is especially prevalent in the elderly, with up to 50% of people older than 65 suffering some degree of glucose intolerance. Hispanics, African Americans, and some Native Americans have a higher rate of diabetes than the white population. The Pima, a Native American tribe, have adult diabetes rates of 20% to 50%.

The far-reaching and devastating physical, social, and economic consequences of diabetes include the following:

- In the United States, diabetes is the leading cause of new blindness among 25- to 74-year-olds and the leading cause of nontraumatic amputations.
- Thirty percent of patients beginning dialysis each year have diabetes.
- Diabetes is the third leading cause of death by disease, mostly because of the high rate of coronary artery disease among people with diabetes.
- Hospitalization rates for people with diabetes are 2.4 times greater for adults and 5.3 times greater for children than for the general population.

The economic cost of diabetes continues to rise because of increasing health care costs and an aging population. Half of all people with diabetes older than 65 are hospitalized each year, and severe and life-threatening complications often contribute to the increased rates of hospitalization. Costs related to diabetes are estimated to be almost $99 billion annually, including direct medical care expenses and indirect costs attributable to disability and premature death (Centers for Disease Control and Prevention, 1997).

Treatment plans for patients with diabetes have as their primary goals control of blood glucose levels and prevention of acute and long-term complications. Thus, the nurse who cares for these patients must assist the patient to develop self-care management skills.

CLASSIFICATION OF DIABETES

There are several different types of diabetes mellitus; they may differ in cause, clinical course, and treatment. The major classifications of diabetes are:

- **Type 1** (previously referred to as insulin-dependent diabetes mellitus
- **Type 2** (previously referred to as non–insulin-dependent diabetes mellitus)
- Diabetes mellitus associated with other conditions or syndromes
- Gestational diabetes mellitus (GDM) (Expert Committee on the Diagnosis and Classification of Diabetes Mellitus, 1998)

The terms "insulin-dependent diabetes" and "non–insulin-dependent diabetes" and their acronyms (IDDM and NIDDM, respectively) are no longer recommended because they have resulted in classification of patients on the basis of the treatment of their diabetes rather than the underlying etiology. Use of Roman numerals (type I and type II) to distinguish between the two types has been changed to type 1 and type 2 to reduce confusion (Expert Committee on the Diagnosis and Classification of Diabetes Mellitus, 1998).

Approximately 5% to 10% of people with diabetes have type 1 diabetes in which the insulin-producing pancreatic beta cells are destroyed by an autoimmune process. As a result, insulin injections are needed to control the blood glucose levels. Type 1 diabetes is characterized by an acute onset, usually before age 30.

Humalog (insulin lispro): an analog of insulin that is the result of switching the amino acid sequence of lycine and proline on the beta chain of insulin; results in a rapid-acting product with a peak-action time of 10 to 50 minutes and a duration of 3 to 5 hours

insulin: a hormone secreted by the beta cell of the islets of Langerhans of the pancreas that is necessary for the metabolism of carbohydrate, protein, and fats; a deficiency of insulin results in diabetes mellitus

impaired fasting glucose (IFG), impaired glucose tolerance (IGT): a metabolic stage intermediate between normal glucose homeostasis and diabetes; not clinical entities in their own right but risk factors for future diabetes and cardiovascular disease

ketone: a highly acidic substance that forms as a result of the breakdown of free fatty acids by the liver when insulin is absent, resulting in diabetic ketoacidosis

nephropathy: a long-term complication of diabetes in which the kidney cells are damaged; characterized by microalbuminuria in early stages and progressing to end-stage renal disease in the late stages, requiring treatment with dialysis or renal transplant

neuropathy: a long-term complication of diabetes resulting from damage to the nerve cell. Can be "peripheral" motor or sensory deficits or "autonomic," in which internal organ function is affected

retinopathy: a long-term complication of diabetes in which the microvascular system of the eye is damaged. Can be background, nonproliferative, or proliferative

sulfonylurea: a classification of oral antidiabetic medication for the treatment of type 2 diabetes; enhances insulin secretion and insulin action. Examples include glipizide (Glucotrol), glyburide (Micronase), glimepiride (Amaryl)

thiazolidinedione: a class of oral antidiabetic medications that reduce insulin resistance in target tissues, enhancing insulin action without directly stimulating insulin secretion. An example is troglitazone (Rezulin)

type 1 diabetes: a metabolic disorder characterized by an absence of insulin production and secretion due to the autoimmune destruction of the beta cells of the islets of Langerhans in the pancreas. Must always be treated with insulin injections. Formerly called insulin-dependent or type I

type 2 diabetes: a metabolic disorder characterized by the relative deficiency of insulin production and a decrease in insulin action. Onset is usually insidious, and family history is common. Amenable to treatment with diet, exercise, oral antidiabetic medications, and insulin. Formerly called non–insulin-dependent diabetes or type II

urine testing: testing urine for glucose is no longer recommended (see self-blood glucose monitoring). Urine testing for ketones is recommended for the patient with type 1 diabetes who is feeling ill or has a blood glucose result exceeding 240 mg/dL (13.2 mmol/L)

Approximately 90% to 95% of people with diabetes have type 2 diabetes. Type 2 diabetes results from a decreased sensitivity to insulin (called insulin resistance) or from a decreased amount of insulin produced. Type 2 diabetes is first treated with diet and exercise. If elevated glucose levels persist, diet and exercise are supplemented with oral hypoglycemic agents. In some individuals with type 2 diabetes, oral agents do not control hyperglycemia, and insulin injections are required. In addition, some individuals who usually can control their type 2 diabetes with diet, exercise, and oral agents may require insulin injections during periods of acute physiologic stress (eg, illness or surgery). Type 2 diabetes occurs most frequently in people who are older than 30 years and obese.

Diabetes complications may develop in any person with type 1 or type 2 diabetes, not only in patients who take insulin. Some patients with type 2 diabetes who are treated with oral medications may have the impression that they do not *really* have diabetes or that they simply have "borderline" diabetes. They may believe that, compared with diabetic patients who require insulin injections, their diabetes is not a serious problem. It is important for the nurse to emphasize to these individuals that they *do* have diabetes and not a borderline problem with sugar (glucose). (Borderline diabetes is classified as **impaired glucose tolerance** [IGT] or **impaired fasting glucose** [IFG] and refers to a condition in which blood glucose levels fall between normal and those levels considered diagnostic for diabetes.)

Table 37-1 summarizes the major classifications of diabetes, current terminology, old labels, and major clinical characteristics. It is important to recognize that this classification system is dynamic in two ways. First, research findings suggest that there are many differences among individuals within each category. Second, except for those with type 1 diabetes, patients may move from one category to another. For example, a woman with gestational diabetes may, after delivery, move into the type 2 category. These types also differ in their etiology, clinical course, and management.

OVERVIEW OF PHYSIOLOGY AND PATHOPHYSIOLOGY

Normal Physiology

Insulin is secreted by beta cells, which are one of four types of cells in the islets of Langerhans in the pancreas. Insulin is an anabolic, or storage, hormone. When a meal is eaten, insulin secretion increases and moves glucose from the blood into muscle, liver, and fat cells. In those cells, insulin has the following effects:

- Transports and metabolizes glucose for energy
- Stimulates storage of glucose in the liver and muscle (in the form of glycogen)
- Enhances storage of dietary fat in adipose tissue
- Accelerates transport of amino acids (derived from dietary protein) into cells

Insulin also inhibits the breakdown of stored glucose, protein, and fat.

During fasting periods (between meals and overnight), the pancreas continuously releases a small amount of insulin; another pancreatic hormone called glucagon (which is secreted by the alpha cells of the islets of Langerhans) is released when blood glucose levels decrease. The insulin and the glucagon together maintain a constant level of glucose in the blood by stimulating the release of glucose from the liver.

Initially, the liver produces glucose through the breakdown of glycogen (glycogenolysis). After 8 to 12 hours without food, the liver forms glucose from the breakdown of noncarbohydrate substances, including amino acids (gluconeogenesis).

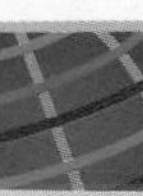

TABLE 37•1 Classification of Diabetes Mellitus and Related Glucose Intolerances

Current Classification	Previous Classifications	Clinical Characteristics and Clinical Implications
Type 1: Insulin-dependent diabetes mellitus (IDDM) (5%–10% of all diabetes)	Juvenile diabetes Juvenile-onset diabetes Ketosis-prone diabetes Brittle diabetes	Onset any age, but usually young (<30 yrs) Usually thin at diagnosis; with recent weight loss Etiology includes genetic, immunologic, or environmental factors (eg, virus). Often have islet cell antibodies Often have antibodies to insulin even before insulin treatment Little or no endogenous insulin Need insulin to preserve life Ketosis-prone when insulin absent Acute complication of hyperglycemia: diabetic ketoacidosis
Type 2: Non–insulin-dependent diabetes (NIDDM) (90%–95% of all diabetes: obese—80% of type 2; nonobese—20% of type 2)	Adult-onset diabetes Maturity-onset diabetes Ketosis-resistant diabetes Stable diabetes	Onset any age, usually over 30 years Usually obese at diagnosis Causes include obesity, heredity, or environmental factors. No islet cell antibodies Decrease in endogenous insulin, or increased with insulin resistance Most patients can control blood glucose through weight loss if obese. Oral antidiabetic agents may improve blood glucose levels if dietary modification and exercise are unsuccessful. May need insulin on a short- or long-term basis to prevent hyperglycemia Ketosis rare, except in stress or infection Acute complication: hyperglycemic hyperosmolar nonketotic syndrome
Diabetes mellitus associated with other conditions or syndromes	Secondary diabetes	Accompanied by conditions known or suspected to cause the disease: pancreatic diseases, hormonal abnormalities, drugs such as corticosteroids and estrogen-containing preparations Depending on the ability of the pancreas to produce insulin, the patient may require treatment with oral antidiabetic agents or insulin.
Gestational diabetes	Gestational diabetes	Onset during pregnancy, usually in the second or third trimester. Due to hormones secreted by the placenta, which inhibit the action of insulin Above-normal risk for perinatal complications, especially macrosomia (abnormally large babies) Treated with diet and, if needed, insulin to strictly maintain normal blood glucose levels. Occurs in about 2%–5% of all pregnancies Glucose intolerance transitory but may recur: • In subsequent pregnancies • 30%–40% will develop overt diabetes (usually type 2) within 10 years (especially if obese) Risk factors include obesity, age older than 30 years, family history of diabetes, previous large babies (over 9 lb). Screening tests (glucose challenge test) should be performed on ALL pregnant women between 24 and 28 weeks' gestation.
Impaired glucose tolerance	Borderline diabetes Latent diabetes Chemical diabetes Subclinical diabetes Asymptomatic diabetes	Oral glucose tolerance test value between 140 mg/dL (7.7 mmol/L) and 200 mg/dL (11 mmol/L) Impaired fasting glucose is defined as a fasting plasma glucose between 110 mg/dL (6 mmol/L) and 126 mg/dL (7 mmol/L). 29% eventually develop diabetes Above-normal susceptibility to atherosclerotic disease Renal and retinal complications usually not significant May be obese or nonobese; obese should reduce weight Should be screened for diabetes periodically
Previous abnormality of glucose tolerance (PrevAGT)	Latent diabetes Prediabetes	Current normal glucose metabolism Previous history of hyperglycemia (eg, during pregnancy or illness) Periodic blood glucose screening after age 40 if there is a family history of diabetes or if symptomatic Encourage ideal body weight, because loss of 10–15 lbs may improve glycemic control.
Potential abnormality of glucose tolerance (PotAGT)	Prediabetes	No history of glucose intolerance Increased risk of diabetes if: • Positive family history • Obesity • Mother of babies over 9 lbs at birth • Member of certain Native American Indian tribes with high prevalence of diabetes (eg, Pima) Screening and weight advice as in PrevAGT

Pathophysiology

Type 1 Diabetes

Type 1 diabetes is characterized by destruction of the pancreatic beta cells. It is thought that a combination of genetic, immunologic, and possibly environmental (eg, viral) factors contributes to beta cell destruction.

The interaction of genetic, immunologic, and environmental factors in the etiology of type 1 diabetes is the subject of continuing research. Although the events that lead to beta cell destruction are not fully understood, it is generally accepted that a genetic susceptibility is a common underlying factor in the development of type 1 diabetes. People do not inherit type 1 diabetes itself; rather, they inherit a genetic predisposition, or tendency, toward developing type 1 diabetes. This genetic tendency has been found in people with certain HLA (human leukocyte antigen) types. HLA refers to a cluster of genes responsible for transplantation antigens and other immune processes. Ninety-five percent of Caucasians with type 1 diabetes exhibit specific HLA types (DR3 or DR4). The risk of developing type 1 diabetes is increased three to five times in people who have one of these two HLA types. The risk is increased 10 to 20 times in people who have both DR3 and DR4 HLA types (as compared with the general population).

There is also evidence of an autoimmune response in type 1 diabetes. This is an abnormal response in which antibodies are directed against normal tissues of the body, responding to these tissues as if they are foreign. Autoantibodies against islet cells and against endogenous (internal) insulin have been detected in people at the time of diagnosis and even several years before the development of clinical signs of type 1 diabetes. Research is being conducted to evaluate the effect of immunosuppressive agents on the progression of disease in people with newly diagnosed type 1 diabetes or people with prediabetes (those with detectable antibodies but no clinical symptoms of diabetes). Other research is examining the protective effect of small doses of insulin on beta cell function.

In addition to genetic and immunologic components, environmental factors that may initiate destruction of the beta cell are being investigated. For example, it has been proposed that certain viruses or toxins may precipitate the autoimmune process that leads to beta cell destruction.

Regardless of the specific etiology, the destruction of the beta cells results in unchecked glucose production by the liver and fasting hyperglycemia. In addition, glucose derived from food cannot be stored in the liver but instead remains in the bloodstream and contributes to postprandial (after meals) hyperglycemia. If the concentration of glucose in the blood exceeds the renal threshold for glucose, usually 180 to 200 mg/dL (9.9 to 11.1 mmol/L), the kidneys may not reabsorb all of the filtered glucose; the glucose then appears in the urine (glucosuria). When excess glucose is excreted in the urine, it is accompanied by excessive loss of fluids and electrolytes. This is called osmotic diuresis.

Because insulin normally inhibits glycogenolysis (breakdown of stored glucose) and gluconeogenesis (production of new glucose from amino acids and other substrates), in people with insulin deficiency, these processes occur unrestrained and contribute further to hyperglycemia. In addition, fat breakdown occurs, resulting in an increased production of **ketone** bodies, which are the byproducts of fat breakdown.

Nursing Alert *Ketone bodies are acids that disturb the acid–base balance of the body when they accumulate in excessive amounts. The resulting diabetic ketoacidosis (DKA) may cause signs and symptoms such as abdominal pain, nausea, vomiting, hyperventilation, fruity odor of the breath, and, if left untreated, altered level of consciousness, coma, and even death. Initiation of insulin treatment, along with fluid and electrolytes as needed, rapidly improves the metabolic abnormalities and resolves symptoms of hyperglycemia and DKA. Diet and exercise with frequent monitoring of blood glucose levels are also important components of therapy.*

Type 2 Diabetes

The two main problems related to insulin in type 2 diabetes are insulin resistance and impaired insulin secretion. Insulin resistance refers to a decreased sensitivity of the tissues to insulin. Normally, insulin binds to special receptors on cell surfaces and initiates a series of reactions involved in glucose metabolism. In type 2 diabetes, these intracellular reactions are diminished, thus rendering insulin less effective at stimulating glucose uptake by the tissues (Fig. 37-1). The exact mechanisms that lead to insulin resistance and impaired insulin secretion in type 2 diabetes are unknown, although genetic factors are thought to play a role.

To overcome insulin resistance and to prevent the buildup of glucose in the blood, increased amounts of insulin must be secreted to maintain the glucose level at a normal or slightly elevated level. However, if the beta cells cannot keep up with the increased demand for insulin, the glucose level rises, and type 2 diabetes develops.

Despite the impaired insulin secretion that is characteristic of type 2 diabetes, there is enough insulin present to prevent the breakdown of fat and the accompanying production of ketone bodies. Therefore, DKA does not occur in type 2 diabetes. Uncontrolled type 2 diabetes may, however, lead to another acute problem, called hyperglycemic hyperosmolar nonketotic syndrome (HHNS) (see later discussion).

Type 2 diabetes occurs most commonly in people older than 30 years who are obese. Because it is associated with a slow (over years), progressive glucose intolerance, the onset of type 2 diabetes may go undetected for many years. If symptoms are experienced, they are frequently mild and may include fatigue, irritability, polyuria, polydipsia, skin wounds that heal poorly, vaginal infections, or blurred vision (if glucose levels are very high).

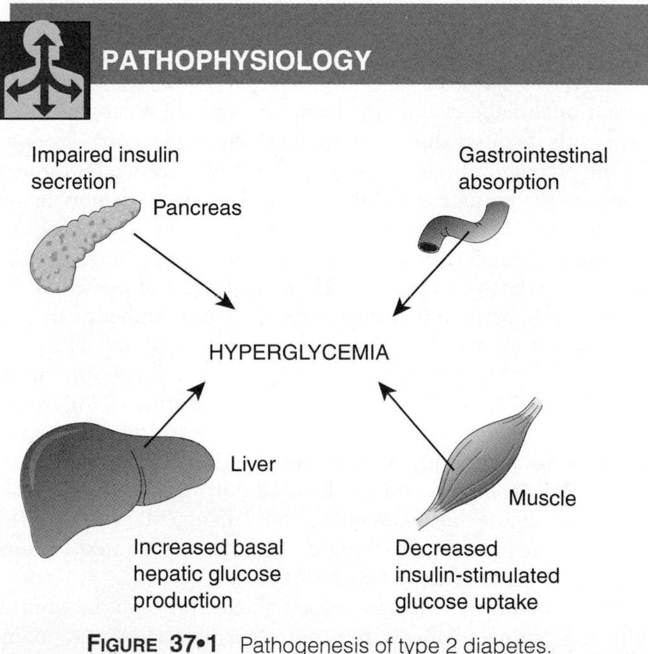

FIGURE 37•1 Pathogenesis of type 2 diabetes.

Risk Factors for DIABETES MELLITUS

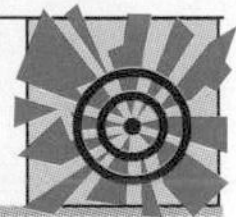

Family history of diabetes (ie, parents or siblings with diabetes)
Obesity (ie, ≥20% over desired body weight or BMI ≥27 kg/m^2)
Race/ethnicity (eg, African Americans, Hispanic Americans, Native Americans, Asian Americans, Pacific Islanders)
Age ≥45 years
Previously identified impaired fasting glucose or impaired glucose tolerance
Hypertension (≥140/90 mm Hg)
HDL cholesterol level ≤35 mg/dL (0.90 mmol/L) and/or triglyceride level ≥ 250 mg/dL (2.8 mmol/L)
History of gestational diabetes or delivery of babies over 9 lbs

Used with permission of American Diabetes Association. (1998). Report of the Expert Committee on the Diagnosis and Classification of Diabetes Mellitus. *Diabetes Care, 21* (Suppl 1), S5–S19.

For most patients (approximately 75%), type 2 diabetes is detected incidentally (eg, when routine laboratory tests are performed). One consequence of undetected diabetes is that long-term diabetes complications (eg, eye disease, peripheral neuropathy, peripheral vascular disease) may have developed before the actual diagnosis of diabetes is made.

Because insulin resistance is associated with obesity, the primary treatment of type 2 diabetes is weight loss. Exercise is also important in enhancing the effectiveness of insulin. Oral antidiabetic agents may be added if diet and exercise are not successful in controlling blood glucose levels. If maximum doses of a single category of oral agents fail to reduce glucose levels to satisfactory levels, additional oral agents may be used. Insulin may be added to oral agent therapy, or patients may move to insulin therapy entirely. Some patients require insulin on an ongoing basis, and a few may require insulin on a temporary basis during periods of acute physiologic stress, such as illness or surgery.

Gestational Diabetes

Gestational diabetes is defined as any degree of glucose intolerance with its onset during pregnancy. Hyperglycemia develops during pregnancy because of the secretion of placental hormones. Selective screening for diabetes during pregnancy is now being recommended for women between the 24th and 28th weeks of gestation who meet one or more of the following criteria: 25 years of age or older; younger than 25 years of age and obese; family history of diabetes in first-degree relatives; or member of an ethnic/racial group with a high prevalence of diabetes (eg, Hispanic American, Native American, Asian American, African American, or Pacific Islander) (Gestational Diabetes Mellitus, 1998). Initial management includes dietary modification and blood glucose monitoring. If hyperglycemia persists, insulin is prescribed. Oral antidiabetic agents should not be used during pregnancy. Goals for blood glucose during pregnancy are 105 mg/dL (5.8 mmol/L) or less before meals and 120 mg/dL (6.7 mmol/L) or less 2 hours after meals (Gestational Diabetes Mellitus, 1998).

After delivery of the infant, blood glucose levels in the woman with gestational diabetes return to normal. However, many women who have had gestational diabetes develop type 2 diabetes

NURSING RESEARCH

Determining the Impact of Body Image on Weight Loss Practices and Satisfaction

Anderson, L., Janes, G., & Zeimer, D. (1997). Diabetes in urban African Americans: Body image, satisfaction with size, and weight change attempts. *Diabetes Educator, 23*(3), 301–308.

Purpose

Being overweight is a risk factor for the development of type 2 diabetes as well as for complications of diabetes. The prevalence of overweight among African American men and women with diabetes is substantially higher than among African Americans without diabetes. Body image, the way individuals picture their bodies in their minds, and satisfaction with that image have been identified as possible factors in overweight as well as in efforts at weight control. This study was conducted to assess these factors in African Americans because of lack of information about them. The purposes of this study were to compare perceptions by status of weight and gender about current body size, desired body size, and what a designated important other sees as the subject's desired body size; to examine how current perceptions of body size relate to satisfaction with size and attempts to alter weight; and to explore the relationships between satisfaction with body size and the variables of self-rated health, mood control, and chance health locus of control.

Study Sample and Design

Subjects in a convenience sample of 370 African Americans (224 women and 146 men) with diabetes (90.8% of whom had type 2 diabetes) completed a body image survey; body size silhouettes were shown to the participants, who were asked to identify the one that looked most like their body. In addition, the participants were asked to identify the body size they want to look like, the dietitian wants them to look like, and the most important person in their life wants them to look like. Overweight was defined as a BMI 27.3 or more for women and 27.8 or more for men.

Findings

Ratings in overweight women showed that desired body size was significantly larger than the size dietitians might desire ($p < 0.0001$). Similar results were found in men who were overweight. Of those classified as overweight, about 13% of women and 21% of men expressed satisfaction with their current body size. Those who expressed less satisfaction with their body size were more likely to report that they were trying to change their weight than those who were satisfied with their body size.

Nursing Implications

It was expected at the beginning of this study that an individual's body image as well as satisfaction with that image would be important in determining whether that person believed weight control was important. The findings of this study were consistent with that expectation. Moreover, most patients believed that dietitians expected them to achieve a body size even smaller than their personal desired body size. It is important to understand patients' perception of the goals set for them. They may perceive them as unrealistic and not pursue the goals from the start. It is important to communicate with patients to ensure that the goals understood by both professionals and patients are one and the same. In this case, weight control is an extremely important goal in the treatment of type 2 diabetes, and every effort needs to be made to convey the importance of this point to patients.

later in life. Therefore, all women who have had gestational diabetes should be counseled to maintain their ideal body weight and to exercise regularly to reduce their risk for type 2 diabetes.

CLINICAL MANIFESTATIONS

Clinical manifestations of diabetes include the "three P's": polyuria, polydipsia, and polyphagia. Polyuria (increased urination) and polydipsia (increased thirst) occur as a result of the excess loss of fluid associated with osmotic diuresis. The patient also experiences polyphagia (increased appetite) resulting from the catabolic state induced by insulin deficiency and the breakdown of proteins and fats. Other symptoms include fatigue and weakness, sudden vision changes, tingling or numbness in hands or feet, dry skin, sores that are slow to heal, and recurrent infections. The onset of type 1 diabetes may also be associated with nausea, vomiting, or abdominal pains.

ASSESSMENT AND DIAGNOSTIC FINDINGS

The presence of abnormally high blood glucose levels is the criterion on which the diagnosis of diabetes is based. **Fasting plasma glucose** (FPG) levels of 126 mg/dL (7.0 mmol/L) or more or random plasma glucose levels of more than 200 mg/dL (11.1 mmol/L) on more than one occasion are diagnostic of diabetes.

The oral glucose tolerance test and the intravenous glucose tolerance test are no longer recommended for routine clinical use. See Chart 37-1 for the American Diabetes Association's diagnostic criteria for diabetes mellitus (Expert Committee on the Diagnosis and Classification of Diabetes Mellitus, 1998).

In addition to the assessment and diagnostic evaluation performed to diagnose diabetes, ongoing specialized assessment of the known diabetic and evaluation for complications in the newly diagnosed diabetic patient are important components of care.

CHART 37•1 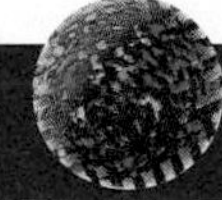 **Criteria for the Diagnosis of Diabetes Mellitus**

1. Symptoms of diabetes plus casual plasma glucose concentration greater than or equal to 200 mg/dL (11.1 mmol/L). Casual is defined as any time of day without regard to time since last meal. The classic symptoms of diabetes include polyuria, polydipsia, and unexplained weight loss.

or

2. Fasting plasma glucose greater than or equal to 126 mg/dL (7.0 mmol/L). Fasting is defined as no caloric intake for at least 8 hours.

or

3. 2-hour postload glucose greater than or equal to 200 mg/dL (11.1 mmol/L) during an oral glucose tolerance test. The test should be performed as described by the World Health Organization, using a glucose load containing the equivalent of 75 g anhydrous glucose dissolved in water.

In the absence of unequivocal hyperglycemia with acute metabolic decompensation, these criteria should be confirmed by repeat testing on a different day. The third measure is not recommended for routine clinical use.

Used with permission of American Diabetes Association. (1998). Report of the Expert Committee on the Diagnosis and Classification of Diabetes Mellitus. *Diabetes Care, 21* (Suppl 1), S5–S19.

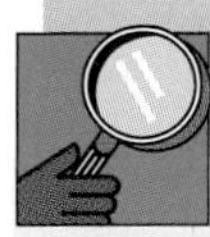

ASSESSMENT THE DIABETIC PATIENT

History

Symptoms of hyperglycemia
Symptoms of hypoglycemia
  Frequency, timing, severity, resolution
Home blood glucose monitoring results
Status of chronic complications
  Nephropathy: most recent microalbuminuria or 24-hour urine collection
  Retinopathy: symptoms, most recent ophthalmologic evaluation
  Neuropathy: symptoms
  Macrovascular disease: symptoms
Dietary compliance
Exercise regimen

Physical Examination

Blood pressure
Weight
Funduscopic exam
Feet
  Lesions and evidence of infection
  Pulses
Neurologic examination
  Vibratory and pinprick sensation
  Deep tendon reflexes

Laboratory Examination

$HgbA_{1c}$ (every 3 months)
Microalbuminuria or 24-hour urine collection (annually)
Fasting lipids (annually)

Referrals

Ophthalmology
Podiatry

Source: Lieberman, S. (1996). Diabetes mellitus. In M. Fishman et al. (Eds.), *Medicine* (4th ed.). Philadelphia: Lippincott-Raven.

Parameters that should be regularly assessed are discussed in "Assessment: The Diabetic Patient."

Gerontologic Considerations

Elevated blood glucose levels appear to be age-related and occur in both men and women throughout the world. Elevation of blood glucose appears in the fifth decade of life and increases in frequency with advancing age. When elderly people with overt diabetes are excluded from the statistics, approximately 10% to 30% of elderly people have age-related hyperglycemia.

The question then arises whether age-related hyperglycemia is part of the normal aging process and benign, or pathologic and requiring therapeutic intervention. Several studies have suggested that the hyperglycemia is pathologic because it leads to macrovascular complications.

The cause of age-related changes in carbohydrate metabolism is still not resolved. Apparently, delayed absorption from the gastrointestinal tract is not a factor. Other possibilities include poor diet, physical inactivity, a decrease in the lean body mass in which ingested carbohydrate may be stored, altered insulin secretion, and insulin resistance.

MANAGEMENT

The main goal of diabetes treatment is to normalize insulin activity and blood glucose levels to reduce the development of the vascular and neuropathic complications. The importance of tight control of blood glucose was demonstrated by the **Diabetes Control and Complications Trial** (DCCT), a 10-year prospective clinical trial conducted from 1983 to 1993 that was designed to determine the impact of intensive glucose control on the development and progression of complications such as **retinopathy**, **nephropathy**, and **neuropathy**. A cohort of 1441 people with type 1 diabetes was randomly assigned to conventional treatment (one or two insulin injections per day) or intensive treatment (three or four insulin injections per day or insulin pump therapy). End-point data were collected, and the results demonstrated that the risk for developing retinopathy was reduced by 76% and the incidences of microalbuminuria and albuminuria, early signs of nephropathy, were reduced by 39% and 54%, respectively. Further, the incidence of neuropathy was decreased by 60% through control of serum glucose levels to normal or near-normal levels. On the basis of these results, it is now recommended that all patients with diabetes strive to achieve glucose control to reduce their risks for complications.

The major adverse effect of intensive therapy was a threefold increase in the incidence of severe **hypoglycemia** (severe enough to require assistance from another person), coma, or seizure. Because of these adverse effects, intensive therapy must be initiated with caution and must be accompanied by intensive education of the patient and family and by responsible behavior on the part of the patient. Careful screening of patients is a key step in initiating intensive therapy. There are other situations that preclude the initiation of very tight control of blood glucose (see discussion of insulin in this chapter).

A study conducted in the United Kingdom and reported in 1998 supported the results of the DCCT in type 2 diabetes and demonstrated a decrease in complications in patients with type 2 diabetes who received intensive therapy when compared to those who received conventional therapy (United Kingdom Prospective Diabetes Study Group [UKPD], 1998).

Therefore, the therapeutic goal for diabetes management is to achieve normal blood glucose levels (euglycemia) without hypoglycemia and without seriously disrupting the patient's usual lifestyle and activity. There are five components of management for diabetes (Fig. 37-2):

- Nutrition management
- Exercise
- Monitoring
- Pharmacologic therapy
- Education

Treatment varies through the disease course because of changes in lifestyle and physical and emotional status as well as advances in treatment methods resulting from research. Therefore, diabetes management involves constant assessment and modification of the treatment plan by health professionals as well as daily adjustments in therapy by the patient. Although the health care team directs the treatment, it is the patient who is faced with the daily charge of managing the intricacies of a complex therapeutic regimen. For this reason, patient and family education is an essential component of diabetes treatment—equal in importance to other components of the regimen.

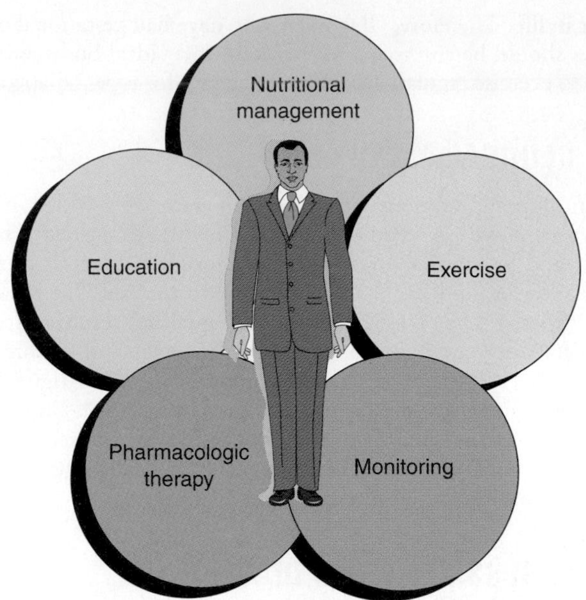

FIGURE 37•2 The five components of diabetes management.

Nutrition Management

Diet and weight control constitute the foundation of diabetes management. Nutritional management of the patient with diabetes is geared toward the following goals:

- Providing all the essential food constituents (eg, vitamins, minerals)
- Achieving and maintaining a reasonable weight
- Meeting energy needs
- Preventing wide daily fluctuations in blood glucose levels with blood glucose levels as close to normal as is safe and practical
- Decreasing serum lipid levels, if elevated

For patients who require insulin to help control blood glucose levels, maintaining as much consistency as possible in the amount of calories and carbohydrates eaten at different meal times is important for control of blood glucose. In addition, consistency in the approximate time intervals between meals, with the addition of snacks if necessary, helps in the prevention of hypoglycemic reactions and in overall blood glucose control.

For obese patients (especially those with type 2 diabetes), weight loss is the key to the treatment of diabetes. Although there are variations in the definitions of overweight and obesity, overweight is generally accepted to be a body mass index (BMI) of 25 to 30; obesity is defined as 20% above ideal body weight or a BMI greater than 30. BMI is a weight-to-height ratio calculated by dividing body weight (in kilograms) by the square of the height (in meters). Calculation of BMI is discussed in more detail in Chapter 5.

For obese patients in general, weight loss is the major preventive factor for the development of diabetes. Obesity is associated with an increased resistance to insulin and is one of the main etiologic factors associated with type 2 diabetes. Some obese patients with type 2 diabetes who require insulin or oral agents for control of blood glucose may be able to reduce or eliminate the need for medication through weight loss. As small a weight loss as 10% of total weight can significantly improve blood glucose levels. For obese diabetic patients who do not take insulin, consistency of meal content or timing is not as critical. Rather, the major focus is on decreasing the overall number of calories eaten. However, meals should not be skipped. Spacing food throughout the day places more manageable demands on the pancreas.

Long-term adherence to the meal plan is one of the most challenging aspects of diabetes management. For obese patients, it may be more realistic to restrict calories only moderately. For those who have lost weight, maintaining the weight loss is often difficult. To assist these patients in incorporating new dietary habits into their lifestyles, behavioral therapy, group support, and ongoing nutrition counseling are encouraged.

For all diabetic patients, the meal plan must take into consideration the patient's food preferences, lifestyle, usual eating times, and ethnic and cultural background. For patients using intensive insulin therapy regimens, there may be a greater flexibility in the timing and content of meals by allowing adjustments for changes in eating and exercise habits.

Meal Planning

CALORIE REQUIREMENTS

The first step in preparing a meal plan is to obtain a thorough diet history to identify the patient's eating habits and lifestyle. It is also necessary to assess the need for weight loss, gain, or maintenance. In most instances, the person with type 2 diabetes requires weight reduction. The most important objective in the dietary management of diabetes is control of total calorie intake to attain or maintain a reasonable body weight and control of blood glucose levels. Success of this alone is often associated with reversal of hyperglycemia in type 2 diabetes. However, achieving this goal is not always easy.

Calorie-controlled diets can be used by first calculating the individual's calorie requirements. Age, gender, height, and weight are used in the Harris-Benedict formula to determine basal energy expenditure, reflecting minimal energy needs. An activity factor is then factored in to provide the actual number of calories required for weight maintenance. To promote a 1- to 2-pound weight loss per week, 500 to 1000 calories are subtracted from the daily total. The calories are distributed into carbohydrates, proteins, and fats, and a meal plan can then be developed.

The 1995 Exchange Lists for Meal Planning are presented to the patient using the appropriate amount of calories with strict diet adherence as the goal. Unfortunately, calorie-controlled diets are often confusing and difficult to comply with: they require patients to measure precise portions and to eat specific foods and amounts at each meal and snack. In this instance, developing a meal plan based on the individual's usual eating habits and lifestyle is often a more realistic approach to glucose control and weight loss or weight maintenance. Both instances require the patient to work closely with a registered dietitian to assess current eating habits and to achieve realistic, individualized goals.

In a young patient with type 1 diabetes, priority should be given to providing a diet with enough calories to maintain normal growth and development. Some patients may be underweight at the onset of type 1 diabetes because of rapid weight loss from severe hyperglycemia. The goal with these patients initially may be to provide a higher-calorie diet to regain lost weight.

CALORIE DISTRIBUTION

A diabetic meal plan also focuses on the percentage of calories to come from carbohydrates, proteins, and fats. There are two main types of carbohydrates—complex and simple. Starches such as bread, cereal, rice, and pasta are complex carbohydrates; fruit and sugars are examples of simple carbohydrates. In general, carbohydrate foods have the greatest effect on blood glucose levels because they are more quickly digested than other foods and are converted into glucose rapidly. Several decades ago it was recommended that diabetic diets contain more calories from protein and fat foods than from carbohydrates to reduce postmeal increases in blood glucose levels. However, more recently it has been found that complex carbohydrates are absorbed more gradually from the gastrointestinal tract and cause less of a rise in the blood glucose level than initially thought. In addition, diets that contain fewer calories from carbohydrates contain increased calories from fats—a problem when trying to reduce the cardiovascular disease commonly associated with diabetes.

The caloric distribution currently recommended is higher in carbohydrates than in fat and protein. However, research into the appropriateness of a higher-carbohydrate diet in patients with decreased glucose tolerance is ongoing, and recommendations may be changed accordingly. Currently, the American Diabetes and American Dietetic Associations recommend that for all levels of caloric intake, 50% to 60% of calories be derived from carbohydrates, 20% to 30% from fat, and the remaining 10% to 20% from protein. These recommendations are also consistent with those of the American Heart Association and American Cancer Society.

Carbohydrates are made up of sugars and starches. There is little scientific evidence to support the belief that simple carbohydrates such as sucrose promote a greater degree of blood glucose rise compared to complex carbohydrates or starches (eg, rice, pasta, or bread). Thus, the latest nutrition guidelines recommend that all carbohydrates be eaten in moderation to avoid high postprandial blood glucose levels (American Diabetes Association, *Exchange Lists for Meal Planning*, 1995). Simple carbohydrates such as sucrose are not eliminated from the diet but should be eaten in moderation (up to 10% of total calories) because these foods are typically high in fat and lack vitamins, minerals, and fiber.

Carbohydrate counting is a new nutritional tool used for blood glucose management because carbohydrates are the main nutrients in food that influence blood glucose levels. This method provides flexibility in food choices, can be less complicated to understand than the diabetic food exchange list, and allows more accurate management with multiple daily injections (insulin before each meal). However, if carbohydrate counting is not used in combination with other meal-planning techniques, weight gain can result. There are a variety of methods used to count carbohydrates. When developing a diabetic meal plan using carbohydrate counting, all food sources should be considered. Once digested, 100% of carbohydrates are converted to blood glucose. However, approximately 50% of protein foods (meat, fish, and poultry) are also converted to glucose.

One method of carbohydrate counting includes counting grams of carbohydrates. This is typically used for those with type 1 diabetes who need to be more accurate while on an insulin regimen. Usually, a dose of 1 to 2 units of fast-acting insulin covers 15 g of carbohydrate consumed. Bread, milk, and fruit are counted as 15 g of carbohydrate. Although nonstarchy vegetables and meats also convert to carbohydrate and are counted as 5 g of carbohydrate per serving, this is typically not factored in because it makes the calculations too complex. However, if target goals are not reached by counting carbohydrates alone, protein will be factored into the calculations. This is especially true if the meal consists of only meat, fish, and nonstarchy vegetables.

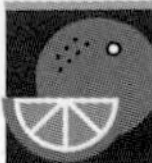

TABLE 37•2 **Summary of Sample Menus Based on the Exchange Lists**

Exchanges	Sample Lunch #1	Sample Lunch #2	Sample Lunch #3
2 starch	2 slices bread	Hamburger bun	1 cup cooked pasta
3 meat	2 oz sliced turkey and 1 oz lowfat cheese	3 oz lean beef patty	3 oz boiled shrimp
1 vegetable	Lettuce, tomato, onion	Green salad	½ cup plum tomatoes
1 fat	1 tsp mayonnaise	1 tbsp salad dressing	1 tsp olive oil
1 fruit	1 medium apple	1¼ cup watermelon	1¼ cup fresh strawberries
"Free" items (optional)	Iced tea	Diet soda	Ice water with lemon
	Mustard, pickle, hot pepper	1 tbsp catsup, pickle, onions	Garlic, basil

An alternative to calculating grams of carbohydrate is measuring servings or choices. This method is used more often with those with type 2 diabetes. It is similar to the food exchange list and emphasizes portion control of total servings of carbohydrate at meals and snacks. One carbohydrate serving is equivalent to 15 g of carbohydrate. Examples of one serving are a 2-inch apple and one slice of bread. Vegetables and meat are counted as one third of a carbohydrate serving.

Although carbohydrate counting is now more commonly used for blood glucose management with type 1 and type 2 diabetes, it is not a perfect system. All carbohydrates, to some extent, may affect the blood glucose to different degrees, regardless of equivalent serving size.

The recommendations regarding fat content of the diabetic diet include both reduction in the total percentage of calories from fat sources to less than 30% of the total calories and limitation of the amount of saturated fats to 10% of total calories. In addition, limiting the total intake of dietary cholesterol to less than 300 mg/day is recommended. These recommendations may help in the reduction of risk factors, such as elevated serum cholesterol levels, which are associated with the development of coronary artery disease, the leading cause of death and disability among people with diabetes.

The meal plan may include the use of some nonanimal sources of protein (eg, legumes, whole grains) to help in the reduction of saturated fat and cholesterol intake. In addition, recommendations for the amount of protein intake may be reduced in patients with early signs of renal disease.

FIBER

The use of fiber in diabetes has received increased attention as researchers study the effects on diabetes of a high-carbohydrate, high-fiber diet. This type of diet plays a role in lowering total cholesterol and low-density lipoprotein cholesterol in the blood. Increasing fiber in the diet may also improve blood glucose levels, leading to a decrease in the need for exogenous insulin.

There are two classifications of dietary fibers: soluble and insoluble. Soluble fiber—in foods such as legumes, oats, and some fruits—plays more of a role in lowering blood glucose and lipid levels than does insoluble fiber. However, the clinical significance of this effect is probably small (American Association of Diabetes Educators, 1998).

The mechanism of action of soluble fiber is thought to be related to the formation of a gel in the gastrointestinal tract. This gel slows the emptying of the stomach and the movement of food through the upper digestive tract. The potential glucose-lowering effect of fiber may be caused by the slower rate of glucose absorption from food that contains soluble fiber.

Insoluble fiber is found in whole-grain breads and cereals and in some vegetables. This type of fiber plays more of a role in increasing stool bulk and preventing constipation. Both insoluble and soluble fibers increase satiety, which is helpful for weight loss.

One risk involved in suddenly increasing fiber intake is that it may require adjusting the dosage of insulin or oral agents to prevent hypoglycemia. Other problems may include abdominal fullness, nausea, diarrhea, increased flatulence, and constipation if fluid intake is inadequate. If amounts of fiber are added to or increased in the meal plan, it should be done gradually and in consultation with a dietitian. The 1995 Exchange Lists for Meal Planning is an excellent guide for increasing fiber intake. Food choices high in fiber within the vegetable, fruit, and starch/bread exchanges are highlighted in the lists.

It appears that adding more fiber to the meal plan is beneficial. However, research is ongoing to determine how fiber works, which fibers are best, and the amount of fiber that is optimal for blood glucose and lipid control.

Food Classification Systems

To teach diet principles and to help patients in meal planning, several systems have been developed in which foods are organized into groups with common characteristics, such as number of calories, composition of foods (ie, amount of protein, fat, or carbohydrate in the food), or effect on blood glucose levels.

EXCHANGE LISTS

A common tool in use is the Exchange Lists for Meal Planning (American Diabetes Association, 1995). There are six main exchange lists: bread/starch, vegetable, milk, meat, fruit, and fat. Foods included on one list (in the amounts specified) contain equal numbers of calories and are approximately equal in grams of protein, fat, and carbohydrate. Patients are given meal plans (tailored to their individual needs and preferences) based on a recommended number of choices from each exchange list. Foods on one list may be interchanged with one another, allowing the patient to choose a variety while maintaining as much consistency as possible in the nutrient content of foods eaten. Table 37-2 presents three sample lunch menus that are interchangeable in terms of carbohydrate, protein, and fat content.

Information on combination foods such as pizza, chili, and chow mein is now available in the exchange list information from the American Dietetic Association. In addition, exchanges for a variety of foods, including convenience packaged foods, desserts, snack foods, and foods from fast-food restaurants are available. Some food manufacturing companies publish exchange lists that describe their products. For more nutrition information, contact the American Diabetes Association, 1660 Duke St., Alexandria, VA 22314; 800-ADA-DISC. Web sites for the American Diabetes Association and the American Dietetic Association can be found at the end of this chapter.

THE FOOD GUIDE PYRAMID

The Food Guide Pyramid, another tool used to develop meal plans, has replaced the basic four food groups. It is commonly used for patients with type 2 diabetes who have a difficult time complying with a calorie-controlled diet. The food pyramid consists of six food groups: (1) bread, cereal, rice, and pasta; (2) fruits; (3) vegetables; (4) meat, poultry, fish, dry beans, eggs, and nuts; (5) milk, yogurt, and cheese; and (6) fats, oils, and sweets (see Chap. 5). The pyramid shape was chosen to emphasize that the foods in the largest area, the base of the pyramid (starches, fruits, and vegetables), are lowest in calories and fat and highest in fiber and should make up the basis of the diet. For those with diabetes, as well as for the general population, 50% to 60% of the daily caloric intake should be from these three groups. As one moves up the pyramid, foods higher in fat (particularly saturated fat) are illustrated; these foods should account for a smaller percentage of the daily caloric intake. The very top of the pyramid illustrates fats, oils, and sweets, foods that should be used sparingly by people with diabetes to obtain weight and blood glucose control and to reduce the risk for cardiovascular disease.

The Food Guide Pyramid can be used to teach patients how to control the portions of foods and to emphasize which foods contain carbohydrate, protein, and fat. Menu planning should include meals with all three types of nutrients, emphasizing complex carbohydrates (starches) and limiting simple sugars and fat.

GLYCEMIC INDEX

One of the main goals of diet therapy in diabetes is to avoid sharp, rapid increases in blood glucose levels after food is eaten. The term "glycemic index" is used to describe how much a given food raises the blood glucose level compared with an equivalent amount of glucose. Studies of the glycemic index of certain carbohydrates have raised questions about a food's effect on blood glucose levels. Although more research is necessary, the following guidelines can be followed when making dietary recommendations:

- Combining starch foods with protein- and fat-containing foods tends to slow their absorption and lower the glycemic response.
- Eating foods that are raw and whole in general results in a lower glycemic response than eating chopped, puréed, or cooked foods.
- Eating whole fruit instead of drinking juice decreases the glycemic response, as fiber in the fruit slows absorption.
- When adding foods with simple sugars to the diet, a lower glycemic response may result if these foods are eaten with other more slowly absorbed foods.

Patients can create their own glycemic index by monitoring their blood glucose level after ingesting a particular food. This can help patients improve blood glucose levels through individualized manipulation of the diet. Many patients who use frequent monitoring of blood glucose levels can use this information to adjust their insulin doses for variations in food intake.

Other Dietary Concerns

ALCOHOL CONSUMPTION

The ingestion of alcohol by diabetic patients need not be completely restricted. It is important, however, for patients and health care professionals to be aware of the potential adverse effects of alcohol specific to diabetes.

In general, the same precautions regarding the use of alcohol by the general public should be applied to patients with diabetes. Moderation in the amount of alcohol consumed is recommended. The main danger with the use of alcohol by a diabetic patient is hypoglycemia. This is especially true for patients who take insulin. Alcohol may decrease the normal physiologic reactions in the body that produce glucose (gluconeogenesis). Thus, if a diabetic patient takes alcohol on an empty stomach, there is an increased likelihood that hypoglycemia will develop. In addition, excessive alcohol intake may impair a person's ability to recognize and treat hypoglycemia and to follow a prescribed meal plan to prevent hypoglycemia.

For the person with type 2 diabetes treated with chlorpropamide (Diabinese), a potential side effect of alcohol consumption is a disulfiram (Antabuse) type of reaction. Depending on the amount of alcohol consumed, the person taking chlorpropamide may experience facial flushing, warmth, headache, nausea, vomiting, sweating, or thirst within minutes of consuming alcohol. This reaction seems to be less common with other sulfonylurea agents.

In addition to these immediate potential effects, alcohol consumption may also lead to excessive weight gain (because of the high caloric content of alcohol), hyperlipidemia, and (especially if mixed drinks and liqueurs are consumed) elevated glucose levels.

Patient teaching regarding alcohol intake must emphasize moderation in the amount of alcohol consumed; lower-calorie or less sweet drinks, such as light beer or dry wine, and the intake of food along with alcohol are advised. For type 2 diabetic patients especially, incorporating the calories from alcohol into the overall meal plan is important for weight control.

SWEETENERS

The use of sweeteners is acceptable for patients with diabetes, especially if it assists in overall dietary adherence. Moderation in the amount of sweetener used is encouraged to avoid potential adverse effects. There are two main types of sweeteners: nutritive and non-nutritive. The nutritive sweeteners contain calories, and the non-nutritive sweeteners have few or no calories in the amounts normally used.

Nutritive sweeteners include fructose (fruit sugar), sorbitol, and xylitol. They are not calorie-free; they provide calories in amounts similar to those in sucrose (table sugar). They cause less elevation in blood sugar levels than sucrose and are often used in "sugar-free" foods. They may have a laxative effect (sorbitol).

Non-nutritive sweeteners have minimal or no calories. They are used in food products and are also available for table use. They produce minimal or no elevation in blood sugar levels and have been approved by the Food and Drug Administration as safe for people with diabetes. Saccharin contains no calories. Aspartame (NutraSweet) is packaged with dextrose; it contains 4 calories per packet and loses sweetness with heat. Acesulfame-K (Sunnette) is also packaged with dextrose; it contains 1 calorie per packet.

The Food and Drug Administration has recently approved a new sweetener to be used in a variety of food products. Sucralose is a non-nutritive, high-intensity sweetener that is about 600 times sweeter than sugar. It is approved for use in baked goods, nonalcoholic beverages, chewing gum, coffee, confections, frostings, and frozen dairy products.

MISLEADING FOOD LABELING

Foods labeled "sugarless" or "sugar-free" may still provide calories equal to those of the equivalent sugar-containing products if they are made with nutritive sweeteners. Thus, for weight loss, these products may not always be useful. In addition, patients must not consider them "free" foods to be eaten in unlimited quantity, because they may elevate blood glucose levels.

Foods labeled "dietetic" are not necessarily reduced-calorie foods. They may be lower in sodium or have other special dietary uses. Patients are advised that foods labeled "dietetic" may still contain significant amounts of sugar or fat.

Patients must also be taught to read the labels of "health foods"—especially snacks—because they often contain sugar products such as honey, brown sugar, and corn syrup. In addition, these supposedly healthy snacks frequently contain saturated vegetable fats (eg, coconut or palm oil), hydrogenated vegetable fats, or animal fats, which may be contraindicated in the patient with an elevated blood lipid level.

Health Teaching About Diet

The clinical dietitian uses various educational tools, teaching materials, and approaches to meal planning. Initial education addresses the importance of consistency in eating habits, the relationship of food and insulin, and the provision of an individualized meal plan. Follow-up education then focuses on more in-depth management skills, such as eating at restaurants, reading food labels, and adjusting the meal plan for exercise, illness, and special occasions. The nurse plays an important role in communicating pertinent information to the dietitian and reinforcing the patient's understanding.

For some patients, learning to use the exchange system may be too difficult. This may be related to limitations in the patient's intellectual level or to emotional issues, such as difficulty accepting the diagnosis of diabetes or feelings of deprivation and undue restriction in eating. It is important to simplify information as much as possible and to provide opportunities for practice and repetition of information. In addition, it should be emphasized that using the exchange system (or any food classification system) provides a new way of thinking about food rather than a completely new way of eating.

Exercise

Exercise is extremely important in the management of diabetes because of its effects on lowering blood glucose and reducing cardiovascular risk factors. Exercise lowers blood glucose by increasing the uptake of glucose by body muscles and by improving insulin utilization. It also improves circulation and muscle tone. Resistance training can increase lean muscle mass, thereby increasing the resting metabolic rate. These effects are useful in diabetes in relation to losing weight, easing stress, and maintaining a feeling of well-being. Exercise also alters blood lipids, increasing levels of high-density lipoproteins and decreasing total cholesterol and triglyceride levels. This is especially important to the person with diabetes because of the increased risk of cardiovascular disease.

However, patients with blood glucose levels of more than 250 mg/dL (14 mmol/L) who have ketones in their urine should not begin exercising until the urine ketone test is negative and the blood glucose level is closer to normal. Exercising with elevated blood glucose levels causes increased secretions of glucagon, growth hormone, and catecholamines. The liver then releases more glucose, resulting in an increase in blood glucose.

The physiologic decrease in circulating insulin that normally occurs with exercise cannot occur in patients treated with insulin. Initially, the patient who requires insulin should be taught to eat a 15-g carbohydrate snack (a fruit exchange) or a snack of complex carbohydrate with a protein before engaging in moderate exercise, to prevent unexpected hypoglycemia. The exact amount of food needed varies from person to person and should be determined by blood glucose monitoring. Some patients find that they do not require a preexercise snack if they exercise within 1 to 2 hours after a meal. Other patients may require extra food regardless of the timing of exercise. If extra food is required, it need not be deducted from the regular meal plan.

Another potential problem for patients who take insulin is hypoglycemia that occurs many hours after exercise. To avoid postexercise hypoglycemia, especially after strenuous exercise, the patient may need to eat a snack at the end of the exercise session and at bedtime and monitor the blood glucose level more frequently. In addition, it may be necessary to have the patient reduce the dosage of insulin that peaks at the time of exercise. Patients who are capable, knowledgeable, and responsible can learn to adjust their own insulin doses. Others need specific instructions on what to do when they exercise.

Patients participating in extended periods of exercise should test their blood glucose levels before, during, and after the exercise period, and they should eat carbohydrate snacks as needed to maintain blood glucose levels. Other participants or observers should be aware that the person exercising has diabetes, and they should know what assistance to give if severe hypoglycemia occurs.

In obese people with type 2 diabetes, exercise in addition to dietary management both improves glucose metabolism and enhances loss of body fat. Exercise coupled with weight loss improves insulin sensitivity and may decrease the need for insulin or oral agents. Eventually, the patient's glucose tolerance may return to normal. The type 2 diabetic patient who is not taking insulin or an oral agent may not need extra food before exercise.

People with diabetes should be taught to exercise at the same time (preferably when blood glucose levels are at their peak) and in the same amount each day. Regular daily exercise, rather than sporadic exercise, should be encouraged. Exercise recommendations must be altered as necessary for patients with diabetic complications such as retinopathy, autonomic neuropathy, sensorimotor neuropathy, and cardiovascular disease; these disorders are discussed later in this chapter. Increased blood pressure associated with exercise may aggravate diabetic retinopathy and increase the risk of a hemorrhage into the vitreous or retina. In patients with ischemic heart disease, there is a risk of triggering angina or a myocardial infarction. Avoidance of trauma to the lower extremities is especially important in the patient with numbness related to neuropathy.

In general, a slow, gradual increase in the length of the exercise period is encouraged. For many patients, walking is a safe and beneficial form of exercise that requires no special equipment (except for proper shoes) and can be performed anywhere. People with diabetes should discuss an exercise program with their physician before undertaking it.

If the patient is older than 30 years and has two or more of the risk factors for heart disease, an exercise stress test is recommended. Risk factors for heart disease include hypertension, obesity, high cholesterol levels, abnormal resting electrocardiogram, sedentary

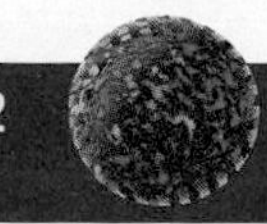

CHART 37•2 General Precautions for Exercise in Diabetics

- Use proper footwear and, if appropriate, other protective equipment.
- Avoid exercise in extreme heat or cold.
- Inspect feet daily after exercise.
- Avoid exercise during periods of poor metabolic control.

lifestyle, smoking, and a family history of heart disease. General guidelines for exercise in diabetes are presented in Chart 37-2.

Gerontologic Considerations

Physical activity that is consistent and realistic is beneficial to the elderly person with diabetes. Advantages include a decrease in hyperglycemia, a general sense of well-being, and the use of ingested calories, resulting in weight reduction. Because there is an increased incidence of cardiovascular problems in the elderly, a pattern of gradual, consistent exercise should be planned that does not exceed the patient's physical capacity. Physical impairment from other chronic diseases must also be considered. In some cases a physical therapy evaluation may be warranted with the goal of determining exercises specific to the patient's needs and abilities. Tools such as the "Armchair Fitness" video may be helpful.

Monitoring Glucose and Ketones

Self-Monitoring of Blood Glucose

Frequent **self-monitoring of blood glucose** (SMBG) enables people with diabetes to adjust the treatment regimen to obtain optimal blood glucose control. This allows for detection and prevention of hypoglycemia and hyperglycemia and plays a crucial role in normalizing blood glucose levels, which may reduce the risk of long-term diabetic complications.

Various methods are available for SMBG. Most of them involve obtaining a drop of blood from the fingertip, applying the blood to a special reagent strip, and allowing the blood to stay on the strip for a specific amount of time (usually 45 to 60 seconds, as specified by the manufacturer). The meter gives a digital readout of the blood glucose value.

Newer blood glucose monitors have eliminated the step of blood removal from the strip. The strip is placed in the meter first, before blood is applied to it. Once the blood is placed on the strip, it remains there for the duration of the test. The meter automatically displays the blood glucose level after a short time (less than 1 minute). One of the newest products uses a glucose sensor cartridge onto which the blood is placed. These new types of meters tend to give blood glucose results in a shorter period and have automatic timers that do not need to be activated by the user.

Meters have been developed that can be used by patients with visual impairments. They have audio components that assist the patient in performing the test and obtaining the result.

ADVANTAGES AND DISADVANTAGES OF SMBG SYSTEMS

It is very important that the method used by patients be matched to their skill level. Factors affecting SMBG performance include visual acuity, fine motor coordination, cognitive ability, comfort with technology, willingness, and cost.

Visual methods are the least expensive and require less equipment. However, they require the ability to distinguish colors and to be exact in timing the procedures; further, they involve subjective interpretation of the results. Monitoring blood glucose using meters is recommended because meters have become much less expensive and less technique-dependent, making results more accurate.

Older meters that require removal of blood from the reagent strip may still be in use by some patients; these procedures have more steps that must be performed in an exact sequence. However, they allow for double-checking the results through visual reading of the strips. The newer generation of meters that do not require removal of blood from the strip generally are simpler to use. However, most of them do not provide a backup method for visually assessing the meter results. Figure 37-3 illustrates a system for glucose monitoring.

A potential hazard of all methods of SMBG is that the patient may obtain and report erroneous blood glucose values as a result of using incorrect techniques. Some common sources of error include:

- Improper application of blood (eg, drop too small)
- Improper cleaning and maintenance of meters (eg, allowing dust or blood to accumulate on the optic window)
- Damage to the reagent strips by heat or humidity; use of outdated strips

The nurse plays an important role in providing initial education in SMBG techniques. Equally important is evaluating the techniques of patients who are experienced in self-monitoring. Patients should be discouraged from purchasing SMBG products from stores or catalogs that do not provide direct education. Every 6 to 12 months, patients should conduct a comparison of their meter with a simultaneous laboratory-measured blood glucose level in their physician's office. The accuracy of the meter and strips should also be assessed with control solutions specific to that meter whenever a new vial of strips is used or whenever the validity of the readings is in doubt.

CANDIDATES FOR SMBG

Blood glucose monitoring is a useful procedure for all people with diabetes. It is a cornerstone of treatment for any intensive insulin therapy regimen (including two to four injections per day or insulin pumps) and for managing diabetes in the pregnant woman. It is also highly recommended for patients with:

- Unstable diabetes
- A tendency for severe ketosis or hypoglycemia

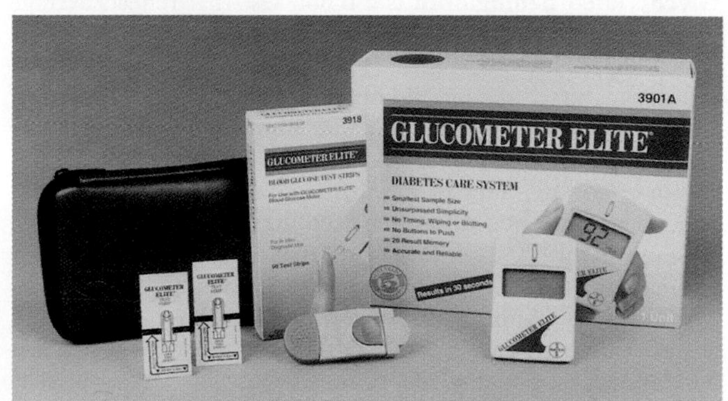

FIGURE 37•3 Example of blood glucose monitors.

- Hypoglycemia without warning symptoms
- Abnormal renal glucose thresholds

For patients not taking insulin, SMBG is helpful for monitoring the effectiveness of exercise, diet, and oral agents. It can also help to motivate patients to continue with treatment. For type 2 diabetic patients, SMBG should also be recommended during periods of suspected hyperglycemia (eg, illness) or hypoglycemia (eg, unusual increased activity levels).

FREQUENCY OF SMBG

For most patients who require insulin, testing two to four times per day is recommended (usually before meals and at bedtime). For patients who take insulin before each meal, testing at least three times per day is required for determining each insulin dose. Patients not receiving insulin may be instructed to assess their blood glucose levels at least two or three times per week, including a 2-hour postprandial test. For all patients, testing is recommended whenever hypoglycemia or hyperglycemia is suspected.

INTERPRETATION OF SMBG RESULTS

Patients should be instructed to keep a record or log book of blood glucose results so they can begin to see patterns emerge. Testing is done at the peak action time of the medication to evaluate the need for dosage adjustments. To evaluate basal insulin and determine bolus insulin doses, testing is performed before meals. To titrate bolus insulin doses, regular or lispro, testing is done 2 hours postprandially. Patients with type 2 diabetes are encouraged to test before and 2 hours after the largest meal of the day. Patients who take insulin at bedtime or who are on an insulin infusion pump must also test at 3 AM once a week to document that the blood glucose level is not decreasing overnight.

If a patient is unwilling or cannot afford to test frequently, then once or twice a day may be sufficient if the patient varies the time of day to test (eg, before breakfast one day, before lunch the next day).

A tendency to discontinue SMBG may be seen in patients who were never instructed on how to use the results for altering their treatment regimen. Instructions vary according to the patient's understanding and the physician's philosophy of diabetes management. At the very least, patients should be given parameters for calling the physician. Patients using intensive insulin therapy regimens may be instructed in the use of algorithms (rules or decision trees) for changing the insulin doses based on patterns of values greater or less than the target range.

Glycosylated Hemoglobin

Glycosylated hemoglobin is a blood test that reflects average blood glucose levels over a period of approximately 2 to 3 months. When blood glucose levels are elevated, glucose molecules attach to hemoglobin in the red blood cell. The longer the amount of glucose in the blood remains above normal, the more glucose binds to the red blood cell, and the higher the glycosylated hemoglobin level. This complex (the hemoglobin attached to the glucose) is permanent and lasts for the life of the red blood cell, approximately 120 days. If near-normal blood glucose levels are maintained, with only occasional increases in blood glucose, the overall value will not be greatly elevated. However, if the blood glucose values are consistently high, then the test result will also be elevated. If patients report mostly normal results of self-glucose monitoring but the glycosylated hemoglobin is high, there may be errors in the methods used for glucose monitoring, errors in recording results, or frequent elevations in glucose levels at times during the day when the patient is not usually monitoring the blood.

There are various tests that measure the same thing but have different names, including hemoglobin A_{1C} and hemoglobin A_1. The normal values differ slightly from test to test and from laboratory to laboratory and normally range from 4% to 6%. Values within the normal range indicate consistently near-normal blood glucose levels, a goal made easier by SMBG.

Urine Testing for Glucose

Before the availability of SMBG methods, **urine glucose testing** was the only method available for day-to-day monitoring of diabetes. Today its use is limited to patients who cannot or will not perform blood glucose testing.

The general procedure involves applying urine to a reagent strip or tablet and matching colors on the strip with a color chart at the end of a specified period. The disadvantages of urine testing include the following:

- Results do not reflect the blood glucose level at the time of the test.
- The renal threshold for glucose is 180 to 200 mg/dL (9.9 to 11.1 mmol/L), far above target blood glucose levels.
- It is impossible to detect hypoglycemia, because a "negative" urine glucose result may occur when blood glucose ranges from 0 to 180 mg/dL (9.9 mmol/L) or higher.
- Patients may have a false sense of being in good control when results are always negative.
- Various medications (eg, aspirin, vitamin C, some antibiotics) may interfere with test results.
- In the elderly and in patients with kidney disease, the renal threshold (the level of blood glucose at which glucose starts to appear in the urine) is raised; thus, false-negative readings may occur at dangerously elevated glucose levels.

The advantages of urine glucose testing are that it is less expensive than SMBG and it is not invasive.

Urine Testing for Ketones

Ketones (or ketone bodies) in the urine signal that control of type 1 diabetes is deteriorating, and the risk of DKA is high. When there is almost no effective insulin available, the body starts to break down stored fat for energy. Ketone bodies are byproducts of this fat breakdown, and they accumulate in the blood and urine. The only method available for self-testing of ketone bodies by patients is urine testing.

The most commonly used method to detect ketonuria is to use a urine dipstick (Ketostix or Chemstrip uK), which measures one type of ketone body. The reagent pad on the strip turns purplish when ketones are present. (One of the ketone bodies is called acetone, and this term is frequently used interchangeably with the term "ketones.") There are also strips available that measure both glucose and ketones (Keto-Diastix or Chemstrip uGK). Large amounts of ketones may depress the color development of the glucose test area.

Urine ketone testing should be performed whenever patients with type 1 diabetes have glucosuria or persistently elevated blood glucose levels (more than 240 mg/dL or 13.2 mmol/L for two testing periods in a row), and during illness and pregnancy.

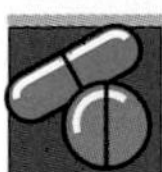

TABLE 37•3 **Categories of Insulin**

Time Course	Agent	Onset	Peak	Duration	Indications
Rapid-acting	Humalog	10–15 min	1 h	3 h	Used for rapid reduction of glucose level, to treat postprandial hyperglycemia, and/or to prevent nocturnal hypoglycemia
Short-acting	Regular ("R")	½–1 h	2–3 h	4–6 h	Usually administered 20–30 minutes before a meal; may be taken alone or in combination with longer-acting insulin
Intermediate-acting	NPH (neutral protamine Hagedorn) Lente ("L")	3–4 h	4–12 h	16–20 h	Usually taken after food
Long-acting	Ultralente ("UL")	6–8 h	12–16 h	20–30 h	Used primarily to control fasting glucose level

Pharmacologic Therapy

Insulin Therapy

As stated earlier, insulin is secreted by the beta cells of the islets of Langerhans and works to lower blood glucose after meals by facilitating the uptake and utilization of glucose by muscle, fat, and liver cells.

In type 1 diabetes, the body loses the ability to produce insulin. Thus, exogenous insulin must be administered on a long-term basis. In type 2 diabetes, insulin may be necessary on a long-term basis to control glucose levels if diet and oral agents have failed. In addition, some patients whose type 2 diabetes is usually controlled by diet alone or by diet and an oral agent may require insulin temporarily during illness, infection, pregnancy, surgery, or some other stressful event.

Frequently, insulin injections are taken two times per day (or even more often) to control blood glucose. Because the insulin dose required by the individual patient is determined by the level of glucose in the blood, accurate monitoring of blood glucose levels is essential. Self-monitoring of blood glucose levels has become the cornerstone of insulin therapy.

INSULIN PREPARATIONS

A number of insulin preparations are available. They vary according to three main characteristics: time course of action, species (source), and manufacturer.

Time Course. Insulins may be grouped into several categories based on the onset, peak, and duration of action (Table 37-3). (Human insulin preparations have a shorter duration of action than insulin from animal sources: the presence of animal proteins causes an immune response, resulting in binding of animal insulin and slowing its availability.)

Rapid-acting insulins such as **Humalog** (insulin lispro) are blood glucose-lowering agents whose effect is more rapid and of shorter duration than regular insulin. Humalog has an onset of 10 to 15 minutes, a peak action of 1 to 2 hours after injection, and a duration of 3 hours. Because of its rapid action, patients should be instructed not to wait the usual 30 minutes after injection to eat. Because of the short duration of action of Humalog, patients with type 1 diabetes also require a long-acting insulin to maintain glucose control.

Short-acting insulins, called regular insulin (marked R on the bottle), have an onset of 30 minutes to 1 hour; peak, 2 to 3 hours; and duration, 4 to 6 hours. Another name for regular insulin is crystalline zinc insulin (CZI). Regular insulin is clear in appearance and is usually administered 20 to 30 minutes before a meal, either alone or in combination with a longer-acting insulin.

Intermediate-acting insulins, called NPH insulin (neutral protamine Hagedorn) or Lente insulin, have an onset of 3 to 4 hours; peak, 4 to 12 hours; and duration, 16 to 20 hours. Both intermediate-acting insulins are similar in their time course of action and are white and cloudy in appearance. If NPH or Lente insulin is taken alone, it is not critical that it be taken a half-hour before the meal. It is important, however, for the patient to have eaten some food around the time of the onset and peak of these insulins.

Long-acting insulins, called Ultralente insulin, are sometimes referred to as peakless insulins because they tend to have a long, slow, sustained action rather than sharp, definite peaks in action. The onset of long-acting human insulin is 6 to 8 hours; peak, 12 to 16 hours; and duration, 20 to 30 hours.

The nurse may find that different sources list differing numbers of hours for the onset, peak, and duration of action of the main types of insulin, and patients' responses may vary (ie, larger doses prolong onset, duration, and peak). The nurse should focus on which meals—and snacks—are being "covered" by which insulin doses. In general, the rapid- and short-acting insulins are expected to cover meals immediately after the injection; the intermediate-acting insulins are expected to cover subsequent meals; and the long-acting insulins provide a relatively constant level of insulin and act as a basal insulin.

Species (Source). In the past, all insulins were obtained from beef (cow) and pork (pig) pancreases. "Human insulins" are now widely available. They are produced by recombinant DNA technology. In the near future, animal insulin will no longer be available.

Manufacturer. The two manufacturers of insulin in the United States are the Lilly and Novo Nordisk companies. The insulins made by the different companies are usually interchangeable, provided the concentration (eg, U-100), species (eg, human), and type (eg, NPH) of insulin are the same. Human insulins made by different companies have different brand names. Therefore, a

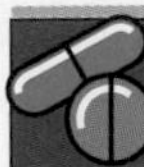

TABLE 37•4 Insulin Preparations Available in the United States

Manufacturer	Product	Species Source	Type
Rapid-Acting			
Lilly	Humalog (insulin analog)	Biosynthetic	Lispro
Short-acting			
Lilly	Iletin II	Beef or pork	Regular
Lilly	Humulin Regular	*	Regular
Novo Nordisk	Regular	Pork	Regular
Novo Nordisk	Purified Pork Regular	Pork	Regular
Novo Nordisk	Novolin R	*	Regular
Novo Nordisk	Velosulin	*	Regular
Intermediate-Acting			
Lilly	Iletin I NPH	Pork	NPH
Lilly	Iletin II NPH	Beef or pork	NPH
Lilly	Humulin NPH	*	NPH
Novo Nordisk	NPH	Beef	NPH
Novo Nordisk	Purified Pork N	Pork	NPH
Novo Nordisk	Novolin N	*	NPH
Lilly	Iletin II Lente	Beef or pork	Lente
Lilly	Humulin L	*	Lente
Novo Nordisk	Lente	Beef	Lente
Novo Nordisk	Purified Pork L	Pork	Lente
Novo Nordisk	Novolin L	*	Lente
Long-Acting			
Lilly	Humulin U	*	Ultralente
Mixed			
Lilly	Humulin 70/30, 50/50	*	70% NPH/30% Reg; 50% NPH/50% Reg
Novo Nordisk	Novolin 70/30	*	70% NPH/30% Reg

*Biosynthetic human; in the near future all insulins will be made from a recombinant DNA process in a laboratory.

patient taking 20 units human NPH insulin may be using either Humulin N or Novolin N. A more complete list of the available insulins appears in Table 37-4.

INSULIN REGIMENS

Insulin regimens vary from one to four injections per day. Usually there is a combination of a short-acting insulin and a longer-acting insulin. The normally functioning pancreas continuously secretes small amounts of insulin during the day and night. In addition, whenever blood glucose rises after ingestion of food, there is a rapid burst of insulin secretion in proportion to the glucose-raising effect of the food. The goal of all but the simplest, one-injection insulin regimens is to mimic this normal pattern of insulin secretion as closely as possible in response to food intake and activity patterns. Table 37-5 describes several different insulin regimens and the advantages and disadvantages of each.

Patients can be taught to use the results of SMBG to vary the insulin doses. This allows patients more flexibility in the timing and content of meals and exercise periods. However, complex insulin regimens require a strong level of commitment, intensive education, and close follow-up by the health care team. In addition, patients aiming for normal blood glucose levels run the risk of more hypoglycemic reactions.

The type of regimen used by any particular patient varies according to a number of factors. For example, patient knowledge, willingness, goals, health status, and finances all may affect decisions regarding insulin treatment. In addition, the physician's philosophy about blood glucose control and the availability of equipment and support staff may influence decisions regarding insulin therapy. There are two general approaches to insulin therapy.

Conventional Regimen. One approach is to simplify the insulin regimen as much as possible, with the aim of avoiding the acute complications of diabetes (hypoglycemia and symptomatic hyperglycemia). With this type of simplified regimen (eg, one or two injections per day), patients may frequently have blood glucose levels well above normal. The exception is the patient who never varies meal patterns and activity levels. This approach would be appropriate for the terminally ill, the frail elderly with limited self-care abilities, or any patient who is completely unwilling or unable to engage in the self-management activities that are part of a more complex insulin regimen.

Intensive Regimen. The second approach is to use a more complex insulin regimen (three or four injections per day) to achieve as much control over blood glucose levels as is safe and practical. The results of the DCCT (1993) and the UKPDS studies (1998) have demonstrated that maintaining blood glucose levels as close to normal as possible prevents or slows the progression of long-term diabetic complications. Another reason for using a more complex insulin regimen is to allow patients more flexibility to change their insulin doses from day to day in accordance with changes in their eating and activity patterns and as needed for variations in the prevailing glucose level.

Although the DCCT found that intensive treatment (three or four injections of insulin per day) reduced the risk of complications, not all people with diabetes are candidates for very tight control of blood glucose. Those who may not be candidates include:

- People with autonomic neuropathy (disease of the autonomic nerves) that causes them to have hypoglycemic

(text continues on page 991)

Table 37•5 Insulin Regimens

Schematic Representation	Description	Advantages	Disadvantages
Normal pancreas 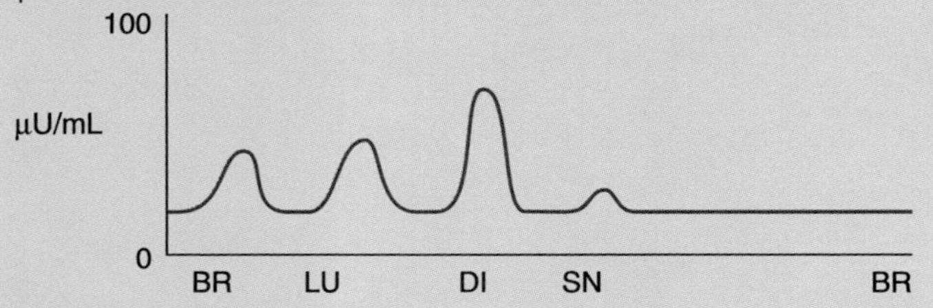 100 µU/mL 0 BR LU DI SN BR	Insulin release increases when blood glucose levels rise and continues at a low steady rate between meals.		
One injection per day 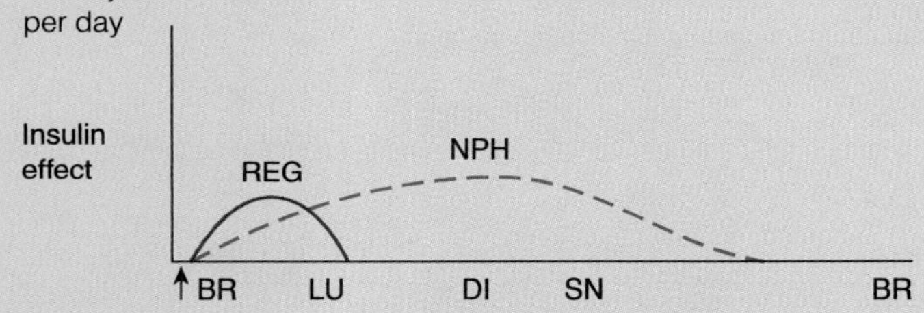 Insulin effect REG NPH BR LU DI SN BR	Before breakfast: • NPH* or • NPH with regular	Simple regimen	Difficult to control fasting blood glucose if effects of NPH do not last Afternoon hypoglycemia may result from attempts to control fasting glucose level by increasing NPH dose
Two injections per day 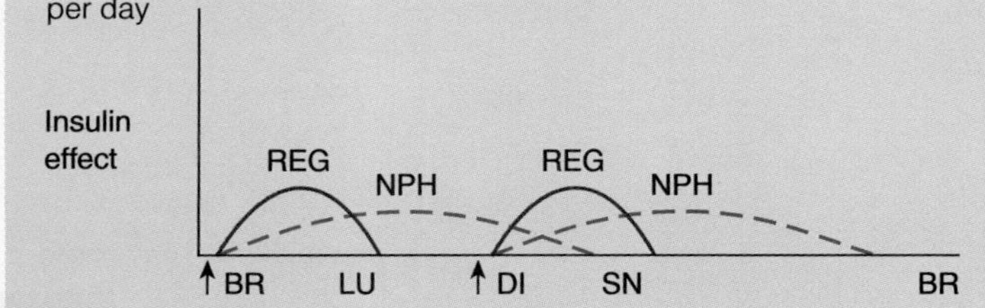 Insulin effect REG NPH REG NPH BR LU DI SN BR	Before breakfast and dinner: • NPH or • NPH with regular or • Premixed (N and R) insulin	Simplest regimen that attempts to mimic normal pancreas	Need relatively fixed schedule of meals and exercise Cannot independently adjust NPH or regular if premixed insulin is used

(continued)

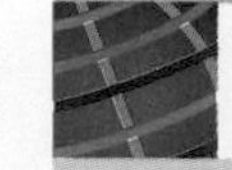

TABLE 37•5 Insulin Regimens *(Continued)*

Schematic Representation	Description	Advantages	Disadvantages
Three or four injections per day Insulin effect: REG, REG, REG, NPH; ↑BR, ↑LU, ↑DI, SN, BR Insulin effect: REG, REG, REG, ULTRALENTE; ↑BR, ↑LU, ↑DI, SN, BR	Regular before each meal with: • NPH at dinner or • NPH at bedtime or • Ultralente one or two times per day	More closely mimics normal pancreas than two-injection regimen Each premeal dose of regular insulin decided independently More flexibility with meals and exercise	Requires more injections than other regimens Requires multiple blood glucose tests on a daily basis Requires intensive education and follow-up
Insulin pump Insulin effect: BOLUS; REG, REG, REG, REG; BASAL RATE; BR, LU, DI, SN, BR	Uses ONLY regular insulin infused at continuous, low rate called *basal rate* (commonly 0.5–1.5 units/hour) and premeal *bolus doses* activated by pump wearer	Most closely mimics normal pancreas Decreases unpredictable peaks of intermediate- and long-acting insulins Increases meal and exercise flexibility	Requires intensive training and frequent follow-up Potential for mechanical problems Requires multiple blood glucose tests on a daily basis Potential increase in expenses (depending on insurance coverage)

*Where NPH appears, Lente insulin may also be used (however, the rate of absorption of regular insulin may be decreased when mixed with Lente preparations). BR, breakfast; LU, lunch; DI, dinner; SN, snack; ↑ indicates insulin injection.

unawareness. Because of autonomic neuropathy, these patients do not experience symptoms of hypoglycemia and therefore are at increased risk for developing severe hypoglycemia. Target goals for glucose levels may need to be raised in these patients.

- Patients who have recurring severe hypoglycemia. Target goals for glucose levels should be raised in the interest of patient safety.
- Patients with permanent, irreversible complications of diabetes (blindness from retinopathy or end-stage renal disease). The rationale is that the risks associated with intensive treatment regimens may outweigh the benefits. An exception is the patient who has received a kidney transplant because of nephropathy and chronic renal failure; this patient should be on an intensive regimen to preserve function of the new kidney.
- Patients with cerebrovascular and cardiovascular complications. It is feared that an occurrence of severe hypoglycemia may trigger another cerebrovascular or cardiovascular event in patients with significant preexisting vascular changes.
- Patients who do not take responsibility for their care. Failure to take responsibility for self-care increases the risk of severe hypoglycemia as a result of poor decision making.

It is very important for patients to be involved in the decision regarding which insulin regimen to use. Patients need to compare the potential benefits of different regimens with the potential costs (eg, time involved, number of injections or fingersticks for glucose testing, amount of record-keeping). There are no set guidelines as to which insulin regimen should be used for which patients. It must not be assumed that an elderly patient or a patient with visual impairment should automatically be given a simplified regimen. Likewise, it must not be assumed that all young people will want to be involved in a complex treatment regimen.

Nurses play an important role in educating patients about the availability of different approaches to insulin therapy. Nurses should refer patients to diabetes specialists or diabetes education centers for further training and education in the various insulin treatment regimens.

COMPLICATIONS OF INSULIN THERAPY

Local Allergic Reactions. A local allergic reaction in the form of redness, swelling, tenderness, and induration or a 2- to 4-cm wheal may appear at the site of injection 1 to 2 hours after the injection is administered. These reactions usually occur during the beginning stages of therapy and disappear with continued use of insulin. These allergic reactions are becoming less frequent because of the increased purity of insulins. The physician may prescribe an antihistamine to be taken 1 hour before the injection if such a local reaction occurs.

Use of alcohol to cleanse the skin is no longer recommended; however, patients who have learned this technique often continue to use it. They should be cautioned to allow the skin to dry after cleansing with alcohol. If the skin is not allowed to dry before injection, the alcohol may be carried into the tissues, resulting in a localized reddened area.

Systemic Allergic Reactions. Systemic allergic reactions to insulin are rare. First, there is an immediate local skin reaction that gradually spreads into generalized urticaria. The treatment is desensitization, with small doses of insulin administered in gradually increasing amounts. These rare reactions are occasionally associated with generalized edema or anaphylaxis.

Insulin Lipodystrophy. Lipodystrophy refers to a localized reaction, in the form of either lipoatrophy or lipohypertrophy, occurring at the site of insulin injections. Lipoatrophy is loss of subcutaneous fat and appears as slight dimpling or more serious pitting of subcutaneous fat. The use of human insulin has almost eliminated this disfiguring complication.

Lipohypertrophy, the development of fibrofatty masses at the injection site, is caused by the repeated use of an injection site. If insulin is injected into scarred areas, absorption may be delayed. This is one reason why rotation of injection sites is so important. The patient should avoid injecting insulin into these areas until the hypertrophy disappears.

Insulin Resistance. Most patients at one time or another have some degree of insulin resistance. This may occur for various reasons, the most common being obesity, which can be overcome by weight loss. Clinical insulin resistance has been defined as a daily insulin requirement of 200 units or more. In most diabetic patients taking insulin, immune antibodies develop and bind the insulin, thereby decreasing the insulin available for use. All animal insulins, as well as human insulins to a lesser degree, cause antibody production in humans.

Very few of these patients develop high levels of antibodies. Many of these patients give a history of insulin therapy interrupted for several months or more. Treatment consists of administering a purer insulin preparation; occasionally, prednisone is needed to block the production of antibodies. This may be followed by a gradual reduction in insulin requirement. Therefore, patients need to monitor themselves for hypoglycemia.

Morning Hyperglycemia. An elevated blood glucose level on arising in the morning may be caused by an insufficient level of insulin due to several causes: the dawn phenomenon, the Somogyi effect or insulin waning. The dawn phenomenon is characterized by a relatively normal blood glucose level until approximately 3 AM, when blood glucose levels begin to rise. The phenomenon is thought to result from nocturnal surges in growth hormone secretion that create a greater need for insulin in the early morning hours in patients with type 1 diabetes. It must be distinguished from insulin waning (the progressive increase in blood glucose from bedtime to morning), or the Somogyi effect (nocturnal hypoglycemia followed by rebound hyperglycemia). Insulin waning is frequently seen if the evening NPH dose is administered before dinner and is prevented by moving the evening dose of NPH insulin to bedtime.

It is often difficult to tell from the patient's history which of these causes is responsible for morning hyperglycemia. To determine the cause, the patient must be awakened once or twice during the night to test blood glucose levels. Testing the blood glucose level at bedtime, at 3 AM, and on awakening provides information that can be used in making adjustments in insulin to avoid morning hyperglycemia caused by the dawn phenomenon. Table 37-6 summarizes the differences among insulin waning, the dawn phenomenon, and the Somogyi effect.

ALTERNATIVE METHODS OF INSULIN DELIVERY

Insulin Pens. These devices use small (150- to 300-unit) prefilled insulin cartridges that are loaded into a penlike holder. A disposable needle is attached to the device for insulin injection. Insulin is delivered by dialing in a dose or pushing a button for

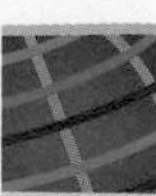

TABLE 37•6 Causes of Morning Hyperglycemia

Characteristic	Treatment
Insulin Waning	
Progressive rise in blood glucose from bedtime to morning	Increase evening (predinner or bedtime) dose of intermediate- or long-acting insulin, or institute a dose of insulin before the evening meal if one is not already in use.
Dawn Phenomenon	
Relatively normal blood glucose until about 3 AM, when the level begins to rise	Change time of injection of evening intermediate-acting insulin from dinnertime to bedtime.
Somogyi Effect	
Normal or elevated blood glucose at bedtime, a decrease at 2–3 AM to hypoglycemic levels, and a subsequent increase caused by the production of counterregulatory hormones	Decrease evening (predinner or bedtime) dose of intermediate-acting insulin, or increase bedtime snack.

every 1- or 2-unit increment administered. People using these devices still need to insert the needle for each injection; however, they do not need to carry insulin bottles or to draw up insulin before each injection. These devices are most useful for patients who need to inject only one type of insulin at a time (eg, premeal regular insulin three times a day and bedtime NPH insulin) or who can use the premixed insulins. These pens are convenient for those who administer insulin before dinner if eating out rather than at home.

Jet Injectors. As an alternative to needle injections, jet injection devices deliver insulin through the skin under pressure in an extremely fine stream. These devices are more expensive than other alternative devices mentioned above and require thorough training and supervision when first used. In addition, patients should be cautioned that absorption rates, peak insulin activity, and insulin levels may be different when changing to a jet injector. (Insulin administered by jet injector is usually absorbed faster.) Bruising has occurred in some patients with use of the jet injector.

Insulin Pumps. **Continuous subcutaneous insulin infusion** involves the use of small, externally worn devices that closely mimic the functioning of the normal pancreas. Insulin pumps contain a 3-mL syringe that is attached to a long (24- to 42-in), thin, narrow-lumen tube with a needle or Teflon catheter attached to the end (Figs. 37-4 and 37-5). The patient inserts the needle or Teflon catheter into the subcutaneous tissue (usually on the abdomen) and secures it with tape or a transparent dressing. The needle or Teflon catheter is changed at least every 3 days. The pump is then worn either on a belt or in a pocket. Some women keep the pump tucked into the front or side of the bra or wear it on a garter belt on the thigh.

The pump uses regular insulin; although lispro is frequently administered by insulin pump, studies are currently examining its use by this route. Insulin is delivered by the pump in two

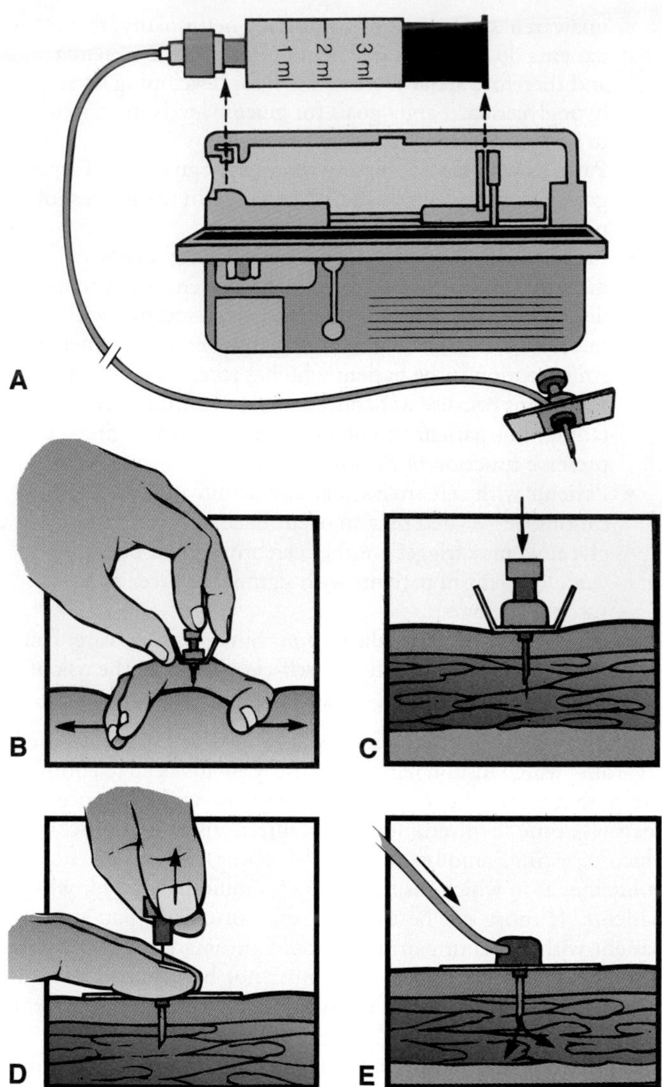

FIGURE 37•4 (A) Diagram of an insulin pump showing syringe in place inside pump and connection of pump via tubing to needle site. (B–E) Actual insertion site before, during, and after the needle and catheter have been inserted.

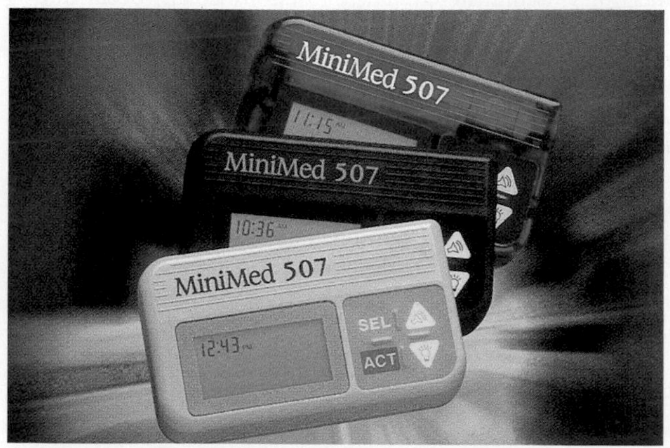

FIGURE 37•5 MiniMed insulin pump.

different ways. First, there is a continuous basal rate of insulin that infuses typically at a rate of 0.5 to 2.0 units/hour. Before each meal, the patient activates the pump (by pushing buttons) to deliver a bolus dose of insulin. The patient can decide on the amount of insulin bolus to infuse based on blood glucose levels and anticipated food intake and activity level.

There has been debate in the diabetes literature as to whether insulin pumps offer better control of blood glucose than other multiple-dose regimens (eg, three or four injections per day). One advantage of insulin pumps is that patients do not have to use intermediate- or long-acting insulins, which may have unpredictable peaks of action and may therefore cause unexpected swings in blood glucose. Some of the other advantages of insulin pumps include increased flexibility in lifestyle (in terms of timing and amount of meals, exercise, and travel) and, for some patients, improved blood glucose control.

A disadvantage of insulin pumps is that unexpected disruptions in the flow of insulin from the pump may occur if the tubing or needle becomes occluded, if the supply of insulin runs out, or if the battery is depleted, increasing the risk of DKA. Another disadvantage is the potential for infection at needle insertion sites. Hypoglycemia may occur with insulin pump therapy; however, this is usually related to the lowered blood glucose levels many patients achieve rather than to a specific problem with the pump itself. The tight diabetic control associated with the use of an insulin pump may increase the incidence of hypoglycemia unawareness because of the gradual decline in serum glucose level from levels greater than 70 mg/dL (3.9 mmol/L) to those less than 60 mg/dL (3.3 mmol/L).

Some patients may find that having to wear the pump virtually 24 hours per day is an inconvenience. However, it can easily be disconnected, per patient preference, for limited periods (eg, for showering, exercise, or sexual activity).

Insulin pump candidates must be willing to assess blood glucose levels multiple times daily while on pump therapy. In addition, they must be psychologically stable and open about having diabetes, because the insulin pump is often a visible sign to others and a constant reminder to the patient that he or she has diabetes. Most important, patients using insulin pumps must have extensive education in the use of the insulin pump and in self-management of blood glucose and insulin doses. They must work closely with a team of health care professionals who are experienced in insulin pump therapy—specifically, a diabetologist/endocrinologist, a dietitian, and a **certified diabetes educator**.

Many insurance policies cover the cost of pump therapy; if it is not covered, the extra expense of the pump and associated supplies may be a deterrent for some patients.

Implantable and Inhalant Insulin Delivery. Research into mechanical delivery of insulin has involved implantable insulin pumps that can be externally programmed according to blood glucose test results. Clinical trials with these devices are in progress. In addition, there is research into the development of implantable devices that both measure the blood glucose level and deliver insulin as needed.

Research into nasal delivery of insulin has demonstrated this method of administration to be less effective and less consistent than hoped.

Transplantation. Transplantation of the whole pancreas or a segment of the pancreas is being performed on a limited population (mostly diabetic patients receiving kidney transplantations simultaneously). One main issue regarding pancreatic transplantation is weighing the risks of antirejection medications against the advantages of pancreas transplantation. Another approach under investigation is the implantation of insulin-producing pancreatic islet cells. This latter approach involves a less extensive surgical procedure and a potentially lower incidence of immunogenic problems. However, thus far independence from exogenous insulin has been limited to 2 years after transplantation of islet cells.

Oral Antidiabetic Agents

Oral antidiabetic agents may be effective for type 2 diabetic patients who cannot be treated by diet and exercise alone; however, they cannot be used during pregnancy. In the United States, oral antidiabetic agents include the sulfonylureas, biguanides, alpha glucosidase inhibitors, thiazolidinediones, and meglitinides (Table 37-7).

SULFONYLUREAS

The **sulfonylureas** exert their primary action by directly stimulating the pancreas to secrete insulin. Therefore, a functioning pancreas is necessary for these agents to be effective, and they cannot be used in patients with type 1 diabetes. An additional important action of these agents, unrelated to a direct pancreatic effect, is to improve insulin action at the cellular level. They may also directly decrease glucose production by the liver. The sulfonylureas can be divided into first- and second-generation categories (see Table 37-7).

The most common side effects of these medications are gastrointestinal symptoms and dermatologic reactions. Hypoglycemia may occur when an excessive dose of a sulfonylurea is used or when meals are omitted or delayed, food intake is decreased, or activity is increased. Because of the prolonged hypoglycemic effects of these agents (especially chlorpropamide), some patients need to be hospitalized for treatment of oral agent–induced hypoglycemia. Another side effect of chlorpropamide is a disulfiram (Antabuse) type of reaction when alcohol is ingested (see section on alcohol for more information). Some medications may directly interact with sulfonylureas, potentiating their hypoglycemic effects (eg, sulfonamides, chloramphenicol, clofibrate, phenylbutazone, and bisohydroxycoumarin). In addition, certain medications may independently affect blood glucose levels, thereby indirectly interfering with these agents. Medications that may increase glucose levels include potassium-losing diuretics, corticosteroids, estrogen compounds, and diphenylhydantoin (Dilantin). Medications that may cause hypoglycemia include salicylates, propranolol, monoamine oxidase inhibitors, and pentamidine.

The second-generation sulfonylureas have the advantage of a shorter half-life and excretion by both the kidney and the liver. This makes these medications safer to use in the elderly, where accumulation of the medication causing recurring hypoglycemia can be a problem.

BIGUANIDES

Another category of oral antidiabetic agents is the biguanides. Metformin (Glucophage) produces its antidiabetic effects by facilitating insulin's action on peripheral receptor sites. Therefore, it can be used only in the presence of insulin. Biguanides have no effect on pancreatic beta cells. Biguanides used in combination with sulfonylurea agents may enhance the glucose-lowering effect more than either medication used alone. Lactic acidosis is a potential serious complication of biguanide therapy; the patient must be monitored closely when therapy is initiated or when dosage changes. Medications that may interact with

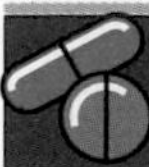

TABLE 37•7 **Oral Antidiabetic Agents Used in the United States**

Generic (Trade) Name	Tablet Size (mg)	Usual Daily Dose (mg)	Maximum Dose (mg)	Duration of Action (h)
First-Generation Sulfonylureas				
acetohexamide (Dymelor)	250–500	250–1500 (D)	1500	12–24
chlorpropamide (Diabinese)	100, 250	100–500 (S)	750	60
tolazamide (Tolinase)	100, 250, 500	100–750 (D)	1000	12–24
tolbutamide (Orinase)	250, 500	500–2000 (D)	3000	6–12
Second-Generation Sulfonylureas				
glipizide (Glucatrol)	5, 10	5–25 (D)	40	10–24
glipizide (Glucatrol XL)	5, 10	5 (S)	10	24
glyburide (Micronase)	1.25, 2.5, 5	2.5–10 (D)	20	12–24
glimepiride (Amaryl)	1, 2, 4	1–2 (S)	8	24
Biguanides				
metformin (Glucophage)	500	1500 (D)	2500	8
Alpha Glucosidase Inhibitors				
acarbose (Precose)	50, 100	1500 (D)	2500	8
Thiazolidinediones				
troglitazone (Rezulin)	200, 400	200–400 (S)	600	—
Meglitinides				
repaglinide (Prandin)	0.5, 1, 2	0.5–4	16	2

(D), divided dose; (S), single dose.

biguanides include anticoagulants, corticosteroids, diuretics, and oral contraceptives. Metformin is contraindicated in patients with renal impairment (serum creatinine level more than 1.4) or those at risk for renal dysfunction (eg, those with acute myocardial infarction). Renal function studies should be done periodically to ensure that function is not impaired. Metformin should not be administered for 2 days before any diagnostic testing that may require use of a contrast agent. Both of these situations increase the risk for lactic acidosis.

ORAL ALPHA GLUCOSIDASE INHIBITORS

Acarbose (Precose) is a member of this drug category, which is used in managing type 2 diabetes. **Alpha glucosidase inhibitors** work by delaying the absorption of glucose in the intestinal system, resulting in a lower postprandial blood glucose level. As a consequence of plasma glucose reduction, hemoglobin A_{1C} levels drop. In contrast to the sulfonylureas, acarbose does not enhance insulin secretion, nor is it systemically absorbed. It can be used with dietary treatment as monotherapy or in conjunction with sulfonylureas, thiazolidinediones, or meglitinides. When it is used in conjunction with sulfonylureas or meglitinides, hypoglycemia may occur. The patient must be advised that if hypoglycemia occurs, sucrose absorption will be blocked and treatment for hypoglycemia should be in the form of glucose, such as glucose tablets. The advantage of oral alpha glucosidase inhibitors is that they are not systemically absorbed and are safe to use. Their side effects are diarrhea and flatulence. These may be minimized by starting at a very low dose and increasing it gradually. Because acarbose works on food absorption, it must be taken immediately before a meal, making compliance a potential problem.

THIAZOLIDINEDIONES

Troglitazone (Rezulin) is an oral diabetes medication indicated for patients with type 2 diabetes who take insulin injections and whose blood glucose control is inadequate (hemoglobin A_{1C} level more than 8.5%). It has also been approved as a first-line agent to treat type 2 diabetes, in conjunction with diet. The mechanism of action of the **thiazolidinediones** is to enhance insulin action at the receptor site without increasing insulin secretion from the beta cells of the pancreas. This agent may affect liver function; therefore, liver function studies must be performed at baseline and at frequent intervals (monthly for the first 12 months of treatment, and quarterly thereafter). This medication can also cause resumption of ovulation in perimenopausal anovulatory women, putting them at risk for pregnancy. Women should be informed of this.

MEGLITINIDES

Repaglinide (Prandin) is an oral glucose-lowering agent of the class of oral agents called meglitinides. Repaglinide lowers the blood glucose level by stimulating the release of insulin from the beta cells of the pancreas. Its effectiveness depends on the presence of functioning beta cells. Therefore, repaglinide is contraindicated in patients with type 1 diabetes. Repaglinide has a fast action and a short duration. It should be taken before each meal to stimulate the release of insulin in response to that meal. Doses range from 0.5 mg to a maximum of 4 mg. It is also indicated for use in combination with metformin in patients whose hyperglycemia cannot be controlled by exercise, diet, and either metformin or repaglinide alone. The principal side effect of repaglinide is hypoglycemia; however, this side effect is less than for sulfonylureas because of the short half-life of the medication (approximately 1 hour). Patients should be taught the signs and symptoms of hypoglycemia and should know that the medication should not be taken if the patient does not eat a meal. Repaglinide is supplied in 0.5-, 1-, and 2-mg tablets.

It is important for patients to understand that oral agents are prescribed as an addition to (and not as a substitute for) other treatment modalities, such as diet and exercise. Use of oral antidiabetic medications may need to be halted temporarily and insulin prescribed if hyperglycemia develops that is attributable to infection, trauma, or surgery.

If, as time goes on, a patient's blood glucose values that were once responsive to oral antidiabetic agents no longer respond to these agents or combination of agents, the patient is then treated with insulin. Approximately half of all patients who initially use oral antidiabetic agents eventually require insulin. This is referred to as a secondary failure. Primary failure occurs when the blood glucose level remains high a month after initial medication use.

Using a combination of oral agents with insulin has been proposed as a treatment for some patients with type 2 diabetes. However, the effectiveness of this approach has not yet been demonstrated. Because the mechanisms of action vary (Fig. 37-6), the effect may be enhanced using multidose, multiple medications (Inzucchi et al., 1998). Use of multiple medications with different mechanisms of action is very common today.

Education

Diabetes mellitus is a chronic illness requiring a lifetime of special self-management behaviors. Because diet, physical activity, and physical and emotional stress can affect diabetic control, patients must learn to balance a multitude of factors. Not only must patients learn daily self-care skills to avoid acute fluctuations in blood glucose, but they must also incorporate into their lifestyle many preventive behaviors for avoidance of long-term diabetic complications. The diabetic patient must become knowledgeable about nutrition, medication effects and side effects, exercise, disease progression, prevention strategies, monitoring techniques, and medication adjustment. In addition, he or she must learn the skills associated with monitoring and managing diabetes and must incorporate many new activities into his or her daily routine. An appreciation for the knowledge and skills that diabetic patients must acquire can help the nurse in providing effective patient education and counseling. Education strategies and specific topics are addressed in the following section.

NURSING MANAGEMENT

Nursing management of the diabetic patient can involve treatment of a wide variety of physiologic problems, depending on the individual patient's health status and whether or not the patient is newly diagnosed or seeks care for an unrelated health problem. Nursing management of the newly diagnosed patient and the patient with diabetes as a secondary diagnosis is presented in subsequent sections. Because all diabetic patients must master the concepts and skills necessary for long-term management of diabetes and its potential complications, a solid educational foundation is necessary for competent self-care and is an ongoing focus of nursing care.

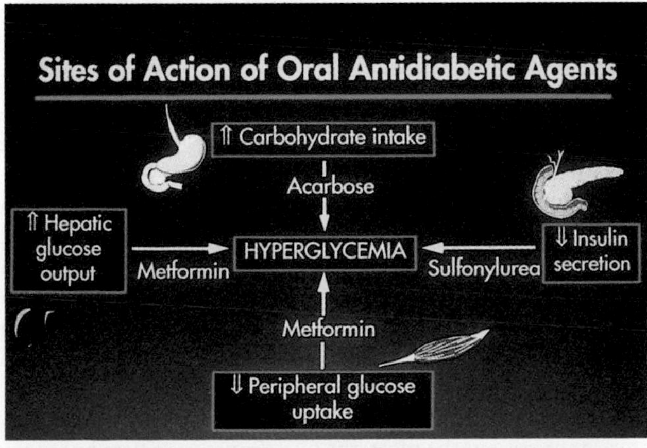

FIGURE 37•6 Sites of action of oral antidiabetic medications.

Developing a Diabetic Teaching Plan

Changes in the health care delivery system as a whole have had a major impact on diabetes education and training. Patients with new-onset diabetes have much shorter hospital stays or may be managed completely on an outpatient basis. There has been a proliferation of outpatient diabetes education and training programs with increasing support of third-party reimbursement. For some patients, however, exposure to diabetes education during hospitalization may be the only opportunity for learning skills of self-management and prevention of complications.

Many hospitals employ nurses who specialize in diabetes education and management. However, because of the large number of diabetic patients who are admitted to every unit of a hospital, the staff nurse plays a vital role in identifying diabetic patients, assessing self-care skills, providing basic education, reinforcing the teaching provided by the specialist, and referring patients for follow-up care after discharge. Diabetes patient education programs that have achieved "recognition status" (ie, they have been peer reviewed by the American Diabetes Association as meeting National Standards for Diabetes Education) can seek reimbursement for education.

Organizing Information

There are various schemes for organizing and prioritizing the vast amount of information that must be taught to diabetic patients. In addition, many hospitals and outpatient diabetes centers have devised written guidelines, care plans, and documentation forms (often based on guidelines from the American Diabetes Association) that may be used to document and evaluate diabetes teaching. A general approach is to organize information and skills into two main types: basic, initial, or "survival" skills and information, and in-depth (advanced) or continuing education.

SURVIVAL SKILLS

This information must be taught to any patient with newly diagnosed type 1 diabetes or any type 2 diabetic patient receiving insulin for the first time. This basic information is literally what the patient must know to survive—that is, to avoid severe hypoglycemic or acute hyperglycemic complications after discharge. Categories of survival information include:

1. Simple pathophysiology
   a. Basic definition of diabetes (having a high blood glucose level)
   b. Normal blood glucose ranges
   c. Effect of insulin and exercise (decrease glucose)
   d. Effect of food and stress, including illness and infections (increase glucose)
   e. Basic treatment approaches
2. Treatment modalities
   a. Insulin administration
   b. Diet information (food groups; timing of meals)
   c. Monitoring of blood glucose, urine ketones
3. Recognition, treatment, and prevention of acute complications
   a. Hypoglycemia
   b. Hyperglycemia

NURSING RESEARCH

Identifying Ethical Conflicts in Diabetes Care

Redman, B., & Fry, S. (1996). Ethical conflicts reported by registered nurse/certified diabetes educators. *Diabetes Educator, 23*(3), 219–224.

Purpose

The purpose of this pilot study was to identify types of ethical conflicts experienced by a group of registered nurses certified as diabetes educators (RN/CDEs) in their practice and to examine demographic, educational, and practice-setting factors associated with ethical conflicts.

Study Sample and Design

The Moral Conflict Questionnaire, an open-ended questionnaire designed to elicit descriptions of ethical conflicts encountered in clinical practice, was used in data collection. Respondents were asked to describe an ethical conflict they had encountered in practice and to identify what the conflict was for them.

A sample of RN/CDE members of the American Association of Diabetes Educators in one geographic area were contacted by mail and asked to participate in the study. Data were obtained from 50 of the 130 subjects initially considered eligible for the study. Of these 50, 43 RN/CDEs reported encountering ethical conflicts in their clinical practice; a total of 46 ethical conflicts were reported and described.

Content analysis was used to analyze the ethical conflicts, which were classified as conflicts with medical practice, institutional policies and expected roles, patient choices, health policy, and researcher vs. practitioner roles. Self-reported conflicts were analyzed according to practice context, ethical principles involved, and how the conflict was experienced.

Findings

The majority of conflicts reported were experienced as "moral dilemmas" where two or more moral principles apply but support mutually inconsistent courses of action. Other conflicts were of "moral distress" (ie, the nurse knew what to do but institutional constraints, lack of authority, or lack of access made it impossible to pursue the right course of action). The majority (75%) of the ethical conflicts were a result of disagreement with the medical care received by the patient. The most frequent resolution was for the RN/CDE to empower the patient to change the practice context.

Nursing Implications

The role of the RN/CDE in the care and education of the diabetic patient has become more important due to the results of the Diabetes Control and Complications Trial (DCCT), which strongly suggest that the care of the patient be provided by a team of health professionals. The RN/CDE is often the educator of the patient in self-management skills. Many times the RN/CDE is the member of the health care team who is most familiar with new monitoring equipment and new products; the RN/CDE promotes high-quality diabetes care based on the American Diabetes Association Standards of Medical Care. Team members need to communicate with each other to resolve ethical conflicts. Awareness of possible ethical conflicts and development of strategies to resolve those conflicts foster communication between health care team members and improve care of the person with diabetes.

4. Pragmatic information
   a. Where to buy and store insulin, syringes, glucose-monitoring supplies
   b. When and how to reach the physician

Newly diagnosed type 2 diabetic patients also need to learn this basic information. Most of the emphasis is initially placed on diet. For patients started on oral sulfonylureas, it is also very important to teach about hypoglycemia. If the diabetes has gone undetected for many years, the patient may already be experiencing some of the chronic diabetic complications. Thus, for some patients with newly diagnosed type 2 diabetes, the basic diabetes teaching must include information on preventive skills such as foot care and eye care (eg, planning yearly or more frequent examinations by the ophthalmologist and understanding that retinopathy is largely asymptomatic until the advanced stages).

It is important for patients to realize that once they master the basic skills and information, further diabetes education must be pursued. Acquiring in-depth and advanced diabetes knowledge occurs throughout the patient's lifetime both informally (through experience and sharing of information with other people with diabetes) and formally (through programs of continuing education).

IN-DEPTH/CONTINUING EDUCATION

This involves teaching more detailed information related to survival skills (eg, learning to vary diet and insulin and preparing for travel) as well as learning preventive measures for avoiding long-term diabetic complications. These preventive measures include:

- Foot care
- Eye care
- General hygiene (eg, skin care, oral hygiene)
- Risk factor management (control of blood pressure and blood lipids, normalizing blood glucose levels)

More advanced continuing education may include alternative methods for insulin delivery, such as the insulin pump, and algorithms or rules for evaluating and adjusting insulin doses. For example, patients can be taught to increase or decrease insulin doses based on a several-day pattern of blood glucose levels.

The amount of advanced diabetes education to be provided depends on the patient's interest and ability. However, learning preventive measures (especially foot care and eye care) is mandatory and vital for reducing the occurrence of amputations and blindness in the diabetic population.

Assessing Readiness to Learn

Before initiating diabetes education, it is important to assess the patient's (and family's) readiness to learn. When patients are first diagnosed with diabetes (or first told of their need for insulin), they go through various stages of the grieving process. These stages may include shock and denial, depression, negotiation, anger, and acceptance. The amount of time it takes for patients and family members to work through the grieving process varies from patient to patient. They may experience helplessness, guilt, altered body image, loss of self-esteem, and concern about the future. The nurse must assess the patient's coping strategies and reassure patients and families that feelings of depression and shock are normal.

Asking the patient and family about their major concerns or fears is an important way to learn about any misinformation that may be contributing to anxiety. Some common misconceptions regarding diabetes and its treatment are listed in Table 37-8. Simple, direct information should be provided to dispel misconceptions. More in-depth information can be provided once survival skills are mastered.

After dispelling misconceptions or answering questions that concern the patient the most, the nurse must use a firm but caring approach to focus attention on concrete survival skills. Because

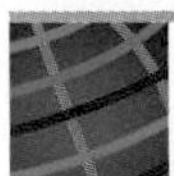

TABLE 37•8 **Misconceptions Related to Diabetes and its Treatment**

Misconception	Nurse's Response
Diabetes is caused by eating too much sugar.	Once diabetes develops, eating too much sugar can cause the glucose level to rise. However, diabetes develops initially as the result of a decrease in the amount of insulin in the body or a decrease in the ability of insulin to control the blood glucose level. These problems are *not* caused by eating too much sugar. In type 1 diabetes, in which the pancreatic beta cells produce little or no insulin, various factors contribute to beta cell damage, including genetics, a defect in the immune system, or an external factor (eg, a virus). In type 2 diabetes, the body is resistant to the effect of insulin. The amount of insulin released by the beta cells is not enough to overcome this insulin resistance, and hyperglycemia results. Insulin resistance and decreased insulin release are *not* caused by eating too much sugar. Two factors that do contribute to the development of type 2 diabetes are obesity and a family history of diabetes.
Sugar is found only in dessert foods.	There are several different types of sugars (simple carbohydrates) that increase blood glucose levels. Dessert foods often contain sucrose, one type of sugar. Many other packaged foods (eg, flavored yogurt, cereals, canned beans, sauces, salad dressing, "health food bars") also contain some form of sugar. Patients should be instructed to check labels for sources of sugar such as corn syrup, dextrose, brown sugar, honey. Fruit and fruit juices also contain sugar. Even if the juice is labeled "unsweetened" or "no sugar added," there is still natural fruit sugar in the product, which causes elevations in the glucose level.
The only diet change needed in the treatment of diabetes is to stop eating sugar.	First, it is important for the patient to realize that it is not feasible (nor advisable) to remove *all* sources of sugar from the diet. There are nutritious foods (such as fruit) that contain some form of sugar and should be included in the meal plan. In addition, recent research has shown that increasing the amount of simple sugars (including table sugar) in the diabetic meal plan may not adversely affect glucose levels. For patients requiring insulin, the meal plan includes limiting concentrated sweets as well as maintaining consistency in time intervals between meals. In addition, patients need to learn to adjust the insulin dose if there are variations in the amount of food eaten or in the carbohydrate content of meals. For patients receiving oral antidiabetic agents, it is important to avoid skipping meals and to limit intake of sugars. If the patient is obese, the meal plan emphasizes limiting total calories, which is best achieved by decreasing the fat content of meals.
Once insulin injections are started (for treatment of type 2 diabetes), they can never be discontinued.	During periods of acute stress (eg, illness, infection, or surgery) or when receiving certain medications that cause elevations in blood glucose, some patients with type 2 diabetes require insulin. If the diabetes had previously been well controlled with diet alone or diet with oral antidiabetic agents, the patient should be able to resume previous methods for control of diabetes when the stress is resolved. In addition, insulin is sometimes used to control blood glucose levels in obese type 2 diabetic patients who have been unsuccessful at weight loss. If the patient can lose weight after insulin therapy is initiated, the insulin doses may be tapered and the patient may be able to switch to diet and exercise alone or with oral antidiabetic agents for control of blood glucose. (For patients with type 1 diabetes, insulin is needed on an ongoing basis. For thin patients with type 2 diabetes, once insulin has to be started, it is usually required permanently).
If increasing doses of insulin are needed to control the blood glucose, the diabetes must be getting "worse."	Explain to the patient that unlike other medications that are given in standard doses, there is not a standard dose of insulin that is effective for all patients. Rather, the dose must be adjusted according to blood glucose test results. If the initial insulin dose prescribed for the patient does not adequately decrease the glucose level, the patient may assume that he or she has a "bad" case of diabetes or that the diabetes is getting worse. It is important to instruct patients that many different factors may affect the ability of insulin to lower the glucose, including obesity, puberty, pregnancy, illness, and certain medications. In addition, to avoid hypoglycemia, physicians frequently initiate insulin therapy with smaller dosages than will eventually be needed. The doses are then increased in small increments until blood glucose levels are in the desired range.
Insulin causes blindness (or other diabetic complications).	When patients have a diabetic acquaintance in whom the initiation of insulin therapy happened to coincide with the onset of diabetic complications, the patient may view insulin as the cause of complications such as blindness or amputation. In these situations, the acquaintance probably had type 2 diabetes that was no longer controllable with diet and oral hypoglycemic agents. It must be explained to the patient that factors such as elevated blood glucose (and not insulin therapy) contribute to some of the diabetic complications. Further, emphasize that insulin is a natural hormone that is present in every person's body, helps control blood glucose levels, and definitely does *not* cause long-term complications of diabetes.
Insulin must be injected directly into the vein.	When patients first learn that one area used for insulin injections on the arm, they may envision inserting the needle directly into a vein in the antecubital area, as in blood withdrawal. The patient must be reassured that insulin is injected into the fat tissue on the *back* of the arm (or on the abdomen, thigh, or hip) and that the needle is much shorter than that used for venipuncture.

(*continued*)

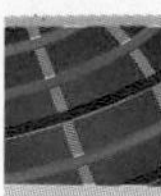

TABLE 37•8 Misconceptions Related to Diabetes and its Treatment *(Continued)*

Misconception	Nurse's Response
There is extreme danger in injecting insulin if there are any air bubbles in the syringe.	Patients may have a fear of dying if air bubbles are injected with a syringe. (This may be related to the misconception that insulin is injected directly into the vein.) Reassure patients that the main danger in having air bubbles in the insulin syringe is that the amount of insulin being injected is less than the required dosage. It is often difficult to remove every small "champagne" bubble from the syringe. The patient should be reassured that injection of insulin when these bubbles are present will not cause harm.
Urine and blood glucose testing are interchangeable (ie, they provide the same information).	Explain to the patient that directly testing the blood is the most accurate method of measuring the glucose level. The *urine* glucose test, which measures the amount of glucose that has "spilled" into the urine since the bladder was last emptied, is only an indirect way of determining the glucose level in the *blood.* The kidneys will not allow sugar to spill into the urine until the blood glucose reaches a level about 180 to 200 mg/dL (10 to 11.1 mmol/L). Therefore, the urine will test negative for glucose when the *blood* glucose is at any level between 0 and 200 mg/dL. Hypoglycemia cannot be detected with urine testing, nor can the blood glucose level be strictly controlled.
Blood glucose levels remain the same throughout the day.	Explain to patients that there is normally a variation in blood glucose levels, with the lowest levels before meals and the highest levels 1 to 2 hours after eating. The goal of the diabetes treatment plan is to minimize wide swings in glucose levels, not to eliminate the normal variations.

Pearce, M. A., Rosenberg, C. S., & Davidson, M. B. (1991). Patient education. In M. B. Davidson (Ed.), *Diabetes Mellitus: Diagnosis and Treatment* (3rd ed.). New York: Churchill Livingstone.

of the immediate need for multiple new skills, teaching is initiated as soon as possible after diagnosis. For patients who are in the hospital, there is not usually the luxury of waiting until the patient feels ready to learn. Short hospital stays necessitate initiation of survival skill education as early as possible in the hospital stay. This gives the patient the opportunity to practice skills with supervision by the nurse before discharge. Follow-up by home health nurses is often necessary for reinforcement of survival skills.

A major goal of patient teaching is an educated consumer. The patient is informed about the wide variations in the prices of medications and supplies and about the importance of comparing prices.

Determining Teaching Methods

Maintaining flexibility in teaching approaches is important. Teaching skills and information in a logical sequence is not always the most helpful for patients. For example, many patients are focused on their fear of the injection. Before they learn how to draw up, purchase, store, and mix insulins, they should be taught to insert the needle and inject insulin (or practice with saline). Numerous demonstrations by the nurse or practice injections before the patient (or family) gives the first injection may actually increase the patient's anxiety and fear of self-injection. Once they have actually performed the injection, most patients are more prepared to hear and to comprehend other information. (If the patient then wants to practice further using a pillow or an orange, that would be appropriate.) Thus, having the patient self-inject first or having the patient perform a fingerstick for glucose monitoring first may enhance learning to draw up the insulin or to operate the glucose monitor.

Various tools can be used to aid in teaching. Many of the companies that manufacture products for diabetes self-care also provide booklets and videotapes to assist in patient teaching. It is important to use a variety of written handouts that match the patient's learning needs (including different languages, low-literacy information, large print). Patients can be encouraged to continue learning about diabetes care by participating in activities sponsored by local hospitals and diabetes organizations. In addition, there are magazines geared toward people with diabetes that provide information on all aspects of diabetes management.

Ample opportunity should be provided for the patient and family to practice skills under supervision (including self-injection, self-testing, meal selection, verbalization of symptoms, and treatment of hypoglycemia). Once skills have been mastered, participation in ongoing support groups may assist patients in incorporating new habits and maintaining adherence to the treatment regimen.

Teaching the Experienced Diabetic Patient

The nurse should continue to assess the skills of patients who have had diabetes for many years, because it has been estimated that up to 50% of patients may make errors in self-care skills. Assessment of these patients must include direct observation of skills, not just asking patients to describe self-care behaviors. In addition, these patients must be fully aware of preventive measures related to foot care, eye care, and risk factor management. If patients are experiencing long-term diabetic complications for the first time, they may go through the grieving process again. Some of these patients may have a renewed interest in diabetes self-care in the hope of delaying further complications. Other patients may be overwhelmed by feelings of guilt and depression. The patient is encouraged to discuss feelings and fears related to complications; appropriate information regarding diabetic complications is provided by the nurse.

Teaching Self-Administration of Insulin

Insulin injections are administered into the subcutaneous tissue with the use of special insulin syringes. A variety of syringes and injection-aid devices are available. Refer to Chart 37-3 and the related Patient Education and Home Care information for a summary of important information to include and evaluate when teaching patients about insulin.

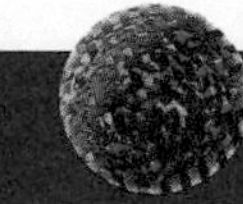

CHART 37•3 Outcome Criteria for Determining Effectiveness of Self-Injection of Insulin Education

Equipment

Insulin

1. Identifies information on label of insulin bottle:
    - Type (eg, NPH, regular, 70/30)
    - Species (human, biosynthetic, pork)
    - Manufacturer (Lilly, Novo Nordisk)
    - Concentration (eg, U-100)
    - Expiration date
2. Checks appearance of insulin:
    - Clear or milky white
    - Checks for flocculation (clumping, frosted appearance)
3. Identifies where to purchase and store insulin:
    - Indicates approximately how long bottle will last (1,000 units per bottle U-100 insulin)
    - Indicates how long opened bottles can be used

Syringes

1. Identifies concentration (U-100) marking on syringe
2. Identifies size of syringe (eg, 100-unit, 50-unit, 30-unit)
3. Describes appropriate disposal of used syringe

Preparation and Administration of Insulin Injection

1. Draws up correct amount and type of insulin
2. Properly mixes two insulins if necessary
3. Inserts needle and injects insulin
4. Describes site rotation:
    - Demonstrates injection with all anatomic areas to be used
    - Describes pattern for rotation, such as using abdomen only or using certain areas at the same time of day
    - Describes system for remembering site locations, such as horizontal pattern across the abdomen as if drawing a dotted line

Knowledge of Insulin Action

1. Lists prescription:
    - Type and dosage of insulin
    - Timing of insulin injections
2. Describes approximate time course of insulin action:
    - Identifies long- and short-acting insulins by name
    - States approximate time delay until onset of insulin action
    - Identifies need to delay food until 15 to 30 minutes after the injection (indicated when injecting regular insulin)
    - Knows that longer time delays are safe when blood glucose level is high, and time delays may need to be shortened when blood glucose level is low

Incorporation of Insulin Injections Into Daily Schedule

1. Recites proper order of premeal diabetes activities:
    - May use mnemonic device such as the word "tie," which helps the patient remember the order of activities ("t" = test [blood glucose], "i" = insulin injection, "e" = eat)
    - Describes daily schedule, such as test, insulin, eat, before breakfast and dinner; test and eat, before lunch and bedtime
2. Describes information regarding hypoglycemia:
    - Symptoms: shakiness, sweating, nervousness, hunger, weakness
    - Causes: too much insulin, too much exercise, not enough food
    - Treatment: 10 to 15 g simple carbohydrate, such as two or three glucose tablets, 1 tube glucose gel, 0.5 to 1 cup juice
    - After initial treatment, follow with snack including starch and protein, such as cheese and crackers, milk and crackers, half sandwich.
3. Describes information regarding prevention of hypoglycemia:
    - Avoid delays in meal timing.
    - Eat a meal or snack approximately every 4 to 5 hours (while awake).
    - Do not skip meals.
    - Increase food intake before exercise.
    - Check blood glucose regularly.
    - Change insulin doses only with medical supervision.
    - Carry a form of fast-acting sugar at all times.
    - Wear a medical identification bracelet.
    - Teach family, friends, coworkers about signs and treatment of hypoglycemia.
    - Have family, roommates, traveling companions learn to use injectable glucagon for severe hypoglycemic reactions.
4. Regular follow-up for evaluation of diabetes control:
    - Keeps written record of blood glucose, insulin doses, hypoglycemic reactions, variations in diet
    - Keeps all appointments with health professionals
    - Sees physician regularly (usually two to four times per year)
    - States how to contact physician in case of emergency
    - States when to call physician to report variations in blood glucose levels

Equipment

INSULIN

Short-acting insulins are clear in appearance, and longer-acting insulins are cloudy and white. The longer-acting insulins must be mixed (gently inverted or rolled in the hands) before use.

Some sources specify that insulin bottles in use be refrigerated, and others simply suggest that insulin be kept at room temperature. There is agreement that extremes of temperature are to be avoided; thus, insulin should not be allowed to freeze and should not be kept in direct sunlight or in a hot car. Before injection, it is recommended that insulin be at room temperature (which may require rolling it in the hands or removing it from a refrigerator for a time before the injection). If a vial of insulin will be used up in 1 month, it may be kept at room temperature.

Insulin bottles should also be assessed for flocculation, which is a frosted, whitish coating inside the bottle of intermediate- or long-acting insulins. This occurs most commonly with human insulins that are not refrigerated. If a frosted, adherent coating is present, some of the insulin is bound and should not be used.

SYRINGES

Syringes must be matched with the insulin concentration (eg, U-100). Currently, three sizes of U-100 insulin syringes are available:

- 1-mL (cc) syringes that hold 100 units
- 0.5-mL syringes that hold 50 units
- 0.3-mL syringes that hold 30 units

The concentration of insulin used in the United States is U-100; that is, there are 100 units per milliliter (or cubic centimeter). Syringe size varies. The use of small syringes allows patients who require small amounts of insulin to measure and draw up the amount of insulin accurately. Patients who require large amounts of insulin would use larger syringes. Although there is a U-500 (500 units/mL) concentration of insulin available by special order

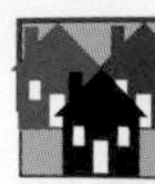

Patient Education and Home Care

Self-Injection of Insulin

1. With one hand, stabilize the skin by spreading it or pinching up a large area.

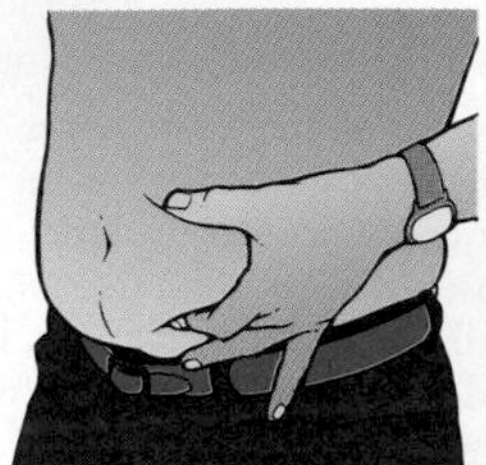

Pinching the skin

2. Pick up syringe with the other hand and hold it as you would a pencil. Insert needle straight into the skin.*

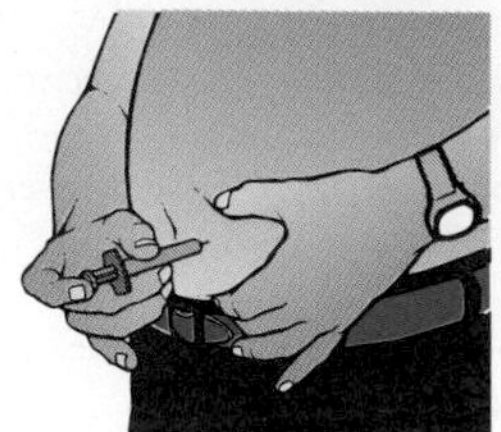

Inserting the needle into the skin

3. To inject the insulin, push the plunger all the way in.

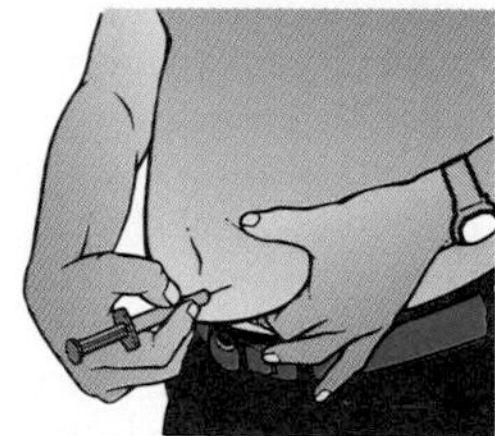

Injecting the insulin

4. Pull needle straight out of skin. Press cotton ball over injection site for several seconds.

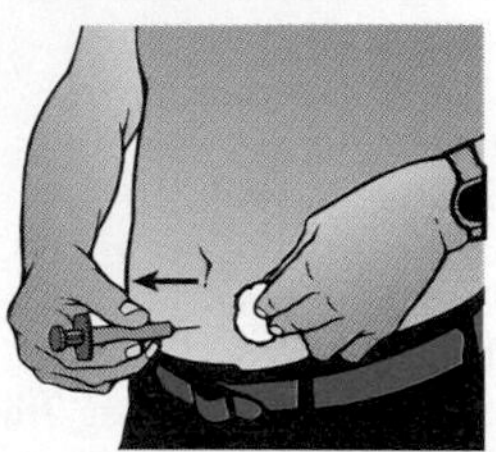

Removing the needle and holding cotton ball over site

5. Use disposable syringe only once and discard into hard plastic container (with a tight-fitting top) such as an empty bleach or detergent container.†

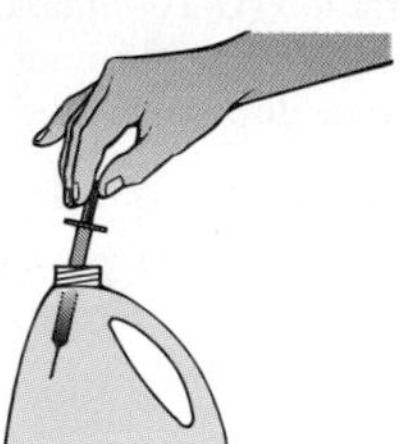

Disposing of syringe

* Some patients may be taught to insert the needle at a 45 degree angle.

† Some studies suggest that it may be safe to reuse disposable syringes.

for patients who have severe insulin resistance and require massive doses of insulin, it is rarely used.

Most insulin syringes have a 27- to 29-gauge needle that is approximately 0.5 inch long. The smaller syringes are marked in 1-unit increments and may be easier to use for patients with visual deficits or patients taking very small doses of insulin. The 1-mL syringes are marked in 2-unit increments. A small disposable insulin needle (29- to 30-gauge, 8 mm long) is now available for very thin patients and children.

Preparing the Injection

MIXING INSULINS

When rapid- or short-acting insulins are to be given simultaneously with longer-acting insulins, they are usually mixed together in the same syringe. There is some question as to whether the two insulins are stable if the mixture is kept in the syringe for more than 5 to 15 minutes. This may depend on the ratio of the insulins as well as the time between mixing and injecting. Some research studies have suggested that when mixing regular insulin with long-acting insulin, there is a binding reaction that slows the action of the regular insulin. This may also occur to a greater degree when mixing regular insulin with one of the Lente insulins. Patients are advised to consult their health care professional for advice on this matter. The most important issue is that patients be consistent in how they prepare their insulin injections from day to day.

There are varying opinions regarding which type of insulin (short- or longer-acting) should be drawn up into the syringe first when they are going to be mixed. Most of the printed materials from pharmaceutical companies recommend drawing up the regular insulin first. The most important issues are, again, that patients be consistent in technique so as not to draw up the wrong dose accidentally or the wrong type of insulin, and that patients not inject one type of insulin into the bottle containing a different type of insulin.

For patients who have difficulty mixing insulins, two options are available: they may use a premixed insulin, or they may have prefilled syringes prepared. Premixed insulins are available in several different ratios of NPH insulin to regular insulin. The ratio of 70/30 (70% NPH and 30% regular insulin in one bottle) is the most common and is available as Novolin 70/30 (Novo Nordisk) and Humulin 70/30 (Lilly). Other ratios available include 80/20, 60/40, and 50/50. The appropriate initial dosage of premixed insulin must be calculated so that the ratio of NPH to regular insulin most closely approximates the separate doses needed.

For patients who can inject insulin but who have difficulty drawing up a single or mixed dose, syringes can be prefilled with the help of home care nurses or family and friends. A 3-week supply of insulin syringes may be prepared and kept in the refrigerator. The prefilled syringes should be kept flat or with the needle in an upright position to avoid clogging of the needle.

WITHDRAWING INSULIN

Most (if not all) of the printed materials available on insulin dose preparation instruct patients to inject air into the bottle of insulin equivalent to the number of units of insulin to be withdrawn. The rationale behind this is to prevent the formation of a vacuum inside the bottle, which would make it difficult to withdraw the proper amount of insulin.

Some nurses specializing in diabetes have found that some patients (who have been taking insulin for many years) have stopped injecting air before withdrawing the insulin. These patients found that the extra step was not necessary for accurately drawing up the insulin doses. Most patients find it easier to withdraw the insulin by eliminating the step and report no difficulty in preparing the proper insulin dose.

Eliminating this step (or alternating it by, for instance, injecting a syringe full of air into the vial once per week) facilitates the teaching process for some patients learning to draw up insulin for the first time. Some patients become confused with the sequence of steps involved in injecting air into two separate bottles in two different amounts before drawing up a mixed dose. For many individuals, including the elderly, simplifying the procedure for preparing insulin injections may have a major positive impact on maintaining independence in daily living.

As with other variations in insulin injection technique, the most important factors are that the patient maintain consistency in the procedure and that the nurse be flexible when teaching new patients or assessing the skills of experienced patients.

Administering the Injection

SELECTING AND ROTATING THE SITE

The four main areas for injection are the abdomen, arms (posterior surface), thighs (anterior surface), and hips (Fig. 37-7). Insulin is absorbed faster when injected into certain areas. The speed of absorption is greatest in the abdomen and decreases progressively in the arm, thigh, and hip.

Systematic rotation of injection sites within an anatomic area is recommended to prevent localized changes in fatty tissue (lipodystrophy). In addition, to promote consistency in insulin absorption, patients should be encouraged to use all available injection sites within one area rather than randomly rotating sites from area to area. For example, some patients almost exclusively use the abdominal area, administering each injection 0.5 to 1 inch away from the previous injection. Another approach to rotation is always to use the same area at the same time of day. For example, patients may inject morning doses into the abdomen and evening doses into the arms or legs.

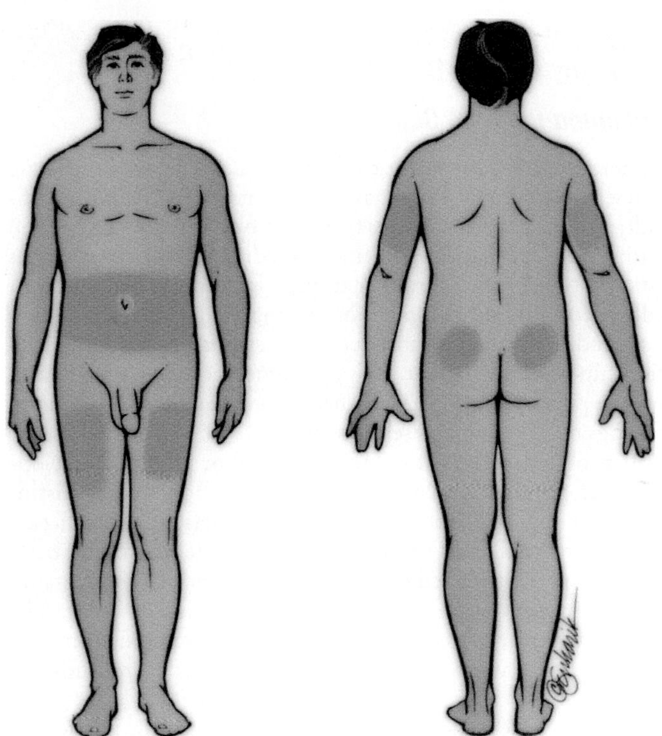

FIGURE 37•7 Suggested areas for insulin injection.

A few general principles apply to all rotation patterns. First, patients should try not to use the same site more than once in 2 to 3 weeks. In addition, if the patient is planning to exercise, insulin should not be injected into the limb that will be exercised, because it will be absorbed faster, and this may result in hypoglycemia.

In the past, patients were taught to rotate injections from one area to the next (eg, injecting once in the right arm, then once in the right abdomen, then once in the right thigh). Patients who still use this system must be taught to avoid repeated injections into the same site within an area. However, as previously stated, it is preferable for the patient to use the same anatomic area at the same time of day consistently; this reduces day-to-day variation in blood glucose levels because of different absorption rates.

INSERTING THE NEEDLE

There are varying approaches to insertion of the needle for insulin injections. The correct technique is based on the need for the insulin to be injected into the subcutaneous tissue. Injection that is too deep (eg, intramuscular) or too shallow may affect the rate of absorption of the insulin. Aspiration (inserting the needle and then pulling back on the plunger to assess for blood being drawn into the syringe) is generally not recommended with self-injection of insulin. Many patients who have been using insulin for an extended period have eliminated this step from their insulin injection routine with no apparent adverse effects.

Promoting Home and Community-Based Care

Teaching Patients Self-Care

Adherence to the therapeutic plan is the most important self-care concept the patient must master. Patients who are having difficulty adhering to the diabetes treatment plan must be approached with a sense of caring and understanding. Using scare tactics (such as threats of blindness or amputation if the patient does not adhere to the treatment plan) or making the patient feel guilty is not productive and may interfere with establishing a trusting relationship with the patient. Using judgmental terms, such as asking the patient if he or she has cheated on the diet, only promotes feelings of guilt and low self-esteem.

If problems exist with glucose control or with the development of preventable complications, it is important to distinguish among nonadherence, knowledge deficit, and self-care deficit. It should not be assumed that problems with diabetes management are related to nonadherence. The patient may simply have forgotten or never learned certain information. The problem may be correctable simply through providing complete information and ensuring that the patient comprehends the information.

If knowledge deficit is not the problem, certain physical or emotional factors may be impairing the patient's ability to perform self-care skills. For example, decreased visual acuity may impair the patient's ability to administer insulin accurately, measure the blood glucose level, or inspect the skin and feet. In addition, decreased joint mobility (especially in the elderly) impairs the ability to inspect the bottom of the feet. Emotional factors such as denial of the diagnosis or depression may impair the patient's ability to carry out multiple daily self-care measures. In other circumstances, family, personal, or work problems and issues may be of higher priority to the patient. The patient facing competing demands for time and attention may benefit from assistance in establishing priorities.

It is also important to assess the patient for infection or emotional stress that may lead to elevated blood glucose levels despite adherence to the treatment regimen.

The following approaches by the nurse are helpful for promoting self-care management skills:

- Address any underlying factors (eg, knowledge deficit, self-care deficit, illness) that may affect diabetic control.
- Simplify the treatment regimen if it is too difficult for the patient to follow.
- Adjust the treatment regimen to meet patient requests (eg, adjust diet or insulin schedule to allow increased flexibility in meal content or timing).
- Establish a specific plan or contract with the patient with simple, measurable goals.
- Provide positive reinforcement of self-care behaviors performed instead of focusing on behaviors that were neglected (eg, positively reinforce blood glucose tests that were performed instead of focusing on the number of missed tests).
- Help the patient to identify personal motivating factors rather than focusing on wanting to please the doctor or nurse.
- Encourage the patient to pursue life goals and interests; discourage an undue focus on diabetes.

Continuing Care

As discussed, continuing care of the diabetic patient is critical in managing and preventing complications. The degree to which the client interacts with health care providers to obtain ongoing care depends on many factors. Age, socioeconomic level, existing complications, type of diabetes, and comorbid conditions all may dictate the frequency of follow-up visits. Many patients with diabetes may be seen by home health nurses for diabetic education, wound care, insulin preparation, or assistance with glucose monitoring. Even patients who achieve excellent glucose control and have no complications can expect to see their primary care provider at least twice a year for ongoing evaluation.

In addition to follow-up care with health professionals, participation in support groups is encouraged for those who have had diabetes for many years as well as those who are newly diagnosed. Such participation may assist the patient and family in coping with changes in lifestyle that occur with the onset of diabetes and with its complications. Those who participate in support groups often have an opportunity to share valuable information and experiences and to learn from others. Support groups provide an opportunity for discussion of strategies to deal with diabetes and its management and to clarify and verify information with the nurse or other health care professionals. Participation in support groups may help patients and their families to become more knowledgeable about diabetes and its management and may promote adherence to the management plan.

ACUTE COMPLICATIONS OF DIABETES

There are three major acute complications of diabetes related to short-term imbalances in blood glucose: hypoglycemia, diabetic ketoacidosis (DKA), and hyperglycemic hyperosmolar nonketotic syndrome (HHNS) (also known as hyperglycemic hyperosmolar nonketotic coma).

Hypoglycemia (Insulin Reactions)

Hypoglycemia (abnormally low blood glucose level) occurs when the blood glucose falls to less than 50 to 60 mg/dL (2.7 to 3.3 mmol/L). It can be caused by too much insulin or oral hypoglycemic agents, too little food, or excessive physical activity. Hypoglycemia may occur at any time of the day or night. It often occurs before meals, especially if meals are delayed or snacks are omitted. For example, midmorning hypoglycemia may occur when the morning regular insulin is peaking, whereas hypoglycemia that occurs in the late afternoon coincides with the peak of the morning NPH or Lente insulin. Middle-of-the-night hypoglycemia may occur because of peaking evening or predinner NPH or Lente insulins, especially in patients who have not eaten a bedtime snack.

Clinical Manifestations

The clinical manifestations of hypoglycemia may be grouped into two categories: adrenergic symptoms and central nervous system symptoms.

In mild hypoglycemia, as the blood glucose level falls, the sympathetic nervous system is stimulated, resulting in a surge of adrenalin. This causes symptoms such as sweating, tremor, tachycardia, palpitation, nervousness, and hunger.

Home Care Teaching Checklist: The Person With Newly Diagnosed Diabetes

At the conclusion of the program, the patient or caregiver will be able to:	Patient	Caregiver
• State the importance of diabetes survival skills.	✔	✔
• Explain underlying pathology of diabetes.	✔	✔
• State normal range of blood glucose.	✔	✔
• Identify factors that cause hyper- and hypoglycemia.	✔	✔
• Describe the major modalities used to control diabetes (diet, exercise, monitoring, medication, education).	✔	✔
• Demonstrate proper technique for drawing up and injecting insulin (including mixing two types of insulin if necessary).	✔	✔
• State dose and timing of injections, peak action and duration of insulin.	✔	✔
• Explain insulin injection rotation plan and its rationale.	✔	✔
• State dose, timing, peak action and duration of prescribed oral agents.	✔	✔
• Describe where to purchase and store insulin, syringes, and glucose monitoring supplies.	✔	✔
• Identify classification of food groups (depending on system used).	✔	✔
• State appropriate schedule for eating snacks and meals.	✔	✔
• Select appropriate foods on menus and identify foods that may be substituted for one another on the meal plan.	✔	
• Demonstrate proper technique for monitoring blood glucose.	✔	
• Describe strategies to be used to treat hypoglycemic episodes.	✔	✔
• Use proper technique for disposing of needles used for blood glucose monitoring and insulin injections.	✔	
• Demonstrate proper technique for urine ketone testing (for patients with type 1 diabetes), and verbalize appropriate times to assess for ketones.	✔	
• Identify community, outpatient resources for obtaining further diabetes education.	✔	
• Identify signs and symptoms of hypoglycemia.	✔	✔
• Describe appropriate treatment of hypoglycemia.	✔	✔
• Identify factors that may cause hypoglycemia.	✔	✔
• State strategies that minimize risk for hypoglycemia.	✔	✔
• State rationale for wearing medical identification and carrying a source of simple carbohydrate at all times.	✔	
• Identify signs and symptoms of hyperglycemia.	✔	✔
• Describe appropriate treatment of hyperglycemia.	✔	✔
• Identify factors that may cause hyperglycemia.	✔	✔
• Identify rules for sick-day management.	✔	✔
• Identify appropriate circumstances for contacting physician.	✔	✔

In moderate hypoglycemia, the fall in blood glucose level deprives the brain cells of needed fuel for functioning. Signs of impaired function of the central nervous system may include inability to concentrate, headache, lightheadedness, confusion, memory lapses, numbness of the lips and tongue, slurred speech, impaired coordination, emotional changes, irrational or combative behavior, double vision, and drowsiness. Any combination of these symptoms (in addition to adrenergic symptoms) may occur with moderate hypoglycemia.

In severe hypoglycemia, central nervous system function is so impaired that the patient needs the assistance of another person for treatment of hypoglycemia. Symptoms may include disoriented behavior, seizures, difficulty arousing from sleep, or loss of consciousness.

Assessment and Diagnostic Findings

Hypoglycemic symptoms may occur suddenly and unexpectedly. The combination of symptoms varies considerably from person to person. To some degree, this may be related to the actual level to which the blood glucose drops or to the rate at which it is dropping. For example, patients who usually have a blood glucose level in the hyperglycemic range (eg, in the 200s or greater) may feel hypoglycemic (adrenergic) symptoms when their blood glucose quickly drops to 120 mg/dL (6.6 mmol/L) or less. Conversely, patients who frequently have a glucose level in the low range of normal may be asymptomatic when the blood glucose slowly falls to less than 50 mg/dL (2.7 mmol/L).

Another factor contributing to altered hypoglycemic symptoms is a decreased hormonal (adrenergic) response to hypoglycemia. This occurs in some patients who have had diabetes for many years. It may be related to one of the chronic diabetic complications—autonomic neuropathy (see section on hypoglycemic unawareness). As the blood glucose level falls, the normal surge in adrenalin does not occur. The patient does not feel the usual adrenergic symptoms, such as sweating and shakiness. The hypoglycemia may not be detected until moderate or severe central nervous system impairment occurs. These patients must perform SMBG on a frequent regular basis, especially before driving or engaging in other potentially dangerous activities.

Gerontologic Considerations

In the elderly, hypoglycemia is a particular concern for many reasons:

- Elderly people frequently live alone and may not recognize the symptoms of hypoglycemia.
- With decreasing renal function, it takes longer for oral hypoglycemic agents to be excreted by the kidneys.

- Skipping meals may occur because of decreased appetite or financial limitations.
- Decreased visual acuity may lead to errors in insulin administration

Medical Management

Immediate treatment must be given when hypoglycemia occurs. The usual recommendation is for 10 to 15 g of a fast-acting simple carbohydrate (such as the following) orally:

- Three or four commercially prepared glucose tablets
- 4 to 6 oz of fruit juice or regular soda
- 6 to 10 Life Savers or other hard candies
- 2 to 3 teaspoons of sugar or honey

It is not necessary to add sugar to juice, even if it is labeled as unsweetened juice. The fruit sugar in juice contains enough simple carbohydrate to raise the blood glucose level. Adding table sugar to juice may cause a sharp increase in the blood glucose level, and the patient may experience hyperglycemia for hours after treatment.

If circumstances permit testing, the blood glucose level should be retested in 15 minutes and retreated if it is less than 70 to 75 mg/dL (3.8 to 4 mmol/L).

If the symptoms persist more than 10 to 15 minutes after initial treatment, the treatment is repeated even if testing of blood glucose is not possible. Once the symptoms resolve, a snack containing protein and starch (eg, milk or cheese and crackers) is recommended unless the patient plans to eat a regular meal or snack within 30 to 60 minutes.

It is important for diabetic patients (especially those receiving insulin) to carry some form of simple sugar with them at all times. There are many different commercially prepared glucose tablets and gels that patients may find convenient to carry. If the patient has a hypoglycemic reaction and does not have any of the recommended emergency foods available, any available food (preferably a simple carbohydrate food) should be eaten.

Patients are encouraged to refrain from eating high-calorie, high-fat dessert foods (eg, cookies, cakes, donuts, ice cream) to treat hypoglycemia. The high fat content of these foods may slow the absorption of the glucose, and the hypoglycemic symptoms may not resolve as quickly as they would with the intake of simple carbohydrates. The patient may subsequently eat more of the foods when symptoms do not resolve rapidly. This in turn may cause very high blood glucose levels for several hours after the reaction and may also contribute to weight gain.

Patients who feel unduly restricted by their meal plan may view hypoglycemic episodes as a time to reward themselves with desserts. It may be more prudent to teach these patients to incorporate occasional desserts into the meal plan. This may make it easier for them to limit their treatment of hypoglycemic episodes to simple (low-calorie) carbohydrates such as juice or glucose tablets.

For patients who are unconscious and cannot swallow, an injection of glucagon 1 mg can be administered either subcutaneously or intramuscularly. Glucagon is a hormone produced by the alpha cells of the pancreas that stimulates the liver to release glucose (through the breakdown of glycogen, the stored glucose). It is packaged as a powder in 1-mg vials and must be mixed with a diluent before being injected. After injection of glucagon, it may take up to 20 minutes for the patient to regain consciousness. A simple sugar followed by a snack should be given to the patient on awakening to prevent recurrence of hypoglycemia (because the duration of the action of 1 mg of glucagon is brief [its onset is 8 to 10 minutes and its action lasts 12 to 27 minutes]), and to replenish liver stores of glucose. Some patients experience nausea after the administration of glucagon. The patient should be instructed to notify the physician after severe hypoglycemia has occurred.

Glucagon is sold by prescription only and should be part of the emergency supplies kept available by patients with diabetes who require insulin. Family members, neighbors, or coworkers should be instructed in the use of glucagon. This is especially true for patients who receive little or no warning of hypoglycemic episodes.

In the hospital or emergency department, patients who are unconscious or cannot swallow may be treated with 25 to 50 mL 50% dextrose in water (D_{50}), administered intravenously. The effect is usually seen within minutes. Patients may complain of a headache and of pain at the injection site. Assuring patency of the intravenous line used for injection of 50% dextrose is essential because hypertonic solutions such as 50% dextrose are very irritating to the vein.

Promoting Home and Community-Based Care

TEACHING PATIENTS SELF-CARE

Hypoglycemia is prevented by a consistent pattern of eating, administering insulin, and exercising. Between-meal and bedtime snacks may be needed to counteract the maximum insulin effect. In general, the patient should cover the time of peak activity of insulin by eating a snack and by taking additional food when physical activity is increased. Routine blood glucose tests are performed so that changing insulin requirements may be anticipated and the dosage adjusted.

Because unexpected hypoglycemia may occur, all patients treated with insulin should wear an identification bracelet or tag stating that they have diabetes.

Patients and family members must be instructed about the potential symptoms of hypoglycemia. Family members especially must be made aware that any subtle (but unusual) change in behavior may be an indication that hypoglycemia is occurring. They should be taught to encourage and even insist that the person with diabetes assess blood glucose levels if hypoglycemia is suspected. Some patients (when hypoglycemic) become very resistant to testing or eating and become angry at family members trying to treat the hypoglycemia. Family members must be taught to persevere and to understand that the hypoglycemia can cause irrational behavior.

Some patients with autonomic neuropathy or those taking beta blockers such as propranolol for the treatment of hypertension or cardiac dysrhythmias may not experience the typical symptoms of hypoglycemia. It is very important for these patients to perform blood glucose tests on a frequent and regular basis.

Type 2 diabetes patients who take oral sulfonylurea agents may also develop hypoglycemia (especially those taking chlorpropamide, which is a long-lasting oral hypoglycemic agent).

Diabetic Ketoacidosis

DKA is caused by an absence or markedly inadequate amount of insulin. This results in disorders in the metabolism of carbohydrate, protein, and fat. The three main clinical features of DKA are:

- Hyperglycemia
- Dehydration and electrolyte loss
- Acidosis

When insulin is lacking, the amount of glucose entering the cells is reduced and glucose production by the liver increases. Both fac-

PATHOPHYSIOLOGY

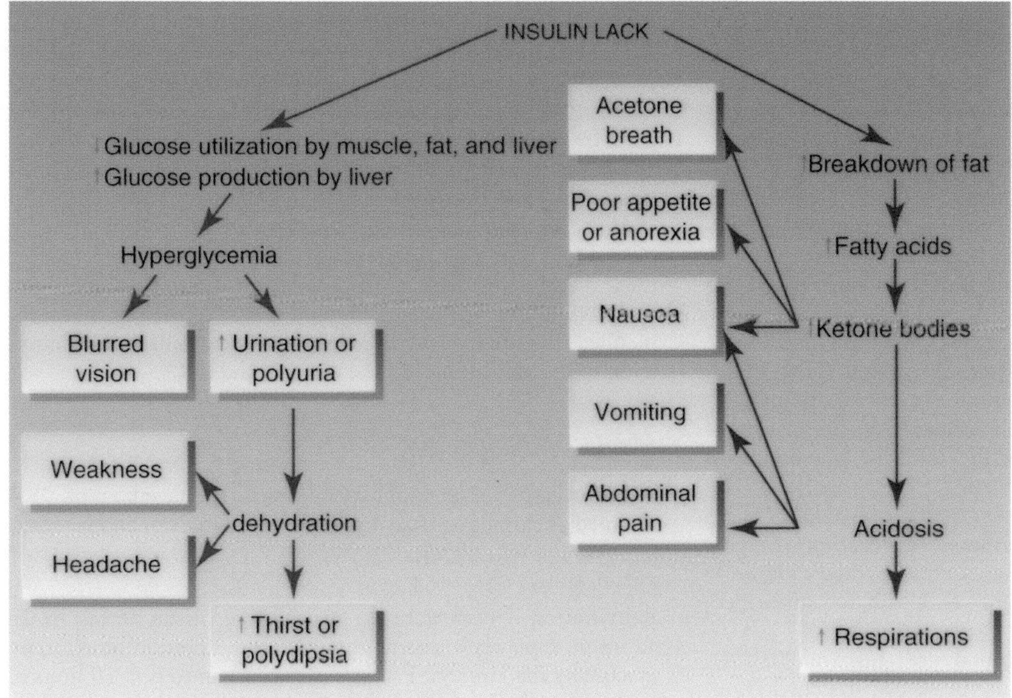

FIGURE 37•8 Abnormal metabolism that causes signs and symptoms of diabetic ketoacidosis: ↑, increased; ↓, decreased. Pearce, M. A., Rosenberg, C. S., & Davidson, M. D. (1991). Patient education. In M.B. Davidson (ed), *Diabetes mellitus: Diagnosis and treatment* (3rd ed.). New York: Churchill Livingstone.

tors lead to hyperglycemia. In an attempt to rid the body of the excess glucose, the kidneys excrete the glucose along with water and electrolytes (eg, sodium and potassium). This osmotic diuresis, which is characterized by excessive urination (polyuria), leads to dehydration and marked electrolyte loss. Patients with severe DKA may lose an average of 6.5 liters of water and up to 400 to 500 mEq each of sodium, potassium, and chloride over a 24-hour period.

Another effect of insulin deficiency is the breakdown of fat (lipolysis) into free fatty acids and glycerol. The free fatty acids are converted into ketone bodies by the liver. In DKA there is excessive production of ketone bodies because of the lack of insulin that would normally prevent this from occurring. Ketone bodies are acids; when they accumulate in the circulation, this leads to metabolic acidosis.

Three main causes of DKA are:

- Decreased or missed dose of insulin
- Illness or infection
- Undiagnosed and untreated diabetes (may be the initial manifestation of diabetes)

A decrease in insulin may result from an insufficient dosage of insulin prescribed or from insufficient insulin being administered by the patient. Errors in insulin dosage may be made by patients who are ill and who assume that if they are eating less or if they are vomiting, they must decrease their insulin doses. (Because illness [especially infections] may cause increased blood glucose levels, patients do not need to decrease their insulin doses to compensate for decreased food intake when ill and may even need to increase the insulin dose.)

Other potential causes of decreased insulin include patient error in drawing up or injecting insulin (especially in patients with visual impairments), intentional skipping of insulin doses (especially in adolescents with diabetes who are having difficulty coping with diabetes or other aspects of their lives), or equipment problems (eg, occlusion of insulin pump tubing).

Illness and infections are associated with insulin resistance. In response to physical (and emotional) stresses, there is an increase in the level of "stress" hormones—glucagon, epinephrine, norepinephrine, cortisol, and growth hormone. These hormones promote glucose production by the liver and interfere with glucose utilization by muscle and fat tissue, counteracting the effect of insulin. If insulin levels are not increased during times of illness and infection, hyperglycemia may progress to DKA.

Clinical Manifestations

The signs and symptoms of DKA are outlined in Figure 37-8. The hyperglycemia of DKA leads to polyuria and polydipsia (increased thirst). In addition, patients may experience blurred vision, weakness, and headache. Patients with marked intravascular volume depletion may have orthostatic hypotension (drop in systolic blood pressure of 20 mm Hg or more on standing). Volume depletion may also lead to frank hypotension with a weak, rapid pulse.

The ketosis and acidosis characteristic of DKA lead to gastrointestinal symptoms such as anorexia, nausea, vomiting, and abdominal pain. The abdominal pain and physical findings on examination can be so severe that it resembles an acute abdominal disorder that requires surgery. Patients may have acetone breath (a fruity odor), which occurs with elevated ketone levels. In addition, hyperventilation (with very deep, but not labored, respirations) may occur. These Kussmaul respirations represent the body's attempt to decrease the acidosis, counteracting the effect of the ketone buildup.

Mental status changes in DKA vary widely from patient to patient. Patients may be alert, lethargic, or comatose, most likely depending on the plasma osmolarity (concentration of osmotically active particles).

Assessment and Diagnostic Findings

Blood glucose levels may vary from 300 to 800 mg/dL (16.6 to 44.4 mmol/L). Some patients have lower glucose values, and others have values of 1000 mg/dL (55.5 mmol/L) or more (usually depending on the degree of dehydration). The severity of DKA is not necessarily related to the blood glucose level. Some patients may have severe acidosis with blood glucose levels in the range of the high 100s to low 200s (5.5 to 11.1 mmol/L), whereas others may have no evidence of DKA despite blood glucose levels of 400 to 500 mg/dL (22.2 to 27.7 mmol/L).

Evidence of ketoacidosis is reflected in low serum bicarbonate (0 to 15 mEq/L) and low pH (6.8 to 7.3) values. A low PCO_2 level (10 to 30 mm Hg) reflects respiratory compensation (Kussmaul respirations) for the metabolic acidosis. Accumulation of ketone bodies (which precipitates the acidosis) is reflected in blood and urine ketone measurements.

Sodium and potassium levels may be low, normal, or high, depending on the amount of water loss (dehydration). Despite the plasma concentration, there has been a marked total body depletion of these (and other) electrolytes. Ultimately, these electrolytes will need to be replaced.

Elevated levels of creatinine, blood urea nitrogen (BUN), hemoglobin, and hematocrit may also be seen with dehydration. After rehydration, continued elevation in the serum creatinine and BUN levels will be present in the patient with underlying renal insufficiency.

Prevention

For prevention of DKA related to illness, patients must be taught "sick day" rules for managing their diabetes when ill. The most important issue to teach patients is not to eliminate insulin doses when nausea and vomiting occur. Rather, they should take their usual insulin dose (or previously prescribed special "sick day" doses) and then attempt to consume frequent small portions of carbohydrates (including foods usually avoided, such as juices, regular sodas, and gelatin). Drinking fluids every hour is important to prevent dehydration. Blood glucose and urine ketones must be assessed every 3 to 4 hours.

If the patient cannot take fluids without vomiting, or if elevated glucose or ketone levels persist, the physician must be contacted. Patients are taught to have available foods for use on sick days. In addition, a supply of urine test strips (for ketone testing) and blood glucose test strips should be available. Patients must know how to contact their physician 24 hours a day.

Diabetes self-management skills (including insulin administration and blood glucose testing) should be assessed to ensure that an accidental error in insulin administration or blood glucose testing did not occur. Psychological counseling is recommended for patients and family members if an intentional alteration in insulin dosing was the cause of the DKA.

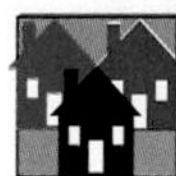

PATIENT EDUCATION AND HOME CARE
Guidelines to Follow During Periods of Illness ("Sick Day Rules")

- Take insulin or oral antidiabetic agents as usual.
- Test blood glucose and test urine ketones every 3 to 4 hours.
- Report elevated glucose levels (greater than 300 mg/dL [16.6 mmol/L] or as otherwise specified) or urine ketones to the physician.
- Insulin-requiring patients may need supplemental doses of regular insulin every 3 to 4 hours.
- If usual meal plan cannot be followed, substitute soft foods (eg, ⅓ cup regular gelatin, 1 cup cream soup, ½ cup custard, 3 squares graham crackers) six to eight times per day.
- If vomiting, diarrhea, or fever persists, take liquids (eg, ½ cup regular cola or orange juice, ½ cup broth, 1 cup Gatorade) every ½ to 1 hour to prevent dehydration and to provide calories.
- Report nausea, vomiting, and diarrhea to the physician, because extreme fluid loss may be dangerous.
- For patients with type 1 diabetes, inability to retain oral fluids, may warrant hospitalization to avoid diabetic ketoacidosis and possibly coma.

Medical Management

In addition to treatment of hyperglycemia, management of DKA is aimed at correcting dehydration, electrolyte loss, and acidosis.

DEHYDRATION

Rehydration is important for maintaining tissue perfusion. In addition, fluid replacement enhances the excretion of excessive glucose by the kidneys. Patients may need up to 6 to 10 liters of intravenous fluid to replace fluid losses caused by polyuria, hyperventilation, diarrhea, and vomiting.

Initially, 0.9% normal saline is administered at a very high rate, usually 0.5 to 1 L per hour for 2 to 3 hours. Hypotonic normal saline (0.45%) may be used for patients with hypertension or hypernatremia or those at risk for congestive heart failure. After the first few hours, 0.45% normal saline is the fluid of choice for continued rehydration, if the blood pressure is stable and the sodium level is not low. Moderate to high rates of infusion (200 to 500 mL per hour) may continue for several more hours. When the blood glucose level reaches 300 mg/dL (16.6 mmol/L) or less, the intravenous fluid may be changed to D_5W to prevent a precipitous decline in the blood glucose level.

Monitoring fluid volume status involves frequent measurements of vital signs (including monitoring for orthostatic changes in blood pressure and heart rate), lung assessment, and monitoring intake and output. Initial urine output will lag behind intravenous fluid intake as dehydration is corrected. Plasma expanders may be necessary to correct severe hypotension that does not respond to intravenous fluid treatment. Monitoring for signs of fluid overload is especially important for older patients, those with renal impairment, or those at risk for congestive heart failure.

ELECTROLYTE LOSS

The major electrolyte of concern during treatment of DKA is potassium. Although the initial plasma concentration of potassium may be low, normal, or even high, there is a major loss of potassium from body stores and an intracellular to extracellular shift of potassium. Further, the level of potassium drops during the course of treatment of DKA as potassium reenters the cells; therefore, it must be monitored frequently.

Some of the factors related to the treatment of DKA that reduce the serum potassium concentration include:

- Rehydration, which leads to increased plasma volume and subsequent decreases in the concentration of serum potas-

sium. Rehydration also leads to increased urinary excretion of potassium.
- Insulin administration, which enhances the movement of potassium from the extracellular fluid into the cells

Cautious but timely potassium replacement is vital to avoid dysrhythmias that may occur with hypokalemia. Up to 40 mEq per hour may be needed for several hours. Because extracellular potassium levels drop during DKA treatment, potassium must be infused even if the plasma potassium level is normal. As DKA resolves, the potassium replacement rate is decreased. For safety, the nurse makes sure that:

- There are no signs of hyperkalemia on the electrocardiogram (tall, peaked [or tented] T waves).
- The laboratory values of potassium are normal or low.
- The patient is urinating (ie, no renal shutdown).

Frequent (every 2 to 4 hours initially) electrocardiogram readings and laboratory measurements of potassium are necessary during the first 8 hours of treatment. Potassium replacement is withheld only if hyperkalemia is present or if the patient is not urinating. However, because the potassium level may drop quickly due to rehydration and insulin treatment, potassium replacement must begin once potassium levels drop to normal.

ACIDOSIS

Ketone bodies (acids) accumulate as a result of fat breakdown. The acidosis that occurs in DKA is reversed with insulin, which inhibits fat breakdown, thereby stopping acid buildup.

Insulin is usually infused intravenously at a slow, continuous rate (eg, 5 units per hour). Hourly blood glucose values must be measured. Dextrose is added to intravenous fluids, such as normal saline (NS) solution (eg, D_5NS or $D_5$0.45NS), when blood glucose levels reach 250 to 300 mg/dL (13.8 to 16.6 mmol/L) to avoid too rapid a drop in the blood glucose level.

Various intravenous mixtures of regular insulin may be used. The nurse must convert hourly rates of insulin infusion (frequently ordered as "units per hour" to intravenous drip rates. For example, if 100 units of regular insulin is mixed in 500 mL 0.9% NS, then 1 unit of insulin equals 5 mL. Thus, an initial insulin infusion rate of 5 units per hour would equal 25 mL per hour. The insulin is often infused separately from the rehydration solutions to allow frequent changes in the rate and content of rehydration solutions.

When mixing the insulin drip, it is important to flush the insulin solution through the entire intravenous infusion set and to discard the first 50 mL of fluid. Insulin molecules adhere to the glass and plastic of intravenous infusion sets; thus, the initial fluid may contain a decreased concentration of insulin.

Insulin must be infused continuously until subcutaneous administration of insulin resumes. Any interruption in administration may result in the reaccumulation of ketone bodies and worsening acidosis. Even if blood glucose levels are dropping to normal, the insulin drip must not be stopped. Rather, the rate or concentration of the dextrose infusion should be increased.

Blood glucose levels are usually corrected before the acidosis is corrected. Thus, intravenous insulin may be continued for 12 to 24 hours, until the serum bicarbonate level improves (to at least 15 to 18 mEq/L) and until the patient can eat.

In general, bicarbonate infusion to correct severe acidosis is avoided during treatment of DKA because it precipitates further, sudden (and potentially fatal) decreases in serum potassium levels. Continuous insulin infusion is usually sufficient for reversing DKA.

Nursing Management

Nursing care of the patient with DKA focuses on monitoring fluid and electrolyte status as well as blood glucose levels, administering fluids, insulin, and other medications, and preventing other complications such as fluid overload. Urine output is monitored to ensure adequate renal function before potassium is administered to avoid hyperkalemia. The patient's ECG is monitored for dysrhythmias indicating abnormal potassium levels. Vital signs, arterial blood gases and other clinical findings are recorded on a flow sheet. The nurse documents the laboratory values and the frequent changes in fluids and medications that are prescribed and monitors the patient's responses.

As the patient recovers, the nurse reassesses the factors that may have led to DKA and teaches the patient and family strategies to prevent its recurrence. If indicated, the nurse initiates a referral for home care to ensure the patient's continued recovery.

Hyperglycemic Hyperosmolar Nonketotic Syndrome

HHNS is a serious condition in which hyperosmolarity and hyperglycemia predominate, with alterations of the sensorium (sense of awareness). At the same time, ketosis is minimal or absent. The basic biochemical defect is lack of effective insulin (ie, insulin resistance). The patient's persistent hyperglycemia causes osmotic diuresis, resulting in losses of water and electrolytes. To maintain osmotic equilibrium, water shifts from the intracellular fluid space to the extracellular fluid space. With glucosuria and dehydration, hypernatremia and increased osmolarity occur.

This condition occurs most often in older people (ages 50 to 70) with no known history of diabetes or with mild type 2 diabetes. HHNS can be traced to a precipitating event, such as an acute illness (eg, pneumonia or stroke), medications that provoke insulin dependency (thiazides), or treatments, such as dialysis. The patient's history includes days to weeks of polyuria with adequate fluid intake. What distinguishes HHNS from DKA is that ketosis and acidosis do not occur in HHNS partly because of differences in insulin levels. In DKA no insulin is present, and this promotes the break-down of stored glucose, protein, and fat, which leads to the production of ketone bodies and ketoacidosis. In HHNS the insulin level is too low to prevent hyperglycemia (and subsequent osmotic diuresis), but high enough to prevent fat breakdown. Patients with HHNS do not have the ketosis-related gastrointestinal symptoms that lead them to seek medical attention. Instead, they may tolerate polyuria and polydipsia until neurologic changes or an underlying illness (or family members or others) prompt them to seek treatment. Because of possible delays in therapy, hyperglycemia and dehydration may be more severe in HHNS.

Clinical Manifestations

The clinical picture of HHNS is one of hypotension, profound dehydration (dry mucous membranes, poor skin turgor), tachycardia, and variable neurologic signs (eg, alteration of sensorium, seizures, hemiparesis). The mortality rate ranges from 5% to 30%, usually related to an underlying illness.

Assessment and Diagnostic Findings

Diagnostic assessment includes a range of blood work, including blood glucose, electrolytes, BUN, complete blood count, serum osmolality, and arterial blood gas analysis. The blood glucose level is usually 600 to 1200 mg/dL, and the osmolality exceeds 350 mOsm/kg. Electrolyte and BUN assessment supports the clinical picture of severe dehydration. Mental status changes, focal neurologic deficits, and hallucinations are common secondary to the cerebral dehydration that results from extreme hyperosmolality. Postural hypotension accompanies the dehydration.

Medical Management

The overall approach to the treatment of HHNS is similar to that of DKA: fluid replacement, correction of electrolyte imbalances, and insulin administration. Because of the increased age of the typical patient with HHNS, close monitoring of volume and electrolyte status is important for prevention of congestive heart failure and cardiac dysrhythmias. Fluid treatment is started with 0.9% or 0.45% NS, depending on the sodium level and the severity of volume depletion. Central venous or arterial pressure monitoring guides fluid replacement. Potassium is added to intravenous fluids when urinary output is adequate and is guided by continuous electrocardiographic monitoring and frequent laboratory determinations of potassium.

Extremely elevated blood glucose levels drop as the patient is rehydrated. Insulin plays a less crucial role in the treatment of HHNS because it is not needed for reversal of acidosis, as in DKA. Nonetheless, insulin is usually administered at a continuous low rate to treat hyperglycemia, and dextrose is added to replacement fluids (as in DKA) when the glucose level decreases to the range of 250 to 300 mg/dL range (13.8 to 16.6 mmol/L).

Other therapeutic modalities are determined by the underlying illness of the patient and the results of continuing clinical and laboratory evaluation. Treatment is continued until metabolic abnormalities are corrected and neurologic symptoms clear. It may take 3 to 5 days for neurologic symptoms to resolve; thus, treatment of HHNS usually continues well beyond the time when metabolic abnormalities are resolved.

After recovery from HHNS, many patients can control their diabetes with diet alone or with diet and oral antidiabetic agents. Insulin may not be needed once the acute hyperglycemic complication is resolved.

NURSING PROCESS: THE PATIENT NEWLY DIAGNOSED WITH DIABETES MELLITUS

Assessment

The history and physical assessment focus on the signs and symptoms of prolonged hyperglycemia and on physical, social, and emotional factors that may affect the patient's ability to learn and perform diabetes self-care activities.

The patient is interviewed and asked for a description of symptoms that preceded the diagnosis of diabetes, such as polyuria, polydipsia, polyphagia, skin dryness, blurred vision, weight loss, vaginal itching, and nonhealing ulcers. The blood glucose and, for patients with type 1 diabetes, urine ketone levels are measured.

Patients with type 1 diabetes are assessed for signs of DKA, including ketonuria, Kussmaul respirations, orthostatic hypotension, and lethargy. The patient is questioned about symptoms of DKA, such as nausea, vomiting, and abdominal pain. Laboratory values are monitored for metabolic acidosis (ie, decreased pH and decreased bicarbonate level) and for electrolyte imbalance.

Patients with type 2 diabetes are assessed for signs of HHNS, including hypotension, altered sensorium, seizures, and decreased skin turgor. Laboratory values are monitored for hyperosmolarity and electrolyte imbalance.

If the patient exhibits signs and symptoms of DKA or HHNS, nursing care first focuses on treatment of these acute complications, as outlined in previous sections. Once these complications are resolving, nursing care then focuses on long-term management of diabetes, as discussed in this section.

The patient is assessed for physical factors that may impair his or her ability to learn or perform self-care skills, such as:

- Visual deficits (the patient is asked to read numbers or words on the insulin syringe, menu, newspaper, or written teaching materials)
- Deficits in motor coordination (the patient is observed eating or performing other tasks or handling a syringe or finger-lancing device)
- Neurologic deficits (eg, due to stroke) (from history in chart; the patient is assessed for aphasia or decreased ability to follow simple commands)

The nurse evaluates the patient's social situation for factors that may influence the diabetes treatment and education plan, such as:

- Decreased literacy (may be evaluated while assessing for visual deficits by having the patient read from teaching materials)
- Limited financial resources or lack of health insurance
- Presence or absence of family support
- Typical daily schedule (patient is asked about timing and number of usual daily meals, work and exercise schedule, plans for travel)

The patient's emotional status is assessed through observation of general demeanor (eg, withdrawn, anxious) and body language (eg, avoids eye contact). The patient is asked about major concerns and fears about diabetes; this allows the nurse to assess for any misconceptions or misinformation regarding diabetes. Coping skills are assessed by asking how the patient has dealt with difficult situations in the past.

Diagnosis

Nursing Diagnoses

Based on the assessment data, the patient's major nursing diagnoses may include the following:

- Risk for fluid volume deficit related to polyuria and dehydration
- Altered nutrition related to imbalance of insulin, food, and physical activity
- Knowledge deficit about diabetes self-care skills/information
- Potential self-care deficit related to physical impairments or social factors
- Anxiety related to loss of control, fear of inability to manage diabetes, misinformation related to diabetes, fear of diabetes complications

Collaborative Problems/Potential Complications

Based on assessment data, potential complications may include:

- Fluid overload, pulmonary edema, congestive heart failure
- Hypokalemia

- Hyperglycemia and ketoacidosis
- Hypoglycemia
- Cerebral edema

Planning and Goals

The major goals for the patient may include maintenance of fluid and electrolyte balance, optimal control of blood glucose levels, reversal of weight lost, ability to perform (survival) diabetes skills and self-care activities, decreased anxiety, and absence of complications.

Nursing Interventions

Maintaining Fluid and Electrolyte Balance

Intake and output are measured. Intravenous fluids and electrolytes are administered as prescribed, and oral fluid intake is encouraged. Laboratory values of serum electrolytes (especially sodium and potassium) are monitored. The patient's vital signs are monitored for signs of dehydration (tachycardia, orthostatic hypotension).

Improving Nutritional Intake

The diet is planned with the control of glucose as the primary goal; however, it must also take into consideration the patient's lifestyle, cultural background, activity level, and food preferences. An appropriate caloric intake is necessary if the patient is to achieve and maintain the desired body weight. The patient is encouraged to eat full meals and snacks as prescribed per diabetic diet. Arrangements are made with the dietitian for extra snacks before increased physical activity. It is important for the nurse to ensure that insulin orders are altered as needed for delays in eating because of diagnostic and other procedures.

Reducing Anxiety

The nurse provides emotional support and sets aside time to talk with the patient who wishes to express feelings, cry, or ask questions about this new diagnosis. Any misconceptions the patient or family may have regarding diabetes are dispelled (see Table 37-8). The patient and family are assisted to focus on learning self-care behaviors. The patient is encouraged to perform the skills that are feared most and must be reassured that once a skill such as self-injection or lancing a finger for glucose monitoring is performed for the first time, anxiety will decrease. Positive reinforcement is given for the self-care behaviors attempted, even if the technique is not yet completely mastered.

Improving Self-Care

Patient teaching (discussed earlier in the Nursing Management section and below) is the major strategy used to prepare the patient for self-care. Special equipment is used for instruction on diabetes survival skills, such as a magnifying glass for insulin preparation or an injection-aid device for insulin injection. Low-literacy information is used as needed. The family is also taught so that they can assist in diabetes management by, for instance, prefilling syringes or monitoring the blood glucose level. The diabetes specialist is consulted regarding various blood glucose monitors and other equipment for use with patients with physical impairments. The patient is assisted in identifying community resources for education and supplies as needed. Other members of the health care team are informed about variations in the timing of meals and the work schedule (eg, if patient works at night or in the evenings and sleeps during the day) so that the diabetes treatment regimen can be adjusted accordingly.

Monitoring and Managing Potential Complications

FLUID OVERLOAD

Fluid overload can occur because of the administration of a large volume of fluid at a rapid rate that is often required to treat the patient with DKA or HHNS. This risk is increased in elderly patients and in those with preexisting cardiac disease. To avoid fluid overload and resulting congestive heart failure and pulmonary edema, the nurse monitors the patient closely during treatment by measuring vital signs at frequent intervals. Central venous pressure monitoring and hemodynamic monitoring may be initiated to provide additional measures of the patient's fluid status. Physical examination focuses on assessment of cardiac rate and rhythm, breath sounds, venous distention, skin turgor, and urine output. The nurse monitors fluid intake and keeps careful records of intravenous and other fluid intake, along with urine output measurements. The patient is monitored for orthostatic hypotension secondary to dehydration.

HYPOKALEMIA

As previously described, hypokalemia is a potential complication during the treatment of DKA as potassium is lost from body stores. Low potassium levels may result from rehydration, increased urinary excretion of potassium, and movement of potassium from the extracellular fluid into the cells with insulin administration. Prevention of hypokalemia includes cautious replacement of potassium; before its administration, however, it is important to ensure that the patient's kidneys are functioning. Because of the adverse effects of hypokalemia on cardiac function, monitoring of the cardiac rate, cardiac rhythm, electrocardiogram, and serum potassium levels is essential.

HYPERGLYCEMIA AND KETOACIDOSIS

Although the hyperglycemia and ketoacidosis that may have led to the new diagnosis of diabetes may be resolved, the patient is at risk for their subsequent recurrence. Therefore, blood glucose levels and urine ketones are monitored, and medications (insulin, oral antidiabetic agents) are administered as prescribed. The patient is monitored for signs and symptoms of impending hyperglycemia and ketoacidosis; if they occur, insulin and intravenous fluids are administered.

HYPOGLYCEMIA

Hypoglycemia may occur if the patient skips or delays meals or does not follow the prescribed diet or greatly increases the amount of exercise without modifying diet and insulin.

Also, the hospitalized patient or outpatient who fasts in preparation for diagnostic testing is at risk for hypoglycemia. Juice or glucose tablets are used for treatment of hypoglycemia. The patient is encouraged to eat full meals and snacks as prescribed per diabetic diet. If hypoglycemia is a recurrent problem, the patient's total therapeutic regimen should be reevaluated.

Because of the risk of hypoglycemia, it is important for the nurse to review with the patient its signs and symptoms, possible causes, and measures to prevent and treat it. The importance of having readily available information regarding diabetes is stressed by the nurse.

CEREBRAL EDEMA

Although the cause of cerebral edema is unknown, it is thought to be caused by correcting hyperglycemia too rapidly, resulting in fluid shifts. Cerebral edema can be prevented by gradual reduction in the blood glucose level. Use of an hourly flow sheet is initiated to enable close monitoring of the patient's blood glucose level, serum electrolyte levels, urine output, mental status, and neurologic signs. Precautions are taken to minimize activities that could increase intracranial pressure.

Promoting Home and Community-Based Care

TEACHING PATIENTS SELF-CARE

The patient is taught survival skills, including simple pathophysiology; treatment modalities (insulin administration, monitoring of blood glucose and, for type 1 diabetes, urine ketones, and diet); recognition, treatment, and prevention of acute complications (hypoglycemia and hyperglycemia); and pragmatic information (where to obtain supplies, when to call the physician). If the patient has signs of long-term diabetes complications at the time of diagnosis of diabetes, teaching about appropriate preventive behaviors (eg, foot care or eye care) should be included at this time.

CONTINUING CARE

Follow-up education is arranged with a home care nurse or an outpatient diabetes education center. This is particularly important for the patient who has had difficulty coping with the diagnosis, the patient who has limitations that may affect his or her ability to learn or to carry out the management plan, or the patient without any family or social supports. Referral to social services and community resources (eg, centers for the visually impaired) may be needed, depending on the patient's financial circumstances and physical limitations. The importance of self-monitoring and of monitoring and follow-up by primary care providers is reinforced, and the patient is reminded about the importance of keeping follow-up appointments.

Evaluation

Expected Outcomes

Expected outcomes may include:

1. Achieves fluid and electrolyte balance
   a. Demonstrates intake and output balance
   b. Exhibits electrolyte values within normal limits
   c. Exhibits vital signs that remain stable with resolution of orthostatic hypotension and tachycardia
2. Achieves metabolic balance
   a. Avoids extremes of glucose levels (hypoglycemia or hyperglycemia)
   b. Demonstrates rapid resolution of hypoglycemic episodes
   c. Avoids further weight loss (if applicable) and begins to approach desired weight
3. Demonstrates/verbalizes diabetes survival skills, including:
   a. Simple pathophysiology
      i. Defines diabetes as a condition in which high blood glucose levels are present
      ii. States normal blood glucose range
      iii. Identifies factors that cause the blood glucose level to fall (insulin, exercise)
      iv. Identifies factors that cause the blood glucose level to rise (food, illness, and infections)
      v. Describes the major treatment modalities: diet, exercise, monitoring, medication, education
   b. Treatment modalities
      i. Demonstrates proper technique for drawing up and injecting insulin (including mixing two types of insulin if necessary)
      ii. States dose and timing of injections, peak action and duration of insulin
      iii. Verbalizes insulin injection rotation plan
      iv. States dose, timing, peak action and duration of prescribed oral agents
      v. Verbalizes understanding of classification of food groups (depending on system used)
      vi. Verbalizes appropriate schedule for eating snacks and meals
      vii. Orders appropriate foods on menus and identifies foods that may be substituted for one another on the meal plan
      viii. Demonstrates proper technique for monitoring blood glucose, including using finger-lancing device; obtaining large, hanging drop of blood; applying blood properly to strip; removing blood from strip at appropriate interval (if necessary); obtaining value of blood glucose; and recording blood glucose value. If meter is used, patient can calibrate and clean meter, change batteries, identify alarms and warnings on meter, and use control solutions to validate strips.
      ix. Demonstrates proper technique for disposing of needles used for blood glucose monitoring and insulin injections (discarding needles into hard plastic container such as empty bleach or detergent container or medical waste containers)
      x. Demonstrates proper technique for urine ketone testing (for patients with type 1 diabetes) and verbalizes appropriate times to assess for ketones (when ill or when blood glucose test results are repeatedly and inexplicably more than 250 to 300 mg/dL [13.8 to 16.6 mmol/L])
      xi. Identifies community, outpatient resources for obtaining further diabetes education
   c. Acute complications (hypoglycemia and hyperglycemia)
      i. Verbalizes symptoms of hypoglycemia (shakiness, sweating, headache, hunger, numbness or tingling of lips or fingers, weakness, fatigue, difficulty concentrating, change of mood) and dangers of untreated hypoglycemia (seizures and coma)
      ii. Identifies appropriate treatment of hypoglycemia, including 10 to 15 g simple carbohydrate (eg, two to four glucose tablets, 4 to 6 oz juice or soda, 2 to 3 teaspoons sugar, or 6 to 10 hard candies, such as Life Savers) followed by a snack of protein and carbohydrate (eg, cheese and crackers or milk), or by a regularly scheduled meal

iii. Identifies potential causes of hypoglycemia (too much insulin, delayed or decreased food intake, increased physical activity)
iv. Verbalizes preventive behaviors, such as frequent monitoring of blood glucose when daily schedule is changed and eating a snack before exercise
v. Verbalizes importance of wearing medical identification and carrying a source of simple carbohydrate at all times.
vi. Verbalizes symptoms of prolonged hyperglycemia (increased thirst and urination)
vii. Verbalizes rules for sick day management

d. Pragmatic information
i. Describes where to purchase and store insulin, syringes, and glucose monitoring supplies
ii. Identifies appropriate circumstances for calling the physician (when ill, when glucose levels repeatedly exceed a certain level [per physician guidelines], or when skin wounds fail to heal)
iii. Identifies name and phone number to reach physician or other member of health care team 24 hours per day

4. Absence of complications
a. Exhibits normal cardiac rate and rhythm and normal breath sounds
b. Exhibits jugular venous pressure and distention within normal limits
c. Exhibits blood glucose and urine ketone levels within normal limits
d. Exhibits no manifestations of hypoglycemia or hyperglycemia
e. Shows improved mental status without signs of cerebral edema
f. States measures to prevent occurrence of complications.

LONG-TERM COMPLICATIONS OF DIABETES

There has been a steady decline in the number of deaths of diabetic patients attributable to ketoacidosis and infection but an alarming rise in the number of deaths from cardiovascular and renal complications. Long-term complications are becoming more common as more people live longer with diabetes. The long-term complications of diabetes can affect almost every organ system of the body. The general categories of chronic diabetic complications are:

- Macrovascular disease
- Microvascular disease
- Neuropathy.

The specific causes and pathogenesis of each type of complication are still being investigated. It appears, however, that increased levels of blood glucose may play a role in neuropathic disease, microvascular complications, and risk factors contributing to macrovascular complications. Hypertension may also be a major contributing factor, especially in macrovascular and microvascular diseases.

Long-term complications are seen in both type 1 and type 2 diabetes, usually not occurring within the first 5 to 10 years of the diagnosis. Renal (microvascular) disease is more prevalent among type 1 diabetic patients, and cardiovascular (macrovascular) complications are more prevalent among older type 2 diabetic patients.

Macrovascular Complications

Diabetic macrovascular complications result from changes in the medium to large blood vessels. Blood vessel walls thicken, sclerose, and become occluded by plaque. Eventually, blood flow becomes blocked. These atherosclerotic changes are indistinguishable from atherosclerotic changes in people without diabetes, but they tend to occur more often and at an earlier age in diabetes. Coronary artery disease, cerebrovascular disease, and peripheral vascular disease are the three main types of macrovascular complications that occur more frequently in the diabetic population.

Myocardial infarction is twice as common in diabetic men and three times as common in diabetic women. There is also an increased risk for complications resulting from myocardial infarction and an increased likelihood of a second myocardial infarction. Some studies suggest that coronary artery disease may account for 50% to 60% of all deaths in patients with diabetes. One unique feature of coronary artery disease in patients with diabetes is that the typical ischemic symptoms may be absent. Thus, patients may not experience the early warning signs of decreased coronary blood flow and may have "silent" myocardial infarctions. These silent myocardial infarctions may be discovered only as changes on the electrocardiogram. This lack of ischemic symptoms may be secondary to autonomic neuropathy (see below).

Cerebral blood vessels are similarly affected by accelerated atherosclerosis. Occlusive changes or the formation of an embolus elsewhere in the vasculature that lodges in a cerebral blood vessel can lead to transient ischemic attacks and strokes. People with diabetes have twice the risk of developing cerebrovascular disease, and studies suggest there may be a greater likelihood of death from cerebrovascular disease in patients with diabetes. In addition, recovery from a stroke may be impaired in patients who have elevated blood glucose levels at the time of and immediately after a stroke. Because symptoms of cerebrovascular disease may be quite similar to symptoms of acute diabetic complications (HHNS or hypoglycemia), it is very important to assess the blood glucose level (and treat abnormal levels) of patients reporting these symptoms before extensive diagnostic testing for cerebrovascular disease is initiated.

Atherosclerotic changes in the large blood vessels of the lower extremities are responsible for the increased incidence (two to three times higher than in nondiabetic people) of occlusive peripheral arterial disease in diabetic patients. Signs and symptoms of peripheral vascular disease include diminished peripheral pulses and intermittent claudication (pain in the buttock, thigh, or calf during walking). The severe form of arterial occlusive disease in the lower extremities is largely responsible for the increased incidence of gangrene and subsequent amputation in diabetic patients. Neuropathy and impairments in wound healing also play a role in diabetic foot disease (see below).

Role of Diabetes in Macrovascular Diseases

Diabetes researchers continue to investigate the relation between diabetes and macrovascular diseases. The main feature unique to diabetes is an elevated blood glucose level; however, a direct link has not been found between hyperglycemia and atherosclerosis. Although it may be tempting to attribute the increased prevalence of macrovascular diseases to the increased prevalence of certain risk factors among diabetic patients (eg, obesity, increased triglyceride levels, hypertension), a higher-than-expected rate of macrovascular diseases exists among patients with diabetes when compared with nondiabetic patients with the same risk factors. Thus, diabetes itself is seen as an independent risk factor for the development of accelerated atherosclerosis. Other potential factors that may play a role in diabetes-related atherosclerosis include platelet and clotting factor abnormalities, decreased flexibility of red blood cells, decreased oxygen release, changes in the arterial wall related to hyperglycemia, and possibly hyperinsulinemia.

Medical Management

Management of macrovascular complications involves prevention and treatment of the commonly accepted risk factors for atherosclerosis. Diet and exercise are important in managing obesity, hypertension, and hyperlipidemia. In addition, the use of medications to control hypertension and hyperlipidemia may be indicated. Smoking cessation is strongly encouraged. There is some evidence that elevated triglyceride levels may improve with control of blood glucose levels. As stated previously, close control of blood glucose levels can significantly reduce the incidence of complications.

When macrovascular complications do occur, treatment is the same as with nondiabetic patients. In addition, patients may require increased amounts of insulin or may need to switch from oral antidiabetic agents to insulin during illnesses.

Microvascular Complications and Diabetic Retinopathy

Although macrovascular atherosclerotic changes are seen in both diabetic and nondiabetic patients, the microvascular changes are unique to diabetes. Diabetic microvascular disease (or microangiopathy) is characterized by capillary basement membrane thickening. The basement membrane surrounds the endothelial cells of the capillary. Researchers postulate that increased blood glucose levels react through a series of biochemical responses to thicken the basement membrane to several times its normal thickness.

Two places where impaired capillary function may have devastating effects are the microcirculation of the retina of the eyes and the kidneys. Diabetic retinopathy is the leading cause of blindness in people between 20 and 74 years of age in the United States. Similarly, about one in every four individuals starting dialysis has diabetic nephropathy.

People with diabetes are subject to multiple visual complications (Table 37-9). The eye pathology referred to as diabetic retinopathy is caused by changes in the small blood vessels in the retina (Fig. 37-9). The retina is the area of the eye that receives images and sends information about the images to the brain. It is richly supplied with blood vessels of all kinds—small arteries and veins, arterioles, venules, and capillaries. There are three main stages of retinopathy: nonproliferative (background) retinopathy, preproliferative retinopathy, and proliferative retinopathy.

As many as 90% of diabetic patients (with poorly controlled blood glucose) develop clinical evidence of background retinopathy within 5 to 15 years of the diagnosis of diabetes. Changes in the microvasculature include microaneurysms, intraretinal hemorrhage, hard exudates, and focal capillary closure. Most of these patients have no visual impairments and have little risk of developing blindness in the future. A complication of nonproliferative retinopathy, macular edema, occurs in approximately 10% of people with type 1 and type 2 diabetes and may lead to visual distortion and loss of central vision.

TABLE 37•9 Ocular Complications of Diabetes

Eye Disorder	Characteristics
Retinopathy	Deterioration of the small blood vessels that nourish the retina
Background	Early stage, asymptomatic retinopathy. Blood vessels within the retina develop microaneurysms that leak fluid, causing swelling and forming deposits (exudates). In some cases, macular edema causes distorted vision.
Preproliferative	Represents increased destruction of retinal blood vessels
Proliferative	Abnormal growth of new blood vessels on the retina. New vessels rupture, bleeding into the vitreous and blocking light. Ruptured blood vessels in the vitreous form scar tissue, which can pull on and detach the retina.
Cataracts	Opacity of the lens of the eye; cataracts occur at an earlier age in patients with diabetes
Lens changes	The lens of the eye can swell when blood glucose levels are elevated. For some patients, visual changes related to lens swelling may be the first symptoms of diabetes. It may take up to 2 months of improved blood glucose control before hyperglycemic swelling subsides and vision stabilizes. Therefore, patients are advised not to change eyeglass prescriptions during the 2 months after discovery of hyperglycemia.
Extraocular muscle palsy	This may occur as a result of diabetic neuropathy. The involvement of various cranial nerves responsible for ocular movements may lead to double vision. This usually resolves spontaneously.
Glaucoma	Results from occlusion of the outflow channels by new blood vessels. Glaucoma may occur with slightly higher frequency in the diabetic population.

An advanced form of background retinopathy, preproliferative retinopathy, is considered a precursor to the more serious proliferative retinopathy. In preproliferative retinopathy, there are more widespread vascular changes and loss of nerve fibers. Epidemiologic evidence suggests that 10% to 50% of patients with preproliferative retinopathy will develop proliferative retinopathy within a short time (possibly as little as 1 year). As with background retinopathy, if visual changes occur during the preproliferative stage, they are usually caused by macular edema.

Proliferative retinopathy represents the greatest threat to vision. Proliferative retinopathy is characterized by the proliferation of new blood vessels growing out of the retina into the vitreous. These new vessels are prone to bleeding. The visual loss associated with proliferative retinopathy is caused by this vitreous hemorrhage and/or retinal detachment. The vitreous is normally clear, allowing light to be transmitted to the retina. When there is a hemorrhage, the vitreous becomes clouded and cannot transmit light, resulting in loss of vision. Another consequence of vitreous hemorrhage is that resorption of the blood in the vitreous

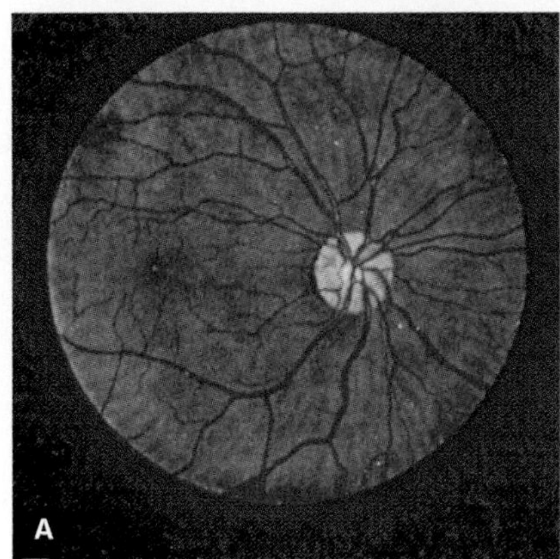

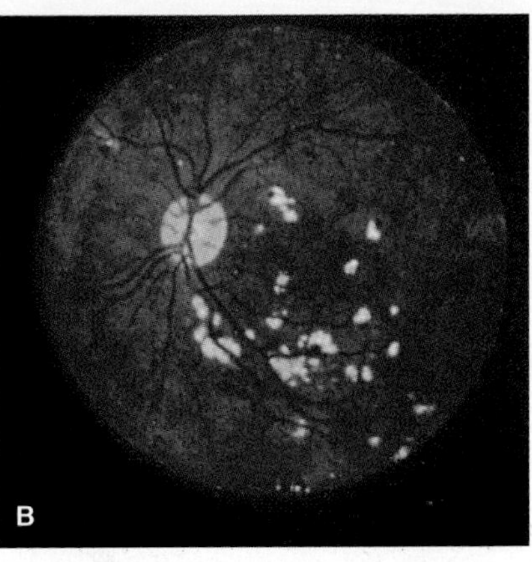

FIGURE 37•9 Diabetic retinopathy. (**A**) In the fundus photograph of a normal eye, the light circular area over which a number of blood vessels converge is the optic disc, where the optic nerve meets the back of the eye. (**B**) The fundus photograph of a patient with diabetic retinopathy shows characteristic waxy-looking retinal lesions, microaneurysms of the vessels, and hemorrhages. Fuller, J., & Schaller-Ayers, J. (1994). *Health assessment: A nursing approach* (2nd ed.). Philadelphia: J. B. Lippincott. Courtesy of American Optometric Association.

leads to the formation of fibrous scar tissue. This scar tissue may place traction on the retina, resulting in retinal detachment and subsequent visual loss.

Clinical Manifestations

Retinopathy is a painless process. In nonproliferative and preproliferative retinopathy, blurry vision secondary to macular edema occurs in some patients, although many patients are asymptomatic. Even patients with a significant degree of proliferative retinopathy and some hemorrhaging may not experience major visual changes. However, symptoms indicative of hemorrhaging include floaters or cobwebs in the visual field, or sudden visual changes including spotty or hazy vision, or complete loss of vision.

Assessment and Diagnostic Findings

Diagnosis is by direct visualization with an ophthalmoscope or with a technique known as fluorescein angiography. Fluorescein angiography can document the type and activity of the retinopathy. It is a technique in which a dye is injected into an arm vein. The dye is carried to various parts of the body through the blood, but especially through the vessels of the retina of the eye. This technique allows the ophthalmologist, using special instruments, to see the retinal vessels in bright detail and gives useful information that cannot be obtained with just an ophthalmoscope.

Side effects of this diagnostic procedure may include nausea during the dye injection; yellowish, fluorescent discoloration of the skin and urine lasting 12 to 24 hours; and occasional allergic reactions, usually manifested by hives or itching. Generally, however, it is a safe diagnostic procedure. Patient preparation includes explaining:

- The steps of the procedure
- The fact that the procedure is painless
- The potential side effects
- The type of information the technique can provide
- That the flash of the camera may be slightly uncomfortable for a short time

Medical Management

The first focus of management is on primary and secondary prevention. The results of the DCCT (1993) demonstrated that maintenance of blood glucose to a normal or near-normal level through intensive insulin therapy decreased the risk for development of retinopathy by 76% when compared with conventional therapy in patients without preexisting retinopathy. The progression of retinopathy was decreased by 54% in patients with very mild to moderate nonproliferative retinopathy at the time of initiation of treatment.

For advanced cases, the main treatment of diabetic retinopathy is argon laser photocoagulation. The laser treatment destroys leaking blood vessels and areas of neovascularization. For patients at increased risk for hemorrhaging, panretinal photocoagulation may significantly reduce the rate of progression to blindness. Panretinal photocoagulation involves the systematic application of multiple (more than 1000) laser burns throughout the retina (except in the macular region). This stops the widespread growth of new vessels and hemorrhaging of damaged vessels. The role of "mild" panretinal photocoagulation (with only a third to a half as many laser burns) in the early stages of proliferative retinopathy or in patients with preproliferative changes is being investigated. For macular edema, focal photocoagulation is used to apply smaller laser burns to specific areas of microaneurysms in the macular region. This may reduce the rate of visual loss from macular edema by 50%.

Photocoagulation treatments are usually performed on an outpatient basis, and most patients can return to their usual activities by the next day. For some patients, limitations may be placed on activities involving weight bearing or bearing down. For most patients, the treatment does not cause intense pain, although they may report varying degrees of discomfort. Usually an anesthetic eye drop is all that is needed during the treatment. A few patients may experience slight visual loss, loss of peripheral vision, or impairments in adaptation to the dark. For most patients, however, the risk of slight visual changes from the laser treatment itself is much less than the potential for loss of vision from progression of retinopathy.

When a major hemorrhage into the vitreous occurs, the vitreous fluid becomes mixed with blood and prevents light from passing through the eye; this can cause blindness. A vitrectomy is a surgical procedure in which vitreous humor filled with blood or fibrous tissue is removed with a special drill-like instrument and replaced with saline or another liquid. A vitrectomy is performed on patients who already have visual loss and in whom the vitreous hemorrhage has not cleared on its own after 6 months. The purpose is to restore useful vision; recovery to near-normal vision is not usually expected.

Studies continue into other ways to slow the progression of diabetic retinopathy. These include:

- Control of hypertension
- Control of blood glucose
- Cessation of smoking

Nursing Management

Nursing management of patients with diabetic retinopathy or other eye disorder involves implementing the individual plan of care and providing patient education. Education focuses on prevention through regular ophthalmologic examinations and blood glucose control, self-management of eye care regimens, and adjustment to impaired vision. Nursing care for the patient with low vision or loss of vision is discussed in detail in Chapter 54.

PROMOTING HOME AND COMMUNITY-BASED CARE

Teaching Patients Self-Care. In all forms of therapy for retinopathy, something is destroyed in the process of saving vision. The facts must be presented to the patient and family as honestly as possible. The course of the retinopathy may be long and stressful. In teaching and counseling the patient, it is important to stress the following:

- Retinopathy may appear after many years of diabetes, and its appearance does not necessarily mean that the diabetes is on a downhill course.
- The odds for maintaining vision are in the patient's favor, especially with adequate control of glucose levels and blood pressure.
- Frequent eye examinations are the best way to preserve vision, because they allow for the detection of any retinopathy.

Some additional points to keep in mind when the patient with diabetes has some type of visual impairment include the following:

- Visual impairment can be a shock. A person's response to vision loss depends on personality, self-concept, and coping mechanisms.
- As in any loss, blindness and its acceptance by the patient occur in stages; some patients may learn to accept blindness in a rather short period, and others may never accept it.
- Although retinopathy occurs bilaterally, the severity may differ in the two eyes.
- Many of the chronic complications of diabetes occur simultaneously. For example, a blind diabetic patient may also have peripheral neuropathy and may experience impairment of manual dexterity and tactile sensation.

Continuing Care. Continuing care for the patient with impaired vision because of diabetic changes depends on the severity of the impairment and the effectiveness of the patient's coping in response to the impairment. The importance of careful diabetes management is emphasized as one means of slowing the progression of visual changes. The patient is reminded of the need to see the ophthalmologist regularly. If eye changes are progressive and unrelenting, the patient needs to be prepared for inevitable blindness. Therefore, consideration is given to making referrals for teaching the patient Braille and for training with a guide dog. Family members are also taught how to assist the patient to remain as independent as possible despite decreasing visual acuity.

Referral for home care may be indicated for some patients, particularly those who live alone, those not coping well, and those who have other health problems or complications of diabetes that may interfere with their ability to perform self-care. During home visits, the nurse can assess the patient's home environment and his or her ability to manage diabetes despite visual impairments.

Medical management and nursing care of patients with visual disturbances are discussed in detail in Chapter 54.

Nephropathy

Nephropathy, or renal disease secondary to diabetic microvascular changes in the kidney, is a common complication of diabetes. People with diabetes account for approximately 25% of patients with end-stage renal disease requiring dialysis or transplantation each year in the United States. People with diabetes have a 20% to 40% chance of developing renal disease.

Patients with type 1 diabetes frequently show initial signs of renal disease after 15 to 20 years, whereas patients with type 2 diabetes develop renal disease within 10 years of the diagnosis of diabetes. Many of these patients with type 2 diabetes may have had diabetes for many years before it was diagnosed and treated.

There is no reliable method to predict whether a person will develop renal disease. The DCCT (1993) results showed that intensive treatment of diabetes with a goal of achieving a hemoglobin A_{1C} as close to the nondiabetic range as possible reduced the occurrence of early signs of nephropathy, such as microalbuminuria, by 39%, and albuminuria by 54%.

Evidence suggests that soon after the onset of diabetes, and especially if the blood glucose levels are elevated, the kidney's filtration mechanism is stressed, allowing blood proteins to leak into the urine. As a result, the pressure in the blood vessels of the kidney increases. It is thought that the elevated pressure serves as the stimulus for the development of nephropathy. Various medications and diets are being tested to prevent these complications.

Clinical Manifestations

Most of the signs and symptoms of renal dysfunction in the person with diabetes are similar to those seen in patients without diabetes. (See Chap. 41 for the management of patients with renal disorders.) Also, as renal failure progresses, the catabolism (breakdown) of both exogenous and endogenous insulin decreases, and frequent hypoglycemic episodes may result. Insulin needs change as a result of changes in the catabolism of insulin, and also as a result of changes in diet related to the treatment of nephropathy. The stress of renal disease affects self-esteem, family relationships, marital relations, and virtually all aspects of daily life. As renal function decreases, the patient commonly has multiple-system failure (eg, declining visual acuity, impotence, foot ulcerations, congestive heart failure, and nocturnal diarrhea).

Assessment and Diagnostic Findings

One of the most important blood proteins that leaks into the urine is albumin. Small amounts may leak undetected for years. Of patients with microalbuminuria, clinical nephropathy eventually develops in more than 85%. However, if microalbuminuria is not present, nephropathy develops in fewer than 5%.

Early microalbuminuria may also be discovered in a 24-hour urine sample. The urine should be checked annually for microalbuminuria. If the microalbuminuria level exceeds 30 mg/24 hours on two consecutive tests, an angiotensin-converting enzyme (ACE) inhibitor should be prescribed. ACE inhibitors lower blood pressure and reduce microalbuminuria and therefore protect the kidney. This preventive strategy should be part of the standard of care for the person with diabetes. Carefully designed low-protein diets also appear to reverse early leakage of small amounts of protein from the kidney.

When a urine dipstick test reads consistently positive for significant amounts of albumin, the patient is tested for serum creatinine and BUN levels. At this point in the development of renal disease, diagnostic testing for cardiac or other systemic problems may also be required. Some of the tests involve injection of special dyes that are not easily cleared by the damaged kidney. Therefore, the value of the diagnostic test must be weighed against the potential risks.

Hypertension often develops in patients (both diabetic and nondiabetic) who are in the early stages of renal disease. However, essential hypertension occurs in up to 50% of all individuals with diabetes (for unknown reasons); thus, it should not be assumed that someone with diabetes who has hypertension also has renal disease. Other diagnostic criteria must also be present.

Medical Management

In addition to achieving and maintaining near-normal blood glucose levels, management for all patients with diabetes should include careful attention to the following:

- Control of hypertension (the use of ACE inhibitors, such as captopril, because control of hypertension may also decrease or delay the onset of early proteinuria)
- Prevention or vigorous treatment of urinary tract infections
- Avoidance of nephrotoxic substances
- Adjustment of medications as renal function changes
- Low sodium diet
- Low protein diet

In renal failure, two types of treatment are available: dialysis (hemodialysis or peritoneal dialysis) and transplantation from a relative or a cadaver. Hemodialysis for the patient with diabetes is similar to that for patients without the disease (see Chap. 40). Because hemodialysis creates additional stress on patients with cardiovascular disease, it may not be indicated in certain patients. In addition, it is extremely intrusive into a patient's life.

Continuous ambulatory peritoneal dialysis is being used by an increasing number of patients with diabetes, mainly because of the independence it allows patients. In addition, insulin can be mixed into the dialysate, which may result in better blood glucose control and end the need for insulin injections. However, these patients may require more insulin because the dialysate contains glucose. Major risks of peritoneal dialysis are infection and peritonitis.

Renal disease is frequently accompanied by advancing retinopathy that may require laser treatments and surgery. Severe hypertension also worsens eye disease because of the additional stress it places on the blood vessels. Patients being treated by hemodialysis who require eye surgery may be changed to peritoneal dialysis and have their hypertension aggressively controlled for several weeks before surgery. The rationale for this change is that hemodialysis requires anticoagulants that can increase the risk of bleeding after the surgery, and peritoneal dialysis minimizes pressure changes in the eyes.

The success rate for kidney transplantation in patients with diabetes has improved. In medical centers performing large numbers of transplants, the chances are 75% to 80% that the transplanted kidney will continue to function in the patient with diabetes for at least 5 years. Like the original kidneys, transplanted kidneys in patients with diabetes can eventually be damaged if blood glucose levels are consistently high after the transplantation. Therefore, monitoring blood glucose levels frequently and adjusting insulin levels in diabetic patients with transplanted kidneys are essential for long-term success. Pancreas transplants are sometimes attempted when a kidney transplant is performed. Pancreatic transplants have not been successful enough to be performed alone because of the risks associated with immunosuppression.

The mortality rate for diabetic patients undergoing dialysis is higher than that in nondiabetic patients undergoing dialysis and is closely related to the severity of cardiovascular problems.

Diabetic Neuropathies

Diabetic neuropathy refers to a group of diseases that affect all types of nerves, including peripheral (sensorimotor), autonomic, and spinal nerves. The disorders appear to be clinically diverse and depend on the location of the affected nerve cells. The prevalence increases with the age of the patient and the duration of the disease and may be as high as 50% in patients who have had diabetes for 25 years.

Elevated blood glucose levels over a period of years have been implicated in the etiology of neuropathy. The pathogenesis of neuropathy may be attributed to either a vascular or a metabolic mechanism or both, but their relative contributions have yet to be determined. Capillary basement membrane thickening and capillary closure may be present. In addition, there may be demyelinization of the nerves, which is thought to be related to hyperglycemia. Nerve conduction is disrupted when there are aberrations of the myelin sheaths. Control of serum glucose levels to normal or near-normal levels was shown in the DCCT (1993) to decrease the incidence of neuropathy by 60%.

The two most common types of diabetic neuropathy are sensorimotor polyneuropathy and autonomic neuropathy. Cranial mononeuropathies, for example those affecting the oculomotor nerve, also occur in diabetes, especially among the elderly (see Table 37-9).

Sensorimotor polyneuropathy is a diabetic neuropathy also called peripheral neuropathy. It most commonly affects the distal portions of the nerves, especially the nerves of the lower extremities. It affects both sides of the body symmetrically and may spread in a proximal direction.

Clinical Manifestations

Initial symptoms include paresthesias (prickling, tingling, or heightened sensation) and burning sensations (especially at night). As the neuropathy progresses, the feet become numb. In addition, a decrease in proprioception (awareness of posture and movement of the body and of position and weight of objects in relation to the body) and a decreased sensation of light touch may lead to an unsteady gait. Decreased sensations of pain and temperature place patients with neuropathy at increased risk for injury and undetected foot infections. Deformities of the foot may also occur, with neuropathy-related joint changes producing Charcot joints. These joint deformities result from the abnormal weight distribution on joints due to lack of proprioception.

On physical examination, a decrease in deep tendon reflexes and vibratory sensation is found. For patients who have few or no symptoms of neuropathy, these physical findings may be the only indication of neuropathic changes. For patients with signs or symptoms of neuropathy, it is important to rule out other possible neuropathies, including alcohol-induced or vitamin-deficiency neuropathies.

Medical Management

The results of the DCCT (1993) demonstrate that intensive insulin therapy and control of blood glucose levels delay the onset and slow the progression of neuropathy.

Pain, particularly of the lower extremities, is a disturbing symptom in some people with neuropathy secondary to diabetes. For some patients, neuropathic pain spontaneously resolves within 6 months. For other patients, pain persists for many years. Various approaches to pain management can be tried. These include analgesics (preferably nonopioid); tricyclic antidepressants; phenytoin or carbamazepine (anticonvulsants); mexiletine (an antiarrhythmic); or transcutaneous electrical nerve stimulation.

The use of aldose reductase inhibitors is under study to determine whether they block the damaging effects of hyperglycemia. The topical medication capsaicin (Axscain) also has been shown in preliminary reports to decrease lower extremity neuropathic pain. Studies of the role of this topical medication in neuropathy continue.

Autonomic Neuropathy

Neuropathy of the autonomic nervous system results in a broad range of dysfunctions affecting almost every organ system of the body.

Clinical Manifestations

CARDIOVASCULAR

Three manifestations of autonomic neuropathy are a fixed, slightly tachycardic heart rate; orthostatic hypotension; and silent, or painless, myocardial ischemia and infarction.

GASTROINTESTINAL

Delayed gastric emptying may occur with the typical symptoms of early satiety, bloating, nausea, and vomiting. In addition, there may be unexplained wide swings in blood glucose levels related to inconsistent absorption of the glucose from ingested foods secondary to the inconsistent gastric emptying. "Diabetic" constipation or diarrhea (especially nocturnal diarrhea) may occur as a result.

URINARY

Urinary retention, a decreased sensation of bladder fullness, and other urinary symptoms of neurogenic bladder result from autonomic neuropathy. Patients with a neurogenic bladder are predisposed to developing urinary tract infections. This is especially true in patients with poorly controlled diabetes, because hyperglycemia impairs resistance to infection.

ADRENAL GLAND (HYPOGLYCEMIC UNAWARENESS)

Autonomic neuropathy of the adrenal medulla is responsible for diminished or absent adrenergic symptoms of hypoglycemia. Patients may report that they no longer feel the typical shakiness, sweating, nervousness, and palpitations associated with hypoglycemia. Strict blood glucose monitoring, including frequent SMBG, is recommended for these patients. Their inability to detect and treat these warning signs of hypoglycemia puts them at risk for developing dangerously low blood glucose levels. Therefore, their goals for blood glucose levels may need to be adjusted to reduce the risk for hypoglycemia.

SUDOMOTOR NEUROPATHY

This neuropathic condition refers to a decrease or absence of sweating (anhidrosis) of the extremities, with a compensatory increase in upper body sweating. Dryness of the feet increases the risk for the development of foot ulcers.

SEXUAL DYSFUNCTION

Sexual dysfunction, especially impotence in men, is a complication of diabetes. The effects of autonomic neuropathy on female sexual functioning are not well documented. Reduced vaginal lubrication has been mentioned as a possible neuropathic effect; however, research studies to address this and other potential female sexual dysfunctions are ongoing.

Impotence, inability of the penis to become rigid and sustain an erection (or difficulty in doing so), occurs with greater frequency in diabetic men than in nondiabetic men of the same age. It is important for the nurse and patient to realize, however, that in diabetic men neuropathy is not the only cause of impotence. Medications such as antihypertensives, psychological factors, and other medical conditions (eg, vascular insufficiency) that may affect nondiabetic men also play a role in impotence in diabetic men.

Some men with autonomic neuropathy have normal erectile function and can experience orgasm but do not ejaculate. Retrograde ejaculation occurs, in which seminal fluid is propelled backward through the posterior urethra and into the urinary bladder. Examination of the urine confirms the diagnosis because of the large number of active sperm present. Fertility counseling is necessary for couples attempting conception.

Medical Management

Management strategies depend on the patient's symptoms. There is no treatment for painless cardiac ischemia, and the prognosis is poor. Detection, however, is important so that education about avoiding strenuous exercise can be provided. Orthostatic hypotension may respond to a diet high in sodium, the discontinuation of medications that impede autonomic nervous system responses, the use of sympathomimetic and other agents (eg, caffeine) that stimulate an autonomic response, and the use of lower body elastic garments that maximize venous return and prevent pooling of blood in the extremities.

Treatment of delayed gastric emptying includes a low-fat diet, frequent small meals, close blood glucose control, and use of agents that increase gastric motility (eg, metoclopramide, bethanechol). Treatment of diabetic diarrhea may include bulk-forming laxatives or antidiarrheal agents. Constipation is treated with a high-fiber diet and adequate hydration; medications, laxatives, and enemas may be necessary when constipation is severe.

Management of the patient with a neurogenic bladder is discussed in Chapter 40. Treatment of sudomotor dysfunction focuses on education about skin care and heat intolerance. Erectile dysfunction is discussed in Chapter 45.

Foot and Leg Problems in Diabetes

From 50% to 75% of lower extremity amputations are performed on people with diabetes. As many as 50% of these amputations are thought to be preventable, provided patients are taught preventive foot care measures and practice preventive foot care on a daily basis.

Three diabetic complications contribute to the increased risk of foot infections:

- Neuropathy: Sensory neuropathy leads to loss of pain and pressure sensation, and autonomic neuropathy leads to increased dryness and fissuring of the skin (secondary to decreased sweating). Motor neuropathy results in muscular atrophy, which may lead to changes in the shape of the foot.
- Peripheral vascular disease: Poor circulation of the lower extremities contributes to poor wound healing and the development of gangrene.
- Immunocompromise: Hyperglycemia impairs the ability of specialized leukocytes to destroy bacteria. Thus, in poorly controlled diabetes, there is a lowered resistance to certain infections.

The typical sequence of events in the development of a diabetic foot ulcer begins with a soft tissue injury of the foot, formation of a fissure between the toes or in an area of dry skin, or formation of a callus (Fig. 37-10). Injuries are not felt by the patient with an insensitive foot and may be thermal (eg, from using heating pads, walking barefoot on hot concrete, or testing bath water with the foot), chemical (eg, burning the foot while using caustic agents on calluses, corns, or bunions), or traumatic (eg, injuring skin while cutting nails, walking with an undetected foreign object in the shoe, or wearing ill-fitting shoes and socks).

If the patient is not in the habit of thoroughly inspecting both feet on a daily basis, the injury or fissure may go unnoticed until a serious infection has developed. Drainage, swelling, redness (from cellulitis) of the leg, or gangrene may be the first sign of foot problems that the patient notices. Treatment of foot ulcers involves bed rest, antibiotics, and débridement. In addition, controlling glucose levels, which tend to increase when infections occur, is important for promoting wound healing. In patients with peripheral vascular disease, foot ulcers may not heal because of the decreased ability of oxygen, nutrients, and antibiotics to reach the injured tissue. Amputation may be necessary to prevent the spread of infection.

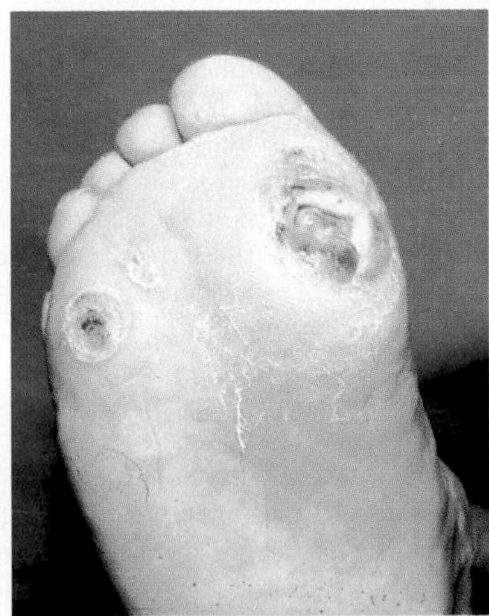

FIGURE 37•10 Neuropathic ulcers occur on pressure points in areas with diminished sensation in diabetic polyneuropathy. Pain is absent (and therefore the ulcer may go unnoticed).

Foot assessment and foot care instructions are most important when dealing with patients who are at high risk for developing foot infections. Some of the high-risk characteristics include:

- Duration of diabetes more than 10 years
- Age older than 40 years
- History of smoking
- Decreased peripheral pulses
- Decreased sensation
- Anatomic deformities or pressure areas (eg, bunions and calluses)
- History of previous foot ulcers or amputation

Nursing Management

Teaching patients proper foot care is a nursing intervention that can prevent costly, painful, and debilitating complications. Preventive foot care includes properly bathing, drying, and lubricating the feet; care must be taken not to allow moisture (water or lotion) to accumulate between the toes. Feet must be inspected on a daily basis for any redness, blisters, fissures, calluses, or ulcerations. For patients with visual impairment or decreased joint mobility (especially the elderly), use of a mirror to inspect the bottom of the feet or instruction of a family member in foot inspection may be necessary. The interior surfaces of shoes should be inspected for any rough spots or foreign objects. Visual and manual inspection of the feet on a daily basis is important. Feet should be examined on a regular basis by a podiatrist, physician, or nurse. Patients with pressure areas, such as calluses, or patients with thick toenails should see the podiatrist routinely for treatment of calluses and trimming of nails.

Patients should be taught to wear well-fitting, closed-toe shoes. Podiatrists can provide patients with inserts (orthotics) to remove pressure from pressure points on the foot. New shoes should be broken in slowly (ie, worn for 1 to 2 hours initially, with gradual increases in the length of time worn) to avoid blister formation. High-risk behaviors should be avoided, such as walking barefoot, using heating pads on the feet, wearing open-toed shoes, and shaving calluses. Toenails should be trimmed straight across and sharp corners filed to follow the contour of the toe (American Association of Diabetes Educators, 1998). If patients have visual deficits or thickened toenails, a podiatrist should cut the nails. Patients should be counseled about strategies to reduce risk factors, such as smoking and elevated blood lipids, that contribute to peripheral vascular disease. Blood glucose control is important for avoiding decreased resistance to infections and for preventing diabetic neuropathy.

The patient may be referred by the physician to a wound care center for management of persistent wounds of the feet or legs. Many wound care centers provide diabetes education; however, the patient needs to discuss recommendations for treating wounds with his or her own physician, as well as raising any questions about diabetes management.

SPECIAL ISSUES IN DIABETES

The Patient With Diabetes Undergoing Surgery

During periods of physiologic stress, such as surgery, blood glucose levels tend to rise as a result of an increase in the level of stress hormones (epinephrine, norepinephrine, glucagon, cortisol, and growth hormone). If hyperglycemia is not controlled during

PATIENT EDUCATION AND HOME CARE

Foot Care Tips

1. Take care of your diabetes.
   - Work with your health care team to keep your blood sugar within a good range.
2. Check your feet every day.
   - Look at your bare feet every day for cuts, blisters, red spots, and swelling.
   - Use a mirror to check the bottoms of your feet or ask a family member for help if you have trouble seeing.
3. Wash your feet every day.
   - Wash your feet in warm, not hot, water every day.
   - Dry your feet well. Be sure to dry between the toes.
4. Keep the skin soft and smooth.
   - Rub a thin coat of skin lotion over the tops and bottoms of your feet, but not between your toes.
5. Smooth corns and calluses gently.
   - Use a pumice stone to smooth corns and calluses.
6. Trim your toenails each week or when needed.
   - Trim your toenails straight across and file the edges with an emery board or nail file.
7. Wear shoes and socks at all times.
   - Never walk barefoot.
   - Wear comfortable shoes that fit well and protect your feet.
   - Feel inside your shoes before putting them on each time to make sure the lining is smooth and there are no objects inside.
8. Protect your feet from hot and cold.
   - Wear shoes at the beach or on hot pavement.
   - Wear socks at night if your feet get cold.
9. Keep the blood flowing to your feet.
   - Put your feet up when sitting.
   - Wiggle your toes and move your ankles up and down for 5 minutes, 2 or 3 times a day.
   - Do not cross your legs for long periods of time.
   - Do not smoke.
10. Check with your doctor.
    - Have your doctor check your bare feet and find out whether you are likely to have serious foot problems. Remember that you may not feel the pain of an injury.
    - Call your doctor right away if a cut, sore, blister, or bruise on your foot does not begin to heal after one day.
    - Follow your doctor's advice about foot care.

---

surgery, the resulting osmotic diuresis may lead to excessive loss of fluids and electrolytes. Type 1 diabetic patients also risk developing ketoacidosis during periods of stress.

Hypoglycemia is also a concern in diabetic patients undergoing surgery. This is especially a concern during the preoperative period if surgery is delayed beyond the morning in a patient who received a morning injection of intermediate-acting insulin.

There are various approaches to managing glucose control during the perioperative period. Frequent capillary glucose monitoring of the diabetic patient is essential throughout the preoperative and postoperative periods, regardless of the method used for glucose control.

For patients who usually take insulin, one half to two thirds of the usual morning dose (either intermediate-acting insulin alone or both short- and intermediate-acting insulins) may be administered subcutaneously in the morning before surgery. The remainder is then administered after surgery. Another approach with subcutaneous insulin is to divide the total number of units of insulin taken daily into four equal doses of regular insulin. These are then administered at 6-hour intervals. Neither of these approaches provides the control achieved by intravenous administration of insulin and dextrose.

The use of intravenous insulin and dextrose has become more widespread with the increased availability of meters for intraoperative glucose monitoring. The morning of surgery, all subcutaneous insulin doses are usually withheld (unless the blood glucose level is elevated—for example, more than 200 mg/dL [11.1 mmol/L], in which case a small dose of subcutaneous regular insulin may be prescribed).

The blood glucose level is controlled during surgery with the intravenous infusion of regular insulin, which is balanced by an infusion of dextrose. The insulin and dextrose infusion rates are adjusted according to frequent (hourly) capillary glucose determinations. After surgery, the insulin infusion may be continued until the patient can eat. If intravenous insulin is discontinued, subcutaneous regular insulin may be administered at set intervals (every 4 to 6 hours), or intermediate-acting insulin may be administered every 12 hours with supplemental regular insulin as necessary until the patient is eating and the usual pattern of insulin dosing is resumed.

The nurse caring for a diabetic patient who is receiving intravenous insulin must carefully monitor the insulin infusion rate and blood glucose levels. Intravenous insulin has a much shorter duration of action than subcutaneous insulin. Thus, if the infusion is interrupted or discontinued, hyperglycemia will develop rapidly (within 1 hour in type 1 diabetes and within a few hours in type 2 diabetes). The nurse must ensure that subcutaneous insulin is administered 30 minutes before discontinuing the intravenous insulin infusion.

Type 2 diabetic patients who do not usually take insulin may require insulin during the perioperative period to control blood glucose elevations. Patients who are taking chlorpropamide, a long-acting oral antidiabetic agent, may be instructed to discontinue the oral agent 24 to 48 hours before surgery. Some of these patients may resume their usual regimen of diet and oral agent during the recovery period. Other patients (who are probably not well controlled with diet and an oral antidiabetic agent before surgery) need to continue with insulin injections after discharge.

For type 2 diabetic patients who are undergoing minor surgery but who do not normally take insulin, glucose levels may remain stable provided no dextrose is infused during the surgery. After surgery, they may require small doses of regular insulin until the usual diet and oral agent are resumed.

During the postoperative period, diabetic patients must also be closely monitored for cardiovascular complications because of the increased prevalence of atherosclerosis in patients with diabetes, wound infections, and skin breakdown (especially in the patient with decreased pain sensation in the extremities caused by neuropathy). Maintaining adequate nutrition and blood glucose control promotes wound healing.

Management of Hospitalized Diabetic Patients

At any one time, 10% to 20% of general medical-surgical patients in the hospital have diabetes. This number may increase as the elderly make up a greater proportion of the population. Although some hospitals may have a specialized diabetic/metabolic unit, typically diabetic patients are admitted to all units of the hospital.

Often diabetes is not the primary medical diagnosis, yet problems with the control of diabetes frequently result from changes in the patient's normal routine or from illness or surgery. Some of the main issues pertinent to nursing care of the hospitalized diabetic patient are presented in the following section.

Self-Care Issues

All patients admitted to the hospital must relinquish control of some aspects of their daily care to the hospital staff. For the diabetic patient who is actively involved in diabetes self-management (especially insulin dose adjustment), relinquishing control over meal timing, insulin timing, and insulin dosage may be particularly difficult. The patient may fear hypoglycemia and express much concern over possible delays in receiving attention from the nurse if hypoglycemic symptoms occur.

It is important for the nurse to acknowledge the patient's concerns and to involve the patient as much as possible in the plan of care. If the patient disagrees with certain aspects of the nursing or medical care related to diabetes, the nurse must communicate this to other members of the health care team and, where appropriate, make changes in the plan to meet the patient's needs.

Hyperglycemia During Hospitalization

Hyperglycemia may occur in the hospitalized patient as a result of the original illness that led to the need for hospitalization. In addition, a number of other factors may contribute to hyperglycemia, such as:

- Changes in the usual treatment regimen (eg, increased food, decreased insulin, decreased activity)
- Medications (eg, glucocorticoids such as prednisone, which are used in the treatment of a variety of inflammatory disorders)
- Intravenous dextrose, which may be part of the maintenance fluids or may be used for the administration of antibiotics and other medications
- Overly vigorous treatment of hypoglycemia
- Mismatched timing of meals and insulin (eg, postmeal hyperglycemia may occur if regular insulin is administered immediately before or even after meals)

Nursing action to correct some of these factors is important for the avoidance of unnecessary hyperglycemia. Assessment of the patient's usual home routine is important. The nurse should try to approximate as much as possible the home schedule of insulin, meals, and activities. Monitoring blood glucose levels and obtaining orders for extra doses of insulin (at times when insulin is usually taken by the patient) are important nursing functions. Insulin doses must not be withheld when blood glucose levels are normal.

Regular insulin is usually needed to avoid postmeal hyperglycemia (even in the patient with normal premeal glucose levels), and NPH insulin does not peak until many hours after the dose is given. Intravenous antibiotics should be mixed in normal saline (if possible) to avoid excess infusion of dextrose (especially in the patient who is eating). It is important to avoid overly vigorous treatment of hypoglycemia, which may lead to hyperglycemia. Treatment of hypoglycemia should be based on the established hospital protocol (usually 10 to 15 g carbohydrate in the form of juice, glucose tablets, or, if necessary, 0.5 to 1 ampule of 50% dextrose administered intravenously). Adding extra sugar to the juice is unnecessary. If the initial treatment does not increase the glucose level adequately, the same treatment may be repeated.

Hypoglycemia During Hospitalization

Hypoglycemia in a hospitalized patient is usually the result of too much insulin or delays in eating. Specific examples include:

- Overuse of "sliding scale" regular insulin, particularly as a supplement to regularly scheduled, twice-daily short- and intermediate-acting insulins
- Lack of dosage change when dietary intake is changed (eg, in the patient taking nothing by mouth)
- Overly vigorous treatment of hyperglycemia (eg, giving too-frequent successive doses of regular insulin before the time of peak insulin activity is reached) so that there is an accumulated effect
- Delayed meal after administration of Lispro insulin (patient should eat within 15 minutes of administration)

Nurses must assess the pattern of glucose values and avoid giving doses of insulin that repeatedly lead to hypoglycemia. Successive doses of subcutaneous regular insulin should be administered no more frequently than every 3 to 4 hours. For patients receiving NPH or Lente insulin before breakfast and dinner, the nurse must use caution in administering supplemental doses of regular insulin at lunch and bedtime. Hypoglycemia may occur when two insulins peak at similar times (eg, morning NPH peaks with lunchtime regular insulin and may lead to late-afternoon hypoglycemia, and dinnertime NPH peaks with bedtime regular insulin and may lead to nocturnal hypoglycemia). To avoid hypoglycemic reactions caused by delayed food intake, the nurse should arrange for a snack to be given to the patient if meals are going to be delayed because of procedures, physical therapy, or other activities.

Common Alterations in Diet

Dietary modifications common during hospitalization require special consideration when the patient has diabetes.

NPO (NOTHING BY MOUTH)

For the patient who must have nothing by mouth in preparation for a diagnostic or surgical procedure, the nurse must ensure that the usual insulin dosage has been changed. These changes may include eliminating the regular insulin and giving a decreased amount (eg, half the usual dose) of intermediate-acting NPH or Lente insulin. Another approach is to use frequent (every 3 to 4 hours) dosing of regular insulin only. Intravenous dextrose may be administered to provide calories and to avoid the development of hypoglycemia.

Even when no food is taken, glucose levels may rise as a result of hepatic glucose production, especially in type 1 and lean type 2 diabetic patients. Further, in type 1 diabetes, complete elimination of the insulin dose may lead to the development of DKA. Thus, administering insulin to the type 1 diabetic patient who is receiving nothing by mouth is an important nursing action.

For type 2 diabetic patients taking insulin, DKA does not develop when insulin doses are eliminated because the patient's own pancreas produces some insulin. Thus, skipping the insulin dose altogether when the patient has type 2 diabetes (and is receiving intravenous dextrose) may be safe.

For patients who receive nothing by mouth for extended periods, glucose testing and insulin administration should be performed at regular intervals, usually two to four times per day. Insulin regimens for the patient who is fasting for an extended period may include NPH insulin every 12 hours (with regular insulin added to the NPH, depending on the results of glucose testing) or regular insulin only every 4 to 6 hours. These patients should receive dextrose infusions to provide some calories and limit ketosis.

To prevent these problems resulting from the need to withhold food, diagnostic tests and procedures and surgery should be scheduled early in the morning if possible.

CLEAR LIQUID DIET

When the diet is advanced to include clear liquids, the diabetic patient will be receiving more simple carbohydrate foods, such as juice and gelatin desserts, than are usually included in the diabetic diet. It is important for hospitalized patients to maintain their nutritional status as much as possible to promote healing. Thus, the use of reduced-calorie substitutes such as diet soda or diet gelatin desserts would not be appropriate when the only source of calories is clear liquids. Simple carbohydrates, when eaten alone, cause a rapid rise in blood glucose levels; thus, it is important to try to match peak times of insulin with peaks in glucose. If a patient was receiving insulin at regular intervals while receiving nothing by mouth, the scheduled times for glucose tests and insulin injections must be changed to match meal times.

ENTERAL TUBE FEEDINGS

Tube feeding formulas contain more simple carbohydrates and less protein and fat than the typical diabetic diet. This results in increased levels of glucose in the diabetic patient receiving tube feedings. It is important that insulin doses be administered at regular intervals (eg, NPH every 12 hours or regular insulin every 4 to 6 hours) when tube feedings are administered at a continuous rate. If insulin is administered at routine (prebreakfast and predinner) times, hypoglycemia during the day may result from patients receiving more insulin without more calories, and hyperglycemia may occur during the night when feedings continue but insulin action decreases.

A common cause of hypoglycemia in patients receiving continuous tube feedings and insulin is inadvertent or purposeful discontinuation of the feeding. The nurse must discuss with the medical team any plans for temporarily discontinuing the tube feeding (eg, when the patient is away from the unit). Planning ahead may allow alterations to be made in the insulin dose, or it may allow for intravenous dextrose to be administered. In addition, if problems with the tube feeding develop unexpectedly (eg, the patient pulls out the tube, the tube clogs, or the feeding is discontinued when residual gastric contents are found), the nurse must notify the physician, assess blood glucose levels more frequently, and administer intravenous dextrose if indicated.

TOTAL PARENTERAL NUTRITION

The diabetic patient receiving TPN may receive both intravenous insulin (added to the TPN container) and subcutaneous intermediate- or short-acting insulins. If the patient is receiving continuous TPN, the blood glucose level should be monitored and insulin administered at regular intervals. If the TPN is infused over a limited number of hours, subcutaneous insulin should be administered so that peak times of insulin action coincide with times of TPN infusion.

Hygiene

The nurse caring for a hospitalized diabetic patient must focus attention on oral hygiene and skin care. Because diabetic patients are at increased risk for periodontal disease, it is important for the nurse to assist patients with daily dental care. The patient may also require assistance in keeping the skin clean and dry—especially in areas of contact between two skin surfaces (eg, groin, axilla, and, in obese women, under the breasts), where chafing and fungal infections tend to occur.

For the bedridden diabetic patient, nursing care must emphasize the prevention of skin breakdown at pressure points. The heels are particularly susceptible to breakdown because of loss of sensation of pain and pressure associated with sensory neuropathy.

Feet should be cleaned, dried, lubricated (but not between the toes), and inspected frequently. If the patient is in the supine position, pressure on the heels can be alleviated by elevating the lower legs on a pillow, with the heels hanging over the edge of the pillow. When the patient is seated in a chair, the feet should be positioned so that pressure is not placed on the heels. If the patient has a foot ulcer, it is important to provide preventive foot care to the unaffected foot as well as to carry out special care of the affected foot.

As always, every opportunity should be taken to teach the patient about diabetes self-management, including daily oral, skin, and foot care. Female diabetic patients should also be instructed about measures for the avoidance of vaginal infections, which occur more frequently when blood glucose levels are elevated. Patients often take their cues from the nurse and realize the importance of daily personal hygiene if this is emphasized during their hospitalization.

Stress

As mentioned earlier, physiologic stress, such as infections and surgery, contribute to hyperglycemia and may precipitate DKA or HHNS. Emotional stress may have a negative impact on diabetic control as well. An increase in stress hormones leads to an increase in glucose levels, especially when the intake of food and insulin remains unchanged. In addition, during periods of emotional stress, the person with diabetes may alter the usual pattern of meals, exercise, and medication. This contributes to hyperglycemia or even hypoglycemia (eg, in the patient taking insulin or oral antidiabetic agents who stops eating in response to stress).

People who have diabetes must be made aware of the potential deterioration in diabetic control that can accompany emotional stress. They must be encouraged to try to adhere to the diabetes treatment plan as much as possible during times of stress. In addition, learning strategies for minimizing stress and coping with stress when it does occur are important aspects of diabetes education.

Gerontologic Considerations

People with diabetes are living longer; therefore, both type 1 and type 2 diabetes are seen more frequently in the elderly population. Regardless of the type or duration of diabetes, the goals of diabetes treatment may need to be altered when caring for the elderly. The focus is on quality-of-life issues, such as maintaining independent functioning and promoting general well-being. Although striving for strict blood glucose control may not be safe or appropriate, prolonged symptomatic hyperglycemia should be avoided.

Some elderly patients cannot manage a detailed diabetes treatment plan, but the nurse must not assume that all patients older than a certain age can adhere only to the simplest regimen. Although the goal may be simply to avoid hypoglycemia and symptomatic hyperglycemia, certain patients may prefer more complex regimens that allow more flexibility in meals and daily schedule. As with all people with diabetes, individualization of the treatment plan with frequent follow-up by the health care team is important.

Some of the barriers to learning and self-care that may be seen in the elderly include decreased vision, hearing loss, memory deficits, decreased mobility and fine motor coordination, increased tremors, depression and loneliness, decreased financial resources, and limitations related to other medical illnesses.

Assessing patients for these barriers as well as discussing any misconceptions or folk beliefs regarding the cause and treatment of diabetes is important in setting up a diabetes treatment plan and educational activities. Presenting brief, simplified instructions with ample opportunity for practice of skills is important. The use of special devices such as a magnifier for the insulin syringe, an insulin pen, or a mirror for foot inspection is helpful. If necessary, family members and other community resources are called on to assist with diabetes survival skills. If possible, it is preferable to teach patients or family members to test blood glucose at home, because urine glucose tests are usually less accurate in the elderly as a result of the increased renal threshold and the increased frequency of renal and urinary problems. Frequent evaluation of self-care skills (insulin administration, blood glucose monitoring, foot care, diet planning) is essential, especially in patients with deteriorating vision and memory.

Dietary adherence is difficult for some elderly patients because of decreased appetite, poor dentition, and decreased physical and financial ability to prepare meals. In addition, patients may be unwilling to change long-standing dietary habits. Altering the meal plan to incorporate these eating habits or other limitations may be necessary.

Nursing Alert *Careful monitoring for diabetes complications must not be neglected in the elderly. Hypoglycemia is especially dangerous because it may go undetected and result in falls. Dehydration is a concern in patients who have chronically elevated blood glucose levels. Assessment for long-term complications—especially eye and foot problems—is important. Avoiding blindness and amputation through early detection and treatment of retinopathy and foot ulcers may mean the difference between institutionalization and continued independent living for the elderly person with diabetes.*

GERONTOLOGIC CONSIDERATIONS

Factors in Elderly Patients That May Affect Diabetes and Its Management

Sensory changes
- Decreased vision
- Decreased smell
- Taste changes
- Decreased proprioception
- Diminished thirst

Gastrointestinal changes
- Dental problems
- Appetite changes
- Delayed gastric emptying
- Decreased bowel motility

Activity/exercise pattern changes
- More sedentary

Renal function changes
- Decreased function
- Decreased drug clearance

Affective/cognitive changes
- Medications/meals omitted or taken erratically

Socioeconomic factors
- Fad diets
- Loneliness/living alone
- Lack of money/lack of support system

Chronic diseases
- Hypertension
- Arthritis
- Neoplasms
- Acute/chronic infections

Potential drug interactions
- Use of another person's medications
- Consulting multiple physicians for different illnesses
- Alcohol use/abuse

NURSING PROCESS: THE PATIENT WITH DIABETES AS A SECONDARY DIAGNOSIS

People with diabetes frequently seek medical attention for problems not directly related to blood glucose control. However, during the course of treatment for the primary medical diagnosis, blood glucose control may worsen. In addition, the only opportunity for some patients with diabetes to update their knowledge about diabetes self-care and prevention of complications is during the time of hospitalization. Therefore, it is important for the nurse caring for the patient with diabetes to focus attention on diabetes, regardless of the primary problem. Further, control of blood glucose levels is important because hyperglycemia impairs resistance to certain infections and contributes to impaired wound healing.

Assessment

Assessment of the patient with diabetes with a primary problem such as cardiac disease, renal disease, cerebrovascular disease, peripheral vascular disease, surgery, or any other type of illness is the same as that for a nondiabetic patient and is described in other chapters. In addition to nursing assessment for the primary problem, assessment of the patient with diabetes must also focus on hypoglycemia and hyperglycemia, skin breakdown, and diabetes self-care skills, including survival skills and measures for prevention of long-term complications.

The patient is assessed for hypoglycemia and hyperglycemia with frequent blood glucose monitoring (usually ordered before meals and at bedtime) and with monitoring for signs and symptoms of hypoglycemia or prolonged hyperglycemia (including DKA or HHNS), as described in previous sections.

Careful assessment of the skin, especially at pressure points and on the lower extremities, is important. The skin is assessed for dryness, cracks, skin breakdown, and redness. The patient is asked about symptoms of neuropathy, such as tingling and pain or numbness of the feet. Deep tendon reflexes are assessed.

Assessment of diabetes self-care skills is performed as early as possible to determine whether the patient requires further diabetes teaching. The nurse observes the patient preparing and injecting the insulin, monitoring blood glucose, and performing foot care.

(Simply questioning the patient about these skills without actually observing performance of the skills is not sufficient.) Knowledge about diet can be assessed with the help of the dietitian through direct questioning and review of patient choices on the menu. The patient is questioned regarding signs, treatment, and prevention of hypoglycemia and hyperglycemia. The patient's knowledge of risk factors for macrovascular disease, including hypertension, increased lipids, and smoking, is assessed. The patient is questioned regarding the date of the last eye examination (including dilation of the pupil).

Diagnosis

Nursing Diagnoses

Based on the assessment data, the patient's major nursing diagnoses may include:

- Altered nutrition related to increase in stress hormones (caused by primary medical problem) and imbalances in insulin, food, and physical activity
- Risk for impaired skin integrity related to immobility and lack of sensation (caused by neuropathy)
- Potential knowledge deficit about diabetes self-care skills (caused by lack of basic diabetes education or lack of continuing in-depth diabetes education)

Collaborative Problems/Potential Complications

Based on the assessment data, potential complications may include:

- Inadequate control of blood glucose levels
- Development of acute complications of diabetes because of inadequate control of blood glucose levels

Planning and Goals

The major goals for the patient may include improved nutritional status, maintenance of skin integrity, ability to perform basic diabetes self-care skills as well as preventive care for the avoidance of chronic diabetes complications, and absence of complications.

Nursing Interventions

Improving Nutritional Status

The patient's diet is planned with the primary goal of glucose control; however, the dietary prescription must also consider the patient's primary health problem in addition to lifestyle, cultural background, activity level, and food preferences. If alterations are needed in the patient's diet because of the primary health problem (eg, gastrointestinal problems), alternative strategies to ensure adequate nutritional intake must be implemented. The patient's nutritional intake is monitored carefully along with blood glucose, urine ketones, and daily weight. Blood glucose records are assessed for patterns of hypoglycemia and hyperglycemia at the same time of day, and findings are reported to the physician for alteration in insulin orders. In the patient with prolonged elevated blood glucose levels, laboratory values and the patient's physical condition are monitored for signs of DKA or HHNS.

Maintaining Skin Care

The skin is assessed daily for dryness or breaks in skin. The feet are cleaned with warm water and soap. Excessive soaking of the feet is avoided. The feet are dried thoroughly, especially between the toes, and lotion is applied to the entire foot except between the toes. For bedridden patients (especially those with a history of neuropathy), the heels are elevated off the bed with a pillow placed under the lower legs and the heels resting over the edge of the pillow. Dermal ulcers are treated as indicated and prescribed. The nurse promotes optimal blood glucose control in patients with skin breakdown.

Monitoring and Managing Potential Complications

Inadequate control of blood glucose levels may hinder the patient's recovery from the immediate health problem. Blood glucose levels are monitored, and insulin is administered as prescribed. It is important for the nurse to ensure that insulin orders are modified as needed to compensate for changes in the patient's schedule or eating pattern. Treatment is given for hypoglycemia (with oral glucose) or hyperglycemia (with supplemental regular insulin no more often than every 3 to 4 hours). Blood glucose records are assessed for patterns of hypoglycemia and hyperglycemia at the same time of day, and findings are reported to the physician for modification in insulin orders. In the patient with prolonged elevated blood glucose levels, laboratory values and the patient's physical condition are monitored for signs of DKA or HHNS.

Development of acute complications of diabetes secondary to inadequate control of blood glucose levels may be associated with other health care problems because of changes in activity level and diet and physiologic alterations related to the primary health problem itself. Therefore, the patient must be monitored for acute complications (hyperglycemia, hypoglycemia) and measures must be implemented for their prevention and early treatment.

Promoting Home and Community-Based Care

TEACHING PATIENTS SELF-CARE

Even if the patient has had diabetes for many years, it is important to assess the patient's knowledge and adherence to the plan of care. It may be necessary to plan and implement a teaching plan that includes basic information about diabetes, its cause and symptoms, and acute and chronic complications and their treatment. The nurse requests that the patient give repeated return demonstrations of skills that were not performed correctly during the initial assessment. The patient is taught self-care activities for the prevention of long-term complications, including foot care, eye care, and risk factor management.

CONTINUING CARE

The patient who is hospitalized for another health problem may require referral for home care for that problem or if gaps in his or her knowledge about self-care are uncovered. In either case, the home care nurse can use this opportunity to assess the patients's knowledge about diabetes management and the patient's and family's ability to carry out that management. Teaching provided in the hospital, clinic, office, or diabetes education center is reinforced by the nurse. The home care environment is assessed to determine its adequacy for self-care and for safety.

During home care visits, the nurse assesses the patient for signs and symptoms of long-term complications and assesses the patient's and family's techniques in blood glucose monitoring, insulin administration, and food selection.

Evaluation

Expected Outcomes

Expected outcomes may include:

1. Achieves optimal control of blood glucose
   a. Avoids extremes of hypoglycemia and hyperglycemia
   b. Takes steps to resolve rapidly any hypoglycemic episodes
2. Maintains skin integrity
   a. Demonstrates intact skin without dryness and cracking
   b. Avoids ulcers caused by pressure and neuropathy
3. Demonstrates/verbalizes diabetes survival skills and preventive care
   a. Treatment modalities
      i. Demonstrates proper technique for administering insulin and assessing blood glucose
      ii. Demonstrates appropriate knowledge of diet through proper menu selections and identification of pattern used for selection of foods at home
      iii. Verbalizes signs, appropriate treatment, and prevention of hypoglycemia and hyperglycemia
   b. Foot care
      i. Inspects feet (using mirror if necessary to see bottom of foot), including inspection for cracks between toes
      ii. Washes feet with warm water and soap; dries feet thoroughly
      iii. Applies lotion to entire foot except between toes
      iv. Verbalizes behaviors that decrease the risk of foot ulcers, including: wearing shoes at all times; using hand or elbow, not foot, to test temperature of bath water; avoiding use of heating pad on feet; wearing cotton socks; avoiding constrictive shoes; wearing new shoes for brief periods; avoiding home remedies for treatment of corns and calluses; having feet examined at every appointment with the physician; and consulting a podiatrist for regular nail care if necessary
   c. Prevention of eye disease
      i. Verbalizes need for yearly or more frequent thorough eye examinations by an ophthalmologist (starting at 5 years after diagnosis for type 1 diabetes or the year of diagnosis for type 2 diabetes)
      ii. Relates that retinopathy usually does not cause change in vision until serious damage to the retina has occurred
      iii. Relates that early laser treatment along with good control of blood glucose and blood pressure may prevent visual loss from retinopathy
      iv. Identifies hypoglycemia and hyperglycemia as two causes of temporary blurred vision
   d. Controlling macrovascular risk factors
      i. Smoking cessation
      ii. Limitation of fats and cholesterol
      iii. Control of hypertension
      iv. Exercise
      v. Regular monitoring of renal function
4. Absence of complications
   a. Maintains blood glucose and urine ketones within normal limits
   b. Experiences no signs or symptoms of hypoglycemia or hyperglycemia
   c. Identifies signs and symptoms of hypoglycemia or hyperglycemia
   d. Reports appearance of symptoms so that treatment can be initiated

Critical Thinking Exercises

1.
A diabetic diet has been prescribed for a newly diagnosed diabetic patient. Compare and contrast the modifications that would be made in the diet in the following situations: (1) the patient is a pregnant woman; (2) the patient is a devout Muslim; (3) the patient is a 65-year-old woman with osteoporosis.

2.
A patient is brought to the emergency department by his coworkers because he has become drowsy and has developed slurred speech over the last hour. You learn that he has diabetes and takes insulin, but no other medical information is available. Describe how you would gather additional assessment data to help you distinguish between hypoglycemia and hyperglycemia. Before conducting an in-depth history or physical examination, the physician administers glucose to the patient. How would you explain the rationale for administering glucose before the definitive cause of the patient's symptoms is identified?

3.
Your patient has had diabetes for many years and has not adhered to a treatment regimen as prescribed. He states to you, "What's the use? I'm going to die from the complications of diabetes anyway." What is your response to him ? What is the next step for him?

4.
Your patient has diabetes and blood glucose monitoring is recommended. What areas of assessment are important in choosing a blood glucose monitoring system for him? Determine a plan for teaching blood glucose monitoring to him.

References and Selected Readings

BOOKS

American Association of Diabetes Educators. (1998). *A core curriculum for diabetes educators* (2nd ed.).

American Diabetes Association. (1995). *Exchange lists for meal planning.*

American Diabetes Association. (1995). *The health professional's guide to diabetes and exercise.*

American Diabetes Association. (1997). *Diabetes education goals.*

American Diabetes Association. (1998). *Intensive diabetes management.*

American Diabetes Association. (1998). *Medical management of pregnancy complicated by diabetes.*

American Diabetes Association. (1998). *Physician's guide to insulin-dependent (type 1) diabetes: Diagnosis and treatment.*

American Diabetes Association. (1998). *Physician's guide to non–insulin-dependent (type 2) diabetes: Diagnosis and treatment.*

Centers for Disease Control and Prevention. (1997). *National diabetes fact sheet: National estimates and general information on diabetes in the United States.* Atlanta: U.S. Department of Health and Human Services, Centers for Disease Control and Prevention.

Dunning, T. (1994). *Care of people with diabetes: A manual of nursing practice.* Boston: Blackwell.

Jovanic-Peterson, L. (1995). *Medical management of pregnancy complicated by diabetes.* Alexandria, VA: American Diabetes Association.

Kozak, G. P., et al. (1995). *Management of diabetic foot problems.* Philadelphia: W. B. Saunders.

Tilton, M. C. (1997). Diabetes and amputation. In M. L. Sipski & C. J. Alexander (Eds.), *Sexual function in people with disability and chronic illness: A health professional's guide.* Gaithersburg, MD: Aspen Publishers.

U.S. Department of Health and Human Services. (1995). *Healthy people 2000: National health promotion and disease prevention objectives. Midcourse review and 1995 revisions.* Washington, DC: U.S. Government Printing Office.

JOURNALS

Asterisks indicate nursing research articles.

General

Ahroni, J. H. (1998). Diabetes education and the primary care provider. *Nurse Practitioner Forum, 9*(2), 66–68.

American Diabetes Association. (1998). Clinical practice recommendations. *Diabetes Care,* Jan 21(Suppl 1), 1–98.

American Diabetes Association. (1998). Screening for type 2 diabetes. *Diabetes Care,* Jan 21(Suppl 1), 520–522.

American Diabetes Association. (1998). Report of the Expert Committee on the Diagnosis and Classification of Diabetes Mellitus. *Diabetes Care,* Jan 21(Suppl 1), S5.

American Diabetes Association. (1998). Economic consequences of diabetes mellitus in the U.S. in 1997. *Diabetes Care, 21*(2), 296–309.

*Anderson, L., Janes, G., Zeimer, D., & Phillips, L. (1997). Diabetes in urban African Americans: Body image, satisfaction with size, and weight change attempts. *Diabetes Educator, 23*(3), 301–308.

Bak, L., Heard, K., & Kearny, G. (1996). Tube feeding your diabetic patient safely. *American Journal of Nursing, 96*(12), 47–49.

Berry, R., Mohn, K. R., & Holzmeister, L. A. (1995). Monitoring diabetes therapy. *Home Healthcare Nurse, 13*(1), 39–42.

Bohannon, N. J. (1999). Coronary artery disease and diabetes. *Postgraduate Medicine, 105*(2), 66–68, 71–72, 77–80.

CDC Diabetes Cost-Effectiveness Study Group. (1998). The cost-effectiveness of screening for type 2 diabetes. *Journal of the American Medical Association, 280,* 1757–1763.

Dagazon, C. (1995). Coping, diabetes and the older African-American. *Nursing Outlook, 43*(6), 254–259.

Dewey, C. M., & Riley, W. J. (1999). Have diabetes, will travel. *Postgraduate Medicine, 105*(2), 111–113, 117–118, 124–126.

Dyck, B. (1998). Clinical update. Diabetes update with a cardiac perspective. *Progress in Cardiovascular Nursing, 13*(2), 28–31, 36.

Funnell, M. M. (1999). Care of the nursing-home resident with diabetes. *Clinics in Geriatric Medicine, 15*(2), 413–422.

Funnell, M. M., Arnold, M. S., Fogler, J., Merritt, J. H., & Anderson, I. A. (1998). Participation in a diabetes education and care program: Experience from the diabetes care for older adults project. *Diabetes Educator, 24*(2), 163–167.

Genuth, S., Palmer, J., & Zimmerman, B. R. (1999). New diagnostic criteria for diabetes. *Patient Care Nurse Practitioner, Diabetes Supplement,* 2–6.

Goldstein, I., et al. (1998). Oral sildenafil in the treatment of erectile dysfunction. *New England Journal of Medicine, 338*(20), 1397–1404.

Guay, A. T. (1998). Treatment of erectile dysfunction in men with diabetes. *Diabetes Spectrum, 11*(2), 101–111.

Ingersoll, G. M. (1998). Research update. Applying experimental methods to diabetes education research and evaluation. *Diabetes Educator, 24*(6), 751–754.

Leontos, C., Wong, F., Gallivan, J., & Lising, M. (1998). Recommendations for diabetes care. National Diabetes Education Program: Opportunities and challenges. *Journal of the American Dietetic Association, 98*(1), 73–75.

Lipton, R. B., Losey, L. M., Giachello, A., Mendex, J., & Giotti, M. H. (1998). Attitudes and issues in treating Latino patients with Type 2 diabetes. Views of healthcare providers. *Diabetes Educator, 24*(1), 67–71.

MacLean, D., & Lo, R. (1998). The non-insulin-dependent diabetic: Success and failure in compliance. *Australian Journal of Advanced Nursing, 15*(4), 33–42.

*Marrero, D., Guare, J., Vandegriff, J., & Fineberg, N. (1997). Fear of hypoglycemia in the parents and adolescents with diabetes: Maladaptive or healthy response? *Diabetes Educator, 23*(3), 281–286.

Martin, W. (1999). Oral health and the older diabetic. *Clinics in Geriatric Medicine, 15*(2), 339–350.

Morris, D. B. (1998). Professional development. Developing a patient education program: Overcoming physician resistance. *Diabetes Educator, 24*(1), 41–42.

*Redman, B., & Fry, S. (1996). Ethical conflicts reported by registered nurse/certified diabetes educators. *Diabetes Educator, 23*(3), 219–224.

Rendell, M. S., et al. (1999). Sildenafil for treatment of erectile dysfunction in men with diabetes. *Journal of the American Medical Association, 281*(5), 421–426.

Stanley, K. (1998). Nutrition Update. Assessing the nutritional needs of the geriatric patient with diabetes. *Diabetes Educator, 24*(1), 29–30.

Sullivan, E. D., & Joseph, D. H. (1998). Struggling with behavior changes: A special case for clients with diabetes. *Diabetes Educator, 24*(1), 72–77.

Taub, L. F. M. (1998). The ADA's clinical practice recommendations in action. *American Journal of Nursing, 98*(10), 16B, C, F.

Testa, M. A., & Simonson, D. C. (1998). Health economic benefits and quality of life during improved glycemic control in patients with type 2 diabetes mellitus. *Journal of the American Medical Association, 280*(17), 1490–1496.

Vanelli, M., Chairi, G., Ghizzoni, L., Costi, G., Giacalone, T., & Chiarelli, F. (1999). Effectiveness of a prevention program for diabetic ketoacidosis in children: An 8 year study in schools and private practices. *Diabetes Care, 22*(1), 7–9.

*Wang, C., & Fenske, M. (1996). Self-care of adults with non–insulin-dependent diabetes mellitus: Influence of family and friends. *Diabetes Educator, 22*(5), 465–470.

Weiss, R. (1999). Communication strategies. Diabetics learn while they shop in disease-management program. *Health Progress, 80*(1), 68.

Complications

Aljahlan, M., Lee, K. C., & Toth, E. (1999). Limited joint mobility in diabetes. *Postgraduate Medicine, 105*(2), 99–101, 105–106.

Beckwith, S. (1999). Complications in diabetes: Measures to reduce the risks. *Community Nurse, 4*(12), 24–26.

DCCT Research Group. (1991). Epidemiology of severe hypoglycemia in the Diabetes Control and Complications Trial. *American Journal of Medicine, 90,* 450–459.

DCCT Research Group. (1993). The effect of intensive treatment of diabetes on the development and progression of long-term complications in insulin-dependent diabetes mellitus. *New England Journal of Medicine, 329*(14), 977–986.

Fore, W. W. (1995). Non–insulin-dependent diabetes mellitus. The prevention of complications. *Medical Clinics of North America, 79*(2), 287–298.

Freeland, B. S. (1998). Diabetic ketoacidosis. *American Journal of Nursing, 98*(8), 52.

Frykberg, R. G. (1998). The team approach in diabetic foot management. *Advances in Wound Care: The Journal for Prevention and Healing, 11*(2), 71–77.

Goldstein, L., et al. (1998). Oral sildenafil in the treatment of erectile dysfunction. *New England Journal of Medicine, 338*(20), 1397–1404.

Grinslade, S., & Buck, E. A. (1999). Diabetic ketoacidosis: Implications for the medical-surgical nurse. *Medsurg Nursing, 8*(1), 37–45.

Halpin-Landry, J. E., & Goldsmith, S. (1999). Feet first: Diabetes care. *American Journal of Nursing, 99*(2), 26–34.

Harman, K. (1999). Focus on feet to reduce risk from diabetes. *Practice Nurse, 17*(2), 91, 94, 96.

*Hathaway, D. K., Cashion, A. K., Wicks, M. N., Milstead, E. J., & Gaber, A. O. (1998). Cardiovascular dysautonomia of patients with end-stage renal disease and type 1 or type 2 diabetes. *Nursing Research, 47*(3), 171–179.

Hernandes D. (1998). Hospitalization can exacerbate devastating complications of type II diabetes, including retinopathy, neuropathy, and nephropathy. *American Journal of Nursing, 98*(6), 27–31.

Kitabchi, A. E., & Wall, B. M. (1995). Diabetic ketoacidosis. *Medical Clinics of North America, 79*(1), 9–37.

Klein, R. (1995). Hyperglycemia and microvascular disease in diabetes. *Diabetes Care, 18*(2), 258–268.

Klein, R., & Klein, B. (1998). Relation of glycemic control to diabetic complications and health outcomes. *Diabetes Care, 21*(Suppl 3), C39–C43.

Lorber, D. (1995). Nonketotic hypertonicity in diabetes mellitus. *Medical Clinics of North America, 79*(1), 39–52.

Maffeo, R. (1996). Helping families cope with type I diabetes. *American Journal of Nursing, 96*(6), 36–39.

Nathan, D. M. (1995). Inferences and implications. Do results from the Diabetes Control and Complications Trial apply in NIDDM? *Diabetes Care, 18*(2), 251–257.

Ramsey, S. D., Newton, K., Blough, D., et al. (1999). Incidence, outcomes, and cost of foot ulcers in patients with diabetes. *Diabetes Care, 22*(3), 382–387.

Rendell, M. S., Rajfer, J., Wicker, P. A., & Smith, M. D. (1999). Sildenafil for treatment of erectile dysfunction in men with diabetes: A randomized controlled trial. Sildenafil Diabetes Study Group. *Journal of American Medical Association, 281*(5), 421–426.

Service, F. J. (1995). Hypoglycemia. *Medical Clinics of North America, 79*(1), 1–8.
Setter, S. M., Baker, D. E., Campbell, R. K., & Johnson, S. B. (1999). Sildenafil (Viagra) for the treatment of erectile dysfunction in men with diabetes. *Diabetes Educator, 25*(1), 79–80, 83–84, 87 passim.
Smitherman, K. O., & Peacock, J. E. Jr. (1995). Infectious emergencies in patients with diabetes mellitus. *Medical Clinics of North America, 79*(1), 53–77.
Spollett, G. (1997). Diet strategies in the treatment of non–insulin-dependent diabetes mellitus. *Lippincott's Primary Care Practice, 1*(3), 295.

Management

American Dietetic Association. (1999). Position of the American Dietetic Association: Medical nutrition therapy and pharmacotherapy. *Journal of the American Dietetic Association, 99*(2), 227–230.
Bode, B., Steed, R., & Davidson, P. (1996). Reduction in severe hypoglycemia with long-term, continuous subcutaneous insulin infusion in type 1 diabetes. *Diabetes Care, 19*(4), 324–327.
Boland, E., Ahern, J., & Grey, M. (1998). A primer on the use of insulin pumps in adolescents. *Diabetes Educator, 24*(1), 78–87.
Boland, E., & Savoye, M. (1997). Nutrition strategies for adolescents with insulin independent diabetes mellitus. *Lippincott's Primary Care Practice, 1*(3), 270–284.
Cooper, J. W. (1998). Oral agent treatment of diabetes mellitus in older adults. *Annals of Long Term Care, 6*(3), 414–422.
Draso, J., & Peterson, A. (1996). Type II diabetes—exploring treatment options. *American Journal of Nursing, 96*(11), 45–50.
Emilien, G., Maloteaux, J. M., & Ponchon, M. (1999). Pharmacological management of diabetes: Recent progress and future perspective in daily drug treatment. *Pharmacology and Therapeutics, 81*(1), 37–51.
Fleming, D. R. (1999). Challenging traditional insulin injection practices. *American Journal of Nursing, 99*(2), 72–74.
Inzucchi, S. E., et al. (1998). Efficacy and metabolic effects of metformin and troglitazone in type II diabetes mellitus. *New England Journal of Medicine, 338*(13), 867–872.
Jacobson, A. F. (1999). Saving limbs with Semmes-Weinstein monofilament. *American Journal of Nursing, 99*(2), 76.
King, D. E., Peragello-Dittko, V., Polonsky, W. H., Prochaska, J. O., & Vinicor, F. (1998). Strategies for improving self-care: Diabetes treatment moves forward. *Patient Care, 32*(3), 91–92, 95–99, 103–104.
Lavin-Thompson, J. (1997). Insulin pump therapy. *Lippincott's Primary Care Practice, 1*(5), 519–526.
O'Neill, S. (1999). How to achieve effective diabetes management. *Nursing Times, 95*(1), 53–54.
Reed, R. L., & Mooradian, A. D. (1998). Management of diabetes mellitus in the nursing home. *Annals of Long Term Care, 6*(3), 100–107.
Reynolds, H. R. (1998). Recipe for success. Medical nutrition therapy in diabetes care. *Advance for Nurse Practitioners, 6*(7), 46–49.
Schlater, A. L. (1998). Diabetes in older persons: Special considerations. *Western Journal of Medicine, 168*(6), 532–533.
Sengewald, J. M. (1999). Update on diabetes medications. *Journal of Emergency Nursing, 25*(1), 28–30.
Swenson, K., & Brackenridge, B. (1998). Lispro insulin for improved glucose control in obese patients with Type 2 diabetes. *Diabetes Spectrum, 11*(1), 13–15.
United Kingdom Prospective Diabetes Study Group. (1998). Intensive blood glucose control with sulfonylureas or insulin compared with conventional treatment and risk of complications with type 2 diabetes. *Lancet, 352,* 837–853.

Patient and Family Education

Clement, S. (1995). Diabetes self management education. *Diabetes Care, 18*(8), 1204–1214.

Pregnancy and Gestational Diabetes

American Diabetes Association. (1998). Gestational diabetes mellitus (position statement). *Diabetes Care, 21*(Suppl 1), S60–S61.
Niesen, K. M., & Ra, M. J. (1994). Pregnancy complicated by diabetes mellitus, superimposed preeclampsia, and adult respiratory distress syndrome: A case study. *Critical Care Nursing Clinics of North America, 6*(4), 841–854.

Resources

AGENCIES

American Association of Diabetes Educators, 444 N. Michigan Ave., Suite 1240, Chicago, IL 60611; 1-800-832-6874; www.diabetesnet.com/aade.html
American Diabetes Association; 1660 Duke St., Alexandria, VA 22314; 1-800-232-3472; www.diabetes.org
American Dietetic Association, 216 W. Jackson Boulevard, Chicago, IL 60606; 1-800-877-1600
American Foundation for the Blind, 15 W. 16th St., New York, NY 10011; 1-800-232-5463
Centers for Disease Control and Prevention: www.cdc.gov/diabetes
Juvenile Diabetes Foundation International, 120 Wall St., 19th Floor, New York, NY 10005; 1-800-JDF-CURE, 1-800-223-1138; www.jdfcure.com.
Medic Alert Foundation International, 2323 Colorado St., Turlock CA 95381-1009; 209-668-3333
National Library Services for the Blind and Physically Handicapped, 1291 Taylor St., NW, Washington DC 20542; 202-287-5100
National Diabetes Information Clearinghouse, 1 Information Way, Bethesda, MD 20892; 1-800-GETWELL, 301-654-3327; www.niddk.nih.gov

JOURNALS FOR PATIENTS

Diabetes Forecast, American Diabetes Association, Membership Center, PO Box 2055, Harlan, IA 51593-0238
Diabetes in the News, Ames Center for Diabetes Education, Miles Inc, PO Box 3105, Elkhart, IN 46515
Diabetes Self-Management, PO Box 51125, Boulder, CO 80321-1125
Living Well With Diabetes, Diabetes Center, 13911 Ridgedale Dr., Suite 250, Minnetonka, MN 55343

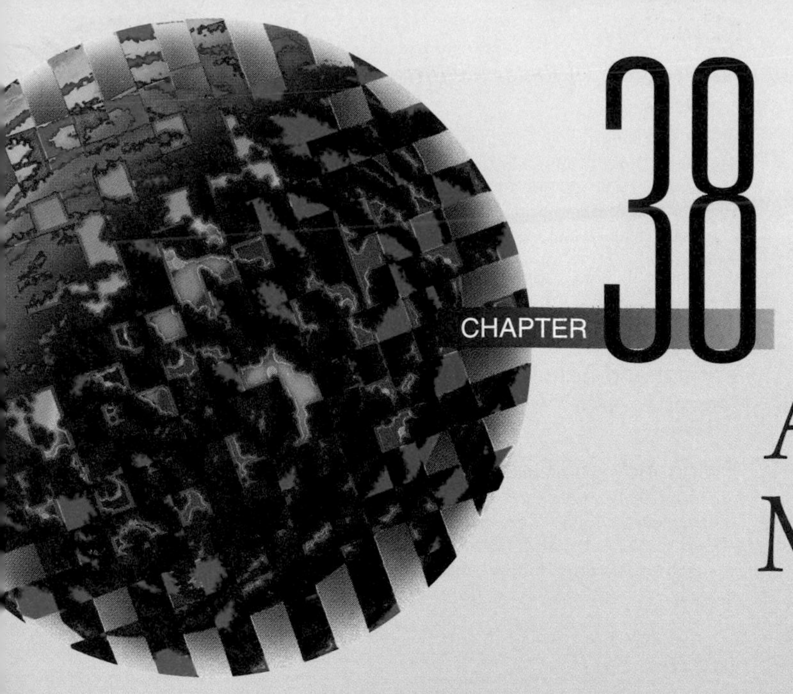

Assessment and Management of Patients With Endocrine Disorders

Learning Objectives

On completion of this chapter, the learner will be able to:

1. Describe the functions of each of the endocrine glands and their hormones.
2. Identify the diagnostic tests used to determine alterations in function of each of the endocrine glands.
3. Compare hypothyroidism and hyperthyroidism: their causes, clinical manifestations, management, and nursing interventions.
4. Develop a plan of nursing care for the patient undergoing thyroidectomy.
5. Compare hyperparathyroidism and hypoparathyroidism: their causes, clinical manifestations, management, and nursing interventions.
6. Compare Addison's disease with Cushing's syndrome: their causes, clinical manifestations, management, and nursing interventions.
7. Use the nursing process as a framework for care of patients with adrenal insufficiency.
8. Use the nursing process as a framework for care of patients with Cushing's syndrome.
9. Identify the teaching needs of patients requiring corticosteroid therapy.
10. Differentiate between acute and chronic pancreatitis.
11. Use the nursing process as a framework for care of patients with acute pancreatitis.
12. Describe the metabolic effects of surgical treatment of tumors of the pancreas.

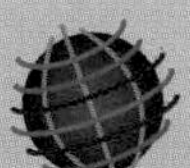

Body systems are controlled by both the nervous system and the interconnected network of glands known as the endocrine system. Disorders of the endocrine system are common and have the potential to affect the function of every organ system in the body. Understanding the function of each of the endocrine glands and the consequences of hypofunction and hyperfunction of each gland enables the nurse to anticipate physiologic changes and to plan interventions to address them. Nursing interventions essential in the management of endocrine disorders are carried out in every setting from the intensive care unit to the outpatient setting and the home.

GLOSSARY

acromegaly: disease process resulting from excessive secretion of somatotropin causing progressive enlargement of peripheral body parts, commonly the face, head, hands, and feet

Addison's disease: chronic adrenocortical insufficiency secondary to destruction of the adrenal glands

addisonian crisis: acute adrenocortical insufficiency; characterized by acute hypotension, cyanosis, fever, nausea and vomiting, and the classic signs of shock; precipitated by stress or abrupt withdrawal of therapeutic glucocorticoids

adrenalectomy: surgical removal of one or both adrenal glands.

adrenocorticotropic hormone (ACTH): hormone secreted by the anterior pituitary, essential for growth and development

amylase: pancreatic enzyme; aids in the digestion of carbohydrates

androgen: hormone secreted by the adrenal cortex; stimulates activity of accessory male sex organs and development of male sex characteristics

adrenogenital syndrome: masculinization in women, feminization in men, or premature sexual development in children; result of abnormal secretion of adrenocortical hormones, especially androgen

basal metabolic rate: method of measuring the body's energy expenditure by recording the rate of oxygen intake and consumption per minute.

calcitonin: a hormone secreted by the parafollicular cells of the thyroid gland; participates in calcium regulation

cholecystokinin-pancreozymin (CCK-PZ): hormone; major stimulus for digestive enzyme secretion; stimulates contraction of the gallbladder

Chvostek's sign: induced spasm of the facial muscles produced by sharply tapping over the facial nerve in front of the parotid gland and anterior to the ear; causes spasm or twitching of the mouth, nose, and eye; suggestive of latent tetany in patients with hypocalcemia

corticosteroids: hormones produced by the adrenal cortex or their synthetic equivalents; also referred to as adrenocortical hormone and adrenocorticosteroid; consists of glucocorticoids, mineralocorticoids, and androgens

cretinism: stunted body growth and mental development appearing during the first year of life as a result of congenital hypothyroidism

Cushing's syndrome: group of symptoms produced by an excess of free circulating cortisol from the adrenal cortex; characterized by truncal obesity, "moon face," acne, abdominal striae, and hypertension

diabetes insipidus: condition in which abnormally large volumes of dilute urine are excreted as a result of deficient production of vasopressin

dilutional hyponatremia: sodium deficiency developed as a result of fluid retention; associated with excessive ADH secretion in patients with SIADH

dwarfism: generalized limited growth; condition caused by insufficient secretion of growth hormone during childhood

endocrine: secreting internally; hormonal secretion of a ductless gland

euthyroid: normal thyroid hormone production

exocrine: secreting externally; hormonal secretion from excretory ducts

exophthalmos: abnormal protrusion of one or both eyeballs; produces a startled expression; usually due to hyperthyroidism (bilateral) or tumor (unilateral)

glucocorticoids: Steroid hormones (ie, cortisol, cortisone, and corticosterone) secreted by the adrenal cortex in response to ACTH; produce a rise of liver glycogen and blood sugar.

Graves' disease: a form of hyperthyroidism; also called Basedow's or Parry's disease; characterized by a diffuse goiter, exophthalmos

goiter: enlargement of the thyroid gland; usually caused by an iodine-deficient diet

Hashimoto's disease: Thyroiditis characterized by high levels of antimicrosomal antibodies; most common cause of hypothyroidism in the United States; also known as chronic lymphocytic thyroiditis or autoimmune thyroiditis

hormones: chemical transmitter substances produced in one organ or part of the body and carried by the bloodstream to other cells or organs on which they have a specific regulatory effect; produced mainly by endocrine glands (ie, pituitary, thyroid, gonads)

hypophysectomy: surgical removal or destruction of all or part of the pituitary gland

lipase: pancreatic enzyme; aids in the digestion of fats

mineralocorticoids: steroid of the adrenal cortex; influences sodium and potassium

myxedema: severe form of hypothyroidism characterized by an accumulation of mucopolysaccharides in subcutaneous and other interstitial tissue; masklike expression, puffy eyelids, hair loss in the eyebrows, thick lips, and a broad tongue

negative feedback: Regulating mechanism whereby return of the input product or signal higher than the setpoint results in a decrease of future output

oxytocin: hormone secreted by the posterior pituitary; causes myometrial contraction at term and milk release during lactation

pancreaticojejunostomy: joining of the pancreatic duct to the jejunum by side-to-side anastomosis; allows drainage of the pancreatic secretions into the jejunum

pancreatitis: inflammation of the pancreas; may be acute or chronic

pheochromocytoma: chromaffin cell tumor, usually benign, located in the adrenal medulla; characterized by secretion of catecholamines resulting in hypertension, severe headache, profuse sweating, visual blurring, anxiety, and nausea

radioimmunoassay: measurement of hormone or other substance using radioisotope-labeled antigen

secretin: hormone responsible for inciting secretion of pancreatic juice; also used as an aid in diagnosing pancreatic exocrine disease and in obtaining desquamated pancreatic cells for cytologic examination

somatostatin: somatotropin release–inhibiting factor; inhibits release of somatotropin by the anterior lobe of the pituitary gland; also released by delta cells in the pancreas causing inhibition of glucagon and insulin release in the gastrointestinal tract

steatorrhea: frothy, foul-smelling stools with a high fat content; results from impaired digestion of proteins and fats due to a lack of pancreatic juice in the intestine

syndrome of inappropriate antidiuretic hormone (SIADH): excessive secretion of antidiuretic hormone (ADH) from the pituitary gland despite subnormal serum osmolality; occurs with oat cell carcinoma of the lung and other malignant tumors that produce ADH

thyroid-stimulating hormone (TSH): released from the pituitary gland; causes stimulation of the thyroid gland resulting in release of T_3 and T_4

thyroid storm: severe life-threatening form of hyperthyroidism precipitated by stress; usually of abrupt onset; characterized by high fever, extreme tachycardia, and altered mental state

thyroidectomy: surgical removal of all or part of the thyroid gland; called chemical thyroidectomy when antithyroid drugs are used to decrease or eliminate thyroid function

thyroiditis: inflammation of the thyroid gland; may lead to chronic hypothyroidism or resolve spontaneously

GLOSSARY

thyrotoxicosis: condition produced by excessive endogenous or exogenous thyroid hormone

thyroxine (T_4): thyroid hormone; active iodine compound formed and stored in the thyroid; deiodinated in peripheral tissues to form triiodothyronine (T_3); maintains body metabolism in a steady state

triiodothyronine (T_3): thyroid hormone; formed and stored in the thyroid; released in smaller quantities, biologically more active and faster onset of action than thyroxine (T_4); widespread effect on cellular metabolism, influences every major organ system

Trousseau's sign: carpopedal spasm induced when blood flow to the arm is occluded using a blood pressure cuff or tourniquet, causing ischemia to the distal nerves; suggestive sign for latent tetany in hypocalcemia

trypsin: pancreatic enzyme; aids in digestion of proteins

vasopressin: antidiuretic hormone secreted by the posterior pituitary; causes contraction of smooth muscle, particularly blood vessels

Zollinger-Ellison tumor: hypersecretion of gastric acid that produces peptic ulcers as a result of a non–beta cell tumor of the pancreatic islets

ANATOMIC AND PHYSIOLOGIC OVERVIEW

The endocrine system has far-reaching effects in the human body because of its links with the nervous system and the immune system. For example, the hormones secreted by the endocrine system are affected in large part by structures in the central nervous system, such as the hypothalamus. Other structures located in the brain, such as the pituitary gland, are endocrine glands that influence the function of a large number of other endocrine glands. The effects of hormones secreted by the endocrine system affect the nervous system and are in turn mediated by the nervous system. For example, the adrenal medulla secretes a number of substances (ie, norepinephrine and epinephrine) that act as neurotransmitters. The immune system also interacts closely with the endocrine system. It responds to the introduction of foreign agents by means of chemicals (eg, interleukins, interferons) and is regulated by hormones secreted by the adrenal cortex.

In addition to the hormones secreted by the major endocrine glands, other tissues produce hormones that are secreted into body fluids and act on nearby cells and tissues. For example, the gastrointestinal mucosa produces hormones (eg, gastrin, enterogastrone, secretin, and cholecystokinin) that are important in the digestive process. Erythropoietin, a hormone that stimulates the bone marrow to produce red blood cells, is produced by the kidneys. The white blood cells produce cytokines that actively participate in inflammatory and immune responses.

Hormones are important in regulation of the internal environment of the body and affect every aspect of life. Some hormones target specific tissues; for example, adrenocorticotropic hormone (ACTH) or corticotropin is secreted by the anterior pituitary gland and targets the adrenal cortex to increase the secretion of the hormones of the adrenal cortex (ie, glucocorticoids, mineralocorticoids, and androgens). Other hormones affect a wide variety of cells and tissues of the body. Thyroid hormone is one example; thyroid hormone affects metabolic activity of cells throughout the body.

Glands of the Endocrine System

The **endocrine** glands include the pituitary, thyroid, parathyroids, adrenals, pancreatic islets, ovaries, and testes (Fig. 38-1). These glands, which secrete their products directly into the bloodstream, are differentiated from **exocrine** glands, such as sweat glands, which secrete through ducts onto epithelial surfaces or into the gastrointestinal tract. The hypothalamus is the link between the nervous system and the endocrine system.

Function and Regulation of Hormones

The chemical substances secreted by the endocrine glands are called **hormones.** Hormones help to regulate organ function in concert with the nervous system. This dual regulatory system, in which rapid action by the nervous system is balanced by slower hormonal action, permits precise control of organ functions in response to varied changes within and outside the body. Table 38-1 lists the major hormones, their target tissue, and some of their properties.

The endocrine glands are composed of secretory cells arranged in minute clusters (acini). No ducts are present, but the glands have a rich blood supply, so that the hormones they produce enter the bloodstream rapidly. In the healthy physiologic state, the concentration in the bloodstream of most hormones is maintained at a relatively constant level. When the hormone concentration rises, further production of that hormone is inhibited. When the hormone concentration falls, the rate of production of that hormone increases. This mechanism for regulation of hormone concentration in the bloodstream is called **negative feedback**, which is important in the regulation of many biologic processes.

Classification and Action of Hormones

Hormones are classified as steroid hormones (such as hydrocortisone), peptide or protein hormones (such as insulin), and amine hormones (such as epinephrine). These different classes of hormones act on the target tissues by different mechanisms. Hormones can alter the function of the target tissue by interacting with chemical receptors located either on the cell membrane or in the interior of the cell.

Peptide and protein hormones interact with receptor sites on the cell surface, which results in the stimulation of the intracellular enzyme adenyl cyclase. This results in increased production of cyclic 3′,5′-adenosine monophosphate (cyclic AMP). The cyclic AMP inside the cell alters enzyme activity. Thus, cyclic AMP is the "second messenger" that links the peptide hormone at the cell surface to a change in the intracellular environment. Some of the protein and peptide hormones may also act by changing membrane permeability. These hormones act within seconds or

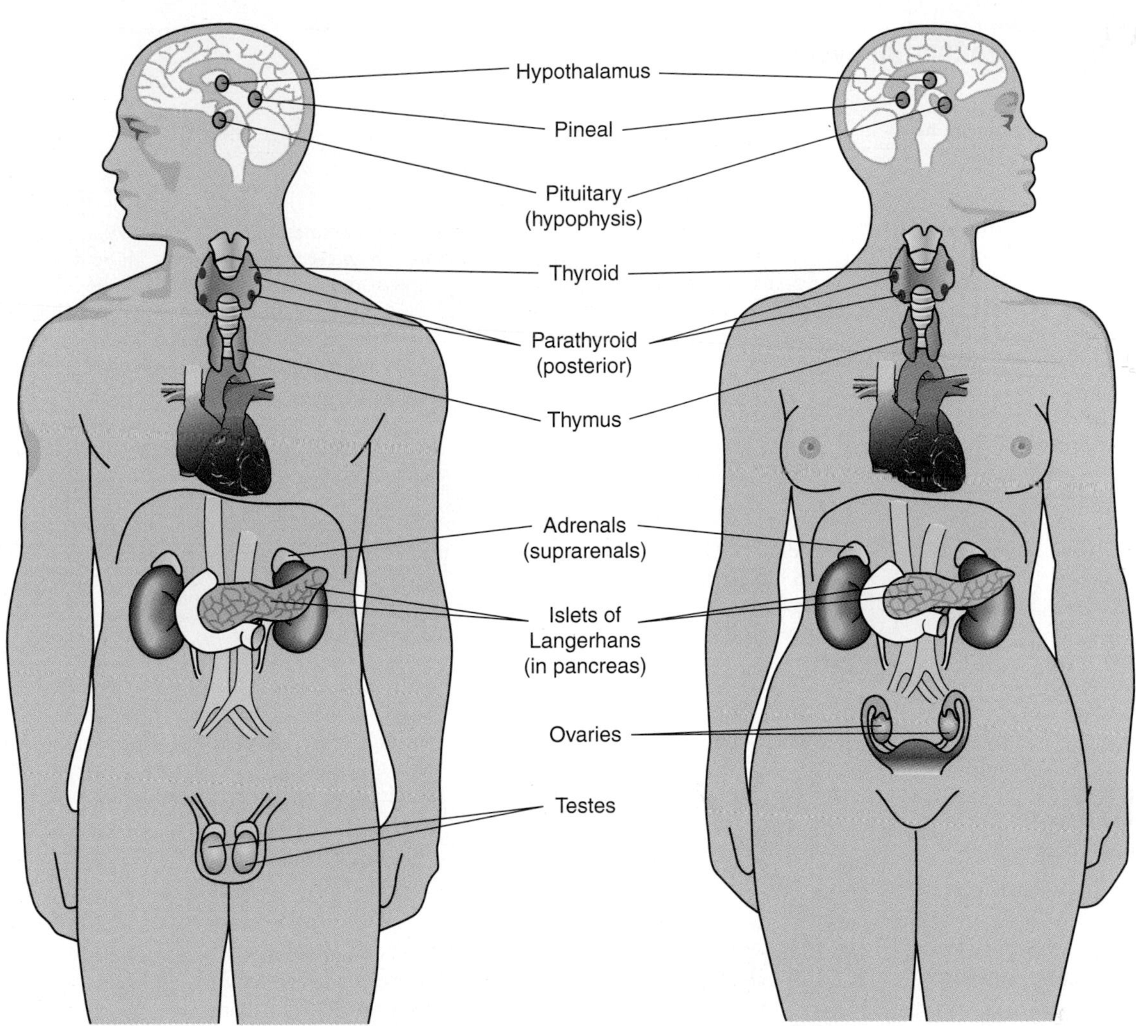

FIGURE 38•1 Major hormone-secreting glands of the endocrine system.

minutes. The mechanism of action for amine hormones is similar to that for peptide hormones.

Steroid hormones, because of their smaller size and higher lipid solubility, penetrate the cell membranes and interact with intracellular receptors. This steroid–receptor complex modifies cell metabolism and formation of messenger ribonucleic acid (RNA) from deoxyribonucleic acid (DNA). The messenger RNA then stimulates protein synthesis within the cell. Steroid hormones, because they exert their action by the modification of protein synthesis, require several hours to exert their effects.

ASSESSMENT

Health History and Clinical Manifestations

Because of the widespread effects of the endocrine system on the body, a wide variety of signs and symptoms may occur with endocrine disorders. Although specific endocrine disorders are often accompanied by specific clinical symptoms, other more general manifestations may occur with a number of endocrine disorders. Changes in energy level and fatigue are common to many endocrine imbalances. During the health history, the patient is asked about fatigue and changes in usual fatigue and energy levels; the patient is also asked about the effects these changes have had on ability to carry out usual activities of daily life. The patient is asked about changes in heat and cold tolerance. Recent changes in weight—increased or decreased—may occur with changes in adrenal and thyroid disorders and may be a result of changes in fat distribution or fluid loss or retention. Changes in sexual function and secondary sex characteristics may occur with any number of endocrine disorders and are assessed by obtaining a sexual history. Changes in mood, memory, and ability to concentrate and altered sleep patterns are assessed by asking the patient or family about these changes because they are very common in endocrine disorders. Other symptoms that occur with specific endocrine disorders are discussed with each of those disorders.

Physical Assessment

The patient is observed for obvious changes in appearance that may indicate endocrine dysfunction. For example, changes in the texture of the skin are common with both hypofunction and hyperfunction of the thyroid gland. Eye changes may occur with exophthalmos of hyperthyroidism and Graves' disease. Changes in physical appearance (ie, appearance of facial hair in women, "moon face," "buffalo hump," thinning of the skin, obesity of the trunk and thinness of the extremities, increased size of the feet and hands, edema) may signify disorders of the thyroid, adrenal cortex or pituitary gland.

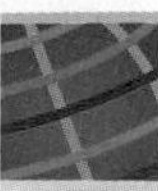

TABLE 38•1 Endocrine System in Summary

Endocrine Gland and Hormone	Principal Site of Action	Principal Processes Affected
Pituitary Gland		
Anterior Lobe		
Growth hormone (somatotropin)	General	Growth of bones, muscles, and other organs
Thyroid-stimulating (TSH)	Thyroid	Growth and secretory activity of thyroid gland
Adrenocorticotropin (ACTH)	Adrenal cortex	Growth and secretory activity of adrenal cortex
Follicle-stimulating (FSH)	Ovaries	Development of follicles and secretion of estrogen
	Testes	Development of seminiferous tubules, spermatogenesis
Luteinizing (LH) or interstitial cell stimulating	Ovaries	Ovulation, formation of corpus luteum, secretion of progesterone
	Testes	Secretion of testosterone
Prolactin or lactogenic (luteotropin)	Mammary glands and ovaries	Secretion of milk; maintenance of corpus luteum
Melanocyte-stimulating	Skin	Pigmentation
Beta-lipotropin		
Posterior Lobe		
Antidiuretic (vasopressin)	Kidney	Reabsorption of water; water balance
	Arterioles	Blood pressure
Oxytocin	Uterus	Contraction
	Breast	Expression of milk
Pineal Gland		
Melatonin	Gonads	Sexual maturation
Thyroid Gland		
Thyroxine and triiodothyronine	General	Metabolic rate; growth and development; intermediate metabolism
Calcitonin	Bone	Inhibits bone resorption; lowers blood level of calcium
Parathyroid Glands		
Parathormone	Bone, kidney, intestine	Promotes bone resorption; increases absorption of calcium; raises blood calcium level
Adrenal Glands		
Cortex		
Mineralocorticoids (eg, aldosterone)	Kidney	Reabsorption of sodium; elimination of potassium
Glucocorticoids (eg, cortisol)	General	Metabolism of carbohydrate, protein, and fat; response to stress; anti-inflammatory
Sex hormones	General	Preadolescent growth spurt
Medulla		
Epinephrine	Cardiac muscle, smooth muscle, glands	Emergency functions: same as stimulation of sympathetic nervous system
Norepinephrine	Organs innervated by sympathetic nervous system	Chemical transmitter substance; increases peripheral resistance
Islet Cells of Pancreas		
Insulin	General	Lowers blood sugar; utilization and storage of carbohydrate; decreases gluconeogenesis
Glucagon	Liver	Raises blood glucose; glycogenolysis
Somatostatin	General	Lowers blood glucose by interfering with release of growth hormone and glucagon
Testes		
Testosterone	General	Development of secondary sex characteristics
	Reproductive organs	Development and maintenance; normal function
Ovaries		
Estrogens	General	Development of secondary sex characteristics
	Mammary glands	Development of duct system
	Reproductive organs	Maturation and normal cyclic function
Progesterone	Mammary glands	Development of secretory tissue
	Uterus	Preparation for implantation; maintenance of pregnancy
Gastrointestinal Tract		
Gastrin	Stomach	Production of gastric juice
Enterogastrone	Stomach	Inhibits secretion and motility
Secretin	Liver and pancreas	Production of bile; production of watery pancreatic juice (rich in $NaHCO_3$)
Pancreozymin	Pancreas	Production of pancreatic juice rich in enzymes
Cholecystokinin	Gallbladder	Contraction and emptying

Vital signs are measured during the physical assessment and compared with previous values if known. Elevated blood pressure may occur with hyperfunction of the adrenal cortex or tumor of the adrenal medulla. Decreased blood pressure may occur with hypofunction of the adrenal cortex. Other specific physical assessment findings are discussed with each endocrine disorder.

DIAGNOSTIC EVALUATION

Although a wide variety of diagnostic tests can be used in the diagnostic workup of a patient in whom an endocrine disorder is suspected, three major categories of diagnostic tests are common: blood tests, urine tests, and stimulation and suppression tests.

Blood tests may be employed to determine hormone blood levels. For example, in a patient thought to have a thyroid disorder, serum levels of thyroid-stimulating hormone (TSH) and thyroid hormone provide information about the nature of the thyroid disorder (hypofunction or hyperfunction of the thyroid gland) and the site of the disorder: the thyroid gland itself or the pituitary or hypothalamus. Other diagnostic blood tests assess the patient for the presence of antibodies or the effect of the hormone on other substances (eg, the effect of insulin on blood glucose levels). Radioimmunoassay tests may be employed as well.

Urine tests may be used to measure the amount of hormone or the end products of hormones excreted by the kidneys. One-time specimens may be obtained, or in some disorders, 24-hour urine specimens are collected, to measure hormones or their metabolites. For example, urinary levels of free catecholamines (norepinephrine, epinephrine, and dopamine) may be measured in patients with suspected tumors of the adrenal medulla (pheochromocytoma).

Stimulation and suppression tests may also be used to diagnose endocrine disorders. Stimulation tests may be used to determine how an endocrine gland responds to the administration of stimulating hormones that are normally produced or released by the hypothalamus or pituitary gland. If the endocrine gland responds to this stimulation, the specific disorder may be in the hypothalamus or pituitary. If the endocrine gland fails to respond to this stimulation, this information is helpful in identifying the problem as being in the endocrine gland itself. Suppression tests may be used to determine whether negative feedback mechanisms that normally control secretion of hormones from the hypothalamus or pituitary gland are intact.

Specific blood tests, urine tests, and stimulation and suppression tests are discussed with the specific endocrine disorders that follow.

THE PITUITARY GLAND

The pituitary gland, or the hypophysis, is a round structure about 1.27 cm (½ inch) in diameter located on the inferior aspect of the brain. It has been referred to as the master gland of the endocrine system because it secretes hormones that control the secretion of hormones by other endocrine glands (Fig. 38-2). The pituitary itself is controlled by the hypothalamus, an adjacent area of the brain connected to the pituitary by the pituitary stalk. The pituitary gland is divided into the anterior, intermediate, and posterior lobes.

Posterior Pituitary

The important hormones secreted by the posterior lobe of the pituitary gland are **vasopressin** (antidiuretic hormone [ADH]) and **oxytocin**. These hormones are synthesized in the hypothalamus and travel from the hypothalamus to the posterior pituitary gland for storage. The primary function of vasopressin is to control the excretion of water by the kidney. Vasopressin secretion is stimulated by an increase in the osmolality of the blood or by a decrease in blood pressure. The primary functions of oxytocin are to facilitate milk ejection during lactation and to increase the force of uterine contractions during labor and delivery. Oxytocin secretion is stimulated during pregnancy and at the time of childbirth.

Anterior Pituitary

The major hormones of the anterior pituitary gland are follicle-stimulating hormone (FSH), luteinizing hormone (LH), prolactin, **adrenocorticotropic hormone** (ACTH), thyroid-stimulating hormone (TSH), and growth hormone. The secretion of each of these major hormones is controlled by releasing factors (RF) secreted by the hypothalamus. These releasing factors reach the anterior pituitary by way of the bloodstream in a special circulation called the pituitary portal blood system. Other hormones include melanocyte-stimulating hormone and beta-lipotropin; the function of lipotropin is poorly understood.

The hormones released by the anterior pituitary enter the general circulation and are transported to their target organs. TSH, ACTH, FSH, and LH have as their main function the release of hormones from other endocrine glands. Prolactin acts on the breast to stimulate milk production. Growth hormone has widespread effects on many target tissues and is discussed later. The other hormones that stimulate other organs and tissues are discussed in conjunction with their target organs.

Growth hormone, also referred to as somatotropin, is a protein hormone that increases protein synthesis in many tissues, increases the breakdown of fatty acids in adipose tissue, and increases the glucose level in the blood. These actions of somatotropin are essential for normal growth, although other hormones, such as thyroid hormone and insulin, are required as well. The secretion of growth hormone is increased by stress, exercise, and low blood glucose levels. The half-life of growth hormone activity in the blood is 20 to 30 minutes. It is largely inactivated in the liver.

Insufficient secretion of growth hormone during childhood results in generalized limited growth and **dwarfism**. Conversely, oversecretion during childhood results in gigantism, with a person reaching 7 or even 8 feet tall. Excess growth hormone in adults results in deformities of bone and soft tissue and enlargement of viscera but no increase in height. This condition is known as acromegaly.

Abnormal Pituitary Function

Abnormalities of pituitary function are caused by oversecretion or undersecretion of any of the hormones produced or released by the gland. Abnormalities of the anterior and posterior portions of the gland may occur independently. Oversecretion (hypersecretion) most commonly involves ACTH or growth hormone, resulting in **Cushing's syndrome** or **acromegaly,** respectively.

Undersecretion (hyposecretion) commonly involves all of the anterior pituitary hormones and is termed panhypopituitarism. In this condition, the thyroid gland, the adrenal cortex, and the gonads atrophy because of loss of the trophic stimulating hormones.

The most common disorder related to posterior lobe dysfunction is **diabetes insipidus**, a condition in which abnormally large volumes of dilute urine are excreted as a result of deficient production of vasopressin.

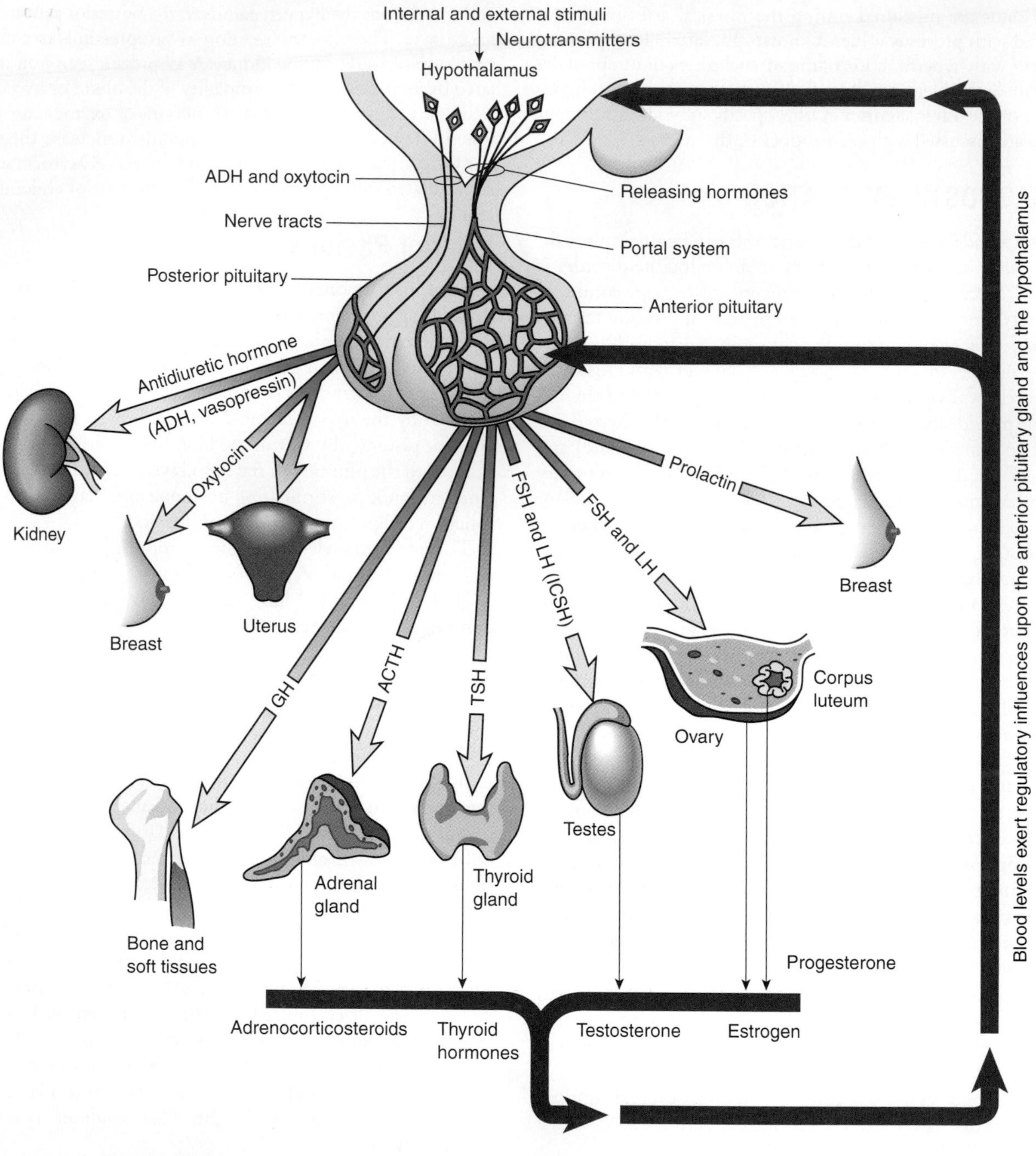

FIGURE 38•2 The pituitary gland, the relationship of the brain to pituitary action, and the hormones secreted by the anterior pituitary and the posterior pituitary.

Hypopituitarism

Hypofunction of the pituitary gland (hypopituitarism) can result from disease of the pituitary gland itself or of the hypothalamus; however, the result is essentially the same. Hypopituitarism may result from destruction of the anterior lobe of the pituitary gland. Panhypopituitarism (Simmonds' disease) is total absence of all pituitary secretions and is rare. Postpartum pituitary necrosis (Sheehan's syndrome) is another uncommon cause of failure of the anterior pituitary. It is more likely to occur in women with severe blood loss, hypovolemia, and hypotension at the time of delivery.

Hypopituitarism is also a complication of radiation therapy to the head and neck area. The total destruction of the pituitary gland by trauma, tumor, or vascular lesion removes all stimuli that are normally received by the thyroid, the gonads, and the adrenal glands. The result is extreme weight loss, emaciation, atrophy of all endocrine glands and organs, hair loss, impotence, amenorrhea, hypometabolism, and hypoglycemia. Coma and death occur without replacement of the missing hormones.

Pituitary Tumors

Pituitary tumors are usually not malignant, although their location and effects on hormone production by target organs can cause life-threatening effects. Tumors of the pituitary gland are of three principal types, representing an overgrowth of (1) eosinophilic cells, (2) basophilic cells, or (3) chromophobic cells (ie, cells with no affinity for either eosinophilic or basophilic stains).

Eosinophilic tumors, if they develop early enough in life, result in gigantism. The person thus affected may be more than 7 feet tall and large in all proportions, yet so weak and lethargic that he or she can hardly stand. If the disorder begins during adult life, the excessive skeletal growth occurs only in the feet, the hands, the superciliary ridge, the molar eminences, the nose, and the chin, giving rise to the clinical picture called acromegaly. Enlargement, however, involves all tissues and organs of the body. Many of these patients suffer from severe headaches and visual disturbances because the tumors exert pressure on the optic nerves. Assessment of central vision and visual fields may indicate loss of color discrimination, diplopia (double vision), or blindness of a portion of a field of vision. Decalcification of the skeleton, muscular weakness, and endocrine disturbances, similar to those occurring in patients with hyperthyroidism, also are associated with tumors of this type.

Basophilic tumors give rise to Cushing's syndrome with features largely attributable to hyperadrenalism, including masculinization and amenorrhea in females, truncal obesity, hypertension, osteoporosis, and polycythemia.

Chromophobic tumors, which constitute 90% of pituitary tumors, usually produce no hormones but destroy the rest of the pituitary gland, causing hypopituitarism. Patients with this disease are often obese and somnolent, exhibiting fine, scanty hair; dry, soft skin; pasty complexion; and small bones. They also experience headaches, loss of libido, and visual defects progressing to blindness. Other symptoms include polyuria, polyphagia, a lowering of the **basal metabolic rate**, and a subnormal body temperature.

Assessment and Diagnostic Findings

Diagnostic evaluation may include careful history and physical examination, including assessment of visual acuity and visual fields. Computed tomography (CT) scanning and magnetic resonance imaging (MRI) are used to diagnose the presence and extent of pituitary tumors. Serum levels of pituitary hormones may be obtained along with measurements of hormones of target organs (eg, thyroid, adrenal) to assist in diagnosis if other information is inconclusive.

Medical Management of Acromegaly or Pituitary Tumors

Surgical removal of the pituitary tumor through a transsphenoidal approach is considered the treatment of choice. Stereotactic radiation therapy, which requires use of a neurosurgical-type stereotactic frame, may be used to deliver external-beam radiation therapy precisely to the pituitary tumor with minimal effect on normal tissue. Other treatments include conventional radiation therapy, bromocriptine (dopamine antagonist), and octreotide (synthetic analog of somatostatin). These medications inhibit production or release of growth hormone and may bring about marked improvement of symptoms. Octreotide may also be used preoperatively to improve the patient's clinical condition and to shrink the tumor.

HYPOPHYSECTOMY

Hypophysectomy, or removal of the pituitary gland, may be performed for treatment of primary tumors of the pituitary gland. It is the treatment of choice in patients with Cushing's syndrome due to excessive production of ACTH by a tumor of the pituitary gland. Hypophysectomy may also be performed on occasion as a palliative measure to relieve bone pain secondary to metastasis of malignant lesions of the breast and prostate.

Several approaches can be used to remove or destroy the pituitary. It can be surgically removed through the transfrontal, subcranial, or oronasal–transsphenoidal approaches; or it can be destroyed by irradiation or cryosurgery. (See Chap. 57 for the transsphenoidal approach to the removal of a pituitary tumor and for the nursing management of a patient undergoing cranial surgery.)

The absence of the pituitary gland alters the function of many parts of the body. Menstruation ceases, and infertility occurs after total or nearly total ablation of the pituitary gland. Replacement therapy with corticosteroids and thyroid hormone is necessary; therefore, patient teaching is imperative and is discussed later in this chapter.

Diabetes Insipidus

Diabetes insipidus is a disorder of the posterior lobe of the pituitary gland due to a deficiency of vasopressin, the ADH. It is characterized by great thirst (polydipsia) and large volumes of dilute urine. It may be secondary to head trauma, brain tumor, or surgical ablation or irradiation of the pituitary gland. It may also occur with infections of the central nervous system (meningitis, encephalitis) or tumors (eg, metastatic disease, lymphoma of the breast or lung). Another cause of diabetes insipidus is failure of the renal tubules to respond to ADH; this nephrogenic form may be related to hypokalemia, hypercalcemia, and a variety of medications (eg, lithium, demeclocycline).

Clinical Manifestations

Without the action of vasopressin on the distal nephron of the kidney, an enormous daily output of very dilute, water-like urine with a specific gravity of 1.001 to 1.005 occurs. The urine contains no abnormal substances, such as glucose and albumin. Because of the intense thirst, the patient tends to drink 4 to 40 liters of fluid daily, with a special craving for cold water. In the hereditary form of diabetes insipidus, the primary symptoms may begin at birth. In adults, it may have an abrupt onset or an insidious onset.

The disease cannot be controlled by limiting the intake of fluids because loss of high volumes of urine continues even without fluid replacement. Attempts to restrict fluids cause the patient to experience an insatiable craving for fluid and to develop hypernatremia and severe dehydration.

Assessment and Diagnostic Findings

The fluid deprivation test is carried out in which fluids are withheld for 8 to 12 hours or until 3% to 5% of the body weight is lost. The patient is weighed frequently during the test. Plasma and urine osmolality studies are performed at the beginning and end of the test. The inability to increase specific gravity and osmolality of the urine is characteristic of diabetes insipidus. The patient with diabetes insipidus continues to excrete large volumes of urine with low specific gravity and experiences weight loss, rising serum osmolality, and elevated serum sodium levels. The patient's condition needs to be monitored frequently during the test, and the test is terminated if the patient develops problems such as tachycardia, excessive weight loss, or hypotension.

Other diagnostic procedures include concurrent measurements of plasma levels of vasopressin and plasma and urine osmolality; a trial of desmopressin (synthetic vasopressin); and intravenous infusion of hypertonic saline.

When the diagnosis is confirmed and the cause is not obvious (eg, head injury), the patient is carefully assessed for the presence of tumors that may be causing the disorder.

Medical Management

The objectives of therapy are (1) to replace vasopressin (which is usually a long-term therapeutic program), (2) to ensure adequate fluid replacement, and (3) to search for and correct the underlying intracranial pathology. Nephrogenic causes require different management approaches.

VASOPRESSIN REPLACEMENT

Desmopressin (DDAVP), synthetic vasopressin without the vascular effects of natural ADH, is particularly valuable because it has a longer duration of action and fewer adverse effects than other preparations previously used to treat the disease. It is administered intranasally; the patient sprays the solution into his or her nose through a flexible calibrated plastic tube. Two to four administrations daily appear to control the symptoms. The agent lypressin (Diapid) is a short-acting agent that is absorbed through the nasal mucosa into the blood; however, its duration may be too short for patients with severe disease. The patient should be observed for chronic rhinopharyngitis if the intranasal route of administration is used.

Another form of therapy is the intramuscular administration of ADH, vasopressin tannate in oil, used when the intranasal route is not possible. It is administered every 24 to 96 hours. The vial of medication should be warmed or shaken vigorously before administration. The injection is administered in the evening, so that maximum results are obtained during sleep. Abdominal cramps are a side effect of this medication. Rotation of injection sites is necessary to prevent lipodystrophy.

PHARMACOTHERAPY TO CONSERVE FLUID

Clofibrate, a hypolipidemic agent, has been found to have an antidiuretic effect on patients with diabetes insipidus who have some residual hypothalamic vasopressin. Chlorpropamide (Diabinese) and thiazide diuretics are also used in mild forms of the disease because they potentiate the action of vasopressin. The patient receiving chlorpropamide should be warned of the possibility of hypoglycemic reactions.

TREATMENT OF NEPHROGENIC CAUSES

If the diabetes insipidus is renal in origin, the previously described treatments are ineffective. Thiazide diuretics, mild salt depletion, and prostaglandin inhibitors (ibuprofen, indomethacin, and aspirin) are used to treat the nephrogenic form of diabetes insipidus.

Nursing Management

The patient with possible diabetes insipidus needs encouragement and support if undergoing studies for a possible cranial lesion. The patient and family are instructed about follow-up care and emergency measures. Specific verbal and written instructions are given about administration of the medications, and opportunity is provided for return demonstration. The patient is also advised to wear a medical identification bracelet and to carry medication and information about this disorder at all times. Caution must be used with administration of vasopressin if coronary artery disease is present because it causes vasoconstriction.

Syndrome of Inappropriate Antidiuretic Hormone Secretion

The **syndrome of inappropriate antidiuretic hormone secretion** (SIADH) includes excessive ADH secretion from the pituitary gland even in the face of subnormal serum osmolality. Patients with this disorder cannot excrete a dilute urine. They retain fluids and develop a sodium deficiency (**dilutional hyponatremia**). SIADH is often of nonendocrine origin; that is, the syndrome may occur in patients with bronchogenic carcinoma in which malignant lung cells synthesize and release ADH. SIADH has also occurred with severe pneumonia, pneumothorax, and other disorders of the lungs in addition to malignant tumors that affect other organs.

Disorders of the central nervous system, such as head injury, brain surgery or tumor, and infection, are thought to produce SIADH by direct stimulation of the pituitary gland. Some medications (vincristine, phenothiazines, tricyclic antidepressants, thiazide diuretics, and others) and nicotine have been implicated in SIADH; they either directly stimulate the pituitary gland or increase the sensitivity of renal tubules to circulating ADH.

This syndrome is generally managed by eliminating the underlying cause if possible and restricting the patient's fluid intake. Because retained water is slowly excreted through the kidneys, the extracellular fluid volume contracts, and the serum sodium concentration gradually increases toward normal. Diuretics (eg, furosemide [Lasix]) may be used along with fluid restriction if severe hyponatremia is present.

Close monitoring of fluid intake and output, daily weight, urine and blood chemistries, and neurologic status is indicated for the patient at risk for SIADH. Supportive measures and explanations of procedures and treatments assist the patient to deal with this disorder.

THE THYROID GLAND

The thyroid gland is a butterfly-shaped organ located in the lower neck anterior to the trachea (Fig. 38-3). It consists of two lateral lobes connected by an isthmus. The gland is about 5 cm long and 3 cm wide and weighs about 30 g. The blood flow to the thyroid, per gram of gland tissue, is very high (about 5 mL/min/g of thyroid), about five times the blood flow to the liver. This reflects the high metabolic activity of the thyroid gland. The thyroid gland produces three hormones: **thyroxine** (T_4) and **triiodothyronine** (T_3), which are referred to collectively as thyroid hormone, and **calcitonin.**

Thyroid Hormone

Two separate hormones produced by the thyroid gland make up thyroid hormone: thyroxine and triiodothyronine. These hormones are amino acids that have the unique property of containing iodine molecules bound to the amino acid structure. T_4 contains

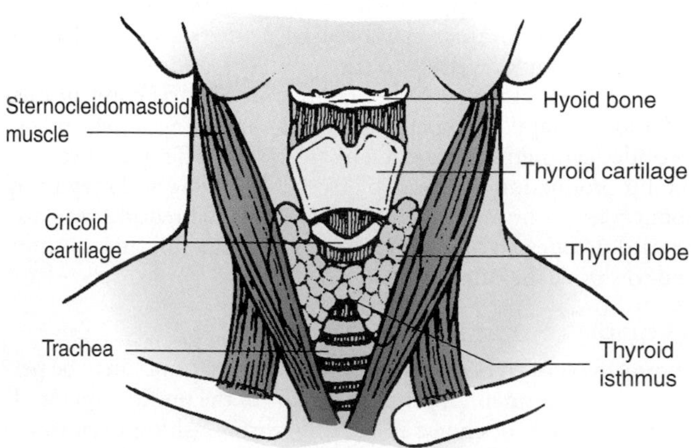

FIGURE 38•3 The thyroid gland and surrounding structures. From Weber, J.W. & Kelley, J. (1998). *Health assessment in nursing.* Philadelphia: Lippincott-Raven.

four iodine atoms in each molecule, and T_3 contains only three. These hormones are synthesized and stored bound to proteins in the cells of the thyroid gland until needed for release into the bloodstream. About 75% of bound thyroid hormone is bound to thyroxine-binding globulin (TBG); the remaining bound thyroid hormone is bound to thyroid-binding prealbumin and albumin.

Iodine Uptake and Metabolism

Iodine is essential to the thyroid gland for synthesis of its hormones. In fact, the major use of iodine in the body is by the thyroid, and the major derangement in iodine deficiency is alteration of thyroid function. Iodide is ingested in the diet and absorbed into the blood in the gastrointestinal tract. The thyroid gland is extremely efficient in taking up iodide from the blood and concentrating it within the cells. There, iodide ions are converted to iodine molecules, which react with tyrosine (an amino acid) to form the thyroid hormones.

Regulation of Thyroid Function

The secretion of T_3 and T_4 by the thyroid gland is under the control of **thyroid-stimulating hormone** (TSH or thyrotropin) from the anterior pituitary gland. TSH controls the rate of thyroid hormone release. In turn, the release of TSH is determined by the level of thyroid hormones in the blood. If thyroid hormone concentration in the blood decreases, release of TSH increases, which causes increased output of T_3 and T_4. This is an example of negative feedback. Thyrotropin-releasing hormone (TRH), secreted by the hypothalamus, exerts a modulating influence on the release of TSH from the pituitary. Environmental factors, such as a decrease in temperature, may lead to increased secretion of TRH and thereby result in elevated secretion of thyroid hormones. Figure 38-4 shows the hypothalamic-pituitary-thyroid axis, which regulates thyroid hormone production.

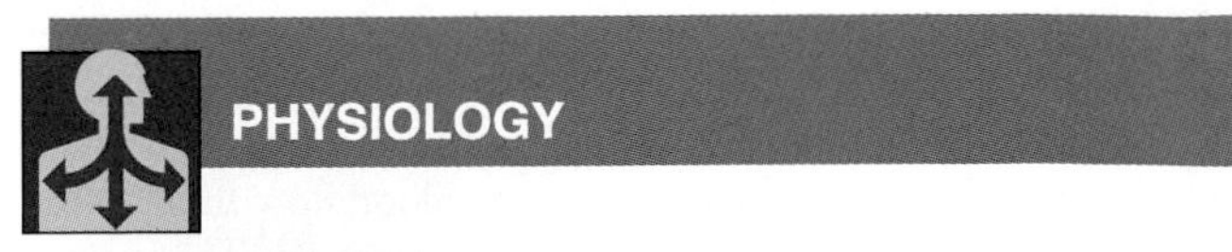

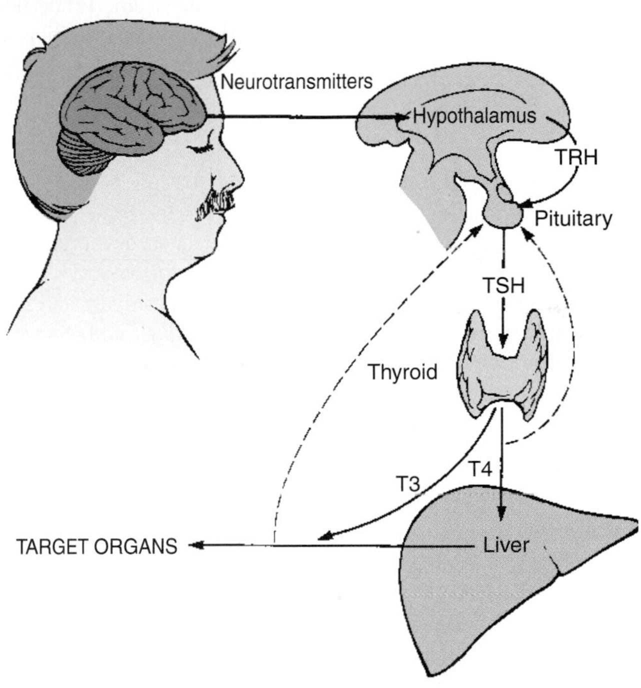

FIGURE 38•4 The hypothalamic-pituitary-thyroid axis. Thyrotropin releasing hormone (TRH) from the hypothalamus stimulates the pituitary gland to secrete thyroid-stimulating hormone (TSH). TSH stimulates the thyroid to produce thyroid hormone (T_3 and T_4). High circulating levels of T_3 and T_4 inhibit further TSH secretion and thyroid hormone production through a negative feedback mechanism (*dashed lines*).

Function of Thyroxine and Triiodothyronine

The primary function of the thyroid hormones is to control the cellular metabolic activity. T_4, a relatively weak hormone, maintains body metabolism in a steady state. T_3 is about five times as potent as T_4 and has a more rapid metabolic action. These hormones accelerate metabolic processes by increasing the level of specific enzymes that contribute to oxygen consumption and altering the responsiveness of tissues to other hormones. The thyroid hormones influence cell replication and are important in brain development. Thyroid hormone is also necessary for normal growth. The thyroid hormones, through their widespread effects on cellular metabolism, influence every major organ system.

Calcitonin

Calcitonin, or thyrocalcitonin, is another important hormone secreted by the thyroid gland. It is secreted in response to high plasma levels of calcium, and it reduces the plasma level of calcium by increasing its deposition in bone.

Examination of the Thyroid Gland

The thyroid gland is inspected and palpated routinely on all patients. Inspection begins with identification of landmarks. The lower neck region between the sternocleidomastoid muscles is inspected for swelling or asymmetry. The patient is instructed to extend the neck slightly and swallow. Thyroid tissue rises normally with swallowing. The thyroid is then palpated for size, shape, consistency, symmetry, and the presence of tenderness.

The examiner may examine the thyroid from an anterior or a posterior position. The thyroid can be effectively palpated from a position behind the patient, with both hands encircling the patient's neck (see Fig. 38-3). The thumbs are rested on the nape of the patient's neck, while the index and middle fingers palpate for the thyroid isthmus and the anterior surfaces of the lateral lobes. When palpable, the isthmus is perceived as firm and of a rubber band consistency.

The left lobe is examined by positioning the patient with the neck flexed slightly forward and to the left. The thyroid cartilage is then displaced to the left with the fingers of the right hand. This maneuver displaces the left lobe deep into the sternocleidomastoid muscle, where it can be more easily palpated. The left lobe is then palpated by placing the left thumb deep into the posterior area of the sternocleidomastoid muscle, while the index and middle fingers exert opposite pressure in the anterior portion of the muscle. Having the patient swallow during the maneuver may assist the examiner to locate the thyroid as it ascends in the neck. The procedure is reversed to examine the right lobe. The isthmus is the only portion of the thyroid that is normally palpable. If a patient has a very thin neck, two thin, smooth, nontender lobes may also be palpable.

If the thyroid gland is enlarged on palpation, auscultation over both lobes with the diaphragm of the stethoscope is performed. Auscultation identifies the localized audible vibration of a bruit. This abnormal finding indicates increased blood flow through the thyroid gland and necessitates referral to a physician. Tenderness, enlargement, and nodularity within the thyroid also require referral for additional evaluation (Table 38-2).

Tests of Thyroid Function

Several thyroid tests are available and may be necessary to give a complete and accurate picture of thyroid function. The most widely used tests for thyroid dysfunction are serum immunoassay for TSH and free thyroxine (FT_4). Third-generation immunometric assay (IMA) tests are 100 times more sensitive than earlier **radioimmunoassay** (RIA) methods for measuring TSH. Assays for FT_4 are the first choice for evaluating thyrometabolic status and have largely replaced measurements of total thyroxine (T_4), resin T_3 uptake (RT_3U), and free thyroxine index (FT_4I).

Thyroid-Stimulating Hormone

Measurement of serum TSH concentration using third-generation methods is the single best screening test of thyroid function in outpatients because of its high sensitivity. The ability to detect minute changes in serum TSH makes it possible to distinguish subclinical thyroid disease from euthyroid states in patients with low or high normal values. Values above the normal range of 0.38 to 6.15 μU/mL are indicative of primary hypothyroidism, and low values indicate hyperthyroidism. When the TSH is normal, there is a 98% chance that FT_4 is also normal. Measurement of TSH is also used for monitoring thyroid hormone replacement therapy and for differentiating between disorders of the thyroid gland itself and disorders of the pituitary or hypothalamus. Current recommendations suggest TSH screening every 5 years for adults older than 35 years of age and routinely for adults older than 60 years of age (Braverman, Dworkin, & MacIndoe, 1997).

Serum Free Thyroxine

The test most commonly used to confirm an abnormal TSH is FT_4. FT_4 is a direct measurement of free (unbound) thyroxine, the only metabolically active fraction of T_4. The range of FT_4 in serum is normally between 0.9 and 1.7 ng/dL (11.5 to 21.8 pmol/L). When measured by dialysis method, FT_4 is not affected by variation in protein binding and is the procedure of choice for following the changes in T_4 secretion during treatment of hyperthyroidism. Measurement of FT_4 by immunoassay technique is less reliable because it may be affected by medication, illness, or changes in protein binding. An estimate (or index) of FT_4 can also be calculated by multiplying total T_4 by T_3 resin uptake.

Serum T_3 and T_4

Measurement of total T_3 or T_4 includes protein-bound and free hormone levels that occur in response to TSH secretion. T_4 is 80% bound to TBG. T_3 is bound less firmly. Only 0.03% of T_4 and 0.3% of T_3 is unbound. Any factor that alters binding proteins also changes the T_4 and T_3 levels. Serious systemic illnesses, medications (eg, oral contraceptives, steroids, phenytoin, salicylates), and protein wasting as a result of nephrosis and use of androgens may interfere with accurate test results. Normal range for T_4 is between 4.5 and 11.5 μg/dL (58.5 to 150 nmol/L). Although serum T_3 and T_4 levels generally increase or decrease together, the T_3 level appears to be a more accurate indicator of hyperthyroidism, which causes a greater rise in T_3 than T_4 levels. The normal range for serum T_3 is 70 to 220 ng/dL (1.15 to 3.10 nmol/L).

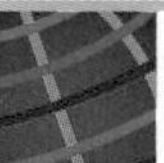

TABLE 38•2 **Summary of Findings on Physical Examination of the Thyroid Gland**

Physical Finding	Differential Diagnosis	Special Features
Single nodule	Autonomously functioning adenoma	Opposite lobe not palpable
	Adenoma or adenomatous nodule	Rubbery, firm; tenderness suggests recent hemorrhage or infarction
	Cancer	Usually hard; may have associated lymph node enlargement or vocal cord palsy
	Hyperplasia secondary to unilobar agenesis	Opposite lobe not palpable
Multiple nodules	Multinodular goiter	
	Hashimoto's thyroiditis	Firm lobes or irregular surface misinterpreted as multiple nodules
Diffuse goiter	Graves' disease	Bruit or thrill; pyramidal lobe
	Hashimoto's thyroiditis	Irregular surface; pyramidal lobe; rubbery or firm; occasionally tender; fibrous variant may be hard
	Subacute thyroiditis	Unilateral or bilateral tenderness; often hard
	Painless (silent) thyroiditis	Small to medium size; no bruit
	Thyroid lymphoma	Rapidly growing goiter, particularly in setting of preexisting Hashimoto's thyroiditis
	Multinodular goiter	Nodules may be hidden within gland and may become apparent with thyroid hormone suppression
Tenderness	Subacute thyroiditis	Unilateral or bilateral; tenderness often severe
	Hemorrhagic or infarcted adenoma	Discrete nodule with tenderness
	Hashimoto's thyroiditis	Mild tenderness
	Cancer	Irregular, firm thyroid nodule with chronic tenderness

T_3 Resin Uptake Test

The T_3 resin uptake test is an indirect measure of unsaturated TBG. Its purpose is to determine the amount of thyroid hormone bound to TBG and the number of available binding sites. This provides an index of the amount of thyroid hormone already present in the patient's circulation. Normally, TBG is not fully saturated with thyroid hormone, and additional binding sites are available to combine with radioiodine-labeled T_3 added to the patient's blood specimen. The normal T_3 uptake value is 25% to 35% (relative uptake fraction, 0.25 to 0.35), which indicates that about one third of the available sites of TBG are occupied by thyroid hormone. If the number of free or unoccupied binding sites is low, as in hyperthyroidism, the T_3 uptake is greater than 35% (0.35). If the number of available sites is high, as occurs in hypothyroidism, the test results are less than 25% (0.25).

T_3 uptake is useful in the evaluation of thyroid hormone levels in patients who have received diagnostic or therapeutic doses of iodine. The test results may be altered by the use of estrogens, androgens, salicylates, phenytoin, anticoagulants, or steroids.

Thyroid Antibodies

Autoimmune thyroid diseases include both hypothyroid and hyperthyroid conditions. Results of testing by immunoassay techniques for antithyroid antibodies, specifically antimicrosomal antibodies, are positive in chronic autoimmune thyroid disease (90%), Hashimoto's thyroiditis (100%), Graves' disease (80%), and other organ-specific autoimmune disease, such as lupus erythematosus and rheumatoid arthritis. Antithyroid antibody titers are normally present in 5% to 10% of the population and increase with age.

Thyroglobulin

Thyroglobulin (Tg), a precursor for T_3 and T_4, can be measured reliably in the serum by radioimmunoassay. Levels of Tg are elevated in most thyroid disorders, thereby limiting its diagnostic value. Clinically, it is used to detect persistence or recurrence of thyroid carcinoma.

Radioactive Iodine Uptake

The radioactive iodine uptake test measures the rate of iodine uptake by the thyroid gland. The patient is administered a tracer dose of iodine-123 (^{123}I) or another radionuclide, and a count is made over the thyroid with use of a scintillation counter, which detects and counts the gamma rays released from the breakdown of ^{123}I in the thyroid. It measures the proportion of the administered dose present in the thyroid gland at a specific time after its administration. It is a simple test and provides reliable results. It is affected by the patient's intake of iodide or thyroid hormone; therefore, a careful preliminary clinical history is essential in evaluating results. Normal values vary from one geographic region to another and with the intake of iodine. Patients with hyperthyroidism exhibit a high uptake of the ^{123}I (in some patients, up to 90%), whereas patients with hypothyroidism exhibit a very low uptake. This test is also used to determine what dose of ^{123}I should be administered to treat a patient with hyperthyroidism.

Fine-Needle Aspiration Biopsy

Using a small-gauge needle for sampling thyroid tissue is a safe and accurate method of detecting malignancy. It is often the initial test for evaluation of thyroid masses. Results are reported as (1) negative (benign), (2) positive (malignant), (3) indeterminant (suspicious), and (4) inadequate (nondiagnostic).

Thyroid Scan, Radioscan, or Scintiscan

Similar to the radioactive iodine uptake test, in a thyroid scan, a scintillation detector or gamma camera moves back and forth across the area to be studied in a series of parallel tracks, and a visual image is made of the distribution of radioactivity in the area being scanned. Although ^{123}I has been the most commonly used isotope, several other radioactive isotopes, including technetium-99m (^{99m}Tc) pertechnetate, thallium, and americium, are also used.

Scans are helpful in determining location, size, shape, and anatomic function of the thyroid gland, particularly when thyroid tissue is substernal or large. Identifying areas of increased function ("hot" areas) or decreased function ("cold" areas) can assist in diagnosis. Although most areas of decreased function are not malignancies, lack of function increases the likelihood of malignancy, particularly if only one nonfunctioning area is present. Scanning of the entire body, to obtain the total-body profile, may be carried out in a search for a functioning thyroid metastasis.

Other Diagnostic Tests

Other diagnostic tests and assessment procedures that are useful in the detection and diagnosis of thyroid disorders or effects of thyroid disease include the Achilles tendon reflex time (measures period of contraction and relaxation of Achilles tendon reflex), serum cholesterol levels, electrocardiogram (ECG), muscle enzyme studies (alanine transaminase [ALT] or serum glutamic-pyruvic transaminase [SGPT], lactic acid dehydrogenase [LDH], and creatine kinase [CK]). Ultrasound, CT scanning, and MRI may be used to clarify or confirm results of other diagnostic studies.

Nursing Implications of Thyroid Tests

When thyroid tests are scheduled, it is necessary to determine whether the patient has taken medications or agents that contain iodine because these may alter the results of some of the scheduled tests. Iodine-containing medications include contrast agents and those used to treat thyroid disorders. Other less obvious sources of iodine are topical antiseptics, multivitamin preparations, and food supplements frequently found in health food stores; cough syrups; and amiodarone, an antidysrhythmic agent. Other medications that may affect test results are estrogens, salicylates, amphetamines, chemotherapeutic agents, antibiotics, corticosteroids, and mercurial diuretics. The patient should be asked about the use of these medications, and their use should be noted on the laboratory requisition. Chart 38-1 gives a partial list of agents that may interfere with accurate testing of thyroid gland function.

Abnormalities of Thyroid Function

Inadequate secretion of thyroid hormone during fetal and neonatal development results in stunted physical and mental growth (**cretinism**) because of general depression of metabolic activity. In adults, hypothyroidism manifests as lethargy, slow mentation, and generalized slowing of body functions.

Oversecretion of thyroid hormones (hyperthyroidism) is manifested by a greatly increased metabolic rate. Many of the other characteristics of hyperthyroidism result from the increased response to circulating catecholamines (epinephrine and norepinephrine). Hypothyroidism and hyperthyroidism are discussed in detail in the following sections of this chapter.

CHART 38•1 Partial List of Medications That May Alter Thyroid Test Results

Estrogens	Opiates
Sulfonylureas	Androgens
Corticosteroids	Salicylates
Iodine	Lithium
Propranolol	Amiodarone
Cimetidine	Clofibrate
5-Fluorouracil	Furosemide
Diphenylhydantoin	Diazepam
Heparin	Danazol
Chloral hydrate	Dopamine antagonists
X-ray contrast agents	Propylthiouracil

Oversecretion of thyroid hormones is usually associated with an enlarged thyroid gland (**goiter**). Goiter also commonly occurs with iodine deficiency. In this latter condition, lack of iodine results in low levels of circulating thyroid hormones, which causes increased release of TSH; the elevated TSH causes overproduction of thyroglobulin and hypertrophy of the thyroid gland.

The term **euthyroid** refers to thyroid hormone production that is within normal limits.

Hypothyroidism

Hypothyroidism results from suboptimal levels of thyroid hormone. Thyroid deficiency can affect all body functions and can range from mild, subclinical forms to **myxedema**, an advanced form.

The most common cause of hypothyroidism in adults is autoimmune thyroiditis (**Hashimoto's disease**), in which the immune system attacks the thyroid gland (Streff & Pachucki-Hyde, 1996). Symptoms of hyperthyroidism may later be followed by those of hypothyroidism and myxedema. Hypothyroidism also commonly occurs in patients with previous hyperthyroidism who have been treated with radioiodine, surgery, or antithyroid medications. It occurs most frequently in older women. Radiation therapy for treatment of head and neck cancer can also cause hypothyroidism in older men; therefore, testing of thyroid function is recommended for all patients who receive such treatment. Other causes of hypothyroidism are presented in Chart 38-2.

Types of Hypothroidism

More than 95% of patients with hypothyroidism have *primary* or *thyroidal hypothyroidism,* which refers to dysfunction of the thyroid gland itself. When thyroid dysfunction is caused by failure of the pituitary gland, the hypothalamus, or both, it is known as *central hypothyroidism.* It may be referred to as *pituitary* or *secondary hypothyroidism* if caused entirely by pituitary disorder, and *hypothalamic* or *tertiary hypothyroidism* if attributable to a disorder of the hypothalamus resulting in inadequate secretion of TSH because of decreased stimulation by TRH. When thyroid deficiency is present at birth, the condition is known as cretinism. In such instances, the mother may also suffer from thyroid deficiency.

The term myxedema refers to the accumulation of mucopolysaccharides in subcutaneous and other interstitial tissue; although myxedema occurs in long-standing hypothyroidism, the term is used appropriately only to describe the extreme symptoms of severe hypothyroidism.

Clinical Manifestations

Early symptoms of hypothyroidism are nonspecific, but extreme fatigue makes it difficult for the person to complete a full day's work or participate in usual activities. Reports of hair loss, brittle nails, and dry skin are common, and numbness and tingling of the fingers may occur. On occasion, the voice may become husky, and the patient may complain of hoarseness. Menstrual disturbances occur, such as menorrhagia or amenorrhea, in addition to loss of libido. Hypothyroidism affects women five times more frequently than men and occurs most often between 30 and 60 years of age.

Severe hypothyroidism results in a subnormal temperature and pulse rate. The patient usually begins to gain weight even without an increase in food intake, although severely hypothyroid patients may be cachectic. The skin becomes thickened because of an accumulation of mucopolysaccharides in the subcutaneous tissues (the origin of the term myxedema). The hair thins and falls out; the face becomes expressionless and masklike. The patient often complains of being cold even in a warm environment.

At first, the patient may be irritable and may complain of fatigue, but as the condition progresses, the emotional responses are subdued. The mental processes become dulled, and the patient appears apathetic. Speech is slow, the tongue enlarges, and hands and feet increase in size. The patient frequently complains of constipation. Deafness may also occur.

Advanced hypothyroidism may produce personality and cognitive changes characteristic of dementia. Inadequate ventilation and sleep apnea can occur with severe hypothyroidism. Pleural effusion, pericardial effusion, and respiratory muscle weakness may also occur.

Severe hypothyroidism is associated with an elevated serum cholesterol level, atherosclerosis, coronary artery disease, and poor left ventricular function. The patient with advanced hypothyroidism is hypothermic and abnormally sensitive to sedatives, opioids, and anesthetic agents. Therefore, these medications are administered only with extreme caution.

CHART 38•2 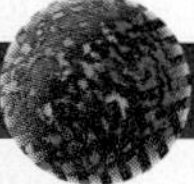 **Causes of Hypothyroidism**

- Chronic lymphocytic thyroiditis (Hashimoto's thyroiditis)
- Atrophy of thyroid gland with aging
- Therapy for hyperthyroidism
  - Radioactive iodine (^{131}I)
  - Thyroidectomy
- Medications
  - Lithium
  - Iodine compounds
  - Antithyroid medications
- Radiation to head and neck for treatment of head and neck cancers, lymphoma
- Infiltrative diseases of the thyroid (amyloidosis, scleroderma)
- Iodine deficiency and iodine excess

Patients with unrecognized hypothyroidism who are undergoing surgery are at increased risk for intraoperative hypotension and postoperative congestive heart failure and altered mental status.

Myxedema coma describes the most extreme, severe stage of hypothyroidism, in which the patient is hypothermic and unconscious. Myxedema coma may follow increasing lethargy, progressing to stupor and then coma. Undiagnosed hypothyroidism may be precipitated by infection or other systemic disease or by use of sedatives or opioid analgesics. The patient's respiratory drive is depressed, resulting in alveolar hypoventilation, progressive CO_2 retention, narcosis, and coma. These symptoms, along with cardiovascular collapse and shock, require aggressive and intensive therapy if the patient is to survive. Even with early vigorous therapy, however, mortality is high.

Gerontologic Considerations

Most patients with primary hypothyroidism are 40 to 70 years of age and present with long-standing mild to moderate hypothyroidism. About 98% or 99% of hypothyroidism in older adults is primary hypothyroidism (Braverman, 1997). The higher prevalence of hypothyroidism in elderly people may be related to alterations in immune function with age. Despite the high incidence of thyroid dysfunction in elderly people, however, the incidence of undiagnosed or misdiagnosed thyroid disease is far greater in elderly people than in younger patients. Regular screening of TSH levels is recommended for people older than 60 years of age because they are at high risk for hypothyroidism (Braverman, Dworkin, & MacIndoe, 1997).

The signs and symptoms of hypothyroidism are often atypical in elderly people; the elderly patient may have few or no symptoms until the dysfunction is severe. Depression, apathy, or decreased mobility or activity may be the major initial symptom. In all patients with hypothyroidism, the effects of analgesics, sedatives, and anesthetic agents are prolonged; particular caution is necessary in administering these agents to elderly patients because of concurrent changes in liver and renal function.

Medical Management

THYROID HORMONE REPLACEMENT

The primary objective in management of hypothyroidism is to restore a normal metabolic state by replacing the missing hormone. Synthetic levothyroxine (Synthroid or Levothroid) is the preferred preparation for treating hypothyroidism and suppressing nontoxic goiters. The dosage for hormone replacement is based on the patient's serum TSH concentration. Desiccated thyroid is used less frequently because it often results in transient elevated serum concentrations of T_3, with occasional symptoms of hyperthyroidism. If replacement therapy is adequate, the symptoms of myxedema disappear, and normal metabolic activity is resumed.

SUPPORTIVE THERAPY

In severe hypothyroidism and myxedema coma, management includes maintaining vital functions. Arterial blood gases may be measured to determine carbon dioxide retention and to guide the use of assisted ventilation to combat hypoventilation. Pulse oximetry may also be helpful in monitoring oxygen saturation levels. Fluids are administered cautiously because of the danger of water intoxication. Application of external heat (ie, heating pads) is avoided because it increases oxygen requirements and may lead to vascular collapse. If hypoglycemia is evident, concentrated glucose may be prescribed to provide glucose without precipitating fluid overload. Thyroid hormone (usually Synthroid) is administered intravenously until consciousness is restored if myxedema has progressed to myxedema coma. The patient is then continued on oral thyroid hormone therapy. Because of an associated adrenocortical insufficiency, corticosteroid therapy may be necessary.

PREVENTION OF CARDIAC DYSFUNCTION

Any patient who has had hypothyroidism for a long period is almost certain to have elevated serum cholesterol levels, atherosclerosis, and coronary artery disease. As long as metabolism is subnormal and the tissues, including the myocardium, require relatively little oxygen, a reduction in blood supply is tolerated without overt symptoms of coronary artery disease. When thyroid hormone is administered, however, the oxygen demand increases, but oxygen delivery cannot be increased unless, or until, the atherosclerosis improves. This occurs very slowly, if at all. The occurrence of angina is the signal that the oxygen needs of the myocardium exceed its blood supply. Angina or dysrhythmias may occur when thyroid replacement is initiated because thyroid hormones enhance the cardiovascular effects of catecholamines.

Nursing Alert *The nurse must monitor for myocardial ischemia or infarction, which may occur in response to therapy in patients with severe, long-standing hypothyroidism or myxedema coma.*

The nurse must also be alert for signs of angina, especially during the early phase of treatment, and if detected, it must be reported and treated at once to avoid a fatal myocardial infarction. Obviously, the administration of thyroid hormone must be discontinued immediately, and later, when it can be resumed safely, thyroid hormone replacement should be prescribed cautiously at a lower dosage and under the close observation of the physician and the nurse.

COMPLICATIONS: MEDICATION INTERACTIONS

Precautions must be taken during the course of therapy because of the interaction of thyroid hormones with other medications. Thyroid hormones may increase blood glucose levels, which may necessitate adjustment in doses of insulin or oral antidiabetic agents. The effects of thyroid hormone may be increased by phenytoin and tricyclic antidepressants. Thyroid hormones may also increase the pharmacologic effects of digitalis glycosides, anticoagulants, and indomethacin, requiring careful observation and assessment by the nurse for side effects of these agents. Bone loss may also occur with thyroid therapy.

Nursing Alert *Severe untreated hypothyroidism is characterized by an increased susceptibility to all hypnotic and sedative agents.*

Even in small doses, these medications may induce profound somnolence, lasting far longer than anticipated. Moreover, they are likely to cause respiratory depression, which can easily be fatal because of decreased respiratory reserve and alveolar hypoventilation. If their use is necessary, the dose is one half or one third that ordinarily prescribed in patients of similar age and weight with normal thyroid function. If these medications must be used, the patient must be monitored closely for signs of impending narcosis (stupor-like condition) or respiratory failure.

GERONTOLOGIC CONSIDERATIONS

In the elderly patient with mild to moderate hypothyroidism, thyroid hormone replacement must be started with low doses and increased very gradually to prevent serious cardiovascular and neurologic side effects. Angina, for example, may occur with rapid thyroid replacement in the presence of coronary artery disease secondary to the hypothyroid state. Congestive heart failure and tachydysrhythmias may worsen during the transition from the hypothyroid state to the normal metabolic state. Dementia may become more apparent during early thyroid hormone replacement in the elderly patient.

Elderly patients with severe hypothyroidism and atherosclerosis may also become confused and agitated if their metabolic rates are raised too quickly. Marked clinical improvement follows the administration of hormone replacement; such medication must be continued for life, even though signs of hypothyroidism disappear during a 3- to 12-week period.

Myxedema and myxedema coma generally occur exclusively in patients older than 50 years of age. The high mortality rate of myxedema coma mandates immediate intravenous administration of high doses of thyroid hormone as well as supportive care.

Nursing Management

MODIFYING ACTIVITY

The patient with hypothyroidism experiences decreased energy and moderate to severe lethargy. As a result, the risk for the complications from immobility increases. The patient's ability to exercise and participate in activities is further limited by the changes in cardiovascular and pulmonary status secondary to hypothyroidism. A major role of the nurse is assisting with care and hygiene while encouraging the patient to participate in activities within established tolerance levels to prevent complications of immobility.

MONITORING PHYSICAL STATUS

The patient's vital signs and cognitive level are monitored closely to detect deterioration of physical and mental status, signs and symptoms indicating that treatment has resulted in the metabolic rate exceeding the ability of the cardiovascular and pulmonary systems to respond, and continued limitations or complications of myxedema.

Nursing Alert *Medications are administered to the patient with hypothyroidism very cautiously because of altered metabolism and excretion and depressed metabolic rate and respiratory status.*

PROMOTING PHYSICAL COMFORT

The patient often experiences chilling and extreme intolerance to cold, even if the room temperature feels comfortable or hot to others. Extra clothing and blankets are provided, and the patient is protected from drafts. Use of heating pads and electric blankets is avoided because of the risk of peripheral vasodilation, further loss of body heat, and vascular collapse. Additionally, the patient could be burned by these items without being aware of it because of delayed responses and decreased mental status.

PROVIDING EMOTIONAL SUPPORT

The patient with moderate to severe hypothyroidism may experience severe emotional reactions to changes in appearance and body image and the frequent delay in diagnosis. The nonspecific, early symptoms may produce negative reactions by family members and friends, and the patient may have been labeled by family and friends as mentally unstable, uncooperative, or unwilling to participate in self-care activities.

As hypothyroidism is treated successfully and symptoms subside, the patient may experience depression and guilt as a result of the progression and severity of symptoms that occurred. The patient and family are informed that the symptoms and inability to recognize them are common and part of the disorder itself. The patient and family may require assistance and counseling to deal with the emotional concerns and reactions that result.

PROMOTING HOME AND COMMUNITY-BASED CARE

Teaching Patients Self-Care. Because most hypothyroidism treatment takes place at home, the patient and family require information and instruction that will enable them to monitor the patient's condition and response to therapy. The patient is instructed about the desired actions and side effects of medications and about how and when to take prescribed medications. The importance of continuing to take medications as prescribed even after symptoms improve is stressed to the patient. Because of the slowed mental processes that occur with hypothyroidism, it is important that a family member also be informed and instructed about treatment goals, medication schedules, and side effects that are to be reported to the physician. Written instructions and guidelines are provided for the patient and family.

Dietary instruction is provided to promote weight loss once medication has been initiated and to promote return of normal bowel patterns. The patient and family are often very concerned about the changes they have observed as a result of the hypothyroid state. It is often reassuring to the patient and family to be informed that many of the symptoms will disappear with effective treatment. See the Home Care Teaching Checklist: The Patient With Hypothyroidism (Myxedema).

Continuing Care. The patient with hypothyroidism and myxedema coma is in need of considerable follow-up and health care. Before hospital discharge, arrangements are made to ensure that the patient returns to an environment that will promote adherence to the prescribed treatment plan. Assistance in devising a schedule or record ensures accurate and complete administration of medications. The importance of continued thyroid hormone replacement and periodic follow-up testing is reinforced, and the patient and family members are instructed about the signs of overmedication and undermedication.

If indicated, a referral is made for home care. The home care nurse assesses the patient's progress toward recovery and ability to cope with the recent changes along with the patient's physical and cognitive status, the patient's and family's understanding of the importance of long-term medication therapy as prescribed, and compliance with the medication schedule and recommended follow-up tests and appointments. Subtle signs and symptoms that may indicate either inadequate or excessive thyroxine hormone are documented and reported to the patient's primary health care provider.

The gerontologic patient requires periodic follow-up monitoring of serum TSH levels because poor compliance with therapy may occur or the patient may take the medications erratically. A careful history may identify the need for further teaching about the importance of the medication. Because of the prevalence of hypothyroidism, testing of serum TSH levels in elderly people every 5 years has been recommended (Braverman, Dworkin, & MacIndoe, 1997).

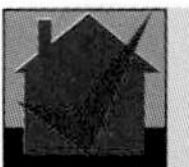

HOME CARE TEACHING CHECKLIST: THE PATIENT WITH HYPOTHYROIDISM (MYXEDEMA)

At the completion of the program, the patient or caregiver will be able to:

	Patient	Caregiver
• State present and potential effects of hypothyroidism on the body	✔	✔
• State precipitating factors and interventions for complications (hyperthyroidism, myxedema coma)	✔	✔
• Explain the purpose, dose, route, schedule, side effects, and precautions of prescribed medication (synthetic thyroid hormone)	✔	✔
• State that compliance with medical regimen is lifelong	✔	✔
• State the need to avoid extreme cold temperature until condition is stable	✔	✔
• State importance of regular follow-up visits with health care provider	✔	✔
• Identify dietary strategies to promote weight reduction and prevent constipation (high fiber, low calorie, adequate fluid intake)	✔	✔
• State potential for menstrual irregularities and family planning need for women	✔	✔
• State the importance of avoiding infection	✔	✔
• Identify changes in personality as related to hypothyroidism	✔	✔
• Identify areas of activity limitations and impact on lifestyle	✔	✔

Nursing care of the patient with hypothyroidism and myxedema is summarized in Plan of Nursing Care 38-1.

Hyperthyroidism

Hyperthyroidism is the second most prevalent endocrine disorder after diabetes mellitus. **Graves' disease**, the most common type of hyperthyroidism, results from an excessive output of thyroid hormones caused by abnormal stimulation of the thyroid gland by circulating immunoglobulins. It affects women eight times more frequently than men and peaks in incidence in the third to fifth decades (Kennedy & Caro, 1996); it may appear after an emotional shock, stress, or an infection, but the exact significance of these relationships is not understood. Other common causes of hyperthyroidism include thyroiditis and excessive ingestion of thyroid hormone.

Clinical Manifestations

Patients with well-developed hyperthyroidism exhibit a characteristic group of signs and symptoms (sometimes referred to as **thyrotoxicosis**). Their presenting symptom is often nervousness. They are often emotionally hyperexcitable, irritable, and apprehensive; they cannot sit quietly; they suffer from palpitations; and their pulse is abnormally rapid at rest as well as on exertion. They tolerate heat poorly and perspire unusually freely; the skin is flushed continuously, with a characteristic salmon color, and is likely to be warm, soft, and moist. Elderly patients, however, may report dry skin and diffuse pruritus. A fine tremor of the hands may be observed. Patients may exhibit **exophthalmos** (bulging eyes), which produces a startled facial expression.

Other manifestations include an increased appetite and dietary intake, progressive weight loss, abnormal muscular fatigability and weakness (difficulty in climbing stairs and rising from a chair), amenorrhea, and changes in bowel function. The pulse rate ranges constantly between 90 and 160 beats/min; the systolic, but characteristically not the diastolic, blood pressure is elevated; atrial fibrillation may occur; and cardiac decompensation in the form of congestive heart failure is common, especially in elderly patients. Osteoporosis and fracture are also associated with hyperthyroidism.

Cardiac effects may include sinus tachycardia or dysrhythmias, increased pulse pressure, and palpitations; it has been suggested that these changes may be related to increased sensitivity to catecholamines or to changes in neurotransmitter turnover. Myocardial hypertrophy and heart failure may occur if the hyperthyroidism is severe and untreated.

The course of the disease may be mild, characterized by remissions and exacerbations and terminating with spontaneous recovery in the course of a few months or years. Conversely, it may progress relentlessly, with the untreated person becoming emaciated, intensely nervous, delirious, even disoriented; eventually, the heart fails.

Symptoms of hyperthyroidism may occur with release of excessive amounts of thyroid hormone as a result of inflammation after irradiation of the thyroid or destruction of thyroid tissue by tumor. Such symptoms may also occur with excessive administration of thyroid hormone for treatment of hypothyroidism. Long-standing use of thyroid hormone in the absence of close monitoring may be a cause of symptoms of hyperthyroidism. It is also likely to result in premature osteoporosis, particularly in women.

Assessment and Diagnostic Findings

The thyroid gland invariably is enlarged to some extent. It is soft and may pulsate; a thrill often can be palpated, and a bruit is heard over the thyroid arteries. These are signs of greatly increased blood flow through the thyroid gland. In advanced cases, the diagnosis is made on the basis of the symptoms and an increase in serum T_4 and an increased ^{123}I, or ^{125}I uptake by the thyroid in excess of 50%.

Gerontologic Considerations

Although hyperthyroidism is much less common in elderly people than hypothyroidism, patients older than 60 years of age account for 10% to 15% of the cases of thyrotoxicosis (Kennedy & Caro, 1997). Although some older patients develop typical signs and symptoms of thyrotoxicosis, in most, an atypical picture is present, which is often subclinical in nature.

Elderly patients commonly present with vague and nonspecific signs and symptoms, making disorders hard to detect. Symptoms, such as tachycardia, fatigue, mental confusion, weight loss, change in bowel habits, and depression, can be attributed to age and other illnesses common to elderly people. The major symptoms of hypothyroidism may be depression and apathy, often accompanied by significant weight loss; one fourth of affected elderly patients

(*text continues on page 1044*)

38•1 PLAN OF NURSING CARE

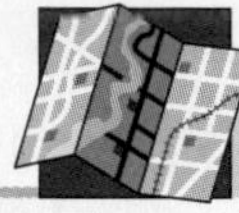

Care of the Patient With Hypothyroidism

Nursing Diagnosis: Activity intolerance related to fatigue and depressed cognitive process
Goal: Increased participation in activities and increased independence

Nursing Interventions	Rationale	Expected Outcomes
1. Promote independence in self-care activities. a. Space activities to promote rest and exercise as tolerated. b. Assist with self-care activities when patient is fatigued. c. Provide stimulation through conversation and nonstressful activities. d. Monitor patient's response to increasing activities.	1. Encouragement needed in fatigued, often depressed patient. a. Encourages activities while allowing time for adequate rest. b. Permits patient to participate to the extent possible in self-care activities. c. Promotes interest without overly stressing the patient. d. Guards against over- and underexertion by the patient.	• Participates in self-care activities • Reports decreased level of fatigue • Displays interest and awareness in environment • Participates in activities and events in environment • Participates in family events and activities • Reports no chest pain, increased fatigue, or breathlessness with increased level of activity

Nursing Diagnosis: Altered body temperature
Goal: Maintenance of normal body temperature

Nursing Interventions	Rationale	Expected Outcomes
1. Provide extra layer of clothing or extra blanket. 2. Avoid and discourage use of external heat source (eg, heating pads, electric or warming blankets) 3. Monitor patient's body temperature and report decreases from patient's baseline value. 4. Protect from exposure to cold and drafts.	1. Minimizes heat loss. 2. Reduces risk of peripheral vasodilation and vascular collapse. 3. Detects decreased body temperature and onset of myxedema coma. 4. Increases patient's level of comfort and decreases further heat loss.	• Experiences relief of discomfort and cold intolerance • Maintains baseline body temperature • Reports adequate feeling of warmth and lack of chilling • Uses extra layer of clothing or extra blanket • Explains rationale for avoiding external heat source

Nursing Diagnosis: Constipation related to depressed gastrointestinal function
Goal: Return of normal bowel function

Nursing Interventions	Rationale	Expected Outcomes
1. Encourage increased fluid intake within limits of fluid restriction. 2. Provide foods high in fiber. 3. Instruct patient about foods with high water content. 4. Monitor bowel function. 5. Encourage increased mobility within patient's exercise tolerance. 6. Encourage patient to use laxatives and enemas sparingly.	1. Promotes passage of soft stools. 2. Increases bulk of stools and more frequent bowel movements. 3. Provides rationale for patient to increase fluid intake. 4. Permits detection of constipation and return to normal bowel pattern. 5. Promotes evacuation of the bowel. 6. Minimizes patient's dependence on laxatives and enemas and encourages normal pattern of bowel evacuation.	• Reports normal bowel function • Identifies and consumes foods high in fiber • Drinks recommended amount of fluid each day • Participates in gradually increasing exercises • Uses laxatives as prescribed and avoids excessive dependence on laxatives and enemas

Nursing Diagnosis: Knowledge deficit about the therapeutic regimen for lifelong thyroid replacement therapy
Goal: Knowledge and acceptance of the prescribed therapeutic regimen

Nursing Interventions	Rationale	Expected Outcomes
1. Explain rationale for thyroid hormone replacement 2. Describe desired effects of medication to patient.	1. Provides rationale for patient to use thyroid hormone replacement as prescribed. 2. Provides encouragement to patient by identifying improved physical status and well-being that will occur with thyroid hormone therapy.	• Describes therapeutic regimen correctly • Explains rationale for thyroid hormone replacement • Identifies positive outcomes of thyroid hormone replacement • Administers medication to self as prescribed

(continued)

38•1

PLAN OF NURSING CARE

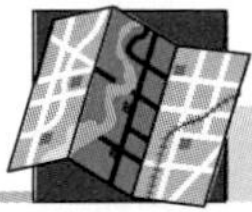

Care of the Patient With Hypothyroidism (*continued*)

Nursing Interventions	Rationale	Expected Outcomes
3. Assist patient to develop schedule and checklist to ensure self-administration of thyroid replacement. 4. Describe signs and symptoms of over- and underdose of medication. 5. Explain the necessity for long-term follow up to patient and family.	3. Increases assurance that medication will be taken as prescribed. 4. Serves as check for patient to determine if therapeutic goals are met. 5. Increases likelihood that hypo- or hyperthyroidism will be detected and treated.	• Identifies adverse side effects that should be reported promptly to physician: recurrence of symptoms of hypothyroidism and occurrence of symptoms of hyperthyroidism • Restates need for periodic/long-term follow-up visits to physician
Nursing Diagnosis: Ineffective breathing pattern related to depressed ventilation **Goal:** Improved respiratory status and maintenance of normal breathing pattern		
1. Monitor respiratory rate, depth, pattern; pulse oximetry and arterial blood gases. 2. Encourage deep breathing, coughing, and use of incentive spirometry. 3. Administer medications (hypnotics and sedatives) with caution. 4. Maintain patent airway through suction and ventilatory support if indicated (see Chap. 22 for care of patients requiring mechanical ventilation).	1. Identifies patient's baseline to monitor further changes and evaluate effectiveness of interventions. 2. Prevents atelectasis and promotes adequate ventilation. 3. Patients with hypothyroidism are *very* susceptible to respiratory depression with use of hypnotics and sedatives. 4. Use of an artificial airway and ventilatory support may be necessary with respiratory depression.	• Shows improved respiratory status and maintenance of normal breathing pattern • Demonstrates normal respiratory rate, depth, and pattern • Takes deep breaths, coughs and uses incentive spirometry when encouraged • Demonstrates normal breath sounds without adventitious sounds on auscultation • Explains rationale for cautious use of medications • Cooperates with suction procedure and ventilator when necessary
Nursing Diagnosis: Altered thought processes related to depressed metabolism and altered cardiovascular and respiratory status **Goal:** Improved thought processes		
1. Orient patient to time, place, date, and events around him or her. 2. Provide stimulation through conversation and nonthreatening activities. 3. Explain to patient and family that change in cognitive and mental functioning is a result of disease process. 4. Monitor cognitive and mental processes and response of these to medication and other therapy.	1. Provides reality orientation to patient. 2. Provides stimulation within patient's level of tolerance for stress. 3. Reassures patient and family about the cause of the cognitive changes and that a positive outcome is possible with appropriate treatment. 4. Permits evaluation of the effectiveness of treatment.	• Shows improved cognitive functioning • Identifies time, place, date, and events correctly • Responds when stimulated • Responds spontaneously as treatment becomes effective • Interacts spontaneously with family and environment • Explains that change in mental and cognitive processes is a result of disease processes • Takes medications as prescribed to prevent decrease in cognitive processes
Collaborative Problem: Myxedema and myxedema coma **Goal:** Absence of complications		
1. Monitor patient for increasing severity of signs and symptoms of hypothyroidism: a. Decreased level of consciousness; dementia b. Decreased vital signs (blood pressure, respiratory rate, temperature, pulse rate) c. Increasing difficulty in awakening or arousing patient	1. Extreme hypothyroidism may lead to myxedema, myxedema coma and slowing of all body systems if untreated.	• Exhibits reversal of myxedema and myxedema coma • Responds appropriately to questions and surroundings • Vital signs return to normal or near-normal ranges • Respiratory status improves with adequate spontaneous ventilatory effort • Reports no episodes of angina or other indicators of cardiac insufficiency

(*continued*)

38•1

PLAN OF NURSING CARE 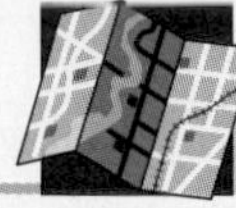 Care of the Patient With Hypothyroidism (*continued*)

Nursing Interventions	Rationale	Expected Outcomes
2. Assist in ventilatory support if respiratory depression and failure occur.	2. Ventilatory support is necessary to maintain adequate oxygenation and maintenance of an airway.	• Experiences minimal or no complications caused by immobility
3. Administer prescribed medications (eg, thyroxine) with extreme caution.	3. The slow metabolism and atherosclerosis of myxedema may result in angina with administration of thyroxine.	
4. Turn and reposition patient at intervals.	4. Minimizes risks associated with immobility.	
5. Avoid use of hypnotic, sedative, and analgesic agents.	5. Altered metabolism of these agents greatly increases the risks of their use in myxedema.	

experience constipation. In addition, the patient may report cardiovascular symptoms and difficulty climbing stairs or rising from a chair because of muscle weakness. New or worsening congestive heart failure or angina is more likely to occur in elderly than in younger patients. The elderly patient may experience a single manifestation, such as atrial fibrillation, anorexia, or weight loss. These signs and symptoms may mask the underlying thyroid disease.

Spontaneous remission of hyperthyroidism is rare in elderly patients. Measurement of TSH is indicated in elderly patients with unexplained physical or mental deterioration.

Medical Management

Treatment of hyperthyroidism is directed toward reducing thyroid hyperactivity to provide effective symptomatic relief and remove the cause of important complications.

Three forms of treatment are available for treating hyperthyroidism and controlling excessive thyroid activity: (1) irradiation, involving the administration of the radioisotope ^{123}I or ^{131}I for destructive effects on the thyroid gland; (2) pharmacotherapy, employing antithyroid medications that interfere with the synthesis of thyroid hormones and other agents that control manifestations of hyperthyroidism; and (3) surgery, with removal of most of the thyroid gland. Treatment depends on the cause of the hyperthyroidism and may require a combination of therapeutic approaches.

RADIOACTIVE IODINE THERAPY

The goal of treatment with radioactive iodine (^{123}I or ^{131}I) is to destroy the overactive thyroid cells. Use of radioactive iodine is the most common treatment in elderly patients. Almost all the iodine that enters and is retained in the body becomes concentrated in the thyroid gland. Therefore, radioactive isotope of iodine is concentrated in the thyroid gland, where it destroys thyroid cells without jeopardizing other radiosensitive tissues. During a period of weeks or months, thyroid cells exposed to the radioactive iodine are destroyed, resulting in reduction of the hyperthyroid state and inevitably hypothyroidism.

The patient is instructed what to expect of this tasteless, colorless radioiodine, which may be administered by the radiologist. A single oral dose of the agent is administered, based on 80 to 160 μCi/g estimated thyroid weight. The patient is observed for signs of **thyroid storm**. About 70% to 85% of patients are cured by one dose of radioactive iodine. An additional 10% to 20% require two doses; rarely is a third dose necessary. Use of an ablative dose of radioactive iodine initially causes an acute release of thyroid hormone from the thyroid gland and may cause an increase of symptoms. Propranolol is useful in controlling these symptoms.

After treatment with radioactive iodine, the patient is followed closely until the euthyroid state is reached. In 3 to 4 weeks, symptoms of hyperthyroidism subside. Because the incidence of hypothyroidism after this form of treatment is very high (ie, more than 90% at 10 years), close follow-up is required to evaluate thyroid function. Thyroid hormone replacement is necessary; small doses are usually prescribed, with the dose gradually increased over a period of months (up to about 1 year) until the FT_4 and TSH levels stabilize within normal ranges.

Radioactive iodine has been used in toxic adenomas and multinodular goiter and in most varieties of thyrotoxicosis (rarely permanently successful) and is preferred for treating patients beyond the childbearing years with diffuse toxic goiter. It is contraindicated in pregnancy and in nursing mothers because radioiodine crosses the placenta and is secreted in breast milk. A major advantage of treatment with radioactive iodine is that it avoids many of the side effects associated with antithyroid medications. However, many patients and their families fear medications that are radioactive. Because of this fear about radioactive substances, many patients elect to take antithyroid medications rather than radioactive iodine.

PHARMACOLOGIC THERAPY

The objective of pharmacotherapy is to inhibit one or more stages in hormone synthesis or hormone release; another goal may be to reduce the amount of thyroid tissue, with resulting decreased thyroid hormone production.

Antithyroid agents effectively block the utilization of iodine by interfering with the iodination of thyrosine and the coupling of iodothyrosines in the synthesis of thyroid hormones. This prevents the synthesis of thyroid hormone. The most commonly used medications are propylthiouracil (Propacil, PTU) or methimazole (Tapazole), until the patient is euthyroid (ie, neither hyperthyroid nor hypothyroid). These medications block extrathyroidal conversion of T_4 to T_3. Because antithyroid medications do not interfere with release or activity of previously formed thyroid hormones, it may take several weeks for relief of symptoms, at which time the maintenance dose is established, followed by a gradual withdrawal of the medication over the next several months.

Therapy is determined on the basis of clinical criteria, including changes in pulse rate, pulse pressure, body weight, size of the goiter, and results of laboratory studies of thyroid function.

Toxic complications of antithyroid medications are relatively uncommon; nevertheless, the importance of periodic follow-up is emphasized because medication sensitization, fever, rash, urticaria, or even agranulocytosis and thrombocytopenia (decrease in granulocytes and platelets) may develop. With any sign of infection, especially pharyngitis and fever or the occurrence of mouth ulcers, the patient is advised to stop the medication, notify the physician immediately, and undergo hematologic studies. Rash, arthralgias, and fever occur in 5% of patients. Agranulocytosis is the most serious toxic side effect and occurs in 1 of every 200 patients. Its incidence is higher in patients older than 40 years of age. It generally occurs within the first 3 months of therapy but may occur up to 1 year after it is started.

Patients taking antithyroid medications are instructed not to use decongestants for nasal stuffiness because they are poorly tolerated. Antithyroid medications are contraindicated in late pregnancy because they may produce goiter and cretinism in the fetus.

Thyroid hormone may occasionally be administered with antithyroid medications to put the thyroid gland at rest. In this approach, hypothyroidism from excess antithyroid medication is avoided, as is stimulation of the thyroid gland by TSH. Thyroid hormone is available as desiccated thyroid, thyroglobulin (Proloid), and levothyroxine sodium (Synthroid). These are slow-acting preparations that take about 10 days to achieve their full effect. Liothyronine sodium (Cytomel) has a more rapid onset, and its action is of short duration.

ADJUNCTIVE THERAPY

Iodine or iodide compounds, once the only therapy available for patients with hyperthyroidism, are no longer used as the sole method of treatment. Such compounds decrease the release of thyroid hormones from the thyroid gland and reduce the vascularity and size of the thyroid. Compounds such as potassium iodide, Lugol's solution, and saturated solution of potassium iodide (SSKI) may be used in combination with antithyroid agents or beta-adrenergic blockers to prepare the patient with hyperthyroidism for surgery. These agents reduce the activity of the thyroid hormone and the vascularity of the thyroid gland, making the surgical procedure safer. Solutions of iodine and iodide compounds are more palatable in milk or fruit juice and are administered through a straw to prevent staining of the teeth. These compounds reduce the metabolic rate more rapidly than antithyroid medications, but their action does not last as long.

Nursing Alert *Patients receiving these medications should be observed for the development of goiter and should be cautioned against use of over-the-counter medications that contain iodides and can increase the response to iodide therapy. Cough medications, expectorants, bronchodilators, and salt substitutes may contain iodide and should be avoided by the patient receiving iodide therapy.*

Beta-adrenergic blocking agents have become a *very* important part of management of hyperthyroidism to control the sympathetic nervous system effects. For example, propranolol is used to control nervousness, tachycardia, tremor, anxiety, and heat intolerance. The patient continues taking propranolol until the FT_4 is within the normal range and the TSH level is approaching normal.

SURGICAL MANAGEMENT

Surgery to remove thyroid tissue was once the primary method of treating hyperthyroidism; today, surgery is reserved for special circumstances, for example, in pregnant women allergic to antithyroid medications, patients with large goiters, or patients who are unable to take antithyroid agents.

The surgical removal of about five sixths of the thyroid tissue (subtotal thyroidectomy) practically ensures a prolonged remission in most patients with exophthalmic goiter. Before surgery, propylthiouracil is administered until signs of hyperthyroidism have disappeared. Alternatively, a beta-adrenergic blocking agent (propranolol) may be used to reduce the heart rate; however, use of these medications does not create a euthyroid state. Iodine (Lugol's solution or potassium iodide) may be prescribed in an effort to reduce blood loss; however, the effectiveness of this is unknown. Patients receiving iodine medication must be monitored for evidence of iodine toxicity (iodism), which requires immediate withdrawal of the medication. Symptoms of iodism include swelling of the buccal mucosa, excessive salivation, coryza, and skin eruptions.

Surgery for treatment of hyperthyroidism is performed soon after the patient's thyroid function has returned to normal (4 to 6 weeks).

GERONTOLOGIC CONSIDERATIONS

The use of radioactive iodine is generally recommended for treatment of thyrotoxicosis in elderly patients unless an enlarged thyroid gland is pressing on the airway. The hypermetabolic state of thyrotoxicosis must be controlled by antithyroid medications before radioactive iodine is administered because radiation may precipitate thyroid storm by increasing the release of hormone from the thyroid gland. Thyroid storm, if it occurs, has a mortality rate of 10% in elderly patients.

The use of beta-adrenergic blocking agents may be indicated to decrease the cardiovascular and neurologic signs and symptoms of thyrotoxicosis. These agents must be used with extreme caution to minimize adverse effects on cardiac function that may produce congestive heart failure.

If antithyroid agents are used, the patient must be monitored closely because elderly patients are more likely to develop granulocytopenia. The dosage of other medications to treat other chronic illnesses in elderly patients may need modification because of the altered rate of metabolism in hyperthyroidism.

Relapse Rate and Risk for Hyperthyroidism After Treatment

None of the treatments for thyrotoxicosis is without side effects, and all three forms of treatment (ie, radioactive iodine therapy, antithyroid medications, and surgery) share the same complications: relapse or recurrent hyperthyroidism and permanent hypothyroidism. The rate of relapse is increased in patients who had very severe disease, a long history of dysfunction, ocular and cardiac symptoms, large goiter, and relapse after previous treatment.

The relapse rate after radioactive iodine therapy is dependent on the dose used in treatment. Patients receiving a lower dose of radioactive iodine are more likely to require subsequent treatment than those being treated with a higher dose. Hypothyroidism occurs in almost 80% of patients at 1 year and in 90% to 100% by 5 years for both the multiple low-dose and single high-dose methods.

Although rates of relapse and the occurrence of hypothyroidism vary, relapse with antithyroid medications is about 45% by 1 year after completion of therapy and almost 75% by 5 years later. Discontinuation of antithyroid medications before therapy is complete usually results in relapse within 6 months in most patients. The incidence of relapse with subtotal thyroidectomy is 19% at 18 months; an incidence of hypothyroidism of 25% has been reported at 18 months after surgery. The risk for these complications illustrates the importance of long-term follow-up of patients treated for hyperthyroidism.

Thyroid Storm (Thyrotoxic Crisis)

Thyroid storm (thyrotoxic crisis) is a form of severe hyperthyroidism, usually of abrupt onset and characterized by high fever (hyperpyrexia), extreme tachycardia, and altered mental state, which frequently appears as delirium. Thyroid storm is a life-threatening condition and is usually precipitated by stress, such as injury, infection, thyroidal and nonthyroid surgery, tooth extraction, insulin reaction, diabetic acidosis, pregnancy, digitalis intoxication, abrupt withdrawal of antithyroid medications, extreme emotional stress, or vigorous palpation of the thyroid. These factors can precipitate thyroid storm in the partially controlled or completely untreated hyperthyroid patient.

Current methods of diagnosis and treatment for hyperthyroidism have greatly decreased the incidence of thyroid storm, making it uncommon today.

Although thyroid crisis may be difficult to identify, the following signs are suggestive: (1) tachycardia (more than 130 beats/min), (2) temperature above 38.5°C (101.3°F), (3) exaggerated symptoms of hyperthyroidism, and (4) disturbances of a major system, for example, gastrointestinal (weight loss, diarrhea, abdominal pain), neurologic (psychosis, somnolence, coma), or cardiovascular (edema, chest pain, dyspnea, palpitations).

Untreated thyroid storm is almost always fatal, but with proper treatment, the mortality rate is reduced substantially.

MEDICAL MANAGEMENT

The immediate objectives are to reduce body temperature and heart rate and to prevent vascular collapse. Measures to reduce the temperature include a hypothermia mattress or blanket, ice packs, a cool environment, hydrocortisone, and acetaminophen (Tylenol).

Nursing Alert *Salicylates are not used because they displace thyroid hormone from binding proteins and worsen the hypermetabolism.*

Humidified oxygen is administered to improve tissue oxygenation and meet the high metabolic demands. Arterial blood gas levels or pulse oximetry may be used to monitor respiratory status. Intravenous fluids containing dextrose are administered to replace liver glycogen stores that have been decreased in the hyperthyroid patient.

PTU or methimazole is administered to impede formation of thyroid hormone and block conversion of T_4 to T_3, the more active form of thyroid hormone. Hydrocortisone is prescribed to treat shock or adrenal insufficiency. Iodine is administered to decrease output of T_4 from the thyroid gland. For cardiac problems such as atrial fibrillation, dysrhythmias, and congestive heart failure, sympatholytic agents may be administered. Propranolol, in combination with digitalis, has been effective in reducing severe cardiac symptoms.

Nursing Alert *The patient with thyroid storm or crisis is critically ill and requires astute observation and aggressive and supportive nursing care during and after the acute stage of illness.*

NURSING PROCESS: THE PATIENT WITH HYPERTHYROIDISM

Assessment

The health history and examination focus on the occurrence of symptoms related to accelerated or exaggerated metabolism. These include the patient's and family's report of irritability and increased emotional reaction and the impact that these changes have had on the patient's interaction with family, friends, and coworkers. The history includes other stressors and the patient's ability to cope with stress.

Nutritional status and the presence of symptoms are assessed. The occurrence of symptoms related to excessive output of the nervous system, and changes in vision and the appearance of the eyes are noted. The patient's cardiac status is assessed and monitored periodically. The heart rate, blood pressure, heart sounds, and peripheral pulses are assessed.

Because of the likelihood of emotional changes related to hyperthyroidism, the patient's emotional state and psychological status are evaluated. The patient is assessed for irritability, anxiety, sleep disturbances, apathy, and lethargy, all of which may occur with hyperthyroidism. The patient's family may provide information about recent changes in the patient's emotional status.

Diagnosis

Nursing Diagnoses

Based on all the assessment data, the major nursing diagnoses of the patient with hyperthyroidism include the following:

- Altered nutrition related to exaggerated metabolic rate, excessive appetite, and increased gastrointestinal activity
- Ineffective coping related to irritability, hyperexcitability, apprehension, and emotional instability
- Disturbance in self-esteem related to changes in appearance, excessive appetite, and weight loss
- Altered body temperature

Collaborative Problems/Potential Complications

Based on assessment data, potential complications may include the following:

- Thyrotoxicosis or thyroid storm
- Hypothyroidism

Planning and Goals

The goals for the patient may be improved nutritional status, improved coping ability, improved self-esteem, maintenance of normal body temperature, and absence of complications.

Nursing Interventions

Improving Nutritional Status

Hyperthyroidism affects all body systems, including the gastrointestinal system. The patient's appetite is increased but may be satisfied by several well-balanced meals of small size, even up to six meals a day. Foods and fluids are selected to replace fluid lost through diarrhea and diaphoresis and to control diarrhea that results from increased peristalsis. Rapid movement of food through the gastrointestinal tract may result in nutritional imbalance and further weight loss. To reduce diarrhea, highly seasoned foods and stimulants, such as coffee, tea, cola, and alcohol, are discouraged. High-calorie, high-protein foods are encouraged. A quiet atmosphere during mealtime may aid digestion. The patient's weight and dietary intake are recorded to monitor nutritional status.

Enhancing Coping Measures

The patient with hyperthyroidism needs reassurance that the emotional reactions being experienced are a result of the disorder and that with effective treatment those symptoms will be controlled. Because of the negative effect these symptoms have on family and friends, they too need reassurance that these symptoms are expected to disappear with treatment.

It is important to use a calm, unhurried approach with the patient. Additionally, stressful experiences are minimized; therefore, if hospitalized, the patient is not placed in a room with very ill or talkative patients. The environment is kept quiet and uncluttered. Noises, such as loud music, conversation, and equipment alarms, are minimized. Relaxing activities are encouraged if they do not overstimulate the patient.

If thyroidectomy is planned, the patient is likely to be apprehensive and anxious about the surgery. The patient is informed that pharmacologic therapy is necessary to prepare the thyroid gland for surgical treatment. The nurse encourages the patient to take the medications as prescribed. Because of hyperexcitability and shortened attention span, the patient may require repetition of this information and written instructions.

Improving Self-Esteem

The hyperthyroid patient is likely to experience changes in appearance, appetite, and weight. These factors, along with the patient's inability to cope well with family and the illness, may result in loss of self-esteem. The nurse conveys an understanding of the patient's concern about these problems and assists the patient to develop effective coping strategies. The patient and family are informed that these changes are a result of the dysfunction of the thyroid gland and are in fact out of the person's control.

If changes in appearance are very disturbing to the patient, mirrors may be covered or removed. In addition, family members and personnel are reminded to avoid bringing these changes to the patient's attention. The nurse explains to the patient and family that most of these changes are expected to disappear with effective treatment.

If the patient experiences eye changes secondary to hyperthyroidism, eye care and protection may become necessary. The patient may need instructions about correct instillation of eye drops or ointment prescribed to soothe the eyes and protect the exposed cornea.

The patient may be embarrassed by the need to eat large meals. Therefore, the nurse arranges for the patient to eat alone if desired and avoids commenting on the large dietary intake of the patient, at the same time making sure that the patient receives sufficient food.

Maintaining Normal Body Temperature

The patient with hyperthyroidism frequently finds a normal room temperature too warm because of an exaggerated metabolic rate and heat production. The environment should be maintained at a cool, comfortable temperature and bedding and clothing changed as needed. Cool baths and cool or cold fluids may provide relief. The reason for the patient's discomfort and the importance of providing a cool environment are explained to the family and staff.

Monitoring and Managing Potential Complications

The patient with hyperthyroidism is monitored closely for signs and symptoms that may be indicative of thyroid storm. Cardiac and respiratory function are assessed by measuring vital signs and cardiac output, ECG monitoring, arterial blood gases, and pulse oximetry. Assessment continues when treatment is initiated because of the potential side effects treatment has on cardiac function. Oxygen is administered to prevent hypoxia, to improve tissue oxygenation, and to meet the high metabolic demands. Intravenous fluids may be necessary to maintain blood glucose levels and to replace lost fluids. Antithyroid medications (PTU or methimazole) may be prescribed to reduce thyroid hormone levels. In addition, propranolol and digitalis may be prescribed to treat cardiac symptoms. If shock develops, strategies to treat shock must be implemented (see Chap. 14).

Hypothyroidism is likely to occur with any one of the treatments used to treat hyperthyroidism. Therefore, the patient must be monitored periodically. Most patients feel a greatly improved sense of well-being after treatment of hyperthyroidism and often fail to continue to take prescribed thyroid replacement therapy. Therefore, an important part of patient and family teaching is instruction about the importance of continued therapy indefinitely after discharge and a discussion of the consequences of failing to take medication.

Promoting Home and Community-Based Care

TEACHING PATIENTS SELF-CARE

The patient with hyperthyroidism is taught how and when to take prescribed medication. Additionally, the patient is instructed about the role of the medication in the broader therapeutic plan. Because of the hyperexcitability and decreased attention span associated with hyperthyroidism, a written plan is provided for the patient's use at home. The type and amount of information given depend on the patient's stress and anxiety levels. The patient and family members receive verbal and written information about the actions and possible side effects of the medications. Adverse effects that should be reported if they occur are pointed out to the patient and family. See the Home Care Teaching Checklist: The Patient With Hyperthyroidism.

If a total or subtotal thyroidectomy is anticipated, the patient is informed about what to expect. This information, however, is repeated as the time of surgery approaches. The patient is advised to avoid those stressful situations that may precipitate thyroid storm.

CONTINUING CARE

Referral for home care, if indicated, allows the home care nurse to assess the home and family environment and the patient's and family's understanding of the importance of adhering to the therapeutic regimen and the recommended follow-up monitoring. The nurse reinforces to the patient and family the importance of long-term follow-up because of the risk for hypothyroidism after thyroidectomy or treatment with antithyroid medications or radioactive iodine. The nurse also assesses the patient for changes indicating return to normal thyroid function and signs and symptoms of hyperthyroidism and hypothyroidism.

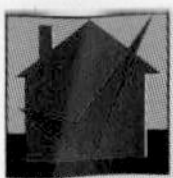

HOME CARE TEACHING CHECKLIST: THE PATIENT WITH HYPERTHYROIDISM

At the completion of the program, the patient or caregiver will be able to:

	Patient	Caregiver
• State present and potential effects of hyperthyroidism on the body	✔	✔
• State precipitating factors and interventions for complications (hypothyroidism, thyroid storm)	✔	✔
• State the purpose, dose, route, schedule, side effects, and precautions of prescribed medications (propylthiouracil, radioactive iodine)	✔	✔
• State the need to contact health care provider before taking over-the-counter medications	✔	✔
• State need for regular follow-up visits with health care provider	✔	✔
• Identify the need for planned rest periods and methods to improve sleep patterns	✔	✔
• Identify the need for increased dietary intake until weight stabilizes	✔	✔
• Identify areas of physical and emotional stress	✔	✔
• State that emotional lability is part of disease process	✔	✔
• Describe the potential benefits and risks of surgical intervention or radioactive iodine therapy	✔	✔
• Identify potential for menstrual irregularities, increased risk for osteoporosis, and family planning need for women	✔	✔
• State need to wear medical identification and carry medical information card	✔	✔

Evaluation

Expected Outcomes

Expected outcomes may include:

1. Improves nutritional status
   a. Reports adequate dietary intake and decreased feelings of hunger
   b. Identifies high-calorie, high-protein foods; identifies foods to be avoided
   c. Avoids use of alcohol and other stimulants
   d. Reports decreased episodes of diarrhea
2. Demonstrates effective coping methods in dealing with family, friends, and coworkers
   a. Explains reasons for irritability and emotional instability
   b. Avoids stressful situations, events, and people
   c. Participates in relaxing, nonstressful activities
3. Achieves increased self-esteem
   a. Verbalizes feelings about self and illness
   b. Describes feelings of frustration and loss of control to others
   c. Describes reasons for increased appetite
4. Maintains normal body temperature
5. Absence of complications
   a. Serum thyroid hormone and TSH levels are within normal limits
   b. Identifies signs and symptoms of thyroid storm and hypothyroidism
   c. Vital signs and results of ECG, arterial blood gases, and pulse oximetry within normal limits
   d. States importance of regular follow-up and lifelong maintenance of prescribed therapy

Thyroiditis

Thyroiditis is inflammation of the thyroid gland; it can be acute, subacute, or chronic in nature. Each type of thyroiditis is characterized by inflammation, fibrosis, or lymphocytic infiltration of the thyroid gland.

Acute Thyroiditis

Acute thyroiditis is a rare disorder caused by infection of the thyroid gland by bacteria, fungi, mycobacteria, or parasites. *Staphylococcus aureus* and other staphylococci are the most common causes. Infection typically causes anterior neck pain and swelling, fever, dysphagia, and dysphonia. Pharyngitis or pharyngeal pain is often present. Examination may reveal warmth, erythema (redness), and tenderness of the thyroid gland. Treatment of acute thyroiditis includes antimicrobial agents and fluid replacement. Surgical incision and drainage may be needed if an abscess is present.

Subacute Thyroiditis

Subacute thyroiditis may be subacute granulomatous thyroiditis (deQuervain's thyroiditis) or painless thyroiditis (silent thyroiditis or subacute lymphocytic thyroiditis).

Subacute granulomatous thyroiditis is an inflammatory disorder of the thyroid gland that predominantly affects women 40 to 50 years of age (Falk, 1997). It presents as a painful swelling in the anterior neck that lasts 1 to 2 months and then disappears spontaneously without residual effect. It often follows a respiratory infection. The thyroid enlarges symmetrically and may be painful. The overlying skin is often reddened and warm. Swallowing may be difficult and uncomfortable. Irritability, nervousness, insomnia, and weight loss—manifestations of hyperthyroidism—are common, and many patients experience chills and fever as well.

The purpose of treatment is to control the inflammation. In general, nonsteroidal anti-inflammatory drugs (NSAIDs) are used to relieve neck pain. Acetylsalicylic acid (aspirin) is avoided if symptoms of hyperthyroidism occur because it displaces thyroid hormone from its binding sites and increases the amount of circulating hormone. Beta-blocking agents may be used to control symptoms of hyperthyroidism; antithyroid agents, which block the synthesis of T_4 and T_3, are not effective in thyroiditis because the associated thyrotoxicosis results from the release of stored thyroid hormones rather than from their increased synthesis. In more severe cases, oral corticosteroids may be prescribed to reduce swelling and relieve pain; however, they do not usually affect the underlying cause. In some cases, temporary hypothyroidism may develop and may necessitate thyroid hormone therapy. Follow-up monitoring is necessary to document the patient's return to a euthyroid state.

Painless thyroiditis (subacute lymphocytic thyroiditis) often occurs in the postpartum period and is thought to be an autoimmune process. Symptoms of hyperthyroidism or hypothyroidism are possible. Treatment is directed at symptoms, and yearly follow-up is recommended to determine the patient's need for treatment of subsequent hypothyroidism.

Chronic Thyroiditis (Hashimoto's Disease)

Chronic thyroiditis, which occurs most frequently in women 30 to 50 years of age, has been termed Hashimoto's disease, or chronic lymphocytic thyroiditis; its diagnosis is based on the histologic appearance of the inflamed gland. In contrast to acute thyroiditis, the chronic forms are usually not accompanied by pain, pressure symptoms, or fever, and thyroid activity is usually normal or low rather than increased.

Cell-mediated immunity may play a significant role in the pathogenesis of thyroiditis, and there may be a genetic predisposition to it. If untreated, the disease runs a slow, progressive course, leading eventually to hypothyroidism.

The objective of treatment is to reduce the size of the thyroid gland and prevent hypothyroidism. Thyroid hormone therapy is prescribed to reduce thyroid activity and the production of thyroglobulin. If hypothyroid symptoms are present, thyroid hormone is prescribed. Surgery may be required if pressure symptoms persist.

Thyroid Tumors

Tumors of the thyroid gland are classified on the basis of being benign or malignant, the presence or absence of associated thyrotoxicosis, and the diffuse or irregular quality of the glandular enlargement. If the enlargement is sufficient to cause a visible swelling in the neck, the tumor is referred to as a goiter.

Goiter

All grades of goiter are encountered, from those that are barely visible to those producing disfigurement. Some are symmetric and diffuse; others are nodular. Some are accompanied by hyperthyroidism, in which case they are described as *toxic;* others are associated with a euthyroid state and are called *nontoxic* goiters.

ENDEMIC (IODINE-DEFICIENT) GOITER

The most common type of goiter, encountered chiefly in geographic regions where the natural supply of iodine is deficient (eg, the Great Lakes areas of the United States), is the so-called simple or colloid goiter. In addition to being caused by an iodine deficiency, simple goiter may be caused by an intake of large quantities of goitrogenic substances in patients with unusually susceptible glands. These substances include excessive amounts of iodine or lithium, which is used in treating bipolar disorders.

Simple goiter represents a compensatory hypertrophy of the thyroid gland, caused by stimulation by the pituitary gland. The pituitary gland produces thyrotropin or TSH, a hormone that controls the release of thyroid hormone from the thyroid gland. Its production increases if there is subnormal thyroid activity, as when insufficient iodine is available for production of the thyroid hormone. Such goiters usually cause no symptoms, except for the swelling in the neck, which may result in tracheal compression when excessive.

Many goiters of this type recede after iodine imbalance is corrected. Supplementary iodine, such as SSKI, is prescribed to suppress the pituitary's thyroid-stimulating activity. When surgery is recommended, risk for postoperative complications is minimized by ensuring a preoperative euthyroid state by treatment with antithyroid medications and iodide to reduce the size and vascularity of the goiter.

Simple or endemic goiter can be prevented by providing children in iodine-poor regions with iodine compounds. If the mean iodine intake is less than 40 μg/day, the thyroid gland hypertrophies. The World Health Organization recommends that salt be iodized to a concentration of 1 part in 100,000, which is adequate for the prevention of endemic goiter. In the United States, salt is iodized to 1 part in 10,000. The introduction of iodized salt has been the single most effective means of preventing goiter in at-risk populations.

NODULAR GOITER

Some thyroid glands are nodular because of areas of hyperplasia (overgrowth). No symptoms may arise as a result of this condition, but, not uncommonly, these nodules slowly increase in size, with some descending into the thorax, where they cause local pressure symptoms. Some nodules become malignant, and some are associated with a hyperthyroid state. Thus, the patient with many thyroid nodules may eventually require surgery.

Thyroid Cancer

Cancer of the thyroid is much less prevalent than other forms of cancer; however, it accounts for 90% of endocrine malignancies. According to the American Cancer Society (1999), about 18,000 new cases of thyroid cancer are diagnosed each year. Women account for 13,500 of the new cases and men, 4600. About 700 women and 500 men die annually from this malignancy. There are several types of cancer of the thyroid gland; the type determines the course and prognosis (Table 38-3).

External radiation of the head, neck, or chest in infancy and childhood increases the risk of thyroid carcinoma. Between 1940 and 1960, radiation therapy was occasionally used to shrink enlarged tonsillar and adenoid tissue, to treat acne, or to reduce an enlarged thymus. For people exposed to external radiation in childhood, there appears to be an increased incidence in thyroid cancer 5 to 40 years after irradiation. Consequently, people who underwent such treatment should consult a physician, request an isotope thyroid scan as part of the evaluation, follow recommended treatment of abnormalities of the gland, and continue with annual checkups.

ASSESSMENT AND DIAGNOSTIC FINDINGS

Lesions that are single, hard, and fixed on palpation or associated with cervical lymphadenopathy suggest malignancy. Thyroid function tests may be helpful in evaluating thyroid nodules and masses; however, their results are rarely conclusive. Needle biopsy of the thyroid gland is used as an outpatient procedure to make a diagnosis of thyroid cancer, to differentiate cancerous thyroid nodules from noncancerous nodules, and to stage the cancer if detected. The procedure is safe and usually requires only a local anesthetic. Patients who undergo the procedure are followed closely, however, because cancerous tissues may be missed during the procedure. A second type of aspiration or biopsy uses a large-bore needle rather than the fine needle used in standard biopsy; it may be used when

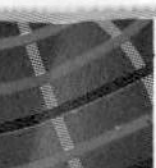

TABLE 38•3 Types of Thyroid Cancers

Type of Thyroid Cancer	Incidence (%)	Characteristics
Papillary adenocarcinoma	70	Most common and least aggressive Asymptomatic nodule in a normal gland Starts in childhood or early adult life, remains localized Metastasizes along the lymphatics if untreated More aggressive in the elderly
Follicular adenocarcinoma	15	Appears after 40 years of age Encapsulated; feels elastic or rubbery on palpation Spreads through the bloodstream to bone, liver, and lung Prognosis is not as favorable as for papillary adenocarcinoma
Medullary	5	Appears after 50 years of age Occurs as part of multiple endocrine neoplasia (MEN) Hormone-producing tumor causing endocrine dysfunction symptoms Metastasizes by lymphatics and bloodstream Moderate survival rate
Anaplastic	5	50% of anaplastic thyroid carcinomas occur in patients older than 60 years Hard, irregular mass that grows quickly and spreads by direct invasion to adjacent tissues May be painful and tender Survival for patients with anaplastic cancer is usually less than 6 months
Thyroid lymphoma	5	Appears after age 40 years May have history of goiter, hoarseness, dyspnea, pain, and pressure Good prognosis

the results of the standard biopsy are inconclusive or with rapidly growing tumors. Additional diagnostic studies include ultrasound, MRI, CT scans, thyroid scans, radioactive iodine uptake studies, and thyroid suppression tests.

MEDICAL MANAGEMENT

The treatment of choice of thyroid carcinoma is surgical removal. Total or near-total thyroidectomy is performed when possible. Modified neck dissection or more extensive radical neck dissection is performed if there is lymph node involvement. Efforts are made to spare parathyroid tissue to reduce the risk for postoperative hypocalcemia and tetany. After surgery, ablation procedures are carried out with radioactive iodine to eradicate residual thyroid tissue if the tumor is radiosensitive. Radioactive iodine also maximizes the chance of discovering thyroid metastasis at a later date if total-body scans are carried out.

After surgery, thyroid hormone is administered in suppressive doses to lower the levels of TSH to a euthyroid state. If remaining thyroid tissue is inadequate to produce sufficient thyroid hormone, thyroxine is required permanently.

Radiation to the thyroid or tissues of the neck may be administered by several routes, including oral administration of radioactive iodine and external administration of radiation therapy. The patient who receives external sources of radiation therapy is at risk for mucositis, dryness of the mouth, dysphagia, redness of the skin, anorexia, and fatigue (see Chap. 15 for discussion of these side effects of radiation.) Chemotherapy is infrequently used to treat thyroid cancer.

Patients whose thyroid cancer is detected early and who are appropriately treated usually do very well. Papillary cancer, the most common and least aggressive tumor, has a 10-year survival rate greater than 90%. Long-term survival is also common in follicular cancer, a more aggressive form of thyroid cancer (Noble, 1996). Continued thyroid hormone therapy and periodic follow-up, however, are important to ensure the patient's well-being.

Postoperatively, the patient is instructed to take exogenous thyroid hormone to prevent the occurrence of hypothyroidism. Later follow-up includes clinical assessment for recurrence of nodules or masses in the neck and signs of hoarseness, dysphagia, or dyspnea. Total-body scans are performed 2 to 4 months after surgery to detect residual thyroid tissue or metastatic disease. Thyroid hormones are stopped for about 6 weeks before the tests. Care must be taken to avoid iodine-containing foods and contrast agents. A repeat scan is done 1 year after the initial surgery. If measurements are stable, a final scan is obtained in 3 to 5 years.

FT_4, TSH, serum calcium, and phosphorus levels are monitored to determine whether the thyroid hormone supplementation is adequate and to note whether calcium balance is maintained.

Although local and systemic reactions to radiation may occur and may include neutropenia or thrombocytopenia, these complications are rare when radioactive iodine is used. Patients who undergo surgery that is combined with radioiodine have a higher survival rate than those undergoing surgery alone. Patient teaching emphasizes the importance of taking prescribed medications and following recommendations for follow-up monitoring. The patient who is undergoing radiation therapy is also instructed in assessment and management of side effects of treatment.

Radiation-Induced Thyroid Damage and Cancer

The thyroid gland has a very efficient mechanism to remove iodine from the bloodstream and concentrate or "trap" it for subsequent synthesis of thyroid hormone. The effectiveness of this mechanism to concentrate iodide is reflected in a concentration of iodide 20 to 40 times the concentration of iodide in the plasma.

If milk and other food sources become contaminated with radioactivity as a result of a nuclear detonation or a nuclear power plant accident, the radioactive iodide would become concentrated in the thyroid gland at very high concentration and would irradiate the thyroid gland, increasing the risk for thyroid gland cancer.

Therefore, in communities exposed to increased radioactivity, attempts have been made to block the uptake of radioactive iodide by flooding or saturating the thyroid gland with nonradioactive iodide.

Administration of SSKI or other iodide preparations as soon as possible after exposure almost completely inhibits thyroid absorption of the radioactive iodide and promotes rapid excretion of any that is absorbed.

Thyroidectomy

Partial or complete thyroidectomy may be carried out as primary treatment of thyroid carcinoma, hyperthyroidism, or hyperparathyroidism. The type and extent of the surgery depend on the diagnosis, goal of surgery, and prognosis.

If the patient is undergoing surgery for treatment of hyperthyroidism, he or she is treated with appropriate medications to return the thyroid hormone levels and metabolic rate to normal and to reduce the risk for thyroid storm and hemorrhage during the postoperative period. Medications that may prolong clotting (eg, aspirin) are stopped several weeks before surgery to minimize the risk for postoperative bleeding.

Nursing Management

PROVIDING PREOPERATIVE CARE

Important preoperative goals are to gain the confidence of the patient and to reduce anxiety. Often, the patient's home has been made tense by the patient's restlessness, irritability, and nervousness secondary to hyperthyroidism. Efforts are necessary to protect the patient from such tension and stress to avoid precipitating thyroid storm. If the patient reports increased stress when with family or friends, suggestions are made to limit contact with them. Quiet and relaxing forms of recreation or occupational therapy may be helpful.

The patient is instructed about the importance of a diet high in carbohydrate and protein foods. A high daily caloric intake is necessary because of the increased metabolic activity and rapid depletion of glycogen reserves. Supplementary vitamins, particularly thiamine and ascorbic acid, may be prescribed. The patient is reminded to avoid tea, coffee, cola, and other stimulants.

Preoperative Preparation. If diagnostic testing is performed before surgery, the patient is informed of the purpose of the test and the preoperative preparations that can be expected to reduce anxiety. In addition, special efforts are made to ensure a good night's rest preceding surgery, although many patients are admitted to the hospital on the day of surgery.

Preoperative teaching includes demonstrating to the patient how to support the neck with the hands after surgery to prevent stress on the incision; that is, raising the elbows and placing the hands behind the neck provide support and reduce strain and tension on the neck muscles and the surgical incision.

PROVIDING POSTOPERATIVE CARE

The patient is moved and turned carefully to support the head and avoid tension on the sutures. The most comfortable position is the semi-Fowler's position with the head elevated and supported by pillows. Analgesics are administered as prescribed for pain. The nurse should anticipate apprehension in the patient and inform him or her that oxygen will assist breathing and provide humidity.

Intravenous fluids are administered during the immediate postoperative period; water may be given by mouth as soon as nausea subsides. Usually, there is a little difficulty in swallowing; initially, cold fluids and ice may be taken better than other fluids. Often, patients prefer a soft diet to a liquid diet in the immediate postoperative period.

The surgical dressings are assessed periodically and reinforced when necessary. When the patient is in a recumbent position, the sides and the back of the neck as well as the anterior dressing must be observed for bleeding. In addition to monitoring the pulse and the blood pressure for any indication of internal bleeding, it is also important to be alert for complaints of sensation of pressure or fullness at the incision site. Such symptoms may indicate hemorrhage and hematoma formation subcutaneously and should be reported.

Difficulty in respiration occurs as a result of edema of the glottis, hematoma formation, or an injury to the recurrent laryngeal nerve. This complication requires that an airway be inserted. Therefore, a tracheostomy set is kept at the patient's bedside at all times, and the surgeon is summoned at the first indication of respiratory distress. If the respiratory distress is due to hematoma formation, surgical evacuation is required.

The patient is advised to talk as little as possible, but when the patient does speak, any voice changes are noted because they might indicate injury to the recurrent laryngeal nerve, which lies just behind the thyroid next to the trachea.

An overbed table may be used to provide easy access to those materials and items that are needed frequently, such as paper tissues, water pitcher and glass, and a small emesis basin. These are kept within easy reach, so that the patient will not need to turn the head to reach for them. It is also convenient to use this table when vapor-mist inhalations are prescribed for the relief of excessive mucous secretions.

The patient is usually permitted out of bed as soon as possible and is encouraged to eat foods that are easily eaten. A well-balanced, high-calorie diet is prescribed to promote weight gain. Sutures or skin clips are usually removed on the second day. The patient may be discharged from the hospital the day of surgery or soon afterward if the postoperative course is uncomplicated.

MONITORING AND MANAGING POTENTIAL COMPLICATIONS

Hemorrhage, hematoma formation, edema of the glottis, and injury to the recurrent laryngeal nerve are complications that have been reviewed previously. Occasionally, in thyroid surgery, the parathyroid glands may be injured or removed, producing a disturbance of the calcium metabolism of the body. As the blood calcium level falls, hyperirritability of the nerves occurs, with spasms of the hands and feet and muscular twitchings. This group of symptoms is termed tetany, and its appearance should be reported at once because laryngospasm, although rare, may occur and obstruct the patient's airway. Tetany of this type is usually treated by the intravenous administration of calcium gluconate. This calcium abnormality may be temporary after thyroidectomy.

PROMOTING HOME AND COMMUNITY-BASED CARE

Teaching Patients Self-Care. The patient may be discharged the evening of surgery or within 1 or 2 days. Therefore, the patient and family need to be knowledgeable about the signs and symptoms of complications that may occur and those that should be reported. Strategies are suggested for managing postoperative pain at home and for increasing humidification. The necessity for rest, relaxation, and nutrition is explained to both the patient and the family. The patient is permitted to resume former activities and responsibilities completely once recovered from surgery.

Continuing Care. If indicated, a referral to home care is made; a visit by the home care nurse enables assessment of the patient's recovery from surgery. Additionally, the surgical incision is assessed, and instruction about limiting activities that put strain on the incision and sutures is reinforced. Family responsibilities and factors relating to the home environment that produce emotional tension have often been implicated as precipitating causes of thyrotoxicosis. A home visit provides an opportunity to evaluate these factors and to suggest ways to improve the home and family environment. Specific instructions are given regarding follow-up visits to the physician or the clinic, which are important for monitoring the patient's thyroid status.

THE PARATHYROID GLANDS

The parathyroid glands, normally four in number, are situated in the neck, embedded in the posterior aspect of the thyroid gland (Fig. 38-5). These small glands are easily overlooked and can be removed accidentally at the time of thyroid surgery. Inadvertent surgical removal is the most common cause of hypoparathyroidism.

Parathormone, the protein hormone from the parathyroid glands, regulates calcium and phosphorus metabolism. Increased secretion of parathormone results in increased calcium absorption from the kidney, the intestine, and bones, thereby raising the blood calcium level. Some actions of this hormone are increased by the presence of vitamin D. Parathormone also tends to lower the blood phosphorus level.

Excess parathormone can result in markedly elevated levels of serum calcium, a potentially life-threatening situation. When the product of serum calcium and serum phosphorus (calcium × phosphorus) rises, calcium phosphate may precipitate in various organs of the body and cause tissue calcification.

The output of parathormone is regulated by the serum level of ionized calcium. Increased serum calcium results in decreased parathormone secretion, forming a negative feedback system.

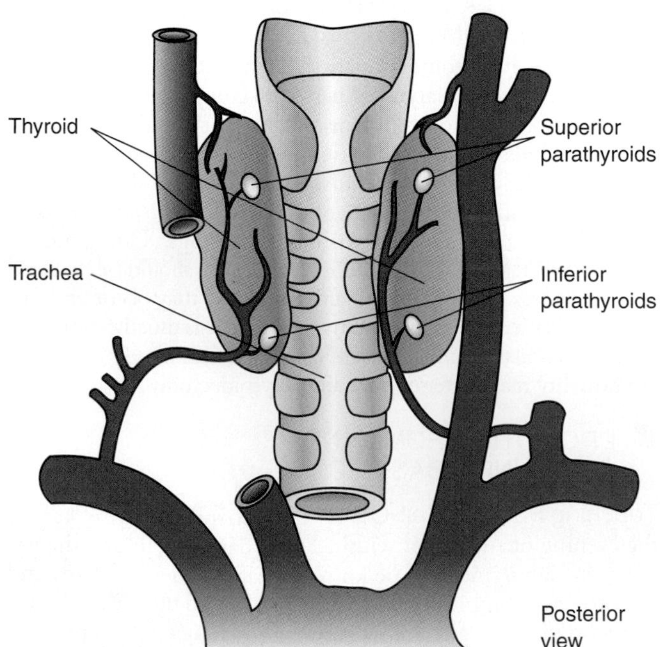

FIGURE 38•5 The parathyroid glands are located behind the thyroid gland. The parathyroids may be embedded in the thyroid tissue.

Hyperparathyroidism

Hyperparathyroidism, which is caused by overproduction of parathyroid hormone by the parathyroid glands, is characterized by bone decalcification and the development of renal stones containing calcium.

Primary hyperparathyroidism occurs two to four times more often in women than in men and is most frequently seen in patients between 60 and 70 years of age. About 100,000 new cases of hyperparathyroidism are detected each year in the United States (NIH Consensus Statement, 1990; Wilson, Foster, Kronenberg, & Larsen, 1998). Incidence of the disease is rare in children younger than 15 years of age and increases 10-fold between the ages of 15 and 65 years. Half of patients currently diagnosed with hyperparathyroidism do not have symptoms.

Secondary hyperparathyroidism with similar manifestations occurs in patients with chronic renal failure and so-called renal rickets as a result of phosphorus retention, increased stimulation of the parathyroid glands, and increased parathyroid hormone secretion.

Clinical Manifestations

The patient may have no symptoms or may experience signs and symptoms resulting from involvement of several body systems. Apathy, fatigue, muscular weakness, nausea, vomiting, constipation, hypertension, and cardiac dysrhythmias, may occur—all attributable to an increased concentration of calcium in the blood. Psychological manifestations may vary from emotional irritability and neurosis to psychoses caused by the direct effect of calcium on the brain and nervous system. An increase in calcium produces a decrease in the excitation potential of nerve and muscle tissue.

The formation of stones in one or both kidneys, related to the increased urinary excretion of calcium and phosphorus, is one of the important complications of hyperparathyroidism and occurs in 55% of patients with primary hyperparathyroidism. Renal damage results from the precipitation of calcium phosphate in the renal pelvis and parenchyma, resulting in renal calculi (kidney stones), obstruction, pyelonephritis, and renal failure.

Musculoskeletal symptoms accompanying hyperparathyroidism may result from demineralization of the bones or bone tumors composed of benign giant cells resulting from overgrowth of osteoclasts. The patient may develop skeletal pain and tenderness, especially of the back and joints; pain on weight bearing; pathologic fractures; deformities; and shortening of body stature. Bone loss attributable to hyperparathyroidism increases the risk for fracture.

The incidence of peptic ulcer and pancreatitis is increased with hyperparathyroidism and may be responsible for many of the gastrointestinal symptoms that occur.

Assessment and Diagnostic Findings

Primary hyperparathyroidism is diagnosed by persistent elevation of serum calcium levels and an elevated level of parathormone. Radioimmunoassays for parathormone are sensitive and differentiate primary hyperparathyroidism from other causes of hypercalcemia in more than 90% of patients with elevated serum calcium levels. An elevated serum calcium level alone is a nonspecific finding because serum levels may be altered by diet, medications, and renal and bone changes. Bone changes may be detected on x-ray or bone scan in advanced disease. The double antibody parathyroid hormone test is used to distinguish between primary hyperparathyroidism and malignancy as a cause of hypercalcemia. Ultrasound, MRI, thallium scan, and fine-needle biopsy have been used to evaluate the function of the parathyroids and to localize parathyroid cysts, adenomas, or hyperplasia.

Complications of Hyperparathyroidism: Hypercalcemic Crisis

Acute hypercalcemic crisis can occur in hyperparathyroidism. This occurs with extreme elevation of serum calcium levels. Serum calcium levels higher than 15 mg/dL (3.7 mmol/L) result in neurologic, cardiovascular, and renal symptoms that can be life-threatening.

Treatment includes rehydration with large volumes of intravenous fluids, diuretic agents to promote renal excretion of excess calcium, and phosphate therapy to correct hypophosphatemia and decrease serum calcium levels by promoting calcium deposit in bone and reducing gastrointestinal absorption of calcium. Cytotoxic agents (mithramycin), calcitonin, and dialysis may be used in emergency situations to decrease serum calcium levels quickly. The patient in acute hypercalcemic crisis requires close monitoring for life-threatening complications and reversal of serum calcium levels.

A combination of calcitonin and corticosteroids has been administered in emergencies to reduce the serum calcium level by increasing calcium deposition in bone. Other agents that may be administered to decrease serum calcium levels include bisphosphonates (eg, etidronate [Didronel], pamidronate).

The patient requires expert assessment and care to minimize complications and reverse the life-threatening hypercalcemia. Medications are administered with care, and attention is given to fluid balance to promote return of normal fluid and electrolyte balance. Supportive measures are necessary for the patient and family.

Medical Management

The insidious onset and chronic nature of hyperparathyroidism and its diverse and often vague symptoms may result in depression and frustration. The family may have considered the patient's illness to be psychosomatic. An awareness of the course of the disorder and an understanding approach by the nurse may help the patient and family to deal with their reactions and feelings. The recommended treatment of primary hyperparathyroidism is the surgical removal of abnormal parathyroid tissue. In some patients without symptoms and with only mildly elevated serum calcium levels and normal renal function, surgery may be delayed and the patient followed closely for worsening of hypercalcemia, the deterioration of bone, renal impairment, or the development of kidney stones (renal calculi).

HYDRATION THERAPY

Because kidney involvement is possible, patients with hyperparathyroidism are at risk for renal calculi. Therefore, a fluid intake of 2000 mL or more is encouraged to help prevent calculus formation. Cranberry juice is suggested because it may lower urinary pH. It can be added to juices and ginger ale for variety. The patient is instructed to report other manifestations of renal calculi, such as abdominal pain and hematuria. Thiazide diuretics are avoided because they decrease the renal excretion of calcium and further elevate serum calcium levels. Because of the risk of hypercalcemic crisis, the patient is instructed to avoid dehydration and seek immediate health care if conditions that commonly produce dehydration (ie, vomiting, diarrhea) occur.

MOBILITY

Mobility of the patient, with walking or use of a rocking chair, is encouraged as much as possible because bones subjected to normal stress give up less calcium. Bed rest increases calcium excretion and risk for renal calculi. Oral phosphates lower the serum calcium level in some patients. Long-term use is not recommended because of risk for ectopic calcium phosphate deposits in soft tissues.

DIET AND MEDICATIONS

Nutritional needs are met, but the patient is advised to avoid a diet with restricted or excess calcium. If the patient has a coexisting peptic ulcer, specifically prescribed antacids and protein feedings are necessary. Because anorexia is common, efforts are made to improve the patient's appetite. Prune juice, stool softeners, and physical activity, along with increased fluid intake, help to offset constipation, which is common postoperatively.

Nursing Management

The nursing management of the patient undergoing parathyroidectomy is essentially the same as that of a patient undergoing thyroidectomy. However, the previously described precautions about dehydration, immobility, and diet are particularly important in the patient awaiting and recovering from parathyroidectomy. Although not all parathyroid tissue is removed during surgery in an effort to control the calcium–phosphorus balance, the patient must be monitored closely to detect symptoms of tetany, which may be an early postoperative complication. Most patients quickly regain function of the remaining parathyroid tissue and experience only mild, transient postoperative hypocalcemia. In patients with significant bone disease or bone changes, a more prolonged period of hypocalcemia should be anticipated. The patient and family are reminded about the importance of follow-up to ensure return of serum calcium levels to normal. See the Home Care Teaching Checklist: The Patient With Hyperparathyroidism.

Hypoparathyroidism

The most common cause of hypoparathyroidism is inadequate secretion of parathyroid hormone after interruption of the blood supply or surgical removal of parathyroid gland tissue during thyroidectomy, parathyroidectomy, or radical neck dissection. Atrophy of the parathyroid glands of unknown cause is a less common cause of hypoparathyroidism.

Pathophysiology

Symptoms of hypoparathyroidism are caused by a deficiency of parathormone that results in elevated blood phosphate (hyperphosphatemia) and decreased blood calcium (hypocalcemia) levels. In the absence of parathormone, there is decreased intestinal absorption of dietary calcium and decreased resorption of calcium from bone and through the renal tubules. Decreased renal excretion of phosphate causes hypophosphaturia, and low serum calcium levels result in hypocalciuria.

Home Care Teaching Checklist: The Patient With Hyperparathyroidism

At the completion of the program, the patient or caregiver will be able to:

	Patient	Caregiver
• State present and potential effects of hyperparathyroidism on the body	✔	✔
• State precipitating factors and interventions for complications	✔	✔
• State importance of regular follow-up visits with health care provider	✔	✔
• Describe potential benefits and risks of parathyroidectomy	✔	✔
• State the purpose, dose, route, schedule, side effects, and precautions of prescribed medications (loop diuretics, phosphate, calcitonin, mithramycin)	✔	✔
• State the need to contact health care provider before taking over-the-counter medication containing calcium	✔	✔
• State need to take pain medications on a scheduled basis	✔	✔
• Describe nonpharmacologic methods of pain management	✔	✔
• Identify safety hazards and methods of injury prevention	✔	✔
• Identify areas of activity limitations and impact on lifestyle	✔	✔
• State need for increased fluid intake and diet low in calcium and vitamin D	✔	✔

Clinical Manifestations

Hypocalcemia causes irritability of the neuromuscular system and contributes to the chief symptom of hypoparathyroidism, tetany–a general muscular hypertonia, with tremor and spasmodic or uncoordinated contractions occurring with or without efforts to make voluntary movements. In latent tetany, there is numbness, tingling, and cramps in the extremities, and the patient complains of stiffness in the hands and feet. In overt tetany, the signs include bronchospasm, laryngeal spasm, carpopedal spasm (flexion of the elbows and wrists and extension of the carpophalangeal joints), dysphagia, photophobia, cardiac dysrhythmias, and seizures. Other symptoms include anxiety, irritability, depression, and even delirium. ECG changes and hypotension may also occur.

Assessment and Diagnostic Findings

Latent tetany is suggested by a positive **Trousseau's sign** or a positive **Chvostek's sign**. **Trousseau's sign** is positive when carpopedal spasm is induced by occluding the blood flow to the arm for 3 minutes with use of a blood pressure cuff. **Chvostek's sign** is positive when a sharp tapping over the facial nerve just in front of the parotid gland and anterior to the ear causes spasm or twitching of the mouth, nose, and eye.

The diagnosis is often difficult because of vague symptoms, such as aches and pains. Therefore, laboratory studies are especially helpful. Tetany develops at serum calcium levels of 5 to 6 mg/dL (1.2 to 1.5 mmol/L) or lower. Serum phosphate levels are increased, and x-rays of bone show increased density. Calcification is detected on x-rays of subcutaneous or paraspinal basal ganglia of the brain.

Medical Management

The goal of therapy is to raise the serum calcium level to 9 to 10 mg/dL (2.2 to 2.5 mmol/L) and to eliminate the symptoms of hypoparathyroidism and hypocalcemia. When hypocalcemia and tetany occur after a thyroidectomy, the immediate treatment is to administer calcium gluconate intravenously. If this does not decrease neuromuscular irritability and seizure activity immediately, sedatives, such as pentobarbital, may be administered.

Parenteral parathormone can be administered to treat acute hypoparathyroidism with tetany. The high incidence of allergic reactions to injections of parathormone, however, limits its use to acute episodes of hypocalcemia. The patient receiving parathormone is monitored closely for allergic reactions and changes in serum calcium levels.

Because of neuromuscular irritability, the patient with hypocalcemia and tetany requires an environment that is free of noise, sudden drafts, bright lights, or sudden movement. Tracheostomy or mechanical ventilation may become necessary, along with bronchodilating medications, if the patient develops respiratory distress.

Therapy for the patient with chronic hypoparathyroidism is determined after serum calcium levels are obtained. A diet high in calcium and low in phosphorus is prescribed. Although milk, milk products, and egg yolk are high in calcium, they are restricted because they also contain high levels of phosphorus. Spinach is also avoided because it contains oxalate, which would form insoluble calcium substances. Oral tablets of calcium salts, such as calcium gluconate, may supplement the diet. Aluminum hydroxide gel or aluminum carbonate (Gelusil, Amphojel) is also administered after meals to bind phosphate and promote its excretion through the gastrointestinal tract.

Variable dosages of a vitamin D preparation—dihydrotachysterol (AT 10 or Hytakerol), ergocalciferol (vitamin D_2), cholecalciferol (vitamin D_3)—are usually required and enhance calcium absorption from the gastrointestinal tract.

Nursing Management

Nursing management of the patient with possible *acute* hypoparathyroidism includes the following:

- Care of postoperative patients having thyroidectomy, parathyroidectomy, and radical neck dissection is directed toward detecting early signs of hypocalcemia and anticipating signs of tetany, seizures, and respiratory difficulties.
- Calcium gluconate is kept at the bedside with equipment necessary for intravenous administration. If the patient has cardiac problems, is subject to dysrhythmias, or is receiving digitalis, calcium gluconate is administered slowly and cautiously.
- Calcium and digitalis increase systolic contraction; furthermore, they potentiate each other. This may produce potentially fatal dysrhythmias. Consequently, the cardiac patient requires continuous cardiac monitoring and careful assessment.

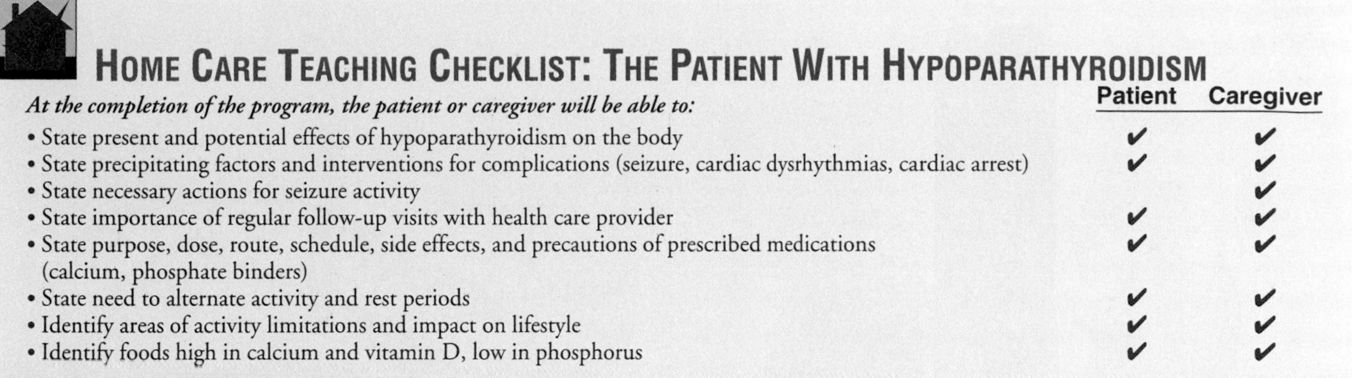

HOME CARE TEACHING CHECKLIST: THE PATIENT WITH HYPOPARATHYROIDISM

At the completion of the program, the patient or caregiver will be able to:	Patient	Caregiver
• State present and potential effects of hypoparathyroidism on the body	✔	✔
• State precipitating factors and interventions for complications (seizure, cardiac dysrhythmias, cardiac arrest)	✔	✔
• State necessary actions for seizure activity		✔
• State importance of regular follow-up visits with health care provider	✔	✔
• State purpose, dose, route, schedule, side effects, and precautions of prescribed medications (calcium, phosphate binders)	✔	✔
• State need to alternate activity and rest periods	✔	✔
• Identify areas of activity limitations and impact on lifestyle	✔	✔
• Identify foods high in calcium and vitamin D, low in phosphorus	✔	✔

An important aspect of nursing care is teaching about medications and diet therapy. The patient needs to know the reason for high calcium and low phosphate intake and the symptoms of hypocalcemia and hypercalcemia and should contact the physician immediately if these symptoms occur. See the Home Care Teaching Checklist: The Patient With Hypoparathyroidism.

THE ADRENAL GLANDS

There are two adrenal glands in the human, each attached to the upper portion of a kidney. Each adrenal gland is, in reality, two endocrine glands with separate, independent functions. The adrenal medulla at the center of the gland secretes catecholamines, and the outer portion of the gland, the adrenal cortex, secretes **corticosteroids** (Fig. 38-6). The secretion of hormones from the adrenal cortex is regulated by the hypothalamic-pituitary-adrenal axis. The hypothalamus secretes corticotropin-releasing hormone (CRH), which in turn stimulates the pituitary gland to secrete ACTH. ACTH then stimulates the adrenal cortex to secrete glucocorticoid hormone (cortisol). Increased levels of the adrenal hormone then inhibit the production or secretion of CRH and ACTH. This system is an example of a negative feedback mechanism.

Adrenal Medulla

The adrenal medulla functions as part of the autonomic nervous system. Stimulation of preganglionic sympathetic nerve fibers, which travel directly to the cells of the adrenal medulla, causes release of the catecholamine hormones epinephrine and norepinephrine. About 90% of the secretion of the human adrenal medulla is epinephrine (also called adrenaline). Catecholamines regulate metabolic pathways to promote catabolism of stored fuels to meet caloric needs from endogenous sources. The major effects of epinephrine release are to prepare to meet a challenge (fight-or-flight response). Secretion of epinephrine causes decreased blood flow to tissues that are not needed in emergency situations, such as the gastrointestinal tract, and causes increased blood flow to those tissues that are important for effective fight or flight, such as cardiac and skeletal muscle. Catecholamines also induce release of free fatty acids, increase the basal metabolic rate, and elevate the blood glucose level.

Adrenal Cortex

A functioning adrenal cortex is necessary for life, although survival in its absence is possible by appropriate replacement with exogenous adrenocortical hormones. The three kinds of steroid hormones produced by the adrenal cortex are **glucocorticoids**, the prototype of which is hydrocortisone; **mineralocorticoids**, mainly aldosterone; and sex hormones, mainly **androgens** (male sex hormones).

Glucocorticoids

The glucocorticoids are given their name because they have an important influence on glucose metabolism; increased hydrocortisone secretion results in elevated blood glucose levels. However, the glucocorticoids have major effects on the metabolism of almost all organs of the body. Glucocorticoids are secreted from the adrenal cortex in response to the release of ACTH from the anterior lobe of the pituitary gland. This system represents an example of negative feedback. The presence of glucocorticoids in the blood inhibits the release of corticotropin-releasing factor from the hypothalamus and also inhibits ACTH secretion from the pituitary. The resultant decrease in ACTH secretion causes diminished release of glucocorticoids from the adrenal cortex.

Glucocorticoids (in the form of corticosteroids) are frequently administered to inhibit the inflammatory response to tissue injury and suppress allergic manifestations. Their side effects include development of diabetes mellitus, osteoporosis, peptic ulcer, increased protein breakdown resulting in muscle wasting and poor wound healing, and redistribution of body fat.

The presence of large amounts of exogenously administered glucocorticoids in the blood inhibits release of ACTH and endogenous glucocorticoids. Because of this, the adrenal cortex can atrophy. If exogenous glucocorticoid administration is suddenly discontinued, adrenal insufficiency results because of the inability of the atrophied cortex to respond adequately.

Mineralocorticoids

Mineralocorticoids exert their major effects on electrolyte metabolism. They act principally on renal tubular and gastrointestinal epithelium to cause increased sodium ion absorption in exchange for excretion of potassium or hydrogen ions. Aldosterone secretion is only minimally influenced by ACTH. It is primarily secreted in response to the presence of angiotensin II in the bloodstream. Angiotensin II is a substance that elevates the blood pressure by constricting arterioles. Its concentration is increased when renin is released from the kidney in response to decreased perfusion pressure. The resultant increased aldosterone levels promote sodium reabsorption by the kidney and the gastrointestinal tract, which tends to restore blood pressure to normal. The release of aldosterone is also increased by hyperkalemia.

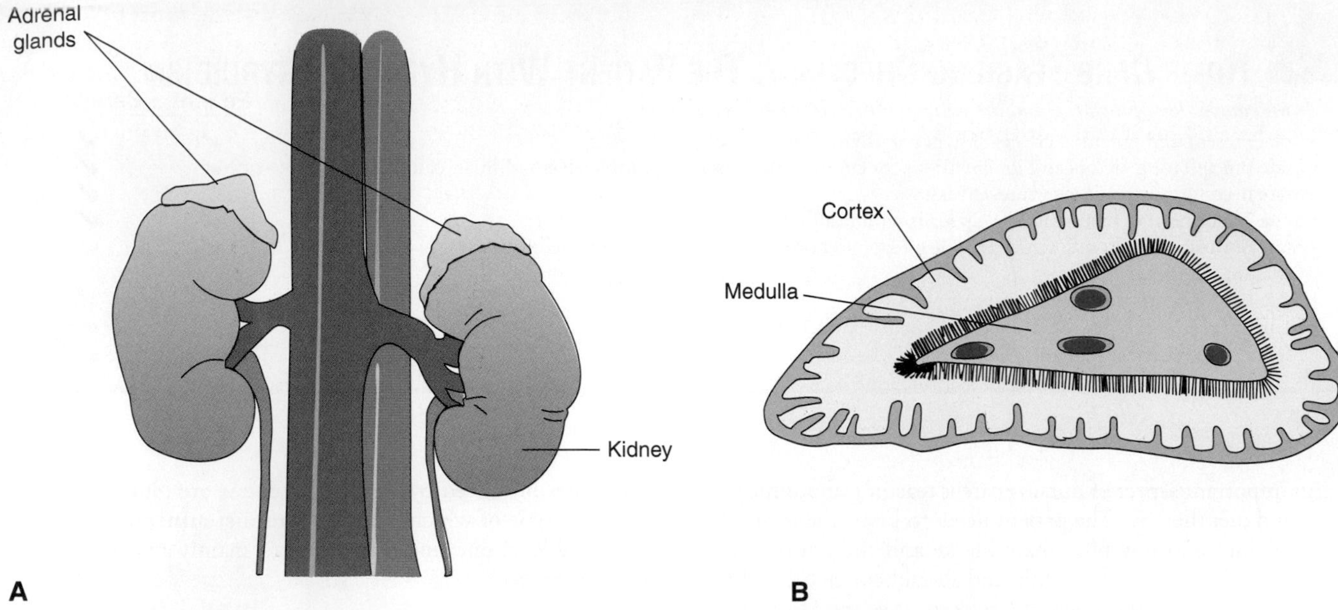

FIGURE 38•6 (**A**) The adrenal glands sit on top of each kidney. (**B**) Each gland is composed of the outer cortex and the inner medulla. Each area secretes specific hormones. The adrenal medulla secretes catecholamines, epinephrine, and norepinephrine; the adrenal cortex secretes glucocorticoids, mineralocorticoids, and sex hormones. From Porth, C. (1998). *Pathophysiology: Concepts of altered health states* (5th ed.). Philadelphia: Lippincott Raven.

Aldosterone is the primary hormone for the long-term regulation of sodium balance.

Adrenal Sex Hormones (Androgens)

Androgens, the third major type of steroid hormones produced by the adrenal cortex, exert effects similar to those of male sex hormones. The adrenal gland may also secrete small amounts of some estrogens, or female sex hormones. Secretion of adrenal androgens is controlled by ACTH. When secreted in normal amounts, the adrenal androgens probably have little effect, but when secreted in excess, in certain inborn enzyme deficiencies, masculinization may result. This is termed the adrenogenital syndrome.

Pheochromocytoma

Pheochromocytoma is a tumor that is usually benign and originates from the chromaffin cells of the adrenal medulla. In 90% of patients (Ram, 1996), the tumor arises in the medulla; in the remaining patients, it occurs in the extra-adrenal chromaffin tissue located in or near the aorta, ovaries, spleen, or other organs. Pheochromocytoma may occur at any age, but its peak incidence is between ages 20 and 50 years (Burton, 1997). It affects men and women equally. Because of the high incidence of pheochromocytoma in family members, the patient's family should be alerted and screened for this tumor. Ten percent of the tumors are bilateral, and 10% are malignant.

Pheochromocytoma is the cause of high blood pressure in 0.09% to 2.2% of patients with hypertension (Ram, 1996). Although it is uncommon, it is one form of hypertension that is usually cured by surgery; without detection and treatment, it is usually fatal. Pheochromocytoma may occur in the familial form as part of multiple endocrine neoplasia type II; therefore, it should be considered a possibility in patients with medullary thyroid carcinoma and parathyroid hyperplasia or tumor.

Clinical Manifestations

The nature and severity of symptoms of functioning tumors of the adrenal medulla depend on the relative proportions of epinephrine and norepinephrine secretion. The typical triad of symptoms includes headache, diaphoresis, and palpitations (Burton, 1997). Hypertension and other cardiovascular disturbances are common. The hypertension may be intermittent or persistent. Only half of patients with pheochromocytoma, however, have sustained or persistent hypertension. If the hypertension is sustained, it may be difficult to distinguish from other causes of hypertension. Other symptoms may include tremor, headache, flushing, and anxiety. Hyperglycemia may result from conversion of liver and muscle glycogen to glucose by epinephrine secretion; insulin may be required to maintain normal blood glucose levels.

The clinical picture in the paroxysmal form of pheochromocytoma is usually characterized by acute, unpredictable attacks, lasting seconds or several hours; during these attacks, the patient is extremely anxious, tremulous, and weak. The patient may experience headache, vertigo, blurring of vision, tinnitus, air hunger, and dyspnea. Other symptoms include polyuria, nausea, vomiting, diarrhea, abdominal pain, and a feeling of impending doom. Palpitations and tachycardia are common. Blood pressures as high as 350/200 mm Hg have been recorded. Such blood pressure elevations are life-threatening and may cause severe complications, such as cardiac dysrhythmias, dissecting aneurysm, stroke, and acute renal failure. Postural hypotension occurs in 70% of patients with untreated pheochromocytoma.

Assessment and Diagnostic Findings

Pheochromocytoma is suspected if signs of sympathetic nervous system overactivity occur in association with marked elevation of blood pressure. These signs can be associated with the "five Hs": *h*ypertension, *h*eadache, *h*yperhidrosis (excessive sweating), *h*ypermetabolism, and *h*yperglycemia (Ram, 1996). Presence of these signs has a 93.8% specificity and a 90.9% sensitivity for pheochromocytoma. Absence of hypertension excludes pheochromocytoma with a 99% certainty (Noble, 1996). Paroxysmal symptoms of pheochromocytoma commonly develop in the fifth decade of life.

Measurements of urine and plasma levels of catecholamines are the most direct and conclusive tests for overactivity of the adrenal medulla. Measures of urinary catecholamine metabolites (metanephrines [MN] and vanillylmandelic acid [VMA]) or free catecholamines are the standard diagnostic tests used in the diagnosis of pheochromocytoma. A 24-hour specimen of urine is collected for determining free catecholamines, MN, and VMA; the use of combined tests increases the diagnostic accuracy of testing. A number of medications and foods (eg, coffee, tea, bananas, chocolate, vanilla, aspirin) may alter the results of these tests; therefore, careful instructions to avoid restricted items must be followed by the patient. Urine collected over a 2- or 3-hour period after an attack of hypertension can be assayed for catecholamine content.

Total plasma catecholamine (norepinephrine and epinephrine) concentration is measured with the patient supine and at rest for 30 minutes. To prevent elevation of catecholamine levels by the stress of venipuncture, a butterfly needle, scalp vein needle, or venous catheter may be inserted 30 minutes before the blood specimen is obtained.

Factors that may elevate catecholamine levels must be controlled to obtain valid results; these factors include consumption of coffee or tea, use of tobacco, emotional and physical stress, and use of many prescription and over-the-counter medications (ie, amphetamines, nose drops or sprays, decongestants, and bronchodilators).

Normal plasma values of epinephrine are 100 pg/mL (590 pmol/L); normal values of norepinephrine are generally less than 100 to 550 pg/mL (590 to 3240 pmol/L). Values of epinephrine greater than 400 pg/mL (2180 pmol/L) or norepinephrine values greater than 2000 pg/mL (11,800 pmol/L) are considered diagnostic of pheochromocytoma; values that fall between normal values and those diagnostic of pheochromocytoma indicate the need for further testing.

A clonidine suppression test may be performed if the results of plasma and urine tests of catecholamines are inconclusive. Clonidine (Catapres) is a centrally acting, antiadrenergic medication that suppresses the release of neurogenically mediated catecholamines. The suppression test is based on the principle that catecholamine levels are normally increased through the activity of the sympathetic nervous system; in pheochromocytoma, increased catecholamine levels result from diffusion of excess catecholamines into the circulation, bypassing normal storage and release mechanisms. Therefore, in patients with pheochromocytoma, clonidine does not suppress release of catecholamines.

The results of the test are considered normal if 2 to 3 hours after a single oral dose of clonidine, the total plasma catecholamine value decreases at least 40% from the patient's baseline (Ram, 1996). Patients with pheochromocytoma exhibit no change in catecholamine levels. False-positive results, however, may occur in patients with primary hypertension.

Imaging studies, such as CT scans, MRI, and ultrasound, may also be carried out to localize the pheochromocytoma and to determine whether more than one tumor is present. Use of ^{131}I-metaiodobenzylguanidine (MIBG) scintigraph may be required to determine the location of the pheochromocytoma and to detect metastatic sites outside the adrenal gland. MIBG is a specific isotope for catecholamine-producing tissue. It has been helpful in identifying tumors not detected by other tests or procedures. MIBG scintigraphy is a noninvasive, safe procedure that has increased the accuracy of diagnosis of adrenal tumors.

Other diagnostic studies may focus on evaluation of function of other endocrine glands because of the association of pheochromocytoma in some patients with other endocrine tumors.

Medical Management

During an episode or attack of hypertension, tachycardia, anxiety, and the other symptoms of pheochromocytoma, the patient is placed on bed rest with the head of the bed elevated to promote an orthostatic decrease in blood pressure.

PHARMACOLOGIC THERAPY

The patient may be moved to the intensive care unit for close monitoring of ECG changes and careful administration of alpha-adrenergic blocking agents (eg, phentolamine [Regitine]) or smooth muscle relaxants (eg, sodium nitroprusside [Nipride]) to lower the blood pressure quickly.

Phenoxybenzamine (Dibenzyline), a long-acting alpha-blocker, may be used when the patient's blood pressure is stable to prepare the patient for surgery. Beta-adrenergic blocking agents, such as propranolol (Inderal) may be used in patients with cardiac dysrhythmias or those not responsive to alpha-blockers. Alpha-adrenergic and beta-adrenergic blocking agents must be used with caution because patients with pheochromocytoma may have increased sensitivity to them. Still other medications that may be used preoperatively are catecholamine synthesis inhibitors, such as alpha-methyl-*p*-tyrosine (metyrosine). These are occasionally used when the effects of catecholamines are not reduced by adrenergic blocking agents.

SURGICAL MANAGEMENT

The definitive treatment of pheochromocytoma is surgical removal of the tumor, usually with **adrenalectomy**. Bilateral adrenalectomy may be necessary if tumors of both adrenal glands are present. Preliminary patient preparation includes effective control of blood pressure and blood volumes. Usually, this is carried out over 7 to 10 days. Phentolamine or phenoxybenzamine (Dibenzyline) may be used safely without causing undue hypotension. Other medications (metyrosine [Demser] and prazosin [Minipress]) have been used to treat pheochromocytoma. The patient needs to be well hydrated before, during, and after surgery to prevent hypotension.

Manipulation of the tumor during surgical excision may cause release of stored epinephrine and norepinephrine with marked increases in blood pressure and changes in heart rate. Therefore, use of sodium nitroprusside (Nipride) and alpha-adrenergic blocking agents may be required during and after surgery. Exploration of other possible sites of tumor is frequently undertaken to ensure removal of all tumor. As a result, the patient is subject to the stress and effects of a long surgical procedure, which may increase the risk of hypertension postoperatively.

Corticosteroid replacement is required if bilateral adrenalectomy has been necessary. Corticosteroids may also be necessary for the first few days or weeks after removal of a single adrenal gland. Intravenous administration of corticosteroids (methylprednisolone sodium succinate [Solu-Medrol]) may begin the evening before surgery and continue during the early postoperative period to prevent adrenal insufficiency. Oral preparations of corticosteroids (prednisone) will be prescribed after the acute stress of surgery diminishes.

Hypotension and hypoglycemia may occur in the postoperative period because of the sudden withdrawal of excessive amounts of catecholamines. Therefore, careful attention is directed toward monitoring and treating these changes. Blood pressure is expected to return to normal with treatment; however, one third of patients may continue to be hypertensive after surgery (Burton, 1997). This may result if all pheochromocytoma tissue has not been removed, if pheochromocytoma recurs, or if the blood vessels have been damaged by severe and prolonged hypertension. Several days after surgery, urine and plasma levels of catecholamines and their metabolites are measured to determine whether surgery has been successful.

Nursing Management

The patient who has undergone surgery to treat pheochromocytoma has experienced a stressful preoperative and postoperative course and may remain fearful of repeated attacks. Although it is usually expected that all pheochromocytoma tissue has been removed, there is a possibility that other sites were undetected and that attacks may recur. The patient is monitored for several days in the intensive care unit with special attention given to ECG changes, arterial pressures, fluid and electrolyte balance, and blood glucose levels. Several intravenous lines are inserted for administration of fluids and medications.

PROMOTING HOME AND COMMUNITY-BASED CARE

Teaching Patients Self-Care. During the preoperative and postoperative phases of care, the patient is informed about the importance of follow-up monitoring to ensure that pheochromocytoma does not recur undetected. After adrenalectomy, use of corticosteroids may be needed. Therefore, the patient is instructed about their purpose, the medication schedule, and the risks of skipping doses or stopping their administration abruptly.

The patient and family are taught how to measure the patient's blood pressure and when to notify the physician about changes in blood pressure. Additionally, they are instructed verbally and in writing about the procedure for collecting 24-hour urine specimens to monitor urinary catecholamines levels.

Continuing Care. A follow-up visit from a home care nurse may be indicated to assess the patient's postoperative recovery, surgical incision, and compliance with the medication schedule. Previous teaching about management and monitoring is reinforced. The home care nurse also obtains blood pressure measurements and assists the patient in preventing or dealing with problems that may result from long-term use of corticosteroids.

Because of the risk of recurrence of hypertension, periodic checkups are required, especially in young patients and in patients whose families have a history of pheochromocytoma. The patient is scheduled for periodic follow-up appointments to observe for return of normal blood pressure and plasma and urine levels of catecholamines.

The adrenal cortex is necessary for life. Adrenocortical secretions make it possible for the body to adapt to stress of all kinds. Without the adrenal cortex, severe stress causes peripheral circulatory failure, shock, and prostration. Life would be maintained only with nutritional, electrolyte, and fluid replacement and replacement of adrenocortical hormones.

Adrenocortical Insufficiency (Addison's Disease)

Pathophysiology

Addison's disease, or adrenocortical insufficiency, results when adrenal cortex function is inadequate to meet the patient's need for cortical hormones. Autoimmune or idiopathic atrophy of the adrenal glands is responsible for 80% of cases of Addison's disease (Gumowski & Loughran, 1996). Other causes include surgical removal of both adrenal glands or infection of the adrenal glands. Tuberculosis (TB) and histoplasmosis are the most common infections that destroy adrenal gland tissue. Although autoimmune destruction has replaced TB as the principal cause of Addison's disease, TB should be considered in the diagnostic workup because of its increasing incidence. Inadequate secretion of ACTH from the pituitary gland also results in adrenal insufficiency because of decreased stimulation of the adrenal cortex.

The symptoms of adrenocortical insufficiency may also result from the sudden cessation of exogenous adrenocortical hormonal therapy, which suppresses the body's normal response to stress and interferes with normal feedback mechanisms. Treatment with daily administration of corticosteroids for 2 to 4 weeks may suppress function of the adrenal cortex; therefore, adrenal insufficiency should be considered in any patient who has been treated with corticosteroids.

Clinical Manifestations

Addison's disease is characterized by muscular weakness; anorexia; gastrointestinal symptoms; fatigue; emaciation; dark pigmentation of the skin, knuckles, knees, elbows, and mucous membranes; hypotension; and low blood glucose, low serum sodium, and high serum potassium levels. Mental status changes such as depression, emotional lability, apathy, and confusion are present in 60% to 80% of patients (Gumowski & Loughran, 1996). In severe cases, the disturbance of sodium and potassium metabolism may be marked by depletion of the sodium and water and severe, chronic dehydration.

With disease progression and acute hypotension, the patient develops **addisonian crisis**, which is characterized by cyanosis, fever, and the classic signs of shock: pallor, apprehension, rapid and weak pulse, rapid respirations, and low blood pressure. In addition, the patient may complain of headache, nausea, abdominal pain, and diarrhea and show signs of confusion and restlessness. Even slight overexertion, exposure to cold, acute infections, or a decrease in salt intake may lead to circulatory collapse, shock, and death if untreated. The stress of surgery or dehydration resulting from preparation for diagnostic tests or surgery may precipitate an addisonian or hypotensive crisis.

Assessment and Diagnostic Findings

Although the clinical manifestations presented appear specific, the onset of Addison's disease usually occurs with nonspecific symptoms. The diagnosis is confirmed by laboratory test results. Laboratory findings include decreased blood glucose and sodium (hypoglycemia and hyponatremia) levels, increased serum potassium (hyperkalemia) level, and an increased white blood cell count (leukocytosis).

The diagnosis is confirmed by low levels of adrenocortical hormones in the blood or urine and decreased serum cortisol levels.

If the adrenal cortex is destroyed, baseline values are low, and ACTH administration fails to cause the normal rise in plasma cortisol and urinary 17-hydroxycorticosteroids. If the adrenal gland is normal but not stimulated properly by the pituitary, a normal response to repeated dosages of exogenous ACTH is seen, but no response follows the administration of metyrapone, which stimulates endogenous ACTH.

Medical Management

Immediate treatment is directed toward combating shock: restoring blood circulation, administering fluids and corticosteroids, monitoring vital signs, and placing the patient in a recumbent position with the legs elevated. Hydrocortisone (Solu-Cortef) is administered intravenously and followed with 5% dextrose in normal saline. Vasopressor amines may be required if hypotension persists.

Antibiotics may be administered if infection has precipitated adrenal crisis in a patient with chronic adrenal insufficiency. Additionally, the patient is assessed closely to identify other factors, stressors, or illnesses that led to the acute episode.

Oral intake may be initiated as soon as tolerated by the patient. Gradually, intravenous fluids are decreased when oral fluid intake is adequate to prevent hypovolemia.

If the adrenal gland does not regain function, the patient needs lifelong replacement of corticosteroids and mineralocorticoids to prevent recurrence of adrenal insufficiency and to prevent addisonian crisis in times of stress and illness. Additionally, the patient probably needs to supplement dietary intake with added salt during times of gastrointestinal losses of fluids through vomiting and diarrhea.

Nursing Management

ASSESSING THE PATIENT

The health history and examination focus on the presence of symptoms of fluid imbalance and on the patient's level of stress. The blood pressure and pulse rate are obtained as the patient moves from a lying to a standing position to detect inadequate fluid volume. Additionally, the patient's skin color and turgor are assessed for changes related to chronic adrenal insufficiency and hypovolemia. The patient is assessed for weight changes, muscle weakness, and fatigue. The patient and family are asked about the onset of illness or stress that may have precipitated the acute crisis.

MONITORING FOR ADDISONIAN CRISIS

The patient at risk is monitored for signs and symptoms indicative of addisonian crisis. These symptoms are often the manifestations of shock: hypotension; rapid, weak pulse; rapid respiratory rate; pallor; and extreme weakness. The patient with addisonian crisis is at risk for circulatory collapse and shock (see Chap. 14 for management of the patient in shock); therefore, physical and psychological stressors must be avoided. These include exposure to cold, overexertion, infection, and emotional distress.

The patient with addisonian crisis requires immediate treatment with intravenous administration of fluid, glucose, and electrolytes, especially sodium; replacement of missing corticosteroids; and vasopressors. During acute addisonian crisis, exertion on the patient's part is avoided; therefore, the nurse anticipates the patient's needs and takes measures to meet those needs.

Careful monitoring of the patient's symptoms, vital signs, weight, and fluid and electrolyte status is essential to monitor the patient's progress and return to a precrisis state. To reduce risk of future episodes of addisonian crisis, efforts are made to identify and reduce factors that may have led to the crisis.

RESTORING FLUID BALANCE

The patient's skin turgor, mucous membranes, and weight are assessed to provide information about fluid balance and adequacy of the patient's hormone replacement. The patient is instructed to report increased thirst, which may indicate impending fluid imbalance. Lying, sitting, and standing blood pressures also provide information about the patient's fluid status. A decrease in systolic pressure (20 mm Hg or more) may be indicative of depletion of fluid volume, especially if accompanied by symptoms. The patient is encouraged to consume foods and fluids that will assist in restoring and maintaining fluid and electrolyte balance. Along with the dietitian, the nurse assists the patient to select foods high in sodium during gastrointestinal disturbances and very hot weather.

The nurse instructs the patient and family to administer hormone replacement as prescribed and to modify the dosage during illness and other stressful occasions. Written and verbal instructions are provided about the administration of mineralocorticoid (Florinef) or glucocorticoid (prednisone) as prescribed.

IMPROVING ACTIVITY TOLERANCE

Until the patient's condition is stabilized, precautions are taken to avoid unnecessary activity and stress that could precipitate another hypotensive episode. Efforts are made to detect signs of infection or the presence of other stressors. Even minor events or stressors may be excessive in the presence of adrenal insufficiency. During the acute crisis, a quiet, nonstressful environment is maintained. All activities (eg, bathing, turning) are carried out *for* the patient. All procedures are explained to the patient and family to reduce anxiety. The nurse explains the rationale for minimizing stress during the acute crisis. The patient is assisted to increase activity gradually.

PROMOTING HOME AND COMMUNITY-BASED CARE

Teaching Patients Self-Care. Because of the need for lifelong replacement of adrenal cortex hormones to prevent addisonian crises, the patient and family members receive explicit verbal and written instructions about the rationale for replacement therapy and proper dosage. Additionally, they are instructed about how to modify the medication dosage and increase salt intake in times of illness, very hot weather, and other stressful situations. The patient is also instructed about modifying diet and fluid intake to help maintain fluid and electrolyte balance.

The patient and family are frequently provided with a syringe and a vial of injectable steroid, such as Solu-Cortef, for use in emergencies, and are given careful instruction about how and when to use it. The patient is instructed to inform other health care providers, such as dentists, about the use of steroids, to wear a medical alert bracelet, and to carry information about the need for steroids at all times. If the patient with Addison's disease requires surgery, careful administration of fluids and corticosteroids is necessary before, during, and after surgery to prevent addisonian crisis.

The patient and family need to know the signs of excessive or insufficient hormone replacement. The development of edema or weight gain may signify *too high* a dose of hormone; postural hypotension (decrease in systolic blood pressure, lightheadedness, dizziness on standing) and weight loss frequently signify *too low* a dose. See the Home Care Teaching Checklist: The Patient With Adrenal Insufficiency (Addison's Disease).

Continuing Care. Although most patients are able to return to job and family responsibilities soon after hospital discharge, others are unable to do so because of concurrent illnesses or incomplete

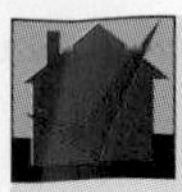

HOME CARE TEACHING CHECKLIST: THE PATIENT WITH ADRENAL INSUFFICIENCY (ADDISON'S DISEASE)

At the completion of the program, the patient or caregiver will be able to:	Patient	Caregiver
• State present and potential effects of adrenal insufficiency on the body	✔	✔
• State warning signs of adrenal crisis and need for emergency care	✔	✔
• Explain components of an emergency kit and indications for their use; demonstrate how to use them	✔	✔
• State strategies for dealing with stress and avoiding adrenal crisis	✔	✔
• State the purpose, dose, route, schedule, side effects, and precautions of prescribed medications (corticosteroid replacement)	✔	✔
• State that compliance with medical regimen is lifelong	✔	✔
• State importance of regular follow-up visits with health care provider	✔	✔
• Recognize the need for dosage adjustment during times of stress	✔	✔
• State need to wear medical alert identification and carry medical information card	✔	✔
• State need to notify health care providers about disease before treatment or procedure	✔	✔
• State need to avoid strenuous activity in hot, humid weather	✔	✔
• State need for increased fluid intake and salt with excessive perspiration	✔	✔
• State need for high-carbohydrate, high-protein diet with adequate sodium intake	✔	✔
• Identify areas of activity limitations and impact on lifestyle	✔	✔

recovery from the episode of adrenal insufficiency. In these circumstances, a referral for home care enables the home care nurse to assess the patient's recovery, monitor hormone replacement, and assess stress in the home. Additionally, the nurse assesses the patient's and family's knowledge about medication therapy and dietary modifications. A home visit also allows the nurse to assess the patient's plans for follow-up visits to the clinic or physician's office.

Cushing's Syndrome

Cushing's syndrome results from excessive, rather than deficient, adrenocortical activity. The syndrome may result from excessive administration of corticosteroids or ACTH or from hyperplasia of the adrenal cortex.

Pathophysiology

Cushing's syndrome may be caused by several mechanisms, including a tumor of the pituitary gland that produces ACTH and stimulates the adrenal cortex to increase its hormone secretion despite adequate amounts being produced. Primary hyperplasia of the adrenal glands in the absence of a pituitary tumor is less common. Administration of corticosteroids or ACTH may also produce Cushing's syndrome. Another less common cause of Cushing's syndrome is the ectopic production of ACTH by malignancies; bronchogenic carcinoma is the most common type of these malignancies. Regardless of the cause, the normal feedback mechanisms that control the function of the adrenal cortex become ineffective, and the usual diurnal pattern of cortisol is lost. The signs and symptoms of Cushing's syndrome are primarily a result of oversecretion of glucocorticoids and androgens (sex hormones), although mineralocorticoid secretion may also be affected.

Clinical Manifestations

When overproduction of the adrenal cortical hormone occurs, arrest of growth, obesity, and musculoskeletal changes occur along with glucose intolerance.

The classic picture of Cushing's syndrome in the adult is that of central-type obesity, with a fatty "buffalo hump" in the neck and supraclavicular areas, a heavy trunk, and relatively thin extremities. The skin is thin, fragile, and easily traumatized; ecchymoses (bruises) and striae develop. The patient complains of weakness and lassitude. Sleep is disturbed because of altered diurnal secretion of cortisol.

Excessive protein catabolism occurs, producing muscle wasting and osteoporosis. Kyphosis, backache, and compression fractures of the vertebrae may result. Retention of sodium and water occurs as a result of increased mineralocorticoid activity, producing hypertension and congestive heart failure.

The patient develops a "moon-faced" appearance and may experience increased oiliness of the skin and acne. There is increased susceptibility to infection. Hyperglycemia or overt diabetes may develop. The patient may also report weight gain, slow healing of minor cuts, and bruises.

Females between the ages of 20 to 40 years are five times more likely than males to develop Cushing's syndrome (Davis-Martin, 1996). In females of all ages, virilization may occur as a result of excess androgens. Virilization is characterized by the appearance of masculine traits and the recession of feminine traits. There is an excessive growth of hair on the face (hirsutism), the breasts atrophy, menses cease, the clitoris enlarges, and the patient's voice deepens. Libido is lost in males and females.

Changes occur in mood and mental activity; psychosis may develop on occasion. Distress and depression are common and are increased by the severity of the physical changes that occur with this syndrome. If Cushing's syndrome is a consequence of pituitary tumor, visual disturbances may occur because of pressure of the growing tumor on the optic chiasm. Chart 38-3 summarizes the changes associated with Cushing's syndrome.

Assessment and Diagnostic Findings

Indicators of Cushing's syndrome include an increase in serum sodium and blood glucose levels and a decreased serum concentration of potassium, a reduction in the number of blood eosinophils, and a disappearance of lymphoid tissue. Measurements of plasma and urinary cortisol levels are obtained. Several blood samples may be collected to determine whether the normal diurnal variation in plasma levels is present. This variation is frequently absent in adrenal dysfunction. If several blood samples are required, it is

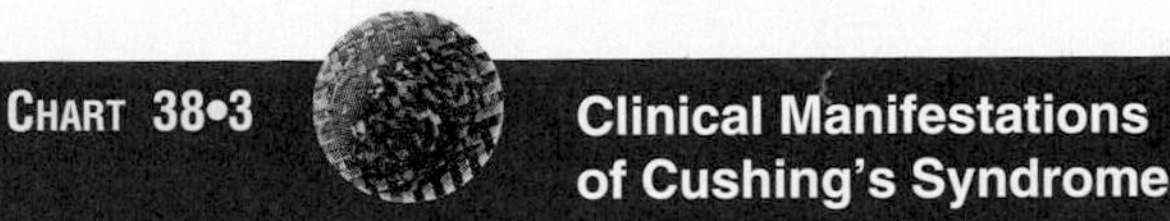

CHART 38•3 Clinical Manifestations of Cushing's Syndrome

Ophthalmic
- Cataracts
- Glaucoma

Cardiovascular
- Hypertension
- Congestive heart failure

Endocrine/Metabolic
- Truncal obesity
- Moon face
- Buffalo hump
- Sodium retention
- Hypokalemia
- Metabolic alkalosis
- Hyperglycemia
- Menstrual irregularities
- Impotence
- Negative nitrogen balance
- Altered calcium metabolism
- Adrenal suppression

Immune Function
- Decreased inflammatory responses
- Impaired wound healing
- Increased susceptibility to infections

Skeletal
- Osteoporosis
- Spontaneous fractures
- Aseptic necrosis of femur
- Vertebral compression fractures

Gastrointestinal
- Peptic ulcer
- Pancreatitis

Muscular
- Myopathy
- Muscle weakness

Dermatologic
- Thinning of skin
- Petechiae
- Ecchymoses
- Striae
- Acne

Psychiatric
- Mood alterations
- Psychoses

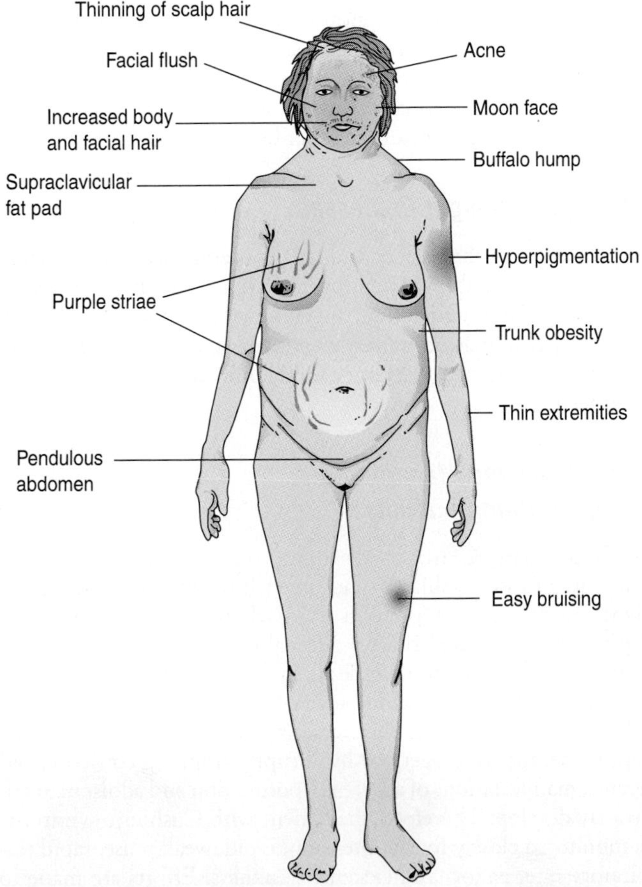

essential that they be collected at the times specified and that the time of collection be noted on the requisition slip.

An overnight dexamethasone suppression test is the most widely used screening test for diagnosis of pituitary and adrenal causes of Cushing's syndrome and can be performed on an outpatient basis (Noble, 1996). Dexamethasone (1 mg) is administered orally at 11:00 PM, and a plasma cortisol level is obtained at 8:00 AM the next morning. Suppression of cortisol to less than 5 mg/dL indicates that the hypothalamic-pituitary-adrenal axis is functioning properly. Stress, obesity, depression, and medications such as antiseizure agents, estrogen, and rifampin can falsely elevate the results. Other diagnostic studies include a 24-hour urinary free cortisol level and a high-dose or low-dose dexamethasone suppression test. High-dose and low-dose suppression tests are similar to the overnight test but vary in dosage and timing.

Measurement of plasma ACTH by radioimmunoassay is used in conjunction with the high-dose suppression test to distinguish pituitary tumors from ectopic sites of ACTH production as the cause of Cushing's syndrome. Elevation of both ACTH and cortisol level is indicative of pituitary or hypothalamic disease. Low ACTH with a high cortisol level is indicative of adrenal disease. A CT scan, ultrasound, or MRI may be performed to localize adrenal tissue and detect tumors of the adrenal gland.

Medical Management

In cases in which Cushing's syndrome is caused by pituitary tumors rather than tumors of the adrenal cortex, treatment is directed at the pituitary gland. Surgical removal of the tumor by transsphenoidal hypophysectomy is the treatment of choice and has a 90% success rate. Radiation of the pituitary gland has also been successful, although it may take several months for control of symptoms. Adrenalectomy is the treatment of choice in patients with primary adrenal hypertrophy.

Postoperatively, symptoms of adrenal insufficiency may begin to appear 12 to 48 hours after surgery because of reduction of the high levels of circulating adrenal hormones. Temporary replacement therapy with hydrocortisone may be necessary for several months until the adrenal glands begin to respond normally to the body's needs. If both adrenal glands have been removed (bilateral adrenalectomy), lifetime replacement of adrenal cortex hormones is necessary.

Adrenal enzyme inhibitors (ie, metyrapone, aminoglutethimide, mitotane, ketoconazole) may be used to reduce hyperadrenalism if the syndrome is caused by ectopic ACTH secretion by a tumor that cannot be totally eradicated. Close monitoring is necessary because symptoms of inadequate adrenal function may result and because of possible side effects of these medications.

If Cushing's syndrome is a result of the administration of corticosteroids, an attempt is made to reduce or taper the medication to the minimum dose needed to treat the underlying disease process (eg, autoimmune and allergic diseases and rejection of transplanted organs). Frequently, alternate-day therapy decreases the symptoms of Cushing's syndrome and allows recovery of the adrenal glands' responsiveness to ACTH.

NURSING PROCESS: THE PATIENT WITH CUSHING'S SYNDROME

Assessment

The health history and examination focus on the effects on the body of high concentrations of adrenal cortex hormones and on the inability of the adrenal cortex to respond to changes in cortisol and aldosterone levels. The history includes information about the patient's level of activity and ability to carry out routine and self-care activities. The patient's skin is observed and assessed for trauma, infection, breakdown, bruising, and edema. Changes in physical appearance are noted, and the patient's responses to these changes are elicited. The nurse assesses the patient's mental function, including mood, responses to questions, awareness of environment, and level of depression. The patient's family is often a good source of information about gradual changes in the patient's physical appearance as well as emotional status.

Diagnosis

Nursing Diagnoses

Based on all the assessment data, the major nursing diagnoses of the patient with Cushing's syndrome include the following:

- Risk for injury related to weakness
- Risk for infection related to altered protein metabolism and inflammatory response
- Self-care deficit related to weakness, fatigue, muscle wasting, and altered sleep patterns
- Impaired skin integrity related to edema, impaired healing, and thin and fragile skin
- Body image disturbance related to altered physical appearance, impaired sexual functioning, and decrease in activity level
- Altered thought processes related to mood swings, irritability, and depression

Collaborative Problems/Potential Complications

Based on assessment data, potential complications may include the following:

- Addisonian crisis
- Adverse effects of adrenocortical activity

Planning and Goals

The patient's major goals include decreased risk for injury, decreased risk for infection, increased ability to carry out self-care activities, improved skin integrity, improved body image, improved mental function, and absence of complications.

Nursing Interventions

Decreasing Risk for Injury

A protective environment is established to prevent falls, fractures, and other injuries to bones and soft tissues. The patient who is very weak may require assistance from the nurse in ambulating to prevent falls or bumping into sharp corners of furniture. Foods high in protein, calcium, and vitamin D are recommended to minimize muscle wasting and osteoporosis. Referral to a dietitian may assist the patient in selecting appropriate foods that are also low in sodium and calories.

Decreasing Risk for Infection

Unnecessary exposure to others with infections is avoided. The patient is assessed frequently for subtle signs of infection because the anti-inflammatory effects of corticosteroids may mask the common signs of inflammation and infection.

Preparing the Patient for Surgery

The patient is prepared for adrenalectomy, if indicated, and postoperative care (see later discussion in this chapter). If Cushing's syndrome is a result of a pituitary tumor, a transsphenoidal hypophysectomy may be performed. Diabetes mellitus and peptic ulcer are common in the patient with Cushing's syndrome; therefore, management includes blood glucose monitoring and assessment of stools for blood and appropriate intervention if indicated.

Encouraging Rest and Activity

Weakness, fatigue, and muscle wasting make it difficult for the patient with Cushing's syndrome to carry out normal activities. Yet moderate activity should be encouraged to prevent complications of immobility and promote increased self-esteem. Insomnia often contributes to the patient's fatigue. Rest periods are planned and spaced throughout the day. Efforts are made to promote a relaxing, quiet environment for rest and sleep.

Promoting Skin Integrity

Meticulous skin care is necessary to avoid traumatizing the patient's fragile skin. Use of adhesive tape is avoided because it can irritate the skin and tear the fragile tissue when the tape is removed. The skin and bony prominences are assessed frequently, and the patient is encouraged and assisted to change positions frequently to prevent skin breakdown.

Improving Body Image

If the cause of Cushing's syndrome can be treated successfully, the major physical changes disappear in time. The patient may benefit from discussion of the effect the changes have had on self-concept and relationships with others. Weight gain and edema may be modified by a low-carbohydrate, low-sodium diet. A high-protein intake may reduce some of the other bothersome symptoms.

Improving Thought Processes

Explanations to the patient and family members about the cause of emotional instability are important in helping them cope with the mood swings, irritability, and depression that may occur. Psychotic behavior may occur in a few patients and should be reported. The nurse encourages the patient and family members to verbalize their feelings.

Monitoring and Managing Potential Complications

ADDISONIAN CRISIS

The patient with Cushing's syndrome whose symptoms are treated by withdrawing corticosteroids or by adrenalectomy or removing a pituitary tumor is at risk for adrenal hypofunction and addisonian crisis. If the function of the adrenal cortex has been suppressed by high levels of circulating adrenal hormones, atrophy of the adrenal cortex is likely. If the circulating hormone level is decreased rapidly because of surgery or by abruptly stopping corticosteroid agents, manifestations of adrenal hypofunction and addisonian crisis may develop. Therefore, the patient with Cushing's syndrome is monitored closely for hypotension, rapid, weak pulse, rapid respiratory rate, pallor, and extreme weakness. Efforts are made to identify factors that may have led to the episode of crisis.

The patient with Cushing's syndrome who experiences highly stressful events, such as trauma or emergency surgery, is at increased risk for addisonian crisis because of long-term suppression of the adrenal cortex. The patient may require intravenous administration of fluid and electrolytes and corticosteroids before, during, and after treatment or surgery. If addisonian crisis occurs, the patient is treated for circulatory collapse and shock (see Chap. 14 for management of the patient in shock).

ADVERSE EFFECTS OF ADRENOCORTICAL ACTIVITY

Fluid and electrolyte status is assessed by monitoring laboratory values and the patient's daily weight. Because of the increased risk for glucose intolerance and hyperglycemia, blood glucose monitoring is initiated, and elevated blood glucose levels are reported to the physician, so that treatment can be prescribed if indicated.

Promoting Home and Community-Based Care

TEACHING PATIENTS SELF-CARE

The patient with Cushing's syndrome and the patient's family require teaching and support to enable them to prevent problems associated with the syndrome and to manage those that cannot be prevented. Therefore, the nurse presents information about Cushing's syndrome verbally and in writing. If the disorder is a result of corticosteroid use for treatment of a chronic disease, the patient and family need to understand that stopping the corticosteroid use abruptly and without medical supervision is likely to result in adrenal insufficiency and reappearance of symptoms of the chronic disease. The nurse emphasizes the need to ensure an adequate supply of the corticosteroid because running out of the medication and skipping doses can precipitate addisonian crisis. Refer to the later discussion, Therapeutic Uses of Corticosteroids, for more information. See the Home Care Teaching Checklist: The Patient With Cushing's Syndrome.

The need for dietary modifications to ensure adequate calcium intake, without increasing the risk for hypertension, hyperglycemia, and weight gain, is stressed to the patient and family. The patient and family may be taught to monitor blood pressure, blood glucose levels, and weight. Wearing a medical alert bracelet and notifying other health providers (eg, dentist) are important to alert others that the patient has Cushing's syndrome.

CONTINUING CARE

The need for continuing follow-up depends on the origin and duration of the disease and its management. The patient who has been treated by adrenalectomy or removal of a pituitary tumor requires close monitoring to ensure that adrenal function has returned to normal and to ensure adequacy of circulating adrenal hormones. The patient who requires continued corticosteroid therapy is monitored to ensure understanding of the medications and the need for a dose that treats the underlying disorder while minimizing the side effects. Home care referral may be indicated to ensure a safe environment that minimizes stress and risk for falls and other side effects. The home care nurse assesses the patient's physical and psychological status and reports changes to the physician. The nurse also assesses the patient's understanding of the medication regimen and the patient's compliance with the regimen and reinforces previous teaching about the medications and the importance of taking them as prescribed. The nurse also emphasizes the importance of regular medical follow-up, side effects and toxic effects of medications, and the need to wear medical identification with Addison's and Cushing's disease.

Evaluation

Expected Outcomes

Expected outcomes may include:

1. Decreases risk for injury
   a. Is free of fractures or soft tissue injuries
   b. Is free of ecchymotic areas
2. Decreases risk for infection
   a. Experiences no temperature elevation, redness, pain, or other signs of infection and inflammation
   b. Avoids contact with others who have infections
3. Increases participation in self-care activities
   a. Plans activities and exercises to allow alternating periods of rest and activity
   b. Reports improved well-being
   c. Is free of complications of immobility
4. Attains/maintains skin integrity
   a. Has intact skin, without evidence of breakdown or infection
   b. Shows evidence of decreased edema in extremities and trunk

HOME CARE TEACHING CHECKLIST: THE PATIENT WITH CUSHING'S SYNDROME

At the completion of the program, the patient or caregiver will be able to:	Patient	Caregiver
• State present and potential effects of Cushing's syndrome on the body	✔	✔
• Identify signs and symptoms of excessive and insufficient adrenal hormone	✔	✔
• State the relationship between adrenal hormones, emotional state, and stress	✔	✔
• Identify methods for managing labile emotions	✔	✔
• State protective skin care measures and use of protective devices and practices	✔	✔
• State the importance of regular follow-up visits with primary health care provider	✔	✔
• State the purpose, dose, route, schedule, side effects, and precautions for prescribed medications (adrenocortical inhibitors)	✔	✔
• Identify need to wear medical alert identification and carry medical information card	✔	✔
• State importance of compliance with medical regimen	✔	✔
• State the need to contact health care provider before taking over-the-counter medications	✔	✔
• Identify foods high in potassium and low in sodium, calories, and carbohydrates	✔	✔
• Identify areas of activity limitations and impact on lifestyle	✔	✔

   c. Changes position frequently and inspects bony prominences daily
5. Achieves improved body image
   a. Verbalizes feelings about changes in appearance, sexual function, and activity level
   b. States that physical changes are a result of excessive corticosteroids
6. Exhibits improved mental functioning
7. Absence of complications
   a. Exhibits normal vital signs and weight and is free of symptoms of addisonian crisis
   b. Identifies signs and symptoms of adrenocortical hypofunction that should be reported and measures to take in case of severe illness and stress
   c. Identifies strategies to minimize complications of Cushing's syndrome
   d. Complies with recommendations for follow-up appointments

Primary Aldosteronism

The principal action of aldosterone is to conserve body sodium. Under the influence of this hormone, the kidneys excrete less sodium and more potassium and hydrogen. Excessive production of aldosterone, which occurs in some patients with functioning tumors of the adrenal gland, causes a distinctive pattern of biochemical changes and a corresponding set of clinical manifestations that are diagnostic of this condition.

Clinical Manifestations

Patients with aldosteronism exhibit a profound decline in the serum levels of potassium (hypokalemia) and hydrogen ions (alkalosis), as demonstrated by an increase in pH and serum bicarbonate level. The serum sodium level is normal or elevated depending on the amount of water reabsorbed with the sodium. Hypertension is the most prominent and almost universal sign of aldosteronism, although it is the primary cause in only 1% of cases of hypertension (Gumowski & Loughran, 1996).

Hypokalemia is responsible for the variable muscle weakness, cramping, and fatigue in patients with aldosteronism, as well as an inability on the part of the kidneys to acidify or concentrate the urine. Accordingly, the urine volume is excessive, leading to polyuria. Serum, by contrast, becomes abnormally concentrated, contributing to excessive thirst (polydipsia) and arterial hypertension. A secondary increase in blood volume and possible direct effects of aldosterone on nerve receptors, such as the carotid sinus, are other factors producing the hypertension.

Hypokalemic alkalosis may decrease the ionized serum calcium level and predispose the patient to tetany and paresthesias. Trousseau's and Chvostek's signs can be used to assess neuromuscular irritability before overt paresthesia and tetany occur. Glucose intolerance may occur because hypokalemia interferes with insulin secretion from the pancreas.

Assessment and Diagnostic Findings

In addition to a high or normal serum sodium level and low serum potassium level, diagnostic studies indicate high serum aldosterone levels and low serum renin levels. The measurement of aldosterone excretion rate after salt loading is a useful diagnostic test for primary aldosteronism. The renin-aldosterone stimulation test and bilateral adrenal venous sampling are useful in differentiating the cause of primary aldosteronism.

Medical Management

Treatment of primary aldosteronism usually involves surgical removal of the adrenal tumor through adrenalectomy. Hypokalemia resolves for all patients after surgery, but hypertension may persist. Spironolactone may be prescribed to control hypertension.

Adrenalectomy

Adrenalectomy may be used in treating adrenal tumors, primary Cushing's syndrome, and aldosteronism. For adrenal tumors, all of the endocrine disturbances associated with a hypersecreting tumor of the adrenal cortex or medulla can be relieved completely by surgical removal of the involved gland.

Adrenalectomy is performed through an incision in the flank or the abdomen. In general, the postoperative care resembles that for other abdominal surgery; however, the patient is susceptible to fluctuations in adrenocortical hormones and requires administration of corticosteroids, fluids, and other agents to maintain blood pressure and prevent acute complications. If the adrenalectomy is bilateral, replacement of corticosteroids will be lifelong; if one adrenal gland is removed, replacement therapy may be temporarily necessary because of suppression of the remaining adrenal gland by high levels of adrenal hormones. A normal serum glucose level is maintained with insulin, appropriate intravenous fluids, and dietary modifications.

Nursing management in the postoperative period includes frequent assessment of vital signs to detect early signs and symptoms of adrenal insufficiency and crisis or hemorrhage. The patient's stress and anxiety level can be reduced by explaining all treatments and procedures, providing comfort measures, and providing rest periods.

Corticosteroid Therapy

Corticosteroids are used extensively for adrenal insufficiency and are also widely used in suppressing inflammation and autoimmune reactions, controlling allergic reactions, and reducing the rejection process in transplantation. Commonly used corticosteroids are listed in Table 38-4. Their anti-inflammatory and antiallergy actions make corticosteroids effective in treating rheumatic or

TABLE 38•4 Commonly Used Corticosteroid Preparations

Generic Names	Trade Names
hydrocortisone	Cortisol, Cortef, Hydrocortone, Solu-Cortef
cortisone	Cortone, Cortate, Cortogen
dexamethasone	Decadron, Dexameth, Deronil, Delalone, Dexasone, Dexone, Hexadrol
prednisone	Meticorten, Deltasone, Orasone, Panasol, Novo-prednisone
prednisolone	Meticortelone, Delta-Cortef, Prelone, Predalone
methylprednisolone	Medrol, Solu-Medrol, Meprolone
triamcinolone	Aristocort, Kenacort, Kenalog, Cenocort, Azmacort, Aristospan
beclomethasone	Beconase, Beclovent, Vanceril, Vancenase, Propaderm
betamethasone	Celestone, Betameth, Betnesol, Betnelan

connective tissue diseases, such as rheumatoid arthritis and systemic lupus erythematosus. They are also frequently used in treatment of asthma, multiple sclerosis, and other autoimmune disorders.

High doses appear to allow patients to tolerate high degrees of stress. Such antistress action may be caused by the ability of corticosteroids to aid circulating vasopressor substances in keeping the blood pressure elevated, or it may be caused by other effects, such as the maintenance of the serum glucose level.

Side Effects

Although the synthetic corticosteroids are safer for some patients because of relative freedom from mineralocorticoid activity, most natural and synthetic corticosteroids produce similar kinds of side effects. The dose required for anti-inflammatory and antiallergy effects also produces metabolic effects, pituitary and adrenal gland suppression, and changes in the function of the central nervous system. Thus, although corticosteroids are highly effective therapeutically, they may also be very dangerous. Dosages of these medications are frequently altered to allow high concentrations when absolutely necessary and then tapered in an attempt to avoid undesirable effects. This requires that patients be closely observed for side effects and that the dose be reduced when high doses are no longer required. Suppression of the adrenal cortex may persist up to a year after a course of corticosteroids of only 2 weeks' duration.

Therapeutic Uses of Corticosteroids

The dosage of corticosteroids is determined by the nature and chronicity of the illness as well as the patient's other medical problems. Rheumatoid arthritis, bronchial asthma, and multiple sclerosis are chronic disorders that corticosteroids do not cure; however, these medications may be useful when other measures do not provide adequate control of symptoms or to treat acute exacerbations.

In such situations, the adverse effects of corticosteroids are weighed against the current problems of the patient. These medications may be used for a period but then should be gradually reduced or tapered as the patient's symptoms subside.

The nurse plays an important role in providing encouragement and understanding during the times the patient may experience recurrence of symptoms and apprehension about these while taking smaller doses.

ACUTE CONDITIONS

Acute flare-ups and crises are treated with large doses of corticosteroids, as in emergency treatment for bronchial obstruction in status asthmaticus and shock from septicemia caused by gram-negative bacteria. Other measures, such as anti-infective agents or medications, are also used with corticosteroids to treat shock and other major symptoms.

At times, corticosteroids are continued past the acute flare-up stage for the purpose of preventing serious complications.

EYE TREATMENT

A different problem exists when corticosteroids are used in treating eye infections. Outer eye infection can be treated by topical application of eye drops because these do not cause systemic toxicity. However, long-term application may cause an increase in intraocular pressure, which may lead to glaucoma in some patients. In some patients, prolonged use of corticosteroids may lead to cataract formation.

DERMATOLOGIC DISORDERS

Topical administration of corticosteroids in the form of creams, ointments, lotions, and aerosols is especially effective in many dermatologic disorders. It may be more effective in some conditions to use occlusive dressings around the affected part, so that maximum absorption of the medication is achieved. Penetration and absorption are also increased if the medication is applied when the skin is hydrated or moist (eg, immediately after bathing).

Absorption of topical agents varies with body location. For example, absorption is greater through the layers of skin on the scalp, face, and genital area than on the forearm; as a result, use of topical agents on these sites increases the risk for side effects of the medication. The availability of over-the-counter topical corticosteroids increases the risk for side effects in patients who are unaware of their potential risks. Excessive use of these agents, especially on large surface areas of inflamed skin, can lead to decreased therapeutic effects and increased side effects.

DOSAGE SCHEDULE

Attempts have been made to determine the best time to administer pharmacologic doses of steroids. When the patient's symptoms have been controlled on a 6-hour or 8-hour program, a once-daily or every-other-day schedule may be implemented. In keeping with the natural secretion of cortisol, the best time of the day for the total steroid dose is in the early morning from 7:00 to 8:00 AM. Large-dose therapy at 8:00 AM, when the gland is most active, produces maximal suppression of the gland. A large 8:00-AM dose is more physiologic because it allows the body to escape effects of the steroids from 4:00 PM to 6:00 AM, when serum levels are normally low, hence minimizing cushingoid effects. If symptoms of the disorder being treated are successfully suppressed, alternate-day therapy is helpful in reducing pituitary-adrenal suppression in patients requiring prolonged therapy. Some patients report discomfort associated with symptoms of their primary illness on the second day; therefore, it is important to explain to patients that this regimen is necessary to minimize side effects and suppression of adrenal function.

TAPERING OF CORTICOSTEROIDS

Corticosteroid dosages are reduced gradually (tapered) to allow normal adrenal function to return and to prevent steroid-induced adrenal insufficiency. Up to 1 year or more after use of corticosteroids, the patient is at risk for adrenal insufficiency in times of stress. For example, if surgery for any reason is necessary, the patient is likely to require intravenous corticosteroids during and after surgery to reduce the risk for acute adrenal crisis. Patients receiving corticosteroids must have an adequate supply of medication on hand, so that they do not miss a scheduled dose and increase their risk for adrenal insufficiency.

Table 38-5 provides an overview of the effects of corticosteroid therapy and their nursing implications.

THE PANCREAS

The pancreas, located in the upper abdomen, has both exocrine (digestive enzymes) and endocrine gland functions. In contrast to endocrine glands, exocrine glands empty their secretions through a duct to their site of utilization rather than directly into the bloodstream.

Exocrine Pancreas

The secretions of the exocrine portion of the pancreas are collected in the pancreatic duct, which joins the common bile duct and enters the duodenum at the ampulla of Vater. Surrounding the

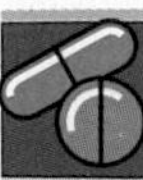

TABLE 38•5 Side Effects of Corticosteroid Therapy and Implications for Practice

Side Effects	Collaborative Interventions
Cardiovascular Effects	
Hypertension Thrombophlebitis Thromboembolism Accelerated atherosclerosis	Monitor for elevated blood pressure Assess for positive Homans' signs Remind patient to avoid positions and situations that restrict blood flow (eg, crossing legs, prolonged sitting in same position, prolonged trips by car or plane without moving or changing position) Encourage foot and leg exercises when recumbent Encourage low sodium intake Encourage limited intake of fat
Immunologic Effects	
Increased risk of infection and masking of signs of infection	Assess for subtle signs of infection and inflammation Encourage patient to avoid exposure to others with upper respiratory infection Monitor patient for fungal infections Encourage hand washing
Eye Changes	
Glaucoma Corneal lesions	Encourage frequent eye examinations Refer patient to ophthalmologist if changes in visual acuity are detected
Musculoskeletal Effects	
Muscle wasting Poor wound healing Osteoporosis with vertebral compression fractures, pathologic fractures of long bones, aseptic necrosis of head of the femur	Encourage high protein intake Encourage diet high in calcium and vitamin D or calcium and vitamin D supplementation if indicated Take measures to avoid falls and other trauma Use caution in moving and turning patient Encourage postmenopausal women on corticosteroids to consider hormone replacement therapy, unless contraindicated Instruct patient to rise slowly from bed or chair to avoid falling due to postural hypotension
Metabolic Effects	
Alterations in glucose metabolism Steroid withdrawal syndrome	Monitor blood glucose levels at periodic intervals Instruct patient about medications, diet, and exercise prescribed to control blood glucose level Report signs of adrenal insufficiency Administer corticosteroids and mineralocorticoids as prescribed Monitor fluid and electrolyte balance Administer fluids and electrolytes as prescribed Instruct patient about importance of taking corticosteroids as prescribed without abruptly stopping therapy Encourage patient to obtain and wear a medical identification bracelet Advise patient to notify all health care providers (eg, dentists, etc.) about need for corticosteroid therapy
Changes in Appearance	
Moon face Weight gain Acne	Encourage caloric restriction Assure patient that most changes in appearance are temporary and will disappear if and when corticosteroid therapy is no longer necessary

ampulla is the sphincter of Oddi, which partially controls the rate at which secretions from the pancreas and the gallbladder enter the duodenum.

The secretions of the exocrine pancreas are digestive enzymes high in protein content and an electrolyte-rich fluid. The secretions are very alkaline because of their high concentration of sodium bicarbonate and are capable of neutralizing the highly acid gastric juice that enters the duodenum. The enzyme secretions include **amylase**, which aids in the digestion of carbohydrates; **trypsin**, which aids in the digestion of proteins; and **lipase**, which aids in the digestion of fats. Other enzymes that promote the breakdown of more complex foodstuffs are also secreted.

The secretion of these exocrine pancreatic juices is stimulated by hormones originating in the gastrointestinal tract. **Secretin** is the major stimulus for increased bicarbonate secretion from the pancreas, and the major stimulus for digestive enzyme secretion is the hormone **cholecystokinin-pancreozymin** (CCK-PZ). The vagus nerve also influences exocrine pancreatic secretion.

Endocrine Pancreas

The islets of Langerhans, the endocrine part of the pancreas, are collections of cells embedded in the pancreatic tissue. They are composed of alpha, beta, and delta cells. The hormone produced by the beta cells is called insulin, the alpha cells secrete glucagon, and the delta cells secrete **somatostatin.**

Insulin

A major action of insulin is to lower blood glucose by permitting entry of the glucose into the cells of the liver, muscle, and other tissues, where it is either stored as glycogen or used for energy. Insulin also promotes the storage of fat in adipose tissue and the synthesis of proteins in various body tissues. In the absence of insulin, glucose is not able to enter the cells and is excreted in the urine. This condition, called diabetes mellitus, can be diagnosed by high levels of glucose in the blood and urine. In diabetes mellitus, stored fats and protein are used for energy instead of glucose, with consequent loss of body mass. (Diabetes mellitus is discussed in detail in Chap. 37.) The rate of insulin secretion from the pancreas is normally regulated by the level of glucose in the blood.

Glucagon

The effects of glucagon (opposite to those of insulin) are chiefly to raise the blood glucose by converting glycogen to glucose in the liver. Glucagon is secreted by the pancreas in response to a decrease in the level of blood glucose.

Somatostatin

Somatostatin exerts a hypoglycemic effect by interfering with release of growth hormone from the pituitary and glucagon from the pancreas, both of which tend to raise blood glucose levels.

Endocrine Control of Carbohydrate Metabolism

Glucose for body energy needs is derived by metabolism of ingested carbohydrates and also from proteins by the process of gluconeogenesis. Glucose can be stored temporarily in the liver, muscles, and other tissues in the form of glycogen. The endocrine system controls the level of blood glucose by regulating the rate at which glucose is synthesized, stored, and moved to and from the bloodstream. Through the action of hormones, blood glucose is normally maintained at about 100 mg/dL (5.5 mmol/L). Insulin is the primary hormone that lowers the blood glucose level. Hormones that raise the blood glucose level are glucagon, epinephrine, adrenocorticosteroids, growth hormone, and thyroid hormone.

The pancreas has both endocrine and exocrine functions, and these functions are interrelated. The major exocrine function is to facilitate digestion through secretion of enzymes into the proximal duodenum. Secretin and CCK-PZ are hormones from the gastrointestinal tract that aid in the digestion of food substances by controlling the secretions of the pancreas. Additionally, neural factors also influence pancreatic enzyme secretion. Considerable dysfunction of the pancreas must occur before enzyme secretion decreases and protein and fat digestion becomes impaired. Pancreatic enzyme secretion is normally 1500 to 2500 mL/day.

Gerontologic Considerations

There is little change in the size of the pancreas with age. There is, however, an increase in fibrous material and some fatty deposition in the normal pancreas in patients older than 70 years of age. Additionally, some localized arteriosclerotic changes occur with age. Studies have suggested a decreased pancreatic secretion rate (decreased lipase, amylase, and trypsin) and bicarbonate output in older patients. Some impairment of normal fat absorption occurs with increasing age, possibly because of delayed gastric emptying and pancreatic insufficiency. Decreased calcium absorption may also occur. These changes require care in interpreting diagnostic tests in the normal elderly person and in providing dietary counseling.

Pancreatitis

Pancreatitis (inflammation of the pancreas) is a serious disorder of the pancreas that can range in severity from a relatively mild self-limiting disorder to a rapidly fatal disease that does not respond to any treatment. Acute pancreatitis can be a medical emergency associated with a high risk for life-threatening complications and mortality, whereas chronic pancreatitis is often undetected until 80% to 90% of the exocrine and endocrine tissue is destroyed (Amann, DiMagno, & Rubin, 1997).

Several theories exist about the cause and mechanism of pancreatitis, which is generally described as the autodigestion of the pancreas. Generally, these theories state that the pancreatic duct becomes obstructed, accompanied by hypersecretion of the exocrine enzymes of the pancreas. These enzymes enter the bile duct, where they are activated and, together with bile, back up (reflux) into the pancreatic duct, causing pancreatitis.

The most basic classification system used to describe or categorize the various stages and forms of pancreatitis is currently under revision. The most basic system divides pancreatitis into acute or chronic forms.

Acute Pancreatitis

Acute pancreatitis ranges from a mild, self-limiting disorder to a severe, rapidly fatal disease that does not respond to any treatment. Mild acute pancreatitis (formerly termed interstitial or edematous pancreatitis) is characterized by edema and inflammation confined to the pancreas. Minimal organ dysfunction is present, and return to normal usually occurs within 6 months. Although this is considered the milder form of pancreatitis, the patient is acutely ill and at risk for shock, fluid and electrolyte disturbances, and sepsis. Severe acute pancreatitis (formerly termed necrotizing or hemorrhagic pancreatitis) is characterized by a more widespread and complete enzymatic digestion of the gland. The tissue becomes necrotic, and the damage extends into the retroperitoneal tissues. Local complications consist of pancreatic cysts or abscesses and acute fluid collections in or near the pancreas. Systemic complications, such as acute respiratory distress syndrome, shock, disseminated intravascular coagulopathy, and pleural effusion, can increase the mortality rate to 50% or higher (Amann, DiMagno, & Rubin, 1997).

Pathophysiology

Acute pancreatitis, or inflammation of the pancreas, is brought about by the digestion of this organ by its own enzymes, principally trypsin. Eighty percent of patients with acute pancreatitis have biliary tract disease; however, only 5% of patients with gallstones develop pancreatitis. Gallstones enter the common bile duct and lodge at the ampulla of Vater, obstructing the flow of pancreatic juice or causing a reflux of bile from the common bile duct into the pancreatic duct, thus activating the powerful enzymes within the pancreas. Normally, these remain in an inactive form until the pancreatic juice reaches the lumen of the duodenum.

Long-term alcohol use is a common cause of acute episodes of pancreatitis, but the patient usually has had undiagnosed chronic pancreatitis before the first episode of acute pancreatitis occurs. Other less common causes of pancreatitis include bacterial or viral infection, with pancreatitis a complication of mumps virus. Spasm and edema of the ampulla of Vater, resulting from duodenitis, can probably produce pancreatitis. Blunt abdominal trauma, peptic ulcer disease, ischemic vascular disease, hyperlipidemia, hypercalcemia, and the use of corticosteroids, thiazide diuretics, and oral contraceptives have been associated with an increased incidence of pancreatitis. Acute pancreatitis may follow surgery on or near the pancreas or after instrumentation of the pancreatic duct. Acute idiopathic pancreatitis may be responsible for 10% to 15% of cases of acute pancreatitis (DiPiro et al., 1997). In addition, there is a small incidence of hereditary pancreatitis.

The mortality rate of patients with acute pancreatitis is high (10%) because of shock, anoxia, hypotension, or fluid and electrolyte imbalances. Attacks of acute pancreatitis may result in complete recovery, may recur without permanent damage, or may progress to chronic pancreatitis. The patient admitted to the hospital with a diagnosis of pancreatitis is acutely ill and needs expert nursing and medical care.

Clinical Manifestations

Severe abdominal pain is the major symptom of pancreatitis that brings the patient to medical care. Abdominal pain and tenderness and back pain result from irritation and edema of the inflamed pancreas that stimulate the nerve endings. Increased tension on the pancreatic capsule and obstruction of the pancreatic ducts also contribute to the pain. Typically, the pain occurs in the midepigastrium. Pain is frequently acute in onset, occurring 24 to 48 hours after a very heavy meal or alcohol ingestion, and it may be diffuse and difficult to locate. It is generally more severe after meals and is unrelieved by antacids. Pain may be accompanied by abdominal distention, a poorly defined, palpable abdominal mass, and decreased peristalsis. Pain caused by pancreatitis is frequently accompanied by vomiting that does not relieve the pain or nausea.

The patient appears acutely ill. Abdominal guarding is present. A rigid or boardlike abdomen may develop and is generally an ominous sign. The abdomen may, however, remain soft in the absence of peritonitis. Ecchymosis (bruising) in the flank or around the umbilicus may indicate severe pancreatitis. Nausea and vomiting are common in acute pancreatitis. The emesis is usually gastric in origin but may also be bile stained. Fever, jaundice, mental confusion, and agitation also may occur.

Hypotension is typical and reflects hypovolemia and shock caused by loss of large amounts of protein-rich fluid into the tissues and peritoneal cavity. The patient may develop tachycardia, cyanosis, and cold, clammy skin in addition to hypotension. Acute renal failure is common.

Respiratory distress and hypoxia are common, and the patient may develop diffuse pulmonary infiltrates, dyspnea, tachypnea, and abnormal blood gas values. Myocardial depression, hypocalcemia, hyperglycemia, and disseminated intravascular coagulopathy may also occur with acute pancreatitis.

Assessment and Diagnostic Findings

The diagnosis of acute pancreatitis is based on a history of abdominal pain, the presence of known risk factors, physical examination findings, and diagnostic findings. Serum amylase and lipase levels are used in making the diagnosis of acute pancreatitis. Peak levels of serum amylase are reached in 24 hours, with a rapid fall to normal levels within 48 to 72 hours; serum lipase rises after 48 hours and remains elevated for 5 to 7 days. Urinary amylase levels also become elevated and remain elevated longer than serum amylase levels. The white blood cell count is usually elevated; hypocalcemia is present in many patients and appears to be correlated with the severity of pancreatitis. Transient hyperglycemia and glucosuria and elevated serum bilirubin levels occur in some patients with acute pancreatitis.

Other laboratory results that may be elevated in acute pancreatitis and used to determine its severity include fibrinogen, C-reactive protein, trypsinogen activation peptide, and polymorphonuclear elastase.

X-rays of the abdomen and chest may be obtained to differentiate pancreatitis from other disorders that may cause similar symptoms and to detect pleural effusions. Ultrasound and contrast-enhanced CT scans are used to identify an increase in the diameter of the pancreas and to detect pancreatic cysts, abscesses, or pseudocysts.

Hematocrit and hemoglobin levels are used to monitor the patient for bleeding. Peritoneal fluid that may be obtained through paracentesis or peritoneal lavage may contain increased levels of pancreatic enzymes.

The stools of patients suffering with pancreatic disease are often bulky, pale, and foul smelling. Fat content varies between 50% and 90% in pancreatic disease; normally, the fat content is 20%.

Endoscopic retrograde cholangiopancreatography (ERCP) is rarely used in the diagnostic evaluation of acute pancreatitis, but it may be valuable in the treatment of gallstone pancreatitis.

Several predictors of the severity of pancreatitis and its prognosis have been identified and are listed in Chart 38-4.

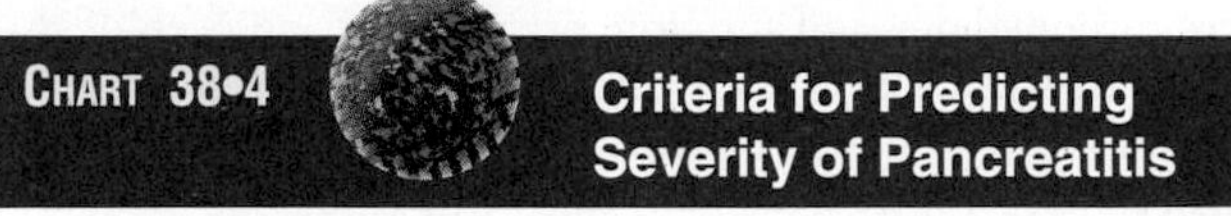

CHART 38•4
Criteria for Predicting Severity of Pancreatitis

Criteria on Admission

Age >55 years
WBC >16,000 mm^3
Serum glucose >200 mg/dL (>11.1 mmol/L)
Serum LDH >350 IU/L (>350 U/L)
SGOT (AST) >250 U/ml (120 U/L)

Criteria Within 48 Hours

Fall in hematocrit >10% (>0.10)
BUN increase >5 mg/dL (>1.7 mmol/L)
Serum calcium <8 mg/dL (<2.0 mmol/L)
Base deficit >4 mEq/L (>4 mmol/L)
Fluid retention or sequestration >6 L
PO_2 <60 mm Hg

2 or fewer signs: 1% mortality
Presence of 3 or more = severe pancreatitis
3–4 signs: 15% mortality
5–6 signs: 40% mortality
>6 signs: 100% mortality

Adapted from Wilson, C., & Imrie, C. W. (1991). Current concepts in the management of pancreatitis. *Drug, 41*(3), 360.

Medical Management

Management of the patient with acute pancreatitis is symptomatic and directed toward preventing or treating complications. All oral intake is withheld to inhibit pancreatic stimulation and secretion of pancreatic enzymes. Total parenteral nutrition (TPN) is usually an important part of therapy, particularly in debilitated patients, because of the metabolic stress associated with acute pancreatitis. Nasogastric suction may be used to relieve nausea and vomiting, to decrease painful abdominal distention and paralytic ileus, and to remove hydrochloric acid, so that it does not enter the duodenum and stimulate the pancreas.

PAIN MANAGEMENT

Adequate pain medication is essential during the course of acute pancreatitis to provide sufficient pain relief and minimize the patient's restlessness, which may stimulate pancreatic secretion further. Morphine and morphine derivatives are avoided because they cause spasm of the sphincter of Oddi. Antiemetics may be prescribed to prevent vomiting.

INTENSIVE CARE

Correction of fluid and blood loss and low albumin levels are necessary to maintain fluid volume and prevent renal failure. The patient is usually acutely ill and is monitored in the intensive care unit where hemodynamic monitoring and arterial blood gas monitoring are initiated. Antibiotics may be prescribed if infection is present; insulin may be required if significant hyperglycemia occurs.

RESPIRATORY CARE

Aggressive respiratory care is indicated because of the high risk for elevation of the diaphragm, pulmonary infiltrates and effusion, and atelectasis. Hypoxemia occurs in a significant number of patients with acute pancreatitis even with normal x-ray findings. Respiratory care may range from close monitoring of arterial blood gases to use of humidified oxygen to intubation and mechanical ventilation.

BILIARY DRAINAGE

Placement of biliary drains (for external drainage) and stents (indwelling tubes) in the pancreatic duct through endoscopy has been performed to reestablish drainage of the pancreas. This has resulted in decreased pain and increased weight gain.

SURGICAL INTERVENTION

Although often risky because the acutely ill patient is a poor surgical risk, surgery may be performed to assist in the diagnosis of pancreatitis (diagnostic laparotomy), to establish pancreatic drainage, or to resect or débride a necrotic pancreas. The patient who undergoes pancreatic surgery may have multiple drains in place postoperatively as well as a surgical incision that is left open and is irrigated and repacked every 2 to 3 days to remove necrotic debris (Fig. 38-7).

POSTACUTE MANAGEMENT

Antacids may be used when acute pancreatitis begins to resolve. Oral feedings low in fat and protein are initiated gradually. Caffeine and alcohol are eliminated from the diet. If the episode of pancreatitis occurred during treatment with thiazide diuretics, corticosteroids, or oral contraceptives, these medications are discontinued. Follow-up of the patient may include ultrasound, x-rays , or ERCP to determine whether the pancreatitis is resolving and to assess for abscesses and pseudocysts. ERCP may also be used to identify the cause of acute pancreatitis if it is in question and for endoscopic sphincterotomy and removal of gallstones from the common bile duct.

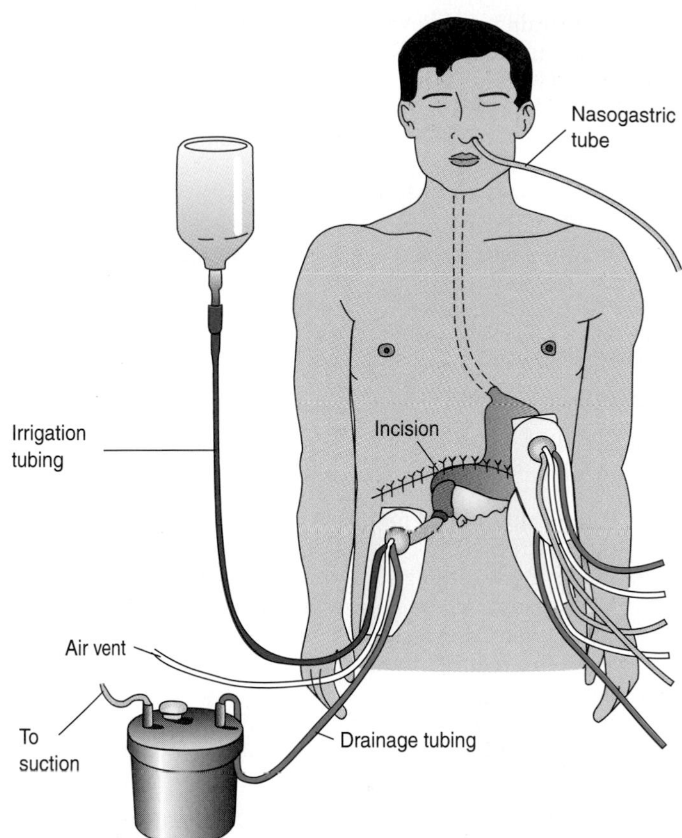

FIGURE 38•7 Multiple sump tubes are used after pancreatic surgery. Triple-lumen tubes consist of ports that provide tubing for irrigation, air venting, and drainage.

GERONTOLOGIC CONSIDERATIONS

Acute pancreatitis affects people of all ages; however, the mortality rate associated with acute pancreatitis increases with advancing age. In addition, the pattern of complications changes with age. Younger patients tend to develop local complications, and the incidence of multiple organ failure increases with age, possibly as a result of progressive decreases in physiologic function of major organs with increasing age. Close observation of major organ function (ie, lungs, kidneys) is indicated, and aggressive treatment is necessary to reduce mortality from acute pancreatitis in the elderly.

NURSING PROCESS: THE PATIENT WITH ACUTE PANCREATITIS

Assessment

The health history focuses on the presence and character of the patient's abdominal pain and discomfort. The presence of pain, its location, its relationship to eating and to alcohol consumption, and the effectiveness of pain relief measures are assessed. The patient's nutritional and fluid status and history of gallbladder attacks and alcohol use are also assessed. A history of gastrointestinal problems, including nausea, vomiting, diarrhea, and passage of fatty stools, is elicited. The abdomen is assessed for pain, tenderness, guarding, and bowel sounds; the presence of a boardlike or soft abdomen is noted. Respiratory status, respiratory rate and pattern, and breath sounds are assessed. Normal and adventitious breath sounds and abnormal findings on chest percussion, including dullness at the bases of the lungs and abnormal tactile fremitus, are documented.

The emotional and psychological status of the patient and family and their coping are assessed because they are often anxious about the severity of the patient's symptoms and the acuity of illness.

Diagnosis

Nursing Diagnoses

Based on all the assessment data, the major nursing diagnoses of the patient with acute pancreatitis include the following:

- Pain (acute) related to inflammation, edema, distention of the pancreas, and peritoneal irritation
- Ineffective breathing pattern related to severe pain, pulmonary infiltrates, pleural effusion, and atelectasis
- Altered nutritional status: less than body requirements related to reduced food intake and increased metabolic demands
- Impaired skin integrity related to poor nutritional status, bed rest, and multiple drains and surgical wound

Collaborative Problems/Potential Complications

Based on assessment data, potential complications that may occur include the following:

- Fluid and electrolyte disturbances
- Necrosis of the pancreas
- Shock and multiple organ dysfunction

Planning and Goals

The major goals for the patient include relief of pain and discomfort, improved respiratory function, improved nutritional status, maintenance of skin integrity, and absence of complications.

Nursing Interventions

Relieving Pain and Discomfort

Because the pathologic process responsible for pain is autodigestion of the pancreas, the objectives of therapy are to relieve pain and to decrease secretion of the enzymes of the pancreas. The pain of acute pancreatitis is often very severe, necessitating the liberal use of analgesics. Meperidine (Demerol) is the medication of choice; morphine sulfate is avoided because it causes spasm of the sphincter of Oddi. Oral feedings are withheld to decrease the formation and secretion of secretin. The patient is maintained on parenteral fluids and electrolytes to restore and maintain fluid balance. Nasogastric suction is used to remove gastric secretions and to relieve abdominal distention. The nurse provides frequent oral hygiene and care to decrease discomfort from the nasogastric tube and relieve dryness of the mouth.

The acutely ill patient is maintained on bed rest to decrease the metabolic rate and reduce the secretion of pancreatic and gastric enzymes. If the patient experiences increasing severity of pain, this is reported to the physician because the patient may be experiencing hemorrhage of the pancreas, or the dose of analgesic may be inadequate.

The patient with acute pancreatitis often has a clouded sensorium because of severe pain, fluid and electrolyte disturbances, and hypoxia. Therefore, frequent and repeated but simple explanations are offered about the need for withholding fluid intake and about maintenance of gastric suction and bed rest.

Improving Breathing Pattern

The patient is maintained in a semi-Fowler's position to decrease pressure on the diaphragm by a distended abdomen and to increase respiratory expansion. Frequent changes of position are necessary to prevent atelectasis and pooling of respiratory secretions. Pulmonary assessment and monitoring of pulse oximetry or arterial blood gases are essential to detect changes in respiratory status, so that early treatment can be initiated. The patient is instructed in techniques of coughing and deep breathing to improve respiratory function and is encouraged and assisted to cough and deep breathe every 2 hours.

Improving Nutritional Status

The patient with acute pancreatitis is not permitted food and oral fluid intake; however, it is important to assess the patient's nutritional status and to note factors that alter the patient's nutritional requirements (eg, temperature elevation, surgery, drainage). Laboratory test results, daily weights, and anthropometric measures are useful in monitoring the patient's nutritional status.

TPN may be prescribed. In addition to administering TPN, the nurse monitors the patient's serum glucose levels every 4 to 6 hours. As the patient's acute symptoms subside, oral feedings are reintroduced gradually. Between acute attacks, the patient receives a diet high in carbohydrates and low in fat and proteins. Heavy meals are avoided, as are alcoholic beverages.

Improving Skin Integrity

The patient is at risk for skin breakdown because of poor nutritional status, enforced bed rest, and restlessness, which may result in pressure ulcers and breaks in tissue integrity. In addition, the patient who has undergone surgery, has had multiple drains inserted, or has an open surgical incision is at risk for skin breakdown and infection. The wound, drainage sites, and skin are assessed carefully for signs of infection, inflammation, and breakdown. Wound care is carried out as prescribed, and precautions are taken to protect intact skin from contact with drainage. Consultation with an enterostomal therapist is often helpful in identifying appropriate skin care devices and protocols. The patient is turned every 2 hours; use of specialty beds may be indicated to prevent skin breakdown.

Monitoring and Managing Potential Complications

Fluid and electrolyte disturbances are common complications because of nausea, vomiting, movement of fluid from the vascular compartment to the peritoneal cavity, diaphoresis, fever, and the use of gastric suction. The patient's fluid and electrolyte status is assessed by noting skin turgor and moistness of mucous membranes. The patient is weighed daily, and fluid intake and output are carefully measured, including urine output, nasogastric secretions, and diarrhea. In addition, the patient is assessed for other factors that may affect fluid and electrolyte status, including increased body temperature and wound drainage. The nurse assesses the patient for the presence of ascites and measures abdominal girth daily if ascites is suspected.

Intravenous fluids are administered and may be accompanied by infusion of blood and albumin to maintain the patient's blood volume and to prevent or treat shock. Emergency medications are kept readily available because of the risk of circulatory collapse and shock. Decreased blood pressure and reduced urine output are reported promptly because they may indicate hypovolemia and shock or renal failure. Low serum calcium and magnesium levels may occur and require prompt treatment.

Pancreatic necrosis is a major cause of morbidity and mortality in patients with acute pancreatitis. The patient who develops necrosis is at risk for hemorrhage, septic shock, and multiple organ failure. The patient may undergo diagnostic procedures to confirm pancreatic necrosis; surgical débridement or insertion of multiple drains may be performed. The patient with pancreatic necrosis is usually critically ill and requires expert medical and nursing management, including hemodynamic monitoring in the intensive care unit.

In addition to careful monitoring of the patient's vital signs and other signs and symptoms, the nurse is responsible for administering prescribed fluids, medications, and blood products; assisting with supportive management, such as use of a ventilator; preventing additional complications; and attending to the patient's physical and psychological care.

Shock and multiple organ failure may occur with acute pancreatitis. Hypovolemic shock may occur as a result of hypovolemia and sequestering of fluid in the peritoneal cavity. Hemorrhagic shock may occur with hemorrhagic pancreatitis. Septic shock may occur with bacterial infection of the pancreas. Cardiac dysfunction may occur as a result of fluid and electrolyte disturbances, acid–base imbalances, and release of toxic substances into the circulation.

The patient must be monitored closely for early signs of neurologic, cardiovascular, renal, and respiratory dysfunction. The nurse must be prepared to respond quickly to rapid changes in the patient's status, treatments, and therapies. Additionally, the patient's family needs to be kept informed about the status and progress of the patient and must be allowed some time to spend with the patient. (Management of the patient in shock is discussed in detail in Chap. 14).

Promoting Home and Community-Based Care

TEACHING PATIENTS SELF-CARE

The patient who has experienced and survived an episode of acute pancreatitis has been acutely ill. A prolonged period is needed to regain strength and return to previous level of activity. The patient is often still weak and debilitated weeks or months after an acute episode of pancreatitis. Because of the severity of the acute illness, the patient may not recall many of the explanations and instructions given during the acute phase. As a result, these often need to be repeated and reinforced. The patient is instructed about those factors implicated in the onset of acute pancreatitis and about the need to avoid high-fat foods, heavy meals, and alcohol. The patient and family receive verbal and written instructions about signs and symptoms of acute pancreatitis and possible complications that should be reported promptly to the physician.

If acute pancreatitis is a result of biliary tract disease, such as gallstones and gallbladder disease, additional explanations are needed about required dietary modifications. If the pancreatitis is a result of alcohol abuse, the patient needs to be reminded of the importance of eliminating *all* alcohol.

CONTINUING CARE

A referral for home care is often indicated; this enables the nurse to assess the patient's physical and psychological status and compliance with the therapeutic regimen. The nurse also assesses the home situation and reinforces instructions about fluid and nutrition intake and avoidance of alcohol.

When the acute attack has subsided, some patients may be inclined to return to their previous drinking habits. Specific information about resources and support groups that may be of assistance in avoiding alcohol in the future is provided to the patient and his family. Referral to Alcoholics Anonymous or other appropriate support groups is essential.

A summary of nursing management of the patient with acute pancreatitis is provided in Plan of Nursing Care 38-2.

Evaluation

Expected Outcomes

Expected outcomes may include:

1. Reports relief of pain and discomfort
   a. Uses analgesics and anticholinergics as prescribed, without overuse
   b. Maintains bed rest as prescribed
   c. Avoids alcohol to decrease abdominal pain
2. Experiences improved respiratory function
   a. Changes position in bed frequently
   b. Coughs and takes deep breaths at least every hour
   c. Demonstrates normal respiratory rate and pattern, full lung expansion, normal breath sounds
   d. Demonstrates normal body temperature and absence of respiratory infection
3. Achieves nutritional and fluid and electrolyte balance
   a. Reports decrease in number of episodes of diarrhea
   b. Identifies and consumes high-carbohydrate, low-protein foods
   c. Explains rationale for eliminating alcohol intake
   d. Maintains adequate fluid intake within prescribed guidelines
   e. Exhibits adequate urine output
4. Exhibits intact skin
   a. Skin is without breakdown or infection
   b. Drainage is adequately contained
5. Absence of complications
   a. Demonstrates normal skin turgor, moist mucous membranes, normal serum electrolyte levels
   b. Exhibits stabilization of weight, with no increase in abdominal girth
   c. Exhibits normal neurologic, cardiovascular, renal, and respiratory function

Chronic Pancreatitis

Chronic pancreatitis is an inflammatory disorder characterized by progressive anatomic and functional destruction of the pancreas. As cells are replaced by fibrous tissue with repeated attacks of pancreatitis, pressure within the pancreas increases. The end result is mechanical obstruction of the pancreatic and common bile ducts and the duodenum. Additionally, there is atrophy of the epithelium

(*text continues on page 1074*)

38•2

PLAN OF NURSING CARE

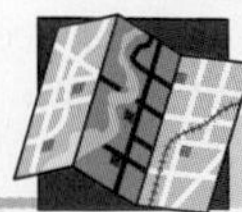

Care of the Patient With Acute Pancreatitis

Nursing Interventions	Rationale	Expected Outcomes
Nursing Diagnosis: Severe pain and discomfort related to edema, distention of the pancreas, and peritoneal irritation		
Goal: Relief of pain and discomfort		
1. Administer meperidine (Demerol) frequently, as prescribed, based on patient's level of pain and discomfort.	1. Meperidine acts by depressing the central nervous system and thereby increasing the patient's pain threshold. Morphine is avoided because it produces spasm of the sphincter of Oddi.	• Reports relief of pain • Moves and turns without increasing pain and discomfort • Rests comfortably and sleeps for increasing periods
2. Assess pain level before and after administration of analgesic.	2. Assessment and control of pain are important because restlessness increases body metabolism, which stimulates the secretion of pancreatic and gastric enzymes.	• Reports less frequent episodes of pain, discomfort, and cramping
3. Report unrelieved pain or increasing intensity of pain.	3. Pain may increase pancreatic enzymes and may also indicate pancreatic hemorrhage.	
4. Assist the patient to assume positions of comfort; turn and reposition every 2 hours.	4. Frequent turning relieves pressure and assists in preventing pulmonary and vascular complications.	
Goal: Reduction of stimulation of the pancreas		
1. Administer anticholinergic medications as prescribed.	1. Anticholinergic medications reduce gastric and pancreatic secretion.	• Reports relief of pain, discomfort, and abdominal cramping
2. Withhold oral intake.	2. Pancreatic secretion is increased by food and fluid intake.	• Takes no fluid and food during acute phase • Maintains bed rest
3. Maintain the patient on bed rest.	3. Bed rest decreases body metabolism and thus reduces pancreatic and gastric secretions.	• Identifies rationale for fluid and dietary restrictions and use of nasogastric drainage
4. Maintain continuous nasogastric drainage. a. Measure gastric secretions at specified intervals. b. Observe and record color and viscosity of gastric secretions. c. Ensure that the nasogastric tube is patent to permit free drainage.	4. Nasogastric suction removes gastric contents and prevents gastric secretions from entering the duodenum and stimulating the secretin mechanism. Decompression of the intestines (if intestinal intubation is used) also assists in relieving respiratory distress.	• Cooperates with insertion of nasogastric tube and suction
Goal: Relief of discomfort associated with nasogastric drainage		
1. Use water-soluble lubricant around external nares.	1. Prevents irritation of nares.	• Exhibits intact skin and tissue of nares at site of nasogastric tube insertion
2. Turn patient at intervals; avoid pressure or tension on nasogastric tube	2. Relieves pressure of tube on esophageal and gastric mucosa.	• Reports no pain or irritation of nares or oropharynx
3. Give oral hygiene and gargling solutions without alcohol.	3. Relieves dryness and irritation of oropharynx.	• Exhibits moist, clean mucous membranes of mouth and nasopharynx
4. Explain rationale for use of nasogastric drainage.	4. Assists patient to cope with the drainage, nasogastric tube, and suction.	• States that thirst is relieved by oral hygiene • Identifies rationale for nasogastric tube and suction
Nursing Diagnosis: Altered nutrition: Less than body requirements related to inadequate dietary intake, impaired pancreatic secretions, increased nutritional needs secondary to acute illness, and increased body temperature		
Goal: Improvement in nutritional status		
1. Assess current nutritional status and increased metabolic requirements.	1. Alteration in pancreatic secretions interferes with normal digestive processes. Acute illness, infection, and fever increase metabolic needs.	• Maintains normal body weight • Demonstrates no additional weight loss • Maintains normal serum glucose levels

(continued)

38•2 PLAN OF NURSING CARE

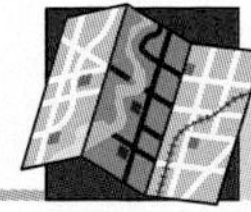

Care of the Patient With Acute Pancreatitis (*continued*)

Nursing Interventions	Rationale	Expected Outcomes
2. Monitor serum glucose levels and give insulin as prescribed.	2. Impairment of endocrine function of the pancreas leads to increased serum glucose levels.	• Reports decreasing episodes of vomiting and diarrhea • Reports return of normal stool characteristics and bowel pattern • Consumes foods high in carbohydrate, low in fat and protein • Explains rationale for high-carbohydrate, low-fat, low-protein diet • Eliminates alcohol from diet • Explains rationale for limiting coffee intake and avoiding spicy foods • Participates in Alcoholics Anonymous or other counseling approach
3. Administer intravenous fluid and electrolytes and parenteral nutrition as prescribed.	3. Parenteral administration of fluids, electrolytes, and nutrients is essential to provide fluids, calories, electrolytes, and nutrients when oral intake is prohibited.	
4. Provide high-carbohydrate, low-protein, low-fat diet when tolerated.	4. These foods increase caloric intake without stimulating pancreatic secretions beyond the ability of the pancreas to respond.	
5. Instruct patient to eliminate alcohol and refer to Alcoholics Anonymous if indicated.	5. Alcohol intake produces further damage to pancreas and precipitates attacks of acute pancreatitis.	
6. Counsel patient to avoid excessive use of coffee and spicy foods.	6. Coffee and spicy foods increase pancreatic and gastric secretions.	

Nursing Diagnosis: Ineffective breathing pattern related to splinting from severe pain, pulmonary infiltrates, pleural effusion, and atelectasis
Goal: Improvement in respiratory function

Nursing Interventions	Rationale	Expected Outcomes
1. Assess respiratory status (rate, pattern, breath sounds), pulse oximetry, and arterial blood gases.	1. Acute pancreatitis produces retroperitoneal edema, elevation of the diaphragm, pleural effusion, and inadequate lung ventilation. Intra-abdominal infection and labored breathing increase the body's metabolic demands, which further decreases pulmonary reserve and leads to respiratory failure.	• Demonstrates normal respiratory rate and pattern and full lung expansion • Demonstrates normal breath sounds and absence of adventitious breath sounds • Demonstrates normal arterial blood gases and pulse oximetry • Maintains semi-Fowler's position when in bed • Changes position in bed frequently • Coughs and takes deep breaths at least every hour • Demonstrates normal body temperature • Exhibits no signs or symptoms of respiratory infection or impairment • Is alert and responsive to environment
2. Maintain semi-Fowler's position.	2. Decreases pressure on diaphragm and allows greater lung expansion.	
3. Instruct and encourage patient to take deep breaths and to cough every hour.	3. Taking deep breaths and coughing will clear the airways and reduce atelectasis.	
4. Assist patient to turn and change position every 2 hours.	4. Changing position frequently assists aeration and drainage of all lobes of the lungs.	
5. Reduce the excessive metabolism of the body. a. Administer antibiotics as prescribed. b. Place patient in an air-conditioned room. c. Administer nasal oxygen as required for hypoxia. d. Use a hypothermia blanket if necessary.	5. Pancreatitis produces a severe peritoneal and retroperitoneal reaction that causes fever, tachycardia, and accelerated respirations. Placing the patient in an air-conditioned room and supporting the patient with oxygen therapy decrease the workload of the respiratory system and the tissue utilization of oxygen. Reduction of fever and pulse rate decreases the metabolic demands on the body.	

Collaborative Problem: Fluid and electrolyte disturbances, hypovolemia, shock
Goal: Improvement in fluid and electrolyte status, prevention of hypovolemia and shock

Nursing Interventions	Rationale	Expected Outcomes
1. Assess fluid and electrolyte status (skin turgor, mucous membranes, urine output, vital signs, hemodynamic parameters)	1. The amount and type of fluid and electrolyte replacement are determined by the status of the blood pressure, the laboratory evaluations of serum electrolyte and blood urea nitrogen levels, the urinary volume, and the assessment of the patient's condition.	• Exhibits moist mucous membranes and normal skin turgor • Exhibits normal blood pressure without evidence of postural (orthostatic) hypotension • Excretes adequate urine output • Exhibits normal, not excessive, thirst

(*continued*)

38•2

PLAN OF NURSING CARE

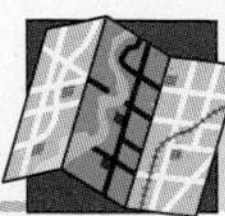

Care of the Patient With Acute Pancreatitis (*continued*)

Nursing Interventions	Rationale	Expected Outcomes
2. Assess sources of fluid and electrolyte loss (vomiting, diarrhea, nasogastric drainage, excessive diaphoresis).	2. Electrolyte losses occur from nasogastric suctioning, severe diaphoresis, emesis, and as a result of the patient's being in a fasting state.	• Maintains normal pulse and respiratory rate • Remains alert and responsive • Exhibits normal arterial pressures and blood gases • Exhibits normal electrolyte levels • Exhibits no signs or symptoms of calcium deficit (eg, tetany, carpopedal spasm) • Exhibits no additional losses of fluids and electrolytes through vomiting, diarrhea, or diaphoresis • Reports stabilization of weight • Demonstrates no increase in abdominal girth • Demonstrates no fluid wave on palpation of the abdomen • Demonstrates stable organ function without manifestations of failure
3. Combat shock if present. a. Administer corticosteroids as prescribed to those who do not respond to conventional treatment. b. Evaluate the amount of urinary output. Attempt to maintain this at 50 mL/h.	3. Extensive acute pancreatitis may cause peripheral vascular collapse and shock. Blood and plasma may be lost into the abdominal cavity, and, therefore, there is a decreased blood and plasma volume. The toxins from the bacteria of a necrotic pancreas may cause shock.	
4. Administer intravenous electrolytes (sodium, potassium, chloride) as prescribed.	4. Patients with hemorrhagic pancreatitis lose large amounts of blood and plasma, which decreases effective circulation and blood volume.	
5. Administer plasma, albumin, and blood products as prescribed.	5. Replacement with blood, plasma or albumin, assists in ensuring effective circulating blood volume.	
6. Keep a supply of intravenous calcium gluconate readily available.	6. Calcium may be prescribed to prevent or treat tetany.	
7. Assess abdomen for ascites formation: a. Measure abdominal girth daily. b. Weigh patient daily. c. Palpate abdomen for fluid wave	7. During acute pancreatitis, plasma may be lost into the abdominal cavity, which diminishes the blood volume.	
8. Monitor for manifestations indicating multiple organ failure: neurologic, cardiovascular, renal, and respiratory dysfunction.	8. All body systems may fail if pancreatitis is severe and treatment is ineffective.	

of the ducts, inflammation, and destruction of the secreting cells of the pancreas.

Alcohol consumption in Western societies and malnutrition worldwide are the major causes of chronic pancreatitis. Excessive and prolonged consumption of alcohol is the major etiologic factor for cases in Western society (Ammann, 1997). The incidence of pancreatitis is 50 times greater in alcoholics than in the nondrinking population. Long-term alcohol consumption causes hypersecretion of protein in pancreatic secretions, resulting in protein plugs and calculi within the pancreatic ducts. Alcohol also has a direct toxic effect on the cells of the pancreas. Damage to these cells is more likely to occur and to be more severe in patients whose diets are poor in protein content and either very high or very low in fat.

Clinical Manifestations

The incidence of chronic pancreatitis is increased in adult men and is characterized by recurring attacks of severe upper abdominal and back pain, accompanied by vomiting. Attacks are often so painful that opioids, even in large doses, do not provide relief. As the disease progresses, recurring attacks of pain are more severe, more frequent, and of longer duration. Some patients experience continuous severe pain; others have a dull, nagging constant pain. The risk of dependence on opioids is increased in pancreatitis because of the chronic nature and severity of the pain.

Weight loss is a major problem in chronic pancreatitis; more than 75% of patients experience significant weight loss, usually caused by decreased dietary intake secondary to anorexia or fear that eating will precipitate another attack. Malabsorption occurs late in the disease when as little as 10% of pancreatic function remains. As a result, digestion, especially of proteins and fats, is impaired. The stools become frequent, frothy, and foul smelling because of impaired fat digestion, which results in stools with a high fat content. This condition is referred to as **steatorrhea.** As the disease progresses, calcification of the gland may occur, and calcium stones may form within the ducts.

Assessment and Diagnostic Findings

ERCP is the most useful study in the diagnosis of chronic pancreatitis. It provides detail about the anatomy of the pancreas and of the pancreatic and biliary ducts. It is also helpful in obtaining tissue for analysis and in differentiating pancreatitis from other conditions, such as carcinoma. A CT scan or ultrasound is helpful to detect the presence of pancreatic cysts.

A glucose tolerance test evaluates pancreatic islet cell function, information necessary for making decisions about surgical resection of the pancreas. An abnormal glucose tolerance test indicative of diabetes may be present. In contrast to the patient with acute pancreatitis, serum amylase levels and the white blood cell count may not be significantly elevated.

Management

The management of chronic pancreatitis depends on its probable cause in each patient. Nonsurgical approaches may be indicated for the patient who refuses surgery, who is a poor surgical risk, or whose disease and symptoms do not warrant surgical intervention. Treatment is directed toward prevention and management of acute attacks, the relief of pain and discomfort, and management of exocrine and endocrine insufficiency of pancreatitis.

Management of abdominal pain and discomfort is similar to that of acute pancreatitis; however, the focus is usually on the use of nonopioid methods to manage pain. The physician, nurse, and dietitian emphasize to the patient and family the importance of avoiding alcohol and other foods that the patient has found tend to produce abdominal pain and discomfort. The fact that no other treatment is likely to relieve pain if the patient continues to consume alcohol is stressed to the patient.

Diabetes mellitus resulting from dysfunction of the pancreatic islet cells is treated with diet, insulin, or oral hypoglycemic agents. The hazard of severe hypoglycemia with alcohol use is stressed to the patient and family members. Pancreatic enzyme replacement is indicated in the patient with malabsorption and steatorrhea.

SURGICAL MANAGEMENT

Surgery is generally carried out to relieve abdominal pain and discomfort, to restore drainage of pancreatic secretions, and to reduce the frequency of acute attacks of pancreatitis. The surgery performed depends on the anatomic and functional abnormalities of the pancreas, including the location of disease within the pancreas, the presence of diabetes, exocrine insufficiency, biliary stenosis, and pseudocysts of the pancreas. Other factors taken into consideration in determining whether surgery is to be performed and what procedure is indicated include continued use of alcohol and the ability of the patient to manage the endocrine or exocrine changes that are expected after surgery.

Pancreaticojejunostomy with a side-to-side anastomosis or joining of the pancreatic duct to the jejunum allows drainage of the pancreatic secretions into the jejunum. Pain relief occurs by 6 months in more than 80% of the patients who undergo this procedure, but pain returns in a substantial number of patients as the disease itself progresses.

Patients who undergo surgery may experience increased weight gain and improved nutritional status; this may result from reduction in pain associated with eating rather than from correction of malabsorption. Other surgical procedures may be performed for different degrees and types of disease, ranging from revision of the sphincter of the ampulla of Vater, to internal drainage of a pancreatic cyst into the stomach, to insertion of a stent, to wide resection or removal of the pancreas.

Autotransplantation or implantation of the patient's pancreatic islet cells has been attempted to preserve the endocrine function of the pancreas. Testing and refinement of this procedure continue in an effort to improve outcomes. Morbidity and mortality after these surgical procedures are high because of the poor physical condition of the patient before surgery and the concomitant occurrence of cirrhosis.

Despite these surgical procedures, the patient is likely to continue to have pain and impaired digestion secondary to pancreatitis unless alcohol is avoided completely.

Pancreatic Cysts

As a result of the local necrosis that occurs at the time of acute pancreatitis, collections of fluid may form in the vicinity of the pancreas. These become walled off by fibrous tissue and are called pancreatic pseudocysts. They are the most common type of pancreatic cysts. Other, less common cysts occur as a result of congenital anomalies or are secondary to chronic pancreatitis or trauma to the pancreas.

Diagnosis of pancreatic cysts and pseudocysts is made by ultrasound, CT scan, and ERCP. ERCP may be used to define the anatomy of the pancreas and to evaluate the patency of pancreatic drainage. Pancreatic pseudocysts may be of considerable size. Because of their location behind the posterior peritoneum, when they enlarge, they impinge on and displace the stomach or the colon, which are adjacent. Eventually, through pressure or secondary infection, they produce symptoms, requiring that they be drained.

Management

CYST DRAINAGE

Drainage into the gastrointestinal tract or through the skin and abdominal wall may be established. In the latter instance, the drainage is likely to be profuse and destructive to tissue because of the enzyme contents. Hence, steps must be taken to protect the skin near the drainage site to prevent excoriation. Ointments protect the skin, provided that they are applied before excoriation takes place. Another method involves the constant aspiration of digestive juice from the drainage tract by means of a suction apparatus, so that skin contact with the digestive enzymes is avoided. This method requires expert nursing attention to be sure that the suction tube does not become dislodged and suction is not interrupted. Consultation with an enterostomal therapist is indicated to identify appropriate strategies to maintain drainage and protect the patient's skin.

SURGICAL MANAGEMENT

When chronic pancreatitis develops as a result of gallbladder disease, the obstruction is treated by surgery to explore the common duct and remove the stones; usually, the gallbladder is removed at the same time. In addition, an attempt is made to improve the drainage of the common bile duct and the pancreatic duct by dividing the sphincter of Oddi, a muscle that is located at the ampulla of Vater (this surgical procedure is known as a sphincterotomy). Nursing care after such surgery is similar to that indicated after other biliary tract surgery. A T tube usually is placed in the common bile duct, requiring a drainage system to collect the bile postoperatively.

General Pancreatic Tumors

The incidence of pancreatic cancer has been steadily increasing for the past 20 to 30 years, especially in nonwhite men. It is the fourth leading cause of cancer deaths in the United States and occurs most frequently in the fifth to seventh decades of life (McEwen, Sanchez, Rosario, & Allen, 1996; American Cancer Society, 1999). Cigarette smoking, exposure to industrial chemicals or toxins in the environment, and a diet high in fat, meat, or both, are associated with pancreatic cancer, although their role is not completely clear. The risk for pancreatic cancer increases as the extent of cigarette smoking increases. Diabetes mellitus, chronic pancreatitis, and hereditary pancreatitis are also associated with pancreatic cancer. The pancreas can also be the site of metastasis from other tumors.

Cancer may arise in any portion of the pancreas (in the head, the body, or the tail), producing clinical manifestations that vary, depending on the location of the lesion and whether functioning, insulin-secreting pancreatic islet cells are involved. Tumors that originate in the head of the pancreas, the most common location, give rise to a distinctive clinical picture. Functioning islet cell tumors, whether benign (adenoma) or malignant (carcinoma), are responsible for the syndrome of hyperinsulinism. With these exceptions, the symptoms are nonspecific, and patients usually do not seek medical attention until late in the disease; 80% to 85% of patients have advanced, unresectable tumor when first detected. In fact, pancreatic carcinoma has only a 3% survival rate at 5 years regardless of the stage of disease at diagnosis or treatment (McEwen et al., 1996).

Clinical Manifestations

Pain, jaundice, or both are present in more than 90% of patients and, along with weight loss, are considered classic signs of pancreatic carcinoma and may not appear until the disease is far advanced. Other signs include rapid, profound, and progressive weight loss as well as vague upper or midabdominal pain or discomfort that is unrelated to any gastrointestinal function and is often difficult to describe.

Such discomfort radiates as a boring pain in the midback and is unrelated to posture or activity. Patients with pancreatic carcinoma often find that they get some relief by sitting hunched forward; pain is often accentuated by lying supine. Pain is often progressive and severe, requiring the use of opioids. It is often more severe at night.

Malignant cells from pancreatic cancer are often shed into the peritoneal cavity, increasing the likelihood of metastasis. The formation of ascites is common.

An important sign, when present, is the onset of symptoms of insulin deficiency: glucosuria, hyperglycemia, and abnormal glucose tolerance. Thus, diabetes may be an early sign of carcinoma of the pancreas. Meals often aggravate epigastric pain, which usually occurs before the appearance of jaundice and pruritus. Gastrointestinal x-rays may demonstrate deformities in adjacent viscera caused by the impinging pancreatic mass.

Assessment and Diagnostic Findings

Ultrasound and CT scan are used to identify the presence of pancreatic tumors. ERCP has become a major diagnostic procedure used in the diagnosis of pancreatic carcinoma. Cells obtained during ERCP are sent to the laboratory for examination.

Percutaneous fine-needle aspiration biopsy of the pancreas is used to diagnose pancreatic tumors and to confirm the diagnosis in patients whose tumors are not resectable, eliminating the stress and postoperative pain of ineffective surgery. In this procedure, a needle is inserted through the anterior abdominal wall into the pancreatic mass, guided by CT scan, ultrasound, ERCP, or other imaging techniques. The aspirated material is examined for malignant cells. Although percutaneous biopsy is a valuable diagnostic tool, it has some potential drawbacks: a false-negative result if small tumors are missed and seeding of cancer cells along the needle track. Low radiation to the site may be used before the biopsy to reduce the risk of seeding.

Percutaneous transhepatic cholangiography is another procedure that may be performed to identify obstructions of the biliary tract by a pancreatic tumor.

Several tumor markers (eg, CA 19-9, CEA, DU-PAN-2) are being used in the diagnostic workup, but they are nonspecific for pancreatic carcinoma. These tumor markers are useful as indicators of disease progression (McEwen et al., 1996).

Angiography, CT scan, and laparoscopy may be performed to determine whether the tumor can be successfully removed surgically.

Medical Management

The surgical procedure is usually extensive if carried out to remove resectable localized tumors. However, definitive surgical treatment (ie, total excision of the lesion) is often not possible because of the extensive growth when the tumor is finally diagnosed and the probable widespread metastases—especially to the liver, lungs, and bones. More often, treatment is limited to palliative measures.

Although pancreatic tumors may be resistant to standard radiation therapy, the patient may be treated with radiation and chemotherapy (fluorouracil). Gemcitabine hydrochloride, an antineoplastic agent that disrupts and inhibits DNA synthesis, has recently been approved for use in patients with advanced or metastatic pancreatic cancer. If the patient undergoes surgery, intraoperative radiation therapy (IORT) may be used to deliver a high dose of radiation to the tumor with minimal injury to other tissues. IORT may also be helpful in relief of pain. Interstitial implantation of radioactive sources has also been used, although the rate of complications is high. A large biliary stent inserted percutaneously or by endoscopy may be used to relieve jaundice.

Nursing Management

Pain management and attention to nutritional requirements are important nursing measures to improve the patient's level of comfort. Skin care and nursing measures are directed toward relief of pain and discomfort associated with jaundice, anorexia, and profound weight loss. Specialty mattresses have been beneficial and protect the bony prominences from pressure. Pain associated with pancreatic cancer may be severe and may require liberal use of opioids; patient-controlled analgesia should be considered in the patient with severe, escalating pain.

PROMOTING HOME AND COMMUNITY-BASED CARE

Teaching Patients Self-Care. The specific patient and family teaching indicated varies with the stage of the patient's disease and the treatment choices made by the patient. If the patient elects chemotherapy, teaching is focused on prevention of side effects and complications of the agents used. If surgery was performed to relieve obstruction and establish biliary drainage, teaching addresses management of the drainage system and monitoring for complications. The family is instructed about changes in the patient's status that should be reported to the physician.

Continuing Care. A referral for home care is indicated to assist the patient and family to deal with the physical problems and discomforts associated with pancreatic cancer and the psychological impact of the disease. The home care nurse assesses the patient's physical status, fluid and nutritional status, skin integrity, and adequacy of pain management. Strategies to prevent skin breakdown and to relieve pain, pruritus, and anorexia are discussed with the patient and family. Palliative care (hospice services) is discussed with the patient and family and arranged in an effort to relieve patient discomfort, assist with care, and comply with the patient's end-of-life decisions and wishes.

Tumors of the Head of the Pancreas

Tumors in this region of the pancreas obstruct the common bile duct where the duct passes through the head of the pancreas to join the pancreatic duct and empty at the ampulla of Vater into the duodenum. Obstructed flow of bile produces jaundice, clay-colored stools, and dark urine. The tumors producing the obstruction may arise from the pancreas, from the common bile duct, or from the ampulla of Vater.

Clinical Manifestations

Malabsorption of nutrients and fat-soluble vitamins may result from obstruction by the tumor to entry of bile in the gastrointestinal tract. Abdominal discomfort or pain and pruritus may be noted along with anorexia, weight loss, and malaise. If these signs and symptoms are present, cancer of this part of the pancreas is suspected.

The jaundice of this disease must be differentiated from that due to a biliary obstruction caused by a gallstone in the common duct, which is usually intermittent and appears typically in obese patients, most often women, who have had previous symptoms of gallbladder disease.

Assessment and Diagnostic Findings

Diagnostic studies may include duodenography, angiography by hepatic or celiac artery catheterization, pancreatic scanning, percutaneous transhepatic cholangiography, ERCP, and percutaneous needle biopsy of the pancreas. Results of a biopsy of the pancreas may aid in the diagnosis.

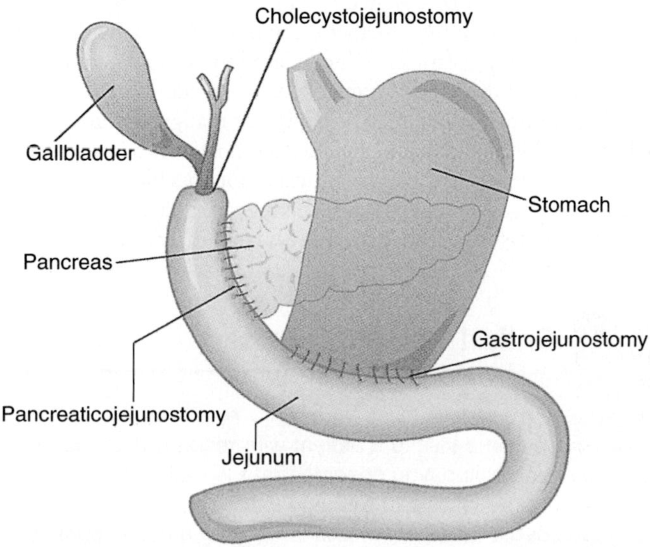

FIGURE 38•8 Pancreatoduodenectomy (Whipple's procedure or resection). End result of the resection of the carcinoma of the head of the pancreas or the ampulla of Vater. The common duct is sutured to the end of the jejunum, and the remaining portion of the pancreas and the end of the stomach are sutured to the side of the jejunum.

Medical Management

Before extensive surgery can be performed, a fairly long period of preparation is often necessary because the patient's nutritional and physical condition is often very compromised. Various liver and pancreatic function studies are performed. A diet high in protein is often prescribed with pancreatic enzymes. Preoperative preparation includes adequate hydration, correction of prothrombin deficiency with vitamin K, and treatment of anemia to minimize postoperative complications. Administration of TPN and blood component therapy is frequently required.

A biliary-enteric shunt may be performed to relieve the jaundice and, perhaps, to provide time for a thorough diagnostic evaluation. Total pancreatectomy (removal of the pancreas) may be performed. A pancreatoduodenectomy (Whipple's procedure or resection) is used for potentially curable cancer of the head of the pancreas (Fig. 38-8). It involves removal of the gallbladder, distal portion of the stomach, duodenum, and head of the pancreas, and anastomosis of the remaining pancreas, stomach, and common duct to the jejunum. The result is removal of the tumor, allowing flow of bile into the jejunum. When excision of the tumor cannot be performed, the jaundice may be relieved by diverting the bile flow into the jejunum by anastomosing the jejunum to the gallbladder, a procedure known as cholecystojejunostomy. (Whipple's resection has also been carried out to relieve the pain of chronic pancreatitis.)

The postoperative management of patients who have undergone a pancreatectomy or a pancreatoduodenectomy is similar to the management of patients after extensive gastrointestinal and biliary surgery. The patient's physical status is often less than optimal, increasing the risk for postoperative complications. The mortality rate after these procedures has improved because of advances in nutritional support and improved surgical techniques. Hemorrhage, vascular collapse, and hepatorenal failure remain the major complications of these extensive surgical procedures.

Nursing Management

Preoperatively and postoperatively, the nursing care is directed toward promoting patient comfort, preventing complications, and assisting the patient to return to and maintain as normal and comfortable a life as possible. The patient is monitored closely in the intensive care unit after surgery, has multiple intravenous and arterial lines in place for fluid and blood replacement as well as for monitoring arterial pressures, and is on a mechanical ventilator in the immediate postoperative period. Careful attention is given to changes in the patient's vital signs, arterial blood gases and pressures, pulse oximetry, laboratory values, and urine output.

Although the patient's physiologic status is the focus of the health care team in the immediate postoperative period, the patient's psychological and emotional state must be considered along with that of the family. The psychosocial considerations are based on the fact that the patient has undergone major and risky surgery and is critically ill; thus, anxiety and depression may affect the patient's recovery. The immediate and long-term outcome of this extensive surgical resection is uncertain, and the patient and family require emotional support and understanding in the critical and stressful preoperative and postoperative periods.

PROMOTING HOME AND COMMUNITY-BASED CARE

Teaching Patients Self-Care. The patient who has undergone this extensive surgery requires careful and thorough preparation for self-care at home. The patient and family are instructed about the need for modifications in the diet because of malabsorption and hyperglycemia resulting from the surgery. They are instructed about the continuing need for pancreatic enzyme replacement and a low-fat diet.

Strategies to relieve pain and discomfort are taught to the patient and family along with strategies to care for drains, if present, and the surgical incision. Patient and family members may require instruction about use of patient-controlled analgesia, TPN, wound care, skin care, and management of drainage. The signs and symptoms of complications are described verbally and in writing, and the patient and family are instructed about those indicators of complications that should be reported promptly.

Discharge of the patient to a long-term care setting may be warranted after surgery as extensive as pancreatectomy or pancreatoduodenectomy, particularly if the patient's preoperative status was not optimal. Efforts are made to communicate to the long-term care staff about the teaching that has been provided, so that instructions can be clarified and reinforced. During the recovery or long-term care phase of care, the patient and family receive further instructions about care that they will carry out at home.

Continuing Care. A referral for home care may be indicated when the patient returns home. The home care nurse assesses the patient's physical and psychological status and the ability of the patient and family to manage needed care. The home care nurse provides needed physical care and monitors the adequacy of pain management. In addition, the patient's nutritional status is assessed, and use of TPN is monitored. The use of hospice services is discussed with the patient and family, and referral is made if indicated.

Pancreatic Islet Tumors

The pancreas contains the islets (islands) of Langerhans—small nests of cells that secrete directly into the bloodstream and, therefore, are part of the endocrine system. The secretion, insulin, is essential for metabolism of glucose. Diabetes mellitus (see Chap. 37) is the result of deficient secretion of insulin.

At least two types of tumors of the pancreatic islet cells are known: those that secrete insulin (insulinoma) and those in which insulin secretion is not increased ("nonfunctioning" islet cell cancer).

Insulinomas produce hypersecretion of insulin and cause an excessive rate of glucose metabolism. The resulting hypoglycemia may produce symptoms of weakness, mental confusion, and seizures. These symptoms may be relieved almost immediately by oral or intravenous administration of glucose. The 5-hour glucose tolerance test is helpful in diagnosing insulinoma and in distinguishing it from other causes of hypoglycemia.

Surgical Management

When diagnosis of a tumor of the islet cells has been made, surgical treatment with removal of the tumor is usually recommended. The tumors may be benign adenomas, or they may be malignant. Their complete removal usually results in almost immediate relief of symptoms. In some patients, symptoms may not be produced by simple hypertrophy of this tissue rather than a tumor of the islet cells. In such cases, a partial pancreatectomy—removal of the tail and part of the body of the pancreas—is performed.

Nursing Management

In preparing the patient for surgery, the nurse must be alert for symptoms of hypoglycemia and be ready to administer glucose as prescribed, if symptoms occur. Postoperatively, the nursing management is the same as that after other upper abdominal surgical procedures, with special emphasis on monitoring serum glucose levels.

Hyperinsulinism

Hyperinsulinism results from the overproduction of insulin by the pancreatic islets. Symptoms resemble those of excessive doses of insulin and are attributable to the same mechanism—an abnormal reduction in blood glucose levels. Clinically, it is characterized by episodes during which the patient experiences unusual hunger, nervousness, sweating, headache, and faintness; in severe cases, seizures and episodes of unconsciousness may occur. The findings at the time of surgery or at autopsy may indicate hyperplasia (overgrowth) of the islets of Langerhans or a benign or malignant tumor involving the islets and capable of producing large amounts of insulin (see preceding discussion). Occasionally, tumors of nonpancreatic origin produce an insulin-like material that can cause severe hypoglycemia that may be responsible for seizures coinciding with blood glucose levels too low to sustain normal brain function (ie, below 30 mg/dL [1.6 mmol/L]).

All the symptoms that accompany spontaneous hypoglycemia are relieved by the oral or parenteral administration of glucose. Surgical removal of the hyperplastic or neoplastic tissue from the pancreas offers the only successful method of treatment. About 15% of patients with spontaneous or functional hypoglycemia eventually develop diabetes mellitus.

Ulcerogenic (Zollinger-Ellison) Tumors

Some tumors (**Zollinger-Ellison tumors**) of the islets of Langerhans are associated with a hypersecretion of gastric acid that produces ulcers in the stomach, duodenum, and jejunum. The hypersecretion is so great that even after partial gastric resection, enough acid is produced to cause further ulceration. When a marked tendency to develop gastric and duodenal ulcers is noted, an ulcerogenic tumor of the islets of Langerhans is considered.

These tumors, which may be benign or malignant, are treated, when possible, by excision. Frequently, however, because of extension beyond the pancreas, removal is not possible. In many patients, a total gastrectomy may be necessary to reduce the secretion of gastric acid sufficiently to prevent further ulceration.

Critical Thinking Exercises

1. During a home visit to a patient with recently diagnosed diabetes mellitus, you observe that the patient's grandmother is slow to respond to others, seems depressed and lethargic, and is wearing a heavy coat in the warm house. You suspect that she might have a severe hypothyroid condition. Describe how you would proceed in this situation, how you would determine what actions to take, and how you would prioritize your actions.

2.
Your patient is beginning antithyroid medication to control her hyperthyroidism. Her husband has been very concerned about her irritability, rapid mood swings, and weight loss. How would you explain to him the reasons for his wife's symptoms and the rationale for the medication being prescribed?

3.
Your patient has been receiving corticosteroids for treating a chronic disease. She has been admitted for an emergency hysterectomy. Based on your knowledge of the effects of the long-term use of corticosteroids, how would you focus your assessment and management strategies of this patient in the postoperative period?

4.
Corticosteroids have been prescribed for your patient, and it is expected that she will take them for at least 1 month. How would you instruct her to minimize complications of corticosteroid use?

5.
A 57-year-old patient has a history of alcoholism and cirrhosis. He is admitted to your unit with a diagnosis of acute pancreatitis. Describe nursing care for this patient, and compare and contrast care with and without the additional diagnosis of pancreatitis.

References and Selected Readings

BOOKS

American Cancer Society. (1999). *Cancer facts and figures.* Atlanta: American Cancer Society.

Bardin, C. W. (1997). *Current therapy in endocrinology and metabolism.* St. Louis: C. V. Mosby.

Braverman, L. E. (Ed.). (1997). *Diseases of the thyroid.* Totowa, NJ: Humana Press.

Conn, P. M., & Melmed, S. (Eds.). (1997). *Endocrinology: Basic and clinical principles.* Totowa, NJ: Humana Press.

DiPiro, J. T. et al. (Eds.). (1997). *Pharmacotherapy: A pathophysiologic approach.* Stamford, CT: Appleton & Lange.

Falk, S. A. (Ed.). (1997). *Thyroid disease: Endocrinology, surgery, nuclear medicine, and radiotherapy.* Philadelphia: Lippincott-Raven.

Greenspan, F. S., & Strewler, G. J. (Eds.). (1997). *Basic and clinical endocrinology.* Stamford, CT: Appleton & Lange.

Kelley, W. N. (Ed.). (1997). *Textbook of internal medicine.* Philadelphia: Lippincott-Raven.

Noble, J. (Ed.). (1996). *Textbook of primary care medicine.* St. Louis: C. V. Mosby.

Robin, N. I. (1996). *Endocrinology and metabolic disease.* New York: Parthenon.

Rupert, S. D., Kernicki, J. G., & Dolan, J. T. (1996). *Dolan's critical care nursing.* Philadelphia: F. A. Davis.

Tierney, L. M., McPhee, S. J., & Papadakis, M. A. (1998). *Current medical diagnosis and treatment.* Stamford, CT: Appleton & Lange.

Wierman, M. E. (Ed.). (1997). *Diseases of the pituitary: Diagnosis and treatment.* Totowa, NJ: Humana Press.

Wilson, J. D., Foster, D. W., Kronenberg, H. M., & Larsen, P. R. (1998). *Williams textbook of endocrinology.* Philadelphia: W. B. Saunders.

JOURNALS

General

Barton-Burk, M. (1999). Gemcitabine: A pharmacologic and clinical overview. *Cancer Nursing, 22*(2), 176–183.

Bello, C. E., & Garrett, S. D. (1999). Therapeutic issues in oral glucocorticoid use. *Lippincott's Primary Care Practice, 3*(3), 333–341.

Loriaux, T. C. (1996). Endocrine assessment: Red flags for those on the front lines. *Nursing Clinics of North America, 31*(4), 695–713.

Rusterholtz, A. (1996). Interpretation of diagnostic laboratory tests in selected endocrine disorders. *Nursing Clinics of North America, 31*(4), 715–724.

Skelly, A. H. (1997). Endocrine disorders. *Lippincott's Primary Care Practice, 1*(5), 459–473.

Winger, J. M., & Hornick, T. (1996). Age-associated changes in the endocrine system. *Nursing Clinics of North America, 31*(4), 782–784.

Adrenal Disorders

Alberio, L., & Lammle, B. (1998). Current concepts: Primary aldosteronism. *New England Journal of Medicine, 339*(25), 1828–1834.

Baker, J. T. (1997). Adrenal disorders: A primary care approach. *Lippincott's Primary Care Practice, 1*(5), 527–535.

Burton, M. (1997). Pheochromocytoma. *American Journal of Nursing, 97*(11), 57

Clayton, L. H., & Dilley, K. B. (1998). Cushing's syndrome. *American Journal of Nursing, 98*(7), 40–41.

Cronin, C. C., Callaghan, N., Kearney, P. J., Murnaghan, D. J., & Shanahan, F. (1997). Addison disease in patients treated with glucocorticoid therapy. *Archives of Internal Medicine, 157*(4), 456–458

Davis-Martin, S. (1996). Pearls for practice: Disorders of the adrenal glands. *Journal of the American Academy of Nurse Practitioners, 8*(7), 323–326.

Ganguly, A. (1998). Current concepts: Primary aldosteronism. *New England Journal of Medicine, 339*(25), 1828–1834.

Gavaghan, M. (1997). Surgical treatment of pheochromocytomas. *AORN Journal, 65*(6), 1043–1068.

Gumowski, J., & Loughran, M. (1996). Diseases of the adrenal gland. *Nursing Clinics of North America, 31*(4), 747–767.

O'Donnel, M. (1997). Addisonian crisis. *American Journal of Nursing, 97*(3), 41.

Ram, C. V. S. (1996). Hypertension: When to suspect underlying pheochromocytoma or aldosteronism. *Consultant, 36*(1), 147–153.

Roberts, A. (1995). The adrenal glands. *Nursing Times, 91*(45), 34–37.

Roberts, A. (1995). The adrenal gland 2. *Nursing Times, 91*(50), 31–33.

Roberts, A. (1995). The adrenal gland 3. *Nursing Times, 92*(2), 31–33.

Streeten, D. H., Anderson, G. H., & Bonaventura, M. (1996). The potential for serious consequences from misinterpreting normal responses to the rapid adrenocorticotropin test. *Journal of Clinical Endocrinology and Metabolism, 81*(1), 285–290.

Pancreatic Disorders

Ammann, R. W. (1997). A clinically based classification system for alcoholic chronic pancreatitis: Summary of an international workshop on chronic pancreatitis. *Pancreas, 15*(4), 402–408.

Aronson, B. S. (1999). Update on acute pancreatitis. *MedSurg Nursing, 8*(1), 9–16.

Banks, P. A. (1996). Practice guidelines in acute pancreatitis. *American Journal of Gastroenterology, 92*(3), 377–386.

Baron, T. H., & Morgan, D. E. (1999). Acute necrotizing pancreatitis. *New England Journal of Medicine, 340*(18), 1412–1417.

Coyne, P. J. (1998). Assessing and treating the pain of pancreatitis. *American Journal of Nursing, 98*(11), 14, 16.

Finlay, T. (1996). Making sense of the care of patients with pancreatitis. *Nursing Times, 92*(32), 38–39.

Kitagawa, M., Naruse, S., Ishiguro, H., Nakae, Y., Kondo, T., & Hayakawa, T. (1997). Evaluating exocrine function tests for diagnosing chronic pancreatitis. *Pancreas, 15*(4), 402–408.

McClave, S. A., Green, L. M., Snider, H. L., Makk, L. J., Cheadle, W. G., Owens, N. A., Dukes, L. G., & Goldsmith, L. J. (1997). Comparison of the safety of early enteral vs parenteral nutrition in mild acute pancreatitis. *Journal of Parenteral and Enteral Nutrition, 21*(1), 14–20.

McEwen, D. R., Sanchez, M. M., Rosario, A., & Allen, W. E. (1996). Managing patients with pancreatic cancer. *AORN Journal, 64*(5), 716–735.

Meissner, J. E. (1997). Caring for patients with pancreatitis. *Nursing, 27*(10), 50–51.

Noone, J. (1995). Acute pancreatitis: An Orem approach to nursing assessment and care. *Critical Care Nursing, 15*(4), 27–37.

Parathyroid Disorders

Elasy, T. A., & Skelly, A. H. (1997). Patient with hyperparathyroidism. *Lippincott's Primary Care Practice, 1*(5), 563–566.

Locker, F. G. (1996). Hormonal regulation of calcium homeostasis. *Nursing Clinics of North America, 31*(4), 797–803.

Lovell, C. L. (1997). Clinical consult: Obtaining accurate PTH readings. *ANNA Journal, 24*(2), 280, 290.

National Institutes of Health Consensus Statement. (1999). Diagnosis and management of asymptomatic primary hyperparathyroidism, *8*(7), 1–18.

Pituitary Disorders

Counsell, C. M., Gilbert, M., & Snively, C. (1996). Challenging diagnosis: Management of the patient with a pituitary tumor resection. *Dimensions of Critical Care Nursing, 15*(2), 75–81.

Mitchell, A., Steffenson, N., & Davenport, K. (1997). Hypopituitarism due to traumatic brain injury: A case study. *Critical Care Nurse, 17*(4), 34–51.

Romeo, J. H. (1996). Hyperfunction and hypofunction in the anterior pituitary. *Nursing Clinics of North America, 31*(4), 769–778.

Thyroid Disorders

Bauer, D. C., & Brown, A. N. (1996). Sensitive thyrotropin and free thyroxine testing in outpatients: Are both necessary? *Archives of Internal Medicine, 156*(20), 2333–2337.

Braverman, L. E., Dworkin, H. J., & MacIndoe, J. H. (1997). Thyroid disease: When to screen, when to treat. *Patient Care, 31*(6), 18–47.

Bunevicius, R., et al. (1999). Effects of thyroxine as compared with thyroxine plus triiodothyronine in patients with hypothyroidism. *New England Journal of Medicine, 11*(6), 424–429.

Chabon, S. L. (1997). Identification and evaluation of thyroid nodules. *Lippincott's Primary Care Practice, 1*(5), 499–504.

Danese, M. D., Powe, N. R., Sawin, C. T., & Ladenson, P. W. (1996). Screening for mild thyroid failure at the periodic health examination: A decision and cost-effectiveness analysis. *Journal of the American Medical Association, 276*(4), 285–292.

Dong, B. J., Hauck, W. W., Gambertoglio, J. G., Gee, L., White, J. R., Bubp, J. L., & Greenspan, F. S. (1997). Bioequivalence of generic and brand name levothyroxine products in the treatment of hypothyroidism. *Journal of the American Medical Association, 277*(15), 1205–1213.

Drake, D. K. (1997). Thyroid hormone replacement. *Lippincott's Primary Care Practice, 1*(5), 550–554.

Gilkison, C. R. (1997). Thyrotoxicosis: Recognition and management. *Lippincott's Primary Care Practice, 1*(5), 485–498.

Hennessey, J. V. (1996). Diagnosis and management of thyrotoxicosis. *American Family Physician, 54*(4), 1315–1324.

Kaiser, F. E. (1995). Thyroid function tests: Use and interpretation. *Clinics in Geriatric Medicine, 11*(2), 171–177.

Kennedy, J. W., & Caro, J. F. (1996). The ABCs of managing hyperthyroidism in the older patient. *Geriatrics, 51*(5), 22–32.

Klee, G. G., & Hay, I. D. (1997). Biochemical testing of thyroid function. *Endocrinology and Metabolism Clinics of North America, 26*(4), 763–775.

Lindsay, R. S., & Toft, A. D. (1997). Hypothyroidism. *Lancet, 347*(9049), 413–417.

McKennis, A., & Waddington, C. (1997). Nursing interventions for potential complications after thyroidectomy. *ORL; Head and Neck Nursing, 15*(1), 27–35.

Nordyke, R. A., et al. (1997). Alternative sequences of thyrotropin and free thyoxine assays for routine thyroid testing. Quality and cost. *Archives of Internal Medicine, 158*(3), 266–272.

Singer, P. A., Cooper, D. S., Levy, E. G., Ladenson, P. W., Braverman, L. E., Daniels, G., Greenspan, F. S., McDougall, I. R., & Nikolai, T. F. (1995). Treatment guidelines for patients with hyperthyroidism and hypothyroidism. *Journal of the American Medical Association, 273*(10), 808–812.

Streff, M. M., & Pachucki-Hyde, L. C. (1996). Management of the patient with thyroid disease. *Nursing Clinics of North America, 31*(4), 779–796.

UNIT 9

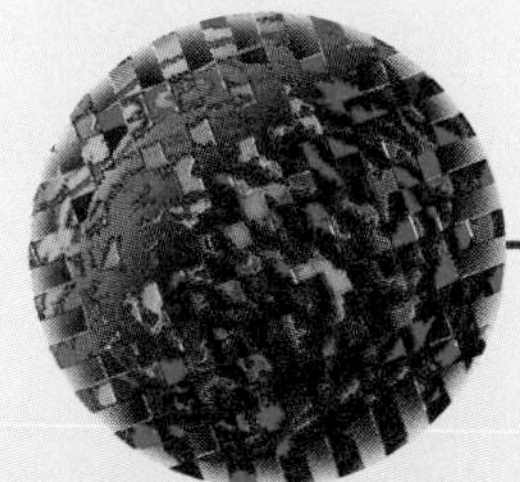

Urinary and Renal Function

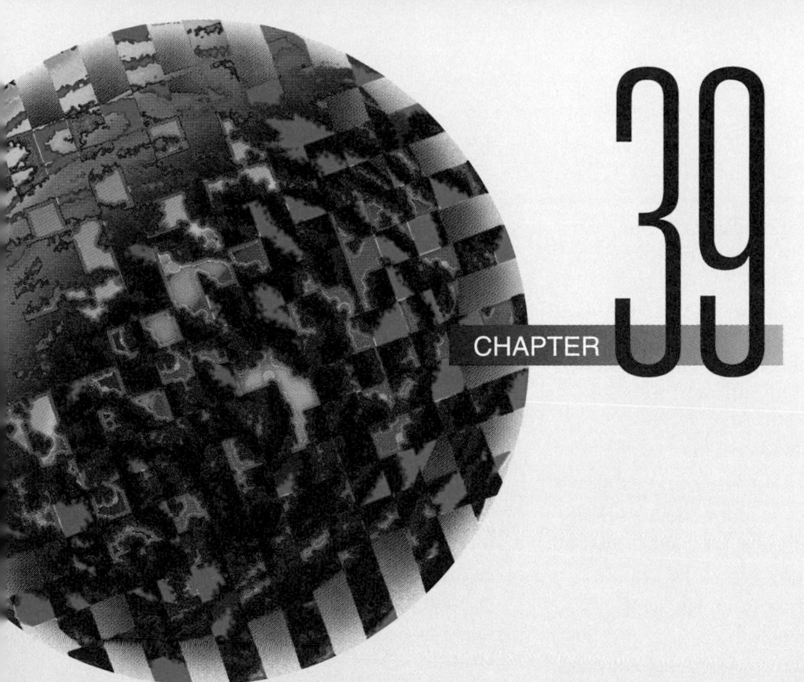

Assessment of Urinary and Renal Function

Learning Objectives

On completion of this chapter, the learner will be able to:

1. Discuss the role of the kidney in regulating fluid and electrolyte balance, acid–base balance, and blood pressure.
2. Use assessment parameters for determining the status of renal and urinary function.
3. Describe diagnostic tests used to determine renal and urinary function.
4. Initiate education and preparation for patients undergoing assessment of the urinary-renal system.

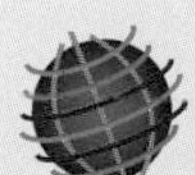

Renal and urinary function is essential to life. Dysfunction of the kidneys and urinary tract are common and may occur at any age and with varying levels of severity. Assessment of kidney and urinary tract function is part of every health examination and necessitates an understanding of the anatomy and physiology of the system as well as of the effect of changes in the system on other physiologic functions.

GLOSSARY

aldosterone: hormone synthesized and released from adrenal cortex; causes sodium reabsorption by the kidney

antidiuretic hormone (ADH): hormone secreted by the posterior pituitary gland; causes increased water reabsorption by the kidney

anuria: total urine output less than 50 mL in 24 hours

bacteriuria: bacteria in the urine; bacterial count higher than 100,000 colonies/mL

clearance: volume of plasma that can be cleared of a specific solute (eg, creatinine) by the kidneys, expressed in milliliters per minute

creatinine: endogenous waste product of muscle energy metabolism

dysuria: painful or difficult urination

frequency: voiding more frequently than every 3 hours

glomerulus: tuft of capillaries forming part of the nephron through which filtration occurs

glomerular filtration rate (GFR): volume of plasma filtered at the glomerulus into the kidney tubules each minute, expressed in milliliters per minute; normal is approximately 120 mL/min

hematuria: red blood cells in the urine

micturition: urination or voiding

nephron: structural and functional unit of the kidney responsible for urine formation

nocturia: awakening at night to urinate

oliguria: total urine output less than 400 mL in 24 hours

osmolality: number of particles dissolved per kilogram of urine; expression of the degree of concentration of the urine

osmolarity: number of particles per liter of urine; expression of the degree of concentration of the urine

proteinuria: protein in the urine

pyuria: white blood cells in the urine

specific gravity: reflects weight of particles dissolved in the urine; expression of degree of concentration of the urine

tubular reabsorption: movement of a substance from the kidney tubules into the blood in the peritubular capillaries or vasa recta

tubular secretion: movement of substances from blood in the peritubular capillaries or vasa recta into the kidney tubule

urea nitrogen: nitrogenous end product of protein metabolism

urinary incontinence: involuntary loss of urine

vesicoureteral reflux: backflow of urine from bladder into the ureters

ANATOMIC AND PHYSIOLOGIC OVERVIEW

The urinary system is composed of the kidneys, ureters, bladder, and urethra. A thorough understanding of the urinary system and renal physiology is necessary both to assess and to plan and implement appropriate nursing care for healthy patients and those with renal or urinary dysfunction.

Anatomy of the Kidneys and Urinary System

Excretory, regulatory, and secretory functions are performed by the urinary system, the structures of which precisely maintain the internal chemical environment of the body.

Kidneys

The kidneys are located retroperitoneally (behind and outside the peritoneal cavity) on the posterior wall of the abdomen from the 12th thoracic vertebra to the 3rd lumbar vertebra (Fig. 39-1). An adult kidney weighs between 120 and 170 g (about 4.5 oz) and is 12 cm (about 4.5 inches) long, 6 cm wide, and 2.5 cm thick. The kidneys are well protected by the ribs, muscles, fascia, perirenal fat, and renal capsule, which surrounds each kidney.

The kidney consists of two distinct regions, the outer cortex and inner medulla (see Fig. 39-1). The cortex contains the glomeruli, proximal and distal tubules, and cortical collecting ducts and their adjacent peritubular capillaries. The medulla resembles pyramids because of the long loops of Henle and the medullary collecting ducts and their corresponding capillaries, known as the vasa recta.

The hilum is the concave portion of the kidney through which the renal artery enters and the renal vein exits. The renal artery (arising from the abdominal aorta) divides into smaller and smaller vessels, eventually forming the afferent arteriole. The afferent arteriole branches to form the **glomerulus**, which is the capillary bed responsible for glomerular filtration. Blood leaves the glomerulus through the efferent arteriole and flows back to the inferior vena cava through a network of capillaries and veins.

Each kidney is composed of about 1 million **nephrons,** the functional units of the kidney. Each kidney is capable of providing adequate renal function if the opposite kidney is damaged or becomes nonfunctional. The nephron consists of a glomerulus containing afferent and efferent arterioles, Bowman's capsule, proximal tubule, loop of Henle, distal tubule, and collecting ducts (Fig. 39-2). Collecting ducts converge into papillae, which empty into the minor calices, which drain into three major calices that open directly into the renal pelvis.

Nephrons are structurally divided into two types: cortical and juxtamedullary. Cortical nephrons are found in the cortex of the kidney, and juxtamedullary nephrons sit adjacent to the medulla. The juxtamedullary nephrons are distinguished by their long loops of Henle and the vasa recta, long capillary loops that dip into the medulla of the kidney.

The glomerulus is composed of three filtering layers: the capillary endothelium, the basement membrane, and the epithelium. The glomerular membrane normally allows filtration of fluid and small molecules yet limits passage of larger molecules, such as blood cells and albumin.

Ureters, Bladder, and Urethra

Urine, which is formed within the nephrons, flows into the ureter, a long fibromuscular tube that connects each kidney to the bladder. The urinary bladder is a muscular, hollow sac located just behind the pubic bone and can hold about 300 to 500 mL of urine. The urethra arises from the bladder; in the male, it passes through the penis, and in the female, it opens just anterior to the vagina. In the male, the prostate gland, which lies just below the bladder neck, surrounds the urethra posteriorly and laterally. The external urinary sphincter is a round, voluntary muscle that controls the initiation of urination.

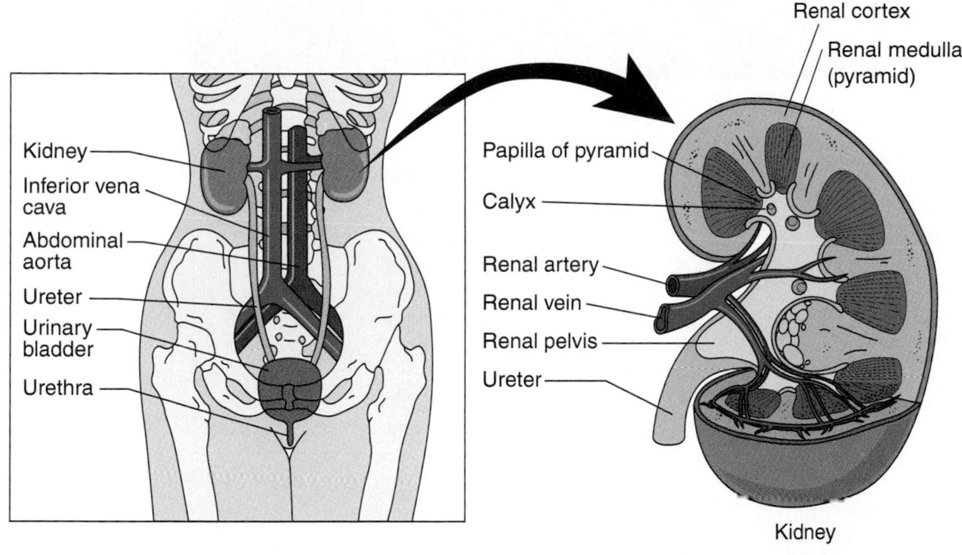

FIGURE 39•1 The urinary tract includes the kidneys (enlargement at right), ureters, and bladder. Adapted from Willis, M.C. (1996). *Medical terminology: The language of healthcare.* Baltimore: Williams & Wilkins.

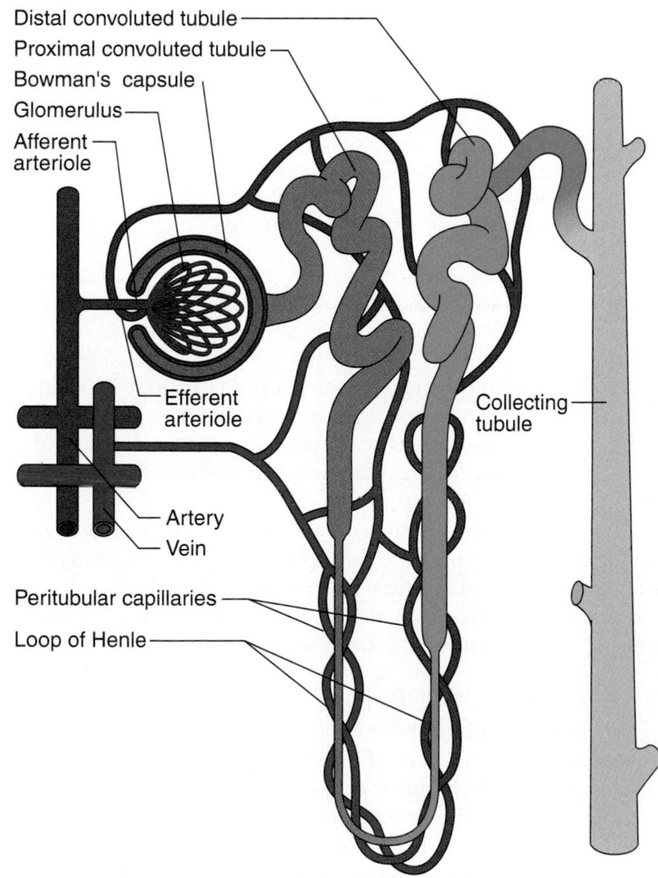

FIGURE 39•2 Representation of a nephron. Each kidney has about 1 million nephrons, which take two forms: cortical and juxtamedullary. Cortical nephrons are located in the cortex of the kidney; juxtamedullary nephrons are adjacent to the medulla. Adapted from Willis, M.C. (1996). *Medical terminology: The language of healthcare.* Baltimore: Williams & Wilkins.

Functions of the Kidneys

The kidneys and urinary system perform a variety of essential excretory, regulatory, and secretory roles, as outlined in Chart 39-1. These functions include urine formation, excretion of waste products, regulation of electrolyte excretion, regulation of acid excretion, regulation of water excretion, and autoregulation of blood pressure.

Urine Formation

Urine is formed in the nephrons through a complex three-step process: glomerular filtration, **tubular reabsorption**, and **tubular secretion.** Figure 39-3 illustrates the three processes of urine formation and typical values of water and electrolytes associated with each process. The various substances normally filtered by the glomerulus, reabsorbed by the tubules, and excreted in the urine include sodium, chloride, bicarbonate, potassium, glucose, urea, creatinine, and uric acid. Within the tubule, some of these substances are selectively reabsorbed into the blood. Other substances are secreted from the blood into the filtrate as

CHART 39•1 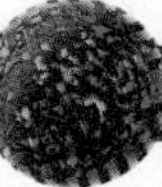 **Functions of the Kidney**

- Urine formation
- Excretion of waste products
- Regulation of electrolytes
- Regulation of acid–base balance
- Control of water balance
- Control of blood pressure
- Renal clearance
- Regulation of red blood cell production
- Synthesis of vitamin D to active form
- Secretion of prostaglandins

PHYSIOLOGY

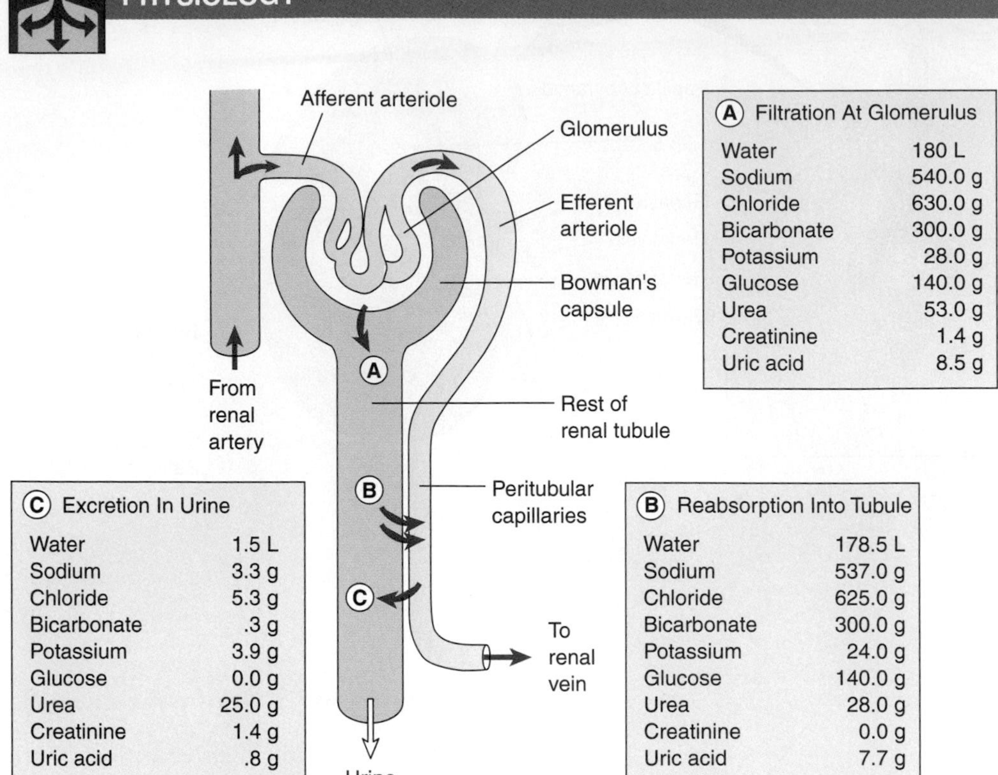

(A) Filtration At Glomerulus	
Water	180 L
Sodium	540.0 g
Chloride	630.0 g
Bicarbonate	300.0 g
Potassium	28.0 g
Glucose	140.0 g
Urea	53.0 g
Creatinine	1.4 g
Uric acid	8.5 g

(B) Reabsorption Into Tubule	
Water	178.5 L
Sodium	537.0 g
Chloride	625.0 g
Bicarbonate	300.0 g
Potassium	24.0 g
Glucose	140.0 g
Urea	28.0 g
Creatinine	0.0 g
Uric acid	7.7 g

(C) Excretion In Urine	
Water	1.5 L
Sodium	3.3 g
Chloride	5.3 g
Bicarbonate	.3 g
Potassium	3.9 g
Glucose	0.0 g
Urea	25.0 g
Creatinine	1.4 g
Uric acid	.8 g

FIGURE 39•3 Urine is formed in the nephrons in a three-step process: filtration, reabsorption, and excretion. Water, electrolytes, and other substances, such as glucose and creatinine, are filtered by the glomerulus, reabsorbed in the renal tubule, and excreted in the urine. Typical normal volumes of these substances during the steps of urine formation appear above. Wide variations may occur in the values depending on diet.

it travels down the tubule. Some substances, such as glucose, are normally completely reabsorbed in the tubule and do not appear in the urine. Amino acids and glucose are usually filtered at the glomerulus and reabsorbed so that neither is excreted in the urine. Glucose, however, appears in the urine (glycosuria) if the glucose concentration in the blood and glomerular filtrate exceeds the ability of the tubules to reabsorb the glucose. Normally, glucose is completely reabsorbed when its concentration in the blood is less than 200 mg/dL (11 mmol/L). In diabetes, when the blood glucose levels exceed the kidneys' reabsorption capacity, glucose appears in the urine. Glycosuria is also common in pregnancy.

Protein molecules are also generally not found in the urine; however, low-molecular-weight proteins (globulins and albumin) may periodically be excreted in small amounts. Transient **proteinuria** in amounts less than 150 mg/dL is considered normal and does not require further evaluation (Ali, 1997). Persistent proteinuria usually signifies damage to the glomeruli.

GLOMERULAR FILTRATION

The normal blood flow through the kidneys is about 1200 mL/min. As blood flows into the glomerulus from an afferent arteriole, filtration occurs. The filtered fluid, also known as *filtrate* or *ultrafiltrate,* then enters the renal tubules. Under normal conditions, about 20% of the blood passing through the glomeruli is filtered into the nephron, amounting to about 180 L/day of filtrate. The filtrate normally consists of water, electrolytes, and other small molecules because water and small molecules are allowed to pass, whereas larger molecules stay in the bloodstream.

Efficient filtration depends on an adequate blood flow maintaining a consistent pressure through the glomerulus. Many factors can alter this blood flow and pressure, including hypotension, decreased oncotic pressure in the blood, and increased pressure in the renal tubules from an obstruction.

TUBULAR REABSORPTION AND TUBULAR SECRETION

The second and third steps of urine formation occur in the renal tubules and are called tubular reabsorption and tubular secretion. In tubular reabsorption, a substance moves from the filtrate back into the peritubular capillaries or vasa recta. In tubular secretion, a substance moves from the peritubular capillaries or vasa recta into tubular filtrate. Of the 180 liters (45 gallons) of filtrate produced each day by the kidneys, 99% is reabsorbed into the bloodstream, resulting in 1000 to 1500 mL of urine each day. Most reabsorption occurs in the proximal tubule, although reabsorption occurs along the entire tubule. Reabsorption and secretion in the tubule frequently involve passive and active transport and may require the use of energy.

Filtrate becomes concentrated in the distal tubule and collecting ducts under the influence of **antidiuretic hormone** (ADH) and becomes urine that then enters the kidney pelvis.

Excretion of Waste Products

The kidney functions as the main excretory organ of the body, eliminating the body's metabolic waste products. The major waste product of protein metabolism is *urea,* of which about 25 to 30 g is produced and excreted daily. All of this urea must be excreted in the urine or it will accumulate in body tissues. Other waste products of metabolism that must be excreted are creatinine, phosphates, and sulfates. Uric acid, formed as a waste product of purine metabolism, is also eliminated in the urine.

Regulation of Electrolyte Excretion

When the kidneys are functioning normally, the volume of electrolytes excreted per day is exactly equal to the amount ingested. For example, the average American daily diet contains between 6 and 8 g each of sodium chloride (salt) and potassium chloride, and nearly all of this is excreted in the urine.

SODIUM

More than 99% of the water and sodium filtered at the glomeruli is reabsorbed into the blood by the time the urine leaves the body. Water from the filtrate follows the reabsorbed sodium to maintain osmotic balance. By regulating the amount of sodium (and therefore water) reabsorbed, the kidney can regulate the volume of body fluids.

Sodium excreted in excess of the amount ingested results in dehydration; sodium excreted in an amount less than that ingested results in fluid retention.

The regulation of the amount of sodium excreted depends on **aldosterone,** a hormone synthesized and released from the adrenal cortex. In the presence of increased aldosterone in the blood, less sodium is excreted in the urine because aldosterone fosters renal reabsorption of sodium.

Release of aldosterone from the adrenal cortex is largely under the control of angiotensin II. Angiotensin II levels are in turn controlled by renin, an enzyme that is released from specialized cells in the kidneys (Fig. 39-4). This complex system is activated when pressure in the renal arterioles falls below normal levels, as occurs with shock and dehydration or when there is decreased sodium chloride delivery to the tubules. Activation of this system increases the retention of water and expansion of intravascular fluid volume.

POTASSIUM

Potassium is the most abundant intracellular ion, with about 98% of the total-body potassium located intracellularly. To maintain a normal potassium balance in the body, the kidneys are responsible for excreting more than 90% of the total daily potassium intake. Several factors influence potassium loss through the kidneys.

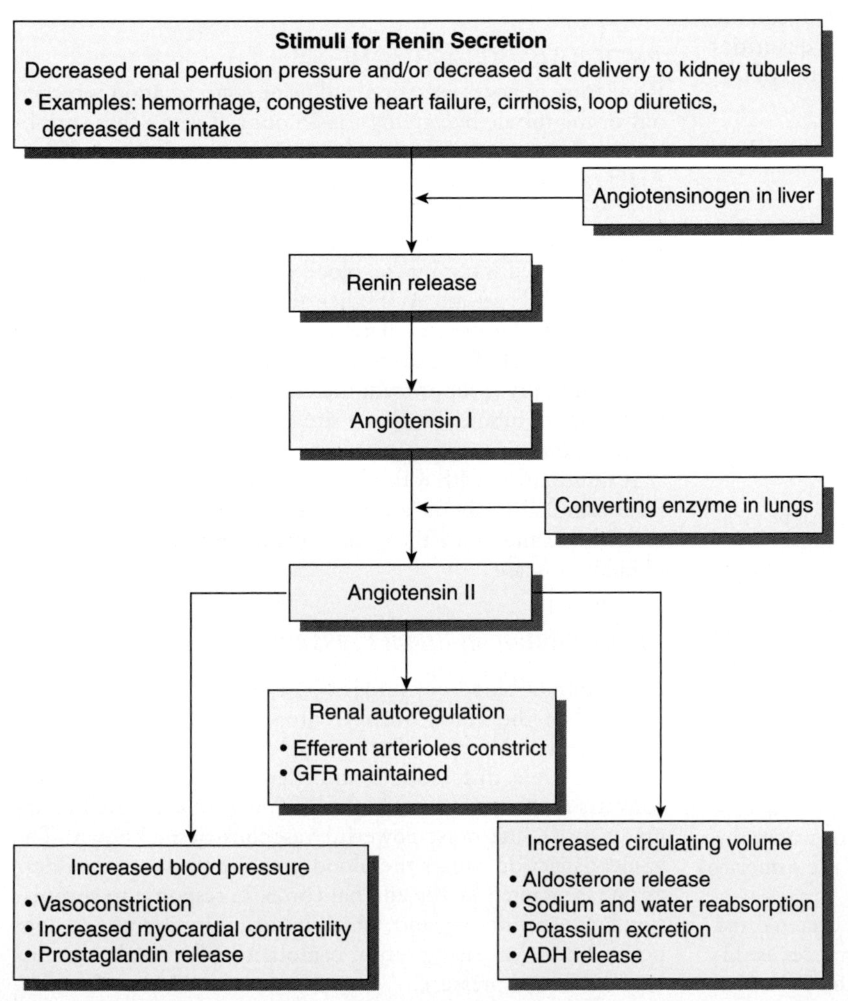

FIGURE 39•4 Renin–angiotensin system. GFR, glomerular filtration rate; ADH, antidiuretic hormone.

Aldosterone causes potassium excretion by the kidney, in contrast to its effects on sodium described previously. Acid–base balance, the amount of dietary potassium intake, and the flow rate of the filtrate in the distal tubule also influence the amount of potassium secreted into the urine.

Retention of potassium is the most life-threatening effect of renal failure.

Regulation of Acid Excretion

The catabolism or breakdown of proteins results in the production of acid compounds, in particular phosphoric and sulfuric acids. The normal daily diet also includes a certain amount of acid materials. Unlike carbon dioxide (CO_2), phosphoric and sulfuric acids are nonvolatile and cannot be eliminated by the lung. Because accumulation of these acids in the blood would lower its pH (making the blood more acidic) and inhibit cell function, they must be excreted in the urine. A person with normal kidney function excretes about 70 mEq of acid each day. The kidney is able to excrete some of this acid directly into the urine until the urine pH reaches 4.5, which is 1000 times more acidic than blood.

More acid, however, usually needs to be eliminated from the body than can be excreted directly as free acid in the urine. These excess acids are bound to chemical buffers so they can be excreted in the urine. Two important chemical buffers are phosphate ions and ammonia (NH_3). When buffered with acid, ammonia becomes ammonium (NH_4). Phosphate is present in the glomerular filtrate, and ammonia is produced by the cells of the renal tubules and secreted into the tubular fluid. Through the buffering process, the kidney is able to excrete large quantities of acid in a bound form without further lowering the pH of the urine.

Regulation of Water Excretion

Regulation of the amount of water excreted is also an important function of the kidney. With a large intake of water or fluid, a large volume of dilute urine must be excreted. Conversely, with a low fluid intake, the urine that is excreted is concentrated. A person normally ingests about 1 to 2 liters of water per day, and normally all but 400 to 500 mL of this fluid intake is excreted in the urine. The remainder is lost from the skin, from the lungs during breathing, and in the feces.

OSMOLALITY

The degree of dilution or concentration of the urine can be measured in terms of **osmolality,** the number of particles (electrolytes and other molecules) dissolved per kilogram of urine. The filtrate in the glomerular capillary normally has the same osmolality as the blood, with a value of about 300 mOsm/L (300 mmol/L). As the filtrate passes through the tubules and collecting ducts, the osmolality may vary from 50 to 1200 mOsm/L, reflecting the maximal diluting and concentrating abilities of the kidney.

When a person is dehydrated or retaining fluid, less water is excreted, and proportionately more particles are present in the urine, giving the urine a concentrated appearance and a high osmolality. When a person excretes a large volume of water, the particles are diluted. The urine appears dilute and the osmolality is low.

Certain substances can alter the volume of water excreted and are described as *osmotically active.* When these substances are filtered, they pull water across the glomerulus and tubules and increase the volume of urine. Glucose and proteins are two examples of osmotically active molecules.

Normal urine osmolality ranges between 300 and 1100 mOsm/kg; after a 12 hour fluid restriction, urine osmolality normally ranges from 500 to 850 mOsm/kg. This wide range of normal makes the test valuable only when the kidneys' concentrating and diluting abilities are questioned.

URINE SPECIFIC GRAVITY

Urine **specific gravity** is another measurement of the kidney's ability to concentrate urine. It compares the weight of urine (weight of particles) to the weight of distilled water, which has a specific gravity of 1.000. Specific gravity can be measured by several methods:

- Multiple-test dipstick (most common method), with a specific reagent area for specific gravity
- Urinometer (least accurate method), in which urine is placed in a small cylinder, and the urinometer is floated in the urine; a specific gravity reading is obtained at the meniscus level of the urine
- Refractometer, an instrument used in a laboratory setting, which measures differences in speed of light passing through air and the urine sample

Normal urine specific gravity is 1.010 to 1.025 when fluid intake is normal. Factors that may interfere with an accurate urine specific gravity reading include radiopaque contrast agents, glucose, and proteins. Cold urine specimens may also produce a false high reading.

ANTIDIURETIC HORMONE

Regulation of water excretion and urine concentration is carried out in the tubule by varying the amount of water that is reabsorbed. The amount of water that is reabsorbed is controlled by ADH (also known as *vasopressin*).

ADH is a hormone that is secreted by the posterior part of the pituitary gland in response to changes in osmolality of the blood. With decreased water intake, blood osmolality tends to rise and stimulate ADH release. ADH then acts on the kidney, increasing reabsorption of water and thereby returning the osmolality of the blood to normal. With excess water intake, the secretion of ADH by the pituitary is suppressed; therefore, less water is reabsorbed by the kidney tubule. This latter situation leads to increased urine volume (*diuresis*).

A dilute urine with a fixed specific gravity (about 1.010) or fixed osmolality (about 300 mOsm/L) indicates an inability to concentrate and dilute the urine, a common early manifestation of kidney disease.

Autoregulation of Blood Pressure

Regulation of blood pressure is also a function of the renal system. When the blood pressure drops, a hormone known as *renin* is secreted by specialized juxtaglomerular cells near the afferent arteriole, distal tubule, and efferent arteriole. An enzyme converts renin to angiotensin I, which is then converted to angiotensin II, the most powerful vasoconstrictor known. The vasoconstriction causes the blood pressure to increase. Aldosterone is secreted by the adrenal cortex in response to stimulation by the pituitary gland, which in turn is in response to poor perfusion or increasing serum osmolality. The result is an increase in blood pressure.

Renal Clearance

Renal **clearance** refers to the ability of the kidneys to clear solutes from the plasma.

A test of renal clearance is used to evaluate how well the kidney performs this important excretory function. Clearance depends on several factors: rate of filtration of the substance across the glomerulus, how much of the substance is reabsorbed along the tubules, and how much of the substance is secreted into the tubules. It is possible to measure the renal clearance of any substance, but the one measure that is particularly useful is the creatinine clearance.

Creatinine is an endogenous waste product of skeletal muscle that is filtered at the glomerulus, passed through the tubules with minimal change, and excreted in the urine. Hence, creatinine clearance is a good measure of the **glomerular filtration rate** (GFR). To calculate creatinine clearance, a 24-hour urine specimen is collected. Midway through the collection, the serum creatinine level is measured. The following formula is then used to calculate the creatinine clearance:

$$\frac{\text{Volume of urine (mL / min)} \times \text{urine creatinine (mg / dL)}}{\text{Serum creatinine (mg/dL)}}$$

The normal adult GFR is about 100 to 120 mL/min (1.67 to 2.0 mL/sec).

Creatinine clearance is an excellent measure of renal function; as renal function declines, creatinine clearance decreases.

Other Kidney Functions

The kidneys are also responsible for several other regulatory functions. When the kidneys sense a decrease in the oxygen tension in renal blood flow, they release erythropoietin. Erythropoietin stimulates the bone marrow to produce red blood cells, thereby increasing the amount of hemoglobin available to carry oxygen. The kidneys are also responsible for the final conversion of inactive vitamin D to its active form, 1,25-dihydroxycholecalciferol. Vitamin D is necessary for maintaining normal calcium balance in the body. The kidneys also produce prostaglandin E_2 (PGE_2) and prostacyclin (PGI_2), which have a vasodilatory effect and are important in maintaining renal blood flow.

Functions of the Ureters, Bladder, and Urethra

Urine formed by the kidney flows from the renal pelvis through the ureter and into the bladder. This movement is facilitated by peristaltic waves (occurring about one to five times per minute) from contraction of the smooth muscle in the ureter wall. There are no sphincters between the ureters and the bladder, whereas there is a sphincter in the urethra.

Storage of Urine

The bladder is the reservoir for urine. Reflux of urine from the bladder is normally prevented by the unidirectional nature of the peristaltic waves and because each ureter enters the bladder at an oblique angle. With overdistention of the bladder, however, the elevated pressure in the bladder can be transmitted back through the ureters, leading to ureteral distention and possible reflux or backup of urine. This can lead to kidney infection (pyelonephritis) and kidney damage from the elevated pressure (hydronephrosis).

Normally, the pressure in the bladder is low, even as the urine accumulates, because the bladder's smooth muscle adapts to the increased stretch. The first sensations of bladder filling ordinarily occur when about 100 to 150 mL of urine is present in the bladder. In most cases, a desire to void occurs when the bladder contains about 200 to 300 mL of urine. A marked sense of fullness usually occurs when the bladder contains 400 mL of urine.

Voiding

Controlled voiding is influenced by muscle and nerves. Voluntary control is a learned behavior and not present at birth.

MUSCLE CONTROL

Voiding of urine is controlled by contraction of the *external urethral sphincter.* This muscle is under voluntary control and is innervated by nerves from the sacral area of the spinal cord. When a person wants to urinate, the external urethral sphincter relaxes, and the *detrusor muscle* (bladder smooth muscle) contracts and expels the urine from the bladder through the urethra. The pressure generated in the bladder during urination (**micturition**) is about 50 to 150 cm H_20. Urine remaining in the urethra drains by gravity in the female and is expelled by voluntary muscle contractions in the male.

NEURAL CONTROL

Contraction of the detrusor muscle is regulated by a reflex involving the parasympathetic nervous system, specifically in the sacral portion of the spinal tract. The sympathetic nervous system plays no essential part in micturition but does prevent semen from entering the bladder during ejaculation.

If the pelvic nerves to the bladder and sphincter are destroyed, voluntary control and reflex urination are abolished, and the bladder becomes overdistended with urine. If the spinal pathways from the brain to the urinary system are destroyed (eg, after a spinal cord injury), reflex contraction of the bladder is maintained but voluntary control over the process is lost. In both these situations, the muscle of the bladder can contract and expel urine, but the contractions are generally insufficient to empty the bladder completely, and *residual urine* (urine left in the bladder after voiding) remains. Normally, residual urine amounts to no more than 50 mL.

ASSESSMENT

Collecting data about previous health problems or diseases provides useful information to the health care team when evaluating the patient's current renal or urologic problem. Obtaining a comprehensive health history, which includes an assessment of risk factors, is the first step in assessing a patient with a renal or urologic dysfunction. A variety of diseases or clinical situations can place a patient at increased risk for developing renal or urologic problems; risk factors for specific diseases are further discussed in Chapter 41.

Health History and Clinical Manifestations

Obtaining a urologic health history requires excellent communication skills, because many patients are embarrassed about or uncomfortable discussing genitourinary functions or symptoms. It is important to use language the patient can understand and to avoid medical terminology. It is also important to review risk factors, particularly in at-risk populations, such as older adults.

Risk Factors for Various Renal or Urologic Disorders

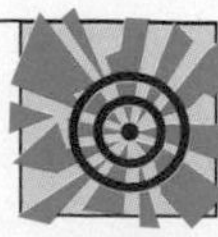

Risk Factor	Possible Renal or Urologic Disorder
Childhood diseases: "strep throat" impetigo, nephrotic syndrome	Chronic renal failure
Advanced age	Incomplete emptying of bladder, leading to urinary tract infection
Instrumentation of urinary tract, cystoscopy, catheterization	Urinary tract infection, incontinence
Immobilization	Kidney stone formation
Occupational, recreational, or environmental exposure to chemicals (plastics, pitch, tar, rubber)	Acute renal failure
Diabetes mellitus	Chronic renal failure, neurogenic bladder
Hypertension	Renal insufficiency, chronic renal failure
Systemic lupus erythematosus	Nephritis, chronic renal failure
Gout, hyperparathyroidism, Crohn's disease	Kidney stone formation
Sickle cell anemia, multiple myeloma	Chronic renal failure
Benign prostatic hypertrophy	Obstruction to urine flow, leading to frequency, oliguria, anuria
Radiation therapy to pelvis	Cystitis, fibrosis of ureter, or fistula in urinary tract
Recent pelvic surgery	Inadvertent trauma to ureters or bladder
Obstetric injury, tumors	Incontinence
Spinal cord injury	Neurogenic bladder, urinary tract infection, incontinence

For example, elderly women often have incomplete emptying of the bladder with urinary stasis, which may result in urinary tract infection. Prostatic enlargement in the elderly male patient causes urethral obstruction, which can result in renal failure and urinary tract infections. When obtaining the health history, the nurse should inquire about the following:

- The patient's chief concern or reason for seeking health care; onset of problem; effect on patient's quality of life
- The location, character, and duration of pain, if present, and its relationship to voiding; factors that precipitate pain, and those that relieve it
- History of urinary tract infections, including past treatment or hospitalization for urinary tract infection
- Fever or chills
- Previous renal or urinary diagnostic tests or use of indwelling urinary catheters
- Symptoms of voiding disorders:
  - Dysuria, when it occurs during voiding (at initiation or termination of voiding)
  - Hesitancy; straining; pain during or after urination
  - Urinary incontinence (stress incontinence, urge incontinence, overflow incontinence, functional incontinence)
- History of any of the following:
  - Hematuria, or change in color or volume of urine
  - Nocturia and its date of onset
  - Renal calculi (kidney stones), passage of stones or gravel in urine
- Female patients: number and type (vaginal or cesarean) of deliveries; use of forceps; vaginal infection, discharge, or irritation; contraceptive practices
- Presence or history of genital lesions or sexually transmitted diseases
- Habits: use of tobacco, alcohol, or recreational drugs
- Any prescription and over-the-counter medications (including those prescribed for renal or urinary problems)

A thorough medication history is especially important for elderly patients, for whom the increased occurrence of chronic illness often necessitates polypharmacy (concurrent use of multiple medications). Aging affects the way the body absorbs, metabolizes, and excretes drugs, thus placing the elderly patient at risk for adverse effects, including compromised renal function.

Other key information to obtain while gathering the health history includes an assessment of the patient's psychosocial status, level of anxiety, perceived threats to body image, available support systems, and sociocultural patterns. Obtaining this information during the initial and subsequent nursing assessments enables the nurse to uncover special needs, misunderstandings, lack of knowledge, and need for patient teaching.

The following signs and symptoms are particularly suggestive of urinary tract disease: pain, changes in voiding, and gastrointestinal symptoms. Dysfunction of the kidney can produce a complex array of symptoms throughout the body.

Pain

Genitourinary pain is usually caused by distention of some portion of the urinary tract because of obstructed urine flow or inflammation and swelling of tissues. Severity of pain is related to the sudden onset rather than the amount of distention.

Table 39-1 summarizes the various types of genitourinary pain, characteristics of the pain, associated signs and symptoms, and possible causes. Many times, however, kidney disease is not accompanied by pain. It tends to be diagnosed because of other symptoms that cause a patient to seek health care. Examples of these symptoms include pedal edema, shortness of breath, and changes in urinary elimination.

Changes in Voiding

Voiding (micturition) is normally a painless function occurring five to six times daily and occasionally once at night. The average person voids 1200 to 1500 mL of urine in 24 hours, although this varies depending on fluid intake, sweating, environmental temperature, vomiting, or diarrhea. Common problems associated with voiding include frequency, urgency, dysuria, hesitancy, incontinence, enuresis, polyuria, oliguria, and hematuria. These problems and others are described in Table 39-2.

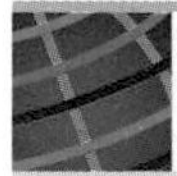

TABLE 39•1 **Identifying Characteristics of Genitourinary Pain**

Type	Location	Character	Associated Signs and Symptoms	Possible Etiology
Kidney	Costovertebral angle, may extend to umbilicus	Dull constant ache; if sudden distention of capsule, pain is severe, sharp, stabbing, and colicky in nature	Nausea and vomiting, diaphoresis, pallor, signs of shock	Acute obstruction, kidney stone, blood clot, acute pyelonephritis, trauma
Bladder	Suprapubic area	Dull, continuous pain, may be intense with voiding, may be severe if bladder full	Urgency, pain at end of voiding, painful straining	Overdistended bladder, infection, interstitial cystitis; tumor
Ureteral	Costovertebral angle, flank, lower abdominal area, testis, or labium	Severe, sharp, stabbing pain, colicky in nature	Nausea and vomiting, paralytic ileus	Ureteral stone, edema or stricture, blood clot
Prostatic	Perineum and rectum	Vague discomfort, feeling of fullness in perineum, vague back pain	Suprapubic tenderness, obstruction to urine flow; frequency, urgency, dysuria, nocturia	Prostatic cancer, acute or chronic prostatitis
Urethral	Male: along penis to meatus; female: urethra to meatus	Pain variable, most severe during and immediately after voiding	Frequency, urgency, dysuria, nocturia, urethral discharge	Irritation of bladder neck, infection of urethra, trauma, foreign body in lower urinary tract

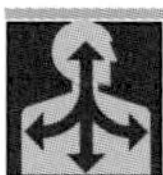

TABLE 39•2 **Problems Associated With Changes in Voiding**

Problem	Definition	Possible Etiology
Frequency	Frequent voiding—more than every 3 hours	Infection, obstruction of lower urinary tract leading to residual urine and overflow, anxiety, diuretics, benign prostatic hyperplasia, urethral stricture, diabetic neuropathy
Urgency	Strong desire to void	Infection, chronic prostatitis, urethritis, obstruction of lower urinary tract leading to residual urine and overflow, anxiety, diuretics, benign prostatic hyperplasia, urethral stricture, diabetic neuropathy
Dysuria	Painful or difficult voiding	Lower urinary tract infection, inflammation of bladder or urethra, acute prostatitis, stones, foreign bodies, tumors in bladder
Hesitancy	Delay, difficulty in initiating voiding	Benign prostatic hyperplasia, compression of urethra, outlet obstruction, neurogenic bladder
Nocturia	Excessive urination at night	Decreased renal concentrating ability, heart failure, diabetes mellitus, incomplete bladder emptying, excessive fluid intake at bedtime, nephrotic syndrome, cirrhosis with ascites
Incontinence	Involuntary loss of urine	External urinary sphincter injury, obstetric injury, lesions of bladder neck, detrusor dysfunction, infection, neurogenic bladder, medications, neurologic abnormalities
Enuresis	Involuntary voiding during sleep	Delay in functional maturation of central nervous system (bladder control usually achieved by 5 years of age), obstructive disease of lower urinary tract, genetic factors, failure to concentrate urine, urinary tract infection, psychological stress
Polyuria	Increased volume of urine voided	Diabetes mellitus, diabetes insipidus, diuretics, excess fluid intake, lithium toxicity, certain types of kidney disease (hypercalcemic and hypokalemic nephropathy)
Oliguria	Urine output less than 400 mL/day	Acute or chronic renal failure (see Chap. 41), inadequate fluid intake
Anuria	Urine output less than 50 mL/day	Acute or chronic renal failure (see Chap. 41), complete obstruction
Hematuria	Red blood cells in the urine	Cancer of genitourinary tract, acute glomerulonephritis, renal stones, renal tuberculosis, blood dyscrasia, trauma, extreme exercise, rheumatic fever, hemophilia, leukemia, sickle cell trait or disease
Proteinuria	Abnormal amounts of protein in the urine	Acute and chronic renal disease, nephrotic syndrome, vigorous exercise, heat stroke, severe heart failure, diabetic nephropathy, multiple myeloma

Gastrointestinal Symptoms

Gastrointestinal symptoms may occur with urologic conditions because of shared autonomic and sensory innervation and renointestinal reflexes. The anatomic relation of the right kidney to the colon, duodenum, head of the pancreas, common bile duct, liver, and gallbladder may cause gastrointestinal disturbances. The proximity of the left kidney to the colon (splenic flexure), stomach, pancreas, and spleen may also result in intestinal symptoms. The most common symptoms include nausea, vomiting, diarrhea, abdominal discomfort, and abdominal distention. Urologic symptoms can mimic disorders such as appendicitis, peptic ulcer disease, or cholecystitis, thus making diagnosis difficult.

Physical Assessment

Because renal dysfunction affects all body systems, a head to toe assessment is indicated, with emphasis on the urinary tract specifically.

Direct palpation may help determine the size and mobility of the kidneys. The correct position for palpation of the kidney is presented in Figure 39-5. It may be possible to feel the smooth, rounded lower pole of the kidney between the hands; the right kidney is felt more easily than the left kidney because it is somewhat lower than the left one.

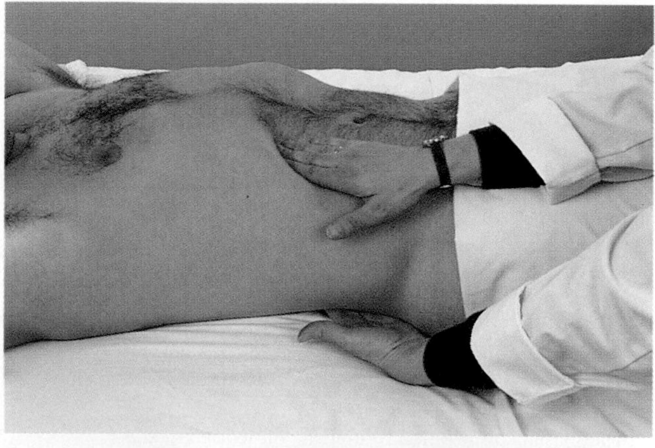

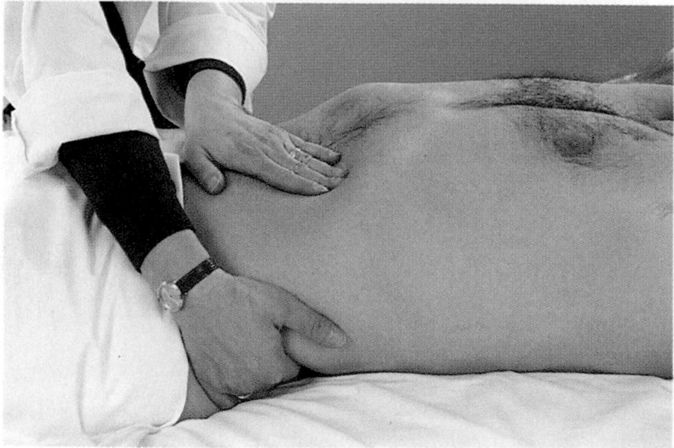

FIGURE 39•5 Technique for palpating the right kidney (*top*). One hand is placed under the patient's back with the fingers under the lower rib. The palm of the other hand is placed anterior to the kidney with fingers above the umbilicus. The hand on top is pushed forward as the patient inhales deeply. The left kidney (*bottom*) is palpated similarly with the nurse reaching over to the patient's left side and placing the right hand beneath the patient's lower left rib. From Weber, J.W., & Kelley, J. (1998). *Health assessment in nursing.* Philadelphia: Lippincott-Raven.

Renal disease may produce tenderness over the costovertebral angle, which lies where the 12th or bottom rib joins the spine. Auscultation of the abdomen (just slightly to the right and left of midline in both upper quadrants) is performed to assess for *bruits* (low-pitched murmur sounds that indicate renal artery stenosis or an aortic aneurysm).

The bladder may be percussed if it contains more than 150 mL of urine. To percuss the bladder, start at the midline just above the umbilicus and percuss downward. The top of the bladder is located under the area where the sound changes from tympanic to dull. The bladder, which cannot be palpated unless it is moderately distended, feels like a smooth, firm, round mass rising out of the abdomen, usually at midline (Fig. 39-6).

To detect prostatic hyperplasia, which is a common cause of urinary difficulty in older men, the prostate gland is palpated by digital rectal examination as part of a man's regular physical examination after age 40. (see Chap. 45). The inguinal area is examined for enlarged nodes, an inguinal or femoral hernia, and a varicocele. In women, the vulva, urethra, and vagina are examined.

The patient is also assessed for edema and changes in body weight. Edema may be observed, particularly in the face and dependent parts of the body, such as the feet and sacral areas, and is suggestive of fluid retention. An increase in body weight often accompanies edema. A 1-kg weight gain equals 1000 mL of gained fluid.

DIAGNOSTIC EVALUATION

Urinalysis

Urinalysis provides important clinical information on kidney function and helps diagnose other nonrenal diseases. Appropriate evaluation of any abnormalities can assist in detecting serious underlying diseases. Routine admission and preoperative screening urinalysis have become controversial because they do not generally produce abnormal findings or define the need for treatment.

Urine examinations include the following:

- Observation of urine color (Table 39-3)
- Assessment of urine clarity and odor
- Measurement of urine pH and specific gravity
- Tests to detect protein, glucose, and ketone bodies in the urine (proteinuria, glucosuria, and ketonuria, respectively)
- Microscopic examination of the urine sediment after centrifuging to detect red blood cells (hematuria), white blood cells, casts (cylindruria), crystals (crystalluria), pus (pyuria), and bacteria (bacteriuria)

Significance of Findings

Several abnormalities produce no symptoms; among them are hematuria and proteinuria, which may be detected during a routine urinalysis using a dipstick. Normally, about 1 million red blood cells pass into the urine daily; this is equivalent to one to three red blood cells per high power field. Hematuria (more than three red blood cells per high power field) can develop from an abnormality anywhere along the genitourinary tract. Common causes include acute infection (cystitis, urethritis, prostatitis), renal calculi, and neoplasm. Hematuria can also be caused by systemic disorders, such as bleeding disorders; malignant lesions; and medications, such as warfarin and heparin. Although hematuria is initially diagnosed by a dipstick test, further microscopic evaluation is necessary.

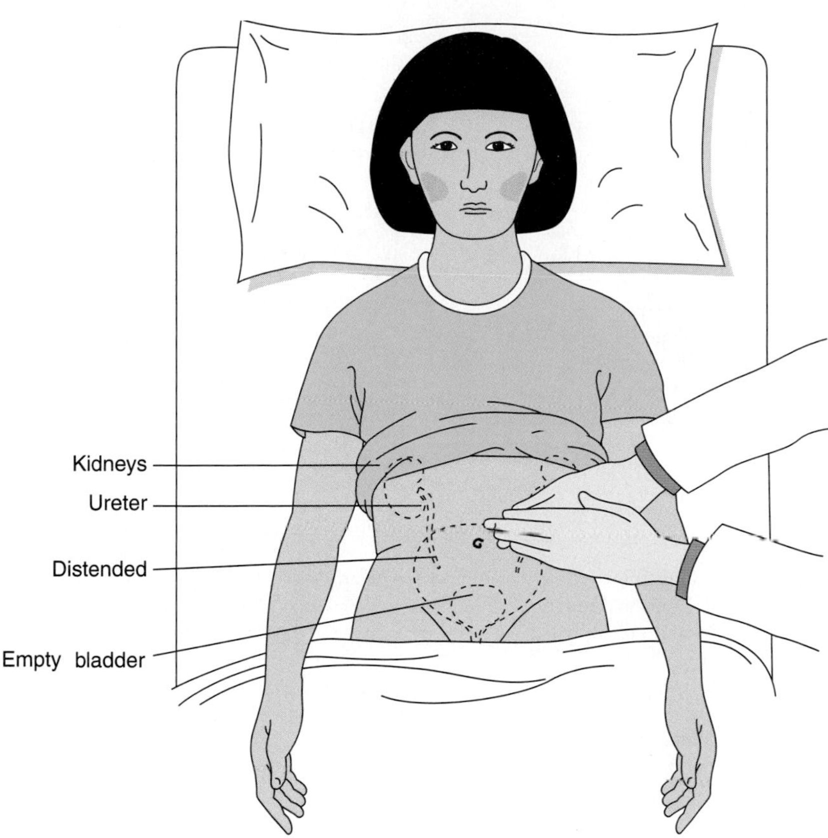

FIGURE 39•6 Palpation of the bladder.

TABLE 39•3 **Changes in Urine Color and Possible Causes**

Urine Color	Possible Cause
Colorless to pale yellow	Dilute urine due to diuretics, alcohol consumption, diabetes insipidus, glycosuria, excess fluid intake, renal disease
Yellow to milky white	Pyuria, infection, vaginal creams
Bright yellow	Multiple vitamin preparations
Pink to red	Hemoglobin breakdown, red blood cells, gross blood, menses, bladder or prostate surgery, beets, blackberries, medications (phenytoin, rifampin, phenothiazine, cascara, senna products)
Blue, blue green	Dyes, methylene blue, *Pseudomonas* species organisms, medications (amitriptyline, triamterene, phenylsalicylate)
Orange to amber	Concentrated urine due to dehydration, fever, bile, excess bilirubin or carotene, medications (phenazopyridium HCl, nitrofurantoin, sulfasalazine, ducosate calcium, thiamine)
Brown to black	Old red blood cells, urobilinogen, bilirubin, melanin, porphyrin, extremely concentrated urine due to dehydration, medications (cascara, metronidazole, iron preparations, quinine, senna products, methyldopa, nitrofurantoin)

Protein in the urine (proteinuria) may be a benign finding or can signify serious disease. Occasional loss of up to 150 mg/day of protein in the urine, primarily albumin and Tamm-Horsfall protein, is considered normal and usually does not require further evaluation. A dipstick examination, which can detect from 30 to 1000 mg/dL of protein, should be used as a screening test only because the results are affected by urine concentration, pH, hematuria, and radiocontrast materials. Because dipstick analysis does not detect protein concentrations of less than 30 mg/dL, the test cannot be used for early detection of diabetic nephropathy. Microalbuminuria (excretion of 20 to 200 mg/dL of protein in the urine) is an early sign of diabetic nephropathy. Common benign causes of transient proteinuria are fever, hard exercise, and prolonged standing.

Persistent proteinuria may be caused by glomerular diseases, malignancies, collagen diseases, diabetes mellitus, preeclampsia, hypothyroidism, congestive heart failure, and medications, such as nonsteroidal anti-inflammatory drugs (NSAIDs), angiotensin-converting enzyme inhibitors, and heavy metals.

Renal Function Tests

Renal function tests are used to evaluate the severity of kidney disease and to assess the patient's clinical progress. These tests also provide information on the effectiveness of the kidney in carrying out excretory function. Renal function test results may be within normal limits until the glomerular filtration rate is reduced to less than 50% of normal. Renal function can be assessed most accurately if several tests are performed and their results analyzed together. Common tests of renal function include renal concentration tests, creatinine clearance, and serum creatinine and blood **urea nitrogen** levels. Table 39-4 describes the purpose and normal ranges for each of these tests. Other helpful tests for evaluating renal function are serum electrolyte measurements.

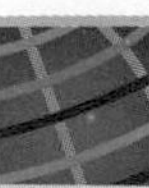

TABLE 39•4 **Tests of Renal Function**

Test	Purpose	Normal Values
Renal Concentration Tests		
Specific gravity	Evaluates ability of kidneys to concentrate solutes in urine.	Specific gravity, 1.010–1.025
Urine osmolality	Concentrating ability is lost early in kidney disease; hence, these test findings may disclose early defects in renal function.	Urine osmolality, 300–900 mOsm/kg/24 h, 50–1200 mOsm/kg random sample
24-Hour Urine Test		
Creatinine clearance	Detects and evaluates progression of renal disease. Test measures volume of blood cleared of endogenous creatinine in 1 minute, which provides an approximation of the glomerular filtration rate. Sensitive indicator of renal disease used to follow progression of renal disease.	Measured in mL/minute/1.73 m^2 *Age* / *Male* / *Female* Under 30: 88–146 / 81–134 30–40: 82–140 / 75–128 40–50: 75–133 / 69–122 50–60: 68–126 / 64–116 60–70: 61–120 / 58–110 70–80: 55–113 / 52–105
Serum Tests		
Creatinine level	Measures effectiveness of renal function. Creatinine is end product of muscle energy metabolism. In normal function, level of creatinine, which is regulated and excreted by the kidneys, remains fairly constant in body.	0.6–1.2 mg/dL (50–110 μmol/L)
Urea nitrogen (blood urea nitrogen [BUN])	Serves as index of renal function. Urea is nitrogenous end product of protein metabolism. Test values are affected by protein intake, tissue breakdown, and fluid volume changes.	7–18 mg/dL Patients over age 60 years: 8–20 mg/dL
BUN to creatinine ratio	Evaluates hydration status. An elevated ratio is seen in hypovolemia; a normal ratio with an elevated BUN and creatinine is seen with intrinsic renal disease.	About 10:1

X-rays and Other Imaging Modalities

Kidney, Ureter, and Bladder Studies

An x-ray study of the abdomen or kidney, ureters, and bladder (KUB) may be performed to delineate the size, shape, and position of the kidneys and to reveal any abnormalities, such as calculi (stones) in the kidneys or urinary tract, hydronephrosis (distention of the pelvis of the kidney), cysts, tumors, or kidney displacement by abnormalities in surrounding tissues.

Ultrasonography

Ultrasonography is a noninvasive procedure that uses sound waves passed into the body through a transducer to detect abnormalities of internal tissues and organs. Structures of the urinary system create characteristic ultrasonographic images. Abnormalities, such as fluid accumulation, masses, congenital malformations, changes in organ size, or obstructions, can be identified. During the test, the lower abdomen and genitalia may need to be exposed for the procedure. Ultrasonography requires a full bladder. Therefore, fluid intake should be encouraged before the procedure. Because of its sensitivity, ultrasonography has replaced many other diagnostic tests as the initial diagnostic procedure.

Bladder Ultrasonography

Bladder ultrasonography is a noninvasive method of measuring the volume of urine in the bladder. It may be indicated for the following situations: urinary frequency, inability to void after removal of an indwelling urinary catheter, measurement of postvoiding residual urine volume, inability to void postoperatively, and assessment of the need for catheterization during the initial stages of an intermittent catheterization training program. Portable, battery-operated devices are available for use at the bedside. The scan head is placed on the patient's abdomen and directed toward the bladder. The device automatically calculates and displays the bladder volume.

Computed Tomography and Magnetic Resonance Imaging

Computed tomography (CT) and magnetic resonance imaging (MRI) are noninvasive techniques that provide excellent cross-sectional views of the kidney and urinary tract. They are used in evaluating genitourinary masses, nephrolithiasis, chronic renal infections, renal or urinary tract trauma, metastatic disease, and soft tissue abnormalities. The nurse should explain to the patient that radiation exposure is minimal and a sedative may be prescribed. Claustrophobia is often a problem, especially with MRI imaging. Patient preparation for the MRI includes removal of any metallic objects, such as jewelry or clothing with metallic clasps. Patients should keep credit cards away from the MRI area because of their magnetic strips. MRI is contraindicated in patients with pacemakers, surgical clips, or any metallic objects anywhere in the body. Occasionally, an oral or intravenous radiopaque contrast material is used in CT scanning to enhance visualization. Nursing care guidelines for patient preparation and test precautions for any imaging procedure requiring a contrast agent (also called a *contrast medium)* are explained in Guideline 39-1.

39•1
GUIDELINES FOR

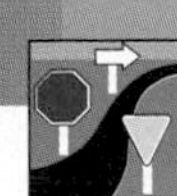

PATIENT CARE DURING UROLOGIC TESTING WITH CONTRAST AGENTS

For some patients, contrast agents are nephrotoxic and allergenic. The following guidelines can help the nurse and other caregivers respond quickly in the event of a problem.

Nursing Actions for Room Preparation

- Have emergency equipment and medications available in case the patient has an anaphylactic reaction to the contrast agent. Emergency supplies include epinephrine, corticosteroids, vasopressors; oxygen; and airway and suction equipment.

Nursing Actions for Patient Preparation

- Obtain the patient's allergy history with emphasis on allergy to iodine, shellfish, or other seafood because many contrast agents contain iodine.
- Notify physician and radiologist if the patient is allergic or suspected to be allergic to iodine.
- Obtain health history. (Contrast agents should be used with caution in older adult patients and other patients who have diabetes mellitus, multiple myeloma, renal insufficiency, or volume depletion.)
- Inform the patient that he or she may experience a temporary feeling of warmth, flushing of the face, and an unusual taste (seafood) sensation in the mouth when the contrast agent is infused.

Nuclear Scans

Nuclear scans require injection of a radioisotope (technetium-99m–labeled compound or iodine-131 hippurate) into the circulatory system, which is then monitored as it moves throughout the blood vessels of the kidneys. A scintillation camera is placed posterior to the kidney with the patient in a supine, prone, or seated position. Hypersensitivity to the radioisotope is rare. The technetium scan provides information about kidney perfusion; the hippurate scan provides information about kidney function.

Nuclear scans are indicated to evaluate acute and chronic renal failure, renal masses, and blood flow before and after kidney transplantation. The radioisotope is injected at a specified time before the study to achieve the proper concentration in the kidneys. After the procedure is completed, the patient is encouraged to drink fluids to promote excretion of the radioisotope by the kidneys.

Intravenous Urography

Intravenous urography includes various specific tests, such as excretory urography, intravenous pyelography, and infusion drip pyelography. An intravenous pyelogram, or intravenous urogram, shows the kidneys, ureter, and bladder. A radiopaque contrast agent is administered intravenously. A *nephrotomogram* may be carried out as part of the study to visualize different layers of the kidney and the diffuse structures within each layer and to differentiate solid masses or lesions from cysts in the kidneys or urinary tract.

Intravenous urography is conducted as part of the initial assessment of any suspected urologic problem, especially lesions in the kidneys and ureters. It also provides a rough estimate of renal function. After the contrast agent (sodium diatrizoate or meglumine diatrizoate) is administered intravenously, multiple serial x-rays are obtained to visualize drainage structures.

Infusion drip pyelography requires an intravenous infusion of a large volume of a dilute contrast agent to opacify the renal parenchyma and completely fill the urinary tract. This method of examination is useful when prolonged opacification of the drainage structures is desired so that *tomograms* (body-section radiography) can be made. Images are obtained at specified intervals after the start of the infusion. These images show the filled and distended collecting system. The patient preparation is the same as for excretory urography, except that fluids are not restricted.

Retrograde Pyelography

In retrograde pyelography, ureteral catheters are advanced through the ureters into the renal pelvis by means of cystoscopy. Contrast agent is then injected. Retrograde pyelography is usually performed if intravenous urography provides inadequate visualization of the collecting systems. It may also be used before extracorporeal shock-wave lithotripsy or in patients with urologic cancer who need follow-up and are allergic to intravenous contrast agents. Possible complications include infection, hematuria, and perforation of the ureter. Retrograde pyelography is used less frequently because of improved techniques in excretory urography.

Cystography

Cystography aids in evaluating **vesicoureteral reflux** (backflow of urine from the bladder into one or both ureters) and assesses for bladder injury. A catheter is inserted into the bladder, and a contrast agent is instilled to outline the bladder wall. Leakage of contrast agent through a small bladder perforation due to bladder injury may occur but is usually harmless. Cystography can also be performed in conjunction with simultaneous pressure recordings inside the bladder.

Voiding Cystourethrography

Voiding cystourethrography uses fluoroscopy to visualize the lower urinary tract and examine urine storage in the bladder. It is commonly used as a diagnostic tool to identify vesicoureteral reflux (between bladder and ureter). A urethral catheter is inserted, and a contrast agent is instilled into the bladder. When the bladder is full and the patient feels the urge to void, the catheter is removed, and the patient voids. *Retrograde urethrography* is always performed before urethral catheterization if urethral trauma is suspected, in which a contrast agent is injected retrograde into the urethra.

Renal Angiography

A renal angiogram, or renal arteriogram, provides an image of the renal arteries. The femoral (or axillary) artery is pierced with a needle, and a catheter is threaded up through the femoral and iliac arteries into the aorta or renal artery. A contrast agent is injected to opacify the renal arterial supply. Angiography is used to evaluate renal blood flow in suspected renal trauma, to differentiate renal cysts from tumors, and to evaluate hypertension. It is used preoperatively for renal transplantation. Before the procedure, a laxative may be prescribed to evacuate the colon so that unobstructed x-rays can be obtained. Injection sites (groin for femoral approach or axilla for axillary approach) may be shaved. The peripheral pulse sites (radial, femoral, dorsalis pedis) are marked for easy access during postprocedural assessment. The patient is informed that there may be a brief sensation of heat along the course of the vessel when the contrast agent is injected.

After the procedure, the patient's vital signs are monitored until stable. If the axillary artery was the site of the injection, blood pressure measurements are taken on the opposite arm. The puncture site is examined for swelling and hematoma formation. Peripheral pulses are palpated, and the color and temperature of the involved extremity are noted and compared with those of the uninvolved extremity. Cold compresses may be applied to the injection site to decrease edema and pain. Possible complications include hematoma formation, arterial thrombosis or dissection, false aneurysm formation, and altered renal function.

Urologic Endoscopic Procedures

Endourology or endoscopic procedures can be performed in one of two ways: (1) by a cystoscope inserted into the urethra, or (2) percutaneously through a small incision. Endourologic procedures are indicated for large kidney stones or abnormal anatomy of the upper urinary tract. They may also be used for biopsy of the kidneys or after failed extracorporeal shock-wave lithotripsy.

Cystoscopic Examination

The cystoscopic examination is used to visualize the urethra and bladder directly. The cystoscope, which is inserted through the urethra into the bladder, has a self-contained optical lens system that provides a magnified, illuminated view of the bladder (Fig. 39-7). The use of a high-intensity light and interchangeable lenses allows excellent visualization and permits still and motion pictures to be taken. The cystoscope is manipulated to allow complete visualization of the urethra and bladder as well as the ureteral orifices and prostatic urethra. Small ureteral catheters can be passed through the cystoscope, allowing assessment of the ureters and the pelvis of each kidney.

The cystoscope also permits the urologist to obtain a urine specimen from each kidney to evaluate its function. Cup forceps can be inserted through the cystoscope for biopsy. Calculi may be removed from the urethra, bladder, and ureter using cystoscopy. Before the procedure, a sedative may be administered. A topical anesthetic is instilled into the urethra by the urologist before the cystoscope is inserted. Alternatively, spinal or general anesthesia may be used.

NURSING INTERVENTIONS

The nurse describes the procedure to the patient and family to prepare them and to allay fears. The patient is usually kept NPO (nothing by mouth) for several hours before the procedure.

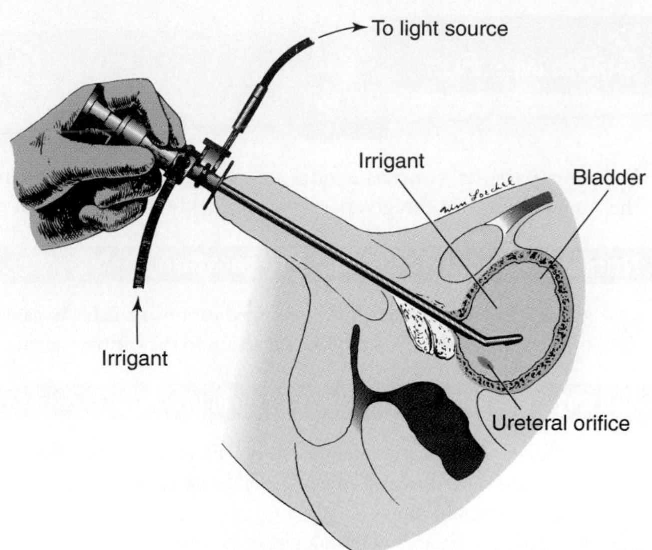

FIGURE 39•7 Cystoscopic examination. A cystoscope is introduced into the bladder. The upper cord is an electric line for the light at the distal end of the cystoscope. The lower tubing leads from a reservoir of sterile irrigant that is used to inflate the bladder.

Postprocedural management is directed at relieving any possible discomfort resulting from the examination. Some burning on voiding, blood-tinged urine, and urinary frequency from trauma to the mucous membrane may occur after cystoscopic examination. Moist heat to the lower abdomen and warm sitz baths are helpful in relieving pain and promoting muscle relaxation.

After cystoscopic examination, the patient with obstructive pathology may experience urinary retention as a result of edema caused by the instrumentation. The nurse carefully monitors the patient with prostatic hyperplasia for urinary retention. Warm sitz baths and relaxant medications help to relieve retention; catheterization, however, may be necessary. The nurse monitors the patient for signs and symptoms of urinary tract infection. Edema of the urethra secondary to local trauma may obstruct urine flow; therefore, the patient is monitored for signs and symptoms of obstruction.

Biopsy

Renal and Ureteral Brush Biopsy

Brush biopsy techniques provide specific information when abnormal x-ray findings of the ureter or renal pelvis raise questions about whether the defect is a tumor, a stone, a blood clot, or an artifact. First, a cystoscopic examination is conducted. Then, a ureteral catheter is introduced, followed by a biopsy brush that is passed through the catheter. The suspected lesion is brushed back and forth to obtain cells and surface tissue fragments for histologic analysis.

After the procedure, intravenous fluids may be administered to help clear the kidneys and prevent clot formation. Urine may contain blood (usually clearing in 24 to 48 hours) from oozing at the brushing site. Postoperative renal colic occasionally occurs and responds to analgesics.

Kidney Biopsy

Biopsy of the kidney is used in diagnosing and evaluating the extent of kidney disease. Indications for biopsy include unexplained acute renal failure, persistent proteinuria or hematuria, transplant rejection, and glomerulopathies. A small section of renal cortex is obtained either percutaneously through the skin and into the renal tissue or by open biopsy through a small flank incision. Before the biopsy is carried out, coagulation studies are conducted to identify any risk for postbiopsy bleeding. Contraindications to a kidney biopsy include bleeding tendencies, uncontrolled hypertension, and a solitary kidney.

PROCEDURE

The patient may be placed on a fasting regimen 6 to 8 hours before the test. An intravenous line is established. A urine specimen is obtained and saved for comparison with the postbiopsy specimen. If a needle biopsy is to be performed, the patient is instructed to hold his or her breath (to prevent movement of the kidney) while the needle is being inserted.

The sedated patient is placed in a prone position with a sandbag under the abdomen. The skin at the biopsy site is infiltrated with a local anesthetic agent. The biopsy needle is introduced just inside the renal capsule of the outer quadrant of the kidney. The location of the needle may be confirmed by fluoroscopy or by ultrasound, in which case a special probe is used. With open biopsy, a small incision is made over the kidney and allows direct visualization of the kidney. Preparation for an open biopsy is similar to that for any major abdominal surgery.

POSTBIOPSY NURSING INTERVENTIONS

After the specimen is obtained, pressure is applied to the biopsy site. The patient may be kept in a prone position immediately after biopsy and on bed rest for 6 to 8 hours to minimize the risk of bleeding.

MONITORING AND MANAGING POTENTIAL COMPLICATIONS

Potential postbiopsy complications include persistent hematuria, fistula or aneurysm formation, or laceration of organs or blood vessels adjacent to the kidney. The nurse monitors the patient closely for hematuria, which may appear soon after biopsy. The kidney is a highly vascular organ, and about one fourth of the entire cardiac output circulates through it in about 1 minute. The passage of the biopsy needle punctures the kidney capsule, and bleeding can occur in the perirenal space. Usually, the bleeding subsides on its own, but a large amount of blood can accumulate in this space in a short period of time without noticeable signs until cardiovascular collapse is evident. The following nursing interventions follow a kidney biopsy:

- Monitor vital signs every 5 to 15 minutes for the first hour to detect early signs of bleeding, and then with decreasing frequency as indicated.
- Be alert for signs and symptoms suggestive of bleeding, including a rise or fall in blood pressure, tachycardia, anorexia, vomiting, and the development of a dull, aching discomfort in the abdomen.
- Report any symptoms of backache, shoulder pain, or dysuria immediately.

Flank pain may occur but usually represents bleeding into the muscle rather than around the kidney. Colicky pain similar to that of ureteral colic may develop when a clot is present in the ureter and may cause excruciating, sharp flank pain that radiates to the groin.

All urine voided by the patient is inspected for evidence of bleeding and compared with the prebiopsy specimen and subsequent voiding samples. If bleeding persists, as indicated by an enlarging hematoma, palpating or manipulating the abdomen is avoided.

Hematocrit and hemoglobin levels are obtained within 8 hours to assess for changes; decreasing levels may indicate bleeding. Usually, the fluid intake is maintained at 3000 mL/day unless the patient has renal insufficiency. If bleeding occurs, the patient is prepared for blood component therapy and surgical intervention to control the hemorrhage, which may necessitate surgical drainage or, rarely, nephrectomy (removal of kidney).

PATIENT TEACHING

Because delayed hemorrhage can occur several days after biopsy, the patient is instructed to avoid strenuous activity, sports, and heavy lifting for at least 2 weeks. The physician or clinic is to be notified if any of the following occur: flank pain, hematuria, lightheadedness and fainting, rapid pulse, or any other signs and symptoms of bleeding.

Urodynamic Tests

Urodynamic tests provide an accurate evaluation of voiding problems, thus assisting the health care provider with diagnosis. Urodynamic studies are useful in evaluating urinary retention of unknown cause, the effects of medications on bladder function, neuropathic bladder dysfunction, incontinence, bladder outlet obstruction, and recurrent urinary tract infections. (See Before and After Urodynamic Testing, which outlines patient education for all basic urodynamic tests.) The following urodynamic test procedures and measurements are the most common.

Uroflowmetry (flow rate) is the record of the volume of urine passing through the urethra per time unit (milliliters per second). The flow rate reflects the combined activity of the detrusor muscle, bladder neck, and urethral function. Because this test is dependent on the amount voided, the patient is instructed to arrive for the test with a normal strong urge to void, but not to be overfull.

A *cystometrogram* (CMG) is a graphic recording of the pressures in the bladder. It is the major diagnostic portion of urodynamic testing and is divided into two portions: filling and emptying of the urinary bladder. During the procedure, the amount of fluid instilled into the bladder, the patient's sensations of bladder fullness and urge to void, the degree of straining or hesitancy, and amount, size, and force of the urinary stream are recorded. These are then compared with the pressures measured in the bladder during bladder filling and voiding. A retention catheter is passed through the urethra into the bladder. The residual volume is measured, and the catheter is left in place. The urethral catheter is connected to a water manometer, and sterile solution is allowed to flow into the bladder, usually at the rate of 1 mL/sec. The patient informs the examiner when the first desire to void is felt, and again when the bladder feels full. The degree of bladder filling at these points is recorded. The pressures above the zero level at the symphysis pubis are measured, and the pressures and volumes within the bladder are plotted and recorded.

A *urinary pressure-flow study*, presently considered the standard urodynamic test, is performed immediately after the filling phase of the CMG and simultaneously with the voiding CMG. Bladder pressure, urine flow, and sphincter electromyography are measured simultaneously. This allows for a detailed picture of the voiding dysfunction.

Electromyography involves the placement of electrodes in the pelvic floor musculature or anal sphincter to evaluate neuro-

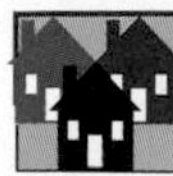

PATIENT EDUCATION AND HOME CARE

Before and After Urodynamic Testing

In preparing the patient for urodynamic testing, the nurse instructs the patient about how urodynamic procedures are performed, what is expected of the patient, and what the patient might feel afterward. The nurse reassures the patient that staff will be present during the procedure, but privacy and comfort will be maintained. Additional information for the patient follows:

- An in-depth interview will be conducted. Questions related to your urologic symptoms and voiding habits will be asked by the staff.
- You will be asked to describe sensations felt during the procedure.
- During the procedure, you might be asked to change positions, for example, from supine to sitting or standing.
- You may be asked to cough or perform Valsalva maneuver (bear down) during the procedure.
- You will probably need to have one or two urethral catheters inserted so that bladder pressure and bladder filling can be measured. Another catheter may be placed in the rectum or vagina to measure abdominal pressure.
- You may also have electrodes (surface, wire, or needle) placed in the perianal area for electromyography. This may be uncomfortable initially during insertion and later during position changes.
- Your bladder will be filled through the urethral catheter one or more times during the procedure.
- After the procedure, you may experience urinary frequency, urgency, or dysuria from the urethral catheters. Avoid caffeinated, carbonated, and alcoholic beverages after the procedure because these can further irritate the bladder. These symptoms usually decrease or subside by the day after the procedure.
- You might notice a slight hematuria (blood-tinged urine) right after the procedure (especially in men with benign prostatic hyperplasia). Drinking fluids will help to clear the hematuria.
- If the urinary meatus is irritated, a warm sitz bath may be helpful.
- Be alert for signs of a urinary tract infection after the procedure. Contact your physician if you experience fever, chills, lower back pain, or continued dysuria and hematuria.
- If you receive an antibiotic medication before the procedure, you should continue taking the complete course of medication after the procedure. This is a measure to prevent infection.

muscular function of the lower tract. It is usually performed at the same time as the CMG.

The *video fluorourodynamic study* is considered the optimal urodynamic evaluation. This test combines a study of the filling and voiding phases of the CMG and the electromyogram with a simultaneous visualization of the lower urinary tract, allowing for a complete and detailed assessment of the voiding dysfunction.

The *urethral pressure profile* measures the amount of urethral pressure along the length of the urethra needed to maintain continence. Gas and fluid are instilled through a catheter that is withdrawn while the pressures along the urethral wall are obtained.

A new urodynamic test is *Valsalva's leak-point pressure test,* which assesses internal sphincter function. While in a sitting or standing position, the patient is asked to cough or perform Valsalva's maneuver until urine leakage occurs. Before this test is performed, it is important to determine if the patient is prone to vasovagal reactions and to alert the aerodynamicist. The patient is also instructed to alert the aerodynamicist if dizziness or lightheadedness are experienced during the procedure.

NURSING IMPLICATIONS

Regardless of the extent or type of their renal or urinary tract dysfunction, all patients undergo tests to assess the function of the renal and urinary tract. Even those who have had these tests repeatedly in the past are apprehensive about the procedures and the results. Patients frequently feel discomfort and embarrassment about a previously private and personal function: voiding. Although health care providers deal routinely with voiding in the course of providing care, these assessments are not routine to patients.

Other considerations for nurses caring for patients undergoing renal-urinary testing include the patient's age or other life span issues; the impact of diagnostic findings, nursing diagnoses, interventions, and outcomes; and the need for teaching.

Gerontologic Considerations

Renal and urinary tract function changes with age. The glomerular filtration rate decreases with age, beginning between ages 35 and 40 years. A yearly decline of about 1 mL/min continues thereafter. Tubular function, including reabsorption and concentrating ability, is also reduced with increasing age. Although renal function usually remains adequate despite these changes, renal reserve is decreased and may reduce the kidneys' ability to respond effectively to drastic or sudden physiologic changes.

Structural or functional abnormalities that occur with aging may prevent complete emptying of the bladder due to increased collagen in the bladder wall or secondary to prostatic enlargement. Vaginal and urethral tissues atrophy and become thinner in aging women due to decreased estrogen levels. In addition, a decreased blood supply to the urogenital tissues may cause urethral and vaginal irritation.

Preparation of the elderly patient for diagnostic tests must be managed carefully to prevent dehydration that might precipitate renal failure in a patient with marginal renal reserve. Limitations in mobility in elderly patients may affect their ability to void adequately or to consume adequate fluids. Patients may limit their own fluid intake to minimize the frequency of voiding or the risk of incontinence; teaching the patient and family about the dangers of an inadequate fluid intake is an important role of the nurse caring for the elderly patient.

Nursing Diagnosis

Potential nursing diagnoses for the patient undergoing assessment of urinary or renal function include the following:

- Knowledge deficit about the procedures and diagnostic tests
- Pain related to renal infection, edema, obstruction, or bleeding along the urinary tract, or to invasive diagnostic procedures
- Fear related to possible diagnosis of serious illness, altered renal function, and embarrassment secondary to discussion of urinary function and invasion of genitalia

Planning, Implementation, and Evaluation

The goals, nursing interventions and rationale, and expected outcomes are discussed in greater detail in Plan of Nursing Care 39-1. Patient and family education are essential to help the patient understand the purpose of the procedure and what to expect before, during, and after it. Pertinent home care considerations can be discussed at this time.

39•1

PLAN OF NURSING CARE

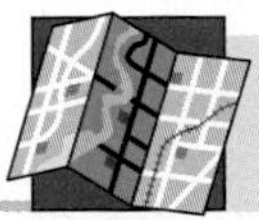

Care of the Patient Undergoing Diagnostic Testing of the Renal-Urologic System

Nursing Diagnosis: Knowledge deficit about procedures and diagnostic tests
Goal: Patient demonstrates understanding of the procedure and tests and expected behaviors.

Nursing Interventions	Rationale	Expected Outcomes
1. Assess patient's level of understanding of planned diagnostic tests.	1. Provides basis for teaching and gives indication of patient's perception of tests	• States rationale for planned diagnostic tests and what tasks and behaviors are expected during the procedure • Complies with urine collection, fluid modifications, or other procedures required for diagnostic evaluation • Restates in own words results of diagnostic tests • Asks for clarification of terms and procedures • Explains rationale for follow-up care • Participates in follow-up care
2. Provide a factual description of tests in language the patient can understand.	2. Understanding what is expected enhances patient compliance and cooperation.	
3. Assess patient's understanding of test results after their completion.	3. Apprehension may interfere with patient's ability to understand information and results provided by health care team.	
4. Reinforce information provided to patient about test results and implications for follow-up care.	4. Provides opportunity for patient to clarify information and anticipate follow-up care	

Nursing Diagnosis: Pain related to infection, edema, obstruction, or bleeding along urinary tract or to invasive diagnostic tests
Goal: Patient reports decrease in pain and absence of discomfort.

Nursing Interventions	Rationale	Expected Outcomes
1. Assess level of pain: dysuria, burning on urination, abdominal or flank pain, bladder spasm.	1. Provides baseline for evaluation of interventions and progression of dysfunction	• Reports decreasing levels of pain • Reports absence of local symptoms • States ability to start and stop urinary stream without discomfort • Consumes increased fluid intake if indicated • Uses sitz bath as indicated • Identifies signs and symptoms to be reported to the health care provider • Takes medications as prescribed • Does not delay in emptying bladder • Uses appropriate hygienic measures, avoids use of bubble bath, uses appropriate hygiene after bowel movements
2. Encourage fluid intake (unless contraindicated).	2. Promotes dilute urine and flushing of the lower urinary tract	
3. Encourage warm sitz baths.	3. Relieves local discomfort and promotes relaxation	
4. Report increased pain to physician.	4. May indicate progression or recurrence of dysfunction, or untoward signs (eg, bleeding, calculi)	
5. Administer analgesics and antispasmodics for pain and spasm as prescribed.	5. May be prescribed for pain or spasm	
6. Assess voiding patterns and hygiene practices and provide instructions about recommended voiding patterns and hygienic practices.	6. Delayed emptying of the bladder and poor hygiene may contribute to pain secondary to renal or urinary tract dysfunction.	

Nursing Diagnosis: Fear related to potential alteration in renal function and embarrassment secondary to discussion of urinary function and invasion of genitalia.
Goal: Patient appears relaxed and reports decreased fear and anxiety.

Nursing Interventions	Rationale	Expected Outcomes
1. Assess patient's level of fear and apprehension.	1. A high level of fear or apprehension can interfere with learning and cooperation.	• Appears relaxed with a low level of fear or apprehension • States rationale for tests and procedures in a calm, relaxed manner • Maintains usual privacy and modesty • Discusses own urinary tract dysfunction using correct terminology without overt indications of embarrassment or discomfort • Relates fears and concerns • Shows correct understanding of procedures and possible outcomes • Appears relaxed with low level of fear and apprehension
2. Explain all procedures and tests to patient.	2. Knowledge about what is expected helps reduce fear and apprehension.	
3. Provide privacy and respect patient's modesty by closing doors and keeping patient covered. Keep urinal and bedpan covered and out of sight.	3. Communicates that you are aware of and accept patient's need for privacy and modesty	
4. Use correct terminology in a factual manner when questioning patient about urinary tract dysfunction.	4. Conveys that you are comfortable discussing patient's urinary dysfunction and symptoms with patient	
5. Assess patient's fears about perceived changes associated with tests and other procedures.	5. May reveal unfounded fears and misinterpretation that can be alleviated by correct understanding	
6. Instruct patient in relaxation techniques.	6. May promote relaxation and assist the patient in coping with uncertainty about outcomes	

Promoting Home and Community-Based Care

Teaching Patients Self-Care

Many of the procedures and tests used to evaluate renal and urinary tract function are carried out in outpatient or short-procedure settings. Therefore, postprocedural care is often provided by family members or other caregivers in the home. Thus, they need clear explanations about the procedures and tests, what to do to prepare for them, and what precautions, if any, will need to be taken after the procedures and tests. The patient and family members are provided with verbal and written explanations about monitoring that may be necessary at home and are instructed about steps to take if complications occur.

Continuing Care

Follow-up telephone calls made to the patient and family provide an opportunity for them to ask questions and to report on the patient's status. Teaching is reinforced, and the patient is reminded of the importance of follow-up appointments with primary health care providers.

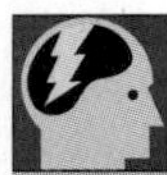

Critical Thinking Exercises

1. After a closed renal biopsy for diagnostic purposes, your patient reports a backache. You also notice that the patient's urinal contains about 300 mL of bright red blood. Based on your knowledge of the risks associated with renal biopsy, explain how you would focus your assessment and nursing care.
2. Your patient is scheduled for a series of urodynamic tests as part of a workup for incontinence. You know that a patient who understands the purpose of the test and what to expect during the procedure will be able to cooperate more while the test is being done. Describe how you would teach this patient, and discuss the details of the explanations you would give.

References and Selected Readings

BOOKS

Agency for Health Care Policy and Research, Public Health Service, U.S. Department of Health and Human Services. (1996). *Urinary incontinence in adults: Acute and chronic management.* Clinical Practice Guideline (AHCPR Pub. No. 96-0682). Washington, DC: U.S. Government Printing Office.

Bickley, L. S. & Hoekelman, R. A. (1999). *Bates' guide to physical examination and history taking* (7th ed.). Philadelphia: Lippincott Williams & Wilkins.

Copstead, L. (1995). *Perspectives on pathophysiology.* Philadelphia: W. B. Saunders.

Fischbach, F. (1996). *A manual of laboratory and diagnostic tests* (5th ed.). Philadelphia: Lippincott-Raven.

Greenberg, A. (1998). *Primer on kidney diseases* (2nd ed.). San Diego: Academic Press.

Karlowicz, K. (1995). *Urologic nursing: Principles and practice.* Philadelphia: W. B. Saunders.

Lancaster, L. (1995). *American Nephrology Nurses Association core curriculum for nephrology nursing* (3rd ed.). Pitman, NJ: American Nephrology Nurses' Association.

Levine, D. (1997). *Caring for the renal patient* (3rd ed.). Philadelphia: W. B. Saunders.

Metheny, N. (1996). *Fluid and electrolyte balance: Nursing considerations* (3rd ed.). Philadelphia: Lippincott-Raven.

Parker, J. (1998). *Contemporary nephrology nursing.* Pitman, NJ: Anthony J. Janetti, Inc.

Palmer, M. (1996). *Urinary continence: Assessment and promotion.* Gaithersburg, MD: Aspen.

Walsh, P., Retik, A., Vaughan, E., & Wein, A. (1997). *Campbell's urology* (7th ed.). Philadelphia: W. B. Saunders.

JOURNALS

Ahmed, Z., & Lee, J. (1997). Asymptomatic urinary abnormalities: Hematuria and proteinuria. *Medical Clinics of North America, 81*(3), 639–651.

Ali, H. (1997). Proteinuria: How much evaluation is appropriate? *Postgraduate Medicine, 101*(4), 173–180.

Fishbane, S. (1996). Overused tests in nephrology. *Patient Care, 28*(5), 113–114.

Hassan, A. (1996). Renal disease in the elderly: Distinctive disorders, tailored treatments. *Postgraduate Medicine, 100*(6), 44–57.

Lash J. & Gardner, C. (1997). Effects of aging and drugs on normal renal function. *Coronary Artery Disease, 8,* 489–494.

Lesko, J., & Johnston, J. (1997). Oliguria. *American Association of Critical Care Nurses Clinical Issues, 8*(3), 459–468.

Morrison, G. (1996). Work-up of the patient with sudden oliguria. *Hospital Medicine, 32*(8), 22–30.

Seaman, S. (1995). Renal physiology. II. Fluid and electrolyte regulation. *Neonatal Network, 14*(5), 5–11.

Seidmon, E. (1997). Office diagnosis of microscopic hematuria: Methodology and clinical significance. *Hospital Medicine, 33*(1), 22–26.

Stark, J. (1998). Interpretation of BUN and serum creatinine. An interactive exercise. *Critical Care Clinics of North America, 10*(4), 491–496.

Steiner, R. (1996). Common misperceptions in diagnosing and managing renal problems. *Hospital Medicine, 32*(6), 15–21.

Wozniak-Petrofsky, J. (1996). Urodynamics for the primary care nurse. *Geriatric Nursing, 17*(3), 115–119.

Wozniak-Petrofsky, J. (1997). Urodynamic tests: Client preparation, assessment, and follow-up. *Nurse Practitioner, 22*(3), 70–91.

Zauderer, B. (1996). Age-related changes in renal function. *Critical Care Nursing Quarterly, 19*(2), 34–40.

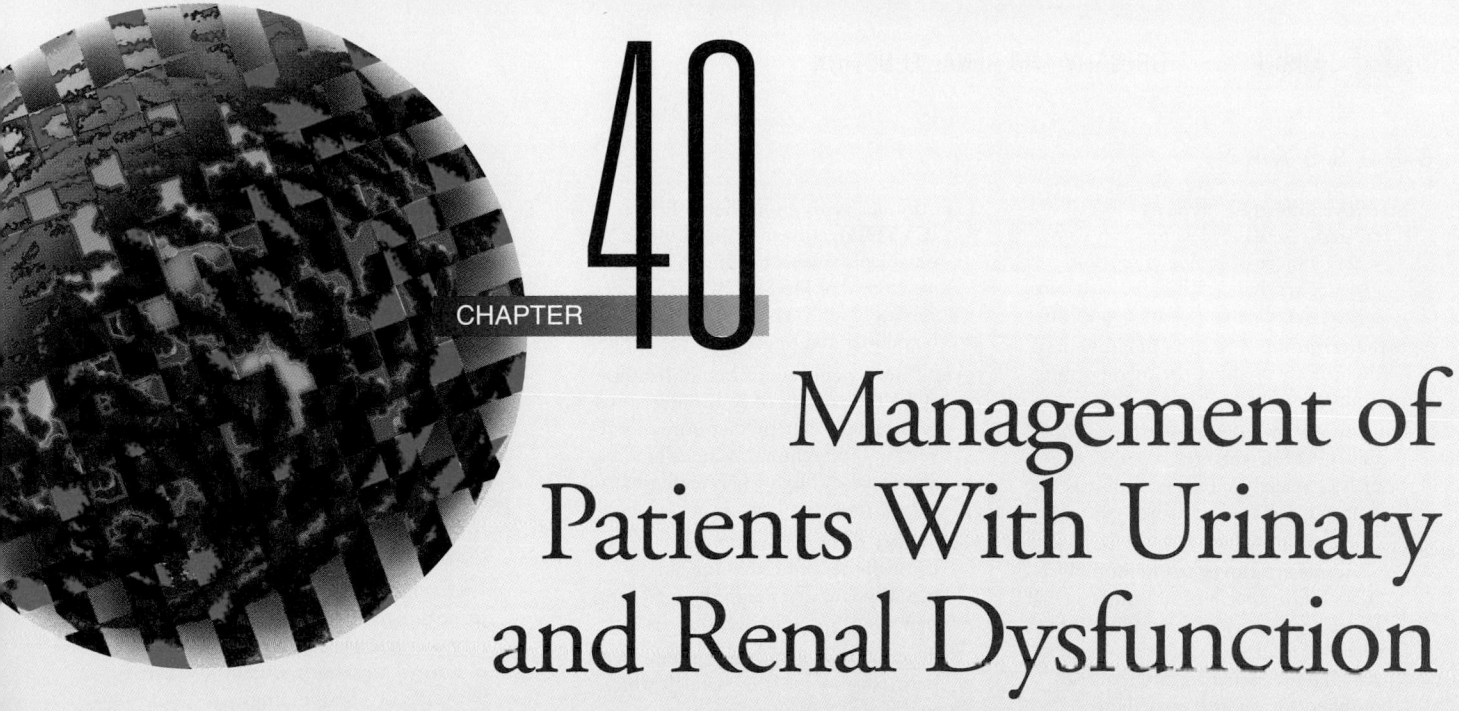

Management of Patients With Urinary and Renal Dysfunction

Learning Objectives

On completion of this chapter, the learner will be able to:

1. Describe the sequence of events leading to urinary tract infection in a patient with an indwelling urinary catheter.
2. Outline the principles of management of a patient with an indwelling urinary catheter.
3. Compare and contrast urinary retention and urinary incontinence: their causes, clinical manifestations, complications, and management.
4. Implement appropriate nursing management techniques for patients with urinary retention or urinary incontinence.
5. Compare and contrast hemodialysis and peritoneal dialysis in terms of underlying principles, procedures, complications, and nursing considerations.
6. Describe nursing management of the hospitalized dialysis patient.
7. Use the nursing process as a framework for care of patients undergoing kidney surgery.

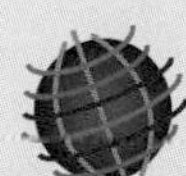

Patients with disorders of the kidneys or lower urinary tract often exhibit similar problems regardless of the underlying disorder. This chapter provides an overview of common problems experienced by patients, such as fluid and electrolyte imbalances and dysfunctional voiding patterns. Interdisciplinary medical and surgical management strategies (eg, catheterization, dialysis, and surgery) for a wide array of renal and urologic diseases and disorders are also discussed.

GLOSSARY

arteriovenous graft: type of surgically created vascular access for dialysis by which a piece of biologic, semibiologic, or synthetic graft material is connected to the patient's artery and vein

catheterization: insertion of a tube into the urinary bladder; the tube permits drainage of urine

continuous ambulatory peritoneal dialysis (CAPD): method of peritoneal dialysis whereby a patient performs four to five complete dialysis exchanges or cycles throughout the day

continuous arteriovenous hemodialysis (CAVHD): a form of continuous renal replacement therapy that results in removal of fluid and waste products; arterial blood is circulated through a hemofilter (surrounded by dialysis cleaning fluid) and returned to the patient through a venous catheter

continuous arteriovenous hemofiltration (CAVH): a form of continuous renal replacement therapy that primarily results in fluid removal; arterial blood is circulated through a hemofilter and returned to the patient through a venous catheter

continuous cyclic peritoneal dialysis (CCPD): method of peritoneal dialysis in which a peritoneal dialysis machine (cycler) automatically performs dialysis exchanges, usually while the patient sleeps

continuous renal replacement therapy (CRRT): variety of methods used to replace normal kidney function by circulating the patient's blood through a hemofilter

continuous venovenous hemodialysis (CVVHD): a form of continuous renal replacement therapy that results in removal of fluid and waste products; venous blood is circulated through a hemofilter and returned to the patient

continuous venovenous hemofiltration (CVVH): a form of continuous renal replacement therapy that primarily results in fluid removal; venous blood is circulated through a hemofilter and returned to the patient

dialysate: dialysis solution that circulates through the artificial kidney in hemodialysis and through the peritoneal membrane in peritoneal dialysis

dialyzer: artificial kidney; contains semipermeable membrane through which particles of a certain size can pass

diffusion: movement of solutes (waste products) from an area of high concentration to an area of lower concentration

fistula: type of vascular access for dialysis; created by surgically connecting an artery to a vein

hemodialysis: circulation of the patient's blood through an artificial kidney to remove waste products and excess fluid

nephrostomy: procedure by which a tube is inserted through the skin and subcutaneous tissue into the pelvis of the kidney for drainage

neurogenic bladder: bladder dysfunction that results from a disorder or dysfunction of the nervous system

osmosis: movement of water through a semipermeable membrane from an area of lower solute concentration to an area of higher solute concentration

overflow incontinence: involuntary urine loss associated with overdistention of the bladder

peritoneal dialysis: form of dialysis in which the patient's own peritoneal membrane is used as the semipermeable membrane for exchange of fluid and solutes

peritonitis: inflammation of the peritoneal membrane that lines the peritoneal cavity

reflex incontinence: involuntary loss of urine due to hyperreflexia or involuntary urethral relaxation in the absence of normal sensations, usually associated with micturition (voiding)

residual urine: urine that remains in the bladder after voiding

suprapubic catheter: a urinary catheter that is inserted through a suprapubic incision into the bladder

stress incontinence: involuntary loss of urine through an intact urethra as a result of a sudden increase in intra-abdominal pressure

ultrafiltration: process by which water is removed from the blood by means of a pressure gradient between the patient's blood and the dialysate

urge incontinence: involuntary loss of urine associated with urgency

urinary incontinence: involuntary or uncontrolled loss of urine from the bladder

FLUID AND ELECTROLYTE IMBALANCES IN RENAL DISORDERS

Patients with renal disorders commonly experience fluid and electrolyte imbalances and require astute assessment and close monitoring for signs of potential problems. A key monitoring tool, the fluid intake–output chart, is kept to monitor and record important fluid parameters, including the amount of fluid taken in (orally or parenterally), the volume of urine excreted, other fluid losses (diarrhea, vomiting, excessive sweating), and any change in weight.

These records are essential for determining the patient's daily fluid allowance and indicating signs of fluid overload or deficit. The patient whose fluid intake exceeds the ability of the kidneys to excrete fluid is said to have a fluid overload. If fluid intake is inadequate, the patient is said to be volume depleted and may show signs and symptoms of fluid volume deficit.

Nursing Alert *The most accurate indicator of fluid loss or gain in an acutely ill patient is weight. An accurate daily weight must be obtained and recorded. A 1-kg weight gain is equal to 1000 mL of retained fluid.*

Clinical Manifestations

The signs of common fluid and electrolyte disturbances that may occur in patients with renal disease are listed in Table 40-1. The nurse should continually assess, monitor, and inform appropriate members of the health care team of the presence of any of these signs. General management strategies for each imbalance are also listed. Dialysis as a management strategy is discussed in greater depth later in this chapter (see also Chap. 13 on fluid and electrolyte disturbances).

DYSFUNCTIONAL VOIDING PATTERNS

Urinary Retention

Urinary retention is the inability to empty the bladder completely during attempts to void. Chronic urinary retention often leads to overflow incontinence (from pressure of retained urine in the bladder) or residual urine. **Residual urine** is urine that remains in the bladder after voiding.

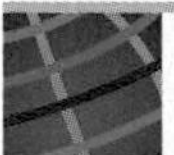

TABLE 40•1 Common Fluid and Electrolyte Disturbances in Renal Disease

Disturbance	Manifestations	General Management Strategies
Fluid volume deficit	Acute weight loss >5%, decreased skin turgor, dry mucous membranes, oliguria or anuria, increased hematocrit, BUN increased out of proportion to creatinine, hypothermia	Fluid challenge, fluid replacement orally or parenterally
Fluid volume excess	Acute weight gain >5%, edema, crackles, shortness of breath, decreased blood urea nitrogen, decreased hematocrit, distended neck veins	Fluid and sodium restriction, diuretics, dialysis
Sodium deficit	Nausea, malaise, lethargy, headache, abdominal cramps, apprehension, seizures	Diet, normal saline or hypertonic saline solutions
Sodium excess	Dry, sticky mucous membranes, thirst, rough dry tongue, fever, restlessness, weakness, disorientation	Fluids, diuretics, dietary restriction
Potassium deficit	Anorexia, abdominal distention, ileus, muscle weakness, ECG changes, dysrhythmias	Diet, oral or parenteral potassium replacement therapy
Potassium excess	Diarrhea, colic, nausea, irritability, muscle weakness, ECG changes	Dietary restriction, diuretics, IV glucose, insulin and sodium bicarbonate, cation exchange resin, calcium gluconate, dialysis
Calcium deficit	Abdominal and muscle cramps, stridor, carpopedal spasm, hyperactive reflexes, tetany, positive Chvostek's or Trousseau's sign, tingling of fingers and around mouth, ECG changes	Diet, oral or parenteral calcium salt replacement
Calcium excess	Deep bone pain, flank pain, muscle weakness, depressed deep tendon reflexes, constipation, nausea and vomiting, confusion, impaired memory, polyuria, polydipsia, ECG changes	Fluid replacement, etidronate, pamidronate, mithramycin, calcitonin, glucocorticoids, phosphate salts
Bicarbonate deficit	Headache, confusion, drowsiness, increased respiratory rate and depth, nausea and vomiting, warm, flushed skin	Bicarbonate replacement, dialysis
Bicarbonate excess	Depressed respirations, muscle hypertonicity, dizziness, tingling of fingers and toes	Fluid replacement if volume depleted; ensure adequate chloride
Protein deficit	Chronic weight loss, emotional depression, pallor, fatigue, soft flabby muscles	Diet, dietary supplements, hyperalimentation, albumin
Magnesium deficit	Dysphagia, muscle cramps, hyperactive reflexes, tetany, positive Chvostek's or Trousseau's sign, tingling of fingers, dysrhythmias, vertigo	Diet, oral or parenteral magnesium replacement therapy
Magnesium excess	Facial flushing, nausea and vomiting, sensation of warmth, drowsiness, depressed deep tendon reflexes, muscle weakness, respiratory depression, cardiac arrest	Calcium gluconate, mechanical ventilation, dialysis
Phosphorus deficit	Deep bone pain, flank pain, muscle weakness and pain, paresthesias, apprehension, confusion, seizures	Diet, oral or parenteral phosphorus supplementation therapy
Phosphorus excess	Tetany, tingling of fingers and around mouth, muscle spasms, soft tissue calcification	Diet restriction, phosphate binders, normal saline solution, IV dextrose solution, and insulin

Urinary retention can occur in any postoperative patient, particularly in those who have undergone surgery on the perineal or anal regions that resulted in reflex spasm of the sphincters. General anesthesia reduces bladder muscle innervation, and thus the urge to void is suppressed.

Pathophysiology

Urinary retention may result from diabetes, prostatic enlargement, urethral pathology (infection, tumor, calculus), trauma (pelvic injuries), pregnancy, or neurologic disorders (cerebrovascular accident, spinal cord injury, multiple sclerosis).

Some medications cause urinary retention, either by inhibiting contractility of the bladder or by increasing bladder outlet resistance. Examples of medications that promote urinary retention by inhibiting contractility are anticholinergics (atropine sulfate, dicyclomine hydrochloride), antispasmodics (oxybutynin chloride, belladonna, and opium suppositories), and tricyclic antidepressants (imipramine, doxepin). Medications that increase bladder outlet resistance include alpha-adrenergics (ephedrine sulfate, pseudoephedrine), beta-adrenergic blockers (propranolol), and estrogens.

Assessment and Diagnostic Findings

Assessment for urinary retention is multifaceted. The signs and symptoms of urinary retention may easily be overlooked. The following questions serve as a guide in assessment:

- What were the time and volume of the last voiding?
- Is the patient passing small amounts of urine frequently?
- Is the patient dribbling urine?
- Does the patient complain of pain or discomfort in the lower abdomen? (Discomfort may be relatively mild if the bladder distends slowly.)
- Is there a rounded swelling arising out of the pelvis (which could indicate retention and a distended bladder)?

- Is there dullness on percussion in the suprapubic region (possibly indicating retention and a distended bladder)?
- Are there other indicators of urinary retention, such as restlessness and agitation?

The patient may verbalize an awareness of bladder fullness and a sensation of incomplete bladder emptying. The nurse also assesses for signs and symptoms of urinary tract infection, such as hematuria and dysuria. A series of urodynamic studies, described in Chapter 39, may be performed to identify the specific type of bladder dysfunction and to aid in determining appropriate treatment. A voiding diary may be completed by the patient to provide a written record of the amount of voided urine and the frequency of voiding.

Complications

Urinary retention can lead to chronic infection. Infections that are unresolved predispose the patient to calculi, pyelonephritis, and sepsis. Eventual deterioration of the kidney can also occur if large volumes of urine are retained, causing backward pressure on the upper urinary tract. In addition, leakage of urine can lead to perineal skin breakdown, especially if regular hygienic measures are neglected.

Nursing Management

Management strategies are instituted to prevent overdistention of the bladder and to treat infection or correct obstruction. Many problems, however, can be prevented by careful nursing assessment and appropriate nursing interventions. The nurse should explain why normal voiding is not occurring and monitor urine output closely. The nurse should also provide reassurance about the temporary nature of retention and successful management strategies.

PROMOTING NORMAL URINARY ELIMINATION

Nursing measures to encourage voiding include providing privacy, ensuring an environment and a position conducive to voiding, and assisting the patient to use the bathroom or commode rather than a bedpan. This provides a more natural setting for voiding. The male patient may stand beside the bed while using the urinal; most men find this position more comfortable and natural.

Additional measures include application of warmth to relax the sphincters (ie, sitz baths, warm compresses to the perineum, showers), hot tea, and encouragement and reassurance. Simple trigger techniques may also be used, such as turning on the water faucet while trying to void. Other examples of trigger techniques are stroking the abdomen or inner thighs, suprapubic tapping, and dipping the patient's hands in warm water. A combination of techniques may be necessary to initiate voiding.

After surgery, the prescribed analgesic should be administered because pain in the incisional area can make voiding difficult.

PROMOTING URINARY ELIMINATION

When the patient cannot void, **catheterization** is used to prevent overdistention of the bladder (see later discussion of neurogenic bladder and catheterization). In the case of prostatic obstruction, attempts at catheterization (by the urologist) may not be successful, requiring that a **suprapubic catheter** be inserted. After restoration of urinary drainage, bladder retraining is initiated for the patient who is unable to void spontaneously.

To promote voiding in chronic urinary retention, Credé's method is used to assist bladder emptying. This involves gentle massage of the bladder in a downward direction toward the pubic area during and after urination. The method is often used along with intermittent catheterization in patients with neurogenic bladder as in multiple sclerosis or spinal cord injury.

Urinary Incontinence

Urinary incontinence is the involuntary or uncontrolled loss of urine from the bladder. More than 13 million adults in the United States suffer from urinary incontinence (Agency for Health Care Policy and Research [AHCPR], 1996). However, urinary incontinence still remains widely underdiagnosed and underreported. Patients may be too embarrassed to seek help, often ignoring or concealing symptoms. Many patients resort to the use of absorbent pads or other devices without having their condition properly diagnosed and treated. Health care providers must be alert to subtle cues of urinary incontinence and stay informed about current management strategies.

The costs of care for patients with urinary incontinence are estimated to be more than $11.2 billion annually in the community and $5.2 billion in nursing homes (AHCPR, 1996). The psychosocial costs of urinary incontinence are also enormous: embarrassment, loss of self-esteem, and social isolation are common outcomes. Urinary incontinence in elderly patients often decreases their ability to maintain an independent lifestyle. This increases dependence on caregivers and often leads to institutionalization.

Urinary incontinence affects people of all ages but is particularly common in elderly people. It has been reported that more than half of all nursing home residents have urinary incontinence. Although urinary incontinence is not a normal consequence of aging, age-related changes in the urinary tract predispose the older person to incontinence.

Urinary incontinence is often regarded as a condition occurring in older multiparous women, but it is also common in young, nulliparous women, especially during high-impact vigor-

Risk Factors for
URINARY INCONTINENCE

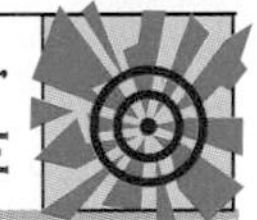

Pregnancy: vaginal delivery, episiotomy
Menopause
Genitourinary surgery
Pelvic muscle weakness
Incompetent urethra due to trauma or sphincter relaxation
Immobility
High-impact exercise
Diabetes mellitus
Stroke
Age-related changes in the urinary tract
Morbid obesity
Cognitive disturbances: dementia, Parkinson's disease
Medications: diuretics, sedatives, hypnotics, opioids
Caregiver or toilet unavailable

ous activity. Age, gender, and number of previous vaginal deliveries are established risk factors and explain, in part, the increased incidence in women. Urinary incontinence is a symptom with many possible causes.

Clinical Manifestations: Types of Incontinence

Stress incontinence is the involuntary loss of urine through an intact urethra as a result of a sudden increase in intra-abdominal pressure (sneezing, coughing, or changing position). It mostly affects women and can be the result of obstetric injury, lesions of the bladder neck, extrinsic pelvic disease, fistulas, detrusor dysfunction, and a variety of other conditions. It may also result from congenital conditions (eg, extrophy of the bladder, ectopic ureter).

Urge incontinence is an involuntary loss of urine associated with urgency. The patient is aware of the need to void but is unable to reach a toilet in time. In many cases, uninhibited contraction of the bladder is a concomitant factor. This may occur in the patient with neurologic dysfunction that impairs inhibition of bladder contraction, or in the patient with local symptoms of irritation from urinary tract infection or bladder tumors.

Reflex incontinence is the loss of urine due to hyperreflexia or involuntary urethral relaxation in the absence of normal sensations usually associated with voiding. This commonly occurs in paraplegic patients because they have no sensory awareness of the need to void.

Overflow incontinence is an involuntary urine loss associated with overdistention of the bladder. The bladder cannot empty normally and becomes overdistended. Despite frequent urine loss, the bladder never empties. Overflow incontinence may be caused by neurologic abnormalities (ie, spinal cord lesions) or by factors that obstruct the outflow of urine (ie, medications, tumors, strictures, and prostatic hyperplasia). Neurogenic bladder is discussed separately in the next section.

Functional incontinence refers to those instances in which the function of the lower urinary tract is intact but in which other factors, such as severe cognitive impairment, make it difficult for the patient to identify the need to void (eg, Alzheimer's dementia) or in which physical impairments make it difficult or impossible for the patient to reach the toilet in time for voiding.

Some patients have several types of urinary incontinence. This mixed incontinence is usually a combination of stress and urge incontinence.

Only with appropriate recognition of the problem, assessment, and referral for diagnostic evaluation and treatment can the outcome of incontinence be determined. *All* people with incontinence should be considered for evaluation and treatment.

Assessment and Diagnostic Findings

Once incontinence is recognized, a thorough history is necessary. This includes a detailed description of the problem and a history of medication use. The patient's voiding history, a diary of fluid intake and voiding, and bedside tests (ie, postvoiding residual urine volume, stress maneuvers) may be used to help determine the type of urinary incontinence. Extensive urodynamic tests may be performed and are described in Chapter 39. Urinalysis and urine culture are performed to identify hematuria (from infection, cancer, or kidney stone), glycosuria (causes polyuria), pyuria, and bacteriuria (infection), all of which may identify transient causes of urinary incontinence.

CHART 40•1 Causes of Transient Incontinence: DIAPPERS

Delirium
Infection of urinary tract
Atrophic vaginitis, urethritis
Pharmacologic agents (anticholinergics, sedatives, alcohol, analgesics, diuretics, muscle relaxants, adrenergic agents)
Psychological factors (depression, regression)
Excessive urine production (increased intake, diabetes insipidus, diabetic ketoacidosis)
Restricted activity
Stool impaction

Successful management depends on the type of urinary incontinence and its causes. Urinary incontinence may be transient or reversible (Chart 40-1) if the underlying cause is successfully treated and the patient's voiding pattern reverts to normal. Management of urinary incontinence not considered transient or reversible falls into three categories: pharmacologic, surgical, and behavioral.

Medical Management

Treatment for urinary incontinence depends on the underlying causative factors. Before appropriate treatment can be initiated, however, the problem must be identified and the causative factors identified.

BEHAVIORAL THERAPY

Behavioral strategies are attempted first. These include timed or habit voiding and bladder retraining, which may involve biofeedback using electromyography and manometry. The behavioral strategies are largely carried out, coordinated and monitored by the nurse.

PHARMACOLOGIC THERAPY

Pharmacologic therapy works best when used as an adjunct to behavioral interventions. Anticholinergics (oxybutynin, dicyclomine) inhibit contraction of the bladder and are considered first-line medications for urge incontinence. Several of the tricyclic antidepressants (imipramine, doxepin, desipramine, and nortriptyline) also decrease bladder contractions as well as increase bladder neck resistance. Stress incontinence may be treated using pseudoephedrine and phenylpropanolamine, ingredients found in over-the-counter decongestants. Estrogen (taken orally, transdermally, or topically) has been shown to be beneficial for all types of urinary incontinence. Estrogen decreases obstruction to urine flow by restoring the mucosal, vascular, and muscular integrity of the urethra.

SURGICAL MANAGEMENT

Surgical correction may be indicated in patients who have not achieved continence using behavioral and pharmacologic therapy. Surgical options vary according to the underlying anatomy and the physiologic problem. Most procedures involve lifting and stabilizing the bladder or urethra to restore the normal urethrovesical angle or to lengthen the urethra.

Women with stress incontinence may have an anterior vaginal repair, retropubic suspension, or needle suspension to reposition the urethra. Procedures to compress the urethra and increase re-

NURSING RESEARCH

Behavioral Strategies and Urinary Incontinence

Bear, M., Dwyer, J.W., Benveneste, D., Jett, K., & Dougherty, M. (1997). Home-based management of urinary incontinence: A pilot study with both frail and independent elders. *Journal of Wound, Ostomy and Continence Nursing, 24*(3),163–171.

Purpose

Urinary incontinence (UI) affects between 15% and 35% of people over 60 years of age who live in the community. This quasi-experimental study tested the effectiveness of known behavioral techniques in the home setting to improve the management of urinary incontinence.

Study Sample and Design

Study participants were women aged 55 years or older with involuntary urine loss twice a week or more and 1 g/day or more; negative urinalysis; residual urine volume of less than 75 mL; and a history of stress, urge, or mixed incontinence. Patients were recruited in several ways: through formation of a community-based advisory board, newspaper and radio advertisements, and mass mailings.

Data were collected by means of a bladder diary for recording fluid intake, voidings, episodes of UI, and activity during UI episodes. A pad test of urine loss was used as a measure; patients received a supply of weighed and packaged incontinence pads, which were returned after use and weighed again.

Participants who responded to the recruitment efforts were screened by telephone interview for eligibility. A home visit was then made, during which time demographic and background information and health history were obtained and mental and functional competence and degree of assistance needed with activities of daily living were assessed. In addition, instructions about the pad test and bladder diary were provided. A second home visit was made 1 week later to complete the pad test, complete additional testing, and pick up the bladder diary and pad test. Women were then randomly assigned to either a control group or a treatment group. The control group received a final home visit, during which time the bladder diary and pad test results were reviewed with the patient. The treatment group participated in behavioral management of continence (BMC), which consisted of several phases: self-monitoring, a scheduled regimen for voiding, and pelvic muscle exercise biofeedback. Progression of subjects through the phases was determined by their participation in these techniques.

Findings

A decrease in frequency and volume of urine loss was recorded for women who completed the BMC program. The initial mean urine loss of all patients was 66 g/day. The treatment group had a 34% decrease in frequency of UI episodes and a 33% decrease in volume of urine loss at the 6-month follow-up. The control group had a 28% increase in the frequency of UI episodes and 22% increase in urine loss at the 6-month follow-up. The researchers concluded that behavioral techniques are effective in treating urinary incontinence. However, the researchers noted that although frail elderly adults were targeted for this study, few were willing or able to participate in the study because of the study's demands.

Nursing Implications

Nurses working with older adults in all settings need to be alert for signs of incontinence and to screen and assess at-risk patients. Identification of the type of incontinence and the cause can then be made so that appropriate treatment, including behavioral techniques, can be instituted.

---

sistance to urine flow include sling procedures and placement of periurethral bulking agents.

A modified artificial sphincter that uses a silicone-rubber balloon as a self-regulating pressure mechanism is also being used to close the urethra. Electronic stimulation of the pelvic floor by means of a miniature pulse generator with electrodes mounted on an intra-anal plug is another method of controlling stress incontinence.

Men with overflow and stress incontinence may have a transurethral resection done to relieve symptoms of prostatic enlargement. An artificial sphincter can be used after prostatic surgery for sphincter incompetence (Fig. 40-1). After surgery, periurethral bulking agents (collagen) can also be injected into the periurethral area to increase compression of the urethra.

Nursing Management

Nursing management begins with the principles that incontinence is not an inevitable part of illness or aging and that it is often reversible and treatable regardless of age.

A program of timed or habit voiding, in which the bladder is emptied before it fills to maximum capacity, is initiated. The goal is to keep the patient dry by having the patient void at regular intervals on a regular schedule. Bladder retraining, which has also been successful, involves teaching the patient to inhibit urinary urgency and gradually to increase the interval between voidings.

The nurse may instruct and encourage the patient to practice pelvic muscle exercises, known as Kegel exercises (see Chap. 43). These exercises strengthen the muscles of the pelvic floor, thereby improving urethral resistance and urinary control. Kegel exercises need to be performed 30 to 80 times a day for at least 6 weeks to be effective. Elderly patients may need to exercise for an even longer time to strengthen the pelvic floor muscles. Kegel exercises are helpful for women with stress incontinence and for men who have undergone prostate surgery.

An adjunct to the Kegel exercises are vaginal cone retention exercises, in which cones of varying weight are inserted intravaginally twice a day. The patient tries to retain the cone for 15 minutes by contracting the pelvic muscles.

For behavioral therapy to be effective, the nurse must provide support and encouragement as it is easy for the patient to become discouraged if therapy does not improve the level of continence quickly.

GERONTOLOGIC CONSIDERATIONS

If nurses and other health care providers accept incontinence as an inevitable part of illness or aging or consider it irreversible and untreatable at any age, it cannot be treated successfully. Collaborative, interdisciplinary efforts are essential in assessing and effectively treating urinary incontinence.

PROMOTING HOME AND COMMUNITY-BASED CARE

Modifications in the home environment and general measures that are often effective in treating urinary incontinence may be simple ones. In adapting the home environment for easy, safe ac-

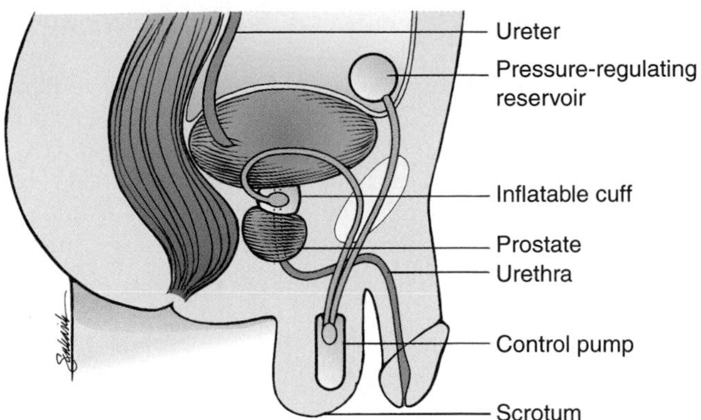

FIGURE 40•1 Male artificial urinary sphincter. An inflatable cuff is inserted surgically around the urethra or neck of the bladder. To empty the bladder, the cuff is deflated by squeezing the control pump located in the scrotum.

cess to the bathroom, the patient may need to remove barriers, such as throw rugs or other objects, from the route. Other modifications that the nurse may recommend include installing support bars in the bathroom and placing a bedpan or urinal within easy reach. Leaving a light on in the darkened bedroom and bathroom and wearing clothing that is easy to remove when using the toilet are additional recommendations (see the accompanying Patient Education and Home Care guidelines).

Neurogenic Bladder

Neurogenic bladder dysfunction results from a lesion of the nervous system. It may be caused by spinal cord injury, spinal tumor, herniated vertebral disk, multiple sclerosis, congenital anomalies (spina bifida, myelomeningocele), infection, and diabetes mellitus.

Pathophysiology

There are two types of neurogenic bladder: spastic or reflex bladder and flaccid bladder.

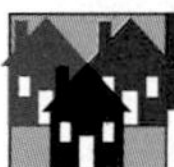

PATIENT EDUCATION AND HOME CARE

Strategies for Managing Urinary Incontinence

The following recommendations are reviewed with patients who are coping with urinary incontinence:

- Increase your awareness of the amount and timing of all fluid intake.
- Avoid taking diuretics after 4 PM.
- Avoid bladder irritants, such as caffeine, alcohol, and aspartame (NutraSweet).
- Take steps to avoid constipation: drink adequate fluids, eat a well-balanced diet high in fiber, exercise regularly, and take stool softeners if recommended.
- Void regularly, 5 to 8 times a day (about every 2 to 3 hours):
    - First thing in the morning
    - Before each meal
    - Before retiring to bed
    - Once during night if necessary
- Perform all pelvic floor muscle exercises as prescribed, every day.
- Stop smoking (smokers usually cough frequently, which increases incontinence).

Spastic or reflex bladder is the most common type and is caused by any lesion of the spinal cord above the voiding reflex arc (upper motor neuron lesion). The result is a loss of conscious sensation and cerebral motor control. A spastic bladder empties on reflex, with minimal or no controlling influence to regulate its activity.

Flaccid bladder is caused by a lower motor neuron lesion, often resulting from trauma. This form of neurogenic bladder has increasingly been recognized as a problem in patients with diabetes mellitus. The bladder continues to fill and becomes greatly distended, and overflow incontinence occurs. The bladder muscle does not contract forcefully at any time. Because sensory loss may accompany a flaccid bladder, the patient feels no discomfort.

Assessment and Diagnostic Findings

Evaluation for neurogenic bladder involves measurement of fluid intake, urinary output, and residual urine volume; urinalysis; and assessment of sensory awareness of bladder fullness and degree of motor control. Comprehensive urodynamic studies are also performed.

Complications

The most common complication of neurogenic bladder is infection from urinary stasis and catheterization. Urolithiasis (stones in the urinary tract) may develop from urinary stasis, infection, and demineralization of bone from prolonged immobilization. Renal failure can also occur from vesicoureteral reflux (backward flow of retained urine from the bladder into the ureters) with eventual hydronephrosis (collection of urine in the renal pelvis) and atrophy of the kidney. Indeed, renal failure is the major cause of death of patients with neurologic impairment of the bladder.

Medical Management

The problems resulting from neurogenic bladder disorders vary considerably from patient to patient and are a major challenge to the health care team. There are several long-term objectives appropriate for all types of neurogenic bladders:

- Preventing overdistention of the bladder
- Emptying the bladder regularly and completely
- Maintaining urine sterility with no stone formation
- Maintaining adequate bladder capacity without reflux

Specific interventions include continuous, intermittent, or self-catheterization (discussed later in this chapter), use of an external condom-type catheter, a diet low in calcium (to prevent calculi), and encouragement of mobility and ambulation. A liberal fluid intake is encouraged to reduce the urinary bacterial count, reduce stasis, decrease the concentration of calcium in the urine, and minimize the precipitation of urinary crystals and subsequent stone formation.

Use of timed or habit voiding is also considered. For example, a 2-hour voiding schedule may be established to prevent overdistention. A bladder retraining program may be effective in treating a spastic bladder.

PHARMACOLOGIC THERAPY

Parasympathomimetic medications, such as bethanechol (Urecholine), may help to increase the contraction of the detrusor muscle.

SURGICAL MANAGEMENT

In some cases, surgery may be carried out to correct bladder neck contractures or vesicoureteral reflux or to perform some type of urinary diversion procedure.

OTHER STRATEGIES

In patients with a urologic disorder or with marginal kidney function, care must be taken to ensure that urinary drainage is adequate and that kidney function is preserved. When urine cannot be eliminated naturally and must be drained artificially, catheters may be inserted directly into the bladder, the ureter, or the renal pelvis. Catheters vary in size, shape, length, material, and configuration. The type of catheter used depends on its purpose.

Indwelling Catheterization. Catheterization is performed to achieve the following:

- Relieve urinary tract obstruction
- Assist with postoperative drainage in urologic and other surgeries
- Provide a means to monitor accurate urinary output in critically ill patients
- Allow urinary drainage in patients with neurogenic bladder dysfunction and urinary retention
- Prevent urinary leakage in patients with stage III to IV pressure ulcers

A patient should be catheterized only if absolutely necessary because catheterization commonly leads to urinary tract infection. In addition, urinary catheters have been associated with a number of other complications, such as bladder spasms, urethral strictures, and pressure necrosis.

Closed Drainage Systems. When an indwelling catheter cannot be avoided, a closed drainage system is essential. This drainage system is designed to prevent any disconnections, thereby reducing the risk of contamination. One common system consists of an indwelling catheter, a connecting tube, and a collecting bag with an antireflux chamber emptied by a drainage spout. Another common system has a triple-lumen indwelling urethral catheter attached to a closed sterile drainage system. With the triple-lumen catheter, urinary drainage occurs through one channel. The retention balloon of the catheter is inflated with water or air through the second channel, and the bladder is continuously irrigated with sterile irrigating solution through the third channel. Triple-lumen catheters are commonly used after transurethral prostate surgery.

An indwelling catheter can lead to infection. Bacterial colonization (bacteriuria) occurs within 2 weeks in half of catheterized patients and within 4 to 6 weeks in almost all patients after insertion of a catheter—even if recommendations for infection control and catheter care are followed carefully.

The urinary tract is the most common site of nosocomial infection, accounting for greater than 40% of the total number of cases reported by hospitals and affecting about 600,000 patients each year (Winn, 1996). Most urinary tract infections follow instrumentation of the urinary tract, usually catheterization. The pathogens responsible for catheter-associated urinary tract infections include *Escherichia coli* and *Klebsiella, Proteus, Pseudomonas, Enterobacter, Serratia,* and *Candida* species. Many of these organisms are part of the patient's endogenous or normal bowel flora or are acquired through cross-contamination by patients or health care personnel or through exposure to nonsterile equipment.

Catheters impede most of the natural defenses of the lower urinary tract by obstructing the periurethral ducts, by irritating the bladder mucosa, and by providing an artificial route for organisms to enter the bladder. Organisms may be introduced from the urethra into the bladder during catheterization, or they may migrate along the epithelial surface of the urethra or external surface of the catheter.

The spout of the urinary drainage bag often becomes contaminated when opened to drain the bag. Bacteria enter the urinary drainage bag, multiply rapidly, and then migrate to the drainage tubing, catheter, and bladder. Scanning electron microscopy has demonstrated that the internal surfaces of catheters and drainage systems are often colonized by thick layers (biofilms) of organisms (Riley et al., 1995; Stickler, Morris, & Williams, 1996).

Nursing Management

ASSESSING THE PATIENT AND THE CATHETER SYSTEM

For patients with indwelling catheters, the drainage system is assessed to ensure that it provides adequate urinary drainage. The color, odor, and volume of urine are also monitored. An accurate record of the patient's fluid intake and urine output provides essential information about the adequacy of renal function and urinary drainage.

The nurse observes the catheter to make sure that it is properly anchored to prevent pressure on the urethra at the penoscrotal junction in male patients and to prevent tension and traction on the bladder in both male and female patients.

Patients at high risk for urinary tract infection from catheterization need to be identified and monitored carefully. These include women, older adults, and patients who are debilitated, malnourished, chronically ill, immunosuppressed, or diabetic. They are observed for signs and symptoms of urinary tract infection: cloudy malodorous urine, hematuria, fever, chills, anorexia, and malaise. The area around the urethral orifice is observed for drainage and excoriation. Urine cultures provide the most accurate means of assessing for infection.

Bladder ultrasonography is now available for noninvasive measurement of bladder volume. A portable bladder scan can be performed to assess the volume of urine in the bladder, the degree of bladder emptying, and therefore, the need for catheterization.

GERONTOLOGIC CONSIDERATIONS

Elderly patients with an indwelling catheter may not exhibit the usual or typical signs and symptoms of infection. Therefore, any subtle change in physical condition or mental status must be considered a possible indication of infection and must be promptly investigated because sepsis may occur before the infection is diagnosed. Figure 40-2 summarizes the sequence of events leading to infection and leakage of urine that often follow long-term use of an indwelling catheter in elderly patients.

PREVENTING INFECTION

Certain principles of care are essential to prevent infection in patients with a closed urinary drainage system. The catheter is a foreign body in the urethra and produces a reaction in the urethral mucosa with some urethral discharge. Vigorous cleaning of the meatus while the catheter is in place is discouraged, however, because the cleaning action can move the catheter to and fro, increasing the risk of infection. To remove obvious encrustations from the external catheter surface, the area can be washed gently with soap during the daily bath. The catheter is anchored as securely as possible to prevent it from moving in the urethra. Encrustations arising from urinary salts may serve as a nucleus for stone formation; however, using silicone catheters results in significantly less crust formation.

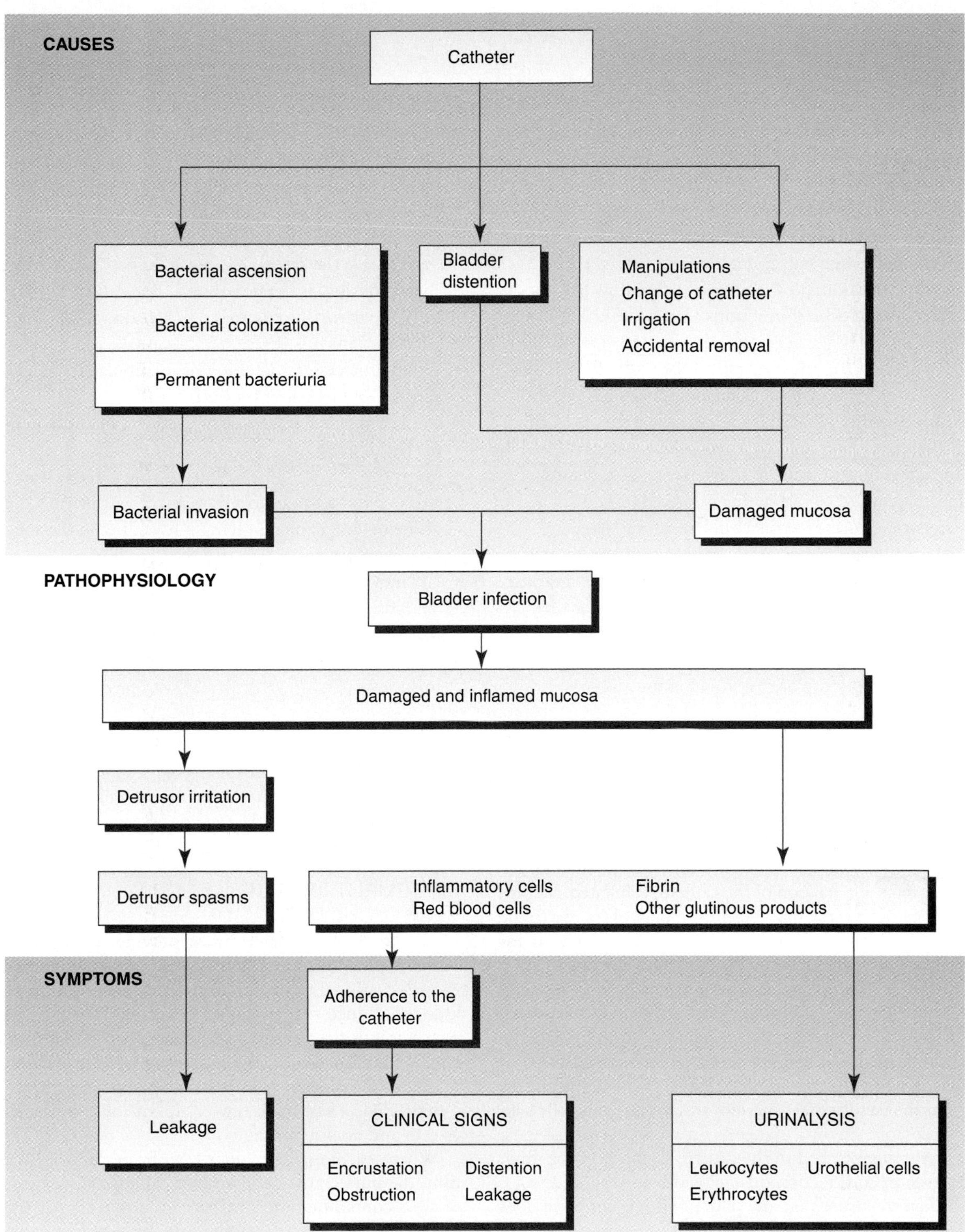

FIGURE 40•2 Pathophysiology and symptoms of bladder infection in long-term catheterized patients.

A liberal fluid intake, within limits of the patient's cardiac and renal reserve, and an increased urine output must be ensured to flush the catheter and to dilute urinary substances that might form encrustations.

Nursing Alert *Hand washing is essential when going from one patient to another to provide care and before and after handling any part of the catheter or drainage system.*

Urine cultures are obtained as prescribed or indicated in monitoring for infection; many catheters have an aspiration (puncture) port from which a specimen can be obtained.

Controversy exists about the usefulness of taking cultures and treating bacteriuria in patients who have symptoms of infection and who have indwelling catheters. Bacteriuria is considered to be inevitable, and overtreatment may lead to resistant strains of bacteria.

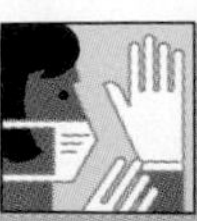

Health Promotion and Illness Prevention

Preventing Infection in the Catheterized Patient

- Use scrupulous aseptic technique during insertion of the catheter. Use a preassembled, sterile, closed urinary drainage system.
- To prevent contamination of the closed system, *never* disconnect the tubing. The drainage bag must *never* touch the floor. The bag and collecting tubing are changed if contamination occurs, if urine flow becomes obstructed, or if tubing junctions start to leak at the connections.
- If the collection bag must be raised above the level of the patient's bladder, clamp the drainage tube. This prevents backflow of contaminated urine into the patient's bladder from the bag.
- Ensure a free flow of urine to prevent infection. Improper drainage occurs when the tubing is kinked or twisted, allowing pools of urine to collect in the tubing loops.
- To reduce the risk of bacterial proliferation, empty the collection bag at least every 8 hours through the drainage spout—more frequently if there is a large volume of urine.
- Avoid contamination of the drainage spout. A receptacle in which to empty the bag is provided for each patient.
- Never irrigate the catheter routinely. If the patient is prone to obstruction from clots or large amounts of sediment, use a three-way system with continuous irrigation.
- Never disconnect the tubing to obtain urine samples, to irrigate the catheter, or to ambulate or transport the patient.
- Never leave the catheter in place longer than is necessary.
- Avoid routine catheter changes. The catheter is changed only to correct problems such as leakage, blockage, or encrustations.
- Avoid unnecessary handling or manipulation of the catheter by the patient or staff.
- Wash hands before and after handling the catheter, tubing, or drainage bag.
- Wash the perineal area with soap and water at least twice a day; avoid a to-and-fro motion of the catheter. Dry the area well, but avoid applying powder because it may irritate the perineum.
- Monitor the patient's voiding when the catheter is removed. The patient must void within 8 hours; if unable to void, the patient may require catheterization with a straight catheter.
- Obtain a urine specimen for culture at the first sign of infection.

MINIMIZING TRAUMA

Trauma to the urethra can be minimized by (1) using a catheter of the appropriate size, (2) lubricating the catheter adequately with a water-soluble jelly during insertion, and (3) inserting the catheter far enough into the bladder to prevent trauma to the urethral tissues when the retention balloon of the catheter is inflated. Manipulation of the catheter is the most common cause of trauma to the bladder mucosa in the catheterized patient. Infection then inevitably occurs when urine invades the damaged mucosa.

The catheter is secured properly to prevent it from moving, causing traction on the urethra, or being accidentally removed, and care is taken to ensure that the catheter position permits the patient leg movement. In male patients, the drainage tube (not the catheter) is taped laterally to the thigh to prevent pressure on the urethra at the penoscrotal junction, which can eventually lead to the formation of a urethrocutaneous fistula. In female patients, the drainage tubing attached to the catheter is taped to the thigh to prevent tension and traction on the bladder.

Care is taken to ensure that any patient who is confused does not accidentally remove the catheter with the retention balloon still inflated. This could cause bleeding and considerable injury to the urethra.

RETRAINING THE BLADDER

The bladder does not fill and contract when a catheter is in place; therefore, it eventually loses some of its tone (atony). When this occurs and the catheter is removed, the patient may be unable to contract the detrusor muscle and empty the bladder. When discontinuing a catheter that has been in place for a prolonged period, bladder retraining should be initiated to develop bladder tone and thus prevent retention (see Chap. 10 and Bladder Retraining After Indwelling Catheterization).

Prolonged use of an indwelling catheter should be avoided; intermittent catheterization used in place of an indwelling catheter for an extended period may decrease or prevent bladder atony.

IMPLEMENTING INTERMITTENT SELF-CATHETERIZATION

Intermittent self-catheterization provides periodic drainage of urine from the bladder. By promoting drainage and eliminating excessive residual urine, intermittent catheterization protects the kidneys, reduces urinary tract infections, and improves continence. It is the treatment of choice in spinal cord injury and other neurologic disorders, such as multiple sclerosis, when the ability to empty the bladder is impaired. Self-catheterization promotes independence, results in few complications, and enhances self-esteem and quality of life.

When teaching the patient how to perform self-catheterization, the nurse must use aseptic technique to minimize the risk of cross-contamination. The patient, however, may use a "clean" (nonsterile) technique at home, where the risk of cross-contamination is reduced. One of three cleaning methods is usually recommended for cleaning urinary catheters at home: povidone-iodine (Betadine), bleach, or hydrogen peroxide solution. The catheter is thoroughly rinsed with tap water after soaking in the cleaning solution. It must dry before reuse.

Teaching emphasizes the importance of frequent catheterization and emptying of the bladder at the prescribed time irrespective of the circumstances. (If the bladder becomes overdistended, blood flow through the bladder wall decreases, and the risk of infection increases.) The most common cause of incontinence in patients who self-catheterize is a mismatch between a high fluid intake and infrequent catheterization.

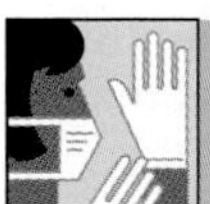

HEALTH PROMOTION AND ILLNESS PREVENTION
Bladder Retraining After Indwelling Catheterization

- Instruct the patient to drink a measured amount of fluid from 8 AM to 10 PM to avoid bladder overdistention. Offer no fluids (except sips) after 10 PM.
- At specified times, ask the patient to void by applying pressure over the bladder, tapping the abdomen, or stretching the anal sphincter with a finger to trigger the bladder.
- Immediately after the voiding attempt, catheterize the patient to determine the amount of residual urine.
- Measure the volumes of urine voided and obtained by catheterization.
- Palpate the bladder at repeated intervals to assess for distention.
- Instruct the patient without usual sensation to be alert for any signs that indicate a full bladder, such as perspiration, cold hands or feet, and feelings of anxiety.
- Lengthen the intervals between catheterizations as the volume of residual urine decreases. Catheterization is usually discontinued when the volume of residual urine is at an acceptable level.

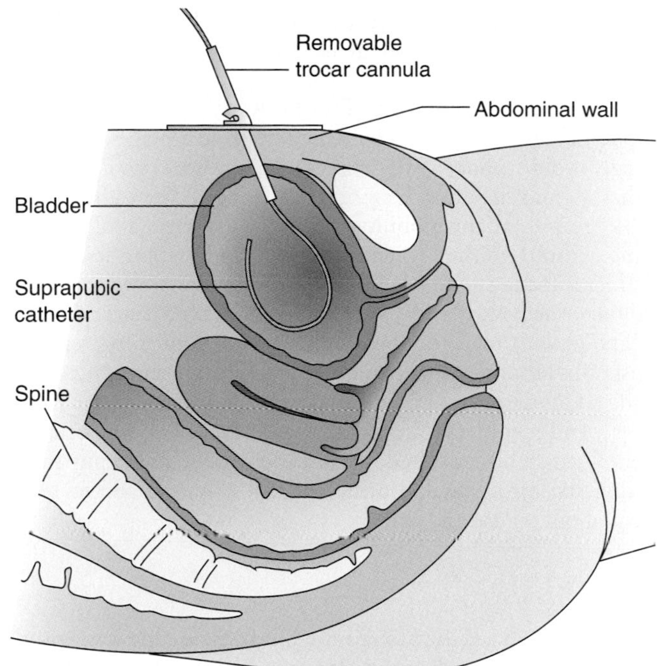

FIGURE 40•3 Suprapubic bladder drainage. A trocar cannula is used to puncture the abdominal and bladder walls. The catheter is threaded through the trocar cannula, which is then removed, leaving the catheter in place. The catheter is secured by tape or sutures to prevent accidental removal.

The female patient assumes a Fowler's position and uses a mirror to help locate the urinary meatus. The nurse teaches her to catheterize herself by inserting a catheter 7.5 cm (3 inches) into the urethra in a downward and backward direction. The male patient, in a Fowler's or sitting position, is taught to lubricate the catheter and retract the foreskin of the penis with one hand while grasping the penis and holding it at a right angle to the body. (This maneuver straightens the urethra and makes it easier to insert the catheter.) The catheter is inserted 15 to 25 cm (6 to 10 inches) until the urine begins to flow. After removal, the catheter is cleaned, rinsed, and wrapped in a paper towel or placed in a plastic bag or case. Patients following this routine should consult a primary health care provider at regular intervals to assess urinary function and the occurrence of complications.

If the patient cannot perform intermittent self-catheterization, a family member may be taught to carry out the procedure at regular intervals during the day.

Another self-catheterization option is creation of the Mitrofanoff umbilical appendicovesicostomy, which provides easy access to the bladder. The technique involves surgically closing the bladder neck and using the appendix to gain access to the bladder from outside the body. A submucosal tunnel is created with the appendix; one end of the appendix is brought to the skin and used as a stoma, and the other end is tunneled into the bladder.

Other Management: Suprapubic Bladder Drainage

Suprapubic bladder drainage is a method of establishing drainage from the bladder by inserting a catheter or tube into the bladder through a suprapubic (above the pubis) incision or puncture (Fig. 40-3). It may be a temporary measure to divert the flow of urine from the urethra when the urethral route is impassable (because of injuries, strictures, prostatic obstruction), after gynecologic or other abdominal surgery when bladder dysfunction is likely to occur, and occasionally after pelvic fractures. Suprapubic catheters may also be used long term for female patients with urethral destruction secondary to long-term indwelling urethral catheters.

IMPLEMENTING THE PROCEDURE

To facilitate insertion of the suprapubic catheter, the patient is placed in a supine position and the bladder is distended by administering oral or intravenous fluids or by instilling sterile saline solution into the bladder through a urethral catheter. These measures make it easier to locate the bladder. The suprapubic area is prepared as for surgery and the puncture site located about 5 cm (2 in) above the symphysis pubis. The surgeon enters the bladder through an incision or through a puncture made by a small trocar (sharp pointed instrument), then threads the catheter or suprapubic drainage tube into the bladder, secures the tube with sutures or tape, and covers the area around the catheter with a sterile dressing. The catheter is connected to a sterile closed drainage system, and the tubing is secured to prevent tension on the catheter.

MAINTAINING DRAINAGE

Suprapubic bladder drainage may be maintained continuously for several weeks. When the patient's ability to void is to be tested, the catheter is clamped for 4 hours, during which time the patient attempts to void. After the patient voids, the catheter is unclamped, and the residual urine (the amount of urine remaining) is measured. If the amount of residual urine is less than 100 mL on two separate occasions (morning and evening), the catheter is usually removed. If the patient complains of pain or discomfort, however, the suprapubic catheter is usually left in place until the patient can void successfully. When a suprapubic catheter remains in place indefinitely, it is changed regularly at 6- to 12-week intervals. Studies of the effectiveness of these strategies are needed.

ADVANTAGES AND DISADVANTAGES

Suprapubic drainage offers patients certain advantages. They can usually void sooner after surgery than those with urethral catheters, and they may be more comfortable. The catheter provides greater patient mobility, permits measurement of residual urine without urethral instrumentation, and presents less risk of bladder infection. The suprapubic catheter is removed when it is no longer necessary, and a sterile dressing is placed over the site.

The patient requires liberal amounts of fluid to prevent encrustation around the catheter. Other problems encountered include the formation of bladder stones, acute and chronic infections, and problems in collecting urine. An enterostomal therapist may be consulted to assist the patient and family in selecting the most suitable urine collection system and to teach them about its use and care.

DIALYSIS

Dialysis is a process used to remove fluid and uremic waste products from the body when the kidneys are unable to do so. It may also be used in treating patients with intractable (not responsive to treatment) edema, hepatic coma, hyperkalemia, hypercalcemia, hypertension, and uremia. Methods of therapy include hemodialysis, **continuous renal replacement therapy** (CRRT; discussed later), and various forms of peritoneal dialysis. The need for dialysis may be acute or chronic.

Acute dialysis is indicated when there is a high and rising level of serum potassium, fluid overload, or impending pulmonary edema, increasing acidosis, pericarditis, and severe confusion. It may also be used to remove certain medications or other toxins (poisoning or medication overdose) from the blood.

Chronic or maintenance dialysis is indicated in chronic renal failure, known as end-stage renal disease (ESRD), in the following instances: the occurrence of uremic signs and symptoms affecting all body systems (nausea and vomiting, severe anorexia, increasing lethargy, mental confusion), hyperkalemia, fluid overload not responsive to diuretics and fluid restriction, and a general lack of well-being. In addition, a pericardial friction rub is an urgent indication for dialysis in patients with chronic renal failure.

Patients with no renal function have been maintained for a number of years by dialysis. Successful kidney transplantation eliminates the need for dialysis. Although the costs of dialysis are usually reimbursable, limitations on the patient's ability to work resulting from illness and dialysis usually impose a great financial burden on patients and families.

The decision to initiate dialysis is one that should be reached after thoughtful discussion among the patient, family, physician, and others as appropriate. Overwhelming issues are associated with the need for dialysis and often require drastic changes in lifestyle. The nurse can assist the patient and family by answering their questions, clarifying information, and supporting their decision.

Hemodialysis

Hemodialysis is the most commonly used method of dialysis. More than 120,000 patients currently receive therapy in the United States (Roberts et al., 1996). It is used for patients who are acutely ill and require short-term dialysis (days to weeks) and for patients with ESRD who require long-term or permanent therapy. A dialyzer or artificial kidney serves as a synthetic, semipermeable membrane, replacing the renal glomeruli and tubules as the filter for the impaired kidneys.

For patients with chronic renal failure, hemodialysis prevents death, although it does not cure renal disease and does not compensate for loss of the kidneys' endocrine or metabolic activities. Patients receiving hemodialysis must undergo treatment for the rest of their lives (usually three times a week for at least 3 to 4 hours per treatment) or until they undergo successful kidney transplantation. Patients are placed on chronic dialysis when they require dialysis therapy for survival and for control of uremic symptoms. The trend in managing ESRD is to initiate treatment before the signs and symptoms associated with uremia become severe.

Principles Underlying Hemodialysis

The objectives of hemodialysis are to extract toxic nitrogenous substances from the blood and to remove excess water. In hemodialysis, the blood, laden with toxins and nitrogenous wastes, is diverted from the patient to a machine, a dialyzer, in which the blood is cleansed and then returned to the patient.

Diffusion, osmosis, and ultrafiltration are the processes at work in hemodialysis. The toxins and wastes in the blood are removed by **diffusion**; that is, they move from an area of greater concentration in the blood to an area of lesser concentration in the dialysate. The **dialysate** is a solution composed of all the important electrolytes in their ideal extracellular concentrations. The electrolyte level in the blood can be brought under control by properly adjusting the dialysate bath. The semipermeable membrane impedes the diffusion of large molecules, such as red blood cells and proteins.

Excess water is removed from the blood by **osmosis**, in which water moves from an area of higher solute concentration (blood) to lower solute concentration (the dialysate bath). **Ultrafiltration** is defined as water moving under high pressure to an area of lower pressure. This process is much more efficient at water removal than is osmosis. Ultrafiltration is accomplished by applying negative pressure or a suctioning force to the dialysis membrane. Because patients with renal disease usually cannot excrete water, this force is necessary to remove fluid to achieve fluid balance.

The body's buffer system is maintained using a dialysate bath composed of bicarbonate (most common) or acetate, which is metabolized to form bicarbonate. The anticoagulant heparin is administered to keep blood from clotting in the dialysis circuit. Cleansed blood is returned to the body. By the end of the dialysis treatment, many waste products have been removed, electrolyte balance has been restored toward normal, and the buffer system has been replenished.

Equipment: Dialyzers

Most **dialyzers**, or artificial kidneys, are either flat-plate dialyzers or hollow-fiber artificial kidneys that contain thousands of tiny cellophane tubules that act as semipermeable membranes. The blood flows through the tubules while a solution, the dialysate, circulates around the tubules. The exchange of wastes from the blood to the dialysate occurs through the semipermeable membrane of the tubules (Fig. 40-4).

Dialyzers have undergone changes in technology. As stated earlier, most dialyzers are either flat-plate dialyzers or hollow-fiber dialyzers. The difference lies in performance and biocompatibility. Biocompatibility refers to the ability of the dialyzer to accomplish its objectives without causing hypersensitive, allergic,

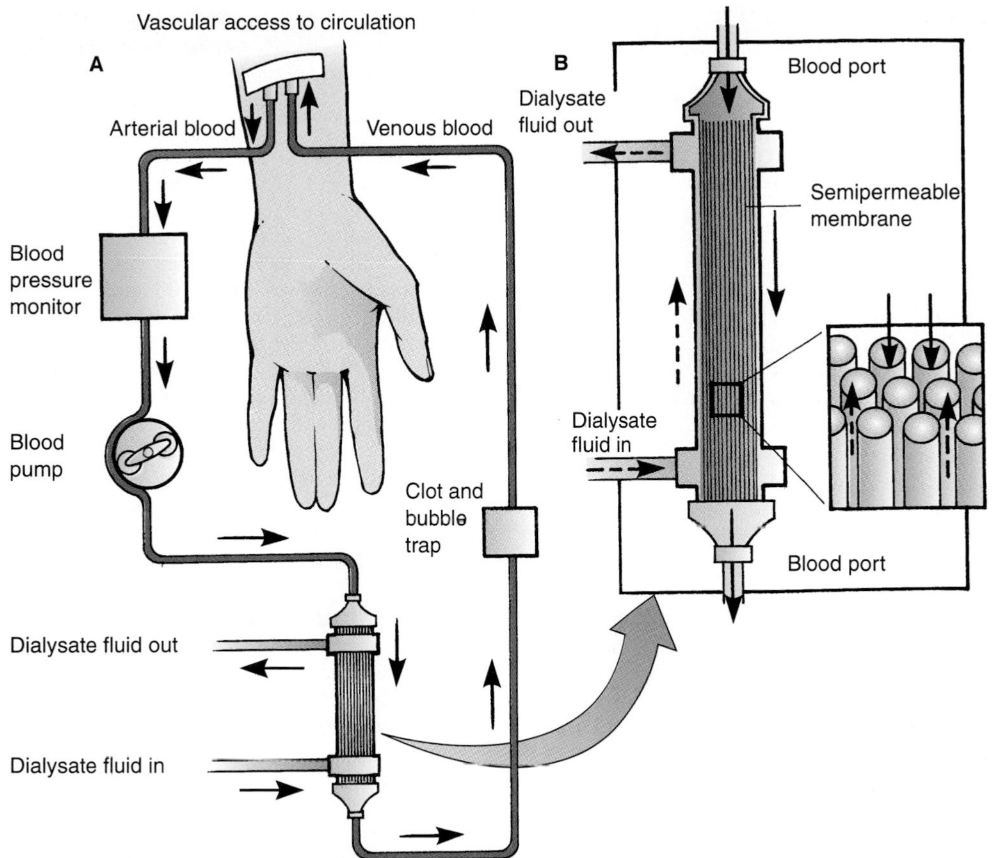

FIGURE 40•4 Hemodialysis system. (**A**) Blood from an artery is pumped into (**B**) a dialyzer where it flows through the cellophane tubes, which act as the semipermeable membrane (*inset*). The dialysate, which has the same chemical composition as the blood except for urea and waste products, flows in around the tubules. The waste products in the blood diffuse through the semipermeable membrane into the dialysate.

or adverse reactions. Some dialyzers remove middle-weight molecules at a faster rate and ultrafiltrate at higher rates. This is thought to reduce neuropathy of the lower extremities, a complication of long-term hemodialysis. In general, the more efficient the dialyzer, the higher the cost.

Another technologic advance is high-flux dialysis, which uses newer, highly permeable membranes that increase the clearance of low- and mid-molecular-weight molecules. These special membranes are used with higher than traditional rates of flow for the blood entering and exiting the dialyzer (500 to 800 mL/min). High-flux dialysis requires the use of precise volumetric ultrafiltration control systems, and not every dialysis unit has the capability of performing this type of dialysis. High-flux dialysis increases the efficiency of treatments while shortening their duration and reducing the need for heparin.

Vascular Access

Blood can be removed, cleaned, and returned to the body at rates between 200 and 800 mL/min; first, however, access to the patient's circulation must be established. Several kinds of access are available.

SUBCLAVIAN, INTERNAL JUGULAR, AND FEMORAL CATHETERS

Immediate access to the patient's circulation for acute hemodialysis is achieved by inserting a double-lumen or multilumen catheter into the subclavian, internal jugular, or femoral vein. Although this method of vascular access is not without risks (eg, hematoma, pneumothorax, infection, thrombosis of the subclavian vein, inadequate flow), it can often be used for several weeks. The catheters are removed when no longer needed because the patient's condition has improved or another type of access has been established. Double-lumen, cuffed catheters may also be surgically inserted into the subclavian vein of patients requiring a central venous catheter for dialysis over a longer term (Fig. 40-5).

FISTULA

A more permanent access, known as a **fistula**, is created surgically (usually in the forearm) by joining (anastomosis) an artery to a vein, either side to side or end to side (Fig. 40-6). Needles are inserted into the vessel to obtain blood flow adequate to pass through the dialyzer. The arterial segment of the fistula is used for arterial flow and the venous segment for reinfusion of the dialyzed blood. The fistula takes 4 to 6 weeks to mature before it is ready for use. This gives time for healing and for the venous segment of the fistula to dilate to accommodate two large-bore (14- or 16-gauge) needles. The patient is encouraged to perform exercises to increase the size of these vessels (ie, squeezing a rubber ball for forearm fistulas) and thereby accommodate the large-bore needles used in hemodialysis.

GRAFT

An **arteriovenous graft** can be created by subcutaneously interposing a biologic, semibiologic, or synthetic graft material be-

NURSING RESEARCH

Vascular Access in Older Hemodialysis Patients

Culp, K., Taylor, L., & Hulme, P.A. (1996). Geriatric hemodialysis patients: A comparative study of vascular access. *American Association of Nephrology Nurses Journal, 23*(6), 583–592.

Purpose

Elderly adults constitute the fastest growing age group in the population with end-stage renal disease (ESRD). Vascular access in this population is crucial in the successful hemodialysis treatment of chronic renal failure. Although access problems are more common in the elderly, no previous study examined the problems specific to vascular access in the elderly.

Study Sample and Design

This study compared vascular access in 136 hemodialysis patients aged 65 years or older with 131 hemodialysis patients younger than age 65 years.

Patients were recruited from 26 of 46 randomly selected dialysis facilities in a network of dialysis centers in four Midwestern states.

On initiation of the first hemodialysis treatment, patients were entered in the study and followed for 1 year. Type and location of the access, date of its surgical placement, date of first cannulation of the access for treatment, and a short summary of the hemodialysis prescription and laboratory values were recorded. At the end of the first year, data were summarized; access failure, diagnostic or therapeutic procedures performed during the year on the vascular access, and occurrence of other problems with the access were recorded and analyzed.

Findings

Younger patients (under 65 years of age) received more arteriovenous fistulas (AVFs) than those aged 65 years and older, who received more arteriovenous grafts (polytetrafluorethylene, or PTFE). The researchers suggested that increased use of PTFE grafts in the older group was due to the higher incidence of peripheral vascular disease in this age group. Patients who were 65 years of age or older with a PTFE graft experienced a higher rate of venous access thrombosis (VAT) than those in the same age group with an AVF. The use of oral anticoagulants did not reduce the risk of VAT for the age 65 years or older group but did so in the group younger than age 65 years. The researchers suggested that the effectiveness of oral anticoagulants in reducing risk of VAT may be related to the type of access rather than the age of the patient and this finding may be due to the greater number of older patients with a PTFE graft than younger patients.

Nursing Implications

The results of this study will assist nurses working with older hemodialysis patients when assessing and monitoring the vascular access. Early detection of VAT is essential so that nonsurgical methods may be used to maintain patency of the vascular access. Measures to ensure patency of the access, such as vigilance in monitoring blood pressures and rotating needle puncture sites, are essential components of care. Given the growing number of elderly patients on hemodialysis, the nurse must be alert to the unique problems of this patient population and their vascular access.

tween an artery and vein (see Fig. 40-6*B*). The most commonly used synthetic graft material is expanded polytetrafluoroethylene. Usually, a graft is created when the patient's own vessels are not suitable for a fistula. Patients with compromised vascular systems (eg, from diabetes) often need to have a graft to undergo hemodialysis. Grafts are usually placed in the forearm, upper arm, or upper thigh. Infection and thrombosis are the most common complications of arteriovenous grafts.

Nursing Alert *Failure of the permanent dialysis access (fistula or graft) accounts for most hospital admissions of patients undergoing long-term hemodialysis, making protection of the access a priority.*

Complications of Hemodialysis

Although hemodialysis can prolong life indefinitely, it does not alter the natural course of the underlying kidney disease, nor does it completely replace kidney function. The patient is subject to a number of problems and complications. One leading cause of death among patients undergoing chronic hemodialysis is atherosclerotic cardiovascular disease. Disturbances of lipid metabolism (hypertriglyceridemia) appear to be accentuated by hemodialysis. Congestive heart failure, coronary heart disease and anginal pain, stroke, and peripheral vascular insufficiency may occur and may incapacitate the patient. Anemia and fatigue contribute to diminished physical and emotional well-being, lack of energy and drive, and loss of interest. Gastric ulcers and other gastrointestinal problems occur from the physiologic stress of chronic illness, medication, and related problems. Disturbed calcium metabolism leads to renal osteodystrophy that produces bone pain and fractures. Other problems include fluid overload associated with congestive heart failure, malnutrition, infection, neuropathy, and pruritus.

Complications of dialysis treatment may include the following:

- Hypotension may occur during the treatment as fluid is removed. Nausea and vomiting, diaphoresis, tachycardia, and dizziness are common signs of hypotension.
- Painful muscle cramping occurs, usually late in dialysis as fluid and electrolytes rapidly leave the extracellular space.
- Exsanguination may occur if blood lines separate or dialysis needles accidentally dislodge.
- Dysrhythmias may result from electrolyte and pH changes or from removal of antiarrhythmic medications during dialysis.
- Air embolism is rare but can occur if air enters the patient's vascular system.
- Chest pain may occur because of anemia or in patients with arteriosclerotic heart disease.
- Dialysis disequilibrium results from cerebral fluid shifts. Manifestations include headache, nausea and vomiting, restlessness, decreased level of consciousness, or seizures; it is more likely to occur in acute renal failure or when blood urea nitrogen levels are very high (exceeding 150 mg/dL).

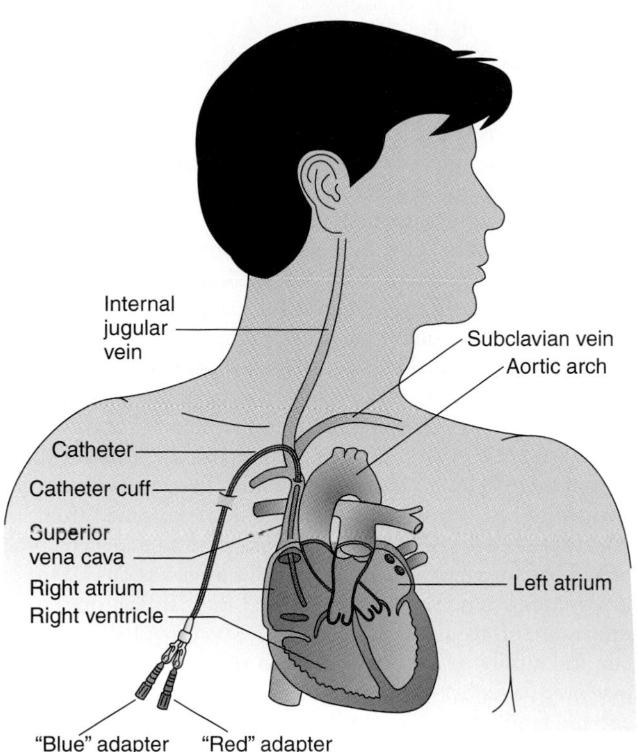

FIGURE 40•5 Double-lumen, cuffed hemodialysis catheter used in acute hemodialysis. The red adapter is attached to a blood line through which blood is pumped from the patient. After the blood passes through the dialyzer (artificial kidney), it returns to the patient through the blue adapter.

Long-Term Management

During dialysis, the patient, the dialyzer, and the dialysate bath require constant monitoring to detect the numerous potential complications, such as air embolism, inadequate or excessive ultrafiltration (hypotension, cramping, vomiting), blood leaks, contamination, and access complications. The nurse in the dialysis unit has an important role in monitoring, supporting, assessing, and educating the patient. Nursing care of the patient and maintenance of the access device are discussed under care of the hospitalized dialysis patient.

Pharmacologic Therapy

Just as many medications normally are excreted wholly or in part by the kidneys, many medications are excreted during hemodialysis. Patients who are on hemodialysis and who require medications (eg, cardiac glycosides, antibiotics, antiarrhythmic agents, antihypertensive agents) are monitored closely to ensure that blood and tissue levels of these medications are maintained without toxic accumulation.

Because some medications are removed from the blood during dialysis, the physician may need to adjust the dosage. Medications that are bound to protein are not removed during dialysis. Removal of other medication metabolites depends on the weight and size of the molecule.

All medications and their dosages must be evaluated carefully in patients receiving dialysis. Antihypertensive therapy, often part of the dialysis patient's regimen, is one example in which communication, teaching, and evaluation can make a difference in patient outcomes. The patient must know when to take and when not to take the medication. For example, if antihypertensive medications are taken on a dialysis day, a hypotensive effect may occur during dialysis, causing dangerously low blood pressure. Many medications that are taken once daily can be held until after the dialysis treatment.

Nutritional and Fluid Therapy

When damaged kidneys are unable to excrete end products of metabolism, these substances accumulate in the patient's serum as toxins. The resulting symptoms, collectively known as uremic symptoms, affect every body system. The more toxins that accumulate, the more severe the symptoms.

Diet is an important factor for patients on hemodialysis because of the effects of uremia. Goals of nutritional therapy are to minimize uremic symptoms and fluid and electrolyte imbalances; to maintain good nutritional status through adequate protein, calories, vitamin, and mineral intake; and to enable the patient to eat a palatable and enjoyable diet. Restricting dietary protein decreases the accumulation of nitrogenous wastes, reduces uremic symptoms, and may even postpone the initiation of dialysis for a few months. Restriction of fluid is also part of the dietary prescription because fluid accumulation may occur, leading to weight gain, congestive heart failure, and pulmonary edema.

With the initiation of hemodialysis, the patient's dietary intake can be improved but usually still requires some restriction of protein, sodium, potassium, and fluid intake. Protein intake is restricted to about 1 g/kg ideal body weight per day; therefore, protein must be of high biologic quality and composed of the essential amino acids to prevent poor protein use and to maintain a positive nitrogen balance. Examples of foods high in biologic protein content include eggs, meat, milk, poultry, and fish. The usual sodium restriction is 2 to 3 g/day while fluids are restricted to an amount equal to the urine output plus 500 mL/day. The goal for hemodialysis patients is to keep their interdialytic (between dialysis treatments) weight gain under 1.5 kg. The degree of potassium restriction (average, 1.5 to 2.5 g/day) depends

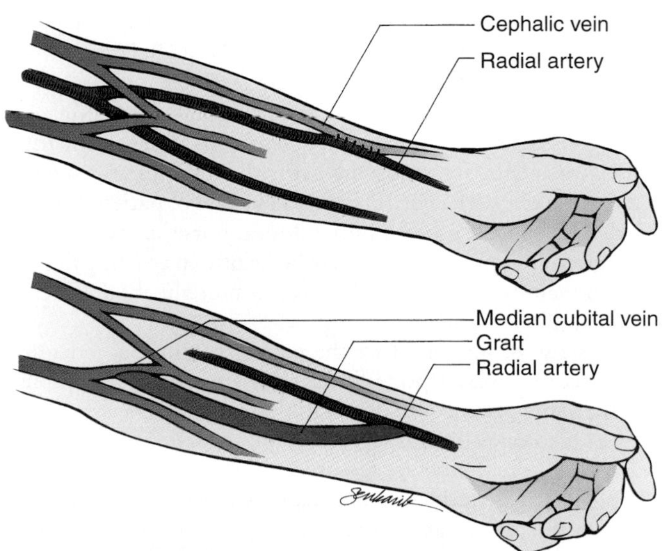

FIGURE 40•6 An internal arteriovenous fistula (*top*) is created by a side-to-side anastomosis of the artery and vein. A graft (*bottom*) can also be established between the artery and vein.

on the amount of residual renal function and the frequency of dialysis.

The dietary restriction is a disturbing and unwelcome change in lifestyle for many patients with chronic renal failure. Patients often feel stigmatized in social situations because there may be few food selections available for their diet. If the restrictions are ignored, life-threatening complications, such as hyperkalemia and pulmonary edema, may result. Thus, the patient may feel punished for responding to basic human drives to eat and drink. The nurse who encounters a patient with symptoms or complications resulting from dietary indiscretion must avoid speaking to the patient in harsh, judgmental, or punitive tones.

Nursing Management

Patients requiring long-term hemodialysis are often concerned about the unpredictability of the illness and the disruption of their lives. They often have financial problems, difficulty holding a job, waning sexual desire and impotence, depression from being chronically ill, and fear of dying. Younger patients worry about marriage, having children, and the burden that they bring to their families. A regimented lifestyle necessitated by the frequent dialysis treatments and restrictions in food and fluid intake is often demoralizing to the patient and family.

MEETING PSYCHOSOCIAL NEEDS

Dialysis alters the lifestyle of the patient and family. The amount of time required for dialysis and physician visits and being chronically ill can create conflict, frustration, guilt, and depression. It may be difficult for the patient, spouse, and family to express anger and negative feelings.

The nurse needs to give the patient and family the opportunity to express any feelings of anger and concern over the limitations imposed by the disease and treatment as well as possible financial problems and job insecurity. If anger is not expressed, it may be directed inward and lead to depression, despair, and attempts at suicide (the incidence of suicide is increased in dialysis patients); although if the anger is projected outward to other people, it may destroy already threatened family relationships.

Although normal in this situation, these feelings are often profound and overwhelming. Counseling and psychotherapy may be necessary. Depression may require treatment with antidepressive agents. Referring the patient and family to a mental health provider with specific expertise in care of patients receiving dialysis may also be helpful. Clinical nurse specialists, psychologists, and social workers may be helpful in assisting the patient and family to deal with the changes brought about by renal failure and its treatment.

The sense of loss faced by the patient cannot be underestimated because every aspect of what once was a normal life is disrupted. Some patients use denial to deal with the overwhelming array of medical problems (eg, infections, hypertension, anemia, neuropathy). Staff who are tempted to label the patient as noncompliant must consider the impact of renal failure and its treatment on the patient and family and coping strategies that they may use. The nurse assists the patient to identify effective and safe coping strategies to deal with these ever-present problems and fears.

PROMOTING HOME AND COMMUNITY-BASED CARE

Teaching Patients Self-Care. The task of preparing a patient for hemodialysis is challenging. Often the patient does not fully comprehend the impact of dialysis, and learning needs may go unrecognized. Good communication between the dialysis staff (in the hospital and outpatient clinic), unit staff, and home care nurses is essential for providing sound, continuous care.

Assessment is conducted to identify the learning needs of the patient and family members. In many cases, the patient is home before learning needs and readiness to learn can be thoroughly evaluated; therefore, hospital-based nurses, dialysis staff, and home care nurses must work together to provide appropriate teaching that meets the patient's and family's changing needs and readiness to learn.

The diagnosis of chronic renal failure and the need for dialysis often overwhelm the patient and family. In addition, many patients with ESRD have depressed mentation, shortened attention span, decreased level of concentration, and altered perceptual states. Therefore, teaching must occur in brief sessions (10 to 15 minutes), and time should be provided for clarification, repetition, and reinforcement. Time must also be provided for the patient and family to ask questions and receive clarification. The nurse needs to convey a nonjudgmental attitude to enable the patient and family to discuss options and their feelings about those options. Team conferences are helpful for sharing information and providing every team member the opportunity to discuss the needs of the patient and family.

Teaching Patients About Hemodialysis. Although most patients who require hemodialysis undergo the procedure in an outpatient satellite setting, home hemodialysis is an option for some. Home hemodialysis requires a highly motivated patient who is willing to take responsibility for the procedure and is able to adjust each treatment to meet the body's changing needs. It also requires the commitment and cooperation of a partner to assist the patient. Often, the patient is not comfortable consuming the time of another and does not wish to subject family members to the feeling that their home is being turned into a clinic.

The decision to use home hemodialysis should never be forced on the patient by the health care team. This endeavor requires many significant changes in the home and family. Whether to perform home hemodialysis must be the patient's and family's decision.

The patient undergoing home hemodialysis and the caregiver who will assist must be trained to prepare, operate, and disassemble the dialysis machine; maintain and clean the equipment; administer medications (eg, heparin) into the machine lines; and handle emergency problems (hemodialysis dialyzer rupture, electrical or mechanical problems, hypotension, shock, and seizures). Because home hemodialysis places primary responsibility for the treatment on the patient and the assistant, it is essential that they understand and can competently perform all aspects of the hemodialysis procedure.

Before initiating home hemodialysis, an extensive assessment is made to evaluate the home environment, household and community resources, and the ability and willingness of the patient and family to carry out this treatment. The home is surveyed to see if electrical outlets, plumbing facilities, and storage space are adequate. Modifications may be needed to enable the patient and assistant to perform dialysis safely and to deal with unexpected emergencies.

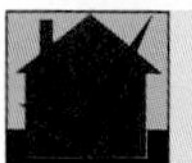

HOME CARE TEACHING CHECKLIST: HEMODIALYSIS

At the completion of the program, the patient or caregiver will be able to:	Patient	Caregiver
• Discuss renal failure and its effects on the body.	✔	✔
• Describe the cause of renal failure and why hemodialysis is necessary.	✔	✔
• Describe the basic principles of hemodialysis.	✔	✔
• Discuss common problems that may occur during hemodialysis and their prevention and management.	✔	✔
• Demonstrate knowledge about what medications are prescribed and the reason for their use, potential side effects, guidelines on when to notify physician, and the schedule of medications on dialysis and nondialysis days.	✔	✔
• Acknowledge dietary and fluid restrictions, rationale, and consequences of noncompliance.	✔	✔
• Describe commonly measured laboratory values, results, and implications.	✔	✔
• List guidelines for prevention and detection of fluid overload, meaning of "dry" weight, and how to weigh self.	✔	✔
• Demonstrate circulatory access care, how to check patency, signs and symptoms of infection, prevention of complications.	✔	✔
• Discuss strategies for detection, management, and relief of pruritus, neuropathy, and other complications of renal failure.	✔	✔
• Develop strategies to manage or reduce anxiety and maintain independence.	✔	✔
• Coordinate financial arrangements for dialysis and strategies to identify and obtain resources.	✔	✔

Periodic visits by the home care nurse are essential once home dialysis is initiated to evaluate the adherence of the patient and assistant to recommended techniques, to assess for complications, to reinforce previous teaching, and to provide reassurance.

Continuing Care. Like the Life Options Rehabilitation Advisory Council, an interdisciplinary group that focuses on the rehabilitation of renal patients, the health care team's goal for patients with chronic renal failure is to maximize their vocational potential, functional status, and quality of life. To facilitate renal rehabilitation, appropriate follow-up and monitoring by members of the health care team (physicians, dialysis nurses, social workers, psychologist, home care nurses, and others as appropriate) are essential to identify problems early so that prompt attention can be provided. Many patients with chronic renal failure can resume relatively normal lives, doing the things that are important to them: traveling, exercising, working, or actively participating in family activities. If appropriate interventions are available early in the course of dialysis, the potential for better health improves, and the patient can remain active in family and community life. Chart 40-2 outlines the essential elements identified by the Life Options Advisory Council for the rehabilitation of dialysis patients. Outcome goals for renal rehabilitation include employment for those able to work; improved physical functioning of all patients; improved understanding about adaptation and options for living well; increased control over the effects of kidney disease and dialysis; and resumption of activities enjoyed before dialysis.

Continuous Renal Replacement Therapies

Several types of continuous renal replacement therapy (CRRT) are available and are widely used in critical care units. CRRT may be indicated for patients who have acute or chronic renal failure and who are too clinically unstable for conventional hemodialysis, for patients with fluid overload secondary to oliguric (low urinary output) renal failure, or for patients whose kidneys are unable to handle their acute high metabolic or nutritional needs. CRRT does not produce rapid fluid shifts, does not require dialysis machines or dialysis personnel to carry out the procedures, and can be initiated quickly in hospitals without dialysis facilities.

CRRTs have several similarities to hemodialysis, including the need for access to the patients' circulation and the need for blood to pass through an artificial filter. A hemofilter (an extremely porous blood filter containing a semipermeable membrane) is used in all methods of CRRT. Types of CRRT are described next.

Continuous Arteriovenous Hemofiltration

Continuous arteriovenous hemofiltration (CAVH) was first used in 1977 to treat fluid overload. Blood is circulated through a small-volume, low-resistance filter by the patient's own arterial pressure rather than that of the blood pump used in hemodialysis. Blood flows from an artery (usually by an arterial catheter in the femoral

CHART 40•2 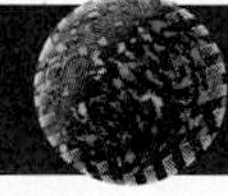 **The Five E's: Bridges to Renal Rehabilitation**

Encouragement: Patients, families, and staff need encouragement to adopt a positive attitude toward rehabilitation.

Education: Patients need to understand their disease. They need to learn strategies for successful adaptation to dialysis and how to maximize functional status, among many other subjects. Parents, staff, and employers require education about the many positive life options of dialysis patients.

Exercise: Exercise is critical to rehabilitation, just as with heart disease. Many levels of activity to fit the different abilities of renal patients are helpful, from vigorous workouts to stretching exercises.

Employment: The primary goal is to allow dialysis patients to keep their current jobs whenever possible. If not possible, vocational rehabilitation counseling should be used.

Evaluation: Systematic evaluation of rehabilitation outcomes is necessary to identify and measure which interventions have made an impact.

Adapted from Life Options Rehabilitation Advisory Council (1994). *Renal rehabilitation: Bridging the barriers.* Madison, WI: Medical Education Institute.

artery) to a hemofilter. A pressure gradient is necessary for optimal filtration; cannulation of the femoral artery and vein provides the necessary gradient (difference) in arterial and venous pressures. The filtered blood then returns to the patient's circulation through a venous catheter. Intravenous fluids may be administered to replace fluid removed by the procedure. With CAVH, there is no concentration gradient, so only filtration of fluid occurs. Electrolytes are eliminated only as they are pulled along and removed with the fluid. Ultrafiltrate is collected in a drainage bag, measured, and discarded. CAVH is usually set up and initiated by trained dialysis staff and then maintained and monitored by critical care personnel.

Continuous Arteriovenous Hemodialysis

Continuous arteriovenous hemodialysis (CAVHD) has many of the characteristics of CAVH but offers the advantage of a concentration gradient to facilitate faster clearance of urea. This is accomplished by the circulation of dialysate on one side of a semipermeable membrane. The blood flow through the system depends on the patient's arterial pressure, as in CAVH; a blood pump is not used as it is in standard hemodialysis. CAVHD is usually set up and initiated by trained dialysis staff and then maintained and monitored by critical care personnel.

Continuous Venovenous Hemofiltration

Continuous venovenous hemofiltration (CVVH) is increasingly being used in managing acute renal failure. Blood from a double-lumen venous catheter is pumped (using a small blood pump) through a hemofilter and then returned to the patient through the same catheter (Fig. 40-7). CVVH provides continuous slow fluid removal (ultrafiltration); therefore, hemodynamic effects are mild and better tolerated by unstable patients. CVVH has several other benefits over CAVH in that no arterial access is required and critical care nurses can set up the system, initiate, maintain, and terminate therapy.

Continuous Venovenous Hemodialysis

Continuous venovenous hemodialysis (CVVHD) is similar to CVVH. Blood is pumped from a double-lumen venous catheter through a hemofilter and returned to the patient through the same catheter. In addition to the benefits of ultrafiltration, CVVHD uses a concentration gradient to facilitate removal of uremic toxins. Therefore, no arterial access is required, hemodynamic effects are usually mild, and the system can be set up, initiated, maintained, and terminated by critical care nurses.

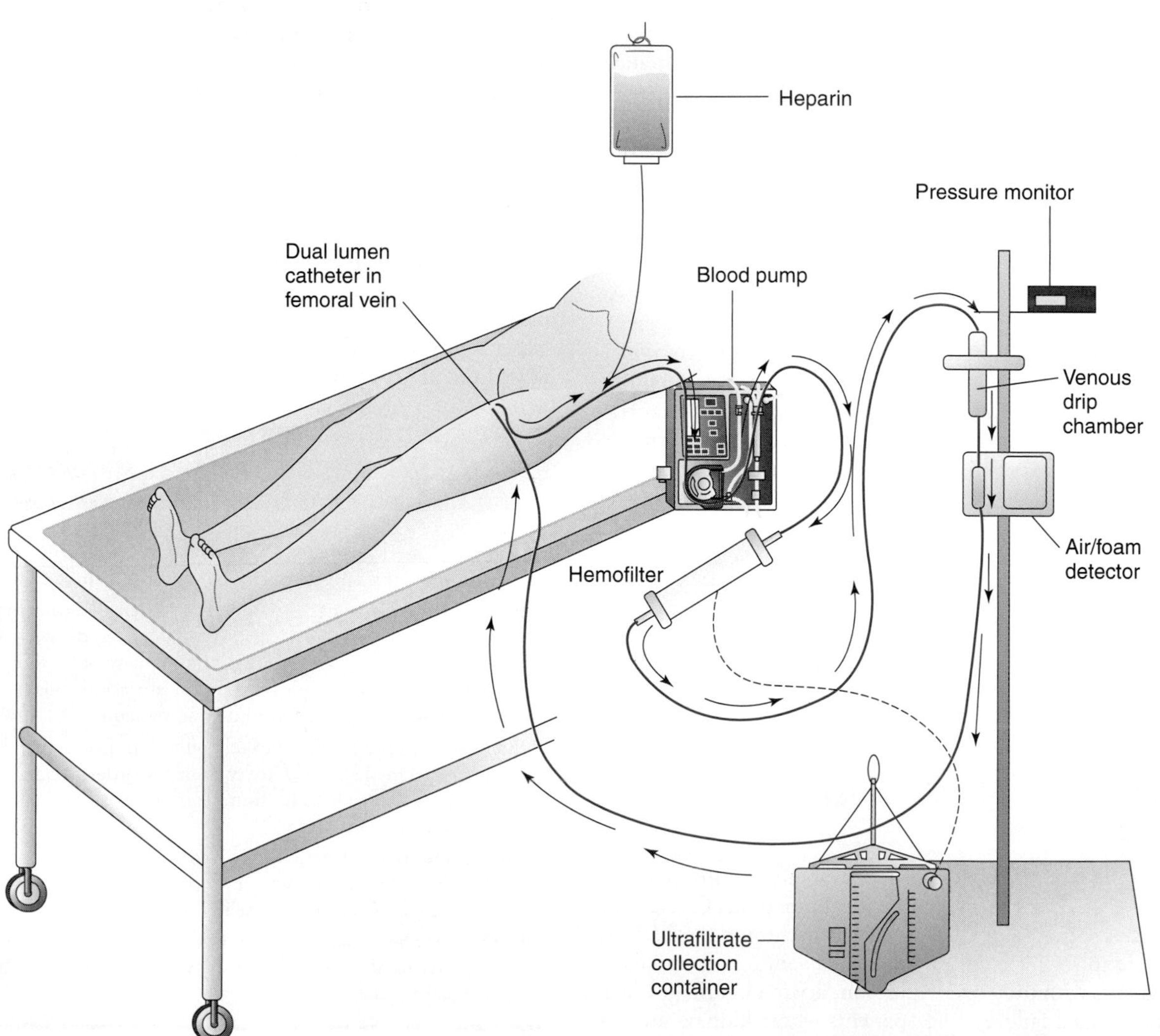

FIGURE 40•7 Continuous venovenous hemofiltration (CVVH) removes fluid (ultrafiltrate) slowly from the blood.

Peritoneal Dialysis

The goals of **peritoneal dialysis** are to remove toxic substances and metabolic wastes and to reestablish normal fluid and electrolyte balance. Peritoneal dialysis may be the treatment of choice for patients with renal failure who are unable or unwilling to undergo hemodialysis or renal transplantation. Patients who are susceptible to the rapid fluid, electrolyte, and metabolic changes that occur during hemodialysis experience fewer of these problems with the slower rate of peritoneal dialysis. Therefore, patients with diabetes or cardiovascular disease, many older patients, and those who may be at risk of side effects of systemic use of heparin would be likely candidates for peritoneal dialysis. Additionally, severe hypertension, congestive heart failure, and pulmonary edema not responsive to usual treatment regimens have been successfully treated with peritoneal dialysis.

Peritoneal dialysis can be performed using several different approaches: acute, intermittent peritoneal dialysis; **continuous ambulatory peritoneal dialysis** (CAPD), and **continuous cyclic peritoneal dialysis** (CCPD). These three methods are discussed in further detail in later sections of this chapter. As with other forms of treatment, the decision to begin peritoneal dialysis is made by the patient and family in consultation with the physician.

Principles Underlying Peritoneal Dialysis

In peritoneal dialysis, the peritoneum, a serous membrane that covers the abdominal organs and lines the abdominal wall, serves as the semipermeable membrane. The surface of the peritoneum constitutes body surface area of about 22,000 cm^2. An appropriate sterile dialysate is introduced into the peritoneal cavity through an abdominal catheter at intervals (Fig. 40-8). Urea and creatinine, metabolic end products normally excreted by the kidneys, are cleared from the blood by diffusion and osmosis as waste products move from an area of higher concentration (the peritoneal blood supply) to an area of lower concentration (the peritoneal cavity) across a semipermeable membrane (the peritoneal membrane). Urea is cleared at a rate of 15 to 20 mL/min, whereas creatinine is removed more slowly. It usually takes 36 to 48 hours to achieve with peritoneal dialysis what hemodialysis accomplishes in 6 to 8 hours. Ultrafiltration (water removal) occurs in peritoneal dialysis through an osmotic gradient created by adding dextrose to the dialysate.

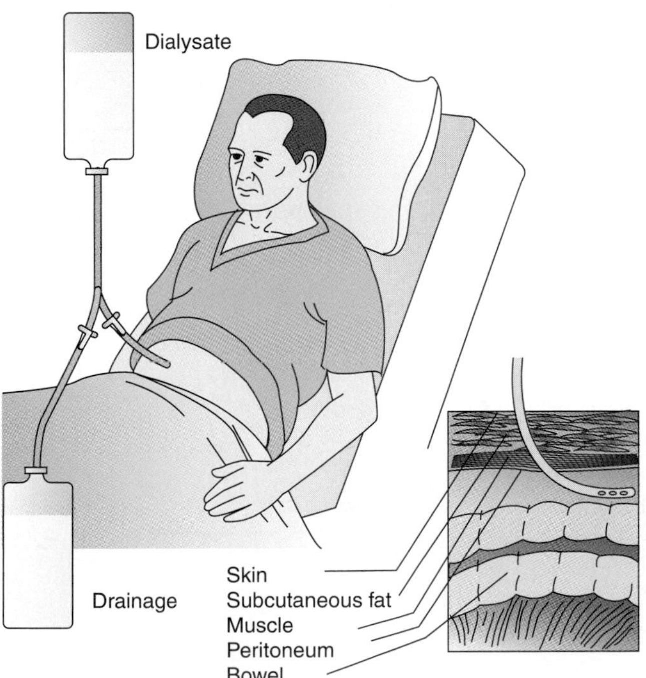

FIGURE 40•8 In peritoneal dialysis and in acute intermittent peritoneal dialysis, dialysate is infused into the peritoneal cavity by gravity, after which the clamp on the infusion line is closed. After a dwell time (when the dialysate is in the peritoneal cavity), the drainage tube is unclamped and the fluid drains from the peritoneal cavity, again by gravity. A new container of dialysate is infused as soon as drainage is complete. The duration of the dwell time depends on the type of peritoneal dialysis.

Peritoneal Dialysis Procedure

The patient about to undergo peritoneal dialysis may be acutely ill, thus requiring short-term treatment to correct severe disturbances in fluid and electrolyte status, or may be a patient with chronic renal failure who will receive ongoing treatments.

PREPARATION OF THE PATIENT

The nurse's preparation of the patient and family for peritoneal dialysis is dependent on the patient's physical and psychological status, level of alertness, previous experience with dialysis, and understanding of and familiarity with the procedure.

The nurse explains the procedure to the patient and obtains signed consent for the procedure. Baseline vital signs, weight, and serum electrolyte levels are recorded. The patient is encouraged to empty the bladder and bowel to reduce the risk of puncturing internal organs. The nurse also assesses the patient's anxiety about the procedure and provides support and instruction. Broad-spectrum antibiotics may be administered to prevent infection. If the peritoneal catheter will be inserted in the operating room, this is explained to the patient and family.

PREPARATION OF THE EQUIPMENT

In addition to assembling the equipment for peritoneal dialysis, the nurse consults with the physician to determine the concentration of dialysate to be used and the medications to be added to it. Heparin may be added to prevent blood clotting and resultant occlusion of the peritoneal catheter. Potassium chloride may be prescribed to prevent hypokalemia. Antibiotics may be added to treat peritonitis. Insulin may be added for diabetic patients; a larger than normal dose may be needed, however, because about 10% of the insulin binds to the dialysate container. All medications are added immediately before the solution is instilled. Aseptic technique is crucial.

Before medications are added, the dialysate is warmed to body temperature to prevent patient discomfort and abdominal pain and to dilate the vessels of the peritoneum to increase urea clearance. Solutions that are too cold cause pain and vasoconstriction and reduce clearance. Solutions that are too hot burn the peritoneum. Dry heating is recommended (heating cabinet, incubator, or heating pad). Although it does not change the pH or chemistry of the dialysate, microwave heating should be used with caution because it causes hot spots in the solution bag, especially in the medication port. Mixing the solution after microwave heating helps to distribute the heated solution evenly.

Immediately before initiating dialysis, the nurse assembles the administration set and tubing. The tubing is filled with the prepared dialysate to reduce the amount of air entering the catheter and peritoneal cavity, which could increase abdominal discomfort and interfere with instillation and drainage of the fluid.

INSERTION OF THE CATHETER

Ideally, the peritoneal catheter is inserted in the operating room to maintain surgical asepsis and minimize risk of contamination. In some circumstances, however, the catheter is inserted by the physician at the patient's bedside under strict asepsis.

A rigid stylet catheter is inserted for acute peritoneal dialysis use only. Before the procedure, the skin is prepared with a local antiseptic to reduce skin bacteria and the risk of contamination and infection. The physician anesthetizes the site with a local anesthetic before making a small incision or stab wound in the lower abdomen, 3 to 5 cm below the umbilicus. Because this area is relatively free of large blood vessels, little bleeding occurs. A trocar is used to puncture the peritoneum as the patient tightens the abdominal muscles by raising his or her head. The catheter is threaded through the trocar and positioned. Previously prepared dialysate is infused into the peritoneal cavity, pushing the omentum (peritoneal lining extending from the abdominal organs) away from the catheter. The physician may then secure the catheter with a pursestring suture and apply antibacterial ointment and a sterile dressing over the site.

Catheters for long-term use (Tenckhoff, Swan, Cruz) are usually made of silicone and are radiopaque to permit visualization on x-ray. These catheters have three sections: (1) an intraperitoneal section, with numerous openings and an open tip to let dialysate flow freely; (2) a subcutaneous section that passes from the peritoneal membrane and tunnels through muscle and subcutaneous fat to the skin; and (3) an external section for connection to the dialysate system. Most of these catheters have two cuffs composed of Dacron polyester. The cuffs stabilize the catheter, limit movement, prevent leaks, and provide a barrier against microorganisms. One cuff is placed just distal to the peritoneum, and the other cuff is placed subcutaneously. The subcutaneous tunnel (5 to 10 cm long) further protects against bacterial infection (Fig. 40 9).

PERFORMING THE EXCHANGE

Peritoneal dialysis involves a series of exchanges or cycles. An exchange is defined as the infusion, dwell, and drainage of the dialysate. This cycle is repeated throughout the course of the dialysis. The dialysate is infused by gravity into the peritoneal cavity. About 5 to 10 minutes are usually required to infuse 2 L of fluid. The prescribed dwell, or equilibration, time allows diffusion and osmosis to occur. Diffusion of small molecules, such as urea and creatinine, occurs maximally in the first 5 to 10 minutes of the dwell time. At the end of the dwell time, the drain portion of the exchange begins. The tube is unclamped, and the solution drains from the peritoneal cavity by gravity through a closed system. Drainage is usually completed in 10 to 30 minutes. The drainage fluid is normally colorless or straw-colored and should not be cloudy. Bloody drainage may be seen in the first few exchanges after insertion of a new catheter but should not occur after that time. The entire exchange (infusion, dwell time, and drainage) takes from 1 to 4 hours depending on the prescribed dwell time. The number of cycles or exchanges and their frequency are prescribed based on the patient's physical status and acuity of illness.

The removal of excess water during peritoneal dialysis is achieved by using a hypertonic dialysate with a high dextrose

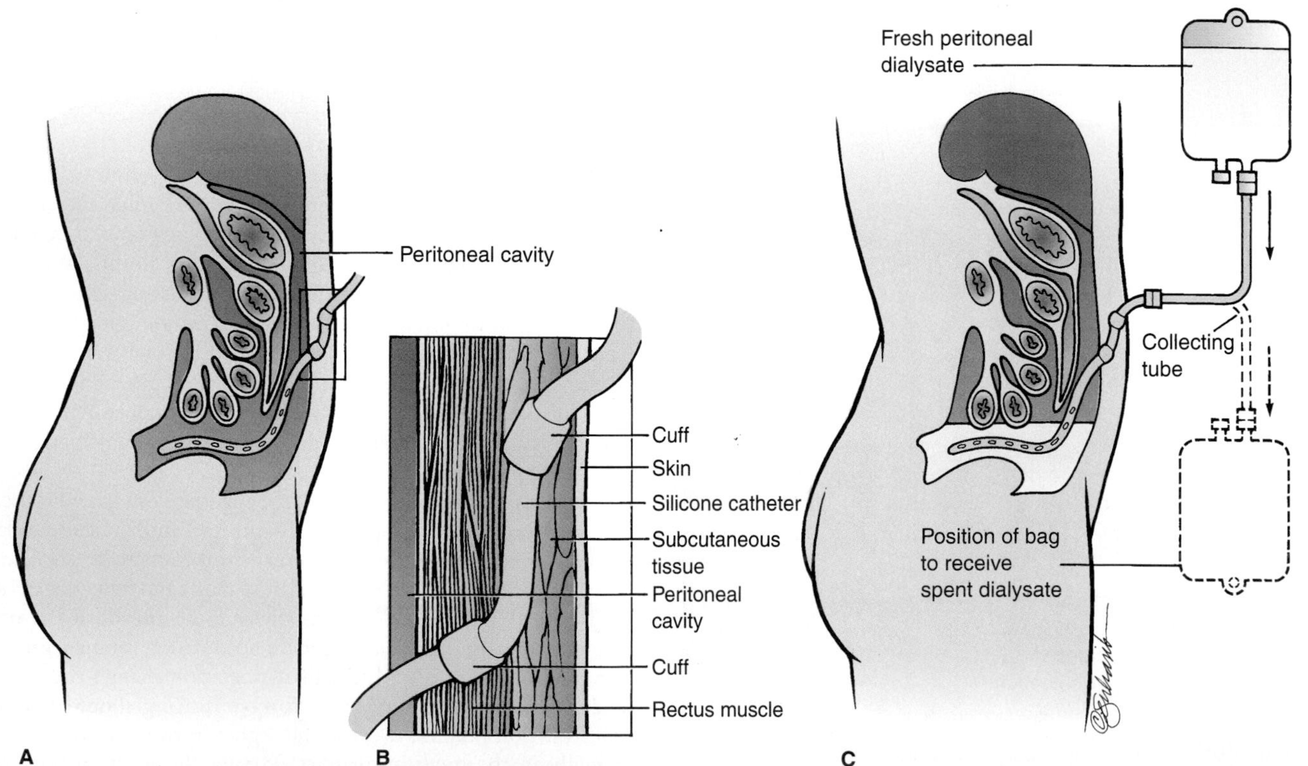

FIGURE 40•9 Continuous ambulatory peritoneal dialysis. (**A**) The peritoneal catheter is implanted through the abdominal wall. (**B**) Dacron cuffs and a subcutaneous tunnel provide protection against bacterial infection. (**C**) Dialysate flows by gravity into the peritoneal catheter and then into the peritoneal cavity. The fluid drains by gravity and is then discarded. Additional solution is then infused into the peritoneal cavity until the next drainage period. Dialysis thus continues on a 24-hour-a-day basis during which the patient is free to move around and engage in his or her usual activities.

concentration that creates an osmotic gradient. Dextrose solutions of 1.5%, 2.5%, and 4.25% are available in several volumes, from 500 mL to 3000 mL, allowing the dialysate selection to fit the patient's tolerance, size, and physiologic needs. The higher the dextrose concentration, the greater the osmotic gradient and the more water removed. Selection of the appropriate solution is based on the patient's fluid status.

Complications of Peritoneal Dialysis

Peritoneal dialysis is not without complications. Most are minor, but several, if unattended, can have serious consequences.

PERITONITIS

Peritonitis (inflammation of the peritoneum), the most common and most serious complication, occurs in 60% to 80% of patients on long-term peritoneal dialysis. The average peritonitis rate in long-term therapy is now less than one episode per patient per year. Most peritonitis episodes result from contamination caused by *Staphylococcus epidermidis.* These episodes result in mild symptoms and have a good prognosis. Peritonitis caused by *Staphylococcus aureus*, however, has a higher morbidity rate, has a more serious prognosis, and runs a longer course. Gram-negative organisms may originate in the bowel, particularly when there is more than one organism in the peritoneal fluid and when the organisms are anaerobic.

Peritonitis is characterized by cloudy dialysate drainage, diffuse abdominal pain, and rebound tenderness. Hypotension and other signs of shock may occur if *S. aureus* is the responsible organism.

The patient with peritonitis may be treated as an inpatient or outpatient (most common), depending on the severity of the infection and the patient's clinical status. Initially, one to three rapid exchanges with a 1.5% dextrose solution without added medications are completed to wash out mediators of inflammation and to reduce abdominal pain. Drainage fluid is examined for cell count, and Gram's stain and culture are used to identify the organism and guide treatment. Antibiotics (aminoglycosides or cephalosporins) are usually added to subsequent exchanges until the Gram's stain or culture results are available for appropriate antibiotic determination. Intraperitoneal administration of antibiotics is as effective as intravenous administration. Heparin (500 to 1000 U/L) may also be added to the dialysate to prevent fibrin clot formation. Antibiotic therapy continues for 10 to 14 days. Careful calculation of the antibiotic dosage helps prevent nephrotoxicity and further compromise of renal function.

Peritonitis that is unresolved after 4 days of appropriate therapy necessitates catheter removal. The patient is maintained on hemodialysis for about 1 month before a new catheter is inserted. In patients with fungal peritonitis, the peritoneal catheter should be removed if there is no response to therapy in 4 to 7 days. Tunnel infections and fecal peritonitis also mandate catheter removal. Systemic antibiotics should continue for 5 to 7 days after catheter removal.

Regardless of which organism causes peritonitis, the patient with peritonitis loses large amounts of protein through the peritoneum. Acute malnutrition and delayed healing may result. Therefore, attention must be given to detecting and promptly treating the infections.

LEAKAGE

Leakage of dialysate through the catheter site may occur immediately after the catheter is inserted. Usually, the leak stops spontaneously if dialysis is withheld for several days to give the incision and exit site time to heal. During this time, it is important to reduce factors that might delay healing, such as undue abdominal muscle activity and straining during bowel movement. Leakage through the exit site or into the abdominal wall can occur for months or years after catheter placement. In many cases, leakage can be avoided by using small volumes (100 to 200 mL) of dialysate, gradually increasing the volume up to 2000 mL.

BLEEDING

A bloody effluent (drainage) may be observed occasionally, especially in young, menstruating women. (The hypertonic fluid pulls blood from the uterus, through the opening in the fallopian tubes, and into the peritoneal cavity.) Bleeding is common during the first few exchanges after a new catheter insertion because some blood exists in the abdominal cavity from the procedure. In many cases, no cause can be found for the bleeding, although catheter displacement from the pelvis has been associated occasionally with bleeding. Some patients have had bloody effluent after an enema or from minor trauma. Invariably, bleeding stops after 1 or 2 days and requires no specific intervention. More frequent exchanges during this time may be necessary to prevent obstruction of the catheter by blood clots.

LONG-TERM COMPLICATIONS

Other complications that may occur with long-term peritoneal dialysis include abdominal hernias (incisional, inguinal, diaphragmatic, and umbilical), probably resulting from continuously increased intra-abdominal pressure. The persistently elevated intra-abdominal pressure also aggravates symptoms of hiatal hernia and of hemorrhoids.

Hypertriglyceridemia commonly affects patients undergoing long-term peritoneal dialysis, suggesting that this therapy may accelerate atherogenesis. Cardiovascular disease remains a major cause of death in this population of patients. Low back pain and anorexia from fluid in the abdomen and a constant sweet taste related to absorption of glucose may also occur.

Mechanical problems occasionally occur and may interfere with instillation or drainage of the dialysate. Formation of clots in the peritoneal catheter and constipation are factors that may contribute to these problems.

Acute Intermittent Peritoneal Dialysis

Indications for acute intermittent peritoneal dialysis, a variation of peritoneal dialysis, include uremic symptoms (nausea, vomiting, fatigue, altered mental status), fluid overload, acidosis, and hyperkalemia. Although peritoneal dialysis is not as efficient as hemodialysis in removing solute and fluid, it permits a more gradual change in the patient's fluid volume status and in waste product removal. Therefore, it may be the treatment of choice for the hemodynamically unstable patient. It can be carried out manually (the nurse warms, spikes, and hangs each container of dialysate) or by a cycler machine. Exchange times range from 30 minutes to 2 hours. A common routine is hourly exchanges consisting of a 10-minute infusion, a 30-minute dwell time, and a 20-minute drain time.

Maintaining the peritoneal dialysis cycle is a nursing responsibility. Strict aseptic technique is maintained when changing solution containers and emptying drainage containers. Vital signs, weight, intake and output, laboratory values, and patient status are monitored frequently. The nurse uses a flow sheet to document each exchange and records vital signs, dialysate concentration, medications added, exchange volume, dwell time, dialysate fluid balance for the exchange (fluid lost or gained), and cumulative fluid balance. The nurse also carefully assesses skin turgor and mucous membranes to evaluate fluid status and monitor for edema.

If the peritoneal fluid does not drain properly, the nurse can facilitate drainage by turning the patient from side to side or raising the head of the bed. The catheter should never be pushed in. Other measures to promote drainage include checking the patency of the catheter by inspecting for kinks, closed clamps, or an air lock. The nurse always monitors for complications, including peritonitis, bleeding, respiratory difficulty, and leakage of peritoneal fluid. Abdominal girth may be measured periodically to determine if the patient is retaining large amounts of dialysis solution. Additionally, the nurse must ensure that the peritoneal dialysis catheter remains secure and that the dressing remains dry. Physical comfort measures, frequent turning, and skin care are provided. The patient and family are educated about the procedure and are kept informed about progress (fluid loss, weight loss, laboratory values). Emotional support and encouragement are given to the patient and family during this stressful and uncertain time.

Continuous Ambulatory Peritoneal Dialysis

CAPD is a form of dialysis used for many patients with ESRD. CAPD is performed at home by the patient or a trained caregiver, who may be a family member. It allows the patient reasonable freedom and control of his or her daily activities.

PRINCIPLES UNDERLYING CAPD

CAPD works on the same principles as other forms of peritoneal dialysis: diffusion and osmosis. Less extreme fluctuations in the patient's laboratory results occur with CAPD than with intermittent peritoneal dialysis or hemodialysis because the dialysis is constantly in progress. The serum electrolyte levels usually remain in the normal range.

CAPD PROCEDURE

The patient performs exchanges four to five times a day, 24 hours a day, 7 days a week at intervals scheduled throughout the day (before meals and bedtime). After infusing the dialysate into the peritoneal cavity through the catheter (about 10 minutes), the patient can fold the bag and tuck it underneath the clothing during the dwell time. This provides the patient with some freedom and reduces the number of connections and disconnections necessary at the catheter end of the tubing, thereby reducing the risk of contamination and peritonitis.

The longer the dwell time, the better the clearance of middle-sized molecules. It is thought that these molecules may be significant uremic toxins. At the end of the dwell time, the dialysate is drained from the peritoneal cavity by unfolding the empty bag, opening the clamp, and placing the bag lower than the abdomen near the floor. This allows the peritoneal fluid to drain out by gravity. When drainage ends, the patient repeats the procedure by spiking a new bag containing dialysate and infusing the solution into the peritoneal cavity. New systems are available that allow the catheter to be clamped, disconnected, and capped, thus allowing the patient freedom from wearing an empty dialysate bag. Before the next exchange, however, an empty drainage bag must be attached to permit drainage of the dwell solution.

COMPLICATIONS

To reduce the risk of peritonitis, the patient takes meticulous care to avoid contaminating the catheter, fluid, or tubing and accidentally disconnecting the catheter from the tubing. The catheter is protected from manipulation, and the catheter entry site is meticulously cared for according to a standardized protocol.

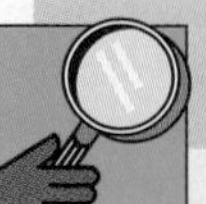

ASSESSMENT
SUITABILITY FOR CAPD

Although CAPD is not suitable for all patients with end-stage renal disease (ESRD), it is a viable therapy for those who can perform self-care and exchanges and who can fit therapy into their own routines. Often, patients on CAPD report having more energy and feeling healthier. Nurses can be instrumental in helping patients with ESRD find the dialysis therapy that best suits their lifestyle. Those considering CAPD need to investigate the advantages and disadvantages along with the indications and contraindications for this form of therapy.

Advantages

- Freedom from a dialysis machine
- Control over daily activities
- Opportunities to avoid dietary restrictions, increase fluid intake, raise serum hematocrit values, improve blood pressure control, avoid venipuncture, and gain a sense of well-being.

Disadvantages

- Continuous dialysis 24 hours a day, 7 days a week

Indications

- Patient's willingness, motivation, and ability to perform dialysis at home
- Strong family or community support system (essential for success), particularly if the patient is an older adult
- Special problems with long-term hemodialysis, such as dysfunctional or failing vascular access devices, excessive thirst, severe hypertension, postdialysis headaches, and severe anemia requiring frequent transfusion
- Interim therapy while awaiting kidney transplantation
- ESRD secondary to diabetes because hypertension, uremia, and hyperglycemia are easier to manage with CAPD than with hemodialysis

Contraindications

- Adhesions from previous surgery (adhesions reduce clearance of solutes) or systemic inflammatory disease
- Chronic backache and preexisting disk disease, which could be aggravated by the continuous pressure of dialysis fluid in the abdomen
- Risk of complications, for example, in patients receiving immunosuppressive medications, which impede healing of the catheter site, and in patients with a colostomy, ileostomy, nephrostomy, or ileal conduit because of the risk of peritonitis. The risk for complications is not an absolute contraindication for CAPD therapy.
- Diverticulitis because CAPD has been associated with rupture of the diverticulum
- Severe arthritis or poor hand strength necessitating assistance in performing the exchange. However, blind or partially blind patients and those with other physical limitations can learn to perform CAPD.

Nursing Management

In addition to the complications of peritoneal dialysis previously described, patients who elect CAPD may experience altered body image because of the abdominal catheter and the bag and tubing. Waist size increases from 1 to 2 inches (or more) with fluid in the abdomen. This affects clothing selection as well as patients' feeling of "being fat." Body image may be so altered that patients do not want to look at or care for the catheter for days or weeks. The nurse may arrange for the patient to talk with other patients who have adapted well to CAPD. Although some patients have no psychological problems with the catheter—they think of it as their lifeline and as a life-sustaining device—other patients feel they are doing exchanges all day long and have no free time, particularly in the beginning. They may experience depression because they feel overwhelmed with the responsibility of self-care.

Patients undergoing CAPD may also experience altered sexuality patterns and sexual dysfunction. The patient and partner may be reluctant to engage in sexual activities, partly because of the catheter being psychologically "in the way" of sexual performance. The peritoneal catheter, drainage bag, and about 2 L of dialysate may interfere with the patient's sexual function and body image as well. Although these problems may resolve with time, some problems may warrant special counseling. The nurse who asks the patient if there are any concerns related to sexuality and sexual function often provides the patient with a welcome opportunity to discuss these issues and a first step toward their resolution.

PROMOTING HOME AND COMMUNITY-BASED CARE

Teaching Patients Self-Care. Patients are taught as inpatients or outpatients to perform CAPD once they are medically stable. Training usually takes 5 days to 2 weeks. Patients are taught according to their own learning ability and knowledge level, and only as much at one time as they can handle without feeling uncomfortable or becoming overwhelmed. Education topics for the patient and family who will be performing peritoneal dialysis at home are described in the Home Care Teaching Checklist.

Because of protein loss with continuous peritoneal dialysis, patients are instructed to eat a high-protein, well-balanced diet. They are also encouraged to increase their fiber intake daily to help prevent constipation, which can impede flow of dialysate into or out of the peritoneal cavity. Often, patients gain from 3 to 5 pounds within a month of initiation of CAPD, so they may be asked to limit their carbohydrate intake to avoid an excessive amount of weight gain. Potassium, sodium, and fluid restrictions are not usually needed. Patients commonly lose about 2 L of fluid over and above the 8 L of dialysate infused into the abdomen during a 24-hour period, permitting a normal fluid intake even in an anephric patient (a patient without kidneys).

Continuing Care. Follow-up care through phone calls, patient visits to the outpatient department, and continuing home care assists patients in the transition to home and promotes their active participation in their own health care. Patients often depend on checking with the nurse to see if they are making the right choices about dialysate or control of blood pressure, or simply to discuss a problem.

Patients may be seen by the CAPD team as outpatients once a month or more if needed. The exchange procedure is evaluated at that time to see that strict aseptic technique is being used. The tubing used to instill the dialysate may be changed by the CAPD nurse every 4 to 8 weeks. Long-life tubing now lasts up to 6 months before tubing changes are necessary. Infrequent tubing changes decrease the risk of possible contamination. Blood chemistry values are followed closely to make certain the therapy is adequate for the patient.

If a referral is made for home care, the home care nurse assesses the home environment and suggests modifications needed to accommodate the equipment and facilities needed to carry out CAPD effectively. In addition, the nurse assesses the patient's and family's understanding of CAPD and their use of safe technique in performing CAPD. Additional assessments include checking for changes related to renal disease, complications such as peritonitis,

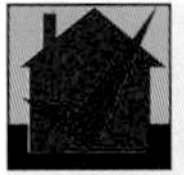

HOME CARE TEACHING CHECKLIST: PERITONEAL DIALYSIS (CAPD OR CCPD)

At the completion of the program, the patient or caregiver will be able to:	Patient	Caregiver
• Discuss basic information about normal kidney function.	✔	✔
• Discuss basic information about the disease process.	✔	✔
• Discuss the basic principles of peritoneal dialysis.	✔	✔
• Demonstrate catheter and exit site care.	✔	✔
• Demonstrate measurement of vital signs and weight measurement.	✔	✔
• Discuss monitoring and management of fluid balance.	✔	✔
• Discuss basic principles of aseptic technique.	✔	✔
• Demonstrate the CAPD exchange procedure using aseptic technique (CCPD patients should also demonstrate exchange procedure in case of failure or unavailability of cycling machine).	✔	✔
• Demonstrate cycler set-up procedure and maintenance if on CCPD.	✔	✔
• Discuss complications of peritoneal dialysis; prevention, recognition, and management of complications.	✔	✔
• Demonstrate procedure for adding medications to the dialysis solution.	✔	✔
• Demonstrate procedure for obtaining sterile dialysis fluid samples.	✔	✔
• Discuss routine laboratory work needed and implications of results.	✔	✔
• Discuss dietary restrictions.	✔	✔
• Discuss medications: name of medications, their actions, potential side effects, and when to contact physician.	✔	✔
• Discuss ordering, storage, and inventory of dialysis supplies.	✔	✔
• Describe plan for follow-up continuing care.	✔	✔
• Demonstrate maintenance of home dialysis records.	✔	✔
• Describe actions in case of emergency.	✔	✔

and treatment-related problems such as congestive heart failure, inadequate drainage, and weight gain or loss. The nurse continues to reinforce and clarify teaching about CAPD and renal disease and assesses the patient's and family's progress in coping with the procedure.

Continuous Cyclic Peritoneal Dialysis

CCPD combines overnight intermittent peritoneal dialysis with a prolonged dwell time during the day. The peritoneal catheter is connected to a cycler machine every evening, and the patient receives three to five 2-L exchanges during the night. In the morning, the patient caps off the catheter after infusing 1 to 2 L of fresh dialysate. This dialysate remains in the abdominal cavity until the tubing is reattached to the cycler machine at bedtime. The patient is able to sleep because the machine is very quiet, and extra-long tubing allows the patient to move and turn normally during sleep.

CCPD has a lower infection rate than other forms of peritoneal dialysis because of fewer opportunities for contamination with bag changes and tubing disconnections. It also allows the patient to be free of exchanges throughout the day, making it possible to work more freely and carry out activities of daily living.

Special Considerations: Care of the Hospitalized Dialysis Patient

Whether undergoing hemodialysis or peritoneal dialysis, the patient may be hospitalized for treatment of complications related to the dialysis treatment, the underlying renal disorder, or health problems not related to renal dysfunction or its treatment.

Nursing Management

PROTECTING THE VASCULAR ACCESS

When the hemodialysis patient is hospitalized for any reason, care must be taken to protect the vascular access from damage. The nurse assesses the vascular access for patency and takes precautions to ensure that the extremity with the vascular access is not used for blood pressure measurements or for obtaining blood specimens; tight dressings, restraints, or jewelry over the vascular access are to be avoided as well.

The bruit or "thrill" over the venous access site must be evaluated at least every 8 hours. Absence of a palpable thrill or audible bruit may indicate blockage or clotting in the access device. Clotting can occur if the patient has an infection anywhere in the body (serum viscosity is increased) or if the blood pressure has dropped. When blood flow is reduced through the access for any reason (hypotension, application of blood pressure cuff or tourniquet), clotting of the access can occur. Infection of the vascular access can also occur. The nurse observes for signs and symptoms of infection, such as redness, swelling, drainage from the site, and fever. Patients with renal disease are more prone to infection; therefore, infection control measures must be used for *all* procedures.

TAKING PRECAUTIONS DURING INTRAVENOUS THERAPY

When the patient needs intravenous therapy, the rate of administration must be as slow as possible and should be strictly controlled by a volumetric infusion pump. Because dialysis patients cannot excrete water, indiscriminate use of intravenous therapies can result in pulmonary edema. Accurate intake and output records are essential.

MONITORING SYMPTOMS OF UREMIA

As metabolic end products accumulate, uremic symptoms worsen. Patients whose metabolic rate accelerates (those on steroid medications or total parenteral nutrition, those with infections or bleeding disorders, those undergoing surgery) accumulate waste products more quickly and may require daily dialysis. These same patients are more likely to experience complications than other dialysis patients.

DETECTING CARDIAC AND RESPIRATORY COMPLICATIONS

Cardiac and respiratory assessment must be conducted frequently. As fluid builds up, congestive heart failure and pulmonary edema develop. Crackles in the bases of the lungs may indicate pulmonary edema.

Pericarditis may result from the accumulation of uremic toxins. If not detected and treated promptly, this serious complication may progress to pericardial effusion and cardiac tamponade. Pericarditis is detected by the patient's report of substernal chest pain (if the patient is able to communicate), low-grade fever (often overlooked), and pericardial friction rub. A pulsus paradoxus (a decrease in blood pressure of more than 10 mm Hg during inspiration) is often present. When pericarditis progresses to effusion, the friction rub disappears, heart sounds become distant and muffled, electrocardiographic waves show very low voltage, and the pulsus paradoxus worsens.

The effusion may progress to life-threatening cardiac tamponade, noted by narrowing of the pulse pressure in addition to muffled or inaudible heart sounds, crushing chest pain, dyspnea, and hypotension. Although pericarditis, pericardial effusion, and cardiac tamponade can be detected by chest x-ray, they should also be detected through astute nursing assessment. Because of their clinical significance, assessment of the patient for cardiac complications is a priority.

CONTROLLING ELECTROLYTE LEVELS AND DIET

Electrolyte alterations are common, and potassium changes are the most deadly. All intravenous solutions and medications to be administered are evaluated for their electrolyte content. Serum laboratory values are assessed daily. If blood transfusions are required, they may be administered during hemodialysis if possible so that excess potassium can be removed. The patient's dietary intake must also be monitored. The patient's frustrations related to dietary restrictions typically increase if the hospital food is unappetizing. The nurse needs to recognize that this may lead to dietary indiscretion and hyperkalemia.

MANAGING DISCOMFORT AND PAIN

Complications such as pruritus and pain secondary to neuropathy must be managed. Antihistamines, such as diphenhydramine hydrochloride (Benadryl), are commonly used, and analgesic medications may be prescribed. Because elimination of metabolites of medications occurs through dialysis rather than through renal excretion, however, medication dosages often require adjustment. Keeping the skin clean and well moisturized using bath oils, superfatted soap, and creams or lotions helps to promote comfort and reduce itching. Teaching the patient to keep the nails trimmed to avoid scratching and excoriation and to rub lotion into the skin instead of scratching also promotes comfort.

MONITORING BLOOD PRESSURE

Hypertension in renal failure is common. It is usually the result of fluid overload and, in part, to oversecretion of renin. Many dialysis patients receive some form of antihypertensive therapy and require intense teaching about its purpose and side effects. The trial-and-error approach that may be necessary to identify the most effective antihypertensive agent and dosage may confuse or alarm the patient if no explanation is provided. Antihypertensive medication must be withheld on dialysis days to avoid hypotension due to the combined effect of the dialysis and the medication.

PREVENTING INFECTION

Patients with ESRD commonly have low white blood cell counts (and decreased phagocytic ability), low red blood cell counts (anemia), and impaired platelet function. Together, these pose a high risk for infection and potential for bleeding after even minor trauma. Infection prevention and control are essential because the incidence of infection is high. Infection of the vascular access site and pneumonia are common.

CARING FOR THE CATHETER SITE

Patients receiving CAPD are usually well versed in caring for the catheter site; however, the patient's hospital stay should be an opportunity to assess compliance with recommended catheter care and to correct any misperceptions or deviations from correct technique. Recommended daily or three to four times weekly routine catheter site care is often performed when showering or bathing. The exit site should not be submerged in bath water. The most common cleaning method is soap and water; liquid soap is recommended. During care, the nurse and patient need to make sure that the catheter remains secure to avoid tension and accidental trauma. The patient may wear a gauze or semi-transparent dressing over the exit site.

ADMINISTERING MEDICATIONS

The medications prescribed for any dialysis patient must be closely monitored to avoid those that are toxic to the kidneys and that may threaten remaining renal function. All medications must be monitored, and alterations in dosages may be necessary to prevent either toxic effects on the kidney or overdosage because of impaired renal excretion. Care must be taken to evaluate all problems and symptoms reported by the patient without attributing them to renal failure or to dialysis therapy.

PROVIDING PSYCHOLOGICAL SUPPORT

Patients undergoing dialysis for a while may begin to reevaluate their status, the treatment modality, their satisfaction with life, and the impact of these factors on their families and support systems. Nurses must provide opportunities for these patients to express their feelings and reactions and to explore possible options.

The decision to begin dialysis does not require that dialysis be continued indefinitely, and it is not uncommon for patients to consider discontinuing treatment. These feelings and reactions must be taken seriously, and the opportunity should be provided to discuss them with the dialysis team as well as with a psychologist, psychiatrist, psychiatric nurse, trusted friend, or member of the clergy. The patient's informed decision about discontinuing treatment, after thoughtful deliberation, should be respected.

KIDNEY SURGERY

A patient may undergo surgery of the kidney to remove obstructions (tumors or calculi); to insert a tube for draining the kidney (nephrostomy, ureterostomy); or to remove the kidney involved in unilateral kidney disease, renal carcinoma, or kidney transplantation.

Preoperative Considerations

Surgery of the kidney is performed only after a thorough evaluation of current renal function. Patient preparation to ensure that optimal renal function is maintained is mandatory. Fluids are encouraged to promote increased excretion of waste products before surgery, unless contraindicated because of preexisting renal or cardiac dysfunction. If kidney infection is present preoperatively, wide-spectrum antimicrobial agents may be prescribed to prevent bacteremia. Antibiotics must be given with extreme care because many are toxic to the kidneys. Coagulation studies (prothrombin time, partial thromboplastin time, platelet count) may be indicated if the patient has a history of bruising and bleeding. The general preoperative preparation is similar to that described in Chapter 16.

Because patients facing kidney surgery are often apprehensive, the nurse encourages the patient to recognize and express any feelings of anxiety. Confidence is reinforced by establishing a relationship of trust and by providing expert care. Patients faced with the prospect of losing a kidney may think that they will be dependent on dialysis for the rest of their life. It is important to teach the patient and family that normal function may be maintained by a single healthy kidney.

Perioperative Concerns

Renal surgery requires a variety of patient positions to expose the operative site adequately. Three surgical approaches are common: flank, lumbar, and thoracoabdominal (Fig. 40-10). During surgery, plans are carried out for managing altered urinary drainage and drainage systems. Plans may include inserting a **nephrostomy** or other drainage tube or using ureteral stents.

Postoperative Management

Because the kidney is a highly vascular organ, hemorrhage and shock are the chief complications of renal surgery. Fluid and blood component replacement is frequently necessary in the immediate postoperative period to treat intraoperative blood loss.

Abdominal distention and paralytic ileus are fairly common after renal and ureter surgery and are thought to be due to a reflex paralysis of intestinal peristalsis and manipulation of the colon or duodenum during surgery. Abdominal distention is relieved by decompression through a nasogastric tube (see Chap. 35 for treatment of paralytic ileus). Oral fluids are permitted when the passage of flatus is noted.

If infection occurs, antibiotics are prescribed based on identification of the causative organism by culture. The toxic effects that antibiotics have on the kidneys (nephrotoxicity) must be kept in mind when assessing the patient. Low-dose heparin therapy may be initiated postoperatively to prevent thromboembolism in patients who had any type of urologic surgery.

Drainage Tubes

Almost all patients undergoing kidney and urologic surgery, as well as patients with other kidney and urologic disturbances, have drains, tubes, or catheters in place. All catheters and tubes must be kept patent (ie, draining) to prevent obstruction by blood clots, which can cause infection, kidney damage, or severe pain (similar to renal colic) from passing along the ureter.

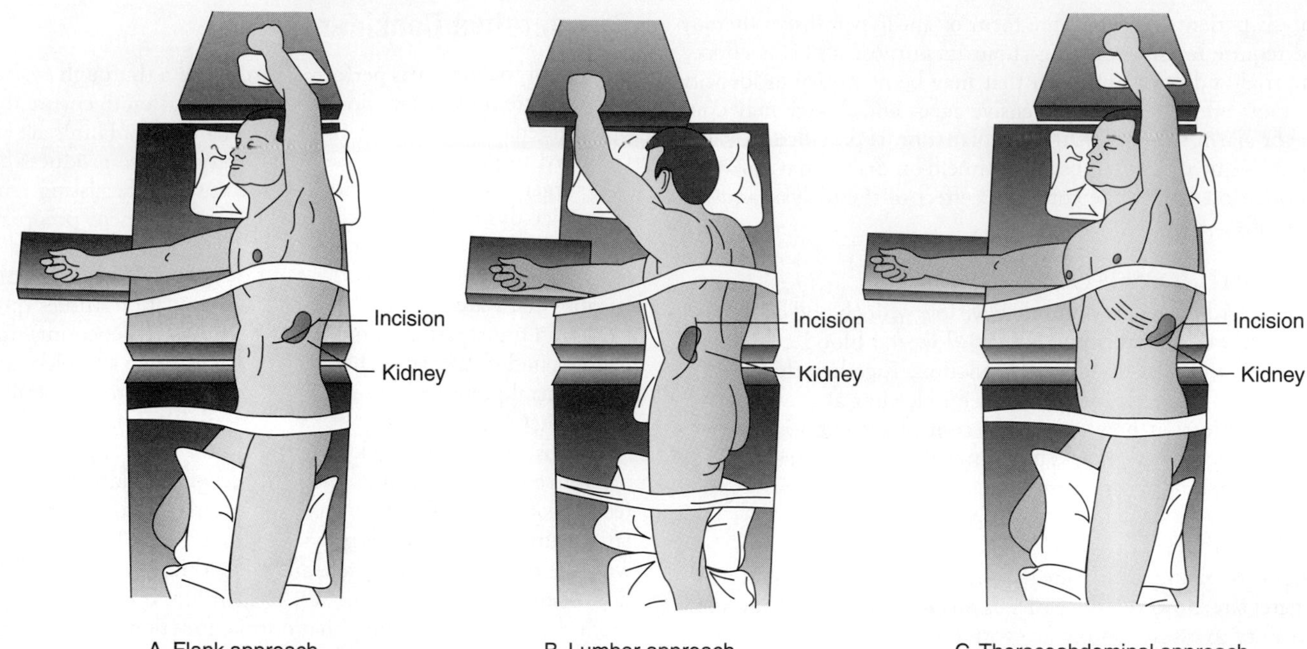

FIGURE 40•10 Patient positioning and incisional approaches (**A**, flank; **B**, lumbar; **C**, thoracoabdominal) for kidney surgery are associated with significant postoperative discomfort.

Nephrostomy Drainage

A nephrostomy tube is inserted directly into the kidney for temporary or permanent urinary diversion. It can be inserted either percutaneously or through a surgical incision. A single tube or a self-retaining U loop or circular nephrostomy tube may be used and is attached to a closed drainage system or to a urostomy appliance. Nephrostomy drainage may be required to provide drainage from the kidney after surgery or to bypass an obstruction in the ureter or lower urinary tract. Permanent nephrostomy tubes are usually changed every 3 months.

Percutaneous nephrostomy is the insertion of a tube through the skin into the pelvis of the kidney. This procedure is performed to provide external drainage of urine from an obstructed ureter, to create a route for inserting a ureteral stent (see following discussion), to dilate strictures, to close fistulas, to administer medications, to allow insertion of a brush biopsy instrument and nephroscope, or to perform selected surgical procedures.

The skin site is prepared and anesthetized, and the patient is asked to inhale and hold his or her breath while a spinal needle is advanced into the renal pelvis. Urine is aspirated for culture, and a contrast agent may be injected into the pyelocalyceal system. An angiographic catheter guide wire is introduced through the needle to the kidney. The needle is withdrawn and the tract dilated by the passage of tubes or guide wires. The nephrostomy tube is introduced and positioned within the kidney or ureter, fixed by skin sutures, and connected to a closed drainage system.

Before a percutaneous nephrostomy tube is inserted, the patient should receive a broad-spectrum antibiotic to prevent infection. In addition, bleeding disorders and uncontrolled hypertension should be corrected before the procedure. Anticoagulants and aspirin are discontinued and bleeding study results (prothrombin time, partial thromboplastin time, platelet count) should be normal before starting the procedure. These measures decrease the chance of the patient developing a perirenal hematoma or renal hemorrhage. Guideline 40-1 describes postsurgical nursing care of the patient

40•1 GUIDELINES FOR PATIENT CARE AFTER A NEPHROSTOMY

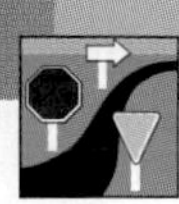

- Assess for possible complications: bleeding at nephrostomy site (main complication) or hematuria, fistula formation, infection.
- Ensure unobstructed drainage of nephrostomy tube or catheter. Obstruction causes pain, trauma, pressure, infection, and stress on suture lines.
- If tube dislodges, report immediately. The surgeon must replace tube immediately to prevent the opening from contracting.
- *Never* clamp a nephrostomy tube, which could cause obstruction and resultant pyelonephritis.
- *Never* irrigate a nephrostomy tube without specific orders.
- Encourage fluid intake to promote natural flushing of the kidney and nephrostomy tube.
- Measure urine output from the nephrostomy tube. If both kidneys have a tube in place, measure output from each tube separately.

with a nephrostomy tube (also see the accompanying Patient Education and Home Care display).

Ureteral Stents

A ureteral stent is a self-retaining tubular device designed to be placed within the ureter that helps maintain the position and caliber of the ureter during healing. Stents are used to maintain urine flow in patients with ureteral obstruction (from edema, stricture, fibrosis, calculi, tumors), to divert urine, to promote healing, and to maintain the caliber and patency of the ureter after surgery (Fig. 40-11). Stents are usually removed 4 to 6 weeks after surgery, in an outpatient setting without the need for general anesthesia or risk of ureteral injury.

The stent, usually made of soft, flexible silicone, may be inserted through a cystoscope or nephrostomy tube or by open surgery. Complications include infection, inflammation secondary to a foreign body in the genitourinary tract, tube encrustation, bleeding or clot obstruction within the stent, and migration or dislodgement of the stent.

Newer stent designs avoid some of these problems. The double-J ureteral stent has a J-shaped curve molded into each end, which prevents upward or downward migration. This stent can be used in place of a nephrostomy for short- or long-term urinary drainage. The double-pigtail ureteral stent has a pigtail coil at each end, which permits placement of the upper coil (pigtail) in the renal pelvis, with the lower coil at the ureteral orifice. The coils prevent the stent from moving and allow free body movement.

Nursing interventions related to the care of a patient with ureteral stents include monitoring for bleeding, observing and measuring urine output, assessing for signs of urinary tract infection or retroperitoneal infection from leakage of urine, and monitoring for stent displacement, which is evidenced by colicky pain and a decrease in urine output. An indwelling stent usually induces local ureteral reaction, including mucosal edema, which can cause temporary obstruction of the ureter and intense pain.

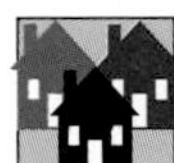

PATIENT EDUCATION AND HOME CARE

Caring for the Nephrostomy Tube at Home

The following recommendations are reviewed with patients going home with a percutaneous nephrostomy tube:

- Drink at least 8 glasses of water a day (unless otherwise directed by the physician).
- Avoid kinking, clamping, or twisting the nephrostomy tube.
- Always keep the drainage bag below the waist.
- During the day, connect the nephrostomy tube to a leg bag and wear it under clothing. At night, connect it to a large bedside drainage bag.
- When connecting to the leg bag or large drainage bag, be sure to clean the ends of the nephrostomy tube and connecting tube with alcohol.
- Change the dressing around the nephrostomy tube at least once a week. It may be changed daily if preferred.
- Avoid getting the dressing wet during showering or bathing.
- Clean the drainage tube and bag daily after each use with warm soapy water. Rinse well to remove the soap. The bag may be disinfected and deodorized using a solution of 1 tablespoon bleach and 2 cups water.
- Notify the physician immediately if the nephrostomy tube comes out, if large amounts of urine leak around the tube, if urine volume decreases, or if fever, back pain, or cloudy, foul-smelling urine develops.

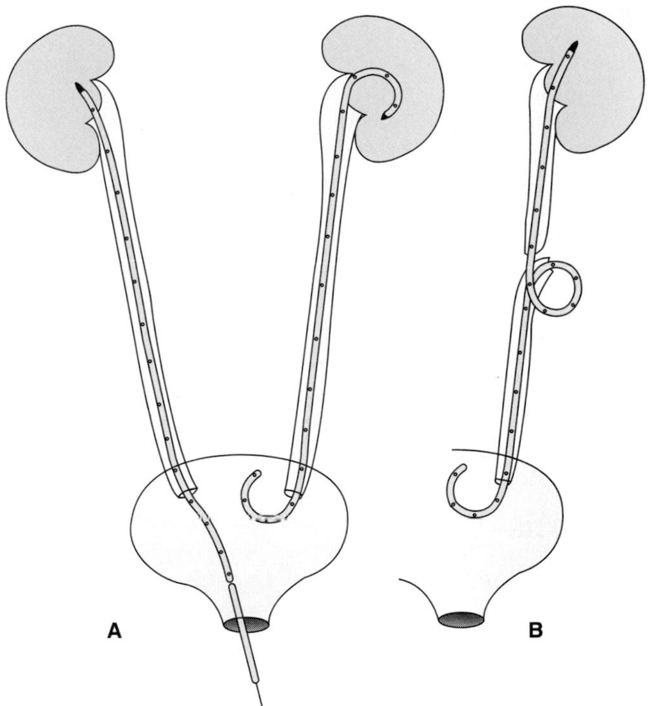

FIGURE 40•11 Ureteral stents. (**A**) Retrograde passage of ureteral stent. The double-J ureteral stent is shaped to resist migration. The proximal J hooks into the lower calix or renal pelvis, and the distal J curves into the bladder. (**B**) Open surgical placement of double-J stent before ureteral anastomosis. Courtesy of Medical Engineering Corporation, Racine, Wisconsin.

NURSING PROCESS: THE PATIENT UNDERGOING KIDNEY SURGERY

Assessment

Immediate care of the postoperative patient who has undergone surgery of the kidney includes assessment of all body systems. The patient's respiratory and circulatory status, pain level, fluid and electrolyte status, and patency and adequacy of urinary drainage systems are assessed.

Respiratory Status

As with any surgery, use of anesthesia increases the risk of respiratory complications. Noting the location of the surgical incision assists the nurse in anticipating respiratory problems and pain. The patient's respiratory status is assessed by monitoring the rate, depth, and pattern of respirations. The location of the surgical incision frequently causes pain on inspiration and coughing; therefore, the patient tends to splint the chest wall and take shallow respirations. Auscultation is performed to assess normal and adventitious breath sounds.

Circulatory Status and Blood Loss

The vital signs and arterial or central venous pressure are monitored. Skin color and temperature and urine output provide information about the adequacy of circulatory status. The surgical incision and drainage tubes are observed frequently to aid in detecting unexpected blood loss and hemorrhage.

Pain

Pain is a major problem for the patient postoperatively because of the location of the surgical incision and the patient's position on the operating table to permit adequate access to the kidney. The location and severity of pain are assessed before and after administration of analgesics. Abdominal distention, which increases the patient's discomfort, is also noted.

Urinary Drainage

The patient's urine output and drainage from tubes inserted during surgery are monitored for amount, color, and type or characteristics. Decreased or absent drainage is reported promptly to the physician because it may indicate obstruction that could cause pain, infection, and disruption of the suture lines.

Diagnosis

Nursing Diagnoses

Based on the history and assessment data and the type of surgical procedure performed, some major nursing diagnoses for the patient include the following (additional diagnoses and interventions appear in the Plan of Nursing Care 40-1):

- Risk for ineffective airway clearance related to the location of the surgical incision
- Risk for ineffective breathing pattern related to surgical incision and anesthesia
- Pain related to the location of the surgical incision, the position assumed on the operating table during surgery, and abdominal distention
- Urinary retention related to pain, immobility, and anesthesia

Collaborative Problems/Potential Complications

Based on assessment data, potential complications that may develop include the following:

- Bleeding
- Pneumonia
- Infection
- Fluid disturbances (deficit or excess)
- Deep vein thrombosis (DVT)

Planning and Goals

The major goals for the patient may include maintenance of effective airway clearance and breathing pattern, maintenance of cardiac output, relief of pain and discomfort, maintenance of urinary elimination, maintenance of fluid balance, and absence of complications.

Nursing Interventions

Maintaining Airway Clearance and Breathing Patterns

The surgical approaches to the kidney predispose the patient to respiratory complications and paralytic ileus. If the pleural cavity has been entered during surgery, a pneumothorax may occur, necessitating insertion of a chest tube. The incision is generally close to the diaphragm, and with a substernal incision, the nerves may be stretched and bruised. These factors can lead to pain and limited chest movement during inspiration; breathing patterns are altered or ineffective when the chest cannot fully expand. If the patient cannot generate an effective cough, either because of incisional pain and restricted movement or as a result of anesthesia, ineffective airway clearance may result.

Adequate use of analgesic medications is necessary to relieve pain so that the patient is able to take deep breaths and cough. When the analgesia is administered at regular, frequent intervals, the patient is able to perform deep-breathing and coughing exercises more effectively. The incentive spirometer may be used to help maximize lung inflation. The patient is encouraged to cough after each deep breath to loosen secretions.

Relieving Pain

In addition to incisional pain, the patient may experience pain and discomfort from distention of the renal capsule (by tumor or blood clot), ischemia (from occlusion of blood vessels), and stretching of the intrarenal blood vessels. The patient also frequently experiences muscular aches and pains resulting from the position assumed on the operating table, which places anatomic and physiologic stresses on the body. Massage, moist heat, and analgesic medications provide relief. Patient-controlled analgesia may be effective in ensuring pain control and the ability of the patient to ambulate, cough, and breathe deeply (see Chap. 12 for discussion of patient-controlled analgesia).

Promoting Urinary Elimination

The nurse closely monitors the patient's urine output and drainage to identify complications and to preserve and protect the patient's remaining kidney function (by preventing obstruction and infection). The output from each urinary drainage tube is recorded separately; very accurate output measurements are essential in monitoring renal function and ensuring the patency of the urinary drainage system.

Strict asepsis is used during manipulation of the drainage catheter and tube. Hand washing is mandatory before and after touching any parts of the system. Use of closed drainage systems is essential to avoid contamination of the system and infection. The urinary drainage is monitored closely for changes in volume, color, odor, and constituents. Urinalysis and urine cultures are indicated to follow the patient's progress. Care is taken to be sure that the collection bag is suspended below the patient's bladder to prevent reflux of urine into the urinary tract. The bag must be kept off the floor to prevent contamination.

Most urinary drainage systems do not require routine irrigation. If irrigation is necessary and prescribed, however, it should be performed carefully, with the use of sterile solution; with minimal pressure, consistent with the physician's instructions; and with strict asepsis without interruption of the closed drainage system.

Monitoring and Managing Potential Complications

Bleeding is a major complication of kidney surgery. If undetected and untreated, bleeding can result in hypovolemia and hemorrhagic shock. The nurse's role is to observe for these complications, to report their signs and symptoms, and to administer prescribed parenteral fluids and blood and blood components if complications

(text continues on page 1131)

40•1

PLAN OF NURSING CARE 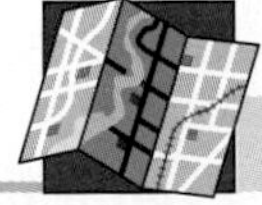

Care of the Patient Undergoing Kidney Surgery

Nursing Diagnosis: Risk for ineffective airway clearance related to pain of high abdominal or flank incision, abdominal discomfort, and immobility; risk for ineffective breathing pattern related to high abdominal incision

Goal: Relief of pain and discomfort

Nursing Interventions	Rationale	Expected Outcomes
1. Administer analgesics as prescribed.	1. Pain relief enables patient to take deep breaths and cough.	• Takes deep breaths and coughs adequately when encouraged and assisted • Exhibits respiratory rate of 12–18 breaths/min • Exhibits normal breath sounds without adventitious sounds • Exhibits full thoracic excursion without shallow respirations • Uses incentive spirometer with encouragement • Splints own incision while taking deep breaths and coughing • Reports progressively less pain and discomfort with coughing and deep breaths • Exhibits normal blood gases and chest x-ray • Exhibits normal body temperature with no signs of atelectasis or pneumonia on assessment
2. Splint patient's incision with hands or pillow to assist patient in coughing.	2. Splints incision and promotes adequate cough and prevention of atelectasis	
3. Assist patient to change positions frequently.	3. Promotes drainage and inflation of all lobes of the lungs	
4. Encourage use of incentive spirometer if indicated or prescribed.	4. Encourages adequate deep breaths	
5. Assist with and encourage early ambulation.	5. Mobilizes pulmonary secretions	

Nursing Diagnosis: Pain and discomfort related to surgical incision, positioning, and stretching of muscles during kidney surgery

Goal: Relief of pain and discomfort

Nursing Interventions	Rationale	Expected Outcomes
1. Assess patient's level of pain.	1. Provides baseline for later assessment of pain-relief strategies	• Reports relief of severe pain and discomfort • Takes analgesia as prescribed • States rationale for use of moist heat and massage • Exercises aching muscles within recommendations • Gradually increases physical activity and exercise • Uses distraction, relaxation exercises, and imagery for pain relief • Exhibits absence of behavioral manifestations of pain and discomfort (eg, restlessness, perspiration, verbal expressions of pain) • Participates in deep-breathing and coughing exercises
2. Administer analgesics as prescribed.	2. Promotes pain relief	
3. Apply moist heat and massage to areas with muscular aches and discomfort.	3. Promotes relaxation and relief of muscle pain and discomfort	
4. Splint patient's incision with hands or pillow during movement or deep breathing and coughing exercises.	4. Minimizes sensation of pulling or tension on incision and provides sense of support to the patient	
5. Assist and encourage early ambulation.	5. Promotes resumption of muscle activity exercise	

Nursing Diagnosis: Fear and anxiety related to diagnosis, outcome of surgery, and alteration in urinary function

Goal: Reduction of fear and anxiety

Nursing Interventions	Rationale	Expected Outcomes
1. Assess patient's anxiety and fear before surgery if possible.	1. Provides a baseline for postoperative assessment	• Verbalizes reactions and feelings to staff • Shares reactions and feelings with family or partner
2. Assess patient's knowledge about procedure and expected surgical outcome preoperatively.	2. Provides a basis for further teaching	

(continued)

40•1 PLAN OF NURSING CARE 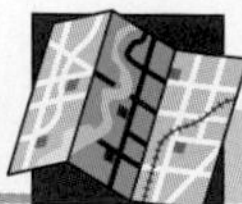

Care of the Patient Undergoing Kidney Surgery (*continued*)

Nursing Interventions	Rationale	Expected Outcomes
3. Evaluate the meaning alterations have for patient and family or partner.	3. Enables understanding of patient's reactions and responses to expected and unexpected results of surgery	• Grieves appropriately for self and for changes in role and function • Identifies information needed to promote own adaptation and coping
4. Encourage patient to verbalize reactions, feelings, and fears.	4. Affirms patient's understanding of and ultimate resolution of feelings and fears	• Participates in activities and events in immediate environment
5. Encourage patient to share feelings with spouse or partner.	5. Enables patient and partner to receive mutual support and reduces sense of isolation from each other	• Accepts visit from support person or participates in support group
6. Offer and arrange for visit from member of support group (eg, ostomy group, if indicated).	6. Provides support from another person who has encountered the same or a similar surgical procedure and an example of how others have coped with the alteration	• Identifies support person from own experience and peer group

Nursing Diagnosis: Altered patterns of urinary elimination related to urinary drainage; high risk for infection related to urinary drainage

Goal: Maintenance of urinary elimination; infection-free urinary tract

Nursing Interventions	Rationale	Expected Outcomes
1. Assess urinary drainage system immediately.	1. Provides basis for further assessment and action	• Exhibits adequate urinary output and patent drainage system
2. Assess adequacy of urinary output and patency of drainage system.	2. Provides baseline	• Exhibits urine output consistent with fluid intake
3. Use asepsis and hand washing when providing care and manipulating drainage system.	3. Prevents or reduces risk of contamination of urinary drainage system	• Demonstrates normal laboratory values: blood urea nitrogen, creatinine, urine specific gravity, and osmolality
4. Maintain closed urinary drainage system.	4. Reduces risk of bacterial contamination and infection	• Exhibits sterile urine on urine culture • Exhibits clear, dilute urine without debris or encrustation in the drainage system
5. If irrigation of the drainage system is necessary, use gloves and sterile irrigating solution and a closed drainage and irrigation system.	5. Permits irrigation when necessary while maintaining closed drainage system, minimizing risk of infection	• States rationale for avoiding manipulation of catheter, drainage, or irrigation system • Exhibits normal placement of urinary stent or ureteral catheters until removed by physician
6. If irrigation is necessary and prescribed, it is carried out gently with sterile saline and the prescribed amount of irrigating fluid.	6. Maintains patency of the catheter or drainage system and prevents sudden increases in pressure in the urinary tract that may cause trauma, pressure on sutures or urinary tract structures, and pain	• Maintains closed urinary drainage system • Exhibits normal body temperature without signs or symptoms of urinary tract infection
7. Assist patient in turning and moving in bed and when ambulating to prevent displacement or accidental removal of urinary stent or ureteral catheters if in place.	7. Prevents trauma from accidental displacement of urinary stent or ureteral catheter necessitating repeated instrumentation of the urinary tract (eg, cystoscopy) to replace them	• Cleans catheter with soap and water • Consumes adequate fluid intake (6–8 glasses of water or more per day unless contraindicated) • Urinary drainage system remains in place until removed or discontinued by physician
8. Observe urine color, volume, odor, and constituents.	8. Provides information about adequacy of urine output, condition and patency of drainage system, and debris in urine	• Maintains urinary drainage system without infection or obstruction
9. Minimize trauma and manipulation of catheter, drainage system, and urethra.	9. Reduces risk of contamination of drainage system and eliminates site of bacterial invasion	• Maintains urinary diversion as instructed • Maintains self-care so that environment is odor free
10. Clean catheter gently with soap during bath; avoid to-and-fro movement of catheter.	10. Removes debris and encrustations without causing trauma or contamination of urethra	• States rationale for close follow-up and maintains recommended schedule of appointments with health care providers
11. Anchor drainage tube.	11. Prevents movement or slipping of drainage tube, minimizing trauma and contamination of urethra or catheter	

(*continued*)

40•1 **PLAN OF NURSING CARE** 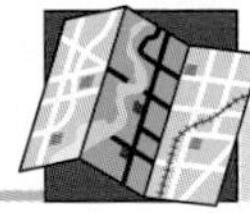 **Care of the Patient Undergoing Kidney Surgery (*continued*)**

Nursing Interventions	Rationale	Expected Outcomes
12. Maintain adequate fluid intake.	12. Promotes adequate urinary output and prevents urinary stasis	
13. Assist with and encourage early ambulation while ensuring placement of urinary drainage system.	13. Minimizes cardiovascular and pulmonary complications while preventing loss, dislodging, or disruption of drainage system	
14. If patient is to be discharged with urinary drainage system (catheter) in place or a urinary diversion, instruct patient and family member in care.	14. Knowledge and understanding of the drainage system or urinary diversion are essential to prevent infection and other complications	

Nursing Diagnosis: Risk for fluid volume excess or deficit related to surgical fluid loss, altered urinary output, parenteral fluid administration

Goal: Normal fluid balance will be maintained.

Nursing Interventions	Rationale	Expected Outcomes
1. Weigh patient daily.	1. Daily weight is the most sensitive indicator of fluid loss or gain.	• Patient's weight will be within 2–3 pounds of normal.
2. Take accurate intake and output measurements.	2. Detects fluid retention due to poor cardiac or renal output.	• Intake that exceeds output will be detected early.
3. Place all parenteral therapy on an infusion pump.	3. Ensures that the patient does not accidentally receive excess or insufficient intravenous fluids.	• The exact amount of solution is infused with no adverse effects resulting from overinfusion or underinfusion.
4. Monitor amount and characteristics of urine.	4. Assists in early detection of possible complications of surgery or tube insertion early.	• Urine is clear and absent of blood, pus, or any foreign substances.
5. Monitor vital signs: temperature, pulse, respiration, and blood pressure.	5. When fluid volume or cardiac output is altered, vital signs will be affected.	• Temperature, pulse, respiration, and blood pressure are normal.
6. Auscultate heart and lungs every shift.	6. When fluid volume is increased because of poor cardiac or renal output, fluid will accumulate in the lungs. Also, heart sounds will change as congestive heart failure develops. Frequent auscultation will ensure early detection.	• Normal heart and lung sounds are present.

occur. Monitoring of the patient's vital signs, skin condition, urinary drainage system, surgical incision, and level of consciousness is necessary to detect evidence of bleeding, decreased circulating blood, and fluid volume and cardiac output. Frequent monitoring of vital signs (initially monitored at least at hourly intervals) and urinary output is necessary for early detection of these complications.

If bleeding goes undetected or is late in being detected, the patient may have lost significant amounts of blood and may experience hypoxemia. In addition to hypovolemic (hemorrhagic) shock, this type of blood loss may precipitate a myocardial infarction or transient ischemic attack. Bleeding may be suspected when the patient experiences fatigue and when urine output is less than 30 mL per hour. As bleeding persists, late signs of hypovolemia, such as cool skin, flat neck veins, and change in level of consciousness or responsiveness occur. Transfusions of blood component products are indicated along with surgical repair of the bleeding vessel.

Pneumonia may be prevented through use of an incentive spirometer, adequate pain control, and early ambulation. Early signs of pneumonia include fever, increased heart and respiratory rates, and the development of adventitious breath sounds.

Prevention of infection is the rationale for use of asepsis when changing dressings and during meticulous care of catheters, other drainage tubes, central venous catheters, and intravenous catheters for administration of fluids. Insertion sites are monitored closely for signs of inflammation: redness, drainage, heat, and pain. Special care must be taken to prevent urinary tract infection, which is associated with use of indwelling urinary catheters. Catheters and other invasive tubes are removed as soon they are no longer needed.

Antibiotic agents are often administered postoperatively to prevent infection. If antibiotic agents are prescribed, the patient's serum creatinine and blood urea nitrogen levels must be monitored closely because many antibiotics are toxic to the kidney or can accumulate to toxic levels if renal function is decreased.

Prevention of fluid imbalance is a critical component of care for the patient undergoing kidney surgery. Both fluid loss and fluid excess are possible after renal surgery. Fluid loss may occur during surgery, as a result of excessive urinary drainage that occurs with removal of obstruction, or if diuretics are used for any reason. It can also occur with gastrointestinal losses: with diarrhea resulting from antibiotic use or with nasogastric drainage.

When postoperative intravenous therapy is inadequate to match the output or fluids lost, a fluid deficit results. Fluid excess or overload may result from cardiac effects of anesthesia, administration of excessive amounts of fluids, or the patient's inability to excrete fluid because of changes in renal function. Decreased urine output must be recognized as an indication of fluid excess.

Astute assessment skills must be used to detect early signs of fluid excess (such as weight gain, pedal edema, urine output below 30 mL/h, and slightly elevated pulmonary wedge pressure, if available) before those symptoms become severe (appearance of adventitious breath sounds, shortness of breath).

Fluid excess may be treated with fluid restriction and administration of furosemide (Lasix) or other diuretics. If renal insufficiency is present, these medications may not result in removal of excess fluid; therefore, dialysis may be necessary to prevent congestive heart failure and pulmonary edema.

DVT may occur postoperatively because of surgical manipulation of the iliac vessels during surgery. Elastic stockings are applied, and the patient is monitored closely for signs and symptoms of DVT and encouraged to exercise the legs. Heparin may be administered postoperatively to reduce the risk of DVT. Specific nursing interventions for the patient undergoing kidney surgery are presented in the Plan of Nursing Care.

Promoting Home and Community-Based Care

TEACHING PATIENTS SELF-CARE

If the patient has a drainage system in place, measures are taken to be sure that both patient and family understand the importance of maintaining the system correctly at home and preventing infection. Verbal and written instructions and guidelines are provided to the patient and family at the time of hospital discharge. The patient may be asked to demonstrate management of the drainage system to ensure understanding. The importance of strategies to prevent postoperative complications (urinary tract infection and obstruction, DVT, atelectasis, and pneumonia) is stressed to the patient and family. Those signs, symptoms, problems, and questions that should be referred to the physician or other primary health care provider are reviewed by the nurse with the patient and family.

CONTINUING CARE

The need for postoperative assessment and care after renal surgery continue regardless of setting: the patient's home, subacute care, outpatient clinic or office, or rehabilitation setting. Referral of the patient for home care is indicated for the patient going home with a urinary drainage system in place. During the home visit, the home care nurse reviews the specific instructions and guidelines given to the patient at hospital discharge. The nurse assesses the patient's ability to carry out the instructions and guidelines in the home and answers questions that the patient or family may have about management of the drainage system and of the surgical incision. Additionally, the home care nurse assesses the patient's vital signs and assesses for infection and obstruction of the urinary tract, adequacy of pain control, and compliance with recommendations. The home care nurse encourages adequate fluid intake and increasing levels of activity. Those signs, symptoms, problems, and questions that should be referred to the physician or other primary health care providers are reviewed by the nurse with the patient and family. If the patient has a drainage tube in place, the nurse assesses the site and patency of the system and monitors the patient for any signs and symptoms of complications, such as DVT, bleeding, or pneumonia.

Evaluation

Expected Outcomes

Expected outcomes may include:

1. Achieves effective airway clearance
   a. Exhibits clear and normal breath sounds, normal respiratory rate, and unrestricted thoracic excursion
   b. Performs deep-breathing exercises, coughs every 2 hours, and uses the incentive spirometer as directed
   c. Demonstrates normal temperature and vital signs
2. Reports progressive decrease in pain
   a. Requires analgesics at less frequent intervals
   b. Turns, coughs, and takes deep breaths as suggested
   c. Ambulates progressively
3. Maintains urinary elimination
   a. Demonstrates unobstructed urine flow from drainage tubes
   b. Exhibits normal fluid and electrolyte balance (normal skin turgor, serum electrolytes within normal range, absence of symptoms of imbalances)
   c. Reports no increase in pain, tenderness, or pressure at drainage site
   d. Exhibits cautious handling of own drainage system
   e. Washes hands before and after handling drainage system, and handles it only when necessary
   f. States rationale for use and maintenance of a closed drainage system
4. Participates in self-care activities
5. Experiences absence of complications
   a. Demonstrates normal vital signs and arterial and central venous pressures, normal skin turgor, temperature, and color
   b. Exhibits no signs or symptoms of bleeding, shock, or hypovolemia (eg, decreased urine output, restlessness, rapid pulse)
   c. Exhibits no signs of infection (eg, fever or pain) or evidence of DVT (tenderness or redness of calves)
   d. Maintains normal fluid balance, without rapid weight gain or loss
   e. Has clear breath sounds; no shortness of breath
   f. Excretes urine at a rate of at least 30 mL/h

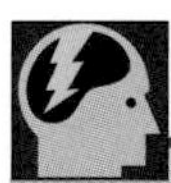

Critical Thinking Exercises

1. A 65-year-old woman comes to the clinic complaining that she loses urine whenever she coughs. She wears a panty liner every day because she is not sure when an accident may occur. She asks if there is anything that can be done to help this problem. Discuss your response to the patient. Include what she can anticipate regarding a diagnostic workup, treatment plan, and patient education strategies.

2. You are a staff nurse in an outpatient dialysis facility. The local nephrologist is sending a young man to the clinic today who will need dialysis in the near future. The physician has asked you to teach the patient and his wife about his dialysis options. Describe how you would develop a teaching plan to explain the different types of dialysis, their goals, and the level of involvement on the part of the patient and family. How would you modify your approach if the patient is so distraught that he does not seem to hear what you are saying?

3.

A patient who is treated with hemodialysis is admitted to the hospital for an elective nephrectomy in preparation for a kidney transplantation. How would your preoperative and postoperative care be modified by the patient's renal failure and the need for dialysis? What differences in your plan of care would be appropriate if the patient is treated with CAPD?

4.

You are the evening charge nurse in an extended care facility. An elderly woman is admitted from the local hospital after fracturing her hip. The staff nurse admitting the patient tells you the patient has urinary incontinence. The nurse intends to contact the physician to get an order for an indwelling catheter. What would be an appropriate response to the staff nurse? Describe the plan of care you would recommend for this patient.

References and Selected Readings

BOOKS

Agency for Health Care Policy and Research, Public Health Service, Department of Health and Human Services. (1996). *Urinary incontinence in adults.* Clinical Practice Guideline (AHCPR 96-0682). Washington, DC: U.S. Government Printing Office, 1996.

Bates, B. (1995). *A guide to physical examination and history taking* (6th ed.). Philadelphia: J.B. Lippincott.

Karlowicz, K. (1995). *Urologic nursing: Principles and practice.* Philadelphia: J. B. Lippincott.

Lancaster, L. (1995). *Core curriculum for nephrology nursing* (3rd ed.). Pitman, NJ: Anthony J. Janetti.

Levine, D. (1997). *Caring for the renal patient* (3rd ed.). Philadelphia: W. B. Saunders.

Life Options Rehabilitation Advisory Council. (1994). *Renal rehabilitation: Bridging the barriers.* CITY: Madison, WI: Medical Education Institute.

Marshall, F. (1996). *Textbook of operative urology.* Philadelphia: W. B. Saunders.

Meeker, M., & Rothrock, J. (1995). *Alexander's care of the patient in surgery.* St. Louis: Mosby–Year Book.

Methany, N. (1996). *Fluid and electrolyte balance: Nursing considerations* (2nd ed.). Philadelphia: J. B. Lippincott, 1996.

National Institutes of Health. (1995). *Morbidity and mortality of dialysis.* NIH Consensus Statement, Nov 1–3:1–33.

Palmer, M. (1996). *Urinary continence: Assessment and promotion.* Gaithersburg, MD: Aspen.

JOURNALS

Asterisks indicate nursing research articles.

General

Barger, M. & Woolner, B. (1995). Assessment and management of genitourinary tract disorders. *Journal of Nurse-Midwifery, 40*(2), 231–245.

Fuse, H., et al. (1996). Measurement of residual urine volume using a ultrasound instrument. *International Urology and Nephrology, 28*(5), 633–637.

Lewis, N. A. (1995). Implementing a bladder ultrasound program. *Rehabilitation Nursing, 20*(4), 215–217.

Meiner, S., Levy, R., & Mueth, E. (1996). Behavioral management of altered patterns of urinary elimination in women. *MedSurg Nursing, 5*(1), 11–22.

Moore, D. A., & Edwards, K. (1997). Using a portable bladder scan to reduce the incidence of nosocomial urinary tract infections. *MedSurg Nursing, 6*(1), 39–43.

Palmer, M. H. (1997). Pelvic muscle rehabilitation: Where do we go from here? *Journal of Wound, Ostomy, and Continence Nursing, 24*(2), 98–105.

Dialysis

Bellomo, R., Ronco, C., & Mehta, R. (1996). Nomenclature for continuous renal replacement therapies. *American Journal of Kidney Diseases, 28*(5), S2–S7.

Berkoben, M., & Schwab, S. (1995). Maintenance of permanent hemodialysis vascular access patency. *American Nephrology Nurses Association Journal, 22*(1), 17–23.

*Blake, C. W., & Courts, N. (1996). Coping strategies and styles of hemodialysis patients by gender. *American Nephrology Nurses Association Journal, 23*(5), 477–484.

Brunier, G. (1995). Peritonitis in patients on peritoneal dialysis: A review of pathophysiology and treatment. *American Nephrology Nurses Association Journal, 22*(6), 575–585.

Brunier, G. (1996). Care of the hemodialysis patient with a new permanent vascular access: Review of assessment and teaching. *American Nephrology Nurses Association Journal, 23*(6), 547–557.

*Culp, K., Taylor, L., & Hulme, P. (1996). Geriatric hemodialysis patients: A comparative study of vascular access. *American Nephrology Nurses Association Journal, 23*(6), 583–592.

Forni, L. G., & Hilton, P. J. (1997). Continuous hemofiltration in the treatment of acute renal failure. *New England Journal of Medicine, 336*(18), 1303–1309.

Gilman, C. M. (1997). Continuous venovenous hemofiltration: A cost effective therapy for the pediatric patient. *American Nephrology Nurses Association Journal, 24*(3), 337–341.

Grandstaff, M. (1996). Rehabilitation and dialysis: A collaborative program. *Rehabilitation Nursing, 21*(3), 148–151.

Henderson, L. W. (1996). Dialysis in the 21st century. *American Journal of Kidney Diseases, 28*(6), 951–957.

Johnson, C., et al. (1996). Working with noncompliant and abusive dialysis patients: Practical strategies based on ethics and the law. *Advances in Renal Replacement Therapy, 3*(1), 77–86.

Leapman, S. B., et al. (1996). The arteriovenous fistula for hemodialysis access: Gold standard or archaic relic? *American Surgeon, 62*(8), 652–656.

McConnell, E. A. (1995). Maintaining a peritoneal dialysis catheter. *Nursing, 25*(5), 26.

Mehta, R. L. (1997). Continuous renal replacement therapies in the acute renal failure setting: Current concepts. *Advances in Renal Replacement Therapy, 4*(2), 81–92.

Ouwendyk, M., & Helferty, M. (1996). Central venous catheter management: How to prevent complications. *American Nephrology Nurses Association Journal, 23*(6), 572–577.

*Pressly, K. B. (1995). Psychosocial characteristics of CAPD patients and the occurrence of infectious complications. *American Nephrology Nurses Association Journal, 22*(6), 563–573.

Roberts, A. B., et al. (1996). Graft surveillance and angioplasty prolongs dialysis graft patency. *Journal of the American College of Surgeons, 185*(5), 486–492.

Sciarini, P., & Dungan, J. (1996). A holistic protocol for management of fluid volume excess in hemodialysis patients. *American Nephrology Nurses Association Journal, 23*(3), 299–305.

Stark, J. (1997). Dialysis choices: Turning the tide in acute renal failure. *Nursing, 27*(2), 41–46.

Swartz, R. D., Boyer, C. L., & Messana, J. M. (1997). Central venous catheters for maintenance hemodialysis: A cautionary approach. *Advances in Renal Replacement Therapy, 4*(3), 275–284.

Szczepanik, M. E. (1995). Assessment and selection considerations: ESRD patient and family education materials and media. *Advances in Renal Replacement Therapy, 2*(3), 207–216.

Wolfson, M., et al. (1995). Difficulty accepting lifestyle limitations after abrupt onset of end-stage renal disease. *Advances in Renal Replacement Therapy, 2*(3), 246–254.

Urinary Catheters

Fiers, S. (1995). Management of the long-term indwelling catheter in the home setting. *Journal of Wound, Ostomy, and Continence Nursing, 22*(3), 140–144.

Hunt, G. M., Oakeshort, P., & Whitaker, R. H. (1996). Intermittent catheterization: Simple, safe, and effective but underused. *British Medical Journal, 7022*(312), 103–107.

*Kurtz, M. J., Van Zandt, K., & Burns, J. L. (1995). Comparison study of home catheter cleaning methods. *Rehabilitation Nursing, 20*(4), 212–217.

*Kurtz, M. J., Van Zandt, K., & Sapp, L. R. (1996). A new technique in independent intermittent catheterization: The Mitrofanoff catheterizable channel. *Rehabilitation Nursing, 21*(6), 311–314.

McConnell, E. A. (1995). Clinical do's and don't: How to remove an indwelling urinary catheter. *Nursing, 25*(1), 22.

McConnell, E. A. (1995). Clinical do's and don't: Inflating an indwelling urinary catheter balloon. *Nursing, 25*(12), 13.

Moore, K. N., & Rayome, R. G. (1995). Problem solving and troubleshooting: The indwelling catheter. *Journal of Wound, Ostomy, and Continence Nursing, 22*(5), 242–247.

Moore, K. N. (1995). Intermittent self-catheterization: Research-based principles. *British Journal of Nursing, 4*(18), 1057–1060.

Pomfret, I. (1996). Catheters: Design, selection and management. *British Journal of Nursing, 5*(4), 245–251.

Riley, D. K., et al. (1995). A large randomized clinical trial of a silver-impregnated urinary catheter: Lack of efficacy and staphylococcal superinfection. *American Journal of Medicine, 98*(4), 349–356.

Stickler, B. J., Morris, N. S., & Williams T. J. (1996). An assessment of the ability of a silver-releasing device to prevent bacterial contamination of urethral catheter drainage systems. *British Journal of Urology, 78*(4), 579–587.

Sylora, J. A., et al. (1997). Intermittent self-catheterization by quadriplegic patients via a catheterizable mitrofanoff channel. *Journal of Urology, 157*(1), 48–50.

White, M. C., & Ragland, K. E. (1995). Urinary catheter-related infections among home care patients. *Journal of Wound, Ostomy, and Continence Nursing, 22*(6), 286–290.

Wilson, M., & Coates, D. (1996). Infection control and urinary drainage bag design. *Professional Nurse, 11*(4), 245–252.

Winn, C. (1996). Basing catheter care on research principles. *Nursing Standard, 10*(18), 38–40.

Woollons, S. (1996). Urinary catheters for long-term use. *Professional Nurse, 11*(12), 825–832.

Urinary Incontinence

*Baer, M., et al. (1997). Home-based management of urinary incontinence: A pilot study with both frail and independent elders. *Journal of Wound, Ostomy, and Continence Nursing, 24*(3), 163–171.

*Chiverton, P. A., et al. (1996). Psychological factors associated with urinary incontinence. *Clinical Nurse Specialist, 10*(5), 229–233.

*Connor, P. A., & Kooker, B. M. (1996). Nurses' knowledge, attitudes, and practices in managing urinary incontinence in the acute care setting. *Med-Surg Nursing, 5*(2), 87–117.

Gallo, M. L., Fallon, P. J., & Staskin, D. R. (1997). Urinary incontinence: Steps to evaluation, diagnosis, and treatment. *Nurse Practitioner, 22*(2), 21–44.

Gallo, M. L., Hancock, R., & Davila, G. W. (1997). Clinical experience with a balloon-tipped urethral insert for stress urinary incontinence. *Journal of Wound, Ostomy, and Continence Nursing, 24*(1),51–57.

Gray, M., & Burns, S. B. (1996). Continence management. *Critical Care Nursing Clinics of North America, 8*(1), 29–38.

Pearson, B. D., & Kelber, S. K. (1996) Urinary incontinence: Treatments, interventions and outcomes. *Clinical Nurse Specialist, 10*(4), 177–184.

Rackley, R. R., & Appell, R. A. (1997) Evaluation and medical management of female urinary incontinence. *Cleveland Clinic Journal of Medicine, 64*(1), 82–92.

Resnick, N. M., Blaivas, J. G., & Ostergard, D. R. (1995). Practical pointers on urinary incontinence. *Patient Care, 29*(16), 103–132.

Sampselle, C. M., et al. (1997). Continence for women: Evidence-based practice. *Journal of Obstetrics, Gynecology, and Neonatal Nursing, 26*(4), 375–385.

Yim, P. S., & Peterson, A. S. (1996). Urinary incontinence: Basic types and their management in older patients. *Postgraduate Medicine, 99*(5), 137–150.

Resources

AGENCIES

American Association of Nephrology Nurses, North Woodbury Road, Box 56, Pitman, NJ 08071; 1-609-589-2187; www.inurse.com~ANNA.

American Kidney Fund, 6110 Executive Blvd., Suite 1010, Rockville, MD 20852; 1-800-638-8299; www.arbon.com/kidney.

American Association of Kidney Patients, 100 South Ashley Dr., Suite 280, Tampa, FL 33602; 1-800-749-2257; www.aakp.org.

National Association for Continence, P.O. Box 8310, Spartanburg, SC 29305-8310; 1-800-BLADDER; www.nafc.org.

National Institute of Diabetes and Digestive and Kidney Diseases, National Institutes of Health, Bethesda, MD 20892; www.niddk.nih.gov.

National Kidney and Urologic Diseases Information Clearinghouse, Box NKUDIC, 9000 Rockville Pike, Bethesda, MD 20892; 1-301-654-4415; www.nkudic@aerie.com.

National Kidney Foundation, 30 East 33rd St., New York, NY 10016; 1-800-622-9010; www.kidney.org.

National Kidney Patients Association, 804 Second Street Pike, Southampton, PA 18966; 1-215-953-8883; www.nkf.org.

North American Society for Dialysis and Transplantation, c/o Wadi N. Suki, MD, 6550 Fannin, Suite 1273, Houston, TX 77030; 1-713-790-3275.

The Simon Foundation for Continence, P.O. Box 815, Wilmette, IL 60091; 1-800-23SIMON.

Wound, Ostomy and Continence Nurses Society, 1500 S. Coast Highway, Suite 201, Laguna Beach, CA 94651; 1-888-224WOCN; www.wocn.org.

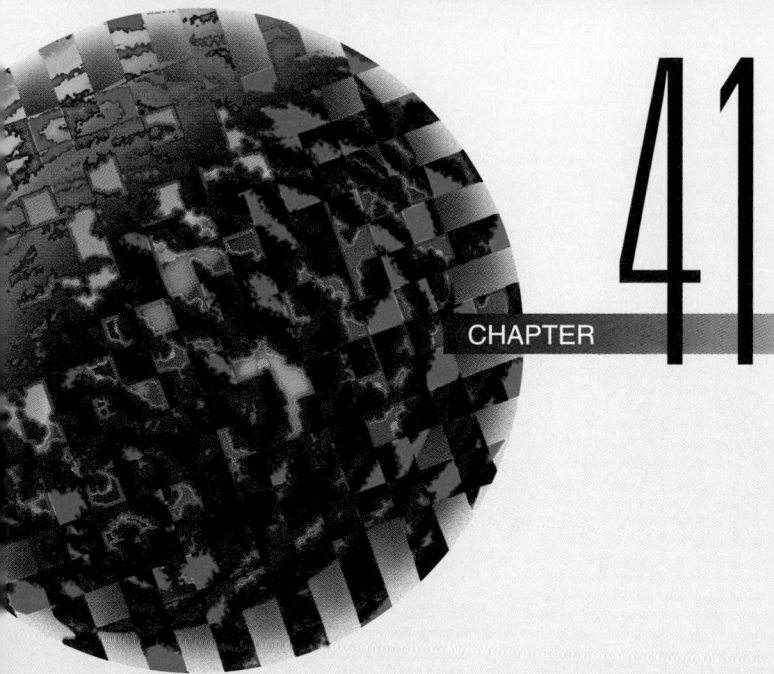

Management of Patients With Urinary and Renal Disorders

Learning Objectives

On completion of this chapter, the learner will be able to:

1. Identify factors contributing to urinary tract infections.
2. Develop a teaching plan for the patient with urinary tract infection.
3. Compare and contrast pyelonephritis, glomerulonephritis, and the nephrotic syndrome: causes, pathophysiologic changes, clinical manifestations, management, and nursing care.
4. Describe causes of acute renal failure and chronic renal failure.
5. Use the nursing process as a framework for the care of patients with acute renal failure.
6. Use the nursing process as a framework for the care of patients with chronic renal failure.
7. Develop a postoperative nursing care plan and teaching plan for the patient undergoing kidney transplantation.
8. Describe management strategies for renal calculi (kidney stones).
9. Develop a teaching plan for the patient undergoing treatment for renal calculi (kidney stones).
10. Formulate preoperative and postoperative nursing diagnoses for the patient undergoing surgery for urinary diversion.
11. Describe interstitial cystitis and its physical and psychological effects on the patient.

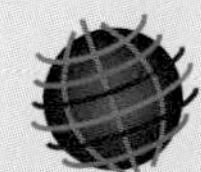

Disorders of the urinary tract and kidneys range from easily treated infections to life-threatening disorders that necessitate organ replacement or long-term treatment with dialysis. Recent advances in pharmacotherapeutics and technology have improved the diagnostic and treatment possibilities for these disorders. Additionally, those disorders that once required surgical intervention and prolonged recuperation can be treated today with noninvasive, nonsurgical techniques.

GLOSSARY

acute tubular necrosis: type of acute renal failure in which there is actual damage to the kidney tubules

bacteriuria: more than 10^5 colonies of bacteria per milliliter urine

continent urinary diversion (Koch, Indiana, Charleston pouch): transplantation of the ureters to a segment of bowel with construction of an effective continence mechanism or valve

cutaneous ureterostomy: procedure in which the distal ureter is detached from the bladder, brought through the abdominal wall, and attached to an opening in the skin

cystectomy: removal of the urinary bladder

cystitis: inflammation of the urinary bladder

end-stage renal disease (ESRD): progressive, irreversible deterioration in renal function that results in retention of uremic waste products

glomerulonephritis: inflammation of the glomerular capillaries

ileal conduit: transplantation of the ureters to an isolated section of the terminal ileum and bringing one end of the ureters to the abdominal wall

interstitial cystitis: inflammation of the bladder wall that eventually causes disintegration of the lining and loss of bladder elasticity

interstitial nephritis: inflammation of the renal interstitial tissue, often due to drugs or chemicals

nephrosclerosis: hardening, or sclerosis, of the arteries of the kidney due to prolonged hypertension

nephrostomy: insertion of a catheter into the renal pelvis by an incision in the flank or by percutaneous placement of a catheter into the kidney

nephrotic syndrome: disorder characterized by proteinuria, edema, hypoalbuminuria, and hyperlipidemia

prostatitis: inflammation of the prostate gland

pyelonephritis: inflammation of the renal pelvis

pyuria: white blood cells in the urine

urethritis: inflammation of the urethra

ureterosigmoidostomy: transplantation of the ureters into the sigmoid colon, allowing urine to flow through the colon and out the rectum

ureterovesical or vesicoureteral reflux: backward flow of urine from the bladder into one or both ureters

urethrovesical reflux: backward flow of urine from the urethra into the bladder

urinary casts: protein plugs secreted by damaged kidney tubules

INFECTIONS OF THE URINARY TRACT

Urinary tract infections (UTIs) are caused by pathogenic microorganisms in the urinary tract (the normal urinary tract is sterile above the urethra). UTIs are generally classified as infections involving the upper or the lower urinary tract (Chart 41-1).

Lower UTIs include **cystitis** (inflammation of the urinary bladder), **prostatitis** (inflammation of the prostate gland), and **urethritis** (inflammation of the urethra). Upper UTIs are much less common and include acute or chronic **pyelonephritis** (inflammation of the renal pelvis), **interstitial nephritis** (inflammation of the kidney), and renal abscesses. Upper and lower UTIs are further classified as uncomplicated or complicated, depending on other patient-related conditions, for example, whether the UTI is recurrent and the duration of the infection. Most uncomplicated UTIs are community acquired and occur in young women. Complicated UTIs usually occur in patients (male and female) with urologic abnormalities or recent catheterization and are often hospital acquired.

UTI is one of the most common reasons patients seek health care, accounting for about 7 million patient visits a year (Bacheller & Bernstein, 1997). Most cases occur in women, with one of every five women in the United States developing a UTI sometime during her lifetime. The urinary tract is the most common site of nosocomial infection, accounting for greater than 40% of the total number reported by hospitals and affecting about 600,000 patients each year (Winn, 1996). In most of these hospital-acquired UTIs, instrumentation of the urinary tract or catheterization is the precipitating cause. More than 250,000 cases of acute pyelonephritis occur in the United States each year, with 100,000 of these patients requiring hospitalization (Kunin, 1997).

Lower Urinary Tract Infections

Several mechanisms maintain the sterility of the bladder: the physical barrier of the urethra, urine flow, ureterovesical junction competence, various antibacterial enzymes and antibodies, and antiadherent effects mediated by the mucosal cells of the bladder. Abnormalities or dysfunctions of these mechanisms are contributing factors to lower UTIs.

Pathophysiology

For infection to occur, bacteria must gain access to the bladder, attach to and colonize the epithelium of the urinary tract to avoid being washed out with voiding, evade host defense mechanisms, and initiate inflammation. Most UTIs result from fecal organisms that ascend from the perineum to the urethra and the bladder and then adhere to the mucosal surfaces.

BACTERIAL INVASION OF THE URINARY TRACT

By increasing the normal slow shedding of bladder epithelial cells (resulting in bacteria removal), the bladder can clear itself of even large numbers of bacteria. Glycosaminoglycan (GAG), a hydrophilic protein, normally exerts a nonadherent protective effect against various bacteria. The GAG molecule attracts water molecules, forming a water barrier that serves as a defensive layer between the bladder and the urine. GAG may be impaired by certain agents (cyclamate, saccharin, aspartame, and tryptophan metabolites). The normal bacterial flora of the vagina and urethral area also interfere with adherence of *Escherichia coli* (the most common microorganism causing UTI). Urinary immunoglobulin A (IgA) in the urethra may also provide a barrier to bacteria.

REFLUX

An obstruction to free-flowing urine is a problem known as **urethrovesical reflux**, which is the reflux (backward flow) of urine from the urethra into the bladder (Fig. 41-1). With coughing, sneezing, or straining, the bladder pressure rises, which may force urine from the bladder into the urethra. When the pressure returns to normal, the urine flows back into the bladder, bringing into the bladder bacteria from the anterior portions of the urethra. Urethrovesical reflux is also caused by dysfunction of the bladder neck or urethra. The urethrovesical angle and urethral closure pressure may be altered with menopause, increasing the incidence of infection in postmenopausal women.

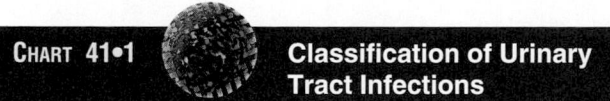

CHART 41•1 Classification of Urinary Tract Infections

Urinary tract infections (UTIs) are classified according to location: either the lower urinary tract (which includes the bladder and structures below the bladder) or the upper urinary tract (which includes the kidneys and ureters).

Lower UTI

Cystitis, prostatitis, urethritis

Upper UTI

Acute pyelonephritis, chronic pyelonephritis, renal abscess, interstitial nephritis, perirenal abscess

Uncomplicated Lower or Upper UTI

Community-acquired infection; common in young women

Complicated Lower or Upper UTI

Often nosocomial (acquired in the hospital) and related to catheterization; occurs in patients with urologic abnormalities, pregnancy, immunosuppression, diabetes mellitus, obstructions

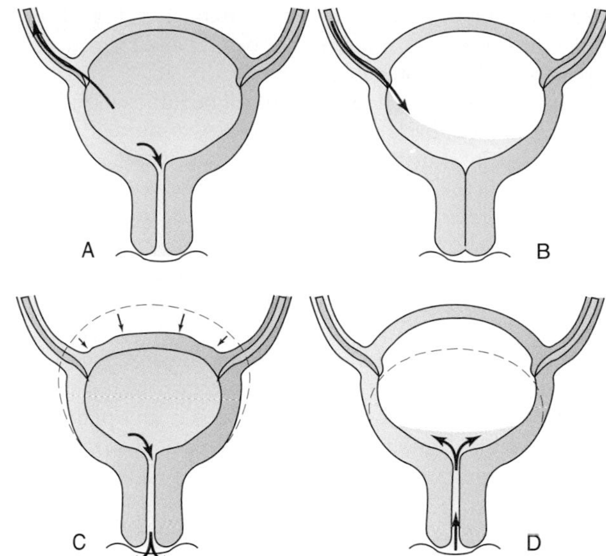

FIGURE 41•1 Mechanisms of ureterovesical and urethrovesical reflux may cause urinary tract infection. **Ureterovesical reflux:** With failure of the ureterovesical valve, urine moves up the ureters during voiding (**A**) and flows into the bladder when voiding stops (**B**). This prevents complete emptying of the bladder. It also leads to urinary stasis and contamination of the ureters with bacteria-laden urine. **Urethrovesical reflux:** With coughing and straining, bladder pressure rises, which may force urine from the bladder into the urethra (**C**). When bladder pressure returns to normal, the urine flows back to the bladder (**D**), which introduces bacteria from the urethra to the bladder.

Ureterovesical or **vesicoureteral reflux** refers to the backward flow of urine from the bladder into one or both ureters (see Fig. 41-1). Normally, the ureterovesical junction prevents urine from traveling back into the ureter. The ureters are tunneled into the bladder wall so that a small portion of the ureter is compressed by the bladder musculature during normal voiding. When the ureterovesical valve is impaired because of congenital causes or ureteral abnormalities, the bacteria may reach and eventually destroy the kidneys.

UROPATHOGENIC BACTERIA

Bacteriuria is generally defined as more than 10^5 colonies of bacteria per milliliter of urine. Because urine samples (especially in women) are commonly contaminated by bacteria normally present in the urethral area, a bacterial count exceeding 10^5 colonies/mL of clean-catch midstream urine is the measure that distinguishes true bacteriuria from contamination. In men, contamination of the collected urine sample occurs less frequently; hence, bacteriuria can be defined as 10^4 colonies/mL urine.

The organisms most frequently responsible for UTIs are those normally found in the lower gastrointestinal tract: *E. coli* accounts for 80% to 90% of uncomplicated UTIs, whereas *Staphylococcus saprophyticus* accounts for another 10% to 15%. Other organisms responsible for UTIs include *Enterococcus* species, *Proteus mirabilis, Pseudomonas aeruginosa,* and *Klebsiella* and *Enterobacter* species.

Risk Factors for URINARY TRACT INFECTION

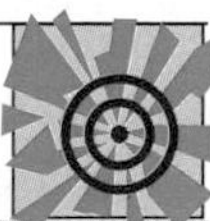

General risk factors for urinary tract infection (UTI) include the following:

- Inability or failure to empty the bladder completely
- Obstructed urinary flow, possibly from congenital anomalies, urethral strictures, contracture of the bladder neck, bladder tumors, calculi (stones) in the ureters or kidneys, compression of the ureters, and neurologic abnormalities
- Decreased natural host defenses or immunosuppression
- Instrumentation of the urinary tract (eg, catheterization, cystoscopic procedures)
- Inflammation or abrasion of the urethral mucosa
- Contributing conditions (certain populations of patients are more prone to UTIs than others); including those with:
  - Diabetes mellitus (increased urinary glucose levels create an infection-prone environment in the urinary tract)
  - Pregnancy, neurologic disorders, gout, and other altered states characterized by incomplete emptying of the bladder and urinary stasis

ROUTES OF INFECTION

There are three well-recognized routes by which bacteria enter the urinary tract: up the urethra *(ascending infection),* through the bloodstream, *(hematogenous spread),* or by means of a fistula from the intestine *(direct extension).*

The most common route of infection is transurethral, in which bacteria (often from fecal contamination) colonize the periurethral area and subsequently enter the bladder by means of the urethra. In women, the short urethra offers little resistance to the movement of uropathogenic bacteria. Sexual intercourse or massage of the urethra forces the bacteria up into the bladder. This accounts for the increased incidence of UTIs in sexually active women. Bacteria may also enter the urinary tract by means of the blood (hematogenous spread) from a distant site of infection or through direct extension by way of a fistula from the intestinal tract.

Clinical Manifestations

A variety of signs and symptoms are associated with UTI. About half of all patients found to have bacteriuria have no symptoms. Signs and symptoms of uncomplicated lower UTI (cystitis) include frequent pain and burning on urination, frequency, urgency, nocturia, incontinence, and suprapubic or pelvic pain. Hematuria and back pain may also be present.

Signs and symptoms of upper UTI (pyelonephritis) include fever, chills, flank or low back pain, nausea and vomiting, headache, malaise, and painful urination. Physical examination reveals pain and tenderness in the area of the costovertebral angles (CVA), which are the angles formed on each side of the body by the bottom rib of the rib cage and the vertebral column (Fig. 41-2).

In patients with complicated UTIs, such as those with indwelling catheters, symptoms can range from asymptomatic bacteriuria to a gram-negative sepsis with shock. Complicated UTIs often are due to a broader spectrum of organisms, have a lower response rate to treatment, and tend to recur. Many catheter-associated UTIs are asymptomatic; however, any patient who suddenly develops signs and symptoms of septic shock should be evaluated for urosepsis.

Assessment and Diagnostic Findings

Various tests help confirm the UTI diagnosis. Among them are colony counts, cellular findings, and urine culture results.

COLONY COUNTS

UTI is diagnosed by bacteria in the urine. A colony count of at least 10^5 colony-forming units (CFU) per milliliter of urine on a clean-catch midstream or catheterized specimen is a major criterion for infection. However, UTI and subsequent sepsis have occurred with lower bacterial colony counts. About one third of women with symptoms of acute infections have negative midstream urine culture results and may go untreated if 10^5 CFU/mL is used as the criterion for infection. The presence of *any* bacteria in specimens obtained by suprapubic needle aspiration of the urinary bladder or catheterization is considered indicative of infection.

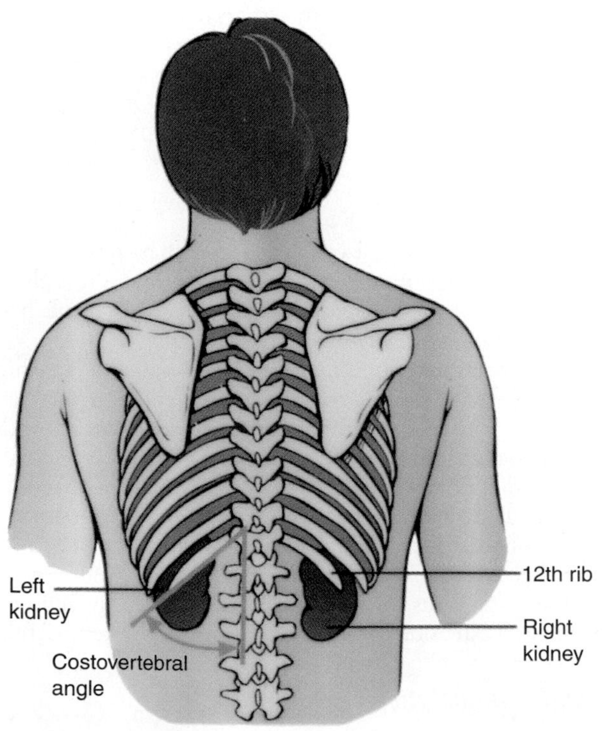

FIGURE 41•2 Location of the costovertebral angle.

CELLULAR FINDINGS

Microscopic hematuria (greater than four red blood cells [RBCs] per high-power field) is present in about half of patients with acute infection. Pyuria (greater than 4 white blood cells [WBCs] per high-power field) occurs in all patients with UTI; however, it is not specific for bacterial infection. Pyuria can also be seen with kidney stones, interstitial nephritis, and renal tuberculosis.

URINE CULTURES

Urine cultures remain the gold standard in documenting a UTI and can identify the specific organism present. Because of the high probability that the organism in young women with their first UTI is *E. coli,* cultures are often omitted. The following groups of patients should have urine cultures obtained when bacteriuria is present:

- All men (because of likelihood of structural or functional abnormalities)
- All children
- Women with a history of compromised immune function or renal problems
- Patients with diabetes mellitus
- Patients who have undergone recent instrumentation (including catheterization) of the urinary tract
- Patients who were hospitalized recently
- Patients with prolonged or persistent symptoms
- Patients with three or more UTIs in past year
- Pregnant women

TESTING METHODS

Multistrip dipstick testing for WBCs, known as the leukocyte esterase test, and nitrites (Griess nitrate reduction test) are common. If the leukocyte esterase test is positive, it is assumed that the patient has pyuria (WBCs in the urine) and should be treated. The Griess nitrate reduction test is considered positive if bacteria that reduce normal urinary nitrates to nitrites are present.

Tests for sexually transmitted diseases (STDs) may be performed because acute urethritis caused by sexually transmitted organisms (ie, *Chlamydia trachomatis, Neisseria gonorrhoeae,* and herpes simplex) or acute vaginitis infections (caused by *Trichomonas* or *Candida* species) may be responsible for symptoms similar to those of UTI. Therefore, evaluation for STDs may be performed (see Chap. 64).

Historically, intravenous pyelography (IVP) was used to detect abnormalities in patients at high risk for complicated or recurring UTI. Today, diagnostic studies, such as computed tomography (CT) and ultrasonography, are preferred detection methods for several reasons: CT scans may detect areas of pyelonephritis or abscesses; ultrasonography is extremely sensitive for detecting obstruction, abscesses, tumors, and cysts. Transrectal ultrasonography (to assess the prostate and bladder) is the procedure of choice for men with recurrent or complicated UTIs. An IVP may be indicted to visualize the ureters or to detect strictures or stones and is necessary for an accurate diagnosis of reflux nephropathy. It is generally accepted that the first episode of UTI in women does not require urologic evaluation (Bacheller & Bernstein, 1997; Hooten & Stamm, 1997).

Gerontologic Considerations

The incidence of bacteriuria in elderly adults differs from that in younger adults. Bacteriuria increases with age and disability, and women are affected more frequently than men. UTI is the

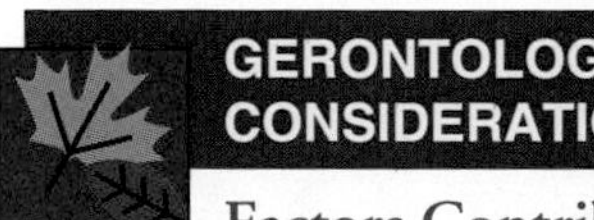

GERONTOLOGIC CONSIDERATIONS

Factors Contributing to Urinary Tract Infection in Older Adults

- High incidence of chronic illness
- Frequent use of antimicrobial agents
- Presence of infected pressure ulcers
- Immobility and incomplete emptying of bladder
- Use of a bedpan rather than a commode or toilet

most common cause of acute bacterial sepsis in patients older than 65 years of age, in whom gram-negative sepsis carries a mortality rate exceeding 50%.

In the elderly population at large, structural abnormalities and neurogenic bladder secondary to strokes or autonomic neuropathy of diabetes may prevent complete emptying of the bladder and increase the risk for UTI. When indwelling catheters are used, the risk for UTI rises dramatically as two or more different strains of bacteria can be found in urine of catheterized patients, in the urine itself, and on the surface of the catheter. Elderly women often have incomplete emptying of the bladder and urinary stasis. In the absence of estrogen, postmenopausal women are susceptible to colonization and increased adherence of bacteria to the vagina and urethra. Oral or topical estrogen is used to restore the glycogen content of vaginal epithelial cells and an acidic pH for some postmenopausal women with recurrent cystitis.

The antibacterial activity of prostatic secretions that protects men from bacterial colonization of the urethra and bladder decreases with aging. Although UTIs are rare in men, the prevalence of infection in men older than 50 years of age approaches that of women in the same age group. The dramatic rise in UTI in men as they age is due largely to prostatic hyperplasia or carcinoma, strictures of the urethra, and neuropathic bladder. The use of catheterization or cystoscopy in evaluation or treatment may contribute further to UTI. The incidence of bacteriuria rises in men with confusion, dementia, or bowel or bladder incontinence. The most common cause of recurrent UTI in the elderly male patient is chronic bacterial prostatitis. Transurethral resection of the prostate gland may help to reduce its incidence (see Chap. 45).

In institutionalized elderly patients, such as those in nursing homes, infecting pathogens are often resistant to many antibiotics. Factors that may contribute to UTI in elderly nursing home patients include: high incidence of chronic illness; frequent use of antimicrobial agents; infected pressure ulcers; immobility and incomplete emptying of bladder; and use of a bedpan rather than a commode or toilet.

Diligent hand washing, careful perineal care, and frequent toileting may decrease the incidence of UTIs in nursing home patients. The organisms responsible for UTIs in the institutionalized elderly may differ from those found in patients residing in the community; this is thought to be due in part to the frequent use of antibiotics by patients in nursing homes. *E. coli* is the most common organism seen in elderly patients in the community or hospital. Patients with indwelling catheters, however, are more likely to be infected with *Proteus, Klebsiella, Pseudomonas,* or *Staphylococcus* species. Patients who have been previously treated with antibiotics may be infected with *Enterococcus* species.

Nursing Alert *Elderly patients often lack the typical symptoms of UTI and sepsis. Although frequency, urgency, and dysuria may occur, nonspecific symptoms, such as altered sensorium, lethargy, anorexia, new incontinence, hyperventilation, and low-grade fever, may be the only clues. Frequent reinfections are common in older adults.*

Medical Management

Management of UTIs typically involves drug therapy and patient education. The nurse is a key figure in teaching the patient about medication regimens and infection prevention measures.

Patients in institutional settings may require 7 to 10 days of medication for the treatment to be effective. Controversy continues about the need for treatment of asymptomatic bacteriuria in the institutionalized elderly patient because resulting antibiotic-resistant organisms and sepsis may be greater threats to the patient. Most experts now recommend withholding antibiotics unless symptoms develop (Nguyen, Smith, & Leidich, 1997; Nicolle, 1997). Treatment regimens, however, are generally the same as those for younger adults, although age-related changes in intestinal absorption of medications and decreased renal function and hepatic flow may necessitate alterations in the antimicrobial regimen. Renal function must be monitored and the dosage of medications altered accordingly.

ACUTE PHARMACOLOGIC THERAPY

The ideal treatment of UTI is an antibacterial agent that effectively eradicates bacteria from the urinary tract with minimal effects on fecal and vaginal flora, thereby minimizing the incidence of vaginal yeast infections. (Yeast vaginitis occurs in as many as 25% of patients treated with antimicrobial agents that affect vaginal flora. Yeast vaginitis often causes more symptoms and is more difficult and costly to treat than the original UTI.) Additionally, the antibacterial agent should be affordable and should produce few side effects and low resistance. Because the organism in initial, uncomplicated UTIs in women is most likely *E. coli* or other fecal flora, the agent should be effective against these organisms. Various treatment regimens have been used successfully to treat uncomplicated lower UTIs in women: single-dose administration, short-course (3 to 4 days) medication regimens, or 7- to 10-day therapeutic courses. The trend is toward a shortened course of antibiotic therapy for uncomplicated UTIs because about 80% of cases are cured after 3 days of treatment (Barry, Ebell, & Hickner, 1997).

Commonly used medications include trimethoprim-sulfamethoxazole (TMP-SMZ, Bactrim, Septra) and nitrofurantoin (Macrodantin). Occasionally, medications such as ampicillin or amoxicillin are used, but *E. coli* has developed resistance to these agents. Trimethoprim-sulfamethoxazole is considered the medication of choice because it is most effective at reducing the number of fecal, vaginal, and periurethral bacteria.

Nitrofurantoin should not be used in patients with renal insufficiency because it is ineffective at glomerular filtration rates (GFRs) of less than 50 mL/min and may cause peripheral neuropathy. Pyridium, a urinary analgesic, may be prescribed to relieve the discomfort associated with the infection.

Regardless of the regimen prescribed, the patient is instructed to take *all* the doses prescribed, even if relief of symptoms occurs promptly. Longer medication courses are indicated for men, pregnant women, and women with pyelonephritis and with other types of complicated UTIs. In pregnant women, amoxicillin, ampicillin, or an oral cephalosporin is used for 7 to 10 days.

LONG-TERM PHARMACOLOGIC THERAPY

Although brief pharmacologic treatment of UTI for 3 days is usually adequate in women, infection recurs in about 20% of women treated for uncomplicated UTI (Bacheller & Bernstein, 1997). Infections that recur within 2 weeks after therapy (referred to as a *relapse*) do so because organisms of the original offending strain remain in the vagina. Relapses suggest that the source of bacteriuria may be the upper urinary tract or that initial treatment was inadequate or administered for too short a time. Recurrent infections in men are usually due to persistence of the same organism; further evaluation and treatment are indicated.

Reinfection of the female patient with new bacteria is the reason for more than 90% of recurrent UTIs in women. If the diagnostic evaluation reveals no structural abnormalities in the urinary tract, the woman with recurrent UTIs may be instructed to begin treatment on her own whenever symptoms occur and to contact the health care provider only when symptoms persist, fever occurs, or the number of treatment episodes exceeds four in a 6-month period. This patient may be taught to use dip-slide culture devices to detect bacteria.

If infection recurs after completing antimicrobial therapy, another short course (3 to 4 days) of full-dose antimicrobial therapy followed by a regular bedtime dose of antimicrobial medication may be prescribed. If there is no recurrence, medication is taken every other night for 6 to 7 months. Other options include a dose of an antimicrobial medication after sexual intercourse, a dose at bedtime, or a dose every other night or three times per week. Long-term use of antimicrobial agents decreases the risk of reinfection and may be indicated in patients with recurrent infections.

If recurrence is caused by persistent bacteria from preceding infections, the cause (ie, kidney stone, abscess), if known, must be treated. After treatment and sterilization of the urine, low-dose preventive therapy (trimethoprim with or without sulfamethoxazole) each night at bedtime is often prescribed.

NURSING PROCESS: THE PATIENT WITH LOWER URINARY TRACT INFECTION

Nursing care of the patient with lower UTI focuses on treating the underlying infection and preventing its recurrence.

Assessment

A history of signs and symptoms related to UTI is obtained from the patient with a suspected UTI. The presence of pain, frequency, urgency, and hesitancy and changes in urine are assessed, documented, and reported. The patient's usual pattern of voiding is assessed to detect factors that may predispose the patient to UTI. Infrequent emptying of the bladder, the association of symptoms of UTI with sexual intercourse, contraceptive practices, and personal hygiene are assessed. The patient's knowledge about prescribed antimicrobial medications and preventive health care measures is also assessed. Additionally, the patient's urine is assessed for volume, color, concentration, cloudiness, and odor, all of which are altered by bacteria in the urinary tract.

Diagnosis

Nursing Diagnoses

Based on the assessment data, the nursing diagnoses may include the following:

- Pain related to inflammation and infection of the urethra, bladder, and other urinary tract structures
- Knowledge deficit related to factors predisposing the patient to infection and recurrence, detection and prevention of recurrence, and pharmacologic therapy

Collaborative Problems/Potential Complications

Based on assessment data, potential complications may include the following:

- Renal failure due to extensive damage of kidney
- Sepsis

Planning and Goals

Major goals for the patient may include relief of pain and discomfort; increased knowledge of preventive measures and treatment modalities; and absence of complications.

Nursing Interventions

Relieving Pain

Pain associated with UTI is quickly relieved once effective antimicrobial therapy is initiated. Antispasmodic agents may also be useful in relieving bladder irritability and pain. Aspirin and applying heat to the perineum help relieve pain and spasm. The patient is encouraged to drink liberal amounts of fluids (water is the best choice) to promote renal blood flow and to flush the bacteria from the urinary tract. Urinary tract irritants (eg, coffee, tea, citrus, spices, colas, alcohol) are avoided. Frequent voiding (every 2 to 3 hours) is encouraged to empty the bladder completely because this can significantly lower urine bacterial counts, reduce urinary stasis, and prevent reinfection.

Monitoring and Managing Potential Complications

Early recognition of UTI and prompt treatment are essential to prevent recurrent infection and the possibility of complications, such as renal failure and sepsis. The goal of treatment is to prevent infection from progressing and causing permanent renal damage and renal failure. Thus, the patient must be taught to recognize early signs and symptoms, to test for bacteriuria, and to initiate treatment as prescribed. Appropriate antimicrobial therapy, liberal fluid intake, frequent voiding, and hygienic measures are commonly prescribed for managing UTI. The patient is instructed to notify the physician if fatigue, nausea, vomiting, or pruritus occurs. Periodic monitoring of renal function (creatinine clearance, blood urea nitrogen [BUN] and serum creatinine levels) may be indicated for patients with repeated UTI. If extensive renal damage does occur, dialysis may be necessary.

Patients with UTI, especially catheter-associated infection, are at increased risk for gram-negative sepsis. Indwelling catheters should be avoided if at all possible and removed at the earliest opportunity. If an indwelling catheter is necessary, however, specific nursing interventions are initiated to prevent infection. These include the following:

- Using strict aseptic technique during insertion of the smallest catheter possible
- Securing the catheter with tape to prevent movement
- Frequently inspecting urine color, odor, and consistency
- Performing meticulous daily perineal care with soap and water
- Maintaining a closed system
- Using the catheter's port to obtain specimens (see Chap. 40)

Careful assessment of vital signs and level of consciousness may warn of impending sepsis. Blood cultures that are positive for infection and elevated WBC counts are reported to the physician. At the same time, appropriate antibiotic therapy and increased fluid intake are prescribed (intravenous antibiotic therapy and fluids may be required). Preventing sepsis is key because the mortality rate for gram-negative sepsis is significant, especially in elderly patients.

Promoting Home and Community-Based Care

TEACHING PATIENTS SELF-CARE

In helping patients learn about and prevent or manage a recurrent UTI, the nurse needs to implement teaching that meets individual patient needs. For a detailed discussion of patient teaching interventions, see Preventing Recurrent Urinary Tract Infections.

Evaluation

Expected Outcomes

Expected outcomes may include:

1. Experiences relief of pain
   a. Reports absence of pain, urgency, dysuria, or hesitancy on voiding
   b. Takes analgesics and antibiotic agents as prescribed
2. Explains UTIs and their treatment
   a. Demonstrates knowledge of preventive measures and prescribed treatments
   b. Drinks 8 to 10 glasses of fluids daily
   c. Voids every 2 to 3 hours
   d. Voids urine that is clear and odorless
3. Experiences no complications
   a. Reports no symptoms of infection or renal failure (nausea, vomiting, fatigue, pruritus)
   b. Has normal BUN and serum creatinine levels, negative urine and blood cultures
   c. Exhibits normal vital signs and temperature; no signs of sepsis
   d. Maintains adequate urine output more than 30 mL/h

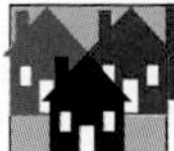

PATIENT EDUCATION AND HOME CARE

Preventing Recurrent Urinary Tract Infections

An objective of teaching about recurrent urinary tract infections (UTIs) is their prevention. Health-related behaviors that help prevent recurrent UTIs include implementing careful personal hygiene, increasing fluid intake to promote voiding and dilution of urine, urinating regularly and more frequently, and adhering to the therapeutic regimen.

Hygiene

- Shower rather than bathe in tub because bacteria in the bath water may enter the urethra.
- After each bowel movement, clean the perineum and urethral meatus from front to back. This will help reduce concentrations of pathogens at the urethral opening and, in women, the vaginal opening.

Fluid Intake

- Drink liberal amounts of fluids daily to flush out bacteria.
- Avoid coffee, tea, colas, alcohol, and other fluids that are urinary tract irritants.

Voiding Habits

- Void every 2 to 3 hours during the day and completely empty the bladder. This prevents overdistention of the bladder and compromised blood supply to the bladder wall. Both predispose the patient to UTI. Precautions expressly for women include the following:
  Void immediately after sexual intercourse.
  Take the prescribed single dose of an oral antimicrobial agent after sexual intercourse.

Therapy

- Take medication *exactly* as prescribed.
- If bacteria continue to appear in the urine, long-term antimicrobial therapy may be required to prevent colonization of the periurethral area and recurrence of infection. The medication should be taken after emptying the bladder just before going to bed to ensure adequate concentration of the medication during the overnight period.
- For recurrent infection, consider acidification of the urine through ascorbic acid (vitamin C), 1000 mg daily, or cranberry juice.
- If prescribed, test urine for bacteria with recommended test devices, such as dip-slides (Microstix), as follows:
  1. Wash around the urethral meatus several times, using different washcloths.
  2. Collect a midstream urine specimen.
  3. Remove a slide from its container, dip it into the urine sample, and return it to the container.
  4. Incubate the slide at room temperature according to product directions.
  5. Read the results by comparing the slide with the colony density chart that comes with the product.
  6. Begin therapy as directed, and complete the full prescribed course of medication.
  7. Notify the health care provider if fever occurs or if signs and symptoms persist.
- Consult the health care provider regularly for follow-up, recurrence of symptoms, or infections nonresponsive to treatment.

Upper Urinary Tract Infection: Acute Pyelonephritis

Pyelonephritis is a bacterial infection of the renal pelvis, tubules, and interstitial tissue of one or both kidneys. Upper UTIs are associated with antibody coating of the bacteria in the urine. (This occurs in the renal medulla; when the bacteria are excreted in the urine, the immunofluorescent test can detect the antibody coating.) Bacteria reach the bladder by means of the urethra and ascend to the kidney. Although the kidneys receive 20% to 25% of the cardiac output, bacteria rarely reach the kidney from the blood. Less than 3% of cases are due to hematogenous spread.

Pyelonephritis is frequently secondary to ureterovesical reflux, in which an incompetent ureterovesical valve allows the urine to back up (reflux) into the ureters (see Fig. 41-1). Urinary tract obstruction (which increases the susceptibility of the kidneys to infection), bladder tumors, strictures, benign prostatic hyperplasia, and urinary stones are among other causes. Pyelonephritis may be acute or chronic.

Patients with acute pyelonephritis usually have enlarged kidneys with interstitial infiltrations of inflammatory cells. Abscesses may be noted on the renal capsule and at the corticomedullary junction. Eventually, atrophy and destruction of tubules and the glomeruli may result. When pyelonephritis becomes chronic, the kidneys become scarred, contracted, and nonfunctioning.

Clinical Manifestations

The patient with acute pyelonephritis appears acutely ill with chills and fever, leukocytosis, bacteriuria and pyuria, flank pain, and CVA tenderness. In addition, symptoms of lower urinary tract involvement, such as dysuria and frequency, are common.

Assessment and Diagnostic Findings

An ultrasound or a CT scan study may be performed to locate any obstruction in the urinary tract. Relief of obstruction is essential to save the kidney from destruction. An IVP is rarely indicated during acute pyelonephritis because findings are normal in up to 75% of patients (Papanicolaou & Pfister, 1996). Radionuclide imaging with gallium citrate and indium-111–labeled WBCs may be useful to identify occult sites of infection that may not be visualized on CT scan or ultrasound. Urine culture and sensitivity tests are performed to determine the causative organism so that appropriate antimicrobial agents can be prescribed.

Medical Management

Patients with acute uncomplicated pyelonephritis are usually treated as outpatients if they are not dehydrated, not experiencing nausea or vomiting, and not showing signs or symptoms of sepsis. In addition, they must be responsible and reliable to ensure that all medications are taken as prescribed. Other patients, including all pregnant women, should be hospitalized for at least 2 or 3 days of parenteral therapy. Oral agents may be substituted once the patient is afebrile and showing clinical improvement.

Pharmacologic Therapy

For outpatients, a 2-week course of antibiotics is recommended because renal parenchymal disease is more difficult to eradicate than bladder mucosal infections. Commonly prescribed agents include trimethoprim-sulfamethoxazole, ciprofloxacin, gentamicin with or without ampicillin, or a third-generation cephalosporin.

A possible problem in acute pyelonephritis treatment is a chronic or recurring symptomless infection persisting for months or years. After the initial antibiotic regimen, the patient may need antibiotic therapy for up to 6 weeks if evidence of a relapse is seen. A follow-up urine culture is done 2 weeks after completion of antibiotic therapy to document clearing of the infection.

Upper Urinary Tract Infection: Chronic Pyelonephritis

Repeated bouts of acute pyelonephritis may lead to chronic pyelonephritis. Evidence suggests that chronic pyelonephritis is now a less common cause of **end-stage renal disease** (ESRD).

Clinical Manifestations

The patient with chronic pyelonephritis usually has no symptoms of infection unless an acute exacerbation occurs. Noticeable signs and symptoms may include fatigue, headache, poor appetite, polyuria, excessive thirst, and weight loss. Persistent and recurring infection may produce progressive scarring of the kidney, with renal failure the end result.

Assessment and Diagnostic Findings

The extent of the disease is assessed by intravenous urogram and measurements of creatinine clearance and BUN and creatinine levels. Bacteria, if detected in the urine, is eradicated if possible.

Complications

Complications of chronic pyelonephritis include ESRD (from progressive loss of nephrons secondary to chronic inflammation and scarring), hypertension, and formation of kidney stones (from chronic infection with urea-splitting organisms).

Pharmacologic Therapy

The choice of an antimicrobial agent is based on which pathogen is identified through urine culture. If the urine cannot be made bacteria free, nitrofurantoin or trimethoprim-sulfamethoxazole may be used to suppress bacterial growth. Impaired renal function alters the excretion of antimicrobial agents and necessitates careful monitoring of renal function, especially if the medications are potentially toxic to the kidneys.

Nursing Management

The patient may require hospitalization or may be treated as an outpatient. When the patient is hospitalized, fluid intake and output are carefully measured and recorded. Unless contraindicated, fluids are encouraged (3–4 L/day) to dilute the urine, decrease burning on urination, and prevent dehydration. The nurse assesses the patient's temperature every 4 hours and administers antipyretics and antibiotics as prescribed. Often the patient is more comfortable on bedrest during the acute phase of the illness.

Patient teaching focuses on prevention of urinary tract infections by consuming an adequate fluid intake, emptying the bladder regularly, and performing recommended perineal hygiene.

PRIMARY GLOMERULAR DISEASES

A variety of diseases can affect the glomerular capillaries, including acute and chronic **glomerulonephritis**, rapidly progressive glomerulonephritis, and **nephrotic syndrome**. In all of these disorders, the glomerular capillaries are primarily involved. Antigen–antibody complexes form in the blood and become trapped in the glomerular capillaries (the filtering portion of the kidney), inducing an inflammatory response. IgG, the major immunoglobulin (antibody) found in the blood, can be detected in the glomerular capillary walls. The major clinical manifestations of glomerular injury include proteinuria, hematuria, decreased GFR, and alterations in excretion of sodium (leading to edema and hypertension).

Acute Glomerulonephritis

Glomerulonephritis is an inflammation of the glomerular capillaries. Acute glomerulonephritis is primarily a disease of children older than 2 years of age; however, it can occur at nearly any age.

Pathophysiology

In most cases of acute glomerulonephritis, there is a history of a group A beta-hemolytic streptococcal infection of the throat preceding the onset of glomerulonephritis by 2 to 3 weeks. It may also follow impetigo (infection of the skin) and acute viral infections (upper respiratory infections, mumps, varicella zoster virus, Epstein-Barr virus, hepatitis B, and human immunodeficiency virus infection). In some patients, antigens outside the body (eg, medications, foreign serum) initiate the process, resulting in the complexes being deposited in the glomeruli. In other patients, the kidney tissue itself serves as the inciting antigen (Fig. 41-3).

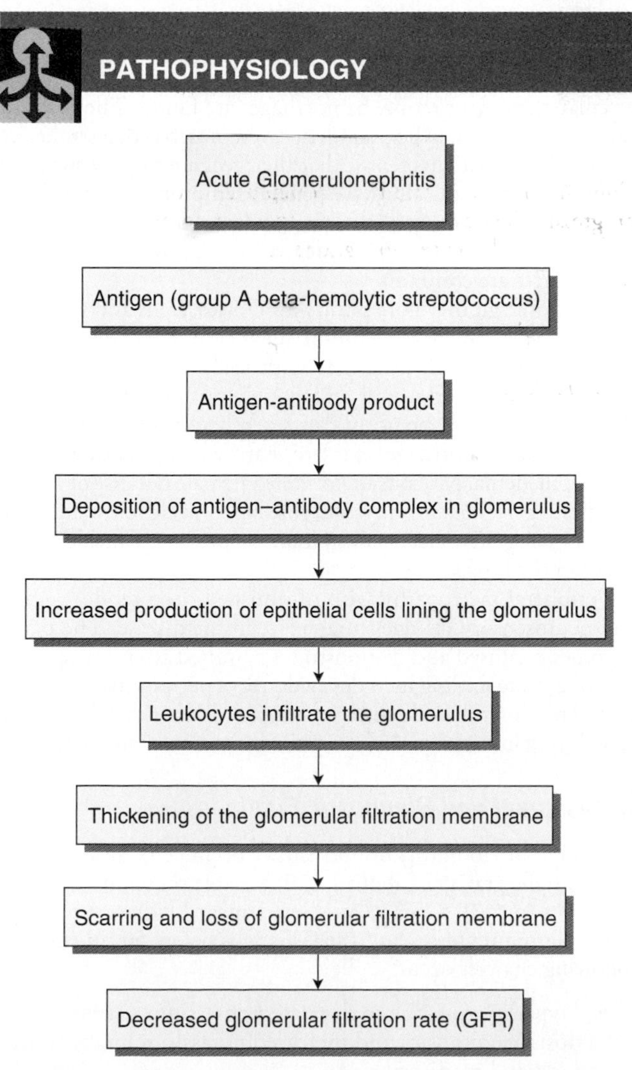

FIGURE 41•3 Sequence of events in acute glomerulonephritis.

Clinical Manifestations

The primary presenting feature of acute glomerulonephritis is hematuria (blood in the urine), which may be microscopic (identifiable through microscopic examination) or macroscopic or gross (visible to the eye). The urine may appear cola-colored because of RBCs and protein plugs or casts. (RBC casts indicate glomerular injury.) Glomerulonephritis may be so mild, however, that hematuria is discovered incidentally through a routine microscopic urinalysis, or the disease may be so severe that the patient has acute renal failure with oliguria. Acute glomerulonephritis typically has an abrupt onset preceded by a latent period between the streptococcal infection and the first indications of renal involvement averaging 10 days.

Proteinuria, primarily albumin, which is present, is due to increased permeability of the glomerular membrane. BUN and serum creatinine levels may rise as urine output drops. The patient may be anemic primarily from fluid retention.

Some degree of edema and hypertension is noted in 75% of patients (Glassock, Cohen, & Adler, 1996). In the more severe form of the disease, the patient also complains of headache, malaise, and flank pain. Tenderness over the CVA is common. Elderly patients may have evidence of circulatory overload with dyspnea, engorged neck veins, cardiomegaly, and pulmonary edema. Atypical symptoms include confusion, somnolence, and seizures, which are often confused with symptoms of a primary neurologic disorder.

Assessment and Diagnostic Findings

In acute glomerulonephritis, the kidneys become large, swollen, and congested. All renal tissues—glomeruli, tubules, and blood vessels—are affected to varying degrees. Electron microscopy and immunofluorescent analysis of the immune mechanism help identify the nature of the lesion; however, a kidney biopsy may be needed for definitive diagnosis.

Serial determinations of antistreptolysin O or anti-DNase B titers are usually elevated in poststreptococcal glomerulonephritis. Serum complement levels may be decreased but generally return to normal within 2 to 8 weeks. More than half of patients with IgA nephropathy (the most common type of primary glomerulonephritis) have an elevated serum IgA and a normal complement level.

If the patient improves, the amount of urine increases, and the urinary protein and sediment diminish. Usually, more than 90% of children recover. The percentage of recovery for adults is not well established but is probably about 70%. Some patients become severely uremic within weeks and require dialysis for survival. Others, after a period of apparent recovery, insidiously develop chronic glomerulonephritis.

Complications

Complications of acute glomerulonephritis include hypertensive encephalopathy, congestive heart failure, and pulmonary edema. Hypertensive encephalopathy is considered a medical emergency, and therapy is directed toward reducing the blood pressure without impairing renal function.

Rapidly progressive glomerulonephritis is a rapid and progressive decline in renal function. Without treatment, it results in ESRD in a matter of weeks or months. Signs and symptoms are similar to those of acute glomerulonephritis (hematuria and proteinuria), but the course of the disease is more severe and rapid. Crescent-shaped cells accumulate in Bowman's space, disrupting the filtering surface. Plasma exchange (plasmapheresis) and treatment with high-dose steroids and cytotoxic agents have been used to reduce the inflammatory response. Dialysis is initiated in acute glomerulonephritis if manifestations of uremia are severe. With aggressive treatment, the prognosis for patients with rapidly progressive glomerulonephritis is greatly improved.

Medical Management

Management consists primarily of treating symptoms, attempting to preserve kidney function, and treating complications promptly.

Pharmacologic therapy depends on the cause of acute glomerulonephritis. If residual streptococcal infection is suspected, penicillin is the agent of choice; however, other antibiotics may be prescribed. Corticosteroids and immunosuppressive agents may be prescribed for patients with rapidly progressive acute glomerulonephritis but in most cases of poststreptococcal acute glomerulonephritis, these medications are of no value and may actually worsen the fluid retention and hypertension.

Dietary protein is restricted when renal insufficiency and nitrogen retention (elevated BUN) develop. Sodium is restricted when the patient has hypertension, edema, and congestive heart failure. Loop diuretics and antihypertensive agents may be prescribed to control hypertension. Prolonged bedrest has little value and does not improve or alter long-term outcomes.

Nursing Management

Although most patients with acute uncomplicated glomerulonephritis are treated as outpatients, nursing care is important no matter what the setting. In a hospital setting, carbohydrates are given liberally to provide energy and reduce the catabolism of protein. Intake and output are carefully measured and recorded. Fluids are given according to the patient's fluid losses and daily body weight. Insensible fluid loss through the respiratory and gastrointestinal tracts (500 to 1000 mL) is considered when estimating fluid loss. Diuresis begins about 1 week after the onset of symptoms with a decrease in edema and blood pressure. Proteinuria and microscopic hematuria may persist for many months, and some patients may go on to develop chronic glomerulonephritis.

Other nursing interventions focus primarily on patient education for safe and effective self-care at home.

PROMOTING HOME AND COMMUNITY-BASED CARE

Teaching Patients Self-Care. Patient education is directed toward maintaining kidney function and preventing complications. Fluid and diet restrictions must be reviewed with the patient to avoid worsening of edema and hypertension. The patient is instructed to notify the physician if symptoms of renal failure occur (eg, fatigue, nausea, vomiting, diminishing urinary output) or at the first sign of any infection. Information is given verbally and in writing.

Continuing Care. The importance of follow-up evaluations of blood pressure, urinalysis for protein, and serum BUN and creatinine levels to determine if the disease has progressed is stressed to the patient. A referral to the home care nurse may be indicated and provides an opportunity for careful assessment of the patient's progress and detection of the onset of early symptoms of renal insufficiency. If corticosteroids, cytotoxic agents, or antibiotics are prescribed, the home care nurse or nurse in the outpatient setting uses the opportunity to review the dosage, desired actions, and side effects of medications and the precautions to be followed.

Chronic Glomerulonephritis

Pathophysiology

Chronic glomerulonephritis may be due to repeated episodes of acute glomerulonephritis, hypertensive nephrosclerosis, hyperlipidemia, chronic tubulointerstitial injury, or hemodynamically mediated glomerular sclerosis. The kidneys are reduced to as little as one fifth their normal size (consisting largely of fibrous tissue). The cortex shrinks to a layer 1 to 2 mm in thickness or less. Bands of scar tissue distort the remaining cortex, making the surface of the kidney rough and irregular. Numerous glomeruli and their tubules become scarred, and the branches of the renal artery are thickened. The result is severe glomerular damage that results in ESRD.

Clinical Manifestations

The symptoms of chronic glomerulonephritis are variable. Some patients with severe disease have no symptoms at all for many years. Their condition may accidentally be discovered when hypertension or elevated BUN and serum creatinine levels are discovered. The diagnosis may be suggested during a routine eye examination when vascular changes or retinal hemorrhages are found. The first indication of disease may be a sudden, severe nosebleed, a stroke, or a seizure. Many patients report that their feet are slightly swollen at night. Most patients also have general symptoms, such as loss of weight and strength, increasing irritability, and an increased need to urinate at night (nocturia). Headaches, dizziness, and digestive disturbances are common.

As chronic glomerulonephritis progresses, signs and symptoms of renal insufficiency and chronic renal failure may develop. The patient appears poorly nourished with a yellow-gray pigmentation of the skin and periorbital and peripheral (dependent) edema. Blood pressure may be normal or severely elevated. Retinal findings include hemorrhage, exudate, narrowed tortuous arterioles, and papilledema. Mucous membranes are pale because of anemia. Cardiomegaly, a gallop rhythm, distended neck veins, and other signs of congestive heart failure may be present. Crackles can be heard in the lungs.

Peripheral neuropathy with diminished deep tendon reflexes and neurosensory changes occurs late in the disease. The patient becomes confused and demonstrates a limited attention span. An additional late finding includes evidence of pericarditis with a pericardial friction rub and pulsus paradoxus (difference in blood pressure during inspiration and expiration of greater than 10 mm Hg).

Assessment and Diagnostic Findings

A number of laboratory abnormalities occur. Urinalysis reveals a fixed specific gravity of about 1.010, variable proteinuria, and urinary casts (protein plugs secreted by damaged kidney tubules). As renal failure progresses and the GFR falls below 50 mL/min, the following changes occur:

- Hyperkalemia due to decreased potassium excretion, acidosis, catabolism, and increased potassium intake from food and medications.
- Metabolic acidosis from decreased acid secretion by the kidney and inability to regenerate bicarbonate

- Anemia secondary to decreased erythropoiesis (production of RBCs)
- Hypoalbuminemia with edema secondary to protein loss through damaged glomerular membrane
- Increased serum phosphorus level due to decreased renal excretion of phosphorus
- Decreased serum calcium level (calcium binds to phosphorus to compensate for elevated serum phosphorus levels)
- Hypermagnesemia from decreased excretion and inadvertent ingestion of antacids containing magnesium
- Impaired nerve conduction due to electrolyte abnormalities and uremia

Chest x-rays may show cardiac enlargement and pulmonary edema. The electrocardiogram may be normal or may indicate left ventricular hypertrophy associated with hypertension and signs of electrolyte disturbances, such as tall, tented (or peaked) T waves associated with hyperkalemia.

Medical Management

Symptoms guide the course of treatment for the patient with chronic glomerulonephritis. If the patient has hypertension, the blood pressure is reduced with sodium and water restriction, antihypertensives, or both. Weight is monitored daily, and diuretics are prescribed to treat fluid overload. Proteins of high biologic value (dairy products, eggs, meats) are provided to promote good nutritional status. Adequate calories are also important to spare protein for tissue growth and repair. UTIs must be treated promptly to prevent further renal damage.

Initiation of dialysis is considered early in the course of the disease to keep the patient in optimal physical condition, prevent fluid and electrolyte imbalances, and minimize the risk of complications of renal failure. The course of dialysis is smoother if treatment begins before the patient develops significant complications.

Nursing Management

If the patient is hospitalized or eligible for home visits, the nurse observes for changes in fluid and electrolyte status and for signs of deterioration of renal function. Changes in fluid and electrolyte status and in cardiac and neurologic status are reported promptly to the physician. Anxiety levels are often extremely high for both the patient and family. Throughout the course of the disease and treatment, the nurse gives emotional support by providing opportunities for the patient and family to verbalize their concerns, have their questions answered, and explore their options.

PROMOTING HOME AND COMMUNITY-BASED CARE

Teaching Patients Self-Care. The nurse has a major role in teaching the patient and family about the prescribed treatment plan and the risks of noncompliance. Instructions to the patient include explanations and scheduling for follow-up evaluations: blood pressure, urinalysis for protein and casts, and blood studies of BUN and creatinine levels. If long-term dialysis is needed, the patient and family are taught about the procedure, how to care for the access site, dietary restrictions, and other necessary lifestyle modifications. See Chapter 40 for a detailed checklist of teaching topics for the dialysis patient.

Periodic hospitalization, visits to the outpatient clinic or office, and home care referrals provide the nurse in each setting with the opportunity for careful assessment of the patient's progress and continued education about problems to report to the primary health care provider. Reportable problems include worsening signs of renal failure, such as nausea, vomiting, and diminished urine output. Specific teaching may include explanations about recommended diet and fluid modifications and medications (purpose, desired effects, side effects, dosage, and administration schedule).

Continuing Care. Periodic evaluation of creatinine clearance and serum BUN and creatinine levels is carried out to assess residual renal function and the need for dialysis or transplantation. If dialysis is initiated, the patient and family will require considerable assistance and support in dealing with therapy and its long-term implications. See Chapter 40 for a discussion of dialysis. (Kidney transplantation is discussed later in this chapter.)

Nephrotic Syndrome

Nephrotic syndrome is a primary glomerular disease characterized by the following:

- Marked increase in protein in the urine (proteinuria)
- Decrease in albumin in the blood (hypoalbuminemia)
- Edema
- High serum cholesterol and low-density lipoproteins (hyperlipidemia)

The syndrome is apparent in any condition that seriously damages the glomerular capillary membrane and results in increased glomerular permeability.

Pathophysiology

Nephrotic syndrome is characterized by the loss of plasma protein, particularly albumin, in the urine. Although the liver is capable of increasing the production of albumin, it is unable to keep up with the daily loss of albumin through the kidneys. Thus, hypoalbuminemia results (Fig. 41-4).

The nephrotic syndrome can occur with almost any intrinsic renal disease or systemic disease that affects the glomerulus. Although generally considered a disorder of childhood, nephrotic syndrome does occur in adults, including the elderly. Causes include chronic glomerulonephritis, diabetes mellitus with intercapillary glomerulosclerosis, amyloidosis of the kidney, systemic lupus erythematosus, multiple myeloma, and renal vein thrombosis.

Clinical Manifestations

The major manifestation of nephrotic syndrome is edema. It is usually soft and pitting and is most commonly found around the eyes (periorbital), in dependent areas (sacrum, ankles, and hands), and in the abdomen (ascites). Other symptoms, including as malaise, headache, irritability, and fatigue, are common.

Assessment and Diagnostic Findings

Proteinuria (predominately albumin) exceeding 3 to 3.5 g/day is sufficient for diagnosis of nephrotic syndrome. Protein electrophoresis and immunoelectrophoresis may be performed on the urine to categorize the type of proteinuria. The urine may also contain increased numbers of WBCs as well as granular and epithelial casts. Needle biopsy of the kidney may be performed for histologic examination of renal tissue to confirm the diagnosis.

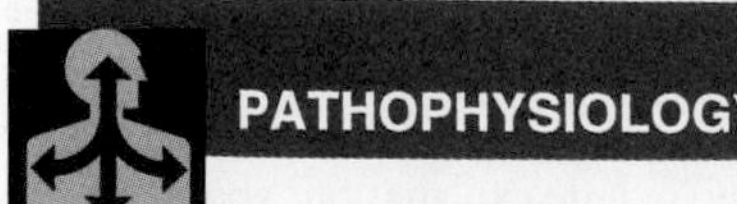

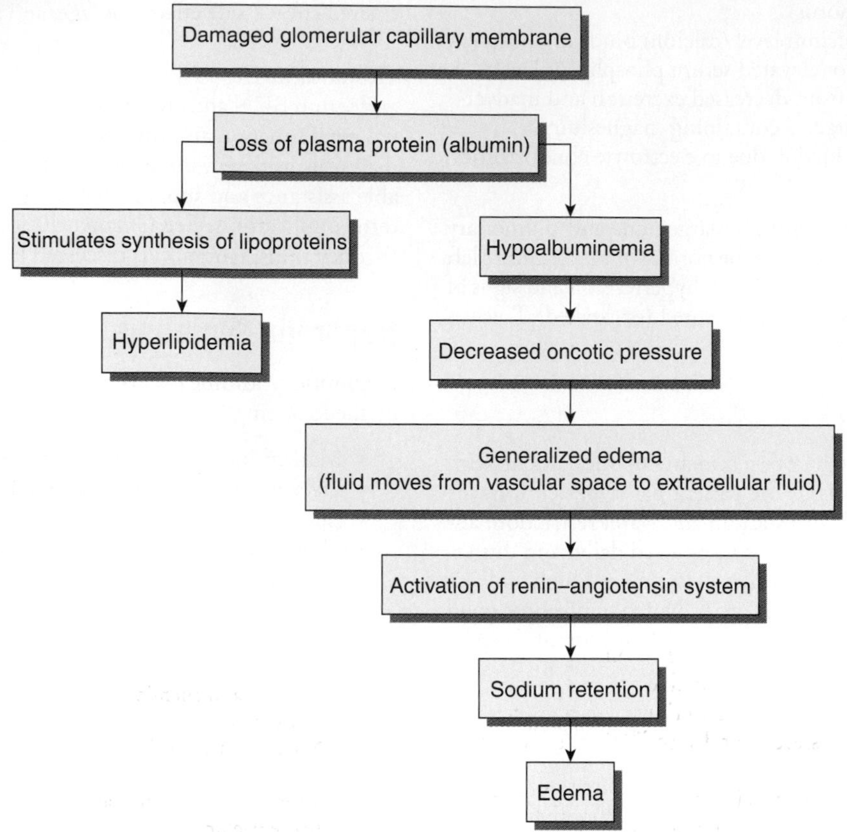

FIGURE 41•4 Sequence of events, in nephrotic syndrome.

Complications

Complications of nephrotic syndrome include infection (due to a deficient immune response), thromboembolism (especially of the renal vein), pulmonary emboli, acute renal failure (due to hypovolemia), and accelerated atherosclerosis (due to hyperlipidemia).

Medical Management

The objective of management is to preserve renal function. Diuretics may be prescribed for the patient with severe edema; however, caution must be used because of the risk of reducing the plasma volume to the point of impaired circulation with subsequent prerenal acute renal failure. The use of angiotensin-converting enzyme (ACE) inhibitors in combination with diuretics often reduces the degree of proteinuria but may take 4 to 6 weeks to be effective.

Other medications used in treating nephrotic syndrome include antineoplastic agents (cyclophosphamide [Cytoxan]) or immunosuppressive agents (azathioprine [Imuran], chlorambucil [Leukeran], or cyclosporine). It may be necessary to repeat treatment with corticosteroids if relapse occurs. Treatment of the associated hyperlipidemia is controversial. The usual medications used to treat hyperlipidemia are often ineffective or have serious consequences, including muscle injury.

The patient may be placed on a low sodium, liberal potassium, low saturated-fat diet. Protein intake should be about 0.8 g/kg/day with emphasis on high biologic proteins (dairy products, eggs, meats).

Nursing Management

In the early stages, the nursing management is similar to that of the patient with acute glomerulonephritis, but as the disease worsens, management is similar to that of the patient with chronic renal failure (see the section that follows). The patient who is receiving corticosteroids or cyclosporine requires instructions about the medications and signs and symptoms that warrant reporting to the physician. Dietary instructions may also be necessary.

RENAL FAILURE

Renal failure results when the kidneys are unable to remove the body's metabolic wastes or perform their regulatory functions. The substances normally eliminated in the urine accumulate in the body fluids as a result of impaired renal excretion and lead to a disruption in endocrine and metabolic functions as well as fluid, electrolyte, and acid–base disturbances. Renal failure is a systemic disease and is a final common pathway of many different kidney and urinary tract diseases. Each year, an estimated 50,000 Americans die from irreversible kidney failure.

Acute Renal Failure

Pathophysiology

Acute renal failure is a sudden and almost complete loss of kidney function (decreased GFR) over a period of hours to days. Although acute renal failure is often thought of as a problem seen only in hospitalized patients, it may occur in the outpatient setting as well. Acute renal failure manifests as either oliguria, anuria, or normal urine volume. *Oliguria* (less than 400 mL/day of urine) is the most common clinical situation seen in acute renal failure; *anuria* (less than 50 mL/day of urine) and normal urine output are not as common.

Regardless of the volume of urine excreted, the patient with acute renal failure experiences rising serum creatinine and BUN levels and retention of other metabolic waste products (*azotemia*) normally excreted by the kidneys.

CATEGORIES OF ACUTE RENAL FAILURE

Three major categories of conditions cause acute renal failure: prerenal (hypoperfusion of kidney), intrarenal (actual damage to kidney tissue), and postrenal (obstruction to urine flow).

- Prerenal conditions occur as a result of impaired blood flow that leads to *hypoperfusion* of the kidney and a drop in the GFR. Common clinical situations are volume-depletion states (hemorrhage or gastrointestinal losses), impaired cardiac performance (myocardial infarction, congestive heart failure, or cardiogenic shock), and vasodilation (sepsis or anaphylaxis).
- Intrarenal causes of acute renal failure are the result of actual *parenchymal damage* to the glomeruli or kidney tubules. Conditions such as burns, crush injuries, and infections, as well as nephrotoxic agents, may lead to **acute tubular necrosis** and cessation of renal function. With burns and crush injuries, myoglobin (a protein released from muscle when injury occurs) and hemoglobin are liberated, causing renal toxicity, ischemia, or both. Severe transfusion reactions may also cause intrarenal failure; hemoglobin is released through hemolysis, filters through the glomeruli and becomes concentrated in the kidney tubules to such a degree that precipitation of hemoglobin occurs. Medications may also predispose a patient to intrarenal damage, especially nonsteroidal anti-inflammatory drugs (NSAIDs) and ACE inhibitors. These medications interfere with the normal autoregulatory mechanisms of the kidney and may cause hypoperfusion and eventual ischemia.
- Postrenal causes of acute renal failure are usually the result of an *obstruction* somewhere distal to the kidney. Pressure rises in the kidney tubules; eventually, the GFR decreases. Common causes of acute renal failure are summarized in Chart 41-2.

Although the exact pathogenesis of acute renal failure and oliguria is not always known, many times there is a clear-cut underlying problem. Some of these factors may be reversible if identified and treated promptly, before kidney function is impaired. This is true of the following conditions that reduce blood flow to the kidney and impair kidney function: (1) hypovolemia; (2) hypotension; (3) reduced cardiac output and congestive heart failure; (4) obstruction of the kidney or lower urinary tract by tumor, blood clot, or kidney stone; and (5) bilateral obstruction of the renal arteries or veins. If these conditions are treated and corrected before the kidneys are permanently damaged, the increased BUN and creatinine levels, oliguria, and other signs associated with acute renal failure may be reversed.

CHART 41•2 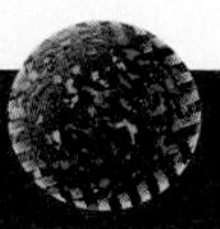 **Causes of Acute Renal Failure**

Prerenal Failure

- Volume depletion resulting from:
  - Hemorrhage
  - Renal losses (diuretics, osmotic diuresis)
  - Gastrointestinal losses (vomiting, diarrhea, nasogastric suction)
- Impaired cardiac efficiency resulting from:
  - Myocardial infarction
  - Congestive heart failure
  - Dysrhythmias
  - Cardiogenic shock
- Vasodilation resulting from:
  - Sepsis
  - Anaphylaxis
  - Antihypertensive medications or other drugs that cause vasodilation

Intrarenal Failure

- Prolonged renal ischemia resulting from:
  - Pigment nephropathy (associated with the breakdown of blood cells containing pigments that in turn occlude kidney structures)
  - Myoglobinuria (trauma, crush injuries, burns)
  - Hemoglobinuria (transfusion reaction, hemolytic anemia)
- Nephrotoxic agents such as
  - Aminoglycoside antibiotics (gentamicin, tobramycin)
  - Radiopaque contrast agents
  - Heavy metals (lead, mercury)
  - Solvents and chemicals (ethylene glycol, carbon tetrachloride, arsenic)
  - Nonsteroidal anti-inflammatory drugs (NSAIDs)
  - Angiotensin-converting enzyme inhibitors (ACE inhibitors)
- Infectious processes such as:
  - Acute pyelonephritis
  - Acute glomerulonephritis

Postrenal failure

- Urinary tract obstruction, including:
  - Calculi (stones)
  - Tumors
  - Benign prostatic hyperplasia
  - Strictures
  - Blood clots

PHASES OF ACUTE RENAL FAILURE

There are four clinical phases of acute renal failure: an initiation period, a period of oliguria, a period of diuresis, and a period of recovery.

The *initiation period* begins with the initial insult and ends when oliguria develops. The *period of oliguria* is accompanied by a rise in the serum concentration of substances usually excreted by the kidneys (urea, creatinine, uric acid, organic acids, and the intracellular cations—potassium and magnesium). The minimum amount of urine needed to rid the body of normal metabolic waste

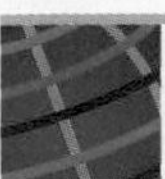

TABLE 41•1 **Comparing Types of Acute Renal Failure**

Characteristics	Types: PRERENAL	INTRARENAL	POSTRENAL
Etiology	Hypoperfusion	Parenchymal damage	Obstruction
Blood urea nitrogen value	Increased (out of normal 20 : 1 proportion to creatinine)	Increased	Increased
Creatinine	Increased	Increased	Increased
Urine output	Decreased	Varies, often decreased	Varies, may be decreased, or sudden anuria
Urine sodium	Decreased to <20 mEq/L	Increased to >40 mEq/L	Varies, often decreased to 20 mEq/L or less
Urinary sediment	Normal, few hyaline casts	Abnormal casts and debris	Usually normal
Urine osmolality	Increased to 500 mOsm	About 350 mOsm similar to serum	Varies, increased or equal to serum
Urine specific gravity	Increased	Low normal, 1.010	Varies

products is 400 mL. It is in this phase that uremic symptoms first appear and that life-threatening conditions such as hyperkalemia develop.

Some patients can have a decrease in renal function with increasing nitrogen retention, yet actually excrete normal amounts of urine (2 L/day or more). This is the nonoliguric form of renal failure and occurs predominantly after nephrotoxic antibiotics are administered to the patient; it may occur with burns, traumatic injury, and use of halogenated anesthesia.

In the *period of diuresis*, the third phase, the patient experiences a gradually increasing urinary output, which signals that glomerular filtration has started to recover. Laboratory values stop rising and eventually begin a downward trend. Although the volume of urinary output may reach normal or elevated levels, renal function may still be markedly abnormal. Uremic symptoms may still be present. Therefore, the need for expert medical and nursing management continues. The patient must be observed closely for dehydration during this phase; if dehydration occurs, the uremic symptoms are likely to increase.

The *period of recovery* signals the improvement of renal function and may take 3 to 12 months. Laboratory values return to the patient's normal level. Although there is often a permanent 1% to 3% reduction in the GFR, it is not clinically significant.

Clinical Manifestations

Almost every system of the body is affected when there is failure of the normal renal regulatory mechanisms. The patient may appear critically ill and lethargic, with persistent nausea, vomiting, and diarrhea. The skin and mucous membranes are dry from dehydration, and the breath may have the odor of urine (uremic fetor). Central nervous system manifestations include drowsiness, headache, muscle twitching, and seizures. Table 41-1 summarizes common clinical findings for all three categories of acute renal failure.

Assessment and Diagnostic Findings

CHANGES IN URINE

The urinary output varies (scanty to normal volume), hematuria may be present, and the urine has a low specific gravity (1.010, compared with a normal value of 1.015 to 1.025). Patients with prerenal azotemia have a decreased amount of sodium in the urine (below 20 mEq/L) and normal urinary sediment. Those patients with intrarenal azotemia usually have urinary sodium levels greater than 40 mEq/L with casts and other cellular debris. Urinary casts are mucoproteins secreted by the renal tubules whenever inflammation is present.

INCREASED BLOOD UREA NITROGEN AND CREATININE LEVELS (AZOTEMIA)

The BUN level rises steadily at a rate dependent on the degree of catabolism (breakdown of protein), renal perfusion, and protein intake. Serum creatinine rises in conjunction with glomerular damage. Serum creatinine levels are useful in monitoring kidney function and disease progression.

HYPERKALEMIA

With a decline in the GFR, the patient is unable to excrete potassium normally. Patients with oliguria and anuria are at greater risk for hyperkalemia than those without oliguria. Protein catabolism results in the release of cellular potassium into the body fluids, causing severe hyperkalemia (high serum K^+ levels). Hyperkalemia may lead to dysrhythmias and cardiac arrest. Sources of potassium include normal tissue catabolism, dietary intake, blood in the gastrointestinal tract, or blood transfusion and other sources (intravenous infusions, potassium penicillin, and extracellular shift in response to metabolic acidosis).

METABOLIC ACIDOSIS

Patients with acute oliguria cannot eliminate the daily metabolic load of acid-type substances produced by the normal metabolic processes. In addition, normal renal buffering mechanisms fail. This is reflected by a fall in the serum CO_2-combining power and blood pH. Thus, progressive metabolic acidosis accompanies renal failure.

CALCIUM AND PHOSPHORUS ABNORMALITIES

There may be an increase in serum phosphate concentrations; serum calcium levels may be low in response to decreased absorption of calcium from the intestine and as a compensatory mechanism for the elevated serum phosphate levels.

ANEMIA

Anemia inevitably accompanies acute renal failure due to reduced erythropoietin production, uremic gastrointestinal lesions, reduced RBC life span, and blood loss, usually from the gastrointestinal

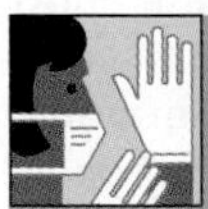

HEALTH PROMOTION AND ILLNESS PREVENTION

Interventions to Prevent Acute Renal Failure

1. Provide adequate hydration to patients at risk for dehydration:
   - Surgical patients before, during, and after surgery
   - Patients undergoing intensive diagnostic studies requiring fluid restriction and contrast agents, (eg, barium enema, intravenous pyelograms), especially elderly patients who may not have adequate renal reserve
   - Patients with neoplastic disorders or disorders of metabolism (ie, gout) and those receiving chemotherapy.
2. Prevent and treat shock promptly with blood and fluid replacement.
3. Monitor central venous and arterial pressures and hourly urine output of critically ill patients to detect the onset of renal failure as early as possible.
4. Treat hypotension promptly.
5. Continually assess renal function (urine output, laboratory values) when appropriate.
6. Take precautions to ensure that the appropriate blood is administered to the correct patient in order to avoid severe transfusion reactions, which can precipitate renal failure.
7. Prevent and treat infections promptly. Infections can produce progressive renal damage.
8. Pay special attention to wounds, burns, and other precursors of sepsis.
9. Give meticulous care to patients with indwelling catheters to prevent infections from ascending in the urinary tract. Remove catheters as soon as possible.
10. To prevent toxic drug effects, closely monitor dosage, duration of use, and blood levels of all medications metabolized or excreted by the kidneys.

tract. With the parenteral form of erythropoietin (Epogen) now available, anemia is not the major problem it once was.

Prevention

A careful history is obtained to determine whether the patient has been taking potentially nephrotoxic antibiotic agents or has been exposed to environmental toxins. The kidneys are especially susceptible to the adverse effects of medications for several reasons. They receive a large blood flow (25% of the cardiac output at rest, and the entire blood volume circulates through the kidneys about 14 times a minute); therefore, the kidneys are repeatedly exposed to substances in the blood. In addition, the kidney is the major excretory organ for many toxic substances, and during the normal urine concentration process, these substances increase in concentration and can be toxic to the kidneys. Therefore, in patients taking potentially nephrotoxic medications (aminoglycosides, gentamicin, tobramycin, colistimethate, polymyxin B, amphotericin B, vancomycin, amikacin, cyclosporine), renal function should be monitored closely. Ideally, blood should be drawn for determining baseline and monitoring serum BUN and creatinine levels by 24 hours after initiation of medication therapy and at least twice a week while the patient is receiving these medications.

Any agent that reduces renal blood flow (eg, chronic analgesic use) may cause renal insufficiency. Chronic analgesic use, particularly with NSAIDs, may cause interstitial nephritis and papillary necrosis. Patients with congestive heart failure or cirrhosis with ascites are at particular risk for NSAID-induced renal failure. Increased age, preexisting renal disease, and the administration of several nephrotoxic agents simultaneously increase the risk for kidney damage.

Management of acute renal failure is expensive and complex, and even when optimal, the mortality rate remains high. Therefore, prevention of acute renal failure is key.

Medical Management

The kidney has a remarkable ability to recover from insult. Therefore, the objectives of treatment of acute renal failure are to restore normal chemical balance and prevent complications until repair of renal tissue and restoration of renal function can take place. A search is made to identify, treat, and eliminate any possible cause of damage. Prerenal azotemia is treated by optimizing renal perfusion, whereas postrenal failure is treated by relieving the obstruction. Treatment of intrarenal azotemia is supportive, with removal of causative agents, aggressive management of prerenal and postrenal failure, and avoidance of associated risk factors. Shock and infection, if present, are treated. Overall, medical management includes maintaining fluid balance, avoiding fluid excesses, or possibly, performing dialysis.

Maintenance of fluid balance is based on daily body weight, serial measurements of central venous pressure, serum and urine concentrations, fluid losses, blood pressure, and the clinical status of the patient. The parenteral and oral intake and the output of urine, gastric drainage, stools, wound drainage, and perspiration are calculated and are used as the basis for fluid replacement. The insensible fluid lost through the skin and lungs and produced through the normal metabolic processes is also considered in fluid management.

Fluid excesses can be detected by the clinical findings of dyspnea, tachycardia, and distended neck veins. The lungs are auscultated for signs of moist crackles. Because pulmonary edema may be caused by excessive administration of parenteral fluids, extreme caution must be used to prevent fluid overload. The development of generalized edema is assessed by examining the presacral and pretibial areas several times daily. Mannitol, furosemide, or ethacrynic acid may be prescribed to initiate a diuresis and prevent or minimize subsequent renal failure.

Adequate blood flow to the kidneys in patients with prerenal causes of acute renal failure may be restored by intravenous fluids or blood-product transfusions. If acute renal failure is caused by hypovolemia secondary to hypoproteinemia, an infusion of albumin may be prescribed. Dialysis may be initiated to prevent serious complications of acute renal failure, such as hyperkalemia, severe metabolic acidosis, pericarditis, and pulmonary edema. Dialysis corrects many biochemical abnormalities; allows for liberalization of fluid, protein, and sodium intake; diminishes bleeding tendencies; and may help wound healing. Hemodialysis, peritoneal dialysis, or any of the new continuous renal replacement therapies may be performed. These forms of dialysis are discussed in Chapter 40, which presents treatment modalities for patients with renal dysfunction.

PHARMACOLOGIC THERAPY

Because hyperkalemia is the most life-threatening of the fluid and electrolyte disturbances, the patient is monitored for hyperkalemia through serial serum electrolyte levels (potassium value more than 5.5 mEq/L; SI: 5.5 mmol/L), electrocardiogram changes (tall, tented, or peaked T waves), and changes in clinical status.

The elevated potassium levels may be reduced by administering ion-exchange resins (sodium polystyrene sulfonate [Kayexalate]) orally or by retention enema. Kayexalate works by exchanging a sodium ion for a potassium ion in the intestinal tract. Sorbitol is often administered in combination with Kayexalate to induce a diarrhea-type effect (it induces water loss in the gastrointestinal tract).

If a retention enema is administered (the colon is the major site for potassium exchange), a rectal catheter with a balloon may be used to facilitate retention if necessary. The patient should retain the resin 30 to 45 minutes to promote potassium removal. Afterward, a cleansing enema may be prescribed to remove the Kayexalate resin as a precaution against fecal impaction.

Nursing Alert *A patient with a high and rising level of serum potassium often requires immediate dialysis.*

Nursing Alert *Intravenous glucose and insulin or calcium gluconate may be used as emergency and temporary measures to treat hyperkalemia. Glucose and insulin drive potassium into the cells, thereby lowering serum potassium levels temporarily. Potassium will move out of the cells and rise again to a dangerous level unless removed by dialysis. The administration of calcium gluconate helps protect the heart from the effects of the high potassium levels.*

Nursing Alert *Sodium bicarbonate may be administered to elevate the plasma pH. Sodium bicarbonate increases the pH, which causes potassium to move into the cell, and the result is lowering of the patient's serum potassium level. This is short-term therapy and is used with other long-term measures, such as dietary restriction and dialysis.*

Nursing Alert *All external sources of potassium (foods, salt substitutes, medications) are eliminated or reduced.*

Because many medications are eliminated through the kidneys, medication dosages must be reduced when acute renal failure is present. Examples of commonly used medications that require adjustment are antibiotics (especially aminoglycosides), digoxin, ACE inhibitors, and medications containing magnesium.

Many medications have been used in patients with acute renal failure in an attempt to improve patient outcomes. Diuretics are often used for management of volume status. They have not been shown, however, to hasten the recovery from acute renal failure.

Low-dose dopamine (1 to 3 μg/kg) is often used to dilate the renal arteries through stimulation of dopaminergic receptors; however, research has not definitely demonstrated that dopamine prevents acute renal failure or improves outcome in patients with established renal failure.

One new promising medication is atrial natriuretic peptide, which inhibits sodium and water absorption and dilates the afferent arteriole, thus improving blood flow to the glomerulus (Brenner, 1996).

Correction of Acidosis and Elevated Phosphate Levels.

When severe acidosis is present, the arterial blood gases or serum bicarbonate levels (CO_2-combining power) must be monitored because the patient may require sodium bicarbonate therapy or dialysis. If respiratory problems develop, appropriate ventilatory measures must be instituted. The patient's elevated serum phosphate level may be controlled with phosphate-binding agents (aluminum hydroxide). These agents help prevent a continuing rise in serum phosphate levels by decreasing absorption of phosphate from the intestinal tract.

NUTRITIONAL THERAPY

Acute renal failure causes severe nutritional imbalances as a result of inadequate intake (from nausea and vomiting), impaired glucose use and protein synthesis, and increased tissue catabolism. The patient is weighed daily and can be expected to lose 0.2 to 0.5 kg (0.5 to 1 lb) daily if the nitrogen balance is negative (ie, the patient is receiving caloric intake that is less than caloric requirements). If the patient gains or does not lose weight or develops hypertension, fluid retention should be suspected.

Dietary proteins are limited to about 1 g/kg during the oliguric phase to minimize protein breakdown and to prevent accumulation of toxic end products. Caloric requirements are met with high-carbohydrate meals because carbohydrates have a protein-sparing effect (ie, in a high-carbohydrate diet, protein is not used for meeting energy requirements but is "spared" for growth and tissue healing). Foods and fluids containing potassium and phosphorus (bananas, citrus fruits and juices, coffee) are restricted. Potassium intake is usually restricted to 40 to 60 mEq/day, and sodium is usually restricted to 2 g/day. The patient may require total parenteral nutrition (see Chap. 33).

The oliguric phase of acute renal failure may last from 10 to 20 days and is followed by the diuretic phase, at which time urinary output begins to increase, signaling that kidney function is returning. Blood chemistry evaluations are made to determine the amounts of sodium, potassium, and water needed for replacement, along with assessment for overhydration or underhydration.

After the diuretic phase, the patient is placed on a high-protein, high-calorie diet and is encouraged to resume activities gradually.

Nursing Management

The nurse has an important role in caring for the patient with acute renal failure. In addition to directing attention to the patient's primary disorder (which may be a factor in the development of acute renal failure), the nurse monitors the patient for complications, participates in emergency treatment of fluid and electrolyte imbalances, assesses the patient's progress and response to treatment, and provides physical and emotional support. Additionally, the nurse keeps family members informed about the patient's condition, assists them in understanding the treatments, and provides psychological support. Although the development of acute renal failure may be the most life-threatening problem, the nurse must continue to include in the plan of care those nursing measures indicated for the patient's primary disorder (eg, burns, shock, trauma, obstruction of the urinary tract).

MONITORING FLUID AND ELECTROLYTE BALANCE

The serious fluid and electrolyte imbalances that can occur with acute renal failure require the nurse to monitor closely the patient's serum electrolyte levels and physical indicators of these complications during all phases of the disorder. Hyperkalemia is the most immediate life-threatening imbalance seen in acute renal failure. Parenteral fluids, all oral intake, and all medications are screened carefully to ensure that hidden sources of potassium are not inadvertently administered or consumed. Intravenous solutions must be carefully selected according to the patient's fluid and electrolyte status. The patient's cardiac function and musculoskeletal status are monitored closely for changes suggestive of hyperkalemia.

The patient's fluid status is monitored by careful attention to fluid intake (intravenous medications should be administered in the smallest volume possible), urine output, the presence of edema, distention of the jugular veins, alterations in heart sounds and breath sounds, and increasing difficulty in breathing. Accurate daily weights, as well as intake and output records, are essential.

Indicators of deterioration of fluid and electrolyte status are reported immediately to the physician, and preparation is made for emergency treatment. Hyperkalemia is treated with glucose and insulin, calcium gluconate, cation-exchange resins (Kayexalate), or dialysis. Fluid and other electrolyte disturbances are often treated with hemodialysis, peritoneal dialysis, or other continuous renal replacement therapies.

REDUCING METABOLIC RATE

The nurse also directs attention to reducing the patient's metabolic rate during the acute stage of renal failure to reduce catabolism and the subsequent release of potassium and accumulation of endogenous waste products (urea and creatinine). Bed rest may be indicated to reduce exertion and the metabolic rate during the most acute stage of the disorder. Fever and infection, both of which increase the metabolic rate and catabolism, are prevented or treated promptly.

PROMOTING PULMONARY FUNCTION

Attention is given to pulmonary function, and the patient is assisted to turn, cough, and take deep breaths frequently to prevent atelectasis and respiratory infection. Drowsiness and lethargy may prevent the patient from moving and turning without encouragement and assistance.

PREVENTING INFECTION

Asepsis is essential with invasive lines and catheters to minimize the risk of infection and increased metabolism. An indwelling urinary catheter is avoided if possible because of the high risk for UTI associated with its use.

PROVIDING SKIN CARE

The patient's skin may be dry or susceptible to breakdown as a result of edema; therefore, meticulous skin care is important. Additionally, excoriation and itching of the skin may result from the deposit of irritating toxins in the patient's tissues. Massaging bony prominences, turning the patient frequently, and bathing the patient with cool water are often comforting and prevent skin breakdown.

PROVIDING SUPPORT

The patient with acute renal failure requires treatment with hemodialysis, peritoneal dialysis, or other continuous renal replacement therapies to prevent serious complications (see Chap. 40); the length of time that these treatments are necessary varies with the cause and extent of damage to the kidneys. The patient and family will need assistance, explanation, and support during this time. The purpose and rationale of the treatments is explained to the patient and family by the physician. High levels of anxiety and fear, however, may necessitate repeated explanation and clarification by the nurse. The family members may initially be afraid to touch and talk to the patient during the procedure but should be encouraged and assisted to do so.

Although many of the nurse's functions are devoted to the technical aspects of the procedure, the psychological needs and concerns of the patient and family cannot be ignored. Continued assessment of the patient for complications of acute renal failure and of its precipitating cause is essential.

Chronic Renal Failure (End-Stage Renal Disease)

Chronic renal failure, or ESRD, is a progressive, irreversible deterioration in renal function in which the body's ability to maintain metabolic and fluid and electrolyte balance fails, resulting in *uremia* or *azotemia* (retention of urea and other nitrogenous wastes in the blood).

The incidence of ESRD has increased at a rate of almost 8% per year for the past 5 years, with about 258,000 patients being treated in the United States (U.S. Renal Data System, 1998).

ESRD may be caused by systemic diseases, such as diabetes mellitus (leading cause); hypertension; chronic glomerulonephritis; pyelonephritis; obstruction of the urinary tract; hereditary lesions, such as in polycystic kidney disease; vascular disorders; infections; medications; or toxic agents. Environmental and occupational agents that have been implicated in chronic renal failure include lead, cadmium, mercury, and chromium. Dialysis or kidney transplantation eventually becomes necessary for patient survival.

Pathophysiology

As renal function declines, the end products of protein metabolism (which are normally excreted in urine) accumulate in the blood. Uremia develops and adversely affects every system in the body. The greater the buildup of waste products, the more severe the symptoms.

There are three well-recognized stages of chronic renal disease: reduced renal reserve, renal insufficiency, and ESRD (Chart 41-3).

The rate of decline in renal function and progression of chronic renal failure is related to the underlying disorder, to the urinary excretion of protein, and to the presence of hypertension. The disease tends to progress more rapidly in patients who excrete signif-

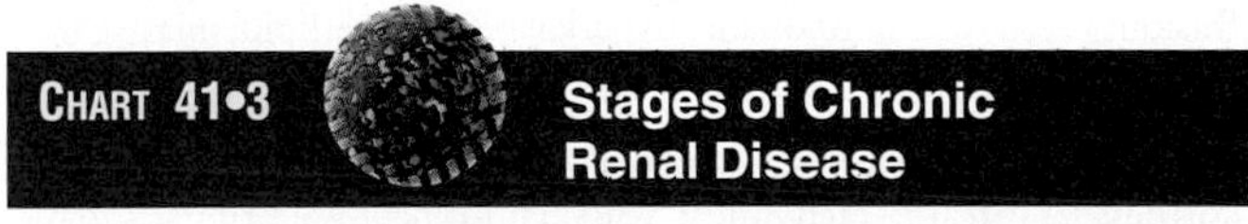

CHART 41•3 Stages of Chronic Renal Disease

Stage 1

Reduced renal reserve, characterized by a 40% to 75% loss of nephron function. The patient usually does not have symptoms because the remaining nephrons are able to carry out the normal functions of the kidney.

Stage 2

Renal insufficiency occurs when 75% to 90% of nephron function is lost. At this point, the serum creatinine and blood urea nitrogen rise, the kidney loses its ability to concentrate urine and anemia develops. The patient may report polyuria and nocturia.

Stage 3

End-stage renal disease (ESRD), the final stage of chronic renal failure, occurs when there is less than 10% nephron function remaining. All of the normal regulatory, excretory, and hormonal functions of the kidney are severely impaired. ESRD is evidenced by elevated creatinine and blood urea nitrogen levels as well as electrolyte imbalances. Once the patient reaches this point, dialysis is usually indicated. Many of the symptoms of uremia are reversible with dialysis.

icant amounts of protein or have elevated blood pressure than in those without these conditions.

Clinical Manifestations

Because virtually every body system is affected by the uremia of chronic renal failure, patients exhibit a number of signs and symptoms. The severity of these signs and symptoms is dependent in part on the degree of renal impairment, other underlying conditions, and the patient's age.

CARDIOVASCULAR MANIFESTATIONS

Hypertension (due to sodium and water retention or from activation of the renin–angiotensin–aldosterone system), congestive heart failure and pulmonary edema (due to fluid overload), and pericarditis (due to irritation of the pericardial lining by uremic toxins) are among the cardiovascular problems manifested in ESRD.

DERMATOLOGIC SYMPTOMS

Severe itching (pruritus) is common. Uremic frost, the deposit of urea crystals on the skin, is uncommon today because of early and aggressive treatment of ESRD with dialysis.

OTHER SYSTEMIC MANIFESTATIONS

Gastrointestinal symptoms are common and include anorexia, nausea, vomiting, and hiccups. Neurologic changes, including altered levels of consciousness, inability to concentrate, muscle twitching, and seizures, have been observed. The precise mechanisms for many of these diverse manifestations have not been identified. It is generally thought, however, that the accumulation of uremic waste products is the probable cause. Chart 41-4 summarizes the signs and symptoms often seen in chronic renal failure.

Assessment and Diagnostic Findings

GLOMERULAR FILTRATION RATE

Decreased GFR can be detected by obtaining a 24-hour urine analysis for creatinine clearance. As glomerular filtration decreases (due to nonfunctioning glomeruli), the creatinine clearance value decreases, whereas the serum creatinine and BUN levels increase. Serum creatinine is the more sensitive indicator of renal function because of its constant production in the body. The BUN is affected not only by renal disease but also by protein intake in the diet, catabolism (tissue and RBC breakdown), hyperalimentation, and medications such as corticosteroids.

CHART 41•4 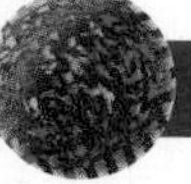 **Signs and Symptoms of Chronic Renal Failure**

Neurologic

Weakness and fatigue; confusion; inability to concentrate; disorientation; tremors; seizures; asterixis; restlessness of legs; burning of soles of feet; behavior changes

Integumentary

Gray-bronze skin color; dry, flaky skin; pruritus; ecchymosis; purpura; thin, brittle nails; coarse, thinning hair

Cardiovascular

Hypertension; pitting edema (feet, hands, sacrum); periorbital edema; pericardial friction rub; engorged neck veins; pericarditis; pericardial effusion; pericardial tamponade; hyperkalemia; hyperlipidemia

Pulmonary

Crackles; thick, tenacious sputum; depressed cough reflex; pleuritic pain; shortness of breath; tachypnea; Kussmaul-type respirations; uremic pneumonitis; "uremic lung"

Gastrointestinal

Ammonia odor to breath "uremic fetor"; metallic taste; mouth ulcerations and bleeding; anorexia, nausea, and vomiting; hiccups; constipation or diarrhea; bleeding from gastrointestinal tract

Hematologic

Anemia; thrombocytopenia

Reproductive

Amenorrhea; testicular atrophy; infertility; decreased libido

Musculoskeletal

Muscle cramps; loss of muscle strength; renal osteodystrophy; bone pain; bone fractures; foot drop

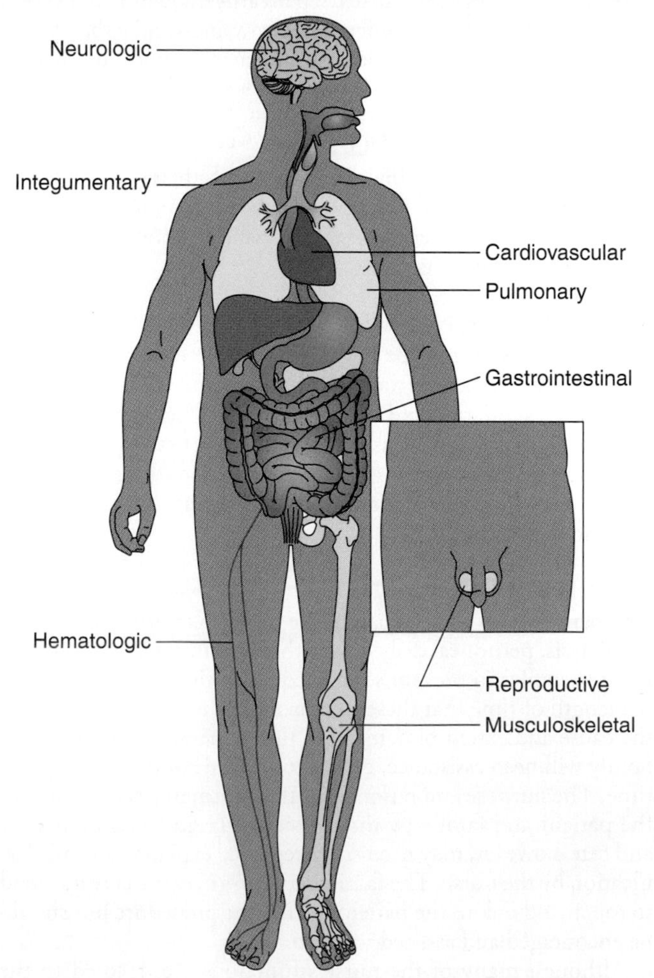

SODIUM AND WATER RETENTION

The kidney is unable to concentrate or dilute the urine normally in ESRD. Appropriate responses by the kidney to changes in the daily intake of water and electrolytes, therefore, do not occur. Some patients retain sodium and water, increasing the risk for edema, congestive heart failure, and hypertension. Hypertension may also result from activation of the renin–angiotensin–aldosterone axis and the concomitant increased aldosterone secretion. Other patients have a tendency to lose salt and run the risk of developing hypotension and hypovolemia. Episodes of vomiting and diarrhea may produce sodium and water depletion, which worsens the uremic state.

ACIDOSIS

With advanced renal disease, metabolic acidosis occurs because the kidney is unable to excrete increased loads of acid. Decreased acid secretion primarily results from inability of the kidney tubules to secrete ammonia (NH_3) and to reabsorb sodium bicarbonate (HCO_3^-). There is also decreased excretion of phosphates and other organic acids.

ANEMIA

Anemia develops as a result of inadequate erythropoietin production, the shortened life span of RBCs, nutritional deficiencies, and the patient's tendency to bleed, particularly from the gastrointestinal tract. Erythropoietin, a substance normally produced by the kidney, stimulates bone marrow to produce RBCs. In renal failure, erythropoietin production decreases, and profound anemia results, producing fatigue, angina, and shortness of breath.

CALCIUM AND PHOSPHORUS IMBALANCE

Another major abnormality seen in chronic renal failure is a disorder in calcium and phosphorus metabolism. The body's serum calcium and phosphate levels have a reciprocal relationship in the body: as one rises, the other decreases. With decreased filtration through the glomerulus of the kidney, there is an increase in the serum phosphate level and a reciprocal or corresponding decrease in the serum calcium level. The decreased serum calcium level causes increased secretion of parathormone from the parathyroid glands. In renal failure, however, the body does not respond normally to the increased secretion of parathormone, and, as a result, calcium leaves the bone, often producing bone changes and bone disease. In addition, the active metabolite of vitamin D (1,25-dihydroxycholecalciferol) normally manufactured by the kidney decreases as renal failure progresses. *Uremic bone disease,* often called *renal osteodystrophy,* develops from the complex changes in calcium, phosphate, and parathormone balance.

Complications

Potential complications of chronic renal failure that concern the nurse and that necessitate a collaborative approach to care include the following:

- *Hyperkalemia* due to decreased excretion, metabolic acidosis, catabolism, and excessive intake (diet, medications, fluids)
- *Pericarditis,* pericardial effusion, and pericardial tamponade due to retention of uremic waste products and inadequate dialysis
- *Hypertension* due to sodium and water retention and malfunction of the renin–angiotensin–aldosterone system
- *Anemia* due to decreased erythropoietin, decreased RBC life span, bleeding in the gastrointestinal tract from irritating toxins, and blood loss during hemodialysis
- *Bone disease* and *metastatic calcifications* due to retention of phosphorus, low serum calcium levels, abnormal vitamin D metabolism, and elevated aluminum levels

Gerontologic Considerations

Changes in kidney function with normal aging increase the susceptibility of elderly patients to kidney dysfunction and renal failure. Because alterations in renal blood flow, glomerular filtration, and renal clearance increase the risk of medication-associated changes in renal function, precautions are indicated with all medications. This is because of the frequent use of multiple-prescription and over-the-counter medications by elderly patients. The incidence of systemic diseases, such as atherosclerosis, hypertension, cardiac failure, diabetes, and cancer, increases with advancing age, predisposing older adults to renal disease associated with these disorders. Therefore, nurses in all settings need to be alert for signs and symptoms of renal dysfunction in elderly patients.

With age, the kidney is less able to respond to acute fluid and electrolyte changes. Therefore, acute problems need to be prevented if possible or recognized and treated quickly to avoid kidney damage. When the elderly patient must undergo extensive diagnostic tests, or when new medications (eg, diuretics) are added, precautions must be taken to prevent dehydration, which can compromise marginal renal function and lead to acute renal failure.

The elderly patient may develop atypical and nonspecific signs of disturbed renal function and fluid and electrolyte imbalances. Recognition of these problems is further hampered by their association with previously existing disorders and the misconception that they are normal changes of aging.

ACUTE RENAL FAILURE IN OLDER ADULTS

The incidence of acute renal failure is increasing in older, hospitalized patients. About half of patients who develop acute renal failure during hospitalization for a medical or surgical problem are older than 60 years of age. Evidence also demonstrates that acute renal failure is often seen in the community setting (Mindell & Chertow, 1997). Nurses in the ambulatory setting need to be cognizant of the risk for acute renal failure in their elderly patients, especially those undergoing diagnostic testing or procedures that can result in dehydration. The mortality rate is slightly higher for acute renal failure in elderly patients than for in younger counterparts.

The etiology of acute renal failure in older adults includes prerenal causes, such as dehydration, and intrarenal causes, such as nephrotoxic agents (medications, contrast agents). Diabetes mellitus increases the risk for contrast agent-induced renal failure because of preexisting renal insufficiency and the imposed fluid restriction needed for many tests. Suppression of thirst, enforced bed rest, unavailable drinking water, and confusion all contribute to the older patient's failure to consume adequate fluids and lead to subsequent dehydration and compromise of already decreased renal function.

CHRONIC RENAL FAILURE IN OLDER ADULTS

Historically, the age of patients developing ESRD steadily rose each year, but it appears to have stabilized since 1993, at a mean age of 60 years. About 44% of all patients with ESRD are older than 65 years of age (U.S. Renal Data System, 1998). In the past, rapidly progressive glomerulonephritis, membranous glomerulonephritis, and nephrosclerosis have been the most common causes of chronic renal failure in the elderly. Today, however, diabetes mellitus and hypertension are the leading causes of chronic renal failure in the elderly. Other common causes of chronic renal failure in the elderly population are interstitial nephritis and urinary tract obstruction (Brenner, 1996). The signs and symptoms of renal disease in the elderly are commonly nonspecific. The occurrence of symptoms of other disorders (congestive heart failure, dementia) can mask the symptoms of renal disease and delay or prevent diagnosis and treatment. The patient often complains of signs and symptoms of nephrotic syndrome, such as edema and proteinuria.

Hemodialysis and peritoneal dialysis have been used effectively in treating elderly patients. Although there is no single age limitation for renal transplantation, concomitant disorders (ie, coronary artery disease, peripheral vascular disease) have made it a less common treatment for the elderly. The outcome, however, is comparable to that of younger patients. Some elderly patients elect not to participate in these management strategies.

Conservative management, including nutritional therapy, fluid control, and medications, such as phosphate binders, may be considered in patients who are not suitable for or elect not to participate in dialysis or transplantation.

Medical Management

The goal of management is to maintain kidney function and homeostasis for as long as possible. All factors that contribute to ESRD and all factors that are reversible (eg, obstruction) are identified and treated. Management is accomplished primarily with medications and diet therapy, although dialysis may also be needed.

PHARMACOLOGIC THERAPY

Complications can be prevented or delayed by administering prescribed antihypertensives, erythropoietin (Epogen), iron supplements, phosphate-binding agents, and calcium supplements. It is also essential that the patient receive adequate dialysis treatments to decrease the level of uremic waste products in the blood.

Antacids. Hyperphosphatemia and hypocalcemia are treated with aluminum-based antacids that bind dietary phosphorus in the gastrointestinal tract. However, concerns about the potential long-term toxicity of aluminum and the association of high aluminum levels with neurologic symptoms and osteomalacia have led some physicians to prescribe calcium carbonate in place of high doses of aluminum-based antacids. This medication also binds dietary phosphorus in the intestinal tract and permits the use of smaller doses of antacids. Both calcium carbonate and phosphorus-binding antacids must be administered with food to be effective. Magnesium-based antacids must be avoided to prevent magnesium toxicity.

Antihypertensive and Cardiovascular Agents. Hypertension is managed by intravascular volume control and a variety of antihypertensive medications. Congestive heart failure and pulmonary edema may also require treatment with fluid restriction, low sodium diets, diuretics, inotropic agents such as digitalis or dobutamine, and dialysis. The metabolic acidosis of chronic renal failure usually produces no symptoms and requires no treatment; however, sodium bicarbonate supplements or dialysis may be needed to correct the acidosis if it causes symptoms.

Anticonvulsants. Neurologic abnormalities may occur and require that the patient be observed for early evidence of slight twitching, headache, delirium, or seizure activity. If seizures occur, the onset of the seizure is recorded along with the type, duration, and general effect on the patient. The physician is notified immediately. Intravenous diazepam (Valium) or phenytoin (Dilantin) is usually administered to control seizures. The side rails of the bed may be padded to protect the patient. The nursing management of the patient with seizures is discussed in Chapter 57.

Erythropoietin. Anemia associated with chronic renal failure is treated with recombinant human erythropoietin (Epogen). Anemic patients (hematocrit less than 30%) present with nonspecific symptoms, such as malaise, general fatigability, and decreased activity tolerance. Epogen therapy is initiated to achieve a hematocrit of 33% to 38%, which generally alleviates the symptoms of anemia. Epogen is administered either intravenously or subcutaneously three times a week. It may take 2 to 6 weeks for the hematocrit to rise; therefore, Epogen is not indicated for patients who need immediate correction of severe anemia. Adverse effects seen with Epogen therapy include hypertension (especially during early stages of treatment), increased clotting of vascular access sites, seizures, and depletion of body iron stores.

The patient receiving Epogen may experience influenza-like symptoms with initiation of therapy; these tend to subside with repeated doses. Management involves adjustment of heparin to prevent clotting of the dialysis lines during hemodialysis treatments, frequent monitoring of hematocrit, and periodic assessment of serum iron and transferrin levels. Because adequate stores of iron are necessary for an adequate response to erythropoietin, supplementary iron may be prescribed. In addition, the patient's blood pressure and serum potassium level are monitored to detect hypertension and rising serum potassium levels, which may occur with therapy and the increasing RBC mass. The occurrence of hypertension requires initiation or adjustment of the patient's antihypertensive therapy. Hypertension that cannot be controlled is a contraindication to recombinant erythropoietin therapy.

Patients who have received Epogen have reported decreased levels of fatigue, an increased feeling of well-being, better tolerance of dialysis, higher energy levels, and improved exercise tolerance. Additionally, this therapy has decreased the need for transfusion and its associated risks (infectious disease, antibody formation, and iron overload).

NUTRITIONAL THERAPY

Dietary intervention is necessary with deterioration of renal function and includes careful regulation of protein intake, fluid intake to balance fluid losses, sodium intake to balance sodium losses, and some restriction of potassium. At the same time, adequate caloric intake and vitamin supplementation must be ensured. Protein is restricted because urea, uric acid, and organic acids—the breakdown products of dietary and tissue proteins—accumulate rapidly in the blood when there is impaired renal clearance. The allowed protein must be of high biologic value (dairy products, eggs, meats). High-biologic-value proteins are those that are complete proteins and supply the essential amino acids necessary for growth and cell repair.

Usually, the fluid allowance is 500 to 600 mL more than the previous day's 24-hour urine output. Calories are supplied by carbohydrates and fat to prevent wasting. Vitamin supplementation is necessary because a protein-restricted diet does not give the necessary complement of vitamins. Additionally, the patient on dialysis may lose water-soluble vitamins from the blood during the dialysis treatment.

OTHER THERAPY: DIALYSIS

Hyperkalemia is usually prevented by ensuring adequate dialysis treatments with potassium removal and careful monitoring of all medications, both oral and intravenous, for their potassium content. The patient is placed on a potassium-restricted diet. Occasionally, Kayexalate, administered orally, may be needed.

The patient with increasing symptoms of chronic renal failure is referred to a dialysis and transplantation center early in the course of progressive renal disease. Dialysis is usually initiated when the patient cannot maintain a reasonable lifestyle with conservative treatment. The details of dialysis treatment can be found in Chapter 40.

Nursing Management

The patient with chronic renal failure requires astute nursing care to avoid the complications of reduced renal function and the stresses and anxieties of dealing with a life-threatening illness.

Examples of potential nursing diagnoses for these patients include the following:

- Fluid volume excess related to decreased urine output, dietary excesses, and retention of sodium and water
- Altered nutrition: less than body requirements related to anorexia, nausea and vomiting, dietary restrictions, and altered oral mucous membranes
- Knowledge deficit regarding condition and treatment regimen
- Activity intolerance related to fatigue, anemia, retention of waste products, and dialysis procedure
- Self-esteem disturbance related to dependency, role changes, changes in body image, and sexual dysfunction

Nursing care is directed toward assessing fluid status and identifying potential sources of imbalance, implementing a dietary program to ensure proper nutritional intake within the limits of the treatment regimen, and promoting positive feelings by encouraging increased self-care and greater independence. It is extremely important to provide explanations and information to the patient and family concerning ESRD, treatment options, and potential complications. A great deal of emotional support is needed by the patient and family because of the numerous changes experienced. Specific interventions, along with rationale and evaluation criteria, are presented in more detail in Plan of Nursing Care 41-1.

PROMOTING HOME AND COMMUNITY-BASED CARE

Teaching Patients Self-Care. The nurse plays an extremely important role in teaching the patient with ESRD. Because of the extensive teaching needed, the home care nurse, dialysis nurse, and nurse in the outpatient setting all provide ongoing education and reinforcement while monitoring the patient's progress and compliance with the treatment regimen.

A nutritional referral and explanations of nutritional needs are helpful because of the numerous dietary changes required. The patient is taught how to check the vascular access device for patency and how to take such precautions as avoiding venipunctures and blood pressure measurements on the arm with the access device.

Additionally, the patient and family require considerable assistance and support in dealing with the need for dialysis and its long-term implications. For instance, they need to know what problems to report to the health care provider, including the following:

- Worsening signs of renal failure (nausea, vomiting, change in normal urine output [if any], ammonia odor on breath)
- Signs of hyperkalemia (muscle weakness, diarrhea, abdominal cramps)
- Signs and symptoms of access problems (clotted fistula or graft, infection)

The above-mentioned signs of worsening renal failure, in addition to increasing BUN and serum creatinine levels, may be indicative of a need to alter the dialysis prescription. The dialysis clinic nurses also provide ongoing education and support at each dialysis treatment visit.

Continuing Care. The importance of follow-up examinations and treatment is stressed to the patient and family because of changing physical status, renal function, and dialysis requirements. Referral for home care provides the home care nurse with the opportunity to assess the patient's environment, emotional status, and the coping strategies used by the patient and family to deal with the changes in family roles often associated with chronic illness.

The home care nurse also assesses the patient for increasing signs of renal failure and complications resulting from the primary renal disorder, the resulting renal failure, and compliance with treatment strategies (eg, dialysis, medications, dietary restrictions). Many patients need ongoing education and reinforcement on the multiple dietary restrictions required, including fluid, sodium, potassium, and protein restriction.

KIDNEY TRANSPLANTATION

Kidney transplantation has become the treatment of choice for most patients with ESRD. During the past 40 years, more than 380,000 kidney transplantations have been performed worldwide, and more than 169,000 have been performed in the United States (Cecka & Terasaki, 1996). Patients choose kidney transplantation for a variety of reasons, such as the desire to avoid dialysis or to improve their sense of well-being and the wish to lead a more normal life. Additionally, the cost of maintaining a successful transplantation is one third the cost of treating a dialysis patient.

Kidney transplantation involves transplanting a kidney from a living donor or human cadaver to a recipient who has ESRD (Chart 41-5). Kidney transplants from well-matched living donors who are related to the patient (those with compatible ABO and HLA antigens) are slightly more successful than those from cadaver donors. A nephrectomy of the patient's own native kidneys may be performed before transplantation. The transplanted kidney is placed in the patient's iliac fossa anterior to the iliac crest. The ureter of the newly transplanted kidney is transplanted into the bladder or anastomosed to the ureter of the recipient (Fig. 41-5).

Preoperative Management

Preoperative management goals include bringing the patient's metabolic state to a level as close to normal as possible. A complete physical examination is performed to detect and treat any conditions that could cause complications after transplantation. Tissue typing, blood typing, and antibody screening are performed to determine compatibility of the tissues and cells of the donor and recipient. Other diagnostic tests must be completed to identify conditions requiring treatment before transplantation. The lower urinary tract is studied to assess bladder neck function and to detect ureteral reflux.

The patient must be free of infection at the time of renal transplantation because after surgery the patient will receive medications to prevent transplant rejection. These medications suppress the immune response, leaving the patient immunosuppressed and at risk for infection. Therefore, the patient is evaluated and

(text continues on page 1159)

41•1 **PLAN OF NURSING CARE**

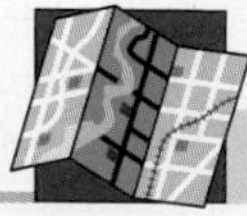

The Patient With Chronic Renal Failure

Nursing Diagnosis: Fluid volume excess related to decreased urine output, dietary excesses, and retention of sodium and water
Goal: Maintenance of ideal body weight without excess fluid

Nursing Interventions	Rationale	Expected Outcomes
1. Assess fluid status: a. Daily weight b. Intake and output balance c. Skin turgor and presence of edema d. Distention of neck veins e. Blood pressure, pulse rate, and rhythm f. Respiratory rate and effort	1. Assessment provides baseline and ongoing database for monitoring changes and evaluating interventions.	• Demonstrates no rapid weight changes • Maintains dietary and fluid restrictions • Exhibits normal skin turgor without edema • Exhibits normal vital signs • Exhibits no neck vein distention • Reports no difficulty breathing or shortness of breath • Performs oral hygiene frequently • Reports decreased thirst • Reports decreased dryness of oral mucous membranes
2. Limit fluid intake to prescribed volume	2. Fluid restriction will be determined on basis of weight, urine output, and response to therapy.	
3. Identify potential sources of fluid: a. Medications and fluids used to take medications: oral and intravenous b. Foods	3. Unrecognized sources of excess fluids may be identified.	
4. Explain to patient and family rationale for restriction	4. Understanding promotes patient and family cooperation with fluid restriction.	
5. Assist patient to cope with the discomforts resulting from fluid restriction	5. Increasing patient comfort promotes compliance with dietary restrictions.	
6. Provide or encourage frequent oral hygiene	6. Oral hygiene minimizes dryness of oral mucous membranes.	

Nursing Diagnosis: Altered nutrition; less than body requirements related to anorexia, nausea, vomiting, dietary restrictions, and altered oral mucous membranes
Goal: Maintenance of adequate nutritional intake

Nursing Interventions	Rationale	Expected Outcomes
1. Assess nutritional status: a. Weight changes b. Anthropometric measures c. Laboratory values (serum electrolyte, BUN, creatinine, protein, transferrin, and iron levels)	1. Baseline data allow for monitoring of changes and evaluating interventions.	• Consumes protein of high biologic value • Chooses foods within dietary restrictions that are appealing • Consumes high-calorie foods within dietary restrictions • Explains in own words rationale for dietary restrictions and relationship to urea and creatinine levels • Takes medications on schedule that does not produce anorexia or feeling of fullness • Consults written lists of acceptable foods • Reports increased appetite at meals • Exhibits no rapid increases or decreases in weight • Demonstrates normal skin turgor without edema; healing and acceptable plasma albumin levels
2. Assess patient's nutritional dietary patterns: a. Diet history b. Food preferences c. Calorie counts	2. Past and present dietary patterns can be considered in planning meals.	
3. Assess for factors contributing to altered nutritional intake: a. Anorexia, nausea, or vomiting b. Diet unpalatable to patient c. Depression d. Lack of understanding of dietary restrictions e. Stomatitis	3. Information about other factors that may be altered or eliminated to promote adequate dietary intake is provided.	
4. Provide patient's food preferences within dietary restrictions.	4. Increased dietary intake is encouraged.	
5. Promote intake of high biologic value protein foods: eggs, dairy products, meats.	5. Complete proteins are provided for positive nitrogen balance needed for growth and healing.	
6. Encourage high-calorie, low-protein, low-sodium, and low-potassium snacks between meals.	6. Reduces source of restricted foods and proteins and provides calories for energy, sparing protein for tissue growth and healing.	
7. Alter schedule of medications so that they are not given immediately before meals.	7. Ingestion of medications just before meals may produce anorexia and feeling of fullness.	

41•1 **PLAN OF NURSING CARE**

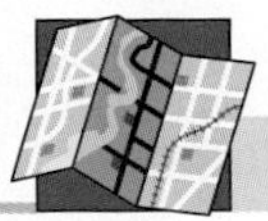

The Patient With Chronic Renal Failure (*continued*)

Nursing Interventions	Rationale	Expected Outcomes
8. Explain rationale for dietary restrictions and relationship to kidney disease and increased urea and creatinine levels.	8. Promotes patient understanding of relationships between diet and urea and creatinine levels to renal disease.	
9. Provide written lists of foods allowed and suggestions for improving their taste without use of sodium or potassium.	9. Lists provide a positive approach to dietary restrictions and a reference for patient and family to use when at home.	
10. Provide pleasant surroundings at mealtimes.	10. Unpleasant factors that contribute to patient's anorexia are eliminated.	
11. Weigh patient daily.	11. Allows monitoring of fluid and nutritional status.	
12. Assess for evidence of inadequate protein intake: a. Edema formation b. Delayed healing c. Decreased serum albumin levels	12. Inadequate protein intake can lead to decreased albumin and other proteins, edema formation, and delay in healing.	

Nursing Diagnosis: Knowledge deficit regarding condition and treatment
Goal: Increased knowledge about condition and related treatment

Nursing Interventions	Rationale	Expected Outcomes
1. Assess understanding of cause of renal failure, consequences of renal failure, and its treatment: a. Cause of patient's renal failure b. Meaning of renal failure c. Understanding of renal function d. Relationship of fluid and dietary restrictions to renal failure e. Rationale for treatment (hemodialysis, peritoneal dialysis, trasplantation)	1. Provides baseline for further explanations and teaching.	• Verbalizes relationship of cause of renal failure to consequences • Explains fluid and dietary restrictions as they relate to failure of kidney's regulatory functions • States in own words relationship of renal failure and need for treatment • Asks questions about treatment options, indicating readiness to learn • Verbalizes plans to continue as normal a life as possible • Uses written information and instructions to clarify questions and seek additional information
2. Provide explanation of renal function and consequences of renal failure at patient's level of understanding and guided by patient's readiness to learn.	2. Patient can learn about renal failure and treatment as he or she becomes ready to understand and accept the diagnosis and consequences.	
3. Assist patient to identify ways to incorporate changes related to illness and its treatment into lifestyle.	3. Patient can see that his or her life does not have to revolve around the disease.	
4. Provide oral and written information as appropriate about: a. Renal function and failure b. Fluid and dietary restrictions c. Medications d. Reportable problems, signs, and symptoms e. Follow-up schedule f. Community resources g. Treatment options	4. Provides patient with information that can be used for further clarification at home.	

Nursing Diagnosis: Activity intolerance related to fatigue, anemia, retention of waste products, and dialysis procedure
Goal: Participation in activity within tolerance

Nursing Interventions	Rationale	Expected Outcomes
1. Assess factors contributing to fatigue: a. Anemia b. Fluid and electrolyte imbalances c. Retention of waste products d. Depression	1. Indications of severity of fatigue are provided.	• Participates in increasing levels of activity and exercise • Reports increased sense of well-being • Alternates rest and activity • Participates in selected self-care activities

(*continued*)

41•1 PLAN OF NURSING CARE

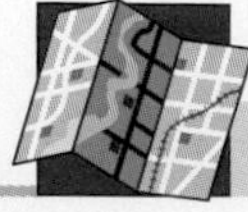

The Patient With Chronic Renal Failure (*continued*)

Nursing Interventions	Rationale	Expected Outcomes
2. Promote independence in self-care activities as tolerated; assist if fatigued.	2. Promotes improved self-esteem	
3. Encourage alternating activity with rest.	3. Promotes activity and exercise within limits and adequate rest.	
4. Encourage patient to rest after dialysis treatments.	4. Adequate rest is encouraged after dialysis treatments, which are exhausting to many patients.	

Nursing Diagnosis: Self-esteem disturbance related to dependency, role changes, change in body image, and change in sexual function
Goal: Improved self-concept

Nursing Interventions	Rationale	Expected Outcomes
1. Assess patient's and family's responses and reactions to illness and treatment.	1. Provides data about problems encountered by patient and family in coping with changes in life.	• Identifies previously used coping styles that have been effective and those no longer possible due to disease and treatment (alcohol or drug use; extreme physical exertion) • Patient and family identify and verbalize feelings and reactions to disease and necessary changes in their life • Seeks professional counseling, if necessary, to cope with changes resulting from renal failure • Reports satisfaction with method of sexual expression
2. Assess relationship of patient and significant family members.	2. Identifies strengths and supports of patient and family.	
3. Assess usual coping patterns of patient and family members.	3. Coping patterns that may have been effective in past may be potentially destructive in view of restrictions imposed by disease and treatment.	
4. Encourage open discussion of concerns about changes produced by disease and treatment: a. Role changes b. Changes in lifestyle c. Changes in occupation d. Sexual changes e. Dependence on health care team	4. Encourages patient to identify concerns and steps necessary to deal with them.	
5. Explore alternate ways of sexual expression other than sexual intercourse.	5. Alternative forms of sexual expression may be acceptable.	
6. Discuss role of giving and receiving love, warmth, and affection.	6. Sexuality means different things to different people, depending on stage of maturity.	

Collaborative Problems: Hyperkalemia; pericarditis, pericardial effusion, and pericardial tamponade; hypertension; anemia; bone disease and metastatic calcifications
Goal: Patient experiences an absence of complications

Hyperkalemia

Nursing Interventions	Rationale	Expected Outcomes
1. Monitor serum potassium levels and notify physician if level greater than 5.5 mEq/L.	1. Hyperkalemia causes detrimental and potentially life-threatening changes in the body.	• Patient has normal potassium level • Experiences no muscle weakness or diarrhea • Exhibits normal ECG pattern • Vital signs are within normal limits
2. Assess patient for muscle weakness, diarrhea, ECG changes (tall-tented T waves and widened QRS).	2. Cardiovascular signs and symptoms are characteristic of hyperkalemia.	

Pericarditis, Pericardial Effusion, and Pericardial Tamponade

Nursing Interventions	Rationale	Expected Outcomes
1. Assess patient for fever, chest pain, and a pericardial friction rub (signs of pericarditis) and, if present, notify physician.	1. About 30%–50% of chronic renal failure patients develop pericarditis due to uremia; fever, chest pain, and a pericardial friction rub are classic signs.	• Has strong and equal peripheral pulses • Absence of a paradoxical pulse • Absence of pericardial effusion or tamponade on cardiac ultrasound • Patient has normal heart sounds
2. If patient has pericarditis, assess for the following every 4 hours: a. Paradoxical pulse >10 mm Hg b. Extreme hypotension c. Weak or absent peripheral pulses d. Altered level of consciousness e. Bulging neck veins	2. Pericardial effusion is a common fatal sequela of pericarditis. Signs of an effusion include a paradoxical pulse (>10 mm Hg drop in blood pressure during inspiration) and signs of shock due to compression of the heart by a large effusion. Cardiac tamponade exists when the patient is severely compromised hemodynamically.	

41•1 PLAN OF NURSING CARE 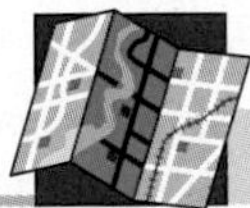 The Patient With Chronic Renal Failure (*continued*)

Nursing Interventions	Rationale	Expected Outcomes
3. Prepare patient for cardiac ultrasound to aid in diagnosis of an effusion and tamponade.	3. Cardiac ultrasound is useful in visualizing pericardial effusions and cardiac tamponade.	
4. If cardiac tamponade develops, prepare patient for emergency pericardiocentesis.	4. Cardiac tamponade is a life-threatening condition, with a high mortality rate. Immediate aspiration of fluid from the pericardial space is essential.	
Hypertension		
1. Monitor and record blood pressure as indicated.	1. Provides objective data for monitoring. Elevated levels may indicate noncompliance.	• Blood pressure within normal limits • Reports no headaches, visual problems, or seizures • Edema is absent • Demonstrates compliance with dietary and fluid restrictions
2. Administer antihypertensive medications as prescribed.	2. Antihypertensive medications play a key role in treatment of hypertension associated with chronic renal failure.	
3. Encourage compliance with dietary and fluid restriction therapy.	3. Adherence to diet and fluid restrictions and dialysis schedule prevents excess fluid and sodium accumulation.	
4. Teach patient to report signs of fluid overload, vision changes, headaches, edema, or seizures.	4. These are indications of inadequate control of hypertension and need to alter therapy.	
Anemia		
1. Monitor RBC count, hemoglobin, and hematocrit levels as indicated.	1. Provides assessment of degree of anemia.	• Patient has a normal color without pallor • Exhibits hematology values within acceptable limits • Experiences no bleeding from any site
2. Administer medications as prescribed, including iron and folic acid supplements, Epogen, and multivitamins.	2. RBCs need iron, folic acid, and vitamins to be produced. Epogen stimulates the bone marrow to produce RBC.	
3. Avoid drawing unnecessary blood specimens.	3. Anemia is aggravated by drawing numerous specimens.	
4. Teach patient to prevent bleeding: avoid vigorous nose blowing and contact sports, and use a soft toothbrush.	4. Bleeding from anywhere in the body worsens anemia.	
5. Administer blood component therapy as indicated.	5. Blood component therapy may be needed if the patient has symptoms.	
Bone Disease and Metastatic Calcifications		
1. Administer the following medications as prescribed: phosphate binders, calcium supplements, vitamin D supplements.	1. Chronic renal failure causes numerous physiologic changes affecting calcium, phosphorus, and vitamin D metabolism.	• Exhibits serum calcium, phosphorus, and aluminum levels within acceptable ranges • Exhibits no symptoms of hypocalcemia • Has no bone demineralization on bone scan • Discusses importance of maintaining activity level and exercise program
2. Monitor serum lab values as indicated (calcium, phosphorus, aluminum levels) and report abnormal findings to physician.	2. Hyperphosphatemia, hypocalcemia, and excess aluminum accumulation are common in chronic renal failure.	
3. Assist patient with an exercise program.	3. Bone demineralization increases with immobility.	

treated for any infections, including gingival (gum) disease and dental caries.

A psychosocial evaluation is conducted to assess the patient's ability to adjust to the transplant, coping styles, social history, social support available, and financial resources. A history of psychiatric illness is important to ascertain because psychiatric conditions are often aggravated by the corticosteroids needed for immunosuppression after transplantation.

Hemodialysis is often performed the day before the scheduled transplantation procedure to optimize the patient's physical status.

Preoperative Nursing Interventions

The nursing aspects of preoperative management are similar to those for patients undergoing other elective abdominal surgery. Preoperative teaching can be done in a variety of settings, including the outpatient preadmission area, the hospital, or the transplantation clinic during the preliminary workup phase. Patient teaching addresses postoperative pulmonary hygiene, pain management options, dietary restrictions, intravenous and arterial lines, tubes (indwelling catheter and possibly a nasogastric tube),

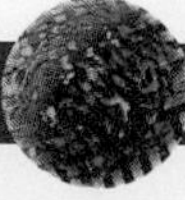

CHART 41•5 Organ Donation

An inadequate number of available kidneys remains the greatest limitation to treating patients with end-stage renal disease successfully. For those interested in donating a kidney, the National Kidney Foundation provides written information describing the organ donation program and a card specifying the organ to be donated in the event of death.

The organ donation card is signed by the donor and two witnesses and should be carried by the donor at all times. Procurement of an adequate number of kidneys for potential recipients is still a major problem, despite national legislation that requires relatives of deceased patients or patients declared brain-dead to be asked if they would consider organ donation.

In some states in the United States, drivers can indicate their desire to be organ donors on their driver's license application or renewal.

and early ambulation. The patient who receives a kidney from a living related donor may be concerned about the donor and how the donor will tolerate the surgical procedure.

Most patients have been on dialysis for months or years before transplantation. Many have waited months to years for a kidney transplant and are very anxious about the surgery, possible rejection, and the need to return to dialysis. Helping the patient to deal with these concerns is part of the nurse's role in preoperative management, as is teaching the patient about what to expect after surgery.

Postoperative Management

The goal of care is to maintain homeostasis until the transplanted kidney is functioning well. The patient whose kidney functions immediately has a more favorable prognosis than the patient whose kidney does not.

Immunosuppressive Therapy

The survival of a transplanted kidney depends on the ability to block the body's immune response to the transplanted kidney. To overcome or minimize the body's defense mechanism, immunosuppressive medications, such as azathioprine (Imuran), corticosteroids (prednisone), cyclosporine, and OKT-3 (a monoclonal antibody), are administered.

Cyclosporine is now available in a microemulsion form (Neoral), which delivers the medication more reliably, thus producing a steady-state serum concentration. Prograf (formerly called FK-506) is similar to cyclosporine and about 100 times more potent. Mycophenolate (RS-61433) was recently approved by the U.S. Food and Drug Administration (FDA) solely for the prevention of renal transplant rejection. It may be used in patients who have failed the standard corticosteroid pulse therapy or OKT-3. Antilymphocyte globulin is occasionally used to modify the immune response. Plasmaleukapheresis, lymph drainage, and cyclophosphamide (Cytoxan) are other methods of immunosuppression, but they are rarely used.

Doses of immunosuppressive agents are gradually tapered over a period of several weeks, depending on the patient's immunologic response to the transplant. The patient will, however, take some form of antirejection medication for the entire time that he or she has the transplanted kidney.

Rejection Concerns

Renal graft rejection and failure may occur within 24 hours (hyperacute), within 3 to 14 days (acute), or after many years (chronic). It is not uncommon for acute rejection to occur during the first year after transplantation. Ultrasound may be used to detect enlargement of the kidney, whereas percutaneous renal biopsy (most reliable) and x-ray techniques are used to evaluate transplant rejection. If the body rejects the transplanted kidney, the patient needs to return to dialysis. The rejected kidney may

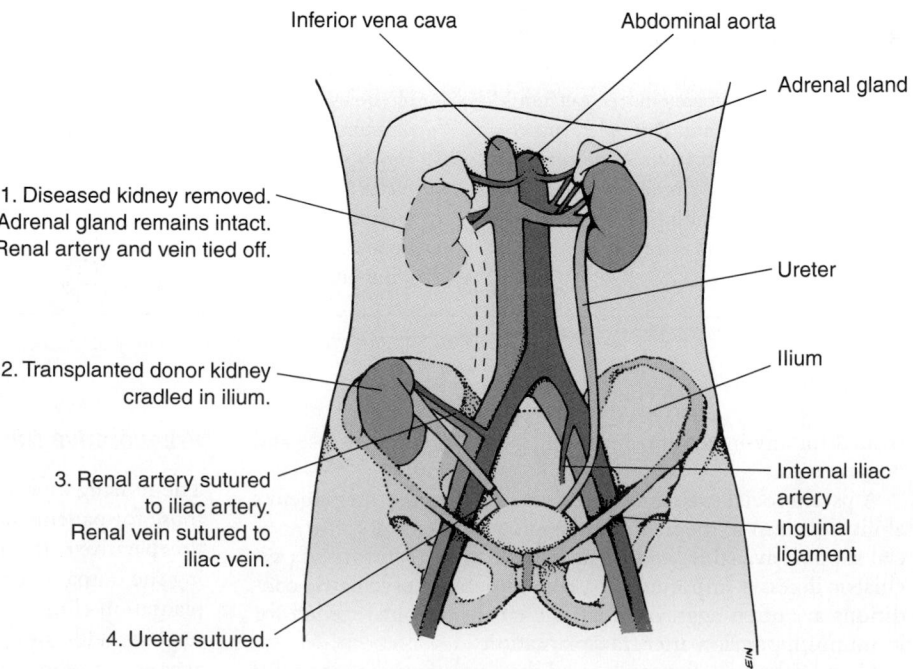

Inferior vena cava
Abdominal aorta
Adrenal gland
1. Diseased kidney removed. Adrenal gland remains intact. Renal artery and vein tied off.

Ilium
2. Transplanted donor kidney cradled in ilium.
3. Renal artery sutured to iliac artery. Renal vein sutured to iliac vein.
Internal iliac artery
Inguinal ligament
4. Ureter sutured.

FIGURE 41•5 Renal transplantation: (**1**) The diseased kidney may be removed and the renal artery and vein tied off. (**2**) The transplanted kidney is placed in the iliac fossa. (**3**) The renal artery of the donated kidney is sutured to the iliac artery, and the renal vein is sutured to the iliac vein. (**4**) The ureter of the donated kidney is sutured to the bladder or to the patient's ureter.

or may not be removed, depending on when the rejection occurs (acute versus chronic) and the risk for infection if the kidney is left in place.

Postoperative Nursing Interventions

ASSESSING FOR REJECTION AND PREVENTING INFECTION

After kidney transplantation, the nurse assesses the patient for signs and symptoms of transplant rejection: oliguria, edema, fever, increasing blood pressure, weight gain, and swelling or tenderness over the transplanted kidney or graft. Patients receiving cyclosporine may not exhibit the usual signs and symptoms of acute rejection. In these patients, the only sign may be an asymptomatic rise in the serum creatinine level (more than a 20% rise is considered acute rejection).

The results of blood chemistry tests (BUN and creatinine) and leukocyte and platelet counts are monitored closely because immunosuppression depresses the formation of leukocytes and platelets. The patient is closely monitored for infection because of susceptibility to impaired healing and infection related to immunosuppressive therapy and complications of renal failure.

***Nursing Alert** A distinction must be made between infection and rejection because impaired renal function and fever are evidence of both infection and rejection, and their treatments differ.*

Immunosuppressive medications of the past made the transplant recipient more vulnerable to opportunistic infections (candidiasis, cytomegalovirus, *Pneumocystis carinii* pneumonia) and infection with other relatively nonpathogenic viruses, fungi, and protozoa, which can be a major hazard. Cyclosporine therapy has reduced the incidence of opportunistic infections because it selectively exerts its effect, sparing T cells that protect the patient from life-threatening infections.

The nurse ensures that the patient is protected from exposure to hospital staff, visitors, and other patients who have active infections. Careful hand washing is imperative; face masks may be worn by hospital staff and visitors to reduce the risk of transmitting infectious agents while the patient is receiving high doses of immunosuppressive medications.

About 75% of kidney transplant recipients have at least one episode of infection in the first year after the transplantation because of the immunosuppressive therapy (Peddi & First, 1997). Infections remain a major cause of death at all points in time for kidney transplant recipients.

***Nursing Alert** Clinical manifestations of infection include shaking chills, fever, rapid heartbeat and respirations (tachycardia and tachypnea), and either an increase or a decrease in WBCs (leukocytosis or leukopenia).*

Infection may be introduced through the urinary tract, the respiratory tract, the surgical site, or other sources. Urine cultures are performed frequently because of the high incidence of bacteriuria during both the early and the late stages of transplantation. Any type of wound drainage should be viewed as a potential source of infection because drainage is an excellent culture medium for bacteria. Catheter and drain tips may be cultured when removed by cutting off the tip of the catheter or drain (using aseptic technique) and placing the cut portion in a sterile container to be taken to the laboratory for culture.

Monitoring Urinary Function

The vascular access for hemodialysis is monitored to ensure patency and to evaluate for evidence of infection. After successful renal transplantation, the vascular access device may clot, possibly from improved coagulation with the return of renal function. Hemodialysis may be necessary postoperatively to maintain homeostasis until the transplanted kidney is functioning well.

A kidney from a living donor related to the patient usually begins to function immediately after surgery and may produce large quantities of dilute urine. A kidney from a cadaver donor may undergo acute tubular necrosis and, therefore, may not function for 2 or 3 weeks, during which anuria, oliguria, or polyuria may be present. During this stage, the patient may experience significant changes in fluid and electrolyte status. Therefore, careful monitoring is indicated. The output from the urinary catheter (connected to a closed drainage system) is measured every hour. Intravenous fluids are administered on the basis of urine volume and serum electrolyte levels and as prescribed by the physician. Hemodialysis may be required if fluid overload and hyperkalemia occur.

MONITORING AND MANAGING POTENTIAL COMPLICATIONS

Gastrointestinal ulceration and steroid-induced bleeding may occur. Fungal colonization of the gastrointestinal tract (especially the mouth) and urinary bladder may occur secondary to corticosteroid and antibiotic therapy. Closely monitoring the patient and notifying the physician about the occurrence of complications are important nursing interventions.

RECOGNIZING PSYCHOLOGICAL CONCERNS

The rejection of a transplanted kidney remains a matter of great concern to the patient, the patient's family, and the supporting health care team for many months. The fears of kidney rejection and the complications of immunosuppressive therapy (Cushing's syndrome, diabetes, capillary fragility, osteoporosis, glaucoma, cataracts, acne) place tremendous psychological stresses on the patient. Anxiety and uncertainty about the future and difficult posttransplantation adjustment are often sources of stress for the patient and family.

PROMOTING HOME AND COMMUNITY-BASED CARE

Teaching Patients Self-Care. The nurse works closely with the patient and family to be sure that they understand the need for continuing the immunosuppressive therapy as prescribed. Additionally, the patient and family are instructed to assess for and report signs of rejection of the transplanted kidney, signs of infection, or significant side effects of the immunosuppressive agents. These include decreased urine output; weight gain; malaise; fever; respiratory distress; tenderness over the transplanted kidney; anxiety; depression; changes in eating, drinking, or other habit patterns; and changes in blood pressure readings. The patient is instructed to inform other health care providers (eg, dentist) about the kidney transplant and the use of immunosuppressive agents.

Continuing Care. The patient is advised that follow-up care after transplantation is a lifelong necessity. Individual verbal and written instructions are provided concerning diet, medication, flu-

NURSING RESEARCH

Stressors in Renal Transplant Recipients

Fallon, M., Gould, D., & Wainwright, S. P. (1997). Stress and quality of life in the renal transplant patient: A preliminary investigation. *Journal of Advanced Nursing 25*(3), 562–570.

Historically, few studies have addressed quality of life in renal transplant patients, despite evidence that even with a well-functioning transplant, patients continue to experience stressors associated with a chronic illness. The purpose of this study was to explore patients' perceptions of stress and quality of life at various points of time after renal transplantation.

Purpose

The study objectives were to identify specific stressors affecting first-time renal transplant patients; to compare and contrast the stress experienced by patients at various time periods after transplantation; and to explore the patients' perceptions of their quality of life at different time intervals post transplant. Data were collected at 6 months, between 1 and 5 years, and 5 years or more after transplantation.

Study Sample and Design

The study sample consisted of 30 adults who were patients at a renal transplantation clinic. Two instruments were used in the study to obtain information on stress experienced and perceived quality of life. The Kidney Transplant Recipient Stress Scale (KTRSS) was slightly modified by deleting questions about costs of health care for the individual patient because the study was conducted in the United Kingdom where the government is responsible for the costs of all health care. The modified KTRSS addressed physical and psychological health, family relationships, employment, and body image. In addition, patients were asked to rate their quality of life as a whole before and after receiving a transplant; a 5-point Likert scale was used with a score of 1 = poor quality of life and a score of 5 = highest possible quality of life.

Findings

Scores on the KTRSS indicated that patients in the 1- to 5-year post-transplantation group had the highest overall stress scores. In the physical and psychological health category, the most commonly selected stressor for all groups was the possibility of rejection. Patients in the first 6-month group also identified injury to the new kidney, lack of information, and risk of infection as stressors.

Patients in the 1- to 5-year posttransplantation group identified limitations in physical activity and risk of infection as great stressors. Patients in the greater than 5 years category mentioned lack of information and changes in self, such as moodiness, as stressors. In the family relationship category, patients in the 1- to 5-year group had the highest stress scores of all three groups. In the employment and daily activities category, all three groups identified fear of repeated hospitalizations as the major stressor.

In the body image category, the 1- to 5-year group scored highest with changes in body appearance and weight gain as the most distressing stressors. Despite these stressors, all three groups reported a significantly better quality of life after the renal transplantation, with patients in the first 6 months and those 5 years after transplantation having the most significant changes.

Nursing Implications

Despite the small sample size, the results of this study can assist nurses working with renal transplant patients to work with patients to develop strategies to cope with the demands of living with a renal transplant after they return home and begin assuming family responsibilities. Further study is needed to examine the experiences of this population in greater depth and with a larger sample. In addition, tools to measure quality of life in renal transplant patients need to be developed and tested.

ids, daily weight, daily measurement of urine, management of intake and output, prevention of infection, resumption of activity, and avoidance of contact sports in which the transplanted kidney may be injured. Because of the risk of other potential complications, the patient is followed closely. Cardiovascular disease is now the major cause of late morbidity and mortality after transplantation, due in part to the increasing age of transplantation patients. An additional problem is possible malignancy; patients receiving long-term immunosuppressive therapy have been found to develop cancers more frequently than the general population.

The National Association of Kidney Patients (listed at the end of this chapter) is a nonprofit organization that serves the needs of those with kidney disease. It has many helpful suggestions for patients and family members learning to cope with dialysis and transplantation.

UROLITHIASIS

Urolithiasis refers to stones (calculi) in the urinary tract. Stones are formed in the urinary tract when urinary concentrations of substances such as calcium oxalate, calcium phosphate, and uric acid increase. This is referred to as supersaturation and is dependent on the amount of substance, ionic strength, and pH of the urine.

Pathophysiology

Stones can also form when there is a deficiency of substances that normally prevent crystallization in the urine, such as citrate, magnesium, nephrocalcin, and uropontin. The fluid volume status of the patient (stones tend to occur more often in dehydrated patients) is another factor playing a key role in stone development.

Calculi may be found anywhere from the kidney to the bladder. They vary in size from minute granular deposits, called sand or gravel, to bladder stones as large as an orange. The different sites of calculi formation in the urinary tract are shown in Figure 41-6.

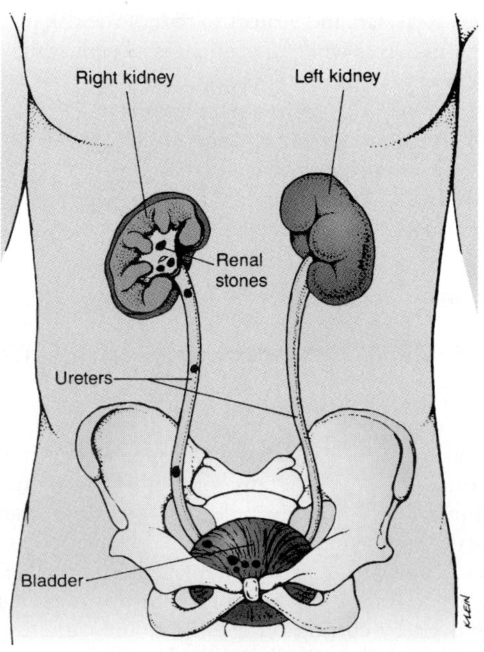

FIGURE 41•6 Various sites of calculi formation in the urinary tract (urolithiasis).

Certain factors favor the formation of stones, including infection, urinary stasis, and periods of immobility (slows renal drainage and alters calcium metabolism).

Causes of *hypercalcemia* (high serum calcium) and *hypercalciuria* (high urine calcium) include the following:

- Hyperparathyroidism
- Renal tubular acidosis
- Cancers
- Granulomatous diseases (sarcoidosis, tuberculosis), which may cause increased vitamin D production by the granulomatous tissue
- Excessive intake of vitamin D
- Excessive intake of milk and alkali
- Myeloproliferative diseases (leukemia, polycythemia vera, multiple myeloma), which produce an unusual proliferation of blood cells from the bone marrow

These factors promote increased calcium concentrations in blood and urine, causing precipitation of calcium and formation of stones (about 75% of all renal stones are calcium based).

For stones containing uric acid, struvite, or cystine, a thorough physical examination and metabolic workup are indicated because of associated disturbances contributing to the stone formation. Uric acid stones (5% to 10% of all stones) may be seen in patients with gout or myeloproliferative disorders. Struvite stones account for 15% of urinary calculi and form in persistently alkaline, ammonia-rich urine caused by the presence of urease-splitting bacteria such as *Proteus, Pseudomonas, Klebsiella, Staphylococcus*, or *Mycoplasma* species. Predisposing factors for struvite stones (commonly called *infection stones*) include neurogenic bladder, foreign bodies, and recurrent UTIs. Cystine stones (1% to 2% of all stones) occur exclusively in patients with a rare inherited defect in renal absorption of cystine (an amino acid).

Urinary stone formation may also occur with inflammatory bowel disease and in patients with an ileostomy or bowel resection because these patients absorb more oxalate. Some medications that are known to cause stones in some patients include antacids, acetazolamide (Diamox), vitamin D, laxatives, and high doses of aspirin. In many patients, however, no cause may be found.

Urinary stones account for about 328,000 hospital admissions each year. Stone disease occurs predominantly in the third to fifth decades of life and affect men more than women. About half of patients with a single renal stone have another episode within 5 years (Begun et al., 1997). Most stones contain calcium or magnesium in combination with phosphorus or oxalate. Most stones are radiopaque and can be detected by radiographic studies.

Clinical Manifestations

The clinical manifestations of stones in the urinary tract depend on the presence of obstruction, infection, and edema. When the stones block the flow of urine, obstruction develops, producing an increase in hydrostatic pressure and distending the renal pelvis and proximal ureter. Infection (pyelonephritis and cystitis with chills, fever, and dysuria) can occur from constant irritation by the stone. Some stones cause few, if any, symptoms while slowly destroying the functional units (nephrons) of the kidney; others cause excruciating pain and discomfort.

Stones in the renal pelvis may be associated with an intense, deep ache in the costovertebral region. Hematuria is often seen; pyuria may also be noted. Pain originating in the renal area radiates anteriorly and downward toward the bladder in the female and toward the testis in the male. If the pain suddenly becomes acute, with tenderness over the costovertebral area, and nausea and vomiting appear, the patient is having an episode of renal colic. Diarrhea and abdominal discomfort may occur. These gastrointestinal symptoms are due to renointestinal reflexes and the anatomic proximity of the kidneys to the stomach, pancreas, and large intestines.

Stones lodged in the ureter (ureteral obstruction) cause acute, excruciating, colicky, wavelike pain, radiating down the thigh and to the genitalia. Often, the patient has a desire to void, but little urine is passed, and it usually contains blood because of the abrasive action of the stone. This group of symptoms is called *ureteral colic*. Colic is mediated by prostaglandin-E_2, a substance that increases ureteral contractility and renal blood flow and that leads to increased intraureteral pressure and pain. In general, the patient spontaneously passes stones 0.5 to 1 cm in diameter. Stones larger than 1 cm in diameter usually must be removed or fragmented so that they can be removed or passed spontaneously.

Stones lodged in the bladder usually produce symptoms of irritation and may be associated with UTI and hematuria. If the stone obstructs the bladder neck, there is urinary retention. If infection is associated with the presence of a stone, the condition is far more serious, with sepsis threatening the patient's life.

Assessment and Diagnostic Findings

The diagnosis is confirmed by kidneys, ureter, bladder (KUB) x-rays, ultrasound, intravenous urography, or retrograde pyelography. Blood chemistries and a 24-hour urine test for measurement of calcium, uric acid, creatinine, sodium, pH, and total volume are part of the diagnostic workup. Dietary and medication histories and family history of renal stones are obtained to identify factors predisposing the patient to the formation of stones.

When stones are recovered (stones may be freely passed by the patient or removed through special procedures), chemical analysis is carried out to determine their composition. Stone analysis can provide a clear indication of the underlying disorder. For example, calcium oxalate or calcium phosphate stones usually indicate disorders of oxalate or calcium metabolism, whereas urate stones suggest a disturbance in uric acid metabolism.

Medical Management

The basic goals of management are to eradicate the stone, to determine the stone type, to prevent nephron destruction, to control infection, and to relieve any obstruction that may be present.

The immediate objective of treatment of renal or ureteral colic is to relieve the pain until its cause can be eliminated. Opioid analgesics are administered to prevent shock and syncope that may result from the excruciating pain. NSAIDs may be as effective as other analgesics in treating renal stone pain. They provide specific pain relief because they inhibit the synthesis of prostaglandin-E_2.

Hot baths or moist heat to the flank areas may also be useful. Unless the patient is vomiting or suffering from congestive heart failure or any other condition requiring fluid restriction, fluids are encouraged. This increases the hydrostatic pressure behind the stone, assisting it in its downward passage. A high, around-the-clock fluid intake reduces the concentration of urinary crystalloids, dilutes the urine, and ensures a high urine output.

Nutritional therapy plays an important role in preventing renal stones. Fluid intake is the mainstay of most medical therapy for renal stones. Unless contraindicated, any patient with renal stones should drink at least eight 8-ounce glasses of water daily to keep the urine dilute. A urine output exceeding 2 liters a day is advisable.

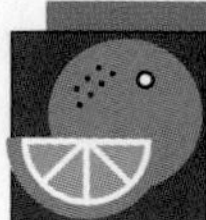

NUTRITION

Dietary Recommendations for Prevention of Kidney Stones

- Restricting protein to 60 g/day is recommended to decrease urinary excretion of calcium and uric acid.
- A sodium restriction of 3–4 g/day is recommended. Table salt and high-sodium foods should be reduced because sodium competes with calcium for reabsorption in the kidneys.
- Low-calcium diets are not generally recommended, except for true absorptive hypercalciuria. Evidence shows that limiting calcium, especially in women, can lead to osteoporosis and does not prevent renal stones.
- Oxalate-containing foods (spinach, strawberries, rhubarb, tea, peanuts, wheat bran) may be restricted.

Calcium Stones. Historically, patients with calcium-based renal stones were advised to restrict calcium in their diet. Recent evidence, however, has questioned the advisability of this practice, except for patients with type II absorptive hypercalciuria (half of all patients with calcium stones), in whom stones are clearly due to excess dietary calcium. Current research supports a liberal fluid intake along with a dietary restriction of protein and sodium. It is thought that a high-protein diet is associated with increased urinary excretion of calcium and uric acid, thereby causing a supersaturation of these substances in the urine. Similarly, a high sodium intake has been shown in some studies to increase the amount of calcium in the urine. The urine may be acidified by use of medications such as ammonium chloride or acetohydroxamic acid (Lithostat) (Saklayen, 1997; Singal & Denstedt, 1997).

Cellulose sodium phosphate (Calcibind) may be effective in preventing calcium stones. It binds calcium from food in the intestinal tract, reducing the amount of calcium absorbed into the circulation. If increased parathormone production (resulting in increased serum calcium levels in blood and urine) is a factor in the formation of stones, therapy with thiazide diuretics may be beneficial in reducing the calcium loss in the urine and lowering the elevated parathormone levels.

Uric Acid Stones. For uric acid stones, the patient is placed on a low-purine diet to reduce the excretion of uric acid in the urine. Foods high in purine (shellfish, anchovies, asparagus, mushrooms, and organ meats) are avoided, and other proteins may be limited. Allopurinol (Zyloprim) may be prescribed to reduce serum uric acid levels and urinary uric acid excretion. The urine is alkalinized. For cystine stones, a low-protein diet is prescribed, the urine is alkalinized, and penicillamine is administered to reduce the amount of cystine in the urine.

Oxalate Stones. For oxalate stones, a dilute urine is maintained, and the intake of oxalate is limited. Many foods contain oxalate; however, only certain foods have been proved to increase the urinary excretion of oxalate significantly. These include spinach, strawberries, rhubarb, chocolate, tea, peanuts, and wheat bran.

SURGICAL MANAGEMENT

If the stone is not passed spontaneously or complications occur, treatment modalities may include surgical, endoscopic, or other procedures, for example, ureteroscopy, extracorporeal shock wave lithotripsy (ESWL), or endourologic (percutaneous) stone removal.

Ureteroscopy (Fig. 41-7) involves first visualizing the stone and then destroying it. Access to the stone is accomplished by inserting a ureteroscope into the ureter and then inserting a laser, electrohydraulic lithotriptor, or ultrasound device through the ureteroscope to fragment and remove the stones. A stent may be inserted and left in place for 48 hours or more after the procedure to keep the ureter patent. Hospital stays are generally brief, and some patients can be treated as outpatients.

ESWL is a noninvasive procedure used to break up stones in the calyx of the kidney (see Fig. 41-7*B*). After the stones are fragmented to the size of grains of sand, the remnants of the stones are spontaneously voided. In ESWL, a high-energy amplitude of pressure, or shock wave, is generated by the abrupt release of energy and transmitted through water and soft tissues. When the shock wave encounters a substance of different intensity (a renal stone), a compression wave causes the surface of the stone to fragment. Repeated shock waves focused on the stone eventually reduce it to many small pieces. These small pieces are excreted in the urine, usually without difficulty.

The need for anesthesia for the procedure depends on the type of lithotriptor used, which determines the number and intensity of shock waves delivered. An average treatment comprises between 1000 and 3000 shocks. The first-generation lithotriptors required use of either regional or general anesthesia.

Although the shock waves usually do not damage other tissue, discomfort from the multiple shocks may occur. The patient is observed for obstruction and infection resulting from blockage of the urinary tract by stone fragments. All urine is strained after the procedure; voided gravel or sand is sent to the laboratory for chemical analysis. Several treatments may be necessary to ensure disintegration of stones. Although lithotripsy is a costly treatment, it has decreased length of hospital stay and expense because an invasive surgical procedure to remove the renal stone is avoided.

Endourologic methods of stone removal (see Fig. 41-7*C*) may be used to extract renal calculi that are unable to be removed by other procedures. A percutaneous **nephrostomy** or a percutaneous nephrolithotomy (which are similar procedures) may be performed, and a nephroscope is introduced through the dilated percutaneous tract into the renal parenchyma. Depending on its size, the stone may be extracted with forceps or by a stone retrieval basket. Alternatively, an ultrasound probe may be introduced through the nephrostomy tube. Then, ultrasonic waves are used to pulverize the stone. Small stone fragments and stone dust are irrigated and suctioned out of the collecting system. Larger stones may be further reduced by ultrasonic disintegration and then removed with forceps or a stone retrieval basket.

Electrohydraulic lithotripsy is a similar method in which an electrical discharge is used to create a hydraulic shock wave to break up the stone. A probe is passed through the cystoscope, and the tip of the lithotriptor is placed near the stone. The strength of the discharge and pulse frequency can be varied. This procedure is performed under topical anesthesia. After the stone is extracted, the percutaneous nephrostomy tube is left in place for a time to ensure that the ureter is not obstructed by edema or blood clots. The most common complications are hemorrhage, infection, and urinary extravasation. After the tube is removed, the nephrostomy tract closes spontaneously.

Chemolysis, stone dissolution using infusions of chemical solutions (eg, alkylating agents, acidifying agents) for the purpose of

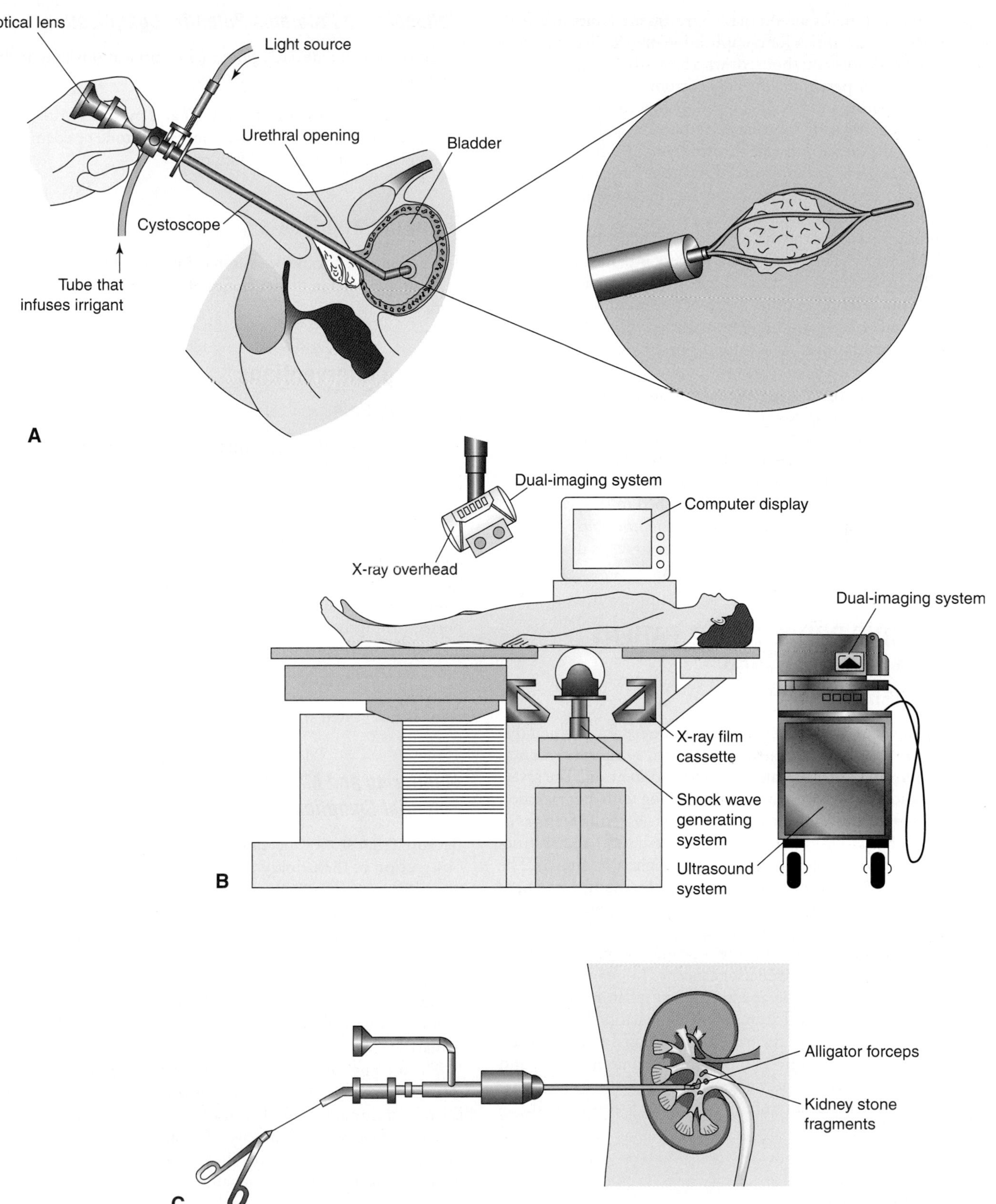

FIGURE 41•7 Methods of treating renal stones. (**A**) During a cystoscopy, which is used for removing small renal stones located close to the bladder, a ureteroscope is inserted into the ureter to visualize the stone. The stone is then fragmented or captured and removed. (**B**) Extracorporeal shock wave lithotripsy (ESWL) is used for most symptomatic nonpassable upper urinary tract stones. Electromagnetically generated shock waves are focused over the area of the renal stone. The high-energy dry shock waves pass through the skin and fragment the stone. (**C**) Percutaneous nephrolithotomy is used to treat larger stones. A percutaneous tract is formed and a nephroscope is inserted through it. Then the stone is extracted or pulverized.

dissolving the stone, is an alternative treatment sometimes used in patients who are at risk for complication of other types of therapy, who refuse other methods, or who have stones (struvite) that dissolve easily. A percutaneous nephrostomy is performed, and the warm irrigating solution is allowed to flow continuously onto the stone. The irrigating solution exits the renal collecting system by means of the ureter or the nephrostomy tube. The pressure inside the renal pelvis is monitored during the procedure. Several of these treatment modalities may be used in combination to ensure successful removal of the stones.

Surgical removal was the major mode of therapy before the advent of lithotripsy. Today, however, surgery is performed in only 1% to 2% of patients. Surgical intervention is indicated if the stone does not respond to other forms of treatment. It may also be performed to correct anatomic abnormalities within the kidney to improve urinary drainage. If the stone is in the kidney, the surgery performed may be a *nephrolithotomy* (incision into the kidney with removal of the stone) or a *nephrectomy*, if the kidney is nonfunctional secondary to infection or hydronephrosis. Stones in the kidney pelvis are removed by a *pyelolithotomy*, those in the ureter by *ureterolithotomy*, and those in the bladder by *cystotomy*. If the stone is in the bladder, an instrument may be inserted through the urethra into the bladder, and the stone is crushed in the jaws of this instrument. Such a procedure is called a *cystolithalopaxy*.

Nursing management following kidney surgery is discussed in Chapter 40.

NURSING PROCESS: THE PATIENT WITH RENAL STONES

Assessment

The patient with suspected renal stones is assessed for pain and discomfort as well as the presence of associated symptoms, such as nausea, vomiting, diarrhea, and abdominal distention. The severity and location of pain are determined, along with any radiation of the pain. Nursing assessment also includes observing for signs of UTI (chills, fever, dysuria, frequency, and hesitancy) and obstruction (frequent urination of small amounts, oliguria, or anuria). The urine is observed for the presence of blood and is strained for stones or gravel. The history focuses on factors that predispose the patient to urinary tract stones or that may have precipitated the current episode of renal or ureteral colic. Predisposing factors include family history of stones, the presence of cancer or bone marrow disorders or the use of chemotherapeutic agents, inflammatory bowel disease, or a diet high in calcium or purines. Factors that may precipitate stone formation in the patient predisposed to renal calculi include episodes of dehydration, prolonged immobilization, and infection. The patient's knowledge about renal stones and measures to prevent their occurrence or recurrence is also assessed.

Diagnosis

Nursing Diagnoses

Based on the assessment data, the nursing diagnoses in the patient with renal stones may include the following:

- Pain related to inflammation, obstruction, and abrasion of the urinary tract
- Knowledge deficit regarding prevention of recurrence of renal stones

Collaborative Problems/Potential Complications

Based on assessment data, potential complications may include the following:

- Infection and sepsis (from UTI and pyelonephritis)
- Obstruction of the urinary tract by a stone or edema with subsequent acute renal failure

Planning and Goals

The major goals for the patient may include relief of pain and discomfort, prevention of recurrence of renal stones, and absence of complications.

Nursing Interventions

Relieving Pain

Immediate relief of severe pain from renal or ureteral colic is accomplished with opioid analgesics (intravenous or intramuscular administration may be prescribed to provide rapid relief) or nonsteroidal anti-inflammatory agents (ketorolac is the only FDA-approved intramuscular agent). The patient is encouraged and assisted to assume a position of comfort. If activity brings some pain relief, the patient is assisted to ambulate. The patient's pain is monitored closely, and increases in severity are reported promptly to the physician so that relief can be provided and additional treatment initiated. The patient is prepared for other treatment (eg, lithotripsy, percutaneous stone removal, ureteroscopy, or surgery) if severe pain is unrelieved and the stone is not passed spontaneously.

Monitoring and Managing Potential Complications

Because renal stones increase the risk for infection, sepsis, and obstruction of the urinary tract, the patient is instructed to report decreased urine volume and bloody or cloudy urine. The total urine output and patterns of voiding are monitored. Increased fluid intake is encouraged to prevent dehydration and increase hydrostatic pressure within the urinary tract to promote passage of the stone. If the patient is unable to take adequate fluids orally, intravenous fluids are prescribed. Ambulation is encouraged as a means of moving the stone through the urinary tract.

The nursing care of patients with calculi requires frequent observation to detect the spontaneous passage of a stone. All urine is strained through gauze because uric acid stones may crumble. Any blood clots passed in the urine should be crushed and the sides of the urinal and bedpan inspected for clinging stones. The patient is instructed to report any sudden increases in pain immediately because of the possibility of a stone fragment obstructing a ureter. Analgesic medications are administered as prescribed for the relief of pain and discomfort.

The patient's vital signs, including temperature, are monitored closely to detect early signs of infection. UTIs may be associated with renal stones due to an obstruction from the stone or from the stone itself. All infections should be treated with the appropriate antibiotic agents before stone dissolution.

Promoting Home and Community-Based Care

TEACHING PATIENTS SELF-CARE

Because the risk of recurring renal stones is high, the nurse provides education about the causes of kidney stones and ways to prevent their recurrence. The patient is encouraged to follow a regimen to avoid further stone formation. One facet of prevention is to maintain a *high fluid intake* because stones form more readily in concentrated urine. A patient who has shown a tendency to form stones should drink enough fluid to excrete greater than 2000 mL of urine every 24 hours (preferably 3000 to 4000 mL), should adhere to the prescribed diet, and should avoid sudden increases in environmental temperatures, which may cause a fall in urinary volume. Occupations and activities that produce excessive sweating can lead to severe temporary dehydration; therefore, fluid intake should be increased. Sufficient fluids should be taken in the evening to prevent urine from becoming too concentrated at night.

Urine cultures may be performed every 1 to 2 months the first year and periodically thereafter. Recurrent UTI is treated vigorously. Because prolonged immobilization slows renal drainage and alters calcium metabolism, increased mobility is encouraged whenever possible. In addition, excessive ingestion of vitamins (especially vitamin D) and minerals is discouraged.

If lithotripsy, percutaneous stone removal, ureteroscopy, or other surgical procedures for stone removal have been performed, the patient is instructed about the signs and symptoms of complications that need to be reported to the physician. The importance of follow-up to assess kidney function and to ensure the successful eradication or removal of all kidney stones is emphasized to the patient and family.

If the patient underwent ESWL, the nurse must provide instructions for home care and necessary follow-up. The patient is encouraged to increase fluid intake to assist in the passage of stone fragments, which may occur for 6 weeks to several months after the procedure. The patient and family are instructed about signs and symptoms that indicate the occurrence of complications, such as fever, decreasing urinary output, and pain. It is also important to tell the patient to expect hematuria (it is anticipated in all patients), but it should disappear within 4 to 5 days. If the patient has a stent in the ureter, hematuria may be expected until it is removed. The patient is instructed to notify the physician if nausea or vomiting, a temperature greater than 38°C (about 101°F), or pain unrelieved by the prescribed medication occurs. The patient is also informed that a bruise may be observed on the treated side of the back.

CONTINUING CARE

The patient is monitored closely in follow-up care to ensure that treatment has been effective and that no complications, such as obstruction, infection, renal hematoma, or hypertension, have developed. During the patient's visits to the clinic or physician's office, the nurse has the opportunity to assess the patient's understanding of ESWL and possible complications. Additionally, the nurse has the opportunity to assess the patient's understanding of factors that increase the risk for recurrence of renal calculi and strategies to reduce those risks

The patient's ability to monitor urinary pH and interpret the results is assessed during follow-up visits to the clinic or physician's office. Because of the high risk for recurrence, the patient with renal stones needs to understand the signs and symptoms of stone formation, obstruction, and infection and the importance of reporting these signs promptly. If medications are prescribed for the prevention of stone formation, the actions and importance of the medications are explained to the patient.

Evaluation

Expected Outcomes

Expected outcomes may include:

1. Reports relief of pain
2. States increased knowledge of health-seeking behaviors to prevent recurrence
   a. Consumes increased high fluid intake (at least eight 8-ounce glasses of fluid per day)
   b. Participates in appropriate activity
   c. Consumes diet prescribed to reduce dietary factors predisposing to stone formation
   d. Recognizes symptoms to be reported to health care provider (fever, chills, flank pain, hematuria)
   e. Monitors urinary pH as directed
   f. Takes prescribed medication as directed to reduce stone formation
3. Experiences no complications
   a. Reports no signs or symptoms of sepsis or infection
   b. Voids 200 to 400 mL per voiding of clear urine without RBCs
   c. Experiences absence of dysuria, frequency, and hesitancy
   d. Maintains normal body temperature.

GENITOURINARY TRAUMA

Various types of injuries of the flank, back, or upper abdomen may result in trauma to the kidney, ureter, bladder, or urethra. Trauma to the kidney accounts for about half of all cases of genitourinary trauma.

Renal Trauma

Normally, the kidneys are protected by the rib cage and musculature of the back posteriorly and by a cushion of abdominal wall and viscera anteriorly. They are highly mobile and are "fixed" only at the renal pedicle (stem of renal blood vessels and the ureter). With

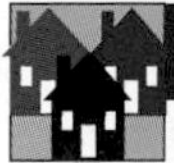

PATIENT EDUCATION AND HOME CARE

Avoiding Recurrent Renal Stones

1. Follow prescribed diet closely.
2. During the day, drink fluids (ideally water) every 1 to 2 hours.
3. Drink two glasses of water at bedtime and an additional glass at each nighttime awakening to prevent urine from becoming too concentrated during the night.
4. Avoid activities that cause excessive sweating and dehydration.
5. Avoid sudden increases in environmental temperatures that may cause excessive sweating and dehydration.
6. Contact primary health care provider at the first sign of a urinary tract infection.

traumatic injury, the kidney can be thrust against the lower ribs, resulting in contusion and rupture. Rib fractures or fractures of the transverse process of the upper lumbar vertebrae may be associated with renal contusion or laceration. Injuries may be blunt (automobile and motorcycle crashes, falls, athletic injuries, assaults) or penetrating (gunshot wounds, stabbings). Failure to wear seat belts contributes to the incidence of renal trauma in motor vehicle crashes. Up to 80% of patients with renal trauma have associated injuries of other internal organs.

Renal trauma may be classified by the mechanism of injury: blunt or penetrating. Blunt renal trauma accounts for 80% to 90% of all renal injuries; penetrating renal trauma accounts for the remaining 10% to 20%. Blunt renal trauma is classified into one of four groups, as follows:

- *Contusion:* bruises or hemorrhages under the renal capsule; capsule and collecting system intact
- *Minor laceration:* superficial disruption of the cortex; renal medulla and collecting system are not involved
- *Major laceration:* parenchymal disruption extending into cortex and medulla, possibly involving the collecting system
- *Vascular injury:* tears of renal artery or vein

The most common renal injuries are contusions, lacerations, ruptures, and renal pedicle injuries or small internal lacerations of the kidney (Fig. 41-8). The kidneys receive half of the blood flow from the abdominal aorta; therefore, even a fairly small renal laceration can produce massive bleeding. About 70% of patients are in shock when admitted to the hospital.

Clinical manifestations include pain, renal colic (due to blood clots or fragments obstructing the collecting system), hematuria, mass or swelling in the flank, ecchymoses, and lacerations or wounds of the lateral abdomen and flank. Hematuria is the most common manifestation of renal trauma; its presence after trauma suggests renal injury. There is no relationship between the degree of hematuria and the degree of injury. Hematuria may not occur, or it may be detectable only on microscopic examination. Signs and symptoms of hypovolemia and shock are likely with significant hemorrhage.

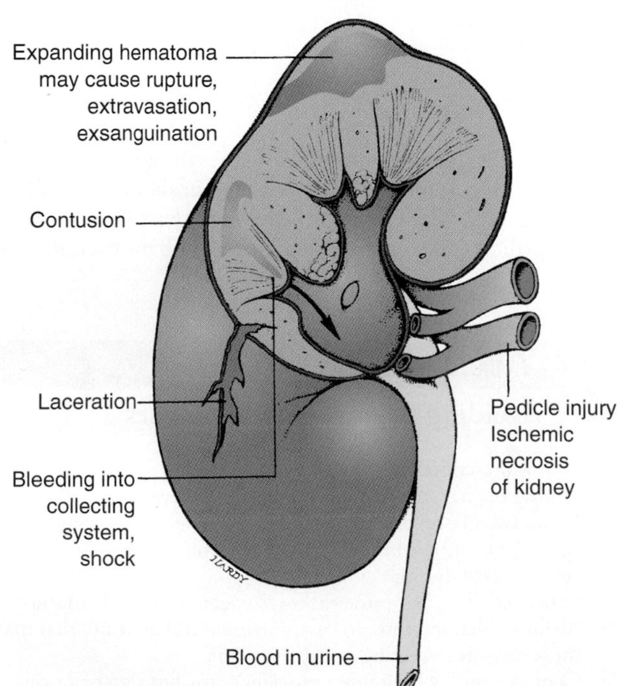

FIGURE 41•8 Types and pathophysiologic effects of renal injuries: contusions, lacerations, rupture, and pedicle injury.

Ureteral Trauma

Penetrating trauma and unintentional injury during surgery are the major causes of trauma to the ureters. Gunshot wounds account for 95% of ureteral injuries, which may range from contusions to complete transection. Unintentional injury to the ureter may occur during gynecologic or urologic surgery.

There are no specific signs or symptoms of ureteral injury; many traumatic injuries are discovered during exploratory surgery. If the ureteral trauma is not detected and urine leakage continues, fistulas are likely to develop.

Intravenous urography detects 90% of ureteral injuries and can be performed on the operating table in patients undergoing emergent surgery. Surgical repair with placement of stents (to divert urine away from the anastomoses) is usually necessary.

Bladder Trauma

Injury to the bladder may occur with pelvic fractures and multiple trauma or from a blow to the lower abdomen when the bladder is full. Blunt trauma may result in contusion evident as an ecchymosis—a large, discolored bruise resulting from escape of blood into the tissues and involving a segment of the bladder wall—or in rupture of the bladder extraperitoneally, intraperitoneally, or both. Complications from these injuries include hemorrhage, shock, sepsis, and extravasation of blood into the tissues, which must be treated promptly.

Urethral Trauma

Urethral injuries usually occur with blunt trauma to the lower abdomen or pelvic region. Many patients also have associated pelvic fractures. A classic triad of symptoms include blood at the urinary meatus, an inability to void, and a distended bladder.

Medical Management

The goals of management in patients with genitourinary trauma are to control hemorrhage, pain, and infection; to preserve and restore renal function; and to maintain urinary drainage. In **renal trauma**, all urine is saved and sent to the laboratory for analysis to detect RBCs and to evaluate the course of bleeding. Hematocrit and hemoglobin levels are monitored closely; decreasing values indicate hemorrhage.

The patient is monitored for oliguria and signs of hemorrhagic shock because a pedicle injury or shattered kidney can lead to rapid exsanguination (lethal blood loss). An expanding hematoma may cause rupture of the kidney capsule. To detect hematoma, the area around the lower ribs, upper lumbar vertebrae, flank, and abdomen is palpated for tenderness. A palpable flank or abdominal mass with local tenderness, swelling, and ecchymosis suggests renal hemorrhage. The area of the original mass can be outlined with a marking pencil so that the examiner can evaluate the area for change.

Renal trauma is often associated with other injuries to the abdominal organs (liver, colon, small intestines); therefore, the patient is assessed for skin abrasions, lacerations, and entry and exit wounds of the upper abdomen and lower thorax because these may be associated with renal injury.

With renal trauma, such as a contusion of the kidney, healing may take place with conservative measures. If the patient has microscopic hematuria and a normal intravenous urogram, outpatient management is possible. If gross hematuria or a minor laceration is present, the patient is hospitalized and kept on bed rest until hematuria clears. Antimicrobial medications may be prescribed to prevent infection from perirenal hematoma or urinoma (a cyst containing urine). Patients with retroperitoneal hematomas may develop low-grade fever as absorption of the clot takes place.

Surgical Management

In *renal trauma*, any sudden change in the patient's condition may indicate hemorrhage and requires surgical intervention.

Nursing Alert *The patient's vital signs, urine output, and level of consciousness are monitored to detect evidence of bleeding and shock. Opioid analgesia is avoided because this may mask accompanying abdominal symptoms.*

Nursing Alert *The patient is prepared for surgery in cases of increasing pulse rate, hypotension, and impending shock.*

Depending on the patient's condition and the nature of the injury, major lacerations may be treated through surgical intervention or conservatively (bed rest, no surgery). Vascular injuries require immediate exploratory surgery because of the high incidence of involvement of other organ systems and the serious complications that may result if these injuries are untreated. The patient is often in shock and requires aggressive fluid resuscitation. The damaged kidney may have to be removed (nephrectomy).

Early postoperative complications (within 6 months) include rebleeding, perinephritic abscess formation, sepsis, urine extravasation, and fistula formation. Other complications include stone formation, infection, cysts, vascular aneurysms, and loss of renal function. Hypertension is a complication of any renal surgery but usually is a late complication of renal injury.

In *bladder trauma*, treatment for rupture of the bladder involves immediate exploratory surgery and repair of the laceration, suprapubic drainage of the bladder and the perivesical space (around the bladder), and insertion of an indwelling urinary catheter. In addition to the usual care following urologic surgery, the drainage systems (suprapubic, indwelling urethral catheter, and perivesical drains) are closely monitored to ensure adequate drainage until healing takes place. The patient with a ruptured bladder may have gross bleeding for several days after repair.

In *urethral trauma*, unstable patients who need monitoring of urinary output may need a suprapubic catheter inserted.

Nursing Alert *Urethral catheterization should not be attempted if blood is seen at the urinary meatus until an emergency retrograde urethrogram can be performed.*

The patient is catheterized after the urethrogram is performed to minimize the risk of urethral disruption and extensive, long-term complications, such as stricture, incontinence, and impotence.

Surgical repair may be performed immediately or at a later time. Delayed surgical repair tends to be the favored procedure because it is associated with fewer long-term complications, such as impotence, strictures, and incontinence. After surgery, an indwelling urinary catheter may remain in place for up to 1 month.

Nursing Management

The patient with genitourinary trauma (particularly renal trauma) should be assessed frequently during the first few days after injury to detect flank and abdominal pain, muscle spasm, and swelling over the flank.

PROMOTING HOME AND COMMUNITY-BASED CARE

Teaching Patients Self-Care. Patients who have had surgery to repair traumatic injury are instructed about care of the incision and the importance of an adequate intake. In addition, instructions about changes that should be reported to the physician, such as fever, hematuria, flank pain, or any signs of decreasing kidney function, are provided. Guidelines for increasing activity gradually, lifting, and driving are also provided in accordance with physician's prescription.

Continuing Care. Follow-up nursing care includes monitoring the blood pressure to detect hypertension and advising the patient to restrict activities for about 1 month after trauma to minimize the incidence of delayed or secondary bleeding. The patient should be advised to schedule periodic follow-up assessments of renal function (creatinine clearance, serum BUN and creatinine analyses). If a nephrectomy was done as a result of the trauma, the patient is advised to wear medical identification.

RENAL TUMORS

Cancer of the kidney accounts for about 2% of all cancers in adults in the United States. It affects almost twice as many men as women. The most common type of renal tumor is renal cell or renal adenocarcinoma, accounting for more than 85% of all kidney tumors (Landis et al., 1999). These tumors may metastasize early to the lungs, bone, liver, brain, and contralateral kidney. One-third of patients have metastatic disease at the time of diagnosis.

Clinical Manifestations

Many renal tumors produce no symptoms and are discovered on a routine physical examination as a palpable abdominal mass. The classic triad of signs and symptoms, which occur in only 10% of patients, includes hematuria, pain, and a mass in the flank. The usual sign that first calls attention to the tumor is painless hematuria, which may be either intermittent and microscopic or continuous and gross. There may be a dull pain in the back from back pressure produced by compression of the ureter, extension of the tumor into the perirenal area, or hemorrhage into the kidney tissue. Colicky pains occur if a clot or mass

Risk Factors for RENAL CANCER

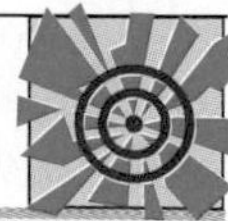

- Gender: Affects men more than women
- Tobacco use
- Occupational exposure to industrial chemicals, such as petroleum products, heavy metals, and asbestos
- Obesity
- Unopposed estrogen therapy
- Polycystic kidney disease

of tumor cells passes down the ureter. Symptoms from metastasis may be the first manifestation of renal tumor and may include unexplained weight loss, increasing weakness, and anemia.

Assessment and Diagnostic Findings

The diagnosis of a renal tumor may require intravenous urography, cystoscopic examination, nephrotomograms, renal angiograms, ultrasonography, or CT scan. These tests may be exhausting for patients already debilitated by the systemic effects of a tumor as well as for elderly patients and those who are anxious about the diagnosis and outcome. The nurse assists the patient to prepare physically and psychologically for these procedures and monitors carefully for signs of dehydration and exhaustion.

Medical Management

The goal of management is to eradicate the tumor before metastasis occurs.

SURGICAL MANAGEMENT

A *radical nephrectomy* is the preferred treatment if the tumor can be removed. This includes removal of the kidney (and tumor), adrenal gland, surrounding perinephric fat and Gerota's fascia, and lymph nodes. Radiation therapy, hormonal therapy, or chemotherapy may be used along with surgery. Immunotherapy may also be helpful. For patients with bilateral tumors or cancer of a functional single kidney, nephron-sparing surgery (partial nephrectomy) may be considered. Favorable results have been achieved in patients with small local tumors and a normal contralateral kidney.

Renal Artery Embolization. In patients with metastatic renal carcinoma, the renal artery may be occluded to deny a blood supply to the tumor and thus kill the tumor cells. Several days after angiographic studies are completed, a catheter is advanced into the renal artery, and embolizing materials (Gelfoam, autologous blood clot, steel coils) are injected into the artery and carried with the arterial blood flow to occlude the tumor vessels mechanically. This decreases the local blood supply, making removal of the kidney (nephrectomy) easier. It also stimulates an immune response because infarction of the renal cell carcinoma releases tumor-associated antigens that enhance the patient's response to metastatic lesions. The procedure may also reduce the number of tumor cells entering the venous circulation during surgical manipulation.

After renal artery embolization and tumor infarction, a characteristic symptom complex called *postinfarction syndrome* occurs, lasting 2 to 3 days. The patient has pain localized to the flank and abdomen, elevated temperature, and gastrointestinal complaints. Pain is treated with parenteral analgesics, and acetaminophen is administered to control fever. Antiemetics, restriction of oral intake, and intravenous fluids are used to treat the gastrointestinal complaints.

PHARMACOLOGIC THERAPY

Many different pharmacologic substances (also called systemic therapy) have been tested in renal cell carcinoma. No chemotherapeutic agent has been found that produces a response adequate to justify its use. However, some success in treating renal tumors with biologic response modifiers has been reported.

Patients may be treated with interleukin-2 (IL-2), a protein that regulates cell growth. This may be used alone or in combination with lymphokine-activated killer cells, which are WBCs that have been stimulated by IL-2 to increase their ability to kill cancer cells. Interferon, another biologic response modifier, appears to have a direct antiproliferative effect on renal tumors. The study of these biologic agents and new biologic response modifiers is a priority because nearly half of all patients with renal cell carcinoma die within 5 years of diagnosis (Motzer, Bander, & Nanus, 1996; Landis et al., 1999).

Nursing Management

The patient with a renal tumor usually undergoes extensive diagnostic and therapeutic procedures, including surgery, radiation therapy, and medication (or systemic) therapy. After surgery, the patient usually has catheters and drains in place to maintain a patent urinary tract, to remove drainage, and to permit accurate measurement of urine output. Because of the location of the surgical incision, the position of the patient during surgery, and the nature of the surgical procedure, pain and muscle soreness are common.

The patient requires frequent analgesia during the postoperative period and assistance with turning. Turning, coughing, use of incentive spirometry, and taking deep breaths are encouraged to prevent atelectasis and other pulmonary complications. The patient and family require assistance and support to cope with the diagnosis and uncertainties about the prognosis. (See the discussion in this chapter of postoperative care of the patient undergoing surgery of the kidney; see also Chapter 15 for care of the oncology patient.)

PROMOTING HOME AND COMMUNITY-BASED CARE

Teaching Patients Self-Care. The patient is taught to inspect and care for the incision and perform other general postoperative care. Additionally, the patient learns about activity and lifting restrictions, driving, and use of pain medications. Instructions are provided about follow-up care and when to notify the physician about problems (fever, breathing difficulty, wound drainage, blood in the urine, pain or swelling of the legs).

The patient is encouraged to eat a well-balanced diet and to drink adequate amounts of liquids to avoid constipation and to maintain an adequate urine volume. Education and emotional support are provided related to the disease process, treatment plan, and continuing care because many patients are concerned about the loss of the other kidney, the need for dialysis, or the recurrence of cancer.

Continuing Care. Follow-up care is essential to detect signs of metastases and to reassure the patient and family about the patient's status and well-being. The patient who has had surgery for renal carcinoma should have a yearly physical examination and chest x-ray because late metastases are not uncommon. All subsequent symptoms should be evaluated with possible metastases in mind.

If follow-up chemotherapy is necessary, the patient and family are informed about the entire treatment plan or chemotherapy protocol, what to expect with each visit, and how to notify the physician. Periodic evaluation of remaining renal function (creatinine clearance, serum BUN and creatinine levels) may also be carried out periodically. A home care nurse may provide care in the home, monitoring the patient's status and psychological well-being and coordinating other services and resources needed by the patient.

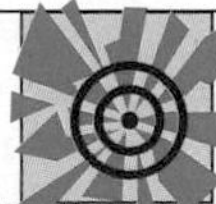

Risk Factors for
BLADDER CANCER

- Cigarette smoking: risk proportional to number of packs smoked daily and number of years of smoking.
- Environmental carcinogens: dyes, rubber, leather, ink, or paint
- Recurrent or chronic bacterial infection of the urinary tract
- Bladder stones
- High urinary pH
- High cholesterol intake
- Pelvic radiation therapy
- Cancers arising from the prostate, colon, and rectum in males

CANCER OF THE BLADDER

Cancer of the urinary bladder is more common in people aged 50 to 70 years. It affects men more than women (3:1) and is more common in whites than in African Americans. Statistics indicate that bladder tumors account for nearly 1 in 25 cancers diagnosed in the United States. There are two forms of bladder cancer: superficial (which tends to recur) and invasive. About 80% to 90% of all bladder cancers are transitional cell (which means they arise from the transitional cells of the bladder); the remaining types of tumors are squamous cell and adenocarcinoma (Kaufman & Shipley, 1997).

The predominant cause of bladder cancer today is cigarette smoking. Cancers arising from the prostate, colon, and rectum in males and from the lower gynecologic tract in females may metastasize to the bladder.

Clinical Manifestations

Bladder tumors usually arise at the base of the bladder and involve the ureteral orifices and bladder neck. Visible, painless hematuria is the most common symptom of bladder cancer. Infection of the urinary tract is a common complication, producing frequency, urgency, and dysuria. Any alteration in voiding or change in the urine, however, may indicate cancer of the bladder. Pelvic or back pain may occur with metastasis.

Assessment and Diagnostic Findings

Diagnostic evaluation includes cystoscopy (mainstay of diagnosis), excretory urography, CT scan, ultrasonography, and bimanual examination with the patient anesthetized. Biopsies of the tumor and adjacent mucosa are the definitive diagnostic procedures.

Transitional cell carcinomas and carcinomas in situ shed recognizable cancer cells. Cytologic examination of fresh urine and saline bladder washings provide information about the patient's prognosis, especially for those at high risk for recurrence of primary bladder tumors.

Medical Management

Treatment of bladder cancer depends on the grade of the tumor (based on the degree of cellular differentiation), the stage of tumor growth (the degree of local invasion and the presence or absence of metastasis), and the multicentricity (having many centers) of the tumor. The patient's age and physical, mental, and emotional status are considered when determining treatment modalities.

SURGICAL MANAGEMENT

Transurethral resection or *fulguration* (cauterization) may be performed for simple papillomas (benign epithelial tumors). These procedures, described in more detail in Chapter 45, eradicate the tumors through surgical incision or electrical current with the use of instruments inserted through the urethra. After this bladder-sparing surgery, intravesical administration of bacillus Calmette-Guèrin (BCG) is the treatment of choice.

Management of superficial bladder cancers presents a challenge because there are usually widespread abnormalities in the bladder mucosa. The entire lining of the urinary tract, or urothelium, is at risk because carcinomatous changes can occur in the mucosa of the bladder, renal pelvis, ureter, and urethra. About 25% to 40% of superficial tumors recur after transurethral resection or fulguration. Patients with benign papillomas should undergo cytology and cystoscopy periodically for the rest of their lives because aggressive malignancies may develop from these tumors.

A simple **cystectomy** (removal of the bladder) or a radical cystectomy is performed for invasive or multifocal bladder cancer. Radical cystectomy in men involves removal of the bladder, prostate, and seminal vesicles and immediate adjacent perivesical tissues. In women, radical cystectomy involves removal of the bladder, lower ureter, uterus, fallopian tubes, ovaries, anterior vagina, and urethra. It may include removal of pelvic lymph nodes. Removal of the bladder requires a urinary diversion procedure.

PHARMACOLOGIC THERAPY

Chemotherapy with a combination of methotrexate, 5-fluorouracil, vinblastine, doxorubicin (Adriamycin), and cisplatin has been effective in producing partial remission of transitional cell carcinoma of the bladder in some patients. Intravenous chemotherapy may be accompanied by radiation therapy.

Topical chemotherapy (intravesical chemotherapy or instillation of antineoplastic agents into the bladder resulting in contact of the agent with the bladder wall) is considered when there is high risk for recurrence, when cancer in situ is present, or when tumor resection has been incomplete. Topical chemotherapy delivers a high concentration of medication (thiotepa, doxorubicin, mitomycin, ethoglucid, and BCG) to the tumor to promote tumor destruction. BCG is now considered the most effective intravesical agent for recurrent bladder cancer because it enhances the body's immune response to cancer.

The patient is allowed to eat and drink before the instillation procedure, but once the bladder is full, the patient must retain the intravesical solution for 2 hours before voiding. At the end of the procedure, the patient is encouraged to void and to drink liberal amounts of fluid to flush the medication from the bladder.

RADIATION THERAPY

Radiation of the tumor may be performed preoperatively to reduce microextension of the neoplasm and viability of tumor cells, thus reducing the chances that the cancer may recur in the immediate area or spread through the circulatory or lymphatic systems. Radiation therapy is also used in combination with surgery or to control the disease in patients with an inoperable tumor.

The transitional cell variety of bladder cancer responds poorly to chemotherapy. Cisplatin, doxorubicin, and cyclophosphamide have been administered in various doses and schedules and appear most effective.

Bladder cancer may also be treated by direct infusion of the cytotoxic agent through the bladder's arterial blood supply to achieve a higher concentration of the chemotherapeutic agent with fewer systemic toxic effects. For more advanced bladder cancer or for patients with intractable hematuria (especially after radiation therapy), a large, water-filled balloon placed in the bladder produces tumor necrosis by reducing the blood supply of the bladder wall (hydrostatic therapy). The instillation of formalin, phenol, or silver nitrate relieves hematuria and strangury (slow and painful discharge of urine) in some patients.

INVESTIGATIONAL THERAPY

The application of photodynamic techniques in treating superficial bladder cancer is under investigation. This procedure involves systemic injection of a photosensitizing material (hematoporphyrin), which the cancer cell picks up. A laser-generated light then changes the hematoporphyrin in the cancer cell into a toxic medication. This process is being investigated for patients in whom intravesical chemotherapy or immunotherapy has failed.

URINARY DIVERSIONS

Urinary diversion procedures are performed to divert urine from the bladder to a new exit site, usually through a surgically created opening (stoma) in the skin. These procedures are primarily performed when a bladder tumor necessitates removal of the entire bladder (cystectomy). Urinary diversion has also been used in managing pelvic malignancy, birth defects, strictures, and trauma to ureters and urethra, neurogenic bladder, chronic infection causing severe ureteral and renal damage, and intractable interstitial cystitis and as a last resort in managing incontinence.

Controversy exists about the best method of establishing permanent diversion of the urinary tract. New techniques are frequently introduced in an effort to improve patient outcomes and quality of life. The age of the patient, condition of the bladder, body build, degree of obesity, degree of ureteral dilation, status of renal function, and patient's learning ability and willingness to participate in postoperative care are all taken into consideration when determining the appropriate surgical procedure.

The extent to which the patient accepts urinary diversion depends to a large degree on the location or position of the stoma, whether the drainage device (pouch or bag) establishes a watertight seal to the skin, and the patient's ability to manage the pouch and drainage apparatus. Paying attention to these considerations helps to promote a positive outcome.

There are two categories of urinary diversion: cutaneous urinary diversion, in which urine drains through an opening created in the abdominal wall and skin (Fig. 41-9), and **continent urinary diversion**, in which a portion of the intestine is used to create a new reservoir for urine (Fig. 41-10).

Cutaneous Urinary Diversions

Ileal Conduit (Ileal Loop)

The **ileal conduit**, the oldest of the urinary diversion procedures, is considered the gold standard because of the low number of complications and surgeons' familiarity with the procedure. In an ileal conduit, the urine is diverted by implanting the ureter into a 12-cm loop of ileum that is led out through the abdominal wall. This loop of ileum is a simple conduit (passageway) for urine from the ureters to the surface. A loop of the sigmoid colon may also be used. An ileostomy bag is used to collect the urine. The resected (cut) ends of the remaining intestine are anastomosed (connected) to provide an intact bowel.

Stents, usually made of thin, pliable tubing, are placed in the ureters to prevent occlusion secondary to postsurgical edema. The bilateral ureteral stents allow urine to drain from the kidney to the stoma and provide a method for accurate measurement of urine output. They may be left in place 10 to 21 days postoperatively. Jackson-Pratt tubes or other types of drains are inserted to prevent the accumulation of fluid in the space created by removal of the bladder.

After surgery, a skin barrier and a transparent, disposable urinary drainage bag are applied around the conduit and connected to drainage. A custom-cut appliance is used until the edema subsides and the stoma shrinks to normal size. The clear bag allows the stoma to be visualized and the patency of the stent and the urinary output to be monitored. The ileal bag drains urine constantly (not feces). The appliance (bag) usually remains in place as long as it is watertight; it is changed when necessary to prevent leakage of urine.

Complications that may follow placement of an ileal conduit include wound infection or wound dehiscence, urinary leakage, ureteral obstruction, hyperchloremic acidosis, small bowel obstruction, ileus, and stomal gangrene. Delayed complications include ureteral obstruction, contraction or narrowing of the stoma (stomal stenosis), renal deterioration due to chronic reflux, pyelonephritis, and renal calculi.

Nursing Management

In the immediate postoperative period, urine volumes are monitored hourly. An output below 30 mL/h may indicate dehydration or an obstruction in the ileal conduit with possible backflow or leakage from the ureteroileal anastomosis. Throughout the patient's hospitalization, the nurse monitors the patient closely for complications, reports signs and symptoms of them promptly, and intervenes quickly to prevent their progression.

PROMOTING URINARY OUTPUT

A catheter may be inserted through the urinary conduit if prescribed to monitor for possible stasis or residual urine from a constricted stoma. Urine may drain through the bilateral ureteral stents as well as around the stents. If the ureteral stents are not draining, the nurse may be instructed to irrigate them with 5 to 10 mL of sterile normal saline solution. It is important to avoid any tension on the stents because this may dislodge them. Hematuria may be noted in the first 48 hours after surgery but usually resolves spontaneously.

PROVIDING STOMA AND SKIN CARE

Because the patient requires specialized care, a consultation is initiated with an enterostomal therapist or clinical nurse specialist in skin care. The stoma is inspected frequently for color and viability. A healthy stoma is beefy red. A change from this normal color to a dark purplish color suggests that the vascular supply may be compromised. If cyanosis and a compromised blood supply persist, surgical intervention may be necessary. The stoma is not sensitive to touch, but the skin around the stoma becomes very sensitive if urine or the appliance irritates it. The skin is inspected for (1) signs of irritation and bleeding of the stomal mucosa, (2) encrustation and skin irritation around the stoma (from alkaline urine coming in contact with exposed skin), and (3) wound infections.

TESTING URINE AND CARING FOR THE OSTOMY

Moisture in bed linens or clothing or the odor of urine around the patient should alert the nurse to the possibility of leakage from the appliance, potential infection, or a problem in hygienic management. Because severe alkaline encrustation can accumulate rapidly around the stoma, the urine pH is kept below 6.5.

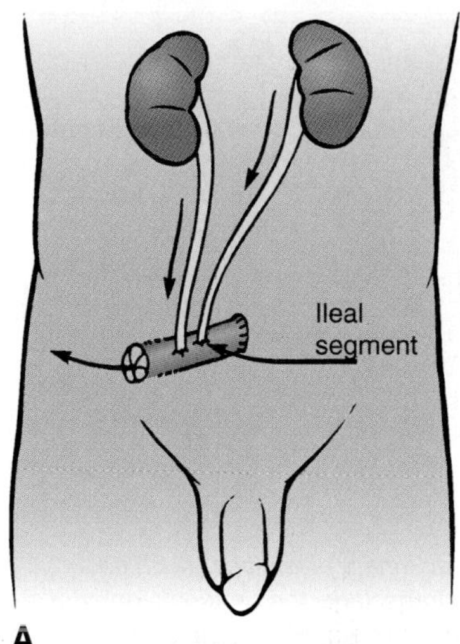

A

Conventional ileal conduit. The surgeon transplants the ureters to an isolated section of the terminal ileum (ileal conduit), bringing one end to the abdominal wall. The ureter may also be transplanted into the transverse sigmoid colon (colon conduit) or proximal jejunum (jejunal conduit).

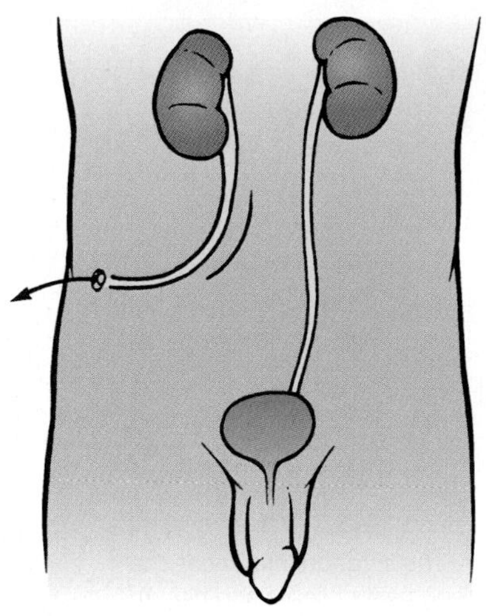

B

Cutaneous ureterostomy. The surgeon brings the detached ureter through the abdominal wall and attaches it to an opening in the skin.

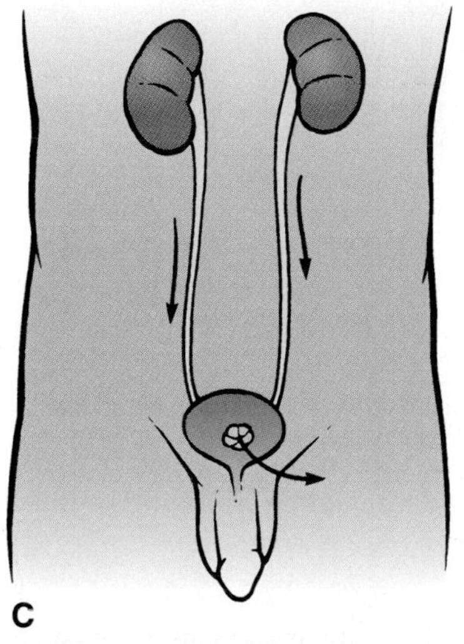

C

Vesicostomy. The surgeon sutures the bladder to the abdominal wall and creates an opening (stoma) through the abdominal and bladder walls for urinary drainage.

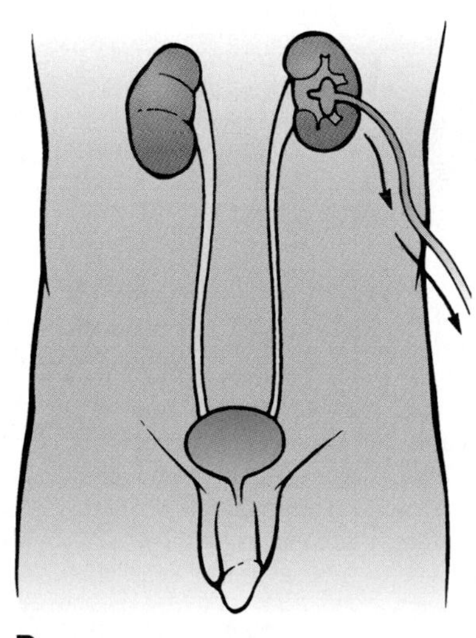

D

Nephrostomy. The surgeon inserts a catheter into the renal pelvis via an incision into the flank or, by percutaneous catheter placement, into the kidney.

FIGURE 41•9 Types of cutaneous diversions include (**A**) the conventional ileal conduit; (**B**) cutaneous ureterostomy, (**C**) vesicostomy, and (**D**) nephrostomy.

Urine pH can be determined by testing the urine draining from the stoma, not from the collecting appliance. A properly fitted appliance is essential to prevent exposure of the peristomal skin (skin around the stoma) to urine. If the urine is foul smelling, the stoma is catheterized, if prescribed, to obtain a urine specimen for culture and sensitivity testing.

ENCOURAGING FLUIDS AND RELIEVING ANXIETY

Because mucous membrane is used in forming the conduit, the patient may excrete a large amount of mucus mixed with urine. This causes many patients to feel anxious. To help relieve this anxiety, the nurse reassures the patient that this is a normal occurrence after an ileal conduit procedure. The nurse encourages adequate fluid intake to flush the ileal conduit and decrease the accumulation of mucus.

SELECTING THE OSTOMY APPLIANCE

Various urine collection appliances are available, and the nurse is instrumental in selecting an appropriate one. The urinary appliance may consist of one or two pieces and may be disposable (usually used once and discarded) or reusable. The choice of appliance is determined by the location of the stoma and by the patient's normal activity, manual dexterity, visual deficits, body

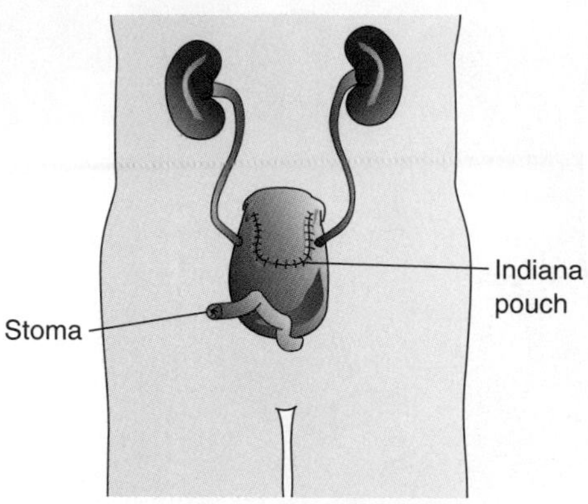

A
Indiana pouch. The surgeon introduces the ureters into a segment of ileum and cecum. Urine is drained periodically by inserting a catheter into the stoma.

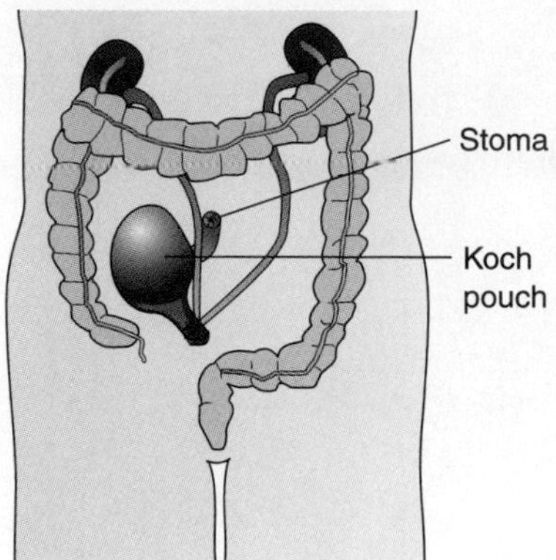

B
Continent ileal urinary diversions (Koch pouch). The surgeon transplants the ureters to an isolated segment of small bowel, ascending colon, or ileocolonic segment and develops an effective continence mechanism or valve. Urine is drained by inserting a catheter into the stoma.

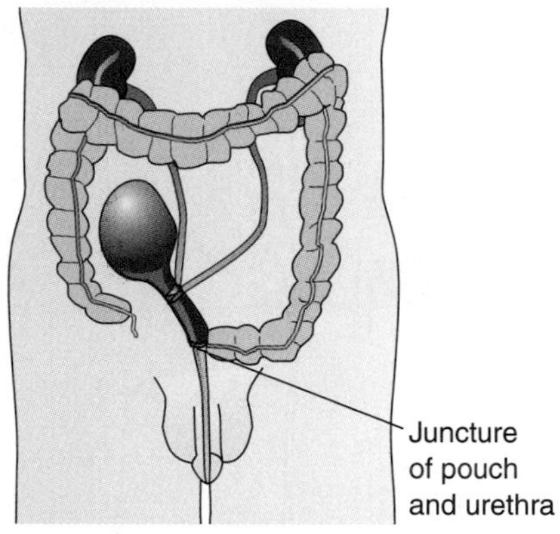

C
In male patients, the *Koch pouch* can be modified by attaching one end of the pouch to the urethra, allowing more normal voiding. The female urethra is too short for this modification.

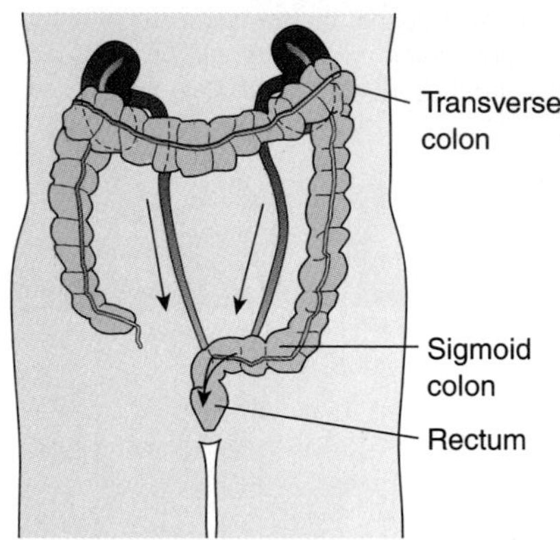

D
Ureterosigmoidostomy. The surgeon introduces the ureters into the sigmoid, thereby allowing urine to flow through the colon and out of the rectum.

FIGURE 41•10 Types of continent urinary diversions include (**A**) the Indiana pouch, (**B** and **C**) the Koch pouch, also called a continent ileal diversion, and (**D**) a ureterosigmoidostomy.

build, economic resources, and preference. A reusable appliance has a faceplate that is attached to the skin surface with cement or adhesive. Either reusable pouches or disposable pouches may be used with the reusable faceplate. Disposable appliances have the advantages of having a surface that is already prepared for application to the skin and of being lightweight and easy to conceal. A skin barrier must be used to protect the skin from excoriation due to exposure to the urine.

PROMOTING HOME AND COMMUNITY-BASED CARE

Teaching Patients Self-Care. Patient education begins in the hospital but continues into the home setting because patients are being discharged within days of surgery. The nurse teaches the patient how to assess and manage the urinary diversion as well as how to deal with body image changes. An enterostomal therapist is invaluable in consulting with the nurse on various aspects of care and patient education.

Changing the Appliance. The patient and family are taught to apply and change the appliance so that they are comfortable carrying out the procedure proficiently. Ideally, the appliance system is changed before the system leaks and at a time that is convenient for the patient. Many patients find early morning most convenient because the urine output is reduced. A variety of appliances are available; an average collecting appliance lasts 3 to 7 days before leakage occurs.

Regardless of the type of appliance used, a skin barrier is essential to protect the skin from irritation and excoriation. To maintain peristomal skin integrity, a skin barrier or leaking pouch is never patched with tape to prevent accumulation of urine under the skin barrier or faceplate. The patient is instructed to avoid moisturizing soaps when cleaning the area because they interfere with adhesion of the pouch. Because the degree to which the stoma protrudes is not the same in all patients, there are various accessories and custom-made appliances to solve individual problems. Guidelines for applying reusable and disposable systems are presented in Guideline 41-1.

41•1 Guidelines For 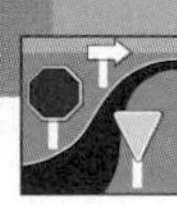 Changing a Leg Bag Collection Device

A patient who wears a leg bag urine collection device (for example a patient with a nephrostomy) will need to change the drainage system and leg bag regularly. Some general guidelines to follow:

1. Gather the supplies: gloves, alcohol wipes, and new leg bag urine collection device.
2. Wash hands and put on gloves.
3. According to the manufacturer's directions, disconnect and dispose of the old collection system.
4. Unwrap the alcohol wipe and cleanse the collection connectors.
5. Maintaining aseptic technique, connect the ends of the new drainage system (near right).
6. Secure the new bag with the leg straps supplied (far right).

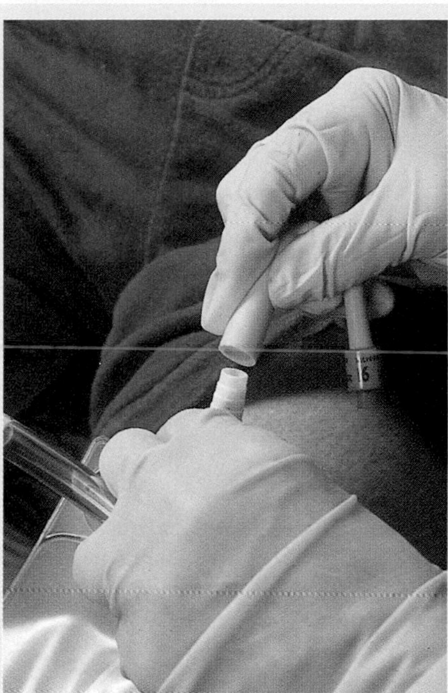

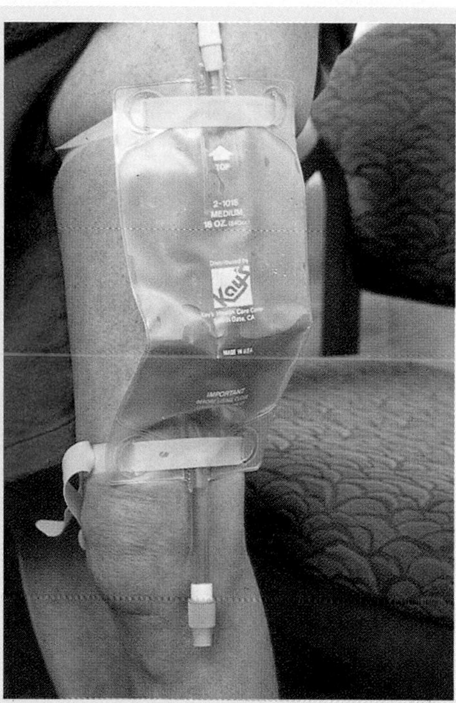

Controlling Odor. The patient is instructed to avoid foods that give the urine a strong odor (eg, asparagus, cheese, eggs). Today, most appliances contain odor barriers, but a few drops of liquid deodorizer or diluted white vinegar may be introduced through the drain spout into the bottom of the pouch with a syringe or eyedropper to reduce odors. Ascorbic acid by mouth helps acidify the urine and suppress urine odor. Patients should be cautioned about putting aspirin tablets in the pouch to control odor because they may ulcerate the stoma. Also, the patient is reminded that odor will develop if the pouch is worn too long and not cared for properly.

Managing the Ostomy Appliance. The patient is instructed to empty the pouch by means of a drain valve when it is one-third full because the weight of the urine will cause the pouch to separate from the skin if filled more. Some patients prefer wearing a leg bag attached with an adapter to the drainage apparatus. To promote uninterrupted sleep, a collecting bottle and tubing (one unit) are snapped onto an adapter that connects to the ileal appliance. A small amount of urine is left in the bag when the adapter is attached to prevent the bag from collapsing against itself. The tubing may be threaded down the pajama leg to prevent kinking. The collecting bottle and tubing are rinsed daily with cool water and once a week with a 3:1 solution of water and white vinegar.

Cleaning and Deodorizing the Appliance. Usually, the reusable appliance is rinsed in warm water and soaked in a 3 : 1 solution of water and white vinegar or a commercial deodorizing solution for 30 minutes. It is rinsed with tepid water and air-dried away from direct sunlight. (Hot water and exposure to direct sunlight dry the pouch and increase the incidence of cracking.) After drying, the appliance may be powdered with cornstarch and stored. Two appliances are necessary—one to be worn while the other is air-drying.

Continuing Care. Follow-up care is essential to determine how the patient has adapted to the body image changes and lifestyle changes. Referral for home care is indicated to determine how well the patient and family are coping with the changes necessitated by altered urinary drainage. The home care nurse assesses the patient's physical status and emotional response to urinary diversion. Additionally, the nurse assesses the ability of the patient and family to manage the urinary diversion and appliance, reinforces previous teaching, and provides additional information (eg, community resources, sources of ostomy supplies, insurance coverage for supplies).

As the postoperative edema subsides, the home care nurse assists in determining the appropriate changes needed in the ostomy appliance. The stoma opening is recalibrated every 3 to 6 weeks for the first few months postoperatively. The correct appliance size is determined by measuring the widest part of the stoma with a ruler. The permanent appliance should be no more than 1.6 mm (1/16 inch) larger than the diameter of the stoma and the same shape as the stoma to prevent contact of the skin with drainage.

The nurse encourages the patient and family to contact the United Ostomy Association and local ostomy association for visits, reassurance, and practical information. In addition, the local division of the American Cancer Society can provide medical equipment and supplies and other resources for the patient who has undergone ostomy surgery for cancer.

The home care nurse also assesses the patient for potential long-term complications, such as ureteral obstruction, stomal stenosis, hernias, or deterioration of renal function, and reinforces previous teaching about these complications.

The nurse also needs to remind the patient who has had surgery for carcinoma to have a yearly physical examination and chest x-ray to assess for metastases. Periodic evaluation of remaining renal function (creatinine clearance, serum BUN and creatinine levels) is also essential. Long-term monitoring for anemia is performed to identify a vitamin B_{12} deficiency that may occur when a significant portion of the terminal ileum is removed. This may take several years to develop and can be successfully treated with vitamin B_{12} injections.

Cutaneous Ureterostomy

A **cutaneous ureterostomy** (see Fig. 41-9), in which the ureters are directed through the abdominal wall and attached to an opening in the skin, is used for selected patients with ureteral obstruction (advanced pelvic cancer); for poor-risk patients, because it requires less extensive surgery than other urinary diversion procedures; and for patients who have had previous abdominal irradiation.

A urinary appliance is fitted immediately after surgery. The management of the patient with a cutaneous ureterostomy is similar to the care of the patient with an ileal conduit, although the stomas are usually flush with the skin or retracted.

Other Cutaneous Urinary Diversions

Other cutaneous urinary diversions are used less frequently and are most often used to bypass obstructions. Suprapubic bladder drainage (cystostomy) and nephrostomy are discussed further in Chapter 40.

Continent Urinary Diversions

Continent Ileal Urinary Reservoir (Indiana Pouch)

The most common continent urinary diversion is the Indiana pouch, created for patients whose bladder is removed or can no longer function (neurogenic bladder). The Indiana pouch uses a segment of the ileum and cecum to form the reservoir for urine (see Fig. 41-10*A*). The ureters are tunneled through the muscular bands of the intestinal pouch and anastomosed. The reservoir is made continent by narrowing the efferent portion of the ileum and sewing the terminal ileum to the subcutaneous tissue, forming a continent stoma flush with the skin. The pouch is sewed to the anterior abdominal wall around a cecostomy tube. Urine can collect in the pouch until a catheter is inserted and the urine is drained.

The pouch must be drained at regular intervals by a catheter to prevent absorption of metabolic waste products from the urine, reflux of urine to the ureters, and UTIs. Postoperative nursing care of the patient with a continent ileal urinary pouch is similar to nursing care of the patient with an ileal conduit. However, these patients usually have additional drainage tubes (cecostomy catheter from the pouch, stoma catheter exiting from the stoma, ureteral stents, Penrose drain, as well as a urethral catheter), as depicted in Figure 41-11. All drainage tubes must be carefully monitored for patency and amount and type of drainage. The cecostomy tube is irrigated two to three times daily to remove mucus from the pouch and prevent blockage.

Other variations of continent urinary reservoirs include the Kock pouch (U-shaped pouch is constructed of ileum, with a nipple-like one-way valve; see Fig. 41-10*B* and *C*) and the Charleston pouch (uses the ileum and ascending colon as the pouch, with the appendix and colon junction serving as the one-way valve mechanism). With both of these methods, the pouch must be drained at regular intervals by a catheter.

Ureterosigmoidostomy

Ureterosigmoidostomy, another form of continent urinary diversion, is an implantation of the ureters into the sigmoid colon (see Fig. 41-10*D*). It is usually performed in patients who have had extensive pelvic irradiation, previous small bowel resection, or coexisting small bowel disease.

After surgery, voiding occurs from the rectum (for life), and an adjustment in lifestyle will be necessary because of urinary frequency (as often as every 2 hours). Drainage has a consistency equivalent to watery diarrhea, and the patient has some degree of nocturia. Patients usually need to plan activities around the fre-

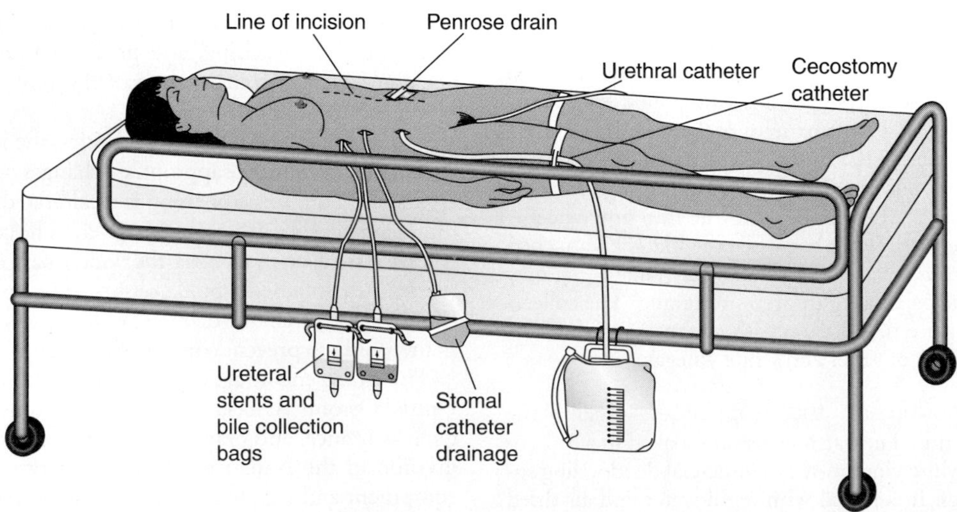

FIGURE 41•11 After surgery to create a continent ileal urinary reservoir (Indiana pouch), the patient will have many drains and catheter devices in place. In actual practice, the patient would be covered with a drape or gown.

quent need to urinate, which in turn may affect the patient's social life. Patients have the advantage, however, of urinary control without having to wear an external appliance.

Nursing Management

In addition to the usual preoperative regimen, the patient may be placed on a liquid diet for several days preoperatively to reduce residue in the colon. Antibiotic agents (neomycin, kanamycin) are administered for bowel disinfection. Ureterosigmoidostomy requires a competent anal sphincter, adequate renal function, and active renal peristalsis. The degree of anal sphincter control may be determined by assessing the patient's ability to retain enemas.

The postoperative regimen initially includes placing a catheter in the rectum to drain the urine and prevent reflux of urine into the ureters and kidneys. The tube is taped to the buttocks, and special skin care is given around the anus to prevent excoriation. Irrigations of the rectal tube may be prescribed, but force is never used because of the danger of introducing bacteria into the newly implanted ureters.

MONITORING FLUID AND ELECTROLYTES

In ureterosigmoidostomy, larger areas of the bowel mucosa are exposed to urine and electrolyte reabsorption. As a result, electrolyte imbalance and acidosis may occur. Potassium and magnesium in the urine may cause diarrhea. Fluid and electrolyte balance is maintained in the immediate postoperative period by closely monitoring the patient's serum electrolyte levels and administering appropriate intravenous infusions. Acidosis may be prevented by placing the patient on a low chloride diet supplemented with sodium potassium citrate.

The patient should be instructed never to wait longer than 2 to 3 hours before emptying urine from the intestine. This keeps rectal pressure low and minimizes the absorption of urinary constituents from the colon. It is essential to teach the patient about the symptoms of UTI: fever, flank pain, and frequency.

RETRAINING THE ANAL SPHINCTER

After the rectal catheter is removed, the patient learns to control the anal sphincter through special sphincter exercises. At first, urination is frequent. With reassurance and encouragement and the passage of time, the patient gains greater control and learns to differentiate between the need to void and the need to defecate.

PROMOTING DIETARY MEASURES

Specific dietary instructions include avoidance of gas-forming foods (flatus can cause stress incontinence and offensive odors). Other ways to avoid gas are to avoid chewing gum, smoking, and any other activity that involves swallowing air. Salt intake may be restricted to prevent hyperchloremic acidosis. Potassium intake is increased through foods and medication because potassium may be lost in acidosis.

MONITORING AND MANAGING POTENTIAL COMPLICATIONS

Pyelonephritis (upper UTI) due to reflux of bacteria from the colon is fairly common. Long-term antibiotic therapy may be prescribed to prevent infection. A late complication is adenocarcinoma of the sigmoid colon, possibly from cellular changes due to exposure of colonic mucosa to urine.

Other Urinary Diversion Procedures

Variations on urinary diversion surgical procedures are devised frequently in an effort to identify and perfect procedures that will improve patient outcomes and reduce the incidence of postoperative problems. These include cecal, patched cecal, and Mainz reservoirs. These techniques involve isolating a part of the large intestine to form a reservoir for urine and creating an abdominal stoma. Another surgical procedure, the Camey procedure, uses a portion of the ileum as a bladder substitute. In this procedure, the isolated ileum serves as the reservoir for urine; it is anastomosed directly to the portion of the remaining urethra after cystectomy. This procedure permits emptying of the bladder through the urethra. The Camey procedure, however, applies only to men because the entire urethra is removed when a cystectomy is performed in women.

NURSING PROCESS: THE PATIENT UNDERGOING URINARY DIVERSION SURGERY

Preoperative Assessment

The following are key preoperative nursing assessment concerns:

- Cardiopulmonary function assessments are performed because patients undergoing cystectomy (excision of the urinary bladder) are usually older people who may not be able to tolerate a lengthy, complex surgical procedure.
- A nutritional status assessment is important because of possible poor nutritional intake related to the patient's underlying health problems.
- Learning needs are assessed to evaluate the patient and the family's understanding of the procedure and the changes in physical structure and function that result from the surgery. The patient's self-concept and self-esteem are assessed, in addition to methods for coping with stress and loss. The patient's mental status, manual dexterity and coordination, and preferred method of learning are noted because they affect postoperative self-care.

Preoperative Nursing Diagnosis

Based on the assessment data, the preoperative nursing diagnoses for the patient undergoing urinary diversion surgery may include the following:

- Anxiety related to anticipated losses associated with the surgical procedure
- Altered nutrition, less than body requirements related to inadequate nutritional intake
- Knowledge deficit about the surgical procedure and postoperative care

Preoperative Planning and Goals

The major goals for the patient may include relief of anxiety, improved preoperative nutritional status, and increased knowledge about the surgical procedure, expected outcomes, and postoperative care.

Preoperative Nursing Interventions

Relieving Anxiety

The threat of cancer and removal of the bladder create fears related to body image and security. The patient faces problems in adapting to an external appliance, a stoma, a surgical incision, and altered toileting habits. The male patient must also adapt to sexual impotency. (A penile implant is considered if the patient is a candidate for the procedure.) Women also fear altered appearance, body image, and self-esteem. A supportive approach, both physical and psychosocial, is needed and includes assessing the patient's self-concept and manner of coping with stress and loss; helping the patient to identify ways to maintain a lifestyle and independence with as few changes as possible; and encouraging the patient to express fears and anxieties about the ramifications of the upcoming surgery. A visitor from the Ostomy Visitation Program of the American Cancer Society can provide emotional support and make adaptation easier both before and after surgery.

Ensuring Adequate Nutrition

In addition to cleansing the bowel to minimize fecal stasis, decompress the bowel, and minimize postoperative ileus, a low residue diet is prescribed and antibiotic medications are administered to reduce pathogenic flora in the bowel and to reduce the risk of infection. Because the patient undergoing a urinary diversion procedure for cancer may be severely malnourished, due to the tumor, radiation enteritis, and anorexia, enteral or total parenteral nutrition may be prescribed to promote healing. Adequate preoperative hydration is imperative to ensure urine flow during surgery and to prevent hypovolemia during the prolonged surgical procedure.

Explaining Surgery and Its Aftermath

An enterostomal therapist is invaluable in preoperative teaching and in planning postoperative care. Explanations of the surgical procedure, the appearance of the stoma, the rationale for preoperative bowel preparation, the reasons for wearing a collection device, and the anticipated effects of the surgery on sexual functioning are part of patient teaching. The placement of the stoma site is planned preoperatively with the patient standing, sitting, or lying down to locate the stoma away from bony prominences, skin creases, and fat folds. The stoma should also be placed away from old scars, the umbilicus, and the belt line.

For ease of self-care, the patient must be able to see and reach the site comfortably. The site is marked with indelible ink so that it can be located easily during surgery. The patient is assessed for allergies or sensitivity to tape or adhesives. (Patch testing of certain appliances may be necessary before the ostomy equipment is selected.) It may be helpful to have the patient practice wearing an appliance partially filled with water before surgery.

Preoperative Evaluation

To measure the effectiveness of care, the nurse evaluates the preoperative patient's anxiety level and nutritional status as well as his or her knowledge and expectations of surgery.

Expected Outcomes

Expected outcomes may include:

1. Exhibits reduced anxiety about surgery and expected losses
   a. Verbalizes fears with health care team and family
   b. Expresses positive attitude about outcome of surgery
2. Exhibits adequate nutritional status
   a. Maintains adequate intake prior to surgery
   b. Maintains body weight
   c. States rationale for enteral or parenteral nutrition if needed
   d. Exhibits normal skin turgor, moist mucous membranes, adequate urine output, and absence of excessive thirst

NURSING RESEARCH

Study of Postdiversional Adjustment

Raleigh, E., Berry, M., & Montie, J. (1995). A comparison of adjustments to urinary diversions: A pilot study. *Journal of Wound, Ostomy and Continence Nursing. 22*(1), 58–63.

Cystectomy with urinary diversion is a common treatment for patients with bladder cancer. Two types of urinary diversions often created postcystectomy include an incontinent diversion (the standard ileal conduit) or a continent diversion (a neobladder connected to the patient's urethra).

Purpose

The purpose of this exploratory study was to examine adjustments reported by male patients who had either an ileal conduit or neobladder surgery.

Study Sample and Design

The study sample consisted of 23 men (mean age, 66.8 ± 7.58 years) who had a cystectomy; 12 had ileal conduits, and 11 had neobladders. Time since surgery ranged from 10.6 months to 30.4 months with a mean of 18 ± 5.92 months. The demographic characteristics of the two groups were similar. Participants completed the Sickness Impact Profile (SIP), which assessed home management, mobility, social interaction, work, recreation, and pasttimes. In addition, ileal conduit patients were asked questions about potential problems with this type of urinary diversion. Neobladder patients were asked specific questions about continuing incontinence, a commonly identified clinical problem.

Findings

The most difficult adjustment reported by the neobladder group was to incontinence, followed by impotence. The ileal conduit group reported overall fewer adjustment problems. The most common problem identified by this group was pouch management. Of the 21 patients who responded to questions about sexual function, all reported impotence; only 12 patients recalled being told about a specialist in management of sexual dysfunction.

Patients were also asked about what motivated them to choose the type of urinary diversion and the most influential factors in their decision. The surgeon and enterostomal nurse were identified most frequently. All patients stated that they would choose the same procedure again if they had to choose again. There were no significant differences between the two groups on the SIP scores. However, both groups identified several normal activities being restricted as a result of their urinary diversion, including reduced work around the house, limited activity in public and social settings, and decreased sexual activity. Overall, patients generally reported good adjustment to the surgery, although some problems continued.

Nursing Implications

This study has implications for nursing practice, despite its small sample. The nurse has an important role in providing education, counseling, and support as the patient facing urinary diversion weighs the decision about the procedure. Providing the opportunity for the patient to talk to an enterostomal therapist is also extremely helpful for these patients. Postoperatively, the nurse can assist patients with incontinence and pouch management through education and support. Again, the enterostomal nurse is an invaluable asset for patients with urinary incontinence. Lastly, nurses can play a role in assisting patients in regard to sexual dysfunction by providing support and assistance with obtaining sexual rehabilitation therapy.

3. Demonstrates knowledge about the surgical procedure and postoperative course
   a. Identifies limitations expected after surgery
   b. Discusses expected immediate postoperative environment (tubes, machines, nursing surveillance)
   c. Practices deep breathing, coughing, and foot exercises

Postoperative Assessment

The role of the nurse in the immediate postoperative period is to prevent complications and to assess the patient carefully for any signs and symptoms of such complications. The catheters and any drainage devices are monitored closely. Urine volume, patency of the drainage system, and color of the drainage are assessed. A sudden decrease in urine volume or increase in drainage is reported promptly to the physician because these may indicate obstruction of the urinary tract, inadequate blood volume, or bleeding. In addition, the patient's needs for pain control are assessed.

Postoperative Diagnosis

Nursing Diagnoses

- Risk for impaired skin integrity related to problems in managing the urine collection appliance
- Pain related to surgical incision
- Body image disturbance related to urinary diversion
- Potential for sexual dysfunction related to structural and physiologic alterations
- Knowledge deficit about management of urinary function

Collaborative Problems/Potential Complications

Potential complications may include the following:

- Peritonitis due to disruption of anastomosis
- Stomal ischemia and necrosis due to compromised blood supply to stoma
- Stoma retraction and separation of mucocutaneous border due to tension or trauma

Postoperative Planning and Goals

The major goals for the patient may include maintaining peristomal skin integrity, increasing self-esteem, developing appropriate coping mechanisms to accept and deal with altered urinary function and sexuality, increasing knowledge about management of urinary function, and preventing potential complications.

Postoperative Nursing Interventions

Postoperative management focuses on monitoring urinary function, preventing postoperative complications (infection and sepsis, respiratory complications, fluid and electrolyte imbalances, fistula formation, and urine leakage), and promoting patient comfort. Catheters or drainage systems are observed, and urine output is monitored carefully. A nasogastric tube is inserted during surgery to decompress the gastrointestinal tract and to relieve pressure on the intestinal anastomosis. It is usually kept in place for several days after surgery. As soon as bowel function resumes, as indicated by bowel sounds, the passage of flatus, and a soft abdomen, oral fluids are permitted. Until that time, intravenous fluids and electrolytes are administered. The patient is assisted to ambulate as soon as possible to prevent complications of immobility.

Maintaining Peristomal Skin Integrity

Strategies to promote skin integrity begin with reducing and controlling those factors that increase the patient's risk for poor nutrition and poor healing. As indicated previously, meticulous skin care and management of the drainage system are provided by the nurse until the patient is able to manage them and is comfortable doing so. Care is taken to keep the drainage system intact to protect the skin from exposure to drainage. Supplies must be readily available to manage the drainage in the immediate postoperative period. Consistency in implementing the skin care program throughout the postoperative period will result in maintenance of skin integrity and patient comfort. Additionally, maintenance of skin integrity around the stoma will enable the patient and family to adjust more easily to the alterations in urinary function and will help them to learn skin care techniques.

Relieving Pain

Analgesic medications are administered liberally postoperatively to relieve pain and promote comfort, thereby allowing the patient to turn, cough, and do deep-breathing exercises. Patient-controlled analgesia and administration of analgesic agents regularly around the clock are two options that may be used to ensure adequate pain relief. A pain-intensity scale is used to judge the adequacy of the medication and the approach to pain management.

Improving Body Image

The patient's ability to cope with the changes associated with the surgery depends to some degree on body image and self-esteem before the surgery and the support and reaction of others. Allowing the patient to express concerns and anxious feelings can help, especially in adjusting to the changes in toileting habits. The nurse can also help improve the patient's self-concept by teaching the skills needed to be independent in managing the urinary drainage devices. Education about ostomy care is conducted in a private setting to encourage the patient to ask questions without fear of embarrassment. Explaining why the nurse must wear gloves when performing ostomy care can prevent the patient from misinterpreting the use of gloves as a sign of aversion to the stoma.

Exploring Sexuality Issues

Patients who experience altered sexual function as a result of the surgical procedure may mourn this loss. Encouraging the patient and partner to share their feelings about this loss with each other and acknowledging the importance of sexual function and expression may assist the patient and partner to seek sexual counseling and to explore alternative ways of expressing sexuality. A visit from another "ostomate" who is functioning fully in society and family life may also assist the patient and family in recognizing that full recovery is possible.

Monitoring and Managing Potential Complications

Complications are not unusual because of the complexity of the surgery, the underlying reason (cancer, trauma) for urinary diversion procedures, and the patient's frequently less than optimal nutritional status. Complications may include the usual postoperative complications (eg, respiratory problems, such as atelectasis, fluid and electrolyte imbalances) as well as breakdown of the anastomoses, sepsis, fistula formation, fecal or urine leakage, and skin irritation. If these occur, the patient will remain hospitalized for an extended length of time and will probably require total parenteral nutrition, gastrointestinal decompression by means of nasogastric suction, and further surgery. The goals of management are to establish drainage, provide adequate nutrition for healing to occur, and prevent sepsis.

Peritonitis. Peritonitis can occur postoperatively if urine leaks at the anastomosis. Signs and symptoms include abdominal pain and distention, muscle rigidity with guarding, nausea and vomiting, paralytic ileus (absence of bowel sounds), fever, and leukocytosis.

Urine output must be monitored closely because a sudden decrease in amount with a corresponding increase in drainage from the incision or drains may indicate urine leakage. In addition, the urine drainage device is observed for leakage. The pouch is changed if a leak is observed. Small leaks in the anastomosis may seal themselves, but surgery may be needed for larger leaks.

Vital signs (blood pressure, pulse and respiratory rates, temperature) are monitored. Changes in vital signs, as well as increasing pain, nausea and vomiting, and abdominal distention, are reported to the physician and may indicate peritonitis.

Stoma Ischemia and Necrosis. The stoma is monitored because stomal ischemia and necrosis can result from tension on the mesentery blood vessels, twisting of the bowel segment (conduit) during surgery, or arterial insufficiency. The new stoma must be inspected at least every 4 hours to assess the adequacy of its blood supply. The stoma should be red or pink. If the blood supply to the stoma is compromised, the color changes to purple, brown, or black. These changes are reported immediately to the physician. The physician or enterostomal therapist may insert a small, lubricated tube into the stoma and shine a flashlight into the lumen of the tube to assess for superficial ischemia or necrosis. A necrotic stoma requires surgical intervention. If the ischemia is superficial, the dusky stoma is observed and may slough its outer layer in several days.

Stoma Retraction and Separation. Stoma retraction and separation of the mucocutaneous border can occur as a result of trauma or tension on the internal bowel segment used for creation of the stoma. In addition, mucocutaneous separation can occur if the stoma does not heal as a result of accumulation of urine on the stoma and mucocutaneous border. Using a collection drainage pouch with an antireflux valve is helpful because the valve prevents urine from pooling on the stoma and mucocutaneous border. Meticulous skin care to keep the area around the stoma clean and dry promotes healing. If a separation of the mucocutaneous border occurs, surgery is not usually needed. The separated area is protected by applying karaya powder, stoma adhesive paste, and a properly fitted skin barrier and pouch. By protecting the separation, healing is promoted. If the stoma retracts back into the peritoneum, surgical intervention is mandatory.

If surgery is needed to manage these complications, the nurse provides explanations to the patient and family. The need for additional surgery is usually perceived as a setback by the patient and family. Emotional support of the patient and family is provided along with physical preparation of the patient for surgery.

Promoting Home and Community-Based Care

TEACHING PATIENTS SELF-CARE

Adequate supplies and complete instruction are necessary to enable the patient and a family member to develop competence and confidence in their skills. Written and verbal instructions are provided, and the patient is encouraged to contact the nurse or physician with follow-up questions. Follow-up telephone calls from the nurse to the patient and family after the patient's discharge may provide added support. Follow-up visits and reinforcement of correct skin care and appliance management techniques also promote skin integrity. Specific techniques for managing the appliance are described in Using Urinary Diversion Collection Appliances.

A major postoperative objective is to assist the patient to achieve the highest level of independence and self-care possible. The primary nurse and enterostomal therapist work closely with the patient and family to instruct and assist them in all phases of managing the ostomy. The patient is encouraged to participate in decisions regarding the type of collecting appliance and the time of day to change the appliance. The patient is assisted and encouraged to look at and touch the stoma early to overcome any fears. The patient and family need to know the characteristics of a normal stoma, as follows:

- Pink and moist, like the inside of the mouth
- Insensitive to pain because it has no nerve endings
- Vascular and may bleed when cleaned

Additionally, if a segment of the gastrointestinal tract was used to create the urinary diversion, mucus may be visible in the urine. By learning what is normal, the patient and family become familiar with what signs and symptoms they should report to the physician or nurse and what problems that they can handle themselves.

Information provided to the patient and the extent of involvement in self-care are determined by the patient's physical recovery and ability to accept and acquire the knowledge and skill needed for independence. Verbal and written instructions are provided, and the patient is given the opportunity to practice and demonstrate the skills needed to manage urinary drainage.

CONTINUING CARE

Follow-up care is essential to determine how the patient has adapted to the body image changes and lifestyle adjustments. Visits from a home care nurse are important to assess the patient's adaptation to the home setting and management of the ostomy. Teaching and reinforcement may assist the patient and family to cope with altered urinary function. It is also necessary to assess for long-term complications that may occur, such as pouch leakage or rupture, stone formation, stomal stenosis, deterioration in renal function, or incontinence. The following procedures are recommended for patients with a continent urinary diversion: pouch-o-gram (x-rays taken after a radioactive agent is instilled into the pouch) between 3 and 6 months, 9 and 12 months, 24 months, then every other year; renal function tests (BUN, serum creatinine) 1 month, 3 months, 6 months, then twice yearly; and pouchoscopy (endoscopic examination of the pouch) every year starting 5 to 7 years after surgery (Rowland, 1995). The patient who has had surgery for carcinoma should have a yearly physical examination and chest x-ray to assess for metastases.

Long-term monitoring for anemia is performed to identify vitamin B_{12} deficiency that may occur when a significant portion of the terminal ileum is removed. This may take several years to develop and can be successfully treated with vitamin B_{12} injections. The patient and family are informed of the United Ostomy Association and any local ostomy support groups to provide ongoing support, assistance, and education.

Postoperative Evaluation

Expected Outcomes

Expected outcomes may include:

1. Maintains skin integrity
   a. Maintains intact peristomal skin and demonstrates skill in managing drainage system and appliance

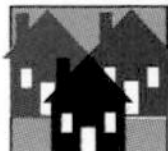

PATIENT EDUCATION AND HOME CARE

Using Urinary Diversion Collection Appliances

Applying a Reusable Pouch System

1. Gather all necessary supplies.
2. Prepare new appliance according to the manufacturer's directions.
   - Apply double-faced adhesive disk that has been properly sized to fit the reusable pouch faceplate. Remove paper backing and lay pouch aside. *or:*
   - Apply thin layer of contact cement to one side of the reusable pouch faceplate. Lay pouch aside.
3. Remove soiled pouch gently. Lay aside to clean later.
4. Clean peristomal skin with small amount of soap and water. Rinse thoroughly and dry. If a film of soap remains on the skin and the site does not dry, the appliance will not adhere adequately.
5. Use a wick (rolled gauze pad or tampon) on top of the stoma to absorb urine and keep the skin dry throughout the appliance change.
6. Inspect peristomal skin (skin around stoma) for irritation.
7. A skin protector wipe or barrier ring may be applied before centering the faceplate opening directly over the stoma.
8. Position appliance over stoma and press gently into place.
9. If desired, use a pouch cover or apply cornstarch under the pouch to prevent perspiration and skin irritation.
10. Clean soiled pouch and prepare for reuse.

Applying a Disposable Pouch System

1. Gather all necessary supplies.
2. Measure stoma and prepare an opening in the skin barrier about an ⅛-inch larger than the stoma and the same shape as the stoma.
3. Remove paper backing from skin barrier and set aside.
4. Gently remove old appliance and set aside.
5. Clean peristomal skin with warm water and dry thoroughly.
6. Inspect peristomal skin (skin around stoma) for irritation.
7. Use a wick (rolled gauze pad or tampon) on top of the stoma to absorb urine and keep the skin dry during the appliance change.
8. Center opening of skin barrier over stoma and apply with firm, gentle pressure to attain a watertight seal.
9. If using a two-piece system, snap pouch onto the flanged wafer that adheres to skin.
10. Close drainage tap or spout at bottom of pouch.
11. A pouch cover can be used or cornstarch applied under pouch to prevent perspiration and skin irritation.
12. Apply hypoallergenic tape around the skin barrier in a picture-frame manner.
13. Dispose of soiled appliance.

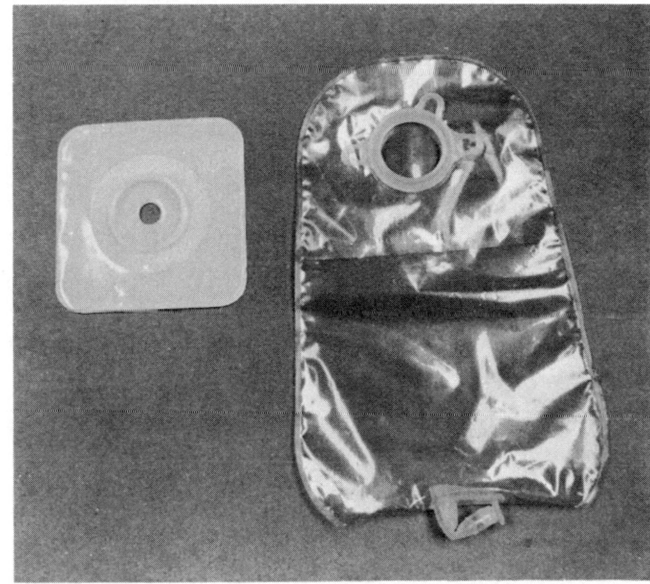

   b. Reports absence of pain or discomfort in peristomal area
   c. States actions to take if skin excoriation occurs
2. Exhibits increased knowledge about managing urinary function
   a. Participates in managing urinary system and skin care
   b. Verbally describes anatomic alteration due to surgery
   c. Revises daily routine to accommodate urinary drainage management
   d. Identifies potential problems, reportable signs and symptoms, and subsequent measures to take
3. Exhibits improved self-concept as evidenced by the following:
   a. Voices acceptance of urinary diversion, stoma, and appliance
   b. Demonstrates increasingly independent self-care, including hygiene and grooming
   c. States acceptance of support and assistance from family members, health care providers, and other ostomates
4. Copes with sexuality issues
   a. Verbalizes concern about possible alterations in sexuality and sexual function
   b. Reports discussion of sexual concerns with partner and appropriate counselor
5. Demonstrates knowledge needed for self-care
   a. Performs self-care and proficient management of urinary diversion and appliance
   b. Asks questions relevant to self-management and prevention of complications
   c. Identifies signs and symptoms needing care of contact physician or other health care providers
6. Absence of complications as evidenced by the following:
   a. Reports absence of pain or tenderness in abdomen
   b. Has temperature within normal range
   c. Reports no urine leakage from incision or drains
   d. Has urine output within desired volume limits
   e. Maintains stoma that is red or pink, moist, and appropriately "budded"
   f. Has intact and healed stomal border

OTHER RENAL AND URINARY TRACT DISORDERS

Nephrosclerosis

Nephrosclerosis is hardening, or sclerosis, of the arteries of the kidney due to prolonged hypertension. This causes decreased blood flow to the kidney and patchy necrosis of the renal parenchyma. Eventually, fibrosis occurs, and glomeruli are destroyed.

Pathophysiology

There are two forms of nephrosclerosis: malignant (accelerated) and benign. Malignant nephrosclerosis is often associated with malignant hypertension (diastolic blood pressure higher than 130 mm Hg). It usually occurs in young adults, and men are affected twice as often as women. The disease process progresses rapidly. Without dialysis, more than half of patients die from uremia in a matter of a few years. Benign nephrosclerosis is usually found in older adults and is often associated with atherosclerosis and hypertension.

Assessment and Diagnostic Findings

Symptoms are rare early in the disease, even though the urine usually contains protein and occasional casts. Renal insufficiency and associated signs and symptoms occur late in the disease.

Medical Management

Treatment of nephrosclerosis is aggressive antihypertensive therapy.

Hydronephrosis

Hydronephrosis is dilation of the renal pelvis and calyces of one or both kidneys due to an obstruction.

Pathophysiology

Obstruction to the normal flow of urine causes the urine to back up, resulting in increased pressure in the kidney. If the obstruction is in the urethra or the bladder, the back pressure affects both kidneys, but if the obstruction is in one of the ureters because of a stone or kink, only one kidney is damaged.

Partial or intermittent obstruction may be caused by a renal stone that has formed in the renal pelvis but has moved into the ureter and blocked it. The obstruction may be due to a tumor pressing on the ureter or to bands of scar tissue resulting from an abscess or inflammation near the ureter that pinches it. The disorder may be due to an odd angle of the ureter as it leaves the renal pelvis or to an unusual position of the kidney, favoring a ureteral twist or kink. In elderly men, the most common cause is urethral obstruction at the bladder outlet by an enlarged prostate gland. Hydronephrosis can also occur in pregnancy because of the enlarged uterus.

Whatever the cause, as the urine accumulates in the renal pelvis, it distends the pelvis and its calyces. In time, atrophy of the kidney results. As one kidney undergoes gradual destruction, the other kidney gradually enlarges (compensatory hypertrophy). Ultimately, renal function is impaired.

Clinical Manifestations

The patient may not have symptoms if the onset is gradual. Acute obstruction may produce aching in the flank and back. If infection is present, dysuria, chills, fever, tenderness, and pyuria may occur. Hematuria and pyuria may be present. If both kidneys are affected, signs and symptoms of chronic renal failure may develop.

Medical Management

The goals of management are to identify and correct the cause of the obstruction, to treat infection, and to restore and conserve renal function. To relieve the obstruction, the urine may have to be diverted by nephrostomy (see Chap. 40) or another type of diversion. The infection is treated with antibiotic agents because residual urine in the calyces leads to infection and pyelonephritis. The patient is prepared for surgical removal of obstructive lesions (calculus, tumor, obstruction of the ureter). If one kidney is severely damaged and its function is destroyed, nephrectomy (removal of the kidney) may be performed.

Urethritis

Urethritis, inflammation of the urethra, is usually an ascending infection and may be classified as gonococcal (see Chap. 64) or nongonococcal. Both conditions may be present in the same patient. Gonococcal and nongonococcal urethritis are the most common STDs occurring in men in developed countries.

Gonococcal urethritis is caused by *N. gonorrhoeae* and is transmitted by sexual contact. In men, inflammation of the meatal orifice occurs with burning on urination. A purulent urethral discharge appears 3 to 14 days (or longer) after sexual exposure, although the disease may be asymptomatic in up to 10% of men. The infection involves the tissues around the urethra, causing periurethritis, prostatitis, epididymitis, and urethral stricture. Sterility may occur as a result of vasoepididymal obstruction. Gonorrhea in women is frequently not diagnosed and reported because a urethral discharge is not always present and the disease may be asymptomatic. Treatment of gonorrhea is discussed and patient education information is provided in Chapter 64.

Nongonococcal urethritis is usually caused by *C. trachomatis* or *Ureaplasma urealyticum*. Male patients with symptoms usually complain of mild to severe dysuria and scant to moderate urethral discharge. Nongonococcal urethritis requires prompt antibiotic treatment with tetracycline or doxycycline. In patients who do not respond or who are allergic to the tetracyclines, erythromycin may be substituted. Follow-up care is necessary to make certain that a cure is achieved. All sexual partners of patients with nongonococcal urethritis should be examined for STDs and treated.

Renal Abscess

Renal abscesses may be localized to the renal cortex (renal carbuncle) or extend into the fatty tissue around the kidney (perinephric abscess). The incidence of renal abscesses ranges from 1 to 10 cases per 10,000 hospital admissions.

Pathophysiology

A renal abscess may be caused by an infection of the kidney (pyelonephritis) or may occur as a hematogenous (spread through the bloodstream) infection originating elsewhere in the body. Offending organisms include *Staphylococcus* and *Proteus* species and *E. coli.* Occasionally, infection spreads from adjacent areas, such as with diverticulitis or appendicitis.

Clinical Manifestations

The manifestations of a perinephritic abscess often are acute in onset, with chills, fever, leukocytosis, dull ache or palpable mass in the flank, abdominal pain with guarding, and costovertebral angle tenderness on palpation. The patient usually appears seriously ill.

Assessment and Diagnostic Findings

The patient with a renal abscess may report a recent history of a cutaneous boil or carbuncle and may complain of malaise, fever, chills, anorexia, weight loss, and a dull pain over the kidney. Leukocytosis and sterile urine (no microorganisms seen because the infection does not extend into the urinary collection system) are present with renal abscesses localized to the renal cortex.

Management

Small localized abscesses are usually cured by intravenous antibiotics alone but may require incision and drainage. Perinephritic abscesses require percutaneous drainage of the abscess. Culture and sensitivity tests are performed, and appropriate antibiotic therapy is prescribed. Drains are usually inserted and left in the perinephric space until all significant drainage has ceased. Because the drainage is often profuse, frequent changes of the outer dressings may be necessary. As in treating an abscess in any site, the patient is monitored for sepsis, fluid intake and output, and general response to treatment. Surgery may be indicated for extensive perinephritic abscesses.

Tuberculosis of the Kidney and Genitourinary Tract

Pathophysiology

Tuberculosis of the kidney and urinary tract is caused by the organism *Mycobacterium tuberculosis* and is relatively rare in developed countries. The organism usually travels from the lungs by means of the bloodstream to the kidneys. On arrival in the kidney, the microorganism may lie dormant for years. After the organism reaches the kidney, a low-grade inflammation and the characteristic tubercles are seen. If the organism continues to multiply, the tubercles enlarge to form cavities, with eventual destruction of parenchymal tissue. The organism spreads down the urinary tract into the bladder and may also infect the prostate, epididymis, and testicles in men.

Clinical Manifestations

At first, the symptoms of renal tuberculosis are mild; there is usually a slight afternoon fever, weight loss, night sweats, loss of appetite, and general malaise. Hematuria (microscopic or gross) and pyuria may be present. Pain, dysuria, and urinary frequency, when they occur, are due to bladder involvement. Cavity formations and calcifications may be noted on an intravenous urogram.

Assessment and Diagnostic Findings

A search for tuberculosis elsewhere in the body is conducted when tuberculosis of the kidney or urinary tract is found. The patient is asked about possible exposure to tuberculosis. Three or more clean-catch, first-morning urine specimens are obtained for culture for *M. tuberculosis*. The erythrocyte sedimentation rate is usually elevated and is helpful in monitoring response to treatment.

Medical Management

The goal of treatment is to eradicate the offending organism. Combinations of ethambutol, isoniazid, and rifampin are used to delay the emergence of resistant organisms. Shorter-course chemotherapy (4 months) has been effective in eradicating the organism and in penetrating renal tissue. Surgical intervention may be necessary to treat obstruction and to remove an extensively diseased kidney. Because renal tuberculosis is a manifestation of a systemic disease, all measures to promote the general health of the patient are taken, including proper nutrition, adequate rest, and good hygiene practices. A scrotal support may be used by male patients for genital swelling.

Nursing Management

For the most part, nursing interventions focus on patient education to promote effective self-care at home and to prevent active recurrence or transmission of disease.

PROMOTING HOME AND COMMUNITY-BASED CARE

Teaching Patients Self-Care. Patient education is provided about prescribed medications—taking them properly, recognizing side effects, and understanding the importance of completing the course of therapy. Instructions are provided about the nature of tuberculosis; its cause, spread, and treatment; and necessary follow-up care. Men are instructed to use condoms during sexual intercourse to prevent spread of the organisms and to abstain from intercourse during treatment for penile or urethral tuberculosis. The patient is encouraged to maintain a healthy lifestyle with a well-balanced diet, adequate amounts of liquids, and exercise.

Continuing Care. Follow-up care is essential to reinforce the importance of taking medications exactly as prescribed (many patients do not take them correctly). The patient is counseled about the need for follow-up examinations (urine cultures, intravenous urograms), usually for 1 year. Treatment is reinstituted if a relapse occurs and the tubercle bacilli again invade the genitourinary tract. Ureteral stenosis or bladder contractures are complications that may develop during healing; therefore, the patient is monitored for these.

Urethral Strictures

A urethral stricture is a narrowing of the lumen of the urethra as a result of scar tissue and contraction.

Pathophysiology

Common causes of strictures are urethral injury (caused by insertion of surgical instruments during transurethral surgery, indwelling catheters, or cystoscopic procedures), straddle injuries, and injuries associated with automobile crashes, untreated gonorrheal urethritis, and congenital abnormalities.

Assessment and Diagnostic Findings

The patient reports that the force and volume of the urinary stream is diminished, and symptoms of urinary infection and retention occur. Stricture causes urine to back up, resulting in cystitis, prostatitis, and pyelonephritis.

Prevention

An important element of prevention is to treat all urethral infections promptly. Prolonged urethral catheter drainage should be avoided and utmost care taken in any type of instrumentation involving the urethra, including catheterization.

Medical Management

Treatment may include gradual dilation of the narrowed area (with metal sounds or bougies) or surgery (internal urethrotomy). If the stricture prevents the passage of a catheter, the urologist uses several small filiform bougies in search of the opening. When one bougie passes beyond the stricture into the bladder, it is fixed in place, and urine drains from the bladder. The opening then can be dilated, bypassing a larger sound (a dilating instrument), with the filiform then acting as a guide. After dilation, hot sitz baths and nonopioid analgesics are administered to control pain. Antibiotic medications are prescribed for several days after dilation to prevent infection.

Surgical excision or urethroplasty may be necessary for severe cases. A suprapubic cystostomy may be necessary in some patients. The postoperative treatment for cystostomy is described earlier in this chapter.

Renal Cysts

Renal cysts are abnormal, fluid-filled sacs that arise from the kidney tissue. They may be genetic in origin, acquired, or associated with a host of unrelated conditions. Cysts of the kidney may be single or multiple (polycystic), involving one or both kidneys. Polycystic disease of the adult is inherited as an autosomal dominant trait and affects men and women equally.

Clinical Manifestations

The kidney gradually enlarges, with signs and symptoms becoming apparent in the fourth or fifth decade of life. The patient reports abdominal or lumbar pain. Hematuria, hypertension, palpable renal masses, and recurrent UTIs are additional manifestations. Renal insufficiency and failure usually develop in the end stages.

Assessment and Diagnostic Findings

Polycystic renal disease is also associated with cystic diseases of other organs (liver, pancreas, spleen) and aneurysms of the cerebral arteries. It has long been recognized that patients on long-term dialysis (both hemodialysis and peritoneal dialysis) develop multiple cysts on their nonfunctioning kidneys. Many of these cysts contain cancer cells. Diagnosis of renal cysts is confirmed either by intravenous urography or CT scan.

Management

Because there is no specific treatment for polycystic renal disease, care of the patient is directed toward relief of pain, symptoms, and complications. Hypertension and UTIs are treated aggressively. Dialysis (see Chap. 40) is initiated when signs of renal insufficiency and failure occur. Genetic counseling is part of management because polycystic kidney disease is a hereditary disease. The patient is advised to avoid sports and occupations that present a risk for trauma to the kidney. Simple cysts of the kidney usually occur unilaterally and differ clinically and pathophysiologically from polycystic kidney disease. The cyst may be drained percutaneously.

Congenital Anomalies

Congenital anomalies of the kidney are not uncommon. Occasionally, there is fusion of the two kidneys, forming what is called a "horseshoe" kidney. One kidney may be small and deformed and is often nonfunctioning. The patient may have a double ureter or congenital stricture of the ureter. Treating these anomalies is necessary only if they cause symptoms, but it is essential to determine that the other kidney is present and functioning before surgery is undertaken.

Interstitial Cystitis

Interstitial cystitis is an ill-defined bladder disorder sometimes referred to as urethral or painful bladder syndrome. It has been defined as an inflammation of the bladder wall that eventually causes disintegration of the lining and loss of bladder elasticity. The disorder occurs mostly in women 40 to 50 years of age but can affect any age or race and either gender. Almost half a million people in the United States are affected by the disease.

Pathophysiology

The cause of interstitial cystitis is unknown, although there is some suggestion of an inflammatory or autoimmune basis. Suggested causes include penetration of urinary irritants into the urothelium or suburothelial tissues due to a defect in the barrier between the urine and bladder wall mucosa.

Clinical Manifestations

Interstitial cystitis is characterized by severe, irritable voiding symptoms (urinary frequency, nocturia, urgency, suprapubic pressure, pain with bladder filling) and a markedly diminished bladder capacity. Some patients may have to void more than 60 times a day. More than 60% of patients with interstitial cystitis report painful intercourse.

Assessment and Diagnostic Findings

The diagnosis of interstitial cystitis is complicated for many reasons. Diagnosis is made by the process of exclusion because there are no definitive diagnostic criteria. As a result, several years may pass, and patients see an average of four to five physicians before the definitive diagnosis is made. The lack of more specific diagnostic criteria does not mean that this is a psychologically based disease; rather, it is a physical disorder with psychological consequences. Many patients have difficulty coping with the lack of a diagnosis, the inability of health care professionals to provide an explanation for their symptoms, and the persistence of symptoms.

Patient health history, symptoms, signs, cystoscopy, urodynamic studies, histology, and laboratory test findings contribute to the diagnosis. A micturition chart or diary with recordings of the frequency of voiding and the volume of each voiding for at least 48 to 72 hours may also aid in diagnosis. Biopsy and x-ray studies, such as urography, cystography, skeletal and pelvic x-ray, ultrasound, and CT scans, are obtained to exclude other conditions that could cause similar symptoms. The only abnormal radiographic finding characteristic of interstitial cystitis is a small bladder, although this may not be present. Urine cultures, cytology, residual volume, and flow rate are usually normal in patients with interstitial cystitis. The urine, however, contains both RBCs and WBCs, even though it is sterile (no bacteria).

Cystoscopy is performed, and special procedures are carried out during cystoscopy to make a diagnosis of interstitial cystitis. Interstitial cystitis is characterized by pinpoint petechial hemorrhages that develop throughout the mucosa of the bladder. These areas often coalesce to become hemorrhagic spots (referred to as *Hunner's ulcers*) on the bladder mucosa that bleed when the bladder is distended under general anesthesia (an important diagnostic criterion). Unlike other causes of painful bladder syndrome, interstitial cystitis may progress to contraction of the bladder with diminished bladder volume.

Medical Management

Treatment strategies include use of tricyclic antidepressants (doxepin and amitriptyline) that, through their central and peripheral anticholinergic actions, may decrease the excitability of smooth muscle in the bladder.

PHARMACOLOGIC THERAPY

Intrabladder instillation of various compounds (ie, silver nitrate, dimethyl sulfoxide, oxychlorosene [Clorpactin]), may provide relief. About 50% of patients respond favorably to intravesical instillation of dimethyl sulfoxide. Antispasmodics, such as oxybutynin (Ditropan), and urinary mucosal anesthetics, such as phenazopyridine (Pyridium), may be useful. In 1996, the FDA approved the use of a bladder protectant, pentosan polysulfate sodium (Elmiron), which is given orally. Intravesical heparin has some effect in decreasing symptoms in half of patients. Patients must be able to self-catheterize to instill the heparin on a daily basis initially, then three to four times weekly.

OTHER THERAPY

Other treatment includes transcutaneous electrical nerve stimulation, destruction of ulcers with laser photoirradiation, and bladder removal with urinary diversion in severe cases (Burrell & Hurm, 1999).

Nursing Management

Often the patient with symptoms of interstitial cystitis has experienced symptoms for a prolonged time. These symptoms prevent the patient from carrying out normal activities of daily living. The patient has usually been treated by a number of health care providers, often with little relief of symptoms. As a consequence, the patient may feel depressed, anxious, distrustful, and skeptical about proposed treatments.

In such situations, the nurse assesses the effectiveness of the patient's ability to cope with the disorder and provides psychological support. The nurse must convey a sense of acceptance to the patient and acknowledge the severity of the symptoms and their effect on the patient's lifestyle. The nurse also teaches the patient about diagnostic tests and treatment regimens.

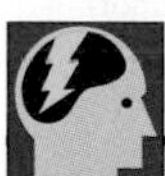

Critical Thinking Exercises

1. Your patient tells you that she is very discouraged because she has had repeated episodes of UTI during the past 3 years. How would you focus your assessment to assist in uncovering factors associated with these infections? Describe the teaching program you would devise to help the patient reduce the incidence of infection.

2. You are working in the emergency department and are caring for a patient who has severe renal colic from a kidney stone. Discuss nursing care of this patient, including pain management strategies. The patient passes the kidney stone and is going to be discharged home. Describe the teaching program you would devise to help the patient obtain the necessary follow-up treatment and prevent recurrence of any kidney stones.

3. Your patient is scheduled for a cystectomy and urinary diversion. Describe how you would meet the emotional and health education needs of the patient if (a) the patient is a 32-year-old woman who was recently married; (b) the patient is a 74-year-old man with limited vision and poor hygiene habits.

4. You are caring for two patients in the same room. One is a diabetic patient in acute renal failure after receiving intravenous contrast dye. The other patient has ESRD from hypertension. Compare and contrast management of each patient, and discuss your different priorities of care for each.

References and Selected Readings

BOOKS

American Cancer Society. (1999). *Facts and Figures.* Atlanta, GA: Author.

Brenner, B. (Ed.). (1996). *Brenner & Rector's: The kidney* (5th ed.). Philadelphia: W. B. Saunders.

Greenberg, A. (1998). *Primer on kidney diseases* (2nd ed.). San Diego: Academic Press.

Karlowicz, K. (1995). *Urologic nursing: Principles and practice.* Philadelphia: W. B. Saunders.

Kunin, C. (1997). *Urinary tract infections: Detection, prevention, and management.* Baltimore: Williams & Wilkins.

Levine, D. (1997). *Caring for the renal patient.* Philadelphia: W. B. Saunders.

Noble, J. (Ed.). (1996). *Textbook of primary care medicine.* St. Louis: C. V. Mosby.

Nolan, M. T., & Augustine, S. M. (1995). *Transplantation nursing: Acute and long-term management.* Norwalk: CT, Appleton & Lange.

Parker, J. (1998). *Contemporary nephrology nursing.* Pitman, NJ: Anthony J. Janetti, Inc.

U.S. Renal Data System. (1998). *USRDS 1998 annual data report.* Bethesda: National Institutes of Health, National Institute of Diabetes and Digestive and Kidney Diseases.

Walsh, P., Retik, A., Vaughan, E., & Wein, A. (1997). *Campbell's urology* (7th ed.). Philadelphia: W. B. Saunders.

JOURNALS

Asterisks indicate nursing research articles.

General

Ali, H. (1996). Renal disease in the elderly: Distinctive disorders, tailored treatments. *Postgraduate Medicine,* 100(6), 44–63.

American Cancer Society. (1997). Cancer statistics 1997. *CA: A Cancer Journal for Clinicians, 47*(1), 8–9.

Brown, W., & Schmitz, P. (1998). Acute and chronic kidney disease. *Clinics in Geriatric Medicine, 14*(2), 211–233.

Byers, J., & Goshorn, J. (1995). How to manage diuretic therapy. *American Journal of Nursing, 95*(2), 38–44.

Solomon, R. (1995). Strategies to delay renal deterioration. *Patient Care 29*(3), 50–57.

Acute Renal Failure

Choudhury, D., & Ahmed, Z. (1997). Drug-induced nephrotoxicity. *Medical Clinics of North America, 81*(3), 705–717.

Craig, M. (1998). Applications in continuous venous to venous hemofiltration: Interactive case studies in the adult patient. *Critical Care Clinics of North America, 10*(2), 209–214.

Dillon, J. (1999). Continuous renal replacement therapy or hemodialysis for acute renal failure? *International Journal of Artificial Organs, 22*(3), 125–127.

Dirkes, S. (1997). A dialysis alternative more nurses can run. *RN, 60*(5), 20–26.

Edelstein, C., Ling, H., Wangsiripaisan, A., & Schrier, R. (1997). Emerging therapies for acute renal failure. *American Journal of Kidney Diseases, 30*(5), S89–S95.

Headrick, C. (1998). Adult/Pediatric CVVH: The pump, the patient, the circuit. *Critical Care Nursing Clinics of North America, 10*(2), 197–207.

Humes, H. (1999). Limiting acute renal failure. *Hospital Practice, 34*(1), 31–48.
Ikizler, T., & Himmelfarb, J. (1997). Nutrition in acute renal failure patients. *Advances in Renal Replacement Therapy, 4*(2), 54–63.
Kelly, M. (1997). Clinical snapshot: Acute renal failure. *American Journal of Nursing, 97*(3), 32–33.
Lesko, J., & Johnston, J. (1997). Oliguria. *AACN Clinical Issues, 8*(3), 459–468.
McAlpine, L. (1998). CAVH: Principles and practical applications. *Critical Care Clinics of North America, 10*(2), 179–189.
Mindell, J., & Chertow, G. (1997). A practical approach to acute renal failure. *Medical Clinics of North America, 81*(3), 731–747.
Pastan, S., & Bailey, J. (1998). Dialysis therapy. *New England Journal of Medicine, 338*(20), 1428–1437.
Perazella, M. (1999). Crystal-induced acute renal failure. *American Journal of Medicine, 106*(4), 459–465.
Racusen, L. (1997). Pathology of acute renal failure: Structure/function correlations. *Advances in Renal Replacement Therapy, 4*(2), 3–16.
Rodriguez, D., & Lewis, S. (1997). Nutritional management of patients with acute renal failure. *ANNA Journal, 24*(2), 232–243.
Stark, J. (1998). Acute renal failure: Focus on advances in acute tubular necrosis. *Critical Care Clinics of North America, 10*(2), 159–170.
Stewart, C., & Barnett, R. (1997). Acute renal failure in infants, children, and adults. *Critical Care Clinics, 13*(3), 575–590.
Yucha, C., & Shapiro, J. (1997). Acute renal failure: Recognition and prevention. *Lippincott's Primary Care Practice, 1*(4), 388–398.

Chronic Renal Failure

Adler, S. (1996). New interventional strategies for diabetic nephropathy. *Hospital Medicine, 32*(1), 23–27.
Baer, C. (1998). Care of the chronically ill chronic renal failure patient. *Critical Care Nursing Clinics of North America, 10*(4), 433–448.
Fishbane, S., & Maesaka, J. (1997). Iron management in end-stage renal disease. *American Journal of Kidney Disease, 29*(3), 319–333.
Golder, R., Delmez, J., & Klahr, S. (1996). Bone disease in long-term dialysis. *American Journal of Kidney Disease, 28*(6), 918–923.
Herzog, C. (1999). Acute myocardial infarction in patients with end-stage renal disease. *Kidney International Supplement, 71*, S130–S133.
Kelly, M. (1996). Clinical snapshot: Chronic renal failure. *American Journal of Nursing, 96*(1), 36–37.
Kobrin, S., & Aradhye, S. (1997). Preventing progression and complications of renal disease. *Hospital Medicine, 33*(11), 11–12, 17–18, 20, 29–31, 35–36, 39–40.
Lapuz, M. (1997). Diabetic nephropathy. *Medical Clinics of North America, 81*(3), 679–687.
Maroni, B., & Mitch, W. (1997). Role of nutrition in the prevention of progression of renal disease. *Annual Review of Nutrition, 17*, 435–455.
Materson, B., & Preston, R. (1997). Prevention of diabetic nephropathy. *Hospital Practice, 32*(2), 129–140.
Maxwell, P., & Fitzpatrick, R. (1998). End stage renal failure and assessment of health related quality of life. *Quality Health Care, 7*(4), 182.
Mendelssohn, D. (1999). Pre end-stage renal disease care: Opportunities and challenges. *Peritoneal Dialysis International, 19*(2), 113–114.
Sosa-Guerrero, S., & Gomez, N. (1997). Dealing with end-stage renal disease. *American Journal of Nursing, 97*(10), 44–50.
Turner, L., et al. (1997). Dietary management in the patient with chronic renal failure. *American Journal of Nursing, 97*(9), 16B–16H.
Winchester, J., & Rakowski, T. (1998). End-stage renal disease and its management in older adults. *Clinics in Geriatric Medicine, 14*(2), 255–265.

Disorders of the Kidney

Glassock, R. (1998). Glomerular disease in the elderly population. *Geriatric Nephrology and Urology, 8*(3), 149–154.
Jenette, J., & Falk, R. (1997). Diagnosis and management of glomerular diseases. *Medical Clinics of North America, 81*(3), 653–677.
Kenae, W., & Eknoyan, G. (1999). Proteinuria, albuminuria, risk, assessment, detection, elimination (PARADE): A position paper of the National Kidney Foundation. *American Journal of Kidney Disease, 33*(5), 1004–1010.
King, L. R. (1995). Hydronephrosis: When is obstruction not obstruction? *Urologic Clinics of North America, 22*(1), 31–42.
Kluth, D., & Rees, A. (1999). New approaches to modify glomerular inflammation. *Journal of Nephrology, 12*(2), 66–75.
Montseny, J. J., et al. (1995). The current spectrum of infectious glomerulonephritis: Experience with 76 patients and review of the literature. *Medicine, 74*(2), 63–73.
Muirhead, N. (1999). Management of idiopathic membranous nephropathy: Evidence-based recommendations. *Kidney International Supplement, 70*, S47–S55.

Interstitial Cystitis

Burrell, M., & Hurm, R. (1999). Care of the patient with interstitial cystitis: Current theories and management. *Journal of Perianesthesia Nursing, 14*(1), 17–22.
Kaufman, M., All, A., Hall, N., & Clark, J. (1997). Caring for the patient with interstitial cystitis. *MedSurg Nursing, 6*(4), 203–208.
Messing, E. (1999). Interstitial cystitis-a light at the end of the tunnel. *Journal of Urology, 161*(6), 1797.

Kidney Transplantation

Cecka, J., & Terasaki, P. (1997). Living donor kidney transplants: Superior success rates despite histoincompatibilities. *Transplant Proceedings, 29*(1-2), 203.
deMattos, A., Olyaei, A., & Bennett, W. (1996). Pharmacology of immunosuppressive medications used in renal diseases and transplantation. *American Journal of Kidney Diseases, 28*(5), 631–667.
Fallon, M., Gould, D., & Wainwright, S.P. (1997). Stress and quality of life in the renal transplant patient: A preliminary investigation. *Journal of Advanced Nursing, 25* (3), 562–570.
Giuliano, K. (1997). Organ transplants: Tackling the tough ethical questions. *Nursing, 27*(5), 34–39.
Newton, S. (1999). Renal transplant recipients' and their physicians' expectations regarding return to work posttransplant. *ANNA Journal, 26*(2), 227–232.
Orlowski, J. (1999). Advances in kidney transplantation: Renal failure in the United States. *Disease of the Month, 45*(5), 185–194.
Peddi, V., & First, M. (1997). Primary care of patients with renal transplants. *Medical Clinics of North America, 81*(3), 767–785.
Vella, J., & Sayegh, M. (1997). Maintenance pharmacological immunosuppressive strategies in renal transplantation. *Postgraduate Medicine, 73*(86), 386–390.

Renal Calculi

Balaji, K., & Menon, M. (1997). Mechanism of stone formation. *Urologic Clinic of North America, 24*(1), 1–11.
Begun, F., et al. (1997). Patient evaluation: Laboratory and imaging studies. *Urologic Clinic of North America, 24*(1), 97–115.
Craig, S. (1996). It's a kidney stone . . . or is it? *Emergency Medicine*, May 2, 122.
Curhan, G., et al. (1996). A prospective study of the intake of vitamins C and B_6, and the risk of kidney stones in men. *Journal of Urology, 155*(6), 1847–1851.
Goldfarb, S., & Coe, F. (1999). Beverages, diet, and prevention of kidney stones. *American Journal of Kidney Disease, 33*(2), 398–403.
Goshorn, J. (1996). Kidney stones. *American Journal of Nursing, 96*(9), 40–41.
Krieger, J., et al. (1996). Dietary and behavioral risk factors for urolithiasis: Potential implications for prevention. *American Journal of Nursing, 28*(2), 195–201.
McDonald, M., & Stoller, M. (1997). Urinary stone disease: A practical guide to metabolic evaluation. *Geriatrics, 52*(5), 38–56.
Pak, C. (1999). Medical prevention of renal stone disease. *Nephron, 81*(1), 60–65.
Renner, C., & Rassweiler, J. (1998). Treatment of renal stones by extracorporeal shock wave lithotripsy. *Nephron, 81*(1), 71–81.
Saklayen, M. (1997). Medical management of nephrolithiasis. *Medical Clinics of North America, 81*(3), 785–799.
Singal, R., & Denstedt, J. (1997). Contemporary management of ureteral stones. *Urologic Clinic of North America, 24*(1), 59–70.
Tawfiek, E., & Bagley, D. (1999). Management of upper urinary tract calculi with ureteroscopic techniques. *Urology, 53*(1), 25–31.
Trivedi, B. (1996). Nephrolithiasis: How it happens and what to do about it. *Postgraduate Medicine, 100*(6), 63–77.

Renal Trauma

Carpio, F., & Moray, A. (1999). Radiographic staging of renal injuries. *World Journal of Urology, 17*(2), 66–70.
Ghali, A., El Malik, E., Ibrahim, A., Ismail, G., & Rashid, M. (1999). Ureteric injuries: Diagnosis, management and outcomes. *Journal of Trauma, 46*(1), 150–158.
Meng, M., Brandes, S., & McAninch, J. (1999). Renal trauma: Indications and techniques for surgical exploration. *World Journal of Urology, 17*(2), 71–77.
Moray, A., & Carroll, P. (1997). Evaluation and management of adult bladder trauma. *Contemporary Urology, 9*(7), 13–22.

Tumors of the Urinary Tract and Urinary Diversion

Benson, M., & Olsson, C. (1999). Continent urinary diversion. *Urologic Clinics of North America, 26*(1), 125–147.

Bradley, M., & Pupiales, M. (1997). Essential elements of ostomy care. *American Journal of Nursing, 97*(7), 38–46.

Guinan, P., et al. (1995). Renal cell carcinoma: Tumor size, stage and survival. *Journal of Urology, 153*(3), 901–903.

Hart, S., et al. (1999). Quality of life after radical cystectomy for bladder cancer in patients with an ileal conduit, cutaneous or urethral kock pouch. *Journal of Urology, 162*(1), 77–81.

Hartmann, J., & Bokemeyer, C. (1999). Chemotherapy for renal cell carcinoma. *Anticancer Research, 19*(2C), 1541–1543.

Jimenez-Cruz, J., et al. (1997). Intravesical immunoprophylaxis in recurrent superficial bladder cancer (stage T1): Multicenter trial comparing bacille Calmette-Guèrin and interferon-alpha. *Urology, 50*(4), 529–534.

Kaufman, D., & Shipley, W. (1997). Organ-sparing treatment of bladder cancer: An innovative approach. *American Family Physician, 55*(4), 1257–1262.

Kelly, L., & Miaskowski, C. (1996). An overview of bladder cancer: Treatment and nursing implications. *Oncology Nursing Forum, 23*(3), 459–468.

Landis, S., Murray, T., Bolden, S., & Wingo, P. (1999). Cancer statistics, 1999. *CA, 49*(1), 8–31.

Lange, P., et al. (1996). Superficial bladder cancer: Treatment and future options. *Contemporay Urology, 7*(4), 61–74.

Motzer, R., Bander, N., & Nanus, D. (1996). Renal-cell carcinoma. *New England Journal of Medicine, 335*(12), 865–875.

Mundy, A. (1999). Metabolic complications of urinary diversion. *Lancet, 353*(9167), 1813–1814.

Schnitz-Drager, B., & Muller, M. (1998). Intravesical treatment of bladder cancer: Current problems and needs. *Urology International, 61*(4), 199–205.

Zinman, L. (1999). Changing concepts in orthotopic urinary diversion. *Journal of Urology, 161*(6), 1807–1808.

Urinary Tract Infections

Bacheller, C., & Bernstein, J. (1997). Urinary tract infections. *Medical Clinics of North America, 81*(3), 719–729.

Barry, H., Ebell, M., & Hickner, J. (1997). Evaluation of suspected urinary tract infection in ambulatory women: A cost-utility analysis of office-based strategies. *Journal of Family Practice, 44*(1), 49–60.

Dembrey, L., & Andriole, V. (1997). Renal and perirenal abscesses. *Infectious Disease Clinics of North America, 11*(3), 663–678.

D'Epiro, P. (1997). Complicated UTI: Underlying disorders and their treatment. *Patient Care, 31*(7), 196–208.

Duffield, P. (1996). Managing urinary tract infections. 2. Caring for children and the elderly. *American Journal of Nursing, 96*(10), 16I–16J.

Goldaber, K. (1997). Urinary tract infection during pregnancy. *Hospital Medicine, 33*(5), 14–24.

Hooton, T., & Stamm, W. (1997). Diagnosis and treatment of uncomplicated urinary tract infection. *Infectious Disease Clinics of North America, 11*(3), 551–574.

*Jackson, B., & Hicks, L. (1997). Effect of cranberry juice on urinary pH in older adults. *Home Healthcare Nurse, 15*(3), 199–202.

Maher, L. (1997). Complicated UTI: Targeting the pathogens. *Patient Care, 31*(7), 212–223.

Marchiondo, K. (1998) A new look at urinary tract infection. *American Journal of Nursing, 3*(3), 4–38.

Newland, J. A. (1998) Cystitis in women. *American Journal of Nursing, 98*(1), 16AAA.

Nguyen, A., Smith, D., & Leidich, R. (1997). Does your elderly patient have asymptomatic bacteriuria or urinary tract infection? *Nursing Home Medicine, 5*(3), 97–102.

Nicolle, L. (1997). Asymptomatic bacteriuria in the elderly. *Infectious Disease Clinics of North America* 1997 Sept; 11(3):647-659.

Orenstein, R., & Wong, E. (1999). Urinary tract infections in adults. *American Family Physician, 59*(5), 1225–1237.

Papanicolaou, N., & Pfister, R. (1996). Acute renal infections. *Radiologic Clinics of North America, 34*(5), 965–995.

Pewitt, E., & Schaeffer, A. (1997). Urinary tract infection in urology, including acute and chronic prostatitis. *Infectious Disease Clinics of North America, 11*(3), 623–645.

Rigby, D. (1998). Urinary tract infections: The hidden cause. *Community Nurse, 4*(5), 30–32.

Ronald, A., & Harding G. (1997). Complicated urinary tract infections. *Infectious Disease Clinics of North America, 11*(3), 583–591.

Ryals, J., Vetrosky, D., & White, G. (1997). Protocols: Urinary tract infections. *Lippincott's Primary Care Practice, 1*(4), 442–445.

Stapleton, A., & Stamm, W. (1997). Prevention of urinary tract infection. *Infectious Disease Clinics of North America, 11*(3), 719–731.

Suchinski, G., et al. (1999). Treating urinary tract infections in the elderly. *Dimensions of Critical Care Nursing, 18*(1), 21–27.

Wood, C., & Abrutyn, E. (1998). Urinary tract infection in older adults. *Clinics in Geriatric Medicine, 14*(2), 267–283.

Resources

American Association of Kidney Patients, 100 South Ashley Dr., Suite 280, Tampa, FL 33602; 1-800-749-2257; www.aakp.org

American Association of Nephrology Nurses, North Woodbury Road, Box 56, Pitman NJ 08071; 1-609-589-2187; www.inurse.com/~ANNA

American Cancer Society, 1599 Clifton Rd. NE, Atlanta, GA 30329; 1-800-ACS-2345; www.cancer.org

American Kidney Fund, 6110 Executive Blvd., Suite 1010, Rockville, MD 20852; 1-800-638-8299; www.arbon.com/kidney

Interstitial Cystitis Association, PO Box 1553, Madison Square Garden Station, New York, NY 10159; 1-212-979-6057; www.ichelp.com

National Association for Patients on Hemodialysis and Transplantation, 211 East 43rd Street, Suite 301, New York, NY 10017; 1-212-867-4486

National Kidney Foundation, 30 East 33rd St., New York, NY 10016; 1-212-889-2210, www.kidney.org

National Kidney and Urologic Disorders Information Clearinghouse, Box NKUDIC, 9000 Rockville Pike, Bethesda, MD, 20892; 1-301-468-6345; www.mkudic@aerie.com

United Ostomy Association, 36 Executive Park, Suite 120, Irvine, CA 92714-6744; 1-800-826-0826; www.uoa.org

Wound, Ostomy and Continent Nurses Society (WOCN), 2755 Bristol Street, Suite 110, Costa Mesa, CA 92626; 1-714-476-0268; www.wocn.org

UNIT

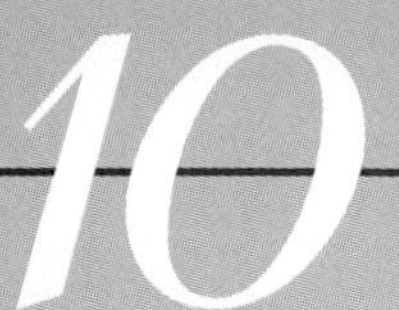

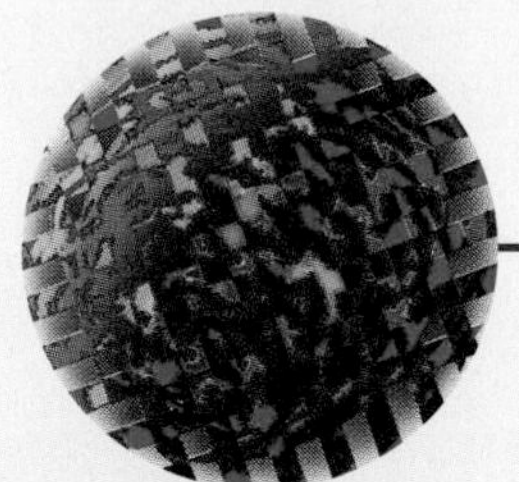

Reproductive Function

CHAPTER 42

Assessment and Management: Problems Related to Female Physiologic Processes

Learning Objectives

On completion of this chapter, the learner will be able to:

1. Describe female reproductive function.
2. Describe approaches to effective sexual assessment.
3. Describe indicators of domestic violence and abuse of women and methods of identification and treatment of a women who is a survivor of abuse.
4. Identify the diagnostic examinations and tests used to determine alteration in female reproductive function and describe the nurse's role during these examinations and procedures.
5. Identify factors that cause disturbances of menstruation and related nursing implications.
6. Describe nursing care for patients with premenstrual syndrome.
7. Develop a teaching plan for women experiencing menopause.
8. Describe methods of contraception and implications for health care and education.
9. Describe the nursing management of the patient having an abortion.
10. Describe the causes and management of infertility.
11. Use the nursing process to plan for the care of patients with ectopic pregnancies.

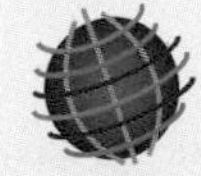

Women's health is a unique and growing specialty of health care. In addition to understanding normal female anatomy and physiology, the nurse needs to understand the physical, developmental, psychological, and social influences on women's health and health care. Health assessment, maintenance, and promotion across the life span must incorporate preconception care, effects of pregnancy on health, and disease entities that affect women. Because women use the health care system more often than men and make up the majority of health care workers, addressing women's health needs and concerns will improve quality and access for all people.

GLOSSARY

adnexa: term used to describe the fallopian tubes and ovaries together

amenorrhea: absence of menstrual flow

androgens: hormones produced by the ovaries and adrenals that affect many aspects of female health, including follicle development, libido, oiliness of hair and skin, and hair growth

cervix: bottom (inferior) part of uterus that is located in the vagina

chandelier sign: pain on movement of the cervix; associated with pelvic infection

corpus luteum: site of a follicle that changes after ovulation to produce progesterone

cystocele: weakness of the anterior vaginal wall allowing the bladder to intrude into the mucosa

dysmenorrhea: painful menstruation

dyspareunia: difficult or painful sexual intercourse

endometriosis: condition in which endometrial tissue seeds in other areas of the pelvis; may produce dysmenorrhea or infertility

endometrium: lining of the uterus

estrogen: female hormone that develops and maintains the female reproductive system

follicle-stimulating hormone (FSH): hormone released by the pituitary gland to stimulate estrogen production and ovulation

fornix: upper part of the vagina

fundus: body of the uterus

graafian follicle: cystic structure that develops on the ovary as ovulation begins

hymen: tissue that may cover the vaginal opening partially or completely before vaginal penetration

introitus: opening to the vagina on the perineum

luteal phase: stage in the menstrual cycle in which the endometrium becomes thicker and more vascular

luteinizing hormone (LH): hormone that stimulates progesterone production

menarche: beginning of menstrual function

menstruation: sloughing and discharge of the lining of the uterus if conception does not take place

osteoporosis: a disorder in which bones lose density and become porous and fragile

ovaries: almond-shaped reproductive organs that produce eggs at ovulation and play a major role in hormone production

ovulation: discharge of a mature ovum from the ovary

perimenopause: period from first signs of menopause to beyond cessation of menses

polyp: growth of tissue on the cervix or endometrial lining; usually benign

progesterone: hormone produced by the corpus luteum

proliferative phase: stage in the menstrual cycle before ovulation when the endometrium proliferates

rectocele: weakness of the posterior vaginal wall allowing rectal cavity to intrude into the submucosa of the vagina

secretory phase: stage of the menstrual cycle in which the endometrium becomes thickened, more vascular, and edematous

uterine prolapse: relaxation of pelvic tone allowing the cervix and uterus to descend into the lower vagina

ROLE OF NURSES IN WOMEN'S HEALTH

As their presence in the labor market has increased, women have faced key changes in their roles, lifestyles, and family patterns. Moreover, they have encountered environmental hazards and stress, prompting them to focus greater attention on health and health-promoting practices. As a result, some women are taking greater interest in and responsibility for their own health care.

Other changes over the years have included delaying pregnancy and childbearing until well after a career is established. Various methods of contraception have made this option possible. As women exercise greater control over their health care options, nurses are becoming more knowledgeable about preventive care for women, particularly with regard to their unique needs. The nurse encourages women to determine their own health goals and behaviors, teaches about health and illness, offers interventional strategies, and provides support, counseling, and ongoing monitoring. Areas of special interest in health promotion include the following:

- Personal hygiene
- Strategies for detecting and preventing disease, especially sexually transmitted diseases (STDs), including human immunodeficiency virus (HIV) infection
- Issues related to sexuality and sexual function, such as contraception; preconceptional, prenatal, and postnatal care; and menopause

Nurses who promote healthful ways of living also need to model that lifestyle for their patients.

An important role of the nurse is promoting positive practices and behaviors related to the reproductive and sexual health of each patient, including the following:

- Providing information about scheduling regular examinations to promote health, detect health problems at an early stage, assess problems related to gynecologic and reproductive function, and discuss questions or concerns related to sexual function and sexuality
- Providing an open, nonjudgmental environment, which is crucial if the patient is to feel comfortable discussing personal issues. The nurse must convey understanding and sensitivity when discussing these issues and must assess their effects on the patient and the patient's partner.
- Recognizing signs and symptoms of abuse and screening all patients in a private and safe environment

ANATOMIC AND PHYSIOLOGIC OVERVIEW

Anatomy of the Female Reproductive System

The female reproductive system consists of external and internal structures. Other anatomic structures that affect the female reproductive system include the hypothalamus and pituitary gland of the endocrine system.

External Genitalia

The external genitalia (the vulva) include two thick folds of tissue called the labia majora and two smaller lips of delicate tissue called the labia minora, which lie within the labia majora. The upper portions of the labia minora unite, forming a partial covering for the clitoris, a highly sensitive organ composed of erectile tissue. Between the labia minora, below and posterior to the clitoris, is the urinary meatus. This is the external opening of the female ure-

External female genitalia.

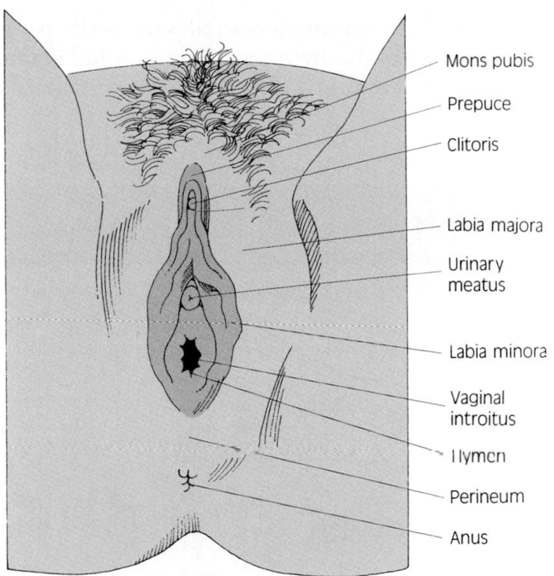

FIGURE 42•1 External female genitalia.

thra and is about 3 cm (1.5 inches) long. Below this orifice is a larger opening, the vaginal orifice, or **introitus** (Fig. 42-1). On each side of the vaginal orifice is a vestibular (Bartholin's) gland, a bean-sized structure that empties its mucous secretion through a small duct. The opening of the duct lies within the labia minora, external to the **hymen**. The tissue between the external genitalia and the anus is the fourchette. All of the tissue that makes up the external female genitalia is called the perineum.

Internal Reproductive Structures

The internal structures consist of the vagina, uterus, ovaries, and fallopian or uterine tubes (Fig. 42-2).

VAGINA

The vagina, a canal lined with mucous membrane, is 7.5 to 10 cm (3 to 4 inches) long and extends upward and backward from the vulva to the cervix. Anterior to it are the bladder and the urethra, and posterior to it lies the rectum. The anterior and posterior walls of the vagina normally touch each other. The upper part of the vagina, the **fornix,** surrounds the **cervix** (the narrow neck of the uterus).

UTERUS

The uterus, a pear-shaped muscular organ, is about 7.5 cm (3 inches) long and 5 cm (2 inches) wide at its upper part. Its walls are about 1.25 cm (0.5 inch) thick. The size of the uterus varies, depending on parity (number of viable births) and uterine abnormalities (eg, fibroids, which are a type of tumor that may distort the uterus). A nulliparous woman (one who has not completed a pregnancy to the stage of fetal viability) usually has a smaller uterus than a multiparous woman (one who has completed two or more pregnancies to the stage of fetal viability). The uterus lies posterior to the bladder and is held in position by several ligaments. The round ligaments extend anteriorly and laterally to the internal inguinal ring and down the inguinal canal, where they blend with the tissues of the labia majora. The broad ligaments are folds of peritoneum extending from the lateral pelvic walls and enveloping the fallopian tubes. The uterosacral ligaments extend posteriorly to the sacrum. The uterus has two parts: the cervix, which projects into the vagina, and a larger upper part, the **fundus** or body, which is covered posteriorly and partly anteriorly by peritoneum. The triangular inner portion of the fundus narrows to a small canal in the cervix that has constrictions at each end, referred

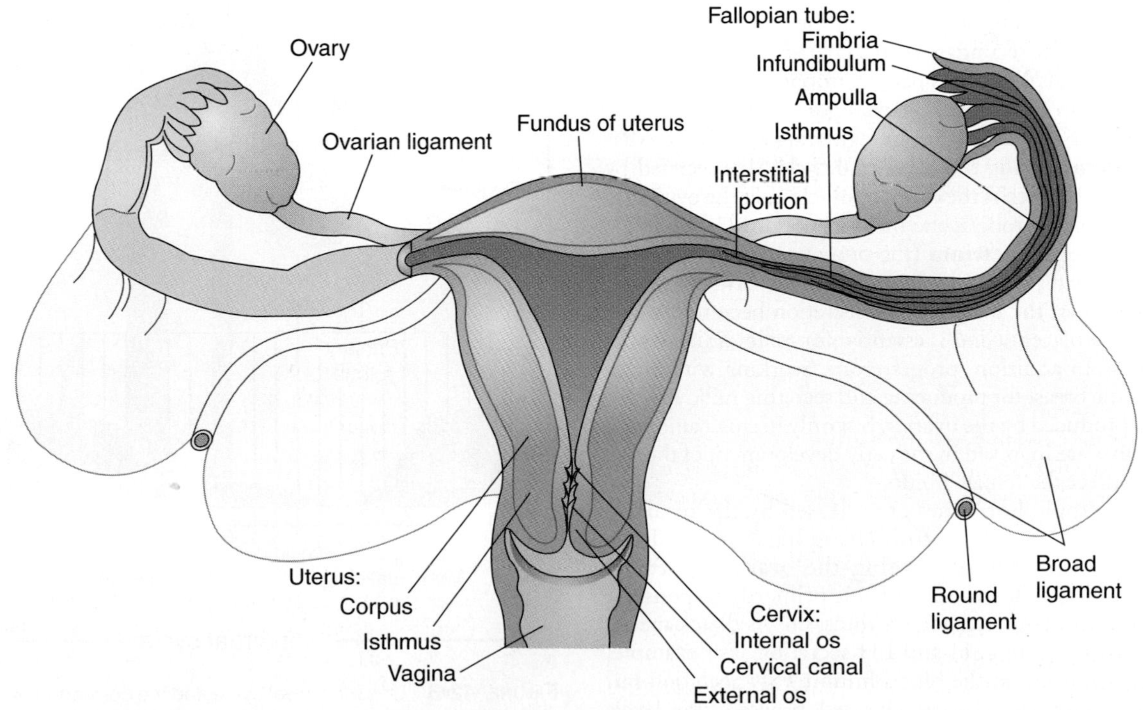

FIGURE 42•2 Internal female reproductive structures.

to as the external os and internal os. The upper lateral parts of the uterus are called the cornua. From here, the oviducts or fallopian (or uterine) tubes extend outward, and their lumina are internally continuous with the uterine cavity.

OVARIES

The **ovaries** lie behind the broad ligaments, behind and below the fallopian tubes. They are oval bodies about 3 cm (1.2 inches) long. At birth, they contain thousands of tiny egg cells, or ova. The ovaries and the fallopian tubes together are referred to as the **adnexa.**

Function of the Female Reproductive System

Ovulation

At puberty (usually between the 12th and 14th years), the ova begin to mature. During a period known as the follicular phase, an ovum enlarges as a type of cyst called a **graafian follicle** until it reaches the surface of the ovary, where rupture occurs. The ovum (or oocyte) is discharged into the peritoneal cavity. This periodic discharge of matured ovum is referred to as **ovulation.** The ovum usually finds its way into the fallopian tube, where it is carried to the uterus. If it meets a spermatozoon, the male reproductive cell, a union occurs and conception takes place. After the discharge of the ovum, the cells of the graafian follicle undergo a rapid change. Gradually, they become yellow (**corpus luteum**) and produce progesterone, a hormone that prepares the uterus for receiving the fertilized ovum. Ovulation usually occurs midway between menstrual periods.

The Menstrual Cycle

The menstrual cycle is a complex process involving the reproductive and endocrine systems. The ovaries produce steroid hormones, predominantly estrogens and progesterone. Several different **estrogens** are produced by the ovarian follicle, which consists of the developing ovum and its surrounding cells. The most potent of the ovarian estrogens is estradiol. Estrogens are responsible for developing and maintaining the female reproductive organs and the secondary sexual characteristics associated with the adult female. Estrogens play an important role in breast development and in monthly cyclic changes in the uterus.

Progesterone is also important in regulating the changes that occur in the uterus during the menstrual cycle. It is secreted by the corpus luteum, which is the ovarian follicle after the ovum has been released. Progesterone is the most important hormone for conditioning the **endometrium** (the mucous membrane lining the uterus) in preparation for implantation of the fertilized ovum. If pregnancy occurs, the progesterone secretion becomes largely a function of the placenta and is essential for maintaining a normal pregnancy. In addition, progesterone, working with estrogen, prepares the breast for producing and secreting milk. **Androgens** are also produced by the ovaries, but only in small amounts. These hormones are involved in the early development of the follicle and also affect the female libido.

Two gonadotropic hormones are released by the pituitary gland: FSH and LH. **Follicle-stimulating hormone** (FSH) is primarily responsible for stimulating the ovaries to secrete estrogen. **Luteinizing hormone** (LH) is primarily responsible for stimulating the progesterone production. Feedback mechanisms, in part, regulate FSH and LH secretion. For example, elevated estrogen levels in the blood inhibit FSH secretion but promote LH secretion, whereas elevated progesterone levels inhibit LH secretion. In addition, gonadotropin-releasing hormone (GnRH) from the hypothalamus affects the rate of FSH and LH release.

Secretion of ovarian hormones follows a cyclic pattern that results in changes of the uterine endometrium and in **menstruation** (Fig. 42-3; Table 42-1). This cycle is typically 28 days in

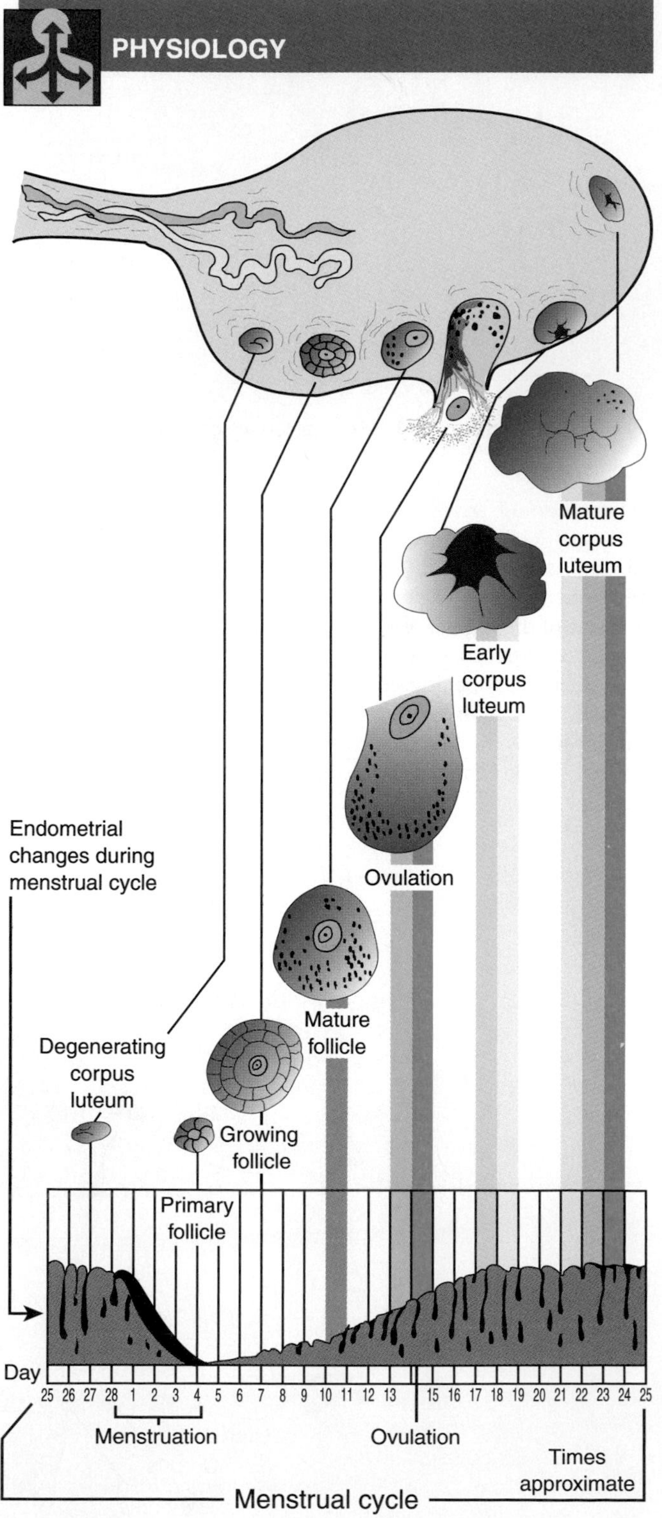

FIGURE 42•3 One menstrual cycle and the corresponding changes in the endometrium.

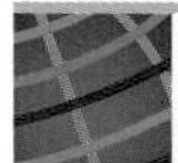

TABLE 42•1 **Hormonal Changes During the Menstrual Cycle**

(Times approximate)

Phase	Menstrual	Follicular	Ovulation	Luteal	Premenstrual
DAYS	1 2 3 4 5 6 7 8	9 10 11 12 13 14	15 16 17	18 19 20 21 22 23 24 25	26 27 28 1 2
Ovary					
	Degenerating corpus luteum; beginning follicular development	Growth and maturation of follicle	Ovulation	Active corpus luteum	Degenerating corpus luteum
Estrogen Production					
	Low	Increasing	High	Declining, then a secondary rise	Decreasing
Progesterone Production					
	None	Low	Low	Increasing	Decreasing
FSH Production					
	Increasing	High, then declining	Low	Low	Increasing
LH Production					
	Low	Low, then increasing	High	High	Decreasing
Endometrium					
	Degeneration and shedding of superficial layer. Coiled arteries dilate, then constrict again	Reorganization and proliferation of superficial layer	Continued growth	Active secretion and glandular dilation; highly vascular; edematous	Vasoconstriction of coiled arteries; beginning degeneration

length, but there are many normal variations. In the **proliferative phase** at the beginning of the cycle (just after menstruation), FSH output increases, stimulating estrogen secretion. This causes the endometrium to thicken and become more vascular. In the **secretory phase** near the middle portion of the cycle (day 14 in a 28-day cycle), LH output increases, stimulating ovulation. Under the combined stimulus of estrogen and progesterone, the endometrium reaches the peak of its thickening and vascularization.

If the ovum has been fertilized, estrogen and progesterone levels remain high, and the complex hormonal changes of pregnancy follow. If the ovum has not been fertilized, FSH and LH output diminishes; estrogen and progesterone secretion falls rapidly; the ovum disintegrates; and the endometrium, which has become thick and congested, becomes hemorrhagic. The product consisting of old blood, mucus, and endometrial tissue is discharged through the cervix and into the vagina. After the menstrual flow stops, the cycle begins again; the endometrium proliferates and thickens from estrogenic stimulation, and ovulation recurs.

Menopausal Period

The menopausal period marks the end of a woman's reproductive capacity. It usually occurs between the ages of 45 and 52 years but may occur in some women as early as 42 or as late as 55 years of age. The median age is 51. Menopause is not a pathologic phenomenon but a normal part of aging and maturation. Menstruation ceases, and because the ovaries are no longer active, the reproductive organs become smaller. No more ova mature; therefore, no ovarian hormones (estrogen) are produced. (An artificial menopause may occur earlier if the ovaries are surgically removed or are destroyed by radiation.) Besides changes in the reproductive system that reduce estrogen levels, multifaceted changes occur throughout the woman's body. These changes include neuroendocrinologic, biochemical, and metabolic alterations related to aging.

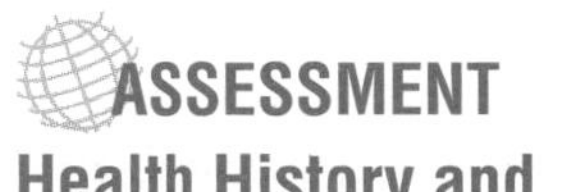

ASSESSMENT

Health History and Clinical Manifestations

In addition to obtaining a general health history, the nurse asks about past illness and experiences that are specific to women's health. Data should be collected about the following:

- Menstrual history (including **menarche**, length of cycles, length and amount of flow, presence of cramps or pain, bleeding between periods or after intercourse, bleeding after menopause)
- History of pregnancies (number of pregnancies, outcomes of pregnancies)
- History of exposure to medications (diethylstilbestrol [DES], immunosuppressive agents, others)
- Pain with menses (**dysmenorrhea**), pain with intercourse (**dyspareunia**), pelvic pain
- History of vaginal discharge and odor or itching
- History of problems with urinary function (ie, frequency or urgency); may be related to STDs or pregnancy
- History of problems with bowel or bladder control
- Sexual history
- History of sexual abuse or physical abuse
- History of surgery or other procedures on structures of reproductive tract (including female genital mutilation or female circumcision)

In collecting data related to reproductive health, the nurse is in a unique position to teach patients about normal physiologic processes, such as menstruation and menopause, and to assess possible abnormalities. Many problems experienced by young or middle-aged women can be corrected easily. If allowed to go untreated, however, they may result in anxiety and health problems. Issues related to sexuality and sexual function are typically brought to the attention of the health care provider who sees the woman for gynecologic care; any nurse, however, should consider these issues to be part of routine health assessment.

Sexual History

A sexual assessment includes both subjective and objective data. Health and sexual histories, physical examination findings, and laboratory results are all part of the database. The purpose of a sexual history is to obtain information that provides a picture of the woman's sexuality and sexual practices and promotes sexual health. The sexual history enables the patient to discuss sexual matters openly and to discuss sexual concerns with an informed health professional. This information can be obtained with the health history after the gynecologic-obstetric or genitourinary history is completed. By incorporating the sexual history into the general health history, the nurse can move from areas of lesser sensitivity to areas of greater sensitivity after establishing initial rapport.

Sexual history taking becomes a dynamic process reflecting an exchange of information between the patient and the nurse and provides the opportunity to clarify myths and explore areas of concern that the patient may not have felt comfortable discussing in the past. In obtaining a sexual history, the nurse must not assume sexual preference until clarified. When asking about sexual health, the nurse also cannot assume that patients are married or unmarried. Asking a woman to label herself as single, married, widowed, or divorced may be seen as an outdated inquiry by many women. Asking about a partner or about current meaningful relationships may be a less offensive way to initiate a sexual history.

Nurses can begin by explaining the purpose of obtaining a sexual history (eg, "I ask all my patients about their sexual health. May I ask you some questions about this?"). History taking continues by inquiring about present sexual activity and sexual orientation (eg, "Are you presently having sex with a man, a women, or both?"). Inquiries about possible sexual dysfunction may include, "Are you having any problems related to your current sexual activity?" Problems may be related to medication, life changes, or onset of physical or emotional illness. Patients can be asked about their thoughts on what is causing the current problem.

Risk for STDs can be assessed by asking about number of partners in the past year or in the patient's lifetime. An open-ended question related to the patient's need for further information should be included (eg, "Do you have any questions or concerns about your sexual health?").

Young women may be apprehensive about irregular periods, may be concerned about STDs, or may need contraception. They may want information on using tampons, emergency contraception, or issues related to pregnancy. Perimenopausal women may have concerns about dryness and burning with intercourse after menopause. Women of any age may have concerns about orgasm or anorgasmia (lack of orgasm).

There is a growing number of women entering the United States health care system who underwent female genital mutilation (FGM) before emigrating to this country. Because FGM can affect sexual function, menstrual hygiene, and bladder function, the possibility of FGM may be included in the sexual history, particularly for women from those cultures and countries where its practice is common.

Domestic Violence and Abuse

Nurses need to be aware of the prevalence of abuse and violence directed against women in our society. Abuse can be physical, emotional-psychological, or sexual. Battering is related to the need to maintain control of the relationship and involves fear of one partner by another and control by threats, intimidation, and physical abuse. Violence is rarely a one-time occurrence in a relationship. It usually continues and escalates in severity. This is an important point to emphasize when a woman states that her partner has hurt her but has promised to change. Batterers can change, but not without extensive counseling and motivation. If a woman states that she is being hurt, sensitive care is required (Guideline 42-1). Because more than 6 million women experience domestic violence each year, battered women are encountered daily in nursing practice. By knowing about this major public health problem, being alert to abuse-related problems, and learning how to elicit information from women about abuse in their lives, nurses can offer intervention for a problem that might otherwise go undetected. Asking each woman about violence in her life in a safe environment (ie, a private room with the door closed) is part of a comprehensive assessment and universal screening.

The Abuse Assessment Screen has been found effective in eliciting the presence of abuse and should be included in the health history of all women. The Abuse Assessment Screen consists of the following three questions:

1. In the past year, have you been hit, slapped, kicked, or otherwise physically hurt by someone?
2. If pregnant, since you have been pregnant, have you been hit, slapped, kicked, or otherwise physically hurt by someone?
3. Have you ever been forced into sexual activity?

No specific signs or symptoms are diagnostic of battering; however, nurses may see an injury that does not fit the account of how it happened (eg, a bruise on the side of the upper arm from "walking into a door"). Manifestations of abuse may involve suicide attempts, drug and alcohol abuse, frequent emergency department visits, vague pelvic pain, and depression. However, there may be no obvious signs or symptoms.

Incest and Childhood Sexual Abuse

Because more than one in five women are incest survivors, nurses must be aware that many women have experienced childhood sexual abuse. It has been reported that female victims of incest have more health problems and undergo more surgery than women who were not victimized. Victims of childhood sexual abuse are reported to experience more chronic depression, posttraumatic stress disorder, morbid obesity, marital instability, gastrointestinal problems, and headaches as well as greater use of health care services than do nonvictims. Nurses should be prepared to offer support and referral to psychologists, community resources, and self-help groups. Women who have experienced rape or sexual abuse frequently have difficulty with pelvic examinations, labor, pelvic or breast irradiation, or any treatment or examination that involves hands-on treatment or requires removal of clothing.

Rape and Sexual Assault

Sexual assault occurs every 6 minutes in the United States. Men, women, and children may be victims. Sexual assault nurse examiners often perform the painstaking collection of forensic evi-

42•1 GUIDELINES FOR MANAGING REPORTED DOMESTIC ABUSE

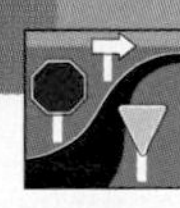

Action	Rationale
1. Reassure the woman that she is not alone.	Many women are hurt by their partners, and nurses see them daily.
2. Express your belief that no one should be hurt, that abuse is the fault of the batterer and is against the law.	Let the woman know that no one deserves to be abused.
3. Assure the woman that her information is confidential, although it does become part of her medical record. (However, **if children are suspected of being abused or are being abused, the law requires that this be reported to the authorities.**)	Women are often afraid that their information will be reported to the police or protective services and their children may be taken away.
4. Document the woman's statement of abuse and take photographs of any visible injuries *if* written formal consent has been obtained. (Emergency departments usually have a camera available if one is not on the nursing unit.)	Provide documentation of injuries that may be needed for later legal or criminal proceedings.
5. Provide teaching: • Inform the woman that shelters are available to ensure safety for her and her children. (Lengths of stay in shelters vary by state but are often up to 2 months. Staff often assist with housing, jobs, and the emotional upheaval that accompanies the break-up of the family.) Provide list of shelters. • Inform woman that violence gets worse, not better. • If the woman chooses to go to a shelter, let her make the call. • If she chooses to return to the abuser, remain nonjudgmental and provide information that will make her safer than she was before disclosing her situation. • Make sure that she has a 24-hour hotline telephone number that provides information and support (Spanish translation and a device for the deaf are also available); police number, and 911. • Assist her to set up a safety plan in case she decides to return home. (A safety plan is an organized plan for departure with packed bags and important papers hidden in a safe spot.)	These options may be life saving for the woman and her children.

dence that is needed for criminal evidence. Oral, anal, and genital tissue is examined for evidence of trauma, semen, or infection. Saliva, hair, and fingernail evidence is also collected. Cultures are obtained for STDs, and prophylactic antibiotics are prescribed. An emergency contraception medication may be provided. Emotional counseling is provided, and follow-up treatment visits are arranged. The rape trauma syndrome defines the emotional reaction to sexual assault and may consist of shock, sleep disturbances, nightmares, flashbacks, anxiety, anger, mood swings, and depression. It is important for victims-survivors to discuss the experience and to obtain professional counseling.

Screening for abuse, rape, and violence should be part of routine assessment because some women do not report or seek treatment for sexual assault. Often, the assailant is a partner, husband, or date. Nurses may encounter women with infections or pregnancies related to sexual assault that were not effectively treated.

Physical Assessment

An annual breast and pelvic examination is important for all women who are 18 years of age or older and for those who are sexually active, regardless of age. The patient deserves understanding and support because of the emotional and physical considerations associated with gynecologic examinations. Women may be sensitive or embarrassed by the usual questions asked by a gynecologic or women's health care provider. Because gynecologic conditions are of a personal and private nature to most women, such information is shared only with those directly involved in patient care (as is true with all patient information).

Throughout the examination, the nurse explains procedures to be performed. This not only encourages the woman to relax but also provides an opportunity for her to ask questions and minimizes the negative reactions that many women associate with gynecologic examinations.

The first pelvic examination is often anxiety producing for women; the nurse can alleviate many of these feelings with explanations and teaching (Chart 42-1). Before the examination begins, the nurse instructs the patient to void. At this time, a urine specimen may be obtained if such tests are part of the total assessment. Voiding ensures patient comfort and eases the examination because a full bladder can make palpation of pelvic organs uncomfortable for the patient and difficult for the examiner.

Positioning

Although several positions may be used for the pelvic examination, the supine lithotomy position is used most commonly, although the upright lithotomy position in which the woman assumes a

CHART 42•1 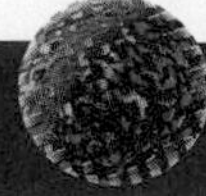 **Patient Education: The Pelvic Examination**

The nurse should explain the following to the patient:

- A pelvic examination includes assessment of the appearance, size, and shape of the vulva, vagina, uterus, and ovaries to ensure reproductive health and absence of illness.
- A pelvic examination should never hurt. Women often describe a feeling of fullness or pressure but should not feel pain. Some women who are very tense feel discomfort, so relaxation is important.
- It is normal to feel uncomfortable and apprehensive.
- A narrow, warmed speculum will be inserted to visualize the cervix.
- A Papanicolaou (Pap) smear will be performed and should not be uncomfortable.
- The patient may watch the examination with a mirror if she chooses.
- The examination is brief and usually takes no longer than 5 minutes.
- Draping will be used to minimize exposure (despite appropriate draping, most women feel uncomfortable or embarrassed during the examination).

semisitting posture may also be used. This position offers several advantages:

- It is more comfortable for some women.
- It allows better eye contact between patient and examiner.
- It may provide an easier means for the examiner to carry out the bimanual examination.
- It enables the woman to use a mirror to see her anatomy (if she chooses) to visualize any conditions that require treatment or to learn about using certain types of contraceptive methods.

In the supine lithotomy position, the patient lies on the table with her feet on foot rests; she is encouraged to relax so that her buttocks are positioned at the edge of the examination table, and she is asked to relax and spread her thighs as widely apart as possible.

If the patient is too ill, disabled, or neurologically impaired to lie on a table with stirrups, Simms' position may be used. In Simms' position, the patient lies on her left side with her right leg bent at a 90-degree angle. The right labia may be retracted for adequate access to the vagina. Other positions for pelvic examination for disabled women make the examination easier for women and their clinicians.

The following equipment is obtained and readily available: a good light source; a vaginal speculum; clean examination gloves; lubricant, spatula, cytobrush, glass slides, fixative solution or spray; and diagnostic testing supplies for screening for occult rectal blood if the woman is older than 40 years of age.

Inspection

When the patient is prepared, the examiner inspects the labia majora and minora, noting epidermal tissue of the labia majora, with hair follicles characteristic of skin that fades to the pink mucous membrane of the vaginal introitus. In the nulliparous woman, the labia minora come together at the opening of the vagina. In women who have delivered children vaginally, the labia minora may gape, and vaginal tissue may protrude.

To identify such protrusions, the examiner asks the patient to "bear down." Trauma to the anterior vaginal wall during childbirth may have resulted in incompetency of musculature, so that a bulge caused by the bladder intruding into the submucosa of the anterior vaginal wall (**cystocele**) may be seen. Childbirth trauma may also have affected the posterior vaginal wall, so that a bulge caused by rectal cavity protrusion (**rectocele**) may be seen. Moreover, the cervix may descend under pressure through the vaginal canal and be seen at the introitus. This is called **uterine prolapse** (see Chap. 43 for a discussion of these structural changes).

The introitus should be free of superficial mucosal lesions. The labia minora may be separated by the fingers of the gloved hand and the lower part of the vagina palpated. In virginal women, a hymen of variable thickness may be felt circumferentially within 1 or 2 cm of the vaginal opening. The hymenal ring usually permits the insertion of one finger. Rarely, the hymen totally occludes the vaginal entrance (imperforate hymen.)

In nonvirginal women, a rim of scar tissue representing the remnants of the hymenal ring may be felt circumferentially around the vagina near its opening. The greater vestibular glands (Bartholin's glands) lie between the labia minora and the remnants of the hymenal ring. An abscess of the Bartholin's gland can cause discomfort and requires incision and drainage.

Speculum Examination

Assorted sizes of the bivalved speculum are available in metal or plastic. (Metal specula are soaked, scrubbed, and sterilized between patients. Some clinicians prefer plastic specula that permit singular use.) Either should be warmed with a heating pad or warm water to make insertion more comfortable for the patient. The speculum is not lubricated because commercial lubricants interfere with cervical cytology (Papanicolaou [Pap] smear) findings. The metal speculum has two setscrews. One, along the handle and holding the two valves of the speculum together, is kept tightened. The setscrew that holds the thumb rest in place is loosened. The speculum is grasped in the dominant hand, with the thumb against the back of the thumb rest to keep the tips of the valves closed.

The speculum is rotated slightly counterclockwise, and the vaginal orifice is held open by the thumb and the forefinger of the gloved nondominant hand by some examiners. Other examiners find that straight insertion of a speculum with downward pressure on the vagina is more comfortable for the patient.

The speculum is gently inserted into the posterior portion of the introitus and slowly advanced to the top of the vagina; this should not be painful or uncomfortable for the woman. The tip of the speculum may then be elevated and the speculum rotated to a transverse position. The speculum is then slowly opened, and the setscrew of the thumb rest is tightened to hold the speculum open (Fig. 42-4).

CERVIX

The cervix is inspected. In nulliparous women, the cervix usually is 2 to 3 cm wide and smooth. Women who have borne children may have a laceration, usually transverse, giving the cervical os a "fishmouth" appearance. Moreover, epithelium from the endocervical canal may have grown onto the surface of the cervix, appearing as beefy red surface epithelium circumferentially around the os. Occasionally, the cervix of a woman whose mother took DES has a hooded appearance (a peaked aspect superiorly or a ridge of tissue surrounding it) and is evaluated by colposcopy when identified.

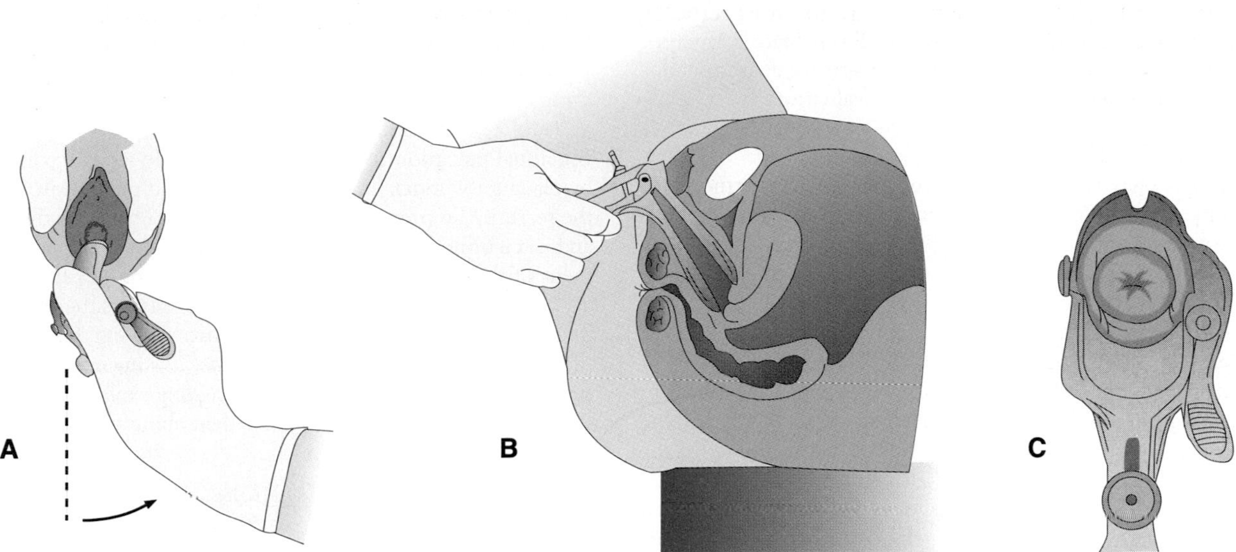

FIGURE 42•4 Technique for speculum examination of the vagina and cervix. (**A**) The labia are spread apart with a gloved left hand, while the speculum is grasped in the right hand and turned counterclockwise before being inserted into the vagina. Once the speculum is inserted, the blades are then spread apart (**B**) to reveal the cervical os (**C**).

ABNORMAL GROWTH

Malignant changes may not be obviously differentiated from the rest of the cervical mucosa. Small, benign cysts may appear on the cervical surface. These are usually bluish or white and are called nabothian cysts. A **polyp** of endocervical mucosa may protrude through the os and usually is dark red. Polyps can cause irregular bleeding; they are rarely malignant and usually are removed easily in an office or clinic setting. A carcinoma may appear as a cauliflower-like growth that bleeds easily when touched. Blueness of the cervix is a sign of early pregnancy (Chadwick's sign).

PAPANICOLAOU SMEAR

During the pelvic examination, a Pap smear is obtained by rotating a small wooden spatula at the os, followed by a cervical brush rotated in the os. The tissue obtained is spread on a glass slide and sprayed or fixed immediately, or inserted into a liquid.

A specimen of any purulent material appearing at the cervical os is obtained for culture. A sterile applicator is used to obtain the specimen, which is immediately placed in an appropriate medium for transfer to a laboratory. In patients at high risk for infection, routine cultures for gonococcal and chlamydial organisms are recommended because of the high incidence of both diseases and the high risk for pelvic infection, fallopian tube damage, and subsequent infertility.

Vaginal discharge, which may be normal or a result of vaginitis, may be present. Discharge caused by bacteria (bacterial vaginosis, or BV) usually appears gray and purulent. Discharge caused by *Trichomonas* species infection is usually frothy, copious, and malodorous. Discharge caused by *Candida* species infection is thick and white-yellow and has a cottage-cheese appearance. See Table 42-2 for a summary of characteristics of vaginal discharge found in different conditions.

The vagina is inspected as the examiner withdraws the speculum. It is smooth in young girls and thickens after puberty, with many rugae (folds) and redundancy in the epithelium. In menopausal women, the vagina thins and has fewer rugae because of decreased estrogen.

Bimanual Palpation

To complete the pelvic examination, the examiner performs a bimanual examination from a standing position. The examination is performed with the forefinger and middle finger of the gloved and lubricated hand. These fingers are placed in the vaginal orifice, while the other fingers are held tightly out of the way, with the

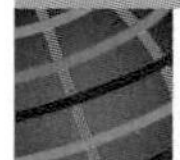

TABLE 42•2 **Characteristics of Vaginal Discharge**

Cause of Discharge	Symptoms	Odor	Consistency/Color
Physiologic	None	None	Mucus/white
Candida species infection	Itching, irritation	Yeast odor or none	Thin to thick, curdlike/white in color
Bacterial vaginosis	Odor	Fishy, often noticed after intercourse	Thin/grayish or yellow in color
Trichomonas species infection	Irritation, odor	Malodorous	Copious, often frothy/yellow-green
Atrophic	Vulvar or vaginal dryness	Occasional mild malodor	Usually scant and mucoid/may be blood tinged

thumb completely adducted. The fingers are advanced vertically along the vaginal canal, and the vaginal wall is palpated. Any firm part of the vaginal wall may represent old scar tissue from childbirth trauma but may also require further evaluation.

CERVICAL PALPATION

The cervix is palpated and assessed for its consistency, mobility, size, and position. The normal cervix is uniformly firm but not hard. Softening of the cervix is a finding in early pregnancy. Hardness may reflect invasion by a neoplasm. Normally, the cervix and uterus are freely movable.

Pain on gentle movement of the cervix is called a positive **chandelier sign** or positive cervical motion tenderness (+CMT) and usually indicates a pelvic infection. Fixation of the uterus in the pelvis may be a sign of **endometriosis** or malignancy. The body of the uterus is normally twice the diameter and twice the length of the cervix, curving anteriorly toward the abdominal wall. Some women have a retroverted or retroflexed uterus, which tips posteriorly toward the sacrum, whereas others have a uterus that is neither anterior nor posterior but is midline.

UTERINE PALPATION

To palpate the uterus, the examiner places the opposite hand on the abdominal wall halfway between the patient's umbilicus and the pubis and presses firmly toward the vagina (Fig. 42-5). Movement of the abdominal wall causes the body of the uterus to descend, and the pear-shaped organ becomes freely movable between the abdominal examining hand and the examining fingers of the pelvic examining hand. Uterine size, mobility, and contour can be estimated through palpation.

ADNEXAL PALPATION

Next, the right and left adnexal areas are palpated to evaluate the fallopian tubes and ovaries. The fingers of the hand examining the pelvis are moved first to one side, then to the other, while the hand palpating the abdominal area is moved correspondingly to either side of the abdomen and downward. The adnexa (ovaries and fallopian tubes) are trapped between the two hands and palpated for an obvious mass, tenderness, and mobility. Commonly, the ovaries are slightly tender and the patient is informed that slight discomfort on palpation is normal.

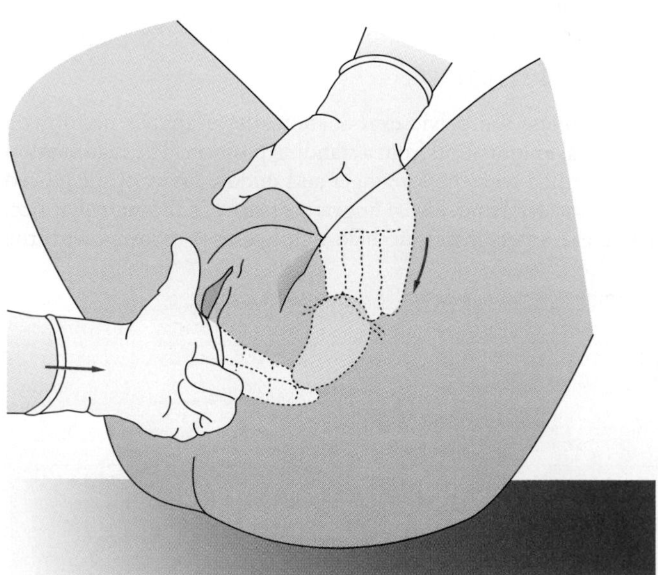

FIGURE 42•5 Technique for the bimanual examination of the pelvis.

VAGINAL AND RECTAL PALPATION

Bimanual palpation of the vagina and cul-de-sac is accomplished by placing the index finger in the vagina and the middle finger in the rectum. To prevent cross-contamination between the vaginal and rectal orifices, the examiner puts on new gloves. A gentle movement of these fingers toward each other compresses the posterior vaginal wall and the anterior rectal wall and assists the examiner in identifying the integrity of these structures. During this procedure, the patient may sense an urge to defecate. The nurse needs to assure the patient that this will not occur. Ongoing explanations are provided to reassure and educate the patient about the procedure.

Gerontologic Considerations

Frequent examinations can help in preventing problems of the reproductive tract in aging women. Often, older women do not have regular gynecologic examinations; and some who have delivered their children at home have never had a pelvic examination. Some regard it as an embarrassing and unpleasant procedure. An important role of the nurse is to encourage an annual pelvic examination for all women. The nurse can make the examination a time for education and reassurance, rather than a time of embarrassment.

Perineal pruritus is a common symptom in older women and should be evaluated because it may indicate a possible disease process (diabetes or malignancy). It may also indicate vulvar dystrophy, a thickened or whitish discoloration of perineal tissue that needs biopsy to rule out abnormal cells suggesting cancer. Topical cortisone and hormone creams may be prescribed for symptomatic relief.

With relaxing pelvic musculature, uterine prolapse and relaxation of the vaginal walls can occur. Appropriate evaluation and surgical repair can provide relief if the patient is a candidate for surgery. After surgery, the patient needs to know that tissue repair and healing may require additional time. Pessaries, latex devices that provide support, are often used if surgery is contraindicated. They are fitted by a health care provider and may reduce discomfort and pressure. Use of a pessary requires the patient to have routine gynecologic examinations to monitor for irritation or infection.

DIAGNOSTIC EVALUATION

Cytologic Test for Cancer (Papanicolaou Smear)

The Pap smear is performed to detect cervical cancer. Before 1940, cervical cancer was the most common cause of cancer death in women. Dr. George Papanicolaou discovered the value of examining exfoliated cells for malignancy in the 1930s. Due to the effectiveness of the Pap smear as a screening method, cervical cancer is now less common than breast or ovarian cancer.

Cervical secretions are gently removed from the cervical os (Fig. 42-6), transferred to a glass slide, and "fixed" immediately by immersing the slide in or spraying it with a fixative. The patient should be instructed not to douche before this examination to avoid washing away cellular material. The Pap smear should be performed when the patient is not menstruating because blood usually interferes with an accurate interpretation. The proper technique for obtaining a cervical specimen for cytologic study is

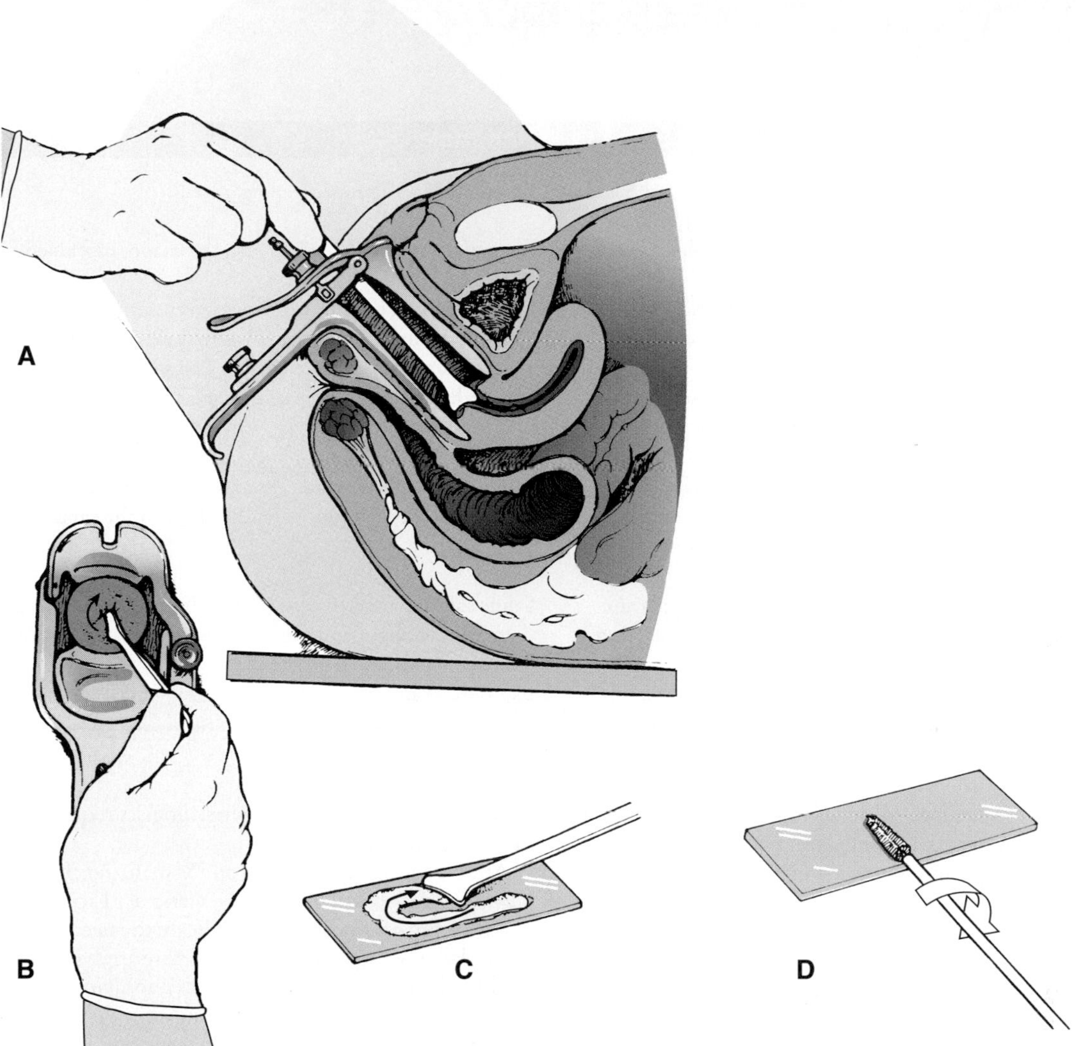

FIGURE 42•6 Method of using a wooden Ayre spatula to obtain cervical secretions for cytology. (**A**) Speculum in place and the Ayre spatula in position at the cervical os. (**B**) The tip of the spatula is placed in the cervical os and the spatula rotated 360 degrees, firmly but nontraumatically. (**C**) Cellular material clinging to the spatula is then smeared smoothly on a glass slide, which is promptly placed in a fixative solution. (**D**) Cytobrush is rotated in the cervical os and rolled onto a glass slide.

described in Guideline 42-2. False-negative Pap smear results occur mostly from sampling errors or improper technique.

Initially, the Papanicolaou classification of cytologic findings was a numeric range from class I to class V, with I being normal and V being malignant. A more descriptive classification system has been developed, using the following terms: normal; inflammation; atypia (not typical); koilocytosis (a change in cells affected by human papillomavirus [HPV]); mild, moderate, or severe dysplasia; and invasive carcinoma.

Other terminology includes the following categories: low-grade squamous intraepithelial lesion (LGSIL), which is equivalent to cervical intraepithelial neoplasia (CIN) type I and to mild and moderate changes related to exposure to HPV. High-grade squamous intraepithelial lesion (HGSIL) equates to CIN III, severe dysplasia, and carcinoma in situ (CIS). These terms are seen on Pap smear findings and encompass all precursors to invasive carcinoma of the cervix. These diagnostic terms are described more fully in Table 42-3.

Pap smears that reveal mild inflammation or atypical squamous cells are usually repeated in 3 to 6 months, with findings often returning to normal. Patients are apprehensive because many women incorrectly assume that an abnormal Pap smear means cancer. If a specific infection is causing inflammation, it is treated appropriately, and the Pap smear is repeated.

Recently, Pap smears have been scrutinized for quality interpretation. Some Pap smears are now evaluated by the cytotechnologist and by computer review (Papnet). This double review is the option of the patient and usually costs more than a normal Pap smear. Newer methods of fixation (eg, Thin Prep) are also available, in which a plastic broomlike device is rotated in the

42•2 Guidelines For Obtaining an Optimal Pap Smear

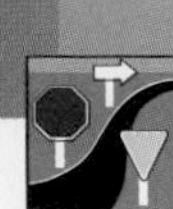

Technique	Rationale
1. Do not obtain a Pap smear if the woman is menstruating or has other frank bleeding (exception: high suspicion of neoplasia).	Blood obscures a proper reading of cells.
2. If performing more than one test (eg, Pap and GC), obtain the Pap smear first.	By performing the Pap smear first, the chance of a bloody smear is avoided.
3. Label frosted end of slide with patient's name in pencil.	Ink may rub off or blur. Labeling prevents improper identification.
4. Put on gloves before gently inserting unlubricated speculum. (Speculum may be moistened with warm water.)	Gloves provide protection and warm water prevents discomfort. Lubricants may obscure cells on Pap smear.
5. Place longer end of the Ayre spatula in cervical canal and rotate in a full circle to obtain a sample from the exocervix. Spread the material obtained onto the Pap smear slide.	This technique will obtain a sampling of exocervix and squamocolumnar junction.
6. Insert a cytobrush 2 cm into the cervical canal and rotate 180 degrees. Roll the brush onto the Pap smear slide. (Thin prep paps are not spread onto a slide. The spatula and brush are placed in a bottle of fixative and swirled.)	This obtains endocervical cells and may sample cells from the squamocolumnar junction if it is high in the canal.
7. In women who have had a hysterectomy, use a cotton applicator moistened with saline solution to obtain a sampling of cells from the vaginal cuff or posterior vagina.	Saline solution prevents drying, which makes interpretation difficult for the cytologist and prevents absorption of cells into the cotton, increasing the yield on the slide.
8. Immediately spray slide or place thin prep Pap into solution.	Exposure to air or light causes distortion of cells.

os and then placed in a fixative solution to release the material collected. Because false-negative results still occur (up to 20%), yearly Pap smears are important.

Colposcopy and Cervical Biopsy

All suspicious Pap smears should be evaluated by colposcopy. The colposcope is an optical instrument, a portable microscope (magnification from 10 to 25 times) that allows the examiner to visualize the cervix and obtain a sample of abnormal tissue for analysis. Nurse practitioners and gynecologists require special training in this diagnostic technique.

After inserting a speculum and visualizing the cervix and vaginal walls, the examiner applies acetic acid to the cervix. Subsequent abnormal findings that indicate the need for biopsy include leukoplakia (white plaque visible before applying acetic acid), acetowhite tissue (white epithelium after applying acetic acid), punctation (dilated capillaries occurring in a dotted or stippled pattern), mosaicism (a tilelike pattern), and atypical vascular patterns.

An endocervical curettage (ECC) may be performed during colposcopy if a problem is suspected based on Pap smear findings. This analysis of tissue from the cervical canal is used to determine whether abnormal changes have occurred in the cervical canal. If these biopsy specimens show premalignant cells or cervical intraepithelial neoplasia, the patient usually needs cryotherapy, laser therapy, or a cone biopsy (excision of an inverted tissue cone from the cervix).

Table 42•3 Interpretation of Pap Smears

Interpretation	Numeric System	Bethesda Classification
Negative (normal)	Class I	Negative (normal)
Probably negative	Class II	Infection Reactive and reparative changes Squamous cell abnormalities
Suspicious	Class III	Low-grade squamous intraepithelial lesion (LGSIL), mild dysplasia
More suspicious	Class IV	High-grade squamous intraepithelial lesion (HGSIL) or carcinoma in situ (CIS): moderate or severe dysplasia
Malignant	Class V	Squamous cell carcinoma

Cryotherapy and Laser Therapy

Cryotherapy (freezing cervical tissue with nitrous oxide) and laser treatment are used in the outpatient setting. Cryotherapy may result in cramping and occasional feelings of faintness (vasovagal response). A watery discharge is normal for a few weeks after the procedure as the cervix heals. With laser therapy, a slice of cervix is removed.

Cone Biopsy

If the ECC findings indicate abnormal changes or if the lesion extends into the canal, the patient may undergo a cone biopsy. This can be performed surgically or with a procedure called LEEP (loop electrosurgical excision procedure), which uses a laser beam.

Usually performed in the outpatient setting, LEEP is associated with a high success rate in removal of abnormal cervical tissue and has a low incidence of complications. The gynecologist excises a small amount of cervical tissue, and the pathologist examines the borders of the specimen to determine if they are free of disease. A patient anesthetized for a surgical cone biopsy is advised to rest for 24 hours after the procedure and to leave any vaginal packing in place until the physician removes it (usually the next day). The patient is instructed to report any excessive bleeding.

Guidelines regarding postoperative sexual activity, bathing, and other activities are provided by the nurse or the physician. Because open tissue may be potentially exposed to HIV and other pathogens, the patient is usually cautioned to use condoms when resuming sexual activity until healing is complete and verified at follow-up.

Endometrial (Aspiration) Smears and Biopsy

A tissue sample obtained directly from the endometrium is an accurate method of diagnosing cellular changes in the endometrium.

Endometrial biopsy, a common method of obtaining endometrial tissue, is performed during the gynecologic pelvic examination, when indicated, as an outpatient procedure. Usually, it can be performed without anesthesia; however, a paracervical block is effective if required. In this procedure, the examiner may apply a tenaculum (a clamplike instrument that stabilizes the uterus) after the pelvic examination and then inserts a thin, hollow, flexible suction tube (pipelle or sampler) through the cervix into the uterus.

Endometrial biopsy is a tolerable and accurate outpatient method for evaluating the endometrium and is usually indicated in cases of midlife irregular bleeding, postmenopausal bleeding, and infertility (to identify changes in the uterine lining after ovulation). Women who are bleeding irregularly while receiving hormone replacement therapy or who are taking tamoxifen and have any bleeding are usually advised to undergo endometrial biopsy.

Dilation and Curettage

During a dilation and curettage (D & C), which may be diagnostic (explains the cause of irregular bleeding) or therapeutic (often temporarily stops irregular bleeding), the cervical canal is widened with a dilator and the uterine endometrium is scraped with a curette. The purpose of the procedure is to secure endometrial or endocervical tissue for cytologic examination, to control abnormal uterine bleeding, and as a therapeutic measure for incomplete abortion.

Because this procedure is usually carried out under anesthesia and requires surgical asepsis, it is usually performed in the operating room. However, it may also take place in the outpatient setting with the patient receiving a local anesthetic, supplemented with diazepam (Valium), midazolam (Versed), or meperidine (Demerol). The patient who receives these medications is carefully monitored until fully recovered.

The nurse provides an explanation of the procedure as well as physical and psychological preparation, informing the patient about what the procedure involves and what to expect in the way of postoperative discomfort and bleeding. The perineum is not shaved, but the patient is instructed to void before the procedure. The patient is placed in the lithotomy position, the cervix is dilated with an instrument, and endometrial scrapings are obtained by a curette. A perineal pad is placed over the perineum after the procedure, and evidence of excessive bleeding is reported. No restrictions are placed on dietary intake. If pelvic discomfort or low back pain occurs, mild analgesics usually provide relief. The physician indicates when sexual intercourse may be safely resumed. To reduce the risk of infection and bleeding, most physicians advise no vaginal penetration for 2 weeks.

Endoscopic Examinations

Laparoscopy (Pelvic Peritoneoscopy)

A laparoscopy involves inserting a laparoscope (a tube about 10 mm wide and similar to a small periscope) into the peritoneal cavity through a 2-cm (0.75-inch) incision below the umbilicus to allow visualization of the pelvic structures (Fig. 42-7). Laparoscopy may be used for diagnostic purposes (eg, in cases of pelvic pain when no cause can be found) or treatment. Laparoscopy also facilitates minor surgical procedures, such as tubal sterilization, ovarian biopsy, and lysis of adhesions (scar tissue that can cause pelvic discomfort). A surgical instrument (intrauterine sound or cannula) may be positioned inside the uterus to permit manipulation or movement during laparoscopy, affording better visualization.

A better view of the pelvic, lower abdominal, and visceral contents is obtained by injecting a prescribed amount of carbon dioxide intraperitoneally into the cavity. Called insufflation, this technique separates the intestines from the pelvic organs. If the patient is undergoing sterilization, the fallopian or uterine tubes may be electrocoagulated and a segment removed for histologic verification. (Clips are an alternative device for occluding tubes.) After the laparoscopy is completed, the laparoscope is withdrawn, carbon dioxide is allowed to escape through the outer cannula, the small skin incision is closed with sutures or a clip, and the incision is covered with an adhesive bandage.

The patient is carefully monitored for several hours to detect any untoward signs indicating bleeding, injury, or possible burns from the coagulator. These complications, however, rarely occur, making laparoscopy a cost-effective and safe short-stay procedure.

Hysteroscopy

Hysteroscopy (transcervical intrauterine endoscopy) allows direct visualization of all parts of the uterine cavity by means of a lighted optical instrument. The procedure is best performed about 5 days after menstruation stops in the estrogenic phase of the menstrual cycle. The vagina and vulva are cleaned, and a paracervical anesthetic block is performed. The instrument used for the procedure, a hysteroscope, is passed into the cervical canal and advanced 1 or 2 cm under direct vision. Uterine-distending fluid (normal saline solution or 5% dextrose in water) is infused through the instrument to dilate the uterine cavity and enhance visibility.

Hysteroscopy is most commonly indicated as an adjunct to a D & C and laparoscopy in cases of infertility, unexplained bleeding, retained intrauterine device (IUD), and recurrent early pregnancy loss. Treatment for some conditions (eg, fibroid tumors) can be accomplished during this procedure. Hysteroscopy is contraindicated in patients with cervical or endometrial carcinoma or acute pelvic inflammation. Endometrial ablation (destruction of the uterine lining) is performed with a hysteroscope and laser beam in cases of severe bleeding that do not respond to other therapies. Performed in an outpatient setting, this rapid procedure is an alternative to hysterectomy for some patients.

Other Diagnostic Procedures

Many diagnostic procedures are helpful in evaluating pelvic conditions. These may include x-rays, barium enemas, gastrointestinal x-ray series, intravenous urography, and cystography studies. Additionally, because the uterus, ovaries, and fallopian tubes are near the kidneys, ureters, and bladder, urologic diagnostic stud-

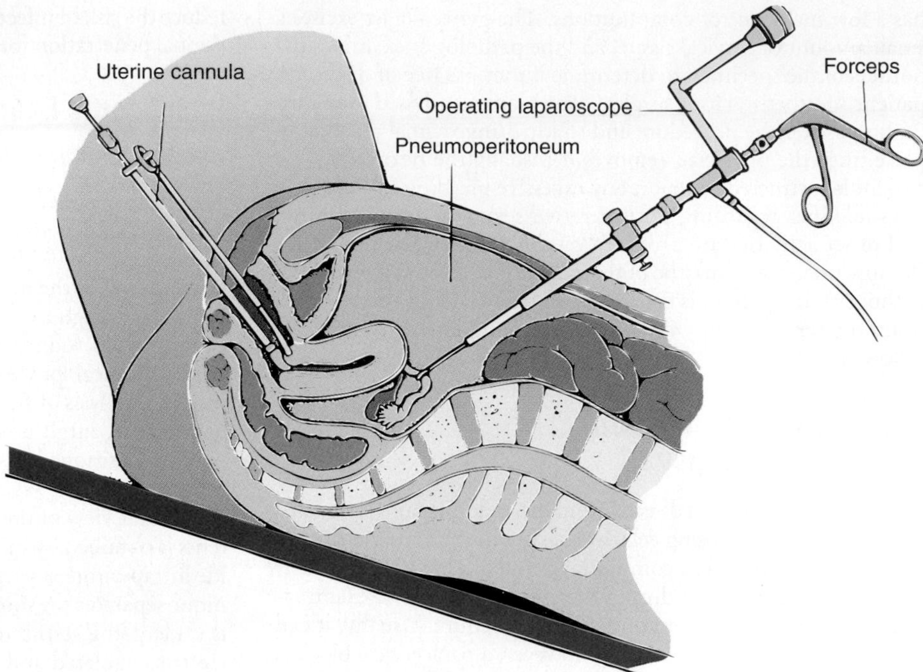

FIGURE 42•7 Laparoscopy. The laparoscope (*right*) is inserted through a small incision in the abdomen. A forceps is inserted through the scope to grasp the fallopian tube. To improve the view, a uterine cannula (*left*) is inserted into the vagina to push the uterus upward. Insufflation of gas creates an air pocket (pneumoperitoneum), and the pelvis is elevated (note the angle), which forces the intestines higher in the abdomen.

ies, such as the KUB (kidney, ureter, and bladder) and pyelogram are used, as are angiography and radioisotope scanning, if needed. Other diagnostic procedures include hysterosalpingography and computed tomography (CT) scan.

Hysterosalpingography or Uterotubography

Hysterosalpingography (HSP) is an x-ray study of the uterus and the fallopian tubes after injection of an x-ray contrast agent. The diagnostic procedure is performed to evaluate infertility or tubal patency and to detect any abnormal condition in the uterine cavity. Sometimes, the procedure may be therapeutic because the flowing contrast agent flushes debris or loosens adhesions.

The procedure requires placing the patient in the lithotomy position and exposing the cervix with a bivalved speculum. A cannula is then inserted into the cervix, and the contrast agent is injected into the uterine cavity and the fallopian tubes. X-rays are taken to show the path and the distribution of the contrast agent.

In preparation for HSP, the intestinal tract is cleansed with cathartics and an enema so that gas shadows do not distort the x-ray findings. An analgesic may be prescribed. Some patients experience nausea, vomiting, cramps, and faintness. After the test, the patient may need to wear a perineal pad for several hours because the radiopaque agent may stain clothing.

Computed Tomography Scan

CT scanning has several advantages over ultrasonography (described subsequently), even though it involves radiation exposure and is more costly. It is more effective with an obese patient or a patient with a distended bowel. A CT scan can also demonstrate a tumor and any extension into the retroperitoneal lymph nodes and skeletal tissue, although it has limited value in diagnosing other gynecologic abnormalities.

Ultrasonography

Ultrasonography (or ultrasound) is a useful adjunct to the physical examination, particularly in the obstetric patient or the patient with abnormal pelvic examination findings. It is a simple procedure based on sound wave transmission that uses pulsed ultrasonic waves at frequencies exceeding 20,000 Hz (formerly, cycles per second). The transducer, which is placed in contact with the abdomen (abdominal scan) or a vaginal probe (vaginal ultrasound), converts mechanical energy into electrical impulses, which in turn are amplified and recorded on an oscilloscope screen while a photograph or video recording of the patterns is taken. The entire procedure takes about 10 minutes and involves no ionizing radiation and no discomfort other than a full bladder, which is necessary for good visualization during an abdominal scan. (A vaginal ultrasound or sonogram does not require a full bladder.) Saline may be instilled into the uterus (saline infusion sonogram [SIS]) to help delineate endometrial polyps or fibroids.

Magnetic Resonance Imaging

Magnetic resonance imaging (MRI) produces patterns that are finer and more definitive than other imaging procedures without exposing the patient to radiation. The MRI, however, is more costly.

MANAGEMENT OF NORMAL AND ALTERED FEMALE PHYSIOLOGIC PROCESSES

Many health concerns of women are related to normal changes or abnormalities of the menstrual cycle. Many result from women's lack of understanding of the menstrual cycle, developmental changes, and factors that may affect the pattern of the menstrual cycle. Informing and educating women about the menstrual cycle and changes over time are important aspects of the nurse's role in providing quality care to women. Teaching should begin early, so that menstruation and the lifelong changes in the menstrual cycle can be anticipated and accepted as a normal part of life.

Menstruation

The flow of blood, menstruation, occurs about every 28 days during the reproductive years, although normal cycles can vary from 21 to 42 days. The flow period usually lasts from 4 to 5 days, during which time 50 to 60 mL, or 4 to 12 teaspoons, of blood is lost.

Management

A perineal pad is generally used to absorb menstrual discharge; deodorant-treated pads are available, but some women are allergic or sensitive to the deodorants. Tampons are also used extensively; there is no significant evidence of untoward effects from their use, provided that there is no difficulty in inserting them. However, tampons should not be used for more than 4 to 6 hours, nor should superabsorbent tampons be used because of the association with toxic shock syndrome (see Chap. 43 for more about this syndrome). If a tampon is hard to remove, the vagina feels dry, or the tampon shreds when removed, less absorbent tampons should be used. If the string breaks or retracts, a woman is instructed to squat in a comfortable position, insert one finger into the vagina, try to locate the tampon, and remove it. If the woman feels uncomfortable attempting this maneuver or if she cannot remove the tampon, she should consult a health care provider.

Psychosocial Considerations

Girls who are approaching menarche (the onset of menstruation) should be instructed about the normal process of the menstrual cycle before it occurs. Psychologically, it is much healthier to refer to this event as a "period" rather than as "being sick." With adequate nutrition, rest, and exercise, most women feel little discomfort, although some report breast tenderness and a feeling of fullness 1 or 2 days before menstruation begins. Others report fatigue and some discomfort in the lower back, legs, and pelvis on the first day and temperament or mood changes. Slight deviations from a usual healthful pattern of daily living are considered normal, but excessive deviation may require evaluation.

Cultural Considerations

Menstruation may be viewed and managed differently among cultures. Some women believe that it is detrimental to change a pad or tampon too frequently; they think that allowing the discharge to accumulate increases the flow, which is considered desirable. Other opinions influenced by culture also deserve consideration. For example, some women believe they are vulnerable to illness during menstruation. Others feel it is harmful to swim, shower, receive a hair permanent, get teeth filled, or eat certain foods during menstruation. They may also avoid using contraception.

In such situations, the nurse is in a position to provide women with accurate information in an accepting and culturally sensitive manner. The objective is to be mindful of these unexpressed, deep-rooted beliefs and to provide correct information with care. Aspects of gynecologic problems cannot always be expressed easily. The nurse needs to convey confidence and openness as well as offer sound advice to facilitate communication.

Perimenopause

Perimenopause is the period extending from the first signs of menopause—usually hot flashes, vaginal dryness, and irregular menses—to beyond the complete cessation of menses (1 year from last menstrual period).

Nursing Management

The following facts about perimenopause must be considered by the nurse when caring for or educating the patient during the perimenopause period:

- Sexuality, fertility, contraception, and STDs may be of concern to perimenopausal women.
- Unintended pregnancy is possible if effective contraception is not used.
- Oral contraceptives may provide perimenopausal women with some protection against uterine cancer, ovarian cancer, anemia, pregnancy, and fibrocystic breast changes as well as relief from perimenopausal symptoms. (Women who smoke and who are age 35 years or older should not take oral contraceptives because of an increased risk for cardiovascular disease.)
- About 16% of cases of breast cancer occur in this group of women, so breast self-examinations (BSEs), routine physical examinations, and mammograms are essential.

Because cardiovascular disease is the leading cause of death in older women, diet and exercise are important topics of patient education, as is hormone replacement therapy (HRT). HRT may protect women from heart disease and osteoporosis. Currently, long-term clinical trials are underway to evaluate this. Various health options should be discussed with female patients before menopause, that is, during the perimenopause.

Menopause

Menopause is described as the physiologic cessation of menses associated with declining ovarian function, during which reproductive function diminishes and ends. Postmenopause is the period beginning from about 1 year after menses cease and beyond. Menopause is associated with some atrophy of breast tissue and genital organs, loss in bone density, and vascular changes.

Menopause starts gradually and is usually signaled by changes in menstruation. The monthly flow may increase, decrease, become irregular, and finally cease. Often, the interval between periods lasts longer; a lapse of several months between periods is not uncommon.

Changes signaling menopause begin to occur as early as the late 30s when ovulation occurs less frequently, estrogen levels fluctuate, and FSH levels rise in an attempt to stimulate estrogen production.

Clinical Manifestations

Because of the hormonal changes described previously, some women notice irregular menses, breast tenderness, and mood changes long before menopause occurs. The hot or warm flashes and night sweats reported by some women are directly attributable to hormonal changes. Hot flashes, which denote vasomotor instability, may vary in intensity from a barely perceptible warm feeling to a sensation of extreme warmth accompanied by profuse sweating, causing discomfort, sleep disturbances, subsequent fatigue, and embarrassment.

Other physical changes may include possible atrophic changes and decreased bone density (**osteoporosis**), resulting in decreased stature and bone fractures. About 1.2 million new fractures due to osteoporosis occur yearly in the United States. The entire genitourinary system is affected by the reduced estrogen level. Changes in the vulvovaginal area may include a gradual thinning of pubic hair and a slow shrinkage of the labia. Vaginal secretions decrease, and the woman may report dyspareunia (discomfort during intercourse). The vaginal pH rises during menopause, predisposing the woman to bacterial infections (atrophic vaginitis). Discharge, itching, and a sensation of vulvar burning may result.

Psychological Considerations

Women's reactions and feelings related to loss of reproductive capacity may vary. For women with grown families and traditional values, menopause may result in feelings ranging from role confusion to feelings of sexual and personal freedom. Other women may be relieved that the childbearing phase of their lives is over. Different circumstances affect the response of each woman and must be considered on an individual basis. Nurses need to be aware of and sensitive to all possibilities and take their cues from the patient.

Management

As stated earlier, menopause may be characterized by decreased vaginal secretions, hot flashes, changes in the urinary tract, and mood swings. Decreased vaginal lubrication may cause dyspareunia (discomfort during intercourse) in the menopausal woman; it may be prevented by added lubrication with a water-soluble lubricant (eg, K-Y jelly, Replens, Astro-Glide, or contraceptive foam or jelly). Vaginal cream containing estrogen or an estrogen-containing vaginal ring is often prescribed.

Women approaching menopause often have many concerns related to hormone replacement. Many would prefer to be "as natural as possible," whereas others want to begin hormone replacement as soon as possible. Some have concerns based on their family history of heart disease, osteoporosis, or breast cancer. Currently, there is no right or wrong approach. Each woman must be evaluated individually. Her concerns and feelings should be discussed with her primary health care provider so that she can make an informed decision about managing menopausal symptoms.

PHARMACOLOGIC THERAPY

The changes in lipid metabolism that occur during menopause have adverse effects on women, placing them at increased risk for atherosclerosis, angina, coronary artery disease, and osteoporosis. HRT may reduce the risk of these conditions and of myocardial infarction as well. Additionally, HRT reduces or eliminates persistent and severe hot flashes. Preliminary results of the Post-menopausal Estrogen/Progestin Interventions (PEPI) trial reveal that estrogen alone or in combination with a progestin improves lipoproteins and lowers fibrinogen levels. Unopposed estrogen, however, is not recommended for women who have not had a hysterectomy because it is associated with endometrial hyperplasia (Writing Group of the PEPI Trial, 1995). In addition to its role in possible prevention of heart disease, HRT may help prevent osteoporosis, a disease characterized by low bone mass and microarchitectural deterioration of bone tissue leading to enhanced bone fragility and increased risk for fracture. Other factors that increase a women's risk for osteoporosis include a thin body frame, race (white or Asian), family history of osteoporosis, nulliparity, early menopause, moderate to heavy alcohol ingestion, smoking, caffeine use, sedentary lifestyle, and a diet low in calcium. Women should be advised to remain active or to begin an exercise program of weight-bearing activity, such as walking; to take a calcium supplement; to decrease or stop smoking; and to discuss the appropriateness of HRT with their primary health care provider. Current studies are evaluating the effect of hormone replacement on risk for Alzheimer's disease and dementia. The Women's Health Initiative is a large National Institutes of Health study that is following more than 160,000 women for 10 years, evaluating the effects of hormone replacement on heart disease, breast cancer, and osteoporosis.

Many women do not take hormones because of past negative publicity or fear of cancer. Some dislike the possibility of resumption of vaginal bleeding. Economics may also be a factor. Nursing assessment should address methods that women are taking to promote their own health in the perimenopausal period.

The decision to take HRT is often a difficult one, especially because research studies needed for women to make a well-informed decision are still incomplete. Current HRT usually consists of estrogen and progesterone. In the past, however, treatment with estrogen alone increased the incidence of uterine cancer. Adding progestin, a synthetic form of progesterone, to the regimen reduced this risk. Progestins are not prescribed for the woman who has had her uterus removed.

HRT is contraindicated in women with a history of breast cancer, except in some cases when the cancer is not dependent on estrogen and when menopausal symptoms are disruptive.

HRT is also contraindicated in women with a history of vascular thrombosis, active liver disease or chronically impaired liver function, some cases of uterine cancer, and undiagnosed abnormal vaginal bleeding. The risk of thromboembolic phenomena is slightly elevated in women taking HRT, and that risk is highest in the first year of use. Women taking HRT should be taught the signs and symptoms of deep vein thrombosis (DVT) or pulmonary embolism and should be instructed to report their occurrence immediately. Nurses should check for leg redness, tenderness, chest pain, and shortness of breath in patients who take HRT.

Regular follow-up care, including a yearly physical examination and mammogram, is recommended for women taking HRT. An endometrial biopsy is indicated for women with any irregular bleeding during treatment.

There are several different approaches for use of hormone replacement. Some women take both estrogen and progestin daily; others take estrogen for 25 consecutive days each month, with progestin taken in cycles (eg, 10 to 14 days of the month). Progestin is taken to prevent proliferation of the uterine lining and hyperplasia in women who have not had their uterus removed. Estrogen patches, which are replaced once or twice weekly, are another option but require an oral progestin along with them.

Vaginal treatment with estrogen cream or an estradiol vaginal ring (Estring) may be used for vaginal dryness or atrophic vaginitis. An estradiol vaginal ring is a small, flexible ring that slowly releases estrogen vaginally in small doses over 3 months.

Women who take hormones for 25 days often experience bleeding after completion of the progestin. Other women take estrogen and progesterone every day and usually experience no bleeding. They occasionally have irregular spotting, which should be evaluated by their primary health care provider.

Some women feel apprehensive about HRT and the lack of complete data about its long-term effects. These women may benefit from learning about alternatives to HRT (including diet, vitamins, and exercise). However, they need to know that these approaches to menopause have not been examined thoroughly through research.

Selective estrogen receptor modulators (SERMS), such as raloxifene (Evista), also provide an alternative to hormone replacement for the treatment of osteoporosis. These medications may not provide the same amount of heart and bone protection but do not appear to increase the risk for breast cancer. They may increase hot flashes. No long-term studies exist on these medications because of their recent development. Tamoxifen is also in this family of medications. Table 42-4 compares HRT and SERMS.

Nonhormonal medications, including alendronate (Fosamax) and calcitonin, for treatment of osteoporosis have given women another option in avoiding this major health problem. See Chapter 62 for more discussion of osteoporosis.

Vitamin B_6 in doses of less than 200 mg has been found to relieve some distressing symptoms. Vitamin E has been effective in decreasing hot flashes for many women. Some women are interested in alternative treatments (eg, natural estrogens and progestins, black cohosh, ginseng, dong quai, and several other herbal preparations); however, very little scientific data exist about the safety or effectiveness of these remedies. Assessment of menopausal patients should include their use of complementary and alternative therapy and supplements.

BEHAVIORAL STRATEGIES

Regular physical exercise, including weight-bearing exercise, raises the heart rate, increases high-density lipoprotein (HDL) levels, preserves bone content, and helps to maintain bone mass. It may also reduce stress, enhance well-being, and improve self-image. Loss of muscle tissue is mediated by exercise; weight-bearing exercise (eg, walking, jogging, bicycling) at least four times a week is recommended.

NUTRITIONAL THERAPY

Women should also be encouraged to decrease caloric intake, decrease fat, and increase whole grains, fiber, fruit, and vegetables. Women of all ages are urged to include high calcium food in their diets daily. For example, 1cup of milk contains about 300 mg of calcium and 1 cup of nonfat yogurt provides 415 mg of calcium. Other sources of dietary calcium include most green, leafy vegetables, seafood, and calcium-fortified foods.

Calcium supplementation may be helpful in preventing bone loss and the morbidity associated with osteoporosis. Bones serve as a storehouse of the body's calcium, and bone density decreases with age. When calcium levels in the blood are low, the bones give up calcium to maintain homeostasis. Women of all age groups take in less than the recommended amount of calcium. The average calcium intake is 300 to 500 mg/day, whereas the amount recommended is 1300 mg/day for adolescents and young adults; 1000 mg/day for adults 19 to 50 years of age; 1200 mg/day for adults 51 years of age and older, including menopausal women taking HRT; and 1500 mg/day for women who are menopausal and not taking HRT.

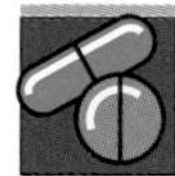

TABLE 42•4 Comparison of the Effects of Hormone Replacement Therapy (HRT) and Selective Estrogen Receptor Modulators (SERMS)

Effect	HRT	SERMS
Bleeding	May be irregular	None
Breast cancer	Risk may increase	Risk may decrease
Uterine cancer	No increase if combined with progesterone	No data No data
Dementia	Possible benefit	No data
Vaginal dryness	Improves	No change
Hot flashes	Prevents	Increases
Cardiovascular disease risk	Probable benefit (studies in process)	No data
Triglycerides	Increases	No effect
HDL cholesterol	Increases	Little change
LDL cholesterol	Reduces	Reduces
Fractures	Reduces	No data but probably no effect
Bone density	Increases	Slight increase, less effect than HRT

Nursing Management

Nurses can encourage women to view menopause as a natural change resulting in freedom from menses and symptoms related to hormonal changes. No relationship exists between menopause and mental health problems; however, social changes that usually coincide with menopause (eg, adolescent or grown children, ill partners, and dependent or ill parents) may produce stress.

Measures should be taken to promote general health. The nurse can explain to the patient that cessation of menses is a physiologic function that is rarely accompanied by nervous symptoms or illness. The current expected life span after menopause for the average woman is 30 to 35 years, which may encompass as many years as the childbearing phase of her life. Menopause is not a complete change of life, however. Normal sexual urges continue, and women retain their usual response to sex long after menopause. Many women enjoy better health after the menopause than before; this is especially true for those who have experienced dysmenorrhea. The individual woman's evaluation of herself and her worth, now and in the future, is likely to affect her emotional reaction to menopause.

Premenstrual Syndrome

Premenstrual syndrome (PMS) is a combination of symptoms that occur before the menses and subside with the onset of menstrual flow (Chart 42-2). This syndrome is experienced by many women before the onset of each menstrual cycle. The cause is unknown, but several theories suggest estrogen excess or progesterone deficit in the **luteal phase** of the menstrual cycle. Another theory holds that unidentified hormones cause symptoms at the time of menstrual changes. Still other theories point to beta-endorphin activity, serotonin deficiency, progesterone withdrawal, fluid retention, elevated prolactin levels, abnormal prostaglandin metabolism, and disturbance of the hypothalamic-pituitary-ovarian axis. Dietary factors may play a role because carbohydrates may affect serotonin.

Clinical Manifestations

Major symptoms include headache, fatigue, low back pain, painful breasts, and a feeling of abdominal fullness. General irritability, mood swings, fear of losing control, binge eating, and crying spells may also occur. Symptoms vary widely from one woman to another and from one cycle to the next in the same person. Great variability is found in the degree of symptoms, and up to 150 symptoms have been described. As many as 40% of women are affected to some degree, but only 2% to 3% are severely affected. Many women are not bothered at all, whereas some experience severe and disabling symptoms.

A generally stressful life and problematic relationships may be related to the intensity of physical symptoms. Some women report moderate to severe life disruption secondary to PMS that negatively affects their interpersonal relationships. PMS may also be a factor in reduced productivity, work-related accidents, and absenteeism.

HOME CARE TEACHING CHECKLIST: THE WOMAN APPROACHING MENOPAUSE

At the completion of the program, the patient or caregiver will able to:	Patient	Caregiver
• Describe menopause as a normal period in a woman's life.	✔	
• State that fatigue and stress may worsen hot flashes.	✔	
• State that a nutritious diet and weight control will enhance physical and emotional well-being.	✔	
• State the importance of exercising for 30 minutes three to four times a week to maintain good health.	✔	
• Describe involvement in outside activities as beneficial in reducing anxiety and tension.	✔	
• Identify the following as changes that often occur in midlife: departure of children, aging, dependence of parents, possible loss of loved ones.	✔	
• Describe this phase of life as having the potential for intellectual growth, personal accomplishment, and initiation of new activities.	✔	
• State the following points about sexual activity:		
• Frequent sexual activity helps to maintain the elasticity of the vagina.	✔	
• Contraception is advised until 1 year passes without menses.	✔	
• Safer sex is important at any age.	✔	
• Sexual functioning may be enhanced at midlife.	✔	
• Identify the importance of an annual physical examination to screen for problems and to promote general health.	✔	
• Identify strategies and methods to prevent or manage the following problems:		
• Itching or burning of vulvar areas: see primary health care provider to rule out dermatologic abnormalities and, if appropriate, to obtain a prescription for a lubricating or hormonal cream.	✔	
• Dyspareunia (painful intercourse): use a water-soluble lubricant, such as K-Y Jelly, Astro-Glide, Replens, hormone cream, or contraceptive foam.	✔	
• Decreased perineal muscle tone and bladder control: practicing Kegel exercises daily (contract the perineal muscles as though stopping urination; hold for 5–10 seconds and release; repeat frequently during the day).	✔	
• Dry skin: use mild emollient skin cream and lotions to prevent dry skin.	✔	
• Weight control: join a weight-reduction support group such as *Weight Watchers* or a similar group if appropriate, or consult a registered dietitian for consultation to counteract the tendency to gain weight, particularly around the hips, thighs, and abdomen.	✔	
• Osteoporosis: observe recommended calcium and vitamin D intake, including calcium supplements, if indicated, to slow the process of osteoporosis.	✔	
• Risk for urinary tract infection (UTI): drink 6 to 8 glasses of water daily and take vitamin C (500 mg) as a possible way to reduce the incidence of UTI related to atrophic changes of the urethra.	✔	
• Vaginal bleeding: report any bleeding after 1 year of no menses to a primary health care provider immediately, no matter how minimal.	✔	

Identifying the time when these symptoms occur helps in determining the diagnosis. Symptoms recur regularly at the same phase of each menstrual cycle, usually 1 week to a few days before menses, and subside once the menstrual flow starts.

Medical Management

With no single treatment or known cure for PMS, women are encouraged to chart their own symptoms, so that they can possibly anticipate and, therefore, cope with them. Exercise is encouraged for all patients. Most researchers agree that caffeine, high-fat foods, and refined sugars should be avoided. Alternative therapies that women have used include vitamins B_6 and E, calcium, magnesium, and oil of evening primrose capsules. No studies have been performed to evaluate the effectiveness of these therapies.

PHARMACOLOGIC THERAPY

Pharmacologic remedies include selective serotonin reuptake inhibitors (eg, Prozac), gonadotropin-releasing hormone agonists, prostaglandin inhibitors (eg, ibuprofen and anaprox), and antianxiety agents (eg, Xanax). Some clinicians prescribe analgesics, diuretics, and natural and synthetic progesterones, although long-term risks of progesterone use are unknown. Many women find over-the-counter carbohydrate products useful; they provide complex carbohydrates along with vitamins and minerals. Ratios of serum levels of tryptophan to other amino acids are elevated in patients who use this aid. It may relieve psychological symptoms and food cravings.

Nursing Management

The nurse should establish rapport with the patient and obtain a health history, noting the time when symptoms began and their nature and intensity. The nurse then determines whether the onset of symptoms occurs before or shortly after the menstrual flow begins. Additionally, the nurse can show the patient how to develop a chart to record the timing and intensity of symptoms. A nutritional history is also elicited to determine if the diet is high in salt, caffeine, or alcohol or low in essential nutrients.

The patient's goals may include reduction of anxiety (mood swings, crying, binge eating, fear of losing control), ability to cope with day-to-day stressors and relationships with family and co-workers, and increased knowledge about PMS with improved use of control measures.

Positive coping measures are facilitated. Partners can be advised to assist by offering support and increased involvement with child care. The patient can try to plan her working time to accommodate the days she will be less productive because of PMS. The

CHART 42•2 Causes, Manifestations, and Treatment of Premenstrual Syndrome

Cause

Unknown; may be related to hormonal changes combined with other factors (diet, stress, and lack of exercise)

Physical Symptoms

- Fluid retention (eg, bloating, breast tenderness)
- Weight gain
- Sleep disturbances
- Migraine headaches with menstruation
- Backache
- Vertigo
- Nausea, vomiting, or diarrhea
- Acne
- Food cravings
- Constipation

Emotional Symptoms

- Irritability, mood changes, emotional lability
- Hostility, depression, anxiety
- Lethargy

Treatment

- Use of social support and family resources
- Nutritious diet consisting of whole grains, fruit, and vegetables; increased water intake
- Decreased intake of caffeine, salt, sweets, and alcohol
- Multivitamins, B complex, and vitamin B_6
- Initiation/maintenance of exercise program
- Stress reduction techniques
- Antidepressants and other antianxiety agents

nurse encourages exercise, meditation, imagery, and creative activities to reduce stress. The nurse also encourages the patient to take medications as prescribed and provides instructions about the desired effects of the medications. Enrolling in a PMS group that meets to discuss problems may help the patient learn that others recognize and understand what she is experiencing.

The nurse assesses the patient for suicidal, uncontrollable, and violent behavior. Any suggestions of suicidal tendencies must be evaluated by psychiatric consultation immediately. Uncontrollable behavior may lead to violence toward family members. If abuse of children or other members of the patient's family is suspected, reporting protocols are implemented and followed. Referral is made for immediate psychiatric or psychological care and counseling.

Dysmenorrhea

Primary dysmenorrhea is painful menstruation, with no identifiable pelvic pathology. It occurs at the time of menarche or shortly thereafter. It is characterized by crampy pain that begins before or shortly after onset of menstrual flow and continues for 48 to 72 hours. Pelvic examination findings are normal. Dysmenorrhea is thought to result from excessive production of prostaglandins, which causes painful contraction of the uterus and arteriolar vasospasm. Psychological factors, such as anxiety and tension, may also contribute to dysmenorrhea. As women grow older, dysmenorrhea often decreases and frequently completely resolves after childbirth.

In secondary dysmenorrhea, pelvic pathology exists, such as endometriosis, tumor, or pelvic inflammatory disease (PID). Patients with secondary dysmenorrhea frequently have pain that occurs several days before menses, with ovulation, and occasionally with intercourse.

Assessment and Diagnostic Findings

A complete pelvic examination is performed to rule out possible abnormalities, such as strictures of the cervix or vagina, an imperforate hymen, or other conditions, such as endometriosis, PID, adenomyosis, and fibroid uterus. A laparoscopy is usually required to identify organic causes.

Management

In *primary dysmenorrhea*, the reason for the discomfort is explained, and the patient is assured that menstruation is a normal function of the reproductive system. If the patient is young and accompanied by her mother, the mother may also need reassurance. Many young women expect to have painful periods if their mothers did. The discomfort of cramps can be treated once anxiety and concern over its cause are dispelled by adequate explanation. Symptoms usually subside with appropriate medication. Aspirin, a mild prostaglandin inhibitor, may be taken at recommended doses every 4 hours. Other useful prostaglandin antagonists include ibuprofen (Motrin), naproxen (Alleve, Anaprox, Naprosyn), and mefenamic acid (Ponstel). If one medication does not provide relief, another may be recommended. Usually, these medications are well tolerated, but some women experience gastrointestinal side effects. Contraindications include allergy, peptic ulcer history, sensitivity to aspirin-like medications, asthma, and pregnancy. Low-dose oral contraceptives provide relief in more than 90% of patients and are indicated in woman with dysmenorrhea who are sexually active but not desirous of pregnancy.

The patient is encouraged to continue her usual activities and to increase physical exercise because exercise provides a neurophysiologic basis for relief. Taking analgesics before cramps start, in anticipation of discomfort, is advised.

Management of *secondary dysmenorrhea* is directed at diagnosis and treatment of the underlying cause (eg, endometriosis or PID). Analgesics used for primary dysmenorrhea may be part of the management of secondary dysmenorrhea due to endometriosis.

Amenorrhea

Amenorrhea (absence of menstrual flow) is a symptom of a variety of disorders and dysfunctions. Primary amenorrhea (delayed menarche) refers to those instances when a young woman older than 16 years of age has not begun to menstruate but otherwise shows evidence of sexual maturation, or when a young woman has neither begun to menstruate nor shows development of secondary sex characteristics by 14 years of age. Amenorrhea may be of considerable concern but is usually due to minor variations in body build, heredity, environment, and physical, mental, and emotional development.

The nurse provides an opportunity for the patient to express her concerns and anxiety about this problem because the patient may feel that she is different from her peers. A complete physical examination, careful health history, and simple laboratory studies help to rule out possible causes, such as physiologic disorders, metabolic or endocrine difficulties, and systemic diseases. Treatment is directed toward correcting any abnormalities.

Secondary amenorrhea (an absence of menses for three cycles or 6 months after a normal menarche) may be caused by pregnancy, tension, emotional upset, or stress. In an adolescent, secondary amenorrhea is usually caused by minor emotional upset related to being away from home, attending college, tension from schoolwork, or interpersonal problems. The second most common cause, however, is pregnancy, so a pregnancy test is almost always indicated.

Secondary nutritional disturbances may also be factors. Obesity can result in anovulation and subsequent amenorrhea. Eating disorders, such as anorexia and bulimia, are characterized by lack of menses because a lack of body fat and caloric intake affects hormonal function. Competitive and serious female athletes typically experience amenorrhea and are frequently placed on HRT to prevent bone loss related to low estrogen levels. On occasion, a pituitary or thyroid dysfunction may cause amenorrhea. These dysfunctions can be treated successfully by treatment of the underlying endocrine disorder. Infrequent periods or oligomenorrhea may be related to thyroid disorders, polycystic ovarian syndrome, or premature ovarian failure. Again, evaluation by a primary health care provider is necessary.

Abnormal Uterine Bleeding

Dysfunctional uterine bleeding is abnormal bleeding that does not have a known organic cause. This can occur at any age but is most common at opposite ends of the reproductive life span. Adolescents account for 20% of these cases as their pituitary-ovarian axis matures. Perimenopausal women account for 50% because of their decreasing ovarian hormone production. The remaining causes are often related to cysts, obesity, or hypothalamic dysfunction. Uterine or vaginal bleeding may be a normal phenomenon (as in menstruation) or may be a manifestation of a major, life-threatening disorder. Vaginal bleeding that is atypical in time or in amount must be evaluated.

Menorrhagia

Menorrhagia is defined as prolonged or excessive bleeding at the time of the regular menstrual flow. In early life, the cause is usually related to endocrine disturbance, whereas in later life, it usually results from inflammatory disturbances, tumors of the uterus, or hormonal imbalance. Emotional disturbances may also affect bleeding.

The nurse encourages a woman with menorrhagia to see her primary health care provider and to describe the amount of bleeding by pad count and saturation (ie, absorbency of perineal pad or tampon and number saturated hourly). Persistent heavy bleeding can result in anemia.

Metrorrhagia

Metrorrhagia, vaginal bleeding between regular menstrual periods, is probably the most significant form of menstrual dysfunction because it may signal cancer, benign tumors of the uterus, or other gynecologic problems. This condition warrants early diagnosis and treatment. Although bleeding between menstrual periods by a woman taking oral contraceptives is usually not serious, irregular bleeding by a woman taking HRT should be evaluated. Menometrorrhagia is heavy vaginal bleeding between and during periods and requires evaluation.

Postmenopausal Bleeding

Bleeding 1 year after menses cease at menopause must be investigated, and a malignant condition must be considered unless proved otherwise. An endometrial biopsy or a D & C is indicated. A vaginal ultrasound is used in postmenopausal bleeding to measure the thickness of the endometrial lining. The uterine lining in postmenopausal women should be thin because of low estrogen levels. A lining that is thicker than 5 mm usually warrants evaluation by endometrial biopsy.

MANAGEMENT OF NORMAL AND ALTERED FEMALE REPRODUCTIVE FUNCTION

Dyspareunia

Dyspareunia, defined as difficult or painful intercourse, is increasing in incidence and can be superficial, deep, primary, or secondary. This problem can be embarrassing for women to discuss because they often believe that it is their problem if their partner is not experiencing any discomfort. Dyspareunia may occur at the beginning, during, or after intercourse and may be related to injury during childbirth, lack of lubrication, a history of incest, endometriosis, pelvic infection, vaginal atrophy with menopause, gastrointestinal disorders, fibroids, urinary tract infection, STDs, or vulvodynia (vulvar pain that affects women of all ages without any discernible physical cause). Because dyspareunia is often due to lack of vaginal lubrication, use of vaginal lubricants can be suggested. Depending on the cause of dyspareunia, antidepressants may be prescribed in selected patients, and surgery to expand or repair the vaginal opening is occasionally needed. Interferon may be used for vulvodynia related to HPV, an STD that has been found to occasionally cause vulvar pain.

Contraception

More than half of the 6 million yearly pregnancies in the United States are unintended. More than 1 million occur in teenagers. The U.S. teen pregnancy rate is twice as high as that in England, Wales, and Canada and more than nine times as high as that in the Netherlands and Japan. Adolescents are more likely to experience higher levels of pregnancy complications and are more prone to have low-birthweight babies. Teen mothers are less likely to obtain a high school diploma and are more likely to live in poverty.

Many women who are sexually active or who are considering becoming sexually active can benefit from learning about contraception. Fewer unwanted pregnancies may reduce the number of abortions, abused children, stressed family units, and consequences of infant mortality and morbidity. It is important that women receive unbiased and nonjudgmental information, understand the benefits and risks of each method, learn about alternatives and how to use them, and receive positive reinforcement and acceptance of their own individual choice.

Nurses involved in helping patients make contraceptive choices need to listen, educate, spend time answering questions, and assist patients in choosing the method they prefer. Methods and prac-

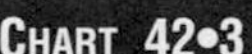
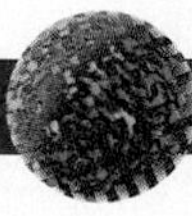

CHART 42•3 Comparison of Sterilization Methods

Vasectomy

Advantages

- Highly effective
- Relieves the female of the contraceptive burden
- Inexpensive in the long run
- Permanent
- Highly acceptable procedure to most clients
- Very safe
- Quickly performed

Disadvantages

- Expensive in the short term
- Serious long-term effects suggested (although currently unproved)
- Permanent (although reversal is possible, it is expensive, requires a highly technical and major surgery, and its results cannot be guaranteed)
- Regret in 5%–10% of patients
- No protection against STDs, including HIV
- Not effective until sperm remaining in the reproductive system are ejaculated

Laparoscopic Tubal Sterilization

Advantages

- Low incidence of complications
- Short recovery
- Leaves small scar
- Quickly performed

Disadvantages

- Permanent
- Reversibility difficult and expensive
- Sterilization procedures technically difficult
- Requires surgeon, operating room (aseptic conditions), trained assistants, medications, surgical equipment
- Expensive at the time performed
- If failure, high probability of ectopic pregnancy
- No protection against STDs, including HIV

tices to prevent unwanted or unplanned pregnancies and births are described in subsequent sections of this chapter.

Abstinence

Abstinence, or celibacy, is the only completely effective means of preventing pregnancy. This may not be a desired or available option for many women because of cultural expectations and their own and their partner's values and sexual needs.

Sterilization

Sterilization by bilateral tubal occlusion or vasectomy is the most effective means of contraception after abstinence. Both procedures must be considered permanent because neither method is easily reversible. Women and men who choose these methods should be certain that they have completed their childbearing, no matter how the circumstances in their life may change. Often, decisions are made that may be regretted at a later point. Some gynecologists suggest a waiting period to ensure that the patient is certain about a potentially irreversible decision.

See Chapter 45 for a discussion of vasectomy (male sterilization).

TUBAL LIGATION

Female sterilization is performed as a same-day surgical procedure. The procedure is carried out by laparoscopy with the patient receiving a general or local anesthetic. The laparoscope, a small periscope-like optical instrument, is inserted through a small umbilical incision. Carbon dioxide is introduced to lift other abdominal organs away from the tubal area. The fallopian tubes are visualized and ligated, thereby disrupting their patency. Despite a 99% effectiveness rate, any woman who has missed a period should still be tested for pregnancy because ectopic and intrauterine pregnancies, although rare, may occur. Ovulatory and menstrual function are not affected by sterilization, although some women report heavier menstrual bleeding and more cramping after tubal ligation. Vasectomy and laparoscopic tubal ligation are compared in Chart 42-3.

Before undergoing tubal ligation, the patient should be informed that an IUD, if present, will be removed. If the patient is taking oral contraceptives, she usually continues up to the time of the procedure. Postoperatively, women may experience some abdominal or shoulder discomfort for a few days, related to the carbon dioxide gas and the manipulation of organs. The woman is instructed to report any of the following: heavy bleeding, fever, and pain that persists or increases. The patient also needs to be informed that for 2 weeks she is to avoid intercourse, strenuous exercise, and lifting. Risks with the procedure are minimal and are more often related to anesthesia than to the surgery itself.

Oral Contraceptives

Oral contraceptive preparations of synthetic estrogen and progesterone block ovarian stimulation by preventing the release of follicle-stimulating hormone (FSH) from the anterior pituitary gland. In the absence of FSH, a follicle does not ripen, and ovulation does not occur. This is the mechanism of action of oral contraceptives. Progestins (synthetic forms of progesterone) suppress the luteinizing-hormone surge, prevent ovulation, and also render the cervical mucus impenetrable to sperm. Synthetic estrogens and progestin, found in the many oral contraceptive variations available, differ in androgenic activity.

BENEFITS AND RISKS

In general, no definite long-term undesirable effects have been observed with prolonged oral contraceptive use. Resumption of normal menses is delayed 2 to 3 months in about 20% of oral contraceptive users. Fetal anomalies do not appear to be a concern, and normal reproductive tract function and fertility are restored after oral contraceptives are discontinued. However, most health care providers recommend that the woman use a barrier contraceptive method for 1 to 2 months after stopping the pill before becoming

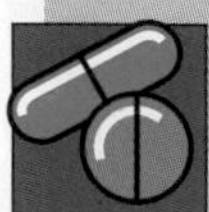

PHARMACOLOGY

Comparison of Oral Contraceptives

There are two kinds of oral contraceptives: *combined* and *progestin only.* The difference lies in the estrogen. The result of both types of medications is a lighter than normal menstrual flow after the contraceptives are taken for 21 days and then stopped for 7 days. The flow is actually withdrawal bleeding from discontinuing hormones because a normal period occurs only with ovulation. Most women using oral contraceptives take the combination medication.

Combined Preparations

- Each dose contains estrogen and progestin.
- Biphasic preparations are available; they contain a constant amount of estrogen with an increase in the progestin on day 10.
- Triphasic preparations are available; they provide varying low doses of estrogen along with progesterone during the 21-day cycle. This variation provides an effective contraceptive that mimics the normal cycle and has enough progesterone to prevent ovulation and spotting.

Progestin-Only "Mini" Preparations

- Each dose contains progestin only (estrogen is not contained in a progestin-only preparation)
- Preparation provides less protection against conception than combined preparations
- About 40% of women taking progestin only have ovulatory cycles.
- Progestin only is useful for women who have had estrogen-related side-effects on combination pills (eg, headaches, hypertension, leg pain, chloasma or skin discoloration, weight gain, or nausea)
- Progestin-only preparations are useful for lactating women who need a hormonal contraceptive method.

pregnant so that the accurate date of the last menstrual period is available to date the pregnancy. Some of the benefits of using oral contraceptives include a reduction in the incidence of benign breast disease, uterine and ovarian cancers, anemia, and pelvic infection.

Nursing Alert *Patients need to be aware that oral contraceptives protect them from pregnancy but not from STDs or HIV infection. In addition, sex with multiple partners or sex without a condom may also result in chlamydial and other infections, including HIV.*

A few patients experience adverse reactions when using oral contraceptives. These include nausea, depression, headache, weight gain, leg cramps, and breast soreness. Usually, these symptoms subside after 3 or 4 months. Because such symptoms are sometimes related to sodium and water retention caused by estrogen, a smaller dose of the hormone or a different hormonal combination, along with salt reduction in the diet, may alleviate the problem. Many patients experience spotting in the first month on the pill or if they take the pill irregularly, so they need to be reassured and advised to take a pill every 24 hours. See the accompanying description of the benefits and risks of oral contraceptive use.

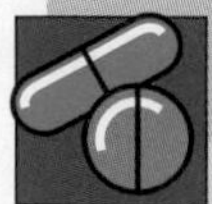

PHARMACOLOGY

Benefits and Risks of Oral Contraceptives

Benefits

- Decreased cramps and bleeding
- Regular bleeding cycle
- Decreased incidence of anemia
- Decrease in acne with some formulations
- Protection from uterine and ovarian cancer
- Decreased incidence of ectopic pregnancy
- Protection from benign breast disease
- Decreased incidence of pelvic infection

Risks

- Rare in healthy women
- Bothersome side effects (eg, breakthrough bleeding, breast tenderness)
- Nausea, weight gain, mood changes
- Small increased risk of developing blood clots, stroke, or heart attack, related more to smoking than to oral contraceptive use alone
- Increased incidence of benign liver tumors
- No protection from STDs (possible increased risk with unsafe sex)

CONTRAINDICATIONS

Absolute contraindications include current or past thromboembolic disorder, cerebrovascular disease, or artery disease; known or suspected breast cancer; known or suspected current or past estrogen-dependent neoplasia; pregnancy; current or past benign or malignant liver tumor; impaired liver function; congenital hyperlipidemia; and undiagnosed abnormal vaginal bleeding.

Relative contraindications include hypertension, bile-induced jaundice, acute phase of mononucleosis, and sickle cell disease. Women older than age 35 years who smoke are at risk for cardiac problems and should not use oral contraceptives. Occasionally, neuro-ocular complications arise, but a cause-and-effect relationship has not been established. If visual disturbances occur, oral contraceptives should be discontinued.

Some gynecologists allow patients with migraine headaches to take oral contraceptives so long as the headaches do not worsen with use or so long as the patient has no neurologic symptoms. (A young woman who has blurred vision with a migraine will probably be discouraged from taking oral contraceptives.) Diabetes is also problematic, although some diabetes specialists allow their patients to use oral contraceptives with careful glucose monitoring. Leiomyomas (fibroid tumors) of the uterus can enlarge with oral contraceptive use. Patients with this condition are advised and monitored carefully, or if fibroids enlarge, they discontinue oral contraceptives and choose other contraceptive methods.

Implant Contraceptive

The Norplant system is a reversible, low-dose, progestin-only contraceptive device consisting of six soft Silastic capsules that are implanted under the skin of the woman's upper arm. The implant releases the progestin levonorgestrel over 5 years, thereby inhibiting ovulation. Contraindications to using this system are

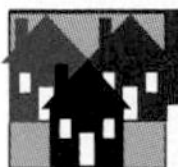

PATIENT EDUCATION AND HOME CARE

Using Oral Contraceptives

- Use condoms to protect against sexually transmitted diseases.
- Take pill at exactly the same time every day.
- Stop smoking or cut down on smoking.
- Report the following symptoms immediately:

  A – abdominal pains
  C – chest pains
  H – headaches
  E – eye problems (blurred vision or spots)
  S – severe leg pains

acute liver disease or liver tumors, pregnancy, unexplained vaginal bleeding, breast cancer, or a history of thrombophlebitis or pulmonary embolism.

Common side effects include irregular bleeding, weight gain, acne, hair growth, and hair loss. If patients are aware of these disadvantages and side effects, they are more likely to tolerate the implant and continue using it. The patient should report headaches or visual symptoms to a health care provider because rare instances of idiopathic intracranial hypertension have been associated with the implant. Papilledema must be ruled out if headaches occur.

Insertion, a minor surgery that is relatively painless, is performed under aseptic conditions in an outpatient setting such as an office or clinic. A small incision is made in the inner upper arm after the patient receives a local anesthetic. The Norplant capsules are inserted within the first 7 days of the menstrual cycle to avoid the possibility of a preexisting pregnancy. The contraceptive effect occurs within 24 hours and lasts for 5 years. Insertion usually takes about 15 minutes. Although the implants can be removed at any time, it can be a more difficult and lengthy procedure because tissue encapsulates the implants. Women who have regular bleeding with a Norplant are at higher risk for pregnancy and should be counseled to have a pregnancy test if the regular bleeding stops.

Depo-Provera

An intramuscular injection of Depo-Provera, a long-acting progestin, every 3 months effectively inhibits ovulation and provides a reliable and convenient contraceptive method. It can be used by lactating women and those with hypertension, liver disease, migraine headaches, heart disease, and hemoglobinopathies. Women who use this method must be prepared for irregular or no bleeding. With continued use, irregular bleeding episodes and spotting decrease, and amenorrhea usually occurs.

Potential disadvantages include irregular or heavy menstrual bleeding, bloating, headaches, hair loss, decreased sex drive, weight loss, or weight gain. In women discontinuing this method, fertility may be delayed; therefore, other methods of contraception may be more appropriate for the woman who wishes to conceive within a year of discontinuing contraception.

Depo-Provera is contraindicated in pregnancy, abnormal vaginal bleeding of unknown cause, breast or pelvic cancer, or sensitivity to synthetic progestin. The long-term effects on the infant of a nursing mother who uses Depo-Provera are unknown but are thought to be negligible; breast cancer and osteoporosis risks are being studied, and the endometrial cancer risk is decreased. Depo-Provera does not protect against STDs.

Intrauterine Device

An IUD is a small plastic device, usually T-shaped, that is inserted into the uterine cavity to prevent pregnancy. A string attached to the IUD is visible and palpable at the cervical os. An IUD prevents conception by causing a local inflammatory reaction, which is toxic to spermatozoa and blastocysts. The IUD does not destroy fertilized eggs, as some people believe.

One type of IUD, the Progestasert, releases progestin and is replaced each year. The progestin may decrease cramping during menses, but patients using this type of IUD have a slightly higher pregnancy rate than those using copper-bearing IUDs. Another available IUD is the Paraguard, a copper-bearing IUD that is effective for 8 years. Copper has an antispermatic effect.

The IUD method is effective over a long time, appears to have no systemic effects, and reduces the possibility of patient error. This reversible method of birth control is as effective as oral contraceptives and more effective than barrier methods.

Disadvantages include possible excessive bleeding, cramps, and backaches and a slight risk of tubal pregnancy, pelvic infection, displacement of the device, and, rarely, perforation of the cervix and uterus. If a pregnancy occurs with an IUD in place, the device is removed immediately to avoid infection. Spontaneous abortion (miscarriage) may occur on removal. An IUD method is not usually used in women who have not had children because the nulliparous uterus may be too small to tolerate it. Women with multiple partners, women with heavy or crampy periods, or those with a history of ectopic pregnancy or pelvic infection are encouraged to use other methods. Some clinicians prescribe antibiotics after inserting an IUD to prevent PID because risk for its occurrence is increased in the first 20 days after IUD insertion. After that, the risk is relatively low. PID is usually manifested by pain, discharge, and bleeding.

Mechanical Barriers

DIAPHRAGM

The diaphragm is an effective contraceptive device, consisting of a round, flexible spring (50 to 90 mm wide) covered with a dome-like latex rubber cup. A spermicidal (contraceptive) jelly or cream is used to coat the concave side of the diaphragm before it is inserted deep into the vagina, covering the cervix. The diaphragm is a spermicide holder; the spermicide inhibits spermatozoa from entering the cervical canal. The diaphragm is not felt by the user or her partner when properly fitted and inserted. Because women vary in size, diaphragms are designed to fit the individual, making it necessary for the woman's diaphragm to be sized and fitted by an experienced clinician. The woman is instructed in using and caring for the device. A return demonstration ensures that the woman can insert the diaphragm correctly and that it covers the cervix.

Each time that the woman uses the diaphragm, she should examine it carefully. By holding it up to a bright light, she can ensure that no pinpoint holes, cracks, or tears have occurred. Spermicidal jelly or cream is applied, and the diaphragm is then positioned to cover the cervix completely. The diaphragm should remain in place at least 6 hours (but no more than 12 hours) after coitus. Additional spermicide is applied if more than 6 hours have passed before intercourse occurs and before each act of intercourse. On removal, the diaphragm is cleansed thoroughly with mild soap and water, rinsed, and dried before it is stored in its original container.

Disadvantages include allergic reactions in those who are sensitive to latex and an increased incidence of urinary tract infections.

Toxic shock syndrome has been reported in some women who have used diaphragms.

CERVICAL CAP

The cervical cap is much smaller (22 to 35 mm) than the diaphragm and covers only the cervix; it is used with a spermicide. If a woman can feel her cervix, she can usually learn to use a cervical cap. The chief advantage is that the cap may be left in place for 2 days.

Although convenient to use, the cervical cap may cause cervical irritation; therefore, before fitting a cap, most clinicians obtain a Pap smear and repeat the smear after 3 months. The cap can stay in place for 48 hours and does not require additional spermicide for repeated acts of intercourse.

FEMALE CONDOM

The female condom was developed to provide women with protection from STDs and HIV as well as pregnancy. The female condom (Reality) consists of a cylinder of polyurethane enclosed at one end by a closed ring that covers the cervix and at the other end by an open ring that covers the perineum (Fig. 42-8). Advantages include some degree of protection from STDs (ie, HPV, herpes simplex virus, and HIV). Disadvantages include the inability to use with some coital positions (ie, standing).

SPERMICIDES

Spermicides are available over the counter as foams, gels, inserts, and on condoms. Spermicides are effective, relatively inexpensive chemical contraceptives when used with condoms. When used alone, spermicide is better than no contraception at all, can be used without a partner's cooperation, and may provide protection from gonorrhea and chlamydia. Burning, a rash, or irritation can develop in either partner and is usually temporary. Changing to another brand often alleviates the problem.

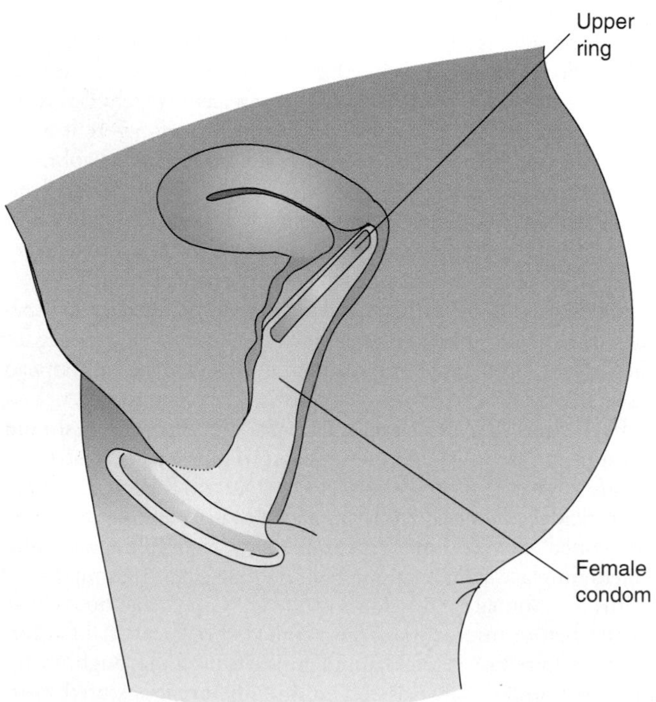

FIGURE 42•8 Female condom. The upper ring keeps the condom in place.

MALE CONDOM

The male condom is an impermeable, snug-fitting cover applied to the erect penis before it enters the vaginal canal. The tip of the condom is pinched while being applied to leave space for ejaculate. If no space is left, ejaculation may cause a tear or hole in the condom and reduce its effectiveness. The penis, with the condom held in place, is removed from the vagina while still erect to prevent the ejaculate from leaking.

The condom is an effective method when used with contraceptive foam. The latex condom also creates a barrier against transmission of STDs, especially gonorrhea, chlamydial infection, and HIV. Natural condoms, however, (those made from animal tissue) do not protect against HIV infection. The nurse needs to reassure women that they have a right to insist on their male partner using a condom and a right to refuse sex without condoms, although women in abusive relationships may increase their risk by doing so. Some women are buying condoms to be certain that one is available. Nurses should be familiar and comfortable with instructions about using a condom because many women need to know about this way of protecting themselves from HIV and other STDs.

During patient teaching about barrier methods of contraception, nurses need to consider the possibility of latex allergy for themselves and their patients. Contact dermatitis is often the first symptom of latex allergy. Swelling and itching can also occur. Possible warning signs include oral itching after blowing up a balloon or eating bananas or fruits with pits (eg, apricots or avocados). Because many contraceptives are made of latex, patients who experience burning or itching while using a latex contraceptive are instructed to see their primary health care provider. Natural condoms (those made from animal tissues) are an alternative. In addition, the female condom is made from polyurethane rather than latex, and a male polyurethane condom (Avanti) is available.

Coitus Interruptus

Coitus interruptus, withdrawing the penis from the vagina before ejaculation, requires careful control by the male and is a frequently used contraceptive method. Some of the uncertainty and unreliability of this method results from the possible presence of sperm in preejaculatory fluid. Many men and women are unaware of this fact and need to be informed that withdrawal is considered an ineffective contraceptive method.

Rhythm and Natural Methods

Natural family planning is any method of conception regulation that is based on awareness of signs and symptoms of fertility during a menstrual cycle. The advantages of natural contraceptive methods include the following: (1) they are not hazardous to a person's health, (2) they are inexpensive, and (3) they are approved by some religions. The disadvantages are that they require discipline by the couple, who must monitor the menstrual cycle and abstain from sex during the fertile phase. The rhythm method of contraception can be difficult to use because it relies on the woman determining her time of ovulation and on avoiding intercourse during the fertile period. The fertile phase (which requires sexual abstinence) is estimated to occur about 14 days before menstruation, although it may occur between the 10th and 17th days. Spermatozoa can fertilize an ovum up to 72 hours after intercourse, and the ovum can be fertilized for 24 hours after leaving the ovary. The pregnancy rate with the rhythm method is about 40% yearly.

According to some researchers, a woman who carefully determines her "safe period," based on a precise recording of menstrual dates for at least 1 year, and who follows a carefully worked out formula may achieve 80% protection. A long abstinence period during each cycle is required. These prerequisites require more time and control than many couples have. Changes in cervical mucus and basal body temperature due to hormonal changes related to ovulation form the scientific basis of this method for the symptothermal method of ovulatory timing.

Courses in natural family planning are offered at many Catholic hospitals and some family planning clinics.

Ovulation detection methods (eg, Ovulindex) are available in most pharmacies. The presence of the enzyme guaiacol peroxidase in cervical mucus signals ovulation 6 days beforehand and also affects mucal viscosity. Test kits are available over the counter and are easy to use and reliable, but they can be expensive. Ovulation prediction kits are more effective for planning conception than for avoiding it.

Emergency Contraception

DOSAGE OF ESTROGEN–PROGESTIN

A properly timed, adequate dosage of estrogen or estrogen and a progestin after intercourse without birth control, or when a method has failed, can prevent pregnancy by inhibiting or delaying ovulation. This method does not interrupt an established pregnancy. Nurses should be aware of this option and the indications for its use. This method obviously is not suitable for long-term contraception because it is not as effective as daily oral contraception or other reliable methods used regularly. but it is valuable in emergency situations such as rape, a defective or torn condom or diaphragm, or other "mishaps" that may occur during intercourse.

Usually, a small dose of oral contraceptives (ie, levonorgestrol and ethinyl estradiol) is given and repeated in 12 hours. This method must be used not more than 72 hours after intercourse. Nausea is a common side effect that can be minimized by taking the medication with meals and with an antiemetic medication. Other side effects, such as breast soreness and irregular bleeding, may occur but are transient. Any patient using this method should be advised of the 1.6% failure rate and counseled about other contraceptive methods. Emergency contraception is related to luteal phase dysfunction, producing an endometrium that is out of phase. There are no known contraindications to the use of this method (Glasier & Baird, 1998).

The nurse reviews instructions for taking pills based on the medication regimen prescribed. If the woman is breastfeeding, a progestin-only formulation is prescribed. To avoid exposing the infant to synthetic hormones through breast milk, she can manually express milk and bottle feed for 24 hours after treatment.

The woman's next menstrual period may begin a few days earlier or a few days later than expected, and she needs to be informed of this. The patient must return for a pregnancy test if she has not had a menstrual period in 3 weeks and should be offered another visit to provide a regular method of contraception if she does not have one currently. This method may also be dispensed by pharmacists without a prescription in some states. See the list of resources at the end of this chapter for more information on this method.

POSTCOITAL INTRAUTERINE DEVICE INSERTION

Postcoital IUD insertion is another form of emergency contraception; it involves insertion of a copper-bearing IUD within 5 days of exposure in women who want this method of contraception; however, it may be inappropriate for some women or if other contraindications exist. The mechanism of action is unknown but is thought to interfere with fertilization. The patient may experience discomfort on insertion and heavier, crampier periods. Contraindications include a confirmed or suspected pregnancy or any contraindication to regular copper IUD use. The patient must be informed that the insertion of an IUD may disrupt a pregnancy that is already present.

NURSING MANAGEMENT

Patients who use emergency contraception may be anxious, embarrassed, and lacking information about birth control. Nurses must be supportive and nonjudgmental and provide accurate information and appropriate patient teaching. If a patient repeatedly uses this method of birth control, she should be informed that the failure rate with this method is higher than with a regularly used method. A toll-free telephone information service (1-888-Not-2-Late) operates 24 hours a day in English and Spanish and provides information and referrals to health care providers.

Abortion

Interruption of pregnancy or expulsion of the product of conception before the fetus is viable is called abortion. The fetus is generally considered to be viable any time after the fifth to sixth month of gestation. The term premature labor is used when a woman experiences labor after this point in the pregnancy.

Spontaneous Abortion

It is estimated that 1 of every 5 to 10 conceptions results in spontaneous abortion. Most of these occur because of an abnormality in the fetus that makes survival impossible. Other causes may include systemic diseases, hormonal imbalance, or anatomic abnormalities. If a pregnant woman experiences bleeding and cramping, a threatened abortion is diagnosed because an actual abortion is usually imminent. Spontaneous abortion occurs most commonly in the second or third month of gestation.

There are various kinds of spontaneous abortion, depending on the nature of the process (threatened, inevitable, incomplete, or complete). In a threatened abortion, the cervix does not dilate. With bed rest and conservative treatment, the abortion may be prevented. If it cannot, an inevitable abortion is imminent. If some—but not all—of the tissue is passed, the abortion is referred to as incomplete. However, if the fetus and all related tissue are spontaneously evacuated, the abortion is complete.

HABITUAL ABORTION

Habitual or recurrent abortion is defined as successive, repeated, spontaneous abortions of unknown cause. As many as 60% of abortions may result from chromosomal anomalies. After two consecutive abortions, patients are referred for genetic counseling and testing, and other conditions that are possible causes are explored. If bleeding occurs in these patients, conservative measures, such as bed rest and administering progesterone to support the endometrium, are tried in an attempt to save the pregnancy. Supportive counseling is crucial in this stressful condition. Bed rest, sexual abstinence, a light diet, and no straining on defecation are recommended in an effort to prevent spontaneous abortion. If infection is suspected, antibiotics may be prescribed.

In the condition known as incompetent or dysfunctional cervix, the cervix dilates painlessly in the second trimester of pregnancy, often resulting in a spontaneous abortion. In such cases, a surgical procedure called the cervical cerclage may be used to prevent the cervix from dilating prematurely. The procedure involves placing a pursestring suture around the cervix at the level of the internal os. Bed rest is usually advised to keep the weight of the uterus off the cervix.

The patient and her health care providers, including those in community health agencies, must be informed that such a suture is in place in this high-risk pregnancy. About 2 to 3 weeks before term or the onset of labor, the suture is cut. Delivery is usually by cesarean section.

MEDICAL MANAGEMENT

After a spontaneous abortion, all tissue passed vaginally is saved for examination. The patient and all personnel caring for her are alerted to save any discharged material. In the rare case of heavy bleeding, the patient may require transfusions and fluid replacement. An estimate of the bleeding volume can be determined by recording the number of perineal pads and the degree of saturation over 24 hours. When an incomplete abortion occurs, oxytocin may be prescribed to cause uterine contractions before dilation and evacuation (D & E) or uterine suctioning.

NURSING MANAGEMENT

Because patients experience loss and anxiety, emotional support and understanding are important aspects of nursing care. The response of the woman who desperately wants a baby is very different from that of the woman who does not want to be pregnant but may be frightened by the possible consequences of an abortion.

The nurse must be aware that the woman having a spontaneous abortion often will experience a grieving period. The grieving may be delayed or unresolved and may cause other problems until the grief reaction has been resolved. The many reasons for a delayed grief reaction include the following: friends may not have known the woman was pregnant; the woman may not have seen the lost fetus and can only imagine the gender, size, and characteristics of the child who never developed; there is usually no burial service; and those who know about the loss (family, friends, caregivers) may encourage denial by rarely talking about the loss or by discouraging the woman from crying.

In any event, providing opportunities for the patient to talk and express her emotions not only helps but also provides clues for the nurse in planning more specific care. Those closest to the woman are encouraged to give emotional support and to allow her to talk and freely express her grief. Unresolved grief may manifest itself in persistent vivid memories of the events surrounding the loss, persistent sadness or anger, and episodes of overwhelming emotion when recalling the loss. Dysfunctional grief may require the assistance of a skilled therapist.

Elective Abortion

A voluntary termination of pregnancy (TOP) is called an elective abortion and is usually performed by skilled health care providers. In 1973, the Supreme Court in Roe v. Wade ruled that decisions about abortion reside with a woman and her physician in the first trimester. During the second trimester, the state may regulate practice in the interest of a woman's health, and during the final weeks of pregnancy may choose to protect the life of the fetus, except when necessary to preserve the life or health of the woman. Legislation has been passed to increase access to clinics and to prevent violence toward those who work in abortion facilities.

The rate of abortion has decreased slightly since 1980. However, it has increased among the following groups of females: unmarried whites under age 15 years, unmarried nonwhites between the ages of 15 and 19 years, and married nonwhites between the ages of 20 and 24 years. The U.S. rates of abortion are among the highest in the industrialized Western world. These numbers point out the need for nurses to provide family planning education and counseling.

Elective abortions may be carried out in many different ways (see Chart 42-4).

MEDICAL MANAGEMENT

Before the procedure is performed, the patient's fears, feelings, and options are explored with her by a nurse or counselor trained in pregnancy counseling. After the patient's choice is identified (ie, continuing pregnancy and parenthood; continuing pregnancy followed by adoption; or terminating pregnancy by abortion), a pelvic examination is performed to determine uterine size. Laboratory studies before an abortion must include a pregnancy test to confirm the pregnancy, the hematocrit value to rule out anemia, an Rh determination, and an STD screen. A patient with anemia may need an iron supplement, and an Rh-negative patient may require RhoGAM to prevent isoimmunization. Before the procedure, all patients should be screened for STDs to prevent introducing pathogens upward through the cervix during the procedure.

NURSING MANAGEMENT

Patient teaching is an important aspect of care for women who elect to terminate a pregnancy. A woman undergoing elective abortion is informed about the procedure, what it entails, and the expected course after the procedure. The patient is scheduled for a follow-up appointment 2 weeks after the procedure and is instructed in recognizing and reporting signs and symptoms of complications (ie, fever, heavy bleeding, or pain).

Available contraceptive methods for postponing or preventing pregnancy are reviewed with the patient at this time. Effectiveness depends on the method used and the extent to which the correct instructions for use are followed by the woman and her partner. The woman who has used any method of birth control should be assessed for her understanding of the method and its potential side effects and her satisfaction with the method. If the patient was not using contraception, the nurse explains all methods, benefits, and risks and assists the patient in making a contraceptive choice after abortion. An increasingly important related teaching issue is the need to use barrier contraceptive devices (ie, condoms) for protection against transmission of STDs and HIV infection.

Psychological support is another important aspect of nursing care. Nurses need to be aware that women terminate pregnancies for many reasons. Some women terminate pregnancies because of severe genetic defects. Infertility patients may elect to undergo selective termination if they become pregnant with multiple fetuses. In pregnancies with multiple gestation, adverse outcomes are directly proportional to the number of fetuses in the uterus. Multifetal reductions are specialized procedures that are stressful and difficult for the parents who are experiencing this situation. Therefore, psychological support and understanding are required. The care of women undergoing termination of pregnancy is stressful, and assistance needs to be provided in a safe and nonjudgmental way. Nurses have the right to refuse to participate in a procedure that is against their religious beliefs but are professionally obligated not to impose their beliefs on their patients.

Nursing Alert *In cases of septic abortion when unskilled attempts are made to end a pregnancy, the methods usually include administering large amounts of various toxic agents (effects are toxic, and the uterus is never fully evacuated) or performing a curettage with the associated risks of uterine rupture, hemorrhage,*

CHART 42•4 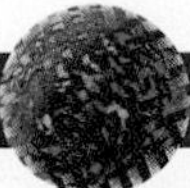 Types of Elective Abortions

Dilation and Evacuation or Suction Curettage

- The cervix is dilated manually with instrumentation or by a laminaria.
- A uterine aspirator is introduced.
- Suction is applied, and tissue is removed from the uterus.

Hypertonic Saline Injection

- A small amount of amniotic fluid is removed and replaced by hypertonic saline solution.
- Osmotic insult occurs, and uterine contractions result in evacuation of the contents of the uterus.
- This method is contraindicated in women with cardiac disease.
- Although rare, serious complications can occur, including cardiovascular collapse, cerebral edema, pulmonary edema, renal failure, and disseminated intravascular coagulopathy (DIC).

Prostaglandins

- Prostaglandins are introduced into amniotic fluid or by vaginal suppository or intramuscular injection in later pregnancy.
- Strong uterine contractions begin within 4 hours and usually result in abortion.
- Gastrointestinal side effects (eg, nausea, vomiting, diarrhea, and abdominal cramping) and fever can occur.

Laminaria

- Laminaria tents are made from a species of seaweed or from synthetic material and are shaped into tampon-like forms with a string on one end.
- When placed in the cervix, the highly hygroscopic tent swells three to five times its original diameter within 4 to 5 hours, causing dilation. Evacuation of the fetus is accomplished by instrumentation.
- Discomfort and slight cramping may occur, and the patient is at risk for low-grade endometritis (inflammation of the endometrium).
- This method requires one visit for insertion of the preparation and a return visit 4 to 6 hours later.
- An alternative agent is Lamicel, a synthetic polyethylene sponge impregnated with magnesium sulfate and compressed into a rod. It works more rapidly than the laminaria tent.

Mifepristone

- Mifepristone (formerly known as RU-486) is a progesterone antagonist that prevents implantation of the ovum.
- Administered orally within 10 days of an expected menstrual period, mifepristone produces a medical abortion in most patients.
- Combined with a prostaglandin suppository, mifepristone causes abortion in up to 95% of patients.
- Prolonged bleeding may occur.

Methotrexate

- Methotrexate has also been used to terminate pregnancy because it is a teratogen that is lethal to the fetus. It has been found to have minimal risk and few side effects in the woman. Its low cost may provide an alternative for some women.

Misoprostol

- Misoprostol is a synthetic prostaglandin analog that produces cervical effacement and uterine contractions.
- Inserted vaginally, misoprostol is effective in terminating a pregnancy in about 75% of cases.
- When combined with methotrexate or RU-486, misoprostol's effectiveness rate is higher than 75%.

Hysterotomy

- A hysterotomy is a miniature cesarean section.
- This surgical procedure is infrequently used as a method for terminating pregnancy.

or infection. If a woman who has had a septic abortion receives proper medical attention early enough and is treated with broad-spectrum antibiotics, the prognosis is excellent. Fluid and blood component replacement may be required before careful attempts are made to evacuate the uterus.

Infertility

Infertility is defined as a couple's inability to achieve pregnancy after 1 year of unprotected intercourse. Primary infertility refers to a couple who has never had a child. Secondary infertility means that at least one conception has occurred but currently the couple cannot achieve a pregnancy. In the United States, infertility is a major medical and social problem affecting 9% to 25% of the reproductive-aged population.

Pathophysiology

Possible causes of infertility include uterine displacement by tumors, congenital anomalies, and inflammation. For an ovum to become fertilized, the vagina, fallopian tubes, cervix, and uterus must be patent, and the mucosal secretions of the cervix must be receptive to sperm. Semen and cervical secretions are alkaline, whereas normal vaginal secretion is acidic. Often, more than one factor may be responsible for the problem. Identifying the possible causes may require the services of a gynecologist, urologist, and endocrinologist.

Assessment and Diagnostic Findings

Careful evaluation includes physical examination, endocrinologic investigation, and consideration of psychosocial factors. Three complete histories (one of each partner and one of the couple), physical examination, and laboratory studies are performed on both partners to rule out such causative factors as previous STDs, anomalies, injuries, tuberculosis, mumps orchitis, impaired sperm production, endometriosis, DES, or antisperm antibodies. Five factors are considered basic to infertility: (1) ovarian, (2) tubal, (3) cervical, (4) uterine, and (5) seminal conditions.

OVARIAN FACTOR

Studies performed to determine if there is regular ovulation and if progestational endometrium is adequate for implantation include a basal body temperature chart for at least four cycles, an endometrial biopsy, and serum progesterone level.

TUBAL FACTOR

Hysterosalpingography is an x-ray study used to rule out uterine or tubal abnormalities. Laparoscopy permits direct visualization of the tubes and other pelvic structures and can assist in identifying conditions that may interfere with fertility (eg, endometriosis).

CERVICAL FACTOR

Cervical mucus can be examined at ovulation and after intercourse to determine whether proper changes occur that promote sperm penetration and survival. A postcoital cervical mucus test (Sims-Huhner test) is performed between 2 and 8 hours after intercourse. Cervical mucus is aspirated with a medicine dropper–like instrument. Aspirated material is placed on a slide and examined under the microscope for the presence and viability of sperm cells.

The woman is instructed not to bathe or douche between coitus and the examination.

UTERINE FACTOR

Fibroids, polyps, and congenital malformations are possible problems in this category. Their presence may be determined by pelvic examination, hysteroscopy, and hysterosalpingography.

SEMINAL FACTOR

After 2 to 3 days of sexual abstinence, a specimen of ejaculate is collected in a clean container, kept warm, and examined within 1 hour for the number of sperm (density), percentage of moving forms, quality of forward movement (forward progression), and morphology (shape and form). From 2 to 6 mL of watery alkaline semen is normal; a normal count is 60 million to 100 million sperm/mL, although the incidence of impregnation is lessened only when the count drops below 20 million sperm/mL. A normal semen analysis should show the following:

- Volume—1.5 to 5 mL
- Density—more than 20 million/mL
- Motility to 60%
- Forward progression to more than 2 (scale, 1 to 4)
- Morphology—more than 60% normal forms
- No sperm clumping, significant red or white blood cells, or thickening of seminal fluid (hyperviscosity)

MISCELLANEOUS FACTORS

Males are also affected by varicoceles, varicose veins around the testicle, which are found in 40% of men evaluated for possible infertility. Retrograde ejaculation or ejaculation into the bladder is assessed by urinalysis after ejaculation.

Blood tests for male partners may include measuring testosterone; FSH and LH (both of which are involved in maintaining testicular function); and prolactin levels and antisperm antibodies (treated with corticosteroids).

Immunologic factors also are being investigated. Some cases of recurrent early pregnancy loss or recurrent natural abortion are the result of an abnormal response by the woman to antigens on fetal or placental tissues. Some women have been treated with infusions of their partner's lymphocytes with some success, but this treatment remains experimental, and the long-term effects are unknown. In a number of cases, no cause of the infertility can be identified.

Medical Management

Infertility is often difficult to treat because it frequently results from a combination of factors. Statistics show that many couples undergoing an infertility evaluation conceive without the cause of infertility coming to light. Likewise, although some couples undergo all tests, the cause of the problem may remain undiscovered. Between these extremes, many problems, both simple and complex, can be discovered and corrected.

Therapy may require surgery to correct a malfunction or anomaly, hormonal supplements, attention to proper timing, and recognition and correction of psychological or emotional factors.

PHARMACOLOGIC THERAPY

Pharmacologically induced ovulation is undertaken when women do not ovulate on their own or ovulate irregularly. Various medications are used, depending on the primary cause of infertility.

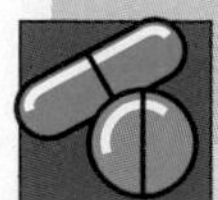

PHARMACOLOGY

Medications That Induce Ovulation

Clomid

Clomid is used when the hypothalamus is not stimulating the pituitary gland to release FSH and LH. This medication stimulates follicles in the ovary. It is usually taken for 5 days beginning on the fifth day of the menstrual cycle. Ovulation should occur 4 to 8 days after the last dose. Patients receive instructions about timing intercourse to facilitate fertilization.

Pergonal

Pergonal, a combination of FSH and LH, is used for women with deficiencies in these hormones. Pergonal stimulates the ovaries, so monitoring by ultrasound and hormone levels is essential because overstimulation may occur.

Metrodin

Metrodin, containing FSH with a small amount of LH, is used in some disorders (ie, polycystic ovarian syndrome) to stimulate follicle growth. Clomid is then used to stimulate ovulation.

Chorionic Gonadotropin

Chorionic gonadotropin is used to stimulate release of the egg from the ovary and may be used in combination with the above medications.

ARTIFICIAL INSEMINATION

Depositing or introducing semen into the female genital tract by artificial means is called artificial insemination. If the sperm cannot penetrate the cervical canal normally, artificial insemination, using the partner's semen (AIH, or artificial insemination with sperm from the husband or partner) may be considered. In azoospermia (lack of sperm in the semen), semen from carefully selected donors may be used (AID, or artificial insemination with sperm from donor).

Indications for using artificial insemination include: (1) the male's inability to deposit semen in the vagina, which may be due to premature ejaculation, pronounced hypospadias (a displaced male urethra), or dyspareunia (painful intercourse experienced by the woman); (2) inability of semen to be transported from the vagina to the uterine cavity, which is usually due to faulty chemical conditions and which may occur with an abnormal cervical discharge; and (3) a single woman's desire to have a child.

Insemination With Partner's Semen. Certain conditions need to be established before semen is transferred to the vagina. The woman must have no abnormalities of the genital system, the tubes must be patent, and ova must be available. In the male, sperm need to be normal in shape, amount, motility, and endurance. The time of ovulation in the woman should be determined as accurately as possible, so that the 2 or 3 days during which fertilization is possible each month can be used. Fertilization seldom occurs from a single insemination. Usually, insemination is attempted between the tenth and seventeenth days of the cycle; three different attempts may be made during one cycle. Semen is collected by masturbation; alternatively, a perforated sheath is worn over the penis during intercourse by couples who object to masturbation. Withdrawal and using condoms for sperm collection are considered unsatisfactory by many infertility specialists because some sperm may be lost or adversely affected.

Insemination With Donor's Semen. When the sperm of the woman's partner is defective or absent or when there is a risk of transmitting a genetic disease, donor sperm may be used. Safeguards are put in place to reduce legal, ethical, emotional, and religious problems. Written consent is obtained to protect all parties involved, including the woman, the donor, and the resulting child.

The donor, selected on the basis of close resemblance to the husband both physically and intellectually, should have no family history of epilepsy, diabetes, or known genetic defects. He should also have negative test results for syphilis and HIV. Preferably, precautions should be taken, so that the donor is not known to the recipient and vice versa.

The woman may have been given Clomid and Pergonal to stimulate ovulation before insemination. Ultrasonographs and blood studies of varying hormone levels are used to pinpoint the best time for insemination. The recipient is placed in the lithotomy position on the examination table, a speculum is inserted, and the vagina and cervix are swabbed with a cotton-tipped applicator to remove any excess secretions. Semen is drawn into a sterile syringe, and a cannula is attached. The semen is then directed to the external os. If this is contraindicated, the semen may be inserted directly into the uterus (intrauterine insemination). In this procedure, the sperm are washed before insertion to remove biochemicals and to select the most active sperm. This is indicated when mucus is inadequate, when antibodies are present, or when sperm count is low. After the careful withdrawal of the syringe, the patient remains in a supine position for 30 minutes.

The success rate for artificial insemination varies. Three to six inseminations may be required over 2 to 4 months. Because artificial insemination is likely to be a stressful and difficult situation for couples, nursing support and strategies to promote coping are crucial.

IN VITRO FERTILIZATION

In vitro fertilization (IVF) involves ovarian stimulation, egg retrieval, fertilization, and embryo transfer. This procedure is accomplished by first stimulating the ovary to produce multiple eggs or ova, usually with medications because pregnancy success rates are greater with more than one early embryo. Many different protocols exist for inducing ovulation with one or more agents. Patients are carefully selected and evaluated, and cycles are carefully monitored by using ultrasound and assessing estradiol levels. At the appropriate time, the ova are recovered by transvaginal ultrasound retrieval. Sperm and eggs are coincubated for up to 36 hours, and the embryos are transferred about 48 hours after retrieval. Implantation should occur in 3 to 5 days.

Gamete intrafallopian transfer (GIFT) is a variation of IVF and is the treatment of choice for patients with ovarian failure. Success rates vary from 20% to 30%. The ovaries are stimulated with gonadotropin derivatives, and follicles are observed with vaginal ultrasound. Once the oocyte is mature, it is retrieved by laparoscopy or transvaginally with ultrasound guidance. The oocyte (unfertilized egg) is removed and drawn into a catheter, where it is mixed with sperm that was obtained shortly before the oocyte retrieval. The most motile fraction of sperm is selected by a washing process. The oocyte and sperm are than inserted into the fallopian tube, where fertilization occurs. The latter method avoids anesthesia. GIFT is the technique of choice for nontubal causes of infertility and for older infertile women.

The most common indications for IVF and GIFT are irreparable tubal damage, endometriosis, immunologic problems, unexplained infertility, inadequate sperm, and exposure to DES.

OTHER REPRODUCTIVE TECHNOLOGIES

Two other techniques that are used in infertility are zygote intrafallopian transfer (ZIFT) and intracytoplasmic sperm injection (ICSI). In ZIFT, an egg is retrieved vaginally, guided by ultrasound while the patient is under light anesthesia. The egg is fertilized in vitro and transferred to the fallopian tube at the pronuclear stage before cell division the following day. At least one functioning fallopian tube is necessary in this procedure. In ICSI, an ovum is retrieved as described previously, and a single sperm is injected through the zona pellucida, through the egg membrane, and into the cytoplasm of the oocyte. The fertilized egg is then transferred back to the donor. These techniques are used when couples have not achieved fertilization in previous IVF cycles or when men have very few motile sperm in their ejaculate. ICSI is the treatment of choice in severe male factor infertility.

Women who cannot produce their own eggs (ie, premature ovarian failure) have the option of using the eggs of a donor after stimulation of the donor's ovaries. The recipient also receives hormones in preparation for these procedures. Couples may also choose this modality if the female partner has a genetic disorder that may be passed on to children.

Nursing Management

Nursing interventions appropriate when working with couples during infertility evaluations include the following: assist in reducing stress in the relationship, encourage cooperation, protect privacy, foster understanding, and refer the couple to appropriate resources when necessary. Because infertility workups are expensive, time-consuming, invasive, stressful, and not always successful, couples need support in working together to deal with this endeavor.

Couples involved in infertility and reproductive technology require education and support to cope with anxiety because these procedures are stressful, time-consuming, and expensive. Resolve, Inc., an organization that provides information and group support for infertile patients, is a nonprofit self-help group originated by a nurse who experienced difficulty conceiving. The literature on infertility that is produced by this group is an important resource for patients and professionals. Most areas across the country have local support groups. More information can be obtained by writing to Resolve, Inc. (see the address at the end of this chapter). A healthy lifestyle (ie, proper diet, regular exercise and stress reduction techniques) may increase the chance of success in treating infertility. Smoking is strongly discouraged because it has an adverse effect on assisted reproduction. These aspects of health maintenance and disease prevention are now being emphasized in many infertility programs.

Ectopic Pregnancy

Ectopic pregnancy occurs in about 1 of 79 to 100 pregnancies. It occurs when a fertilized ovum (a blastocyst) becomes implanted on any tissue other than the uterine lining (eg, the fallopian tube, ovary, abdomen, or cervix; Fig. 42-9). The highest incidence of ectopic implantation occurs in the fallopian tube.

Possible causes include salpingitis, peritubal adhesions (after pelvic infection, endometriosis, appendicitis), structural abnormalities of the fallopian tube (rare and usually related to DES exposure), previous ectopic pregnancy (after one ectopic pregnancy, the risk of recurrence is 7% to 15%), previous tubal

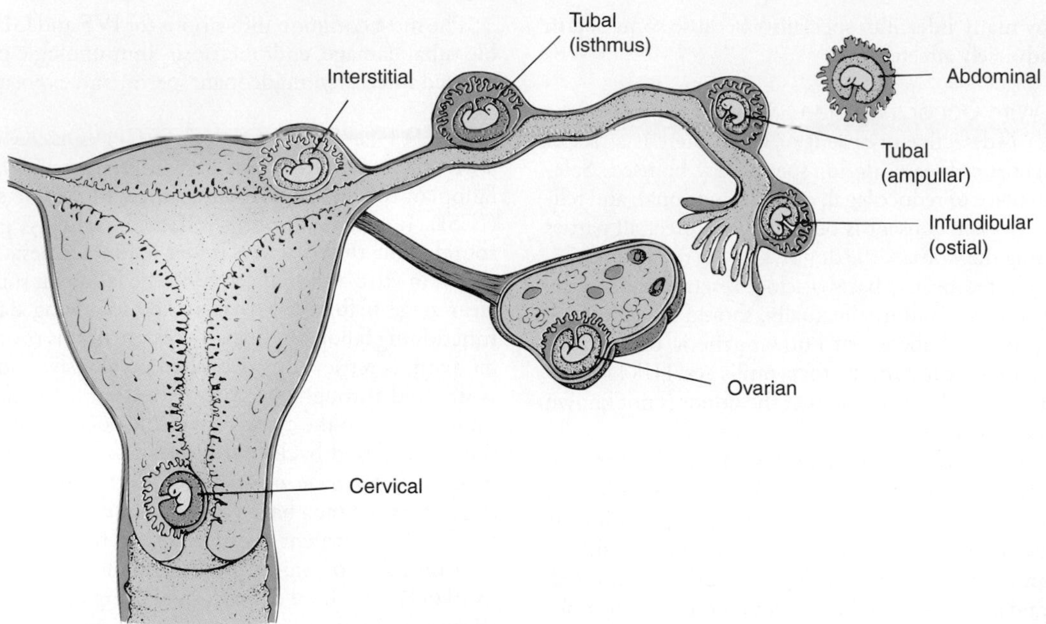

FIGURE 42•9 Sites of ectopic pregnancy.

surgery, multiple previous induced abortions (particularly if followed by infection), tumors that distort the tube, and IUD and progestin-only contraceptives. PID appears to be the major risk factor for ectopic pregnancy. Improved antibiotic therapy for PID usually prevents total tubal closure but may leave a stricture or narrowing, predisposing the woman to ectopic implantation. The odds of recurrent ectopic pregnancy are three times higher if an infectious pathology was the cause of the first one. If a woman has a second ectopic pregnancy, assisted reproduction is considered.

The rate of tubal pregnancies has increased in disproportion to population growth. Ectopic pregnancies are being diagnosed sooner and more often because of advanced diagnostic techniques. Moreover, they are being treated conservatively before emergency rupture and hemorrhage occur. It may be that the increased numbers result from better diagnostic techniques. Conservative treatment makes ectopic pregnancy less life-threatening than previously, but this condition persists as the second leading cause of maternal mortality in the United States.

Clinical Manifestations

Signs and symptoms vary, depending on whether tubal rupture has occurred. Delay in menstruation from 1 to 2 weeks followed by slight bleeding (spotting) or a description of a slightly abnormal period suggests the possibility of an ectopic pregnancy. Symptoms may begin late, with vague soreness on the affected side, probably due to uterine contractions and distention of the tube. Typically, the patient experiences sharp, colicky pain. Most patients experience pelvic or abdominal pain and some spotting or bleeding. Gastrointestinal symptoms, dizziness, or lightheadedness are common. The patient frequently thinks the abnormal bleeding is a menstrual period, especially if a recent period occurred and was normal.

If implantation occurs in the fallopian tube, the tube becomes more and more distended and can rupture if the ectopic pregnancy remains undetected for 4 to 6 weeks or longer after conception. When the tube ruptures, the ovum is discharged into the abdominal cavity.

When tubal rupture occurs, the woman experiences agonizing pain, dizziness, faintness, and nausea and vomiting. These symptoms are related to peritoneal reaction to blood escaping from the tube. Air hunger and symptoms of shock may occur, and the signs of hemorrhage—rapid and thready pulse, decreased blood pressure, subnormal temperature, restlessness, pallor, and sweating—are evident. Later, the pain becomes generalized in the abdomen and radiates to the shoulder and neck because of accumulating intraperitoneal blood that irritates the diaphragm.

Assessment and Diagnostic Findings

During vaginal examination, a large mass of clotted blood that has collected in the pelvis behind the uterus or a tender adnexal mass may be palpable. If an ectopic pregnancy is suspected, the patient is evaluated by sonogram and the beta portion of human chorionic gonadotropin (hCG) levels. If the ultrasound results are inconclusive, the beta-hCG test is repeated to evaluate the rate of rise in the level. The levels of hCG (the diagnostic hormone of pregnancy) double in early normal pregnancies every 3 days, but are reduced in abnormal or ectopic pregnancies. A less than normal increase is cause for suspicion. Urine tests for pregnancy are not helpful in ectopic pregnancies.

Ultrasound can detect a pregnancy between 5 and 6 weeks from the last menstrual period. Detectable fetal heart movement outside the uterus on ultrasound is firm evidence of an ectopic pregnancy. On occasion, an ultrasound study is not definitive, and diagnosis must be made with combined diagnostic aids (hCG level, ultrasound, pelvic examination, and clinical judgment). Ultrasound with Doppler flow studies, in which color indicates perfusion, are helpful.

Occasionally, the clinical picture makes the diagnosis relatively easy. However, when clinical signs and symptoms are questionable, which is often the case, other aids have value. Laparoscopy is used most often because the physician can visually note an unruptured tubal pregnancy and thereby circumvent the risk of its rupture.

Medical Management

SURGICAL MANAGEMENT

When surgery is performed early, almost all patients recover rapidly; if tubal rupture occurs, mortality increases. The type of surgery is determined by the size and extent of local tubal damage. Conservative surgery would include "milking" an ectopic pregnancy from the tube. A resection of the involved fallopian tube with end-to-end anastomosis may be effective. Some surgeons attempt to salvage the tube with a salpingostomy, which involves opening and evacuating the tube and controlling bleeding. More extensive surgery includes removing the tube alone (salpingectomy) or with the ovary (salpingo-oophorectomy). Depending on the amount of blood lost, blood component therapy and treatment of shock may be necessary before and during surgery. Methotrexate, a chemotherapeutic agent and folic acid antagonist, is used after surgery to treat any remaining tissue, as indicated by a persistent or rising beta-hCG level. The beta-hCG study is repeated 2 weeks after surgery to ensure a falling level.

PHARMACOLOGIC THERAPY

Another option is using methotrexate without surgery. Because this medication stops the pregnancy from progressing by interfering with DNA synthesis and the multiplication of cells, it interrupts early, small unruptured tubal pregnancies. Patients must be hemodynamically stable, have no active renal or hepatic disease, have no evidence of thrombocytopenia or leukopenia, and have a very small unruptured tubal pregnancy on ultrasound. The medication is given intramuscularly or intravenously. Leucovorin is usually not needed to reduce side effects. Complete blood count (CBC), blood typing, and tests of renal function are conducted to monitor the patient. The patient is advised to refrain from alcohol, intercourse, and vitamins with folic acid until the pregnancy is resolved because these may exacerbate the adverse side effects of methotrexate. Abdominal pain may occur within 5 to 10 days and may indicate termination of the pregnancy, This requires careful assessment by the health care provider. Serum levels of hCG are monitored carefully, and these levels should gradually decrease. Ultrasonography may also be used for monitoring. Side effects of methotrexate include stomatitis and diarrhea, bone marrow suppression, impaired liver function, dermatitis, and pleuritis.

NURSING PROCESS: THE PATIENT WITH AN ECTOPIC PREGNANCY

Assessment

The health history includes the menstrual pattern and any (even slight) bleeding since the patient's last menstrual period (LMP). The nurse elicits the patient's description of pains and their location. The nurse asks the patient whether any sharp, colicky pains have occurred. Then the nurse notes whether pain radiates to the shoulder and neck, possibly caused by rupture and pressure on the diaphragm.

The nurse monitors vital signs, level of consciousness, and nature and amount of vaginal bleeding. If possible, the nurse assesses how the woman is coping with the loss of a pregnancy.

Diagnosis

Nursing Diagnoses

Based on the assessment data, the patient's major nursing diagnoses may include the following:

- Pain related to the progression of the tubal pregnancy
- Grieving related to the loss of pregnancy and effect on future pregnancies
- Knowledge deficit related to the treatment and effect on future pregnancies

Collaborative Problems/Potential Complications

Based on the assessment data, major complications may include the following:

- Hemorrhage
- Shock

Planning and Goals

The major goals of the patient may include relief of pain; acceptance and resolution of grief and pregnancy loss; increased knowledge about ectopic pregnancy, its treatment, and its outcome; and absence of complications.

Nursing Interventions

Relieving Pain

The abdominal pain associated with ectopic pregnancy may be described as cramping or severe continuous pain. If the patient is to have surgery, preanesthetic medications may provide pain relief. Postoperatively, analgesic agents are administered liberally; this promotes early ambulation and enables the patient to cough and take deep breaths.

Supporting the Grieving Process

Patients' distress levels vary. If the pregnancy is wanted, loss may or may not be expressed verbally by the patient and her partner. The impact may not be fully realized until much later. The nurse should be available to listen and provide support. The patient's partner, if appropriate, should participate in this process. Even if the pregnancy was unplanned, a loss has been experienced, and a grief reaction may follow. Severe and persistent psychological distress may require referral for psychological counseling.

Monitoring and Managing Potential Complications

Potential complications of ectopic pregnancy are hemorrhage and shock. Careful assessment is essential to detect the development of these complications. Continuous monitoring of vital signs, level of consciousness, amount of bleeding, and the patient's intake and output provides information about the possibility of hemorrhage and the need to prepare for intravenous therapy. Bed rest is indicated. Hematocrit, hemoglobin, and blood gas levels are monitored to assess hematologic status and adequacy of tissue perfusion. Significant deviations in these laboratory values are reported immediately, and the patient is prepared for possible surgery. Blood component therapy may be required if blood loss has been rapid and extensive. If hypovolemic shock occurs, the treatment is directed toward reestablishing tissue perfusion and adequate blood volume. See Chapter 14 for a discussion of the intravenous fluids and medications used in treating hypovolemic shock.

Promoting Home and Community-Based Care

TEACHING PATIENTS SELF-CARE

If the patient has experienced life-threatening hemorrhage and shock, these complications must be addressed and treated before in-depth teaching can begin. At this time, the patient's attention is focused on the crisis and not on learning. Therefore, it may be later that the patient begins to ask questions about what has happened and why certain procedures were performed. Procedures are explained in terms that a distressed and apprehensive patient can understand. The patient's partner is included in teaching and explanations when possible. After the patient recovers from postoperative discomforts, it may be more appropriate to address any questions and concerns that the patient and her partner may have, including the effect of this pregnancy on future pregnancies. Patients should be advised that ectopic pregnancies may recur. Reviewing signs and symptoms with the patient and instructing her to report an abnormal menstrual period promptly are important. Patient teaching is based on the needs of the patient and her partner and must take into consideration their distress and grief. The patient is informed about possible complications and instructed to report early signs and symptoms.

CONTINUING CARE

Because of the risk of subsequent ectopic pregnancies, the patient is advised to seek preconception counseling before considering future pregnancies and to seek early prenatal care. Psychological support and counseling may be advisable for women and their partners to assist them to deal with the loss of the pregnancy.

Evaluation

Expected Outcomes

Expected outcomes may include:

1. Experiences relief of pain
   a. Reports a decrease in pain and discomfort
   b. Ambulates as prescribed, performs coughing and deep breathing
2. Begins to accept loss of pregnancy and expresses grief by verbalizing feelings and reactions to loss
3. Verbalizes an understanding of the causes of ectopic pregnancy
4. Experiences no complications
   a. Exhibits no signs of bleeding, hemorrhage, or shock
   b. Has decreased amounts of discharge (on perineal pad)
   c. Has normal skin color and turgor
   d. Exhibits stable vital signs and adequate urine output
   e. Levels of beta-hCG return to normal

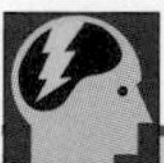

Critical Thinking Exercises

1. A 35-year-old woman is having a complete physical examination for the first time since she was sexually assaulted 4 years ago. She is very apprehensive about pelvic exams. How would you approach the history and physical examination with her?

2. You are a nurse practitioner in a neighborhood clinic. Upon performing a pelvic examination on a 15-year-old, you discover that she is pregnant. Her father, who has brought her for the examination because she has missed two menstrual periods, asks you the results of the examination. How would you respond to the patient's father if he insists that his daughter is not sexually active? How would you discuss the results of the examination with the patient?

3. A 47-year-old woman tells you that she believes she is perimenopausal. She has read a great deal about menopause, its effect on women's health, and the risks associated with hormone replacement therapy. She asks you for your advice and recommendations about measures to maintain health, including the use of hormone therapy. How would you respond to her request? How would you modify your recommendation if she had a strong family history of breast cancer?

4. A 23-year old woman has been admitted to the hospital with possible ectopic pregnancy. What emergency management strategies would you anticipate and which nursing measures would you plan for the patient's hospital stay and long-term recovery? Include the rationale for your decisions.

5. During a checkup at the clinic where you work, a 35-year-old lesbian patient tells you that she has met a new partner and is not concerned about sexual risks of STDs because of her sexual orientation. How would you address the educational needs of this patient?

References and Selected Readings

BOOKS

Allen, K. M., & Phillips, J. M. (1997) *Women's health across the lifespan: A comprehensive perspective.* Philadelphia: Lippincott-Raven.

American College of Obstetricians and Gynecologists. (1996). *Guidelines for women's health care.* Washington, DC: ACOG.

American Medical Association. (1998). *Essential guide to menopause.* New York: Pocket Books.

Committee on Health Care for Underserved Women, American College of Obstetricians and Gynecologists. (1998). Washington, DC.

Cowan, B. D., & Seifer, D. B. (1997). Clinical reproductive medicine. Philadelphia: Lippincott-Raven.

Dickey, R. (1998). *Managing contraceptive pill patients* (12th ed.). Durant, OK: Creative Infomatics.

Hatcher, R., et al. (1998). *Contraceptive technology* (17th ed.). New York: Ardent Media.

Jansen, R. (1997). *Overcoming infertility: A compassionate resource for getting pregnant.* New York: W. H. Freeman.

Johnson, C., Johnson, B., Murray, J., & Apgar, B. (1996). *Women's health care handbook.* Philadelphia: Hanley and Belfus.

Lethbridge, D. J., & Hanna, K. M. (1997). *Promoting effective contraceptive use.* New York: Springer.

Lobo, R. A., et al. (1997). *Mishell's textbook of infertility, contraception, and reproductive endocrinology* (4th ed.). Malden, MA: Blackwell Scientific.

Moore, A., Furniss, K., & Garner, C. (July 1997). *Acute onset menopause: A self study module.* (An educational module provided by AWHONN and NANPRH and published by MPE communications.)

Northrup, C. (1998). *Women's bodies, women's wisdom: Creating physical and emotional health and healing.* New York: Bantam.

Nosek, M. A. et al. (1997). Center for Research on Women with Disabilities. (1997) *National study of women with physical disabilities: Final report.* Houston, TX: Baylor College of Medicine Department of Physical Medicine and Rehabilitation.

Rainsbury, P. A., & Viniker, D. A. (1997). *Practical guide to reproductive medicine.* New York: Parthenon.

Seibel, M. M. (1997). *Infertility: A comprehensive text* (2nd ed.). Stamford, CT: Appleton & Lange.

Sipski, M., & Alexander, C. (Eds.). (1997). *Sexual function in people with disability and chronic illness: A health professional's guide.* Gaithersburg, MD: Aspen.

Stewart, D. E., & Robinson, G. E. (1997). *A clinician's guide to menopause.* Washington, DC: Health Press International.

Strasburger, V. C., & Brown, R. T. (1998). *Adolescent medicine: A practical guide.* Philadelphia: Lippincott-Raven.

Woods, J., & Woods, J. E. (Eds.). (1998). *Loss during pregnancy or in the newborn period: Principles of care with clinical cases and analyses.* Pittman, NJ: Janetti Publishing.

JOURNALS

Asterisks indicate nursing research articles.

General

Alteneder, R., & Hartzell, D. (1997). Addressing couples' sexuality concerns during the childbearing years: Use of the PLISSIT Model. *Journal of Obstetric, Gynecologic, and Neonatal Nursing, 26*(6), 651–659.

Borum, M., et al. (1998). Women's health issues. *Medical Clinics of North America, 82*(2), 189–401.

*Estok, P., & Rudy, E. (1996). The relationship between eating disorders and running in women. *Research in Nursing & Health, 19*(5), 377–387.

Finan, S. (1997). Promoting healthy sexuality: Guidelines for early through older adulthood. *Nurse Practitioner, 22*(12), 54–64.

Foulks, M. (1998). The Papanicolaou smear: Its impact on the promotion of women's health. *Journal of Obstetric, Gynecologic, and Neonatal Nursing, 27*(4), 367–373.

Gibeau, A. (1998). Female genital mutilation: When a cultural practice generates clinical and ethical dilemmas. *Journal of Obstetric, Gynecologic, and Neonatal Nursing, 27*(1), 85–91.

*Golding, J. (1996). Sexual assault history and limitations in physical functioning in two general population samples. *Research in Nursing & Health, 19*(1), 33–44.

Heller, D., Westhoff, J., Gordon, R., & Katz, A. (1996). The relationship between perineal cosmetic talc usage and ovarian talc particle burden. *American Journal of Obstetrics and Gynecology, 174*(5), 1507–1510.

Jones, K., Lehr, S., & Hewell, S. (1997). Dyspareunia: Three case reports. *Journal of Obstetric, Gynecologic, and Neonatal Nursing, 26*(1), 19–23.

Kass, A. B. (1997). Complementary health care in the U.S.: Role of the NP. *Contemporary Nurse Practitioner, 2*(2), 22–30.

*Keller, M., Duerst, B., & Zimmerman, J. (1996). Adolescents' views of sexual decision making. *Image—The Journal of Nursing Scholarship, 28*(2), 125–130.

Muscari, M. E. (1999). Adolescent health: The first gynecologic exam. *American Journal of Nursing, 99*(1), 66–67.

Saunders, C. (1998). The active woman: Special health concerns. *Patient Care, 32*(12), 184–186, 189, 193–195.

Schuster, M., Bell, R., & Kanuse, D. (1996). The sexual practices of adolescent virgins: Genital sexual activities of high school students who have never had vaginal intercourse. *American Journal of Public Health, 86*(11), 1570–1576.

Smith-Bindman, R., et al. (1998). Endovaginal ultrasound to exclude endometrial cancer and other endometrial abnormalities. *Journal of the American Medical Association, 280*(17), 1510–1517.

Sjeldestad, F., Hadgu, A., & Eriksson, N. (1990). Epidemiology of repeat ectopic pregnancy: A population-based cohort study. *Obstetrics and Gynecology, 91*(1), 129–135.

Walker, L., & Tinkle, M. (1996). Toward an integrative science of women's health. *Journal of Obstetric, Gynecologic, and Neonatal Nursing, 25*(5), 379–381.

*Wilbur, J. E., et al.(1998). Women's physical activity patterns: Nursing implications. *Journal of Obstetric, Gynecologic, and Neonatal Nursing, 27*(4), 383–392.

Abortion

*Bryar, S. (1997). One day you're pregnant and one day you're not: Pregnancy interruption for fetal anomalies. *Journal of Obstetric, Gynecologic, and Neonatal Nursing, 26*(5), 559–566.

Evins, G., et al. (1996). Prevalence of domestic violence among women seeking abortion services. *Women's Health Issues, 6*(4), 204–210.

*Hutti, M. (1998). A study of miscarriage: Development and validation of the Perinatal Grief Intensity Scale. *Journal of Obstetric, Gynecologic, and Neonatal Nursing, 27*(5), 547–555.

Assessment of Function and Dysfunction of Female Reproductive Function

Appleby, J. (1995). Management of the abnormal Papanicolaou smear. *Medical Clinics of North America, 72*(2), 345–360.

Stewart, E., & Nowak, R. (1998). New concepts in the treatment of uterine leiomyomas. *Obstetrics and Gynecology, 92*(4), 624–627.

Warner, P. H., Rowe, T., & Whipple, B. (1999). Shedding light on the sexual history. *American Journal of Nursing, 99*(6):34–40.

Wathen, P.I., Henderson, M. C., & Witz, C. A. (1995). Abnormal uterine bleeding. *Medical Clinics of North America, 79*(2), 329–323.

Conception Control

Chez, R., & Chapin, J. (1997). Emergency contraception. *Lifelines, 1*(5), 28–32.

Cockey, C. (1997). Preventing teen pregnancy: It's time to stop kidding around. *Lifelines,* (3), 32–40.

Cody, M. M. (1998). New developments in contraception: What's happening. *Clinical Excellence for Nurse Practitioners, 2*(3), 146.

Glasier, A., & Baird, D. (1998). The effects of self-administering emergency contraception. *New England Journal of Medicine, 339*(1), 1–4.

Grimes, D. (Ed.). (1997). Reproductive health issues for adolescents. *The Contraception Report, 8*(3), 2–16

Grimes, D. (Ed.). (1997). Future barrier methods and microbicides. *The Contraception Report, 8*(1), 2–13.

Haws, J., Butta, P., & Girvin, S. (1997). A comprehensive and efficient process for counseling patients desiring sterilization. *Nurse Practitioner, 22*(6), 52–66.

*Hutchinson, M. (1998). Something to talk about: Sexual risk communication between young women and their partners. *Journal of Obstetric, Gynecologic, and Neonatal Nursing, 27*(2), 127–133.

Kaunitz, A., & Jordan, C. (1997). Two long acting hormonal contraceptive options. *Contemporary Nurse Practitioner, 2*(2), 10–21.

Kjos, S. (1997). Contraception for women at risk: The case for the intrauterine device. *Contemporary Obstetrics and Gynecology, 42*(11), 105–24.

Nokes, K., & Brown, J. (1997). Teaching about the female condom. *Holistic Nurse Practitioner, 11*(2), 1–8.

Reifsnider, E. (1997). On the horizon: New options for contraception. *Journal of Obstetric, Gynecologic, and Neonatal Nursing, 26*(1), 91–100.

Ward-Morgan, K., & Deneris, A. (1997). Emergency contraception: Preventing unintended pregnancy. *Nurse Practitioner, 22*(11), 34–48.

Wysocki, S. (1998). Improving patient success with oral contraceptives: The importance of counseling. *Nurse Practitioner, 23*(4), 51–52, 55–56, 59–60, 62.

Ectopic Pregnancy

Ander, D., & Ward, K. (1997). Medical management of ectopic pregnancy: The role of methotrexate. *Journal of Emergency Medicine, 15*(2), 177–182.

Maiolatesi, C., & Peddicord, K. (1996). Methotrexate for nonsurgical treatment of ectopic pregnancy: Nursing implications. *Journal of Obstetric, Gynecologic, and Neonatal Nursing, 25*(3), 205–208.

Minnick-Smith, K., & Cook, F. (1997). Current treatment options for ectopic pregnancy. *MCN: American Journal of Maternal Child Nursing, 22*(1), 21–25.

Patton, C. M. (1999). Ectopic pregnancy. *Journal of Nursing, 99*(7): 39.

Powell, M., & Spellman, J. (1996). Medical management of the patient with an ectopic pregnancy. *Journal of Perinatal and Neonatal Nursing, 9*(4), 31–43.

Infertility

Greenfeld, D. (1997). Infertility and assisted reproductive technology: the role of the perinatal social worker. *Social Work in Health Care, 24*(3–4), 39–46.

Hoxsey, R., & Rinehart, J. (1997). Infertility and subsequent pregnancy. *Clinics in Perinatology, 24*(2), 321.

Kennedy, H. P. (1998). Enabling conception and pregnancy. *Journal of Nurse Midwifery, 43*(3), 190–207.

Palermo, G., Colomber, L., and Rosenwaks, Z. (1996). ICSI: A new treatment for male factor infertility. *Contemporary Obstetrics and Gynecology,* January, 23–34.

Palermo, G., Cohen, J., Rosenwaks, Z. (1997). Intracytoplasmic sperm injection: A powerful tool to overcome fertilization failure. *Fertility and Sterility, 67*(3), 583–584.

Palermo, G., Colombrero, L., Schattman, G., et al. (1996). Evolution of pregnancies and initial followup of newborns delivered after intracytoplasmic sperm injection. *Journal of the American Medical Association, 276*(23), 1893–1897.

Stotland, N., & Stotland, N. (1997). When your patient demands a baby. Primary care update for OB/GYNs. *4*(5), 175–179.

Tesslelr, S., & Peipert, J. (1997). Perceptions of contraceptive effectiveness and health effects of oral contraception. *Women's Health Issue, 7*(6), 400–406.

Menstruation, Perimenopause, and Menopause

*Aber, C. S., Arathuzik, D., & Righter, A. R. (1998). Women's perceptions and concerns about menopause. *Clinical Excellence for Nurse Practitioners, 2*(4), 232–238.

Chez, R., & Jonas, W. (1997). Complementary and alternative medicine: Part II, clinical studies in gynecology. *Obstetrical and Gynecological Survey, 52*(11), 709–716.

Colditz, G. A., et al. (1995). The use of estrogens and progestins and the risk of breast cancer in postmenopausal women. *New England Journal of Medicine, 332*(24), 1589–1593.

Diesner, J. (1998). A review of estrogen replacement therapy use in the prevention and treatment of Alzheimer disease. *Primary Care Update for OB/GYNs, 5*(1), 50–53.

Fogel, C. (1997). Endocrine causes of amenorrhea. *Lippincott's Primary Care Practice, 1*(5), 507–18.

Goss, G. L. (1998). Osteoporosis in women. *Nursing Clinics of North America, 33*(4), 573–582.

Hooker, R. (1998). Management of established osteoporosis. *Primary Care Practice, 2*(1), 32–37.

Kaplan, H., & Abisla, M. (1997). In transition: Empowering your menopausal patients. *Advance for Nurse Practitioners, 5*(6), 28–33.

Katz, T. (1997). Homeopathic treatment during the menopause. *Complementary Therapy in Nurse Midwifery, 3*(2), 46–50.

Kwandala, S. (1998). Primary care of the perimenopausal woman. *Primary Care Update for OB/GYNs, 5*(1), 43–49.

McGee, C. (1997). Secondary amenorrhea leading to osteoporosis: Incidence and prevention. *Nurse Practitioner, 22*(5), 38–64.

MacPherson, K. (1997). Menopause on the Internet: Building knowledge and community on line. *Advances in Nursing Science, 20*(1), 66–78.

Mehring, P. (1997). Dysfunctional uterine bleeding. *Advances for Nurse Practitioners, 5*(11), 27–32.

Norman, D. (1997). Variations on Traditional HRT. *Advances for Nurse Practitioners, 5*(11), 34–37.

Norwitz, E. (1997). Managing the menopause without estrogen. *Female Patient, 22*(2), 62

*Perez, J. M. (1997). Development of the Menopause Symptom List: A factor analytic study of menopause associated symptoms. *Women & Health, 25*(1), 53–69.

Peters, S. (1998). Menopause: A new era. *Advances for Nurse Practitioners, 6*(7), 61–64.

Rabin, D. (1998). Understanding why women won't take HRT. *Contemporary Obstetrics and Gynecology, 43*(1), 133–141.

*Rothert, L., et al.(1997). An educational interview as decision support for menopausal women. *Research in Nursing & Health, 20*(5), 337–387.

Rousseau, M. (1997). Dietary prevention of osteoporosis. *1*(3), 307–319.

Scura, K., & Whipple, B. (1997). How to provide better care for the postmenopausal woman. *American Journal of Nursing, 97*(4), 36–43.

Smith, A., & Hughes, P. L. (1998). The estrogen dilemma. *American Journal of Nursing, 98*(4), 17–20.

*Woods, N., Lentz, M., Mitchell, E. J., Heitkemper, M., & Shaver, J. (1997). PMS after 40: Persistence of a stress related symptom pattern. *Research in Nursing & Health, 20*(4), 329–340.

*Woods, N., & Mitchell, E. (1997). Pathways to depressed mood for midlife women: Observations from the Seattle Midlife health study. *Research in Nursing & Health, 20*(2), XX. 3

Writing Group of the PEPI Trial. (1995). Effects of estrogen or estrogen/progestin regimens on heart disease risk factors in postmenopausal women. *Journal of the American Medical Association, 273*(3), 199–207.

Premenstrual Syndrome

Morse, G. (1997). Effect of positive reframing and social support on perception of perimenstrual changes among women with premenstrual syndrome. *Health Care for Women International, 18*(2), 175–193.

Peters, S. (1997). The puzzle of premenstrual syndrome. *Advances for Nurse Practitioners, 5*(10), 41–79.

Ransom, S., et al. (1998). Premenstrual syndrome: Systematic diagnosis and individualized therapy. *Physician SportsMedicine, 26*(4), 35–40, 43, 104.

Sayegh, R., et al. (1995). The effect of a carbohydrate-rich beverage on mood, appetite, and cognitive function in women with premenstrual syndrome. *Obstetrics and Gynecology, 86*(4 Pt 1), 520–528.

Ugarizza, D., et al. (1998). Premenstrual syndrome: Diagnosis and intervention (consumer/patient teaching materials). *Nurse Practitioner, 23*(9), 40, 45, 49–50.

Violence, Physical and Sexual Assault

Burgess, A., & Fawcett, J. (1996). The comprehensive sexual assault assessment tool. *Nurse Practitioner, 21*(4), 66–76.

Clark, S., & Gioro, S. (1998). Nurses, indirect trauma and prevention. *Image—The Journal of Nursing Scholarship, 30*(1), 85–87.

Curry, M., Perin, N. & Wall, E. (1998). Effects of abuse on maternal complications and birth weight in adult and adolescent women. *Obstetrics and Gynecology, 92*(4), 530–534.

Davison, J. (1997). Domestic violence: The nursing response. *Professional Nurse, 12*(9), 632–634.

*Dickson, F., & Tutty, L. M. (1996). The role of public health nurses in responding to abused women. *Public Health Nursing, 13*(4), 263–268.

Erickson, R. A., & Hart, S. J. (1998). Domestic violence: Legal, practice, and educational issues. *MedSurg Nursing, 7*(3), 142–147, 164.

Hawkins, J. (1998). Domestic violence: Do we care enough? *Clinical Excellence for Nurse Practitioners, 2*(3), 131–132.

Lathrop, A. (1998). Pregnancy resulting from rape. *Journal of Obstetric, Gynecologic, and Neonatal Nursing, 27*(1), 25–32.

*McFarlane, J., Parker, J. B., Soeken, K., Silva, C., & Reel, S. (1998). Safety behaviors of abused women after an intervention during pregnancy. *Journal of Obstetric, Gynecologic, and Neonatal Nursing, 27*(1), 64–69.

McGrath, M., Hogan., J., & Peipert, J. (1998). A prevalence survey of abuse and screening for abuse in urgent care patients. *Obstetrics and Gynecology, 91*(4), 511–514.

Nieves-Khouw, F. (1997). Recognizing victims of physical and sexual abuse. *Critical Care Nursing Clinics of North America, 9*(2), 141–148.

Rickert, V., & Wiemann, C. (1998). Date rape: Office based solutions. *Contemporary Obstetrics and Gynecology, 43*(3), 133–152.

Shea, C. A., Mahoney, M., & Lacey, J. M. (1997). Breaking through the barriers to domestic violence intervention. *American Journal of Nursing, 97*(6), 26–34.

Resources

American College of Obstetricians and Gynecologists (ACOG), 409 12th St. SW, P.O. Box 96920, Washington, DC 20090-6920; www.acog.org

Association of Women's Health, Obstetrical and Neonatal Nurses-AWHONN (formerly NAACOG), 2000 L Street NW, Suite 740, Washington, DC 20036; www.awhonn.org

Department of Adolescent Health, American Medical Association, 515 North State St., Chicago, IL 60610; Adolescent Health on Line at http://www.ama-assn.org

D.E.S. Action, Long Island Jewish Medical Center, New Hyde Park, NY 11040; www.lij.edu/lij homepage ns.htmL.

Emergency Contraception; 1-888-Not-2-Late; http://opr.princeton.edu/ec

National Coalition Against Domestic Violence, P.O. Box 18749, Denver, CO 80218-0749

National Association of Nurse Practitioners in Reproductive Health (NANPRH), 1090 Vermont Ave., Washington, DC 20005; www.nurse.org/nanprh

Nursing Network on Violence Against Women, c/o Dan Sheridan, 14980 SW 103rd Ave., Tigard, OR 97224

Planned Parenthood Federation of America, 810 Seventh Ave., New York, NY 10019; 1-212-541-7800; www.plannedparenthood.org

Resolve National Headquarters, 5 Water St., Arlington, MA 02174; www.resolve.org

Serono Symposia (Clinical information on infertility), 100 Longwater Circle, Norwell, MA 02061; www.springer-NY.com/serosym/serono.htm

Sexuality Information and Education Council of the United States, 130 W. 42nd Street, Suite 350, New York, NY 10036; 1-212-819-9770; www.siecus.org

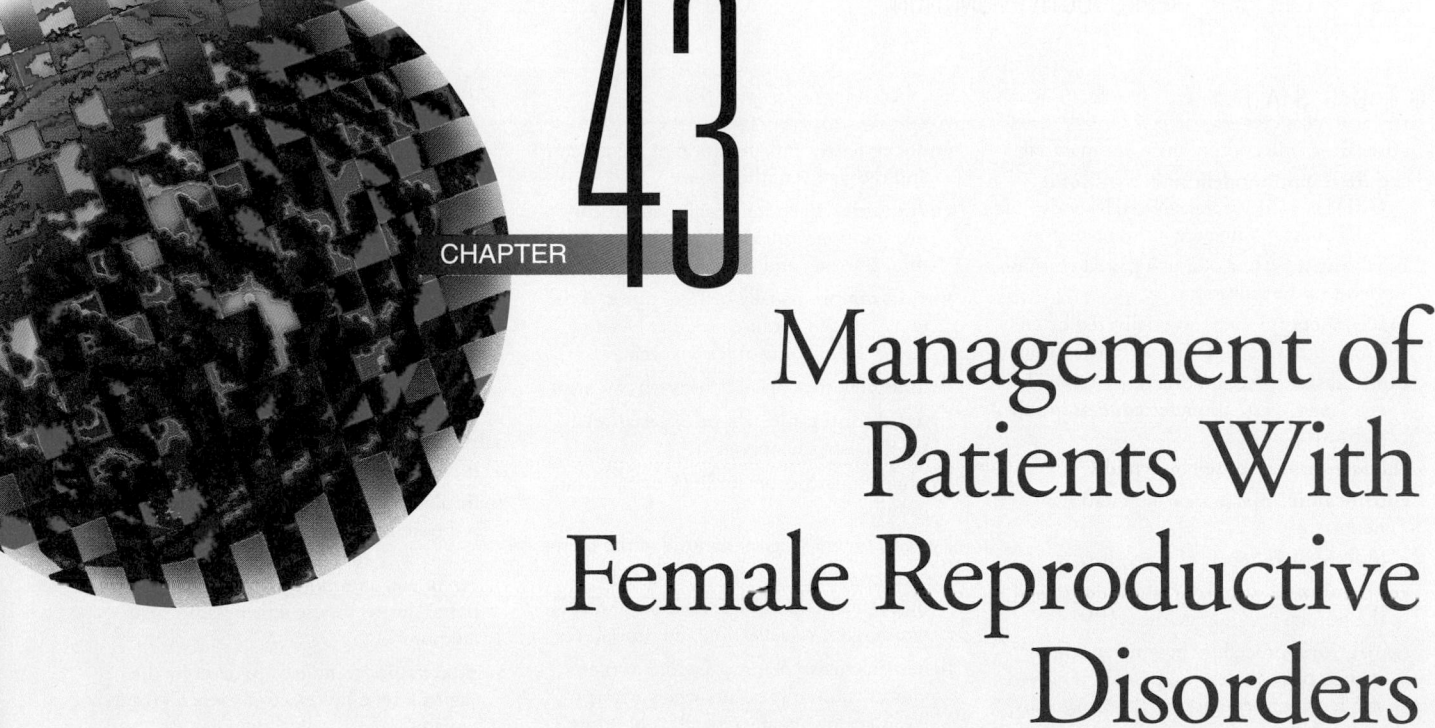

Management of Patients With Female Reproductive Disorders

Learning Objectives

On completion of this chapter, the learner will be able to:

1. Compare the various types of vaginal infections and the risk factors associated with each.
2. Develop an educational program for the patient with a vaginal infection.
3. Use the nursing process as a framework for care of the patient with a vulvovaginal infection.
4. Use the nursing process as a framework for care of the patient with genital herpes.
5. Describe nursing implications for preventing and managing toxic shock syndrome and the rationale for each intervention.
6. Use the nursing process as a framework for caring for the patient with toxic shock syndrome.
7. Discuss the signs and symptoms, management, and nursing care implications of malignant disorders of the female reproductive tract.
8. Use the nursing process as a framework for care of the patient undergoing hysterectomy.
9. Describe indications for a wide excision of the vulva, or vulvectomy, and the preoperative and postoperative nursing interventions.
10. Compare nursing interventions indicated for the patient undergoing radiation therapy and chemotherapy for cancer of the female reproductive tract.

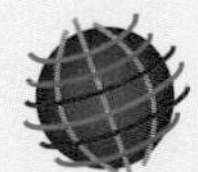

Disorders of the female reproductive system are common. Some disorders are self-limited and cause only minor inconvenience to women; others are life-threatening and require immediate attention and long-term therapy. Many disorders are managed by the patient at home, whereas others require hospitalization and surgical interventions. All disorders require understanding and skill in patient teaching on the part of the nurse. The nurse must also be sensitive to women's concerns and their possible lack of comfort in discussing and dealing with these disorders.

GLOSSARY

abscess: a collection of purulent material

acquired immunodeficiency syndrome (AIDS): a disease transmitted by body fluids that results in impaired immune response

Bartholin's cyst: a cyst in a paired vestibular gland in the vulva

brachytherapy: radiation delivered by an internal device placed close to the tumor

candidiasis: infection caused by *Candida* species or yeast; also referred to as monilial vaginitis

chancre: lesion caused by syphilis

choriocarcinoma: a type of gestational neoplasm

colporrhaphy: repair of the vagina

condylomata: warty growths indicative of the human papillomavirus (HPV)

conization: procedure in which a cone-shaped piece of cervical tissue is removed as a result of detection of abnormal cells; also called cone biopsy; a colposcopically directed biopsy

cryotherapy: destruction of tissue by freezing (eg, with liquid nitrogen)

cystocele: bulging of the bladder into the vagina

dermoid cyst: ovarian tumor of undefined origin that consists of undifferentiated embryonal cells

Doderlein's bacilli: one component of normal vaginal flora

douche: rinsing the vaginal canal with fluid

dysplasia: term related to abnormal cell changes found on Pap smear reports

endocervicitis: inflammation of the mucosa and the glands of the cervix

endometriosis: endometrial tissue in abnormal locations; causes pain with menstruation, scarring, and possible infertility

fibroid tumor: usually benign tumor of the uterus that may cause irregular bleeding, also called myoma or leiomyoma

fistula: abnormal opening between two organs

hydatidiform mole: a type of gestational trophoblastic neoplasm

hyphae: microscopic findings that indicate monilia

hysterectomy: surgical removal of the uterus

laparoscope: surgical device inserted through a periumbilical incision to facilitate surgical visualization and procedures

lichen sclerosis: benign disorder of the vulva that usually occurs when estrogen levels are low; characterized by bleeding and itching

liposomal therapy: chemotherapy delivered in a liposome, a nontoxic drug carrier

loop electrocautery excision procedure (LEEP): procedure in which laser energy is used to remove a portion of cervical tissue after abnormal biopsy findings

mucopurulent cervicitis (MCP): inflammation of the cervix with exudate; almost always related to a chlamydial infection

oophorectomy: surgical removal of an ovary

pelvic exenteration: major surgical procedure in which pelvic organs are removed

pelvic inflammatory disease (PID): infection of uterus and fallopian tubes, usually from a sexually transmitted disease

perineorrhaphy: surgical repair of perineal lacerations

rectocele: bulging of the rectum into the vagina

salpingo-oophorectomy: removal of the ovary and its fallopian tube (removal of the fallopian tube alone is a salpingectomy)

salpingitis: inflammation of the fallopian tube

toxic shock syndrome (TSS): an infrequent but potentially life-threatening infection caused by a toxin produced by *Staphylococcus aureus;* commonly associated with, but not exclusive to, use of superabsorbent tampons

vaginal vault: term used to describe the vagina after a hysterectomy when no cervix remains

vaginitis: inflammation of the vagina, usually secondary to infection

vestibulitis: inflammation causing pain with intercourse or dyspareunia

vulvar dystrophy: thickening or lesions of the vulva; usually causes itching and requires biopsy to exclude malignancy

vulvectomy: removal of the tissue of the vulva

vulvitis: inflammation of the vulva, usually secondary to infection or irritation

vulvodynia: painful condition that affects the vulva

INFECTIOUS DISORDERS

The vaginal area of the female reproductive system is protected against infection by its normally low pH (3.5 to 4.5), which is maintained by the actions of **Doderlein's bacilli** (a part of the normal vaginal flora) and the hormone estrogen. The risk of infection rises if a woman's resistance is reduced by stress or illness, if the pH is altered, or if a pathogen is introduced.

Vulvovaginal Infections

Vulvovaginal infections are common problems, and nurses have an important role in providing information that may prevent their occurrence. To prevent these infections, women need to understand their own anatomy and vulvovaginal hygienic measures. In addition, continued research into causes and treatments is needed, along with better ways to encourage growth of Doderlein's bacillus.

The epithelium of the vagina is highly responsive to estrogen, which induces glycogen formation. The subsequent breakdown of glycogen into lactic acid produces a low vaginal pH. When estrogen decreases during lactation and menopause, glycogen also decreases. With reduced glycogen formation, infections may occur. In addition, as estrogen production ceases during the perimenopausal and postmenopausal periods, the vagina and labia may atrophy (thin), making the vaginal area more susceptible to infection. When patients are treated with antibiotics, the normal vaginal flora are reduced. This results in altered pH and growth of organisms. Other potential factors that may initiate infections include sexual intercourse with an infected partner and wearing tight, nonabsorbent, and heat-retaining clothing.

Vulvitis, Vulvodynia, and Nonspecific Vaginitis

Vulvitis (inflammation of the vulva) may occur with other disorders, such as diabetes, dermatologic problems, poor hygiene, or sexually transmitted diseases (STDs), or it may be secondary to a specific vaginitis.

Vulvodynia, or intense burning and inflammation of the vulva, is a puzzling disorder that typically disrupts the lives of the women who are affected. It may be related to a high level of calcium oxalate crystals in the urine. With proper diet, symptoms may abate. This condition can coexist with chronic interstitial cystitis, an irritation of the bladder. Treatment with tricyclic antidepressants has been effective for some patients with this disorder.

Vaginitis (inflammation of the vagina) occurs when *Candida* or *Trichomonas* species or other bacteria invade the vagina. The

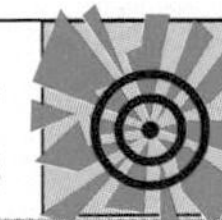

Risk Factors for VULVOVAGINAL INFECTIONS

Premenarche
Pregnancy
Perimenopause
Poor personal hygiene
Tight undergarments
Synthetic clothing
Frequent douching
Allergies
Oral contraceptives
Broad-spectrum antibiotics
Diabetes mellitus
Low estrogen levels
Intercourse with infected partner
Oral–genital contact (yeast can inhabit the mouth and intestinal tract)
HIV infection

normal white vaginal discharge, which may occur in slight amounts during ovulation or just before the onset of menstruation, becomes more profuse when vaginitis occurs. Urethritis may accompany vaginitis because of the proximity of the urethra to the vagina. Discharge that occurs with vaginitis may produce itching, odor, redness, burning, or edema, which may be aggravated by voiding and defecation. After the causative organism has been identified, appropriate treatment (discussed later) is prescribed. This may include oral medication or local medication that may be dispensed into the vagina from a tube with an applicator. Hydrocortisone ointment or cream may be applied externally, as prescribed, for symptomatic relief of itching or perineal irritation.

Candidiasis

Vulvovaginal **candidiasis** is a fungal or yeast infection caused by strains of *Candida* (Table 43-1). *Candida albicans* accounts for most cases, but other strains, such as *Candida glabrata*, may also be implicated. This organism is a normal inhabitant of the mouth, throat, large intestine, and vagina; it propagates in areas that are warm and moist, such as mucous membranes and tissue folds. This condition occurs in some patients who have been receiving antibiotic therapy. These medications decrease bacteria, thereby altering natural protective organisms usually present in the vagina. Clinical infection may occur during pregnancy, with a systemic condition such as diabetes mellitus or human immunodeficiency virus (HIV) infection, or in a patient taking corticosteroids or oral contraceptives.

Clinical Manifestations

Clinical manifestations include a vaginal discharge that causes pruritus (itching) and possible irritation. The discharge may be watery, or thick and tenacious with white, cottage cheese–like particles. A burning sensation, which may follow urination, may result from excoriation from scratching. Symptoms are usually more severe just before menstruation and are usually less responsive to treatment during pregnancy. Diagnosis is made by microscopic identification of spores and **hyphae** on a glass slide prepared from a discharge specimen mixed with potassium hydroxide.

Medical Management

The goal of management is to eliminate symptoms. Treatments include antifungal agents, such as miconazole (Monistat), nystatin (Mycostatin), clotrimazole (Gyne-Lotrimin), and terconazole (Terazol) cream. These agents are inserted into the vagina with an applicator at bedtime and may be applied to the vulvar area for pruritus. There are 1-night, 3-night, or 7-night treatment courses available. Oral medication is also available (fluconazole [Diflucan]). Fluconazole is given in a one-pill dose; relief should be noted within 3 days.

Vaginal creams are available without a prescription; however, patients are cautioned to use these creams only if they are certain that they have a yeast or monilial infection. Many patients use these remedies for problems other than yeast infections. If the patient is uncertain about the cause of her symptoms or has not obtained relief after using these creams, she is instructed to seek health care promptly.

Bacterial Vaginosis

Bacterial vaginosis is caused by an overgrowth of bacteria normally found in the vagina (see Table 43-1). It is characterized by an odor that patients describe as fishlike and particularly noticeable after sexual intercourse or during menstruation as a result of a rise in the vaginal pH. It is usually accompanied by a heavier-than-normal discharge.

Bacterial vaginosis can occur throughout the menstrual cycle and does not produce any local discomfort or pain. More than half of women with bacterial vaginosis do not notice any symptoms. Discharge, if noticed, is gray to yellowish white. The fishlike odor can be detected readily by adding a drop of potassium hydroxide to a glass slide with a sample of vaginal discharge, which releases amines. Under the microscope, vaginal cells are coated with bacteria and are described as "clue cells." The pH of the discharge is usually above 4.7 because of the amines that result from enzymes from anaerobes. Lactobacilli, a natural host defense, are usually absent. Bacterial vaginosis is usually not a serious condition, but it has been associated with premature labor, endometritis, and recurrent urinary tract infection.

Medical Management

Metronidazole, administered orally twice a day for 1 week, is effective; a vaginal gel is also available. Clindamycin (Cleocin) vaginal cream is equally effective. If the infection recurs, some practitioners treat the woman's sexual partner.

Trichomoniasis

Trichomonas vaginalis is a flagellated protozoan that causes a common, usually sexually transmitted vaginitis. It may be transmitted by an asymptomatic carrier who harbors the organism in the urogenital tract (see Table 43-1).

Clinical Manifestations

Clinical manifestations include a vaginal discharge that is thin (sometimes frothy), yellow to yellow-brown, malodorous, and very irritating. An accompanying vulvitis may result, with intense vulvovaginal burning and itching. Diagnosis is made by microscopic detection of the pear-shaped, mobile, flagellate organisms. Inspection with a speculum often reveals vaginal and cervical erythema (redness) with multiple small petechiae ("strawberry spots").

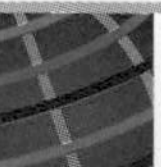

TABLE 43•1 **Vaginal Infections**

Infection	Cause	Clinical Manifestations	Management Strategies
Candidiasis	*Candida albicans, glabrata,* or *tropicalis*	Inflammation of vaginal epithelium, producing itching, reddish irritation White, cheeselike discharge clinging to epithelium	Eradicate the fungus by administering an antifungal agent. Frequently used brand names of vaginal creams and suppositories are Monistat, Femstat, Terazol, and Gyne-Lotrimin. Review other causative factors (ie, antibiotic therapy, nylon underwear, tight clothing, pregnancy, oral contraceptives). Assess for diabetes and HIV infection in patients with recurrent monilia.
Gardnerella-associated bacterial vaginosis	*Gardnerella vaginalis* and vaginal anaerobes	Usually no edema or erythema of vulva or vagina Gray-white to yellow-white discharge clinging to external vulva and vaginal walls	Administer metronidazole, with instructions about avoiding alcohol while taking this medication. If infection is recurrent, treat partner.
Trichomonas vaginalis vaginitis (STD)	*Trichomonas vaginalis*	Inflammation of vaginal epithelium, producing burning and itching Frothy yellow-white or yellow-brown vaginal discharge	Remove exudate, relieve inflammation, restore acidity, and reestablish normal bacterial flora: provide oral metronidazole for patient and partner.
Bartholinitis (infection of greater vestibular gland)	*Escherichia coli* *Trichomonas vaginalis* Staphylococcus Streptococcus Gonococcus	Erythema around vestibular gland Swelling and edema Abscessed vestibular gland	Drain the abscess; provide antibiotic therapy; excise gland of patients with chronic bartholinitis.
Cervicitis: acute and chronic	Chlamydia Gonorrhea Streptococcus Many pathogenic bacteria	Profuse purulent vaginal discharge Backache Urinary frequency and urgency	Determine the cause: perform cytologic examination of cervical smear and appropriate cultures. Eradicate the gonococcus, if present: penicillin (as directed) or spectinomycin or tetracycline, if patient is allergic to penicillin. Tetracycline, doxycycline (Vibramycin) to eradicate chlamydia. Eradicate other causes: cervical cauterization.
Atrophic vaginitis	Lack of estrogen; glycogen deficiency	Discharge and irritation with alkaline pH of vaginal secretions	Provide topical vaginal estrogen therapy; improve nutrition if necessary; relieve dryness through use of moisturizing medications.

Medical Management

The most effective treatment for trichomoniasis is metronidazole (Flagyl). Both partners receive a one-time loading dose or a smaller dose three times a day for 1 week. The one-time dose is more convenient; consequently, compliance tends to be greater. The week-long treatment has occasionally been noted to be more effective. Some patients complain of an unpleasant but transient metallic taste when taking metronidazole. Nausea and vomiting, as well as a hot, flushed feeling occur when this medication is taken with an alcoholic beverage. In view of these possible side effects, the patient is strongly advised to refrain from alcohol while taking the medication.

Additionally, intercourse should be avoided unless a condom is used. Metronidazole therapy is contraindicated in patients with some blood dyscrasias or central nervous system diseases, in the first trimester of pregnancy, and in women who are breastfeeding. Because metronidazole may diminish white blood cell production, it is usually not prescribed without examination.

GERONTOLOGIC CONSIDERATIONS

After menopause, the vaginal mucosa becomes thinner and may atrophy. This condition can be complicated by infection from pyogenic bacteria, resulting in atrophic vaginitis (see Table 43-1). Leukorrhea (vaginal discharge) may cause itching and burning. Management is similar to that for bacterial vaginosis if bacteria are present. Estrogenic hormones, either taken orally or inserted into the vagina in a cream form, can also be effective in restoring the epithelium.

NURSING PROCESS: THE PATIENT WITH A VULVOVAGINAL INFECTION

Assessment

The woman with vulvovaginal symptoms should be examined as soon as possible after onset of symptoms. She is instructed not to **douche** because doing so removes the vaginal discharge needed to make the diagnosis. The area is observed for erythema, edema, excoriation, and discharge. Each of the infection-producing organisms produces its own characteristic discharge and effect (see Table 43-1). The patient is asked to describe any discharge and other symptoms, such as odor, itching, or burning. Dysuria often occurs as a result of local irritation of the urinary meatus. A urinary tract infection may need to be ruled out by obtaining a urine specimen for culture and sensitivity testing.

Factors contributing to irritation or infection include the following:

- Physical and chemical phenomena, such as constant moisture from tight or synthetic clothing, perfumes and powders, soaps, bubble bath, a soiled perineal area, and feminine hygiene products
- Psychogenic factors (eg, stress, fear of STDs, abuse)
- Medical conditions or endocrine factors, such as a predisposition to vulvar involvement in a patient who has diabetes, is elderly, or is chronically ill
- Medications, such as antibiotics, which may alter the vaginal flora and allow an overgrowth of monilial organisms

The nurse may prepare a vaginal smear (wet mount) to assist in diagnosing the infection. A common method for preparing the smear is to collect vaginal secretions with an applicator and place the secretions on two separate glass slides. A drop of saline solution is added to one slide, and a drop of 10% potassium hydroxide is added to another slide for examination under a microscope. If bacterial vaginosis is present, the slide with normal saline solution added shows epithelial cells dotted with bacteria ("clue cells"). If *Trichomonas* species is present, small motile cells are seen. In the presence of yeast, the potassium hydroxide slide reveals typical characteristics. Discharge associated with bacterial vaginosis produces a strong odor when mixed with potassium hydroxide. This is called a positive "whiff test."

Nursing Diagnosis

Based on the nursing assessment and other data, the patient's major nursing diagnoses may include the following:

- Pain, discomfort, and distress related to burning, odor, or itching from the infectious process
- Anxiety related to stressful symptoms
- Risk for reinfection or spread of infection
- Knowledge deficit about proper hygiene and preventive measures

Planning and Goals

The major goals for the patient may include relief of pain and discomfort; reduction of anxiety related to stress symptoms; prevention of reinfection or infection of sexual partner; and acquisition of knowledge about methods for preventing vulvovaginal infections and managing self-care.

Nursing Interventions

Relieving Pain

The nurse may need to reinforce instructions for warm perineal irrigations that can provide comfort and also clean the infected area if indicated. Irrigations may be recommended after urination or defecation. Additionally, a sitz bath may be taken either in a tub or by using a small disposable unit that fits over the toilet seat. If the patient's upper thighs are chafed, a dusting of cornstarch powder may alleviate discomfort.

Reducing Anxiety

Although vulvovaginal infections are upsetting and require treatment, they are not life-threatening. The patient who experiences such an infection, however, may be anxious and fearful about the significance of symptoms and possible causes. Explaining the cause of symptoms may reduce anxiety related to fear of more serious illness. Discussing ways to help prevent vulvovaginal infections may help the patient adopt specific strategies to decrease infection and the related symptoms.

Preventing Reinfection or Spread of Infection

One of the basic goals of treatment is to reduce tissue irritation caused by scratching or wearing tight clothing. The area needs to be kept clean by daily bathing and adequate cleaning after voiding and defecation. When teaching the patient about medications, such as suppositories, and devices, such as applicators to dispense cream or ointment, the nurse may demonstrate the procedure by using a plastic model of the pelvis and vagina. The nurse should also stress the importance of hand washing before and after each administration of medication. To prevent the medication from escaping from the vagina, the patient should recline for 30 minutes after it is inserted. If seepage of medication occurs, a perineal pad may be worn.

When medications such as antibiotics are prescribed for any infection, the nurse instructs the patient about usual precautions related to using these agents. If vaginal itching occurs, the patient can be reassured that this is usually not an allergic reaction but may be a yeast or monilial infection resulting from altered vaginal bacteria. Treatment for monilial infection is prescribed.

Promoting Home and Community-Based Care

TEACHING PATIENTS SELF-CARE

Vulvovaginal conditions are treated on an outpatient basis, unless the patient has other medical problems. Patient teaching, tact, and reassurance are important aspects of nursing care. Women may express embarrassment, guilt, or anger if they are concerned that the infection may be serious or may have been acquired from a sex partner. In some instances, treatment plans may include the partner.

In addition to reviewing ways of relieving discomfort and preventing reinfection, the nurse assesses each patient's learning needs relative to the immediate problem. The patient needs to know the characteristics of normal as opposed to abnormal discharge. Questions often arise about douching. Normally, douching and use of feminine hygiene sprays are unnecessary because daily baths or showers and proper cleaning after voiding and defecating keep the perineal area clean. Douching has a tendency to eliminate normal flora, reducing the body's ability to ward off infection. In addition, repeated douching may result in vaginal epithelial breakdown and chemical irritation and has been associated with other pelvic disorders.

Therapeutic douching, however, may be recommended and prescribed to reduce unpleasant, abnormal odors; to remove excessive discharge; to change the pH (such as vinegar douches); and to serve as an antiseptic irrigating solution. The procedure is reviewed with the patient, as is the care and cleaning of equipment, so that it is properly disinfected. In the case of recurrent yeast infections, the perineum should be kept as dry as possible. Loose-fitting cotton instead of tight-fitting synthetic, nonabsorbent, heat-retaining underwear is recommended.

Evaluation

Expected Outcomes

Expected outcomes may include:

1. Experiences reduced pain and discomfort
   a. Cleans the perineum as instructed
   b. Reports that itching is relieved
   c. Maintains urine output within normal limits and without dysuria
2. Experiences relief of anxiety
3. Remains free from infection
   a. Has no signs of inflammation, pruritus, odors, or dysuria
   b. Notes that vaginal discharge appears normal (thin, clear, nonfrothy)
4. Participates in self-care
   a. Takes medication as prescribed
   b. Wears absorbent underwear
   c. Avoids unprotected sexual intercourse
   d. Douches only as prescribed

Human Papillomavirus

Human papillomavirus (HPV) infection is sexually transmitted. Several different strains exist, some of which are associated with cervical abnormalities, including dysplasia and cancer. The most common strains, 6 and 11, usually cause warty growths, called **condylomata,** on the vulva. These are often visible or may be palpable by the patient. Condylomata are rarely premalignant but are an outward manifestation of the virus. Strains 6 and 11 are associated with a low risk for cervical cancer. Some strains may not cause condylomata but affect the cervix, resulting in abnormal Papanicolaou (Pap) smear results. For example, strains 16, 18, 33, and 35 affect the cervix only, causing nearly invisible cervical changes that may appear as koilocytosis on Pap smear or abnormal smear results. These strains are associated with a higher risk for cervical cancer.

The incidence of HPV in young sexually active college women is high. Risk factors include being sexually active, being of Hispanic or African descent, having multiple sex partners, and having sex with a partner who has or has had multiple partners. High alcohol consumption is a risk factor because it impairs careful decision making, judgment, and self-care.

Medical Management

Treatment includes use of trichloroacetic acid, podophyllin, interferon, chemotherapeutic agents, electrocautery, and laser therapy. Topical agents, such as podofilox (Condylox), are applied by the patient to external lesions. Treatment usually eradicates perineal warts or condylomata. However, they may resolve spontaneously without treatment and may also recur.

Patients with HPV should have regular Pap smears, possibly every 6 months for several years, because of the propensity of HPV to cause **dysplasia** (changes in cervical cells).

Women are often exposed to this virus by a partner who is unknowingly a carrier. Condoms prevent some but not all transmission because transmission occurs during skin-to-skin contact in areas not covered by condoms. In many cases, patients are angry about having warts or HPV and do not know who infected them because the incubation period can be long, and partners may have no symptoms. Acknowledging the emotional distress that occurs when an STD is diagnosed is often helpful to the patient.

Herpesvirus Type 2 Infection (Herpes Genitalis, Herpes Simplex Virus)

Herpes genitalis is a viral infection that causes herpetic lesions (blisters) on the cervix, vagina, and external genitalia. It is an STD but may also be transmitted asexually from wet surfaces or by self-transmission (ie, touching a cold sore and then touching the genital area). The initial infection is usually very painful and lasts about 1 week. Recurrences are less painful and usually produce minor itching and burning. Some patients have few or no recurrences, whereas others may have frequent bouts. Recurrences are associated with stress, sunburn, dental work, or inadequate rest or nutrition. The incidence of herpes infection has increased fivefold since the late 1970s among white teenagers and young people in their 20s. About one in five Americans has this condition (Sacks et al., 1996). The prevalence of other STDs has decreased slightly, possibly due to increased condom use, but herpes can be transmitted by contact with skin not covered by a condom. Transmission is possible even when the carrier does not have symptoms. Lesions increase vulnerability to HIV infection and other STDs.

Pathophysiology

Of the known herpesviruses, six affect humans: (1) herpes simplex type 1 (HSV-1), which usually causes "cold sores" of the lips; (2) herpes simplex type 2 (HSV-2), or genital herpes; (3) varicella zoster, or shingles; (4) Epstein-Barr virus; (5) cytomegalovirus; and (6) human B-lymphotrophic virus. HSV-2 appears to be the cause of about 80% of genital and perineal lesions; HSV-1 may cause about 20%.

There is considerable overlap between HSV-1 and HSV-2, which are clinically indistinguishable. Close human contact by the mouth, oropharynx, mucosal surface, vagina, or cervix appears necessary to acquire the infection. Other susceptible sites are skin lacerations and conjunctivae. Usually, the virus is killed at room temperature by drying. When viral replication diminishes, the virus ascends the peripheral sensory nerves and remains inactive in the nerve ganglia. Another outbreak may occur when the host is subjected to stress. In pregnant women with active herpes, babies delivered vaginally may become infected with the virus. There is a risk for fetal morbidity and mortality if this occurs; therefore, a cesarean delivery may be performed if the virus recurs near the time of delivery.

Clinical Manifestations

Itching and pain accompany the process as the infected area becomes red and swollen (edematous). The vesicular state often appears as a blister, which later coalesces, ulcerates, and encrusts. In women, the labia is the usual primary site, although the cervix, vagina, and perianal skin may be affected. In men, the glans penis, foreskin, or penile shaft are typically affected sites. Influenzalike symptoms may occur 3 or 4 days after the lesions appear. Inguinal lymphadenopathy (swollen lymph nodes in the groin), minor temperature elevation, malaise, headache, myalgia (aching muscles), and dysuria (pain on urination) are often noted. Pain is evident during the first week and then decreases. The lesions subside in about 2 weeks unless secondary infection occurs.

Rarely, complications may arise from extragenital spread, such as to the buttocks, upper thighs, or even the eyes as a result of touching lesions and then touching other areas. Patients should be advised to wash their hands after contact with lesions. Other potential problems are aseptic meningitis and severe emotional stress related to the diagnosis.

Medical Management

There is no cure for HSV-2 infection, but treatment is aimed at relieving the symptoms. Management goals are preventing the spread of infection, making the patient comfortable, decreasing potential health risks, and initiating a counseling and education program. Acyclovir (Zovirax), valcyclovir (Valtrex), and famciclovir (Famvir) are antiviral agents that can suppress symptoms and alter the course of the infection. Acyclovir is available for topical, oral, and intravenous use. Other antiviral agents are also available. All of them are effective at reducing the duration of lesions and preventing recurrences. Resistance and long-term side effects do not appear to be major problems. Recurrent episodes are much milder than the initial episode.

NURSING PROCESS: THE PATIENT WITH A GENITAL HERPESVIRUS INFECTION

Assessment

The health history and a physical and pelvic examination are important in establishing the nature of the infectious condition. Additionally, the patient is assessed for risk for STDs. The perineum is inspected for painful lesions. Inguinal nodes are assessed because they often are enlarged and tender during an HSV occurrence.

Nursing Diagnosis

Based on the assessment data, the patient's major nursing diagnoses may include the following:

- Pain related to the genital lesions
- Risk for recurrence of infection or spread of infection
- Anxiety and distress related to the disease
- Knowledge deficit about the disease and about methods of avoiding spread and preventing recurrences

Planning and Goals

The major goals for the patient may include relief of pain and discomfort, control of infection and its spread, relief of anxiety, knowledge of and adherence to the treatment regimen, and self-care and knowledge about implications for the future.

Nursing Interventions

Relieving Pain

The lesions are to be kept clean, and proper hygienic practices are advocated. Sitz baths ease discomfort and voiding. The patient's clothing should be clean, loose, soft, and absorbent. Aspirin and other analgesics are usually effective in controlling pain. Occlusive ointments and powders are avoided because they prevent the lesions from drying.

If there is considerable pain and malaise, bed rest may be required. The patient is encouraged to increase fluid intake, to be alert for possible bladder distention, and to contact her primary health care provider immediately if unable to void because of discomfort. Painful voiding may occur if urine comes in contact with the herpes lesions. Discomfort with voiding can be reduced by pouring warm water over the vulva or by sitz baths. When oral acyclovir or other antiviral agents are prescribed, the patient is instructed about when to take the medication and what side effects to note, such as rash and headache. Rest, fluids, and a nutritious diet are recommended to promote recovery.

Promoting Home and Community-Based Care

TEACHING PATIENTS SELF-CARE

Genital herpes causes physical pain and emotional distress. Usually, the patient is upset on learning the diagnosis. Therefore, when counseling the patient, the nurse should explain the causes of the condition and the manner in which it can be managed. Questions are encouraged because they may indicate that the patient is receptive to learning.

The nurse can provide reassurance that the lesions will heal and that recurrences can be minimized by adopting a healthful lifestyle and by taking prescribed medications. Self-care measures for the person with genital herpes are listed in the accompanying Home Care Teaching Checklist.

Evaluation

Expected Outcomes

Expected outcomes may include:

1. Experiences a reduction in pain and discomfort
2. Keeps infection under control by practicing proper hygienic techniques and taking medication as prescribed
3. Acquires knowledge about genital herpes and how to control and minimize recurrences

Toxic Shock Syndrome

Toxic shock syndrome (TSS), a condition first identified in the late 1970s, is caused by a toxin produced by strains of the bacterium *Staphylococcus aureus* in susceptible patients. This infrequent condition is associated with menstruating women (although about half of TSS cases are not related to menstruation). The incidence of TSS in menstruating women is 6 to 7 per 100,000. Other risk factors that may predispose a woman to TSS include chronic vaginal infection, pelvic infection, lung abscess, surgical wound infection, soft tissue infection, postpartum and gynecologic infections, use of intravenous (or injectable) drugs, and use of superabsorbent tampons. Using barrier methods of contraception (eg, diaphragm) has also been implicated, whereas using oral contraceptives appears to reduce the risk. TSS has occurred after various clinical infections and may be missed initially if diagnosticians associate it only with menstruation. The rate of recurrence is 30%. Most recurrences develop in the first 2 months after the initial illness and may occur during menstruation.

Clinical Manifestations

In an otherwise healthy person, the onset of TSS occurs with a sudden fever (temperature as high as 38.9°C [102°F]), chills, malaise, and muscle pain. Vomiting, diarrhea, hypotension, headache, and

HOME CARE TEACHING CHECKLIST: THE PATIENT WITH GENITAL HERPES

At the completion of the program, the patient or caregiver will be able to:	Patient	Caregiver
• State that herpes is transmitted mainly by direct contact.	✔	✔
• State that abstinence from sex is required for a brief period (intercourse is avoided during treatment, but other options such as hand-holding and kissing are acceptable).	✔	✔
• State that intercourse during a herpes outbreak not only increases the risk of transmission but also increases the likelihood of contracting HIV and other STDs.	✔	✔
• State that transmission is possible even in the absence of active lesions.	✔	✔
• State that condoms and use of nonoxynol 9 may provide some protection against viral transmission.	✔	✔
• Explain that women with herpes can have children, but that obstetricians or midwives should be informed of the condition so that it is appropriately monitored.	✔	✔
• Describe appropriate hygienic practices of cleanliness (hand washing, perineal cleanliness, gentle washing of lesions with mild soap and running water and lightly drying lesions) and importance of avoiding occlusive ointments, strong perfumed soaps, or bubble bath.	✔	✔
• State that control of the condition may require changes in sexual behavior and use of medications.	✔	✔
• Describe strategies to avoid self-infection (ie, avoid touching lesions during an outbreak).	✔	
• Explain rationale for avoiding self-infection (ie, lesions can become infected from germs on the hand, and the virus from the lesion can be transmitted from the hand to another area of the body or another person).	✔	✔
• Describe health promotion strategies: wear loose, comfortable clothing; eat a balanced diet; get adequate rest and relaxation.	✔	
• State rationale for avoiding exposure to the sun (can cause recurrences and skin cancer).	✔	✔
• Identify importance of taking medications as prescribed, keeping follow-up appointments with health care provider, and reporting recurrences (may not be as severe as the initial episode).	✔	✔
• Describe possible benefits of joining a group to share solutions and experiences and hear about newer treatments, such as HELP (Herpetics Engaged in Living Productively).	✔	

signs suggesting early septic shock may develop. A red, macular rash similar to a sunburn (diffuse, macular erythroderma) often occurs. In some patients, this rash appears first on the torso; in others, it is first seen on the hands (palms and fingers) and feet (soles and toes). Inflammation of mucous membranes also may occur. In 7 to 10 days, it may desquamate (become scaly or peel). Myalgia and dizziness are common.

Assessment and Diagnostic Findings

Urine output decreases, and the blood urea nitrogen level increases, often resulting in disorientation. Results of laboratory studies also reveal leukocytosis and elevated bilirubin. Uncontrollable hypotension and disseminated intravascular coagulopathy (DIC) may also occur. The clinical picture of shock (described in Chapter 14) results. Respiratory distress may develop as a result of pulmonary edema. If adult respiratory distress syndrome occurs, the outlook becomes grave. About 2% to 3% of patients with TSS die of complications.

Medical Management

The patient is placed on bed rest, and the treatment plan is directed primarily at controlling the infection with antibiotics and restoring circulating blood volume. Antibiotic therapy is based on the results of blood, urine, and other cultures. In cases of respiratory distress, oxygen therapy is instituted; if signs of acidosis appear, sodium bicarbonate is administered. Calcium is prescribed for hypocalcemia. A Swan-Ganz catheter (for monitoring pulmonary artery pressure) and intravenous dopamine may be used to manage shock. The entire treatment plan, including strategies directed toward emotional and psychological concerns, is adjusted according to each patient's condition, which may vary from mild to acute.

NURSING PROCESS: THE PATIENT WITH TOXIC SHOCK SYNDROME

Assessment

Because TSS has been associated with menstruation, the health history is directed toward determining whether the patient used tampons recently, which type (absorbency) she used, how long she retained a single tampon before changing it, and whether she noted any problems when inserting the tampon, which may have injured the vaginal tissue. Because diaphragms have also been implicated in TSS, a history of their use is also obtained.

Diagnosis

Nursing Diagnoses

Based on the assessment data, the patient's major nursing diagnoses may include the following:

- Anxiety related to the severity and suddenness of the symptoms and to concerns about recovery
- Fluid volume deficit related to vomiting and diarrhea
- Fatigue related to severity of illness and of shock, prolonged immobility, excessive nutritional demands, and stress
- Knowledge deficit about risk factors and behaviors

Collaborative Problems/Potential Complications

Based on assessment data, potential complications may include the following:

- DIC
- Septic shock

Planning and Goals

The major goals for the patient may include reduction of anxiety and emotional stress, maintenance of fluid balance, decreased level of fatigue, acquisition of relevant knowledge, and absence of complications.

Nursing Interventions

Relieving Anxiety

The patient who experiences TSS is usually frightened by the severity and suddenness of the symptoms. Additionally, she feels apprehensive about her own survival and recovery. Providing emotional support and reassurance usually reduces anxiety and apprehension. During the early phases of TSS, the patient is kept informed about diagnostic procedures and treatments. As the patient begins to recover, she is provided with the opportunity to participate in her own care when possible and to take an active role in decision making. Extending that support to the family also often helps to alleviate the patient's anxiety.

Improving Fluid Volume Status

Because of vomiting and diarrhea, the patient is at risk for fluid volume deficit. Therefore, the nurse closely monitors the patient's fluid intake and output and assesses the patient for clinical manifestations of fluid deficit (rapid pulse, decreased blood pressure, decreased skin turgor, dry mucous membranes). The nurse administers intravenous and oral fluids as prescribed and carefully documents changes in fluid status, body weight, intake, and output. If vomiting and diarrhea persist, the nurse collaborates with the physician about administering antiemetics and antidiarrheal agents.

The patient with a fluid volume deficit is often thirsty and uncomfortable. Comfort measures (eg, frequent oral hygiene) are important for the patient's comfort and well-being.

Decreasing Fatigue

Because the patient with TSS has been seriously ill and may have experienced shock, prolonged immobility, and excessive nutritional demands and stress, recovery may be slow and prolonged. The patient may report extreme generalized fatigue or lack of stamina. Nursing interventions include efforts to assist the patient with self-care and to increase stamina and resume usual activities gradually. A nutritious diet is important to counteract weight loss. The patient's weight and caloric intake are monitored and dietary supplements are provided if necessary. An exercise and activity program to build stamina is planned in collaboration with the patient and the physical therapist.

Monitoring and Managing Potential Complications

Closely monitoring and documenting vital signs and arterial blood gas levels provide valuable information about the patient's physical status. The nurse notes skin changes and fluid intake and loss; these data assist in evaluating hydration and kidney function. The patient is often critically ill and is cared for in the intensive care unit to facilitate constant monitoring and an immediate response to the onset of complications.

DIC has been observed in patients with TSS, making it essential for the nurse to observe the patient for hematomas, petechiae, oozing from needle and infusion sites, cyanosis, and coolness of the nose, fingertips, and toes. Additionally, the patient must be observed for and protected from injury. The nurse also assists in managing DIC by promptly administering prescribed medications.

Because of the likelihood of severe shock, the patient must be monitored closely for changes in vital signs, level of consciousness, and laboratory values. The patient's response to prescribed medications and fluids is also evaluated. See Chapter 14 for further description of management of shock.

Promoting Home and Community-Based Care

TEACHING PATIENTS SELF-CARE

The long time required for recovery from TSS necessitates that the patient be prepared to increase participation in self-care activities gradually. The patient and caregiver need instructions about detection and prevention of complications associated with immobility. The nurse also explains the possible causes of TSS and steps to take to prevent its recurrence. Because use of tampons during menstruation has been linked with TSS, women who have had TSS should not use tampons. If a diaphragm is used, it should not be left in place longer than 8 to 10 hours. Using the diaphragm or cervical cap during menses or in the first 3 months postpartum is also discouraged. The risk of developing TSS increases any time a woman bleeds vaginally (ie, during menses and postpartum). Because of the risk of TSS, all women who use tampons should be informed that they must be changed frequently (every 4 hours) and inserted carefully to avoid abrasions (applicators with rough edges should be avoided). Use of superabsorbent tampons is not recommended.

CONTINUING CARE

In some circumstances, the patient may need assistance with home care while recovering. The home care nurse uses the home visit to assess the patient's physical and emotional status and recovery from TSS. The nurse reinforces previous teaching and encourages and assists the patient to increase activity gradually. The nurse also reinforces the importance of keeping follow-up appointments with the primary health care provider.

Evaluation

Expected Outcomes

Expected outcomes may include:

1. Exhibits reduced anxiety and emotional stress
2. Is free of fluid loss and imbalance
   a. Does not experience vomiting and diarrhea
   b. Takes adequate fluids
   c. Maintains blood pressure and pulse rate within normal limits
   d. Exhibits normal skin turgor
3. Reports decreased fatigue level
4. Demonstrates knowledge of risk factors for TSS and avoids use of tampons and diaphragms
5. Reports absence of complications

a. Has normal arterial blood gas and coagulation studies
b. Exhibits no manifestations of infection, sepsis, or shock
c. Exhibits normal vital signs (blood pressure, pulse, and temperature)

Endocervicitis and Cervicitis

Endocervicitis is an inflammation of the mucosa and the glands of the cervix that may occur when organisms gain access to the cervical glands after intercourse and, less often, after procedures such as abortion, intrauterine manipulation, or vaginal delivery. If untreated, the infection may extend into the uterus, fallopian tubes, and pelvic cavity. Inflammation can irritate the cervical tissue, resulting in spotting or bleeding and **mucopurulent cervicitis** (MCP).

Chlamydia and Gonorrhea

Chlamydia and gonorrhea are the most common causes of endocervicitis, although mycoplasma may also be involved. Chlamydia, with about 4 million cases occurring yearly in the United States, is most commonly found in young, sexually active people with more than one partner and is transmitted through sexual intercourse. It may cause pelvic infections and sterility. Chlamydial infections of the cervix often produce no symptoms, although cervical discharge, dyspareunia, dysuria, and bleeding may occur. Other complications include conjunctivitis and perihepatitis. If a pregnant woman is infected, stillbirth, neonatal death, and premature labor may occur.

Chlamydial infection and gonorrhea often coexist. As many as 25% of females who have chlamydial infections also have gonorrhea. The inflamed cervix that results from this infection may leave a woman more vulnerable to HIV transmission from an infected partner. In males, urethritis and epididymitis may occur. Diagnosis can be confirmed by culture, smear, or other methods, using a swab to obtain a sample of cervical discharge or penile discharge from the patient's partner. Self tests for at-home use may be a cost-effective and time-saving option for patients in the future.

Medical Management

The Centers for Disease Control and Prevention (CDC) recommend treating chlamydia with doxycycline for 1 week or with a single dose of azithromycin. Partners should also be treated. Pregnant women are cautioned not to take tetracycline because of potential adverse effects on the fetus. In these cases, erythromycin may be prescribed. Results are usually good if treatment begins early. Possible complications from delayed treatment are tubal disease, ectopic pregnancy, pelvic inflammatory disease (PID), and infertility.

Cultures for chlamydia and other STDs should be taken from all patients who are victims of sexual assault when they first seek medical attention and are treated prophylactically. Cultures should then be repeated in 2 weeks.

Nursing Management

All sexually active women may be at risk for chlamydia, gonorrhea, and other STDs, including HIV. Nurses can assist patients in assessing their own risk. Recognition of risk is a first step before changes in behavior occur. Patients should be discouraged from assuming that a partner is "safe." Nonjudgmental attitudes, educational counseling, and role playing may all be helpful (Hutchinson, 1998).

Because chlamydia, gonorrhea, and other STDs may have a serious effect on future health and fertility and because many STDs can be prevented by the use of condoms, spermicides, and discriminatory choice of partners, the nurse has a major role in discussion of sex that is as safe as possible. Exploring options with patients, determining their use of safer sex practices and their knowledge deficits, and correcting misinformation may prevent morbidity and mortality.

PROMOTING HOME AND COMMUNITY-BASED CARE

Teaching Patients Self-Care. Nurses can educate women and help them to develop sexual communication skills and to initiate dialogue about sex with partners. Communicating with partners about sex, risk, postponing intercourse, and using safer sex behaviors, including use of condoms, may be lifesaving. Some young women report having sex with someone but not being comfortable enough to discuss sexual risk issues. Nurses can pose the question, "If you are uncomfortable talking about sex with this person, how do you feel about having a sexual relationship with this person?"

Pelvic Infection (Pelvic Inflammatory Disease)

Pelvic inflammatory disease (PID) is an inflammatory condition of the pelvic cavity that may involve the uterus (endometritis), fallopian tubes (**salpingitis**), ovaries (oophoritis), pelvic peritoneum, or pelvic vascular system. Infection, which may be acute, subacute, recurrent, or chronic and localized or widespread, is usually caused by bacteria but may be attributed to a virus, fungus, or parasite. Gonorrheal and chlamydial organisms are the most likely causes. Mycoplasma has also been implicated. This condition can result in the fallopian tubes becoming narrowed and scarred, which increases the risk for ectopic pregnancy (fertilized eggs become trapped in the tube), infertility, recurrent pelvic pain, tubo-ovarian **abscess** and recurrent disease. Rupture of a tubo-ovarian abscess has a 5% to 10% mortality rate and usually necessitates a complete hysterectomy. About 1 million women are diagnosed with PID each year in the United States; most are younger than 25 years of age, and one fourth of them have serious sequelae (ie, infertility, ectopic pregnancy, or chronic pelvic pain).

Pathophysiology

The exact pathogenesis of PID has not been determined, but it is presumed that organisms usually enter the body through the vagina, pass through the cervical canal, colonize the endocervix, and move upward into the uterus. Under various conditions, the organisms may proceed to one or both fallopian tubes and ovaries and into the pelvis. In bacterial infections that occur after childbirth or abortion, pathogens are disseminated directly through the tissues that support the uterus by way of the lymphatics and blood vessels (Fig. 43-1). In pregnancy, the increased blood supply required by the placenta provides more pathways for infection. These postpartum and postabortion infections tend to be unilateral. Infections can cause perihepatic inflammation when the organism invades the peritoneum.

In gonorrheal infections, the gonococci pass through the cervical canal and into the uterus, where the environment, especially

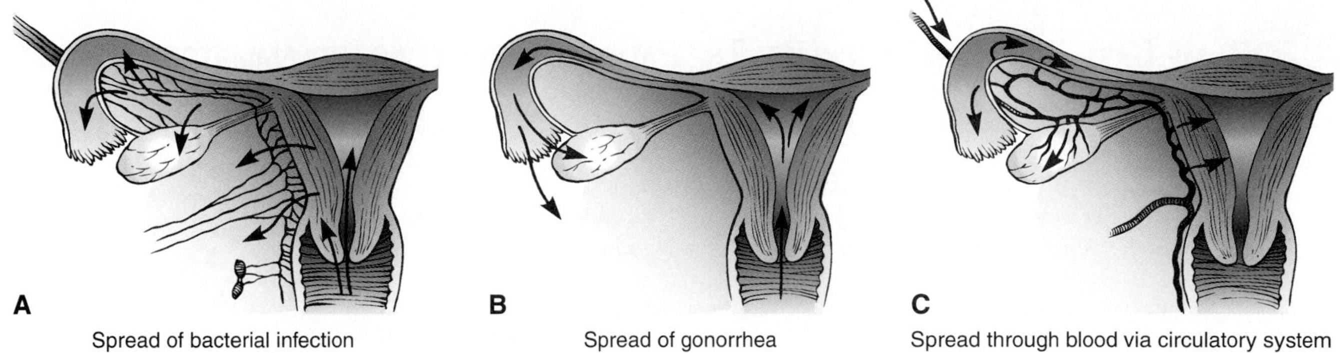

FIGURE 43•1 Pathway by which microorganisms spread in pelvic infections. (**A**) Bacterial infection spreads up the vagina into the uterus and through the lymphatics. (**B**) Gonorrhea spreads up the vagina into the uterus and then to the tubes and ovaries. (**C**) Bacterial infection can reach the reproductive organs through the bloodstream (hematogenous spread).

during menstruation, allows them to multiply rapidly and spread to the fallopian tubes and into the pelvis (see Fig. 43-1*B*). The infection is usually bilateral. In rare instances, some diseases (eg, tuberculosis) gain access to the reproductive organs by way of the bloodstream from the lungs (see Fig. 43-1*C*). One of the most common causes of salpingitis (inflammation of the fallopian tube) is chlamydia, possibly accompanied by gonorrhea.

Pelvic infection is most commonly caused by sexual transmission but can also occur with invasive procedures such as endometrial biopsy, surgical abortion, hysteroscopy, or IUD insertion. Bacterial vaginosis, a vaginal infection, may predispose women to pelvic infection. Risk factors include early age at first intercourse, multiple sexual partners, frequent intercourse, intercourse without condoms, sex with a partner with an STD, and a history of STDs or previous pelvic infection.

Clinical Manifestations

Symptoms of pelvic infection usually begin with vaginal discharge, lower abdominal pelvic pain, and tenderness that occurs after menses. Pain usually increases during voiding or defecation. Other symptoms include fever, general malaise, anorexia, nausea, headache, and possibly vomiting. On pelvic examination, intense tenderness may be noted on palpation of the uterus or movement of the cervix (cervical motion tenderness). Symptoms may be acute and severe or low grade and subtle.

Complications

Pelvic or generalized peritonitis, abscesses, strictures, and fallopian tube obstruction may develop. Obstruction may cause an ectopic pregnancy in the future if a fertilized egg cannot pass a tubal stricture, or scar tissue may occlude the tubes, resulting in sterility. Adhesions are common, often result in chronic pelvic pain, and eventually may require removal of the uterus, fallopian tubes, and ovaries. Other complications include bacteremia with septic shock and thrombophlebitis with possible embolization.

Medical Management

The patient is placed on broad-spectrum antibiotic therapy. Women with mild infections may be treated as outpatients, but hospitalization may be necessary at times. Intensive therapy includes bed rest, intravenous fluids, and intravenous antibiotic therapy. If the patient has abdominal distention or ileus, nasogastric intubation and suction are initiated. Carefully monitoring vital signs and symptoms assists in evaluating the status of the infection. Treating sexual partners is necessary to prevent reinfection.

Nursing Management

Infection takes its toll, both physically and emotionally. The patient may feel well one day and experience vague symptoms and discomfort the next. She may also suffer from constipation and menstrual difficulties.

The hospitalized patient is maintained on bed rest and is usually placed in the semi-Fowler's position to facilitate dependent drainage. Accurate recording of vital signs and the characteristics and amount of vaginal discharge is necessary as a guide to therapy.

The nurse minimizes the transmission of infection to others by carefully handling perineal pads with gloves, discarding the soiled pad according to hospital guidelines for disposal of biohazardous material, and carefully washing hands with a germicidal soap.

PROMOTING HOME AND COMMUNITY-BASED CARE

Teaching Patients Self-Care. The patient must be informed of the need for precautions and must be encouraged to take part in procedures to prevent contaminating others and protecting herself from reinfection. If a partner is not well known or has had other sexual partners recently, use of condoms may prevent life-threatening infection and its sequelae. If reinfection occurs or if the infection spreads, symptoms may include abdominal pain, nausea and vomiting, fever, malaise, malodorous purulent vaginal discharge, and leukocytosis. Patient teaching consists of explaining how pelvic infections occur, how they can be controlled and avoided, and their signs and symptoms. Guidelines and instructions provided to the patient are summarized in the accompanying Home Care Teaching Checklist.

All patients who have had PID need to be informed of the signs and symptoms of ectopic pregnancy—pain, abnormal bleeding, delayed menses, faintness, dizziness, and shoulder pain—because they are prone to this complication. (See Chapter 42 for a discussion of ectopic pregnancy.)

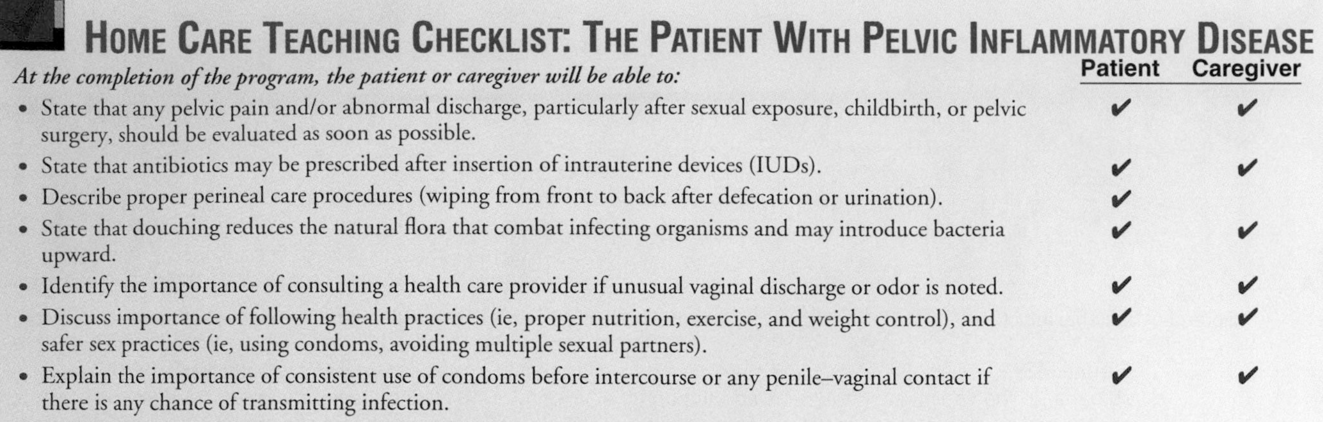

HOME CARE TEACHING CHECKLIST: THE PATIENT WITH PELVIC INFLAMMATORY DISEASE

At the completion of the program, the patient or caregiver will be able to:	Patient	Caregiver
• State that any pelvic pain and/or abnormal discharge, particularly after sexual exposure, childbirth, or pelvic surgery, should be evaluated as soon as possible.	✔	✔
• State that antibiotics may be prescribed after insertion of intrauterine devices (IUDs).	✔	✔
• Describe proper perineal care procedures (wiping from front to back after defecation or urination).	✔	
• State that douching reduces the natural flora that combat infecting organisms and may introduce bacteria upward.	✔	✔
• Identify the importance of consulting a health care provider if unusual vaginal discharge or odor is noted.	✔	✔
• Discuss importance of following health practices (ie, proper nutrition, exercise, and weight control), and safer sex practices (ie, using condoms, avoiding multiple sexual partners).	✔	✔
• Explain the importance of consistent use of condoms before intercourse or any penile–vaginal contact if there is any chance of transmitting infection.	✔	✔
• State that a gynecologic examination should be performed at least once a year.	✔	✔

Human Immunodeficiency Virus Infection and Acquired Immunodeficiency Syndrome

Any discussion of vulvovaginal infections must include the topic of HIV and **acquired immunodeficiency syndrome** (AIDS), described in Chapter 48.

Increasing incidence of HIV infection and AIDS is occurring in women. Females represent the fastest growing segment of the AIDS epidemic. Most are in the reproductive age group, and more than 70% are African American or Hispanic. More than half are intravenous (or injecting) drug users, whereas the other half have been exposed through sexual contact with HIV-infected partners. Women who exchange sex for drugs are at high risk, as are women who engage in anal intercourse. Heterosexual transmission is the leading cause of new HIV infection in women. Women are nine times more likely to get HIV from men than men are from women. Factors that may account for this difference include a higher quantity of HIV in semen as compared with vaginal secretions, a larger inoculum on ejaculation, retention of HIV-infected semen in the vagina, and traumatic microscopic mucosal injury during intercourse. The presence of genital ulcers or a friable cervix increases risk. Intercourse during menses may also increase risk. Additionally, any break in skin integrity increases the possibility of infection (eg, a herpetic lesion or syphilitic **chancre** could provide a portal of entry). Nurses need to inform women about the dangers of unprotected sex.

Syphilis appears to accelerate in HIV-positive patients and proceeds directly from primary to tertiary disease in some patients. Chlamydia is associated with a high risk for HIV (which may be related to inflammatory changes of the cervix, providing entry sites). HIV-positive women have a higher rate of HPV, and this risk increases as their CD4 cell count decreases. Infections with HPV and HIV together increase the risk of malignant transformation and cervical cancer. This risk also increases as the CD4 cell count decreases. Thus, women with HIV infection should have frequent Pap smears. HIV-positive women also appear to have larger and more painful herpes lesions with more recurrences, probably related to immunosuppression from their disease. Treatment with acyclovir is appropriate for such patients. HSV may often result in pneumonitis, esophagitis, and disseminated skin involvement in this population. Candidiasis also occurs frequently in this population; oral candidiasis may signal a rapidly advancing disease. About 42% of HIV-infected women have gynecologic disorders, including candidiasis, PID, anogenital warts, and cervical dysplasia.

Women with HIV must be counseled about safer sex. Consistent use of condoms with an HIV-infected partner can keep seroconversion rates to about 1%, but inconsistent use results in an annual 7.2% seroconversion. Because there is a 25% to 30% chance of perinatal transmission, decisions to conceive or to use contraception must be informed decisions based on teaching and care. (The use of antiretroviral agents by pregnant women has been shown to decrease perinatal transmission of HIV infection significantly. Therefore, the use of agents during pregnancy must also be discussed.) For those who choose to avoid conception, condoms and a spermicidal agent or condoms with oral contraceptives are possible choices. The risk of transmitting the virus to or from a partner will decrease with either choice.

Women who are at risk for HIV should be offered testing after informed consent by a trained nurse or counselor. Because patients may be reluctant to discuss risk-taking behavior, routine screening should be offered to all women. Early detection permits early treatment to delay progression of the disease. The nurse's role in education about HIV and prevention of HIV infection and AIDS is crucial.

STRUCTURAL DISORDERS

Fistulas of the Vagina

A **fistula** is an abnormal, tortuous opening between two internal hollow organs or between an internal hollow organ and the exterior of the body. The name of the fistula indicates the two areas that are connected abnormally: a vesicovaginal fistula is an opening between the bladder and the vagina, and a rectovaginal fistula is an opening between the rectum and the vagina (Fig. 43-2). Fistulas may occur congenitally. In adults, however, breakdown usually occurs because of tissue damage resulting from injury sustained during surgery, vaginal delivery, radiation therapy, or disease processes, such as carcinoma.

Clinical Manifestations

Symptoms depend on the specific defect. For example, in the patient with a vesicovaginal fistula, urine escapes continuously into the vagina. With a rectovaginal fistula, there is fecal inconti-

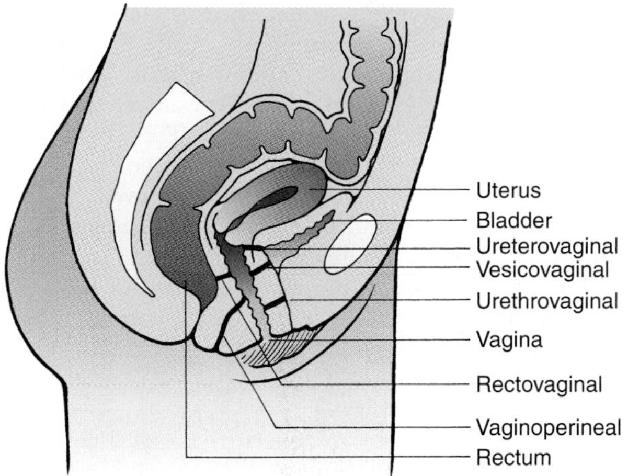

FIGURE 43•2 Common sites for vaginal fistulas. *Vesicovaginal*—bladder and vagina. *Urethrovaginal*—urethra and vagina. *Vaginoperineal*—vagina and perineal area. *Ureterovaginal*—ureter and vagina. *Rectovaginal*—rectum and vagina.

nence, and flatus is discharged through the vagina. The combination of fecal discharge with a leukorrhea results in malodor that is difficult to control.

Methylene blue dye helps delineate the course of the fistula. In vesicovaginal fistula, the dye is instilled into the bladder and appears in the vagina. After a negative methylene blue test result, indigo carmine is injected intravenously; the appearance of the dye in the vagina indicates a ureterovaginal fistula. Cystoscopy may then be used to determine the exact location.

Medical Management

The goal is to eliminate the fistula and to treat infection and excoriation. Frequently, a fistula heals without surgical intervention. If the primary care provider determines that a fistula will heal without surgical intervention, care is planned to relieve discomfort, prevent infection, and improve the patient's self-concept and self-care abilities. Measures to effect healing include proper nutrition, cleansing douches and enemas, rest, and administration of prescribed intestinal antibiotics. A rectovaginal fistula heals faster when the patient follows a low-residue diet and when the affected tissue drains properly. Warm perineal irrigations and controlled heat-lamp treatments are effective in promoting healing.

Sometimes, a fistula does not heal on its own and cannot be surgically repaired. Effective care to assist the woman whose fistula cannot be repaired must be planned and implemented on an individual basis. Cleanliness, frequent sitz baths, and deodorizing douches are required, as are perineal pads and protective undergarments. Meticulous skin care is necessary to prevent excoriation. Applying bland creams or lightly dusting with cornstarch may be soothing. Additionally, attending to the patient's social and psychological needs is an essential aspect of care. If the patient will have a fistula repaired surgically, preoperative treatment of any existing vaginitis is important to ensure success. Usually, the vaginal approach is used for repairing vesicovaginal and urethrovaginal fistulas, and the abdominal approach for repairing fistulas higher in the abdomen. Fistulas that are difficult to repair or that are very large may require surgical repair with a urinary or fecal diversion.

Because fistulas usually are related to obstetric or surgical trauma, occurrence in a patient without previous vaginal delivery or a history of surgery must be evaluated carefully. Crohn's disease or lymphogranuloma venereum may be possible causes. Despite the best surgical intervention, fistulas may recur. After surgery, medical follow-up continues for at least 2 years to monitor for a possible recurrence.

Cystocele, Rectocele, Enterocele, and Lacerations of the Perineum

Cystocele is a downward displacement of the bladder toward the vaginal orifice (Fig. 43-3). It usually results from injury and strain during childbirth. The condition usually appears some years later when genital atrophy associated with aging occurs, but younger, multiparous, premenopausal women are also affected.

Rectocele and perineal lacerations may affect the muscles and tissues of the pelvic floor and may occur during childbirth. Because of muscle tears below the vagina, the rectum may pouch upward, thereby pushing the posterior wall of the vagina forward. This structural abnormality is called a rectocele. At times, the lacerations may extend, completely severing the fibers of the anal sphincter (complete tear). An enterocele is a protrusion of the intestinal wall into the vagina.

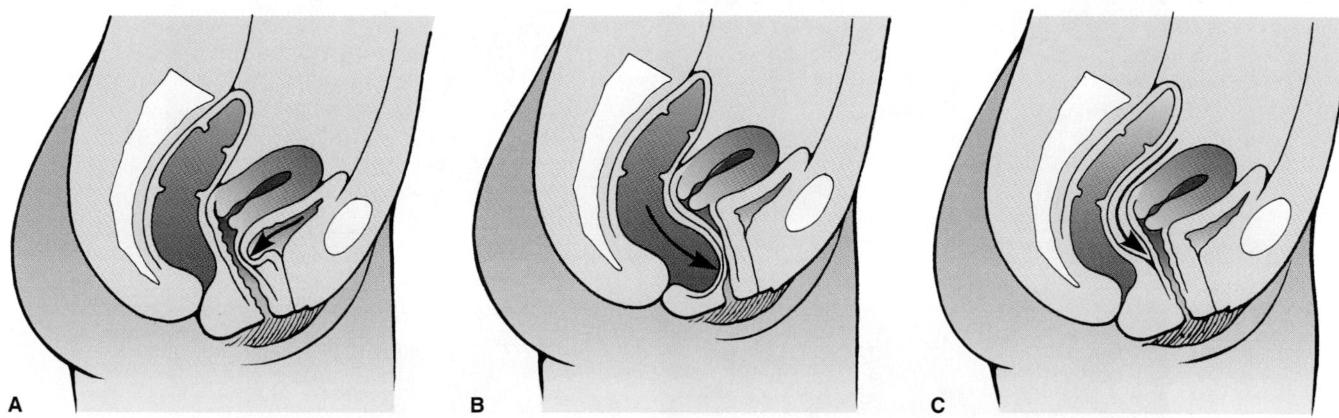

FIGURE 43•3 Diagrammatic representation of the three most common types of pelvic floor relaxation: (**A**) cystocele, (**B**) rectocele, and (**C**) enterocele. *Arrows* depict sites of maximum protrusion.

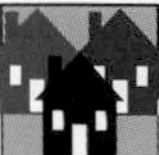

PATIENT EDUCATION AND HOME CARE

Performing Kegel (Pelvic Muscle) Exercises

Purposes: To strengthen and maintain the tone of the pubococcygeal muscle, which supports the pelvic organs; reduce or prevent stress incontinence and uterine prolapse; enhance sensation during sexual intercourse; and hasten postpartum healing

1. Become aware of pelvic muscle function by "drawing in" the perivaginal muscles and anal sphincter as if to control urine or defecation, but not contracting the abdominal, buttock, or inner thigh muscles.
2. Sustain contraction of the muscles for up to 10 seconds, followed by at least 10 seconds of relaxation.
3. Perform these exercises 30–80 times a day.

Training and exercise should be individualized for each patient.

Clinical Manifestations

Because a cystocele causes the anterior vaginal wall to bulge downward, the patient may report a sense of pelvic pressure, fatigue, and urinary problems, such as incontinence, frequency, and urgency. Back pain and pelvic pain may occur as well.

The symptoms of rectocele resemble those of cystocele, with one exception—instead of urinary symptoms, the patient may experience rectal pressure. Constipation, uncontrollable gas, and fecal incontinence may occur in patients with complete tears.

Medical Management

Kegel exercises, which involve contracting or tightening the vaginal muscles, are prescribed to help strengthen these weakened muscles. The exercises are more effective in the early stages of a cystocele. Kegel exercises are easy to do and are recommended for all women, including those with strong pelvic floor muscles.

If surgery is contraindicated or refused, a pessary may be prescribed, especially for mild problems. This device is inserted into the vagina and positioned to keep an organ, such as the bladder, uterus, or intestine, properly aligned when a cystocele, rectocele, or prolapse has occurred. Pessaries are usually ring shaped or doughnut shaped and are made of various materials, such as rubber or plastic (Fig. 43-4). The size and type are selected and fitted by a gynecologic health care provider. The patient can be taught to remove it at bedtime and reinsert it upon waking. If it remains in place, the patient should have it removed, examined, and cleaned by her health care provider at prescribed intervals. At this checkup, vaginal walls are examined for pressure points or signs of irritation. Normally, the patient experiences no pain, discomfort, or discharge with a pessary, but if chronic irritation occurs, alternative measures may be needed.

SURGICAL MANAGEMENT

In many cases, surgery helps to correct structural abnormalities. The procedure to repair the anterior vaginal wall is called anterior **colporrhaphy**, repair of a rectocele is called a posterior colporrhaphy, and repair of perineal lacerations is called a **perineorrhaphy**. These repairs are frequently performed laparoscopically, resulting in short hospital stays and good outcomes. A **laparoscope** is inserted through small abdominal incisions, the pelvis is visualized, and surgical repairs are performed.

Altered Positions and Uterine Prolapse

Usually, the uterus and the cervix lie at right angles to the long axis of the vagina and with the body of the uterus inclined slightly forward. The uterus is normally freely movable upon examination. Individual variations may result in an anterior, middle, or posterior uterine position. A backward positioning of the uterus, known as retroversion and retroflexion, may give rise to such symptoms as backache or pelvic pressure (Fig. 43-5). Most retrograde positions, however, cause no symptoms. Asymptomatic retroversion of the uterus occurs in about 20% of women and is a variant of normal. Women need to be reassured that a uterus that "tips back" is not a problem and that no treatment is needed.

If the structures that support the uterus weaken (typically from childbirth), the uterus may work its way down the vaginal canal

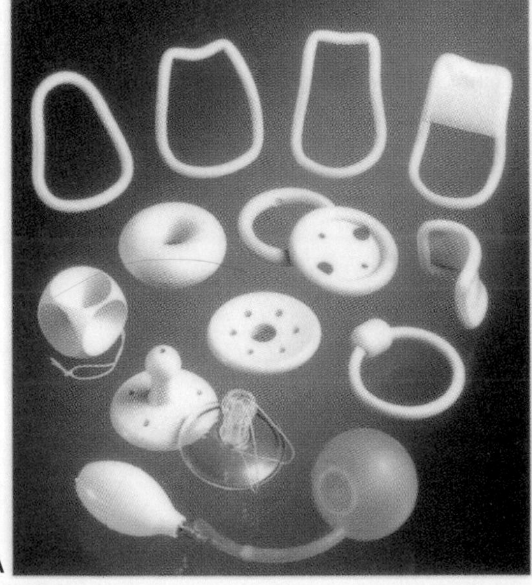

A

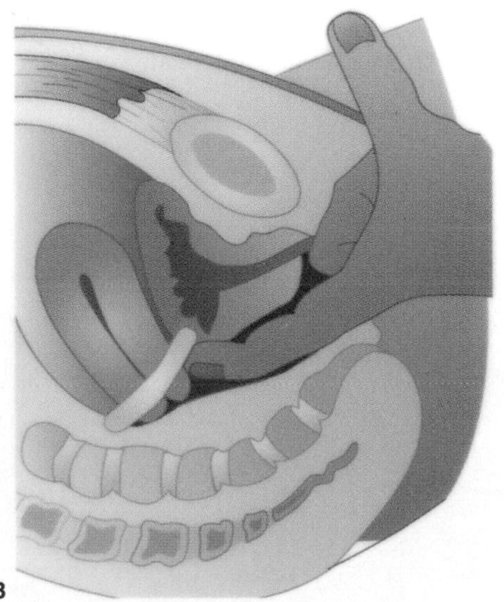

B

FIGURE 43•4 Examples of pessaries. (**A**) Various shapes and sizes of pessaries available. (**B**) Insertion of one type of pessary.

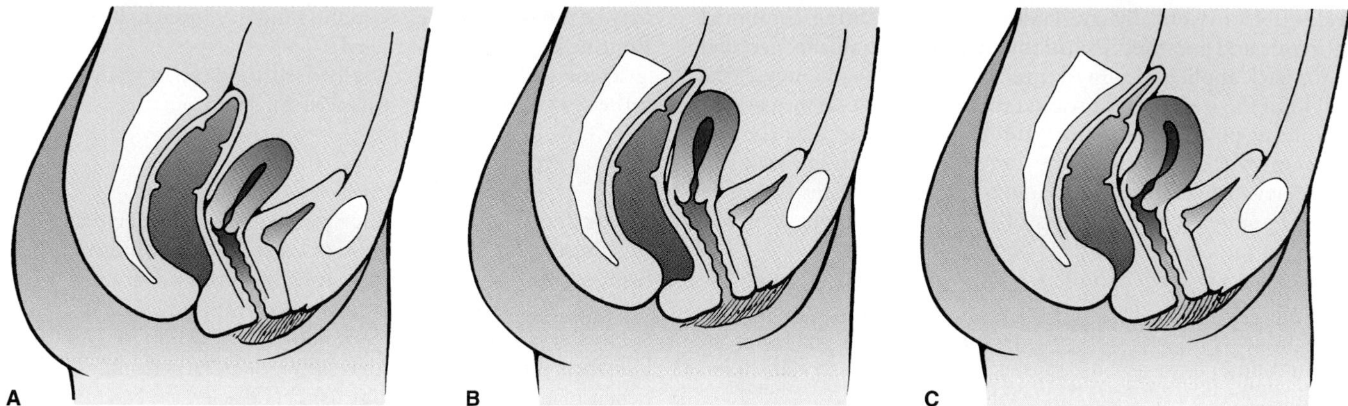

FIGURE 43•5 Positions of the uterus. (**A**) The most common position of the uterus detected on palpation. (**B**) In *retroversion* the uterus turns posteriorly as a whole unit. (**C**) In *retroflexion* the fundus bends posteriorly above the cervical end.

(prolapse) and even appear outside the vaginal orifice (procidentia) (Fig. 43-6). As the uterus descends, it may pull the vaginal walls and even the bladder and rectum with it. Symptoms include pressure and urinary problems (incontinence or retention) from displacement of the bladder. The problems are aggravated when the woman coughs, lifts a heavy object, or stands for a long time. Normal activities, even walking up stairs, may aggravate the problem. The woman with such symptoms is encouraged to seek medical attention because time will not correct the problem.

Medical Management

Surgery is the treatment of choice. The uterus is sutured back into place and repaired to strengthen and tighten the muscle bands. In postmenopausal women, the uterus may be removed (hysterectomy). For elderly women or those who are too ill to withstand the strain of surgery, pessaries may be the treatment of choice.

Nursing Management

IMPLEMENTING PREVENTIVE MEASURES

Some problems related to "relaxed" pelvic muscles (cystocele, rectocele, and uterine prolapse) may be prevented. During pregnancy, early visits to the health care provider permit early detection of potential problems. During the postpartum period, the woman can be taught to perform Kegel exercises to strengthen the muscles that support the uterus.

Delays in obtaining evaluation and treatment may result in complications such as infection, cervical ulceration, cystitis, and hemorrhoids. The nurse, therefore, encourages the patient to obtain prompt treatment for these structural disorders.

IMPLEMENTING PREOPERATIVE NURSING CARE

Before surgery to correct uterine position, the patient needs to know the extent of the proposed surgery, the expectations for the postoperative period, and the effect of surgery on future sexual function. In addition, the patient having a rectocele repair needs to know that before surgery, a laxative and a cleansing enema may be prescribed. A perineal shave may be prescribed as well.

The patient is usually placed in a lithotomy position for surgery, with special attention given to moving both legs in and out of the stirrups simultaneously to prevent muscle strain and excess pressure on the legs and thighs. Other preoperative interventions are similar to those described in Chapter 16.

INITIATING POSTOPERATIVE NURSING CARE

Immediate postoperative goals include preventing infection and pressure on any existing suture line. This may require perineal care and may preclude using dressings. The patient is encouraged to void within a few hours after surgery for cystocele and complete tear. If the patient does not void within this period and reports discomfort or pain in the bladder region after 6 hours, she will need to be catheterized. Some physicians prefer to leave an indwelling catheter in place for 2 to 4 days. Therefore, some women may return home with a catheter in place. Various other bladder care methods are described in Chapter 18. After each voiding or bowel movement, the perineum is cleansed with warm, sterile saline solution and dried with sterile absorbent material if a perineal incision has been made.

After an external perineal repair, several methods are used in caring for the sutures. In one method, the sutures are left alone until healing occurs (in 5 to 10 days). Thereafter, daily vaginal douches with sterile saline solution may be administered during recovery. In another method—the wet method—small, sterile saline douches are administered twice daily, beginning on the day after surgery and continuing throughout recovery. A heat lamp or hair dryer may be used to help dry the area and promote

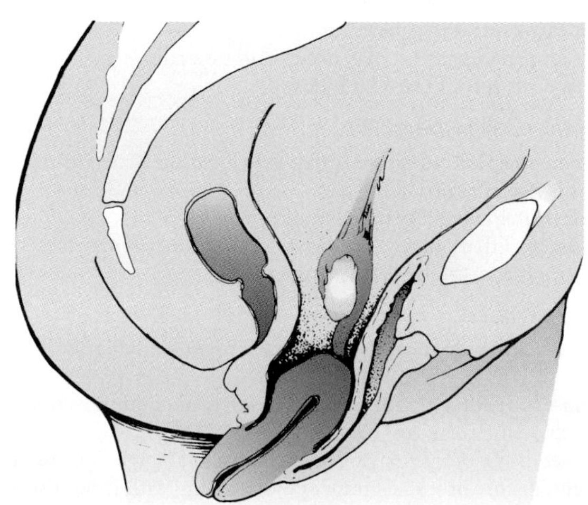

FIGURE 43•6 Complete prolapse of the uterus through the introitus.

healing. Commercially available sprays containing combined antiseptic and anesthetic solutions are soothing and effective, and an ice pack applied locally may relieve discomfort. However, the weight of the ice bag must rest on the bed and not on the patient.

Routine postoperative care is similar to that given after abdominal surgery. The patient is positioned in bed, with the head and knees elevated slightly. The patient may go home the day of or day after surgery; the duration of hospital stay depends on the surgical approach.

After surgery for a complete perineal laceration (through the rectal sphincter), special care and attention are required. The bladder is drained through the catheter to prevent strain on the sutures. Throughout recovery, stool-softening agents are administered nightly after the patient begins a soft diet.

PROMOTING HOME AND COMMUNITY-BASED CARE

Teaching Patients Self-Care. Predischarge instructions include information pertaining to the gynecologist's postoperative instructions related to douching, using mild laxatives, performing exercise as recommended, and avoiding lifting heavy objects or standing for prolonged periods. The patient is reminded to return to the gynecologist for a follow-up visit and to consult with the physician about safely resuming sexual intercourse.

The patient is instructed to report any pelvic pain, unusual discharge, inability to carry out personal hygiene, and vaginal bleeding. She is advised to continue with perineal exercises, which are recommended for muscle strength and tone.

BENIGN TUMORS AND CONDITIONS

Vulvar Cysts

Bartholin's cyst results from obstruction of a duct in one of the paired vestibular glands located in the posterior third of the vulva, near the vestibule. This cyst is the most common of vulvar tumors. A simple cyst may be asymptomatic, but an infected cyst or an abscess may cause discomfort. Infection may be due to a gonococcal organism, *Escherichia coli,* or *Staphylococcus aureus* and can cause an abscess with or without involving the inguinal lymph nodes. Skene's duct cysts may result in pressure, dyspareunia, altered urinary stream and pain, especially if infection is present. Vestibular cysts, located inferior to the hymen, may also occur.

Medical Management

The usual treatment for Bartholin's cyst is incision and drainage followed by antibiotic therapy. If a cyst is asymptomatic, treatment is unnecessary. Moist heat or sitz baths may promote drainage and resolution. If surgery is necessary, a Word Bartholin gland catheter is usually used. This catheter, a short latex stem with an inflatable bulb at the distal end, creates a tract that preserves the gland and allows for drainage. A nonopioid analgesic may be administered before this outpatient procedure. A local anesthetic agent is injected, and the cyst is incised or lanced and cleaned out with normal saline; the catheter is inserted and inflated with 2 to 3 mL of water. The catheter stem is then tucked into the vagina to allow freedom of movement. The catheter is left in place for 4 to 6 weeks until the tract reepithelializes. The patient is informed that discharge should be expected as the catheter allows drainage of the cyst. She is instructed to contact her primary health care provider if pain occurs because the bulb may be too large for the cavity and fluid may need to be removed. Routine hygiene is encouraged.

Skene's duct cysts can be excised or drained with a Word catheter. Vestibular cysts are excised if symptomatic.

Vulvar Dystrophy

Vulvar **dystrophy** is a condition found in older women that causes dry, thickened skin on the vulva or slightly raised, whitish papules, fissures, or macules. Symptoms usually consist of varying degrees of itching, but some patients have no symptoms. A few patients with vulvar cancer have associated dystrophy. Biopsy with careful follow-up is the standard intervention. Benign dystrophies include lichen planus, simplex chronicus, lichen sclerosis, squamous cell hyperplasia, vulvar vestibulitis, and other dermatoses (Chart 43-1).

Medical Management

Topical corticosteroids (ie, hydrocortisone suppositories) are the usual treatment for lichen planus. Topical progesterones, testosterones, and estrogens have been tried, but corticosteroids are the most effective treatment for lichen sclerosis. Their use is decreased as symptoms abate. Topical corticosteroids are effective in treating squamous cell hyperplasia. Treatment is often complete in 2 to 3 weeks; this condition is not likely to recur after treatment is complete. Research is ongoing for treatment for vulvar vestibulitis, but local topical treatments, topical estrogens, steroids, and interferon have been used. Biofeedback is also used.

If malignant cells are detected on biopsy, local excision, laser therapy, local chemotherapy, and immunologic treatment are

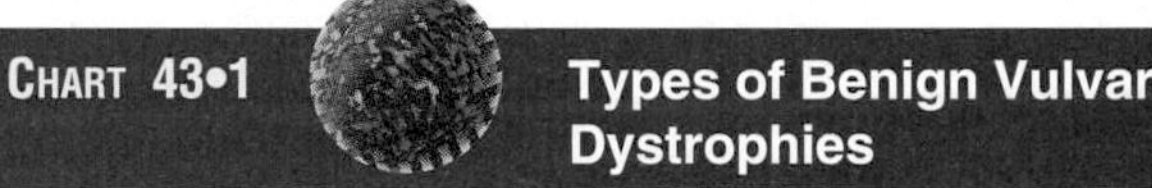

Lichen Planus and Simplex Chronicus

- Chronic vulvar and vaginal disorders that are diagnosed by biopsy
- May appear as mild inflammation or as severe erosion
- Result in redness, lesions, pain, and dyspareunia

Lichen Sclerosis

- A benign epithelial disorder that is most common in prepubertal and postmenopausal females
- A familial tendency toward this condition may exist
- Epithelial thinning, edema, and fibrosis occur, and the vulva appears white and paper thin.
- Bleeding and pruritus may occur, and intercourse may be difficult
- Diagnosis is confirmed by biopsy

Squamous Cell Hyperplasia

- A benign epithelial disorder that may look like lichen sclerosus but is not inflamed
- Causes itching and plaquelike excoriated skin
- Must be differentiated from vulvar intraepithelial neoplasia or carcinoma in situ by biopsy

Vulvar Vestibulitis

- An inflammatory process associated with vulvodynia and possibly interstitial cystitis
- Causes pain during and after intercourse; discomfort may also preclude intercourse
- Onset of symptoms may be related to vaginal infection, laser treatment, history of sexual abuse or overwashing with irritant soaps
- Examination reveals redness, inflammation, and tenderness

used. Vulvectomy is avoided, if possible, to spare the patient from the stress of disfigurement and possible sexual dysfunction.

Nursing Management

Key nursing responsibilities for patients with vulvar dystrophies focus on teaching. Important topics include hygiene and self-monitoring for signs and symptoms of complications.

PROMOTING HOME AND COMMUNITY-BASED CARE

Teaching Patients Self-Care. Instructions for patients with benign vulvar dystrophies include the importance of maintaining good personal hygiene and keeping the vulva dry. Lanolin or hydrogenated vegetable oil is recommended for relief of dryness. Sitz baths may help but should not be overused because dryness may result or increase. The patient is instructed to notify her primary health care provider about a persistent ulcer because biopsy may be necessary to rule out possible squamous cell carcinoma.

By encouraging all patients to perform genital self-examinations regularly and have any itching, lesions, or unusual symptoms assessed by a health care provider, nurses can help prevent complications and progression of vulvar lesions.

Ovarian Cysts

The ovary is a common site for cysts, which may be simple enlargements of normal ovarian constituents, the graafian follicle, or corpus luteum, or they may arise from abnormal growth of the ovarian epithelium.

Dermoid cysts are tumors that are thought to arise from parts of the ovum that normally disappear with ripening (maturation). Their origin is undefined, and they consist of undifferentiated embryonal cells. They grow slowly and are found during surgery to contain a thick, yellow, sebaceous material arising from the skin lining. Hair, teeth, bone, and many other tissues are found in a rudimentary state within these cysts. Dermoid cysts are only one type of lesion that may develop. Many other types can occur, and treatment usually depends on the type.

The patient may or may not report acute or chronic abdominal pain. Symptoms of a ruptured cyst mimic various acute abdominal emergencies, such as appendicitis or ectopic pregnancy. Larger cysts may produce abdominal swelling and exert pressure on adjacent abdominal organs.

Polycystic ovary syndrome, a complex endocrine disorder involving a disorder in the hypothalamic-pituitary and ovarian network or axis resulting in anovulation, occurs in women of childbearing age. Symptoms are related to androgen excess. Irregular periods resulting from lack of regular ovulation, obesity, and hirsutism may be presenting complaints. Cysts form in the ovaries because the hormonal milieu is unable to cause ovulation on a regular basis. Onset may occur at menarche or later. When pregnancy is desired, medications to stimulate ovulation are often effective. Women with polycystic ovary syndrome may develop insulin resistance and may be at higher risk for cardiac disorders in later life.

Medical Management

The treatment of large ovarian cysts is usually surgical removal. For cysts that are small and appear to be fluid-filled or physiologic in a young, healthy patient, however, oral contraceptives may be used to suppress ovarian activity and resolve the cyst. Oral contraceptives are also usually prescribed to treat polycystic ovary syndrome. About 98% of lesions that occur in women aged 29 years and younger are benign. In women older than 50 years of age, only half of these cysts are benign. The postoperative nursing care after surgery to remove an ovarian cyst is similar to that after abdominal surgery, with one exception. The marked decrease in intra-abdominal pressure resulting from removal of a large cyst usually leads to considerable abdominal distention. This complication may be prevented to some extent by applying a snug-fitting abdominal binder.

Some surgeons discuss the option of a hysterectomy when a woman is undergoing a bilateral ovary removal because of a suspicious mass because it may increase life expectancy, avoid a later second surgery, and save on health care costs. It is preventive in that future cancer is avoided, as is benign disease that might require hysterectomy. Patient preference is a priority in determining its appropriateness.

Benign Tumors of the Uterus: Fibroids (Leiomyomas and Myomas)

Myomatous or **fibroid tumors** of the uterus are almost always benign (99.5%). They arise from the muscle tissue of the uterus and can be found in the lining, muscle wall, and outside surface of the uterus. They are common, occurring in about 20% of white women and 40% to 50% of African American women. They develop slowly in women between the ages of 25 and 40 years and may become large. Fibroids may cause no symptoms, or they may produce abnormal vaginal bleeding. Other symptoms are due to pressure on the surrounding organs and include pain, backache, constipation, and urinary problems. Menorrhagia (excessive bleeding) and metrorrhagia (irregular bleeding) may occur because fibroids may distort the uterine lining.

Medical Management

The treatment of uterine fibroids depends to a large extent on their size, symptoms, and location. The patient with minor symptoms is observed closely. If she plans to have children, treatment is as conservative as possible. As a rule, large tumors that produce pressure symptoms should be removed. The uterus may be removed (hysterectomy) if symptoms are bothersome and childbearing is completed (see later discussion of nursing care for a patient having a hysterectomy). A small tumor or tumors may be removed in a procedure known as a myomectomy; laser surgery is often used.

Several new alternatives to hysterectomy have been developed for the treatment of excessive bleeding because of fibroids. In one approach, a portion of the uterine lining is destroyed by heated water circulated through a balloon that is inserted into the uterus. This procedure takes about 30 minutes; a sedative and local anesthesia are all that are required. A catheter is passed through the cervix into the uterus, and the catheter balloon is then filled with sterile fluid. The fluid is heated to 87°C, and the heated balloon remains in the uterus for 8 minutes. It is then deflated and removed. The most common side effects are cramping after the procedure and a watery discharge for 2 to 4 weeks as endometrial tissue is sloughed. A small amount of endometrium may remain, so some women may continue to menstruate and some may become pregnant; therefore, women should be informed about this possibility.

Fibroids usually shrink and disappear during menopause when estrogen is no longer produced. Medications (eg, leuprolide

[Lupron]) that induce medical menopause may be prescribed to shrink the tumors. This medical treatment consists of monthly injections, which may cause hot flashes and vaginal dryness. This treatment is usually short term (ie, before surgery).

Endometriosis

In **endometriosis**, a benign lesion or lesions with cells similar to those lining the uterus grow aberrantly in the pelvic cavity outside the uterus. Often, extensive endometriosis may cause few symptoms, whereas an isolated lesion may produce severe symptoms. Between 3 and 5 million women in the United States are affected by this disorder. It appears to be increasing in incidence and is a major cause of infertility. In order of frequency, pelvic endometriosis involves the ovary, uterosacral ligaments, cul-de-sac, rectovaginal septum, uterovesical peritoneum, cervix, outer surface of the uterus, umbilicus, laparotomy scar tissue, hernial sacs, and appendix.

Endometriosis has been diagnosed more frequently as a result of the increased use of laparoscopy. Before laparoscopy, major surgery was necessary before a diagnosis could be made. There is a high incidence among patients who bear children late and among those who have fewer children. In countries where tradition favors early marriage and early childbearing, endometriosis is rare. There also appears to be a familial predisposition to endometriosis; it is more common in women whose close female relatives are affected. Other factors that may suggest increased risk include a shorter menstrual cycle less than every 27 days, flow longer than 7 days, outflow obstruction, and younger age at menarche. Characteristically, endometriosis is found in young, nulliparous women between the ages of 25 and 35 years.

Pathophysiology

Misplaced endometrial tissue responds to and depends on ovarian hormonal stimulation. During menstruation, this ectopic tissue bleeds—mostly into areas having no outlet—which causes pain and adhesions. The lesions are typically small, puckered, and brown or blue-black, indicating concealed bleeding.

Endometrial tissue contained within an ovarian cyst has no outlet for the bleeding; this formation is referred to as a pseudocyst or chocolate cyst. Adhesions, cysts, and scar tissue may result, causing pain and infertility.

The more popular theories regarding the origin of endometrial lesions are the transplantation theory and the metaplasia theory. The transplantation theory suggests that a backflow of menses (retrograde menstruation) transports endometrial tissue to ectopic sites through the fallopian tubes. Transplantation of tissue can also occur during surgery if endometrial tissue is transferred inadvertently by way of surgical instruments. Endometrial tissue can also be spread by lymphatic or venous channels. The metaplasia theory relates to retained remnants of embryonic epithelial tissue, which during growth may be transformed into endometrial tissue by means of outside stimuli. Endometriosis may result from a combination of these factors.

Clinical Manifestations

Symptoms vary with the location of endometrial tissue. Usually, the chief symptom is a type of dysmenorrhea, unlike typical uterine cramps. The patient complains of a deep-seated aching in the lower abdomen, vagina, posterior pelvis, and back that occurs 1 or 2 days before the menstrual cycle and lasts 2 or 3 days. Some patients, however, have no pain. Abnormal uterine bleeding may occur and dyspareunia (painful intercourse) may also be evident in sexually active women. Excess prostaglandin released from the cells that are shed may contribute to nausea and diarrhea.

Assessment and Diagnostic Findings

A health history, including an account of the menstrual pattern, is necessary to elicit specific symptoms. On bimanual pelvic examination, fixed tender nodules may be detected and uterine mobility may be limited, indicating adhesions. Laparoscopic examination confirms the diagnosis and helps to stage the disease. In stage 1, the patient has superficial or minimal lesions; stage 2, mild involvement; stage 3, moderate involvement; and stage 4, deep involvement and dense adhesions, with obliteration of the cul-de-sac.

Medical Management

Treatment depends on the patient's symptoms and desire for pregnancy and the extent of the disease. If the woman does not have symptoms, routine examination may be all that is required. Other therapy for varying degrees of symptoms may be palliation, hormone administration, or surgery. Pregnancy alleviates symptoms because neither ovulation nor menstruation occurs.

PHARMACOLOGIC THERAPY

Palliative measures include use of medications, such as analgesics and prostaglandin inhibitors, for pain. Hormonal therapy is effective in suppressing endometriosis and relieving dysmenorrhea (menstrual pain). Oral contraceptives are used frequently. Side effects that may occur with oral contraceptives include fluid retention, weight gain, or nausea. These can usually be managed by changing brands or formulations. Depo-Provera, an injectable progesterone contraceptive, may also be used.

Several types of hormonal therapy are also available in addition to the oral contraceptives. A synthetic androgen, danazol (Danocrine), causes atrophy of the endometrium and subsequent amenorrhea. The medication inhibits the release of gonadotropin with minimal overt sex hormone stimulation. The drawbacks of this medication are that it is expensive and may cause troublesome side effects, such as fatigue, depression, weight gain, oily skin, decreased breast size, mild acne, hot flashes, and vaginal atrophy. Another gonadotropin-releasing hormone (GnRH) agonist, or GnRH blocker, known as Synarel, decreases estrogen production and causes subsequent amenorrhea. It is administered by nasal spray twice a day for 6 months. Side effects are related to low estrogen levels (eg, hot flashes and vaginal dryness). Leuprolide, another medication, is injected monthly to suppress hormones, induce an artificial menopause, and, thereby, avoid menstrual effects and relieve endometriosis. Some clinicians prescribe a combination of therapies. Most women continue treatment despite side effects, and symptoms diminish for 80% to 90% of women with mild to moderate endometriosis.

Hormonal medications are not used, however, in patients with a history of abnormal vaginal bleeding, liver, heart, or kidney disease. Possible bone loss from the antiestrogen effects of some of these treatment methods is being studied.

SURGICAL MANAGEMENT

If conservative measures are not helpful, surgery may be necessary to relieve pain and enhance the possibility for pregnancy. The procedure selected depends on the individual patient.

Laparoscopy may be used to fulgurate (cut with high-frequency current) endometrial implants and to release adhesions. Laser surgery is another option made possible by laparoscopy. Laser therapy vaporizes or coagulates the endometrial implants, thereby destroying this tissue. Other surgical options include laparotomy, abdominal hysterectomy, oophorectomy, bilateral **salpingo-oophorectomy,** and appendectomy. For women older than 35 years of age or those willing to sacrifice reproductive capability, total hysterectomy is an option.

Nursing Management

The health history and physical examination focus on specific symptoms (eg, pain) and when and how long they have been bothersome, the effect of prescribed medications, and the woman's reproductive preferences. This information helps in determining the treatment plan. Explaining the various diagnostic procedures may help to alleviate the patient's anxiety. Patient goals include relief of pain, dysmenorrhea, dyspareunia, and avoidance of infertility.

As the treatment plan progresses, the woman with endometriosis and her partner may find that pregnancy is not easily possible, and the psychosocial impact of this realization must be recognized and addressed. Alternatives, such as in vitro fertilization or adoption, may be discussed at an appropriate time and referrals offered.

The nurse's role in patient education is to dispel myths and encourage the patient to seek care if dysmenorrhea or abnormal bleeding patterns occur. The Endometriosis Association (listed at the end of this chapter) is a helpful resource for patients seeking further information and support for this condition, which can cause disabling pain and severe emotional distress.

Adenomyosis

In adenomyosis, the tissue that lines the endometrium invades the uterine wall. The incidence is highest in women from 40 to 50 years of age. Symptoms include hypermenorrhea (excessive and prolonged bleeding), acquired dysmenorrhea, polymenorrhea (abnormally frequent bleeding), and premenstrual staining. Physical examination findings on palpation include an enlarged, firm, and tender uterus. Treatment depends on the severity of bleeding and pain. Hysterectomy may offer greater relief than more conservative therapies.

MALIGNANT CONDITIONS

Malignant tumors of the female reproductive system (excluding breast cancer) occur in 274,000 women and are estimated to kill more than 27,100 women in the United States each year. The number of new cases each year and the number of deaths resulting from these cases for specific types of reproductive system cancer include the following (American Cancer Society, 1999):

- Cervical cancer (estimates do not include in situ cancers): 12,800 new cases, 4800 deaths
- Uterine cancer: 37,400 new cases, 6400 deaths
- Ovarian cancer: 25,200 new cases, 14,500 deaths
- Other genital cancers: 5600 new cases, 1500 deaths
- Carcinoma in situ: 45,000 new cases

Although some cancers are difficult to detect or prevent, yearly pelvic examination with a Pap smear is a painless and relatively inexpensive method of early detection. Health care providers can encourage women to follow this health practice by providing nonstressful examinations that are educational and supportive and offer an opportunity for the patient to ask questions and clarify misinformation. If more women understood that the pelvic examination and Pap smear do not have to be uncomfortable or embarrassing, early detection rates would undoubtedly improve, and lives would be saved.

Cancer of the Cervix

Carcinoma of the cervix is predominantly squamous cell cancer (10% are adenocarcinomas). During the past 20 years, invasive cervical cancer has decreased from 14.2 cases per 100,000 women to 7.8 cases per 100,000 women. It is less common than it once was because of early detection by Pap smear. However, it is still the third most common female reproductive cancer and affects about 13,000 women in the United States every year (American Cancer Society, 1999). Cervical cancer occurs most commonly in women between the ages of 30 and 45 years, but it can occur as early as age 18 years. Risk factors vary from multiple sex partners to smoking to chronic cervical infection.

Clinical Manifestations

Early cervical cancer rarely produces symptoms. When symptoms, such as discharge, irregular bleeding, or bleeding after sexual intercourse, occur, the disease may be advanced. The vaginal discharge in advanced cervical cancer increases gradually and becomes watery and, finally, dark and foul smelling from necrosis and infection of the tumor. The bleeding, which occurs at irregular intervals, between periods (metrorrhagia), or after menopause, may be slight (just enough to spot the undergarments) and occurs usually after mild trauma or pressure (such as intercourse, douching, or bearing down during defecation). As the disease continues, the bleeding may persist and increase.

As the cancer advances, it may invade the tissues outside the cervix, including the lymph glands anterior to the sacrum. In one third of patients with invasive cervical cancer, the disease involves the fundus. The nerves in this region may be affected, producing excruciating pain in the back and the legs that is relieved only by large doses of opioid analgesia. If the disease progresses, it often produces extreme emaciation and anemia, usually accompanied by fever due to secondary infection and abscesses in the ulcerating mass, and by fistula formation.

Assessment and Diagnostic Findings

Diagnosis may be made on the basis of abnormal Pap smear results, followed by biopsy results identifying severe dysplasia (cervical intraepithelial neoplasia type III [CIN III], HGSIL, or carcinoma in situ; see below). HPV infections are usually implicated in these conditions. Biopsy results may indicate carcinoma in situ. Carcinoma in situ is technically classified as severe dysplasia and is defined as cancer that has extended through the full thickness of the epithelium of the cervix, but not beyond. This is often referred to as preinvasive cancer.

In its very early stages, invasive cervical cancer is found microscopically by Pap smear. In later stages, pelvic examination may reveal a large, reddish growth or a deep, ulcerating lesion. The patient may report spotting or a bloody discharge.

When the patient has been diagnosed with invasive cervical cancer, clinical staging estimates the extent of the disease, so that treatment can be planned more specifically and prognosis rea-

Risk Factors for CERVICAL CANCER

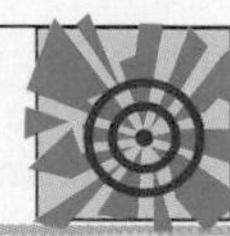

Risk Factors

Sexual activity:
- Multiple sex partners
- Early (younger than 20) sexarche at first intercourse (exposure of the vulnerable young cervix to potential carcinogens from a partner)
- Early childbearing

Exposure to human papillomavirus (more than 90% of cases; American Cancer Society, 1998)
HIV infection
Smoking
Exposure to diethylstilbestrol (DES) in utero.
Low socioeconomic status (may be related to early marriage and early childbearing)
Nutritional deficiencies (folate, beta-carotene, and vitamin C levels are lower in women with cervical cancer than in women without it)
Chronic cervical infection

Preventive Measures

Regular pelvic examinations and Pap tests for all women, especially older women past childbearing age (decrease the chance of dying from cervical cancer from 1 in 250 to 1 in 2000 women)
Education related to reproductive health and safer sex
Smoking cessation

sonably predicted. The International Classification adopted by the International Federation of Gynecology and Obstetrics (Table 43-2) is the most widely used staging system; the TNM (tumor, nodes, and metastases) classification is also used in describing cancer stages. In this system, T refers to the extent of the primary tumor, N to lymph node involvement, and M to metastasis, or spread of the disease.

Signs and symptoms are evaluated, and x-rays, laboratory tests, and special examinations, such as punch biopsy and colposcopy, are performed. Depending on the stage of the cancer, other tests and procedures may be performed to determine the extent of disease and appropriate treatment. These tests include dilation and curettage (D & C), computed tomography (CT) scan, magnetic resonance imaging (MRI), intravenous urogram (IVU), cystogram, and barium x-ray studies.

Medical Management

PRECURSOR OR PREINVASIVE LESIONS

When precursor lesions, such as LGSIL (CIN I and II or mild to moderate dysplasia) are found by colposcopy and biopsy, careful monitoring by frequent Pap smears or conservative treatment is possible. Conservative treatment may consist of **cryotherapy** (freezing with nitrous oxide) or laser therapy. A **loop electrocautery excision procedure** (LEEP) may also be used to remove abnormal cells. A thin wire loop with laser is used to cut away a thin layer of cervical tissue. LEEP is an outpatient procedure, is usually performed in a doctor's office, and takes only a few minutes. Analgesia is given before the procedure, and a local anesthetic is injected into the area. This procedure allows the pathologist to examine the removed tissue sample to determine if the borders of the tissue are disease free. Also called a cone biopsy, **conization** (removing a cone-shaped portion of the cervix) is performed when biopsy findings demonstrate CIN III or HGSIL, equivalent to severe dysplasia and carcinoma in situ.

If preinvasive cervical cancer (*carcinoma in situ*) occurs when a woman has completed childbearing, a hysterectomy is usually recommended. If a woman has not completed childbearing and invasion is less than 1 mm, a cone biopsy may be sufficient. Frequent subsequent periodic examinations are performed to monitor for recurrence.

Patients who have precursor or premalignant lesions need reassurance that they do not have cancer. However, the importance of close follow-up is emphasized because the condition, if untreated for a long time, may progress to cancer. Patients with cervical cancer in situ also need to know that this is usually a slow-growing and nonaggressive type of cancer that is not expected to recur after appropriate treatment.

INVASIVE CANCER

Treatment of invasive cervical cancer depends on the stage of the lesion, the patient's age and general health, and the judgment and experience of the physician. Surgery and radiation treatment (intracavitary and external) are most often used. When tumor invasion is less than 3 mm, a hysterectomy is often sufficient. Invasion exceeding 3 mm usually requires a radical hysterectomy with pelvic node dissection and aortic node assessment. Stage 1B1 tumors are treated with radical hysterectomy and radiation. Stage 1B2 tumors (Chart 43-2) are treated individually because no single correct course has been determined, and many variable options may be seen clinically. Frequent follow-up after surgery by gynecologic oncologists is imperative because the risk of recurrence is 35% after treatment for invasive cervical cancer. Recurrence usually occurs within the first 2 years. Recurrences are often in the upper quarter of the vagina, and ureteral obstruction may be a sign. Weight loss, leg edema, and pelvic pain may be signs of lymphatic obstruction and metastasis.

Radiation is often part of treatment to reduce recurrent disease and may be delivered by an external beam or by **brachytherapy** (method by which the radiation source is placed near the tumor). Low-dose-rate brachytherapy reduces the rate of local recurrence and is the most commonly used technique. High-dose-rate brachytherapy is increasing in use, but more studies are needed to determine its long-term effects and complications. Serum tumor markers are being studied to determine benefit.

Cisplatin, carboplatin, and paclitaxel (Taxol) are chemotherapeutic agents commonly used to treat advanced cervical cancer. They are often used in combination with radiation therapy, surgery, or both. Studies are ongoing to find the best approach to treat advanced cervical cancer.

Some patients with recurrences of cervical cancer are considered for **pelvic exenteration**, in which a large portion of the pelvic contents is removed. Unilateral leg edema, sciatica, and ureteral obstruction indicate likely disease progression. Patients with these symptoms are not considered candidates for this major surgical procedure. Surgery is often complex because it is performed close to the bowel, bladder, ureters, and great vessels. Complications can be considerable and include pulmonary emboli, pulmonary edema, myocardial infarction, cerebral vascular accident, hemorrhage, sepsis, small bowel obstruction, fistula formation, urinary obstruction of ileal conduit, bladder dysfunction, and pyelonephritis, most often in the first 18 months. Vein constriction must be avoided postoperatively. Patients with varicose

TABLE 43•2 International Classification of Carcinoma of the Uterine Cervix

Stage of Lesion	Size and Description
Preinvasive	
Stage 0	**Carcinoma in situ; cancer limited to epithelial layer; no evidence of invasion**
Invasive	
Stage I	**Carcinoma strictly confined to cervix**
Stage Ia	Microinvasive; identified only microscopically
Stage Ia1	Invasion no greater than 3 mm in depth and no wider than 7 mm
Stage Ia2	Invasion > 3 mm and no greater than 5 mm and no wider than 7 mm
Stage Ib	Clinical lesions confined to cervix or preclinical lesions > stage Ia
Stage Ib1	Clinical lesions no greater than 4 cm in size
Stage Ib2	Clinical lesions > 4 cm in size
Stage II	**Carcinoma extends beyond the cervix but not onto the pelvic wall**
Stage IIa	Vaginal extension only (not illustrated)
Stage IIb	Paracervical extension with or without vaginal involvement
Stage III	**Carcinoma extends to one or both pelvic walls** Involves lower third of vagina. One or both ureters obstructed by the tumor on IV urogram
Stage IIIa	No extension onto the pelvic wall
Stage IIIb	Extension onto the pelvic wall or hydronephrosis or nonfunctioning kidney, or both
Stage IV	**Extension of carcinoma beyond the true pelvis** Clinical involvement of the mucosa of the bladder or rectum
Stage IVa	Spread of carcinoma to adjacent organs
Stage IVb	Spread to distant organs

Examples

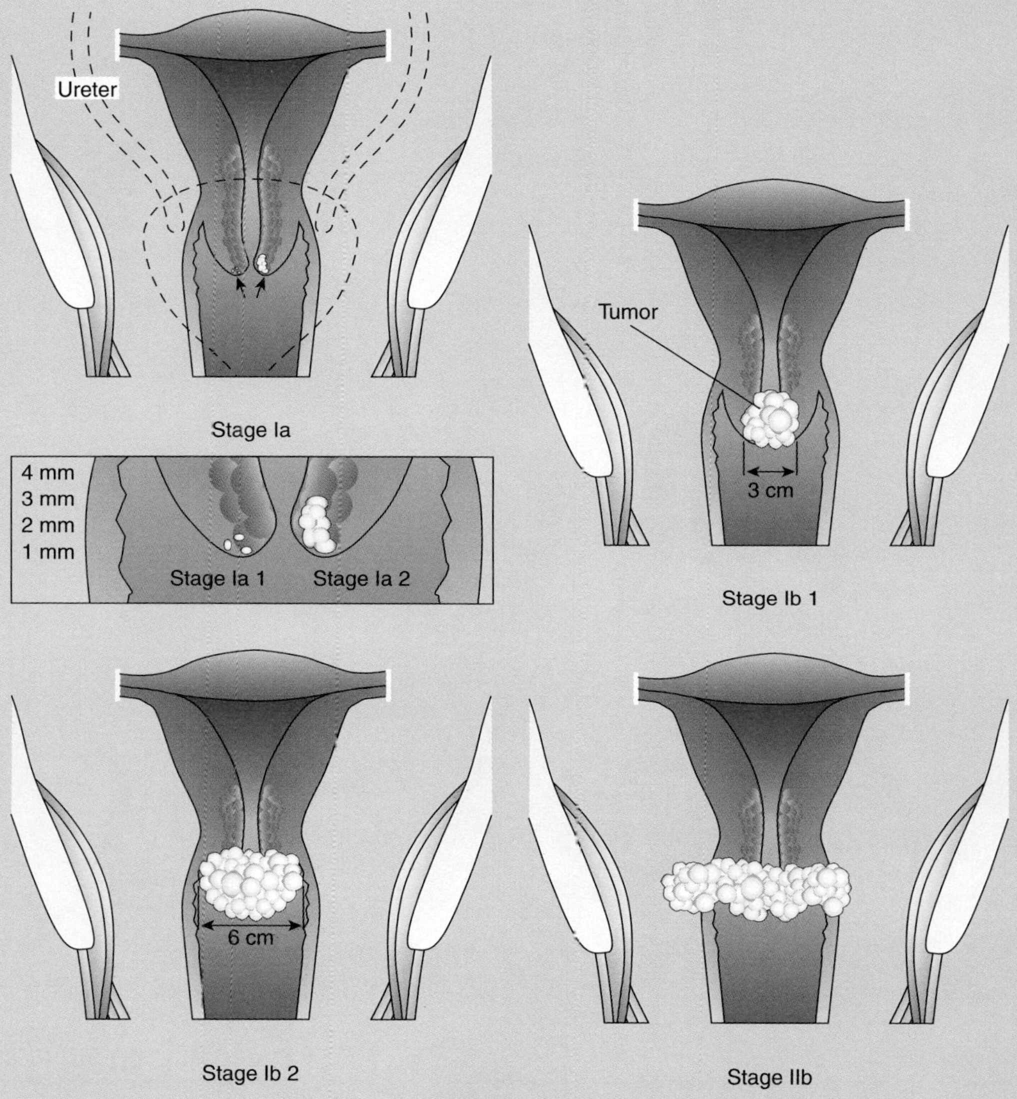

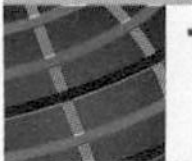

TABLE 43•2 International Classification of Carcinoma of the Uterine Cervix *(Continued)*

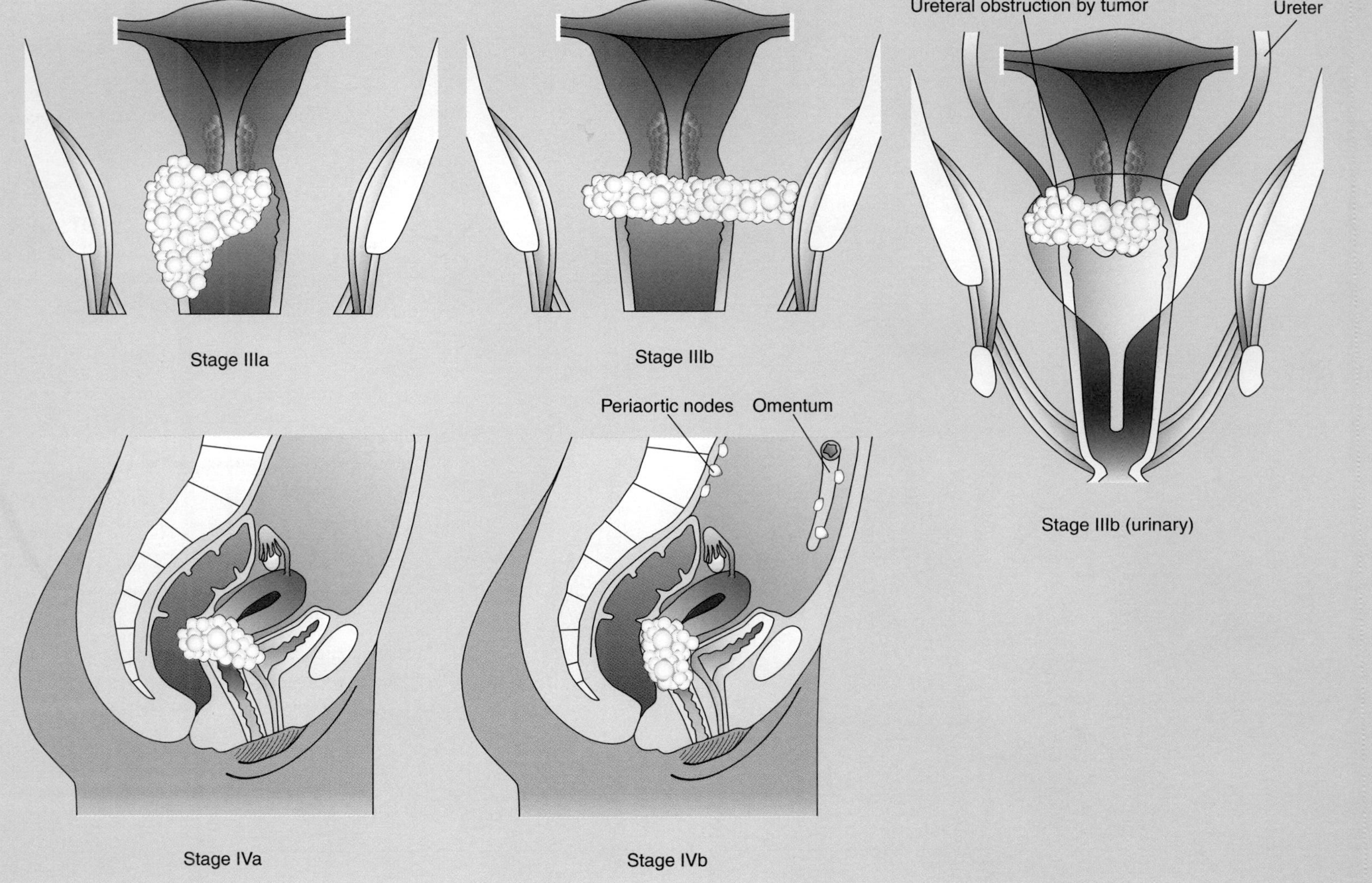

Stage IIIa
Stage IIIb
Ureteral obstruction by tumor
Ureter
Stage IIIb (urinary)
Periaortic nodes
Omentum
Stage IVa
Stage IVb

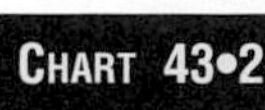 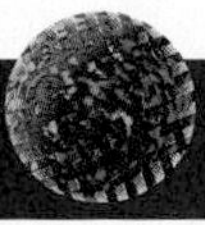

CHART 43•2 Surgical Procedures for Cervical Cancer

Surgical procedures that may be carried out to treat cervical cancer include the following:

Total hysterectomy—removal of the uterus, cervix, and ovaries

Radical hysterectomy—removal of the uterus, adnexa, proximal vagina, and bilateral lymph nodes through an abdominal incision (*Note:* "radical" indicates that an extensive area of the paravaginal, paracervical, parametrial, and uterosacral tissues is removed with the uterus.)

Radical vaginal hysterectomy—vaginal removal of the uterus, adnexa, and proximal vagina

Bilateral pelvic lymphadenectomy—removal of the common iliac, external iliac, hypogastric, and obturator lymphatic vessels and nodes

Pelvic exenteration—removal of the pelvic organs, including the bladder or rectum and pelvic lymph nodes, and construction of diversional conduit, colostomy, and vagina

veins or a history of thromboembolic disease may be treated prophylactically with heparin. Pneumatic compression stockings are prescribed. Nursing care of these patients is complex and requires coordination and care by experienced health care professionals. Mortality from this surgery is less than 10% and is continuing to decline.

Hydatidiform Mole

Hydatidiform mole is a type of gestational trophoblastic neoplasm that occurs in 1 in 1000 pregnancies. Delayed menses with spotting is the most common sign. Preeclampsia, a pregnancy-related complex of symptoms that includes edema, hypertension, and proteinuria, may occur. Treatment consists of suction curettage followed by serial beta-human chorionic gonadotropin levels, which usually take about 2½ months to return to normal. This condition may recur. **Choriocarcinoma** is another gestational neoplasm that usually occurs in the postpartum period.

Cancer of the Uterus (Endometrium)

Cancer of the uterine endometrium (fundus or corpus) has increased in incidence, partly because people are living longer and because reporting is more accurate. About 37,400 cases are estimated to occur annually, with 6400 deaths (American Cancer Society, 1999). Most uterine cancers are adenocarcinomas, originating in the lining of the uterus. After breast, colorectal, and lung cancer, endometrial cancer is the fourth most common cancer in women and the most common pelvic neoplasm. Among prominent risk factors are older age and increased weight.

Assessment and Diagnostic Findings

All women should be encouraged to have annual checkups, including a gynecologic examination. If they are experiencing bleeding, women who are taking hormone replacement therapy (HRT) without progesterone may be monitored by regular endometrial aspiration or biopsy to rule out hyperplasia, a possible precursor of endometrial cancer. Ultrasonography can also measure the thickness of the endometrium. A biopsy or aspiration is diagnostic.

Risk Factors for **UTERINE CANCER**

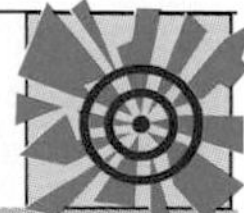

- Age: at least 55 years; median age, 61 years
- Postmenopausal bleeding
- Obesity because of increased estrone levels (related to excess weight) resulting from conversion of androstenedione to estrone in body fat, which exposes the uterus to unopposed estrogen
- Unopposed estrogen therapy (estrogen used without progesterone, which offsets the risk of unopposed estrogen) (PEPI, 1995).
- Other: nulliparity, truncal obesity, late menopause (after 52 years of age) and, possibly, use of tamoxifen

Medical Management

Treatment consists of total hysterectomy (discussed later in this chapter) and bilateral salpingo-oophorectomy. Depending on the stage, preoperative and postoperative treatments may include intracavitary radiation or external pelvic radiation. Recurrent cancer usually occurs inside the **vaginal vault** or in the upper vagina, and metastasis usually occurs in lymph nodes or the ovary. Recurrent lesions in the vagina are treated with surgery and radiation. Recurrent lesions beyond the vagina are treated with hormonal therapy or chemotherapy. Progestin therapy is used frequently. Patients should be prepared for such side effects as nausea, depression, rash, or mild fluid retention with this therapy.

Cancer of the Vulva

Primary cancer of the vulva represents 3% to 5% of all gynecologic malignancies and is seen mostly in postmenopausal women, although its incidence in younger women is increasing. The median age for cancer limited to the vulva is 44 years, whereas the median age for invasive vulvar cancer is 61 years. The incidence is higher in women with hypertension, obesity, and diabetes. More whites than nonwhites are afflicted. Squamous cell carcinoma accounts for most primary vulvar tumors. Less common are Bartholin's gland cancer, basal cell carcinoma, and malignant melanoma. Little is known about what causes this disease; however, possible increased risk may be related to chronic vulvar irritation and vulvar disorders.

Clinical Manifestations

Long-standing pruritus and soreness are the most common symptoms of vulvar cancer, but many patients have no symptoms. Itching occurs in half of all patients with vulvar malignancy. Bleeding, foul-smelling discharge, and pain may also be present and are usually signs of advanced disease. Cancerous lesions of the vulva are visible and accessible and grow relatively slowly. Early lesions appear as a chronic dermatitis; later, the patient may note a lump that continues to grow and becomes a hard, ulcerated, cauliflower-like growth. Biopsy should be performed on any vulvar lesion that persists, ulcerates, or fails to heal quickly with proper therapy.

The nurse is in an ideal position to encourage a woman to perform vulvar self-examination regularly. Using a mirror, the patient can see what constitutes normal female anatomy and learn about changes that should be reported (eg, lesions, ulcers, masses, and persistent itching). The nurse must urge women to seek health care if they notice anything abnormal because this is one of the most curable of all malignant conditions.

Medical Management

Vulvar intraepithelial lesions are preinvasive and are also called vulvar carcinoma in situ. They may be treated by local excision, laser vaporization, chemotherapeutic creams (ie, 5-fluorouracil), or cryosurgery.

When invasive vulvar carcinoma exists, primary treatment may include wide excision or removal of the vulva (**vulvectomy**). An effort is made to individualize treatment, depending on the extent of the disease. A wide excision is performed only if lymph nodes are normal. More pervasive lesions require vulvectomy with deep pelvic node dissection. Vulvectomy is very effective at prolonging life but is frequently followed by complications (ie, scarring, wound breakdown, leg swelling, vaginal stenosis, or rectocele). To reduce complications, only necessary tissue is removed.

Radiation is used to treat unresectable tumors or cancer that has spread to the lymph nodes. If a widespread area is involved or the disease is advanced, a radical vulvectomy with bilateral groin dissection may be performed. Antibiotic and heparin prophylaxis may be prescribed preoperatively and continued postoperatively to prevent infection, deep vein thrombosis (DVT), and pulmonary emboli.

NURSING PROCESS: THE PATIENT UNDERGOING VULVAR SURGERY

Assessment

The health history is a valuable tool for establishing rapport with the patient. The reason for the patient seeking health care is apparent. What the nurse can tactfully elicit is the reason a delay, if any, occurred, in seeking health care, for example, because of modesty, economics, denial, neglect, or fear (abusive partners sometimes prevent women from seeking health care). The patient's health habits are identified, and her receptivity to learning is evaluated. Psychosocial factors are also assessed. Preoperative preparation and psychological encouragement begin at this time.

Diagnosis

Nursing Diagnoses

Based on all the assessment data, the patient's major nursing diagnoses may include the following:

- Anxiety related to the diagnosis and surgery
- Alteration in skin integrity related to the wound and drainage
- Pain related to surgical incision and subsequent wound care
- Sexual dysfunction related to change in body part
- Self-care deficit related to lack of understanding of perineal care and general health status

Collaborative Problems/Potential Complications

Based on assessment data, potential complications may include the following:

- Wound infection and sepsis
- DVT
- Hemorrhage

Planning and Goals

The major goals for the patient may include acceptance of and preparation for surgical intervention, relief of pain, maintenance of skin integrity, recovery of optimal sexual function, ability to perform adequate and appropriate self-care, and absence of complications.

Preoperative Nursing Interventions

Relieving Anxiety

The patient must be allowed time to talk and ask questions. Fear often decreases when a woman of childbearing age who is to undergo wide excision of the vulva or vulvectomy learns that the possibility for subsequent sexual relations is good and that pregnancy is possible after a wide excision. The nurse must know what information the physician has given to the patient about the surgery to reinforce that information and address the patient's questions and concerns.

Preparing Skin for Surgery

Skin preparation may include cleansing the lower abdomen, inguinal areas, upper thighs, and vulva with a detergent germicide for several days before the surgical procedure.

Postoperative Nursing Interventions

Relieving Pain

Because of the wide excision, the patient may experience severe pain and discomfort even with minimal movement. Inadequate pain relief will inhibit the patient's mobility and increase the likelihood of complications. Therefore, analgesics are administered preventively (ie, around the clock at designated times) to relieve pain and increase the patient's comfort level. Patient-controlled analgesia may be used to provide pain relief and promote patient comfort. Careful positioning using pillows usually increases comfort, as do soothing back rubs. A low Fowler's position or, occasionally, a pillow placed under the knees will reduce pain by relieving tension on the incision; however, efforts must be made to avoid pressure behind the knees, which increases the risk for DVT. Positioning the patient on her side, with pillows between her legs and against the lumbar region, provides comfort and reduces tension on the surgical wound.

Improving Skin Integrity

The patient may be confined to bed for several days to promote healing of the surgical and donor sites (if skin grafts were used). A pressure-reducing mattress is used to prevent pressure ulcers. Moving from one position to another requires time; use of an overbed trapeze bar may help the patient to move herself more easily. Ambulation may be attempted on the second day.

The extent of the surgical incision and the type of dressing are considered when choosing strategies to promote skin integrity. Intact skin needs to be protected from drainage and moisture, and dressings must be changed as needed to ensure patient comfort, to perform wound care and irrigation (if prescribed), and to permit observation of the surgical site. When the patient returns from the operating room, perineal dressings are more likely to remain in place and be comfortable if a T-binder is used.

A skin graft from the buttocks may have been performed if the edges of the excision could not be approximated, and drains may have been put in place as well. A pressure stent may be applied to the grafted site to promote adhesion. Nursing care includes monitoring for suppuration (accumulation of purulent material) under the graft and assisting the patient to keep the perineal area clean and dry.

The wound is cleansed daily with warm, normal saline irrigations or other antiseptic solutions as prescribed. A transparent dressing or Xeroform gauze may be in place over the wound to minimize exposure to the air and subsequent pain. The appearance of the surgical site and the characteristics of drainage are assessed and documented. After the dressings are removed, a bed cradle may be used to keep the bed linens away from the surgical site. The nurse must protect the patient from exposure when visitors arrive or someone else enters the room.

Supporting Positive Sexuality and Sexual Function

The patient who undergoes vulvar surgery usually experiences concerns about the effects of the surgery on her body image, sexual attractiveness, and functioning. Establishing a trusting nurse–patient relationship is important for the patient to feel comfortable expressing her concerns and fears. The patient is encouraged to share and discuss her concerns with her sexual partner.

Because alterations in sexual sensation and functioning depend on the extent of surgery, the nurse needs to know about any structural and functional changes resulting from the surgery. Consulting with the surgeon will clarify which changes to expect, and referring the patient and her partner to a sex counselor may help them address these changes and resume satisfying sexual activity.

Monitoring and Managing Potential Complications

INFECTION

The location and extent of the incision put the patient at risk for infection and sepsis. The patient is monitored closely for local and systemic signs and symptoms of infection: purulent drainage, redness, increased pain, fever, and an increased white blood cell count. The nurse assists in obtaining tissue specimens for culture if infection is suspected, and administers antibiotics as prescribed. Hand washing, always a crucial infection-preventing measure, is of particular importance whenever there is an extensive area of exposed tissue. Catheters, drains, and dressings are handled carefully and with gloves to avoid cross-contamination. A low-residue diet prevents straining on defecation and wound contamination. Sitz baths are discouraged after a wide excision because of the risk for infection.

DEEP VEIN THROMBOSIS

The patient is at risk for DVT because of the positioning required during surgery, postoperative edema, and the usually prolonged immobility needed to promote healing. Elastic pressure stockings are applied, and the patient is encouraged and reminded to perform ankle exercises to minimize venous pooling, which leads to DVT. The patient is encouraged and assisted in changing position by using the overhead trapeze. Pressure behind the knees is avoided when positioning the patient because this may increase venous pooling. The patient is assessed for signs and symptoms of DVT (leg pain, positive Homans' sign) and pulmonary embolism (chest pain, tachycardia, dyspnea). Fluid intake is encouraged to prevent dehydration, which also increases the risk for DVT.

HEMORRHAGE

The extent of the surgical incision and possibly wide excision of tissue increase the risk of postoperative bleeding and hemorrhage. Although the pressure dressings that are applied after surgery minimize the risk, the patient must be monitored closely for signs of hemorrhage and resulting hypovolemic shock. These signs may include decreased blood pressure, increased pulse rate, decreased urine output, decreased mental status, and cold, clammy skin.

If hemorrhage and shock occur, interventions include fluid replacement, blood component therapy, and vasopressor medications. Laboratory results (eg, hematocrit and hemoglobin levels) and hemodynamic monitoring are used to assess the patient's response to treatment. Depending on the specific cause of hemorrhage, the patient may be returned to the operating room. The patient who experiences hemorrhage is anxious and apprehensive. Providing brief explanations of the procedures being performed and offering reassurance that the problem has been identified and is being taken care of contribute to reducing the anxiety and fears of the patient and her family.

Promoting Home and Community-Based Care

TEACHING PATIENTS SELF-CARE

Preparing the patient for hospital discharge begins before hospital admission. The patient and family are informed about what to expect during the immediate postoperative and recovery periods. Posthospital care requires giving complete instructions to a family member or significant other who will help care for the patient at home and to the home care nurse who will provide follow-up care. Depending on the changes resulting from the surgery, the patient and her family may need instruction about wound care, urinary catheterization, and possible complications. The patient is encouraged to share her concerns and to assume increasing responsibility for her own care. She is encouraged and assisted in learning to care for the surgical wound.

CONTINUING CARE

Shortened hospital stays may result in the patient's discharge during the early postoperative recovery stage. Thus, home care referral or discharge to a subacute facility may be indicated. During this phase, the patient's physical status and psychological responses to the surgery are assessed. Additionally, the patient is assessed for complications and healing of the surgical site. During home visits, the patient's environment is assessed to determine if modifications are needed to facilitate patient care. The home care nurse uses the home visit to reinforce previous teaching and to assess the patient's and the family's understanding and adherence to the prescribed treatment strategies. Follow-up phone calls by the nurse to the patient between home visits are usually reassuring to the patient and family, who may be responsible for performing complex care procedures. Communication between the nurse involved in the patient's immediate postoperative care and the home care nurse is essential to ensure continuity of care.

Evaluation

Expected Outcomes

Expected outcomes may include:

1. Adjusts to the trauma of the surgical experience
   a. Uses available resources in coping with and alleviating emotional stress
   b. Asks questions related to postoperative expectations

   c. Demonstrates willingness to discuss alternative approaches to sexual expression
2. Obtains pain relief
   a. Reports progressive decline in pain and discomfort
   b. Assumes position of comfort
3. Maintains skin integrity
   a. States rationale for use of a special mattress or other device
   b. Uses overhead trapeze to change position frequently
   c. Exhibits healing of surgical site without excoriated skin
   d. Cares for incision and surgical site as instructed
4. Exhibits positive outlook about sexuality and sexual functioning
   a. Verbalizes concerns and anxieties about sexual functioning
   b. Discusses options and alternative approaches to sexual intercourse
5. Increases participation in self-care activities
   a. Demonstrates self-care activities as instructed
   b. Identifies signs and symptoms of complications that should be reported to the nurse or physician
   c. Properly cleans the surgical site after voiding and defecation
6. Experiences no complications
   a. Is free of any signs and symptoms of infection: has normal vital signs (temperature, blood pressure, pulse rate); has no purulent discharge
   b. Identifies activities to prevent DVT: avoids crossing legs or sitting with pressure against knees; exercises ankles and legs
   c. Exhibits no signs or symptoms of DVT (leg pain, redness, edematous or swollen extremities)
   d. Demonstrates no signs or symptoms of hemorrhage

Cancer of the Vagina

Cancer of the vagina usually results from metastasized choriocarcinoma or from cancer of the cervix or adjacent organs (such as the uterus, vulva, bladder, or rectum). Primary cancer of the vagina is uncommon.

Risk factors include previous cervical cancer, in utero exposure to diethylstilbestrol (DES), previous vaginal or vulvar cancer, previous radiation therapy, history of HPV, or pessary use. Any patient with previous cervical cancer should be examined regularly for vaginal lesions.

Before 1970, vaginal cancer occurred primarily in postmenopausal women. In the 1970s, it was shown that maternal ingestion of DES affected female offspring who were exposed in utero. Benign genital tract abnormalities have occurred in some of these young women. Vaginal adenosis (abnormal tissue growth) may also occur. The risk for clear cell tumor related to DES exposure is 0.14 to 1.4 in 1000 women. Colposcopy is indicated for all women exposed to this medication in utero. If colposcopic examination discloses adenosis or a significant cervical lesion, follow-up is essential.

Vaginal pessaries, used to support prolapsed tissues, have been associated with vaginal cancer only if the devices were not cared for properly (ie, regularly cleaned and the vagina examined by a health care professional) because pessaries can be a source of chronic irritation.

Patients often do not have symptoms but may report slight bleeding after intercourse, spontaneous bleeding, vaginal discharge, pain, and urinary or rectal symptoms (or both). Diagnosis is often by Pap smear of the vagina.

Medical Management

Treatment of early lesions may be local excision or administration of a chemotherapeutic cream (ie, 5-fluorouracil applied with a tampon or a diaphragm). Cotton balls placed at the introitus lessen spillage which otherwise can result in perineal irritation. Laser therapy is becoming a common treatment option in early vaginal and vulvar cancer. Radiation is another treatment option and is delivered by external beam to the pelvis, by vaginal intracavitary radiation using a tandem and colpostats, or by interstitial vaginal implants using an obturator and vaginal template. For a tumor located in the lower third of the vagina, radical node dissection is followed by radiation.

Encouraging close follow-up by health care providers is the prime focus of nursing interventions with women who were exposed to DES in utero and who are at an age when sexuality and all its ramifications, including pregnancy, are significant. Because DES was used only from the 1940s to the 1970s, the incidence will decrease with each subsequent year. Emotional support for mothers and daughters is essential. For young women who have had vaginal reconstructive surgery, specific vagina-dilating procedures may be initiated and taught. Water-soluble lubricants are helpful in reducing painful intercourse (dyspareunia). If a lesion requiring treatment develops, all aspects and effects of radiation therapy, chemotherapy, or surgery need to be explored on an individual basis.

Cancer of the Fallopian Tubes

Malignancies of the fallopian tube are rare and are the least common type of genital cancer. Symptoms include a profuse, watery discharge and a colicky lower abdominal pain or abnormal vaginal bleeding. An enlarged fallopian tube may be found on examination. Surgery followed by radiation therapy is the usual treatment.

Cancer of the Ovary

Ovarian cancer is a very distressing disease to patients and health care providers because its silent onset and lack of warning symptoms usually result in advanced disease by the time of diagnosis. It causes more deaths than any other cancer of the female reproductive system. An estimated 25,200 new cases and 14,500 deaths occur annually (American Cancer Society, 1999). About 75% of cases are detected at a late stage.

The ovary is a common site of primary as well as metastatic lesions from other cancers. Most cases affect women between the ages of 50 and 59 years. The incidence of ovarian cancer is highest in industrialized countries, except for Japan, where its incidence is low.

A woman with ovarian cancer has a threefold to fourfold increased risk for breast cancer, and women with breast cancer have an increased risk for ovarian cancer. No definitive causative factors have been determined, but oral contraceptives appear to provide a protective effect. Heredity may play a part, and many physicians advocate biannual pelvic examinations for women having one or two relatives with ovarian cancer. Despite careful examination, ovarian tumors are often difficult to detect because they are usually deep in the pelvis. No early screening mechanism exists at present, although tumor markers are being explored. Transvaginal ultrasound and Ca-125 antigen testing are helpful in those at high risk for this condition. Tumor-associated antigens are helpful in follow-up care after diagnosis and treatment, but not in early general screening.

CHART 43•3 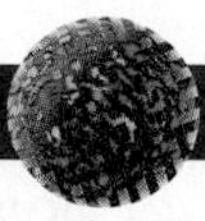 **Stages of Ovarian Cancer**

I—Growth limited to the ovaries
II—Growth involves one or both ovaries with pelvic extension
III—Growth involves one or both ovaries with metastases outside the pelvis or positive retroperitoneal or inguinal nodes
IV—Growth involves one or both ovaries with distant metastases

Advances in our knowledge of genetics are changing the approaches to detecting and treating breast and ovarian cancer. Some families have specific genes that predispose them to various cancers. BRCA-1 is a genetic mutation that results in an increased risk for breast and ovarian cancer. BRCA-2 is another genetic mutation that may result in increased risk for both female and male breast cancers and for ovarian cancer. Other mutations are also under study. Testing for susceptibility is in the early stages at centers that have expertise in genetics, testing, and counseling. Testing is indicated when a family history of three or more cases of closely related members includes premenopausal breast cancer or ovarian cancer.

One member with cancer is tested, and if positive, other members without cancer may undergo testing. Much more needs to be learned about the risks associated with some mutations, reliability of testing, and efficacy of follow-up. Confidentiality and insurance risk are ethical issues that need clarification. Because there are no primary methods of preventing breast or ovarian cancer, emotional distress is also a problem. Patients with concerns about their family history should be referred to a cancer genetics center to obtain information and testing, if indicated.

Risk factors also include nulliparity, infertility, and anovulation. Older age is a major risk factor because the incidence of this disease peaks in the eighth decade of life. Survival rates depend on the stage of the cancer at diagnosis.

Clinical Manifestations

Fifteen percent of all new cases of ovarian tumors have low malignancy potential. These borderline tumors resemble ovarian cancer but have much more favorable outcomes. Women diagnosed with this type of cancer tend to be younger, in their early 40s. Parity, lactation, and oral contraceptive use appear to be protective, while use of talc powder in the perineal region may increase risk. Symptoms are nonspecific and include increased abdominal girth, pelvic pressure, and pelvic pain. Surgical staging is individual because many women with this diagnosis are of reproductive age and may even be pregnant. A conservative surgical approach is now used. The affected ovary is removed, but the uterus and the contralateral ovary may remain. Adjuvant therapy may not be warranted for these tumors.

Ovarian cancer is often silent, but enlargement of the abdomen from an accumulation of fluid is the most common sign. Other signs and symptoms include abdominal pain, ascites, change in bowel habits, back pain, bladder changes that are similar to symptoms of stress urinary incontinence, dyspareunia, gastroesophageal reflux and postprandial reflux, irregular menses, increasing premenstrual tension, heavy menstrual flow (menorrhagia) with breast tenderness, early menopause, abdominal discomfort, dyspepsia, pelvic pressure, and urinary frequency. These symptoms are typically vague, but any woman with gastrointestinal symptoms and without a known diagnosis must be evaluated with ovarian cancer in mind. Flatulence, fullness after a light meal, and increasing abdominal girth are significant symptoms.

The combination of two major clues—a long history of ovarian dysfunction and vague, undiagnosed, persistent gastrointestinal symptoms—should alert the nurse to the possibility of early ovarian malignancy. A palpable ovary in a woman who has gone through menopause is investigated because ovaries normally become smaller and less palpable after menopause.

Assessment and Diagnostic Findings

Any enlarged ovary must be investigated. Pelvic examination does not detect early ovarian cancer, and pelvic imaging techniques are not always definitive. About 75% of ovarian cancers have metastasized by the time of diagnosis; about 60% have spread beyond the pelvis. Of the many different ovarian cancer cell types, epithelial tumors constitute 90%. Germ cell tumors and stromal tumors make up the other 10%.

Medical Management

SURGICAL MANAGEMENT

Surgical removal is the treatment of choice; the preoperative workup includes barium enema, proctosigmoidoscopy, upper gastrointestinal series, chest x-rays, and intravenous urography. Staging the tumor is important to direct treatment (Chart 43-3). A total abdominal hysterectomy with removal of the fallopian tubes and ovaries and the omentum (bilateral salpingo-oophorectomy and omentectomy) is the standard procedure for early disease.

PHARMACOLOGIC THERAPY

Chemotherapy often follows surgery, usually with cyclophosphamide, cisplatin, carboplatin, or paclitaxel. Hexamethylmelamine, ifosfamide, bone marrow transplantation, and peripheral blood stem cell support may also be used. Paclitaxel and cisplatin are most often used because of their excellent clinical benefits and manageable toxicity. Leukopenia, neurotoxicity, and fever may occur.

Paclitaxel, an agent derived from the Pacific yew tree, works by causing microtubules within the cells to gather and prevents the breakdown of these threadlike structures. In general, cells cannot function when they are clogged with microtubules and cannot divide. Because this medication often causes leukopenia, the patient may need to take granulocyte colony-stimulating factor as well.

Paclitaxel is contraindicated in patients with hypersensitivity to medications formulated in polyoxyethylated castor oil and in patients with baseline neutropenia. Adverse cardiac effects are also associated with paclitaxel; hence, this agent is not used in patients with cardiac disorders. Hypotension, dyspnea, angioedema, and urticaria indicate severe reactions that usually occur soon after the first and second doses are administered. The nurse must be prepared to assist in treating anaphylaxis. The patient should be prepared for inevitable hair loss.

Cisplatin is used frequently in chemotherapeutic treatment of ovarian cancer, both alone and in combination with other agents, and in intraperitoneal applications. Patients may require bone marrow transplantation or stem cell transplantation to treat ovarian cancer. Care for these patients is described in Chapter 15. Intraperitoneal chemotherapy with cisplatin may provide a promising mode of treatment. Other new drugs include topotecan, irinotecan, gemcitabine, vinorelbine, liposomal doxorubicin (Doxil), and docetaxel.

Liposomal therapy, delivery of chemotherapy in a liposome, allows the highest possible dose of chemotherapy to the tumor target with a reduction in adverse effects. Liposomes are used as drug carriers because they are nontoxic, biodegradable, easily available, and relatively inexpensive. This encapsulated chemotherapy allows increased duration of action and better targeting. The encapsulation of doxorubicin lessens the incidence of nausea, vomiting, and alopecia. The patient must be monitored for myelosuppression. Gastrointestinal and cardiac effects may also occur. These medications are administered by oncology nurses as a slow intravenous infusion over 60 to 90 minutes.

Genetic engineering and identification of cancer genes may make gene therapy a future possibility. Radiation may be helpful and is more useful in some types of ovarian cancer than others.

After adjunct therapies are completed, a second-look laparotomy may be performed in some clinical centers to evaluate the treatment results and to obtain multiple tissue samples for biopsy. Occasionally, catheters are left in place if radioactive agents are to be used postoperatively. Chemotherapy is the most common form of treatment in advanced disease.

Nursing Management

Nursing measures include those related to the patient's various treatment plan, be it surgery, radiation, chemotherapy, or palliation. Emotional support, comfort measures, and information, plus attentiveness and caring, are meaningful aids to this patient and her family.

Nursing interventions after pelvic surgery to remove the tumor are similar to those of other abdominal surgeries. If ovarian cancer occurs in a young woman and the tumor is unilateral, it is removed. Childbearing, if desired, is encouraged in the near future. After childbirth, surgical reexploration may be performed, and the remaining ovary may be removed. If both ovaries are involved, surgery is performed, and chemotherapy follows.

Patients with advanced ovarian cancer may develop ascites and pleural effusion. Nursing care may include administering intravenous therapy to alleviate fluid and electrolyte imbalances, initiating total parenteral nutrition (TPN) to provide adequate nutrition, providing postoperative care after intestinal bypass to alleviate an obstruction, and providing pain relief and managing drainage tubes. These conditions are complex and often require assistance and support from an oncology nurse specialist.

HYSTERECTOMY

A total **hysterectomy** involves removing the uterus and the cervix. This procedure is performed for many conditions other than cancer, including dysfunctional uterine bleeding; endometriosis; nonmalignant growths on the uterus, cervix, and adnexa; problems of pelvic relaxation and prolapse; and irreparable injury to the uterus. Malignant conditions often require a total abdominal hysterectomy and bilateral salpingo-oophorectomy (removal of fallopian tubes and ovaries).

Laparoscopically assisted hysterectomy is performed by some physicians with excellent results and rapid recovery. This method is used only for vaginal hysterectomy and is performed as a short-stay procedure or ambulatory surgery in carefully selected patients. Patients have a short hospital stay and a low incidence of postoperative infection.

The number of hysterectomies in the United States per year has stabilized at 600,000, despite an increase in the number of baby-boomers who have reached the age when this procedure is likely to be performed. The rate may be stabilizing because women often seek second opinions, and the number of therapeutic options (ie, laser therapy and medications to shrink fibroid tumors) has increased.

Preoperative Management

The physical preparation of a patient undergoing a hysterectomy differs little from that of a patient undergoing a laparotomy. Usually, the lower half of the abdomen and the pubic and perineal regions are carefully shaved and cleaned with soap and water (some surgeons do not require that the patient be shaved). The intestinal tract and the bladder need to be empty before the patient is taken to the operating room to prevent contamination and accidental injury to the bladder or intestinal tract. An enema and antiseptic douche may be prescribed the evening before surgery. Preoperative medications administered before surgery may help the patient relax.

Postoperative Management

The principles of general postoperative care for abdominal surgery apply, with particular attention given to peripheral circulation to prevent thrombophlebitis and DVT (noting varicosities, promoting circulation with leg exercises, and using elastic pressure stockings). Major risks are infection and hemorrhage. In addition, because the surgical site is close to the bladder, voiding problems may occur, particularly after a vaginal hysterectomy.

Edema or nerve trauma may cause temporary loss of bladder tone (bladder atony), and an indwelling catheter may be used. During surgery, the handling of the bowel may cause ileus and interfere with bowel functioning.

NURSING PROCESS: THE PATIENT UNDERGOING A HYSTERECTOMY

Assessment

The health history and the physical and pelvic examination are obtained, and laboratory studies are performed. Additional assessment data include the patient's psychosocial responses because the need for a hysterectomy may elicit strong emotional reactions and fears. If the hysterectomy is performed to remove a malignant tumor, anxiety related to fear of cancer and its consequences adds to the stress of the patient and her family. These women may be at greater risk for psychological symptoms, physical symptoms, postmenopausal syndrome, and increased use of health care postoperatively. Other women note improved physical and mental health after hysterectomy.

Diagnosis

Nursing Diagnoses

Based on all the assessment data, the patient's major nursing diagnoses may include the following:

- Anxiety related to the diagnosis of cancer, fear of pain, possible perception of loss of femininity, and disfigurement
- Body image disturbance related to altered fertility and fears about sexuality and relationships with partner and family

- Pain related to surgery and other adjuvant therapy
- Knowledge deficit of the perioperative aspects of hysterectomy and self-care

Collaborative Problems Potential Complications

Based on assessment data, potential complications may include the following:

- Hemorrhage
- DVT
- Bladder dysfunction

Planning and Goals

The major goals for the patient may include relief of anxiety, acceptance of loss of the uterus, absence of pain or discomfort, increased knowledge of self-care requirements, and absence of complications.

Nursing Interventions

Relieving Anxiety

Anxiety stems from several factors: unfamiliar environment, the effects of surgery on body image and reproductive ability, fear of pain and other discomfort, and, possibly, feelings of embarrassment about exposure of the genital area in the perioperative period. Conflicts between medical treatment and religious beliefs may arise as well. In such cases, the nurse needs to determine what the experience means to the patient and how to assist her in expressing her feelings. Throughout the surgical experience, explanations are given about physical preparations and procedures that are performed.

Improving Body Image

The patient may have strong emotional reactions to having a hysterectomy and strong personal feelings related to the diagnosis, views of significant others who may be involved (family, partner), religious beliefs, and fears about prognosis. Concerns may surface (such as the inability to have children and the effect on femininity), as may questions about the effects of surgery on sexual relationships, function, and satisfaction. The patient needs reassurance that she will still have a vagina and that she can experience sexual intercourse after a temporary postoperative abstinence while tissues heal. Information that sexual satisfaction and orgasm arise from clitoral stimulation rather than from the uterus reassures many women. Most women note some change in sexual feelings after hysterectomy, but they vary in intensity. In some cases, the vagina is shortened by surgery, and this may affect sensitivity or comfort.

Moreover, when hormonal balance is upset, as usually occurs in reproductive system disturbances, the patient may experience depression and heightened emotional sensitivity to people and situations. The nurse needs to approach and evaluate each patient individually in light of these factors. The nurse who exhibits interest, concern, and willingness to listen to the patient's fears will assist in the patient's progress throughout the surgical experience.

Relieving Pain

A hysterectomy may be performed abdominally or vaginally. The surgeon makes this decision based on the diagnosis and the size of the uterus. An abdominal approach is used when the patient has cancer or when the uterus is enlarged. Resultant pain and abdominal discomfort are common. Analgesics are administered as prescribed to relieve pain and promote movement and ambulation.

To relieve discomfort from abdominal distention, a nasogastric tube may be inserted before the patient leaves the operating room, especially if excessive handling of the viscera was required or if a large tumor was removed. Its excision could cause edema because of the sudden release of pressure. In the postoperative period, fluids and food may be restricted for 1 or 2 days. If the patient has abdominal distention or flatus, a rectal tube and applications of heat to the abdomen may be prescribed. When abdominal auscultation reveals resumption of bowel sounds signaling peristalsis, the patient can receive additional fluids and a soft diet. Ambulation facilitates the return of normal peristalsis.

Monitoring and Managing Potential Complications

HEMORRHAGE

Vaginal bleeding and hemorrhage may occur after hysterectomy. To detect these complications early, the nurse counts the perineal pads used, assesses the extent of saturation with blood, and monitors the patient's vital signs. Abdominal dressings are monitored for drainage if an abdominal surgical approach was used. In preparation for hospital discharge, the nurse gives guidelines for activity restrictions to promote healing and to prevent postoperative bleeding.

DEEP VEIN THROMBOSIS

Because of positioning during surgery, postoperative edema, and immobility, the patient is at risk for DVT and pulmonary embolus. To minimize the risk, elastic stockings are applied. Additionally, the patient is encouraged and assisted to change positions frequently, although pressure under the knees is avoided. The nurse assists the patient to ambulate early in the postoperative period, and the patient is encouraged to exercise her legs and feet while in bed. Additionally, the nurse assesses for DVT or phlebitis (leg pain, redness, warmth, positive Homans' sign) and pulmonary embolism (chest pain, tachycardia, dyspnea). Because the patient may be discharged within 1 or 2 days of surgery, she is instructed to avoid prolonged sitting in a chair with pressure at the knees, sitting with crossed legs, and immobility.

BLADDER DYSFUNCTION

Because of possible difficulty in voiding postoperatively, an indwelling catheter may be inserted before or during surgery and is left in place in the immediate postoperative period. If a catheter is in place, it is usually removed shortly after the patient begins to ambulate. After the catheter is removed, the patient's urinary output is monitored; additionally, the abdomen is assessed for distention. If the patient does not void within a prescribed time, measures are initiated to encourage voiding (eg, assisting the patient up to the bathroom, pouring warm water over the perineum). If the patient cannot void, catheterization may be necessary.

Promoting Home and Community-Based Care

TEACHING PATIENTS SELF-CARE

Information provided to the patient is tailored according to her needs. She must know, however, what limitations or restrictions, if any, to expect. She is instructed to check the surgical incision daily and to contact her primary health care provider if redness or purulent discharge appears. She is informed that her periods are now over but that she may have a slightly bloody discharge for a few days, after which time, if bleeding recurs, it should be reported immediately. The patient is instructed about the importance of an adequate oral intake and of maintaining bowel and urinary tract function. The patient is informed that postoperative fatigue may occur but that it should gradually decrease.

The patient should resume activities gradually. This does not mean sitting for long periods because doing so may cause blood to pool in the pelvis, increasing the risk for thromboembolism. The nurse explains that showers are preferable to tub baths to reduce the possibility of infection and to avoid the dangers of injury from getting in and out of the bathtub. The patient is instructed to avoid straining, lifting, having sexual intercourse, or driving until her physician permits her to resume these activities. Vaginal discharge, foul odor, excessive bleeding, any leg redness or pain, or an elevated temperature should be reported to her primary health care provider promptly. The nurse should be familiar with information given to the patient by the surgeon regarding resumption of sexual intercourse.

CONTINUING CARE

Follow-up telephone contact provides the nurse with the opportunity to determine whether the patient is recovering without problems and to answer any questions that may have arisen. The patient is reminded about postoperative follow-up appointments. If the patient's ovaries were removed, HRT may be considered unless contraindications exist. The patient is reminded to discuss HRT and alternative therapies with her primary care provider.

Evaluation

Expected Outcomes

Expected outcomes may include:

1. Experiences decreased anxiety
2. Accepts changes related to surgery
    a. Discusses changes resulting from surgery with her partner
    b. Verbalizes understanding of her disorder and the treatment plan
    c. Displays minimal depression or sadness
3. Experiences minimal pain and discomfort
    a. Reports relief of abdominal pain and discomfort
    b. Ambulates without pain
4. Verbalizes knowledge and understanding of self-care
    a. Practices deep-breathing, turning, and leg exercises as instructed
    b. Increases activity and ambulation daily
    c. Reports adequate fluid intake and adequate urinary output
    d. Identifies reportable symptoms
    e. Schedules and keeps follow-up appointments
5. Experiences no complications
    a. Has minimal vaginal bleeding and exhibits normal vital signs
    b. Ambulates early
    c. Notes no chest or calf pain and no redness, tenderness, or swelling in the extremities
    d. Reports no urinary problems or abdominal distention

RADIATION THERAPY

Radiation is usually the treatment of choice for squamous cell carcinoma of the cervix, depending on the stage of the cancer. In uterine and ovarian cancers, however, radiation is usually an adjunct to surgery. When radiation is the definitive treatment of cervical cancer, a combination of external pelvic irradiation and internal (intracavitary) irradiation may be used. Only in the earliest microinvasive carcinomas of the cervix is intracavitary irradiation used alone. Cure rates exceeding 85% can be expected with cervical cancer limited to the cervix alone. As the disease extends into the parametrium, the cure rate drops to about 65%. Once the disease extends to the pelvic sidewalls, however, perhaps only one third of patients are cured, although many more benefit from the palliative effects of radiation (ie, reduction in tumor bulk and control of infection, pain, and bleeding).

Side Effects of Radiation Therapy

Radiation side effects are cumulative and tend to appear when the total dose exceeds the body's natural capacity to repair the damage caused by radiation. Radiation enteritis, resulting in diarrhea and abdominal cramping, and radiation cystitis, manifested by urinary frequency, urgency, and dysuria, may occur. These effects are manifestations of the normal tissues' response to radiation therapy. Occasionally, severe reactions require interrupting treatment until normal tissue repair occurs.

The radiation oncologist and nurse must carefully inform the patient in advance of possible side effects and implement management strategies when they occur. Such measures include dietary control (restricting the amount of fiber, roughage, and lactose) and the use of antispasmodic medications. The purpose of a low-residue diet is to prevent frequent bowel movements and to avoid blockage resulting from possible constriction of the gastrointestinal tract. An oncologic nutritionist may be consulted.

Evaluating the patient's (and family's) physical, emotional, and learning needs is part of the nursing assessment before and during treatment. Information overload, along with anxiety that impairs learning, must be anticipated.

Any method of therapy requires adequate preparation, education, and emotional support. The patient who has been adequately prepared, supported, and educated before treatment through expert nursing care will find it easier to cope with the rigors and stress of cancer and its treatment.

Methods of Radiation Therapy

Several approaches are used to deliver radiation to the female reproductive system; these include intraoperative radiation therapy (IORT), internal (intracavitary) irradiation, and intracavitary brachytherapy. The cervix and uterus lend themselves naturally to internal irradiation because they can serve as a receptacle for radioactive sources.

Intraoperative Radiation Therapy

IORT allows radiation to be applied directly to the affected area during surgery. An electron beam is directed at the disease site. This direct-view irradiation may be used when para-aortic nodes are involved or for unresectable (inoperable) or partially resectable neoplasms. Benefits include accurate beam direction (which precisely limits the radiation to the tumor) and the ability during treatment to block sensitive organs from radiation. IORT is usually combined with external-beam irradiation preoperatively or postoperatively.

Internal (Intracavitary) Irradiation

The patient receives an anesthetic and is examined, after which specially prepared applicators are inserted into the endometrial cavity and vagina. These devices are not loaded with radioactive material until the patient returns to her room. X-rays are obtained to verify the precise relationship of the applicator to the normal pelvic anatomy and to the tumor. Only when this step is completed does the radiation oncologist load the applicators with predetermined amounts of radioactive material. This procedure, called afterloading, allows for precise control of the radiation exposure received by the patient, with minimal exposure of the physician, nurse, and other health care personnel. A patient undergoing internal radiation treatment remains isolated in a private room until the application is completed. Adjacent rooms may need to be evacuated and a lead shield placed at the doorway to the patient's room.

Of the various applicators developed for intracavitary treatment, some are inserted into the endometrial cavity and endocervical canal as multiple small irradiators (eg, Heyman's capsules). Others consist of a central tube (a tandem or intrauterine "stem") placed through the dilated endocervical canal into the uterine cavity, which remains in a fixed relationship with the irradiators placed in the upper vagina on each side of the cervix (vaginal ovoids) (Fig. 43-7).

When the applicator is inserted, an indwelling urinary catheter is also inserted. Vaginal packing is inserted to keep the applicator in place and to keep other organs, such as the bladder and rectum, as far from the radioactive source as possible. The objective of the internal treatment is to maintain the distribution of internal radiation at a fixed dosage throughout the application. Such applications usually last 24 to 72 hours, depending on dose calculations made by the radiation physicist.

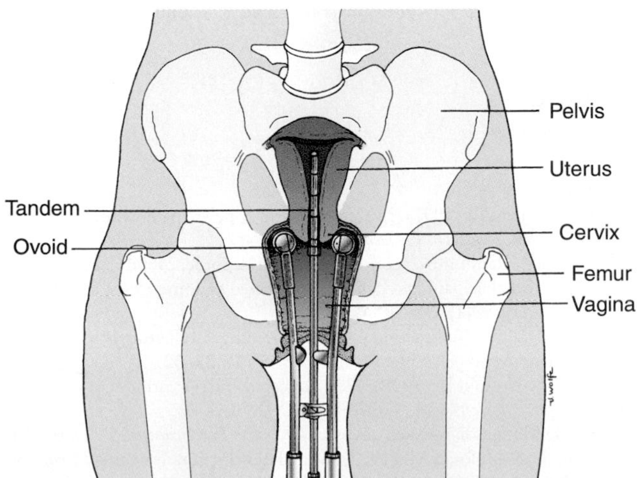

FIGURE 43•7 Placement of tandem and ovoids for internal radiation therapy. © J. Wolfe.

Automated high-dose-rate intracavitary brachytherapy systems have been developed that allow outpatient radiation therapy. Treatment time is shorter, thereby decreasing patient discomfort. Staff exposure to radiation is also avoided. Isotopes of radium and cesium are used for intracavitary irradiation.

Nursing Considerations

Various radioactive elements are used in intracavitary therapy. Regardless of the specific agent used, diligent nursing care must be provided. The patient is carefully observed, and care is provided; however, the nursing staff must minimize radiation exposure to themselves as much as possible by applying the principles of time, distance, and shielding, as follows:

- Minimize amount of time near a radioactive source
- Maximize distance from radioactive source
- Use required shielding to minimize exposure

Nurses who are or may be pregnant should not be involved in the immediate care of such patients. Visits to the patient should have a specific purpose. To minimize radiation exposure, the nurse remains as far away from the radiation source as possible (ie, at the entrance to the room) but makes special efforts to provide some time for discussing the patient's anxieties and fears.

The nurse needs to explain that during the treatment, the patient must stay on absolute bed rest. She may move from side to side with her back supported by a pillow, and the head of the bed may be raised to 15 degrees. She should be encouraged to practice deep-breathing and coughing exercises and to flex and extend the feet to stretch the calf muscles, promoting circulation and venous return. Elastic pressure stockings are important. Back care, though appreciated by the patient, needs to be performed within the minimal time allowed at the bedside.

Nursing Priorities

Of the many nursing concerns, primary concerns involve providing the patient with emotional support and physical comfort and not dislodging the applicator. Although the radiation oncologist takes steps to secure the internal applicator in place, and nursing personnel need not be preoccupied with the fear that the applicator will be prematurely extruded, they should monitor to see that the applicator or the radioactive sources have not been dislodged. Should this happen, the nurse should avoid touching the radioactive object and notify the Radiation Safety Department at once.

Usually, the patient receives a low-residue diet to prevent frequent bowel movements. In addition, a urinary catheter will be in place and must be inspected frequently to ensure that it drains properly. The chief hazard of improper drainage is that the bladder may become distended and its walls exposed to radiation. Although perineal care is not performed at this time, any profuse discharge should be reported immediately to the radiation oncologist or gynecologic surgeon.

Additional nursing interventions include observing the patient for temperature elevation, nausea, and vomiting. These symptoms should be reported because they may indicate such complications as infection or perforation.

Patient teaching includes informing the patient that abdominal fullness, cramping, backache, and the urge to void are normal feelings during therapy. Severe pain should not be experienced. Administering mild opioids, muscle relaxants, or sedatives may be helpful. The Radiation Safety Department will give specific safety precautions to those who will be in contact with the patient, including health care providers and family. Nurses caring for the patient will receive directions about safe times and distances related to care provisions to ensure that their occupational exposure is *as low as reasonably achievable* (ALARA). Other instructions vary but may include the following:

- Film badges or pocket ion chambers are worn to monitor exposure.
- Rubber gloves are needed to dispose of any soiled matter that may be contaminated. (These gloves, however, do not provide protection from sealed radiation sources.)
- Specific laundry and housekeeping directions are provided.
- The patient is restricted to her room and allowed no visitors who are or may be pregnant or who are younger than 18 years of age.
- A discharge survey is usually performed by Radiation Safety Department personnel before the patient leaves the room to ensure that all sources of radiation have been removed.

Applicator Removal

The radiation oncologist calculates precisely the radiation dose. At the end of the prescribed period, the nurse may be requested to assist the physician in removing the applicator. Because the sources are afterloaded, they can be removed by the physician in the same manner as they were inserted. This does not require local or general anesthesia and is performed in the patient's room. Medicating the patient with a mild sedative may be required, however, before removing the applicator.

Posttreatment Care

Progressive ambulation is recommended after any period of enforced bed rest. Diet may be offered as tolerated. The patient may shower as soon as she wishes but should be instructed not to douche after removal of the applicator. Because the cervix may have been dilated, any chance of bacterial contamination should be minimized.

Both before and after treatment, nurses caring for patients undergoing radiation therapy need to assess any possible misconceptions about this mode of treatment that the patient and family may have. The oncology clinical nurse specialist may be a valuable resource for information and problem-solving assistance, if necessary. Resources for further clinical and patient information are listed at the end of Chapter 15.

Critical Thinking Exercises

1.
Your 24-year-old patient has received a diagnosis of genital HPV and is very upset, stating that her boyfriend lied to her when he told her that she was his first sexual partner. What approach would you take to assist her in learning about HPV and coping with her feelings related to her relationship?

2.
How would you explain Kegel exercises to a woman? How would your explanation differ if the woman understands little English?

3.
Your 54-year-old patient is scheduled for surgery to treat cervical cancer. In discussing with her the strategies to prevent postoperative complications, you realize that her husband believes they will never be able to have sexual relations again. What approach would you take in discussing this with the patient and with her husband?

4.
During a routine pelvic examination, a suspicious vulvar lesion is detected in a 70-year-old patient. What treatment options are likely, and what are the implications for the preoperative and postoperative phases of nursing care and for home care?

References and Selected Readings

BOOKS

Agency for Health Care Policy and Research. (1994). *Management of cancer pain: Clinical practice guideline Number 9.* Washington, DC: U.S. Department of Health and Human Services, Public Health Service.

American Cancer Society. (1999). *Cancer facts and figures, 1999.* Atlanta: American Cancer Society.

Centers for Disease Control and Prevention. (1998). *1998 Guidelines for treatment of sexually transmitted diseases.* Atlanta: U.S. Department of Health and Human Services.

Carlson, K., Eisenstat, S., & Ziporyn, J. T. (1996). *The Harvard guide to women's health.* Cambridge, MA: Harvard University Press.

DiSaia, P., & Creasman, W. (1997). *Clinical gynecological oncology.* St. Louis: C. V. Mosby.

Emans, J., Laufer, M., & Goldstein, D. (1998). *Pediatric and adolescent gynecology* (4th ed.). Philadelphia: Lippincott-Raven.

Holland, J., Frei, E., Bast, R., et al. (1997). *Cancer medicine.* Baltimore: Williams & Wilkins.

Miaskowsi, C. (Ed.). (1995). *Oncology nursing.* Albany: Delmar Publishers.

Nichols, D. H., & Sweeney, P. J. (1995). *Ambulatory gynecology.* Philadelphia: Lippincott-Raven.

O'Hara, M. W. (1995). *Psychological aspects of women's reproductive health.* New York: Springer.

U.S. Department of Health and Human Services, (1994). *Put prevention into practice: Clinician's handbook of preventive services.* Washington, DC: Public Health Services.

JOURNALS

Asterisks indicate nursing research articles.

General

Hewitt, G, Brown, R. (1997). Evaluating chronic pelvic pain in adolescents. *Contemporary Adolescent Gynecology, 3*(1), 10–17.

Ling, F. (1999). Randomized controlled trial of depot leuprolide in patients with chronic pelvic pain and clinically suspected endometriosis. *Obstetrics and Gynecology, 93*(1), 51–58.

Mehring, P. (1997). Dysfunctional uterine bleeding: Evaluating this common complaint. *Advance for Nurse Practitioners, 5*(11), 27–32.

Stewart, E., & Nowak, R. (1998). New concepts in the treatment of uterine leiomyomas. *Obstetrics and Gynecology, 92*(4), 624–627.

Stine, K. (1997). Lesbian issues. *Advance for Nurse Practitioners, 5*(11), 60–62.

Vermilion, S., & Holmes, M. (1997). Sexual dysfunction in women. *Primary Care Update for ObGyns, 4*(6), 234–240.

Wathen, P. I., Henderson, M. C., & Witz, C. A. (1995). Abnormal uterine bleeding. *Medical Clinics of North America, 79*(2), 329–344.

Benign Tumors and Pelvic Conditions

(1997). Vulvar nonneoplastic epithelial disorders. *ACOG Educational Bulletin,* No. 241, October.

Richart, R. (moderator). (1997). Current management of genital warts. *Contemporary Obstetrics and Gynecology, 42*(11), 74–103.

Stringer, N., et al. (1997). Power morcellation technique for laparoscopic myoma removal. *Contemporary Obstetrics and Gynecology, 42*(12), 36–45.

Cervical Cancer

Appleby, J. (1995). Management of the abnormal Papanicolaou smear. *Medical Clinics of North America, 79*(2), 345–360.

Chapman, G. (1997). Patterns of cervical carcinoma in women of advanced age. *Journal of the National Medical Association, 89,* 801–804.

Cheng, W. (1998). Preoperative ultrasound study in predicting lymph node metastasis for endometrial cancer patients. *Gynecologic Oncology, 71*(3), 424–427.

Colletta, L. (1997). HPV in women with HIV. *Advance for Nurse Practitioners, 5*(10), 16–21.

Finan, M., & Kline, R. (1998). Controversies in the management of stage 1b cervical cancer. *Contemporary Obstetrics and Gynecology, 43*(4), 77–100.

Goodman, M. (1997). Diet, body size, physical activity and the risk of endometrial cancer. *Cancer Research, 57*(22), 5077–5085.

Higgins, P., & Smith, P. (1997). Assessing cervical cancer risk. *Lifelines, 1*(6), 43–48.

Hudson, L. (1998). Cancer of the cervix and the perioperative nurse. *AORN Journal, 11*(1), 33–35.

(1996). Cervical cancer. *National Institutes of Health Consensus Statement,* April 1–3, *14*(1), 1–38.

Neilson, A., et al. (1998). Women's lay knowledge of cervical cancer/cervical screening: Accounting for non-attendance at cervical screening clinics. *Journal of Advanced Nursing, 28*(3), 571–575.

Sankaranarayanan, R. (1998). Visual inspection of the uterine cervix after the application of acetic acid in the detection of cervical carcinoma and its precursors. *Cancer 83*(10), 2150–2156.

Shepherd, J. C., & Fried, R. A. (1995). Preventing cervical cancer: The role of the Bethesda system. *American Family Physician, 51*(2), 434–440, 443–444.

Vonka, V., et al. (1999). Prospective study of cervical neoplasia: Presence of HPV antibodies. *International Journal of Cancer, 80*(3), 339–444.

Hysterectomy

Grover, C., Kupperman, M., Kahn, J., & Washington, A. (1996). Concurrent hysterectomy at bilateral salpingo-oophorectomy: Benefits, risks and costs. *Obstetrics and Gynecology, 88*(6), 907–913.

Helmkamp, B. F., et al. (1997). Radical hysterectomy: Current Management Guidelines. *American Journal of Obstetrics and Gynecology, 177*(2), 372–374.

*Lambden, J., Bellamy, G., Ogburn-Russell, L., Preece, C., Moore, S., Pein, T., Croop, J., Culbert, G., et al. (1997). Women's sense of well being before and after hysterectomy. *Journal of Gynecologic and Neonatal Nursing, 25*(5), 540–550.

Ovarian Cancer

Drake, J. (1998). Diagnosis and management of adnexal masses. *American Family Physician, 57*(10), 2471–2376.

Eltabbakh, G. (1997). Telomerase in gynecologic cancers. *Obstetrics and Gynecology, 90*(6), 1015–1018.

Lessick, M., Wickham, R., Rehwaldt, M. (1997). Breast and ovarian cancer: Genetics update and implications for nursing. *MedSurg Nursing, 6*(6), 341–349.

Mackey, S. E., & Creasman, W. T. (1995). Ovarian cancer screening. *Journal of Clinical Oncology, 13*(3):783–793.

(1994). Ovarian cancer: Screening, treatment, and follow-up. *National Institutes of Health Consensus Statement, 12*(3), 1–30.

Oriel, K., Hartenback, E., & Remington, P. (1999). Trends in United States ovarian cancer mortality. *Obstetrics and Gynecology, 93*(1), 30–33.

Qazi, F., & McGuire, W. P. (1995). The treatment of epithelial ovarian cancer. *CA: A Cancer Journal for Clinicians, 45*(2), 88–101.

Rosenthal, A., et al. (1998). Ovarian cancer screening. *Seminars in Oncology, 25*(3), 315–325.

Sharpless, N., & Seiden, M. (1998). Advanced ovarian cancer: Recent progress and current challenges. *Contemporary Obstetrics and Gynecology, 43*(4), 133–137.

Teneriello, M. G., & Park, R. C. (1995). Early detection of ovarian cancer. *CA: A Cancer Journal for Clinicians, 45*(2), 71–87.

Pelvic Disorders

Ivey, J. (1997). The adolescent with pelvic inflammatory disease: Assessment and management. *Nurse Practitioner: American Journal of Primary Health Care, 22*(2):78, 81–82, 84 passim.

Kelsey, B., Freeman, S. (1996). Identifying and treating pelvic inflammatory disease. *American Journal of Nursing, 96*(Suppl 11), 17–22.

Padian, N. S., & Washington, A. E. (1994). Pelvic inflammatory disease: A brief overview. *Annals of Epidemiology 4*(2), 128–132.

Quan, M. (1994). Pelvic inflammatory disease: Diagnosis and management. *Journal of the American Board of Family Practice, 7*(2), 110–123.

Soper, D. E. (1994). Pelvic inflammatory disease. *Infectious Disease Clinics of North America, 8*(4), 821–840.

Prolapse and Pessaries

Fritzinger, K., Newman, D., & Dinkin, E. (1997). Use of a pessary for management of pelvic organ prolapse. *Primary Care Practice, 1*(4), 431–436.

Newman, D. (1997). Pelvic Muscle (Kegel) exercises. *Primary Care Practice, 1*(4), 446.

Norman, D. (1997). Estrogen androgen therapy. *Advances for Nurse Practitioners, 5*(11), 34–37.

Reproductive Malignancy

Brown, A., et al. (1999). Cost-effectiveness of three methods to enhance the sensitivity of Papanicolaou testing. *Journal of the American Medical Association, 282*(4), 347–353.

Ferreira, S. (1998). CIN diagnosis: Emotional impact and nursing implications. *Clinical Excellence in Nursing Practice, 2*(4), 218–224.

Rajaram, S. (1998). Nonadherence to follow-up treatment of an abnormal pap smear: A case study. *Cancer Nursing 21*(5), 342–348.

Roland, P. (1997). Outpatient management of abnormal pap smears: A decision analysis. *Contemp Obstetrics and Gynecology, 42*(12), 47–52.

Woods, N. F. (1995). Cancer research: Future agendas for women's health. *Seminars in Oncology Nursing, 11*(2), 137–142.

Yarbro, C. (Ed.). (1995). Effects of cancer on women. *Seminars in Oncology Nursing, 11*(2), 78–147.

Sexually Transmitted Diseases

Andrist, L. (1997). Genital herpes: Overcoming barriers to diagnosis and treatment. *American Journal of Nursing, 97*(10): 16AAA–DDD (nurse practitioner edition).

Bonny, A., & Biro, F. (1997). Recognizing and treating STDs in the adolescent. *Contemporary Obstetrics and Gynecology, 42*(11), 37–57.

Goldenberg, W., Andrews, W., & Yuan, A. (1997). Sexually transmitted diseases and adverse outcomes of pregnancy. *Clinics in Perinatology,* 24(1):23–41.

Hutchinson, M. K. (1998). Something to talk about: Sexual risk communication between young women and their partners. *Journal of Gynecologic and Neonatal Nursing, 27*(2), 127–133.

Larkin, J., Ison, M. Toney, J., & Brokamp, K. (1997). Recognizing HIV in women. *Infections in Medicine,* February, 124–137.

Polaneczky, M., Quigley, C., Pollock, L., Dulko, D., & Witkin, S. (1998). Use of self-collected vaginal specimens for detection of *Chlamydia trachomatis* infection. *Obstetrics and Gynecology, 91*(3), 375–378.

Sacks, S., et al. (1996). Patient-initiated twice daily oral ganciclovir for early recurrent genital herpes. *Journal of the American Medical Association, 276*(1), 44–49.

Sipes, C. (1995). Guidelines for assessing HIV in women. *MCN: American Journal of Maternal Child Nursing, 20*(1), 29–33.

Structural Disorders

Holley, R. L. (1994). Enterocele: A review. *Obstetrical and Gynecological Survey, 49*(4), 284–293.

Richardson, A., Saye, W., Miklos, J. (1997). Repairing paravaginal defects laparoscopically. *Contemporary Obstetrics and Gynecology, 42*(11), 125–130.

Toxic Shock Syndrome

Hanrahan, S. N. (1994). Historical review of menstrual shock syndrome. *Women and Health, 21*(2–3), 141–165.

Darmstadt, D. (1998). Toxic shock syndrome: Diagnosis in adolescents–scarlet fever and its relatives. *Contemporary Pediatrics, 15*(2), 44–52.

Vulvar Cancer

Benedet, J., Miller, D., Ehlen, T., & Bertrand, M. (1997). Basal cell carcinoma of the vulva: Clinical features and treatment results in 28 patients. *Obstetrics and Gynecology, 90,* 765–768.

Finn, M. (1997). Advanced vulvar carcinoma. *Gynecological and Oncological Nursing, 7*(1), 47–48.

Hall, D. (1996). Lichen sclerosus: Early diagnosis is the key to treatment. *Nurse Practitioner, 21,* 57–62.

Vulvovaginal Infections

Andrist, L. (1997). Genital herpes: Overcoming barriers to diagnosis and treatment. *American Journal of Nursing, 97*(10), 16AAA–16DDD.

Goode, M. A., Grauer, K., & Gums, J. G. (1994). Infectious vaginitis: Selecting therapy and preventing recurrence. *Postgraduate Medicine, 96*(6), 85–88, 91–98.

Krohn, M. (1997). Screening tests for vaginitis. *Contemporary Obstetrics and Gynecology, 42*(12), 11–21.

Selleck, C. (1997). Identifying and treating bacterial vaginosis. *American Journal of Nursing, 97*(9), 16AAA–16DDD.

Sobel, J. D., et al. Single oral dose fluconazole compared with conventional clotrimazole topical therapy of *Candida vaginitis.* Fluconazole Vaginitis Study Group. *American Journal of Obstetrics and Gynecology, 172*(4 Pt 1), 1263–1268.

Resources

AGENCIES

American Cancer Society, 1599 Clifton Road NE, Atlanta, GA 30329; 1-800-ACS-2345; www.cancer.org

American Social Health Association, PO Box 13827, Research Triangle Park, NC 27709

Herpes Hotline at 1-919-361-8488

Endometriosis Association, 8585 N. 76th Place, Milwaukee, WI 53223; 1-800-992-3636

Herpetics Engaged in Living Productively (HELP), 260 Sheridan Avenue, Palo Alto, CA 94306

Resolve Inc. (Infertility), 5 Water Street, Arlington, MA 02174; 1-617-643-2424

Medscape: www.medscape.com (look under Women's Health)

The Cancer Journey: Issues for Survivors. A leader's guide and videotape available from the National Cancer Institute (1-800-4-CANCER)

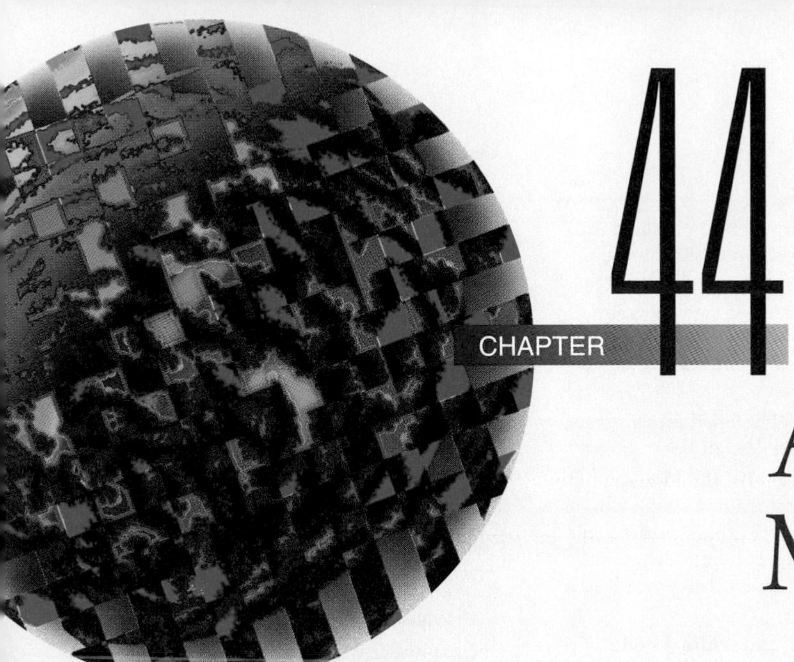

CHAPTER 44

Assessment and Management of Patients With Breast Disorders

Learning Objectives

On completion of this chapter, the learner will be able to:

1. Develop a teaching plan for breast self-examination for patients and consumer groups.
2. Describe diagnostic tests used to detect breast disorders.
3. Use the nursing process as a framework for care of the patient with cancer of the breast.
4. Compare the therapeutic usefulness of chemotherapy, surgery, and radiation therapy in treating breast cancer.
5. Describe the physical, psychosocial, and rehabilitative needs of the patient who has had breast surgery for the treatment of breast cancer.

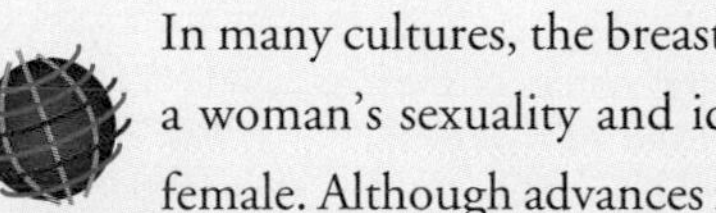

In many cultures, the breast plays a significant role in a woman's sexuality and identification of herself as female. Although advances in the diagnosis and treatment of breast disorders are changing the prognosis for breast disease and cancer, women's responses to possible breast disease include fear of disfigurement, loss of sexual attractiveness, and fear of death. The woman with breast disease may undergo diagnostic testing, surgery, radiation therapy, chemotherapy, and hormonal therapy. Thus, nurses caring for patients with breast disease must have an in-depth understanding of these treatment modalities and expert assessment and clinical skills to address physical and psychological needs of patients facing breast disorders and their families.

GLOSSARY

atypical hyperplasia: abnormal increase in the number of cells in a specific area within the ductal or lobular areas of the breast; this abnormal proliferation increases the risk for cancer

benign proliferative breast disease: various types of noncancerous, yet atypical, breast tissue that increase the risk for breast cancer

BRCA-1: a gene on chromosome 17 that, when damaged or mutated, places a woman at greater risk for breast or ovarian cancer or both, compared with women who do not have the mutation

BRCA-2: a gene on chromosome 17 that, when damaged or mutated, places a woman at greater risk for breast cancer (though less so than BRCA-1), compared with women who do not have the mutation

breast conservation therapy: surgery to remove a breast tumor and a margin of tissue around the tumor without removing any other part of the breast; may include an axillary lymph node dissection, or radiation therapy, or both

breast self-examination (BSE): a technique for checking one's own breasts for lumps or suspicious changes

ductal carcinoma in situ (DCIS): cancer cells that start in the ductal system of the breast but have not penetrated the surrounding tissue

estrogen and progesterone receptor assay: a test to determine whether the breast tumor is nourished by hormones, providing information useful in making a prognosis and determining treatment

fibrocystic breast changes: a term used to describe certain benign changes within the breast, typically associated with palpable nodularity, lumpiness, swelling, or pain

fine-needle aspiration (FNA): the removal of fluid for diagnostic analysis from a cyst or cells from a mass using a needle and syringe

galactography: the use of mammography after an injection of a radiopaque dye to diagnose problems within the ductal system of the breast

gynecomastia: overdeveloped breast tissue typically seen in adolescent boys

lobular carcinoma in situ (LCIS): an atypical change and proliferation of the lobular cells of the breast; previously considered a premalignant condition but now considered a marker of increased risk for invasive breast cancer

lymphatic mapping and sentinel node biopsy: a procedure using radiopaque dye and nuclear medicine procedures to identify and analyze the first draining lymph node from the breast within the axillary region

lymphedema: chronic swelling of an extremity due to interrupted lymphatic circulation, typically from an axillary dissection

mammography: an x-ray of the breast, and the principal method of screening and detection of breast cancer in women

mammoplasty: a surgical procedure to reconstruct or change the size or shape of the breast; can be done for reduction or augmentation

mastalgia: breast pain, usually related to hormonal fluctuations or irritation of a nerve

mastitis: inflammation or infection of the breast

medullary carcinoma: a special type of infiltrating breast cancer in which the tumor is well defined with obvious boundaries

modified radical mastectomy: removal of the breast tissue, nipple–areola complex, and portion of the axillary lymph nodes

Paget's disease: a form of breast cancer that begins in the ductal system and involves the nipple, areola, and surrounding skin

prophylactic mastectomy: the removal of the breast to reduce risk or to prevent the development of breast cancer; generally done for women considered at high risk

stereotactic biopsy: a computer-guided method of core needle biopsy useful when masses in the breast cannot be felt but can be visualized using mammography

surgical biopsy: a procedure in which tissue samples or the entire specimen is removed for examination under a microscope by a pathologist

tissue expander with permanent implant: a series of surgical procedures used to reconstruct the breast after a mastectomy; involves stretching the skin and muscle before inserting the permanent implant

total mastectomy: removal of the breast tissue and nipple–areola complex, typically used as one type of treatment for DCIS

transverse rectus abdominous myocutaneous flap (TRAM flap): a method of breast reconstruction in which adipose tissue and muscle from the lower abdomen along with their circulatory structures are transferred to the mastectomy site

ultrasonography: an imaging method using high-frequency sound waves to diagnose whether masses are solid or fluid filled

wire needle localization: a procedure used to perform a breast biopsy when the lump is difficult to palpate but can be visualized using mammography; a wire is placed into the breast under mammographic visualization, and the surgeon then removes the tissue surrounding the wire

ANATOMIC AND PHYSIOLOGIC OVERVIEW

In males and females, the breasts are the same until puberty, when estrogen and other hormones initiate breast development in females. This development usually occurs at about the age of 10 years and continues until about 16 years of age, although the range is wide and can vary from 9 to 18 years. Stages of breast development are described as Tanner stages 1 through 5, after the physician who initiated the classification of adolescent breast changes. Stage 1 describes a prepubertal breast. Stage 2 is breast budding, the first sign of puberty in a female. Stage 3 involves further enlargement of breast tissue and the areola (a darker tissue ring around the nipple), and stage 4 occurs when the nipple and areola form a secondary mound on top of breast tissue. Stage 5 is the continued development of a larger breast with a single contour.

The breast contains glandular (parenchyma) and ductal tissue, along with fibrous tissue that binds the lobes together and fatty tissue in and between the lobes. These paired mammary glands are located between the second and sixth ribs over the pectoralis major muscle from the sternum to the midaxillary line. An area of breast tissue, called the tail of Spence, extends into the axilla. Cooper's ligaments, which are fascial bands, support the breast on the chest wall. Figure 44-1 shows the anatomy of the fully developed breast.

Each breast consists of 12 to 20 cone-shaped lobes that are made up of lobules containing clusters of acini, small structures ending in a duct. All of the ducts in each lobule empty into an ampulla, which then opens onto the nipple after narrowing. About 85% of the breast is fat.

ASSESSMENT

Health History and Clinical Manifestations

When assessing a patient who describes a breast problem, the nurse should ask the woman when she noted the problem and how long it has been present. Other questions include: Is pain associated with the symptom, and can you feel any areas in your breast which are of concern? What are your **breast self-examination** (BSE) practices? Have you had a mammogram or any other screening or

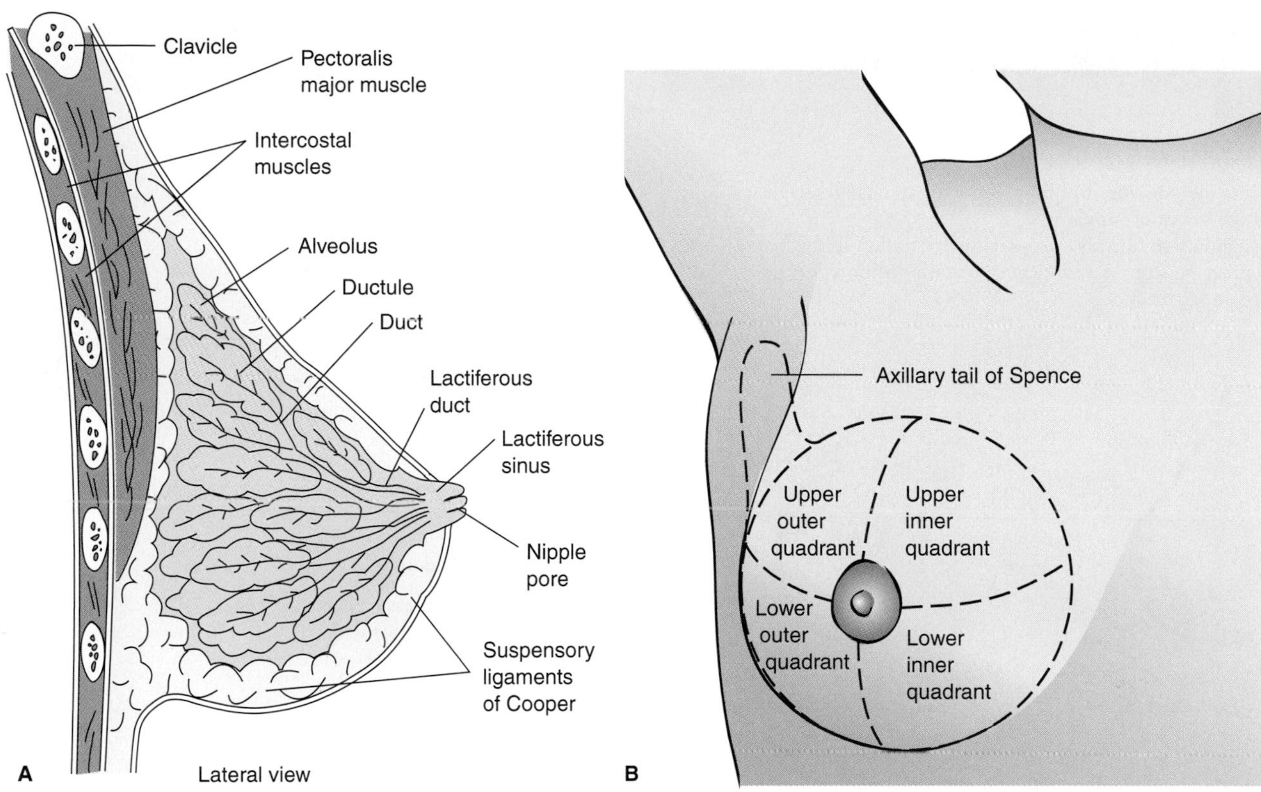

FIGURE 44•1 (**A**) Anatomy of the breast. (**B**) Areas of breast, including the tail of Spence. Adapted from Weber, J.W., & Kelley, J. (1998). *Health assessment in nursing.* Philadelphia: Lippincott-Raven.

diagnostic tests? If so, when? What follow-up recommendations have been made?

The woman is asked about her reproductive history because of its relationship to risk for breast disorders. Questions should include the woman's age at menarche, last menstrual period, cycle regularity, and use of oral contraceptives or other hormone products. Other necessary information includes her history of pregnancies, live births, abortions, or miscarriages, and breastfeeding. If the patient is postmenopausal, her age at menopause and any symptoms she experienced and current or previous use of hormone replacement therapy are also addressed.

General health assessment includes the patient's use of tobacco and alcohol. Her medical and surgical history is important to obtain along with any family history of diseases, particularly cancer. Social information, such as marital status, occupation, and the availability of resources and support persons, should also be elicited.

Psychosocial Implications of Breast Disease

Because of the significant role of the breast in women's sexuality, responses to any actual or suspected disease may include fear, anxiety, and depression. Specific responses may include fears of disfigurement, loss of sexual attractiveness, abandonment by partner, and death. These fears may cause some women to delay seeking health care for evaluation of a possible breast problem. Alternatively, some women's anxiety or fear regarding breast cancer may cause them to seek the services of a health care provider for the slightest change or problem.

In response to these reactions, the nurse's role is to identify the patient's concerns, anxieties, and fears. Patient education and psychosocial support become key nursing interventions. Assessment of the woman's concerns related to breast care and her responses to a potential problem is important whether the problem is benign or a potential malignancy. Nurses can help women through the potentially frightening visit to the primary health care provider or surgeon. Because of underlying fears about a breast problem, anxiety management is a valuable intervention, and the nurse's calm, caring demeanor, along with astute listening skills and concrete direction and guidance, can decrease a woman's anxiety during the process.

Physical Assessment: Female Breast

Examination of the female breast can be conducted during any general physical or gynecologic examination or whenever the patient suspects, reports, or fears breast disease. A clinical breast examination is recommended at least every 3 years for women between the ages of 20 and 40 years, and then annually. A thorough breast examination, including instruction in BSE, takes at least 10 minutes or more.

Inspection

Examination begins with inspection. The patient disrobes to the waist and sits in a comfortable position facing the examiner. The breasts are inspected for size and symmetry. A slight variation in the size of each breast is common and generally a normal finding. The skin is inspected for color, venous pattern, and thickening or edema. Erythema (redness) may indicate benign local inflammation or superficial lymphatic invasion by a neoplasm. A prominent venous pattern can signal increased blood supply required by a tumor. Edema and pitting of the skin may result from a neoplasm blocking lymphatic drainage and giving the skin an orange-peel appearance (peau d'orange), a classic sign of advanced breast cancer. (Examples of abnormal breast findings can be found in Abnormal Breast Findings).

ASSESSMENT
ABNORMAL BREAST FINDINGS

Retraction Signs

- Signs include skin dimpling, creasing, or changes in the contour of the breast or nipple
- Secondary to fibrosis or scar tissue formation in the breast
- Retraction signs may appear only with position changes or with breast palpation.

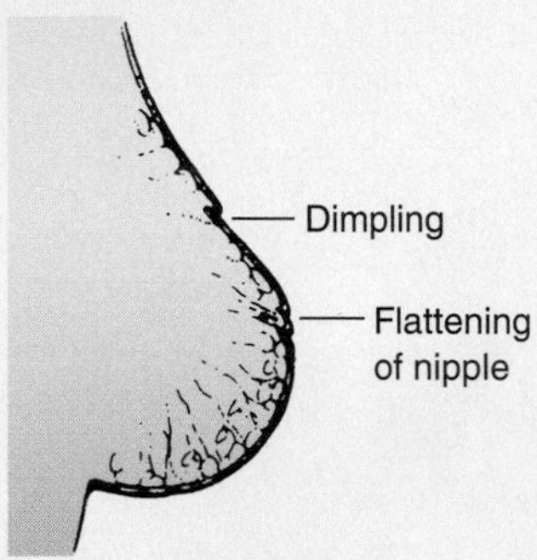

Retraction signs

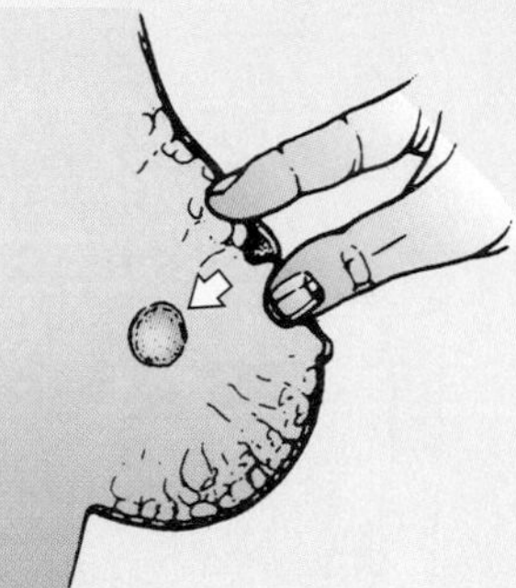

Retraction with compression

Breast Cancer Mass (Malignant Tumor)

- Usually occurs as a single mass (lump) in one breast
- Usually nontender
- Irregular shape
- Firm, hard, embedded in surrounding tissue
- Referral and biopsy indicated for definitive diagnosis

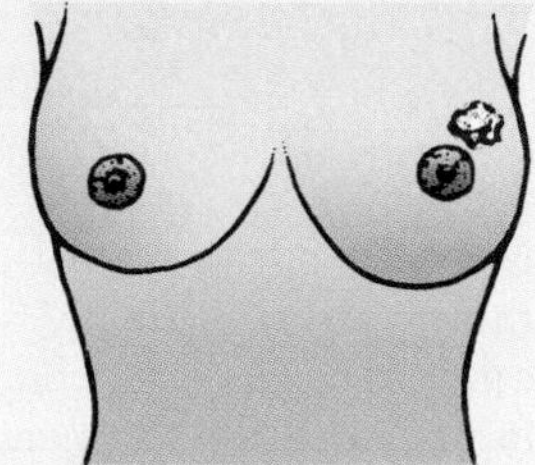

Breast cancer mass

Breast Cyst (Benign Mass of Fibrocystic Disease)

- Occur as single or multiple lumps in one or both breasts
- Usually tender (omitting caffeine reduces tenderness); tenderness increases during premenstrual period
- Round shape
- Soft or firm, mobile
- Referral and biopsy indicated for definitive diagnosis, especially for first mass; later masses may be evaluated over time by a specialist

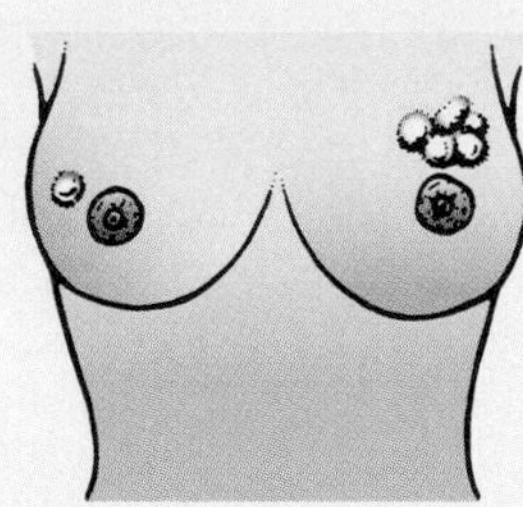

Breast cysts

Fibroadenoma (Benign Breast Lump)

- Usually occurs as a single mass in women aged 15–35 years
- Usually nontender
- May be round or lobular
- Firm, mobile, and not fixed to breast tissue or chest wall
- No premenstrual changes
- Referral and biopsy indicated for definitive diagnosis

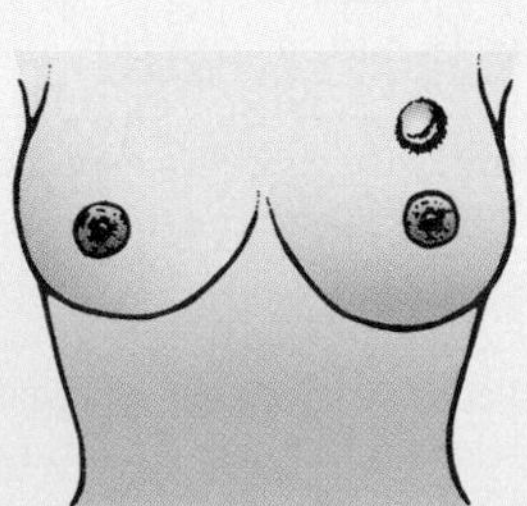

Fibroadenoma

Increased Venous Prominence

- Associated with breast cancer if unilateral
- Unilateral localized increase in venous pattern associated with malignant tumors
- Normal with breast enlargement associated with pregnancy and lactation if bilateral and bilateral symmetry

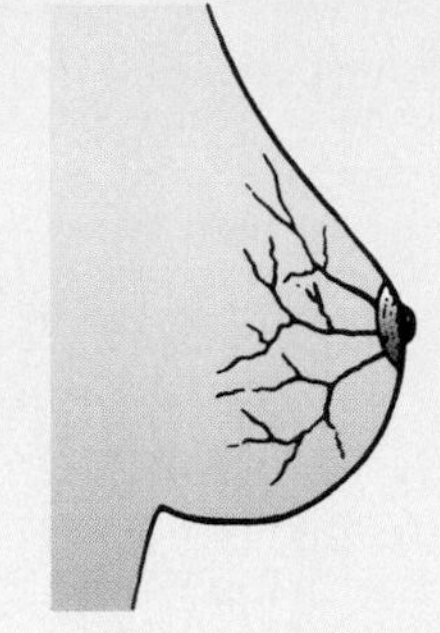

Increased venous prominence

Peau d'Orange (Edema)

- Associated with breast cancer
- Caused by interference with lymphatic drainage
- Breast skin has orange peel appearance
- Skin pores enlarge
- May be noted on the areola
- Skin becomes thick, hard, immobile
- Skin discoloration may occur

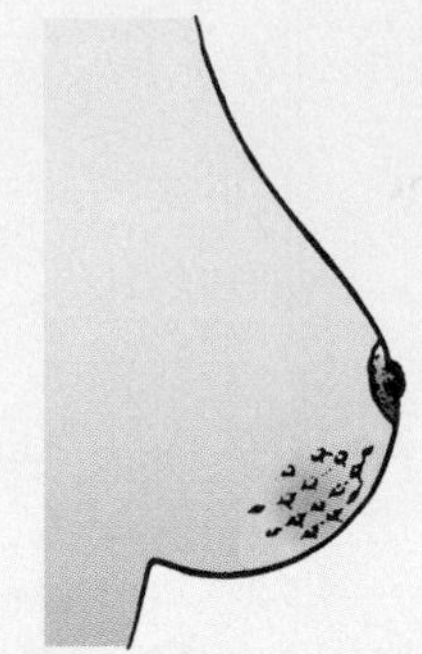

Peau d'orange

Nipple Inversion

- Considered normal if longstanding
- Associated with fibrosis and malignancy if recent development

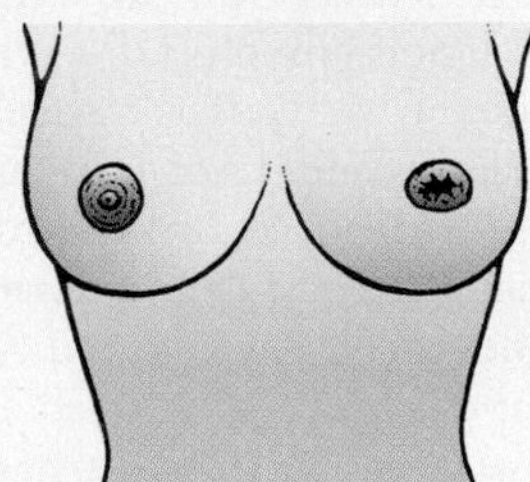

Nipple inversion

Acute Mastitis (Inflammation of the Breasts)

- Associated with lactation but may occur at any age
- Nipple cracks or abrasions noted
- Breast skin reddened and warm to touch
- Tenderness
- Systemic signs include fever and increased pulse

Paget's Disease (Malignancy of Mammary Ducts)

- Early signs: erythema of nipple and areola
- Late signs: thickening, scaling, and erosion of the nipple and areola

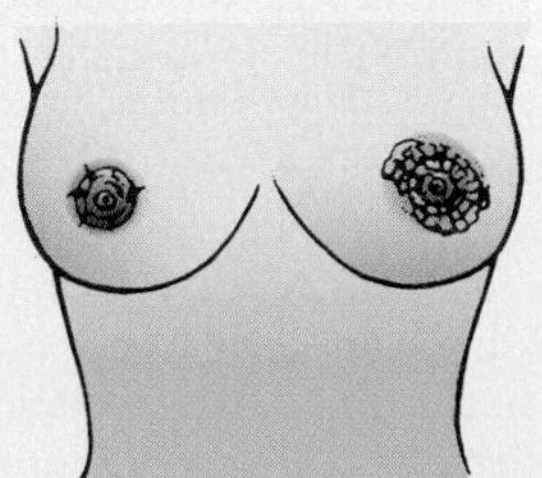

Paget's disease

Although the appearance of the nipple–areola complex varies greatly between patients, for individual women, the two are generally similar in size and shape. Inversion of one or both is not uncommon and is a significant finding only when of recent origin. Ulceration, rashes, or spontaneous nipple discharge requires evaluation. To elicit a dimpling or retraction that may otherwise go undetected, the examiner instructs the patient to raise both arms overhead. This maneuver normally elevates both breasts equally. Next, the patient is instructed to place her hands at her waist and push in. These movements, causing contraction of the pectoral muscles, do not normally alter the breast contour or nipple direction. Any dimpling or retraction during these position changes may suggest a potential malignancy. The clavicular and axillary regions are inspected for swelling, discoloration, lesions, or enlarged lymph nodes.

Palpation

Palpation of the axillary and clavicular areas is easily performed with the patient seated. To examine the axillary lymph nodes, the examiner gently abducts the patient's arm from the thorax. The patient's left forearm is grasped gently and supported with the examiner's left hand. The right hand is then free to palpate the axillae and note any lymph nodes that may be lying against the thoracic wall. The flat parts of the fingertips are used to gently palpate the areas of the central, lateral, subscapular, and pectoral nodes (Fig. 44-2). Normally, these lymph nodes are not palpable, but if they are enlarged, their size, location, mobility, consistency, and tenderness are noted. The breasts are also palpated with the patient sitting in an upright position.

The patient is then assisted to a supine position. Before the breast is palpated, the patient's shoulder is elevated by a small pillow to balance the breast on the chest wall (Fig. 44-3). Failure to do this allows the breast tissue to slip laterally, and a breast mass may be missed in this thickened tissue. Light, systematic palpation includes the entire surface of the breast and the axillary tail. The examiner may choose to proceed in a clockwise direction following imaginary concentric circles from the outer limits of the breast toward the nipple. Other acceptable methods are to palpate from each number on the face of the clock toward the nipple in a clockwise fashion or along imaginary vertical lines on the breast.

During palpation, the examiner notes tissue consistency, patient reported tenderness, or masses. If a mass is detected, it is described by its location (eg, left breast, 2 cm from the nipple at 2-o'clock position). Size, shape, consistency, border delineation, and mobility are included in the description. Finally, the areola around the nipple is gently compressed to detect any discharge or secretion.

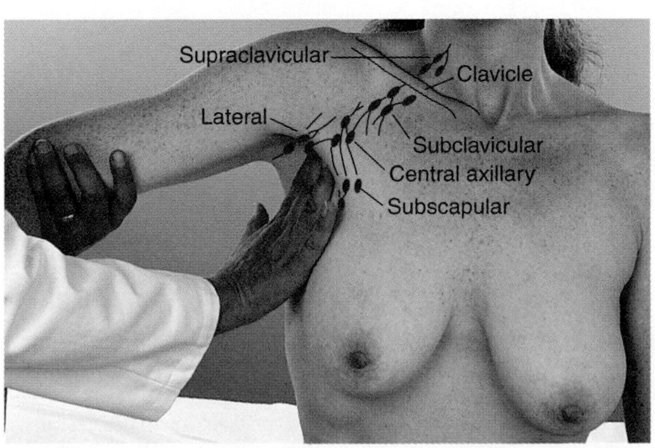

FIGURE 44•2 Palpating axillary nodes in breast examination.

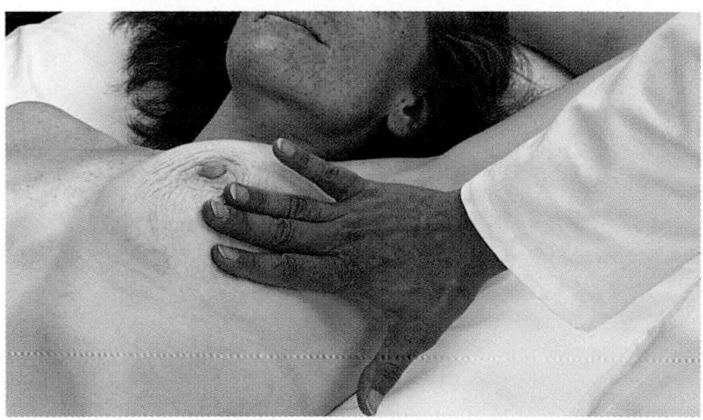

FIGURE 44•3 Breast examination with the woman in a supine position. The entire surface of the breast is palpated from the outer edge of the breast to the nipple. From Weber, J.W., & Kelley, J. (1998). *Health assessment in nursing*. Philadelphia: Lippincott-Raven.

The breast tissue of the adolescent is usually firm and lobular, whereas that of postmenopausal women is more likely to feel thinner and more granular. During pregnancy and lactation, the breasts are firmer and larger, with lobules that are more distinct. Hormonal changes cause the areola to darken. Cysts are commonly found in menstruating women and are usually well defined and freely movable. Premenstrually, cysts may be larger and more tender. Malignant tumors, on the other hand, tend to be hard, of pencil eraser consistency, poorly defined, fixed to the skin or underlying tissue, and usually nontender. A physician should evaluate any abnormalities detected during inspection and palpation.

Physical Assessment: Male Breast

Because breast cancer can occur in men, examination of the male breast and axillae is an important part of physical assessment. The nipple and areola are inspected for masses. Most cancers in men are found at a later stage, possibly because men are not aware of their risk for developing breast cancer. Treatment of breast cancer in males is similar as well.

Gynecomastia (overdeveloped mammary glands in the male) is differentiated from the soft, fatty enlargement of obesity by the firm enlargement of glandular tissue beneath and immediately surrounding the areola. The same procedure for palpating the female axillae is used when assessing the male axillae.

DIAGNOSTIC EVALUATION

Breast Self-Examination

BSE instruction can be performed during assessment as part of the physical examination; it can be taught in any setting either to individuals or groups. Instructions about BSE are provided to men if they have a family history of breast cancer because these men may be at higher risk for male breast cancer.

Variations in breast tissue occur during the menstrual cycle, pregnancy, and menopause. Therefore, normal changes must be distinguished from those that may signal disease. Most women notice increased tenderness and lumpiness before their menstrual period; therefore, BSE is best performed after menses (day 5 to day 7, counting the first day of menses as day 1), when less fluid is retained. Also, many women have grainy-textured breast tissue, but these areas are usually less nodular after menses.

Because women themselves detect many breast cancers, priority is given to teaching all women how and when to examine their breasts. It is estimated that only 25% to 30% of women perform BSE proficiently and regularly each month. Younger women, who have normal lumps in their breasts, find it particularly difficult to perform BSE because they have a harder time distinguishing normal from abnormal lumps and are not sure of what they are feeling due to the density of their breast tissue. Even women who perform BSE may delay seeking medical attention because of fear, economic factors, lack of education, reluctance to act if no pain is involved, psychological factors, and modesty.

Women should begin practicing BSE at the time of their first gynecologic examination, which usually occurs in their late teens or early 20s. All health care providers, aware of these implications, should encourage women to examine their own breasts and teach them to recognize early changes that may indicate problems. The nurse plays a pivotal role in preventive education. Almost all settings lend themselves to teaching, providing information, and encouraging appropriate care for prevention, detection, and treatment of breast problems. An individual teaching session with the patient can increase frequency of performance of self-examination.

A lesson in BSE should include the following: optimal timing for BSE (5 to 7 days after menses begin for premenopausal women and once monthly for postmenopausal women), a demonstration of examination techniques, a review of what normal breast tissue feels like, a discussion on identification of breast changes, and a return demonstration on the patient and a breast model. Patients who have had breast surgery for the treatment of breast cancer are carefully instructed to examine themselves for any nodules or changes in their breasts or along the chest wall that may indicate a recurrence of the disease.

Films or videos about BSE, shower cards, and pamphlets can be obtained from local chapters of the American Cancer Society. The National Cancer Institute in Bethesda, Maryland, offers a program that teaches nurses to instruct patients in BSE and also provides teaching aids. The National Alliance for Breast Cancer Organizations, a clearinghouse for lay materials on breast cancer education, is another resource.

Mammography

Mammography is a breast-imaging technique that can detect nonpalpable lesions and assist in diagnosing palpable masses. The procedure takes about 20 minutes and can be performed in a hospital radiography department or independent imaging center. Two views are taken of each breast: a craniocaudal view and a mediolateral oblique view. For these views, the breast is mechanically compressed from top to bottom and side to side. Women may experience some fleeting discomfort because maximum compression is necessary for proper visualization. The current mammograms are compared with previous mammograms, and any changes indicate a need for further investigation. Mammography may detect a breast tumor before it is clinically palpable (ie, smaller than 1 cm); however, it has limitations and is not foolproof. A false-negative rate ranging between 5% and 10% applies, generally greater in younger women with greater density of breast tissue. Some patients have very dense breast tissue, making it difficult to detect lesions with mammography.

Patients scheduled for a mammogram may voice concern about exposure to radiation. The radiation exposure is equivalent to about 1 hour of exposure to sunlight, so patients would have to have many mammograms in a year to increase their cancer risk. The benefits of this test outweigh the risks. Because the quality of mammography varies widely from one setting to the next, it is important for women to find accredited breast care centers that produce reliable mammograms.

Current mammographic screening guidelines from the American Cancer Society recommend a mammogram every year starting at the age of 40 years. A baseline mammogram should be obtained after the age of 35 years and by the age of 40. Younger women who are identified as at a higher risk for breast cancer by family history should seek the opinion of a breast specialist about when to begin screening mammograms. Several studies suggest that screening for high-risk women should begin about 10 years before the age of diagnosis of the family member with breast cancer (Bilimoria & Morrow, 1995; Vogel, 1996). In families with a history of breast cancer, a downward shift in age of diagnosis of about 10 years is seen (eg, grandmother diagnosed with breast cancer at age 48, mother diagnosed with breast cancer at age 38, then daughter should begin screening at age 28) (Benedict, Goon, Hoomani, & Holder, 1997). Nurses need to provide teaching about screening guidelines for women in the general population and those at high risk, so that these women can make informed choices about screening.

Screening mammography combined with physical examination and BSE have demonstrated effectiveness in reducing overall mortality from breast cancer by 30% among women between the ages of 50 and 69 years. More recent long-term studies of women aged 40 to 49 years suggest a similar benefit in this younger age group, although this remains an issue of controversy (Feig, 1997; Harris & Leininger, 1995). Despite the decreased mortality associated with mammographic screening, it has not been used equitably across the U.S. population. Some studies indicate that nearly 75% of women have had a mammogram during their lifetime, yet only 40% continue to follow current screening guidelines. Women with fewer resources (eg, elderly, poor, minority women, women without health insurance) often do not have the means to undergo mammography or the resources for follow-up treatment when positive lesions are detected. Recent studies have shown that social support contributes to adherence to mammographic screening guidelines (Lierman et al., 1994; McCance, Mooney, Field, & Smith, 1996). Many nurses direct their efforts to educating women about the benefits of mammography. Working to overcome barriers to screening mammography, especially among the elderly, is an important nursing intervention in the community, and nurses have an important role in the development of educational materials targeted to specific literacy levels and ethnic groups.

Galactography

Galactography is a mammographic diagnostic procedure that involves injection of less than 1 mL of radiopaque material through a cannula inserted into a ductal opening on the areola, followed by a mammogram. It is performed when the patient has a bloody nipple discharge on expression, spontaneous nipple discharge, or a solitary dilated duct noted on mammography. These symptoms may be indicative of a benign lesion or a cancerous one.

Ultrasonography

Ultrasonography (ultrasound) is used in conjunction with mammography to distinguish fluid-filled cysts from other lesions. A transducer is used to transmit high-frequency sound waves through

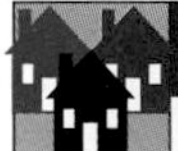

Patient Education and Home Care

Breast Self-Examination (BSE)

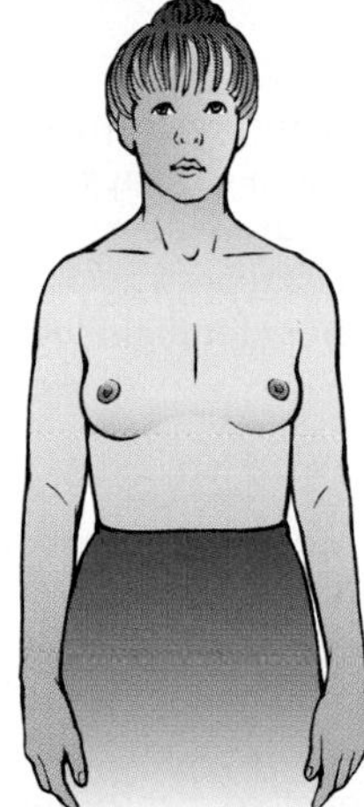

Step 1

1. Stand before a mirror.
2. Check both breasts for anything unusual.
3. Look for discharge from the nipple, puckering, dimpling, or scaling of the skin.

The next two steps are done to check for any changes in the contour of your breasts. As you do them, you should be able to feel your muscles tighten.

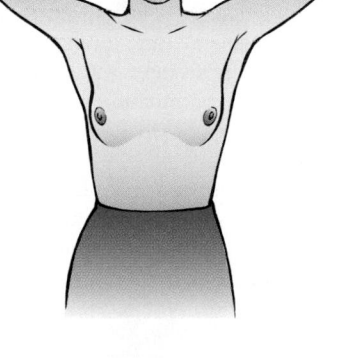

Step 2

1. Watch closely in the mirror as you clasp your hands behind your head and press your hands forward.
2. Note any change in the contour of your breasts.

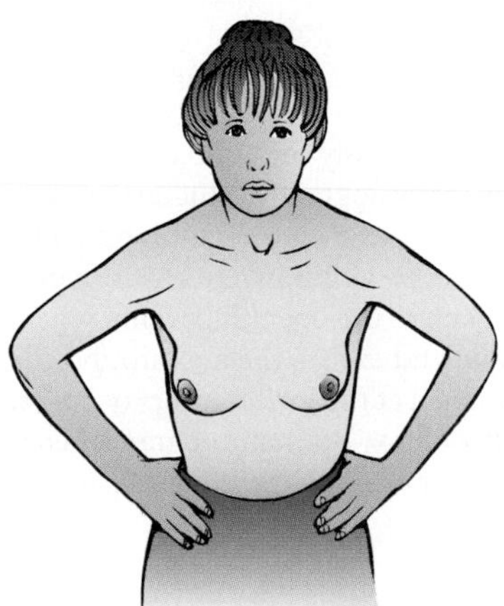

Step 3

1. Next, press your hands firmly on your hips and bow slightly toward the mirror as you pull your shoulders and elbows forward.
2. Note any change in the contour of your breasts.

Some women do the next part of the examination in the shower. Your fingers will glide easily over soapy skin, so you can concentrate on feeling for changes inside the breast.

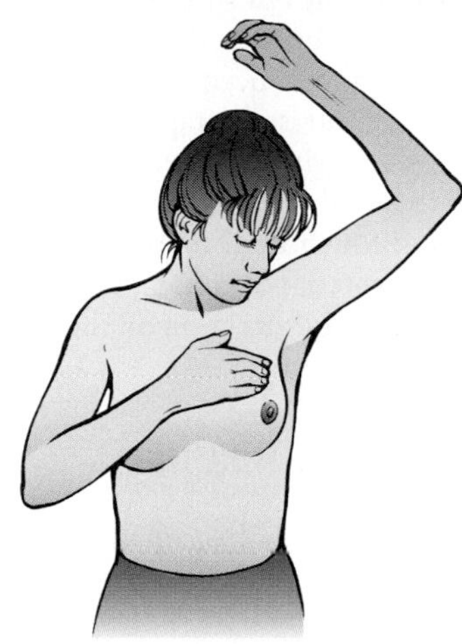

Step 4

1. Raise your left arm.
2. Use 3 or 4 fingers of your right hand to feel your left breast firmly, carefully, and thoroughly.
3. Beginning at the outer edge, press the flat part of your fingers in small circles, moving the circles slowly around the breast.
4. Gradually work toward the nipple.
5. Be sure to cover the whole breast.
6. Pay special attention to the area between the breast and the underarm, including the underarm itself.
7. Feel for any unusual lumps or masses under the skin.
8. If you have any spontaneous discharge during the month—whether or not it is during your BSE—see your doctor.
9. Repeat the examination on your right breast.

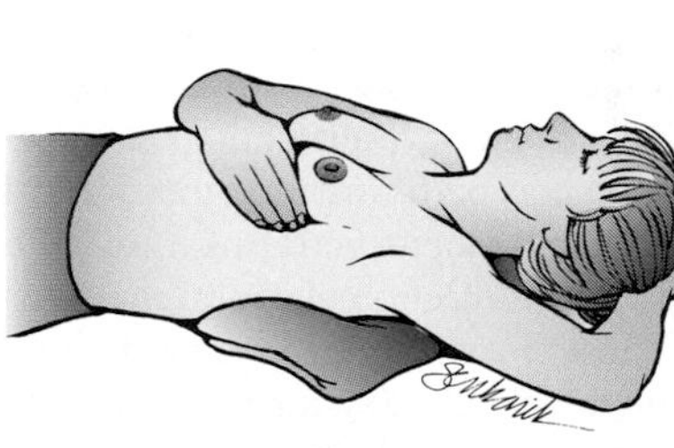

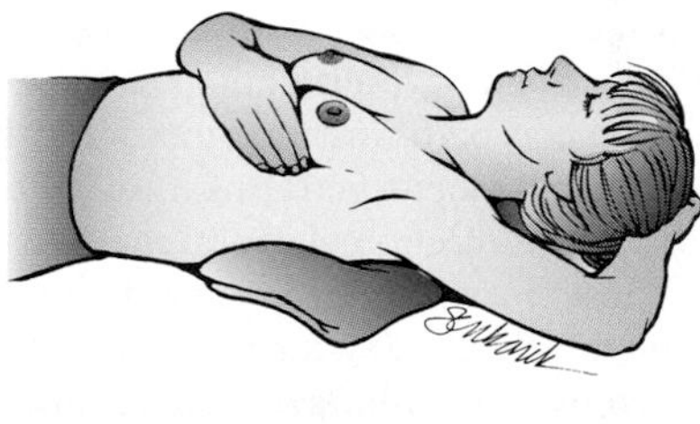

Step 5

1. Step 4 should be repeated lying down.
2. Lie flat on your back with your left arm over your head and a pillow or folded towel under your left shoulder. (This position flattens your breast and makes it easier to check.)
3. Use the same circular motion described above.
4. Repeat on your right breast.

Adapted from U.S. Department of Health and Human Services, Public Health Service, *What you need to know about breast cancer.* Bethesda, MD: National Institutes of Health.

the skin and into the breast, and an echo signal is measured. The echo waves are interpreted electronically and then displayed on a screen. This technique is 95% to 99% accurate in diagnosing cysts but does not definitively rule out a malignant lesion.

For women with dense breasts, the introduction of screening ultrasound examinations has been researched during this past decade. The addition of ultrasonography to breast cancer screening can increase the sensitivity of screening for this population of women, who tend to be either young or on hormone replacement therapy. The largest study showed an increase in cancer detection by 17% with the addition of screening ultrasonography. Further research will help provide information on the usefulness of ultrasound as a screening modality.

Magnetic Resonance Imaging

Magnetic resonance imaging (MRI) of the breast is a promising tool for use in diagnosing breast conditions. It is a highly sensitive, although not specific, test and serves as an adjunct to mammography. A coil is placed around the breast, and the patient is placed inside the MRI machine for about 2 minutes. An injection of gadolinium, a contrast dye, is given intravenously. MRI of the breast can be helpful in determining the exact size or presence of multiple foci of a lesion more precisely than mammography. It also can determine if a lesion is fixed to the chest wall more precisely than a computed tomography scan. Other uses include identifying occult (undetectable) breast cancer, determining tumor response to chemotherapy, and determining the integrity of saline or silicone breast implants. The cost of breast MRI, however, is prohibitive; therefore, it is not currently used for routine screening.

Procedures for Tissue Analysis

Fine-Needle Aspiration

Fine-needle aspiration (FNA) is an outpatient procedure usually initiated when mammography, ultrasonography, or palpation detects a lesion. A surgeon performs the procedure when there is a palpable lesion, or a radiologist performs it under x-ray guidance for nonpalpable lesions. Injection of a local anesthetic may or may not be used, but most times, the surgeon or radiologist inserts a 21- or 22-gauge needle attached to a syringe into the site to be sampled. The syringe is then used to withdraw tissue or fluid into the needle. This cytologic material is spread on a slide and sent to the laboratory for analysis. FNAs can be performed less expensively than other diagnostic methods, and results are usually available quickly, although this diagnostic test is often not 100% accurate, and the false-negative rate is substantial. False-negative or false-positive results are possible, and clinical follow-up depends on level of suspicion about the breast lesion.

Stereotactic Biopsy

Stereotactic biopsy, also an outpatient procedure, is performed for nonpalpable lesions found on mammography. The patient lies prone on a special table, and the breast is positioned through an opening in the table and compressed for a mammogram. The lesion to be sampled is then located with the aid of a computer. Next, a local anesthetic is injected into the entry site on the breast, a core needle is inserted, and samples of the tissue are taken for pathologic examination. If the lesion is small, a clip is placed at the site of the biopsy, so that a specific area can be visualized again as another mammography is performed. This technique allows accurate diagnosis and often allows the patient to avoid a surgical biopsy, although some patients may end up needing a surgical biopsy depending on the pathologic diagnosis.

Surgical Biopsy

Surgical biopsy is the most common outpatient surgical procedure. It is important to note that 8 out of 10 lesions on biopsy are benign. The procedure is usually done using local anesthesia, conscious (or monitored) sedation, or both. The biopsy involves excising the lesion and sending it to the laboratory for pathologic examination.

EXCISIONAL BIOPSY

Excisional biopsy is the usual procedure for any palpable breast mass. The entire lesion with a margin of surrounding tissue is removed. This type of biopsy may also be referred to as a lumpectomy. Depending on the clinical situation, a frozen section (a small piece of the mass or lesion is given a provisional diagnosis by the pathologist) may be done at the time of the biopsy, so that the surgeon can provide the patient with a diagnosis in the recovery room.

INCISIONAL BIOPSY

Incisional biopsy is performed when tissue sampling alone is required, and this is done both to confirm a diagnosis and to determine hormonal receptor status. Complete excision of the area may not be possible or immediately beneficial to the patient, depending on the clinical situation. This procedure is often performed in women with locally advanced breast cancer or in cancer patients with a suspicion of recurrent disease, whose treatment may depend on the tumor's estrogen and progesterone receptor status. These receptors are identified during pathologic examination of the tissue.

TRU-CUT CORE BIOPSY

In Tru-Cut core biopsy, the surgeon uses a special large-lumen needle to remove a core of tissue. This procedure is used when a tumor is relatively large and close to the skin surface and the surgeon strongly suspects that the lesion is a carcinoma. If cancer is diagnosed, the tissue is also tested for hormone receptor status.

WIRE NEEDLE LOCALIZATION

Wire needle localization is a technique used when mammography detects minute, pinpoint calcifications (indicating a potential malignancy) or nonpalpable lesions and a biopsy is necessary. A long, thin wire is inserted, usually painlessly, through a needle before the excisional biopsy under mammographic guidance to ensure that the wire tip designates the area to undergo biopsy. The wire remains in place after the needle is withdrawn to ensure a precise biopsy. The patient is then taken to the operating room, where the surgeon follows the wire down and excises the area around the wire tip. The tissue removed is x-rayed at the time of the procedure; these specimen x-rays, along with follow-up mammograms taken several weeks later (after the site has healed), verify that the area of concern was located and removed.

OVERVIEW OF BREAST CONDITIONS AND DISEASES

Not all disorders of the breast are cancerous. Some disorders are structural, such as fissure, or infection related, such as mastitis. Some conditions may progress from a benign to a malignant condition, such as benign proliferative breast disease; and some problems are clearly cancer of various kinds in various stages.

CONDITIONS AFFECTING THE NIPPLE

Fissure

A fissure is a longitudinal ulcer that tends to develop in breast-feeding women. If the nipple becomes irritated, a painful, raw area may form and become a site of infection. Daily washing with water, massage with breast milk or lanolin, and exposure to air are helpful. Breastfeeding can continue with a nipple shield, if necessary. If the fissure is severe or extremely painful, the woman is advised to stop breastfeeding; a breast pump can be used until the breastfeeding can be resumed. Persistent ulceration requires further diagnostic and therapeutic approaches. Guidance with breast-feeding from a nurse or lactation consultant may be helpful because nipple irritation can result from improper positioning (ie, the infant has not grasped the areola fully).

Breast Discharge

Breast discharge in a woman who is not lactating may be related to many causes. Carcinoma, papilloma, pituitary adenoma, cystic breasts, and various medications can result in a discharge of fluid from the nipple. Oral contraceptives, pregnancy, hormone replacement therapy, chlorpromazine-type medications, and frequent breast stimulation may be contributing factors. In some athletic women, breast discharge may occur during running or aerobic exercises. Breast discharge should be evaluated by the patient's health care provider, but it is not often a cause for alarm. One in three women have clear discharge on expression, which is usually normal. Causes for concern are green discharge, which usually indicates infection, and brown or red discharge, which is indicative of a problem. Spontaneous discharge should *always* be evaluated because it is not normal, unless a woman is lactating. The discharge is examined for fat globules to determine if it is breast milk. It is also tested for occult blood because malignancy must be considered.

Bleeding or Bloody Nipple Discharge

At times, a bloody discharge may be produced when pressure is placed on one area at the edge of the areola. Although a bloody discharge can signal a malignancy, it usually results from a wart-like, benign epithelial tumor or papilloma growing in one of the large collecting ducts just at the edge of the areola or in an area of cystic disease. Bleeding occurs with any trauma, and the blood collects in the duct until it is pressed out at the nipple. Treatment includes excision of the duct with the papilloma. Such a lesion is usually benign, but it should be evaluated histologically after it is removed to rule out malignancy.

BREAST INFECTIONS

Mastitis

Mastitis is an inflammation or infection of breast tissue and occurs most commonly in breastfeeding women, although it may also occur in nonlactating women. The infection may result from a transfer of microorganisms to the breast by the patient's hands or those of others or from a breastfed infant with an oral, eye, or skin infection. Mastitis may also be caused by bloodborne organisms. As inflammation progresses, an infection of the ducts results, causing milk to stagnate in one or more of the lobules. The breast texture becomes tough or doughy, and the patient complains of dull pain in the infected region.

A nipple that is discharging purulent material, serum, or blood needs to be investigated.

Treatment consists of antibiotics and local heat. A broad-spectrum antibiotic may be prescribed for 7 to 10 days. The patient should wear a snug bra and perform personal hygiene carefully. Adequate rest and hydration are important aspects of management.

Lactational Abscess

A breast abscess may develop as a consequence of acute mastitis. In such a case, the area affected becomes tender and red. Purulent matter can usually be expressed from the nipple, and incision and drainage are usually required. At the time of drainage, specimens are obtained for culture.

BENIGN CONDITIONS OF THE BREAST

Benign breast lesions include fibrocystic changes, fibroadenomas, and cysts.

Fibrocystic Breast Changes

Fibrocystic breast changes occur as ducts dilate and cysts form. This condition occurs most commonly in women between the ages of 30 and 50 years. Although the cause is unknown, estrogen appears to be a factor because cysts usually disappear after menopause. Cystic areas often fluctuate in size, depending on the menstrual cycle. They are usually larger premenstrually and smaller postmenstrually because of the retention of fluid in the days preceding the menstrual period. The cysts may be painless or may become very tender premenstrually. Occasionally, a patient may report breast pain, which is usually intermittent and can be shooting or a dull ache (see Table 44-1 for a description of various breast masses). Breast pain (**mastalgia**) is usually related to hormonal fluctuations and their effect on the breasts or is stimulated by irritation of a nerve in the chest wall from an activity such as weight-training.

Medical Management

If pain and tenderness are severe, danazol (Danocrine) may be prescribed; this agent has an antiestrogenic effect, therefore decreasing breast pain and nodularity. Danazol is used only in severe cases because of its potential side effects, which include flushing, vaginitis, and androgenic changes (virilization).

Nursing Management

The nurse may recommend that the patient wear a supportive bra both day and night for a week except during bathing, decrease salt and caffeine intake, and take ibuprofen (Motrin) as needed for its anti-inflammatory actions. Vitamin E supplements or oil of evening primrose (an over-the-counter herbal preparation) may also be helpful, but this recommendation is based on anecdotal information from patients, not on research.

If diuretics or oral contraceptives are prescribed, the patient should know that symptoms usually recur after these medications are discontinued. Patients should also be reassured that breast pain is rarely indicative of cancer in its early stages. If the pain is not relieved after menses begin, however, the woman should see her primary health care provider.

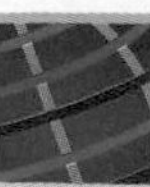

TABLE 44•1 Variations in Breast Masses

The most common breast masses are due to fibrocystic changes, fibroadenomas, or malignancy. Biopsy is usually needed for confirmation, but the following characteristics are diagnostic clues:

Characteristics	Fibrocystic Changes	Fibroadenomas	Malignancy
(Illustrations show how the lump may feel because it is usually not visible.)			
Age	30–60 years, regress after menopause except with estrogen therapy	Puberty to menopause	30–90 years; most common, 40–80 years
Number	Single or multiple	Usually single	Usually single
Shape	Round	Round, disk, or lobular	Irregular or stellate
Consistency	Soft to firm, usually elastic	Usually firm	Firm or hard
Mobility	Mobile	Mobile	May be fixed to skin or underlying tissues
Tenderness	Usually tender	Usually nontender	Usually nontender
Retraction signs	Absent	Absent	May be present

Fibroadenomas

Fibroadenomas are firm, round, movable, benign tumors of the breast that usually affect women in their late teens to late 30s. These masses are nontender and are sometimes removed for diagnostic certainty.

Other Benign Conditions

Cystosarcoma phyllodes is a fibroepithelial lesion that tends to grow rapidly. It is rarely malignant and is surgically excised. If it is malignant, mastectomy may follow. Fat necrosis is a rare condition of the breast that is often related to trauma from a blow; however, it may be indistinguishable from carcinoma and the entire mass is usually excised.

Gigantomastia or macromastia (overly large breasts) is a problem for some women. Weight loss and various medications have been tried to little avail. Reduction mammoplasty (discussed later in this chapter) is an elective procedure for the patient who is physically or emotionally distressed by this condition. Superficial thrombophlebitis of the breast (Mondor's disease) is an uncommon condition that is usually associated with pregnancy, trauma, or breast surgery. Pain and redness occur as a result of a superficial thrombophlebitis in the vein that drains the outer part of the breast. The mass is usually linear, tender, and erythematous. Treatment consists of analgesics and heat.

Benign Proliferative Breast Disease

The two most common diagnoses of **benign proliferative breast disease** found on biopsy are atypical hyperplasia and lobular carcinoma in situ. Both of these diagnoses increase a woman's risk for the development of breast cancer. **Atypical hyperplasia** is an abnormal increase in the ductal or lobular cells in the breast and is usually found incidentally in mammographic abnormalities. Atypical hyperplasia increases a woman's risk for breast cancer about 10% to 20% over a period of 10 years; the risk is greater for premenopausal women and decreases significantly after menopause. **Lobular carcinoma in situ** (LCIS) is usually an incidental finding in breast tissue because it cannot be seen on mammography and does not form a palpable lump. Historically, LCIS was considered a premalignant condition, and treatment consisted of a bilateral prophylactic mastectomy; however, current research indicates that LCIS is a marker for the risk for invasive breast cancer, which can either be ductal or lobular in origin and can develop in either breast. LCIS increases a woman's risk for breast cancer by about 30% to 40% over a period of 25 years, and the risk does not diminish with time.

Medical Management

After a woman has been diagnosed with a benign proliferative condition, such as atypical hyperplasia or LCIS, she has the choice of three treatment options: long-term surveillance (observation), bilateral prophylactic mastectomy (a risk-reducing surgical procedure), or chemoprevention (using a medication to decrease risk and possible development of breast cancer). Each of these options may be offered by a breast specialist, usually associated with a comprehensive breast center. Most choose surveillance and attempt to modify certain risk factors, such as diet, exercise, and alcohol consumption. For some women, however, prophylactic mastectomy may be an option (see discussion later in this chapter); or taking tamoxifen (Nolvadex) may be an option for others. Tamoxifen has recently been shown to decrease the incidence of invasive breast cancer for high-risk women by 45% (Wickerham, 1998). The risks and benefits of each of these options must be explained, so that women can carefully choose an option.

MALIGNANT CONDITIONS OF THE BREAST

Breast cancer is a major health problem in the United States. Its overall incidence rose by 54% between 1950 and 1990. In the 1990s, the incidence leveled off and stabilized (American Cancer Society, 1999).

At present, there is no cure for breast cancer. Between 1990 and 1994, the mortality rate for breast cancer decreased by 5.6%, the largest short-term decline in more than 40 years, suggesting that the combination of early detection and better systemic treatment options is producing an effect on overall survival.

Current statistics indicate that a woman's lifetime risk for developing breast cancer is 1 in 8. This risk, however, is not the same for all age groups. For example, the risk for developing breast cancer by the age of 35 years is 1 in 622; the risk for developing breast cancer by the age of 60 years is 1 in 24. According to the American Cancer Society, more than 175,000 cases of breast cancer are diagnosed each year, with an estimated 43,300 deaths. About 1% of these cancers occur in men. Women who are diagnosed with early-stage localized breast cancer have a 5-year survival rate of 97%. By the year 2000, nearly 2 million women in the United States will have been affected by breast cancer during the decade, with more than 460,000 dying of the disease in the 1990s (American Cancer Society, 1999).

Carcinoma in Situ (Noninvasive)

In situ carcinoma of the breast is being detected more frequently with the widespread use of screening mammography. The incidence of in situ carcinoma has increased markedly over the past 2 decades, reflecting the increased use of screening mammography. In situ carcinoma now accounts for 20% to 25% of diagnosed breast cancer cases. This disease is characterized by the proliferation of malignant cells within the ducts and lobules, without invasion into the surrounding tissue; therefore, it is a noninvasive form of cancer and is considered stage 0 breast cancer. There are two types of in situ carcinoma: ductal and lobular.

Ductal Carcinoma in Situ

Ductal carcinoma in situ (DCIS), the more common of the two types, is divided histologically into two major subtypes: comedo and noncomedo, but there are many different forms of noncomedo DCIS. Because DCIS has the capacity to progress to invasive cancer, the most traditional treatment is total or simple mastectomy (removal of the breast only), with a cure rate of 98% to 99%. The use of breast-conserving surgery for invasive cancer led to the use of **breast conservation therapy** (limited surgery followed by radiation) for patients with DCIS, and this option is appropriate for localized lesions. About half of cases of DCIS are now being treated with breast conservation therapy; however, the rate of local recurrence is 15% to 20%. In some cases, lumpectomy alone may be an option, but this is usually decided on a case-by-case basis.

Lobular Carcinoma in Situ

LCIS is characterized by proliferation of cells within the breast lobules. LCIS is usually an incidental finding discovered on pathologic evaluation of a breast biopsy for a breast change noted during physical examination or on screening mammography, is commonly associated with multicentric disease, and is rarely associated with invasive cancer. Historically, treatment was bilateral total mastectomy; current thinking that LCIS is a marker of increased risk for the development of an invasive cancer (rather than an actual malignancy) has changed this approach. Long-term surveillance is one appropriate option. Another option is a bilateral prophylactic mastectomy to decrease risk, and current research (Hartmann et al., 1999) suggests that a 90% reduction in risk is possible with this option (prophylactic mastectomy is discussed in more detail at the end of this chapter). The other treatment option for LCIS is chemoprevention. In the fall of 1998, the U.S. Food and Drug Administration (FDA) approved the use of tamoxifen (Nolvadex) as a chemopreventive agent for women at high risk; however, as with any drug, tamoxifen has both benefits and risks, along with possible side effects.

Invasive Carcinoma

Infiltrating Ductal Carcinoma

Infiltrating ductal carcinomas are the most common histologic type and account for 75% of all breast cancers. These tumors are notable because of their hardness on palpation. They usually metastasize to the axillary nodes. Prognosis is poorer than for other cancer types.

Infiltrating Lobular Carcinoma

Infiltrating lobular carcinoma is rare and accounts for 5% to 10% of breast cancers. These tumors typically occur as an area of ill-defined thickening in the breast, as compared with the infiltrating ductal types. They are most often multicentric; that is, several areas of thickening may occur in one or both breasts. Infiltrating ductal and infiltrating lobular carcinomas usually spread to bone, lung, liver, or brain, whereas lobular carcinomas may metastasize to meningeal surfaces or other unusual sites.

Medullary Carcinoma

Medullary carcinoma constitutes about 6% of breast cancers and grows in a capsule inside a duct. This type of tumor can become large, but the prognosis is often favorable.

Mucinous Cancer

Mucinous cancer accounts for about 3% of breast cancers. A mucin producer, it is also slow growing; thus, it has a more favorable prognosis than many other types.

Tubular Ductal Cancer

Tubular ductal cancer is rare, accounting for only 2% of cancers. Because axillary metastases are uncommon with this histology, prognosis is usually excellent.

Inflammatory Carcinoma

Inflammatory carcinoma is a rare type of breast cancer (1% to 2%) that produces symptoms that are different from those of other breast cancers. The localized tumor is tender and painful; the breast is abnormally firm and enlarged. The skin over it is red and dusky. Often, edema and nipple retraction occur. These symptoms rapidly grow more severe and usually prompt the woman to seek health care sooner than the woman with a small breast mass. The disease can spread to other parts of the body rapidly; chemotherapeutic agents play a major role in attempting to control the progression of this disease. Radiation and surgery are also used to control spread.

Paget's Disease

Paget's disease of the breast is a less common type of breast cancer. A scaly lesion and burning and itching around the nipple–areola complex are frequent symptoms. The neoplasm is ductal and may be in situ alone or may also have invasive cancer cells. Often, a tumor mass cannot be palpated underneath the nipple where this disease arises. Mammography may be the only diagnostic test that detects the tumor, but results of the mammography are often negative, making biopsy of the lesion the only definitive test.

CURRENT RESEARCH IN BREAST CANCER

Because of the incidence, significant mortality rates, and lack of a cure, breast cancer survivors, advocates, and activists have brought social and political attention to this disease and put it in the national spotlight. Activists have demanded and obtained increased federal funding for a national breast cancer program aimed at finding a cure.

Chemoprevention

Preventing the development of cancer through the use of drugs is a relatively new and exciting area of research. In April 1998, the results of the Breast Cancer Prevention Trial were released to the general public. This nationwide, randomized, double-blind, placebo-controlled clinical trial evaluated tamoxifen (Nolvadex) versus a placebo in more than 13,000 women considered to be at high risk for the development of breast cancer. Those women who received tamoxifen had a 45% reduction in the incidence of breast cancer (Fisher, 1998). These results suggested that tamoxifen was an effective chemopreventive agent. Much attention has been focused on this medication, and it is now available with FDA approval for high risk women. Clinicians are still unclear, however, about who should receive the medication, and no consensus exists at present. Nurses can provide information to patients on the benefits, risks, and possible side effects of tamoxifen to help women in considering this option.

Another agent that shows promise for chemoprevention is raloxifene (Evista). This medication is FDA approved for the prevention of osteoporosis; however, in the studies done, incidental findings indicated that fewer of those women who received raloxifene developed breast cancer. This has led to the hypothesis that this drug may also be an effective chemopreventive agent. Presently, researchers are embarking on the initiation of another nationwide, randomized, clinical trial, the Study of Raloxifene and Tamoxifen, which will compare these two agents in postmenopausal women for the prevention of breast cancer. Twenty-two thousand women are needed for this trial; thus, results will not be available for a number of years.

PROPHYLACTIC MASTECTOMY

Some women who are at high risk for breast cancer may elect to undergo **prophylactic mastectomy**. This procedure can reduce the risk for cancer by 90% (Hartmann et al., 1999), so a more appropriate term for this surgery is "risk-reducing" mastectomy. The procedure, performed by a breast surgeon, consists of a **total mastectomy** (removal of breast tissue only). Possible candidates are women with a strong family history of breast cancer, a diagnosis of LCIS or atypical hyperplasia, a diagnosis of BRCA-1 or BRCA-2 gene mutation, an extreme fear of cancer ("cancerphobia"), or previous cancer in one breast. Many women opt for immediate reconstruction with the mastectomy.

Women need to understand that this surgery is elective and not emergent. To be sure the she understands the implications of surgery, the woman should be offered a consultation with a plastic surgeon, a genetic counseling session, and a psychological evaluation. Women who make an informed decision tend to demonstrate more satisfaction with the cosmetic results.

Nursing interventions for the woman considering a risk-reducing mastectomy include ensuring that the patient has information about reconstructive options and providing referrals to the plastic surgeon, genetic counselor, and psychological counselor. For many women, who need time to think over the procedure, the nurse can be helpful in answering questions about the procedure and its possible implications and in assisting the patient to decide whether the surgery is an appropriate option. It may sometimes be appropriate for the woman considering this option to talk with a woman who has had the procedure.

BREAST CANCER

There is no single, specific cause of breast cancer; rather, a combination of hormonal, genetic, and, possibly, environmental events may contribute to its development.

Etiology

Hormones produced by the ovaries have an important role in breast cancer. Two key ovarian hormones—estradiol and progesterone—are altered in the cellular environment by a variety of factors, and these may affect growth factors for breast cancer.

HORMONES

The role of hormones and their relationship to breast cancer remain controversial. Research suggests that a relationship exists between estrogen exposure and the development of breast cancer. In laboratory studies, tumors grow much faster when exposed to estrogen, and epidemiologic research suggests that women who have longer exposure to estrogen have a higher risk for breast cancer. Early menarche, nulliparity, childbirth after 30 years of age, and late menopause are known but minor risk factors. The assumption is that these factors are all associated with prolonged exposure to estrogen because of menstruation. The theory is that each cycle (which has high levels of endogenous estrogen) provides the cells of the breast another chance to mutate, increasing the chance for cancer to develop. Estrogen itself, however, does not cause breast cancer but is associated with its development.

GENETICS

Growing evidence indicates that genetic alterations are associated with the development of breast cancer. These genetic alterations include changes or mutations in normal genes and the influence of proteins that either promote or suppress the development of breast cancer. Genetic alterations may be somatic (acquired) or germline (inherited). To date, two gene mutations have been identified that may play a role in the development of breast cancer. A mutation in the **BRCA-1** gene has been linked to the development of breast and ovarian cancer, whereas a mutation in the **BRCA-2** gene identifies risk for breast cancer but less so for ovarian (Baron & Borgen, 1997). These gene mutations may also play a role in the development of colon, prostate, and pancreatic cancer, but this is far from clear at present. It has been estimated that 1 of 600 women in the general population has either a BRCA-1 or BRCA-2 gene mutation. For women who carry either mutation, the risk for developing breast cancer can range from 20% to 90%.

At present, only 5% to 10% of all breast cancers are estimated to be associated with the BRCA-1 or BRCA-2 gene mutations. It is thought, however, that breast cancer is genetic and that up to 80% of women diagnosed with breast cancer before the age of 50 years have a genetic component to their disease. This is believed to be linked to either unidentified BRCA-1 or BRCA-2 carriers or less penetrating genes that have yet to be identified through genetics research. Interpretation of a woman's risk for either BRCA-1 or BRCA-2 should be interpreted with caution and with an exhaustive look at all her other risk factors; this is usually carried out by a genetics counselor.

Abnormalities in either of the two genes can be identified by a blood test; however, women should be counseled about the risks and benefits before actually undergoing genetic testing. The risks and benefits of a positive or negative result should be explored. Treatment options for a positive result are either long-term surveillance, bilateral prophylactic mastectomy, or chemoprevention with tamoxifen, as discussed previously. A positive result can cause tremendous anxiety and fear, unleash potential discrimination in employment and insurability, and cause a woman to search for answers that may not be available. A negative result can produce survivor guilt in a person with a strong family history of cancer. For these women, the risk for breast cancer is similar to that of the general population, routine screening guidelines should be followed. The decision to pursue genetic testing has to be made carefully, and women should be asked what they will do differently after they know the results. Furthermore, because testing is relatively new and health care providers have yet to determine a true benefit from a positive or negative result, genetic testing should be done under the auspices of clinical research protocols to protect the patient (because these data are kept separate from the patient's medical record). Nurses play a role in educating patients and their family members about the implications of genetic testing.

Risk Factors

Although there are no specific known causes of breast cancer, researchers have identified a cluster of risk factors. These factors are important in helping to develop prevention programs. One must bear in mind, however, that nearly 60% of women diagnosed with breast cancer have no identifiable risk factors other than their hormonal environment. Thus, all women are considered at risk for developing breast cancer during their lifetime. Nonetheless, identifying risk factors provides a means for identifying women who may benefit from increased surveillance and early treatment. In addition, further research into risk factors will help in developing effective strategies to prevent or modify breast cancer in the future.

A high-fat diet was once thought to increase the risk of breast cancer. Epidemiologic studies of American and Japanese women showed a fivefold difference in the rate of breast cancer between the two groups, with the American women having the greater incidence. Japanese women who migrated to the United States were shown to have breast cancer rates similar to their white counterparts. Recent cohort studies show only weak or inconclusive relationships between high-fat diet and breast cancer (Greenwald & McDonald, 1997). Because fat is implicated in colon cancer

Risk Factors for BREAST CANCER

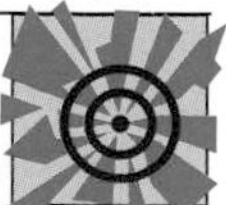

BRCA-1 or BRCA-2 genetic mutation
- Women with gene mutation have a 50% to 90% for developing breast cancer and a 50/50 possibility of developing breast cancer before 50 years of age

Increasing age
- Greatest risk for breast cancer occurs after age 50.

Personal or family history of breast cancer
- Risk of developing breast cancer in the other breast increases about 1% per year.
- Risk increases twofold if first-degree female relatives (sister, mother, or daughter) had breast cancer
- Risk increases if the mother was affected with cancer before 60 years of age.
- Risk increases four to six times if breast cancer occurred in two first-degree relatives.

Early menarche
- Menses beginning before 12 years of age.

Nulliparity and late maternal age at first birth
- Women having their first child after 30 years of age have twice the risk for breast cancer as women having first child before 20 years of age.

Late menopause
- Menopause after 55 years of age but women with bilateral oophorectomy before 35 years of age have one third the risk.

History of benign proliferative breast disease
- Risk doubles in women with benign tumors with proliferative epithelial changes; risk quadruples with atypical hyperplasia or LCIS.

Exposure to ionizing radiation between puberty and 30 years of age.
- Risk doubles; exposure to radiation causes potential aberrations while the breast cells are developing.

Obesity
- Weak risk among obese postmenopausal women: estrogen is stored in body adipose tissue, and dietary fat increases pituitary prolactin, thus increasing estrogen production. Obese women diagnosed with breast cancer have a higher mortality rate, which may be related to these hormonal influences or perhaps a delayed diagnosis.

Hormone replacement therapy
- Reported risk for breast cancer related to hormone replacement therapy varies.
- Older women taking estrogen supplements for more than 5 years *may* have an increased risk; addition of progesterone to estrogen replacement decreases the incidence of endometrial cancer, but it does not decrease the risk of breast cancer.

Alcohol intake
- As a risk factor, alcohol use remains controversial; however, a slightly increased risk is found in women who consume even one drink daily. The risk doubles among women drinking three drinks daily. In countries where wine is consumed daily (eg, France and Italy), the rate is slightly higher. Some research findings suggest that young women who drink alcohol are more vulnerable in later years.

and heart disease, however, women may benefit from efforts to lower overall caloric intake of fat.

Oral contraceptives were once thought to increase the risk for breast cancer. Currently, no association is thought to exist between the use of birth control pills and the development of breast cancer in women in the general population. However, no data exist on their effect on women considered to be at high risk.

The role of tobacco and smoking in breast cancer remains unclear. Most studies suggest that smoking does not increase a woman's risk for breast cancer. Some studies, however, do suggest that smoking increases the risk for breast cancer and that the earlier a woman begins smoking, the higher her risk. Smoking does increase the risk for lung cancer, which is the leading cause of death in women with cancer (breast cancer is second). Smoking cessation is part of a healthy lifestyle, and nurses have a key role in providing women with information about smoking cessation programs.

Silicone breast implants can be associated with fibrous capsular contraction, and some women and medical professionals have claimed an association with certain immune disorders. There is no evidence, however, that breast implants are associated with an increased risk of breast cancer.

Protective Factors

Certain factors may be protective in relation to the development of breast cancer. Regular, vigorous exercise has been shown to decrease risk, perhaps because it can delay menarche, suppress menstruation, and, like pregnancy, reduce the number of ovulatory menstrual cycles. Also, exercise decreases body fat, where estrogens are stored and produced from other steroid hormones. Thus, decreased body fat can decrease extended exposure to estrogen. Breastfeeding is also thought to decrease risk because it prevents the return of menstruation, again decreasing exposure to endogenous estrogen. Having had a full-term pregnancy before the age of 30 years is also thought to be protective. Protective hormones are released after delivery of the fetus, with the purpose of reverting to normal the proliferation of cells in the breast that occur with pregnancy.

Clinical Manifestations

Breast cancers occur anywhere in the breast, but most are found in the upper outer quadrant where most breast tissue is located. Generally, the lesions are nontender rather than painful, fixed rather than mobile, and hard with irregular borders rather than encapsulated and smooth. Complaints of diffuse breast pain and tenderness occurring at the time of menstruation are usually associated with benign breast disease. Marked pain at presentation, however, may be associated with breast cancer in the later stages.

With the increased use of mammography, more women are seeking treatment at an earlier stage of disease. These women may have no symptoms and no palpable lump, but abnormal lesions are detected on mammography. Unfortunately, many women with advanced disease seek initial treatment only after ignoring symptoms. For example, they may seek attention for dimpling or for a peau d'orange (orange-peel) appearance of the skin—a condition caused by swelling that results from obstructed lymphatic circulation in the dermal layer. Nipple retraction and lesions fixed to the chest wall may also be evident. Involvement of the skin is manifested by ulcerating and fungating lesions. These classic signs and symptoms characterize breast cancer in the late stages. A high index of suspicion should be maintained with any breast abnormality and should be promptly evaluated.

Assessment and Diagnostic Findings

Techniques to determine the histology and tissue diagnosis of breast cancer include FNA, excisional (or open) biopsy, incisional biopsy, needle localization, core biopsy, and stereotactic biopsy (described previously). In addition to the staging criteria described below, other pathologic features and prognostic tests are used to identify different patient groups that may benefit from adjuvant treatment. Histologic examination of the cancer cells helps determine the prognosis and leads to a better understanding of how the disease progresses.

Breast Cancer Staging

Staging involves classifying breast cancer according to the extent of disease (Fig. 44-4). Staging of any cancer is important because it helps the health care team identify and recommend the best treatment available, offer a prognosis, and compare the results of various treatment regimens. Several diagnostic tests and procedures are performed in the staging of the disease. These may include chest x-rays, bone scans, and liver function tests. Clinical staging involves the physician's approximation of the size of the breast tumor and estimation of axillary node involvement by physical examination (palpable nodes may indicate progression of the disease) and mammography. After the diagnostic workup and the definitive surgical treatment are carried out, the breast cancer is staged according to the TNM system, which evaluates the size of the tumor, number of nodes involved, and evidence of distant metastasis (Table 44-2). Pathologic staging based on histology provides information for a more accurate prognosis. Table 44-3 lists typical treatment guidelines by staging at diagnosis (see following management section for details regarding the types of treatment listed in Table 44-3).

Prognosis

Several features of breast tumors contribute to the prognosis. Generally, the smaller the tumor, the better the prognosis. Carcinoma of the breast is not a pathologic entity that develops overnight. It starts with a genetic alteration in a single cell. It can take about 16 doubling times for a carcinoma to become 1 cm or larger, at which point it becomes clinically apparent. Assuming that it takes at least 30 days for each doubling time, it would take a minimum of 2 years for a carcinoma to become palpable. This concept is important for nurses in teaching and counseling patients because once breast cancer is diagnosed, women have a safe period of several weeks to make a decision regarding treatment.

The prognosis also depends on whether the cancer has spread. For example, the overall 5-year survival rate is greater than 97% when the tumor is confined to the breast. When the cancer cells have spread to the regional lymph nodes, however, the overall 5-year survival rate falls to 77%. The 5-year survival rate for women diagnosed with metastatic disease is 21%. At diagnosis, about 37% of patients have evidence of regional or distant spread or metastasis. The most common route of regional spread is to the axillary lymph nodes. See Table 44-4 for a description of the relationship between positive axillary lymph nodes and the risk for breast cancer recurrence. Other sites of lymphatic spread include the internal mammary and supraclavicular nodes (Fig. 44-5). Distant metastasis can affect any organ, but the most common sites are the bone (71%), lungs (69%), liver (65%), pleura (51%), adrenals (49%), skin (30%), and brain (20%) (Tyler, 1998).

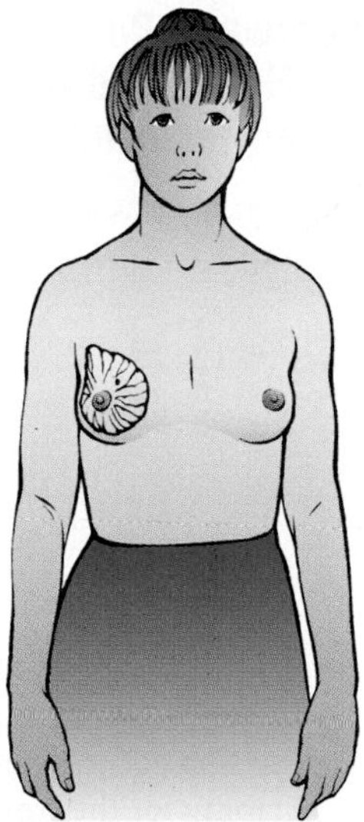

Stage I: Tumors are less than 2 cm in diameter and confined to breast.

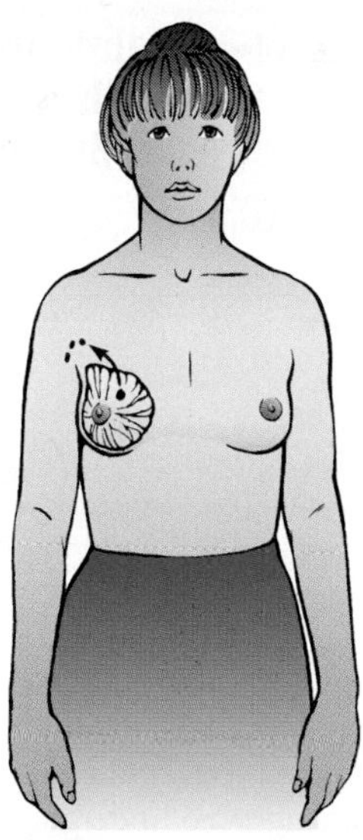

Stage II: Tumors are less than 5 cm, or tumors are smaller with mobile axillary lymph node involvement.

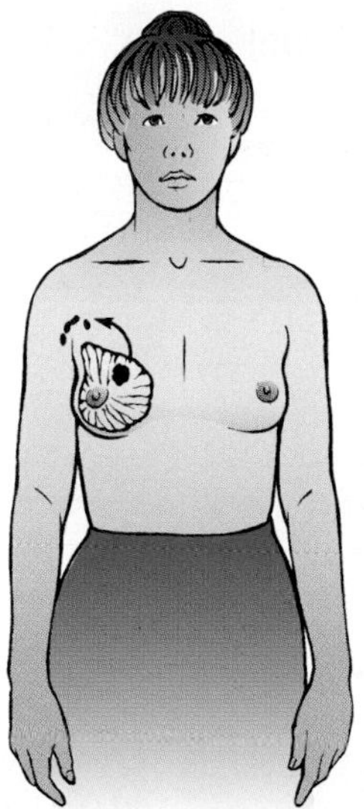

Stage IIIa: Tumors are greater than 5 cm, or tumors are accompanied by enlarged axillary lymph nodes fixed to one another or to adjacent tissue.

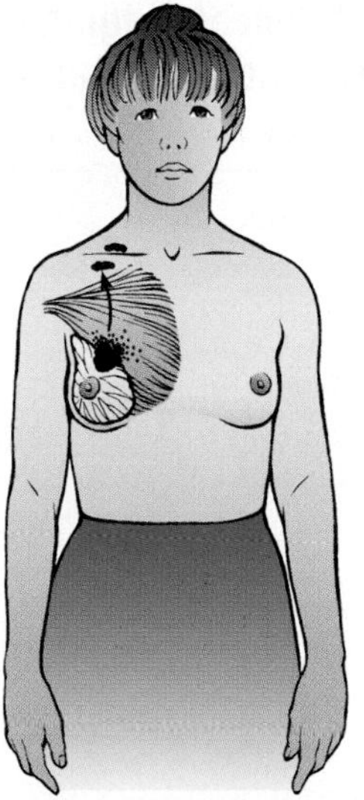

Stage IIIb: More advanced lesions with satellite nodules, fixation to the skin or chest wall, ulceration, edema, or with supraclavicular or intraclavicular nodal involvement.

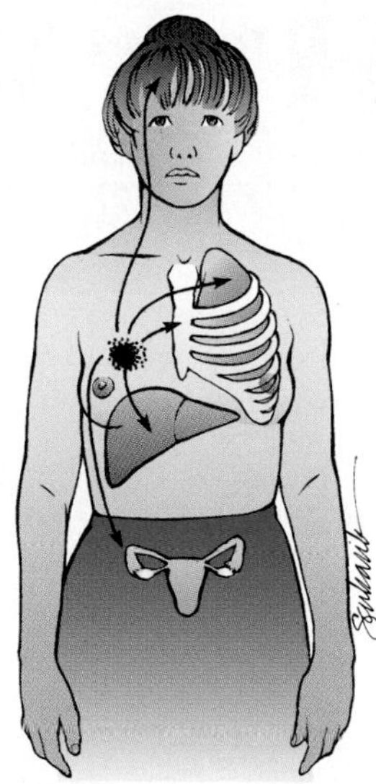

Stage IV: All tumors with distant metastases.

FIGURE 44•4 Stages of breast cancer.

In addition to tumor size, nodal involvement, evidence of metastasis, and histologic type, other measures help in determining prognosis. The presence of estrogen and progesterone receptor proteins indicates a retention of regulatory controls of the mammary epithelium. Presence of both receptor proteins is associated with an improved prognosis; their absence is associated with a poorer prognosis. Similarly, a tumor with a high degree of differentiation is associated with a better prognosis than a poorly differentiated anaplastic tumor. The assessment of a tumor's proliferative rate (S-phase fraction) and DNA content (ploidy) by laboratory assay may help to determine prognosis because these two factors are strongly correlated with other prognostic factors, and research is ongoing to examine how helpful these two factors may actually be. Tumors classified as diploid (normal DNA content) are associated with a better prognosis than are tumors classified as aneuploid (abnormal DNA content).

Medical Management

CHANGING APPROACHES

In 1990, the National Institutes of Health Consensus Development Conference on Breast Cancer issued its third statement on the management of breast cancer. Based on results of worldwide data, surgery that conserved the breast (such as lumpectomy), along with radiation therapy, was found to result in a survival rate equal to that of modified radical mastectomy. In addition, recommendations were made for systemic treatment, with chemotherapy based on the patient's menopausal status and the presence of hormone receptors. For a premenopausal woman without involvement of the lymph nodes, adjuvant chemotherapy was recommended if the woman was at high risk for recurrence. For a postmenopausal woman without involvement of the lymph nodes, adjuvant chemotherapy was not recommended regardless of hormonal receptor status. For premenopausal women with involvement of the nodes, adjuvant chemotherapy was recommended. In a postmenopausal woman, hormone therapy was recommended if the woman had estrogen-receptor–positive tumors. The section on hormonal therapy later in this chapter describes this in more depth.

In 1991, the National Cancer Institute issued a clinical alert that altered the recommendations of the 1990 Consensus Development Conference Statement. This alert recommended that all premenopausal, node-negative women at high risk for recurrent disease receive adjuvant chemotherapy. This clinical alert was issued before results of clinical trials were published, thus creating some confusion among clinicians and patients alike. Nevertheless, the current management of breast cancer is based on local or systemic treatment and on the individual characteristics of the patient and the disease.

Decisions regarding local treatment with either mastectomy or breast-conserving surgery with radiation still vary widely. Mastectomy is still performed in many cases, and rates for breast-conserving surgery are higher in metropolitan areas with teaching and research hospitals and medical centers. In the past, women have not routinely been presented with the option of breast-conserving surgery by their physicians, and in many instances, insurance reimbursement patterns favor mastectomy. Thus, women have not uniformly had the opportunity to exercise informed choice in their options for local treatment, but this is changing as women become more knowledgeable about breast cancer and its treatment. A second opinion regarding treatment options is usually helpful to women diagnosed with breast cancer.

SURGICAL MANAGEMENT

The main goal of surgical treatment is to eradicate the local presence of the cancer. The procedures most often used for the local management of invasive breast cancer are mastectomy with or without reconstruction and breast-conserving surgery combined

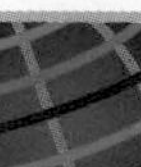

TABLE 44•2 Breast Cancer Staging by Tumor, Nodes, and Metastasis

Stage	Tumor	Nodes	Metastasis
0	Tis	N0	M0
I	T1	N0	M0
IIA	T0	N1	M0
	T1	N1	M0
	T2	N0	M0
IIB	T2	N1	M0
	T3	N0	M0
IIIA	T0	N2	M0
	T1	N2	M0
	T2	N2	M0
	T3	N1	M0
	T3	N2	M0
IIIB	T4	Any N	M0
	Any T	N3	M0
IV	Any T	Any N	M1

Key:

PRIMARY TUMOR (T)

T0	No evidence of primary tumor
Tis	Carcinoma in situ: intraductal carcinoma, lobular carcinoma in situ, or Paget's disease of the nipple with no tumor
T1	Tumor ≤ 2 cm in greatest dimension
T2	Tumor > 2 cm but not > 5 cm in greatest dimension
T3	Tumor > 5 cm in greatest dimension
T4	Tumor of any size with direct extension to chest wall or skin

REGIONAL LYMPH NODES (N)

N0	No regional lymph node metastasis
N1	Metastasis to movable ipsilateral axillary lymph node(s)
N2	Metastasis to ipsilateral axillary lymph node(s) fixed to one another or to other structures
N3	Metastasis to ipsilateral internal mammary lymph node(s)

DISTANT METASTASIS (M)

M0	No distance metastasis
M1	Distant metastasis (includes metastasis to ipsilateral supraclavicular lymph node(s))

Adapted from American Joint Committee on Cancer. *Manual for staging of cancer* (5th ed.). Philadelphia: J. B. Lippincott, 1997.

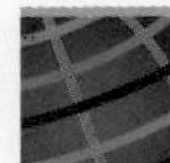

TABLE 44•4 Relationship Between Positive Axillary Lymph Nodes and Risk for Breast Cancer Recurrence*

No. of Positive Axillary Lymph Nodes	Risk for Breast Cancer Recurrence (%)
0	<10
1–3	12–20
4–9	30–35
>10	>50

*At 5 years' follow-up.

with radiation therapy. These procedures are described as follows. (The array of surgical treatment options are summarized in Table 44-5). For patients who undergo total mastectomy for the treatment of DCIS or as prophylactic surgery for the treatment for LCIS, the nursing care is similar to that of a modified radical mastectomy (described later in the text). However, total mastectomy does not involve the removal of axillary lymph nodes; therefore, mobility of the arm on the affected side is regained much quicker, and there is no risk for lymphedema. Women still face the same psychosocial issues involving the diagnosis of cancer and the loss of the breast, and the nurse needs to address these in a similar manner.

Modified Radical Mastectomy. **Modified radical mastectomy** is removal of the entire breast tissue along with axillary lymph nodes. The pectoralis major and pectoralis minor remain intact. Before surgery, the surgeon plans an incision that will provide maximum opportunity to remove the tumor and the affected nodes. At the same time, efforts are made to avoid a scar that will be visible and restrictive. An objective of surgical treatment is to maintain or restore normal function to the hand, arm, and shoulder girdle on the affected side. Skin flaps and tissue are handled meticulously to ensure proper viability, hemostasis, and drainage. If reconstructive surgery is planned, a consultation is made with a plastic surgeon before the mastectomy is performed.

After the tumor is removed, bleeding points are ligated, and the skin is closed over the chest wall. Skin grafting is performed if the skin flaps are too small to close the wound. A nonadherent dressing (Adaptic) may be applied and covered by a pressure

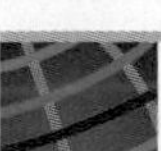

TABLE 44•3 Breast Cancer Treatment Guidelines by Stage at Diagnosis

Stage	Tumor	Surgery	Chemotherapy	Radiation
0	DCIS	TM or lumpectomy	Not necessary	For lumpectomy
I	0–2 cm	BCT or MRM	For tumor size >1 cm	For BCT
II	2–5 cm	BCT or MRM	Regimen depends on tumor size and nodal status	For BCT
III	>5 cm	MRM	Postoperative and possibly preoperative	To chest wall and possibly axillae after MRM
IV	Metastatic disease	Possible lumpectomy or MRM	To control progression and/or palliation	To control progression and/or palliation

DCIS, ductal carcinoma in situ; TM, total mastectomy; BCT, breast conservation treatment (lumpectomy and axillary dissection); MRM, Modified radical mastectomy

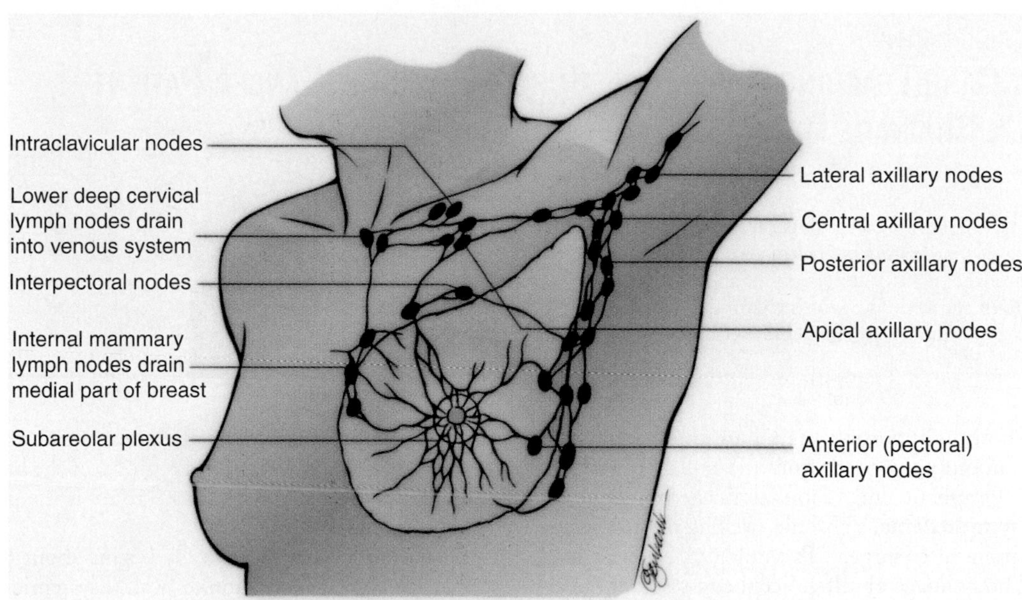

FIGURE 44•5 Lymphatic drainage of the breast.

dressing. Two drainage tubes may be placed in the axilla and beneath the superior skin flap, and portable suction devices may be used; these remove the blood and lymph fluid that collect after surgery. The dressing may be held in place by wide elastic bandages or a surgical bra.

TABLE 44•5 Surgical Treatment of Breast Cancer

Surgical Procedure	Description
Breast conserving procedures: Lumpectomy Wide excision Partial mastectomy Segmental mastectomy Quadrantectomy	Relatively synonymous terms to describe removal of varying amounts of breast tissue, including the malignant tissue and some surrounding tissue to ensure clear margins; axillary lymph nodes are also removed with these procedures, if the cancer was of the invasive type
Axillary lymph node dissection	Removal of some or all fat-enmeshed axillary lymph nodes for determination of extent of disease spread; the single most important determinant for prognosis and for need for adjuvant treatment
Total mastectomy	Removal of the breast tissue only; this procedure is generally done for the treatment of carcinoma in situ, typically ductal
Modified radical mastectomy	Removal of the breast tissue and an axillary lymph node dissection; the pectoralis major and minor muscles remain intact
Radical mastectomy	Removal of the breast tissue along with pectoralis major and minor muscles in conjunction with an axillary lymph node dissection

Breast-Conserving Surgery. Breast-conserving surgery consists of lumpectomy, wide excision, partial or segmental mastectomy, or quadrantectomy (resection of the involved breast quadrant) and removal of the axillary nodes (axillary lymph node dissection) for tumors with an invasive component, followed by a course of radiation therapy to treat residual, microscopic disease.

The goal of breast conservation is to remove the tumor completely with clear margins, while achieving an acceptable cosmetic result. The axillary lymph nodes are also removed through a separate semicircular shaped incision under the hair-bearing portion of the axillae. A drain is inserted into the axillae through a separate stab wound to remove blood and lymph fluid. A dressing is applied over the breast and under the arm and is secured with wide elastic bandages or a surgical bra. Survival rates after breast-conserving surgery are equivalent to those after modified radical mastectomy. The risk for local recurrence, however, is greater, at 1% per year after surgery. If the patient experiences a local recurrence, standard treatment is a completion or salvage mastectomy, in which the rest of the breast tissue is removed. Survival rates after this procedure are equivalent to those after mastectomy, but because the skin has been irradiated, choices for reconstruction remain limited, and women should be informed of this possibility at the time of diagnosis and when considering their treatment options.

Postoperative Issues. Postoperatively, the care of the patient undergoing a modified radical mastectomy or breast-conserving surgery is similar because both involve an alteration to the breast and removal of lymph nodes from the axillary region. As with any surgical patient, the immediate focus is recovery from general anesthesia and pain management. In addition, the patient who has had breast surgery may experience both physical and psychological effects. Possible complications include the accumulation of blood (hematoma) at the incision site, infection, and late accumulation of serosanguineous fluid (seroma) after drain removal. Most patients who undergo breast surgery are discharged home with a drainage collection device in place. The nurse teaches the patient and family members to manage the drainage system.

Nerve trauma with resultant phantom breast sensations, numbness, tingling, or burning sensations may also occur and may per-

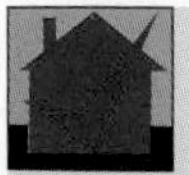

Home Care Teaching Checklist: Surgical Breast Cancer Patient With a Drainage Device

At the completion of the program, the patient or caregiver will be able to:

	Patient	Caregiver
• Demonstrate how to empty and measure fluid from the drainage device	✔	✔
• Demonstrate how to strip or milk clots through the tubing of the drainage device	✔	✔
• State observations that require contacting the physician or nurse (eg, sudden drainage color change, sudden cessation of drainage, signs or symptoms of an infection)	✔	✔
• Care for the drain site as per surgeon's recommendation	✔	✔
• Identify when the drain is ready for removal (usually when draining less than 30 mL for a 24-hour period)	✔	✔

sist for a period of months or possibly years after surgery. Impaired arm and shoulder mobility can result from the axillary dissection. The disruption of lymphatic and venous drainage can leave the patient at risk for **lymphedema**, a chronic swelling of the affected extremity, at any point after surgery. Psychological sequelae may include an altered body image or self-concept as a result of the alteration or loss of the breast. Other major psychosocial concerns include the uncertainty about the future, fear of recurrence, and the effects of breast cancer and its treatment on family and work roles.

Lymphatic Mapping and Sentinel Node Biopsy. A new procedure is being investigated for its use in patients undergoing breast surgery for the treatment of invasive breast cancer. About 55% of patients who undergo an axillary lymph node dissection to determine the extent of the disease have negative nodes. The use of **lymphatic mapping and sentinel node biopsy** may change the way these patients are treated because it may provide the same prognostic information as the axillary dissection. At the time of surgery, a radiocolloid or blue dye is injected into the tumor site; the patient then undergoes the surgical procedure. The surgeon uses a handheld probe to locate the sentinel node (the primary drainage site from the breast), excises it, and has it examined by the pathologist. In theory, if the sentinel node is negative for metastatic breast cancer, axillary dissection is not needed, thus sparing the patient the sequelae of the procedure (presence of a surgical drain, altered mobility of the extremity, paresthesias, and the risk for lymphedema). If the sentinel node is positive, the patient undergoes the standard axillary dissection. Reported results of this technique suggest a success rate of more than 90% in correctly identifying the sentinel node and correctly predicting axillary metastases (Krag et al., 1998).

Nursing issues for this new procedure in relation to patients with breast cancer focus on informing patients about the expectations and possible implications. Because patients with a negative node are spared the axillary dissection, they are discharged home the same day. Research is needed on the technique's sequelae, however. Questions to be addressed include: Do patients experience similar sensations in the affected arm as those who had an axillary dissection? Do patients demonstrate impaired mobility? Do these patients develop axillary seromas after the procedure? What is the risk for lymphedema? These issues depend on the anatomic location of the sentinel node and the extent of exploration needed by the surgeon to excise the node. To answer these questions, nursing research and further clinical experience with the procedure are needed.

RADIATION THERAPY

After breast-conserving surgery, a course of external-beam radiation therapy usually follows excision of the tumor mass to decrease the chance of local recurrence and to eradicate any residual microscopic cancer cells. Radiation treatment is necessary to obtain results equal to those of removal of the breast. If radiation therapy is contraindicated, mastectomy is the patient's only option (Chart 44-1).

Radiation treatment typically begins about 6 weeks after the surgery to allow the incision to heal. If systemic chemotherapy is indicated, radiation therapy usually begins after completion of the chemotherapy. External-beam irradiation provided by a linear accelerator using photons is delivered on a daily basis over 5 to 7 weeks to the entire breast region. In addition, a concentrated radiation dose or "boost" is administered to the primary site by means of electrons. Before radiation therapy begins, patients undergo a planning session for radiation treatment that will serve as the model for daily treatments. Small permanent ink markings are used to identify breast tissue to be irradiated. Patients need reassurance about the procedure and specific self-care instructions related to side effects and their management.

Postoperative radiation after mastectomy is not common today but is still used in certain cases: when tumors have spread regionally (chest wall involvement, numerous positive nodes, or large tumors [>5 cm]). Occasionally, patients who have had a mastectomy may require radiation treatment to the chest wall, and this generally occurs after completion of a course of systemic chemotherapy. Treatment usually consists of a course of external-beam irradiation to the area for a period of several weeks, but the time frame is determined by the radiation oncologist. Some studies suggest that for high-risk premenopausal women who receive chest wall irradiation after mastectomy, survival may be enhanced.

Postirradiation Reaction. Generally, radiation therapy is well tolerated. Side effects are temporary and usually consist of mild to moderate skin reaction and fatigue. The fatigue that occurs

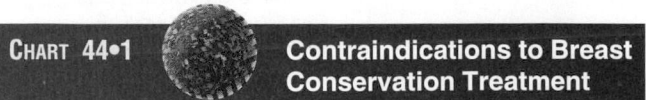

Note: Breast conservation treatment includes both surgery and radiation.

Absolute Contraindications

- First or second trimester of pregnancy
- Presence of multicentric disease in the breast
- Prior radiation to the breast or chest region

Relative Contraindications

- History of collagen vascular disease
- Large tumor-to-breast ratio
- Tumor beneath nipple

with radiation usually occurs about 2 weeks after treatment and may last for several weeks after the treatments are completed. Fatigue can be depressing, as can the frequent trips to the radiation oncology unit or department for treatment. The patient needs to be reassured that the fatigue is normal and not a sign of recurrence. Rare complications of radiation therapy to the breast include pneumonitis, rib fracture, and breast fibrosis.

Postirradiation Nursing Management. Self-care instructions for patients receiving radiation are based on maintaining skin integrity during and after radiation therapy:

- Use mild soap with minimal rubbing
- Avoid perfumed soaps or deodorants
- Use hydrophilic lotions (Lubriderm, Eucerin, Aquaphor) for dryness
- Use nondrying, antipruritic soap (Aveeno) if itching occurs
- Avoid tight clothes, underwire bras, excessive temperatures, and ultraviolet light

Patients may note increased redness and, rarely, skin breakdown at the "booster site" (tissue site that received concentrated radiation). Important aspects of follow-up care include teaching patients to minimize exposure of the treated area to the sun for 1 year and reassurance that minor twinges and shooting pain in the breast are normal reactions after radiation treatment.

CHEMOTHERAPY

Chemotherapy is administered to eradicate the micrometastatic spread of the disease. An overview of chemotherapy is presented in Chapter 15. Although chemotherapy is generally initiated after breast surgery, no single standard exists for the sequencing of systemic chemotherapy and radiation therapy. Ongoing clinical trials may help to determine which treatment sequence produces the best outcomes.

Chemotherapy regimens for breast cancer combine several agents to increase tumor cell destruction and to minimize medication resistance. The chemotherapeutic agents most often used in combination are cytoxan (C), methotrexate (M), fluorouracil (F), and doxorubicin (Adriamycin) (A). Paclitaxel (Taxol) (T) has been recently introduced into the adjuvant chemotherapy setting, and the data from clinical trials show promising results. The combination regimen of CMF or CAF is a common treatment protocol. AC, ACT (AC given first followed by T), or ATC (all three agents given together) are other regimens that may be used (Hortobagyi, 1998). Decisions regarding the chemotherapeutic protocol are based on the patient's age, physical status, disease status, and whether she is participating in a clinical trial. Chemotherapy treatment modalities are summarized in Table 44-6.

Reactions to Chemotherapy. Anticipatory anxiety is a common response among patients facing chemotherapy. Today, however, side effects can be managed well, with many women continuing their daily work and routine schedules. This has occurred in large measure because of the meticulous educational and psychological preparation provided to patients and their families by the oncology nurses, oncologists, social workers, and other members of the health care team. The other factor is the availability of medication regimens that can alleviate the side effects of nausea and vomiting.

Common physical side effects of chemotherapy for breast cancer include nausea, vomiting, taste changes, alopecia (hair loss), mucositis, dermatitis, fatigue, weight gain, and bone marrow suppression. In addition, premenopausal women may experience temporary or permanent amenorrhea leading to sterility.

Less common side effects include hemorrhagic cystitis and conjunctivitis. Although its cause is unknown, weight gain of more than 10 pounds occurs in about half of all patients. Aerobic exercise and its anxiety-alleviating effects may be helpful to decrease weight gain and elevate the patient's mood. Side effects may vary with the chemotherapeutic agent used. CMF is generally well tolerated with only minimal side effects. Doxorubicin can be toxic to tissue if it infiltrates the vein, so it is usually diluted and infused through a large vein. Nausea and vomiting can occur. Antiemetics and tranquilizers may provide relief, as may visual imagery and relaxation exercises. Doxorubicin and paclitaxel usually cause alopecia, so obtaining a wig before hair loss occurs may prevent some of the associated emotional trauma. The patient needs reassurance that new hair will grow when treatment is completed, although the color and texture of the hair may differ. It is helpful to provide a list of wig suppliers in the patient's geographic region and to become familiar with creative ways to use scarves and turbans to minimize patient discomfort with hair loss. The American Cancer Society offers a program known as "Look Good, Feel Better" that provides useful tips for applying cosmetics during chemotherapy.

Nursing Management in Chemotherapy. Nurses working with patients receiving chemotherapy play an important role in assisting those who have difficulty with the side effects of treatment. Encouraging the use of medications to limit nausea, vomiting, and mouth sores reduces discomfort during chemotherapy. Also, some patients may receive granulocyte colony-stimulating factor (G-CSF), a synthetic growth-stimulating factor injected subcutaneously daily for 10 days, which boosts the white blood cell count to prevent nadir fever (a fever that occurs with infection when the patient's blood cell counts are at their lowest level) and infections. The nurse instructs the patient and family on injection technique and about symptoms that require follow-up with a physician.

Taking time to explain side effects and possible solutions may alleviate some of the anxiety of women who feel uncomfortable asking questions. The more informed a patient is about side effects of chemotherapy and how to manage them, the better she can anticipate and deal with them.

Chemotherapy may negatively affect the patient's self-esteem, sexuality, and sense of well-being. Combined with the stress of a potentially life-threatening diagnosis, these changes can be overwhelming. Because many women are distressed by financial concerns and time spent away from the family, nursing support and teaching can avert serious emotional distress during treatment. Important aspects of nursing care include communication, facilitating support groups, encouraging patients to ask questions, and promoting the patient's trust in health care providers. Adequate time must be scheduled for clinical appointments to allow for patient discussion and questions. Most women with breast cancer today are treated in a multidisciplinary environment, and referrals to nutrition, social work, psychiatry, or pastoral care can assist in dealing with many of the issues of cancer treatment. In addition, numerous community supports and advocacy groups are available to these patients and their families.

HORMONAL THERAPY

Decisions about hormonal therapy for breast cancer are based on the outcome of an **estrogen and progesterone receptor assay** of tumor tissue taken during the initial biopsy. The tissue requires special handling by laboratory technicians with expertise in proper assessment techniques. Normal breast tissue contains receptor

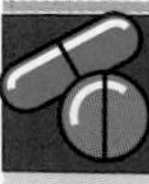

TABLE 44•6 Chemotherapy and Hormonal Therapy for Breast Cancer

Type of Treatment	Goals of Therapy	Possible Side Effects	Nursing Interventions
Chemotherapy	Destroy neoplastic cells Decrease or prevent metastasis		
doxorubicin (Adriamycin) (A)		ECG changes, tachycardia, nausea, vomiting, stomatitis, hair loss, severe cellulitis if infiltration occurs	*Nausea & vomiting:* Administer antiemetics as prescribed; monitor fluid intake and output *Anorexia:* Assist patient and family to identify appetizing foods; provide frequent small meals if better tolerated than three regular meals; refer to dietitian for assistance in planning palatable, nutritious meals
cytoxan (C)		Nausea, vomiting, anorexia, menstrual abnormalities, hemorrhagic cystitis	
methotrexate (M)		Stomatitis, CNS changes, hair loss	*Stomatitis:* Avoid commercial mouth washes; use baking soda, salt and water rinses, or oral anesthetic agents
5-fluorouracil (F)		CNS changes, neurotoxicity, nausea, vomiting, constipation, stomatitis	*Hair loss:* Avoid brushing, blow drying, frequent shampooing; encourage use of turbans and scarves; encourage patient to obtain wig before hair loss occurs
paclitaxel (Taxol) (T)		Hypersensitivity, peripheral neuropathy, nausea, vomiting, diarrhea, stomatitis, hair loss	*CNS changes:* Monitor for weakness, malaise, fatigue, seizures, change in cognitive status; assist with activities of daily living if fatigue and malaise occur
Combination therapy: CMF CAF AC ACT			*Neurotoxicity:* Monitor deep tendon reflexes, assess gait and muscle strength, monitor for changes in sensory function *Fluid retention:* Monitor weight, fluid intake and output, skin turgor *Cardiac changes:* Monitor ECG, cardiac rate and rhythm; notify physician of dysrhythmias *Hypercalcemia:* Monitor serum calcium levels, monitor cardiac rate and rhythm *Constipation:* Monitor bowel function; consider that constipation may be indicative of neurotoxicity; administer softeners, laxatives as prescribed; encourage adequate intake of fluids and fiber *Anxiety:* Administer tranquilizers as prescribed; encourage use of strategies to minimize anxiety (imagery, relaxation)
Hormonal Therapy			
Androgens fluorymesterone (Halotestin)	Suppress estrogens	Masculinization, fluid retention, cholestatic jaundice, hypercalcemia	*Hormonal instability:* Observe for changes (hot flashes, vaginal bleeding, flare); facial hirsutism, deepening of voice; fluid retention, Cushing's syndrome (fullness of face, lower extremity edema, weight gain); increased blood pressure; assess for thrombophlebitis; monitor serum calcium levels; educate patient on symptom management of hot flashes and assure patient that most changes are temporary
Estrogens diethystilbestrol (DES)	Suppress FSH and LH	Nausea, vomiting, anorexia, dizziness, headache	
Corticosteroids prednisone	Suppress estrogen production by the adrenals and decrease urinary estrogen metabolites	Cushing's syndrome: fullness of face, weight gain, edema of lower extremities	
Antihormonal agents tamoxifen (Nolvadex)	Estrogen antagonist; effective in decreasing risk for cancer recurrence in postmenopausal women and as a palliative treatment for recurrent cancer	Weight gain, hot flashes, nausea, anorexia, lethargy	

(continued)

TABLE 44•6 **Chemotherapy and Hormonal Therapy for Breast Cancer** *(Continued)*

Type of Treatment	Goals of Therapy	Possible Side Effects	Nursing Interventions
megesterol acetate (Megace)	Progestational agent; may decrease number of estrogen receptors in breast tissue	Weight gain, hot flashes, vaginal bleeding, increased blood pressure, peripheral edema, depression, tumor flare	
aminoglutethimide (Cytadren)	Enzyme antagonist that inhibits estrogen synthesis	CNS changes: dizziness, clumsiness, drowsiness, depression, headache	
anastrozole (Arimedex)	Aromatase inhibitor; blocks production of estrogen in peripheral tissues	Asthenia, nausea, headache, hot flashes, back pain	

* This listing of medications, side effects, and nursing interventions is not meant to be exhaustive but is rather a sample of frequently used chemotherapeutic agents for breast cancer.
FSH, follicle-stimulating hormone; LH, luteinizing hormone.

sites for estrogen. However, only about one third of breast cancers are estrogen dependent, or ER-positive (ER+). An ER+ assay indicates that tumor growth depends on estrogen supply; therefore, measures that reduce hormone production may limit the progression of the disease, and these receptors can be considered prognostic indicators. ER+ tumors may grow more slowly than those that do not depend on estrogen, or are ER negative (ER–). A value less than 3 fmol/mg is considered negative. Values of 3 to 10 are questionable, and values greater than 10 are considered positive. The greater the value, the more beneficial the anticipated effect from hormone suppression can be. Patients with both estrogen and progesterone positive (PR+) tumors generally have a more favorable prognosis than patients with tumors that are ER– and PR–. Most progesterone receptive tumors also have a positive estrogen receptor status. The loss of progesterone receptors can be a sign of advancing disease. Premenopausal women and perimenopausal women are more likely to have non–hormone-dependent lesions. Postmenopausal women are likely to have hormone-dependent lesions.

Hormonal therapy may include surgery to remove endocrine glands (eg, the ovaries, pituitary, or adrenal glands) with the goal of suppressing hormone secretion. Oophorectomy (removal of the ovaries) is one treatment option for premenopausal women with estrogen-dependent tumors. Tamoxifen is the primary hormonal agent used in breast cancer treatment today. Arimedex, Megace, diethylstilbestrol (DES), fluoxymesterone (Halotestin), and aminoglutethimide (Cytadren) are other hormonal agents used to suppress hormone-dependent tumors. All of these agents may be associated with menopausal symptoms, such as vasomotor changes. Hypercalcemia may also occur and may necessitate discontinuing the agent. Each type of hormonal agent is described in Table 44-6.

BONE MARROW TRANSPLANTATION

Bone marrow transplantation (BMT) involves removing bone marrow from the patient and then administering high-dose chemotherapy. The patient's bone marrow, spared from the effects of chemotherapy, is then reinfused intravenously. This highly specialized procedure is usually performed in specialized transplantation centers, and specific patient preparation, education, and support must be given throughout the treatment course.

Because chemotherapy and radiation therapy dosage are limited by the degree of their toxicity to the bone marrow, BMT is increasingly being used. Studies have indicated that autologous BMT induces a response in 50% to 80% of women, 30% of whom have a complete response for several years. Initially, mortality rates were high with autologous BMT, because of sepsis. The use of growth factors to stimulate the bone marrow, however, has led to an overall decline in mortality. BMT is described more fully in Chapter 15.

INVESTIGATIONAL THERAPY: THE FUTURE

Research is underway to develop chemotherapeutic agents that modify multidrug resistance and agents that enhance or modify standard chemotherapy. Research in breast cancer treatment includes the following areas: peripheral stem cell transplants, oncogenes (tumor genes that control cell growth), growth factors (substances released by cancer cells to make the environment more

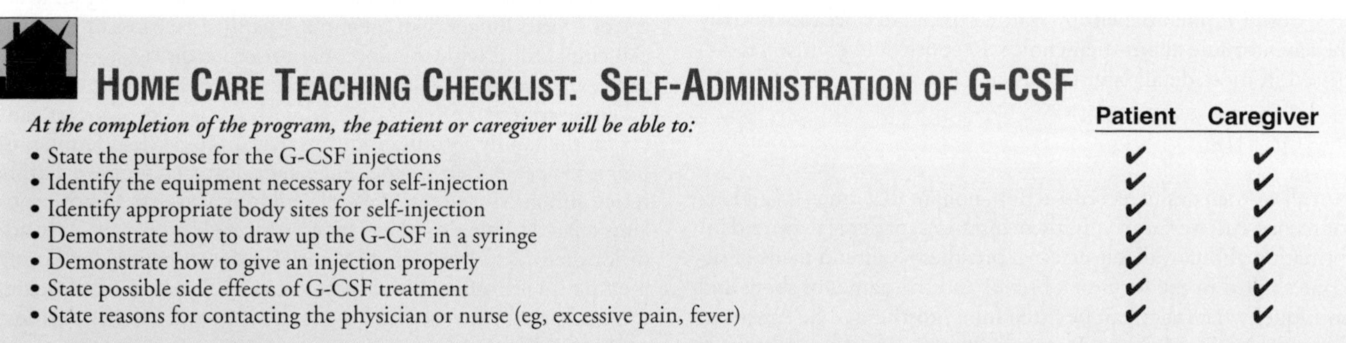

HOME CARE TEACHING CHECKLIST: SELF-ADMINISTRATION OF G-CSF

At the completion of the program, the patient or caregiver will be able to:

	Patient	Caregiver
• State the purpose for the G-CSF injections	✔	✔
• Identify the equipment necessary for self-injection	✔	✔
• Identify appropriate body sites for self-injection	✔	✔
• Demonstrate how to draw up the G-CSF in a syringe	✔	✔
• Demonstrate how to give an injection properly	✔	✔
• State possible side effects of G-CSF treatment	✔	✔
• State reasons for contacting the physician or nurse (eg, excessive pain, fever)	✔	✔

conducive to growth), monoclonal antibodies (synthetic antibodies that fight cancer cells), biologic response modifiers (substances that help increase the body's immune system response), and vaccine studies.

One new treatment modality that shows promise has been the introduction of trastuzumab (Herceptin). This monoclonal antibody was engineered from mouse antibodies and closely resembles a human antibody. Herceptin binds with the Her2 protein, and this protein regulates cell growth, thus inhibiting tumor cell growth. For women with metastatic breast cancer, about 25% to 30% of tumors overproduce Her2, and this monoclonal antibody can slow growth and possibly stimulate the immune response. In the fall of 1998, the FDA approved this agent for the treatment of women with metastatic breast cancer. Research is ongoing, but the addition of this agent to traditional chemotherapy has shown improvement in survival rates in clinical trials. Further research and clinical experience will demonstrate the potential of this drug in the treatment of women with breast cancer.

SPECIAL ISSUES IN BREAST CANCER MANAGEMENT

Reconstructive Surgery

After mastectomy, some women may elect to have reconstructive surgery, which provides considerable psychological benefit. Support groups and informational classes provide education and peer support for those patients who are candidates for and interested in breast reconstruction. Some concerns that women may have about reconstructive surgery are cost, safety, and timing—whether to undergo reconstruction immediately (at the time of mastectomy) or delay it (6 months to 1 year after surgery). Cost to the patient may vary depending on her health insurance, but because reconstruction is considered rehabilitative surgery, it is often covered.

In regard to safety, there are the usual surgical risks of infection, potential reaction to anesthesia, and the potential risk of a cosmetically unsatisfactory result. Reconstructive surgery is contraindicated if a woman has locally advanced, metastatic, or inflammatory breast cancer. Otherwise, most women with either in situ or early-stage breast cancer are candidates for immediate reconstruction. Breast reconstruction does not interfere with systemic treatment, nor does it affect the risk of the cancer recurring.

If a woman decides to have reconstructive surgery at the time of mastectomy, she avoids future surgery, although the total operative time increases. Some women find that immediate reconstruction lessens the feelings of loss and disfigurement. Occasionally, reconstruction cannot be performed because skin and muscles are too tight. Loose, supple skin and subcutaneous tissue with a sufficient blood supply contribute to reconstructive success. Some women benefit by waiting until later because initially they are not sure about their choice. Reconstructive surgery is discussed in more detail later in this chapter.

Prosthetics

Not all women desire reconstruction, nor are all women candidates for reconstructive surgery. In these instances, patients may need information about available external prostheses (a mold made of silicone shaped in the form of a breast) and the names of shops and boutiques where they can be fitted for a prosthesis. The American Cancer Society's Reach to Recovery Program can provide women with names and addresses of local establishments where they can be fitted. Women should be encouraged to find a place that provides a comfortable, supportive atmosphere and employs a certified prosthetics consultant. Generally, medical supply shops are not recommended because they often do not have the appropriate resources to ensure proper fit of a prosthesis.

Before discharge from the hospital, the nurse usually provides the patient with a temporary cotton fluff, which can be worn until the surgical incision is well healed (4 to 6 weeks). At that time, the woman can be fitted for a prosthesis. Insurance generally covers the cost of a prosthesis and the special bras that hold it in place. Women should be encouraged to wear the prosthesis because it provides a sense of psychological restoration and wholeness. The prosthesis also assists the woman in resuming proper posture because it helps to balance the weight of the remaining breast.

Quality of Life and Breast Cancer

Despite current treatment, there has been only a slight overall improvement in survival for breast cancer patients. Consequently, quality-of-life considerations have become important issues in treatment and recovery. Quality of life is a multidimensional construct that includes functional (self-care) status, social and family functioning, and psychological and spiritual well-being. These parameters are important indicators of how well a patient is functioning after diagnosis and treatment.

Breast cancer is the most frequently investigated cancer in quality-of-life studies. Early psychosocial studies emphasized that the loss of the breast was the single most important factor in women's adjustment, especially in Western cultures. Thus, it is not surprising that studies of women's adjustment to breast cancer found similar results. A growing body of research, however, indicates that concerns related to uncertainty about the future, day-to-day issues occurring in work and family relationships, and demands of illness are more important factors in adjusting to having breast cancer than the loss of the breast alone. For example, younger women are more vulnerable to issues of psychosocial adjustment than many older women. They worry about their jobs and whether they will be able to keep their health care benefits. They are concerned about their work productivity and career advancement. They face many family concerns related to whether they can have children, whether they will live to see their children grow up, and whether their disease will recur and incapacitate them. Middle-aged women worry about their disease in relation to their family and work. They also worry about their aging parents and whether they will be able to care for them in the future. They are increasingly concerned about their daughters' risk for breast cancer. Older women are more vulnerable to chronic health problems. Living an average of 6 years longer than men, older women face loss of their social circles, deal with the potential for other diseases, and worry about whether they will have resources to pay for medications.

These concerns are intertwined with the effects of breast cancer on the family. Studies indicate that up to 35% of families of breast cancer patients experience significant changes in family functioning. More than 25% of children also experience problems related to their mothers' breast cancer (Hilton, 1994). In addition, families shoulder substantial costs in caring for family members with advanced breast cancer. These out-of-pocket, unreimbursed expenses include lost wages and salaries and lost opportunities.

When faced with any life-threatening illness, spiritual and existential concerns usually surface. Patients with breast cancer often express the need to talk about the uncertainties of their future and their hope and faith that they will be able to manage whatever crisis or challenge comes their way.

Pregnancy and Breast Cancer

From 2% to 5% of breast cancers occur in relation to pregnancy. The potent hormones released during pregnancy (1000 times greater than those during a menstrual cycle) stimulate changes in breast tissue. Thus, detecting masses is more difficult during pregnancy. An important aspect of health promotion is to encourage BSE throughout pregnancy.

If a mass is found during pregnancy, ultrasound is the preferred diagnostic method because it involves no exposure to radiation, although mammography with appropriate shielding, FNA, and biopsy may also be indicated. Treatment is basically the same as in other women, although radiation is contraindicated in pregnancy. Some oncologists begin chemotherapy as early as the 16th week of pregnancy because fetal organs are already formed at this point. If systemic treatment is necessary, a cesarean section may be performed as soon as safety of the fetus allows. If aggressive disease is detected early in pregnancy and chemotherapy is advised, termination of the pregnancy is an issue that some patients must face. If a mass is found while a woman is breastfeeding, she is urged to stop breastfeeding to allow the breast to involute (return to its baseline state) before any type of surgery is performed.

After a woman has completed treatment for breast cancer, she may consider having children. In this case, individual issues must be addressed, including the patient and her partner's desire for children and family, disease and prognostic concerns, age, fertility and infertility issues, and social, financial, ethical, and quality-of-life issues. Although recommendations vary, most women are advised to wait 2 years before becoming pregnant after completing treatment for breast cancer. Most retrospective studies indicate that pregnancy after treatment for breast cancer does not appear to increase the risk of the disease recurring (Dow, Harris, & Roy, 1994; Surbone & Petrek, 1997); however, prospective studies are needed to confirm this. Counseling, providing accurate information, and active listening and caring are important nursing interventions when patients are involved in making difficult personal decisions about treatment options, childbearing, or terminating pregnancy.

NURSING PROCESS: THE PATIENT WITH BREAST CANCER

Assessment

The health history includes an assessment of the patient's reaction to the diagnosis and her ability to cope with it. Pertinent questions include the following:

- How is the patient responding to the diagnosis?
- What coping mechanisms does she find most helpful?
- What psychological or emotional supports does she have and use?
- Is there a partner, family member, or friend available to assist her in making treatment choices?
- What are the most important areas of information she needs?
- Is the patient experiencing any discomfort?

Diagnosis

Preoperative Nursing Diagnoses

Based on the health history and other assessment data, the patient's major preoperative nursing diagnoses may include the following:

- Knowledge deficit about breast cancer and treatment options
- Anxiety related to cancer diagnosis
- Fear related to specific treatments, body image changes, or possible death
- Risk for ineffective coping (individual or family) related to the diagnosis of breast cancer and related treatment options
- Decisional conflict related to treatment options

Postoperative Nursing Diagnoses

Based on the health history and other assessment data, the patient's major postoperative nursing diagnoses may include the following:

- Pain related to surgical procedure
- Impaired skin integrity due to surgical incision
- Risk for infection related to surgical incision and presence of surgical drain
- Body image disturbance related to loss or alteration of the breast related to the surgical procedure
- Self-care deficit related to partial immobility of upper extremity on operative side
- Sensory/perceptual alterations (kinesthetic) related to sensations in affected arm, breast, or chest wall
- Risk for impaired adjustment related to the diagnosis of cancer, surgical treatment, and fear of death
- Risk for sexual dysfunction related to loss of body part, change in self-image, and fear of partner's responses
- Knowledge deficit: drain management after breast surgery
- Knowledge deficit: arm exercises to regain mobility of affected extremity
- Knowledge deficit: hand and arm care after an axillary lymph node dissection

Collaborative Problems/Potential Complications

Based on the assessment data, potential complications may include the following:

- Lymphedema
- Infection
- Hematoma formation

Planning and Goals

The major goals for the patient may include increased knowledge about the disease and its treatment; reduction of preoperative and postoperative fears, anxiety, and emotional stress; improvement of decision-making ability; pain management; maintenance of skin integrity; improved self-concept; improved sexual function; and the absence of complications.

Preoperative Nursing Interventions

Explaining Breast Cancer and Treatment Options

The patient confronting the diagnosis of breast cancer reacts with feelings of fear, dread, and anxiety. In view of the usually overwhelming emotional reactions to the diagnosis, the patient must be given time to absorb the significance of the diagnosis and any information that will help her to evaluate available treatment options.

The nurse caring for the woman who has just received a diagnosis of breast cancer needs to be knowledgeable about current treatment options and able to discuss them with the patient. The nurse should be aware of the information that has been given to the patient by the physician to answer specific questions the patient may have.

Information about the surgery, the location and extent of the tumor, and postoperative treatments involving radiation therapy and chemotherapy are details that the patient needs to help her make decisions. As appropriate, the nurse discusses uses of medications, the extent of treatment, management of side effects, possible reactions after treatment, frequency and duration of treatment, and treatment goals with the patient. Methods to compensate for physical changes related to mastectomy are also discussed and planned (eg, prostheses and plastic surgery). The amount and timing of the information provided are based on the patient's responses, coping ability, and readiness to learn.

Reducing Fear and Anxiety and Improving Coping Ability

The patient's emotional preparation begins when the tentative diagnosis of cancer is made. Patients who have lost close relatives to breast cancer (or any cancer) may have difficulty coping with the possible diagnosis of breast cancer because memories of loss and death can emerge during their own crisis.

The patient may have the diagnostic procedure performed in the surgeon's office or in the hospital when she is admitted for ambulatory or same-day surgery for a biopsy. Fears and concerns are common and are discussed with the patient. If she will undergo a mastectomy, information about various resources and options are made available. Such services include prostheses, reconstructive surgery, and groups such as Reach to Recovery. Discussion with a plastic surgeon about the various options for reconstructive surgery can be invaluable as a source of information and support.

The nurse provides anticipatory teaching and counseling at each stage of the process and identifies sensations that can be expected during additional diagnostic procedures. The nurse also discusses the implications of each treatment option and how it may affect various aspects of the patient's treatment course and lifestyle. The patient is introduced to other members of the oncology team (eg, radiation oncologist, medical oncologist, oncology nurse, and social worker) and acquainted with the role of each in her care. After the treatment plan has been established, the nurse needs to promote preoperative physical, psychological, social, and nutritional well-being. The patient usually prefers to be active in her care and decision making. Some women find it helpful and reassuring to talk to a breast cancer survivor, someone who has completed treatment and has been trained as a volunteer to talk with newly diagnosed patients.

Promoting Decision-Making Ability

At times, a patient may demonstrate behavior that indicates she cannot make a decision about treatment. Careful guidance and supportive counseling are the interventions the nurse can use to help such a patient. Also, encouraging the patient to take one step of the treatment process at a time can be helpful. The advanced practice nurse or oncology social worker can be helpful for patients and family members in discussing some of the personal issues that may arise in relation to treatment. Some patients may need a mental health consultation before surgery to assist them in the entire process of coping with the diagnosis and impending treatment. Such patients may have had a history of psychiatric problems or demonstrate behavior that leads the surgeon or nurse to initiate a referral to the psychiatrist, psychologist, or psychiatric clinical nurse specialist.

Postoperative Nursing Interventions

Relieving Pain and Discomfort

Ongoing nursing assessment of pain and discomfort is important because patients experience differing degrees of pain intensity. Some women may have more generalized pain and discomfort of the chest wall, affected breast, or affected arm. Moderate elevation of the involved extremity is one means of relieving pain because it decreases tension on the surgical incision, promotes circulation, and prevents venous congestion in the affected extremity. Intravenous or intramuscular opioid analgesics are another method to manage pain in the initial postoperative phase. After the patient is taking fluids and food and the anesthesia has cleared sufficiently (usually by the next morning), oral analgesics can be effective in relieving pain. Patient teaching before discharge to home then becomes important in managing discomfort after surgery because pain intensity varies widely. Patients should be encouraged to take analgesics (opioid or nonopioid analgesics such as acetaminophen) before exercises or at bedtime and also to take a warm shower twice daily (usually allowed on the second postoperative day) to alleviate discomfort that comes from referred muscle pain.

Maintaining Skin Integrity and Preventing Infection

In the immediate postoperative period, the patient will have a snug but not tight dressing or a surgical bra packed with gauze over the surgical site and one or more drainage tubes in place. A particular concern is preventing fluid from accumulating under the chest wall incision or in the axillae by maintaining the patency of the surgical drains. The dressings and drains should be inspected for bleeding and the extent of drainage monitored regularly.

If a hematoma develops, it usually occurs within the first 12 hours after surgery; thus, monitoring the incision is important postoperatively. The development of a hematoma could cause necrosis of the surgical flaps, although this complication is rare in breast surgery patients. If either of these complications occur, the surgeon should be notified, and the patient should have an ace wrap placed around the incision and an ice pack applied. Initially, the fluid in the surgical drain appears bloody, but it gradually changes to a serosanguinous and then a serous fluid during the next several days. The drain is usually left in place for 7 to 10 days and is then removed after the output is less than 30 mL in a 24-hour period. The patient is discharged home with the drains in place; therefore, teaching of the patient and family is important to ensure correct management of the drainage system (see the Home Care Teaching Checklist: Surgical Breast Cancer Patients With a Drainage Device).

Dressing changes present an opportunity for the nurse and patient to discuss the incision, particularly how it looks and feels and the progressive changes in its appearance. The nurse explains the care of the incision, sensations to expect, and the possible signs and symptoms of an infection. Generally, the patient may shower on the second postoperative day and wash the incision and drain site with soap and water to prevent infection. A dry dressing should be applied to the incision each day for 7 days. The patient needs to know that sensation is decreased in the operative area because the nerves were disrupted during surgery and that gentle care is needed to avoid injury. After the incision is completely healed (usually 4 to 6 weeks), lotions or creams may be applied to the area to increase skin elasticity. After the incision is fully healed, the patient may again use deodorant on the affected side, although many women note that they no longer perspire as much as before the surgery. During teaching sessions for incision care, the nurse can address the patient's perception of the body image changes and physical alteration of the breast. Using the term "incision" rather than "scar" reduces feelings of deformity.

Reducing Stress and Improving Coping Skills

Patients may initially be uncomfortable looking at the surgical incision. No matter how prepared a patient may be, the actual site of her own incision may still be difficult to view. Exploring this sensitive area must be a careful nursing action, and cues provided by the patient must be respected and sensitively handled. Privacy is a consideration when assisting the woman to view her incision fully for the first time and allows the patient to express her feelings safely to the nurse. Asking the patient what she perceives, acknowledging her feelings, and allowing her to express her emotions are important nursing actions. Explaining that her feelings are a normal response to breast cancer surgery may be reassuring to the patient.

Ongoing assessment of the patient's support systems is important, and the patient's spouse or partner may need guidance, support, and education as well. In addition, the patient may benefit from a wide network of available community resources, including the American Cancer Society's Reach to Recovery, advocacy groups, or a spiritual advisor. Encouraging the patient to discuss issues and concerns with other patients who have had breast cancer may help her to understand that her feelings are normal and that other women who have had breast cancer can provide invaluable support and understanding.

Another important aspect of nursing care includes answering questions and addressing the patient's concerns about treatment options that may follow surgery. After the actual surgery has been completed, thoughts about what lies in the future in terms of additional treatment are normal, and this topic can cause understandable anxiety. Refocusing the patient on the recovery from surgery, while addressing her concerns and answering her questions, can be helpful. Being knowledgeable about the plan of care and encouraging the patient to ask questions of the appropriate members of the health care team will also promote coping during recovery.

Promoting Participation in Care

Ambulation is encouraged when the patient is free of postanesthesia nausea and is tolerating fluids. The nurse supports the patient on the nonoperative side. Exercises (hand, shoulder, arm, and respiratory) are initiated on the second postoperative day, although instruction occurs on the first postoperative day. The goals of the exercise regimen are to increase circulation and muscle strength, prevent joint stiffness and contractures, and restore full range of motion. Hand exercises are also important for the same reasons.

Postmastectomy exercises are usually performed three times daily for 20 minutes at a time until full range-of-motion is restored (generally 4 to 6 weeks). Showering before exercising loosens stiff muscles, and taking an analgesic 30 minutes before beginning exercise increases the abilities of the patient to comply with the regimen. Also, self-care activities, such as brushing the teeth, washing the face, and combing and brushing the hair are physically and emotionally therapeutic because they aid in restoring arm function and a sense of normalcy for the patient.

The nurse encourages the patient to use the muscles in both arms and to maintain proper posture. If a patient is favoring or splinting the affected side, or not standing up straight, any exercise will be ineffective. If a patient has skin grafts, a tense, tight surgical incision, or immediate reconstruction, exercises may need to be prescribed specifically and introduced gradually. Most patients find that after the drain is removed, range of motion returns quickly if they have been compliant with their exercise programs.

Patients are instructed regarding activity limitations while healing postoperatively. Generally, heavy lifting is avoided, although normal household and work-related activities are promoted to maintain muscle tone. Driving may begin after the drain is removed and when the patient has full range-of-motion and is no longer taking opioid analgesics. General guidelines for activity focus on gradually introducing previous activities (eg, bowling, weight-training) when fully healed, although checking with the physician beforehand is usually indicated.

Transient edema in the affected extremity is common during the healing period, and women are encouraged to elevate the arm above the level of the heart on a pillow for 45 minutes at a time three times daily to promote circulation. Performing the prescribed exercises also assists in reducing the transient edema. Prevention of lymphedema is taught to patients before discharge. Hand and arm care after an axillary lymph node dissection focuses on the prevention of injury or trauma to the affected extremity, which increases the likelihood of developing lymphedema.

Managing Postoperative Sensations

Because nerves in the skin are cut during breast surgery, patients experience a variety of sensations. Common sensations are tightness, pulling, burning, and tingling along the chest wall, in the axilla, and along the inside aspect of the upper arm. They tend to become more noticeable and increase as the patient begins to heal. They usually persist for several months up to a year and then begin to diminish. Explaining to the patient that this is a normal part of healing helps to reassure her that these sensations are not indicative of a problem. Performing the exercises may decrease the sensations. Acetaminophen (Tylenol), taken as needed, also assists in managing the discomfort. Many breast surgery patients report these sensations as one of the most bothersome aspects of having the surgery.

Improving Sexual Function

Most breast surgery patients are physically allowed to engage in sexual activity once discharged from the hospital. However, any change in the patient's body image and self-esteem or the partner's response may increase the couple's anxiety level and may affect sexual function. Some partners may have difficulty looking at the incision, whereas others appear to be unaffected and comfortable. Either response affects the patient's self-image, sexuality, and acceptance. Open discussion and clear communication

Patient Education and Home Care
Postmastectomy Exercises

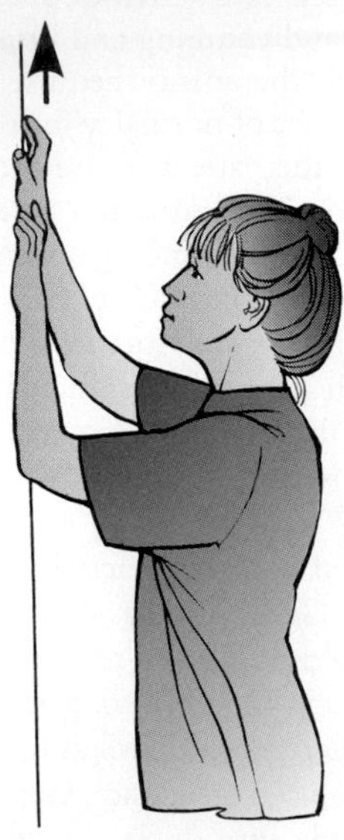

1. *Wall handclimbing.* Stand facing the wall with feet apart and toes as close to the wall as possible. With elbows slightly bent, place the palms of the hand on the wall at shoulder level. By flexing the fingers, work the hands up the wall until arms are fully extended. Then reverse the process, working the hands down to the starting point.

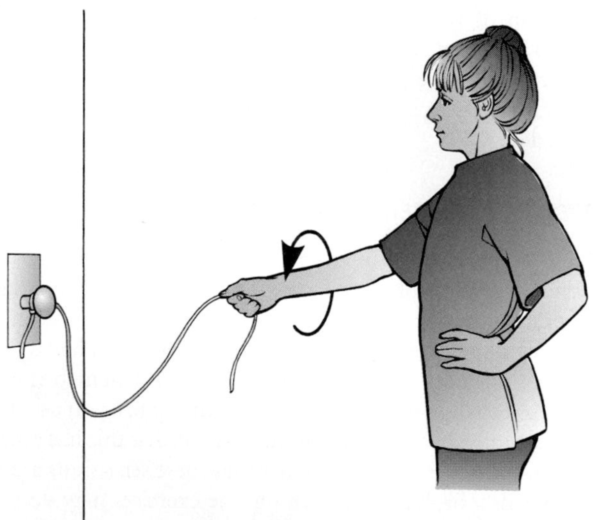

2. *Rope turning.* Tie a light rope to a doorknob. Stand facing the door. Take the free end of the rope in the hand on the side of surgery. Place the other hand on the hip. With the rope-holding arm extended and held away from the body (nearly parallel with the floor), turn the rope, making as wide swings as possible. Begin slowly at first; speed up later.

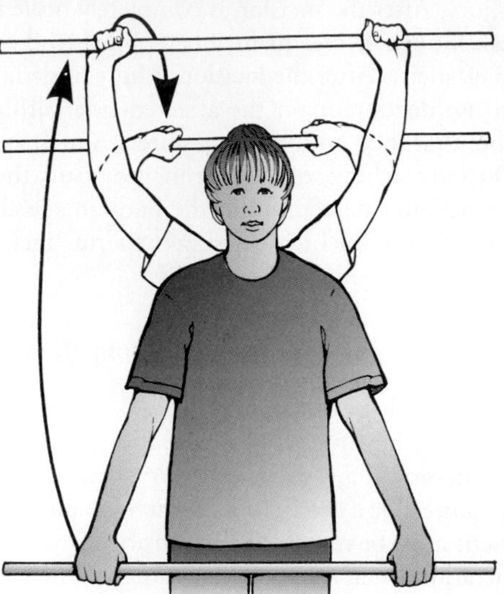

3. *Rod or broomstick lifting.* Grasp a rod with both hands, held about 2 feet apart. Keeping the arms straight, raise the rod over the head. Bend elbows to lower the rod behind the head. Reverse maneuver, raising the rod above the head, then return to the starting position.

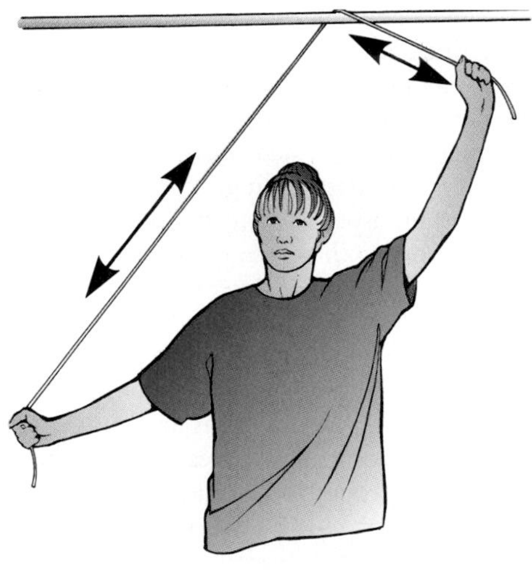

4. *Pulley tugging.* Toss a light rope over a shower curtain rod or doorway curtain rod. Stand as nearly under the rope as possible. Grasp an end in each hand. Extend the arms straight and away from the body. Pull the left arm up by tugging down with the right arm, then the right arm up and the left down in a see-sawing motion.

about how the patient sees herself and about possible decreased libido related to fatigue, anxiety, or nausea may help to clarify issues for her and her partner. Encouraging discussion about fears, needs, and desires may reduce the couple's stress. Suggestions regarding varying the time of day for sexual activity (when the patient is less tired) or assuming positions that are most comfortable can be helpful, as are alternative options (eg, hugging, kissing, manual stimulation) for expressing affection.

Most patients and their partners adjust with minimal difficulty if they openly discuss their issues and concerns; however, if prob-

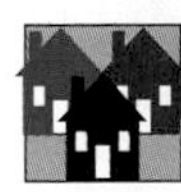

PATIENT EDUCATION AND HOME CARE

Hand and Arm Care After Axillary Dissection

- Avoid blood pressures, injections, and blood draws in affected extremity
- Use sunscreen (higher than 15 SPF) for extended exposure to sun
- Apply insect repellent to avoid bug bites
- Wear gloves for gardening
- Use cooking mitt for removing objects from oven
- Avoid cutting cuticles; push them back during manicures
- Use electric razor only for shaving armpit
- Avoid lifting objects greater than 5–10 pounds
- If a trauma or break in the skin occurs, wash the area with soap and water, and apply an over-the-counter antibacterial ointment (Bacitracin or Neosporin).
- Observe the area and extremity for 24 hours; if redness, swelling, or a fever occurs, call the surgeon or nurse.

lems develop or persist regarding sexual function after surgery for the treatment of breast cancer, referral to one of the psychosocial resources (psychologist, psychiatrist, or psychiatric clinical nurse specialist, social worker, or sex therapist) can be helpful for the woman and her partner.

Monitoring and Managing Potential Complications

LYMPHEDEMA

Lymphedema can occur any time after an axillary lymph node dissection. Lymphedema results if functioning lymphatic channels are inadequate to ensure a return flow of lymph fluid to the general circulation. After removal of axillary nodes, collateral or auxiliary circulation must take over their function. Transient edema in the postoperative period occurs until this collateral circulation has fully assumed functioning for the removed nodes, which generally occurs within a month's time by moving and exercising the affected arm. Patients need reassurance that this transient swelling is not lymphedema. Education about how to prevent lymphedema is an important part of hand and arm care after an axillary dissection. Lymphedema occurs in about 10% to 20% of patients who undergo an axillary dissection. Risk factors for lymphedema are increasing age, obesity, presence of extensive axillary disease, radiation treatment, and injury or infection to the extremity. Patients should follow these guidelines to prevent injury to the affected extremity because lymphedema is subsequently associated with a trauma of some type.

If lymphedema occurs, the patient should contact the surgeon or nurse to discuss management because she may need a course of antibiotics or specific exercises to decrease the swelling. Emphasis should be placed on early intervention because lymph-

NURSING RESEARCH

Postoperative Lymphedema

Carter, B. J. (1997). Women's experiences of lymphedema. *Oncology Nursing Forum, 24*(5), 875–882.

Purpose

The purpose of this descriptive qualitative study was to describe the experiences of women with lymphedema after breast cancer treatment because few studies have examined the impact of lymphedema on women's lives. Breast cancer survivors with lymphedema experience more functional impairment and psychosocial distress than survivors without lymphedema, and this can be related to the fact that lymphedema is visible and difficult to hide with clothing, impairs mobility, and can cause discomfort. Moreover, the development of lymphedema becomes a reminder of the breast cancer's impact on the woman's life, and it can be managed with various treatments, but is never truly cured.

Study Sample and Design

The 10 women comprising the sample ranged in age from 36 to 75 years. They were from an urban community, were white, married, and from middle to upper socioeconomic groups. Mean survival time from the cancer was 7 years, and the mean onset of lymphedema was 4 years. The women had completed their treatment for stage I or II breast cancer at least 1 year before the study and had developed lymphedema at least 2 months after surgery. They were interviewed twice.

The first interview focused on a description of the participants' experience at the time of lymphedema onset and treatment. The second interview, done 1 week later, attempted to gain an understanding of the participants' experience with long-term management as well as the impact of the lymphedema on their lives.

Findings

Analysis of the data from the interviews revealed themes related to the experience of lymphedema: (1) abandoned by medicine, (2) concealing the imperfect image, and (3) living the interrupted life.

Because lymphedema could not be entirely eliminated through medical treatments, these women demonstrated distress. They felt that their physicians were insensitive to their needs because they provided only vague suggestions and no concrete ways to treat or manage their symptoms. The women also described difficulty in finding information and treatment centers for lymphedema despite being in an urban community. This resulted in women feeling abandoned by medicine. The women described being very self-conscious about their physical appearance and went to great lengths to conceal the swollen arm, avoiding bathing suits, low-cut dresses, and short or tight-sleeved outfits. Furthermore, they avoided usual activities so as not to have to show their "unsightly" arm. Because the condition required special care, women experienced the lymphedema as a constant reminder of the disease that forced them to modify their intimate, work, and social habits. Thus, they considered their lives to be interrupted.

Nursing Implications

In providing care, all women who have had breast cancer and have been treated with an axillary dissection should be instructed preoperatively and postoperatively about the incidence of lymphedema after treatment (about 15%), the risk factors (increasing age, obesity, radiation treatment, and infection), and care of the hand and arm to prevent infection (the major causative factor). Teaching should emphasize early treatment of lymphedema to provide optimal management, and specific resources should be identified, so that women know whom to contact and where to go for evaluation and treatment. Psychosocial support is also a key nursing intervention for these women. Validating their feelings, normalizing them, and allowing them to verbalize them can assist these women in coping with the development and management of lymphedema. Further research is needed to document the incidence and possible causes of lymphedema, assess women's coping with the condition, and explore its effect on functional abilities, psychosocial status, and quality of life.

edema can be manageable if treated early; however, if allowed to progress without any treatment, the swelling can become painful and difficult to reverse. Management consists of arm elevation with the elbow above the shoulder, and the hand higher than the elbow, along with specific exercises, such as hand pumps. A referral to a physical therapist or rehabilitation specialist may be necessary for a custom-made elastic sleeve, exercises, manual lymph drainage, or a special pump to decrease swelling.

HEMATOMA FORMATION

Hematoma formation may occur after either mastectomy or breast conservation. The nurse monitors the surgical site for excessive swelling and monitors the drainage device, if present. Gross swelling or output from the drain may indicate hematoma formation, and the surgeon should be notified promptly. Depending on the surgeon's assessment, an ace wrap may be applied for compression of the surgical site along with ice packs for 24 hours, or the patient may be returned to surgery to identify the source of bleeding. The nurse monitors the site, provides reassurance to the patient that this complication is rare but does occur, and that she will be assisted through its management. A calm demeanor on the part of the nurse helps prevent feelings of anxiety and panic on the part of the patient.

INFECTION

Infection follows breast surgery in about 1 in 100 patients. Infection can occur for a variety of reasons, including concurrent conditions (diabetes, immune disorders, advanced age) and exposure to pathogens. In addition, cellulitis may occur after breast surgery. Before discharge, patients are taught to monitor for signs and symptoms of infection (redness, foul-smelling drainage, temperature greater than 100.4°F) and to contact the surgeon or nurse to arrange to be evaluated. Treatment consists of oral or intravenous antibiotics for 1 or 2 weeks depending on the severity of the infection. Cultures are taken of any foul-smelling discharge. Infections are a serious threat to women who have had breast reconstruction because they may lose the breast mound if the infection persists; there is a risk of lymphedema in women who develop an infection and have had an axillary lymph node dissection.

Promoting Home and Community-Based Care

TEACHING PATIENTS SELF-CARE

Patients who undergo breast surgery receive a tremendous amount of information before and after surgery. Additional teaching is necessary to prepare the patient and family to manage aspects of care after home discharge. Even though the ambulatory care nurse prepares the patient for what to expect postoperatively, the details often appear less important to the patient in light of the diagnosis of breast cancer. Thus, teaching may need to be repeated and reinforced postoperatively. Most patients are discharged in 1 or 2 days after the surgery with the drains in place. The nurse assesses the patient's readiness to assume self-care and focuses on teaching the patient incision care; signs to report, such as an infection; pain management; arm exercises; hand and arm care; and management of the drainage system at home. Family members may be included in the discharge teaching, and many women find it reassuring and helpful to have another person assist them with management of the drainage system. The nurse reinforces teaching by telephone follow-up and during postoperative visits in the office.

CONTINUING CARE

Referral for home care may be indicated to assist the patient and family caregiver with postoperative care at home. The home care nurse assesses the patient's incision and drainage system, physical and psychological status, adequacy of pain management, and adherence to the exercise plan. In addition, the home care nurse reinforces previous teaching and communicates important physiologic findings or psychosocial issues to the patient's primary care provider, nurse, or surgeon.

Follow-up visits to the physician after diagnosis and treatment of breast cancer depend on the individual and on postoperative treatments, stage of disease at time of diagnosis, late effects from cancer, and the patient's adaptation. Visits every 3 months for 2 years, followed by every 6 months up to 5 years, may be then extended to annual examinations, depending on the patient's progress and the physician's preference. A disease-free state for as long as possible is the goal. Patients are also encouraged to do BSE on the remaining breast (and operative side if breast-conserving surgery was done) and the chest wall (after mastectomy) between appointments with the primary health care provider as part of self-care because the risk for cancer in the remaining breast (or recurrence in the operative breast) is about 1% per year after the original diagnosis.

Preoperative Evaluation

Expected Outcomes

Expected outcomes may include:

1. Exhibits knowledge about diagnosis and treatment options
   a. Asks relevant questions about diagnosis and available treatments
   b. States rationale for surgery and other treatment options
   c. Describes advantages and disadvantages of treatment options
2. Verbalizes willingness to deal with anxiety and fears related to the diagnosis and the effects of surgery on self-image and sexual functioning
3. Demonstrates ability to cope with diagnosis and treatment
   a. Verbalizes feelings appropriately and recognizes normalcy of mood lability
   b. Proceeds with treatment in timely fashion
   c. Discusses impact of diagnosis and treatment on family and work
4. Demonstrates ability to make decisions regarding treatment options in timely fashion

Postoperative Evaluation

Expected Outcomes

Expected outcomes may include:

1. Reports that pain has decreased and states pain and discomfort management strategies are effective
2. Exhibits clean, dry, and intact surgical incisions without signs of inflammation or infection
3. Lists the signs and symptoms of infection to be reported to the nurse or surgeon
4. Verbalizes feelings regarding change in body image

5. Participates actively in self-care activities
   a. Performs exercises as prescribed
   b. Participates in self-care activities as prescribed
6. Recognizes that postoperative sensations are normal and identifies management strategies
7. Discusses meaning of the diagnosis, surgical treatment, and fears (especially of death) appropriately
8. Discusses issues of sexuality and resumption of sexual relations
9. Demonstrates knowledge of postdischarge recommendations and restrictions
   a. Describes follow-up care and activities
   b. Demonstrates appropriate care of the incisions and drainage system
   c. Demonstrates arm exercises and describes exercise regimen and activity limitations during postoperative period
   d. Describes care of affected arm and hand and lists indications to contact the surgeon or nurse
10. Experiences no complications
    a. Identifies signs and symptoms of reportable complications (ie, redness, heat, pain, edema)
    b. Describes side effects of chemotherapy and strategies to cope with possible side effects
    c. Explains how to contact appropriate health care providers in case of complications

Care of the patient with breast cancer is summarized in Plan of Nursing Care 44-1.

Recurrent Breast Cancer

The recurrence of breast cancer can be very difficult for patients and their family members. Depending on the clinical presentation, progression of the disease can have different meanings. Generally, the longer the disease-free interval for the patient, the better the prognosis. Local recurrence either in the affected breast or along the chest wall can be treated, generally with surgery, radiation, or hormonal manipulation, although a metastatic disease workup may be in order to look for further evidence of disease. Although metastatic spread of the breast cancer (to the bone, lungs, brain, or liver) cannot be cured, a variety of treatments are available (chemotherapy, radiation treatment, hormonal manipulation, or possibly some form of surgery). In some patients, metastases progress very slowly, and life functioning is generally not affected, whereas in others, disease progresses rapidly despite treatment, and death from the complications of metastatic disease is inevitable.

The patient with advanced breast cancer is monitored closely for signs that the tumor has recurred or that metastasis has occurred. The following studies are conducted to monitor for spread of disease: metastatic x-ray series (chest, skull, long bones, and pelvis); liver function tests (alkaline phosphatase, SGOT, SGPT, lactate dehydrogenase); mammogram of contralateral breast and ipsilateral breast (if breast-conserving surgery was originally performed); and bone, liver, and brain imaging. In half of all patients with recurrent disease, the cancer reappears locally (on the chest wall or in the conserved breast) or regionally in the remaining lymph nodes, and in one fourth, other organs become involved. Bone metastasis is the most common site for spread of the disease, usually involving the hips, spine, ribs, or pelvis. Other sites for metastatic spread are the brain, lungs, and liver.

Medical Management

Regression or relief of the symptoms is the goal of nursing and medical management, and quality of survival time is an important focus of nursing intervention. Assessing the patient's physical and psychosocial status is a challenge for the nurse. Information from family members and significant others is valuable and should be included in planning care for the patient with advanced disease.

Palliative treatment, if indicated, is also an important aspect of care. Comfort and a pain-free existence, even if the disease cannot be eradicated, enhance the quality of remaining life. Palliative surgery may be offered if the patient has a fungating or necrotic tumor in the breast; the most common procedure is a modified radical mastectomy. In patients with bone metastases that cause pain or produce pathologic fractures, reparative or restorative surgery may also be an option; however, this may not be indicated depending on the patient's medical status and personal choices. Hospice and home health care may be indicated as alternatives. Regardless, specific arrangements for these services should be discussed and planned early, before the actual need arises, to decrease patient distress. Severe anxiety and depression may occur. Treatment modes vary and depend on the patient's condition, the modalities available, and the patient's preferences for end-of-life care. Chapter 15 provides more information on the general care of the patient with advanced cancer, including hospice care.

RECONSTRUCTIVE BREAST SURGERY

Because the breast plays such an important part in self-image of many women, any perceived abnormality may lead to a request for surgical intervention, such as **mammoplasty** (plastic surgery of the breast in which size, shape, or position is altered). Variations in the size of the breasts are a common reason for women to seek information about reconstructive breast surgery. Reduction mammoplasty is performed to reduce the size of the breast, whereas augmentation mammoplasty is performed to increase the size of the breast. Other women desire surgery to reconstruct their breasts after mastectomy. There are several different procedures used for this type of reconstructive surgery. In addition, some women choose to undergo prophylactic mastectomy if they are at high risk for breast cancer. This type of mastectomy is included within this discussion because it is considered elective.

Reduction Mammoplasty

Reduction mammoplasty is usually performed on women who have breast hypertrophy (excessively large breasts). If the enlargement occurs early in life, it is called virginal breast hypertrophy. The condition is usually bilateral but may affect just one breast. Hypertrophy in later life almost always affects both breasts.

Tenderness, diffuse pain, and fatigue are common complaints of women with hypertrophy. Premenstrual tenderness and pain are marked. The weight of the enlarged breasts causes a dragging sensation in the shoulder, and support is commonly futile, despite use of the most supportive bra. Many women have deep grooves in their shoulders from the weight borne by bra straps. Poor posture, discomfort, and embarrassment when wearing bathing suits and participating in athletic events may limit the woman's social life. As a result, insecurity may develop from poor self-image.

After a surgical or plastic surgery consultation, a reduction mammoplasty may be performed under general anesthesia. One approach is an incision in the skin of the anterior breast in the

44•1

Plan of Nursing Care

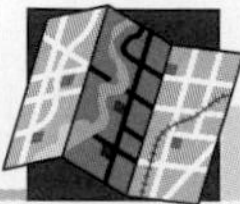

Care of the Patient With Breast Cancer

Nursing Diagnosis: Fear and ineffective coping related to the diagnosis of breast cancer, its treatment, and prognosis
Goal: Reduction of emotional stress, fear, and anxiety

Nursing Interventions	Rationale	Expected Outcomes
1. Begin emotional preparation of the patient (and partner) as soon as she is informed of tentative diagnosis.	1. This enables the patient to initiate coping responses.	• Displays reduced emotional stress and anxiety and exhibits an ability to cope with the problem
2. Assess a. Personal experience with and knowledge about breast cancer b. Coping mechanisms in crisis c. Support systems d. Emotional reaction to diagnosis	2. These factors strongly affect the patient's behavior and ability to deal with the diagnosis, surgery, and follow-up treatment. If a patient has lost close relatives or friends to breast cancer, she will probably react differently from a patient who has friends surviving with an excellent quality of life.	• Participates in the treatment plan and asks questions relating to the best choice for her particular needs • States that anger, anxiety, depression, denial, and withdrawal are normal reactions. • Responds positively to the information she has received
3. Inform the patient of recent research and new treatment modalities for breast cancer.	3. Increasing options and improved results both statistically and cosmetically greatly reduce the fear and promote acceptance of the treatment plan.	• Describes the value of social support of family, friends, and women who have had breast surgery in coping with a stressful experience
4. Describe the experiences the patient will face and encourage her questions.	4. Fear of the unknown decreases.	• Is aware that partner has been advised and prepared with regard to supportive role.
5. Acquaint her with available resources to facilitate her recovery.	5. The information about new prosthetics, reconstruction specialists, and other resources confirms that a great deal of attention is being given to newer treatment methods for breast cancer.	• Reads literature provided

Nursing Diagnosis: Disturbance in self-concept related to nature of surgery and side effects of radiation and/or chemotherapy
Goal: Realistic adaptation to changes that will occur relative to treatment modalities

Nursing Interventions	Rationale	Expected Outcomes
1. Confirm with the physician the nature of the treatment anticipated.	1. This sets the basis for a cooperative therapeutic plan that will prevent conflicting information from reaching the patient.	• Decides on the treatment plan after discussion with physician and family • Verbalizes that grief must run its course
2. Explain that it is normal to experience grief at the loss of a body part.	2. With this understanding, the patient can then be free to move to the next level of coping.	• Uses her support system effectively; plans future activities with them • Eventually looks at her incision site and participates in dressing changes
3. Encourage visits by loved ones and understanding friends.	3. Support systems that are meaningful to the patient are more endurable than those from relative strangers.	• Expresses an understanding of the long-term benefits of chemotherapy/radiation (if prescribed) even though there may be uncomfortable side effects
4. Explain that it is normal not to want herself or partner to view the incision (do not refer to this as a "scar"); further reinforce the fact that each day the site will look better.	4. This reduces the feeling that she will never be able to adjust to her altered body.	
5. Discuss the use of prosthesis, reconstruction possibilities, and clothing adjustment as realistic and attainable expectations.	5. The emphasis on the positive and the availability of adaptations will enhance her self-concept and promote positive acceptance of the treatment plan.	

Nursing Diagnosis: Pain related to tissue trauma from incision(s)
Goal: Absence of pain and discomfort

Nursing Interventions	Rationale	Expected Outcomes
1. Assess intensity, nature, and location of pain.	1. Provides baseline to assess effectiveness of pain-relief measures.	• Reports when pain is worsening and accepts prescribed pain medication
2. Administer analgesia by IM, oral, or IV route as prescribed.	2. Promotes pain relief.	• Adjusts her position to relieve discomfort; uses small pillows effectively

(continued)

44•1 **Plan of Nursing Care**

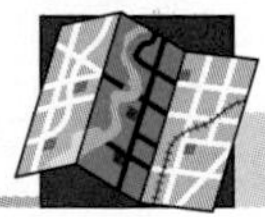

Care of the Patient With Breast Cancer (*continued*)

Nursing Interventions	Rationale	Expected Outcomes
3. Collaborate with physician about use of patient-controlled analgesia (PCA).	3. Patient-controlled analgesia results in pain relief and increased comfort and maintains patient's sense of control.	• Exercises frequently; moves affected arm gently and shows progress in moving from passive to active exercises
4. Explain that analgesics are available for pain relief.	4. Analgesics and opioids can interrupt nerve pathways to the brain and spinal cord.	• Describes home-related activities that will provide the required range of motion of the affected arm
5. Proper body positioning will promote comfort, such as semi-Fowler's position and elevation of the arm of the affected side.	5. Stress on the incision site is reduced; gravity reduces fluid accumulation in the arm. (Squeezing ball and wrist flexion begin in first 24 hours.)	• Relates procedures to follow if accidental injury is sustained • Orders medical identification tags when arm lymphedema is diagnosed
6. Promote passive and then active exercises of the hand, arm, and shoulder of the affected side.	6. This will stimulate circulation, promote neurovascular competence, and prevent stasis and subsequent stiffening of the shoulder girdle.	
7. Encourage protection and the avoidance of anything that can break through the skin barrier to impose stress on the arm and shoulder (cuts, burns, strong detergents, infections, carrying a heavy bag or purse).	7. Impaired circulation and weakened muscles are vulnerable to sudden or prolonged stress.	
8. Suggest application of an effective cream several times a day.	8. This practice will keep the skin healthy, intact, pliable, and resistant to breakdown.	
9. Instruct patient to contact the physician if the arm or incision site becomes painful, swollen, or red.	9. Early treatment of possible infection or injury will avoid further discomfort and complications.	
10. Suggest wearing a medical identification tag if there is a potential for injury or edema.	10. A recognized medical identification tag will serve as a precaution against injury to the affected arm.	

Nursing Diagnosis: Self-care deficit related to partial immobility of upper extremity on side of breast surgery
Goal: Avoidance of impaired mobility and achievement of self-care to the fullest possible level

Nursing Interventions	Rationale	Expected Outcomes
1. Encourage patient's active participation in postoperative care.	1. Patient involvement enhances and facilitates the recovery process.	• Participates in dressing change; expresses interest in working with rehabilitative team, including physical therapist
2. Encourage patient's socialization, particularly with others who have successfully recovered in similar circumstances.	2. Humans thrive more effectively when they are able to relate to others socially.	• Expresses concern about her appearance and accepts suggestions from rehabilitation support groups
3. Make progressive modifications in the patient's exercise program as dictated by comfort and tolerance levels.	3. There is lessened strain on tissues; improvement is consistent.	• Participates in self-care (ie, dressing, bathing, grooming)
4. Provide positive reinforcement when ingenuity and creativity are in evidence, such as an attractive hair style or make-up application.	4. Psychological well-being complements the effects of optimal physical good health.	• Verbalizes anticipation and enjoyment of partner's visits and relates her progress

Nursing Diagnosis: Possible sexual dysfunction related to loss of body part and fear of partner's reaction to this loss
Goal: Identification of alternative satisfying/acceptable sexual experiences

Nursing Interventions	Rationale	Expected Outcomes
1. Become comfortable in discussing sexuality; display a caring, nonjudgmental, supportive attitude.	1. The patient will easily sense insincerity, insecurity, lack of knowledge, and inexperience. Nurses new to this area can obtain assistance from the oncology clinical nurse specialist.	• Responds by conveying trust and a desire to obtain assistance; asks appropriate questions. • Includes partner in discussion of issues that concern both. • Verbalizes concerns about sexuality issues

(*continued*)

44•1 **Plan of Nursing Care**

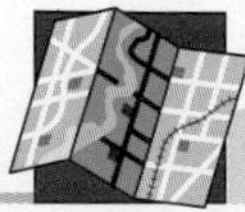

Care of the Patient With Breast Cancer (*continued*)

Nursing Interventions	Rationale	Expected Outcomes
2. Encourage, at the appropriate time, both partners to discuss their concerns; this can be done before and after major treatment.	2. The patient will not feel that she is alone in facing problems that may concern both partners.	• Accepts the incision site as evidenced by assisting with dressings and using an appropriate prescribed emollient such as cocoa butter • Expresses awareness that any adjustments take time but that with patience and understanding, the desired goals can be approached and possibly reached
3. Arrange for privacy when discussing personal problems with the patient.	3. Sensitive personal problems are not revealed when people not close to the patient are present.	
4. Describe the incision site and its appearance to the partner before partner actually sees it.	4. Partner will know what to expect and not likely register shock in front of the patient.	
5. Emphasize that behavioral changes take time and should not be interpreted as rejection.	5. Undergoing any surgery takes time for acceptance, recuperation, and perhaps altered lifestyle.	

Collaborative Problem: Infection, injury, lymphedema, neurovascular deficits
Goal: Avoidance of complications

Nursing Interventions	Rationale	Expected Outcomes
1. Encourage elevation of the arm, if not contraindicated, with each joint positioned higher than the more proximal joint.	1. Edema is reduced and there is less pressure on the nerves and blood vessels; pain and discomfort are reduced.	• Demonstrates positioning pillows so that proper elevation of arm is maintained • Describes strategies for avoiding injury and infection • Gradually moves the arm freely so that hair combing and "climbing the wall" can be achieved with no discomfort. Avoids the discomfort of a frozen shoulder • Acquires good health habits and avoids complications
2. Instruct patient to avoid injury, strenuous activity, or infection.	2. These can produce fluid accumulation and compromise the neurovasculature of the arm.	
3. Describe and demonstrate exercises in a step-up fashion from simple to more complex.	3. A graduated exercise program will improve muscle tone and hasten full range of activities with avoidance of impairment, such as a frozen shoulder.	
4. Recommend physical therapy and a weight-reduction program if indicated.	4. Properly prescribed activities and exercise plus diet modification are general health measures that enhance well-being and reduce risk for complications.	

shape of a keyhole or an anchor if a great amount of tissue needs to be removed. Another approach is through an incision around the areola complex. The surgeon then removes the excess tissue and transplants the nipple to a new location. Skin edges are approximated with sutures, and the nipple is secured with sutures. Drains are placed in the incision where they remain for 1 to 2 days. Simple gauze dressings are applied, without pressure.

Postoperative Nursing Management

After mammoplasty, usual postoperative care is indicated. Patients are ambulatory fairly quickly and typically describe their surgery as nontraumatic, possibly because of the relief they experience. Hypertrophy does not recur, but if the patient gains weight, the breasts may enlarge. The newly transplanted nipple most likely becomes scab covered. As the nipple regains a new blood supply, the scab falls off, and the appearance approximates normal. Lactation may be impossible after this type of surgery, although half of women who have this surgery can breastfeed successfully. Sensory changes, such as numbness, are normal after this surgery but resolve after several months, although there may be diminished sensation in the nipples that can persist. Feelings postoperatively may be a mixture of euphoria, relief, sorrow over loss of a body part, and anxiety over these feelings. Providing reassurance is an important nursing measure.

Augmentation Mammoplasty

Augmentation mammoplasty is requested frequently by women desiring larger or fuller breasts. It is performed through an incision along the undermargin of the breast, in the axilla, or at the border of the areola. The breast is then elevated, and a pocket is formed between the breast and the chest wall into which various types of synthetic materials are inserted to enlarge and uplift the breast. The subpectoral approach is preferred because it interferes less with clinical breast examinations or mammography than do subglandular implants. These procedures may be performed on an outpatient basis with local anesthesia. Infection is an immediate complication that can occur and may require subsequent removal of the implant. A delayed complication, which usually occurs years after the surgery, is a capsular contracture (scar formation around the implant); further surgery may be needed to correct this problem.

Saline implants are typically used for augmentation mammography. Silicone implants have been used in the past; however, because of the reported systemic complications associated with their use, they have been removed from the market. They are now available only to women enrolled in controlled clinical trials designed to study specific safety questions. Long-term risks associated with their use are also being studied. Women with breast implants need to be aware that accurate mammograms are more difficult, and they should seek radiologists at specialized breast centers who are familiar with reading mammograms of women who have breast implants.

Reconstructive Procedures After Mastectomy

When a woman undergoes a mastectomy (either total or modified radical) for the treatment of breast cancer, she may desire to have immediate reconstruction at the time of surgery, or delayed reconstruction may be an option at a later point after all treatments have been completed. About 75% of women with breast cancer undergoing mastectomy elect immediate reconstruction. A consultation with the surgeon may assist women in deciding whether reconstruction is something that they desire at the time of surgery. It is important for women to understand that reconstruction does not interfere with the treatment of their breast cancer, and they should also understand that although a good cosmetic result can be obtained, the reconstructed breast will never be what they once had. Another key point for women to understand is that reconstruction is a three-stage process that occurs over a period of months: the first is creation of the breast mound, the second is achieving symmetry with the contralateral breast, and the third is creation of the nipple–areola complex (described later). Women who undergo reconstruction with realistic expectations tend to be more pleased with the cosmetic result. Also, women who have mastectomy with immediate reconstruction may demonstrate a more positive adjustment afterward.

The choice of the surgical procedure is based on the patient's wishes, the condition of the overlying skin and underlying muscle, and any previous scars that may be present because they may limit possible reconstructive options. Another important factor is any secondary medical conditions that may affect the healing process (eg, hypertension, diabetes mellitus, tobacco use, or obesity).

Tissue Expanders With Permanent Implants

One method of reconstruction is the **tissue expander with permanent implant** (Fig. 44-6). After the surgeon has completed the mastectomy, the plastic surgeon creates a pocket inside the pectoralis muscle and inserts a partially filled Silastic expander and a drainage device. Then, over a period of weeks, the patient comes to the office for injections of additional saline into the expander through a port that is under the skin; this temporary expander stretches the skin and muscle. When the implant is fully expanded (usually one third larger than the other breast to create a natural crease and droop to match the contralateral breast), the patient has the temporary implant exchanged for a permanent implant. This is usually done as outpatient surgery. It may be done 4 to 6 months later to allow the tissue to soften and become more pliable before the permanent implant is inserted.

Postoperative care is similar to that of the patient undergoing breast surgery, although more discomfort can be expected due to the additional surgery. Nausea may take longer to clear because there was a greater period under general anesthesia. Patients receive instruction just as any other surgical breast cancer patient would, but usually they are not allowed to shower until the drain is removed.

Tissue Transfer Procedures

Another method of reconstruction is using the patient's own tissue and transferring it to the mastectomy site. These flap surgeries can use the **transrectus abdominal myocutaneous flap** (TRAM flap) (Fig. 44-7), gluteal muscle, or latissimus dorsi muscle (Fig. 44-8). The plastic surgeon transfers the muscle flap with attached circulatory structures, skin, and fatty tissue, rotates it to the operative site, and molds it to create a mound that simulates the breast. These procedures are far more extensive and involves greater operative time (about 8 to 10 hours total time for the mastectomy and reconstruction) and duration of general anesthesia than does the tissue expander procedure. The risk for potential complications is greater (infection, bleeding, flap necrosis), but the benefits are a more natural-looking breast and avoidance of synthetic material. The recovery period is greater, and activity restrictions are different due to the cut muscles.

The TRAM flap is the most commonly used tissue transfer procedure, and postoperative care involves drain management and monitoring the operative site for changes in circulation. During

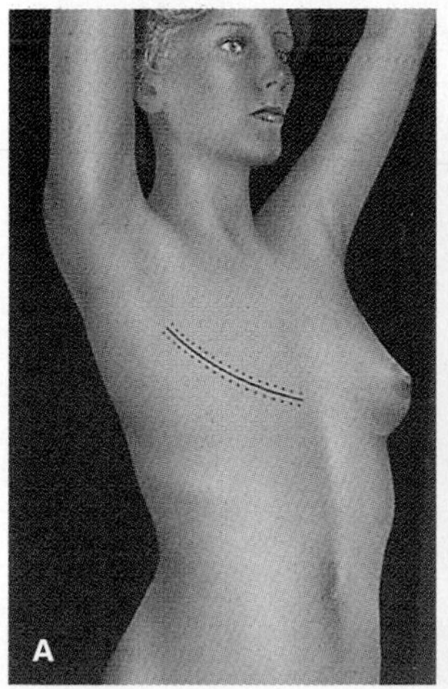

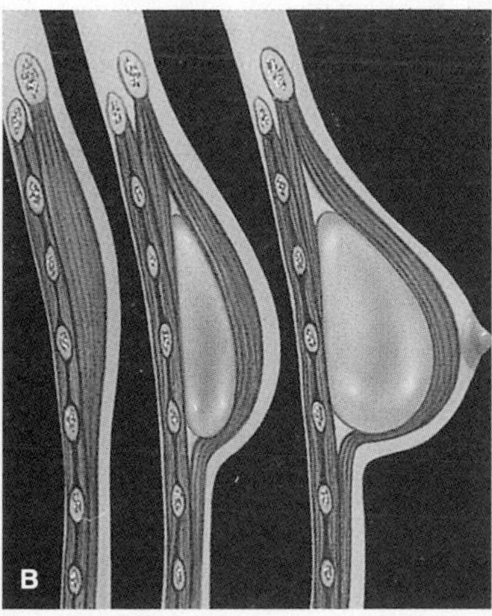

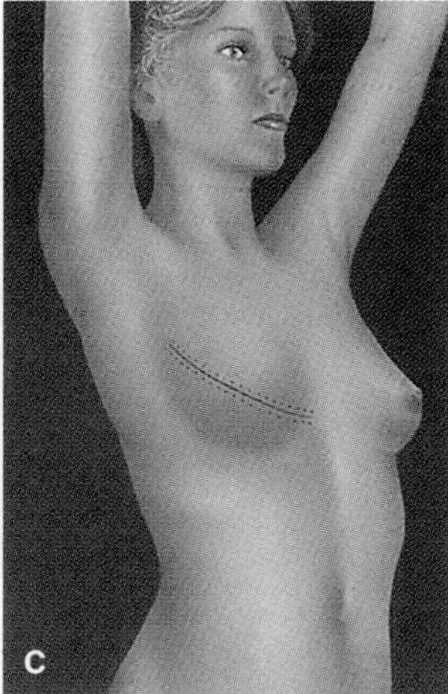

FIGURE 44•6 Breast reconstruction with tissue expander. (**A**) After mastectomy, a tissue expander is inserted to prepare for reconstruction. (**B**) The expander is gradually filled with saline solution through a tube to stretch the skin enough to accept an implant beneath the chest muscle. (**C**) The breast mound is restored. Although permanent, scars will fade with time. The nipple and areola are reconstructed later. Courtesy of American Society of Plastic and Reconstructive Surgeons, Arlington Heights, Illinois.

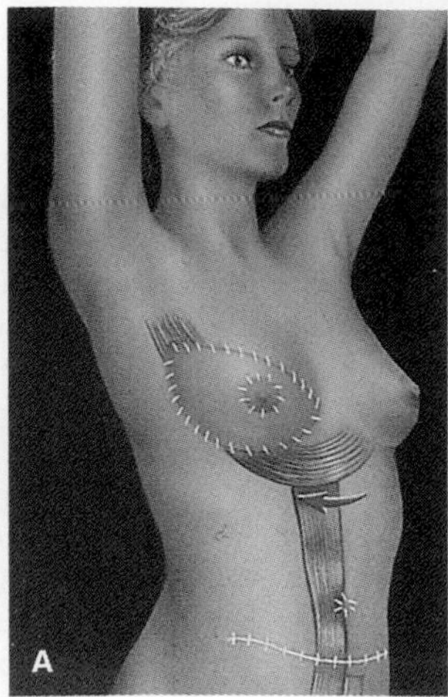

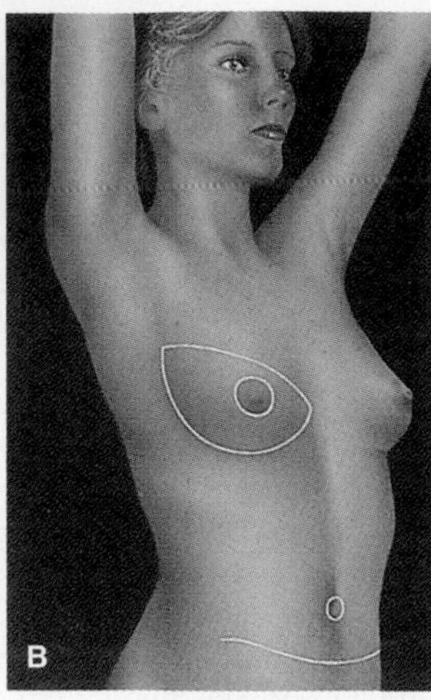

FIGURE 44•7 Breast reconstruction: TRAM flap. (**A**) The flap of the transrectus abdominal muscle is tunneled through the abdomen to the breast area. In some cases a breast implant may not be needed if enough skin and muscle can be transferred. (**B**) Scarring will fade substantially over time. Courtesy of American Society of Plastic and Reconstructive Surgeons, Arlington Heights, Illinois.

the immediate postoperative period, patients are more limited in their activity and are at greater risk for respiratory complications, so that pulmonary hygiene is essential. Measures to reduce tension on the incisions include elevating of the bed by 30 degrees and flexing the patient's knees to reduce tension on an abdominal incision. Antiemetics are administered to control nausea and vomiting, and analgesics are administered to reduce pain and discomfort. Assessing circulation by observing the color and temperature of the newly constructed breast area is an important nursing function. Mottling or an obvious decrease in skin temperature is reported to the surgeon immediately. Excessive drainage should also be reported.

During ambulation, the patient usually protects the surgical incision by splinting. Gradually, she will achieve a more upright position. The patient is instructed to avoid tight and underwire bras until the surgeon indicates that no injury will result. Elevating the arms above the shoulder and lifting more than 5 pounds of weight are avoided for 1 month after surgery to avoid stress on the incision.

Nipple–Areola Reconstruction

After the breast mound has been created and the site has healed, some women choose to have a nipple–areola reconstruction. This consists of minor surgical procedures carried out either in the physician's office or as outpatient surgery. A nipple is created using a skin graft from the inner thigh or labia because this skin has darker pigmentation than the skin on the reconstructed breast. After the nipple graft has healed, the areolar complex is usually completed with micropigmentation (tattooing). The surgeon is usually able to match the reconstructed nipple–areola complex with that of the contralateral breast for an acceptable cosmetic result.

DISEASES OF THE MALE BREAST

Gynecomastia

Gynecomastia, or overdeveloped breast tissue, is the most common breast condition in the male. Adolescent boys can be affected by this condition because of hormones secreted by the testes. Gynecomastia usually subsides in 1 or 2 years, but it can occur before or after puberty and at times in elderly men. It is usually unilateral and presents as a firm, tender mass underneath the areola. In adult men, gynecomastia may be diffuse and related to medications (ie, digitalis, reserpine, ergotamine, ranitidine, and phenytoin). Pain and tenderness are initial symptoms. Treatment depends on the individual's feelings and preference. Observation is acceptable because it may resolve on its own; surgical removal of the tissue through an incision around the areola is another option. Liposuction of the tissue done by a plastic surgeon is another option and yields a positive cosmetic result.

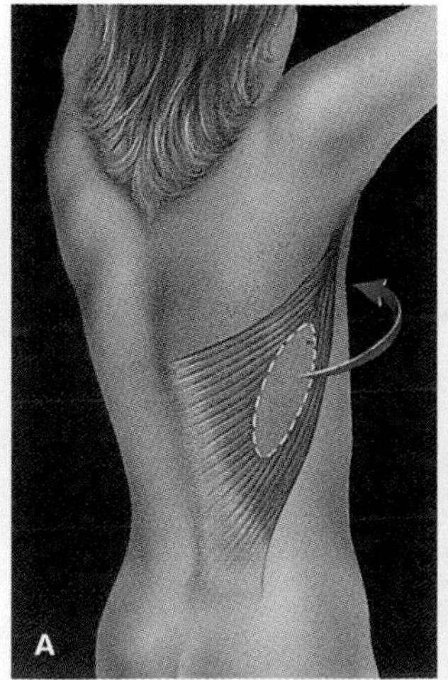

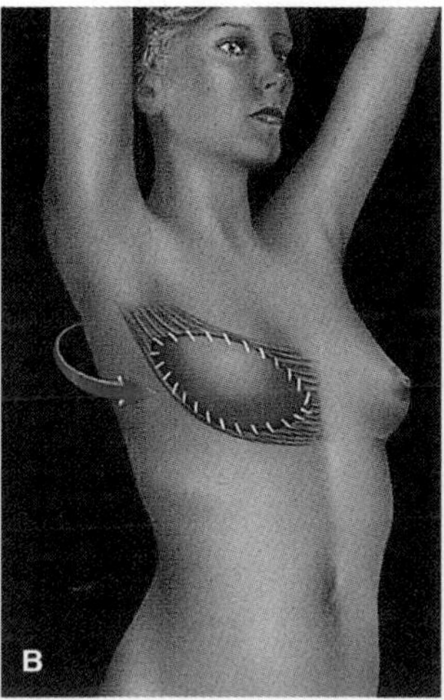

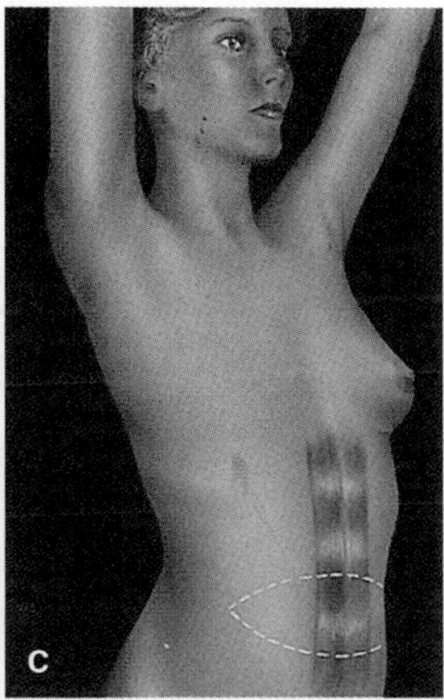

FIGURE 44•8 Breast reconstruction: latissimus dorsi flap. (**A**) Tissue taken from the back is tunneled to the front of the chest wall to support the reconstructed breast. (**B**) The transported tissue forms a flap that can hold a breast implant if there is not enough tissue to form a breast mound or (**C**) tissue may be taken from the abdomen and tunneled to the breast or surgically transplanted to form a new breast mound. Courtesy of American Society of Plastic and Reconstructive Surgeons, Arlington Heights, Illinois.

Male Breast Cancer

Cancer of the male breast accounts for 1% of all breast cancers. Symptoms can include a painless lump beneath the areola, nipple retraction, nipple discharge, or skin ulceration. Diagnostic tests and treatment modalities are similar to those used for women. The average age of the patient at the time of diagnosis is 60 years, but it can occur in younger men, especially if there is a genetic link to the disease, because there may be a relationship to BRCA-2 in men with breast cancer. Risk factors may include history of mumps orchitis, radiation exposure, and Klinefelter's syndrome (a chromosomal condition reflecting decreased testosterone levels).

Detection usually occurs well into the disease because cancer of the breast is not a common concern among men. Therefore, treatment generally consists of a modified radical mastectomy. If the pectoralis muscles are involved, a radical mastectomy is indicated. Radiation therapy may be used postoperatively. Prognosis varies depending on the stage of disease at the time of diagnosis. Bone and soft tissue are usually the most common sites of advanced disease and metastasis. Orchidectomy (removal of the testes), adrenalectomy (removal of the adrenal gland), and hypophysectomy (removal of the pituitary gland) may be used in advanced disease, but antihormonal agents are preferable because they are less invasive and disfiguring.

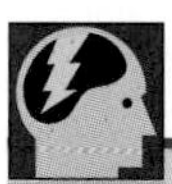

Critical Thinking Exercises

1. Your 35-year-old patient has just been diagnosed with breast cancer. Her mother, aunt, and one of her sisters have all had breast cancer. She is very worried about her own children's well-being and future. Describe the teaching program you feel is indicated for this patient and her children.

2. A 42-year-old woman reports to you that she has never had a mammogram and is afraid to have one done. How would you respond to her, and what teaching would you provide?

3. Two of your patients have undergone surgery for the treatment of breast cancer. One had a lumpectomy and axillary lymph node dissection; the other had a modified radical mastectomy. How would your nursing assessment and management of these two patients differ?

4. A 40-year-old woman is scheduled for a modified radical mastectomy and indicates that she is confused about the various types of breast reconstruction procedures. How would you instruct her about the differences, including the advantages and disadvantages of each and the postoperative course of each?

5. When you ask your patient about her pattern of doing BSE, she states that she does not know how to do it. Describe the teaching approach you would use to teach her. How would your approach differ if the patient did not speak English? What modifications would you make if the patient previously had a mastectomy?

References and Selected Readings

BOOKS

American Cancer Society. (1999). *Cancer facts and figures 1999.* Atlanta: American Cancer Society.

American Cancer Society. (1999). *Cancer statistics 1999.* Atlanta: American Cancer Society.

Baum, M., Saunders, C., & Meredith, S. (1994). *Breast cancer: A guide for every woman.* New York: Oxford University Press.

Berger, K. J., & Bostwick, J. III. (1994). *A woman's decision: Breast care, treatment and reconstruction.* St. Louis: Quality Medical Publisher.

Bickley, L. S., & Hoekelman, R. A. (1999). *Bates' guide to physical examination and history taking* (7th ed.). Philadelphia: Lippincott, Williams & Wilkins.

Bland, K. I., & Copeland, E. M. III (Eds.). (1998). *The breast: Comprehensive management of benign and malignant diseases.* Philadelphia: W. B. Saunders.

Dow, K. H. (1996). *Contemporary issues in breast cancer.* Boston: Jones & Bartlett.

Elston, C. W., & Ellis, I. O. (1998). *The breast.* New York: Churchill Livingstone.

Fentiman, I. S. (1998). *Detection and treatment of breast cancer.* London: M. Dunitz.

Fogel, C., & Lauver, D. (1990). *Sexual health promotion.* Philadelphia: W. B. Saunders.

Greenwald, P., Kramer, B. S., & Weed, D. L. (1995). *Cancer prevention and control.* New York: Marcel Dekker.

Groenwald, S. (1997). *Cancer nursing: Principles and practices.* Sudbury, MA: Jones & Bartlett.

Harris, J. R., Lippman, M. E., Morrow, M., & Hellman, S. (1996). *Diseases of the breast.* Philadelphia: Lippincott-Raven.

Holland, J. C. (1998) *Psycho-oncology.* New York, Oxford University Press.

Kavenaugh, J. J., et al. (1998). *Cancer in women.* Malden, MA: Blackwell Scientific.

Love, S. M. (1995). *Dr. Susan Love's breast book.* Reading, MA: Addison-Wesley.

Mansel, R. E. (Ed.). (1994). *Recent developments in the study of benign breast disease.* Proceedings of the 5th International Symposium on Benign Breast Disease. New York: Parthenon.

Miaskowsi, C. (Ed.). (1995). *Oncology nursing.* Albany: delmar Publishers.

Moore, G. (Ed.). (1997). *Women and cancer: A gynecologic oncology nursing perspective.* Boston: Jones & Bartlett.

O'Grady, L. F. (1995). *A practical approach to breast disease.* Boston: Little, Brown.

Packer, S. H., & Jobe, W. E. (1993). *Percutaneous breast biopsy.* New York: Raven Press.

Powell, D. E., & Stelling, C. B. (1994). *The diagnosis and detection of breast disease.* St. Louis: C. V. Mosby.

JOURNALS

Asterisks indicate nursing research articles.

General

Ashley, B. (1998). Mastalgia. *Lippincott's Primary Care Practice, 2*(2), 189–193.

*Benedict, S., Williams, R. D., & Baron, P. L. (1994). Recalled anxiety: From discovery to diagnosis of a benign breast mass. *Oncology Nursing Forum, 21*(10), 1723–1727.

Capriotti, T. (1998). Drug discoveries on the road to preventing breast cancer. *MedSurg Nursing, 7*(5), 304–307.

*Deane, K. A., & Degner, L. F. (1997). Determining the information needs of women after breast biopsy procedures. *AORN Journal, 65*(4), 767–776.

Hartmann, L. C., et al. (1999). Efficacy of bilateral prophylactic mastectomy in women with a family history of breast cancer. *New England Journal of Medicine, 340*(2), 77–84.

Hortobagyi, G. N. (1998). Treatment of breast cancer. *New England Journal of Medicine, 339*(14), 974–983.

Krag, D., et al. (1998). The sentinel node in breast cancer: A multicenter validation study. *New England Journal of Medicine, 339*(14), 941–946.

*Lauver, D., & Tak, Y. (1995). Optimism and coping with a breast cancer symptom. *Nursing Research, 44*(4), 202–207.

Morrison, C. (1998). The significance of nipple discharge: Diagnosis and treatment regimes. *Lippincott's Primary Care Practice, 2*(2), 129–140.

*Northouse, L. L., et al. (1995). Emotional distress reported by women and husbands prior to a breast biopsy. *Nursing Research, 44*(4), 196–201.

*Northouse, L. L., Tocco, K. M., & West, P. (1997). Coping with a breast biopsy: How healthcare professionals can help women and their husbands. *Oncology Nursing Forum, 24*(3), 473–480.

Osborne, C. K. (1998). Tamoxifen in the treatment of breast cancer. *New England Journal of Medicine, 339*(22), 1609–1618.

Ziegfeld, C. R. (1998). Differential diagnosis of a breast mass. *Lippincott's Primary Care Practice, 2*(2), 121–128.

Breast Cancer Risk and Prevention

Appling, S. (1996). One in nine: Risks and prevention strategies for breast cancer. *MedSurg Nursing, 5*(1), 62–64.

Bilimoria, M., & Morrow, M. (1995). The woman at increased risk for breast cancer: Evaluation and management strategies. *CA: A Cancer Journal for Clinicians, 45*(5), 263–278.

Canty, L. (1997). Breast cancer risk: Protective effect of an early first full-term pregnancy versus increased risk of induced abortion. *Oncology Nursing Forum, 24*(6), 1025–1031.

Fisher, B., & Constantino, J. (1997). Highlights of the NSABP breast cancer prevention trial. *Cancer Control, 4*(1), 78–86.

Fisher, B., Constantino, J. P., Wickerham, D. L., et al. (1998). Tamoxifen for prevention of breast cancer. Report of the National Surgical Adjuvant Breast and Bowel Project P-1 Study. *Journal of National Cancer Institute, 90*(18), 1371–1388.

Gagnon, P., et al. (1996). Perception of breast cancer risk and psychological distress in women attending a surveillance program. *Psycho-Oncology, 5,* 259–269.

Greenwald, P., & McDonald, S. S. (1997). Cancer prevention: The roles of diet and chemoprevention. *Cancer Control, 4*(2), 118–127.

Gross, R. E. (1998). Women at high risk for breast cancer. *American Journal of Nursing, 98*(4), 55–58.

Gross, R. E., Van Zee, K. J., & Heerdt, A. S. (1997). The special surveillance breast program: A model of intervention for women at high risk for breast cancer. *Journal of the New York State Nurses Association, 28*(4), 9–12.

Swan, D. K., & Ford, B. (1997). Chemoprevention of cancer: Review of the literature. *Oncology Nursing Forum, 24*(4), 719–727.

Thune, I., Brenn, T., Lund, E., & Gaard, M. (1997). Physical activity and the risk of breast cancer. *New England Journal of Medicine, 336*(18), 1269–1275.

*Walcott-McQuigg, J. A., Logan, B., & Smith, E. (1994). Prevention health practices of African American women. *Journal of the National Black Nurses Association, 7*(1), 25–35.

Wickerham, D. L. (1998). *Breast cancer prevention trial technical report.* Pittsburgh: National Surgical Adjuvent Breast and Bowel Project.

Woods, N. F. (1996). Cancer risk controversies: Women's exposure to exogenous ovarian hormones. *Oncology Nursing Updates: Patient Treatment and Support, 2*(1), 1–16.

Vogel, V. (1996). Assessing women's potential risk of developing breast cancer. *Oncology, 10*(10), 1451–1461.

Vogel, V., & Parker, L. S. (1997). Ethical issues of chemoprevention clinical trials. *Cancer Control, 4*(2), 142–149.

Cancer

Baron, R. H., & Walsh, A. (1995). Nine facts everyone should know about breast cancer. *American Journal of Nursing, 95*(7), 29–33.

Ganz, P. A. (1995). Advocating for the woman with breast cancer. *CA: A Cancer Journal for Clinicians, 45*(2), 114–126.

*Gray, R. E., et al. (1998). The information needs of well, longer-term survivors of breast cancer. *Patient Education and Counseling, 33*(3), 245–255.

Gross, R. E., & Major, M. (1997). Treatment options for breast cancer. *Gynecologic Oncology Nursing, 7*(1), 13–22.

Haas, B. K. (1997). The effect of managed care on breast cancer detection, treatment, and research. *Nursing Outlook, 45,* 167–172.

Harris, J., et al. (1992). Breast cancer, Part 1. *New England Journal of Medicine, 327*(5), 319–327. Part 2. 1992 Aug 6; 327(6):390-397. Part 3. 1992 Aug 13; 327(7):473-480.

Harris, J., et al. (1992). Breast cancer, Part 2. *New England Journal of Medicine, 327*(6), 390–397.

Harris, J., et al. (1992). Breast cancer, Part 3. *New England Journal of Medicine, 327*(7), 473–480.

Jaiyesimi, I., et al. (1992). Carcinoma of the male breast. *Annals of Internal Medicine, 117*(9), 771–777.

*Kilpatrick, M. G., Kristjanson, I. J., & Tataryn, D. J. (1998). Measuring the information needs of husbands of women with breast cancer: Validity and reliability of the Family Inventory of Needs-Husbands. *Oncology Nursing Forum, 25*(8), 1347–1351.

Knobf, M. T. (1994). Treatment options for early stage breast cancer. *MedSurg Nursing, 3*(4), 249–259, 328.

Knobf, M. T. (1994). Decision-making for primary breast cancer treatment. *MedSurg Nursing, 3*(3), 169–175, 180.

National Institutes of Health. (1990). Consensus statement: Treatment of early stage breast cancer. 8(6), 1–19.

*Pierce, P. (1993). Deciding on breast cancer treatment: A description of decision behavior. *Nursing Research, 42*(1), 22–28.

Samarel, N., et al. (1999). A resource kit for women with breast cancer: development and evaluation. *Oncology Nursing Forum, 26*(3):611–8.

Shea, B., Kleban, R., & Knauer, C. J. (1991). Breast cancer rehabilitation. *Seminars in Surgical Oncology, 7,* 326–330.

Snyder, G. M., Sielsch, E. C., & Reville, B. (1998). The controversy of hormone replacement therapy in breast cancer survivors. *Oncology Nursing Forum, 25*(4): 699–706.

Stommel, M., Given, C. W., & Given, B. (1991). The cost of cancer home care to families. *Cancer, 71*(5), 1867–1874.

Wagner, J. L., et al. (1995). Carcinoma of the male breast: Update 1994. *Medical and Pediatric Oncology, 24*(2), 123–132.

Weber, E. S. (1997). Questions and answers about breast cancer diagnosis. *American Journal of Nursing, 97*(10), 34–38.

Winchester, D. P., & Cox, J. D. (1998). Standards for diagnosis and management of invasive breast carcinoma. *CA: A Cancer Journal for Clinicians, 48*(2), 83–107.

Winchester, D. P., & Strom, E. A. (1998). Standards for the diagnosis and management of ductal carcinoma in situ (DCIS) of the breast. *CA: The Cancer Journal for Clinicians, 48*(2), 108–128.

*Woo, B., et al. (1998). Differences in fatigue by treatment methods in women with breast cancer. *Oncology Nursing Forum, 25*(5):915–920.

*Wyatt, G. K., & Friedman, L. L. (1998). Physical and psychosocial outcomes of midlife and older women following surgery and adjuvant therapy for breast cancer. *Oncology Nursing Forum, 25*(4):761–768.

Chemotherapy

*Berger, A. M. (1998). Patterns of fatigue and activity and rest during adjuvant breast cancer chemotherapy. *Oncology Nursing Forum, 25*(1), 51–62.

Boothe, V. A., et al. (1994). Tamoxifen in the treatment and prevention of breast cancer. *Cancer Practice, 2*(5), 334–342.

Foelber, R. (1998). Autologous stem cell transplant plus interleukin-2 for breast cancer: Review and nursing management. *Oncology Nursing Forum, 25*(3), 563–568.

Jaiyesimi, I. A., et al. (1995). Use of tamoxifen for breast cancer: Twenty-eight years later. *Journal of Clinical Oncology, 13*(2), 513–529.

Pasacretta, J. V., & McCorkle, R. (1998). Providing accurate information to women about tamoxifen therapy for breast cancer: Current indications, effects, and controversies. *Oncology Nursing Forum, 25*(9), 1577–1583.

Recht, A., et al. (1996). The sequencing of chemotherapy and radiation therapy after conservative surgery for early-stage breast cancer. *New England Journal of Medicine, 334*(21), 1356–1361.

Tyler, T. (1998). The medical management of breast cancer. *Lippincott's Primary Care Practice, 2*(2), 176–183.

Wasaff, B. (1997). Current status of hormonal treatments for metastatic breast cancer in postmenopausal women. *Oncology Nursing Forum, 24*(9), 1515–1520.

*Young-McCaughan, S. (1997). The impact of chemotherapy and endocrine therapy on sexual functioning in women with breast cancer. *Innovations in Breast Cancer Care, 2*(3), 50–62.

Genetics

Audrain, J., et al. (1998). Psychological distress in women seeking genetic counseling for breast-ovarian cancer risk: The contributions of personality and appraisal. *Annals of Behavioral Medicine, 19*(4), 370–377.

Baron, R. H., & Borgen, P. I. (1997). Genetic susceptibility for breast cancer: Testing and primary prevention options. *Oncology Nursing Forum, 23*(4), 461–468.

Biesecker, B. B. (1997). Psychological issues in cancer genetics. *Seminars in Oncology Nursing, 13*(2), 129–134.

Bove, C. M., Fry, S. T., & MacDonald, D. J. (1997). Presymptomatic and predisposition testing: Ethical and social considerations. *Seminars in Oncology Nursing, 13*(2), 135–140.

Calzone, K. A. (1997). Genetic predisposition testing: Clinical implications for oncology nurses. *Oncology Nursing Forum, 24*(4), 712–718.

*Geller, G., et al. (1998). Decision-making about breast cancer susceptibility testing: How similar are the attitudes of physicians, nurse practitioners, and at-risk women? *Journal of Clinical Oncology, 16*(8), 2868–2876.

Hughes, K. S., & Roche, C. A. (1996). How do we apply genetic testing for breast cancer susceptibility to clinical practice? *Journal of Surgical Oncology, 62,* 155–157.

Lessick, M., Wickham, R., & Rehwaldt, M. (1997). Breast and ovarian cancer: Genetic update and implications for nursing. *MedSurg Nursing, 6*(6), 341–352.

McCance, K. J., et al. (1998). Evaluating the genetic risk of breast cancer. *Nurse Practitioner, 23*(8), 14–16.

Schrag, D., Kuntz, K. M., Garber, E., & Weeks, J. C. (1997). Decision analysis: Effects of prophylactic mastectomy and oophorectomy on life expectancy among women with BRCA1 and BRCA2 mutations. *New England Journal of Medicine, 335*(20), 1401–1408.

Geriatric Considerations

Fanciosa, D., & Shaw, S. L. J. (1994). Breast cancer and benign breast disease in men. *Nurse Practitioner Forum, 5*(1), 56–58.

Hecht, J. R., & Winchester, D. J. (1994). Male breast cancer. *American Journal of Clinical Pathology, 102*(4 Suppl 1), S25–S30.

Lymphedema

*Carter, B. J. (1997). Women's experiences with lymphedema. *Oncology Nursing Forum, 24*(5), 875–882.

Humble, C. A. (1995). Lymphedema: Incidence, pathophysiology, management, and nursing care. *Oncology Nursing Forum, 22,* 1503–1509.

Marcks, P. (1997). Lymphedema: Pathogenesis, prevention, and treatment. *Cancer Practice, 5,* 32–38.

Price, J., & Purtell, J. R. (1997). Prevention and treatment of lymphedema after breast cancer. *American Journal of Nursing, 97*(9), 34–37.

Plastic Surgery and Breast Reconstruction

Bostwick, J. (1995). Breast reconstruction following mastectomy. *CA: A Cancer Journal for Clinicians, 45,* 289–304.

Carlson, G. W. (1994). Breast reconstruction: Surgical options and patient selection. *Cancer, 74*(Suppl 1), 436–439.

Fowler, M. E. (1994). Body contouring surgery. *Nursing Clinics of North America, 29*(4), 753–761.

Giomuso, C. B., & Suster, V. (1994). Free flap breast reconstruction. *MedSurg Nursing, 3*(1), 9–24.

Harden, J. T., & Girard, N. (1994). Breast reconstruction using an innovative flap procedure. *AORN Journal, 60*(2), 184–192.

Mangan, M. A. (1994). Current concepts in breast reconstruction. *Nursing Clinics of North America, 29*(4), 763–776.

*Neill, K. M., Armstrong, N., & Burnett, C. B. (1998). Choosing reconstruction after mastectomy: A qualitative analysis *Oncology Nursing Forum, 24*(4), 743–750.

Oberle, K., & Allen, M. (1994). Breast augmentation surgery: A woman's health issue. *Journal of Advanced Nursing, 20*(5), 844–852.

Schumann, D. (1994). Health risks for women with breast implants. *Nurse Practitioner: American Journal of Primary Health Care, 19*(7), 19–20, 23–25, 29–30.

Slavin, S. A., et al. (1998). Skin-sparing mastectomy and immediate reconstruction: Oncologic risks and aesthetic results in patients with early-stage breast cancer. *Plastic and Reconstructive Surgery, 102*(1), 49–62.

Pregnancy and Breast Cancer

Baron, R. H. (1994). Dispelling the myths of pregnancy-associated breast cancer. *Oncology Nursing Forum, 21*(3), 507–512.

Collichio, F. A., Agnello, R., & Staltzer, J. (1998). Pregnancy after breast cancer: From psychological issues through conception. *Oncology, 12*(5), 759-765.

*Dow, K. H., Harris, J. R., & Roy, C. (1994). Pregnancy after breast-conserving surgery and radiation therapy for breast cancer. *Journal of the National Cancer Institute, 16,* 131–137.

Friedland, D. M., et al. (1997). Adjuvant chemotherapy for breast cancer in pregnancy: Can recommendations be made with confidence. *Seminars in Oncology, 24*(2), 25–37.

Petrek, J. A. (1994). Breast cancer during pregnancy. *Cancer, 74*(Suppl 1), 518–531.

Preftakes, D. K. (1994). Breast cancer and pregnancy: Implications for perinatal care and fetal outcomes. *Journal of Perinatal and Neonatal Nursing, 7*(4), 31–41.

Surbone, A., & Petrek, J. A. (1997). Childbearing issues in breast carcinoma survivors. *Cancer, 79*(1), 1271–1278.

Psychological Aspects of Breast Cancer and Its Treatment

*Cohen, M. Z., Kahn, D. I., & Steeves, R. H. (1998). Beyond body image: The experience of breast cancer. *Oncology Nursing Forum, 25*(5), 835–841.

*Dow, K. H., et al. (1999). The meaning of quality of life in cancer survivorship. *Oncology Nursing Forum, 25*(3), 519–528.

*Ferrell, B. R., et al. (1998). Quality of life in breast cancer survivors: Implications for developing support services. *Oncology Nursing Forum, 25*(5), 887–895.

Girouard, S. A. (1996). Special needs of women whose mothers died of breast cancer. *Innovations in Breast Cancer Care, 1*(4), 77–79.

*Gross, R. E., Burnett, C. B., & Borelli, M. (1996). Coping responses to the diagnosis of breast cancer in postmastectomy patients. *Cancer Practice, 4*(5), 204–211.

*Hilton, B. A. (1994). Family communication patterns in coping with early breast cancer. *Western Journal of Nursing Research, 16*(4), 366–391.

*Kirkpatrick, M. G., et al. (1998). Information needs of husbands of women with breast cancer. *Oncology Nursing Forum, 25*(9), 1595–1601.

Oktay, J. S. (1998). Psychosocial aspects of breast cancer. *Lippincott's Primary Care Practice, 2*(2), 149–159.

*Pasacreta, J. V. (1997). Depressive phenomena, physical symptom distress, and functional status among women with breast cancer. *Nursing Research, 46*(4), 214–221.

Saleeba, A. K., Weitzner, M. A., & Meyers, C. A. (1996). Subclinical psychological distress in long-term survivors of breast cancer: A preliminary communication. *Journal of Psychosocial Oncology, 14*(1), 83–93.

Segar, M. L., et al. (1998). The effect of aerobic exercise on self-esteem and depressive and anxiety symptoms among breast cancer survivors. *Oncology Nursing Forum, 25*(1), 107–113.

Van der Pompe, G., Antoni, M., Visser, A., & Garssen, B. (1996). Adjustment to breast cancer: The psychobiological effects of psychosocial interventions. *Patient Education and Counseling, 28*(2), 209–219.

Walker, L. G., & Eremin, O. (1996). Psychological assessment and intervention: Future prospects for women with breast cancer. *Seminars in Surgical Oncology, 12,* 76–83.

Radiation Therapy

*Johnson, J. E., Fieler, V. K., Wlasowicz, G. S., Mitchell, M. L., & Jones, L. S. (1997). The effects of nursing care guided by self-regulation theory on coping with radiation therapy. *Oncology Nursing Forum, 24*(6), 1041–1050.

*Kolcaba, K., & Fox, C. (1999). The effects of guided imagery on comfort of women with early stage breast cancer undergoing radiation therapy. *Oncology Nursing Forum, 26*(1), 67–72.

*Mock, V., et al. (1997). Effects of exercise on fatigue, physical functioning, and emotional distress during radiation therapy for breast cancer. *Oncology Nursing Forum, 24*(6), 991–1000.

Overgaard, M., et al. (1997). Postoperative radiotherapy in high-risk premenopausal women with breast cancer who receive adjuvant chemotherapy. *New England Journal of Medicine, 337*(14), 949–955.

*Porock, D., et al. (1998). Predicting the severity of radiation skin reactions in women with breast cancer. *Oncology Nursing Forum, 26*(6), 1019–1029.

Screening, Breast Self-Examination, and Mammography

Barron, C. R., Houfek, J. F., & Foxall, M. J. (1997). Coping style, health beliefs and breast self-examination. *Issues in Mental Health Nursing, 18*(4), 331–350.

*Benedict, S., Goon, G., Hoomani, J., & Holder, P. (1997). Breast cancer detection by daughters of women with breast cancer. *Cancer Practice, 5*(4), 213–219.

Brown, L. W., & Williams, R. D. (1994). Culturally sensitive breast cancer screening programs for older black women. *Nurse Practitioner: American Journal of Primary Health Care, 19*(3), 21, 25–26, 31.

Cole, C. F. (1998). Issues in breast imaging. *Lippincott's Primary Care Practice, 2*(2), 141–148.

Deinger, M. J., & Llewellyn, J. (1995). Increasing compliance with breast self-examination. *MedSurg Nursing, 4*(5), 359–366.

Feig, S. A. (1997). Increased benefit from shorter screening mammography intervals for women ages 40-49 years. *Cancer, 80*(11), 2035–2039.

Gail, M. H., & Rimer, B. K. (1998). Risk-based recommendations for mammographic screening for women in their forties. *Journal of Clinical Oncology, 16*(9), 3105–3114.

Harris, R., & Leininger, L. (1995). Clinical strategies for breast cancer screening: Weighing and using the evidence. *Annals of Internal Medicine, 122*(7), 539–547.

*Lauver, D. (1994). Care-seeking behavior with breast cancer symptoms in Caucasian and African-American women. *Research in Nursing & Health, 17*(6), 421–431.

*Lauver, D. R., et al. (1999). Engagement in breast cancer screening behaviors. *Oncology Nursing Forum, 26*(3):545–554.

*Lierman, L. M., et al. (1994). Effects of education and support on breast self examination in older women. *Nursing Research, 43*(3), 158–163.

*Lierman, L. M., et al. (1994). Using social support to promote breast self examination performance. *Oncology Nursing Forum, 21*(6), 1051–1057.

McCance, K. L., Mooney, K. H., Field, R., & Smith, K. R. (1996). Influence of others in motivating women to obtain cancer screening. *Cancer Practice, 4*(3), 141–155.

*Miller, A. M., & Champion, V. L. (1996). Mammography in older women: One-time and three-year adherence to guidelines. *Nursing Research, 45*(4), 239–245.

National Institutes of Health. (1997). Consensus statement: Breast cancer screening for women ages 40–49. *15*(1), 1–35.

Stratton, B., et al. (1994). Breast self exam proficiency. *Journal of Woman's Health, 3*(3), 185–195.

Sternberger, C. (1994). Breast self-examination: How nurses can influence performance. *MedSurg Nursing, 3*(5), 367–371.
Vogel, V. (1993). Mammographic screening in younger women. *Female Patient, 18*(5), 21–27.

Surgical Treatment of Breast Cancer

Barnwell, J. M., et al. (1998). Sentinel node biopsy in breast cancer. *Annals of Surgical Oncology, 5*(2), 126–130.
Baron, R. H. (1999). Sentinel lymph node biopsy in breast cancer and the role of the oncology nurse. *Clinical Journal of Oncology Nursing, 3*(1), 17–22.
Burke, C. C., Zabka, C. L., McCarver, K. J., & Singletary, S. E. (1997). Patient satisfaction with 23-hour "short-stay" observation following breast cancer surgery. *Oncology Nursing Forum, 24,* 645–651.
Dell, D. D. (1997). Common questions about ductal carcinoma in situ. *American Journal of Nursing, 97*(5), 61–65.
Gazet, J. C. (1996). Future prospects in limited surgery for early breast cancer. *Seminars in Surgical Oncology, 12,* 39–45.
Gross, R. E. (1998). Current issues in the surgical treatment of early stage breast cancer. *Clinical Journal of Oncology Nursing, 2*(2), 55–63.
Hetelekidis, S., Schnitt, S. J., Morrow, M., & Harris, J. R. (1995). Management of ductal carcinoma i in situ. *CA: A Cancer Journal for Clinicians, 45,* 244–253.
Johnson, J. R. (1994). Caring for the woman who's had a mastectomy. *American Journal of Nursing, 94*(5), 25–31.
Moore, M. P., & Kinne, D. W. (1995). The surgical management of primary invasive breast cancer. *CA: A Cancer Journal for Clinicians, 45,* 279–288.
O'Hea, B. J., et al. (1998). Sentinel node biopsy in breast cancer: Initial experience at Memorial Sloan-Kettering Cancer Center. *Journal American College of Surgeons, 186*(4), 423–427.
Reintgen, D., et al. (1997). The role of selective lymphadenectomy in breast cancer. *Cancer Control, 4,* 211–225.
Small, W., & Morrow, M. (1997). Local management of primary breast cancer. *Cancer Control, 4,* 201–210.
Solin, L. J., et al. (1996). Fifteen-year results of breast conserving surgery and definitive breast irradiation for the treatment of ductal carcinoma in situ of the breast. *Journal of Clinical Oncology, 14,* 754–763.
Strozzo, M. D. (1998). An overview of surgical management of stage I and stage II breast cancer for the primary care provider. *Lippincott's Primary Care Practice, 2*(2), 160–169.
Veronesi, U., et al. (1997). Sentinel-node biopsy to avoid axillary dissection in breast cancer with clinically negative lymph-nodes. *Lancet, 349,* 1864–1867.

Resources

AGENCIES

American Cancer Society, 1599 Clifton Road, NE, Atlanta, GA 30329-4251; 1-404-320-3333; www.cancer.org (extensive professional and patient literature is available, including booklets on reconstruction, radiation, and chemotherapy)
American Cancer Society Breast Health Department, 19 West 56th Street, New York, NY 10019; 1-212-586-8700; www.cancer.org
American Society of Plastic and Reconstructive Surgeons, 444 East Algonquin Avenue, Arlington Heights, IL 60006; 1-800-635-0635; www.plasticsurgery.org
National Alliance of Breast Cancer Organizations, 1180 Avenue of the Americas, 2nd Floor, New York, NY 10036; 1-212-719-0154; Email: nabco@aol.com
National Breast Cancer Coalition, 1707 L Street NW, Suite 1060, Washington, DC 20036; 1-202-296-7477; www.natlbcc.org (This activist group has raised funds and consciousness levels regarding breast cancer and was instrumental in obtaining funds for research on prevention.)
National Cancer Institute, Public Inquiry Section, Office of Cancer Communications, National Cancer Institute, Building 31, Room 10 A 24, Bethesda, MD 20892; 1-800-422-6237; www.cancernet.nci.nih.gov (Patient materials can be ordered on the following topics: biopsies, treatment options, mastectomy, radiation, chemotherapy, reconstruction, diet, and clinical trials.)
National Lymphedema Network, 2211 Post Street, Suite 404, San Francisco, CA 94115; 1-800-541-3259; Email: lymphnet@hooked.net
Oncology Nursing Society, 501 Holiday Drive, Pittsburgh, PA 15220-2749; 1-412-921-7373; www.ons.org
Reach to Recovery Program—I Can Cope Program. (Information available through local American Cancer Society chapters.)
Susan G. Komen Breast Cancer Foundation, 5005 LBJ Freeway, Suite 370, Dallas, TX 75244; 1-800-I'M AWARE (1-800-462-9273); www.komen.org
Y-ME Breast Cancer Support Program, 212 West Van Buren Street, Chicago, IL 60607; 1-800-221-2141; www.y-me.org

WEBSITES

cancernet.nci.gov (produced jointly by the International Cancer Information Center, NCI, and the Office of Cancer Communications)
mskcc.org (information on Memorial Sloan-Kettering Cancer Center's programs and services for the prevention, cure, and control of cancer)
nysernet.org/bcic (serves as a clearinghouse for information on breast cancer)
oncolink.upenn.edu (University of Pennsylvania's educational resource for patients with cancer)
access.digex.net/~mkragen/index.html (a guide to cancer resources);
cancercareinc.org (produced by Cancer Care, Inc., an organization supported through educational grants and private contributions that provides telephone services and sponsors free teleconferenced seminars in addition to its Web-based services)

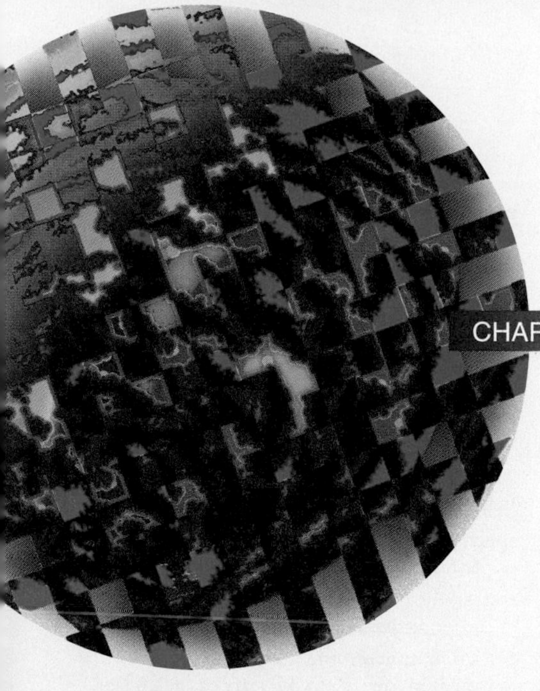

CHAPTER 45

Assessment and Management: Problems Related to Male Reproductive Processes

Learning Objectives

On completion of this chapter, the learner will be able to:

1. Describe structures and function of the male reproductive system.
2. Discuss nursing assessment of the male reproductive system and identify diagnostic tests that complement assessment.
3. Discuss the causes and management of male sexual dysfunction.
4. Compare the types of prostatectomy with regard to advantages and disadvantages.
5. Use the nursing process as a framework for care of the patient undergoing prostatectomy.
6. Describe the nursing management of patients with testicular cancer.
7. Describe the various conditions affecting the penis, including pathophysiology, clinical manifestations, and management.

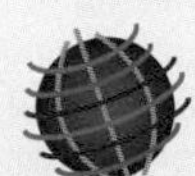

Disorders of the male reproductive system include a wide variety of conditions that usually affect both the urinary and reproductive systems. Because these disorders focus on the genitalia and in some instances sexuality, the patient may experience anxiety and embarrassment. Nursing care must incorporate the recognition of the patient's need for privacy with his need for education. This requires an openness to discuss critical and sensitive issues with the patient as well as effective assessment, management, and communication on the part of the nurse.

GLOSSARY

benign prostatic hyperplasia (BPH)**:** noncancerous enlargement or hypertrophy of the prostate; BPH is the most common pathologic condition in older men and the second most common cause of surgical intervention in men older than 60 years of age

Bowen's disease: a form of squamous cell carcinoma in situ of the penile shaft

circumcision: excision of the foreskin, or prepuce, of the glans penis

cryosurgery of the prostate: localized treatment of the prostate by application of freezing temperatures

cryptorchidism: most common congenital defect characterized by failure of the testes to descend into the scrotum

epididymitis: infection of the epididymis that usually descends from an infected prostate or urinary tract; also may develop as a complication of gonorrhea

erectile dysfunction: also called *impotence;* the inability to either achieve or maintain an erection sufficient to accomplish sexual intercourse

human papillomavirus (HPV)**:** virus that causes an infection that is increasing in prevalence; HPV infection manifests as genital condylomas, or genital warts; increases the risk for genitourinary cancer in men and their sexual partners

hydrocele: a collection of fluid, generally in the tunica vaginalis of the testis, although it also may collect within the spermatic cord

nocturia: urination during the night

orchiectomy: surgical removal of one of the testes

orchitis: inflammation of the testes (testicular congestion) caused by pyogenic, viral, spirochetal, parasitic, traumatic, chemical, or unknown factors

penile cancer: represents about 0.5% of malignancies in men in the United States; can involve the glans, the body of the penis, the urethra, and regional or distant lymph nodes

penis: male organ for copulation and for urination; consists of a glans penis, a body, and a root

Peyronie's disease: buildup of fibrous plaques in the sheath of the corpus cavernosum causing curvature of the penis when it is erect

phimosis: the condition in which the foreskin is constricted, so that it cannot be retracted over the glans; can occur congenitally or from inflammation and edema

priapism: an uncontrolled, persistent erection of the penis occurring from either neural or vascular causes, including medications, sickle cell thrombosis, leukemic cell infiltration, spinal cord tumors, and tumor invasion of the penis or its vessels

prostate cancer: the most common cancer in men; risk factors include increasing age, African American race, and possibly higher-fat diet; the genetic association of prostate cancer and the increased incidence within families is still being investigated

prostate gland: gland that lies just below the neck of the bladder, surrounds the urethra, and is traversed by the ejaculatory duct, a continuation of the vas deferens; produces a secretion that is chemically and physiologically suitable to the needs of the spermatozoa in their passage from the testes

prostate-specific antigen (PSA)**:** produced by the prostate gland and measured in a blood specimen; PSA levels are increased with prostate cancer; the PSA test is used in combination with digital rectal examinations to detect prostate cancer

prostatism: the obstructive and irritative symptom complex, which includes increased frequency and hesitancy in starting urination, a decrease in the volume and force of the urinary stream, acute urinary retention, and recurrent urinary tract infections

prostatitis: an inflammation of the prostate gland caused by infectious agents (bacteria, fungi, mycoplasma) or by various other problems (eg, urethral stricture, prostatic hyperplasia)

spermatogenesis: production of sperm in the testes

testes: the ovoid sex glands encased in the scrotum; the testes produce sperm

testicular cancer: the most common cancer in men 15 to 35 years of age and the second most common malignancy in those 35 to 39 years of age; its cause is unknown

testosterone: male sex hormone secreted by the testes, induces and preserves the male sex characteristics

transurethral resection of the prostate (TUR or TURP)**:** resection of the prostate through endoscopy; the surgical and optical instrument is introduced directly through the urethra to the prostate, and the gland is then removed in small chips with an electrical cutting loop

varicocele: an abnormal dilation of the veins of the pampiniform venous plexus in the scrotum (the network of veins from the testis and the epididymis, which constitute part of the spermatic cord)

vasectomy: also called male sterilization; the ligation and transection of part of the vas deferens, with or without removal of a segment of the vas to prevent the passage of the sperm from the testes

ANATOMIC AND PHYSIOLOGIC OVERVIEW

In the male, several organs serve as parts of both the urinary tract and the reproductive system. Disorders in the male reproductive organs may interfere with the functions of one or both of these systems. As a result, diseases of the male reproductive system are usually treated by a urologist. The structures in the male reproductive system are the testes, the vas deferens (ductus deferens) and the seminal vesicles, the penis, and certain accessory glands, such as the prostate gland and Cowper's gland (bulbourethral gland) (Fig. 45-1).

Testicular Development

The **testes** are formed in the embryo within the abdominal cavity near the kidney. During the last month of fetal life, they descend posterior to the peritoneum and pierce the abdominal wall in the groin. Later, they progress along the inguinal canal into the scrotum. In this descent, they are accompanied by blood vessels, lymphatics, nerves, and ducts, which support the tissue and make up the spermatic cord. This cord extends from the internal inguinal ring through the abdominal wall and the inguinal canal to the scrotum. As the testes descend into the scrotum, a tubular extension of peritoneum accompanies them. Normally, this tissue is obliterated, the only remaining portion being that which covers the testes, the tunica vaginalis. (When this peritoneal process is not obliterated but remains open into the abdominal cavity, a potential sac remains, into which abdominal contents may enter to form an indirect inguinal hernia.)

The testes are encased in the scrotum, which keeps them at a slightly lower temperature than the rest of the body to facilitate **spermatogenesis** (production of sperm). The testes consist of numerous seminiferous tubules in which the spermatozoa form.

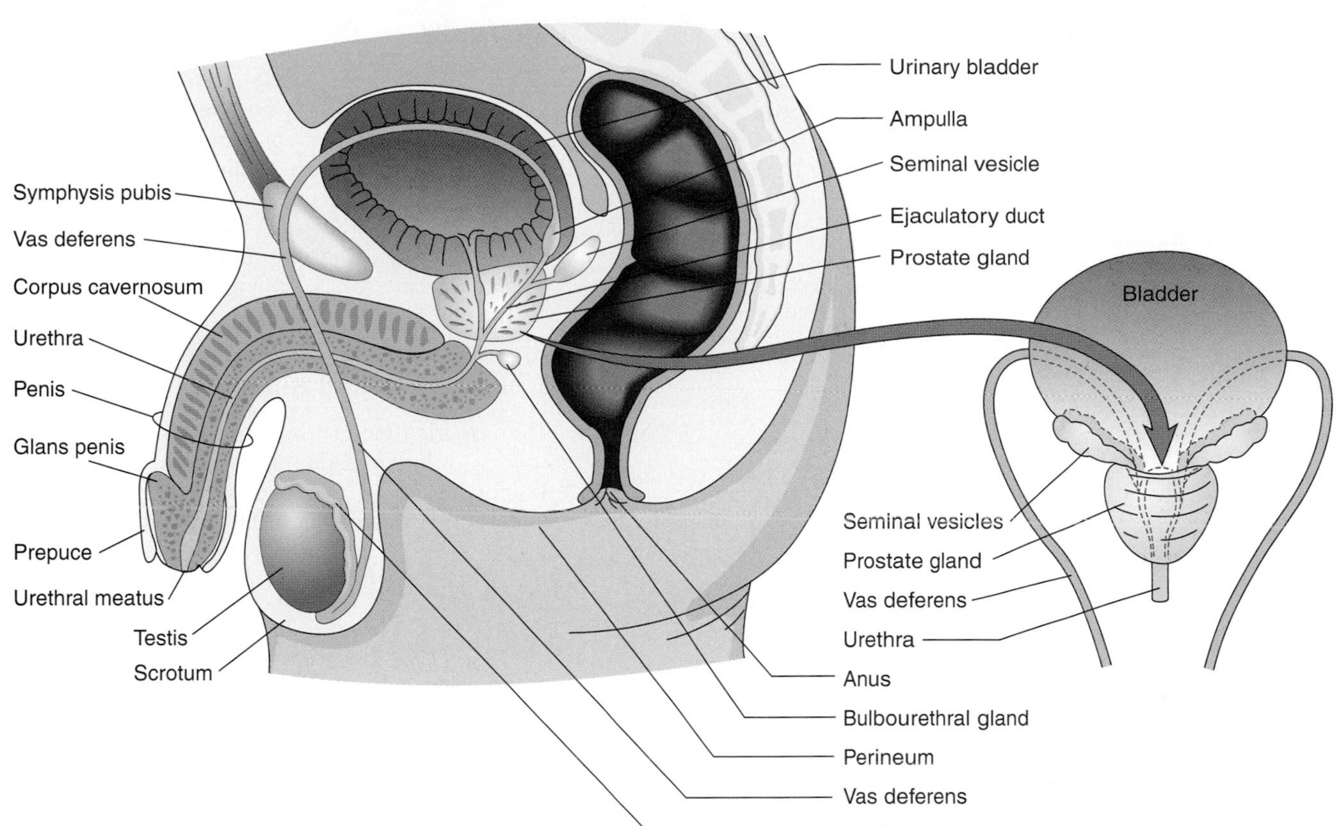

FIGURE 45•1 Organs of the male reproductive system. Adapted from Willis, M.C. (1996). *Medical terminology: The language of health care.* Baltimore: Williams & Wilkins.

Collecting tubules transmit the spermatozoa into the epididymis, a hoodlike structure lying on the testes and containing winding ducts that lead into the vas deferens. This firm, tubular structure passes upward through the inguinal canal to enter the abdominal cavity behind the peritoneum. It then extends downward toward the base of the bladder. An outpouching from this structure is the seminal vesicle, which acts as a reservoir for testicular secretions. The tract is continued as the ejaculatory duct, which passes through the prostate gland to enter the urethra. Testicular secretions take this pathway when they exit the penis during ejaculation.

Glandular Function

The testes have a dual function: the formation of spermatozoa from the germinal cells of the seminiferous tubules and the secretion of the male sex hormone **testosterone,** which induces and preserves the male sex characteristics.

The **prostate gland** lies just below the neck of the bladder. It surrounds the urethra and is traversed by the ejaculatory duct, a continuation of the vas deferens. This gland produces a secretion that is chemically and physiologically suitable to the needs of the spermatozoa in their passage from the testes.

Cowper's gland lies below the prostate within the posterior aspect of the urethra. This gland empties its secretions into the urethra at the time of ejaculation, providing lubrication. The **penis** has a dual function: it is the organ for copulation and for urination. Anatomically, it consists of a glans penis, a body, and a root. The glans penis is the soft, rounded portion at the distal end of the penis. The urethra, the tube that carries urine, opens at the tip of the glans. The glans is naturally covered or protected by elongated penile skin—the foreskin—which may be retracted to expose the glans. However, many men have had the foreskin removed (circumcision). The body of the penis is composed of erectile tissues containing numerous blood vessels that become distended, leading to an erection during sexual excitement. The urethra, which passes through the penis, extends from the bladder through the prostate to the distal end of the penis.

ASSESSMENT

Health History and Clinical Manifestations

To assess sexual function in the male, the health history focuses on sexual function as well as manifestations of sexual dysfunction. In addition, the patient is asked about changes in urinary function and symptoms that may occur with an obstruction caused by an enlarged prostate gland. The patient is asked about his usual state of health and any recent changes in general physical and sexual activity. Any symptoms or changes in function are explored fully and described in detail. Factors that may affect sexual functioning (eg, stress; physical disease; use of medications, drugs, or alcohol) are identified.

Physical Assessment

In addition to the customary aspects of the physical examination, two essential components address disorders of the male genital or reproductive system: the digital rectal examination and the testicular examination.

Digital Rectal Examination

The digital rectal examination (DRE) is recommended as part of the regular health checkup for every man older than 40 years of age; it is invaluable in screening for cancer of the prostate gland. The DRE enables the examiner to assess the size, shape, and consistency of the prostate gland (Fig. 45-2). Tenderness of the prostate gland on palpation and the presence and consistency of any nodules are noted. Although having this examination may be embarrassing for the patient, it is an important screening tool.

Testicular Examination

The male genitalia are inspected for abnormalities and palpated for masses. The scrotum is palpated carefully for nodules, masses, or inflammation. Examining the scrotum can reveal such disorders as hydrocele, hernia, or tumor of the testis. The penis is inspected and palpated for ulcerations, nodules, signs of inflammation, and discharge. The testicular examination provides an excellent opportunity to instruct the patient about techniques for testicular self-examination and its importance in early detection of **testicular cancer** (discussed later in this chapter).

DIAGNOSTIC EVALUATION

Diagnostic studies that relate to the male reproductive organs and to the ability to participate in sexual activity may be performed. They include the following.

Prostate-Specific Antigen Test

The prostate gland produces a substance known as **prostate-specific antigen (PSA)**, which is measured in a blood specimen and which increases with prostate cancer. The PSA test and DRE are used to detect prostate cancer.

Ultrasonography

Transrectal ultrasound studies (TRUS) may be performed in patients with abnormalities detected by DRE or those with elevated PSA levels. After DRE, a lubricated, condom-covered, rectal probe transducer is inserted into the rectum along the anterior wall. Water may be introduced to the condom to aid in transmission of sound waves to the prostate during the ultrasound study. TRUS may be used in detecting nonpalpable prostate cancers and in staging localized prostate cancer. Needle biopsies of the prostate are commonly guided by TRUS.

Prostate Fluid or Tissue Analysis

Specimens of prostatic fluid or tissue may be obtained for culture when disease or inflammation of the prostate gland is suspected. A biopsy of the prostate gland may be necessary to obtain tissue for histologic examination. This may be performed at the time of prostatectomy or by means of a perineal or transrectal needle biopsy.

Tests of Male Sexual Function

If the patient is unable to engage satisfactorily in sexual intercourse, a detailed history is obtained. Nocturnal penile tumescence tests may be conducted in a sleep laboratory to monitor changes in penile circumference (using a mercury strain gauge placed around the penis) during sleep; the test results help to identify the cause of erectile dysfunction. Arterial blood flow to the penis is measured with the Doppler probe. Nerve conduction tests and psychological evaluations are also part of the diagnostic workup and are usually conducted by a specialized team of health care providers.

DISORDERS OF MALE SEXUAL FUNCTION

Erectile Dysfunction

Erectile dysfunction, also called impotence, is the inability to achieve or maintain an erection sufficient to accomplish intercourse. The man may report decreased frequency of erections, in-

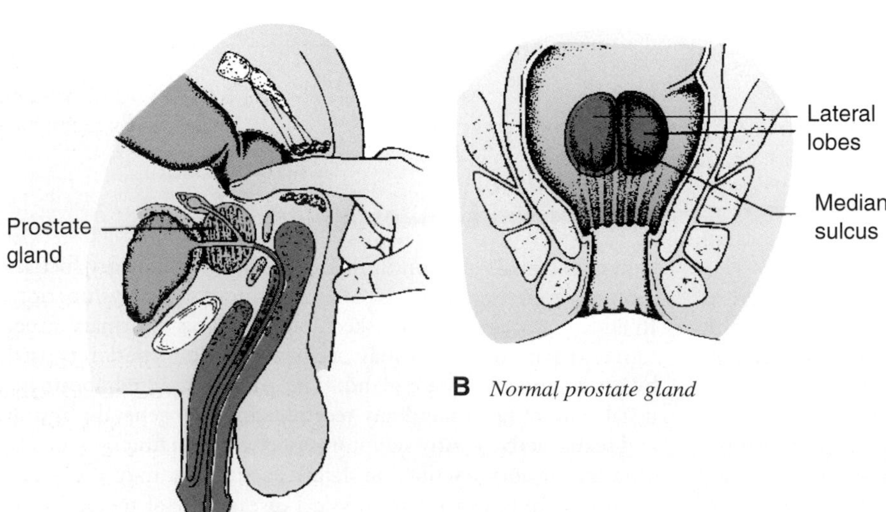

FIGURE 45•2 (**A**) Palpation of the prostate gland during digital rectal examination (DRE) enables the examiner to assess the size, shape, and texture of the gland. (**B**) The prostate is round, with a palpable median sulcus or groove separating the two lobes. It should feel rubbery and free of nodules and masses.

ability to achieve a firm erection, or rapid detumescence (subsiding of erection). Incidence ranges from 25% to 50% in men older than 65 years of age. The physiology of erection and ejaculation is complex and involves sympathetic and parasympathetic components. At the time of erection, pelvic nerves carry parasympathetic impulses that dilate the smaller blood vessels of the region and increase blood flow to the penis, expanding the corpora cavernosa.

Erectile dysfunction has both psychogenic and organic causes. Psychogenic causes include anxiety, fatigue, depression, and cultural pressure to perform sexually. Research suggests, however, that organic impotence may account for more impotence than previously realized. Organic causes include occlusive vascular disease, endocrine disease (diabetes, pituitary tumors, hypogonadism with testosterone deficiency, hyperthyroidism, and hypothyroidism), cirrhosis, chronic renal failure, genitourinary conditions (radical pelvic surgery), hematologic conditions (Hodgkin's disease, leukemia), neurologic disorders (neuropathies, parkinsonism), trauma to the pelvic or genital area, alcohol, medications (psychoactive agents, anticholinergics) and drug abuse.

Assessment and Diagnostic Findings

Diagnosis of erectile dysfunction requires a sexual and medical history; an analysis of presenting symptoms; a physical examination, including a neurologic examination; a detailed assessment of all medications, alcohol, and drugs used; and various laboratory studies. Nocturnal penile tumescence tests are conducted in sleep laboratories to monitor changes in penile circumference. In healthy men, nocturnal penile erections closely parallel rapid-eye-movement sleep in occurrence and duration. Organically impotent men show inadequate sleep-related erections that correspond to their waking performance. The nocturnal penile tumescence test can help to determine whether erectile impotence has an organic or psychological cause. Arterial blood flow to the penis is measured by means of a Doppler probe. In addition, nerve conduction tests and extensive psychological evaluations are carried out.

Medical Management

Treatment, which depends to some extent on the cause, can be medical, surgical, or both (Table 45-1). Nonsurgical therapy includes treating associated conditions, such as alcoholism, and readjusting hypertensive agents or other medications. Endocrine therapy may be instituted for erectile dysfunction secondary to hypothalamic-pituitary-gonadal dysfunction and may reverse the condition. Insufficient penile blood flow may be treated with vascular surgery. Patients with erectile dysfunction from psychogenic causes are referred to a health care provider or therapist specializing in sexual dysfunction. Patients with erectile dysfunction secondary to organic causes may be candidates for penile implants.

PENILE IMPLANTS

Penile implants are available in two types: the semirigid rod and the inflatable prosthesis. The semirigid rod (such as the Small-Carrion prosthesis) leaves the man with a permanent semierection. The inflatable prosthesis simulates natural erections and natural flaccidity. Complications after implantation include infection, erosion of the prosthesis through the skin (more common with the semirigid rod than with the inflatable prosthesis), and persistent pain, which may require removal of the implant. Cystoscopic surgery, such as **transurethral resection of the prostate** (TUR, also TURP) is more difficult with a semirigid rod than with the inflatable prosthesis. Factors to consider in choosing a prosthesis are the patient's activities of daily living and social activities and the expectations of the patient and his partner. Ongoing counseling for the patient and his partner is usually necessary to help them in adapting to the prosthesis.

NEGATIVE-PRESSURE DEVICES

Negative-pressure (vacuum) devices may also be used to induce an erection. A plastic cylinder is placed over the flaccid penis, and negative pressure is applied. When an erection is attained, a constriction band is placed around the base of the penis to maintain the erection. Although many men find this method satisfactory, others experience premature loss of penile rigidity or pain when applying suction or during intercourse.

PHARMACOLOGIC THERAPY

Pharmacologic measures to induce erections include injecting vasoactive agents, such as alprostadil, papaverine, and phentolamine, directly into the penis. Complications include **priapism** (a persistent abnormal erection) and development of fibrotic plaques at the injection sites. Alprostadil is also formulated in a gel pellet that can be inserted into the urethra to create an erection. Sildenafil (Viagra) is an oral medication for erectile dysfunction (Goldstein et al., 1998). When it is taken about 1 hour before sex, erections can occur with stimulation and last for about 60 minutes. Despite the effectiveness of this medication, it does have side effects. These may include headache, flushing, and dyspepsia. Sildenafil is contraindicated in patients who take organic nitrates and should be used with caution in patients with retinopathy, especially those with diabetic retinopathy.

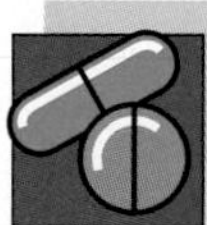

PHARMACOLOGY

Classes of Medications Associated With Erectile Dysfunction

- Antipsychotics: haloperidol (Haldol)
- Anticholinergics and phenothiazines: prochlorperazine (Compazine)
- Anxiolytics, sedative hypnotics, and tranquilizers: lorazepam (Ativan), triazolam (Halcion)
- Antiadrenergics and antihypertensives: guanethidine (Ismelin), clonidine (Catapres)
- Thiazide diuretics: hydrochlorothiazide (HydroDIURIL)
- Tricyclic antidepressants: amitriptyline (Elavil)

Nursing Management

The nurse needs to be aware that the ability to satisfy a partner and personal satisfaction are common concerns of patients. People with illness and disabilities may need the assistance of a sex therapist to find, implement, and integrate their sexual beliefs and behaviors into a healthy and satisfying lifestyle. The nurse can

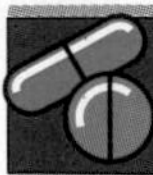

Table 45•1 Treatments for Erectile Dysfunction

Method	Description	Advantages and Disadvantages	Duration
Penile implants • Semi-rigid rod • Inflatable Penile implant	Surgically implanted into corpus cavernosum	Reliable Requires surgery Healing takes up to 3 weeks Subsequent cystoscopic surgery is difficult Semirigid rod results in permanent semierection	Indefinite Inflatable prosthesis: saline returns from penile receptacle to reservoir
Negative-pressure (vacuum) devices Penile vacuum pump	Induction of erection with vacuum; maintained with constriction band around base of penis	Few side effects Cumbersome to use before intercourse Vasocongestion of penis can cause pain or numbness	To prevent penile injury, constriction band must not be left in place for longer than 1 hour
Pharmacologic therapy • Injection (alprostadil, papaverine, phentolamine) Penile injection	Smooth muscle relaxant causing blood to flow into penis	Firm erections are achievable in more than 50% of cases Pain at injection site; plaque formation, risk of priapism	Injection 20 minutes before intercourse Erection can last up to 1 hour

(continued)

TABLE 45•1 Treatments for Erectile Dysfunction *(Continued)*

Method	Description	Advantages and Disadvantages	Duration
• Urethral suppository (alprostadil) Penile suppository	Smooth muscle relaxant causing blood to flow into penis	May be used twice a day Not recommended with pregnant partners	Inserted 10 minutes before intercourse Erection can last up to 1 hour
• Oral medication (sildenafil [Viagra]) VIAGRA Oral medication	Smooth muscle relaxant causing blood to flow into penis	Can cause headache and diarrhea Contraindicated for men taking organic nitrates Used with caution in patients with retinopathy, especially diabetic retinopathy	Taken orally 1 hour before intercourse Stimulation is required to achieve erection Erection can last 1 hour

inform patients that support groups for men with erectile dysfunction and their partners have been established. Information about Impotence Anonymous and I-Anon for their partners can be found at the end of this chapter.

Ejaculation Problems

Premature ejaculation occurs when a man cannot voluntarily control the ejaculatory reflex and, once aroused, reaches orgasm before or shortly after intromission. It is the most common dysfunction in men. Inhibited or retarded ejaculation is the involuntary inhibition of the ejaculatory reflex. The varying responses include occasional ejaculation through intercourse or self-stimulation or the complete inability to ejaculate under any circumstances.

Treatment modalities for ejaculation problems depend on the nature and severity of the problem. Behavioral therapies may be indicated for people with premature ejaculation; these therapies often involve the man and his sexual partner. Homework assignments are often given to the couple to encourage them to identify their sexual needs and to communicate those needs with each other. In some cases, pharmacologic and behavioral therapy together may be effective.

Disability (ie, spinal cord injury, multiple sclerosis), surgery (prostatectomy), and medications are the most common causes of inhibited ejaculation. Chemical, vibratory, and electrical stimulation have been used with some success. Treatment is usually multidisciplinary in approach and addresses the physical and psychological factors that are often involved in inhibited ejaculation. (Ducharme & Gill, 1997).

For men with retrograde ejaculation, the urine may be collected after ejaculation and sperm collected from the urine for use in artificial insemination. In men with spinal cord injury, electroejaculation may be used to produce sperm for artificial insemination.

Effects of trauma, chronic illness, and physical disability on sexual function can be profound. In addition to the effect of psychogenic factors, physical changes associated with illness and injury can potentially impair sexual function.

INFECTIONS OF THE MALE GENITOURINARY TRACT

Acute uncomplicated cystitis in adult men is uncommon but is occasionally noted in men whose sexual partner has vaginal infection with *Escherichia coli.* Asymptomatic bacteriuria may also

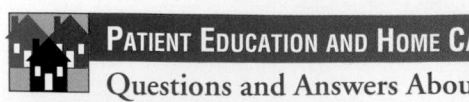

PATIENT EDUCATION AND HOME CARE

Questions and Answers About Viagra

What is Viagra?

It is a pill that is taken by mouth to restore erectile function in men with impotence. Viagra will not restore desire or sex drive.

How Does Viagra Work?

Viagra works by relaxing the penis, thus increasing the efficiency of the erection. The enzyme that the medication specifically works on is a type 5 phosphodiesterase (PDE-5), which is found almost exclusively in the penis.

How Do I Take Viagra?

Take 1 hour before intercourse. The peak action occurs between 30 and 120 minutes. *You must have sexual stimulation to create the erection.* If you fall asleep or need to go out in public, you will have no erection if you have no stimulation.

What Happens If I Don't Have Stimulation in the First Hour?

The beneficial effect can be seen as late as 8 hours, but most of the effectiveness is within the first 4 hours.

How Often May I Use Viagra?

The recommended frequency is once a day. If you take it more than once a day, you may experience back and leg aches as well as nausea and vomiting. Taking Viagra more than once a day will not improve its effects. You may take it 7 days a week if you desire, but it does not build up in your blood. Remember, only take it when you want to have intercourse.

What Are the Side Effects of Viagra?

Mild headache—but not bad enough to prevent taking the drug or enjoying its effects

Facial flushing—your face may get red

Indigestion—very mild upset stomach, which can be severe if you take more than one pill a day

Runny nose

Visual disturbance ("blue haze")—a transient, or temporary change in your vision that makes everything appear blue for about an hour; this will happen if you take more than the highest dose available (100 mg).

Are There Any Interactions With Other Medications?

You should not take Viagra if you are taking any nitrate medications:

Nitroglycerin	Isordil
Nitro-bid	Ismo
Any nitro medication	Indur

If you are unsure about your medications, it is important that you ask your doctor or pharmacist. You do not need to worry about blood pressure medications or diabetic medications.

Can I Use Viagra with MUSE or Penile Injections?

The use of Viagra with other forms of therapy has not been tested and should be avoided.

Is There More Than One Dose of Viagra?

The doses available are 25 mg, 50 mg, and 100 mg. Your first prescription will be for two tablets of each dose. Use the 25-mg dose first. If the 25-mg dose does not work, then try the 50-mg tablet. If this is not strong enough, then try the 100-mg tablet. *Do not take more than one tablet per day of any one dose.* When you find a dose that works for you, call your physician or provider, and a long-term prescription will be sent to you.

Used with permission of John Rieke, MD, Virginia Mason Division of Radiation Oncology.

occur from genitourinary manipulation, catheterization, or instrumentation. Urinary tract infections in the male are discussed in Chapter 41.

Sexually transmitted diseases (STDs) are increasing in men and women. STDs are most common in young, sexually active people, with the incidence higher in men than women. STDs affect people from all walks of life—from all social, educational, economic, and racial backgrounds. Several diseases are classified as STDs: urethritis (gonococcal and nongonococcal), genital ulcers (genital herpes infections, primary syphilis, chancroid, granuloma inguinale, and lymphogranuloma venereum), genital warts, scabies, pediculosis pubis, molluscum contagiosum, hepatitis and enteric infections, proctitis, and acquired immunodeficiency syndrome (AIDS). Trichomoniasis is an STD that is thought to increase susceptibility to human immunodeficiency virus (HIV) infection; it is associated with nonchlamydial, nongonococcal urethritis.

Treatment of STDs must be targeted to the patient as well as his sexual partner and sometimes the unborn child. A thorough history that includes a sexual history is crucial to identify patients at risk and to direct care and teaching. It is essential that the partners of men with STDs also be examined, treated, and counseled to prevent reinfection and complications in the partners and to limit the spread of the disease. Sexual abstinence during treatment and recovery is advised to prevent the treatment of STDs. Using condoms and spermicides containing nonoxynol 9 for at least 6 months after completion of treatment is recommended to decrease transmission of human papillomavirus (HPV) infections as well as other STDs, including HIV infection. Because patients with one STD may also have another STD, it is important to examine and test for other STDs. See Chapters 48 and 64 for more detailed discussions of HIV infection and AIDS and other STDs.

CONDITIONS OF THE PROSTATE

Prostatitis

Prostatitis is an inflammation of the prostate gland caused by infectious agents (bacteria, fungi, mycoplasma) or by various other problems (eg, urethral stricture, prostatic hyperplasia). *E. coli* is the most commonly isolated organism. Microorganisms are usually carried to the prostate from the urethra. Prostatitis may be classified as bacterial or abacterial, depending on the presence or absence of microorganisms in the prostatic fluid.

Clinical Manifestations

The symptoms of prostatitis may include perineal discomfort, burning, urgency, frequency, and pain with or after ejaculation. Prostatodynia (pain in the prostate) is manifested by pain on voiding or perineal pain without evidence of inflammation or bacterial growth in the prostatic fluid.

Acute bacterial prostatitis may produce sudden fever and chills and perineal, rectal, or low back pain. Urinary symptoms, such as dysuria, frequency, urgency, and nocturia (urination during the night), may occur. Some patients, however, do not have symptoms. Chronic bacterial prostatitis is a major cause of relapsing urinary tract infection in men. Symptoms are usually mild, consisting of frequency, dysuria, and occasionally urethral discharge. High temperature and chills are uncommon.

Complications of prostatitis may include swelling of the prostate gland and urinary retention. Other complications include epididymitis, bacteremia, and pyelonephritis.

Assessment and Diagnostic Findings

Diagnosis of prostatitis requires a careful history, culture of prostatic fluid or tissue, and, occasionally, a histologic examination of the tissue. To locate the source of a lower genitourinary infection (bladder neck, urethra, prostate), it is necessary to collect a divided urinary specimen for segmental urine culture. After cleaning the glans penis and retracting the foreskin (if present), the patient voids 10 to 15 mL of urine into a container. This represents urethral urine. Without interrupting the urinary stream, he collects 50 to 75 mL of urine in a second container; this represents bladder urine.

If the patient does not have acute prostatitis, the physician immediately performs a prostatic massage and collects any prostatic fluid that is expressed into a third container. If it is not possible to collect prostatic fluid, the patient voids a small quantity of urine. The specimen may contain the bacteria present in the prostatic fluid. Urinalysis after prostate examination commonly reveals many white blood cells.

Medical Management

The goal of therapy for acute bacterial prostatitis is to avoid the complications of abscess formation and septicemia. A broad-spectrum antibiotic agent (to which the causative organism is sensitive) is administered for 10 to 14 days. Intravenous administration of the agent may be necessary to achieve high serum and tissue levels. The patient is encouraged to remain on bed rest to alleviate symptoms quickly. Comfort is promoted with analgesics (to relieve pain), antispasmodics and bladder sedatives (to relieve bladder irritability), sitz baths (to relieve pain and spasm), and stool softeners (to prevent pain from straining).

Chronic bacterial prostatitis is difficult to treat because most antibiotics diffuse poorly from the plasma into the prostatic fluid. Nevertheless, antibiotics may be prescribed, including trimethoprim-sulfamethoxazole (TMP-SMZ), tetracycline, minocycline, and doxycycline. Continuous therapy with low-dose antibiotics to suppress the infection may also be indicated. The patient is advised that the urinary tract infection may recur and is instructed to recognize its symptoms. In addition, treatment for chronic prostatitis may include reducing the retention of prostatic fluid by ejaculation through sexual intercourse or masturbation. Other treatments include antispasmodics, sitz baths, stool softeners, and evaluation of sexual partners to reduce the possibility of cross-infection. The treatment of nonbacterial prostatitis is directed toward relieving symptoms.

Nursing Management

If the patient experiences symptoms of acute prostatitis (fever, severe pain and discomfort, or inability to urinate, malaise), he may be hospitalized for intravenous antibiotic therapy. The nursing management includes administration of prescribed antibiotics and provision of comfort measures, including prescribed analgesics and sitz baths.

The patient with chronic prostatitis is usually treated on an outpatient basis and needs to be instructed about the importance of continuing antibiotic therapy.

PROMOTING HOME AND COMMUNITY-BASED CARE

Teaching Patients Self-Care. The nurse instructs the patient to complete the prescribed course of antibiotics. Hot sitz baths (10 to 20 minutes) may be taken several times daily. Fluids are encouraged to satisfy thirst but are not "forced" because an effective medication level must be maintained in the urine. Foods and liquids that have diuretic action or that increase prostatic secretions, such as alcohol, coffee, tea, chocolate, cola, and spices, should be avoided. During periods of *acute* inflammation, sexual arousal and intercourse should be avoided.

To minimize discomfort, the patient should avoid sitting for long periods. Medical follow-up is necessary for at least 6 months to 1 year because prostatitis caused by the same or different organisms can recur.

Benign Prostatic Hyperplasia (Enlarged Prostate)

In many patients older than 50 years of age, the prostate gland enlarges, extending upward into the bladder and obstructing the outflow of urine by encroaching on the vesical orifice. This condition is known as **benign prostatic hyperplasia (BPH)**, the enlargement, or hypertrophy, of the prostate. BPH is the most common pathologic condition in older men and the second most common cause of surgical intervention in men older than 60 years of age.

Clinical Manifestations

Examination reveals a prostate that is large, rubbery, and nontender. The cause is uncertain, but evidence suggests that hormones initiate hyperplasia of the supporting stromal tissue and the glandular elements in the prostate. The hypertrophied lobes may obstruct the vesical neck or prostatic urethra, causing incomplete emptying of the bladder and urinary retention. As a result, a gradual dilation of the ureters (hydroureter) and kidneys (hydronephrosis) can occur. Urinary tract infections may result from urinary stasis, because some urine remains in the urinary tract and serves as a medium for infective organisms.

Assessment and Diagnostic Findings

The obstructive and irritative symptom complex (referred to as **prostatism**) includes increased frequency of urination, nocturia, urgency, hesitancy in starting urination, abdominal straining with urination, a decrease in the volume and force of the urinary stream, interruption of the urinary stream, dribbling (in which urine dribbles out after urination), a sensation that the bladder has not completely emptied, acute urinary retention (when more than 60 mL of urine remain in the bladder after urination), and recurrent urinary tract infections. Ultimately, azotemia (accumulation of nitrogenous waste products) and renal failure can occur with chronic urinary retention and large residual volumes. Generalized symptoms may also be noted, including fatigue, anorexia, nausea, vomiting, and epigastric discomfort. Other disorders producing similar symptoms include urethral stricture, prostate cancer, neurogenic bladder, and urinary bladder stones.

A physical examination with DRE and diagnostic studies may be performed to determine the degree to which the prostate is enlarged, the presence of any changes in the bladder wall, and the efficiency of renal function. These tests may include urinalysis and urodynamic studies to assess urine flow. Renal function tests, including serum creatinine levels, may be performed to determine if there is renal impairment from prostatic back-pressure and to evaluate renal reserve. Complete blood studies are performed. Because hemorrhage is a major complication of prostate surgery, all clotting defects must be corrected. A high percentage of patients with BPH have cardiac or respiratory complications, or both, because of their age; therefore, cardiac and respiratory function are also assessed.

Medical Management

The treatment plan depends on the cause of BPH, the severity of the obstruction, and the condition of the patient. If a patient's admission is as an emergency because he cannot void, he is immediately catheterized. The ordinary catheter may be too soft and pliable to advance through the urethra into the bladder. In such cases, a thin wire called a stylet is introduced (by a urologist) into the catheter to prevent the catheter from collapsing when it encounters resistance. In severe cases, metal catheters with a pronounced prostatic curve may be used. Sometimes, an incision is made into the bladder (a suprapubic cystostomy) to provide drainage.

Although prostatectomy (described later in the chapter) to remove the hyperplastic prostatic tissue is frequently performed, other treatment options are available. These include "watchful waiting," transurethral incision of the prostate (TUIP), balloon dilation, alpha-blockers, 5-alpha-reductase inhibitors, transurethral laser resection, transurethral needle ablation, and microwave thermotherapy (Agency for Health Care Policy and Research [AHCPR], 1994; Reilly, 1997). Watchful waiting is the appropriate treatment for many patients because the likelihood of progression of the disease or the development of complications is unknown. Patients are monitored periodically for severity of symptoms, physical findings, laboratory testing, and diagnostic urologic tests.

Alpha$_1$-adrenergic receptor blockers (eg, terazosin) relax smooth muscle of the bladder neck and prostate. Although the long-term efficacy of these agents is not known, they do reduce symptoms in many patients. Research into the long-term usefulness of these agents is ongoing (AHCPR, 1994).

Because the hormonal component of BPH has been identified, one method of treatment involves hormonal manipulation with antiandrogen agents, such as finasteride (Proscar). In clinical studies, 5-alpha-reductase inhibitors such as finasteride have been effective in preventing the conversion of testosterone to dihydrotestosterone. With decreased levels of dihydrotestosterone, suppression of glandular cell activity and decreases in prostate size have been demonstrated. Side effects of these medications include gynecomastia (breast enlargement), erectile dysfunction, and flushing.

With ultrasound guidance, resection of the prostate can be accomplished with lasers. The treated tissue either vaporizes or becomes necrotic and sloughs. This treatment is delivered in the outpatient setting and generally results in less postoperative bleeding than a traditional surgical prostatectomy.

Transurethral needle ablation uses low-level radio frequencies to produce localized heat to destroy prostate tissue while sparing the urethra, nerves, muscles, and membranes. The radio frequencies are delivered by thin needles placed into the prostate gland from a catheter. The body then reabsorbs the dead tissue.

Microwave thermotherapy applies heat to the hypertrophied prostatic tissue. A transurethral probe is inserted into the urethra, and microwaves are carefully directed to the prostate tissue. A water-cooling system helps to minimize damage to the urethra and decreases the discomfort from the procedure. The tissue becomes necrotic and sloughs.

Cancer of the Prostate

Cancer of the prostate is the most common cancer in men (other than nonmelanoma skin cancer) and the second most common cause of cancer deaths in American men older than 55 years of age (American Cancer Society, 1999). In African American men, **prostate cancer** is the most prevalent cancer overall; its incidence is almost twice that of the general population of men, and the death rate is about three times greater. About 1 in 5 men in the United States develop prostate cancer. An estimated 180,000 new cases of prostate cancer are diagnosed each year, and 37,000 men who already have it die from it each year (American Cancer Society, 1999). Risk factors include increasing age and possibly a high-fat diet. The genetic association of prostate cancer and the increased incidence within families is still being investigated. The growth of the prostate gland depends on the presence of androgenic hormones, such as testosterone. Because dihydrotestosterone is an important promoter of prostate cancer, medications such as finasteride are being advocated as a means of preventing

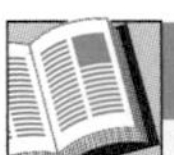

NURSING RESEARCH

Prostate Cancer Education

Collins, M. (1997). Increasing prostate cancer awareness in African American men. *Oncology Nursing Forum, 24* (1), 91–95.

Purpose

Prostate cancer is the leading cause of cancer in men. African American men are twice as likely as the general population of men to be diagnosed with prostate cancer and three times as likely to die from the disease. This study evaluated an educational approach to increase prostate cancer awareness in African American men.

Study Sample and Design

A convenience sample of 75 African American men aged 23 to 88 years of age who attended health screenings, health fairs, and other community-based meetings participated in the study. Before and after an educational program, participants completed a seven-item questionnaire about prostate cancer incidence, risk factors, and detection. The questionnaire was based on patient education materials from the American Cancer Society. The percentage of items answered correctly was calculated. A brief educational session was provided outlining incidence, risk factors, and detection of prostate cancer.

Findings

The scores increased from 23% correct on the pretest to 64% correct on the posttest (following the educational intervention). The three most frequently missed questions in the pretest addressed urinary frequency as an early symptom of prostate cancer, the incidence of prostate cancer in African American men, and the increased risk for prostate cancer among African American men. These questions were also the most frequently missed in the posttest.

Nursing Implications

The results of this study indicate that a brief educational intervention can be effective in increasing knowledge and awareness of prostate cancer in African American men. Because of the increased risk of prostate cancer in this population, it is important to provide education about prostate cancer to improve early detection endeavors. Further research is needed to determine if the increased knowledge is retained and if educational efforts that result in increased knowledge about prostate cancer have an effect on the participation of African American men in screening for prostate cancer.

prostate cancer from developing by inhibiting prostatic cell proliferation and killing prostatic cancer cells.

Clinical Manifestations

Cancer of the prostate in its early stages rarely produces symptoms. The symptoms that develop from urinary obstruction occur late in the disease. This cancer tends to vary in its course. If the neoplasm is large enough to encroach on the bladder neck, signs and symptoms of urinary obstruction occur, namely, difficulty and frequency of urination, urinary retention, and decreased size and force of the urinary stream. Prostatic cancer commonly metastasizes to bone and lymph nodes. Symptoms related to metastases include backache, hip pain, perineal and rectal discomfort, anemia, weight loss, weakness, nausea, and oliguria (decreased urine output). Hematuria may result from the cancer invading the urethra or bladder, or both. Unfortunately, these symptoms may be the first overt indications of prostate cancer.

Assessment and Diagnostic Findings

When prostate cancer is detected at an early stage, the likelihood of cure is high. Every man older than 40 years of age should have a DRE as part of his regular health checkup. Routine repeated rectal palpation of the gland (preferably by the same examiner) is important because early cancer may be felt as a nodule within the substance of the gland or as an extensive hardening in the posterior lobe. The more advanced lesion is "stony hard" and fixed. DRE also provides useful clinical information about the rectum, anal sphincter, and quality of stool.

The diagnosis of prostate cancer is confirmed by a histologic examination of tissue removed surgically by transurethral resection, open prostatectomy, or transrectal needle biopsy. Fine-needle aspiration is a quick, painless method of obtaining prostate cells for cytologic examination. The procedure is helpful for determining the stage of disease as well.

Most prostate cancers are diagnosed when a man seeks medical attention for symptoms of a urinary obstruction or after abnormalities are found by DRE. Incidentally detected cancer with transurethral resection of the prostate for clinically benign disease and prostatism occurs in 10% to 20% of patients. Rarely do patients have other signs and symptoms, such as azotemia (nitrogen compounds in the blood), weakness, anemia, or bone pain.

PSA, a neutral serine protease, is produced by the normal and neoplastic ductal epithelium of the prostate and secreted into the glandular lumen. A simple blood test can detect and measure PSA levels. The concentration of PSA in the blood is proportional to the total prostatic mass. Although the PSA level indicates the presence of prostate tissue, it does not necessarily indicate malignancy. PSA testing is routinely used to monitor the patient's response to cancer therapy and to detect local progression and early recurrence of prostate cancer. The combination of DRE and PSA testing appears to be a cost-effective method for detecting prostate cancer. The American Cancer Society recommends that beginning at 50 years of age, annual DRE and measurement of PSA level be offered to men who have a life expectancy of at least 10 years and to younger men who are at high risk.

Transrectal ultrasound (TRUS) studies are indicated for men who have elevated PSA levels and abnormal DRE findings. TRUS studies help in detecting nonpalpable prostate cancers and assist with staging localized prostate cancer. Needle biopsies of the prostate are commonly guided by TRUS.

Other tests include bone scans to detect metastatic bone disease, skeletal x-rays to identify osteoblastic metastases, excretory urography to detect changes caused by ureteral obstruction, renal function tests, and computed tomography (CT) scans or lymphangiography to identify metastases in the pelvic lymph nodes. Monoclonal antibody–based imaging techniques can also be used to detect prostate cancer cells in lymph nodes and other parts of the body.

Sexual Complications

Men with prostate cancer commonly experience sexual dysfunction before the diagnosis is made. Each treatment (see discussion that follows) for prostate cancer further increases the incidence of sexual problems. With nerve-sparing radical prostatectomy, the chance of recovering erections is better for men who are younger and in whom both neurovascular bundles are spared. Hormonal therapy also affects the central nervous system mechanisms that mediate sexual desire and arousability.

The prevalence rate of erectile dysfunction after definitive radiation therapy is about 25%. Researchers have found that men with borderline function before radiation therapy were more likely to experience impotence after therapy than men who had full erections and engaged in intercourse several times a month (Zinreich et al., 1990).

Medical Management

Treatment is based on the stage of the disease and the patient's age and symptoms. Partin and associates (1997) combined PSA level with clinical stage and the pathologic grade of the tumor to create a nomogram to predict pathologic stage of localized prostate cancer. This nomogram can be useful in making treatment decisions and predicting treatment outcomes. Table 45-2 summarizes the staging system used for prostate cancer. Nursing care of the patient with cancer of the prostate is summarized in Plan of Nursing Care 45-1.

SURGICAL MANAGEMENT

A radical prostatectomy (removal of the prostate and seminal vesicles) still remains the standard surgical procedure for patients who have early-stage, potentially curable disease and a life expectancy of 10 years or more. Sexual impotence follows radical prostatectomy, and 5% to 10% of patients have various degrees of urinary incontinence.

RADIATION THERAPY

If prostate cancer is detected in its early stage, the treatment may be curative radiation therapy—either teletherapy with a linear accelerator or interstitial irradiation (implantation of radioactive seeds of iodine or palladium), also referred to as brachytherapy. Teletherapy involves about 6 to 7 weeks of daily (5 days/week) radiation treatments. Interstitial seed implantation is performed with anesthesia. About 80 to 100 seeds are placed with ultrasound guidance. The patient returns home after the procedure. Exposure of others to radiation is minimal. Close contact with pregnant women and infants is avoided. Radiation safety guidelines include straining urine for seeds and using a condom during sexual intercourse for 2 weeks after implantation.

Side effects, which usually are transitory, include inflammation of the rectum, bowel, and bladder (proctitis, enteritis, and cystitis), due to their proximity to the prostate and the radiation

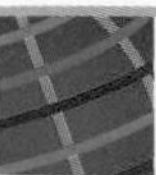

TABLE 45•2 **Staging Cancer of the Prostate**

Stage	Tumor	Nodes	Metastasis	Histopathologic Grade
I	T1	N0	M0	G2, 3–4
II	T2	N0	M0	Any G
III	T3	N0	M0	Any G
IV	T4 or any T	N0–N3	M0 or M1	Any G

Primary Tumor (T)
T0 = No evidence of primary tumor
T1 = Clinically inapparent tumor not palpable or visible by imaging
T2 = Tumor confined within the prostate
T3 = Tumor extends through the prostatic capsule
T4 = Tumor is fixed or invades adjacent structures other than the seminal vesicles

Regional Lymph Nodes (N)
N0 = No regional lymph node metastasis
N1 = Metastasis in a single lymph node ≤ 2 cm in greatest dimension
N2 = Metastasis in a single lymph node > 2 cm but not > 5 cm in greatest dimension or multiple lymph node metastasis, none > 5 cm
N3 = Metastasis in a lymph node > 5 cm greatest dimension

Distant Metastasis (M)
M0 = No distant metastasis
M1 = Distant metastasis

Histopathologic Grade (G)
G1 = Well differentiated
G2 = Moderately differentiated
G3–4 = Poorly differentiated or undifferentiated

Adapted from *AJCC cancer staging handbook* (5th ed). (1997). Philadelphia: Lippincott Williams & Wilkins.

doses. Irritation of the bladder and urethra from radiation therapy can cause pain during ejaculation until the irritation subsides. There is a greater preservation of sexual potency, however, with radiation therapy than with surgery. For locally advanced prostate cancer, hormonal treatments before and during radiation therapy are frequently used to improve local control and disease-free survival.

HORMONAL THERAPY

Hormonal therapy is one method used to control rather than cure prostate cancer. In the early 1940s, it was determined that most prostate cancers were androgen dependent and could be controlled by androgen withdrawal. Hormonal therapy for advanced prostate cancer suppresses all androgenic stimuli to the prostate by decreasing the circulating plasma testosterone levels or interrupting the conversion to or binding of dihydrotestosterone. As a result, the prostatic epithelium atrophies (decreases). This effect is accomplished either by **orchiectomy** (removal of the testes) or by administering medications.

Orchiectomy effectively lowers plasma testosterone levels because about 93% of circulating testosterone is of testicular origin (7% is from adrenal glands). As a result, the testicular stimulus required for continued prostatic growth is completely removed and results in prostatic atrophy. Although orchiectomy does not cause the side effects associated with other hormonal therapies, it carries a significant emotional impact.

Estrogen therapy, usually in the form of diethylstilbestrol (DES), has long been used to inhibit the gonadotropins responsible for testicular androgenic activity, thereby removing the androgenic hormone that promotes the growth of the malignancy. DES relieves symptoms of advanced prostate cancer, reduces tumor size, decreases pain from metastatic nodules, and promotes an improved sense of well-being. However, DES significantly increases the risk for thromboembolism, pulmonary embolism, myocardial infarction, and stroke. Other side effects of estrogen therapy include impotence, decreased libido, difficulties in achieving orgasm, decreased sperm production, and gynecomastia (enlargement of breasts in men).

Newer hormonal therapies include the luteinizing hormone–releasing hormone (LH-RH) agonists and antiandrogen agents, such as flutamide. LH-RH suppresses testicular androgen, whereas flutamide causes adrenal androgen suppression. Cyproterone acetate is a synthetic progesterone derivative that provides effective, competitive inhibition of androgens at the target cells. In contrast to estrogen, the newer hormonal agents have a lower incidence of cardiovascular side effects, gynecomastia, and decreased sexual function. Hot flushing can occur with orchiectomy or LH-RH agonist therapy (eg, leuprolide [Lupron], goserelin [Zoladex]) because these agents increase hypothalamic activity, which stimulates the thermoregulatory centers of the body.

OTHER THERAPIES

Cryosurgery of the prostate gland is used to ablate prostate cancer in patients who could not physically tolerate surgery or in those with recurrence of prostate cancer. Transperineal probes are inserted into the prostate with ultrasound guidance to freeze the tissue directly. Chemotherapy, such as doxorubicin, cisplatin, and cyclophosphamide, may also be used.

Keeping the urethral passage patent may require repeated transurethral resections. When this is impractical, catheter drainage is instituted by way of the suprapubic or transurethral route.

Because about half of affected patients have locally advanced tumors or evidence of metastatic disease at the time they first seek treatment, palliative measures are indicated. Although cures are unlikely with advanced prostate cancer, many men survive for long intervals apparently free of metastatic disease. If prostate cancer metastasizes to the bones, these bone lesions can be very painful. Opioid and nonopioid medications are used to control the pain. In addition, external-beam radiation therapy can be delivered to skeletal lesions to relieve pain. Radiopharmaceuticals, such as strontium-89 and samarium-153, can also be intravenously injected to treat multiple sites of bone metastases. Antiandrogen therapies are used in an effort to reduce the circulating androgens. If the antiandrogen therapies are not effective, medications such as prednisone and mitoxantrone have been effective in reducing pain and improving quality of life. With advanced prostate cancer, blood transfusions are administered to maintain adequate hemoglobin levels when bone marrow is replaced by tumor.

The Patient Undergoing Prostate Surgery

Prostate surgery may be indicated for the patient with BPH or prostate cancer. The preoperative objectives before prostate surgery are to assess the patient's general health status and to establish optimum renal function. Prostate surgery should be performed before acute urinary retention develops and damages the upper urinary tract and collecting system or, in the case of prostate cancer, before cancer progresses.

(*text continues on page 1313*)

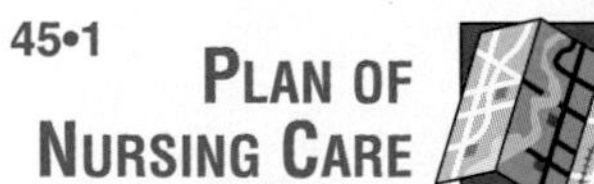

45•1 PLAN OF NURSING CARE

The Patient With Prostate Cancer

Nursing Interventions	Rationale	Expected Outcomes
Nursing Diagnosis: Anxiety related to concern and lack of knowledge about the diagnosis, treatment plan, and prognosis **Goal:** Reduced stress and improved ability to cope		
1. Obtain health history to determine the following: a. Patient's concerns b. His level of understanding of his health problem c. His past experience with cancer d. Whether he knows his diagnosis of malignancy and its prognosis e. His support systems and coping methods	1. Nurse clarifies information and facilitates patient's understanding and coping.	• Appears relaxed • States that anxiety has been reduced or relieved • Demonstrates understanding of illness and treatment when questioned • Engages in open communication with others
2. Provide education about diagnosis and treatment plan: a. Explain in simple terms what diagnostic tests to expect, how long they will take, and what will be experienced during each test. b. Review treatment plan and allow patient to ask questions.	2. Helping the patient to understand the diagnostic tests and treatment plan will help decrease his anxiety and promote cooperation.	
3. Assess his psychological reaction to his diagnosis/prognosis and how he has coped with past stresses.	3. This information provides clues in determining appropriate measures to facilitate coping.	
4. Provide information about institutional and community resources for coping with prostate cancer: social services, support groups, community agencies	4. Institutional and community resources can help the patient and family cope with the illness and treatment on an ongoing basis.	
Nursing Diagnosis: Urinary retention related to urethral obstruction secondary to prostatic enlargement or tumor and loss of bladder tone due to prolonged distention/retention **Goal:** Improved pattern of urinary elimination		
1. Determine patient's usual pattern of urinary function.	1. Provides a baseline for comparison and goal to work toward.	• Voids at normal intervals • Reports absence of frequency, urgency, or bladder fullness • Displays no palpable suprapubic distention after voiding • Maintains balanced intake and output
2. Assess for signs and symptoms of urinary retention: amount and frequency of urination, suprapubic distention, complaints of urgency and discomfort.	2. Voiding 20 to 30 mL frequently and output less than intake suggests retention.	
3. Catheterize patient to determine amount of residual urine.	3. Determines amount of urine remaining in bladder after voiding	
4. Initiate measures to treat retention: a. Encourage assuming normal position for voiding. b. Recommend using Valsalva maneuver. c. Administer prescribed cholinergic agent. d. Monitor effects of medication.	4. Promotes voiding a. Usual position provides relaxed conditions conducive to voiding. b. Valsalva maneuver exerts pressure to force urine out of bladder. c. Stimulates bladder contraction. d. If unsuccessful, another measure may be required.	
5. Consult with physician regarding intermittent or indwelling catheterization; assist with procedure as required.	5. Catheterization will relieve urinary retention until the specific cause is determined; it may be an obstruction that can be corrected only surgically.	

(continued)

45•1 PLAN OF NURSING CARE 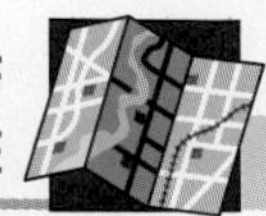 **The Patient With Prostate Cancer (*continued*)**

Nursing Interventions	Rationale	Expected Outcomes
6. Monitor catheter function; maintain sterility of closed system; irrigate as required.	6. Adequate functioning of catheter is to be ensured to empty bladder and to prevent infection.	
7. Prepare patient for surgery if indicated.	7. Surgical removal of obstruction may be necessary.	

Nursing Diagnosis: Knowledge deficit related to the diagnosis of: cancer, urinary difficulties, and treatment modalities
Goal: Understanding of the diagnosis and ability to care for self

Nursing Interventions	Rationale	Expected Outcomes
1. Encourage communication with the patient.	1. This is designed to establish rapport and trust.	• Discusses his concerns and problems freely • Asks questions and shows interest in his condition • Describes activities that help or hinder recovery • Identifies ways of attaining/maintaining bladder control • Demonstrates satisfactory technique and understanding of catheter care • Lists signs and symptoms that must be reported should they occur
2. Review the anatomy of the involved area.	2. Orientation to one's anatomy is basic to understanding its function.	
3. Be specific in selecting information that is relevant to the patient's particular treatment plan.	3. This is based on the treatment plan; as it varies with each patient, individualization is desirable.	
4. Identify ways to reduce pressure on the operative area after prostatectomy. a. Avoid prolonged sitting (in a chair, long automobile rides), standing, walking. b. Avoid straining, such as during exercises, bowel movement, lifting, and sexual intercourse.	4. This is to prevent bleeding; such precautions are in order for 6 to 8 weeks postoperatively.	
5. Familiarize patient with ways of attaining/maintaining bladder control.	5. These measures will help control frequency and dribbling and aid in preventing retention.	
a. Encourage urination every 2 to 3 hours; discourage voiding when supine.	a. By sitting or standing, patient is more likely to empty his bladder.	
b. Avoid drinking cola and caffeine beverages; urge a cutoff time in the evening for drinking fluids to minimize frequent voiding during the night.	b. Spacing the kind and amount of liquid intake will help to prevent frequency.	
c. Describe perineal exercises to be performed every hour.	c. Exercises will assist him in starting and stopping the urinary stream.	
d. Develop a schedule with patient that will fit into his routine.	d. A schedule will assist in developing a workable pattern of normal activities.	
6. Demonstrate catheter care; encourage his questions; stress the importance of position of urinary receptacle.	6. By requiring a return demonstration of care, collection, and emptying of the device, he will become more independent and also can prevent backflow of urine, which can lead to infection.	

Nursing Diagnosis: Altered nutrition: less than body requirements related to decreased oral intake because of anorexia, nausea, and vomiting brought on by cancer or its treatment
Goal: Maintain optimal nutritional status

Nursing Interventions	Rationale	Expected Outcomes
1. Assess the amount of food eaten.	1. This assessment will help determine nutrient intake.	• Responds positively to his favorite foods • Assumes responsibility for his oral hygiene • Notes increase in weight after improved appetite
2. Routinely weigh patient.	2. Weighing the patient on the same scale under similar conditions can help monitor changes in weight.	
3. Elicit patient's explanation of why he is unable to eat more.	3. His explanation may present easily corrected practices.	

45•1

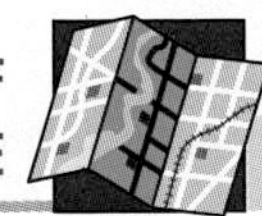

PLAN OF NURSING CARE The Patient With Prostate Cancer (*continued*)

Nursing Interventions	Rationale	Expected Outcomes
4. Cater to his individual food preferences (eg, avoiding foods that are too spicy or too cold).	4. He will be more likely to consume larger servings if food is palatable and appealing.	
5. Recognize effect of medication or radiation therapy on appetite.	5. Many chemotherapeutic agents and radiation therapy promote anorexia.	
6. Inform patient that alterations in taste can occur.	6. Aging and the disease process can reduce taste sensitivity. In addition, smell and taste can be altered as a result of the body's absorption of byproducts of cellular destruction (brought on by malignancy and its treatment).	
7. Use measures to control nausea and vomiting. a. Administer prescribed antiemetics, around the clock if necessary. b. Provide oral hygiene after vomiting episodes. c. Provide rest periods after meals.	7. Prevention of nausea and vomiting can stimulate appetite.	
8. Provide frequent small meals and a comfortable and pleasant environment.	8. Smaller portions of food are less overwhelming to the patient.	
9. Assess patient's ability to obtain and prepare foods.	9. Disability or lack of social support can hinder the patient's ability to obtain and prepare foods.	
Nursing Diagnosis: Sexual dysfunction related to effects of therapy: chemotherapy, hormonal therapy, radiation therapy, surgery **Goal:** Ability to resume/enjoy modified sexual functioning		
1. Determine from nursing history what effect patient's medical condition is having on his sexual functioning.	1. Usually decreased libido and, later, impotence may be experienced.	• Describes the reasons for changes in sexual functioning • Discusses with appropriate health care personnel alternative approaches and methods of sexual expression • Includes partner in discussions related to changes in sexual function
2. Inform patient of the effects of prostate surgery, orchiectomy (when applicable), chemotherapy, irradiation, and hormonal therapy on sexual function.	2. Treatment modalities may alter sexual function, but each is evaluated separately with regard to its effect on a particular patient.	
3. Include his partner in developing understanding and in discovering alternative, satisfying close relations with each other.	3. Often the bonds between a couple are strengthened with new appreciation and support that had not been evident before the current illness.	
Nursing Diagnosis: Pain related to progression of disease and treatment modalities **Goal:** Relief of pain		
1. Evaluate nature of patient's pain, its location and intensity using pain rating scale.	1. Determining nature and causes of pain and its intensity helps to select proper relief modality and provide baseline for later comparison.	• Reports relief of pain • Expects exacerbations, reports their quality or intensity, and obtains relief • Uses pain relief strategies appropriately and effectively • Identifies strategies to avoid complications of analgesic use
2. Avoid activities that aggravate or worsen pain.	2. Bumping the bed is an example of an action that can intensify the patient's pain.	
3. Because pain is usually related to bone metastasis, ensure that patient's bed has a bed board on a firm mattress. Also, protect the patient from falls/injuries.	3. This will provide added support and is more comfortable. Protecting the patient from injury protects him from additional pain.	

(*continued*)

45•1

PLAN OF NURSING CARE 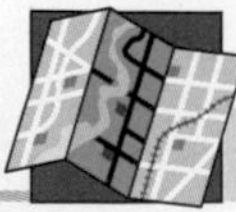

The Patient With Prostate Cancer (*continued*)

Nursing Interventions	Rationale	Expected Outcomes
4. Provide support for affected extremities.	4. More support, coupled with reduced movement of the part, helps in pain control.	
5. Prepare patient for radiation therapy if prescribed.	5. Radiation therapy may be effective in controlling pain.	
6. Administer analgesics or opioids at regularly scheduled intervals as prescribed.	6. Analgesics alter perception of pain and provide comfort. Regularly scheduled analgesics around the clock rather than PRN provide more consistent pain relief.	
7. Initiate bowel program to prevent constipation.	7. Opioid analgesics and inactivity contribute to constipation.	

Nursing Diagnosis: Impaired physical mobility and activity intolerance related to tissue hypoxia, malnutrition, and exhaustion and to spinal cord or nerve compression from metastases
Goal: Improved physical mobility

Nursing Interventions	Rationale	Expected Outcomes
1. Assess for factors causing limited mobility (eg, pain, hypercalcemia, limited exercise tolerance).	1. This information offers clues to the cause; if possible, cause is treated.	• Achieves improved physical mobility • Relates that short-term goals are encouraging him because they are attainable
2. Provide pain relief by administering prescribed medications.	2. Analgesics/opioids allow the patient to increase his activity more comfortably.	
3. Encourage use of assistive devices: cane, walker.	3. Support may offer the security needed to become mobile.	
4. Involve significant others in helping patient with range-of-motion exercises, positioning, and walking.	4. Assistance from partner or others encourages patient to repeat activities and achieve goals.	
5. Provide positive reinforcement for achievement of small gains.	5. Encouragement stimulates improvement of performance.	
6. Assess nutritional status.	6. See Nursing Diagnosis: Altered nutrition: less than body requirements.	

Collaborative Problems: Hemorrhage, infection, bladder neck obstruction
Goal: Absence of complications

Nursing Interventions	Rationale	Expected Outcomes
1. Alert the patient to changes that may occur (after discharge) and that need to be reported:	1. Certain changes signal beginning complications, which call for nursing and medical interventions.	• Experiences no bleeding or passage of blood clots • Reports no pain around the catheter • Experiences normal frequency or urination • Reports normal urinary output • Maintains bladder control
a. Continued bloody urine; passing blood clots	a. Hematuria with or without blood clot formation may occur postoperatively.	
b. Pain; burning around the catheter	b. Indwelling urinary catheters may be a source of infections.	
c. Frequency of urination	c. Urinary frequency may be caused by urinary tract infections or by bladder neck obstruction, resulting in incomplete voiding.	
d. Diminished urinary output	d. Bladder neck obstruction decreases the amount of urine that is voided.	
e. Increasing loss of bladder control	e. Urinary incontinence may be a result of urinary retention.	

Surgical Procedures

Several approaches are used to remove the hypertrophied portion of the prostate gland: transurethral resection (TUR) of the prostate, suprapubic prostatectomy, perineal prostatectomy, and retropubic prostatectomy (Table 45-3). In these approaches, the surgeon removes all hyperplastic tissue, leaving behind only the capsule of the prostate. The transurethral approach is a closed procedure; the other three are open procedures (ie, a surgical incision is required). The specific procedure performed depends on the underlying disorder, the patient's age and physical status, and patient preference.

TRANSURETHRAL RESECTION

TUR is the most common procedure and can be carried out through endoscopy. The surgical and optical instrument is introduced directly through the urethra to the prostate, which can then be viewed directly. The gland is removed in small chips with an electrical cutting loop (Fig. 45-3**A**). This procedure, which requires no incision, may be used for glands of varying size and is ideal for patients who have small glands and those who are considered poor surgical risks.

This approach usually requires an overnight hospital stay. Strictures are more frequent, and repeated procedures may be necessary because the residual prostatic tissue can grow back. TUR rarely causes erectile dysfunction, but it may cause retrograde ejaculation because removing the prostatic tissue at the bladder neck can cause the seminal fluid to flow backward into the bladder rather than forward through the urethra during ejaculation.

SUPRAPUBIC PROSTATECTOMY

Suprapubic prostatectomy is one method of removing the gland through an abdominal incision. An incision is made into the bladder, and the prostate gland is removed from above (see Fig. 45-3**B**). Such an approach can be used for a gland of any size, and few complications occur, although blood loss may be greater than with other methods. Another disadvantage is the need for an abdominal incision, with the concomitant hazards of any major abdominal surgical procedure.

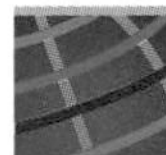

TABLE 45•3 Comparing Surgical Approaches for Treatment of Prostate Disorders

The surgical approach of choice depends on (1) the size of the gland, (2) the severity of the obstruction, (3) the age of the patient, (4) the condition of patient, and (5) the presence of associated diseases.

Surgical Approach	Advantages	Disadvantages	Nursing Implications
Transurethral Resection (TUR or TURP) (removal of prostatic tissue by instrument introduced through urethra)	Avoids abdominal incision Safer for surgical-risk patient Shorter hospitalization and recovery periods Lower morbidity rate Causes less pain	Requires highly skilled surgeon Recurrent obstruction, urethral trauma, and stricture may develop Delayed bleeding may occur	Monitor for hemorrhage Observe for symptoms of urethral stricture (dysuria, straining, weak urinary stream).
Open Surgical Removal			
Suprapubic approach	Technically simple Offers wide area of exploration Permits exploration for cancerous lymph nodes Allows more complete removal of obstructing gland Permits treatment of associated bladder lesions	Requires surgical approach through the bladder Control of hemorrhage difficult Urine may leak around the suprapubic tube Recovery may be prolonged and uncomfortable	Monitor for indications of hemorrhage and shock. Give meticulous aseptic care to the area around suprapubic tube.
Perineal approach	Offers direct anatomic approach Permits gravity drainage Particularly effective for radical cancer therapy Allows hemostasis under direct vision Low mortality rate Lower incidence of shock Ideal for very old, frail, and poor-surgical-risk patient with large prostate	Higher postoperative incidence of impotence and urinary incontinence Possible damage to rectum and external sphincter Restricted operative field Greater potential for infection	Avoid using rectal tubes or thermometers and enemas after perineal surgery. Use drainage pads to absorb excess urinary drainage. Provide foam rubber ring for patient comfort in sitting. Anticipate urinary leakage around the wound for several days after the catheter is removed.
Retropubic approach	Avoids incision into the bladder Permits surgeon to see and control bleeders Shorter recovery period Less bladder sphincter damage	Cannot treat associated bladder disease Increased incidence of hemorrhage from prostatic venous plexus; pubic osteitis	Monitor for hemorrhage. Anticipate posturinary leakage for several days after removing the catheter.
Transurethral Incision (TUIP)	Results comparable to TURP Lower incidence of erectile dysfunction No bladder neck contracture Lower incidence of retrograde ejaculation	Requires highly skilled surgeon Recurrent obstruction and urethral trauma Delayed bleeding	Monitor for hemorrhage.

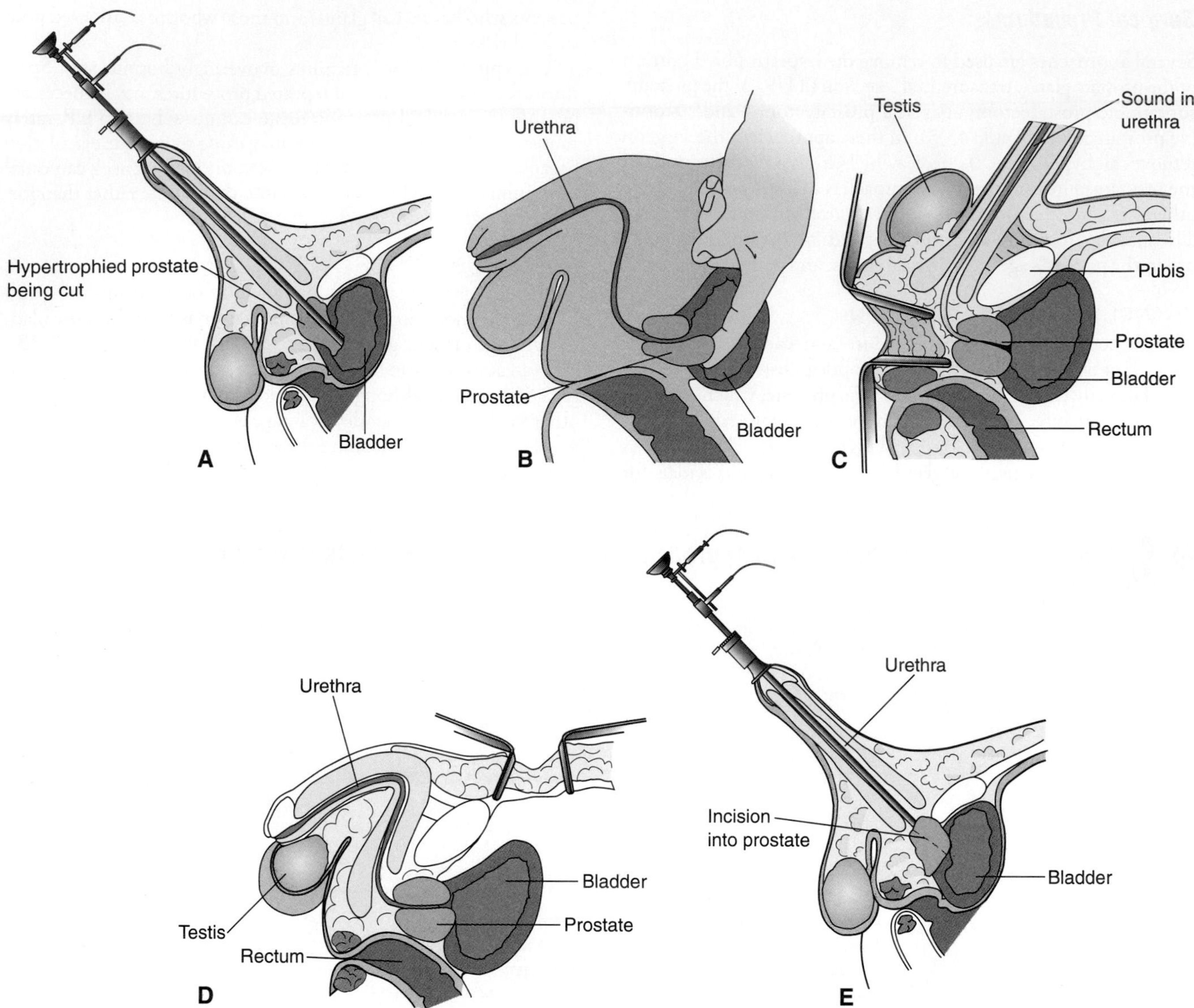

FIGURE 45•3 Prostate surgery procedures. (**A**) Transurethral resection (TUR). A loop of wire connected with a cutting current is rotated in the cystoscope to remove shavings of prostate at the bladder orifice. (**B**) Suprapubic prostatectomy. With an abdominal approach, the prostate is shelled out of its bed. (**C**) Perineal prostatectomy. Two retractors on the left spread the perineal incision to provide a view of the prostate. (**D**) Retropubic prostatectomy is performed through a low abdominal incision. Note two abdominal retractors and *arrow* pointing to the prostate gland. (**E**) Transurethral incision of prostate (TUIP) involves one or two incisions into the prostate to reduce pressure on the urethra.

PERINEAL PROSTATECTOMY

Perineal prostatectomy involves removing the gland through an incision in the perineum (see Fig. 45-3**C**). This approach is practical when other approaches are not possible and is useful for an open biopsy. Postoperatively, the wound may easily become contaminated because the incision is near the rectum. Moreover, incontinence, impotence, and rectal injury are more likely complications of this surgery.

RETROPUBIC PROSTATECTOMY

Retropubic prostatectomy is another technique and is more common than the suprapubic approach. The surgeon makes a low abdominal incision and approaches the prostate gland between the pubic arch and the bladder without entering the bladder (see Fig. 45-3**D**). This procedure is suitable for large glands located high in the pelvis. Although blood loss can be better controlled and the surgical site is easier to visualize, infections can readily start in the retropubic space.

TRANSURETHRAL INCISION OF THE PROSTATE

TUIP is another procedure used in treating BPH. An instrument is passed through the urethra (see Fig. 45-3**E**). One or two incisions are made in the prostate and prostate capsule to reduce the prostate's pressure on the urethra and to reduce urethral constriction. TUIP is indicated when the prostate gland is small (30 g or less) and would be effective treatment for many cases of BPH. The TUIP procedure can be performed on an outpatient basis and has a lower complication rate than other invasive prostate procedures (AHCPR, 1994).

Complications

Complications associated with a prostatectomy depend on the type of surgery and include hemorrhage, clot formation, catheter obstruction, and sexual dysfunction. All prostatectomies carry a risk of impotence because of potential damage to the pudendal nerves. In most instances, sexual activity may be resumed in 6 to 8 weeks, the time required for the prostatic fossa to heal. During ejaculation, the seminal fluid goes into the bladder and is excreted with the urine. (The anatomic changes in the posterior urethra lead to retrograde ejaculation.) A vasectomy may be performed during surgery to prevent infection from spreading from the prostatic urethra through the vas and into the epididymis.

After total prostatectomy (usually for cancer), impotence almost always results. For the patient who does not want to give up sexual activity, options are available to create penile erections for sexual intercourse. These options include prosthetic penile implants, negative-pressure (vacuum) devices, and pharmacologic interventions (see earlier discussion in this chapter).

NURSING PROCESS: THE PATIENT UNDERGOING PROSTATECTOMY

Assessment

The nurse assesses how the underlying disorder (benign prostatic hyperplasia or prostate cancer) has affected the patient's lifestyle. Has he been reasonably active for his age? What is his presenting urinary problem (described in the patient's words)? Has he experienced decreased force of urinary flow, decreased ability to initiate voiding, urgency, frequency, nocturia, dysuria, urinary retention, hematuria? Does the patient report associated problems, such as back pain, flank pain, and lower abdominal or suprapubic discomfort? If he reports such discomfort, possible causes may include infection, retention, and, possibly, renal colic.

The nurse obtains further information about the patient's family history of cancer and heart or kidney disease, including hypertension. Has he lost weight? Does he appear pale? Can he raise himself out of bed and return to bed without assistance? Is he able to perform usual activities of daily living? This information will help in determining how soon he will return to normal activities after prostatectomy.

Diagnosis

Based on the assessment data, the patient's major nursing diagnoses may include the following:

Preoperative Nursing Diagnoses

- Anxiety about surgery and its outcome
- Pain related to bladder distention
- Knowledge deficit about factors related to the disorder and the treatment protocol

Postoperative Nursing Diagnoses

- Pain related to the surgical incision, catheter placement, and bladder spasms
- Knowledge deficit about postoperative care and management

Collaborative Problems/Potential Complications

Based on the assessment data, the potential complications may include the following:

- Hemorrhage and shock
- Infection
- Deep vein thrombosis
- Catheter obstruction

Planning and Goals

The major *preoperative* goals for the patient may include reduced anxiety and learning about his prostate disorder and the perioperative experience. The major *postoperative* goals may include correction of fluid volume disturbances, relief of pain and discomfort, ability to perform self-care activities, and absence of complications.

Preoperative Nursing Interventions

Reducing Anxiety

The nurse familiarizes the patient with the hospital environment and initiates measures to reduce anxiety. Communication is established about his understanding of the problem and what the physician has already told him. Because the patient may be sensitive and embarrassed to discuss problems related to the genitalia and issues of sexuality, the nurse provides privacy and establishes a trusting and professional relationship. Guilt feelings often surface if the patient falsely assumes a cause-and-effect relationship between sexual practices and his current problems. His verbalization of feelings and concerns is encouraged. The nurse clarifies the nature of the surgery and expected postoperative outcomes.

Relieving Discomfort

If signs and symptoms of discomfort are apparent, the patient is placed on bed rest, analgesic agents are administered, and measures to relieve anxiety are initiated. The nurse monitors the patient's voiding patterns, watches for bladder distention, and assists with catheterization. An indwelling catheter is inserted if the patient has continuing urinary retention or if laboratory test results indicate azotemia (accumulation of nitrogenous waste products in the blood). The catheter can help to decompress the bladder gradually over several days, especially if the patient is elderly and hypertensive and has diminished renal function or an excessive amount of urinary retention that has existed for many weeks. For a few days after the bladder begins draining, the blood pressure may fluctuate, and renal function may decline. If the patient cannot tolerate a urinary catheter, he is prepared for a cystostomy (see Chapters 40 and 41).

Providing Instruction

A convenient time is established for the patient (ensuring his privacy) to review the anatomy of the affected parts and how they function in relation to the urinary and reproductive systems, with diagrams and other teaching aids, if indicated. The nurse explains what will take place as the patient is prepared for diagnostic tests and then for surgery (depending on the kind of prostatectomy planned). The nurse describes the type of incision, which varies with the type of surgical approach (directly over the bladder, low on the abdomen, or in the perineal area; in the case of a transurethral procedure, no incision will be made).

The patient is informed about the type of urinary drainage system that is expected, the type of anesthesia, and the recovery room procedure. The amount of information is based on the patient's needs and questions. Procedures expected during the immediate perioperative period are explained, questions are answered, and support is provided. In addition, the patient is instructed about postoperative use of medications for pain management.

Preparing the Patient

When the patient is scheduled for a prostatectomy, the preparation described in Chapter 16 is provided. Elastic pressure stockings are applied before surgery and are particularly important for prevention of deep vein thrombosis if the patient is placed in a lithotomy position during surgery. A preoperative enema may prevent postoperative straining, which can induce postoperative bleeding.

Postoperative Nursing Interventions

Relieving Pain

After a prostatectomy, the patient is assisted to dangle his legs from the side of the bed on the day of surgery. The next morning, the patient is assisted to ambulate. If pain occurs, the cause and location must be determined. It may be related to the incision; it may be the result of excoriation of the skin at the catheter site; it may be in the flank area, indicating a kidney problem; or it may be due to bladder spasms. Bladder irritability can initiate bleeding and result in clot formation, leading to urinary retention.

When patients are experiencing bladder spasms, they may note an urgency to void, a feeling of pressure or fullness in the bladder, and bleeding from the urethra around the catheter. Medications that relax the smooth muscles can help to ease the spasms, which can be intermittent and severe. Warm compresses to the pubis or sitz baths may relieve the spasms.

The nurse monitors the drainage tubing and irrigates the system as prescribed to relieve any obstruction that may cause discomfort. Usually, the catheter is irrigated with 50 mL of irrigating fluid at a time. It is important to make sure that the same amount is recovered in the drainage receptacle. Securing the catheter drainage tubing to the leg or abdomen can help to decrease tension on the catheter and prevent bladder irritation. Discomfort may be caused by dressings that are too snug, too saturated with drainage, or improperly placed. Analgesics are administered as prescribed.

When ambulatory, the patient is encouraged to walk but not to sit for prolonged periods because this increases intra-abdominal pressure and the possibility of discomfort and bleeding. Prune juice and stool softeners are provided to ease bowel movements and to prevent excessive straining. An enema, if prescribed, is administered with caution to avoid possible rectal perforation.

Monitoring and Managing Potential Complications

After prostatectomy, the patient is monitored for major complications, such as hemorrhage, infection, deep vein thrombosis, and catheter obstruction.

HEMORRHAGE

The immediate dangers after a prostatectomy are bleeding and shock. This risk is increased with BPH because a hyperplastic prostate gland is very vascular. Bleeding may occur from the prostatic bed. Bleeding may also result in the formation of clots, which then obstruct the flow of urine. The drainage normally begins as reddish pink and then clears to a light pink within 24 hours after surgery.

- Bright red bleeding with increased viscosity and numerous clots usually indicates arterial bleeding. Venous blood appears darker and less viscous.
- Arterial hemorrhage usually requires surgical intervention (eg, suturing of bleeders or transurethral coagulation of bleeding vessels), whereas venous bleeding may be controlled by applying prescribed traction to the catheter, so that the balloon holding the catheter in place applies pressure to the prostatic fossa.

Nursing management includes strategies to stop the bleeding and to prevent or reverse hemorrhagic shock. If blood loss is extensive, fluids and blood component therapy may be administered. If hemorrhagic shock occurs, treatments described in Chapter 14 are initiated.

Nursing interventions include close monitoring of the patient's vital signs, administering medication, intravenous fluids, and blood component therapy that are prescribed; maintaining an accurate record of intake and output; and careful monitoring of drainage to ensure adequate urine flow and patency of the drainage system. The patient who experiences hemorrhage and his family are often anxious and benefit from explanations and reassurance about the event and about procedures that are performed.

INFECTION

After perineal prostatectomy, the surgeon usually changes the dressing on the first postoperative day. Further dressing changes may become the nurse's responsibility. Careful aseptic technique is used because the possibility for infection is great. Dressings can be held in place by a double-tailed, T-binder bandage or a padded athletic supporter. The tails cross over the incision to give double thickness, and then each tail is drawn up on either side of the scrotum to the waistline and fastened.

Rectal thermometers, rectal tubes, and enemas are avoided because of the risk for injury to and bleeding in the prostatic fossa. After the perineal sutures are removed, the perineum is cleansed as indicated. A heat lamp may be directed to the perineal area to promote healing. The scrotum is protected with a towel while the heat lamp is in use. Sitz baths are also used to promote healing.

Urinary tract infections and epididymitis are possible complications after prostatectomy. The patient is assessed for their occurrence; if they occur, the nurse administers antibiotics as prescribed.

Because the risk for infection continues after a patient's discharge from the hospital, the patient and family need to be instructed to monitor for signs and symptoms of infection. These include fever, chills, sweats, myalgias, dysuria, urinary frequency, and urgency. Patients and families are instructed to contact their urologist if these symptoms occur.

DEEP VEIN THROMBOSIS

Patients undergoing prostatectomy have a high incidence of deep vein thrombosis (DVT) and pulmonary embolism. Thus, the physician may prescribe prophylactic (preventive) low-dose heparin therapy. The nurse assesses the patient frequently after surgery for manifestations of DVT and applies elastic stockings to reduce the risk for DVT and pulmonary embolism. Nursing and medical management of DVT and pulmonary embolism are detailed in Chapters 28 and 21, respectively. The patient who is receiving heparin must be closely monitored for excessive bleeding. Elastic pressure stockings may be used to prevent DVT.

OBSTRUCTED CATHETER

After a TUR, the catheter must drain well; an obstructed catheter produces distention of the prostatic capsule and resultant hemorrhage. Furosemide (Lasix) may be prescribed to promote urination and initiate postoperative diuresis, thereby helping to keep the catheter patent.

The nurse observes the lower abdomen to ensure that the catheter has not become blocked. An overdistended bladder presents a distinct, rounded swelling above the pubis.

The drainage bag, dressings, and incisional site are examined for bleeding. The color of the urine is noted and documented; a change in color from pink to amber indicates reduced bleeding. Blood pressure, pulse, and respirations are monitored and compared with baseline preoperative vital signs to detect hypotension. The nurse also observes the patient for restlessness, cold sweats, pallor, any drop in blood pressure, and an increasing pulse rate.

Drainage of the bladder may be accomplished by gravity through a closed sterile drainage system. A three-way drainage system is useful in irrigating the bladder and preventing clot formation (Fig. 45-4). Continuous irrigation may be used with TUR. Some urologists leave an indwelling catheter attached to a dependent drainage system. Gentle irrigation of the catheter may be prescribed to remove any obstructing clots.

If the patient complains of pain, the tubing is examined. The drainage system is irrigated, if indicated and prescribed, to clear any obstruction before an analgesic is administered. Usually, the catheter is irrigated with 50 mL of irrigating fluid at a time. The amount of fluid recovered in the drainage bag must equal the amount of fluid injected. Overdistention of the bladder is avoided because it can induce secondary hemorrhage by stretching the coagulated blood vessels in the prostatic capsule.

The nurse maintains an intake and output record, including the amount of fluid used for irrigation.

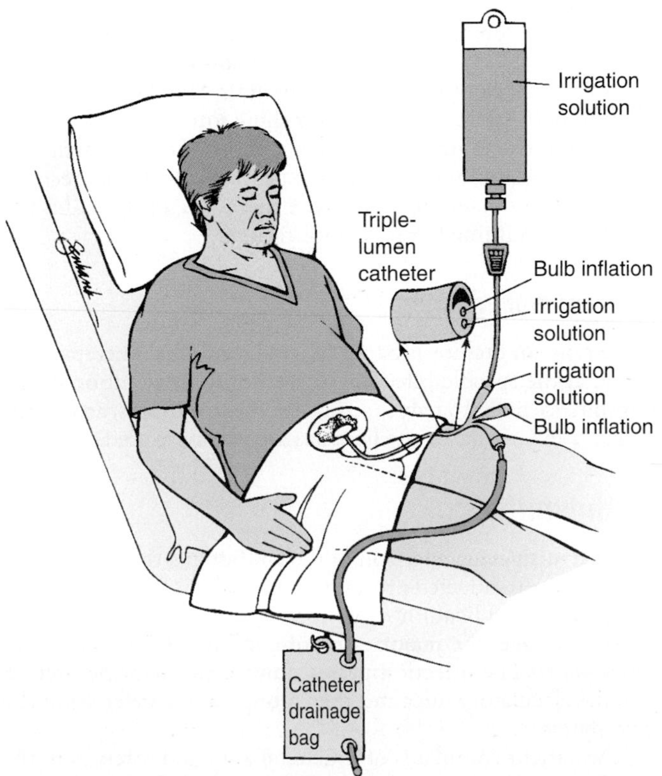

FIGURE 45•4 A three-way system for bladder irrigation.

The drainage tube (not the catheter) is taped to the shaved inner thigh to prevent traction on the bladder. If a cystostomy catheter is in place, it is taped to the abdomen. The nurse explains the purpose of the catheter to the patient and assures him that the urge to void results from the presence of the catheter and from bladder spasms. He is cautioned not to pull on the catheter because this causes bleeding and subsequent catheter blockage, which leads to urinary retention.

COMPLICATIONS WITH CATHETER REMOVAL

After the catheter is removed (usually when the urine appears clear), urine may leak around the wound for several days in patients who have undergone perineal, suprapubic, and retropubic surgery. The cystostomy tube may be removed before or after the urethral catheter is removed. Some urinary incontinence may occur after catheter removal, and the patient is informed that this is likely to subside in time.

Promoting Home and Community-Based Care

TEACHING PATIENTS SELF-CARE

The patient undergoing prostatectomy may be discharged within several days. Length of hospitalization depends on the type of prostatectomy performed. Patients undergoing a perineal prostatectomy are hospitalized for 3 to 5 days. If a retropubic or suprapubic prostatectomy is performed, the length of hospital stay is from 5 to 7 days. The patient and family require instructions about how to manage the drainage system, how to assess for complications, and how to promote recovery. Verbal and written instructions are provided about the need to maintain the drainage system and to monitor urinary output, about wound care, and about strategies to prevent complications, such as infection, bleeding, and thrombosis. They are informed about signs and symptoms that should be reported to the physician (eg, blood in urine, decreased urine output, fever, change in wound drainage, calf tenderness).

As the patient recovers and drainage tubes are removed, he may show signs of discouragement and depression because he cannot regain bladder control immediately. Moreover, urinary frequency and burning may occur after the catheter is removed. Teaching the following exercises may help the patient regain urinary control:

- Tense the perineal muscles by pressing the buttocks together; hold this position; relax. This exercise can be performed 10 to 20 times each hour while sitting or standing.
- Try to interrupt the urinary stream after starting to void; wait a few seconds and then continue to void.

Perineal exercises should continue until the patient gains full urinary control. The patient is instructed to urinate as soon as he feels the *first* urge to do so. It is important for the patient to know that regaining urinary control is a gradual process, that he may continue to "dribble" after being discharged from the hospital, but that the dribbling should gradually diminish (within up to 1 year). Lining underwear with absorbent pads can help to minimize embarrassing stains on clothing. The urine may be cloudy for several weeks after surgery but should clear as the prostate area heals.

While the prostatic fossa heals (6 to 8 weeks), the patient should avoid activities that produce Valsalva effects (straining at stool, heavy lifting) because this increases venous pressure and may produce hematuria. He should avoid long motor trips and strenuous exercise, which increase the tendency to bleed. He should also know that spicy foods, alcohol, and coffee may cause bladder dis-

HOME CARE TEACHING CHECKLIST: POSTPROSTATECTOMY CARE

At the completion of the program, the patient or caregiver will be able to:

	Patient	Caregiver
• Demonstrate appropriate measures to control postoperative pain and discomfort.	✔	✔
• Demonstrate appropriate care of urinary catheter and collection receptacle.	✔	✔
• Demonstrate appropriate wound care.	✔	✔
• Demonstrate performance of perineal muscle exercises to facilitate bladder control.	✔	
• Demonstrate increased activity and ambulation.	✔	
• Identify activities to avoid, such as lifting heavy objects.	✔	
• Identify signs and symptoms of complications that should be reported to surgeon	✔	✔

comfort. The patient is cautioned to drink enough fluids to avoid dehydration, which increases the tendency for a blood clot to form and obstruct the flow of urine. Signs of complications, such as bleeding, passage of blood clots, a decrease in the urinary stream, urinary retention, or urinary tract infection symptoms, are to be reported to the physician.

CONTINUING CARE

Referral for home care may be indicated if the patient is elderly or, has other health problems, if the patient and family are unable to provide care in the home, or if the patient lives alone without available supports. The home care nurse assesses the patient's physical status (cardiovascular and respiratory status, fluid and nutritional status, patency of the urinary drainage system, wound and nutritional status) and provides catheter and wound care, if indicated. The nurse reinforces previous teaching and assesses the ability of the patient and family to manage required care. The home care nurse encourages the patient to ambulate and to carry out perineal exercises as prescribed. The patient may need to be reminded that return of bladder control may take time.

Evaluation

Expected Preoperative Outcomes

Expected preoperative outcomes may include:

1. Demonstrates reduced anxiety
2. States that pain and discomfort are decreased
3. Relates understanding of the surgical procedure and postoperative course and practices perineal muscle exercises and other techniques useful in facilitating bladder control

Expected Postoperative Outcomes

Expected postoperative outcomes may include:

1. Relates relief of discomfort
2. Participates in self-care measures
    a. Increases activity and ambulation daily
    b. Produces urine output within normal ranges and consistent with intake
    c. Performs perineal exercises and interrupts urinary stream to promote bladder control
    d. Avoids straining and lifting heavy objects
3. Is free of complications
    a. Maintains vital signs within normal limits
    b. Exhibits wound healing, without signs of inflammation or hemorrhage
    c. Maintains acceptable level of urinary elimination
    d. Maintains optimal drainage of catheter and other drainage tubes

CONDITIONS AFFECTING THE TESTES AND ADJACENT STRUCTURES

Undescended Testis (Cryptorchidism)

Cryptorchidism is a congenital condition characterized by failure of the testis to descend into the scrotum. One or both testes may be absent. The testis may be located in the abdominal cavity or inguinal canal. If the testis does not descend as the boy matures, a surgical procedure known as orchiopexy is performed to position it properly. An incision is made over the inguinal canal, and the testis is brought down and anchored in the scrotum.

Orchitis

Orchitis is an inflammation of the testes (testicular congestion), caused by pyogenic, viral, spirochetal, parasitic, traumatic, chemical, or unknown factors. Mumps is one such factor. Mumps vaccination is recommended for postpubertal men who have not been infected. When postpubertal men contract mumps, about one in five develops some form of orchitis 4 to 7 days after the jaw and neck swell. The testis may show some atrophy. In past years, sterility and impotence often resulted. Today, a man who has never had mumps and who is exposed to the disease receives gamma-globulin immediately; the disease is likely to be less severe, with minimal or no complications.

Medical Management

If the cause of orchitis is bacterial, viral, or fungal, therapy is directed at the specific infecting organism. Rest, elevation of the scrotum, ice packs to reduce scrotal edema, antibiotics, analgesics, and anti-inflammatory medications are recommended.

Epididymitis

Epididymitis is an infection of the epididymis that usually descends from an infected prostate or urinary tract. It may also develop as a complication of gonorrhea. In men younger than 35 years of age, the major cause of epididymitis is *Chlamydia trachomatis.* The infection passes upward through the urethra and the ejaculatory duct and then along the vas deferens to the epididymis.

The patient complains of unilateral pain and soreness in the inguinal canal along the course of the vas deferens and then develops pain and swelling in the scrotum and the groin. The epididymis becomes swollen and extremely painful; the patient's temperature is elevated. The urine may contain pus (pyuria) and bacteria (bacteriuria), and the patient may experience chills and fever.

Medical Management

If the patient is seen within the first 24 hours after onset of pain, the spermatic cord may be infiltrated with a local anesthetic agent to relieve pain. If the epididymitis is from a chlamydial infection, the patient and his sexual partner must be treated with antibiotics. The patient is observed for abscess formation as well. If no improvement occurs within 2 weeks, an underlying testicular tumor should be considered. An epididymectomy (excision of the epididymis from the testis) may be performed for patients with recurrent, incapacitating episodes of epididymitis or for those with chronic, painful conditions. With long-term epididymitis, the passage of sperm may be obstructed. If the obstruction is bilateral, infertility may result.

Nursing Management

The patient is placed on bed rest, and the scrotum is elevated with a scrotal bridge or folded towel to prevent traction on the spermatic cord and to promote venous drainage and relieve pain. Antimicrobials are administered as prescribed until the acute inflammation subsides. Intermittent cold compresses to the scrotum may help ease the pain. Later, local heat or sitz baths may help resolve the inflammation. Analgesics are administered for pain relief as prescribed.

The nurse instructs the patient to avoid straining, lifting, and sexual stimulation until the infection is under control. He should continue taking analgesics and antibiotics as prescribed and using ice packs if necessary to relieve discomfort. He needs to know that it may take 4 weeks or longer for the epididymis to return to normal.

Testicular Cancer

Testicular cancer is the most common cancer in men 15 to 35 years of age and the second most common malignancy in men 35 to 39 years of age. An estimated 7600 men are diagnosed with testicular cancer each year (Landis et al., 1998). Such cancers are classified as germinal or nongerminal. Germinal tumors arise from the germinal cells of the testes (seminomas, teratocarcinomas, choriocarcinomas, yolk sac carcinomas, and embryonal carcinomas); nongerminal tumors arise from epithelium (Leydig cell tumors and Sertoli cell tumors). Ninety-five percent of all testicular cancers are germinal, with about 40% of these being seminomas. Seminomas tend to remain localized, whereas nonseminomatous tumors are fast growing. The cause of testicular tumors is unknown, but cryptorchidism, infections, and genetic and endocrine factors appear to play a part in their development.

The risk for testicular cancer is 35 times greater in men with any type of undescended testis than in the general population of men (Hussey, 1994). Prenatal exposure to DES may also be a risk factor. In the 1950s and early 1960s, DES was frequently used by women to prevent miscarriages and premature deliveries. Testicular tumors tend to metastasize early, spreading from the testis to the lymph nodes in the retroperitoneum and to the lungs.

Clinical Manifestations

The symptoms appear gradually with a mass or lump on the testicle and generally painless enlargement of the testis. The patient may complain of heaviness in the scrotum, inguinal area, or lower abdomen. Backache (from retroperitoneal node extension), pain in the abdomen, loss of weight, and general weakness may result from metastasis. The enlargement of the testis without pain is a significant diagnostic finding.

Assessment and Diagnostic Findings

Monthly testicular self-examinations (TSEs) are effective in detecting testicular cancers. Teaching men to perform TSE is an important health promotion intervention for early detection of this disease.

Human chorionic gonadotropin and alpha-fetoprotein are tumor markers that may be elevated in patients with testicular cancer. (Tumor markers are substances synthesized by the tumor cells and released into the circulation in abnormal amounts.) Newer immunocytochemical techniques can help identify the cells that apparently produce these markers. Tumor marker levels in the blood are used for diagnosis, staging, and monitoring the response to treatment. Other diagnostic tests include intravenous urography to detect any ureteral deviation caused by a tumor mass; lymphangiography to assess the extent of tumor spread to the lymphatic system; and CT scan of the chest, abdomen, and pelvis to determine the extent of the disease in the lungs, retroperitoneum, and pelvis.

Medical Management

Testicular cancer is one of the most curable solid tumors. The goals of management are to eradicate the disease and achieve a cure. Treatment selection is based on the cell type and the anatomic extent of the disease. The testis is removed by orchiectomy through an inguinal incision with a high ligation of the spermatic cord. A gel-filled prosthesis can be implanted to offset the absence of one testis. After unilateral orchiectomy for testicular cancer, most patients experience no impairment of endocrine function. Other patients, however, have decreased hormonal levels, suggesting that the unaffected testis is not functioning at normal levels. Retroperitoneal lymph node dissection (RPLND) to prevent lymphatic spread of the cancer may be performed after orchiectomy. Although normal libido and orgasm are usually unimpaired after RPLND, the patient may develop ejaculatory dysfunction with resultant infertility. Thus, sperm banking before surgery may be considered.

Postoperative irradiation of the lymph nodes from the diaphragm to the iliac region is used in treating seminomas and is only delivered to the affected side. The other testis is shielded from radiation to preserve fertility. Radiation is also used for patients who do not respond to chemotherapy or for whom lymph node surgery is not recommended.

Testicular carcinomas are highly responsive to chemotherapy. Chemotherapy with cisplatin and other agents, such as vinblastine, bleomycin, dactinomycin, and cyclophosphamide, results in a high percentage of complete remission. Good results may be obtained by combining different types of treatment, including surgery, radiation therapy, and chemotherapy. Even with disseminated testicular cancer, the prognosis is favorable, and the disease is probably curable because of advances in diagnosis and treatment.

Patient Education and Home Care

Testicular Self-Examination

Testicular self-examination (TSE) is to be performed once a month. The test is neither difficult nor time-consuming. A convenient time is usually after a warm bath or shower when the scrotum is more relaxed.

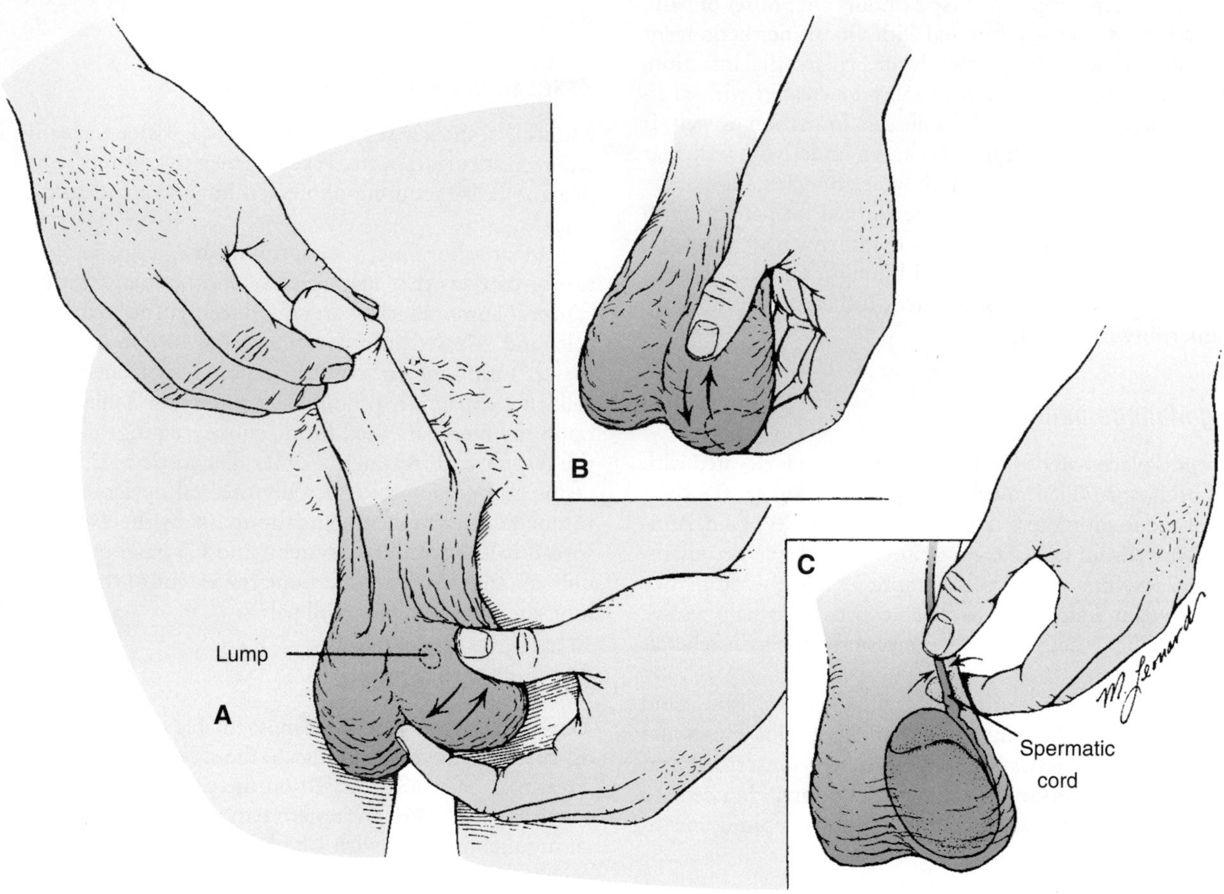

1. Use both hands to palpate the testis. The normal testicle is smooth and uniform in consistency.
2. With the index and middle fingers under the testis and the thumb on top, roll the testis gently in a horizontal plane between the thumb and fingers (**A**).
3. Feel for any evidence of a small lump or abnormality.
4. Follow the same procedure and palpate upward along the testis (**B**).
5. Locate and palpate the epididymis (**C**), a cord-like structure on the top and back of the testicle that stores and transports sperm. Also locate and palpate the spermatic cord.
6. Repeat the examination for the other testis, epididymis, and spermatic cord. It is normal to find that one testis is larger than the other.
7. If you find any evidence of a small, pea-like lump or if the testis is swollen (possibly from an infection or tumor), consult your physician.

A patient with a history of one testicular tumor has a greater chance of developing subsequent tumors. Follow-up studies include chest x-rays, excretory urography, radioimmunoassay of human chorionic gonadotropins and alpha-fetoprotein levels, and examination of lymph nodes to detect recurrent malignancy.

Nursing Management

Because the patient may have difficulty coping with his condition, issues related to body image and sexuality should be addressed. He needs encouragement to maintain a positive attitude during what may be a long course of therapy. He also needs to know that radiation therapy will not necessarily prevent him from fathering children, nor does unilateral excision of a tumor necessarily decrease virility.

Hydrocele

A **hydrocele** is a collection of fluid, generally in the tunica vaginalis of the testis, although it may also collect within the spermatic cord. The tunica vaginalis becomes widely distended with fluid. Hydrocele can be differentiated from a hernia by transillumination; hydrocele transmits light, whereas a hernia does not. Hydrocele may be acute or chronic. Acute hydrocele may occur in association with acute infectious diseases of the epididymis or as a result of local injury or systemic infectious diseases, such as mumps. The cause of chronic hydrocele is unknown.

Usually, therapy is not required. Treatment is necessary only if the hydrocele becomes tense and compromises testicular circulation or if the scrotal mass becomes large, uncomfortable, or embarrassing. In the surgical treatment of hydrocele, an incision is made through the wall of the scrotum down to the distended tunica vaginalis. The sac is resected or, after being opened, is sutured together to collapse the wall. Postoperatively, the patient wears an athletic supporter for comfort and support. The major complication is hematoma in the loose scrotal tissues.

Varicocele

A **varicocele** is an abnormal dilation of the veins of the pampiniform venous plexus in the scrotum (the network of veins from the testis and the epididymis that constitute part of the spermatic cord). Varicoceles usually occur in the veins on the upper portion of the left testicle in adults. In some men, a varicocele has been associated with infertility. Few, if any, subjective symptoms may be produced by the enlarged spermatic vein, and no treatment is required unless fertility is a concern. Symptomatic varicocele (pain, tenderness, and discomfort in the inguinal region) is corrected surgically by ligating the external spermatic vein at the inguinal area. An ice pack may be applied to the scrotum for the first few hours after surgery to relieve edema. The patient then wears a scrotal supporter.

Vasectomy

Vasectomy, or male sterilization, is the ligation and transection of part of the vas deferens, with or without removal of a segment of the vas deferens. To prevent the passage of the sperm from the testes, the vas deferens is exposed through a surgical opening in the scrotum or by use of a sharp, curved hemostat (Fig. 45-5). The severed ends are occluded with ligatures or clips, or the lumen of each vas deferens is sealed by cautery. The spermatozoa, which are manufactured in the testes, cannot travel up the vas deferens after this surgery.

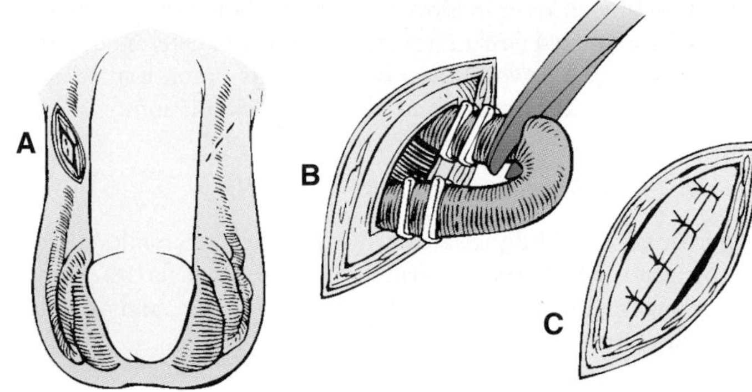

FIGURE 45•5 A vasectomy is a resection of the vas deferens to prevent passage of sperm from the testes to the urethra during ejaculation. (**A**) An incision or small puncture is made to expose the vas deferens. (**B**) The vas deferens is isolated and severed. (**C**) The severed ends are occluded with ligatures or clips, or the lumen of each vas is sealed by electrocautery and the incision is sutured closed. (Suturing may not be required if a puncture approach has been used.)

Because seminal fluid is manufactured predominantly in the seminal vesicles and prostate gland, which are unaffected by vasectomy, no noticeable decrease occurs in the amount of ejaculate even though it contains no spermatozoa. Because the sperm cells have no exit, they are reabsorbed into the body. This procedure has no effect on sexual potency, erection, ejaculation, or production of male hormones and provides no protection against sexually transmitted diseases.

Couples who worry about pregnancy resulting from contraceptive failure often report a decrease in concern and an increase in spontaneous sexual arousal after vasectomy. Concise and factual preoperative explanations may minimize or relieve the patient's concerns related to masculinity. Although a relationship between vasectomy and autoimmune disorders and prostatic cancer has been suggested, there is no clinical evidence of either.

The patient is advised that he will be sterile but that potency will not be altered after a bilateral vasectomy. As with any surgical procedure, a surgical consent form must be signed. On rare occasions, a spontaneous reanastomosis of the vas deferens occurs, making it possible to impregnate a partner.

Complications of vasectomy include scrotal ecchymoses and swelling, superficial wound infection, vasitis (inflammation of the vas deferens), epididymitis or epididymo-orchitis, hematomas, and spermatic granuloma. A spermatic granuloma is an inflammatory response to the collection of sperm leaking into the scrotum from the severed end of the proximal vas deferens. This can initiate recanalization of the vas deferens, making pregnancy of the partner possible.

Nursing Management

Ice bags are applied intermittently to the scrotum for several hours after surgery to reduce swelling and to relieve discomfort. The nurse advises the patient to wear cotton, jockey-type briefs for added comfort and support. He may become greatly concerned about the discoloration of the scrotal skin and superficial swelling. These are temporary conditions that occur frequently after vasectomy and may be relieved by sitz baths.

Sexual intercourse may be resumed as desired, although fertility remains for a varying time after vasectomy until the spermatozoa stored distal to the severed vas deferens have been evacuated. Other methods of contraception should be used until infertility is confirmed by an examination of ejaculate. Some physicians examine a specimen 4 weeks after the vasectomy to determine sterility; others examine two consecutive specimens 1 month apart; and still others consider a patient sterile after 36 ejaculations.

Vasovasostomy (Sterilization Reversal)

Microsurgical techniques are used to reverse vasectomies (vasovasostomy), which restores patency to the vas deferens. Many men have sperm in their ejaculate after a reversal, and 40% to 75% can impregnate a partner.

Banking Sperm

Storing fertile semen in a sperm bank *before* a vasectomy is an option for men who face an unforeseen life event that may cause them to want to father a child at a later time. The success rate in achieving pregnancy with frozen sperm is uncertain, and legal problems related to using stored sperm make this an ongoing issue.

CONDITIONS AFFECTING THE PENIS

Hypospadias and Epispadias

Hypospadias and epispadias are congenital anomalies of the urethral opening. In hypospadias, the urethral opening is a groove on the underside of the penis. In epispadias, the urethral opening is on the dorsum. These anatomic abnormalities may be repaired by various types of plastic surgery, usually when the boy is very young.

Phimosis

Phimosis, a condition in which the foreskin is constricted so that it cannot be retracted over the glans, can occur congenitally or from inflammation and edema. With the trend away from routine circumcision of newborns, the child and adult require early instruction in cleansing the prepuce. In adults who do not clean the preputial area, normal secretions accumulate, causing subsequent inflammation (balanitis), which can lead to adhesions and fibrosis. The thickened secretions become encrusted with urinary salts and calcify, forming calculi in the prepuce. In elderly men, penile carcinoma may develop. Phimosis is corrected by circumcision (see later discussion).

Paraphimosis is a condition in which the foreskin is retracted behind the glans and, because of narrowness and subsequent edema, cannot be returned to its usual position (covering the glans). Paraphimosis is treated by firmly compressing the glans to reduce its size and then pushing the glans back while simultaneously moving the prepuce forward (manual reduction). Circumcision is usually indicated after the inflammation and edema subside.

Cancer of the Penis

Cancer of the penis occurs in men older than 60 years of age and represents about 0.5% of malignancies in men in the United States. In some countries, however, the incidence is 10%. Cancer of the penis rarely occurs in circumcised males. It appears on the skin of the penis as a painless, wartlike growth or ulcer. Cancer of the penis can involve the glans, the coronal sulcus under the prepuce, the corporal bodies, the urethra, and regional or distant lymph nodes. **Bowen's disease** is a form of squamous cell carcinoma in situ of the penile shaft. Typically, a man delays seeking treatment for more than a year, probably because of guilt, embarrassment, or ignorance.

Prevention

Circumcision in infancy almost eliminates the possibility of **penile cancer** because chronic irritation and inflammation of the glans penis predispose to penile tumors. In uncircumcised men, personal hygiene is an important preventive measure.

Medical Management

Smaller lesions involving only the skin may be controlled by excision. Topical chemotherapy with 5-fluorouracil cream may be one option in selected patients. Radiation therapy is used to treat small squamous cell carcinomas of the penis or for palliation in advanced tumors or lymph node metastasis. Partial penectomy (removal of the penis) is preferred to total penectomy if possible; about 40% of patients can then participate in sexual intercourse and stand for urination. The shaft of the penis can still respond to sexual arousal with an erection and has the sensory capacity for orgasm and ejaculation. Total penectomy is indicated when the tumor is not amenable to conservative treatment. After a total penectomy, the patient may still experience orgasm with stimulation of the perineum and scrotal area.

Priapism

Priapism is an uncontrolled, persistent erection of the penis that causes the penis to become large, hard, and painful. It occurs from either neural or vascular causes, including sickle cell thrombosis, leukemic cell infiltration, spinal cord tumors, and tumor invasion of the penis or its vessels. This condition may result in gangrene and often results in impotence, whether treated or not.

Priapism is a urologic emergency. The goal of therapy is to improve venous drainage of the corpora cavernosa to prevent ischemia, fibrosis, and impotence. The initial treatment is directed at relieving the erection and includes bed rest and sedation. The corpora may be irrigated with an anticoagulant, which allows stagnant blood to be aspirated. Shunting procedures to divert the blood from the turgid corpora cavernosa to the venous system (corpora cavernosa–saphenous vein shunt) or into the corpus spongiosum–glans penis compartment may be attempted.

Peyronie's Disease

Peyronie's disease involves the buildup of fibrous plaques in the sheath of the corpus cavernosum. These plaques are not visible when the penis is relaxed. When erect, however, curvature of the penis occurs that can be painful and can make sexual intercourse difficult or impossible. Peyronie's disease primarily occurs in middle-aged and older men. Although the plaques may shrink over time, surgical removal of the plaques may be necessary.

Urethral Stricture

Urethral stricture is a condition in which a section of the urethra is narrowed. It can occur congenitally or from a scar along the urethra. Traumatic injury to the urethra, for example, from instrumentation or infections, can result in strictures. Treatment involves dilation of the urethra or, in severe cases, urethrotomy (surgical removal of the stricture).

Circumcision

Circumcision is the excision of the foreskin, or prepuce, of the glans penis. It is usually performed in infancy. In adults, it is part of the treatment for phimosis, paraphimosis, and recurrent infections of the glans and foreskin and may be performed at the personal desire of the patient.

Postoperatively, a petrolatum (Vaseline) gauze dressing is applied and changed as indicated. The patient is observed for bleeding. Because a considerable amount of pain may occur after circumcision, analgesics are administered as needed.

GERONTOLOGIC CONSIDERATIONS

As men age, the prostate gland enlarges, prostate secretion decreases, the scrotum hangs lower, the testes become smaller and more firm, and pubic hair becomes sparser and stiffer. Changes in gonadal function include a decline in plasma testosterone levels and reduced production of progesterone. Other changes include decreasing sexual function, slower sexual responses, increased incidence of genitourinary tract cancer, and urinary incontinence for various reasons.

Male reproductive capability is maintained with advancing age. Although degenerative changes occur in the seminiferous tubules, spermatogenesis (production of sperm) continues. Sexual function, however, involving libido (desire) and potency, decreases. Vascular problems cause about half of cases of impotence in men older than 50 years of age.

Hypogonadism occurs in up to one fourth of older men. The relationship of hypogonadism to impotence is uncertain. This decline is more evident in men older than 70 years but is also noted in men in their 60s. In older men, the sexual response slows. Erection takes longer in men older than 50 years of age, and full erections may not be attained until orgasm. Sexual function is affected by several factors, such as psychological problems, illnesses, and medications. In general, the sexual act takes longer. In older men, ejaculatory control increases; however, if erection is partially lost, there may be difficulty in attaining a full erection again, and resolution may occur without orgasm. Sexual activity is closely correlated with the man's sexual activity of his earlier years; if he was more active than average as a young man, he will most likely continue to be more active than average in his later years.

Cancers of the kidney, bladder, prostate, and penis all have increased incidence in men older than 50 years of age. DRE and screening tests for hematuria and may uncover a higher percentage of malignancies at earlier stages.

Urinary incontinence in the elderly man may have many causes, including medications and age-related conditions, such as neurologic diseases or benign prostatic hyperplasia (also referred to as hypertrophy and called an enlarged prostate by the lay public). Diagnostic tests are performed to exclude reversible causes of urinary incontinence. For some patients with severe incontinence, augmentation cystoplasty (repair of the bladder) with the placement of an artificial urinary sphincter may help alleviate this problem.

Critical Thinking Exercises

1.
A 49-year-old man tells you he has been informed by his physician that he has an elevated PSA level but that he does not understand its significance or what action he should take. How would you respond to his statement? What factors you would consider in formulating your response?

2.
One of your patients, a 50-year-old man with long-standing diabetes, asks you about Viagra. What information and teaching approach would you give to him about Viagra? How would your approach differ if the patient is a 32-year-old patient with a spinal cord injury? If your patient is a 68-year-old man with coronary artery disease?

3.
You are caring for two patients who have undergone prostatectomy. One has had a TUR; the other has undergone an open surgical approach to remove the prostate. How would your care differ for these two patients? How would your assessment be directed to detect possible complications?

4.
A 28-year-old man is seeking treatment for his sixth episode of STD. In addition to assisting with medical management and follow-up, what other interventions would you consider for this patient?

5.
During a routine physical examination, a 23-year-old man indicates that he does not perform TSE and does not know how to do so. Develop a teaching plan to instruct him in this examination. How would you modify the plan and approach if the patient is unable to understand English? If the patient has severely impaired vision?

References and Selected Readings

BOOKS

Agency for Health Care Policy and Research. (1994). *Benign prostatic hyperplasia: Diagnosis and treatment.* Clinical Practice Guidelines No. 8. AHCPR Publication No. 94-0582. Bethesda, MD: U.S. Department of Health and Human Services.

American Cancer Society. (1999). *Cancer facts and figures,* Atlanta: American Cancer Society.

Bosl, G. J., Bajorin, D. F., Scheinfeld, J., & Motzer, R. J. (1997). Cancer of the testis. In DeVita, V. T., Hellman, S., & Rosenberg, S. A. (Eds.). *Cancer principles and practice of oncology* (5th ed.). Philadelphia: Lippincott-Raven.

Bruner, D. W., & Iwamoto, R. R. (1999). Altered sexual health. In Yarbro, C. H., Frogge, M. H., & Goodman, M. (Eds.). *Cancer symptom management.* (2nd ed.). Boston: Jones & Bartlett.

Ducharme, S. H., & Gill, K. M. (1997). Management of other male sexual dysfunctions. In Sipski, M. L., & Alexander, C. J. *Sexual function in people with disability and chronic illness.* Gaithersburg, MD: Aspen.

Hellstrom, W. J. G. (1997). Male infertility and sexual dysfunction. New York: Springer.

Hinman, F. (Ed.). (1998). *Atlas of urologic surgery* (2nd ed.). Philadelphia: W. B. Saunders.

Karlowicz, K. A. (Ed.). (1995). *Urologic nursing: Principles and practice.* Philadelphia: W. B. Saunders.

Lipshultz, L. I., & Howards, S. S. (Ed.). (1997). *Infertility in the male* (3rd ed.). St. Louis: C. V. Mosby.

Marshall, F. F. (Ed.). (1996). *Textbook of operative urology.* Philadelphia: W. B. Saunders.

Oesterling, J. E., Fuks, Z., Lee, C. T., & Scher, H. I. (1997). Cancer of the prostate. In DeVita, V. T., Hellman, S., & Rosenberg, S. A. (Eds.). *Cancer principles and practice of oncology* (5th ed.). Philadelphia: Lippincott-Raven.

Retik, A. B., Vaughn, E. D., & Walsh, P. C. (Eds.). (1997). *Campbell's urology* (8th ed.). Philadelphia: W. B. Saunders.

Sipski, M. L., & Alexander, C. J. (Eds.). (1997). *Sexual function in people with disability and chronic illness: A health professional's guide.* Gaithersburg, MD: Aspen.

Thomas, G. M., & Williams, S. D. (1998). Testis. In Perez, C. A., & Brady, L. W. (Eds.). *Principles and practices of radiation oncology* (3rd ed.). Philadelphia: Lippincott-Raven.

JOURNALS

Asterisks indicate nursing research articles.

General

Millon-Underwood, S., & Sanders, E. (1990). Factors contributing to health promotion behaviors among African-American men. *Oncology Nursing Forum, 17*(5), 707–712.

Vetrosky, D. (1997). Prostatitis. *Primary Care Practice, 1*(4), 437–441.

Assessment of Function and Dysfunction of Male Reproductive Function

Feldman, H. A., et al. (1994). Impotence and its medical and psychological correlates: Results of the Massachusetts male aging study. *Journal of Urology, 151*(1), 54–61.

Goldstein, I., et al. (1998). Oral sildenafil in the treatment of erectile dysfunction. *New England Journal of Medicine, 338*(20), 1397–1404.

Klingman, L. (1999). Assessing the male genitalia. *American Journal of Nursing, 99*(7), 47–50.

Lewis, J. H. (1993). Nursing management for patients using external vacuum devices: A unique opportunity. *Urology Nursing, 13*(3), 80–85.

National Institutes of Health Consensus Development Panel on Impotence. (1993). Impotence. *Journal of the American Medical Association, 270*(1), 83–90.

O'Keefe, M., & Hunt, D. K. (1995). Assessment and treatment of impotence. *Medical Clinics of North America, 79*(2), 415–434.

Padma-Nathan, H., et al. (1997). Treatment of men with erectile dysfunction with transurethral alprostadil. Medical Urethral System for Erection (MUSE) Study Group. *New England Journal of Medicine, 336*(1), 1–7.

Smith, D. B., & Babaian, R. J. (1992). The effects of treatment for cancer on male fertility and sexuality. *Cancer Nursing, 15*(4), 271–275.

Sundaram, C. P., et al. (1997). Long-term follow-up of patients receiving injection therapy for erectile dysfunction. *Urology, 49*(6), 932–935.

Benign Prostatic Hyperplasia

Barry M. J., et al. (1997). The natural history of patients with benign prostatic hyperplasia as diagnosed by North American urologists. *Journal of Urology, 157*(1), 10–15.

Gerber, G. S. (1995). Lasers in the treatment of benign prostatic hyperplasia. *Urology, 45*(2), 193–199.

Gormley, G. J., et al. (1992). The effect of finasteride in men with benign prostatic hyperplasia. *New England Journal of Medicine, 327*(17), 1185–1191.

Keetch D. W., et al. (1995). Cryosurgical ablation of the prostate. *AORN Journal, 61*(5), 807–813.

Ramsey, E. W., et al. (1997). A novel transurethral microwave thermal ablation system to treat benign prostatic hyperplasia: Results of a prospective multicenter clinical trial. *Journal of Urology, 158*(1), 112–119.

Reilly, N. J. (1997). Benign prostatic hyperplasia in older men. *Lippincott's Primary Care Practice, 1*(4), 421–430.

Infertility

Baker, H. W. (1994). Male infertility. *Endocrinology and Metabolism Clinics of North America, 23*(4), 783–793.

Howards, S. S. (1995). Treatment of male infertility. *New England Journal of Medicine, 332*(5), 312–317.

Prostate Cancer

Ahlering, T., et al. (1996). Practice guidelines for prostate cancer. *Cancer Journal from Scientific American, 2*(Suppl 3A), S77–S86.

Altman, G. B., & Lee, C. A. (1996). Strontium-89 for treatment of painful bone metastasis from prostate cancer. *Oncology Nursing Forum, 23*(3), 523–527.

Bolla, M., et al. (1997). Improved survival in patients with locally advanced prostate cancer treated with radiotherapy and goserelin. *New England Journal of Medicine, 337*(5), 295–300.

Brenner, Z. R., & Krenzer, M. E. (1995). Update on cyrosurgical ablation for prostate cancer. *American Journal of Nursing, 95*(4), 44–48.

Cash, J. C., & Dattoli, M. J. (1997). Management of patients receiving transperineal palladium-103 prostate implants. *Oncology Nursing Forum, 24*(8), 1361–1367.

Cher, M. L., & Carroll, P. R. (1995). Screening for prostate cancer. *Western Journal of Medicine, 162*(3), 235–242.

Coley, C. M., et al. (1997). Early detection of prostate cancer. I. Prior probability and effectiveness of tests. American College of Physicians. *Annals of Internal Medicine, 126*(5), 394–406.

Coley, C. M., et al. (1997). Early detection of prostate cancer. II. Estimating the risks, benefits, and costs. American College of Physicians. *Annals of Internal Medicine, 126*(6), 468–479.

*Collins, M. (1997). Increasing prostate cancer awareness in African American men. *Oncology Nursing Forum, 24*(1), 91–95.

Cotter, V. T. (1998). Prostate cancer: Examining the risks and benefits of screening. *Advance for Nurse Practitioners, 6*(7), 51–53.

*Davison, B. J., et al. (1995). Information and decision-making preferences of men with prostate cancer. *Oncology Nursing Forum, 22*(9), 1401–1408.

*Esper, P., et al. (1999). Quality-of-life evaluation in patients receiving treatment for advanced prostate cancer. *Oncology Nursing Forum, 26*(1), 107–112.

*Gelfand, D. E., et al. (1995). Digital rectal examinations and prostate cancer screening: Attitudes of African American men. *Oncology Nursing Forum, 22*(8), 1253–1263.

Gerard, M. J., & Frank-Stromborg, M. (1998). Screening for prostate cancer in asymptomatic men: Clinical, legal, and ethical implications. *Oncology Nursing Forum, 25*(9), 1561–1569.

Greco, K. E., & Kulawiak, L. (1994). Prostate cancer prevention: Risk reduction through life-style, diet, and chemoprevention. *Oncology Nursing Forum, 21*(9), 1504–1511.

Haas, G. P., & Sakr, W. A. (1997). Epidemiology of prostate cancer. *CA: A Cancer Journal for Clinicians, 47*(5), 273–287.

Held, J. L., et al. (1994). Cancer of the prostate: Treatment and nursing implications. *Oncology Nursing Forum, 21*(9), 1517–1529.

Herr, H. W. (1997). Quality of life in prostate cancer patients. *CA: A Cancer Journal for Clinicians, 47*(4), 207–217.

Kaps, E. C. (1994). The role of the support group, "Us Too." *Cancer, 74*(7 Suppl), 2188–2189.

Krongrad, A., et al. (1997). Survival after radical prostatectomy. *Journal of the American Medical Association, 278*(1), 44–46.

Landis, S. H., et al. (1998). Cancer statistics, 1998. *CA: A Cancer Journal for Clinicians, 48,* 6–29.

Lazzaro, M., & Thompson, M. (1997). Update on prostate cancer screening. *Lippincott's Primary Care Practice, 1*(4), 408–418.

McKee, J. M. (1994). Cues to action in prostate cancer screening. *Oncology Nursing Forum, 21*(7), 1171–1176.

Mettlin, C. (1997). National patterns of prostate cancer detection and treatment. The American Cancer Society National Prostate Cancer Detection Project. *CA: A Cancer Journal for Clinicians, 47*(5), 365–272.

Middleton, R. G. (1996). The management of clinically localized prostate cancer: guidelines from the American Urological Association. *CA: A Cancer Journal for Clinicians, 46*(4), 249–253.

*O'Rourke, M. E., & Germino, B. B. (1998). Prostate cancer treatment decisions: A focus group exploration. *Oncology Nursing Forum, 25*(1), 97–104.

Partin, A. W., et al. (1997). Combination of prostate-specific antigen, clinical stage, and Gleason score to predict pathological stage of localized prostate cancer: A multi-institutional update. *Journal of the American Medical Association, 277*(18), 1445–1451.

Pilepich, M. V., et al. (1995). Androgen deprivation with radiation therapy compared with radiation therapy alone for locally advanced prostatic carcinoma: A randomized comparative trial of the Radiation Therapy Oncology Group. *Urology, 45*(4), 616–623.

Ragde, H., et al. (1997). Interstitial iodine-125 radiation without adjuvant therapy in the treatment of clinically localized prostate carcinoma. *Cancer, 80*(3), 442–453.

Society of Surgical Oncology. (1997). Prostate cancer surgical practice guidelines. *Oncology, 11*(6), 907–912.

Sodee, D. B., et al. (1996). Preliminary imaging results using In-111 labeled CYT-356 (Prostascint) in the detection of recurrent prostate cancer. *Clinical Nuclear Medicine, 21*(10), 759–767.

Travis, M., & Gwozdz, D. T. (1993). Nursing case management for patients with TURP. *Urology Nursing, 13*(2), 48–54.

von Eschenbach, A., et al. (1997). American Cancer Society guideline for the early detection of prostate cancer: Update 1997. *CA: A Cancer Journal for Clinicians, 47*(5), 261–264.

Waxman, E. S. (1993). Sexual dysfunction following treatment for prostate cancer: Nursing assessment and interventions. *Oncology Nursing Forum, 20*(10), 1567–1571.

*Yarbro, C. H., & Ferrans, C. E. (1998). Quality of life of patients with prostate cancer treated with surgery or radiation therapy. *Oncology Nursing Forum, 25*(4), 685–693.
*Zimmerman, S. M. (1997). Factors influencing Hispanic participation in prostate cancer screening. *Oncology Nursing Forum, 24*(3), 499–504.
Zinreich, E. S., et al. (1990). Pre and posttreatment evaluation of sexual function in patients with adenocarcinoma of the prostate. *International Journal of Radiation Oncology, Biology, Physics, 19*(3), 729–732.

Testicular Cancer

*Brodsky, M. S. (1995). Testicular cancer survivors' impressions of the impact of the disease on their lives. *Qualitative Health Research, 5*(1), 78–96.
Hawkins, C., & Miaskowski, C. (1996). Testicular cancer: A review. *Oncology Nursing Forum, 23*(8), 1203–1211.
Higgs, D. J. (1990). The patient with testicular cancer: Nursing management of chemotherapy. *Oncology Nursing Forum, 17*(2), 243–249.

Resources

AGENCIES

American Cancer Society, 1599 Clifton Road, NE, Atlanta, GA 30326; 1-800-ACS-2345; www.cancer.org
American Foundation for Urologic Disease, Prostate Cancer Support Network, 300 West Pratt, Suite 401, Baltimore, MD 21201-2463; 1-800-828-7866
Impotence Anonymous and I-Anon, Impotence World Association, P.O. Box 410, Bowie, MD 20718-0410; 1-800-669-1603
National Cancer Institute, Office of Cancer Communications, Building 31, Room 10A24, Bethesda, MD 20892; 1-800-4-CANCER
Prostate Cancer At-A-Glance-Centers for Disease Control: www.cdc.gov/nccd-php/dcpc/prostate/pros95.htm
The Prostate Cancer InfoLink: www.cp,ed.com/prostate
US Too International, Inc., Prostate Cancer Survivor Support Group, 930 North York Road, Suite 50, Hinsdale, Illinois 60521-2993; 1-800-80-US-TOO; www.ustoo.com

PATIENT RESOURCES

Marks, S. (1995). *Prostate and cancer: A family guide to diagnosis, treatment and survival.* Fisher Books, Tucson, AZ.
Rous, S. (1995). *The prostate book* (2nd ed.). New York: W. W. Norton.
Schover, L. R. (1988). *Sexuality and cancer: For the man who has cancer, and his partner.* Atlanta: American Cancer Society.
Walsh, P. C., & Worthington, J. F. (1995). *The prostate: A guide for men and the women who love them.* Baltimore: The Johns Hopkins University Press.

UNIT

11

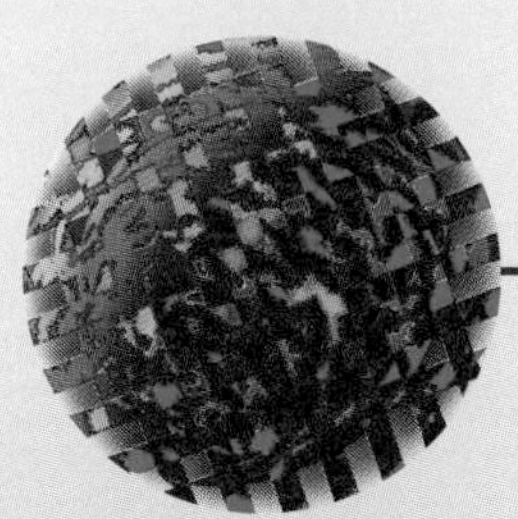

Immunologic Function

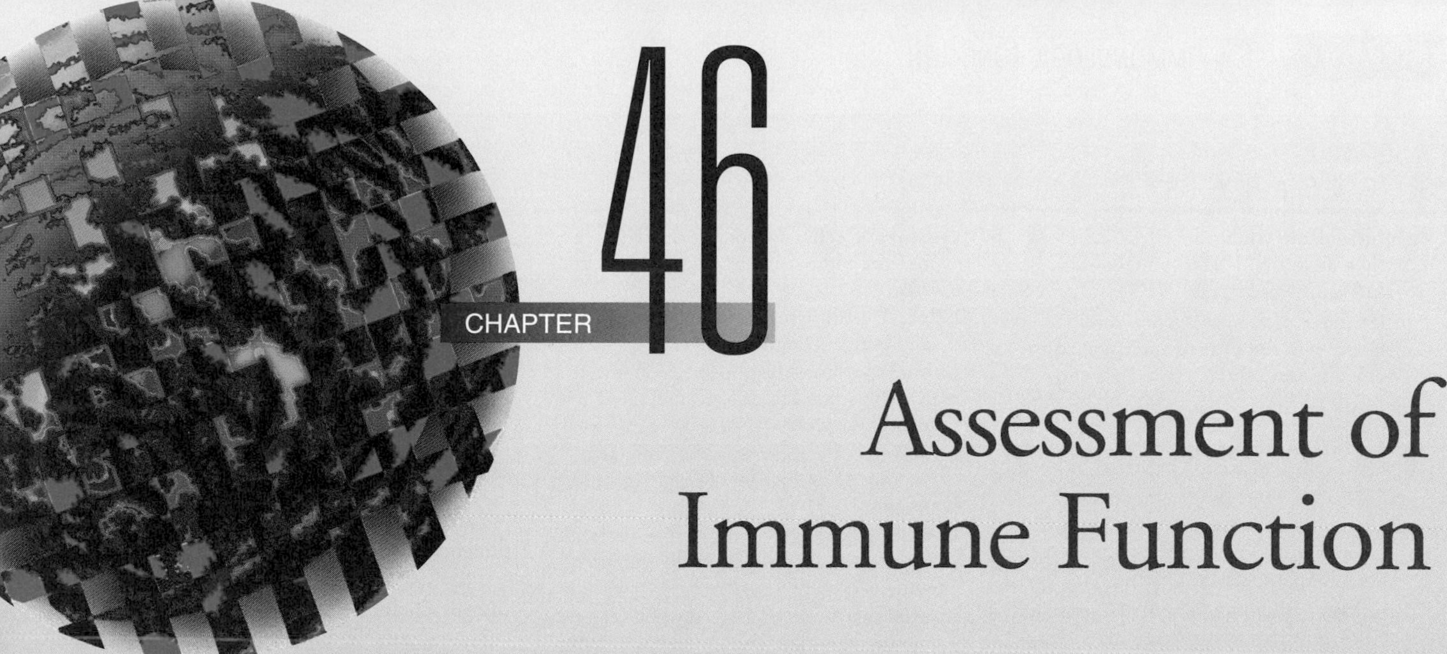

CHAPTER 46

Assessment of Immune Function

Learning Objectives

On completion of this chapter, the learner will be able to:

1. Describe the body's general immune responses.
2. Discuss the stages of the immune response.
3. Differentiate between cellular and humoral immune responses.
4. Describe the effects of the following variables on function of the immune system: age, gender, nutrition, psychoneuroimmunology, concurrent illness, cancer, medications, and radiation.
5. Use assessment parameters for determining the status of immune function.

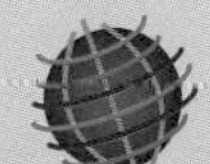

The immune system functions as the body's defense mechanism against invasion. The term **immunity** refers to the body's specific protective response to an invading foreign agent or organism. Immune function is affected by age and by a variety of other factors, such as central nervous system function, emotional status, medications, the stress of illness, trauma, and surgery. Dysfunctions involving the immune system occur across the life span. Many are genetically based; others are acquired. The term **immunopathology** refers to the study of diseases resulting from dysfunctions within the immune system. Disorders of the immune system may stem from excesses or deficiencies of immunocompetent cells, alterations in the function of these cells, immunologic attack on self-antigens, or inappropriate or exaggerated responses to specific antigens (Table 46-1).

To gain insight into immunopathology and the growing number of immunologic-based disorders and to assess and care for people with immunologic disorders, the nurse needs a sound knowledge base of the immune system and how it functions.

GLOSSARY

agglutination: clumping effect occurring when an antibody acts as a cross-link between two antigens

antibody: a protein substance developed by the body in response to and interacting with a specific antigen

antigen: substance that induces the production of antibodies

B cells: cells that are important in producing circulating antibodies

cellular immune response: the immune system's third line of defense involving the attack of pathogens by T cells

complement: series of enzymatic proteins in the serum that, when activated, destroy bacteria and other cells

cytokines: generic term for nonantibody proteins that act as intercellular mediators, as in the generation of immune response

cytotoxic T cells: leukocytes that lyse cells infected with virus; also play a role in graft rejection

helper T cells: lymphocytes that attack foreign invaders (antigens) directly

humoral immune response: the immune system's second line of defense; often termed the *antibody response*

immunity: the body's specific protective response to an invading foreign agent or organism

immunopathology: study of diseases resulting in dysfunctions within the immune system

interferons: proteins formed when cells are exposed to viral or foreign agents; capable of activating other components of the immune system

lymphokines: substances released by sensitized lymphocytes when they contact specific antigens

memory cells: responsible for recognizing antigens from previous exposure and mounting an immune response

natural killer cells (NK cells)**:** lymphocytes that defend against microorganisms and malignant cells

null lymphocytes: lymphocytes that destroy antigens already coated with the antibody.

opsonization: the coating of antigen–antibody molecules with a sticky substance to facilitate phagocytosis

phagocytic cells: cells that engulf, ingest, and destroy foreign bodies or toxins

phagocytic immune response: the immune system's first line of defense involving white blood cells that have the ability to ingest foreign particles

suppressor T cells: lymphocytes that decrease B-cell activity to a level at which the immune system is compatible with life

ANATOMIC AND PHYSIOLOGIC OVERVIEW

Anatomy of the Immune System

Essentially, the system is made up of the bone marrow, the white blood cells (WBCs) produced by the bone marrow, and the lymphoid tissues. Lymphoid tissues include the thymus gland, the spleen, the lymph nodes, the tonsils and adenoids, and similar tissues in the gastrointestinal, respiratory, and reproductive systems (Fig. 46-1).

Bone Marrow

The bone marrow is the production site of the WBCs involved in immunity (Fig. 46-2): the B lymphocytes (B cells) and the T lymphocytes (T cells). B lymphocytes mature in the bone marrow

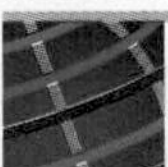

TABLE 46•1 Immune System Disorders

Disorder	Description
Autoimmunity	Normal protective immune response paradoxically turns against or attacks the body, leading to tissue damage
Hypersensitivity	Body produces inappropriate or exaggerated responses to specific antigens
Gammopathies	Immunoglobulins are overproduced
Immune deficiencies	
Primary	Deficiency results from improper development of immune cells or tissues, usually with a genetic basis
Secondary	Deficiency results from some interference with an already developed immune system

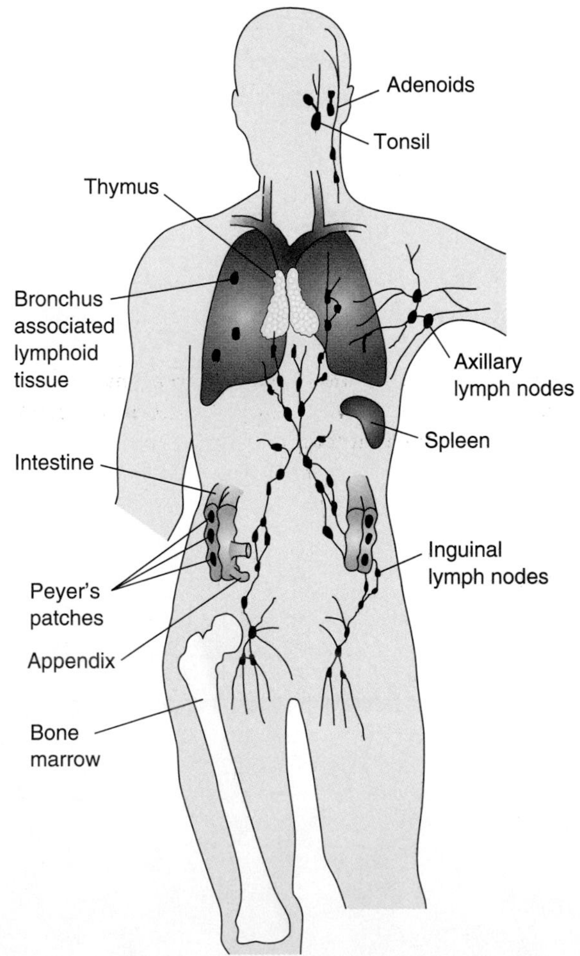

FIGURE 46•1 Structures in the normal immune system. From Porth, C. M. (1998). *Pathophysiology: Concepts of altered health states* (5th ed.). Philadelphia: Lippincott Williams & Wilkins.

PHYSIOLOGY

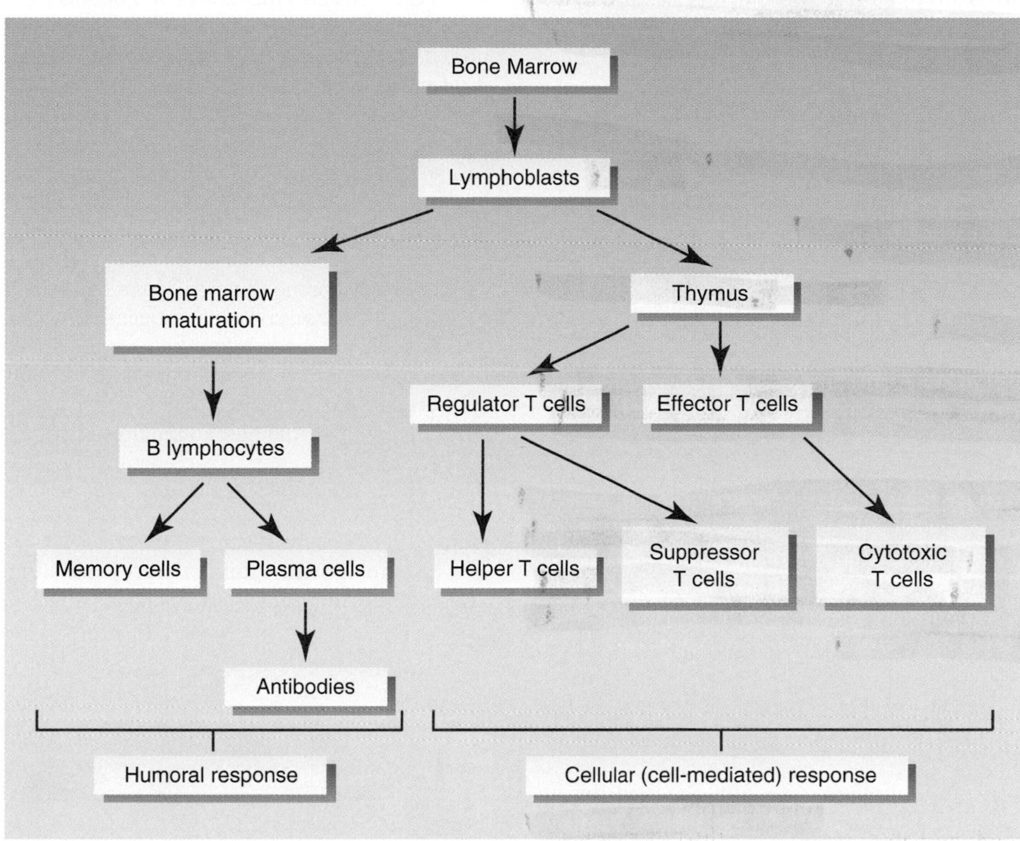

FIGURE 46•2 Development of cells of the immune system.

and then enter the circulation. T lymphocytes move from the bone marrow to the thymus, where they mature into several kinds of cells capable of different functions.

Lymphoid Tissues

The spleen, composed of red and white pulp, acts somewhat like a filter. The red pulp is the site where old and injured red blood cells are destroyed. The white pulp contains concentrations of lymphocytes. The lymph nodes are distributed throughout the body. They are connected by lymph channels and capillaries, which remove foreign material from the lymph before it enters the bloodstream. The lymph nodes also serve as centers for immune cell proliferation. The remaining lymphoid tissues, such as the tonsils and adenoids and other mucoid lymphatic tissues, contain immune cells that defend the body against microorganisms.

Immune Function: Defenses and Responses

There are two general types of immunity: natural and acquired. Natural immunity is a nonspecific immunity present at birth. Acquired or specific immunity develops after birth. Although each type of immunity plays a distinct role in defending the body against harmful invaders, the various components usually act in an interdependent manner.

Natural Immunity

Natural immunity provides a nonspecific response to any foreign invader, regardless of the invader's composition. The basis of natural defense mechanisms is merely the ability to distinguish between friend and foe or "self" and "nonself." Such natural mechanisms include physical and chemical barriers, the action of WBCs, and inflammatory responses.

PHYSICAL AND CHEMICAL BARRIERS

Physical barriers include intact skin and mucous membranes, which prevent pathogens from gaining access to the body, and the cilia of the respiratory tract along with coughing and sneezing responses, which act to filter and clear pathogens from the upper respiratory tract before they can invade the body further. Chemical barriers, such as acidic gastric juices, enzymes in tears and saliva, and substances in sebaceous and sweat secretions, act in a nonspecific way to destroy invading bacteria and fungi. Viruses are countered by other means, such as interferon. **Interferon**, one type of biologic response modifier, is a nonspecific viricidal protein naturally produced by the body and capable of activating other components of the immune system.

WHITE BLOOD CELL ACTION

WBCs, or leukocytes, participate in both the natural and the acquired immune responses. Granular leukocytes, or granulocytes (so called because of granules in their cytoplasm), fight invasion by foreign bodies or toxins by releasing cell mediators, such as histamine, bradykinin, and prostaglandins, and engulfing the foreign bodies or toxins. Granulocytes include neutrophils, eosinophils, and basophils.

Neutrophils (also called polymorphonuclear leukocytes, or PMNs, because their nuclei have multiple lobes) are the first cells to arrive at the site where inflammation occurs. *Eosinophils* and *basophils*, other types of granulocytes, increase in number during allergic reactions and stress responses. Nongranular leukocytes include *monocytes* or *macrophages* (referred to as histiocytes when they enter tissue spaces) and *lymphocytes*. Monocytes also function as **phagocytic cells**, engulfing, ingesting, and destroying greater numbers and quantities of foreign bodies or toxins than granulocytes. Lymphocytes, consisting of B cells and T cells, play major roles in humoral and cell-mediated immune responses.

INFLAMMATORY RESPONSE

The inflammatory response is a major function of the natural (nonspecific) immune system elicited in response to tissue injury or invading organisms. Chemical mediators assist this response by minimizing blood loss, walling off the invading organism, activating phagocytes, and promoting formation of fibrous scar tissue and regeneration of injured tissue. (The inflammatory response is discussed in detail later.)

Acquired Immunity

Acquired immunity—immunologic responses acquired during life but not present at birth—usually develops as a result of immunization (vaccination) or contracting a disease, both of which generate a protective immune response. Weeks or months after exposure to the disease or vaccine, the body produces an immune response that is sufficient to defend against the disease upon reexposure to it.

The two types of acquired immunity are known as active and passive. In *active acquired immunity*, the immunologic defenses are developed by the person's own body. This immunity generally lasts many years or even a lifetime.

Passive acquired immunity is temporary immunity transmitted from another source that has developed immunity through previous disease or immunization. For example, gamma-globulin and antiserum, obtained from the blood plasma of people with acquired immunity, are used in emergencies to provide immunity to diseases when the risk for contracting a specific disease is great and there is not enough time for a person to develop adequate active immunity. Both types of acquired immunity involve humoral and cellular (cell-mediated) immunologic responses (described later in this chapter).

Response to Invasion

When the body is invaded or attacked by bacteria, viruses or other pathogens, it has three means of defending itself:

- The phagocytic immune response
- The humoral or antibody immune response
- The cellular immune response

The first line of defense, the **phagocytic immune response**, involves the WBCs (granulocytes and macrophages), which have the ability to ingest foreign particles. These cells move to the point of attack, where they engulf and destroy the invading agents. A second protective response, the **humoral immune response** (sometimes called the antibody response), begins with the B lymphocytes, which can transform themselves into plasma cells that manufacture antibodies. These antibodies, highly specific proteins, are transported in the bloodstream and attempt to disable the invaders. The third mechanism of defense, the **cellular immune response,** also involves the T lymphocytes, which can turn into special cytotoxic (or killer) T cells that can attack the pathogens themselves.

The part of the invading or attacking organism that is responsible for stimulating antibody production is called an **antigen** (or an immunogen). For example, an antigen can be a small patch of proteins on the outer surface of the microorganism. A single bacterium, even a single large molecule, such as a toxin (diphtheria or tetanus toxin), may have several such antigens, or *markers,* on its surface, thus inducing the body to produce a number of different antibodies. Once produced, an antibody is released into the bloodstream and carried to the attacking organism. There it combines with the antigen, binding with it like an interlocking piece of a jigsaw puzzle (Fig. 46-3). There are four well-defined stages in an immune response: recognition, proliferation, response, and the effector stage.

RECOGNITION STAGE

The immune system's ability to recognize antigens as foreign, or nonself, is the initiating event in any immune response. The body

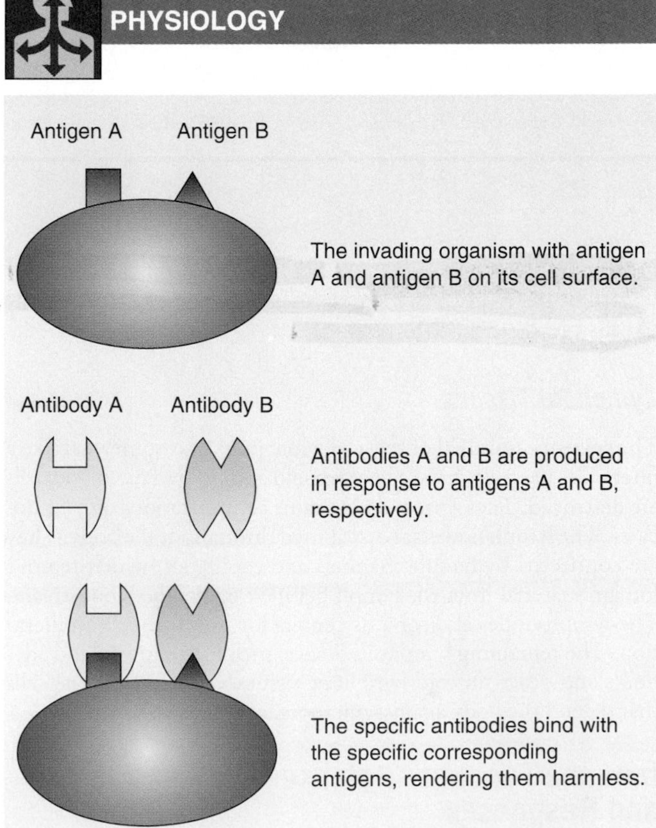
PHYSIOLOGY
Antigen A
Antigen B
The invading organism with antigen A and antigen B on its cell surface.
Antibody A
Antibody B
Antibodies A and B are produced in response to antigens A and B, respectively.
The specific antibodies bind with the specific corresponding antigens, rendering them harmless.

FIGURE 46•3 Antibody specificity. Antibodies are produced by B-cell lymphocytes to bind with specific antigens.

must first recognize invaders as foreign before it can react to them. The body accomplishes recognition using lymph nodes and lymphocytes for surveillance. Lymph nodes are widely distributed internally and externally near the body's surfaces. They continuously discharge small lymphocytes into the bloodstream. These lymphocytes patrol the tissues and vessels that drain the areas served by that node.

Lymphocytes are found in the lymph nodes and in the circulating blood. The volume of lymphocytes in the body is impressive. These lymphocytes recirculate from the blood to lymph nodes and from the lymph nodes back into the bloodstream, in a never-ending series of patrols. Some circulating lymphocytes can survive for decades. Some of these small, hardy cells maintain their solitary circuits for the lifetime of the person.

The exact way in which circulating lymphocytes recognize antigens on foreign surfaces is not known; however, theorists think that recognition depends on specific receptor sites on the surface of the lymphocytes. Macrophages play an important role in helping the circulating lymphocytes process the antigens. When foreign materials enter the body, a circulating lymphocyte comes into physical contact with the surfaces of these materials. Upon contact, the lymphocyte, with the help of macrophages, either removes the antigen from the surface or in some way picks up an imprint of its structure, which comes into play with subsequent reexposure to the antigen.

In a streptococcal throat infection, for example, the streptococcal organism gains access to the mucous membranes of the throat. A circulating lymphocyte moving through the tissues of the neck comes in contact with the organism. The lymphocyte, familiar with the surface markers on the cells of its own body, recognizes the antigens on the microbe as different (nonself) and the streptococcal organism as antigenic (foreign). This triggers the second stage of the immune response—proliferation.

PROLIFERATION STAGE

The circulating lymphocyte containing the antigenic message returns to the nearest lymph node. Once in the node, the sensitized lymphocyte stimulates some of the resident dormant T and B lymphocytes to enlarge, divide, and proliferate. T lymphocytes differentiate into cytotoxic (or killer) T cells, whereas B lymphocytes produce and release antibodies. Enlargement of the lymph nodes in the neck in conjunction with a sore throat is one example of the immune response.

RESPONSE STAGE

In the response stage, the changed lymphocytes function either in a humoral or a cellular fashion. The production of antibodies by the B lymphocytes in response to a specific antigen begins the humoral response. *Humoral* refers to the fact that the antibodies are released into the bloodstream and so reside in the plasma (fluid fraction of the blood).

With the initial cellular response, the returning sensitized lymphocytes migrate to areas of the lymph node (other than those areas containing lymphocytes programmed to become plasma cells). Here, they stimulate the residing lymphocytes to become cells that will attack microbes directly rather than through the action of antibodies. These transformed lymphocytes are known as cytotoxic (killer) T cells. The T stands for *thymus,* signifying that during embryologic development of the immune system, these T lymphocytes spent time in the thymus of the developing fetus, where they were genetically programmed to become T lymphocytes rather than the antibody-producing B lymphocytes. Viral rather than bacterial antigens induce a cellular response. This response is manifested by the increasing number of T lymphocytes (lymphocytosis) seen in the blood smears of people with viral illnesses, such as infectious mononucleosis. (Cellular immunity is discussed in further detail later in this chapter.)

Most immune responses to antigens involve both humoral and cellular responses, although one usually predominates. For example, during transplantation rejection, the cellular response predominates, whereas in the bacterial pneumonias and sepsis, the humoral response plays the dominant protective role (Chart 46-1).

EFFECTOR STAGE

In the effector stage, either the antibody of the humoral response or the cytotoxic (killer) T cell of the cellular response reaches and couples with the antigen on the surface of the foreign invader. The coupling initiates a series of events that in most instances results in the total destruction of the invading microbes or the complete neutralization of the toxin. The events involve an interplay of antibodies (humoral immunity), complement, and action by the cytotoxic T cells (cellular immunity). Figure 46-4 summarizes the stages of the immune response.

Humoral Immune Response

The humoral response is characterized by production of antibodies by the B lymphocytes in response to a specific antigen. Although the B lymphocyte is ultimately responsible for the production of antibodies, both the macrophages of natural immunity and the special T-cell lymphocytes of cellular immunity are involved in recognizing the foreign substance and in producing antibodies.

ANTIGEN RECOGNITION

Several theories exist about the mechanisms by which the B lymphocytes recognize the invading antigen and respond by producing antibodies. This is probably because the B lymphocytes recognize invading antigens in more than one way and respond in several ways as well. Additionally, the B lymphocytes appear to respond to

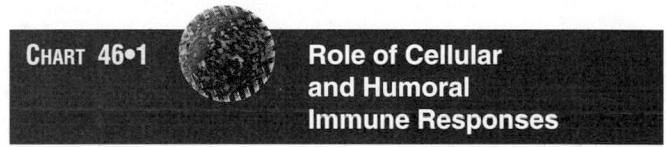

CHART 46•1 Role of Cellular and Humoral Immune Responses

Whereas B-cell antibodies are distinctive components of the humoral immune response, cytotoxic T cells are distinguishing components of the cellular immune response. Some specific roles of B cells and T cells are as follows:

Humoral Responses (B Cells)

- Bacterial phagocytosis and lysis
- Anaphylaxis
- Allergic hay fever and asthma
- Immune complex disease
- Bacterial and some viral infections

Cellular Responses (T Cells)

- Transplant rejection
- Delayed hypersensitivity (tuberculin reaction)
- Graft-versus-host disease
- Tumor surveillance or destruction
- Intracellular infections
- Viral, fungal, and parasitic infections

PHYSIOLOGY

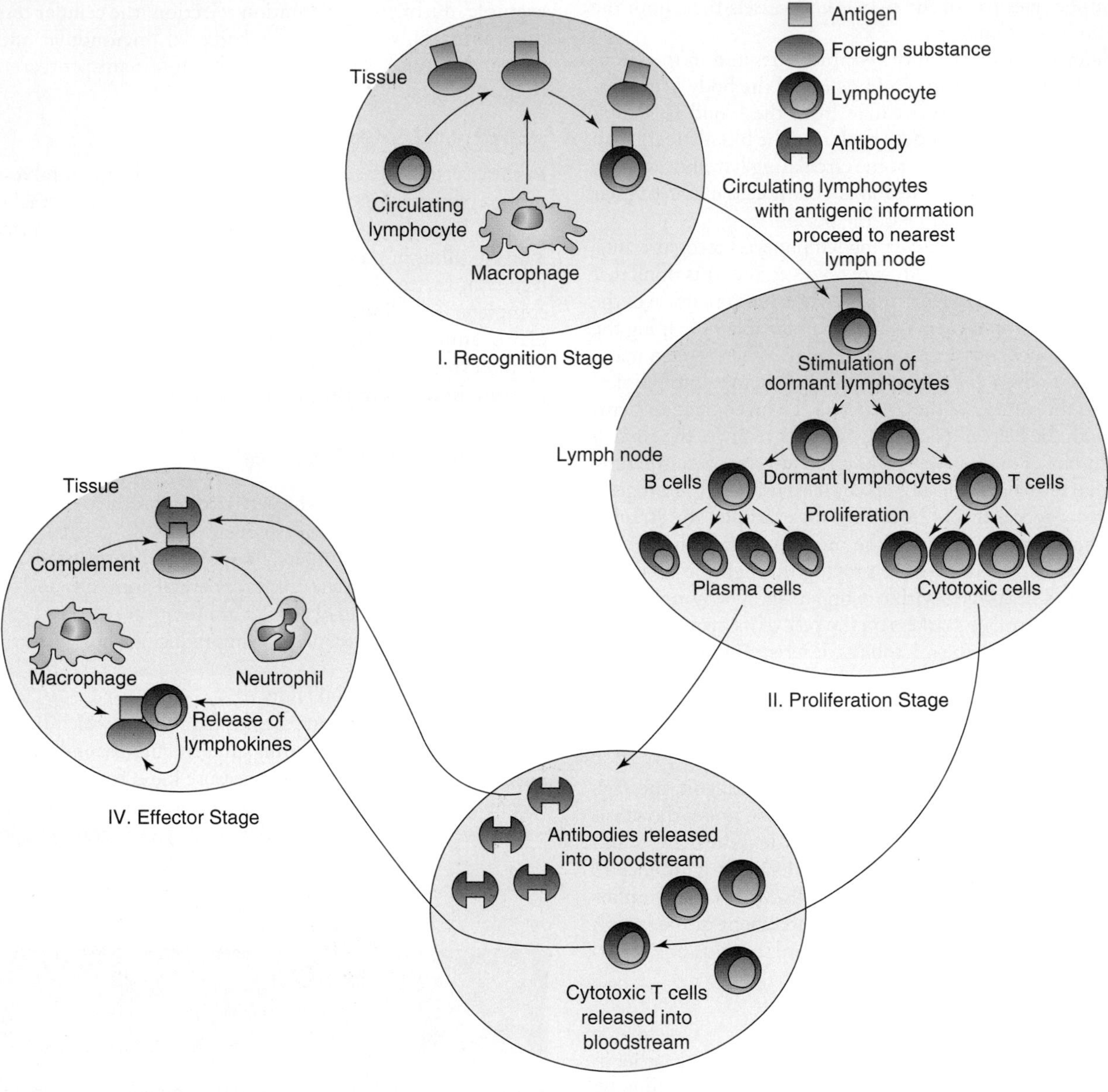

FIGURE 46•4 Stages of the immune response. (**I**) In the *recognition stage,* antigens are recognized by circulating lymphocytes and macrophages. (**II**) In the *proliferation stage,* the dormant lymphocytes proliferate and differentiate into cytotoxic (killer) T cells or B cells responsible for formation and release of antibodies. (**III**) In the *response stage* the cytotoxic T cells and the B cells perform cellular and humoral functions, respectively. (**IV**) In the *effector stage,* antigens are destroyed or neutralized through the action of antibodies, complement, macrophages, and cytotoxic T cells.

some antigens by triggering antibody formation directly. In response to other antigens, however, they need the assistance of T cells to trigger antibody formation.

T cells (or T lymphocytes), part of a surveillance system dispersed throughout the body, recycle through the general circulation, tissues, and lymphatic system. With the assistance of macrophages, the T lymphocytes are believed to recognize the antigen of a foreign invader. The T lymphocyte picks up the antigenic message, or "blueprint," of the antigen and returns to the nearest lymph node with that message.

Production of B Lymphocytes. B lymphocytes stored in the lymph nodes are subdivided into thousands of clones, each responsive to a single group of antigens having almost identical characteristics. When the antigenic message is carried back to the lymph node, specific clones of the B lymphocyte are stimulated to enlarge, divide, proliferate, and differentiate into plasma cells capable of producing specific antibodies to the antigen. Other B lymphocytes differentiate into B lymphocyte clones with a memory for the antigen. These memory cells are responsible for the more exaggerated and rapid immune response in a person who is repeatedly exposed to the same antigen.

ROLE OF ANTIBODIES

Antibodies are large proteins called *immunoglobulins* because they are found in the globulin fraction of the plasma proteins. Each antibody molecule consists of two subunits, each of which contains a light and a heavy peptide chain (Fig. 46-5). The subunits are held together by a chemical link composed of disulfide bonds. Each subunit has a portion that serves as a binding site for a specific antigen referred to as the *Fab fragment.* This site provides the "lock" portion that is highly specific for an antigen. An additional portion, known as the *Fc fragment,* allows the antibody molecule to take part in the complement system.

Antibodies defend against foreign invaders in several ways, and the type of defense employed depends on the structure and composition of both the antigen and the immunoglobulin. The antibody molecule has at least two combining sites, or Fab fragments. One antibody can act as a cross-link between two antigens, causing them to bind or clump together. This clumping effect, referred to as **agglutination,** helps clear the body of the invading organism by facilitating phagocytosis. Some antibodies assist in removing offending organisms through **opsonization.** In this process, the antigen–antibody molecule is coated with a sticky substance that also facilitates phagocytosis.

Antibodies also promote the release of vasoactive substances, such as histamine and slow-reacting substance, two of the chemical mediators of the inflammatory response. In addition, antibodies are involved in activating the complement system.

Types of Immunoglobulins.

The body can produce five different types of immunoglobulins. (Immunoglobulins are commonly designated by the abbreviation Ig.) Each of the five types, or classes, is identified by a specific letter of the alphabet (IgA, IgD, IgE, IgG, and IgM). Classification is based on the chemical structure and biologic role of the individual immunoglobulin. The following list summarizes some outstanding characteristics of the immunoglobulins:

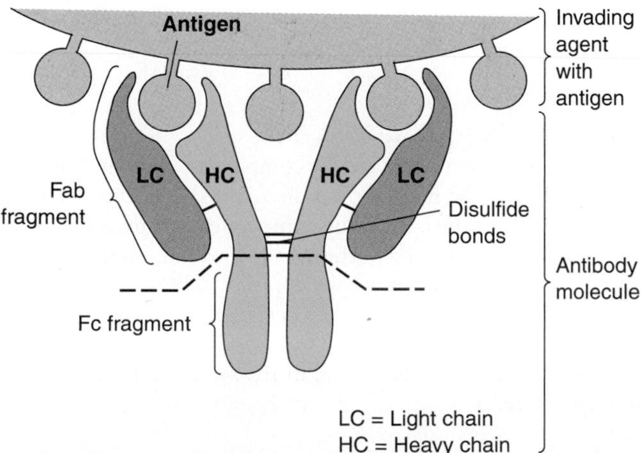

FIGURE 46•5 An antibody molecule. The Fab fragment serves as the binding site for a specific antigen. The Fc fragment initiates classic complement activation.

IgG (75% of Total Immunoglobulin)

- Appears in serum and tissues (interstitial fluid)
- Assumes major role in bloodborne and tissue infections
- Activates complement system
- Enhances phagocytosis
- Crosses placenta

IgA (15% of Total Immunoglobulin)

- Appears in body fluids (blood, saliva, tears, breast milk, and pulmonary, gastrointestinal, prostatic, and vaginal secretions)
- Protects against respiratory, gastrointestinal, and genitourinary infections
- Prevents absorption of antigens from food
- Passes to neonate in breast milk for protection

IgM (10% of Total Immunoglobulin)

- Appears mostly in intravascular serum
- Appears as the first immunoglobulin produced in response to bacterial and viral infections
- Activates complement system

IgD (0.2% of Total Immunoglobulin)

- Appears in small amounts in serum
- Possibly influences B-lymphocyte differentiation, but plays unclear role

IgE (0.004% of Total Immunoglobulin)

- Appears in serum
- Takes part in allergic and some hypersensitivity reactions
- Combats parasitic infections

ANTIGEN–ANTIBODY BINDING

The portion of the antigen involved in binding with the antibody is referred to as the antigenic determinant. The binding of the Fab fragment (antibody-binding site) to the antigenic determinant can be likened to a lock-and-key situation (Fig. 46-6). The most efficient immunologic responses occur when the antibody and antigen fit exactly. Poor fit can occur with an antibody that was produced in response to a different antigen. This phenomenon is known as *cross-reactivity.* For example, in acute rheumatic fever, the antibody produced against *Streptococcus pyogenes* in the upper respiratory tract may cross-react with the patient's heart tissue, leading to heart valve damage.

Cellular Immune Response

Whereas the B lymphocytes are responsible for humoral immunity, the T lymphocytes (or T cells) are primarily responsible for cellular immunity. These lymphocytes spend time in the thymus, where they are programmed to become T cells rather than antibody-producing B lymphocytes. Several types of T cells exist, each with designated roles in the defense against bacteria, viruses, fungi, parasites, and malignant cells. T cells attack foreign invaders directly rather than by producing antibodies.

Cellular reactions are initiated by the binding of an antigen with an antigen receptor located on the surface of a T cell. This may occur with or without the assistance of macrophages. The T cells then

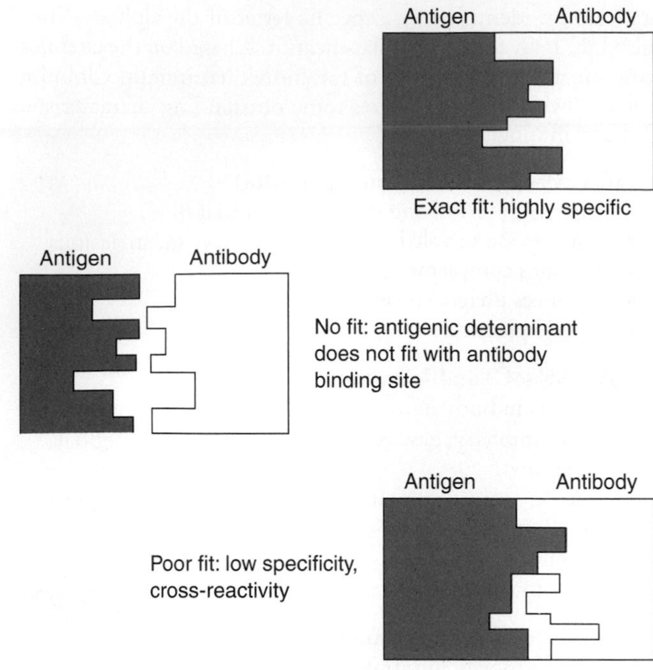

FIGURE 46•6 Antigen–antibody binding. (*Top*) A highly specific antigen–antibody complex. (*Middle*) No match and therefore, no immune response. (*Bottom*) Poor fit or match with low specificity; antibody reacts to antigen with similar characteristics, producing cross-reactivity.

carry the antigenic message, or blueprint, to the lymph nodes, where the production of other T cells is stimulated. Some T cells remain in the lymph nodes and retain a memory for the antigen. Other T cells migrate from the lymph nodes into the general circulatory system and ultimately to the tissues, where they remain until they either come in contact with their respective antigens or die.

ROLE OF T LYMPHOCYTES

Two major categories of effector T cells are helper T cells and cytotoxic T cells. These cells participate in destroying foreign organisms. Other T cells include suppressor T cells and memory T cells. T cells interact closely with B cells, indicating that humoral and cellular immune responses are not separate, unrelated processes but rather branches of the immune response that can and do affect each other.

Helper T cells (helper T_4 cells) are activated upon recognition of antigens and stimulate the rest of the immune system. When activated, helper T cells secrete **cytokines** that attract and activate B cells, cytotoxic T cells, natural killer cells, macrophages, and other cells of the immune system. Separate subpopulations of helper T cells produce different types of cytokines and determine whether the immune response will be the production of antibodies or a cell-mediated immune response. Helper T_1 cells produce **lymphokines,** one category of cytokines. These lymphokines activate other T cells (interleukin-2, or IL-2), natural and cytotoxic T cells (interferon-gamma), and other inflammatory cells (tumor necrosis factor). Helper T_2 cells produce IL-4 and IL-5, lymphokines that activate B cells to grow and differentiate (Table 46-2).

Cytotoxic T cells (killer T cells) attack the antigen directly by altering the cell membrane and causing cell lysis (disintegration) and releasing cytolytic enzymes and cytokines. Lymphokines can recruit, activate, and regulate other lymphocytes and WBCs. These cells then assist in destroying the invading organism. Delayed-type hypersensitivity is an example of an immune reaction that protects the body from antigens through the production and release of lymphokines and is discussed in more detail later.

Another type of cell, **suppressor T cells**, has the ability to decrease B-cell production, thereby keeping the immune response at a level that is compatible with health (eg, sufficient to fight infection adequately without attacking the body's healthy tissues). **Memory T cells** are responsible for recognizing antigens from previous exposure and mounting an immune response (Table 46-3).

ROLES OF NULL LYMPHOCYTES AND NATURAL KILLER CELLS

Null lymphocytes and natural killer (NK) cells are other lymphocytes that assist in combating organisms. These are distinct from B cells and T cells and lack the usual characteristics of B cells and T cells. **Null lymphocytes**, a subpopulation of lymphocytes, destroy antigens already coated with antibody. These cells have special Fc receptor sites on their surfaces that allow them to couple with the Fc end of antibodies (antibody-dependent, cell-mediated cytotoxicity).

Natural killer cells, another subpopulation of lymphocytes, defend against microorganisms and some types of malignant cells. NK cells are capable of directly killing invading organisms and producing cytokines. The helper T cells contribute to the differentiation of null and NK cells.

Complement System

Circulating plasma proteins, which are made in the liver and activated when an antibody couples with its antigen, are known as **complement**. These proteins interact sequentially with one another in a cascade or "falling domino" effect. This complement cascade alters the cell membranes on which antigen and antibody complex form, permitting fluid to enter the cell and leading eventually to cell lysis and death. In addition, activated complement molecules attract macrophages and granulocytes to areas of antigen–antibody reactions. These cells continue the body's defense by devouring the antibody-coated microbes and by releasing bacterial agents.

Complement plays an important role in the immune response. Destruction of an invading or attacking organism or toxin is not achieved merely by the binding of the antibody and antigens; it also requires activation of complement, the arrival of killer T cells, or the attraction of macrophages.

CLASSIC PATHWAY OF COMPLEMENT ACTIVATION

There are two ways to activate the complement system. One, the classic pathway (the first method discovered), involves the reaction of the first of the circulating complement proteins (C_1) with the receptor site of the Fc portion of an antibody molecule after formation of an antigen–antibody complex. The activation of the first complement component then activates all the other components in the following sequence: C_4, C_2, C_3, C_5, C_6, C_7, C_8, and C_9. (The components are named in the sequence in which they were discovered.)

ALTERNATE PATHWAY OF COMPLEMENT ACTIVATION

The alternative method of complement activation occurs without the formation of antigen–antibody complexes. This alternate path-

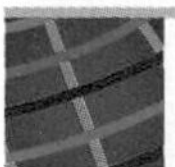

TABLE 46•2 **Cytokines and Their Biologic Effects**

Cytokine*	Action
Interleukin-1	Promotes differentiation of T and B cells, natural killer (NK) cells, and null cells
Interleukin-2	Stimulates growth of T cells and special activated killer lymphocytes (known as lymphocyte-activated killer cells—LAK cells)
Interleukin-3	Stimulates growth of mast cells and other blood cells
Interleukin-4	Stimulates growth of T and B cells, mast cells, and macrophages
Interleukin-5	Stimulates antibody responses
Interleukin-6	Stimulates growth and function of B cells and antibodies
Interleukin-7	Stimulates growth of pre-B, CD4, and CD8, T cells and activates mature T cells
Interleukin-8	Promotes chemotaxis and activation of neutrophils
Interleukin-9	Stimulates growth and proliferation of T cells
Interleukin-10	Inhibits interferon-gamma and mononuclear cell inflammation
Interleukin-11	Promotes induction of acute-phase proteins
Interleukin-12	Introduces helper T cells
Interleukin-13	Inhibits mononuclear phagocyte inflammation and promotes differentiation of B cells
Interleukin-16	Promotes chemotaxis CD4 T cells and eosinophils
Permeability factor	Increases vascular permeability, allowing white cells into area
Interferon	Interferes with viral growth, stopping the spread of viral infection
Migration inhibitory factor	Suppresses movement of macrophages, keeping macrophages in area of foreign cells
Skin reactive factor	Induces inflammatory response
Cytotoxic factor (lymphotoxin)	Kills certain antigenic cells
Macrophage chemotactic factor	Attracts macrophages into the area
Lymphocyte blastogenic factor	Stimulates more lymphocytes, recruiting additional lymphocytes into the area
Macrophage aggregation factor	Causes clumping of macrophages and lymphocytes
Macrophage activation factor	Allows macrophages to adhere to surfaces more readily
Proliferation inhibitor factor	Inhibits growth of certain antigenic cells
Cytophilic antibody	Binds to an Fc receptor on macrophages, thereby permitting macrophages to bind to antigens
Tumor necrosis factor (alpha)	Stimulates inflammation, wound healing, and tissue remodeling
Tumor necrosis factor (beta)	Mediates inflammation and graft rejection

* Cytokines are biologically active substances released by cells to regulate growth and function of other cells within the immune system. Lymphocytes produce lymphokines, and monocytes and macrophages produce monokines. This table lists some of the cytokines that play a role in immune system functioning.

way can be initiated by the release of bacterial products, such as endotoxins. When complement is activated through this pathway, the process bypasses the first three components (C_1, C_4, and C_2) and begins with C_3. Whatever the method of activation, however, once activated, the complement destroys cells by altering or damaging the cell membrane of the antigen, by chemically attracting phagocytes to the antigen (chemotaxis), and by rendering the antigen more vulnerable to phagocytosis (opsonization). The complement system enhances the inflammatory response by releasing vasoactive substances.

This response is usually therapeutic and can be lifesaving if the cell attacked by the complement system is a true foreign invader, such as a streptococcal or staphylococcal organism. If that cell however, is in reality part of the person—a cell of the brain or liver, the tissue lining the blood vessels, or the cells of a transplanted organ or skin graft, for example—the result can be devastating disease and even death. The result of the immune response—the vigorous attack on any material identified as foreign, the deadliness of the struggle—is obvious in the purulent material, or pus (the remains of microbes, granulocytes, macrophages, T-cell lymphocytes, plasma proteins, complement, and antibodies), that accumulates in wound infections and abscesses.

Role of Interferons

Biologic response modifiers, such as the interferons, are currently under investigation to determine their roles in the immune system and their potential therapeutic effects in disorders characterized by disturbed immune responses. Interferons have antiviral and antitumor properties. In addition to responding to viral infection, they are produced by T lymphocytes, B lymphocytes, and macrophages in response to antigens. They are thought to modify the immune response by suppressing antibody production and cellular immunity. They also facilitate the cytolytic role of macrophages and NK cells. Interferons are undergoing extensive testing to evaluate their effectiveness in treating tumors and acquired immunodeficiency syndrome (AIDS). Some interferons are already used to treat immune-related disorders, such as multiple sclerosis.

ASSESSMENT

An assessment of immune function begins with a health history and physical examination. The history should contain information about the patient's age along with information about past and present conditions and events that may provide clues to the status of the patient's immune system. Areas to be addressed

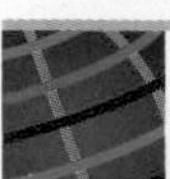

TABLE 46•3 Lymphocytes Involved in Immune Responses

Cell Type	Function	Type of Immune Response
B cell	Produces antibodies or immunoglobulins (IgA, IgD, IgE, IgG, IgM)	Humoral
T cell		Cellular
Helper T4	Attacks foreign invaders (antigens) directly Initiates and augments inflammatory response	
Helper T_1	Increases activated cytotoxic T cells	
Helper T_2	Increases B-cell antibody production	
Suppressor T	Suppresses the immune response	
Memory T	Remembers contact with an antigen and on subsequent exposures mounts an immune response	
Cytotoxic T (killer T)	Lyses cells infected with virus; plays a role in graft rejection	
Non-T or B lymphocytes		Nonspecific
Null cells	Destroys antigens already coated with antibody	
Natural killer (NK) (granular lymphocyte)	Defends against microorganisms and some types of malignant cells; produces cytokines	

include nutrition; infections and immunizations; allergies; disorder and disease states, such as autoimmune disorders, cancer, and chronic illnesses; surgery; medications; and blood transfusions. Physical assessment includes palpation of the lymph nodes and examination of the skin, mucous membranes, and respiratory, gastrointestinal, genitourinary, cardiovascular, and neurosensory systems.

Health History

Age

With the health history, the patient's age is obtained. People at the extremes of the lifespan are more likely to develop problems related to immune system functioning than are those in their middle years.

GERONTOLOGIC CONSIDERATIONS

Frequency and severity of infections are increased in elderly people, possibly from a decreased ability to respond adequately to invading organisms. Both the production and the function of T and B lymphocytes may be impaired. The incidence of autoimmune diseases also increases with aging, possibly from a decreased ability of antibodies to differentiate between self and nonself. Failure of the surveillance system to recognize mutant, or abnormal, cells may be responsible for the high incidence of cancer associated with increasing age.

Declining function of various organ systems associated with increasing age also contributes to impaired immunity. Decreased gastric secretions and motility allow normal intestinal flora to proliferate and produce infection, causing gastroenteritis and diarrhea. Decreased renal circulation, filtration, absorption, and excretion contribute to risk for urinary tract infections. Moreover, pros-tatic enlargement and neurogenic bladder can impede urine passage and subsequently bacterial clearance through the urinary system. Urinary stasis, common in elderly people, permits the growth of organisms. Exposure to tobacco and environmental toxins impairs pulmonary function. Prolonged exposure to these agents decreases the elasticity of lung tissue, the effectiveness of cilia, and the ability to cough effectively. These impairments hinder the removal of infectious organisms and toxins, increasing the elderly person's susceptibility to pulmonary infections and cancers.

Finally, with aging, the skin becomes thinner and less elastic. Peripheral neuropathy and the accompanying decreased sensation and circulation may lead to stasis ulcers, pressure ulcers, abrasions, and burns. Impaired skin integrity predisposes the aging person to infection from organisms that are part of normal skin flora.

Nutrition

Adequate nutrition is essential for optimal functioning of the immune system. Vitamin intake, essential for DNA and protein synthesis, if inadequate may lead to protein-calorie deficiency and subsequently to impaired immune function. Vitamins also help in the regulation of cell proliferation and maturation of immune cells. Excess or deficiency of trace elements (ie, copper, iron, manganese, selenium, or zinc) in the diet generally suppresses immune function.

Fatty acids are the building blocks that make up the structural components of cell membranes. Lipids are precursors of vitamins A, D, E, and K as well as cholesterol. Both excess and deficiency of fatty acids have been found to suppress immune function.

Depletion of protein reserves results in atrophy of lymphoid tissues, depression of antibody response, reduction in the number of circulating T cells, and impaired phagocytic function. As a result, susceptibility to infection is greatly increased. During periods of infection and serious illness, nutritional requirements may be exaggerated further, potentially contributing to depletion of protein, fatty acid, vitamin, and trace elements and an even greater risk of impaired immune response and sepsis.

Infection and Immunization

The patient is asked about immunizations (including those received recently and those received in childhood) and the usual childhood diseases. Known past or present exposure to tuberculosis is assessed, and the dates and results of any tuberculin tests (purified protein derivative [PPD] or tine test) and chest x-rays are obtained. Recent patient exposure to any infections and the exposure dates are elicited. A history of past and present infections and the dates and types of treatments that were used, along with a history of any multiple persistent infections, fevers of unknown origin, lesions or sores, or any type of drainage, are obtained.

Allergy

The patient is asked about history of any allergies, including types of allergens (pollens, dust, plants, cosmetics, food, medications, vaccines), the symptoms experienced, and seasonal variations in occurrence or severity in the symptoms. A history of testing and treatments that the patient has received or is currently receiving for these allergies and the effectiveness of the treatments is obtained. All medication and food allergies are listed on an allergy alert sticker and placed on the front of the patient's health record or chart to alert others to the possibility of these allergies. Continued assessment for potential allergic reactions in this patient is vital.

Disorders and Diseases

AUTOIMMUNE DISORDERS

In general, autoimmune disorders are more common in females than in males. This is believed to be the result of the activity of the sex hormones. The ability of sex hormones to modulate immunity has been well established. There is evidence that estrogen modulates the activity of T lymphocytes (especially suppressor cells), whereas androgens act to preserve IL-2 production and suppressor cell activity. The effects of sex hormones on B cells are less pronounced. Estrogen activates the autoimmune-associated B-cell population that expresses the CD5 marker (an antigenic marker on the B cell). Estrogen tends to enhance immunity, whereas androgen tends to be immunosuppressive.

The patient is asked about any autoimmune disorders, such as lupus erythematosus, rheumatoid arthritis, or psoriasis. The onset, severity, remissions and exacerbations, functional limitations, treatments that the patient has received or is currently receiving, and the effectiveness of the treatments are described.

NEOPLASTIC DISEASE

A history of cancer in the patient is obtained, along with the type of cancer and date of diagnosis. Dates and results of any cancer screening tests are also obtained.

Immunosuppression contributes to the development of cancers; however, cancer itself is immunosuppressive. Large tumors can release antigens into the blood, and these antigens combine with circulating antibodies and prevent them from attacking the tumor cells. Furthermore, tumor cells may possess special blocking factors that coat tumor cells and prevent destruction by killer T lymphocytes. During the early development of tumors, the body may fail to recognize the tumor antigens as foreign and subsequently fail to initiate destruction of the malignant cells. Hematologic cancers, such as leukemia and lymphoma, are associated with altered production and function of WBCs and lymphocytes.

All treatments that the patient has received or is currently receiving, such as radiation or chemotherapy, are recorded. Radiation destroys lymphocytes and decreases the population of cells required to replace them. The size or extent of the irradiated area determines the extent of immunosuppression. Whole-body irradiation may leave the patient totally immunosuppressed. Chemotherapy also destroys immune cells and causes immunosuppression.

A family history of cancer is obtained. If there is a family history of cancer, the type of cancer, age of onset, and relationship (maternal or paternal) of the patient to the affected family member is noted.

CHRONIC ILLNESS AND SURGERY

The health assessment includes a history of chronic illnesses, such as diabetes mellitus, renal disease, or chronic obstructive pulmonary disease. The onset and severity of illnesses, as well as treatment that the patient is receiving for the illness, are obtained. Chronic illness may contribute to immune system impairments in various ways. Renal failure is associated with a deficiency in circulating lymphocytes. In addition, immune defenses may be altered by acidosis and uremic toxins. In diabetes, an increased incidence of infection has been associated with vascular insufficiency, neuropathy, and poor control of serum glucose levels. Recurrent respiratory tract infections are associated with chronic obstructive pulmonary disease as a result of altered inspiratory and expiratory function and ineffective airway clearance. Additionally, a history of surgical removal of the spleen, lymph nodes, or thymus or a history of organ transplantation is noted because these conditions may place the patient at risk for impaired immune function.

SPECIAL PROBLEMS

Conditions such as burns and other forms of injury and infection may contribute to altered immune system function. Major burns or other factors cause impaired skin integrity and compromise the body's first line of defense. Loss of large amounts of serum with burn injuries depletes the body of essential proteins, including immunoglobulins. The physiologic and psychological stressors associated with surgery or injury stimulate cortisol release from the adrenal cortex; increased serum cortisol also contributes to suppression of normal immune responses.

Medications and Blood Transfusions

A listing of past and present medications is obtained. In large doses, antibiotics, corticosteroids, cytotoxic agents, salicylates, nonsteroidal anti-inflammatory drugs, and anesthetics can cause immune suppression (Table 46-4).

A history of single or multiple blood transfusions is obtained because previous exposure to foreign antigens through transfusion may be associated with abnormal immune function. Additionally, although the risk of exposure to the human immunodeficiency virus (HIV) is extremely low in patients who report having had a blood transfusion after 1985 (the year that testing of blood for HIV was initiated in the United States), a risk still exists.

Lifestyle and Other Factors

Like any other body system, the immune system functions depend on the function of other body systems. A detailed history of smoking, alcohol consumption, dietary intake and nutritional status, amount of perceived stress, and occupational or residential exposure to radiation or pollutants is obtained. Poor nutritional status, smoking, excessive consumption of alcohol, and exposure to environmental radiation and pollutants have been associated with impaired immune function and are assessed in the patient history.

PSYCHONEUROIMMUNOLOGIC FACTORS

Evidence from clinical observations and studies in humans and animals indicates that the immune response is regulated and modulated in part by neuroendocrine influences. Lymphocytes and

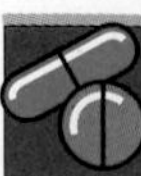

TABLE 46•4 Selected Medications and Effects on the Immune System

Drug Classification (and Examples)	Effects on the Immune System
Antibiotics (in large doses)	***Bone Marrow Suppression***
chloramphenicol (Chloromycetin)	Leukopenia, aplastic anemia
dactinomycin (Cosmogen)	Agranulocytosis, neutropenia
gentamicin sulfate (Garamycin)	Agranulocytosis, granulocytosis
penicillins	Agranulocytosis
streptomycin	Leukopenia, neutropenia, pancytopenia
vancomycin	Transient leukopenia
Antithyroid Drugs	
propylthiouracil	Agranulocytosis, leukopenia
Nonsteroidal Anti-Inflammatory Drugs (NSAIDs) (in large doses)	***Inhibit Prostaglandin Synthesis or Release***
aspirin	Agranulocytosis
ibuprofen	Leukopenia, neutropenia
indomethacin	Agranulocytosis, leukopenia,
phenylbutazone	Pancytopenia, agranulocytosis, aplastic anemia
Adrenal Corticosteroids	***Immunosuppression***
prednisone	
Antineoplastic Agents (Cytotoxic Agents)	***Immunosuppression***
alkylating agents	
cyclophosphamide (Cytoxan)	Leukopenia, neutropenia
mechlorethamine HCl (Mustargen)	Agranulocytosis, neutropenia
cyclosporine	Leukopenia, inhibits T-cell function
Antimetabolites	***Immunosuppression***
fluorouracil (pyrimidine antagonist)	Leukopenia, eosinophilia
methotrexate (folic acid antagonist)	Leukopenia, aplastic bone marrow
mercaptopurine (6-MP) (purine antagonist)	Leukopenia, pancytopenia

macrophages have receptors capable of responding to neurotransmitters and endocrine hormones. Lymphocytes can produce and secrete adrenocorticotropic hormone and endorphin-like compounds. Neurons in the brain, especially in the hypothalamus, can recognize prostaglandins, interferons, and interleukins as well as histamine and serotonin, which are released during the inflammatory process. Like all other biologic systems functioning in the interest of homeostasis, the immune system is integrated with other psychophysiologic processes and is subject to regulation and modulation by the brain.

Conversely, the immune processes can affect neural and endocrine function, including behavior. Thus, the interaction of the nervous system and immune system appears to be bidirectional. Growing evidence indicates that measurable immune system parameters can be influenced by biobehavioral strategies involving self-regulation. Examples of these strategies are relaxation and imagery techniques, biofeedback, humor, hypnosis, and conditioning.

Physical Examination

On physical examination, the patient's skin and mucous membranes are assessed for lesions, dermatitis, purpura (subcutaneous bleeding), urticaria, inflammation, or any discharge. Additionally, any signs of infection are noted. The patient's temperature is recorded, and the patient is observed for chills and sweating. The anterior and posterior cervical, axillary, and inguinal lymph nodes are palpated for enlargement; if palpable nodes are detected, the location, size, consistency, and reports of tenderness upon palpation are noted. Joints are assessed for tenderness and swelling and for limited range of motion. The patient's respiratory, cardiovascular, gastrointestinal, genitourinary, and neuro-sensory status is evaluated for signs and symptoms indicative of immune dysfunction. The patient's nutritional status, level of stress, and coping ability are also assessed along with his or her age and any functional limitations (fatigue and endurance).

ASSESSMENT
INDICATIONS OF IMMUNE DYSFUNCTION

Respiratory System

- Changes in respiratory rate
- Cough (dry or productive)
- Abnormal lung sounds (wheezing, crackles, ronchi)
- Rhinitis
- Hyperventilation
- Bronchospasm

Cardiovascular System

- Hypotension
- Tachycardia
- Dysrhythmia
- Vasculitis
- Anemia

Gastrointestinal System

- Hepatosplenomegaly
- Colitis
- Vomiting
- Diarrhea

Genitourinary System

- Frequency and burning on urination
- Hematuria
- Discharge

Neurosensory System

- Cognitive dysfunction
- Hearing loss
- Visual changes
- Headaches and migraines
- Ataxia
- Tetany

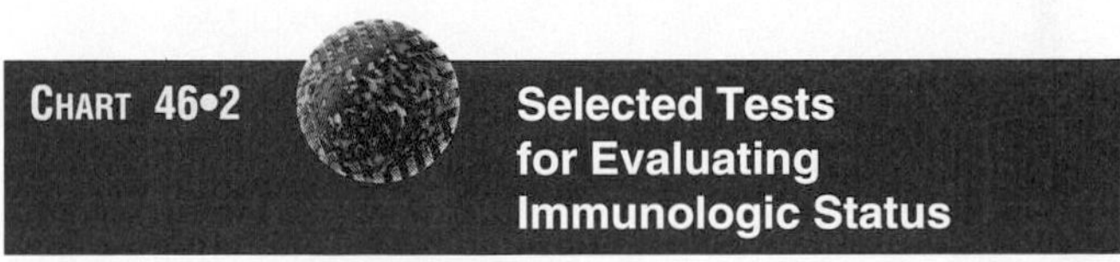

CHART 46•2 Selected Tests for Evaluating Immunologic Status

Various laboratory tests may be ordered to assess immune system activity or dysfunction. The studies assess leukocytes and lymphocytes, humoral immunity, cellular immunity, phagocytic cell function, complement activity, hypersensitivity reactions, specific antigen-antibodies, or HIV infection.

Leukocytes and Lymphocyte Tests

- White blood cell count and differential
- Bone marrow biopsy

Humoral (Antibody-Mediated) Immunity Tests

- B-cell quantification with monoclonal antibody
- In vivo immunoglobulin synthesis with T-cell subsets
- Specific antibody response
- Total serum globulins and individual immunoglobulins (by electrophoresis, immunoelectrophoresis, single radial immunodiffusion, nephelometry, isohemagglutinin techniques)

Cellular (Cell-Mediated) Immunity Tests

- Total lymphocyte count
- T-cell and T-cell subset quantification with monoclonal antibody
- Delayed hypersensitivity skin test
- Cytokine production
- Lymphocyte response to mitogens, antigens, and allogenic cells
- Helper and suppressor T-cell functions

Phagocytic Cell Function Tests

- Nitroblue tetrazolium reductase assay

Complement Component Tests

- Total serum hemolytic complement
- Individual complement component titrations
- Radial immunodiffusion
- Electroimmunoassay
- Radioimmunoassay
- Immunonephelometric assay
- Immunoelectrophoresis

Hypersensitivity Tests

- Scratch test
- Patch test
- Intradermal test
- Radioallergosorbent test (RAST)

Specific Antigen-antibody Tests

- Radioimmunoassay
- Immunoflorescence
- Agglutination
- Complement fixation test

HIV infection Tests

- Enzyme-linked immunosorbent assay (ELISA)
- Western blot
- CD4 and CD8 cell counts
- P24 antigen test
- Polymerase chain reaction (PCR)

DIAGNOSTIC EVALUATION

A series of blood tests and skin tests and a bone marrow biopsy may be performed to evaluate the patient's immune competence. Specific laboratory and diagnostic tests are discussed in greater detail along with specific disease processes in subsequent chapters in this unit. Laboratory and diagnostic tests used to evaluate immune competence are summarized in Chart 46-2.

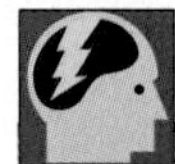

Critical Thinking Exercises

1. A 20-year-old college student who has been sexually active for 3 years asks if you think it is a good idea for her to be tested for HIV infection. How would you respond to her, and what recommendations would you give and why?
2. Your patient is an 68-year-old woman who is hospitalized with a fractured hip. Her long-standing rheumatoid arthritis has been treated with anti-inflammatory medications and corticosteroids periodically for the last 30 years. Describe the parameters you would use to assess her immune function. How would altered immune function affect your care?

References and Selected Readings

BOOKS

Eisenhauer, L., Nichols, L. W., Spencer, R. T., & Bergen, F. W. (1998). *Clinical pharmacology and nursing management* (5th ed.). Philadelphia: Lippincott-Raven.

Elgert, K. D. (1996). *Immunology: Understanding the immune system.* New York: Wiley-Liss.

Hyde, R. M. (1995). *Immunology* (3rd ed.). Baltimore: Williams & Wilkins.

Levinson, W., & Jawet, E. (1996). *Medical microbiology and immunology.* Stamford, CT: Appleton & Lange.

Melvoi, R. W. (1997). Review of immunology. In Patterson, R., Grammer, L. C., & Greenberger, P. A. (Eds.). *Allergic diseases diagnosis and management* (5th ed.). Philadelphia: Lippincott-Raven.

Roitt, I. (1997). *Essential immunology* (9th ed.). London: Blackwell Scientific.

Roitt, I., Brostoff, J., & Male, D. (1996). *Immunology* (4th ed.). St. Louis: C. V. Mosby.

Sheehan, C. (1997). *Clinical immunology principles and laboratory diagnosis* (2nd ed.). Philadelphia: Lippincott-Raven.

JOURNALS

Ballow, M., & Nelson, R. (1997). Immunopharmacology: Immunomodulation and immunotherapy. *Journal of the American Medical Association, 278*(22), 2008–2017.

Costa, J. J., Weller, P. F., & Galli, S. J. (1997). The cells of the allergic response: Mast cells, basophils, and eosinophils. *Journal of the American Medical Association, 278*(22), 1815–1834.

deShazo, R. D. (1997). Future trends in allergy and immunology. *Journal of the American Medical Association, 278*(22), 2024–2025.

Fleisher, T. A. (1997). Introduction to diagnostic laboratory immunology. *Journal of the American Medical Association, 278*(22), 1823–1834.

Huston, D. P. (1997). The biology of the immune system. *Journal of the American Medical Association, 278*(22), 1804–1822

Luster, A. D. (1998). Chemokines—Chemotactic cytokines that mediate inflammation. *New England Journal of Medicine, 338*(7), 436–445.

Stadtmauer, G., & Cunningham-Rundies, C. (1997). Outcome analysis and cost assessment in immunologic disorders. *Journal of the American Medical Association, 278*(22), 2018–2023.

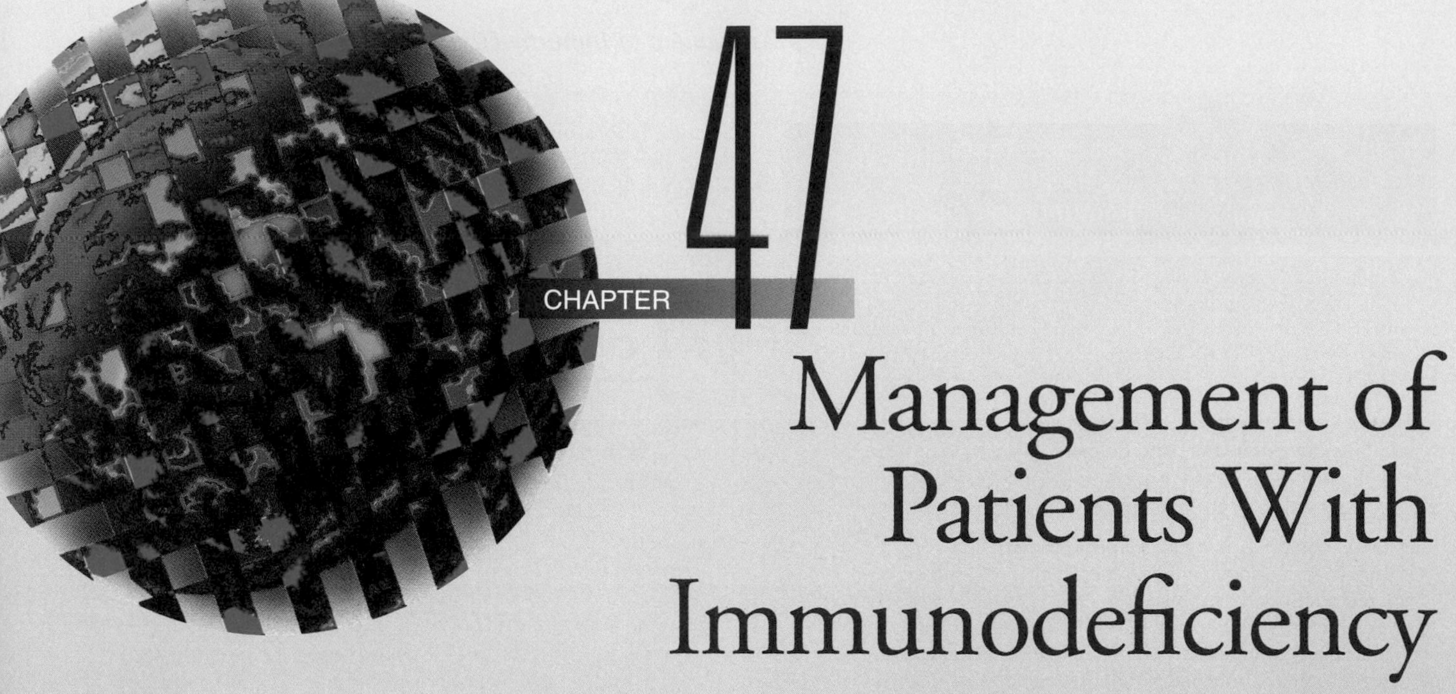

CHAPTER 47

Management of Patients With Immunodeficiency

Learning Objectives

On completion of this chapter, the learner will be able to:

1. Compare the different types of primary immunodeficiency disorders, addressing causes, clinical manifestations, management, possible complications, and available treatments.
2. Discuss the possible management of patients with immunodeficiency disorders.
3. Describe the nursing management of the patient with an immunodeficiency.
4. Identify the teaching points necessary for a patient with an immunodeficiency.

Immunodeficiency disorders may be caused by a defect or deficiency in phagocytic cells, B lymphocytes, T lymphocytes, or the complement system. The specific symptoms and their severity, age of onset, and prognosis depend on the immune system components affected and their degree of functional impairment. Regardless of the underlying cause, the cardinal symptoms of immunodeficiency include chronic or recurrent severe infections, infections caused by unusual organisms or organisms that are normal body flora, poor response to treatment of infections, and chronic diarrhea. In addition, the patient is susceptible to a variety of secondary disorders.

Immunodeficiencies may be classified as either primary or secondary and by the components of the immune system that are affected. Knowledge of the immune system and of the possibility of secondary disorders, skillful assessment and management, coupled with sensitivity and responsiveness to the learning needs of the patient and caregiver, provide the essential elements for effective nursing care.

GLOSSARY

agammaglobulinemia: disorder marked by an almost complete lack of immunoglobulins or antibodies

angioneurotic edema: condition marked by development of urticaria and an edematous area of skin, mucous membranes, or viscera

ataxia: uncoordinated muscle movement

ataxia-telangiectasia: autosomal recessive disorder affecting T- and B-cell immunity primarily seen in children and resulting in a degenerative brain disease

hypogammaglobulinemia: lack of one or more of the five immunoglobulins; caused by B-cell deficiency

immunocompromised host: person with a secondary immunodeficiency and associated immunosuppression

Nezelof's syndrome: disorder involving lack of a thymus gland and subsequent B-cell deficiencies in combination with increased, decreased, or normal immunoglobulins

panhypoglobulinemia: general lack of immunoglobulins in the blood

severe combined immunodeficiency disease (SCID): disorder involving a complete absence of humoral and cellular immunity resulting from an X-linked or autosomal genetic abnormality

telangiectasia: vascular lesions caused by dilated blood vessels

thymic hypoplasia: T-cell deficiency that occurs when the thymus gland fails to develop normally during embryo-genesis; also known as DiGeorge's Syndrome.

Wiscott-Aldrich syndrome: immunodeficiency characterized by thrombocytopenia and the absence of T- and B-cells

PRIMARY IMMUNODEFICIENCIES

Primary immunodeficiencies, rare disorders with genetic origins, are seen primarily in infants and young children. Symptoms usually develop early in life after protection from maternal antibodies decreases. Without treatment, infants and children with these disorders seldom survive to adulthood. These disorders may involve one or more components of the immune system. Symptoms of immune deficiency diseases are related to the role that the deficient component normally plays (Table 47-1).

Phagocytic Dysfunction

Clinical Manifestations

Phagocytic cell disorders are manifested by an increased incidence of opportunistic bacterial and fungal infections. People with hyperimmunoglobulinemia E (HIE) syndrome, formerly known as Job's syndrome, also develop fungal infections from *Candida* organisms and viral infections from herpes simplex or herpes zoster virus. These patients experience recurrent furunculosis, cutaneous abscesses, chronic eczema, bronchitis, pneumonia, chronic otitis media, and sinusitis. In HIE syndrome, white blood cells are unable to produce an inflammatory response to the skin infections; this results in deep-seated cold abscesses, which lack the classic signs and symptoms of inflammation (redness, heat, and pain).

Assessment and Diagnostic Findings

Diagnosis is based on the history, signs and symptoms, and laboratory analysis of the cytocidal activity of the phagocytic cells by the nitroblue tetrazolium reductase test.

Medical Management

Management of phagocytic cell disorders includes treating bacterial infections with prophylactic antibiotic therapy. In patients with HIE syndrome, additional treatment for fungal and viral infections may be needed. Granulocyte transfusions, although used, are seldom successful because of the short half-life of the cells. Treatment with granulocyte-macrophage colony-stimulating factor (GM-CSF) or granulocyte colony-stimulating factor (G-CSF) may prove successful because these proteins draw non-lymphoid stem cells from the bone marrow and hasten their maturation.

B-Cell Deficiencies

Two types of inherited B-cell deficiencies exist. The first type results from lack of differentiation of B-cell precursors into mature B cells. As a result, plasma cells are lacking, and the germinal centers from all lymphatic tissues disappears, leading to a complete lack of antibody production against invading bacteria, viruses, and other pathogens. Infants born with this disorder suffer from severe infections starting soon after birth. This syndrome is called sex-linked **agammaglobulinemia** (Bruton's disease) because all antibodies disappear from the patient's plasma.

The second type of B-cell deficiency results from a lack of differentiation of B cells into plasma cells. Only diminished antibody production occurs with this disorder. Although plasma cells are the most vigorous producers of antibodies, affected patients have normal lymph follicles and many B lymphocytes that produce some antibodies. This syndrome, called **hypogammaglobulinemia,** is a frequently occurring immunodeficiency. Thus, it is also called common variable immunodeficiency (CVID), a term that encompasses a variety of defects ranging from immunoglobulin A (IgA) deficiency, in which only the plasma cells that produce IgA are lacking, to the other extreme, in which there is severe **panhypoglobulinemia** (general lack of immunoglobulins in the blood).

CVID, the most common primary immunodeficiency seen in adulthood, affects both males and females equally. Although this disease can occur at any age, its onset is most often in the second decade of life.

Clinical Manifestations

More than half of patients with CVID develop pernicious anemia. Lymphoid hyperplasia of the small intestine and spleen and gastric atrophy detected by biopsy of the stomach are common findings. Other autoimmune diseases, such as arthritis and hypothyroidism, frequently develop in patients with CVID. CVID must be distinguished from secondary immunodeficiency diseases caused by protein-losing enteropathy, nephrotic syndrome, or burns.

Patients with CVID are susceptible to infections with encapsulated bacteria, such as *Haemophilus influenza, Streptococcus pneumoniae,* and *Staphylococcus aureus.* Frequent respiratory tract infections typically lead to chronic progressive bronchiectasis and pulmonary failure. Commonly, infection with *Giardia lamblia* occurs. Opportunistic infections with *Pneumocystis carinii,* however, are seen only in patients who have a concomitant deficiency in T-cell immunity.

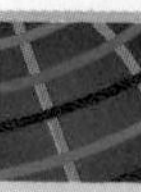

TABLE 47•1 Selected Primary Immunodeficiency Disorders

Immune Component	Disorder	Major Symptoms	Treatment
Phagocytic cells	Hyperimmunoglobulinemia E (HIE) syndrome	Bacterial, fungal, and viral infections; deep-seated cold abscesses	Antibiotic therapy and treatment for viral and fungal infections Granulocyte-macrophage colony-stimulating factor (GM-CSF); granulocyte colony-stimulating factor (G-CSF)
B lymphocytes	Sex-linked agammaglobulinemia (Bruton's disease)	Severe infections soon after birth	Passive pooled plasma or gamma-globulin
	Common variable immunodeficiency (CVID)	Bacterial infections, infection with *Giardia lamblia*	IV gamma-globulin Metronidazole (Flagyl) Quinacrine HCl (Atabrine)
		Pernicious anemia	Vitamin B_{12}
		Chronic respiratory infections	Antimicrobial therapy
	Immunoglobulin A (IgA) deficiency	Predisposition to recurrent infections, adverse reactions to blood transfusions or gamma-globulin, autoimmune diseases, hypothyroidism	None
	IgC_2 deficiency	Heightened incidence of infectious diseases	Pooled gamma-globulin
T lymphocytes	Thymic hypoplasia (DiGeorge's syndrome)	Recurrent infections; hypoparathyroidism; hypocalcemia, tetany, convulsions; congenital heart disease; possible renal abnormalities; abnormal facies	Thymus graft
	Chronic mucotaneous candidiasis	*Candida albicans* infections of mucous membrane, skin, and nails; endocrine abnormalities (hypoparathyroidism, Addison's disease)	Antifungal agents: Topical: miconazole Oral: clotrimazole, ketoconazole IV: amphotericin B
B and T lymphocytes	Ataxia-telangiectasia	Ataxia with progressive neurologic deterioration; telangiectasia (vascular lesions); recurrent infections; malignancies	Antimicrobial therapy; management of presenting symptoms; fetal thymus transplant, IV gamma-globulin
	Nezelof's syndrome	Severe infections; malignancies	Antimicrobial therapy; IV gamma-globulin, bone marrow transplantation; thymus transplantation; thymus factors
	Wiscott-Aldrich syndrome	Thrombocytopenia, resulting in bleeding; infections; malignancies	Antimicrobial therapy; splenectomy with continuous antibiotic prophylaxis; IV gamma-globulin and bone marrow transplantation
	Severe combined immunodeficiency disease (SCID)	Overwhelming severe fatal infections soon after birth (also includes opportunistic infections)	Antimicrobial therapy; IV gamma-globulin and bone marrow transplantation
	Angioneurotic edema	Episodes of edema in various parts of the body, including respiratory tract and bowels	Pooled plasma, androgen therapy
Complement system	Paroxysmal nocturnal hemoglobinuria (PNH)	Lysis of erythrocytes due to lack of decay-accelerating factor (DAF) on erythrocytes	None

Assessment and Diagnostic Findings

The diagnosis of CVID is based on the history of bacterial infections, quantification of B-cell activity, and reported signs and symptoms. The number of B lymphocytes and the total and specific immunoglobulin levels are measured. Total serum globulin level alone is an inadequate measure because a compensatory overproduction of one globulin may mask the loss of a missing globulin or one present in very low amounts. Antibody titers to confirm successful childhood vaccination are determined by specific serologic tests. Previous successful childhood immunization indicates that B cells were functioning adequately earlier in life. If the patient exhibits signs and symptoms suggestive of pernicious anemia, hemoglobin and hematocrit levels are also obtained.

Medical Management

Patients with CVID may need replacement therapy with intravenous gamma-globulin. Those who are receiving adequate treatment with intravenous gamma-globulin usually do not require prophylactic antibiotics unless they also have chronic respiratory disease. Antimicrobial therapy is prescribed for respiratory infections to prevent complications such as pneumonia, sinusitis, and otitis media. Intestinal infestation with *G. lamblia* is treated with a 7-day course of metronidazole (Flagyl) or a 7-day course of quinacrine hydrochloride (Atabrine). Patients with pernicious anemia receive parenteral injections of vitamin B_{12} at monthly intervals.

T-Cell Deficiencies

Pathophysiology

Because the T cells play a regulatory role in immune system function, the loss of T-cell function is usually accompanied by some loss of B-cell activity.

DiGeorge's syndrome, or **thymic hypoplasia**, is a T-cell deficiency that occurs when the thymus gland fails to develop normally during embryogenesis.

Chronic mucocutaneous candidiasis with or without endocrinopathy is a disorder associated with a selective defect in T-cell immunity thought to be caused by an autosomal recessive inheritance. Affecting both men and women, it is considered an autoimmune disorder in which the thymus and other endocrine glands are involved in the autoimmune process. The disease causes extensive morbidity resulting from endocrine dysfunction.

Clinical Manifestations

Infants born with DiGeorge's syndrome have hypoparathyroidism with resultant hypocalcemia resistant to standard therapy, congenital heart disease, abnormal facies, and possibly, renal abnormalities. These infants, susceptible to yeast, fungal, protozoan, and viral infections, are particularly susceptible to childhood diseases (chickenpox, measles, and rubella), which are usually severe and may be fatal.

The initial presentation of chronic mucocutaneous candidiasis may be either chronic candidal infection or idiopathic endocrinopathy. Patients may survive to the second or third decade of life. Problems may include hypocalcemia and tetany secondary to hypofunction of the parathyroid glands. Hypofunction of the adrenal cortex (Addison's disease) is the major cause of death in these patients, possibly developing suddenly and without any history of previous symptoms.

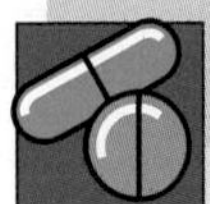

PHARMACOLOGY

Managing a Gamma-Globulin Infusion

Previously available only for intramuscular injection, gamma-globulin can now be administered for replacement therapy as an IV infusion in greater, more effective doses without painful side effects.

How Supplied

Gamma-globulin is supplied in a 5% solution or a lyophilized powder with a reconstituting diluent prepared from Cohn fraction II obtained from pools of 1,000 to 10,000 donors. Currently, a number of different IV preparations are approved for use and have been shown to be effective and safe by the Food and Drug Administration.

Dosage

The optimal dose is that determined by the patient's response. In most instances, an IV dose of 100 to 400 mg/kg of body weight is given once monthly or more frequently to ensure adequate serum IgG levels.

Adverse Effects

- Complaints of flank pain, shaking chills, and tightness in the chest, terminating with a slight rise in body temperature
- Hypotension (possible with severe reactions)
- Anaphylactic reactions

Guidelines for Nursing Management

- Weigh the patient before treatment.
- Obtain vital signs before, during, and after treatment.
- Administer the prescribed pretreatment prophylactic aspirin or IV antihistamine, such as diphenhydramine (Benadryl).
- Be aware that prednisone may be used to prevent possible severe reactions.
- Administer the IV infusion at a slow rate, not to exceed 3 mL/minute.
- Assess the patient for adverse reactions, including the early signs of anaphylactic shock; prepare to slow the infusion rate if necessary.
- Be aware that patients with low gamma-globulin levels have more severe reactions than those with normal levels (e.g., patients who receive gamma-globulin for thrombocytopenia or Kawasaki disease).
- Keep in mind that patients who have an immunoglobulin A (IgA) deficiency have IgE antibodies to IgA, which requires administration of plasma or immunoglobulin replacement from IgA-deficient patients. Because all IV gamma-globulin preparations contain some IgA, they may cause an anaphylactic reaction in patients with IgE anti-IgA antibodies.
- Remember that the risk for transmission of hepatitis, HIV, or other known viruses is extremely low.

Assessment and Diagnostic Findings

The status of T cells can be evaluated by peripheral blood lymphocyte counts. Because T cells constitute 65% to 85% of peripheral blood lymphocytes, lymphopenia may signify a T-cell deficit. Dermal sensitization of the patient or stimulation of the patient's

T cells in vitro may be done to evaluate whether the T cells are capable of producing the expected responses.

Medical Management

Systemic infections with *Candida* organisms usually do not occur; however, chronic skin and mucous membrane candidal infections are difficult to treat. Often, patients with severe candidal infection of the skin and mucous membranes develop severe psychological problems. Topical treatment with various antifungal agents has been tried but with little success. Topical miconazole therapy has been used in some patients with positive results. Additionally, courses of intravenous amphotericin B have been beneficial in some patients, but use of this medication is limited because of its renal toxicity. Use of oral clotrimazole and ketoconozole have also been beneficial.

Combined B-Cell and T-Cell Deficiencies

Ataxia-telangiectasia is an autosomal recessive disorder affecting both T- and B-cell immunity. In 40% of patients with this disease, a selective IgA deficiency exists. IgA and IgG subclass deficiencies, along with IgE deficiencies, have been identified. Variable degrees of T-cell deficiencies are observed and become more severe with advancing age. The disease involves the neurologic, vascular, endocrine, and immune systems.

Nezelof's syndrome is thought to be caused by a genetic recessive characteristic. Infants born with Nezelof's syndrome do not have a thymus gland and have various degrees of B-cell immunodeficiency associated with various combinations of increased, decreased, or normal immunoglobulin levels.

Both B and T cells are missing in **severe combined immunodeficiency disease** (SCID). There is a complete absence of humoral as well as cellular immunity caused by an X-linked or autosomal genetic abnormality. In some instances, sporadic forms of the disease occur. **Wiscott-Aldrich syndrome** is a variation of SCID compounded by thrombocytopenia (loss of platelets). The prognosis is generally poor because most affected infants develop overwhelming fatal infections.

Clinical Manifestations

The onset of **ataxia** (uncoordinated muscle movement) and **telangiectasia** (vascular lesions caused by dilated blood vessels) usually occurs in the first 4 years of life. Many patients, however, may remain symptom free for 10 years or longer. As patients approach the second decade of life, morbidity with chronic lung disease, mental retardation, neurologic symptoms, and physical disability becomes severe. Long-term survivors develop progressive deterioration of immunologic and neurologic functions. Some affected patients have reached the fifth decade of life. The primary causes of death in these patients are overwhelming infection and lymphoreticular or epithelial cancer.

Infants with Nezelof's syndrome are highly susceptible to viral, bacterial, fungal, and protozoan infection; they also have a high incidence of malignant disease.

Medical Management

Treatment of ataxia-telangiectasia includes early management of infections with antimicrobial therapy, management of chronic lung disease with postural drainage and physical therapy, and management of other presenting symptoms. Other treatments include transplantation of fetal thymus tissue and intravenous administration of gamma-globulin.

Treatment options under investigation for SCID include bone marrow transplantation, intravenous immunoglobulin replacement, administration of thymus-derived factors, and thymus gland transplantation. As treatment improves, an increased number of those who previously would have died in infancy may live to adulthood.

Deficiencies of the Complement System

Improved techniques to identify the individual components of the complement system have led to a steady increase in the number of deficiencies identified. C2 and C3 component deficiencies result in diminished resistance to bacterial infections. **Angioneurotic edema** is caused by an inherited deficiency of the inhibitor of C1 esterase, which opposes the release of inflammatory mediators. A deficiency of this inhibitor results in frequent episodes of urticaria and edema in various parts of the body.

Patients with paroxysmal nocturnal hemoglobinuria (PNH) lack decay-accelerating factor (DAF), found on erythrocytes (red blood cells). DAF normally protects the erythrocytes from lysis (disintegration). In PNH, the complement component C3b accumulates on the CR1 molecule on the erythrocyte, acts as a binding site for the late-acting component, and allows lysis to occur.

SECONDARY IMMUNODEFICIENCIES

Secondary immunodeficiencies are more common than primary deficiencies and frequently occur as a result of underlying disease processes or from the treatment of these diseases. Common causes of secondary immunodeficiencies include malnutrition, chronic stress, burns, uremia, diabetes mellitus, certain autoimmune disorders, certain viruses, exposure to immunotoxic medications and chemicals, and self-administration of recreational drugs and alcohol. Acquired immunodeficiency syndrome (AIDS) is the most common secondary immunodeficiency disorder; it is discussed in detail in Chapter 48. Patients with secondary immunodeficiencies have immunosuppression and are often referred to as **immunocompromised hosts.**

Medical Management

Management of secondary immunodeficiencies includes diagnosing and treating the underlying disease process. Interventions include eliminating the contributing factors, treating the underlying condition, and using sound principles of infection control.

Nursing Management

Nursing management of immunocompromised patients includes a careful assessment of the patient's immune status. Because the immunocompromised patient is at high risk for infection, assessment focuses on history of past infections, particularly the type and frequency of infection; signs and symptoms of any current skin, respiratory, gastrointestinal, or genitourinary infection; and level of knowledge of the disease and measures that prevent infection. Assessment also focuses on nutritional status; stress level and coping skills; use of alcohol, drugs, or tobacco; and general hygiene, all of which may affect immune function.

Nursing care is directed toward reducing the patient's risk for infection, assisting with medical measures aimed at treating infec-

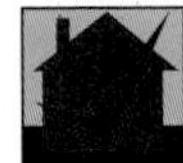

Home Care Teaching Checklist: Infection Prevention for the Patient With Immunodeficiency

At the completion of the program, the patient or the caregiver will be able to:	Patient	Caregiver
• Identify signs and symptoms of infection to report to the health care provider, such as fever, chills; wet or dry cough; breathing problems; white patches in the mouth; swollen glands; nausea; vomiting; persistent abdominal pain; persistent diarrhea; problems with urination; red, swollen, or draining wounds; sores or lesions on the body; and persistent vaginal discharge with or without itching.	✔	✔
• Demonstrate correct handwashing procedure.	✔	✔
• State rationale for thorough handwashing before eating, after using the bathroom, and before and after performing health care procedures.	✔	✔
• State rationale for use of cream and emollients to prevent or manage dry, chaffed, or cracked skin.	✔	✔
• Demonstrate recommended personal hygiene in bathing and foot care to prevent bacterial and fungal diseases.	✔	✔
• State rationale for avoiding contact with people who have known illness or who have recently been vaccinated.	✔	✔
• Verbalize understanding of ways to maintain a well-balanced diet and adequate calories.	✔	✔
• State the reason for avoiding the eating of raw fruits and vegetables, cooking all foods thoroughly, and immediately refrigerating all leftover food.	✔	✔
• Identify the rationale for frequent cleaning of kitchen and bathroom surfaces with disinfectant.	✔	✔
• Identify rationale and benefits of avoiding alcohol, tobacco, and unprescribed medications.	✔	✔
• State rationale for taking prescribed medications as directed.	✔	✔
• Verbalize ways to cope with stress successfully, plans for regular exercise, and rationale for obtaining adequate rest.	✔	✔

tion, improving the patient's nutritional status, and maintaining bowel and bladder function. Other aspects of nursing care include assisting the patient in managing stress and in adopting a lifestyle that enhances immune system function.

The nurse monitors the patient for signs and symptoms of infection: fever; chills; cough with or without sputum; shortness of breath; difficulty breathing; difficulty swallowing; white patches in the oral cavity; swollen lymph glands; nausea; vomiting; persistent diarrhea; frequency, urgency, or pain on urination; redness, swelling, or drainage from skin wounds; lesions on the face, lips, or perianal area; persistent vaginal discharge with or without perianal itching; and persistent abdominal pain.

The nurse also monitors laboratory values (ie, white blood cell count and differential cell count) for changes indicating infection. Culture and sensitivity reports from wound drainage, lesions, sputum, stool, urine, and blood are monitored to identify pathogenic organisms and appropriate antimicrobial therapy.

Interventions are initiated to reduce the risk for preventable infections. These include washing hands carefully, encouraging the patient to cough and perform deep-breathing exercises at regular intervals, and protecting the integrity of the skin and mucous membranes. All health care personnel must use strict aseptic technique when performing invasive procedures, such as dressing changes, venipunctures, and bladder catheterizations. Changes in laboratory results and subtle changes in clinical status must be reported to the physician because the immunocompromised patient may not develop typical signs and symptoms of infection.

PROMOTING HOME AND COMMUNITY-BASED CARE

Teaching Patients Self-Care. The patient and the caregivers are instructed about the signs and symptoms indicative of infection. They are also alerted to actions to take if they occur—for example, contacting the health care provider and initiating prescribed therapy. The patient and caregiver need instruction about any prophylactic medication regimen, including dosage, indications, times, actions, and side effects. The patient is instructed about the importance of avoiding others with infections and avoiding crowds. The patient and family also need to learn about other ways to prevent infection.

If the patient is to receive gamma-globulin infusion therapy at home, the patient will need information about expected benefits and outcomes of the treatment and expected adverse reactions and their management. Patients who can perform self-infusion at home are instructed in sterile technique, medication dosages, administration rate, and detection and management of adverse reactions.

Home Care Teaching Checklist: Home Infusion of Gamma-Globulin

At the completion of the program, the patient or caregiver will be able to:	Patient	Caregiver
• Identify the benefits and expected outcome of IV gamma-globulin.	✔	✔
• Demonstrate how to check for patency of IV access device.	✔	✔
• Demonstrate how to prepare the IV infusion of gamma-globulin.	✔	✔
• Demonstrate how to infuse IV gamma-globulin.	✔	✔
• Demonstrate how to clean and maintain IV equipment.	✔	✔
• Identify side effects and adverse effects of IV gamma-globulin.	✔	✔
• State rationale for prophylactic use of aspirin and an antihistamine before treatment begins.	✔	✔
• Verbalize understanding of emergency measures for anaphylactic shock.	✔	✔

Continuing Care. The importance of follow-up appointments is emphasized to the patient and family. Additionally, they are urged to notify the primary health care provider about early signs and symptoms of infection, including any subtle changes, because typical signs and symptoms of infection and inflammation may not occur because of the immunodeficiency. The importance of continuing disease prevention strategies is stressed. These strategies need to be followed for the duration of the patient's lifetime.

If the patient's treatment includes gamma-globulin and the patient or family is unable to administer it, a referral for home care or for an infusion service may be warranted.

Critical Thinking Exercises

1. Gamma-globulin infusions have been prescribed for your patient, who has an immunodeficiency. He tells you that he is very fearful that he may contract HIV infection or AIDS from the infusion. How would you respond to these fears and concerns?

2. During a home care visit to a patient who is immunocompromised, you note spoiled food in the kitchen, dirty dishes and countertops, an unclean bathroom, and the presence of several cats and dogs. Explain the course of action you would take to ensure a safe environment for your patient.

3. Describe the teaching plan you would use to instruct a patient with an immunodeficiency disorder about prevention and management of infection. How would you modify your approach if the patient understood little English? If the patient was unable to read?

References and Selected Readings

BOOKS

Antel, P., Birnbaum, G., & Hartung, H. P. (1998). *Clinical neuroimmunology.* Malden, MA: Blackwell Scientific.

Bradley, J., & McCluskey, J. (Eds.) (1997). *Clinical immunology.* New York: Oxford University Press.

Datiles, T. B., & Humphry R. L. (1997). Immune deficiency. In C. Sheehan (Ed.). *Principles and laboratory diagnosis* (2nd ed.) Philadelphia: Lippincott-Raven.

Delves, P. J. (1998). *Encyclopedia of immunology* (2nd ed.). San Diego: Academic Press.

Eales, L. J. (1997). *Immunology for life scientists. A basic introduction: A student-centered learning approach.* New York: John Wiley & Sons.

Hyde, R. M. (1995). *Immunology* (3rd ed.). Baltimore: Williams & Wilkins.

Kuhn, M. A. (1998). *Pharmacotherapeutics: A nursing process approach* (4th ed.). Philadelphia: F. A. Davis.

Levenson, W., & Jawetz, E. (1996). *Medical microbiology and immunology* (4th ed.). Stamford, CT: Appleton & Lange.

Miaskowski, C. (1997). *Oncology nursing: An essential guide for patient care.* Philadelphia: W. B. Saunders.

Nakamura, R. M., et al. (Eds.) (1998). *Clinical diagnostic immunology: Protocols in quality assurance and standardization.* Malden, MA: Blackwell Scientific.

Roitt, I., Brostoff, J., & Male, D. K. (Eds.). (1998). *Immunology* (5th ed.). St. Louis: C. V. Mosby.

Stites, D. P., Terr, A. I., & Parslow, T. G. (Eds.) (1997). *Medical immunology* (9th ed.). Stamford, CT: Appleton & Lange.

Weir, D. M., & Steward, J. (1997). *Immunology* (8th ed.). New York: Churchill Livingstone.

Virella, G. (Ed.). (1998). *Introduction to medical immunology* (4th ed.). New York: Marcel Dekker.

JOURNALS

Alcoser, P. W., & Burchett, B. A. (1999). Bone marrow transplantation. Immune system suppression and reconstitution. *American Journal of Nursing, 99*(6), 26–31.

Ballow, M., & Nelson, R. (1997). Immunopharmacology: Immunomodulation and immunotherapy. *Journal of the American Medical Association, 278*(22), 2008–2017.

Berkman, S. A., Lee, M. L., & Gale, R. P. (1990). Clinical uses of intravenous immunoglobulins. *Annals of Internal Medicine, 112,* 278–292.

Buckley, R. H., Schiff, S. E., Schiff, R. I., et al. (1999). Hematopoietic stem-cell transplantation for the treatment of severe combined immunodeficiency. *New England Journal of Medicine, 340*(7), 508–516.

Costa, J. J., Weller, P. F., & Galli, S. J. (1997). The cells of the allergic response: Mast cells, basophils, and eosinophils. *Journal of the American Medical Association, 278*(22), 1815–1834.

deShazo, R. D. (1997). Future trends in allergy and immunology. *Journal of the American Medical Association, 278*(22), 2024–2025.

DiJulio, J. (1991). Hematopoiesis: An overview. *Oncology Nursing Forum, 18*(2), 3–6.

Fleisher, T. A. (1997). Introduction to diagnostic laboratory immunology. *Journal of the American Medical Association, 278*(22), 1823–1834.

Hall, R. A., Salhany, K. E., Lebel, E., Bavaria, J. E., & Kaiser, L. R. (1995). Fungal pulmonary abscess in an adult secondary to hyperimmunoglobulin E (Job's) syndrome. *Annals of Thoracic Surgery, 59*(3), 759–61.

Huston, D. P. (1997). The biology of the immune system. *Journal of the American Medical Association, 278*(22), 1804–1822.

Khan, G. A., & Bank, N. (1994). An adult patient with hyperimmunoglobulinemia E (Job's) syndrome, end-stage renal disease and repeated episodes of peritonitis. *Clinical Nephrology, 41*(4), 233–236.

Puck, J. M. (1997). Primary immunodeficiency diseases. *Journal of the American Medical Association, 278*(22), 1835–1841.

Smith, J. K., Krishnaswamy, G. H., Dykes, R., Reynolds, S., & Berk, S. L. (1997). Clinical manifestations of IgE hypogammaglobulinemia. *Annals of Allergy, Asthma, and Immunology, 78*(3), 313–18.

Stadtmauer, G., & Cunningham-Rundies, C. (1997). Outcome analysis and cost assessment in immunologic disorders. *Journal of the American Medical Association, 278*(22), 2018–2023.

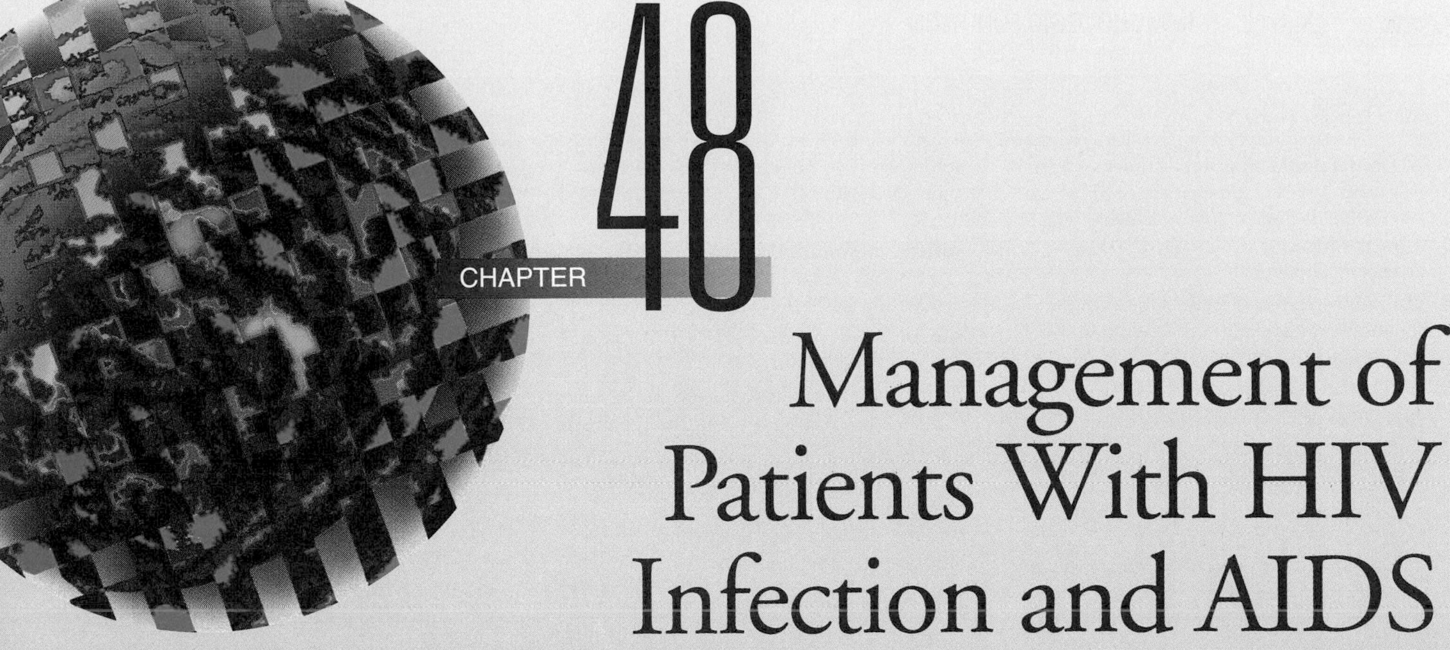

Management of Patients With HIV Infection and AIDS

Learning Objectives

On completion of this chapter, the learner will be able to:

1. Describe the pathophysiology of HIV infection.
2. Describe the modes of transmission of HIV infection.
3. Explain the physiology underlying the clinical manifestations of HIV infection.
4. Describe the management of patients with HIV infection.
5. Describe nursing diagnoses common to patients with AIDS.
6. Discuss the nursing interventions appropriate for patients with HIV infection and AIDS.
7. Use the nursing process as a framework for care of the patient with AIDS.

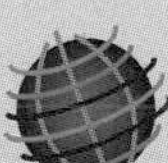

Although progress has been made in treating HIV infection and AIDS, nevertheless, the virus remains a critical public health issue in all communities across the country and around the world. Prevention, early detection, and aggressive treatment remain important aspects of care for people with HIV infection and AIDS. Nurses in all settings encounter people with this disease; thus, nurses need an understanding of the disorder, knowledge of the physical and psychological consequences associated with its diagnosis, and expert assessment and clinical management skills to provide optimal care for people with HIV infection and AIDS.

GLOSSARY

AIDS dementia complex: clinical syndrome caused by HIV and characterized by a progressive decline in cognitive behavioral and motor functions; also called HIV encephalopathy

alpha-interferon: protein substance that has antiviral and antitumor activity

B-cell lymphoma: common malignancy occurring in patients with HIV/AIDS

candidiasis: yeast infection of skin or mucous membrane

cervical intraepithelial neoplasia (CIN): cellular change that is frequently a precursor to cervical cancer

colony-stimulating factors: substances naturally produced by the body to stimulate growth and production of red and white blood cells

Cryptococcus neoformans: fungus that causes an opportunistic infection in patients with HIV/AIDS

cytomegalovirus: a species-specific herpes virus that may cause retinitis in people with HIV/AIDS

HIV encephalopathy: an abnormal condition of the structure or function of the tissues of the brain

enzyme-linked immunosorbant assay (ELISA): a blood test that confirms the presence of antibodies to HIV

helper T4 lymphocyte: cell that becomes infected with HIV; also known as a CD4+ cell

human immunodeficiency virus (HIV): retrovirus responsible for causing HIV infection and AIDS

human papillomavirus (HPV): virus that causes venereal warts

Kaposi's sarcoma: malignancy that involves the epithelial layer of blood and lymphatic vessels

***Mycobacterium avium* complex (MAC):** one of several acid fast bacilli that commonly causes a respiratory illness but can also infect other body systems

opportunistic infection: an infection caused by various organisms, such as fungi and bacteria, that occurs in immunocompromised patients

p24 antigen: blood test that measures viral core protein

peripheral neuropathy: demyelinating disorders associated with pain and numbness in the extremities, weakness, and deep tendon reflexes

***Pneumocystis carinii* pneumonia (PCP):** a lung cell infection caused by an organism thought to be a protozoan but structurally believed to be a fungus based on its structure

polymerase chain reaction (PCR): blood test used to detect HIV RNA or proviral DNA

progressive multifocal leukoencephalopathy (PML): demyelinating central nervous system disorder affecting the oligodendroglia

protease inhibitor: medication that inhibits the function of protease, an enzyme needed for HIV replication

retrovirus: a virus that carries genetic material in RNA instead of DNA and contains reverse transcriptase

reverse transcriptase: enzyme that transforms single-stranded RNA into a double-stranded DNA

wasting syndrome: protein-energy malnutrition with profound involuntary weight loss exceeding 10% of baseline body weight

Western blot assay: a blood test that identifies antibodies to HIV

HIV INFECTION AND AIDS

Acquired immunodeficiency syndrome (AIDS) is defined as the most severe form of a continuum of illnesses associated with **human immunodeficiency virus** (HIV) infection. Manifestations of HIV infection range from mild abnormalities in the immune response without overt signs and symptoms to profound immunosuppression associated with various life-threatening infections and malignancies.

In the fall of 1982, the Centers for Disease Control and Prevention (CDC) issued a case definition of AIDS after the first 100 cases were reported. Since then, the CDC has revised the case definition twice (in 1987 and 1993). The most prevalent type of HIV is referred to as HIV-1. There are two other strains of HIV, HIV-2, and HIV-3. Unless otherwise indicated, HIV-1 is the infectious agent discussed in this chapter.

As of January 1999, there were 688,200 reported cases of AIDS and 410,800 deaths from AIDS in adults, adolescents, and children in the United States. In January 1993, the surveillance definition of AIDS was expanded to include conditions that occur earlier in the course of HIV infection, resulting in an increase in the number of cases of AIDS being reported. Data indicate an increased incidence of HIV infection in the heterosexual population, especially on the East Coast. AIDS has reached epidemic proportions in other parts of the world.

Analysis of the sociodemographic and exposure categories indicates that as of January 1999, African Americans and Hispanics accounted for 54.7% of all cases of AIDS; non-Hispanic whites accounted for 44.2%; and Asians, Pacific Islanders, Native Americans, and Alaskan natives accounted for 1.0%. African Americans and Hispanics account for about 50% of cases in men, 76.7% of cases in women, and 81.4% of cases in children. This disproportionate representation may be related to injecting drug use, having sex with an injecting drug user, and a lack of access to health care and education.

Large urban areas continue to report more cases of AIDS than rural areas because of a higher incidence of injecting drug use and high-risk sexual practices. HIV is predominantly an infection of young people, with most cases involving people between ages 17 and 55 years. However, it has also been reported in elderly men and women.

AIDS is the second leading cause of death for Americans between ages 25 and 44 and the leading cause of death for African American men and women in this age group. About half of all new HIV infections in the USA are among young people under age 25, with most being infected through sexual transmission. In women, ages 13 to 24, about 49% are infected heterosexually and 13% are infected via injecting drug use. As AIDS increases among people in the childbearing years, the number of children with HIV is expected to increase.

Pathophysiology

HIV belongs to a group of viruses known as **retroviruses,** which indicates that the virus carries its genetic material in ribonucleic acid (RNA) rather than deoxyribonucleic acid (DNA). HIV-1 is

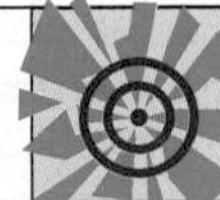

Risk Factors for HIV INFECTION AND AIDS

In the United States, most people with AIDS have engaged in high-risk behaviors, such as the following:

- Male homosexual relations
- Intravenous (IV) (or injection) drug use (the term *intravenous drug user* [IDU] has been replaced by the term *injecting drug user*). This term includes people who inject illicit drugs intravenously as well as those who inject drugs intradermally. This method is sometimes referred to as "skin popping."
- Heterosexual relations with an HIV-infected partner or a partner who is at high risk for infection because of IV (injecting) drug use
- Sexual relations with infected individuals

Also at risk are people who received blood or blood products contaminated with HIV (especially before blood screening was instituted in 1985) and children born to mothers with HIV infection.

a virus surrounded by a glycoprotein envelope. This envelope contains RNA in a truncated bullet-shaped protein core composed of viral proteins p24 and p17. Knobs that protrude through the viral wall consist of the protein gp120 anchored to the protein gp41. The outer viral glycoprotein gp120 and gp41 are essential for binding HIV-1 to the CD4-positive (CD4+) T lymphocyte.

CD4+ cells include monocytes, macrophages, and **helper T4 lymphocytes,** the most numerous of these cells. (In HIV infection, the T4 cell count determines the degree of immune suppression and refers in this circumstance only to the CD4+ T cells). The CD4+ cell plugs into a port on the gp120 protein of the virus. The gp120 uses a sugar "cloak" and other hidden structures to avoid triggering the human immune system. The connection of gp120 with the CD4+ cell causes the gp120 to change shape. Now the virus is able to attach to another one of the CD4+ cell's surface proteins, called a chemokine, that brings the virus and CD4+ cell closer together. Once the gp120 connects to the chemokine, the CD4+ cell opens holes in its membrane, and the virus inserts two identical strands of RNA into the helper T4 cell. Using an enzyme known as **reverse transcriptase,** HIV reprograms the genetic materials of the infected T4 cell to make double-stranded DNA. This DNA is incorporated in the T4 cell nucleus as a provirus, and permanent infection is established.

Infection of monocytes and macrophages appears to be persistent and does not result in significant cell death. These cells serve as reservoirs for HIV, allowing the virus to hide from the immune system and to be transported throughout the system to infect a variety of body tissues. Most of these tissues either contain the CD4+ molecule or have the ability to produce it. Studies show that after the initial infection, about 25% of lymph node cells are also infected with HIV.

Viral replication, occurring primarily in lymphoid tissues, is ongoing throughout the course of HIV infection. The HIV replication cycle is restricted to this stage until the infected cell is activated. Activation of the infected cell may be achieved by antigens, mitogens, select cytokines (tumor necrosis factor-alpha or interleukin-1), or virus gene products of such viruses as **cytomegalovirus** (CMV), Epstein-Barr virus, herpes simplex virus, and hepatitis. Consequently, whenever the infected T4 cell is activated, HIV replication and budding occur, and the T4 cell is destroyed. Newly formed HIV is then released into the blood plasma and infects other CD4+ cells (Fig. 48-1).

Studies suggest that the immune system in HIV infection is more active than previously thought, as evidenced by the production of as many as 2 billion CD4+ lymphocytes daily. The entire population of peripheral CD4+ cells turns over every 15 days (Ho et al., 1995).

The rate of HIV production is thought to be associated with the health status of the infected person. If the person is not fighting another infection, HIV reproduction may proceed slowly. HIV reproduction appears to accelerate, however, when the person is combating another infection or when the immune system is stimulated. This may explain the latent period exhibited by some people after infection with HIV. For example, some may remain symptom-free for many years. However, a large portion of infected people (up to 80% to 90%) go on to develop symptomatic HIV disease or AIDS within 10 years of infection.

In the immune response, several important roles are played by the T4 lymphocyte: recognition of foreign antigens, activation of antibody-producing B lymphocytes, stimulation of cytotoxic T lymphocytes, production of lymphokines, and defense against parasitic infections. When T4 lymphocyte function is impaired, organisms that do not usually cause disease have the opportunity to invade and cause serious illness. Infections that develop as a result of immune system impairment are referred to as **opportunistic infections.**

General Transmission

HIV-1 is transmitted by way of body fluids that contain HIV-1 or CD4+ T lymphocytes. These fluids include serum, seminal fluid, vaginal secretions, amniotic fluid, and breast milk (ie, HIV may be transmitted in utero from mother to child and later through breast milk). Some recent strains of HIV-1 have height-

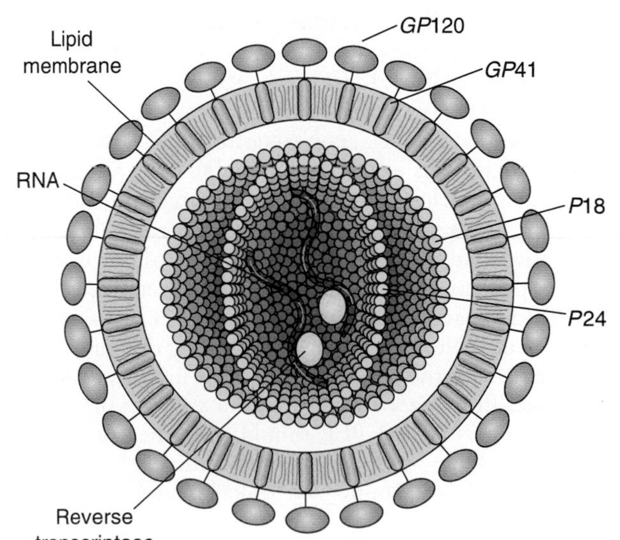

FIGURE 48•1 Structure of the HIV-1 virus. A glycoprotein envelope surrounds the virus, which carries its genetic material in RNA. Knobs, consisting of protein gp120 and gp41, protrude from the envelope. These proteins are essential for binding the virus to the CD4+ T lymphocyte. From Porth, C. (1998). *Pathophysiology: Concepts of altered health states* (5th ed.). Philadelphia: Lippincott Williams & Wilkins.

ened virulence and infectious ability. People with a high viral load (a large number of HIV-1 in their body fluids) have an increased ability to infect people exposed to their body secretions.

In male homosexuals, *anal intercourse or manipulation* increases the risk for trauma to the rectal mucosa. Subsequently, the chance of exposure to the virus through body secretions increases. Increased frequency of these practices and sex with multiple partners also contribute to the spread of this disease. *Heterosexual intercourse* with people who have HIV infection is a mode of transmission that continues to increase.

Transmission by *injection drug use* occurs through direct blood exposure to contaminated needles and syringes. Although the amount of blood in a syringe is relatively small, the cumulative effect of repeatedly sharing contaminated equipment leads to an increased risk of transmission.

Blood and blood products, including those used by persons with hemophilia, can transmit HIV to recipients. However, the risk associated with transfusions has been reduced as a result of voluntary self-deferral, serologic testing, heat treating of clotting factor concentrates, and more effective virus inactivation methods. In the past, blood donor screening tests detected antibodies to HIV-1 and HIV-2 even though few HIV-2 infections had been reported in the United States. In August 1995, the Food and Drug Administration (FDA) recommended that all donated blood and plasma be screened for HIV-1 p24 antigen because the antigen can be detected in the blood much earlier than antibodies. Donor screening with HIV-1 p24 antigen is expected to reduce the number of undetected infectious donations. Unfortunately, some infectious donations will still be missed. It takes about 3 weeks (window period is about 5 to 10 days) after HIV infection for the HIV-1 p24 antigen to test positive. Blood donated during the window period will be infectious but will test negative.

Transmission to Health Care Providers

The incidence of HIV for health care workers who are exposed to HIV through *needle-stick injury* is estimated to be about 0.3%. Large-scale studies of exposed health care workers continue to be conducted by the CDC and other groups.

POSTEXPOSURE PROPHYLAXIS FOR HEALTH CARE PROVIDERS

Although the effectiveness of postexposure prophylaxis in response to health care workers' exposure to blood or body fluids infected with HIV is inconclusive, the CDC (1998) recommends that all health care providers who have sustained a significant exposure be counseled and offered anti-HIV postexposure prophylaxis (PEP), if appropriate. Some clinicians are presently considering using PEP for patients exposed to HIV from high-risk sexual behavior or possible contact through injecting drug use. There is controversy about the use of PEP in these instances because of concern that PEP may be substituted for safer sex practices and safer drug injection use. PEP should never be considered an acceptable method of primary HIV prevention.

The medications recommended for PEP are those used to treat established HIV infection. The preferred regimen is treatment with reverse transcriptase inhibitors, zidovudine (AZT), and lamivudine (Epivir, 3TC). An alternative two-drug regimen includes the reverse transcriptase inhibitors stavudine (Zerit, d4T) and didanosine (Videx, dd1). If the source patient has advanced HIV infection and a high viral load or has previously been treated with any of the drugs in the previous two-medication treatment regimens, the CDC recommends adding either nelfinavir (Viracept) or indinavir (Crixivan), both of which are **protease inhibitors**.

Ideally, prophylaxis needs to start within hours of exposure. Therapy started more than 72 hours after exposure is thought to be of no benefit and therefore is not recommended. The recommended course of PEP therapy involves taking the prescribed medications at least twice a day for a total of 4 weeks. (For more information, refer to other sections in this chapter for specific information on viral load testing, antiviral drug therapy, and adverse effects.)

People who choose PEP must be ready for the temporary side effects of the medications and must be willing to face the unknown long-term risks because HIV often becomes resistant to the medications used to treat it. If the person becomes infected despite use of PEP, viral drug resistance may reduce future treatment options. The cost of PEP is also of concern; the cost of a two- or three-drug regimen for several months of therapy ranges from $500 to more than $1000. In addition to the cost of the medications are the costs of concomitant testing and counseling. Health insurance may or may not cover the costs of medications, laboratory fees, or counseling.

Prevention of Transmission

Epidemiologic evidence indicates that HIV is transmitted only through intimate sexual contact, parenteral exposure to infected blood or blood products, and perinatal transmission from mother to neonate. Studies of nonsexual household contacts of AIDS patients and of nonsexual person-to-person contact that generally occurs in the workplace have not demonstrated any increased risk for transmission of AIDS through such contact.

In the interest of public health in 1985, however, the CDC and the Surgeon General of the United States issued recommendations for preventing transmission of HIV. The guidelines, entitled "Universal Blood and Body Fluids Precautions" or Universal Precautions (UP), were intended to prevent parenteral, mucous membrane, and nonintact skin exposures of health care providers to bloodborne pathogens of all patients regardless of HIV status. These guidelines applied to health care workers in all settings as well as to family members and friends providing care in the home.

In 1987, another system, called Body Substance Isolation (BSI), was used by some institutions as an alternative to UP. BSI offered an even broader isolation strategy to reduce the risk of disease transmission to patients and health care workers alike, and eliminated the need for health care workers to identify particular body fluids.

STANDARD PRECAUTIONS

In 1996, efforts were made to standardize procedures and reduce risk of exposure further through development of *Standard Precautions* (SP). Standard Precautions incorporate the major features of UP (transmission of bloodborne pathogens) and BSI (transmission of pathogens from moist body substances) and applies them to all patients receiving care in hospitals regardless of their diagnosis or presumed infectious status (Guideline 48-1). SP applies to blood; all body fluids, secretions, and excretions, except sweat, regardless of whether they contain visible blood; nonintact skin; and mucous membranes (Hospital Infection Control Practices Advisory Committee [HICPAC], 1996, p. 64).

The primary goal of SP is to prevent the transmission of nosocomial infection. The first tier, referred to as SP, was developed to reduce the risk for all recognized or unrecognized sources of infec-

(*text continues on page 1354*)

48•1 Guidelines For Standard Precautions

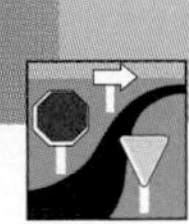

The following guidelines were developed to prevent the transmission of infection during patient care for all patients regardless of known or unknown infectious status.

Hand Washing

- Wash hands after touching blood, body fluids, secretions, excretions, and contaminated items whether or not gloves are worn.
- Wash hands immediately after gloves are removed, between patient contacts, and when otherwise indicated to avoid transfer of microorganisms to other patients or environments.
- Wash hands between tasks and procedures on the same patient to prevent cross-contamination of different body sites.
- Use a plain (nonantimicrobial) soap for routine hand washing.
- Use an antimicrobial agent or waterless antiseptic agent for specific circumstances (control of outbreaks or hyperendemic infections). (See Contact Precautions.)

Gloves

- Wear clean, nonsterile gloves when touching blood, body fluids, secretions, excretions, and contaminated items.
- Put on clean gloves just before touching mucous membranes and nonintact skin.
- Change gloves between tasks and procedures on the same patient after contact with materials that may contain a high concentration of microorganisms.
- Remove gloves promptly after use, before touching noncontaminated items and environmental surfaces, and before going to another patient.
- Wash hands immediately after removing gloves.

Mask, Eye Protection, Face Shield

- Wear a mask and eye protection or a face shield to protect mucous membranes of the eyes, nose, and mouth during procedures and patient care activities that are likely to generate splashes or sprays of blood, body fluids, secretions, or excretions.

Gown

- Wear a clean, nonsterile gown to protect skin and prevent soiling of clothing during procedures and patient care activities that are likely to generate splashes or sprays of blood, body fluids, secretions, or excretions.
- Select a gown that is appropriate for the activity and amount of fluid likely to be encountered.
- Remove a soiled gown as promptly as possible and wash hands to prevent the transfer of microorganisms to other patients or environments.

Patient Care Equipment

- Handle used patient care equipment soiled with blood, body fluids, secretions, and excretions in a manner that prevents skin and mucous membrane exposures, contamination of clothing, and transfer of microorganisms to other patients and environments.
- Ensure that reusable equipment is not used for the care of another patient until it has been cleaned and reprocessed appropriately.
- Ensure that single-use items are discarded properly.

Environmental Control

- Ensure that the hospital has adequate procedures for the routine care, cleaning, and disinfection of environmental surfaces, beds, bed rails, bedside equipment, and other frequently touched surfaces.
- Ensure that procedures are being followed.

Linen

- Handle, transport, and process used linen soiled with blood, body fluids, secretions, and excretions in a manner that prevents skin and mucous membrane exposures and contamination of clothing and that avoids transfer of microorganisms to other patients and environments.

(continued)

48•1
GUIDELINES FOR 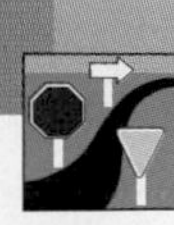 STANDARD PRECAUTIONS *(Continued)*

Occupational Health and Bloodborne Pathogens

- Take care to prevent injuries when using needles, scalpels, and other sharp instruments or devices:
  - When handling sharp instruments after procedures
  - When cleaning used instruments
  - When disposing of used needles
- Never recap used needles or otherwise manipulate them by using both hands or use any technique that involves directing the point of the needle toward any part of the body.
- Use either a one-handed scoop technique or a mechanical device designed for holding the needle sheath.
- Do not remove used needles from disposable syringes by hand and do not bend, break, otherwise manipulate used needles by hand.
- Place used disposable syringes and needles, scalpel blades, and other sharp items in appropriate puncture-resistant containers as close as practical to the area in which the items were used.
- Place reusable syringes and needles in a puncture-resistant container for transport to the reprocessing area.
- Use mouthpieces, resuscitation bags, or other ventilation devices as an alternative to mouth-to-mouth resuscitation methods in areas where the need for resuscitation is predictable.

Patient Placement

- Place a patient who contaminates the environment or who does not or cannot be expected to assist in maintaining appropriate hygiene or environmental control in a private room.
- If a private room is not available, consult with infection control professionals regarding patient placement or other alternatives.

Adapted from (1996) Guideline for Isolation Precautions in Hospitals. *Infection Control and Hospital Epidemiology, 17,* 53–80.

tions in hospitals. A second tier for infection control precautions for specified conditions, called Transmission-Based Precautions, was designed for use in addition to SP for patients with documented or suspected infections involving highly transmissible pathogens. The three types of Transmission-Based Precautions are referred to as Airborne Precautions, Droplet Precautions, and Contact Precautions. They can be used singularly or in combination, but they are always to be used in addition to SP.

Clinical Manifestations

The clinical manifestations of AIDS are widespread and may affect virtually any organ system. Diseases associated with HIV infection and AIDS result from infections, malignancies, or the direct effect of HIV on body tissues. The following discussion is limited to the most common clinical manifestations and effects of severe HIV infection.

RESPIRATORY MANIFESTATIONS

Shortness of breath, dyspnea (labored breathing), cough, chest pain, and fever are associated with various opportunistic infections, such as those caused by *Pneumocystis carinii*, *Mycobacterium avium-intracellulare* (MAI), CMV, and *Legionella* species. The most common infection in people with AIDS is ***Pneumocystis carinii* pneumonia** (PCP), one of the first opportunistic diseases described in association with AIDS.

Pneumocystis carinii Pneumonia. PCP is the initial manifestation of AIDS in 60% of patients. Without prophylactic therapy, PCP will develop in 80% of all HIV-infected individuals. *P. carinii* was originally classified as a protozoan; however, studies and analysis of its ribosomal RNA structure suggest that it is a fungus. Its structure and antimicrobial sensitivity are very different from other disease-causing fungi. PCP causes disease only in immunocompromised hosts invading and proliferating within the pulmonary alveoli, with resultant consolidation of the pulmonary parenchyma.

The clinical presentation of PCP in the patient with AIDS is generally less acute than in people who are immunosuppressed as a result of other conditions. The time between the onset of symptoms and the actual documentation of disease may be weeks to months. Patients with AIDS initially develop nonspecific signs and symptoms, such as fever, chills, nonproductive cough, shortness of breath, dyspnea, and occasionally chest pain. PCP may be present despite the absence of crackles. Arterial oxygen concentrations in patients breathing room air may be mildly decreased, indicating minimal hypoxemia.

Untreated, PCP eventually progresses and causes significant pulmonary impairment and, ultimately, respiratory failure. A few patients have a dramatic onset and fulminant course involving severe hypoxemia, cyanosis, tachypnea, and altered mental status. Respiratory failure can develop within 2 to 3 days of initial symptoms.

PCP can be diagnosed definitively by identifying the organism in lung tissue or bronchial secretions. This is accomplished by such procedures as sputum induction, bronchial-alveolar lavage, and transbronchial biopsy (by fiberoptic bronchoscopy).

Mycobacterium avium Complex. ***Mycobacterium avium* complex** (MAC) disease is a leading bacterial infection in people with AIDS. Organisms belonging to MAC include *M. avium*, *M. intracellulare*, and *M. scrofulaceum*. MAC, comprising a group of acid-fast bacilli, usually causes respiratory infection but is also commonly found in the gastrointestinal (GI) tract, lymph nodes, and bone marrow. Most patients with AIDS have widespread disease at the time of diagnosis and are usually debilitated. MAC infections are associated with rising mortality rates.

Tuberculosis. HIV-associated *Mycobacterium tuberculosis* tends to occur in injecting drug users and other groups with a preexisting high prevalence of tuberculosis (TB) infection. Unlike other opportunistic infections, tuberculosis tends to occur early in the course of HIV infection, usually preceding a diagnosis of AIDS. This early occurrence is associated with the development of caseating granulomas (dry, cheeselike masses of granulation tissue), which should raise the suspicion of a diagnosis of TB. At this stage, TB responds well to antituberculosis therapy.

TB that occurs late in HIV infection is characterized by absence of a tuberculin skin test response because the compromised immune system can no longer respond to the TB antigen. In the later stages of HIV infection, TB is associated with dissemination to extrapulmonary sites, such as the central nervous system, bone, pericardium, stomach, peritoneum, and scrotum. Multiple drug-resistant strains of the bacillus have now emerged and are often associated with noncompliance with antituberculosis therapy.

GASTROINTESTINAL MANIFESTATIONS

The GI manifestations of AIDS include loss of appetite, nausea, vomiting, oral and esophageal candidiasis, and chronic diarrhea. Diarrhea is a problem in 50% to 90% of all AIDS patients. In some instances, GI symptoms may be related to the direct effect of HIV on the cells lining the intestines. Some of the enteric pathogens that occur most frequently, identified by stool cultures or intestinal biopsy, include *Cryptosporidium muris, Salmonella* species, *Isopora belli, Giardia lamblia*, CMV, *Clostridium difficile*, and *M. avium-intracellulare*. In patients with AIDS, the effects of diarrhea can be devastating in terms of profound weight loss (more than 10% of body weight), fluid and electrolyte imbalances, perianal skin excoriation, weakness, and inability to perform the usual activities of daily living.

Oral Candidiasis. Oral **candidiasis**, a fungal infection, occurs in nearly all patients with AIDS and AIDS-related conditions. Commonly preceding other life-threatening infections, it is characterized by creamy-white patches in the oral cavity. When untreated, oral candidiasis will progress to involve the esophagus and stomach. Associated signs and symptoms include difficult and painful swallowing and retrosternal pain. Some patients also develop ulcerating oral lesions and are particularly susceptible to dissemination of candidiasis to other body systems.

Wasting Syndrome. **Wasting syndrome** is part of the case definition for AIDS. Diagnostic criteria include profound involuntary weight loss exceeding 10% of baseline body weight and either chronic diarrhea for more than 30 days or chronic weakness and documented intermittent or constant fever in the absence of any concurrent illness that could explain these findings. This protein-energy malnutrition is multifactorial. In some AIDS-associated illnesses, patients experience a hypermetabolic state in which excessive calories are burned and lean body mass is lost. This state is similar to that seen in sepsis and trauma and can lead to organ failure. A distinction between cachexia (wasting) and malnutrition or between cachexia and simple weight loss is important because the metabolic derangement seen in wasting syndrome may not be modified by nutritional support alone (Fig. 48-2).

Anorexia, diarrhea, GI malabsorption, and lack of nutrition in chronic disease all contribute to wasting syndrome. Progressive tissue wasting, however, may occur with only modest GI involvement and without diarrhea. Tumor necrosis factor (TNF) and interleukin-1 (IL-1) are cytokines that play important roles in AIDS-related wasting syndrome. Both act directly on the hypothalamus to cause anorexia. Cytokine-induced fever accelerates the body's metabolism by 14% for every 1°F increase in temperature. TNF causes inefficient use of lipids by reducing enzymes that are needed for fat metabolism, whereas IL-1 triggers the release of amino acids from muscle tissue. People with AIDS generally experience increased protein metabolism in relation to fat metabolism, which results in significant decreases in lean body mass due to muscle and protein breakdown.

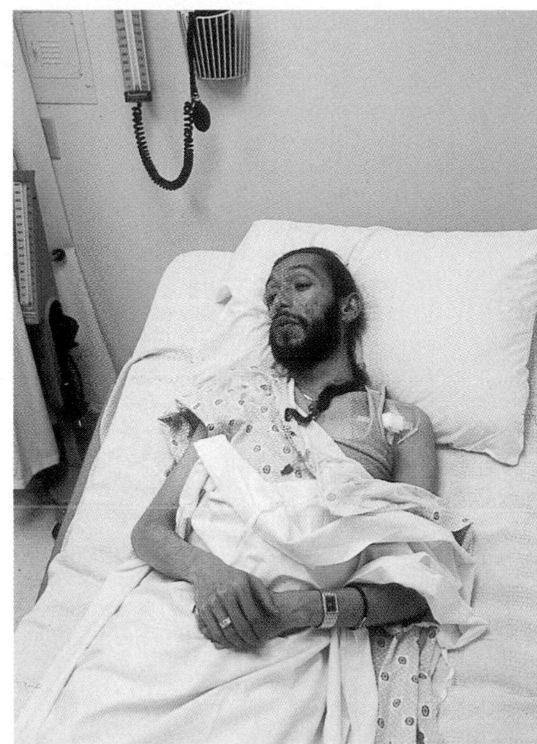

FIGURE 48•2 The wasting syndrome of AIDS.

Hypertriglyceridemia, seen in people with AIDS and attributed to chronically elevated cytokine levels, can persist in people with AIDS for months without tissue wasting and loss of lean body mass. It is believed that infections and sepsis lead to transient rises in TNF, IL-1, and other cell mediators above the chronically elevated levels generally seen. These transient rises in TNF and IL-1 trigger muscle wasting.

ONCOLOGIC MANIFESTATIONS

Patients with AIDS have a higher than usual incidence of cancer, possibly related to HIV stimulation of developing cancer cells or to the immune deficiency allowing cancer-causing substances, such as viruses, to transform susceptible cells into malignant cells. Kaposi's sarcoma, certain types of B-cell lymphomas, and invasive cervical carcinoma are included in the CDC classification of AIDS-related malignancies. Carcinomas of the skin, stomach, pancreas, rectum, and bladder also occur more frequently than expected in people with AIDS.

Kaposi's Sarcoma. **Kaposi's** (pronounced KA-po-sheez) **sarcoma** (KS), the most common HIV-related malignancy, is a disease involving the endothelial layer of blood and lymphatic vessels. When first noted in 1872 by Dr. Moritz Kaposi, KS characteristically presented as lower-extremity skin lesions in elderly men of Eastern European ancestry. This form, referred to as *classic*

Kaposi's sarcoma, was slow to progress and easily treated. An *endemic* form of KS, found in children and young men in equatorial Africa, is more virulent than the classic form.

Acquired KS occurs in patients who are treated with immunosuppressive agents and commonly occurs in patients who have undergone organ transplantation. In such patients, acquired KS usually resolves once the dose of the immunosuppressive medication is decreased or discontinued. In people with AIDS, *epidemic* KS is most often seen in male homosexuals and bisexuals. Although the histopathology of all forms of KS is virtually identical, the clinical manifestations differ with AIDS-related KS, which exhibits a more variable and aggressive course, ranging from localized cutaneous lesions to disseminated disease involving multiple organ systems.

Cutaneous lesions appearing anywhere on the body are usually brownish pink to deep purple. They may be flat or raised and surrounded by ecchymoses (hemorrhagic patches) and edema (Fig. 48-3). Rapid development of lesions involving large areas of skin is associated with extensive disfigurement. The location and size of some lesions can lead to venous stasis, lymphedema, and pain. Ulcerative lesions disrupt skin integrity and increase patient discomfort and susceptibility to infection. The most common sites of visceral involvement include the lymph nodes, GI tract, and lungs. Involvement of internal organs may eventually lead to organ failure, hemorrhage, infection, and death.

Diagnosis of KS is confirmed by biopsy of suspected lesions. Prognosis depends on the extent of the tumor, presence of constitutional symptoms, and CD4+ count. Death may result from tumor progression. More often, however, it results from other complications of HIV infection.

B-Cell Lymphomas. **B-cell lymphomas** are the second most common malignancy occurring in people with AIDS. Lymphomas associated with AIDS usually differ from those occurring in the general population. Patients with AIDS are generally much younger than the usual population affected by non-Hodgkin's lymphoma (NHL). In addition, AIDS-related lymphomas tend to develop outside the lymph nodes, most commonly in the brain, bone marrow, and GI tract. These types of lymphomas are characteristically of a higher grade, indicating aggressive growth and resistance to treatment. The course of AIDS-related lymphomas includes multiple sites of organ involvement and complications related to developing opportunistic infections. Although aggressive combination chemotherapy is frequently successful in NHL not associated with HIV infection, it is less successful in people with AIDS because of the severe hematologic toxicity and complications of opportunistic infections that occur from treatment.

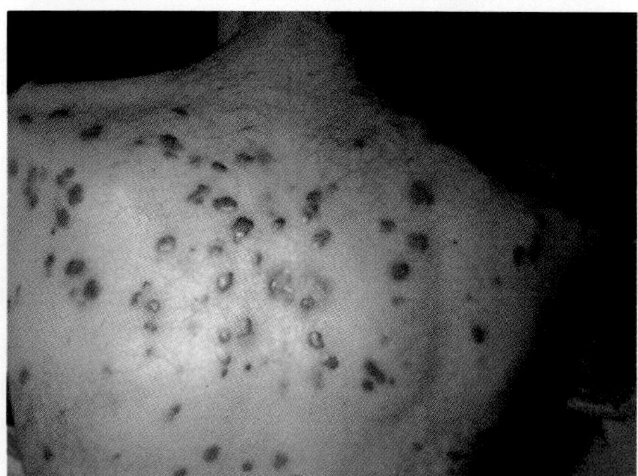

FIGURE 48•3 Lesions of the AIDS-related Kaposi's sarcoma. Whereas some patients may have lesions that remain flat, others experience extensively disseminated, raised lesions with edema. From DeVita, V. T. Jr., Hellman, S., & Rosenberg, S. (Eds.). (1997). *AIDS: Etiology, diagnosis, treatment, and prevention* (4th ed.). Philadelphia: Lippincott-Raven.

NEUROLOGIC MANIFESTATIONS

An estimated 80% of all patients with AIDS experience some form of neurologic involvement during the course of HIV infection. Many neuropathologic disorders are underreported because patients may have neurologic involvement without overt signs or symptoms. Neurologic complications involve central, peripheral, and autonomic functions.

Neurologic dysfunction results from the direct effects of HIV on nervous system tissue, opportunistic infections, primary or metastatic neoplasms, cerebrovascular changes, metabolic encephalopathies, or complications secondary to therapy. Immune system response to HIV infection in the central nervous system includes inflammation, atrophy, demyelination, degeneration, and necrosis.

HIV Encephalopathy. **HIV encephalopathy** is also referred to as **AIDS dementia complex** (ADC). This condition occurs in at least two thirds of patients with AIDS. It is a clinical syndrome characterized by a progressive decline in cognitive, behavioral, and motor functions. Substantial evidence exists that ADC is a direct result of HIV infection. HIV has been found in the brain and cerebrospinal fluid (CSF) of patients with ADC. The brain cells infected by HIV are predominantly the CD4+ cells of monocyte-macrophage lineage. HIV infection is thought to trigger the release of toxins or lymphokines that result in cellular dysfunction or interference with neurotransmitter function rather than cellular damage.

Signs and symptoms may be subtle and difficult to distinguish from fatigue, depression, or the adverse effects of treatments for infections and malignancies. Early manifestations include memory deficits, headache, difficulty with concentration, progressive confusion, psychomotor slowing, apathy, and ataxia. Later stages include global cognitive impairments, delay in verbal responses, a vacant starelike affect, spastic paraparesis, hyperreflexia, psychosis, hallucinations, tremor, incontinence, seizures, mutism, and death.

Confirming the diagnosis of HIV encephalopathy may be difficult. Extensive neurologic evaluation includes a computed tomography (CT) scan, which may indicate diffuse cerebral atrophy and ventricular enlargement. Other tests that may detect abnormalities include magnetic resonance imaging (MRI), analysis of CSF through lumbar puncture, and brain biopsy.

Cryptococcus neoformans. A fungal infection, ***Cryptococcus neoformans*** is the fourth most common opportunistic infection among patients with AIDS and the third most common infectious agent causing neurologic disease. Cryptococcal meningitis is characterized by symptoms such as fever, headache, malaise, stiff neck, nausea, vomiting, mental status changes, and seizures. Diagnosis is confirmed by CSF analysis.

Progressive Multifocal Leukoencephalopathy. **Progressive multifocal leukoencephalopathy** (PML) is a demyelinating central nervous system disorder that affects the oligodendroglia and that occurs in about 3% of AIDS patients. Clinical manifestations often begin with mental confusion and rapidly progress to include blindness, aphasia, paresis (slight paralysis), and death.

Other Neurologic Disorders. Other common infections involving the nervous system include *Toxoplasma gondii,* CMV, and *M. tuberculosis.* Additional neurologic manifestations include both central and peripheral neuropathies. Vascular myelopathy is a degenerative disorder affecting lateral and posterior columns of the spinal cord, resulting in progressive spastic paraparesis, ataxia, and incontinence. HIV-related **peripheral neuropathy** is thought to be a demyelinating disorder; it is associated with pain and numbness in the extremities, weakness, diminished deep tendon reflexes, orthostatic hypotension, and impotence.

DEPRESSIVE MANIFESTATIONS

The prevalence of depression among people with HIV infection is unknown. The causes of depression are multifactorial and may include a history of preexisting mental illness, neuropsychiatric disturbances, and psychosocial factors. Depression also occurs in people with HIV infection in response to the physical symptoms, including pain and weight loss, and the lack of someone to talk with about their concerns. People with HIV/AIDS who are depressed may experience irrational guilt and shame, loss of self-esteem, feelings of helplessness and worthlessness, and suicidal ideation.

INTEGUMENTARY MANIFESTATIONS

Cutaneous manifestations are associated with HIV infection and the accompanying opportunistic infections and malignancies. KS, described previously, and opportunistic infections, such as herpes zoster and herpes simplex, are associated with painful vesicles that disrupt skin integrity. *Molluscum contagiosum* is a viral infection characterized by deforming plaque formation. Seborrheic dermatitis is associated with an indurated, diffuse, scaly rash involving the scalp and face. Patients with AIDS may also exhibit a generalized folliculitis associated with dry, flaking skin or atopic dermatitis, such as eczema or psoriasis. Up to 60% of patients treated with trimethoprim-sulfamethoxazole (TMP-SMZ) for PCP develop a drug-related rash that is pruritic with pinkish red macules and papules. Regardless of the origin of these rashes, patients experience discomfort and are at increased risk for additional infection from disrupted skin integrity.

ENDOCRINE MANIFESTATIONS

Endocrine manifestations of HIV infection are not completely understood. At autopsy, endocrine glands show infiltration and destruction from opportunistic infections or neoplasms. Endocrine function may also be affected by therapeutic agents, although most people with HIV infection do not have clinical evidence of endocrine dysfunction.

MANIFESTATIONS SPECIFIC TO WOMEN

Persistent, recurrent vaginal candidiasis may be the first sign of HIV infection in women. Past or present genital ulcer disease is a risk factor for the transmission of HIV infection. Women with HIV infection are more susceptible to and have increased rates and recurrence of genital ulcer disease and venereal warts. Ulcerative sexually transmitted diseases (STDs), such as chancroid, syphilis, and herpes, are more severe in women with HIV infection. **Human papillomavirus** (HPV) causes venereal warts and is a risk factor for **cervical intraepithelial neoplasia** (CIN), a cellular change that is frequently a precursor to cervical cancer. Women with HIV are 10 times more likely to develop CIN than are those not infected with HIV. There is a strong association between abnormal Papanicolaou smears and HIV seropositivity. HIV-seropositive women with cervical carcinoma present with a more advanced stage of disease and have more persistent and recurrent disease and a shorter interval to recurrence and death than women who do not have HIV infection.

A significant percentage of women who require hospitalization for pelvic inflammatory disease (PID) have HIV infection. Women with HIV are at increased risk for PID, and the inflammation associated with PID may potentiate the transmission of HIV infection. Moreover, women with HIV appear to have a higher incidence of menstrual abnormalities, including amenorrhea or bleeding between periods, than women without HIV infection. The failure of health care providers to consider HIV infection in women may lead to a later diagnosis, thereby denying women appropriate treatment. (Disorders of the female reproductive system are discussed in Chap. 43.)

Assessment and Diagnostic Findings

The HIV diagnosis is based on clinical history, identification of risk factors, physical examination, laboratory evidence of immune dysfunction, identification of HIV antibodies, signs and symptoms, and infections and malignancies included in the CDC classification system for HIV infection. This classification system categorizes HIV infection and AIDS in adults and adolescents on the basis of clinical conditions associated with HIV infection and CD4+ T-cell counts. The classification system, which is presented in Table 48-1, groups clinical conditions into one of three categories denoted as A, B, or C.

Clinical category A consists of one or more listed conditions without any of the conditions listed in categories B or C. Category B consists of symptomatic conditions in HIV-infected patients that are not included in the conditions listed in category C. These conditions must also meet one of the following criteria: (1) the condition is due to HIV infection or a defect in cellular immunity, and (2) the condition must be considered to have a clinical course or require management that is complicated by HIV infection. If an individual was once treated for a category B condition and has not developed a category C disease but is now symptom free, that person's illness would be considered category B. Category C includes clinical conditions listed in the AIDS surveillance case definition. Once a person has had a category C condition, that person will remain in category C.

The CD4+ T-cell counts cover three ranges, which guide management of HIV-infected patients. Although the revised classification emphasizes CD4+ T-cell counts, it allows for CD4+ percentages (percentage of CD4+ T cells of total lymphocytes). The CD4+ percentage is less subject to variation on repeated measurements than is the absolute CD4+ T-cell count. Data correlating the natural history of HIV infection with the CD4+ percentage, however, have not been as consistently available as data on absolute CD4+ T-cell counts. This current classification system is more inclusive of clinical conditions experienced by people with HIV infection.

LABORATORY TESTS AND SPECIAL CONSIDERATIONS

Before an HIV test is performed, the meaning of the test and possible test results are explained, and informed consent for the test is obtained from the patient. When results of the HIV antibody testing are received, they are carefully explained to the patient. All

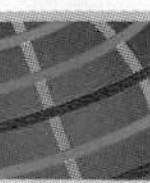

TABLE 48•1 Classification System for HIV Infection and Expanded AIDS Surveillance Case Definition for Adolescents and Adults

Diagnostic Categories	Clinical Categories		
CD4+ T-CELL CATEGORIES	A ASYMPTOMATIC, ACUTE (PRIMARY) HIV OR PGL	B SYMPTOMATIC, NOT (A) OR (C) CONDITIONS	C AIDS-INDICATOR CONDITIONS
(1) ≥500/μL	A1	B1	C1
(2) 200–499/μL	A2	B2	C2
(3) <200/μL AIDS-indicator T-cell count	A3	B3	C3

As of January 1, 1993, people with AIDS-indicator conditions (clinical category C) and those in categories A3 or B3 were considered to have AIDS.

Clinical Category A

Includes one or more of the following in an adult or adolescent with confirmed HIV infection and without conditions in clinical categories B and C:

- Asymptomatic HIV infection
- Persistent generalized lymphadenopathy (PGL)
- Acute (primary) HIV infection with accompanying illness or history of acute HIV infection

Clinical Category B

Examples of conditions in clinical category B include, but are not limited to, the following:

- Bacillary angiomatosis
- Candidiasis, oropharyngeal (thrush), or vulvovaginal (persistent, frequent, or poorly responsive to therapy)
- Cervical dysplasia (moderate or severe)/cervical carcinoma in situ
- Constitutional symptoms, such as fever (38.5°C) or diarrhea exceeding 1 month in duration
- Hairy leukoplakia, oral
- Herpes zoster (shingles), involving at least two distinct episodes or more than one dermatome
- Idiopathic thrombocytopenic purpura
- Listeriosis
- Pelvic inflammatory disease, particularly if complicated by tubo-ovarian abscess
- Peripheral neuropathy

Clinical Category C

Examples of conditions in adults and adolescents include the following:

- Candidiasis of bronchi, trachea, or lungs; esophagus
- Cervical cancer, invasive
- Coccidioidomycosis, disseminated or extrapulmonary
- Cryptococcosis, extrapulmonary
- Cryptosporidiosis, chronic intestinal (exceeding 1 month's duration)
- Cytomegalovirus disease (other than liver, spleen, or lymph nodes)
- Cytomegalovirus retinitis (with loss of vision)
- Encephalopathy, HIV-related
- Herpes simplex: chronic ulcer(s) (exceeding 1 month's duration); or bronchitis, pneumonitis, or esophagitis
- Histoplasmosis, disseminated or extrapulmonary
- Isosporiasis, chronic intestinal (exceeding 1 month's duration)
- Kaposi's sarcoma
- Lymphoma, Burkitt's (or equivalent term); immunoblastic (or equivalent term); primary, of brain
- *Mycobacterium avium* complex or *M. kansasii,* disseminated or extrapulmonary
- *Mycobacterium tuberculosis,* any site (pulmonary or extrapulmonary)
- *Mycobacterium,* other species or unidentified species, disseminated or extrapulmonary
- *Pneumocystis carinii* pneumonia
- Pneumonia, recurrent
- Progressive multifocal leukoencephalopathy
- *Salmonella* septicemia, recurrent
- Toxoplasmosis of brain
- Wasting syndrome due to HIV

Adapted from Centers for Disease Control, U.S. Department of Health and Human Services. (1992). 1993 revised classification system for HIV infection and expanded surveillance case definition for AIDS among adolescents and adults. *MMWR CDC Recommendations and Reports, 41* (RR 17),1–19.

test results are kept confidential. Education and counseling about the test results and disease transmission are essential.

Patients whose test results are seronegative may develop a false sense of security, possibly resulting in continued high-risk behaviors or feelings that they are immune to the virus. They may need ongoing counseling to help them modify high-risk behaviors and to return for repeated testing. Other patients may experience anxiety regarding the uncertainty of their status.

Patients' psychological responses to seropositive test results may include feelings of panic, depression, and hopelessness. The social and interpersonal consequences of a positive test result can be devastating. Patients may lose their sexual partners or their health insurance because of disclosure; they may experience discrimination in employment and housing as well as social ostracism. For these reasons and others, patients who test positive may need ongoing counseling as well as referrals for social, financial, medical, and psychological support services.

Since the discovery of HIV in 1983, scientists have learned much about its characteristics and pathogenicity. Based on this knowledge, diagnostic tests, some still investigational, have been developed. Laboratory tests are now used to diagnose HIV and to monitor disease progression and response to treatment in the HIV-infected person. Table 48-2 summarizes laboratory tests used to diagnose HIV infection and to track its progression.

HIV Antibody Tests. When an individual is infected with HIV, the immune system responds by producing antibodies against the virus. Antibodies generally develop within 3 to 12 weeks of exposure but may take as long as 6 to 14 months. This helps to explain why a person may be infected but not test positive initially. Unfortunately, the antibodies for HIV are ineffective and unable to halt the development of HIV infection. The ability to document HIV antibodies in the blood has permitted screening of blood products and has facilitated diagnostic evaluations of indi-

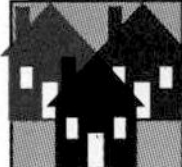

Patient Education and Home Care
HIV Test Results: Implications for Patients

HIV antibody is produced in response to HIV infection. Because seropositivity does not diagnose or confirm AIDS or project future illness, HIV test results must be interpreted cautiously. Some considerations for patients follow.

Interpretation of Positive Test Results

- Antibodies to HIV are present in the blood (the patient has been infected with virus, and the body has produced antibodies).
- HIV is probably active in the body, and the patient should assume that he or she can transmit the virus to others.
- Despite HIV infection, the patient does not necessarily have AIDS.
- The patient may not necessarily get AIDS in the future.
- The patient is not immune to AIDS (the antibodies do not indicate immunity).

Interpretation of Negative Test Results

- Antibodies to HIV are not present in the blood at this time, which can mean that the patient has not been infected with HIV or, if infected, the body has not produced antibodies (which takes from 3 weeks to 6 months or longer).
- The patient should continue taking precautions. The test result does not mean that the patient is immune to the virus, nor does it mean the patient is not infected (it just means that the body may not have produced antibodies yet).

viduals with HIV infection. In 1985, the FDA licensed an HIV antibody assay for all blood and plasma donations.

Three tests are used to confirm the presence of antibody to HIV and to assist in diagnosing HIV infection. The **enzyme-linked immunosorbent assay** (ELISA) test identifies antibodies directed specifically against HIV. The ELISA test does not establish a diagnosis of AIDS. Rather, it indicates that the person has been exposed to or infected with HIV. People whose blood contains antibodies for HIV are said to be seropositive.

The **Western blot assay** is another test that can identify HIV antibodies and is used to confirm seropositivity as identified by the ELISA. Indirect immunofluorescence assay (IFA) is being used by some physicians instead of the Western blot to confirm seropositivity. The advantage of the IFA is that it is rapid, is easy to perform, and requires minimal skill. Another test, the radioimmunoprecipitation assay (RIPA), detects HIV protein rather than antibody.

Home Testing. Home-based testing for HIV infection first proposed in 1985 was not approved by the FDA until 1995. The test, which entails collecting a blood sample on a test card and mailing the card to a laboratory for HIV antibody testing, was withdrawn because of lack of consumer demand. People using the product found that the cost of the kit and laboratory fees were not covered by insurance and were costlier than having the test performed by their health care provider. Several home test kits are available, but only Home Access HIV-1 Test System, from Home Access Health Corp., Hoffman Estates, Illinois, 1-800-HIV-TEST has been approved. Because false-positive test results are possible, any positive result should be confirmed with follow-up blood testing. Those who use home test kits need to know that test results may be negative in the early stages of infection because the body has not yet produced antibodies to HIV.

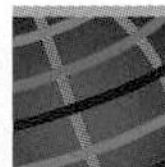

Table 48•2 Selected Laboratory Tests for Diagnosing and Tracking HIV and Assessing Immune Status

Test	Findings in HIV Infection
HIV Antibody Tests	
Enzyme-linked immunosolvent assay (ELISA)	• Positive test result must be confirmed by Western blot
Western blot	• Positive
Indirect immunofluorescence assay (IFA)	• Positive test result must be confirmed by Western blot
Radioimmunoprecipitation assay (RIPA)	• Positive, more sensitive and specific than Western blot
HIV Tracking	
p24 antigen	• Positive for free viral protein
Polymerase chain reaction (PCR)	• Detection of HIV RNA or DNA
Branch DNA (bDNA)	• Detection of HIV RNA
Nucleic acid sequence–based amplification (NASBA)	• Detection of HIV RNA
Peripheral blood mononuclear cell (PBMC) culture for HIV-1	• Positive when two consecutive assays detect reverse transcriptase or p24 antigen in increasing magnitude
Quantitative cell culture	• Measures viral load within cells
Quantitative plasma culture	• Measures viral load by free infectious virus in the plasma
β_2 microglobulin	• Protein is increased with disease progression
Serum neopterin	• Increased levels seen with disease progression
Immune Status	
Number of CD4+ cells	• Decreased
Percentage of CD4+ cells	• Decreased
CD4:CD8 ratio	• Decreased CD4:CD8 ratio
WBC count	• Normal to decreased
Immunoglobulin levels	• Increased
CD4 cell function tests	• T4 cells have decreased ability to respond to antigen
Skin test sensitivity reaction	• Decreased to absent

Testing should be done often if they engage in unprotected sex or injecting drug use.

HIV Tracking. Direct determination of HIV presence and activity is used to track the progression of the disease as well as response to treatment. The **p24** (viral core protein) **antigen** capture assay is highly specific for HIV-1. The levels of p24 antigens in people with asymptomatic HIV infection are very low; however, people with measurable titers of p24 progress to AIDS much sooner. The p24 antigen capture assay has been used along with other tests, such as the CD4+, to evaluate the treatment effects of antiviral agents.

In clinical drug trials, processes called target amplifications, which quantify HIV RNA or DNA levels in the plasma, are replacing p24 antigen capture assays. Target amplification methods include reverse transcriptase **polymerase chain reaction** (RT PCR) or nucleic acid sequence-based amplification (NASBA). A signal amplification method is branched DNA (bDNA). More sensitive versions of these assays are in development. Currently, these tests are used to track viral load and response to treatment for HIV infection.

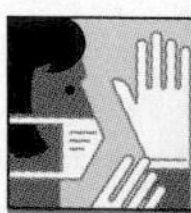

HEALTH PROMOTION AND ILLNESS PREVENTION
Safer Sex and Safer Behaviors

- Practice abstinence.
- Reduce the number of sexual partners to one.
- Always use latex condoms with a water-soluble lubricant containing the spermicide nonoxynol 9.
- Do not reuse condoms.
- Do not use cervical caps or diaphragms without using a condom as well.
- Always use dental dams for oral female genital or anal stimulation.
- Avoid anal intercourse because this practice may injure tissues.
- Avoid manual–anal intercourse (fisting).
- Do not ingest urine or semen.
- Avoid having sex with people who are injecting drug users.
- Engage in nonpenetrative sex such as body massage, social kissing (dry), mutual masturbation, fantasy, and sex films.
- If female, avoid pregnancy if you or your sexual partner is HIV seropositive.
- Inform prospective sexual partners of your HIV-positive status.
- Notify previous and present sexual partners if you learn that you are HIV seropositive.
- If HIV seropositive, do not have unprotected sex with another HIV-seropositive person because cross-infection with another HIV strain can increase the severity of the disease.
- Do not share needles, razors, toothbrushes, sex toys, or other blood-contaminated articles.
- If HIV seropositive, do not donate blood, plasma, body organs, or sperm.

PCR is also used to detect HIV in high-risk seronegative people before the development of antibodies, to confirm a positive ELISA, to screen neonates, and to determine the exact strain of virus that is present. One disadvantage of the PCR is that false-positive test results can occur if the reagents used in the test are contaminated.

HIV culture or quantitative plasma culture and plasma viremia are additional tests that measure viral burden. Other tests may be performed to monitor immune status or to monitor the progression of HIV disease.

Prevention of Disease

Until an effective vaccine is developed (discussed later in this chapter), preventing HIV by eliminating or reducing risk behaviors is essential. Primary prevention efforts through effective educational programs are vital for control and prevention. AIDS is not transmitted by casual contact.

PREVENTIVE EDUCATION

Effective educational programs have been initiated to educate the public regarding safer sexual practices to decrease the risk of transmitting HIV-1 infection to sexual partners. Latex condoms with a water-soluble lubricant containing the spermicide nonoxyl 9 should be used during vaginal or anal intercourse. Nonlatex condoms are available for people with latex allergy. A condom should be used for oral contact with the penis, and dental dams should be used for oral contact with the vagina or rectum.

Other teaching topics include the importance of avoiding sexual practices that might cut or tear the lining of the rectum or penis and avoiding sexual contact with multiple partners or people who are known to be HIV positive or injecting drug users. In addition, people who are HIV positive or use injecting drugs should be instructed not to donate blood or share drug equipment with others.

RELATED REPRODUCTIVE EDUCATION

Because HIV in women usually occurs during the childbearing years, family planning issues need to be addressed. Attempts to achieve pregnancy by couples in which one partner has HIV and the other does not expose the unaffected partner to the virus. Efforts at artificial insemination using processed semen from an HIV-infected partner are underway. Studies are needed because HIV has been found in spermatozoa of patients with AIDS, with possible HIV replication in the male germ cell. Women considering pregnancy need to have adequate information about the risks of transmitting HIV infection to themselves, their partner, and their future children and about the benefits of antiretroviral agents in reducing perinatal HIV transmission. In addition, other than abstinence, the condom has been the only method that has proved to decrease the sexual risk of transmission of HIV infection.

Certain contraceptive methods may pose additional health risks for women. Estrogen in oral contraceptives may increase a women's risk for HIV infection. In addition, women infected with HIV using estrogen oral contraceptives have shown increased shedding of HIV in vaginal and cervical secretions. The intrauterine contraceptive device (IUD) may also increase the risk for HIV transmission because the device's string may serve as a means to transmit HIV infection. In addition, it also can cause penile abrasions. The female condom is as effective in preventing pregnancy as other barrier methods, such as the diaphragm and the male condom. Unlike the diaphragm, the female condom is also effective in preventing the transmission of HIV infection and STDs. The female condom has the distinction of being the first barrier method that can be controlled by women (see Chap. 42).

Gerontologic Considerations

More than 10% of all AIDS cases in the United States have occurred in people aged 50 years or older. Of this percentage, 25% are 60 years of age or older. HIV infection in the elderly may be underreported and underdiagnosed because health care professionals erroneously believe that older people are not at risk for HIV infection. Many older adults are sexually active but do not use condoms, viewing them only as a means of unneeded birth control and not considering themselves at risk for HIV infection. Sexual expression in the elderly population is not limited to heterosexual partners. Many older homosexual men who grew up and lived in an era when disclosure of their sexual orientation was not acceptable have lost long-time partners. Thus, they may turn to younger males for sexual gratification. Older adults may also be injecting drug users or may have received HIV-infected blood through transfusions before 1985. As a result, they may be at risk for HIV infection.

Normal age-related changes include a reduction in immune system function similar to that of HIV infection. Older adults are normally at greater risk for infections, cancer, and autoimmune disorders. Many older adults also experience the loss of loved ones, resulting in depression and bereavement, factors that are also associated with depressed immune function. HIV-related dementia in the older adult may imitate Alzheimer's disease and may be misdiagnosed. As with anyone at risk for HIV infection, the elderly patient needs educational programs that address HIV infection prevention.

HIV as a Chronic Illness

Earlier diagnosis and treatment of opportunistic infections and antiviral therapy are thought to be responsible for a dramatic improvement in survival of people with AIDS since the early years of the epidemic; thus, HIV infection is now being described as a chronic disorder.

People with chronic disability resulting from HIV infection frequently experience fatigue, decreased endurance, weight loss, edema, blindness, and swallowing difficulties leading to various degrees of functional impairment. Many people with HIV infection experience neurologic involvement resulting in dementia, hemiplegia, spastic paraparesis, painful neuropathies, and proximal and distal muscle weakness. In addition to medical and nursing management, many people with chronic HIV infection need the rehabilitation services of occupational, physical, and speech therapists.

Almost all AIDS patients develop at least one opportunistic infection during the course of the disease. Although many infections are successfully treated, some patients never fully recover and are at increased risk for a second infection or cancer. Treatment is often complicated by the debilitating signs and symptoms of HIV/AIDS, which include unexplained fatigue, headache, profuse night sweats, unexplained weight loss, dry cough, shortness of breath, extreme weakness, diarrhea, and persistent lymphadenopathy. Chronic illness develops when opportunistic diseases and the symptoms of HIV/AIDS do not resolve. The effects of chronic illness—decreased energy, increased expenses, change in lifestyle, repeated and prolonged hospitalizations—can be devastating.

Patients who progress to the terminal phases of HIV/AIDS are usually severely immunocompromised. Multiple local and disseminated infections involving several organ systems are common. Many people become profoundly malnourished as a result of impaired oral intake, GI malabsorption, and the effects of opportunistic diseases. Pulmonary, renal, and hepatic failure may develop as a result of infection or malignancy. Skin breakdown related to immobility, profuse diarrhea, and progression of KS is common. Neurologic impairments may progress to coma and eventually death.

Patients in the advanced stages of HIV/AIDS usually cannot work, maintain current roles or relationships, or care for themselves independently. Death occurs because there is no known effective treatment for the opportunistic diseases or the patient no longer responds to standard therapy.

Medical Management

Medical management efforts encompass several approaches, including treatment of HIV-associated infections and malignancies, arresting HIV replication through antiviral agents, and augmentation and restoration of the immune system by using immunomodulators. Supportive care is needed because of the debilitating effects of HIV infection and AIDS, including malnutrition, skin breakdown, immobility, and altered mental status.

ANTIRETROVIRAL THERAPY

In 1998, the CDC recommended that all people who have advanced or symptomatic HIV infection receive aggressive antiviral therapy. Initiation of therapy in those with asymptomatic infection is much more complex, and virologic, immunologic, and social factors must be considered. In general, therapy should be offered to all people whose CD4+ T-cell count is less than 500/mm^3. The strength of the recommendation should be based on the person's willingness to accept therapy and the prognosis for AIDS-free survival. People who have more than 500/mm^3. CD4+ T cells can be observed for progression to AIDS or offered therapy. In this case, the risk of progression to AIDS should be based on levels of HIV viral load and CD4+ cell count. Ideally, viral load and CD4+ count should be measured twice before initiating therapy or changing the antiviral regimen.

Once antiretroviral therapy is initiated, treatment should be aggressive. Viral suppression is the goal. Initially, highly active antiretroviral therapy (HAART) consisting of a triple-drug regimen—a protease inhibitor and two non-nucleoside reverse transcriptase inhibitors—is recommended. Drawbacks of HAART are difficulty with adherence to the regimen, the need for taking multiple medications on different dosing schedules, and risk for drug interactions. The duration of therapy in acute HIV infection is unknown, but may continue for several years or for life.

Combination therapy is now the standard of care for patients who can tolerate it. Initially, zidovudine (AZT) was used with one of the other reverse transcriptase inhibitors. As new drugs are developed, the number of combinations continue to increase. Safety and efficacy data on many of the combination therapies are limited. Use of three- and four-drug combination regimens has become more widespread, starting earlier in the course of infection, with careful monitoring by quantitative viral load measures. In some patients receiving three-drug regimens, viral load levels are so low that they are no longer measurable. Future therapy may be individualized based on the viral strain and resistance to antiretroviral drugs (Table 48-3).

IMMUNOMODULATOR THERAPY

Combating AIDS requires not only agents that will inhibit viral growth but also agents that will restore or augment the damaged immune system. Low-dose oral **alpha-interferon** is being studied for its antiviral properties and its ability to stimulate macrophages and T-cell lymphocytes. Parenteral alpha-interferon is also being used to treat cutaneous KS. Other substances being evaluated for their role in macrophage and lymphocyte stimulation include IL-2, inosine pranobex (Isoprinosine), diethyldithiocarbamate (DTC), lentinan, and granulocyte-macrophage **colony-stimulating factor** (G-CSF). G-CSF, along with erythropoietin, is being used to reverse anemia and neutropenia caused by zidovudine therapy.

Many of these substances cause a flulike reaction that includes fevers, chills, arthralgias, myalgias, and headache. In addition, some agents cause nausea, vomiting, elevated liver enzymes, neutropenia, confusion, and behavioral changes.

VACCINES

Since it was first discovered, researchers have been working to develop a vaccine for HIV. A vaccine is a substance that triggers the production of antibodies to destroy the offending organism.

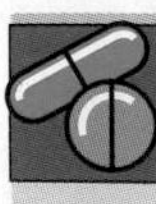

TABLE 48•3 Antiretroviral Agents

Drug	Uses	Comments
Nucleoside Reverse Transcriptase Inhibitors (NRTIs)		
Inhibit viral reverse transcriptase and prevent reproduction of HIV by mimicking one of the molecular substances used by HIV to build DNA for new virus particles. By altering the structural components of the DNA chain, new virus production is inhibited.		
zidovudine (ZDV, Retrovir; formerly called AZT)	Approved for use for severe HIV infection/AIDS, for use in HIV before profound immunosuppression occurs, and for use in HIV-positive pregnant women to reduce the risk of perinatal transmission. *Note:* Research (Hirsch, D'Aguila, & Kaplan, 1997) demonstrates benefits to be time limited and most effective in combination with other antiretroviral drugs.	• Side effects include bone marrow toxicity, dose-limiting anemia, and neutropenia requiring discontinuation of medication *Note:* Granulocyte colony-stimulating factor (G-CSF) and epoetin alfa (human recombinant erythropoietin [Epogen, Procrit]) are effective in treating neutropenia and anemia associated with zidovudine use. The body produces colony-stimulating factors to stimulate growth and production of red and white blood cells. • Other side effects are nausea, GI upset, fevers, chills, aches, and headache. Less common are confusion, somnolence, and seizures. • Zidovudine may be discontinued if the patient needs treatment for opportunistic infections, lymphomas, and other malignancies because treatments for these conditions may cause hematologic toxicity. • Regular examinations, assessment, and management of side effects are indicated. • Medication costs may prompt referrals for financial counseling.
didanosine (ddI, Videx)	Shows promise as an alternative to zidovudine *Note:* Therapy with didanosine either alone or combined with zidovudine resulted in a survival benefit when compared with therapy with zidovudine alone (Hirsch, D'Aquila, & Kaplan, 1997)	• For adequate absorption, administer medication on an empty stomach or 30 minutes before or 1 to 2 hours after a meal. • The major dose-limiting toxicities associated with ddI are life-threatening pancreatitis and peripheral neuropathy. Other toxicities include diarrhea, restlessness, and increased serum uric acid levels (in high-dose therapy). • Nausea, diarrhea, confusion, seizures, headache, electrolyte abnormalities, and cardiac dysrhythmias are additional side effects.
zalcitabine (ddC, HIVID)	Because the HIV virus mutates rapidly and drug resistance occurs, zalcitabine is best used for combination therapy to control HIV.	• Severe peripheral neuropathy can occur with high doses. • Other toxicities include GI intolerance and mucosal ulcerations. • In treating AIDS-related encephalopathy, ddC does not penetrate the spinal fluid and thus is not as effective as zidovudine.
stavudine (d4T, Zerit)	For patients with advanced HIV infection who are unresponsive to other antiviral agents or who cannot tolerate their side effects	• Major adverse effects include peripheral neuropathy, suppression of bone marrow, myalgia, and hepatotoxicity. Peripheral neuropathy is signaled by pain, burning, aching, weakness, or other changes in sensation. These signs and symptoms should be reported.
lamivudine (3TC, Epivir)	Useful with zidovudine; active against hepatitis B	• Slight increase in headaches and side effects similar to those associated with zidovudine; rarely, mania and psychosis.
abacavir (ABC, Zigan)	Combined with ZDV and 3TC, which seems to suppress plasma viral load	• Side effects include hypersensitivity (can be fatal), fever, rash, nausea and vomiting, malaise, loss of appetite, lactic acidosis with rare but fatal liver changes.
efavirenz (Sustiva)	Inhibits HIV production	• Side effects include rash, CNS symptoms (insomnia or somnolence, dizziness, hallucinations, confusion, amnesia, distractibility, agitation), increased transaminase levels.
Non-nucleoside Reverse Transcriptase Inhibitors (NNRTIs)		
Bind directly to reverse transcriptase acting at the same site in the HIV life cycle as the reverse transcriptase inhibitors		
nevirapine (Viramune)	Inhibits HIV production	• Side effects include rash, fever, and thrombocytopenia (NNRTIs). • Resistance to the beneficial effects of this medication emerges rapidly when used alone. • Do not coadminister with protease inhibitors because interaction reduces the serum concentration of protease inhibitor.
delavirdine (Rescriptor)	Inhibits HIV production	• Side effects include rash. • Resistance to the beneficial effects of this medication emerges rapidly when used alone. • Do not coadminister with protease inhibitors because interaction reduces the serum concentration of protease inhibitor.

(*continued*)

TABLE 48•3 Antiretroviral Agents *(Continued)*

Drug	Uses	Comments
Protease Inhibitors (PIs) Inhibit the function of protease, an enzyme needed for HIV replication and production of infectious virions. PIs act at a later point in the HIV life cycle than the reverse transcriptase inhibitors. Inhibition of HIV-1 protease results in noninfectious virus particles with reduced reverse transcriptase activity. Because these agents inhibit virus replication in a different way than reverse transcriptase inhibitors, they show promise in combination with reverse transcriptase inhibitors. They have high potency and low toxicity.		
saquinavir (Fortovace)	Approved by FDA for use in combination with nucleoside reverse transcriptase inhibitors.	• Least potent and best tolerated of all the PIs • Mild GI discomfort; must be taken within 2 hours after a full meal (*Note:* Blood levels of the drug after a high-calorie, high-fat meal were two times higher than those after a low-calorie, low-fat meal [Phillips, 1996]). • Preparation formulated with lactose may cause diarrhea.
ritonavir (Norvir)	Approved for clinical use in combination with other established antiretroviral therapy to effect a significant drop in the viral load and an increase in the CD4+ count	• Nausea and GI distress; tingling in hands and feet • Ritonavir can interact with other medications to increase their plasma concentrations (eg, antidepressants, sedatives, hypnotics, calcium-channel blockers, and analgesics). Because ritonavir is formulated with alcohol, it cannot be administered with disulfiram (Antabuse) or metronidazole, which would result in disulfiram reaction (including nausea and vomiting, flushing headache, hyperventilation and dyspnea, palpitations and chest pain, confusion, and anxiety). • Other side effects include diarrhea, abdominal pain, and anorexia. Significant common GI effects may often be prevented or minimized by starting with a low dose and increasing the dose. Sometimes, nausea can be controlled by taking the medication with a high-fat meal.
indinavir (Crixivan)	Used in combination with other antiretroviral agents to reduce HIV counts	• The most potent anti-HIV activity of currently available PIs, but viral strains develop resistance after a few weeks in most patients. • A virus resistant to indinavir is likely to be cross-resistant to ritonavir. • Side effects include asymptomatic hyperbilirubinema and kidney stones (nephrolithiasis) composed of precipitated drug. Kidney function is unaffected but pain management may be needed because kidney stones can cause great discomfort. *Note:* Kidney stones may be prevented by drinking at least six 8-ounce glasses of water daily, including a full glass of water with each dose of indinavir (although stones may still occur despite increased fluid intake). • Dose reduction is not recommended even though the drug can be halted for a few days. • Indinavir must be taken every 8 hours on an empty stomach or with a very light meal to ensure adequate absorption. This schedule and fluid requirements make this medication regimen difficult to follow.
nelfinavir (Viracept)	Used with other antiretroviral agents to reduce HIV counts	• Side effects include diarrhea, hyperglycemia, fat distribution and lipid abnormalities, possible bleeding in hemophiliacs

Most vaccines activate the humoral arm of the immune system, which stimulates the production of protective antibodies. In addition to antibodies, B lymphocytes take the form of memory B cells. These cells do not produce antibodies immediately but respond vigorously to subsequent exposure. Vaccines that stimulate the cellular arm of the immune system are being developed. Many HIV vaccine researchers are working on this type of vaccine because those designed to generate antibodies to HIV have failed to elicit an immune response against strains of the virus.

Since 1995, there have been a variety of vaccines under study using different strategies to prevent HIV infection in animals and humans. Some researchers are exploring whether different immunization schedules, different schedules of boosters, or a combination of several vaccines will result in stronger or more durable responses.

At present, there is no evidence that vaccination against HIV is possible. Many strains of HIV with distinctly different structures have been identified from different parts of the world. It is not known if these differences will hamper the development of effective vaccines. No protective vaccines are ready for large-scale testing in humans. Extensive research is directed toward development of a vaccine using live attenuated (weakened) HIV virus.

MEDICATIONS FOR HIV-RELATED INFECTIONS

General Infections. TMP-SMZ (Bactrim, Septra) is an antibacterial agent for treating various organisms causing infection. Patients with AIDS who are treated with TMP-SMZ experience a high incidence of adverse effects, such as fever, rashes, leukopenia, thrombocytopenia, and renal dysfunction. Recently, desensitization for TMP-SMZ drug-related reactions has been successful. Intravenous administration in patients with normal GI function has not been found to be more advantageous.

Pneumocystis carinii Pneumonia. In the past several years, there have been many advances in the treatment of PCP. TMP-SMZ, the drug of choice for PCP in patients with AIDS and in immunocompromised patients without HIV infection, is available in both intravenous and oral preparations.

Pentamidine, an antiprotozoal medication, is used as an alternative agent for combating PCP. If adverse effects develop or if patients do not improve clinically when treated with TMP-SMZ, the health care provider may recommend pentamidine. Intramuscular administration is avoided because of the potential for painful sterile abscess formation. Also, intravenous pentamidine may cause severe hypotension if it is administered too rapidly. Other adverse effects include impaired glucose metabolism (with frank diabetes mellitus), renal damage, hepatic dysfunction, and neutropenia. Initially, the success of aerosolized pentamidine (AP) led to its use as a treatment for mild to moderate PCP. However, it has proved to be less effective and more costly than TMP-SMZ, and early relapses are common. Because of these limitations, the inhalant form of pentamidine is usually reserved for patients with mild to moderate PCP who are intolerant of other treatments. The combination of TMP-SMZ and pentamidine has shown no additional benefit and is avoided because of the cumulative toxic effects that may result.

The combination of oral trimethoprim (Proloprim, Trimpex) and dapsone (Avlosulfon, DDS) has proved highly effective for treating mild to moderate PCP. Other medications being evaluated as rescue therapy for patients who fail to respond to conventional therapy include intravenous clindamycin (Cleosin HCl), oral primaquine, trimetrexate, hydroxynapthoquinone, and atovaquone (Mepron). Some patients with moderate to severe PCP benefit from systemic corticosteroids; however, there are no data to justify the use of corticosteroids for mild PCP or rescue therapy.

Mycobacterium avium Complex. Treatment for MAC infections involves multidrug regimens administered over a prolonged period. Combination therapy with two to five agents is presently recommended. The most commonly used agents include clarithromycin (Biaxin), azithromycin (Zithromax), rifampin, (Rifadin, Rimactane), rifabutin (Mycobutin), clofazimine (Lamprene), ethambutal (Myambutal), ciprofloxacin (Cipro), and amikacin. There is limited consensus regarding the optimal regimen. Many patients take clarithromycin or azithromycin with one or more other agents to minimize toxicity or drug interactions. Rifabutin has been shown to be effective in preventing MAC in patients with HIV infection who have CD4+ cell counts of 200/mm^3 or less. Because of the likelihood of development of resistant strains, monotherapy is discouraged.

Meningitis. Current primary therapy for cryptococcal meningitis is intravenous amphotericin B with or without oral flucytosine or fluconazole (Diflucan). Serious potential adverse effects of amphotericin B include anaphylaxis, renal and hepatic impairment, electrolyte imbalances, anemia, fevers, and rigors. Intrathecal administration of amphotericin B has been used in place of or in combination with intravenous administration in patients who have failed to respond to the latter. Until fluconazole, a new antifungal agent, was approved and used for lifelong suppressive therapy, frequent relapses and high mortality rates often necessitated prolonged therapy with amphotericin B. In some instances, the patient continues to receive intravenous amphotericin in the home setting. Oral fluconazole is used as suppressive therapy when the CSF tests negative for the organism. This medication is less toxic and better tolerated than amphotericin B.

Cytomegalovirus Retinitis. Retinitis caused by CMV is a leading cause of blindness in patients with AIDS. Two antiviral agents, ganciclovir and foscarnet (Foscavir) offer effective treatment but not a cure for CMV retinitis. Because ganciclovir and foscarnet do not kill the virus but rather control its growth, they must be given for the remainder of the patient's life. Relapse rates of the two agents are similar. Discontinuation of the medication is associated with the relapse of retinitis within 1 month. Initially, ganciclovir is given intravenously (based on body weight) every 12 hours for 2 to 3 weeks. Maintenance therapy is given once a day for 5 to 7 days each week to prevent relapse. Initially, foscarnet is given intravenously every 8 hours for 2 to 3 weeks. Maintenance therapy is given over 2 to 3 hours five times per week. Either may be prescribed for home administration once long-term venous access is established. In some patients, CMV retinitis progresses despite treatment.

A common adverse reaction to ganciclovir is severe neutropenia, which limits the concomitant use of zidovudine. For patients who cannot tolerate systemic ganciclovir because of severe neutropenia, infection at the venous access site, or the need to take zidovudine, intravitreal injections of ganciclovir have been effective. Zidovudine can be given with foscarnet. Common adverse reactions to foscarnet are nephrotoxicity, including acute renal failure, and electrolyte imbalances, including hypocalcemia, hyperphosphatemia, and hypomagnesemia, which can be life-threatening. Other common adverse effects include seizures, GI disturbances, anemia, phlebitis at the infusion site, and low back pain. Possible bone marrow suppression (producing a decrease in white blood cell and platelet counts), oral candidiasis, and liver and renal impairments require close patient monitoring.

Cidofovir is a systematic agent used for the intravenous treatment of CMV retinitis. Because of its long intracellular half-life, it can be administered less frequently. Initial treatment with cidofovir is given once a week for 2 weeks followed by maintenance doses once every other week. It can be given to patients with AIDS with newly diagnosed CMV retinitis as well as those whose disease has relapsed on ganciclovir or foscarnet. The major toxicity is renal damage. To prevent renal damage, it is given with concomitant saline hydration and probenecid. Probenecid inhibits active renal tubular secretion of ionic drugs, such as cidofovir. Before the day of infusion, blood and urine tests are obtained to measure serum creatinine and urine protein values. The cidofovir dosage is reduced if the serum creatinine levels increase, and the medication may be discontinued if the urine protein levels increase. Patients with advanced HIV infection often receive other nephrotoxic medications for treatment of other opportunistic infections and cancer. Therefore, these medications must be administered with great caution. Examples of these drugs are amikacin, gentamicin, tobramycin, amphotericin B, foscarnet, nonsteroidal anti-inflammatory drugs (NSAIDs), pentamidine, and vancomycin. Careful assessment, patient teaching, and outpatient monitoring are needed.

Other Infections. Acyclovir and foscarnet are being used to treat encephalitis caused by herpes simplex or herpes zoster. Pyrimethamine (Daraprim) and sulfadiazine or clindamycin

(Cleosin HCl) are used both for treatment and for lifelong suppressive therapy for *Toxoplasmosis gondii.* Esophageal or oral candidiasis is treated topically with clotrimazole (Mycelex) oral troches or nystatin suspension. Chronic refractory infection with candidiasis (thrush) or esophageal involvement is treated with ketoconazole or fluconazole.

ANTIDIARRHEAL THERAPY

Although many forms of infectious diarrhea respond to treatment, it is not unusual for the infections to recur and become a chronic problem for the patient. Therapy with octreotide acetate (Sandostatin), a synthetic analog of somatostatin, has been shown to be effective in managing chronic severe diarrhea. High concentrations of somatostatin receptors have been found in the GI tract and other tissues. Somatostatin inhibits many physiologic functions, including GI motility and intestinal secretion of water and electrolytes.

MEDICATION THERAPY FOR NUTRITIONAL DISORDERS

Appetite stimulants have been successfully used in patients with AIDS-related anorexia. Megestrol acetate (Megace), a synthetic oral progesterone preparation used to treat breast cancer, promotes significant weight gain and inhibits cytokine IL-1 synthesis. In patients with HIV infection, it increases body weight primarily by increasing body fat stores. Dronabinol (Marinol), synthetic tetrahydrocannabinol (THC), the active ingredient in marijuana, has been used to relieve nausea and vomiting associated with cancer chemotherapy. Preliminary results show that after beginning Marinol therapy, almost all patients with HIV infection experience a modest weight gain. The effects on body composition are unknown.

CHEMOTHERAPY

Kaposi's Sarcoma. Management of KS is usually difficult because of the variability of symptoms and the organ systems involved. KS is rarely life-threatening except when there is pulmonary or GI involvement. The treatment goal is reduction of symptoms by decreasing the size of the skin lesions, reducing discomfort associated with edema and ulcerations, and controlling symptoms associated with mucosal or visceral involvement. No one treatment has been shown to increase survival. Localized treatment includes surgical excision of the lesions or application of liquid nitrogen to local skin lesions and injections of intraoral lesions with dilute vinblastine. Injection of intraoral lesions has been associated with local pain and skin irritation. To date, the most effective chemotherapy regimen appears to be ABV (doxorubicin [Adriamycin], bleomycin, and vincristine). However, significant myelosuppression occurs in 40% to 50% of patients on this regimen, with a 30% increase in the incidence of opportunistic infections.

Radiation therapy is effective as a palliative measure to relieve localized pain due to tumor mass (especially in the legs) or for KS lesions that are in sites such as the oral mucosa, conjunctiva, face and soles of the feet.

Interferon is known for its antiviral and antitumor effects. Patients with cutaneous KS treated with alpha-interferon have experienced tumor regression and improved immune system function. Positive responses have been observed in 30% to 50% of patients, with the best responses seen in those with limited disease and no opportunistic infections. Alpha-interferon is administered by either the intravenous, intramuscular, or subcutaneous route. Patients may self-administer interferon at home or receive it in an outpatient setting.

Lymphoma. Successful treatment of AIDS-related lymphomas has been limited because of the rapid progression of these malignancies. Combination chemotherapy and radiation therapy regimens may produce an initial response, but the response is usually short-lived. Because standard regimens for non-AIDS lymphomas have been ineffective, many clinicians suggest that AIDS-related lymphomas be studied as a separate group in clinical trials.

ANTIDEPRESSANT THERAPY

Treatment for depression in people with HIV infection involves psychotherapy integrated with pharmacology. If depressive symptoms are severe and of sufficient duration, treatment with antidepressants may be initiated. Antidepressants, such as imipramine (Tofranil), desipramine (Norpramin), and fluoxetine (Prozac), may be used because these medications also alleviate the fatigue and lethargy that are associated with depression. A psychostimulant, such as methylphenidate (Ritalin), may be used in low doses in patients with neuropsychiatric impairment. Electroconvulsive therapy may be considered an option for patients with severe depression that has not responded to pharmacologic interventions.

NUTRITIONAL THERAPY

Malnutrition increases the risk for infection and may also increase the incidence of opportunistic infections. Nutrition therapy should be integrated into the overall management plan and should be tailored to meet the nutritional needs of the patient, from oral diet to enteral tube feedings through parenteral nutritional support if needed. As with all patients, a balanced diet is essential for the patient with HIV infection. Calorie counts should be obtained for all patients with AIDS with unexplained weight loss to evaluate nutritional status and to initiate appropriate therapy. The goal is to maintain the patient's ideal weight and, when necessary, to increase weight.

Oral supplements may be used to supplement diets deficient in calories and protein. Ideally, oral supplements should be lactose free (many people with HIV infection are lactose intolerant), high in calories and easily digestible protein, low in fat with the fat easily digestible, palatable, inexpensive, and tolerated without causing diarrhea. Advera is a nutritional supplement that has been developed specifically for people with HIV infection and AIDS. Parenteral nutrition is the final option because of the costs and associated risks, including infections.

Alternative Management (Therapies)

Traditional Western medicine focuses on the treatment of disease. These treatments or interventions are taught in medical schools and are used by physicians in the care of patients. Alternative therapies are often viewed as unconventional and unorthodox treatments or interventions not traditionally taught in medical schools. Alternative therapy stresses the need to treat the whole person, recognizing the interaction of the body, mind, and spirit. What is considered to be an alternative therapy in one culture may actually be a traditional therapy in another. The use of alternative therapy in HIV infection and AIDS has resulted from disillusionment with standard medical treatment, which to date has provided no cure. Used with traditional therapies, alternative therapies may improve the patient's overall well-being.

Alternative therapies can be divided into four categories:

- *Spiritual or psychological therapies* may include humor, hypnosis, faith healing, guided imagery, and positive affirmations.
- *Nutritional therapies* may include vegetarian or macrobiotic diets, vitamin C or beta-carotene supplements, and turmeric, which contains curcumin, a food spice supplement. Chinese herbs, such as traditional herbal mixtures, as well as compound Q (a Chinese cucumber extract) and *Monmordica charantia* (bitter melon), which is given as an enema, are also used.
- *Drug and biologic therapies* include medicines not approved by the FDA. Examples of these include *N*-acetylcysteine, pentoxifylline (Trental), and 1-chloro-2, 4-dinitrobenzene. Also included in this category are oxygen therapy, ozone therapy, and urine therapy.
- *Treatment with physical forces and devices* may include acupuncture, acupressure, massage therapy, reflexology, therapeutic touch, yoga, and crystals.

Although there is insufficient research on the effects of alternate therapy, there is a growing body of literature reporting benefits in area of nutrition, exercise, psychosocial treatment, and Chinese medicine. Clinical trials are in progress to examine the effect of Chinese herbal treatments of HIV-associated symptoms related to inadequate nutrition, such as fatigue, nausea, vomiting, painful or difficult swallowing, altered taste sensation, and diarrhea. At the present time, there are no definitive study results that indicate that these treatments are effective, but some look as though they may be show some promise.

Many patients who use these alternative therapies do not always report their use to their health care providers. To obtain a complete health history, the nurse should ask questions about their use of alternative therapies. Patients may need to be encouraged to report their use to their primary health care provider. Problems may arise when patients are using alternative therapies while they are participating in clinical drug trials. They may have significant adverse side effects, making it difficult to assess the effects of the medications in the clinical trial. The nurse needs to become familiar with the potential adverse side effects of alternative therapies. The nurse who suspects that the alternative therapy is causing a side effect needs to discuss this with the patient, the alternative therapy provider, and the primary health care provider. It is important for the nurse to view alternative therapies with an open mind and to try to understand the importance of this treatment to the patient. Doing so will improve communication with the patient and reduce conflict, so that all involved in care can meet the patient's needs.

Supportive Care

Patients who are weak and debilitated as a result of chronic illness associated with HIV infection typically require many kinds of supportive care. Nutritional support may be as simple as providing assistance in obtaining or preparing meals. For patients with more advanced nutritional impairment that results from decreased intake, wasting syndrome, or GI malabsorption associated with diarrhea, parenteral feedings, such as total parenteral nutrition, may be required. Imbalances that result from nausea, vomiting, and profuse diarrhea often necessitate intravenous fluid and electrolyte replacement.

Skin breakdown associated with KS, perianal skin excoriation, and immobility is managed with thorough and meticulous skin care involving regular turning, cleansing, and applying medicated ointments and dressings.

Pain associated with skin breakdown, abdominal cramping, peripheral neuropathy, or KS is managed by analgesics given at regular intervals around the clock. Relaxation and guided imagery may be helpful in reducing pain and anxiety in some patients.

Pulmonary symptoms, such as dyspnea and shortness of breath, may be related to infection, KS, or fatigue. For these patients, oxygen therapy, relaxation training, and energy conservation techniques may be helpful. Patients with severe respiratory dysfunction may require mechanical ventilation. Before placing a patient on mechanical ventilation, the procedure is explained to the patient and the caregiver. The patient may elect not to be placed on mechanical ventilation, and the patient's wishes should be followed. Ideally, the patient has prepared an advanced directive identifying preferences for treatments and end-of-life care, including hospice care. If the patient has not identified preferences in advance, treatment options are described, so that the patient can make informed decisions and have those wishes respected.

NURSING PROCESS: THE PATIENT WITH AIDS

The nursing care of patients with AIDS is challenging because of the potential for any organ system to be the target of infections or cancers. In addition, this disease is complicated by many emotional, social, and ethical issues. The plan of care for the patient with AIDS is individualized to meet the needs of the patient (Plan of Nursing Care 48-1). Care includes many of the interventions and concerns cited previously in the supportive care section.

Assessment

Nursing assessment includes identification of potential risk factors, including a history of risky sexual practices and injecting drug use. The patient's physical status and psychological status are assessed. All factors affecting immune system functioning are thoroughly explored.

Nutritional Status

Nutritional status is assessed by obtaining a dietary history and identifying factors that may interfere with oral intake, such as anorexia, nausea, vomiting, oral pain, or difficulty swallowing. In addition, the patient's ability to purchase and prepare food is assessed. Weight, anthropometric measurements, and blood urea nitrogen (BUN), serum protein, albumin, and transferrin levels provide objective measurements of nutritional status.

Skin Integrity

The skin and mucous membranes are inspected daily for evidence of breakdown, ulceration, or infection. The oral cavity is monitored for redness, ulcerations, and the presence of creamy-white patches indicative of candidiasis. Assessment of the perianal area for excoriation and infection in those patients with profuse diarrhea is important. Wounds are cultured to identify infectious organisms.

(*text continues on page 1371*)

48•1

PLAN OF NURSING CARE

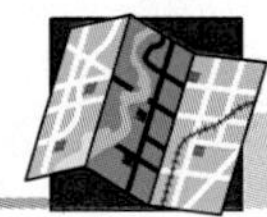

Care of the Patient With AIDS

Nursing Diagnosis: Diarrhea related to enteric pathogens or HIV infection
Goal: Resumption of usual bowel habits

Nursing Interventions

1. Assess patient's normal bowel habits.
2. Assess for diarrhea: frequent, loose stools; abdominal pain or cramping, volume of liquid stools, and exacerbating and alleviating factors.
3. Obtain stool cultures and administer antimicrobial therapy as prescribed.
4. Initiate measures to reduce hyperactivity of bowel:
   a. Maintain food and fluid restrictions as prescribed.
   b. Discourage smoking.
   c. Avoid bowel irritants such as fatty or fried foods, raw vegetables, and nuts. Offer small, frequent meals.
5. Administer anticholinergic antispasmodics and opioids or other medications as prescribed.
6. Maintain fluid intake of at least 3 L unless contraindicated.

Rationale

1. Provides baseline for evaluation.
2. Detects changes in status, quantifies loss of fluid, and provides basis for nursing measures.
3. Identifies pathogenic organism; therapy targets specific organism.
4. Promotes bowel rest, which may decrease acute episodes.
   a. Reduces stimulation of bowel.
   b. Eliminates nicotine which acts as bowel stimulant.
   c. Prevents stimulation of bowel and abdominal distention and promotes adequate nutrition.
5. Decreases intestinal spasms and motility.
6. Prevents hypovolemia.

Expected Outcomes

- Exhibits return to normal bowel patterns
- Reports decreasing episodes of diarrhea and abdominal cramping
- Identifies and avoids foods that irritate the gastrointestinal tract
- Appropriate therapy is initiated as prescribed
- Exhibits normal stool cultures
- Maintains adequate fluid intake
- Maintains body weight and reports no additional weight loss
- States rationale for avoiding smoking
- Enrolls in program to stop smoking
- Uses medication as prescribed
- Maintains adequate fluid status
- Exhibits normal skin turgor, moist mucous membranes, adequate urine output, and absence of excessive thirst

Nursing Diagnosis: Risk for infection related to immunodeficiency
Goal: Absence of infection

Nursing Interventions

1. Monitor for infection: fever, chills, and diaphoresis; cough; shortness of breath; oral pain or painful swallowing; creamy-white patches in oral cavity; urinary frequency, urgency, or dysuria; redness, swelling, or drainage from wounds; vesicular lesions on face, lips, or perianal area.
2. Teach patient or caregiver about need to report possible infection.
3. Monitor white blood cell count and differential.
4. Obtain cultures of wound drainage, skin lesions, urine, stool, sputum, mouth, and blood as prescribed. Administer antimicrobial therapy as prescribed.
5. Instruct patient in ways to prevent infection:
   a. Clean kitchen and bathroom surfaces with disinfectants.
   b. Clean hands thoroughly after exposure to body fluids.
   c. Avoid exposure to others' body fluids or sharing eating utensils.
   d. Turn, cough, and deep breathe, especially when activity is decreased.
   e. Maintain cleanliness of perianal area.

Rationale

1. Allows for early detection of infection, essential for prompt initiation of treatment. Repeated and prolonged infections contribute to patient's debilitation.
2. Allows early detection of infection.
3. Identifies elevated WBC possibly associated with infection.
4. Assists in determining offending organism to initiate appropriate treatment.
5. Minimizes exposure to infection and transmission of HIV infection to others.

Expected Outcomes

- Identifies reportable signs and symptoms of infection
- Reports signs and symptoms of infection if present
- Exhibits and reports absence of fever, chills, and diaphoresis
- Exhibits normal (clear) breath sounds without adventitious breath sounds
- Maintains weight
- Reports adequate energy level without excessive fatigue
- Reports absence of shortness of breath and cough
- Exhibits pink, moist oral mucous membranes without fissures or lesions
- Takes appropriate therapy as prescribed
- Experiences no infection
- States rationale for strategies to avoid infection
- Modifies activities to reduce exposure to infection or infectious persons
- Practices "safer sex"
- Avoids sharing eating utensils and toothbrush
- Exhibits normal body temperature

(continued)

48•1

PLAN OF NURSING CARE

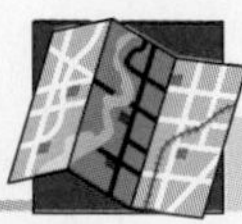

Care of the Patient With AIDS (*continued*)

Nursing Interventions

f. Avoid handling pet excreta or cleaning litter boxes, bird cages, or aquariums.
g. Cook meat and eggs thoroughly.

6. Maintain aseptic technique when performing invasive procedures such as venipunctures, bladder catheterizations, and injections.

Rationale

6. Prevents hospital-acquired infections.

Expected Outcomes

- Uses recommended techniques to maintain cleanliness of skin, skin lesions, and perianal area
- Has others handle pet excreta and cleanup
- Uses recommended cooking techniques

Nursing Diagnosis: Ineffective airway clearance related to *Pneumocystis carinii* pneumonia, increased bronchial secretions, and decreased ability to cough related to weakness and fatigue

Goal: Improved airway clearance

Nursing Interventions

1. Assess and report signs and symptoms of altered respiratory status, tachypnea, use of accessory muscles, cough, color and amount of sputum, abnormal breath sounds, dusky or cyanotic skin color, restlessness, confusion, or somnolence.
2. Obtain sputum sample for culture prescribed. Administer antimicrobial therapy as prescribed.
3. Provide pulmonary care (cough, deep breathing, postural drainage, and vibration) every 2 to 4 hours.
4. Assist patient in attaining semi- or high-Fowler's position.
5. Encourage adequate rest periods.
6. Initiate measures to decrease viscosity of secretions:
   a. Maintain fluid intake of at least 3 L per day unless contraindicated.
   b. Humidify inspired air as prescribed.
   c. Consult with physician concerning use of mucolytic agents delivered through nebulizer or IPPB treatment.
7. Perform tracheal suctioning as needed.
8. Administer oxygen therapy as prescribed.
9. Assist with endotracheal intubation; maintain ventilator settings as prescribed.

Rationale

1. Indicates abnormal respiratory function.
2. Aids in identification of pathogenic organisms.
3. Prevents stasis of secretions and promotes airway clearance.
4. Facilitates breathing and airway clearance.
5. Maximizes energy expenditure and prevents excessive fatigue.
6. Facilitates expectoration of secretions; prevents stasis of secretions.
7. Removes secretions if patient is unable to do so.
8. Increases availability of oxygen.
9. Maintains ventilation.

Expected Outcomes

- Maintains normal airway clearance:
  Respiratory rate <20 breaths/min
  Unlabored breathing without use of accessory muscles and flaring nares (nostrils)
  Skin color pink (without cyanosis)
  Alert and aware of surroundings
  Arterial blood gas values normal
  Normal breath sounds without adventitious breath sounds
- Begins appropriate therapy
- Takes medication as prescribed
- Reports improved breathing
- Maintains clear airway
- Coughs and takes deep breaths every 2–4 hours as recommended
- Demonstrates appropriate positions and practices postural drainage every 2–4 hours
- Reports reduced breathing difficulty when in semi- or high-Fowler's position
- Practices energy-conserving strategies and alternates rest with activity
- Demonstrates reduction in thickness (viscosity) of pulmonary secretions
- Reports increased ease in coughing up sputum
- Uses humidified air or oxygen as prescribed and indicated
- Indicates need for assistance with removal of pulmonary secretions
- Understands need for and cooperates with endotracheal intubation and use of a mechanical ventilator
- Verbalizes concerns about respiratory difficulty, intubation, and mechanical ventilation

---

Nursing Diagnosis: Altered nutrition, less than body requirement, related to decreased oral intake

Goal: Improvement of nutritional status

Nursing Interventions

1. Assess for malnutrition with height, weight, age, BUN, serum protein, and albumin, transferrin levels, hemoglobin, hematocrit, cutaneous anergy, and anthropometric measurements.

Rationale

1. Provides objective measurement of nutritional status.

Expected Outcomes

- Identifies factors limiting oral intake and uses resources to promote adequate dietary intake
- Reports increased appetite
- States understanding of nutritional needs

(*continued*)

48•1

Plan of Nursing Care — Care of the Patient With AIDS (*continued*)

Nursing Interventions	Rationale	Expected Outcomes
2. Obtain dietary history, including likes and dislikes and food intolerances.	2. Defines need for nutritional education; helps individualize interventions.	• Identifies ways to reduce factors that limit oral intake
3. Assess factors that interfere with oral intake.	3. Provides basis and directions for interventions.	• Rests before meals • Eats in pleasant, odor-free environment
4. Consult with dietitian to determine patient's nutritional needs.	4. Facilitates meal planning.	• Arranges meals to coincide with visitors' visits
5. Reduce factors limiting oral intake:	5. Address factors limiting intake.	• Reports increased dietary intake
a. Encourage patient to rest before meals.	a. Minimizes fatigue, which can decrease appetite.	• Uses oral hygiene before meals • Takes analgesics before meals as prescribed
b. Plan meals so that they do not occur immediately after painful or unpleasant procedures.	b. Decreases noxious stimuli.	• Identifies ways to increase protein and caloric intake • Identifies foods high in protein and calories
c. Encourage patient to eat meals with visitors or others when possible.	c. Limits social isolation.	• Consumes foods high in protein and calories • Reports decreased rate of weight loss.
d. Encourage patient to prepare simple meals or to obtain assistance with meal preparation if possible.	d. Limits energy expenditure.	• Maintains adequate intake • States rationale for enteral or parenteral nutrition if needed
e. Serve small, frequent meals: 6 per day.	e. Prevents overwhelming patient.	• Demonstrates skill in preparing alternate sources of nutrition
f. Limit fluids 1 hour before meals and with meals.	f. Reduces satiety.	
6. Instruct patient in ways to supplement nutrition: consume protein-rich foods (meat, poultry, fish) and carbohydrates (pasta, fruit, breads).	6. Provides additional proteins and calories.	
7. Consult with physician and dietitian about alternative feeding (enteral or parenteral nutrition).	7. Provides nutritional support if patient is unable to take sufficient amounts by mouth.	
8. Consult with social worker or community liaison about financial assistance if patient cannot afford food.	8. Increases availability of resources and nutrition.	

Nursing Diagnosis: Knowledge deficit related to means of preventing HIV transmission
Goal: Increased knowledge concerning means of preventing disease transmission

Nursing Interventions	Rationale	Expected Outcomes
1. Instruct patient, family, and friends about routes of transmission of HIV.	1. Knowledge about disease transmission can help prevent spread of disease; may also alleviate fears.	• Patient, family, and friends state means of transmission • Reports and demonstrates practices to reduce exposure of others to HIV
2. Instruct patient, family, and friends about means of preventing transmission of HIV:	2. Reduces transmission risk	• Avoids intravenous drug use
a. Avoid sexual contact with multiple partners, and use precautions if sexual partner's HIV status is not certain.	a. The risk of infection increases with the number of sexual partners, male or female, and sexual contact with those who engage in high-risk behaviors.	• Demonstrates knowledge of safer sexual practices • Identifies means of preventing disease transmission
b. Use condoms during sexual intercourse (vaginal, anal, oral–genital); avoid mouth contact with the penis, vagina, or rectum; avoid sexual practices that can cause cuts or tears in the lining of the rectum, vagina, or penis.	b. Risk of HIV transmission is reduced.	• States that sexual partners are informed about positive HIV antibodies in blood • Avoids IV injection drug use and sharing of drug equipment with others
c. Avoid sex with prostitutes and others at high risk.	c. Many prostitutes are infected with HIV through sexual contact with multiple partners or intravenous/injection drug use.	
d. Do not use intravenous drugs; if addicted and unable or unwilling to	d. Clean needles and syringes are the only way to prevent HIV transmission for	

(*continued*)

48•1

PLAN OF NURSING CARE

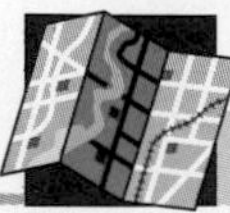

Care of the Patient With AIDS (*continued*)

Nursing Interventions	Rationale	Expected Outcomes
change behavior, use clean needles and syringes.	those who continue to use drugs. Taking precautions is important for those who are antibody positive to prevent transmitting HIV.	
e. Women who may have been exposed to AIDS through sexual or drug practices should consult with a physician before becoming pregnant; consider use of antiretroviral agents if pregnant.	e. AIDS can be transmitted from mother to child in utero; antiretroviral agents during pregnancy significantly reduce perinatal transmission of HIV.	

Nursing Diagnosis: Social isolation related to stigma of the disease, withdrawal of support systems, isolation procedures, and fear of infecting others

Goal: Decreased sense of social isolation

Nursing Interventions	Rationale	Expected Outcomes
1. Assess patient's usual patterns of social interaction.	1. Establishes basis for individualized interventions.	• Shares with others the need for valued social interaction • Demonstrates interest in events, activities, and communication • Verbalizes feelings and reactions to diagnosis, prognosis, and life changes • Identifies modes of transmission of AIDS • States ways of preventing transmission of AIDS virus to others while maintaining contact with valued friends and relatives • Reveals AIDS diagnosis to others when appropriate • Identifies resources (ie, family, friends, and support groups) • Uses resources when appropriate • Accepts offers of assistance and support • Reports decreased sense of isolation • Maintains contacts with those of importance to him or her • Develops or continues hobbies that effectively serve as diversion or distraction
2. Observe for behaviors indicative of social isolation, such as decreased interaction with others, hostility, noncompliance, sad affect, and stated feelings of rejection or loneliness.	2. Promotes early detection of social isolation which may be manifested in several ways.	
3. Provide instruction concerning modes of transmission of HIV.	3. Provides accurate information, corrects misconceptions, and alleviates anxiety.	
4. Assist patient to identify and explore resources for support and positive mechanisms for coping (eg, contact with family, friends, AIDS task force).	4. Enables mobilization of resources and supports.	
5. Allow time to be with patient other than for medications and procedures.	5. Promotes feelings of self-worth and provides social interaction.	
6. Encourage participation in diversional activities such as reading, television, or hand crafts.	6. Provides distraction.	

Collaborative Problems: Opportunistic infections; impaired breathing; wasting syndrome and fluid and electrolyte imbalances; adverse reaction to medications

Goal: Absence of complications

Opportunistic Infections

Nursing Interventions	Rationale	Expected Outcomes
1. Monitor vital signs.	1. Changes in vital signs such as increases in pulse rate, respirations, blood pressure, and temperature may indicate infection.	• Exhibits stable vital signs • Experiences control of infection • Identifies signs and symptoms correctly and experiences no complications • Identifies signs and symptoms that are reportable to the physician • Takes medications as prescribed
2. Collect laboratory specimens and monitor test results.	2. Smears and cultures can identify causative agents such as bacteria, fungi and protozoa, and sensitivity studies can identify antibiotics or other medications effective against the causative agent.	
3. Instruct the patient and caregiver about signs and symptoms of infection and the need to report them early.	3. Early recognition of symptoms facilitates prompt treatment and avoids extra complications.	

(*continued*)

48•1

PLAN OF NURSING CARE 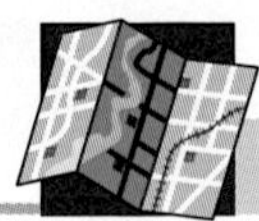

Care of the Patient With AIDS (*continued*)

Nursing Interventions	Rationale	Expected Outcomes
Impaired Breathing		
1. Monitor respiratory rate and pattern.	1. Rapid shallow breathing, diminished breath sounds, and shortness of breath may indicate respiratory failure resulting in hypoxia.	• Maintains stable respiratory rate and pattern within the normal limits • Exhibits no adventitious lung sounds; normal breath sounds • Has stable pulse rate and blood pressure within normal limits, and exhibits no evidence of hypoxia • Oxygen saturation levels within acceptable range
2. Auscultate the chest for breath sounds and abnormal lung sounds.	2. Crackles and wheezes may indicate fluid in the lungs, which disrupts respiratory function and alters the blood's oxygen-carrying capacity.	
3. Monitor pulse rate, blood pressure, and oxygen saturation levels.	3. Changes in pulse rate, blood pressure, and oxygen levels may indicate the development of respiratory or cardiac failure.	
Wasting Syndrome and Fluid and Electrolyte Disturbances		
1. Monitor weight and laboratory values for nutritional status.	1. Weight loss, malnutrition, and anemia are common in HIV infection and increase risk for superinfection.	• Maintains stable weight • Eats a nutritious diet • Attains and maintains hemoglobin, hematocrit, and ferritin levels within normal limits • Sustains fluid–electrolytes balance within normal limits • Exhibits no signs and symptoms of dehydration
2. Monitor intake and output and laboratory values for fluid and electrolyte imbalance (potassium, sodium, calcium, phosphorus, magnesium, and zinc).	2. Chronic diarrhea, inadequate oral intake, vomiting and profuse sweating deplete electrolytes. Small intestine inflammation may impair the absorption of fluids and electrolytes.	
3. Monitor for and report signs and symptoms of dehydration.	3. Fluid loss results in decreased circulating volume leading to tachycardia, dry skin and mucous membranes, poor skin turgor, elevated urine specific gravity, and thirst. Early detection allows early treatment.	
Reactions to Medications		
1. Monitor for drug interactions.	1. People with HIV infection receive many medications for HIV and for disease complications. Using medications concurrently with zidovudine may cause hepatic and hematologic abnormalities. Early detection of drug interaction is necessary to prevent complications.	• Experiences no serious side effects or complications from medications • Correctly describes medication regimen and complies with therapy
2. Monitor for and promptly report side effects from antiretroviral agents.	2. Side effects from antiretroviral agents can be life-threatening. Serious side effects include anemia, pancreatitis, peripheral neuropathy, mental confusion, and persistent nausea and vomiting. Corrective measures need to be instituted.	
3. Instruct the patient and caregiver in the medication regimen.	3. Knowledge of the medication purpose, (correct administration, side effects, and strategies to manage of prevent side effects) promotes safety and greater compliance with treatment.	

Respiratory Status

Respiratory status is assessed by monitoring the patient for cough, sputum production, shortness of breath, orthopnea, tachypnea, and chest pain. The presence and quality of breath sounds are also investigated. Other measures of pulmonary function include chest x-rays, arterial blood gas values, pulse oximetry, and pulmonary function test results.

Neurologic Status

Neurologic status is determined by assessing the patient's level of consciousness; orientation to person, place, and time; and the occurrence of memory lapses. Mental status is assessed as early as possible to provide a baseline for monitoring changes in behavior. The patient is also assessed for sensory deficits (visual changes, headache, or numbness and tingling in the extremities)

ASSESSMENT
MENTAL STATUS IN HIV INFECTION

Assessment	Function	Selected Descriptors
Appearance	Physical characteristics, grooming, dress	Obese, cachectic, emaciated, poor eye contact, clean, disheveled, inappropriate dress for weather, slumped posture
Behavior	Motor activity	Restless, agitated, lethargic, hyperactive, rigid, repetitive
Speech	Verbal communication	Intelligible, clear, slurred, rapid, slowed, pressured, repetitive, perseveration, mute
Mood	General feeling tone	Friendly, fearful, hostile, euphoric, despondent, labile
Affect	Emotional expression	Appropriate, bizarre, flat, blunted, apathetic, overly dramatic
Cognition	Memory and orientation	Oriented (to time, place, and person); confused; disoriented; distractible; short attention span, intact remote and immediate memory, forgetful
Comprehension	Intellectual functioning	Able to abstract, concrete, poor judgment, lacks insight, unable to compute, lacks general knowledge, able to learn
Thought process	Expression of thoughts	Goal oriented, tangential, delusional, looseness of associations, confabulation, obsessive, ritualistic
Perception	Perspective of world	Presence of auditory, visual, olfactory, or kinesthetic hallucinations

and motor involvement (altered gait, paresis, or paralysis) and seizure activity.

Fluid and Electrolyte Balance

Fluid and electrolyte status is assessed by examining the skin and mucous membranes for turgor and dryness. Increased thirst, decreased urine output, low blood pressure or a decrease in systolic blood pressure between 10 and 15 mm Hg with a concurrent rise in pulse rate when the patient sits up or stands, weak and rapid pulse, and urine specific gravity of 1.025 or more may indicate dehydration. Electrolyte imbalances, such as decreased serum sodium, potassium, calcium, magnesium, and chloride, typically result from profuse diarrhea. The patient is assessed for signs and symptoms of electrolyte depletion, including decreased mental status (see Assessment box above), muscle twitching, muscle cramps, irregular pulse, nausea and vomiting, and shallow respirations.

Knowledge Level

The patient's level of knowledge about the disease and the modes of disease transmission is evaluated. In addition, the level of knowledge of family and friends is assessed. The patient's psychological reaction to the diagnosis of HIV infection or AIDS is important to explore. Reactions vary among patients and may include denial, anger, fear, shame, withdrawal from social interactions, and depression. It is often helpful to gain an understanding of how the patient has dealt with illness and major life stress in the past. The patient's resources for support are also identified.

Use of Alternative Therapies

Many patients who use these alternative therapies do not always report their use to their health care providers. To obtain a complete health history, the nurse should ask questions about use of alternative therapies. Patients may need to be encouraged to report their use to their primary health care provider. Problems may arise when patients are using alternative therapies while they are participating in clinical drug trials or receiving complex or multiple medications. They may have significant adverse side effects, making it difficult to assess the effects of the medications in the clinical trial or the patient's regimen of medications. The nurse needs to become familiar with the potential adverse side effects of alternative therapies. The nurse who suspects that the alternative therapy is causing a side effect needs to discuss this with the patient, the alternative therapy provider, and the primary health care provider. It is important for the nurse to view alternative therapies with an open mind and to try to understand the importance of this treatment to the patient. Doing so will improve communication with the patient and reduce conflict, so that all involved in care can meet the patient's needs.

Diagnosis

Nursing Diagnoses

The list of potential nursing diagnoses is extensive because of the complex nature of this disease. Based on assessment data, however, major nursing diagnoses for the patient may include the following:

- Impaired skin integrity related to cutaneous manifestations of HIV infection, excoriation, and diarrhea
- Diarrhea related to enteric pathogens or HIV infection
- Risk for infection related to immunodeficiency
- Activity intolerance related to weakness, fatigue, malnutrition, impaired fluid and electrolyte balance, and hypoxia associated with pulmonary infections
- Altered thought processes related to shortened attention span, impaired memory, confusion, and disorientation associated with HIV encephalopathy
- Ineffective airway clearance related to PCP, increased bronchial secretions, and decreased ability to cough related to weakness and fatigue
- Pain related to impaired perianal skin integrity secondary to diarrhea, KS, and peripheral neuropathy
- Altered nutrition: less than body requirements related to decreased oral intake
- Social isolation related to stigma of the disease, withdrawal of support systems, isolation procedures, and fear of infecting others
- Anticipatory grieving related to changes in lifestyle and roles and to unfavorable prognosis
- Knowledge deficit related to HIV infection, means of preventing HIV transmission, and self-care

Collaborative Problems/Potential Complications

Based on the assessment data, possible complications may include the following:

- Opportunistic infections
- Impaired breathing or respiratory failure
- Wasting syndrome and fluid and electrolyte imbalance
- Adverse reaction to medications

Planning and Goals

Goals for the patient may include achievement and maintenance of skin integrity, resumption of usual bowel habits, absence of infection, improved activity tolerance, improved thought processes, improved airway clearance, increased comfort, improved nutritional status, increased socialization, expression of grief, increased knowledge regarding disease prevention and self-care, and absence of complications.

Nursing Interventions

Promoting Skin Integrity

The skin and oral mucosa are assessed routinely for changes in appearance, location and size of lesions, and evidence of infection and breakdown. The patient is encouraged to maintain a balance between rest and mobility whenever possible. Patients who are immobile are assisted to change position every 2 hours. Devices such as alternating-pressure mattresses and low-air loss beds are used to prevent skin breakdown. Patients are encouraged to avoid scratching, to use nonabrasive, nondrying soaps, and to apply nonperfumed skin moisturizers to dry skin surfaces. Regular oral care is also encouraged.

Medicated lotions, ointments, and dressings are applied to affected skin surfaces as prescribed. Adhesive tape is avoided. Skin surfaces are protected from friction and rubbing by keeping bed linens free of wrinkles and avoiding tight or restrictive clothing. Patients with foot lesions are advised to wear white cotton socks and shoes that do not cause the feet to perspire. Antipruritics, antibiotics, and analgesics are administered as prescribed.

The patient's perianal region is assessed frequently for impairment of skin integrity and infection. The patient is instructed to keep the area as clean as possible. The perianal area is cleaned after each bowel movement with nonabrasive soap and water to prevent further excoriation and breakdown of the skin and infection. If the area is very painful, soft cloths or cotton sponges may prove to be less irritating than washcloths. In addition, sitz baths or gentle irrigation may facilitate cleaning and promote comfort. The area is dried thoroughly after cleaning. Topical lotions or ointments may be prescribed to promote healing. Wounds are cultured if infection is suspected, so that the appropriate antimicrobial treatment can be initiated. Debilitated patients may require assistance in maintaining hygienic practices.

Promoting Usual Bowel Habits

The patient's bowel patterns are assessed for the occurrence of diarrhea. The nurse monitors frequency and consistency of stools and reports of abdominal pain or cramping associated with bowel movements. Factors that exacerbate frequent diarrhea are also assessed. The quantity and volume of liquid stools are measured to document fluid volume losses. Stool cultures are obtained to identify pathogenic organisms.

The patient is counseled about ways to decrease diarrhea. The physician may recommend restriction of oral intake to rest the bowel during periods of acute inflammation associated with severe enteric infections. As the patient's dietary intake is increased, foods that act as bowel irritants, such as raw fruits and vegetables, popcorn, carbonated beverages, spicy foods, and foods of extreme temperatures, should be avoided. Small, frequent meals help to prevent abdominal distention. The physician may prescribe medications, such as anticholinergic antispasmodics or opioids, which decrease diarrhea by decreasing intestinal spasms and motility. Antidiarrheal agents that are administered on a regular schedule may be more beneficial and effective than administering them on an as-needed (PRN) basis. Antibiotics and antifungal agents may also be prescribed to combat pathogens identified by stool cultures.

Preventing Infection

The patient and caregivers are instructed to monitor for signs and symptoms of infection. These include fever; chills; night sweats; cough with or without sputum production; shortness of breath; difficulty breathing; oral pain or difficulty swallowing; creamy-white patches in the oral cavity; unexplained weight loss; swollen lymph nodes; nausea; vomiting; persistent diarrhea; frequency, urgency, or pain on urination; headache; visual changes or memory lapses; redness, swelling, or drainage from skin wounds; and vesicular lesions on the face, lips, or perianal area. The nurse also monitors laboratory values that indicate infection, such as the white blood cell count and differential. The physician may decide to culture specimens of wound drainage, skin lesions, urine, stool, sputum, mouth, and blood to identify pathogenic organisms and the most appropriate antimicrobial therapy. The patient is instructed to avoid others with active infections (ie, URIs).

Improving Activity Tolerance

Activity tolerance is assessed by monitoring the patient's ability to ambulate and perform activities of daily living. Patients may be unable to maintain usual levels of activity because of weakness, fatigue, shortness of breath, dizziness, and neurologic involvement. Assistance in planning daily routines that maintain a balance between activity and rest may be necessary. In addition, patients benefit from instructions about energy conservation techniques, such as sitting while washing or while preparing meals. Personal items that are frequently used should be kept within the patient's reach. Measures such as relaxation and guided imagery may be beneficial because they decrease anxiety that contributes to weakness and fatigue.

Collaboration with other members of the health care team may uncover other factors associated with increasing fatigue and strategies to address them. For example, if fatigue is related to anemia, administering epoetin alfa (Epogen) as prescribed may relieve fatigue and increase activity tolerance.

Maintaining Thought Processes

The patient is assessed for alterations in mental status that may be related to neurologic involvement, metabolic abnormalities, infection, side effects of treatment, and coping mechanisms. Manifestations of neurologic impairment may be difficult to distinguish from psychological reactions to HIV infection, such as anger and depression.

Family members are instructed to speak to the patient in simple, clear language and give the patient sufficient time to respond to questions. Family members are instructed to orient the patient to the daily routine by talking about what is taking place during daily activities. They are encouraged to provide the patient with a regular daily schedule for medication administration, grooming, meal times, bedtimes, and awakening times. Posting the schedule in a prominent area (ie, on the refrigerator), providing nightlights for the patient's bedroom and bathroom, and planning safe leisure activities allow the patient to maintain a regular routine in a safe manner. Activities that the patient previously enjoyed are encouraged. These should be easy to accomplish and fairly short in duration. The nurse encourages the family to remain calm and not to argue with the patient while protecting the patient from injury. Around-the-clock supervision may be necessary, and strategies can be implemented to prevent the patient from engaging in potentially dangerous activities, such as driving, using the stove, or mowing the lawn. Strategies for improving or maintaining functional abilities and for providing a safe environment are used for patients with HIV encephalopathy (Guideline 48-2).

Improving Airway Clearance

Respiratory status, including rate, rhythm, use of accessory muscles, and breath sounds; mental status; and skin color must be assessed at least daily. Any cough and the quantity and characteristics of sputum are documented. Sputum specimens are analyzed for infectious organisms. Pulmonary therapy (coughing, deep breathing, postural drainage, percussion, and vibration) is provided as often as every 2 hours to prevent stasis of secretions and to promote airway clearance. Because of weakness and fatigue, many patients require assistance in attaining a position (such as a high-Fowler's or semi-Fowler's position) that facilitates breathing

48•2 Guidelines For Care of the Patient With HIV Encephalopathy

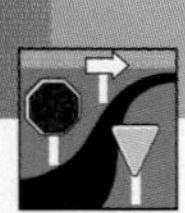

Altered Thought Processes

- Assess mental status and neurologic functioning.
- Monitor for drug interactions, infections, electrolyte imbalance, and depression.
- Frequently orient the patient to time, place, person, reality, and the environment.
- Use simple explanations.
- Teach the patient to perform tasks in incremental steps.
- Provide memory aids (clocks and calendars).
- Provide memory aids for medication administration.
- Post activity schedule.
- Give positive feedback for appropriate behavior.
- Teach caretakers how to orient patient to time, place, person, reality, and the environment.
- Encourage the patient to designate a responsible person to assume power of attorney.

Sensory Perceptual Alterations

- Assess sensory impairment.
- Decrease amount of stimuli in the patient's environment.
- Correct inaccurate perceptions.
- Provide reassurance and safety if the patient displays fear.
- Provide a feeling of security and stability in the patient's environment.
- Teach caregivers how to recognize inaccurate sensory perceptions.
- Teach caregivers techniques to correct inaccurate perceptions.
- Teach the patient and caregivers to report any changes in the patient's vision to the patient's health care provider.

Risk for Injury

- Assess the patient's level of anxiety, confusion, or disorientation.
- Assess the patient for delusions or hallucinations.
- Remove potentially dangerous objects from the patient's environment.
- Structure the environment for safety (ensure adequate lighting, avoid clutter, provide bed rails if needed).
- Supervise smoking.
- Do not let the patient drive a car if confusion is present.
- Instruct the patient and caregiver in home safety.
- Provide assistance as needed for ambulation and in getting in and out of bed.
- Pad headboard and side rails if the patient has seizures.

Self-Care Deficit

- Encourage performing activities of daily living within the patient's level of ability.
- Encourage independence but intervene if the patient cannot perform an activity.
- Show or demonstrate how to perform any activity that the patient is having difficulty accomplishing.
- Keep strict records of food and fluid intake.
- Weigh patient weekly.
- Encourage the patient to eat, and offer nutritious meals, snacks, and adequate fluids.
- If patient is incontinent, establish a routine toileting schedule.
- Teach caregivers how to meet the patient's self-care needs.

and airway clearance. Adequate rest is essential to maximize the patient's energy expenditure and prevent excessive fatigue. The patient's fluid volume status is evaluated, so that adequate hydration can be maintained. Unless contraindicated by renal or cardiac disease, an intake of 3 L of fluid daily is encouraged. Humidified oxygen may be prescribed, and nasopharyngeal or tracheal suctioning, intubation, and mechanical ventilation may be necessary to maintain adequate ventilation.

Relieving Pain and Discomfort

The patient is assessed for the quality and severity of pain associated with impaired perianal skin integrity, the lesions of KS, and peripheral neuropathy. In addition, the effects of pain on elimination, nutrition, sleep, affect, and communication are explored, along with exacerbating and relieving factors. Cleaning the perianal area as previously described can promote comfort. Topical anesthetics or ointments may be prescribed. Use of soft cushions or foam pads may increase comfort while sitting. The patient is instructed to avoid foods that act as bowel irritants. Antispasmodics and antidiarrheal preparations may be prescribed to reduce discomfort and frequency of bowel movements. If necessary, systemic analgesics may also be prescribed.

Pain from KS is frequently described as a sharp, throbbing pressure and heaviness if lymphedema is present. Pain management may include using NSAIDs and opioids plus nonpharmacologic approaches such as relaxation techniques. When NSAIDs are used in patients receiving zidovudine, hepatic and hematologic status needs to be monitored.

The patient with pain related to peripheral neuropathy frequently describes it as burning, numbness, and "pins and needles." Pain management measures may include opioids, tricyclic antidepressants, and elastic stockings to equalize pressure. Tricyclic antidepressants have been found helpful in controlling the symptoms of neuropathic pain. They also potentiate the actions of opioids and can be used to relieve pain without increasing the dose of the opioid.

Improving Nutritional Status

Nutritional status is assessed by monitoring weight; dietary intake; anthropometric measurements; and serum albumin, BUN, protein, and transferrin levels. The patient is also assessed for factors that interfere with oral intake, such as anorexia, oral and esophageal candidal infection, nausea, pain, weakness, fatigue, and lactose intolerance. Based on the results of assessment, the nurse can implement specific measures to facilitate oral intake. The dietitian is consulted to determine the patient's nutritional requirements.

Control of nausea and vomiting with antiemetic medications administered on a regular basis may increase the patient's dietary intake. Inadequate food intake resulting from pain caused by mouth sores or a sore throat may be managed by administering prescribed opioids and viscous lidocaine (rinse the mouth and swallow). Additionally, the patient is encouraged to eat foods that are easy to swallow and to avoid rough, spicy, or sticky food items and foods that are excessively hot or cold. Oral hygiene before and after meals is encouraged.

When fatigue and weakness interfere with intake, the patient is encouraged to rest before meals. If the patient is hospitalized, meals should be scheduled so that they do not occur immediately after painful or unpleasant procedures. The patient with diarrhea and abdominal cramping is encouraged to avoid foods that stimulate intestinal motility and abdominal distention, for example, fiber-rich food or lactose if the patient is lactose intolerant. The patient is instructed about ways in which to enhance the nutritional value of meals. The addition of eggs, butter, margarine, and fortified milk (powdered skim milk is added to milk to increase the caloric content) to gravies, soups, or milkshakes can provide additional calories and protein. Commercial supplements, such as puddings, powders, milkshakes, and Advera (a nutritional product specifically designed for people with HIV infection or AIDS), may also be useful. Patients who cannot maintain nutritional status through oral intake may require enteral or parenteral feedings.

Decreasing the Sense of Isolation

People with AIDS are at risk for double stigmatization. They have what society refers to as "a dread disease," and they may have a lifestyle that differs from what is considered acceptable by many people. Many people with AIDS are young adults at a developmental stage usually associated with establishing intimate relationships and personal and career goals and having and raising children. Their focus changes as they are faced with a disease that threatens their life expectancy with no cure. In addition, they may be forced to reveal hidden lifestyles or behaviors to family, friends, coworkers, and health care providers. As a result, people with HIV infection may be overwhelmed with emotions such as anxiety, guilt, shame, and fear. They also may be faced with multiple losses, such as rejection by family and friends and loss of sexual partners, family, and friends; financial security; normal roles and functions; self-esteem; privacy; ability to control bodily functions; ability to interact meaningfully with the environment; and sexual functioning. Some patients may harbor feelings of guilt because of their chosen lifestyle or because of the possibility of having infected others in current or previous relationships. Other patients may feel anger toward sexual partners who transmitted the virus.

Infection-control measures used in the hospital or at home may further contribute to the patient's emotional isolation. Any or all of these stressors may cause the patient with AIDS to withdraw both physically and emotionally from social contact.

Nurses are in a key position to provide an atmosphere of acceptance and understanding of people with AIDS and their families and partners. A patient's usual level of social interaction is assessed as early as possible to provide a baseline for monitoring changes in behavior indicative of social isolation (eg, decreased interaction with staff or family, hostility, noncompliance). Patients are encouraged to express feelings of isolation and loneliness with the assurance that these feelings are not unique or abnormal.

Providing information about how to protect themselves and others may help patients avoid social isolation. Patients, family, and friends must be assured that AIDS is not spread through casual contact. Educating ancillary personnel, nurses, and physicians will help to reduce factors that might contribute to patients' feelings of isolation. Patient care conferences that address the psychosocial issues associated with AIDS may help sensitize nurses to patients' needs.

Coping With Grief

The nurse can help patients verbalize feelings and explore and identify resources for support and mechanisms for coping, especially when the patient is grieving through anticipated losses.

Patients are encouraged to maintain contact with family and friends and to use local or national AIDS support groups and hotlines. If at all possible, losses are identified and dealt with. The patient is encouraged to maintain interaction with family, friends, or coworkers and to continue usual activities whenever possible. Consultations with mental health counselors are useful for many patients.

Monitoring and Managing Potential Complications

Patients who are immunosuppressed are at risk for opportunistic infections. Therefore, anti-infective agents may be prescribed and laboratory tests obtained to monitor their effect. Signs and symptoms of opportunistic infections, including fever, malaise, difficulty breathing, nausea or vomiting, diarrhea, difficulty swallowing, and any occurrences of swelling or discharge, should be reported.

RESPIRATORY FAILURE

Impaired breathing is a major complication that increases the patient's discomfort and anxiety and may lead to respiratory failure and cardiac failure. The patient's respiratory rate and pattern are monitored and the lungs auscultated for abnormal breath sounds. The patient is instructed to report shortness of breath and increasing difficulty in carrying out usual activities. Pulse rate and rhythm, blood pressure, and oxygen saturation are monitored. Suctioning and oxygen therapy may be prescribed to ensure an adequate airway and to prevent hypoxia. Mechanical ventilation may be necessary for a patient who cannot maintain adequate ventilation as a result of pulmonary infection, fluid and electrolyte imbalance, or respiratory muscle weakness. Arterial blood gas values are used to guide ventilator settings. If the patient is intubated, a method must be established to allow communication with the nurse and others. Attention must be given to assisting the patient on mechanical ventilation to cope with the stress associated with intubation and ventilator assistance. The possible need for mechanical ventilation in the future should be discussed early in the course of the disease, when the patient is able to make his or her desires about treatment known. The use of mechanical ventilation should be consistent with the patient's decisions about end-of-life treatment.

CACHEXIA AND WASTING

Wasting syndrome and fluid and electrolyte disturbances, including dehydration, are common complications of HIV infection and AIDS. The patient's nutritional and electrolyte status is evaluated by monitoring weight gains or losses, skin turgor, ferritin levels, hemoglobin and hematocrit values, and electrolyte levels. Fluid and electrolyte status is monitored on an ongoing basis; fluid intake and output and urine specific gravity may be monitored daily if the patient is hospitalized with complications. The patient's skin is assessed for dryness and adequate turgor. Vital signs are monitored for decreased systolic blood pressure or increased pulse rate upon sitting or standing. Signs and symptoms of electrolyte disturbances, such as muscle cramping, weakness, irregular pulse, decreased mental status, nausea, and vomiting, are documented and reported to the physician. Serum electrolyte values are monitored and abnormalities reported.

The nurse helps the patient select foods that will replenish electrolytes, such as oranges and bananas (potassium) and cheese and soups (sodium). A fluid intake of 3 L or more, unless contraindicated, is encouraged to replace fluid lost with diarrhea and measures to control diarrhea are initiated. If fluid and electrolyte imbalances persist, the nurse may administer intravenous fluids and electrolytes as prescribed. Effects of parenteral therapy are monitored.

SIDE EFFECTS OF MEDICATIONS

Adverse reactions are of concern in patients who receive many medications to treat HIV infection or its complications. Many medications can cause severe toxic effects. Information about the purpose of the medications; their correct administration; side effects, including those that should be reported immediately to the physician or nurse practitioner; and strategies to manage or prevent side effects are provided. Signs and symptoms of side effects that should be reported immediately include the following:

- For zidovudine (AZT, Retrovir)—headache, fever, fatigue, rash, muscle pain, severe upper abdominal pain, and shortness of breath
- For didanosine (ddI, Videx)—diarrhea, upper abdominal pain, persistent nausea and vomiting, pain, tingling, or numbness, difficulties breathing, and mental confusion
- For dideoxycytidine (ddC, Hivid)—mouth sores, rashes, itching, upper abdominal pain, persistent nausea and vomiting, numbness or tingling, mental confusion, and seizures
- For stavudine—numbness, pain, or tingling of the extremities
- For lamivudine (3TC, Epivir)—similar to zidovudine plus mania, psychosis, and confusion
- For saquinavir—occasionally diarrhea if formulated with lactose
- For ritinovir—nausea, vomiting, diarrhea, abdominal pain, and anorexia
- For indinivir—asymptomatic hyperbilirubinemia and nephrolithiasis.
- For nevirapine (Viramune)—rash, fever, thrombocytopenia
- For delavirdine (Rescriptor)—rash

Other medications that may be required include but are not limited to opioids, tricyclics, and NSAIDs for pain relief; medications for treatment of opportunistic infections; antihistamines (diphenhydramine) for relief of pruritus (itching); acetaminophen or aspirin for management of fever; and antiemetics for control of nausea and vomiting. Use of many of these medications concurrently may cause many drug interactions including hepatic and hematologic abnormalities. Therefore, careful laboratory monitoring for these abnormalities is warranted.

Promoting Home and Community-Based Care

TEACHING PATIENTS SELF-CARE

Patients, families, and friends are instructed about the routes of transmission of AIDS. The nurse discusses precautions to prevent transmitting HIV, including using condoms during vaginal or anal intercourse; using dental dams or avoiding oral contact with the penis, vagina, or rectum; avoiding sexual practices that might cut or tear the lining of the rectum, vagina, or penis; and avoiding sexual contact with multiple partners, individuals known to be HIV infected, people who use illicit injectable drugs, and sexual partners of people who inject drugs.

Patients and their families or caregivers must receive instructions about how to prevent disease transmission, including handwashing techniques, and in methods for safely handling of items soiled with body fluids. Caregivers in the home are taught how to administer medications, including intravenous preparations.

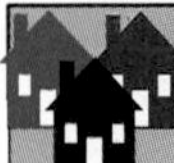

PATIENT EDUCATION AND HOME CARE
The Right Way to Use a Male Condom

1. Put on a new condom before any kind of sex.
2. Hold the condom by the tip to squeeze out the air.

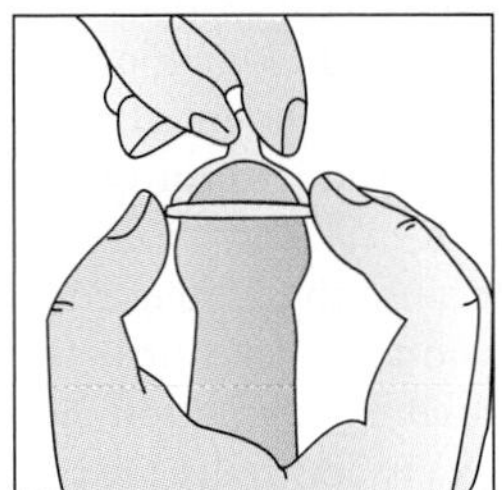

3. Unroll the condom all the way over the erect penis.

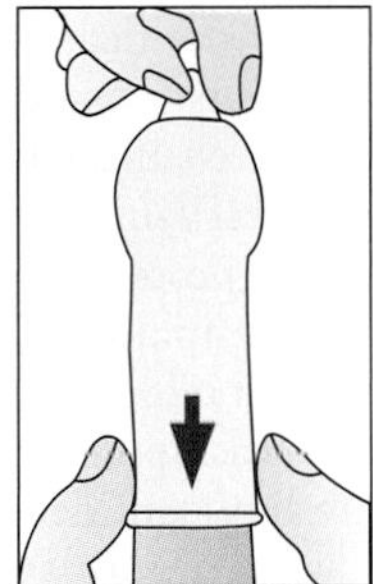

4. Have sex.
5. Hold the condom so it cannot come off the penis.
6. Pull out.
7. Use a new condom if you want to have sex again or if you want to have sex in a different place (eg, in the anus and then in the vagina).

*Keep condoms cool and dry. Never use skin lotions, baby oil, petroleum jelly, or cold cream with condoms. The oil in these products will cause the condom to break. You may use products made with water (like K-Y jelly or glycerin).

The medication regimens used for patients with HIV infection and AIDS are often complex and expensive. Patients receiving combination therapies for treatment of HIV infection and its complications require careful teaching about the importance of taking medications as prescribed and explanations and assistance in fitting the medication regimen into their lives.

Guidelines about infection and infection control, follow-up care, diet, rest, and activity are also necessary. Patient teaching also includes strategies to avoid infection. The importance of personal hygiene is emphasized. Kitchen and bathroom surfaces should be cleaned regularly with disinfectants to prevent fungal and bacterial growth. Patients with pets are instructed to have another person clean areas soiled by animals, such as bird cages and litter boxes. If this is not possible, the patient should use gloves to clean up after pets. Patients are advised to avoid exposure to others who are sick or who have been recently vaccinated. Patients with AIDS and their sexual partners are *strongly* urged to avoid exposure to body fluids during sexual activities and to use condoms for any form of sexual intercourse. Intravenous/injection drug use is *strongly* discouraged because of the risk to the patient of other infections and transmission of HIV infection to others. Patients who are already infected by HIV are also urged to avoid exposure to bodily fluids (through sexual contact or intravenous/injection drug use) to prevent exposure to other HIV strains. The importance of avoiding smoking and maintaining a balance between diet, rest, and exercise is also emphasized.

If the patient requires enteral or parenteral feedings, instruction is provided to patients and families about how to administer such feedings to the patient at home. Home care nurses provide ongoing teaching and support for the patient and family.

Both the patient and the caregivers require support and guidance in coping with AIDS.

Patients who are HIV positive or who inject drugs are instructed not to donate blood. Injecting drug users who are unwilling to stop using drugs are advised to avoid sharing drug equipment with others.

HOME CARE TEACHING CHECKLIST: ADHERING TO MEDICATION THERAPY FOR HIV

At the completion of the program, the patient or caregiver will be able to:	Patient	Caregiver
• Verbalize knowledge of each medication name.	✔	✔
• State the action of each medication.	✔	✔
• State the correct times that medications are to be taken.	✔	✔
• Identify special guidelines to follow when taking medications (eg, with meals, on an empty stomach, medications that are not to be taken together).	✔	✔
• Demonstrate method of keeping track of the medication regimen.	✔	✔
• Identify specific laboratory tests that are necessary for the prescribed medication regimen.	✔	✔
• List expected side effects of each medication.	✔	✔
• Identify side effects that should be reported to health care giver.	✔	✔
• Explain the importance of and necessity for compliance with prescribed medication regimen.	✔	✔
• State need for use of parenteral route for medications.	✔	✔
• Demonstrate correct disposal of parenteral medication according to Standard Precautions guidelines.	✔	✔
• Demonstrate correct administration of IM, SC, or IV medications.	✔	✔
• Demonstrate correct use of syringes or IV equipment.	✔	✔
• Discuss with the health care worker any problems that he or she is having with side effects and compliance.	✔	✔
• Report any episodes of noncompliance with the medication regimen.	✔	✔

CONTINUING CARE

Many people with AIDS remain in their community and continue their usual daily activities, whereas others are unable to continue employment or maintain their preexisting level of independence. Families or caregivers may need assistance in providing supportive care.

Community health nurses, home care nurses, and hospice nurses are in an excellent position to provide the support and guidance so often needed in the home setting. As hospital costs continue to rise and insurance coverage continues to decline, the complexity of home care continues to increase. Home care nurses are key in the administration of parenteral antibiotics, chemotherapy, and nutrition in the home.

During visits to the patient at home, the nurse assesses the patient's physical and emotional status and home environment. The patient's adherence to the therapeutic regimen is assessed, and strategies are suggested to assist with adherence. The patient is assessed for progression of disease and for adverse side effects of medications. Previous teaching is reinforced, and the importance of keeping follow-up appointments is stressed.

Complicated wound care or respiratory care may be required in the home. Patients and families are seldom able to meet these skilled care needs without assistance. Nurses may refer patients to many community programs located in towns and cities throughout the country. These programs offer a range of services for patients, friends, and families, including help with housekeeping, grooming, and meals; transportation and shopping; individual and group therapy; support for caregivers; telephone networks for the homebound; and legal and financial assistance. These services are typically provided by both professional and nonprofessional volunteers. A social worker may be consulted to identify sources of financial support, if needed.

Home care and hospice nurses are increasingly called on to provide physical and emotional support to patients and families as patients with AIDS enter the terminal stages of disease. This support takes on special meaning when people with AIDS lose friends and when family members fear the disease or feel anger concerning their lifestyle. The nurse encourages the patient and family to discuss end-of-life decisions and to assure that care is consistent with those decisions and that all comfort measures are employed and that the patient is treated with dignity at all times.

Evaluation

Expected Outcomes

Expected outcomes may include:

1. Maintains skin integrity
2. Resumes usual bowel habits
3. Experiences no infections
4. Maintains adequate level of activity tolerance
5. Maintains usual level of thought processes
6. Maintains effective airway clearance
7. Experiences increased sense of comfort, less pain
8. Maintains adequate nutritional status
9. Experiences decreased sense of social isolation
10. Progresses through grieving process
11. Reports increased understanding of AIDS and participates in self-care activities as possible
12. Remains free of complications

EMOTIONAL AND ETHICAL CONCERNS FOR NURSES

Nurses in all settings will be called on to provide care for patients with HIV infection. In doing so, they encounter not only the physical challenges of this epidemic but also emotional and ethical concerns. The concerns raised by health care professionals involve issues such as fear of contagion, responsibility for giving care, values clarification, confidentiality, developmental stages of patients and caregivers, and poor prognostic outcomes.

Many patients with HIV infection have engaged in "stigmatized" behaviors. Because these behaviors challenge some traditional religious and moral values, nurses may feel reluctant to provide care for these patients. In addition, health care providers may still have fear and anxiety about disease transmission despite education concerning infection control and the low incidence of transmission to health care providers (see Ethics and Related Issues). Nurses are encouraged to examine their personal beliefs and use the process of values clarification to approach controversial issues. The American Nurses Association's Code for Nurses can also be used to help resolve ethical dilemmas that might affect the quality of care given to HIV-infected patients.

Nurses are responsible for protecting the patient's right to privacy by safeguarding confidential information. Inadvertent disclosure of confidential patient information may result in personal, financial, and emotional hardships for HIV-infected individuals. The controversy surrounding confidentiality concerns identifying the circumstances when information can be disclosed to others. Health care team members need accurate patient information to conduct assessment, planning, implementation, and evaluation of patient care. Failure to disclose HIV status could compromise the quality of patient care. Sexual partners of HIV-infected patients should know about the potential for infection and the need to engage in safer sex practices as well as the potential need for testing and medical care. Nurses are advised to discuss concerns about confidentiality with nurse administrators and physicians to identify the most appropriate courses of action.

AIDS has had a high mortality rate. Advances in antiretroviral and multidrug therapy have demonstrated promise in slowing or controlling disease progression. It is not known whether current treatment regimens will remain effective because viral drug resistance has developed with most previous medications. Most nurses have never faced an epidemic in which almost all patients will experience serious illness and die during the usual course of the disease process. Nurses may struggle with the value and meaning of their professional roles as they witness repeated instances of deterioration. Exposure to so many deaths in a population that is at the same developmental stage as many nurses can create feelings of stress. Contributing to this stress are personal fears of contagion or disapproval of the patient's lifestyle and behaviors. Unlike cancer or other diseases, AIDS is associated with controversies challenging our legal and political systems as well as religious and personal beliefs. Nurses who feel stressed and overburdened may experience physical and mental distress in the form of fatigue, headache, changes in appetite and sleep patterns, helplessness, irritability, apathy, negativity, and anger.

Many strategies have been used by nurses to cope with stress associated with caring for AIDS patients. Education and provision of up-to-date information help to alleviate apprehension and prepare nurses to deliver safe, high-quality patient care. Interdisciplinary meetings allow participants to support one another and still provide comprehensive patient care. Staff support groups

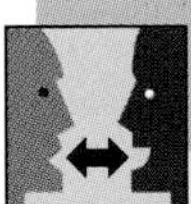

ETHICS AND RELATED ISSUES

Revealing One's HIV Status

Should all people who are infected with HIV be required to reveal this status to all their sexual and or needle-sharing contacts?

Situation

The human immunodeficiency virus (HIV) causes HIV infection, which progresses to AIDS, a disease that is currently incurable and ultimately fatal. Many HIV-positive people are aware that they carry the virus but refuse to share this information with others, especially their sexual partners or injecting drug contacts. Because sexual contacts and needle-sharing partners are at risk for developing the disease, would a policy that requires notification of contacts infringe on the liberty and privacy of the known HIV infected person?

Dilemma

The person's right to privacy conflicts with notifying all people who are contacts either through sexual or needle-sharing behavior (autonomy versus justice). The person's right to privacy conflicts with society's need to contain the deadly virus and stem a deadly epidemic (autonomy versus justice).

Discussion

What arguments would you offer in favor of notifying all the person's contacts?

What arguments would you offer against notifying all or some of the person's contacts?

Each state has various laws that pertain to whether contacts can be notified and who is responsible for notifying contacts. Is there a law for contact notification in the state in which you live? If there is such a law in your state, who is the individual that is to be responsible for contact notification?

What would you do if the person responsible for contact notification refuses to do so based on his own beliefs for confidentiality of HIV infection status?

give nurses an opportunity to problem-solve and explore values and feelings about caring for AIDS patients and their families; they also provide a forum for grieving. Other sources of support include nursing administrators, peers, and spiritual leaders.

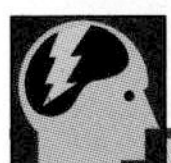

Critical Thinking Exercises

1.
A patient tells you that he and his sexual partner are both HIV positive. He informs you that because they both have HIV infection already, they do not practice safe sex. How would you respond to this, and what approach would you use to educate the patient and his partner?

2.
You are making a home visit to a patient with HIV encephalopathy. Describe the aspects of the home environment you would assess to ensure safety and adequate care.

3.
You are the nurse manager of a medical-surgical unit. A new graduate working on your unit accidentally sticks herself with a needle during a resuscitation effort. She tells you that she is frightened about the possible consequences of this. What actions should you take as nurse manager? What do you tell the new graduate about possible risks and consequences related to her needlestick?

4.
The wife of a patient hospitalized with AIDS asks you directly, "Does my husband have AIDS?" Explain how you would respond to her and why you decided on this course of action.

5.
You are caring for a 24-year-old woman who is HIV positive. During your conversation with her, she tells you that she and her husband are considering having a child. She asks you what you think of this idea. How would you respond to her? What information would you consider in your response?

References and Selected Readings

BOOKS

Agency for Health Care Policy and Research. (1994). *Evaluation and management of early HIV infection.* Clinical Practice Guideline No. 7. U.S. Department of Health and Human Services (Pub. No. 94-0572). Washington, DC.

Antel, P., Birnbaum, G., & Hartung, H. P. (1998). *Clinical neuroimmunology.* Malden, MA: Blackwell Scientific.

Bardana, E. J. Jr., Montanaro, A. (1997). *Indoor air pollution and health.* New York: Marcel Dekker.

Bennett, J. V., & Brachman, P. S. (Eds.). (1998). *Hospital infections* (4th ed.). Philadelphia: Lippincott-Raven.

Bradley, J., & McCluskey, J. (Eds.). (1997). *Clinical immunology.* New York: Oxford University Press.

Centers for Disease Control and Prevention. (1998). Appendix-First-line drugs for HIV postexposure prophylaxis (PEP). *MMWR CDC Recommendation and Reports, 47*(RR-7), 29–30.

Delves, P. J. (1998). *Encyclopedia of immunology* (2nd ed.). San Diego: Academic Press.

DeVita, V. T., Hellman, S., Rosenberg, S. A., Curran, J., Essex, M., & Fauci, A. S. (Eds.). (1997). *AIDS etiology, diagnosis, treatment and prevention* (4th ed.). Philadelphia: Lippincott-Raven.

Eales, L. J. (1997). *Immunology for life scientists. A basic introduction: A student-centered learning approach.* New York: John Wiley & Sons.

Faden, R. R., & Kass, N. E. (Eds.) (1996). *HIV, AIDS, and childbearing: Public policy, private lives.* New York: Oxford University Press.

Fahey, J. L., & Flemmig, D. S. (Eds.). (1997). *AIDS/HIV reference guide for medical professionals* (4th ed.). Baltimore: Williams & Wilkins.

Fauci, A. S., & Pantaleo, G (Eds.). (1997). *Immunopathogenesis of HIV infection.* New York: Springer.

Frank, S., Esch, J. F., & Margeson, N. E. (1998). Mandatory HIV testing of newborns. The impact on women. *American Journal of Nursing, 98*(10), 49–51.

Gupta, S. (1996). *Immunology of HIV infection.* New York: Plenum Medical Book Co.

International Perinatal HIV Group. (1999). The mode of delivery and the risk of vertical transmission of human immunodeficiency virus type I. *New England Journal of Medicine, 340*(13), 977–987.

Jones, S. G., & Baggett, T. H. (1999). Clinical update: New drugs for HIV/AIDS. *MedSurg Nursing, 8*(2), 108–112.

Kay, A. B. (1997). *Allergy and allergic diseases.* Malden, MA: Blackwell Scientific.

Kirton, C. A., Ferri, R. S., & Eleftherakis, V. (1999). Primary care and case management of persons with HIV/AIDS. *Nursing Clinics of North America, 34*(1), 71–94.

Lane, N. E. (1997). *AIDS, allergy, and rheumatology.* Totowa, NJ: Humana Press.

Levy, J. A. (1998). *HIV and the pathogenesis of AIDS* (2nd ed.). Washington, DC: ASM Press.

Mantell, J. E., DiVittis, A. T., & Auerbach, M. I. (1997). *Evaluating HIV prevention interventions.* New York: Plenum Press.

Miaskowski, C. (1997). *Oncology nursing: An essential guide for patient care.* Philadelphia: W. B. Saunders.

Muma, R. D. (1997). *HIV manual for health care professionals* (2nd ed.). Stamford, CT: Appleton & Lange.

Nakamura, R. M., et al. (Ed.). (1998). *Clinical diagnostic immunology: Protocols in quality assurance and standardization.* Malden, MA: Blackwell Scientific.

Pizzo, P. A., & Wilfert, C. M. (1998). *Pediatric AIDS: The challenge of HIV infection in infants, children, and adolescents* (3rd ed.). Baltimore: Williams & Wilkins.

Porche, D. J. (1999). State of the art antiretroviral and prophylactic treatment in HIV/AIDS. *Nursing Clinics of North America, 34*(1), 95–112.

Powderly, W. G. (1997). *Manual of HIV therapeutics.* Philadelphia: Lippincott-Raven.

Powell, J. (1996). *AIDS and HIV-related diseases: An educational guide for professionals and the public.* New York: Insight Books.

Roitt, I., Brostoff, J., & Male, D. K. (Eds.). (1998). *Immunology* (5th ed.). St. Louis: C. V. Mosby.

Ropka, M., & Williams, A. (1998). *HIV nursing and symptom management.* Sudbury, MA: Jones & Bartlett.

Said, G., et al. (1997). *Neurological complications of HIV and AIDS.* Philadelphia: W. B. Saunders.

Sande, M. A., & Volberding, P. A. (Eds.). (1997). *The medical management of AIDS* (5th ed.). Philadelphia: W. B. Saunders.

Sherman, D. W. (1999). HIV/AIDS Update. *Nursing Clinics of North America, 34*(1), 1–237.

Spach, D. H., & Hooton, T. M. (Ed.). (1996). *The HIV manual: A guide to diagnosis and treatment.* New York: Oxford University Press.

Stephenson, J. (1998). Medical news and perspectives AIDS vaccine moves into phase 3 trials. *Journal of the American Medical Association, 289*(1), 8–9.

Stites, D. P., Terr, A. I., & Parslow, T. G. (Eds.). (1997). *Medical immunology* (9th ed.). Stamford, CT: Appleton & Lange.

Ungvarski, P. J., & Flaskerud, J. H. (Eds.). (1999). *HIV/AIDS: A guide to primary care management* (4th ed.). Philadelphia: W. B. Saunders.

Virella, G. (Ed.). (1998). *Introduction to medical immunology* (4th ed.). New York: Marcel Dekker.

Weir, D. M., & Steward, J. (1997). *Immunology* (8th ed.). New York: Churchill Livingstone.

Williams, A. B. (1999). Adherance to a highly active antiretroviral therapy. *Nursing Clinics of North America, 34*(1), 113–129.

Wormser, G. P. (1998). *AIDS and other manifestations of HIV infection* (3rd ed.). Philadelphia: Lippincott-Raven.

JOURNALS

Asterisks indicate nursing research articles.

Anastasi, J. K., & Sun, V. (1996). Controlling diarrhea in the HIV patient. *American Journal of Nursing, 96*(8), 35–42.

Baltimore, D., & Heilman, C. (1998), HIV vaccines: Prospects and challenges. *Scientific American, 279*(1), *July,* 98–103.

Branson, B. M. (1998). Home sample collection tests for HIV infection. *Journal of the American Medical Association, 280*(19), 1699–1701.

Brennan, C., & Porche, D. J. (1997). HIV immunopathogenesis. *Journal of the Association of Nurses in AIDS Care, 8*(4), 7–22.

Brown, M. A. (1997). Knowledge generation for the HIV-affected family. *Image: A Journal of Nursing Scholarship, 29*(3), 269–274.

Buchbinder, S. (1998). Avoiding infection after HIV exposure. *Scientific American, 279*(1) *July,* 104–105.

Carpenter, C. C. J., et al. (1997). Antiretroviral therapy for HIV infection in 1997: Updated recommendations of the international AIDS society—USA panel. *Journal of the American Medical Association, 277*(24), 1962–1969.

Carpenter, C. C. J., et al. (1998). Antiretroviral therapy for HIV infection in 1998. Updated recommendations of the International AIDS Society—USA Panel. *Journal of the American Medical Association, 280*(1), 78–86.

Casey, K. M. (1997). Malnutrition associated with HIV/AIDS. Part Two: Assessment and interventions. *Journal of the Association of Nurses in AIDS Care, 8*(5), 39–48.

Collier, A. C., et al. (1996). Treatment of human immunodeficiency virus infection with saquinavir, zidovudine and zalcitabine. *New England Journal of Medicine, 334*(16), 1011–1017.

Centers for Disease Control and Prevention, U.S. Department of Health and Human Services. (1998). *HIV/AIDS Surveillance Report, 10*(2), 1–43.

Centers for Disease Control and Prevention. (1998). Public health service guidelines for the management of health-care worker exposure to HIV and recommendations for postexposure prophylaxis. *MMWR CDC Recommendations and Reports, 47*(RR-7), 1–28.

Centers for Disease Control and Prevention, U.S. Department of Health and Human Services. (1998). Report of the NIH panel to define principles of therapy of HIV infection and guidelines for the use of antiretroviral agents in HIV infected adults and adolescents. *MMWR CDC Recommendations and Reports, 24*(RR-5), 1–82.

Centers for Disease Control and Prevention. (1996). U.S. public health service guidelines for testing and counseling blood and plasma donors for human immunodeficiency virus type-I antigen. *MMWR CDC Recommendations and Reports, 45*(RR-2), 1–8.

Centers for Disease Control and Prevention, U.S. Department of Health and Human Services. (1992). 1993 revised classification system for HIV infection and expanded surveillance case definition for AIDS among adolescents and adults. *MMWR CDC Recommendations and Reports, 41*(RR-17), 1–19.

D'Aquila, R. T., et al. (1996). Nevirapine, zidovudine, and diadanosine compared with zidovudine and didanosine in patients with HIV-1 infection. *Annals of Internal Medicine, 124*(12), 1019–1030.

Dwyer, J. T., et al. (1995). The use of unconventional remedies among HIV-positive men living in California. *Journal of the Association of Nurses in AIDS Care, 6*(1), 17–28.

Evans, B. M. (1999). Complementary therapies and HIV infection. *American Journal of Nursing, 99*(2), 42–45.

Fleishman, J. H. (1997). Utilization of home care among people with HIV infection. *Health Services Research, 32*(2), 155–175.

Frank, S., Esch, J. F., & Margeson, N. E. (1998). Mandatory HIV testing of newborns: The impact on women. *American Journal of Nursing, 98*(10), 49–51.

Frick, P. A., Gal, P., Lane, T. W., & Sewell, P. C. (1998). Antiretroviral medication compliance in patients with AIDS. *AIDS Patient Care and STDs, 12*(6), 463–470.

Hammer, S. M. (1996). Advances in antiretroviral therapy and viral load monitoring. *AIDS, 10*(Suppl 3), S1–S11.

Harvath, T. A., et al. (1995). Dementia-related behaviors in Alzheimer's disease and AIDS. *Journal of Psychosocial Nursing and Mental Health Services, 33*(1), 35–39.

Havlir, D. V., & Barnes, P. F. (1999). Tuberculosis in patients with human immunodeficiency virus infection. *New England Journal of Medicine, 340*(5), 367–372.

Hirschfeld, S. (1998). Pain as a complication of HIV disease. *AIDS Patient Care and STDs, 12*(2), 91–108.

Ho, D. D., et al. (1995). Rapid removal of plasma virons and CD4 lymphocytes in HIV infection. *Nature, 373*(6510), 123–126.

Hofbauer, L. C., & Heufelder, A. E. (1996). Endocrine implications of human immunodeficiency virus infection. *Medicine, 75*(5), 262–278.

Holzemer, W. L., Henry, S. B., & Reilly, C. A. (1998). Assessing and managing pain in AIDS care: The patient perspective. *Journal of the Association of Nurses in AIDS Care, 9*(1), 22–30.

Hospital Infection Control Practices Advisory Committee. (1996). Guidelines for isolation precautions in hospitals. *Infection Control and Hospital Epidemiology, 47*(1), 53–80.

Jemmott, J. B. III, Jemmott, L. S., & Fong, G. T. (1998). Abstinence and safer sex HIV risk-reduction interventions for African American adolescents: A randomized controlled trial. *Journal of the American Medical Association, 279*(19), 1529–1536.

Jones, S. G, Holloman, F., & Coffin, D. (1998). Body temperature alterations in hospitalized HIV/AIDS patients. *MedSurg Nursing, 7*(4), 217–225.

Kahn, J. O., & Walker, B. D. (1998). Acute human immunodeficiency virus type I infection. *New England Journal of Medicine, 339*(1), 33–39.

Katzenstein, D. A. (1997). Adherence as a particular issue with protease inhibitors. *Journal of the Association of Nurses in AIDS Care, 8*(Suppl), 10–17.

Katzenstein, D. A., et al. (1997). HIV therapeutics: Confronting adherence. *Journal of the Association of Nurses in AIDS Care, 8*(Suppl), 46–58.

Keithley, J. K., & Swanson, B. (1998). Minimizing HIV/AIDS malnutrition. *MedSurg Nursing, 7*(5), 256–267.

Klaus, B. D. (1994). Late manifestations of HIV infection and AIDS. *Nurse Practitioner: American Journal of Primary Health Care, 19*(6), 4–5.

Kosko, D. A. (1997). Dermatologic manifestations of human immunodeficiency virus disease. *Lippincott's Primary Care Practice, 1*(1), 50–61.

Kwong, P. D., Wyatt, R., Robinson, J., Sweet, R. W., Sodroski, J., & Hendrickson, W. A. (1998). Structure of an HIV gp 120 envelope glycoprotein in complex with the CD4 receptor and a neutralizing antibody. *Nature, 393,* 648–659.

*Lauver, D., et al. (1995). HIV risk status and preventive behaviors among 17,619 women. *Journal of Obstetric, Gynecologic, and Neonatal Nursing, 24*(1), 33–39.

Lin, H. J., Haywood, M., & Hollinger, F. B. (1996). Application of commercial kit for detection of PCR products to quantification of human immuno-

deficiency virus type 1 RNA and proviral DNA. *Journal of Clinical Microbiology, 34*(2), 329–333.
Lisanti, P., & Zwolski, K. (1997). Understanding the devastation of AIDS. *American Journal of Nursing, 97*(7), 27–35.
Lyons, C. (1997). HIV drug adherence: Special situations. *Journal of the Association of Nurses in AIDS Care, 8*(Suppl), 29–36.
MacIntyre, R. C., & Holzemer, W. L. (1997). Complementary and alternative medicine and HIV/AIDS. II. Selected literature review. *Journal of the Association of Nurses in AIDS Care, 8*(2), 25–38.
Martin, M. A., & Kane, C. (1997). Nursing considerations in the use of cidofovir for CMV retinitis in patients with AIDS: Report of a roundtable meeting. *Journal of the Association of Nurses in AIDS Care, 8*(5), 66–74.
Melroe, N. H., Stawarz, K. E., Simpson, J., & Kenry, W. K. (1997). HIV RNA quantitation: Marker of HIV infection. *Journal of the Association of Nurses in AIDS Care, 8*(5), 31–38.
Morris, N. J. (1996). Depression and HIV+ disease: A critical review. *Journal of the American Psychiatric Nursing Association, 2*(5), 154–163.
National Institutes of Health. (1997). Interventions to prevent HIV risk behaviors. *NIH Consensus Statement, 15*(2), 1–41.
Pahwa, S., & Morales, M. (1998). Interleukin-2 therapy in HIV infection. *AIDS Patient Care and STDs, 3*(12), 187–197.
Perelson, A. S., Neuman, A. U., Markowitz, M., Leonard, T. M., & Ho, D. D. (1996). HI1 dynamics in vivo: Viron clearance rate, infected cell life-span and viral generation time. *Science, 271,* 1582–1586.
Portillo, C. J., et al. (1996). American Academy of Nursing's HIV/AIDS nursing care summit: The final synthesis. *Nursing Outlook, 44*(5), 229–234.
Phillips, P. (1997). No plateau for HIV/AIDS epidemic in US women. *Journal of the American Medical Association, 227*(22), 1747–1749.
Ratcliffe, J., Gibb, D., Sculpher, M. J., & Briggs, A. H. (1998). Prevention of mother-to-child transmission of HIV-I infection: Alternative strategies and their cost-effectiveness. *AIDS, 12*(11), 1381–1387.
Rosenbert, P. S., & Biggar, R. J. (1998). Trends in HIV incidence among young adults in the United States. *Journal of the American Medical Association, 279*(23), 1894–1899.
Saag, M. S. (1998). Strategies for long-term patient management. *AIDs Patient Care and STDs, 12*(7), 533–536.
Saag, M. S., et al. (1996). HIV viral load markers in clinical practice. *Nature Medicine, 2*(6), 625–629.
*Sowell, R. L., Phillips, K. D., & Grier, J. (1998). Restructuring life to face the future: The perspective of men after a positive response to protease inhibitor therapy. *AIDS Patient Care and STDs, 12*(1), 33–41.
*Sowell, R. L., & Misener, T. R. (1997). Decisions to have a baby by HIV-infected women. *Western Journal of Nursing Research, 19*(1), 56–70.
Stetz, K. M., & Brown, M. A. (1997). Taking care: Caregiving to persons with cancer and AIDS. *Cancer Nursing, 20*(1), 12–22.
*Taylor, C. A., Keller, M. L., & Egan, J. J. (1997). Advice from affected persons about living with human papillomavirus infection. *Image: A Journal of Nursing Scholarship, 29*(1), 27–32.
Ungvarski, P. J. (1997). Adherence to prescribed HIV-1 protease inhibitors in the home setting. *Journal of the Association of Nurses in AIDS Care, 8*(Suppl), 37–45.
Ungvarski, P. J., & Rottner, J. E. (1997). Errors in prescribing HIV-1 protease inhibitors. *Journal of the Association of Nurses in AIDS Care, 8*(4), 55–61.
*Vitiello, M. A., & Smeltzer, S. C. (1999). HIV, pregnancy and zidovudine: What do women know? *Journal of the Association of Nurses in AIDS Care, 10*(4), 41–47.
Walsek, C., Zafonte, M., & Bowers, J. M. (1997). Nutritional issues and HIV/AIDS: Assessment and treatment strategies. *Journal of the Association of Nurses in AIDS Care, 8*(6), 71–80.
Webb, A. A., Bower, D. A., & Gill, S. (1997). Satisfaction with nursing care: A comparison of patients with HIV/AIDS infectious diseases, and medical diagnoses. *Journal of the Association of Nurses in AIDS Care, 8*(2), 39–46.
Wei, X., et al. (1995). Viral dynamics in human immunodeficiency virus type I infection. *Nature, 373*(6510), 117–122.
Williams, A. (1997). Antiretroviral therapy: Factors associated with adherence. *Journal of the Association of Nurses in AIDS Care, 8*(Suppl), 18–23.
Williams, A. B. (1997). New horizons: Antiretroviral therapy. *Journal of the Association of Nurses in AIDS Care, 8*(4), 26–38.
Wyatt, R., Kwong, P. D., Desjardins, E., Sweet, R. W., Robinson, J., Hendrickson, W. A., & Sodroski, J. G. (1998). The antigenic structure of the HIV gp120 envelope glycoprotein. *Nature, 393,* 705–711.
Zelenetz, P. D., & Epstein, M. E. (1998). HIV in the elderly. *AIDS Patient Care and STDs, 12*(4), 255–262.

Resources

BOOKS

Bartlett, J. G., & Finbeiner, A. K. (1998). *The guide to living with HIV infection* (4th ed.). Baltimore: Johns Hopkins University Press.
Cohen, M. R. (1998). *The HIV wellness sourcebook: An East/West guide to living well with HIV/AIDS and related conditions.* New York: H. Holt.
Houts, P. S. (Ed.). (1998). *Home care guide for HIV and AIDS: For family and friends giving care at home.* Philadelphia: American College of Physicians.

AGENCIES

AIDS Action Council, 875 Connecticut NW, Suite 700, Washington, DC 20003; 1-202-986-1300; Fax 1-202-986-1345; www.aidsaction.org
AIDS Clinical Trials Information Service, P.O. 621, Rockville, MD 20849-6421; 1-800-874-2572 (1-800-TRIALS-A); *Hearing impaired,* 1-800-243-7012; Fax 1-301-519-6616; www.actis.org
American Foundation for AIDS Research, 120 Wall St., New York, NY 10005; 1-212-806-1600; 1-212-806-1601; www.amfar@amfar.org
American Red Cross National Headquarters, HIV/AIDS Education, 8111 Gatehouse Rd., Falls Church, VA 22042; 1-703-206-7180; Fax 1-703-206-7754; www.redcross.org (or local Red Cross)
American Social Health Association, P.O. Box 13827, Research Triangle Park, NC 27709; 1-919-361-8400, Fax 1-919-361-8425; www.afhastd.org
CDC National AIDS Hotline, P.O. Box 12827, Research Triangle Park, NC 27709; 1-800-342-AIDS; *Spanish,* 1-800-344-7432; *Hearing impaired,* 1-800-243-7889; www.ashstd.org
CDC Prevention Network Analytical Science Inc., 8401 Colesville Rd., Suite 200, Silver Spring, MD 20910; 1-301-562-1000; Fax 1-301-562-1001; www.cdcnpin.org
Gay Men's Health Crisis Network, 1209 West 20th St., New York, NY 10011; 1-212-807-6655
Hemophilia and AIDS/HIV Network for the Dissemination of Information, The National Hemophilia Foundation, 116 West 32nd St., 11th Floor, New York, NY 10001; 1-212-328-3700; 1-800-42-HANDI; Fax 1-212-328-3777; www.hemophilia.org
Mothers of AIDS Patients (MAP), c/o Barbara Peabody, 3403 E St., San Diego, CA 92102; 1-619-234-3432
National Association of People With AIDS, 1413 K Street, N.W., 7th Floor, Washington, DC 20005; 1-202-898-0414; Fax 1-202-898-0435; www.natwa.org
National Council of Churches/AIDS Task Force and Minority Task Force, 475 Riverside Dr., Room 572, New York, NY 10115; 1-212-870-242, 1-212-749-1214

AIDS EDUCATION AND TRAINING CENTERS (ETCs)

Central Office

AIDS ETC Program, 5600 Fishers Lane, Room 9A-39, Rockville, MD 20857; 1-301-443-6364; Fax 1-301-433-9887; contact for information about local ETC.

AIDS HOTLINES

CDC AIDS Hotline:
English: 1-800-342-AIDS (2437)
Spanish: 1-800-344-7432
TDY Service for the Deaf: 1-800-243-7889
HIV Telephone Consultation Service: 1-800-933-3413
American Foundation for AIDS Research: 1-800-39AMFAR (392-6327)
AIDS Treatment News: 1-800-TREAT 1-2 (873-2812)
AIDS Clinical Trials Information Service (ACTIS): 1-800-TRIALS-A (874-2572)
Drug Abuse Hotline 1-800-662-HELP (4357)
National Hemophilia Foundation (212) 328-3700
Hemophilia and AIDS/HIV Network for Dissemination of Information (HANDI) 1-800-42-HANDI (424-2634)
National Pediatric HIV Resource Center 1-800-362-0071
National Association of People with AIDS 1-202-898-0414
National Sexually Transmitted Disease Hotline/American Social Health Association: 1-800-227-8922

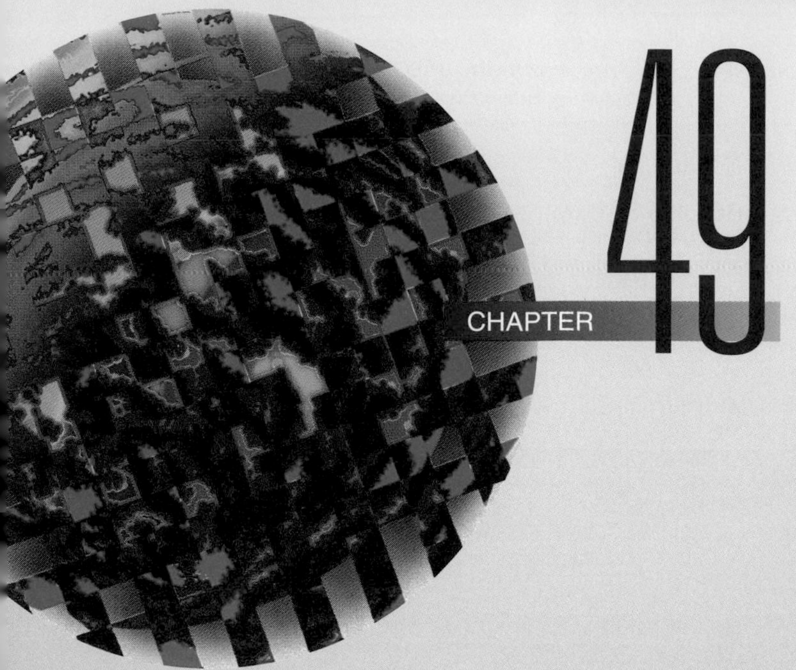

Assessment and Management of Patients With Allergic Disorders

Learning Objectives

On completion of this chapter, the learner will be able to:

1. Explain the physiologic events involved with allergic reactions.
2. Describe the types of hypersensitivity.
3. Describe the management of patients with allergic disorders.
4. Describe measures to prevent and manage anaphylaxis.
5. Use the nursing process as a framework for care of the patient with allergic rhinitis.
6. Discuss the different allergic disorders according to type.
7. Describe the prevention and management of anaphylaxis.

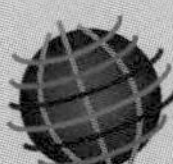

The human body is menaced by a host of potential invaders—**allergens** as well as microbial organisms—that constantly threaten its surface defenses. After penetrating those defenses, these allergens and organisms compete with the body for its nutrients and, if allowed to flourish unimpeded, disrupt its enzyme systems and destroy its vital tissues. To protect against these agents, the body is equipped with an elaborate defense system.

The epithelial cells coating the skin and making up the lining of the respiratory, gastrointestinal, and genitourinary tracts provide the first line of defense. The structure and continuity of these surfaces and the resistance to penetration are initial deterrents to invaders.

One of the most effective defense mechanisms is the body's capacity to equip itself rapidly with weapons (*antibodies*) individually designed to meet each new invader, namely, specific protein *antigens.* Antibodies react with antigens in a variety of ways: (1) by coating the antigens' surfaces if they are particular substances, (2) by neutralizing the antigens if they are toxic, and (3) by precipitating the antigens out of solution if they are dissolved.

The antibodies prepare the antigens so that the phagocytic cells of the blood and the tissues can dispose of them. In some cases, however, the body produces inappropriate or exaggerated responses to specific antigens, and the result is an allergic or **hypersensitivity** disorder.

GLOSSARY

allergen: substance that causes manifestations of allergy

allergy: inappropriate and often harmful immune system response to substances that are normally harmless

anaphylaxis: clinical response to an immediate immunologic reaction between a specific antigen and antibody

angioneurotic edema: condition characterized by urticaria and diffuse swelling of the deeper layers of the skin

antibody: protein substance developed by the body in response to and interacting with a specific antigen

antigen: substance that induces the production of antibodies

antihistamine: medication that opposes the action of histamine

atopic dermatitis: type I hypersensitivity involving inflammation of the skin evidenced by itching, redness, and a variety of skin lesions

B lymphocyte: cells that are important in producing circulating antibodies

bradykinin: polypeptide that stimulates nerve fibers and causes pain

eosinophil: granular leukocyte

erythema: diffuse redness of the skin

hapten: incomplete antigen

histamine: substance in the body that causes increased gastric secretion, dilation of capillaries, and constriction of the bronchial smooth muscle

hypersensitivity: abnormal heightened reaction to a stimulus of any kind

immunoglobulins: a family of closely related proteins capable of acting as antibodies

leukotrienes: a group of chemical mediators that initiate the inflammatory response

lymphokines: substances released by sensitized lymphocytes when they contact specific antigens

mast cell: connective tissue cells that contain heparin and histamine in their granules

prostaglandins: unsaturated fatty acids that have a wide assortment of biologic activity

rhinitis: inflammation of the nasal mucosa

serotonin: chemical mediator that acts as a potent vasoconstrictor and bronchoconstrictor

T lymphocyte: cells that can cause graft rejection, kill foreign cells, or suppress production of antibodies

urticaria: hives

ALLERGIC REACTION: PHYSIOLOGIC OVERVIEW

An *allergic reaction* is a manifestation of tissue injury resulting from interaction between an antigen and an antibody. **Allergy** is an inappropriate and often harmful response of the immune system to normally harmless substances. In this case, the substance is termed an allergen.

When the body is invaded by an **antigen**, usually a protein that the body's defenses recognize as foreign, a series of events occurs in an attempt to render the invader harmless, destroy it, and remove it from the body. When lymphocytes respond to the antigen, **antibodies** (protein substances that protect against antigens) are produced. Common allergic reactions occur when the immune system of a susceptible person responds aggressively to a substance that is normally harmless (eg, dust, weeds, pollen, dander). Chemical mediators released in allergic reactions may produce symptoms ranging from mild to life-threatening.

The many cells and organs of the immune system secrete various substances important in the immune response. These parts of the immune system must work together to ensure adequate defense against invaders (ie, virus, bacteria, other foreign substances) without destroying the body's own tissues by an overly aggressive reaction.

Function and Production of Immunoglobulins

Antibodies formed by lymphocytes and plasma cells in response to an immunogenic stimulus constitute a group of serum proteins called **immunoglobulins**. Grouped into five classes as IgE, IgD, IgG, IgM, and IgA, these can be found in the lymph nodes, tonsils, appendix, and Peyer's patches of the intestinal tract or circulating in the blood and lymph. Antibodies of the IgM, IgG, and IgA classes have definite and well-established protective functions. These include neutralization of toxins and viruses and precipitation, agglutination, and lysis of bacteria and other foreign cellular material. (See Chap. 46 for further discussion of these functions.)

Immunoglobulins of the IgE class are involved in allergic disorders and some parasitic infections, evidenced by elevation of IgE levels. IgE-producing cells are located in the respiratory and intestinal mucosa. Two or more IgE molecules bind together to an allergen and trigger **mast cells** or basophils to release chemical mediators, such as histamine, serotonin, kinins, slow-reacting substance of anaphylaxis (SRS-A), and the neutrophil factor, which produces allergic skin reactions, asthma, and hay fever.

Antibodies combine with antigens in a special way, likened to keys fitting into a lock. Antigens (the keys) only fit certain antibodies (the locks). Hence, the term *specificity* refers to the specific reaction of an antibody to an antigen. There are many variations and complexities in these patterns.

Antibody molecules are *bivalent;* that is, they have two combining sites. Therefore, the antibody easily becomes a cross-link between two antigen groups, causing them to clump together (*agglutination*). By this action, foreign invaders are cleared from the bloodstream. Agglutination is the means for determining blood group in laboratory tests.

Role of B Cells

The B cell, or **B lymphocyte**, is programmed to produce one specific antibody. On encountering a specific antigen, a B cell stimulates production of plasma cells, the site of antibody production. The result is the outpouring of antibodies for the purpose of destroying and removing the antigen.

Role of T Cells

The *T cell,* or **T lymphocyte,** assists the B cells in producing antibodies. T cells secrete substances known as **lymphokines,** which encourage cell growth, promote cell activation, direct the flow of cell activity, destroy target cells, and stimulate the macrophages. Macrophages present the antigen to the T cells and initiate the immune response. They also digest antigens and assist in removing cells and other debris.

Function of Antigens

Antigens are divided into two groups: complete protein antigens and low-molecular-weight substances. Complete protein antigens, such as animal dander, pollen, and horse serum, stimulate a complete humoral response. (See Chap. 46 for a discussion of humoral immunity.) Low-molecular-weight substances, such as medications, function as **haptens** (incomplete antigens), binding to tissue or serum proteins to produce a carrier complex that initiates an antibody response.

In an allergic reaction, the production of antigen-specific IgE antibodies requires active communication between macrophages, T cells, and B cells. When the allergen is absorbed through the respiratory tract, gastrointestinal tract, or skin, allergen sensitization occurs. The macrophage processes the antigen and presents it to the appropriate T cell. B cells that are influenced by the T cell mature into an allergen-specific IgE immunoglobulin-secreting plasma cell that synthesizes and secretes antigen-specific IgE antibody.

Function of Chemical Mediators

Mast cells, which have a major role in IgE-mediated immediate hypersensitivity, are located in the skin and mucous membranes. When mast cells are stimulated by antigens, powerful chemical mediators are released that cause a sequence of physiologic events resulting in symptoms of immediate hypersensitivity (Fig. 49-1). There are two types of chemical mediators: primary, which are preformed and found in mast cells or basophils, and secondary, which are inactive precursors formed or released in response to primary mediators. The most prevalent known primary and secondary mediators are described next. (Table 49-1 on page 1385 summarizes the actions of primary and secondary chemical mediators.)

Primary Mediators

HISTAMINE

Histamine plays an important role in the immune response. These effects include contraction of bronchial smooth muscle, resulting in wheezing and bronchospasm; dilation of small venules and constriction of larger vessels, causing erythema (redness), edema, and urticaria; and increased secretion of gastric and mucosal cells, resulting in diarrhea. Histamine action results from stimulation of histamine-1 (H_1) and histamine-2 (H_2) receptors found on different types of lymphocytes, particularly T-lymphocyte suppressor cells and basophils. H_1 receptors are found predominantly on bronchiolar and vascular smooth muscle cells. H_2 receptors are found on gastric parietal cells.

Certain medications are categorized by their action at these receptors. Diphenhydramine (Benadryl) is an example of an **antihistamine**, which is a medication displaying an affinity for H_1 receptors; whereas cimetidine, another pharmacologic agent, targets H_2 receptors to inhibit gastric secretions in peptic ulcer disease.

EOSINOPHIL CHEMOTACTIC FACTOR OF ANAPHYLAXIS

Preformed in the mast cells, this *chemotactic factor*, which affects movement of **eosinophils** (a granular leukocyte) to the site of allergens, is released upon degranulation to inhibit the action of leukotrienes and histamine.

PLATELET-ACTIVATING FACTOR

Platelet-activating factor (PAF) is responsible for initiating platelet aggregation at sites of immediate hypersensitivity reactions. It also causes bronchoconstriction and increased vascular permeability. PAF also activates factor XII, or Hageman factor, which induces the formation of bradykinin.

PROSTAGLANDINS

Prostaglandins, composed of unsaturated fatty acids, produce smooth muscle contraction as well as vasodilation and increased capillary permeability. The fever and pain that occur with inflammation are due, in part, to the prostaglandins.

Secondary Mediators

LEUKOTRIENES

Leukotrienes are chemical mediators that initiate the inflammatory response. One of these substances, slow-reacting substance of anaphylaxis (SRS-A), produces sustained spasm of the bronchioles. Compared with histamine, leukotrienes are 100 to 1000 times more potent in causing bronchospasm. Many manifestations of inflammation can be attributed, in part, to leukotrienes.

BRADYKININ

Bradykinin, a polypeptide, contracts smooth muscles of the bronchi and blood vessels. It causes increased permeability of the capillaries, resulting in edema. Bradykinin stimulates nerve cell fibers and produces pain.

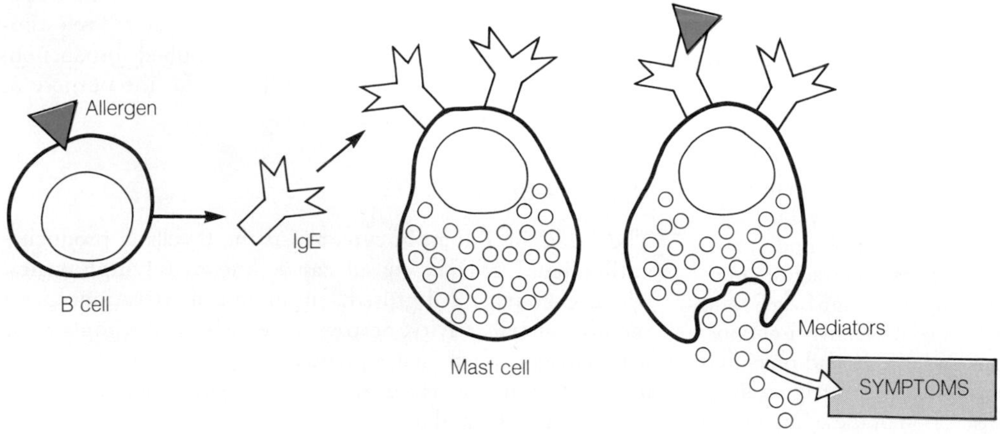

FIGURE 49•1 Allergen triggers B cell to make IgE antibody, which attaches to mast cell. When that allergen reappears, it binds to the IgE and triggers the mast cell to release its chemicals. Courtesy of U.S. Dept. of Health and Human Services, National Institutes of Health.

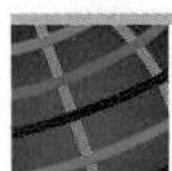

TABLE 49•1 Chemical Mediators of Hypersensitivity

Mediators	Action
Primary Mediators	
(Preformed and found in mast cells or basophils)	
Histamine (preformed in mast cells)	Vasodilation Smooth muscle contraction, increased vascular permeability, increased mucus secretions
Eosinophil chemotactic factor of anaphylaxis (ECF-A) (preformed in mast cells)	Attracts eosinophils
Platelet-activating factor (PAF) (requires synthesis by mast cells, neutrophils, and macrophages)	Smooth muscle contraction Incites platelets to aggregate and release serotonin and histamine
Prostaglandins (chemically derived from arachidonic acid; require synthesis by cells)	D and F series → bronchoconstriction E series → bronchodilation D, E, and F series → vasodilation
Basophil kallikrein (preformed in mast cells)	Frees bradykinin, which causes bronchoconstriction, vasodilation, and nerve stimulation
Secondary Mediators	
(Inactive precursors formed or released in response to primary mediators)	
Bradykinin (derived from precursor kininogen)	Smooth muscle contraction, increased vascular permeability, stimulates pain receptors, increased mucus production
Serotonin (preformed in platelets)	Smooth muscle contraction, increased vascular permeability
Heparin (preformed in mast cells)	Anticoagulant
Leukotrienes (derived from arachidonic acid and activated by mast cell degranulation) C, D, and E or slow-reacting substance of anaphylaxis (SRS-A)	Smooth muscle contraction, increased vascular permeability

SEROTONIN

Serotonin is released during platelet aggregation, acting as a potent vasoconstrictor and causing contraction of bronchial smooth muscle.

Hypersensitivity

A hypersensitivity reaction is an abnormal, heightened reaction to any type of stimuli. It usually does not occur with the first exposure to an allergen. Rather, the reaction follows a reexposure after sensitization in a predisposed individual. Sensitization initiates the humoral response or buildup of antibodies. To promote understanding of the immunopathogenesis of disease, hypersensitivity reactions have been classified into four specific types of reactions (Fig. 49-2). Most allergies are identified as either type I or type IV hypersensitivity reactions.

Anaphylactic (Type I) Hypersensitivity

Type I or anaphylactic hypersensitivity is an immediate reaction beginning within minutes of exposure to an antigen. This reaction is mediated by IgE antibodies rather than IgG or IgM antibodies. Type I hypersensitivity requires previous exposure to the specific antigen. In turn, the plasma cells produce IgE antibodies in the lymph nodes, where helper T cells aid in promoting this reaction. The IgE antibodies bind to membrane receptors on mast cells found in connective tissue and basophils. During reexposure, the antigen binds to adjacent IgE antibodies, activating a cellular reaction that triggers degranulation and the release of chemical mediators (histamine, leukotrienes, and eosinophil chemotactic factor of anaphylaxis [ECF-A]).

Primary chemical mediators are responsible for the symptoms of type I hypersensitivity because of their effects on the skin, lungs, and gastrointestinal tract. When chemical mediators continue to be released, a delayed reaction may occur lasting for up to 24 hours. Clinical symptoms are determined by the amount of the allergen, the amount of mediator released, the sensitivity of the target organ, and the route of allergen entry. Type I hypersensitivity reactions may include both local and systemic anaphylaxis.

Cytotoxic (Type II) Hypersensitivity

A type II, or cytotoxic, hypersensitivity occurs when the system mistakenly identifies a normal constituent of the body as foreign. This reaction may be a result of a cross-reacting antibody, possibly leading to cell and tissue damage. Type II hypersensitivity involves the binding of either IgG or IgM antibody to the cell-bound antigen. The result of antigen–antibody binding is activation of the complement cascade (see Chap. 46) and destruction of the cell to which the antigen is bound.

A type II hypersensitivity reaction is associated with several disorders. For example, in myasthenia gravis, the body mistakenly generates antibodies against normal nerve ending receptors. In Goodpasture's syndrome, antibodies against lung and renal tissue are generated, producing lung damage and renal failure. A type II hypersensitivity reaction resulting in red blood cell destruction is associated with drug-induced immune hemolytic anemia, Rh-hemolytic disease of the newborn, and incompatibility reactions in blood transfusions (see Chap. 30).

Immune Complex (Type III) Hypersensitivity

When these type III complexes are deposited in tissues or vascular endothelium, two factors contribute to injury: the increased amount of circulating complexes and the presence of vasoactive amines. As a result, there is an increase in vascular permeability and tissue injury. The joints and kidneys are particularly susceptible to this type of injury. Type III hypersensitivity is associated with systemic lupus erythematosus, rheumatoid arthritis, serum sickness, certain types of nephritis, and some types of bacterial endocarditis.

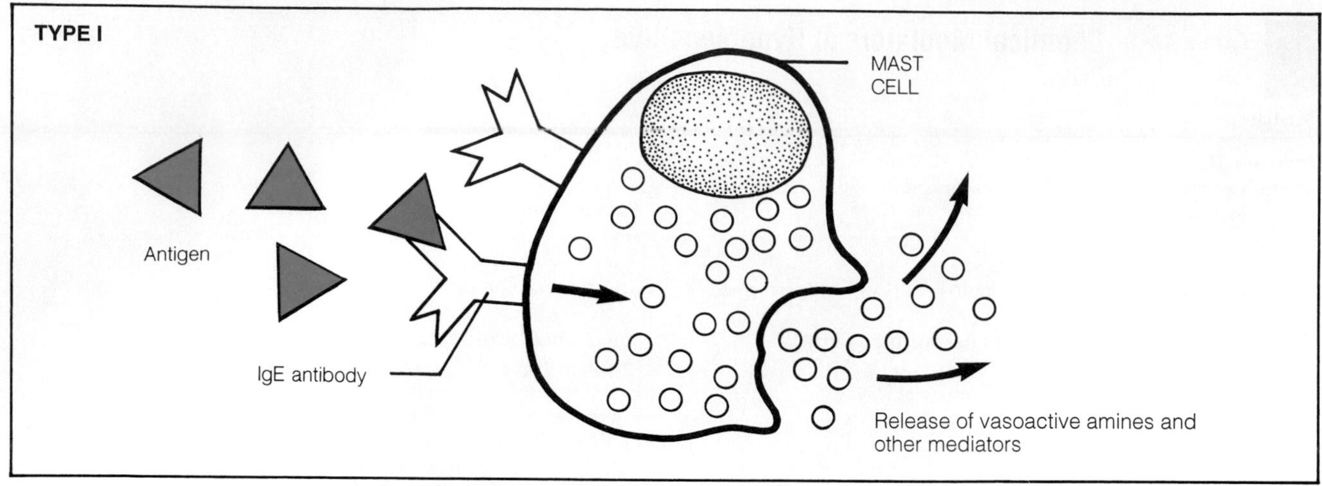

Type I. An anaphylactic reaction is characterized by vasodilation, increased capillary permeability, smooth muscle contraction, and eosinophilia. Systemic reactions may involve laryngeal stridor, angioedema, hypotension, and bronchial, GI, or uterine spasm; local reactions are characterized by hives. Examples of type I reactions include extrinsic asthma, allergic rhinitis, systemic anaphylaxis, and reactions to insect stings.

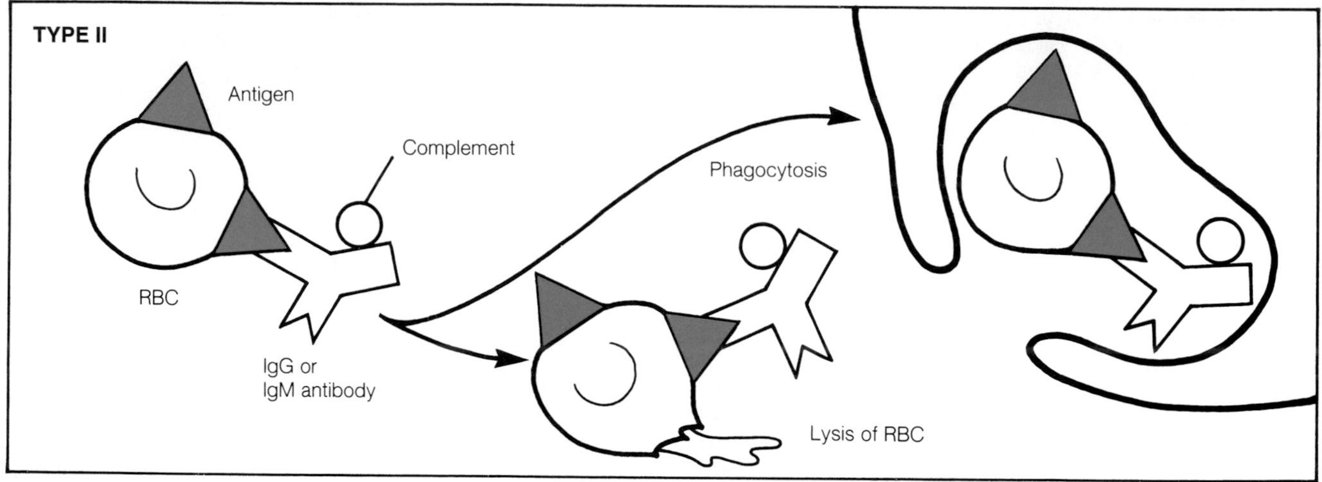

Type II. A cytotoxic reaction, which involves the binding of either the IgG or IgM antibody to a cell-bound antigen, may lead to eventual cell and tissue damage. The reaction is the result of mistaken identity when the system identifies a normal constituent of the body as foreign and activates the complement cascade. Examples of type II reactions are myasthenia gravis, Goodpasture's syndrome, pernicious anemia, hemolytic disease of the newborn, transfusion reaction, and thrombocytopenia.

FIGURE 49•2 Four types of hypersensitivity reactions.

Type III, or immune complex, hypersensitivity involves immune complexes formed when antigens bind to antibodies. These complexes are then cleared from the circulation by phagocytic action. When these complexes are deposited in tissues or the vascular endothelium, however, the volume of circulating complexes increases, and vascular permeability increases. Tissue injury results and affects the joints and kidneys.

Delayed-Type (Type IV) Hypersensitivity

Type IV, or delayed-type hypersensitivity, also known as cellular hypersensitivity, occurs 24 to 72 hours after exposure to an allergen. It is mediated by sensitized T cells and macrophages. An example of this reaction is the effect of an intradermal injection of tuberculin antigen or purified protein derivative (PPD). Sensitized T cells react with the antigen at or near the injection site. Lymphokines are released and attract, activate, and retain macrophages at the site. These macrophages then release lysozymes, causing tissue damage. Edema and fibrin are responsible for the positive tuberculin reaction.

An example of a type IV hypersensitivity reaction is contact dermatitis resulting from exposure to allergens such as cosmetics, adhesive tape, topical medications, medication additives, and plant toxins. The primary exposure results in sensitization. Reexposure causes a hypersensitivity reaction composed of low-molecular-weight molecules (haptens) that bind with proteins or carriers and are then processed by Langerhans' cells in the skin. The symptoms that occur include itching, erythema, and raised lesions.

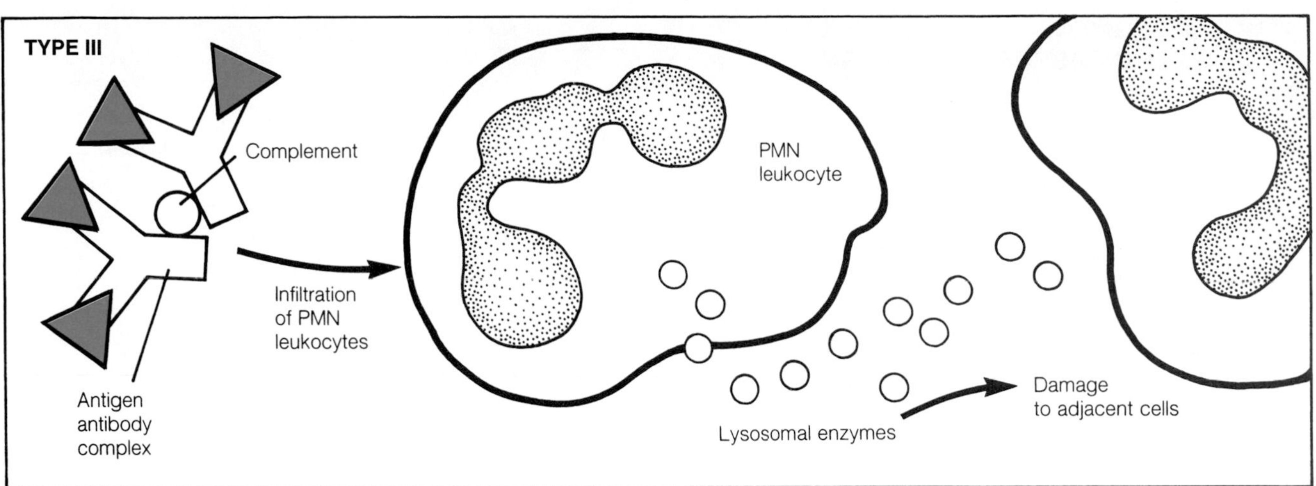

Type III. An immune complex reaction is marked by acute inflammation resulting from formation and deposition of immune complexes. The joints and kidneys are particularly susceptible to this kind of reaction, which is associated with systemic lupus erythematosus, serum sickness, nephritis and rheumatoid arthritis. Some signs and symptoms include urticaria, joint pain, fever, rash, and adenopathy (swollen glands).

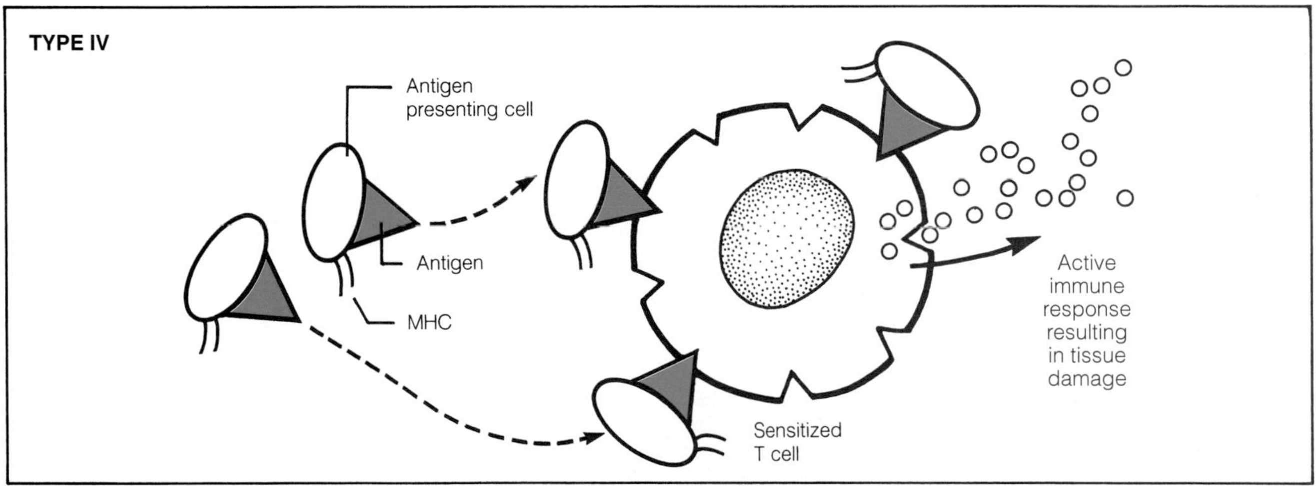

Type IV. A delayed, or cellular, reaction occurs 1 to 3 days after exposure to an antigen. The reaction, which results in tissue damage, involves activity by lymphokines, macrophages, and lysozymes. Erythema and itching are common; a few examples include contact dermatitis, graft-versus-host disease, Hashimoto's thyroiditis, and sarcoidosis.

FIGURE 49•2 *(Continued)*

ASSESSMENT

Health History and Clinical Manifestations

A comprehensive allergy history and a thorough physical examination provide useful data for the diagnosis and management of patients with allergic disorders. An assessment form is useful for obtaining and organizing this information.

The degree of difficulty and discomfort experienced by the patient because of allergic symptoms and the degree of improvement in those symptoms with and without treatment are assessed and documented. The relationship of symptoms to exposure to possible allergens is noted.

DIAGNOSTIC EVALUATION

Diagnostic evaluation of the patient with allergic disorders commonly includes blood tests, smears of body secretions, skin tests, and the radioallergosorbent test (RAST). Results of laboratory blood studies provide supportive data for various diagnostic possibilities; however, they are not the major criteria for the diagnosis of allergic disease.

Complete Blood Count With Differential

The white blood cell (WBC) count is usually normal except during infective states. Eosinophils, granular leukocytes, normally make up 1% to 3% of the total number of WBC. A level between

ASSESSMENT
ALLERGY ASSESSMENT FORM

Name ______ Age ______ Sex ______ Date ______

I. Chief complaint: ______

II. Present illness: ______

III. Collateral allergic symptoms: ______

- Eyes: Pruritus ______ Burning ______ Lacrimation ______
  Swelling ______ Injection ______ Discharge ______
- Ears: Pruritus ______ Fullness ______ Popping ______
  Frequent infections ______
- Nose: Sneezing ______ Rhinorrhea ______ Obstruction ______
  Pruritus ______ Mouth-breathing ______
  Purulent discharge ______
- Throat: Soreness ______ Postnasal discharge ______
  Palatal pruritus ______ Mucus in the morning ______
- Chest: Cough ______ Pain ______ Wheezing ______
  Sputum ______ Dyspnea ______
  Color ______ Rest ______
  Amount ______ Exertion ______
- Skin: Dermatitis ______ Eczema ______ Urticaria ______

IV. Family allergies

V. Previous allergic treatment or testing: ______

Prior skin testing: ______

Medications:
- Antihistamines Improved ______ Unimproved ______
- Bronchodilators Improved ______ Unimproved ______
- Nose drops Improved ______ Unimproved ______
- Hyposensitization Improved ______ Unimproved ______
  - Duration ______
  - Antigens ______
  - Reactions ______
- Antibiotics Improved ______ Unimproved ______
- Corticosteroids Improved ______ Unimproved ______

VI. Physical agents and habits: ______

Bothered by:

Tobacco for ______ years	Alcohol ______	Air cond. ______
Cigarettes ______ packs/day	Heat ______	Muggy weather ______
Cigars ______ per day	Cold ______	Weather changes ______
Pipes ______ per day	Perfumes ______	Chemicals ______
Never smoked ______	Paints ______	Hair spray ______
Bothered by smoke ______	Insecticides ______	Newspapers ______
	Cosmetics ______	

VII. When symptoms occur: ______

Time and circumstances of 1st episode: ______

Prior health: ______

Course of illness over decades: progressing ______ regressing ______

Time of year: ______ Exact dates: ______

- Perennial ______
- Seasonal ______
- Seasonally exacerbated ______

Monthly variations (menses, occupation): ______

Time of week (weekends vs. weekdays): ______

Time of day or night: ______

After insect stings: ______

VIII. Where symptoms occur: ______

Living where at onset: ______

Living where since onset: ______

Effect of vacation or major geographic change: ______

Symptoms better indoors or outdoors: ______

Effect of school or work: ______

Effect of staying elsewhere nearby: ______

Effect of hospitalization: ______

Effect of specific environments: ______

(continued)

ASSESSMENT
ALLERGY ASSESSMENT FORM *(Continued)*

Do symptoms occur around: ____
old leaves ____ hay ____ lakeside ____ barns ____
summer homes ____ damp basement ____ dry attic ____
lawnmowing ____ animals ____ other ____
Do symptoms occur after eating:
cheese ____ mushrooms ____ beer ____ melons ____
bananas ____ fish ____ nuts ____ citrus fruits ____
other foods (list) ____
Home: city ____ rural ____
house ____ age ____
apartment ____ basement ____ damp ____ dry ____
heating system ____
pets (how long) ____ dog ____ cat ____ other ____

Bedroom:	Type	Age	*Living room:*	Type	Age
Pillow	____	____	Rug	____	____
Mattress	____	____	Matting	____	____
Blankets	____	____	Furniture	____	____
Quilts	____	____			
Furniture	____	____			

Anywhere in home symptoms are worse: ____
IX. What does patient think makes symptoms worse? ____
X. Under what circumstances is patient free of symptoms? ____
XI. Summary and additional comments: ____

5% and 15% is nonspecific but does suggest allergic reaction. Other levels are considered moderate and severe, as follows:

Moderate eosinophilia—15% to 40% of blood leukocytes as eosinophils are found in patients with allergic disorders as well as in patients with malignancy, immunodeficiencies, parasitic infections, congenital heart disease, and those receiving peritoneal dialysis.

Severe eosinophilia—50% to 90% of blood leukocytes as eosinophils are found in the idiopathic hypereosinophilic syndrome.

Eosinophil Count

An actual count of eosinophils may be obtained from blood samples or smears of secretions. A total eosinophil count can be obtained from a blood sample by using special diluting fluids that hemolyze erythrocytes and stain the eosinophils. During symptomatic episodes, smears obtained from nasal secretions, conjunctival secretions, and sputum of atopic patients usually reveal eosinophils, indicative of an active allergic response.

Total Serum Immunoglobulin E Levels

High total serum IgE levels support the diagnosis of atopic disease. A normal IgE level, however, does not exclude the diagnosis of an allergic disorder. IgE levels are not as sensitive as the paper radioimmunosorbent test (PRIST) and the enzyme-linked immunosorbent assay (ELISA). Commercial kits are available for IgE determinations. Indications for determining IgE levels include the following:

- Evaluation of immunodeficiency
- Evaluation of drug reactions
- Initial laboratory screening for allergic bronchopulmonary aspergillosis
- Evaluation of allergy among children with bronchiolitis
- Differentiation of atopic and nonatopic eczema
- Differentiation of atopic and nonatopic asthma and rhinitis

Skin Tests

Skin testing entails the simultaneous intradermal injection or superficial application (epicutaneous), of several solutions at separate sites. These solutions contain individual antigens representing an assortment of allergens, including pollen, most likely to be implicated in the patient's disease. Positive reactions (wheal and flare) are clinically significant when correlated with the history, physical findings, and results of other laboratory tests.

Skin tests lend importance to other evidence obtained from the patient's history. They indicate which of several antigens are most likely to provoke symptoms and provide some clue to the intensity of the patient's sensitization. The dosage of the antigen (allergen) injected is also important. Most patients are hypersensitive to more than one pollen. Under testing conditions, they may not react (although they usually do) to the specific pollens that induce their attacks.

In cases of doubt about the validity of the skin tests, a RAST or a provocative challenge test may be performed. If a skin test is indicated, there is a reasonable suspicion that a specific allergen is producing symptoms in an allergic patient. Several precautionary steps, however, must be observed before skin testing:

- Testing is not performed during periods of bronchospasm.
- Epicutaneous tests (scratch or prick tests) are performed before other testing methods in an effort to minimize the risk of systemic reaction.
- Emergency equipment must be readily available to treat anaphylaxis.

Types of Skin Tests

The methods of skin testing include prick skin tests, scratch tests, and intradermal skin testing (Fig. 49-3). After prick or scratch tests, intradermal skin testing is performed with allergens that did not elicit positive reactions. Because a larger antigen challenge is being used, local or systemic reactions could occur if the same antigens that produced positive skin or scratch reactions are used. The patient's back is the most suitable area of the body for skin testing because it permits the performance of many tests. The multi-test applicator is a commercially available device with multiple test heads that allows simultaneous administration of antigens by multiple punctures at different sites.

Interpretation of Skin Test Results

Familiarity with and consistent use of a grading system are essential. The grading system used should be identified on a skin test sheet for later interpretation. A positive reaction, evidenced by the appearance of an urticarial wheal (round, reddened skin elevation) (Fig. 49-4), localized erythema (diffuse redness) in the area of inoculation or contact, or pseudopodia (irregular projection at the end of a wheal) with associated erythema is considered indicative of sensitivity to the corresponding antigen.

There may be false-negative results due to improper technique, outdated allergen solutions, and prior use of medications that suppress skin reactivity. Corticosteroids and antihistamines, including allergy medications, suppress skin test reactivity and should be withheld 48 to 96 hours before testing, depending on the duration of their activity. False-positive skin tests may result from improper preparation or administration of allergen solutions.

Interpretation of positive or negative skin tests must be based on the patient's history, physical examination, and other laboratory results. The following guidelines are used for the interpretation of skin test results:

- Skin tests are more reliable for diagnosing atopic sensitivity in patients with allergic rhinoconjunctivitis than in patients with asthma.
- Positive skin tests correlate highly with food allergy.
- The use of skin tests to diagnose immediate hypersensitivity to medications is limited because metabolites of medications, not the medications themselves, are usually responsible for causing hypersensitivity.

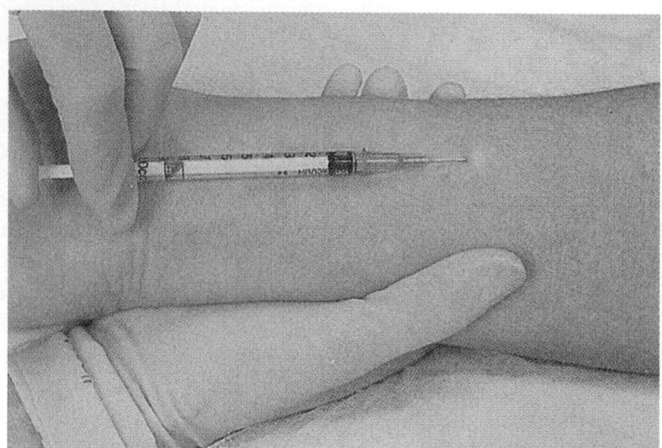

FIGURE 49•3 Intradermal testing. A 0.5-mL or 1-mL sterile syringe with a 26/27 gauge intradermal needle is used to inject 0.02 to 0.03 mL of intradermal allergen. The needle is inserted with the bevel facing upward and the syringe parallel to the skin. The skin is penetrated superficially, and a small amount of the allergen solution is injected to create a bleb (raised area) approximately 5 mm in diameter. A separate sterile syringe and needle are used for each injection. From Taylor, C., Lillis C., & LeMone, P. (1997). Fundamentals of nursing: *The art and science of nursing care* (3rd ed.). Philadelphia; Lippincott-Raven.

Provocative Testing

Provocative testing involves the direct administration of the suspected allergen to the sensitive tissue, such as the conjunctiva, nasal or bronchial mucosa, or gastrointestinal tract (by ingestion of the allergen) with observation of target organ response. This type of testing is helpful in identifying clinically significant allergens in patients with a large number of positive tests. Major disadvantages of this type of testing are the limitation of one antigen per session and the risk of producing severe symptoms, particularly bronchospasm, in patients with asthma.

Radioallergosorbent Test

RAST is a radioimmunoassay that measures allergen-specific IgE. A sample of the patient's serum is exposed to a variety of suspected allergen particle complexes. If antibodies are present, they will combine with radiolabeled allergens.

After the patient's serum is centrifuged, radioimmunoassay detects the allergen-specific IgE antibody. Test results are then compared with control values. In addition to detecting an allergen, RAST indicates the quantity of allergen necessary to evoke an allergic reaction. Values are reported on a scale from 0 to 5. Values of 2+ or greater are considered significant. The major advantages of RAST over other tests include decreased risk of systemic reaction, stability of antigens, and lack of dependence on skin reactivity modified by medications. The major disadvantages include the limited allergen selection, reduced sensitivity as compared with intradermal skin tests, lack of immediately available results, and cost.

ALLERGIC DISORDERS

A type I hypersensitivity response results in *atopic* (allergic) diseases, which affect 10% to 20% of the U.S. population. Genetic factors play a role in susceptibility to these diseases. Disorders characterized as atopic include anaphylaxis, allergic rhinoconjunctivitis, atopic dermatitis, urticaria and angioedema, gastrointestinal allergy, and asthma. Latex allergy may be considered a type I or type IV hypersensitivity reaction. Contact dermatitis is considered a type IV hypersensitivity reaction.

Anaphylaxis

Anaphylaxis is a clinical response to an immediate (type I hypersensitivity) immunologic reaction between a specific antigen and an antibody. The reaction results from IgE antibody.

Pathophysiology

An anaphylactic reaction occurs as follows:

1. An antigen attaches to the IgE antibody fixed to the surface membrane of mast cells and basophils, causing these target cells to become activated.
2. Mast cells and basophils then release mediators, causing vascular changes, including activation of platelets, eosinophils, and neutrophils and the coagulation cascade.

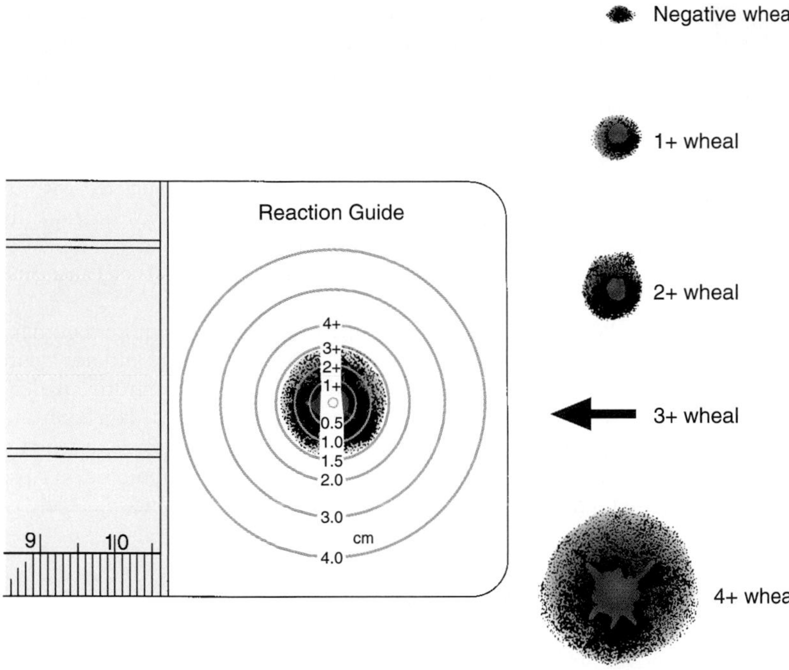

FIGURE 49•4 Interpretation of reactions: Negative = wheal soft with minimal erythema. 1+ = wheal present (5–8 mm) with associated erythema. 2+ = wheal (7–10 mm) with associated erythema. 3+ = wheal (9–15 mm) slight pseudopodia possible with associated erythema. 4+ = wheal (12 mm+) with pseudopodia and diffuse erythema.

An anaphylactoid (anaphylaxis-like) reaction is clinically similar to anaphylaxis; however, it is not mediated by antigen–antibody interactions. Rather, it results from substances that act directly on the mast cells or tissues, causing the release of mediators. An anaphylactoid reaction may occur with medications, food, exercise, and cytotoxic antibody transfusions. The reaction may be local or systemic. Local reactions usually involve urticaria and angioedema at the site of the antigen exposure. Although possibly severe, anaphylactoid reactions are rarely fatal. Systemic reactions occur within about 30 minutes of exposure involving cardiovascular, respiratory, gastrointestinal, and integumentary organ systems.

Clinical Manifestations

The major signs and symptoms of anaphylactic reactions may be categorized as mild, moderate, and severe systemic reactions.

Mild systemic reactions consist of peripheral tingling and a sensation of warmth, possibly accompanied by a fullness in the mouth and throat. Nasal congestion, periorbital swelling, pruritus, sneezing, and tearing of the eyes can also be expected. Onset of symptoms begins within the first 2 hours of exposure.

Moderate systemic reactions may include flushing, warmth, anxiety, and itching in addition to any of the above symptoms. More serious reactions include bronchospasm and edema of the airways or larynx with dyspnea, cough, and wheezing. The onset of symptoms is the same as for a mild reaction.

Severe systemic reactions have an abrupt onset with the same signs and symptoms described above. These, however, progress rapidly to bronchospasm, laryngeal edema, severe dyspnea, and cyanosis. Dysphagia (difficulty swallowing), abdominal cramping, vomiting, diarrhea, and seizures can also occur. Rarely, cardiac arrest and coma result.

Prevention

Prevention is the single most important aspect for the patient at risk for anaphylaxis. People sensitive to insect bites and stings, those who have experienced food or medication reactions, and those who have experienced idiopathic or exercise-induced anaphylactic reactions should always carry an emergency kit that contains epinephrine. The Epipen from Center Laboratories is a commercially available first-aid device that delivers premeasured doses of 0.3 mg (Epipen) and 0.15 mg (Epipen Jr.) of epinephrine (Fig. 49-5). The autoinjection system requires no preparation, and the self-administration technique is uncomplicated. The patient must be given an opportunity to demonstrate the correct

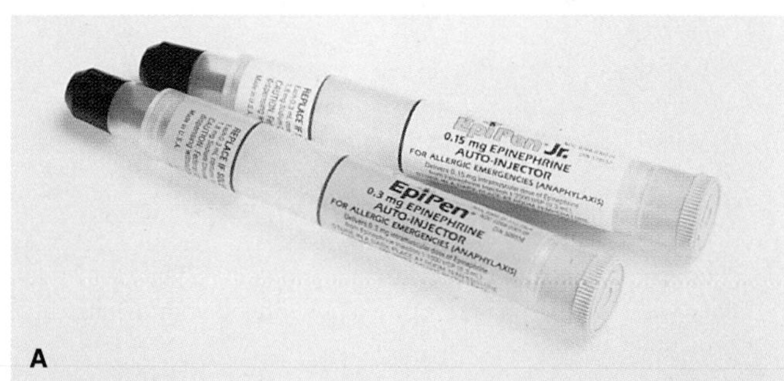

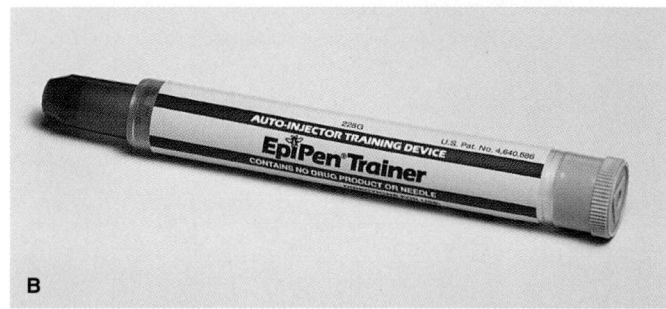

FIGURE 49•5 (**A**) The Epipen and Epipen Jr. Autoinjectors are commercially available first-aid devices that administer premeasured doses of epinephrine. (**B**) An Epipen training device is available for patients to practice correct self-injection technique. Courtesy of Center Laboratories, Port Washington, New York.

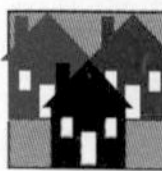

Patient Education and Home Care
Self-Administration of Epinephrine

The patient is taught how to inject epinephrine in the event of an anaphylactic reaction. The patient should be encouraged to practice this technique using a training device.

1. Carefully uncap the Epipen device, holding it so that the injecting end is upright.

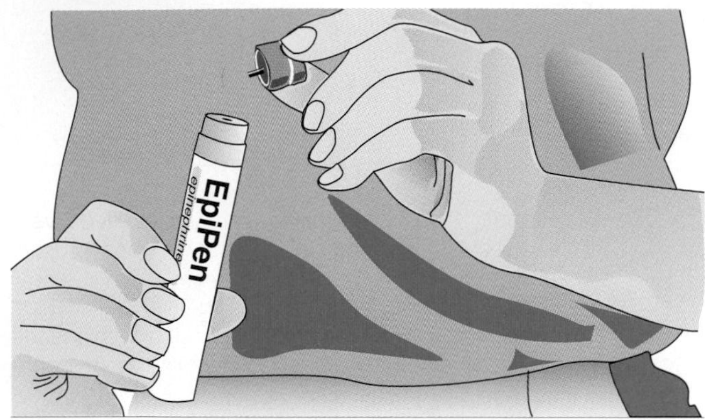

2. Position the device at the middle portion of the thigh.

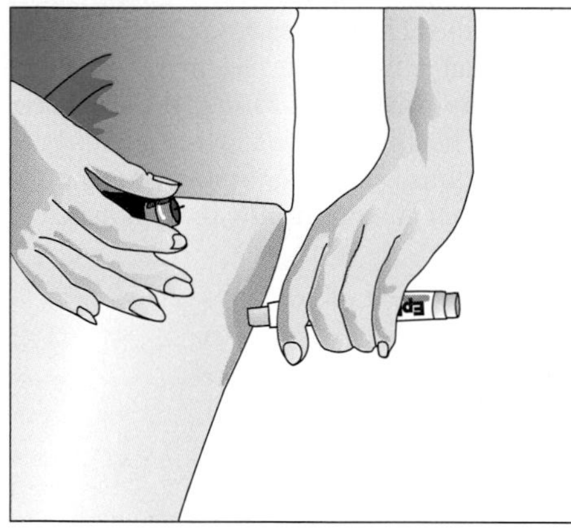

3. Push the device into the thigh as far as possible. The Epipen device will autoinject a premeasured dose of epinephrine into the subcutaneous tissue.

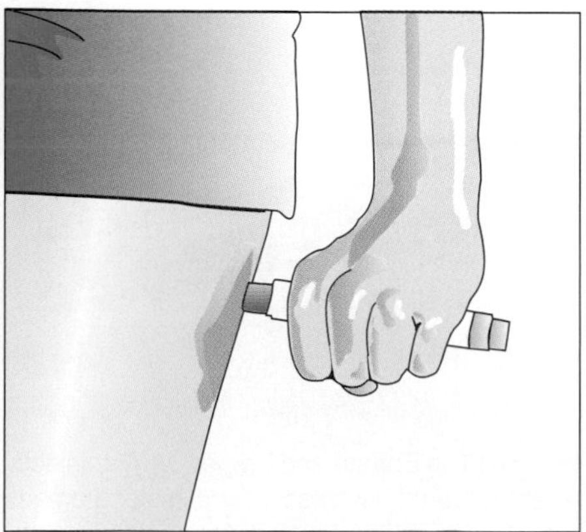

technique for use. An Epipen training device is available to assist in this effort. Verbal and written information about the emergency kit, as well as strategies to avoid exposure to threatening allergens, is also provided.

A careful patient history of any sensitivity to suspected antigens must be obtained before administering any medication, particularly in parenteral form, because this route is associated with the most severe anaphylaxis. Patients who are predisposed to anaphylaxis should wear some form of identification, such as a medical alert bracelet, naming allergies to medications, food, and other substances.

People who are allergic to insect venom may require venom immunotherapy, which is used as a control measure and not a cure. Insulin-allergic diabetic patients and penicillin-sensitive patients may require desensitization. Desensitization is based on controlled anaphylaxis, with a gradual release of mediators. Patients who undergo desensitization are cautioned that there should be no lapses in therapy because this may lead to the reappearance of an allergic reaction when the medication is reinstituted.

Medical Management

Management depends on the severity of the reaction. Initially, respiratory and cardiovascular function are evaluated. If the patient is in cardiac arrest, cardiopulmonary resuscitation is instituted. Oxygen is provided in high concentrations during cardiopulmonary resuscitation or when a patient is cyanotic, dyspneic, or wheezing. Epinephrine, in a solution of 1 : 1000 dilution, is given subcutaneously in the upper extremity or thigh and may be followed by a continuous intravenous infusion. Antihistamines and corticosteroids may also be given to prevent recurrences of the reaction and to treat urticaria and angioedema. To maintain blood pressure and normal hemodynamic status, volume expanders and vasopressor agents are given. In people with episodes of bronchospasm or a history of bronchial asthma or chronic obstructive pulmonary disease, aminophylline and corticosteroids may also be administered to improve airway patency and function. In cases in which hypotension is unresponsive to vasopressors, intravenous administration of glucagon may be used for its acute inotropic and chronotropic effects. Patients with severe reactions are observed closely for 12 to 14 hours. Because of the potential for recurrence, patients with even mild reactions must be educated concerning this risk.

Allergic Rhinitis

Allergic **rhinitis** (inflammation of nasal mucosa; hay fever, chronic allergic rhinitis, pollinosis) is the most common form of respiratory allergy presumed to be mediated by an immediate (type I hypersensitivity) immunologic reaction affecting about 8% to 10% of the U.S. population (20% to 30% of adolescents). When untreated, many complications may result, such as allergic asthma, chronic nasal obstruction, chronic otitis media with hearing loss, anosmia (absence of the sense of smell), and, in children, orofacial dental deformities. Early diagnosis and adequate treatment are essential.

Because allergic rhinitis is induced by airborne pollens or molds, it is characterized by the following seasonal occurrences:

Early spring—tree pollen (oak, elm, poplar)

Early summer—rose pollen (rose fever), grass pollen (Timothy, red-top)

Early fall—weed pollen (ragweed)

Each year, attacks begin and end at about the same time. Airborne mold spores require warm, damp weather. Although there is no rigid seasonal pattern, these spores appear in early spring, are rampant during the summer, and taper off and disappear by the first frost.

Pathophysiology

Sensitization begins by ingestion or inhalation of an antigen. On reexposure, the nasal mucosa reacts by the slowing of ciliary action, edema formation, and leukocyte (primarily eosinophil) infiltration. Histamine is the major mediator of allergic reactions in the nasal mucosa. Tissue edema results from vasodilation and increased capillary permeability.

Clinical Manifestations

Typical signs and symptoms of allergic rhinitis include nasal congestion; clear, watery nasal discharge; intermittent sneezing; and nasal itching. Itching of the throat and soft palate is common. Drainage of nasal mucus into the pharynx initiates multiple attempts to clear the throat and results in a dry cough or hoarseness. Headache, pain over the paranasal sinuses, and epistaxis can accompany allergic rhinitis. The symptoms of this chronic condition depend on environmental exposure and intrinsic host responsiveness.

Assessment and Diagnostic Findings

Diagnosis of seasonal allergic rhinitis is based on history, physical examination, and diagnostic test results. Diagnostic tests include nasal smears, peripheral blood counts, total serum IgE, epicutaneous and intradermal testing, RAST, food elimination and challenge, and nasal provocation tests. Results indicative of allergy as the cause of rhinitis include increased IgE and eosinophil levels and positive reactions on allergen testing. False-positive and false-negative responses to these tests, particularly skin testing and provocation tests, may occur.

Medical Management

The goal of therapy is to provide relief from symptoms. Therapy may include one or all of the following interventions: avoidance therapy, pharmacotherapy, and immunotherapy. Oral instruction must be reinforced by written information to provide the patient with permanent reminders. A knowledge of general concepts regarding assessment and therapy in allergic diseases is important.

PHARMACOLOGIC THERAPY

Antihistamines. Antihistamines, now classified as H_1-receptor antagonists (or H_1-blockers) are used in managing mild allergic disorders. H_2-receptor antagonists are used to treat gastric and duodenal ulcers. H_1-blockers bind selectively to H_1 receptors, preventing the actions of histamines at these sites. They do not prevent the release of histamine from mast cells or basophils. The H_1-antagonists have no effect on H_2-receptors, but they do have the ability to bind to nonhistaminic receptors. The ability of certain antihistamines to bind to and block muscarinic receptors underlies several of the prominent anticholinergic side effects of these medications.

Oral antihistamines, which are readily absorbed, are most effective when given at the first occurrence of symptoms because they prevent the development of new symptoms by blocking the actions of histamine at the H_1-receptors. The effectiveness of these medications is limited to certain patients with hay fever, vasomotor rhinitis, urticaria (hives), and mild asthma. They are rarely effective in other conditions or in any severe conditions.

Antihistamines are the major class of medications prescribed for the symptomatic relief of allergic rhinitis. The major side effect is sedation. Additional side effects include nervousness, tremors, dizziness, dry mouth, palpitations, anorexia, nausea, and vomiting. They are contraindicated during the third trimester of pregnancy; for nursing mothers and newborns; in children and elderly people; and in patients whose conditions can be aggravated by muscarinic blockade (ie, asthma, urinary retention, open-angle glaucoma, hypertension, and prostatic hyperplasia).

Newer antihistamines are called second-generation or nonsedating H_1-receptor antagonists. Unlike first-generation H_1-receptor antagonists, they do not cross the blood–brain barrier and do not bind to cholinergic, serotonin, or alpha-adrenergic receptors. They bind to peripheral rather than central nervous system H_1-receptors, causing less sedation.

Although no more potent than their predecessors, they are more expensive than traditional antihistamines. They are generally well tolerated. However, astemizole (Hismanal) has been associated with fatal cardiac dysrhythmias, usually as a result of overdosage or interaction with many other medications. Its use is contraindicated in patients with liver disorders. Because of these risks, its use has decreased (Table 49-2).

Adrenergic Agents. Adrenergic agents, vasoconstrictors of mucosal vessels, are used topically (nasal and ophthalmic) in addition to the oral route. The topical route (drops and sprays) causes fewer side effects than oral administration; however, the use of drops and sprays should be limited to a few days to avoid rebound congestion. Adrenergic nasal decongestants are used for the relief of nasal congestion when applied topically to the nasal mucosa. They activate the alpha-adrenergic receptor sites on the smooth muscle of the nasal mucosal blood vessels, reducing local blood flow, fluid exudation, and mucosal edema. Topical ophthalmic drops are used for symptomatic relief of eye irritations due to allergies. Potential side effects include hypertension, dysrhythmias, palpitations, central nervous system stimulation, irritability, tremor, and tachyphylaxis (acceleration of hemodynamic status). Examples of adrenergic decongestants and their routes of administration are found in Table 49-3.

Mast Cell Stabilizers. Intranasal cromolyn sodium (Nasalcrom) is a spray that acts by stabilizing the mast cell membrane, thus inhibiting the release of histamine and other mediators of the allergic response. Cromolyn is used prophylactically before exposure to allergens or therapeutically in chronic allergic rhinitis. This spray is as effective as antihistamines but less effective than intranasal corticosteroids in the treatment of seasonal allergic rhinitis. Patients must be informed that the beneficial effects of the medication may take a week or so to develop. The medication is of no benefit in the treatment of nonallergic rhinitis. Adverse effects are usually mild (ie, sneezing, local stinging, and burning sensations).

Corticosteroids. Intranasal corticosteroids are indicated in more severe cases of allergic and perennial rhinitis that cannot be

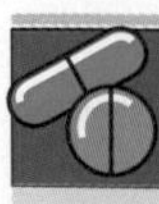

TABLE 49•2 Chemical Classes of H_1 Antihistamines

Classification and Example	Major Side Effects	Nursing Implications
Sedating		
Ethanolamines Ex: diphenhydramine (Benadryl)	Drowsiness, confusion	Teach patient to avoid alcohol, driving, or engaging in any hazardous activities until CNS response to drug treatment is stabilized.
	Dry mouth, nausea, vomiting	Suggest sucking on hard candy or ice chips for relief of dry mouth.
	Photosensitivity	Encourage use of sunscreen and hat while outdoors.
	Urinary retention	Assess for urinary retention; monitor urinary output.
Piperazines Ex: hydroxyzine (Atarax)	Dulls mental alertness; drowsiness	Teach patient to avoid alcohol, driving, or engaging in any hazardous activities until CNS response to drug treatment is stabilized.
	Dry mouth	Suggest sucking on hard candy or ice chips for relief of dry mouth.
Alkylamines Ex: chlorpheniramine (Chlor-Trimeton)	Less CNS depression than other groups; best class for daytime use	Teach patient to avoid alcohol, driving, or engaging in any hazardous activities until CNS response to drug treatment is stabilized.
Ethylenediamines Ex: tripelennamine (PBZ)	Gastrointestinal upset	Administer medication with food or milk to decrease GI distress. Increase fluid intake.
	Drowsiness	Teach patient to avoid alcohol, driving, or engaging in any hazardous activities until CNS response to drug treatment is stabilized.
	Palpitations	Instruct patient to sit and relax a few minutes before activity.
Phenothiazines Ex: promethazine (Phenergan)	Heavy sedation and drowsiness	Teach patient to avoid alcohol, driving, or engaging in any hazardous activities until CNS response to drug treatment is stabilized.
	Nasal congestion	Encourage use of humidification at home.
	Hypotension	Instruct patient to rise from a sitting position slowly.
cetirizine (Zyrtec)	Drowsiness, dry mouth	Teach patient to avoid alcohol, driving, or engaging in any hazardous activities until CNS response to drug treatment is stabilized.
Nonsedating		
loratadine (Claritin)	Gastrointestinal upset	Counsel patient to take the medication on an empty stomach.
fexofenadine (Allegra)	Occasional drowsiness and fatigue	Teach patient to avoid alcohol, driving, or engaging in any hazardous activities until CNS response to drug treatment is stabilized.
astemizole (Hismanal)	Cardiac dysrhythmias, potential cardiac arrest	Teach patient not to exceed the prescribed dose; teach patient to notify all physicians that he/she is taking Hismanal and is unable to take many other medications concurrently. Use with extreme caution.
	Nausea, diarrhea, and abdominal pain	Teach patient to take medication at least 2 hours after a meal or have no food for 1 hour after taking the medication because of decreased or poor medication absorption.
	Increased appetite and weight gain	Counsel patient to monitor weight and report increase in appetite and weight to physician.
	Dizziness	Teach patient to avoid hazardous activity, stop medication, and notify physician as dizziness may signal impending cardiac dysrhythmia.

controlled by more conventional medications, such as decongestants, antihistamines, and intranasal cromolyn. These medications include beclomethasone (Beconase, Vancenase); budesonide (Rhinocort); dexamethasone (Decadron Phosphate Turbinaire); flunisolide (Nasalide); fluticasone (Cutivate, Flonase); and triamcinolone (Nasacort).

Because of their anti-inflammatory actions, these medications are equally effective in preventing or suppressing the major symptoms of allergic rhinitis. Corticosteroids are administered by metered-spray devices. If the nasal passages are blocked, a topical decongestant can be used to clear the passages before the administration of the intranasal corticosteroid. Patients must be aware that full benefit may not be achieved for several days to 2 weeks. Adverse effects of intranasal corticosteroids are mild and include drying of the nasal mucosa and burning and itching sensations caused by the vehicle used to administer the medication. Systemic effects are more likely with dexamethasone. Recommended use of this medication is limited to 30 days. Beclometha-

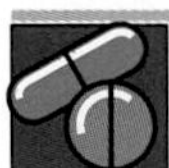

TABLE 49•3 **Adrenergic Decongestants and Their Routes of Administration**

Adrenergic Decongestant	Trade Name	Route of Administration
naphazoline hydrochloride	Privine	Topical
oxymetazoline hydrochloride	Afrin, Dristan long-lasting, Neo-Synephrine 12 hour, Sinex long-lasting	Topical
phenylephrine hydrochloride	Neo-Synephrine	Topical
phenylpropanolamine hydrochloride	Propagest	Oral
pseudoephedrine hydrochloride	Sudafed	Oral
tetrahydrozoline hydrochloride	Collyrium, Murine Plus, Visine	Topical ophthalmic and nasal preparations
xylometazoline hydrochloride	Neo-Synephrine II, Otrivin	Topical

sone, budesonide, flunisolide, fluticasone, and triamcinolone are deactivated rapidly after absorption, so that they do not achieve significant blood levels. Corticosteroids suppress host defenses. Thus, they must be used with caution in people with tuberculosis or untreated bacterial infections of the lungs.

Oral and parenteral corticosteroids are used when conventional therapy has failed and symptoms are severe and of short duration. They can control symptoms of allergic reactions, such as hay fever, medication-induced allergies, and allergic reactions to insect stings. Because the response to corticosteroids is delayed, they have little or no value in acute therapy for severe reactions, such as anaphylaxis. Patients who receive corticosteroids must be cautioned not to stop taking the medication suddenly or without specific instructions from the physician. The patient is also instructed about side effects, which include fluid retention, weight gain, hypertension, gastric irritation, glucose intolerance, and adrenal suppression.

IMMUNOTHERAPY

Immunotherapy is indicated only when IgE hypersensitivity (type I hypersensitivity) is demonstrated to specific inhalant allergens that the patient cannot avoid (house dust, pollens). Goals of immunotherapy include reducing the level of circulating IgE, increasing the level of blocking antibody IgG, and reducing mediator cell sensitivity. Immunotherapy has been most effective for ragweed pollen; however, treatment for grass, tree pollen, cat, and house dust mite allergens has also been effective.

Correlation of a positive skin test with a positive allergy history is an indication for immunotherapy if the allergen cannot be avoided. The value has been fairly well established in instances of allergic rhinitis and bronchial asthma that are clearly due to sensitivity to one of the common pollens, molds, or house dust. Although immunotherapy is referred to as a "hypersensitization" procedure, the effects are most likely attributable to the opposite process (ie, immunization). This procedure appears to stimulate the production of a new antibody with the capacity to neutralize the allergy-provoking properties of the responsible allergen.

Although helpful in most patients, immunotherapy does not cure the condition. Before immunotherapy is initiated, the patient must understand what to expect and the importance of continuing therapy for several years. When skin tests are performed, the results are correlated with clinical manifestations; treatment is based on the patient's needs rather than on skin tests.

The most common method of treatment is the serial injection of one or more antigens that are selected in each particular case on the basis of skin tests. This method provides a simple and efficient technique for identifying IgE antibodies to specific antigens. Specific treatment consists of injecting extracts of the pollens or mold spores that cause symptoms in a particular patient. Injections begin with very small amounts and are gradually increased, usually at weekly intervals, until a maximum tolerated dose is attained. Maintenance "booster" injections are given at 2- to 4-week intervals, frequently for a period of several years, before maximum benefit is achieved.

There are three methods of injection therapy: coseasonal, preseasonal, and perennial. When treatment is given on a *coseasonal basis*, therapy is initiated during the season in which the patient experiences symptoms. This method has been proved ineffective and thus is used less frequently. Also, there is increased risk of systemic reactions. *Preseasonal therapy* injections are given 2 to 3 months before symptoms are expected, allowing time for hyposensitization to occur. This treatment is discontinued after the season begins. *Perennial therapy* is administered all year round, usually on a monthly basis, and is the preferred method because it has more effective, longer-lasting results.

Nursing Alert *A possibility exists that the injection of an allergen may induce systemic reactions. Therefore, the injection is given only in a setting (ie, physician's office, clinic) where epinephrine is immediately available.*

Because of the dangers involved, injections should not be given by a lay person or by the patient. The patient remains in the office or clinic for a minimum of 30 minutes after the injection has been given and is observed for possible systemic symptoms. If a large, local swelling develops at the injection site, the next dose should *not* be increased because this may be a warning sign of a possible systemic reaction.

Therapeutic failure is evident when a patient does not experience a decrease of symptoms within 12 to 24 months, develop an increase in tolerance to known allergens, and decrease the use of medications to reduce symptoms. Potential causes of treatment failure include misdiagnosis of allergies, inadequate doses of allergen, newly developed allergies, and inadequate environmental controls.

AVOIDANCE THERAPY

In avoidance therapy, every attempt is made to remove those allergens that act as precipitating factors. Simple measures and environmental controls are often effective in decreasing symptoms. Examples of these include use of air conditioners, air cleaners, humidifiers and dehumidifiers, and smoke-free environments.

NURSING PROCESS: THE PATIENT WITH ALLERGIC RHINITIS

Assessment

The examination and history of the patient reveal sneezing, often in paroxysms, thin and watery nasal discharge, itching eyes and nose, lacrimation, and occasionally headache. The nursing history includes a personal or family history of allergy. The allergy assessment identifies the nature of antigens, seasonal changes in symptoms, and medication history. The nurse also obtains subjective data about how the patient feels just before symptoms become obvious, such as the occurrence of pruritus, breathing problems, and tingling sensations. In addition to these symptoms, hoarseness, wheezing, hives, rash, erythema, and edema are noted. Any relationship between emotional problems or stress and the triggering of allergy symptoms is assessed.

Diagnosis

Nursing Diagnoses

Based on the assessment data, the patient's major nursing diagnoses may include the following:

- Ineffective breathing pattern related to allergic reaction
- Knowledge deficit about allergy and the recommended modifications in lifestyle and self-care practices
- Impaired individual coping with chronicity of condition and need for environmental modifications

Collaborative Problems/Potential Complications

Based on assessment data, potential complications may include the following:

- Anaphylaxis
- Impaired breathing
- Adverse reactions to medications
- Nonadherence to therapeutic regimen

Planning and Goals

The goals for the patient may include restoration of normal breathing pattern, knowledge about the causes and control of allergic symptoms, improved coping with alterations and modifications, and absence of complications.

Nursing Interventions

Improving Breathing Pattern

The patient is instructed and assisted to modify the environment to reduce the severity of allergic symptoms or to prevent their occurrence. Additionally, the patient is instructed to reduce exposure to people with upper respiratory infections (URIs). If URI occurs, the patient is encouraged to take deep breaths and cough frequently to ensure adequate gas exchange and prevent atelectasis. The patient is instructed to seek medical attention because allergy symptoms along with URI may compromise adequate lung function. Compliance with medications and other treatment regimens is encouraged and reinforced.

Promoting Understanding of Allergy and Control

Instruction for the patient includes discussion of strategies to minimize exposure to allergens, desensitization procedures, and correct use of medications.

Coping with Chronic Disorder

Although allergic reactions are infrequently life-threatening, they require constant vigilance for allergens and modification of the patient's lifestyle or environment to prevent recurrence of symptoms. Allergic symptoms are often present year-round and create discomfort and inconvenience for the patient. Although patients may not feel ill during allergy seasons, they often do not feel well either. The need to be alert for possible allergens in the environment may be tiresome for some patients, placing extra burdens on their ability to lead normal lives. Stress related to these difficulties may in turn increase the frequency or severity of symptoms.

To assist the patient in adjusting to these modifications, the nurse must have an appreciation of the difficulties encountered by the patient. The patient is encouraged to verbalize feelings and concerns in a supportive environment and to identify strategies to deal with them effectively.

Monitoring and Managing Potential Complications

ANAPHYLAXIS AND IMPAIRED BREATHING

Respiratory and cardiovascular functioning can be dangerously altered during allergic reactions owing to the reaction itself or to medications used. Therefore, the patient's respiratory and cardiovascular status is evaluated by monitoring the respiratory rate, assessing for the presence of breathing difficulties or abnormal lung sounds, and monitoring the pulse rate and rhythm, and blood pressure. Vital signs are monitored and recorded regularly or any time the patient complains of symptoms such as itching or difficulty breathing. In the event of signs and symptoms indicative of anaphylaxis, emergency medications and equipment must be available for immediate use.

ADVERSE REACTIONS TO MEDICATIONS

Excessive doses of astemizole or terfenadine can lead to dysrhythmias or cardiac arrest. Adverse signs and symptoms (ie, urticaria, difficulty breathing, dry mouth, palpitations, headaches, or dizziness) should be immediately reported to the physician. Caution must be used with use of these medications.

NONADHERENCE TO THERAPEUTIC REGIMEN

Knowledge of the treatment regimen does not necessarily ensure adherence. Having the patient identify potential barriers and explore acceptable solutions for lifestyle changes needed for effective management of the condition can increase adherence to the treatment regimen.

Promoting Home and Community-Based Care

TEACHING PATIENTS SELF-CARE

The patient is instructed about strategies to minimize exposure to allergens, the actions and adverse effects of medications, and the correct use of medications. The patient should know the names, dose, frequency, actions, and side effects of all medications taken.

Instruction about strategies to control allergic symptoms is based on the individual needs of the patient as determined by the results of tests, the severity of symptoms, and the motivation of the patient and family to deal with the condition. Suggestions for patients sensitive to dust and mold in the home are included in the accompanying Home Care Teaching Checklist: Allergy Management.

If the patient is to undergo desensitization, the nurse reinforces the physician's explanation regarding the purpose and procedure. Instructions are given regarding the series of inoculations, usually given every 2 weeks or every month. These include remaining in the physician's office or the clinic at least 30 minutes after the injection, so that emergency treatment may be given if the patient has a reaction; avoiding rubbing or scratching the injection site; and continuing with the series for the period of time required. In addition, the patient and family are instructed about emergency treatment of severe allergic symptoms.

Because antihistamines often produce drowsiness, the patient is cautioned about this and other side effects of the particular medication. Operating machinery, driving a car, and performing activities requiring intense concentration should be postponed. The patient is also informed about the dangers of drinking alcohol when taking these medications. These medications tend to exaggerate the effects of alcohol.

The patient must be aware of the effects caused by *overuse* of the sympathomimetic agents in nose drops or sprays. A condition referred to as *rhinitis medicamentosa* may result (Fig. 49-6). After topical application of the medication, a rebound period may occur in which the nasal mucous membranes become more edematous and congested than they were before the medication was used. Such a reaction encourages the use of more medication. A cyclical pattern results. The topical agent must be discontinued immediately and completely to correct this problem.

CONTINUING CARE

Follow-up telephone calls to the patient are often reassuring to the patient and family and provide an opportunity for the nurse to answer any questions. The patient is reminded to keep follow-up appointments and is informed about the importance of continuing with treatment.

Evaluation

Expected Outcomes

Expected outcomes may include:

1. Exhibits normal breathing patterns
   a. Demonstrates lungs clear on auscultation
   b. Exhibits absence of adventitious breath sounds (crackles, rhonchi, wheezing)
   c. Demonstrates an effective respiratory rate
   d. Reports no complaints of respiratory distress (shortness of breath, difficulty on inspiration or expiration)
2. Demonstrates knowledge about allergy and strategies to control symptoms
   a. Identifies causative allergens, if known
   b. States methods of avoiding allergen and how to control for indoor and outdoor precipitating factors
   c. Removes from the environment those items that retain dust
   d. Wears a dampened mask if dust or mold may be a problem
   e. Avoids smoke-filled rooms and dust-filled or freshly sprayed areas
   f. Uses air-conditioning for a major part of the day
   g. Takes antihistamines as prescribed; participates in hyposensitization program, if applicable
   h. Describes name, purpose, side effects, and method of administration of prescribed medications

HOME CARE TEACHING CHECKLIST: ALLERGY MANAGEMENT

At the completion of the program, the patient or caregiver will be able to:	Patient	Caregiver
• Verbalize how to maintain a dust-free environment by removing drapes, curtains, and venetian blinds and replacing them with pull shades; covering the mattress with a hypoallergenic cover that can be zipped; and removing rugs and replacing them with wood flooring or linoleum.	✔	✔
• Identify rationale for washing the floor and dusting and vacuuming daily.	✔	✔
• Identify rationale for replacing stuffed furniture with wood pieces that can easily be dusted.	✔	✔
• State rationale for wearing a mask whenever cleaning is being done.	✔	✔
• Identify rationale for avoiding use of tufted bedspreads, stuffed toys, and feather pillows and replacing them with washable cotton material.	✔	✔
• State rationale for avoiding the use of any clothing that causes itching.	✔	✔
• Verbalize ways to reduce dust in the house as a whole by using steam or hot water for heating rather than air and using air filters or air conditioning.	✔	✔
• Verbalize ways to reduce exposure to pollens or molds by identifying seasons of the year when pollen counts are high; wearing a mask at times of increased exposure (windy days and when grass is being cut); and avoiding contact with weeds, dry leaves, and freshly cut grass.	✔	✔
• State rationale for seeking air-conditioned areas at the height of the allergy season.	✔	✔
• State rationale for avoiding sprays and perfumes.	✔	✔
• State rationale for use of hypoallergenic cosmetics.	✔	✔
• State rationale for taking prescribed medications as ordered.	✔	✔
• Identify specific foods that may cause allergic symptoms. (Examples of foods that can cause allergic reactions are fish, nuts, eggs, and chocolate.)	✔	✔
• Develop a list of foods to avoid.	✔	✔

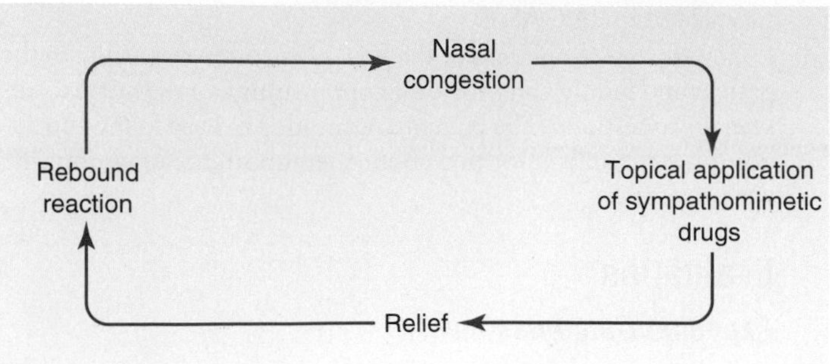

FIGURE 49•6 Rhinitis medicamentosa. This cyclic pattern results from overuse of sympathomimetic nose drops or sprays.

   i. Identifies when to seek immediate medical attention for severe allergic responses
   j. Describes activities that are possible, including ways to maximize these activities without activating the allergies
3. Experiences relief of discomfort while adapting to the inconveniences of an allergy
   a. Relates the emotional aspects of the allergic response
   b. Demonstrates use of measures to cope positively with allergy
4. Remains free of complications
   a. Demonstrates vital signs within normal limits
   b. Reports no symptoms or episodes of anaphylaxis (urticaria, itching, peripheral tingling, fullness in the mouth and throat, flushing, or difficulty swallowing) or coughing, wheezing, or difficulty breathing
   c. Demonstrates correct procedure to self-administer emergency medications to treat severe allergic reaction
   d. Correctly states medication names, dose and frequency of administration, and medication actions
   e. Correctly identifies side effects and untoward signs and symptoms to report to physician
   f. Discusses acceptable lifestyle changes and solutions for identified potential barriers for compliance with treatment and medication regimen

Contact Dermatitis

Contact dermatitis (dermatitis venenata), a type IV delayed hypersensitivity reaction response, is an inflammatory, often eczematous condition caused by a skin reaction to a variety of irritating or allergenic materials. There are four basic types: *allergic, irritant, phototoxic,* and *photoallergic*, described in Table 49-4. Almost any substance can produce contact dermatitis. Poison ivy is probably the most common example; cosmetics, soaps, detergents, and industrial chemicals are frequent offenders. The skin sensitivity may develop after brief or prolonged periods of exposure, and the clinical picture may appear hours or weeks after the sensitized skin has been exposed.

Clinical Manifestations

Symptoms include itching, burning, erythema, skin lesions (vesicles), and edema, followed by weeping, crusting, and finally drying and peeling of the skin. In severe responses, hemorrhagic bullae may develop. Repeated reactions may be accompanied by thickening of the skin and pigmentary changes. Secondary invasion by bacteria may develop in skin abraded by rubbing or scratching. Usually, there are no systemic symptoms unless the eruption is widespread.

Assessment and Diagnostic Findings

The basis of the location of the eruption and history of exposure aid in determining the condition. In cases of obscure irritants or an unobservant patient, however, diagnosis may be extremely difficult, often involving many trial-and-error procedures before the cause is correctly determined. Patch tests on the skin with suspected offending agents may clarify the diagnosis.

Atopic Dermatitis

Atopic dermatitis is a type I immediate hypersensitivity disorder. A family history is common. Incidence of atopic dermatitis is highest in infants and children. Most patients have significant elevations of serum IgE and peripheral eosinophilia. Pruritus and hyperirritability of the skin are the most consistent features of atopic dermatitis and are related to large amounts of histamine in the skin. Excessive dryness of the skin with resultant itching is related to changes in lipid content, sebaceous gland activity, and sweating. In response to stroking, immediate redness appears on the skin and is followed in 15 to 30 seconds by pallor, which persists for 1 to 3 minutes. Lesions develop secondary to the trauma of scratching and appear in areas of increased sweating and hypervascularity. Atopic dermatitis is chronic, with remissions and exacerbations. Treatment must be individualized to the needs of each patient.

Medical Management

Guidelines for treatment include decreasing itching and scratching by wearing cotton fabrics, washing with a mild detergent, humidifying dry heat in winter, maintaining room temperature at 20°C to 22.2°C (68°F to 72°F), using antihistamines such as diphenhydramine (Benadryl), and avoiding animals, dust, sprays, and perfumes. Keeping the skin moisturized with daily baths to hydrate the skin and topical skin moisturizers is encouraged. Topical corticosteroids are used to prevent inflammation, and any infection is treated with antibiotics to eliminate *Staphylococcus aureus* when indicated.

Dermatitis Medicamentosa (Drug Reactions)

Dermatitis medicamentosa, a type I hypersensitivity disorder, is the term applied to skin rashes induced by the internal administration of certain medications. Although individuals react differently to each medication, certain medications tend to induce eruptions of similar types.

In general, drug reactions appear suddenly, have a particularly vivid color, present with characteristics that are more intense than the somewhat similar eruptions of infectious origin, and, with the

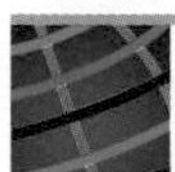

TABLE 49•4 **Types, Testing, and Treatment of Contact Dermatitis**

Type	Etiology	Clinical Presentation	Diagnostic Testing	Treatment
Allergic	Results from contact of skin and allergenic substance. Has a sensitization period of 10–14 days.	Vasodilation and perivascular infiltrates on the dermis Intracellular edema Usually seen on dorsal aspects of hand	Patch testing (contraindicated in acute, widespread dermatitis)	Avoidance of offending material Burow's solution or cool water compress Systemic corticosteroids (prednisone) for 7–10 days Topical corticosteroids for mild cases Oral antihistamines to relieve pruritus
Irritant	Results from contact with a substance that chemically or physically damages the skin on a nonimmunologic basis. Occurs after first exposure to irritant or repeated exposures to milder irritants over an extended time.	Dryness lasting days to months Vesiculation, fissures, cracks Hands and lower arms most common areas	Clinical picture Appropriate negative patch tests	Identification and removal of source of irritation Application of hydrophilic cream or petrolatum to soothe and protect Topical corticosteroids and compresses for weeping lesions Antibiotics for infection and oral antihistamines for pruritus
Phototoxic	Resembles the irritant type but requires sun and a chemical in combination to damage the epidermis.	Similar to irritant dermatitis	Photopatch test	Same as for allergic and irritant dermatitis
Photoallergic	Resembles allergic dermatitis but requires light exposure in addition to allergen contact to produce immunologic reactivity.	Similar to allergic dermatitis	Photopatch test	Same as for allergic and irritant dermatitis

exception of bromide and the iodide rashes, disappear rapidly after the medication is withdrawn. Rashes may be accompanied by systemic or generalized symptoms. Upon discovery of a medication allergy, patients are warned that they have a hypersensitivity to a particular medication and are advised not to take it again. Information identifying the hypersensitivity should be carried with them at all times.

Skin eruptions related to medication therapy suggest more serious hypersensitivities. Frequent assessment and prompt reporting of the appearance of any eruptions are important, so that early treatment can be initiated.

Urticaria and Angioneurotic Edema

Urticaria (hives) is a type I hypersensitive allergic reaction of the skin characterized by the sudden appearance of pinkish, edematous elevations that vary in size and shape, itch, and cause local discomfort. They may involve any part of the body, including the mucous membranes (especially those of the mouth), the larynx (occasionally with serious respiratory complications), and the gastrointestinal tract.

Each hive remains for a period of time, varying from a few minutes to several hours, before disappearing. For hours or days, clusters of these lesions may come, go, and return episodically. If this sequence continues indefinitely, the condition is called *chronic urticaria.*

Angioneurotic edema involves the deeper layers of the skin, resulting in more diffuse swelling rather than the discrete lesions characteristic of hives. On occasion, this reaction may cover the entire back. The skin over the reaction may appear normal but often has a reddish hue. The skin does not pit on pressure, as ordinary edema does. The regions most often involved are the lips, eyelids, cheeks, hands, feet, genitalia, and tongue; the mucous membranes of the larynx, the bronchi, and the gastrointestinal canal may also be affected, particularly in cases of the hereditary type. Swellings may appear suddenly, in a few seconds or minutes, or slowly, in 1 or 2 hours. In the latter case, their appearance is often preceded by itching or burning sensations. Seldom does more than a single swelling appear at one time, although one may develop while another is disappearing. Infrequently, swelling may recur in the same region. Individual lesions usually last from 24 to 36 hours. On rare occasions, swelling may recur with remarkable regularity at intervals of 3 to 4 weeks.

Hereditary Angioedema

Hereditary angioedema, although not an immunologic disorder in the usual sense, is included because of its resemblance to allergic angioedema and because of the seriousness of the condition. Symptoms are due to edema of the skin, the respiratory tract, or the digestive tract. Attacks may be precipitated by trauma or may seem to occur spontaneously.

Clinical Manifestations

When skin is involved, the swelling is usually diffuse, does not itch, and is usually not accompanied by urticaria. Gastrointestinal edema may cause abdominal pain severe enough to suggest the need for surgery. Edema of the upper respiratory tract may cause marked swelling of the uvula and of the larynx, resulting in suffocation. Acute laryngeal edema, the most serious manifestation of this disorder, has caused death by asphyxiation in nearly 20% of these patients.

Medical Management

Attacks usually subside within 3 to 4 days, but during this time, the patient should be observed carefully for signs of laryngeal obstruction, which may necessitate tracheostomy as a life-saving measure. Epinephrine, antihistamines, and corticosteroids are usually used in treatment, but the success of these agents is limited.

Food Allergy

IgE-mediated food allergy, a type I hypersensitivity reaction, occurs in 0.1% to 7.0% of the population. Almost any food can cause allergic symptoms. The most common offenders are nuts (especially peanuts), eggs, milk, soy, wheat, and chocolate.

Clinical Manifestations

Clinical symptoms are classic allergic symptoms (urticaria, atopic dermatitis, wheezing, cough, laryngeal edema, angioedema) and gastrointestinal symptoms (itching; swelling of lips, tongue, and palate; abdominal pain; nausea; cramps; vomiting; and diarrhea).

Assessment and Diagnostic Findings

A careful diagnostic workup is required in any patient with a suspected food hypersensitivity. Included is a detailed allergy history, a physical examination, and pertinent diagnostic tests. When testing for allergy, skin testing is used to identify the source of symptoms and is useful in identifying specific foods as causative agents.

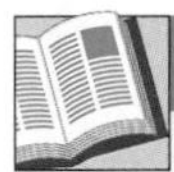

NURSING RESEARCH

Connection Between Food Reactions and Asthma

Emery, N. L., Vollmer, W. L, Buist, A. S., & Osborne, M. L. (1996). Self-reported food reactions and their associations with asthma. *Western Journal of Nursing Research, 18*(6), 643–654.

Purpose

The purposes of this study were to evaluate the types of self-reported food reactions in asthmatic patients and to determine the association between self-reported food reactions and the self-reported severity of asthma and use of asthma health care.

Study Sample and Design

The sample consisted of 914 patients aged 3 to 55 years of age. All subjects were members of a large health maintenance organization (HMO) who had medically diagnosed asthma. At the time of data collection, all subjects had either been hospitalized for asthma during the 4 years before recruitment or had at least two dispensings of antiasthma medications in the year before enrollment in the study.

Baseline cross-sectional data were collected as part of a longitudinal study to describe risk factors for episodes of hospital-based asthma care. Baseline data instruments included questionnaires to collect information about respiratory symptoms and food reactions. Skin prick testing was done to inhalant allergens, and spirometry was done 5 minutes after the administration of two puffs of isoproterenol. These baseline clinical evaluations were conducted at one testing site on all subjects.

Two questionnaires were used to obtain data about respiratory symptoms, characteristics of asthma, demographic factors, tobacco use, allergen exposure, medication use, and reactions to food. Spirometry was performed using standardized methods. The best 1-second forced expiratory volume (FEV_1) and forced vital capacity (FVC) were chosen for analysis. Asthma severity was assessed on a researcher-developed index corresponding to the criteria set by the National Asthma Educational Program guidelines. Both daytime or nocturnal symptoms were given a score, as follows: 0 = once per week or less, 1 = 2 to 6 times per week, and 2 = daily. Oral corticosteroid use was scored as follows: 0 = no corticosteroid use; 1 = sometimes (<50% of the time) during acute attacks; 2 = usually (>50% of the time) during and acute attacks; 3 = daily oral corticosteroids, even without shortness of breath. Spirometry was scored as follows: 0 = FEV_1 >80% of predicted value; 1 = FEV_1 of 60% to 80% of predicted value; 2 = FEV_1 <60% of predicted value. These three scores were summed to give an overall score, which was considered to be an indicator of the severity of asthma. For most analyses, these scores were dicotomized as follows: mild = 0–2; moderate to severe = 3–7.

Findings

Results showed that 414 (45%) of subjects reported adverse reactions to food. The group that reported food reactions was significantly older with a higher proportion of women than the group that reported no food reactions. Subjects reporting food reactions were also more likely to come from a minority background and to report a history of family food allergies. Groups did not differ in terms of household income. Of the 414 subjects reporting food reactions, 131 (32%) reported that they had been previously diagnosed with food allergies. The top five foods causing reactions were milk, red wine, eggs, chocolate, and peanuts.

Overall, the presence of food allergy was significantly associated with greater asthma severity (32% versus 26%; odds ratio [OR] = 1.4; $p = .05$). The presence of food reactions was also significantly associated with a history of hospitalization for asthma (31% versus 22%; OR = 1.6; $p = .004$).

Nursing Implications

A sizable portion of subjects in this study reported food reactions. Food reactions were more common in people with moderate to severe asthma and in those with prior hospitalization for asthma. Those who reported food reactions were more frequently female. The findings suggest that it is important for the nurse to identify patients with food reactions and to optimize their asthma care carefully. Nurses in community, home, and outpatient settings may be able to intervene earlier with these high-risk clients to prevent hospitalization.

HOME CARE TEACHING CHECKLIST: MANAGING FOOD ALLERGIES

At the completion of the program, the patient or caregiver will be able to:

	Patient	Caregiver
• Verbalize understanding of the need to maintain an allergen-free diet.	✔	✔
• Demonstrate reading of food labels to identify hidden allergens in food.	✔	✔
• Identify ways to manage an allergen-free diet when eating away from home.	✔	✔
• State the need to wear a medical alert medallion or bracelet.	✔	✔
• List symptoms of food allergy.	✔	✔
• Demonstrate emergency administration of epinephrine.	✔	✔
• State the importance of prompt treatment and health care follow-up.	✔	✔

Medical Management

Therapy for food hypersensitivity includes elimination of the food responsible for the patient's hypersensitivity. See the checklist about food allergies for more information. Pharmacologic therapy is necessary in patients with uncontrolled exposure to offending foods or patients with multiple food sensitivities not responsive to elimination measures. Medication therapy involves the use of H_1- and H_2-blockers, antihistamines, adrenergic agents, corticosteroids, and cromolyn sodium.

Many food allergies disappear with time, particularly in children. About one third of proven allergies disappear in 1 to 2 years if the patient carefully avoids the offending food.

Serum Sickness

The illness known as serum sickness is an example of an immune complex type III hypersensitivity. It has traditionally resulted from the administration of therapeutic antisera of animal sources for the treatment or prevention of infectious diseases, such as tetanus, pneumonia, rabies, diphtheria, botulism, and venomous snake and black widow spider bites. With the advent of human antitetanus serum and antibiotics, classic serum sickness is much less common now than in previous years. However, various medications (primarily penicillin) may cause a serum sickness–like reaction similar to that caused by foreign sera.

Clinical Manifestations

Symptoms are due to a reaction and immunologic attack on the serum or medication. Antibodies appear to be of the IgE and IgM classes. Early manifestations, beginning 6 to 10 days after the administration of the medication, include an inflammatory reaction at the site of injection of the medication, followed by regional and generalized lymphadenopathy. There is usually a skin rash, which may be urticarial or purpuric. Joints are frequently tender and swollen. Vasculitis may occur in any organ but is most commonly observed in the kidney, resulting in proteinuria and, occasionally, casts in the urine. There may be mild to severe cardiac involvement. Peripheral neuritis may cause temporary paralysis of the upper extremities or may be widespread, causing Guillain-Barré syndrome.

Medical Management

The usual course lasts for several days to a few weeks if untreated, but the patient responds promptly and completely if treated with antihistamines and corticosteroids. Aggressive therapy, including ventilator support, may be necessary if peripheral neuritis and Guillain-Barré syndrome occur.

Latex Allergy

Latex allergy and hypersensitivity were identified as early as 1933. Natural rubber latex is derived from the sap of the *Helva brasilinsis* tree. The conversion of the liquid rubber latex into a finished product is a complicated process that entails the addition of more than 100 chemicals. Latex contains proteins, amino acids, lipids, and many other substances. The proteins in the natural rubber latex (hevea proteins) or the various chemicals that are used in the manufacturing process are thought to be the source of the allergic reactions.

Although the prevalence of latex allergy is not known, since 1989, the number of cases of latex allergy has steadily increased. Reasons for the increase in the number of cases may be either the implementation of universal and now standard precautions whereby health care workers are wearing gloves for a great many more procedures and for longer periods than before the acquired immunodeficiency syndrome (AIDS) epidemic or changes instituted in the manufacturing of gloves to speed up the process to meet the increased demand for gloves.

Populations at risk include health care workers, people with atopic allergies or multiple surgeries, people working in factories manufacturing latex products, females, and persons with spina bifida. Because more food handlers, hairdressers, and auto mechanics are now wearing latex gloves, they may also be at risk for latex allergy. There have been cross-reactions reported in people who are allergic to certain food products, such as kiwis, bananas, pineapples, passion fruits, avocados, and chestnuts.

Routes of exposure to latex products can be cutaneous, percutaneous, mucosal, parenteral, and aerosol. The most frequent source of exposure is cutaneous, which usually involves the wearing of natural latex gloves. Aerosolization of powder from latex gloves can occur when gloves are dispensed from the box or when gloves are removed from the hands. Mucosal exposure can occur from use of latex condoms, catheters, airways, and nipples. Parenteral exposure can occur from intravenous lines or hemodialysis equipment. In addition to latex-derived medical devices, many household items also contain latex. Examples of medical and household items containing latex and a list of alternative products are found in Table 49-5.

Clinical Manifestations

Symptoms of latex allergy can range from mild contact dermatitis to moderately severe symptoms of rhinitis, conjunctivitis, ur-

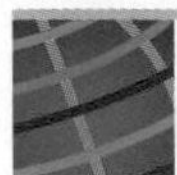

TABLE 49•5 Selected Products Containing Natural Rubber Latex and Latex-Free Alternatives

Products Containing Latex	Alternatives
Hospital Environment	
Ace bandage (brown)	Ace bandage, white all cotton
Adhesive bandages; Band-Aid dressing	Cotton pads and plastic or silk tape
Ambu bag	Neoprene anesthesia kit (King) Clear bags (Respironics, Laerdal)
Elastic pressure stockings	Kendall SCD stockings with stokinette
Blood pressure cuff, tubing and bladder	Single-use nylon or vinyl blood pressure cuffs or wrap with stockinette or apply over clothing
Catheters	All-silicone or vinyl catheters
Catheter leg bag straps	Velcro straps
ECG Pads	Baxter, Red Dot 3M ECG pads
Gloves	Dermaprene, Neoprene, polymer, or vinyl gloves
IV catheters	Jelko, Deseret IV catheters
IV rubber injection ports	Use three-way stopcocks on plastic tubing
Levin tube	Salem sump
Medication vials	Remove rubber stopper
Pads for crutches	Cover with cloth
Prepackaged enema kits	None
Stethoscopes	Place cloth around latex
Syringes—single use (Monoject, B & D)	Terumo syringes
Home Environment	
Balloons	Mylar balloons
Condoms, diaphragms	Polyurethane products, Durex/Avanti and Reality products
Feminine hygiene pad	Kimberly-Clark products

ticaria, and bronchospasm to severe life-threatening anaphylaxis. Delayed-type (type IV) or anaphylactic (type I) hypersensitivities may occur. Clinical manifestations of delayed-type hypersensitivity include symptoms of contact dermatitis, such as pruritus, edema, erythema, vesicles, papules, and crusting and thickening of the skin. Clinical manifestations of anaphylactic hypersensitivity have a rapid onset of symptoms: urticaria, wheezing, dyspnea, laryngeal edema, bronchospasm, tachycardia, angioedema, hypotension, and cardiac arrest.

Irritant dermatitis, caused by the powder in gloves, may occur but is not an allergy to latex. The most common symptoms are erythema and pruritus. These symptoms can be eliminated by changing glove brands or using powder-free gloves.

Medical Management

The only treatment available for latex allergy is the avoidance of latex products. Avoidance of latex products may be impossible because there are so many-latex based products. People who have experienced an anaphylactic reaction should be counseled to wear medical identification and to carry a supply of nonlatex gloves. Antihistamines and an emergency kit containing epinephrine should be provided along with instructions about emergency management of their symptoms. These people should be counseled to notify all health care workers as well as local paramedic and ambulance companies about their allergy. Some people with type I hypersensitivity have warning labels on their car windows to alert police and paramedics of their allergy in case of a car accident. These people should be provided with a list of resources of alternative products and referred to local support groups.

In the working environment, people with type I latex sensitivity may be unable to continue to work in their area of expertise if a latex-free environment is not possible. These people are frequently surgeons, dentists, and operating room or intensive care nurses. Occupational implications for employees with type IV latex sensitivity are usually easier to manage by changing to nonlatex gloves and avoidance of direct contact with latex-based medical equipment.

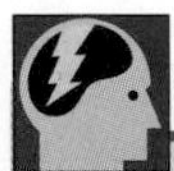

Critical Thinking Exercises

1. During a patient's hospital admission procedure, you inquire about allergies. The patient reports that he is allergic "to everything." Describe the additional information you would obtain from him and how you would document this information on the patient's medical record.

2. Your patient has had a skin test done before a diagnostic test because of the possibility that she is allergic to the contrast agent that will be used for the test. She reports pruritus, tightness in the throat and chest, and a feeling of anxiety. How would you respond to this situation? Describe the medical management you would anticipate and the nursing strategies you expect to carry out.

3. A patient is undergoing extensive diagnostic studies to identify the allergens that are causing her allergic symptoms. What recommendations would you give to her about her home environment? How might you modify those instructions if the patient lives near an industrial area? On a farm? Has small children, each of whom has a favorite pet?

References and Selected Readings

BOOKS

Antel, P., Birnbaum, G., & Hartung, H. P. (1998). *Clinical neuroimmunology.* Malden, MA: Blackwell Scientific.

Bardana, E. J. Jr., Montanaro, A. (1997). *Indoor air pollution and health.* New York: Marcel Dekker.

Bernstein, J. A. (1997). Antihistamines. In: R. Patterson, L. C. Grammer, & P. A. Greenberger. *Allergic diseases: Diagnosis and management* (5th ed.). Philadelphia: Lippincott-Raven.

Booth, B. H. (1997). Diagnosis of immediate hypersensitivity. In: R. Patterson, L. C. Grammer, & P. A. Greenberger. *Allergic diseases: Diagnosis and management* (5th ed.). Philadelphia: Lippincott-Raven.

Bradley, J., & McCluskey, J. (Eds.) (1997). *Clinical immunology.* New York: Oxford University Press.

Delves, P. J. (1998). *Encyclopedia of immunology* (2nd ed.). San Diego: Academic Press.

Ditto, A. M., & Grammer, L. C. (1997). Food allergy. In: R. Patterson, L. C. Grammer, & P. A. Greenberger. *Allergic diseases: Diagnosis and management* (5th ed.). Philadelphia: Lippincott-Raven.

Eales, L. J. (1997). *Immunology for life scientists. A basic introduction: A student-centered learning approach.* New York: John Wiley & Sons.

Eisenhauer, L., Nichols, L. W., Spencer, R. T., & Bergan, F. W. (1998). *Clinical pharmacology and nursing management* (5th ed.). Philadelphia: Lippincott-Raven.

Elgert, K. D. (1996). *Immunology: Understanding the immune system.* New York: Wiley-Liss.

Frank, M. M. (Ed.). (1995). *Samter's immunologic diseases.* Boston: Little, Brown.

Grammar, L. C. (1997). Atopic dermatitis. In: R. Patterson, L. C. Grammer, & P. A. Greenberger. *Allergic diseases: Diagnosis and management* (5th ed.). Philadelphia: Lippincott-Raven.

Grammar, L. C., & Shaughnessy, M. A. (1997). Principles of immunologic management of allergic diseases due to extrinsic antigens. In: R. Patterson, L. C. Grammer, & P. A. Greenberger. *Allergic diseases: Diagnosis and management* (5th ed.). Philadelphia: Lippincott-Raven.

Huot, A. E., & Sheehan, C. (1997). Hypersensitivity. In: C. Sheehan C (Ed.). *Clinical immunology: Principles and laboratory diagnosis* (2nd ed.). Philadelphia: Lippincott-Raven.

Kay, A. B. (1997). Allergy and allergic diseases. Malden, MA: Blackwell Scientific.

Lane, N. E. (1997). *AIDS, allergy, and rheumatology.* Totowa, NJ: Humana Press.

Metzger, W. J. (1997), Urticaria, angioedema, and hereditary angioedema. In: R. Patterson, L. C. Grammer, & P. A. Greenberger. *Allergic diseases: Diagnosis and management* (5th ed.). Philadelphia: Lippincott-Raven.

McGrath, K. G. (1997). Anaphylaxis. In: R. Patterson, L. C. Grammer, & P. A. Greenberger. *Allergic diseases: Diagnosis and management* (5th ed.). Philadelphia: Lippincott-Raven.

Middleton, E. Jr (Ed.). (1998). *Allergy: Principles and practice.* St. Louis: C. V. Mosby.

Nakamura, R. M., et al. (Eds.). (1998). *Clinical diagnostic immunology: Protocols in quality assurance and standardization.* Malden, MA: Blackwell Scientific.

Patterson, R., & Cheriyan, S. (1997). Stevens-Johnson syndrome and erythema multiforme. In: R. Patterson, L. C. Grammer, & P. A. Greenberger. *Allergic diseases diagnosis and management* (5th ed.). Philadelphia: Lippincott-Raven.

Patterson, R., & Harris, K. E. (1997). Idiopathic anaphylaxis. In: R. Patterson, L. C. Grammer, & P. A. Greenberger. *Allergic diseases: Diagnosis and management* (5th ed.). Philadelphia: Lippincott-Raven.

Reisman, R. E. (1997). Allergy to stinging insects. In: R. Patterson, L. C. Grammer, & P. A. Greenberger. *Allergic diseases: Diagnosis and management* (5th ed.). Philadelphia: Lippincott-Raven.

Ricketti, A. J. (1997). Allergic rhinitis. In: R. Patterson, L. C. Grammer, & P. A. Greenberger. *Allergic diseases: Diagnosis and management* (5th ed.). Philadelphia: Lippincott-Raven.

Roitt, I., Brostoff, J., & Male, D. K. (Eds.). (1998). *Immunology* (5th ed.). St. Louis: C. V. Mosby.

Stites, D. P., Terr, A. I., & Parslow, T. G. (Eds.). *Medical immunology* (9th ed.). (1997). Stamford, CT: Appleton & Lange.

Terr, A. I. (1997). Controversial and unproven methods in allergy diagnosis and treatment. In: R. Patterson, L. C. Grammer, & P. A. Greenberger. *Allergic diseases: Diagnosis and management* (5th ed.). Philadelphia: Lippincott-Raven.

Virella, G. (Ed.). (1998). *Introduction to medical immunology* (4th ed.). New York: Marcel Dekker.

Wasserman, S. I. (1997). *Biochemical mediators of allergic reactions.* In: R. Patterson, L. C. Grammer, & P. A. Greenberger. *Allergic diseases: Diagnosis and management* (5th ed.). Philadelphia: Lippincott-Raven.

Weir, D. M., & Steward, J. (1997). *Immunology* (8th ed.). New York: Churchill Livingstone.

Zeiss, C. R., & Pruzansky, J. J. (1997). Immunology of IgE-mediated and other hypersensitivity states. In: R. Patterson, L. C. Grammer, & P. A. Greenberger. *Allergic diseases: Diagnosis and management* (5th ed.). Philadelphia: Lippincott-Raven.

JOURNALS

Asterisks indicate nursing research articles.

Barbarito, C. (1999). Anaphylaxis. *American Journal of Nursing, 99*(1), 33.

Ballow, M., & Nelson, R. (1997). Immunopharmacology: Immunomodulation and immunotherapy. *Journal of the American Medical Association, 278*(22), 2008–2017.

Barton, C. R., & Beeson, M. (1995). Allergic drug reactions. *CRNA: The Clinical Forum for Nurse Anesthetists, 6*(4), 159–165.

Blaylock, B. (1997). Latex allergies: Overview, prevention and implications for nursing care. *Ostomy Wound Management, 43*(3), 46–53.

Bernstein, D. I. (1997). Allergic reactions to workplace allergens. *Journal of the American Medical Association, 278*(22), 1907–1913.

Burt, S. (1998). What you need to know about latex allergy. *Nursing '98, 28*(10), 33–39.

Chang, B. L., Vredevoe, D., & Hirsch, M. (1995). Allergy as a risk factor for nursing care problems in the elderly cancer patient. *Cancer Nursing, 18*(2), 83–88.

Cook, L. S. (1997). Blood transfusion reactions involving an immune response. *Journal of Intravenous Nursing, 20*(1), 5–14.

Costa, J. J., Weller, P. F., & Galli, S. J. (1997). The cells of the allergic response: Mast cells, basophils, and eosinophils. *Journal of the American Medical Association, 278*(22), 1815–1834.

deShazo, R. D. (1997). Future trends in allergy and immunology. *Journal of the American Medical Association, 278*(22), 2024–2025.

deShazo, R. D., & Kemp, S. F. (1997). Allergic reactions to drugs and biologic agents. *Journal of the American Medical Association, 278*(22), 1895–1906.

Donohoe, M. R. (1997). Allergic diseases. *Lippincott's Primary Care Practice, 1*(2), 117–128.

*Emery, N. L., Vollmer, W. M., Buist, A. S., & Osborne, M. L. (1996). Self-reported food reactions and their associations with asthma. *Western Journal of Nursing Research, 18*(6), 643–654.

Galen, B. A. (1997). Rhinitis. *Lippincott's Primary Care Practice, 1*(2), 129–141.

Graft, D. F. (1996). Allergic and nonallergic rhinitis. *Postgraduate Medicine, 100*(2), 64–74.

Gritter, M. (1997). Latex allergy. *Lippincott's Primary Care Practice, 1*(2), 142–151.

Gritter, M. (1998). The latex threat. *American Journal of Nursing, 98*(9), 26–32.

Grzybowski, M., Ownby, D. R., Peyser, P. A., Johnson, C. C., & Schork, M. A. (1996). The prevalence of anti-latex IgE antibodies among registered nurses. *Journal of Allergy and Clinical Immunology, 98*(3), 535–544.

Harkins, L. (1997). Contact dermatitis. *Lippincott's Primary Care Practice, 1*(1), 97–98.

Heffner, D. (1997). Anaphylaxis. *Lippincott's Primary Care Practice, 1*(2), 220–223.

Huss, K., Vessy, J. A., Mason, P., Aschenbrenner, D. S., & Huss, R. W. (1996). Controlling allergies by assessing risks in the home. *Pediatric Nursing, 22*(5), 432–435.

Jackson, D. (1995). Latex allergy and anaphylaxis: What to do? *Journal of Intravenous Nursing, 18*(1), 33–52.

Leung, D. Y. M., Diaz, L. A., DeLeo, V., & Sotor, N. A. (1997). Allergic and immunologic skin disorders. *Journal of the American Medical Association, 278*(22), 1914–1923.

Lilley, L. L., & Gaunci, R. (1999). Cross sensitivities: Medication errors waiting to happen. *American Journal of Nursing, 99*(2), 12.

Maher, J. (1997). Urticaria and angioedema. *Lippincott's Primary Care Practice, 1*(2), 172–182.

Majamaa, H., & Isolauri, E. (1997). Probiotics: A novel approach in the management of food allergy. *Journal of Allergy and Clinical Immunology, 99*(2), 179–185.

Naclerio, R., & Solomon, W. (1997). Rhinitis and inhalant allergens. *Journal of the American Medical Association, 278*(22), 1842–1848.

Pearl, E. R. (1997). Food allergy. *Lippincott's Primary Care Practice, 1*(2), 154–167.

Redman, M. C. (1996). Latex allergy: Recognition and perioperative management. *Journal of Post Anesthesia Nursing, 11*(1), 6–12.

Sampson, H. A. (1997). Food allergy. *Journal of the American Medical Association, 278*(22), 1888–1894.

Smith, L. J. (1995). Diagnosis and treatment of allergic rhinitis. *Nurse Practitioner, 20*(10), 58–66.

Sussman, G. L., & Beezhold, D. H. (1995). Allergy to latex rubber. *Annals of Internal Medicine, 122*(1), 43–46.

Titler, M. G., & Steelman, V. M. (1996). Preventing allergic reactions to latex. *MedSurg Nursing, 5*(2), 111–114, 134.

Weber, R. W. (1997). Immunotherapy with allergens. *Journal of the American Medical Association, 278*(22), 1881–1887.

Young, M. A., & Meyers, M. (1997). Latex allergy considerations for the care of pediatric patients and employee safety. *Nursing Clinics of North America, 32*(1), 169–182.

Resources

ALERT, Inc., Allergy to Latex Education and Resource Team, P.O. Box 13930, Milwaukee, WI 53213; 1-888-97-ALERT (972-5378); www.execpc.com/~alert/

American Academy of Allergy, Asthma and Immunology, 611 E. Wells St., Milwaukee, WI 53202; 1-800-822-2762; Fax: 1-414-276-3349; www.aaaai.org (For a series of patient-oriented pamphlets, Tips to Remember)

American College of Allergy, Asthma and Immunology, 85 W. Algonquin Road, Suite 500, Arlington Heights, IL: 60005; 1-847-427-1200; Fax: 1-847-427-1294; www.allergy.mcg.edu

Asthma and Allergy Foundation of America, 1125 15th St. NW Suite 502, Washington, DC 20005; 1-202-466-7643 ext. 226; Fax: 1-202-466-8940; www.aafa.org

Center Laboratories Division of EM Pharmaceuticals, Inc., 35 Channel Dr., Port Washington, NY 11050; 1-800-223-6837

ELASTIC, Education for Latex Allergy/Support Team & Information Coalition, 196 Pleasant Run Road, West Chester, PA 19380; 1-610-436-4801; netcom.com/~ecbdmd/elastic.html

Food Allergy Network, 10400 Eaton Place, Suite 107, Fairfax, VA 22030-2208; 1-800-929-4040 (to order); 1-703-691-3179 (for questions); Fax: 1-703-691-2713; www.foodallergy.org; E-mail: fan@worldweb.net

Latex Allergy News, 176 Roosevelt Avenue, Torrington, CT 06790; 1-860-482-6869; www.latexallergyhelp.com

Medic Alert Foundation International, P.O. Box 819008, Turlock, CA 95381; 1-800-825-3785; 1-800-344-3226 (for information, service); www.medicalert.org

National Institute for Occupational Safety and Health; 1-800-35-NIOSH (1-356-4674); www.cdc.gov/niosh/latexalt.html

National Institute of Allergy and Infectious Diseases National Institute of Health, Bldg 31. Room 7A50, 31 Center Drive MSC 2520, Bethesda, MD 20892; 1-301-496-5717; Fax: 1-301-402-0120; www.Niaid.nih.gov

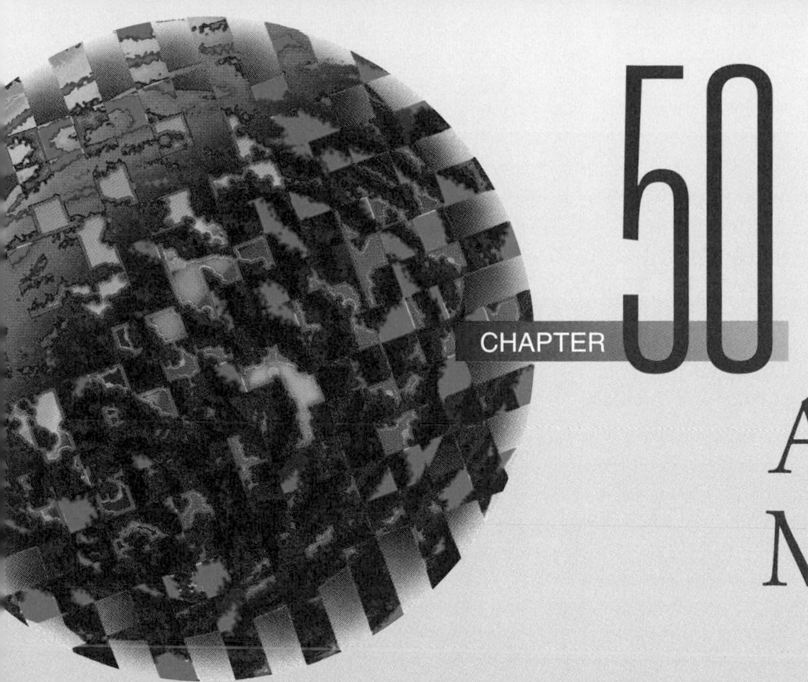

Assessment and Management of Patients With Rheumatic Disorders

Learning Objectives

On completion of this chapter, the learner will be able to:

1. Explain the processes of inflammation and degeneration in the development of rheumatic diseases.
2. Describe the assessment and diagnostic findings that may be evidenced by patients with a suspected diagnosis of rheumatic disease.
3. Discuss appropriate nursing interventions based on nursing diagnoses and collaborative problems that commonly occur with rheumatic disorders.
4. Apply the nursing process as a framework for the care of the patient with a rheumatic disease, such as connective tissue disease or osteoarthritis.
5. Describe the systemic effects of a connective tissue disease.
6. Devise a teaching plan for the patient with newly diagnosed rheumatic disease.

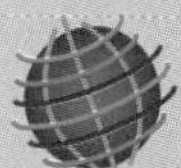

Rheumatic diseases include common disorders such as osteoarthritis (OA) or more rare conditions such as systemic lupus erythematosus (SLE) or scleroderma. These conditions can be life-threatening or merely an inconvenience. The problems caused by the rheumatic diseases not only include the obvious limitations in mobility and activities of daily living but also the subtle systemic effects that can lead to organ failure and death or result in problems such as pain, fatigue, altered self-image, and sleep disturbances. The rheumatic disease may be the patient's primary health problem or a secondary diagnosis. Thus, thorough understanding of rheumatic diseases and their effects on the patient's function and well-being is the key to developing an appropriate plan of care.

GLOSSARY

ankylosis: fixation or immobility of a joint

antibody: a protein substance developed by the body in response to and interacting with a specific antigen

antigen: a substance that induces production of antibodies

arthroplasty: replacement of a joint

cytokines: generic term for nonantibody proteins that act as intercellular mediators, as in the generation of immune response

diarthrodial: a joint with two freely moveable parts

hemarthrosis: bleeding into the joint

joint effusion: the escape of fluid from the blood vessels or lymphatics into the joint cavity

leukotriene: substance produced from arachidonic acid during the inflammatory process that acts as a mediator of inflammation

osteophyte: a bony outgrowth or protuberance; spur

pannus: newly formed synovial tissue infiltrated with inflammatory cells

prostaglandin: substance produced from arachidonic acid during the inflammatory process that acts as a mediator of inflammation

subchondral bone: bony plate that supports the articular cartilage

synovial: pertaining to the joint-lubricating fluid

tophi: accumulation of crystalline deposits in articular surfaces, bones, soft tissue, and cartilage

RHEUMATIC DISEASES

Commonly called arthritis (inflammation of a joint) and thought of as one condition, the rheumatic diseases are actually more than 100 different types of disorders that primarily affect skeletal muscles, bones, ligaments, tendons, and joints of males and females of *all* ages. Some disorders are more likely to occur at a particular time of life or to affect one gender more than the other. Moreover, the onset of these conditions may be acute or insidious, with a course possibly marked by periods of *remission* (a period when disease symptoms are reduced or absent) and *exacerbation* (a period when symptoms occur or increase). Treatment can be very simple, aimed at localized relief, or it can be complex, directed toward relieving systemic effects. Permanent changes may result from the disease.

The rheumatic diseases are classified into 10 categories demonstrating a wide variety of multisystem disorders. Conditions that secondarily may affect the musculoskeletal structure are also included, emphasizing the diversity of the rheumatic diseases.

Pathophysiology

Understanding the normal anatomy and physiology of the **diarthrodial** or **synovial** joints is key to understanding the pathophysiology of the rheumatic diseases. The function of the synovial joints is movement. Each synovial joint has a given range of motion, although each person does not have the same range of motion in the movable joints.

In a normal synovial joint, a smooth, resilient surface for movement is provided by *articular cartilage,* which covers the bone end of the joint. Lining the inner surface of the fibrous capsule is the *synovial membrane,* which secretes fluid into the space between the bones. This synovial fluid functions as a shock absorber and a lubricant, allowing the joint to move freely in the appropriate direction.

The joint is the area most commonly affected by the inflammation and degeneration seen in rheumatic diseases. Despite the diversity of rheumatic diseases, from localized involvement of one joint to systemic, multisystem disorders, they all involve some degree of inflammation and degeneration, which may occur simultaneously. Inflammation is demonstrated in the joints as *synovitis.* In inflammatory rheumatic diseases, the primary process is inflammation as a result of the immune response. Degeneration occurs as a secondary process, resulting from the effect of **pannus** (proliferation of newly formed synovial tissue infiltrated with inflammatory cells). The inflammation is a result of the immune response.

Conversely, in degenerative rheumatic diseases, inflammation occurs as a secondary process. This synovitis is usually milder, is more likely to be seen in advanced disease, and represents a reactive process. The synovitis may be related to the release of free cartilage proteoglycan from the deteriorating articular cartilage, but immunologic factors may also be involved.

INFLAMMATION

Inflammation involves a series of related steps. With the triggering event, the **antigen** stimulus activates monocytes and T lymphocytes (also called T cells). Next, the immunoglobulin antibodies form immune complexes with antigens. Phagocytosis of the immune complexes is initiated, generating an inflammatory reaction (joint swelling, pain, and edema) (Fig. 50-1).

During the next step, the normal immune response deviates. Phagocytosis produces chemicals such as leukotrienes and prostaglandins. **Leukotrienes** contribute to the inflammatory process by attracting other white blood cells to the area. **Prostaglandins** act as modifiers to inflammation. In some cases, they increase inflammation; in other cases, they slow it down. Leukotrienes and prostaglandins produce enzymes, such as collagenase, that break down collagen, a vital part of a normal joint. The release of these enzymes in the joint causes edema, proliferation of synovial membrane and pannus formation, destruction of cartilage, and erosion of bone.

The immunologic inflammatory process begins when antigens are presented to T lymphocytes, leading to a proliferation of T and B cells. B cells are a source for **antibody**-forming cells, or plasma cells. In response to specific antigens, plasma cells produce and release antibodies. Antibodies combine with corresponding antigens to form pairs, or immune complexes. The immune complexes build up and are deposited in synovial tissue or other organs in the body, thereby triggering the inflammatory reaction that can ultimately damage the involved tissue.

The systemic nature of the rheumatic disease category known as the diffuse connective tissue diseases is reflected in the resultant widespread inflammatory process. Although focused in the joints, inflammation also involves other areas. The blood vessels (vasculitis and arteritis), lungs, heart, and kidneys may also be affected by the inflammation. In the joints, this inflammatory response is manifested as pannus extending throughout the joint

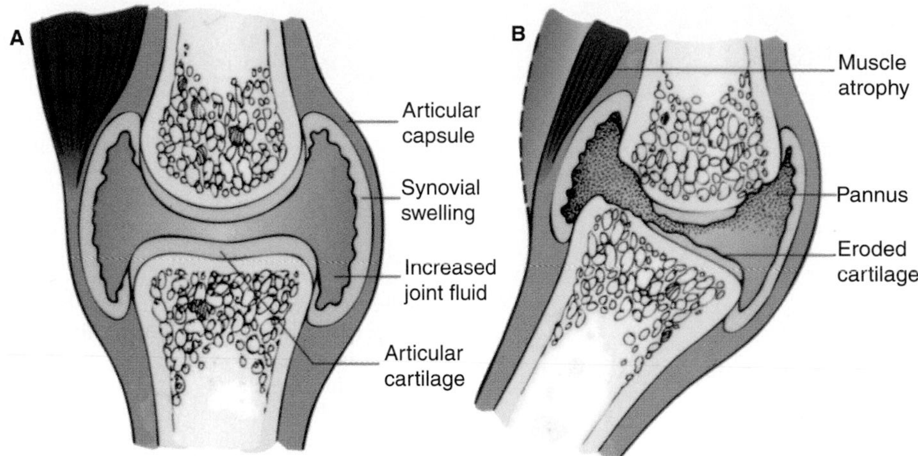

FIGURE 50•1 (**A**) Synovial swelling and fluid accumulation. (**B**) Pannus (a proliferation of synovial tissue), eroded articular cartilage, and joint space narrowing—all of which contribute to muscle atrophy and ankylosis (joint rigidity and immobility).

space and, if persistent, eroding the articular cartilage, causing secondary degenerative changes to the joint.

DEGENERATION

Degeneration of the articular cartilage is caused by a physiologic imbalance between mechanical stress and the ability of the joint tissues to resist that stress. The articular cartilage and bone are normal, but an excessive load (force from the weight of the body) applied to the joints causes the tissues to fail. Or the articular cartilage or bone is defective and thus is unable to withstand a physiologically reasonable load applied to the joint. Defective cartilage or bone may result from genetic and endocrine factors.

Articular cartilage plays two essential mechanical roles in joint physiology. First, the articular cartilage provides a remarkably smooth weight-bearing surface and, with synovial fluid, provides extremely low friction during movement. Second, the cartilage transmits load or pressure to the bone, dissipating the mechanical stress. Specific factors have been implicated in association with degenerative joint changes.

Mechanical Stress. Articular cartilage is highly resistant to wear under conditions of repeated movement. However, repetitive impact loading (velocity at which the force is applied) rapidly leads to joint failure at the cartilage level. When a person walks, three to four times the body weight is transmitted through the knee. A deep knee bend transmits up to nine times the body weight through the patellofemoral joint. As a joint undergoes repeated mechanical stress, the elasticity of the joint capsule, articular cartilage, and ligaments is reduced. The *articular plate* (**subchondral bone**) thins, and its ability to absorb shock decreases. The joint space narrows, accompanied by a loss of stability. When the articular plate disappears, bony spurs (**osteophytes**) form at the edges of the joint surfaces, and the capsule and synovial membranes thicken. The joint cartilage degenerates and atrophies (shrinks), the bones harden and hypertrophy (thicken) at their articular surfaces, and the ligaments calcify. As a result, sterile **joint effusions** (fluid escaping from the blood vessels or lymphatics into the joint cavity) and secondary synovitis may be present (Fig. 50-2).

Altered Lubrication. In addition to the changes in the articular cartilage and subchondral bone, lubrication of the joint is also a factor in joint degeneration. With joint loading (forces carried through the joint), lubrication depends on a film of interstitial fluid squeezed out of the cartilage upon compression of the opposing surfaces of the joint. The mechanisms that normally operate under high-weight loads to produce this lubricating film may be affected.

Immobility. Immobilization of a joint is another factor that can produce degenerative changes in articular cartilage. Although these changes are more marked and appear earlier in areas of contact, they also occur in areas not subject to mechanical compression. Cartilage degeneration due to joint immobility may result from loss of the pumping action of lubrication that occurs with joint movement. By 3 weeks after remobilization of the joint, the cartilage abnormalities are reversed. However, impact exercising (activities such as running) prevents reversal of the atrophy. Instead, slow, gradual range of motion is thought to be very important in preventing cartilage injury.

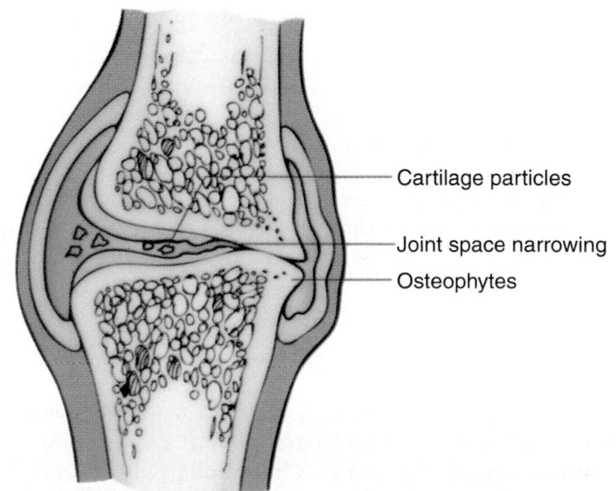

FIGURE 50•2 Joint space narrowing and osteophytes (bone spurs) are characteristic of degenerative changes in joints.

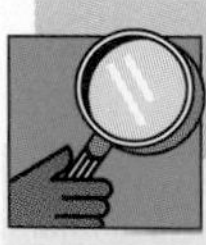

ASSESSMENT
RHEUMATIC DISEASES

In addition to the head-to-toe assessment or systems review, the following are important areas of consideration to be noted when performing the complete physical assessment of a patient with a known or suspected rheumatic disease.

Manifestation	Significance
Skin (inspect and inquire)	
Rash, lesions	• Associated with lupus erythematosus (LE), vasculitides, adverse effect of medication
Increased bruising	• Associated with several rheumatic diseases and adverse effect of medication
Erythema	• Sign of inflammation
Thinning	• Adverse effect of medication
Warmth	• Sign of inflammation
Photosensitivity	• Associated with systemic lupus erythematosus (SLE), dermatomyositis, adverse effect of medication
Hair (inspect and inquire)	
Alopecia or thinning	• Associated with rheumatic diseases or adverse effect of medication
Eye (inspect and inquire)	
Dryness, grittiness	• Associated with Sjögren's syndrome (commonly occurring with rheumatoid arthritis [RA] and LE)
Decreased acuity or blindness	• Associated with temporal arteritis, medication complications
Cataracts	• Adverse effect of medication
Decreased peripheral vision	• Adverse effect of medication
Conjunctivitis, uveitis	• Associated with ankylosing spondylitis (AS) and Reiter's syndrome
Ear (inquire)	
Tinnitus	• Adverse effect of medication
Decreased acuity	• Adverse effect of medication
Mouth (inspect and inquire)	
Buccal, sublingual lesions	• Associated with vasculitis, dermatomyositis, adverse effect of medication
Altered sense of taste	• Adverse effect of medication
Dryness	• Associated with Sjögren's syndrome
Dysphagia	• Associated with myositis
Difficulty chewing	• Associated with decreased range of motion of jaw
Chest (inspect and inquire)	
Pleuritic pain	• Associated with RA and SLE
Decreased chest expansion	• Associated with AS
Activity intolerance (dyspnea)	• Associated with pulmonary hypertension in scleroderma
Cardiovascular system (inspect, inquire, palpate)	
Blanching of fingers on exposure to cold	• Associated with Raynaud's phenomenon
Peripheral pulses	• Deficit may indicate vascular involvement or edema associated with medication effect or rheumatic diseases, especially SLE or scleroderma

Clinical Manifestations

Pain is the symptom of a rheumatic disease that most commonly causes a person to seek medical attention. Other common symptoms include joint swelling, limited movement, stiffness, weakness, and fatigue.

Assessment and Diagnostic Findings

Assessment begins with a general health history, which includes the onset of symptoms and how they evolved, family history, and any other contributing factors. This is followed by a complete physical assessment. Because many of the rheumatic diseases are chronic conditions, the health history should also include information about the patient's perception of the problem, previous treatments and their effectiveness, the patient's support systems, and the patient's current knowledge base and the source of that information.

Assessment for rheumatic diseases combines the physical examination with a functional assessment. Inspection of the patient's general appearance occurs during initial contact. Gait, posture, and general musculoskeletal size and structure are observed. Gross deformities and abnormalities in movement are noted. The symmetry, size, and contour of other connective tissues, such as the skin and adipose tissue, are also noted and recorded. The assessment chart outlines the important areas for consideration during the physical assessment. The functional assessment is a combination of history (what the patient reports that he or she can and cannot do) and examination (observation of activities: the patient demonstrates what he or she can and cannot do, such as dressing and getting in and out of a chair). Observation also includes the adaptations and adjustments the

ASSESSMENT
RHEUMATIC DISEASES *(Continued)*

Manifestation	Significance
Abdomen (inquire and palpate)	
Altered bowel habits	• Associated with scleroderma, spondylosis, ulcerative colitis, decreased physical mobility, medication effect
Nausea, vomiting, bloating pain	• Adverse effect of medication
Weight change	• Associated with RA (decreased), adverse effect of medication (increased or decreased)
Genitalia (inspect and inquire)	
Dryness, itching	• Associated with Sjögren's syndrome
Abnormal menses	• Adverse effect of medication
Altered sexual performance	• Fear of pain (or of pain caused by partner) and limitation of motion may affect sexual mobility
Hygiene	• Poor hygiene may be related to limitations in activities of daily living
Urethritis, dysuria	• Associated with AS and Reiter's syndrome
Lesions	• Associated with vasculitis
Neurologic (inspect and inquire)	
Paresthesias of extremities; abnormal reflex pattern	• Nerve compressions associated with carpal tunnel syndrome, spinal stenosis, etc.
Headaches	• Associated with temporal arteritis, adverse effect of medication
Musculoskeletal (inspect and palpate)	
Joint redness, warmth, swelling, tenderness, deformity—location of first joint involved, pattern of progression, symmetry, acute vs chronic nature	• Signs of inflammation
Joint range of motion	• Decreased range of motion may indicate severity or progression of disease
Surrounding tissue findings	• Extra-articular manifestations
Muscle atrophy, subcutaneous nodules, popliteal cyst	
Muscle strength (grip)	• Muscle strength decreases with increased disease activity

patient may have made (sometimes without awareness), for example, lowering the mouth to the fork rather than raising the fork to the mouth.

The history and physical assessment data are supplemented by supportive or confirming diagnostic test findings. In some instances, tests are used to follow the course of the disease. For example, the erythrocyte sedimentation rate (ESR) reflects inflammatory activity and indirectly the progression or remission of disease. The following tests are most commonly used for patients with rheumatic diseases.

ARTHROCENTESIS

An arthrocentesis (needle aspiration of synovial fluid) may be performed not only to obtain a sample of synovial fluid for analysis but also to relieve pain—usually in the knee or shoulder. Synovial fluid is usually analyzed in cases such as suspected joint infection to determine the presence of inflammatory cells and to identify crystals or the presence of blood, indicating trauma.

After the joint is anesthetized locally, a large-bore needle is inserted into the joint space to obtain a fluid specimen. Because this procedure has the potential for introducing bacteria into the joint, aseptic technique is essential. After the procedure, the patient is observed for signs of infection and **hemarthrosis** (bleeding into the joint).

Normally, synovial fluid is clear, viscous, straw-colored, and scanty in volume with few cells. In inflammatory joint disease, however, the fluid may become cloudy, milky, or dark yellow and may contain numerous inflammatory cells, such as leukocytes (white blood cells) and complement (a plasma protein associated with immunologic reactions). The viscosity is reduced in inflammatory disease, and copious amounts of fluid may be present. Diagnostically a valuable test, obtaining joint fluid in small joints such as the fingers or wrist may be difficult.

X-RAY STUDIES

X-rays are often used in evaluating patients with rheumatic disease. The timing of the x-rays influences their usefulness. It is unlikely that a patient with a 2-month history of joint inflammation will have demonstrable changes on x-ray. Someone with knee crepitus (a grating sound heard on movement), however, will likely show severe joint degeneration. X-rays can also be used to monitor disease activity and progression, demonstrating the loss of cartilage and narrowing of the joint space over time. X-rays can also demonstrate cartilage abnormalities, joint erosions, abnormal bony growth, and osteopenia (decreased bone mineralization).

Arthrography. Arthrography is a diagnostic radiographic technique used to detect connective tissue disorders. A radiopaque substance or air is injected into the joint cavity, especially of the knee or shoulder, to outline the contour of the joint. The joint is then put through passive range of motion while several x-rays are obtained. The radiopaque substance is absorbed systemically, and joint swelling consequently subsides. After the procedure, the patient is observed for signs of infection and hemarthrosis.

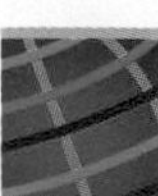

TABLE 50•1 **Common Serum Studies for Rheumatic Diseases**

Test	Normal Value	Significance
Serum		
Creatinine		
Metabolic waste excreted through the kidneys	0.6–1.2 mg/dL (50–110 μmol/L)	Increase may indicate renal damage in SLE, scleroderma, and polyarteritis.
Erythrocyte Sedimentation Rate (ESR)		
Measures the rate at which red blood cells settle out of unclotted blood in 1 hour	Westergren = *Men,* 0–15 mm/h, *Women,* 0–20 mm/h Wintrobe = *Men,* 0–9 mm/h, *Women* 0–15 mm/h	Increase is usually seen in inflammatory CTD. An increase indicates rising inflammation, resulting in clustering of RBCs, which makes them heavier than normal. The higher the ESR, the greater the inflammatory activity.
Hematocrit		
Measures the size, capacity, and number of cells present in blood	*Men:* 45–50 vol/dL *Women:* 40–45 vol/dL	Decrease can be seen in chronic inflammation (anemia of chronic disease); also, blood loss through bowel due to medication.
Red Blood Cell Count		
Measures circulating erythrocytes	*Men:* Average 4.8 million/μL *Women:* Average 4.3 million/μL	Decrease can be seen in RA, SLE.
White Blood Cell Count		
Measures circulating leukocytes	5000–10,000 cells/mm³	Decrease may be seen in SLE.
VDRL (Venereal Disease Research Laboratory)		
Measures antibody to syphilis	Nonreactive	False-positive results are sometimes found with SLE.
Uric Acid		
Measures level of uric acid in serum	2.5–8 mg/dL (0.15–0.5 mmol/L)	Increase is seen with gout.
Serum Immunology		
Antinuclear Antibody (ANA)		
Measures antibodies that react with a variety of nuclear antigens If antibodies are present, further testing determines the type of ANA circulating in the blood (anti-DNA, anti-RNP).	Negative A few healthy adults have a positive ANA	Positive test is associated with SLE, RA, scleroderma, Raynaud's disease, Sjögren's syndrome, necrotizing arteritis. The higher the titer, the greater the inflammation. The pattern of immunofluorescence (speckled, homogeneous, or nucleolar) helps determine the diagnosis.

(continued)

BONE AND JOINT SCANS

A bone scan reflects the degree to which the crystal lattice of bone "takes up" or absorbs a bone-seeking radioactive isotope. An area demonstrating increased uptake, such as a joint, is considered abnormal. A joint scan, the most sensitive study, allows determination of joint damage throughout the body. Because bone and joint scans are not the most cost-effective method for detecting early disease, they are not done routinely at the time of diagnosis.

BIOPSIES

A muscle biopsy, carried out to examine skeletal muscle, is useful in diagnosing myositis. Using local anesthesia under sterile conditions in an outpatient setting or in an operating room, a surgical incision is made to obtain the desired specimen, which is then sent to the laboratory for microscopic analysis. A pressure dressing is applied, and the affected extremity is immobilized for 12 to 24 hours.

An arterial biopsy may be performed to examine a specimen of an arterial wall using a procedure similar to that for a muscle biopsy. Most frequently, the temporal artery is selected, but other arteries may be used as indicated. Arterial biopsy most often confirms inflammation of the vessel wall, or *arteritis*, a type of vasculitis.

A skin biopsy may be performed to confirm inflammatory connective tissue diseases, such as lupus erythematosus or scleroderma. A specimen may be lightly scraped from the patient's skin without causing discomfort. Deeper skin biopsies may need to be carried out when scraping is not sufficient.

BLOOD TESTS

In general, serum laboratory studies in rheumatology are based on the assumption that most rheumatic diseases are autoimmune disorders. Although many of the tests are highly complex and technical, no one test used in isolation sufficiently supports a diagnosis of a rheumatic disease. Some of the most common serum studies are listed with their corresponding normal value ranges and primary indications in Table 50-1. Because many of the tests require special laboratory techniques, they may not be used in every health care facility. The physician determines which tests are necessary, basing this decision on the symptoms, stage of disease, cost, and likely benefit of the test.

TABLE 50•1 Common Serum Studies for Rheumatic Diseases *(Continued)*

Test	Normal Value	Significance
Anti-DNA, DNA binding Titer measurement of antibody to double-stranded DNA	Negative	High titer is seen in SLE; increases in titer may indicate increase in disease activity.
Complement levels—C_3, C_4 *Complement* is a protein substance that binds with antigen–antibody complexes for the purpose of lysis. When the number of complexes increases markedly, complement is used for lysis, thus depleting the amount available in the blood.	C_3: 55–120 mg/dL (550–1200 mg/L) C_4: 11–40 mg/dL (110–400 mg/L)	Decrease may be seen in RA and SLE. Decrease indicates autoimmune and inflammatory activity.
C-Reactive Protein Test (CRP) Shows presence of abnormal glycoprotein due to inflammatory process	Trace 6 μg/mL	A positive reading indicates active inflammation. Often is positive for RA, disseminated lupus erythematosus.
Immunoglobulin Electrophoresis Measures the values of immunoglobulins	IgA 50–300 mg/dL (0.5–3 g/L) IgG 635–1400 mg/dL (6.35–14 g/L) IgM 40–280 mg/dL (0.4–238 g/L)	Increased levels are found in people who have autoimmune disorders.
Rheumatoid Factor (RF) Determines the presence of abnormal antibodies seen in CTD	Negative	Positive titer > 1:80 Present in 80% of those with RA Positive RF may also suggest SLE, Sjögren's syndrome, or mixed CTD. The higher the titer (number at right of colon), the greater the inflammation.
Tissue Typing *HLA-B27 Antigen* Measures presence of HLA antigens, which are used for tissue recognition	Negative	Found in 80%–90% of those with ankylosing spondylitis and Reiter's syndrome.

IMPLICATIONS

Diagnosis of a specific rheumatic disease may or may not be relatively simple and clear-cut. Commonly, observation of clinical signs and symptoms over time is needed to make the diagnosis. The combination of history, assessment and testing, and evolving manifestations of the disease may require explanation and interpretation to the patient with early disease. This is especially true for patients with multisystem rheumatic disease, such as one of the connective tissue diseases.

The presence of crystals or bacteria in the synovial fluid is specifically diagnostic for gout or infectious arthritis, respectively. Diagnosis, however, may be more presumptive in the case of the older person who is thought to have osteoarthrosis (OA) based on single joint involvement, supportive x-ray findings, and no evidence of other disease processes.

Many forms of rheumatic disease can be accurately diagnosed by the primary health care provider. Patients with more complicated signs and symptoms may need referral to a rheumatologist, a physician who specializes in diagnosing and treating rheumatic disease. Patients should know which type of rheumatic disease they have, not just that they have "arthritis" or "arthritis of the knee."

Gerontologic Considerations

Although people of all ages, from infancy through childhood, adolescence, and maturity, may be affected, rheumatic disease is commonly thought of by the patient, family, and society as a whole as an inevitable consequence of aging. Many older people expect and accept the immobility and self-care problems related to the rheumatic diseases and do not seek help, thinking that nothing can be done. Careful diagnosis and appropriate treatment can improve the quality of life for older people. However, the rheumatic diseases do have some special implications for the older adult.

In elderly patients, other medical conditions may take precedence over the rheumatic disease, which commonly becomes a secondary diagnosis and concern. Identifying the effects of the rheumatic disease on the patient's lifestyle, independence, and other chronic or acute conditions is important.

The frequency, pattern of onset, clinical features, severity, and effects on function of the rheumatic disease in elderly patients may be different in very elderly patients. Some of the rheumatic diseases, such as OA, are more prevalent with advancing age. One disease, polymylagia rheumatica, is exclusive to the older person, whereas some disorders may be less severe for elderly people than for younger patients. However, OA, the most prevalent activity-limiting condition among older people, may account for more total disability among elderly patients than many diseases, such as stroke or cancer, that are considered more serious.

In some instances, the age of the patient and coexisting health problems may make diagnosis difficult. A missed diagnosis is not unusual because of the assumption that most older people with joint problems have OA. In addition, it may be difficult to differentiate problems associated with aging from those caused by a rheumatic disease. For example, rheumatoid arthritis (RA) that begins in the later years has been shown to differ prognostically and therapeutically from RA that begins earlier. In the elderly patient with initial RA, onset is more likely to be abrupt. The clinical course, however, does not appear to differ from that of RA with an insidious onset. Moreover, patients with elderly-onset RA are less likely to have subcutaneous nodules or rheumatoid factor at disease onset.

Hip fractures and spinal compression fractures in the elderly are most often related to osteoporosis. For the elderly person who has had a diffuse connective tissue disease, the risk for osteoporosis is increased. Pain, loss of mobility, loss of positive self-image, and increasing morbidity can result from progressive osteoporosis. Thus, treatment for osteoporosis should not be overlooked in this population. Exercise, postural assistance, analgesics, modification of activities of daily living, and psychological support can be useful.

Other conditions, for example, soft tissue problems such as bursitis, usually are not problematic by themselves. When combined with the physiologic processes of aging, however, these conditions may significantly affect the patient's quality of life. In fact, the effects of most forms of rheumatic disease may lead to considerable changes in the individual's lifestyle, possibly threatening independence. Decreased vision and altered balance, often present in elderly people, may be problematic for the patient whose rheumatic disease in the lower extremities affects locomotion. Also, the combination of poor hearing, diminished vision, memory loss, and depression contribute to nonadherence to the treatment regimen in elderly patients. Special techniques for promoting patient safety, self-management, and strategies, including memory aids for medications, may be necessary.

Partly because of the more frequent contact of the elderly with the health care system, overtreatment or inappropriate treatment is possible. Effective exercise programs may not be instituted because of inadequate teaching time and follow-up by a therapist. Complaints of pain may be met with a prescription for an opioid analgesic rather than instructions for rest, use of an assistive device, and local comfort measures, such as heat or cold. Acetaminophen may be appropriate and worth trying before using other medications that pose a greater chance of side effects. Intra-articular corticosteroid injections, with their usual rapid relief of symptoms, may be requested by the patient who is unaware of the consequences of too frequent use.

Pharmacologic treatment of rheumatic disease in older patients is more difficult than that in younger patients. If the medications used have an effect on the senses (hearing, cognition), this effect is intensified in the elderly. The cumulative effect of medications is accentuated because of the physiologic changes of aging. For example, decreased renal function in the elderly alters the metabolism of certain medications, such as nonsteroidal anti-inflammatory drugs (NSAIDs). Elderly patients are more prone to such side effects as gastroduodenal ulceration or bleeding, and they are more likely to use nonprescription remedies, to try many different medications (polypharmacy), and to be more susceptible to unproven treatment methods.

Elderly patients with rheu-matic disease may accept or endure pain, loss of ambulation, and difficulty with activities of daily living unnecessarily. The need to view oneself as capable of managing life independently despite increasing age may take considerable energy. The body image and self-esteem of the elderly person with rheumatic disease, combined with underlying depression, may interfere with the use of assistive devices such as canes. Use of adaptive equipment, such as long-handled reachers or tongs, may be viewed as evidence of aging rather than as a means of increased independence.

The elderly person usually has a lifelong pattern of dealing with stress. Depending on the success of that pattern, the elderly person can often maintain a positive attitude and self-esteem when faced with a rheumatic disease—especially with support.

Medical Management

A treatment program involving the interdisciplinary team, including the patient, is the basis for managing the rheumatic diseases. The chronic nature of most of these diseases mandates that the patient understand the disease, have the information necessary to make good self-management decisions, and be presented with a therapeutic program that is compatible with his or her lifestyle. Table 50-2 outlines the goals and strategies of basic rheumatic disease management.

PHARMACOLOGIC THERAPY

Medications are used with the rheumatic diseases to control inflammation and, in some instances, to modify the disease. Three basic categories of useful medication include the salicylates, NSAIDs, and disease-modifying antirheumatic drugs (DMARDs). Table 50-3 reviews the various medications often used.

Controlling the inflammation related to the disease process will help in managing pain, but this is often a delayed response. Nonopioid medications are often used for pain management, especially early in the treatment program, until other measures can be instituted effectively. Short-term use of low-dose antidepressant medications, such as amitriptyline, may be prescribed to reestablish adequate sleep patterns and better pain management.

NONPHARMACOLOGIC PAIN MANAGEMENT

Nonpharmacologic methods of pain management are important. Methods used include therapeutic heat or cold and devices such as a cane or a wrist splint to protect the joint. A combination of methods may be required because different methods often work better at different times.

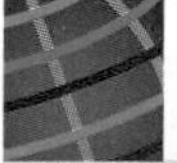

TABLE 50•2 Goals and Strategies for Rheumatic Diseases

Major Goals	Management Strategy
Suppress inflammation and the autoimmune response	Administer medications (anti-inflammatory and disease-modifying agents)
Control pain	Protect joints; ease pain with splints, thermal modalities, relaxation techniques
Maintain or improve joint mobility	Implement exercise programs for joint motion and muscle strengthening
Maintain or improve functional status	Make use of adaptive devices and techniques
Increase patient's knowledge of disease process	Provide and reinforce patient teaching
Promote self-management by patient compatible with the therapeutic regimen	Emphasize compatibility of therapeutic regimen and lifestyle

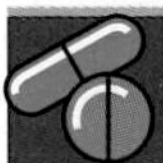

TABLE 50•3 **Medications Used in Rheumatic Diseases**

Medication	Action, Use, and Indication	Nursing Considerations
Salicylates *Acetylated* aspirin *Nonacetylated* choline magnesium trisalicylate (Trilisate) choline salicylate (Arthropan) diflunisal (Dolobid) salsalate (Disalcid) sodium salicylate	*Action:* anti-inflammatory, analgesic, antipyretic Acetylated salicylates are platelet aggregation inhibitors Anti-inflammatory doses will produce blood salicylate levels of 20–30 mg/dL	Administer with meals to prevent gastric irritation. Assess for tinnitus, gastric intolerance, GI bleeding, and purpura. Monitor for possible confusion in the elderly.
Nonsteroidal Anti-inflammatory Drugs (NSAIDs) diclofenac (Voltaren) etodolac (Lodine) flurbiprofen (Ansaid) ibuprofen (Motrin) indomethacin (Indocin) ketoprofen (Orudis, Oruvail) meclofenamate (Meclomen) nabumatone (Relafen) naproxen (Naprosyn) oxaprozin (DayPro) piroxicam (Feldene) sulindac (Clinoril) tolmetin sodium (Tolectin)	*Action:* anti-inflammatory, analgesic, antipyretic, platelet aggregation inhibitor Anti-inflammatory effect occurs 2–4 weeks after initiation All NSAIDs are useful for short-term treatment of acute gout attack NSAIDs are alternative to salicylates for first-line therapy in several rheumatic diseases	Administer NSAIDs with food. Monitor for GI, CNS, cardiovascular, renal, hematologic, and dermatologic adverse effects. Avoid salicylates; use acetaminophen for additional analgesia. Watch for possible confusion in the elderly.
Cox-2 Inhibitors celocoxib (Celebrex) rofecoxib (Vioxx)	*Action:* Inhibits only cyclooxygenase-2 (COX-2) enzymes, which are produced during inflammation and spare COX-1 enzymes, which can be protective to the stomach and kidneys.	Monitoring the same as for other NSAIDs Appropriate for the elderly and patients who are at high risk for gastric ulcers.
Disease-Modifying Antirheumatic Drugs (DMARDs) Antimalarials hydroxychloroquine chloroquine	*Action:* Anti-inflammatory, inhibits lysosomal enzymes Slow acting, onset may take 2–4 months Useful in RA and SLE	Administer concurrently with NSAIDs. Assess for visual changes, GI upset, skin rash, headaches, photosensitivity, bleaching of hair. Emphasize need for ophthalmologic exams (every 6–12 months).
Gold-containing compounds aurothioglucose gold sodium thiomalate auranofin	*Action:* Inhibits T- and B-cell activity, suppresses synovitis during active stage of rheumatoid disease Slow acting, onset may take 3–6 months IM preparations are given weekly for about 6 months, then every 2–4 weeks	Administer concurrently with NSAIDs. Assess for stomatitis, diarrhea, dermatitis, proteinuria, hematuria, bone marrow suppression (decreased WBCs and/or platelets), CBC and urinalysis with every other injection
sulfasalazine	*Action:* Anti-inflammatory, reduces lymphocyte response, inhibits angiogenesis Useful in RA, seronegative spondyloarthropathies	Administer concurrently with NSAIDs. Do not use in patients with allergy to sulfa medications or salicylates. Emphasize adequate fluid intake. Assess for GI upset, skin rash, headache, liver abnormalities, anemia.
penicillamine	*Action:* Anti-inflammatory, inhibits T-cell function, impairs antigen presentation Slow acting, onset may take 2–3 months Useful in RA and systemic sclerosis	Administer concurrently with NSAIDs. Assess for GI irritation, decreased taste, skin rash or itching, bone marrow suppression, proteinuria with CBC, and urinalysis every 2–4 weeks.
Immunosuppressives methotrexate azathioprine cyclophosphamide	*Action:* Immune suppression, effects DNA synthesis and other cellular effects Have teratogenic potential; azathioprine and cyclophosphamide reserved for more aggressive or unresponsive disease Methotrexate is gold standard for RA treatment, also useful in SLE	Assess for bone marrow suppression, GI ulcerations, skin rashes, alopecia, bladder toxicity, increased infections. Monitor CBC, liver enzymes, creatinine every 2–4 weeks. Advise patient of contraceptive measures because of teratogenecity.

(*continued*)

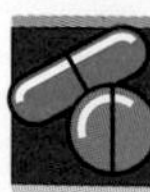

TABLE 50•3 Medications Used in Rheumatic Diseases *(Continued)*

Medication	Action, Use, and Indication	Nursing Considerations
cyclosporine	*Action:* Immunomodulator Used for severe, progressive RA, unresponsive to other DMARDS Used in combination with methotrexate	Assess slow dose titration upward until response noted or toxicity occurs. Assess for toxic effects: bleeding gums, fluid retention, hair growth, tremors. Monitor blood pressure and creatinine every 2 weeks until stable.
Immunomodulators leflunomide (Arava)	*Action:* Inhibits pyrimidine synthesis and inhibits COX-2, so anti-inflammatory. May be used alone or in combination with other DMARDs. Used in moderate to severe RA.	Long half-life; requires loading dose followed by daily administration. Assess for diarrhea, nausea, rash, alopecia. Rapid reduction of serum levels requires Cholestyramine x11days.
etanercept (Enbrel)	*Action:* Binds to tumor necrosis factor, a cytokine involved in inflammatory and immune responses. Used in moderate to severe RA unresponsive to methotrexate. May be used in combination with methotrexate.	Teach patient subcutaneous self-injection to be administered 2x/week. Monitor for injection site reactions. Educate patient about increased potential for infection and to withhold medication if fever occurs.
Corticosteroids prednisone prednisolone hydrocortisone intra-articular injections	*Action:* Anti-inflammatory, analgesic Used for shortest duration, and lowest dose possible to minimize adverse effects Useful for unremitting RA, SLE, PMR, myositis, arteritis Fast acting; onset in days Injections useful for joints unresponsive to NSAIDs	Assess for toxicity: cataracts, GI irritation, hyperglycemia, hypertension, fractures, avascular necrosis, hirsutism, psychosis. Recognize that joints most amenable to injections include ankles, knees, hips, shoulders, and hands. Be aware that repeated injections can cause joint damage.

Exercise and Activity

The ongoing nature of most rheumatic diseases makes it important to maintain and, when possible, improve joint mobility and functional status. The individualized exercise program is crucial to movement. Table 50-4 summarizes the exercises appropriate for patients with rheumatic diseases.

The major challenge for the patient and the care provider is the need to adjust all aspects of treatment according to the activity of the disease. Especially for the patient with an active diffuse connective tissue disease, such as RA or SLE, activity level adjustments may vary from day to day and even within the day itself.

TABLE 50•4 Suggested Exercises to Promote Mobility

Inflammatory Process (Pain)	Recommended Exercise	Patient Performance Level
Acute exacerbation; severe pain	Passive range of motion (ROM)	Unable to perform exercises alone
Subacute; moderate or minimal pain	Active assistive or active ROM within pain tolerance	Can perform with help from another person or an assistive mechanical device
Inactive; remission; minimal pain or absence of pain	Active ROM; isometrics	Can perform alone

NURSING PROCESS: THE PATIENT WITH A RHEUMATIC DISEASE

Assessment

The depth and focus of the nursing assessment depend on several factors. These factors include the health care setting (clinic or office, home, extended care facility, or hospital), the role of the nurse (home care nurse; nurse practitioner; hospital, clinic, or office nurse), and the needs of the patient. The nurse, often the first of the health care team members to come in contact with the patient, is frequently the care provider in the best position to assist with basic care and hygiene. This may enable the nurse to assess the patient's perceptions of the disorder and situation, actions taken to relieve symptoms, plans for treatment, and expectations. The nurse's assessment may lead to identifying problems that can be addressed by nursing interventions and, through collaboration with other team members, to achieving the expected patient outcomes.

The health history and physical assessment focus on current and past symptoms, such as fatigue, weakness, pain, stiffness, fever, or anorexia, and the effects of these symptoms on the patient's lifestyle and self-image. Because the rheumatic diseases affect many body systems, the history and physical assessment include a review and examination of all systems, with particular attention given to those areas most commonly affected, including the musculoskeletal system. (See the assessment chart presented earlier in the chapter.)

The patient's psychological and mental status and social support systems are also assessed, as is the patient's ability to participate in daily activities, comply with the treatment regimen, and manage self-care. The information obtained can give insight into the patient's understanding of the medication regimen and may reveal misuse of medications, noncompliance, or use of unproven remedies. Additional areas assessed include the patient's understanding, motivation, knowledge, coping abilities, past experiences, preconceptions, and fears. The effects of the disease on the patient's self-concept and coping abilities are also assessed. The patient's perception of the condition and its impact influences the decisions, choices, and actions associated with treatment recommendations.

Diagnosis

Nursing Diagnoses

Although many nursing diagnoses are appropriate for the patient with a rheumatic disease, a few of the most common include the following:

- Pain related to inflammation and increased disease activity, tissue damage, fatigue, or lowered tolerance level
- Fatigue related to increased disease activity, pain, inadequate sleep/rest, deconditioning, inadequate nutrition, emotional stress/depression
- Impaired physical mobility related to decreased range of motion, muscle weakness, pain on movement, limited endurance, lack of or improper use of ambulatory devices
- Self-care deficits related to contractures, fatigue, or loss of motion
- Body image disturbance related to physical and psychological changes and dependency imposed by chronic illness
- Ineffective coping related to actual or perceived lifestyle or role changes

Collaborative Problems/Potential Complications

Based on assessment data, potential complications may include the following:

- Adverse effects of medications

Planning and Goals

The major goals for the patient may include relief of pain and discomfort, relief of fatigue, increased mobility, maintenance of self-care, improved body image, effective coping, and absence of complications.

Nursing Interventions

An understanding of the underlying disease process (ie, degeneration or inflammation, including degeneration resulting from inflammation or inflammation resulting from degeneration) guides the nurse's thought processes. In addition, the nurse's knowledge about whether the condition is localized or more widely systemic influences the scope of the nursing activity.

Some rheumatic diseases (eg, OA) are more localized alterations in which control of symptoms such as pain or stiffness is possible. Others (eg, gout) have a known cause and specific treatment to control the symptoms. The diseases that usually present the greatest challenge are those with systemic manifestations, such as the diffuse connective tissue diseases. Plan of Nursing Care 50-1 details the nursing interventions to be considered for each nursing diagnosis.

Relieving Pain and Discomfort

Medications are used on a short-term basis to relieve acute pain. Because the pain may be persistent, nonopioid analgesics, such as acetaminophen, are often used. After administering medications, the nurse needs to reassess pain levels at intervals. With persistent pain, assessment findings should be compared with baseline measurements and evaluations. Additional measures include exploring coping skills and strategies that have worked in the past.

The patient needs to understand the importance of taking medications, such as NSAIDs and disease-modifying drugs, exactly as prescribed to achieve maximum benefits. These benefits include relief of pain as the disease is brought under control. Because disease control and pain relief are delayed, the patient may mistakenly believe the medication is ineffective or may think of the medication as merely "pain pills," taking them only sporadically and failing to achieve control over the disease activity.

A weight reduction program may be recommended to relieve stress on painful joints. Heat applications are also helpful in relieving pain, stiffness, and muscle spasm. Superficial heat may be applied in the form of warm tub baths or showers and warm moist compresses. Paraffin baths (dips), which offer concentrated heat, are helpful to patients with wrist and small-joint involvement. Maximum benefit is achieved within 20 minutes of application. More frequent use for shorter lengths of time is most beneficial. Therapeutic exercises can be carried out more comfortably and effectively after heat has been applied.

In some patients, however, heat may actually increase pain, muscle spasm, and synovial fluid volume. If the inflammatory process is acute, cold applications in the form of moist packs or an ice bag may be tried. Both heat and cold are analgesic to nerve pain receptors and can relax muscle spasms. Safe use of heat and cold must be evaluated and taught, particularly to patients with impaired sensation.

The use of braces, splints, and assistive mobility devices, such as canes, crutches, and walkers, eases pain by limiting movement or stress from weight bearing on painful joints. Acutely inflamed joints can be rested by applying splints to limit motion. Splints also support the joint to relieve spasm. Canes and crutches can relieve stress from inflamed and painful weight-bearing joints while promoting safe ambulation. Cervical collars may be used to support the weight of the head and limit cervical motion. A metatarsal bar or special pads may be put into shoes if foot pain or deformity is present.

Other strategies for decreasing pain include muscle relaxation techniques, imagery, self-hypnosis, and distraction.

Decreasing Fatigue

Fatigue related to rheumatic disease can be both acute (brief and relieved by rest or sleep) and chronic. Chronic fatigue, related to the disease process, is persistent, cumulative, and not eliminated by rest but is influenced by biologic, psychological, social, and personal factors.

Disease-related factors that may influence the amount and severity of fatigue include persistent pain, sleep disturbance, impaired physical activity, and disease duration. Pain increases fatigue by requiring additional physical and emotional energy to deal with it. It may also cause the patient to expend more energy to do tasks in a way that causes less pain. Pain may also interfere with sleep, thereby increasing fatigue level.

Efforts are aimed at modifying and reducing the fatigue. Energy may be regained by using rest periods. Patient needs determine the type of rest and how much is needed. Naps or nighttime sleep can

(text continues on page 1419)

50•1

PLAN OF NURSING CARE 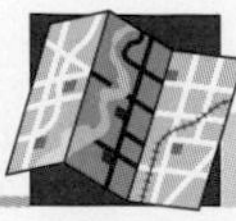

Care of the Patient With a Rheumatic Disease

Nursing Interventions | **Rationale** | **Expected Outcomes**

Nursing Diagnosis: Pain related to inflammation and increased disease activity, tissue damage, or lowered tolerance level
Goal: Improvement in comfort level; incorporation of pain management techniques into daily life

Nursing Interventions	Rationale
1. Provide variety of comfort measures a. Application of heat or cold b. Massage, position changes, rest c. Foam mattress, supportive pillow, splints d. Relaxation techniques, diversional activities	1. Pain may respond to nondrug interventions such as joint protection, exercise, relaxation, and thermal modalities.
2. Administer anti-inflammatory, analgesic, and slow-acting antirheumatic medications as prescribed.	2. Pain of rheumatic disease responds to individual or combination drug regimens.
3. Individualize medication schedule to meet patient's need for pain management.	3. Previous pain experiences and management strategies may be different from those needed for persistent pain.
4. Encourage verbalization of feelings about pain and chronicity of disease.	4. Verbalization promotes coping.
5. Teach pathophysiology of pain and rheumatic disease, and assist patient to recognize that pain often leads to unproved treatment methods.	5. Knowledge of rheumatic pain and appropriate treatment may help patient avoid unsafe, ineffective therapies.
6. Assist in identification of pain that leads to use of unproven methods of treatment.	6. The impact of pain on an individual's life often leads to misconceptions about pain and pain management techniques.
7. Assess for subjective changes in pain.	7. The individual's description of the pain sensation is a more reliable indicator than objective measurements such as change in vital signs, body movement, and facial expression.

Expected Outcomes

- Identifies factors that exacerbate or influence pain response
- Identifies and uses pain management strategies
- Verbalizes decrease in pain
- Reports signs and symptoms of side effects in timely manner to prevent additional problems
- Verbalizes that pain is characteristic of rheumatic disease
- Establishes realistic pain-relief goals
- Verbalizes that pain often leads to the use of nontraditional and unproved self-treatment methods
- Identifies changes in quality or intensity of pain

Nursing Diagnosis: Fatigue related to increased disease activity, pain, inadequate sleep/rest, deconditioning, inadequate nutrition, and emotional stress/depression
Goal: Incorporates as part of daily activities strategies necessary to modify fatigue

Nursing Interventions	Rationale
1. Provide instruction about fatigue	1. The patient's understanding of fatigue will affect his or her actions.
a. Describe relationship of disease activity to fatigue.	a. The amount of fatigue is directly related to the activity of the disease.
b. Describe comfort measures while providing them.	b. Relief of discomfort can relieve fatigue.
c. Develop and encourage a sleep routine (warm bath and relaxation techniques that promote sleep).	c. Effective bedtime routine promotes restorative sleep.
d. Explain importance of rest for relieving systematic, articular, and emotional stress.	d. Different kinds of rest are needed to relieve fatigue and are based on patient need and response.
e. Explain how to use energy conservation techniques (pacing, delegating, setting priorities).	e. A variety of measures can be used to conserve energy.
f. Identify physical and emotional factors that can cause fatigue.	f. Awareness of the various causes of fatigue provides the basis for measures to modify the fatigue.

Expected Outcomes

- Self-evaluates and monitors fatigue pattern
- Verbalizes the relationship of fatigue to disease activity
- Uses comfort measures as appropriate
- Practices effective sleep hygiene and routine
- Makes use of various devices (splints, canes) and methods (bed rest, relaxation techniques) to ease different kinds of fatigue
- Incorporates time management strategies in daily activities
- Uses appropriate measures to prevent physical and emotional fatigue
- Has an established plan to ensure well-paced, therapeutic activity schedule
- Adheres to therapeutic program
- Follows a planned conditioning program

(continued)

50•1 PLAN OF NURSING CARE

Care of the Patient With a Rheumatic Disease (*continued*)

Nursing Interventions	Rationale	Expected Outcomes
2. Facilitate development of appropriate activity/rest schedule. 3. Encourage adherence to the treatment program. 4. Refer to and encourage a conditioning program. 5. Encourage adequate nutrition, including source of iron from food and supplements.	2. Alternating rest and activity conserves energy while allowing most productivity. 3. Overall control of disease activity can decrease the amount of fatigue. 4. Deconditioning resulting from lack of mobility, understanding, and disease activity contributes to fatigue. 5. A nutritious diet can help counteract fatigue.	• Consumes a nutritious diet consisting of appropriate food groups and recommended daily allowance of vitamins and minerals
Nursing Diagnosis: Impaired physical mobility related to decreased range of motion, muscle weakness, pain on movement, limited endurance, lack of or improper use of ambulatory devices **Goal:** Attains and maintains optimal functional mobility		
1. Encourage verbalization regarding limitations in mobility.	1. Mobility is not necessarily related to deformity. Pain, stiffness, and fatigue may temporarily limit mobility. The degree of mobility is not synonymous with the degree of independence. Decreased mobility may influence a person's self-concept and lead to social isolation.	• Identifies factors that interfere with mobility • Describes and uses measures to prevent loss of motion • Identifies environmental (home, school, work, community) barriers to optimal mobility • Uses appropriate techniques and/or assistive equipment to aid mobility • Identifies community resources available to assist in managing decreased mobility
2. Assess need for occupational or physical therapy consultation: a. Emphasize range of motion of affected joints. b. Promote use of ambulatory devices. c. Explain use of safe footwear. d. Use individual appropriate positioning/posture.	2. Therapeutic exercises, proper footwear, and/or assistive equipment may improve mobility. Correct posture and positioning are necessary for maintaining optimal mobility.	
3. Assist to identify environmental barriers.	3. Furniture and architectural adaptations may enhance mobility.	
4. Encourage independence in mobility and assist as needed. a. Allow ample time for activity b. Provide rest period after activity. c. Reinforce principles of joint protection and work simplification.	4. Changes in mobility may lead to a decrease in personal safety.	
5. Initiate referral to community health agency.	5. The degree of mobility may be slow to improve or may not improve with intervention.	
Nursing Diagnosis: Self-care deficits related to contractures, fatigue, or loss of motion **Goal:** Achieves self-care independently or with the use of resources		
1. Assist patient to identify self-care deficits and factors that interfere with ability to perform self-care activities.	1. The ability to perform self-care activities is influenced by the disease activity and the accompanying pain, stiffness, fatigue, muscle weakness, loss of motion, and depression.	• Identifies factors that interfere with the ability to perform self-care activities • Identifies alternative methods for meeting self-care needs • Uses alternative methods for meeting self-care needs • Identifies and uses other health care resources for meeting self-care needs
2. Develop a plan based on the patient's perceptions and priorities on how to establish and achieve goals to meet self-care needs, incorporating joint protection, energy conservation, and work simplification concepts.	2. Assistive devices may enhance self-care abilities. Effective planning for changes must include the patient who must accept and adopt the plan.	

(*continued*)

50•1 **PLAN OF NURSING CARE**

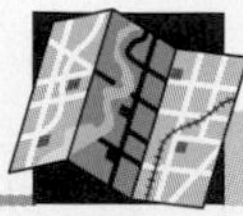

Care of the Patient With a Rheumatic Disease (*continued*)

Nursing Interventions	Rationale	Expected Outcomes
a. Provide appropriate assistive devices. b. Reinforce correct and safe use of assistive devices. c. Allow patient to control timing of self-care activities. d. Explore with the patient different ways to perform difficult tasks or ways to enlist the help of someone else.		
3. Consult with community health care agencies when individuals have attained a maximum level of self-care yet still have some deficits, especially regarding safety.	3. Individuals differ in ability and willingness to perform self-care activities. Changes in ability to care for self may lead to a decrease in personal safety.	

Nursing Diagnosis: Body image disturbance related to physical and psychological changes and dependency imposed by chronic illness
Goal: Achieves a reconciliation between self-concept and the physical and psychological changes imposed by the rheumatic disease

Nursing Interventions	Rationale	Expected Outcomes
1. Help patient identify elements of control over disease symptoms and treatment. 2. Encourage verbalization of feelings, perceptions, and fears. a. Help to assess present situation and identify problems. b. Assist to identify past coping mechanisms. c. Assist to identify effective coping mechanisms.	1. The individual's self-concept may be altered by the disease or its treatment. 2. The individual's coping strategies reflect the strength of his or her self-concept.	• Verbalizes an awareness that changes taking place in self-concept are normal responses to rheumatic disease and other chronic illnesses • Identifies strategies to cope with altered self-concept

Nursing Diagnosis: Ineffective coping related to actual or perceived lifestyle or role changes
Goal: Use of effective coping behaviors for dealing with actual or perceived limitations and role changes

Nursing Interventions	Rationale	Expected Outcomes
1. Identify areas of life affected by disease. Answer questions and dispel possible myths. 2. Develop plan for managing symptoms and enlisting support of family and friends to promote daily function.	1. The effects of disease may be more or less manageable once identified and explored reasonably. 2. By taking action and involving others appropriately, patient develops or draws on coping skills and community support.	• Names functions and roles affected and not affected by disease process • Describes therapeutic regimen and states actions to take to improve, change, or accept a particular situation, function, or role

Collaborative Problems: Complications secondary to effects of medications
Goal: Experiences absence or resolution of complications

Nursing Interventions	Rationale	Expected Outcomes
1. Perform periodic clinical assessment and laboratory evaluation. 2. Instruct in correct self-administration, side effects, and importance of monitoring. 3. Counsel regarding methods to reduce side effects and manage symptoms. 4. Administer medications in modified doses as prescribed if complications occur.	1. Skillful assessment helps detect early symptoms of side effects of medications. 2. The patient needs accurate information about medications and side effects to avoid or manage them. 3. Appropriate identification and early intervention may minimize complications. 4. Modifications may help minimize side effects or other complications.	• Complies with monitoring procedures and experiences minimal side effects • Takes medication as prescribed and lists potential side effects • Identifies strategies to reduce side effects • Reports that side effects or complications have subsided

provide systemic rest. Splints can provide articular rest by limiting motion and stress on the joints. Relaxation techniques can provide emotional rest. Inactivity may lead to deconditioning and fatigue. Therefore, measures to build endurance should be instituted. Conditioning exercises, such as walking, swimming, or biking, require gradual progression of activity and monitoring of disease activity.

Psychosocial factors with an effect on fatigue include depression, learned helplessness, and perceived social support. These factors affect the patient's perception and evaluation of the fatigue. Improvement of functional status can positively affect mood.

Promoting Restorative Sleep

Good quality of sleep is important in helping the patient to cope with pain, minimize physical fatigue, and deal with the changes necessitated by a chronic disease. The sleep of patients whose disease is active (in flare) is frequently reduced in time and fragmented by prolonged awakenings. Stiffness, depression, and medications may also compromise the quality of sleep and increase daytime fatigue. A sleep-inducing routine, medication, and comfort measures may help improve the quality of sleep.

Increasing Mobility

Proper body positioning is essential to minimize stress on inflamed joints and prevent deformities that limit mobility. All joints should be supported in a position of optimal function. When in bed, the patient should lie flat on a firm mattress, with feet positioned against a footboard and with only one pillow under the head because of the risk of dorsal kyphosis. A pillow should not be placed under the knees because this promotes flexion contracture. The patient should lie prone (on the abdomen) several times daily to prevent hip flexion contracture.

Active range-of-motion exercises are encouraged because they prevent joint stiffness. If the patient cannot actively exercise the joints, passive range of motion should be performed.

Measures to reinforce proper body posture and increase mobility include walking erect and using chairs with straight backs. When seated, the patient should rest the feet flat on the floor and the shoulders and hips against the back of the chair.

Care must be taken so that splinting for comfort does not restrict mobility later. The knee is splinted at full extension and the wrist at slight dorsiflexion. Because of the predominant strength of flexor muscles, the joints should not be permitted to "freeze" in positions of flexion. This can be prevented by regularly removing the splint and exercising the joint through a range of motion. Splint modification may be needed when changes occur in joint structure.

Additionally, assistive devices may be necessary for mobility. They should be properly fitted and the patient instructed in their correct and safe use. A cane, long enough to allow for only a slight bend of the elbow, should be held in the hand *opposite* the affected side. Forearm-trough style crutches may be needed to protect the upper extremities if the disease involves the patient's hands and wrists. This is especially important for the patient undergoing rehabilitation after lower extremity joint reconstructive surgery. Assistive devices can mean the difference between dependence and independence in mobility; however, they may also alter the patient's body image, which can become a barrier to compliance with treatment.

Facilitating Self-Care

Adaptive equipment may increase the patient's independence. When introducing adaptive equipment, however, the nurse should be sensitive to the patient's feelings by demonstrating acceptance and positive attitudes about using these devices. The nurse needs to keep in mind that a patient's deformity need not equate with disability. For example, swollen hands may be more limiting than deformed hands. The hospital-based and extended care facility nurse can help preserve the patient's independence in these settings by making available adaptive equipment for eating, toileting, bathing, and dressing. In the home, the nurse can encourage use of these devices. Again, by relieving pain, stiffness, and fatigue, the nurse may increase the patient's ability to perform self-care (see the accompanying Nursing Research chart.)

Improving Body Image

All aspects of the patient's life, including the patient's perception of self, work role, social life, sexual function, and financial status, may be altered because of the unpredictability and uncertainty of the course of a rheumatic disease. Body-image changes may cause social isolation and depression. The nurse and the family need to empathize with the patient's emotional reactions to the disease. Communication should be encouraged, so that the patient and family verbalize feelings, perceptions, and fears related to the disease. The nurse helps the patient and family identify areas in which they have some control over disease symptoms and treatment. The nurse also encourages commitment to the treatment program, which is a key to positive outcomes.

Monitoring and Managing Potential Complications

Medications used for treating rheumatic diseases have the potential for serious and adverse effects. Thus, an important aspect of care is avoiding drug-induced complications. The physician bases the prescribed medication regimen on clinical findings and past medical history, then monitors for side effects with periodic clinical assessments and laboratory testing. The nurse has a major role in working with the physician and pharmacist to help the patient recognize and deal with side effects from medications. These side effects may include gastrointestinal bleeding or irritation, bone marrow suppression, kidney or liver toxicity, increased incidence of infection, mouth sores, rashes, and changes in vision. Other signs and symptoms include bruising, breathing problems, dizziness, jaundice, dark urine, black or bloody stools, diarrhea, nausea and vomiting, and headaches. Systemic and local infections, which can often be masked by high doses of corticosteroids, need close monitoring. (Refer to Table 50-3 for more information about administration considerations.)

Patient instruction also includes teaching techniques of correct self-administration, methods of reducing side effects, and measures to ensure regular monitoring. The nurse can be available for consultation between physician visits. If side effects occur, the medication may need to be stopped or the dose reduced. The patient may experience an increase in symptoms while the complication is being resolved or a new medication is being initiated. In such cases, the nurse's counseling regarding symptom management may relieve potential anxiety and distress.

Promoting Home and Community-Based Care

TEACHING PATIENTS SELF-CARE

Patient teaching is an essential aspect of nursing care of the patient with rheumatic disease to enable the patient to maintain

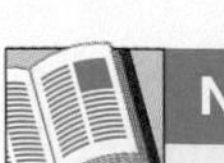

NURSING RESEARCH

Self-Care for Rheumatoid Arthritis

Ailinger, R. L., & Dear, M. R. (1997). An examination of the self-care needs of clients with rheumatoid arthritis. *Rehabilitation Nursing, 22*(3), 135–140.

Purpose

The purpose of this study was to examine changes in self-care needs of people with rheumatoid arthritis (RA) and the effects of age, gender, and changes in health state on their self-care needs. This study used Orem's self-care deficit theory, which addresses self-care and the limitations an individual might experience in performance of self-care activities. Universal self-care requisites (USCR), one of the three types of self-care requisites identified by Orem, include the need for maintenance of sufficient air, food, water, and elimination; a balance between activity and rest; a balance between solitude and social interaction; prevention of hazards to life and well-being; and promotion of normalcy. An individual's self-care system is made up in part of the actions taken to meet the USCRs. RA has the potential for influencing the ways in which individuals meet their USCRs. The researchers hypothesized that age, gender, and health state would affect the ways individuals meet USCR.

Study Sample and Design

This study was part of a larger research project. A descriptive design was used to examine the modifications in USCRs reported by patients with RA. The convenience sample (n = 59) consisted of 47 women and 12 men between 27 and 79 years of age (mean = 52.34; SD = 11.88) with RA. The mean number of years since diagnosis of RA was 14.17 (SD = 9.38).

Study participants' health status (ie, disease severity, function, pain, and duration of illness) was based on a physician's assessment of disease severity, with the disability index and the pain scale of the Health Assessment Questionnaire (HAQ). In addition, participants were personally interviewed about USCRs; they were asked to respond to the question: "Since you have had arthritis, in what ways do you care for yourself differently than before you had it?" Interviews were tape-recorded and transcribed; they were then analyzed by experts on Orem's self-care deficit theory and coded for USCRs.

Findings

Most participants in the study had mild to moderate disease severity with some limitation of function and the presence of pain (mean = 3.95, SD = 2.63) on a 10-point visual analog scale. Results of analysis of the interviews revealed that the most frequently reported USCRs were the maintenance of a balance between activity and rest (83%), promotion of normalcy (66%), prevention of hazards (58%), maintenance of sufficient intake of food (27%), and maintenance of a balance between solitude and social interaction (17%). All study participants reported that RA had affected at least one USCR.

Clients' health state and age, but not their gender, affected USCRs. Participants who had the disease for a longer time reported a greater need for prevention of hazards (ie, falls, muscle strains). There was no significant association with disease severity, functional status, or perception of pain. Younger patients reported fewer changes in the level of normalcy than did older ones. There was no association between age and the number of USCRs participants reported as being affected.

Nursing Implications

Although generalizability of the study is limited by the small sample size, subjects' high educational level, and an environment where they received considerable medical attention and nursing care, the findings suggest that older people with RA may view the effects of the disease as distinct from the usual changes related to the aging process. More attention by careful assessment of patients' attitudes and feelings about normalcy should be paid to the psychological changes that are part of RA patients' experience. Activities that enhance the individual's feelings of normalcy should be encouraged and modifications made to promote them if necessary while simultaneously emphasizing issues of safety. Helping the patient learn how to deal with potential hazards can enhance a sense of competence in managing situations.

Nurses must be aware of the increased need for rest periods for this group of patients as demonstrated in this study by the patient reports. Balancing rest and activity is difficult and highly individualistic. Nurses can help patients by assessing the quality and pattern of rest and offering options for improvement. Activities can be prioritized and delegated as the patient sees necessary and possible. Knowledge about a patient's changes in self-care needs should be integrated into the rehabilitation plan.

as much independence as possible, to take medications accurately and safely, and to use adaptive devices correctly. Patient teaching focuses on the disorder itself, the possible changes related to the disorder, the therapeutic regimen prescribed to treat it, the side effects of medications, strategies to maintain independence and function, and patient safety in the home (see the Home Care Teaching Checklist).

The patient and family are encouraged to verbalize their concerns and ask questions. Pain, fatigue, and depression can interfere with the patient's ability to learn and should be addressed

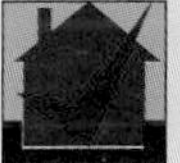

HOME CARE TEACHING CHECKLIST: THE PATIENT WITH RHEUMATIC DISEASE

At the completion of the program, the patient or caregiver will be able to:	Patient	Caregiver
• Explain the nature of the disease and principles of disease management.	✔	✔
• Describe the medication regimen (name of medications, dosage, schedule of administration, precautions, side effects, and desired effects).	✔	✔
• Identify monitoring procedures and strategies that should be implemented.	✔	✔
• Demonstrate accurate and safe self-administration of medications.	✔	✔
• Describe and demonstrate use of pain management techniques.	✔	✔
• Demonstrate use of joint protection techniques in activities of daily living (ADLs).	✔	✔
• Demonstrate ability to perform self-care activities independently or with assistive devices.	✔	
• Demonstrate a safe exercise program.	✔	
• Demonstrate a relaxation technique.	✔	

before initiating a teaching program. Various educational strategies may then be used, depending on the patient's previous knowledge base, interest level, degree of comfort, social or cultural influences, and readiness to learn. The nurse instructs the patient about basic disease management and necessary adaptations in lifestyle. Because suppression of inflammation and autoimmune responses requires the use of anti-inflammatory, disease-modifying antirheumatic and immunosuppressive agents, the patient is taught about prescribed medications, including type, dosage, rationale, side effects, self-administration, and required monitoring procedures. If hospitalized, the patient is encouraged to practice new self-management skills with support from caregivers and significant others. The nurse then reinforces disease management skills during each patient contact. Barriers to compliance are assessed and measures are taken to promote adherence to medications and treatment program.

CONTINUING CARE

Depending on the severity of the disorder and the patient's resources and supports, referral for home care may or not be warranted. However, the patient who is elderly or frail, has a rheumatic disorder that limits function significantly, and lives alone may need a referral for home care.

The impact of rheumatic disease on everyday life is not always evident when the patient is seen in the hospital or an ambulatory care setting. The increased frequency with which nurses see patients in the home provides opportunities for recognizing problems and implementing interventions aimed at improving the quality of life of patients with rheumatic disorders. The patient encountered in the home setting often has a rheumatic disease that is secondary to the primary reason for the visit. In such cases, the problems caused by the rheumatic disease may interfere with the treatment of the primary condition. For example, the patient who is recovering from coronary artery surgery may have been instructed to exercise but is unable or only partially able to do so because of the rheumatic disease. Conversely, treatment of the primary condition may cause or increase problems related to the rheumatic disease. For example, the cardiac patient who has been instructed to walk long distances every day may find that doing so increases the symptoms of OA in the knees.

During home visits, the nurse has the opportunity to assess the patient's home environment and its adequacy for patient safety and management of the disorder. Compliance with the treatment program can be more easily monitored in the home setting where physical and social barriers to adherence are more readily identified. For example, the patient with insulin-dependent diabetes may be unable to fill the syringe accurately or administer the insulin because of impaired joint mobility. Appropriate adaptive equipment needed for increased independence is often identified more readily when the nurse sees how the patient functions in the home. Any barriers to compliance can be identified and appropriate referrals made.

For patients at risk for impaired skin integrity, the home care nurse can closely monitor skin status and also instruct, provide, or supervise the patient and family in preventive skin care measures. The nurse also assesses the patient's need for assistance in the home and supervises home health aides, who may meet many of the needs of the patient with a rheumatic disease. Referrals to physical and occupational therapists may be made as problems are identified and limitations increase. A home care nurse can visit the home to make sure the patient can function as independently as possible despite mobility problems and can safely manage treatments and pharmacotherapy. The patient and family should be alerted to support services such as Meals on Wheels and local Arthritis Foundation chapters.

Because many of the medications to suppress inflammation are injectable, the nurse may administer the medication to the patient or teach self-injection procedure. These frequent contacts allow the nurse to reinforce other disease management techniques.

The nurse also assesses the patient's physical and psychological status, adequacy of symptom management, and adherence to the management plan. Previous teaching is reinforced with emphasis on side effects of medications and changes in physical status indicating disease progression and the need to contact or see the health care provider for reevaluation. Otherwise, patients may wait until their next appointment. The importance of follow-up appointments is emphasized to the patient and family.

Evaluation

Expected Outcomes

Expected outcomes may include:

1. Experiences relief of pain or improved comfort level
   a. Identifies factors that cause or increase pain
   b. Identifies realistic goals for pain relief
   c. Uses pain management strategies safely and effectively
   d. Reports decreased pain and increased comfort level
2. Experiences reduction in level of fatigue
   a. Identifies factors that contribute to fatigue
   b. Verbalizes the relationship of fatigue to disease activity
   c. Schedules periodic rest periods and identifies and uses other measures to prevent or modify fatigue
   d. Reports decreased level of fatigue
3. Increases or maintains level of mobility
   a. Identifies factors that impede mobility
   b. Participates in activities and exercises that promote or maintain mobility
   c. Uses assistive devices appropriately and safely
   d. Demonstrates good body alignment and posture
4. Maintains self-care activities
   a. Participates in self-care activities within capabilities
   b. Uses adaptive equipment and alternative methods to increase participation in self-care activities
   c. Maintains self-care at highest possible level
5. Experiences improved body image
   a. Verbalizes concerns about the impact of rheumatic disease on appearance and function
   b. Sets and achieves meaningful goals
   c. States acceptance of self-worth
   d. Reconciles body image and changes caused by disease
6. Experiences absence of complications
   a. Takes medications as prescribed
   b. States potential side effects of medications and names reportable side effects
   c. Verbalizes understanding of rationale for monitoring
   d. Identifies strategies to reduce risks of side effects

DIFFUSE CONNECTIVE TISSUE DISEASES

Diffuse connective tissue disease (CTD) refers to a group of disorders that are chronic in nature and characterized by diffuse inflammation and degeneration in the connective tissues. These disorders share similar clinical features and may affect some of the same organs. The characteristic clinical course is one of exacerbations and remissions. Although the diffuse CTDs have unknown causes, they are thought to be the result of immunologic abnormalities. The CTDs include RA, SLE, scleroderma, polymyositis (PM), and polymyalgia rheumatica (PMR).

Rheumatoid Arthritis

Pathophysiology

In RA, the autoimmune reaction (Fig. 50-3) primarily occurs in the synovial tissue. Phagocytosis produces enzymes within the joint. The enzymes break down collagen, causing edema, proliferation of the synovial membrane, and ultimately pannus formation. Pannus destroys cartilage and erodes the bone. The consequence is loss of articular surfaces and joint motion. Muscle fibers undergo degenerative changes. Muscle elasticity and contractile power are lost.

Clinical Manifestations

Clinical manifestations of RA vary, usually reflecting the stage and severity of the disease. Joint pain, swelling, warmth, erythema, and lack of function are classic. Palpation of the joints reveals spongy or boggy tissue. Often, fluid can be aspirated from the inflamed joint. Characteristically, the pattern of joint involvement begins with the small joints in the hands, wrists, and feet. As the disease progresses, the knees, shoulders, hips, elbows, ankles, cervical spine, and temporomandibular joints are involved. The onset of symptoms is usually acute. Symptoms are usually bilateral and symmetric. In addition to joint pain and swelling, another classic sign of RA is joint stiffness, especially in the morning, lasting for more than 30 minutes.

In the early stages of disease, even before bony changes occur, limitation in function can occur when there is active inflammation in the joints. Joints that are hot, swollen, and painful are not easily moved. The patient tends to guard or protect these joints through immobilization. Immobilization for extended periods can lead to contractures, creating soft tissue deformity.

Deformities of the hands and feet are common in RA (Fig. 50-4). The deformity may be caused by misalignment resulting from swelling, progressive joint destruction, or the subluxation (partial dislocation) that occurs when a bone slips over another and eliminates the joint space.

RA is a systemic disease with multiple extra-articular features. Most common are fever, weight loss, fatigue, anemia, lymph node enlargement, and Raynaud's phenomenon (cold- and stress-

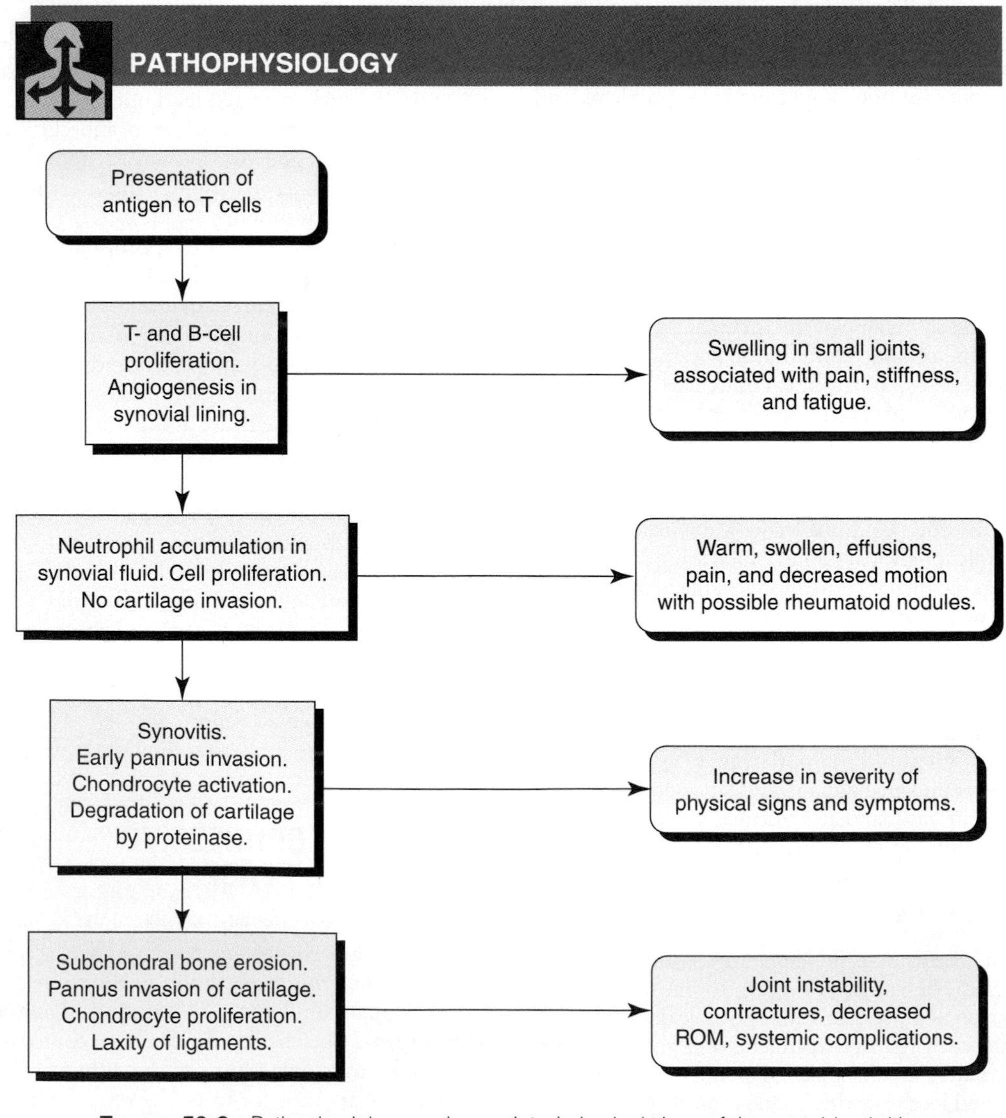

FIGURE 50•3 Pathophysiology and associated physical signs of rheumatoid arthritis.

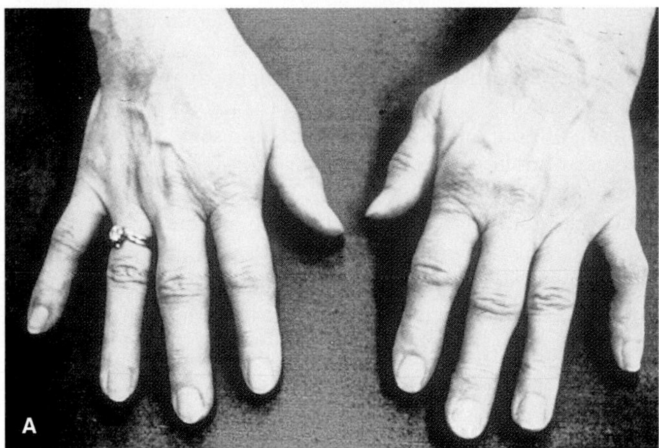

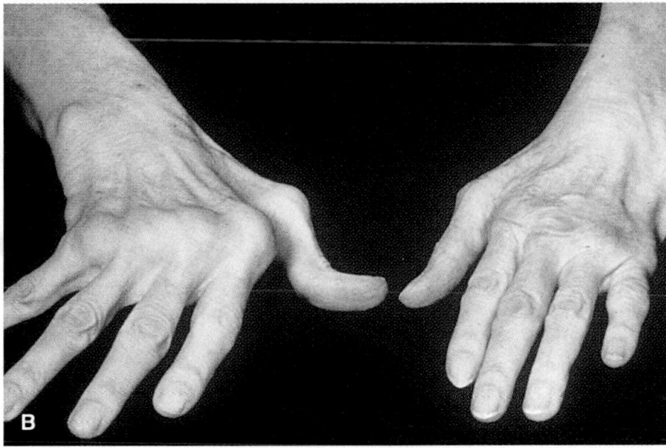

FIGURE 50•4 Rheumatoid arthritis. (**A**) Early. (**B**) Advanced.

induced vasospasm causing episodes of digital blanching or cyanosis). Rheumatoid nodules may be noted in patients who have more advanced RA, developing at some time in up to half of patients (Klippel, 1997). These nodules are usually nontender and movable in the subcutaneous tissue. They usually appear over bony prominences such as the elbow, are varied in size, and can disappear spontaneously. Nodules occur only in individuals who have rheumatoid factor (RF). The nodules often are associated with rapidly progressive and destructive disease. Other extra-articular features include arteritis, neuropathy, scleritis, pericarditis, splenomegaly, and Sjögren's syndrome (dry eyes and dry mucous membranes).

Assessment and Diagnostic Findings

Several factors can contribute to an RA diagnosis: rheumatoid nodules, joint inflammation detected on palpation, and certain laboratory findings. The history and physical examination address manifestations such as bilateral and symmetric stiffness, tenderness, swelling, and temperature changes to the joints. The patient is also assessed for extra-articular changes; these often include weight loss, sensory changes, lymph node enlargement, and fatigue. RF is present in more than 80% of patients with RA; however, its presence alone is not diagnostic of RA. The ESR is significantly elevated with RA. The red blood cell (RBC) count and C_4 complement component are decreased. The C-reactive protein (CRP) and antinuclear antibody (ANA) test results may also be positive. An arthrocentesis shows synovial fluid that is cloudy, milky, or dark yellow and contains numerous inflammatory cells, such as leukocytes and complement.

X-ray studies, performed to help diagnose and monitor the progression of disease, show characteristic bony erosions and narrowed joint spaces occurring later in the disease.

Medical Management

EARLY RHEUMATOID ARTHRITIS

In patients with early RA, treatment begins with education, a balance of rest and exercise, and referral to community agencies for support. Medical management begins with therapeutic doses of salicylates or NSAIDs. When used in full therapeutic dosages, these medications provide both anti-inflammatory and analgesic effects. Taking medications as prescribed to maintain a consistent blood level is necessary to optimize the effectiveness of the anti-inflammatory drug.

A new class of NSAIDs, called COX-2, inhibitors has been approved for treatment of RA. COX (cyclo-oxygenase) is an enzyme involved in the inflammatory process. COX-2 inhibitors block the enzyme involved in inflammation while leaving the enzyme involved in protecting the stomach lining. As a result, COX-2 agents are much less toxic than current NSAIDs.

The trend in management is toward a more aggressive pharmacologic approach earlier in the disease. A window of opportunity for symptom control and improved disease management occurs within the first 2 years of disease onset. Therefore, the disease-modifying antirheumatic agents (antimalarials, gold, penicillamine, or sulfasalazine) are initiated early in treatment. If symptoms appear to be aggressive (ie, early bony erosions as seen on x-rays), methotrexate may be considered. Methotrexate is currently the gold standard in treatment of RA because of its success in improving disease parameters (ie, pain, tender and swollen joints, and quality of life). The goal is to prevent destruction of the joints.

A newer treatment approach for RA is emerging in the area of biologic therapies. Biologic response modifiers are a group of agents that consist of molecules produced by cells of the immune system or by cells that participate in the inflammatory reactions (Pannush & Arend, 1997). This includes monoclonal antibodies, soluble cell-surface receptors, **cytokines** (nonantibody protein acting as intercellular mediators), and lymphocyte vaccines. Antitumor necrosis factor receptors are currently being tested as a potential new treatment for RA. Initial studies have shown favorable results in reduction of symptoms, and the side effects have been mild (Moreland et al., 1997).

Additional analgesia may be prescribed for periods of extreme pain. Opioid analgesics are avoided because of the potential for continuing need for pain relief. Nonpharmacologic pain management techniques (ie, relaxation techniques, heat and cold applications) are taught.

MODERATE, EROSIVE RHEUMATOID ARTHRITIS

For moderate, erosive RA, a formal program with occupational and physical therapy is prescribed to educate the patient about principles of joint protection, pacing activities, work simplification, range of motion, and muscle-strengthening exercises. The patient is encouraged to participate actively in the management program. The medication program is reevaluated periodically, and appropriate changes are made if indicated. Cyclosporine, an immunomodulator, may be added to enhance the disease-modifying effect of methotrexate.

PERSISTENT, EROSIVE RA

For persistent, erosive RA, reconstructive surgery and corticosteroids are often used. Reconstructive surgery is indicated when pain cannot be relieved by conservative measures. Surgical procedures include synovectomy (excision of the synovial membrane), tenorrhaphy (suturing a tendon), arthrodesis (surgical fusion of the joint), and arthroplasty (surgical repair and replacement of the joint). Surgery is not performed during disease flares.

Systemic corticosteroids are used when the patient has unremitting inflammation and pain or needs a "bridging" medication while waiting for the slower disease-modifying antirheumatic agent (eg, methotrexate) to begin working. Low-dose corticosteroid therapy is prescribed for the shortest time necessary (to minimize side effects). Joints that are severely inflamed and fail to respond promptly to the measures outlined previously may be treated by local injection of a corticosteroid.

ADVANCED, UNREMITTING RA

For advanced, unremitting RA, immunosuppressive agents are prescribed because of their ability to affect the production of antibodies at the cellular level. These include high-dose methotrexate, cyclophosphamide, and azathioprine. These medications, however, are highly toxic and can produce bone marrow suppression, anemia, gastrointestinal disturbances, and rashes.

Through all stages of RA, depression and sleep deprivation may require the short-term use of low-dose antidepressant medications, such as amitriptyline, to reestablish an adequate sleep pattern and to manage chronic pain better.

Recently the FDA approved a new medical device for use in treating patients with more severe cases of RA with longstanding disease who have failed on or are intolerant to DMARDs. The device, a protein A Immunoadsorption column (Prosorba), is used in 12 weekly apheresis treatments to bind IgG (ie, circulating immune complex). About 30% who receive the treatments will have 20% improvement in their symptoms.

Nutritional Therapy

Patients with RA frequently experience anorexia, weight loss, and anemia. A dietary history identifies usual eating habits and food preferences. Food selection should include the daily requirements from the basic food groups, with emphasis on foods high in vitamins, protein, and iron for tissue building and repair. For the extremely anorexic patient, small, frequent feedings with increased protein supplements may be prescribed. Some medications (ie, oral corticosteroids) used in RA treatment stimulate the appetite and, when combined with decreased activity, may lead to weight gain. Therefore, patients should be counseled about eating a well-balanced, calorie-restricted diet.

Nursing Management

The nursing care of the patient with RA follows the basic plan of nursing care presented earlier in the chapter. The most common problems for the patient with RA include pain, sleep disturbance, fatigue, and limited motion. The patient with newly diagnosed RA needs information about the disease to make daily self-management decisions and to cope with having a chronic disease.

Systemic Lupus Erythematosus

Pathophysiology

SLE is a result of disturbed immune regulation that causes an exaggerated production of autoantibodies. This immunoregulatory disturbance is brought about by some combination of genetic, hormonal (as evidenced by the usual onset during the childbearing years), and environmental factors (sunlight, thermal burns). Certain medications, such as hydralazine (Apresoline), procainamide (Pronestyl), isoniazid, chlorpromazine, and some anticonvulsants, have been implicated in chemical or drug-induced SLE, as have foods such as alfalfa sprouts.

In SLE, the increase in autoantibody production is thought to result from abnormal suppressor T-cell function, leading to immune complex deposition and tissue damage. Inflammation stimulates antigens which, in turn, stimulate additional antibodies, and the cycle repeats.

Clinical Manifestations

The onset of SLE may be insidious or acute. For this reason, the patient with SLE may remain undiagnosed for many years. Clinical features of SLE involve multiple body systems.

MUSCULOSKELETAL MANIFESTATIONS

The musculoskeletal system's involvement, with arthralgias and arthritis (synovitis), is a common presenting features of SLE. Joint swelling, tenderness, and pain on movement are also common. Frequently, these are accompanied by morning stiffness.

SKIN MANIFESTATIONS

Several different types of skin manifestations may occur in patients with SLE, including subacute cutaneous lupus erythematosus (SCLE), which involves papulosquamous or annular polycyclic lesions, and discoid lupus erythematosus (DLE), which is a chronic rash that has erythematous papules or plaques and scaling, and can cause scarring and pigmentation changes. The most familiar skin manifestation (but occurring in fewer than half of patients with SLE) is an acute cutaneous lesion consisting of a butterfly-shaped rash across the bridge of the nose and cheeks (Fig. 50-5). In some cases of DLE, only skin involvement may occur. In some SLE patients, the initial skin involvement may be the precursor to more systemic involvement. The lesions often worsen during exacerbations (flares) of the systemic disease and possibly are provoked by sunlight or artificial ultraviolet light (Boumpas et al., 1995).

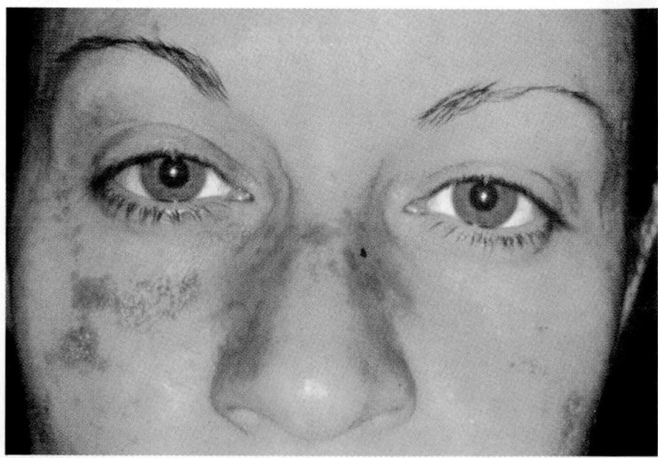

FIGURE 50•5 The characteristic butterfly rash of systemic lupus erythematosus. Courtesy of Drs. S. Wilson and W. Larson, SmithKline Beecham.

Oral ulcers, which may accompany skin lesions, may involve the buccal mucosa or the hard palate. The ulcers occur in crops and are often associated with exacerbations.

CARDIOPULMONARY MANIFESTATIONS

Pericarditis is the most common cardiac manifestation, occurring in up to 30% of patients. It may be asymptomatic and is often accompanied by pleural effusions. Lung and pleural involvement occurs in 20% to 40% of patients, most often manifested by pleuritis or pleural effusions.

VASCULAR AND LYMPHATIC MANIFESTATIONS

The vascular system can be involved, with inflammation of the terminal arterioles. Papular, erythematous, and purpuric lesions develop, possibly on the fingertips, elbows, toes, and extensor surfaces of the forearms or lateral sides of the hand. These lesions may progress to necrosis. Lymphadenopathy occurs in half of all SLE patients at some time during the course of illness.

RENAL MANIFESTATIONS

Renal involvement, usually affecting the glomeruli, occurs in about 32% of patients with SLE. The extent of kidney damage indicates whether renal involvement will be reversible.

NEUROLOGIC AND BEHAVIORAL MANIFESTATIONS

Central nervous system involvement is widespread, encompassing the entire range of neurologic disease. The varied and frequent neuropsychiatric presentations of SLE are now widely recognized. These are generally demonstrated by subtle changes in behavior patterns or cognitive ability. Depression and psychosis are common.

Assessment and Diagnostic Findings

Diagnosis of SLE is based on a complete history, physical examination, and blood tests. In addition to the general assessment performed for a patient with a rheumatic disease, assessment for known or suspected SLE has special features. The skin is inspected for erythematous rashes. Cutaneous erythematous plaques with an adherent scale may be observed on the scalp, face, or neck. Areas of hyperpigmentation or depigmentation may be noted, depending on the phase and type of the disease. The patient should be questioned about skin changes (because these may be transitory) and specifically about sensitivity to sunlight or artificial ultraviolet light. The scalp should be inspected for alopecia and the mouth and throat for ulcerations reflecting gastrointestinal involvement.

Cardiovascular assessment includes auscultation for pericardial friction rub, possibly associated with myocarditis and accompanying pleural effusions. The pleural effusions and infiltrations, which reflect respiratory insufficiency, are demonstrated by abnormal lung sounds. Papular, erythematous, and purpuric lesions developing on the fingertips, elbows, toes, and extensor surfaces of the forearms or lateral sides of the hand that may become necrotic suggest vascular involvement.

Joint swelling, tenderness, warmth, pain on movement, stiffness, and edema may be detected on physical examination. The joint involvement is often symmetric and similar to that found in RA.

Typically, assessment reveals classic symptoms, including fever, fatigue, and weight loss and possibly arthritis, pleurisy, and pericarditis. Interactions with the patient and family may provide further evidence of systemic involvement. The neurologic assessment is directed at identifying and describing any central nervous system problems. The patient and family members are asked about any behavioral changes, including manifestations of neuroses or psychosis. Signs of depression are noted, as are reports of seizures, chorea, or other central nervous system manifestations.

No single laboratory test confirms SLE; rather, serum testing reveals moderate to severe anemia, thrombocytopenia, leukocytosis, or leukopenia and positive antinuclear antibodies. Other diagnostic immunologic tests support but do not confirm the diagnosis. Hematuria may be found on urinalysis.

Medical Management

Treatment of SLE includes management of acute and chronic disease. Although SLE can be life-threatening, advances in its treatment have been a major factor in improvements in patient survival and reduction of disease morbidity (Klippel, 1997). Acute disease requires interventions directed at controlling increased disease activity or exacerbations that may involve any organ system. Disease activity is a composite of clinical and laboratory features that reflect active inflammation secondary to SLE. Management of the more chronic condition involves periodic monitoring and recognition of meaningful clinical changes requiring adjustments in therapy (Ulak, 1995).

The goals of treatment include preventing progressive loss of organ function, reducing the likelihood of acute disease, minimizing disease-related disabilities, and preventing complications from therapy. Management of SLE involves regular monitoring to assess disease activity and therapeutic effectiveness.

PHARMACOLOGIC THERAPY

Medication therapy for SLE is based on the concept that local tissue inflammation is mediated by exaggerated or heightened immune responses, which can vary widely in intensity and require different therapies at different times. The NSAIDs used for minor clinical manifestations are often used along with corticosteroids in an effort to minimize corticosteroid requirements.

Corticosteroids are the single most important medication available for treatment. They are used topically for cutaneous manifestations, in low oral doses for minor disease activity, and in high doses for major disease activity. Intravenous administration of corticosteroids is an alternative to traditional high-dose oral use. Antimalarial medications are effective for managing cutaneous, musculoskeletal, and mild systemic features of SLE. Immunosuppressive agents (alkylating agents and purine analogs) are used because of their effect on immune function. These medications are generally reserved for patients who have serious forms of SLE and who have not responded to conservative therapies (National Institutes of Health, 1998).

Nursing Management

The nursing care of the patient with SLE is based on the basic plan presented earlier in the chapter. The most common problems include fatigue, impaired skin integrity, body image disturbance, and lack of knowledge for self-management decisions. The disease or its treatment may produce dramatic changes in appearance and considerable distress for the patient. The changes and the unpredictable course of SLE necessitate expert assessment skills and nursing care and sensitivity to the psychological reactions of the patient.

NURSING RESEARCH

Psychosocial Variables Affecting Women's Adjustment to Systemic Lupus Erythematosus

Faillia, S., Kuper, B. C., Nick, T. G., & Lee, F. A. (1996). Adjustment of women with systemic lupus erythematosus. *Applied Nursing Research, 9*(2), 87–96.

Purpose

The fluctuation of symptoms associated with systemic lupus erythematosus (SLE) leading to a feeling of helplessness and lack of control was the impetus for this descriptive, correlational study. The researchers examined the influence of psychosocial variables on the adjustment of women with SLE. Two research questions were examined:

1. What relationships exist among the variables of uncertainty, health-related hardiness, hopelessness, social support, and adjustment in women with SLE?
2. What demographic and psychosocial variables predict adjustment in women with SLE?

Study Sample and Design

The convenience sample of 31 women with SLE, 23 to 65 years of age, completed questionnaires relating to perceptions of uncertainty, health-related hardiness, hopelessness, social support, and adjustment. Additionally, demographic data were collected. Ranges, means, and standard deviations of scores were calculated, and Pearson correlations were used to identify relationships among the study variables.

Findings

Scores of the sample on the questionnaires reflected uncertainty yet hopefulness about the illness, health-related hardiness, and ability to adjust to the illness. Total adjustment was not related to any aspect of health-related hardiness. However, several relationships were found to exist between other study variables. Total adjustment had a moderate negative association with hopelessness, whereas several adjustment dimensions (vocation and domestic environment, sexual and extended family relationships, and psychological distress) had a low to moderate negative correlation with hopelessness. Uncertainty and total adjustment had a low-moderate negative association. Scores on several adjustment subscales (health care orientation, domestic environment, extended family relationships, and psychological distress) demonstrated low to low-moderate negative correlations with uncertainty. Only the extended family relations subscale reflected a low positive correlation with total health-related hardiness and its subscale of commitment/challenge. Higher incomes and levels of education were associated with higher levels of adjustment for the domestic environment subscale. Education, health-related hardiness, and the commitment/challenge subscale of health-related hardiness were positively correlated with the extended family relationships subscale of adjustment. A negative relationship existed between hopelessness and health-related hardiness, whereas there was a positive correlation between hopelessness and uncertainty.

Stepwise multiple regression analysis revealed that hopelessness and income were significant predictors of adjustment. These findings show that uncertainty, hopelessness, the commitment/challenge dimension of health-related hardiness, education, and income are associated with adjustment and its dimensions. However, hopelessness is the only psychosocial variable predictive of adjustment. These findings demonstrate the effect of this psychosocial variable on adjustment to SLE; however, generalization of the findings is limited because of the sample size.

Nursing Implications

Based on these findings, nurses should acknowledge the impact of hope when caring for SLE patients. Assisting the individual in identifying elements that foster hope is an important part of the nursing care. These elements might include the presence of meaningful relationships, a sense of one's spirituality, positive memories of the past, access to resources, self-worth, a sense of purpose, and feelings of happiness. The nurse can facilitate the process by encouraging and assisting the individual in fostering these activities. A plan of care that supports hopefulness and establishes realistic goals may allow the individual to perceive SLE as a challenge, to feel optimistic, and to make needed adjustments.

Scleroderma

Pathophysiology

Like other diffuse CTDs, scleroderma has a variable course with remissions and exacerbations. Its prognosis, however, is not as optimistic as that of lupus. The disease commonly begins with skin involvement. Mononuclear cells cluster on the skin and stimulate lymphokines to stimulate procollagen. Insoluble collagen is formed and accumulates excessively in the tissues. Initially, the inflammatory response causes edema formation, with a resulting taut, smooth, and shiny skin appearance. The skin then undergoes fibrotic changes, leading to loss of elasticity and movement. Eventually, the tissue degenerates and becomes nonfunctional. This chain of events, from inflammation to degeneration, also occurs in blood vessels, major organs, and body systems, potentially resulting in death (Klippel, 1997).

Clinical Manifestations

Scleroderma starts insidiously with Raynaud's phenomenon and swelling in the hands. The skin and the subcutaneous tissues become increasingly hard and rigid and cannot be pinched up from the underlying structures. Wrinkles and lines are obliterated. The skin is dry because sweat secretion over the involved region is suppressed. The extremities stiffen and lose mobility. The condition spreads slowly. For years, these changes may remain localized in the hands and the feet. The face appears masklike, immobile, and expressionless, and the mouth becomes rigid.

The changes within the body, although not visible directly, are vastly more important than the visible changes. The left ventricle of the heart is involved, resulting in heart failure. The esophagus hardens, interfering with swallowing. The lungs sustain scarring, impeding respiration. Digestive disturbances occur because of hardening (sclerosing) of the intestinal mucosa. Progressive renal failure may occur.

The patient may manifest a variety of symptoms referred to as the *CREST syndrome.* The letters CREST stand for calcinosis (*c*alcium deposits in the tissues), *R*aynaud's phenomenon, *e*sophageal hardening and dysfunctioning, *s*clerodactyly (scleroderma of the digits), and *t*elangiectasis (capillary dilation that forms a vascular lesion).

Assessment and Diagnostic Findings

Assessment focuses on the sclerotic changes in the skin, contractures in the fingers, and color changes or lesions in the fingertips. Assessment of systemic involvement requires a systems review with special attention to gastrointestinal, pulmonary, renal, and cardiac symptoms. Limitations in mobility and self-care activities should be assessed, along with the impact the disease has had (or will have) on body image.

There is no one conclusive test to diagnose scleroderma. A skin biopsy is performed to identify cellular changes specific to scleroderma. Pulmonary studies show ventilation-perfusion abnormalities. Echocardiography identifies pericardial effusion (often present with cardiac involvement). Esophageal studies demonstrate decreased motility in 75% of patients with scleroderma. Blood tests may detect antinuclear antibodies (ANAs), indicating a connective tissue disorder and possibly distinguishing the subgroup of scleroderma. A positive ANA test result is common in patients with scleroderma. An ANA finding that demonstrates the anticentromere pattern is associated with the CREST syndrome.

Medical Management

Treatment of scleroderma depends on the clinical manifestations. All patients require counseling, during which realistic individual goals may be determined. Support measures include strategies to decrease pain and limit disability. A moderate exercise program is encouraged, to prevent joint contractures. Patients are advised to avoid extreme temperatures and to use lotions to minimize skin dryness.

PHARMACOLOGIC THERAPY

No medication regimen has proved effective in controlling scleroderma; however, various medications can be used to treat the symptoms. Penicillamine has been the most promising medication in decreasing skin thickening, reducing the rate of new visceral organ involvement, and prolonging life. Captopril and other potent antihypertensive agents are effective in controlling hypertensive crises. Anti-inflammatory medications can be used to control arthralgia, stiffness, and general musculoskeletal discomfort. Vasodilators have not proved effective for vascular abnormalities.

Nursing Management

The nursing care of the patient with scleroderma is based on the basic plan of nursing care presented earlier in the chapter. The most common problems of the patient with scleroderma include impaired skin integrity; self-care deficits; altered nutrition, less than body requirements; and body image disturbance. The patient with advanced disease may also have problems with impaired gas exchange, decreased cardiac output, impaired swallowing, and constipation.

Polymyositis

Pathophysiology

PM is classified as autoimmune because autoantibodies are present. However, these antibodies do not cause damage to muscle cells, indicating only an indirect role in tissue damage. The pathogenesis of PM is considered multifactorial. A genetic predisposition is likely. Drug-induced disease is rare but has been reported. Some evidence suggests a viral link.

Clinical Manifestations

The onset of PM varies from sudden with rapid progression to a very slow, insidious onset. Proximal muscle weakness is typically a first symptom. Muscle weakness is usually symmetric and diffuse. Dermatomyositis, a related condition, is most commonly identified by an erythematous smooth or scaly lesion found over the joint surface.

Assessment and Diagnostic Findings

A complete history and physical examination helps to exclude other muscle-related disorders. As with other diffuse connective tissue disorders, no one test confirms PM. An electromyogram is performed to rule out degenerative muscle disease. Muscle biopsy may reveal inflammatory infiltrate in the tissue. Serum studies indicate increased muscle enzyme activity.

Medical Management

Management of PM involves high-dose corticosteroid therapy initially, followed by a gradual dosage reduction over several months as muscle enzyme activity decreases. Patients who do not respond to corticosteroids require the addition of an immunosuppressive agent. For patients who are unresponsive to corticosteroids and immunosuppressive medications (up to 10% of patients), plasmapheresis may be tried. Skin rashes may respond to hydroxychloroquine. Physical therapy is initiated slowly with range-of-motion exercises to maintain joint mobility, followed by gradual strengthening exercises.

Nursing Management

The nursing care of the patient with PM is based on the basic plan of nursing care presented earlier in the chapter. The most frequent problems for the patient with PM include impaired physical mobility, fatigue, self-care deficit, and insufficient knowledge of self-management techniques.

Polymyalgia Rheumatica

Pathophysiology

The underlying mechanism involved with PMR is unknown. This disease occurs predominately in whites, and often in first-degree relatives. An association with the genetic marker HLA-DR4 suggests a familial predisposition. Immunoglobulin deposits in the walls of inflamed temporal arteries also suggest an autoimmune process.

Clinical Manifestations

PMR is characterized by severe proximal muscle discomfort with mild joint swelling. Complaints of severe aching in the neck, shoulder, and pelvic muscles are common. Stiffness is noticeable most often in the morning and after periods of inactivity. Systemic features include low-grade fever, weight loss, malaise, anorexia, and depression. Because PMR generally occurs in people 50 years of age and older, it may be confused with, or disregarded as, an inevitable consequence of aging.

Giant cell arteritis (GSA), sometimes associated with PMR, may cause headaches, changes in vision, and jaw claudication. These symptoms should be evaluated immediately because of the potential for a sudden and permanent loss of vision. PMR and GSA generally run a self-limited course, lasting several months to several years (Stone & Hellmann, 1998).

Assessment and Diagnostic Findings

Assessment focuses on evidence of musculoskeletal tenderness, weakness, and decreased function. Careful attention should be directed toward assessing the head (vision, headaches, and jaw claudication).

Often, diagnosis is difficult because of the lack of specificity of tests. A markedly high ESR is a screening test but is not definitive. Diagnosis is more likely to be made by eliminating other potential diagnoses, but this is highly dependent on the skills and experience of the diagnostician. The dramatic and immediate response to treatment with corticosteroids is considered by some to be diagnostic.

Medical Management

PMR (without GSA) is treated with moderate doses of corticosteroids. NSAIDs are sometimes used for mild disease. For patients with GSA, rapid initiation and strict adherence to a regimen of corticosteroids are essential to avoid the complication of blindness.

Nursing Management

The nursing care of the patient with PMR is based on the basic plan of nursing care presented earlier in the chapter. The most common problems for the patient with PMR include pain and insufficient knowledge of the medication regimen.

DEGENERATIVE JOINT DISEASE (OSTEOARTHRITIS)

OA, also known as degenerative joint disease or osteoarthrosis (even though inflammation may be present), is the most common and frequently disabling of the joint disorders. OA is both overdiagnosed and trivialized; it is frequently overtreated or undertreated. The functional impact of OA on quality of life, especially for elderly patients, is often ignored.

OA has been classified as primary (idiopathic), with no prior event or disease related to the OA, and secondary. The distinction between primary and secondary OA, however, is not always clear.

Increasing age directly relates to the degenerative process in the joint as the ability of the articular cartilage to resist microfracture with repetitive low loads diminishes. OA often begins in the third decade of life and peaks between the fifth and sixth decades. By age 75 years, 85% of the population has either x-ray findings or clinical evidence of OA; only 15% to 25% of these people, however, experience significant symptoms.

Pathophysiology

OA may be thought of as the end result of many pathologies combining in a generalized predisposition to the disease. OA affects the articular cartilage, subchondral bone (the bony plate that supports the articular cartilage), and synovium. A combination of degradation, inflammation, and repair occurs. The basic degenerative process in the joint exemplified in OA is presented in Figure 50-6. Understanding of OA has been greatly expanded beyond what previously was thought of as simply "wear and tear" related to aging. Risk factors for OA are summarized in the accompanying display.

A hereditary subset of OA, known as nodal generalized OA (involving three or more joint groups), has been confirmed (George, Creamer, & Dieppe, 1994). This type of OA involves a primary inflammatory process. Postmenopausal women in the same family have been observed to have a type of OA of the hands

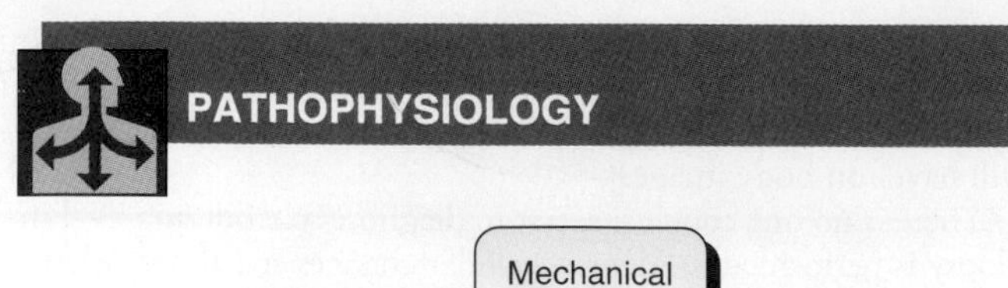

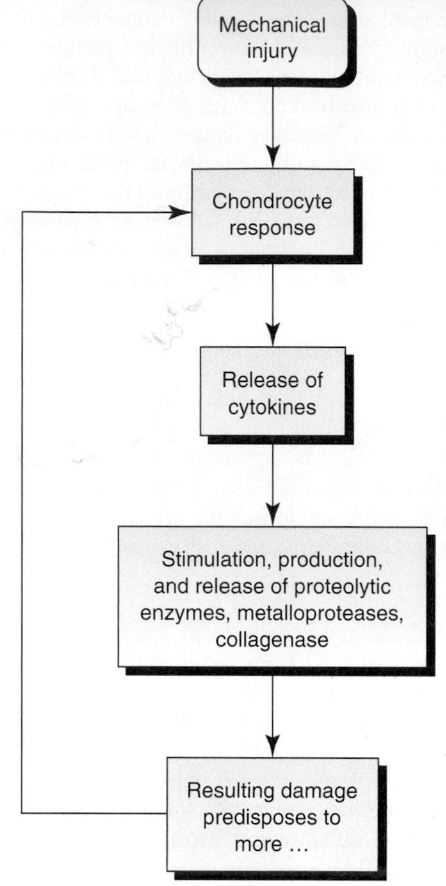

FIGURE 50•6 Pathophysiology of osteoarthritis.

characterized by the presence of nodes at the distal interphalangeal joint and at the proximal interphalangeal joint in the hand.

Congenital and developmental disorders of the hip are well known for predisposing a person to OA of the hip. These include congenital subluxation–dislocation of the hip, acetabular dysplasia, Legg-Calvé-Perthes disease, and slipped capital femoral epiphysis.

Obesity has been associated with OA of the knee in women. This may be due to mechanical stress and misalignment of the knee joint in relationship to the rest of the body because of the diameter of the thighs. Another theory is that mechanically, obesity increases the force across the joint and, therefore, causes cartilage degeneration. Obesity may have a direct effect on cartilage; it has been theorized that a hormone or biologic mediator linked with obesity may cause OA. Obesity is associated with increased subchondral bone mass, which may lead to bony stiffness, making subchondral bone less flexible upon impact loading, transmitting more force to overlying articular cartilage, and thus making it more susceptible to injury.

Obese women have been shown to have OA of the knee four times more often than women of average weight (Oddis, 1996). The question has been raised as to whether obesity precedes OA or is the result of a sedentary lifestyle adopted by symptomatic patients. Recent studies suggest the former. It has also been shown that obesity during young adulthood, when OA is extremely rare,

Risk Factors for
OSTEOARTHRITIS

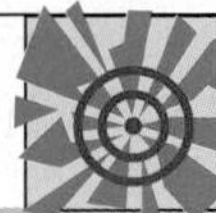

- Increased age
- Genetic disposition
- Gender and hormonal factors
- Obesity
- Mechanical factors
- Prior inflammatory disease

Adapted from Cicuttini, F. M., & Spector, T. D. (1995). Osteoarthritis in the aged. *Drugs and Aging, 6*(5), 409–420.

increases the risk of later OA of the knee. Weight loss in the middle or later years appears to reduce the risk for later OA of the knee. These findings appear to apply more to women than to men, in whom knee injury may be a more important causal agent. Thus, preventing or reducing obesity may be important in preventing OA of the knee.

Mechanical factors, such as joint trauma, sports activities, and occupation, have also been implicated. These factors include cruciate ligament damage and meniscal tears, heavy physical activity, and frequent knee bending.

Clinical Manifestations

The primary clinical manifestations of OA are pain, stiffness, and functional impairment. The pain is due to an inflamed synovium, stretching of the joint capsule or ligaments, irritation of nerve endings in the periosteum over osteophytes, trabecular microfracture, intraosseous hypertension, bursitis, tendinitis, and muscle spasm. Stiffness, which is most commonly experienced in the morning or after awakening, usually lasts less than 30 minutes and decreases with movement. Functional impairment is due to pain on movement and limited motion caused by structural changes in the joints.

Although OA occurs most often in weight-bearing joints (hips, knees, cervical and lumbar spine), the proximal and distal finger joints are also often involved. Characteristic bony nodes may be present; on inspection and palpation, these are usually painless, unless inflammation is present.

Assessment and Diagnostic Findings

Diagnosis of OA is complicated because only 30% to 50% of patients with changes seen on x-rays report symptoms. Physical assessment of the musculoskeletal system reveals tender and enlarged joints. Inflammation, when present, is not the destructive type seen in the connective tissue diseases such as RA. OA is characterized by a progressive loss of the joint cartilage, which appears on x-rays as a narrowing of joint space. In addition, reactive changes occur at the joint margins and on the subchondral bone in the form of osteophytes (or spurs) as the cartilage attempts to regenerate. Neither the presence of osteophytes nor joint space narrowing alone is specific for OA; however, when combined, these are sensitive and specific findings. In early or mild OA, there is only a weak correlation between joint pain and synovitis. Serum studies are not useful in the diagnosis of this disorder.

Medical Management

Although no treatment halts the degenerative process, certain preventive measures can slow the progress if undertaken early enough. These include weight reduction, prevention of injuries, perinatal screening for congenital hip disease, and ergonomic modifications.

Conservative treatment measures include the use of heat, weight reduction, joint rest and avoidance of joint overuse, orthotic devices to support inflamed joints (splints, braces), and isometric and postural exercises. Occupational and physical therapy can help the patient adopt self-management strategies.

PHARMACOLOGIC THERAPY

The pharmacologic regimen is based on newer understanding of the damage from OA caused by the remodeling process and is directed at improving cartilage repair and retarding breakdown. Some studies have raised the possibility that salicylates and some of the NSAIDs may accelerate the progression of cartilage breakdown in OA. Acetaminophen may be as effective as NSAIDs in the symptomatic treatment of OA (Oddis, 1996). Initially, high daily doses of acetaminophen are prescribed along with nonpharmacologic measures of pain relief. Side effects and cost of NSAIDs are greater than those of acetaminophen. If control of joint symptoms is not achieved within a reasonable period, an NSAID is then prescribed. Ongoing reassessment is directed at reducing the dosage or using the NSAID only intermittently at times of joint pain exacerbation. Intra-articular injections of corticosteroids are used cautiously for an immediate, short-term effect when a joint is acutely inflamed.

SURGICAL MANAGEMENT

Surgical management is usually done when pain is intractable and function has been lost. For patients with OA of the knee, which is unresponsive to the traditional methods of pain management, *viscosupplementation* (the reconstitution of synovial fluid viscosity) is a new therapeutic concept that is being used. Hyaluronic acid (Hyalgan, Synvisc), a glycosaminoglycan that acts as a lubricant and shock-absorbing fluid in the joint, may be used in this procedure. Hyaluronic acid stimulates the production of synoviocytes, possibly providing better and more prolonged pain control. A series of three to five weekly intra-articular injections is given. Pain relief may last for 6 months (Kellick et al., 1998).

Tidal irrigation (washing debris from the joint space), arthroscopic débridement, drilling of osteochondral defects, or abrasion arthroplasty (to smooth the joint surface) may reduce pain in the knees of some patients with OA, although their effectiveness has not been demonstrated. For patients with end-stage disease, joint **arthroplasty** (replacement) can relieve pain and restore loss of function. Treatment of OA of the knee accounts for most knee surgery, including most total knee replacements (see Chap. 61 for discussion of knee replacement).

SPONDYLOARTHROPATHIES

The *spondyloarthropathies* are another category of systemic inflammatory disorders of the skeleton. The spondyloarthropathies include ankylosing spondylitis (AS), reactive arthritis, and psoriatic arthritis. Spondyloarthritis is also associated with inflammatory bowel diseases such as regional enteritis (Crohn's disease) and ulcerative colitis.

These rheumatic diseases share several common clinical features. The inflammation tends to occur peripherally at the sites of attachment—at tendons, joint capsules, and ligaments. Periosteal inflammation may be present. Many patients have arthritis of the sacroiliac joints. Onset tends to occur during young adulthood, with the disease affecting men more often than women. There is a strong tendency for these conditions to occur in families. Frequently, the HLA-B27 genetic marker is found.

Medical Management

Medical management focuses on treating pain and maintaining mobility by suppressing inflammation. For the patient with AS, good body positioning and posture are essential, so that if **ankylosis** (fixation) does occur, the patient is in the most functional position. Maintaining range of motion with a regular exercise and muscle-strengthening program is especially important.

PHARMACOLOGIC THERAPY

Salicylates, NSAIDs, and corticosteroids often produce marked improvement in back, skin, and joint symptoms. Methotrexate is also used to control psoriasis as well as joint inflammation.

SURGICAL MANAGEMENT

Surgical management may include total hip replacement. (See Chapter 61 for a discussion of hip replacement.)

Ankylosing Spondylitis

AS affects the cartilaginous joints of the spine and surrounding tissues. Occasionally, the large synovial joints, such as hips, knees, or shoulders, may be involved. AS is usually diagnosed in the second or third decade of life. The disease is not usually as severe in females as in males, in whom the disease is more prevalent and likely to include significant systemic involvement.

Clinical Manifestations

The characteristic feature of AS is back pain. As the disease progresses, ankylosis of the entire spine may occur, leading to respiratory compromise and complications.

Reiter's Syndrome

Reiter's syndrome affects young adult males and is characterized primarily by urethritis, arthritis, and conjunctivitis. Dermatitis and ulcerations of the mouth and penis may also be present. Low back pain is common.

Psoriatic Arthritis

Psoriatic arthritis (PA) is characterized by synovitis, polyarthritis, and spondylitis. One third of patients with psoriasis also have arthritis, making the incidence of PA similar to that of RA. As many as 20% of patients with PA have a severe course of disease, leading to deformity and joint damage. Early treatment is important because most of the damage appears to occur early in the course of the disease.

METABOLIC AND ENDOCRINE DISEASES ASSOCIATED WITH RHEUMATIC DISORDERS

Metabolic and endocrine diseases may be associated with rheumatic disorders. These include biochemical abnormalities (amyloidosis and scurvy), endocrine diseases (diabetes mellitus and acromegaly), immunodeficiency diseases (AIDS), and other hereditary disorders (hypermobility syndromes). The most common conditions, however, are the crystal-induced arthropathies in which crystals, such as monosodium urate (gout) or calcium pyrophosphate (calcium pyrophosphate dihydrate disease [*CPPD*] or pseudogout), are deposited within joints.

Gout

Gout is a heterogeneous group of conditions related to a genetic defect of purine metabolism resulting in hyperuricemia. An oversecretion of uric acid or a renal defect resulting in decreased excretion of uric acid, or a combination of both, occurs.

In *primary hyperuricemia*, elevated serum urate levels or manifestations of urate deposition appear to be consequences of faulty uric acid metabolism. Primary hyperuricemia may be due to severe dieting or starvation, excessive intake of foods that are high in purines (shellfish, organ meats), or heredity. In *secondary hyperuricemia*, gout is a minor clinical feature secondary to any of a number of genetic or acquired processes, including conditions in which there is an increase in cell turnover (leukemia, multiple myeloma, some types of anemias, psoriasis) and an increase in cell breakdown. Altered renal tubular function, either as a major action or as an unintended side effect of certain pharmacologic agents (diuretics such as thiazides and furosemide), low-dose salicylates, and ethanol can contribute to uric acid underexcretion.

Pathophysiology

Hyperuricemia (serum concentration greater than 7 mg/dL (0.4 μmol/L) can but does not always cause monosodium urate crystal deposition. Attacks of gout appear to be related to sudden increases or decreases of serum uric acid levels. When the urate crystals precipitate within a joint, an inflammatory response occurs, and an attack of gout begins. With repeated attacks, accumulations of sodium urate crystals, called **tophi**, are deposited in peripheral areas of the body, such as the great toe, the hands, and the ear. Renal urate lithiasis (kidney stones) with chronic renal disease secondary to urate deposition may develop.

The finding of urate crystals in the synovial fluid of asymptomatic joints suggests that factors other than crystals may be related to the inflammatory reaction. Recovered monosodium urate crystals are coated with immunoglobulins that are mainly immunoglobulin G (IgG). IgG enhances crystal phagocytosis, thereby demonstrating immunologic activity.

Clinical Manifestations

Manifestations of the gout syndrome include acute gouty arthritis (recurrent attacks of severe articular and periarticular inflammation), tophi (crystalline deposits accumulating in articular tissue, osseous tissue, soft tissue, and cartilage), gouty nephropathy (renal impairment), and uric acid urinary calculi. Four stages of gout can be identified: asymptomatic hyperuricemia, acute gouty arthritis, intercritical gout, and chronic tophaceous gout.

Fewer than one in five hyperuricemic patients will at any point develop clinically apparent urate crystal deposition. The subsequent development of gout is directly related to the duration and magnitude of the hyperuricemia. Therefore, the commitment to lifelong pharmacologic treatment of hyperuricemia is deferred until there is an initial attack of gout.

For those hyperuricemic people who are going to develop gout, acute arthritis is the most common early clinical manifestation. The

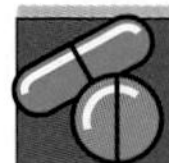

TABLE 50•5 **Medications Used to Treat Gout**

Medication	Actions and Use	Nursing Implications
colchicine	Lowers the deposition of uric acid and interferes with leukocytes and kinin formation, thus reducing inflammation; does not alter serum or urine levels of uric acid; used in acute and chronic management	*Acute management:* Administer when attack first begins; dosage increased until pain relieved or diarrhea develops *Chronic management:* Recognize that prolonged use may decrease vitamin B_{12} absorption; causes gastrointestinal upset in most patients
probenecid (Benemid)	Uricosuric agent Inhibits renal reabsorption of urates and increases the urinary excretion of uric acid; prevents tophi formation	Be alert for nausea, rash, and constipation.
allopurinol (Zyloprim)	Xanthine oxidase inhibitor Interrupts the breakdown of purines before uric acid is formed; inhibits xanthinoxidase because it blocks uric acid formation	Be alert for side effects, including bone marrow depression, vomiting, and abdominal pain.

metatarsophalangeal joint of the big toe is the most commonly affected (75% of patients). The tarsal area, ankle, or knee may also be affected. Less commonly, the wrists, fingers, and elbows may be affected. The acute attack may be triggered by trauma, alcohol ingestion, dieting, medications, surgical stress, or illness. The abrupt onset often occurs at night, awakening the patient with severe pain, redness, swelling, and warmth of the affected joint. Early attacks tend to subside spontaneously over 3 to 10 days even without treatment. The attack is followed by a symptom-free period—the intercritical stage—until the next attack, which may not come for months or years. With time, however, attacks tend to occur more frequently, involve more joints, and last longer.

Tophi are generally first noted an average of 10 years after the onset of gout. Unless urate-lowering agents are used, 70% of patients eventually develop tophaceous deposits after 20 years (Schumacher, 1996). Tophi are generally associated with more frequent and severe inflammatory episodes. Higher serum concentrations of uric acid are also associated with more extensive tophus formation. Tophi most commonly occur in the synovium, olecranon bursa, subchondral bone, infrapatellar and Achilles tendons, subcutaneous tissue on the extensor surface of the forearms, and overlying joints. They have also been found in the aortic walls, heart valves, nasal and ear cartilage, eyelids, cornea, and sclerae. Joint enlargement may cause a loss of joint motion.

Parenchymal compromise and renal stones may occur in patients with gout. The risk for urolithiasis is increased in patients with gout. The incidence of renal stones is two times higher for patients with secondary gout than for those with primary gout. Stone formation is related to the increase in serum uric acid, acidity of the urine, and urinary concentration.

Medical Management

Colchicine (oral or parenteral) or an NSAID, such as indomethacin, is used to relieve an acute attack of gout. Management of hyperuricemia, tophi, joint destruction, and renal problems is usually initiated after the acute inflammatory process has subsided. Uricosuric agents, such as probenecid, correct hyperuricemia and dissolve deposited urate. Allopurinol is also effective, but its use is limited because of the risk of toxicity. When reduction of the serum urate level is indicated, the uricosuric agents are the medications of choice. When the patient has, or is at risk for, renal insufficiency or renal calculi (kidney stones), allopurinol is the medication of choice (Table 50-5).

ARTHRITIS ASSOCIATED WITH INFECTIOUS ORGANISMS

Arthritis, tenosynovitis, and bursitis can be associated with infectious organisms. Some inflammation of joints, tendons, and bursae is directly related to infection caused by bacterial, viral, fungal, or parasitic agents. Bacterial arthritis is the most rapidly destructive form of infectious arthritis. There are two major classes of bacterial arthritis: arthritis caused by *Neisseria gonorrheae* and nongonococcal bacterium. Most prevalent of the nongonococcal agents include *Staphylococcus aureus* and the various streptococcal variants. Less common pathogens are related to syphilis, tuberculosis, leprosy, fungi (particularly coccidiomycosis), mycoplasmas, and viral agents, such as rubella, parvovirus, and hepatitis B.

Clinical Manifestations

The characteristic symptom is acute onset of a warm, swollen joint. Culture of the bacterium from the synovial fluid confirms the diagnosis. This condition is a medical emergency necessitating early diagnosis and appropriate treatment to eliminate the causative organism; otherwise, the joint may be destroyed relatively quickly.

NEOPLASMS AND NEUROVASCULAR, BONE, AND EXTRA-ARTICULAR DISORDERS

Primary neoplasms of joints, tendon sheaths, and bursae are rare. Most neoplasms are benign, arising from the synovium. These benign tumors include lipoma, hemangioma, and fibroma and tumor-like lesions, such as ganglion, bursitis, and synovial cyst. Malignant tumors include primary tumors, such as synovial and bone sarcomas, and secondary involvement as manifestations of joint invasion by leukemia, lymphoma, and myeloma or metastasis. Neoplasms present as back or neck pain.

Neurovascular disorders include the compression syndromes, such as those with peripheral entrapment (carpal tunnel syndrome), radiculopathy, and spinal stenosis. Raynaud's phenomenon or disease and erythromelalgia are also included in this category.

Bone and cartilage disorders include osteoporosis, osteomalacia, hypertrophic osteoarthropathy, diffuse idiopathic skeletal hyperostosis, Paget's disease, osteonecrosis, avascular necrosis, costochondritis, osteolysis or chondrolysis, and biomechanical or anatomic abnormalities. Notably, these conditions involve destruction, infection, or remodeling of bone.

Extra-articular rheumatism is a descriptive term for a group of conditions affecting structures other than the joints. Included are general and regional pain syndromes, low back pain and intervertebral disk disorders, tendonitis and bursitis, and ganglion cysts.

Fibromyalgia, a generalized pain syndrome, is a poorly understood chronic condition characterized by diffuse musculoskeletal aching and pain, fatigue, morning stiffness, and disturbed sleep. Although many patients complain of joint pain and may have some mild joint tenderness, there is no evidence of joint swelling or an inflammatory or degenerative process. Patients do, however, have multiple tender points in specific areas. Disturbances of non-REM sleep, mechanical stresses on the lumbar and cervical spine, emotional distress, and disturbance of central nervous system endorphins and enkephalins are among the hypothesized causes of this disorder. Fibromyalgia is not progressive. The difficulty in diagnosis and the chronic nature of the pain make the nursing care of these patients especially important. Support includes reassurance that although the pain can be severe at times, pain relief is possible, and fibromyalgia is neither deforming nor crippling. Tricyclic antidepressants are used at bedtime to increase the amount of non-REM sleep. The focus is on maintaining activity and helping patients learn to continue activity despite discomfort. A regular conditioning program, such as walking, keeps muscles toned. Relaxation and stress-management techniques are important treatment modalities. Self-management programs, such as those offered through the Arthritis Foundation, can be beneficial.

OTHER DISORDERS

The last category in the classification of the rheumatic diseases is aptly labeled "miscellaneous" disorders because it contains a mix of disorders frequently associated with arthritis and other conditions. These disorders include the direct result of trauma (including internal derangement and loose bodies of joints), pancreatic disease (related to avascular necrosis or osteonecrosis), sarcoidosis (a multisystem disorder particularly of the lymph nodes and lungs), and palindromic rheumatism (an uncommon variety of recurring and acute arthritis and periarthritis with symptom-free periods of days to months that in some may progress to RA). Other conditions include villonodular synovitis, chronic active hepatitis, and drug-related rheumatic syndromes. The nursing interventions related to these varied conditions are specific to the multisystemic problems experienced by the patient. However, the musculoskeletal components should not be neglected nor overlooked.

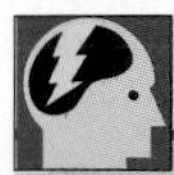

Critical Thinking Exercises

1. You are caring for a 46-year-old woman after a second knee replacement because of RA. She depends on other family members for assistance with most activities because her hands, hips, and knees are severely affected. She tells you that she does not want to be a burden on her family any longer. Explore possible self-care strategies you could suggest she try during her hospitalization and when she is recovering at home.

2. As a nurse in an immunology clinic, you receive a call from a young woman who has just been informed that her sister has been diagnosed with SLE. She is very concerned about her own risks and those of her children for developing this disorder. How would you respond to her concerns and fears?

3. An elderly woman is admitted for surgery to treat suspected cancer of the colon. She has a history of OA. How would you modify your care of this patient because of the OA?

4. An NSAID has been prescribed for your patient because of RA. What instructions and recommendations would you give to the patient to ensure safe administration of this medication? If the patient tells you that she has a hard time remembering whether she has taken her medication, how would you modify or focus your instructions?

References and Selected Readings

BOOKS

Fries, J. F. (1995). *Arthritis: A take care of yourself health guide for understanding your arthritis.* Reading, MA: Addison-Wesley.

Klippel, J. H. (Ed.). (1997). *Primer of rheumatic diseases* (11th ed.). Atlanta: Arthritis Foundation.

Nadler, S. (1997). Arthritis and other connective tissue diseases. In M. L. Sipski & C. J. Alexander (Eds.). (1997). *Sexual function in people with disability and chronic illness* (pp. 261–278). Gaithersburg, MD: Aspen.

Pigg, J. S., Driscoll, P. W., & Caniff, R. (1985). *Rheumatology nursing: A problem-oriented approach.* Albany, NY: Delmar.

Wegener, S. T. (Ed.). *Clinical care in the rheumatic diseases.* Atlanta: American College of Rheumatology.

JOURNALS

Asterisks indicate nursing research articles.

General

Beehrle, D. M., & Evans, D. (1999). A review of NSAID complications: Gastrointestinal and more. *Lippincott's Primary Care Practice, 3*(3), 305–315.

Bello, C. E., & Garrett, S. D. (1999). Therapeutic issues in oral glucocorticoid use. *Lippincott's Primary Care Practice, 3*(3), 333–341.

*Burma, M. R., Rachow, J. W., Kolluri, S., & Saag, K. G. (1996). Methotrexate patient education: A quality improvement study. *Arthritis Care Research, 9*(3), 216–222.

Farhey, Y., & Hess, E. V. (1997). Mixed connective tissue disease. *Arthritis Care Research, 10*(5), 333–342.

Pannush, R. S., & Arend, W. P. (1997). Emerging role of biologic therapies for treatment of rheumatic disease. *Journal of the American Medical Association, 277*(23), 1899–1900.

Polisson, R. (1996). Nonsteroidal anti-inflammatory drugs: Practical and theoretical consideration in their selection. *American Journal of Medicine, 100*(S2A), 2A-31S–2A-36S.

Shmerling, R. H. (1996). Rheumatic disease: Choosing the most useful diagnostic tests. *Geriatrics, 51*(11), 22–32.

Arthritis

*Ailinger, R. L., & Dear, M. R. (1997). An examination of the self-care needs of clients with rheumatoid arthritis. *Rehabilitation Nursing, 22*(3), 135–140.

*Allaire, S. H. (1996). Gender and disability associated with arthritis: Difference and issues. *Arthritis Care Research, 9*(6), 435–440.

*Allaire, S. H., Anderson, J. J., & Meenan, R. F. (1996). Reducing work disability associated with rheumatoid arthritis: Identification of additional risk factors and persons likely to benefit from intervention. *Arthritis Care Research, 9*(5), 349–357.

Bautch, J. C., Malone, D. G., & Vailas, A. C. (1997). Effects of exercise on knee joints with osteoarthritis: A pilot study of biologic markers. *Arthritis Care Research, 10*(1), 48–55.
Cash, J. M., & Wilder, R. L. (1995). Refractory rheumatoid arthritis: Therapeutic options. *Rheumatic Diseases Clinics of North America, 21*(1), 1–18.
Cicuttini, F. M., & Spector, T. D. (1995). Osteoarthritis in the aged. *Drugs and Aging, 6*(5), 409–420.
Crowther, C. L. (1999). COX-2 inhibitors. *Lippincott's Primary Care Practice, 3*(4), 394–396.
Dowdy, S. W., et al. (1996). Gender and psychological well-being of persons with rheumatoid arthritis. *Arthritis Care Research, 9*(6), 449–456.
Fiddler, M. A. (1997). Rheumatoid arthritis and pregnancy: Issues for consideration in clinical management. *Arthritis Care Research, 10*(4), 264–272.
Gerber, L. H., & Hicks, J. E. (1995). Surgical and rehabilitation options in the treatment of the rheumatoid arthritis patient resistant to pharmacologic agents. *Rheumatic Diseases Clinics of North America, 21*(1), 19–39.
Hartzheim, L. A., & Gross, G. L. (1998). Rheumatoid arthritis: A case study. *Nursing Clinics of North America, 33*(4), 595–602.
Hewlett, S., Young, P., & Kirwan, J. (1995). Dissatisfaction, disability, and rheumatoid arthritis. *Arthritis Care Research, 8*(1), 4–9.
Katz, P. P., & Criswell, L. A. (1996). Differences in symptom reports between men and women with rheumatoid arthritis. *Arthritis Care Research, 9*(6), 441–448.
Kellick, K. A., Martins–Richards, J., & Chow, C. (1998). Management of arthritis. *Lippincott's Primary Care Practice, 2*(1), 66–80.
Kirwan, J. R., & lLim, K. K. T. (1996). Low dose corticosteroids in early rheumatoid arthritis: Can these drugs slow disease progression? *Drugs and Aging, 8*(3), 157–161.
Krug, B. (1997). Rheumatoid arthritis and osteoarthritis: A basic comparison. *Orthopaedic Nursing, 16*(5), 73–75.
Lozada, D. M., & Altman, R. D. (1997). Chondroprotection in osteoarthritis. *Bulletin on the Rheumatic Diseases, 46*(7), 5–7.
Mahat, G. (1990). Rheumatoid arthritis. *American Journal of Nursing, 98*(12), 42–43.
Mandell, B. F., & Lipani, J. (1995). Refractory osteoarthritis: Differential diagnosis and therapy. *Rheumatic Diseases Clinics of North America, 21*(1), 163–178.
Moreland, L. W., et al. (1997). Treatment of rheumatoid arthritis with a recombinant human tumor necrosis factor receptor. *New England Journal of Medicine, 337*(3), 141–147.
Oddis, C. V. (1996). New perspectives on osteoarthritis. *American Journal of Medicine, 100*(Suppl 2A), 105–155.
Peck, B. (1998). Rheumatoid arthritis: Early intervention can change outcomes. *Advance for Nurse Practitioners, 6*(7), 34–38, 41.
Pigg, J. S. (1997). Case management of the patient with arthritis. *Orthopaedic Nursing, 16*(2), 33–40.
Ross, C. (1997). A comparison of osteoarthritis and rheumatoid arthritis: Diagnosis and treatment. *Nurse Practitioner, 22*(9), 20–41.
Schumacher, H. R. (1996). Crystal-induced arthritis: An overview. *American Journal of Medicine, 100*(Suppl 2A), 46S–52S.
Semble, E. L. (1995). Rheumatoid arthritis: New approaches for its evaluation and management. *Archives of Physical Medicine and Rehabilitation, 76,* 190–201.

Systemic Lupus Erythematosus

Boumpas, D., et al. (1995). Systemic lupus erythematosus: Emerging concepts. Part 2: Dermatologic and joint disease, the anti-phospholipids antibody syndrome, pregnancy and hormonal therapy, morbidity, mortality, and pathogenesis. *Annals of Internal Medicine, 123*(1), 42–53.
*Failla, S., Kuper, B. C., Nick, T. G., & Lee, F. A. (1996). Adjustment of women with systemic lupus erythematosus. *Applied Nursing Research, 9*(2), 87–96.
Fessler, B. J., & Boumpas, D. T. (1995). Severe major organ involvement in systemic lupus erythematosus: Diagnosis and management. *Rheumatic Diseases Clinics of North America, 21*(1), 81–98.
Johnson, B. (1999). Systemic lupus erythematosus. *American Journal of Nursing, 99*(1), 40–41.
Karasz, A., & Ouellette, S. C. (1995). Rose strain and psychological well-being in women with systemic lupus erythematosus. *Women and Health, 23*(3), 41–57.
National Institutes of Health, National Institute of Arthritis and Musculoskeletal and Skin Diseases. *Handout on Health–Systemic Lupus Erythematosus,* 1998.
Ulak, L. J. (1995). Special nursing considerations for SLE patients. *MedSurg Nursing, 4*(2), 146–148.

Other Specific Rheumatic Diseases

Gordon, S., & Morrison, C. (1998). Fibromyalgia and its primary care implications. *MedSurg Nursing, 7*(4), 207–213, 216.
Halverson, P. B. (1997). The spondyloarthropathies. *Orthopedic Nursing, 16*(4), 21–27.
Legerton, C. W. III, Smith, E. A., & Silver, R. M. (1995). Systemic sclerosis (scleroderma). Clinical management of its major complications. *Rheumatic Diseases Clinics of North America, 21*(1), 203–216.
Simms, R. W. (1996). Fibromyalgia syndrome: Current concepts in pathophysiology, clinical features, and management. *Arthritis Care Research, 9*(4), 315–328.
Smith, W. A. (1998). Fibromyalgia syndrome. *Nursing Clinics of North American, 33*(4), 653–669.
St. Pierre, J. (1998). Understanding fibromyalgia syndrome. *American Journal of Nursing, 98*(10), 17–18.
Stone, J. H., & Hellmann, D. B. (1998). Giant cell arteritis. When to suspect, how to treat. *Women's Health in Primary Care, 1*(4), 333–343.
Viitanen, J. V., & Suni, J. (1995). Management principles of physiotherapy in ankylosing spondylitis: Which treatments are effective? *Physiotherapy, 81*(6), 322–329.
Wilke, W. S., & Hoffman, G. S. (1995). Treatment of corticosteroid-resistant giant cell arteritis. *Rheumatic Diseases Clinics of North America, 21*(1), 59–71.

Resources

Ankylosing Spondylitis Association, 511 N. La Cienge, Suite 216, Los Angeles, CA 90048; 1-800-777-8189
The Arthritis Foundation, 1330 West Peachtree St., Atlanta, GA 30309; 1-404-872-7100 or 1-800-283-7800 (information line); www.arthritis.org
Association of Rheumatology Health Professionals, 60 Executive Park South, Suite 150, Atlanta, GA 30329; 1-404-633-3777; E-mail: awiens@rheumatology.org
Lupus Foundation of America, Inc., 1300 Picard Drive, Suite 200, Rockville, MD 20850-4303; 1-800-558-0121; www.lupus.org/lupus
National Institute of Arthritis and Musculoskeletal and Skin Diseases, National Institutes of Health, Building 31, Room 4C05, 31 Center Drive, Bethesda, MD 20892-2350; 1-301-496-8188, www.nih.gov/niams
Sjögren's Syndrome Foundation, Inc., 333 N. Broadway, Jericho, NY 11753; 1-516-933-6365; www.sjögrens.com
United Scleroderma Foundation, Inc., P.O. Box 399, Watsonville, CA 95077; 1-408-728-2202; www.scleroderma.com

UNIT

12

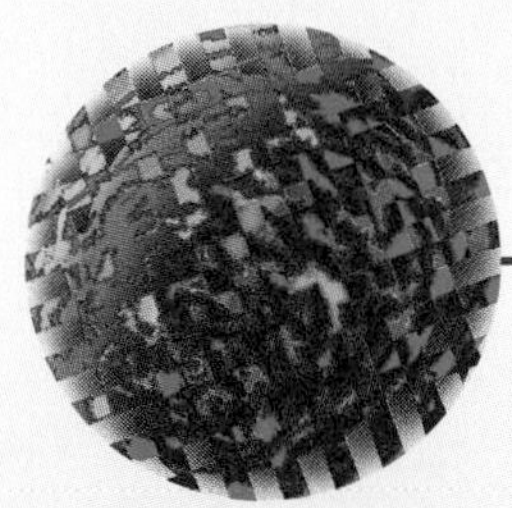

Integumentary Function

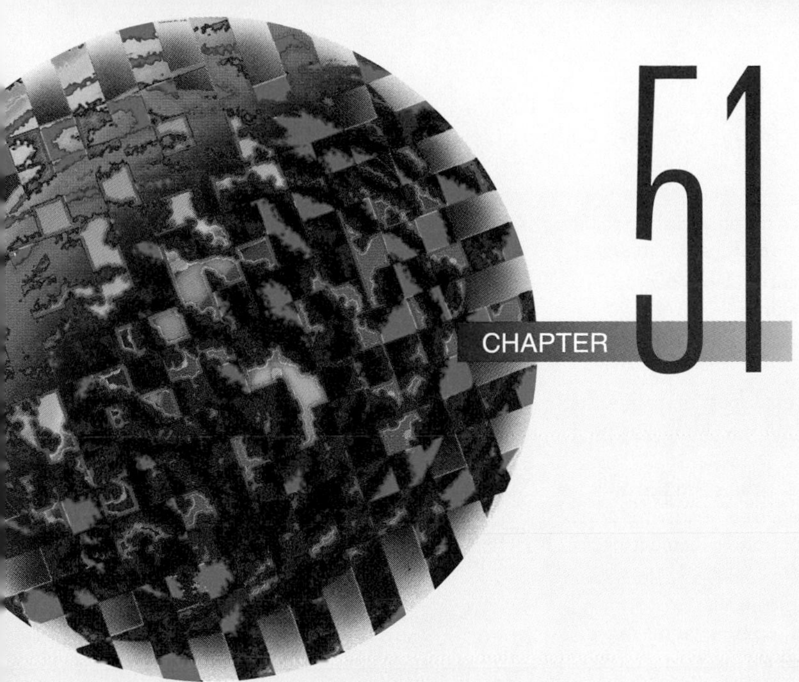

CHAPTER 51

Assessment of Integumentary Function

Learning Objectives

On completion of this chapter, the learner will be able to:

1. Identify the structures and functions of the skin.
2. Differentiate the composition and function of each skin layer: epidermis, dermis, and subcutaneous tissue.
3. Identify and describe primary and secondary skin lesions and their pattern and distribution.
4. Recognize common skin eruptions and manifestations associated with systemic disease.
5. Describe the normal aging process of the skin and skin changes common to elderly patients.
6. List appropriate questions that will help elicit information during an assessment of the skin.
7. Describe the components of physical assessment most useful when examining the skin, hair, and nails.
8. Discuss common skin tests and procedures used in diagnosing skin and related disorders.

Skin problems are encountered frequently in nursing practice. Indeed, skin-related disorders account for up to 10% of all ambulatory patient visits in this country. Because the skin mirrors the general condition of the patient, many systemic conditions may be accompanied by dermatologic manifestations.

The psychological stress of illness or various personal and family problems is commonly exhibited outwardly as dermatologic problems. Any hospitalized patient may suddenly develop itching and a rash secondary to the treatment regimen. In certain systemic conditions, such as hepatitis and cancer, dermatologic manifestations may be the first sign of the disorder.

GLOSSARY

alopecia: the loss of hair from any cause

anagen phase: the active phase of hair growth

erythema: redness of the skin caused by congestion of the capillaries

hirsutism: the condition of having excessive hair growth

hyperpigmentation: increase in the melanin of the skin, resulting in an increase in pigmentation

hypopigmentation: decrease in the melanin of the skin, resulting in a loss of pigmentation

keratin: an insoluble fibrous protein that forms the outer layer of skin

lichenification: a leathery thickening of the skin

Merkel cells: cells of the epidermis that play a role in transmission of sensory messages

melanin: the substance responsible for coloration of the skin

melanocytes: the cells of the skin that produce melanin

petechiae: pinpoint red spots that appear on the skin as a result of blood leakage into the skin

rete ridges: the undulations and furrows that appear at the dermis–epidermis junction and are responsible for cementing the two layers together

sebaceous glands: glands that exist within the epidermis and secrete sebum to keep the skin soft and pliable

sebum: fatty secretion of the sebaceous glands

striae: bandlike streaks on the skin, usually purplish or white

telangiectases: red marks on the skin caused by stretching of the superficial blood vessels

vitiligo: a condition characterized by destruction of the melanocytes in circumscribed areas of the skin, resulting in white patches. It may be localized or widespread

Wood's light: a blue light used for diagnosing skin conditions

ANATOMIC AND PHYSIOLOGIC OVERVIEW

The largest organ system of the body, the skin is indispensable for human life. Skin forms a barrier between the internal organs and the external environment and participates in many vital body functions. The skin is continuous with the mucous membrane at the external openings of the digestive, respiratory, and urogenital systems. Because skin disorders are readily visible, dermatologic complaints are commonly the primary reason for a patient to seek health care.

Anatomy of the Skin

The skin is composed of three layers: the epidermis, the dermis, and the subcutaneous tissue (Fig. 51-1). The epidermis is an outermost layer of stratified epithelial cells composed predominantly of keratinocytes. It ranges in thickness from about 0.1 mm on the

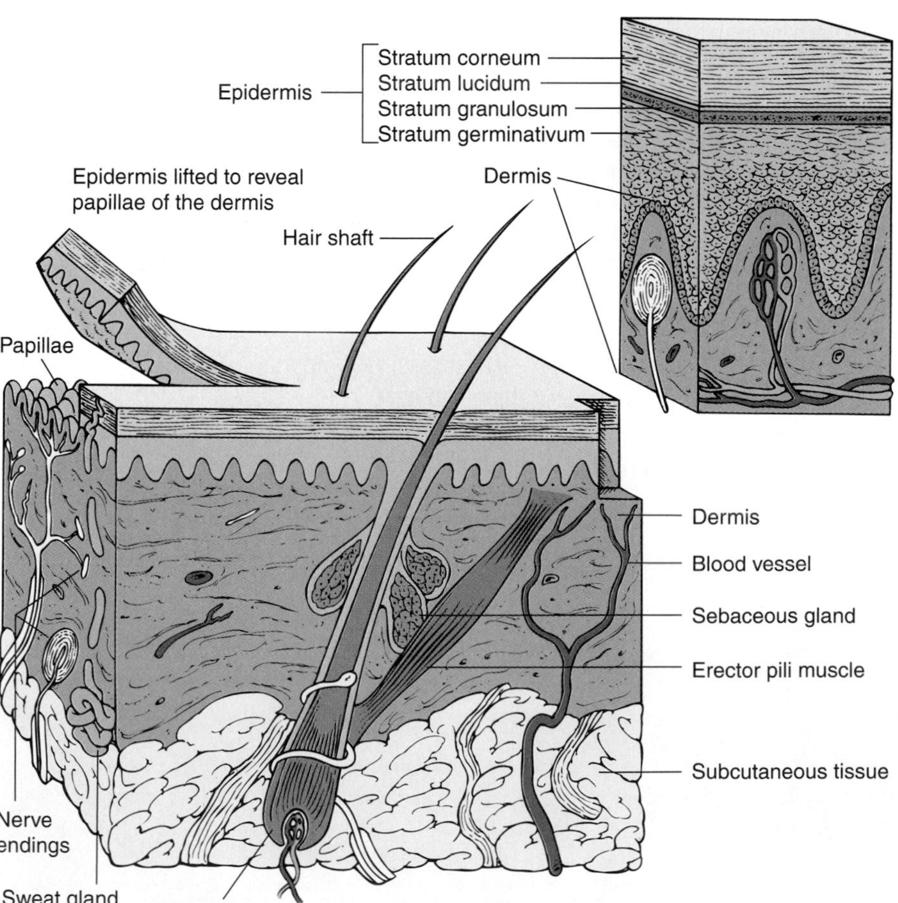

FIGURE 51•1 Anatomic structures of the skin. From Weber, J. W., & Kelley, J. (1998). *Health assessment in nursing.* Philadelphia: Lippincott-Raven.

eyelids to about 1 mm on the palms of the hands and soles of the feet. Four distinct layers compose the epidermis (in order from innermost to outermost)—the stratum germinativum, stratum granulosum, stratum lucidum, and stratum corneum. Each layer becomes more differentiated (mature and with more specific functions) as it rises from the basal stratum germinativum layer to the outermost stratum corneum layer.

The epidermis, which is contiguous with the mucous membranes and the lining of the ear canals, consists of live, continuously dividing cells covered on the surface by dead cells that were originally deeper in the dermis but were pushed upward by the newly developing, more differentiated cells underneath. This external layer is almost completely replaced every 3 to 4 weeks. The dead cells contain large amounts of **keratin**, an insoluble, fibrous protein that forms the outer barrier of the skin and has the capacity to repel pathogens and prevent excessive fluid loss from the body. Keratin is the principal hardening ingredient of the hair and nails.

Melanocytes are the special cells of the epidermis that are primarily involved in producing the pigment **melanin**, which colors the skin and hair. The more melanin, the darker the color. Most of the skin of dark-skinned people and the darker areas of the skin on light-skinned people (eg, the nipple) contain larger amounts of this pigment. Normal skin color depends on race and varies from pale pink to dark brown. Systemic disease affects skin color as well. For example, the skin appears bluish when there is insufficient oxygenation of the blood, yellow-green in people with jaundice, or red or flushed when there is inflammation or fever (Table 51-1).

Production of melanin is controlled by a hormone secreted from the hypothalamus of the brain called melanocyte-stimulating hormone. It is believed that melanin can absorb ultraviolet light in sunlight.

Two other cells are common to the epidermis: Merkel and Langerhans cells. **Merkel cells** are the receptors that transmit stimuli to the axon via a chemical synapse. Langerhans cells are believed to play a significant role in cutaneous immune system reactions. These accessory cells of the afferent immune system process invading antigens and transport the antigens to the lymph system to activate the T lymphocytes.

The epidermis is modified in different areas of the body. It is thickest over the palms of the hands and soles of the feet and contains increased amounts of keratin. The thickness of the epidermis can increase with use and can result in calluses forming on the hands or corns forming on the feet.

The junction of the epidermis and dermis is an area of many undulations and furrows called **rete ridges**. This junction anchors the epidermis to the dermis and permits the free exchange of essential nutrients between the two layers. This interlocking between the dermis and epidermis produces ripples on the surface of the skin. On the fingertips, these ripples are called fingerprints. They are a person's most individual characteristic, and they rarely change.

The dermis makes up the largest portion of the skin, providing strength and structure. It is composed of two layers: papillary and reticular. The papillary dermis lies directly beneath the epidermis and is composed primarily of fibroblast cells capable of producing one form of collagen, a component of connective tissue. The reticular layer lies beneath the papillary layer and also produces collagen and elastic bundles. The dermis is also made up of blood and lymph vessels, nerves, sweat and sebaceous glands, and hair roots. The dermis is often referred to as the "true skin."

The subcutaneous tissue or hypodermis is the innermost layer of the skin. It is primarily adipose tissue, which provides a cushion between the skin layers, muscles, and bones. It promotes skin mobility, molds body contours, and insulates the body. Fat is deposited and distributed according to the person's gender and in part accounts for the difference in body shape between men and women. Overeating results in increased deposition of fat beneath the skin. The subcutaneous tissues and amount of fat deposited are important factors in body temperature regulation.

Hair

An outgrowth of the skin, hair is present over the entire body except for the palms and soles. The hair consists of a root formed in the dermis and a hair shaft that projects beyond the skin. It grows in a cavity called a hair follicle. The proliferation of cells in the bulb of the hair causes the hair to form (see Fig. 51-1).

Hair follicles undergo cycles of growth and rest. The rate of growth varies; beard growth is the most rapid, followed by hair on the scalp, axillae, thighs, and eyebrows. The growth or **anagen** phase may last up to 6 years for scalp hair, whereas the telogen or resting phase is approximately 4 months. During telogen, hair sheds from the body. The hair follicle recycles into the growing phase spontaneously, or it can be induced by plucking out hairs. Growing and resting hair can be found side by side on all parts of the body. About 90% of the 100,000 hair follicles on a normal scalp are in the growing phase at any one time, and 50 to 100 scalp hairs are shed each day.

In certain locations on the body, hair growth is controlled by sex hormones. The most vivid example is the growth of hair on the face (beard and mustache), chest, and back, which is controlled by the male hormones known as androgens.

Hair in different parts of the body serves different functions. The hairs of the eyes (eyebrows and lashes), nose, and ears filter out dust, bugs, and airborne debris. The hair of the skin provides thermal insulation in lower animals. This function is enhanced during cold or fright by piloerection (hairs standing on end), caused by contraction of the tiny erector muscles attached to the hair follicle. The piloerector response that occurs in humans is probably vestigial (rudimentary).

Hair color is supplied by varying amounts of melanin within the hair shaft. Gray or white hair reflects the loss of pigment. Hair quantity and distribution can be affected by endocrine conditions. For example, Cushing's syndrome causes **hirsutism** (excessive hair growth, especially in women); hypothyroidism (underactive thyroid) causes changes in hair texture. In many cases, chemotherapy and radiation therapy cause hair thinning or weakening of the hair shaft, resulting in partial or complete **alopecia** (hair loss) from the scalp as well as from other parts of the body.

Nails

On the dorsal surface of the fingers and toes, a hard, transparent plate of keratin, called the nail, overlies the skin. The nail grows from its root, which lies under a thin fold of skin called the cuticle. The nail protects the fingers and toes by preserving their highly developed sensory function, which promotes certain fine functions, such as picking up small objects.

Nail growth is continuous throughout life, with an average growth of 0.1 mm daily. Growth is faster in fingernails than toenails and tends to slow with aging. Complete renewal of a fingernail takes about 170 days, whereas toenail renewal takes 12 to 18 months.

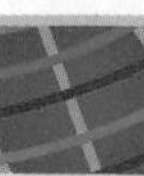

TABLE 51•1 Selected Cutaneous Manifestations of Systematic Diseases

Common cutaneous manifestations of systemic diseases include *pruritus* (itching), which may result from chronic renal disease, scabies, pediculosis (lice), obstructive biliary disease with jaundice, Hodgkin's and non-Hodgkin's lymphoma, or medication reactions; *pallor,* which suggests anemia or a cardiopulmonary disorder; and *skin thickening and hardening,* such as that which occurs with scleroderma and dermatomyositis.

	Manifestation	Systemic Disease
	Plaques and scales on the nose, chin, ears, scalp, malar (cheek) area; telangiectasias (red marks on the skin caused by stretching of the superficial blood vessels)	Connective tissue disorder (such as systemic lupus erythematosis)
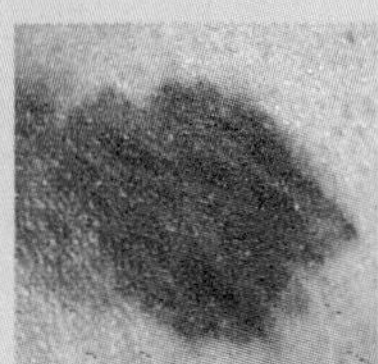 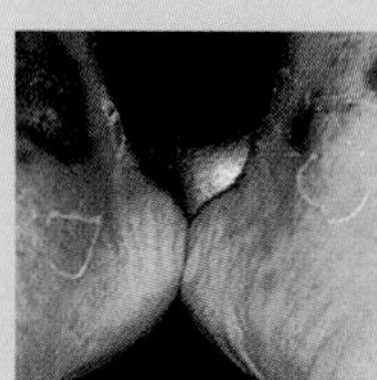	Ecchymosis (bruise) and purpura (bleeding into the skin)	Platelet disorder, vessel fragility
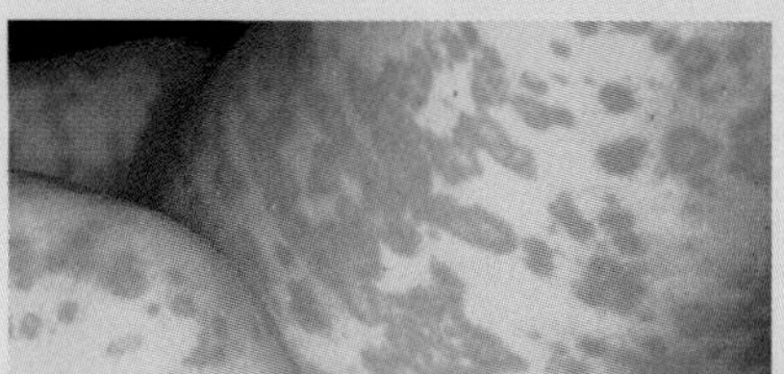	Urticaria (wheals or hives)	Infections, allergic reactions
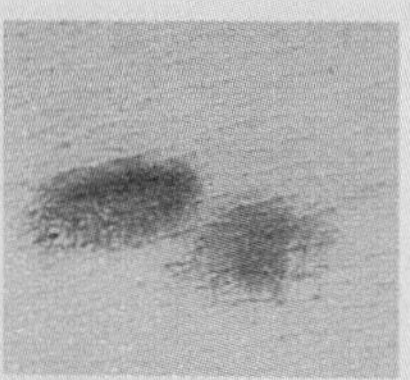 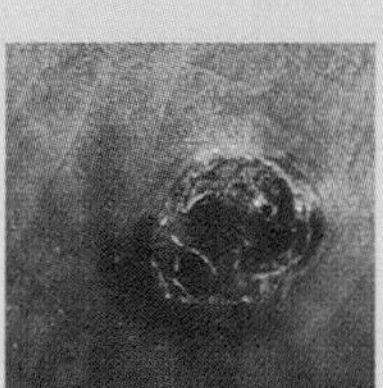	Cutaneous lesions: blue-red or dark brown plaques and nodules	Kaposi's sarcoma
	Macular, tan café-au-lait spots	Neurocutaneous disorders, such as neurofibromatosis (von Recklinghausen's disease)
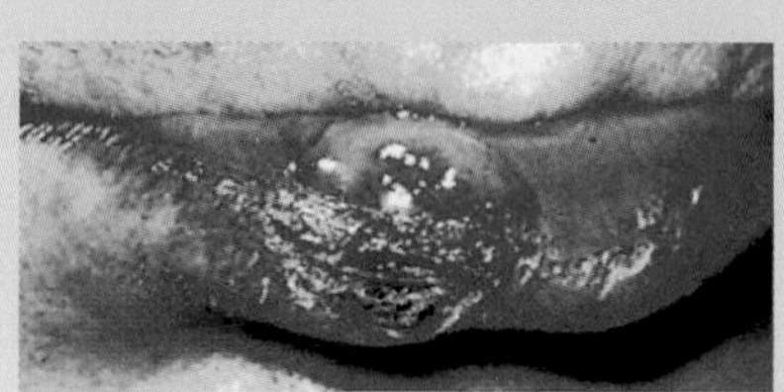	Painless chancre or ulcerated lesion	Syphilis

Glands

There are two types of skin glands—sebaceous glands and sweat glands (see Fig. 51-1). The **sebaceous glands** are associated with hair follicles. The ducts of the sebaceous glands empty **sebum** (an oily secretion) onto the space between the hair follicle and the hair shaft. For each hair there is a sebaceous gland, the secretions of which lubricate the hair and render the skin soft and pliable.

Sweat glands are found in the skin over most of the body surface. They are heavily concentrated in the palms of the hands and soles of the feet. Only the glans penis, the margins of the lips, the external ear, and the nail bed are devoid of sweat glands. Sweat glands are subclassified into two categories: eccrine and apocrine.

The eccrine sweat glands are found in all areas of the skin. Their ducts open directly onto the skin surface. The thin, watery secretion called sweat is produced in the basal coiled portion of the eccrine gland and is released into its narrow duct. Sweat is composed predominantly of water and contains about half of the salt content of the blood plasma. Sweat is released from eccrine glands in response to elevated ambient temperature and elevated body temperature. The rate of sweat secretion is under the control of the sympathetic nervous system. Excessive sweating of the palms and soles, axillae, forehead, and other areas may occur in response to pain and stress.

The apocrine sweat glands are larger, and in contrast to that of the eccrine glands their secretion contains parts of the secretory cells. They are located in the axillae, anal region, scrotum, and labia majora. Their ducts generally open onto hair follicles. The apocrine glands become active at puberty. In women, they enlarge and recede with each menstrual cycle. Apocrine glands produce a milky sweat that is broken down by bacteria to produce the characteristic underarm odor.

Specialized apocrine glands called ceruminous glands are found in the external ear, where they produce cerumen (wax).

Functions of the Skin

Protection

The skin covering most of the body is only about 1 or 2 mm thick, but it provides very effective protection against invasion by bacteria and other foreign matter. The thickened skin of the palms and soles protects against the effects of the constant trauma that occurs in these areas.

The epidermis is the outermost layer of the skin and is composed of several layers of keratanocytes that change character as they migrate to the surface. The stratum corneum, the outer layer of the epidermis, provides the most effective barrier to both epidermal water loss and penetration of environmental factors such as chemicals, microbes, insect bites, and other trauma.

Various lipids are synthesized in the stratum corneum and are the basis for the barrier function of this layer. These are long-chain lipids that are better suited than phospholipids for water resistance. The presence of these lipids in the stratum corneum serves to create a relatively impermeable barrier both for water egress and for the ingress of toxins, microbes, and other substances that come in contact with the surface of the skin.

Some substances do penetrate the skin but meet resistance in trying to move through the channels between the cell layers of the stratum corneum. Microbes and fungi, which are part of the body's normal flora, cannot penetrate unless there is a break in the skin barrier.

The dermal–epidermal junction is the basal layer, which is composed of collagen. The basal layer serves four functions. It acts as a scaffold for tissue organization and a template for regeneration, it provides selective permeability for filtration of serum, it is a physical barrier between different types of cells, and it adheres the epithelium to underlying cell layers.

Sensation

The receptor endings of nerves in the skin allow the body to constantly monitor the conditions of the immediate environment. The primary functions of the receptors in the skin are to sense temperature, pain, light touch, and pressure (or heavy touch). Different nerve endings respond to each of the different stimuli. Although the nerve endings are distributed over the entire body, they are more concentrated in some areas than in others. For example, the fingertips are more densely innervated than the skin on the back.

Water Balance

The stratum corneum (outermost layer of the epidermis) has the capacity to absorb water, thereby preventing an excessive loss of water and electrolytes from the internal body and retaining moisture in the subcutaneous tissues. When skin is damaged, as occurs with a severe burn, large quantities of fluids and electrolytes may be lost rapidly, possibly leading to circulatory collapse, shock, and death.

However, the skin is not completely impermeable to water. Small amounts of water continuously evaporate from the skin surface. This evaporation, called insensible perspiration, amounts to approximately 600 mL daily in a normal adult. Insensible water loss varies with the body and ambient temperature. In a person with a fever, this loss can increase. During immersion in water, the skin can accumulate water up to three or four times its normal weight. A common example of this is the swelling of the skin after prolonged bathing.

Temperature Regulation

The body continuously produces heat as a result of the metabolism of food, which produces energy. This heat is dissipated primarily through the skin. Three major physical processes are involved in loss of heat from the body to the environment. The first process, radiation, is the transfer of heat to another object of lower temperature situated at a distance. The second process, conduction, is the transfer of heat from the body to a cooler object in contact with it. Heat transferred by conduction to the air surrounding the body is removed by the third process, convection, which consists of movement of warm air molecules away from the body.

Evaporation from the skin aids heat loss by conduction. Heat is conducted through the skin into water molecules on its surface, causing the water to evaporate. The water on the skin surface may be from insensible perspiration, sweat, or the environment.

Normally, all of these mechanisms for heat loss are used. When the ambient temperature is very high, however, radiation and convection are ineffective, and evaporation becomes the only means for heat loss.

Under normal conditions, metabolic heat production is exactly balanced by heat loss, and the internal temperature of the body is maintained constant at approximately 37°C (98.6°F). The rate of heat loss depends primarily on the surface temperature of the skin, which is a function of the skin blood flow. Under normal conditions, the total blood circulated through the skin is approximately 450 mL/min, or 10 to 20 times the amount of blood required to provide necessary metabolites and oxygen. Blood flow through these skin vessels is controlled primarily by the sympathetic nervous system. Increased blood flow to the skin results in more heat delivered to the skin and a greater rate of heat loss from the body. In contrast, decreased skin blood flow decreases the skin temperature and helps conserve heat for the body. When the temperature of the body begins to fall, as occurs on a cold day, the blood vessels of the skin constrict, thereby reducing heat loss from the body.

Sweating is another process by which the body can regulate the rate of heat loss. Sweating does not occur until the core body temperature exceeds 37°C, regardless of skin temperature. In extremely hot environments, the rate of sweat production may be as high as 1 L/hr. Under some circumstances (eg, emotional stress), sweating may occur as a reflex and may be unrelated to the need to lose heat from the body.

Vitamin Production

Skin exposed to ultraviolet light can convert substances necessary for synthesizing vitamin D (cholecalciferol). Vitamin D is essential for preventing rickets, a condition that causes bone deformities and results from a deficiency of vitamin D, calcium, and phosphorus.

Immune Response Function

Recent research findings (Demis, 1998) indicate that several dermal cells (Langerhans cells, interleukin-1–producing keratinocytes, and subsets of T lymphocytes) are important components of the immune system. Ongoing research should more clearly define the role of these dermal cells in immune function.

Gerontologic Considerations

The skin undergoes many physiologic changes associated with normal aging. A lifetime of excessive sun exposure, systemic diseases, poor nutrition, and medications can enhance the range of skin problems and the rapidity with which skin problems appear. The outcome is an increasing vulnerability to injury and to certain diseases. Skin problems are common among older people.

Before conducting a skin assessment, the nurse needs to be aware of significant changes that occur with aging. The major changes in the skin of older people include dryness, wrinkling, uneven pigmentation, and various proliferative lesions. Cellular changes associated with aging include a thinning at the junction of the dermis and epidermis. This results in fewer anchoring sites between the two skin layers, so that even minor injury or stress to the epidermis can cause it to shear away from the dermis. This phenomenon of aging may account for the increased vulnerability of aged skin to trauma. With increasing age, the epidermis and dermis thin and flatten, causing wrinkles, sags, and overlapping skin folds (Fig. 51-2).

Loss of the subcutaneous tissue substances of elastin, collagen, and subcutaneous fat diminishes the protection and cushioning of underlying tissues and organs, decreases muscle tone, and results in the loss of the insulating properties of fat.

Cellular replacement slows as a result of aging. As the dermal layers thin, the skin becomes fragile and transparent. The blood supply to the skin also changes with age. Vessels, especially the capillary loops, decrease in number and size. These vascular changes contribute to the delayed wound healing commonly seen in the elderly patient. In addition, both sweat and sebaceous glands decrease in number and functional capacity, leading to dry and scaly skin. Reduced hormonal levels of androgens are thought to contribute to declining sebaceous gland function.

Hair growth gradually diminishes, especially over the lower legs and dorsum of the feet. Thinning is common in the scalp, axilla, and pubic hair. Other functions affected with normal aging include the barrier function, sensory perception, and thermoregulation.

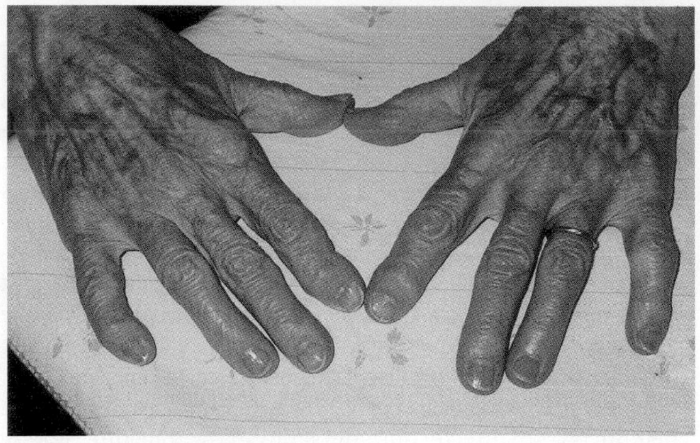

FIGURE 51•2 Hands with wrinkling and overlapping folds common to aging skin.

Photoaging, or damage from excessive sun exposure, has detrimental effects on the normal aging of skin. A lifetime of outdoor work or outdoor activities (construction workers, lifeguards, or sunbathers) without prudent use of sunscreens can lead to profound wrinkling, increased loss of elasticity, mottled pigmented areas, cutaneous atrophy, and benign or malignant lesions.

Many skin lesions are part of normal aging. Recognizing these lesions can help the examiner assist the patient to feel less anxious about changes in skin. Chart 51-1 summarizes some skin lesions that are expected to appear as the skin ages. These are all normal and require no special attention unless the skin becomes infected or irritated.

ASSESSMENT

Health History and Clinical Manifestations

When caring for patients with dermatologic disorders, the nurse obtains important information through the health history and direct observations. The nurse's skill in physical assessment and an understanding of the anatomy and function of the skin can ensure that deviations from normal are recognized, reported, and documented.

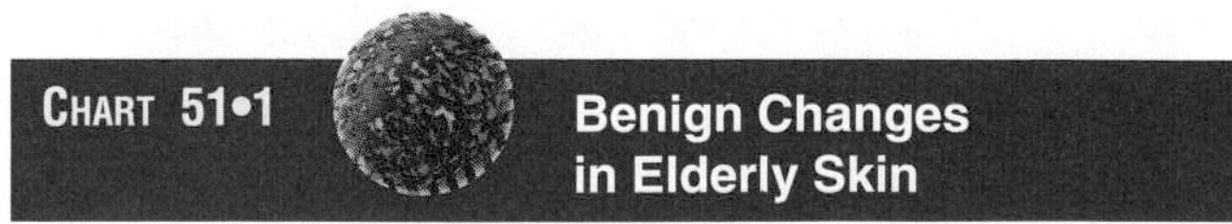

CHART 51•1 Benign Changes in Elderly Skin

- Cherry angiomas (bright red "moles")
- Diminished hair, especially on scalp and pubic area
- Dyschromias (color variations)
  - Solar lentigo (liver spots)
  - Melasma (dark discoloration of the skin)
  - Lentigines (freckles)
- Neurodermatitis (itchy spots)
- Seborrheic keratoses (crusty brown "stuck-on" patches)
- Spider angiomas
- Telangiectasias (red marks on skin caused by stretching of the superficial blood vessels)
- Wrinkles
- Xerosis (dryness)
- Xanthelasma (yellowish waxy deposits on upper eyelids)

During the health history interview, the nurse asks about any family and personal history of skin allergies, allergic reactions to food, medications, chemicals, previous skin problems, and skin cancer. The names of cosmetics, soaps, shampoos, or other personal hygiene products are obtained if there have been any recent skin problems noted with the use of these products. The health history contains specific information about the onset, signs and symptoms, location, and duration of any pain, itching, rashes, or other discomfort experienced by the patient. The accompanying assessment chart lists selected questions typically used in obtaining appropriate information.

Physical Assessment

Assessment of the skin involves the entire skin area, including the mucous membranes, scalp, hair, and nails. The skin is a reflection of a person's overall health, and alterations commonly correspond to disease in other organ systems. Inspection and palpation are the chief procedures used in examining the skin. The room must be well lighted and warm. A penlight may be used to highlight lesions. The patient completely disrobes and is adequately draped. Gloves are always worn during skin examination.

Assessing General Appearance

The general appearance of the skin is assessed by observing color, temperature, moisture, dryness, skin texture (rough or smooth), lesions, vascularity, mobility, and the condition of the hair and nails. Skin turgor, possible edema, and elasticity are assessed by palpation.

Skin color varies from person to person and ranges from ivory to deep brown. The skin of exposed portions of the body, especially in sunny, warm climates, tends to be more pigmented than the rest of the body. The vasodilation effects of fever, sunburn, and inflammation produce a pink or reddish hue to the skin. Pallor is an absence of or a decrease in normal skin tones and vascularity and is best observed in the conjunctivae.

The bluish hue of cyanosis indicates cellular hypoxia and is easily observed in the extremities, nail beds, lips, and mucous membranes. Jaundice, a yellowing of the skin, is directly related to elevations in serum bilirubin and is often noted in the sclerae and mucous membranes (Fig. 51-3).

ASSESSMENT
PATIENT HISTORY: SKIN DISORDERS

Patient history relevant to skin disorders may be obtained by asking the following questions:

When did you first notice this skin problem (also investigate duration and intensity)?
Has it occurred previously?
Are there any other symptoms?
What site was first affected?
What did the rash or lesion look like when it first appeared?
Where and how fast did it spread?
Do you have any itching, burning, tingling, or crawling sensations?
Is there any loss of sensation?
Is the problem worse at a particular time or season?
How do you think it started?
Do you have a history of hay fever, asthma, hives, eczema, or allergies?
Who in your family has skin problems or rashes?
Did the eruptions appear after certain foods were eaten? Which foods?
When the problem occurred, had you recently had alcohol?
What relation do you think there may be between a specific event and the outbreak of the rash or lesion?
What medications are you taking?
What topical medication (ointment, cream, salve) have you put on the lesion (including over-the-counter medications)?
What skin products or cosmetics do you use?
What is your occupation?
What in your immediate environment (plants, animals, chemicals, infections) might be precipitating this problem? Is there anything new, or are there any changes in the environment?
Does anything touching your skin cause a rash?
Is there anything else you wish to talk about in regard to this problem?
How has this affected you (or your life)?

Assessing Patients With Dark Skin

The color gradations that occur in dark-skinned people are largely determined by genetic transmission; they may be described as light, medium, or dark. In dark-skinned people, melanin is produced at a faster rate and in larger quantities than in lighter-skinned people. Healthy, dark skin has a reddish base or undertone. The buccal mucosa, tongue, lips, and nails normally appear pink.

When examining the dark-skinned patient, it is important to have good lighting and to examine the skin and the nail beds as well as the mouth. The degree of pigmentation of the dark-skinned patient's skin may affect the appearance of a lesion. Lesions may be black, purple, or gray instead of the tan or red seen in light-skinned patients.

In general, people with dark skin suffer the same skin conditions as those with light skin. However, they are less likely to have skin cancer and scabies but more likely to have keloid or scar formation and disorders resulting from occlusion or blockage of hair follicles.

Table 51-2 provides an overall view of color changes in light-skinned and dark-skinned people, and the following information provides specific guidelines for assessing dark skin.

ERYTHEMA

Because dark skin tends to assume a purplish-grayish cast when an inflammatory process is present, it may be difficult to detect **erythema** (redness of the skin caused by congestion of capillaries). To determine possible inflammation, the skin is palpated for increased warmth or for smoothness (edema) or hardness. The adjacent lymph nodes are also palpated.

RASH

In instances of pruritus (itching), the patient should be asked to indicate which areas of the body are involved. The skin is then stretched gently to decrease the reddish tone and make the rash stand out. The differences in skin texture are then assessed by running the tips of the fingers lightly over the skin. Usually, the borders of the rash can be felt. The patient's mouth and ears are included in the examination. (Sometimes rubeola, or measles, causes a red cast to appear on the tip of the ears.) Finally, the patient's temperature is assessed and the lymph nodes are palpated.

CYANOSIS

When a person with dark skin is in shock, the skin usually assumes a grayish cast. To detect cyanosis, the areas around the mouth and lips and over the cheekbones and earlobes should be observed. Other indications of decreased tissue perfusion include

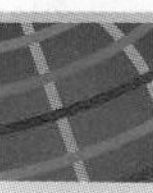

TABLE 51•2 **Color Changes in Light and Dark Skin**

Etiology	Light Skin	Dark Skin
Pallor		
Anemia—decreased hematocrit Shock—decreased perfusion, vasoconstriction	Generalized pallor	Brown skin appears yellow-brown, dull; black skin appears ashen gray, dull (observe areas with least pigmentation: conjunctivae, mucous membranes)
Local arterial insufficiency	Marked localized pallor (lower extremities, especially when elevated)	Ashen gray, dull; cool to palpation
Albinism—total absence of pigment melanin	Whitish pink	Tan, cream, white
Vitiligo—a condition characterized by destruction of the melanocytes in circumscribed areas of the skin. It may be localized or widespread.	Patchy, milky white spots, often symmetric bilaterally	Same
Cyanosis		
Increased amount of unoxygenated hemoglobin: Central—chronic heart and lung disease cause arterial desaturation	Dusky blue	Dark but dull, lifeless. Only severe cyanosis is apparent in skin (observe conjunctiva, oral mucosa, nail beds).
Peripheral—exposure to cold, anxiety	Nail beds dusky	
Erythema		
Hyperemia—increased blood flow through engorged arterial vessels, such as in inflammation, fever, alcohol intake, blushing	Red, bright pink	Purplish tinge, but difficult to see (palpate for increased warmth with inflammation, taut skin, and hardening of deep tissues)
Polycythemia—increased red blood cells, capillary stasis	Ruddy blue in face, oral mucosa, conjunctiva, hands and feet	Well concealed by pigment (observe for redness in lips)
Carbon monoxide poisoning	Bright, cherry red in face and upper torso	Cherry red nail beds, lips, and oral mucosa
Venous stasis—decreased blood flow from area, engorged venules	Dusky rubor of dependent extremities (a prelude to necrosis with pressure ulcer)	Easily masked (use palpation to identify warmth or edema)
Jaundice		
Increased serum bilirubin level, >2–3 mg/100 mL due to liver inflammation or hemolytic disease as occurs after severe burns or some infections	Yellow first in sclera, hard palate, mucous membranes and then over skin	Check sclera for yellow near limbus. Do not mistake normal yellowish fatty deposits in the periphery under eyelids for jaundice. Jaundice best noted in junction of hard and soft palate; also palms.
Carotenemia—increased level of serum carotene from ingestion of large amounts of carotene-rich foods	Yellow-orange tinge in forehead, palms and soles, nasolabial folds, but no yellowing in sclera or mucous membranes	Yellow-orange tinge in palms and soles
Uremia—renal failure causes retained urochrome pigments in the blood	Orange-green or gray overlaying pallor of anemia. May also have ecchymoses and purpura.	Easily masked (rely on laboratory and clinical findings)
Brown-Tan		
Addison's disease—cortisol deficiency stimulates increased melanin production	Bronzed appearance, an "external tan," most apparent around nipples; perineum, genitalia, and pressure points (inner thighs, buttocks, elbows, axillae)	Easily masked (rely on laboratory and clinical findings)
Café-au-lait spots—due to increased melanin pigment in basal cell layer	Tan to light brown, irregularly shaped, oval patch with well-defined borders	

cold, clammy skin, a rapid, thready pulse, and rapid, shallow respirations. When the conjunctivae of the eyelids are examined for **petechiae** (pinpoint red spots that appear on the skin as a result of blood leakage into the skin), it is important not to mistake them for normal melanin deposits.

COLOR CHANGES

Changes in skin color in dark-skinned people are noticeable and usually cause distress to the patient. For example, **hypopigmentation** (a decrease in the melanin of the skin, resulting in a loss of pigmentation), which may be due to **vitiligo** (a condition characterized by destruction of the melanocytes in circumscribed areas of the skin, resulting in white patches), may cause more concern in the dark-skinned person because it is so readily visible. **Hyperpigmentation** (an increase in the melanin of the skin, resulting in increased pigmentation) may occur after disease or injury to the skin. A pigmented nasal crease below the eye may be an external sign of allergy. However, pigmented streaks in the nails are considered normal.

Assessing Skin Lesions

Skin lesions are the most prominent characteristics of dermatologic conditions. They vary in size, shape, and cause and are classified ac-

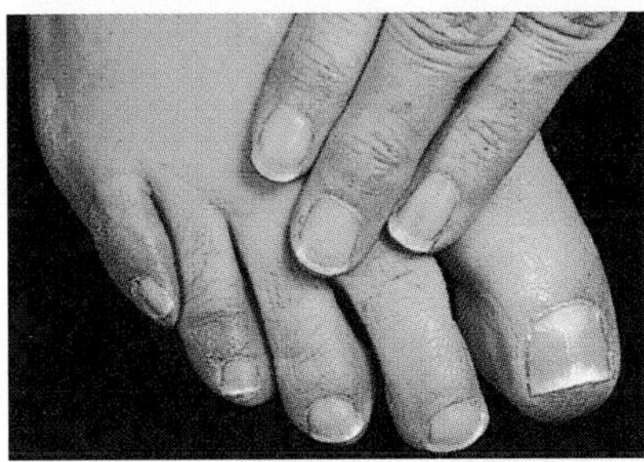
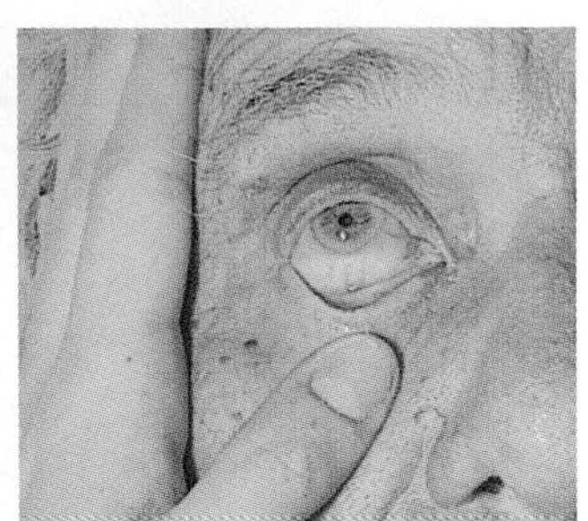

FIGURE 51•3 Examples of skin color changes: the bluish tint of cyanosis (*left*) and the yellow hue of jaundice (*right*).

cording to their appearance and origin. Skin lesions can be described as primary or secondary. Primary lesions are the initial lesions and are characteristic of the disease itself. Secondary lesions result from external causes, such as scratching, trauma, infections, or changes caused by wound healing. Depending on the stage of development, skin lesions are further categorized according to type and appearance (Chart 51-2).

A preliminary assessment of the eruption or lesion should help to identify the type of dermatosis (abnormal skin condition) and indicate whether the lesion is primary or secondary. At the same time, the anatomic distribution of the eruption should be noted, because certain diseases tend to affect certain sites of the body and are distributed in characteristic patterns and shapes (Figs. 51-4 and 51-5). To determine the extent of the regional distribution, the left and right sides of the body should be compared while the color and shape of the lesions are noted. After observation, the lesions are palpated to determine their texture, shape, and border and to see if they are soft or filled with fluid, or hard and fixed to the surrounding tissue.

A metric ruler is used to measure the size of the lesions so that any further extension can be compared with this initial baseline measurement. The dermatosis is then documented on the patient's health record; it should be described clearly and in detail, using precise terminology.

After the characteristic distribution of the lesions has been determined, the following information should be obtained and described clearly and in detail:

- Color of the lesion
- Any redness, heat, pain, or swelling
- Size and location of the involved area
- Pattern of eruption (macular, papular, scaling, oozing, discrete, confluent)
- Distribution of the lesion (symmetric, linear, circular)

If acute open wounds or lesions are found on inspection of the skin, a comprehensive assessment should be made and documented in the medical record. This assessment should address several issues:

- Wound bed: Inspect for necrotic and granulation tissue, epithelium, exudate, color, and odor.
- Wound edges and margins: Observe for undermining (extension of the wound under the surface skin) and evaluate for condition.
- Wound size: Measure in millimeters or centimeters as appropriate to determine diameter and depth of the wound and surrounding erythema.
- Surrounding skin: Assess for color, suppleness and moisture, irritation, scaling, and so forth.

Assessing Vascularity and Hydration

Once the color of the skin has been inspected and lesions have been noted, an assessment of vascular changes in the skin is performed. A description of vascular changes includes location, distribution, color, size, and the presence of pulsations. Common vascular changes include petechiae, ecchymoses, **telangiectases** (red marks on the skin caused by stretching of the superficial blood vessels), angiomas, and venous stars.

Skin moisture, temperature, and texture are assessed primarily by palpation. The elasticity (turgor) of the skin, which decreases in normal aging, may be a factor in assessing the hydration status of a patient.

Assessing the Nails and Hair

NAILS

A brief inspection of the nails includes observation of configuration, color, and consistency. Many alterations in the nail or nail bed reflect local or systemic abnormalities in progress or result from past events (Fig. 51-6). Transverse depressions known as Beau's lines in the nails may reflect retarded growth of the nail matrix secondary to severe illness or, more commonly, local trauma. Ridging, hypertrophy, and other changes may also be visible with local trauma. Paronychia, an inflammation of the skin around the nail, is usually accompanied by tenderness and erythema. The angle between the normal nail and its base is 160 degrees. When palpated, the nail base is usually firm. Clubbing is manifested by a straightening of the normal angle (180 degrees or greater) and a softening of the nail base. This softening is perceived as spongelike when palpated.

HAIR

The hair assessment is carried out by inspecting and palpating. Gloves are worn and the examination room should be well lighted. Separating the hair so that the condition of the skin underneath can be easily seen, the nurse notes color, texture, and distribution. Any abnormal lesions, evidence of itching, inflammation, or signs of infestation (lice or mites) are documented.

Color and Texture. Natural hair color ranges from white to black. Hair color begins to gray as one ages, initially appearing during the third decade of life, when the loss of melanin begins to become apparent. However, it is not unusual for the hair of younger people to turn gray as a result of family hereditary traits. The person with albinism (partial or complete absence of pigmentation) has a genetic predisposition to white hair from birth. The natural state of the hair can be altered by using hair dyes, bleaches, and curling or relaxing products. The types of products used are identified during the assessment.

(*text continues on page 1448*)

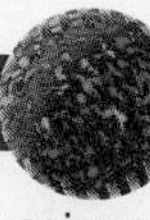

CHART 51•2 Primary and Secondary Skin Lesions

Primary Skin Lesions

Primary skin lesions are original lesions arising from previously normal skin. Secondary lesions can originate from primary lesions.

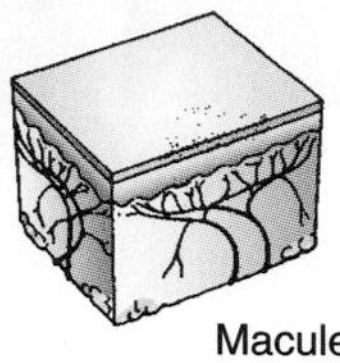

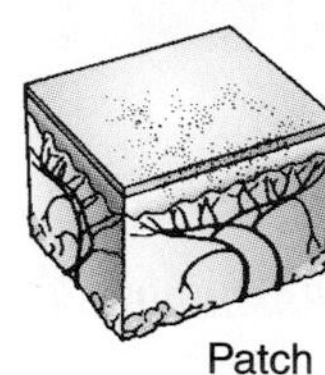

Macule, Patch

- *Macule:* <1 cm, circumscribed border
- *Patch:* >1 cm, may have irregular border
- Flat, nonpalpable skin color change (color may be brown, white, tan, purple, red)

Examples:
Freckles, flat moles, petechia, rubella, vitiligo, port wine stains, ecchymosis

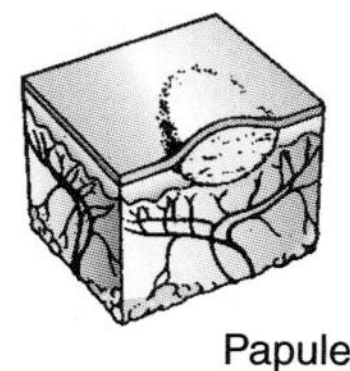

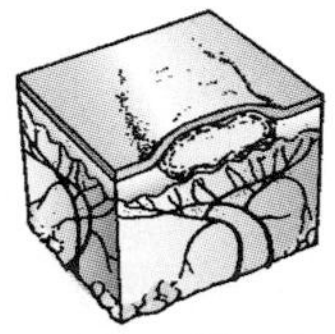

Papule, Plaque

- *Papule:* <0.5 cm
- *Plaque:* >0.5 cm
- Elevated, palpable, solid mass
- Circumscribed border
- Plaque may be coalesced papules with flat top

Examples:
Papules: Elevated nevi, warts, lichen planus
Plaques: Psoriasis, actinic keratosis

Tumor

Nodule, Tumor

- *Nodule:* 0.5–2 cm
- *Tumor:* >1–2 cm
- Elevated, palpable, solid mass
- Extends deeper into the dermis than a papule
- Nodules circumscribed
- Tumors do not always have sharp borders

Examples:
Nodules: Lipoma, squamous cell carcinoma, poorly absorbed injection, dermatofibroma
Tumors: Larger lipoma, carcinoma

Bulla Vesicle

Vesicle, Bulla

- *Vesicle:* <0.5 cm
- *Bulla:* >0.5 cm
- Circumscribed, elevated, palpable mass containing serous fluid

Examples
Vesicles: Herpes simplex/zoster, chickenpox, poison ivy, second-degree burn (blister)
Bulla: Pemphigus, contact dermatitis, large burn blisters, poison ivy, bullous impetigo

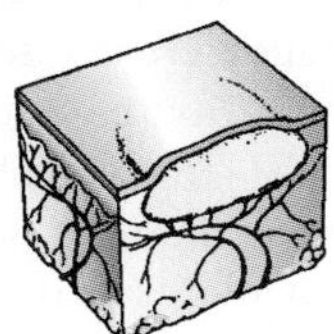

Wheal

- Elevated mass with transient borders
- Often irregular
- Size, color varies
- Caused by movement of serous fluid into the dermis
- Does not contain free fluid in a cavity as, for example, a vesicle

Examples:
Urticaria (hives), insect bites

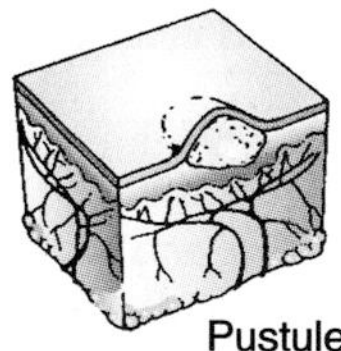

Pustule

- Pus-filled vesicle or bulla

Examples:
Acne, impetigo, furuncles, carbuncles

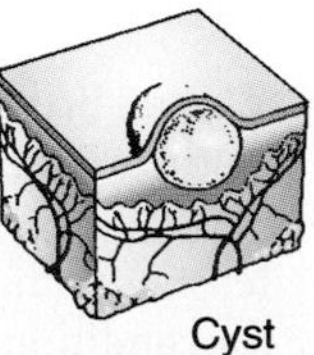

Cyst

- Encapsulated fluid-filled or semisolid mass
- In the subcutaneous tissue or dermis

Examples:
Sebaceous cyst, epidermoid cysts

(*continued*)

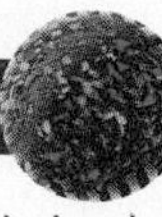

CHART 51•2 Primary and Secondary Skin Lesions *(Continued)*

Secondary Skin Lesions

Secondary skin lesions result from changes in primary lesions.

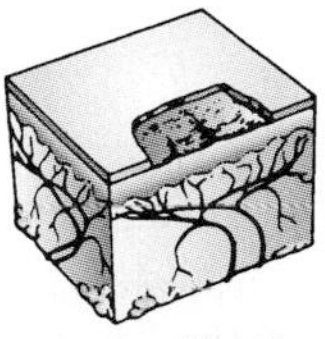
Erosion

Erosion

- Loss of superficial epidermis
- Does not extend to dermis
- Depressed, moist area

Examples:
Ruptured vesicles, scratch marks

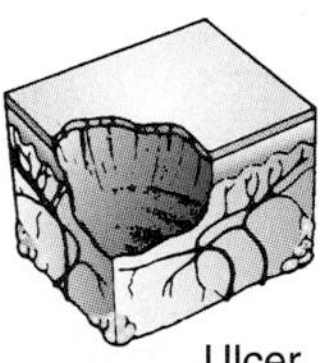
Ulcer

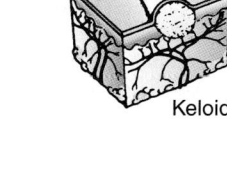

Ulcer

- Skin loss extending past epidermis
- Necrotic tissue loss
- Bleeding and scarring possible

Examples:
Stasis ulcer of venous insufficiency, pressure ulcer

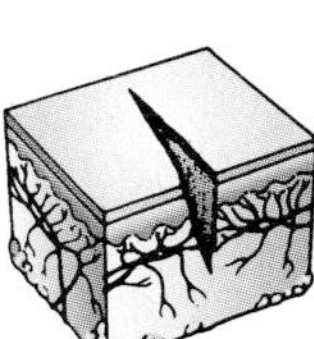
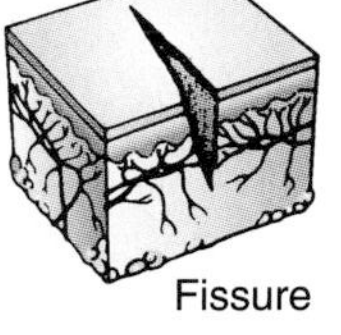
Fissure

Fissure

- Linear crack in the skin
- May extend to dermis

Examples:
Chapped lips or hands, athlete's foot

Scales

Scales

- Flakes secondary to desquamated, dead epithelium
- Flakes may adhere to skin surface
- Color varies (silvery, white)
- Texture varies (thick, fine)

Examples:
Dandruff, psoriasis, dry skin, pityriasis rosea

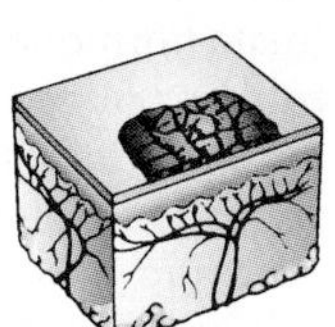
Crust

Crust

- Dried residue of serum, blood, or pus on skin surface
- Large adherent crust is a scab

Examples:
Residue left after vesicle rupture: impetigo, herpes, eczema

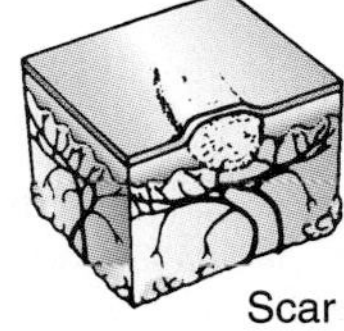
Scar

Scar (Cicatrix)

- Skin mark left after healing of a wound or lesion
- Represents replacement by connective tissue of the injured tissue
- Young scars: red or purple
- Mature scars: white or glistening

Examples:
Healed wound or surgical incision

Keloid

Keloid

- Hypertrophied scar tissue
- Secondary to excessive collagen formation during healing
- Elevated, irregular, red
- Greater incidence in African Americans

Example:
Keloid of ear piercing or surgical incision

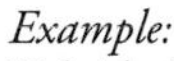

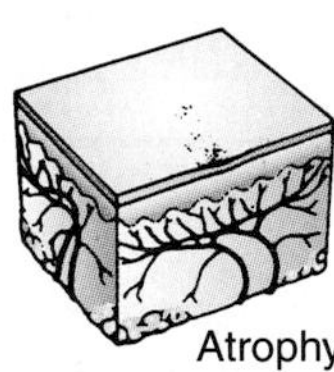
Atrophy

Atrophy

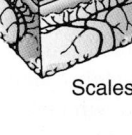

- Thin, dry, transparent appearance of epidermis
- Loss of surface markings
- Secondary to loss of collagen and elastin
- Underlying vessels may be visible

Examples:
Aged skin, arterial insufficiency

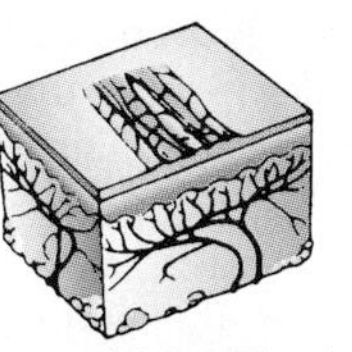
Lichenification

Lichenification

- Thickening and roughening of the skin
- Accentuated skin markings
- May be secondary to repeated rubbing, irritation, scratching

Example:
Contact dermatitis

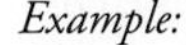

(continued)

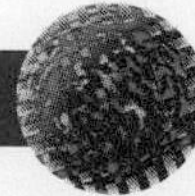

CHART 51•2 Primary and Secondary Skin Lesions *(Continued)*

Vascular Skin Lesions

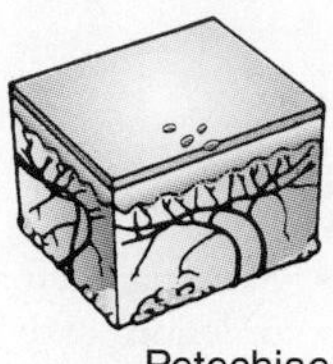

Petechiae

Petechia (*pl.* petechiae)

- Round red or purple macule
- Small: 1–2 mm
- Secondary to blood extravasation
- Associated with bleeding tendencies or emboli to skin

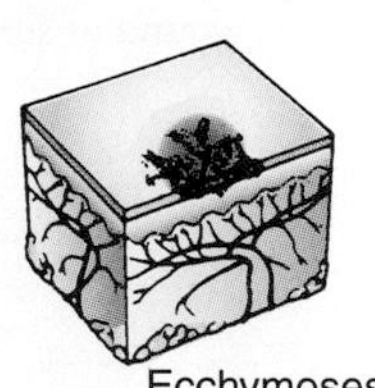

Ecchymoses

Ecchymosis (*pl.* ecchymoses)

- Round or irregular macular lesion
- Larger than petechia
- Color varies and changes: black, yellow, and green hues
- Secondary to blood extravasation
- Associated with trauma, bleeding tendencies

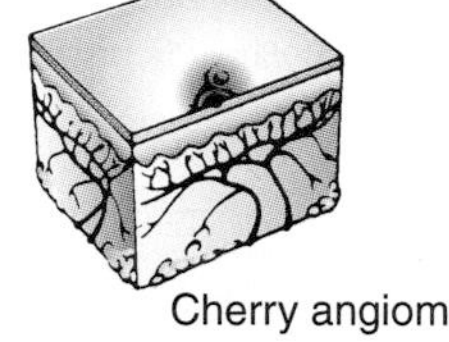

Cherry angioma

Cherry Angioma

- Papular and round
- Red or purple
- Noted on trunk, extremities
- May blanch with pressure
- Normal age-related skin alteration
- Usually not clinically significant

Spider angioma

Spider Angioma

- Red, arteriole lesion
- Central body with radiating branches
- Noted on face, neck, arms, trunk
- Rare below the waist
- May blanch with pressure
- Associated with liver disease, pregnancy, vitamin B deficiency

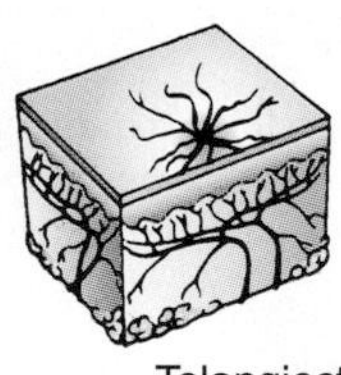

Telangiectasia

Telangiectasia (Venous Star)

- Shape varies: spider-like or linear
- Color bluish or red
- Does not blanch when pressure is applied
- Noted on legs, anterior chest
- Secondary to superficial dilation of venous vessels and capillaries
- Associated with increased venous pressure states (varicosities)

The texture of scalp hair ranges from fine to coarse; silky to brittle; oily to dry; shiny to dull; and straight, curly, or kinky. Dry, brittle hair may result from overuse of hair dyes, hair dryers, and curling irons, or from thyroid dysfunction. Oily hair is usually due to increased secretion from the sebaceous glands close to the scalp. If the patient reports a recent change in hair texture, the underlying reason is pursued; the alteration may arise simply from the overuse of commercial hair products or from changing to a new shampoo.

Distribution. Body hair distribution varies with location. Hair over most of the body is fine, except in the axillae and pubic areas, where it is coarse and develops at puberty. Pubic hair distribution in males forms a diamond shape extending up to the umbilicus. Female pubic hair resembles an inverted triangle. If the pattern found is more characteristic of the opposite gender, further investigation is in order because this may indicate an endocrine problem. Racial differences in hair are expected, such as straight hair in Asians and curly, coarser hair in African-Americans.

Men tend to have more body and facial hair than women. Loss of hair, alopecia, can occur over the entire body or be confined to a specific area. Scalp hair loss may be localized to patchy areas or may range from generalized thinning to total baldness. When assessing scalp hair loss, it is important to investigate the underlying cause with the patient. Patchy hair loss may be from habitual "hair pulling" or from excessive traction on the hair (braiding too tightly); excessive use of dyes, straighteners, and oils; chemotherapeutic agents (doxorubicin or cyclophosphamide); fungus infection; or moles or cancer on the scalp. Regrowth may be erratic, and distribution may never attain the previous thickness.

Hair Loss. The most common cause of hair loss is male pattern baldness, which affects more than half of the male population and is believed to be related to heredity, aging, and androgen (male hormone) levels. Androgen is necessary for male pattern baldness to develop. The pattern of hair loss begins with receding of the hairline in the frontal-temporal area and progresses to gradual thinning and complete loss of hair over the top of the scalp and crown. Figure 51-7 illustrates the usual male pattern hair loss.

Other Changes. Male pattern hair distribution may be seen in some women at the time of menopause, when the hormone estrogen is no longer produced by the ovaries. In women with hirsutism, excessive hair may grow on the face, chest, shoulders, and pubic area. When menopause is ruled out as the underlying

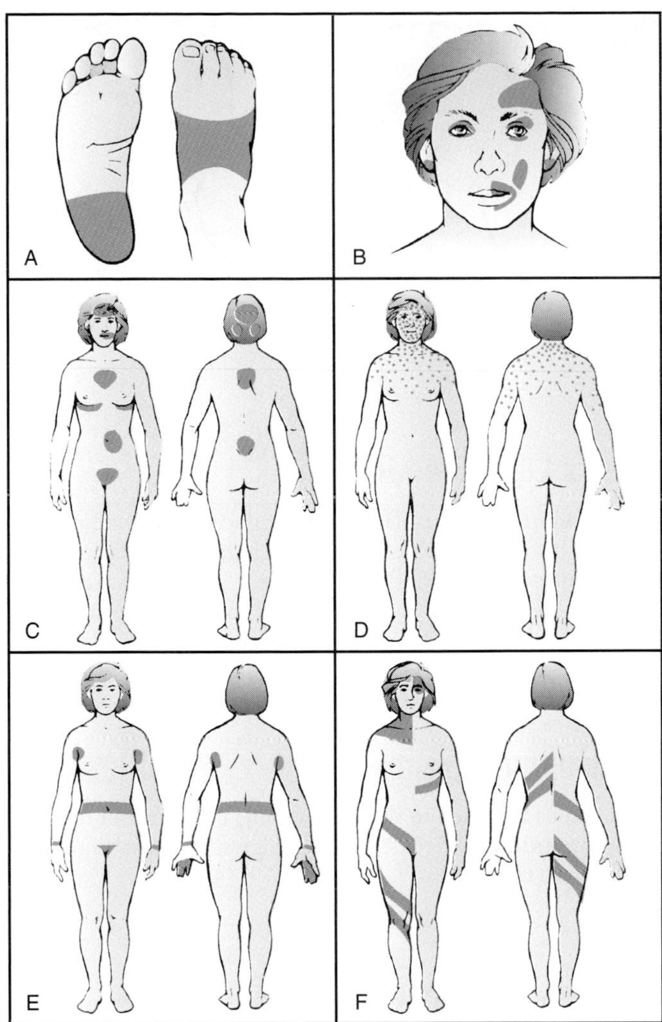

FIGURE 51•4 Anatomic distribution of common skin disorders: (**A**) contact dermatitis (shoes); (**B**) contact dermatitis (cosmetics, perfumes, earrings); (**C**) seborrheic dermatitis; (**D**) acne; (**E**) scabies; (**F**) herpes zoster (shingles).

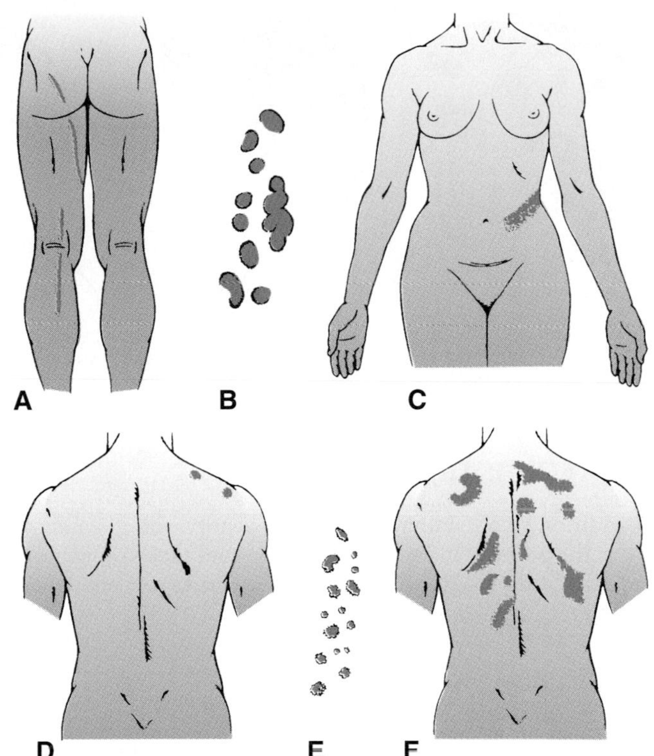

FIGURE 51•5 Skin lesion configurations: (**A**) linear (in a line), (**B**) annular and arciform (circular or arcing), (**C**) zosteriform (linear along a nerve route), (**D**) grouped (clustered), (**E**) discrete (separate and distinct), (**F**) confluent (merged). From Weber, J. W., & Kelley, J. (1998). *Health assessment in nursing.* Philadelphia: Lippincott-Raven.

etiology, hormonal abnormalities related to pituitary or adrenal dysfunction must be pursued.

Because patients with skin conditions can see and feel their problems, they are more likely to be disturbed by their ailments than are patients with other conditions. Skin conditions can lead to disfigurement, isolation, job loss, and economic hardship.

Some conditions may subject the patient to a protracted illness, leading to feelings of depression, frustration, self-consciousness, and rejection. Itching and skin irritation also may be a constant annoyance and are features of most skin diseases. The results of these discomforts may be loss of sleep, anxiety, and depression, all of which reinforce the general distress and fatigue that so frequently accompany skin disorders. In addition, skin diseases often result in concerns related to self-image and interpersonal relationships.

For patients suffering such physical and psychological discomforts, the nurse needs to provide understanding, explanations of the problem, appropriate instructions related to treatment, nursing support, patience, and encouragement. It takes time to help patients gain insight into their problems and resolve their difficulties. It is imperative, therefore, to overcome any aversion that might be felt when caring for patients with unattractive skin disorders. The nurse should show no sign of hesitancy when approaching patients with skin disorders. Such hesitancy only reinforces the psychological trauma of the disorder.

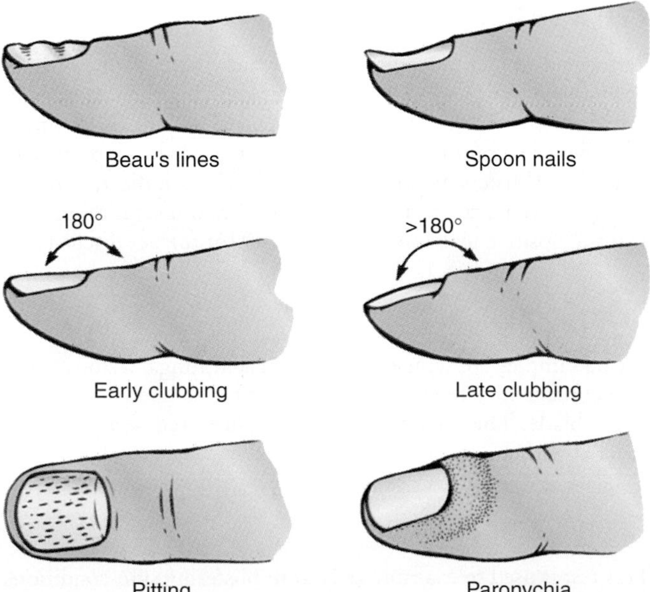

FIGURE 51•6 Common nail disorders. From Weber, J. W., & Kelley, J. (1998). *Health assessment in nursing.* Philadelphia: Lippincott-Raven.

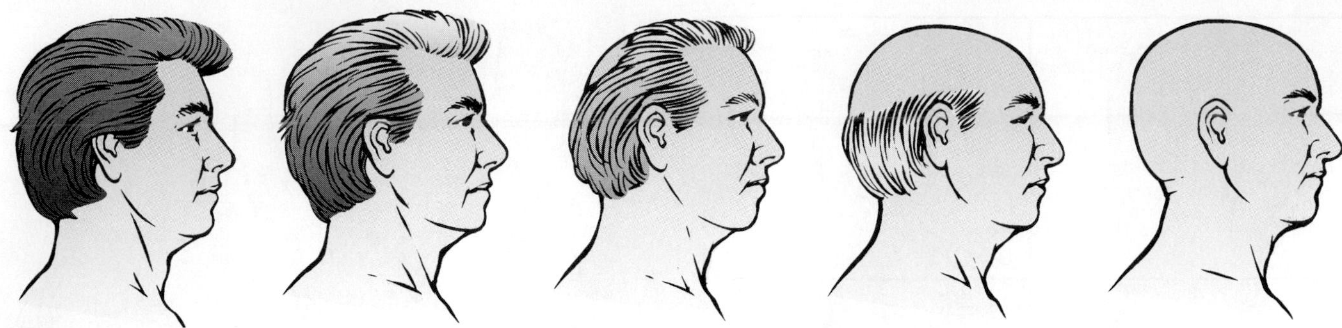

FIGURE 51•7 The progression of male pattern baldness.

DIAGNOSTIC EVALUATION

In addition to obtaining the patient's history, the examiner inspects the primary and secondary lesions and their configuration and distribution. Certain diagnostic procedures may also be used to help identify skin conditions.

Skin Biopsy

Performed to obtain tissue for microscopic examination, a skin biopsy may be obtained by scalpel excision or by a skin punch instrument that removes a small core of tissue. Biopsies are performed on skin nodules, plaques, blisters, and other lesions to rule out malignancy and to establish an exact diagnosis.

Immunofluorescence

Designed to identify the site of an immune reaction, immunofluorescence (IF) testing combines an antigen or antibody with a fluorochrome dye (antibodies can be made fluorescent by attaching them to a dye). IF tests on skin (direct IF test) are techniques to detect autoantibodies directed against portions of the skin. The indirect IF test detects specific antibodies in the patient's serum.

Patch Testing

Performed to identify substances to which the patient has developed an allergy, patch testing involves applying the suspected allergens to normal skin under occlusive patches. The development of redness, fine bumps, or itching is considered a weak positive reaction; fine blisters, papules, and severe itching indicate a moderately positive reaction; and blisters, pain, and ulceration indicate a strong positive reaction. (See Chap. 49 for further discussion.)

Skin Scrapings

Tissue samples are scraped from suspected fungal lesions with a scalpel blade moistened with oil so that the scraped skin adheres to the blade. The scraped material is transferred to a glass slide, covered with a coverslip, and examined microscopically.

Tzanck Smear

This test is used to examine cells from blistering skin conditions, such as herpes zoster, varicella, herpes simplex, and all forms of pemphigus. The secretions from a suspected lesion are applied to a glass slide, stained, and examined.

Wood's Light Examination

Wood's light is a special lamp that produces long-wave ultraviolet rays (black light), which result in a characteristic dark-purple fluorescence. The color of the fluorescent light is best seen in a darkened room, where it is possible to differentiate epidermal from dermal lesions and hypopigmented and hyperpigmented lesions from normal skin. The patient is reassured that the light is not harmful to skin or eyes.

Clinical Photographs

Photographs are taken to show the nature and extent of the skin condition and are used to determine progress or improvement resulting from treatment.

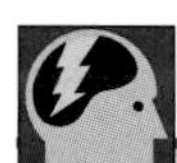

Critical Thinking Exercises

1. An elderly, debilitated patient is to be discharged home to be cared for by her daughter. You know that skin trauma and pressure ulcers can occur if proper care is not carried out. How would you instruct the daughter in preventing these skin problems, especially in someone as old as her mother?
2. An elderly patient complains of very dry, itchy skin. Based on your knowledge of the skin changes that occur in the elderly, how would you proceed to instruct and guide this patient? What if the patient were a 30-year-old mother of two small children? How would you assess this situation, and what factors might you surmise could be causing the dry, itchy skin in a person of this age?

References and Selected Readings

BOOKS

Arndt, K. A., Wintroub, B. U., Robinson, J. K., LeBoit, P. E. (1997). *Primary care dermatology.* Philadelphia: W. B. Saunders.

Demis, D. J. (Ed.). (1998). *Clinical dermatology.* Philadelphia: Lippincott-Raven.

Fitzpatrick, T. B., et al. (1997). *Color atlas & synopsis of clinical dermatology* (3rd ed.). New York: McGraw-Hill.

JOURNALS

Boiko, S. (1997). Diapers and diaper dermatitis. *Dermatology Nursing, 9*(1), 33–47.

Bryant, R. L. (1995). Preventative foot care program: A nursing prospective. *Ostomy/Wound Management, 41*(4), 28–34.

Draelos, Z. D. (1997). Understanding African-American hair. *Dermatology Nursing, 9*(4), 227–231.

Kerstein, M. D. (1997). Wound management update. The scientific basis of healing. *Physician Assistant, 9*(6), 28–51.

McMichael, A. J. (1996). Successful aging in the elderly dermatology patient. *Journal of Geriatric Dermatology, 4*(4), 132–136.

Nicol, N. H., & Baumeister, L. L. (1997). Topical corticosteroid therapy. *Lippincott's Primary Care Practice, 1*(1), 62–69.

Sun-protection behaviors used by adults for their children: U.S., 1997. (1998). *Morbidity and Mortality Weekly Report, 47*(23), 48–52.

Weinstock, M. A., & Rossi, J. S. (1998). The Rhode Island Sun Smart Project: A scientific approach to skin cancer prevention. *Clinical Dermatology, 16*(4), 411–413.

Resources

Alopecia Areata Foundation, P.O. Box 150760, San Rafael, CA 94915-0760; www.keratin.com

American Cancer Society Inc., 777 Third Ave., New York, NY 10017; www.ca.cancer.org

Lupus Foundation, 1300 Piccard Dr., Rockville, MD 20850-4303; www.lupus.org

National Institute of Arthritis, Musculoskeletal and Skin Diseases, National Institutes of Health, Bethesda, MD 20892

National Psoriasis Foundation, 6600 S.W. 92nd Ave., Suite 300, Portland, OR 97223-7195; www.psoriasis.org

Skin Cancer Foundation, 575 Park Ave. S., New York, NY 10016; www.skincancer.org

Vitiligo Foundation, P.O. Box 6337, Tyler, TX 75703; www.dermnet.org.nz

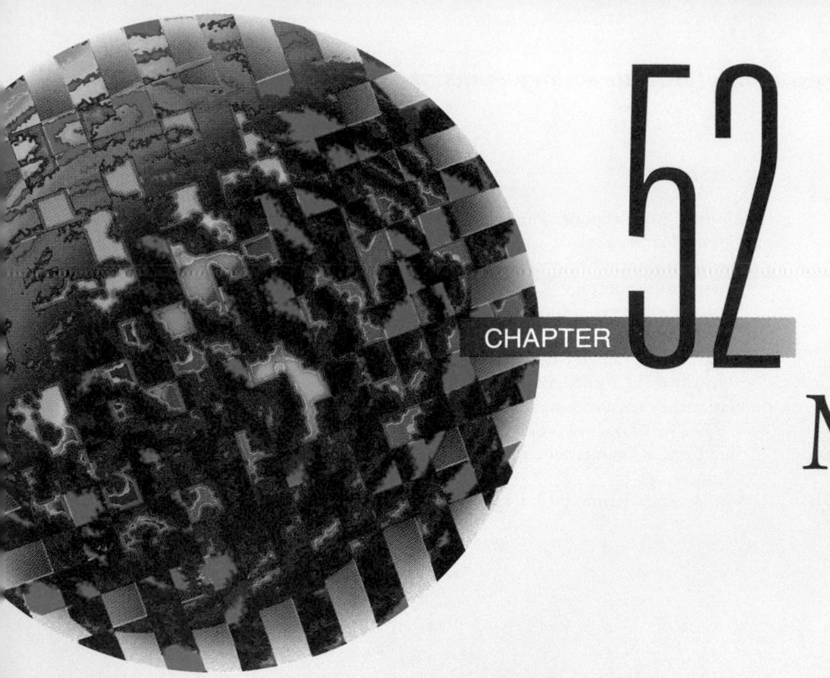

Management of Patients With Dermatologic Problems

Learning Objectives

On completion of this chapter, the learner will be able to:

1. Describe the general management of the patient with an abnormal skin condition.
2. Use the nursing process as a framework for care of the patient with psoriasis.
3. Describe the health education needs of the patient with infections of the skin and parasitic skin diseases.
4. Use the nursing process as a framework for care of patients with noninfectious inflammatory dermatoses.
5. Describe the management and nursing care of the patient with skin cancer.
6. Use the nursing process as a framework for care of the patient with malignant melanoma.
7. Describe characteristics of the various types of Kaposi's sarcoma.
8. Compare the various types of dermatologic and plastic reconstructive surgeries.
9. Use the nursing process as a framework for care of the patient undergoing facial reconstructive surgery.

Nursing care for patients with dermatologic problems includes administering topical and systemic medications, managing wet dressings and other special dressings, and providing therapeutic baths. The four major objectives of therapy are to prevent additional damage, prevent secondary infection, reverse the inflammatory process, and relieve the symptoms.

GLOSSARY

acantholysis: separation of epidermal cells from each other due to damage or abnormality of the intracellular substance

balneotherapy: a bath with therapeutic additives

carbuncle: a localized skin infection involving several hair follicles

cheilitis: dry cracking at the corners of the mouth

comedones: the primary lesions of acne, caused by sebum blockage in the hair follicle

débridement: removal of necrotic or dead tissue by mechanical, surgical, or autolytic means

dermatitis: any inflammation of the skin

dermatosis: any abnormal skin lesion

epidermopoiesis: the development of epidermal cells

furuncle: a localized skin infection of a single hair follicle

hydrophyllic: a material that absorbs moisture

hydrophobic: a material that repels moisture

hygroscopic: absorbs moisture from the air

linaments: lotions with added oil for increased softening of the skin

plasmapheresis: the exchange of plasma by cells

Propionibacterium acnes (P. acnes): bacteria that live on the skin; the primary causative agent of acne

pyodermas: bacterial skin infections

suspensions: liquid preparations in which powder is suspended, requiring shaking before use

tinea: a superficial fungal infection on the skin or scalp

MANAGEMENT OF SKIN CARE FOR PATIENTS WITH SKIN CONDITIONS

Some skin problems are markedly aggravated by soap and water. Therefore, bathing routines are modified according to the condition. Denuded skin, whether the area of desquamation is large or small, is excessively prone to damage by chemicals and trauma. The friction of a towel, if applied with vigor, is sufficient to produce a brisk inflammatory response that causes any existing lesion to flare up and extend.

Protecting the Skin

The essence of skin care and protection in bathing a patient with skin problems is as follows: use a mild, lipid-free soap or soap substitute, rinse the area completely, and blot the area dry with a soft cloth. Avoid deodorant soaps.

Special care is necessary when changing dressings. Pledgets saturated with oil, sterile saline, or another prescribed solution will help loosen crusts, remove exudates, or free an adherent dry dressing.

Preventing Secondary Infection

Potentially infectious skin lesions should be regarded strictly as such, and proper precautions should be observed until the diagnosis is established. Most lesions with pus contain infectious material. The nurse and physician must adhere to universal precautions and wear either clean or sterile gloves when inspecting the skin or changing the dressing. Proper disposal of any contaminated dressing is carried out according to Occupational Safety and Health Administration (OSHA) regulations.

Reversing the Inflammatory Process

The type of skin lesion (oozing, infected, or dry) usually determines the type of local medication or treatment that is prescribed. As a rule, if the skin is acutely inflamed (hot, red, and swollen) and oozing, it is best to apply wet dressings and soothing lotions. In chronic conditions in which the skin surface is dry and scaly, water-soluble emulsions, creams, ointments, and pastes are used. The therapy must be changed as the response indicates. The patient and the nurse should note if the medication or dressings seem to irritate the disorder. The success or failure of skin therapy usually depends on adequate instruction and motivation of the patient and the interest of, and support by, the health care personnel.

DRESSINGS FOR SKIN CONDITIONS

There are three major classifications of dressings for skin conditions: wet, moisture-retentive, and occlusive. During the 1980s and 1990s, new product development quadrupled the available choices for wound care, especially within the moisture-retentive dressing classification. Products classified as moisture-retentive dressings include hydrogels, foams, and alginates. In addition, biologicals and biosynthetics containing collagen and growth factor are being researched and will soon be available. Chart 52-1 lists generic wound care products.

Dressings and Rules of Wound Care

Even with the increased availability of dressings, an appropriate selection can be made if certain principles are maintained, referred to as the five rules of wound care.

CHART 52•1 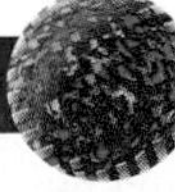 **Wound Care Products**

- adhesives
- adhesive removers
- adhesive skin closures
- adhesive tapes
- alginate dressings
- antibiotics
- antimicrobials
- antiseptics
- bandages
- biosynthetic dressings
- cleansers
- collagen dressings
- composite dressings
- contact layers
- creams or skin protectant pastes
- dressing covers
- enzyme débriding agents
- foam dressings
- gauze dressings
- growth factors
- hydrocolloid dressings
- hydrogel dressings
- leg ulcer wraps, compression bandages or wraps
- lubricating, stimulating sprays
- moisturizers
- moisture barrier ointments
- ointments
- perineal cleansers
- skin sealants
- transparent film dressings
- wound fillers: pastes, powders, beads, etc.
- wound pouches

Rule 1: Categorization

Learn about dressings by generic category and compare new products with those that already make up the category. As hundreds of choices become available, the nurse should become familiar with the generic categories and develop a systematic approach to product selection. The nurse should become familiar with indications, contraindications, and side effects. The best dressing may be created by combining products in different categories to achieve several goals at the same time. These categories will be discussed below.

Rule 2: Selection

Select the safest and most effective, user-friendly, and cost-effective dressing possible. In most cases, nurses carry out the physician's orders for dressings, but they should be prepared to give the physician feedback about the dressing's effect on the wound, ease of use for the patient, and other considerations where applicable.

Rule 3: Change

Change dressings based on patient, wound, and dressing assessment, not on standardized routines. Traditional nursing care plans called for changing dressings on a routine schedule, often three or four times a day.

Nursing Alert *It is now thought that the natural wound-healing process should be disrupted as little as possible. Unless the wound is infected or has heavy discharge, it is common to leave chronic wounds covered for 48 to 72 hours and acute wounds for 24 hours.*

Rule 4: Evolution

As the wound progresses through the phases of wound healing, the dressing protocol is altered to optimize wound healing. It is rare, especially in chronic wounds, that the same dressing material is appropriate throughout the healing process. The rule assumes that the nurse and the patient or family have access to a wide variety of products and knowledge about their use. The nurse teaches the patient or family caregiver about wound care and ensures that the family has access to appropriate dressing choices.

Rule 5: Practice

Practice with dressing material is required for the nurse to learn the performance parameters of the particular dressing. Refining skills of applying appropriate dressings correctly and learning about new dressing products are essential nursing responsibilities. Dressing changes should not be delegated to assistive personnel; these techniques require the knowledge base and assessment skills of professional nurses.

Wet Dressings

Wet dressings (wet compresses applied to the skin) were traditionally used for acute, weeping, inflammatory lesions. They have become almost obsolete in light of the many newer products available for wound care. Wet dressings are sterile or nonsterile (clean), depending on the condition. They are used to reduce inflammation by producing constriction of the blood vessels (thereby decreasing vasodilation and local blood flow in inflammation); to clean the skin of exudates, crusts, and scales; to maintain drainage of infected areas; and to promote healing by facilitating the free movement of epidermal cells across the involved skin so that new granulation tissue forms. Wet dressings can be used for vesicular, bullous, pustular, and ulcerative disorders, as well as for inflammatory conditions.

Before applying these dressings, the nurse washes the hands and puts on sterile or clean gloves. The open dressing requires frequent changes because evaporation is rapid; the closed dressing is changed less frequently. However, there is always a danger that the closed dressing will cause not only softening but actual maceration of the underlying skin. Wet-to-dry dressings are used to remove exudate from erosions or ulcers. The dressing remains in place until it dries. It is then removed without soaking so that crusts, exudate, or pus from the skin lesion will adhere to the dressing and be removed with it.

Moisture-Retentive Dressings

New, commercially produced moisture-retentive dressings can perform the same functions as wet compresses but are more efficient at removing exudate because of their higher moisture-vapor transmission rate; some have reservoirs that can hold excessive exudate. There is also clear evidence that moist wound healing results in wound resurfacing 40% faster than with air exposure. A number of moisture-retentive dressings are already impregnated with saline solution, petrolatum, zinc-saline solution, hydrogel, and antimicrobial agents, thereby eliminating the need to coat the skin to avoid maceration. The main advantages of moisture-retentive dressings over wet compresses include reduced pain, fewer infections, less scar tissue, gentle autolytic débridement, and decreased frequency of dressing changes. Depending on the product used and the type of dermatologic problem encountered, most moisture-retentive dressings may remain in place from 12 to 24 hours; some can remain in place as long as a week (Table 52-1).

Hydrogels are polymers with a 90% to 95% water content. They are available in either impregnated sheets or gel in a tube. Their high moisture content makes them ideal for autolytic débridement of wounds. They are semitransparent, allowing for wound inspection without dressing removal. They are comfortable and soothing for the painful wound. They have no inherent adhesive and require a secondary dressing to keep them in place. Hydrogels are appropriate for superficial wounds with high serous output, such as abrasions, skin graft sites, and draining venous ulcers.

Hydrocolloids are composed of a water-impermeable, polyurethane outer covering separated from the wound by a hydrocolloid material. They are adherent and nonpermeable to water vapor and oxygen. As it evaporates over the wound, water is absorbed into the dressing, which softens and discolors with the increased water content. The dressing can be removed without damage to the wound. As the dressing absorbs water, it produces a foul-smelling, yellowish covering over the wound. This is a normal chemical interaction between the dressing and wound exudate and should not be confused with purulent drainage from the wound. Unfortunately, most of the hydrocolloid dressings are opaque, limiting inspection of the wound without removal of the dressing.

Available in sheets and in gels, hydrocolloids are a good choice for mildly to moderately exudative wounds, as well as acute wounds. Easy to use and comfortable, hydrocolloid dressings promote **débridement** (removal of necrotic or dead tissue by mechanical, surgical, or autolytic means) and formation of granulation tissue. They do not have to be removed for bathing. Most can be left in place for up to 7 days.

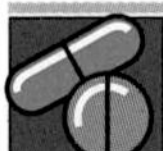

TABLE 52•1 **Quick Guide to Wound Dressing Function and Categories**

Function	Action	Example
Absorption	Absorbs exudate	Alginates, composite dressings, foams, gauze, hydrocolloids, hydrogels
Cleansing	Removes purulent drainage, foreign debris, and devitalized tissue	Wound cleansers
Débridement	*Autolytic;* covers a wound and allows enzymes to self-digest sloughed skin	Absorption beads, pastes, powders; alginates; composite dressings; foams; hydrate gauze; hydrogels; hydrocolloids; transparent films; wound care systems
	Chemical; applied topically to break down devitalized tissue	Enzymatic débridement agents
	Mechanical; removes devitalized tissue with mechanical force	Wound cleansers, gauze (wet to dry)
Hydration	Adds moisture to a wound	Gauze (saturated with saline) solution, hydrogels, wound care systems
Maintain moist environment	Manages moisture levels in a wound and maintains a moist environment	Composites, contact layers, foams, gauze (impregnated or saturated), hydogels, hydrocolloids, transparent films, wound care systems
Manage high-output wounds	Manages excessive quantities of exudate	Pouching systems
Pack or fill dead space	Prevents premature wound closure or fills shallow areas and provides absorption	Absorbant beads, powders, pastes; alginates, composites, foams, gauze (impregnated and non-impregnated)
Protect and cover wound	Provides protection from the external environment	Composites, compression bandages/wraps, foams, gauze dressings, hydrogels, hydrocolloids, transparent film dressings
Protect periwound skin	Prevents moisture and mechanical trauma from damaging delicate tissue around wound	Composites, foams, Hydrocolloids, pouching systems, skin sealants, transparent film dressings
Provide therapeutic compression	Provides appropriate levels of support to the lower extremities in venous stasis disease	Compression bandages, wraps

Foam dressings consist of microporous polyurethane with an absorptive **hydrophyllic** (water-absorbing) surface that covers the wound, plus a **hydrophobic** (water-resistant) backing to block leakage of exudate. They are nonadherent and require a secondary dressing to keep them in place. Moisture is absorbed into the foam layer, decreasing maceration of surrounding tissue. A moist environment is maintained, and removal of the dressing does not damage the wound. The foams are opaque and must be removed for wound inspection. Foams are a good choice for mildly to moderately exudative wounds. They are especially helpful over bony prominences because they provide contoured cushioning.

Calcium alginates are derived from seaweed and consist of tremendously absorbent calcium alginate fibers. They are hemostatic and bioabsorbable and can be used as sheets, mats, or ropes of absorbent material. As the exudate is absorbed, the fibers turn into a viscous hydrogel. They are quite useful in areas where the tissue is more irritated or macerated. The alginate dressing forms a moist pocket over the wound while the surrounding skin stays dry. They also react with wound fluid to form a foul-smelling coating. Alginates work well when packed into a deep cavity, wound, or sinus tract with heavy drainage (Krastner & Kane, 1997). They are nonadherent and require a secondary dressing.

Occlusive Dressings

Occlusive dressings may be commercially produced or made inexpensively from sterile or nonsterile gauze squares or wrap. Occlusive dressings cover topical medication that is applied to a **dermatosis** (abnormal skin lesion). The area is kept airtight by using plastic film (such as plastic wrap). Plastic film is thin and readily adapts to all sizes, body shapes, and skin surfaces. Plastic surgical tape containing a corticosteroid in the adhesive layer can be cut to size and applied to individual lesions. Generally, plastic wrap should be used no more than 12 hours a day.

Nursing Management

A primary nursing responsibility in managing patients with skin conditions is teaching. The nurse, the patient, and appropriate caregivers review how to apply dressings properly at home. In addition to explaining general infection prevention measures, such as washing hands and putting on sterile or clean gloves, and dressing application procedures, the nurse teaches the patient how to recognize signs of healing or infection and actions to take in either case.

PROMOTING HOME AND COMMUNITY-BASED CARE

Teaching Patients Self-Care. To teach the patient to apply the dressing at home, the nurse explains how to wash the affected area and pat it dry, rub medication into the lesion while the skin is moist, cover the area with plastic (eg, Telfa pads, plastic wrap, vinyl gloves, plastic bag), and cover with an elastic bandage, dressing, or paper tape to seal the edges. Dressings should be removed for 12 of every 24 hours to prevent skin thinning (atrophy), striae (bandlike streaks), telangiectasia (small, red lesions caused by dilation of blood vessels), and maceration.

Other forms of dressings used to cover topical medications include soft cotton cloth and stretchable cotton dressings (Surgitube, Tubergauze), which can be used for fingers, toes, hands, and feet. The hands can be covered with disposable polyethylene or vinyl gloves sealed at the wrists; the feet can be wrapped in plastic bags covered by cotton socks. When large areas of the body must be covered, cotton cloth topped by expandable stockinette can be used. Disposable diapers or cloths folded diaper-fashion are useful for dressing the groin and the perineal areas. Axillary dressings can be made of cotton cloth, or a commercially prepared dressing may be used and taped in place or held by dress shields. A turban or plastic shower cap is useful for holding dressings on the scalp. A face mask, made from gauze with holes cut out for the eyes, nose, and mouth, may be held in place with gauze ties looped through holes cut in the four corners of the mask.

THERAPEUTIC BATHS (BALNEOTHERAPY) AND MEDICATIONS

Baths or soaks, known as **balneotherapy**, are useful when large areas are involved; these are used to remove crusts, scales, and old medications and to relieve the inflammation and itching that accompany acute dermatoses. The water temperature should be comfortable, and the bath should not exceed 20 to 30 minutes because of the tendency of baths and soaks to produce skin maceration. Table 52-2 lists the different types of therapeutic baths and their uses.

Topical Pharmacotherapy

Because skin is easily accessible and, therefore, easy to treat, topical medications are often used. High concentrations of some medications can be applied directly to the affected site with little systemic absorption and, therefore, few systemic side effects. However, some medications are readily absorbed through the skin and can produce systemic effects. Because topical preparations may induce allergic contact **dermatitis** (inflammation of the skin) in sensitive patients, any untoward response should be reported immediately and the medication discontinued.

Medicated lotions, creams, ointments, and powders are frequently used to treat skin lesions. In general, moisture-retentive dressings, with or without medication, are used in the acute stage, lotions and creams are reserved for the subacute stage, and ointments are used when inflammation has become chronic and the skin is dry with scaling or lichenification (leathery thickening).

With all types of topical medication, the patient is taught to apply the medication gently but thoroughly and, when necessary, to cover the medication with a dressing to protect clothing. Table 52-3 lists some commonly used topical preparations.

Lotions

Lotions are of two types: suspensions and linaments. **Suspensions** consist of a powder in water, which requires shaking before application, and clear solutions, containing completely dissolved active ingredients. Lotions are usually applied directly to the skin, but a dressing soaked in the lotion can be placed on the affected area. A suspension such as calamine lotion provides a rapid cooling and drying effect as it evaporates, leaving a thin medicinal layer of powder on the affected skin. Lotions are frequently used to replenish lost skin oils or to relieve pruritus. Lotions must be applied every 3 or 4 hours for sustained therapeutic effect. If left in place for a longer period, they may crust and cake on the skin. **Linaments** are lotions with oil added to prevent crusting. They may be used for this purpose. Because lotions are easy to use, therapeutic compliance is generally high.

Powders

Powders usually have a talc, zinc oxide, bentonite, or cornstarch base and are dusted on the skin with a shaker or with cotton sponges. Although their therapeutic action is brief, powders act as **hygroscopic** agents that absorb and retain moisture from the air and reduce friction between skin surfaces and clothing or bedding.

Creams

Creams may be suspensions of oil in water or emulsions of water in oil, with ingredients to prevent bacterial and fungal growth. Both may cause an allergic reaction, such as contact dermatitis. Oil-in-water creams are easily applied and usually are the most cosmetically acceptable to the patient. Although they can be used on the face, they tend to have a drying effect. Water-in-oil emulsions are greasier and are preferred for drying and flaking dermatoses.

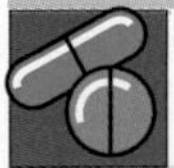

TABLE 52•2 Types of Therapeutic Baths

Bath Solution	Effects and Uses	Nursing Interventions
Water	Same effect as wet dressings	• Fill the tub half full.
Saline	Used for widely disseminated lesions	• Keep the water at a comfortable temperature.
Colloidal (Aveeno, oatmeal)	Antipruritic, soothing	• Do not allow the water to cool excessively.
Sodium bicarbonate (baking soda)	Cooling	• Use a bath mat—*medications added to bath can cause the tub to be slippery.*
Starch	Soothing	• Apply an emollient cream to damp skin after the bath if lubrication is desired.
Medicated tars	Psoriasis and chronic eczema	• Because tars are volatile, the bath area should be well ventilated.
Bath oils	Antipruritic and emollient action; acute and subacute generalized eczematous eruptions	• Dry by gently blotting with a towel.
		• Keep room warm to minimize temperature fluctuations.
		• Encourage the patient to wear light, loose clothing after the bath.

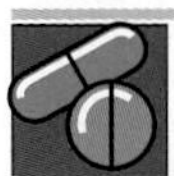

TABLE 52•3 **Common Topical Preparations and Medications**

Preparation	Product Name
Bath preparations	
with tar	Balnetar, Doak Oil, Lavatar
with colloidal oatmeal	Aveeno Oilated Bath Powder
with oatmeal and mineral oil	Aveeno Bath Oil, Nutra Soothe
with mineral oil	Nutraderm Bath Oil, Lubath, Alpha-Keri Bath Oil
Moisturizer creams	Acid Mantle Cream, Curel Cream, Dermasil, Eucerin, Lubriderm, Noxzema Skin Cream
Moisturizer ointments	Aquaphor Ointment, Eutra Swiss Skin Cream, Vaseline Ointment
Topical anesthetics	lidocaine (Xylocaine) of various strengths in the form of spray, ointment, gel; Emla cream (lidocaine 2.5% and prilocaine 2.5%)
Topical antibiotics	bacitracin, Polysporin (bacitracin and polymixin B), Bactroban ointment or cream (mupirocin 2%), erythromycin 2% (Emgel, Eryderm Solution), clindamycin phosphate 1% (Cleocin cream, gel, solution), gentamicin sulfate 1% (Garamycin cream or ointment), 1% silver sulfadiazine cream (Silvadene)

Creams are generally rubbed into the skin by hand. They are used for their moisturizing and emollient effects.

Gels

Gels are semisolid emulsions that become liquid when applied to the skin or scalp. They are cosmetically acceptable to the patient because they are not visible after application, and they are greaseless and nonstaining. The newer water-based gels appear to penetrate the skin more effectively and cause less stinging on application. They are especially useful for acute dermatitis in which there is weeping exudate (eg, poison ivy).

Pastes

Pastes are mixtures of powders and ointments and are used in inflammatory conditions. They adhere to the skin and may be difficult to remove without using an oil (eg, olive oil, mineral oil). Pastes are applied with a wooden tongue depressor or by hand (gloved).

Ointments

Ointments retard water loss and lubricate and protect the skin. They are the preferred vehicle for delivering medication to chronic or localized skin conditions. Ointments are applied with a wooden tongue depressor or by hand (gloved).

Sprays and Aerosols

Spray and aerosol preparations may be used on extensive lesions. They evaporate on contact and are used infrequently.

Corticosteroids

Corticosteroids are widely used in treating dermatologic conditions to provide anti-inflammatory, antipruritic, and vasoconstrictive effects. The patient is taught to apply this medication according to strict guidelines, using it sparingly but rubbing it into the prescribed area thoroughly. Absorption of topical corticosteroid is enhanced when the skin is hydrated or the affected area is covered by an occlusive or moisture-retentive dressing. Inappropriate use of topical corticosteroids can result in both local and systemic side effects, especially when the medication is absorbed through inflamed and excoriated skin, under occlusive dressings, or when used for long periods on sensitive areas. Local side effects may include skin atrophy and thinning, striae, and telangiectasia. Thinning of the skin results from the ability of corticosteroids to inhibit skin collagen synthesis (Arndt et al., 1997). The thinning process can be reversed by discontinuing the medication, but striae and telangiectasia are permanent. Systemic side effects may include hyperglycemia and symptoms of Cushing's syndrome. Caution is required when applying corticosteroids around the eyes because long-term use may cause glaucoma or cataracts. In addition, the anti-inflammatory effect of corticosteroids may mask existing viral or fungal infections.

Concentrated (fluorinated) corticosteroids are never applied on the face or intertriginous areas (axilla and groin) because these areas have a thinner stratum corneum and absorb the medication much more quickly than areas such as the forearm or legs. Persistent use of concentrated topical corticosteroids in any location may produce both acne-like dermatitis, known as steroid-induced acne, and hypertrichosis (excessive hair growth). Because some topical corticosteroid preparations are available without prescription, patients should be cautioned about prolonged and inappropriate use. Table 52-4 lists topical corticosteroid preparations according to potency.

Intralesional Therapy

Intralesional therapy consists of injecting a sterile suspension of medication (usually a corticosteroid) into or just below a lesion. Although this treatment may have an anti-inflammatory effect, local atrophy may result if the medication is injected into subcutaneous fat. Skin lesions treated with intralesional therapy include psoriasis, keloids, and cystic acne. Occasionally, immunotherapeutic and antifungal agents are administered by intralesional therapy.

Systemic Medications

Systemic medications are also prescribed for skin conditions. These include the corticosteroids for short-term therapy for contact dermatitis or for long-term treatment of a chronic dermatosis, such as pemphigus vulgaris. Other frequently used systemic medications include antibiotics, antifungals, antihistamines, sedatives and tranquilizers, analgesics, and cytotoxic agents.

NURSING PROCESS: THE PATIENT WITH AN ABNORMAL SKIN CONDITION

Assessment

The skin is the most visible organ of the body. When a dermatologic condition arises, it is difficult for the patient to ignore it or to conceal it from others. A disease of the skin may arise as a dis-

TABLE 52•4 Potency: Topical Corticosteroids

Potency	Topical Corticosteroid	Preparations
OTC	0.5–0.1% hydrocortisone	cr, lot, oint*
Lowest	dexamethasone 0.1% (Decaderm)	cr, oint, aerosol, gel
	alclometasone 0.05% (Aclovate)	cr, oint
	hydrocortisone 2.5% (Hytone)	cr, lot, oint
Low–medium	desonide 0.05% (DesOwen, Tridesilon)	cr, lot, oint
	fluocinolone acetonide 0.025% (Synalar)	cr, solution
	hydrocortisone valerate 0.2% (Westcort)	cr, solution
	betamethasone valerate 0.1% (Valisone)	cr, oint
	fluticasonepropionate 0.05% (Cutivate)	cr, oint
Medium–high	triamcinolone acetonide 0.1–0.5% (Aristocort)	cr, oint, lot
	fluocinonide 0.05% (Lidex)	cr, oint, gel
	desoximetasone 0.05–0.25% (Topicort)	cr, oint, gel
	fluocinolone 0.2% (Synalar)	cr, oint
	diflorasone diacetate 0.05% (Psorcon)	cr, oint
Very high	clobetasol propionate 0.05% (Temovate)	cr, oint, gel
	betamethasone dipropionate 0.05% (Diprolene)	cr, oint, gel
	halobetasole propionate 0.05% (Ultravate)	cr, oint

*cr, cream; lot, lotion; oint, ointment.

tinct entity unto itself or may be the outward manifestation of an unrelated systemic disease.

The health history and direct observation provide information about the patient's perception of the dermatosis, how it began, what may have precipitated the condition, what relieves the symptoms, and other physical or emotional problems the patient is experiencing. A complete physical examination should be performed. (See Chap. 51 to review the assessment of the integumentary system.)

Diagnosis

Nursing Diagnoses

Based on the assessment data, major nursing diagnoses may include:

- Risk for impaired skin integrity related to changes in the barrier function of the skin
- Pain and itching related to skin lesions
- Sleep pattern disturbance related to pruritus
- Body image disturbance related to unsightly appearance of the skin
- Potential for impaired social interaction related to disturbance in body image
- Knowledge deficit about the treatment regimen
- Potential for anxiety related to mastering treatment plan

Collaborative Problems/Potential Complications

Based on the assessment data, a potential complication may be the following:

- Infection

Planning and Goals

The major goals for the patient may include maintenance of skin integrity, relief of discomfort, promotion of restful sleep, self-acceptance, knowledge about skin care, and avoidance of complications.

Nursing Interventions

Maintaining Skin Integrity

Many people have dry and sensitive skin that is easily irritated. This is especially true of elderly patients. Too much or too vigorous washing and scrubbing can increase the problem. Soaps are also drying and irritating. People with sensitive skin should bathe or be bathed with tepid water with minimal soap, taking care to rinse well and dry by gently patting the skin with a towel. A fragrance-free emollient can be applied to damp skin to trap moisture. Dry air is irritating because it reduces skin moisture; therefore, keeping the environment humidified is also helpful.

Skin problems of the hands are a common complaint. The skin of the back of the hand is thin, accounting for its sensitivity and dryness and its poor tolerance of soaps and detergents. People with this problem should protect the hands from contact with soaps, solvents, detergents, and other chemicals by wearing cotton-lined, heavy-duty vinyl gloves when handling these agents. People with irritations of the hands can be advised to wear white cotton gloves (cosmetic gloves) for dry housework and to minimize contact with water.

In patients with diagnosed skin conditions, the skin should be protected from maceration (excessive hydration of the stratum corneum) when applying wet dressings. Thermal injuries must be prevented as well. The patient with a compromised immune system is at increased risk for cutaneous infection. Plan of Nursing Care 52-1 summarizes nursing interventions for patients with skin problems related to trauma and infection.

Relieving Discomfort

A skin disorder that seems trivial to the observer may cause extreme discomfort to the patient. Cystic lesions, for example, may be tender and painful. Many skin disorders produce itching, making the patient irritable and unable to sleep. Pruritus (itching) is a significant symptom that scratching does not relieve. The patient is advised to keep cool, especially at night, and to avoid taking hot baths or wearing woolen clothing. If itching persists, the patient is advised to see the physician or nurse practitioner, who may prescribe a topical or oral agent.

In providing care for a patient with itching skin lesions, the nurse attempts to discover the cause of discomfort. A sudden onset of generalized rash may indicate a medication allergy. Other causes are discussed in the section below on pruritus.

Nursing interventions appropriate for relieving itching include humidifying the environment, maintaining a cool temperature, removing excess bedding and clothing, and limiting soaps to those made for sensitive skin. The nails are trimmed to decrease skin

(*text continues on page 1462*)

52•1

Plan of Nursing Care 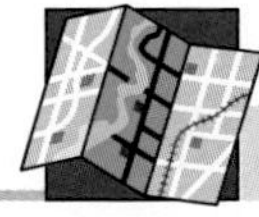 Patients With Dermatoses (Abnormal Skin Conditions)

Nursing Interventions	Rationale	Expected Outcomes
Nursing Diagnosis: Impaired skin integrity related to changes in the barrier function of the skin **Goal:** Maintenance of skin integrity		
1. Protect healthy skin from maceration (excessive hydration of stratum corneum) when applying wet dressings.	1. Maceration of healthy skin can cause skin breakdown and extension of the primary condition.	• Maintains skin integrity • Absence of maceration • No signs of thermal injury • Absence of infection • Applies prescribed topical medication • Takes prescribed medication on schedule
2. Remove moisture from skin by blotting gently and avoiding friction.	2. Friction and maceration play a major role in some skin diseases.	
3. Guard carefully against risks of thermal injuries from excessively hot wet dressings and from subtle heat injuries (heating pads, radiators).	3. Patients with dermatoses may have decreased sensitivity to heat.	
4. Advise patient to use sunscreening agents.	4. Many cosmetic problems and virtually all cutaneous malignancies can be attributed to chronic skin damage.	
Nursing Diagnosis: Pain and itching related to skin lesions **Goal:** Relief of discomfort		
1. Examine area of involvement.	1. Understanding the extent and characteristics of the skin involved helps in planning interventions.	• Achieves relief of discomfort • Verbalizes that itching has been relieved • Demonstrates absence of skin excoriation from scratching • Complies with prescribed treatment • Keeps skin hydrated and lubricated • Demonstrates intact skin; skin regaining healthy appearance
a. Attempt to discover cause of discomfort.	a. Helps to identify appropriate comfort measures.	
b. Record observations in detail, using descriptive terminology.	b. An accurate description of a cutaneous eruption is necessary for diagnosis and treatment. Many skin conditions appear similar but have different etiologies. Cutaneous inflammatory response may be muted in elderly patients.	
c. Anticipate possible allergic reaction; obtain a medication history.	c. A generalized rash, particularly of sudden onset, may indicate a medication allergy.	
2. Control environmental and physical factors.	2. Itching is aggravated by heat, chemicals, and physical irritants.	
a. Keep humidity about 60%; use a humidifier.	a. At low humidity, the skin loses water.	
b. Maintain a cool environment.	b. Coolness deters itching.	
c. Use mild soap for sensitive skin (Dove, Cataphyl, Aveeno).	c. These contain no detergents, dyes, fragrances, or hardening agents.	
d. Remove excess clothing or bedding.	d. Promotes cool environment.	
e. Wash Bed linens and clothing with mild fragrance-free soap.	e. Strong soaps and laundry additives can cause skin irritation.	
f. Stop repeated exposures to detergents, cleansers, and solvents.	f. Any substance that removes water, lipids, or protein from the epidermis alters the skin's barrier function.	
3. Use skin care measures to maintain skin integrity and promote comfort.	3. The skin is an important barrier that must be maintained intact to function properly.	
a. Provide tepid cooling baths or cool dressings for itching.	a. Gradual evaporation of water from dressings cools the skin and relieves pruritus.	
b. Treat dryness (xerosis) as prescribed.	b. Dry skin can produce areas of dermatitis with redness, itching, scaling, and, in more severe forms, swelling, blistering, cracking, and weeping.	
c. Apply skin lotion or cream immediately after bathing.	c. Effective hydration of the stratum corneum prevents compromise of the barrier layer of the skin.	

(continued)

52•1

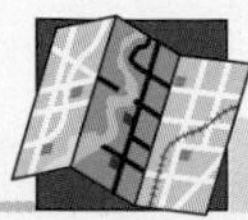

Plan of Nursing Care: Patients With Dermatoses (Abnormal Skin Conditions) (*continued*)

Nursing Interventions	Rationale	Expected Outcomes
d. Keep nails trimmed.	d. Trimming decreases skin damage from scratching.	
e. Apply prescribed topical therapy.	e. This helps to relieve symptoms.	
f. Help the patient accept possibly prolonged treatment.	f. Effective coping measures usually promote comfort.	
g. Advise the patient to refrain from using salves or lotions that are commercially available.	g. The patient's problem may be aggravated by self-medication.	

Nursing Diagnosis: Sleep pattern disturbance related to pruritus
Goal: Achievement of restful sleep

Nursing Interventions	Rationale	Expected Outcomes
1. Prevent and treat dry skin.	1. Nocturnal pruritus interferes with normal sleep.	• Achieves restful sleep • Reports relief of itching • Maintains appropriate environmental conditions • Avoids caffeine in late afternoon and evening • Identifies measures to promote sleep • Experiences satisfactory rest/sleep pattern
a. Advise patient to keep bedroom well ventilated and humidified.	a. Dry air will make skin feel itchy. A comfortable environment promotes relaxation.	
b. Keep skin moisturized.	b. This prevents water loss. Dry, itchy skin can usually be controlled but not cured.	
c. Bathe/shower only as necessary if skin is excessively dry. Use no soap or only mild soap. Apply skin lotion/cream immediately after bathing while skin is damp.	c. These measures preserve skin moisture.	
2. Advise patient of the following measures that may be helpful in promoting sleep:		
a. Keep a regular schedule for sleeping. Go to bed at the same time; get up at the same time.	a. Regularity of sleep schedule is important in maintaining sleep.	
b. Avoid caffeinated drinks in the evening.	b. Caffeine has peak effect 2–4 hours after being consumed.	
c. Exercise regularly, particularly in late afternoon.	c. Exercise at this time appears to have beneficial sleep effect.	
d. Use a bedtime routine or ritual.	d. This eases transition from wakefulness to sleep.	
e. Use an antihistamine at bedtime if prescribed.		

Nursing Diagnosis: Body image disturbance related to unsightly skin appearance
Goal: Development of increasing self-acceptance

Nursing Interventions	Rationale	Expected Outcomes
1. Assess patient for disturbance of self-image (avoidance of eye contact, self-negating verbalizations, expression of disgust about skin condition).	1. Disturbance of body image may accompany any disease or condition that is apparent to the patient. An impression of one's own body has an effect on self-concept.	• Develops increasing acceptance of own body • Follows through and participates in self-care measures • Reports feeling in control of situation • Gives self positive reinforcement • Verbalizes a more healthful self-regard • Appears less self-conscious; is not afraid to socialize and be seen by others • Uses concealing and highlighting techniques to enhance appearance
2. Identify psychosocial stage of development.	2. There is a relationship between development stage, self-image, and the patient's reaction to and understanding of skin condition.	
3. Provide opportunity for expression. Listen (in an open, nonjudgmental way) to expressions of grief/anxiety about changes in body image.	3. The patient needs the experience of being heard and understood.	
4. Assess the patient's concerns and fears. Assist anxious patient to develop insight and identify and cope with problems.	4. This gives health care personnel opportunity to neutralize undue anxiety and restore reality to the situation. Fear is destructive to adaptation.	

(*continued*)

52•1

Plan of Nursing Care 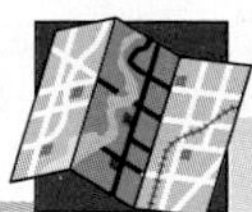 Patients With Dermatoses (Abnormal Skin Conditions) (*continued*)

Nursing Interventions	Rationale	Expected Outcomes
5. Support patient's efforts to improve body image (participation in skin treatments; grooming), develop self-acceptance, socialize with others, and use cosmetics to conceal disfigurement.	5. A positive approach and suggestions about cosmetic techniques are often helpful in promoting self-acceptance and socialization.	
Nursing Diagnosis: Knowledge deficit about skin care and methods of treating skin ailment **Goal:** Understanding of skin care		
1. Determine what the patient knows (understands and misunderstands) about the condition.	1. Provides baseline data for developing the teaching plan.	• Acquires understanding of skin care • Follows treatment as prescribed and can verbalize rationale for measures taken • Carries out prescribed baths, soaks, wet dressings • Uses topical medication appropriately • Understands importance of nutrition to skin health
2. Keep the patient informed; correct misconceptions/misinformation.	2. Patients need to have a sense that there is something they can do. Most patients benefit from explanations and reassurance.	
3. Demonstrate application of prescribed therapy (wet compresses; topical medication).	3. Allows patient the opportunity to visualize the correct way to perform therapies.	
4. Advise the patient to keep skin moist and flexible with hydration and application of skin cream and lotion.	4. The stratum corneum needs water to stay flexible. Application of skin cream or lotion to damp skin prevents dry, rough, cracked, and scaly skin.	
5. Encourage the patient to attain a healthy nutritional status.	5. The appearance of the skin reflects a person's general health. Changes may signal abnormal nutrition.	
Collaborative Problems: Infection **Goal:** Absence of complications		
1. Have a high index of suspicion for an infection in patients with compromised immune systems.	1. Any condition that compromises the immune status increases the risk of cutaneous infection.	• Remains free of infection • Verbalizes skin care measures that promote cleanliness and prevent skin breakdown • Identifies signs and symptoms of infection to report • Identifies adverse effects of medications that should be reported to health care personnel • Participates in skin care measures (eg, dressing changes, soaks)
2. Instruct the patient clearly and in detail about the therapeutic regimen.	2. Effective patient education is dependent on the interpersonal skills of the health professionals and on giving clear instructions reinforced through written instructions.	
3. Apply intermittent wet dressings as prescribed to reduce intensity of inflammation.	3. A wet dressing produces evaporative cooling, causing constriction of superficial cutaneous vessels and thereby decreasing erythema and serum production. Wet dressings help in débridement of vesicles and crusts and control inflammatory processes.	
4. Provide tub baths and soaks as prescribed.	4. Loosens exudates and scales.	
5. Administer prescribed antimicrobial agents.	5. Kills or prevents the growth of the infectious organism.	
6. Use topical medications containing corticosteroids as prescribed and as indicated. a. Observe lesion periodically for changes in response to therapy. b. Instruct the patient about possible adverse effects of long-term use of fluorinated topical corticosteroids.	6. Corticosteroids have an anti-inflammatory action, resulting in part from their ability to induce vasoconstriction of the small vessels in the upper dermis. Extensive prolonged use of topical corticosteroids can lead to antiproliferative effects on epidermal cells (loss of hair in area used).	
7. Advise patient to stop using any skin agent that makes the problem worse.	7. A contact dermatitis or allergic reaction may develop from any ingredient in the medication.	

damage from scratching. Every effort should be made to keep the skin hydrated and moistened to avoid skin breakdown. The patient is advised to avoid using over-the-counter preparations to relieve itching because the skin problem may be increased by irritation or sensitization from self-medication.

Gradual evaporation of water from dressings cools the skin and relieves pruritus. The nurse reinforces teaching and makes sure that the patient understands that normal skin should be protected during the application of wet dressings. The patient is instructed to moisten an adherent dressing before removal to relieve discomfort. When taking therapeutic baths (a form of wet dressing), the patient is advised to limit bathing time to 20 to 30 minutes to prevent skin maceration. Generally, therapeutic baths may be taken twice daily.

Achieving Restful Sleep

Irritation and itching interfere with normal sleep. The following measures to promote sleep are discussed with the patient:

- Keep a regular schedule for sleeping; go to bed at the same time and get up at the same time.
- Avoid caffeinated beverages in the evening.
- Use a bedtime routine or ritual to ease the transition from wakefulness to sleep.
- Use oral antihistamines as prescribed.
- Exercise regularly if there are no physical limitations.

In addition, the bedroom should be well ventilated and humidified. Other measures to promote skin comfort and aid relaxation are found in Plan of Nursing Care 52-1.

Increasing Self-Acceptance

Physical appearance exerts a profound influence in society and in the way people are treated. Preferential treatment is often based on physical attractiveness. Clean and healthy skin is closely correlated with attractiveness and, thereby, one's self-esteem.

Skin diseases can cause emotional suffering and can affect social and business relationships and recreational activities. For example, people with eczema often have difficulty convincing others that their disease is not contagious. Those with flaking and scaling conditions may be wary of meeting new people. Comments from strangers may be difficult to handle. Diminishing self-confidence, excessive fixation on skin defects, and worry about scarring are frequently found in patients with acne. All of these factors can generate negative emotions in the patient.

The nurse must recognize that body image is a complex psychological concept that is related to the mental concept of self and self-esteem. Allowing patients to express their feelings freely provides support and acceptance. Mutual trust and respect between patient and nurse are necessary to promote communication.

Understanding Skin Care

Informed patients are usually less anxious and more cooperative. Thus, teaching them about their condition and its treatment may make them more hopeful, which may reinforce their ability to use their resources effectively.

Self-care, particularly hair and skin care, can make a difference in the way others perceive the patient. Appropriate cosmetics can bring substantial benefits to a person with a chronic skin condition or disfigurement. Referral to an expert cosmetologist to camouflage birthmarks, mottled skin, scars, and chronic dermatitis can be beneficial. People who remain depressed over their condition may benefit from counseling.

Monitoring and Managing Potential Complications

INFECTION

Potentially infected skin lesions should be treated with proper precautions until the diagnosis is established and the infecting organism identified. Keeping the affected area clean and administering medications as prescribed are primary defenses against infection, as is adequate nutrition. The patient should be instructed how to perform daily skin care (including dressing changes, if appropriate) and how to recognize and report general signs and symptoms of infection, such as redness, swelling, pain, pus, and fever.

Promoting Home and Community-Based Care

TEACHING PATIENTS SELF-CARE

Healthy skin reflects one's general health. Principles of good nutrition, exercise, rest, and sleep are emphasized in any teaching program focused on skin care. In addition, preprinted materials are available that describe common dermatologic conditions ranging from acne and warts to postoperative measures, including care of an open wound, suture care, or applying soaks or topical medications.

A patient who is receiving treatment for a skin condition is usually informed by the physician what the skin condition is, its source or cause, and what to expect from treatment. Some patients hear or understand only part of what is being said. Many patients find it helpful to have a relative or friend present, not only for emotional support but also to listen to treatment instructions, which may be lengthy and complex.

Printed information sheets help reinforce instructions. They can be taken home and referred to as needed, and they can answer questions about the condition or incidental queries about such things as skin cancer, sunscreens, or office hours, fees, billing policies, and emergency contact information. Information sheets can be individualized by writing specific or additional information directly on the sheet (eg, how to apply a topical medication, the amount to apply, the size of the area to be treated, and the frequency of application). Potential side effects may be identified and highlighted on the sheet to emphasize their importance.

A major problem encountered in using printed information is the readability level. Information must be written at or near a fifth-grade reading level so that most patients can understand and comply with the instructions. Information should be presented in short sentences, using familiar or common words and large type. Only essential information should be included, without unnecessary detail. This is especially important for elderly patients or those with vision deficits.

Evaluation

Expected Outcomes

Expected outcomes may include:

1. Maintains skin integrity
   a. Indicates absence of skin cracking
   b. Protects skin from contact with irritating substances
   c. Applies emollient to skin as prescribed
2. Achieves relief of discomfort
   a. Uses topical medication and treatments as prescribed
   b. Reports relief of itching

3. Achieves more restful sleep
   a. States is "sleeping better"
   b. Reports an increased feeling of well-being
4. Demonstrates increasing self-acceptance
   a. Voices fewer self-deprecating remarks
   b. Pays attention to appearance
5. Acquires understanding of skin care
   a. Verbalizes rationale of prescribed treatment
   b. Demonstrates ability to perform treatments

PRURITUS

Pruritus (itching) is one of the most common complaints in dermatologic disorders. Itch receptors are unmyelinated, penicillate (brushlike) nerve endings that are found exclusively in the skin, mucous membranes, and cornea. Although pruritus is usually due to primary skin disease with resultant rash or lesions, it may occur without a rash or lesion. This is referred to as essential pruritus, which generally has a rapid onset, may be severe, and interferes with normal daily activities.

Pruritus may be the first indication of a systemic internal disease such as diabetes mellitus, blood disorders, or cancer. Itching may also accompany renal, hepatic, and thyroid diseases (Chart 52-2). Some common oral medications such as aspirin, antibiotics, hormones (estrogens, testosterone, or oral contraceptives), and opioids (morphine or cocaine) may cause pruritus as well. Certain soaps and chemicals, radiation therapy, prickly heat (miliaria), and contact with woolen garments are also associated with pruritus. Pruritus may also be caused by psychological factors, such as excessive stress in family or work situations.

Scratching causes the inflamed cells and nerve endings to release histamine, which produces more pruritus and, in turn, a vicious itch–scratch cycle. If the patient responds to an itch by scratching, the integrity of the skin may be altered, and excoriation, redness, raised areas (wheals), infection, and changes in pigmentation may result. Pruritus usually is more severe at night and is less frequently reported during waking hours, probably because the person is distracted by daily activities. At nighttime, when there are few distractions, the slightest pruritus cannot be easily ignored. Severe itching is debilitating.

Gerontologic Considerations

Pruritus may occur in elderly people, commonly as a result of dry skin.

Medical Management

A thorough history and physical examination usually provides clues to the underlying cause of the pruritus (hay fever, allergy, recent ingestion of a new medication, change of cosmetics or soaps). Once the cause has been identified and removed, treatment of the condition should relieve the pruritus. Signs of infection and environmental clues, such as warm, dry air or irritating bed linens, should be identified. In general, washing with soap and hot water is avoided. Bath oils (eg, Lubath, Alpha-Keri) containing a surfactant that makes the oil mix with bath water may be sufficient for cleaning. However, an elderly patient or a patient with unsteady balance should avoid adding oil because it increases the danger of slipping in the bathtub. In addition, a warm bath with a mild soap followed by application of a bland emollient to moist skin can control xerosis (dry skin). Applying a cold compress, ice cube, or cool agents containing soothing menthol and camphor that constrict blood vessels may also help relieve pruritus.

PHARMACOLOGIC THERAPY

Topical corticosteroids may be beneficial as anti-inflammatory agents to decrease itching. Oral antihistamines are even more effective because they can overcome the effects of histamine release from damaged mast cells. An antihistamine, such as diphenhydramine (Benadryl) or hydroxyzine (Atarax), prescribed in a sedative dose at bedtime is effective in producing a restful and comfortable sleep. Nonsedating antihistamine medications such as fexofenadine (Allegra) should be used to relieve daytime pruritus. Tricyclic antidepressants, such as doxepin (Sinequan), may be prescribed for pruritus of neuropsychogenic origin. If pruritus continues, further investigation of a systemic problem is advised.

Nursing Management

The nurse reinforces the reasons for the prescribed therapeutic regimen and counsels the patient on specific points of care. If baths have been prescribed, the patient is reminded to use tepid (not hot) water and to shake off the excess water and blot between intertriginous (body fold) areas with a towel. Rubbing vigorously with the towel is avoided because this overstimulates the skin and causes more itching. It also removes water from the stratum corneum. Immediately after bathing, the skin should be lubricated with an emollient that traps moisture.

The patient is instructed to avoid situations that cause vasodilation (expansion of the blood vessels). Examples include exposure to an overly warm environment and ingestion of alcohol or hot foods and liquids. All will induce or intensify itching. Using a humidifier is helpful if environmental air is dry and provokes pruritus. Activities that result in perspiration should be limited because sweat may be irritating and may promote general itching. If the patient is troubled at night with itching that interferes with sleep, the nurse can advise wearing cotton clothing next to the skin rather than synthetic materials. The room should be kept cool and humidified. Vigorous scratching is to be avoided and nails should be kept trimmed to prevent skin damage and infec-

CHART 52•2 Systemic Disorders Associated With Generalized Pruritus

Chronic renal disease

Obstructive biliary disease (primary biliary cirrhosis, extrahepatic biliary obstruction, drug-induced cholestasis)

Endocrine disease (thyrotoxicosis, hypothyroidism, diabetes mellitus, mastocytosis, iron deficiency anemia)

Psychiatric disorders (emotional stress, anxiety, neurosis, phobias)

Malignancies (polycythemia vera, Hodgkin's disease, lymphoma, leukemia, multiple myeloma, mycosis fungoides, and cancers of the lung, breast, central nervous system, and gastrointestinal tract)

Neurologic disorders (multiple sclerosis, brain abscess, brain tumor)

Infestations (scabies, lice, other insects)

Pruritus of pregnancy (PUPP [pruritic urticarial papules of pregnancy], cholestasis of pregnancy, pemphigoid of pregnancy)

Folliculitis (bacterial, candidiasis, dermatophyte)

Skin conditions (seborrheic dermatitis, folliculitis, iron deficiency anemia, atopic dermatitis, drug exanthems)

tion. When the underlying cause of pruritus is not known and further testing is required, the nurse explains each test and the expected outcome.

Perianal Itching

Pruritus of the anal and genital regions may be caused by small particles of fecal material lodged in the perianal crevices or attached to anal hairs, or by perianal skin damage caused by scratching, moisture, and decreased skin resistance as a result of corticosteroid or antibiotic therapy. Other possible causes of perianal itching include local irritants such as scabies and lice, local lesions such as hemorrhoids, fungal or yeast infections, and pinworm infestation. Conditions such as diabetes mellitus, anemias, hyperthyroidism, and pregnancy may also result in perianal pruritus.

Nursing Management

The nurse instructs the patient to follow proper hygiene measures and to discontinue home and over-the-counter remedies. The perianal area should be rinsed with lukewarm water and the area blotted dry with cotton balls. Premoistened tissues may be used after defecation.

As part of health teaching, the nurse instructs the patient to avoid bathing in water that is too hot and to avoid using bubble baths, sodium bicarbonate, or detergent soaps, all of which aggravate dryness. To keep the perianal skin as dry as possible, patients should avoid wearing underwear made of synthetic fabrics. Local anesthetic agents should not be used because of possible allergic effects. The patient should also avoid vasodilating agents or stimulants (alcohol, coffee) and mechanical irritants such as rough or woolen clothing. A diet that includes adequate fiber may help maintain soft stools and prevent minor trauma to the anal mucosa.

SECRETORY DISORDERS

The main secretory function of the skin is performed by the sweat glands, which help to regulate body temperature. These glands excrete a fluid, perspiration, which evaporates, thereby cooling the body. The sweat glands are located in various parts of the body and respond to different stimuli. Those on the trunk generally respond to thermal stimulation, those on the palms and soles respond to nervous stimulation, and those in the axillae and on the forehead respond to both kinds of stimulation. Normal sweat has no odor. Body odor is produced by the increase in bacteria on the skin and the interaction of bacterial waste products with the chemicals of perspiration.

As a rule, moist skin is warm and dry skin is cool. However, this is not a hard-and-fast rule. It is not unusual to observe cold sweats, warm, dry skin in a dehydrated patient, and very hot dry skin peculiar to some febrile states.

Normally sweat can be controlled with the use of antiperspirants and deodorants. Most antiperspirants are aluminum salts that block the opening to the sweat duct. Pure deodorants inhibit bacterial growth and block the metabolism of sweat; they have no antiperspirant effect. Fragrance-free deodorants are available for those with sensitive skin (Arndt et al., 1997).

Seborrheic Dermatoses

Seborrhea is excessive production of sebum (secretion of sebaceous glands) in areas where glands are normally found in large numbers (face, scalp, eyebrows, eyelids, at the sides of the nose and upper lip, malar [cheek] regions, ears, axillae, under the breasts, groin, and gluteal crease of the buttocks). Seborrheic dermatitis is a chronic inflammatory disease of the skin with a predilection for areas that are well supplied with sebaceous glands or lie between skin folds, where the bacteria count is high.

Clinical Manifestations

Two forms of seborrheic dermatoses can occur—an oily form and a dry form. Either form may start in childhood and continue throughout life. The oily form appears moist or greasy. There may be patches of sallow, greasy skin, with or without scaling, and slight erythema (redness), predominantly on the forehead, nasolabial fold, beard area, and scalp, and between adjacent skin surfaces in the regions of the axillae, groin, and breasts. Small pustules or papulopustules resembling acne may appear on the trunk. The dry form, consisting of flaky desquamation of the scalp with a profuse amount of fine, powdery scales, is commonly called dandruff. The mild forms of the disease are asymptomatic. When scaling occurs, it is often accompanied by pruritus, which may lead to scratching and secondary complications, such as infection and excoriation.

Seborrheic dermatitis has a genetic predisposition. Hormones, nutritional status, infection, and emotional stress influence its course. The remissions and exacerbations of this condition should be explained to the patient.

Medical Management

Because there is no known cure for seborrhea, the objective of therapy is to control the disorder and allow the skin to repair itself. Seborrheic dermatitis of the body and face may respond to a topically applied corticosteroid cream, which allays the secondary inflammatory response. However, this medication should be used with caution near the eyelids, because it can induce glaucoma and cataracts in predisposed patients. Patients with seborrheic dermatitis may develop a secondary candidal (yeast) infection in body creases or folds. To avoid this, patients should be advised to ensure maximum aeration of the skin and to clean carefully areas where there are creases or folds in the skin. Patients with persistent candidiasis should be evaluated for diabetes.

The mainstay of dandruff treatment is proper, frequent shampooing (daily or at least three times weekly) with medicated shampoos. Two or three different types of shampoo should be used in rotation to prevent the seborrhea from becoming resistant to a particular shampoo. The shampoo is left on at least 5 to 10 minutes. As the condition of the scalp improves, the treatment can be less frequent. Antiseborrheic shampoos include those containing selenium sulfide suspension, zinc pyrithione, salicylic acid/sulfur compounds, and tar shampoo that contains sulfur or salicylic acid.

Nursing Management

A person with seborrheic dermatitis is advised to remove external irritants and to avoid excessive heat and perspiration; rubbing and scratching prolong the disorder. To avoid secondary infections, the patient should air the skin and keep skin folds clean and dry.

Instructions for using medicated shampoos are reinforced for those with dandruff that requires treatment. Frequent shampooing is contrary to some cultural practices; the nurse should be sensitive to these differences when teaching the patient about home care.

The patient is cautioned that seborrheic dermatitis is a chronic problem that tends to wax and wane. The goal is to keep it under control. Patients need to be encouraged to adhere to the treatment program. Those who become discouraged and disheartened by the effect on body image should be treated with sensitivity and an awareness of their need to express their feelings.

Acne Vulgaris

Acne vulgaris is a common follicular disorder affecting susceptible pilosebaceous follicles (hair follicles), most commonly found on the face, neck, and upper trunk. It is characterized by **comedones** (primary acne lesions), both closed comedones (whiteheads) and open comedones (blackheads), as well as papules, pustules, nodules, and cysts.

Acne is the most commonly encountered skin condition in adolescents and young adults between ages 12 and 35. Both genders are affected equally, although with a slightly earlier onset for girls. This may be due to the fact that girls reach pubertal development at a younger age than boys. It becomes more marked at puberty and during adolescence, because at this age the endocrine glands that influence the secretions of the sebaceous glands are functioning at peak activity. Acne appears to stem from an interplay of genetic, hormonal, and bacterial factors. In most cases there is a family history of acne.

Pathophysiology

During childhood, the sebaceous glands are small and virtually nonfunctioning. These glands are under endocrine control, especially the androgens. During puberty, androgens stimulate the sebaceous glands, causing them to enlarge and to secrete a natural oil, sebum, which rises to the top of the hair follicle and flows out onto the skin surface. In adolescents who develop acne, androgenic stimulation produces a heightened response in the sebaceous glands so that acne occurs when accumulated sebum plugs the pilosebaceous ducts. This accumulated material forms comedones.

Clinical Manifestations

The primary lesions of acne are comedones. Closed comedones (whiteheads) are obstructive lesions formed from impacted lipids or oils and keratin that plug the dilated follicle. They are small, whitish papules with minute follicular openings that generally cannot be seen. These closed comedones may evolve into open comedones, in which the contents of the ducts are in open communication with the external environment. Open comedones are termed blackheads. The color of the blackhead results not from dirt, but from an accumulation of lipid, bacterial, and epithelial debris.

Although the exact cause is not known, some closed comedones may rupture, resulting in an inflammatory reaction caused by leakage of follicular contents (sebum, keratin, bacteria) into the dermis. This inflammatory response may result from the action of certain skin bacteria, such as **Propionibacterium acnes,** that live in the hair follicles and break down the triglycerides of the sebum into free fatty acids and glycerin. The resultant inflammation is seen clinically as erythematous papules, inflammatory pustules, and inflammatory cysts. Mild papules and cysts drain and heal on their own without treatment. Deeper papules and cysts may result in scarring of the skin. Acne is usually graded as mild, moderate, or severe based on the number and type of lesions (comedones, papules, pustules, cysts).

Assessment and Diagnostic Findings

The acne diagnosis is based on the history and physical examination, evidence of lesions characteristic of acne, and age. Acne does not occur until puberty. The presence of the typical comedones (whiteheads and blackheads) along with excessively oily skin is characteristic. Oiliness is more prominent in the midfacial area; other parts of the face may appear dry. When there are numerous lesions, some of which are open, the person may exude a distinct sebaceous odor. Female patients may report a history of flare-ups a few days before menses. Biopsy of lesions is seldom necessary for a definitive diagnosis.

Medical Management

The goals of management are to reduce bacterial colonies, decrease sebaceous gland activity, prevent the follicles from becoming plugged, reduce inflammation, combat secondary infection, minimize scarring, and eliminate factors that predispose the person to acne. The therapeutic regimen depends on the type of lesion (comedonal, papular, pustular, cystic).

There is no predictable cure for the disease, but combinations of therapies are available that can control its activity effectively. Topical treatment may be all that is needed to treat mild to moderate lesions as well as superficial inflammatory lesions (papular or pustular).

NUTRITIONAL THERAPY

Although food restrictions have been recommended from time to time in treating acne, diet does not play a major role in therapy. The elimination of a specific food or food product associated with a flare-up of acne, such as chocolate, cola, fried foods, or milk products, should be promoted. Maintenance of good nutrition equips the immune system for effective action against bacteria and infection.

SKIN HYGIENE

In mild cases of acne, washing twice a day with a cleansing soap may be all that is required. These soaps can remove the excessive skin oil and the comedo in most cases. Providing positive reassurance, listening attentively, and being sensitive to the feelings of the patient with acne are essential contributors to the patient's psychological well-being and understanding of the disease and treatment plan. Over-the-counter acne medications contain salicylic acid and benzoyl peroxide, both of which are very effective at removing the sebaceous follicular plugs. However, the skin of some people is sensitive to these products. They can cause irritation or excessive dryness, especially when used with some prescribed topical medications. The patient should be taught to discontinue use of over-the-counter products if severe irritation occurs. Oil-free cosmetics and creams should be chosen. These products are usually designated as useful for acne-prone skin. The duration of treatment depends on the extent and severity of the acne. In severe cases, treatment may extend over years.

TOPICAL PHARMACOLOGIC THERAPY

Benzoyl Peroxide. Benzoyl peroxide preparations are widely used because they produce a rapid and sustained reduction of inflammatory lesions. They depress sebum production and promote breakdown of comedo plugs. They also produce an antibacterial effect by suppressing *P. acnes.* Initially, benzoyl peroxide causes redness and scaling, but generally the skin adjusts quickly to its use. Usually the patient applies a gel of benzoyl peroxide once daily. In many instances this is the only treatment needed. Benzoyl peroxide, benzoyl erythromycin, and benzoyl sulfur combinations are available over the counter and by prescription. Vitamin A acid (tretinoin) applied topically is used to clear the keratin plugs from the pilosebaceous ducts. Vitamin A acid speeds the cellular turnover, forces out the comedones, and prevents new comedones.

The patient should be informed that symptoms may worsen during early weeks of therapy because inflammation may occur during the process. Erythema and peeling are also a frequent result. Improvement may take 8 to 12 weeks. Some patients cannot tolerate this therapy. The patient is cautioned against sun exposure while using this topical medication because it may cause an exaggerated sunburn. Package insert directions should be followed carefully.

Topical Antibiotics. Topical antibiotic treatment for acne is widespread. Topical antibiotics suppress the growth of *P. acnes*, reduce superficial free fatty acid levels, decrease comedones, papules, and pustules, and produce no systemic side effects. Common topical preparations include tetracycline, clindamycin, and erythromycin.

SYSTEMIC PHARMACOLOGIC THERAPY

Antibiotics. Oral antibiotics, such as tetracycline, doxycycline, or minocycline, administered in small doses over a long period are very effective in treating moderate and severe acne, especially when the acne is inflammatory and results in pustules, abscesses, and scarring. Therapy may continue for months to years. The tetracycline family of antibiotics is contraindicated in children younger than age 12 and in pregnant women. Although these medications are considered safe for long-term use in most cases, administration during pregnancy can affect the development of teeth, causing enamel hypoplasia and permanent discoloration of teeth in infants. Side effects of tetracyclines include photosensitivity, nausea, diarrhea, and cutaneous infection in either gender, and vaginitis in women. (In some women, broad-spectrum antibiotics may suppress normal vaginal bacteria and predispose the patient to candidiasis, a fungal infection.)

Oral Retinoids. Synthetic vitamin A compounds (retinoids) are being used with dramatic results in patients with nodular cystic acne unresponsive to conventional therapy. One compound is isotretinoin (Accutane). Isotretinoin is also used for active inflammatory papular pustular acne that has a tendency to scar. Isotretinoin reduces sebaceous gland size and inhibits sebum production. It also causes the epidermis to shed (epidermal desquamation), thereby unseating and expelling existing comedones.

The most common side effect, experienced by almost all patients, is **cheilitis** (inflammation of the lips). Dry and chafed skin and mucous membranes are frequent side effects. These changes are reversible with the withdrawal of the medication. Most important, isotretinoin is teratogenic in humans, meaning that it can have an adverse effect on a fetus, causing central nervous system and cardiovascular defects and structural abnormalities of the face. Therefore, contraceptive measures for women of childbearing age are mandatory during treatment and for about 4 to 8 weeks thereafter. To avoid additive toxic effects, patients are cautioned not to take vitamin A supplements while taking isotretinoin.

Hormone Therapy. Estrogen therapy (progesterone/estrogen preparations) suppresses sebum production and reduces skin oiliness. It is usually reserved for young women when the acne begins somewhat later than usual and tends to flare at certain times in the menstrual cycle. Estrogen in the form of estrogen-dominant oral contraceptive compounds may be administered on a prescribed cyclic regimen. Estrogen is not administered to male patients because of undesirable side effects.

SURGICAL TREATMENT

Surgical treatment of acne consists of comedo extraction, injections of corticosteroids into the inflamed lesions, and incision and drainage of large, fluctuant (moving in palpable waves), nodular cystic lesions. Cryosurgery (freezing with liquid nitrogen) may be used for nodular and cystic forms of acne. Patients with deep scars may be treated with deep abrasive therapy (dermabrasion), in which the epidermis and some superficial dermis are removed down to the level of the scars.

Comedones may be removed with a comedo extractor. The site is first cleaned with alcohol. The opening of the extractor is then placed over the lesion, and direct pressure is applied to cause extrusion of the plug through the extractor.

Removal of comedones leaves erythema, which may take several weeks to subside. Recurrence of comedones after extraction is common because of the continuing activity of the pilosebaceous glands.

Table 52-5 summarizes current treatment modalities for acne vulgaris.

Nursing Management

MONITORING AND MANAGING POTENTIAL COMPLICATIONS

Major nursing activities in caring for patients with acne include education, particularly in proper skin care techniques and managing potential problems related to the skin disorder or therapy.

TABLE 52•5 Commonly Prescribed Treatments of Acne Vulgaris

Kind of therapy	Prescribed Treatment Agent
Topical	benzoyl peroxide wash, gel Benzamycin gel (benzoyl peroxide and erythromycin) Bensulfoid cr (benzoyl peroxide and sulfur) resorcinol (as ingredient in other preparations) salicylic acid (as ingredient in other preparations) sulfur (as ingredient in other preparations) tretinoin (Retin A, Avita) topical antibiotics
Systemic	oral antibiotics (erythromycin, tetracycline, doxycycline, minocin, trimethoprim—sulfamethoxazole) Accutane hormones: corticosteroids high dose for anti-inflammatory action low dose to suppress androgenic action intralesional for anti-inflammatory action antiandrogens oral contraceptives (women only)
Surgical	extraction of comedo contents drainage of pustules and cysts excision of sinus tracts and cysts intralesional corticosteroids for anti-inflammatory action cryotherapy dermabrasion for scars

Treatments listed are common but do not include all available forms of therapy.

Scarring. Prevention of scarring is the ultimate goal of therapy. The chance of scarring increases as the grade of acne increases. Grades III and IV (25 to more than 50 comedones, papules, or pustules) usually require longer-term therapy with systemic antibiotics or isotretinoin. Patients should be warned that discontinuing these medications can exacerbate acne, lead to more flare-ups, and increase the chance of deep scarring. Moreover, manipulation of the comedones, papules, and pustules increases the potential for scarring.

When acne surgery is prescribed to extract deep-seated comedones or inflamed lesions or to incise and drain cystic lesions, the intervention itself may result in further scarring. Dermabrasion, which levels existing scar tissue, has the potential for increasing scar formation as well. In addition, hyper- or hypopigmentation may affect the tissue involved. The patient should be informed of these potential outcomes before electing surgical intervention for acne.

Infection. Female patients receiving long-term antibiotic therapy with tetracycline should be advised to watch for and report signs and symptoms of oral or vaginal candidiasis, a yeastlike fungal infection.

PROMOTING HOME AND COMMUNITY-BASED CARE

Teaching Patients Self-Care. In addition to receiving instructions for taking prescribed medications, patients are instructed to wash the face and other affected areas with mild soap and water twice a day to remove surface oils and prevent obstruction of the oil glands. They are cautioned to avoid scrubbing the face; acne is not caused by dirt and cannot be washed away.

Mild abrasive soaps and drying agents are prescribed to eliminate the oily feeling that troubles many patients. At the same time, patients are cautioned to avoid excessive abrasion because it makes acne worse. Excessive abrasion causes minute scratches on the skin surface and increases possible bacterial contamination. In addition, soap itself can irritate the skin.

All forms of friction and trauma are avoided: propping the hands against the face, rubbing the face, and wearing tight collars and helmets. Patients are instructed to avoid manipulation of pimples or blackheads. Squeezing merely worsens the problem, because a portion of the blackhead is pushed down into the skin, which may cause the follicle to rupture. Because cosmetics, shaving creams, and lotions can aggravate acne, these substances are best avoided unless the patient is advised otherwise. There is no evidence that a particular food can cause or aggravate acne. In general, eating a nutritious diet helps the body maintain a strong immune system.

BACTERIAL INFECTIONS (PYODERMAS)

Also called **pyodermas**, pus-forming bacterial infections of the skin may be primary or secondary. Primary skin infections originate in previously normal-appearing skin and are usually caused by a single organism. Secondary skin infections arise from a preexisting skin disorder or from disruption of the skin integrity from injury or surgery. In either case, several microorganisms may be implicated (eg, *Staphylococcus aureus* or group A streptococci). The most common primary bacterial skin infections are impetigo and folliculitis. Folliculitis may lead to furuncles or carbuncles.

Impetigo

Impetigo is a superficial infection of the skin caused by staphylococci, streptococci, or multiple bacteria. Bullous impetigo, a more deep-seated infection of the skin caused by *S. aureus*, is characterized by the formation of bullae (large fluid-filled blisters) from original vesicles. The bullae rupture, leaving raw, red areas.

The exposed areas of the body, face, hands, neck, and extremities are most frequently involved. Impetigo is contagious and may spread to other parts of the patient's skin or to other members of the family who touch the patient or use towels or combs that are soiled with the exudate of the lesions.

Although impetigo is seen at all ages, it is particularly common among children living in poor hygienic conditions. Often it appears secondary to pediculosis capitis (head lice), scabies (itch mites), herpes simplex, insect bites, poison ivy, or eczema. Chronic health problems, poor hygiene, and malnutrition may predispose an adult to impetigo. Some people have been identified as asymptomatic carriers of *S. aureus,* usually in the nasal passages.

Clinical Manifestations

The lesions begin as small, red macules, which quickly become discrete, thin-walled vesicles that soon rupture and become covered with a loosely adherent honey-yellow crust (Fig. 52-1). These crusts are easily removed to reveal smooth, red, moist surfaces on which new crusts soon develop. If the scalp is involved, the hair is matted, which distinguishes the condition from ringworm.

Medical Management

Systemic antibiotic therapy is the usual treatment. It reduces contagious spread, treats deep infection, and prevents acute glomerulonephritis (kidney infection), which may occur as an aftermath of streptococcal skin diseases. In nonbullous impetigo, benzathine penicillin or oral penicillin may be prescribed. Bullous impetigo is treated with a penicillinase-resistant penicillin (cloxacillin, dicloxacillin). In penicillin-sensitive patients, erythromycin is an effective alternative.

Topical antibacterial therapy (eg, mupirocin) may be prescribed when the disease is limited to a small area. However, topical therapy requires that the medication be applied to the lesions several times daily for a week. The treatment regimen may be impossible for some patients or their caregivers to follow. In addition, topical antibiotics generally are not as effective as systemic therapy in eradicating or preventing the spread of streptococci

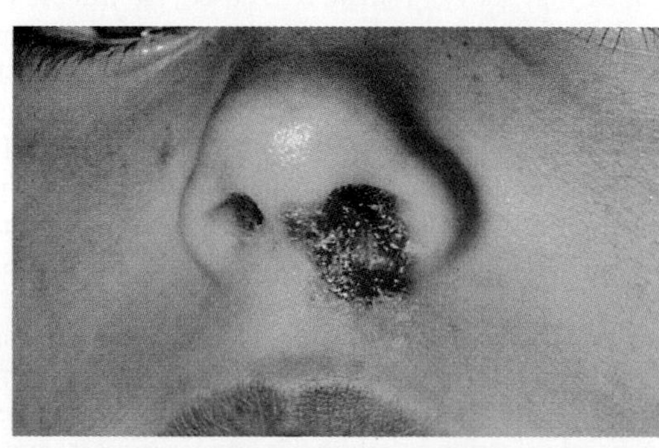

FIGURE 52•1 Impetigo of the nostril.

from the respiratory tract, thereby increasing the risk of developing glomerulonephritis.

When topical therapy is prescribed, lesions are soaked or washed with soap solution to remove the central site of bacterial growth, thus giving the topical antibiotic an opportunity to reach the infected site. After the crusts are removed, a topical medication (eg, polysporin, bacitracin) may be applied. Gloves are worn when providing patient care. An antiseptic solution, such as povidone–iodine (Betadine) or chlorhexidine (Hibiclens), may be used to clean the skin, reduce bacterial content in the infected area, and prevent spread.

Nursing Management

The nurse instructs the patient and family members to bathe at least once daily with bactericidal soap. Cleanliness and good hygiene practices help prevent the spread of the lesions from one skin area to another and from one person to another. Each person should have a separate towel and washcloth. Because impetigo is a contagious disorder, infected people should avoid contact with other infected people until the lesions heal.

Folliculitis, Furuncles, and Carbuncles

Folliculitis is an infection of either bacterial or fungal origin that arises within the hair follicles. Lesions may be superficial or deep. Single or multiple papules or pustules appear close to the hair follicles. Folliculitis commonly affects the beard area of men who shave, and women's legs. Other areas include the axillae, trunk, and buttocks.

Pseudofolliculitis barbae ("shaving bumps") is an inflammatory reaction that occurs predominately on the faces of African American and other curly-haired men. It is caused by shaving. The sharp ingrowing hairs have a curved root that grows at a more acute angle and pierces the skin, provoking an irritative reaction. The only entirely effective treatment is to avoid shaving. Other treatments include using special lotions or antibiotics or using a handbrush to dislodge the hairs mechanically. If the patient must remove facial hair, a depilatory cream or electric razor may be more useful than a straight razor.

A **furuncle** (boil) is an acute inflammation arising deep in one or more hair follicles and spreading into the surrounding dermis. It is a deeper form of folliculitis. (Furunculosis refers to multiple or recurrent lesions.) Furuncles may occur anywhere on the body but are more prevalent in areas subjected to irritation, pressure, friction, and excessive perspiration, such as the back of the neck, the axillae, or the buttocks.

A furuncle may start as a small, red, raised, painful pimple. Frequently, the infection progresses and involves the skin and subcutaneous fatty tissue, causing tenderness, pain, and surrounding cellulitis. The area of redness and induration represents an effort of the body to keep the infection localized. The bacteria (usually staphylococci) produce necrosis of the invaded tissue. The characteristic pointing of a boil follows in a few days. When this occurs, the center becomes yellow or black, and the boil is said to have "come to a head."

A **carbuncle** is an abscess of the skin and subcutaneous tissue that represents an extension of a furuncle that has invaded several follicles and is large and deep-seated. It is usually caused by a staphylococcal infection. Carbuncles appear most commonly in areas where the skin is thick and inelastic. The back of the neck and the buttocks are common sites. In carbuncles, the extensive inflammation frequently is not associated with a complete walling off of the infection, so absorption occurs, resulting in high fever, pain, leukocytosis, and even extension of the infection to the bloodstream.

Furuncles and carbuncles are more likely to occur in patients with underlying systemic diseases, such as diabetes or hematologic malignancies, and in those receiving immunosuppressive therapy for other diseases. Both are more prevalent in hot climates, especially on skin beneath occlusive clothing.

Medical Management

In treating staphylococcal infections, it is important not to rupture or destroy the protective wall of induration that localizes the infection. Therefore, the boil or pimple should never be squeezed.

The follicular disorders (folliculitis, furuncles, carbuncles) are usually caused by staphylococci, although if the immune system is impaired, the causative organisms may be gram-negative bacilli. Systemic antibiotic therapy, selected by sensitivity study, is generally indicated. Oral cloxacillin, dicloxacillin, and flucloxacillin are first-line medications. Cephalosporins and erythromycin are also effective. Bed rest is advised for patients who have boils on the perineum or in the anal region, and a course of systemic antibiotic therapy is indicated to prevent the spread of the infection.

When the pus has localized and is fluctuant, a small incision with a scalpel will speed resolution by relieving the tension and ensuring direct evacuation of the pus and slough. The patient is instructed to keep the draining lesion covered with a dressing.

Nursing Management

Intravenous fluids, fever reduction, and other supportive treatments are indicated for patients who are very ill or suffering with toxicity. Warm, moist compresses increase vascularization and hasten resolution of the furuncle or carbuncle. The surrounding skin may be cleaned gently with antibacterial soap, and an antibacterial ointment may be applied. Soiled dressings are handled according to standard precautions. Nursing personnel should carefully follow isolation precautions to avoid becoming carriers of staphylococci. Disposable gloves are worn when caring for these patients.

Nursing Alert *Nurses must take special precautions in caring for boils on the face, because the skin area drains directly into the cranial venous sinuses. Sinus thrombosis, with fatal pyemia, can develop after manipulating a boil in this location. In addition, the infection can travel through the sinus tract and penetrate the brain cavity, causing brain abscess.*

PROMOTING HOME AND COMMUNITY-BASED CARE

Teaching Patients Self-Care. To prevent and control staphylococcal skin infections (boils, carbuncles), the staphylococcal pathogen must be eliminated from the skin and environment. Efforts must be made to increase the patient's resistance and provide a hygienic environment. If lesions are actively draining, the mattress and pillow should be covered with plastic material and wiped off with disinfectant daily; the bed linens, towels, and clothing should be laundered after each use; and the patient should use an antibacterial soap and shampoo for an indefinite period, often for several months.

Recurrent infection is prevented with the use of prescribed antibiotic therapy (eg, a daily dose of oral clindamycin to be taken continuously for about 3 months). The patient must take the full dose for the time prescribed. The purulent exudate (pus) is a source of reinfection or transmission of infection to caregivers. When the patient has a history of recurrent infections, a carrier state may exist, which should be investigated and treated with an antibacterial cream such as mupirocin.

VIRAL SKIN INFECTIONS

Herpes Zoster

Herpes zoster, also called shingles, is an infection caused by the varicella zoster virus, a member of a group of DNA viruses. (The viruses of chickenpox and herpes zoster are indistinguishable, hence the name varicella zoster.) The disease is characterized by a painful vesicular eruption along the area of distribution of the sensory nerves from one or more posterior ganglia. It is assumed that herpes zoster represents a reactivation of latent varicella (chickenpox) virus and reflects lowered immunity. After a case of chickenpox runs its course, it is thought that the varicella zoster viruses responsible for the outbreak lie dormant inside nerve cells near the brain and spinal cord. Later, when these latent viruses are reactivated, they travel by way of the peripheral nerves to the skin. There, the viruses multiply, creating a red rash of small, fluid-filled blisters. About 10% of adults get shingles during their lifetime, usually after age 50. There is an increased frequency of herpes zoster in patients with weakened immune systems and cancers, especially the leukemias and the lymphomas.

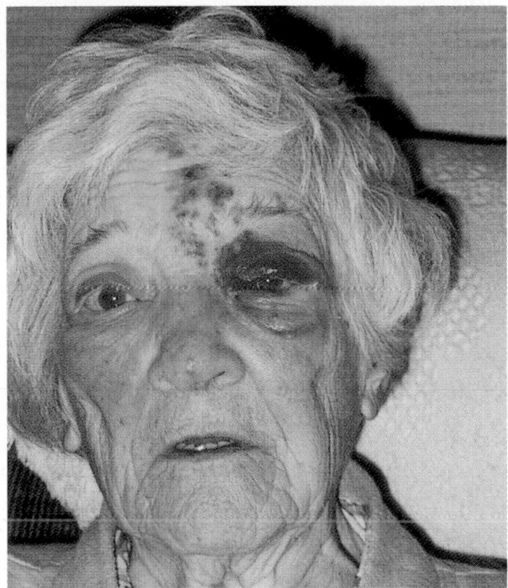

FIGURE 52•2 Herpes zoster (shingles).

Clinical Manifestations

The eruption is usually accompanied or preceded by pain, which may radiate over the entire region supplied by the nerves. The pain may be burning, lancinating (tearing, sharply cutting), stabbing, or aching. Some patients have no pain, but itching and tenderness may occur over the area. At times, malaise and gastrointestinal disturbances precede the eruption. The patches of grouped vesicles appear on the red and swollen skin. The early vesicles, which contain serum, later become purulent, rupture, and form crusts. The inflammation is usually unilateral, involving the thoracic, cervical, or cranial nerves in a bandlike configuration. The blisters are usually confined to a narrow region of the face or trunk (Fig. 52-2). The clinical course varies from 1 to 3 weeks. If an ophthalmic nerve is involved, the patient may have eye pain. Inflammation and a rash on the trunk may cause pain with the slightest touch. The healing time varies from 7 to 26 days.

Herpes zoster in healthy adults is usually localized and benign. However, in immunosuppressed patients the disease may be severe and the clinical course acutely disabling.

Medical Management

The goals of herpes zoster management are to relieve the pain and to reduce or avoid complications. These include infection, scarring, and postherpetic neuralgia and eye complications.

Pain is controlled with analgesics, because adequate pain control during the acute phase helps prevent persistent pain patterns. Systemic corticosteroids are prescribed for patients older than age 50 to reduce the incidence and duration of postherpetic neuralgia (persistent pain of the affected nerve after healing). Healing usually occurs sooner in those who have been treated with corticosteroids. Triamcinolone (Aristocort, Kenacort, Kenalog) injected subcutaneously under painful areas is effective as an anti-inflammatory agent.

There is some evidence that infection is arrested if oral antiviral agents such as acyclovir (Zovirax), valacyclovir (Valtrex), or famciclovir (Famvir) are administered within 24 hours of the initial eruption. Intravenous acyclovir, if started early, is effective in significantly reducing the pain and halting the progression of the disease. In older patients, the pain from herpes zoster may persist as postherpetic neuralgia for months after the skin lesions disappear.

Ophthalmic herpes zoster occurs when an eye is involved. This is considered an ophthalmic emergency, and the patient should be referred to an ophthalmologist immediately to prevent the possible sequelae of keratitis, uveitis, ulceration, and blindness.

People who have been exposed to varicella (chicken pox) either by primary infection or by vaccination are not at risk of infection after exposure to patients with herpes zoster.

Nursing Management

The nurse assesses the patient's discomfort and response to medication and collaborates with the physician to make necessary adjustments to the treatment regimen. The patient is taught how to apply wet dressings or medication to the lesions and to follow proper hand washing techniques to avoid spreading the virus.

Diversionary activities and relaxation techniques are encouraged to ensure restful sleep and to alleviate discomfort. A caregiver may be required to assist with dressings, particularly if the patient is elderly and unable to apply them. Relatives, neighbors, or a community health nurse may need to help with dressing changes and food preparation for patients who cannot care for themselves or prepare nourishing meals.

Herpes Simplex

Herpes simplex is a very common skin infection. There are two types of the causative virus, as identified by viral typing. Generally type I occurs on the mouth and type II in the genital area, but both viral types can be found in both locations. About 85% of adults worldwide are seropositive for herpes type I. The prevalence of type II is lower; type II usually appears at the onset of sexual activity. Serologic testing reveals that many more people are infected than have a history of clinical disease.

Herpes simplex is classified as a true primary infection, a nonprimary initial episode, or a recurrent episode. True primary infection is the initial exposure to the virus. A nonprimary initial episode is the initial episode of either type I or type II in a person previously infected with the other type. Recurrent episodes are subsequent episodes of the same viral type.

Orolabial Herpes

Orolabial herpes, also called fever blisters or cold sores, consists of erythematous-based clusters of grouped vesicles on the lips. A prodrome of tingling or burning, with pain, may precede the appearance of the vesicles by up to 24 hours. Certain triggers, such as sunlight exposure or increased stress, may cause recurrent episodes. Fewer than 1% of people with primary orolabial herpes infections develop herpetic gingivostomatitis. This complication occurs more in children and young adults. The onset is often accompanied by high fever, regional lymphadenopathy, and generalized malaise. Another complication of orolabial herpes is the development of erythema multiforme, an acute inflammation of the skin and mucous membranes with characteristic lesions that have the appearance of targets.

Genital Herpes

Genital herpes, type II, presents with a broad spectrum of clinical signs. Minor infections may produce no symptoms at all; severe primary infections with type I can cause systemic flulike illness. Lesions appear as grouped vesicles on an erythematous base initially involving the vagina, rectum, or penis. New lesions can continue to appear for 7 to 14 days. Lesions are symmetric and usually cause regional lymphadenopathy. Fever and flulike symptoms are common. Typical recurrences begin with a prodrome of burning, tingling, or itching about 24 hours before the vesicles appear. As the vesicles rupture, erosions and ulcerations begin to appear. Severe infections can cause extensive erosions of the vaginal or anal canal.

Complications

Eczema herpeticum is a condition in which patients with eczema contract herpes that spreads throughout the eczematous areas. The same type of spread of herpes may occur in severe seborrhea, scabies, and other chronic skin conditions.

Herpes whitlow is an infection of the pulp of a fingertip with herpes type I or II. There is tenderness and erythema of the lateral fold of the cuticle. Deep-seated vesicles appear within 24 hours.

Most cases of neonatal infection with herpes occur during delivery, by contact of the infant with the mother's active ulcerations. Very rarely, in mothers who have primary infections during pregnancy, intrauterine neonatal infections occur. Fetal anomalies include skin lesions, microcephaly, encephalitis, and intracerebral calcifications.

Assessment and Diagnostic Findings

Herpes simplex infections are confirmed in several ways. Generally the appearance of the skin eruption is strongly suggestive. Both viral cultures and rapid assays are available. The type of test used depends on lesion morphology. Acute vesicular lesions are more likely to react positively to the rapid assay, whereas older, crusted patches are better diagnosed with viral culture. In all cases, it is imperative to obtain enough viral cells for testing. Therefore, careful collection methods are important. All crusts should be gently removed or vesicles gently unroofed. A sterile cotton swab premoistened in viral culture preservative is used to rub the base of the vesicle to obtain a specimen for analysis.

Medical Management

In many patients, recurrent orolabial herpes represents more of a nuisance than a disease. Because sun exposure is a common trigger, those with recurrent orolabial herpes should use a sunscreen liberally on the lips and face. Topical treatment with drying agents may accelerate healing. In more severe outbreaks, or in patients who have identified a trigger, intermittent treatment with acyclovir 200 mg five times a day for 5 days can begin as soon as the earliest symptoms occur.

Treatment of genital herpes depends on the severity, the frequency, and the psychological impact of recurrences and the infectious status of the sexual partner. For people who have mild or rare outbreaks, no treatment may be required. For those who have more severe outbreaks, but for whom outbreaks are still infrequent, intermittent treatment as described for oral lesions can be used. Intermittent treatment reduces the duration of the infection by only 24 to 36 hours, so it should be initiated as early as possible.

Patients who have more than six recurrences a year may benefit from suppressive therapy. Use of acyclovir, valacyclovir, or famciclovir suppresses 85% of recurrences, and 20% of patients are free of recurrences during suppressive therapy. Also, suppressive therapy reduces viral shedding by almost 95%, making the person less contagious. Treatment with suppressive doses of oral antiviral medications prevents recurrent erythema multiforme.

Management of eczema herpeticum is with oral or intravenous acyclovir.

Management of genital herpes in pregnancy is controversial. Routine prenatal cultures do not predict shedding at the time of delivery. The use of scalp electrodes during delivery should be avoided because they increase the risk of infection in the newborn. Because the risk of neonatal herpes is greater in women with their initial episode during pregnancy, suppression should be started in these women to reduce outbreaks during the third trimester. All women with active lesions at the time of delivery undergo cesarean section.

In immunocompromised patients, suppression therapy should be considered. In severe infections of the hospitalized patient, intravenous acyclovir is given.

FUNGAL (MYCOTIC) INFECTIONS

Fungi, tiny representatives of the plant kingdom that feed on organic matter, are responsible for various common skin infections. In some cases, they affect only the skin and its appendages (ie, hair and nails), but in others the internal organs are involved, and this disease may be life-threatening. Superficial infections, however, rarely cause even temporary disability and respond readily to treatment. Secondary infection with bacteria or *Candida* or both may occur.

The most common fungal skin infection is **tinea** (called ringworm because of its characteristic appearance, like a round ring or tunnel under the skin). Tinea infections affect the head, body, groin, feet, and nails. Table 52-6 summarizes the tinea infections.

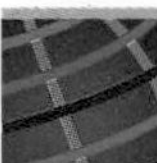

TABLE 52•6 Tinea (Ringworm) Infections

Type and Location	Clinical Manifestations	Treatment
Tinea capitis (head) Contagious fungal infection of the hair shaft	• Common in children • Oval, scaling, erythematous patches • Small papules or pustules on the scalp • Brittle hair that breaks easily	• Griseofulvin for 6 weeks • Shampoo hair 2 or 3 times with Nizoral or selenium sulfide shampoo.
Tinea corporis (body)	• Begins with red macule, which spreads to a ring of papules or vesicles with central clearing • Lesions found in clusters. • Many spread to the hair, scalp, or nails • Very pruritic • An infected pet may be the source.	• Mild conditions: topical antifungal creams • Severe conditions: griseofulvin or terbinafine
Tinea cruris (groin area; "jock itch")	• Begins with small, red scaling patches, which spread to circular elevated plaques • Very pruritic • Clusters of pustules may be seen around borders.	• Mild conditions: topical antifungal creams • Severe conditions: griseofulvin or terbinafine • Soak feet in vinegar and water solution.
Tinea pedis (foot; "athlete's foot")	• Soles of one or both feet have scaling and mild redness with maceration in the toe webs. • More acute infections may have clusters of clear vesicles on dusky base.	• Resistant infections: griseofulvin or terbinafine • Terbinafine daily for 3 months • Itraconazole in pulses of 1 week a month for 3 months
Tinea ungum (toenails; affects about 50% of adults)	• Nails thicken, crumble easily, and lack luster. • Whole nail may be destroyed.	

To obtain a specimen for diagnosis, the lesion is cleaned and a scalpel or glass slide is used to remove scales from the margin of the lesion. The scales are dropped onto a slide to which potassium hydroxide has been added. The diagnosis is made by examining the infected scales microscopically for spores and hyphae or by isolating the organism in culture. Under a Wood's light, a specimen of infected hair appears fluorescent; this may be helpful in diagnosing some cases of tinea capitis.

Tinea Pedis (Athlete's Foot)

Tinea pedis is the most common fungal infection. It is especially prevalent in those who use communal showers or swimming pools (Fitzpatrick et al., 1997).

Clinical Manifestations

Tinea pedis may appear as an acute or chronic infection on the soles of the feet or between the toes. The toenail may also be involved. Lymphangitis and cellulitis occur occasionally when bacterial superinfection occurs. Sometimes a mixed infection involving fungi, bacteria, and yeast occurs.

Medical Management

During the acute (vesicular) phase, soaks of Burow's saline or potassium permanganate solutions are used to remove the crusts, scales, and debris and to reduce the inflammation. Topical antifungal (miconazole, clotrimazole) agents are applied to the infected areas. Topical therapy is continued for several weeks because of the high rate of recurrence.

Nursing Management

Footwear provides a favorable environment for fungi; thus, the causative fungus may be in the shoes or socks. Because moisture encourages the growth of fungi, the patient is instructed to keep the feet as dry as possible, including the areas between the toes. Small pieces of cotton can be placed between the toes at night to absorb moisture. Socks should be made of absorbent cotton, and hosiery should have cotton feet because synthetic material does not absorb perspiration as well as cotton.

For people whose feet perspire excessively, perforated shoes permit better aeration of the feet. Plastic- or rubber-soled footwear should be avoided. Talcum powder or antifungal powder applied twice daily helps to keep the feet dry. Several pairs of shoes should be alternated so that they can dry completely before being worn again.

Tinea Corporis (Ringworm of the Body)

In tinea corporis, the typical ringed lesion appears on the face, neck, trunk, and extremities (Fig. 52-3). Animal varieties (nonhuman variety) are known to cause an intense inflammatory reaction in humans because they are not normally adapted to living on human hosts. Humans make contact with animal varieties through contact with pets or objects that have been in contact with an animal.

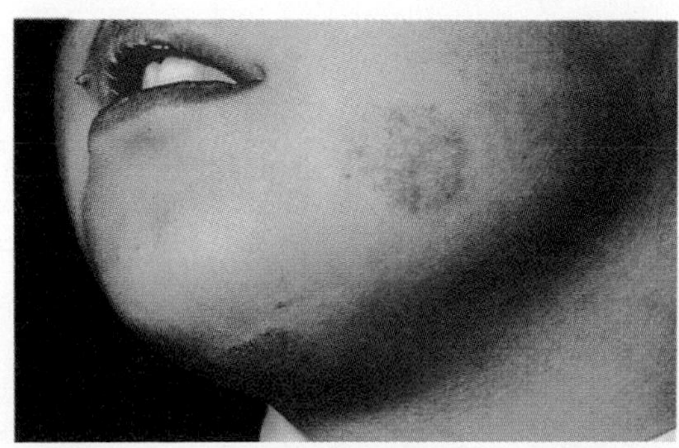

FIGURE 52•3 Tinea corporis (ringworm) of the face.

Medical Management

Topical antifungal medication may be applied to small areas. Oral antifungal agents are used only in extensive cases. Side effects of oral antifungal agents include photosensitivity, skin rashes, headache, and nausea. Newer antifungal agents, including itraconazole, fluconazole, and terbinafine, have been shown to be more effective with fewer systemic side effects than griseofulvin in patients with chronic fungal (dermatophyte) infections.

Nursing Management

The patient is instructed to use a clean towel and washcloth daily. Because fungal infections thrive in heat and moisture, all skin areas and skin folds that retain moisture must be dried thoroughly. Clean cotton clothing should be worn next to the skin.

Tinea Capitis (Ringworm of the Scalp)

Ringworm of the scalp is a contagious fungal infection of the hair shafts and a common cause of hair loss in children. Any child with scaling of the scalp should be considered to have tinea capitis until proven otherwise. Clinically, one or several round, red scaling patches are present. Small pustules or papules may be seen at the edges of such patches. As the hairs in the affected areas are invaded by the fungi, they become brittle and break off at or near the surface of the scalp, leaving bald patches or the classic sign of black dots, which are the broken ends of hairs. Most cases of tinea capitis heal without scarring, so the hair loss is only temporary.

Medical Management

Griseofulvin, an antifungal agent, is prescribed for patients with tinea capitis. Topical agents do not provide an effective cure because the infection occurs within the hair shaft and below the surface of the scalp. However, topical agents can be used to inactivate organisms already on the hair. This minimizes contagion and eliminates the need to clip the hair. Infected hairs break off anyway, and noninfected ones may remain in place. The hair should be shampooed two or three times weekly, and a topical antifungal preparation should be applied to reduce dissemination of the organisms.

Nursing Management

Because tinea capitis is contagious, the patient and family should be advised to set up a hygiene regimen for home use. Each person should have a separate comb and brush and should avoid exchanging hats and other headgear. All infected members of the family and household pets must be examined because familial infections are relatively common.

Tinea Cruris (Ringworm of the Groin)

Tinea cruris ("jock itch") is ringworm infection of the groin, which may extend to the inner thighs and buttock area. It occurs most frequently in young joggers, obese people, and those who wear tight underclothing. The incidence of tinea cruris is increased in people with diabetes.

Medical Management

Mild infections may be treated with topical medication such as clotrimazole, miconazole, or terbinafine for at least 3 to 4 weeks to ensure eradication of the infection. Oral antifungal agents may be required for more severe infections. Heat, friction, and maceration (from sweating) predispose the patient to the infection. The nurse instructs the patient to avoid excessive heat and humidity as much as possible and to avoid wearing nylon underwear, tight-fitting clothing, and a wet bathing suit. The groin area should be cleaned, dried thoroughly, and dusted with a topical antifungal agent, such as tolnaftate (Tinactin) as a preventive measure, because the infection is likely to recur.

Tinea Unguium (Onychomycosis)

Tinea unguium (ringworm of the nails) is a chronic fungal infection of the toenails or, less commonly, the fingernails. It is usually caused by *Trichophyton* species (*T. rubrum, T. mentagrophytes*) or *Candida albicans*. It is usually associated with longtime fungal infection of the feet. The nails become thickened, friable (easily crumbled), and lusterless. In time, debris accumulates under the free edge of the nail. Ultimately, the nail plate separates. Because of the chronicity of this infection, the entire nail may be destroyed.

Medical Management

An oral antifungal agent is prescribed for 6 weeks when the fingernails are involved and 12 weeks when the toenails are involved. Selection of the antifungal agent depends on the causative fungus. Candidal infections are treated with fluconazole (Diflucan) or itraconazole (Sporanox). Griseofulvin is no longer considered effective therapy because of its long treatment course and poor cure rate. Response to oral antifungal agents in treating infections of the toenails is poor at best. Frequently, when the treatment stops, the infection returns.

PARASITIC SKIN INFESTATION

Pediculosis (Lice)

Lice infestation affects people of all ages. Three varieties of lice infest humans: *Pediculus humanus capitis* (head louse), *Pediculus humanus corporis* (body louse), and *Phthirus pubis* (pubic louse or crab louse). Lice are called ectoparasites because they live on the outside of the host's body. They depend on the host for their nourishment, feeding on human blood approximately five times a day. They inject their digestive juices and excrement into the skin, which causes severe itching.

Pediculosis Capitis

Pediculosis capitis is an infestation of the scalp by the head louse. The female louse lays her eggs (nits) close to the scalp. The nits become firmly attached with a tenacious substance to the hair shafts. The young lice hatch in about 10 days and reach maturity in 2 weeks.

Clinical Manifestations

Head lice are found most commonly along the back of the head and behind the ears. The eggs are visible to the naked eye as silvery, glistening oval bodies that are difficult to remove from the hair. The bite of the insect causes intense itching, and the resultant scratching often leads to secondary bacterial infection, such as impetigo or furunculosis. The infestation is more common in children and people with long hair. Head lice may be transmitted directly by physical contact or indirectly by infested combs, brushes, wigs, hats, and bedding.

Medical Management

Treatment involves washing the hair with a shampoo containing lindane (Kwell) or pyrethrin compounds with piperonyl butoxide (RID or R&C Shampoo). The patient is instructed to shampoo the scalp and hair according to the product directions. After the hair is rinsed thoroughly, it is combed with a fine-toothed comb dipped in vinegar to remove any remaining nits or nit shells freed from the hair shafts. These are extremely difficult to remove and may have to be picked off with the fingernails, one by one.

All articles, clothing, towels, and bedding that might have lice or nits should be washed in hot water—at least 54°C (130°F)—or dry-cleaned to prevent reinfestation. Upholstered furniture, rugs, and floors should be vacuumed frequently. Combs and brushes are also disinfected with the shampoo. All family members and close contacts are treated. Complications such as severe pruritus, pyoderma, and dermatitis are treated with antipruritics, systemic antibiotics, and topical corticosteroids.

Nursing Management

The nurse reassures the patient that head lice may infest anyone and are not a sign of uncleanliness. This condition spreads rapidly, so treatment must be started immediately. School epidemics may be managed by having all of the students shampoo their hair on the same night. Students should be warned not to share combs, brushes, or hats. Each family member should be inspected for head lice daily for at least 2 weeks. The patient should be instructed that lindane may be toxic when not used properly.

Pediculosis Corporis and Pubis

Pediculosis corporis is an infestation of the body by the body louse. This is a disease of unwashed people or those who live in close quarters and do not change their clothing.

Pediculosis pubis is extremely common. The infestation is generally localized in the genital region and is transmitted chiefly by sexual contact.

Clinical Manifestations

The areas of the skin chiefly involved are those that come in closest contact with the underclothing (ie, the neck, trunk, and thighs). The body louse lives primarily in the seams of underwear and clothing, to which it clings as it pierces the skin with its proboscis. Its bites cause characteristic minute hemorrhagic points. Widespread excoriation may appear as a result of intense itching and scratching, especially on the trunk and neck. Among the secondary lesions produced are parallel linear scratches and a slight degree of eczema. In long-standing cases, the skin may become thick, dry, and scaly, with dark pigmented areas.

Itching is the most common symptom of pediculosis pubis, particularly at night. In addition, reddish-brown dust (the excretions of the insects) may be found in the patient's underclothing. The pubic crease should be examined with a magnifying glass for lice crawling down a hair shaft or nits cemented to the hair or at the junction with the skin. Infestation by pubic lice may coexist with sexually transmitted diseases (gonorrhea, herpes, syphilis). *Phthirus pubis* may also infest the hairs of the chest, armpit, beard, and eyelashes. Gray-blue macules may sometimes be seen on the trunk, thighs, and axillae as a result of either the reaction of the insects' saliva with bilirubin (converting it to biliverdin) or an excretion produced by the salivary glands of the louse.

Medical Management

The patient is instructed to bathe with soap and water. Then, either lindane (Kwell) or permethrin 5% (Elemite) is applied to affected areas of the skin and to hairy areas, according to the product directions. An alternative topical therapy is an over-the-counter strength of permethrin (1% Nix). If the eyelashes are involved, petrolatum may be thickly applied twice daily for 8 days, followed by mechanical removal of any remaining nits.

Complications, such as severe pruritus, pyoderma, and dermatitis, are treated with antipruritics, systemic antibiotics, and topical corticosteroids. Body lice can transmit epidemic disease in humans, namely rickettsial disease (epidemic typhus, relapsing fever, and trench fever). The causative organism may be in the gastrointestinal tract of the insect and may be excreted on the skin surface of the infested person.

Nursing Management

All family members and sexual contacts must be treated and educated in personal hygiene and methods to prevent or control infestation. The patient and partner must also be scheduled for a diagnostic workup for coexisting sexually transmitted disease. All clothing and bedding should be machine-washed in hot water or dry-cleaned.

Scabies

Scabies is an infestation of the skin by the itch mite *Sarcoptes scabiei.* The disease may be found in people living in substandard hygienic conditions, but it is also common in very clean individuals and among the sexually active. However, infestations are not dependent on sexual activity because the mites frequently involve the fingers, and hand contact may produce infection. In children, overnight stays with friends or the exchange of clothes may be a source of infection. Health care personnel who have prolonged hands-on physical contact with an infected patient may likewise become infected.

The adult female burrows into the superficial layer of the skin and remains there for the rest of her life. With her jaws and the sharp edges of the joints of her forelegs, the mite extends the burrow, laying two or three eggs daily for up to 2 months. She then dies. The larvae (eggs) hatch in 3 to 4 days and progress through larval and nymphal states to form adult mites in about 10 days.

Clinical Manifestations

It takes approximately 4 weeks from the time of contact for the patient's symptoms to appear. The patient complains of severe itching caused by a delayed type of immunologic reaction to the mite or its fecal pellets. During examination, the patient is asked where the itch is most severe. A magnifying glass and a penlight are held at an oblique angle to the skin while a search is made for the small, raised burrows. The burrows may be multiple, straight or wavy, brown or black, threadlike lesions, most commonly observed between the fingers and on the wrists. Other sites are the extensor surfaces of the elbows, the knees, the edges of the feet, the points of the elbows, around the nipples, in the axillary folds, under pendulous breasts, and in or near the groin or gluteal fold, penis, or scrotum. Red pruritic eruptions usually appear between adjacent skin areas. The burrow, however, is not always visible. Any patient with a rash may have scabies.

One classic sign of scabies is the increased itching that occurs at night, perhaps because the increased warmth of the skin has a stimulating effect on the parasite. Also, hypersensitivity to the organism and its products of excretion may contribute to the itching. If the infection has spread, other members of the family and close friends also complain of itching about a month later.

Secondary lesions are quite common and include vesicles, papules, excoriations, and crusts. Bacterial superinfection may result from constant excoriation of the burrows and papules.

Assessment and Diagnostic Findings

The diagnosis is confirmed by recovering *Sarcoptes scabiei* or the mites' byproducts from the skin. A sample of superficial epidermis is scraped off the top of the burrows or papules with a small scalpel blade. The scrapings are placed on a microscope slide and examined through a low-powered microscope to demonstrate the mite at any stage (adult, eggs, egg casings, larva, nymph) and fecal pellets.

Gerontologic Considerations

Although the older patient itches severely, the vivid inflammatory reaction seen in younger people seldom occurs. Scabies may not be recognized in the elderly person; the itching may erroneously be attributed to the dry skin of old age or to anxiety.

Health care personnel in extended-care facilities should wear gloves when providing hands-on care for a patient suspected of having scabies until the diagnosis is confirmed and treatment accomplished. It is advisable to treat all residents, staff, and families of patients at the same time to prevent reinfection.

Medical Management

The patient is instructed to take a warm, soapy bath or shower to remove the scaling debris from the crusts and then to dry thoroughly and allow the skin to cool. A prescription scabicide, such as lindane (Kwell), crotamiton (Eurax), or permethrin 5% (Elimite), is applied thinly to the entire skin from the neck down, sparing only the face and scalp (which are not affected in scabies). The medication is left on for 12 to 24 hours, after which the patient is instructed to wash thoroughly. One application may be curative, but it is advisable to repeat the treatment in 1 week.

Nursing Alert *The patient must understand these instructions, because application of a scabicide immediately after bathing and before the skin dries and cools increases percutaneous absorption of the scabicide and the potential for central nervous system abnormalities such as seizures.*

Nursing Management

The patient should wear clean clothing and sleep between freshly laundered bed linens. All bedding and clothing should be washed in very hot water and dried on the hot dryer cycle, because the mites can survive up to 36 hours in linens. If bed linens or clothing cannot be washed in hot water, dry-cleaning is advised.

After treatment is completed, the patient should apply an ointment, such as a topical corticosteroid, to skin lesions because the scabicide may irritate the skin. The patient's hypersensitivity does not cease on destruction of the mites. Itching may continue for several weeks as a manifestation of hypersensitivity, particularly in atopic (allergic) people. This is not a sign that the treatment has failed. The patient is instructed not to apply more scabicide (because this will cause more irritation and increased itching) and not to take frequent hot showers (because this dries the skin and produces itching). Oral antihistamines such as diphenhydramine (Benadryl) or hydroxyzine (Atarax) can help control the itching.

All family members and close contacts should be treated simultaneously to eliminate the mites. Some scabicides are approved for use in infants and pregnant women. If scabies is sexually transmitted, the patient may require treatment for coexisting sexually transmitted disease. Scabies may also coexist with pediculosis.

CONTACT DERMATITIS

Contact dermatitis is an inflammatory reaction of the skin to physical, chemical, or biologic agents. The epidermis is damaged by repeated physical and chemical irritations. Contact dermatitis may be of the primary irritant type, in which a nonallergic reaction results from exposure to an irritating substance, or it may be allergic (allergic contact dermatitis), resulting from exposure of sensitized people to contact allergens. (Allergic dermatoses are discussed in Chap. 49.) Common causes or irritant dermatitis are soaps, detergents, scouring compounds, and industrial chemicals. Predisposing factors include extremes of heat and cold, frequent contact with soap and water, and a preexisting skin disease.

Clinical Manifestations

The eruptions begin when the causative agent contacts the skin. The first reactions include itching, burning, and erythema, followed soon by edema, papules, vesicles, and oozing or weeping. In the subacute phase, these vesicular changes are less marked, and they alternate with crusting, drying, fissuring, and peeling. If repeated reactions occur, or if the patient continually scratches the skin, lichenification and pigmentation occur. Secondary bacterial invasion may follow.

Medical Management

The objectives of management are to rest the involved skin and protect it from further damage. The distribution pattern of the reaction is determined to differentiate between allergic and irritant contact dermatitis. A detailed history is obtained. Then, the offending irritant is identified and removed. Local irritation should be avoided, and soap is not generally used until healing occurs.

Many preparations are advocated for relieving dermatitis. In general, a bland, unmedicated lotion is used for small patches of erythema (inflamed skin). Cool, wet dressings also are applied over small areas of vesicular dermatitis. Finely cracked ice added to the water often enhances its antipruritic effect.

Wet dressings usually help clear the oozing eczematous lesions. Then, a thin layer of cream or ointment containing a corticosteroid may be used. Medicated baths at room temperature are prescribed for larger areas of dermatitis. In widespread conditions, a short course of systemic corticosteroids may be prescribed.

NONINFECTIOUS INFLAMMATORY DERMATOSES

Psoriasis

Psoriasis is a chronic, noninfectious, inflammatory disease of the skin in which epidermal cells are produced at a rate that is about six to nine times faster than normal. The cells in the basal layer of the skin divide too quickly, and the newly formed cells move so rapidly to the skin surface that they become evident as profuse

Patient Education and Home Care

Strategies for Avoiding Contact Dermatitis

The following precautions may help prevent repeated cases of contact dermatitis. Follow these instructions for at least 4 months after your skin appears to be completely healed.

- Study the pattern and location of your dermatitis and think about which things have touched your skin and which things may have caused the problem.
- Try to avoid contact with these materials.
- Avoid heat, soap, and rubbing, all of which are external irritants.
- Choose bath soaps, laundry detergents, and cosmetics that do not contain fragrance.
- Avoid using a fabric softener dryer sheet (Bounce, Cling). Fabric softeners that are added to the washer may be used.
- Avoid topical medications, lotions, or ointments, except those specifically prescribed for your condition.
- Wash your skin thoroughly immediately after exposure to possible irritants.
- When wearing gloves (for example, for washing dishes or general cleaning), be sure they are cotton-lined. Do not wear them more than 15 or 20 minutes at a time.

scales or plaques of epidermal tissue. The psoriatic epidermal cell may travel from the basal cell layer of the epidermis to the stratum corneum (skin surface) and be cast off in 3 to 4 days, which is in sharp contrast to the normal 26 to 28 days. As a result of the increased number of basal cells and rapid cell passage, the normal events of cell maturation and growth cannot take place. This abnormal process does not allow the normal protective layers of the skin to form.

One of the most common skin diseases, psoriasis affects approximately 2% of the population, appearing more often in people who have a European ancestry (Arndt et al., 1997). It is thought that the condition stems from a hereditary defect that causes overproduction of keratin. Although the primary cause is unknown, a combination of specific genetic makeup and environmental stimuli may trigger the onset of disease. There is some evidence that the cell proliferation is mediated by the immune system. Periods of emotional stress and anxiety aggravate the condition. In addition, trauma, infections, and seasonal and hormonal changes are trigger factors. The onset may occur at any age but is most common between the ages of 15 and 50 years (Arndt et al., 1997). Psoriasis has a tendency to improve and then recur periodically throughout life.

Clinical Manifestations

Lesions appear as red, raised patches of skin covered with silvery scales. The scaly patches are formed by the buildup of living and dead skin resulting from the vast increase in the rate of skin-cell growth and turnover (Fig. 52-4). If the scales are scraped away, the dark-red base of the lesion is exposed, producing multiple bleeding points. These patches are not moist and may or may not be pruritic. One variation of this condition is called guttate psoriasis because the lesions remain about 1 cm wide and are scattered like raindrops over the body. This variation is believed to be associated with a recent streptococcal throat infection. Psoriasis may range in severity from a cosmetic source of annoyance to a physically disabling and disfiguring affliction.

Particular sites of the body tend to be affected most by this condition; they include the scalp, the extensor surface of the elbows and knees, the lower part of the back, and the genitalia. Bilateral symmetry is a feature of psoriasis. In approximately one quarter to one half of patients, the nails are involved, with pitting, discoloration, crumbling beneath the free edges, and separation of the nail plate. When psoriasis occurs on the palms and soles, it can cause pustular lesions, called palmar pustular psoriasis.

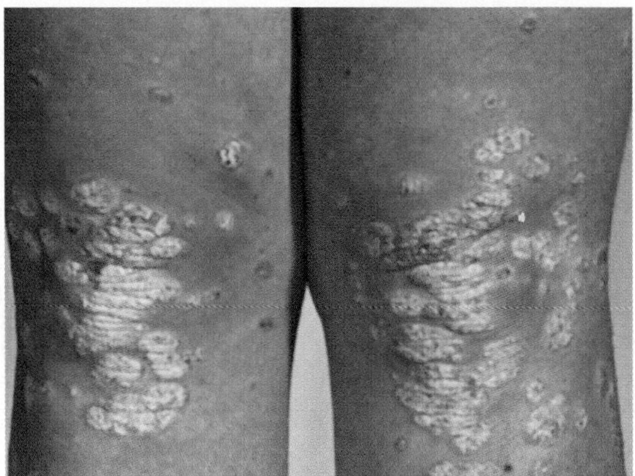

FIGURE 52•4 Psoriasis. Courtesy of Roche Laboratories.

Complications

The disease may be associated with asymmetric rheumatoid factor-negative arthritis of multiple joints. The arthritic development can occur either before or after the skin lesions appear. The relation between arthritis and psoriasis is not understood. Another complication is an exfoliative psoriatic state in which the disease progresses to involve the total body surface, called erythrodermic psoriasis. In this case, the patient is more acutely ill, having fever, chills, and an electrolyte imbalance. Erythrodermic psoriasis often appears in people with chronic psoriasis after infections or after exposure to certain medications, including withdrawal of systemic steroids (Arndt et al., 1997).

Psychological Considerations

Psoriasis may cause despair and frustration for the patient; observers may stare, comment, ask embarrassing questions, or even avoid the person. The disease can eventually exhaust the patient's resources, interfere with his or her job, and make life miserable in general. Teenagers are especially vulnerable to the psychological effects of this ailment. The family, too, is affected, because time-consuming treatments, messy salves, and constant shedding of scales may disrupt home life and cause resentment. The patient's frustrations may be expressed through hostility directed at health care personnel and others.

Assessment and Diagnostic Findings

The presence of the classic plaque-type lesions generally confirms the diagnosis of psoriasis. Lesions tend to change histologically as they progress from early to chronic plaques. Therefore, biopsy of the skin is of little value in diagnosis, and there are no specific blood tests helpful in diagnosing the condition. When in doubt, the health professional should assess for signs of nail and scalp involvement, as well as a positive family history.

TABLE 52•7 Current Treatments for Psoriasis

Topical Agents	Use	Selected Agents
Topical corticosteroids	Mild to moderate lesions	Aristocort, Kenalog, Valisone
	Moderate to severe lesions	Lidex, Psorcon, Cutivate
	Severe lesions	Temovate, Diprolene, Ultravate
	Lesions on face and groin	Aclovate, DesOwen, Hytone 2.5%
Topical nonsteroidals	Mild to severe	Retinoids such as tazarotene (Tazorac) Vitamin D_3 derivative calcipotriene (Dovonex)
Coal tar products	Mild to moderate lesions	Coal tar and salicylic acid ointment (Aquatar, Estar gel, Fototar, Zetar); anthralin (AnthraDerm, Dritho-Cream); Neutrogena T-Derm, Psori Gel)
Medicated shampoos	Scalp lesions	Neutrogena T-Gel, T-Sal, Zetar, Head & Shoulders, Desenex, Selsun Blue, Bakers P&S (emulsifying agent with phenol, saline solution, and mineral oil)
Intralesional therapy	Thick plaques & nails	Kenalog, Cordran-impregnated tape, Fluoroplex
Systemic therapy	Extensive lesions and nails	Methotrexate (Folex, Mexate); hydrourea (Hydrea); retinoic acid (Tegison) (not to be used in women of childbearing age)
	Psoriatic arthritis	Oral gold (auranofin), etrentinate, methotrexate
Photochemotherapy	Moderate to severe lesions	UVA or UVB light with or without topical medications PUVA (combines UVA light with oral psoralens, or topical tripsoralen)

Medical Management

The goals of management are to slow the rapid turnover of epidermis, to promote resolution of the psoriatic lesions, and to control the natural cycles of the disease. There is no known cure.

The therapeutic approach should be one that the patient understands; it should be cosmetically acceptable and not too disruptive of lifestyle. It will involve the commitment of time and effort by the patient and possibly the family. First, any precipitating or aggravating factors are removed. Then an assessment is made of lifestyle, because psoriasis is significantly affected by stress. The patient must also be advised that treatment of severe psoriasis can be time-consuming, expensive, and aesthetically unappealing at times.

The most important principle of psoriasis treatment is gentle removal of scales. This can be accomplished with baths. Oils (such as olive oil, mineral oil, or Aveeno Oilated Oatmeal Bath) or coal tar preparations (Balnetar) can be added to the bath water and a soft brush used to scrub the psoriatic plaques gently. After bathing, the application of emollient creams containing alpha hydroxy acids (Lac-Hydrin, Penederm) or salicylic acid will continue to soften thick scales. The patient and family should be encouraged to establish a regular skin care routine that can be maintained even when the psoriasis is not in an acute stage.

Three types of therapy are standard: topical, intralesional, and systemic (Table 52-7).

TOPICAL PHARMACOLOGIC THERAPY

Topically applied agents are used to slow the overactive epidermis without affecting other tissues. Medications include tar preparations, anthralin, salicylic acid, and corticosteroids. Two new topical treatments introduced within the last few years are a vitamin D preparation, calcipotriene (Dovonex), and a retinoid compound, tazarotene (Tazorac). Treatment with these agents tends to suppress **epidermopoiesis** (the development of epidermal cells) and cause sloughing of the rapidly growing epidermal cells.

Topical formulations include lotions, ointments, pastes, creams, and shampoos. Older treatments, including tar baths and application of tar preparations on involved skin, are rarely used. Tar and anthralin cause irritation of the skin at the sites of application, are malodorous and difficult to apply, and do not give reliable results. Newer preparations that cause less irritation and have more consistent results are becoming more widely used.

Topical corticosteroids may be applied for their anti-inflammatory effect. Choosing the correct strength of corticosteroid for the involved site and choosing the most effective vehicle base are important aspects of topical treatment. In general, high-potency topical corticosteroids should not be used on the face and intertriginous areas, and their use on other areas should be limited to a 4-week course of twice-daily applications. A 2-week break should be taken before repeating treatment with the high-potency corticosteroids. For long-term therapy, moderate-potency corticosteroids are used. On the face and intertriginous areas, only low-potency corticosteroids are appropriate for long-term use (see Table 52-4).

Occlusive dressings may be applied to increase the effectiveness of the corticosteroid. For the hospitalized patient, large plastic bags may be used—one for the upper body (with holes cut out for the head and arms) and one for the lower body (with holes for the legs). This leaves only the extremities to wrap. In some dermatologic units, large rolls of tubular plastic are used (such as the kind used by dry cleaners to cover clean clothes). For patients being treated at home, a plastic vinyl jogging suit may be used. The medication is applied and the suit simply put over it. The hands can be wrapped in gloves, the feet in plastic bags, and the head in a shower cap.

Nursing Alert *When plastic substances are used, the nurse needs to check for flammability. Some thin, plastic films burn slowly (if touched by a lighted cigarette), whereas others burst rapidly into flame. The patient should be cautioned not to smoke while wrapped in plastic dressing.*

When psoriasis involves large areas of the body, topical corticosteroid treatment can become expensive and involve some systemic risk. Some potent corticosteroids, when applied to large areas of the body, have the potential to cause adrenal suppression through percutaneous absorption of the medication. In this event, other treatment modalities (nonsteroidal topical medications or ultraviolet light) may be used instead or in combination to decrease the need for corticosteroids.

Newer nonsteroidal topical preparations are available and effective for many patients. Calcipotriene 0.05% (Dovonex) is a derivative of vitamin D_3. It works to decrease the mitotic turnover of the psoriatic plaques. Its most common side effect is local irritation; thus, the intertriginous areas and face should be avoided when using this medication. Patients should be monitored for symptoms of hypercalcemia. It is available as a cream for use on the body and a solution for the scalp. Calcipotriene is not recommended for use by elderly patients because of their more fragile skin, or in pregnant or lactating women.

The second advance in topical treatment of psoriasis is tazarotene (Tazorac). Tazarotene, a retinoid, causes sloughing of the scales covering psoriatic plaques. As with other retinoids, it causes increased sensitivity to sunlight, so patients should be cautioned to use an effective sunscreen and avoid other photosensitizers (eg, tetracycline, antihistamines). Tazarotene is listed as a category X drug in pregnancy, so a negative result on a pregnancy test should be obtained before initiating this medication and effective contraceptive should be continued during treatment. Side effects of terzarotene include burning, erythema, or irritation at the site of application, and worsening of psoriasis.

INTRALESIONAL THERAPY

Intralesional injections of triamcinolone acetonide (Aristocort, Kenalog-10, Trymex) can be administered directly into highly visible or isolated patches of psoriasis that are resistant to other forms of therapy. Care must be taken to ensure that normal skin is not injected with the medication.

SYSTEMIC THERAPY

Although systemic corticosteroids may cause rapid improvement of psoriasis, their usual risks as well as the risk of triggering a severe flare on withdrawal limit their use. Systemic cytotoxic preparations, such as methotrexate, have been used in treating extensive psoriasis that fails to respond to other forms of therapy. Other systemic medications in current use include hydroxyurea (Hydrea) and cyclosporine A (CyA).

Methotrexate appears to inhibit DNA synthesis in epidermal cells, thereby reducing the turnover time of the psoriatic epidermis. However, the medication can be very toxic, especially to the liver, which can suffer irreversible damage. Thus, laboratory studies must be monitored to ensure that the hepatic, hematopoietic, and renal systems are functioning adequately. Bone marrow suppression is another potential side effect. The patient should avoid drinking alcohol while taking methotrexate, because alcohol ingestion increases the possibility of liver damage. The medication is teratogenic (producing physical defects in the fetus) in pregnant women.

Hydroxyurea also inhibits cell replication by affecting DNA synthesis. The patient is monitored for signs and symptoms of bone marrow depression.

Cyclosporine A, a cyclic peptide used to prevent rejection of transplanted organs, has shown some success in treating severe, therapy-resistant cases of psoriasis. Its use, however, is limited by such side effects as hypertension and nephrotoxicity.

Oral retinoids (synthetic derivatives of vitamin A and its metabolite, vitamin A acid) modulate the growth and differentiation of epithelial tissue. Etretinate is especially useful for severe pustular or erythrodermic psoriasis. Etretinate is a teratogen with a very long half-life; it cannot be used in women who still have childbearing potential.

PHOTOCHEMOTHERAPY

A treatment for severely debilitating psoriasis is the combination of psoralens and ultraviolet-A (PUVA) light therapy. In this treatment, the patient takes a photosensitizing medication (usually 8-methoxypsoralen) in a standard dose and is subsequently exposed to long-wave ultraviolet light as the medication plasma levels peak. (Ultraviolet light is the portion of the electromagnetic spectrum containing wave lengths ranging from 180 to 400 nm.) Although the mechanism of action is not completely understood, it is thought that when psoralens-treated skin is exposed to ultraviolet-A light, the psoralens binds with DNA and decreases cellular proliferation. PUVA is not without its hazards; it has been associated with long-term risks of skin cancer, cataracts, and premature aging of the skin.

The PUVA unit consists of a chamber that contains high-output black-light lamps and an external reflectance system. The exposure time is calibrated according to the specific unit in use and the anticipated tolerance of the patient's skin. The patient is usually treated two or three times a week until the psoriasis clears. An interim period of 48 hours between treatments is necessary because it takes this long for any burns resulting from PUVA therapy to become evident.

After the psoriasis clears, the patient begins a maintenance program. Once little or no disease is active, less potent therapies are used to keep minor flare-ups under control.

Ultraviolet-B (UVB) light therapy is also used to treat generalized plaques. It is used alone or combined with topical coal tar. Side effects are similar to those of PUVA therapy. If access to a light treatment unit is not feasible, the patient can expose himself or herself to sunlight. The risks of all light treatments are similar and include acute sunburn reaction, exacerbation of photosensitive disorders such as lupus, rosacea, and polymorphic light eruption, and other skin changes, such as increased wrinkles, thickening, and possibly an increased risk of skin cancer. Table 52-7 summarizes treatment plans.

NURSING PROCESS: THE PATIENT WITH PSORIASIS

Assessment

The nursing assessment focuses on how the patient is coping with the psoriatic skin condition, the appearance of the normal skin, and the appearance of the skin lesions (see the section Clinical Manifestations above). The major notable manifestations are red, scaling papules that coalesce to form oval, well-defined plaques. Silvery-white scales may also be present. Adjacent skin areas reveal red, smooth plaques with a macerated surface. It is important to examine the areas especially prone to psoriasis: elbows, knees, scalp, gluteal cleft, fingers, and toenails (for small pits).

The nurse should assess the impact of the disease on the patient and the coping strategies used for conducting normal activities and interactions with family and friends. Many patients need reassurance that the condition is not infectious, not a reflection of poor personal hygiene, and not skin cancer.

Diagnosis

Nursing Diagnoses

Based on the nursing assessment data, the patient's major nursing diagnoses may include:

- Knowledge deficit about the disease process and treatment
- Impaired skin integrity related to lesions and inflammatory response
- Body image disturbance related to embarrassment over appearance and self-perception of uncleanliness

Collaborative Problems/Potential Complications

Based on the assessment data, potential complications include:

- Infection
- Psoriatic arthritis

Planning and Goals

Major goals for the patient may include increased understanding of psoriasis and the treatment regimen, achievement of smoother skin with control of lesions, development of self-acceptance, and absence of complications.

Nursing Interventions

Promoting Understanding

The nurse explains with sensitivity that currently there is no cure for psoriasis and that lifetime management is necessary, but that the condition can usually be controlled. The pathophysiology of psoriasis is reviewed, as are the factors that provoke it—irritation or injury to the skin (cut, abrasion, sunburn), current illness (eg, pharyngeal streptococcal infection), and emotional stress. It is emphasized that repeated trauma to the skin as well as an unfavorable environment (eg, cold) or a specific medication (eg, lithium, beta blockers, indomethacin) may exacerbate psoriasis. The patient is cautioned about taking any nonprescription medications because some may aggravate mild psoriasis.

Reviewing and explaining the treatment regimen are essential to ensure compliance. For example, if the patient has a mild condition confined to localized areas, such as the elbows or knees, the application of an emollient to maintain softness and minimize scaling may be all that is required. However, if the patient uses anthralin, the dosage schedule, possible side effects, and problems to report to the nurse or physician need to be explained.

Most patients need a comprehensive plan of care that ranges from using topical medications and shampoos to more complex and lengthy treatment with systemic medications and photochemotherapy, such as PUVA therapy. Patient education materials that include a description of the therapy and specific guidelines are helpful but cannot replace face-to-face discussions of the treatment plan.

Increasing Skin Integrity

To avoid injuring the skin, the patient is advised not to pick at or scratch the affected areas. Measures to prevent dry skin are encouraged because dry skin worsens psoriasis. Too-frequent washing produces more soreness and scaling. Water should be warm, not hot, and the skin should be dried by patting with a towel rather than rubbing. Emollients have a moisturizing effect, providing an occlusive film on the skin surface so that normal water loss through the skin is halted and allowing the trapped water to hydrate the stratum corneum. A bath oil or emollient cleansing agent can comfort sore and scaling skin. Softening the skin can prevent fissures (see Plan of Nursing Care 52-1).

Improving Self-Concept and Body Image

A therapeutic relationship between health care professionals and the patient with psoriasis is one that includes both education and support. Once the treatment regimen is established, the patient should begin to feel more confident and empowered in carrying it out and in using coping strategies that help deal with the altered self-concept and body image brought about by the disease. Introducing the patient to successful coping strategies used by others with psoriasis and making suggestions for reducing or coping with stressful situations at home, school, or work will facilitate a more positive outlook and acceptance of the chronic nature of the disease.

Monitoring and Managing Potential Complications

PSORIATIC ARTHRITIS

The diagnosis of psoriasis, especially when it is accompanied by the complication of arthritis, is usually difficult to make. Psoriatic arthritis involving the sacroiliac and distal joints of the fingers may be overlooked, especially if the patient has the typical psoriatic lesions. However, patients who complain of mild joint discomfort and some pitting of the fingernails may not be diagnosed with psoriasis until the more obvious cutaneous lesions appear.

The complaint of joint discomfort in the patient with psoriasis should be noted and evaluated. The symptoms of psoriatic arthritis can mimic the symptoms of Reiter's disease and ankylosing spondylitis. Therefore, a definitive diagnosis must be made. Treatment of the condition usually involves joint rest, application of heat, and salicylates.

The patient requires education about the care and treatment of the involved joints and the need for compliance with therapy. The incidence of psoriatic arthropathy is not known because the symptoms are so variable. It is believed, however, that when the psoriasis is extensive and a family history of inflammatory arthritis is elicited, the chance that the patient will develop psoriatic arthritis increases substantially. It is recommended that a rheumatologist be consulted to assist in the diagnosis and treatment of the arthropathy.

Promoting Home and Community-Based Care

TEACHING PATIENTS SELF-CARE

Printed patient education materials may be provided to reinforce face-to-face discussions about treatment guidelines and other considerations. For example, the patient and the family caregiver may need to know that the topical agent anthralin will leave a brownish-purple stain on the skin but that the discoloration will subside when anthralin treatment stops. They should also be instructed to cover lesions treated with anthralin (with gauze, stockinette, or other soft coverings) to avoid staining clothing, furniture, or bed linens.

Patients using topical corticosteroid preparations repeatedly on the face and around the eyes should be aware that cataract development is possible. Strict guidelines for applying these medications should be emphasized because overuse can result in skin atrophy, striae (streaks), and medication resistance.

Photochemotherapy (PUVA), which is reserved for moderate to severe psoriasis, produces photosensitization, which means that the skin is sensitive to the sun until methoxsalen has been excreted from the body (in about 6 to 8 hours). Therefore, patients undergoing PUVA treatments should avoid exposure to the sun. If exposure is unavoidable, the skin must be protected with sunscreen and clothing. Gray- or green-tinted wraparound sunglasses should be worn to protect the eyes during and after treatment, and ophthalmologic examinations should be performed on a regular basis.

HOME CARE TEACHING CHECKLIST: THE PATIENT WITH PSORIASIS

At the completion of the program, the patient or caregiver will be able to:

	Patient	Caregiver
• Describe the etiology of psoriasis.	✔	✔
• Describe optimal skin maintenance practices to maintain moisture of skin and prevent infection.	✔	✔
• Demonstrate proper application of prescribed topical medications.	✔	✔
• Describe common side effects of oral medication, if prescribed.	✔	✔
• Demonstrate appropriate therapeutic bath technique, if prescribed.	✔	✔
• Verbalize optimism about condition.	✔	
• Identify a support person with whom to discuss feelings and concerns.	✔	

Nausea, which may be a problem in some patients, is lessened when methoxsalen is taken with food. Lubricants and bath oils may be used to help remove scales and prevent excessive dryness. No other creams or oils are to be used except on areas that have been shielded from ultraviolet light. Contraceptives should be used by sexually active women of reproductive age, because the teratogenic effect of PUVA has not been determined. The patient is kept under constant and careful supervision and is encouraged to recognize unusual changes in the skin.

If indicated, referral may be made to a mental health professional who can help to ease emotional strain and give support. Belonging to a support group may also help patients acknowledge that they are not alone in experiencing life adjustments in response to a visible, chronic disease. The National Psoriasis Foundation publishes periodic bulletins and reports about new and relevant developments in this condition.

Evaluation

Expected Outcomes

Expected outcomes may include:

1. Acquires knowledge and understanding of disease process and its treatment
   a. Describes psoriasis and the prescribed therapy
   b. Verbalizes that trauma, infection, and emotional stress may be trigger factors
   c. Maintains control with appropriate therapy
   d. Demonstrates proper application of topical therapy
2. Achieves smoother skin and control of lesions
   a. Exhibits no new lesions
   b. Keeps skin lubricated and soft
3. Develops self-acceptance
   a. Identifies someone with whom to discuss feelings and concerns
   b. Expresses optimism about outcomes of treatment
4. Experiences no psoriatic arthritis
   a. Has no joint discomfort
   b. Reports control of cutaneous lesions with no extension of disease

Exfoliative Dermatitis

Exfoliative dermatitis is a serious condition characterized by progressive inflammation in which erythema and scaling occur in a more or less generalized distribution. It may be associated with chills, fever, prostration, severe toxicity, and an itchy scaling of the skin. There is a profound loss of stratum corneum (outermost layer of the skin), which causes capillary leakage, hypoproteinemia, and negative nitrogen balance. Because of widespread dilation of cutaneous vessels, large amounts of body heat are lost. Thus, exfoliative dermatitis has a marked effect on the entire body.

Exfoliative dermatitis has a variety of causes. It is considered to be a secondary or reactive process to an underlying skin or systemic disease. It may appear as a part of the lymphoma group of diseases and may actually precede the appearance of lymphoma. Preexisting skin disorders that have been implicated as a cause include psoriasis, atopic dermatitis, and contact dermatitis. It also appears as a severe reaction to many medications, including penicillin and phenylbutazone. The etiology is unknown in approximately 25% of cases.

Clinical Manifestations

This condition starts acutely as either a patchy or a generalized erythematous eruption accompanied by fever, malaise, and occasionally gastrointestinal symptoms. The skin color changes from pink to dark red. After a week, the characteristic exfoliation (scaling) begins, usually in the form of thin flakes that leave the underlying skin smooth and red, with new scales forming as the older ones come off. Hair loss may accompany this disorder. Relapses are common. The systemic effects include high-output congestive heart failure, intestinal disturbances, breast enlargement, elevated levels of uric acid in the blood (hyperuricemia), and temperature disturbances.

Medical Management

The objectives of management are to maintain fluid and electrolyte balance and to prevent infection. The treatment is individualized and supportive and should be initiated as soon as the condition is diagnosed.

The patient may be hospitalized and placed on bed rest. All medications that may be implicated are discontinued. A comfortable room temperature should be maintained because the patient does not have normal thermoregulatory control as a result of temperature fluctuations caused by vasodilation and evaporative water loss. Fluid and electrolyte balance must be maintained because there is considerable water and protein loss from the skin surface. Plasma volume expanders may be indicated.

Nursing Management

Continual nursing assessment is carried out to detect infection. The disrupted, erythematous, moist skin is susceptible to infection and becomes colonized with pathogenic organisms, which produce more inflammation. Antibiotics, prescribed if infection is present, are selected on the basis of culture and sensitivity.

Nursing Alert *The nurse observes the patient for signs and symptoms of congestive heart failure because hyperemia and increased cutaneous blood flow can produce cardiac failure of high-output origin.*

Hypothermia may also occur because increased blood flow in the skin, coupled with increased water loss through the skin, leads to heat loss by radiation, conduction, and evaporation. Changes in vital signs are closely monitored and reported.

As in any acute dermatitis, topical therapy is used to give symptomatic relief. Soothing baths, compresses, and lubrication with emollients are used to treat the extensive dermatitis. The patient is likely to be extremely irritable because of the severe itching. Oral or parenteral corticosteroids may be prescribed when the disease is not controlled by more conservative therapy. When a specific cause is known, more specific therapy may be used. The patient is advised to avoid all irritants in the future, particularly medications.

COMMON BLISTERING DISEASES

Blisters in the skin have many origins, including infections (bacterial, fungal, or viral), allergic contact reactions, metabolic disorders, and immunologically mediated reactions. Some of these have been discussed previously (herpes simplex and zoster, contact dermatitis). Immunologically mediated diseases are autoimmune reactions and represent a defect of IgM, IgE, IgG, and C3. Some of these conditions are life-threatening; others become chronic problems.

Diagnosis is always made by histologic examination of a biopsy specimen by a dermatopathologist. A specimen from the blister and surrounding skin demonstrates **acantholysis** (separation of epidermal cells from each other because of damage to or an abnormality of the intracellular substance). Circulating antibodies may be detected by immunofluorescent studies of the patient's serum.

Pemphigus

Pemphigus is a group of serious diseases of the skin characterized by the appearance of bullae (blisters) of various sizes on apparently normal skin (Fig. 52-5) and mucous membranes. Available evidence indicates that pemphigus is an autoimmune disease involving IgG, an immunoglobulin. It is thought that the pemphigus antibody is directed against a specific cell-surface antigen in epidermal cells. A blister forms from the antigen–antibody reaction. The level of serum antibody is predictive of disease severity. Genetic factors may also play a role in its development, with the highest incidence in those of Jewish or Mediterranean descent. This disorder usually occurs in men and women in middle and late adulthood. This condition may be associated with ingestion of the penicillins and captopril, and with myasthenia gravis.

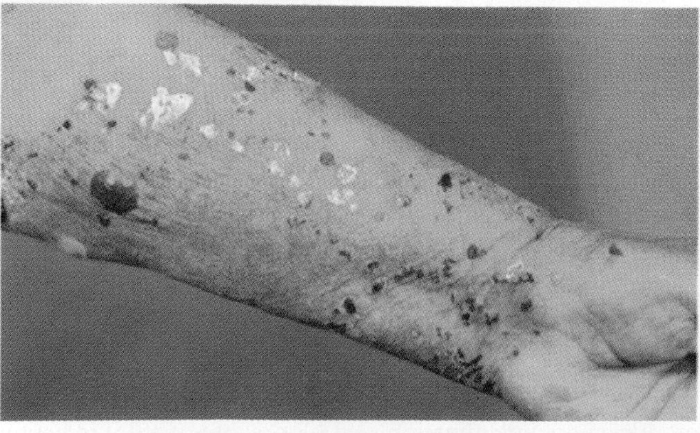

FIGURE 52•5 Pemphigus vulgaris blisters on the forearm.

Clinical Manifestations

Most patients initially present with oral lesions appearing as irregularly shaped erosions that are painful, bleed easily, and heal slowly. The skin bullae enlarge, rupture, and leave large, painful eroded areas that are accompanied by crusting and oozing. A characteristic offensive odor emanates from the bullae and the exuding serum. There is blistering or sloughing of uninvolved skin when minimal pressure is applied (Nikolsky's sign). The eroded skin heals slowly, so that eventually huge areas of the body are involved. Bacterial superinfection is common.

Complications

The most common complications of pemphigus vulgaris arise when the disease process is widespread. Before the advent of corticosteroid and immunosuppressive therapy, patients were very susceptible to secondary bacterial infection. Skin bacteria have relatively easy access to the bullae as they ooze, rupture, and leave denuded areas that are open to the environment. Fluid and electrolyte imbalance results from the loss of both fluid and protein as the bullae rupture. Hypoalbuminemia is common when the disease process includes extensive areas of the body skin surface and mucous membranes.

Medical Management

The goals of therapy are to bring the disease under control as rapidly as possible, to prevent loss of serum and the development of secondary infection, and to promote reepithelization (renewal of epithelial tissue).

Corticosteroids are administered in high doses to control the disease and keep the skin free of blisters. The high dosage level is maintained until remission is apparent. In some cases the corticosteroid therapy must be maintained for life.

Corticosteroids are administered with or immediately after a meal and may be accompanied by an antacid as prophylaxis against gastric complications. Essential to therapeutic management are daily evaluations of body weight, blood pressure, blood glucose levels, and fluid balance. High-dose corticosteroid therapy has its own serious toxic effects (see Chap. 38).

Immunosuppressive agents (azathioprine, cyclophosphamide, gold) may be prescribed to help control the disease and reduce the corticosteroid dose. **Plasmapheresis** (plasma exchange) temporarily decreases the serum antibody level and has been used with variable success, although it is generally reserved for life-threatening cases.

Bullous Pemphigoid

Bullous pemphigoid is an acquired disease of flaccid blisters appearing either on normal or erythematous skin. It appears more often on the flexor surfaces of the arms, legs, axilla, and groin. Oral lesions, if present, are usually transient and minimal. When the blisters break, the skin has shallow erosions that heal fairly quickly. Pruritus can be intense, even before the appearance of the blisters. Bullous pemphigoid is common in the elderly, with peak incidence about age 60. There is no gender or racial predilection, and the disease can be found throughout the world.

Medical Management

Medical treatment includes topical corticosteroids for localized eruptions and systemic corticosteroids for widespread involvement. Systemic prednisone may be continued for months, in alternate-day doses. The patient needs to understand the implications of long-term corticosteroid ingestion, including loss of calcium in bone, cataracts, peptic ulcers, psychotic reactions, increased risk for infection, weight gain from water retention, and the potential for adrenal suppression.

Dermatitis Herpetiformis

Dermatitis herpetiformis is an intensely pruritic, chronic disease that manifests with small tense blisters, distributed symmetrically over the elbows, knees, buttocks, and nape of the neck. It is most common between the ages of 20 and 40 but can appear at any age. Most patients with dermatitis herpetiformis have a subclinical defect in gluten metabolism.

Medical Management

Most patients respond to dapsone (a combination of tetracycline and nicotinamide) and to a gluten-free diet. All patients should be screened for G6PD deficiency, because dapsone can induce severe hemolysis in these individuals. Patients benefit from dietary counseling because the dietary restrictions are lifelong, and a gluten-free diet is often difficult to follow. They need emotional support as they deal with the process of learning new habits and accepting major changes in their life.

Herpes Gestationis

Herpes gestationis is a disease that occurs during or shortly after pregnancy. It shares several clinical features with bullous pemphigoid and despite its name has no relation to the herpes virus. This disease is relatively rare, with an incidence of approximately 1 in every 50,000 pregnancies. It appears in the second or third trimester. It begins with urticarial papules on the abdomen and spreads to the trunk and extremities. It usually resolves within a few weeks of delivery but can recur in subsequent pregnancies, with menses, or with the ingestion of oral contraceptives.

Medical Management

Herpes gestationis is best managed with systemic corticosteroids. There is debate as to whether there is any risk of fetal morbidity or mortality in babies born to mothers with herpes gestationis. As in other blistering diseases, special attention is required to prevent secondary infection.

NURSING PROCESS: THE PATIENT WITH COMMON BLISTERING DISEASES

Assessment

Patients with blistering disorders may experience significant disability. There is constant itching and possible pain in the denuded areas of skin. There may be drainage from the denuded areas, which may be malodorous. Effective assessment and nursing management become a challenge.

Disease activity is monitored clinically by examining the skin for the appearance of new blisters. Areas where healing has occurred may show signs of hyperpigmentation. Particular attention is given to assessing for signs and symptoms of infection.

Diagnosis

Nursing Diagnoses

Based on nursing assessment data, the patient's major nursing diagnoses may include:

- Pain of oral cavity and skin related to blistering and erosions
- Impaired skin integrity related to ruptured bullae and denuded areas of the skin
- Anxiety and ineffective coping related to the appearance of the skin and no hope of a cure
- Knowledge deficit about medications and side effects

Collaborative Problems/Potential Complications

Based on the assessment data, potential complications include:

- Infection and sepsis related to loss of protective barrier of skin and mucous membranes
- Fluid volume deficit and electrolyte imbalance related to loss of tissue fluids

Planning and Goals

The major goals for the patient may include relief of discomfort from lesions, skin healing, reduced anxiety and improved coping capacity, and absence of complications.

Nursing Interventions

Relieving Oral Discomfort

The patient's entire oral cavity may be affected with erosions and denuded surfaces. A necrotic slough may develop over these areas, adding to the patient's discomfort and interfering with food intake. Weight loss and hypoproteinemia may result. Meticulous oral hygiene is important to keep the oral mucosa clean and allow the epithelium to regenerate. Frequent rinsing of the mouth is prescribed to rid the mouth of debris and to soothe ulcerative areas. Commercial mouthwashes are avoided. The lips are kept moist with lanolin, petrolatum, or lip balm. Cool mist therapy helps to humidify environmental air.

Enhancing Skin Integrity

Cool wet dressings or baths are protective and soothing. The patient with painful and extensive lesions should be premedicated with analgesics before skin care is initiated. Patients with large areas of blistering have a characteristic odor that decreases when secondary infection is controlled. After the patient's skin is bathed, it is dried carefully and dusted liberally with nonirritating powder, which enables the patient to move freely in bed. Fairly large amounts are necessary to keep the patient's skin from sticking to the sheets. Tape should never be used on the skin because it may produce more blisters. Hypothermia is common, and measures to keep the patient warm and comfortable are priority nursing activities. The nursing management of patients with bullous skin conditions is similar to that of patients with extensive burns (see Chap. 53).

Reducing Anxiety

Critical to the nursing management of the patient with blistering diseases is the development of a trusting relationship. This encompasses the way the nurse listens, interacts, and demonstrates a warm and caring manner. The patient has legitimate concerns that may be reduced when the health team responds appropriately. The patient is encouraged to express anxieties, discomfort, and feelings of hopelessness freely. This is necessary for specific reassurance to be most effective.

Attention to the psychological needs of the patient requires being available, giving expert nursing care, and educating the patient and the family. Arranging for a family member or a close friend to spend more time with the patient can be supportive. When patients receive information about the disease and its treatment, uncertainty and anxiety are reduced and the patient's capacity to act on his or her own behalf is enhanced. A referral for psychological counseling may be helpful to assist the patient in dealing with fears, anxiety, and depression.

Monitoring and Managing Potential Complications

INFECTION AND SEPSIS

The patient is susceptible to infection because the barrier function of the skin is compromised. Bullae are also susceptible to infection, and sepsis may follow. The skin is kept clean to eliminate debris and dead skin and to prevent infection.

Secondary infection may be accompanied by an offensive odor from skin or oral lesions. *C. albicans* of the mouth (thrush) commonly affects patients receiving high-dose corticosteroid therapy. The oral cavity is inspected daily, and any changes are noted and reported. Oral lesions are slow to heal.

Infection is the leading cause of death in patients with blistering diseases. Particular attention is given to assessing the patient for signs and symptoms of local and systemic infection. Seemingly trivial complaints or minimal changes are investigated, because corticosteroids can mask or alter typical signs and symptoms of infection. The patient's vital signs are taken, and temperature fluctuations are monitored. The patient is observed for chills, and all secretions and excretions are monitored for changes suggesting infection. Results of culture and sensitivity tests are monitored. Antimicrobial agents are administered as prescribed, and response to treatment is noted. Health care personnel must perform effective hand washing and wear gloves.

In the hospitalized patient, environmental contamination is avoided as much as possible by having the housekeeping department dust with a damp cloth and wash the floor with a wet mop. Protective isolation measures and standard precautions may be implemented.

FLUID AND ELECTROLYTE IMBALANCE

Extensive denudation of the skin leads to fluid and electrolyte imbalance because of significant loss of fluids and sodium chloride from the skin. This sodium chloride loss is responsible for many of the systemic symptoms associated with the disease and is treated by intravenous administration of saline solution.

A large amount of protein and blood is lost from the denuded skin areas. Blood component therapy may be prescribed to maintain the blood volume as well as the hemoglobin and plasma protein concentrations. Serum albumin, protein, hemoglobin, and hematocrit values are monitored.

The patient is encouraged to maintain adequate oral fluid intake. Cool, nonirritating fluids are encouraged to maintain hydration. Small, frequent meals or snacks of high-protein, high-calorie foods (Ensure, Sustacal, eggnogs, milkshakes) help maintain nutritional status. Total parenteral nutrition is considered if the patient cannot eat an adequate diet.

Evaluation

Expected Outcomes

Expected outcomes may include:

1. Achieves relief from pain of oral lesions
   a. Identifies therapies that reduce pain
   b. Uses mouthwashes and anesthetic/antiseptic aerosol mouth spray
   c. Drinks chilled fluids at 2-hour intervals
2. Achieves skin healing
   a. States purpose of therapeutic regimen
   b. Cooperates with soaks/bath regimen
   c. Reminds caregivers to use liberal amounts of nonirritating powder on bed linens
3. Is less anxious and better able to cope
   a. Verbalizes concerns about condition, self, and relationships with others
   b. Participates in self-care
4. Experiences no infection
   a. Cultures from bullae, skin, and orifices are negative for pathogenic organisms.
   b. Has no purulent drainage
   c. Shows signs that skin is clearing
   d. Has normal temperature
5. Attains fluid and electrolyte balance
   a. Keeps intake record to ensure adequate fluid intake and normal fluid and electrolyte balance
   b. Verbalizes the rationale for intravenous infusion therapy
   c. Urine output within normal limits
   d. Has serum chemistry and hemoglobin and hematocrit values within normal limits

Toxic Epidermal Necrolysis and Stevens-Johnson Syndrome

Toxic epidermal necrolysis (TEN) and Stevens-Johnson syndrome (SJS) are potentially fatal skin disorders and the most severe form of erythema multiforme. The mortality rate from TEN approaches 30%. Both conditions are triggered by a reaction to medications or are secondary to a viral infection. Antibiotics, anticonvulsants, butazones, and sulfonamides are the most frequent medications implicated in TEN and SJS.

Clinical Manifestations

TEN and SJS are characterized initially by conjunctival burning or itching, cutaneous tenderness, fever, cough, sore throat, headache, extreme malaise, and myalgias (aches and pains). These signs are followed by a rapid onset of erythema (reddening of the skin) involving much of the skin surface and mucous membranes (oral mucosa, conjunctiva, and genitalia). In severe cases of mucosal involvement, there may be danger of damage to the larynx, bronchi, or esophagus from ulcerations. Large, flaccid bullae develop in some areas; in other areas, large sheets of epidermis are shed, exposing the underlying dermis. Fingernails, toenails, eyebrows, and eyelashes may all be shed, along with the surrounding epidermis. The skin is excruciatingly tender, and the loss of skin leaves a weeping surface similar to that of a total-body second-degree burn; thus, the condition is also referred to as scalded skin syndrome.

These conditions occur in all ages and both genders. The incidence is increased in older people, simply because they are usually taking more medications. People with HIV, particularly those with AIDS, as well as others who are immunocompromised are at higher risk for SJS and TEN. Although the incidence of TEN and SJS in the general population is about 3 per million person-years, the risk associated with sulfonamides in HIV-positive individuals may approach 1 per 1000 (Arndt et al., 1997).

Complications

Sepsis and keratoconjunctivitis are complications of TEN and SJS. Unrecognized and untreated sepsis can be life-threatening. Keratoconjunctivitis can impair vision and result in conjunctival retraction, scarring, and corneal lesions.

Assessment and Diagnostic Findings

Histologic studies of frozen skin cells from a fresh lesion and cytodiagnosis of collections of cellular material from a freshly denuded area are performed. A history of ingestion of medications known to precipitate TEN or SJS may verify medication reaction as the underlying cause.

Immunofluorescent studies may be performed to detect atypical epidermal autoantibodies. A genetic predisposition to erythema multiforme has been suggested but is not confirmed for all cases.

Medical Management

The goals of treatment include control of fluid and electrolyte balance, prevention of sepsis, and prevention of ophthalmic complications. Supportive care is the mainstay of treatment.

All nonessential medications are discontinued immediately. If possible, the patient is treated in a regional burn center, because aggressive treatment similar to that given for a severe burn is required. Skin loss may approach 100% of the total body surface area. Surgical débridement or hydrotherapy in a Hubbard tank (a large steel tub) may be performed to remove involved skin.

Tissue samples from the nasopharynx, eyes, ears, blood, urine, skin, and unruptured blisters are obtained for culture to identify the pathogenic organisms. Intravenous fluids are prescribed to maintain fluid and electrolyte balance, especially in the patient who has severe mucosal involvement and who cannot easily swallow nourishment. Because an indwelling intravenous catheter may be the site of infection, however, fluid replacement is carried out by nasogastric tube and then orally as soon as possible.

Initial treatment with systemic corticosteroids is controversial. Some experts argue for early high-dose corticosteroid treatment. However, in most cases, the risk of infection, the complication of fluid and electrolyte balance, the delay in the healing process, and the difficulty in initiating oral corticosteroids early in the course of the disease outweigh the perceived benefits. In patients with TEN thought to result from a medication reaction, corticosteroids may be administered; however, the patient should be closely monitored.

Protecting the skin with topical agents is crucial. Various topical antibacterial and anesthetic agents are used to prevent wound sepsis and to assist with pain management. Systemic antibiotic therapy is employed with extreme caution. Temporary biologic dressings (eg, pigskin, amniotic membrane) or plastic semipermeable dressings (Vigilon) may be used to reduce pain, decrease evaporation, and prevent secondary infection until the epithelium regenerates. Meticulous oropharyngeal and eye care is essential when there is severe involvement of the mucous membranes and the eye.

NURSING PROCESS: THE PATIENT WITH TOXIC EPIDERMAL NECROLYSIS

Assessment

A careful inspection of the skin is made, including its appearance and the extent of involvement. The normal skin is closely observed to determine if new areas of blisters are developing. Seepage from blisters is monitored for amount, color, and odor. Inspection of the oral cavity for blistering and erosive lesions is performed daily; the patient is assessed daily for itching, burning, and dryness of the eyes. The patient's ability to swallow and drink fluids, as well as speak normally, is determined.

The patient's vital signs are monitored, and special attention is given to the presence and character of fever and the respiratory rate, depth, rhythm, and cough. The characteristics and amount of respiratory secretions are noted. Assessment for high fever, tachycardia, and extreme weakness and fatigue is essential because these indicate the process of epidermal necrosis, increased metabolic needs, and possible gastrointestinal and respiratory mucosal sloughing. Urine volume, specific gravity, and color are monitored. The insertion sites of intravenous lines are inspected for signs of local infection. Daily body weights are recorded.

The patient is asked to describe fatigue and pain levels. An attempt is made to evaluate the patient's level of anxiety. The patient's basic coping mechanisms are assessed and effective coping strategies are identified.

Diagnosis

Nursing Diagnoses

Based on the assessment data, the patient's major nursing diagnoses may include:

- Impaired tissue integrity (oral, eye, and skin) related to epidermal shedding
- Fluid volume deficit and electrolyte losses related to loss of fluids from denuded skin
- Risk for altered body temperature (hypothermia) related to heat loss secondary to skin loss
- Pain related to denuded skin, oral lesions, and possible infection
- Anxiety related to the physical appearance of the skin and prognosis

Collaborative Problems/Potential Complications

Based on the assessment data, potential complications include:

- Sepsis
- Conjunctival retraction, scars, and corneal lesions

Planning and Goals

The major goals for the patient may include skin and oral tissue healing, fluid balance, prevention of heat loss, relief of pain, reduced anxiety, and absence of complications.

Nursing Interventions

Maintaining Skin and Mucous Membrane Integrity

The local care of the skin is an important area of nursing management. The skin denudes easily, even when the patient is lifted and turned; it may be necessary to place the patient on a circular turning frame. The nurse applies the prescribed topical agents that reduce the bacterial population of the wound surface. Warm compresses, if prescribed, should be applied gently to denuded areas. The topical antibacterial agent may be used in conjunction with hydrotherapy in a tank, bathtub, or shower. The nurse monitors the patient's condition during the treatment and encourages the patient to exercise the extremities during the hydrotherapy.

The painful oral lesions make oral hygiene difficult. Careful oral hygiene is performed to keep the oral mucosa clean. Prescribed mouthwashes, anesthetics, or coating agents are used frequently to rid the mouth of debris, soothe ulcerative areas, and control foul mouth odor. The oral cavity is inspected several times a day, and any changes are documented and reported. Petrolatum (or prescribed ointment) is applied to the lips.

Attaining Fluid Balance

The vital signs, urine output, and sensorium are observed for indications of hypovolemia. Mental changes from fluid and electrolyte imbalance, sensory overload, or sensory deprivation may occur. Laboratory test results are evaluated, and abnormal results are reported. The patient is weighed daily (with a bed scale if necessary).

The nurse regulates intravenous fluids at prescribed infusion rates and assesses for systemic (overinfusion or underinfusion) and local (infection) complications. Oral lesions may result in dysphagia, making tube feeding or total parenteral nutrition necessary. Prescribed enteral nourishment or enteral supplements can be administered by tube feeding until oral ingestion can be tolerated. A daily calorie count and accurate recording of all intake and output are essential.

Preventing Hypothermia

The patient with TEN is prone to chilling. Dehydration may be made worse by exposing the denuded skin to a continuous current of warm air. The patient is usually sensitive to room temperature changes. Measures implemented for a burn patient, such as cotton blankets, ceiling-mounted heat lamps, or heat shields, are useful in maintaining body temperature. To minimize shivering and heat loss, the nurse should work rapidly and efficiently when large wounds are exposed for wound care. The patient's temperature is carefully monitored.

Relieving Pain

The nurse assesses the patient's pain, its characteristics, any factors that influence the pain, and the patient's behavioral responses. Prescribed analgesics are administered, and the nurse observes and documents pain relief and any side effects. Analgesics are administered before painful treatments are performed. Providing thorough explanations and speaking soothingly to the patient during treatments can allay the anxiety that may intensify pain. Offering emotional support and reassurance and implementing measures that promote rest and sleep are basic in achieving pain control. As the pain diminishes and the patient has more physical and emotional energy, self-management techniques for pain relief, such as progressive muscle relaxation and imagery, may be taught.

Reducing Anxiety

Because the lifestyle of patients with TEN has been abruptly changed to one of complete dependence, an assessment of their emotional state may reveal anxiety, depression, and fear of dying. Patients can be reassured that these reactions are normal. They also need nursing support, honest communication, and hope that their situation can improve. They are encouraged to express their feelings to someone they trust. Listening to their concerns and being readily available with skillful and compassionate care are important anxiety-relieving interventions. Emotional support by a psychiatric nurse, chaplain, psychologist, or psychiatrist may be invaluable for promoting coping during the long recovery period.

Monitoring and Managing Potential Complications

SEPSIS

The major cause of death from TEN is infection, and the most common sites of infection are the skin and mucosal surfaces, lungs, and blood. The organisms most often involved are *S. aureus, Pseudomonas, Klebsiella, Escherichia coli, Serratia,* and *Candida.* Monitoring vital signs closely and noting any adverse changes in respiratory, renal, or gastrointestinal function may quickly detect the beginning of an infection. Strict asepsis is always maintained during routine skin care measures. Hand washing and wearing sterile gloves when carrying out procedures are necessary. When the condition involves a large portion of the body, the patient should be in a private room to prevent possible cross-infection from other patients. Visitors should wear protective garments and wash their hands before and after coming into contact with the patient. People with any infectious disease should not visit the patient until they are no longer a danger to the patient.

CONJUNCTIVAL RETRACTION, SCARS, AND CORNEAL LESIONS

The eyes are inspected daily for signs of itching, burning, and dryness, which may indicate progression of TEN to keratoconjunctivitis, the principal eye complication. Applying a cool, damp cloth over the eyes may relieve burning sensations. The eyes are kept clean and observed for signs of discharge or discomfort, and the progression of symptoms is documented and reported. Administering an eye lubricant, when prescribed, may alleviate dryness and prevent corneal abrasion. Using eye patches or reminding the patient to blink periodically may also counteract dryness. The patient is instructed to avoid rubbing the eyes or putting any medication into the eyes that has not been prescribed or approved by the physician.

Evaluation

Expected Outcomes

Expected outcomes may include:

1. Achieves increasing skin and oral tissue healing
   a. Demonstrates areas of healing skin
   b. Swallows fluids and speaks clearly

2. Attains fluid balance
   a. Demonstrates laboratory values within normal ranges
   b. Maintains urine volume and specific gravity within acceptable range
   c. Shows stable vital signs
   d. Increases intake of oral fluids without discomfort
   e. Gains weight, if appropriate
3. Attains thermoregulation
   a. Registers body temperature within normal range
   b. Reports no chills
4. Reports lessening of pain intensity
   a. Uses analgesics as prescribed
   b. Uses self-management techniques for relief of pain
5. Appears less anxious
   a. Discusses concerns freely
   b. Sleeps for progressively longer periods
6. Experiences no complications, such as sepsis and impaired vision
   a. Body temperature within normal range
   b. Laboratory values within normal ranges
   c. Has no abnormal discharges or signs of infection
   d. Continues to see objects at baseline acuity level
   e. Shows no signs of keratoconjunctivitis

ULCERATIONS

The superficial loss of surface tissue as a result of death of the cells is called an ulceration. A simple ulcer, such as the kind found in a small, superficial, second-degree burn, tends to heal by granulation (new tissue granules) if kept clean and protected from injury. If it is exposed to the air, the serum that escapes will dry and form a scab, under which the epithelial cells will grow and cover the surface completely. Certain diseases cause characteristic ulcers—tuberculous ulcers and syphilitic ulcers are examples.

Ulcers related to problems with arterial circulation are seen in patients with peripheral vascular disease, arteriosclerosis, Raynaud's disease, and frostbite. In these patients, treatment is carried out in conjunction with the arterial disease treatment (see Chap. 28). Nursing management includes use of the dressings discussed at the beginning of this chapter. If nursing interventions are instituted early in the progression of an ulcer, the condition can often be effectively improved. Surgical amputation of an affected limb is a last resort.

BENIGN TUMORS OF THE SKIN

Cysts

Cysts of the skin are epithelium-lined cavities containing fluid or solid material. Epidermal cysts (epidermoid) occur frequently and may be described as slow-growing, firm, elevated tumors found most frequently on the face, neck, upper chest, and back. Removal of the cysts provides a cure.

Pilar cysts (trichilemmal cysts), originally called sebaceous cysts, are most frequently found on the scalp. They originate from the middle portion of the hair follicle and from the cells of the outer hair root sheath. The treatment is surgical removal.

Actinic and Seborrheic Keratoses

Seborrheic keratoses are benign, wartlike lesions of varying size and color, ranging from light tan to black. They are usually located on the face, shoulders, chest, and back and are the most common skin tumors seen in middle-aged and elderly people. They may be cosmetically unacceptable to the patient. A black keratosis may be erroneously diagnosed as malignant melanoma. The treatment is removal of the tumor tissue by excision, electrodesiccation and curettage, or application of carbon dioxide or liquid nitrogen. However, there is no harm in allowing these growths to remain, because there is no medical significance to their presence.

Actinic keratoses are premalignant skin lesions that develop in chronically sun-exposed areas of the body. They appear as rough, scaly patches with underlying erythema. A small percentage of these lesions gradually transform into cutaneous squamous cell carcinoma; thus, they are usually removed either by cryotherapy or shave excision.

Verrucae (Warts)

Warts are common benign skin tumors caused by infection with the human papillomavirus, which belongs to the DNA virus group. All age groups may be affected, but the condition occurs most frequently between ages 12 and 16 years. There are many types of warts.

As a rule, warts are asymptomatic, except when they occur on weight-bearing areas, such as the soles of the feet. They may be treated with locally applied laser therapy, liquid nitrogen, salicylic acid plasters, electrodesiccation, or cantharidin.

Warts occurring on the genitalia and perianal areas are known as condylomata acuminata. They may be transmitted sexually and are treated with liquid nitrogen, cryosurgery, electrosurgery, topically applied trichloracetic acid, and curettage. Most condylomata have no medical significance, but those that affect the uterine cervix predispose the patient to cervical cancer.

Angiomas

Angiomas are benign vascular tumors involving the skin and the subcutaneous tissues. They are present at birth and may occur as flat, violet-red patches (port-wine angiomas) or as raised, bright-red, nodular lesions (strawberry angiomas). The latter tend to involute spontaneously within the first few years of life. Port-wine angiomas, in contrast, usually persist indefinitely. Most patients use masking cosmetics (Covermark or Dermablend) to camouflage the defect. The argon laser is being used on various angiomas with some success. Treatment of strawberry angiomas is more successful if undertaken as soon after birth as possible.

Pigmented Nevi (Moles)

Moles are common skin tumors of various sizes and shades, ranging from yellowish-brown to black. They may be flat, macular lesions or elevated papules or nodules that occasionally contain hair. Most pigmented nevi are harmless lesions. However, in rare cases, malignant changes supervene and a melanoma develops at the site of the nevus. Some authorities believe that all congenital moles should be removed, because they may have a higher incidence of malignant change. However, depending on the quantity and location, this may be impractical. Nevi that show a change in color or size or become symptomatic (itch) or develop irregular borders should be removed to determine if malignant changes have occurred. Moles that occur in unusual places should be examined carefully for any irregularity and for notching of the border and variation in color. Early melanomas may display some redness and irritation and areas of bluish pigmentation where the pigment-containing cells have spread deeper into the skin. Late melanomas have areas of paler color, where pigment cells have stopped producing melanin. Nevi larger than 1 cm should be examined carefully. Excised nevi should be examined histologically.

Keloids

Keloids are benign overgrowths of fibrous tissue at the site of a scar or trauma. They appear to be more common among dark-skinned people. Keloids are asymptomatic but may cause disfigurement and cosmetic concern. The treatment, which is not always satisfactory, consists of surgical excision, intralesional corticosteroid therapy, and radiation.

Dermatofibroma

A dermatofibroma is a common benign tumor of connective tissue that occurs predominantly on the extremities. It is a firm, dome-shaped papule or nodule that may be skin-colored or pinkish-brown. Excisional biopsy is the recommended method of treatment.

Neurofibromatosis (von Recklinghausen's Disease)

Neurofibromatosis is a hereditary condition manifested by pigmented patches (café-au-lait macules), axillary freckling, and cutaneous neurofibromas that vary in size. Developmental changes may occur in the nervous system, muscles, and bone. Malignant degeneration of the neurofibromas occurs in some patients.

SKIN CANCER

Skin cancer is the most common cancer in the United States. If the incidence continues at the present rate, an estimated one of eight fair-skinned Americans will develop skin cancer, especially basal cell carcinoma. Because the skin is easily inspected, skin cancer is readily seen and detected and is the most successfully treated type of cancer.

Exposure to the sun is the leading cause of skin cancer; incidence is related to the total amount of exposure to the sun. Sun damage is cumulative, and harmful effects may be severe by age 20. The increase in skin cancer is probably due to changing lifestyles and the emphasis on sunbathing and related activities, in light of changes in the environment, such as holes in the world's ozone layer. Protective measures should be used throughout life, and nurses need to inform patients about risk factors associated with skin cancer.

Risk Factors for SKIN CANCER

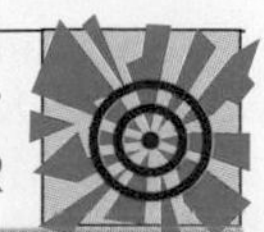

Changes in the ozone layer from the effects of worldwide industrial air pollutants, such as chlorofluorocarbons, have prompted concern that the incidence of skin cancers, especially malignant melanoma, will increase. The ozone layer, a stratospheric blanket of bluish, explosive gas formed by the sun's ultraviolet radiation, varies in depth with the seasons and is thickest at the North and South Poles and thinnest at the equator. Scientists believe that it helps protect the earth from the effects of solar ultraviolet radiation. Proponents of this theory predict an increase in skin cancers as a consequence of changes in the ozone layer. Further research should disclose whether ozone destruction is a viable concern and a potential health hazard. Other skin cancer risk factors follow.

- Fair-skinned, fair-haired, blue-eyed people, particularly those of Celtic origin, with insufficient skin pigmentation to protect underlying tissues
- People who sustain sunburn and who do not tan
- Long-time sun exposure (farmers, fishermen, construction workers)
- Exposure to chemical pollutants (industrial workers in arsenic, nitrates, coal, tar and pitch, oils and paraffins)
- Age (elderly people) and sun-damaged skin
- History of x-ray therapy for acne or benign lesions
- Scars form severe burns; chronic skin irritations
- Immunosuppression
- Genetic factors

Basal Cell and Squamous Cell Carcinoma

The most common types of skin cancer are basal cell carcinoma (BCC) and squamous cell (epidermoid) carcinoma (SCC). The third most common type, malignant melanoma, is discussed separately. Skin cancer is diagnosed by biopsy and histologic evaluation.

Clinical Manifestations

BCC is the most common type of skin cancer. It generally appears on sun-exposed areas of the body and is more prevalent in regions where the population is subjected to intense and extensive exposure to the sun. The incidence is proportional to the age of the patient (average age 60) and the total amount of sun exposure and is inversely proportional to the amount of melanin in the skin.

BCC usually begins as a small, waxy nodule with rolled, translucent, pearly borders; telangiectatic vessels may be present. As it grows, it undergoes central ulceration and sometimes crusting (Fig. 52-6). The tumors appear most frequently on the face. BCC is characterized by invasion and erosion of contiguous (adjoining) tissues. It rarely metastasizes, but recurrence is common. However, a neglected lesion can account for the loss of a nose, an ear, or a lip. Other variants of BCC may appear as shiny, flat, gray, or yellowish plaques.

SCC is a malignant proliferation arising from the epidermis. Although it usually appears on sun-damaged skin, it may arise from normal skin or from preexisting skin lesions. It is of greater concern than BCC because it is a truly invasive carcinoma, metastasizing by the blood or lymphatic system.

Metastases account for 75% of deaths from SCC. The lesions may be primary, arising on both the skin and mucous membranes, or they may develop from a precancerous condition, such as actinic keratosis (lesions occurring in sun-exposed areas), leukoplakia (premalignant lesion of the mucous membrane), or scarred or ulcerated lesions. SCC appears as a rough, thickened, scaly tumor that may be asymptomatic or may involve bleeding (see Fig. 52-6). The border of an SCC lesion may be wider, more infiltrated, and more inflammatory than that of a BCC lesion. Secondary infection can occur. Exposed areas, especially of the upper extremities and of the face, lower lip, ears, nose, and forehead, are common sites.

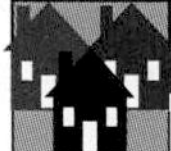

PATIENT EDUCATION AND HOME CARE

Preventing Skin Cancer

Because skin cancer rates are rising, taking preventive measures such as the ones outlined below may help individuals avoid increasing their skin cancer risk.

- Do not try to tan if your skin burns easily, never tans, or tans poorly.
- Avoid unnecessary exposure to the sun, especially during the time of day when ultraviolet radiation (sunlight) is most intense (10 AM to 3 PM).
- Avoid sunburn.
- Apply sunscreen when in the sun; sunscreens block harmful sun rays.
- Use a sunscreen with an SPF of 15 or higher. Sunscreens are rated in strength from 4 (weakest) to 50 (strongest). The SPF indicates the solar protection factor, or how much longer you can stay in the sun before getting burned. Look for sunscreens that protect against both ultraviolet-A (UVA) and ultraviolet-B (UVB) light.
- Reapply water-resistant sunscreens after swimming, if heavily sweating, and every 2 to 3 hours during prolonged periods of sun exposure.
- Avoid oils. Applied before or during sun exposure, oils do not protect against sunlight or sun damage.
- Use a lip balm that contains a sunscreen with the highest SPF number.
- Wear protective clothing, such as a broad-brimmed hat and long sleeves.
- Remember that up to 50% of ultraviolet rays can penetrate loosely woven clothing.
- Remember that ultraviolet light can penetrate a cloud cover, and a sunburn can still occur.
- Do not use sun lamps for indoor tanning, and avoid commercial tanning booths. These rays are just as harmful.
- Teach children to avoid all but modest sun exposure and to use a sunscreen regularly for lifelong protection.

Prognosis

The prognosis for BCC and SCC depends on the incidence of metastases, which is related to the histologic type and the level or depth of invasion. Usually, tumors arising in sun-damaged areas are less invasive and rarely cause death, whereas SCC that arises without a history of sun or arsenic exposure or scar formation appears to have a greater chance for spread. Regional lymph nodes should be evaluated for metastases.

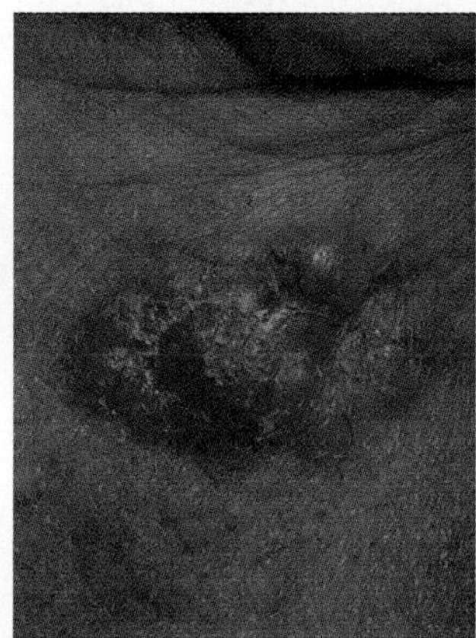

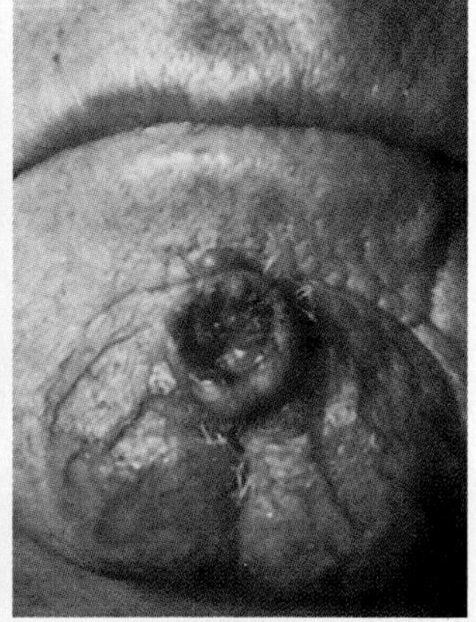

FIGURE 52•6 Basal cell carcinoma (left), squamous cell carcinoma (right).

Medical Management

The goal of treatment is to eradicate the tumor. The treatment method depends on the tumor location, the cell type (location and depth), the cosmetic desires of the patient, the history of previous treatment, whether the tumor is invasive, and the presence or absence of metastatic nodes. The management of BCC and SCC includes surgical excision, Mohs' micrographic surgery, electrosurgery, cryosurgery, and radiation therapy.

SURGICAL MANAGEMENT

The primary goal is to remove the tumor entirely. The best way to maintain cosmetic appearance is to place the incision properly along natural skin tension lines and natural anatomic body lines. In this way, scars are less noticeable. The size of the incision depends on the tumor size and location but usually involves a length-to-width ratio of 3:1.

The adequacy of the surgical excision is verified by microscopic evaluation of sections of the specimen. When the tumor is large, reconstructive surgery with use of a skin flap or skin grafting may be required. The incision is closed in layers to enhance cosmetic effect. A pressure dressing applied over the wound provides support. Infection after a simple excision is uncommon if proper surgical asepsis is maintained.

MOHS' MICROGRAPHIC SURGERY

Mohs' micrographic surgery is the technique that is most accurate and that best conserves normal tissue. When the surgical technique was introduced, the excision followed an application of zinc chloride paste to the tumor (chemosurgery), but currently Mohs' surgery is performed without the initial chemosurgery component. The procedure requires that the tumor be removed layer by layer. The first layer excised includes all evident tumor and a small margin of normal-appearing tissue. The specimen is frozen and analyzed by section to determine if all the tumor has been removed. If not, additional layers of tissue are shaved and examined until all tissue margins are tumor-free. In this manner, only the tumor and a safe normal-tissue margin are removed. Mohs' surgery is the recommended tissue-sparing procedure, with cure rates for BCC and SCC approaching 99%. Thus, it is the treatment of choice and the most effective for tumors around the eyes, nose, upper lip, and auricular and periauricular areas.

ELECTROSURGERY

Electrosurgery is the destruction or removal of tissue by electrical energy. The current is converted to heat, which then passes to the tissue from a cold electrode. Electrosurgery may be preceded by curettage (excising the skin tumor by scraping its surface with a curette). Electrodesiccation is then implemented to achieve hemostasis and to destroy any viable malignant cells at the base of the wound or along its edges. Electrodesiccation is useful for small lesions—smaller than 1 to 2 cm (0.4 to 0.8 in) wide.

This method takes advantage of the fact that the tumor in each instance is softer than surrounding skin and therefore can be outlined by a curette, which "feels" the extent of the tumor. The tumor is removed and the base cauterized. The process is repeated twice. Usually, healing occurs within a month.

CRYOSURGERY

Cryosurgery destroys the tumor by deep-freezing. A thermocouple needle apparatus is inserted into the skin, and liquid nitrogen is directed to the center of the tumor until the tumor base is −40° to −60°C. Liquid nitrogen has the lowest boiling point of all cryogens tried, is inexpensive, and is easy to obtain. The tumor tissue is frozen, allowed to thaw, and then refrozen. The site thaws naturally and then becomes gelatinous and heals spontaneously. Swelling and edema follow the freezing. The appearance of the lesion varies. Normal healing, which may take 4 to 6 weeks, occurs faster in areas with a good blood supply.

RADIATION THERAPY

Radiation therapy is frequently performed for cancer of the eyelid, the tip of the nose, and areas in or near vital structures (eg, facial nerve). It is reserved for older patients, because x-ray changes may be seen after 5 to 10 years and malignant changes in scars may be induced by x-rays 15 to 30 years later.

The patient should be informed that the skin may become red and blistered. A bland skin ointment prescribed by the physician may be applied to relieve discomfort. The patient should also be cautioned to avoid exposure to the sun.

Nursing Management

Because many skin cancers are removed by excision, patients are usually treated in outpatient surgical units. The role of the nurse is to teach the patient about self-care after surgery.

PROMOTING HOME AND COMMUNITY-BASED CARE

Teaching Patients Self-Care. The wound is usually (but not always) covered with a dressing to protect the site from physical trauma, external irritants, and contaminants. The patient is advised when to report for a dressing change or is given written and verbal information on how to change dressings—including the type of dressing to purchase, how to remove dressings and apply fresh ones, and the importance of hand washing before and after the procedure.

The patient is advised to watch for excessive bleeding and tight dressings that compromise circulation. If the lesion is in the perioral area, the patient is instructed to drink liquids through a straw and limit talking and facial movement.

After the sutures are removed, an emollient cream may be used to help reduce dryness. Applying a sunscreen over the wound is advised to prevent postoperative hyperpigmentation if the patient spends time outdoors.

Follow-up examinations should be at regular intervals, usually every 3 months for a year, and should include palpation of the adjacent lymph nodes. The patient should also be instructed to seek treatment for any moles that are subject to repeated friction and irritation, and to watch for indications of potential malignancy in moles as described above. Another point to emphasize is the importance of lifelong follow-up evaluations.

Malignant Melanoma

A malignant melanoma is a malignant neoplasm in which atypical melanocytes (pigment cells) are present in both the epidermis and the dermis (and sometimes the subcutaneous cells). It is the most lethal of all the skin cancers and is responsible for about 2% of all cancer deaths.

It can occur in one of several forms: superficial spreading melanoma, lentigo-maligna melanoma, nodular melanoma, and acral-lentiginous melanoma. These types have certain clinical and histologic features as well as different biologic behaviors. Most melanomas derive *de novo* from cutaneous epidermal melanocytes, but some appear in preexisting nevi (moles) in the skin or develop in the uveal tract of the eye. Melanomas frequently appear simultaneously with cancer of other organs.

The worldwide incidence of melanoma doubles every 10 years, a rise that is probably related to increased recreational sun exposure and better methods of early detection. Peak incidence occurs between ages 20 and 45. The incidence of melanoma is increasing faster than that of almost any other cancer, and the mortality rate is increasing faster than that of any other cancer except lung cancer.

Risk Factors

The etiology of malignant melanoma is unknown, but ultraviolet rays are a strongly suspected cause, based on indirect evidence such as the increased incidence of melanoma in countries near the equator and the increased incidence of melanoma in people younger than age 30 who have used a tanning bed more than 10 times per year. In general, 1 in 100 Caucasians will get melanoma every year (Wachsmuth, 1998). Up to 10% of melanoma patients are members of melanoma-prone families who have multiple changing moles (dysplastic nevi) that are susceptible to malignant transformation. Patients with dysplastic nevus syndrome have been found to have unusual moles, larger and more numerous moles, lesions with irregular outlines, and pigmentation located all over the skin. Microscopic examination of dysplastic moles shows disordered, faulty growth.

Clinical Manifestations

Superficial spreading melanoma occurs anywhere on the body and is the most common form of melanoma. It usually affects middle-aged people and occurs most frequently on the trunk and lower extremities. The lesion tends to be circular, with irregular outer portions. The margins of the lesion may be flat or elevated and palpable (Fig. 52-7). This type of melanoma may appear in a combination of colors, with hues of tan, brown, and black mixed with gray, bluish-black, or white. Sometimes a dull-pink rose color can be seen in a small area within the lesion.

Lentigo-maligna melanomas are slowly evolving, pigmented lesions that occur on exposed skin areas, especially the dorsum of

Risk Factors for MALIGNANT MELANOMA

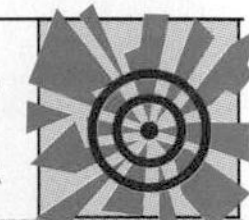

- Fair-skinned or freckled, blue-eyed, light-haired people of Celtic or Scandinavian origin
- People who burn and do not tan or who have a significant history of severe sunburn
- Environmental exposure to intense sunlight (older Americans retiring to the southwestern United States appear to have a higher incidence)
- History of melanoma (personal or family)
- Skin with giant congenital nevi

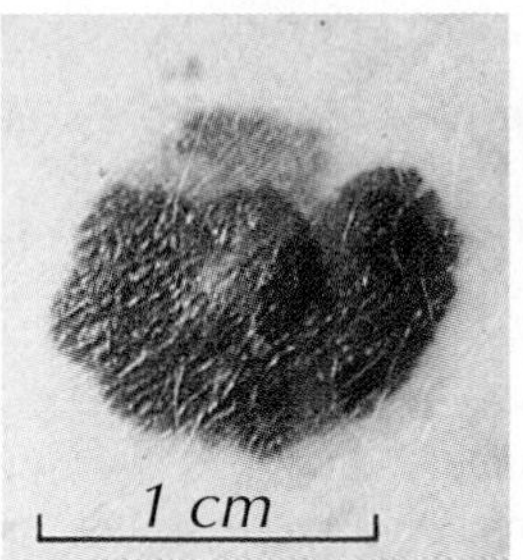

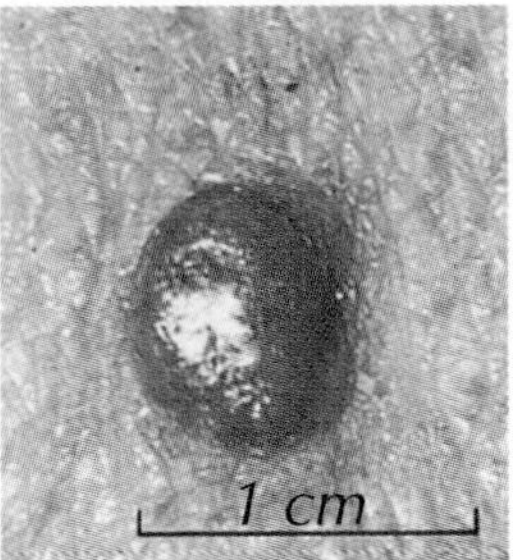

FIGURE 52•7 Two forms of malignant melanoma: superficial spreading (left) and nodular (right). Bickley, L. S., & Hoekelman, R. A. (1999). *Bates' guide to physical examination and history taking* (7th ed.). Philadelphia: Lippincott Williams & Wilkins.

the hand, the head, and neck in elderly people. Often the lesions are present for many years before they are examined by the physician. They first appear as tan, flat lesions and in time undergo changes in size and color.

Nodular melanoma is a spherical, blueberry-like nodule with a relatively smooth surface and a relatively uniform, blue-black color (see Fig. 52-7). It may be dome-shaped with a smooth surface. It may have other shadings of red, gray, or purple. Sometimes nodular melanomas appear as irregularly shaped plaques. The patient may describe this as a blood blister that fails to resolve. A nodular melanoma invades directly into adjacent dermis (vertical growth) and hence has a poorer prognosis.

Acral-lentiginous melanoma is a form of melanoma that occurs in areas not excessively exposed to sunlight and where hair follicles are absent. It is found on the palms of the hands, on the soles, in the nail beds, and in the mucous membranes in dark-skinned people. These melanomas appear as irregular, pigmented macules that develop nodules. They may become invasive early.

Assessment and Diagnostic Findings

Biopsy results confirm the diagnosis of melanoma. An excisional biopsy specimen reveals histologic information on the type, level of invasion, and thickness of the lesion. An excisional biopsy specimen that includes a 1-cm margin of normal tissue and a portion of underlying subcutaneous fatty tissue is sufficient for staging either a melanoma *in situ* or an early, noninvasive melanoma. Incisional biopsy should be performed when the suspicious lesion is too large to remove safely without extensive scarring. Biopsy specimens obtained by shaving, curettage, or needle aspiration are not considered reliable histologic proof of disease.

A thorough history and physical examination should include not only a thorough skin examination but also palpation of regional lymph nodes that drain the lesional area. Because melanoma occurs in families, a positive family history of melanoma is investigated so that first-degree relatives, who may be at high risk for melanoma, can be evaluated for atypical lesions. A chest x-ray, complete blood count, liver function tests, and radionuclide or computed tomography scans are usually ordered once melanoma has been confirmed to stage the extent of disease.

Prognosis

The prognosis for long-term (5-year) survival is considered poor when the lesion is more than 4 mm thick. Patients with melanoma on the hand, foot, or scalp have an increased chance of metastases, which tend to spread to the bone, liver, lungs, spleen, central nervous system, and lymph nodes. Men and elderly patients also have a poorer prognosis (Demis, 1998).

Medical Management

Treatment depends on the level of invasion and the depth of the lesion. Surgical excision is the treatment of choice for small, superficial lesions. Deeper lesions require wide local excision, after which skin grafting may be needed. A regional lymph node dissection is commonly performed to rule out metastasis.

Immunotherapy has had varied success. Immunotherapy modifies immune function and also other biologic responses to cancer. Several forms of immunotherapy offer encouraging results (eg, bacillus Calmette-Guérin [BCG] vaccine, *Corynebacterium paravum*, and levamisole). Some investigational therapies include biologic response modifiers (alpha-interferon, interleukin-2), adaptive immunotherapy (lymphokine-activated killer cells), and monoclonal antibodies directed at melanoma antigens. One of these, proleukin, shows promise in preventing recurrence of melanoma (Demis, 1998). Under investigation is the laboratory assay of tyrosinase, an enzyme believed to be produced only by melanoma cells (Demis, 1998).

MANAGING METASTASES

Current treatments for metastatic melanoma are largely unsuccessful, with cure generally impossible. Further surgical intervention may be performed to debulk the tumor or to remove part of the organ involved (eg, lung, liver, or colon). The rationale for more extensive surgery, however, is for relief of symptoms, not for cure. Chemotherapy for metastatic melanoma may be used; however, few agents (dacarbazine, nitrosoureas, cisplatin) have been effective in controlling the disease.

When the melanoma is located in an extremity, regional perfusion may be used: the chemotherapeutic agent is perfused directly into the area that contains the melanoma. This approach delivers a high concentration of cytotoxic agents while avoiding systemic, toxic side effects. The limb is perfused for 1 hour with high concentrations of the medication at temperatures of 39° to 40°C (102.2° to 104°F) with a perfusion pump. Inducing hyperthermia enhances the effect of the chemotherapy so that a smaller total dose can be used. It is hoped that regional perfusion can control the metastasis, especially if it is used in combination with surgical excision of the primary lesion and with regional lymph node dissection.

NURSING PROCESS: THE PATIENT WITH MALIGNANT MELANOMA

Assessment

Assessment of the patient with malignant melanoma is based on the patient's history and symptoms. The patient is asked specifically about pruritus, tenderness, and pain, which are not features of a benign nevus. The patient is also questioned about changes in preexisting moles or the development of new, pigmented lesions. People at risk are assessed carefully.

A magnifying lens and good lighting are needed for inspecting the skin for irregularity and changes in the mole. Signs that suggest malignant changes are referred to as the ABCDs of moles.

Common sites of melanomas are the skin of the back, the legs (especially in women), between the toes and on the feet, face, scalp, fingernails, and backs of hands. In dark-skinned people, melanomas are most likely to occur in less pigmented sites: palms,

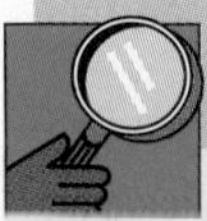

ASSESSMENT
THE ABCDs OF MOLES

A for Asymmetry

- The lesion does not appear balanced on both sides. If an imaginary line were drawn down the middle, the two halves would not look alike.
- The lesion has an irregular surface with uneven elevations (irregular topography) either palpable or visible. A change in the surface may be noted from smooth to scaly.
- Some nodular melanomas have a smooth surface.

B for Irregular Border

- Angular indentations or multiple notches appear in the border
- The border is fuzzy or indistinct, as if rubbed with an eraser.

C for Variegated Color

- Normal moles are usually a uniform light to medium brown. Darker coloration indicates that the melanocytes have penetrated to a deeper layer of the dermis.
- Colors that may indicate malignancy if found together within a single lesion are shades of red, white, and blue; shades of blue are ominous.
- White areas within a pigmented lesion are suspicious.
- Some malignant melanomas, however, are not variegated but are uniformly colored (bluish-black, bluish-gray, bluish-red).

D for Diameter

- A diameter exceeding 6 mm (about the size of a pencil eraser) is considered more suspicious, although this finding without other signs is not significant. Many benign skin growths are larger than 6 mm, whereas some early melanomas may be smaller.

soles, subungual areas, and mucous membranes. Satellite lesions (those situated near the mole) are noted.

Diagnosis

Nursing Diagnoses

Based on the nursing assessment data, the patient's major nursing diagnoses may include:

- Pain related to surgical excision and grafting
- Anxiety and depression related to possible life-threatening consequences of melanoma and disfigurement
- Knowledge deficit about early signs of melanoma

Collaborative Problems/Potential Complications

Based on the assessment data, potential complications that may develop include:

- Metastasis
- Infection of the surgical site

Planning and Goals

The major goals for the patient may include relief of pain and discomfort, reduced anxiety, knowledge of early signs of melanoma, and absence of complications.

Nursing Interventions

Relieving Pain and Discomfort

Surgical removal of melanoma in different locations (head and neck, eye, trunk, abdomen, extremities, central nervous system) presents different challenges, taking into consideration the removal of the primary melanoma, the intervening lymphatic vessels, and the lymph nodes to which metastases may spread. Nursing management of the patient having surgery in these regions is discussed in the appropriate chapters.

Nursing intervention after surgery for a malignant melanoma centers on promoting comfort, because wide excision surgery may be necessary. A split-thickness or full-thickness skin graft may be necessary when large defects are created by surgical removal of a melanoma. Anticipating the need for and administering appropriate analgesic medications are important.

Reducing Anxiety

Psychological support is essential when disfiguring surgery is performed. Support includes allowing patients to express feelings about the seriousness of this cutaneous neoplasm, understanding their anger and depression, and conveying understanding of these feelings. During the diagnostic workup and staging of the depth, type, and extent of the tumor, the nurse answers questions, clarifies information, and helps clarify misconceptions. Learning that they have a melanoma can cause patients considerable fear and anguish. Pointing out patients' resources, past effective coping mechanisms, and social support systems helps them to cope with the problems associated with diagnosis, treatment, and continuing follow-up. The immediate family should be included in all discussions to clarify the information presented, ask questions that the patient might be reluctant to ask, and provide emotional support.

Monitoring and Managing Potential Complications

METASTASIS

The prognosis of malignant melanoma is related to metastasis: the deeper and thicker (more than 4 mm) the melanoma, the greater the likelihood of metastasis. If the melanoma is growing radially (horizontally) and is characterized by peripheral growth with minimal or no dermal invasion, the prognosis is favorable. When the melanoma progresses to the vertical growth phase (dermal invasion), the prognosis is poor. Lesions with ulceration have a poor prognosis. Melanomas of the trunk appear to have a poorer prognosis than those of other sites, perhaps because the network of lymphatics in the trunk permits metastasis to regional lymph nodes.

The role of the nurse in caring for the patient with metastatic disease is holistic. The nurse must be knowledgeable about the most effective current therapies and must deliver supportive care, provide and clarify information about the therapy and the rationale for its use, identify potential side effects of therapy and ways to manage them, and instruct the patient and family about the expected outcomes of treatment. The nurse monitors and documents symptoms that may indicate metastasis: lung (difficulty breathing, shortness of breath, increasing cough), bone (pain, decrease in mobility and function, pathologic fractures), and liver (change in liver enzyme levels, pain, jaundice). Nursing care is planned according to the patient's symptoms.

Although the chance of a cure for malignant melanoma that has metastasized is dismal, the nurse encourages the patient to have hope in the therapy employed while maintaining a realistic perspective about the disease and ultimate outcome. Moreover, the nurse provides time for the patient to express fears and concerns regarding future activities and relationships, offers information about support groups and contact people, and arranges palliative and hospice care (see Chap. 15).

Promoting Home and Community-Based Care

TEACHING PATIENTS SELF-CARE

The best hope of controlling the disease lies in educating patients regarding the early signs of melanoma. Patients at risk are taught to examine their skin and scalp monthly in a systematic manner. The nurse also points out that a key factor in the development of malignant melanoma is exposure to sunlight.

Evaluation

Expected Outcomes

Expected outcomes may include:

1. Experiences relief of pain and discomfort
   a. States pain has lessened and is diminishing
   b. Exhibits healing of surgical scar without heat, redness, or swelling
2. Is less anxious
   a. Expresses fears and fantasies
   b. Asks questions about medical condition
   c. Requests repetition of facts about melanoma
   d. Identifies support and comfort provided by family member or significant other
3. Demonstrates understanding of the means for detecting melanoma
   a. Demonstrates how to conduct self-examination of skin on a monthly basis
   b. Verbalizes the following danger signals of melanoma: change in size, color, shape, or outline of mole, mole surface, or skin around mole
   c. Identifies measures to protect self from exposure to sunlight
4. Experiences absence of metastasis
   a. Recognizes abnormal signs and symptoms that should be reported to physician
   b. Complies with recommended follow-up procedures and prevention strategies

Metastatic Skin Tumors

The skin is an important, although not a common, site of metastatic cancer. All types of cancer may metastasize to the skin, but carcinoma of the breast is the primary source of cutaneous metastases in women. Other sources include cancer of the large intestine, ovaries, and lungs. In men, the most common primary sites are the lungs, large intestine, oral cavity, kidneys, or stomach. Skin metastases from melanomas are found in both genders. The clinical appearance of metastatic skin lesions is not distinctive, except perhaps in some cases of breast cancer in which diffuse, brawny hardening of the skin of the involved breast is seen (cancer *en cuirasses*). In most instances, metastatic lesions occur as multiple cutaneous or subcutaneous nodules of varying size that may be skin-colored or different shades of red.

OTHER MALIGNANCIES OF THE SKIN

Kaposi's Sarcoma

First described by Moritz Kaposi in 1872, Kaposi's sarcoma (KS) has received renewed attention since its association with AIDS. Its occurrence with AIDS involves a more varied and aggressive form of KS than was seen previously. Before the AIDS epidemic, KS was considered a rare malignancy. It was subdivided into three categories: classic KS, African (endemic) KS, and KS associated with immunosuppressant therapy. Classic KS occurs predominantly in men of Mediterranean or Jewish ancestry between ages 40 and 70. Most patients have nodules or plaques on the lower extremities that rarely metastasize beyond the lower extremities. This KS is chronic, relatively benign, and rarely fatal.

African KS affects people predominantly in the eastern half of Africa near the equator. Men are affected more often than women, and children can be affected as well. The disease may resemble classic KS or it may infiltrate and progress to lymphadenopathic forms.

KS associated with immunosuppressive therapy, as in transplant patients, is characterized by local skin lesions and disseminated visceral and mucocutaneous diseases. The greater the degree of immunosuppression, the higher the incidence of KS.

AIDS-related KS was identified in the early 1980s as distinctly different from previously described types of KS. Typically, it is an aggressive tumor that involves multiple body organs. Its presentation resembles that of KS associated with immunosuppressive therapy. Most patients are between ages 20 and 40. Chapter 48 discusses AIDS-related KS.

DERMATOLOGIC AND PLASTIC RECONSTRUCTIVE SURGERY

The word "plastic" comes from a Greek word meaning "to form." Plastic or reconstructive surgery is performed to reconstruct or alter congenital or acquired defects to restore or improve the body's form and function. (Often the terms plastic and reconstructive are used interchangeably.) This type of surgery includes closure of wounds, removal of skin tumors, repair of soft tissue injuries or burns, correction of deformities, and repair of cosmetic defects. Plastic surgery can be used to repair many parts of the body and numerous structures, such as bone, cartilage, fat, fascia, mucous membrane, muscle, nerve, and cutaneous structures. Bone inlays and transplants for deformities and nonunion can be performed, muscle can be transferred, nerves can be reconstructed and spliced, and cartilage can be replaced. As important as any of these measures is the reconstruction of the cutaneous tissues around the neck and the face; this is usually referred to as aesthetic or cosmetic surgery.

Wound Coverage: Grafts and Flaps

Skin Grafts

Skin grafting is a technique in which a section of skin is detached from its own blood supply and transferred as free tissue to a distant (recipient) site. Skin grafting can be used to repair almost any type of wound and is the most common form of reconstructive surgery.

Skin grafts are commonly used to repair defects that result from excision of skin tumors, to cover areas denuded of skin, and to cover wounds in which insufficient skin is available to permit wound closure. They are also used when primary closure of the wound increases the risk of complications or when primary wound closure would interfere with function.

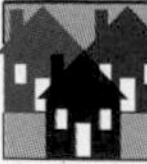

PATIENT EDUCATION AND HOME CARE

How to Examine Your Skin

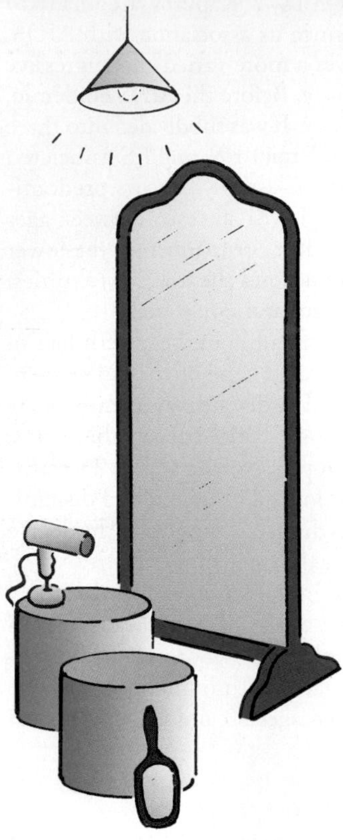

Step 1

Make sure the room is well lighted, and that you have nearby a full-length mirror, a hand-held mirror, a hand-held blow dryer, and two chairs or stools. Undress completely.

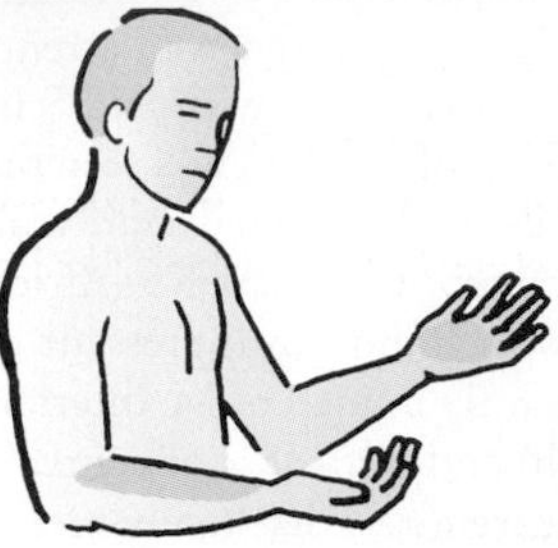

Step 2

Hold your hands with the palms face up, as shown in the drawing. Look at your palms, fingers, spaces between the fingers, and forearms. Then turn your hands over and examine the backs of your hands, fingers, spaces between the fingers, fingernails and forearms.

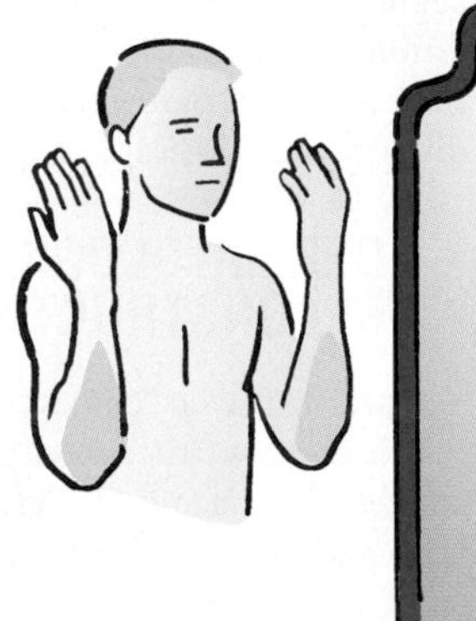

Step 3

Now position yourself in front of the full-length mirror. Hold up your arms, bent at the elbows, with your palms facing you in the mirror, look at the backs of your forearms and elbows.

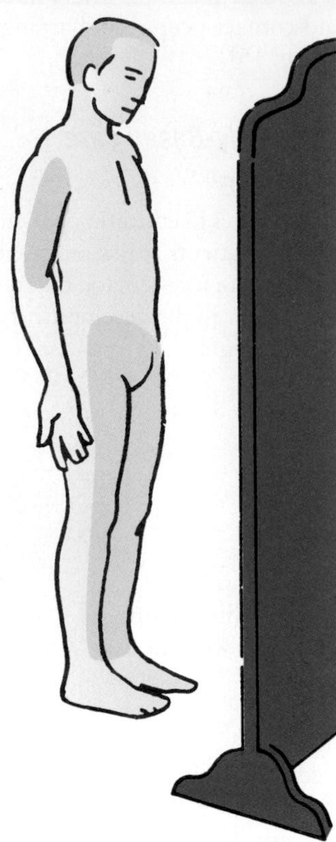

Step 4

Again using the full-length mirror, observe the entire front of your body. In turn, look at your face, neck, and arms. Turn your palms to face the mirror and look at your upper arms. Then look at your chest and abdomen; pubic area; thighs and lower legs.

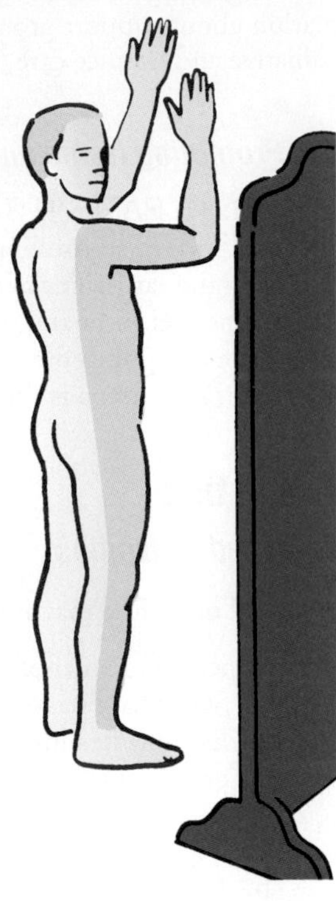

Step 5

Still standing in front of the mirror, lift your arms over your head with the palms facing each other. Turn so that your right side is facing the mirror and look at the entire side of your body, your hands and arms, underarms, sides of your trunk, thighs and lower legs. Then turn, and repeat the process with your left side.

Skin grafts may be classified as autografts, allografts, or xenografts. An autograft is tissue obtained from the patient's own skin. An allograft is tissue obtained from a donor of the same species. These grafts are also called allogeneic or homograft. A xenograft or heterograft is tissue from another species.

Grafts are also referred to by their thickness. A skin graft may be split-thickness (thin, intermediate, or thick) or full-thickness, depending on the amount of dermis included in the specimen. A split-thickness graft can be cut at varying thicknesses and is commonly used to cover large wounds or defects for which a full-thickness graft or flap is impractical (Fig. 52-8). A full-thickness graft consists of epidermis and the entire dermis without the underlying fat. It is used to cover wounds that are too large to be closed directly.

APPLICATION

A graft is obtained by a variety of instruments: razor blades, skin-grafting knives, electric- or air-powered dermatomes, or drum dermatomes. The skin graft is taken from the donor or host site and applied to the desired site, called the recipient site or graft bed.

For a graft to survive and be effective, certain conditions must be met:

1. The recipient site must have an adequate blood supply so that normal physiologic function can resume.

PATIENT EDUCATION AND HOME CARE
How to Examine Your Skin

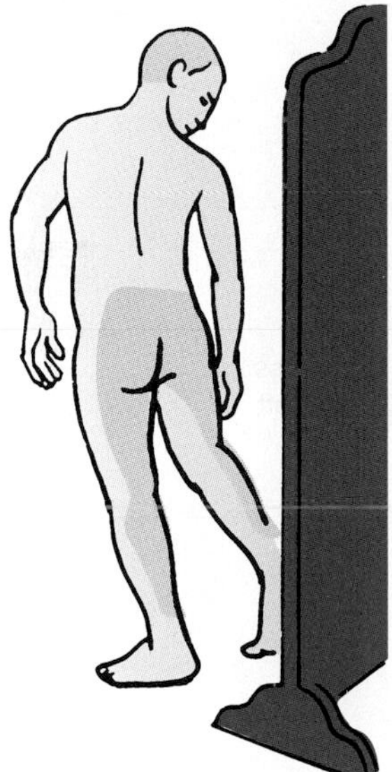

Step 6

With your back toward the full-length mirror, look at your buttocks and the backs of your thighs and lower legs.

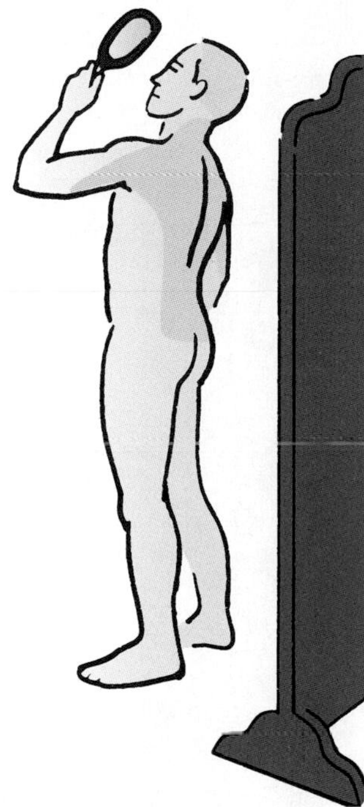

Step 7

Now pick up the hand-held mirror. With your back still to the full-length mirror, examine the back of your neck, and your back and buttocks. Also examine the backs of your arms in this way. Some areas are hard to see, and you may find it helpful to ask your spouse or a friend to assist you.

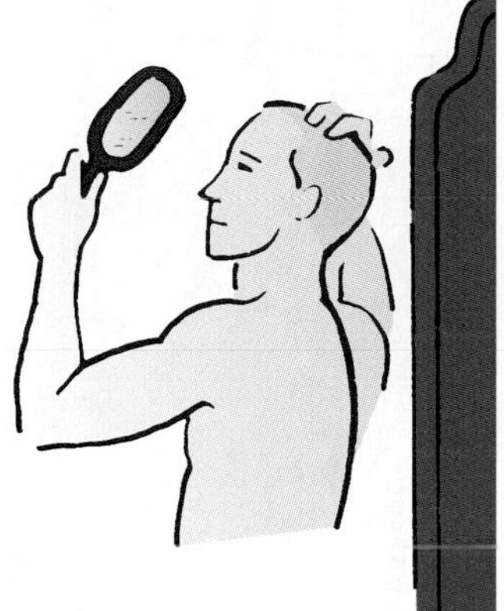

Step 8

Use the hand-held mirror and the full-length mirror to look at your scalp. Because the scalp is difficult to examine, we suggest you also use a hand-held blow dryer turned to a cool setting, to lift the hair from the scalp. While some people find it easy to hold the mirror in one hand and the dryer in the other, while looking in the full-length mirror, many do not. For the scalp examination in particular, then, you might ask your spouse or a friend to assist you.

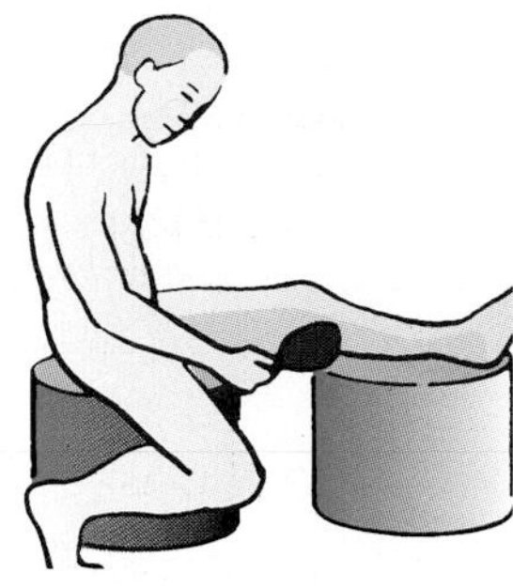

Step 9

Sit down and prop up one leg on a chair or stool in front of you as shown. Using the hand-held mirror, examine the inside of the propped-up leg, beginning at the groin area and moving the mirror down the leg to your foot. Repeat the procedure for your other leg.

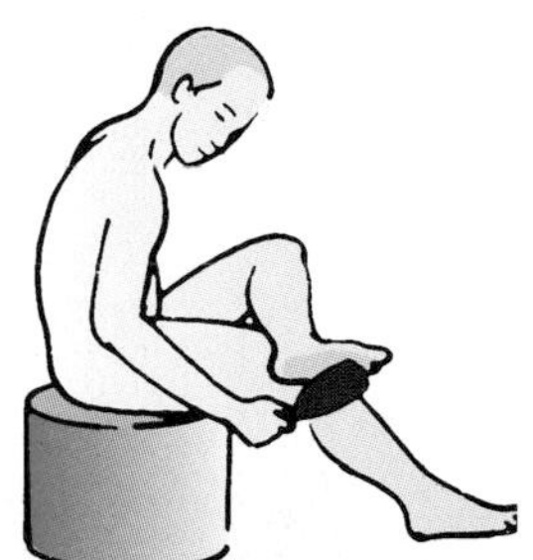

Step 10

Still sitting, cross one leg over the other. Use the hand-held mirror to examine the top of your foot, the toes, toenails, and spaces between the toes. Then look at the sole or bottom of your foot. Repeat the procedure for the other foot.

2. The graft must be in close contact with its bed (to avoid accumulation of blood or fluid);.
3. The graft must be fixed firmly (immobilized) so that it remains in place on the recipient site.
4. The area must be free of infection.

The graft, when applied to the recipient site, may or may not be sutured in place. It may be slit and spread apart to cover a greater area. The process of revascularization (establishing the blood supply) and reattachment of a skin graft to a recipient bed is referred to as a "take."

After a skin graft is put in place, it may be left exposed (in areas that are impossible to immobilize) or covered with a light dressing or a pressure dressing, depending on the area.

NURSING INTERVENTIONS

The nurse instructs the patient to keep the affected part immobilized as much as possible. For a facial graft, strenuous activity must be avoided. A graft on the hand or arm may be immobilized with a splint. When a graft is placed on a lower extremity, the part is kept elevated because the new capillary connections are fragile and excess venous pressure may cause rupture. When ambulation is permitted, the patient wears an elastic stocking to counterbalance venous pressure.

The nurse instructs the patient, family member, or other caregiver to inspect the dressing daily. Unusual drainage or an inflammatory reaction around the wound margin suggests infection and should be reported to the physician. Any fluid, purulent drainage, blood, or serum that has collected is gently evacuated by the sur-

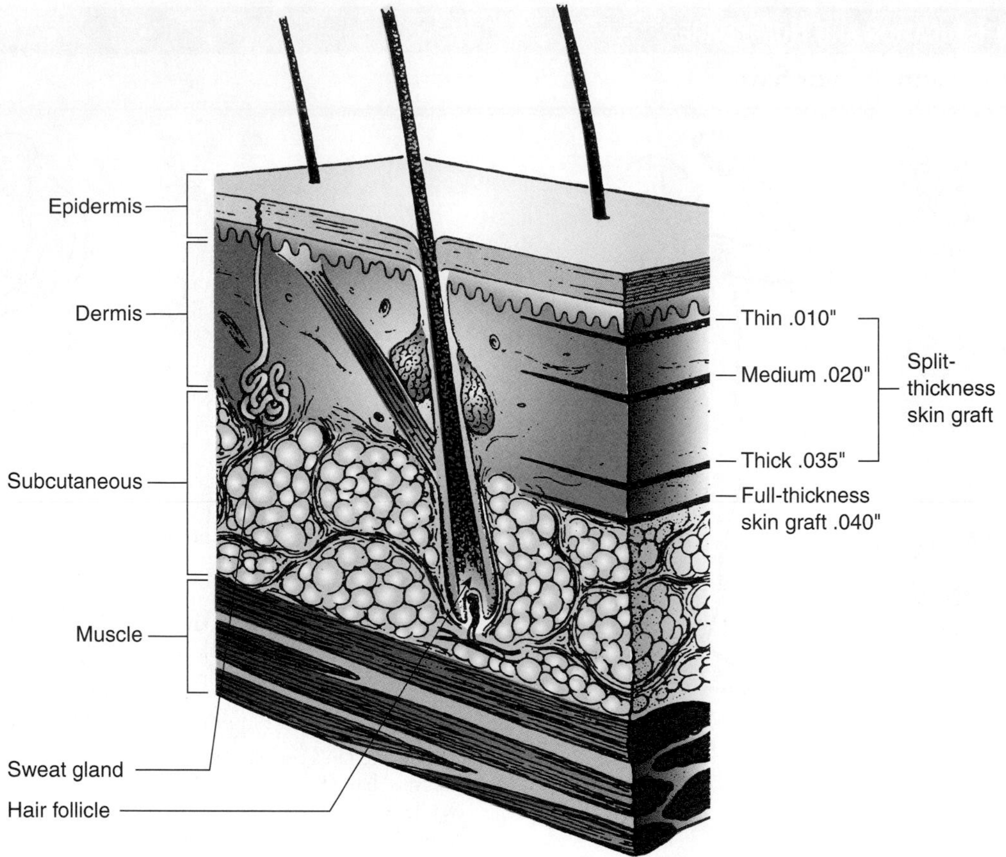

FIGURE 52•8 Layers of skin appropriate for split-thickness and full-thickness graft.

geon, because accumulation of this material would cause the graft to separate from its bed.

When the graft appears pink, it is vascularized. After 2 to 3 weeks, mineral oil or a lanolin cream is massaged into the wound to moisten the graft. Because there may be loss of feeling or sensation in the grafted area for a prolonged period, the application of heating pads and exposure to sun are avoided to prevent burns and further skin trauma.

DONOR SITE

Selection Criteria. The donor site is selected with several criteria in mind:

1. Achieving the closest possible color match in keeping with the amount of skin graft required
2. Matching the texture and hair-bearing qualities
3. Obtaining the thickest possible skin graft without jeopardizing the healing of the donor site (Fig. 52-9)
4. Considering the cosmetic effects of the donor site after healing, so that it is in an inconspicuous location

Donor Site Care. Detailed attention to the donor site is just as important as the care of the recipient area. The donor site heals by reepithelization of the raw, exposed dermis. Usually a single layer of nonadherent, fine-mesh gauze is placed directly over the donor site. Absorbent gauze dressings are then placed on top to absorb blood or serum from the wound. A membrane dressing (such as Op-Site) may be used and provides certain advantages: it is transparent and allows the wound to be observed without dis-

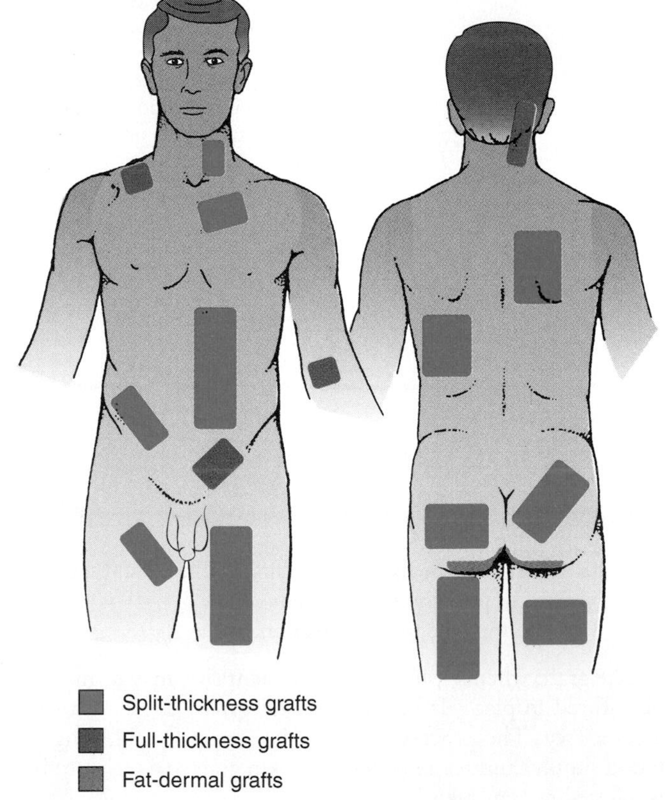

FIGURE 52•9 Common donor skin graft sites. Blue skin areas are appropriate for full-thickness grafts; green areas are used for split-thickness grafts and rose sites are used for fat-dermal grafts.

turbing the dressing, and it permits the patient to shower without fear of saturating the dressing with water.

After healing, the patient is instructed to keep the donor site soft and pliable with cream (lanolin, olive oil). Extremes in temperature, external trauma, and sunlight are to be avoided both for donor sites and grafted areas because these areas are sensitive, especially to thermal injuries.

Flaps

Another form of wound coverage may be provided by flaps. A flap is a segment of tissue that remains attached at one end (called a base or pedicle) while the other end is moved to a recipient area. Its survival depends on functioning arterial and venous blood supplies and lymphatic drainage in its pedicle or base. A flap differs from a graft in that a portion of the tissue is attached to its original site and retains its blood supply. (An exception is the free flap, described below.)

Flaps may consist of skin, mucosa, muscle, adipose tissue, omentum, and bone. They are used for wound coverage and provide bulk, especially when bone, tendon, blood vessels, or nerve tissue is exposed. Flaps are used to repair defects caused by congenital deformity, trauma, or tumor ablation (removal, usually by excision) in an adjacent part of the body.

Flaps offer an aesthetic solution because a flap retains the color and texture of the donor area, is more likely to survive than a graft, and can be used to cover nerves, tendons, and blood vessels. However, several surgical procedures are usually required to advance a flap. The major complication is necrosis of the pedicle or base as a result of failure of the blood supply.

FREE FLAPS

A striking advance in reconstructive surgery is the use of free flaps or free-tissue transfer, achieved by microvascular techniques. A free flap is completely severed from the body and transferred to another site, and it receives early vascular supply from microvascular anastomosis (attachment) with vessels at the recipient site. Thus, the procedure is generally completed in one step, eliminating the need for a series of surgical procedures to move the flap. Microvascular surgery allows surgeons to use a variety of donor sites for tissue reconstruction.

Chemical Face Peeling

Chemical face peeling, a technique that involves applying a chemical mixture to the face for superficial destruction of the epidermis and the upper layers of the dermis, treats fine wrinkles, keratoses, and pigment problems. It is especially useful for wrinkles at the upper and lower lip, forehead, and periorbital areas.

Pretreatment may consist of cleansing the face and hair for several days before the procedure with a hexachlorophene detergent. Pretreatment medication (analgesic and tranquilizer) may be prescribed to alleviate apprehension and control pain. This permits the patient to be sedated yet conscious during the procedure, although some patients request general anesthesia.

The type of chemical used depends on the planned depth of the peel. A phenol-based chemical in an oil–water emulsion is commonly used because it produces a controlled, predictable chemical burn. The chemical is applied systematically to the face with cotton-tipped applicators. The conscious patient feels a burning sensation at this time. A mask of waterproof adhesive may then be applied directly to the skin and molded closely to the contours of the face, thereby acting as an occlusive dressing that increases the chemical penetration and action. (Some surgeons think that equally good results can be obtained with occlusive tape.) After the tape mask is applied, the burning sensation continues and the tape mask remains in place for 12 to 24 hours. Frequent small doses of analgesics and tranquilizers are prescribed to keep the patient comfortable.

Complications

Complications may arise when control of the chemically induced burn cannot be sustained. Complications include pigment changes, infection, milia (small inclusion cysts that disappear after several months), scarring, atrophy, sensitivity changes, and long-term erythema (4 to 5 months) or pruritus.

Nursing Management

Because chemical face peeling is performed in the physician's office or in an outpatient surgical department, most care takes place in the home. After 6 to 8 hours, the face becomes edematous and the eyelids often swell shut. The patient should be reassured that this reaction is expected and normal. The patient is cautioned to move the mouth as little as possible so that the tape continues to adhere to the skin. The head of the bed is elevated, and liquids are administered through a straw. Most of the burning sensation and discomfort subside after the first 12 to 24 hours.

By the second day, the patient may feel moisture under the dressings as serous exudate seeps from the chemically exfoliated skin. Dressings are usually removed 24 to 48 hours after treatment, exposing skin resembling a second-degree burn. The patient may be alarmed by the appearance of the skin and should be reassured. After the tape mask is removed, some surgeons dust the treated skin surface with thymol–iodine powder for its drying and bacteriostatic effects. Application of triple-antibiotic ointment may be substituted in some cases. The skin surface is left uncovered to dry. The patient may be permitted to wash the face with lukewarm water or advised to shower several times daily to help remove any remaining facial crusting. An ointment is prescribed to cover the face and soften and loosen the crust between washings.

The nurse reinforces the physician's explanation that the redness of the skin will gradually subside over the next 4 to 12 weeks. Although a line between treated and untreated skin may be noted, makeup is usually permitted after the first few weeks. The patient is cautioned to avoid direct or reflected sunlight, because the treatment reduces the natural protection of the skin from sun. The skin will probably never tan evenly again. Blotchy pigmentation can occur with exposure to the sun.

Dermabrasion

Dermabrasion is a form of skin abrasion used to correct acne scarring, aging, and sun-damaged skin. A special instrument (motor-driven wire brush, diamond-impregnated disk, serrated wheel) is used in the procedure. The epidermis and some superficial dermis are removed, while enough of the dermis is preserved to allow reepithelization of the treated areas. Results are best in the face because it is rich in intradermal epithelial elements.

Preparation and Procedure

The primary reason for undergoing dermabrasion is to improve appearance. The surgeon explains to the patient what can be expected from dermabrasion. The patient should also be informed about the nature of the postoperative dressing, what discomfort may be experienced, and how long it will be before the tissues look normal.

Dermabrasion may be performed in the physician's office, the operating room, or an outpatient setting. It is performed under local or general anesthesia. During the procedure, some surgeons use refrigerant anesthetics to turn the skin into a numb, solid mass of rigid tissue and to provide a momentarily bloodless surgical field. During and after planing, the area is irrigated with copious amounts of saline solution to remove debris and allow the surgeon to see the area. A dressing impregnated with ointment is usually applied to the abraded surface.

Nursing Management

The nurse instructs the patient about the after-effects of surgery. Edema occurs during the first 48 hours and may cause the eyelids to close. The head of the bed is elevated to hasten fluid drainage. Erythema occurs and can last for weeks or months. After 24 hours, the dressing may be removed if the physician approves. When the serum oozing from the skin begins to gel, the patient applies the prescribed ointment to the face several times a day to prevent hard crusting and to keep the abraded areas soft and flexible. Clear water cleansing or soaking of the face is started with physician approval to remove crusts from the healing skin.

The patient is advised to avoid extreme cold and heat and excessive straining or lifting, which may bruise delicate new capillaries. Direct or reflected sunlight should be avoided for 3 to 6 months and a sunscreen used.

Facial Reconstructive Surgery

Reconstructive procedures on the face are individualized to the patient's needs and desired outcomes. They are performed to repair deformities or restore normal function as much as possible. They may vary from closure of small defects to complicated procedures involving implantation of prosthetic devices to conceal a large defect or reconstruct a lost part of the face (eg, nose, ear, jaw). Each surgical procedure is custom-tailored and involves a variety of incisions, flaps, and grafts.

In correcting a primary defect, the surgeon may have to create a secondary defect. Although the procedure may restore some function, such as eating or talking, the cosmetic or aesthetic results may be limited. The original appearance of a patient who has severe damage to soft tissue and bone structure can seldom be restored. Multiple surgical procedures may be required. The process of facial reconstruction is usually slow and tedious.

NURSING PROCESS: THE PATIENT WITH FACIAL RECONSTRUCTION

Assessment

The face is a part of the body that every person desires to keep at its best or improve, because most human interactions involve the face. When the face loses its appearance and function (eg, by injury or disease), significant emotional reactions often occur. Changes in appearance frequently cause anxiety and depression. Patients with facial changes frequently mourn for the lost part, suffer a loss of self-esteem due to reactions or rejection by others, and withdraw and isolate themselves. Health care personnel can acknowledge that anxiety and depression are appropriate for what the patient is experiencing.

The nurse assesses the patient's emotional responses and identifies strengths as well as usual coping mechanisms to determine how the patient will handle the surgical procedure. Any area in which the patient and family need extra support is identified.

The preoperative assessment determines the extent of disfigurement and improvement that can be anticipated, as well as the patient's understanding and acceptance of these limitations. The nurse is in a better position to reinforce facts and clarify misconceptions once the surgeon has fully informed the patient about the procedure, the functional defects that may result, the possible need for a tracheostomy and/or other prosthesis, and the probability of additional surgery. The nurse instructs the patient about various postoperative measures: intravenous therapy, the use of a nasogastric tube to allow gastric decompression and prevent vomiting, and the frequent and lengthy periods that may be required to care for wounds, flaps, and skin grafts and to change dressings. Extra time is needed when presenting this information to anxious patients because they may not hear, concentrate, or comprehend what is being said.

Diagnosis

Nursing Diagnoses

Based on the nursing assessment data, the patient's major postoperative nursing diagnoses may include:

- Ineffective airway clearance related to tracheobronchial secretions
- Pain related to facial edema and effects of the procedure
- Altered nutrition: Less than body requirements related to altered physiology of oral cavity, drooling, impaired chewing and swallowing, or excision affecting the tongue
- Impaired verbal communication related to trauma/surgery producing anatomic and physiologic abnormalities of speech
- Body image disturbance related to disfigurement
- Altered family processes related to grief reaction and disruption of family life

Collaborative Problems/Potential Complications

Based on the assessment data, potential complications that may develop include:

- Infection

Planning and Goals

The major goals for the patient may include a patent airway and pulmonary function, increased comfort, adequate nutritional status, an effective communication method, positive self-concept, effective family coping, and absence of infection.

Nursing Interventions

Maintaining Airway and Pulmonary Function

The immediate concern after facial reconstruction is maintenance of an adequate airway. If the patient has regained consciousness, mental confusion with combative, anxious behavior is a sign of hypoxia (reduced oxygen supply to tissues). Sedatives or opioids are not prescribed in this situation because they may impair oxygenation. If the patient shows signs of restlessness, the airway is carefully inspected to detect laryngeal edema or accumulation of tracheobronchial mucus. Secretions are suctioned as necessary until the patient can manage the secretions without help. If the patient has a tracheostomy, suctioning is performed with sterile technique to prevent infection and cross-contamination. (See Chap. 22 for care of the patient with a tracheostomy.)

Achieving Comfort and Relieving Pain

Facial edema is an uncomfortable but natural consequence of facial reconstructive surgery. The patient's head and upper torso are kept slightly elevated (if the blood pressure is stable) to help reduce facial edema. Suction catheters attached to closed drainage may be in place to keep the tissue in close apposition and to remove serous discharge. If extensive reconstruction has been performed, the patient's head should be properly aligned and supported so that minimal stress is placed on the suture line.

Mild doses of analgesics are prescribed to control pain. If bone grafts have been used for reconstruction, there is usually considerable pain in the donor area. If the patient has head and neck cancer and increasing levels of pain, more sophisticated nursing management is required (see Chap. 12).

Maintaining Adequate Nutrition

After oral edema and pharyngeal edema diminish, the incisional areas and flaps heal, and the patient can swallow saliva, fluids may be offered. Gradually, soft foods are added as tolerated. If the patient cannot meet nutritional needs by the oral route, total parenteral nutrition (infusion of nutrients, water, and vitamins into the stomach or proximal small intestine through a tube) is initiated. The formula strength and feeding rate are gradually increased until the desired daily caloric level is attained. (See Chap. 33 for nursing management of the patient requiring enteral feedings.) Patients who have had radical surgery for large, encroaching neoplasms may have difficulty resuming eating. Positive nutrition is reflected in weight gain, and nutritional status is monitored by measuring body weight daily and assessing serum protein and electrolyte levels periodically.

Enhancing Communication

Communication problems may range from a minimal problem to the loss of oral speech. Some tumors and injuries require extensive surgery involving the larynx, tongue, and mandible. Paper, pen or pencil, and a firm writing surface should be provided. If the patient cannot write, a pictograph board may be used. Referral to a speech therapist may be necessary for the patient who has undergone structural changes. The family may become frustrated by the patient's inability to communicate. The patient soon senses this, and both parties may withdraw. Allowing the family to vent their feelings and fears (away from the patient) is important.

Improving Self-Concept

Success in rehabilitating the patient undergoing reconstructive surgery depends on the relationships among the patient and the nurse, the physician, and other health care personnel. Mutual trust, respect, and clear lines of communication are essential. Unhurried care provides emotional reassurance and support.

The kinds of dressings worn, the unusual positions to be maintained, and the temporary incapacities experienced can upset the most stable person. Honest reinforcement of the patient's coping improves self-esteem. If prosthetic devices are used, the patient is taught how to use and care for them to gain a sense of greater independence. Once involved in self-care activities, the patient may feel some control over what was previously an overwhelming situation.

Patients with severe disfigurement are encouraged to socialize in the hospital to experience the reactions of others in a more protected environment. Gradually they can widen their sphere of contact. Every effort is made to cover or mask defects. Patients may require support by members of the mental health team to accept their changed appearance.

Promoting Family Coping

The family is informed about the patient's appearance after surgery, the supportive equipment, and the ways that the equipment aids recovery. It is helpful to join the family for a few minutes during their first postoperative visit to help them cope with the changes they will see.

A major role of the nurse is to support the family in their decision to participate (or not to participate) in the patient's treatment. Nursing interventions also include helping the family members communicate by suggesting ways to reduce anxiety and stress and to promote problem solving and decision making. These activities encourage family members and promote growth.

Monitoring and Managing Potential Complications

INFECTION

Secondary infection is a primary concern after reconstructive surgery. The source of infection depends on the location and extent of the procedure, the suture line, and the pedicle flap.

The mouth is inspected to note the location of sutures so that they are not accidentally disturbed during the cleaning process. The mouth is cleaned according to protocol several times daily. Loose blood clots may be removed with gentle swabbing. The patient is advised not to loosen clots with the tongue because this may cause fresh bleeding. The patient is instructed not to use fingers to clean or remove blood clots because this may introduce organisms that cause infection.

The suture line will be under stress for several days after surgery because of edema, increased drainage, and hematoma formation. The nurse assesses the suture line carefully for signs of increased tension and infection (elevated temperature, increasing edema, redness, bleeding, and increased pain) with each dressing change. Dressings may need to be changed many times a day until the drainage begins to decrease. Drainage and edema are expected after reconstructive surgery; however, both should decrease, and the process is hastened by using properly placed, functioning suction devices and elevating the head of the bed about 45 degrees. The nurse inspects the suction devices, empties them promptly, and documents the amount and consistency of drainage, as well as any unusual odor. When drainage is not removed or if saturated dressings are left unchanged for long periods, infection is likely to occur. Strict asepsis must be maintained in wound care.

A pedicle flap used in reconstruction may become a source of infection if its circulation becomes compromised. Poor circulation may result from a hematoma forming beneath the flap and causing increased pressure on the underlying vasculature. The nurse inspects the flap for changes in color and temperature indicative of poor circulation. Signs of necrosis, increased drainage, or an odor may be a warning of an infection and should be reported promptly. Reinforcing preoperative teaching about wound healing, the need for strict sterile technique, good personal hygiene, and the need to restrict movement and stress on the operative site is an important part of the nurse's role in postoperative care and in the prevention of secondary infection.

Evaluation

Expected Outcomes

Expected outcomes may include:

1. Maintains patent airway
   a. Demonstrates respiratory rate within normal limits
   b. Exhibits normal breath sounds
   c. Demonstrates no signs of choking or aspiration
2. Achieves increasing comfort
   a. Reports decreasing pain
   b. Follows instructions on proper positioning
   c. Avoids movements that add stress to the operative site
3. Attains adequate nutrition
   a. Consumes adequate amounts of food and fluids
   b. Maintains weight within normal range or progressively regains weight lost in the early postoperative period
   c. Maintains serum protein and electrolyte levels within normal range
4. Communicates effectively
   a. Uses appropriate aids to enhance communication
   b. Interacts with health care team members, family, and other support people using new communication strategies
5. Develops positive self-image
   a. Expresses positive feelings about surgical changes
   b. Demonstrates increasing independence in self-care activities
   c. Uses prosthetic devices independently (when appropriate)
   d. Verbalizes plans for resuming usual activities (eg, work, recreation)
6. Family members cope with situation
   a. Demonstrate decreasing anxiety and conflict
   b. Verbalize what to expect
7. Experiences no postoperative infection
   a. Demonstrates vital signs within normal limits
   b. Undergoes normal wound healing without signs of infection or sepsis
   c. Lists signs of infection that should be reported
   d. Understands the need for asepsis (sterile procedures) and good personal hygiene

Face Lift

Rhytidectomy (face lift) is a surgical procedure that removes soft tissue folds and minimizes cutaneous wrinkles on the face. It is performed to create a more youthful appearance.

Psychological preparation requires that the patient recognize the limitations of surgery and the fact that miraculous rejuvenation will not occur. The patient is informed that the face may appear bruised and swollen after the dressings are removed and that several weeks may pass before the edema subsides.

The procedure is performed under local or general anesthesia, often in the outpatient setting. The incisions are concealed in natural skin folds and creases and areas hidden by hair. The loose skin, separated from underlying muscle, is pulled upward and backward. Excess skin that overlaps the incision line is removed. Liposuction-assisted rhytidectomy is being performed more frequently. In this procedure, fat is suctioned from the body via a cannula through a small incision.

Nursing Management

The nurse encourages the patient to rest quietly for the first 2 postoperative days until the dressings are removed. The head of the bed is elevated and neck flexion is discouraged to avoid compromising the circulation and the suture line. The patient may feel some tightness of the face and neck due to pressure created by the newly tightened muscles, fascia, and skin. Analgesics may be prescribed to relieve discomfort. A liquid diet may be given by means of straws, and a soft diet is permitted if chewing is not too uncomfortable.

When the dressings are removed, the skin is gently cleaned of crusting and oozing and coated with the prescribed topical ointment. Any hair matted with drainage may be combed with warm water and a wide-toothed comb.

The patient is advised not to lift or bend for 7 to 10 days because this activity may increase edema and provoke bleeding. Activities are gradually resumed. When all sutures are removed, the hair may be shampooed and blown-dry with warm, not hot, air to avoid burning the ears, which may be numb for a while.

The patient needs to know that a face lift will not stop the aging process and that with time, the tissues will resume the downward drift. Some patients have two or more face lifts.

Sudden pain indicates that blood is accumulating underneath the skin flaps; it should be reported to the surgeon immediately. Complications include sloughing of the skin, deformities of the face and neck, and partial facial paralysis. Cigarette smoking has been implicated as a cause of skin slough in some patients.

Laser Treatment of Cutaneous Lesions

Lasers are devices that amplify or generate highly specialized light energy. They can mobilize immense heat and power when focused at close range and are valuable tools in surgical procedures. Several types of lasers (argon laser, carbon dioxide laser, and tunable pulse-dye laser) are used in dermatologic surgery. Each type of laser emits its own wavelength within the color spectrum.

Argon Laser

The argon laser produces a blue-green visible light that is absorbed by vascular tissue and hence is useful in treating vascular lesions: port-wine stains, telangiectases, vascular tumors, and pigmented lesions. The argon beam can penetrate approximately 1 mm of skin and reach the pigmented layer, causing protein coagulation in this area. An immediate effect is that tiny blood vessels under the skin coagulate, causing the area to turn a much lighter color. A crust forms within a few days.

During the procedure, the patient may require local anesthesia (lidocaine) only if the lesion, such as a port-wine stain, is wider than 0.5 cm. Laser beams, regardless of type, are reflected and scattered in all directions during the treatment. Laser radiation is known to be hazardous to the eye. Therefore, the eyes of the patient and all personnel involved in the surgical procedure and those who are within the immediate surgical environment must be protected with orange, argon light-absorbing safety goggles.

NURSING MANAGEMENT

Cold compresses are usually applied over the treatment area for approximately 6 hours to minimize edema, exudate, and loss of capillary permeability. The nurse advises the patient that swelling will subside in 1 to 2 days and will be followed by a crust that will last 7 to 10 days. The nurse instructs the patient to avoid picking at the crust, to apply an antibacterial ointment sparingly until the crust separates, to avoid applying makeup until the wound heals, and to stay out of the sun. Sunscreen is to be used when exposure is unavoidable.

Carbon Dioxide Laser

The carbon dioxide (CO_2) laser emits invisible light in the infrared spectrum that is absorbed at the skin surface because of the high water content of the skin and the long wavelength of the CO_2 light.

As the laser beam strikes tissue, it is absorbed by the intracellular and extracellular water, which vaporizes, destroying the tissue. The CO_2 laser is a precise surgical instrument that vaporizes and excises tissue with minimal damage. Because the beam can seal blood and lymphatic vessels, it creates a dry surgical field that makes many procedures easier and quicker. It is therefore safe to use on patients with bleeding disorders or those receiving anticoagulant therapy. It is useful for removing epidermal nevi, tattoos, certain warts, skin cancer, ingrown toenails, and keloids. Incisions made with the laser beam heal and scar much like those made by a scalpel.

In addition to wearing safety goggles, the patient and personnel wear laser-grade surgical masks to avoid inhaling the byproduct smoke, referred to as a plume.

NURSING MANAGEMENT

Immediately after undergoing CO_2 laser surgery, the treated area turns a charcoal color. The wound is covered with antibacterial ointment and a nonadhesive dressing. The patient is instructed to keep the wound dry except for gentle cleansings with mild soap several times a day. After the skin is cleaned, a prescribed ointment and light dressing are applied.

Because nerve endings and lymphatic vessels are sealed by the laser, less edema and pain follow the laser procedure than conventional surgery. A mild analgesic is sufficient to maintain patient comfort. Wound healing occurs by secondary intention, with granulation tissue appearing within a week; complete healing occurs in several weeks. Sun exposure to the area should be avoided for approximately 6 months. Application of a sunscreen with a solar protection factor (SPF) of at least 15 is recommended. People at high risk for skin cancer from sun exposure may be advised to use a sunscreen with an SPF greater than 15 to block ultraviolet-B as well as ultraviolet-A light.

Pulse-Dye Laser

The tunable pulse-dye laser (varying wavelengths) is the latest laser available for dermatologic surgery. It is especially useful in treating cutaneous vascular lesions (port-wine stains, telangiectasia). Eye protection used for the argon and CO_2 lasers is not sufficient when the pulse-dye laser is in use. Special eyeglasses, such as those made of didymium glass, are required for the patient and all personnel. The procedure is generally painless. For procedures requiring anesthesia, lidocaine without epinephrine is sufficient because local vasoconstriction (which epinephrine induces) is unnecessary.

NURSING MANAGEMENT

The patient should be informed that after treatment, there may be a sensation of stinging in the treated area for several hours. Applying ice to the area and a light antibacterial ointment followed by a nonstick dressing (Telfa) usually eases discomfort.

If crusting occurs, the patient is advised to wash the area gently with soap and water and reapply the antibacterial cream twice daily until the crust disappears. The nurse also advises the patient to avoid wearing makeup until all crust is removed. Sun exposure should be avoided as well; sunscreens with an SPF of 15 or greater should be used for 3 to 4 months after the treatment. Complete removal of the lesion at one session, especially a port-wine stain, is rare. The patient should be informed that several treatments may be necessary.

Critical Thinking Exercises

1. A corticosteroid cream has been prescribed for a patient at a dermatology clinic. The patient expresses relief that he now has a medicine that he can use to relieve his symptoms whenever they occur. How would you caution this patient about the use of this medication, and how would you explain the reasons for these precautions?

2. You are caring for a young man who has had surgery. You notice that his face, arms, and torso are very tan. He states that he does yard work during summer breaks from school and spends time at the beach whenever he can. What type of precautions would you suggest in view of the harmful effects ultraviolet rays can have on the skin?

3. A teenage patient requests a diet to control his acne. How would you explain to this patient the nutritional and dietary considerations associated with acne? What other factors might need to be assessed in counseling this patient?

4. A patient in a home for senior citizens has an ill-defined, red patch on her face, which she says has been present for at least 6 months and bleeds when she washes her face. She tells you that the area is painful and that she has been applying a hydrocortisone cream to it but it is not getting better. How would you assess this situation to determine what course of action to take? Explain your reasoning for deciding how to proceed.

References and Selected Readings

BOOKS

Arndt, K. A., Wintroub, B. U., Robinson, J. K., & LeBoit, P. E. (1997). *Primary care dermatology.* Philadelphia: W. B. Saunders.

Demis, D. J. (Ed.). (1998). *Clinical dermatology.* Philadelphia: Lippincott-Raven.

Fitzpatrick, T. B., et al. (1997). *Color atlas & synopsis of clinical dermatology* (3rd ed.). New York: McGraw-Hill.

Krastner, D., & Kane, D. (1997). *Chronic wounds.* Wayne, PA: Health Management Publications.

Murphy, J. L. (Ed.) (1998). *Nurse practitioner prescribing reference.* New York: Prescribing Reference.

JOURNALS

Bueller, H. A., & Bernhard, J. D. (1998). Review of pruritus therapy. *Dermatology Nursing, 10*(2), 101–107.

Byers, H. R., & Bhawan, J. (1998). Pathologic parameters in the diagnosis and prognosis of primary cutaneous melanoma. *Hematologic and Oncologic Clinics of North America, 12*(4), 717–735.

Crissey, J. T. (1998). Common dermatophyte infections: A simple diagnostic test and current management. *Postgraduate Medicine, 103*(2), 191–205.
Crutchfield, C. E. (1998). The causes and treatment of pseudofolliculitis barbae. *Cutis, 61*(6), 351–356.
Dyall, R., et al. (1998). Heteroclitic immunization induces tumor immunity. *Journal of Experimental Medicine, 188*(9), 1553–1561.
Eichenfield, L. F. (1998). Practical insights on managing pediatric atopic dermatitis. *Skin and Aging,* 30–36.
Goolsby, M. J. (1998). The elusive itch: Assessment, diagnosis, and management of pruritus. *Advance For Nurse Practitioners,* 61–64.
Gritter, M. (1998). The latex threat. *American Jouranl of Nursing, 98*(9), 26–33.
Hautmann, G., & Panconesi, E. (1997). Vitiligo: A psychologically influenced and influencing disease. *Clinical Dermatology, 15*(6), 879–890.
Kempers, S., Katz, H. I., Wildnauer, R., & Green, B. (1998). An evaluation of the effect of an alpha hydroxy acid-blend skin cream in the cosmetic improvement of symptoms of moderate to severe xerosis, epidermolytic hyperkeratosis, and ichthyosis. *Cutis, 61*(6), 347–350.
Koo, J. (1998). How and why to use sequential therapy for psoriasis. *Skin and Aging,* 42–46.
Laffrey, S. C., Bailey, B. J., & Craig, K. K. (1996). Social support and health promotion outcomes of adults with psoriasis. *Dermatology Nursing, 8*(2), 109–119.
Leston, J. M., Garcia, J. V., Santos, A. A., Varela-Centelles, P. I., & Romero, M. A. (1998). Dark oral lesions: Differential diagnosis with oral melanoma. *Cutis, 61*(5), 279–282.
McCowan, C. B. (1998). Systemic lupus erythromatosus. *Journal of the American Academy of Nurse Practitioners, 10*(5), 225–231.
McDonald, L. L., & Smith, M. L. (1998). Diagnostic dilemmas in pediatric/adolescent dermatology: Scaly scalp. *Journal of Pediatric Health Care, 12*(2), 80–84.
Media dissemination of and public response to the ultraviolet index—United States, 1994–1995. (1997). *MMWR, 46*(17), 370–373.
Mercurio, M. G. (1998). Managing the patient with hirsutism. *Hospital Medicine, 34*(9), 45–51.
Nair, S. K., Boczkowski, D., Synder, D., & Gilboa, E. (1997). Antigen-presenting cells pulsed with unfractionated tumor-derived peptides are potent tumor vaccines. *European Journal of Immunology, 26*(3), 589–597.
Nicol, N. H., Ruszkowski, A. M., & Moore, J. A. (1995). Contact dermatitis and the role of patch testing in its diagnosis and management. *Dermatology Nursing* (supplement).
Noble, S. L., Forbes, R. C., & Stamm, P. L. (1998). Diagnosis and management of common tinea infections. *American Family Physician, 58* (1), 163–178.
Nordlund, J. J. (1997). The epidemiology and genetics of vitiligo. *Clinical Dermatology, 15*(6), 875–878.
Phillips, T. J. (1996). Leg ulcer management. *Dermatology Nursing, 8*(5), 333–340.
Pride, M. W., Shuey, S., Grillo-Lopez, A., et al. (1998). Enhancement of cell-mediated immunity in melanoma patients immunized with murine anti-idiopathic monoclonal antibodies that mimic the higher molecular weight proteoglycan antigen. *Clinical Cancer Research, 4*(10), 2363–2370.
Rasmussen, J. E. (1995). Erythema multiforme, Stevens-Johnson syndrome, and toxic epidermal necrolysis. *Dermatology Nursing, 7*(1), 37–43.
Reintgen, D., et al. (1997). Clinical practice guidelines for melanoma. *Journal of the Moffitt Cancer Center, 4*(1), 45–52.
Roberts, J. L. (1997). Androgenic alopecia in men and women: An overview of cause and treatment. *Dermatology Nursing, 9*(6), 379–386.
Ruszkowski, A. M., Nicol, N. H., & Mooree, J. A. (1995). Patch testing basics: Patient selection, application techniques, and guidelines for interpretation. *Dermatology Nursing* (supplement).
Schwartz, R. A., & Janniger, C. K. (1996). Onychomycosis. *Cutis, 57*(2), 67–74.
Scher, R. K., Tulumbas, B., Argo, L. F., Holwell, J. E., Smith, E. B., & Drake, L. A. (1995). The nurse's role in diagnosing and treating onychomycosis. *Dermatology Nursing, 7*(6), 335–347.
Sherertz, E. F., & Byers, S. V. (1997). Common patch test allergens: General guidelines for avoidance. *Dermatology Nursing, 9*(2), 122–126.
Talarico, L. D. (1998). Aging skin: Best approaches to common problems. *Patient Care Nurse Practitioner, 1*(5), 28–40.
Wachsmuth, R. C. (1998). The atypical mole syndrome and predisposition to melanoma. *New England Journal of Medicine, 339*(5), 348–349.
Wolkenstein, P. E., Roujeau, J. C., & Revuz, J. (1998). Drug-induced toxic epidermal necrolysis. *Clinical Dermatology, 16*(3), 399–408.
Woodard, I. (1997). Common warts. *Lippincott's Primary Care Practice, 1*(1), 100–106.

Resources

American Cancer Society, Inc., 777 Third Ave., New York, NY 10017; www.ca.cancer.org
Lupus Foundation, 1300 Piccard Dr., Rockville, MD 29850-4303; www.lupus.org
National Institute of Arthritis, Musculoskeletal and Skin Diseases, National Institutes of Health, Bethesda, MD 29892
National Psoriasis Foundation, 6600 S.W. 92nd Ave, Suite 300, Portland, OR 97223-7195; www.psoriasis.org
Skin Cancer Foundation, 575 Park Ave. S., New York, NY 10016; www.skincancer.org
Vitiligo Foundation, P.O. Box 6337, Tyler, TX 75703; www.dermnet.org.nz

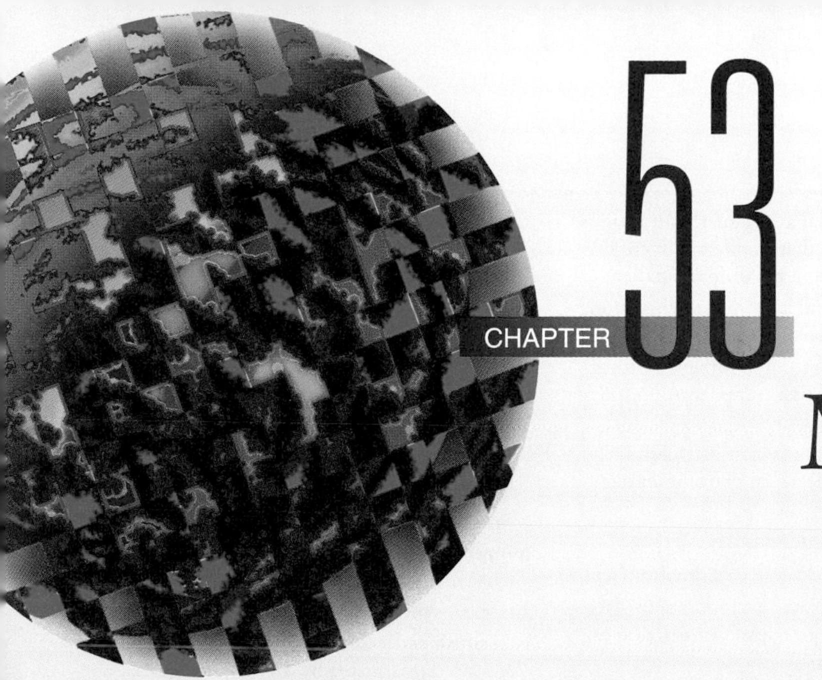

CHAPTER 53

Management of Patients With Burn Injury

Learning Objectives

On completion of this chapter, the learner will be able to:

1. Discuss the classification system used for burn injuries.
2. Describe the local and systemic effects of a major burn injury.
3. Describe the three phases of burn care and the priorities of care for each phase.
4. Compare and contrast the potential fluid and electrolyte alterations of the emergent/resuscitative and acute phases of burn management.
5. Describe the goals of the following aspects of burn wound care and the nurse's role in each: wound cleaning, topical antibacterial therapy, wound dressing, dressing changes, wound débridement, and wound grafting.
6. Describe the nurse's role in the following areas of management: pain management, restrictions of activity and joint motion, psychological support of the patient and family, nutritional support, pulmonary care, and patient and family education.
7. Use the nursing process as a framework for care of the patient during the the rehabilitation phase of burn care.

The nurse who cares for a patient with a burn injury requires a high level of knowledge about the physiologic changes that occur after a burn, as well as astute assessment skills to detect subtle changes in the patient's condition. In addition, the nurse must be able to provide sensitive, compassionate care to patients who are critically ill and must initiate rehabilitation early in the course of care. The nurse must also be able to communicate effectively with burn patients, distraught family members, and members of the entire burn management team. This will ensure quality care, which increases the likelihood of survival and promotes optimal quality of life.

GLOSSARY

Alloderm: processed dermis from human cadaver skin; can be used as dermal layer for skin grafts

autograft: a graft derived from one part of a patient's body and used on another part of that same patient's body

Biobrane: synthetic dressing composed of a nylon, Silastic membrane combined with a collagen derivative

carboxyhemoglobin: a compound of carbon monoxide and hemoglobin, formed in the blood with exposure to carbon monoxide

collagen: a protein present in skin, tendon, bone, cartilage, and connective tissue

contracture: shrinkage of burn scar through collagen maturation

cultured epithelial autografts: autologous epidermal cells that proliferate in culture and then are regrafted onto the patient

dermis: the second layer of skin containing sweat glands, hair follicles, and nerves

débridement: removal of foreign material and devitalized tissue until surrounding healthy tissue is exposed

donor site: the area from which skin is taken to provide a skin graft for another part of the body

epidermis: the outermost layer of skin

eschar: devitalized tissue resulting from a burn

escharotomy: a linear excision made through eschar to release constriction of underlying tissue

excision: surgical removal of tissue

fasciotomy: an incision made through the fascia to release constriction of underlying muscle

heterograft: graft obtained from an animal of a species other than that of the recipient (ie, pigskin); also called a xenograft

homograft: a graft transferred from one human (living or cadaveric) to another human; also called allograft

hydrotherapy: cleansing of wounds through use of bath, shower, shower cart table, or immersion

hypertrophic scar: excessive scar formation that rises above the level of the skin

Integra: synthetic dermal substitute

rule of nines: method for calculating body surface area burned by dividing the body into multiples of nine

INCIDENCE OF BURN INJURY

Approximately 1.25 million people suffer a burn injury in the United States each year. Of this group, 51,000 require acute hospital admissions. About 5,500 people die from burns and related inhalation injuries annually (Bringham & McLoughlin, 1996). One million work days are lost each year due to burn injury (Gordon & Goodwin, 1997). Young children and elderly people are at particularly high risk for burn injury. The skin in people in these two age groups is thin and fragile; therefore, even a limited period of contact with a source of heat can create a full-thickness burn.

Most burn injuries occur in the home, usually in the kitchen while cooking and in the bathroom by means of scalds or by improper use of electrical appliances around water sources (Gordon & Goodwin, 1997). Burn injuries can also occur from work accidents. The National Institute for Burn Medicine, which collects statistical data from burn centers throughout the United States, notes that most patients (75%) are victims of their own actions. Contributing to the statistics are scalds in toddlers, school-age children playing with matches, electrical injury in teenage boys, and smoking in adults combined with the use of drugs and alcohol.

Many burns could have been prevented. Nurses can play an active role in preventing fires and burns by teaching prevention concepts and promoting legislation related to fire safety (Chart 53-1).

There are four major goals relating to burns:

1. Prevention
2. Institution of lifesaving measures for the severely burned person
3. Prevention of disability and disfigurement through early, specialized, individualized treatment
4. Rehabilitation through reconstructive surgery and rehabilitative programs

OUTLOOK FOR SURVIVAL AND RECOVERY

Great strides in research have helped to increase the survival rate of burn victims. Research in areas such as fluid resuscitation, emergent burn treatment, and inhalation injury treatment and changes in wound care practice with early débridement and excision have contributed greatly to the decrease in burn deaths. Very young and very old people have a high risk of death after burn injuries due to immature and stressed immunologic systems and preexisting medical conditions, respectively. Chances of survival are greater in children older than age 5 and in adults younger than age 40. Inhalation injuries in addition to cutaneous burns worsen the prognosis. Outcome depends on the depth and extent of the burn as well as on the preinjury health status and age of the patient.

PATHOPHYSIOLOGY OF BURNS

Burns are caused by a transfer of energy from a heat source to the body. Heat may be transferred through conduction or electromagnetic radiation. Burns are categorized as thermal (which includes electrical burns), radiation, or chemical. Tissue destruction results from coagulation, protein denaturation, or ionization of cellular contents. The skin and the mucosa of the upper airways are the sites of tissue destruction. Deep tissues, includ-

CHART 53•1 Burn Prevention Tips

- Keep all matches and lighters out of the reach of children.
- Never leave children unattended around fire or in bathroom/bathtub.
- Install and maintain smoke detectors in the home.
- Develop and practice a home exit fire drill with all members of the household.
- Set the water heater temperature no higher than 120°F.
- Do not smoke in bed. Do not fall asleep while smoking.
- Do not throw flammable liquids onto an already burning fire.
- Do not use flammable liquids to start fires.
- Do not remove radiator cap from a hot engine.
- Watch for overhead electrical wires and underground wires when working outside.
- Never store flammable liquids near a fire source, such as a pilot light.
- Use caution when cooking.
- Keep a working fire extinguisher in your home.

ing the viscera, can be damaged by electrical burns or through prolonged contact.

The depth of the injury depends on the temperature of the burning agent and the duration of contact with the agent. For example, in the case of scald burns in adults, 1 second of contact with hot tap water at 68.9°C (156°F) may result in a burn that destroys both the **epidermis** and the **dermis**, causing a full-thickness (third-degree) injury. Fifteen seconds of exposure to hot water at 56.1°C (133°F) results in a similar full-thickness injury. Temperatures less than 111°F are tolerated for long periods without injury.

Classification of Burns

Burn injuries are described according to the depth of the injury and the extent of body surface area (BSA) injured.

Burn Depth

Burns are classified according to the depth of tissue destruction as superficial partial-thickness injuries, deep partial-thickness injuries, or full-thickness injuries. See Chapter 51 for a diagram of skin layers; see also Table 53-1. (The categories of superficial partial-thickness, deep partial-thickness, and full-thickness burns are similar to, but not the same as, first-, second-, and third-degree burns.)

In a superficial partial-thickness burn, the epidermis is destroyed or injured and a portion of the dermis may be injured. The wounded skin may be painful and appear red and dry, as in sunburn, or it may blister.

A deep partial-thickness burn involves destruction of the epidermis and upper layers of the dermis and injury to deeper portions of the dermis. The wound is painful, appears red, and exudes fluid. Capillary refill follows tissue blanching. Hair follicles remain intact.

A full-thickness burn involves total destruction of epidermis and dermis and in some cases underlying tissue as well. Wound color ranges widely from white to red, brown, or black. The burned area is painless because nerve fibers are destroyed. The wound appears leathery; hair follicles and sweat glands are destroyed (Fig. 53-1).

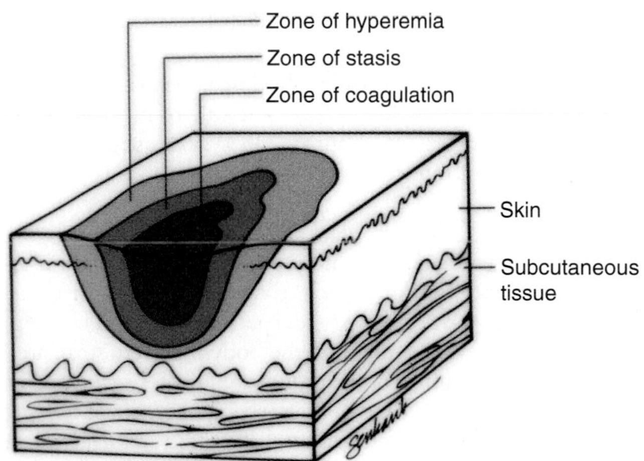

FIGURE 53•1 Zones of burn injury. Each burned area has three zones of injury. The inner zone (known as the area of coagulation, where cellular death occurs), sustains the most damage. The middle area, or zone of stasis, has a compromised blood supply, inflammation and tissue injury. The outer zone—the zone of hyperemia—sustains the least damage.

TABLE 53•1 Characteristics of Burns According to Depth

Depth of Burn and Causes	Skin Involvement	Symptoms	Wound Appearance	Recuperative Course
Superficial Partial-Thickness (Similar to First Degree)				
Sunburn Low-intensity flash	Epidermis; possibly a portion of dermis	Tingling Hyperesthesia (supersensitivity) Pain that is soothed by cooling	Reddened; blanches with pressure; dry Minimal or no edema Possible blisters	Complete recovery within a week; no scarring Peeling
Deep Partial-Thickness (Similar to Second Degree)				
Scalds Flash flame	Epidermis, upper dermis, portion of deeper dermis	Pain Hyperesthesia Sensitive to cold air	Blistered, mottled red base; broken epidermis; weeping surface Edema	Recovery in 2 to 4 weeks Some scarring and depigmentation contractures Infection may convert it to full thickness
Full-Thickness (Similar to Third Degree)				
Flame Prolonged exposure to hot liquids Electric current Chemical	Epidermis, entire dermis, and sometimes subcutaneous tissue; may involve connective tissue, muscle, and bone	Pain free Shock Hematuria (blood in the urine) and possibly hemolysis (blood cell destruction) Possible entrance and exit wounds (electrical burn)	Dry; pale white, leathery, or charred Broken skin with fat exposed Edema	Eschar sloughs Grafting necessary Scarring and loss of contour and function; contractures Loss of digits or extremity possible

The determination of depth takes the following factors into consideration:

- History of how the injury occurred
- Causative agent, such as flame or a scalding liquid
- Temperature of the burning agent
- Duration of contact with the agent
- Thickness of the skin

Extent of Body Surface Area Injured

RULE OF NINES

An estimation of the total BSA involved in a burn is simplified by using the **rule of nines** (Fig. 53-2). The rule of nines is a quick way to calculate the extent of burns. The system assigns percentages in multiples of nine to major body surfaces.

LUND AND BROWDER METHOD

A more precise method of estimating the extent of a burn is the Lund and Browder method, which recognizes that the percentage of BSA of various anatomic parts, especially the head and legs, changes with growth. By dividing the body into very small areas and providing an estimate of the proportion of BSA accounted for by such body parts, one can obtain a reliable estimate of the total BSA burned. The initial evaluation is made on the patient's arrival at the hospital and is revised on the second and third postburn days, because the demarcation usually is not clear until then.

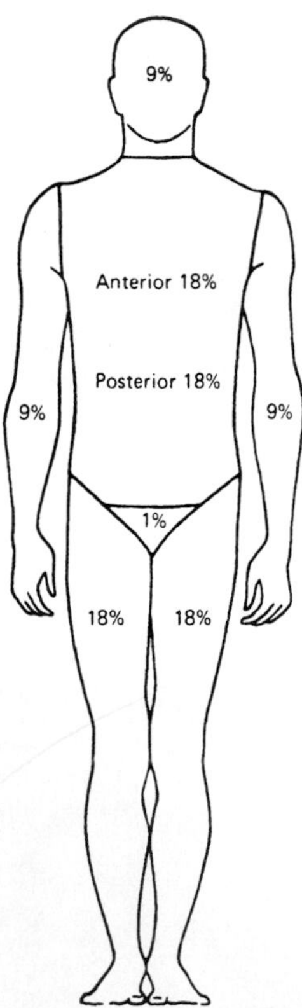

FIGURE 53•2 The Rule of Nines: Estimated percentage of body surface area (BSA) in the adult is arrived at by sectioning the body surface into areas with a numerical value related to nine. (Note: The anterior and posterior head total 9% of BSA). In burn victims, the total estimated percentage of BSA injured is used to calculate the patient's fluid replacement needs.

PALM METHOD

In patients with scattered burns, a method to estimate the percentage of burn is the palm method. The size of the patient's palm is approximately 1% of BSA. The size of the palm can be used to assess the extent of burn injury.

Local and Systemic Responses to Burns

Burns that do not exceed 25% of the total BSA produce a primarily local response, whereas burns that exceed 25% BSA may produce both a local and a systemic response, which is considered a major burn injury.

Pathophysiologic changes resulting from major burns during the initial burn-shock period include tissue hypoperfusion and organ hypofunction secondary to decreased cardiac output, followed by a hyperdynamic and hypermetabolic phase. The incidence, magnitude, and duration of pathophysiologic changes in burns are proportional to the extent of burn injury, with a maximal response seen in burns covering 60% or more BSA.

The initial systemic event after a major burn injury is hemodynamic instability, resulting from loss of capillary integrity and a subsequent shift of fluid, sodium, and protein from the intravascular space into the interstitial spaces. Figure 53-3 illustrates pathophysiologic processes in acute major burns. Hemodynamic instability involves cardiovascular, fluid and electrolyte, blood volume, pulmonary, and other mechanisms.

Cardiovascular Response

Cardiac output decreases before any significant change in blood volume is evident. As fluid loss continues and vascular volume decreases, cardiac output continues to fall and blood pressure drops. This is the onset of burn shock. In response, the sympathetic nervous system releases catecholamines, resulting in an increase in peripheral resistance (vasoconstriction) and an increase in pulse rate. Peripheral vasoconstriction further decreases cardiac output.

Prompt fluid resuscitation maintains the blood pressure in the low-normal range and improves cardiac output. Despite adequate fluid resuscitation, cardiac filling pressures—central venous pressure, pulmonary artery pressure, and pulmonary artery wedge pressure—remain low during the burn-shock period. If inadequate fluid resuscitation occurs, distributive shock will occur (see Chap. 14).

Generally, the greatest volume of fluid leak occurs in the first 24 to 36 hours after the burn, peaking by 6 to 8 hours. As the capillaries begin to regain their integrity, burn shock resolves and fluid returns to the vascular compartment. As fluid is reabsorbed from the interstitial tissue into the vascular compartment, blood volume increases. If renal and cardiac function is adequate, urinary output increases. Diuresis continues for several days to 2 weeks.

As previously noted, in burns involving less than 25% of the total BSA, the loss of capillary integrity and shift of fluid are localized to the burn itself, resulting in blister formation and edema only in the area of injury. Patients with more severe burns develop massive systemic edema. As edema increases in circumferential burns, pressure on small blood vessels and nerves in distal extremities causes an obstruction of blood flow and consequent ischemia. This complication is known as compartment syndrome. The physician may need to perform an **escharotomy**, a surgical incision into the **eschar** (devitalized tissue resulting from a burn), to relieve the constricting effect of the burned tissue.

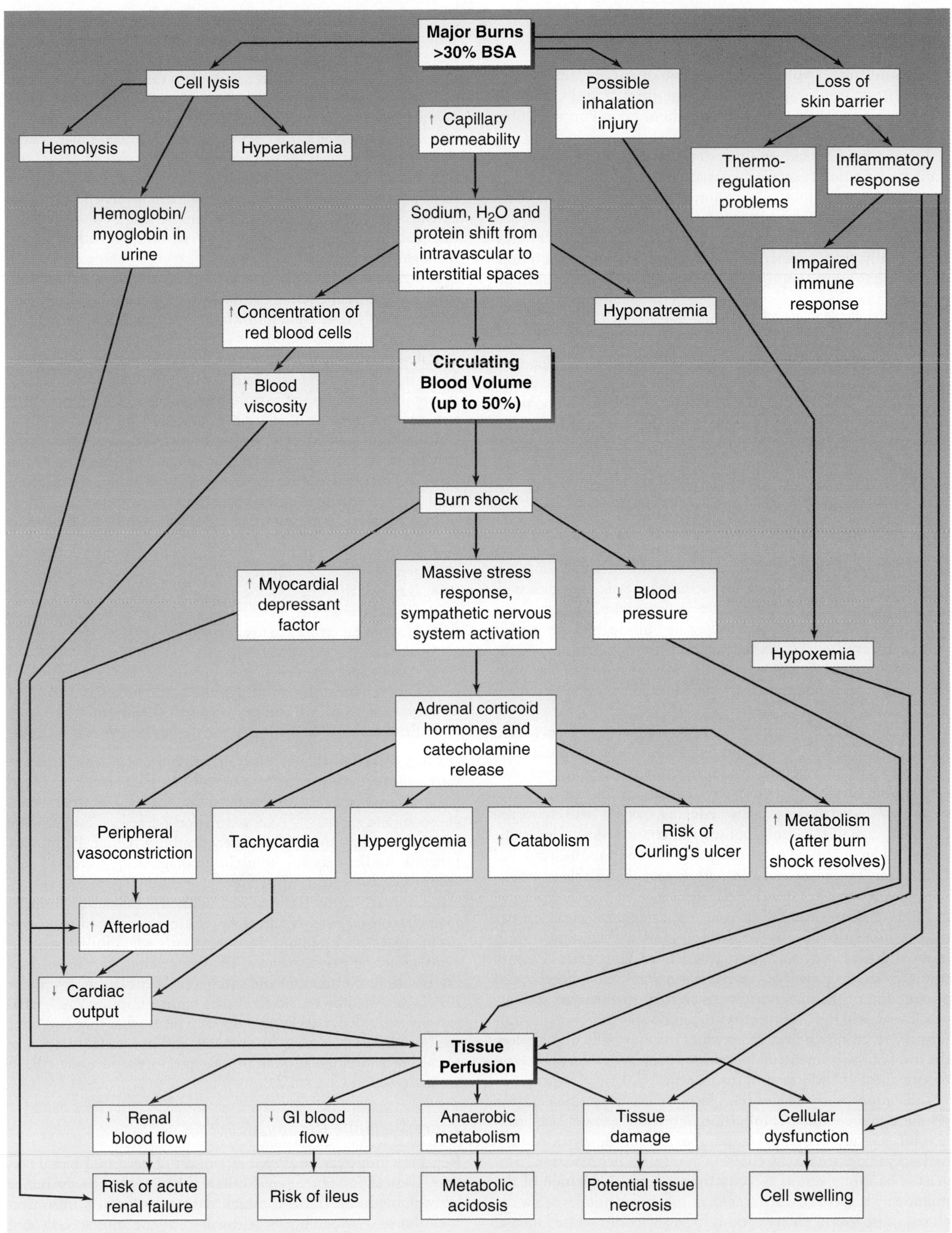

FIGURE 53•3 Overview of physiologic changes that occur after major burn.

Effects on Fluids, Electrolytes, and Blood Volume

Circulating blood volume decreases dramatically during burn shock. In addition, evaporative fluid loss through the burn wound may reach 3 to 5 L or more over a 24-hour period until the burn surfaces are covered.

During burn shock, serum sodium levels vary in response to fluid resuscitation. Usually hyponatremia (sodium depletion) is present. Hyponatremia is also common during the first week of the acute phase, as water shifts from the interstitial to the vascular space.

Immediately after burn injury, hyperkalemia (excessive potassium) results from massive cell destruction. Hypokalemia (potassium depletion) may occur later with fluid shifts and inadequate potassium intake.

At the time of burn injury, some red blood cells may be destroyed and others damaged, resulting in anemia. Despite this, the patient's hematocrit may be elevated due to plasma loss. Blood loss during operative procedures, wound care, and diagnostic studies and ongoing hemolysis further contribute to anemia. Blood transfusions are required periodically to maintain adequate hemoglobin levels for oxygen delivery. Abnormalities in coagulation, including a decrease in platelets (thrombocytopenia) and prolonged clotting and prothrombin times, also occur with burn injury.

Pulmonary Response

Inhalation injury is the leading cause of death in fire victims. It is estimated that half of these deaths could have been prevented with use of a smoke detector. Often, burn victims make it out of a burning home safely. However, once they are outside, they may realize that their loved ones, pets, or valuable items are still inside the burning home. They then reenter the burning home and are overcome with toxic smoke and fumes and become disoriented and/or unconscious.

One third of all burn patients have a pulmonary problem related to the burn injury. Even without pulmonary injury, hypoxia (oxygen starvation) may be present. Early in the postburn period, catecholamine release in response to the stress of the burn injury alters peripheral blood flow, thereby reducing oxygen delivery to the periphery. Later, hypermetabolism and continued catecholamine release lead to increased tissue oxygen consumption, which can lead to hypoxia. To ensure that adequate oxygen is available to the tissues, supplemental oxygen may be needed.

Pulmonary injuries fall into several categories: upper airway injury; inhalation injury below the glottis, including carbon monoxide poisoning; and restrictive defects. Upper airway injury results from direct heat or edema. It is manifested by mechanical obstruction of the upper airway, including the pharynx and larynx. Because of the cooling effect of rapid vaporization in the pulmonary tract, direct heat injury does not normally occur below the level of the bronchus. Upper airway injury is treated by early nasotracheal or endotracheal intubation.

Inhalation injury below the glottis results from inhaling the products of incomplete combustion or noxious gases. These products include carbon monoxide, sulfur oxides, nitrogen oxides, aldehydes, cyanide, ammonia, chlorine, phosgene, benzene, and halogens. The injury results directly from chemical irritation of the pulmonary tissues at the alveolar level. Inhalation injuries below the glottis cause loss of ciliary action, hypersecretion, severe mucosal edema, and possibly bronchospasm. The pulmonary surfactant is reduced, resulting in atelectasis (collapse of alveoli). Expectoration of carbon particles in the sputum is the cardinal sign of this injury.

Carbon monoxide is probably the most common cause of inhalation injury because it is a byproduct of the combustion of organic materials and is therefore present in smoke. The pathophysiologic effects are due to tissue hypoxia, a result of carbon monoxide combining with hemoglobin to form **carboxyhemoglobin**, which competes with oxygen for available hemoglobin-binding sites. The affinity of hemoglobin for carbon monoxide is 200 times greater than that for oxygen. Treatment usually consists of early intubation and mechanical ventilation with 100% oxygen. However, some patients may require only oxygen therapy, depending on the extent of pulmonary injury and edema. Using 100% oxygen is essential to accelerate the removal of carbon monoxide from the hemoglobin molecule.

Restrictive defects arise when edema develops under full-thickness burns encircling the neck and thorax. Chest excursion may be greatly restricted, resulting in decreased tidal volume. In such situations, escharotomy is necessary.

Pulmonary abnormalities are not always immediately apparent. More than half of all burn victims with pulmonary involvement do not initially demonstrate pulmonary signs and symptoms. Any patient with possible inhalation injury must be observed for at least 24 hours for respiratory complications. Airway obstruction may occur very rapidly or develop in hours. Decreased lung compliance, decreased arterial oxygen levels, and respiratory acidosis may occur gradually over the first 5 days after a burn.

Indicators of possible pulmonary damage include the following:

- History indicating that the burn occurred in an enclosed area
- Burns of the face or neck
- Singed nasal hair
- Hoarseness, voice change, dry cough, stridor, sooty sputum
- Bloody sputum
- Labored breathing or tachypnea (rapid breathing) and other signs of reduced oxygen levels (hypoxemia)
- Erythema and blistering of the oral or pharyngeal mucosa

Diagnosis of inhalation injury is an important priority for many burn victims. Serum carboxyhemoglobin levels and arterial blood gas levels are frequently used to assess for inhalation injuries. Bronchoscopy and xenon^{133} (^{133}Xe) ventilation-perfusion scans can also be used to aid diagnosis in the early postburn period. Pulmonary function studies may also be useful in diagnosing decreased lung compliance or obstructed air flow.

Pulmonary complications secondary to inhalation injuries include acute respiratory failure and acute respiratory distress syndrome (ARDS). Respiratory failure occurs when impairment of ventilation and gas exchange is life-threatening. The immediate intervention is intubation and mechanical ventilation. If ventilation is impaired by restricted chest excursion, immediate escharotomy is needed. ARDS may develop in the first few days after the burn injury secondary to systemic and pulmonary responses to the burn and inhalation injury. Respiratory failure and ARDS are discussed in Chapter 21.

Other Systemic Responses

Renal function may be altered as a result of decreased blood volume. Destruction of red blood cells at the injury site results in free hemoglobin in the urine. If muscle damage occurs (eg, from electrical burns), myoglobin is released from the muscle cells and excreted by the kidney. Adequate fluid volume replacement restores renal blood flow, increasing the glomerular filtration rate and urine volume. If there is inadequate blood flow through the kidney, the

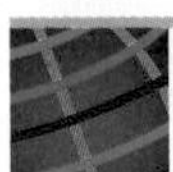

TABLE 53•2 **Phases of Burn Care**

Phase	Duration	Priorities
Emergent or immediate resuscitative	From onset of injury to completion of fluid resuscitation	• First aid • Prevention of shock • Prevention of respiratory distress • Detection and treatment of concomitant injuries • Wound assessment and initial care
Acute	From beginning of diuresis to near completion of wound closure	• Wound care and closure • Prevention or treatment of complications, including infection • Nutritional support
Rehabilitation	From major wound closure to return to individual's optimal level of physical and psychosocial adjustment	• Prevention of scars and contractures • Physical, occupational, and vocational rehabilitation • Functional and cosmetic reconstruction • Psychosocial counseling

hemoglobin and myoglobin occlude the renal tubules, resulting in acute tubular necrosis and renal failure (see Chap. 41).

The immunologic defenses of the body are greatly altered by burn injury. The loss of skin integrity is compounded by the release of abnormal inflammatory factors, altered levels of immunoglobulins and serum complement, impaired neutrophil function, and a reduction in lymphocytes (lymphocytopenia). Immunosuppression places the burn patient at high risk for sepsis.

Loss of skin also results in an inability to regulate body temperature. Burn patients may therefore exhibit low body temperatures in the early hours after injury, but as hypermetabolism resets core temperatures, burn patients become hyperthermic for much of the postburn period, even in the absence of infection.

Two potential gastrointestinal complications may occur: paralytic ileus (absence of intestinal peristalsis) and Curling's ulcer. Decreased peristalsis and bowel sounds are manifestations of paralytic ileus resulting from burn trauma. Gastric distention and nausea may lead to vomiting unless gastric decompression is initiated. Gastric bleeding secondary to massive physiologic stress may be signaled by occult blood in the stool, regurgitation of "coffee ground" material from the stomach, or bloody vomitus. These signs suggest gastric or duodenal erosion (Curling's ulcer).

MANAGEMENT OF THE PATIENT WITH A BURN INJURY

Burn care must be planned according to the burn depth and local response, the extent of the injury, and the presence or absence of a systemic response. Burn care then proceeds through three phases—emergent/resuscitative phase, acute/intermediate phase, and rehabilitation phase. Although priorities exist for each of the phases, the phases overlap, and assessment and management of specific problems and complications are not limited to these phases but take place throughout the course of burn care. The three phases and the priorities for care are summarized in Table 53-2.

Emergent/Resuscitative Phase of Burn Care

On-the-Scene Care

Anyone who encounters a burn victim for the first time may feel overwhelmed. The burned person's appearance can be frightening at first. It can be very difficult not to get caught up with the appearance of the person and concentrate on the burn wounds. However, the burn wound is not the first priority at the scene. The first priority in on-the-scene care for a burn victim is to prevent injury to the rescuer. If needed, fire and emergency medical services should be requested at the first opportunity. Additional emergency procedures are highlighted in Chart 53-2.

AIRWAY, BREATHING, CIRCULATION

Although the local effects of a burn are the most evident, the systemic effects pose a greater threat to life. Therefore, it is important to remember the ABCs of all trauma care during the early postburn period:

- **A**irway
- **B**reathing
- **C**irculation; **C**ervical spine immobilization for all high-voltage electrical injuries and if indicated for other injuries; **C**ardiac monitoring for all electrical injuries for at least 24 hours after cessation of dysrhythmia

Some practitioners include "DEF" in the trauma assessment—**D**isability, **E**xposure, and **F**luid resuscitation (Gordon & Goodwin, 1997).

Nursing Alert *Breathing must be assessed and a patent airway established immediately during the initial minutes of emergency care. Immediate therapy is directed toward establishing an airway and administering humidified 100% oxygen. If such a high concentration of oxygen is not available under emergency conditions, oxygen by mask or nasal cannula is given initially. If qualified personnel and equipment are available and if the victim has severe respiratory distress or airway edema, the rescuers can insert an endotracheal tube and initiate manual ventilation.*

The circulatory system must also be assessed quickly. Apical pulse and blood pressure are monitored frequently. Tachycardia (abnormally rapid heart rate) and slight hypotension are expected in the untreated patient soon after the burn. The neurologic status is assessed quickly in the patient with extensive burns. Often the burn patient is awake and alert initially, and vital information can be obtained at that time. A secondary head-to-toe survey of the patient is carried out to identify other potentially life-threatening injuries. (The **E** and **F** parameters of trauma assessment are discussed in detail later. Preventing shock in a burn patient is imperative.)

CHART 53•2 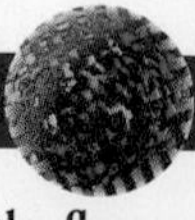 Emergency Procedures at the Burn Scene

- **Extinguish the flames.** When clothes catch fire, the flames can be extinguished if the victim falls to the floor or ground and rolls ("drop and roll"); anything available to smother the flames, such as a blanket, rug, or coat, may be used. Standing still forces the victim to breathe flames and smoke, and running fans the flames. If the burn source is electrical, the electrical source must be disconnected.
- **Cool the burn.** After the flames are extinguished, the burned area and adherent clothing are soaked with *cool* water, briefly, to cool the wound and halt the burning process. Once a burn has been sustained, the application of cool water is the best first-aid measure. Soaking the burn area intermittently in cool water or applying cool towels gives immediate and striking relief from pain and restricts local tissue edema and damage. However, *never* apply ice directly to the burn, *never* wrap burn victims in ice, and *never* use cold soaks or dressings for longer than several minutes; such procedures may worsen the tissue damage and lead to hypothermia in patients with large burns.
- **Remove restrictive objects.** If possible, remove clothing immediately. Adherent clothing may be left in place once cooled. Other clothing and all jewelry should be removed to allow for assessment and to prevent constriction secondary to rapidly developing edema.
- **Cover the wound.** The burn should be covered as quickly as possible to minimize bacterial contamination and decrease pain by preventing air from coming into contact with the injured surface. Sterile dressings are best, but any clean, dry cloth can be used as an emergency dressing. Ointments and salves should *not* be used. Other than the dressing, no medication or material should be applied to the burn wound.
- **Irrigate chemical burns.** Chemical burns resulting from contact with a corrosive material are irrigated immediately. Most chemical laboratories have a high-pressure shower for such emergencies. If such an injury occurs at home, brush off the chemical agent, remove clothes immediately, and rinse all areas of the body that have come in contact with the chemical. Rinsing can occur in the shower or any other source of continuous running water. If a chemical gets in or near the eyes, the eyes should be flushed with cool, clean water immediately. Outcomes for the patient with chemical burns are significantly improved by rapid, sustained flushing of the injury at the scene.

***Nursing Alert** No food or fluid is given by mouth, and the patient is placed in a position that will prevent aspiration of vomitus because nausea and vomiting typically occur due to paralytic ileus resulting from the stress of injury.*

Usually, rescue workers will cool the wound, establish an airway, supply oxygen, and start an intravenous line.

Emergency Medical Management

The patient is transported to the nearest emergency department. The hospital and physician are alerted that the patient is en route to the emergency department so that life-saving measures can be initiated immediately by a trained team.

Initial priorities in the emergency department remain airway, breathing, and circulation. For mild pulmonary injury, inspired air is humidified and the patient is encouraged to cough so that secretions can be removed by suctioning. For more severe situations, it is necessary to remove secretions by bronchial suctioning and to administer bronchodilators and mucolytic agents. If edema of the airway develops, endotracheal intubation may be necessary. Continuous positive airway pressure and mechanical ventilation may also be required to achieve adequate oxygenation.

After adequate respiratory and circulatory status has been established, attention is directed to the burn wound itself. All clothing and jewelry are removed. Flushing of chemical burns with water is continued. The patient is checked for contact lenses; these are removed immediately if chemicals have contacted the eyes or if facial burns have occurred. It is important to validate an account of the burn scenario provided by the patient, witnesses at the scene, and paramedics and to assess for cervical spinal injuries or head injury if the patient was involved in an explosion, a fall, a jump, or an electrical injury.

A history of preexisting diseases, allergies, and medications and the use of drugs, alcohol, and tobacco is obtained at this point to plan the patient's care. A large-bore (16- or 18-gauge) intravenous catheter should be inserted in a nonburned area (if not inserted earlier). Some patients have a central venous catheter so that large amounts of intravenous fluids can be given quickly and central venous pressures can be monitored. If the patient's burn exceeds 25% BSA or if the patient is nauseated, a nasogastric tube should be inserted and connected to suction to prevent paralytic ileus (absence of peristalsis).

The physician evaluates the patient's general condition, assesses the burn, determines the priorities of care, and directs the individualized plan of treatment, which is divided into systemic management and local care of the burned area. Nonsterile gloves, caps, and gowns are worn while assessing the exposed burned areas. Clean technique is maintained while assessing burn wounds.

Assessment of both the extent of BSA burned and the depth of the burn is completed after soot and debris have been gently cleansed from the burn wound. Assessment is repeated frequently throughout burn wound care. Photographs may be taken of the burn areas initially and periodically throughout the treatment. In this way, the healing progress may be determined quickly. Such documentation is invaluable for insurance and legal claims. Clean sheets are placed under and over the patient to protect the area from contamination, maintain body temperature, and decrease pain caused by air currents passing over exposed nerve endings.

An indwelling urinary catheter is inserted to permit more accurate monitoring of urine output and renal function. Baseline height, weight, arterial blood gases, hematocrit, electrolyte values, urinalysis, and chest x-rays are obtained. If the patient has an electrical burn, a baseline electrocardiogram is obtained. Because burns are contaminated wounds, tetanus prophylaxis is administered if the patient's immunization status is not current or is unknown.

Although the major focus of care during the emergent phase is physical stabilization, the nurse must also attend to the patient's and family's psychological needs. Burn injury is a crisis, causing variable emotional responses. The patient's and family's coping abilities and available supports are assessed. Circumstances surrounding the burn injury should be considered when providing care. Individualized psychosocial support must be given to the patient and family. Because the emergent burn patient is usually anxious and in pain, those in attendance should provide reassurance and support, explanations of procedures, and adequate pain medication. Because poor tissue perfusion accompanies burn injuries, only intravenous pain medication (usually morphine) is given. If the patient wishes to see a spiritual advisor, one is notified.

Transfer to a Burn Center

The depth and extent of the burn are considered in determining whether the patient should be transferred to a burn center. Patients with major burns, those who are at the extremes of the age continuum, those with coexisting health problems that may affect recovery, and those with circumstances that increase their risk for acute and long-term complications are transferred to a burn center. Chart 53-3 lists the American Burn Association's criteria for burn center referral after initial assessment and management.

If the patient is to be transported to a burn center, the following measures are instituted before transfer:

1. A secure intravenous line is placed, with fluid infusing at the rate required to attain urine output of at least 30 mL per hour.
2. A patent airway is ensured.
3. Adequate pain relief is attained.
4. Adequate peripheral circulation is established in any burned extremity.
5. Wounds are covered with a clean, dry sheet, and the patient is kept comfortably warm.

Assessments and treatments are documented, and this information is provided to the burn center personnel. The transferring facility must relay accurate intake and output totals to burn center personnel so that adequate fluid resuscitation measures continue.

Management of Fluid Loss and Shock

Next to handling respiratory difficulties, the most urgent need is preventing irreversible shock by replacing lost fluids and electrolytes. As mentioned previously, survival of burn victims depends on adequate fluid resuscitation. Table 53-3 summarizes the fluid and electrolyte changes in the emergent phase of burn care. Intravenous lines and an indwelling catheter must be in place before implementing fluid resuscitation. Baseline weight and laboratory test results are obtained as well. These parameters must be monitored closely in the immediate postburn (resuscitation) period.

FLUID REPLACEMENT

There is no known way to stop fluid from moving into the interstitial spaces, but fluid replacement is possible. The projected fluid requirements for the first 24 hours are calculated by the physician based on the extent of the burn injury. Some combination of fluid categories may be used: colloids (whole blood, plasma, and plasma expanders) and crystalloids/electrolytes (physiologic sodium chloride or lactated Ringer's solution). Adequate fluid resuscitation results in slightly decreased blood volume levels during the first 24 postburn hours and restores plasma levels to normal by the end of 48 hours.

Formulas have been developed for estimating fluid loss based on the estimated percentage of burned BSA and the weight of the patient. Length of time since burn injury occurred is also very important in calculating estimated fluid needs. Formulas must be adjusted so that initiation of fluid replacement reflects time of injury. The formulas are individualized to meet the requirements of each patient. The various formulas are discussed below and summarized in Chart 53-4.

As early as 1978, the NIH Consensus Development Conference on Supportive Therapy in Burn Care established that salt and water are required in burn patients, but that colloid may or may not be useful during the first 24 to 48 postburn hours. The consensus formula provides for the volume of balanced salt solution to be administered in the first 24 hours in a range of 2 to 4 mL/kg per percent burn. Generally, 2 mL/kg/% burn of lactated Ringer's solution may be used initially for adults. This is the most common fluid replacement formula in use today. As with the other formulas, half of the calculated total should be given over the first 8 postburn hours, and the other half should be given over the next 16 hours. The rate and volume of the infusion must be regulated according to the patient's response.

Studies demonstrate that with large burns, there is a failure of the sodium-potassium pump (a physiologic mechanism involved in fluid–electrolyte balance) at the cellular level. Thus, patients with very large burns may need proportionately more milliliters of fluid per percent of burn than those with smaller burns. Also, patients with electrical injury, pulmonary injury, and delayed fluid resuscitation and those who were burned while intoxicated may need additional fluids.

Let us use as an example a 70-kg (about 168 lb) patient with a 50% BSA burn:

1. Consensus formula: 2 to 4 mL/kg/% BSA
2. $2 \times 70 \times 50 = 7000$ mL/24 hours
3. Plan to administer: First 8 hours = 3500 mL, or 437 mL/ hour; next 16 hours = 3500 mL, or 219 mL/hour

Most fluid replacement formulas use isotonic electrolyte solutions. Regardless of which standard replacement formula is used, the patient receives approximately the same fluid volume and sodium replacement during the first 48 hours.

Another fluid replacement method requires hypertonic electrolyte solutions. This method uses concentrated solutions of sodium chloride and lactate (a balanced salt solution) so that the resulting fluid has a concentration of 250 to 300 mEq of sodium. The rationale for this replacement method is that by increasing serum osmolality, fluid will be pulled back into the vascular space

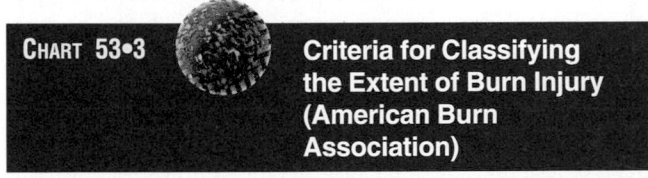

Minor burn injury

- Second-degree burn of <15% total body surface area (TBSA) burn in adults or <10% TBSA in children
- Third-degree burn of <2% TBSA not involving special care areas (eyes, ears, face, hands, feet, perineum, joints)
- Excludes electrical injury, inhalation injury, concurrent trauma, all poor-risk patients (ie, extremes of age, intercurrent disease)

Moderate, uncomplicated burn injury

- Second-degree burns of 15%–25% TBSA in adults or 10%–20% in children
- Third-degree burns of <10% TBSA not involving special care areas
- Excludes electrical injury, inhalation injury, concurrent trauma, all poor-risk patients (ie, extremes of age, intercurrent disease)

Major burn injury

- Second-degree burns of >25% TBSA in adults or 20% in children
- All third-degree burns of ≥10% TBSA
- All burns involving eyes, ears, face, hands, feet, perineum, joints
- All inhalation injury, electrical injury, concurrent trauma, all poor-risk patients

From Hudak, C. M., Gallo, B. M., & Morton, P. G. (1998). *Critical care nursing: A holistic approach* (7th ed.). Philadelphia: Lippincott Williams & Wilkins.

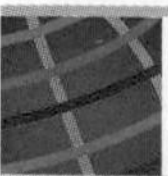

TABLE 53•3 **Fluid and Electrolyte Changes in the Emergent/Resuscitative Phase**

Fluid accumulation phase (shock phase)
Plasma → interstitial fluid (edema at burn site)

Observation	Explanation
Generalized dehydration	Plasma leaks through damaged capillaries.
Reduction of blood volume	Secondary to plasma loss, fall of blood pressure, and diminished cardiac output
Decreased urinary output	Secondary to: Fluid loss Decreased renal blood flow Sodium and water retention caused by increased adrenocortical activity (Hemolysis of red blood cells, causing hemoglobinuria and myonecrosis or myoglobinuria)
Potassium (K^+) excess	Massive cellular trauma causes release of K^+ into extracellular fluid (ordinarily, most K^+ is intracellular).
Sodium (Na^+) deficit	Large amount of Na^+ is lost in trapped edema fluid and exudate and by shift into cells as K^+ is released from cells (ordinarily most Na^+ is extracellular).
Metabolic acidosis (base-bicarbonate deficit)	Loss of bicarbonate ions accompanies sodium loss.
Hemoconcentration (elevated hematocrit)	Liquid blood component is lost into extravascular space.

from the interstitial space. Reduced systemic and pulmonary edema has been reported after administering hypertonic solutions.

Nursing Alert *Formulas are only a guide. The patient's response, evidenced by heart rate, blood pressure, and urine output, is the primary determinant of actual fluid therapy and must be assessed at least hourly. Patient outcomes are improved by optimal fluid resuscitation.*

GOALS OF FLUID REPLACEMENT THERAPY

The total volume and rate of intravenous fluid replacement are gauged by the patient's response. Goals of fluid replacement are a systolic blood pressure exceeding 100 mm Hg, pulse rate less than 110/minute, and urine output of 30 to 50 mL/hour.

Nursing Alert *These parameters are far more important in resuscitation than any formula. Indeed, the patient's individual response is the formula.*

Additional gauges of fluid requirements and response to fluid resuscitation include hematocrit and hemoglobin and serum sodium levels. If the hematocrit and the hemoglobin level decrease or if the urinary output exceeds 50 mL/hour, the rate of intravenous fluid administration may be decreased. The goal is to maintain serum sodium levels in the normal range during fluid replacement.

NURSING PROCESS: CARE DURING THE EMERGENT/RESUSCITATIVE PHASE

Assessment

Assessment data obtained by prehospital providers (rescuers such as emergency medical technicians) are shared with the physician and nurse in the emergency department. Nursing assessment in the emergent phase of burn injury focuses on the major priorities for any trauma patient; the burn wound is a secondary consideration. Aseptic management of the burn wounds and invasive lines continues.

The nurse checks vital signs frequently. Respiratory status is monitored closely. Apical, carotid, and femoral pulses are evaluated. Cardiac monitoring is indicated if the patient has a history of cardiac disease, electrical injury, or respiratory problems, or if the pulse is dysrhythmic or the rate is abnormally slow or rapid.

If all extremities are burned, determining blood pressure may be difficult. A sterile dressing applied under the blood pressure cuff will protect the wound from contamination. Because increasing edema makes blood pressure difficult to auscultate, a Doppler (ultrasound) device or a noninvasive electronic blood pressure device may be helpful. In severe burns, an arterial catheter is used for blood pressure measurement and for collecting blood specimens. Peripheral pulses of burned extremities are checked hourly; the Doppler device is useful for this. Elevation of burned extremities is crucial to decrease edema. Elevation of the lower extremities on pillows and of the upper extremities on pillows or by suspension using intravenous poles may be helpful.

Large-bore intravenous lines and an indwelling urinary catheter are inserted, and the nurse's assessment includes monitoring fluid intake and output. Urine output, an excellent indicator of circulatory status, is monitored carefully and measured hourly. The amount of urine first obtained when the urinary catheter was inserted is recorded. This may assist in determining the extent of preburn renal function and fluid status. Urine specific gravity, pH, and glucose, acetone, protein, and hemoglobin levels are assessed frequently.

Burgundy-colored urine suggests the presence of hemochromogen and myoglobin resulting from muscle damage. This is associated with deep burns caused by electrical injury or prolonged contact with flames. Glucosuria is a common finding in the early postburn hours and results from the release of stored glucose from the liver in response to stress.

Although not responsible for calculating the patient's fluid requirements, the nurse needs to know the maximal volume of fluid the patient should receive. Infusion pumps and rate controllers are used to deliver a complex regimen of prescribed intravenous fluids. Monitoring intravenous therapy is a major nursing responsibility.

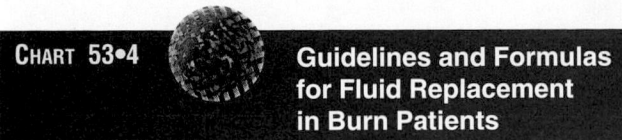

CHART 53•4 Guidelines and Formulas for Fluid Replacement in Burn Patients

Consensus Formula

Lactated Ringer's solution (or other balanced saline solution): 2–4 mL × kg body weight × % body surface area (BSA) burned. Half to be given in first 8 hours; remaining half to be given over next 16 hours.

Evans Formula

1. Colloids: 1 mL × kg body weight × % BSA burned
2. Electrolytes (saline): 1 mL × body weight × % BSA burned
3. Glucose (5% in water): 2000 mL for insensible loss
   Day 1: Half to be given in first 8 hours; remaining half over next 16 hours
   Day 2: Half of previous day's colloids and electrolytes; all of insensible fluid replacement

Maximum of 10,000 mL over 24 hours. Second- and third-degree (partial- and full-thickness) burns exceeding 50% BSA are calculated on the basis of 50% BSA.

Brooke Army Formula

1. Colloids: 0.5 mL × kg body weight × % BSA burned
2. Electrolytes (lactated Ringer's solution): 1.5 mL × kg body weight × % BSA burned
3. Glucose (5% in water): 2000 mL for insensible loss
   Day 1: Half to be given in first 8 hours; remaining half over next 16 hours
   Day 2: Half of colloids; half of electrolytes; all of insensible fluid replacement.

Second- and third-degree (partial- and full-thickness) burns exceeding 50% BSA are calculated on the basis of 50% BSA.

Parkland/Baxter Formula

Lactated Ringers' solution: 4 mL × kg body weight × % BSA burned.
Day 1: Half to be given in first 8 hours; half to be given over next 16 hours
Day 2: Varies. Colloid is added.

Hypertonic Saline Solution

Concentrated solutions of sodium chloride (NaCl) and lactate with concentration of 250–300 mEq of sodium per liter, administered at a rate sufficient to maintain a desired volume of urinary output. Do not increase the infusion rate during the first 8 postburn hours. Serum sodium levels must be monitored closely. Goal: Increase serum sodium level and osmolality to reduce edema and prevent pulmonary complications.

Body temperature, body weight, preburn weight, and history of allergies, tetanus immunization, past medical and surgical problems, current illnesses, and use of medication are assessed. A head-to-toe assessment is performed, focusing on signs and symptoms of concomitant illness, injury, or developing complications. Patients with facial burns should have their eyes examined for potential injury to the corneas. An ophthalmologist is consulted for complete assessment via fluorescent staining.

Assessing the extent of the burn wound continues and is facilitated with anatomic diagrams (described previously). In addition, the nurse works with the physician to assess the depth of the wound and areas of full- and partial-thickness injury. Assessment of the circumstances surrounding the injury is important. Obtaining a history of the burn injury can help to plan the care for the patient. Assessment should include the time of injury, mechanism of burn, whether the burn occurred in a closed space, the possibility of inhalation of noxious chemicals, and any related trauma.

The neurologic assessment focuses on the patient's level of consciousness, psychological status, pain and anxiety levels, and behavior. The patient's and family's understanding of the injury and treatment is assessed as well.

Nursing care of the patient during the emergent/resuscitative phase of burn injury is detailed in the Plan of Nursing Care 53-1.

Acute or Intermediate Phase of Burn Care

The acute or intermediate phase of burn care follows the emergent/resuscitative phase and begins 48 to 72 hours after the burn injury. During this phase, attention is directed toward continued assessment and maintenance of respiratory and circulatory status, fluid and electrolyte balance, and gastrointestinal function. Infection prevention, burn wound care (ie, wound cleaning, topical antibacterial therapy, wound dressing, dressing changes, wound débridement, and wound grafting), pain management, and nutritional support are priorities at this stage and are discussed in detail below.

Airway obstruction caused by upper airway edema can take as long as 48 hours to develop. Changes detected by x-ray and blood gas studies may occur as the effects of resuscitative fluid and the chemical reaction of smoke ingredients with lung tissues become apparent. The patient's arterial blood gas values and other parameters determine the need for intubation or mechanical ventilation.

As capillaries regain integrity, at 48 or more postburn hours, fluid moves from the interstitial to the intravascular compartment and diuresis begins (Table 53-4). If cardiac or renal function is inadequate, for instance in the elderly patient or in the patient with preexisting cardiac disease, fluid overload occurs and symptoms of congestive heart failure may result (see Chap. 27). Early detection allows for early intervention and carefully calculated fluid intake. Vasoactive medications, diuretics, and fluid restriction may be used to support circulatory function and prevent congestive heart failure and pulmonary edema.

Cautious administration of fluids and electrolytes continues during this phase of burn care because of the shifts in fluid from the interstitial to intravascular compartments, losses of fluid from large burn wounds, and the patient's physiologic responses to the burn injury. Blood components are administered as needed to treat blood loss and anemia.

Fever is common in burn patients after burn shock resolves. A resetting of the core body temperature in severely burned patients results in a body temperature a few degrees higher than normal for several weeks after the burn. Bacteremia and septicemia also cause fever in many patients. Acetaminophen (Tylenol) and hypothermia blankets may be required to maintain body temperature in a range of 37.2° to 38.3°C (99° to 101°F) to reduce metabolic stress and tissue oxygen demand.

Central venous, peripheral arterial, or pulmonary artery thermodilution catheters may be required for monitoring venous and arterial pressures, pulmonary artery pressures, pulmonary capillary wedge pressures, or cardiac output. Generally, however, invasive vascular lines are avoided unless essential because they provide an additional port for infection in an already greatly compromised patient.

Infection progressing to septic shock is the major cause of death in patients who have survived the first few days after a major burn. The immunosuppression that accompanies extensive burn injury places the patient at high risk for sepsis. The infection that begins within the burn site may spread to the bloodstream.

(text continues on page 1515)

15•1 PLAN OF NURSING CARE 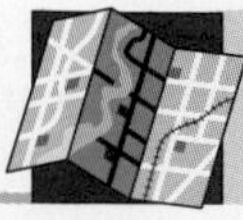

Care of the Patient During the Emergent/Resuscitative Phase of Burn Injury

Nursing Diagnosis: Impaired gas exchange related to carbon monoxide poisoning, smoke inhalation, and upper airway obstruction
Goal: Maintenance of adequate tissue oxygenation

Nursing Interventions	Rationale	Expected Outcomes
1. Provide humidified oxygen.	1. Humidified oxygen provides moisture to injured tissues; supplemental oxygen increases alveolar oxygenation	• Absence of dyspnea • Respiratory rate between 12 and 20 breaths/min • Lungs clear on auscultation • Arterial oxygen saturation >96% by pulse oximetry • Arterial blood gas levels within normal limits
2. Assess breath sounds, and respiratory rate, rhythm, depth, and symmetry. Monitor patient for signs of hypoxia.	2. These factors provide baseline for further assessment and evidence of increasing respiratory compromise.	
3. Observe for the following: a. Erythema or blistering of lips or buccal mucosa b. Singed nostrils c. Burns of face, neck, or chest d. Increasing hoarseness e. Soot in sputum or tracheal tissue in respiratory secretions	3. These signs indicate possible inhalation injury and risk of respiratory dysfunction.	
4. Monitor arterial blood gas values, pulse oximetry readings, and carboxyhemoglobin levels.	4. Increasing PCO_2 and decreasing PO_2 and O_2 saturation may indicate need for mechanical ventilation.	
5. Report labored respirations, decreased depth of respirations, or signs of hypoxia to physician immediately.	5. Immediate intervention is indicated for respiratory difficulty.	
6. Prepare to assist with intubation and escharotomies.	6. Intubation allows mechanical ventilation. Escharotomy enables chest excursion in circumferential chest burns.	
7. Monitor mechanically ventilated patient closely.	7. Monitoring allows early detection of decreasing respiratory status or complications of mechanical ventilation.	

Nursing Diagnosis: Ineffective airway clearance related to edema and effects of smoke inhalation
Goal: Maintain patent airway and adequate airway clearance

Nursing Interventions	Rationale	Expected Outcomes
1. Maintain patent airway through proper patient positioning, removal of secretions, and artificial airway if needed.	1. A patent airway is crucial to respiration.	• Patent airway • Respiratory secretions are minimal, colorless, and thin • Respiratory rate, pattern, and breath sounds normal
2. Provide humidified oxygen.	2. Humidity liquefies secretions and facilitates expectoration.	
3. Encourage patient to turn, cough, and deep breathe. Encourage patient to use incentive spirometry. Suction as needed.	3. These activities promote mobilization and removal of secretions.	

Nursing Diagnosis: Fluid volume deficit related to increased capillary permeability and evaporative losses from the burn wound
Goal: Restoration of optimal fluid and electrolyte balance and perfusion of vital organs

Nursing Interventions	Rationale	Expected Outcomes
1. Observe vital signs (including central venous pressure or pulmonary artery pressure, if indicated) and urine output, and be alert for signs of hypovolemia or fluid overload.	1. Hypovolemia is a major risk immediately after the burn injury. Overresuscitation might cause fluid overload	• Serum electrolytes within normal limits • Urine output between 0.5 and 1.0 mL/kg/hr • Blood pressure higher than 90/60 mm Hg • Heart rate less than 120 beats/min • Exhibits clear sensorium • Voids clear yellow urine with specific gravity within normal limits
2. Monitor urine output at least hourly and weigh patient daily.	2. Output and weight provide information about renal perfusion, adequacy of fluid replacement, and fluid requirement and fluid status.	
3. Maintain IV lines and regulate fluids at appropriate rates, as prescribed.	3. Adequate fluids are necessary to maintain fluid and electrolyte balance and perfusion of vital organs.	

(*continued*)

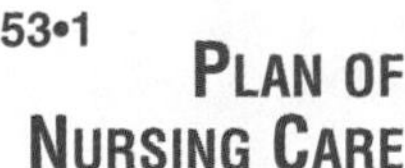
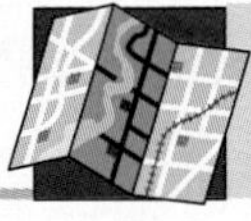

53•1 PLAN OF NURSING CARE

Care of the Patient During the Emergent/Resuscitative Phase of Burn Injury (*continued*)

Nursing Interventions	Rationale	Expected Outcomes
4. Observe for symptoms of deficiency or excess of serum sodium, potassium, calcium, phosphorus, and bicarbonate.	4. Rapid shifts in fluid and electrolyte status are possible in the postburn period.	
5. Elevate head of patient's bed and elevate burned extremities.	5. Elevation promotes venous return.	
6. Notify physician immediately of decreased urine output, blood pressure, central venous, pulmonary artery, or pulmonary artery wedge pressures, or increased pulse rate.	6. Because of the rapid fluid shifts in burn shock, fluid deficit must be detected early so that distributive shock does not occur.	

Nursing Diagnosis: Hypothermia related to loss of skin microcirculation and open wounds
Goal: Maintenance of adequate body temperature

Nursing Interventions	Rationale	Expected Outcomes
1. Provide a warm environment through use of heat shield, space blanket, heat lights, or blankets.	1. A stable environment minimizes evaporative heat loss.	• Body temperature remains 36.1 to 38.3°C (97° to 101°F) • Absence of chills or shivering
2. Work quickly when wounds must be exposed.	2. Minimal exposure minimizes heat loss from wound.	
3. Assess core body temperature frequently.	3. Frequent temperature assessments help detect developing hypothermia.	

Nursing Diagnosis: Pain related to tissue and nerve injury and emotional impact of injury
Goal: Control of pain

Nursing Interventions	Rationale	Expected Outcomes
1. Use pain intensity scale to assess pain level (ie, 1 to 10). Differentiate from hypoxia.	1. Pain level provides baseline for evaluating effectiveness of pain relief measures. Hypoxia can cause similar signs and must be ruled out before analgesic medication is administered.	• States pain level is decreased • Absence of nonverbal cues of pain
2. Administer intravenous opioid analgesics as prescribed. Observe for respiratory depression in the patient who is not mechanically ventilated. Assess response to analgesic.	2. Intravenous administration is necessary because of altered tissue perfusion from burn injury.	
3. Provide emotional support and reassurance.	3. Emotional support is essential to reduce fear and anxiety resulting from burn injury. Fear and anxiety increase the perception of pain.	

Nursing Diagnosis: Anxiety related to fear and the emotional impact of burn injury
Goal: Minimization of patient's and family's anxiety

Nursing Interventions	Rationale	Expected Outcomes
1. Assess patient's and family's understanding of burn injury, coping skills, and family dynamics.	1. Previous successful coping strategies can be fostered for use in the present crisis. Assessment allows planning of individualized interventions.	• Patient and family verbalize understanding of emergent burn care • Able to answer simple questions
2. Individualize responses to the patient's and family's coping level.	2. Reactions to burn injury are extremely variable. Interventions must be appropriate to the patient's and family's present level of coping.	
3. Explain all procedures to the patient and the family in clear, simple terms.	3. Increased understanding alleviates fear of the unknown. High levels of anxiety may interfere with understanding of complex explanations.	
4. Maintain adequate pain relief.	4. Pain increases anxiety.	

(*continued*)

53•1

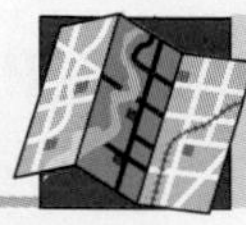

PLAN OF NURSING CARE — **Care of the Patient During the Emergent/Resuscitative Phase of Burn Injury (*continued*)**

Nursing Interventions	Rationale	Expected Outcomes
5. Consider administering prescribed anti-anxiety medications if the patient remains extremely anxious despite nonpharmacologic interventions.	5. Anxiety levels during the emergent phase may exceed the patient's coping abilities. Medication decreases physiologic and psychological anxiety responses.	

Collaborative Problems: Acute respiratory failure, distributive shock, acute renal failure, compartment syndrome, paralytic ileus, Curling's ulcer

Goal: Absence of complications

Nursing Interventions	Rationale	Expected Outcomes
Acute Respiratory Failure		
1. Assess for increasing dyspnea, stridor, changes in respiratory patterns.	1. Such signs reflect deteriorating respiratory status.	• Arterial blood gas values within acceptable limits: PO_2 >80 mm Hg, PCO_2 <50 mm Hg
2. Monitor pulse oximetry, arterial blood gas values for decreasing PO_2 and oxygen saturation, and increasing PCO_2.	2. Such signs reflect decreased oxygenation status.	• Breathes spontaneously with adequate tidal volume
3. Monitor chest x-ray results.	3. X-ray may disclose pulmonary injury.	• Chest x-ray findings normal
4. Assess for restlessness, confusion, difficulty attending to questions, or decreasing level of consciousness.	4. Such manifestations may indicate cerebral hypoxia.	• Absence of cerebral signs of hypoxia
5. Report deteriorating respiratory status immediately to physician.	5. Acute respiratory failure is life-threatening, and immediate intervention is required.	
6. Prepare to assist with intubation or escharotomies as indicated.	6. Intubation allows mechanical ventilation. Escharotomies allow improved chest excursion with respirations.	
Distributive Shock		
1. Assess for decreasing urine output, pulmonary artery and pulmonary artery wedge pressures, blood pressure, and cardiac output, or increasing pulse.	1. Such signs and symptoms may indicate distributive shock and inadequate intravascular volume.	• Urine output between 0.5 and 1.0 mL/kg/hr • Blood pressure within patient's normal range (usually >90/60 mm Hg)
2. Assess for progressive edema as fluid shifts occur.	2. As fluid shifts into the interstitial spaces in burn shock, edema occurs and may compromise tissue perfusion.	• Heart rate within patient's normal range (usually <110/min) • Pressures and cardiac output remain within normal limits
3. Adjust fluid resuscitation in collaboration with the physician in response to physiologic findings.	3. Optimal fluid resuscitation prevents distributive shock and improves patient outcomes.	
Acute Renal Failure		
1. Monitor urine output and blood urea nitrogen (BUN) and creatinine levels.	1. These values reflect renal function.	• Adequate urine output • BUN and creatinine values remain normal
2. Report decreased urine output or increased BUN and creatinine values to physician.	2. These laboratory values indicate possible renal failure.	
3. Assess urine for hemoglobin or myoglobin.	3. Hemoglobin or myoglobin in the urine points to an increased risk of renal failure.	
4. Administer increased fluids as prescribed.	4. Fluids help to flush out hemoglobin and myoglobin from renal tubules, decreasing the potential for renal failure.	
Compartment Syndrome		
1. Assess peripheral pulses hourly with Doppler ultrasound device.	1. Assessment with Doppler device substitutes for auscultation and indicates characteristics of arterial blood flow.	• Absence of paresthesias or symptoms of ischemia of nerves and muscles • Peripheral pulses detectable by Doppler
2. Assess warmth, capillary refill, sensation, and movement of extremity hourly. Compare affected with unaffected extremity.	2. These assessments indicate characteristics of peripheral perfusion.	
3. Remove blood pressure cuff after each reading.	3. Cuff may act as a tourniquet as extremities swell.	
4. Elevate burned extremities.	4. Elevation reduces edema formation.	

(*continued*)

53•1 PLAN OF NURSING CARE 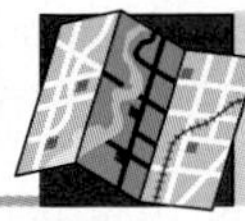

Care of the Patient During the Emergent/Resuscitative Phase of Burn Injury (*continued*)

Nursing Interventions	Rationale	Expected Outcomes
5. Report loss of pulse or sensation or presence of pain to physician immediately.	5. These signs and symptoms may indicate inadequate tissue perfusion.	
6. Prepare to assist with escharotomies.	6. Escharotomies relieve the constriction caused by swelling under circumferential burns and improve tissue perfusion.	
Paralytic Ileus		
1. Maintain nasogastric tube on low intermittent suction until bowel sounds resume.	1. This measure relieves gastric and abdominal distention, also prevents vomiting.	• Absence of abdominal distention • Normal bowel sounds within 48 hours
2. Auscultate for bowel sounds, abdominal distention.	2. As bowel sounds resume, feeding may be slowly initiated. Abdominal distention reflects inadequate decompression.	
Curling's Ulcer		
1. Assess gastric aspirate for pH and blood.	1. Acidic pH indicates need for antacids or histamine blockers. Blood indicates possible gastric bleeding.	• Absence of abdominal distention • Normal bowel sounds within 48 hours • Gastric aspirate and stools do not contain blood
2. Assess stools for occult blood.	2. Blood in stools may indicate gastric or duodenal ulcer.	
3. Administer histamine blockers and antacids as prescribed.	3. Such medications reduce gastric acidity and risk of ulceration.	

Infection Prevention

Despite aseptic precautions and the use of topical antimicrobial agents, the burn wound is an excellent medium for bacterial growth and proliferation. Bacteria such as *Staphylococcus*, *Proteus*, *Pseudomonas*, *Escherichia coli*, and *Klebsiella* find optimal conditions for growth within the burn wound. The burn eschar is a nonviable crust with no blood supply; therefore, neither polymorphonuclear leukocytes or antibodies nor systemic antibiotics can reach the area. Phenomenal numbers of bacteria—more than 1 billion per gram of tissue—may appear and subsequently spread to the bloodstream or release their toxins, which reach distant sites. Fungi such as *Candida albicans* also grow easily in burn wounds.

When the burn wound is healing through spontaneous reepithelialization or is being prepared for skin grafting, it must be protected from sepsis. Burn wound sepsis has these characteristics:

- 10^5 bacteria per gram of tissue
- Inflammation
- Sludging and thrombosis of dermal blood vessels

The primary source of bacterial infection appears to be the patient's intestinal tract. A major secondary source is the environment. Cap, gown, mask, and gloves are worn while caring for the patient with open burn wounds. Clean technique is used when caring directly for burn wounds.

Antibiotics are seldom given prophylactically because of the risk of promoting resistant strains of bacteria. Tissue specimens are taken for culture regularly to monitor colonization of the wound by microbial organisms. These may be swab, surface, or tissue biopsy cultures. Swab or surface cultures are noninvasive, simple, and painless, but data obtained from such cultures apply only to the area sampled; therefore, invasive wound biopsy cultures may be required. Systemic antibiotics are administered when there is documentation of burn wound sepsis or other positive cultures such as urine, sputum, or blood. Sensitivity of the organisms to the prescribed antibiotics should be determined before administration. Several parenteral antimicrobial agents may be given together to treat the infection.

TABLE 53•4 Fluid and Electrolyte Changes in the Acute Phase

Fluid remobilization phase (state of diuresis)
Interstitial fluid → plasma

Observation	Explanation
Hemodilution (decreased hematocrit)	Blood cell concentration is diluted as fluid enters the intravascular compartment; loss of red blood cells destroyed at burn site
Increased urinary output	Fluid shift into intravascular compartment increases renal blood flow and causes increased urine formation.
Sodium (Na^+) deficit	With diuresis, sodium is lost with water; existing serum sodium is diluted by water influx.
Potassium (K^+) deficit (occurs occasionally in this phase)	Beginning on the fourth or fifth postburn day, K^+ shifts from extracellular fluid into cells.
Metabolic acidosis	Loss of sodium depletes fixed base; relative carbon dioxide content increases.

Wound Cleaning

Various measures can be taken to clean the burn wound. **Hydrotherapy** in the form of shower carts, individual showers, and bed baths can be used to clean the wounds. Total immersion hydrotherapy is performed in some settings. Because of the high risk of infection and sepsis, the use of plastic liners and thorough decontamination of hydrotherapy equipment and wound care areas are necessary to prevent cross-contamination. Tap water alone can be used for burn wound cleansing. The temperature of the water is maintained at 37.8°C (100°F), and the temperature of the room should be maintained between 26.6° and 29.4°C (80° to 85°F). Hydrotherapy, in whatever form, should be limited to a 20- to 30-minute period to prevent chilling and additional metabolic stress.

During the bath, the patient is encouraged to be as active as possible. Hydrotherapy provides an excellent opportunity for exercising the extremities and cleaning the entire body. When the patient is removed from the tub after the bath, any residue adhering to the body is washed away with a clear water spray or shower. Unburned areas, including the hair, must be washed regularly as well. At the time of wound cleaning, all skin is inspected for any hints of redness, breakdown, or local infection. Hair in and around the burn area, except the eyebrows, should be clipped short. Intact blisters may be left, but the fluid should be aspirated with a needle and syringe and discarded.

Conscientious management of the burn wound is essential. When nonviable loose skin is removed, aseptic conditions must be established. Wound cleaning is usually performed at least daily in wound areas that are not undergoing surgical intervention. When the eschar begins to separate from the viable tissue beneath (approximately 1.5 to 2 weeks after the burn), more frequent cleaning and débridement may be in order.

After the burn wounds are cleaned, they are gently patted with towels and the prescribed method of wound care is performed. Physician preferences, the skill level of the nursing staff, and resources in terms of number of personnel, supplies, and time must be considered in choosing the best method for a given patient. Whatever the method, the goal is to protect the wound from overwhelming proliferation of pathogenic organisms and invasion of deeper tissues until either spontaneous healing or skin grafting can be achieved.

Patient comfort and ability to participate in the prescribed treatment are also important considerations. Wound care procedures, particularly tub baths, are metabolically stressful. Therefore, the patient is assessed for signs of chilling, fatigue, changes in hemodynamic status, and pain unrelieved by analgesic medications or relaxation techniques.

Topical Antibacterial Therapy

There is general agreement that some form of antimicrobial therapy applied to the burn wound is the best method of local care in extensive burn injury. Topical antibacterial therapy does not sterilize the burn wound; it simply reduces the number of bacteria so that the overall microbial population can be controlled by the body's host defense mechanisms. Topical therapy promotes conversion of the open, dirty wound to a closed, clean one.

Criteria for choosing a topical agent include the following:

- It is effective against gram-negative organisms, *Pseudomonas aeruginosa*, *Staphylococcus aureus*, and even fungi.
- It is clinically effective.
- It penetrates the eschar but is not systemically toxic.
- It does not lose its effectiveness, allowing another infection to develop.
- It is cost-effective, available, and acceptable to the patient.
- It is easy to apply, minimizing nursing care time.

The three most commonly used topical agents are silver sulfadiazine (Silvadene), silver nitrate, and mafenide acetate (Sulfamylon). These agents are described in Table 53-5. Many other top-

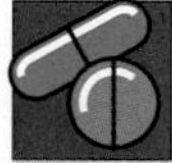

TABLE 53•5 Overview of Topical Antibacterial Agents Used for Burn Wounds

Agent	Indication	Application	Nursing Implications
Silver sulfadiazine 1% (Silvadene) water-soluble cream	• Most bactericidal agent • Minimal penetration of eschar	Apply 1/16-inch layer of cream with a sterile glove 1–3 times daily.	• Watch for leukopenia 2–3 days after initiation of therapy. (Leukopenia usually resolves within 2–3 days.) • Anticipate formation of pseudo-eschar (proteinaceous gel), which is removed easily after 72 hours.
Mafenide acetate 5% to 10% (Sulfamylon) hydrophilic-based cream	• Effective against gram-negative and gram-positive organisms • Diffuses rapidly through eschar • In 10% strength, it is the agent of choice for electrical burns because of its ability to penetrate thick eschar.	Apply thin layer with sterile glove twice a day and leave open as prescribed. Or if the wound is dressed, change the dressing every 6 hours as prescribed.	• Monitor arterial blood gas levels and discontinue as prescribed, if acidosis occurs. Mafenide acetate is a strong carbonic anhydrase inhibitor that may reduce renal buffering and cause metabolic acidosis. • Premedicate the patient with an analgesic before applying mafenide acetate because this agent causes severe burning pain for up to 20 minutes after application.
Silver nitrate 0.5% aqueous solution	• Bacteriostatic and fungicidal • Does *not* penetrate eschar	Apply solution to gauze dressing and place over wound. Keep the dressing wet but covered with dry gauze and dry blankets to decrease vaporization. Remoisten every 2 hours, and redress wound twice a day.	• Monitor serum sodium (Na^+) and potassium (K^+) levels and replace as prescribed. Silver nitrate solution is hypotonic and acts as wick for sodium and potassium. • Protect bed linen and clothing from contact with silver nitrate, which stains everything it touches black.

ical agents are available, including povidone–iodine ointment 10% (Betadine), gentamicin sulfate, nitrofurazone (Furacin), Dakin's solution, acetic acid, miconazole, and chlortrimazole.

No single agent is universally effective. Using different agents at different times in the postburn period may be necessary. Bacteriologic cultures are required to monitor the effect of topical medications. Prudent use and alternation of antimicrobial agents results in less-resistant strains of bacteria, greater effectiveness of the agents, and a decreased risk of sepsis.

Before a topical agent is reapplied, the previously applied topical agent must be thoroughly removed. The number of times the dressings are changed and soaked is planned to promote optimal therapeutic use of the topical agent.

Wound Dressing

When the wound is clean, the burned areas are patted dry and the prescribed topical agent is applied; the wound is then covered with several layers of dressings. A light dressing is used over joint areas to allow for motion (unless the area has a graft there and motion is contraindicated). A light dressing is also applied over areas for which a splint has been designed to conform to the body contour for proper positioning. Circumferential dressings should be applied distally to proximally. If the hand or foot is burned, the fingers and toes should be wrapped individually to promote adequate healing.

Close communication and cooperation among the patient, surgeon, nurse, and other health care team members are essential for optimal burn wound care. Different wound areas on a given patient may require a variety of wound care techniques. Diagrams posted at the bedside are useful to inform staff of the current prescription for wound care, splints to be applied over dressings, and the exercise regimen to be followed before dressings are reapplied.

EXPOSURE METHOD

Occasionally, a wound is treated by exposing it to air. Wound care proceeds in the described manner and a topical agent is applied (mafenide most frequently), but no dressings are applied. The success of the exposure method depends on keeping the immediate environment free of organisms. Some practitioners maintain that everything coming in contact with the patient must be sterile. Linens are sterile; those who come in direct contact with the patient wear masks, caps, sterile gowns, and gloves; and visitors are instructed to wear protective garb and not to touch the bed or hand the patient anything. Other practitioners maintain a clean environment and rely on the efficiency of the topical antibacterial agents to limit burn wound infection.

The patient's room must be maintained at a comfortably warm temperature with 40% to 50% humidity to prevent excessive evaporative fluid losses as well as to maintain the patient's body temperature. A cradle may be placed over the patient to prevent sheets from coming in contact with the burn area, to minimize the effects of air currents (to which a burn patient is unusually sensitive), and to provide some covering.

Generally, small areas such as the face, neck, or perineum may also be effectively treated with the exposure method, while other areas of the wound may be dressed.

OCCLUSIVE METHOD

There is a role for occlusive dressings in treating specific wounds. An occlusive dressing is a thin gauze that is either impregnated with a topical antimicrobial or that is applied after topical antimicrobial application. Occlusive dressings are most often used over areas with new skin grafts. These dressings are applied under sterile conditions in the operating room. Their purpose is to protect the graft, promoting an optimal condition for its adherence to the recipient site. Ideally, these dressings remain in place for 3 to 5 days, at which time they are removed by the physician for examination of the graft.

When these dressings are applied, precautions are taken to prevent two body surfaces from touching, such as fingers or toes, ear and scalp, the areas under the breasts, any point of flexion, or between the genital folds. Functional body alignment positions are maintained by using splints or by careful positioning of the patient.

Dressing Changes

Dressings are changed in the patient's unit, hydrotherapy room, or treatment area approximately 20 minutes after an analgesic is administered. They may also be changed in the operating room after the patient is anesthetized. A mask, hair cover, disposable plastic apron or cover gown, and gloves are worn by health care personnel when removing the dressings. The outer dressings are slit with blunt scissors, and the soiled dressings are removed and disposed of in accordance with established procedures for contaminated materials.

Dressings that adhere to the wound can be removed more comfortably if they are moistened with saline solution or if the patient is allowed to soak for a few moments in the tub. The remaining dressings are carefully and gently removed with forceps or gloved hands. The patient may participate in removing the dressings, providing some degree of control over this painful procedure. The wounds are then cleaned and débrided to remove debris, any remaining topical agent, exudate, and dead skin. Sterile scissors and forceps may be used to trim loose eschar and encourage separation of devitalized skin. During this procedure, the wound and surrounding skin are carefully inspected. The color, odor, size, exudate, signs of reepithelialization, and other characteristics of the wound and the eschar and any changes from the previous dressing change are noted.

Wound Débridement

Débridement, another facet of burn wound care, has two goals:

- To remove tissue contaminated by bacteria and foreign bodies, thereby protecting the patient from invasion of bacteria
- To remove devitalized tissue or burn eschar in preparation for grafting and wound healing

There are three types of débridement—natural, mechanical, and surgical.

NATURAL DÉBRIDEMENT

With natural débridement, the dead tissue separates from the underlying viable tissue spontaneously. After partial- and full-thickness burns occur, bacteria that are present at the interface of the burned tissue and the viable tissue underneath gradually liquefy the fibrils of **collagen** (a protein present in skin, tendon, bone, cartilage, and connective tissue) that hold the eschar in place for the first or second postburn week. Proteolytic and other natural enzymes cause this phenomenon. Using antibacterial topical agents, however, tends to slow down this natural process of eschar separation. It is advantageous to the patient to speed this process through other means, such as mechanical or surgical débridement, thereby reducing the time during which bacterial invasion and other iatrogenic problems may arise.

MECHANICAL DÉBRIDEMENT

Mechanical débridement involves using surgical scissors and forceps to separate and remove the eschar. This technique can be performed by skilled physicians, nurses, or physical therapists and is usually done with daily dressing changes and wound cleaning procedures. Débridement by these means is carried out to the point of pain and bleeding. Hemostatic agents or pressure can be used to stop bleeding from small vessels.

Dressings are also helpful débriding agents. Coarse-mesh dressings applied dry or wet-to-dry (applied wet and allowed to dry) will slowly débride the wound of exudate and eschar when they are removed. Topical enzymatic débridement agents are available to promote débridement of the burn wounds. Because such agents are not antibacterial in themselves, they should be used with topical antibacterial therapy to protect the patient from bacterial invasion.

SURGICAL DÉBRIDEMENT

Surgical débridement is an operative procedure involving either primary **excision** (surgical removal of tissue) of the full thickness of the skin down to the fascia (tangential excision) or shaving the burned skin layers gradually down to freely bleeding, viable tissue. Surgical excision is initiated early in burn wound management. This may be performed a few days after the burn or as soon as the patient is hemodynamically stable and edema has decreased. Ideally, the wound is then covered immediately with a skin graft, if needed, and an occlusive dressing. If the wound bed is not ready for a skin graft at the time of excision, a temporary biologic dressing may be used until a skin graft can be applied during subsequent surgery.

The use of surgical excision carries with it risks and complications, especially with large burns. The procedure creates a high risk of extensive blood loss (as much as 100 to 125 mL of blood per percent BSA excised) and lengthy operating and anesthesia time. However, when conducted in a timely and efficient manner, surgical excision results in shorter hospital stays and possibly a decreased risk of complications from invasive burn wound sepsis.

Grafting the Burn Wound

If wounds are deep (full-thickness) or extensive, spontaneous reepithelialization is not possible. Therefore, coverage of the burn wound is necessary until coverage with a graft of the patient's own skin (**autograft**) is possible. The purposes of wound coverage are to decrease the risk for infection; prevent further loss of protein, fluid, and electrolytes through the wound; and minimize heat loss through evaporation. Several methods of wound coverage are available; some are temporary until grafting with permanent coverage is possible. Wound coverage may use biologic, biosynthetic, synthetic, and autologous methods or a combination of these approaches.

The main areas for skin grafting include the face, for cosmetic and psychological reasons; the hands and other functional areas such as the feet; and areas that involve joints. Grafting permits earlier functional ability and reduces **contractures** (shrinkage of burn scar through collagen maturation). When burns are very extensive, the chest and abdomen may be grafted first to reduce the burn surface.

During wound healing, granulation tissue develops. It fills the space created by the wound, creates a barrier to bacteria, and serves as a bed for epithelial cell growth. Richly vascular granulation tissue is pink, firm, shiny, and free of exudate and debris. It should have a bacterial count of less than 100,000 per gram of tissue to optimize graft take. A preoperative culture is mandatory before autografting, because enzymes of bacteria can dissolve a graft and lead to its failure. Beta-hemolytic streptococci are a major factor in graft failure.

BIOLOGIC DRESSINGS (HOMOGRAFTS AND HETEROGRAFTS)

Biologic dressings have several uses. In extensive burns, they can be lifesaving by providing temporary wound closure and protecting the granulation tissue until autografting is possible. This is common in patients with large areas of burn and little remaining normal skin donor sites. Biologic dressings may also be used to débride untidy wounds after eschar separation. With each biologic dressing change, débridement occurs. Once the biologic dressing appears to be "taking," or adhering to the granulating surface with minimal underlying exudation, the patient is ready for an autograft.

Biologic dressings also provide immediate coverage for clean, superficial burns and decrease the wound's evaporative water and protein loss. They decrease pain by protecting nerve endings and are an effective barrier against water loss and entry of bacteria. When applied to superficial partial-thickness wounds, they seem to speed healing. Biologic materials can be left open or covered. They stay in place for varying lengths of time but are removed in instances of infection or rejection.

Biologic dressings consist of **homografts** (or allografts) and **heterografts** (or xenografts). Homografts are skin obtained from living or recently deceased humans. The amniotic membrane (amnion) from the human placenta may also be used as a biologic dressing. Heterografts consist of skin taken from animals (usually pigs). Most biologic dressings are used as temporary coverings of burn wounds and are eventually rejected because of the body's immune reaction to them as foreign.

Homografts tend to be the most expensive biologic dressings. They are available from skin banks in fresh and cryopreserved (frozen) forms. Homografts are thought to provide the best infection control of all the biologic or biosynthetic dressings available. Revascularization occurs within 48 hours, and the graft may be left in place for several weeks.

Amnion is low in cost and is available in hospitals with burn centers and specialized tissue banks, which obtain and process it in cooperation with obstetric services. However, amnion grafts do not become vascularized by the patient's vessels and can be left in place only briefly.

Pigskin is available from commercial suppliers. It is available fresh, frozen, or lyophilized (freeze-dried) for longer shelf life. Pigskin impregnated with a topical antibacterial such as silver nitrate is also available.

Unlike other biologic dressings, which are eventually rejected by the body, one new biologic dressing that has shown promise for permanent burn wound coverage is **Alloderm**. Alloderm is processed dermis from human cadaver skin, which can be used as the dermal layer for skin grafts. When a **donor site** (the area from which skin is taken to provide a skin graft for another part of the body) is harvested for an autologous skin graft, both the epidermal and dermal layers of skin are removed from the donor site. However, Alloderm provides a permanent dermal layer replacement. Use of Alloderm allows the burn surgeon to harvest a thinner skin graft consisting of the epidermal layer only. The patient's epidermal layer is placed directly over the dermal base (Alloderm). The new graft is then treated according to the burn unit's protocol. Use of Alloderm has resulted in less scarring and contractures with healed grafts; donor sites heal much more quickly than conventional donor sites because only the epidermal layer has been harvested. This is important when donor sites are limited because of extensive burns.

BIOSYNTHETIC AND SYNTHETIC DRESSINGS

Problems with availability, sterility, and cost have prompted the search for biosynthetic and synthetic skin substitutes, which may eventually replace biologic dressings as temporary wound coverings. Currently, the most widely used synthetic dressing is **Biobrane**, which is composed of a nylon, Silastic membrane combined with a collagen derivative. The material is semitransparent and sterile. It has an indefinite shelf life and is less costly than homograft or pigskin. Like biologic dressings, Biobrane protects the wound from fluid loss and bacterial invasion.

Biobrane adheres to the wound fibrin, which binds to the nylon–collagen material. Within 5 days, cells migrate into the nylon mesh. Generally, adherence to the wound surface correlates directly with low bacterial counts. When the Biobrane dressing adheres to the wound, the wound remains stable and the Biobrane can remain in place for 3 to 4 weeks. Biobrane dressings (Fig. 53-4) readily adhere to donor sites and meticulously clean débrided partial-thickness wounds; they will remain until spontaneous epithelialization and wound healing occur. Biobrane can be laid on top of a wide-meshed autograft to protect the wound until the autograft epithelium grows out to close the interstices. As the Biobrane gradually separates, it is trimmed, leaving a healed wound.

Biobrane is also useful for intermediate or long-term closure of a surgically excised wound until an autograft becomes available. Like biologic dressings, Biobrane should not be used over grossly contaminated or necrotic wounds. Removal of Biobrane after several weeks is similar to but easier than removal of a vascularized allograft and leaves a bleeding granulation bed that readily accepts an autograft.

Several other synthetic dressings are available for burn wound care. Op-Site, a thin, transparent, polyurethane elastic film, can be used to cover clean partial-thickness wounds and donor sites. This dressing is occlusive and waterproof but permeable to water vapor and air; this permeability not only provides protection from microbial contamination but also allows for the exchange of gases, which occurs much more quickly in a moist environment. Other synthetic dressings used for burn wounds include Tegaderm, N-Terface, and DuoDerm.

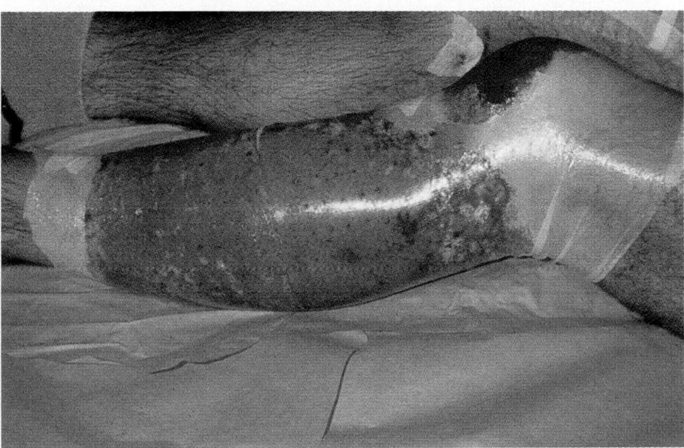

FIGURE 53•4 Biobrane dressing applied to lower extremity partial-thickness burn. Used with permission of Dow Hickam Pharmaceuticals.

Artificial skin (**Integra**) is the newest type of synthetic dressing. A dermal analogue, Integra is composed of two main layers. The epidermal layer, consisting of Silastic, acts as a bacterial barrier and prevents water loss from the dermis. The dermal layer is composed of animal collagen. It interfaces with the open wound surface and allows migration of fibroblasts and capillaries into the material. This "neodermis" becomes a permanent structure. The artificial dermis is biodegraded and resorbed. The epidermal layer is removed 2 to 3 weeks after application and is replaced with the patient's own skin. Contracture has been reported to be minimal, with no hypertrophic scarring. The appearance resembles that of normal skin.

AUTOGRAFTS

Autografts are the ideal means of covering burn wounds because they come from the patient's own skin and thus are not rejected by the patient's immune system. They can be split-thickness, full-thickness, pedicle flaps, or **cultured epithelium**. Full-thickness and pedicle flaps are commonly used for reconstructive surgery, months or years after the initial injury.

Use of cultured epithelium is becoming common at several burn centers. This involves a biopsy of the patient's skin in an unburned area. Keratinocytes are then isolated and epithelial cells are cultured in a laboratory. The original epithelial cell sample can multiply to 10,000 times its original size over 30 days. These cells are then attached to the burn wound. Varying degrees of success have been reported, and results are encouraging.

Split-thickness autografts can be applied in sheets or in postage stamp–like pieces, or they can be expanded by meshing so that they can cover 1.5 to 9 times more than a given donor site area. Skin meshers enable the surgeon to cut tiny slits into a sheet of donor skin, making it possible to cover large areas with smaller amounts of donor skin. These expanded grafts cling to the recipient site more easily than sheet grafts and prevent the accumulation of blood, serum, air, or purulent material under the graft. However, any kind of graft other than a sheet graft will contribute to scar formation as it heals. Using expanded grafts may be necessary in large wounds but should be viewed as a compromise in terms of cosmesis.

If blood, serum, air, fat, or necrotic tissue lies between the recipient site and the graft, there may be partial or total loss of the graft. Infection and mishandling of the graft, as well as trauma during dressing changes, account for most other instances of graft loss. Using split-thickness grafts allows the remaining donor site to retain sweat glands and hair follicles and minimizes donor site healing time.

Care of the Patient With an Autograft.

Occlusive dressings are commonly used initially after grafting to immobilize the graft. Occupational therapists may be helpful in constructing splints to immobilize newly grafted areas to prevent dislodging the graft. Homografts, heterografts, or synthetic dressings may also be used to protect grafts. The graft may be left open with skin staples to immobilize it, which allows close observation of progress.

The first dressing change is usually performed by the surgeon 3 to 5 days after surgery, or earlier in case of purulent drainage or a foul odor. If the graft is dislodged, sterile saline compresses will help prevent drying of the graft until the physician reapplies it.

The patient is positioned and turned carefully to avoid disturbing the graft or putting pressure on the graft site. If an extremity has been grafted, it is elevated to minimize edema. The patient begins exercising the grafted area 5 to 7 days after grafting.

Care of Donor Site. A moist gauze dressing is applied at the time of surgery to maintain pressure and to stop any oozing. A thrombostatic agent such as thrombin or epinephrine may be applied directly to the site as well. The donor site may be treated in several ways, from single-layer gauze impregnated with petrolatum, scarlet red, or bismuth to new biosynthetic dressings such as Biobrane. Donor sites must remain clean, dry, and free from pressure. Ultimately, because a donor site is usually a partial-thickness wound, it will heal spontaneously within 7 to 14 days with proper care; however, the donor site is often painful.

Pain Management

Pain is inevitable during recovery from any burn injury. Management of the often severe pain is one of the most difficult challenges facing the burn team. Many factors contribute to the patient's burn pain experience. These factors include but are not limited to the severity of the patient's pain, the health care provider's pain assessment, the appropriateness and adequacy of pharmacologic treatment of pain, the multiple procedures involved in burn care (ie, wound care, rehabilitative exercises), and appropriate assessment of the effectiveness of pain relief measures. The outstanding features of burn pain are its intensity and long duration. Further, necessary wound care carries with it the anticipation of pain and anxiety. In partial-thickness burns, the nerve endings are exposed, resulting in excruciating pain with exposure to air currents. Although nerve endings are destroyed in full-thickness burns, the margins of the burn wound are hypersensitive to pain, and there is deep pain and pain in adjacent structures. Most severe burns are a combination of partial-thickness and full-thickness burns, resulting in severe pain.

Over a typical burn pain course, there are many peaks and valleys. The primary pain from the burn itself is intense in the initial acute postburn phase. This primary pain gradually subsides. However, for weeks thereafter, until the skin heals or skin grafts are applied and take, the pain level remains high because of treatment-induced pain. Wound cleaning, dressing changes, débridement, and physical therapy are performed often and simultaneously or serially, inflicting intense pain. Even when grafts are applied, making the burn site more comfortable, donor sites are created, which may be intensely painful for several days. Discomfort related to tissue healing, such as itching, tingling, and tightness of contracting skin and joints, adds to the duration, if not the intensity, of pain over weeks or months.

Because pain cannot be eliminated short of complete anesthesia, the goal is to minimize the pain with analgesics before the patient faces wound care procedures. With adequate staff working gently, swiftly, and skillfully, the duration of pain from wound care can be shortened. Bolus doses of opioids, usually morphine, are often provided. Ketamine anesthesia administered intravenously is also used for some wound care procedures in burn units. Sedation with antianxiety mediations such as lorazepam (Ativan) or midazolam (Versed) may be indicated in addition to analgesia.

Patient-controlled analgesia, using both continuous and bolus morphine infusions, and sustained-release oral morphine, given every 12 hours with an additional dose before wound care, have helped burn patients. Self-administered nitrous oxide also helps to make dressing changes more tolerable for patients who have sufficient hand function to hold a mask to their faces intermittently during dressing changes. Early surgical excision with grafting under anesthesia may be the best way to reduce the overall pain experience for burn patients.

Nutritional Support

Hypermetabolism persists after burn injury until wounds are closed, thereby increasing the basal metabolic need by as much as 100%. The goal of nutritional support is to promote a state of positive nitrogen balance. The nutritional support required is based on the patient's preburn status and the extent of total BSA burned.

Several formulas exist for estimating the daily metabolic expenditure and caloric requirements of burn patients. Protein requirements may range from 1.5 to 4.0 g of protein per kilogram of body weight every 24 hours. Lipids are included in the nutritional support of every burn patient because of their importance for wound healing, cellular integrity, and absorption of fat-soluble vitamins. Carbohydrates are included to meet caloric requirements as high as 5,000 calories per day and to spare protein, which is essential for wound healing. The patient also needs adequate vitamins and minerals.

Recent research findings have brought about changes in specific guidelines for estimating energy expenditure during various phases of postburn recovery. The proportions of fat, protein, and carbohydrate are carefully planned for maximal use. Overfeeding can also be detrimental. Therefore, a dietitian familiar with current concepts in nutrition for burn patients should be consulted for all patients with major burns.

Patients lose a great deal of weight during recovery from severe burns. Reserve fat deposits are catabolized, fluids are lost, and caloric intake may be limited. Because burns lower the patient's resistance to infection and disease, the nutritional status must be improved even though the patient has a poor appetite and is weak.

As soon as gastrointestinal function resumes after the patient's condition stabilizes, nutritional support begins. The enteral route is preferred, and many burn patients will tolerate oral fluids and food. In patients with extensive burns, tube feeding may be initiated to ensure a certain number of daily calories. In this case, high-protein, high-caloric snacks and fluids may be offered as supplements to the essential tube feedings. A diet containing semisolid or solid food is usually begun toward the end of the first week, when the patient's tolerance for food improves.

Indications for total parenteral nutrition (TPN) include weight loss greater than 10% of normal body weight, inadequate intake of enteral nutrition due to clinical status, prolonged wound exposure, and malnutrition or debilitated condition before injury. The risk of infection at the site of the central venous catheter required for TPN must be considered. Moreover, the risk of Curling's ulcer continues in the acute phase.

Disorders of Wound Healing

Disorders of wound healing in the burn patient result from excessive abnormal healing or inadequate new tissue formation. **Hypertrophic scarring** and keloid formation result from excessive abnormal healing.

Scars

Hypertrophic scars and wound contractures are more likely to occur if the initial burn injury extends below the level of the deep dermis. Healing of such deep wounds results in the replacement of normal integument with highly metabolically active tissues that lack the normal architecture of the skin. In the collagen layer beneath the epithelium, many fibroblasts proliferate gradually. Myofibroblasts, cells that have the ability to contract, are also present in immature wounds. As the myofibroblasts contract, the collagen fibers, which normally lie in flat bundles, tend to form a wavy pattern. Eventually the collagen bundles take on a supercoiled appearance and collagen nodules develop. The scar becomes very red (because of its hypervascular nature), raised, and hard.

Burn personnel are trained to be proactive in the management of potential scar formation. Compression measures are instituted early in the burn wound treatment. Ace wraps are used initially to help promote adequate circulation, but they can be used as the first form of compression. Scar management occurs mainly in the rehabilitative phase, after the wounds are closed. Hypertrophic scarring may cause severe contracture across involved joints. Therefore, prevention and management of this type of scarring is essential (see "Preventing Hypertrophic Scarring" in the rehabilitation phase discussion). However, these scars are limited to the area of injury and gradually regress over time.

Keloids

A large, heaped-up mass of scar tissue, a keloid, may develop and extend beyond the wound surface. Keloids tend to be found in darkly pigmented people, tend to grow outside of wound margins, and are more likely to recur after surgical excision.

Failure to Heal

Failure of the wound to heal may relate to many factors, including infection and inadequate nutrition. A serum albumin level of less than 2 g/dL is usually a factor in impaired healing in the burn patient.

Contractures

Contractures are another concern as wounds heal. The burn wound tissue shortens because of the force exerted by the fibroblasts and the flexion of muscles in natural wound healing. An opposing force provided by splints, traction, and purposeful movement and positioning must be used to counteract deformity in burns affecting joints.

NURSING PROCESS: BURN CARE DURING THE ACUTE PHASE

Assessment

Continued assessment of the burn patient during the early weeks after the burn focuses on hemodynamic alterations, wound healing, pain and psychosocial responses, and early detection of complications. Assessment of respiratory and fluid status remains the highest priority for detection of potential complications.

The nurse assesses vital signs frequently. Continued assessment of peripheral pulses is essential for the first few postburn days while edema continues to increase, potentially damaging peripheral nerves and restricting blood flow. Observation of the electrocardiogram may give clues to cardiac dysrhythmias resulting from potassium imbalance, preexisting cardiac disease, or the effects of electrical injury or burn shock.

Assessment of residual gastric volumes and pH in the patient with a nasogastric tube is also important and gives clues to early sepsis or the need for antacid therapy. Blood in the gastric fluid or the stools must also be noted and reported.

Assessment of the burn wound requires an experienced eye, hand, and sense of smell. Important wound assessment features include size, color, odor, eschar, exudate, abscess formation under the eschar, epithelial buds (small pearl-like clusters of cells on the wound surface), bleeding, granulation tissue appearance, progress of grafts and donor sites, and quality of surrounding skin. Any significant changes in the wound are reported to the physician, because they usually indicate burn wound or systemic sepsis and require immediate intervention.

Other significant and ongoing assessments focus on pain and psychosocial responses, daily body weights, caloric intake, general hydration, and serum electrolyte and hemoglobin levels and hematocrit. Assessment for excessive bleeding from blood vessels adjacent to areas of surgical exploration and débridement is necessary as well. The Plan of Nursing Care 53-2 provides an outline of nursing activities in the acute phase of burn care.

Diagnosis

Nursing Diagnoses

Based on the assessment data, priority nursing diagnoses in the acute phase of burn care may include the following:

- Fluid volume excess related to resumption of capillary integrity and fluid shift from interstitial to intravascular compartment
- Risk for infection related to loss of skin barrier and impaired immune response
- Altered nutrition, less than body requirements, related to hypermetabolism and wound healing needs
- Impaired skin integrity related to open burn wounds
- Pain related to exposed nerves, wound healing, and treatments
- Impaired physical mobility related to burn wound edema, pain, and joint contractures
- Ineffective individual coping related to fear and anxiety, grieving, and forced dependence on health care providers
- Altered family processes related to burn injury
- Knowledge deficit about the course of burn treatment

Collaborative Problems/Potential Complications

Based on the assessment data, potential complications that may develop in the acute phase of burn care may include:

- Congestive heart failure and pulmonary edema
- Sepsis
- Acute respiratory failure
- ARDS
- Visceral damage (electrical burns)

Planning and Goals

The major goals for the patient may include restoration of normal fluid balance, absence of infection, attainment of anabolic state and normal weight, improved skin integrity, reduction of pain and discomfort, optimal physical mobility, adequate patient and family coping, adequate patient and family knowledge of burn treatment, and absence of complications. Achieving these goals requires a collaborative, interdisciplinary approach to patient management.

Nursing Interventions

Restoring Normal Fluid Balance

To reduce the risk of fluid overload and consequent congestive heart failure, the nurse closely monitors the patient's intravenous and oral fluid intake, using intravenous infusion pumps to minimize the risk of rapid fluid infusion. To monitor changes in fluid status, careful intake and output and daily weights are obtained. Changes in pulmonary artery, wedge, and central venous pressures,

(text continues on page 1526)

53•2

PLAN OF NURSING CARE 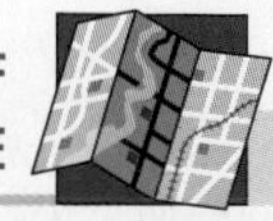 Care of the Patient During the Acute Phase of Burn Injury

Nursing Diagnosis: Fluid volume excess related to resumption of capillary integrity and fluid shift from interstitial to intravascular compartment
Goal: Maintenance of optimal fluid balance

Nursing Interventions	Rationale	Expected Outcomes
1. Monitor vital signs, intake and output, weight. Assess for edema, jugular vein distention (JVD), crackles, increased arterial pressures.	1. These signs reflect fluid status.	• Intake, output, and body weight correlate with expected pattern • Vital signs and arterial pressures remain within designated limits • Urine output increases in response to diuretic and vasoactive medications
2. Notify physician of urine output <30 mL/hr, weight gain, JVD, crackles, increased arterial pressures.	2. These indicate increased fluid volume.	
3. Maintain intravenous fluids on pumps or rate controllers.	3. Regulation prevents accidental fluid bolus.	
4. Administer dopamine or diuretics as prescribed. Assess response.	4. Dopamine increases renal perfusion, which increases urine output. Diuretics promote increased urine formation and urine output and decrease intravascular volume.	

Nursing Diagnosis: Risk for infection related to loss of skin barrier and impaired immune response
Goal: Absence of localized or systemic infection

Nursing Interventions	Rationale	Expected Outcomes
1. Use asepsis in all aspects of patient care: a. Meticulous hand washing before and after patient care. b. Use clean or sterile gloves for wound care. c. Wear isolation gown or protective plastic apron for patient care. d. Wear mask and hair cover when wounds are exposed and during sterile procedures. e. Change invasive lines and tubings as recommended by CDC.	1. Aseptic techniques minimize risk of cross-contamination and spread of bacterial contamination.	• Wound cultures show minimal bacteria • Normal blood, urine, and sputum cultures • Urine output and vital signs within acceptable range • Absence of signs and symptoms of infection and sepsis
2. Screen visitors for respiratory, gastrointestinal, or integumentary infections. Provide isolation gowns for visitors without active infection and instruct in hand washing.	2. Avoiding known infecting agents prevents introduction of additional microorganisms.	
3. Exclude plants and flowers in water from patient's room.	3. Stagnant water is a potential source of bacterial growth.	
4. Inspect wound for signs of infection, purulent drainage, or discoloration.	4. Such signs indicate localized infection.	
5. Monitor white blood cell (WBC) count, culture and sensitivity results.	5. Increased WBC count indicates infection. Culture and sensitivity indicate microorganisms present and appropriate antibiotics to be used.	
6. Administer antibiotics as prescribed.	6. Antibiotics reduce bacteria.	
7. Provide regular linen changes and assist patient with personal hygiene.	7. These measures reduce potential bacterial colonization of burn wound.	
8. Report to physician decreased bowel sounds, tachycardia, decreased blood pressure, decreased urine output, fever, and flushing.	8. These signs may indicate sepsis.	
9. Administer fluids and vasoactive medications as prescribed. Assess response.	9. These agents are used to maintain tissue perfusion in sepsis.	

(*continued*)

53•2 PLAN OF NURSING CARE

Care of the Patient During the Acute Phase of Burn Injury (*continued*)

Nursing Diagnosis: Altered nutrition, less than body requirements, related to hypermetabolism and wound healing
Goal: Attainment of anabolic nutritional status

Nursing Interventions	Rationale	Expected Outcomes
1. Provide high-calorie, high-protein diet; include patient preferences and homemade food. Give nutritional supplements as prescribed.	1. The patient needs sufficient nutrients for wound healing and increased metabolic requirements.	• Gains weight daily after initial loss • Exhibits no signs of protein, vitamin, or mineral deficiencies • Meets required nutritional needs entirely by oral intake • Participates in selection of diet with prescribed nutrients • Serum protein levels within acceptable range
2. Monitor patient's daily weight and calorie count.	2. These measures assist in determining whether dietary needs are being met.	
3. Administer supplemental vitamins and minerals as prescribed.	3. These help meet additional nutritional needs; adequate vitamins and minerals are necessary for wound healing and cellular function.	
4. Administer enteral or total parenteral nutrition per protocol if dietary needs are not met through oral intake.	4. Nutritional techniques ensure that nutritional needs are met.	
5. Report abdominal distention, large gastric residual volumes, or diarrhea to physician.	5. These signs may indicate intolerance of route or type of feeding.	

Nursing Diagnosis: Impaired skin integrity related to open burn wounds
Goal: Demonstration of improved skin integrity

Nursing Interventions	Rationale	Expected Outcomes
1. Clean wounds, body, and hair daily.	1. Daily cleaning reduces potential bacterial colonization.	• Skin is generally intact, and free of signs of infection, pressure, and trauma • Open wounds are pink, reepithelializing, and free of infection • Donor sites are clean and reepithelializing • Healed wounds are soft and smooth • Skin is lubricated and elastic
2. Provide wound care as prescribed.	2. Care promotes wound healing.	
3. Apply topical antibacterial agents and dressing as prescribed.	3. Wound care regimen reduces bacterial colonization and promotes healing.	
4. Prevent pressure, infection, and mobilization of skin grafts.	4. These measures promote graft take and healing.	
5. Provide donor site care.	5. Care promotes healing of donor site.	
6. Provide adequate nutritional support.	6. Adequate nutrition is essential for normal granulation and healing.	
7. Assess wound and graft sites. Report signs of poor healing, poor graft take, or trauma to physician.	7. Early intervention for poor wound healing or graft take is essential. Grafted or healed burn wounds are susceptible to trauma.	

Nursing Diagnosis: Pain related to exposed nerves, wound healing, and treatments
Goal: Reduction or control of pain

Nursing Interventions	Rationale	Expected Outcomes
1. Assess pain level using pain intensity scale. Observe for nonverbal indicators of pain: grimacing, tachycardia, clenched fists.	1. Pain assessment data provide baseline for assessing response to interventions.	• Requests analgesics for specific wound care procedures or physical therapy activities • States pain is minimal • Gives no physiologic or nonverbal cues that pain is moderate or severe • Uses pain control measures such as nitrous oxide, relaxation, imagery, and distraction techniques to assist with coping with pain • Can sleep without being disturbed by pain • Reports skin is comfortable with no itching or tightness
2. Educate the patient about the usual pain trajectory in burn recovery and options for pain control. Allow patient as much control as possible regarding pain management.	2. Knowledge reduces fear of the unknown and provides some measure of control to the patient.	
3. Offer analgesics approximately 20 minutes before painful procedures.	3. Premedication allows time for therapeutic response.	
4. Provide analgesia before pain becomes severe.	4. Pain is more easily controlled before it becomes severe.	
5. Instruct and assist patient in relaxation, imagery, distraction techniques.	5. Nonpharmacologic pain measures provide multiple interventions to decrease pain sensation.	
6. Assess and document the patient's response to interventions.	6. Patient's responses assist in ascertaining best pain control techniques for the patient.	

(*continued*)

53•2 PLAN OF NURSING CARE

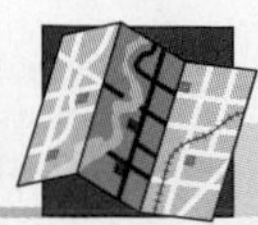

Care of the Patient During the Acute Phase of Burn Injury (*continued*)

Nursing Interventions	Rationale	Expected Outcomes
7. Administer antianxiety and antipruritic agents as indicated.	7. These medications help to increase patient's comfort.	
8. Lubricate healing burn wounds with water- or silica-based lotion.	8. These preparations decrease sensation of skin tightness.	

Nursing Diagnosis: Impaired physical mobility related to burn wound edema, pain, and joint contractures
Goal: Achievement of optimal physical mobility

Nursing Interventions	Rationale	Expected Outcomes
1. Position patient carefully to prevent flexed position in burned areas.	1. Proper positioning reduces risk of flexion contractures.	• Improves range of motion of joints daily • Demonstrates preinjury range of motion of all joints • Absence of signs of periarticular calcification • Participates in activities of daily living
2. Implement range-of-motion (ROM) exercises several times daily.	2. ROM exercises minimize muscle atrophy.	
3. Assist with early sitting and ambulation.	3. Early mobility encourages increased use of muscles.	
4. Use splints and exercise devices recommended by occupational and physical therapists.	4. Such devices encourage activity while maintaining proper position of joints.	
5. Encourage self-care to the extent of the patient's ability.	5. Self-care promotes both independence and increased activity.	

Nursing Diagnosis: Ineffective individual coping related to fear and anxiety, grieving, and forced dependence on health care providers
Goal: Use of appropriate coping strategies to deal with postburn problems

Nursing Interventions	Rationale	Expected Outcomes
1. Assess patient for coping abilities and previous successful coping strategies.	1. Psychosocial data provide baseline for planning care.	• Verbalizes reactions to burns, therapeutic procedures, losses • Identifies coping strategies used previously in stressful situations • Accepts dependency on health care providers during acute illness • Resolves grief over losses resulting from burn injury • Participates in decision making regarding care • Has hopeful attitude toward future
2. Demonstrate acceptance of patient. Provide positive feedback and support.	2. Acceptance encourages self-esteem and continued progress toward independence.	
3. Assist patient to set achievable short-term goals for increased independence in activities of daily living.	3. Short-term goal setting leads to pattern of success for patient. Long-term goals may seem unrealistic or unattainable to patient.	
4. Use multidisciplinary approach to promote mobility and independence.	4. Communication among disciplines provides consistent approach.	
5. Consult with health care team members for assistance with regressive or maladaptive behaviors.	5. Collaboration uses the expertise of others.	

Nursing Diagnosis: Altered family processes related to burn injury
Goal: Achievement of appropriate patient/family processes

Nursing Interventions	Rationale	Expected Outcomes
1. Assess patient and family's perception of impact of burn injury on family functioning.	1. Assessment data provide baseline from which to plan care.	• Patient verbalizes feelings regarding alteration in family interactions • Family can emotionally support the patient during hospitalization • Family states that needs are met
2. Demonstrate willingness to listen. Provide realistic support.	2. Empathetic attitude promotes verbalizing of concerns.	
3. Refer family to social services and other resources as needed.	3. Collaboration assists to address concerns comprehensively.	
4. Explain the burn patient's coping patterns to family. Discuss ways that they can support the patient.	4. Explanations help decrease anxiety about the unknown and promote appropriate intervention by families toward patient.	

Nursing Diagnosis: Knowledge deficit about the course of burn treatment
Goal: Verbalization of understanding of the course of burn treatment by patient and family

Nursing Interventions	Rationale	Expected Outcomes
1. Assess readiness of patient and family to learn.	1. Limit education to patient's and family's ability to process information.	• States rationale for different aspects of treatment

(*continued*)

53•2 PLAN OF NURSING CARE 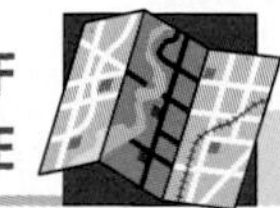

Care of the Patient During the Acute Phase of Burn Injury (*continued*)

Nursing Interventions	Rationale	Expected Outcomes
2. Explore patient and family's previous experience with hospitalization and illness.	2. This information provides a baseline for explanations and indication of patient's and family's expectations.	• States realistic time period for recovery • Patient and family participate in management plans as appropriate
3. Review general course of burn treatment with patient and family.	3. Knowing what to expect prepares patient and family for upcoming events.	
4. Explain importance of patient participation in care for optimal results.	4. This information provides specific direction to patient.	
5. Realistically explain length of time involved in burn recovery.	5. Honesty promotes realistic expectations.	

Collaborative Problems: Congestive heart failure, pulmonary edema, sepsis, acute respiratory failure, ARDS, visceral damage (electrical burns)

Goal: Absence of complications

Nursing Interventions	Rationale	Expected Outcomes
Congestive Heart Failure (CHF) and Pulmonary Edema		
1. Assess for decreased urine output, JVD, or an S_3 or S_4 heart sound.	1. These signs may indicate decreased cardiac output and the onset of CHF.	• Lungs clear to auscultation • Absence of dypsnea, orthopnea, JVD, and S_3 or S_4 heart sounds • Urine output, arterial pressures, and cardiac output within normal limits
2. Monitor for increases in arterial pressures or decrease in cardiac output.	2. Increased pressures indicate increased preload and intravascular volumes. Decreasing cardiac output reflects less oxygen and nutrients available to the tissues and may indicate the onset of CHF.	
3. Assess for crackles on lung auscultation, dypsnea, orthopnea, or decreased oxygenation detected by pulse oximetry or arterial blood gas values.	3. Such signs may indicate progression of CHF to pulmonary edema.	
4. Report the above mentioned signs and symptoms to the physician.	4. Prompt medical intervention is needed.	
5. Position patient with the head of bed up 45° to 90° as tolerated.	5. Elevation facilitates gas exchange.	
6. Administer diuretics as prescribed. Assess patient's response.	6. Diuretics increase urine output and decrease cardiac preload and intravascular volumes.	
Sepsis		
1. Assess for fever, increased pulse, widened pulse pressure, and flushed, dry skin in unburned areas. Watch trends and notify physician if noted.	1. Such signs may indicate impending sepsis.	• Normal blood, sputum, and urine cultures • Absence of tachycardia, widening pulse pressure, and flushed, dry skin in unburned areas
2. Monitor wound and blood cultures and notify physician of positive cultures.	2. Positive cultures indicate infection and possible sepsis.	
3. Administer fluids, vasoactive medications and antibiotics as prescribed. Monitor for therapeutic response. Check that infecting organisms are sensitive to prescribed antibiotics.	3. Antibiotics kill susceptible bacteria. Intravenous fluids and vasoactive medications maintain intravascular volume and blood pressure.	
4. Monitor for therapeutic serum antibiotic levels.	4. Antibiotics are most effective at therapeutic levels. Excessive levels can cause systemic damage.	
Acute Respiratory Failure/ARDS		
1. Assess for respiratory distress, changes in respiratory patterns, or onset of adventitious breath sounds. Report to physician.	1. Such problems indicate possible acute respiratory failure. Pulmonary complications may not appear for 24 to 48 hours after the burn injury.	• Arterial blood gases within normal limits • Normal lung compliance • Absence of respiratory distress • Improved PO_2 level
2. Monitor pulse oximetry and arterial blood gas levels for decreasing oxygen saturation and PO_2. Report to physician.	2. Decreasing oxygenation indicates deteriorating respiratory status. Medical intervention is needed.	

(*continued*)

53•2

PLAN OF NURSING CARE 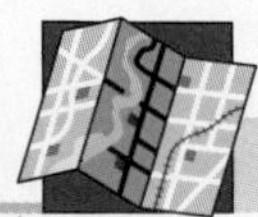

Care of the Patient During the Acute Phase of Burn Injury (*continued*)

Nursing Interventions	Rationale	Expected Outcomes
3. Monitor the mechanically ventilated patient for decreased spontaneous tidal volumes and lung compliance.	3. Respiratory problems reflect increased difficulty with ventilation and may indicate the onset of ARDS.	
4. In collaboration with the physician and respiratory therapist, administer positive end-expiratory pressure and pressure support. Assess patient's response.	4. These measures optimize diffusion of oxygen across the alveolar capillary membrane.	
Visceral Damage (Electrical Burns)		
1. Assess patient for signs of deep pain. Focus on areas between entrance and exit wounds of burn.	1. Pain may reflect visceral damage.	• Absence of visceral organ damage • Stable cardiac rhythm
2. Monitor ECG rhythm.	2. The patient with electrical burns is at risk for dysrhythmias.	
3. Report to the physician any complaints of deep pain or dysrhythmias.	3. Visceral damage requires immediate intervention.	

as well as in blood pressure and pulse rate, are reported to the physician. Low-dose dopamine to increase renal perfusion and diuretics may be prescribed to promote increased urine output. The nurse's role is to administer these medications as prescribed and to monitor the patient's response.

Preventing Infection

A major part of the nurse's role during the acute phase of burn care is detecting and preventing infection. The nurse is responsible for providing a clean and safe environment and for closely scrutinizing the burn wound to detect early signs of infection. Culture results and white blood cell counts are monitored.

Aseptic technique is used for wound care procedures and for any invasive procedures, such as insertion of intravenous lines and urinary catheters or tracheal suctioning. Meticulous hand washing before and after each patient contact is also an essential component of preventing infection.

The nurse protects the patient from sources of contamination, including other patients, staff members, visitors, and equipment. Invasive lines and tubing must be routinely changed according to recommendations of the Centers for Disease Control and Prevention. Tube feeding reservoirs, ventilator circuits, and drainage containers are replaced regularly. Fresh flowers, plants, or fresh fruit baskets are not permitted in the patient's room because of the risk of microorganism growth. Visitors are screened to avoid exposing the immunocompromised burn patient to pathogens.

Patients can inadvertently promote migration of microorganisms from one burned area to another by touching their wounds or dressings. Bed linens also can spread infection through either colonization with wound microorganisms or fecal contamination. Regularly bathing unburned areas and changing linens can help prevent infection.

Maintaining Adequate Nutrition

Oral fluids should be initiated slowly when bowel sounds resume. The patient's tolerance is noted. If vomiting and distention do not occur, fluids may be increased gradually and the patient may advance to a normal diet or to tube feedings.

The nurse collaborates with the dietitian to plan a protein- and calorie-rich diet that is acceptable to the patient. Family members may be encouraged to bring nutritious and favored foods to the hospital. Milkshakes and sandwiches made with meat, peanut butter, or cheese may be offered as snacks between meals and late in the evening. Nutritional supplements such as Ensure or Resource may be offered. Caloric intake must be documented. Vitamin and mineral supplements may be given.

If caloric goals cannot be met by oral feeding, a feeding tube is inserted and used for continuous or bolus feedings of specific formulas. The volume of residual gastric secretions should be checked to ensure absorption. TPN may also be required but should be used only if gastrointestinal function is compromised (see Chap. 33).

Patients should be weighed each day and their weights graphed. This can be used to help them set goals for their own nutritional intake and to monitor weight loss and gain. Ideally, the patient will lose no more than 5% of preburn weight if aggressive nutritional management is implemented.

The patient with anorexia requires encouragement and support from the nurse to increase food intake. The patient's surroundings should be as pleasant as possible at mealtime. Catering to food preferences and offering high-protein, high-vitamin snacks are ways of encouraging the patient to increase his or her intake.

Promoting Skin Integrity

Wound care is usually the single most time-consuming element of burn care after the emergent phase. The physician will prescribe the desired topical antibacterial agents and specific biologic, biosynthetic, or synthetic wound coverings and will plan for surgical excision and grafting. The nurse needs to make astute assessments of wound status, to use creative approaches to wound dressing, and to support the patient during the emotionally distressing and very painful experience of wound care.

The nurse serves as the coordinator of the complex aspects of wound care and dressing changes for the patient. The nurse must be aware of the rationale and nursing implications for the various wound management approaches. Nursing functions include assessing and recording any changes or progress in wound healing and keeping all members of the health care team informed of changes in the wound or treatment. A diagram, updated daily by the nurse responsible for the patient's care, helps to inform all those concerned about the latest wound care procedures in use for the patient.

The nurse also assists the patient and family by instruction, support, and encouragement to take an active part in dressing changes and wound care when appropriate. Discharge planning needs for wound care are anticipated early in the course of burn management, and the strengths of the patient and family are assessed and used in preparing for eventual discharge and home care.

Relieving Pain and Discomfort

Pain is more severe in partial-thickness burns than in full-thickness burns because the nerve endings are not destroyed. Exposed nerve endings are sensitive to cool, moving air; therefore, a covering can help to reduce pain. However, patients with full-thickness burns still have deep pain and pain in the areas surrounding their burns.

Analgesics and antianxiety medications are administered as prescribed. Frequent assessment of pain and discomfort is essential. To increase its effectiveness, analgesic medication is provided before the pain becomes too severe.

Nursing interventions such as teaching the patient relaxation techniques, giving the patient some control over wound care and analgesia, and providing frequent reassurance are helpful. Guided imagery may be effective in altering patients' perceptions of and responses to pain. Other pain-relieving approaches include distraction through video programs or video games; hypnosis, biofeedback, and behavioral modification have also been useful for pain management.

The nurse works quickly to complete treatments and dressing changes to reduce pain and discomfort. The patient is encouraged to take analgesic medications before painful procedures. The patient's response to the medication and other interventions is assessed and documented.

Healing burn wounds are typically described by patients as itchy and tight. Oral antipruritic agents, a cool environment, frequent lubrication of the skin with water or a silica-based lotion, exercise and splinting to prevent skin contracture, and diversional activities all help to promote comfort in this phase.

NURSING RESEARCH

Are Some Pain Assessment Tools Better Than Others?

Gordon, M., Greenfield, E., Marvin, J., Hester, C., & Lauterbach, S. (1998). Use of pain assessment tools: Is there a preference? *Journal of Burn Care and Rehabilitation, 19*(5), 451–454.

Purpose

Pain is a major issue throughout the care of the patient with burns; it has been identified as the leading issue needing nursing research in a Delphi study. Assessment of pain has been identified as a top research priority among nurses involved in burn care. The purpose of this study was to identify preferences for using pain assessment scales among patients with burns.

Study Sample and Design

Forty patients were enrolled in the study. Pain levels were assessed twice each day during two 3-day cycles. Pain was assessed during a time when pain was expected to be lower and again immediately after an activity likely to increase pain. During the first cycle, visual analogue and color scales were used by patients to rate their pain intensity; in the second 3-day cycle, word and faces scales were used for pain assessment. Patients were then asked to identify their preferred pain assessment tool.

Findings

Patients indicated a preference for the faces and color assessment tools rather than the visual analogue and word or adjective (descriptive) scales in use in most burn centers. Further research is needed to assess the impact of using different pain assessment scales on pain management strategies and the effectiveness of pain relief measures.

Nursing Implications

The results of this study suggest the need to examine the pain assessment tools in current use and patient preferences in assessment of pain.

Promoting Physical Mobility

An early priority is to prevent complications resulting from immobility. Deep breathing, turning, and proper repositioning are essential nursing practices to prevent atelectasis and pneumonia, to control edema, and to prevent pressure ulcers and contractures. These interventions are modified to meet the patient's needs. Low air loss and rotation beds may be useful, and early sitting and ambulation are encouraged. Whenever the lower extremities are burned, elastic pressure bandages should be applied before the patient is placed in an upright position. These bandages promote venous return and minimize swelling.

The burn wound is in a dynamic state for a year or more after wound closure. During this time, aggressive efforts must be made to prevent contracture and hypertrophic scarring. Both passive and active range-of-motion exercises are initiated from the day of admission and are continued after grafting, within prescribed limitations. Splints or functional devices may be applied to extremities for contracture control. The nurse monitors the splinted areas for signs of vascular insufficiency and nerve compression.

Strengthening Coping Strategies

In the acute phase of burn care, the patient is facing the reality of the burn trauma and is grieving over obvious losses. Depression, regression, and manipulative behavior are common responses of burn patients. Withdrawal from participation in required treatments and regression must be viewed with an understanding that such behavior helps the patient cope with an enormously stressful event. Much energy goes into maintaining vital physical functions and wound healing in the early postburn weeks, leaving little emotional energy for coping in a more effective manner. Nurses can assist patients to develop effective coping strategies by setting specific expectations for behavior, promoting truthful communication to build trust, helping patients practice appropriate strategies, and giving positive reinforcement when appropriate. Most importantly, the nurse and all members of the health care team must demonstrate acceptance of the patient.

The patient frequently ventilates feelings of anger. At times the anger may be directed inward because of a sense of guilt—perhaps for causing the fire or even for surviving when loved ones perished—or the anger may reach outward toward those who escaped unharmed or to those who are now providing care. One way to help the patient handle these emotions is to enlist someone to whom the patient can vent feelings without fear of retaliation. A nurse, social worker, psychiatric liaison nurse, or clergy member who is not involved in direct care activities may fill this role successfully.

Burn patients are very dependent on health care team members during the long period of acute illness. However, even when physically unable to contribute much to self-care, they can be included in decisions regarding care and encouraged to assert their individuality in terms of preferences and recognition of their unique identities. As patients improve in mobility and strength, the nurse works with them to set realistic expectations for self-care, including self-feeding, assistance with wound care procedures, exercise, and planning for the future. Many patients respond positively to the use of contractual agreements and other strategies that recognize their independence and their specific role as part of the health care team moving toward the goal of self-care.

Supporting Patient and Family Processes

Family functioning is disrupted with burn injury. One of the nurse's responsibilities is to support the patient and family and to address their spoken and unspoken concerns. Family members need to be instructed in ways that they can support the patient as adaptation to burn trauma occurs. The family also needs support by the health care team. The burn injury has tremendous psychological, economic, and practical impact on the patient and family. Referrals for social services or psychological counseling should be made as appropriate. This support continues into the rehabilitation phase.

Burn patients are commonly sent to burn centers far from home. Because burn injuries are not anticipated, family roles are disrupted. Therefore, both the patient and the family need thorough information about the patient's burn care and expected course of treatment. Patient and family education begins at the initiation of burn management. Barriers to learning are assessed and considered in teaching. The preferred learning styles of both the patient and family are assessed. This information is used to tailor teaching activities. It is important to assess the ability of the patient and family to grasp and cope with the information. To reinforce content, verbal information is supplemented by videos, models, or printed materials if available. Patient and family education is a priority in the rehabilitation phase.

Monitoring and Managing Potential Complications

CONGESTIVE HEART FAILURE AND PULMONARY EDEMA

The patient is assessed for fluid overload, which may occur as fluid is mobilized from the interstitial compartment back into the intravascular compartment. If the cardiac and renal systems cannot compensate for the excess vascular volume, congestive heart failure and pulmonary edema may result. The patient is assessed for signs of congestive heart failure, including decreased cardiac output, oliguria, jugular vein distention, edema, and the onset of an S_3 or S_4 heart sound. Increasing central venous, pulmonary artery, and wedge pressures indicate increased fluid volume.

Crackles in the lungs and increased difficulty with respiration may indicate a fluid buildup in the lungs, which is reported promptly to the physician. In the meantime, the patient is positioned comfortably, with the head of the bed raised (if not contraindicated because of other treatments or injuries) to promote lung expansion and gas exchange. Management of this complication includes providing supplemental oxygen, administering intravenous diuretics, carefully assessing the patient's response, and possibly providing vasoactive medications.

SEPSIS

The signs of early systemic sepsis are subtle and require a high index of suspicion and very close monitoring of changes in the patient's status. Early signs of sepsis may include increased temperature, increased pulse rate, widened pulse pressure, and flushed dry skin in unburned areas. As with many observations of the burn patient, one needs to look for patterns or trends in the data. (See Chap. 14 for a more detailed discussion of septic shock.)

Wound and blood cultures are performed as prescribed, and results are reported to the physician immediately. The nurse also observes for early signs of septicemia and promptly intervenes, administering prescribed intravenous fluids and antibiotics to prevent septic shock, a complication with a high mortality rate. Antibiotics must be given as scheduled to maintain proper blood concentrations. Serum antibiotic levels are monitored for evidence of maximal effectiveness, and the patient is monitored for toxic side effects.

ACUTE RESPIRATORY FAILURE AND ACUTE RESPIRATORY DISTRESS SYNDROME

The patient's respiratory status is monitored closely for increased difficulty in breathing, change in respiratory pattern, and onset of adventitious (abnormal) sounds. Typically at this stage, signs and symptoms of injury to the respiratory tract become apparent. Respiratory failure may follow. As described previously, signs of hypoxia (decreased O_2 to the tissues), decreased breath sounds, wheezing, tachypnea, stridor, and sputum tinged with soot (or in some cases containing sloughed tracheal tissue) are among the many possible findings that may develop. Patients receiving mechanical ventilation must be assessed for a decrease in tidal volume and lung compliance. The key sign of the onset of ARDS is hypoxemia while receiving 100% oxygen, decreased lung compliance, and significant shunting. The physician should be notified immediately of deteriorating respiratory status.

Medical management of the patient with acute respiratory failure requires intubation and mechanical ventilation (if not already in use). If ARDS has developed, higher oxygen levels, positive end-expiratory pressure, and pressure support are used with mechanical ventilation to promote gas exchange across the alveolar–capillary membrane.

VISCERAL DAMAGE

The nurse is alert to signs of necrosis of visceral organs due to electrical injury. Tissues affected are usually between the entrance and exit wounds of the electrical burn. All patients with electrical burns should undergo electrocardiographic monitoring, with dysrhythmias being reported to the physician. Careful attention must also be paid to signs or reports of pain related to deep muscle ischemia. To minimize the severity of complications, visceral ischemia must be detected as early as possible. The physician can perform **fasciotomies** to relieve the swelling and ischemia in the muscles and fascia and to promote oxygenation of the injured tissues. Because of the deep incisions involved with fasciotomies, the patient must be monitored carefully for signs of excessive blood loss and hypovolemia.

Evaluation

Expected Outcomes

Expected outcomes may include:

1. Achieves optimal fluid balance
   a. Maintains intake, output, and body weight that correlate with expected pattern

   b. Exhibits vital signs and central venous, pulmonary artery, and wedge pressures within designated limits
   c. Demonstrates increased urine output in response to diuretic and vasoactive medications
   d. Has heart rate less than 110 beats/minute in normal sinus rhythm
2. Has no localized or systemic infection
   a. Has wound culture results showing minimal bacteria
   b. Has normal urine and sputum culture results
3. Demonstrates anabolic nutritional status
   a. Gains weight daily after initial loss secondary to fluid diuresis and no oral intake of food or fluid
   b. Shows no signs of protein, vitamin, or mineral deficiencies
   c. Meets required nutritional needs entirely by oral intake
   d. Participates in selecting diet containing prescribed nutrients
   e. Exhibits normal serum protein levels
4. Demonstrates improved skin integrity
   a. Sustains generally intact skin that remains free of infection, pressure, and injury
   b. Demonstrates remaining open wound areas that are pink, reepithelializing, and free of infection
   c. Demonstrates donor graft sites that are clean and healing
   d. Has healed wounds that are soft and smooth
   e. Demonstrates skin that is lubricated and elastic
5. Has minimal pain
   a. Requests analgesics only for specific wound care procedures or physical therapy activities
   b. Reports minimal pain
   c. Gives no physiologic or nonverbal cues that pain is moderate or severe
   d. Uses pain control measures such as nitrous oxide, relaxation, imagery, and distraction techniques to cope with and alleviate discomfort
   e. Can sleep without being disturbed by pain
   f. Reports skin is comfortable, with no itching or tightness
6. Demonstrates optimal physical mobility
   a. Improves range of motion of joints daily
   b. Demonstrates preinjury range of motion of all joints
   c. Has no signs of calcification around the joints
   d. Participates in activities of daily living
7. Uses appropriate coping strategies to deal with postburn problems
   a. Verbalizes reactions to burns, therapeutic procedures, losses
   b. Identifies coping strategies used effectively in previous stressful situations
   c. Accepts dependency on health care providers during acute phase
   d. Verbalizes realistic view of problems resulting from burn injury and plans for future
   e. Cooperates with health care providers in required therapy
   f. Participates in decision making regarding care
   g. Resolves grief over losses resulting from burn injury and circumstances surrounding injury (eg, death of others, damage to home or other property)
   h. States realistic objectives for plastic surgery, further medical intervention, and results
   i. Verbalizes realistic abilities and goals
   j. Displays hopeful attitude toward future
8. Relates appropriately in patient/family processes
   a. Patient and family verbalize feelings regarding change in family interactions
   b. Family emotionally supports the patient during the hospitalization
   c. Family states that own needs are met
9. Patient and family verbalize understanding of the treatment course
   a. State rationale for different aspects of treatment
   b. State realistic time period for recovery
10. Has no complications
   a. Lungs clear on auscultation
   b. Exhibits no dyspnea or orthopnea and can breathe easily when standing, sitting, and lying down
   c. Exhibits no S_3 or S_4 heart sounds or jugular venous distention
   d. Experiences urine output, central venous, pulmonary artery, and pulmonary artery wedge pressures, and cardiac output within normal limits
   e. Exhibits normal blood, sputum, and urine culture results
   f. Maintains arterial blood gas values within normal limits
   g. Has normal lung compliance
   h. Has no visceral organ damage
   i. Has stable cardiac rhythm

Rehabilitation Phase of Burn Care

Although long-term aspects of burn care are discussed last, rehabilitation begins immediately after the burn has occurred—as early as the emergent period and often extends for years after injury. In the aftermath of the acute stages of injury, the burn patient increasingly focuses on the alterations in self-image and lifestyle that may occur. Wound healing, psychosocial support, and restoring maximal functional activity remain priorities. The focus on maintaining fluid and electrolyte balance and improving nutritional status continues. Reconstructive surgery to improve body appearance and function may be needed.

Burn injuries can have a major impact on quality of life. Changes in physical activity and social, psychological, and employment status may occur. Therefore, psychological and vocational counseling and referral to support groups may be helpful to promote recovery and quality of life. Family members also need support and guidance in assisting the patient to return to optimal health.

Prevention of Hypertrophic Scarring

The wound is in a dynamic state for 1.5 to 2 years after the burn occurs. If appropriate measures are instituted during this active period, the scar tissue loses its redness and softens. Healed areas that are prone to hypertrophic scarring require the patient to wear a pressure garment (Fig. 53-5). These devices are especially useful for partial-thickness wounds that required more than 2 weeks to heal and for the edges of grafted skin. Applying elastic pressure garments loosens collagen bundles and encourages parallel orientation of the collagen to the skin surface, with the disappearance of the dermal nodules. As pressure continues over time, there is a restructuring of the collagen and a decrease in vascularity and cellularity.

The physical therapist, occupational therapist, or a representative of the manufacturer of elastic pressure garments measures the patient for correct fit. While awaiting the arrival of the garment,

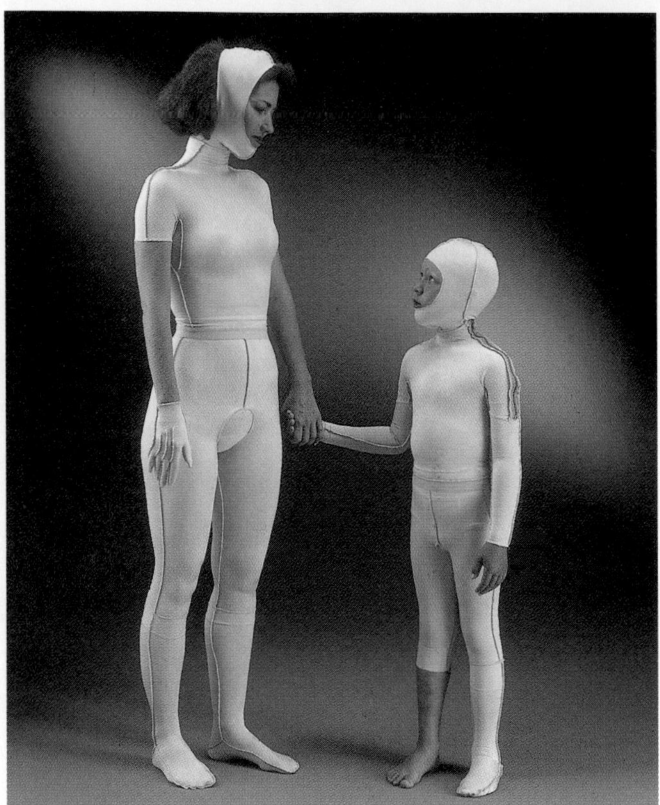

FIGURE 53•5 Elastic pressure garments. Application of pressure garments helps prevent hypertrophic burn scarring. Used with permission of Jobst Institute, Inc., Toledo, Ohio.

soft, tubular, knit elastic pressure bandages can be used to help desensitize the patient's skin, protect healing areas, apply pressure, and promote venous return. Patients must be instructed about the need for lubrication and protection of the healing skin and the need for pressure garments for at least a year after the injury. A program including elastic pressure garments, splints, and exercise under the supervision of an experienced physical and occupational therapy team is recommended for optimal functional and cosmetic results.

NURSING PROCESS: BURN CARE DURING THE REHABILITATION PHASE

Assessment

Information about the patient's educational level, occupation, leisure activities, cultural background, religion, and family interactions is obtained early. The patient's self-concept, mental status, emotional response to the injury and hospitalization, level of intellectual functioning, previous hospitalizations, response to pain and pain relief measures, and sleep pattern are also essential components of a comprehensive assessment. Information about the patient's general self-concept, self-esteem, and coping strategies in the past will be valuable in addressing emotional needs.

Ongoing physical assessments related to rehabilitation goals include range of motion of affected joints, functional abilities in activities of daily living, early signs of skin breakdown from splints or positioning devices, evidence of neuropathies (neurologic damage), activity tolerance, and quality or condition of healing skin. The patient's participation in care and ability to demonstrate self-care in such areas as ambulation, eating, wound cleaning, and applying pressure wraps are documented on a regular basis. In addition to these assessment parameters, specific complications and treatments require additional specific assessments; for example, the patient undergoing primary excision requires postoperative assessment.

Recovery from burn injury involves every system of the body. Therefore, assessment of the burn patient must be comprehensive and continuous. Priorities will vary at different points during the rehabilitation phase. Understanding the pathophysiologic responses to burn injury forms the framework for detecting early progress or signs and symptoms of complications. Early detection leads to early intervention and enhances the potential for successful rehabilitation.

Diagnosis

Nursing Diagnoses

Based on the assessment data, priority nursing diagnoses in the long-term rehabilitation phase of burn care may include the following:

- Activity intolerance related to pain on exercise, limited joint mobility, muscle wasting, and limited endurance
- Body image disturbance related to altered physical appearance and self-concept
- Knowledge deficit about postdischarge home care and follow-up needs

Collaborative Problems/Potential Complications

Based on the assessment data, potential complications that may develop in the rehabilitation phase include:

- Contractures
- Inadequate psychological adaptation to burn injury

Planning and Goals

The major goals for the patient include increased participation in activities of daily living; increased understanding of the injury, treatment, and planned follow-up care; adaptation and adjustment to alterations in body image, self-concept, and lifestyle; and absence of complications.

Nursing Interventions

Promoting Activity Tolerance

Nursing interventions that must be carried out according to a strict regimen and the pain that accompanies movement take their toll on a burn patient. The patient may become confused and disoriented and lack the energy to participate optimally in care. The nurse must schedule care in such a way that each patient has periods of uninterrupted sleep. A good time for planned patient rest is after the stress of dressing changes and exercise, while pain interventions and sedatives may still be effective. This plan must be communicated to family members and other care providers.

Burn patients may have insomnia related to frequent nightmares about the burn injury or to other fears and anxieties about the outcome of the injury. The nurse listens to and reassures the patient and administers hypnotics, as prescribed, to promote sleep.

Reducing metabolic stress by relieving pain, preventing chilling or fever, and promoting physical integrity of all body systems will help the patient conserve energy for therapeutic activities and wound healing.

The nurse incorporates physical therapy exercises in the patient's care to prevent muscle atrophy and to maintain the mobility required for daily activities. The patient's activity tolerance, strength, and endurance will gradually increase if activity occurs over increasingly longer periods. Fatigue, fever, and pain tolerance are monitored and used to determine the amount of activity to be encouraged on a daily basis. Activities such as family visits or recreational or play therapy (eg, video games, radio, TV, or walking to the patient lounge) can provide diversion, improve the patient's outlook, and increase tolerance for physical activity as well.

Improving Body Image and Self-Concept

Burn patients frequently suffer profound losses. These include not only a loss of body image due to disfigurement but also losses of personal property, homes, loved ones, and ability to work. They lack the benefit of anticipatory grief often seen in a patient approaching surgery or a person dealing with the terminal illness of a loved one.

As care progresses, the patient who is recovering from burns becomes aware of daily improvement and begins to exhibit basic concerns: Will I be disfigured? How long will I be in the hospital? What about my job and family? Will I ever be independent again? How can I pay for my care? Was my burn the result of my carelessness? As the patient expresses such concerns, the nurse must take time to listen and to provide realistic support. The nurse can refer patients to a support group, such as those usually available at regional burn centers or through organizations such as the Phoenix Society. Through participation in such groups, patients will meet others with similar experiences and learn to develop coping strategies to help them deal with their losses. Interaction with other burn survivors allows the patient to see that adaptation to the burn injury is possible. If a support group is not available, visits from burn survivors can be helpful to the patient in coping with such a traumatic injury.

A major responsibility of the nurse is to assess constantly the patient's psychosocial reactions. What are the patient's fears and concerns? Does the patient fear loss of control of care, independence, or sanity itself? Is the patient afraid of rejection by family and loved ones? Does he or she fear being unable to cope with pain or physical appearance? Does the patient have concerns about sexual function? Being aware of these anxieties and understanding the basis of the patient's fears enable the nurse to provide support and to cooperate with other members of the health care team in developing a plan to help the patient deal with these feelings.

When caring for burn patients, the nurse needs to be aware that there are prejudices and misunderstandings in society about those who are viewed as different. Opportunities and accommodations available to others are often denied to those who are disfigured. Such amenities include social participation, employment, prestige, various roles, and status. The health care team must actively promote a healthy body image and self-concept in burn survivors so that they can accept or challenge others' perceptions of the disfigured. Survivors themselves must show others who they are, how they function, and how they want to be treated.

The nurse can help patients practice their responses to people who may stare or inquire about their injury once they are discharged from the hospital. The nurse can help patients build self-esteem by recognizing their uniqueness—for example, with small gestures such as providing a birthday cake, combing the patient's hair before visiting hours, sharing information on the availability of a cosmetician to enhance appearance, and teaching the patient ways to direct attention away from a disfigured body to the self within. Consultants such as psychologists, social workers, vocational counselors, and teachers are valuable participants in assisting burn patients to regain their self-esteem.

Monitoring and Managing Potential Complications

CONTRACTURES

With early and aggressive physical and occupational therapy, contractures are rarely a long-term complication. However, surgical intervention is indicated if a full range of motion in the burn patient is not achieved. (See Chap. 10 for a discussion of prevention contractures.)

IMPAIRED PSYCHOLOGICAL ADAPTATION TO THE BURN INJURY

Some patients, particularly those with limited coping skills or psychological function or a history of psychiatric problems before the burn injury, may not achieve adequate psychological adaptation to the burn injury. Psychological counseling or psychiatric referral is made as soon as major coping problems become apparent.

Promoting Home and Community-Based Care

TEACHING PATIENTS SELF-CARE

As the inpatient phase of recovery becomes shorter, the focus of rehabilitative interventions is directed toward outpatient care or care in a rehabilitation center. In the long term, a good deal of care for healed burns will be performed by the patient and others at home. Throughout the phases of burn care, efforts are made to prepare the patient and family for the care that will continue at home. Thus, they are instructed about measures and procedures that they will need to perform. For example, patients commonly have small areas of clean, open wounds that are healing slowly. They are instructed to wash these areas daily with mild soap and water and to apply the prescribed topical agent or dressing.

In addition to instructions about wound care, patients and families require careful written and verbal instructions about prevention of complications, pain management, and nutrition. In addition, information about specific exercises and use of pressure garments and splints is fully reviewed with both the patient and family; written instructions are provided for reference. They are also taught to recognize abnormal signs to report to the physician. All of this information will enable patients to progress successfully through the rehabilitative phase of burn management.

The patient and family also are assisted in planning for the patient's continued care and in identifying and acquiring supplies and equipment that may be needed at home.

CONTINUING CARE

Follow-up care by an interdisciplinary burn care team will be necessary. Preparations should begin during the early stages of care. Patients who receive care in a burn center usually return to a burn clinic or center periodically for evaluation by the burn team, modification of home care instructions, and planning for reconstructive surgery. Other patients receive ongoing care from the general or plastic surgeon who cared for them during the acute phase of their management. Still other patients require the services of a rehabilitation center and may be transferred to such a center for aggressive rehabilitation before going home. Many

HOME CARE TEACHING CHECKLIST: THE PATIENT WITH A BURN INJURY

At the completion of the program, the patient or caregiver will be able to:	Patient	Caregiver
Mental Health		
Identify strategies to promote own mental health; for example:		
• Remember that changes in lifestyle take time.	✔	✔
• Resume previous interests and activities gradually.	✔	
• Take one day at a time to regain physical and mental strength.	✔	
• Be aware of own feelings and fears and discuss them with selected others.	✔	✔
• Expect concerns, frustrations, and depression about changes in appearance.	✔	✔
• Be honest with self, family, and friends about needs, hopes, and fears.	✔	✔
• Realize that emotional adjustment to the burn injury will occur with time.	✔	✔
Burn Skin Precautions and Wound Care		
Identify the following skin precautions and wound care:		
• Wear sun block with the highest SPF possible to protect burned skin from the sun.	✔	
• Avoid further trauma to burned skin; leave unbroken blisters that may form.	✔	✔
• Lubricate healed burned skin with mild lotion (as prescribed); avoid scratching.	✔	
• Wear wide-brimmed hats if face has been burned to protect the area from the sun.	✔	
• Use only mild soap and lotion (ie, products without perfume) on burned areas.	✔	✔
Exercise		
Describe the following guidelines for exercise:		
• Do as much for self as possible.	✔	
• Adhere to the exercise regimen given by the therapist.	✔	
• Participate in exercise every day, several times a day, even when "not feeling like it."	✔	
Nutrition		
Identify the following guidelines for nutrition:		
• Eat a diet high in calories and protein.	✔	
• Drink adequate volume of fluids to prevent constipation associated with use of analgesic medications.	✔	
Pain Management		
Describe the following steps for managing pain:		
• Take analgesic medication as prescribed.	✔	
• Avoid situations that require alertness (analgesics may produce drowsiness).	✔	
• Use analgesic medication as prescribed (30 minutes before painful procedures such as dressing changes).	✔	✔
• Use relaxation and distraction to relieve pain and discomfort.	✔	
Thermoregulation		
Identify strategies to compensate for inability to regulate body temperature:		
• Dress to accommodate cold and hot weather or environment.	✔	
• Avoid extremes of temperature.	✔	
Clothing Considerations		
State the following strategies in selection of clothing to wear:		
• Avoid tight clothing over burned areas.	✔	
• Select white cotton, loose-fitting clothing so that dyes in colored clothes do not irritate healing skin.	✔	
• Wear clothing and gloves to protect healing skin from unnecessary bruises, bumps, and scratches.	✔	
Management of Burn Scar		
Describe the following strategies to manage burn scar:		
• Massage and stretch skin to maintain/increase its elasticity.	✔	✔
• Use lotion for massage as recommended by therapist.	✔	✔
• Wear compression garments 23 hours a day.	✔	
Resumption of Sexual Relations		
Identify the following guidelines regarding resumption of sexual relationships:		
• Realize that resumption of sexual relationships is the rule rather than the exception.	✔	✔
• Expect sensitivity of and around the genital area for several months if these areas were burned.	✔	
• Resume sexual activity slowly; endurance will increase with time.	✔	

Adapted with permission from Orlando Regional Medical Center Burn Unit's *Personal Guide to Burn Care.*

patients require outpatient physical and/or occupational therapy, often several times weekly. It is often the nurse who is responsible for coordinating all aspects of care and ensuring that the patient's needs are met. Such coordination is an important aspect of meeting the challenge of assisting a burn victim to achieve independent functioning.

Burn patients who return home after a severe burn, those who cannot manage their own burn care, and those with inadequate support systems will need referral for home care. During visits to the patient at home, the home care nurse assesses the patient's physical and psychological status as well as the adequacy of the home setting for safe and adequate care. The nurse monitors the patient's progress and adherence to the plan of care and the occurrence of problems that interfere with the patient's ability to carry out the care. During the visit, the nurse assists the patient and family with wound care and exercises. Patients with severe or persistent depression or difficulty adjusting to their social and/or occupational roles are identified and referred to the burn team for possible referral to a psychologist, psychiatrist, or vocational counselor.

The burn team or home care nurse identifies appropriate community resources that may be helpful for the patient and family. Several burn patient support groups and other organizations throughout the United States offer services for burn victims. They provide caring people (often recovered burn victims) who can visit a burn patient in the hospital or home or telephone the patient and family periodically to provide support and counseling about skin care, cosmetics, and problems related to psychosocial adjustment. Such organizations, and many regional burn centers, sponsor group meetings and social functions at which outpatients are welcome. Some also provide school-reentry programs and are active in burn prevention activities. If more information is needed regarding burn prevention, the American Burn Association can help locate the nearest burn center and offer current burn prevention tips (see Chart 53-1).

Evaluation

Expected Outcomes

Expected outcomes may include:

1. Demonstrates activity tolerance required for desired daily activities
   a. Obtains sufficient sleep daily
   b. Reports absence of nightmares or sleep disturbances
   c. Shows gradually increasing tolerance and endurance in physical activities
   d. Can concentrate during conversations
   e. Has energy available to sustain desired daily activities
2. Adapts to altered body image
   a. Verbalizes accurate description of alterations in body image and accepts physical appearance
   b. Demonstrates interest in resources that may improve body appearance and function
   c. Uses cosmetics, wigs, and prostheses as desired to achieve acceptable appearance
   d. Socializes with significant others, peers, and usual social group
   e. Seeks and achieves return to role in family, school, or community as a contributing member
3. Demonstrates knowledge of required self-care and follow-up care
   a. Describes surgical procedures and treatments accurately
   b. Verbalizes detailed plan for follow-up care
   c. Demonstrates ability to perform wound care and prescribed exercises
   d. Returns for follow-up appointments as scheduled
   e. Identifies resource people and agencies to contact for specific problems
4. Exhibits no complications
   a. Demonstrates full range of motion
   b. Shows no signs of withdrawal or depression
   c. Displays no psychotic behaviors

CARE OF BURNS IN THE HOME SETTING

More and more burns are being treated exclusively in outpatient settings, including wound clinics, physicians' offices, or emergency department clinics. The outpatient setting is appropriate for the care of minor burns and most moderate burns. However, a number of factors must be considered in determining the appropriate site of care. These factors include the age of the patient, the extent and depth of the burn, the availability of family support systems and community resources to assist the patient, the patient's adherence to the prescribed plan of care, and the distance from home to the outpatient setting.

Initially, looking at and touching the burn wound may be difficult and even frightening to some family members and patients. However, with encouragement and support, most can handle burn wound care with little need for daily professional care. Instructions, both verbal and written, are given to the patient about burn wound care, pain management strategies, need for adequate nutrition, and the importance of exercise and rest. Instruction is also given about signs and symptoms of infection that should be reported to the physician. The importance of notifying the physician about complications early and of keeping follow-up appointments is emphasized to the patient and family.

GERONTOLOGIC CONSIDERATIONS

Reduced mobility, changes in vision, and decreased sensation in the feet and hands place elderly people at higher risk for burn injury; scalds and flames are the leading causes. These changes also place older people at risk for suffering a severe burn because they have difficulty in extinguishing the fire and removing themselves from the burn source.

Morbidity and mortality rates associated with burns are usually greater in elderly patients than in younger patients. Thinning and loss of elasticity of the skin in the elderly predispose them to a deep injury from a thermal insult that might cause a less severe burn in a younger person. Moreover, chronic illnesses decrease the older person's ability to withstand the multisystem stresses imposed by burn injury. Decreased function of the cardiovascular, renal, and pulmonary systems increases the need to observe closely elderly patients with even relatively minor burns during the emergent and acute phases. Acute renal failure is much more common in elderly patients than in those younger than age 40. The margin of difference between hypovolemia and fluid overload is very small. Suppressed immunologic response, a high incidence of malnutrition, and an inability to withstand metabolic stressors (eg, a cold environment) further compromise the elderly person's ability to heal.

Eschar separation in full-thickness burns is typically delayed in elderly patients, and older patients are frequently poor risks for surgical excision. Therefore, prolonged hospitalization, immobilization, and associated problems may be common. If the elderly patient can tolerate surgery, early excision with skin grafting is the treatment of choice because it decreases the mortality rate in this population.

Nursing Interventions

An important goal of nurses in community and home settings is preventing burn injury among the elderly. Nurses need to assess an elderly patient's ability to perform activities of daily living safely, assist elderly patients and families to modify the environment to ensure safety, and make referrals as needed.

Nursing assessment of the elderly burn patient should include particular attention to pulmonary function, response to fluid resuscitation, and signs of mental confusion or disorientation. A careful history of preburn medications and preexisting illnesses is essential.

Nursing care promotes early mobilization, aggressive pulmonary care, and attention to preventing complications. Because of lowered resistance, burn wound sepsis and lethal systemic septicemia are more likely in elderly patients. Moreover, fever may not be present in the elderly to signal such events. Therefore, surveillance for other signs of infection becomes even more important.

Rehabilitation must take into account preexisting functional abilities and problems, such as arthritis and low activity tolerance. Elderly patients commonly lack family members who can provide home care, so social services and community nursing services must be contacted to provide optimal care and supervision after hospital discharge.

Critical Thinking Exercises

1.
A 62-year-old patient is being treated for partial- and full-thickness burns over 20% of her body. She received these burns in her home 3 days ago. She is becoming confused, is refusing to eat or drink fluids, and is not cooperating with dressing changes. She is afebrile and her vital signs have not changed significantly from her baseline values. Analyze these data and explain why you think these cognitive changes have occurred. Based on your analysis, explain the assessment and management strategies you would implement at this time, and describe the patient outcomes that would indicate that your interventions have been successful.

2.
An 18-year-old has suffered severe burns of the head and neck, necessitating a tracheostomy. It is expected that the burned areas will require extensive skin grafting. Describe the physical and developmental issues you would consider important in the immediate care of this patient, and explain how you would expect these issues to change during the different phases of burn care.

3.
Your patient is expected to be discharged from the hospital after 1 month of treatment for severe burns of the legs. What instructions and recommendations would you give to the patient and family to ensure that his recovery will continue? If this patient lived alone, how would you modify your teaching and discharge planning?

References and Selected Readings

BOOKS

Caine, R. M., & Lefcourt, N. D. (1996). Patients with burns. In J. M. Clochesy, et al. (Eds.), *Critical care nursing* (2nd ed.). Philadelphia: W. B. Saunders.

Carrougher, G. J. (1998). *Burn care and therapy.* St. Louis: Mosby.

Herndon, D. N. (1996). *Total burn care.* Philadelphia: W. B. Saunders.

Hudak, C. M., Gallo, B. M., & Morton, P. G. (1997). *Critical care nursing: A holistic approach.* Philadelphia: Lippincott-Raven.

Molter, N. C., et al. (1997). Burns. In J. Hartshorn, M. Lamborn, & M. L. Noll (Eds.), *Introduction to critical care nursing.* Philadelphia: W. B. Saunders.

JOURNALS

Asterisks indicate nursing research articles.

*Arons, J. A., et al. (1992). The surgical applications and implications of cultured human epidermis: A comprehensive review. *Surgery, 111,* 4–11.

Ashburn, M. A. (1996). Burn pain: The management of procedure-related pain. *Journal of Burn Care and Rehabilitation, 17*(3), 365–371.

Atkinson, A. (1998). Nursing burn wounds on general wards. *Nursing Standard, 12*(41), 58–67.

Brigham, P. A., & McLoughlin, E. (1996). Burn incidence and medical care use in the United States: Estimates, trends, and data sources. *Journal of Burn Care and Rehabilitation, 17*(2), 95–107.

Cortiella, J., & Marvin, J. A. (1997). Management of the pediatric burn patient. *Nursing Clinics of North America, 32*(2), 311–329.

Covington, D. S., et al. (1996). Prognostic indicators in the elderly patient with burn. *Journal of Burn Care and Rehabilitation, 17*(3), 222–230.

Davis, S. T., & Sheeley-Adolphson, P. (1997). Psychosocial interventions: Pharmacologic and psychologic modalities. *Nursing Clinics of North America, 32*(2), 331–342.

*Demling, R. H. (1995). Use of Biobrane in management of scalds. *Journal of Burn Care and Rehabilitation, 16*(3), 329–330.

DeSanti, L., et al. (1998). Development of a burn rehabilitation unit: Impact of burn center length of stay and functional outcome. *Journal of Burn Care and Rehabilitation, 19*(5), 414–419.

Essex, T. L. (1999). Burn tragedy. *Rehabilitation Nursing, 24*(1), 5–6.

*Everett, J. J., et al. (1994). Pain assessment from patients with burns and their nurses. *Journal of Burn Care and Rehabilitation, 15*(2), 194–198.

*Fakhry, S. M., et al. (1995). Regional and institutional variation in burn care. *Journal of Burn Care and Rehabilitation, 16*(1), 86–90.

*Faldmo, L., & Kravitz, M. (1993). Management of acute burns and burn shock resuscitation. *AACN Clinical Issues in Critical Care Nursing, 4*(2), 351–366.

Forjuoh, S. N. (1998). The mechanisms, intensity of treatment, and outcomes of hospitalized burns: Issues for prevention. *Journal of Burn Care and Rehabilitation, 19*(5), 456–460.

Fowler, A. (1998). Nursing management of minor burn injuries. *Nursing Standard, 12*(49), 47–52.

Fratianne, R. B., et al. (1997). Determining when care for burns is futile. *Journal of Burn Care and Rehabilitation, 18*(3), 262–267.

*Gordon, M., et al. (1998). Use of pain assessment instrument tools: Is there a preference? *Journal of Burn Care and Rehabilitation, 19*(5), 451–454.

Gordon, M., & Goodwin, C. W. (1997). Initial assessment, management and stabilization. *Nursing Clinics of North America, 32*(2), 237–249.

Greenfield, E., & Jordan, B. (1996). Advances in burn wound care. *Critical Care Nursing Clinics of North America, 8*(2), 203–215.

Greenfield, E., & McManus, A. T. (1997). Infectious complications: Prevention and strategies for their control. *Nursing Clinics of North America, 32*(2), 297–309.

*Hansbrough, W. (1995). Nursing care of donor sites wounds. *Journal of Burn Care and Rehabilitation, 16*(3), 337–340.

Hedderich, R., & Ness, T. J. (1999). Analgesia for trauma and burns. *Critical Care Clinics, 15*(1), 167–84.

Hermans, M. H. (1998). Results of a survey on the use of different treatment options for partial- and full-thickness burns. *Burns, 24*(6), 539–551.

Jain, S., & Bandi, V. (1999). Electrical and lightning injuries. *Critical Care Clinics, 15*(2), 319–331.

*Jepson, C., Pickett, M., Keane, A., Tax, A., & McCorkle, R. (1996). Experiences of African American and Caucasian women who survive urban residential fires. *Health Care for Women International, 17*(6), 505–513.

*Johnson, J., et al. (1994). Compliance with pressure garment use in burn rehab. *Journal of Burn Care and Rehabilitation, 15*(2), 181–188.

Jordon, B. S., & Harrington, D. T. (1997). Management of the burn wound. *Nursing Clinics of North America, 32*(2), 251–273.

*Keane, A., Jepson, C., Pickett, M., Robinson, L., & McCorkle, R. (1996). Demographic characteristics, fire experiences, and distress of residential fire survivors. *Issues in Mental Health Nursing, 17*(5), 487–501.

*Lewandowski, R., et al. (1993). Burn injuries in the elderly. *Burns, 19*(6), 513–515.

Lim, J. J., Rehmar, S. G., & Elmore, P. (1998). Rapid response: Care of burn victims. *AAOHN Journal, 46*(4), 169–178.

McCain, D., & Sutherland, S. (1998). Nursing essentials: Skin grafts for patients with burns. *American Journal of Nursing, 98*(7), 34–38.

Mertens, D. M., Jenkins, M. E., & Warden, G. D. (1997). Outpatient burn management. *Nursing Clinics of North America, 32*(2), 343–364.

*Molter, N. C. (1993). When is the burn injury healed? Psychosocial implications of care. *AACN Clinical Issues in Critical Care Nursing, 4*(2), 424–432.

Parsons, L. (1997). Office management of minor burns. *Lippincott's Primary Care Practice, 1*(1), 40–49.

Patterson, D. R. (1996). Non-opioid-based approaches to burn pain. *Journal of Burn Care and Rehabilitation, 17*(4), 372–375.

Pessina, M., & Ellis, S. M. (1997). Rehabilitation. *Nursing Clinics of North America, 32*(2), 365–374.

Polko, L. E., & McMahon, M. J. (1998). Burns in pregnancy. *Obstetrical and Gynecological Survey, 53*(1), 50–56.

Ramzy, P. I., Barret, J. P., & Herndon, D. N. (1999). Thermal injury. *Critical Care Clinics, 15*(2), 333–352.

Richard, R., et al. (1997). To splint or not to splint: Past philosophy and present practice. Part III. *Journal of Burn Care and Rehabilitation, 18*(3), 251–254.

Rodriquez, D. J. (1996). Nutrition in patients with severe burns: State of the art. *Journal of Burn Care and Rehabilitation, 17*(1), 62–70.

Rose, J. K., & Herndon, D. N. (1997). Advances in treatment of burn patients. *Burns, 23*(Suppl 1), S19–S23.

*Rue, L. W., et al. (1993). Wound closure and outcome in extensively burned patients treated with cultured autologous keratinocytes. *Journal of Trauma, 34*(5):662–667.

*Rue, L. W., & Cioffi, W. G. (1991). Resuscitation of thermally injured patients. *Critical Care Nursing Clinics of North America, 3*(2), 181–189.

*Saffle, J. R., et al. (1995). Recent outcomes in the treatment of burn injury in the United States: A report form the American Burn Association patient registry. *Journal of Burn Care and Rehabilitation, 16*(3), 219–232.

Schiller, W. R., et al. (1997). Hyperdynamic resuscitation improves survival in patients with life-threatening burns. *Journal of Burn Care and Rehabilitation, 18*(1), 10–16.

*Smith, D. J. (1995). Use of Biobrane in wound management. *Journal of Burn Care and Rehabilitation, 16*(3), 317–320.

Smith, M. A., Munster, A. M., & Spence, R. J. (1998). Burns of the hand and upper limb—a review. *Burns, 24*(6), 493–505.

Staley, R. M., et al. (1996). Functional outcomes for the patient with burn injuries. *Journal of Burn Care and Rehabilitation, 17*(4), 362–368.

*Thurston, N., et al. (1995). Emotional responses of hospitalized patients with burns to débridement during the acute phase. *Journal of Burn Care and Rehabilitation, 6*(3), 269–275.

*Turner, J. G., et al. (1998). The effect of therapeutic touch on pain and anxiety in burn patients. *Journal of Advanced Nursing, 28*(1), 10–20.

Wainright, D., et al. (1996). Clinical evaluation of an acellular allograft dermal matrix in full-thickness burns. *Journal of Burn Care and Rehabilitation, 17*(2), 124–136.

*Walter, P. H. (1993). Burn wound management. *AACN Clinical Issues in Critical Care Nursing, 4*(2), 378–387.

*White, K. M. (1993). Using continuous SVO_2 to assess oxygen supply/demand in the critically ill patient. *AACN Clinical Issues in Critical Care Nursing, 4*(1), 134–147.

Winfree, J., & Barillo, D. J. (1997). Nonthermal injuries. *Nursing Clinics of North America, 32*(2), 275–296.

*Wong, L., & Munster, A. M. (1993). New techniques in burn wound management. *Surgical Clinics of North America, 73*(2), 363–371.

Also see issues of *The Journal of Burn Care and Rehabilitation* and *Burns—The Journal of the International Society for Burn Injuries.*

Resources

Alisa Ann Ruch Burn Foundation, 20944 Sherman Way, Suite 115, Canoga Park, CA 91303; (818) 883-7700; http://www.aarbf.org

American Burn Association, 625 N. Michigan Ave., Suite 1530, Chicago, IL 60611; (800) 548—BURN; http://ameriburn.org

Burn Foundation, 1128 Walnut St., Philadelphia, PA 19107; (215) 629-9200; burnctrs@AOL.com

Burn Institute, 3702 Ruffin Rd. #101, San Diego, CA 92123-1812; (619) 541-2277; http://www.burninstitute.com

Burn Prevention, (610) 481-9810; http://www.burnprevention.org

Fire Fighters Burn Foundation of Westchester-Putnam Counties, N.Y., Inc., P.O. Box 911, Yonkers, NY 10703-0911; fax: (914) 375-0540

Firefighters Pacific Burn Institute, 3101 Stockton Blvd., Sacramento, CA 95820; (916) 739-8525; http://www.ffpbi.org.

Greater Cincinnati Burn Victim Foundation, Cincinnati F. D. Local 48, 213 W. 9th St., Cincinnati, OH 45202; (513) 241-3541.

Integra Life Sciences Corporation, P.O. Box 688, 105 Morgan Lane, Plainsboro, NJ 08536; (800)-654-2873; fax: (609)-799-3297; http://www.integra-ls.com

International Association of Fire Fighters Burn Foundation, 1750 New York Ave., NW, Washington, DC 20006; (202) 737-8484; http://www.iaff.org.

Lifecell Corporation, 3606 Research Forest Dr., The Woodlands, TX 77381; (800)-367-5737; http://www.lifecell.com

National Burn Victim Foundation, 246-A Madisonville Rd., P.O. Box 409, Basking Ridge, NJ 07920; http://www.nbvf.org.

Northern California Burn Council, c/o Andrew McGuire, Director, Trauma Foundation, Trauma Center, Building 1, San Francisco General Hospital, San Francisco, CA 94110

Phoenix Society for Burn Survivors, 11 Rust Hill Rd., Levittown, PA 19056; (215) 946-BURN; (800) 888-BURN; http://www.burns-phoenix-society.org.

UNIT

13

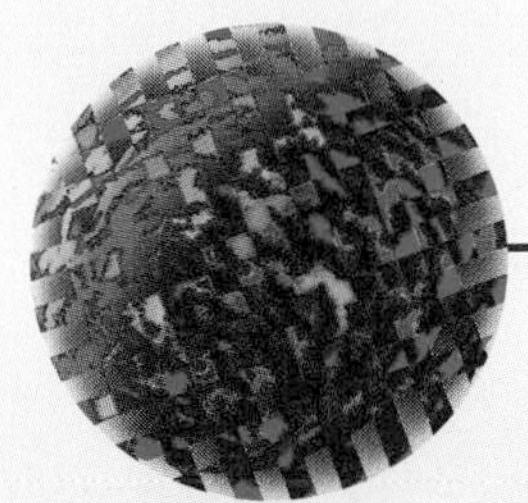

Sensorineural Function

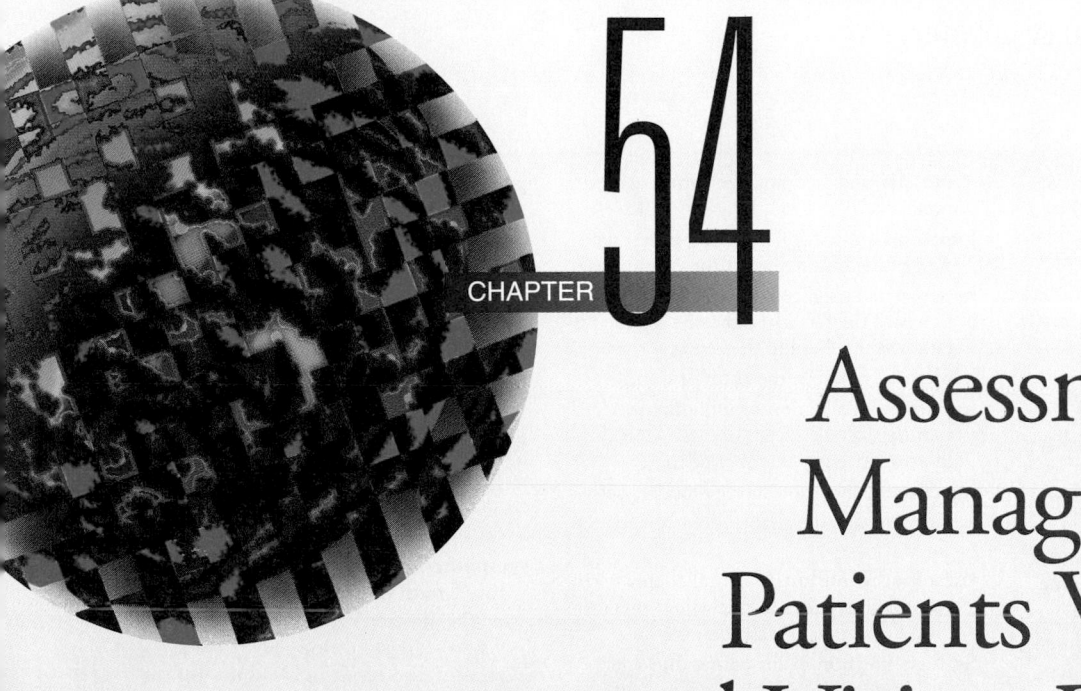

Assessment and Management of Patients With Eye and Vision Disorders

Learning Objectives

On completion of this chapter, the learner will be able to:

1. Identify significant eye structures and describe their functions.
2. Identify diagnostic tests for assessment of vision and evaluation of visual disabilities.
3. Discuss clinical features of ocular disorders, diagnostic assessment and examinations, medical or surgical management, and patient care for all eye conditions in the chapter.
4. Describe therapeutic effects of ophthalmic medications.
5. Define low vision and blindness and differentiate between functional and visual impairment.
6. List and describe low-vision assessment and management strategies.
7. Demonstrate orientation and mobility techniques for low-vision patients in a hospital setting.
8. Demonstrate instillation of eye drops and ointment and punctal occlusion.
9. Discuss general discharge instructions for patients after ocular surgery.

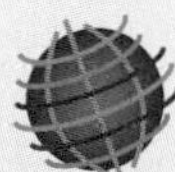

Our ability to see the world clearly can easily be taken for granted. The eye is a sensitive, highly specialized sense organ subject to a variety of disorders, many of which lead to impaired vision. Impaired vision affects an individual's independence in self-care, work and lifestyle choices, sense of self-esteem, safety, ability to interact with society and the environment, and overall quality of life. Many of the leading causes of visual impairment are associated with aging (eg, cataracts, glaucoma, and macular degeneration), and two thirds of the visually impaired population is older than 65 years of age. Younger people are also at risk for eye disorders, particularly traumatic injuries.

Although most people with eye disorders are treated in an ambulatory care setting, many patients under a nurse's care have eye diseases as a comorbid condition. In addition to understanding the prevention, treatment, and consequences of eye disorders, nurses in all settings should assess visual acuity in those at risk (eg, patients who are elderly and those with diabetes or acquired immunodeficiency syndrome [AIDS]), refer patients to eye care specialists as appropriate, implement measures to prevent further visual loss, and help the patient to adapt to impaired vision.

GLOSSARY

accommodation: process whereby the eye adjusts for near distance (eg, reading) by changing the curvature of the lens to focus a clear image on the retina.

anterior chamber: space in the eye bordered anteriorly by the cornea and posteriorly by the iris and pupil

aphakia: absence of the natural lens

astigmatism: refractive error in which light rays are spread over a diffuse area rather than sharply focused on the retina; this condition is due to the differences in the curvature of the cornea and lens

binocular vision: normal ability of both eyes to focus on one object and fuse the two images into one

blindness: inability to see, usually defined as corrected visual acuity of 20/400 or less, or a visual field of no more than 20 degrees in the better eye

chemosis: edema of the conjunctiva

cones: retinal photoreceptor cells essential for visual acuity and color discrimination

diplopia: seeing one object as two; double vision

emmetropia: absence of refractive error

enucleation: complete removal of the eyeball and part of the optic nerve

exenteration: surgical removal of the entire contents of the orbit, including the eyeball and lids

evisceration: removal of the intraocular contents through a corneal or scleral incision; the optic nerve, sclera, extraocular muscles, and at times, the cornea are left intact

hyperemia: "red eye" resulting from dilation of the vasculature of the conjunctiva

hyperopia: farsightedness; a refractive error in which the focus of light rays from a distant object is behind the retina.

hyphema: blood in the anterior chamber

hypopyon: collection of inflammatory cells that have a pale layer appearance in the inferior anterior chamber of the eye

injection: congestion of the blood vessels

keratoconus: cone-shaped deformity of the cornea

keratopathy, bullous: corneal edema with painful blisters in the epithelium due to excessive corneal hydration

limbus: junction of the cornea and sclera

miotic: a medication that causes pupillary constriction

mydriatic: a medication that causes pupillary dilation

myopia: nearsightedness; a refractive error in which the focus of light rays from a distant object is anterior to the retina

neovascularization: growth of abnormal new blood vessels

nystagmus: involuntary oscillation of the eyeball

papilledema: swelling of the optic disc due to increased intracranial pressure

photophobia: ocular pain on exposure to light

posterior chamber: space between the iris and vitreous

proptosis: downward displacement of the eyeball resulting from an inflammatory condition of the orbit or mass within the orbital cavity

ptosis: drooping eyelid

refraction: determination of the refractive errors of the eye and correction by lenses

rods: retinal photoreceptor cells essential for bright and dim light

scotoma: blind or partially blind area in the visual field

strabismus: a condition in which there is deviation from perfect ocular alignment.

sympathetic ophthalmia: an inflammatory condition created in the fellow eye by the affected eye (without useful vision): the condition may become chronic and result in blindness (of the fellow eye)

vitreous: gelatinous material (transparent and colorless) that fills the eyeball behind the lens

Ophthalmic Abbreviations

BCVA: best corrected visual acuity

HM: hand motions

LP: light perception

NLP: no light perception

OD: ocular dexter (right eye)

OS: oculus sinister (left eye)

OU: oculus uterque (each eye)

UCVA: uncorrected visual acuity

V: vision

VA: visual acuity

ANATOMIC AND PHYSIOLOGIC OVERVIEW

Unlike most organs of the body, the eye presents itself for external examination, and its anatomy is more easily assessed than many other body parts (Fig. 54-1).

The eyeball, or globe, sits in a protective bony structure known as the orbit. Lined with muscle, connective, and adipose tissues, the orbit is about 4 cm in height, width, and depth and is shaped roughly like a four-sided pyramid, surrounded on three sides by the sinuses: the ethmoid (medially), the frontal (superiorly), and the maxillary (inferiorly). The optic nerve and the ophthalmic artery enter the orbit at its apex through the optic foramen.

The eyeball is moved though all fields of gaze by the extraocular muscles. The four rectus muscles and two oblique muscles (Fig. 54-2) are innervated by cranial nerves (CN) III, IV, and VI. Ideally, the movements of the two eyes are coordinated, so that the brain perceives a single image.

The anterior portion of the eye is protected by the eyelids, composed of thin elastic skin that covers striated and smooth muscles. The eyelids contain multiple glands, among them sebaceous, sweat, and accessory lacrimal glands, and they are lined with conjunctival material. The upper lid normally covers the uppermost portion of the iris and is innervated by the oculomotor nerve (CN III). The lid margins contain meibomian glands, the inferior and superior puncta, and the eyelashes. The triangular spaces formed by the junction of the eyelids are known as the inner or medial canthus and the outer or lateral canthus. With every blink of the eyes, the lids wash the cornea and conjunctiva with tears.

Tears are vitally important to the health of the anterior segment of the eye. They are formed by the lacrimal gland and the accessory lacrimal glands. A healthy tear is composed of three layers: lipoid, aqueous, and mucoid. If there is a defect in the composition of either of these layers, the integrity of the cornea may be compromised. Tears are secreted in response to reflex or emotional stimuli.

The **conjunctiva,** a mucous membrane, provides a barrier to the external environment and nourishes the eye. The goblet cells of the conjunctiva secrete lubricating mucus. The bulbar conjunctiva covers the sclera, whereas the palpebral conjunctiva lines the inner surface of the upper and lower eyelids. The junction of the two portions is known as the fornix.

The **sclera,** commonly known as the "white of the eye," is a dense fibrous structure that composes the posterior five sixths of the eye (Fig. 54-3). The sclera helps to maintain the shape of the

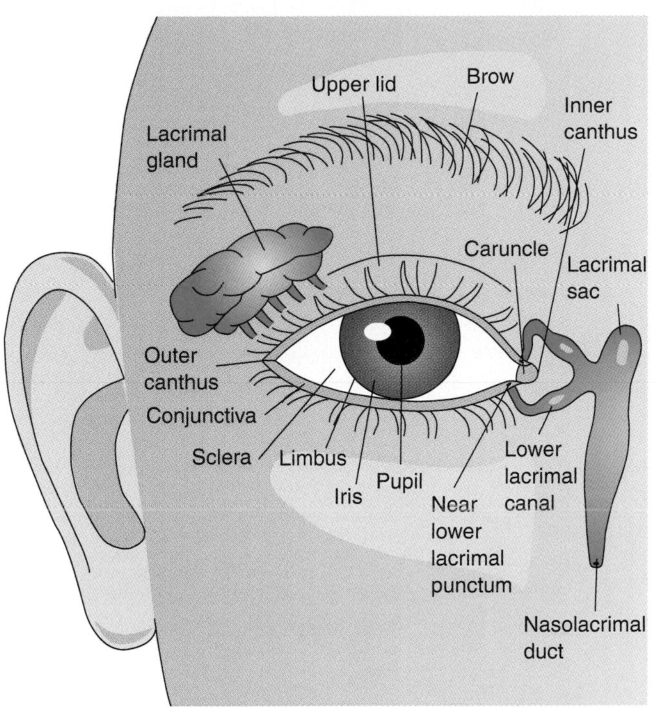

FIGURE 54•1 External structures of the eye and position of the lacrimal structures.

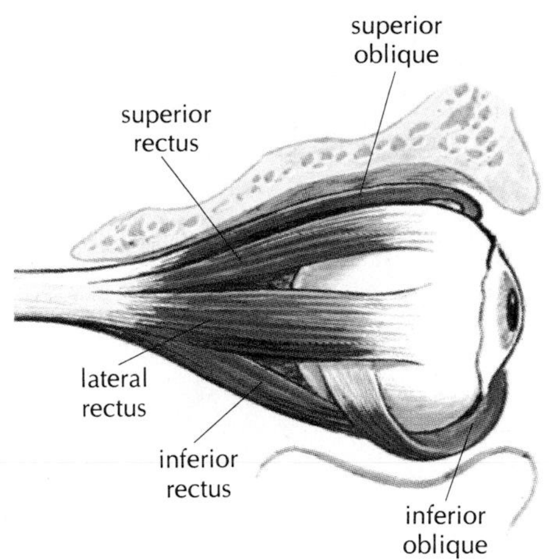

FIGURE 54•2 The extraocular muscles responsible for eye movement. The medial rectus muscle (not shown) is responsible for opposing the movement of the lateral rectus muscle.

eyeball and protects the intraocular contents from trauma. The sclera may have a slightly bluish tinge in young children, a dull white color in adults, and a slightly yellowish color in the elderly. Externally, it is overlaid with conjunctiva, a thin transparent mucous membrane that contains fine blood vessels. The conjunctiva meets the cornea at the **limbus**, on the outermost edge of the iris.

The cornea (Fig. 54-4), a transparent avascular domelike structure, forms the most anterior portion of the eyeball and is the main refracting surface of the eye. It is composed of five layers: the epithelium, Bowman's membrane, the stroma, Descemet's membrane, and the endothelium. The epithelial cells are capable of rapid replication and are completely replaced every 7 days.

Behind the cornea lies the **anterior chamber**, filled with a continually replenished supply of clear aqueous humor, which nourishes the cornea. The aqueous humor is produced by the ciliary body, and its production is related to the intraocular pressure (IOP). Normal pressure is 10 to 21 mm Hg.

The **uvea** consists of the iris, the ciliary body, and the choroid. The iris, or colored part of the eye, is a highly vascularized, pigmented collection of fibers surrounding the pupil. The pupil is a space that dilates and constricts in response to light. Normal pupils are round and constrict symmetrically when a bright light is shown on them. About 20% of the population have pupils that

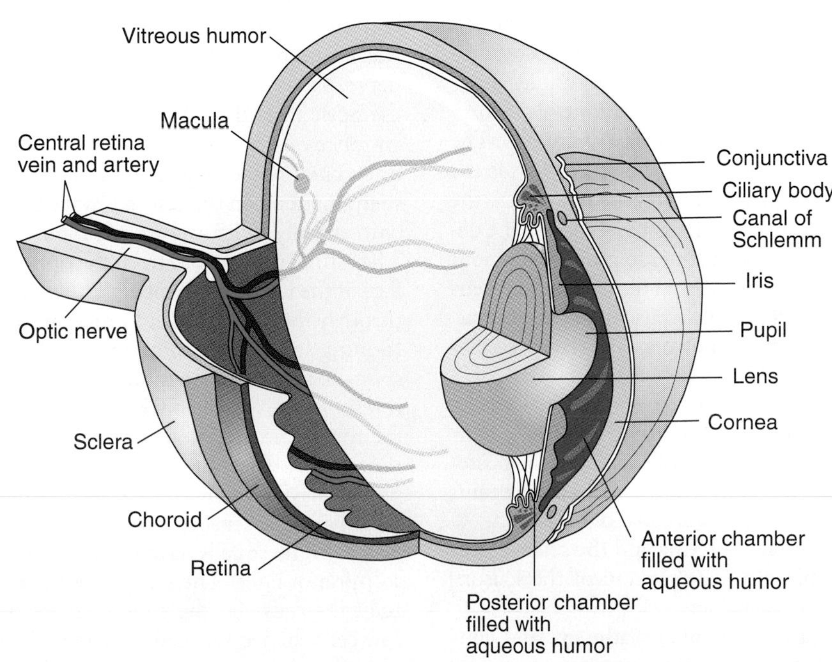

FIGURE 54•3 Three-dimensional cross-section of the eye.

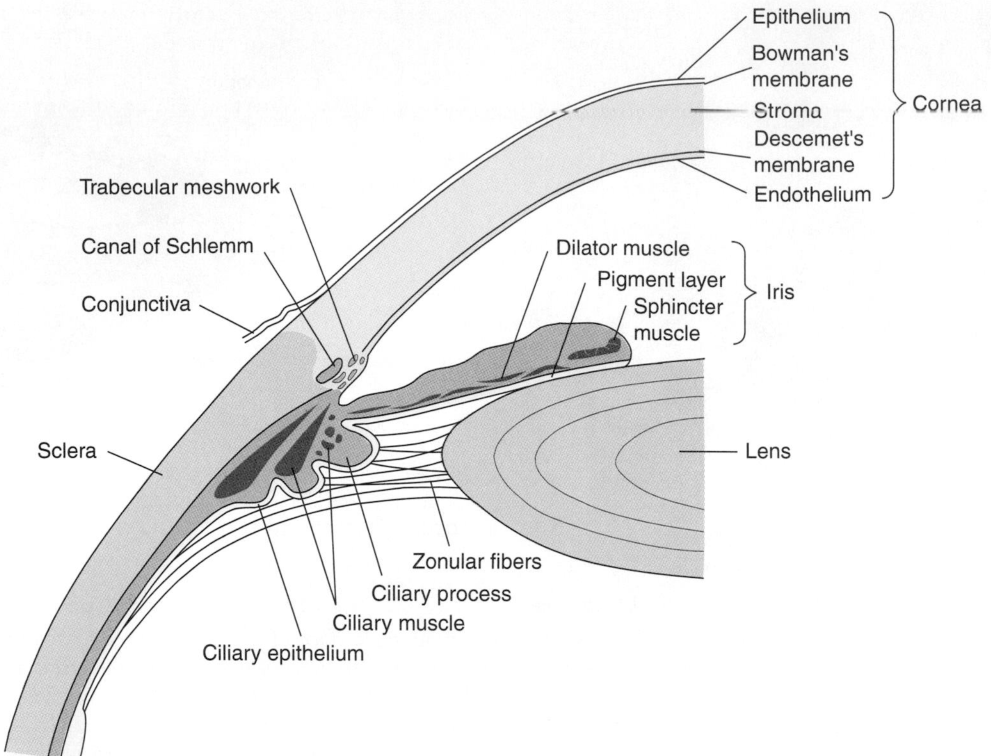

FIGURE 54•4 Internal structures of the eye. From Goldblum, K. (Ed.) (1997). *Core curriculum for ophthalmic nursing, American Society of Ophthalmic Registered Nurses.* Dubuque, IA: Kendall/Hall Publishing.

are slightly unequal in size but that respond equally to light. Dilation and constriction are controlled by the sphincter and dilator pupillae muscles. The dilator muscle is controlled by the sympathetic nervous system, whereas the sphincter muscle is controlled by the parasympathetic nervous system.

Directly behind the pupil and iris lies the lens, a colorless and almost completely transparent biconvex structure held in position by zonular fibers. It is avascular and has no nerve or pain fibers. The lens enables focusing for near vision and refocusing for distance vision. The ability to focus and refocus is called **accommodation**. The lens is suspended behind the iris by the zonules and is connected to the ciliary body. The ciliary body controls accommodation through the zonular fibers and the ciliary muscles. The aqueous humor is anterior to the lens; posterior to the lens is the vitreous humor. All cells formed throughout life are retained by the lens. This makes the cell structure of the lens susceptible to the degenerative effects of aging. The lens continues to grow throughout life, laying down fibers in concentric rings. This gradual thickening eventually results in an increasingly dense core or nucleus, which can then limit accommodative powers. This becomes evident in the fifth decade of life.

The **posterior chamber** is a small space between the vitreous and the iris. Aqueous fluid is manufactured in the posterior chamber by the ciliary body. This aqueous fluid flows from the posterior chamber into the anterior chamber, where it then drains through the trabecular meshwork into the canal of Schlemm.

The choroid is layered between the retina and the sclera and is a vascular tissue, supplying blood to the portion of the sensory retina closest to it.

The ocular fundus is the largest chamber of the eye and contains the vitreous humor, a clear gelatinous substance, mostly water, encapsulated by a hyaloid membrane. The vitreous humor occupies about two thirds of the eye's volume and helps maintain the shape of the eye. As the body ages, the perfect gel-like characteristics are gradually lost, and various cells and fibers cast shadows that the patient perceives as "floaters." The vitreous is in continuous contact with the retina and is attached to the retina by scattered collagenous filaments. The vitreous shrinks and shifts with age.

The innermost surface of the fundus is the retina. The retina is composed of 10 microscopic layers and has the consistency of wet tissue paper. It is neural tissue, an extension of the optic nerve. Viewed through the pupil, the landmarks of the retina are the optic disc, the retinal vessels, and the macula. The point of entrance of the optic nerve into the retina is known as the optic disc. The optic disc is oval or circular, is pink in color, and has sharp margins. In the disc, a physiologic depression or cup is present centrally, with the retinal blood vessels emanating from it. The retinal tissues arise from the optic disc and line the inner surface of the vitreous chamber. The retinal vessels also enter the eye through the optic nerve, branching out through the retina and forming superior and inferior arcades. The area of the retina responsible for central vision is the macula. The rest of the retina is responsible for peripheral vision. In the center of the macula is the fovea, the most sensitive area, which is avascular and is surrounded by the superior and inferior vascular arcades. Two important layers of the retina are the retinal pigment epithelium (RPE) and the sensory retina. A single layer of cells composes the RPE, and these cells have numerous functions, including the absorption of light. The sensory retina contains the photoreceptor cells: the rods and the cones. The rods and cones are long, narrow cells shaped like rods or cones. The **rods** are mainly responsible for night vision or vision in low light, whereas the **cones** provide the best vision for bright light, color vision, and fine detail. Cones are distributed throughout the retina with their greatest concentration in the fovea. Rods are absent in the fovea.

Good visual acuity is not dependent solely on a healthy functioning eyeball but also on an intact visual pathway (Fig. 54-5). This pathway is made up of the retina, optic nerve, optic chiasm, optic tracks, lateral geniculate bodies, optic radiations, and the visual cortex area of the brain. The pathway is an extension of the central nervous system.

The optic nerve is innervated by the second cranial nerve (CN II). Its purpose is to transmit impulses from the retina to the occipital lobe of the brain. The optic nerve head, or optic disc, is the physiologic blind spot in each eye. The optic nerve leaves the eye and then meets the optic nerve from the other eye at the optic chiasm. This anatomic area, the chiasm, is the point at which the nasal fibers from the nasal retina of each eye cross to the opposite side of the brain. The nerve fibers from the temporal retina of each eye remain uncrossed. Therefore, fibers from the right half of each eye, which would be the left visual field, carry impulses to the right occipital lobe. Fibers from the left half of each eye, the right visual field, carry impulses to the left occipital lobe. After the chiasm, these fibers are known as the optic track. The optic track continues on to the lateral geniculate body. The lateral geniculate body leads to the optic radiations and then to the cortex of the occipital lobe of the brain.

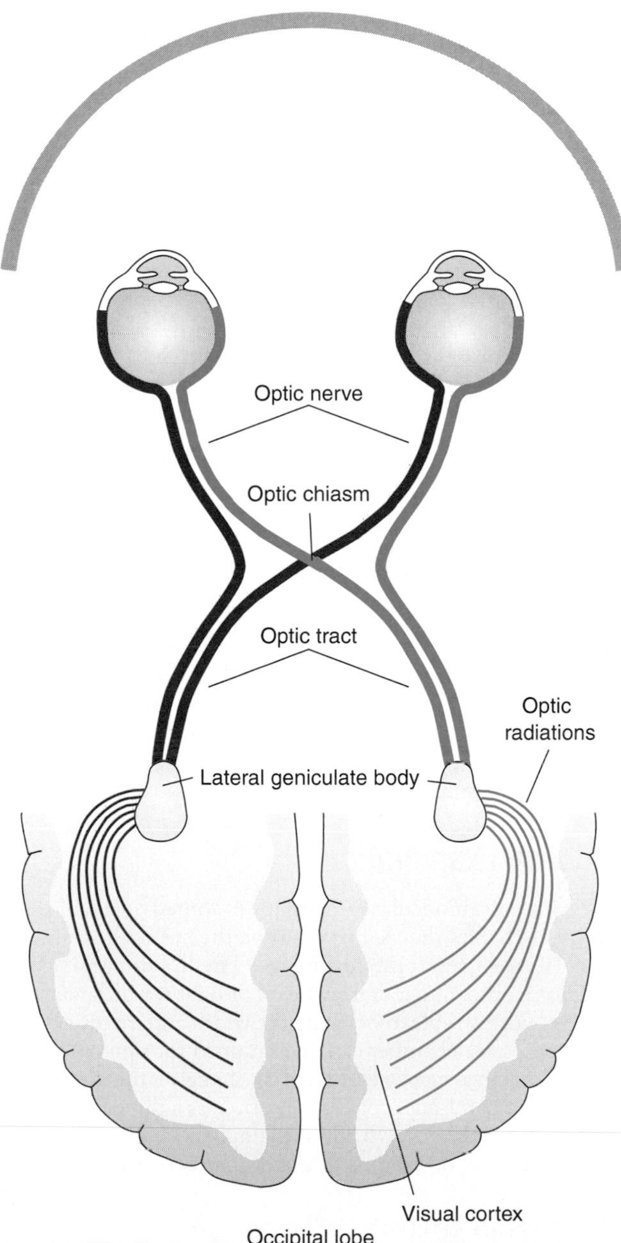

FIGURE 54•5 The visual pathway, from Goldblum, K. (Ed.) (1997). *Core curriculum for ophthalmic nursing, American Society of Ophthalmic Registered Nurses.* Dubuque, IA: Kendall/Hall Publishing.

ASSESSMENT

The health care provider, through careful questioning, can elicit the necessary information that will lead to diagnosis of an ophthalmic condition. Pertinent questions to ask during the interview can be found in the display entitled Taking an Ocular History.

The Ocular Examination

Visual Acuity

After the patient's chief complaint and history have been established, visual acuity should be assessed. This is an essential part of the eye examination and a measure against which all therapeutic outcomes are based. Most health care providers are familiar with the standard Snellen chart. This chart is composed of a series of progressively smaller rows of letters and is used to test distance vision. The fraction 20/20 is considered the standard of normal vision. Most people can see the letters on the line designated as 20/20 from a distance of 20 feet. A person whose vision is 20/200 can see an object from 20 feet away that a person whose vision is 20/20 can see from 200 feet away.

The patient is positioned at the proscribed distance, usually 20 feet, from the chart and is asked to read the smallest line that he or she can see. The patient should wear distance correction (eye glasses or contact lenses) if required, and each eye should be tested separately. The right eye is commonly tested first and then the left. If the patient is unable to read the 20/20 line, he or she is given a pinhole occluder and asked to read again, with the eye in question. A makeshift occluder may be created by making a pinhole in an index card and asking the patient to look through

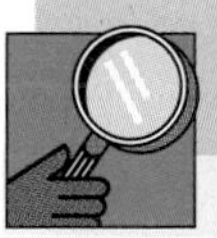

ASSESSMENT
TAKING AN OCULAR HISTORY

What does the patient perceive to be the problem?
Is visual acuity diminished?
Does the patient experience blurred, double, or distorted vision?
Is there pain; is it sharp or dull; is it worse when blinking?
Is the discomfort an itching sensation or more of a foreign body sensation?
Are both eyes affected?
Is there a history of discharge? If so, question color, consistency, odor.
What is the duration of the problem?
Is this a recurrence of a previous condition?
How has the patient self-treated?
What makes the symptoms improve or worsen?
Are there any systemic diseases? What medications are used in their treatment?
What concurrent ophthalmic conditions does the patient have?
Is there an ophthalmic surgery history?
Have other family members had the same symptoms or condition?

the pinhole. Squinting produces the same effect. Patients should be encouraged to read more letters and to guess, if necessary. Often, patients avoid guessing and prefer not to try at all rather than to make a mistake. The patient should be encouraged to read every letter possible.

The visual acuity (VA) is recorded in the following way. If the patient reads all five letters from the 20/20 line with the right eye **(OD)** and three of the five letters on the 20/15 line with the left eye **(OS)**, the examiner writes OD 20/20, OS 20/15-2, or VA 20/20, 20/15-2.

If the patient is unable to read the largest letter on the chart (the 20/200 line), the patient should be moved toward the chart or the chart moved toward the patient, until the patient is able to identify the largest letter on the chart. If the patient can recognize only the letter E on the top line at a distance of 10 feet, the visual acuity would be recorded as 10′/200. If the patient is unable to see the letter E at any distance, the examiner should determine if the patient can count fingers **(CF).** The examiner holds up a random number of fingers and asks the patient to count the number he or she sees. If the patient could correctly identify the number of fingers at 3 feet, the examiner would record CF/3′.

If the patient is unable to count fingers, the examiner raises one hand up and down or moves it side to side and asks in which direction the hand is moving. This level of vision is known as hand motions **(HM)**. A patient who could only perceive light would be described as having light perception **(LP)**. The vision of a patient who is unable to perceive light would be described as no light perception **(NLP)**.

The External Eye Examination

After the visual acuity has been recorded, an external eye examination is performed. The position of the eyelids is noted. Commonly, the upper 2 mm of the iris is covered by the upper lid. The patient is examined for **ptosis** (a lid that is drooping) and for lid retraction (too much of the eye exposed). Sometimes the upper or lower lid turns out, affecting closure. The lid margins and lashes should be without edema, erythema, or lesions. Scaling or crusting is noted. The sclera is inspected at this time. A normal sclera is opaque and white. Lesions on the conjunctiva, discharge, and tearing or blinking are noted.

The room should be darkened so that the pupils can be examined. The pupillary response should be checked with a pen light to be certain that the pupils are equally reactive and regular. A normal pupil is black. An irregular pupil may result from trauma, previous surgery, or a disease process.

The patient's eyes are observed in primary or direct gaze, and any head tilt is noted. A tilt may indicate a cranial nerve palsy. The patient is asked to stare at a target; each eye is covered and uncovered quickly, noting any shift in gaze. The examiner observes for **nystagmus** (oscillating movement of the eyeball). The extraocular movements of the eyes are simply tested by having the patient follow the examiner's finger or hand light through the six cardinal directions of gaze (up and down, right and left, and diagonally). This is especially important when screening patients for ocular trauma or for neurologic disorders.

DIAGNOSTIC EVALUATION

Direct Ophthalmoscopy

A direct ophthalmoscope is a hand-held instrument with varying plus and minus lenses. The lenses can be rotated into place, enabling the examiner to bring the cornea, lens, and retina into focus sequentially. The examiner holds the ophthalmoscope in the right hand and uses the right eye to examine the patient's right eye. The examiner switches to the left hand and left eye when examining the patient's left eye.

During this examination, the room should be darkened, and the patient's eye should be on the same level as the examiner's eye. Both the patient and the examiner should be comfortable. Both should breathe normally. The patient is given a target to gaze on and is encouraged to keep both eyes open and steady.

When the fundus is examined, the vasculature comes into focus first. The veins are larger in diameter than the arteries. The examiner should focus on a large vessel and then follow it toward the midline of the body, which leads to the optic nerve. The central depression in the disc is known as the "cup." The normal cup is about one third of the disc. The size of the physiologic optic cup should be estimated. Are the disc margins sharp, or are they blurred? Do the veins have a silvery or coppery appearance? The periphery of the retina can be examined by having the patient shift his or her gaze. The last area of the fundus to be examined should be the macula because this area is the most light sensitive. The retina of a young person often has a glistening effect. This is sometimes referred to as a cellophane reflex.

The healthy fundus should be free of any lesions. The examiner should look for intraretinal hemorrhages, which may appear as red smudges or, if the patient has hypertension, may look somewhat flame shaped. Lipid may be present in the retina of patients with hypercholesterolemia or diabetes. This lipid has a yellowish appearance. The presence of any soft exudates that have a fuzzy white appearance (also known as cotton-wool spots) should be noted. Microaneurysms may be seen, which look like little red dots. Any nevi should be noted. Drusen (small, hyaline, globular growths), commonly found in macular degeneration, appear to be yellowish in color with indistinct edges. Small drusen have a more distinct edge. The examiner should sketch the fundus and note any abnormalities.

Indirect Ophthalmoscopy

The indirect ophthalmoscope is an instrument commonly used by the ophthalmologist. It produces a bright and intense light. The light source is affixed with a pair of binocular lenses, which are mounted on the examiner's head. The ophthalmoscope is used in conjunction with a hand-held 20-diopter lens. This instrument enables the examiner to see larger areas of the retina, although in an unmagnified state.

Slit-Lamp Examination

The slit lamp is a binocular microscope mounted on a table. This instrument enables the user to examine the eye with magnification of 10 to 40 times the real image. The illumination can be varied from a broad to a narrow beam of light for different parts of the eye. For example, by varying the width and intensity of the light, the anterior chamber can be examined for signs of inflammation. Cataracts may be evaluated by changing the angle of the light. When a hand-held contact lens, such as a three mirror lens, is used in conjunction with the slit lamp, the angle of the anterior chamber may be examined, as may the ocular fundus.

Color Vision Testing

Because alteration in color vision is sometimes indicative of optic nerve problems, color vision testing is often performed in a neuro-ophthalmologic workup. The most common color vision test is performed using Ishihara polychromatic plates. These plates are bound together in a booklet. On each plate of this booklet are dots of primary colors that are integrated into a background of secondary colors. These dots are arranged in simple patterns, such as numbers or geometric shapes. Patients whose color vision has diminished may be unable to identify the hidden shapes.

Amsler Grid

The Amsler grid is a test often used for patients with macular problems, such as macular degeneration. It consists of a geometric grid of identical squares with a central fixation point. The grid should be viewed by the patient wearing normal reading glasses. Each eye is tested separately. The patient is instructed to stare at the central fixation spot on the grid and note if there is any distortion in any of the squares of the grid itself. In patients with macular problems, some of the squares may look faded, or the lines may be wavy. Patients with age-related macular degeneration are commonly given these Amsler grids to take home and encouraged to check them frequently, as often as daily, to pick up any early signs of distortion that may indicate the development of a neovascular choroidal membrane.

Ultrasonography

Lesions in the globe or the orbit may not be directly visible and are evaluated by ultrasound. A probe placed against the eye aims the beam of sound. High-frequency sound waves emitted from a special transmitter are bounced back from the lesion and collected by a receiver that amplifies and displays the sound waves on a special screen. Ultrasonography can be used to identify orbital tumors, retinal detachment, and changes in tissue composition.

Color Fundus Photography

Fundus photography is a technique used to detect and document retinal lesions. The patient's pupils are widely dilated during the procedure, and visual acuity is diminished for about 30 minutes due to retinal "bleaching" by the intense flashing lights.

Fluorescein Angiography

Fluorescein angiography is used to evaluate clinically significant macular edema, document macular capillary nonprofusion, and identify choroidal **neovascularization** (growth of abnormal new blood vessels) in age-related macular degeneration. It is an invasive procedure in which fluorescein dye is injected, usually into an antecubital area vein. Within 10 to 15 seconds, this dye can be seen coursing through the retinal vessels. Over a 10-minute period, a series of black-and-white photographs are taken of the retinal vasculature. Some patients may demonstrate a gold tone to their skin, and the patient's urine will be deep yellow or orange.

Tonometry

Tonometry is used to measure IOP by determining the amount of force necessary to indent or flatten (applanate) a small anterior area of the globe of the eye. The principle involved is that a soft eye is dented more easily than a hard eye. Pressure is measured in millimeters of mercury (mm Hg). High readings indicate that there is high pressure; low readings indicate that there is low pressure.

The three most common types of tonometers are indentation, applanation, and noncontact. The procedure is noninvasive and is usually painless. A topical anesthetic eye drop is instilled in the lower conjunctival sac before measurement.

Gonioscopy

Gonioscopy is used to visualize the angle of the anterior chamber to identify abnormalities in appearance and measurements. The gonioscope uses a refracting lens that can either be direct or indirect. The indirect lens views the mirror image of the opposite anterior chamber angle and can only be used with a slit lamp. The direct gonioscopy lens gives a direct view of the angle and its structures.

Perimetry Testing

Perimetry testing is used to evaluate the field of vision. A visual field is the area or extent of physical space visible to an eye in a given position. Its average extent is 65 degrees upward, 75 degrees downward, 60 degrees inward, and 95 degrees outward when the eye is in the primary gaze (ie, looking straightforward). It is a three-dimensional contour representing areas of relative retinal sensitivity. Visual acuity is sharpest at the very top of the field and declines progressively toward the periphery.

The two methods of perimetric testing are manual and automated perimetry. Manual perimetry involves the use of moving (kinetic) or stationary (static) stimuli or targets. An example of kinetic manual perimetry is the tangent screen. A tangent screen is a black felt material mounted on a wall that has a series of concentric circles dissected by straight lines emanating from the center. It tests the central 30 degrees of the visual field.

The patient is seated 1 to 2 meters from the screen and positioned with the center of the screen at his or her eye level. The patient is allowed to use eyeglasses for the corrected visual acuity. The eye that is not tested is occluded; the patient is asked to look at a fixed point in the center of the screen. A test object is introduced from the periphery at different areas toward the center at 30-degree intervals. The size of the object is dependent on the visual acuity of the patient. For example, smaller objects are used for patients with 20/20 vision than for patients with 20/70 vision. The patient is asked to determine when the object is detected while he or she remains focused on the point at the center of the screen.

Automated perimetry uses stationary targets. Stationary targets are harder to detect than moving targets. The Humphrey field analyzer is an example of an automated perimetry. Light is projected in different areas of a hollow dome in random fashion through the use of a computer. While looking at a telescope opening, the patient presses the button when the stimulus is detected. Automated perimetry has been found to be more accurate than manual perimetry; there is no examiner bias, and the same test can be repeated automatically for verification of results.

IMPAIRED VISION

Refractive Errors

In refractive errors, vision is impaired because a shortened or elongated eyeball prevents light rays from focusing sharply on the retina. Blurred vision due to refractive error can be corrected with eyeglasses and contact lenses. The appropriate eyeglass or contact lens is determined by refraction. **Refraction** ophthalmology consists of placing various types of lenses in front of the patient's eyes to determine which lens best improves the patient's vision.

The depth of the eyeball is important in determining refractive error (Fig. 54-6). Those patients for whom the visual image focuses precisely on the macula and who do not need eye glasses or contact lenses are said to have **emmetropia**. People with **myopia** have deeper eyeballs; the distant visual image focuses in front of, or short of, the retina. These people are nearsighted and are termed myopic and experience blurred distance vision. When people have a shorter depth to their eyes, the visual image focuses beyond the retina; the eyes are more shallow and are termed hyperopic. People who have **hyperopia** are farsighted. These patients experience near vision blurriness, whereas their distance vision is excellent.

Another important cause of refractive error is **astigmatism,** an irregularity in the curve of the cornea. Because this causes a distortion of the visual image, it can mean a decreased acuity of both distance and near vision. A cylinder correction can be built into the eye glasses. Rigid or soft toric contact lenses are appropriate for these patients.

Low Vision and Blindness

Low vision is a general term used to describe a state of visual impairment that requires the use of devices and strategies in addition to corrective lenses to perform visual tasks. Low vision is defined as a best corrected visual acuity **(BCVA)** of 20/70 to 20/200 (Table 54-1). According to some estimates, there are about 2.3 million visually impaired Americans; however, other researchers estimate that 10 million adults have difficulty reading newsprint even with corrective lenses, and 1.6 million cannot see words or letters (McNeil, 1993).

Blindness is defined as a BCVA of 20/400 to no light perception. The clinical definition of absolute blindness is the absence of light perception. Legal blindness is a condition of impaired vision in which an individual has a BCVA that does not exceed 20/200 in the better eye, or whose widest visual field diameter is 20 degrees or less. This definition does not equate with functional ability, nor does it classify the degrees of visual impairment. Legal blindness ranges from an inability to perceive light to some vision remaining. An individual who meets the criteria for legal blindness may obtain government financial assistance. There are more than 900,000 legally blind Americans among the 40-year-old and older age group. African Americans have a higher rate of blindness than do whites.

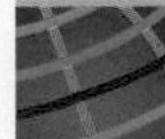

TABLE 54•1 Categories of Visual Impairment

Category of Visual Impairment	Visual Acuity (Best Corrected)
Low vision	
1	6/18 3/10 (0.3) 20/70
2	6/60 1/10 (0.1) 20/200
Blindness	
3	3/60 (finger counting at 3m) 1/20 (0.05) 20/400
4	1/60 (finger counting at 1m) 1/50 (0.02) 5/300
5	No light perception

Visual Field

Patients with a visual field radius no greater than 10 degrees but greater than 5 degrees around central fixation should be placed in category 3, and patients with a field no greater than 5 degrees around central fixation in category 4—even if the central acuity is not impaired.

Adapted from the *International Classification of Diseases,* World Health Organization, 1977 and from Vaughn, D. G., Asbury, T., & Riorda-Eva, P. (Eds.). (1995). *General ophthalmology.* Stamford, CT: Appleton & Lange.

Impaired vision is accompanied by difficulty in performing functional activities. Individuals with visual acuity of 20/80 to 20/100 with a visual field restriction of 60 degrees to greater than 20 degrees can read at a nearly normal level with optical aids. Their visual orientation is near normal but requires increased scanning of the environment (systematic use of head and eye movements). In a visual acuity range of 20/200 to 20/400 with a 20-degree to greater than 10-degree visual field restriction, the individual can read slowly with optical aids. His or her visual orientation is slow, with constant scanning of the environment; individuals in this category have travel vision. Individuals with hand motion vision or no vision may benefit from the use of mobility devices (eg, a long white cane or guide dog) and should be encouraged to learn braille and to use computer aids.

The most common causes of blindness and visual impairment among adults aged 40 years and older are macular degeneration, glaucoma, cataract, diabetic retinopathy, injuries, inflammatory diseases, and genetic disorders (Prevent Blindness America, 1994). Macular degeneration is more prevalent among whites, whereas glaucoma is more prevalent among African Americans. The annual cost of blindness in the United States is estimated at 4 billion dollars.

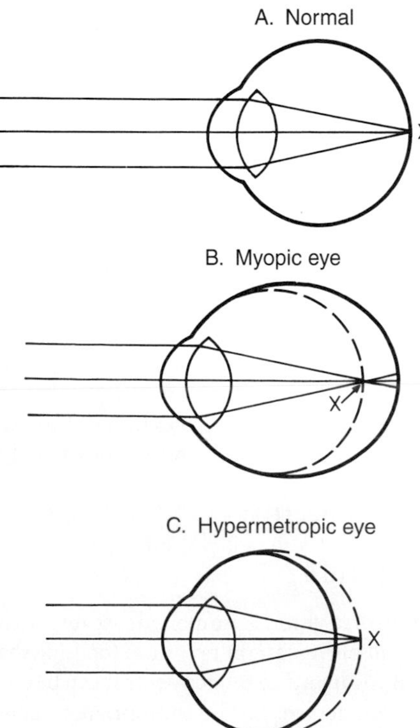

FIGURE 54•6 Eyeball shape determines visual acuity in refractive errors. (**A**) Normal eye. (**B**) Myopic eye. (**C**) Hypermetropic eye.

Low-Vision Assessment

The assessment of low vision includes a thorough history and examinations of distance and near visual acuity, visual field, contrast sensitivity, glare, color perception, and refraction.

PATIENT INTERVIEW

During history taking, the cause and duration of the patient's visual impairment are identified. Patients with diabetic macular edema, for example, typically have fluctuating visual acuity. Patients with macular degeneration have central acuity problems. Central acuity problems result in difficulty in performing activities that require finer vision, such as reading. People with peripheral field defects have more difficulties with mobility. The patient's customary activities of daily living, medication regimen, habits (such as smoking), acceptance of the physical limitations brought about by the visual impairment, and realistic expectations from low-vision aids must also be identified. These aspects of the patient's activities are important indicators for planning care that will include guidelines for safety and referrals to social services.

ASSESSMENT

Distance acuity testing determines the patient's ability to identify letters or symbols of varying sizes at a given distance and is typically measured by the standard Snellen chart or the Lighthouse Distance Visual Acuity chart, a specially designed low-vision visual acuity chart. For children and adults who are not literate, symbols are used instead of letters.

Color testing is used to determine whether the patient has difficulty distinguishing color. Patients with central vision conditions (eg, macular degeneration) have more difficulty identifying colors than those with peripheral vision problems (eg, glaucoma) because central vision identifies color.

Visual field testing (perimetry) helps to identify what parts of the patient's central and peripheral visual fields have useful vision. It is most helpful in detecting the central **scotomas** (blind areas in the visual field) in macular degeneration and the peripheral field defects in glaucoma and retinitis pigmentosa.

Contrast sensitivity testing measures visual acuity in different degrees of contrast. The initial test may take the form of simply turning on the lights while testing the distance acuity. If the patient is able to read better with the lights on, the patient can benefit from magnification.

Glare testing enables the examiner to obtain a more realistic evaluation of the patient's ability to function in his or her environment. Glare can reduce a person's ability to see, especially in patients with cataracts. Devices that test glare, such as the Brightness Acuity Tester, produce three degrees of bright light to create a dazzle effect while the patient is viewing a target, such as Snellen letters on the wall. The lights have been calibrated to imitate certain objects that create glare, such as the brightness of a car's headlights at night.

Management

Managing low vision involves magnification and image enhancement through the use of low-vision aids and strategies, and referrals to social services and community agencies serving the visually impaired. The goals are to enhance visual function and assist patients with low vision to perform customary activities.

Low-vision aids include optical and nonoptical devices. The optical devices include convex lens aids, such as magnifiers and spectacles; telescopic devices; antireflective lenses that diminish glare; and electronic reading systems, such as closed-circuit television and computers with large print. Magnifiers can be handheld or attached to a stand with or without illumination. Telescopic devices can be spectacle telescopes or clip-on or hand-held loupes. Nonoptical aids include large print publications and a variety of writing aids. The types of low-vision aids suggested for performing activities of daily living are listed in Table 54-2.

Strategies that enhance the performance of visual tasks include modification of body movements and illumination and training for independent living skills. Head movements and positions can be modified to place images in functional areas of the visual field. Illumination is an added feature in magnifiers. Adjusting the

TABLE 54•2 Activities Affected by Visual Impairment and Visual Aids

Activity	Optical Aids	Nonoptical Aids
Shopping	Hand magnifier	Lighting, color cues
Fixing a snack	Bifocals	Color cues, consistent storage plan
Eating out	Hand magnifier	Flashlight, portable lamp
Identifying money	Bifocals, hand magnifier	Arrange paper money in wallet compartments
Reading print	High-power spectacle, bifocals, hand magnifier, stand magnifier, closed-circuit television	Lighting, high-contrast print, large print, reading slit
Writing	Hand magnifier, focusable telescope, closed-circuit television	Lighting, bold-tip pen, black ink
Dialing a telephone	Hand magnifier	Large print dial, hand-printed directory
Crossing streets	Telescope	Cane, ask directions
Finding taxis and bus signs	Telescope	
Reading medication labels	Hand magnifier	Color codes, large print
Reading stove dials	Hand magnifier	Color codes, raised dots
Adjusting the thermostat	Hand magnifier	Enlarged print model
Using a computer	Spectacles	High-contrast color, large-print program
Reading signs	Spectacles	Move closer
Watching sporting event	Telescope	Sit in front rows

Adapted from Vaughn, D. G., Asbury, T., & Riorda-Eva, P. (Eds.). (1995). *General ophthalmology.* Stamford, CT: Appleton & Lange.

lighting is helpful with reading and other activities. Simple optical and nonoptical aids are available in low-vision clinics.

Referrals to community agencies may be necessary for low-vision patients living alone who are unable to self-administer their medications. Patients who smoke must be reminded that it may be best to smoke in the presence of a family member as a safety precaution. Community agencies, such as the Lighthouse for the Blind, offer services to low-vision patients that include training in independent living skills and the provision of occupational and recreational activities and a wide variety of assistive devices for vision enhancement and orientation and mobility.

Coping With Blindness

Coping with blindness involves three types of adaptation: emotional, physical, and social. The emotional adjustment to blindness or severe visual impairment determines the success of the physical and social adjustments of the patient. Successful emotional adjustment means acceptance of blindness or severe visual impairment. Effective coping may not occur until the patient recognizes the permanence of the blindness. Clinging to false hopes of regaining vision retards effective adaptation to blindness. A newly blind patient and his or her family undergo the various steps of grieving: denial and shock, anger and protest, restitution, loss resolution, and acceptance. Family members, especially those who live with the patient, also grieve and suffer a loss. Their positive and negative attitudes can translate into corresponding influences on the rehabilitation of the blind patient. In addition to grieving, four other aspects are important to consider: value change, independence–dependence conflict, coping with stigma, and learning to communicate in social settings without visual cues.

SOCIAL MISCONCEPTIONS

Misconceptions about the state of blindness by sighted people result in pity, overprotection, rejection, uneasiness, fear, and revulsion. Misconceptions about blindness are varied. For example, sighted people may believe that blind people are inferior, are totally impaired, no longer have the power of visualization, and lead unhappy lives. The definition of legal blindness does not clarify this misconception because it does not categorize the degrees of visual impairment. The terms visual disability, visual handicap, visual deficit, visual impairment, visual loss, and partial sight are alternative phrases used to describe the impairment of vision. These terms do not provide specific definitions of the degree of blindness or functional impairment.

As a result of the negative perceptions of blindness, blind people may withdraw or, conversely, overcompensate to prove to themselves and others that inadequacy does not exist. The limitations associated with blindness are a result not only of the impairment of vision but also of the misconceptions and negative perceptions of the sighted society.

SPATIAL ORIENTATION AND MOBILITY

Blind people detect and incorporate less information about their environment than sighted people. The information that the blind person relies on is egocentric, sequential, and positional. It is centered on the blind person and his or her relationship to the objects in the environment. For example, the topographic concepts of front, back, left, right, above, and below and measures of distances are most useful in determining the exact position, sequence, and location of objects in relation to the blind person. Although the basis of information received by blind people may be different from that of sighted people, they are able to comprehend spatial concepts.

The goal of orientation and mobility training is to foster independence to a reasonable degree. Certain techniques using auditory and tactile cues are effective when orienting a blind person to his or her environment. Orientation and mobility performance are enhanced by anticipatory information. The spatial representation of the complete composition of the environment (cognitive map) enhances a blind person's independence.

Orientation and mobility training are programs offered by community agencies serving blind and visually impaired individuals. The training includes the use of mobility devices for travel, the long cane, electronic travel aids, dog guides, and orientation aids. The basic orientation and mobility techniques used by a sighted person to assist a blind or visually impaired person to ambulate safely and efficiently are called sighted-guide techniques.

REHABILITATION

Managing blindness in a health care setting consists of an understanding of the emotional dynamics of the loss paradigm and coping with blindness, awareness of the misconceptions of blindness, use of the basic orientation and mobility techniques, inclusion of the family as an important part of care, and early referral for rehabilitation. The physician has the primary responsibility for explaining the inevitability of blindness to the patient and his or her family, when efforts to recover vision have failed. The goal of rehabilitation is to improve the quality of life by teaching skills that will restore independence to a reasonable degree. The ultimate goal is to have blind patients return to the mainstream of society and enjoy satisfying lives. Referrals to community agencies ensure the continuity of care for minimizing the physical, psychological, social, and vocational sequelae of blindness.

Rehabilitation training for the blind includes orientation and mobility training, independent living skills, reading and writing skills (by the use of computers, writing aids, computers, or braille), and the use of assistive devices for enhancing vision, occupational training, and recreational activities. Orientation and mobility training include the use of the long cane, electronic adaptive devices for travel, and dog-guide training. Some rehabilitation agencies offer training that requires blind people to reside in the facility while being trained. Nonresidence training programs typically offer transportation to and from the facility.

Rehabilitation counselors assist visually impaired people to obtain career and vocational opportunities. Most blind people need to undergo counseling and career development interventions before they are ready for career placement.

COMMUNITY PROGRAMS AND SERVICES

In the United States, governmental support of the blind is made possible by the enactment of laws such as the Rehabilitation Act, the Civil Rights Act, and the Americans With Disability Act. Governmental services include the following:

- Income assistance through Social Security Disability Income and Supplemental Security Income
- Health insurance through Medicaid and Medicare programs
- Support services offered by the Division of Blind Services, such as vocational rehabilitation programs that include counseling, vocational training, job placement, rehabilitation centers, vending facility program, and educational, medical, and social services
- Tax exemptions and tax deductions
- Department of Veterans Affairs special programs for visually impaired veterans

The U.S. Postal Service offers reduced postage for braille reading and writing materials and talking books. Private nonprofit organizations, such as The Lighthouse for the Blind, offer rehabilitation training programs. Other organizations, such as the American Foundation for the Blind, also offer services, such as publications about blindness. International organizations, such as the International Agency for the Prevention of Blindness and the World Council for the Welfare of the Blind, sponsor programs to promote global awareness about the eradication of preventable and curable diseases that cause blindness. A complete listing of organizations that serve visually impaired people is provided at the end of this chapter.

CARE OF THE BLIND OR SEVERELY VISUALLY IMPAIRED PATIENT IN THE HOSPITAL SETTING

A patient who is blind or severely visually impaired requires coping strategies for adapting to the environment. The monocular postoperative patient whose functioning eye is restricted by a surgical patch dressing or by postoperative inflammation requires early ambulation just like any postoperative patient. Ambulation is not only for physiologic functioning but also for the patient's effective functioning in the environment within the range of the visual limitations. The mastery of activities of daily living, such as walking to a chair from a bed, require spatial concepts. The patient needs to know where he or she is in relation to the composition of the room environment, the changes that may occur, and how to approach the desired location safely. This requires a collaborative effort between the patient and the nurse, who is the sighted guide.

Patients whose visual impairment is a result of a chronic progressive eye condition, such as those with glaucoma, have better cognitive mapping skills than the suddenly blinded patient. They have developed the use of spatial and topographic concepts early and gradually; hence, the representation of a room layout in memory is easier for them to achieve. Suddenly blinded patients have more difficulty in adjusting to cognitive mapping. The emotional and psychological issues of coping with blindness may hinder readiness to learn and the effectiveness of teaching. These patients require intensive emotional support.

During meals, the patient is oriented to the composition of the meal tray by using the face of a clock. For example, the main course plate may be described as at 12 o'clock or the coffee cup at 3 o'clock. When patients are assisted to move from an erect position to a sitting position, they are asked to feel the seat by letting the back of their legs touch the seat before sitting down. This gives them an idea of their exact position in relation to the chair. The bedside table and the call button must always be within reach. The parts of the call button are explained, and the patient is encouraged to touch and press the buttons or dials until the activity is mastered. The patient must be familiarized with the location of the telephone, water pitcher, and other objects on the bedside table. All articles and furniture must be replaced in the same positions. Introducing oneself upon entering a patient's room is always a polite gesture and helps in the orientation of a blind patient.

At the initial patient contact, the nurse must assess the degree of physical assistance the patient with a visual deficit requires. The nurse should be aware of the importance of technique in providing physical assistance, developing independence, and safety. The readiness of the patient and his or her family to learn must be established before the initiation of orientation and mobility training.

Familiarization to Room Layout. When describing an environment like a room setting, the parts of or objects in a room are described with regard to their direction from the patient (ie, right, left, front, back) and the relationship between them and the distance in measurable terms, such as number of feet. As an illustration, when orienting a patient to a hospital room, the bed may be used as a constant and permanent landmark to serve as a reference point. This reference point helps to maintain a directional orientation relative to significant objects within the room environment.

Movable objects in the room, such as over-bed tables and chairs, are differentiated from the stationary objects, such as large and heavy armchairs, to avoid confusion in the mental mapping of the room environment. The distances of these objects in the room from the reference point of the bed are also described. The nurse may describe the room to a visually impaired patient who is in bed 1 of a two-bed room as follows: "The bedside table is within arm's length toward your right next to the wall, near the head of your bed. Next to your bedside table is the bedside table of the other patient. The other patient's bed is next to this table, about 4 feet from your bed, toward your right. Next to the other bed are the glass windows, which are about 9 feet from your bed, toward your right."

When describing other areas, such as bathrooms, hallways, examination rooms, or elevators, the same technique is used. Touching objects helps to reinforce a representation of the environment in memory. As the nurse guides the patient within the room setting, such as in walking to the bathroom or the examination rooms, a repeated narration to familiarize the patient with the room layout is necessary.

Discharge Planning. The nurse must assess the patient's orientation and mobility skills and skills required for administration of eye medications and other medications, such as insulin injections. Eye drops may be marked for better identification. Insulin syringes may be prefilled and placed in refrigerators for a week's supply or until the next clinic visit. Many patients require referral to social services. Patients with habits that may jeopardize safety, such as smoking, need to be cautioned and assisted in making their environment safe.

GLAUCOMA

Glaucoma is the term used to describe a group of ocular conditions characterized by optic nerve damage. The optic nerve damage is related to increased IOP caused by congestion of aqueous humor in the eye. Glaucoma is one of the leading causes of irreversible blindness in the world and is the leading cause of blindness among adults in the United States. It is estimated that at least 2 million Americans have glaucoma and between 5 and 10 million more are at risk (Margolis and Schachat, 1998). Glaucoma is more prevalent among people older than 40 years of age, and the incidence increases with age. It is also more prevalent among males and in the African American and Asian populations. Currently, there is no cure for glaucoma, but continuing research has shown significant results in successfully controlling this disease.

Aqueous Humor and Intraocular Pressure

Aqueous humor flows between the iris and the lens, nourishing the cornea and lens. Most (90%) of the fluid then flows out of the anterior chamber, draining through the spongy trabecular meshwork into the canal of Schlemm and the episcleral veins

Risk Factors for GLAUCOMA

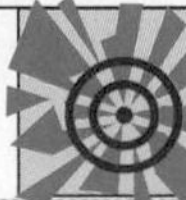

Family history of glaucoma
African American
Age
Diabetes
Cardiovascular disease
Migraine syndromes
Nearsightedness (myopia)
Eye trauma
Prolonged use of topical or systemic corticosteroids

(Fig. 54-7). About 10% of the aqueous fluid exits through the ciliary body into the suprachoroidal space, then drains into the venous circulation of the ciliary body, choroid, and sclera. Unimpeded outflow of aqueous fluid depends on an intact drainage system and an open angle (about 45 degrees) between the iris and the cornea. A narrower angle places the iris closer to the trabecular meshwork, diminishing the angle. The amount of aqueous humor produced tends to decrease with age, in systemic diseases such as diabetes, and in the presence of ocular inflammatory conditions.

IOP is determined by the rate of aqueous production, the resistance encountered by the aqueous humor as it flows out of the passages, and the venous pressure of the episcleral veins that drain into the anterior ciliary vein. When aqueous fluid production and drainage are in balance, the IOP varies between 10 and 21 mm Hg. When aqueous fluid is inhibited from flowing out, pressure builds up within the eye. Fluctuations in IOP may be attributed to time of day, exertion, and food and drugs. It tends to increase with blinking, tight lid squeezing, and upward gazing. Systemic conditions, such as hypertension, and intraocular conditions, such as uveitis and retinal detachments, have been associated with elevated IOP. Exposure to cold weather, alcohol, a fat-free diet, heroin, and marijuana have been found to lower IOP.

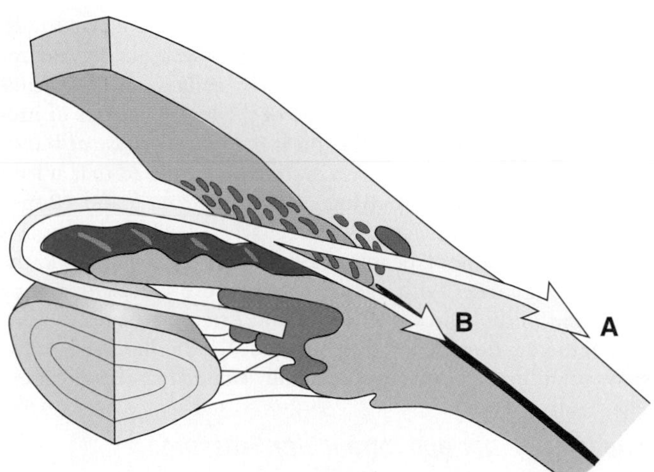

FIGURE 54•7 Normal outflow of aqueous humor. (**A**) Trabecular meshwork. (**B**) Uveoscleral route. From Kanski, J. J. (1994). *Clinical ophthalmology.* Oxford: Butterworth-Heinemann Ltd.

Pathophysiology

There are two accepted theories regarding how increased IOP damages the optic nerve in glaucoma. The *direct mechanical theory* suggests that high IOP damages the retinal layer as it passes through the optic nerve head. The *indirect ischemic theory* suggests that high IOP compresses the microcirculation in the optic nerve head, resulting in cell injury and death. Some glaucomas appear as exclusively mechanical and some are exclusively ischemic types. Typically, most cases are a combination of both.

According to a new theory, nerve cell destruction is due to high levels of the amino acid glutamate (Margolis and Schachat, 1998). This substance stimulates optic nerve cells to send signals to the brain; in toxic levels, the substance may cause overstimulation, resulting in cellular damage. Patients with glaucoma have higher serum levels of the amino acid glutamate than patients without glaucoma.

Regardless of the cause of damage, glaucomatous changes typically evolve through clearly discernible stages. The stages of glaucoma are as follows:

1. *Initiating events:* precipitating factors that include illness, emotional stress, congenital narrow angles, long-term use of corticosteroids, and **mydriatics** (medication causing pupillary dilatation). These events lead to the second stage.
2. *Structural alterations in the aqueous outflow system:* tissue changes and conditions, such as cellular changes caused by factors that affect aqueous humor dynamics. These structural alterations lead to the third stage.
3. *Functional alterations:* conditions such as increased IOP or impaired blood flow. The functional changes lead to the fourth stage.
4. *Optic nerve damage:* atrophy of the optic nerve characterized by loss of nerve fibers and blood supply. The fourth stage inevitably progresses to the fifth stage.
5. *Visual loss:* the progressive loss of vision characterized by visual field defects.

Classification of Glaucoma

As stated previously, glaucoma is not a single entity but rather a group of conditions that share similar characteristics. There are several types of glaucoma. Glaucoma can be *open angle* or *angle closure*, depending on which mechanisms cause the impairment of the aqueous outflow. Glaucoma can also be primary or secondary, depending on whether associated factors contribute to the rise in IOP.

The classification of glaucoma is changing as knowledge about the mechanisms leading to optic nerve damage and consequent loss of vision evolves. Currently, the clinical forms of glaucoma are defined as follows: open-angle glaucomas, angle-closure glaucomas (also called pupillary block), congenital glaucomas, and glaucomas associated with other conditions, such as developmental anomalies, corticosteroid use, and other ocular conditions. For the purposes of this chapter, the two clinical forms of glaucoma commonly encountered in the adult ophthalmologic setting will be presented: open-angle and angle-closure glaucomas. Even though there are several different types of glaucoma, the disease process and treatment patterns are similar. See Table 54-3 for general characteristics of the different types of open-angle and angle-closure glaucomas.

Clinical Manifestations

Although the degree of the manifestations and course of the disease are varied, glaucoma is often called "the silent thief of sight" because most patients initially are not aware they have the disease

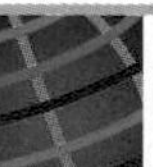

TABLE 54•3 Glaucoma Types, Clinical Manifestation, and Treatment

Types of Glaucoma	Clinical Manifestations	Treatment
Open-Angle Glaucomas		
Usually bilateral, but one eye may be more severely affected than the other. In all three types of open-angle glaucoma, the anterior chamber angle is open and appears normal.		
Chronic open-angle glaucoma (COAG)	Optic nerve damage, visual field defects, IOP >21 mm Hg. May have fluctuating IOPs. Usually no symptoms but possible ocular pain, headache, and halos.	Decrease IOP 20% to 50%. Additional topical and oral agents added as necessary. If medical treatment is unsuccessful, laser trabeculoplasty (LT) can provide a 20% drop in intraocular pressure. Glaucoma filtering surgery if continued optic nerve damage despite drug therapy and LT.
Normal tension glaucoma	IOP ≤ 21 mm Hg. Optic nerve damage, visual field defects.	Treatment similar to COAG, however, the best management for normal tension glaucoma management is yet to be established. Goal is to lower the IOP by at least 30%.
Ocular hypertension	Elevated IOP. Possible ocular pain or headache.	Lower IOP by at least 20%.
Angle-Closure (Pupillary Block) Glaucomas		
Obstruction in aqueous humor outflow due to the complete or partial closure of the angle from the forward shift of the peripheral iris to the trabecula. The obstruction results in an increased IOP.		
Acute angle-closure glaucoma (AACG)	Rapidly progressive visual impairment. periocular pain, conjunctival hyperemia, and congestion. Pain may be associated with nausea, vomiting, bradycardia, and profuse sweating. Reduced central visual acuity, severely elevated IOP, corneal edema. Pupil is vertically oval, fixed in a semi-dilated position, and unreactive to light and accommodation.	Ocular emergency; administration of hyperosmotics, azetazolamide, and topical ocular hypotensive agents, such as pilocarpine and beta-blockers (betaxolol). Possible laser incision in the iris (iridotomy) to release blocked aqueous and reduce IOP. Other eye is also treated with pilocarpine eye drops and/or surgical management to avoid a similar spontaneous attack.
Subacute angle-closure glaucoma	Transient blurring of vision, halos around lights; temporal headaches and/or ocular pain; pupil may be semi-dilated.	Prophylactic peripheral laser iridotomy. Can lead to acute or chronic angle-closure glaucoma if untreated.
Chronic angle-closure glaucoma	Progression of glaucomatous cupping and significant visual field loss; IOP may be normal or elevated; ocular pain and headache.	Management similar to that for COAG: includes laser iridotomy and medications.

until they have experienced visual changes and vision loss. The patient may not seek health care until he or she experiences blurred vision or "halos" around lights, problems focusing, difficulty adjusting eyes in low lighting, loss of peripheral vision, aching or discomfort around the eyes, and headache.

Assessment and Diagnostic Findings

The purpose of a glaucoma workup is to establish the diagnostic category, assess the optic nerve damage, and formulate a treatment plan. The patient's ocular and medical history must be detailed to investigate the history of predisposing factors. There are four major types of examinations used in glaucoma evaluation, diagnosis, and management: tonometry to measure the IOP, ophthalmoscopy to inspect the optic nerve, gonioscopy to examine the filtration angle of the anterior chamber, and perimetry to assess the visual fields.

The changes in the optic nerve significant for the diagnosis of glaucoma are pallor and cupping of the optic nerve disc. The pallor of the optic nerve is due to lack of blood supply that results from cellular destruction. Cupping is characterized by an exaggerated bending of the blood vessels as they cross the optic disc, resulting in an enlarged optic cup that appears more basin-like when compared with a normal cup. The progression of cupping in glaucoma is due to the gradual loss of retinal nerve fibers accompanied by the loss of blood supply, resulting in increased pallor of the optic disc.

As the optic nerve diminishes in the course of glaucoma, visual perception in the area is lost and becomes a defect in the visual field. These localized areas of visual loss (scotomas) represent loss of retinal sensitivity and are measured and mapped by perimetry. The results are mapped on a graph. The perimetry graph representation of the scotomas seen in patients with glaucoma has a distinct pattern that is different from other ocular diseases and is very useful in establishing the diagnosis. The progression of visual field defects caused by glaucoma is shown in Figure 54-8.

Management

The main focus of treatment of any form of glaucoma is prevention of optic nerve damage. This can be achieved through medical therapy, laser or nonlaser surgery, or a combination of these approaches. Lifelong therapy is almost always necessary because glaucoma cannot be cured. Treatment cannot reverse the damage to the optic nerve, but further damage can be controlled. Therefore, the goal of treatment is to maintain an IOP within a range that is unlikely to cause further optic nerve damage.

The initial target for IOP among patients with elevated IOP and those with low-tension glaucoma with progressive visual field loss

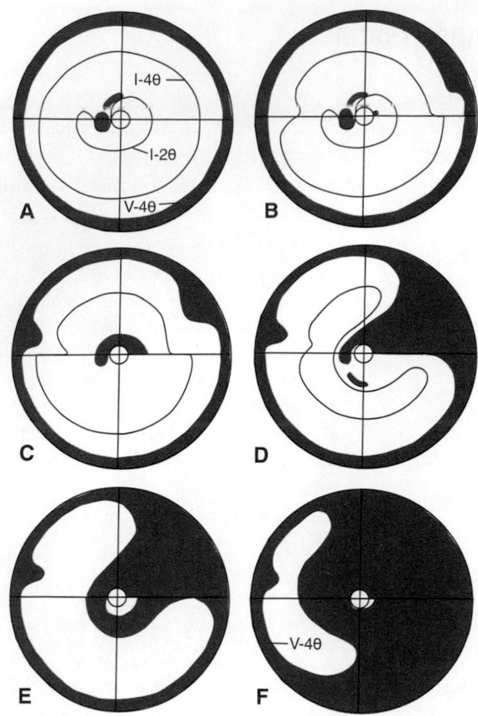

FIGURE 54•8 Progression of glaucomatous visual field defects. A central scotoma at 10 to 20 degrees of fixation near the blind spot is the initial significant finding (**A, B**). As the glaucoma progresses, the scotomas enlarge and deepen, resulting in peripheral field vision loss. (**C**) Defect within 5 degrees of the fixation point nasally; (**D**) peripheral involvement enlarges; (**E**) Ringlike scotoma. Eventually, vision is lost (**F**). The resulting "island of vision" becomes the characteristic visual field appearance of glaucoma and correlates with to the commonly called "tunnel vision" in which peripheral vision is lost. From Kanski, J. J. (1994). *Clinical ophthalmology.* Oxford: Butterworth-Heinemann Ltd.

is typically set at 30% lower than the current pressure. The patient is monitored for the stability of the optic nerve. If there is evidence of progressive damage, the target IOP is again lowered until the optic nerve shows stability.

Treatment is focused on achieving the greatest benefit at the least risk, cost, and inconvenience to the patient. All treatment options have potential complications, especially surgery, which yields the best success rates. In the United States, the more common approach is medical management; surgical management is the last resort. Some ophthalmologists, however, recommend surgery or laser therapy as the initial treatment. In Great Britain, the initial treatment of choice is surgery.

PHARMACOLOGIC THERAPY

Medical management of glaucoma includes the use of both systemic and topical ocular medications that lower IOP. Periodic follow-up examinations are essential to monitor IOP, appearance of the optic nerve, visual fields, and side effects of medications. In deciding to start a patient on a therapeutic regimen, the ophthalmologist follows the principle of delivering efficacy with the least side effects and inconvenience at low cost, which is suitable to the patient's health history, stage of glaucomatous disease, and compliance. Comfort, affordability, convenience, lifestyle, and the patient's personality are factors to consider in the patient's compliance to the medical regimen.

The patient is usually started on the lowest dose of topical medication, then advanced to increased concentrations until the desired IOP level is reached and maintained. Because of their efficacy, minimal dosing (can be used once a day), and low cost, beta-blockers are the preferred initial topical medications. One eye is treated first, with the other eye used as a control in determining the efficacy of the medication; once efficacy has been established, treatment of the fellow eye is started. If IOP is elevated in both eyes, both eyes are treated. When results are not satisfactory, a new medication is substituted. The main markers of the efficacy of the medication in glaucoma control are the lowering of the IOP to the target pressure, the appearance of the optic nerve head, and the visual field.

Several types of ocular medications are currently used to treat glaucoma; these include **miotics** (causing pupillary constriction), adrenergic agonists (sympathomimetics), beta-blockers, alpha$_2$ (adrenergic) agonists, carbonic anhydrase inhibitors, and prostaglandins. Cholinergics (miotics) increase the outflow of the aqueous humor by affecting ciliary muscle contraction and pupil constriction, allowing flow through a larger opening between the iris and the trabecular meshwork. Adrenergic agonists increase aqueous outflow but primarily decrease aqueous production with an action similar to beta-blockers and carbonic anhydrase inhibitors (Table 54-4).

Alpha-adrenergic agonists also decrease aqueous production without altering the outflow. Topical prostaglandin (latanoprost), a potent and efficacious topical ocular hypotensive agent given once a day, increases the aqueous outflow through an alternate drainage system called the uveoscleral pathway located behind the trabecular meshwork. Using latanoprost (Xalatan) as an additive medication to other glaucoma medications can result in significant further pressure reduction.

Combination medications, such as dorzolamide (Dorzopt) and timolol (Cosopt), are more convenient for patients and increase compliance. Hyperosmotic agents produce the most rapid and dramatic decrease in IOP during an acute attack of angle-closure glaucoma. Glycerol or isosorbide can be administered orally; mannitol or urea can be administered intravenously.

Several medications are under investigation for glaucoma control that alter aqueous humor dynamics. These include cannabinoids (marijuana), ethacrynic acid, vasoactive peptides, several types of systemic medications that have hypotensive effects (including phenothiazines), fish oil acids, and new compounds that alter intracellular and extracellular matrix attachments (cytoskeletal agents).

In managing open-angle glaucoma, when there is visual field and optic nerve head damage, medication therapy is indicated to reduce the IOP no matter what the damage level may be. The usual management consists of topical ocular hypotensives, such as beta-blockers (timolol, betaxolol). In ocular hypertension, when there is normal optic nerve and visual field, the ophthalmologist typically starts medication therapy only when the patient is at high risk (IOP of 30 mm Hg or greater) for developing optic nerve damage.

In acute angle-closure glaucoma, immediate medication therapy is necessary to reduce the extremely elevated IOP promptly and to relieve angle closure. Depending on the IOP level, management may start with carbonic anhydrase inhibitors (Diamox) orally and instillation of topical beta-blockers (eg, timolol) or alpha-adrenergic agonists (eg, apraclonidine). If the IOP is unresponsive, oral (glycerol, isosorbide) or intravenous (mannitol, urea) hyperosmotic agents may be used. If the IOP is severely elevated, a surgical procedure may be performed initially. After the IOP is under control, a miotic, such as pilocarpine, is instilled, at least 3 hours after the administration of acetazolamide or timolol, to break the pupillary block and open the angle.

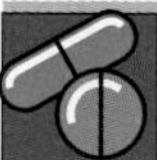

TABLE 54•4 **Medications Used in Managing Glaucoma**

Medication	Action	Side Effects	Nursing Implications
Cholinergics (miotics) (pilocarpine, carbachol)	Increases aqueous fluid outflow by contracting the ciliary muscle and causing miosis (constriction of the pupil) and opening of trabecular meshwork	Periorbital pain, blurry vision, difficulty seeing in the dark	Warn patients about diminished vision in dimly lit areas
Adrenergic agonists (dipivefrin, epinephrine)	Reduces production of aqueous humor and increases outflow	Eye redness and burning; can have systemic effects, including palpitations, elevated blood pressure, tremor, headaches, and anxiety	Teach patients punctal occlusion to limit systemic effects
Beta-blockers (betaxolol, timolol)	Decreases aqueous humor production	Can have systemic effects, including bradycardia, exacerbation of pulmonary disease, and hypotension	Contraindicated in patients with asthma, chronic obstructive pulmonary disease, second- or third-degree heart block, bradycardia, or cardiac failure; teach patients punctal occlusion to limit systemic effects
Alpha-adrenergic agonists (apraclonidine, brimonidine)	Decreases aqueous humor production	Eye redness, dry mouth and nasal passages	Teach patients punctal occlusion to limit systemic effects
Carbonic anhydrase inhibitors (acetazolamide, methazolamide, dorzolamide)	Decreases aqueous humor production	Oral medications (acetazolamide and methazolamide) associated with serious side effects, including anaphylactic reactions, electrolyte loss, depression, lethargy, gastrointestinal upset, impotence, and weight loss; topical form (dorzolamide) side effects include topical allergy	Do not administer to patients with sulfa allergies; monitor electrolyte levels
Prostaglandin analogs (latanoprost)	Increases uveoscleral outflow	Darkening of the iris, conjunctival redness, possible rash	Instruct patients to report any side effects

SURGICAL MANAGEMENT

Laser Surgery. In laser surgery for glaucoma, intense heat is used to create an opening in the anterior chamber angle to facilitate aqueous humor outflow. The ocular structures involved are the trabecular meshwork and the iris. The procedure temporarily creates an exit passage for the blocked aqueous humor, resulting in lower IOP. Laser surgery helps about 80% of patients with glaucoma avoid or delay other surgical interventions. The most common laser surgeries for glaucoma are laser trabeculoplasty and laser iridotomy. Before the procedure, explanation about the nature of the glaucoma condition, laser procedure, risks and possible complications, and postoperative management at home are given to the patient. Because cooperation of the patient is extremely important in any laser surgery procedure, the procedure is contraindicated in uncooperative patients, including children.

In laser trabeculoplasty, about 80 to 100 evenly spaced laser burns are applied to the inner surface of the trabecular meshwork, resulting in scar formation and shrinkage of collagen tissue. Intratrabecular spaces open, and the canal of Schlemm widens, which results in better outflow of aqueous humor. The increased outflow results in decreased IOP levels. Laser trabeculoplasty is indicated when IOP is not adequately controlled despite a maximally tolerated medication regimen, as an adjunct to medication therapy, or to eliminate poorly tolerated medication, such as pilocarpine, in a patient with cataract. This procedure is least effective in patients whose glaucoma is associated with other ocular conditions, in patients with **aphakia** (absence of the natural lens), and in young patients. It is contraindicated in patients in whom the trabecular meshwork cannot be fully visualized because of narrow angles. The most serious known postoperative complication of laser trabeculoplasty is a transient IOP elevation, usually occurring 2 hours after the procedure, that may become persistently elevated. IOP assessment is extremely important in the immediate postoperative period.

In laser iridotomy, an opening in the iris is created by the laser beam as a surgical incision technique, to eliminate the pupillary block. It is indicated in all cases of pupillary block glaucoma. It is contraindicated in patients with corneal edema because the edema limits the ability of the laser beam to focus adequately and to deliver sufficient energy to the iris surface. The edema also increases susceptibility to laser-induced corneal burns. The potential complications of laser iridotomy are burns to the cornea, lens, or retina; transient elevated IOP; closure of the iridotomy; uveitis; and blurring (if the iris surgical site is not beneath the upper lid area). To prevent closure of the iridotomy, pilocarpine is usually prescribed.

Filtering Procedures. The most common surgical procedure for chronic glaucoma is the filtering procedure. An opening or a fistula in the trabecular meshwork is created to allow the drainage of aqueous humor from the anterior chamber to the subconjunctival space into a bleb, thereby bypassing the usual drainage structures. The filtering bleb allows the aqueous to flow and exit to different routes, such as through absorption by the conjunctival vessels or by mixing with tears. It is seen as an elevation in the conjunctiva. Trabeculectomy is the standard technique for filtering procedures that involve the removal of a part of the trabecular meshwork. The most serious complications of filtering procedures include hemorrhage, an extremely low (hypotony) or elevated IOP, uveitis, cataracts, bleb failure, bleb leak, and endophthalmitis.

In glaucoma filtering procedures, unlike other surgical procedures, the goal is to achieve incomplete healing of the surgical wound. The outflow of aqueous in a newly created drainage fistula is circumvented by the granulation of fibrovascular tissue or scar tissue formation on the surgical site. The inhibition of scarring is obtained by the use of antifibrosis agents. The common medications used are antineoplastic agents, such as 5-fluorouracil (5-FU) and mitomycin C. These medications, like all antineoplastic agents, require special handling procedures before, during, and after the surgical procedure. 5-FU can be given intraoperatively during a filtering procedure and as subconjunctival injections during follow-up clinic visits. Mitomycin C, a much more potent medication than 5-FU, is used only intraoperatively.

Drainage Implant Surgery. Drainage implants are devices that maintain the patency of the drainage fistula by draining to an external reservoir. These implants consist of an open tube implanted in the anterior chamber that shunts the aqueous humor to an attached plate in the conjunctival space. The plate serves as an episcleral explant where the aqueous is diverted. A fibrous capsule develops around the episcleral plate and filters the aqueous humor, thereby regulating the outflow and controlling IOP.

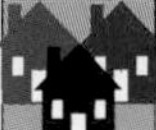

PATIENT EDUCATION AND HOME CARE

Managing Glaucoma

- Know your intraocular pressure measurement and the desired range.
- Be informed about the extent of your vision loss and optic nerve damage.
- Keep a record of your eye pressure measurements and visual field test results to monitor your own progress.
- Review all your medications (including over-the-counter medications) with your ophthalmologist, and mention any side effects each time you visit.
- Ask about potential side effects and drug interactions of your eye medications.
- Ask if generic or cheaper forms of your eye medications are available.
- Review the dosing schedule with your ophthamologist and inform him or her if you have trouble complying with the schedule.
- Participate in the decision-making process. Let your doctor know what dosing schedule works for you and other preferences regarding your eye care.
- Have the nurse observe you instilling eye medication to determine whether you are administering it properly.
- Be aware that glaucoma medications can cause adverse effects if used inappropriately. Eyedrops are to be administered as ordered, not when eyes feel irritated.
- Ask your ophthamologist to send a report to your primary care physician after each appointment.
- Keep all follow-up appointments.

PROMOTING HOME AND COMMUNITY-BASED CARE

Teaching Patients Self-Care. The medical and surgical management of glaucoma retards the progression of glaucoma but does not cure it. Because medication therapy is a lifelong therapeutic regimen, patient education is crucial. The nature of the disease and the importance of strict adherence to the medication regimen must be explained. A thorough patient interview is essential to determine systemic conditions, current systemic and ocular medications, family history, and problems with compliance to glaucoma medications.

The drug interactions of glaucoma-control medications with other medications should be explained. For example, the diuretic effect of acetazolamide has an additive effect to the diuretic effects of other antihypertensive medications and can result in hypokalemia. The effects of glaucoma control medications on vision must also be explained. Miotics and sympathomimetics result in alterations in the focusing of vision; therefore, patients must be advised to be cautious in navigating their surroundings. Refer to the section on ophthalmic medications for information about instilling ocular medication and preventing systemic absorption with punctal occlusion.

Nurses in all settings encounter patients with glaucoma. Even patients with long-standing disease and those with glaucoma as a secondary diagnosis should be assessed for knowledge level and compliance with the therapeutic regimen. Refer to the Patient Education and Home Care display for points to review with glaucoma patients.

Continuing Care. For patients whose glaucoma is severe and in whom functional impairment is apparent, referral to services that assist the patient to enhance performance of customary activities is necessary. The loss of peripheral vision impairs mobility the most. These patients need to be referred to low-vision and rehabilitation services. Patients who meet the criteria for legal blindness, should be referred to agencies that assist in obtaining benefits from federally assisted programs.

Reassurance and emotional support are important aspects of care. A lifelong disease involving a possible loss of sight has psychological, physical, social, and vocational ramifications. The family must be integrated into the plan of care as well. Because the disease has a familial tendency, family members must be encouraged to undergo ophthalmologic examinations at least once every 2 years for the early detection of glaucoma, particularly after 40 years of age.

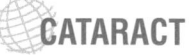

CATARACT

A cataract is a lens opacity or cloudiness (Fig. 54-9). Cataracts rank only behind arthritis and heart disease as a leading cause of disability in older adults. Fifty percent of people between the ages of 65 and 74 years and 70% of those aged 75 years or older have cataracts. In the United States, cataracts are the most common cause of visual impairment and the third most common cause of preventable blindness.

Pathophysiology

Cataracts can develop at any age and may be due to a variety of causes. However, they are most common in later life and are associated with aging. Cataracts can develop in both eyes, although one eye is usually more compromised. Visual impairment normally progresses at the same rate in both eyes, that is, over many years or in a matter of months.

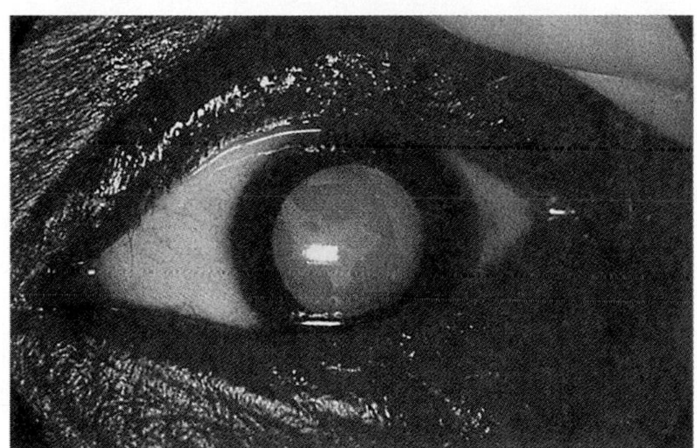

FIGURE 54•9 A cataract is a cloudy or opaque lens. On visual inspection the lens appears gray or milky. From Rubin, E., & Farber, J. L. (1999). *Pathology* (3rd ed.). Philadelphia: Lippincott Williams & Wilkins.

The three most common types of senile cataracts are defined by their location in the lens: nuclear, cortical, and posterior subcapsular. The extent of visual impairment depends on the size, density, and location in the lens. More than one type can be present in one eye.

Nuclear cataract is often associated with myopia. When a cataract progresses over time, the myopia (nearsightedness) worsens. This may be managed temporarily by periodic changes in prescription eyeglasses. This type of cataract generally progress slowly; however, a dense nuclear cataract causes severe blurring of vision.

Cortical cataract involves the anterior, posterior, or equatorial cortex of the lens. A cataract in the equator or periphery of the cortex does not interfere with the passage of light through the center of the lens and has little effect on vision. Cortical cataracts progress at a highly variable rate. Vision is worse in very bright light. Studies show that people with the highest levels of sunlight exposure have twice the risk of developing cortical cataracts than do those with low-level sunlight exposure.

Posterior subcapsular cataract occurs in front of the posterior capsule. It typically develops in younger people and in some cases is associated with prolonged corticosteroid use, inflammation, or trauma. Near vision is diminished, and there is increased sensitivity to glare from bright sunlight and headlights from oncoming cars.

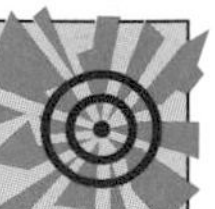

Risk Factors for CATARACT FORMATION

Aging
Loss of lens transparency
Clumping or aggregation of lens protein (which leads to light scattering)
Accumulation of a yellow-brown pigment due to the breakdown of lens protein
Decreased oxygen uptake
Increase in sodium and calcium
Decrease in vitamin C, protein levels, and glutathione (an antioxidant)

Associated Ocular Conditions
Retinitis pigmentosa
Myopia
Retinal detachment and retinal surgery
Infection (ie, herpes zoster, uveitis)
Following drainage surgery

Toxic Factors
Corticosteroids, especially at high doses and in long-term use
Alkaline chemical eye burns, poisoning
Cigarette smoking
Calcium, copper, iron, gold, silver, and mercury, which tend to deposit in the pupillary area of the lens

Nutritional Factors
Reduced levels of antioxidants
Poor nutrition
Obesity

Physical Factors
Dehydration associated with chronic diarrhea, use of purgatives in anorexia nervosa, and use of hyperbaric oxygenation
Blunt trauma, perforation of the lens with a sharp object or foreign body, electric shock
Ultraviolet radiation in sunlight and x-rays

Systemic Diseases and Syndromes
Diabetes mellitus
Down's syndrome
Disorders related to lipid metabolism
Renal disorders
Musculoskeletal disorders

Clinical Manifestations

Painless blurring of vision is characteristic of cataracts. The patient perceives that his or her surroundings have become dimmed, as if glasses are in need of cleaning. Light scattering is common, and the individual experiences a reduction in contrast sensitivity, sensitivity to glare, and reduced visual acuity. Other demonstrable ways in which vision is affected include myopic shift, astigmatism, monocular **diplopia** (double vision), color shift (aging lens becomes progressively more absorbent at the blue end of the spectrum), brunescense (the color values shift to yellow brown), and reduced light transmission.

Assessment and Diagnostic Findings

Decrease in visual acuity is directly proportionate to density of the cataract. The Snellen visual acuity test, ophthalmoscopy, and slit-lamp biomicroscopic examination establish the degree of cataract formation. The degree of lens opacity does not always correlate with the patient's functional status. Some patients are able to perform normal activities despite clinically significant cataracts. Others with a lesser degree of lens opacification have a disproportionate decrease in visual acuity; hence, visual acuity is an imperfect measure of visual impairment.

Medical Management

There is no nonsurgical treatment that cures cataract. Ongoing studies are directed toward investigating ways to retard the progression of cataracts, such as intake of vitamin C and other antioxidants (beta-carotene, vitamin E). In the early stages of cataract development, glasses, contact lenses, strong bifocals, or magnifying lenses may improve vision. Reducing glare with proper light and appropriate positioning of light can facilitate reading. Mydriatics can be used as short-term treatment to dilate the pupil and allow more light to reach the retina. This, however, increases glare.

SURGICAL MANAGEMENT

Less than 15% of people with cataracts suffer vision problems severe enough to require surgery. In general, if reduced vision from cataract does not interfere with normal activities, surgery may not be needed. The patient's functional and visual status should be a primary consideration in deciding when cataract surgery is to be performed. If the patient requires surgery, it is performed on an outpatient basis and usually takes less than an hour. The patient is often discharged in 30 minutes (or less) after surgery. Although complications from cataract surgery are uncommon, they can have significant effects on vision (Table 54-5).

When both eyes have cataracts, one eye is treated at a time, with at least several weeks, preferably months, separating the two operations. Because cataract surgery is performed to improve visual functioning, the delay for the other eye gives time for the patient and the surgeon to evaluate whether the results from the first surgery are adequate enough to preclude the need for a second operation. In addition, the delay provides time for the first eye to recover; if there are any complications, the surgeon may decide to perform the second procedure differently.

Intracapsular Cataract Extraction.

From the late 1800s until the 1970s, the technique of choice for cataract extraction was intracapsular cataract extraction (ICCE). The entire lens (the nucleus, cortex, and capsule) is removed and very fine sutures are used to close the incision. ICCE is not frequently performed today; however, it is indicated when there is a need to remove all of the lens, such as with a subluxated cataract (lens is partially or completely dislocated).

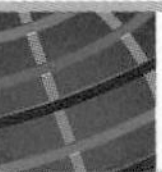

TABLE 54•5 Potential Complications of Cataract Surgery

Complication	Effects	Management and Outcome
Immediate Preoperative		
Retrobulbar hemorrhage: Can result from retrobulbar infiltration of anesthetic agents if the short ciliary artery is located by the injectia	Increased IOP, proptosis, lid tightness, and subconjunctival hemorrhage with or without edema	Emergent lateral canthotomy is performed to stop central retinal perfusion when the IOP is dangerously elevated. If this procedure fails to reduce IOP, a puncture of the anterior chamber with removal of fluid is considered. The patient must be closely monitored for at least a few hours. Postponement of cataract surgery for 2 to 4 weeks is advised. Complications such as iris prolapse, vitreous loss, and choroidal hemorrhage could result in a catastrophic visual outcome.
Intraoperative Complications		
Rupture of the posterior capsule	May result in loss of vitreous	Anterior vitrectomy is required if vitreous loss occurs.
Suprachoroidal (expulsive) hemorrhage: Profuse bleeding into the suprachoroidal space	Extrusion of intraocular contents from the eye or opposition of retinal surfaces	Closure of the incision and administration of a hyperosmotic agent to reduce IOP or corticosteroids to reduce intraocular inflammation. Vitrectomy is performed 1 to 2 weeks later. Visual prognosis is poor; some useful vision may be salvaged on rare occasions.
Early Postoperative Complications		
Acute bacterial endophthalmitis: Devastating complication that occurs in about 1 in 1000 cases; the most common causative organisms are *Staphylococcus epidermitus, S. aureus, Pseudomonas* and *Proteus* species	Characterized by marked visual loss, pain, lid edema, hypopyon, corneal haze, and chemosis	Managed by aggressive antibiotic therapy. Broad-spectrum antibiotics are administered while awaiting culture and sensitivity results. Once results are obtained, the appropriate antibiotics are administered via intravitreal injection. Corticosteroid therapy is also administered.
Late Postoperative Complications		
Suture-related problems	Toxic reactions or mechanical injury from broken or loose sutures	Suture removal relieves the symptoms. Topical corticosteroids are used when the incision is not healed and sutures cannot be removed.
Malposition of the IOL	Results in astigmatism, sensitivity to glare, or appearance of halos	Miotics are used for mild cases, whereas IOL removal and replacement is necessary for severe cases.
Chronic endophthalmitis	Persistent, low-grade inflammation and granuloma	Corticosteroids and antibiotics are administered systemically. If the condition persists, removal of the IOL and capsular bag, vitrectomy, and intravitreal injection of antibiotics are required.
Opacification of the posterior capsule (most common late complication of extracapsular cataract extraction)	Visual acuity is diminished.	YAG laser is used to create a hole in the posterior capsule. Blurred vision is cleared immediately.

Extracapsular Surgery. Extracapsular cataract extraction (ECCE) achieves the intactness of smaller incisional wounds (less trauma to the eye) and maintenance of the posterior capsule of the lens (reducing postoperative complications, particularly aphakic retinal detachment and cystoid macular edema). In ECCE, a portion of the anterior capsule is removed, allowing extraction of the lens nucleus and cortex. The posterior capsule and zonular support are left intact. An intact zonular–capsular diaphragm provides the needed safe anchor for the posterior chamber intraocular lens (IOL). After the pupil has been dilated and the surgeon has made a small incision on the upper edge of the cornea, a viscoelastic substance (clear gel) is injected into the space between the cornea and the lens. This prevents the space from collapsing and facilitates insertion of the IOL.

Phacoemulsification. This method of extracapsular surgery uses an ultrasonic device that liquefies the nucleus and cortex, which are then suctioned out through a tube. The posterior capsule is left intact. Because the incision is even smaller than the standard ECCE, there is more rapid wound healing with early stabilization of refractive error and less astigmatism.

Lens Replacement. After the removal of the crystalline lens, the patient is referred to as aphakic (without lens). The lens, which focuses light on the retina, must be replaced for the patient to see clearly. There are three lens replacement options: aphakic eyeglasses, contact lenses, and IOL implants.

Although aphakic glasses are effective, they are heavy, and objects are magnified by 25%, making them appear closer than they actually are, which causes a disorienting sensation. These thick, heavy glasses also magnify objects unequally, giving a distorting effect; in addition, they tend to limit peripheral vision. There is no chance of **binocular vision** (ability of both eyes to focus on one object and fuse the two images into one) if the other eye is phakic.

Contact lenses are better options than aphakic glasses because they provide patients with almost normal vision. Contact lenses need to be removed on certain occasions; thus, a pair of aphakic glasses is also necessary. Contact lenses are not advisable for patients who have difficulty inserting, removing, and cleaning them. Frequent handling and improper disinfection increase the risk for infection.

Insertion of IOLs during cataract surgery is the usual approach to lens replacement. Because of the inherent disadvantages of aphakic glasses and contact lenses, more than 90% (more than 1 million) of all cataract surgeries in the United States involve IOL implantation. After ICCE, an anterior chamber IOL is implanted in front of the iris. Posterior chamber lenses are generally used in ECCE. They are implanted behind the iris. ECCE and posterior chamber IOL have a lower incidence of complications (ie, hyphema, macular edema, secondary glaucoma, and damage to the corneal endothelium). IOL implantation is contraindicated in patients with recurrent uveitis, proliferative diabetic retinopathy, neovascular glaucoma, or rubeosis iridis. Like any device, IOLs have the potential for complications and can malfunction. Only in wide use since 1977, long-term effects may not yet have emerged.

Nursing Management

PROVIDING PREOPERATIVE CARE

The patient with cataracts should receive the usual preoperative care for ambulatory surgical patients undergoing eye surgery. To reduce the risk for retrobulbar hemorrhage (after retrobulbar injection), any anticoagulation therapy that the patient is receiving is withheld, if medically appropriate. Aspirin should be withheld for 5 to 7 days, nonsteroidal anti-inflammatory drugs (NSAIDs) for 3 to 5 days, and warfarin (Coumadin) until the prothrombin time of 1.5 is almost reached.

Dilating drops are administered every 10 minutes for four doses at least 1 hour before surgery. Additional dilating drops may be administered in the operating room (immediately before surgery) if the operative eye is not fully dilated. Antibiotic, corticosteroid, NSAID drops may be administered prophylactically to prevent postoperative infection and inflammation.

PROVIDING POSTOPERATIVE CARE

After recovery from anesthesia, the patient receives verbal and written instruction regarding how to protect the operative eye, administer medications, recognize signs of complications, and obtain emergency care. Activities to be avoided are discussed.

The nurse explains that there is minimal discomfort after surgery and to take a mild analgesic, such as acetaminophen, as needed. Antibiotic, anti-inflammatory, and corticosteroid eye drops or ointments are prescribed postoperatively.

PROMOTING HOME AND COMMUNITY-BASED CARE

Teaching Patients Self-Care. To prevent accidental rubbing or poking of the eye, the patient wears a protective eye patch for 24 hours after surgery, followed by eyeglasses worn during the day and a metal shield worn at night for 1 to 4 weeks. The nurse instructs the patient and family in how to apply and care for the eye shield. Sunglasses should be worn while outdoors during the day because the operated eye is sensitive to light.

Slight morning discharge, some redness, and a scratchy feeling may be expected for a few days. A clean, damp washcloth may be used to remove slight morning eye discharge. Cataract surgery increases the risk for retinal detachment. The patient must know to notify the surgeon if new floaters (dots) in vision, flashing lights, decrease in vision, pain, or increase in redness occur.

Continuing Care. The eye patch is removed after the first doctor's appointment. Patients may experience blurring of vision for several days to weeks. Sutures left in the eye alter the curvature of the cornea, resulting in temporary blurring and some astigmatism. Vision gradually improves as the eye heals. Patients with IOL implants have visual improvement faster than those waiting for aphakic glasses or contact lenses. Vision is stabilized when the eye is completely healed, usually within 6 to 12 weeks, when final corrective prescription is completed. Visual correction is needed for any remaining nearsightedness or farsightedness (even in patients with IOL implants). With continuous improvement in cataract surgery (ie, smaller incision to reduce postoperative astigmatism and improvement in IOL design and optics), the goal of cataract surgery is transitioning from BCVA to excellent unaided distance vision.

CORNEAL DISORDERS

Corneal Dystrophies

Corneal dystrophies are inherited as autosomal dominant traits and present at about 20 years of age. They are characterized by deposits in the corneal layers. A decrease in vision is due to the irregular corneal surface and the corneal deposits. Corneal endothelial decompensation leads to corneal edema and blurring of vision. Persistent edema leads to **bullous keratopathy**, which is formation of blisters that cause pain and discomfort on rupturing. This condition is usually associated with primary open-angle glaucoma.

A bandage contact lens is used to flatten the bullae, protect the exposed corneal nerve endings, and provide comfort to the patient. Symptomatic treatments, such as hypertonic drops or ointment (5% sodium chloride), may reduce epithelial edema; lowering of IOP will reduce stromal edema as well. Penetrating keratoplasty has a high success rate in advanced cases (refer to section on corneal surgical procedures).

Keratoconus

Keratoconus is a condition characterized by a conical protuberance of the cornea with progressive thinning on protrusion and irregular astigmatism. The condition is hereditary and has a higher incidence in women. The onset occurs at puberty; the condition may progress for more than 20 years and is bilateral. Corneal scarring occurs in severe cases. Blurred vision is a prominent symptom.

Rigid gas-permeable contact lenses correct irregular astigmatism and improve vision. Advances in contact lens design have reduced the need for surgery. Penetrating keratoplasty is indicated when contact lens correction is no longer effective.

Corneal Surgical Procedures

Phototherapeutic Keratectomy

Phototherapeutic keratectomy (PTK) uses a laser to treat diseased corneal tissue by removing or reducing corneal opacities and smoothing the anterior corneal surface to improve functional vision. PTK is a safer, more effective (when indicated) alternative than penetrating or lamellar keratoplasty. PTK is contraindicated in patients with active herpetic keratitis because the ultraviolet rays may reactivate latent virus. Common side effects are induced hyperopia and stromal haze. Complications are delayed reepithelialization (particularly in patients with diabetes) and bacterial keratitis.

Postoperative management consists of oral analgesics for eye pain. Reepithelialization is promoted with either a pressure patch or therapeutic soft contact lens. Antibiotic and corticosteroid ointment and NSAIDs are prescribed postoperatively. Follow-up examinations are required for up to 2 years.

Keratoplasty

Keratoplasty (corneal transplantation or corneal grafting) involves the replacement of the abnormal host tissue with a healthy donor corneal tissue. The graft may be partial thickness (lamellar keratoplasty) or full thickness (penetrating keratoplasty). Common indications are keratoconus, corneal dystrophy, corneal scarring from herpes simplex keratitis, and chemical burns.

The decision to perform penetrating keratoplasty is a joint agreement between the surgeon and the informed patient. The expected visual outcome must be evaluated, and the effects of other ocular conditions must be considered preoperatively. The patient's history should include accurate information about the patient's best visual acuity before the development of the corneal opacification.

The state of the recipient's cornea is a determinant for the success of penetrating keratoplasty. The corneal evaluation includes assessment of the corneal thickness, evaluation of vascularization, size of opacity, and presence of inflammation. Other ocular structures (the lids, conjunctiva), tear film function, and adequacy of blinking also determine the success of the graft. Such conditions as glaucoma, retinal disease, and **strabismus** (deviation in ocular alignment) can negatively influence the outcome. Penetrating keratoplasty requires frequent immediate and subsequent long-term follow-up care.

The success of keratoplasty depends primarily on the viability of the donor endothelium; hence, the corneal tissue must be carefully chosen and meticulously stored. Tissue that is the possible source of disease transmission from donor to recipient or cornea with functionally compromised endothelium is typically not used for grafting (Chart 54-1). Although the age of the donor is not a factor in long-term graft survival, endothelial abnormalities and dysfunction are more common as the eye matures. Surgeons prefer to use corneal tissue from people younger than 65 years of age but older than 2 years of age.

SURGICAL PROCEDURE

The surgeon determines the graft size before the procedure, and the appropriate size is marked on the surface of the cornea. The surgeon prepares the donor cornea and then the recipient bed. The diseased cornea is removed. The donor cornea is placed on the recipient bed and sutured. Sutures are left in place for 12 to 18 months. Potential complications include early graft failure secondary to poor quality of donor tissue, surgical trauma, acute infection, or persistent increased IOP and late graft failure due to rejection.

Nursing Management

Postoperatively, mydriatics are prescribed for 2 weeks, and topical corticosteroids are prescribed for 12 months (daily for 6 months and then tapered). Patients typically describe a sensation of postoperative eye discomfort rather than acute pain.

The patient is instructed about visual rehabilitation and visual improvement. Despite a technically successful corneal graft, the final visual acuity may be disappointing because of the new optical surface that has formed. The surgeon waits for months to allow wound healing before selectively removing sutures. Suturing technique and selective suture removal affect the degree of

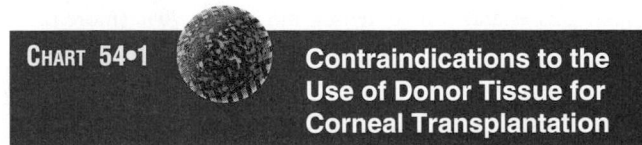

Systemic Disorders

- Death from unknown cause
- Creutzfeldt-Jacob disease
- AIDS and high risk for HIV infection
- Hepatitis
- Eye infection, systemic infection

Intrinsic Eye Disease

- Retroblastoma
- Ocular inflammation
- Malignant tumors of anterior segment
- Disorders of the conjunctiva or corneal surface involving the optical zone of the cornea

History of Eye Trauma

corneal distortion and resultant astigmatism. Correction of the refractive error with eyeglasses or contact lens determines the final visual outcome. It is only after several months that patients start seeing the natural and true colors of their environment. The nurse assesses the patient's support system and his or her ability to comply with long-term follow-up, which includes frequent clinic visits for several months for tapering of topical corticosteroids, selective suture removal, and ongoing evaluation of the graft site and visual acuity. The nurse initiates appropriate referral to community services when indicated.

Graft failure is an ophthalmic emergency. Because it can occur at any time, the primary goal of nursing care is to educate the patient to identify signs and symptoms of graft failure for their lifetime. The early symptoms are blurred vision, discomfort, tearing, or redness of the eye. Decreased vision results after graft destruction. Patients must contact the ophthalmologist as soon as symptoms occur. Treatment of graft rejection is prompt administration of hourly topical corticosteroids and periocular corticosteroid injections. Efforts are directed at preventing immune graft rejection. Systemic immunosuppressive agents may be necessary for severe, resistant cases.

RETINAL DISORDERS

Although the retina is composed of multiple microscopic layers, the two innermost layers, the sensory retina and the RPE, are the most relevant to the discussion of common retinal disorders. Just as the film in a camera captures an image, so does the retina, the neural tissue of the eye. The rods and cones, the photoreceptor cells, are found in the sensory layer of the retina. When they are stimulated by light, an electrical impulse is generated, and the image is transmitted to the brain. Beneath the sensory layer lies the RPE, the pigmented layer.

Retinal Detachment

Retinal detachment refers to the separation of the retinal pigment epithelium (RPE) from the sensory layer. The four types of retinal detachment are rhegmatogenous, traction, a combination of rhegmatogenous and traction, and exudative. Rhegmatogenous detachment is the most common. In this condition, a hole or tear develops in the sensory retina, allowing some of the liquid vitreous to seep through the sensory retina and detach it from the RPE (Fig. 54-10). People at risk for this type of detachment include those with high myopia or aphakia after cataract surgery. Trauma may also play a role in the development of rhegmatogenous retinal detachment. Between 5% and 10% of all rhegmatogenous retinal detachments are associated with proliferative retinopathy, a retinopathy associated with diabetic neovascularization (see Chap. 37).

Tension or a pulling force is responsible for traction retinal detachment. An ophthalmologist must ascertain all of the areas of retinal break and identify and release the scars or bands of fibrous material providing traction on the retina. Generally, patients with this condition have developed fibrous scar tissue from conditions such as diabetic retinopathy, vitreous hemorrhage, or the retinopathy of prematurity. The hemorrhages and fibrous proliferation associated with these conditions exert a pulling force on the delicate retina.

Patients can also have both rhegmatogenous and traction retinal detachment. Exudative retinal detachments are the result of the production of a serous fluid under the retina from the choroid. Conditions such as uveitis or macular degeneration may cause the production of this serous fluid.

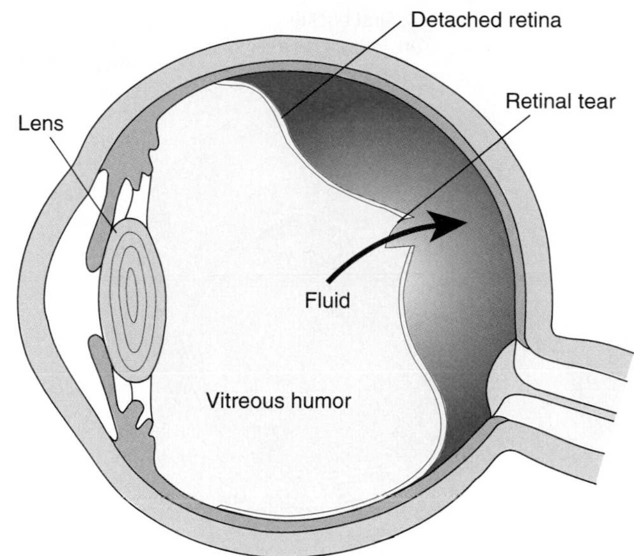

FIGURE 54•10 Retinal detachment.

Clinical Manifestations

Patients may report the sensation of a shade or curtain coming across the vision of one eye, cobwebs, bright flashing lights, or the sudden onset of a great number of floaters. Patients do not complain of pain.

Assessment and Diagnostic Findings

After visual acuity is determined, the patient must have a dilated fundus examination using both an indirect ophthalmoscope and a Goldmann three-mirror examination. This examination is detailed and prolonged and can be very uncomfortable for the patient. Many patients describe this as looking directly into the sun. All retinal breaks, all fibrous bands that may be causing traction on the retina, and all degenerative changes must be identified. A detailed retinal drawing is made by the ophthalmologist.

Management

In rhegmatogenous detachment, an attempt is made to reattach the sensory retina to the RPE surgically. The retinal surgeon compresses the sclera (often with a scleral buckle or a silicone band; Fig. 54-11) to indent the scleral wall from the outside of the eye and bring the two retinal layers in contact with each other. Gas bubbles, silicone oil, or perfluorocarbon and liquids may also be injected into the vitreous cavity to help push the sensory retina up against the RPE. Argon laser photocoagulation or cryotherapy is also used to "spot-weld" small holes.

In traction retinal detachment, a vitrectomy is performed. A vitrectomy is an intraocular procedure in which 1- to 4-mm incisions are made at the pans plana. One incision allows the introduction of a light source (the edoilluminator), and another incision serves as the portal for the vitrectomy instrument. The surgeon dissects preretinal membranes under direct visualization while the retina is stabilized by an intraoperative vitreous substitute. Technologic advances, including the use of operating microscopes, microinstrumentation, irrigating contact lenses, and instruments that combine vitreous cutting, aspiration, and illumination capabilities into one device, have allowed tremendous

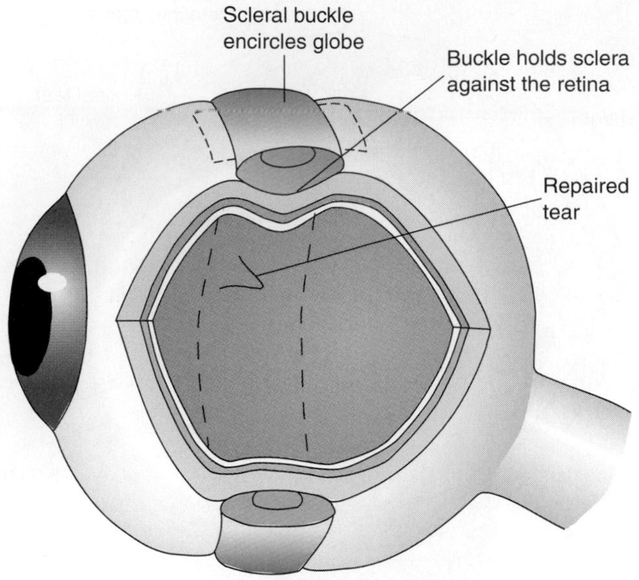

FIGURE 54•11 Scleral buckle.

progress in vitreoretinal surgery. The techniques of vitreoretinal surgery can be used in various procedures, including the removal of foreign bodies, vitreous opacities such as blood, and dislocated lenses and in retinal detachment repair. Traction on the retina may be relieved through vitrectomy and may be combined with scleral buckling to repair retinal breaks. Treatment of macular holes includes vitrectomy, laser photocoagulation, air–fluid–gas exchanges, and the use of growth factor.

PROMOTING HOME AND COMMUNITY-BASED CARE

Teaching Patients Self-Care. If gas as a gas tamponade is used to flatten the retina, the patient may have to be specially positioned to make the gas bubble float into the best position. Some patients must lie face down or on their side for days at a time. Patients and family members should be made aware of these special needs beforehand, so that the patient can be made as comfortable as possible.

Continuing Care. In many cases, vitreoretinal procedures can be performed on an outpatient basis. The patient is seen the next day in follow-up and closely monitored thereafter as required. Patients must be taught about the signs and symptoms of increasing IOP and postoperative infection. Postoperative complications in these patients may include increased IOP, endophthalmitis, the development of other retinal detachments, the development of cataracts, and the loss of turgor of the eye (phthisis).

Retinal Vascular Disorders

Loss of vision can occur from occlusion of a retinal artery or vein. Such occlusions may result from atherosclerosis, cardiac valvular disease, venous stasis, hypertension, or increased blood viscosity.

Central Retinal Vein Occlusion

Blood supply to the ocular fundus is provided by the central retinal artery and vein. Patients who have suffered a central retinal vein occlusion present with decreased visual acuity. This loss of visual acuity may range from mild blurring to vision that is limited to only hand-motion vision.

Direct ophthalmoscopy of the retina reveals optic disc swelling, venous dilation and tortuousness, retinal hemorrhages, cotton-wool spots, and a so-called blood and thunder appearance to the retina. The better the initial visual acuity, the better the general prognosis.

Fluorescein angiography may reveal extensive areas of capillary closure. The patient should be monitored carefully over the ensuing several months for signs of neovascularization and neovascular glaucoma. Laser panretinal photocoagulation may be necessary to treat the abnormal neovascularization. Neovascularization of the iris may cause neovascular glaucoma, which may be difficult to control.

Branch Retinal Vein Occlusion

Some patients with branch retinal vein occlusions are symptom free, whereas others complain of a sudden loss of vision if the macular area is involved. A more gradual loss of vision may occur if there is development of macular edema associated with the branch retinal vein occlusion.

On examination, the ocular fundus appears similar to that found with central retinal vein occlusion; however, only those portions of the retina affected by the obstructive veins show the blood and thunder appearance. The diagnostic evaluation and follow-up are the same as for central retinal vein occlusion. Potential complications are similar. The examiner should bear in mind that there may be other associated conditions, such as glaucoma, systemic hypertension, diabetes mellitus, hyperlipidemia, and hyperviscosity syndrome.

Central Retinal Artery Occlusion

The patient with central retinal artery occlusion presents with a sudden loss of vision. Visual acuity is greatly reduced to counting fingers or perhaps worse, and the field of vision is tremendously restricted. A relative afferent pupillary defect is present. Examination of the ocular fundus reveals a pale retina with a cherry-red spot at the fovea. The retinal arteries are thin, and emboli are occasionally seen in the central retinal artery or its branches.

Central retinal artery occlusion is a true ocular emergency. Various treatment modalities are used, including ocular massage, anterior chamber paracentesis, intravenous administration of hyperosmotic agents such as acetazolamide, and high concentrations of oxygen.

Macular Degeneration

Macular degeneration is the most common cause of visual loss in people older than 60 years of age. Commonly termed age-related macular degeneration (AMD), it is characterized by tiny yellowish spots (drusen) beneath the retina. Most people older than 60 years of age have at least a few small drusen. There is a wide range of visual loss in patients with macular degeneration, but most patients do not experience total blindness. Central vision is generally the most affected; most patients retain peripheral vision (Fig. 54-12). There are two types of AMD: dry type and wet type.

Between 85% and 90% of people with AMD have the dry or nonexudative type in which the outer layers of the retina slowly break down. When these drusen occur outside of the macular area, patients generally have no symptoms. When the drusen occur within the macula, there is a gradual blurring of vision that patients may notice when they try to read. There is no known treatment that can slow or cure this type of AMD.

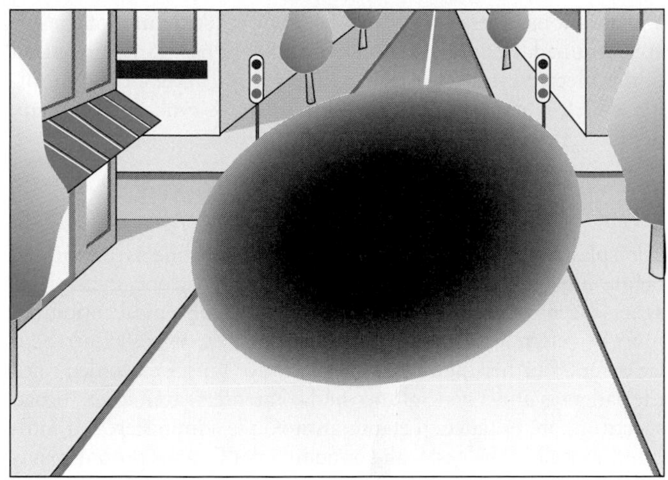

FIGURE 54•12 Visual loss associated with macular degeneration.

The second type of AMD, the wet or exudative type, may have an abrupt onset. Patients complain that straight lines appear crooked and distorted or that letters in words appear broken up. This results from proliferation of abnormal blood vessels growing under the retina, within the choroid layer of the eye. These vessels can leak fluid and blood, raising the retina. Some patients can be treated with the laser to stop the leakage from these vessels. This treatment is not ideal because vision may be affected by the laser treatment and abnormal vessels often grow back after treatment.

Most patients benefit from the use of bright lighting and magnification devices and referral to a low-vision center. Some low-vision centers send representatives into the patient's home or place of employment to evaluate the living and working conditions and make recommendations to improve lighting, thereby improving vision and promoting safety. The home care nurse can make the same assessment and recommendations.

Amsler grids are given to patients to use in their home to monitor for a sudden onset of distortion of vision. These may provide the earliest sign that macular degeneration is getting worse. Patients should be encouraged to use these grids and to look at them several times a week with their glasses on, one eye at a time. If there is a change in the grid, for example, if the lines or squares appear distorted or faded, the patient should be instructed to notify the ophthalmologist immediately and to arrange to be seen promptly.

ORBITAL AND OCULAR TRAUMA

Orbital Trauma

Injury to the orbit is usually associated with a head injury; hence, the patient's general medical condition must first be stabilized before conducting an ocular examination. When the patient is stable, the globe is assessed for soft tissue injury. During inspection, the face is meticulously assessed for possible fractures. Underlying fractures should always be suspected if there is blunt trauma. To establish the extent of ocular injury, visual acuity is assessed as soon as possible, even if it is only a rough estimate. Soft tissue orbital injuries often result in damage to the optic nerve. Major ocular injuries indicated by a soft globe, prolapsing tissue, ruptured globe, hemorrhage, and loss of red reflex require immediate surgical attention.

Soft Tissue Injury and Hemorrhage

The signs and symptoms of soft tissue injury from blunt or penetrating trauma include tenderness, ecchymosis, lid swelling, **proptosis** (downward displacement of the eyeball), and hemorrhage. Closed injuries lead to contusions with subconjunctival hemorrhage, commonly known as "black eye." Blood accumulates in the tissues of the conjunctiva. Hemorrhage may be caused by a soft tissue injury to the eyelid or by an underlying fracture.

Management of soft tissue hemorrhage that is not threatening vision is usually conservative and consists of thorough inspection, cleansing, and repair of wounds; cold compresses are used in the early phase, followed by warm compresses. Hematomas that appear as swollen fluctuating areas may be surgically drained or aspirated; if they are causing significant orbital pressure, they may be surgically evacuated.

Penetrating injuries or severe head blow can result in severe optic nerve damage.

Visual loss can be sudden or delayed and progressive. Immediate loss of vision after an ocular injury is usually irreversible. Delayed visual loss has a better prognosis. Corticosteroid therapy is indicated to reduce optic nerve swelling. Surgery, such as optic nerve decompression, may be performed.

Fractures

Orbital fractures are clearly established by facial x-rays. Depending on the orbital structures involved, orbital fractures can be classified as blow-out, zygomatic or tripod, maxillary, mid-facial, orbital apex, and orbital roof fractures. Blow-out fractures are orbital floor fractures that result from compression of soft tissue and sudden increase in orbital pressure where the force is transmitted to the orbital floor, the area of least resistance.

The inferior rectus and inferior oblique muscles, with their fat and fascial attachments, or the nerve that courses along the inferior oblique may become entrapped, and the globe may be displaced inward (enophthalmos). Computed tomography (CT) scanning can firmly identify the muscle and its auxiliary structures that are entrapped. These fractures are usually caused by blunt small objects, such as a fist, knee, elbow, or tennis or golf balls.

The most common indications for surgical intervention are displacement of bone fragments disfiguring the normal facial contours, interference with normal binocular vision caused by extraocular muscle entrapment, interference with mastication in zygomatic fracture, and obstruction of the nasolacrimal duct. Surgery is usually nonemergent, and a period of 10 to 14 days gives the ophthalmologist time to assess ocular function, especially the extraocular muscles and the nasolacrimal duct. Emergency surgical repair is usually not performed unless the globe is displaced to the maxillary sinus. Operative repair is primarily directed at freeing the entrapped ocular structures and restoring the integrity of the orbital floor. Cosmetic surgery for deformities of the globe and enophthalmos may follow after 4 to 6 months, but successful repair is usually difficult.

Orbital roof fractures are dangerous because of potential complications to the brain. The surgical management of these fractures requires a neurosurgeon and an ophthalmologist.

Foreign Bodies

Foreign bodies that enter the orbit are usually tolerated, except for copper, iron, and vegetative materials such as those from plants or trees, which may cause purulent infection. X-rays and

CT scans identify the foreign body. Careful history taking is important, especially if the foreign body has been in the orbit for a period of time and the incident forgotten. It is important to identify metallic foreign bodies because they prohibit the use of magnetic resonance imaging (MRI) as a diagnostic tool.

After the extent of the orbital damage is assessed, the decision is made between conservative treatment and surgical removal. In general, orbital foreign bodies are usually removed if they are superficial and anterior in location, have sharp edges that may affect adjacent orbital structures, or are composed of copper, iron, or vegetative material. The surgical intervention is directed at prevention of further ocular injury and maintaining the integrity of the affected areas. Cultures are usually obtained, and the patient is placed on prophylactic intravenous antibiotics; these are later changed to oral antibiotics.

Ocular Trauma

Ocular trauma is the leading cause of blindness among children and young adults, especially males. The most common circumstances of ocular trauma are occupational injuries (construction industry), sports (baseball, basketball, racket sports, boxing), weapons (air guns, BB guns), assault, motor vehicle crashes (broken windshields), and war (blast fragments).

For the nonophthalmic practitioner, initial intervention is performed in only two conditions: (1) chemical burns, for which irrigation of the eye with normal saline or even plain tap water must be done immediately; and (2) foreign body, for which no attempt is made to remove the foreign material, small or big, or apply pressure or patch to the injured eye. The eye must be protected using a metal shield if available or a stiff paper cup (Fig. 54-13). All traumatic eye injuries should be properly shielded.

Assessment and Diagnostic Findings

A thorough history is obtained, in particular the patient's ocular history, such as preinjury vision in the affected eye and any past ocular surgery. Details related to the injury that help in the diagnosis and need for further tests include the nature of the ocular injury (ie, blunt or penetrating trauma), the type of activity causing the injury (to determine the nature of the force striking the eye), and whether vision loss was sudden in onset, slow, or progressive. For chemical eye burns, the identity of the chemical agent must be determined and tested for pH (if a sample is available). The corneal surface is examined for foreign bodies, wounds, and abrasions, after which the other external structures of the eye are examined. Pupillary size, shape, and light reaction of the pupil of the affected eye are compared with the other eye. Ocular motility, which is the ability of the eyes to move synchronously up, down, right and left, is also assessed.

Immediate Management

For splash injuries, irrigation with normal saline is performed before further evaluation. In cases of ruptured globe, cycloplegic agents (agents that paralyze the ciliary muscle) or topical antibiotics must be deferred because of potential toxicity to exposed intraocular tissues. Further manipulation of the eye must be avoided until the patient is under general anesthesia. Parenteral antibiotics (broad spectrum) are initiated. Tetanus antitoxin is administered, if indicated, as well as analgesics and antiemetics. (Tetanus prophylaxis is recommended for full-thickness ocular and skin wounds.) Any topical medication (anesthetic, dyes) must be sterile.

Foreign Bodies on the Surface of the Eye and Corneal Abrasions

After removal of a foreign body from the surface of the eye, an antibiotic ointment is applied, and the eye is patched. The eye is examined daily for evidence of infection until the wound is completely healed.

Contact lens wear is a common cause of corneal abrasion. The patient experiences severe pain and **photophobia** (ocular pain on exposure to light). Corneal epithelial defects are treated with antibiotic ointment and a pressure patch to immobilize the lids. It is of utmost importance that topical anesthetic eye drops are not given to a patient for repeated use after corneal injury because this masks further damage, delays healing, and can lead to permanent corneal scarring. Corticosteroids are avoided while the epithelial defect exists.

Penetrating Injuries and Contusions of the Eyeball

Sharp penetrating injury or blunt contusion force can rupture the eyeball. When the eye wall, cornea, and sclera rupture, either rapid decompression or herniation of the orbital contents into adjacent sinuses can occur. In general, blunt traumatic injuries (with an increased incidence of retinal detachment, intraocular tissue avulsion, and herniation) have a worse prognosis than penetrat-

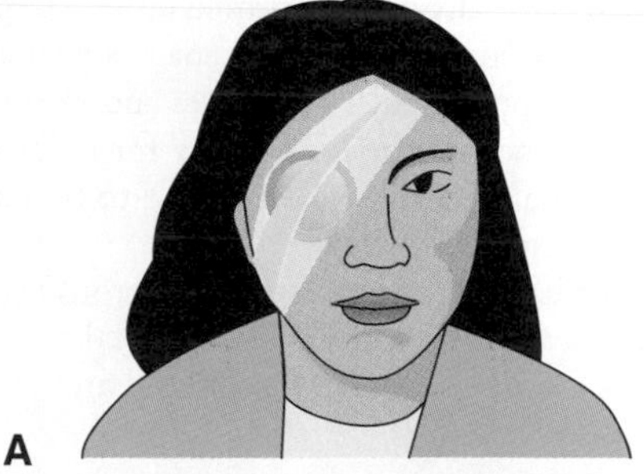

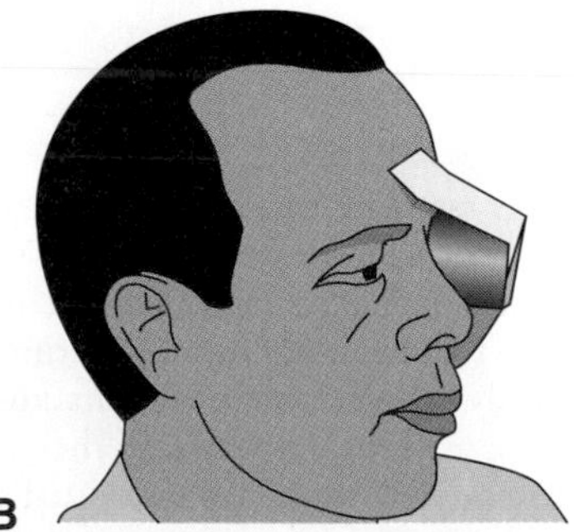

FIGURE 54•13 Two kinds of eye patches. (**A**) Metal shield, (**B**) Stiff paper cup shield (innovative substitute when metal shield is unavailable.) Adapted from MacCumber, M. W. (Ed.). (1997). *Management of ocular injuries and emergencies.* Philadelphia: Lippincott-Raven.

ing injuries. Most penetrating injuries result in marked loss of vision and exhibit the following signs: hemorrhagic **chemosis** (edema of the conjunctiva), conjunctival laceration, shallow anterior chamber with or without an eccentrically placed pupil, **hyphema** (hemorrhage within the chamber), or vitreous hemorrhage.

Hyphema is caused by contusion forces that tear the vessels of the iris and damage the anterior chamber angle. Preventing rebleeding and prolonged increased IOP are the goals of treatment for hyphema. In severe cases in which patient compliance is questionable, the patient is hospitalized with moderate activity restriction. An eye shield is applied. Topical corticosteroids are prescribed to reduce inflammation. An antifibrinolytic agent, aminocaproic acid (Amicar), stabilizes clot formation at the site of hemorrhage. Aspirin is contraindicated.

A ruptured globe and severe injuries with intraocular hemorrhage require surgical intervention. Vitrectomy is performed for traumatic retinal detachments. Primary **enucleation** (complete removal of the eyeball and part of the optic nerve) is considered only if the globe is irreparable with no light perception. It is a general rule that enucleation is performed within 2 weeks of the initial injury (in an eye that has no useful vision after sustaining penetrating injury) to prevent the risk fpr **sympathetic ophthalmia**, an inflammation created in the fellow eye by the affected eye that can result in blindness of the fellow eye.

Intraocular Foreign Bodies

A patient who complains of blurring of vision and discomfort after a history of explosion, striking metal against metal, motor vehicle crash with facial injury, gunshot wound, grinding wheel work, or dental surgery may have an intraocular foreign body (IOFB). IOFB is diagnosed and localized by slit-lamp biomicroscopy and indirect ophthalmoscopy as well as CT or ultrasound. MRI is contraindicated because most foreign bodies are metallic and magnetic. It is important to determine the composition, size, location, and affected eye structures. Every effort should be made to identify the type of IOFB and whether it is magnetic. Iron, steel, copper, and vegetable matter cause intense inflammatory reactions. The incidence of endophthalmitis is also high. If the cornea is perforated, tetanus prophylaxis and intravenous antibiotics are administered. The extraction route (surgical incision) of the foreign body depends on its location and composition and associated ocular injuries. Specially designed IOFB forceps and magnets are used to grasp and remove the foreign body. Any damaged area of the retina is treated to prevent retinal detachment.

Ocular Burns

Alkali, acid, and other chemically active organic substances, such as mace and tear gas, cause chemical burns. Alkali burns (lye, ammonia) result in the most injury because they penetrate the ocular tissues rapidly and continue to cause damage long after the injury is sustained. They also cause an immediate rise in IOP. Acids (bleach, car batteries, refrigerant) generally cause less damage because the precipitated necrotic tissue proteins form a barrier to further penetration and damage. Chemical burns may appear as superficial punctate keratopathy (spotty damage to the cornea), subconjunctival hemorrhage, or complete marbleizing of the cornea.

In chemical burns, every minute counts. Immediate tap water irrigation should be started on site before transport to an emergency department. Only a brief history and examination is done; copious irrigation of the corneal surfaces and conjunctival fornices using normal saline or any neutral solution is done immediately. A local anesthetic is instilled, and a lid speculum is applied to overcome blepharospasm (spasms of the eyelid muscles that result in closure of the lids). Particulate matter must be removed from the fornices using moistened cotton-tip applicators. Minimal pressure is placed on the globe. Irrigation continues until the conjunctival pH normalizes (between 7.3 and 7.6). The pH of the corneal surface is checked by placing a pH paper strip in the fornix. Antibiotics are instilled, and the eye is patched.

The goal of intermediate treatment is to prevent tissue ulceration and promote reepithelialization. Intense lubrication using nonpreserved tears is essential. Reepithelialization is promoted with patching or the use of therapeutic soft lenses. The patient is usually monitored daily for several days. Prognosis depends on the type of injury and adequacy of the irrigation immediately after exposure. Long-term treatment or rehabilitation consists of two phases: (1) restoration of the ocular surface through grafting procedures, and (2) surgical restoration of corneal integrity and optical clarity.

Thermal injury is due to exposure to a hot object (curling iron, tobacco, ash), whereas photochemical injury results from ultraviolet irradiation or infrared exposure (exposure to the reflections from snow, sun gazing, viewing an eclipse of the sun without an adequate filter). These injuries can cause corneal epithelial defect, corneal opacity, conjunctival chemosis and **injection** (congestion of blood vessels), and burns of the eyelids and periocular region. Antibiotics and a pressure patch for 24 hours constitute the treatment of mild injuries. Scarring of the eyelids may require oculoplastic surgery, whereas corneal scarring may require corneal surgery.

Prevention of Eye Injuries

All eye injuries are preventable. Legislative regulation of the workplace requiring protective lenses has been in place in the United States since 1912. Employers must mandate the use of safety glasses and make them available. Noncompliance is the single greatest risk factor in the workplace. In sports, governing bodies and organized leagues must implement specific rules to prevent ocular trauma. Face protectors should be used for field hockey, sports goggles for basketball and racquet ball, and head gear for boxing. Nonpowder firearms, such as air guns and BB guns, must be kept away from children unless they are supervised by responsible adults. Safety goggles should be worn by all military troops in the field to prevent injuries from blast fragments.

INFECTIOUS AND INFLAMMATORY CONDITIONS

Inflammation and infection of eye structures are common. Eye infection is a leading cause of blindness worldwide. Table 54-6 describes selected common infections and their treatment.

Dry Eye Syndrome

Dry eye syndrome, or keratoconjunctivitis sicca, is a condition in which there is deficiency in the production of any of the aqueous, mucin, or lipid tear film components; lid surface abnormalities; or epithelial abnormalities related to systemic diseases, infection or injury, or complications of medications.

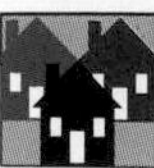

PATIENT EDUCATION AND HOME CARE

Preventing Eye Injuries

In and Around the House

Make sure that all spray nozzles are directed away from you before you press down on the handle.

Read instructions carefully before using cleaning fluids, detergents, ammonia, or harsh chemicals. Wash hands thoroughly after use.

Use grease shields on frying pans to decrease spattering.

Wear special goggles to shield your eyes from fumes and splashes when using powerful chemicals.

Use opaque goggles to avoid burns from sunlamps.

In the Workshop

Protect your eyes from flying fragments, fumes, dust particles, sparks, and splashed chemicals by wearing safety glasses.

Read instructions thoroughly before using tools and chemicals, and follow precautions for their use.

Around Children

Pay attention to age and responsibility level of a child when selecting toys and games. Avoid projectile toys, such as darts and pellet guns.

Supervise children when they are playing with toys or games that can be dangerous.

Teach children the correct way to handle potentially dangerous items, such as scissors and pencils.

In the Garden

Do not let anyone stand on the side or in front of a moving lawn mower.

Pick up rocks and stones before going over them with the lawn mower. These stones can hurl out of the rotary blades and rebound off curbs or walls, causing severe injury to the eye.

Make sure that pesticide spray can nozzles are directed away from your face.

Avoid low-hanging branches.

Around the Car

Before opening the hood of the car, put out all smoking materials and matches. Use a flashlight, not a match or lighter, to look at the battery at night.

Wear goggles when grinding metal or striking metal against metal while performing auto body repair.

When using jumper cables to start the car, wear goggles; make sure the cars are not touching one another; make sure the jumper cable clamps never touch each other; never lean over the battery when attaching cables. *Never* attach a cable to the negative terminal of the dead battery.

In Sports

Wear protective safety glasses, especially for sports such as racquetball, squash, tennis, baseball, and basketball.

Wear protective caps, helmets, or face protectors when appropriate, especially for sports such as ice hockey.

Around Fireworks

Wear eye glasses or safety goggles.

Do not use explosive fireworks.

Never allow children to ignite fireworks.

Do not stand near others when lighting fireworks.

Do not try to relight duds. Douse them in water.

Clinical Manifestations

The most common complaint in dry eye syndrome is a scratchy or foreign body sensation. Other symptoms include itching, excessive mucus secretion, inability to produce tears, burning sensation, redness, pain, and difficulty moving the lids.

Assessment and Diagnostic Findings

Slit-lamp examination shows an absent or interrupted tear meniscus at the lower lid margin, and the conjunctiva is thickened, edematous, hyperemic, and has lost its luster. A tear meniscus is the crescent-shaped edge of the tear film in the lower lid margin. Chronic dry eyes may result in chronic conjunctival and corneal irritation that can lead to corneal erosion, scarring, ulceration, thinning, or perforation that can seriously threaten the loss of vision. Secondary bacterial infection can occur.

Management

Management of dry eye syndrome requires the complete cooperation of the patient in the regimen that needs to be followed at home. It is explained to the patient that the dry eye condition is a long-term problem and that complete abatement of symptoms is unlikely. The management includes hydration and lubrication through tear stimulation, use of artificial tears and lubricants, tear preservation, the preservation of a moist ocular surface, and use of anti-inflammatory medications. Instillation of artificial tears during the day and an ointment at night is the usual regimen. Moisture chambers, such as moisture chamber spectacles or swim goggles, may provide additional relief.

Patients may become hypersensitive to chemical preservatives, such as benzalkonium chloride and thimerosal. For these patients, preservative-free ophthalmic solutions are used. Management of the dry eye syndrome also includes the concurrent treatment of infections, such as chronic blepharitis and acne rosacea, and treating the underlying systemic disease, such as Sjögren's syndrome (an autoimmune disease).

In advanced cases of dry eye syndrome, surgical treatment that includes punctal occlusion, grafting procedures, and lateral tarsorrhaphy (uniting the edges of the lids) are options. Punctal plugs are made of silicone material for the temporary or permanent occlusion of the puncta. This helps preserve the natural tears and prolongs the effects of artificial tears. Short-term occlusion is performed by inserting punctal or silicone rods in all four puncta. If tearing is induced, the upper plugs are removed, and the remaining lower plugs are removed in another week. Permanent occlusion is only performed in severe cases among adults who do not develop tearing after partial occlusion and who have repeated Schirmer's test of 2 mm or less.

Several approaches to dry eye therapy are used with promising results. Increased blinking as an intentional activity reduces exposure of the ocular surface. The use of specially devised glasses with side panels containing wet sponges prevents tear evaporation. For maintaining tear stability, there are new artificial tear preparations that contain hyaluronic acid and high-viscosity methylcellulose. These preparations are viscoelastic agents, making tears as a mucin substitute. The use of topical epidermal growth factor, aldose reductase inhibitor, vitamin A, and immunotherapeutic agents such as cyclosporin and interferon in protecting and maintaining the integrity of the corneal epithelium and conjunctiva are areas of continuing research.

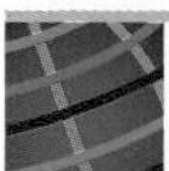

TABLE 54•6 **Common Infections and Inflammatory Disorders of Eye Structures**

Disorder	Description	Management
Hordeolum (sty)	Acute suppurative infection of the glands of the eyelids caused by *Staphylococcus aureus.* The lid is red and edematous with a small collection of pus in the form of an abscess. There is considerable discomfort.	Warm compresses are applied directly to the affected lid area three to four times a day for 10 to 15 minutes. If the condition is not improved after 48 hours, incision and drainage may be indicated. Application of topical antibiotics may be prescribed thereafter.
Chalazion	Sterile inflammatory process involving chronic granulomatous inflammation of the meibomian glands; can appear as a single granuloma or multiple granulomas in the upper or lower eyelids	Warm compresses applied three to four times a day for 10 to 15 minutes may resolve the inflammation in the early stages. Most often, however, surgical excision is indicated. Corticosteroid injection to the chalazion lesion may be used for smaller lesions.
Blepharitis	Chronic bilateral inflammation of the eyelid margins. There are two types: staphylococcal and seborrheic. Staphylococcal blepharitis is usually ulcerative and is more serious due to the involvement of the base of hair follicles. Permanent scarring can result.	The seborrheic type is chronic and is usually resistant to treatment, but the milder cases may respond to lid hygiene and lid scrubs. Staphylococcal blepharitis requires topical antibiotic treatment. Instructions on lid hygiene (to keep the lid margins clean and free of exudates) are given to the patient.
Bacterial keratitis	Infection of the cornea by *S. aureus, Streptococcus pneumoniae,* and *Pseudomonas aeruginosa*	Fortified (high-concentration) antibiotic eyedrops are administered every 30 minutes around the clock for the first few days then every 1–2 hours. Systemic antibiotics may be given. Cycloplegics are given to reduce pain caused by ciliary spasm. Corticosteroid therapy and subconjunctival injections of antibiotics are controversial.
Herpes simplex keratitis	Leading cause of corneal blindness in the United States. Symptoms are severe pain, tearing, and photophobia. The dendritic ulcer has a branching, linear pattern with feathery edges and terminal bulbs at its ends. Herpes simplex keratitis can lead to recurrent stromal keratitis and last up to 12 months with residual corneal scarring.	Many lesions heal without treatment and residual effects. The treatment goal is to minimize the damaging effect of the inflammatory response and eliminate viral replication within the cornea. Penetrating keratoplasty is indicated for corneal scarring and must be performed when the herpetic disease has been inactive for many months.

Conjunctivitis

Conjunctivitis (inflammation of the conjunctiva) is the most common ocular disease worldwide. It is characterized by a pink appearance (hence the common term "pink eye") because of subconjunctival blood vessel hemorrhages.

Clinical Manifestations

General symptoms include foreign body sensation, scratching or burning sensation, itching, and photophobia. Conjunctivitis may be unilateral or bilateral, but the infection usually starts in one eye and then spreads to the other eye by hand contact.

Assessment and Diagnostic Findings

The four main clinical features important to evaluate are the type of discharge (watery, mucoïd, purulent, or mucopurulent), type of conjunctival reaction (follicular or papillary), presence of pseudomembranes or true membranes, and presence or absence of lymphadenopathy (enlargement of the preauricular and submandibular lymph nodes where the eyelids drain). *Pseudomembranes* consist of coagulated exudate that adhere to the surface of the inflamed conjunctiva. *True membranes* form when the exudate adheres to the superficial layer of the conjunctiva, and removal results in bleeding. *Follicles* are multiple slightly elevated lesions, encircled by tiny blood vessels; they look like grains of rice. *Papillae* are hyperplastic conjunctival epithelium in numerous projections that are usually seen as a fine mosaic pattern under slit-lamp examination.

The diagnosis is based on the distinctive characteristics of ocular signs, acute or chronic presentation, and identification of any precipitating events. Positive results of swab smear preparations and cultures confirm the diagnosis.

Types of Conjunctivitis

Conjunctivitis is classified according to its cause. The major causes are microbial infection, allergy, and irritating toxic stimuli. There is a wide spectrum of exogenous microbes that can cause conjunctivitis, including bacteria, viruses, chlamydia, fungus, and parasites. Conjunctivitis can also be a secondary infection of an existing ocular infection or can be a manifestation of a systemic disease.

MICROBIAL CONJUNCTIVITIS

Bacterial conjunctivitis can be acute or chronic. The acute type can develop into a chronic condition. Signs and symptoms can vary from mild to severe. Chronic bacterial conjunctivitis is usually seen in patients with lacrimal duct obstruction, chronic dacryocystitis, and chronic blepharitis. The most common causative microorganisms are *Streptococcus pneumoniae, Haemophilus influenzae,* and *Staphylococcus aureus.*

There is an acute onset of redness, burning, and discharge. There is papillary formation, conjunctival irritation, and injection in the fornices. The exudates are variable but are usually present upon waking in the morning. The eyes may be difficult to open due to the adhesions caused by the exudate. Purulent discharge occurs in severe acute bacterial infections, whereas mucopurulent discharge appears in mild cases. In *gonococcal conjunctivitis,* the symptoms are more acute. The exudate is profuse and purulent, and there is lymphadenopathy. Pseudomembranes may or may not be present.

Viral conjunctivitis (Fig. 54-14) can also be acute and chronic. The discharge is watery, and follicles are prominent. Severe cases include pseudomembranes. The common causative organisms are adenovirus and herpes simplex virus. Conjunctivitis caused by adenovirus is highly contagious. The symptoms include extreme tearing, redness, and foreign body sensation that can involve one or both eyes. The condition is usually preceded by symptoms of upper respiratory infection. Corneal involvement causes extreme photophobia. There is lid edema, ptosis, conjunctival **hyperemia** (dilation of the conjunctival blood vessels), watery discharge, follicles, and papillae. These signs and symptoms vary from mild to severe and may last for 2 weeks. Viral conjunctivitis, although self-limited, tends to last longer than bacterial conjunctivitis.

Epidemic keratoconjunctivitis (EKC) is most often accompanied by preauricular lymphadenopathy and occasionally periorbital pain. There are marked follicular and papillary formations. EKC can lead to keratopathy. EKC is a highly contagious viral conjunctivitis that is easily transmitted from one person to another among household members, school children, and health care workers. The outbreak of epidemics is seasonal, especially during the summer when people frequent swimming pools.

Chlamydial conjunctivitis includes trachoma and inclusion conjunctivitis. *Trachoma* is an ancient disease and is the leading cause of preventable blindness in the world. It is prevalent in areas with hot, dry, and dusty environments and in areas with poor living conditions. It is spread by direct contact or fomites, and the vectors can be insects such as flies and gnats.

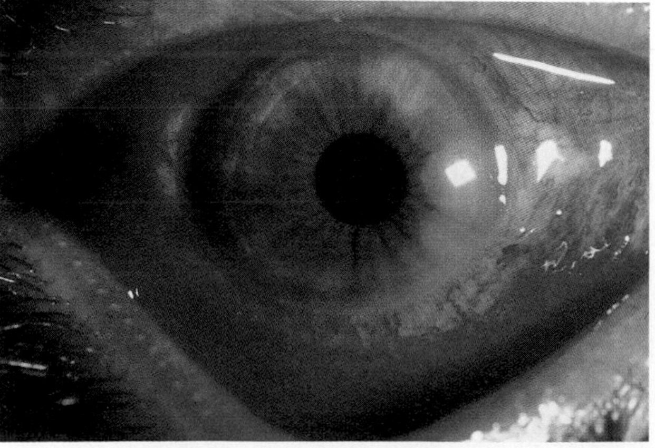

FIGURE 54•14 Conjunctival hyperemia in viral conjunctivitis.

Trachoma is a bilateral chronic follicular conjunctivitis of childhood that leads to blindness during adulthood, if left untreated. The onset in children is usually insidious, but it can be acute or subacute in adults. The initial symptoms include red inflamed eyes, tearing, photophobia, ocular pain, purulent exudates, preauricular lymphadenopathy, and lid edema. Initial ocular signs include follicular and papillary formations. At the middle stage of the disease, there is an acute inflammation with papillary hypertrophy and follicular necrosis, after which trichiasis and entropion begin to develop. The lashes that are turned in rub against the cornea and, after prolonged irritation, cause corneal erosion and ulceration. The late stage of the disease is characterized by scarred conjunctiva, subepithelial keratitis, abnormal vascularization of the cornea (pannus), and residual scars from the follicles that look like depressions in the conjunctiva (called Herbert's pits). Severe corneal ulceration can lead to perforation and, consequently, blindness.

Inclusion conjunctivitis affects sexually active young people who have genital chlamydial infection. Transmission is by oral genital sexual practice or hand-to-eye transmission. It has been reported that indirect transmission has been acquired from inadequately chlorinated swimming pools. The eye lesions usually present a week after exposure and may be associated with a nonspecific urethritis or cervicitis. The discharge is mucopurulent, follicles are present, and there is lymphadenopathy.

ALLERGIC CONJUNCTIVITIS

Immunologic or *allergic conjunctivitis* is a hypersensitivity reaction as a part of allergic rhinitis (hay fever), or it can be an independent allergic reaction. The patient usually has a history of an allergy to pollens and other environmental allergens. There is extreme itching, epiphora (excessive secretion of tears), injection, and most often severe photophobia. The stringlike mucoid discharge is usually associated with rubbing the eyes because of severe itching. *Vernal conjunctivitis* is also known as "seasonal conjunctivitis" because it appears mostly during warm weather. There may be large formations of papillae that have a cobblestone appearance. It is more common in children and young adults. Most affected individuals have a history of asthma or eczema.

TOXIC CONJUNCTIVITIS

Chemical conjunctivitis can be the result of medications, chlorine from swimming pools (more common during the summer), exposure to toxic fumes among industrial workers, or exposure to other irritants such as smoke, hair sprays, and acid and alkalis.

Management

The management of conjunctivitis is dependent on the type. Most types of mild and viral conjunctivitis are self-limiting, benign conditions that may not require treatment and laboratory procedures. For more severe cases, topical antibiotics, eye drops, or ointment are prescribed.

Patients with gonococcal conjunctivitis require urgent antibiotic therapy. If left untreated, this ocular disease can lead to corneal perforation and blindness. The systemic complications can include meningitis and generalized septicemia.

Acute bacterial conjunctivitis is almost always self-limiting. If left untreated, the disease follows a 2-week course with resolution of symptoms. If treated with appropriate antibiotics, it may last for a few days, with the exception of gonococcal and staphylococcal conjunctivitis. Viral conjunctivitis is not responsive to any treatment. Cold compresses may alleviate some symptoms. It is extremely important to remember that viral conjunctivitis, especially EKC, is highly transmissible. Patients must be made aware of the contagious nature of the disease, and adequate instructions must be given.

Proper steps must be taken to avoid nosocomial infections. Frequent hand washing, procedures for environmental cleaning, and disinfection of equipment used for eye examination must be strictly followed at all times. During outbreaks of conjunctivitis caused by adenovirus, it is necessary that, to contain its spread, health care facilities assign specified areas for treating patients with or suspected of having conjunctivitis caused by adenovirus. All forms of tonometry must be avoided unless medically indicated. All multidose medications must be discarded at the end of each day or when contaminated. Infected employees and others must not be allowed to work or attend school until symptoms have resolved, which can take 3 to 7 days.

Patients with allergic conjunctivitis, especially recurrent vernal conjunctivitis, are usually given corticosteroids in ophthalmic preparations. Depending on the severity of the disease, they may be given oral preparations. Use of vasoconstrictors, such as topical epinephrine solution, cold compresses, ice packs, and cool ventilation usually provide comfort.

For trachoma, treatment is usually with broad-spectrum antibiotics administered topically and systemically. Surgical management includes the correction of trichiasis to prevent conjunctival scarring. Adult inclusion conjunctivitis requires a 1-week course of antibiotics. Prevention of reinfection is important, and affected individuals and their sexual partners must be advised to seek evaluation and management for sexually transmitted disease.

For conjunctivitis caused by chemical irritants, the eye must be irrigated immediately and profusely with saline or sterile water.

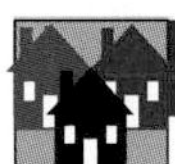

PATIENT EDUCATION AND HOME CARE

Instructions for Patients With Viral Conjunctivitis

Viral conjunctivitis is a highly contagious eye infection. It can easily spread from one person to another. The symptoms can be alarming, but they are not serious. The following information will help you understand this eye condition and how to take care of yourself and/or your family member at home.

- Your eyes will look red and will have watery discharge, and your lids will be swollen for about a week.
- You will experience eye pain, a sandy sensation in your eye, and sensitivity to light.
- Symptoms will resolve after about a week.
- You may use light cold compresses over your eyes for about 10 minutes four to five times a day to soothe the pain.
- You may use artificial tears for the sandy sensation in your eye and mild pain medications such as acetaminophen (Tylenol).
- You need to stay at home. Children must not play outside. You may return to work or school after 7 days when the redness and discharge have cleared. You may obtain a doctor's note from the clinic to return to work or school.
- Do not share towels, linens, makeup, or toys.
- Wash your hands thoroughly with soap and water frequently and before and after you apply artificial tears or cold compresses.
- Use a new tissue every time you wipe the discharge from your eye. You may dampen the tissue with clean water to clean the outside of the eye.
- You may wash your face and take a shower as you normally do.
- Discard all your makeup articles. You must not apply makeup until the disease is over.
- You may wear dark glasses if bright lights bother you.
- If the discharge from your eye turns yellowish and puslike or you experience changes in your vision, you need to return to the health care provider for an examination.

Uveitis

Inflammation of the uveal tract is called uveitis and can affect the iris, the ciliary body, or the choroid. There are two type of uveitis: nongranulomatous and granulomatous.

The most common type of uveitis is the *nongranulomatous type*, which presents as an acute problem with pain, photophobia, and a pattern of conjunctival injection, especially around the cornea. The pupil is small or irregular, and vision is blurred. There may be small, fine precipitates on the posterior corneal surface and cells in the aqueous humor (cell and flare). If severe, a **hypopyon** (an accumulation of pus in the anterior chamber) may occur. The condition may be unilateral or bilateral and may be recurrent. Repeated attacks of nongranulomatous anterior uveitis can cause anterior synechia (the peripheral iris adheres to the cornea and impedes outflow of aqueous humor). The development of posterior synechia (the adherence of the iris and lens) blocks aqueous outflow from the posterior chamber. Secondary glaucoma can result from either anterior or posterior synechia. Cataracts may also occur as a sequela to uveitis.

Granulomatous uveitis can have a more insidious onset and can involve any portion of the uveal tract. It tends to be chronic. Symptoms, such as photophobia and pain, may be minimal. The keratic precipitate may be large and grayish. Vision is markedly and adversely affected. Conjunctival injection is diffuse, and there may be vitreous clouding. In a severe posterior uveitis, such as chorioretinitis, there may be retinal and choroidal hemorrhages.

Management

Because photophobia is a common complaint, patients should wear dark glasses outdoors. Ciliary spasm and synechia are best avoided through mydriasis; cyclogel and atropine are commonly used. Local corticosteroid drops, such as Pred Forte 1% and Flarex 0.1%, taken four to six times a day are also used to decrease inflammation. In very severe cases, systemic corticosteroids, as well as intravitreal corticosteroids, may be used.

If the uveitis is recurrent, a medical workup should be initiated to discover any underlying causes. This evaluation should include a physical examination and complete systems review; diagnostic tests, including a complete blood count, erythrocyte sedimentation rate, antinuclear antibodies (ANA), VDRL, and a Lyme disease titer. Underlying causes include toxoplasmosis, herpes zoster virus, ocular candidiasis, histoplasmosis, herpes simplex virus, tuberculosis, and syphilis.

Orbital Cellulitis

Orbital cellulitis is inflammation of the tissues surrounding the eye and may be secondary to bacterial, fungal, or viral inflammatory conditions of contiguous structures, such as the face, oropharynx, dental structures, or intracranial structures (Fig. 54-15). It can also result from foreign bodies and from a preexisting ocular infection, such as dacryocystitis and panophthalmitis, or from generalized septicemia. Infection of the sinuses is the most frequent cause. Infection originating in the sinuses can spread easily to the orbit through the thin bony walls and foramina or by means of the inter-

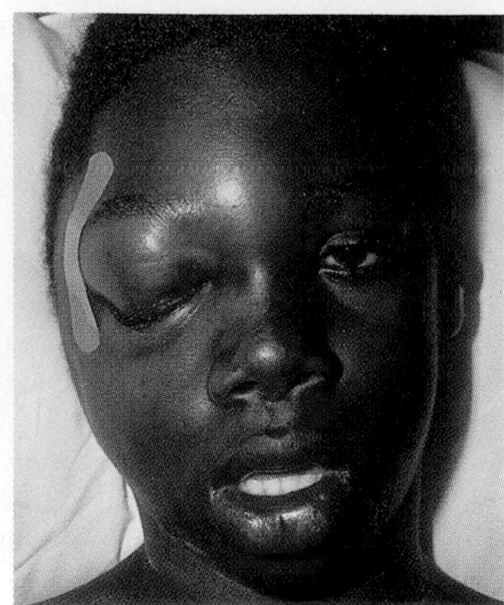

FIGURE 54•15 Orbital cellulitis.

connecting venous system of the orbit and sinuses. In children, ethmoid and maxillary sinuses are the origin of infection from viruses, including influenza. In contrast, the origin of infection in adults is frontal-ethmoid, and predisposing factors include recurrent sinusitis, polyps, allergy, trauma, or recent dental extraction. The most common causative organisms are staphylococci and streptococci in adults and *H. influenzae* in children.

Permanent visual loss can result in orbital cellulitis from the severe intraorbital tension caused by the abscess formation and the impairment of optic nerve function. Because of the orbit's proximity to the brain, orbital cellulitis can lead to life-threatening complications, such as intracranial abscess and cavernous sinus thrombosis.

Orbital cellulitis may progress through five stages. The earliest stage, *periorbital cellulitis,* is characterized by lid swelling with or without generalized malaise and fever. In the next stage, *orbital cellulitis,* the infection has infiltrated the orbit, resulting in edema, congestion, proptosis, and ocular motor and visual impairment. In the worsening stage of *subperiosteal abscess,* the purulent material has filled the subperiosteal space, resulting in displacement of the globe, a fluctuating mass, local tenderness, proptosis, decreased visual acuity, decreased extraocular movement, chemosis, venous congestion of the retinal and choroidal vessels, increasing pain, and increasing IOP. There is marked generalized body malaise and fever. This condition can worsen rapidly.

Without treatment, the condition can progress to the *orbital abscess* stage, which is characterized by marked progression of the cellulitis, resulting in increased proptosis, increased inflammatory signs, ophthalmoplegia, severe visual deficit, and severe systemic toxicity. The symptoms include severe malaise and spiking temperature. If the central nervous system becomes involved, *cavernous sinus thrombosis,* the final stage, may develop. Symptoms include headache, nausea, vomiting, and fever. Ocular symptoms are progressive in severity, and there is decreased ocular movement.

Management

Immediate antibiotic therapy is indicated. In adults, high-dose broad-spectrum systemic antibiotics, such as clindamycin, cefotaxime, cloxacillin, chloramphenicol, and vancomycin, or a combination of any of these, are used. Cultures and Gram-stained smears are obtained. Monitoring changes in visual acuity, degree of proptosis, central nervous system function (nausea, vomiting, fever, level of consciousness), displacement of the globe, extraocular movements, pupillary signs, and the fundus is extremely important in the first 24 to 48 hours to establish accurately the stage and progression of the disease. Management is focused on treatment of the condition, surgical drainage (when necessary), relief of symptoms, and prevention of complications. Consultation with an otolaryngologist is necessary, especially when sinusitis is suspected.

In the event of abscess formation or progressive loss of vision, surgical drainage of the abscess or sinus is indicated. A sinusotomy and antibiotic irrigation are also performed. Patients are discharged with oral antibiotics. Follow-up is extremely important to ensure complete and adequate treatment.

Mucormycosis

With normal body defenses, mucormycosis (a fungal disease) rarely affects healthy individuals. Individuals with uncontrolled diabetes and those who are immunocompromised and debilitated are prone to develop rhino-orbital mucormycosis. The causative organism is a fungus from the *Phycomycetes* species. Naturally found in body orifices, skin, air, food, and fecal material, this organism tends to invade and occlude vessels, compounding the inflammatory process. Necrosis starts at the nasopharyngeal tissues, rapidly spreads to the orbit and then, if not arrested, to the intracranial cavity, resulting in meningitis and brain abscess.

Early diagnosis is extremely important in saving both sight and life. Early orbital symptoms include pain and proptosis. Usually, the patient has sinusitis, pharyngitis, and nasal discharge. CT scan shows displacement of orbital structures adjacent to an opacified sinus with and without bony destruction.

Management

Sample tissues are obtained for culture and smear. The underlying metabolic condition is treated, and surgical intervention is necessary to remove the necrotic tissues, drain the abscess, and irrigate with antifungal antibiotics. The medication of choice is amphotericin B. Caution is required in administering this medication due to its numerous side effects. If the condition is treated early, radical surgery can be avoided. Postsurgical drainage is usually performed. Because of the possible facial deformity from the surgical excisions, alteration in the patient's body image, psychological readiness, and the threat of the disease to life and vision must be addressed. Recurrence of the orbital disease in predisposed patients is common.

ORBITAL AND OCULAR TUMORS

Benign Tumors of the Orbit

Benign tumors can develop from infancy and grow rapidly or slowly and present themselves in later life. Some benign tumors are superficial and are easily identifiable by external presentation, palpation, and x-rays, but some are deep and may require a CT scan for a more thorough precise diagnosis. There can be a significant proptosis, and visual function may be jeopardized.

Benign tumors are masses characterized by the lack of infiltration in the surrounding tissues. Examples are cystic dermoid cysts and mucocele, hemangiomas, lymphangiomas, lacrimal tumors, and neurofibromas.

Management

To prevent recurrence, benign masses are excised completely when possible. Sometimes, excision is difficult because of the involvement of some portions of the orbital bones, such as deep dermoid cysts, in which dissection of the bone is required. Subtotal resection may be indicated in deep benign tumors that intertwine with other orbital structures, such as optic nerve meningiomas. Complete removal of the tumor may endanger visual function.

Benign Tumors of the Eyelids

Benign tumors include a wide variety of neoplasms and increase in frequency with age. Nevi may be unpigmented at birth and may enlarge and darken in adolescence or may never acquire any pigment at all. Hemangiomas are vascular capillary tumors that may be bright superficial strawberry red lesions (strawberry nevus) or bluish and purplish deeper lesions. Milia are small white slightly elevated cysts of the eyelid that, when in multiples, create a blemish. Xanthelasma are yellowish lipoid deposits on both lids near the inner angle of the eye that commonly appear as a result of the aging of the skin or a lipid disorder. Molluscum contagiosum lesions are flat symmetric growths along the lid margin caused by a virus that can result in conjunctivitis and keratitis once the debris gets into the conjunctival sac.

Management

Treatment of benign congenital lid lesions is rarely indicated, except when visual function is affected. Corticosteroid injection to the hemangioma lesion is usually effective, but surgical excision may be performed. Benign lid lesions usually present aesthetic problems rather than visual function problems. Surgical excision, or electrocautery, is primarily performed for cosmetic reasons, except for cases of molluscum contagiosum, in which the surgical intervention is to prevent an infectious process that may ensue.

Benign Tumors of the Conjunctiva

Conjunctival nevus, a congenital benign neoplasm, is a flat, slightly elevated brown spot that becomes pigmented during late childhood or adolescence. This should be differentiated from the pigmented lesion melanosis acquired at middle age, which tends to wax and wane and become malignant melanoma. The keratin- and sebum-containing dermoid cysts are congenital and can be found in the conjunctiva. Dermolipoma is a congenital tumor that presents as a smooth rounded growth in the conjunctiva near the lateral canthus. Papillomas are usually soft with irregular surfaces and appear on the lid margins. Treatment consists of surgical excision.

Malignant Tumors of the Orbit

Rhabdomyosarcoma is the most common malignant primary orbital tumor in childhood, but it can also develop in the elderly. The symptoms of rhabdomyosarcoma include sudden painless proptosis of one eye followed by lid swelling, conjunctival chemosis, and impairment of ocular motility. Imaging of these tumors establishes the size, configuration, location, stage of the disease, and degree of bone destruction and is useful in estimating the field of radiotherapy, if needed. The most common site of metastasis of rhabdomyosarcoma is to the lung.

Management

Management of these primary malignant orbital tumors involves three major therapeutic modalities: surgery, radiotherapy, and adjuvant chemotherapy. The degree of orbital destruction is important in planning the surgical approach. In the orbit, resection often involves removal of the globe. The psychological needs of the patient and family, especially the parents of a pediatric patient, are paramount in planning the management approach.

Malignant Tumors of the Eyelid

Basal cell carcinoma is the most common malignant tumor of the eyelid. Squamous cell carcinoma occurs less frequently but is considered the second most malignant tumor. Malignant melanoma is rare. Malignant eyelid tumors occur more frequently among people with fair complexion who have a history of chronic exposure to the sun.

Basal cell carcinoma appears as a painless nodule that may ulcerate. The lesion is invasive, spreads to the surrounding tissues, and grows slowly but does not metastasize. It usually appears on the lower lid margin near the inner canthus with a pearly white margin. Squamous cell carcinoma of the eyelids may resemble basal cell carcinoma initially because it also grows slowly and painlessly. It tends to ulcerate and invade the surrounding tissues, but it can metastasize to the regional lymph nodes. Malignant melanoma may not be pigmented and can arise from nevi. It spreads to the surrounding tissues and metastasizes to other organs.

Management

Treatment of these carcinomas is by complete excision followed by reconstruction with skin grafting if the surgical excision is extensive. The ocular postoperative site and the graft donor site are monitored for bleeding. Donor graft sites may include the buccal mucosa, the thigh, or the abdomen. The patient is referred to an oncologist for evaluation for the need for radiotherapy treatment and monitoring for metastasis. Early diagnosis and surgical management are the basis of a good prognosis. These conditions have life-threatening consequences, and surgical excisions may result in facial disfigurement. Emotional support and reassurance are important aspects of nursing management.

Malignant Tumors of the Conjunctiva

Conjunctival carcinoma most often grows in the exposed areas of the conjunctiva. The typical lesions are usually gelatinous and whitish due to keratin formation. They grow gradually, and deep invasion and metastasis are rare. Malignant melanoma is rare but may arise from a preexisting nevus or acquired melanosis during middle age. Squamous cell carcinoma is also rare but invasive.

Management

The management is surgical incision. Some benign tumors and most malignant tumors recur. To avoid recurrences, patients usually undergo radiotherapy and cryotherapy after the excision of malignant tumors. Cosmetic disfigurement may result from extensive excision when deep invasion by the malignant tumor is involved.

Ocular Melanoma

This very rare malignant choroidal tumor is often discovered on a retinal examination. In its early stages, it could be mistaken for a nevus. Many ophthalmologists may practice for decades and never encounter this lesion. For this reason, any patient who is suspected of having ocular melanoma should be immediately referred to an ocular oncologist with experience in this diagnosis.

Although many patients do not have symptoms in the early stages, some patients complain of blurred vision or a change in eye color. A number of such tumors have been found in blind, painful eyes. In addition to a complete physical examination to discover any evidence of metastasis (tumor metastasis is to the liver, lung, and breast), retinal fundus photography, fluorescein angiography, and ultrasonography are performed. The diagnosis is confirmed at biopsy after enucleation.

Management

Tumors are classified according to size (small, medium, and large). Very small tumors are generally watched, whereas medium and large tumors require treatment. Treatment consists of radiation, enucleation, or both. Radiation is either by external beam done in repeated doses over several days or through the surgical implantation of a radioactive plaque, which is removed after several days.

SURGICAL PROCEDURES AND ENUCLEATION

Orbital Surgeries

Orbital surgeries may be performed to repair fractures, remove a foreign body, or remove benign or malignant growths. Surgical procedures involving the orbit and lids affect facial appearance (cosmesis). The goals are not only to recover and preserve visual function but also to maintain the anatomic relationship of the ocular structures to cosmesis. During the repair of orbital fractures, the orbital bones are realigned to follow the anatomic positions of facial structures.

Orbital surgical procedures involve working around delicate structures of the eye, such as the optic nerve, retinal blood vessels, and ocular muscles. Complications of orbital surgical procedures may include blindness as a result of damage to the optic nerve and its blood supply. Sudden pain and loss of vision may indicate intraorbital hemorrhage or compression of the optic nerve. Ptosis and diplopia may result from trauma to the extraocular muscles during the surgical procedure, but these conditions typically resolve after a few weeks.

Nursing Management

The head of the patient's bed should be elevated to a comfortable position anywhere from 30 to 45 degrees. Light ice compresses over the periocular area postoperatively are essential to decrease periorbital swelling, facial swelling, and hematoma. The ice compresses are typically applied around the clock for the first 24 to 48 hours. The periocular area may turn to a bluish discoloration due to blood seepage into the tissues during surgery.

Prophylaxis with intravenous antibiotics is the usual postoperative regimen after orbital surgery, especially with repair of orbital fractures and intraorbital foreign body removal. Intravenous corticosteroids are used if there is a concern for optic nerve swelling. Topical ocular antibiotics are typically instilled, and antibiotic ointments are applied externally to the skin suture sites. After the course of intravenous medication, the patient is discharged on oral antibiotics.

Providing comfort, reassurance, and emotional support is an important aspect of care. The patient with periocular and lid swelling, discoloration, and ocular pain needs to be reassured that these symptoms will subside and that there are comfort measures to relieve them. Discharge instructions include medication instructions for antibiotics and mild analgesics, application of cold compresses for periocular and lid swelling, instillation of ocular medications, mobility techniques for monocular vision, available resources in the community for support, and follow-up.

Enucleation

Enucleation is the removal of the entire eye and part of the optic nerve. It may be performed for the following conditions:

- Severe injury resulting in prolapse of uveal tissue or loss of light projection or perception
- An irritated, blind, painful, deformed, or disfigured eye, usually secondary to glaucoma, retinal detachment, or chronic inflammation
- An eye without useful vision that is producing or has created sympathetic ophthalmia in the other eye
- Intraocular tumors that are untreatable by other means

The procedure for enucleation involves the separation and cutting of each of the ocular muscles, dissection of the Tenon's capsule (the fibrous membrane covering the sclera), and the cutting of the optic nerve from the eyeball. The insertion of an orbital implant typically follows, and the conjunctiva is closed. A large pressure dressing is applied over the area.

Evisceration involves the surgical removal of the intraocular contents through an incision or opening in the cornea or sclera. The optic nerve, sclera, extraocular muscles, and at times, the cornea are left intact. The main advantage of evisceration over enucleation is that the final cosmetic result and motility after fitting the ocular prosthesis are enhanced. This procedure would be more acceptable to a patient whose concept of the alteration of body image is severely threatened. The main disadvantage is the strong possibility of sympathetic ophthalmia.

Exenteration is the removal of the eyelids, the eye, and varying amounts of orbital contents. It is indicated in malignancies in the orbit that are life-threatening or when more conservative modalities of treatment have failed or are inappropriate. An example is squamous cell carcinoma of the paranasal sinuses, skin, and conjunctiva with deep orbital involvement. In its most extensive form, exenteration may include the removal of all orbital tissues and resection of the orbital bones.

Orbital implants and conformers (ocular prostheses usually made of silicone rubber) maintain the shape of the eye after enucleation or evisceration to prevent a contracted sunken appearance. The temporary conformer is placed over the conjunctival closure after the implantation of an orbital implant. A conformer is placed after the enucleation or evisceration procedure to protect the suture line, maintain the fornices, prevent contracture of the socket in preparation for the ocular prosthesis, and promote the integrity of the eyelids. When the anophthalmic socket is completely healed, conformers are replaced by prosthetic eyes.

An ocularist is a specially trained and skilled professional who makes prosthetic eyes. After the ophthalmologist is satisfied that the anophthalmic socket is completely healed and is ready for prosthetic fitting, the patient is referred to an ocularist. The healing period is usually 6 to 8 weeks. It is advisable for the patient to have a consultation with the ocularist before the fitting. Obtaining accurate information and verbalizing concerns can lessen anxiety about wearing an ocular prosthesis.

All ocular prosthetics have limitations in their motility. There are two designs of eye prosthesis. The anophthalmic ocular prostheses are used in the absence of the globe. Scleral shells look just like the anophthalmic prosthesis (Fig. 54-16) but are thinner and

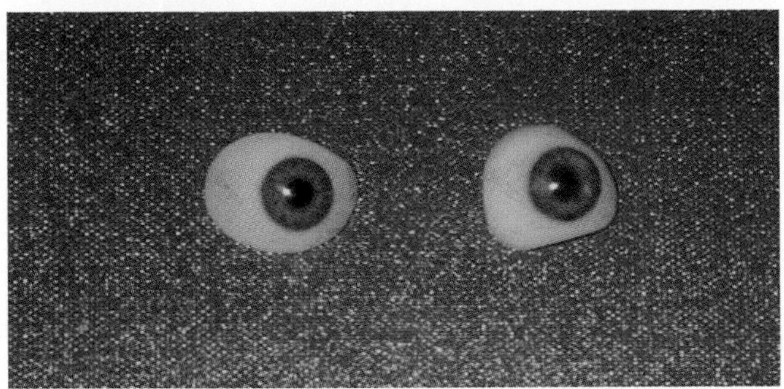

FIGURE 54•16 Eye prostheses. (*Left*) Anophthalmic ocular prosthesis. (*Right*) Scleral shell.

fit over a globe with intact corneal sensation. An eye prosthesis usually lasts about 6 years, depending on the quality of fit, comfort, and cosmetic appearance.

Nursing Management

Removal of an eye has physical, social, and psychological ramifications for any person. The significance of loss of the eye and vision is important for the nurse to understand and address in the plan of care. The patient's psychological preparation should include information about the surgical procedure involved and the availability of ocular prosthetics that will enhance cosmetic appearance. In some cases, patients may opt to see an ocularist before the surgery to discuss the available ocular prosthetics.

The function of orbital implants and conformers must be explained to reassure patients that facial appearance will not be abnormal after these procedures. The patient must be advised that conformers may accidentally fall out of the socket. Should this happen the conformer must be washed, wiped dry, and placed back in the socket. There will be some situations in which eye removal is unexpected, such as severe ocular trauma, leaving no time for the patient and family to prepare for the loss. The nurse's role in giving reassurance and emotional support is crucial.

Patients who undergo eye removal usually have large ocular pressure dressings. The dressing is typically removed after a week, and an ophthalmic topical antibiotic ointment is applied in the socket three times daily. There are times when the dressing loosens and falls off before the scheduled return visit. When this happens, the patient is asked to begin the topical ointment then.

After the removal of an eye, there is a loss of depth perception. Patients must be advised to take extra caution in their mobility to avoid miscalculations that may result in falls. It may take a period of time to adjust to being mobile with monocular vision because there is only one eye that receives visual information. For safety, it may be necessary to turn the head or the body to the side to visualize the environment completely.

PROMOTING HOME AND COMMUNITY-BASED CARE

Teaching Patients Self-Care. Patients need to be taught how to insert, remove, and care for the prosthetic eye. Proper hand washing must be observed before inserting and removing an ocular prosthesis. The fingers are usually sufficient to perform this procedure, but a suction cup may be used if there are problems with manual dexterity. Precautions, such as draping a towel over the sink and closing the sink drain, must be taken to avoid loss of the prosthesis. When instructing patients or family members, a return demonstration is important to assess their level of understanding and ability to perform the procedure.

Before insertion, the inner punctal or outer lateral aspects and the superior and inferior aspects of the prosthesis must be identified by locating the identifying marks, such as a reddish color in the inner punctal area. For people with low vision, other forms of identifying markers are used, such as dots, or notches. The upper lid is raised high enough to create a space; then the prosthesis is slid up underneath and behind the upper eyelid. The lower eyelid is pulled down to aid the prosthesis in place and to have its inferior edge fall back gradually to the lower eyelid. The lower eyelid is checked for correct positioning.

To remove the prosthesis, the patient cups one hand on the cheek to catch the prosthesis, places the forefinger of the free hand against the mid-portion of the lower eyelid, and gazes upward. Gazing upward brings the inferior edge of the prosthesis nearer the inferior eyelid margin. With the finger pushing inward, downward, and laterally against the lower eyelid, the prosthesis slides out and the cupped hand acts as the receptacle.

Continuing Care. An eye prosthesis can be worn and left in place for several months. Hygiene and comfort are usually maintained with daily irrigation of the prosthesis in place with the use of a balanced salt solution, hard contact lens solution, or artificial tears. In the case of dry eye symptoms, the use of ophthalmic ointment lubricants or oil-based drops, such as vitamin E and mineral oil, can be helpful. Removing crusting and mucous discharge that accumulates overnight is performed with the prosthesis in place. Malpositions may occur when wiping or rubbing the prosthesis in the socket. The prosthesis can be turned back in place with the use of clean fingers. Proper wiping of the prosthesis should be a gentle temporal-to-nasal motion to avoid malpositions.

The prosthesis needs to be removed and cleaned when it becomes uncomfortable and when there is increased mucous discharge. The socket should also be rendered free of mucus and inspected for any signs of infection. Any unusual discomfort, irritation, or redness of the globe or eyelids may indicate excessive wear, debris under the shell, or lack of proper hygiene. Any infection or irritation that does not subside needs medical attention.

OCULAR CONSEQUENCES OF SYSTEMIC DISEASE

Diabetic Retinopathy

Of all of the medical disorders that the nurse encounters, diabetes mellitus is one of the most common and one that can have devastating effects on the individual patient. Diabetes affects every system of the body in a deleterious way and consequently affects the patient's family and society in general. Diabetes is the leading cause of new cases of blindness in working-aged people in the United States today. Before the discovery of insulin in the 1920s, diabetic retinopathy was relatively rare. Most people with diabetes did not survive for more than 1 or 2 years; however, with the use of insulin, more and more patients are able to survive and enjoy relatively normal life spans. They are also confronted with the complications of long-term diabetes. One of the most serious complications is retinopathy. Refer to Chapter 37 for a complete discussion of diabetic retinopathy.

Cytomegalovirus Retinitis

There are many ophthalmic complications associated with AIDS. On autopsy, up to 90% of patients have ocular lesions directly related to AIDS. Cytomegalovirus (CMV) is the most common cause of retinal inflammation in patients with AIDS. Forty percent of patients who have CMV retinitis lose their central vision in both eyes by the time of their death.

Early symptoms of CMV retinitis vary from patient to patient. Some patients complain of floaters or a decrease in peripheral vision. Some patients have a paracentral or central scotoma, whereas others have a fluctuation in vision from macular edema. The retina often becomes thin and atrophic and susceptible to retinal tears and breaks.

CMV retinitis generally takes one of three forms: hemorrhagic, brushfire, or granular. In the hemorrhagic type, large areas of white necrotic retina may be seen with associated retinal hemorrhage. The brushfire form appears to have a yellowish white margin, which begins at the edge of burned-out atrophic retina. This retinitis expands and, if untreated, involves the entire retina. The granular form of CMV retinitis consists of white granular lesions in the periphery of the retina, which gradually expand. The white feathery infiltration of the retina destroys sensory retina and leads to necrosis, optic atrophy, and retinal detachment.

Management

Pharmacologic agents available for treatment of CMV retinitis include ganciclovir, foscarnet, and cidofoviar. ISIS 2922 is under investigation.

Ganciclovir is administered intravenously, orally, or intravitreously in the acute stage of CMV retinitis. A surgically implanted intraocular device has provided a new mode of effective ganciclovir administration. This enables a higher, more effective dose of medication to be administered and is well tolerated by patients. This constant intraocular concentration of ganciclovir lasts for about 6 to 10 months before the inserts must be replaced. Once begun, ganciclovir must be given continuously. This very potent medication, when administered systemically, can cause neutropenia, thrombocytopenia, anemia, and elevated serum creatinine levels. Although the surgically implanted sustained release device enables higher concentrations of ganciclovir to reach the CMV retinitis, there are risks and complications associated with the devices, including endophthalmitis, retinal detachment, and hypotony.

Foscarnet inhibits viral DNA replication. It may be the drug of choice when ganciclovir is ineffective. It may be given intravenously or locally by intravitreal injections. The combination of foscarnet and ganciclovir has been more effective then either foscarnet alone or ganciclovir alone. Nephrotoxicity is a problem with systemic foscarnet; therefore, renal function must be monitored carefully.

Cidofovir impedes CMV replication. This medication is given intravenously at a dosage of 5 mg/kg/week for 2 weeks; then a maintenance dose of 5 mg/kg every 2 weeks. Cidofovir has been shown to delay the progression of CMV retinitis significantly. Nephrotoxicity, proteinuria, and increased serum creatinine levels are significant side effects of administration of this medication.

Hypertension-Related Eye Changes

Hypertension, known as the "silent killer," can shorten the life span by as many as 20 years. End-organ damage affects the heart, brain, kidney, and eye. Hypertension may be manifested in one of two forms: either chronic or acute. This differentiation is determined by the rapidity in rise of the blood pressure as well as the degree of elevation. The retinal changes observed with each form are different and have different consequences for the eye.

Chronic hypertension and atherosclerosis go hand in hand, and the associated retinal changes are evidenced by the development of retinal arteriolar changes, such as tortuousness, narrowing, and a change in light reflex. Fundoscopic examination revels a copper or silver coloration of the arterioles and venous compression (arteriovenous nicking) at the atrial and venous crossings. Intraretinal hemorrhages secondary to hypertension appear flame shaped because they occur in the nerve fiber layer of the retina.

Acute hypertension can result from pheochromocytoma, acute renal failure, pregnancy-induced hypertension, and malignant essential hypertension. The retinopathy associated with these crisis states is florid, and the manifestations include cotton-wool spots, retinal hemorrhages, retinal edema, and retinal exudates, often clustered around the macula.

The choroid is also affected by the profound and abrupt rise in blood pressure and resulting vasoconstriction, and ischemia may result in serous retinal detachments and infarction of the retinal pigment epithelium (RPE). Ischemic optic neuropathy and **papilledema** (swelling of the optic disc due to increased IOP) may also result.

CONCEPTS IN OCULAR MEDICATION ADMINISTRATION

The main objective of ocular medication delivery is to maximize the amount of medication that reaches the ocular site of action in sufficient concentration to produce a beneficial therapeutic effect. This is determined by the dynamics of ocular pharmacokinetics: absorption, distribution, metabolism, and excretion.

Topical administration of ocular medications results in only a 1% to 7% absorption rate by the ocular tissues. Ocular absorption involves the entry of a medication into the aqueous humor through the different routes of ocular drug administration. The rate and extent of aqueous humor absorption are determined by the characteristics of the medication and the barriers imposed by the anatomy and physiology of the eye. The natural barriers of absorption that diminish the efficacy of ocular medications include the following:

Limited size of the conjunctival sac. The conjunctival sac can hold only 50 µL, and any excess is wasted. The volume of one eye drop from commercial topical ocular solutions typically ranges from 20 to 35 µL.

Corneal membrane barriers. The epithelial, stromal, and endothelial layers are barriers to absorption.

Blood–ocular barriers. Blood–ocular barriers prevent high ocular tissue concentration of most ophthalmic drugs because they separate the bloodstream from the ocular tissues and keep foreign substances from entering the eye, thereby limiting a medication's efficacy.

Tearing, blinking, and drainage. Increased tear production and drainage due to ocular irritation or an ocular condition may dilute or wash out an instilled eyedrop; blinking facilitates the expulsion of an instilled eyedrop from the conjunctival sac.

The distribution of an ocular medication into the ocular tissues involves the partitioning and compartmentalizing of the medication between the tissues of the conjunctiva, cornea, lens, iris, ciliary body, choroid, and vitreous. Medications penetrate the corneal epithelium by diffusion, either by passing through the cells (intracellular) or by passing between the cells (intercellular). Water-soluble medications (hydrophilic) diffuse through the intracellular route, and fat-soluble medications (lipophilic) diffuse through the intercellular route. Topical administration usually does not reach the retina in significant concentrations. Because the space between the ciliary process and the lens is small, medication diffusion in the vitreous is slow. Therefore, when high therapeutic medication concentration in the vitreous is required, intraocular injection is the choice of delivery to bypass the natural ocular anatomic and physiologic barriers.

Aqueous solutions are the most commonly used ocular medications. They are the least expensive and the least interfering with vision. However, the contact time with the cornea is short because the medication is diluted by tears. Ophthalmic ointments have extended retention time in the conjunctival sac and a higher concentration than eye drops. The major disadvantage of ointments is the blurred vision that results after application. In general, eyelids and eyelid margins are best treated with ointments. The conjunctiva, limbus, cornea, and anterior chamber are treated most effectively with instilled solutions or suspensions. Subconjunctival injection may be necessary for better absorption in the anterior chamber. If high medication concentrations are required in the posterior chamber, intravitreal injections or systemically absorbed medications are considered. Contact lenses and collagen shields soaked in antibiotics have also been used as alternative delivery methods for treating corneal infections. Of all these, the topical route of administration—instillation of eye drops and application of ointments—remains the most common route of administration. Topical instillation allows the medication to be self-administered. It is the least invasive process and produces fewer side effects than other administration methods.

Preservatives that are commonly used in the preparation of ocular medications, such as benzalkonium chloride, prevent the growth of organisms when the sterile medication is opened and enhance the corneal permeability of most medications. Some patients have an allergy to this preservative. This is suspected even if the patient had never before experienced an allergic reaction to the systemic use of the medication in question. Eyedrops without preservatives can be prepared by pharmacists.

Commonly Used Ocular Medications

Common ocular medications include topical anesthetics, mydriatics and cycloplegics, medications that reduce IOP, anti-infectives, corticosteroids, NSAIDS, antiallergy medications, eye irrigants, and lubricants.

Topical Anesthetics

One to two drops of proparacaine hydrochloride (ophthaine 0.5%) and tetracaine hydrochloride (pontocaine 0.5%) are instilled before diagnostic procedures such as tonometry and gonioscopy and in minor ocular procedures such as removal of sutures or conjunctival or corneal scrapings. The nurse must instruct patients not to rub their eyes while anesthetized because this may result in corneal damage. Patients must never be allowed to take topical anesthetics home. Prolonged use can delay wound healing and can lead to permanent corneal opacification and scarring, resulting in visual loss. Topical anesthetic is also applied in eyes with severe pain to allow the patient to open his or her eyes for examination or treatment (eye irrigation for chemical burns). Anesthesia occurs within 20 seconds to 1 minute and lasts 10 to 20 minutes.

Mydriatics and Cycloplegics

Mydriasis, or pupil dilation, is the main objective of the administration of mydriatics and cycloplegics (Table 54-7). These two medications function differently and are used in combination to achieve the maximal dilation that is needed during surgery and fundus examinations to give the ophthalmologist a better view of the internal structures of the eye. Mydriatics potentiate alpha-adrenergic sympathetic effects that result in the relaxation of the ciliary muscle. This causes the pupil to dilate. This sympathetic action alone, however, is not enough to sustain mydriasis because of its short duration of action. The strong light against the eye

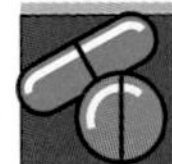

TABLE 54•7 Mydriatics and Cycloplegics

Drug	Available Preparation/ Concentration	Indication/Dosage	Peak: MYDRIASIS	Peak: CYCLOPLEGIA	Recovery Time: MYDRIASIS	Recovery Time: CYCLOPLEGIA
phenylephrine	Solutions (2.5%, 10%)	Given with cycloplegics in pupillary dilation for ophthalmoscopy and surgical procedures every 5–10 minutes ×3 or until fully dilated	10–60 minutes	—	3–6 hours	—
atropine	Ointment (0.5%–2%) Solutions (0.5%–3%)	In glaucoma, uveitis, or after surgery, 2× to 4× daily	30–40 minutes	60–180 minutes	7–10 days	6–12 days
scopolamine	Solution (0.25%)	The same as atropine	20–30 minutes	30–60 minutes	3–7 days	3–7 days
homatropine	Solution (5%–2.5%)	The same as atropine and scopolamine	40–60 minutes	30–60 minutes	1–3 days	1–3 days
cyclopentolate	Solution (0.5%–2%)	Given with mydriatics q 5–10 minutes ×3 or until fully dilated for pupillary dilation in ophthalmoscopy and surgical procedures	30–60 minutes	25–75 minutes	1 day	6 hours to 1 day
tropicamide	Solution (0.25%–1%)		20–40 minutes	20–35 minutes	6 hours	Less than 6 hours

Data on peak and recovery time from *Ophthalmic Drug Facts* by *Facts and Comparisons* (1998), pp. 45 and 49.

during an eye examination also stimulates miosis (pupillary contraction). Cycloplegics are given to paralyze the iris sphincter.

Patients are instructed about the temporary effects of mydriasis on vision, such as glare and the inability to focus properly. Patients may not be able to read and should not drive. The effects of the various mydriatics and cycloplegics can last from 3 hours to several days. Patients are advised to bring sunglasses (most eye clinics provide protective sunglasses) and to have a responsible adult for accompaniment home, if necessary.

Mydriatics and cycloplegics affect the central nervous system. Their effects are most prominent in children and elderly patients; hence, these patients must be assessed closely for symptoms, such as rise in blood pressure, tachycardia, dizziness, ataxia, confusion, disorientation, incoherent speech, and hallucination. These medications are contraindicated in patients with narrow angles or shallow anterior chambers and in patients taking monoamine oxidase inhibitors or tricyclic antidepressants.

Medications Used to Treat Glaucoma

The purpose of the medical therapeutic regimen for glaucoma is the delivery of medications to lower IOP by decreasing aqueous production or increasing aqueous outflow. Because glaucoma calls for long-term, if not lifetime, therapy, patients must be instructed regarding both the ocular and systemic side effects of the medications.

Most antiglaucoma ocular medications affect the accommodation of the lens and limit light entry through a constricted pupil. Focusing and visual acuity may be affected. Factors to consider in selecting glaucoma medications are efficacy, systemic and ocular side effects, tolerability, convenience, and cost. For a more in-depth discussion of glaucoma medications, please refer to the section on glaucoma.

Anti-Infectives

Anti-infective medications include antibiotics, antifungals, and antivirals. Most are available as drops, ointments, or subconjunctival or intravitreal injections. Antibiotics include penicillin, the cephalosporins, aminoglycosides, and fluoroquinolones. The main antifungal agent is amphotericin B. Side effects of amphotericin are serious and include severe pain, conjunctival necrosis, iritis, and retinal toxicity. Antivirals include acyclovir and ganciclovir. They are used to treat ocular infections associated with herpesvirus and cytomegalovirus. Patients receiving ocular anti-infectives are subject to the same side effects and adverse reactions as those receiving oral or parenteral medications.

Corticosteroids and Nonsteroidal Anti-Inflammatory Drugs

The topical preparations of corticosteroids are commonly used in inflammatory conditions of the eyelids, conjunctiva, cornea, anterior chamber, lens, and uvea. In posterior segment diseases that involve the posterior sclera, retina, and optic nerve, the topical agents are less effective; hence, the parenteral and oral routes are preferred. The topical eyedrop preparation is prepared in suspension; the patient is instructed to shake the bottle several times to obtain the maximum therapeutic effect of the medication.

The most common ocular side effects of long-term topical corticosteroid administration are glaucoma, cataracts, susceptibility to infection, impaired wound healing, mydriasis, and ptosis. High IOP may develop, which is reversible once the corticosteroid use is discontinued.

To avoid the side effects of corticosteroids, NSAIDS are used as an alternative in controlling inflammatory eye conditions and postoperatively to reduce inflammation. NSAID therapy in both topical and oral preparations is an important adjunct therapy in the management of patients with uveitis.

Antiallergy Medications

Ocular hypersensitivity reactions, such as allergic conjunctivitis, are extremely common. These conditions are primarily the result of responses to environmental allergens. The allergens are airborne or carried to the eye by the hand or by other means. Allergic reactions may also be a drug-induced sensitivity. Corticosteroids are also commonly used as anti-inflammatory and immunosuppressive agents to control ocular hypersensitivity reaction.

Ocular Irrigating Solutions

Most irrigating solutions are used to cleanse the external lids to maintain lid hygiene, to irrigate the external corneal surface to regain normal pH (such as in chemical burns), to irrigate the corneal surface to eliminate debris, or to inflate the globe intraoperatively. These solutions have various compositions that include sodium, potassium, magnesium, calcium, bicarbonate, glucose, and glutathione (a substance found in the aqueous humor).

Sterile irrigating solutions, such as Dacriose, for lid hygiene are available. Irrigating solutions are safe to use with an intact corneal surface. The corneal surface should not be irrigated in patients with threatening corneal perforation. For patients with severe corneal ulcer, specific orders must be obtained regarding whether it is safe to irrigate the corneal surface or just to cleanse the external lids. Although it is good practice to promote hygiene, prevention of complications must be the primary concern. Normal saline solutions are commonly used to irrigate the corneal surface when chemical burns have occurred.

Lubricants

Lubricants, such as artificial tears, are primarily used to alleviate corneal irritation, such as dry eye syndrome. Artificial tears are topical preparations of methyl or hydroxypropyl cellulose that are prepared as eyedrop solutions, ointments, or ocular inserts. The ocular insert is inserted at the lower conjunctival cul-de-sac once a day. The eyedrops can be instilled as often as every hour, depending on the severity of symptoms of corneal irritation from dry eye syndrome.

Nursing Considerations

The objectives in administering ocular medications are to ensure proper administration to maximize the therapeutic effects and to ensure the safety of the patient by monitoring manifestations of possible systemic and local side effects. The absorption of eyedrops by the nasolacrimal duct is undesirable due to the potential systemic side effects of ocular medications. To diminish systemic absorption and minimize the side effects, it is important to occlude the puncta (Guideline 54-1). This is especially important for patients most vulnerable to medication overdose, including elderly people, children and infants, women who are lactating or are pregnant, and patients with cardiac, pulmonary, hepatic, or renal disease.

A 30-second interval between eyedrop instillations has a 45% rate of wash-out loss. With a 5-minute interval between instilla-

54•1 GUIDELINES FOR INSTILLING EYE MEDICATIONS

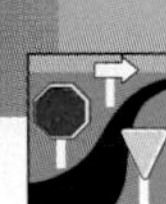

Follow these general guidelines when instilling eye medications:

- Shake suspensions or "milky" solutions to obtain the desired medication level.
- Wash hands thoroughly before and after the procedure.
- Ensure adequate lighting.
- Read the label of the eye medication to make sure it is the correct medication.
- Assume a comfortable position.
- Do not touch the tip of the medication container to any part of the eye or face.
- Hold the lower lid down; do not press on the eyeball. Apply gentle pressure to the cheek bone to anchor the finger holding the lid.

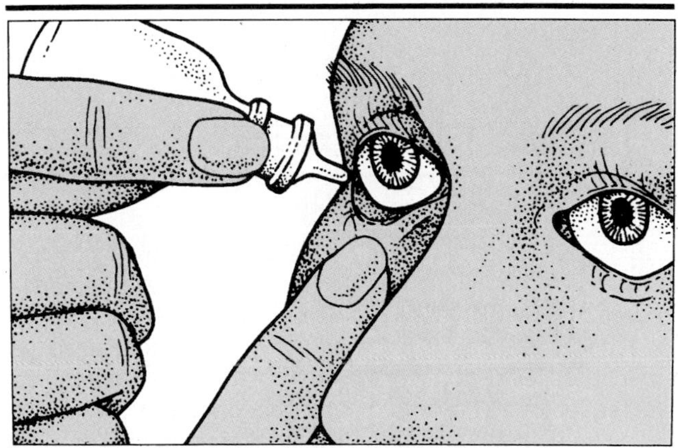

- Instill eye drops before applying ointments.
- Apply a ½-inch ribbon of ointment to the lower conjunctival sac.

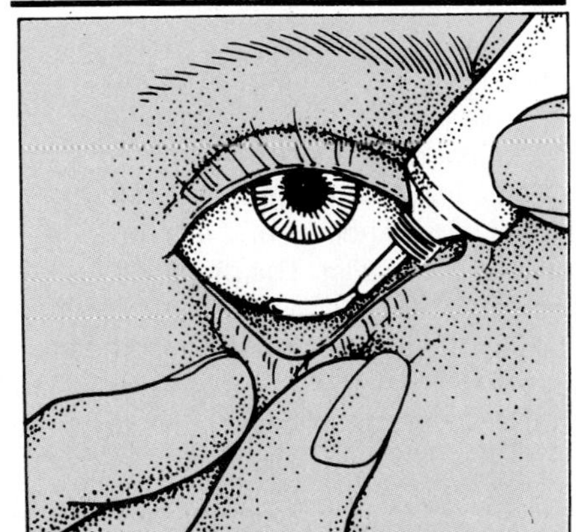

- Keep the eyelids closed, and apply gentle pressure on the inner canthus (punctal occlusion) near the bridge of the nose for about 1–2 minutes immediately after instilling eyedrops.
- Gently pat with clean tissue any excess eyedrops that run on the cheeks.
- Wait 5 to 10 minutes before instilling another eye medication.

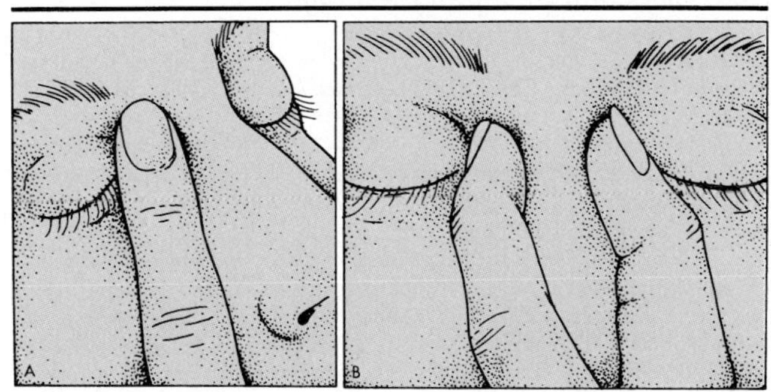

tions, there is no wash-out effect seen on the first eyedrop instilled (Mauger & Craig, 1996), making it important to wait at least 5 minutes between instillations of different drops.

Before the administration of ocular medications, the nurse should warn the patient that blurred vision, stinging, and burning sensation are symptoms that ordinarily occur right after instillation and are temporary. Risk for interactions of the ocular medication with other ocular and systemic medications must be emphasized; therefore, a careful patient interview regarding medications being currently taken must be obtained.

Emphasis must be placed on hand-washing techniques before and after medication instillation. The tip of the eyedrop bottle or the ointment tube must never touch any part of the eye. The medication must be recapped immediately after each use. If patients who instill their own medications are unable to feel the eye drops when they are instilled, the eye medication may be refrigerated because a cold drop is easier to feel. A 5-minute interval between successive eyedrop administration allows adequate drug retention and absorption. The patient or the caregiver at home should demonstrate actual eyedrop or ointment instillation and punctal occlusion.

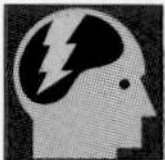

Critical Thinking Exercises

1. During a follow-up telephone call with a nurse after cataract surgery, the patient reports that his eye that was operated on is red and painful and that he cannot see clearly. He states that acetaminophen does not relieve the pain, particularly in the last 12 hours, that the redness has increased over the last 24 hours, and that his vision is hazy and blurred compared with the morning after surgery. What are the implications of these signs and symptoms? What nursing actions are appropriate?
2. A patient who has sustained an eyelid laceration is seen by the emergency department staff and found to have decreased peripheral vision and IOPs of 34 and 38 mm Hg. The ophthalmologist informs the patient of the significance of these findings and arranges for follow-up with a glaucoma specialist. The patient informs the nurse he has been on glaucoma medication for 3 years but stopped taking it 6 months ago because he could not afford the medication. He does not see the need to go to a specialist for follow-up. What nursing actions are appropriate?

References and Selected Readings

BOOKS

Abbott, R. L., & Hwang, D. G. (1997). *Refractive surgery.* Philadelphia: W. B. Saunders.

Brow, A. J., Tripathi, R. C., & Tripathi, B. J. (1997). *Wolff's anatomy of the eye and orbit.* London: Chapman & Hall Medical.

Blasch, B., Wiener, W., & Welsh, R. (Eds.). *Foundations of orientation and mobility.* New York: AFB Press.

Carrol, T. J. (1961). *Blindness: What it is, what it does, and how to live with it.* Boston: Little, Brown.

Cassin, B., & Latif, H. (1995). *Fundamentals for ophthalmic technical personnel.* Philadelphia: W. B. Saunders.

Corn, B., & Koenig, A. (Eds.). (1996). *Foundations of low vision.* New York: AFB Press.

Cullom, R. D. Jr., & Chang, B. (1994). *The Wills eye manual office of emergency room diagnosis and treatment of eye disease.* Philadelphia: J. B. Lippincott.

Fechner, P. J., & Teichman, K. D. (1998). *Ocular therapeutics: Pharmacology and clinical application.* Thorofare, NJ: Slack.

Facts and Comparisons. (1998). *Ophthalmic drug facts.* St. Louis: Facts and Comparisons.

Glaucoma Research Foundation. (1996). *Understanding and living with glaucoma: A reference guide for people with glaucoma and their families.* San Francisco: Glaucoma Research Foundation.

Goldblum, K. (1997). *Core curriculum for ophthalmic nursing.* Dubuque, IA: Kendall/Hunt.

Hersh, P. S., & Wagoner, M. D. (1997). *Excimer laser for corneal disorders.* New York: Thieme.

Hill, E., & Ponder, P. (1976). *Orientation and mobility techniques: A guide for the practitioner.* New York: AFB Press.

The Johns Hopkins School of Medicine, Wilmer Institute. (1998). *Policy and procedure instructions for EKC.* Baltimore: Johns Hopkins Wilmer Institute.

Kanski, J. J. (1994). *Clinical ophthalmology.* Oxford: Butterworth-Heinemann Ltd.

Kanski, J., McAllister, J., & Salmon, J. (1996). *Glaucoma: A color manual of diagnosis and treatment.* Oxford, UK: Butterworth-Heinemann Ltd.

Krachmer, J. H., Mann's, M. J., & Holland E. J. (1997). *Cornea surgery of the cornea and conjunctiva.* St. Louis: C. V. Mosby.

Leibowitz, H. M., & Waring G. O. III. (1998). *Corneal disorders: Clinical diagnosis and management.* Philadelphia: W. B. Saunders.

MacCumber, M. W. (Ed.). (1997). *Management of ocular injuries and emergencies.* Philadelphia: Lippincott-Raven.

Margolis, S., & Schachat, A. P. (1998). *Vision disorders: The Johns Hopkins white papers.* New York: Medletter Associates.

Mauger, T., & Craig, E. (1996). *Mosby's ocular handbook.* St. Louis: Mosby–Year Book.

Moore, J. E., Graves, W., & Patterson, J. B. (Eds.). (1997). *Foundations of rehabilitation counseling with persons who are blind or visually impaired.* New York: AFB Press.

Navarro, V. B., & Tolley, F. M. (1995). Corneal transplantation. In M. T. Nolan, & S. M. Augustine, S. M. (Eds.). *Transplantation nursing: Acute and long term management* (pp. 291–318). Norwalk, CT: Appleton & Lange.

O'Brien, T. (1998). Conjunctivitis. In R. Rakel (Ed). *Conn's Current Therapy* (pp. 67–72). Philadelphia: W. B. Saunders.

Phelps Brown, N., Brow, A. J. (1996). *Lens disorders: A clinical manual of cataract diagnosis.* Oxford, UK: Butterworth-Heinemann Ltd.

Prevent Blindness America. (1994). *Vision problems in the US.* Scaumberg, IL: Prevent Blindness America.

Resources for Rehabilitation. (1996) *Living with low vision: A resource guide for people with sight loss.* Lexington, KY: Resources for Rehabilitation.

Ritch, R., Shields, M., & Krupin, T. (1996). *The glaucomas: Clinical science* (vol. 1-111). St. Louis: C. V. Mosby.

Rootman, J., & Chang, K. W. (1998). *Diseases of the orbit.* Philadelphia: Lippincott-Raven.

Serdarevoc, O. N. (1997). *Refractive surgery: Current techniques and management.* New York: Igaku-Shoin.

Shields, G. (1998). *Textbook of glaucoma.* Baltimore: Williams & Wilkins.

Snell, R. S., & Lemp, M. A. (1998). *Clinical anatomy of the eye* (2nd ed.). Malden, MA: Blackwell Scientific.

Stein, H., Slatt, H., & Stein, R. (1994). *The ophthalmic assistant.* St. Louis: C. V. Mosby.

Stein, H., Slatt, B., & Stein, R. (1992). *A primer in ophthalmology.* St. Louis: C. V. Mosby.

Stewart, W. (1995). *Surgery of the eyelid, orbit, and lacrimal system* (vol. 1–3). San Francisco: American Academy of Ophthalmology.

Tierney, L. M., McPhee, S. J., & Papadakis, M. A. (1998). *Current: Medical diagnosis and treatment.* Norwalk, CT: Appleton & Lange.

Varma, R. (1997). *Essentials of eye care: The Johns Hopkins Wilmer handbook.* Philadelphia: Lippincott-Raven.

Vaughn, D. G., Asbury, T., & Riorda-Eva, P. (Eds.). (1995). *General ophthalmology.* Stamford, CT: Appleton & Lange.

Whitcher, J. (1995). Blindness. In D. Vaughn et al. (Eds). *General ophthalmology* (pp. 396–400). Norwalk, CT: Appleton & Lange.

Wilson, R. P. (Ed.). (1997). *The Yearbook of ophthalmology.* St. Louis: C. V. Mosby.

Wright, K. (Ed.). (1997). *Textbook of ophthalmology,* Baltimore: Williams & Wilkins.

Wu, G. (1995). *Retina: The fundamentals.* Philadelphia: W. B. Saunders.

Zimmerman, G. (1996). Optics and low vision devices. In A. Corn & A. Koenig (Eds.). *Foundations of low vision* (pp. 115–142). New York: AFB Press.

JOURNALS

Abelson, M., Herrin, S., Morrill, K., & Bethke, W. (1997). On the cutting edge: New refractive surgery technology. *Review of Ophthalmology, 3*(2), 68–87.

Adamsons, I. A., Vitale, S., Stark, W. J., & Rubin, G. S. (1996). The association of postoperative subjective visual function with acuity, glare, and contrast sensitivity in patients with early cataract. *Archives of Ophthalmology, 114,* 529–536.

Atwood, J. D. (Ed). (1998). What's new in contact lenses. *Review of Ophthalmology, 5*(5), 115–116.

Azuara-Blanco, A. (1997). Aqueous tube shunts for refractory glaucomas. *Journal of Ophthalmic Nursing and Technology, 16*(3), 103–107.

Bethke, W. (1998). Cataract surgeons move forward. *Review of Ophthalmology, 5*(2), 70–73.

Blecher, M. H. (Ed). (1998). What's new in cataract surgery. *Review of Ophthalmology, 5*(5), 62–65.

Blecher, M. H. (1997). Beyond clear cornea. *Review of Ophthalmology, 4*(4), 72–77.

Cholden, L. (1954). Some psychological problems in the rehabilitation of the blind. *Bulletin of the Menninger Clinic, 18*, 1107–1112.

Diamond, B., & Ross, A. (1945). Emotional adjustment of newly blinded soldiers. *American Journal of Psychiatry, 102*, 367–371.

Eller, A. W. (1998). Cataract surgery in diabetics: What to consider before you operate. *Review of Ophthalmology, 5*(2), 48–53.

Ernest, P. H. (1997). A corneal incision you can be comfortable with. *Review of Ophthalmology, 4*(4), 73–77.

Fishkind, W. J. (1998). A better way to assess cataract patients. *Review of Ophthalmology, 5*(3), 59–66.

Gabelt, B., Kaufman, P. (1998). A rational approach to adding glaucoma medications. *Review of Ophthalmology, 5*(5), 44–54.

Hannush, S. (Ed.). (1998). Refractive surgery moves forward. *Review of Ophthalmology, 5*(5), 96–103.

Hannush, S. (Ed.). (1998). What's new in corneal and external disease. *Review of Ophthalmology, 5*(5), 68–74.

Ionides, A., & Claoue, C. (1996). Resource management of cataract patients: Can visual rehabilitation be achieved in three visits. *Journal of Cataract and Refractive Surgery, 22*, 717–720.

Jampel, H. (1998). Laser trabeculoplasty is the treatment of choice for chronic open-angle glaucoma. *Archives of Ophthalmology, 116*, 240–241.

Lakhanpal, R., Robin, A., Gabelt, B. T., & Kaufman, P. (1998). A global guide to glaucoma medications. *Review of Ophthalmology, 5*(5), 42–57.

Lee, O., & Netland, P. (Ed.). (1998). What's new in glaucoma. *Review of Ophthalmology, 5*(5), 86–95.

Mamalis, N., & Hymas, D. C., (1998). The facts about foldable IOLs. *Review of Ophthalmology, 5*(1), 65–76.

Monroe, L. R. (1998). IOLs: the future of refractive surgery? *Eye Net, 2*(8), 20–21.

Orticio, L. (1994). Do perceptions of blindness affect care? *Journal of Ophthalmic Nursing and Technology, 13*(4), 172–179.

Piegenga, L. W., Matta, C. S., Deitz, M. R., Tauber, J., Irvine, J. W., & Sabates, F. N. (1993). Excimer photorefractive keratectomy for myopia. *Ophthalmology, 100*(9), 1335–1345.

Regillo, C. (Ed.). (1998). What's new in retina. *Review of Ophthalmology, 5*(5), 77–82.

Scherick, K. (1998). How to solve the lens care problem. *Review of Ophthalmology, 5*(1), 57–59.

Steinberg, E. P., Tielach, J. M., & Schein, O. (1994). The VF-14: An index of functional impairment in patients with cataract. *Archives of Ophthalmology, 112*, 630–638.

Steinert, R. F. (1998). How to use the new multifocal IOL. *Review of Ophthalmology, 5*(2), 74–80.

Stonecipher, K. G., & Salz, J. J. (1998). Point-counterpoint: Should we perform bilateral LASIK? *Review of Ophthalmology, 5*(1), 60–76.

West, S. K., & Valmadrid, C. T. (1995). Epidemiology of risk factors for age-related cataract. *Survey of Ophthalmology, 39*(4), 323–334.

Resources

HEALTH INFORMATION ORGANIZATIONS AND SUPPORT GROUPS

American Academy of Ophthalmology, P.O. Box 7424, San Francisco, CA 94120-7424; www.eyenet.org

American Council of the Blind, 1155 15th St. N.W., Suite 720, Washington, DC 20005; www.acb.org

American Optometric Association, 243 North Lindbergh Boulevard, St. Louis, MO 63141; www.aoanet.org/aoanet

Association for Macular Diseases, Inc., 210 East 64th St., New York, NY 10021; www.macular.org

The Foundation Fighting Blindness, Executive Plaza I, Suite 800, 11350 McCormick Road, Hunt Valley, MD 21031-1014; www.blindness.org

Glaucoma Research Foundation, 490 Post St., Suite 830, San Francisco, CA 94102; www.glaucomal.org

The Lighthouse National Center for Vision and Aging, 111 E. 59th St., New York, NY 10022; www.lighthouse.org

National Association for the Visually Handicapped, 22 W. 21st St., 6th Floor. New York, NY 10010; www.navh.org

National Eye Institute Information Office, Bldg. 31, Rm. 6A-32, 31 Center Drive MSC2510, Bethesda, MD 20892-2510; www.nei.nih.gov

Prevent Blindness America, 500 E. Remington Road, Schaumburg, IL 60173; www.prevent-blindness.org

Vision Foundation, 818 Mt. Auburn St., Watertown, MA 02172

Vision World Wide, Inc., 5707 Brockton Dr., Suite 302, Indianapolis, IN 46220-5481; www.netdirect.net/vision-enhancement/

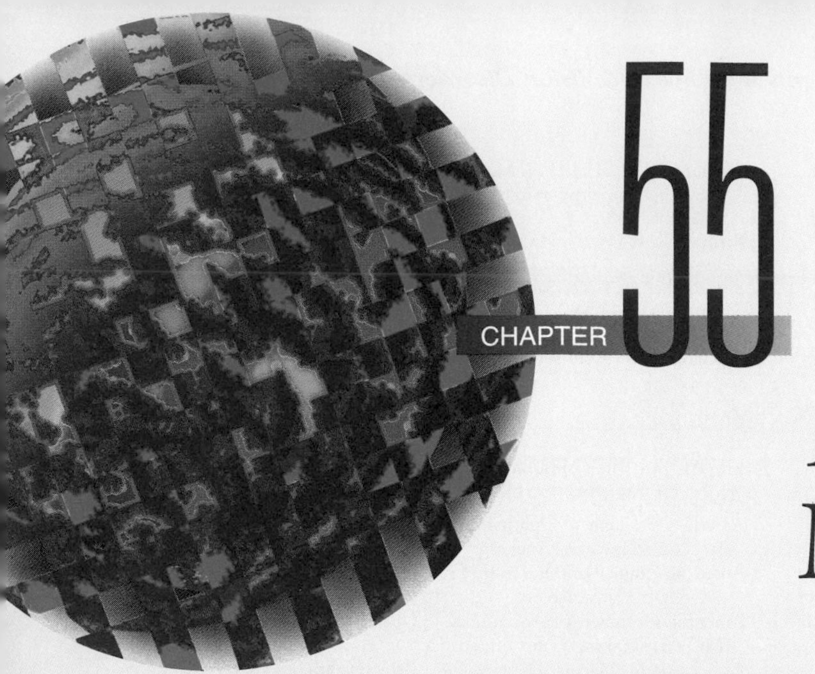

Assessment and Management of Patients With Hearing and Balance Disorders

Learning Objectives

On completion of this chapter, the learner will be able to:

1. Describe methods used to assess hearing and diagnose hearing and balance disorders.
2. List the manifestations that may be exhibited by a person with a hearing disorder.
3. Identify ways to communicate effectively with a person who is hearing-impaired.
4. Differentiate problems of the external ear from those of the middle ear and inner ear.
5. Compare the various types of surgical procedures used for managing middle ear disorders, including appropriate nursing care.
6. Describe the teaching topics that need to be addressed for patients undergoing middle ear and mastoid surgery.
7. Describe the different types of inner ear disorders, including the clinical manifestations, diagnosis, and management.

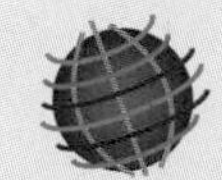

The ear is a sensory organ with dual functions—hearing and balance. The sense of hearing is essential for normal development and maintenance of speech and the ability to communicate with others. Balance, or equilibrium, is essential for maintaining body movement, position, and coordination.

GLOSSARY

acute otitis media: inflammation in the middle ear of short duration (less than 6 weeks)

cholesteatoma: benign tumor of the middle ear and/or mastoid

chronic otitis media: repeated episodes of acute otitis media causing irreversible tissue damage and persistent tympanic membrane perforation

conductive hearing loss: loss of hearing in which efficient sound transmission to the inner ear is interrupted by some obstruction or disease process

dizziness: altered sensation of orientation in space

endolymphatic hydrops: dilation of the endolymphatic space of the inner ear; the pathologic correlate of Ménière's disease

exostoses: small, hard, bony protrusions in the lower posterior bony portion of the ear canal

labyrinthitis: inflammation of the labyrinth of the inner ear

Ménière's disease: condition of the inner ear characterized by a triad of symptoms: episodic vertigo, tinnitus, and fluctuating sensorineural hearing loss

middle ear effusion: fluid in the middle ear without evidence of infection

myringotomy (tympanotomy): incision in the tympanic membrane

nystagmus: involuntary rhythmic eye movement

ossiculoplasty: surgical reconstruction of the middle ear bones to restore hearing

otalgia: sensation of fullness or pain in the ear

otitis externa (external otitis): inflammation of the external auditory canal

otorrhea: drainage from the ear

otosclerosis: a condition characterized by abnormal spongy bone formation around the stapes

presbycusis: progressive hearing loss associated with aging

rhinorrhea: drainage from the nose

sensorineural hearing loss: loss of hearing related to damage of the end organ for hearing and/or cranial nerve VIII

tinnitus: subjective perception of sound with internal origin; unwanted noises in the head or ear

tympanoplasty: surgical repair of the tympanic membrane

vertigo: illusion of movement where the individual or the surroundings are sensed as moving

ADULT HEARING AND BALANCE

The ear is a complex organ. The delicate structure and function make early detection and accurate diagnosis of disorders necessary for preservation of normal hearing and balance. Among the professionals involved in the diagnosis and treatment of these disorders are otolaryngologists, pediatricians, internists, and nurses. Nurses involved in the specialty of otolaryngology can become certified through the Society of Otorhinolaryngology and Head-Neck Nurses, Inc.

This chapter addresses the assessment and management of hearing and balance disorders common to the adult population. The reader is referred to pediatric otolaryngology literature for otologic disorders pertaining to that population.

ANATOMIC AND PHYSIOLOGIC OVERVIEW

The cranium encloses and protects the brain and surrounding structures, providing attachment for various muscles that control head and jaw movements. Eight bones form the cranium: the occipital bone, the frontal bone, two parietal bones, two temporal bones, the sphenoid bone, and the ethmoid bone. Some of these

CHART 55•1 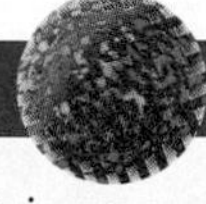 Definition of Terms: Ear Anatomy

Acoustic pertaining to sound or the sense of hearing

Acoustic nerve the division of the eighth cranial (vestibulocochlear) nerve, which goes to the cochlea

Cerumen brown, waxlike secretion found in the external auditory canal

Cochlea the winding, snail-shaped bony tube that forms a portion of the inner ear and contains the organ of Corti, the transducer for hearing

Eustachian tube the 3- to 4-cm tube that extends from the middle ear to the nasopharynx

External auditory canal the canal leading from the external auditory meatus to the tympanic membrane; about 2.5 cm in length

External ear the portion of the ear that consists of the auricle and external auditory canal; it is separated from the middle ear by the tympanic membrane

Incus the second of the three ossicles in the middle ear; it articulates with the malleus and stapes; the anvil

Inner ear the portion of the ear that consists of the cochlea, vestibule, and semicircular canals

Internal auditory canal a canal in the petrous portion of the temporal bone, which houses the facial and vestibulocochlear nerves (cranial nerves VII and VIII)

Malleus the first (most lateral) and largest of the three ossicles in the middle ear; it is connected to the tympanic membrane laterally and articulates with the incus; the hammer

Middle ear the small air-filled cavity in the temporal bone, which contains the three ossicles

Organ of Corti the end organ of hearing located in the cochlea

Ossicle a small bone; there are three in the middle ear, the malleus, incus, and stapes

Oval window a fenestra (aperture) between the vestibule of the inner ear and the middle ear occupied by the base of the stapes

Pinna the outer part of the external ear, which collects and directs sound waves into the external auditory canal; the auricle

Round window a fenestra between the middle ear and the inner ear at the base of the cochlea occupied by the round window membrane

Semicircular canals the superior, posterior, and lateral bony tubes that form part of the inner ear; contain the receptor organs for balance

Stapes the third (most medial) ossicle of the middle ear; it articulates with the incus and its footplate fits into the oval window; the stirrup

Temporal bone a bone on both sides of the skull at its base; composed of the squamous, mastoid, and petrous portions

Tympanic membrane the membrane that separates the middle ear from the external auditory canal

Vestibulocochlear nerve cranial nerve VIII; auditory nerve and vestibular nerve

bones contain sinuses, which are cavities lined with mucous membranes and connected to the nasal cavity. These sinuses, along with the mastoid air cells, reduce the weight of the skull. The ears are located on either side of the cranium at approximately eye level.

Anatomy of the External Ear

The external ear, housed in the temporal bone, includes the auricle (pinna) and the external auditory canal (Fig. 55-1). The external ear is separated from the middle ear by a disklike structure called the tympanic membrane (eardrum).

Auricle

The auricle, attached to the side of the head by skin, is composed mainly of cartilage, except for the fat and subcutaneous tissue in the earlobe. The auricle collects the sound waves and directs vibrations into the external auditory canal.

External Auditory Canal

The external auditory canal is approximately 2.5 cm long. The lateral third is an elastic cartilaginous and dense fibrous framework to which thin skin is attached. The medial two thirds is bone lined with thin skin. The external auditory canal ends at the tympanic membrane.

The skin of the canal contains hair, sebaceous glands, and ceruminous glands, which secrete a brown, waxlike substance called cerumen (ear wax). The ear's self-cleaning mechanism moves old skin cells and cerumen to the outer part of the ear.

Just anterior to the external auditory canal is the temporomandibular joint. The head of the mandible can be felt by placing a fingertip in the external auditory canal while opening and closing the mouth.

Anatomy of the Middle Ear

The middle ear, an air-filled cavity, includes the tympanic membrane laterally and the otic capsule medially. The middle ear cleft lies between the two. The middle ear is connected by the eustachian tube to the nasopharynx and is continuous with air-filled cells in the adjacent mastoid portion of the temporal bone.

The eustachian tube, which is approximately 1 mm wide and 35 mm long, connects the middle ear to the nasopharynx. Normally, the eustachian tube is closed, but it opens by action of the tensor veli palatini muscle when performing the Valsalva maneuver or by yawning or swallowing. The tube serves as a drainage channel for normal and abnormal secretions of the middle ear and equalizes pressure in the middle ear with that of the atmosphere.

Eardrum

The eardrum, about 1 cm in diameter and very thin, is normally pearly gray and translucent. The eardrum consists of three layers of tissue: an outer layer, continuous with the skin of the ear canal; a fibrous middle layer; and an inner mucosal layer, continuous with the lining of the middle ear cavity. Approximately 80% of the eardrum is composed of all three layers and is called the pars tensa. The other 20% of the eardrum lacks the middle layer and is called the pars flaccida. The absence of this fibrous middle layer

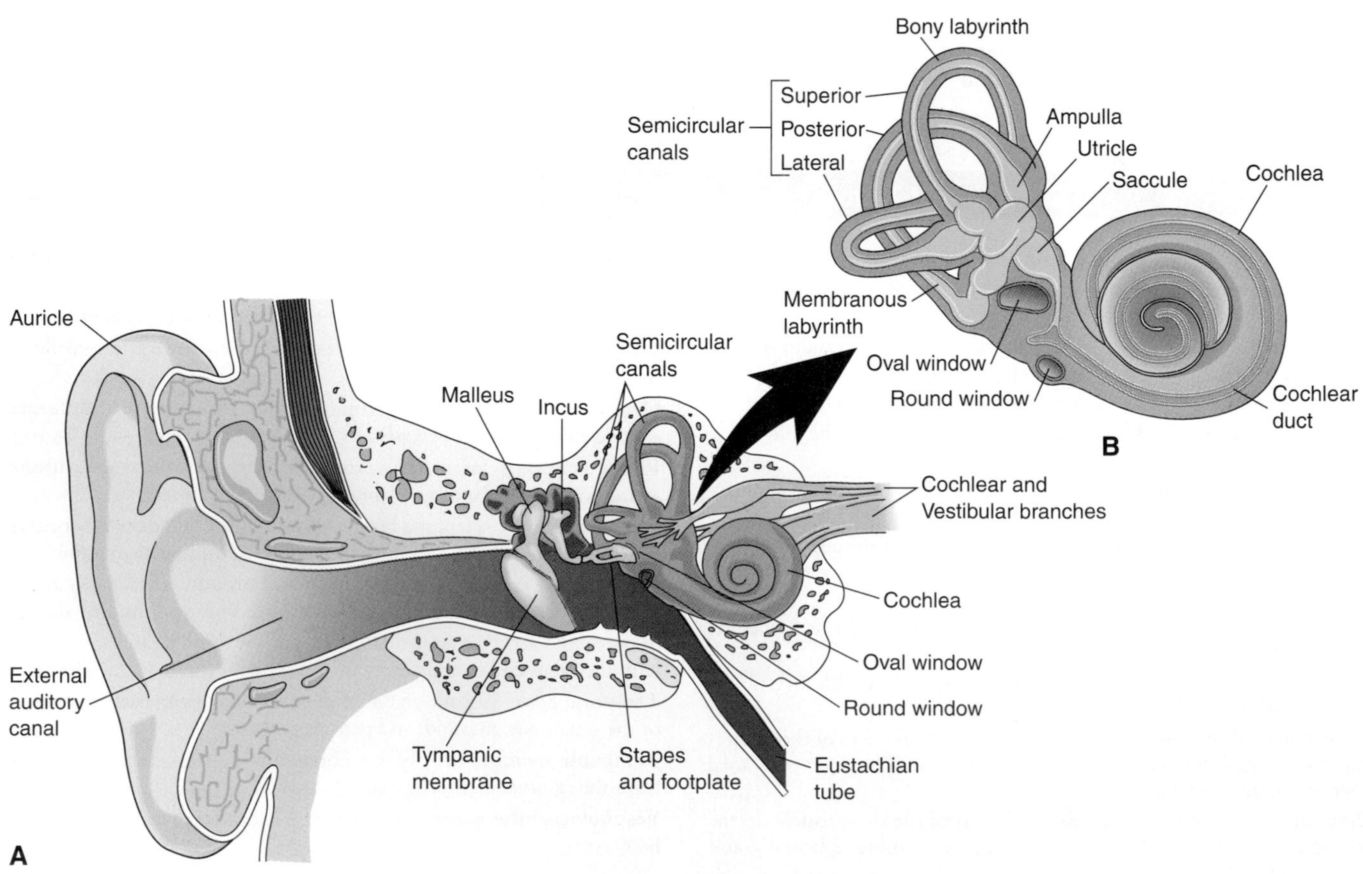

FIGURE 55•1 (**A**) Anatomy of the ear. (**B**) The inner ear.

makes the pars flaccida more vulnerable to pathologic disorders than the pars tensa. Distinguishing landmarks of the eardrum include the annulus, the fibrous border that attaches the eardrum to the temporal bone; the short process of the malleus; the long process of the malleus; the umbo of the malleus, which attaches to the eardrum in the center; the pars flaccida; and the pars tensa.

The eardrum protects the middle ear and conducts sound vibrations from the external canal to the ossicles. The sound pressure is magnified 22 times as a result of transmission from a larger area to a smaller one.

Ossicles

The middle ear contains the three smallest bones (ossicles) of the body: the malleus, incus, and stapes. The ossicles, which are held in place by joints, muscles, and ligaments, assist in the transmission of sound. Two small fenestrae (the oval and round windows), located in the medial wall of the middle ear, separate the middle ear from the inner ear. The footplate of the stapes sits in the oval window, secured by a fibrous annulus, or ring-shaped structure. The footplate transmits sound to the inner ear. The round window, covered by a thin membrane, provides an exit for sound vibrations.

Anatomy of the Inner Ear

The inner ear is housed deep within the temporal bone. The organs for hearing (cochlea) and balance (semicircular canals), as well as cranial nerves VII (facial nerve) and VIII (vestibulocochlear nerve), are all part of this complex anatomy (see Fig. 55-1). The cochlea and semicircular canals are housed in the bony labyrinth. The bony labyrinth surrounds and protects the membranous labyrinth, which is bathed in a fluid called perilymph.

Membranous Labyrinth

The membranous labyrinth is comprised of the utricle, the saccule, the cochlear duct, and the organ of Corti. The membranous labyrinth contains a different fluid called endolymph. The three semicircular canals—posterior, superior, and lateral, which lie at 90 degree angles to one another—contain sensory receptor organs arranged to detect rotational movement. These receptor end organs are stimulated by changes in the rate or direction of an individual's movement. The utricle and saccule are involved with linear movements.

ORGAN OF CORTI

The organ of Corti is located in the cochlea, a snail-shaped, bony tube about 3.5 cm long with two and a half spiral turns. Membranes separate the cochlear duct (scala media) from the scala vestibuli, and the scala tympani from the basilar membrane. The organ of Corti is located on the basilar membrane stretching from the base to the apex of the cochlea. As sound vibrations enter the perilymph at the oval window and travel along the scala vestibuli, they pass through the scala tympani, enter the cochlear duct, and cause movement of the basilar membrane. The organ of Corti, also called the end organ for hearing, transforms mechanical energy into neural activity and separates sounds into different frequencies. This electrochemical impulse travels via the acoustic nerve to the temporal cortex of the brain to be interpreted as meaningful sound. In the internal auditory canal, the cochlear (acoustic) nerve, arising from the cochlea, joins the vestibular nerve, arising from the semicircular canals, utricle, and saccule, to become the vestibulocochlear nerve (cranial nerve VIII). This canal also houses the facial nerve and the blood supply from the ear to the brain.

Function of the Ears

Hearing

Hearing is conducted over two pathways: air and bone. Sounds transmitted by air conduction travel over the air-filled external and middle ear via vibration of the tympanic membrane and ossicles. Sounds transmitted by bone conduction travel directly through bone to the inner ear, bypassing the tympanic membrane and ossicles. Normally, air conduction is the more efficient pathway. However, defects in the tympanic membrane or interruption of the ossicular chain disrupt normal air conduction, which results in a loss of the sound/pressure ratio and subsequently a conductive hearing loss.

SOUND CONDUCTION AND TRANSMISSION

Sound enters the ear through the external auditory canal and causes the tympanic membrane to vibrate. These vibrations transmit sound through the lever action of the ossicles to the oval window as mechanical energy. This mechanical energy is then transmitted through the inner ear fluids to the cochlea, stimulating the hair cells, and is subsequently converted to electrical energy. The electrical energy travels via the vestibulocochlear nerve to the central nervous system, where it is analyzed and interpreted in its final form as sound.

Vibrations transmitted by the tympanic membrane to the ossicles of the middle ear are transferred to the cochlea, lodged in the labyrinth of the inner ear. The stapes rocks, causing vibrations (waves) in fluids contained in the inner ear. These fluid waves, in turn, cause movement of the basilar membrane to occur that then stimulates the hair cells of the organ of Corti, in the cochlea, to move in a wavelike manner. The movements of the membrane set up electrical currents that stimulate the various areas of the cochlea. The hair cells set up neural impulses that are encoded and then transferred to the auditory cortex in the brain, where they are decoded into a sound message.

The footplate of the stapes receives impulses transmitted by the incus and the malleus from the tympanic membrane. The round window, which opens on the opposite side of the cochlear duct, is protected from sound waves by the intact tympanic membrane, thus permitting motion of the inner ear fluids by sound wave stimulation. For example, in the normally intact tympanic membrane, sound waves stimulate the oval window first, and a lag occurs before the terminal effect of the stimulus reaches the round window. This lag phase is changed, however, when a perforation of the tympanic membrane is large enough to allow sound waves to impinge on both the oval and round windows simultaneously. This effect cancels the lag and prevents the maximal effect of inner ear fluid motility and its subsequent effect in stimulating the hair cells in the organ of Corti. The result is a reduction in hearing ability.

Balance and Equilibrium

Body balance is maintained by the cooperation of the muscles and joints of the body (proprioceptive system), the eyes (visual system), and the labyrinth (vestibular system). These areas send their information about equilibrium, or balance, to the brain (cerebellar system) for coordination and perception in the cerebral cortex. The brain obtains its blood supply from the heart and arterial system. A problem in any of these areas, such as arteriosclerosis or impaired vision, can cause a balance disturbance. The vestibular apparatus of the inner ear provides feedback regarding the movements and the position of the head and body in space.

ASSESSMENT

Physical Assessment

The external ear is examined by inspection and direct palpation, and the tympanic membrane is inspected with an otoscope and indirect palpation with a pneumatic otoscope. Until recently, with the advent of middle ear endoscopy, inspection of the middle ear was impossible. Evaluation of gross auditory acuity also is included in every physical examination.

Inspection

Inspection of the external ear is a simple procedure but is often overlooked. The auricle and surrounding tissues should be inspected for deformities, lesions, and discharge as well as size, symmetry, and angle of attachment to the head. Manipulation of the auricle does not normally elicit pain. If this maneuver is painful, acute external otitis is suspected. Tenderness on palpation in the area of the mastoid may indicate acute mastoiditis or inflammation of the posterior auricular node. Occasionally, sebaceous cysts and tophi (subcutaneous mineral deposits) are present on the pinna. A flaky scaliness on or behind the auricle usually indicates seborrheic dermatitis and can be present on the scalp and facial structures as well.

Otoscopic Examination

To examine the external auditory canal and tympanic membrane, the patient's head is tipped away from the examiner. The otoscope is held in one hand while the auricle is grasped with the other hand firmly and pulled upward, backward, and slightly outward (Fig. 55-2). This straightens the canal in the adult, allowing the examiner to visualize the tympanic membrane.

The speculum is gently and slowly inserted into the ear canal, and the examiner's eye is held close to the magnifying lens of the otoscope to visualize the canal and tympanic membrane. The largest speculum that the canal can accommodate (usually 5 mm in an adult) is guided gently down into the canal and slightly forward. Because the distal portion of the canal is bony and covered by a sensitive layer of epithelium, only light pressure may be used without causing pain. Any discharge, inflammation, or foreign body in the external auditory canal is noted.

The healthy tympanic membrane is pearly gray and is positioned obliquely at the base of the canal. The landmarks are identified if visible (see Fig. 55-2): the pars tensa, the umbo, the manubrium of the malleus, and its short process. A slow circular movement of the speculum allows further visualization of the malleolar folds and periphery. The position and color of the membrane as well as any unusual markings or deviations from normal are noted. The presence of fluid, air bubbles, blood, or masses in the middle ear also should be noted.

Proper otoscopic examination of the external auditory canal and tympanic membrane requires that the canal be free of large amounts of cerumen. Cerumen is normally present in the external canal, and small amounts should not interfere with otoscopic examination. If the tympanic membrane cannot be visualized because of cerumen, the cerumen may be removed by gently irrigating the external canal (if there are no contraindications to this). If adherent cerumen is present, a small amount of mineral oil or over-the-counter cerumen softener may be instilled within the ear canal, and the patient is instructed to return for subsequent removal of the cerumen and inspection of the ear. The use of instruments such as a cerumen curette for cerumen removal is reserved for otolaryngologists and nurses with specialized training because of the danger of perforating the tympanic membrane or excoriating the external auditory canal. Cerumen buildup is a common cause of hearing loss and local irritation.

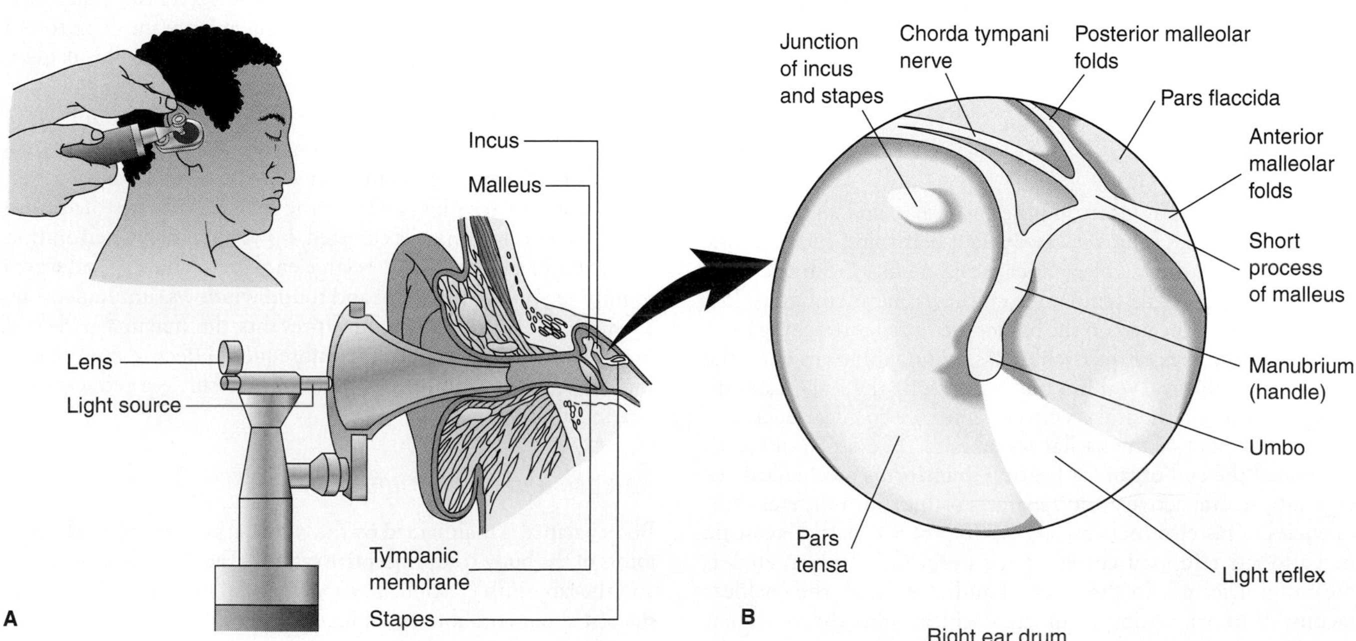

FIGURE 55•2 (**A**) Technique for using the otoscope to see (**B**) the tympanic membrane.

Evaluation of Gross Auditory Acuity

A general estimation of the patient's hearing can be made by assessing his or her ability to hear a whispered phrase or a ticking watch, testing one ear at a time. The Weber and Rinne tests may be used to distinguish conductive loss from sensorineural loss when hearing is impaired. These tests are part of the usual screening physical examination and are useful if a more specific assessment is needed, if hearing loss is detected, or if substantiation of audiometric results is desired.

WHISPER TEST

To exclude one ear from the testing, the examiner covers the untested ear with the palm of the hand. Then the examiner whispers softly from a distance of 1 or 2 feet from the unoccluded ear and out of the patient's sight. The patient with normal acuity can correctly repeat what was whispered.

WEBER TEST

The Weber test uses bone conduction to test lateralization of sound. A tuning fork, set in motion by grasping it firmly by its stem and tapping it on the examiner's knee or hand, is then placed on the patient's head or forehead (Fig. 55-3). The patient is asked to identify whether the sound is heard in the middle of the head, the right ear, or the left ear. A person with normal hearing will hear the sound equally in both ears or describe the sound as centered in the middle of the head. In cases of **conductive hearing loss** (eg, from otosclerosis or otitis media), the sound is heard better in the affected ear. In cases of **sensorineural hearing loss** (resulting from damage to the cochlear or vestibulocochlear nerve), however, the sound lateralizes to the better-hearing ear. The Weber test is useful for detecting unilateral hearing loss.

RINNE TEST

In the Rinne test, the examiner shifts the stem of a vibrating tuning fork between two positions: 2 inches from the opening of the ear canal (air conduction) and against the mastoid bone (bone conduction) (Fig. 55-4). As the position changes, the patient is asked to indicate which tone is louder or when the tone is no longer audible. Normally, sound heard by air conduction is audible longer than sound heard by bone conduction. The Rinne test is useful for distinguishing between conductive and sensorineural hearing losses. With a conductive hearing loss, bone-conducted sound is heard as long as or longer than air-conducted sound, whereas with a sensorineural hearing loss, air-conducted sound is audible longer than bone-conducted sound. In a normal hearing ear, air conduction is louder than bone conduction.

DIAGNOSTIC EVALUATION

Many diagnostic procedures are available to measure the auditory and vestibular systems indirectly. These tests are usually performed by an audiologist who is recognized by the American Speech-Language-Hearing Association with a certificate of clinical competence in audiology.

Audiometry

In detecting hearing loss, audiometry is the single most important diagnostic instrument. Audiometric testing is of two kinds: pure-tone audiometry, in which the sound stimulus consists of a pure or musical tone (the louder the tone before the patient perceives it, the greater the hearing loss), and speech audiometry, in

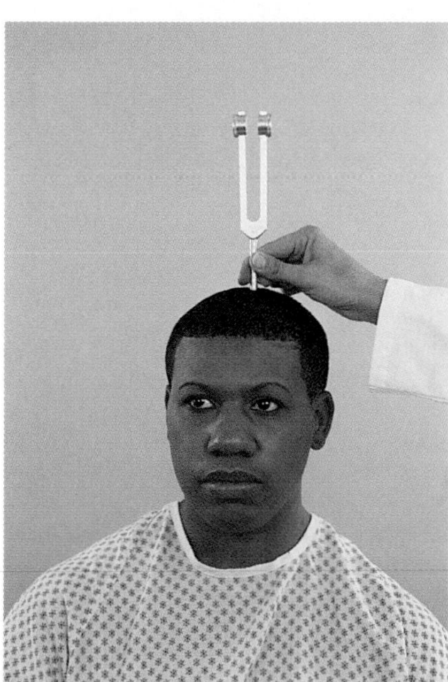

FIGURE 55•3 The Weber test assesses bone conduction of sound. From Weber, J. W., & Kelley, J. (1998). *Health assessment in nursing.* Philadelphia: Lippincott-Raven.

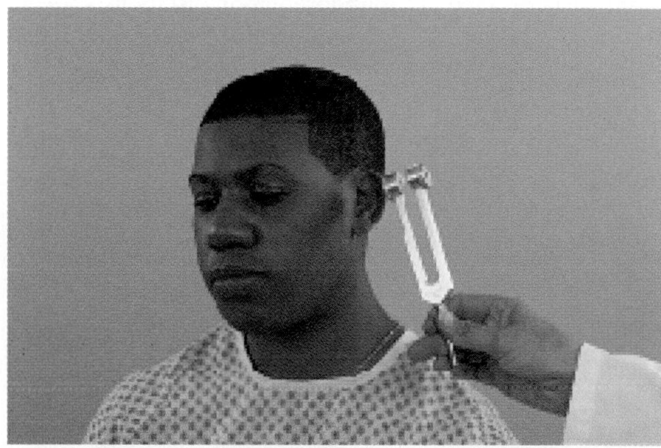

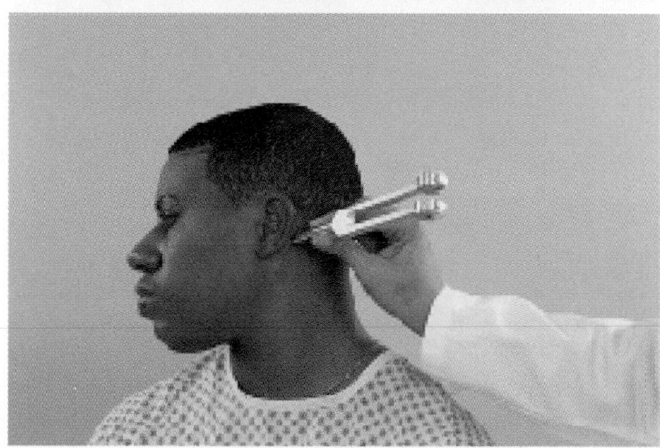

FIGURE 55•4 The Rinne test assesses both air and bone conduction of sound. From Weber, J. W., & Kelley, J. (1998). *Health assessment in nursing.* Philadelphia: Lippincott-Raven.

which the spoken word is used to determine the ability to hear and discriminate sounds and words.

When evaluating hearing, three characteristics are important: frequency, pitch, and intensity. Frequency refers to the number of sound waves emanating from a source per second—cycles per second or hertz (Hz). The normal human ear perceives sounds ranging in frequency from 20 to 20,000 Hz. The frequencies from 500 to 2,000 Hz are important in understanding everyday speech and are referred to as the speech range or speech frequencies. Pitch is the term used to describe frequency; a tone with 100 Hz is considered of low pitch, and a tone of 10,000 Hz is considered of high pitch.

The unit for measuring loudness (intensity of sound) is the decibel (dB), the pressure exerted by sound. Hearing loss is measured in decibels, a logarithmic function of intensity that is not easily converted into a percentage. The critical level of loudness is approximately 30 dB. The shuffling of papers in quiet surroundings is about 15 dB; a low conversation, 40 dB; and a jet plane 100 feet away, about 150 dB. Sound louder than 80 dB is perceived by the human ear to be harsh and can be damaging to the inner ear. Table 55-1 classifies hearing loss based on decibel level. With surgical treatment of patients with hearing loss, the aim is to improve the hearing level to 30 dB or better within the speech frequencies.

With audiometry, the audiologist performs the testing while the patient wears earphones and signals when hearing a tone. When the tone is applied directly over the external auditory canal, air conduction is measured. When the stimulus is applied to the mastoid bone, bypassing the conductive mechanism (the ossicles), nerve conduction is tested. For accuracy, audiometric evaluations are performed in a soundproof room. Responses are plotted on a graph known as an audiogram, which differentiates between conductive and sensorineural hearing loss (Fig. 55-5). Speech discrimination is also measured (Fig. 55-6).

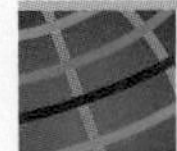

TABLE 55•1 Severity of Hearing Loss

Loss in Decibels	Interpretation
0–15	Normal hearing
>15–25	Slight hearing loss
>25–40	Mild hearing loss
>40–55	Moderate hearing loss
>55–70	Moderate to severe hearing loss
>70–90	Severe hearing loss
>90	Profound hearing loss

Tympanogram

A tympanogram, or impedance audiometry, measures middle ear muscle reflex to sound stimulation, and compliance of the tympanic membrane, by changing the air pressure in a sealed ear canal (Fig. 55-7). Compliance is impaired with middle ear disease.

Auditory Brain Stem Response

The auditory brain stem response is a detectable electrical potential from cranial nerve VIII and the ascending auditory pathways of the brain stem in response to sound stimulation. Electrodes are placed on the patient's forehead. Acoustic stimuli, usually in the form of clicks, are made in the ear. The resulting electrophysio-

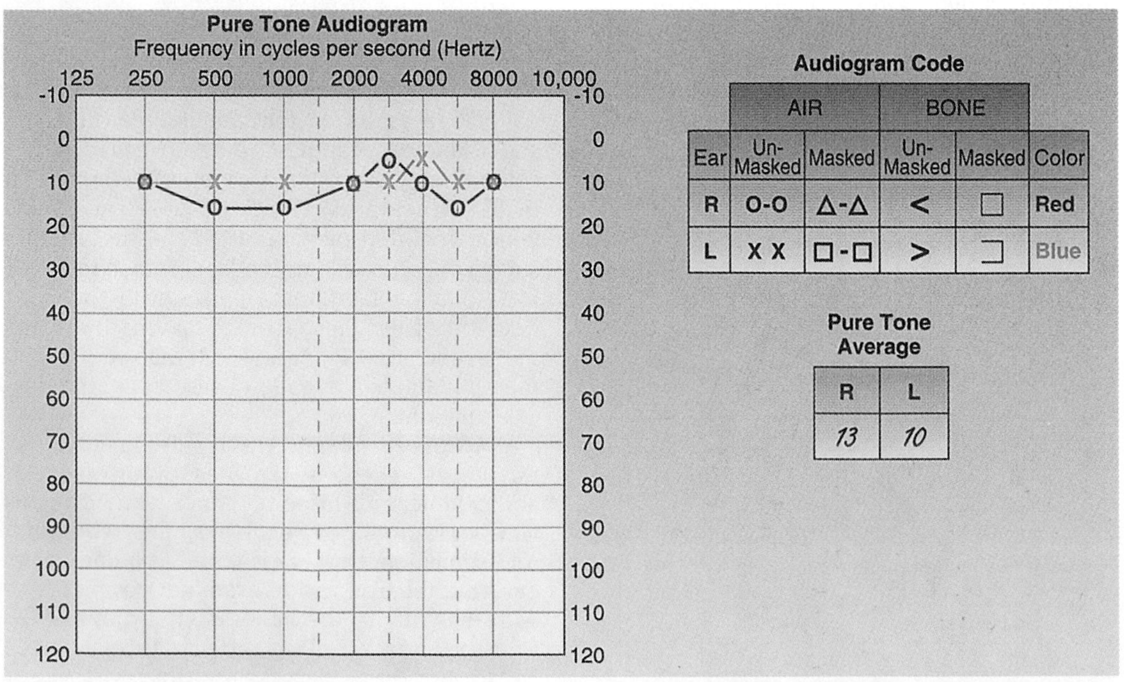

FIGURE 55•5 An audiogram presents a graphic outline of hearing as measured by tones of different pitches ranging from 125 through 8000 cycles per second (cps) or Hertz (Hz). This audiogram shows normal hearing bilaterally. The box on the right indicates the symbols used on an audiogram.

SPEECH HEARING TESTS					
TEST		R	L	BIN	SF
Sp. Reception Threshold (SRT)		10 db	10 db	db	db
Sp. Discrim. Scores	80 db HL	100%	100%	%	%
(PB)	___db HL	%	%	%	%
	___db HL	%	%	%	%

FIGURE 55•6 The speech reception threshold is the sound intensity level at which a patient is just capable of correctly identifying simple speech stimuli. Speech discrimination determines the patient's ability to distinguish different sounds, in the form of words, at a decibel level where sound is heard.

logic measurements can determine at which decibel level a patient hears and whether there are any impairments along the nerve pathways (eg, tumor on cranial nerve VIII).

Electronystagmography

Electronystagmography is the measurement and graphic recording of the changes in electrical potentials created by eye movements during spontaneous, positional, or calorically evoked nystagmus. It is also used to assess the oculomotor and vestibular systems and their corresponding interaction. It helps in diagnosing conditions such as Ménière's disease and tumors of the internal auditory canal or posterior fossa. Any vestibular suppressants, such as sedatives, tranquilizers, antihistamines, or alcohol are withheld for 24 hours before testing.

Platform Posturography

Platform posturography is used to investigate postural control capabilities. The integration of visual, vestibular, and proprioceptive cues (sensory integration) with motor response output and coordination of the lower limbs is tested. The patient stands on a platform, surrounded by a screen, and different conditions such as a moving platform with a moving screen or a stationary platform with a moving screen are presented. The responses from the patient on six different conditions are measured and indicate which of the above mentioned systems may be impaired. Preparation for the testing is the same as for electronystagmography.

Sinusoidal Harmonic Acceleration

Sinusoidal harmonic acceleration, or a rotary chair, is used to assess the vestibulo-ocular system by analyzing compensatory eye movements in response to the clockwise and counterclockwise rotation of the chair. Although such testing cannot identify the side of the lesion in unilateral disease, it helps identify disease and evaluate the course of recovery. The same patient preparation is required as for electronystagmography.

Middle Ear Endoscopy

With the advent of endoscopes with very small diameters and acute angles, the ear can be examined endoscopically. Middle ear endoscopy is performed safely and effectively as an office procedure to evaluate suspected perilymphatic fistula and new-onset conductive hearing loss, the anatomy of the round window before transtympanic treatment of Ménière's disease, and the tympanic cavity before ear surgery to treat chronic middle ear and mastoid infections.

The tympanic membrane is anesthetized topically for about 10 minutes. Then, the external auditory canal is irrigated with sterile normal saline solution. With the aid of a microscope, a tympanotomy is created with a laser beam or a myringotomy knife, so that the endoscope can be inserted into the middle ear cavity. Video and photo documentation can be accomplished.

HEARING LOSS

More than 28 million people in the United States have some form of hearing impairment. Most can be helped with medical or surgical therapies or with a hearing aid. By the year 2050, about one out of every five people in the United States, or almost 58 million people, will be age 55 or older. Of this population, almost half can expect a hearing impairment (NIDCD, 1998).

A conductive hearing loss usually results from an external ear disorder, such as impacted cerumen, or a middle ear disorder, such as otitis media or otosclerosis. In such instances, the efficient transmission of sound by air to the inner ear is interrupted. A sensorineural loss involves damage to the cochlea or vestibulocochlear nerve.

A mixed hearing loss and a functional hearing loss also may occur. The patient with a mixed hearing loss has both a conductive and sensorineural loss, resulting from dysfunction of both air and bone conduction. A functional (or psychogenic) hearing loss is nonorganic and unrelated to detectable structural changes in the hearing mechanisms; it is usually a manifestation of an emotional disturbance.

Clinical Manifestations

Early manifestations of hearing impairment and loss may include tinnitus, increasing inability to hear in groups, and a need to turn up the volume of the television. Hearing impairment can also trigger changes in personality and attitude, the ability to communicate, the awareness of surroundings, and even the ability to protect oneself, thus affecting the person's quality of life. In a classroom, a student with impaired hearing may be disinterested and inattentive and have failing grades. A person at home may feel isolated because of an inability to hear the clock chime, the refrigerator hum, the birds sing, or the traffic pass. A hearing-impaired pedestrian may attempt to cross the street and fail to hear an approaching car. Hearing-impaired people may miss parts of a conversation. Many people are unaware of their gradual hearing impairment. Often it is not the person with the hearing loss, but the people with whom he or she is communicating, who recognize the impairment first.

For various reasons, some people with hearing loss refuse to seek medical attention or wear a hearing aid. Others feel self-conscious wearing a hearing aid. Introspective patients generally ask those with whom they are trying to communicate to let them know whether difficulties in communication exist. These attitudes and behaviors should be taken into account when counseling patients who need hearing assistance. The decision to wear a hearing aid is a personal one that is affected by these attitudes and behaviors.

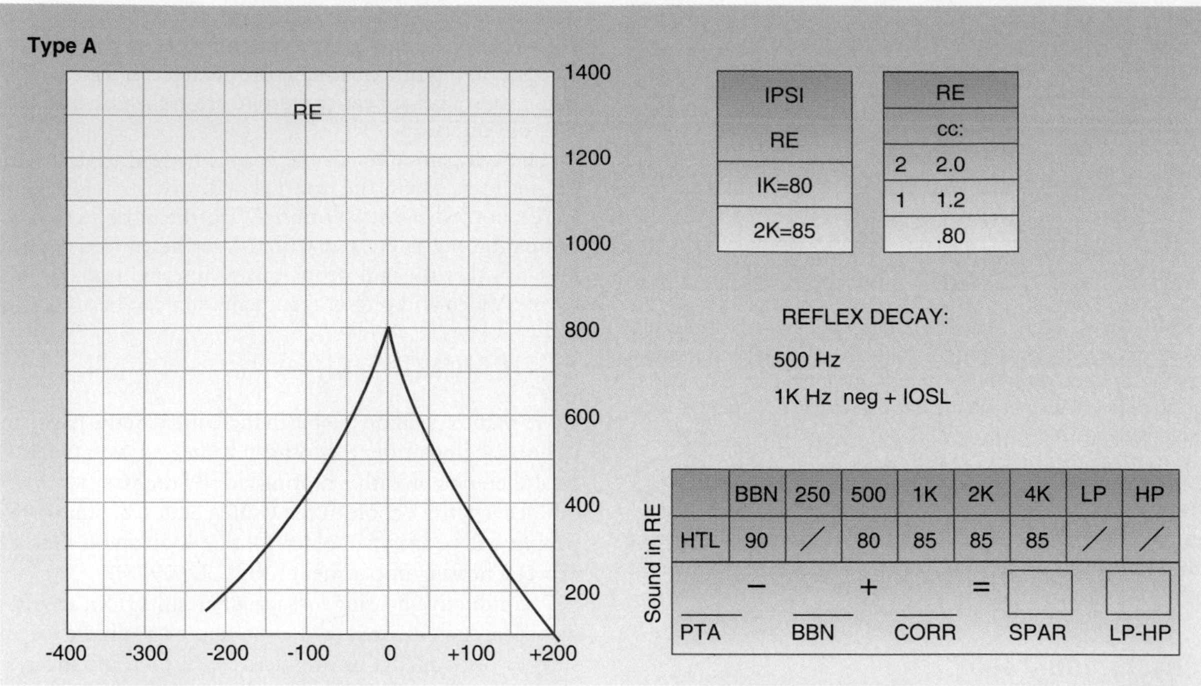

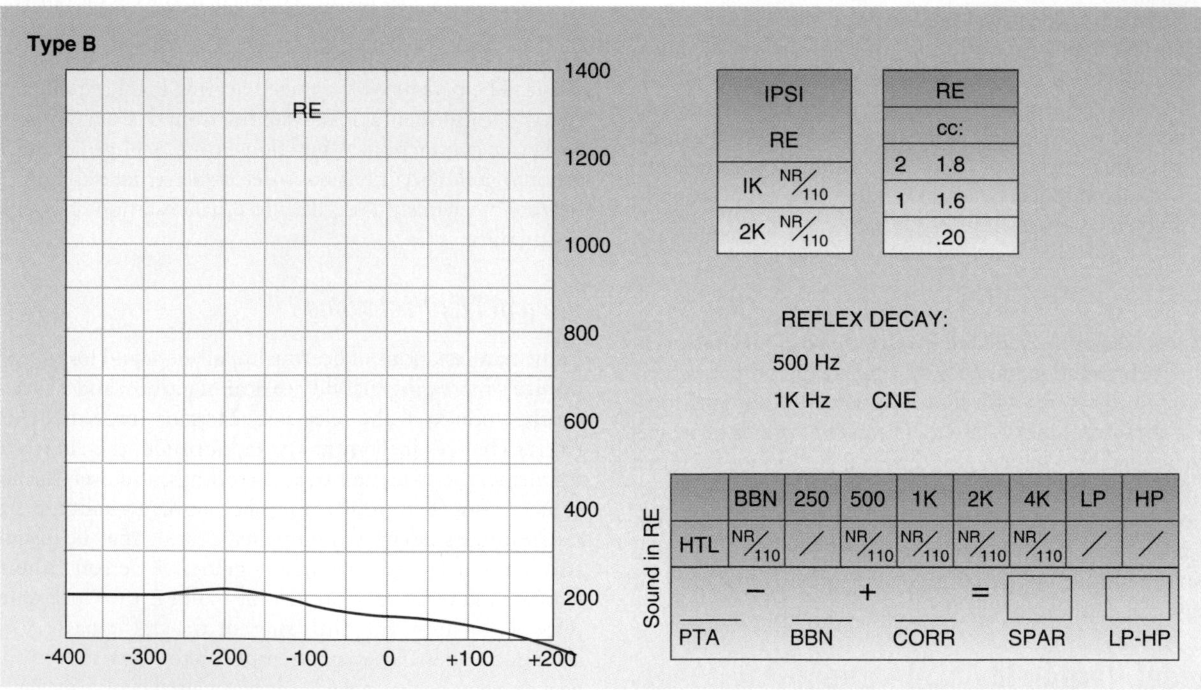

FIGURE 55•7 The typical normal, or type A, tympanogram shows a pressure/compliance curve by changing air pressure in a sealed ear canal. A typical "flat," or type B, tympanogram shows an absence of a pressure/compliance peak and indicates middle ear effusion or massive ossicular fixation.

Prevention

Many environmental factors have an adverse effect on the auditory system and with time result in permanent sensorineural hearing loss. The most common is noise.

Noise (unwanted and unavoidable sound) has been identified as one of the environmental hazards of the 20th century. The sheer volume of noise that surrounds us daily has increased from a simple annoyance into a potentially dangerous source of physical and psychological damage.

In terms of physical impact, loud, persistent noise has been found to cause constriction of peripheral blood vessels, increased blood pressure and heart rate (because of increased secretion of adrenalin), and increased gastrointestinal activity. Additional research is needed to address the overall effects of noise on the human body. It seems certain, however, that a quiet environment

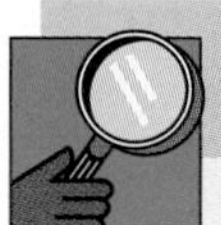

ASSESSMENT
SYMPTOMS OF HEARING LOSS

Speech deterioration The person who slurs words or drops word endings, or produces flat-sounding speech, may not be hearing correctly. The ears guide the voice, both in loudness and pronunciation.

Fatigue If a person tires easily when listening to conversation or to a speech, fatigue may be the result of straining to hear. Under these circumstances, the person may become irritable very easily.

Indifference It is easy for the person who cannot hear what others say to become depressed and disinterested in life in general.

Social withdrawal Not being able to hear what is going on causes the hearing-impaired person to withdraw from situations that might prove embarrassing.

Insecurity Lack of self-confidence and fear of mistakes create a feeling of insecurity in many hearing-impaired people. No one likes to say the wrong thing or do anything that might appear foolish.

Indecision and Procrastination Loss of self-confidence makes it increasingly difficult for a hearing-impaired person to make decisions.

Suspiciousness The hearing-impaired person, who often hears only part of what is being said, may suspect that others are talking about him or her, or that portions of the conversation are deliberately spoken softly so that he or she will not hear them.

False pride The hearing-impaired person wants to conceal the hearing loss and thus often pretends to be hearing when he or she actually is not.

Loneliness and unhappiness Although everyone wishes for quiet now and then, *enforced* silence can be boring and even somewhat frightening. People with a hearing loss often feel isolated.

Tendency to dominate the conversation Many hearing-impaired people tend to dominate the conversation, knowing that as long as it is centered on them and they can control it, they are not so likely to be embarrassed by some mistake.

is more conducive to peace of mind. A person who is ill feels more at ease when noise is kept to a minimum.

The term "noise-induced hearing loss," a preventable disorder, is used to describe hearing loss that follows a long period of exposure to loud noise (eg, heavy machinery, engines, artillery). Acoustic trauma refers to the hearing loss caused by a single exposure to an extremely intense noise, such as an explosion. Usually, noise-induced hearing loss occurs at a high frequency (around 4,000 Hz). However, with continued noise exposure, the hearing loss can become more severe and include adjacent frequencies. The minimum noise level known to cause noise-induced hearing loss, regardless of duration, is about 85 to 90 dB.

Noise exposure is inherent in many jobs (eg, mechanics, printers, pilots, and musicians) as well as in hobbies such as woodworking and hunting. The Occupational Safety and Health Administration requires that workers wear ear protection to prevent noise-induced hearing loss when exposed to noise above the legal limits. There are no medications that protect against noise-induced hearing loss; hearing loss is permanent because the hair cells in the organ of Corti are destroyed. Ear protection against noise is the most effective preventive measure available.

Gerontologic Considerations

About 25% of people between ages 65 and 74 years and 50% of people aged 75 years and older have hearing difficulties. The cause is unknown; linkages to diet, metabolism, arteriosclerosis, stress, and heredity have been inconsistent (Nobel et al., 1995).

With aging, changes occur in the ear that may eventually lead to hearing deficits. Although few changes occur in the external ear, cerumen tends to become harder and drier, posing a greater chance of impaction. In the middle ear, the tympanic membrane may atrophy or become sclerotic. In the inner ear, cells at the base of the cochlea degenerate. A familial predisposition to sensorineural hearing loss is also seen, manifested by a loss in the ability to hear high-frequency sounds, followed in time by the loss of middle and lower frequencies. The term **presbycusis** is used to describe this progressive hearing loss.

In addition to age-related changes, other factors can affect hearing in the elderly population, such as lifelong exposure to loud noises (eg, jets, guns, heavy machinery, circular saws). Certain medications, such as the aminoglycosides and even aspirin, have ototoxic effects when renal changes (eg, in the older person) result in delayed medication excretion. Many older people take quinine for treatment of leg cramps; quinine can cause a hearing loss. Psychogenic factors and other disease processes (eg, diabetes) also may be partially responsible for sensorineural hearing loss.

When a hearing problem occurs, an evaluation is warranted. Even with the best medical care, the person must learn to adjust to varying degrees of hearing loss. Care of elderly patients includes recognizing emotional reactions related to hearing loss, such as suspicion of others because of an inability to hear adequately; frustration and anger, with repeated statements such as, "I didn't hear what you said"; and feelings of insecurity because of the inability to hear the telephone or alarms.

Medical Management

If a hearing loss is permanent or untreatable with medical or surgical intervention, or if the patient elects not to have surgery, aural rehabilitation (discussed at the end of the chapter) may be beneficial.

Nursing Management

The nurse who understands the different types of hearing loss will be more successful in adopting a communication style to fit the patient's needs. Trying to speak in a loud voice to a person who cannot hear high-frequency sounds only makes understanding more difficult. However, strategies such as talking into the less-impaired ear and using gestures and facial expressions can help. See Guideline 55-1.

CONDITIONS OF THE EXTERNAL EAR

Cerumen Impaction

Cerumen (ear wax) normally accumulates in the external canal in varying amounts and colors. Although wax does not usually need to be removed, on occasion impaction can occur, causing **otalgia**, a sensation of fullness or pain in the ear, with or without a hearing loss. Accumulation of cerumen is especially significant in the geriatric population as a cause of hearing deficit. Attempts to clear the external auditory canal with matches, hair pins, and other implements are dangerous because trauma to the skin, infection, or damage to the eardrum can occur.

Management

Cerumen can be removed by irrigation, suction, or instrumentation. Unless the patient has a perforated eardrum or an inflamed external ear (otitis externa), gentle irrigation usually helps remove

55•1 Guidelines For Communicating With the Hearing-Impaired Person

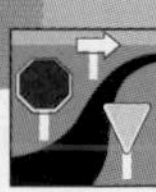

For the hearing-impaired person whose speech is difficult to understand:

- Devote full attention to what the person is saying. Look and listen—do not try to attend to another task while listening.
- Engage the speaker in conversation when it is possible for you to anticipate the replies. This enables you to become accustomed to any peculiarities in speech patterns.
- Try to determine the essential context of what is being said; you can often fill in the details from context.
- Do not try to appear as if you understand if you do not.
- If you cannot understand at all or have serious doubt about your ability to understand what is being said, have the person write the message rather than risk misunderstanding. Having the person repeat the message in speech, after you know its content, also aids you in becoming accustomed to the person's pattern of speech.

For the hearing-impaired person who speech reads:

- When speaking, always face the person as directly as possible.
- Make sure your face is as clearly visible as possible. Locate yourself so that your face is well lighted; avoid being silhouetted against strong light. Do not obscure the person's view of your mouth in any way; avoid talking with any object held in your mouth.
- Be sure the patient knows the topic or subject before going ahead with what you plan to say. This enables the person to use contextual clues in speech reading.
- Speak slowly and distinctly, pausing more frequently than you would normally.
- If you question whether some important direction or instruction has been understood, check to be certain that the patient has the full meaning of your message.
- If for any reason your mouth must be covered (as with a mask) and you must direct or instruct the patient, write the message.

impacted cerumen, particularly if it is not tightly packed in the external auditory canal. For successful removal, the water stream must flow behind the obstructing cerumen to move it first laterally and then out of the canal. To prevent injury, the lowest effective pressure should be used. If the eardrum behind the impaction is perforated, however, water can enter the middle ear, producing acute vertigo and infection. If irrigation is unsuccessful, direct visual, mechanical removal can be performed on a cooperative patient by a trained health care provider.

Instilling a few drops of warmed glycerin, mineral oil, or half-strength hydrogen peroxide into the ear canal for 30 minutes can soften cerumen before its removal. Cerumenolytic agents, such as peroxide in glyceryl (Debrox), are available; however, these compounds may cause an allergic dermatitis reaction. Using any softening solution two or three times a day for several days is generally sufficient. If the cerumen cannot be dislodged by these methods, instruments, such as a cerumen curette, aural suction, and a binocular microscope for magnification, can be used.

Foreign Bodies

Some objects are inserted intentionally into the ear by adults who may have been trying to clean the external canal or relieve itching or by children who introduce the objects for various reasons. Other objects, such as insects, peas, beans, pebbles, toys, and beads enter the ear canal by accident. In either case, the effects may range from no symptoms at all to profound pain and decreased hearing.

Management

Removing a foreign body from the external auditory canal can be quite challenging. The three standard methods for removing foreign bodies are the same as those for removing cerumen: irrigation, suction, and instrumentation. The contraindications for irrigation are the same as well. However, foreign vegetable bodies and insects tend to swell, also contraindicating irrigation. Usually, an insect can be dislodged by instilling mineral oil, which will kill the insect and allow it to be removed.

Attempts to remove any foreign body from the external canal may be dangerous in unskilled hands. The object may be pushed completely into the bony portion of the canal, lacerating the skin and perforating the tympanic membrane. In difficult cases, the foreign body may be extracted in the operating room with the patient under general anesthesia.

External Otitis (Otitis Externa)

External otitis refers to an inflammation of the external auditory canal. Causes may include water in the ear canal (swimmer's ear); trauma to the skin of the ear canal, permitting entrance of organisms into the tissues; and systemic conditions, such as vitamin deficiency and endocrine disorders. Bacterial or fungal infections are most frequently encountered. The most common bacterial pathogens associated with external otitis are *Staphylococcus aureus* and *Pseudomonas* species. The most common fungus isolated in both normal and infected ears is *Aspergillus*. External otitis is often due to a dermatosis such as psoriasis, eczema, or seborrheic dermatitis. Even allergic reactions to hair spray, hair dye, and permanent wave lotions can cause dermatitis, which clears when the offending agent is removed.

Clinical Manifestations

The patient usually reports pain, discharge from the external auditory canal, aural tenderness (usually not present in middle ear infections), and occasionally fever, cellulitis, and lymphadenopathy. Other symptoms may include pruritus and hearing loss or a feeling of fullness. On otoscopic examination, the ear canal is erythematous and edematous. Discharge may be yellow or green and foul-smelling. In fungal infections, the hairlike black spores may even be visible.

Medical Management

The principles of therapy are aimed at relieving the discomfort, reducing the swelling of the ear canal, and eradicating the infection. Patients may require prescription analgesics for the first 48 to 92 hours. If the tissues of the external canal are edematous, a wick should be inserted to keep the canal open so that liquid medications (eg, Burow's solution, antibiotic otic preparations) can be introduced. These medications may be administered by dropper at room temperature. Such medications usually combine antibiotic and corticosteroid agents to soothe the inflamed tissues. For cellulitis or fever, systemic antibiotics may be prescribed. For fungal disorders, antifungal agents are prescribed.

Nursing Management

Nurses need to teach patients not to clean the external auditory canal with cotton-tipped applicators, to avoid swimming, and not to allow water to enter the ear when shampooing or showering. A cotton ball can be covered in a water-insoluble gel such as petroleum jelly and placed in the ear as a barrier to water contamination. Infection can be prevented by using antiseptic otic preparations after swimming (eg, Swim Ear or Ear Dry), unless there is a history of tympanic membrane perforation or a current ear infection.

Malignant External Otitis

A more serious, although rare, external ear infection is malignant external otitis (temporal bone osteomyelitis). This is a progressive, debilitating, and occasionally fatal infection of the external auditory canal, the surrounding tissue, and the base of the skull. *Pseudomonas aeruginosa* is usually the infecting organism in patients with low resistance to infection (eg, patients with diabetes). Successful treatment includes control of the diabetes, administration of antibiotics (usually intravenously), and aggressive local wound care. Standard parenteral antibiotic treatment includes the combination of an antipseudomonal agent and an aminoglycoside, both of which have potentially serious side effects. Because aminoglycosides are nephrotoxic and ototoxic, serum aminoglycoside levels and renal and auditory function must be monitored during therapy. Local wound care includes limited débridement of the infected tissue, including bone and cartilage, depending on the extent of the infection.

Masses of the External Ear

Exostoses are small, hard, bony protrusions found in the lower posterior bony portion of the ear canal; they usually occur bilaterally. The skin covering the exostosis is normal. Many people think exostoses are caused by an exposure to cold water, as in scuba diving or surfing. The usual treatment, if any, is surgical excision.

Malignant tumors also may be found in the external ear. Most common are basal cell carcinomas on the pinna and squamous cell carcinomas in the ear canal. If untreated, squamous cell carcinoma may spread through the temporal bone, causing facial nerve paralysis and hearing loss. Carcinomas must be treated surgically.

Gaping Earring Puncture

This problem results from wearing heavy earrings for a long time or after an infection, or reaction from the earring or other impurities in the earring. One or more gaping punctures may result from wearing more than one earring. Whatever its etiology, this deformity can only be corrected surgically. The edges of the perforation(s) are excised on the lateral and medial surfaces of the earlobe. Next the entire tract is removed, joining the above two incisions and resulting in a much larger defect that is closed separately on each surface. Then, an antibiotic dressing is applied.

CONDITIONS OF THE MIDDLE EAR

Tympanic Membrane Perforation

Perforation of the tympanic membrane is usually caused by infection or trauma. Sources of trauma include skull fracture, explosive injury, or a severe blow to the ear. Less frequently, perforation is caused by foreign objects (eg, cotton-tipped applicators, bobby pins, keys) that have been pushed too far into the external auditory canal. In addition to tympanic membrane perforation, injury to the ossicles and even the inner ear may result from this type of action. Thus, attempts by patients to clear the external auditory canal should be discouraged. During infection, the tympanic membrane can rupture if the pressure in the middle ear exceeds the atmospheric pressure in the external auditory canal.

Medical Management

Although most tympanic membrane perforations heal spontaneously within weeks after rupture, some may take several months to heal. Some perforations persist because scar tissue grows over the edges of the perforation, thus preventing extension of the epithelial cells across the margins and final healing. In the case of a head injury or temporal bone fracture, a patient is observed for evidence of cerebrospinal fluid **otorrhea** or **rhinorrhea**—a clear, watery drainage from the ear or nose, respectively. While healing, the ear must be protected from water.

SURGICAL MANAGEMENT

Perforations that do not heal on their own may require surgery. The decision to perform a **tympanoplasty** (repair of the tympanic membrane) is usually based on the need to prevent potential infection from water entering the ear or the desire to improve the patient's hearing. Performed on an outpatient basis, tympanoplasty may involve a variety of surgical techniques. In all techniques, tissue is placed across the perforation to allow healing. Surgery is usually successful in closing the perforation permanently and improving hearing.

Acute Otitis Media

Acute otitis media is an acute infection of the middle ear, usually lasting less than 6 weeks. The primary cause of acute otitis media is usually *Streptococcus pneumoniae*, *Haemophilus influenzae*, and *Moraxella catarrhalis*, which enter the middle ear after eustachian tube dysfunction caused by obstruction related to upper respiratory infections, inflammation of surrounding structures (eg, sinusitis, adenoid hypertrophy), or allergic reactions (eg, allergic rhinitis). Bacteria can enter the eustachian tube from contaminated secretions in the nasopharynx and the middle ear from a tympanic membrane perforation. A purulent exudate is usually present in the middle ear, resulting in a conductive hearing loss.

Clinical Manifestations

The symptoms of otitis media vary with the severity of the infection. The condition, usually unilateral in adults, may be accompanied by otalgia. The pain is relieved after spontaneous perforation or therapeutic incision of the tympanic membrane. Other symptoms may include drainage from the ear, fever, and hearing loss. On otoscopic examination, the external auditory canal appears normal. The patient reports no pain with movement of the auricle. The tympanic membrane is erythematous and often bulging. Table 55-2 differentiates acute external otitis from acute otitis media.

Medical Management

The outcome of acute otitis media depends on the efficacy of therapy (ie, the prescribed dose of an oral antibiotic and the duration of therapy), the virulence of the bacteria, and the physical status of the patient. With early and appropriate broad-spectrum antibiotic therapy, otitis media may clear up with no serious sequelae. If drainage occurs, an antibiotic otic preparation is usually prescribed. The condition may become subacute (ie, lasting 3 weeks to 3 months), with persistent purulent discharge from the ear. Rarely does permanent hearing loss occur. Secondary complications involving the mastoid and other serious intracranial complications, such as meningitis or brain abscess, although rare, can occur.

SURGICAL MANAGEMENT

An incision in the tympanic membrane is known as **myringotomy** or tympanotomy. The tympanic membrane is numbed with a local anesthetic such as phenol or by iontophoresis (an electrical current flows through a lidocaine-and-epinephrine solution to numb the ear canal and tympanic membrane). The procedure is painless and takes less than 15 minutes. Under microscopic guidance, an incision is made through the tympanic membrane to relieve pressure and to drain serous or purulent fluid from the middle ear.

Normally, this procedure is unnecessary for treating acute otitis media, but it may be performed if pain persists. Myringotomy also allows the drainage to be analyzed (by culture and sensitivity testing) so that the infecting organism can be identified and appropriate antibiotic therapy prescribed. The incision heals within 24 to 72 hours.

If episodes of acute otitis media recur and there is no contraindication, a ventilating, or pressure-equalizing, tube may be inserted. The ventilating tube, which temporarily takes the place of the eustachian tube in equalizing pressure, is retained for 6 to 18 months. The ventilating tube is then extruded with normal skin migration of the tympanic membrane, with the hole healing in nearly every case. Ventilating tubes are more commonly used to treat recurrent episodes of acute otitis media in children than in adults.

Serous Otitis Media

Serous otitis media (**middle ear effusion**) implies fluid, without evidence of active infection, in the middle ear. In theory, this fluid results from a negative pressure in the middle ear caused by eustachian tube obstruction. This condition is found primarily in children. When it occurs in adults, an underlying cause for the eustachian tube dysfunction must be sought. A middle ear effusion is frequently seen in patients after radiation therapy or barotrauma and in patients with eustachian tube dysfunction from a concurrent upper respiratory infection or allergy. Barotrauma results from sudden pressure changes in the middle ear due to changes in barometric pressure, as in scuba diving or airplane descent. A carcinoma (eg, nasopharyngeal cancer) obstructing the eustachian tube should be ruled out in an adult with persistent unilateral serous otitis media.

Clinical Manifestations

Patients may complain of hearing loss, fullness in the ear or a sensation of congestion, and perhaps even popping and crackling noises, which occur as the eustachian tube attempts to open. The tympanic membrane appears dull on otoscopy, and air bubbles may be visualized in the middle ear. Usually, the audiogram shows a conductive hearing loss.

Management

Serous otitis media need not be treated medically unless infection occurs (acute otitis media). If the hearing loss associated with middle ear effusion is a problem for the patient, a myringotomy can be performed and a tube may be placed to keep the middle ear ventilated. Corticosteroids, in small doses, sometimes decrease the edema of the eustachian tube in cases of barotrauma. Decongestants have not proved effective. Performing the Valsalva maneuver, which forcibly opens the eustachian tube by increasing nasopharyngeal pressure, should be encouraged.

Chronic Otitis Media

Chronic otitis media is the result of repeated episodes of acute otitis media causing irreversible tissue pathology and persistent perforation of the tympanic membrane. Chronic infections of

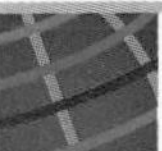

TABLE 55•2 **Clinical Features of Otitis**

Feature	Acute External Otitis	Acute Otitis Media
Otorrhea	May or may not be present	Present if tympanic membrane perforates; discharge is profuse
Otalgia	Persistent, may awaken patient at night	Relieved if tympanic membrane ruptures
Aural tenderness	Present on palpation of auricle	Usually absent
Systemic symptoms	Absent	Fever, upper respiratory infection, rhinitis
Edema of external auditory canal	Present	Absent
Tympanic membrane	May appear normal	Erythema, bulging, may be perforated
Hearing loss	Conductive type	Conductive type

the middle ear not only cause damage to the tympanic membrane but can also destroy the ossicles and involve the mastoid. Before the discovery of antibiotics, infections of the mastoid were life-threatening. Now, the use of medications in acute otitis media has made acute mastoiditis a rare condition.

Clinical Manifestations

Symptoms may be minimal, with varying degrees of hearing loss and the presence of a persistent or intermittent foul-smelling otorrhea. Pain is not usually present except in cases of acute mastoiditis, when the postauricular area is tender to the touch and even erythematous and edematous. Otoscopic evaluation of the tympanic membrane may reveal a perforation, and cholesteatoma can be present as a white mass behind the tympanic membrane or coming through to the external canal from a perforation. **Cholesteatoma** is an ingrowth of the skin of the external layer of the eardrum into the middle ear. The skin forms a sac that fills with degenerated skin and sebaceous materials. The sac can be attached to the structures of the middle ear and/or mastoid. Cholesteatoma, by itself, usually does not cause pain. In cases of chronic otitis media or cholesteatoma, audiometric tests often show a conductive or mixed hearing loss.

Medical Management

Local treatment consists of careful suctioning of the ear under microscopic guidance. Instillation of antibiotic drops or application of antibiotic powder is used to treat a purulent discharge. Systemic antibiotics are usually not prescribed except in cases of acute infection.

SURGICAL MANAGEMENT

Various surgical procedures are used after medical treatments are determined to be ineffective. These include tympanoplasty, ossiculoplasty, and mastoidectomy. Chronic otitis media can cause chronic mastoiditis and lead to the formation of cholesteatoma. It can occur in the middle ear, mastoid cavity, or both, often dictating the type of surgery to be performed. If untreated, cholesteatoma will continue to enlarge, possibly causing damage to the facial nerve and horizontal canal and destruction of other surrounding structures.

Tympanoplasty. The most common surgical procedure for chronic otitis media is a tympanoplasty—surgical reconstruction of the tympanic membrane. Reconstruction of the ossicles may also be required. The purposes of a tympanoplasty are to reestablish middle ear function, close the perforation, prevent recurrent infection, and improve hearing.

There are five types of tympanoplasties. The simplest surgical procedure, type I (myringoplasty), is designed to close a perforation in the tympanic membrane. The other procedures, types II through V, involve more extensive repair of middle ear structures. The structures and the degree of involvement can differ, but all tympanoplasty procedures include restoring the continuity of the sound conduction mechanism.

Tympanoplasty is performed through the external auditory canal, either transcanal or through a postauricular incision. The contents of the middle ear are carefully inspected, and the ossicular chain is evaluated. Ossicular interruption is most frequent in chronic otitis media, but problems of reconstruction can also occur with malformations of the middle ear and ossicular dislocations due to head injuries. Dramatic improvement in hearing can result from closure of a perforation and reestablishment of the ossicles. Surgery is usually performed in an outpatient environment under conscious sedation or general anesthesia.

Ossiculoplasty. Many people use the term tympanoplasty to include **ossiculoplasty**—surgical reconstruction of the middle ear bones to restore hearing. Prostheses, made of materials such as Teflon, stainless steel, and hydroxyapatite, are used to reconnect the ossicles, thereby reestablishing the sound conduction mechanism. However, the greater the damage, the lower the success rate for restoring normal hearing.

Mastoidectomy. The objectives of mastoid surgery are to remove the cholesteatoma, gain access to diseased structures, and create a dry and healthy ear. If possible, the ossicles are reconstructed during the initial surgical procedure. However, on occasion, the extent of the disease dictates that this be performed as part of a planned second-stage operation.

A mastoidectomy is usually performed through a postauricular incision. Infection is eliminated by removing the mastoid air cells. Although infrequently injured, the facial nerve, which runs through the middle ear and mastoid, is at some risk for injury during mastoid surgery. As the patient awakens from anesthesia, any evidence of facial paresis should be reported to the physician. A second mastoidectomy may be necessary to check for recurrent or residual cholesteatoma. The hearing mechanism may be reconstructed at this time. The success rate for correcting this conductive hearing loss is approximately 75%. Surgery is usually performed in an outpatient setting. The patient will have a mastoid pressure dressing, which can be removed 24 to 48 hours after surgery.

NURSING PROCESS: THE PATIENT UNDERGOING MASTOID SURGERY

Although several otologic surgical procedures are performed under conscious sedation, mastoid surgery is performed using general anesthesia.

Assessment

The health history includes a complete description of the ear problem, including infection, otalgia, otorrhea, hearing loss, and vertigo. Data are collected about the duration and intensity of the problem, its causes, and previous treatments. Information is obtained about other health problems and all medications that the patient is taking. In addition, medication allergies and family history of ear disease should be obtained.

Physical assessment includes observation for erythema, edema, otorrhea, lesions, and characteristics, such as odor and color of discharge. The results of the audiogram should be reviewed.

Nursing Diagnosis

Based on the assessment data, the patient's major nursing diagnoses may include the following:

- Anxiety related to surgical procedure, potential loss of hearing, potential taste disturbance, and potential loss of facial movement
- Pain related to mastoid surgery
- Risk for infection related to mastoidectomy, placement of grafts, prostheses, and electrodes, and surgical trauma to surrounding tissues and structures

- Auditory sensory perception alterations related to ear disorder, surgery, or packing
- Risk for trauma related to balance difficulties or vertigo during the immediate postoperative period
- Sensory/perceptual alterations related to potential damage to facial nerve (cranial nerve VII) and chorda tympani nerve
- Impaired skin integrity related to ear surgery, incisions, and graft sites
- Knowledge deficit about mastoid disease, surgical procedure, and postoperative care and expectations

Planning and Goals

The major goals of caring for a patient undergoing mastoidectomy include reduction of anxiety; freedom from pain and discomfort; prevention of infection; stable or improved hearing and communication; absence of injury from vertigo; absence of, or adjustment to, sensory/perceptual alterations; return of skin integrity; and increased knowledge regarding the disease, surgical procedure, and postoperative care.

Nursing Interventions

Reducing Anxiety

Information that the otologic surgeon has discussed with the patient, including anesthesia, the location of the incision (postauricular), and expected surgical results (hearing, balance, taste, facial movement), is reinforced. The patient also is encouraged to discuss any anxieties and concerns about the surgery.

Relieving Pain

Although most patients complain very little about incisional pain after mastoid surgery, they do have some ear discomfort. Aural fullness or pressure after surgery is due to residual blood or fluid in the middle ear. The prescribed analgesic may be taken for the first 24 hours after surgery and then only as needed. The patient is instructed in the use of and side effects of the medication.

A tympanoplasty may also be performed at the time of the mastoidectomy. A wick or external auditory canal packing is used after a tympanoplasty to stabilize the tympanic membrane. Patients should be informed that they may experience intermittent sharp, shooting pains in the ear for 2 to 3 weeks after surgery as the eustachian tube opens and allows air to enter the middle ear.

Preventing Infection

Measures are initiated to prevent infection in the operated ear. The external auditory canal wick, or packing, may be impregnated with an antibiotic solution before instillation. Prophylactic antibiotics are given as prescribed, and the patient is instructed to prevent water from entering the external auditory canal for 6 weeks. A cotton ball or lamb's wool covered with a water-insoluble substance (petroleum jelly) and placed in the ear will usually prevent water contamination. The postauricular incision should be kept dry for 2 days. Signs of infection such as an elevated temperature and purulent drainage are reported. Some serosanguineous drainage from the external auditory canal is normal after surgery.

Improving Hearing and Communication

Hearing in the operated ear may be reduced for several weeks because of edema, accumulation of blood and tissue fluid in the middle ear, and dressings or packing. Measures to improve hearing and communication, such as reducing environmental noise, facing the patient when speaking, speaking clearly and distinctly without shouting, providing good lighting if the patient relies on speech reading, and using nonverbal clues (eg, facial expression, pointing, gestures) and other forms of communication are initiated. Family members or significant others are instructed about effective ways to communicate with the patient. If the patient uses hearing-assistive devices, one can be used in the unaffected ear.

Preventing Injury

Vertigo may occur after mastoid surgery if the semicircular canals or other areas of the inner ear are traumatized. This symptom is relatively uncommon after this type of ear surgery and usually is temporary. Antiemetics or antivertiginous medications (eg, antihistamines) can be prescribed should a balance disturbance or vertigo occur. The patient should be instructed about the expected effects and potential side effects. Safety measures such as assisted ambulation are implemented to prevent falls.

Preventing Altered Sensory Perception

Facial nerve injury is a potential, although rare, complication of mastoid surgery. The patient is instructed to report immediately any evidence of facial nerve (cranial nerve VII) weakness, such as drooping of the mouth on the operated side. A more frequent occurrence is a temporary disturbance in the chorda tympani nerve, a small branch of the facial nerve that runs through the middle ear. Patients will experience a taste disturbance and dry mouth on the side of surgery for several months until the nerve regenerates.

Promoting Wound Healing

The patient is instructed to avoid heavy lifting, straining, exertion, and nose blowing for 2 to 3 weeks after surgery to prevent dislodging the tympanic membrane graft or ossicular prosthesis.

Increasing Knowledge

The patient is informed about the surgery and operating room environment. Discussing postoperative expectations helps to decrease anxiety about the unknown. Postoperative instructions for mastoid surgery vary among otologic surgeons. Therefore, it is important for the nurse to be aware of the surgeon's preferences when teaching the patient.

Promoting Home and Community-Based Care

TEACHING PATIENTS SELF-CARE

Patients require instruction about prescribed medication therapy, such as analgesics, antivertiginous agents, and antihistamines prescribed for balance disturbance. Teaching includes information about the expected effects and potential side effects of the medication. Patients also need instruction about any activity restrictions. Possible complications such as infection, facial nerve weakness, or taste disturbances, including the signs and symptoms to report immediately, should be addressed.

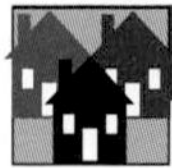

PATIENT EDUCATION AND HOME CARE

Self-Care After Middle Ear or Mastoid Surgery

Postoperative instructions for middle ear and mastoid surgery vary greatly among otolaryngologists. These patient teaching guidelines may require modification for the individual patient.

1. Take antibiotics and other medications as prescribed.
2. Blow nose gently one side at a time for 1 week after surgery.
3. Sneeze and cough with the mouth open for a few weeks after surgery.
4. Check with your health care provider about returning to work (usually 2 to 3 days postoperatively.) Avoid heavy (greater than 25 pounds) lifting, straining, and bending over for a few weeks after surgery.
5. Know that popping and crackling in the operative ear is normal for approximately 3 to 5 weeks after surgery.
6. Be aware that packing in the operated ear, as well as blood and fluid in the middle ear after surgery, will cause a hearing loss. You may also feel that you are talking in a well or hearing echoes.
7. Remember that minor ear discomfort is normal; use the analgesics prescribed. Report any excessive ear pain to the surgeon.
8. Note that some slightly bloody or serosanguineous drainage from the ear is normal after surgery. Report any excessive or purulent ear drainage to the surgeon.
9. Change the cotton ball in the ear as needed.
10. Check with the surgeon for instructions regarding air travel.
11. Avoid getting water in the operated ear for 2 weeks after surgery. You may shampoo the hair 2 to 3 days postoperatively if the ear is protected from water by saturating a cotton ball with petroleum jelly (or some other water-insoluble substance) and placing it in the ear. If the postauricular suture line becomes wet, pat (not rub) the area and cover it with a thin layer of antibiotic ointment.

CONTINUING CARE

Some patients, particularly elderly patients, who have had mastoid surgery may require the services of a home care nurse for a few days after returning home. However, most people find that assistance from a family member or a friend is sufficient. The caregiver and patient are cautioned that the patient may experience some vertigo and will therefore require help with ambulation to avoid falling. Any symptoms of complications are to be reported promptly to the surgeon. The importance of scheduling and keeping follow-up appointments is also stressed.

Evaluation

Expected Outcomes

Expected outcomes may include:

1. Demonstrates reduced anxiety about surgical procedure
   a. Verbalizes and exhibits less stress, tension, and irritability
   b. Verbalizes acceptance of the results of surgery and adjustment to possible hearing impairment
2. Remains free of discomfort or pain
   a. Exhibits no facial grimacing, moaning, or crying, and reports absence of pain
   b. Uses analgesics appropriately
3. Demonstrates no signs or symptoms of infection
   a. Has normal vital signs, including temperature
   b. Demonstrates absence of purulent drainage from the external auditory canal
   c. Describes method for barring water from contaminating packing
4. Exhibits signs that hearing has stabilized or improved
   a. Describes surgical goal for hearing and judges whether the goal has been met
   b. Verbalizes that sounds not heard before surgery are heard now
5. Remains free of injury and trauma secondary to vertigo
   a. Reports absence of vertigo or balance disturbance
   b. Experiences no injury or fall
   c. Modifies environment to avoid falls (eg, night light, no clutter on stairs)
6. Adjusts to or remains free from altered sensory perception
   a. Reports no taste disturbance, mouth dryness, or facial weakness
7. Demonstrates no skin breakdown
   a. Lists ways to prevent dislodging graft or prosthesis
   b. Is aware of limitations in activities and for how long (bathing, lifting, air travel)
8. Verbalizes the reasons for and methods of care and treatment
   a. Shares knowledge with family about treatment protocol
   b. Describes treatment and the time frame for the recovery phase
   c. Discusses the discharge plan formulated with the nurse with regard to rest periods, medication, and activities permitted and restricted
   d. Lists symptoms that should be reported to health care personnel
   e. Keeps follow-up appointments

Otosclerosis

Otosclerosis involves the stapes and is thought to result from the formation of new, abnormal spongy bone, especially around the oval window, with resulting fixation of the stapes. The efficient transmission of sound is prevented because the stapes cannot vibrate and carry the sound as conducted from the malleus and incus to the inner ear. More common in females and frequently hereditary, otosclerosis may be worsened by pregnancy.

Clinical Manifestations

The condition can involve one or both ears and presents as a progressive conductive or mixed hearing loss. The patient may or may not complain of tinnitus. Otoscopic examination usually reveals a normal tympanic membrane. Bone conduction is better than air conduction on Rinne testing. The audiogram confirms a conductive hearing loss or a mixed loss, especially in the low frequencies.

Medical Management

There is no known nonsurgical treatment for otosclerosis. However, some physicians believe the use of Fluorical (a fluoride supplement) can mature the abnormal spongy bone growth. Amplification with a hearing aid also may help.

SURGICAL MANAGEMENT

A stapedectomy, performed through the canal, involves removing the stapes superstructure and part of the footplate and inserting a tissue graft and a suitable prosthesis (Fig. 55-8). Some surgeons elect to remove only a small part of the stapes footplate (stapedotomy).

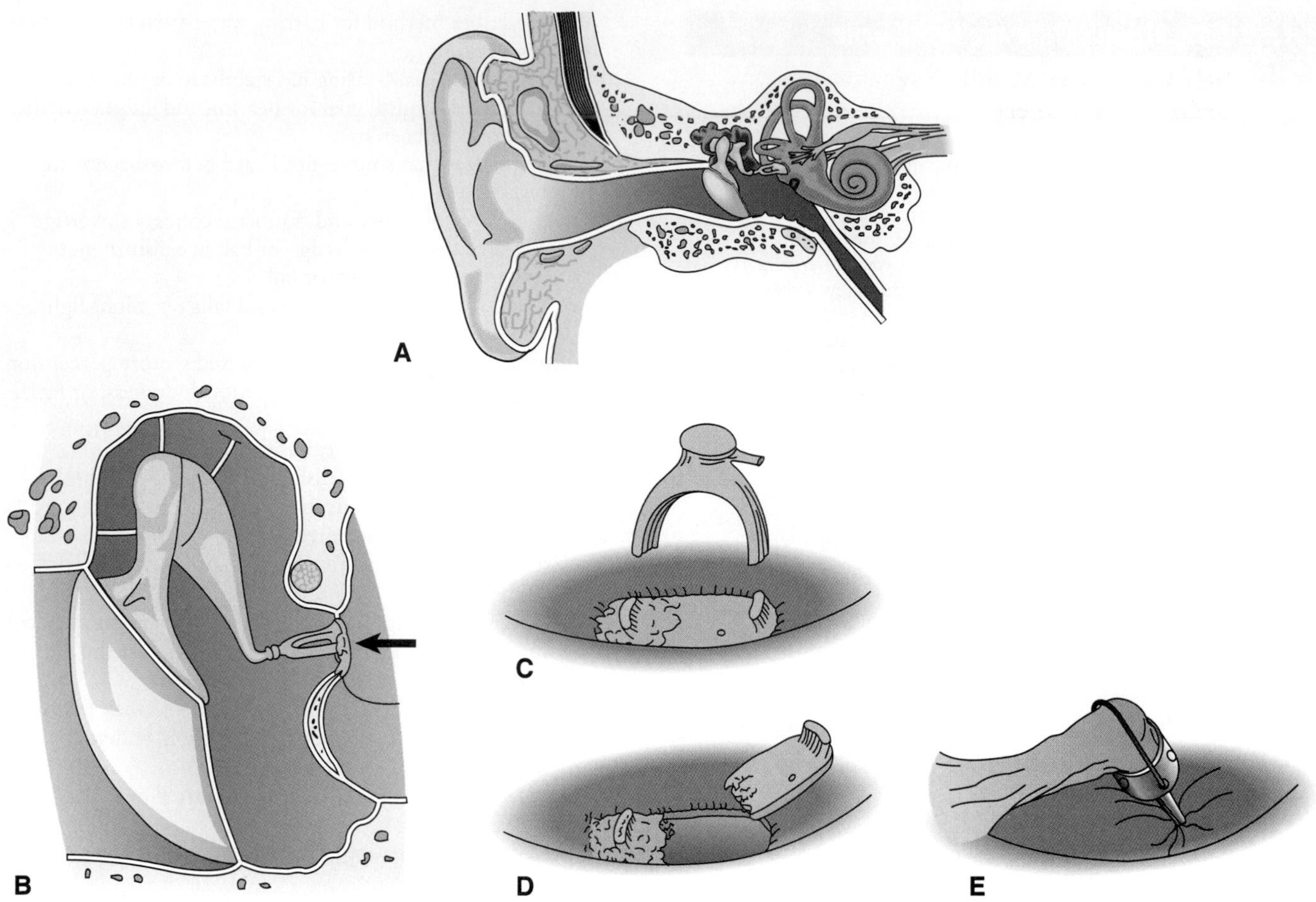

FIGURE 55•8 Stapedectomy for otosclerosis. (**A**) Normal anatomy. (**B**) Arrow points to sclerotic process at the foot of the stapes. (**C**) Stapes broken away surgically from its diseased base. The hole in the footplate provides an area where an instrument can grasp the plate. (**D**) The footplate is removed from its base. Some otosclerotic tissue may remain, and tissue is placed over it. (**E**) Robinson stainless-steel prosthesis in position.

Regardless of the method used, the prosthesis bridges the gap between the incus and the inner ear, providing better sound conduction. Stapes surgery is very successful in improving hearing. Balance disturbance or true vertigo, which rarely occurs in other middle ear surgical procedures, can occur for a short time after stapedectomy.

Middle Ear Masses

Other than cholesteatoma, masses in the middle ear are rare. Glomus jugulare is a tumor that arises from the jugular bulb. A histologically identical tumor that arises from Jacobson's nerve and remains limited to the middle ear is known as a glomus tympanicum. On otoscopy, a red blemish on or behind the tympanic membrane is indicative of a glomus tumor. The treatment for glomus tumors is surgical excision, except in poor surgical candidates, in whom radiation therapy is used.

A facial nerve neuroma is a tumor on cranial nerve VII, the facial nerve. These types of tumors are usually not visible on otoscopic examination but are suspected when a patient presents with a facial nerve paresis. X-ray evaluation is necessary to determine the site of the tumor along the facial nerve. The treatment is surgical removal.

Other less common problems of the middle ear include cholesterin granuloma and tympanosclerosis. Cholesterin granuloma is an immune system reaction to the byproducts of blood (cholesterol crystals) within the middle ear. Tympanosclerosis is a deposit of collagen and minerals within the middle ear that can harden around the ossicles as a result of repeated infection. It can also be found as plaque on the tympanic membrane; this can decrease hearing.

CONDITIONS OF THE INNER EAR

Disorders of balance and the vestibular system involving the inner ear afflict more than 30 million Americans aged 17 or older. Falls secondary to these disorders account for more than 100,000 hip fractures in elderly people each year (NIDCD, 1998).

The term **dizziness** is used frequently by patients and health care providers to describe any altered sensation of orientation in space. **Vertigo** is defined as the misperception or illusion of motion, either of the person or the surroundings. Most people with vertigo describe a spinning sensation or say they feel as though objects are moving around them. Ataxia is the failure of muscular coordination and may be present in patients with vestibular disease. Syncope, fainting, and loss of consciousness are not forms of vertigo, nor are they characteristic of an ear problem; they usually indicate disease in the cardiovascular system.

Nystagmus is an involuntary rhythmic movement of the eyes. Nystagmus occurs normally when a person watches a rapidly moving object (eg, through the side window of a moving car or train). However, pathologically it is an ocular disorder associated with vestibular dysfunction. Nystagmus can be horizontal, vertical, or rotary and can be caused by a disorder in the central or peripheral nervous system.

Motion Sickness

Motion sickness is a disturbance of equilibrium caused by constant motion. For example, it can occur aboard a ship or while riding on a merry-go-round or swing, or even in the back seat of a car.

Clinical Manifestations

The syndrome manifests itself in sweating, pallor, nausea, and vomiting caused by vestibular overstimulation. These manifestations may persist for several hours after the stimulation stops.

Management

Over-the-counter antihistamines used to treat vertigo, such as Dramamine or Bonine, provide some relief. Anticholinergic medications, such as scopolamine patches, may be helpful. These must be replaced every few days. Side effects such as dry mouth and drowsiness occur with these medications, which may prove to be more troublesome than helpful. Potentially hazardous activities such as driving a car or operating heavy machinery should be avoided if the patient experiences drowsiness.

Ménière's Disease

In 1861, a French physician, Prosper Ménière, first described a triad of symptoms involving episodic incapacitating vertigo, tinnitus, and fluctuating sensorineural hearing loss as an ear disease (**Ménière's disease**) and not a central, or brain, disease. Although the etiology of Ménière's disease is unknown, many theories exist, including abnormal hormonal and neurochemical influences on the blood flow to the labyrinth, electrolyte disturbance within labyrinthine fluids, allergic reaction, and autoimmune disorders. Some attribute the impairment of the microvasculature of the inner ear to abnormally high levels of metabolites (glucose, insulin, triglycerides, and cholesterol) in the blood. Ménière's disease is to the ear as glaucoma is to the eye—that is, too much circulating fluid.

Currently, Ménière's disease is thought to represent an abnormal inner ear fluid balance caused by a malabsorption in the endolymphatic sac. However, evidence indicates that many people with Ménière's disease may have a blockage in the endolymphatic duct. Regardless of the cause, **endolymphatic hydrops**, a dilation in the endolymphatic space, develops. Either increased pressure in the system or rupture of the inner ear membranes occurs, producing symptoms of Ménière's disease.

Ménière's disease affects more than 2.4 million people in the United States. More common in adults, it has an average age of onset in the 40s, with symptoms usually beginning between the ages of 20 and 60. However, the disease has been reported in children as young as age 4 and in adults of all ages, up to the 90s. Ménière's disease appears to be equally common in both genders. The right and left ears are affected with equal frequency; the disease occurs bilaterally in about 20% of patients. About 20% of the patients have a positive family history for the disease.

Clinical Manifestations

Ménière's disease involves the following symptoms: fluctuating, progressive sensorineural hearing loss; **tinnitus** or a roaring sound; a feeling of pressure or fullness in the ear; and episodic, incapacitating vertigo, often accompanied by nausea and/or vomiting. The effects of these symptoms range from a minor nuisance to extreme disability, especially if the attacks of vertigo are severe. At the onset of the disease, perhaps only one or two of the symptoms are manifested.

Some clinicians believe that there are two subsets of the disease, known as atypical Ménière's disease: cochlear and vestibular. Cochlear Ménière's disease is recognized as a fluctuating, progressive sensorineural hearing loss associated with tinnitus and aural pressure in the absence of vestibular symptoms or findings. Vestibular Ménière's disease is characterized as the occurrence of episodic vertigo associated with aural pressure with no cochlear symptoms. In some patients, cochlear or vestibular Ménière's disease develops first. In most patients, however, eventually all of the symptoms develop.

Assessment and Diagnostic Findings

Vertigo is usually the most troublesome complaint. A careful history is taken to determine the frequency, duration, severity, and character of the vertigo attacks. Typically, the patient reports that vertigo lasts from minutes to hours, possibly accompanied by nausea and/or vomiting. In addition, patients complain of diaphoresis and a persistent feeling of imbalance or disequilibrium, which may last for days. They may also complain of attacks that awaken them at night. Between attacks, however, they usually feel well. The hearing loss may fluctuate, with tinnitus and aural pressure waxing and waning with changes in hearing. The tinnitus and feeling of aural pressure may occur only during or before attacks, or they may be constant.

Findings of the physical examination are usually normal, with the exception of the evaluation of cranial nerve VIII. Sounds from a tuning fork (Weber test) may lateralize to the ear opposite the hearing loss (the one affected with Ménière's disease). The diagnosis of Ménière's disease is based on the patient's history and results of the audiovestibular diagnostic procedures. Additional laboratory tests and x-rays may be performed to rule out other causes for symptoms (eg, syphilis, autoimmune disease, stroke, or acoustic neuroma). An audiogram typically reveals a sensorineural hearing loss in the affected ear. This can be in the form of a "Pike's Peak" pattern, which looks like a hill or mountain, or it may show a sensorineural loss in the low frequencies. As the disease progresses, the hearing loss increases. The electronystagmogram may be normal or may show reduced vestibular response. There is, however, no absolute diagnostic test.

Medical Management

Most patients with Ménière's disease can be successfully treated with diet and medication therapy. Many patients can control their symptoms by adhering to a low-sodium (2000 mg/day) diet. The amount of sodium is one of many factors that regulate the balance of fluid within the body. Sodium and fluid retention disrupts the delicate balance between endolymph and perilymph in the inner ear. Psychological evaluation may be indicated if the patient is anxious, uncertain, fearful, or depressed.

PHARMACOLOGIC THERAPY

Pharmacologic therapy for Ménière's disease consists of antihistamines such as meclizine (Antivert), which suppress the vestibular system. Tranquilizers such as diazepam (Valium) may be used in acute instances to help control vertigo. However, because of their addiction potential, these agents are not used on a long-term basis. Antiemetics such as promethazine (Phenergan) suppositories help control the nausea and vomiting and also the vertigo because of their antihistamine effect. Diuretic therapy (eg, hydrochlorothiazide) sometimes relieves symptoms by lowering the pressure in the endolymphatic system. Intake of foods containing potassium (eg, bananas, tomatoes, and oranges) is necessary if the patient takes a diuretic that causes potassium loss.

Vasodilators, such as nicotinic acid, papaverine hydrochloride (Pavabid), and methantheline bromide (Banthine), have no scientific basis for alleviating the symptoms, but they are often used in conjunction with other therapies.

SURGICAL MANAGEMENT

Although most patients respond well to conservative therapy, some continue to have disabling attacks of vertigo. If these attacks reduce their quality of life, patients may elect to undergo surgery for relief. However, hearing loss, tinnitus, and aural fullness may continue, because the surgical treatment of Ménière's disease is aimed at eliminating the attacks of vertigo.

Endolymphatic Sac Decompression. Endolymphatic sac decompression, or shunting, theoretically equalizes the pressure in the endolymphatic space. A shunt or drain is inserted in the endolymphatic sac via a postauricular incision. This procedure is favored by many otolaryngologists as a first-line surgical approach to treat the vertigo of Ménière's disease because it is relatively simple and safe and can be performed on an outpatient basis.

Middle and Inner Ear Perfusion. Ototoxic medications, such as streptomycin or gentamicin, can be given to patients by infusion into the middle and inner ear. These medications are used to decrease vestibular function and thus decrease vertigo. The success rate for eliminating vertigo is high, about 85%, but the risk of significant hearing loss is also high. This procedure of inner ear perfusion usually requires an overnight stay in the hospital. After the procedure, many patients have a period of imbalance that lasts several weeks.

Intraotologic Catheters. In an attempt to deliver medication directly to the inner ear, catheters are being developed to provide a conduit from the outer ear to the inner ear. The route of the catheter is from the external ear canal through or around the tympanic membrane, and to the round window niche or membrane. Thus, medicinal fluids can be placed against the round window for a direct route to the inner ear fluids.

Potential uses of these catheters include treatment for sudden hearing loss and various disorders causing intractable vertigo. Future applications may include tinnitus and slowly progressing sensorineural hearing loss. Intratympanic injections of ototoxic medications for round window membrane diffusion can be used to decrease vestibular function. Established surgical techniques can be used for the patient with vertigo who has not responded to medical or physical therapeutic modalities.

Labyrinthectomy. Labyrinthectomy procedures by transcanal and transmastoid approaches are also about 85% successful in eliminating vertigo. However, these procedures destroy the auditory function of the inner ear. Additional complications are associated with these procedures, and some otologists believe that if a patient is to be subjected to these risks (ie, facial nerve injury, cerebrospinal fluid leak, total hearing loss), a potentially more successful procedure such as a vestibular nerve section (sectioning cranial nerve VIII) should be performed.

Vestibular Nerve Section. Vestibular nerve section provides the greatest success rate (approximately 98%) in eliminating the attacks of vertigo. It can be performed by a translabyrinthine (through the hearing mechanism) approach or in a manner that will conserve hearing (suboccipital or middle cranial fossa), depending on the degree of hearing loss. Most patients with incapacitating Ménière's disease have little or no effective hearing anyway. Cutting the nerve actually prevents the brain from receiving input from the semicircular canals. This procedure requires a brief hospital stay. Nursing care for the patient with vertigo is presented in the Plan of Nursing Care 55-1.

Labyrinthitis

Labyrinthitis, an inflammation of the inner ear, can be bacterial or viral in origin. Although rare because of antibiotic therapy, bacterial labyrinthitis usually occurs as a complication of otitis media. The infection can enter the inner ear by penetrating the membranes of the oval or round windows. Viral labyrinthitis is a common medical diagnosis, but little is known about this disorder, which affects both hearing and balance. The most commonly identified viral causes are mumps, rubella, rubeola, and influenza. Viral illnesses of the upper respiratory tract as well as herpetiform disorders of the facial and acoustic nerves (Ramsay Hunt syndrome) also cause labyrinthitis.

Clinical Manifestations

Labyrinthitis is characterized by a sudden onset of incapacitating vertigo, usually with nausea and vomiting, varying degrees of hearing loss, and possibly tinnitus. The first episode is usually the worst; subsequent attacks, which usually occur over a period of several weeks to months, are less severe.

Management

Treatment for bacterial labyrinthitis includes intravenous antibiotic therapy, fluid replacement, and administration of a vestibular suppressant, such as meclizine (Antivert), and antiemetic medications. Treatment for viral labyrinthitis is according to the patient's symptoms.

Vestibular Neuronitis

Vestibular neuronitis is a disorder of the vestibular nerve characterized by severe vertigo with normal hearing. It can be caused by viruses, vascular and demyelinating diseases, and toxins. Many patients have had a previous ear, nose, or throat infection.

The onset is sudden with severe vertigo, often with nausea and vomiting, with no loss of hearing or tinnitus. The first attack is usually the worst, with subsequent attacks of less intensity. Recovery usually occurs without treatment over a period of several weeks to a month. A less common chronic form can persist for months to years.

Benign Paroxysmal Positional Vertigo

Benign paroxysmal positional vertigo is a brief period of incapacitating vertigo that occurs when the position of the patient's head is changed with respect to gravity (typically by placing the

(text continues on page 1599)

55•1

PLAN OF NURSING CARE

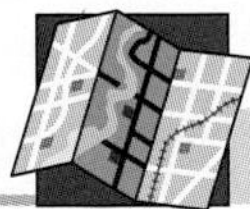

Care of the Patient with Vertigo

Nursing Interventions	Rationale	Expected Outcomes
Nursing Diagnosis: Risk for injury related to altered mobility because of gait disturbance and vertigo **Goal:** Remains free of any injuries associated with imbalance and/or falls		
1. Assess for vertigo, including history, onset, description of attacks, duration, frequency, and any associated ear symptoms (hearing loss, tinnitus, aural fullness). 2. Assess extent of disability in relation to living. 3. Teach or reinforce vestibular/balance therapy as prescribed. 4. Administer, or teach administration of, antivertiginous medications and/or vestibular sedation medication; instruct patient about side effects. 5. Encourage patient to sit down when dizzy. 6. Place pillow on each side of head to restrict movement. 7. Assist patient in identifying aura that suggests an impending attack. 8. Recommend that the patient keep eyes open and stare straight ahead when lying down and experiencing vertigo.	1. History provides basis for interventions. 2. Extent of disability indicates risk of falling. 3. Exercises hasten labyrinthine compensation, which may decrease vertigo and gait disturbance. 4. Alleviates acute symptoms of vertigo 5. Decreases possibility of falling and injury 6. Movement aggravates vertigo. 7. Recognition of aura may trigger the need to take medication before an attack occurs, thereby minimizing the severity of effects. 8. Sensation of vertigo decreases and motion decelerates if eyes are kept in a fixed position.	• Experiences no falls due to balance disturbance • Fear and anxiety are reduced • Performs exercises as prescribed • Takes prescribed medications appropriately • Assumes safe position when dizzy • Keeps head still when dizzy • Identifies a characteristic fullness or sense of pressure in the ear as occurring before a full-blown attack • Reports measures that help reduce vertigo
Nursing Diagnosis: Impaired adjustment related to disability requiring change in lifestyle due to unpredictability of vertigo **Goal:** Modifies lifestyle to decrease disability and exert maximum control and independence within limits posed by chronic vertigo		
1. Encourage patient to identify personal strengths and roles that can still be fulfilled. 2. Provide information about vertigo and what to expect. 3. Include family and significant others in rehabilitative process. 4. Encourage patient to maintain sense of control by making decisions and assuming more responsibility for care.	1. Maximizes sense of regaining control and independence 2. Reduces fear and anxiety 3. Perceived beliefs of significant others are important for patient's adherence to medical regimen. 4. Reinforces positive psychological and social outcomes	• Exerts maximum control of environment and independence within limits imposed by vertigo • Is informed about condition • Family and significant others are included in rehabilitation process • Uses strengths and potentials to engage in the most independent and constructive lifestyle
Nursing Diagnosis: Risk for fluid volume imbalance related to increased fluid output, altered intake, and medications **Goal:** Maintains a normal fluid–electrolyte balance		
1. Assess, or have patient assess, intake and output (including emesis, liquid stools, urine, and diaphoresis). Monitor laboratory values. 2. Assess indicators of dehydration, including blood pressure (orthostasis), pulse, skin turgor, mucous membranes, and level of consciousness. 3. Encourage oral fluids as tolerated; discourage beverages containing caffeine (a vestibular stimulant). 4. Administer, or teach administration of, antiemetics and antidiarrheal medication as prescribed and needed. Instruct patient in side effects.	1. Accurate records provide basis for fluid replacement. 2. Prompt recognition of dehydration allows early intervention. 3. Oral replacement is begun as soon as possible to replace losses. Caffeine may increase diarrhea. 4. Antiemetics reduce nausea and vomiting, reducing fluid losses and improving oral intake. Antidiarrheal medication reduces intestinal motility and fluid losses.	• Laboratory values within normal limits • Alert and oriented; vital signs within normal limits, skin turgor normal; electrolytes normal • Mucous membranes are moist • Vomiting or diarrhea has stopped; usual oral intake resumed

(continued)

55•1 PLAN OF NURSING CARE

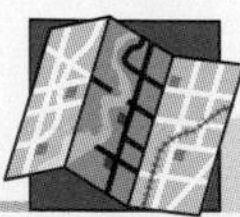

Care of the Patient with Vertigo (*continued*)

Nursing Interventions	Rationale	Expected Outcomes
Nursing Diagnosis: Anxiety related to threat of, or change in, health status and disability effects of vertigo **Goal:** Experiences less or no anxiety		
1. Assess level of anxiety. Help patient identify coping skills used successfully in the past.	1. Guides therapeutic interventions and participation in self-care. Past coping skills can relieve anxiety.	• Fear and anxiety about vertiginous attacks reduced or eliminated
2. Provide information about vertigo and its treatment.	2. Increased knowledge helps to decrease anxiety.	• Acquires knowledge and skills to deal with vertigo
3. Encourage patient to discuss anxieties and explore concerns about vertigo attacks.	3. Promotes awareness and understanding of relationship between anxiety level and behavior	• Feels less tension, apprehension, and uncertainty
4. Teach patient stress management techniques or make appropriate referral.	4. Improved stress management can reduce the frequency and severity of some vertiginous attacks.	• Uses stress management techniques when needed
5. Provide comfort measures and avoid stress-producing activities.	5. Stressful situations may exacerbate symptoms of the condition.	• Avoids upsetting encounters
6. Instruct patient in aspects of treatment regimen.	6. Patient knowledge helps to decrease anxiety.	• Repeats instructions given and verbalizes understanding of treatments
Nursing Diagnosis: Risk for trauma related to balancing difficulties **Goal:** Reduces the risk of trauma by adapting the home environment and by using rehabilitative devises as necessary		
1. Assess for balance disturbance and/or vertigo by taking history and by examination for nystagmus, positive Romberg, and inability to perform tandem Romberg.	1. Peripheral vestibular disorders cause these signs and symptoms.	• Has adapted home environment or uses rehabilitative devices to reduce risk of falling
2. Assist with ambulation when indicated.	2. Abnormal gait can predispose patient to unsteadiness and falls.	• Ambulates with needed assistance
3. Assess for visual acuity and proprioceptive deficits.	3. Balance depends on visual, vestibular, and proprioceptive systems.	• Visual and proprioceptive risks identified
4. Encourage increased activity level with or without use of assistive devices.	4. Increased activity may help retrain balance system.	• Activity level increased
5. Help identify hazards in home environment.	5. Adaptation of home environment can reduce risk of falls during rehabilitative process.	• Home environment free of hazards
Nursing Diagnosis: Ineffective individual coping related to personal vulnerability and unmet expectations stemming from vertigo **Goal:** Develops coping skills necessary to decrease vulnerability and unmet needs and demonstrates effective coping		
1. Assess cognitive appraisal of illness and factors that may be contributing inability to cope.	1. To improve patient's self-image and to enhance coping process	• Copes effectively with vertigo
2. Provide factual information about treatment and future health status.	2. To clarify any misinformation or confusion	• Has acquired knowledge and skills to cope with vertigo
3. Encourage and help patient participate in decision making about adjustments in lifestyle.	3. To help patient regain sense of power and control in self-care with activities of daily living	• Verbalizes less threatening appraisal of situation
4. Encourage patient to maintain diversional or recreational activities, exercise, and social events.	4. Social isolation and avoiding pleasant activities intensify isolation and reduce ability to cope with vertigo.	• Is involved in outside activities
5. Help patient identify personal strengths and develop coping strategies based on previous positive experiences in dealing with stress, and situational supports.	5. To enhance patient's strengths that help maintain hope	• Identifies specific strategies for coping
6. Refer patient to support groups or counseling as indicated.	6. May help patient feel less alone and isolated	• Uses support groups or counseling as appropriate

(*continued*)

55•1 PLAN OF NURSING CARE 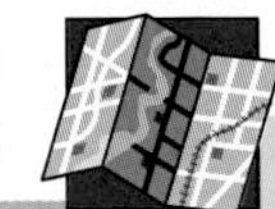 **Care of the Patient with Vertigo (*continued*)**

Nursing Interventions	Rationale	Expected Outcomes
Nursing Diagnosis: Diversional activity deficit related to environmental lack of such activity **Goal:** Engages in diversional activities		
1. Assess level and type of diversional activity to plan appropriate activities. 2. Discuss usual pattern of diversional activities with patient. Suggest opportunities to continue meaningful diversional activities.	1. Boredom may be exhibited as well as depression; helps determine tolerances as well as preferences. 2. To provide information about perceived and actual stressors that influence activity level; to support patient's sense of self-worth and productivity.	• Verbalizes decreased feelings of boredom and appears alert and animated • Seeks realistic opportunities for involvement in diversional activities.
Nursing Diagnosis: Self-care deficit: feeding, bathing/hygiene, dressing/grooming, toileting, related to labyrinth dysfunction and episodes of vertigo **Goal:** Able to care for self		
1. Administer, or teach administration of, antiemetics and other prescribed medications to relieve nausea and vomiting associated with vertigo. 2. Encourage patient to care for bodily needs when free of vertigo. 3. Review diet with patient and caregivers. Offer fluids as necessary.	1. Antiemetics and sedative-type medications depress stimuli in the cerebellum. 2. Spacing activities is important because episodes of vertigo vary in occurrence. 3. Sodium restriction helps improve an inner ear fluid imbalance in some patients, thereby decreasing vertigo. Fluids help prevent dehydration.	• Carries out necessary functions during symptom-free periods. Takes medications to relieve nausea or vomiting. • Carries out daily activities • Accepts dietary plan and reports its effectiveness. • Drinks fluids in sufficient amounts
Nursing Diagnosis: Powerlessness related to illness regimen and being helpless in certain situations due to vertigo/balance disturbance **Goal:** Experiences increased sense of control over life and activities despite vertigo/balance disturbance		
1. Assess patient's needs, values, attitudes, and readiness to initiate activities. 2. Provide opportunities for patient to express feelings (catharsis) about self and illness. 3. Help patient identify previous coping behaviors that were successful.	1. Involving patient in planning activities and care enhances potential for mastery. 2. Expressing feelings increases understanding of individual coping styles and defense mechanisms. 3. Awareness increases understanding of stressors that trigger feeling of powerlessness. Awareness of past successes enhances self-confidence.	• Does not restrict activities unnecessarily due to vertigo • Verbalizes positive feelings about own ability to achieve a sense of power and control • Identifies previous successful coping behaviors

head back with the affected ear turned down). The onset is sudden and followed by a predisposition for positional vertigo, usually for hours to weeks but occasionally for months or years. Severe cases cause vertigo induced by any head movement. The vertigo is accompanied by nausea and vomiting.

A common strategy is to withhold treatment to see whether the condition resolves. Antivertiginous medications usually do not prevent the paroxysmal attacks. Vestibular rehabilitation can be used in the management of vestibular disorders. This strategy promotes active use of the vestibular system through a multidisciplinary team approach including medical and nursing care, stress management, biofeedback, vocational rehabilitation, and physical therapy. A physical therapist prescribes balance exercises that help the brain compensate for the impairment to the balance system.

Ototoxicity

A variety of medications may have adverse effects on the cochlea, vestibular apparatus, or cranial nerve VIII. Only a few, such as aspirin and quinine, cause reversible hearing loss. At high doses, aspirin toxicity also can produce tinnitus. Intravenous medications, especially the aminoglycosides, are the most common cause of ototoxicity and actually destroy the hair cells in the organ of Corti.

To prevent loss of hearing or balance, patients receiving potentially ototoxic medications should be counseled about the side effects of these medications. Patients receiving long-term intravenous antibiotics should be monitored with an audiogram twice a week during therapy.

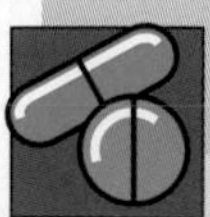

PHARMACOLOGY

Selected Ototoxic Substances

Diuretics
- ethacrynic acid
- furosemide
- acetazolamide

Chemotherapeutic Agents
- cisplatin
- nitrogen mustard

Antimalarials
- quinine
- chloroquine

Anti-inflammatory Agents
- salicylates (aspirin)
- indomethacin

Chemicals
- alcohol
- arsenic

Aminoglycoside Antibiotics
- amikacin
- gentamicin
- kanamycin
- netilmicin
- neomycin
- streptomycin
- tobramycin

Other Antibiotics
- erythromycin
- minocycline
- polymyxin B
- vancomycin

Metals
- gold
- mercury
- lead

Acoustic Neuroma

An acoustic neuroma is a slow-growing, benign tumor of cranial nerve VIII, usually arising from the Schwann cells of the vestibular portion of the nerve. Most acoustic tumors arise within the internal auditory canal and extend into the cerebellopontine angle to press on the brain stem. Acoustic neuromas account for 5% to 10% of all intracranial tumors and seem to occur with equal frequency in men and women at any age, although most occur during middle age. Most acoustic neuromas are unilateral, except in von Recklinghausen's disease (neurofibromatosis or NF-2), in which bilateral tumors occur.

Assessment and Diagnostic Findings

The most common presenting assessment findings in patients with an acoustic neuroma are unilateral tinnitus and hearing loss with or without vertigo or balance disturbance. It is important to note asymmetry in audiovestibular test results so that further workup can be performed to rule out an acoustic neuroma. Magnetic resonance imaging (MRI) with a paramagnetic contrast agent (gadolinium or Magnevist) is the imaging study of choice. If the patient is claustrophobic or cannot tolerate an MRI, or if the scan is unavailable, a computed tomography (CT) scan with contrast dye is performed. However, MRI is more sensitive in delineating a small tumor than is CT.

Management

Surgical removal of acoustic tumors is the treatment of choice because these tumors do not respond well to radiation or chemotherapy. Because treatment of acoustic tumors crosses several specialties, a multidisciplinary treatment approach involving both a neurotologist and a neurosurgeon is used. The objective of the surgery is to remove the tumor while preserving facial nerve function. Most acoustic tumors have damaged the cochlear portion of cranial nerve VIII so that no real serviceable hearing exists before surgery. In these patients, the surgery is performed using a translabyrinthine approach and the hearing mechanism is destroyed. If hearing is still good before surgery, a suboccipital or middle cranial fossa approach to removing the tumor may be used, and intraoperative monitoring of cranial nerve VIII will be performed to save the hearing.

Complications of surgery for acoustic neuroma include facial nerve paralysis, cerebrospinal fluid leak, meningitis, and cerebral edema. Death from acoustic neuroma surgery is very rare.

AURAL REHABILITATION

If hearing loss is permanent or cannot be treated by medical or surgical means, or if the patient elects not to have surgery, aural rehabilitation may be beneficial. The purpose of aural rehabilitation is to maximize the hearing-impaired person's communication skills. Aural rehabilitation includes auditory training, speech reading, speech training, and the use of hearing aids and hearing guide dogs.

Auditory training emphasizes listening skills, so the hearing-impaired person concentrates on the speaker. Speech reading (formerly known as lip reading) can help fill the gaps left by missed or misheard words. Speech training attempts to conserve, develop, and prevent deterioration of current skills.

It is important to identify the type of hearing impairment a person has so that rehabilitative efforts can be directed at his or her particular need. Surgical correction may be all that is necessary to treat and improve a conductive hearing loss (Fig. 55-9). With recent advances in hearing aid technology, amplification for patients with sensorineural hearing loss is more helpful than ever before.

Hearing Aids

A hearing aid is a device through which speech and environmental sounds are received by a microphone, converted to electrical signals, amplified, and reconverted to acoustic signals. Many aids available for sensorineural hearing loss depress the low frequencies, or tones, and enhance hearing for the high frequencies. A general guideline for assessing the patient's need for a hearing aid is a hearing loss exceeding 30 dB in the range of 500 to 2000 Hz in the better-hearing ear.

The evolution in technology has led to the availability of many smaller and more effective hearing aids. It is estimated that 98%

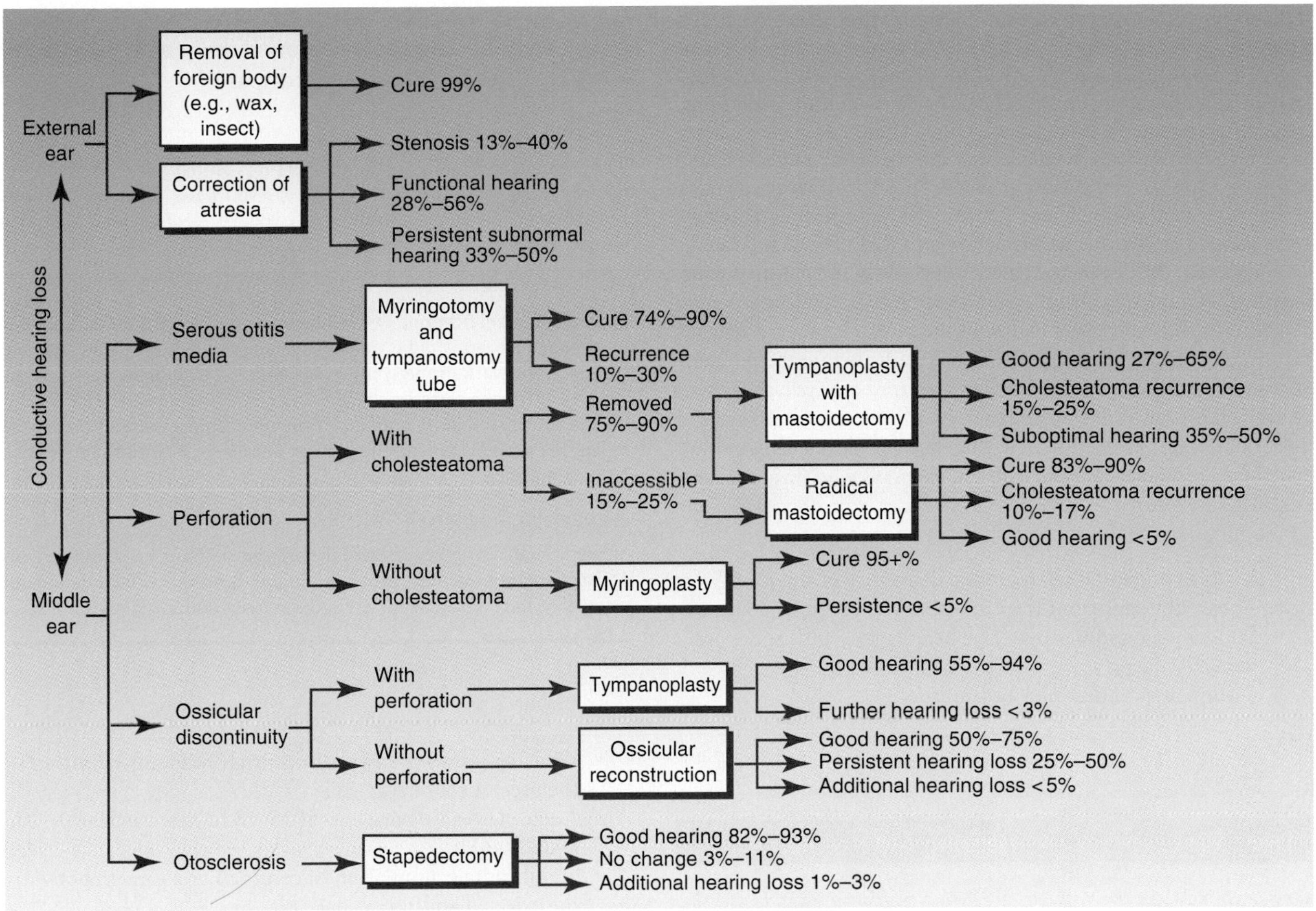

Conductive hearing loss
External ear
Removal of foreign body (e.g., wax, insect) → Cure 99%
Correction of atresia → Stenosis 13%–40%; Functional hearing 28%–56%; Persistent subnormal hearing 33%–50%
Middle ear
Serous otitis media → Myringotomy and tympanostomy tube → Cure 74%–90%; Recurrence 10%–30%
Perforation → With cholesteatoma → Removed 75%–90%; Inaccessible 15%–25%
Tympanoplasty with mastoidectomy → Good hearing 27%–65%; Cholesteatoma recurrence 15%–25%; Suboptimal hearing 35%–50%
Radical mastoidectomy → Cure 83%–90%; Cholesteatoma recurrence 10%–17%; Good hearing <5%
Without cholesteatoma → Myringoplasty → Cure 95+%; Persistence <5%
Ossicular discontinuity → With perforation → Tympanoplasty → Good hearing 55%–94%; Further hearing loss <3%
Without perforation → Ossicular reconstruction → Good hearing 50%–75%; Persistent hearing loss 25%–50%; Additional hearing loss <5%
Otosclerosis → Stapedectomy → Good hearing 82%–93%; No change 3%–11%; Additional hearing loss 1%–3%

FIGURE 55•9 Conductive hearing loss. When a patient presents with this problem, the above flow chart indicates how the diagnosis determines the management of the patient and further predicts the outcome. Jafek, B. W. & Balkany, T. J. Conductive hearing loss. In B. Eiseman (Ed.). *Prognosis of surgical disease.* Philadelphia: W. B. Saunders.

of all hearing aids sold today are either behind-the-ear, in-the-ear, or in-the-canal types (Table 55-3).

A hearing aid should be fitted with the patient's needs foremost (eg, type of hearing loss, manual dexterity) rather than by the brand name, by a certified audiologist licensed to dispense hearing aids. Many states have a consumer protection law that allows the hearing aid to be returned after a trial use if the patient is not completely satisfied.

A hearing aid makes sounds louder, but it does not improve a patient's ability to discriminate words or understand speech.

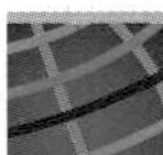

TABLE 55•3 Hearing Aids

Site (and Range of Hearing Loss)	Advantages	Disadvantages
Body (mild–profound)	Separation of receiver and microphone prevents acoustic feedback, allowing high amplification. Generally used in a school setting.	Bulky; requires long wire, which may be cosmetically displeasing; some loss of high-frequency response
Behind the ear (mild–profound)	Larger size permits use of larger components that enable the aid to provide more power and features; most versatile due to size; no long wires	Large size
In the ear (mild–moderately severe)	One-piece custom fit to contour of ear; no tubes or cords; miniature microphone is located in the ear, which is a more natural placement; more cosmetically appealing due to easy concealment	Smaller size limits output; patients who have arthritis or cannot perform tasks requiring good manual dexterity may have difficulty with the small size of aid and/or battery; can require more repair than the behind-the-ear aid
In the canal (mild–moderately severe)	Same as in-the-ear aids; less visible, so more cosmetically pleasing	Even smaller than in-the-ear aids; requires good manual dexterity

Therefore, people who have low discrimination scores on audiogram (ie, 20%) may derive little benefit from a hearing aid. Hearing aids amplify all sounds, including background noise, which may be disturbing to the wearer. Chart 55-2 identifies additional problems associated with hearing aid use. There are, however, computerized hearing aids available that compensate for background noise or allow amplification at certain programmed frequencies rather than at all frequencies. Occasionally, depending on the type of hearing loss, binaural aids (one for each ear) may be indicated.

To protect the health and safety of people with hearing impairments, the Food and Drug Administration has established certain regulations. A medical evaluation of the impairment by a licensed physician must be obtained within 6 months before the purchase of a hearing aid. The written statement from a physician may be waived, however, if the patient (a fully informed adult 18 years of age or older) signs a document to this effect. Children must be evaluated by a physician. Health care professionals who dispense hearing aids are required to refer prospective users to a physician if any of the following otologic conditions are evident:

- Visible congenital or traumatic deformity of the ear
- Active drainage from the ear within the previous 90 days
- Sudden or rapidly progressive hearing loss within the previous 90 days
- Complaints of dizziness or tinnitus
- Unilateral hearing loss that occurred suddenly or within the previous 90 days
- Audiometric air/bone gap of 15 dB or more at 500, 1000, and 2000 Hz
- Significant accumulation of cerumen or a foreign body in the external auditory canal
- Pain or discomfort in the ear

A user instruction brochure is to accompany every hearing aid device. In this brochure, the following information is presented:

- Specification that good health practice requires a medical evaluation before purchasing a hearing aid
- Notification that any of the eight otologic conditions listed above should be investigated by a physician before purchase of a hearing aid
- Instructions for proper use, maintenance, and care of the hearing aid, as well as instructions for replacing or recharging the batteries
- Repair service information
- Description of avoidable conditions that could damage the hearing aid
- List of any known side effects that may warrant physician consultation (eg, skin irritation, accelerated cerumen accumulation)

Implanted Hearing Devices

Three types of implanted hearing devices are either currently available or in the investigational stage: the cochlear implant, the bone conduction device, and the semi-implantable hearing device. Cochlear implants are for patients with little or no hearing. Bone conduction devices, which transmit sound through the skull to the inner ear, are used in patients with a conductive hearing loss if a hearing aid is contraindicated (ie, those with chronic infection). The device is implanted postauricularly under the skin into the

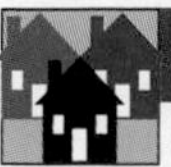

PATIENT EDUCATION AND HOME CARE

Tips for Hearing Aid Care

Cleaning

The earmold is the only part of the hearing aid that may be washed frequently (even daily if necessary) with soap and water. The earmold must be dry before it is snapped into the receiver. The cannula is cleaned with a small pipe cleaner–like device.

Malfunctioning

Inadequate amplification, a whistling noise, or pain from the mold can occur when a hearing aid is not functioning properly. If the hearing aid still does not work properly after checking for malfunctions (eg, Is the switch on? Are the batteries charged and positioned correctly?), the hearing aid dealer should be notified. If the unit requires extended time for repair, the dealer may lend the patient a hearing aid until the repair can be accomplished.

Recognizing Complications

When occluded by a hearing aid, the external auditory canal can become moist. Common medical problems among hearing aid wearers include external otitis and pressure ulcers in the external auditory canal or meatus.

CHART 55•2 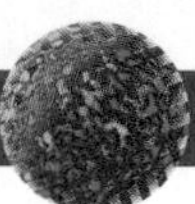 **Hearing Aid Problems**

Whistling Noise
- Loose ear mold:
  - Improperly made
  - Improperly worn
  - Worn out

Improper Aid Selection
- Too much power required in aid, with inadequate separation between microphone and receiver
- Open mold used inappropriately

Inadequate Amplification
- Dead batteries
- Wax in ear
- Wax or other material in mold
- Wires or tubing disconnected from aid
- Aid turned off or volume too low
- Improper mold
- Improper aid for degree of loss

Pain From Mold
- Improperly fitted mold
- Ear skin or cartilage infection
- Middle ear infection
- Ear tumor
- Unrelated causes:
  - Temporomandibular joint
  - Throat or larynx
  - Other

skull, and an external device—worn above the ear, not in the canal—transmits the sound through the skin. Semi-implantable hearing aids, although not yet approved by the Food & Drug Administration except in testing sites, still require the use of an external device. However, research to develop a fully implantable hearing aid continues.

Cochlear Implant

A cochlear implant is an auditory prosthesis used for people with profound sensorineural hearing loss bilaterally who do not benefit from conventional hearing aids. The hearing loss may be congenital or acquired. An implant does not restore normal hearing; rather, it helps the person detect medium to loud environmental sounds and conversation. The implant is designed to provide stimulation directly to the auditory nerve, bypassing the hair cells of the inner ear, which are not functioning. The microphone and signal processor are worn outside the body and transmit electrical stimuli inside the body to the implanted electrodes. The electrical signals stimulate the auditory nerve fibers and then the brain, where they are interpreted.

Candidates for cochlear implant, who are usually at least 1 year old, are selected after careful screening by otologic history, physical examination, audiologic testing, and x-rays and psychological testing. The general criteria for choosing adults who may benefit from a cochlear implant are:

- Profound sensorineural hearing loss in both ears
- Inability to hear and recognize speech well with hearing aids
- No medical contraindication to a cochlear implant or general anesthesia
- Indications that being able to hear would enhance the patient's life

The surgery involves implanting a small receiver in the temporal bone, through a postauricular incision, and placing electrodes into the inner ear (Fig. 55-10). The microphone and transmitter are worn on an external unit. The patient undergoes extensive cochlear rehabilitation with the multidisciplinary team, which includes an audiologist and speech pathologist. Several months may be needed to learn to interpret the sounds heard. Children and adults who lost their hearing before they learned to speak take much longer to acquire speech. There are wide variations of success with cochlear implants, and there is also controversy about their use, especially among the deaf community.

Hearing Guide Dogs

Specially trained dogs are available to assist the person with a hearing loss. People who live alone are eligible to apply for a dog trained by International Hearing Dog, Inc. At home, the dog reacts to the sound of a telephone, a doorbell, an alarm clock, a baby's cry, a knock at the door, a smoke alarm, or an intruder. The dog does not bark but alerts its master by physical contact; the dog then runs to the source of the noise. In public, the dog positions itself between the hearing-impaired person and any potential hazard that the person cannot hear, such as an oncoming vehicle or a loud, hostile person. In many states, a hearing-impaired person with a certified hearing guide dog is legally permitted access to public transportation, public eating places, and stores, including food markets.

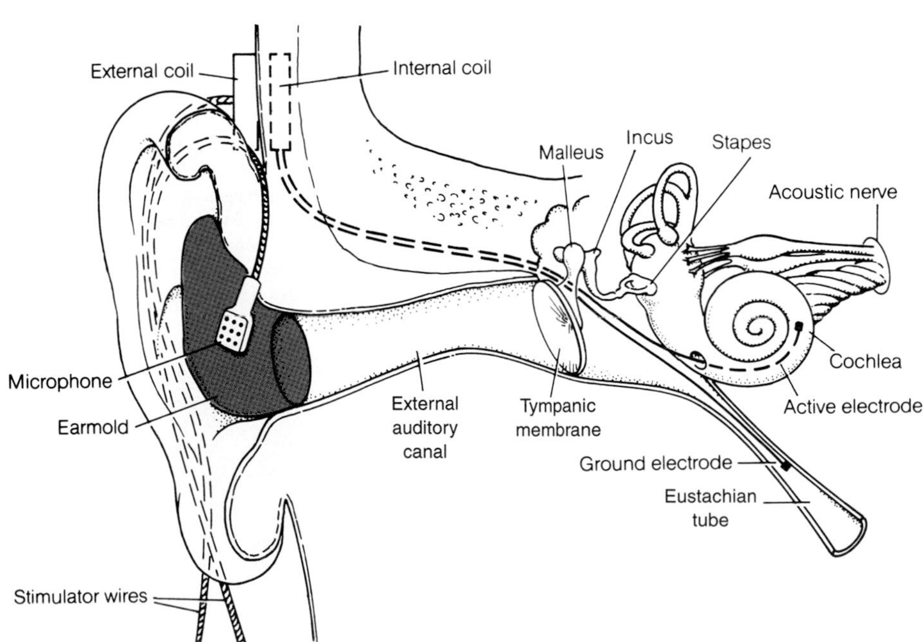

FIGURE 55•10 The cochlear implant. The internal coil has a stranded electrode lead. The electrode is inserted through the round window into the scala tympani of the cochlea. The external coil (the transmitter) is held in alignment with the internal coil (the receiver) by a magnet. The microphone receives the sound. The stimulator wire receives the signal after it has been filtered, adjusted, and modified so that the sound is at a comfortable level for the patient. Sound is passed by the external transmitter to the inner coil receiver by magnetic conduction and is then carried by the electrode to the cochlea.

Critical Thinking Exercises

1.
An elderly patient in an extended care facility appears withdrawn and distrustful of others. She does not participate in conversations with other residents. You suspect that she has a hearing loss. Describe the strategies you would use to assess this patient's hearing. What intervention strategies would you implement if your assessment confirms that the woman has a hearing loss? If your assessment indicates that she does not have a hearing loss?

2.
An antiemetic and a tranquilizer have been prescribed for a patient with Ménière's disease. You realize that safety precautions are indicated. Devise a teaching plan for this patient and explain the reasons behind each part of the plan.

3.
The daughter of an elderly patient complains that her father refuses to use his hearing aid. How would you focus your assessment to gather other pertinent information in determining a plan of action? Describe the patient outcomes you anticipate your interventions will achieve.

References and Selected Readings

BOOKS

Blitzer, A., et al. (Eds.) (1998). *Office-based surgery in otolaryngology.* New York: Thieme.

Harris, L. L., & Huntoon, M. B. (1998). *Core curriculum for otorhinolaryngology and head/neck nursing.* New Smyrna Beach, FL: SOHN.

National Strategic Research Plan of the National Institute on Deafness and Other Communication Disorders (NIDCD). (1998). Narberth, PA: National Institutes of Health.

Schuring, L. T. (1995). Assessment of the ear. In W. J. Phipps et al. (Eds.), *Medical-surgical nursing: Concepts and clinical practice* (5th ed., pp. 2113–2126). St Louis: Mosby.

Schuring, L. T. (1995). Management of persons with problems of the ear. In W. J. Phipps et al. (Eds.), *Medical-surgical nursing: Concepts and clinical practice* (5th ed., pp. 2127–2154). St Louis: Mosby.

Schuring, L. T. (1997). Caring for people with ear, nose, throat, head, and neck disorders. In J. Luckmann (Ed.), *Manual of nursing care* (pp. 795–866). Philadelphia: W. B. Saunders.

Sigler, B. A., & Schuring, L. T. (1993). *Ear, nose, and throat disorders.* St. Louis: Mosby.

Society of Otorhinolaryngology–Head and Neck Nurses, Inc. (1996). *Nursing practice guidelines for care of the otorhinolaryngology—head and neck patient.* New Smyrna Beach, FL: SOHN.

JOURNALS

Asterisks indicate nursing research articles.

Cavenish, R. (1998). Adult hearing loss. *American Journal of Nursing, 98*(8), 50–51.

*Lusk, S. L., et al. (1994). Test of the health promotion model as a causal model of workers' use of hearing protection. *Nursing Research, 43*(3), 151–157.

Nobel, W., Ter-Horst, K., & Byrne, D. (1995). Disabilities and handicaps associated with impaired auditory localization. *Journal of the American Academy of Audiology, 6*(2), 129–140.

Pollock, K. J. (1995). Ménière's disease: A review of the problem. *ORL—Head and Neck Nursing, 13*(2), 10–13.

Resources

Acoustic Neuroma Association, P.O. Box 12402, Atlanta, GA 30355; http://ANAusa.org/

Alexander Graham Bell Association for the Deaf, Inc., 3417 Volta Place, NW, Washington, DC 20007-2778; http://www.agbell.org/index.html

American Academy of Audiology, 8201 Greensboro Dr., Suite 300, McLean, VA 22102; http://www.audiology.com/

American Academy of Facial Plastic and Reconstructive Surgery, 1101 Vermont Ave., NW, Suite 220, Washington, DC 20005-3522; http://www.surgeon.org/contacts/listings/aafprs.htm

American Academy of Otolaryngology–Head and Neck Surgery, One Prince Street, Alexandria, VA 22314-3357; http://www.entnet.org/

American Board of Facial Plastic & Reconstructive Surgery, One Prince Street, Suite 310, Alexandria, VA 22314; http://www.abfprs.org/

American Speech-Language-Hearing Association, 10801 Rockville Pike, Rockville, MD 20852; http://www.asha.org/

American Tinnitus Association, P.O. Box 5, Portland, OR 97207-0005; http://www.ata.org/

International Hearing Dog Inc., 5901 E. 89th Ave., Henderson, CO 80640; http://members.aol.com/ihdi/IHDI.html

National Institute on Deafness and Other Communication Disorders, National Institutes of Health, Building 31, Room 3c35 9000, Rockville Pike, Bethesda, MD 20892; http://www.nih.gov/nidcd/

Self-Help for Hard of Hearing People, 7910 Woodmont Ave., Suite 1200, Bethesda, MD 20814; http://www.shhh.org/

Society of Otorhinolaryngology and Head–Neck Nurses, Inc., 116 Canal Street, Suite A, New Smyrna Beach, FL 32168; http://www.entnet.org/sohn/

Vestibular Disorders Association, P.O. Box 4467, Portland, OR 97208-4467; http://www.teleport.com/~veda/

UNIT

14

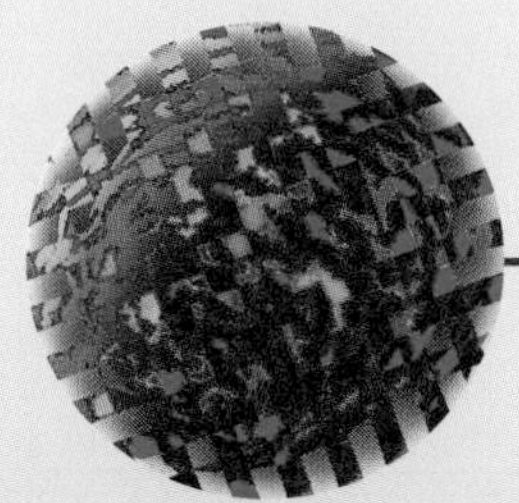

Neurologic Function

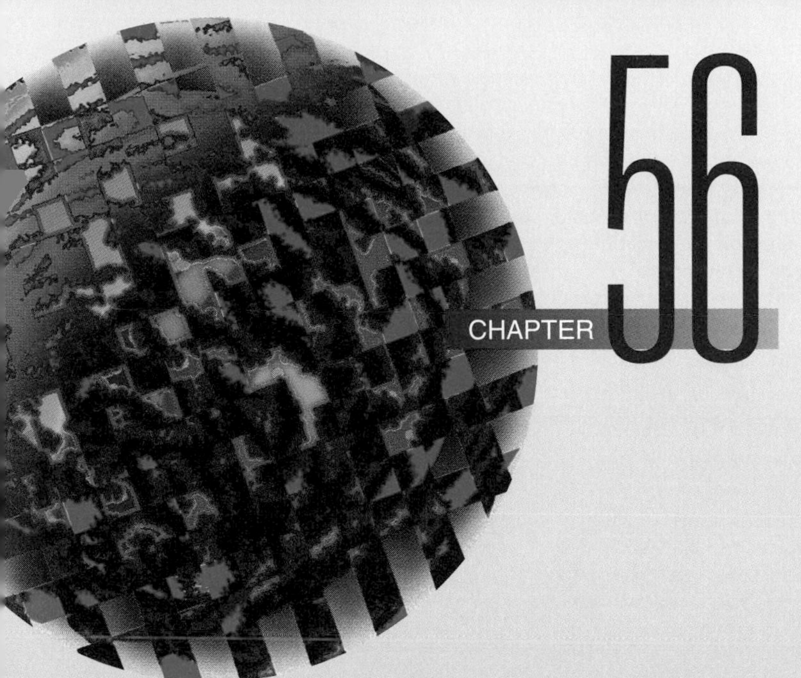

Assessment of Neurologic Function

Learning Objectives

On completion of this chapter, the learner will be able to:

1. Differentiate between pathologic changes that affect motor control and those that affect sensory pathways.
2. Compare the functioning of the sympathetic and parasympathetic nervous systems.
3. Describe the significance of physical assessment to the diagnosis of neurologic dysfunction.
4. Describe changes in neurologic function with aging and their impact on neurologic assessment findings.
5. Describe diagnostic tests used for assessment of neurologic function and the related nursing implications.

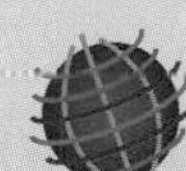

Disorders of the nervous system can occur at any time of life and can vary from mild, self-limiting symptoms to devastating, life-threatening disorders. Assessment of the neurologic system may be very structured and extensive or may focus on specific areas of function. Assessment in either case requires knowledge of the anatomy and physiology of the nervous system and an understanding of the tests and procedures used to diagnose neurologic disorders.

GLOSSARY

agnosia: loss of ability to recognize objects through a particular sensory system; may be visual, auditory, or tactile

aneurysm: a weakening or bulge in an arterial wall

aphasia: loss of the ability to express oneself or to understand language

ataxia: inability to coordinate muscle movements, resulting in difficulty in walking, talking, and performing self-care tasks

Babinski reflex (sign): a reflex action of the toes, indicative of abnormalities in the motor control pathways leading from the cerebral cortex

decerebrate posturing: abnormal posturing with extension and external rotation of the arms and wrists, extension and plantar flexion and internal rotation of the feet

decorticate posturing: abnormal posturing with flexion and internal rotation of the arms and wrists, extension and plantar flexion and internal rotation of the feet

delirium: transient loss of intellectual function, usually due to systemic problems

dementia: organic loss of intellectual function

electroencephalogram (EEG): a method of recording in graphic form, the electrical activity of the brain

electromyogram (EMG): a method of recording, in graphic form, the electrical activity of the muscle

flaccid: limp, floppy, lacking tone

hemiplegia/hemiparesis: weakness/paralysis of one side of the body, or part of it, due to an injury to the motor areas of the brain

infarction: a zone of tissue deprived of blood supply

myelography (myelogram): an x-ray study of the spinal cord after injection of a contrast agent into the subarachnoid space

paraparesis/paraplegia: weakness/paralysis of both legs and the lower part of the trunk

photophobia: inability to tolerate light

position (postural) sense: awareness of position of parts of the body without looking at them

quadriparesis/quadriplegia: a weakness/paralysis that involves all four extremities

reflex: an automatic response to stimuli

spasticity: an abnormal increase in muscle tone, causing the muscles to resist being stretched

tone: tension present in a muscle at rest

ANATOMIC AND PHYSIOLOGIC OVERVIEW

The nervous system is separated into two divisions: the central nervous system (CNS), comprising the brain and spinal cord, and the peripheral nervous system, made up of the cranial and spinal nerves. The peripheral nervous system can be further divided into the somatic or voluntary nervous system, and the autonomic or involuntary nervous system. The function of the nervous system is to control all motor, sensory, autonomic, cognitive, and behavioral activities. The nervous system has approximately 10 million sensory neurons that feed information to the brain about the internal and external environments and 500,000 motor neurons that control the body's muscles and glands. The brain itself contains more than 20 billion nerve cells that link the motor and sensory pathways, monitor the body's processes, respond to the external environment, maintain homeostasis, and direct all psychological, biologic, and physical activity through complex chemical and electrical messages (Johnson, 1997).

Cells of the Nervous System

The basic functional unit of the brain is the neuron (Fig. 56-1). It is composed of a cell body, a dendrite, and axon. The dendrite is a branch-type structure with synapses for receiving electrochemical messages. The axon is a long projection that carries impulses away from the cell body. Nerve cell bodies occurring in clusters are called ganglia or nuclei. A cluster of cell bodies with the same function is called a center (ie, the respiratory center). Neuroglial cells, the second type of nerve cell, support, protect, and nourish neurons.

Neurotransmitters

Neurotransmitters communicate messages from one neuron to another or from a neuron to a specific target tissue. Neurotransmitters are manufactured and stored in synaptic vesicles. When released, the neurotransmitter crosses the synaptic cleft, binds to receptors in the postsynaptic cell membrane, and either excites or inhibits the target cell's activity. There are various types of neurotransmitters; major neurotransmitters are described in Table 56-1 (Hickey, 1997; Johnson, 1997).

The Central Nervous System

Anatomy of the Brain

The brain represents approximately 2% of the total body weight; it weighs approximately 1400 g in an average young adult. In the elderly, the average brain weighs approximately 1200 g. The brain is divided into three major areas: the cerebrum, the brain stem, and the cerebellum. The cerebrum is composed of two hemispheres,

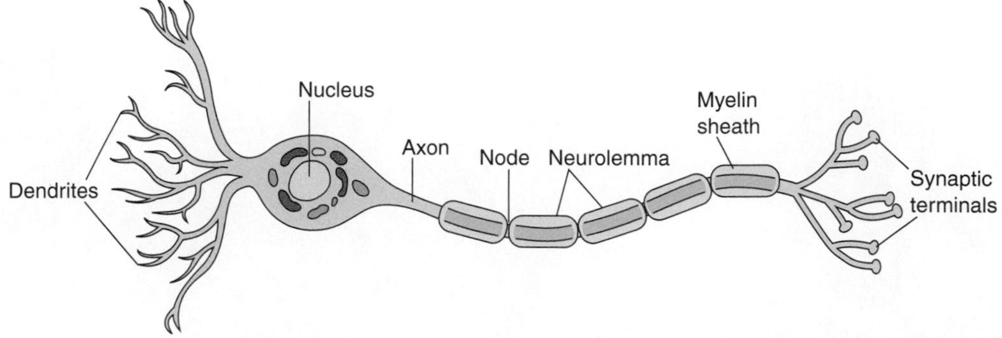

FIGURE 56•1 Neuron. Adapted from Willis, M. C. (1996). *Medical terminology: The language of health-care.* Baltimore: Williams & Wilkins.

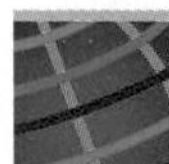

TABLE 56•1 Major Neurotransmitters

Neurotransmitter	Source	Action
Acetylcholine (major transmitter of the parasympathetic nervous system)	Many areas of the brain; autonomic nervous system	Usually excitatory; parasympathetic effects sometimes inhibitory (vagal stimulation of heart)
Serotonin	Brain stem, hypothalamus, dorsal horn of the spinal cord	Inhibitory, helps control mood and sleep, inhibits pain pathways
Dopamine	Substantia nigra and basal ganglia	Usually inhibitory, affects behavior (attention, emotions) and fine movement
Norepinephrine (major transmitter of the sympathetic nervous system)	Brain stem, hypothalamus, postganglionic neurons of the sympathetic nervous system	Usually excitatory; affects mood and overall activity
Gamma-aminobutyric acid (GABA)	Spinal cord, cerebellum, basal ganglia, some cortical areas	Inhibitory; muscle and nerve transmission
Enkephalin, endorphin	Nerve terminals in the spine, brain stem, thalamus and hypothalamus, pituitary gland	Excitatory; pleasurable sensation, inhibits pain transmission

the thalamus, the hypothalamus, and the basal ganglia. Additionally, connections for the olfactory (cranial nerve I) and optic (cranial nerve III) nerves are found in the cerebrum. The brain stem includes the midbrain, pons, medulla, and connections for cranial nerves II and IV through XII. The cerebellum is located under the cerebrum and behind the brain stem (Fig. 56-2).

CEREBRUM

The cerebrum consists of two hemispheres that are incompletely separated by the great longitudinal fissure. This sulcus separates the cerebrum into the right and left hemispheres. The two hemispheres are joined at the lower portion of the fissure by the corpus callosum. The surface of the hemispheres has a wrinkled appearance that is the result of many folded layers or convolutions called gyri, which provide a tremendous increase in the surface area of the brain. The external or outer portion of the cerebrum (the cerebral cortex) is made up of gray matter approximately 2 to 5 mm in depth; it contains billions of neurons/cell bodies, giving it a gray appearance. White matter makes up the innermost layer and is composed of nerve fibers and neuroglia (support tissue) that form tracts or pathways connecting various parts of the brain with one another (transverse and association pathways) and the cortex to

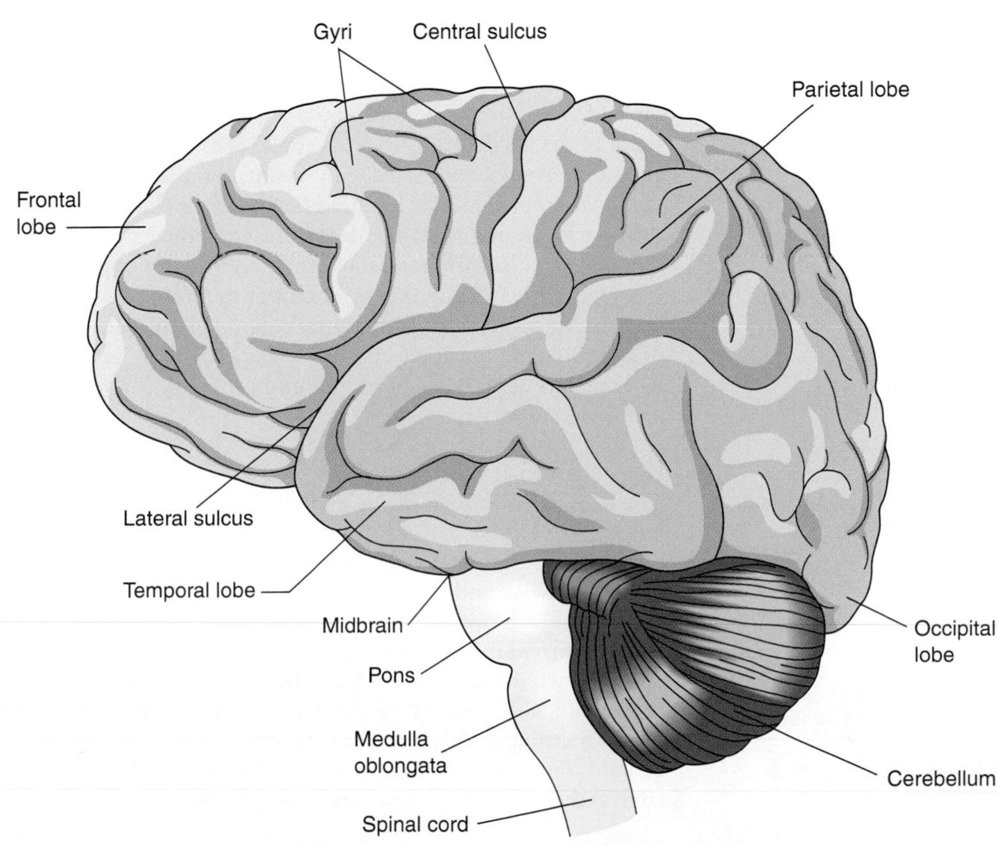

FIGURE 56•2 View of the external surface of the brain, showing lobes and key parts. Adapted from Memmler, R. L., Cohen, B. J., & Wood, D. L. (1996). *The human body in health and disease* (8th ed.). Philadelphia: Lippincott-Raven.

lower portions of the brain and spinal cord (projection fibers). The cerebral hemispheres are divided into pairs of frontal, parietal, temporal, and occipital lobes. The four lobes are as follows (see Fig. 56-2):

Frontal—the largest lobe. This area controls concentration, abstract thought, information storage or memory, and motor function. It also contains Broca's area, a speech association area that participates in word formulation. The frontal lobe is also responsible in large part for an individual's affect, judgment, personality, and inhibitions.

Parietal—a predominantly sensory lobe. It contains the primary sensory cortex, which analyzes sensory information and relays the interpretation of this information to the thalamus and other cortical areas. It is also essential to an individual's awareness of the body in space, as well as orientation in space and spatial relations.

Temporal—contains the auditory receptive areas. Contains a vital area called the interpretive area that provides integration of somatization, visual, and auditory areas and plays the most dominant role of any area of the cortex in cerebration.

Occipital—the posterior lobe of the cerebral hemisphere is responsible for visual interpretation.

The corpus callosum is a thick collection of nerve fibers that connects the two hemispheres of the brain and is responsible for the transmission of information from one side of the brain to the other. Information transferred is sensory, memory, and learned discrimination. Right-handed people and some left-handed people have cerebral dominance on the left side of the brain for verbal, linguistic, arithmetical, calculating, and analytic functions. The nondominant hemisphere is responsible for geometric, spatial, visual, pattern, and musical functions.

The basal ganglia are masses of nuclei located deep in the cerebral hemispheres that are responsible for motor control of fine body movements, including those of the hands and lower extremities.

The thalamus (Fig. 56-3) lies on either side of the third ventricle and acts primarily as a relay station for all sensation except smell. All memory, sensation, and pain impulses pass through this section.

The hypothalamus is located anterior and inferior to the thalamus. The hypothalamus lies immediately beneath and lateral to the lower portion of the wall of the third ventricle. It includes the optic chiasm (the point at which the two optic tracts cross) and the mamillary bodies (involved in olfactory reflexes and emotional response to odors). The infundibulum of the hypothalamus connects it to the posterior pituitary gland. The hypothalamus plays an important role in the endocrine system because it regulates the pituitary secretion of hormones that influence metabolism, reproduction, stress response, and urine production. It works with the pituitary to maintain fluid balance and maintains temperature regulation by promoting vasoconstriction or vasodilation.

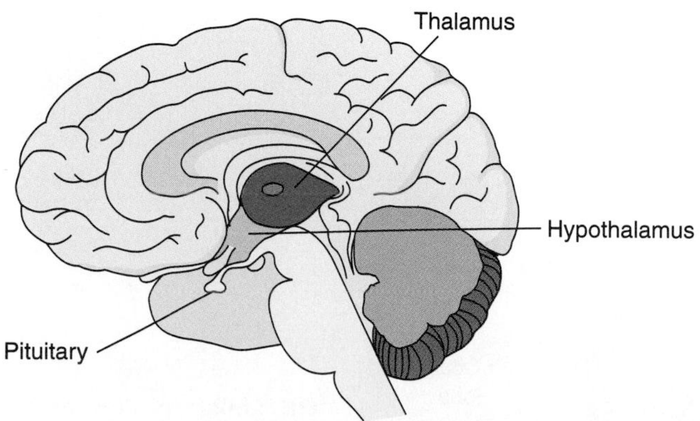

FIGURE 56•3 Diagram showing the thalamus, hypothalamus, and pituitary (hypophysis). Adapted from Memmler, R. L., Cohen, B. J., & Wood, D. L. (1996). *The human body in health and disease* (8th ed.). Philadelphia: Lippincott-Raven.

The hypothalamus is the site of the hunger center and is involved in appetite control. It houses centers that regulate the sleep–wake cycle, blood pressure, aggressive and sexual behavior, and emotional responses (ie, blushing, rage, depression, panic, and fear). The hypothalamus also controls and regulates the autonomic nervous system.

The pituitary gland is located in the sella turcica at the base of the brain and is connected to the hypothalamus. The pituitary is the third most common site for brain tumors in adults; frequently they are detected by physical signs and symptoms that can be traced to the pituitary, such as hormonal imbalance or visual disturbances secondary to pressure on the optic chiasm.

Nerve fibers from all portions of the cortex converge in each hemisphere and exit in the form of tight bundles known as the internal capsule. Having entered the pons and the medulla, each bundle crosses to the corresponding bundle from the opposite side. Some of these axons make connections with axons from the cerebellum, basal ganglia, thalamus, and hypothalamus; some connect with the cranial nerve cells. Other fibers from the cortex and the subcortical centers are channeled through the pons and the medulla into the spinal cord.

Although the various cells in the cerebral cortex are quite similar in appearance, their functions vary widely, depending on location. The topography of the cortex in relation to certain of its functions is shown in Figure 56-4. The posterior portion of each hemisphere (ie, the occipital lobe) is devoted to all aspects of visual perception. The lateral region, or temporal lobe, incorporates the auditory center. The midcentral zone, or parietal zone, posterior to the fissure of Rolando, is concerned with sensation; the anterior portion is concerned with voluntary muscle movements. The large area behind the forehead (ie, the frontal lobes) contains the association pathways that determine emotional attitudes and responses and contribute to the formation of thought processes. Damage to the frontal lobes as a result of trauma or disease is by no means incapacitating from the standpoint of muscular control or coordination, but it affects a person's personality, as reflected by basic attitudes, sense of humor and propriety, self-restraint, and motivations.

BRAIN STEM

The brain stem consists of the midbrain, pons, and medulla oblongata (see Fig. 56-2). The midbrain connects the pons and the cerebellum with the cerebral hemispheres; it contains sensory and motor pathways and serves as the center for auditory and visual reflexes. Cranial nerves III and IV originate in the midbrain. The pons is situated in front of the cerebellum between the midbrain and the medulla and is a bridge between the two halves of the cerebellum, and between the medulla and the cerebrum. Cranial nerves V through VIII connect to the brain in the pons. The pons contains motor and sensory pathways. Portions of the pons also control the heart, respiration, and blood pressure.

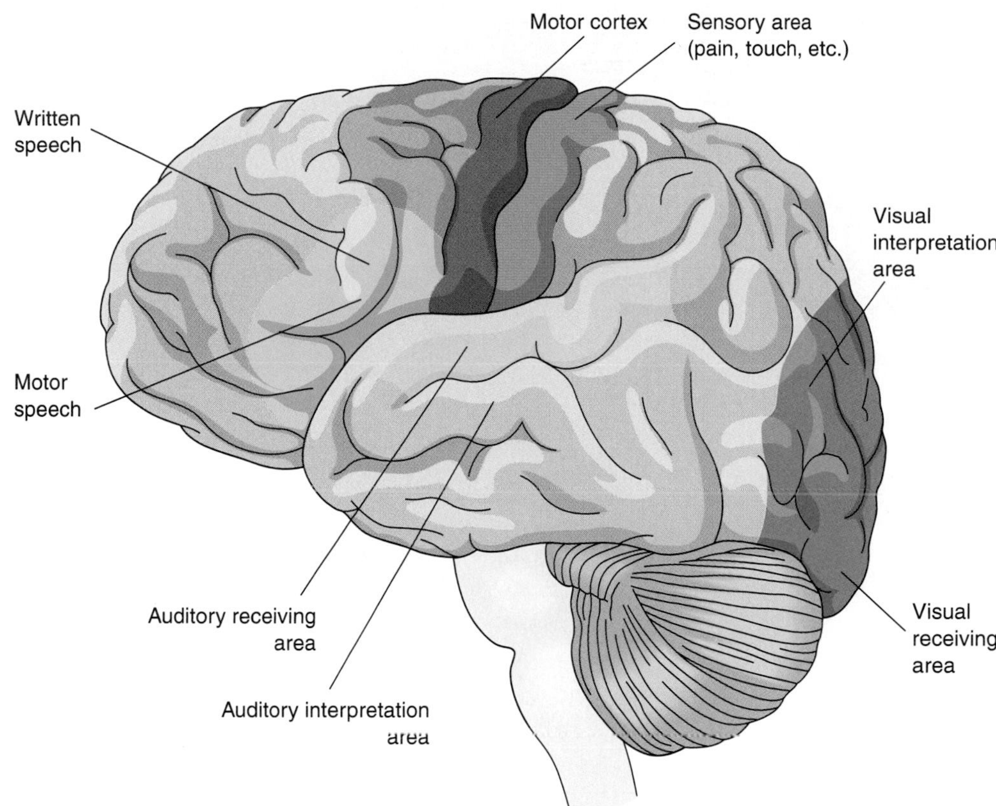

FIGURE 56•4 Functional areas of the cerebral cortex. Adapted from Memmler, R. L., Cohen, B. J., & Wood, D. L. (1996). *The human body in health and disease* (8th ed.). Philadelphia: Lippincott-Raven.

The medulla oblongata transmits motor fibers from the brain to the spinal cord and sensory fibers from the spinal cord to the brain. Most of these fibers cross, or decussate, at this level. Cranial nerves IX through XII connect to the brain in the medulla.

CEREBELLUM

The cerebellum is separated from the cerebral hemispheres by a fold of dura mater, the tentorium cerebelli. The cerebellum has both excitatory and inhibitory actions and is largely responsible for coordination of movement. It also controls fine movement, balance, **position sense** (awareness of where each part of the body is), and integration of sensory input.

Structures Protecting the Brain

The brain is contained in the rigid skull, which protects it from injury. The major bones of the skull are the frontal, temporal, parietal, and occipital bones. These bones join at the suture lines (Fig. 56-5).

Meninges—fibrous connective tissues that cover the brain and spinal cord—provide protection, support, and nourishment to the brain and spinal cord. The layers of the meninges are the dura, arachnoid, and pia mater (Fig. 56-6).

- Dura mater—the outermost layer; covers the brain and the spinal cord. It is tough, thick, inelastic, fibrous, and gray. There are four extensions of the dura: the falx cerebri, which separates the two hemispheres in a longitudinal plane; the tentorium, which is an infolding of the dura that forms a tough membranous shelf; the falx cerebelli, which is between the two lateral lobes of the cerebellum; and the diaphragma sellae, which provides a "roof" for the sella turcica. The tentorium supports the hemispheres and separates them from the lower part of the brain. When excess pressure occurs in the cranial cavity, brain tissue may be compressed against the tentorium or displaced downward, a process called herniation. Between the dura mater and the skull in the cranium, and between the periosteum and the dura in the vertebral column, is the epidural space, a potential space.
- Arachnoid—the middle membrane; an extremely thin, delicate membrane that closely resembles a spider web (hence the name arachnoid). It appears white because it

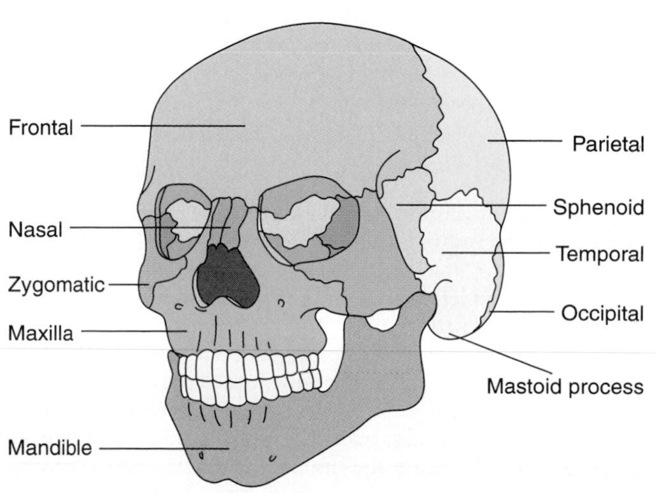

FIGURE 56•5 Bones of the skull.

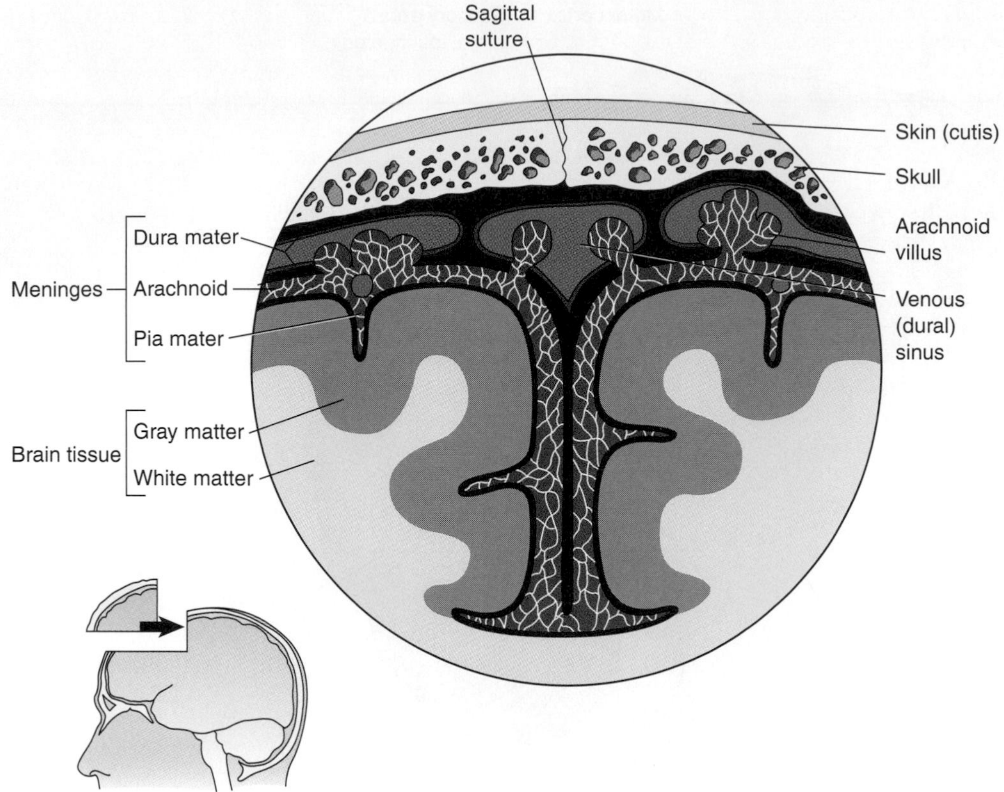

FIGURE 56•6 Meninges and related parts as seen through the frontal section of the top of the head. Adapted from Memmler, R. L., Cohen, B. J., & Wood, D. L. (1996). *The human body in health and disease* (8th ed.). Philadelphia: Lippincott-Raven.

has no blood supply. The arachnoid layer contains the choroid plexus, which is responsible for the production of cerebrospinal fluid (CSF). This membrane also has unique finger-like projections, arachnoid villi, that absorb CSF. In the normal adult, approximately 500 mL of CSF are produced each day; all but 150 mL are absorbed by the villi. When blood enters the system (from, eg, trauma, a ruptured aneurysm, stroke), the villi become obstructed and hydrocephalus (increased size of ventricles) may result. The subdural space is between the dura and the arachnoid layer, and the subarachnoid space is located between the arachnoid and pia layers and contains the CSF.

- Pia mater—the innermost membrane; a thin, transparent layer that hugs the brain closely and extends into every fold of the brain's surface.

Cerebrospinal Fluid

CSF, a clear and colorless fluid with a specific gravity of 1.007, is produced in the ventricles and is circulated around the brain and the spinal cord by the ventricular system. There are four ventricles: the right and left lateral, and the third and fourth ventricles. The two lateral ventricles open into the third ventricle at the interventricular foramen or the foramen of Monro. The third and fourth ventricles connect via the aqueduct of Sylvius. The fourth ventricle supplies CSF to the subarachnoid space and down the spinal cord on the dorsal surface. CSF is returned to the brain and is then circulated around the brain, where it is absorbed by the arachnoid villi.

CSF is produced in the choroid plexus of the lateral, third, and fourth ventricles. The ventricular and subarachnoid system contains approximately 150 mL of fluid; 15 to 25 mL of CSF is located in each lateral ventricle.

The organic and inorganic contents of CSF are similar to those of plasma, but their concentration is somewhat different. CSF is analyzed for protein, glucose, and chloride on routine assay; it may also be tested for immunoglobulins. Normally, CSF has a minimal number of white blood cells and no red blood cells.

Cerebral Circulation

The cerebral circulation receives approximately 15% of the cardiac output, or 750 mL per minute. The brain does not store nutrients and has a high metabolic demand that requires the high blood flow. The brain's blood pathway is unique because it flows against gravity; its arteries fill from below and the veins drain from above. In contrast to other organs that may tolerate decreases in blood flow because of their adequate collateral flow, the brain lacks additional collateral blood flow, which may result in irreversible tissue damage when blood flow is occluded.

ARTERIES

The arterial blood supply to the brain is provided by two internal carotid arteries and two vertebral arteries and their extensive system of branches. The internal carotids arise from the bifurcation of the common carotid and supply much of the anterior circulation of the brain. The vertebral arteries branch from the subclavian arteries, flow back and upward on either side of the cervical vertebrae, and enter the cranium through the foramen magnum. The vertebral arteries join to become the basilar artery at the level of the brain stem; the basilar artery divides to form the two branches of the posterior cerebral arteries. The vertebrobasilar arteries supply most of the posterior circulation of the brain.

At the base of the brain surrounding the pituitary gland, a ring of arteries is formed between the vertebral and internal carotid arterial chains. This ring is called the circle of Willis and is formed from the branches of the internal carotid arteries, anterior and middle cerebral arteries, and anterior and posterior communicating arteries (Fig. 56-7). Functionally, the posterior portion of the circulation and the anterior or carotid circulation usually remain separate. The arteries of the circle of Willis can provide alternative routes of blood flow if one or more of the four vessels supplying it become occluded or are ligated.

The arterial anastomosis along the circle of Willis is a frequent site of aneurysms, which may be congenital or the result of degenerative changes in the vessel wall. **Aneurysms** can be formed when the pressure at a weakened arterial wall causes the artery to balloon out. An aneurysm can press on adjacent cerebral structures, such as the optic chiasm, causing varying visual deficits. If an artery becomes occluded by vasospasm, an embolus, or a thrombus, the neurons distal to the occlusion are deprived of their blood supply and the cells quickly die. The result is a stroke (cerebrovascular accident or **infarction**, "brain attack"). The effects of the occlusion depend on which vessels are involved and which areas of the brain these vessels supply.

VEINS

Venous drainage for the brain does not follow the arterial circulation as in other body structures. The veins of the brain reach the brain's surface and join larger veins. These cross the subarachnoid space and empty into the dural sinuses, which are the vascular channels lying within the tough dura mater. The network of the sinuses carries venous outflow for the brain and empties into the internal jugular vein, which then returns the blood to the heart. Cerebral veins and sinuses are unique because, unlike other veins in the body, they do not have valves to prevent blood from flowing backward.

Blood–Brain Barrier

The CNS is inaccessible to many substances that circulate in the blood (ie, dyes, medications, antibiotics). After being injected into the blood, these substances do not reach the neurons of the CNS because of the blood–brain barrier. This barrier is formed by the endothelial cells of the brain's capillaries, which form continuous tight junctions, creating a barrier to macromolecules and many compounds. The barrier preventing large molecules from entering the CSF is the low permeability of the secretory cells of the choroid plexus. All substances entering the CSF must filter through the capillary membranes of the choroid plexus. Often altered by trauma, cerebral edema, and cerebral hypoxemia, the blood–brain barrier has implications in the treatment and selection of medication for CNS disorders.

Anatomy of the Spinal Cord

The spinal cord and medulla form a continuous structure extending from the cerebral hemispheres and serving as the connection between the brain and the periphery. Approximately 45 cm (18 in) long and about the thickness of a finger, it extends from the foramen magnum at the base of the skull to the lower border of the first lumbar vertebra, where it tapers to a fibrous band called the conus medullaris. Continuing below the second lumbar space are the nerve roots that extend beyond the conus, which are called the cauda equina because they resemble a horse's tail. Like the brain, the spinal cord consists of gray and white matter. Gray matter in the brain is external and white matter is internal; in the spinal cord, gray matter is in the center and is surrounded on all sides by white matter.

The spinal cord is surrounded by the meninges, dura, arachnoid, and pia layers. Between the dura mater and the vertebral canal is the epidural space. The spinal cord is an H-shaped structure with nerve cell bodies (gray matter) surrounded by ascending and descending tracts (white matter) (Fig. 56-8). The lower portion of the H is broader than the upper portion and corresponds to the anterior horns. The anterior horns contain cells that have fibers that form the anterior (motor) root end and that are essential for the voluntary and reflex activity of the muscles they innervate. The thinner posterior (upper horns) portion contains cells with fibers that enter over the posterior (sensory) root end and thus serve as a relay station in the sensory/reflex pathway.

The thoracic region of the spinal cord has a projection from each side at the crossbar of the H of gray matter called the lateral horn. It contains the cells that give rise to the autonomic fibers of

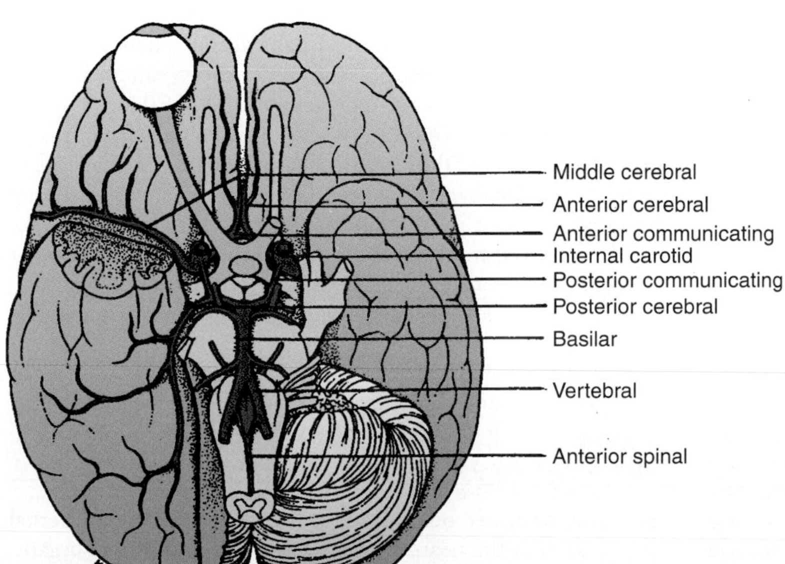

FIGURE 56•7 Arterial blood supply of the brain, including the circle of Willis, as viewed from the ventral surface. From Porth, C. (1998). *Pathophysiology: Concepts of altered health states* (5th ed.). Philadelphia: Lippincott Williams & Wilkins.

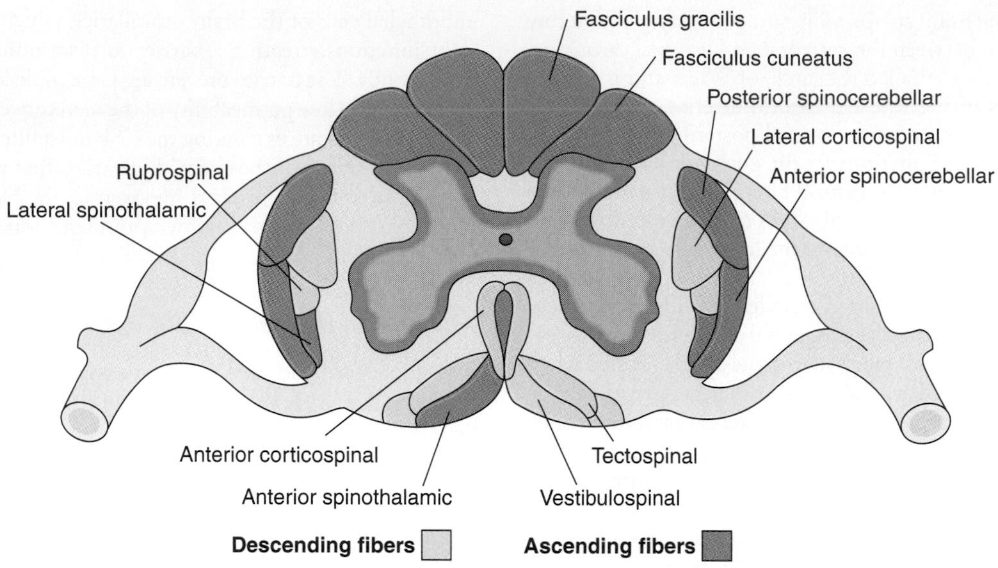

FIGURE 56•8 Cross-sectional diagram of the spinal cord showing major spinal tracts.

the sympathetic division. The fibers leave the spinal cord through the anterior roots in the thoracic and upper lumbar segments.

SENSORY AND MOTOR PATHWAYS: THE SPINAL TRACTS

The white matter of the cord is composed of myelinated and unmyelinated nerve fibers. The fast-conducting myelinated fibers form bundles that also contain glial cells. Fiber bundles with a common function are called tracts. There are six ascending tracts. Two conduct sensation, principally the perception of touch, pressure, vibration, position, and passive motion from the same side of the body. Before reaching the cerebral cortex, these fibers cross to the opposite side in the medulla. Two spinocerebellar tracts conduct sensory impulses from muscle spindles, providing necessary input for coordinated muscle contraction. They ascend essentially uncrossed and terminate in the cerebellum.

There are eight descending tracts, seven of which are engaged in motor function. The two corticospinal tracts conduct motor impulses to the anterior horn cells from the opposite side of the brain and control voluntary muscle activity. The three vestibulospinal tracts descend uncrossed and are involved in some autonomic functions (influence sweating, pupil dilation, and circulation) and involuntary muscle control. The corticobulbar tract conducts impulses responsible for voluntary head and facial muscle movement and crosses at the level of the brain stem. The rubrospinal and reticulospinal tracts conduct impulses involved with involuntary muscle movement.

VERTEBRAL COLUMN

The vertebral column surrounds and protects the spinal cord and normally consists of 7 cervical, 12 thoracic, and 5 lumber vertebrae, as well as the sacrum, a fused mass of five vertebrae. It terminates in the coccyx. Nerve roots exit from the vertebral column through the intervertebral foramina (openings). The vertebrae are separated by disks, except for the first and second cervical, sacral, and coccygeal vertebrae. Each vertebra has a ventral solid body and a dorsal segment or arch, which is posterior to the body. The arch is composed of two pedicles and two laminae supporting seven processes. The vertebral body, arch, pedicles, and laminae all encase the vertebral canal.

The Peripheral Nervous System

The peripheral nervous system includes the cranial nerves, the spinal nerves, and the autonomic nervous system.

Cranial Nerves

There are 12 pairs of cranial nerves that emerge from the lower surface of the brain and pass through the foramina in the skull. Three are entirely sensory (I, II, VIII), five are motor (III, IV, VI, XI, and XII), and four are mixed (V, VII, IX, and X). The cranial nerves are numbered in the order in which they arise from the brain. For example, cranial nerves I and II attach in the cerebral hemispheres, whereas cranial nerves IX, X, XI, and XII attach at the medulla (Fig. 56-9). Most cranial nerves innervate the head, neck, and special sense structures. Table 56-2 lists the names and primary functions of the cranial nerves.

Spinal Nerves

The spinal cord is composed of 31 pairs of spinal nerves: 8 cervical, 12 thoracic, 5 lumbar, 5 sacral, and 1 coccygeal. Each spinal nerve has a ventral root and a dorsal root (Fig. 56-10).

The dorsal roots are sensory and transmit sensory impulses from specific areas of the body known as dermatomes (Fig. 56-11) to the dorsal ganglia. The sensory fiber may be somatic, carrying information about pain, temperature, touch, and position sense (proprioception) from the tendons, joints, and body surfaces; or visceral, carrying information from the internal organs.

The ventral roots are motor and transmit impulses from the spinal cord to the body. These fibers are also either somatic or visceral. The visceral fibers include autonomic fibers that control the cardiac muscles and glandular secretions.

Autonomic Nervous System

The autonomic nervous system regulates the activities of internal organs such as the heart, lungs, blood vessels, digestive organs, and glands. Maintenance and restoration of internal homeostasis

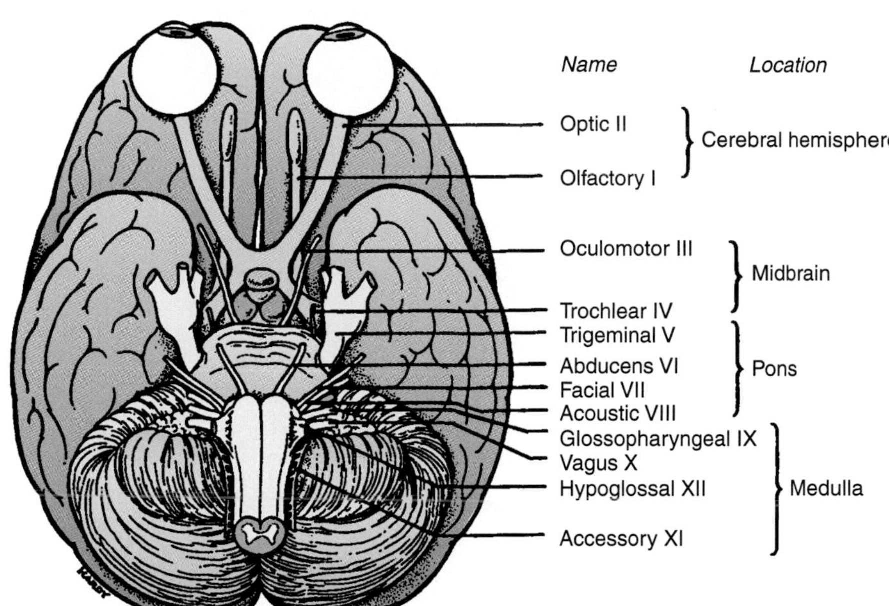

FIGURE 56•9 Diagram of the base of the brain showing entrance or exit of the cranial nerves. The right column indicates the anatomic location of the connection of each cranial nerve to the central nervous system.

is largely the responsibility of the autonomic nervous system. There are two major divisions: the sympathetic and parasympathetic systems, which generally act in opposition to each other. For example, parasympathetic stimulation constricts the pupil; sympathetic stimulation dilates it.

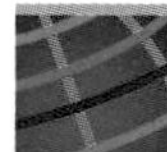

TABLE 56•2 Cranial Nerves

Cranial Nerve	Type	Function
I (olfactory)	Sensory	Sense of smell
II (optic)	Sensory	Visual acuity
III (oculomotor)	Motor	Muscles that move the eye and lid, pupillary constriction, lens accommodation
IV (trochlear)	Motor	Muscles that move the eye
V (trigeminal)	Mixed	Facial sensation, corneal reflex, mastication
VI (abducens)	Motor	Muscles that move the eye
VII (facial)	Mixed	Facial expression and muscle movement, salivation and tearing, taste, sensation in the ear
VIII (vestibulocochlear)	Sensory	Hearing and equilibrium
IX (glossopharyngeal)	Mixed	Taste, sensation in pharynx and tongue, pharyngeal muscles
X (vagus)	Mixed	Muscles of pharynx, larynx, and soft palate; sensation in external ear, pharynx, larynx, thoracic and abdominal viscera; parasympathetic innervation of thoracic and abdominal organs
XI (spinal accessory)	Motor	Sternocleidomastoid and trapezius muscles
XII (hypoglossal)	Motor	Movement of the tongue

The autonomic nervous system innervates most body organs; although usually considered part of the peripheral nervous system, it is regulated by centers in the spinal cord, brain stem, and hypothalamus. The autonomic nervous system has two neurons in a series extending between the centers in the CNS and the organs innervated. The first neuron, the preganglionic neuron, is located in the brain or spinal cord, and its axon extends to the autonomic ganglia. There, it synapses with the second neuron, the postganglionic neuron, located in the autonomic ganglia, and its axon synapses with the target tissue and innervates the effector organ. Its regulatory effects are exerted not on individual cells but on large expanses of tissue and on entire organs. The responses elicited do not appear instantaneously but only after a lag period. These responses are sustained far longer than other neurogenic responses to ensure maximal functional efficiency on the part of receptor organs, such as blood vessels.

The quality of these responses is explained by the fact that the autonomic nervous system transmits its impulses by way of nerve pathways, enhanced by chemical mediators, resembling in this respect the endocrine system. Electrical impulses, conducted through nerve fibers, stimulate the formation of specific chemical agents at

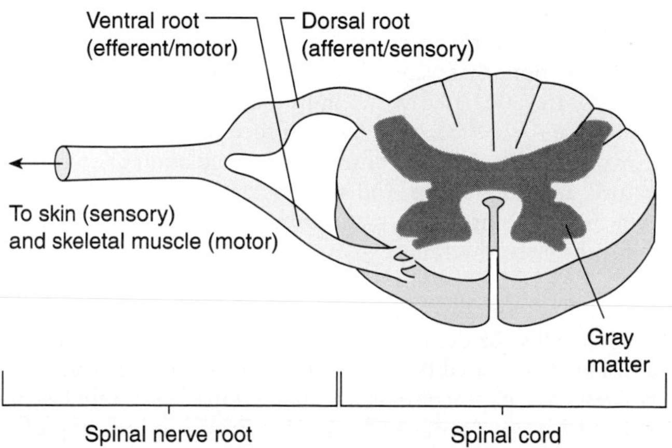

FIGURE 56•10 Cross-section of spinal cord, showing dorsal and ventral roots of a spinal nerve.

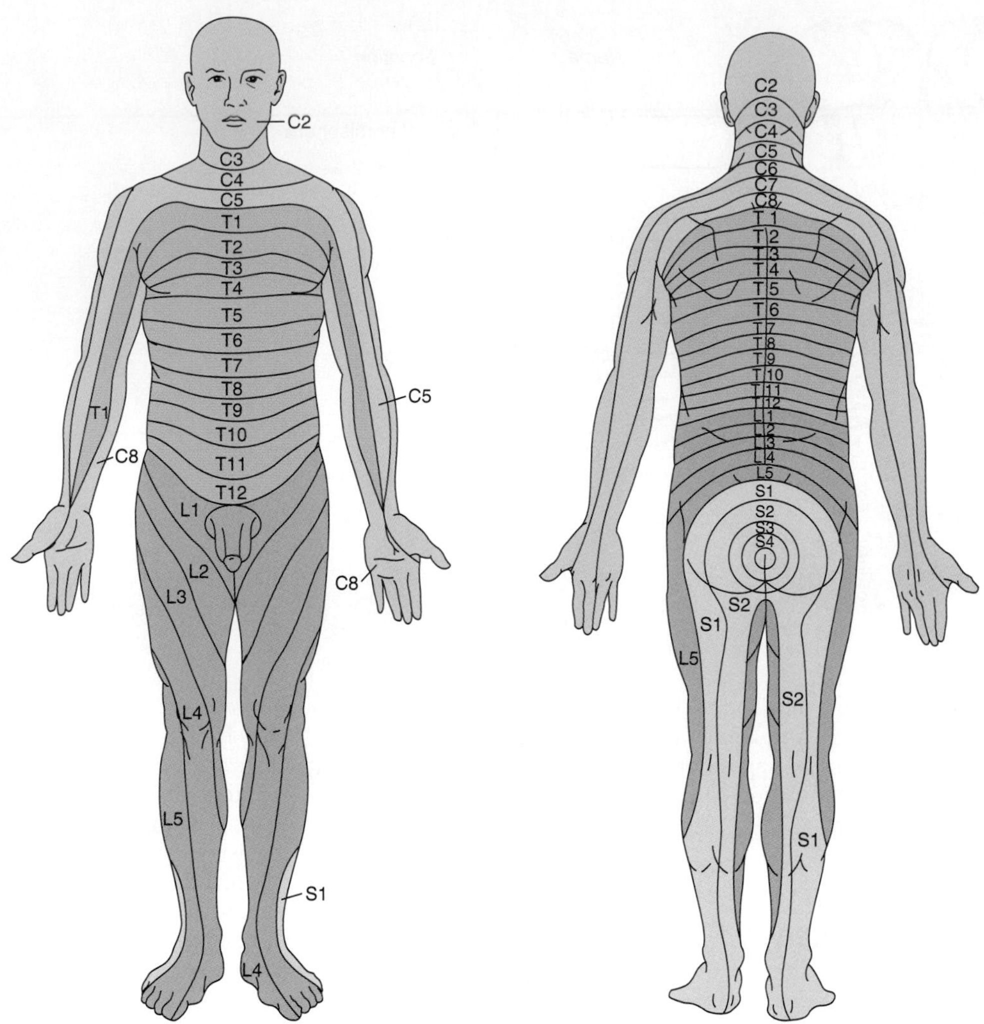

FIGURE 56•11 Dermatome distribution. From Fuller, J., & Schaller-Ayres, J. (1999). *Health assessment: A nursing approach* (3rd ed.). Philadelphia: Lippincott Williams & Wilkins.

strategic locations within the muscle mass; the diffusion of these chemicals is responsible for the contraction.

The hypothalamus is the major subcortical center for the regulation of visceral and somatic activities, with an inhibitory–excitatory role in the autonomic nervous system. The hypothalamus has connections that link the autonomic system with the thalamus, the cortex, the olfactory apparatus, and the pituitary gland. Here reside the mechanisms for the control of visceral and somatic reactions that were originally important for defense or attack, and are associated with emotional states (eg, fear, anger, anxiety); for the control of metabolic processes, including fat, carbohydrate, and water metabolism; for the regulation of body temperature, arterial pressure, and all muscular and glandular activities of the gastrointestinal tract; for control of genital functions; and for the sleep rhythm.

The autonomic nervous system is separated into the anatomically and functionally distinct sympathetic and parasympathetic divisions. Most of the tissues and the organs under autonomic control are innervated by both systems. Sympathetic stimuli are mediated by norepinephrine, and parasympathetic impulses are mediated by acetylcholine. These chemicals produce opposing and mutually antagonistic effects. Both divisions produce stimulatory and inhibitory effects. For example, the parasympathetic division causes contraction (stimulation) of the urinary bladder and a decrease (inhibition) in heart rate, whereas the sympathetic division produces vasoconstriction (stimulation) of blood vessels and dilation (inhibition) of the airways in the lungs. Table 56-3 compares the sympathetic and the parasympathetic effects.

SYMPATHETIC NERVOUS SYSTEM

The sympathetic division of the autonomic nervous system is best known for its role in the body's "fight or flight" response. Under stress conditions from either physical or emotional causes, sympathetic impulses increase greatly. As a result, the bronchioles dilate for easier gas exchange; the heart's contractions are stronger and faster; the arteries to the heart and voluntary muscles dilate, carrying more blood to them; peripheral blood vessels constrict, making the skin feel cool but shunting blood to essential active organs; the pupils dilate; the liver releases glucose for quick energy; peristalsis slows; hair stands on end; and perspiration increases. The sympathetic neurotransmitter is norepinephrine (noradrenaline), and this increase in sympathetic discharge is the same as if the body has been given an injection of adrenalin—hence, the term adrenergic is often used to refer to this division.

Sympathetic neurons are located in the thoracic and the lumbar segments of the spinal cord; their axons, called preganglionic fibers, emerge by way of all anterior nerve roots from the eighth cervical or first thoracic segment to the second or third lumbar segment. A

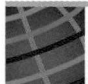

TABLE 56•3 **Autonomic Effects of the Nervous System**

Structure or Activity	Parasympathetic Effects	Sympathetic Effects
Pupil of the Eye	Constricted	Dilated
Circulatory System		
Rate and force of heart beat	Decreased	Increased
Blood vessels		
In heart muscle	Constricted	Dilated
In skeletal muscle	*	Dilated
In abdominal viscera and the skin	*	Constricted
Blood pressure	Decreased	Increased
Respiratory System		
Bronchioles	Constricted	Dilated
Rate of breathing	Decreased	Increased
Digestive System		
Peristaltic movements of digestive tube	Increased	Decreased
Muscular sphincters of digestive tube	Relaxed	Contracted
Secretion of salivary glands	Thin, watery saliva	Thick, viscid saliva
Secretions of stomach, intestine, and pancreas	Increased	*
Conversion of liver glycogen to glucose	*	Increased
Genitourinary System		
Urinary bladder		
Muscular walls	Contracted	Relaxed
Sphincters	Relaxed	Contracted
Muscles of the uterus	Relaxed; variable	Contracted under some conditions; varies with menstrual cycle and pregnancy
Blood vessels of external genitalia	Dilated	*
Integument		
Secretion of sweat	*	Increased
Pilomotor muscles	*	Contracted (gooseflesh)
Adrenal Medullae	*	Secretion of epinephrine and norepinephrine

* *No direct effect.*

From Hickey, J. (1997). *Clinical practice of neurological and neurosurgical nursing* (4th ed.). Philadelphia: Lippincott-Raven.

short distance from the cord, these fibers diverge to join a chain, composed of 22 linked ganglia, that extends the entire length of the spinal column, flanking the vertebral bodies on both sides. Some form multiple synapses with nerve cells within the chain. Others traverse the chain without making connections or losing continuity to join large "prevertebral" ganglia in the thorax, the abdomen, or the pelvis or one of the "terminal" ganglia in the vicinity of an organ, such as the bladder or the rectum (Fig. 56-12). Postganglionic nerve fibers originating in the sympathetic chain rejoin the spinal nerves that supply the extremities and are distributed to blood vessels, sweat glands, and smooth muscle tissue in the skin. Postganglionic fibers from the prevertebral plexuses (eg, the cardiac, pulmonary, splanchnic, and pelvic plexuses) supply structures in the head and neck, thorax, abdomen, and pelvis, respectively, having been joined in these plexuses by fibers from the parasympathetic division.

The adrenal glands, kidneys, liver, spleen, stomach, and duodenum are under the control of the giant celiac plexus, commonly known as the solar plexus. This receives its sympathetic nerve components by way of the three splanchnic nerves, composed of preganglionic fibers from nine segments of the spinal cord (T4 to L1), and is joined by the vagus nerve, representing the parasympathetic division. From the celiac plexus, fibers of both divisions travel along the course of blood vessels to their target organs.

Sympathetic Syndromes. Certain syndromes are distinctive to diseases of the sympathetic nerve trunks. Among these are dilation of the pupil of the eye on the same side as a penetrating wound of the neck (evidence of disturbance of the cervical sympathetic cord); temporary paralysis of the bowel (indicated by the absence of peristaltic waves and the distention of the intestine by gas) after fracture of any one of the lower dorsal or upper lumbar vertebrae with hemorrhage into the base of the mesentery; and the marked variations in pulse rate and rhythm that often follow compression fractures of the upper six thoracic vertebrae.

PARASYMPATHETIC NERVOUS SYSTEM

The parasympathetic nervous system functions as the dominant controller for most visceral effectors. During quiet, nonstressful conditions, impulses from parasympathetic fibers (cholinergic) predominate. The fibers of the parasympathetic system are located in two sections, one in the brain stem and the other from spinal segments below L2. Because of the location of these fibers, the parasympathetic system is referred to as the craniosacral division, as distinct from the thoracolumbar (sympathetic) division of the autonomic nervous system.

The parasympathetic nerves arise from the midbrain and the medulla oblongata. Fibers from cells in the midbrain travel with the third oculomotor nerve to the ciliary ganglia, where postganglionic fibers of this division are joined by those of the sympathetic system, creating controlled opposition, with a delicate balance maintained between the two at all times.

Motor and Sensory Functions of the Nervous System

Motor System Function

The motor cortex, a vertical band within each cerebral hemisphere, governs the voluntary movements of the body. The exact locations within the brain at which the voluntary movements of the muscles of the face, thumb, hand, arm, trunk, and leg originate are known (Fig. 56-13). To initiate muscle movement, these particular cells must send the stimulus down along their fibers. Stimulation of these cells with an electric current will also result in muscle contraction. En route to the pons, the motor fibers converge into a tight bundle known as the internal capsule. A comparatively small injury to the capsule causes paralysis in more muscles than does a much larger injury to the cortex itself.

Within the medulla, the motor axons from the cortex form the motor pathways or tracts, notably the corticospinal or pyramidal tracts. Here, most of these fibers cross (or decussate) to the opposite side, continuing thereafter as the crossed pyramidal tract. The remaining fibers then enter the spinal cord on the original side as the direct pyramidal tract. Each fiber in this tract finally crosses to

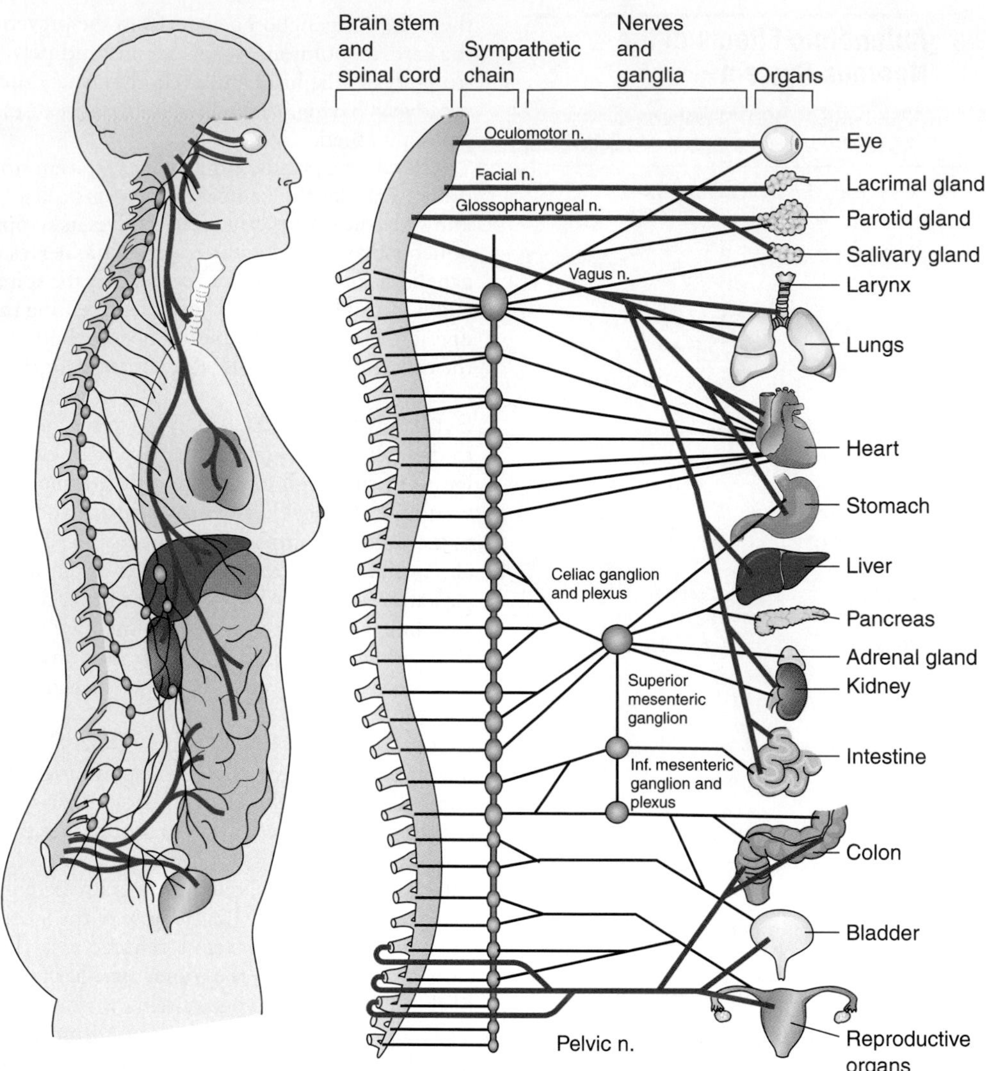

FIGURE 56•12 Anatomy of the autonomic nervous system. Adapted from Memmler, R. L., Cohen, B. J., & Wood, D. L. (1996). *The human body in health and disease* (8th ed.). Philadelphia: Lippincott-Raven.

the opposite side of the cord and terminates within the gray matter of the anterior horn on that side, in proximity to a motor nerve cell. Fibers of the crossed pyramidal tract terminate within the anterior horn and make connections with anterior horn cells on the same side. All of the motor fibers of the spinal nerves represent extensions of these anterior horn cells, with each of these fibers communicating with only one particular muscle fiber.

The motor system is complex, and motor function reflects the integrity of the corticospinal tracts, the extrapyramidal system, and cerebellar function. A motor impulse consists of a two-neuron pathway (described below). The motor nerve pathways are contained in the spinal cord. Some represent the pathways of the so-called extrapyramidal system, establishing connections between the anterior horn cells and the automatic control centers located in the basal ganglia and the cerebellum. Others are components of reflex arcs, forming synaptic connections between anterior horn cells and sensory fibers that have entered adjacent or neighboring segments of the cord.

UPPER AND LOWER MOTOR NEURONS

The voluntary motor system consists of two groups of neurons: upper motor neurons and lower motor neurons. Upper motor neurons originate in the cerebral cortex, the cerebellum, and the brain stem and modulate the activity of the lower motor neurons. Upper motor neuron fibers make up the descending motor pathways and are located entirely within the CNS. Lower motor neurons are located either in the anterior horn of the spinal cord gray matter or within cranial nerve nuclei in the brain stem. Axons of both extend through peripheral nerves and terminate in skeletal muscle. Lower motor neurons are therefore located in both the CNS and the peripheral nervous system.

The motor pathways from the brain to the spinal cord, as well as from the cerebrum to the brain stem, are formed by upper motor neurons. They begin in the cortex of the opposite side of the brain, descend through the internal capsule, cross to the opposite side in the brain stem, descend through the corticospinal tract, and synapse with the lower motor neurons in the cord. The lower motor neurons receive the impulse in the posterior part of the cord and run to the myoneural junction located in the peripheral muscle. The clinical features of lesions of upper and lower motor neurons are discussed in the sections that follow and in Table 56-4.

Upper Motor Neuron Lesions. Upper motor neuron lesions can involve the motor cortex, the internal capsule, the spinal cord, and other structures of the brain through which the cortico-

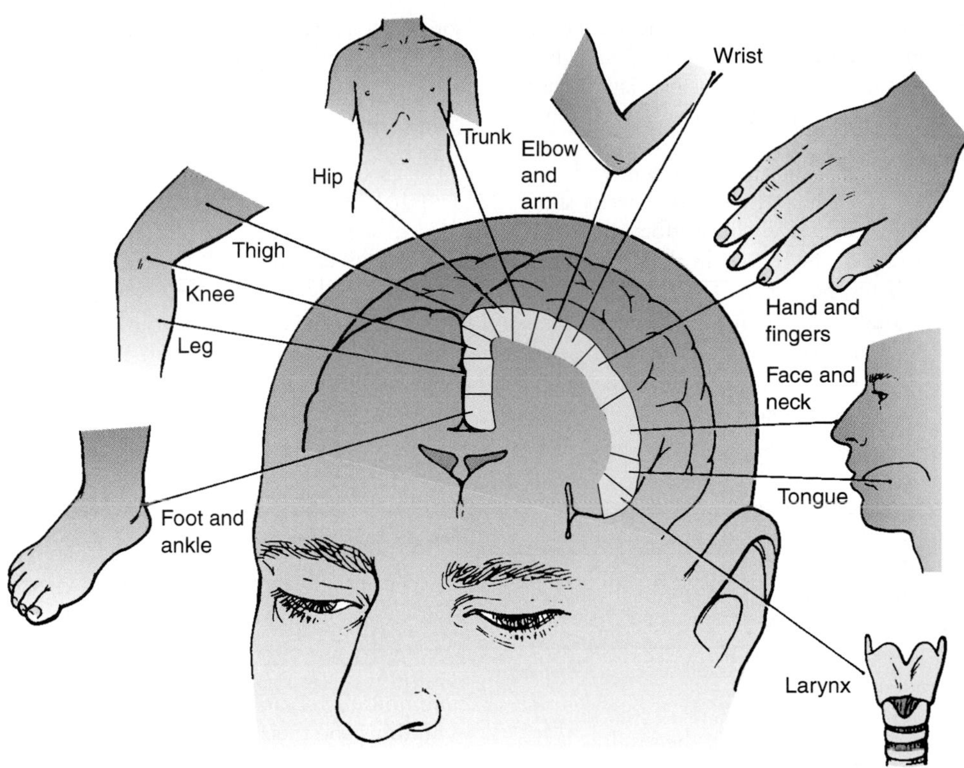

FIGURE 56•13 Diagrammatic representation of the cerebrum, showing locations for motor movements of various portions of the body. From Bullock, B. (1996). *Pathophysiology: Adaptations and alterations in function* (4th ed.). Philadelphia: Lippincott-Raven.

spinal tract descends. If the upper motor neurons are damaged or destroyed, as frequently occurs with stroke or spinal cord injury, paralysis (loss of voluntary movement) results. However, because the inhibitory influences of intact upper motor neurons are now impaired, **reflex** (involuntary) movements are uninhibited, and hence hyperactive deep tendon reflexes, diminished or absent superficial reflexes, and pathologic reflexes such as a Babinski response occur. Severe leg spasms can occur as the result of an upper motor neuron lesion; the spasms result from the preserved reflex arc, which lacks inhibition along the spinal cord below the level of injury.

There is little or no muscle atrophy, and muscles remain permanently tense, exhibiting spastic paralysis or paresis (weakness). Paralysis associated with upper motor neuron lesions usually affects a whole extremity, both extremities, or an entire half of the body. **Hemiplegia** (paralysis of an arm and leg on the same side of the body) can be the result of an upper motor neuron lesion. If hemorrhage, an embolus, or a thrombus destroys the fibers from the motor area in the internal capsule, the arm and the leg of the opposite side become stiff and very weak or paralyzed, and the reflexes are hyperactive. When both legs are paralyzed, the condition is called **paraplegia**. Paralysis of all four extremities is **quadriplegia**.

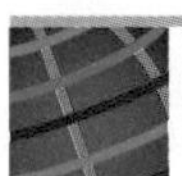

TABLE 56•4 Comparison of Upper Motor Neuron and Lower Motor Neuron Lesions

Upper Motor Neuron Lesions	Lower Motor Neuron Lesions
Loss of voluntary control	Loss of voluntary control
Increased muscle tone	Decreased muscle tone
Muscle spasticity	Flaccid muscle paralysis
No muscle atrophy	Muscle atrophy
Hyperactive and abnormal reflexes	Absent or decreased reflexes

Lower Motor Neuron Lesions. A patient is considered to have lower motor neuron damage if a motor nerve is severed between the muscle and the spinal cord. The result of lower motor neuron damage is muscle paralysis. Reflexes are lost, and the muscle becomes limp and atrophied from disuse. If the patient has injured the spinal trunk and it can heal, use of the muscles connected to that section of the spinal cord may be regained. If the anterior horn motor cells are destroyed, however, the nerves cannot regenerate and the muscles are never useful again. Flaccid paralysis and atrophy of the affected muscles are the principal signs of lower motor neuron disease. Lower motor neuron lesions can be the result of trauma, infection (poliomyelitis), toxins, vascular disorders, congenital malformations, degenerative processes, and neoplasms. Compression of nerve roots by herniated intervertebral disks is a common cause of lower motor neuron dysfunction.

COORDINATION OF MOVEMENT

The smoothness, accuracy, and strength that characterize the muscular movements of a normal person are attributable to the influence of the cerebellum and the basal ganglia.

The cerebellum (see Fig. 56-2), described earlier, is located beneath the occipital lobe of the cerebrum; it is responsible for the coordination, balance, and timing of all muscular movements that originate in the motor centers of the cerebral cortex. Through the action of the cerebellum, the contractions of opposing muscle groups are adjusted in relation to each other to maximal mechanical advantage; muscular contractions can be sustained evenly at the desired tension and without significant fluctuation, and reciprocal movements can be reproduced at high and constant speed, in stereotyped fashion and with relatively little effort.

The basal ganglia, masses of gray matter in the midbrain beneath the cerebral hemispheres, border the lateral ventricles and lie in proximity to the internal capsule. The basal ganglia play an important role in planning and coordinating motor movements and posture. Complex neural connections link the basal ganglia with the cerebral cortex. The major effect of these structures is to inhibit unwanted muscular activity; disorders of the basal ganglia result in exaggerated, uncontrolled movements.

Impaired cerebellar function, which may occur as a result of an intracranial injury or some type of an expanding mass (eg, a hemorrhage, abscess, or tumor), results in loss of muscle tone, weakness, and fatigue. Depending on the area of the brain affected, the patient has different motor symptoms or responses. The patient may demonstrate decorticate, decerebrate, or flaccid posturing, usually as a result of cerebral trauma.

- Decortication (**decorticate posturing**): the result of lesions of the internal capsule or cerebral hemispheres, in which the patient has flexion and internal rotation of the arms and wrists and extension, internal rotation, and plantar flexion of the feet.
- Decerebration (**decerebrate posturing**): the result of lesions at the midbrain; more ominous than decortication. The patient has extension and external rotation of the arms and wrists and extension, plantar flexion, and internal rotation of the feet.
- **Flaccid posturing:** usually the result of lower brain stem dysfunction. The patient has no motor function, is limp, and lacks motor tone.

Flaccidity preceded by decerebration in a patient with cerebral injury indicates severe neurologic impairment, which may precede brain death. However, before the declaration of brain death, the patient must have spinal cord injury ruled out, the effects of all neuromuscular paralyzing agents must have worn off, and any other possible treatable causes of neurologic impairment must be investigated.

Tumors, infection, or abscess and increased intracranial pressure can all affect the cerebellum. Cerebellar signs, such as ataxia, incoordination, and seizures, as well as CSF obstruction and compression of the brain stem may be seen. Signs of increased intracranial pressure, including vomiting, headache, and changes in vital signs and level of consciousness, are especially common when CSF flow is obstructed.

Destruction or dysfunction of the basal ganglia leads not to paralysis but to muscular rigidity, with consequent disturbances of posture and movement. Such patients tend to have involuntary movements. These may take the form of coarse tremors, most often in the upper extremities, particularly in the distal portions; athetosis, movement of a slow, squirming, writhing, twisting type; or chorea, marked by spasmodic, purposeless, irregular, uncoordinated motions of the trunk and the extremities, and facial grimacing. Disorders due to lesions of the basal ganglia include Parkinson's disease, Huntington's disease (see Chap. 59), Wilson's disease (hepatolenticular degeneration), and spasmodic torticollis.

Sensory System Function

INTEGRATING SENSORY IMPULSES

The thalamus, a major receiving and transmitting center for the afferent sensory nerves, is a large structure connected to the midbrain. It lies next to the third ventricle and forms the floor of the lateral ventricle (see Fig. 56-3). The thalamus serves to integrate all sensory impulses except olfaction. It plays a role in the conscious awareness of pain and the recognition of variation in temperature and touch. The thalamus is responsible for the sense of movement and position and the ability to recognize the size, shape, and quality of objects.

RECEIVING SENSORY IMPULSES

Afferent impulses travel from their points of origin to their destinations in the cerebral cortex via the ascending pathways directly, or they may cross at the level of the spinal cord or in the medulla, depending on the type of sensation that is registered. Sensory information may be integrated at the level of the spinal cord or may be relayed to the brain. Knowledge of these pathways is important for neurologic assessment and for understanding symptoms and their relation to various lesions.

The axon of the nerve in which the sensory impulse originates enters the spinal cord by way of the posterior root. Axons conveying sensations of heat, cold, and pain immediately enter the posterior gray column of the cord, where they make connections with the cells of secondary neurons. Pain and temperature fibers cross immediately to the opposite side of the cord and course upward to the thalamus. Fibers carrying sensations of touch, light pressure, and localization do not connect immediately with the second neuron but ascend the cord for a variable distance before entering the gray matter and completing this connection. The axon of the secondary neuron crosses the cord and proceeds upward to the thalamus.

Position and vibratory sensation are produced by stimuli arising from muscles, joints, and bones. These stimuli are conveyed, uncrossed, all the way to the brain stem by the axon of the primary neuron. In the medulla, synaptic connections are made with cells of the secondary neurons, whose axons cross to the opposite side and then proceed to the thalamus.

SENSORY LOSSES

Destruction of a sensory nerve results in total loss of sensation in its area of distribution. Transection of the spinal cord yields complete anesthesia below the level of injury. Selective destruction or degeneration of the posterior columns of the spinal cord is responsible for a loss of position and vibratory sense in segments distal to the lesion, without loss of touch, pain, or temperature perception. A lesion, such as a cyst, in the center of the spinal cord causes dissociation of sensation—loss of pain at the level of the lesion. This occurs because the fibers carrying pain and temperature cross within the cord immediately on entering; thus, any lesion that divides the cord longitudinally divides these fibers. Other sensory fibers ascend the cord for variable distances, some even to the medulla, before crossing, thereby bypassing the lesion and avoiding destruction.

Irritative lesions affecting the posterior spinal nerve roots may cause impairment of tactile sensation, including intermittent severe pain that is referred to their areas of distribution. Tingling of the fingers and the toes can be a prominent symptom of spinal cord disease, presumably due to degenerative changes in the sensory fibers that extend to the thalamus (ie, belonging to the spinothalamic tract).

ASSESSMENT: THE NEUROLOGIC EXAMINATION

The neurologic examination is a systematic process that includes a variety of tests, observations, and assessments designed to evaluate a complex system. Although the neurologic examination is often limited to a simple screening, the examiner must be able to conduct a thorough neurologic assessment when the history or other physical findings warrant it.

The brain and spinal cord cannot be examined as directly as other systems of the body. Thus, much of the neurologic examination is an indirect evaluation that assesses the function of the specific body part or parts controlled or innervated by the nervous system. A neurologic assessment is divided into five components: cerebral function, cranial nerves, motor system, sensory system, and reflexes. As in other parts of the physical assessment, the neurologic examination follows a logical sequence and progresses from higher levels of cortical function to a determination of the integrity of peripheral nerves.

Much of the patient's neurologic function is assessed during the history and during early parts of the physical examination. Much can be learned about speech patterns, mental status, gait, stance, motor power, and coordination during the nurse–patient interaction. The simple act of shaking a patient's hand in greeting can provide useful information to the alert examiner.

Assessing Cerebral Function

Cerebral abnormalities may cause disturbances in communication and intellectual functioning and in patterns of emotional behavior.

Mental Status

An assessment of mental status begins by observing the patient's appearance and behavior, noting the patient's dress, grooming, and personal hygiene. Posture, gestures, movements, facial expressions, and motor activity often provide important information about the patient. The patient's manner of speech and level of consciousness are also assessed. Is the patient's speech clear and coherent? Is the patient alert and responsive, or drowsy and stuporous?

Assessing orientation to time, place, and person assists in evaluating the patient's mental status. Does the patient know what day it is, what year it is, and the name of the president of the United States? Is the patient aware of where he or she is? Is the patient aware of who the examiner is and of his or her purpose for being in the room? Is the capacity for immediate memory intact? (See Chart 11-1: Mini-Mental State Examination [MMSE] in Chap. 11.)

Intellectual Function

A person with an average IQ can repeat seven digits without faltering and can recite five digits backward. The examiner might ask the patient to count backward from 100 or to subtract 7 from 100, then 7 from that, and so forth (called serial 7s). The capacity to interpret well-known proverbs tests abstract reasoning, which is a higher intellectual function; for example, does the patient know what is meant by "the early bird catches the worm"? Often, patients who are toxic or who have destruction of the frontal cortex appear superficially normal until one or more tests of integrative capacity are performed.

Thought Content

During the course of the interview, it is important to assess the patient's thought content. Are the patient's thoughts spontaneous, natural, clear, relevant, and coherent? Does the patient have any fixed ideas, illusions, or preoccupations? What are his or her insights into these thoughts? Preoccupation with death or morbid events, evidence of hallucinations, and paranoid ideation are all important and require further evaluation.

Emotional Status

An assessment of cerebral functioning also includes the patient's emotional status. Is the patient's affect natural and even, or irritable and angry, anxious, apathetic, or euphoric? Does his or her mood fluctuate normally, or does the patient unpredictably swing from joy to sadness during the interview? Is affect appropriate to words and thought content? Are verbal communications consistent with nonverbal cues?

Perception

The examiner may now consider more specific areas of higher cortical function. **Agnosia** is the inability to interpret or recognize objects seen through the special senses. The patient may see a pencil but not know what it is called or what to do with it. The patient may even be able to describe it but not to interpret its function. The patient may experience auditory or tactile agnosia as well as visual agnosia. Each of the dysfunctions implicates a different part of the cortex (Chart 56-1).

Screening for visual and tactile agnosia provides insight into the patient's cortical interpretation ability. The patient is shown a familiar object and asked to identify it by name. Tactile interpretation is easily assessed by placing a familiar object (eg, key, coin) in the patient's hand and having him or her identify it while both eyes are closed.

Motor Ability

Assessment of cortical motor integration is carried out by asking the patient to perform a skilled act (throw a ball, move a chair). Successful performance requires the ability to understand the activity

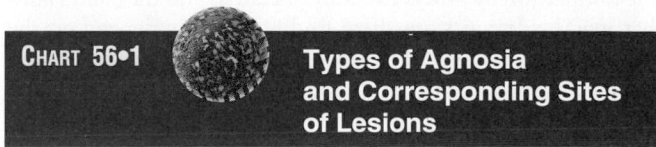

Type of Agnosia	Affected Cerebral Area
Visual	Occipital lobe
Auditory	Temporal lobe (lateral and superior portions)
Tactile	Parietal lobe
Body parts and relationships	Parietal lobe (posteroinferior regions)

CHART 56•2  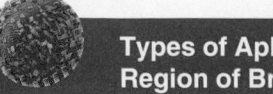 Types of Aphasia and Region of Brain Involved

Type of Aphasia	Brain Area Involved
Auditory-receptive	Temporal lobe
Visual-receptive	Parietal-occipital area
Expressive speaking	Inferior posterior frontal areas
Expressive writing	Posterior frontal area

desired and normal motor strength. Failure signals cerebral dysfunction.

Language Ability

Language function is also assessed. The person with normal neurologic function can understand and communicate in spoken and written language. Does the patient answer questions appropriately? Can he or she read a sentence from a newspaper and explain its meaning? Can the patient write his or her name or copy a simple figure that the examiner has drawn? A deficiency in language function is called **aphasia**. Different types of aphasia result from injury to different parts of the brain (Chart 56-2). Aphasia is discussed in detail in Chapter 57.

Impact on Lifestyle

The nurse includes in the assessment of neurologic function the impact the neurologic impairment has on the patient's lifestyle. Two issues are important in considering the impact of neurologic impairment: first, the limitations imposed by the neurologic deficit on the patient and the patient's role in society, including family and community, and second, a plan of care that will support adaptation to the neurologic deficit within the patient's support system.

Documentation of Findings

Interpretation and documentation of neurologic abnormalities, particularly mental status, should be specific and nonjudgmental. Lengthy descriptions and the use of terms such as "inappropriate" or "demented" should be avoided. Terms such as these often mean different things to different people and are therefore not useful when describing behavior. The examiner records and reports specific observations regarding orientation, level of consciousness, emotional state, or thought content, all of which permit comparison by others over time. Analysis and the conclusions that may be drawn from these findings usually depend on the examiner's knowledge of neuroanatomy, neurophysiology, and neuropathology.

Examining the Cranial Nerves

Table 56-5 describes how to assess the cranial nerves.

Examining the Motor System

A thorough examination of the motor system includes an assessment of muscle size, tone, and strength, coordination, and balance. The patient is instructed to walk across the room while the examiner observes posture and gait. The muscles are inspected, and palpated if necessary, for their size and symmetry. Any evidence of atrophy or involuntary movements (tremors, tics) is noted. Muscle **tone** (the tension present in a muscle at rest) is evaluated by palpating various muscle groups at rest and during passive movement. Resistance to these movements is assessed and documented. Abnormalities in tone include **spasticity** (increased muscle tone), rigidity, and flaccidity.

Muscle Strength

Muscle strength is tested by assessing the patient's ability to flex or extend the extremities against resistance. The function of an individual muscle or group of muscles is evaluated by placing the muscle at a disadvantage. The quadriceps, for example, is a powerful muscle responsible for straightening the leg. Once the leg is straightened, it is exceedingly difficult for the examiner to flex the knee. Conversely, if the knee is flexed and the patient is asked to straighten the leg against resistance, a more subtle disability can be elicited. It is important to compare both sides of the body to detect subtle difference in muscle strength.

Many clinicians use a five-point scale to rate muscle strength. A 5 indicates full power of contraction; 4 indicates fair but not full strength; 3 indicates just sufficient strength to overcome the force of gravity; 2 indicates the ability to move but not to overcome the force of gravity; 1 indicates minimal contractile power; and 0 indicates no contraction whatsoever.

Assessment of muscle strength can be as detailed as necessary. One may quickly test the strength of the proximal muscles of the upper and lower extremities, always comparing both sides. The strength of the finer muscles that control the function of the hand (hand grasp) and the foot (dorsiflexion and plantar flexion) can then be assessed.

Balance and Coordination

Cerebellar influence on the motor system is reflected in balance control and coordination. Coordination in the hands and upper extremities is tested by having the patient perform rapid, alternating movements and point-to-point testing. First, the patient is instructed to pat the thigh as fast as possible with each hand separately. Then the patient is instructed to alternately pronate and supinate the hand as rapidly as possible. Lastly, the patient is asked to touch each of the fingers with the thumb in a consecutive motion. Speed, symmetry, and degree of difficulty are noted.

Point-to-point testing is accomplished by having the patient touch the examiner's extended finger and then his or her own nose. This is repeated several times. This assessment is then carried out with the patient's eyes closed.

Coordination in the lower extremities is tested by having the patient run the heel down the anterior surface of the tibia of the other leg. Each leg is tested in turn. **Ataxia** is defined as incoordination of voluntary muscle action, particularly of the muscle groups used in activities such as walking or reaching for objects. The presence of ataxia or tremors (rhythmic, involuntary movements) during these movements suggests cerebellar disease.

It is not necessary to carry out each of these assessments for coordination. During a routine examination, it is advisable to perform a simple screening of the upper and lower extremities by having the patient perform either rapid, alternating movements or point-to-point testing. When abnormalities are observed, a more thorough examination is indicated.

The Romberg test is a screening test for balance. The patient stands with feet together and arms at the side, first with eyes open and then with both eyes closed for 20 to 30 seconds. The exam-

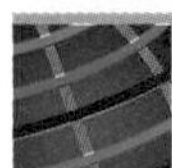

TABLE 56•5 **Assessing Cranial Nerve Function**

Cranial Nerve	Clinical Examination
I (olfactory)	With eyes closed, the patient identifies familiar odors (coffee, tobacco). Each nostril is tested separately.
II (optic)	Snellen eye chart; visual fields; ophthalmoscopic examination
III (oculomotor) IV (trochlear) VI (abducens)	For cranial nerves III, IV, and VI: test for ocular rotations, conjugate movements, nystagmus. Test for pupillary reflexes, and inspect eyelids for ptosis.
V (trigeminal)	Have patient close the eyes. Touch cotton to forehead, cheeks, and jaw. Opposite sides of face are compared. Sensitivity to superficial pain is tested by using the sharp and dull ends of a broken tongue blade. Alternate between the sharp point and the dull end. Patient reports "sharp" or "dull" with each movement. If responses are incorrect, test for temperature sensation. Test tubes of cold and hot water are used alternately. While the patient looks up, *lightly* touch a wisp of cotton against the temporal surface of each cornea. A blink and tearing is a normal response. Have the patient clench the jaw and move it from side to side. Palpate the masseter and temporal muscles, noting strength and equality.
VII (facial)	Observe for symmetry while the patient performs facial movements: smiles, whistles, elevates eyebrows, frowns, tightly closes eyelids against resistance (examiner attempts to open them). Observe face for flaccid paralysis (shallow nasolabial folds). Patient extends tongue. Ability to discriminate between sugar and salt is tested.
VIII (vestibulocochlear)	Whisper or watch-tick test Test for lateralization (Weber) Test for air and bone conduction (Rinne)
IX (glossopharyngeal)	Assess patient's ability to discriminate between sugar and salt on posterior third of the tongue.
X (vagus)	Depress a tongue blade on posterior tongue, or stimulate posterior pharynx to elicit gag reflex. Note any hoarseness in voice. Have patient say "ah." Observe for symmetric rise of uvula and soft palate.
XI (spinal accessory)	Palpate and note strength of trapezius muscles while patient shrugs shoulders against resistance. Palpate and note strength of each sternocleidomastoid muscle as patient turns head against opposing pressure of the examiner's hand.
XII (hypoglossal)	While the patient protrudes the tongue, any deviation or tremors are noted. The strength of the tongue is tested by having the patient move the protruded tongue from side to side against a tongue depressor.

iner stands close to reassure the patient of support if he or she begins to fall. Slight swaying is normal, but a loss of balance is abnormal and is considered a positive Romberg sign. Additional cerebellar tests for balance in the ambulatory patient include hopping in place, alternating knee bends, and heel-to-toe walking (both forward and backward).

Examining the Reflexes

The motor reflexes are involuntary contractions of muscles or muscle groups in response to abrupt stretching near the site of the muscle's insertion. The tendon is struck directly with a reflex hammer or indirectly by striking the examiner's thumb, which is placed firmly against the tendon. Testing these reflexes enables the examiner to assess involuntary reflex arcs that depend on the presence of afferent stretch receptors, spinal synapses, efferent motor fibers, and a variety of modifying influences from higher levels. Common reflexes that may be tested include the deep tendon reflexes (biceps, brachioradialis, triceps, patellar, and ankle reflexes) and superficial or cutaneous reflexes (abdominal reflexes and plantar or Babinski response) (Fig. 56-14).

Technique

A reflex hammer is used to elicit a deep tendon reflex. The handle of the hammer is held loosely between the thumb and index finger, allowing a full swinging motion. The wrist motion is similar to that used during percussion. The extremity is positioned so that the tendon is slightly stretched. This requires a sound knowledge of the location of muscles and their tendon attachments. The tendon is then struck briskly, and the response is compared with that on the opposite side of the body. A wide variation in reflex response may be considered normal; it is more important, however, that the reflexes be symmetrically equivalent. When the comparison is made, both sides should be equivalently relaxed and each tendon struck with equal force.

Valid findings depend on several factors: proper use of the reflex hammer, proper positioning of the extremity, and a relaxed patient. If the reflexes are symmetrically diminished or absent, the examiner may use reinforcement to increase reflex activity. This involves the isometric contraction of other muscle groups. If lower extremity reflexes are diminished or absent, the patient is instructed to lock the fingers together and pull in opposite directions. Having the patient clench the jaw or press the heels against the floor or examining table may similarly elicit more reliable biceps, triceps, and brachioradialis reflexes.

Grading the Reflexes

The absence of reflexes is significant, although ankle jerks (Achilles reflex) may be normally absent in older people. Reflex responses are often graded on a scale of 0 to 4+. A 4+ indicates a hyperactive reflex with sustained clonus; 3+ indicates a hyperactive reflex; 2+ indicates a normal reflex; 1+ indicates a hypoactive reflex; and 0 is an absent reflex. As stated previously, scale ratings are highly subjective. When used, the findings are recorded as a fraction,

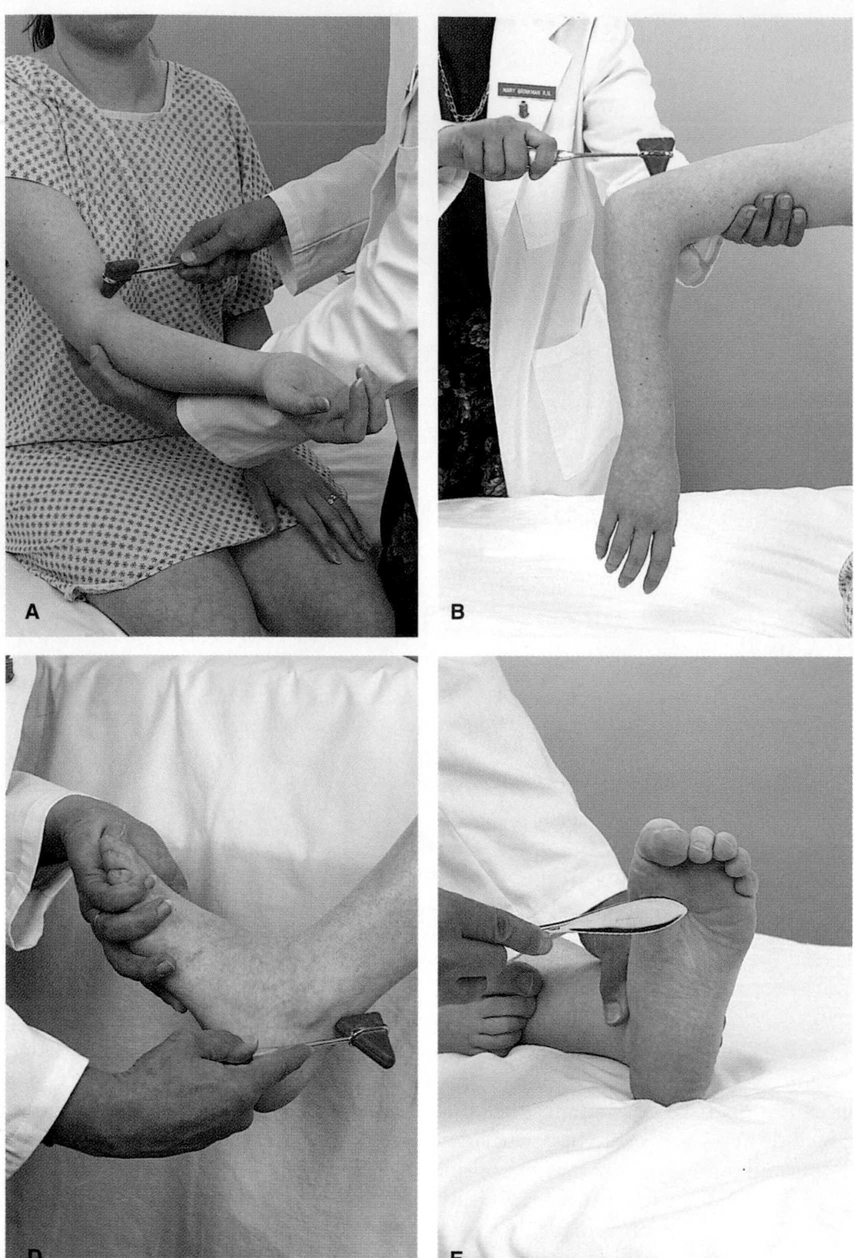

FIGURE 56•14 Techniques for eliciting major reflexes. (**A**) Biceps reflex. (**B**) Triceps reflex. (**C**) Patellar reflex. (**D**) Ankle or Achilles reflex. (**E**) Babinski response. From Weber, J. W., & Kelley, J. (1998). *Health assessment in nursing.* Philadelphia: Lippincott-Raven.

indicating the scale range (eg, 2⁄4). Some examiners prefer to use the terms present, absent, and diminished when describing reflexes.

Biceps Reflex

The biceps reflex is elicited by striking the biceps tendon of the flexed elbow. The examiner supports the forearm with one arm while placing the thumb against the tendon and striking the thumb with the reflex hammer. The normal response is flexion at the elbow and contraction of the biceps (see Fig. 56-14A).

Triceps Reflex

To elicit a triceps reflex, the patient's arm is flexed at the elbow and positioned in front of the chest. The examiner supports the patient's arm and identifies the triceps tendon by palpating 2.5 to 5 cm (1 to 2 in) above the elbow. A direct blow on the tendon normally produces contraction of the triceps muscle and extension of the elbow (see Fig. 56-14B).

Brachioradialis Reflex

With the patient's forearm resting on the lap or across the abdomen, the brachioradialis reflex is assessed. A gentle strike of the hammer 2.5 to 5 cm (1 to 2 in) above the wrist results in flexion and supination of the forearm.

Patellar Reflex

The patellar reflex is elicited by striking the patellar tendon just below the patella. The patient may be in a sitting or a lying position. If the patient is supine, the examiner supports the legs to facilitate relaxation of the muscles. Contraction of the quadriceps and knee extension are normal responses (see Fig. 56-14C).

Ankle Reflex

To elicit an ankle (Achilles) reflex, the foot is dorsiflexed at the ankle and the hammer strikes the stretched Achilles tendon (see Fig. 56-14D). This reflex normally produces plantar flexion. If the examiner cannot elicit the ankle reflex and suspects that the patient cannot relax, the patient is instructed to kneel on a chair or similar elevated, flat surface. This position places the ankles in dorsiflexion and reduces any muscular tension in the gastrocnemius. The Achilles tendons are struck in turn, and plantar flexion is usually demonstrated.

Clonus

When reflexes are very hyperactive, a phenomenon called clonus may be elicited. If the foot is abruptly dorsiflexed, it may continue to "beat" two or three times before it settles into a position of rest. Occasionally, in CNS disease this activity persists, and the foot does not come to rest while the tendon is being stretched but persists in repetitive activity. The unsustained clonus associated with normal but hyperactive reflexes is not considered pathologic. Sustained clonus always indicates the presence of CNS disease and requires further evaluation.

Abdominal Contraction Reflex

Certain superficial reflexes may be elicited by scratching the skin of the abdominal wall or the inside of the thigh in men. The former results in involuntary contraction of the abdominal muscles, and the latter results in retraction of the scrotum.

Babinski Response

A well-known reflex indicative of CNS disease affecting the corticospinal tract is the **Babinski response**. If the lateral aspect of the sole of the foot of a person with an intact CNS is stroked, the toes contract and are drawn together (see Fig. 56-14E). In patients who have CNS disease of the motor system, however, the toes fan out and are drawn back. This is normal in newborns but represents a serious abnormality in adults. Several other reflexes convey similar information. Many of them are interesting but not particularly informative.

Sensory Examination

The sensory system is even more complex than the motor system because sensory modalities are carried in different tracts, located in different portions of the spinal cord. The sensory examination is largely subjective and requires the cooperation of the patient. The examiner should be familiar with dermatomes that represent the distribution of the peripheral nerves that arise from the spinal cord (see Fig. 56-11). Most sensory deficits result from peripheral neuropathy and follow anatomic dermatomes. Exceptions to this include major destructive lesions of the brain; loss of sensation, which may affect an entire side of the body; and the neuropathies associated with alcoholism, which occur in a glove-and-stocking distribution.

Assessment of the sensory system involves tests for tactile sensation, superficial pain, vibration, and position sense (proprioception). Throughout the sensory assessment, the patient's eyes are closed. The cooperation of the patient is encouraged by simple directions and reassurance that the examiner will not hurt or startle the patient.

Tactile sensation is assessed by lightly touching a cotton wisp to corresponding areas on each side of the body. The sensitivity of proximal parts of the extremities is compared with that of distal parts.

Pain and temperature sensations are transmitted together in the lateral part of the spinal cord. Thus, it is not necessary to test for temperature sense in most circumstances. Superficial pain perception can be assessed by determining the patient's sensitivity to a sharp object. The patient is asked to differentiate between the sharp and dull ends of a broken wooden cotton swab or tongue blade; using a safety pin is avoided because it breaks the integrity of the skin. Both the sharp and dull sides of the object are applied with equal intensity at all times, and the two sides are compared.

Vibration and proprioception are transmitted together in the posterior part of the cord. Vibration may be evaluated through the use of a low-frequency (128- or 256-Hertz) tuning fork. The handle of the vibrating fork is placed against a bony prominence, and the patient is asked whether he or she feels a sensation and is instructed to signal the examiner when the sensation ceases. Common locations used to test for vibratory sense include the distal joint of the great toe and the the proximal thumb joint. If the patient does not perceive the vibrations at the distal bony prominences, the examiner progresses upward with the tuning fork until the vibrations are perceived by the patient. As with all measurements of sensation, a side-to-side comparison is made.

Position sense or proprioception may be determined by asking the patient to close both eyes and indicate, as the great toe is alternately moved up and down, in which direction movement has taken place. Vibration and position sense are often lost together, frequently in circumstances in which all others remain intact.

Integration of sensation in the brain is evaluated next. This may be performed by testing two-point discrimination—when the patient is touched with two sharp objects simultaneously, are they perceived as two or as one? If touched simultaneously on opposite sides of the body, the patient should normally report being touched in two places. If only one site is reported, the one not being recognized is said to demonstrate extinction. A good test of higher cortical sensory ability is stereognosis. The patient is instructed to close both eyes and identify a variety of objects (eg, keys, coins) that are placed in one hand by the examiner.

GERONTOLOGIC CONSIDERATIONS

The nervous system of older adults undergoes many changes from the normal aging process and is extremely vulnerable to general systemic illness. Changes throughout the nervous system vary in degree as the person ages. Nerve fibers that connect directly to muscles show little decline in function with age, as do simple neurologic functions that involve a number of connections in the spinal cord. Disease in the elderly often makes it difficult to distinguish normal from abnormal changes.

Structural Changes

Many elderly people assume a flexed posture and display muscle rigidity, tremor, and a slowness in movements. Among the known structural alterations that occur with increasing age are a decrease in brain weight and in the number of synapses. The loss of neurons occurs in select layers and regions of the brain but is not consistent throughout the CNS. Memory loss, particularly for recent events, and slower reaction times may be annoyances to the elderly, and they may require extra time to choose among several responses to a situation.

A number of other neurologic alterations occur with the aging process. For example, the pupillary response becomes more sluggish or may not appear at all if the individual has cataracts. Other changes include diminished or absent Achilles reflexes, loss of strength, and muscle wasting.

Sensory Alterations

Sensory isolation due to visual and hearing loss causes confusion, anxiety, disorientation, misinterpretation, and feelings of inadequacy. Sensory alterations may require modification of the home environment such as large-print reading material or sound enhancement for the telephone, as well as extra orientation to new surroundings. Simple explanations of routines, the location of the bathroom, and how to operate the call bell are just a few examples of information the elderly patient needs when hospitalized.

Temperature Regulation and Pain Perception

Other manifestations of neurologic changes are related to temperature regulation and pain. The elderly patient usually feels cold more easily than heat and may require extra covering when in bed; a room temperature somewhat higher than usual may be desirable. Reaction to painful stimuli may be decreased with age. Because pain is an important warning signal, caution must be used when hot or cold packs are used. The older patient may be burned or suffer frostbite before being aware of any discomfort. Complaints of pain, such as abdominal discomfort or chest pain, may be more serious than the patient's perception might indicate and thus require careful evaluation.

Taste and Smell Alterations

The acuity of the taste buds decreases with age; along with an altered olfactory sense, this may cause a decreased appetite. Extra seasoning often increases food intake as long as it does not cause gastric irritation. A decreased sense of smell due to atrophy of olfactory organs may present a safety hazard, because elderly people living alone may be unable to detect household gas leaks or fires if they occur. Smoke and carbon monoxide detectors, important for all, are critical for the elderly.

Tactile and Visual Alterations

Another neurologic alteration in the elderly patient is the dulling of tactile sensation due to a decrease in the number of areas of the body responding to all stimuli and in the number and sensitivity of sensory receptors. There may be difficulty in identifying objects by touch, and because fewer tactile cues are received from the bottom of the feet, the person may get confused as to body position and location.

These factors, combined with sensitivity to glare, decreased peripheral vision, and a constricted visual field, may result in disorientation, especially at night when there is little or no light in the room. Because the elderly person takes longer to recover visual sensitivity when moving from a light to dark area, night lights and a safe and familiar arrangement of furniture are essential.

Mental Status

Mental status is evaluated while the history is obtained, and areas of judgment, intelligence, memory, affect, mood, orientation, speech, and grooming are assessed. Changes in mental status may be noticed by family members who bring the patient to the attention of the health care provider. Drug toxicity should always be suspected as a causative factor when the patient has a change in mental status. **Delirium** (mental confusion, usually with delusions and hallucinations) is seen in elderly patients who have underlying CNS damage or are experiencing an acute condition such as infection or dehydration. **Dementia** (deterioration of intellectual function) may be reversible and treatable (as in drug toxicity or thyroid disease) or chronic and irreversible. Depression may produce impairment of attention and memory.

Nursing Implications

Nursing care for the patient with an aging nervous system should include the modifications previously described. In addition, patient teaching is also affected because the nurse must understand the altered responses and the changing needs of the elderly patient before beginning to teach.

When caring for the elderly patient, the nurse adapts activities such as preoperative teaching, diet therapy, and instruction about new medications, their timing, and doses to the changes in the aging nervous system. The nurse considers the presence of decline in fine motor movement and failing vision. When using visual materials for teaching or menu selection, adequate lighting without glare, contrasting colors, and large print are used to offset visual difficulties caused by rigidity and opacity of the lens in the eye and slower pupillary reaction.

Procedures and preparations needed for diagnostic tests are explained, taking into account the possibility of impaired hearing and slowed responses in the elderly. Even with hearing loss, the elderly patient often hears adequately if the health care provider uses a low-pitched, clear speaking voice; shouting only makes it harder for the patient to understand the spoken voice. Providing auditory and visual cues aids understanding.

Teaching at an unrushed pace and using reinforcement enhances learning and retention. Material should be short, concise, and concrete. Vocabulary is matched to the patient's ability, and terms are clearly defined. The elderly patient requires adequate time to receive and respond to stimuli, to learn, and to react. These measures allow comprehension, memory, and formation of association and concepts.

DIAGNOSTIC EVALUATION

Computed Tomography Scanning

Computed tomography (CT) makes use of a narrow x-ray beam to scan the head in successive layers. The images provide cross-sectional views of the brain, with distinguishing differences in tissue densities of the skull, cortex, subcortical structures, and ventricles. The brightness of each slice of the brain in the final image is proportional to the degree to which it absorbs x-ray. The image is displayed on an oscilloscope or TV monitor and is photographed and stored digitally.

Lesions in the brain are seen as variations in tissue density differing from the surrounding normal brain tissue. Abnormalities of tissue indicate possible tumor masses, brain infarction, displacement of the ventricles, and cortical atrophy. Whole-body CT scanners allow sections of the spinal cord to be visualized. The injection of a water-soluble iodinated contrast agent into the subarachnoid space through lumbar puncture improves the visualization of the spinal and intracranial contents on these images. The CT scan, along with magnetic resonance imaging (MRI), has largely replaced the myelogram as a diagnostic procedure for the diagnosis of herniated lumbar disks.

CT scanning is usually performed first without contrast material and then with intravenous contrast enhancement. The patient lies on an adjustable table with the head held in a fixed position, while the scanning system rotates around the head and produces cross-sectional images. The patient must lie with the head held perfectly still without talking or moving the face, because head motion will distort the image.

CT scanning is noninvasive and painless and has a high degree of sensitivity for detecting lesions. With advances in CT scanning, the number of disorders and injuries that can be diagnosed is increasing, and the need for invasive diagnostic procedures is decreasing.

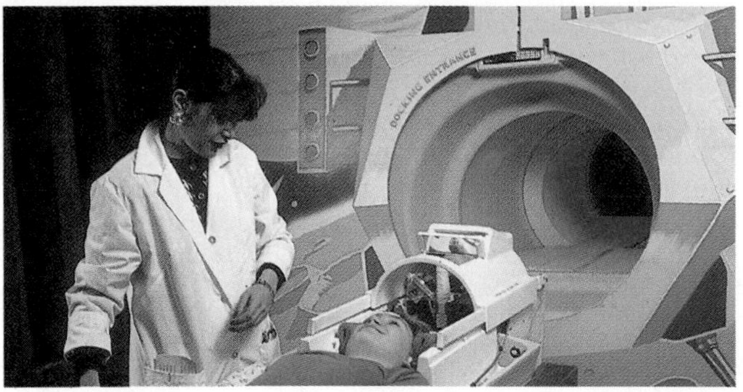

FIGURE 56•15 Technician explains what to expect during MRI.

Positron Emission Tomography

Positron emission tomography (PET) is a computer-based nuclear imaging technique that produces images of actual organ functioning. The patient either inhales a radioactive gas or is injected with a radioactive substance that emits positively charged particles. When these positrons combine with negatively charged electrons (normally found in the body's cells), the resultant gamma rays can be detected by a scanning device that produces a series of two-dimensional views at various levels of the brain. This information is integrated by a computer and gives a composite picture of the brain at work.

PET permits the measurement of blood flow, tissue composition, and brain metabolism. The brain is one of the most metabolically active organs, consuming 80% of the glucose the body uses. PET measures this activity in specific areas of the brain and can detect changes in glucose use.

This test is useful in showing metabolic changes in the brain (Alzheimer's disease), locating lesions (brain tumor, epileptogenic lesions), identifying blood flow and oxygen metabolism in patients with strokes, evaluating new therapies for brain tumors, and revealing biochemical abnormalities associated with mental illness. PET scanning is currently not widely available.

Nursing Interventions

Key nursing interventions include patient preparation, which involves explaining the test and teaching the patient about inhalation techniques and the possible sensations (eg, dizziness, lightheadedness, headache) that may occur. The intravenous injection of the radioactive substance produces similar side effects. Relaxation exercises may reduce anxiety during the test.

Single Photon Emission Computed Tomography

Single photon emission computed tomography (SPECT) is a three-dimensional imaging technique that uses radionuclides and instruments to detect single photons. Gamma photons are emitted from a radiopharmaceutical agent administered to the patient and are detected by a rotating gamma camera or cameras; the image is sent to a minicomputer. This approach allows areas behind overlying structures or background to be viewed, greatly increasing the contrast between normal and abnormal tissue. It is relatively inexpensive, and patient participation time is similar to that of CT scanning.

SPECT is useful in detecting the extent and location of abnormally perfused areas of the brain, thus allowing detection, localization, and sizing of stroke (before it is visible by CT scan), localization of seizure foci in epilepsy, and evaluation of perfusion before and after neurosurgical procedures. Pregnancy and breastfeeding are contraindications to SPECT. Therefore, premenopausal women are advised to practice effective contraception before and for several days after testing, and the woman who is breastfeeding is instructed to stop nursing for the period of time recommended by the nuclear medicine department.

Magnetic Resonance Imaging

MRI uses a powerful magnetic field to obtain images of different areas of the body (Fig. 56-15). Hydrogen nuclei (protons) within the body align like small magnets in a magnetic field. In combination with radiofrequency pulses, the protons emit signals, which are converted to images. MRI has the potential for identifying a cerebral abnormality earlier and more clearly than other diagnostic tests. It can provide information about the chemical changes within cells, thus allowing the clinician to monitor a tumor's response to treatment. It is particularly useful in the diagnosis of multiple sclerosis. MRI does not involve ionizing radiation.

Nursing Interventions

Before the patient enters the room where the MRI is to be performed, all metallic objects and credit cards (the magnetic field can erase them) are removed. A history is obtained to determine the presence of any metal objects inside the patient (eg, aneurysm clips, orthopedic hardware, pacemakers, artificial heart valves, intrauterine devices). These objects could malfunction, be dislodged, or heat up as they absorb energy.

The patient lies on a flat platform that is moved into a tube containing the magnet. The scanning process is painless, but the patient hears loud thumping of the magnetic coils as the magnetic field is being pulsed. Because the MRI scanner is a narrow tube, patients may experience claustrophobia; sedation may be prescribed in these circumstances. Newer versions of MRI machines are less claustrophobic than the earlier devices and are available in some locations. However, the images produced on these machines are not optimal, and the traditional device is preferable.

Patient preparation should include teaching relaxation techniques and informing the patient that he or she will be able to talk to the staff by means of a microphone located inside the scanner.

Cerebral Angiography

Cerebral angiography is an x-ray study of the cerebral circulation with a contrast agent injected into a selected artery. Cerebral angiography is a valuable tool to investigate vascular disease, aneurysms, and arteriovenous malformations. It is frequently performed before craniotomy to assess the patency and adequacy of the cerebral circulation and to determine the site, size, and nature of the pathologic processes.

Most cerebral angiograms are performed by threading a catheter through the femoral artery in the groin and up to the desired vessel. Alternatively, direct puncture of the carotid or vertebral artery or retrograde injection of a contrast agent into the brachial artery may be performed.

Nursing Interventions

The patient should be well hydrated, and clear liquids are usually permitted up to the time of the study. Before going to the radiology department, the patient is instructed to void. The locations of the appropriate peripheral pulses are marked with a felt-tip pen. The patient is instructed to remain immobile during the angiogram process and is told to expect a brief feeling of warmth in the face, behind the eyes, or in the jaw, teeth, tongue, and lips, and a metallic taste when the contrast agent is injected.

After the groin is shaved and prepared, a local anesthetic is administered to prevent pain at the insertion site and to reduce arterial spasm. A catheter is introduced into the femoral artery, flushed with heparinized saline, and filled with contrast agent. Fluoroscopy is used to guide the catheter to the appropriate vessels. During injection of the contrast agent, images are made of the arterial and venous phases of circulation through the brain.

Nursing care after cerebral angiography includes observation for signs and symptoms of altered cerebral blood flow. In some instances, patients may experience major or minor arterial blockage due to embolism, thrombosis, or hemorrhage, producing a neurologic deficit. Signs of such an occurrence include alterations in the level of responsiveness and consciousness, weakness on one side of the body, motor or sensory deficits, and speech disturbances. Therefore, it is necessary to observe the patient frequently for these signs and to report them immediately if they occur.

The injection site is observed for hematoma formation (a localized collection of blood), and an ice bag may be applied intermittently to the puncture site to relieve swelling and discomfort. Because a hematoma at the puncture site or embolization to a distant artery affects the peripheral pulses, these pulses are monitored frequently. The color and temperature of the involved extremity are assessed to detect possible embolism.

Digital Subtraction Angiography

In digital subtraction angiography, x-ray images of the area in question are obtained before and after the injection of a contrast agent. The computer analyzes the differences between the two images and produces an enhanced image of the carotid and vertebral arterial systems. The injection can be given through a peripheral vein.

Myelography

A **myelogram** is an x-ray of the spinal subarachnoid space taken after the injection of a contrast agent into the spinal subarachnoid space through a lumbar puncture. It outlines the spinal subarachnoid space and shows any distortion of the spinal cord or spinal dural sac caused by tumors, cysts, herniated vertebral disks, or other lesions. Water-based agents have replaced oil-based agents; these agents disperse upward through the CSF. Myelography is performed less frequently today because of the sensitivity of CT scanning and MRI.

Nursing Interventions

Because many patients have some misconceptions about this procedure, the nurse clarifies the explanation given by the physician and answers questions. The patient is informed about what to expect during the procedure and is informed that changes in position may be made during the procedure. The meal that would normally be eaten before the procedure is omitted. A sedative may be prescribed to help the patient cope with this rather lengthy test. Patient preparation for lumbar puncture is discussed later in this chapter.

After myelography, the patient lies in bed with the head of the bed elevated 30 degrees to 45 degrees. The patient is advised to remain in bed in the recommended position for 3 hours or as prescribed by the physician. The patient is encouraged to drink liberal amounts of fluid for rehydration and replacement of CSF and to decrease the incidence of postlumbar puncture headache. The blood pressure, pulse, respiratory rate, and temperature are monitored, as well as the patient's ability to void. Untoward signs include headache, fever, stiff neck, **photophobia** (sensitivity to light), seizures, and signs of chemical or bacterial meningitis.

Lumbar Epidural Venography

In lumbar epidural venography, a catheter is inserted percutaneously into the femoral vein and guided into the ascending lumbar vein or internal iliac vein. The contrast agent is injected to fill the epidural veins overlying the disk spaces and to opacify the epidural venous plexus. The procedure may be useful in the diagnosis of herniated lumbar disks not visualized on myelography. It shows deviation or compression of the epidural veins due to a herniated disk or tumor.

The procedure is usually well tolerated, fairly painless, and not associated with arachnoiditis. Lumbar epidural venography and myelography may be performed as complementary diagnostic studies. After the test, the site is observed for evidence of hematoma formation.

Radionuclide Imaging Studies (Brain Scan)

Radionuclide imaging is based on the principle that a radiopharmaceutical agent may diffuse through the blood–brain barrier at a point where the barrier has been disrupted and collect in abnormal cerebral tissue. (Normal brain tissue is relatively impermeable.) There is increased uptake of radioactive material at the site of pathology.

In this procedure, a radioactive agent is injected intravenously. The radioactivity subsequently transmitted through the skull is detected by a scanner that prints out an image, or a gamma camera is used to monitor the passage of the radiopharmaceutical agent through the cerebral circulation to gain information about cerebral blood flow.

A brain scan may be used to evaluate vascular lesions of the brain and meninges, to locate vascular neoplasms and brain tumors, to detect and evaluate stroke and brain abscess, and to follow up surgery or radiation therapy of the brain. Newer techniques permit the evaluation of cerebral circulation during the brain scan. However, CT scans and MRI have replaced traditional radioisotope scanning, and this study is infrequently performed.

Echoencephalography

Echoencephalography is the recording of sound waves reflected by the structures of the brain in response to ultrasound signals created by a transducer positioned over specific areas of the head. Echoencephalography is a rapid and useful technique to determine the position of midline structures of the brain and the distance from the midline to the lateral ventricular wall or the third ventricular wall. Therefore, it is performed to detect a shift of the cerebral midline structures caused by subdural hematoma, intracerebral hemorrhage, massive cerebral infarction, and tumors. It is useful to evaluate hydrocephalus because it can detect dilation of the ventricles.

Noninvasive Carotid Flow Studies

Noninvasive carotid flow studies use ultrasound imagery and Doppler measurements of arterial blood flow to evaluate carotid and deep orbital circulation. These tests are often obtained before arteriography, which carries combined risks of strokes and death (0.5% to 2%). Carotid Doppler, carotid ultrasonography, oculoplethysmography, and ophthalmodynamometry are four common noninvasive vascular techniques that permit evaluation of arterial blood flow and detection of arterial stenosis, occlusion, and plaques.

Nursing Interventions

The procedure is described to the patient. To reduce anxiety, the patient is informed that this is a noninvasive test, that a hand-held transducer will be placed over the neck and orbits of the eyes, and that some type of water-soluble jelly is used on the transducer.

Electroencephalography

An **electroencephalogram** (EEG) represents a record of the electrical activity generated in the brain and is obtained through electrodes applied on the scalp surface or through microelectrodes placed within the brain tissue. It provides physiologic assessment of cerebral activity.

The EEG is a useful test for diagnosing seizure disorders such as the epilepsies and is a screening procedure for coma or organic brain syndrome. Tumors, brain abscesses, blood clots, and infection may cause abnormal patterns in electrical activity. The EEG is also used in making a determination of brain death.

Electrodes are applied to the scalp to record the electrical activity in various regions of the brain. The amplified activity of the neurons between any two of these electrodes is recorded on continuously moving paper; this record is called the encephalogram.

For a baseline recording, the patient lies quietly with both eyes closed. The patient may be asked to hyperventilate for 3 to 4 minutes and then look at a bright, flashing light for photic stimulation. These are activation procedures performed to evoke abnormal electrical discharges, such as seizure potentials. A sleep EEG may be recorded after sedation because some abnormal brain waves are seen only when the patient is asleep. If the epileptogenic area is inaccessible to conventional scalp electrodes, nasopharyngeal electrodes may be used.

Depth recording of EEG is performed by introducing electrodes stereotactically (radiologically placed using instrumentation) into a target area of the brain, as indicated by the patient's seizure pattern and scalp EEG. It is used to identify patients who may benefit from surgical excision of epileptogenic foci.

Special transsphenoidal, mandibular, and nasopharyngeal electrodes can be used, and video recording combined with EEG monitoring and telemetry is used in hospital settings to capture epileptiform abnormalities and their sequelae. Some epilepsy centers provide long-term ambulatory EEG monitoring with portable recording devices.

Nursing Interventions

To increase the chances of recording seizure activity, it is sometimes recommended that the patient be deprived of sleep on the night before the EEG. Tranquilizers and stimulants should be withheld 24 to 48 hours before an EEG, because these medications can alter the EEG wave patterns or mask the abnormal wave patterns of seizure disorders. Coffee, tea, chocolate, and cola drinks are omitted in the meal before the test because of their stimulating effect. The meal is not omitted, however, because an altered blood glucose level can also cause changes in the brain wave patterns.

The patient is informed that the standard EEG takes 45 to 60 minutes, longer for a sleep EEG. At the same time, the patient is assured that the procedure does not cause an electric shock and that the EEG is a diagnostic test and not a form of treatment.

Evoked Potential Studies

In evoked potential studies, electrodes are applied to the scalp and an external stimulus is applied to peripheral sensory receptors to elicit or evoke changes or responses in the brain waves. Evoked changes are detected with the aid of computerized devices that extract the signal, display it on an oscilloscope, and store the data on magnetic tape or disk. These studies are based on the concept that any insult or dysfunction that can alter neuronal metabolism or disturb membrane function may change evoked responses in brain waves. In neurologic diagnosis, they reflect conduction times in the peripheral nervous system. In clinical practice, the visual, auditory, and somatosensory systems are most often tested.

In visual evoked responses, the patient looks at a visual stimulus (flashing lights, a checkerboard pattern on a screen). The average of several hundred stimuli is recorded by EEG leads placed over the occiput. The transit time from the retina to the occipital area is measured using computer-averaging methods.

Auditory evoked responses or brain stem evoked responses are measured by applying an auditory stimulus (a repetitive auditory click) and measuring the transit time up the brain stem into the cortex. Specific lesions in the auditory pathway modify or delay the response.

In somatosensory evoked responses, the peripheral nerves are stimulated (electrical stimulation through skin electrodes) and the transit time up the spinal cord to the cortex is measured and recorded from scalp electrodes.

This test is used to detect a deficit in spinal cord conduction and to monitor cord function during operative procedures. Because myelinated fibers conduct impulses at a higher rate of speed, nerves with an intact myelin sheath record the highest velocity. Demyelination of nerve fibers leads to a decrease in speed of conduction, as found in Guillain-Barré syndrome, multiple sclerosis, and polyneuropathies.

Nursing Interventions

There is no specific patient preparation other than to explain the procedure and to reassure the patient and encourage him or her to relax. The patient is advised to remain perfectly still throughout the recording to prevent artifacts (signals not generated by the brain) that interfere with the recording and interpretation of the test.

Electromyography

An **electromyogram** (EMG) is obtained by introducing needle electrodes into the skeletal muscles to measure changes in the electrical potential of the muscles and the nerves leading to them. The electrical potentials are shown on an oscilloscope and amplified by a loudspeaker so that both the sound and appearance of the waves can be analyzed and compared simultaneously.

Electromyograms are useful in determining the presence of a neuromuscular disorder and myopathies. They help to distinguish weakness due to neuropathy (functional or pathologic changes in the peripheral nervous system) from weakness due to other causes.

Nursing Interventions

The procedure is explained and the patient is warned to expect a sensation similar to that of an intramuscular injection as the needle is inserted into the muscle. The muscles examined may ache for a short time after the procedure.

Nerve Conduction Studies

Nerve conduction studies are performed by stimulation of a peripheral nerve at several points along its course and recording the muscle action potential or the sensory action potential that results. Surface or needle electrodes are placed on the skin over the nerve to stimulate the nerve fibers. This test is useful in the study of peripheral neuropathies.

Lumbar Puncture and Examination of Cerebrospinal Fluid

A lumbar puncture (spinal tap) is carried out by inserting a needle into the lumbar subarachnoid space to withdraw CSF. The test may be performed to obtain CSF for examination, to measure and reduce CSF pressure, to determine the presence or absence of blood in the CSF, to detect spinal subarachnoid block, and to administer antibiotics intrathecally—that is, into the spinal canal—in certain cases of infection.

The needle is usually inserted into the subarachnoid space between the third and fourth or fourth and fifth lumbar vertebrae. Because the spinal cord divides into a sheaf of nerves at the first lumbar vertebra, insertion of the needle below the level of the third lumbar vertebra prevents puncture of the spinal cord.

A successful lumbar puncture requires that the patient be relaxed; an anxious patient is tense, and this may increase the pressure reading. CSF pressure with the patient in a lateral recumbent position is normally 70 to 200 mm H_2O. Pressures of more than 200 mm H_2O are considered abnormal.

A lumbar puncture may be quite risky in the presence of an intracranial mass lesion, because intracranial pressure is decreased by the removal of CSF and the brain may herniate downward through the tentorium and the foramen magnum.

Queckenstedt's Test

A lumbar manometric test (Queckenstedt's test) may be performed by compressing the jugular veins on each side of the neck during the lumbar puncture. The increase in pressure caused by the compression is noted; then the pressure is released and pressure readings are made at 10-second intervals.

Normally, CSF pressure rises rapidly in response to compression of the jugular veins and returns quickly to normal when the compression is released. A slow rise and fall in pressure indicates a partial block due to a lesion compressing the spinal subarachnoid pathways. If there is no pressure change, a complete block is indicated. This test is not performed if an intracranial lesion is suspected.

See Guideline 56-1 for assisting with a lumbar puncture.

Examining the Cerebrospinal Fluid

The CSF should be clear and colorless. Pink, blood-tinged, or grossly bloody CSF may indicate a cerebral contusion, laceration, or subarachnoid hemorrhage. Sometimes with a difficult lumbar puncture, the CSF initially is bloody because of local trauma but then becomes clearer.

Usually, specimens are obtained for cell count, culture, and glucose and protein testing. The specimens should be sent to the laboratory immediately because changes will take place and alter the result if the specimens are allowed to stand. (See Appendix C for the normal values of CSF.)

Postlumbar Puncture Headache

A postlumbar puncture headache, ranging from mild to severe, may appear a few hours to several days after the procedure. This is the most common complication, occurring in 11% to 25% of patients. It is a throbbing bifrontal or occipital headache, dull and deep in character. It is particularly severe on sitting or standing upright but lessens or disappears when the patient lies down.

The headache is caused by the leakage of CSF at the puncture site. The fluid continues to escape into the tissues by way of the needle track from the spinal canal. It is then absorbed promptly by the lymphatics. As a result of this leak, the supply of CSF in the cranium is depleted to a point at which it is insufficient to maintain proper mechanical stabilization of the brain. This leakage of CSF allows settling of the brain when the patient assumes an upright position, producing tension and stretching the venous sinuses and pain-sensitive structures. Both traction and pain are lessened and the leakage is reduced when the patient lies down.

The lumbar puncture headache may be avoided if a small-gauge needle is used and if the patient remains prone after the procedure. When a large volume of fluid (>20 mL) is removed, the patient is positioned prone for 2 hours, then flat in a side-lying position for 2 to 3 hours, and then supine or prone for 6 more hours. Keeping the patient flat overnight may reduce the incidence of headaches.

The postpuncture headache is usually managed by bed rest, analgesics, and hydration. Occasionally, if the postpuncture headache persists, the epidural blood patch technique may be used. Blood is withdrawn from the patient's antecubital vein and injected into the epidural space, usually at the site of the previous spinal puncture. The rationale is that the blood acts as a gelatinous plug to seal the hole in the dura, thus preventing further loss of CSF.

Other Complications of Lumbar Puncture

Herniation of the intracranial contents, spinal epidural abscess, spinal epidural hematoma, and meningitis are rare but serious complications of lumbar puncture. Other complications include temporary voiding problems, slight elevation of temperature, backache or spasms, and stiffness of the neck.

56•1 GUIDELINES FOR ASSISTING WITH A LUMBAR PUNCTURE

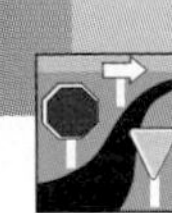

A needle is inserted into the subarachnoid space through the third and fourth or fourth and fifth lumbar interface to withdraw spinal fluid.

Preprocedure

1. Determine whether written consent for the procedure has been obtained.
2. Explain the procedure to the patient and describe sensations that are likely during the procedure (ie, a sensation of cold as the site is cleansed with solution, a needle prick when local anesthetic is injected).
3. Determine whether the patient has any questions or misconceptions about the procedure; reassure the patient that the needle will not enter the spinal cord or cause paralysis.
4. Instruct the patient to void before the procedure.

Procedure (performed by the physician)

1. The patient is positioned on one side at the edge of the bed or examining table with back toward the physician; the thighs and legs are flexed as much as possible to increase the space between the spinous processes of the vertebrae, for easier entry into the subarachnoid space.

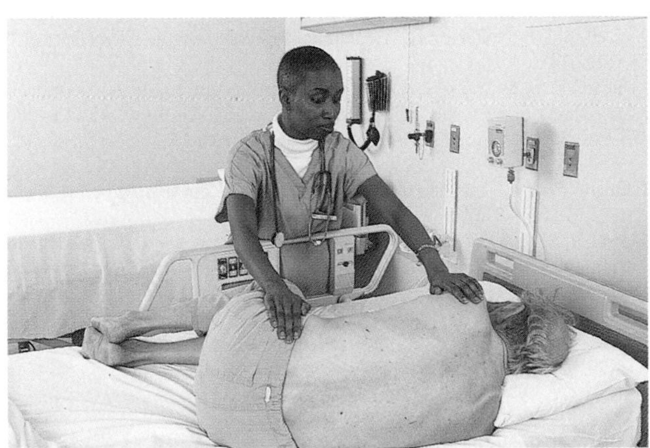

2. A small pillow may be placed under the patient's head to maintain the spine in a horizontal position; a pillow may be placed between the legs to prevent the upper leg from rolling forward.
3. The nurse assists the patient to maintain the position to avoid sudden movement, which can produce a traumatic (bloody) tap.
4. The patient is encouraged to relax and is instructed to breathe normally, because hyperventilation may lower an elevated pressure.
5. The nurse describes the procedure step by step to the patient as it proceeds.
6. The physician cleanses the puncture site with an antiseptic solution and drapes the site.
7. Local anesthetic is injected to numb the puncture site, and then a spinal needle is inserted into the subarachnoid space through the third and fourth or fourth and fifth lumbar interspace.

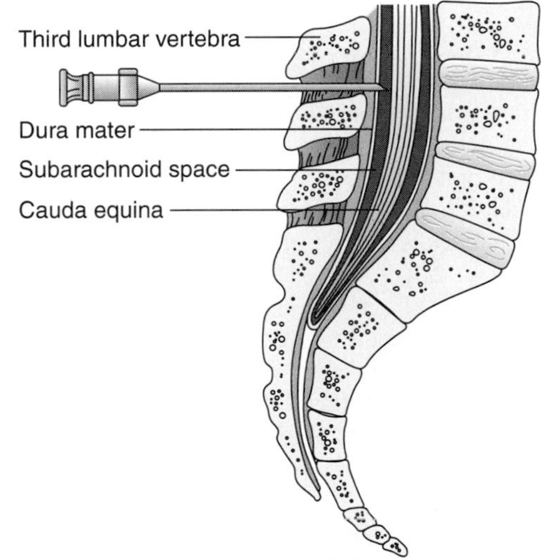

8. A specimen of CSF is removed and usually collected in three test tubes, labeled in order of collection. A pressure reading may be obtained. The needle is withdrawn.
9. A small dressing is applied to the puncture site.
10. The tubes of CSF are sent to the laboratory immediately.

Postprocedure

1. Instruct the patient to lie prone for 2 to 3 hours to separate the alignment of the dural and arachnoid needle punctures in the meninges, to reduce leakage of CSF.
2. Monitor the patient for complications of lumbar puncture; notify physician if complications occur.
3. Encourage increased fluid intake to reduce the risk of postprocedure headache.

Home and Community-Based Care

Teaching Patients Self-Care

Many diagnostic tests that were once performed as part of a patient's hospital stay are now carried out in short-procedure units and outpatient testing settings or units. As a result, the postprocedure care is often provided by family members. Therefore, the patient and family must receive clear verbal and written instructions about precautions to take after the procedure, complications to watch for, and steps to take if complications occur. Because many patients undergoing neurologic diagnostic studies are elderly or have neurologic deficits, provisions must be made to ensure that transportation and postprocedure care and monitoring are available.

Continuing Care

Phoning the patient and family after diagnostic testing enables the nurse to determine whether they have any questions about the procedure or whether the patient had any untoward results. During these calls, teaching is reinforced and the patient and family are reminded to make and keep follow-up appointments.

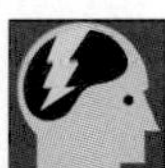

Critical Thinking Exercises

1. Your patient is scheduled to have a lumbar puncture (spinal tap) and says she is afraid that she may end up paralyzed as a result of the procedure. Based on your knowledge of the anatomy and physiology of the CNS, how would you structure your explanation to reassure the patient and dispel her fears?

2. Your patient is to have MRI. How would you explain the test to the patient and the precautions that are needed before the procedure? How would you adjust your approach if the patient has difficulty understanding English? If the patient is elderly and has severe skeletal deformities?

3. A 50-year-old patient is scheduled for several diagnostic tests (MRI, evoked potentials, and lumbar puncture) to determine the cause of a recent onset of sensory and motor symptoms. After the tests, he is expected to go home. He tells you that he lives alone in a small apartment; he knows none of his neighbors. What teaching would be indicated for him? What resources may be needed to enable him to go home as scheduled?

References and Selected Readings

BOOKS

Adams, R., Victor, M., & Ropper, A. (1997). *Principles of neurology* (6th ed.). New York: McGraw-Hill.

Bennett, S. E., & Karnes, J. L. (1998). *Neurological disabilities: Assessment and treatment.* Philadelphia: Lippincott-Raven.

Goetz, C. G., & Pappert, E. J. (1999). *Textbook of clinical neurology.* Philadelphia: W. B. Saunders.

Hickey, J. (1997). *Clinical practice of neurologic and neurosurgical nursing* (4th ed.). Philadelphia: Lippincott-Raven.

Hoeman, S. (Ed.). (1996). *Rehabilitation nursing: Process and application* (2nd ed.). St. Louis: Mosby–Year Book.

Johnson, B. S. (1997). *Psychiatric–mental health nursing: Adaptation and growth* (4th ed.). Philadelphia: Lippincott-Raven.

Katzman, R., & Rowe, J. (1995). *Principles of geriatric neurology.* Philadelphia: F. A. Davis.

Nolan, M. (1995). *Introduction to the neurologic examination.* Philadelphia: F. A. Davis.

Rein, H. (1995). Diagnostic tests for neurologic disorders. In S. M. Tilkian, et al. (Eds.), *Clinical and nursing implications of laboratory tests.* St Louis: Mosby–Year Book.

Simon, R. P., Aminoff, M. J., & Greenberg. (1999). *Clinical neurology.* Stamford, CT: Appleton & Lange.

Weiner, L., Levitt, L. P., Rae-Grant, A., & Weiner, H. L. (1999). *Neurology* (6th ed.). Philadelphia: Lippincott Williams & Wilkins.

JOURNALS

Asterisks indicate nursing research articles.

Barker, E. (1995). Don't dismiss whiplash. *RN, 58*(11), 26–31.

Bauman, S. L. (1993). Mental health assessment of people with HIV. *Journal of Association of Nurses in AIDS Care, 4*(4), 36–44.

Crigger, N., & Forbes, W. (1997). Assessing neurologic function in older patients. *American Journal of Nursing, 97*(3), 37–40.

Darvovic, G. (1997). Assessing pupillary responses. *Nursing, 27*(2), 49.

Ditunno, J. F. Jr., Graziani, V., & Tessler, A. (1997). neurologic assessment in spinal cord injury. *Advances in Neurology, 72*, 325–333.

Dunlap, E. (1993). Extrapyramidal symptoms: A challenge for the consultant. *Clinical Nurse Specialist, 7*(4), 224.

Frizzell, J. (1998). Cerebral angiography. *American Journal of Nursing, 98*(9), 16II–16JJ.

Gallegos, S. J., & Michalec, D. L. (1996). Orthopedic essentials: Neurologic assessment of the orthopedic patient. *Orthopaedic Nursing, 15*(5), 23–29.

Gilman, S. (1998). Imaging of the brain. *New England Journal of Medicine, 338*(12), 812–820.

Gilman, S. (1998). Imaging of the brain, Pt. II. *New England Journal of Medicine, 338*(13), 889–896.

Harrahill, M. (1995). Trauma notebook. Upper extremity nerve assessment: A quick review. *Journal of Emergency Nursing, 21*(4), 360–362.

Jacobs, B. B. (1995). Emergent neurologic events. *Critical Care Nursing Clinics of North America, 7*(3), 427–444.

*Juarez, V. J., & Lyons, M. (1995). Interrater reliability of the Glasgow Coma Scale. *Journal of Neuroscience Nursing, 27*(5), 283–286.

Lehman, L. (1995). The neurologic causes of weakness. *Emergency Medicine, 27*(8), 22–24.

McConnell, E. (1995). What's wrong with this patient? *Nursing, 25*(6), 66–67.

Nance, P., & Hoy, C. (1996). Assessment of the autonomic nervous system. *Physical Medicine and Rehabilitation: State of the Art Reviews, 10*(1), 15–35.

Neal, L. (1997). Is anybody home? Basic neurologic assessment of the home care client. *Home Healthcare Nurse, 15*(3), 156–169.

O'Hanlon-Nichols, T. (1999). Neurologic assessment. *American Journal of Nursing, 99*(6), 44–50.

Pressman, E., Zeidman, S., & Summers, L. (1995). Primary care for women: Comprehensive assessment of the neurologic system. *Journal of Nurse Midwifery, 40*(2), 216–219.

*Rosenberg, D. M., McLaulin, B., Bennett, M., & Mathison, K. (1996). Diagnosing HIV dementia: A retrospective analysis. *Journal of Association of Nurses in AIDS Care, 7*(6), 57–66.

Shpritz, D. (1995). Understanding neurologic assessment. *Journal of Postanesthesia Nursing, 10*(4), 216–219.

Simpson, D., & Tagliati, M. (1994). Neurologic manifestations of HIV infection. *Annals of Internal Medicine, 12*(10), 769–785.

Souder, E., Saykin, A., & Alavi, A. (1995). Multi-modal assessment in Alzheimer's Disease: ADL in relation to PET, MRI and neuropsychology. *Journal of Gerontologic Nursing, 21*(9), 1–13.

Tan, T., & Pomeranz, S. (1995). PET: A new frontier in diagnosis and patient care. *Applied Radiology, 24*(12), 6–18.

*Way, C., & Segatore, M. (1994). Development and preliminary testing of the neurologic Assessment Instrument. *Journal of Neuroscience Nursing, 26*(5), 278–287.

Wooten, C. (1996). The trauma top 10: The top 10 ways to detect deteriorating central neurologic status. *Journal of Trauma Nursing, 3*(1), 25–27.

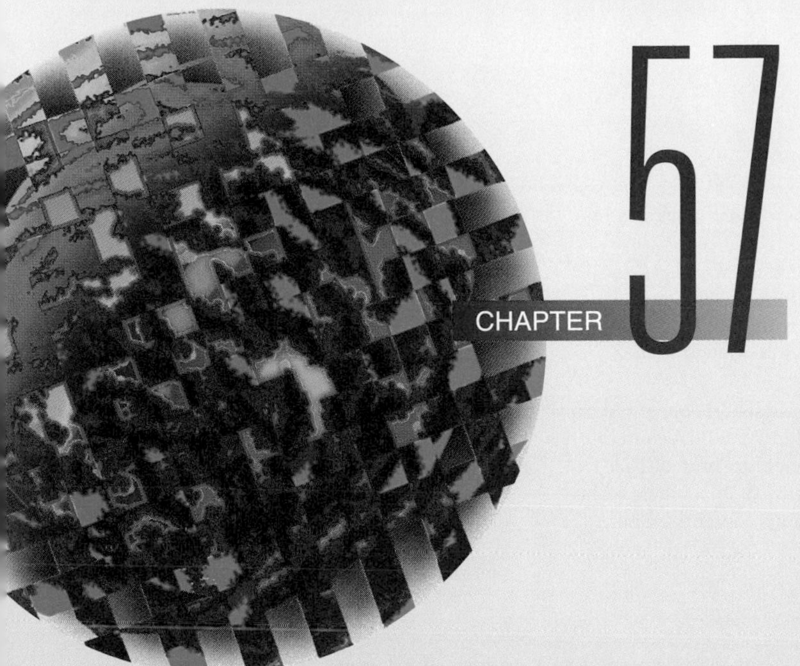

CHAPTER 57

Management of Patients With Neurologic Dysfunction

Learning Objectives

On completion of this chapter, the learner will be able to:

1. Describe the special nursing needs of patients with neurologic dysfunction.
2. Identify the early and late clinical manifestations of increased intracranial pressure.
3. Use the nursing process as a framework for care of the patient with increased intracranial pressure.
4. Describe the multiple needs of the unconscious patient.
5. Use the nursing process as a framework for care of the unconscious patient.
6. Describe the various types of aphasia and the nursing management of the aphasic patient.
7. Identify the risk factors for stroke and related measures for stroke prevention.
8. Compare the various types of stroke: their causes, clinical manifestations, and nursing and medical management.
9. Use the nursing process as a framework for care of the patient with stroke.
10. Use the nursing process as a framework for care of the patient undergoing intracranial surgery.
11. Compare the various types of neurosurgical procedures used to treat intractable pain.

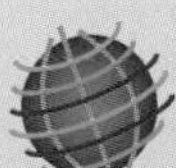

The term "neurologic dysfunction" indicates isolated or system-wide conditions that result from either structural or metabolic compromise of the brain and its environment. Structural causes of neurologic dysfunction include head injury, intracranial hemorrhage, encephalitis, brain abscess, and stroke. The two structural mechanisms by which neurologic dysfunction occurs are related to the expansion of brain tissue in the inflexible cranium. First, increased intracranial pressure (ICP) leads to decreased cerebral perfusion, and second, the expanding brain tissue herniates through the tentorial notch, compressing and damaging the midbrain and brain stem.

Metabolic causes of neurologic dysfunction include sepsis, hypovolemia, myocardial infarction, respiratory arrest, hypoglycemia, electrolyte imbalance, drug and/or alcohol overdose, hypertensive encephalopathy, diabetic ketoacidosis, and hepatic encephalopathy. The mechanisms by which metabolic conditions cause neurologic dysfunction include the accumulation of toxins, causing neurologic depression, and reduced cerebral perfusion from decreased cardiac output, increased ICP, or peripheral vasodilation.

Some structural and metabolic conditions may be treated and corrected with little permanent neurologic impairment; however, many result in permanent dysfunction. Dysfunction may range from slight hand weakness to paralysis, difficulty speaking or swallowing, or total unresponsiveness to any stimuli.

GLOSSARY

akinetic mutism: unresponsiveness to the environment; the patient makes no movement or sound but sometimes opens the eyes

autoregulation: ability of cerebral blood vessels to dilate or constrict to maintain stable cerebral blood flow despite changes in systemic arterial blood pressure

brain death: irreversible loss of all functions of the entire brain, including the brain stem

coma: prolonged state of unconsciousness

Cushing's response: brain's attempt to restore blood flow by increasing arterial pressure to overcome the increased intracranial pressure

Cushing's triad: three classic symptoms—bradycardia, hypertension, and bradypnea—seen with pressure on the medulla as a result of brain stem herniation

Monro-Kellie hypothesis: theory about the dynamic equilibrium of cranial contents; states that because of the limited space for expansion within the skull, an increase in any one of the cranial contents—brain tissue, blood, or CSF—causes a change in the volume of the others by displacing or shifting CSF, increasing the absorption of CSF, or decreasing cerebral blood volume

persistent vegetative state: condition in which the patient is wakeful but devoid of conscious content, without cognitive or affective mental function

unconsciousness: condition of being unresponsive to and unaware of environmental stimuli

Although neuroscience nursing is a specialty requiring an understanding of neuroanatomy, neurophysiology, neurodiagnostic testing, critical care nursing, and rehabilitation nursing, nurses in all settings will care for patients with neurologic dysfunction. Ongoing assessment of the patient's neurologic function and health needs, identification of problems, mutual goal setting, care plan development and implementation (including teaching, counseling, and coordinating activities), and evaluation of the outcomes of care are nursing actions integral to the recovery of the patient. The nurse also collaborates with other members of the health care team to provide essential care, offer a variety of solutions to existing problems, help the patient gain control, and explore the educational and supportive resources available in the community. The goals are to achieve as high a level of function as possible and to enhance the quality of life for the neurologically impaired patient and his or her family.

This chapter discusses care of the patient with increased ICP, one of the major mechanisms resulting in neurologic dysfunction, and care of the unconscious patient. In addition, cerebral vascular disease, a leading source of neurologic impairment, is discussed. Neurosurgery and neurosurgical interventions for pain management are also addressed.

INCREASED ICP

The rigid cranial vault contains brain tissue (1,400 g), blood (75 mL), and cerebrospinal fluid (CSF; 75 mL). The volume and pressure of these three components are usually in a state of equilibrium. The **Monro-Kellie hypothesis** states that because of the limited space for expansion within the skull, an increase in any one of these components causes a change in the volume of the others by displacing or shifting CSF, increasing the absorption of CSF, or decreasing cerebral blood volume. Without such changes, ICP will begin to rise.

Under normal circumstances, minor changes in blood volume and CSF volume occur constantly when there are changes in intrathoracic pressure (coughing, sneezing, straining), posture, and blood pressure, and fluctuations in arterial blood gas levels. The normal ICP is 10 to 20 mm Hg.

Pathophysiology

Increased ICP is a syndrome that affects many patients with acute neurologic conditions because pathologic conditions alter the relation between intracranial volume and pressure. Although an elevated ICP is most commonly associated with head injury, it may be seen as a secondary effect in various other conditions, such as brain tumors, subarachnoid hemorrhage, and toxic and viral encephalopathies. Increased ICP from any cause affects cerebral perfusion, produces distortion, and shifts brain tissue.

DECREASED CEREBRAL BLOOD FLOW

Increased ICP may significantly reduce cerebral blood flow, resulting in ischemia. Mechanisms leading to cell death are illustrated in Figure 57-1. If complete ischemia occurs and lasts for more than 3 to 5 minutes, the brain will be irreversibly damaged. In the early stages of cerebral ischemia, the vasomotor centers are stimulated and the systemic pressure rises to maintain cerebral blood flow. Usually this is accompanied by a slow bounding pulse and respiratory irregularities. These changes in blood pressure, pulse, and respiration are important clinically because they suggest increased ICP.

PATHOPHYSIOLOGY

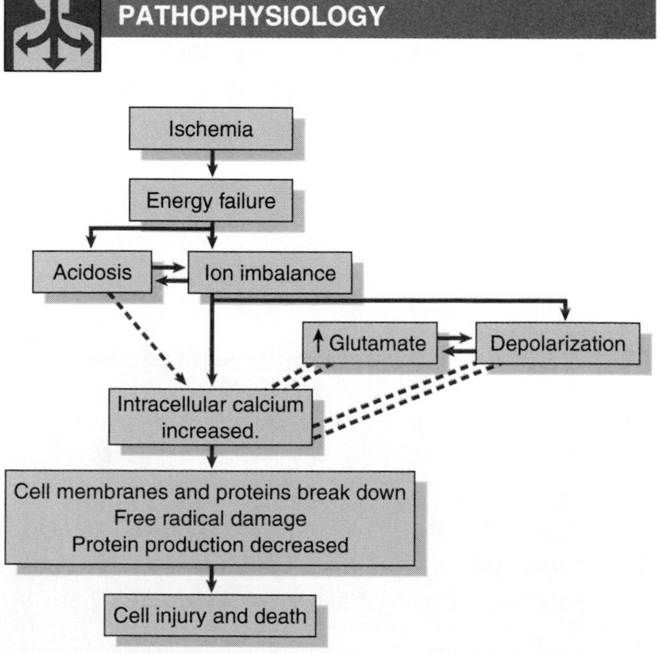

FIGURE 57•1 Processes contributing to ischemic brain cell injury. Courtesy of National Stroke Association, Englewood, Colorado.

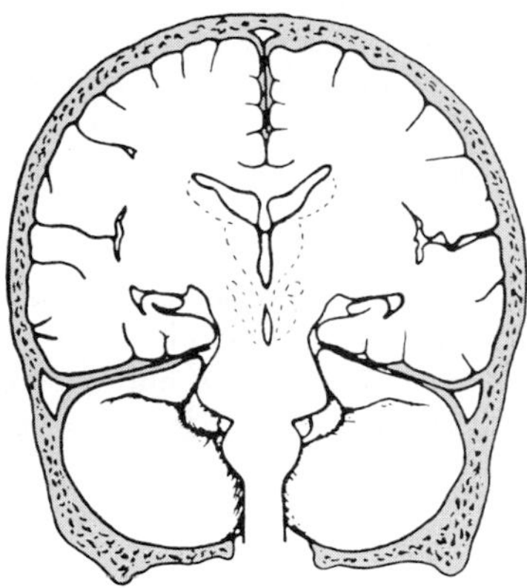

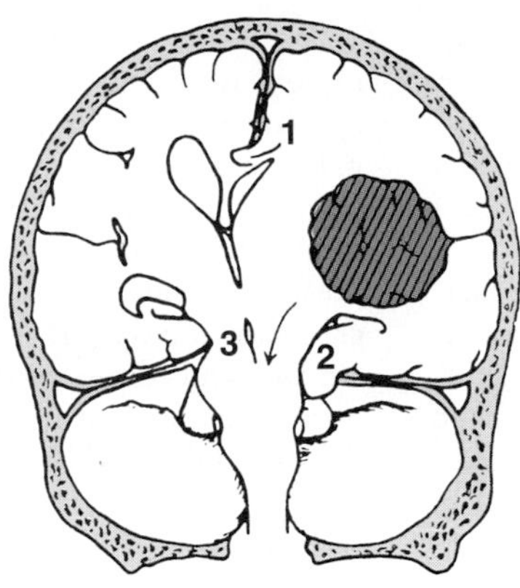

FIGURE 57•2 Cross section of a normal brain (**left**) and a brain with intracranial shifts from supratentorial lesions (**right**). (1) Herniation of the cingulate gyrus under the falx. (2) Herniation of the temporal lobe into the tentorial notch. (3) Downward displacement of the brain stem through the notch.

The concentration of carbon dioxide in the blood and in the brain tissue also has a role in the regulation of cerebral blood flow. A rise in carbon dioxide partial pressure ($PaCO_2$) causes cerebral vasodilation, leading to increased cerebral blood flow and increased ICP; a fall in $PaCO_2$ has a vasoconstricting effect. Decreased venous outflow may also increase cerebral blood volume, thus raising ICP.

CEREBRAL EDEMA

Cerebral edema or swelling occurs when there is an increase in the water content of the brain tissue. Certain brain tumors are associated with the excessive production of antidiuretic hormone, resulting in fluid retention. Even a small tumor may create a great increase in ICP.

CEREBRAL RESPONSE TO INCREASED ICP

Autoregulation refers to the brain's ability to change the diameter of its blood vessels automatically to maintain a constant cerebral blood flow during alterations in systemic blood pressure. The brain can effectively autoregulate its hemodynamics when arterial systolic blood pressure is 60 to 160 mm Hg and ICP is less than 40 mm Hg. When autoregulation fails, cerebral blood flow diminishes, leading to ischemia. Infarction will result if the ischemia is not corrected.

The cerebral perfusion pressure (CPP) is calculated by subtracting the value of the ICP from the mean arterial pressure. The normal CPP is 70 to 100 mm Hg. The autoregulatory mechanism of the brain, once impaired, may cause CPP to be greater than 100 mm Hg or less than 50 mm Hg. Patients with CPP less than 50 mm Hg experience irreversible neurologic dysfunction due to decreased cerebral perfusion, cerebral ischemia, and the resulting **Cushing's response**. Cushing's response (or Cushing's reflex) is seen with a decrease in cerebral blood flow. The brain, in an attempt to restore blood flow, increases arterial pressure to overcome the increased ICP. Reperfusion of the brain will reverse the ischemia that occurred as a result of the hypoperfusion.

Cushing's response should be distinguished from **Cushing's triad** (bradycardia, hypertension, and bradypnea), which ensues once the protective mechanisms are no longer effective. Cushing's triad indicates a potentially terminal event and requires emergent intervention.

At a certain volume or pressure, the ability of the brain to autoregulate becomes ineffective and decompensation begins. In this phase, the patient exhibits a significant change in mental status and vital signs: bradycardia, widening pulse pressure, and respiratory changes (Cushing's triad). At this point, herniation of the brain stem and occlusion of the cerebral blood flow occur if therapeutic intervention is not initiated. Herniation occurs when a portion of brain tissue shifts from an area of high pressure to an area of lower pressure (Fig. 57-2). The herniated tissue exerts pressure on the brain area to which it has herniated or shifted, interfering with the blood supply in that area. Cessation of cerebral blood flow results in cerebral ischemia and infarction, leading to **brain death**.

Clinical Manifestations

When ICP increases to the point at which the brain's ability to adjust has reached its limits, neural function is impaired; this may be manifested by changes in the level of consciousness (LOC) and by abnormal respiratory and vasomotor responses. The level of responsiveness and consciousness is the most important indicator of the patient's condition. See Chart 57-1 for terms related to altered levels of consciousness.

Nursing Alert *The earliest sign of increasing ICP is a change in LOC. Slowing of speech and delay in response to verbal suggestions are early indicators.*

CHART 57•1 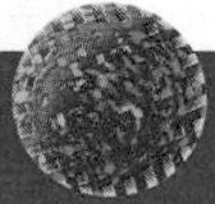 **Terms That Describe Altered Level of Consciousness**

confused: disoriented to time, person, place (progresses from time to person to place); has difficulty following commands, may be agitated or irritable, may hallucinate

lethargic: oriented to time, person, and place but sleeps often; speech and thought processes slowed

obtunded: sleeps almost constantly but is arousable and can follow simple commands; stays awake only with persistent stimulation

stuporous: awakens only to vigorous stimulation such as shaking; responds appropriately to painful stimuli, but verbal responses are incomprehensible

comatose: does not respond to environmental stimuli

light coma: unarousable, no spontaneous movement, withdraws appropriately to painful stimuli; brain stem reflexes (pupillary response, gag, and corneal reflexes) intact

coma: unarousable, withdraws nonpurposefully from painful stimuli; brain stem reflexes may or may not be intact; may exhibit decorticate or decerebrate posturing

deep coma: unarousable, unresponsive to painful stimuli; absent brain stem reflexes; decerebrate posturing

Any sudden change in the patient's condition, such as restlessness (without apparent cause), confusion, or increasing drowsiness, has neurologic significance. These signs may result from compression of the brain due to either swelling from hemorrhage or edema or an expanding intracranial lesion (hematoma or tumor), or a combination of both.

As pressure increases, the patient becomes stuporous, reacting only to loud auditory or painful stimuli. At this stage, serious impairment of brain circulation is probably taking place, and immediate surgical intervention may be required. As neurologic impairment deteriorates further and the patient becomes comatose, abnormal motor responses in the form of decortication, decerebration, or flaccidity are seen (Fig. 57-3). When the coma is profound, with the pupils dilated and fixed and respirations impaired, death is usually inevitable.

Assessment and Diagnostic Findings

Diagnostic studies are used to determine the underlying cause of increased ICP. The patient may undergo cerebral angiography, computed tomography (CT) scanning, magnetic resonance imaging (MRI), or positron emission tomography (PET). Transcranial Doppler studies may provide information about cerebral blood flow. The patient with increased ICP may also undergo electrophysiologic monitoring to monitor cerebral blood flow indirectly. Evoked potential monitoring is accomplished by measuring the electrical potentials produced by nerve tissue in response to external stimulation (auditory, visual, or sensory). Lumbar puncture is avoided in patients with increased ICP because the sudden release of pressure can cause the brain to herniate.

Complications

Complications of increased ICP include brain stem herniation, diabetes insipidus, and syndrome of inappropriate antidiuretic hormone (SIADH).

Brain stem herniation results from an excessive increase in ICP, when the pressure builds in the cranial vault and the brain tissue presses down on the brain stem. This increasing pressure on the brain stem results in the cessation of blood flow to the brain, causing irreversible brain anoxia and brain death.

Diabetes insipidus is the result of decreased secretion of antidiuretic hormone. The patient has excessive urine output. Therapy consists of administration of fluid volume, electrolyte replacement, and vasopressin (desmopressin, DDAVP) therapy. Diabetes insipidus is discussed in more detail in Chapter 38.

SIADH is the result of increased secretion of antidiuretic hormone. The patient becomes volume-overloaded and has decreased urine output. Treatment of SIADH includes fluid restriction and administration of phenytoin to decrease antidiuretic hormone release or lithium to increase free water loss. Further discussion of SIADH is presented in Chapter 38.

Management

Increased ICP constitutes a true emergency and must be treated promptly. Invasive monitoring of ICP is an important component of management, but immediate management to relieve increased ICP involves decreasing cerebral edema, lowering the volume of CSF, or decreasing blood volume, while maintaining cerebral perfusion. These goals are accomplished by administering osmotic diuretics and corticosteroids, restricting fluids, draining CSF, hyperventilating the patient, controlling fever, and reducing cellular metabolic demands.

MONITORING ICP

The purposes of ICP monitoring are to identify increased pressure early in its course (before cerebral damage occurs), quantify the degree of abnormality, initiate appropriate treatment, provide access to CSF for sampling and drainage, and evaluate the effectiveness of treatment. ICP can be monitored by an intraventricular catheter (ventriculostomy), a subarachnoid bolt, an epidural or subdural catheter, or a fiberoptic transducer-tipped catheter placed in the brain tissue or the ventricle (Fig. 57-4).

In ventricular catheter monitoring, a fine-bore catheter is inserted into a lateral ventricle. The catheter is connected by a fluid-filled system to a transducer, which records the pressure in the form of an electrical impulse. In addition to obtaining continuous ICP recordings, the ventricular catheter allows CSF to drain, particularly during acute rises in pressure. The ventriculostomy also can be used to drain the ventricle of blood. Also, continuous drainage of ventricular fluid under pressure control is an effective

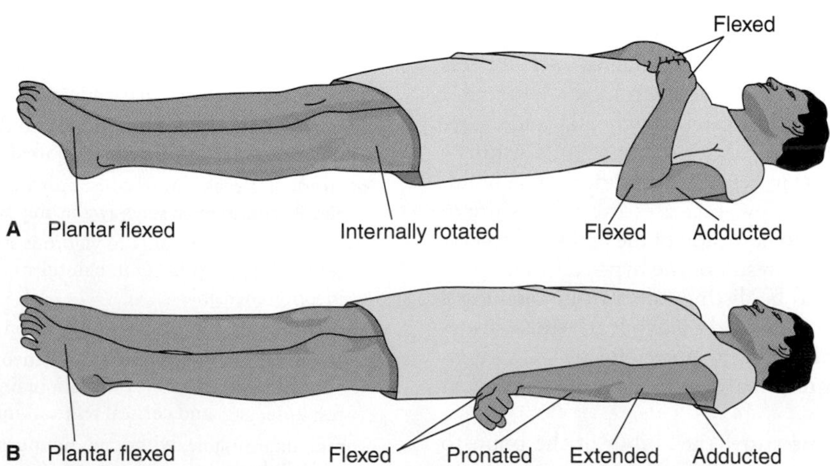

FIGURE 57•3 Abnormal posture responses to stimuli. (**A**) Decorticate posturing, involving adduction and flexion of upper extremities, internal rotation of lower extremities, and plantar flexion of the feet. (**B**) Decerebrate posturing, involving extension and outward rotation of the upper extremities and plantar flexion of the feet.

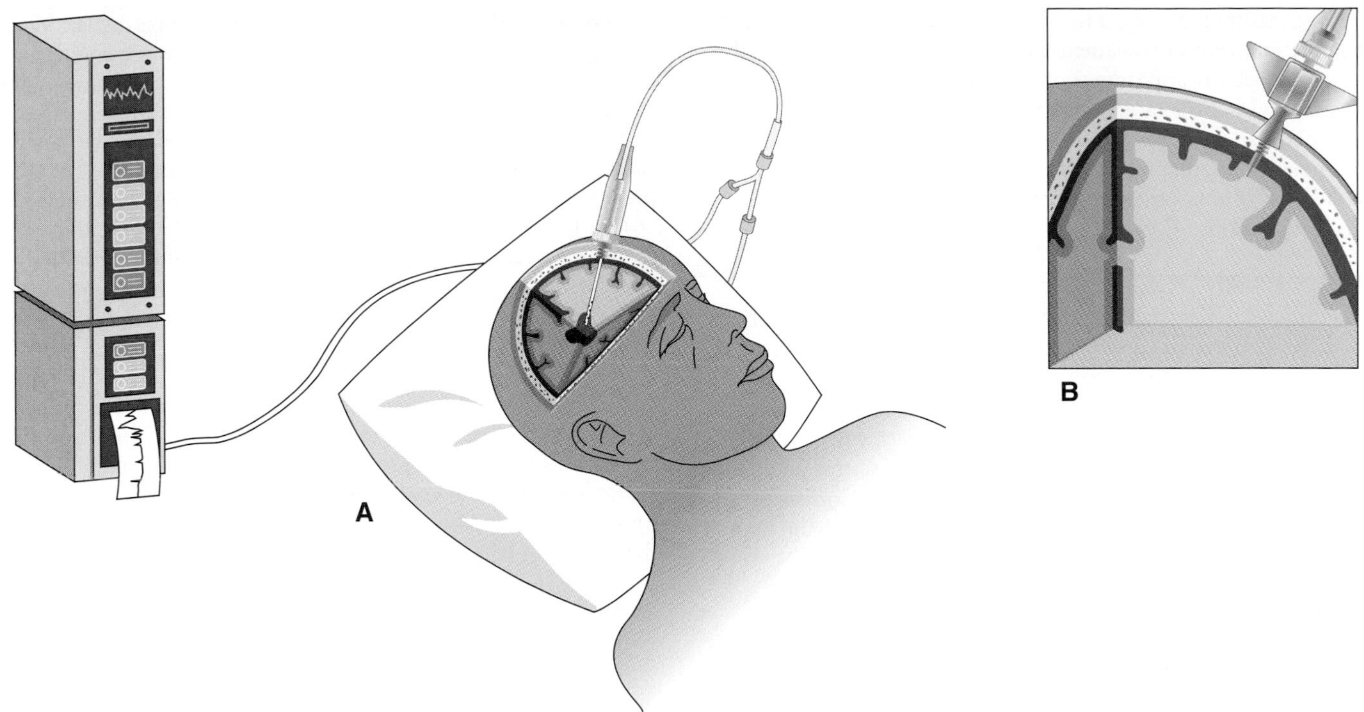

FIGURE 57•4 Current technology allows intracranial pressure to be monitored by (**A**) a fiberoptic, transducer-tipped pressure-temperature ventricular monitoring catheter or (**B**) a ventricular bolt. Such a device connects to a pressure transducer and display system.

method of treating intracranial hypertension. Another advantage of an indwelling ventricular catheter is the route it provides for the intraventricular administration of medications and the instillation of air or a contrast agent for ventriculography. Complications include ventricular infection, meningitis, ventricular collapse, occlusion of the catheter by brain tissue or blood, and problems with the monitoring system.

The subarachnoid screw (or bolt) is a hollow screw inserted through the skull and dura mater into the cranial subarachnoid space. It has the advantage of not requiring a ventricular puncture. The subarachnoid screw is attached to a pressure transducer, and the output is recorded on an oscilloscope. The hollow screw technique has the advantage of avoiding complications from brain shift and small ventricle size. Complications include blockage of the screw by clot or brain tissue, which leads to a loss of pressure tracing and a decrease in accuracy at high ICP readings.

Epidural ICP monitoring uses a pneumatic flow sensor, which functions on a nonelectrical basis. This pneumatic epidural monitoring system has a low incidence of infection and complications and appears to read pressures accurately. Calibration of the system is maintained automatically, and abnormal pressure waves trigger an alarm system. One disadvantage to the epidural catheter is the inability to withdraw CSF for analysis.

A fiberoptic transducer-tipped catheter is becoming widely used as an alternative to standard intraventricular, subarachnoid, and subdural systems. The miniature transducer reflects pressure changes, which are converted to electrical signals in an amplifier and displayed on a digital monitor. The catheter can be inserted into the ventricle, subarachnoid space, subdural space, or brain parenchyma or under a bone flap.

Changes in ICP are indicated by waves of high pressure and troughs of relatively normal pressure. Waveforms are captured and recorded on an oscilloscope. These waves have been classified as A waves (plateau waves), B waves, and C waves (Fig. 57-5). The plateau waves (A waves) are transient, paroxysmal, recurring elevations of ICP that may last from 5 to 20 minutes and range in amplitude from 50 to 100 mm Hg. Plateau waves have clinical significance and indicate changes in vascular volume within the intracranial compartment that are beginning to compromise cerebral perfusion. A waves may increase in amplitude and frequency, reflecting cerebral ischemia and brain damage that can occur before overt signs and symptoms of raised ICP are seen clinically. B waves are of shorter duration (30 seconds to 2 minutes) with smaller

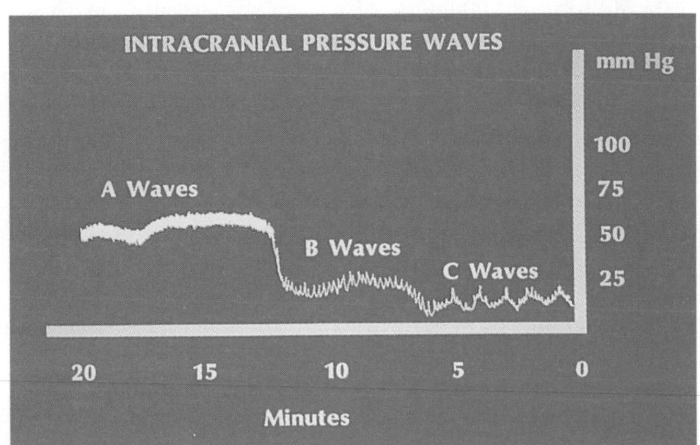

FIGURE 57•5 Intracranial pressure waves. Composite diagram of A (plateau) waves, which indicate cerebral ischemia; B waves, which may indicate intracranial hypertension and variations in the respiratory cycle; and C waves, which relate to variations in systemic arterial blood pressure and respirations.

amplitude (up to 50 mm Hg). They have less clinical significance, but if seen in runs in a patient with depressed consciousness, they may precede the appearance of A waves. B waves may be seen in patients with intracranial hypertension and decreased intracranial compliance. C waves are small, rhythmic oscillations with frequencies of approximately six per minute. They appear to be related to rhythmic variations of the systemic arterial blood pressure and respirations.

DECREASING CEREBRAL EDEMA

Osmotic diuretics (mannitol) may be given to dehydrate the brain and reduce cerebral edema. They act by drawing water across intact membranes, thereby reducing the volume of brain and extracellular fluid. An indwelling urinary catheter is usually inserted to monitor urinary output and to manage the resulting diuresis. When a patient is receiving osmotic diuretics, serum osmolality should be determined to assess hydration status. Corticosteroids (eg, dexamethasone) help reduce edema surrounding brain tumors when a brain tumor is the cause of increased ICP.

MAINTAINING CEREBRAL PERFUSION

The cardiac output is maintained to provide adequate perfusion to the brain. Improvements in cardiac output are made using fluid volume and inotropic agents, such as dobutamine hydrochloride. The effectiveness of the cardiac output is reflected in the CPP, which is maintained at more than 80 mm Hg. A lower CPP would indicate that the cardiac output is insufficient to maintain adequate cerebral perfusion.

REDUCING CSF AND BLOOD VOLUME

CSF drainage is frequently employed because the removal of CSF, with a ventriculostomy drain, may dramatically reduce ICP and restore CPP. Caution should be used in draining CSF because excessive drainage may result in collapse of the ventricles.

Hyperventilation, which results in vasoconstriction, has been used for many years in patients with increased ICP. Recent research has demonstrated that hyperventilation may not be as beneficial as once thought. The reduction in the $PaCO_2$ may result in hypoxia, ischemia, and an increase in cerebral lactate levels. Maintaining the $PaCO_2$ in the range of 30 to 35 mm Hg may prove beneficial. Hyperventilation is indicated in patients whose ICP is unresponsive to conventional therapies to reduce ICP, but it should be used judiciously.

CONTROLLING FEVER

Temperature control is aimed at preventing an elevation of temperature, because fever increases cerebral metabolism and the rate at which cerebral edema forms. Strategies to reduce temperature include administration of antipyretic medications, as prescribed, and use of a cooling blanket. The patient's temperature is monitored closely, and the patient is observed for shivering, which should be avoided because it increases ICP. Chlorpromazine (Thorazine) may be prescribed to control shivering.

REDUCING METABOLIC DEMANDS

Reduction of cellular metabolic demands may also be accomplished through the administration of high doses of barbiturates when the patient is unresponsive to conventional treatment. The mechanism by which barbiturates decrease ICP and protect the brain is uncertain, but the resultant comatose state is thought to reduce the metabolic requirements of the brain, thus providing some protection.

Another method of reducing cellular metabolic demand and improving oxygenation is administration of pharmacologic paralyzing agents (muscle relaxants such as vecuronium bromide [Norcuron]). The patient who receives these agents cannot move; the result is a decrease in cerebral oxygen demand. Because the patient cannot respond or report pain, sedation and analgesia must be provided because the paralyzing agents do not provide either.

Patients receiving barbiturates or pharmacologic paralyzing agents are cared for in a critical care unit and require cardiovascular monitoring, endotracheal intubation, mechanical ventilation, ICP monitoring, and arterial pressure monitoring. Blood and serum barbiturate levels must be monitored.

The level of pharmacologic paralysis can be assessed by the "train of four" procedure or test. This procedure tests the patient's response to four electrical impulses applied to the ulnar nerve 0.5 seconds apart. If the receptors in the neuromuscular junction are not totally saturated—that is, some of the receptors can accept impulses—the patient will demonstrate a twitching movement of the thumb. A patient whose thumb does not twitch is said to be overparalyzed, and the paralyzing agent should be reduced to a level at which the patient has some twitch response.

In addition to the twitch response, other important parameters that must be assessed include blood pressure, heart rate, respiratory rate, and response to ventilator therapy (eg, bucking the ventilator). The level of pharmacologic paralysis is adjusted based on the twitch response and the physical assessment parameters.

NURSING PROCESS: THE PATIENT WITH INCREASED ICP

Assessment

Initial assessment of the patient with increased ICP includes obtaining a history of events leading to the present illness and other subjective data; it may be necessary to obtain this information from family or friends. The neurologic examination should be as complete as the patient's condition allows. It includes an evaluation of mental status, LOC, cranial nerve function, cerebellar function (balance and coordination), reflexes, and motor and sensory function. Because the patient is critically ill, ongoing assessment will probably be more focused, including pupil checks, assessment of selected cranial nerves, frequent measurements of vital signs and intracranial pressure, and use of the Glasgow Coma Scale.

LOC, a sensitive indicator of neurologic function, is assessed frequently based on the criteria identified in the Glasgow Coma Scale: eye opening, verbal response, and motor response. The patient's responses are rated on a scale from 3 to 15. A score of 3 indicates severe impairment of neurologic function; a score of 15 indicates that the patient is fully responsive.

Eye opening indicates the ability of the patient to open his or her eyes to a command. Patients with severe neurologic dysfunction cannot do so. The nurse should assess for periorbital edema, which may prevent the patient from opening the eyes, and document if edema interferes with eye opening.

Verbal response must be carefully evaluated: one cannot assume that because the patient responds, he or she is oriented. The examiner needs to assess the patient's orientation to time, person, and place. Verbal response cannot be evaluated when the patient is intubated, and this should be clearly documented.

Motor response includes spontaneous, purposeful movement (eg, the awake patient can move all four extremities with equal strength), movement only in response to noxious stimuli (eg, pressure), or abnormal posturing. If the patient is not responding to commands, motor response is tested by applying a painful stimulus (firm but gentle pressure) on the supraorbital notch or to the nailbed or by squeezing a muscle. If the patient attempts to push away or withdraw, the response is recorded as purposeful or appropriate ("patient withdraws to painful stimuli"). An inappropriate or nonpurposeful response is random and aimless. Posturing may be decerebrate or decorticate (see Fig. 57-3 and refer to discussion in Chap. 56); the most severe neurologic impairment results in flaccidity. Occasionally, posturing cannot be elicited if the patient has been given pharmacologic paralyzing agents. Body functions (circulation, respiration, elimination, fluid and electrolyte balance) are examined in a systematic manner.

Diagnosis

Nursing Diagnoses

Based on the assessment data, the major nursing diagnoses may include the following:

- Ineffective airway clearance related to accumulation of secretions secondary to depression of level of responsiveness
- Ineffective breathing patterns related to neurologic dysfunction (brain stem compression, structural displacement)
- Altered cerebral tissue perfusion related to the effects of increased ICP
- Risk for fluid volume deficit related to dehydration procedures
- Risk for infection related to ICP monitoring system (fiberoptic or intraventricular catheter)

Other relevant nursing diagnoses could include altered oral mucous membranes related to mouth breathing, absence of pharyngeal reflex, and inability to ingest fluids; risk for impaired skin integrity related to immobility and constraints imposed by ICP monitoring system; impaired tissue integrity (cornea) related to diminished or absent corneal reflex; risk for altered bowel or bladder elimination; and altered family processes related to crisis situation. These diagnoses are discussed below.

Collaborative Problems/Potential Complications

Based on the assessment data, potential complications may include:

- Brain stem herniation
- Diabetes insipidus
- SIADH

Planning and Goals

The goals for the patient may include maintenance of a patent airway, normalization of respiration, adequate cerebral tissue perfusion through reduction in ICP, restoration of fluid balance, absence of infection, and absence of complications.

Nursing Interventions

Maintaining a Patent Airway

The patency of the airway is assessed. If secretions are obstructing the airway, they must be suctioned with care, because transient elevations of ICP occur with suctioning. The patient is hyperoxygenated before and after suctioning to maintain adequate oxygenation. Hypoxia caused by poor oxygenation leads to cerebral ischemia and edema. Coughing is discouraged because coughing and straining also increase ICP. The lung fields are auscultated at least every 8 hours to determine the presence of adventitious sounds or any areas of congestion. Elevating the head of the bed may aid in clearing secretions as well as improving venous drainage of the brain.

Attaining Normal Respiratory Pattern

The patient must be monitored constantly for respiratory irregularities. Increased pressure on the frontal lobes or deep midline structures may result in Cheyne-Stokes respirations, whereas pressure in the midbrain may cause hyperventilation. When the lower portion of the brain stem (the pons and medulla) is involved, respirations become irregular and eventually cease.

When hyperventilation therapy is used to reduce ICP (by causing cerebral vasoconstriction and a decrease in cerebral blood volume), the nurse collaborates with the respiratory therapist in monitoring $PaCO_2$, which is usually maintained at 30 to 35 mm Hg.

Nursing Alert *A neurologic observation record (Fig. 57-6) is maintained, and all observations are made in relation to the patient's baseline condition. Repeated assessments of the patient are made (sometimes minute by minute) so that improvement or deterioration may be noted immediately. If the patient's condition deteriorates, preparations are made for surgical intervention.*

Preserving and Improving Cerebral Tissue Perfusion

In addition to ongoing nursing surveillance, nurses implement strategies to reduce factors contributing to the elevation of ICP (Table 57-1).

Proper positioning helps to reduce ICP. The patient's head is kept in a neutral (midline) position, maintained with the use of a cervical collar if necessary, to promote venous drainage. Slight elevation of the head is maintained to aid in venous drainage unless otherwise prescribed. Extreme rotation of the neck and flexion of the neck are avoided because compression or distortion of the jugular veins increases ICP. Extreme hip flexion is also avoided because this position causes an increase in intra-abdominal and intrathoracic pressures, which can produce a rise in ICP. Relatively minor changes in the patient's position may significantly affect ICP. If monitoring parameters demonstrate that turning the patient raises ICP, rotating beds and turning sheets may be used and the patient's head may be held by the nurse's hands during turning to minimize the stimuli that increase ICP.

The Valsalva maneuver, which can be produced by straining at defecation or even moving in bed, raises ICP and is to be avoided. Stool softeners may be prescribed. If the patient is alert and able to eat, a diet high in fiber may be indicated. Abdominal distention, which increases intra-abdominal and intrathoracic pressure and ICP, should be noted. Enemas and cathartics are avoided if possible. When moving or being turned in bed, the patient can be instructed to exhale (which opens the glottis) to avoid the Valsalva maneuver.

Mechanical ventilation presents unique problems for the patient with increased ICP. Before suctioning, the patient should be preoxygenated and hyperventilated using 100% oxygen on the ventilator. Suctioning should not last longer than 15 seconds. High levels of positive end-expiratory pressure are avoided because they may decrease venous return to the heart and decrease venous drainage from the brain through increased intrathoracic pressure.

(text continues on page 1642)

NURSING NEUROLOGICAL CRITICAL CARE FLOWSHEET

	ADDRESSOGRAPH												
	Date												
	Time												
	Initials												
Level of orientation (✓)	Person, Place, Date												
	Person												
	Place												
	Date												
	No orientation												
Awakens to (✓)	Voice												
	Touch												
	Noxious stimuli												
	Painful stimuli												
	No response												
Best verbal response (✓)	Clear and appropriate												
	Clear and inappropriate												
	Difficulty speaking*												
	Perseveration												
	Aphasic expressive (non-fluent)												
	Aphasic receptive (fluent)												
	Sounds no speech												
	No response												
	ETT/TRACH												
Best motor response (✓)	MAE/purposefully												
	Withdraws and lifts to painful stimuli												
	Moves to painful stimuli												
	Triple flexes (spinal reflex)												
	Decorticates (spinal reflex)												
	Decerebrates (spinal reflex)												
	No response												
Best motor strength upper extremities (✓)	No drifts (R/L)	R / L	R / L	R / L	R / L	R / L	R / L	R / L	R / L	R / L	R / L	R / L	R / L
	Drift (R/L)	R / L	R / L	R / L	R / L	R / L	R / L	R / L	R / L	R / L	R / L	R / L	R / L
	Can only lift forearm (R/L)	R / L	R / L	R / L	R / L	R / L	R / L	R / L	R / L	R / L	R / L	R / L	R / L
	Trace movement of hand or arm (R/L)	R / L	R / L	R / L	R / L	R / L	R / L	R / L	R / L	R / L	R / L	R / L	R / L
	Trace movement of fingers only (R/L)	R / L	R / L	R / L	R / L	R / L	R / L	R / L	R / L	R / L	R / L	R / L	R / L
	No response (R/L)	R / L	R / L	R / L	R / L	R / L	R / L	R / L	R / L	R / L	R / L	R / L	R / L
Best strength lower extremities (✓)	Raises leg off bed (R/L)	R / L	R / L	R / L	R / L	R / L	R / L	R / L	R / L	R / L	R / L	R / L	R / L
	Drags heel on bed and lifts knee (R/L)	R / L	R / L	R / L	R / L	R / L	R / L	R / L	R / L	R / L	R / L	R / L	R / L
	Trace movement of foot or leg (R/L)	R / L	R / L	R / L	R / L	R / L	R / L	R / L	R / L	R / L	R / L	R / L	R / L
	Trace movement of toes only (R/L)	R / L	R / L	R / L	R / L	R / L	R / L	R / L	R / L	R / L	R / L	R / L	R / L
	No response (R/L)	R / L	R / L	R / L	R / L	R / L	R / L	R / L	R / L	R / L	R / L	R / L	R / L
Seizure activity (✓)	No seizure activity												
	With LOC*												
	Without LOC*												
Ataxia (✓)	Gross ataxia												
	Fine motor ataxia												
	Does not apply												
ICP monitoring	Ventriculostomy CC's												
	ICP												
	Not applicable												

***= FURTHER DOCUMENTATION IS REQUIRED TO VALIDATE ASSESSMENT**

FIGURE 57•6 A neurologic assessment flow sheet.

PUPIL GAUGE (mm)

2 3 4 5 6

7 8 9

B=Brisk, S=Sluggish, F=Fixed

ADDRESSOGRAPH

	Date												
	Time												
	Initials												
Incision +/–	Dry and intact												
	Drainage												
Pupils refer to gauge (✓) (+)=Present (–)=Absent	Size (R/L)	R / L	R / L	R / L	R / L	R / L	R / L	R / L	R / L	R / L	R / L	R / L	R / L
	Regular (R/L)	R / L	R / L	R / L	R / L	R / L	R / L	R / L	R / L	R / L	R / L	R / L	R / L
	Irregular* (R/L)	R / L	R / L	R / L	R / L	R / L	R / L	R / L	R / L	R / L	R / L	R / L	R / L
	Reaction (R/L) (B) - (S) - (F)	R / L	R / L	R / L	R / L	R / L	R / L	R / L	R / L	R / L	R / L	R / L	R / L
	Pstosis (R/L) (+) (–)	R / L	R / L	R / L	R / L	R / L	R / L	R / L	R / L	R / L	R / L	R / L	R / L
	Gaze preference (R/L) (+)* (–)	R / L	R / L	R / L	R / L	R / L	R / L	R / L	R / L	R / L	R / L	R / L	R / L
Meningeal signs (+)=Present (–)=Absent	Headache												
	Nuchal rigidity												
	Photophobia												
Visual fields (+)=Present (–)=Absent* NA=Not applicable	Right upper outer												
	Right lower outer												
	Left upper outer												
	Left lower outer												
Nystagmus (+)=Present (–)=Absent	Lateral (R/L)	R / L	R / L	R / L	R / L	R / L	R / L	R / L	R / L	R / L	R / L	R / L	R / L
	Vertical (R/L)	R / L	R / L	R / L	R / L	R / L	R / L	R / L	R / L	R / L	R / L	R / L	R / L
Cranial nerves (+)=Present (–)=Absent	III, IV, VI, Extra occular movements												
	VII – Peripheral facial droop (R/L)	R / L	R / L	R / L	R / L	R / L	R / L	R / L	R / L	R / L	R / L	R / L	R / L
	XII – Tongue deviation (R/L)	R / L	R / L	R / L	R / L	R / L	R / L	R / L	R / L	R / L	R / L	R / L	R / L
	IX – Gag reflex												
	V, VII – Corneal reflex (R/L)	R / L	R / L	R / L	R / L	R / L	R / L	R / L	R / L	R / L	R / L	R / L	R / L
	X, IX – Cough reflex												
	Doll's eyes if appropriate												
Follows commands	Two step verbal command												
	One step verbal command												
	Unable to follow command												

***= FURTHER DOCUMENTATION IS REQUIRED TO VALIDATE ASSESSMENT**

Initials	Signature	Title	Initials	Signature	Title

FIGURE 57•6 *(Continued)*

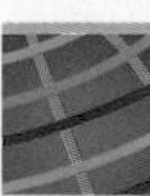

TABLE 57•1 Increased ICP and Interventions

Factor	Physiology	Interventions	Rationale
Cerebral edema	Can be caused by contusion, tumor, or abscess; water intoxication (hypo-osmolality); alteration in the blood–brain barrier (protein leaks into the tissue, causing water to follow)	Administer osmotic diuretics as prescribed (monitor serum osmolality). Maintain head of bed elevated 30 degrees. Maintain alignment of the head.	Promotes venous return Prevents impairment of venous return through the jugular veins
Hypoxia	A decrease in the PaO_2 causes cerebral vasodilation at less than 60 mm Hg.	Maintain PaO_2 greater than 60 mm Hg. Maintain oxygen therapy. Monitor arterial blood gas values. Suction when needed. Maintain a patent airway.	Prevents hypoxia and vasodilation
Hypercapnia (elevated CO_2)	Causes vasodilation	Maintain $PaCO_2$ (normally 25–30 mm Hg) through hyperventilation.	Decreased $PaCO_2$ prevents vasodilation and thus reduces the cerebral blood volume.
Impaired venous return	Increases the cerebral blood volume	Maintain head alignment. Elevate head of bed 30 degrees.	Hyperextension, rotation, or hyperflexion of the neck causes a decreased venous return.
Increase in intrathoracic or abdominal pressure	Increase in these pressures due to coughing, PEEP, Valsalva maneuver causes a decrease in venous return.	Monitor arterial blood gas values and keep PEEP as low as possible. Provide humidified oxygen. Administer cathartics as prescribed.	To keep secretions loose and easy to suction or expectorate Soft bowel movements will prevent straining or Valsalva maneuver.

Nursing activities that raise ICP should be avoided if possible. Spacing nursing interventions may prevent transient increases in ICP. During nursing interventions, the ICP should not rise above 25 mm Hg and should return to baseline levels within 5 minutes. Patients with increased ICP should not demonstrate a significant increase in pressure or change in the ICP waveform. Patients with the potential for a significant increase in ICP should receive sedation or paralyzation before initiation of any nursing activities.

Emotional stress and frequent arousal from sleep are to be avoided. A calm atmosphere is maintained. Environmental stimuli (noise, conversation) should be minimal. Isometric muscle contractions are also contraindicated, because they raise the systemic blood pressure and hence the ICP.

Monitoring Fluid Balance

The administration of various dehydrating agents is part of the treatment protocol. Corticosteroids are used to reduce cerebral edema, and fluids may be restricted. All of these treatment modalities promote the development of dehydration.

The patient's skin turgor, mucous membranes, and serum and urine osmolality are monitored for signs of dehydration. If fluids are given intravenously, the nurse ensures they are administered at a slow to moderate rate with an intravenous infusion pump to prevent too-rapid administration. For the patient receiving mannitol, the nurse observes for the possible development of congestive heart failure and pulmonary edema, because mannitol may cause fluid to shift from the intracellular compartment to the intravascular system.

For patients undergoing dehydrating procedures, vital signs, including blood pressure, must be monitored to assess fluid volume status. An indwelling urinary catheter is usually inserted to permit assessment of renal function and fluid status. During the acute phase, urine output should be monitored every hour. An output greater than 200 mL/hr for 2 consecutive hours may indicate the onset of diabetes insipidus. These patients also need careful oral hygiene because dehydration is associated with mouth dryness. Frequently rinsing the mouth, lubricating the lips, and removing encrustations relieve dryness and promote comfort.

Preventing Infection

Risk for infection is greatest when ICP is monitored with an intraventricular catheter. Most health care facilities have written protocols for managing these systems and maintaining their sterility; strict adherence to them is essential.

The dressing over the ventricular catheter must be kept dry because a wet dressing is conducive to bacterial growth. Aseptic technique is used when managing the system and changing the ventricular drainage bag. The drainage system is also checked for loose connections because they cause leakage and contamination of the CSF as well as inaccurate readings of ICP. The patient is monitored for signs and symptoms of meningitis: fever, chills, nuchal (neck) rigidity, and increasing or persisting headache.

Monitoring and Managing Potential Complications

The primary complication of increased ICP is brain herniation resulting in death. Nursing management is focused on detecting early signs of increasing ICP because medical interventions are usually ineffective once later signs develop. Frequent neurologic assessment and documentation and analysis of trends will reveal the subtle changes that may herald rising ICP, which may be fatal.

DETECTING EARLY INDICATIONS OF INCREASING ICP

The nurse assesses for and immediately reports any of the following early signs or symptoms of increasing ICP:

- Changes in LOC, disorientation, restlessness, increased respiratory effort, purposeless movements, and mental confusion, which are early clinical indications of rising ICP because brain cells responsible for cognition are extremely sensitive to decreased oxygenation
- Pupillary changes and impaired ocular movements, which occur as the increasing pressure displaces the brain against the oculomotor and optic nerves (cranial nerves II, III, IV, and VI) arising from the midbrain and brain stem (see Chap. 56)
- Weakness in one extremity or on one side of the body, which occurs as increasing ICP compresses the pyramidal tracts
- Headache that is constant, increasing in intensity, and aggravated by movement or straining, which occurs as increasing ICP causes pressure and stretching of venous and arterial vessels in the base of the brain

DETECTING LATER SIGNS OF INCREASED ICP

As ICP rises, the patient's condition worsens, as manifested by the following later signs and symptoms:

- LOC continues to deteriorate until the patient is comatose.
- The pulse rate and respiratory rate decrease, and the blood pressure and temperature rise. The pulse pressure (the difference between the systolic and the diastolic pressure) widens. The pulse fluctuates rapidly, varying from bradycardia to tachycardia.
- Altered respiratory patterns develop, including Cheyne-Stokes breathing (rhythmic waxing and waning of rate and depth of respirations alternating with brief periods of apnea) and ataxic breathing (irregular breathing with a random sequence of deep and shallow breaths).
- Projectile vomiting may occur with increased pressure on the reflex center in the medulla.
- Hemiplegia or decorticate or decerebrate posturing develops as pressure on the brain stem increases. Bilateral flaccidity occurs before death ensues.
- Loss of brain stem reflexes, including pupillary, corneal, gag, and swallowing reflexes, is an ominous sign.

MONITORING ICP

Because clinical assessment is not always a reliable guide in recognizing increased ICP, especially in comatose patients, ICP monitoring is an essential part of management. ICP is monitored closely for continuous elevation or significant increase over baseline. The trend of ICP measurements over time is an important indication of the underlying status of the patient. Vital signs are assessed when the increase in ICP is noted.

Strict aseptic technique is used when handling any part of the monitoring system. The insertion site is inspected for signs of infection. Temperature, pulse, and respirations are closely monitored for systemic signs of infection. All connections and stopcocks are checked for leaks, because even small leaks can distort pressure readings.

When ICP is recorded, the transducer is zeroed at a particular reference point, usually 2.5 cm (1 in) above the ear in the supine patient; this point corresponds to the level of the foramen of Monro (Fig. 57-7). (CSF pressure readings depend on the patient's position.) For subsequent pressure readings, the patient's head should be in the same position relative to the transducer. Fiberoptic catheters are zeroed before insertion and do not require further zeroing; they do not require the head of the bed to be at a specific position.

Whenever technology is associated with patient management, the nurse must be certain that the technology remains functioning. The most important concern must be the patient who is attached to the technology. Talking in a soothing tone and gently touching the patient's hand or stroking the cheek may be helpful in reducing emotional stress.

The measurement of ICP is only one parameter of patient assessment, however. Repeated neurologic checks and clinical examinations remain important measures. Astute observation, comparison of findings with previous observations, and interventions can assist in preventing life-threatening elevations of ICP.

MONITORING FOR SECONDARY COMPLICATIONS

The nurse also assesses for other complications of increased ICP. Urine output should be monitored closely. Diabetes insipidus requires fluid and electrolyte replacement, along with the administration of vasopressin to replace and slow the urine output. Serum electrolyte levels should be monitored for replacement. SIADH requires fluid restriction and monitoring of serum electrolyte levels.

Evaluation

Expected Outcomes

Expected outcomes may include:

1. Is free of excessive airway secretions; airway is patent
2. Attains normal respirations
   a. Breathes in a normal pattern
   b. Attains or maintains arterial blood gas values within acceptable range

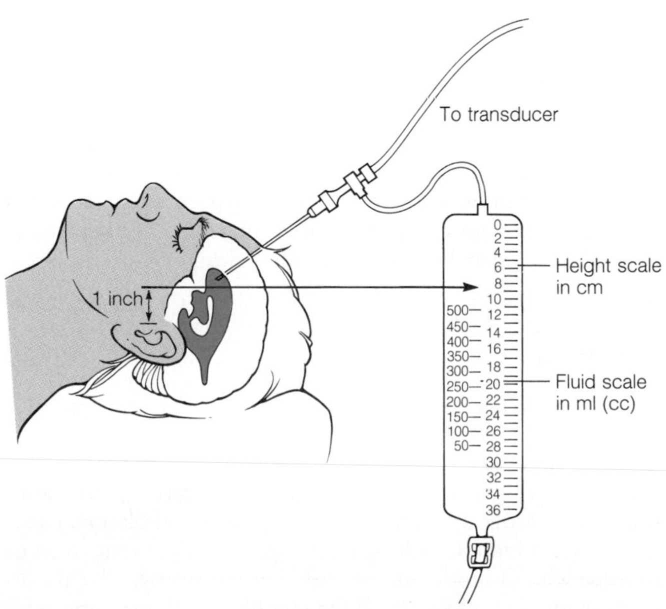

FIGURE 57•7 Location of foramen of Monro for calibration of intracranial pressure monitoring system.

3. Demonstrates improved cerebral tissue perfusion
   a. Becomes increasingly oriented to time, place, and person
   b. Follows verbal commands; answers questions correctly
4. Attains improved fluid balance
   a. Takes fluids orally
   b. Demonstrates serum and urine osmolality values within acceptable range
5. Has no sign of infection
   a. Has no fever
   b. Shows no signs of infection at dressing or arterial, intravenous, and urinary catheter sites
   c. Has no purulent drainage from ventricular drainage system
6. Is free of complications
   a. Has ICP values that remain within normal limits
   b. Demonstrates urine output and serum electrolyte levels within acceptable limits

THE UNCONSCIOUS PATIENT

Unconsciousness is a condition in which the patient is unresponsive to and unaware of environmental stimuli. The term is usually reserved for unresponsiveness of short duration (momentary to several hours). **Coma** is a clinical state of unconsciousness in which the patient is unaware of self or the environment for prolonged periods (days to months or even years). **Akinetic mutism** is a state of unresponsiveness to the environment in which the patient makes no movement or sound but sometimes opens the eyes. **Persistent vegetative state** is a condition in which the patient is described as wakeful but devoid of conscious content, without cognitive or affective mental function. The causes of unconsciousness or coma may be neurologic (head injury, stroke), toxicologic (drug overdose, alcohol intoxication), or metabolic (hepatic or renal failure, diabetic ketoacidosis).

Assessment and Diagnostic Findings

If the patient is comatose and localized signs are severe, it is assumed that neurologic disease is present until proved otherwise. If the patient is comatose and a pupillary light reflex is preserved, a toxic or metabolic disorder is suspected.

Procedures used to evaluate and identify the cause of unconsciousness include scanning, imaging, tomography (eg, CT, MRI, positron emission tomography), and electroencephalography. Laboratory tests include analysis of blood glucose, electrolyte, serum ammonia, and blood urea nitrogen levels, as well as osmolality, calcium level, and prothrombin time. Other studies may evaluate serum ketones and alcohol, drug, and arterial blood gas levels.

Complications

Potential complications for the unconscious patient include respiratory failure, pneumonia, pressure ulcers, and aspiration. Respiratory failure may develop shortly after the patient becomes unconscious. If the patient cannot maintain effective respirations, supportive care is initiated to provide adequate ventilation. Pneumonia is common in patients receiving mechanical ventilation or in those who cannot maintain and clear the airway. The unconscious patient is subject to all the complications associated with immobility, such as pressure sores, venous stasis, musculoskeletal deterioration, and disturbed gastrointestinal functioning. Pressure ulcers may become infected and a source of sepsis. Aspiration of gastric contents or feedings may occur, precipitating the development of pneumonia or occluding the airway.

Medical Management

The first priority of treatment of the unconscious patient is to obtain and maintain a patent airway. The patient may be either orally or nasally intubated, or a tracheostomy may be performed. Until a determination has been made about the patient's ability to breathe on his or her own, a mechanical ventilator is used to maintain adequate oxygenation. An intravenous catheter is inserted to maintain fluid balance, and nutritional support using either a feeding tube or gastrostomy tube should be started. The circulatory status (blood pressure, heart rate) is monitored to ensure that adequate perfusion to the body and brain is maintained.

NURSING PROCESS: THE UNCONSCIOUS PATIENT

Assessment

The nursing assessment of the unconscious patient is essentially the same as for the patient with increased ICP. Table 57-2 summarizes the assessment and the clinical significance of the findings.

Diagnosis

Nursing Diagnoses

Based on the assessment data, the major nursing diagnoses may include the following:

- Ineffective airway clearance related to cranial nerve impairment and/or unconscious state
- Altered protection and risk for injury related to unconscious state
- Risk for fluid volume deficit related to inability to ingest fluids
- Altered oral mucous membranes related to mouth-breathing, absence of pharyngeal reflex, and inability to ingest fluids
- Risk for impaired skin integrity related to immobility
- Impaired tissue integrity of cornea related to diminished or absent corneal reflex
- Ineffective thermoregulation related to damage to hypothalamic center
- Altered urinary elimination (incontinence or retention) related to the unconscious state
- Altered bowel elimination (diarrhea and/or constipation) related to the unconscious state
- Altered family processes related to sudden crisis of unconsciousness

Collaborative Problems/Potential Complications

Based on the assessment data, potential complications may include:

- Respiratory distress or failure
- Pneumonia
- Aspiration
- Pressure ulcer

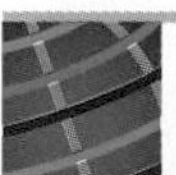

TABLE 57•2 Nursing Assessment of the Unconscious Patient

Examination	Clinical Assessment	Clinical Significance
Level of responsiveness or consciousness	Eye opening; verbal and motor responses; pupils (size, equality, reaction to light)	Obeying commands is a favorable response and demonstrates a return to consciousness.
Pattern of respiration		Disturbances of respiratory center of brain may result in various respiratory patterns.
	Cheyne-Stokes respiration	Suggests lesions deep in both hemispheres; area of basal ganglia and upper brain stem
	Hyperventilation	Suggests onset of metabolic problem or brain stem damage
	Ataxic respiration with irregularity in depth/rate	Ominous sign of damage to medullary center
Eyes		
Pupils (size, equality, reaction to light)	Equal, normally reactive pupils	Suggests that coma is toxic or metabolic in origin
	Equal or unequal diameter	Localizing sign
	Progressive dilation	Indicates increasing ICP
	Fixed dilated pupils	Indicates injury at level of midbrain
Eye movements	Normally, eyes should move from side to side.	Functional and structural integrity of brain stem is assessed by inspection of extraocular movements; usually absent in deep coma.
Corneal reflex	When cornea is touched with a wisp of clean cotton, blink response is normal.	Tests cranial nerves V and VII; localizing sign if unilateral; absent in deep coma
Facial symmetry	Asymmetry (sagging, decrease in wrinkles)	Sign of paralysis
Swallowing reflex	Drooling versus spontaneous swallowing	Absent in coma Paralysis of cranial nerves X and XII
Neck	Stiff neck	Subarachnoid hemorrhage, meningitis
	Absence of spontaneous neck movement	Fracture or dislocation of cervical spine
Response of extremity to noxious stimuli	Firm pressure on a joint of the upper and lower extremity Observe spontaneous movements.	Asymmetric response in paralysis Absent in deep coma
Deep tendon reflexes	Tap patellar and biceps tendons.	Brisk response may have localizing value Asymmetric response in paralysis Absent in deep coma
Pathologic reflexes	Firm pressure with blunt object on sole of foot, moving along lateral margin and crossing to the ball of foot	Flexion of the toes, especially the great toe, is normal except in newborn. Dorsiflexion of toes (especially great toe) indicates contralateral pathology of corticospinal tract (Babinski reflex). Localizing signs
Abnormal posture	Observation for posturing (spontaneous or in response to noxious stimuli)	Deep extensive brain lesion
	Flaccidity with absence of motor response	Seen with cerebral hemisphere pathology and in metabolic depression of brain function
	Decorticate posture (flexion and internal rotation of forearms and hands) Decerebrate posture (extension and external rotation)	Decerebrate posturing indicates deeper and more severe dysfunction than does decorticate posturing; implies brain pathology; poor prognostic sign.

Planning and Goals

The goals of care of the unconscious patient include maintenance of a clear airway, protection from injury, attainment of fluid volume balance, achievement of intact oral mucous membranes, maintenance of normal skin integrity, absence of corneal irritation, attainment of thermoregulation, absence of urinary retention and infection, absence of diarrhea or fecal impaction, maintenance of intact family or support system, and absence of complications.

The quality of nursing care provided for an unconscious patient may literally mean the difference between life and death, because the patient's protective reflexes are impaired. The nurse must assume responsibility for the patient until the basic reflexes return (coughing, blinking, and swallowing) and the patient becomes conscious and oriented. Thus, the major nursing goal is to provide these protective reflexes until the patient regains these functions.

Nursing Interventions

Maintaining the Airway

The most important consideration in managing the unconscious patient is to establish an adequate airway and ensure ventilation. Obstruction of the airway is a risk facing the unconscious patient because the epiglottis and tongue may relax, occluding the oropharynx, or the patient may aspirate vomitus or nasopharyngeal secretions.

- The patient is positioned in a lateral or semiprone position, which permits the jaw and tongue to fall forward and thus facilitates drainage of secretions.
- An unconscious patient should have frequent position changes.
- The accumulation of secretions in the pharynx presents a serious problem. Because the patient cannot swallow and lacks pharyngeal reflexes, these secretions must be removed to eliminate the danger of aspiration.
- Elevating the head of the bed to 30 degrees helps prevent aspiration of secretions.
- The patient requires frequent suctioning and oral hygiene. Suctioning is performed to remove secretions from the posterior pharynx and upper trachea. With the suction turned off, a whistle-tip catheter is lubricated with a water-soluble lubricant and inserted to the desired level. Then the suction is turned on (negative pressure) while the aspirating catheter is withdrawn with a twisting motion of the thumb and forefinger. This twisting maneuver prevents the suctioning end of the catheter from irritating the tracheal or pharyngeal mucosa, because irritation increases secretions and produces mucosal trauma and bleeding. Before and after suctioning, the patient is hyperoxygenated and hyperventilated to prevent hypoxia.
- The chest is auscultated at least every 8 hours for adventitious breath sounds or absence of breath sounds.
- The patient may require intubation and mechanical ventilation. The nurse must maintain the patency of the endotracheal tube or tracheostomy, provide frequent oral care, monitor arterial blood gas measurements, and maintain ventilator settings.
- Chest physiotherapy and postural drainage are initiated to promote pulmonary hygiene, unless contraindicated by the patient's underlying condition.

Protecting the Patient and Maintaining Safety

For the protection of the patient, padded siderails are provided and raised at all times. Care should be taken to prevent injury from invasive lines and equipment, and potential sources of injury should be identified (eg, tight dressings, environmental irritants, damp bedding or dressings, tubes and drains).

Nursing Alert *If the patient begins to emerge from unconsciousness, every measure that is available and appropriate for calming and quieting him or her should be carried out. Any form of restraint is likely to be countered by the patient with resistance, leading to self-injury or to a dangerous increase in ICP. Therefore, physical restraints should be avoided if possible; a written prescription should be obtained if their use is essential for the patient's well-being.*

Protection also encompasses the concept of protecting the patient's dignity during unconsciousness. Simple measures such as providing privacy and speaking to the patient during nursing care activities preserve the patient's humanity. Not speaking negatively about the patient's condition or prognosis is also important, because patients in a light coma may be able to hear. The comatose patient has an increased need for advocacy, and it is the nurse's responsibility to see that these advocacy needs are met.

Maintaining Fluid and Nutritional Balance

The patient is assessed for hydration status; the mucous membranes are examined and the skin is assessed for tissue turgor. Fluid needs are initially met by giving the required fluids intravenously and then by nasogastric or gastrostomy feedings.

Intravenous solutions and blood transfusions for patients with intracranial conditions must be administered slowly. If given too rapidly, they may increase the ICP. The quantity of fluids administered may be restricted to minimize the possibility of producing cerebral edema.

A feeding tube, placed in the duodenum, or a gastrostomy tube may be inserted for the administration of enteral feedings.

Providing Mouth Care

The patient's mouth is inspected for dryness, inflammation, and crusting. The unconscious patient requires conscientious oral care because there is a risk of parotitis if the mouth is not kept scrupulously clean. The mouth is cleansed and rinsed carefully to remove secretions and crusts and to keep the mucous membranes moist. A thin coating of petrolatum on the lips prevents drying, cracking, and encrustations. If the patient has an endotracheal tube, the tube should be moved to the opposite side of the mouth daily to prevent ulceration of the mouth and lips.

Maintaining Skin Integrity

Preventing skin breakdown requires continuing nursing assessment and intervention. Special attention is given to unconscious patients because they are insensitive to external stimuli. This includes a regular schedule of turning to avoid pressure, which can cause breakdown and necrosis of the skin. Turning also provides kinesthetic (sensation of movement), proprioceptive (awareness of position), and vestibular (equilibrium) stimulation. After turning, the patient is carefully repositioned to prevent ischemic necrosis over pressure areas. Dragging the patient up in bed must be avoided, because this creates a shearing force and friction on the skin surface.

Maintaining correct body position is important; equally important is passive exercise of the extremities so that contractures are prevented. The use of splints or foam boots aids in the prevention of footdrop and eliminates the pressure of bedding on the toes. Trochanter rolls supporting the hip joints keep the legs in proper alignment. The arms should be in abduction, the fingers lightly flexed, and the hands in a position of slight supination. Heels and feet should be assessed for pressure areas. Specialty beds, such as fluidized or low-air-loss beds, may be used to decrease pressure on bony prominences.

Preserving Corneal Integrity

Some unconscious patients lie with their eyes open and have inadequate or absent corneal reflexes. The cornea is likely to become irritated or scratched, leading to keratitis and corneal ulcers.

The eyes may be cleansed with cotton balls moistened with sterile normal saline to remove debris and discharge. If artificial tears are prescribed, they may be instilled every 2 hours. Periocular edema (swelling around the eyes) often occurs after cranial surgery. Cold compresses may be prescribed, and care must be exerted to avoid contact with the cornea. Eye patches should be used cautiously because of the potential for corneal abrasion from the cornea coming in contact with the patch.

Achieving Thermoregulation

High fever in the unconscious patient may be caused by infection of the respiratory or urinary tract, drug reactions, or damage to the hypothalamic temperature-regulating center. A slight elevation of temperature may be caused by dehydration. The environment can be adjusted, depending on the patient's condition, to promote a normal body temperature. If body temperature is elevated, a minimum amount of bedding—a sheet or perhaps only a small drape—is used. The room may be cooled to 18.3°C (65°F). However, if the patient is elderly and does not have an elevated temperature, a warmer environment is needed.

Nursing Alert *The body temperature of an unconscious patient is never taken by mouth. Rectal or tympanic (if not contraindicated) temperature measurement is preferred to the less accurate axillary temperature.*

Because of damage to the heat-regulating center in the brain or severe intracranial infection, unconscious patients often develop very high temperatures. Such temperature elevations must be controlled because the increased metabolic demands of the brain will overburden cerebral circulation and oxygenation, resulting in cerebral deterioration. Persistent hyperthermia is indicative of brain stem damage and indicates a poor prognosis.

Reducing body temperature is a major goal in treating some cerebral disorders. It has been shown that body temperatures below normal will decrease cerebral edema, reduce the oxygen and metabolic requirements of the brain, and protect the brain from continued ischemia. If body metabolism can be reduced by lowering body temperature, the collateral circulation in the brain may be able to provide an adequate blood supply to the brain.

Inducing and maintaining hypothermia is a major clinical procedure and requires knowledge and skilled nursing observation and management. It is desirable to begin treatment before the patient's temperature gets too high.

- All bedding over the patient should be removed (with the possible exception of a light sheet or small drape).
- Repeated doses of aspirin or acetaminophen are given as prescribed.
- Cool sponge baths and an electric fan blowing over the patient to increase surface cooling may be helpful.
- The use of a hypothermia blanket and equipment is usually effective in controlling neurogenic hyperthermia.

Frequent temperature monitoring is indicated to assess the patient's response to the therapy and to prevent an excessive decrease in temperature and shivering. Shivering may increase cellular oxygen demands and result in cellular hypoxia; it may also increase ICP by isometric muscle contraction. Chlorpromazine (Thorazine) is administered as prescribed to control shivering.

Preventing Urinary Retention

The unconscious patient is either incontinent or has urinary retention. The bladder is palpated at intervals to determine whether urinary retention is present, because a full bladder may be an overlooked cause of incontinence.

If there are signs of urinary retention, initially an indwelling urinary catheter attached to a closed drainage system is inserted. Because the catheter is a major cause of urinary infection, the patient is observed for fever and cloudy urine. The area around the urethral orifice is inspected for drainage. The urinary catheter is usually removed when the patient has a stable cardiovascular system and if no problems with diuresis, sepsis, or voiding existed before the onset of coma. Although many unconscious patients urinate spontaneously after catheter removal, the patient's bladder should be palpated periodically for urinary retention.

An external catheter (condom catheter) for the male patient and absorbent pads for the female patient can be used for the unconscious patient who can urinate spontaneously although involuntarily. As soon as consciousness is regained, a bladder training program is initiated. The incontinent patient is monitored frequently for skin irritation and skin breakdown. Appropriate skin care is implemented to prevent these complications.

Promoting Bowel Function

The abdomen is assessed for distention by listening for bowel sounds and measuring the girth of the abdomen with a tape measure. There is a risk of diarrhea from infection, antibiotics, and hyperosmolar fluids. Frequent loose stools may also occur with fecal impaction. Commercial fecal collection bags are available for patients with fecal incontinence.

Immobility and lack of dietary fiber may cause constipation. The nurse monitors the number and consistency of bowel movements and performs a rectal examination for signs of fecal impaction. Stool softeners may be prescribed and can be administered with tube feedings. To facilitate bowel emptying, a glycerine suppository may be indicated. The patient may require an enema every other day to empty the lower colon. Enemas may be contraindicated, however, if the Valsalva maneuver increases a compromised ICP.

Providing Sensory Stimulation

Sensory stimulation is provided to help overcome the profound sensory deprivation of the unconscious patient. Efforts are made to maintain the sense of daily rhythm by keeping the usual day and night patterns for activity and sleep. The nurse touches and talks to the patient and encourages family members and friends to do so. Communication is extremely important and includes touching the patient and spending enough time with him or her to become sensitive to his or her needs. It is also important to avoid making any negative comments about the patient's status or prognosis in the patient's presence.

The nurse orients the patient to time and place at least once every 8 hours. Sounds from the patient's home and workplace may be introduced by means of a tape recorder. In addition, family members can read to the patient from a favorite book and may suggest radio and television programs that the patient previously enjoyed as a means of enriching the environment and providing familiar input. When the patient has regained consciousness, videotaped family or social events may assist the patient in recognizing family and friends and allow him or her to be a part of missed events.

Supporting the Family

The family of the unconscious patient may be thrown into a sudden state of crisis and go through the process of severe anxiety, denial, anger, remorse, grief, and reconciliation. To help family members mobilize their own adaptive capacities, nurses can reinforce and clarify information about the patient's condition, permit the family to be involved in the care of their loved one, and listen to and encourage ventilation of feelings and concerns while supporting them in their decision-making process concerning posthospitalization management and placement. Families may benefit from participation in support groups offered through the hospital, rehabilitation facility, or community organizations.

When hope for recovery is no longer possible, the family must confront the death of their loved one. The neurologic patient is often pronounced brain dead before physiologic death occurs. The term "brain death" describes irreversible loss of all functions of the entire brain, including the brain stem. The term may be misleading to the family because although brain function has ceased, the patient appears to be alive while the heart rate and blood pressure are sustained by vasoactive medications, and breathing continues by mechanical ventilation. When discussing a patient who is brain dead with family members, it is important to use the term "dead"; the term "brain dead" may confuse them.

Monitoring and Managing Potential Complications

Pneumonia, aspiration, and respiratory failure are potential complications in any patient who is unconscious and unable to protect the airway or turn, cough, and take deep breaths. The longer the period of unconsciousness, the greater the risk that pulmonary complications will develop.

Vital signs and respiratory function are monitored closely to detect any signs of respiratory failure or distress. Total blood count and arterial blood gas measurements are assessed to determine whether there are adequate red blood cells to carry oxygen and whether ventilation is effective. Chest physiotherapy and suctioning are initiated to prevent respiratory complications such as pneumonia. If pneumonia develops, cultures are obtained to identify the organism so that appropriate antibiotics can be administered.

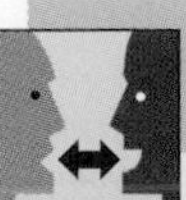

ETHICS AND RELATED ISSUES

Do obligations to patients differ according to health status—for example, if the patient is in a persistent vegetative state or in a coma?

Situation

The family of a 55-year-old woman, who has been diagnosed to be in a persistent vegetative state, wants to withdraw tube feedings and let the patient die. The nursing assistant states that the patient is not brain dead because the patient moves her eyes toward the nursing assistant and has periods of sleep and awakening.

Dilemma

What is the difference between the outcome for persistent vegetative state and coma, and is treatment futile?

Discussion

Is the maintenance of medical treatment morally obligatory in patients in a persistent vegetative state? What is the role of the nursing assistant with regard to making his or her views considered? How can the nurse help the assistant? If treatments are withdrawn, is the health care team committing euthanasia?

The unconscious patient is monitored closely for evidence of impaired skin integrity, and strategies to prevent skin breakdown and pressure ulcers are continued through all phases of care, including hospital, rehabilitation, and home care. Factors that contribute to impaired skin integrity (eg, incontinence, inadequate dietary intake, pressure on bony prominences, edema) are addressed. If pressure ulcers develop, strategies to promote healing are undertaken. Care is taken to prevent bacterial contamination of pressure ulcers, which may lead to sepsis and septic shock. Assessment and management of pressure ulcers are discussed in detail in Chapter 10.

Evaluation

Expected Outcomes

Expected outcomes may include:

1. Maintains clear airway and demonstrates appropriate breath sounds
2. Experiences no injuries
3. Attains/maintains adequate fluid status
   a. Has no clinical signs of dehydration
   b. Demonstrates normal range of serum electrolytes
4. Attains/maintains healthy oral mucous membranes
5. Maintains normal skin integrity
6. Has no corneal irritation
7. Attains or maintains thermoregulation
8. Has no urinary retention
9. Has no diarrhea or fecal impaction
10. Family members cope with crisis
    a. Verbalize fears and concerns
    b. Participate in patient's care and provide sensory stimulation by talking and touching

11. Is free of complications
    a. Has arterial blood gas values within normal range
    b. Displays no signs of pneumonia
    c. Exhibits intact skin over pressure areas

CEREBROVASCULAR DISEASE

Cerebrovascular disease refers to any functional abnormality of the central nervous system that occurs when the normal blood supply to the brain is disrupted. The pathology may involve an artery, a vein, or both. Cerebral circulation can become impaired as a result of partial or complete occlusion of a blood vessel or hemorrhage resulting from a tear in the vessel wall. The blood vessel most frequently associated with cerebrovascular disease is the internal carotid artery.

Vascular disease of the central nervous system may be caused by arteriosclerosis (most common), hypertensive changes, arteriovenous malformations, vasospasm, inflammation, arteritis, or embolism. As a result of vascular disease, blood vessels lose their elasticity, become hardened, and develop atheromatous deposits, or plaques, which may be the source of an embolus. The lumen of the vessel may gradually close, causing impairment of cerebral circulation and ischemia of the brain. If cerebral ischemia is transient, as in a transient ischemic attack (TIA), there is usually no lasting neurologic deficit. Should the ischemic area not receive oxygen, the area will progress to an infarction. Occlusion of a large vessel, however, produces cerebral infarction. The vessel may rupture and produce hemorrhage.

Transient Ischemic Attacks

A TIA is a transient or temporary episode of neurologic dysfunction, commonly manifested by a sudden loss of motor, sensory, or visual function. It may last a few seconds or minutes but does not last longer than 24 hours. Complete recovery usually occurs between attacks. TIAs precede a stroke in 10% of patients. Approximately 20% of patients who have had a TIA will go on to have a stroke within 3 years (Kelley, 1997). A TIA may serve as a warning of impending stroke, which has its greatest incidence in the first month after the first attack. Lack of evaluation and treatment of a patient who has experienced previous TIAs may result in a stroke and irreversible deficits. Some patients may have symptoms that are consistent with a TIA but that last more than 24 hours and resolve within 21 days without any neurologic deficit; this is known as *reversible ischemic neurologic deficits* (RIND).

Risk factors for TIAs include hypertension, Type 1 diabetes mellitus, cardiac disease, history of smoking, family history of strokes, and chronic alcoholism. The symptoms are caused by a temporary impairment of blood flow to a specific region of the brain for various reasons, such as atherosclerosis, obstruction of cerebral microcirculation by a small embolus, a decrease in CPP, or cardiac dysrhythmias.

Clinical Manifestations

The signs and symptoms of a TIA depend on the location of the affected vessel. Interrupted anterior circulation established by the carotid circulation (ophthalmic, middle cerebral, and anterior cerebral arteries) produces lateral signs such as amaurosis fugax (sudden painless loss of vision in one eye), contralateral weakness, or aphasia. *Amaurosis fugax* is due to retinal artery ischemia and occurs without warning. Posterior circulation, which is established by the vertebrobasilar circulation (posterior cerebral and cerebellar arteries), results in focal changes such as vertigo, diplopia, numbness or paresthesias, dysphagia, or ataxia.

Assessment and Diagnostic Findings

A *bruit* (abnormal sound heard on auscultation resulting from interference with normal blood flow) may be heard over the carotid artery. There are diminished or absent carotid pulsations in the neck.

Carotid phonoangiography may be performed; this involves auscultation, direct visualization, and photographic recording of carotid bruits. Oculoplethysmography measures the pulsation in blood flow through the ophthalmic artery. Carotid angiography allows visualization of intracranial and cervical vessels. Digital subtraction angiography is used to define carotid artery obstruction and provides information on patterns of cerebral blood flow.

Medical Management

Patients who are not candidates for surgical intervention may be placed on anticoagulant therapy to prevent future attacks and a possible massive cerebral infarction. Platelet-inhibiting medications (particularly aspirin) are useful in decreasing the occurrence of cerebral infarction in patients who have experienced multiple TIAs. Prevention of future attacks is accomplished through treatment of hypertension and hyperglycemia and cessation of smoking.

SURGICAL MANAGEMENT

Surgical intervention procedures for managing TIAs and preventing stroke are carotid endarterectomy and angioplasty. During angioplasty, a catheter with a balloon is inserted in the artery to compress the plaque against the arterial wall and thereby improve blood flow. A carotid endarterectomy is the removal of an atherosclerotic plaque or thrombus from the carotid artery to prevent stroke in patients with occlusive disease of the extracranial cerebral arteries (Fig. 57-8). Most ischemic strokes are associated with lesions of the extracranial arteries.

Nursing Management

After endarterectomy, a neurologic flow sheet is used to monitor and document neurologic status. The neurosurgeon is notified immediately if a neurologic deficit develops. Formation of a thrombus at the site of the endarterectomy can be suspected if there is a sudden increase in neurologic deficits, such as weakness on one side of the body. The patient should be prepared for reoperation.

The primary complications of carotid endarterectomy are stroke, cranial nerve injuries, infection or hematoma of the wound, and carotid artery disruption. It is important to maintain adequate blood pressure levels in the immediate postoperative period. Hypotension is avoided to prevent cerebral ischemia and thrombosis. Uncontrolled hypertension may precipitate cerebral hemorrhage, edema, hemorrhage at the surgical incision, or disruption of the arterial reconstruction. Sodium nitroprusside is commonly used to reduce the blood pressure to previous levels. Close cardiac monitoring is necessary because these patients have a high incidence of coronary artery disease.

Difficulty in swallowing, hoarseness, or other signs of cranial nerve dysfunction must be assessed. Some swelling in the neck after

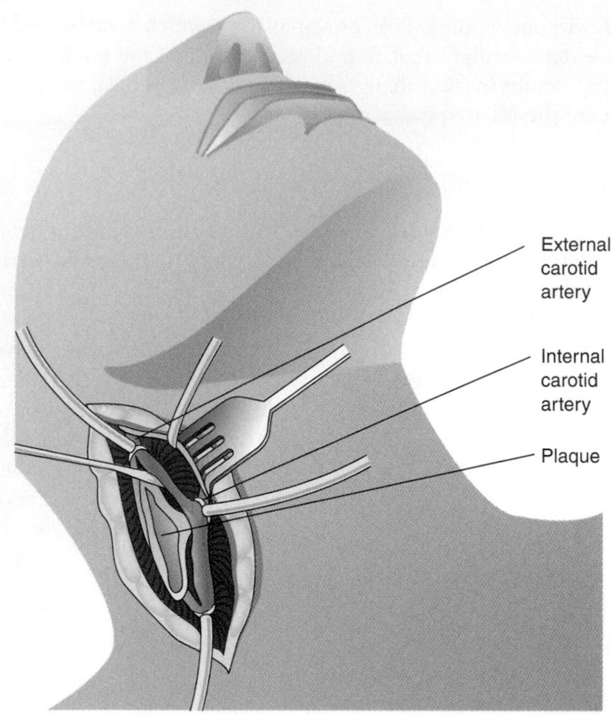

FIGURE 57•8 Plaque, a potential source of emboli in TIA and stroke, is surgically removed from the carotid artery.

surgery is expected; if large enough, however, swelling and hematoma formation can obstruct the airway. Emergency airway supplies, including those needed for a tracheostomy, must be available. Table 57-3 provides more information about complications of carotid surgery.

Stroke (Cerebrovascular Accident)

A stroke, cerebrovascular accident, or what is now being termed "brain attack" is a sudden loss of brain function resulting from disruption of the blood supply to a part of the brain. This event is usually the result of long-standing cerebrovascular disease. The term "brain attack" is being used to suggest to health care practitioners and the public that a stroke is as urgent a health care issue as a heart attack. This change in terms also reflects a similar management strategy in both diseases. Early treatment results in fewer symptoms and less loss of function.

Stroke is the primary neurologic problem in the United States and in the world. Although preventive efforts have brought about a steady decline in its incidence in the last several years, stroke is the third leading cause of death. Approximately 730,000 people will have a stroke, with 160,000 people dying from the stroke each year. The incidence for the first stroke among African Americans is almost twice that of white Americans; African Americans also suffer more extensive physical impairments and are twice as likely to die from stroke than whites (NINDS, 1997; Broderick et al., 1998).

TABLE 57•3 Selected Complications of Carotid Endarterectomy and Nursing Interventions

Complication	Characteristics	Nursing Interventions
Wound hematoma	Occurs in 5.5% of patients. Larger or rapidly expanding hematomas require emergency treatment. If the airway is obstructed by the hematoma, the wound may be opened at the bedside.	Monitor neck discomfort and wound expansion. Report swelling, subjective feelings of pressure in the neck, difficulty breathing.
Hypertension	Poorly controlled hypertension increases the risk of postoperative complications, including hematoma and hyperperfusion syndrome. There is an increased incidence of neurologic impairment and death due to intracerebral hemorrhage. May be related to surgically induced abnormalities of carotid baroreceptor sensitivity.	Risk is highest in the first 48 hours after surgery. Check blood pressure frequently and report deviations from baseline. Observe for and report new onset of neurologic deficits.
Postoperative hypotension	Occurs in approximately 5% of patients. Treated with fluids and low-dose phenylephrine infusion. Usually resolves in 24 to 48 hours. Patients with hypotension should have serial ECGs to rule out myocardial infarction.	Monitor blood pressure and observe for signs and symptoms of hypotension.
Hyperperfusion syndrome	Occurs when cerebral vessel autoregulation fails. Arteries accustomed to diminished blood flow may be permanently dilated; increased blood flow after endarterectomy coupled with insufficient vasoconstriction leads to capillary bed damage, edema, and hemorrhage.	Observe for severe unilateral headache improved by sitting upright or standing.
Intracerebral hemorrhage	Occurs infrequently, but is often fatal (60%) or results in serious neurologic impairment. Can occur secondary to hyperperfusion syndrome. Increased risk with advanced age, hypertension, presence of high-grade stenosis, poor collateral flow, and slow flow in the region of the middle cerebral artery.	Monitor neurologic status and report any changes in mental status or neurologic functioning immediately.

Pathophysiology

Strokes can be divided into two major categories: nonhemorrhagic (85%) and hemorrhagic (15%). A nonhemorrhagic or ischemic stroke usually results from one of three events: (1) thrombosis (a blood clot within a blood vessel of the brain or neck), (2) cerebral embolism (a blood clot or other material carried to the brain from another part of the body), or (3) ischemia (decrease of blood flow to an area of the brain). A hemorrhagic stroke is a cerebral hemorrhage (rupture of a cerebral blood vessel with bleeding into the brain tissue or spaces surrounding the brain). In either type of stoke, the result is an interruption in the blood supply to the brain, causing temporary or permanent loss of movement, thought, memory, speech, or sensation.

ISCHEMIC STROKES

Ischemic strokes are subdivided into five different types: large artery thrombosis (20%), small penetrating artery thrombosis (25%), cardiogenic embolic stroke (20%), cryptogenic (30%) and other (5%).

Large artery thrombotic strokes are due to atherosclerosis of the large blood vessels within the brain. Thrombus formation may also occur, and along with the atherosclerosis there is a decrease in blood supply to the area, resulting in ischemia and infarction.

Small penetrating artery thrombotic strokes affect one or more vessels and are the most common type of ischemic stroke. Small artery thrombotic strokes are also called lacunar strokes because of the cavity that is created once the infarcted brain tissue dissipates.

Cardiogenic embolic strokes are associated with cardiac arrhythmias, usually atrial fibrillation. Emboli originate from the heart and circulate to the cerebral vasculature, resulting in a stroke (most commonly the left middle cerebral artery). Embolic strokes may be prevented with the use of anticoagulation in patients with atrial fibrillation.

The last two classifications of ischemic strokes are cryptogenic strokes, which have no known cause, and other strokes, from causes such as vasospasm, cocaine use, migraines, and coagulopathies.

HEMORRHAGIC STROKES

Hemorrhagic strokes are the result of bleeding into the brain tissue or into a space such as the subarachnoid space (Fig. 57-9). Hemorrhagic strokes can be caused by arteriovenous malformations, aneurysm rupture, certain drugs (eg, anticoagulants and amphetamines), or uncontrolled hypertension. Bleeding can occur in the epidural or subarachnoid spaces or intracerebrally. In diagnosing a hemorrhagic stroke in a patient younger than 40, some clinicians may obtain a toxicology screen for drug use.

Extradural hemorrhage (epidural hemorrhage) is a neurosurgical emergency; this patient requires urgent care. It usually follows skull fracture with a tear of the middle artery or other meningeal artery. The patient must be treated within hours of the injury to survive (see the section on head injury in Chap. 58).

Subdural hemorrhage (excluding acute subdural hemorrhage) is basically the same as an epidural hemorrhage, except that in subdural hematoma usually a bridging vein is torn. Thus, a longer period (longer lucid interval) is required for the hematoma to form and cause pressure on the brain. Some patients may have chronic subdural hemorrhages without exhibiting signs or symptoms. (This is also discussed in the section on head injury in Chap. 58.)

Subarachnoid hemorrhage (hemorrhage in the subarachnoid space) may occur as a result of trauma or hypertension, but the most common cause is a leaking aneurysm in the area of the circle of Willis and congenital arteriovenous malformations of the brain. Any artery within the brain can be the site of an aneurysm. (The treatment of intracranial aneurysms is discussed in Chap. 59.)

Intracerebral hemorrhage, bleeding into the brain substance, is most common in patients with hypertension and cerebral atherosclerosis because degenerative changes from these diseases cause rupture of the vessel. In people younger than 40, intracerebral hemorrhages are usually caused by arteriovenous malformations, hemangioblastomas, and trauma. They also may be due to certain types of arterial pathology, brain tumor, and the use of medications (oral anticoagulants, amphetamines, and a variety of addictive drugs).

The bleeding is usually arterial and occurs most commonly in a portion of the basal ganglia and the adjacent internal capsule and the thalamus. Occasionally, the bleeding ruptures the wall of the lateral ventricle and causes intraventricular hemorrhage, which is frequently fatal.

Clinical Manifestations

A stroke causes a wide variety of neurologic deficits, depending on the location of the lesion (which vessels are obstructed), the size of the area of inadequate perfusion, and the amount of collateral (secondary or accessory) blood flow. The patient may have any of the following general signs or symptoms:

- Numbness or weakness of the face, arm, or leg, especially on one side of the body
- Confusion or change in mental status
- Trouble speaking or understanding speech
- Visual disturbances
- Difficulty walking, dizziness, or loss of balance or coordination
- Sudden severe headache

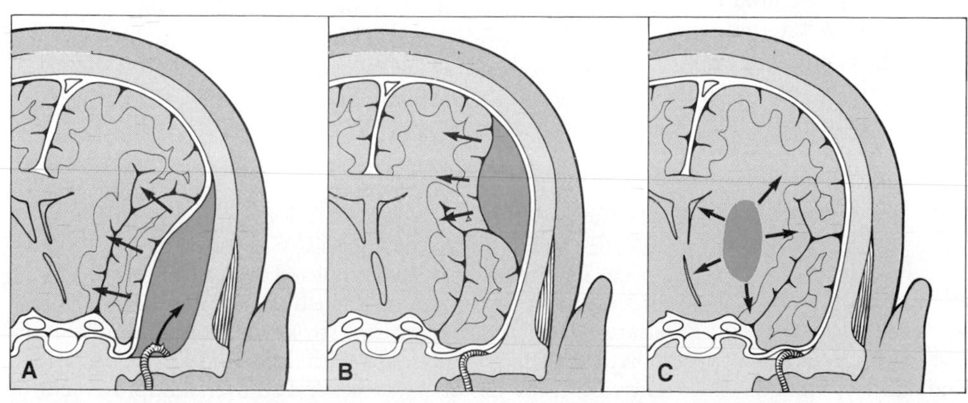

FIGURE 57•9 Cerebral hemorrhage or bleeding. (**A**) Epidural or extradural hematoma—bleeding between the inner skull and the dura, compressing the brain underneath. (**B**) Subdural hematoma—bleeding between the dura mater and arachnoid membrane. (**C**) Intracerebral hemorrhage—bleeding in the brain or the cerebral tissue with displacement of surrounding structures.

After the patient is hospitalized, further evaluation will reveal the extent of the neurologic deficits. Motor, sensory, cranial nerve, cognitive, and other functions may be disrupted. Table 57-4 reviews the neurologic deficits frequently seen in patients with strokes. Table 57-5 compares the symptoms seen in right hemispheric stroke with those seen in left hemispheric stroke.

MOTOR LOSS

Stroke is a disease of the upper motor neurons and results in loss of voluntary control over motor movements. Because the upper motor neurons decussate (cross), a disturbance of voluntary motor control on one side of the body may reflect damage to the upper motor neurons on the opposite side of the brain. The most common motor dysfunction is hemiplegia (paralysis of one side of the body) due to a lesion of the opposite side of the brain. Hemiparesis, or weakness of one side of the body, is another sign.

In the early stage of stroke, the initial clinical features may be flaccid paralysis and loss of or decrease in the deep tendon reflexes. When these deep reflexes reappear (usually by 48 hours), increased tone is observed along with spasticity (abnormal increase in muscle tone) of the extremities on the affected side.

COMMUNICATION LOSS

Other brain functions affected by stroke are language and communication. Stroke is the most common cause of aphasia. Dysfunction of language and communication may be manifested by the following:

- Dysarthria (difficulty in speaking), as demonstrated by poorly intelligible speech caused by paralysis of the muscles responsible for producing speech
- Dysphasia or aphasia (defective speech or loss of speech), which is mainly expressive or receptive
- Apraxia (inability to perform a previously learned action), as may be seen when a patient picks up a fork and attempts to comb his hair with it

PERCEPTUAL DISTURBANCES

Perception is the ability to interpret sensation. Stroke can result in visual-perceptual dysfunctions, disturbances in visual-spatial relations, and sensory loss.

Visual-perceptual dysfunctions are due to disturbances of the primary sensory pathways between the eye and visual cortex. Homonymous hemianopsia (loss of half of the visual field) may occur from stroke and may be temporary or permanent. The affected side of vision corresponds to the paralyzed side of the body. To assess for hemianopsia, the patient is asked to look at the examiner's face. The examiner's finger is placed about 30 cm (12 in) from the patient's ear on the unaffected side and is moved inward toward the patient's field of vision. The patient is asked to indicate when he or she first detects movement of the examiner's finger. Inability to detect movement on one or both sides suggests hemianopsia.

Disturbances in visual-spatial relations (perceiving the relation of two or more objects in spatial areas) are frequently seen in patients with right hemispheric damage.

SENSORY LOSS

Sensory losses from stroke may take the form of slight impairment of touch or may be more severe, with loss of proprioception (ability to perceive position and motion of body parts) as well as difficulty in interpreting visual, tactile, and auditory stimuli.

COGNITIVE IMPAIRMENT AND PSYCHOLOGICAL EFFECTS

If damage has occurred to the frontal lobe, learning capacity, memory, or other higher cortical intellectual functions may be impaired. Such dysfunction may be reflected in a limited attention span, difficulties in comprehension, forgetfulness, and a lack of motivation, which cause these patients to experience frustrations in their rehabilitation programs. Depression is common and may be exaggerated by the patient's natural response to this catastrophic illness. Other psychological problems are common and are manifested by emotional lability, hostility, frustration, resentment, and lack of cooperation.

Assessment and Diagnostic Findings

Any patient with neurologic deficits needs a careful history and a complete physical and neurologic examination. Initial assessment will focus on the patient's ability to maintain a patent airway (due to loss of gag or cough reflexes and altered respiratory pattern), cardiovascular status (including blood pressure, cardiac rhythm and rate, carotid bruit), and gross neurologic losses.

Initial diagnostic tests include a CT scan or MRI to determine whether the stroke is ischemic or hemorrhagic (which determines treatment), electrocardiography, and a carotid ultrasound. Other studies may include cerebral angiography, transcranial Doppler flow studies, and echocardiography.

Prevention

Prevention of stroke is the best possible approach. Steps are taken to alter the predisposing factors that increase a person's risk for stroke. Several methods of preventing strokes have been identified for patients with TIAs or cardiac disease (eg, control of atrial fibrillation, which increases the risk of emboli). Carotid endarterectomy was described previously. The administration of warfarin (Coumadin), an anticoagulant that inhibits clot formation, may prevent both thrombotic and embolic strokes.

Complications

Complications of a stroke include cerebral hypoxia, decreased cerebral blood flow, and extension of the area of injury. Cerebral hypoxia is minimized by providing adequate oxygenation of blood to the brain. Brain function is dependent on available oxygen being delivered to the tissues. Administering supplemental oxygen and maintaining the hemoglobin and hematocrit at acceptable levels will assist in maintaining tissue oxygenation.

Cerebral blood flow is dependent on the blood pressure, cardiac output, and integrity of cerebral blood vessels. Adequate hydration (intravenous fluids) must be ensured to reduce blood viscosity and improve cerebral blood flow. Extremes of hypertension or hypotension need to be avoided to prevent changes in cerebral blood flow and the potential for extending the area of injury.

Medical Management

THROMBOLYTIC THERAPY FOR THE PATIENT WITH AN ISCHEMIC STROKE

In 1995, a 5-year study was completed by the National Institutes of Neurologic Disorders and Stroke (NINDS). This study demonstrated that rapid diagnosis of stroke and initiation of thrombolytic therapy in patients with ischemic stroke lead to a decrease in the size of the stroke and an overall improvement in

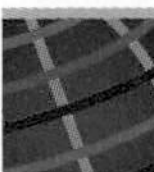

TABLE 57•4 Neurologic Deficits of Stroke: Manifestations and Nursing Implications

Neurologic Deficit	Manifestation	Nursing Implications/Patient Teaching Applications
Visual Field Deficits		
Homonymous hemianopsia (loss of half of the visual field)	• Unaware of persons or objects on side of visual loss • Neglect of one side of the body • Difficulty judging distances	Place objects within intact field of vision. Approach the patient from side of intact field of vision. Instruct/remind the patient to turn head in the direction of visual loss to compensate for loss of visual field. Encourage the use of eyeglasses if available. When teaching the patient, do so within patient's intact visual field.
Loss of peripheral vision	• Difficulty seeing at night • Unaware of objects or the borders of objects	Place objects in center vision. Encourage the use of a cane or other object to identify objects in the periphery of the visual field. Avoid night driving or other risky activities in the darkness.
Diplopia	• Double vision	Explain to the patient the location of an object when placing it near the patient. Consistently place patient care items in the same location.
Motor Deficits		
Hemiparesis	• Weakness of the face, arm, and leg on the same side (due to a lesion in the opposite hemisphere)	Place objects within the patient's reach on the non-affected side. Instruct the patient to exercise and increase the strength on the unaffected side.
Hemiplegia	• Paralysis of the face, arm, and leg on the same side (due to a lesion in the opposite hemisphere)	Encourage the patient to provide range-of-motion exercises to the affected side. Provide immobilization as needed to the affected side. Maintain body alignment in functional position. Exercise unaffected limb to increase mobility, strength, and use.
Ataxia	• Staggering, unsteady gait • Unable to keep feet together; needs a broad base to stand	Support patient during the initial ambulation phase. Provide supportive device for ambulation (walker, cane). Instruct the patient not to walk without assistance or supportive device.
Dysarthria	• Difficulty in forming words	Provide the patient with alternative methods of communicating. Allow the patient sufficient time to respond to verbal communication. Support patient and family to alleviate frustration related to difficulty in communicating.
Dysphagia	• Difficulty in swallowing	Test the patient's pharyngeal reflexes before offering food or fluids. Assist the patient with meals. Place food on the unaffected side of the mouth. Allow ample time to eat.
Sensory Deficits		
Paresthesia (occurs on the side opposite the lesion)	• Numbness and tingling of body parts. • Difficulty with proprioception	Instruct the patient to avoid using this body part as the dominant limb. Provide range of motion to affected areas and apply corrective devices as needed. Place patient care items toward the nonaffected side.
Verbal Deficits		
Expressive aphasia	• Unable to form words that are understandable; may be able to speak in single-word responses	Encourage patient to repeat sounds of the alphabet.
Receptive aphasia	• Unable to comprehend the spoken word; can speak but may not make sense	Speak slowly and clearly to assist the patient in forming the sounds.
Global aphasia	• Combination of both receptive and expressive aphasia	Speak clearly and in simple sentences; use gestures or pictures when able.
Cognitive Deficits		
	• Short- and long-term memory loss • Decreased attention span • Impaired ability to concentrate • Poor abstract reasoning	Reorient patient to time, place, and situation frequently. Use verbal and auditory cues to orient patient. Provide familiar objects (family photographs, favorite objects).

(continued)

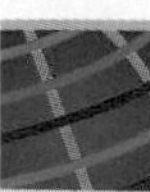

TABLE 57•4 **Neurologic Deficits of Stroke: Manifestations and Nursing Implications** *(Continued)*

Neurologic Deficit	Manifestation	Nursing Implications/Patient Teaching Applications
	• Altered judgment	Use noncomplicated language. Match visual tasks with a verbal cue: holding a toothbrush, simulate brushing of teeth while saying, "I would like you to brush your teeth now." Minimize distracting noises and views when teaching the patient. Repeat and reinforce instructions frequently.
Emotional Deficits	• Loss of self-control • Emotional lability • Decreased tolerance to stressful situations • Depression • Withdrawal • Fear, hostility, and anger • Feelings of isolation	Support patient during uncontrollable outbursts. Discuss with the patient and family that the outbursts are due to the disease process. Encourage patient to participate in group activity. Provide stimulation for the patient. Control stressful situations, if possible. Provide a safe environment. Encourage patient to express feelings and frustrations related to disease process.

functional outcome after 3 months. Patients were given recombinant tissue plasminogen activator (t-PA), a clot-dissolving medication, within 3 hours of the onset of symptoms. Patients with a history of bleeding disorders or those receiving anticoagulant therapy were not candidates for t-PA and were excluded from the study. Results showed that 30% or more of the patients in the experimental group experienced complete or nearly complete recovery (NINDS t-PA Stroke Study Group, 1995).

To realize the full potential of thrombolytic therapy, community education directed at recognizing the symptoms of stroke and obtaining appropriate emergency care is necessary to ensure rapid transport to a hospital and initiation of therapy within the 3-hour time frame. Delays make the patient ineligible for thrombolytic therapy because revascularization of necrotic tissue (which develops after 3 hours) increases the risk of cerebral edema and hemorrhage. After being notified by emergency medical services personnel, the emergency department calls the appropriate staff (neurologist, neuroradiologist, radiology department, nursing staff, and electrocardiogram technician) and informs them of the patient's imminent arrival at the hospital. Many institutions have brain attack teams that respond rapidly, ensuring that treatment occurs within the allotted time frame.

Initial management requires the definitive diagnosis of an ischemic stroke by CT scanning and determination of whether the patient meets all the criteria (Chart 57-2) for t-PA therapy. Once it is determined that the patient's condition is suitable for t-PA therapy, no anticoagulants are to be administered. Before receiving t-PA, the patient should be assessed using the National Institutes of Health Stroke Scale (NIHSS), which contains 42 items evaluating neurologic deficits and is useful in differentiating between ischemic strokes and TIAs.

Thrombolytic Administration. Recombinant t-PA binds to fibrin and converts plasminogen to plasmin, stimulating fibrinolysis of the atherosclerotic lesion. After it is determined that the patient is a candidate for t-PA therapy, the patient is weighed and the dose of t-PA determined. The minimum t-PA dose is 0.9 mg/kg; the maximum dose is 90 mg. The loading dose is 10% of the calculated dose and is administered over 1 minute. The remaining dose is administered over 1 hour via an infusion pump. After the infusion is completed, the line is flushed with 20 mL of normal saline

TABLE 57•5 **Comparison of Left and Right Hemispheric Strokes**

Left Hemispheric Stroke	Right Hemispheric Stroke
Paralysis on right side of body Right visual field defects Aphasia (expressive, receptive, or global) Altered intellectual ability Slow, cautious behavior	Paralysis on left side of body Left visual field defects Spatial-perceptual deficits Increased distractibility Impulsive behavior and poor judgment Lack of awareness of deficits

Risk Factors for **STROKE**

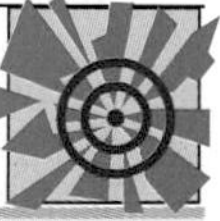

- Hypertension—the major risk factor. Controlling hypertension is the key to preventing stroke.
- Cardiovascular disease—cerebral emboli may originate in the heart.
  - Coronary artery disease
  - Congestive heart failure
  - Left ventricular hypertrophy
  - Rhythm abnormalities (especially atrial fibrillation)
  - Rheumatic heart disease
- High cholesterol
- Obesity
- Elevated hematocrit—increases the risk of cerebral infarction.
- Diabetes—associated with accelerated atherogenesis
- Oral contraceptives (especially with coexisting hypertension, smoking, and high estrogen levels)
- Smoking
- Drug abuse (especially cocaine)
- Alcohol consumption

CHART 57•2 Eligibility Criteria for t-PA Administration

Age 18 years or older
Clinical diagnosis of stroke with NIH stroke scale score under 22
Time of onset of stroke known and is 3 hours or less
BP systolic ≤ 185; diastolic ≤ 110
Not a minor stroke or rapidly resolving stroke
No seizure at onset of stroke
Not taking warfarin (Coumadin)
Prothrombin time ≤ 15 seconds or INR ≤ 1.7
Not receiving heparin during the past 48 hours with elevated partial thromboplastin time
Platelet count ≥ 100,000
Blood glucose level between 50 and 400 mg/dL
No acute myocardial infarction
No prior intracranial hemorrhage, neoplasm, arteriovenous malformation, or aneurysm
No major surgical procedures within 14 days
No stroke or serious head injury within 3 months
No gastrointestinal or urinary bleeding within last 21 days
Not lactating or postpartum ≤ 30 days

solution to ensure that all the medication is administered to the patient.

The patient is admitted to the intensive care unit, where continuous cardiac monitoring is implemented. Vital signs are obtained every 15 minutes for the first 2 hours, every 30 minutes for the next 6 hours, then every hour for 16 hours. The blood pressure should be maintained with the systolic pressure less than 180 mm Hg and the diastolic pressure less than 100 mm Hg. Airway management is instituted based on the clinical condition of the patient and arterial blood gas values.

Bleeding is the most common side effect of t-PA administration, and the patient should be closely monitored for any bleeding (intravenous insertion sites, urinary catheter site, endotracheal tube, nasogastric tube, urine, stool, emesis, other secretions). Administration of thrombolytics in patients with hemorrhagic stroke is contraindicated.

THERAPY FOR PATIENTS NOT RECEIVING T-PA

Not all patients are suitable for t-PA therapy. Other treatments include anticoagulant administration (intravenous heparin or low-molecular-weight heparin) for ischemic strokes and careful maintenance of cerebral hemodynamics to maintain cerebral perfusion. Management of patients with hemorrhagic stroke is focused on management of increased ICP and its associated problems. Interventions during this period include methods to reduce ICP, such as administering an osmotic diuretic, maintaining $PaCO_2$ within the range of 30 to 35 mm Hg, and avoiding hypoxia. Other treatment measures include the following:

- Elevation of the head of the bed to promote venous drainage and to lower increased ICP
- Intubation with an endotracheal tube to establish a secure airway, if necessary
- Continuous electrocardiographic and vital signs monitoring. Systolic pressure should be maintained at less than 180 mm Hg, diastolic pressure at less than 100 mm Hg. Maintaining the blood pressure within this range reduces the potential for additional bleeding or further ischemic damage.
- Neurologic assessment to determine whether the stroke is evolving or whether other acute complications are developing, such as bleeding from anticoagulation or medication-induced bradycardia, resulting in hypotension and subsequent decreases in cardiac output and CPP

Therapy for Complications. Adequate cerebral blood flow is essential for cerebral oxygenation. If cerebral blood flow is inadequate, the amount of oxygen supplied to the brain will decrease and tissue ischemia will result. Therefore, maintaining cardiac output within the normal range of 4 to 8 L/minute, or sometimes greater, can improve the cerebral blood flow and oxygen delivery. Adequate oxygenation begins with pulmonary care, maintenance of a patent airway, and administration of supplemental oxygen as needed. The importance of gas exchange cannot be overemphasized in these patients (see Fig. 57-6 for the components of a neurologic assessment).

NURSING PROCESS: THE PATIENT RECOVERING FROM A STROKE

The acute phase of stroke may last 1 to 3 days, but ongoing monitoring of all body systems is essential as long as the patient requires care. The stroke patient is subject to multiple complications, including deconditioning and other musculoskeletal problems, swallowing difficulties, bowel and bladder dysfunction, inability to perform self-care, and skin breakdown. After the stroke completes, management focuses on the prompt initiation of rehabilitation for any deficits.

Assessment

During the acute phase, a neurologic flow sheet is maintained to reflect the following nursing assessment parameters:

- Change in the level of consciousness or responsiveness as evidenced by movement, resistance to changes of position, and response to stimulation; orientation to time, place, and person
- Presence or absence of voluntary or involuntary movements of the extremities; muscle tone; body posture; and position of the head
- Stiffness or flaccidity of the neck
- Eye opening, comparative size of pupils and pupillary reactions to light, and ocular position
- Color of the face and extremities; temperature and moisture of the skin
- Quality and rates of pulse and respiration; arterial blood gas values as indicated, body temperature, and arterial pressure
- Ability to speak
- Volume of fluids ingested or administered; volume of urine excreted each 24 hours
- Presence of bleeding
- Maintenance of blood pressure within the desired parameters

After the acute phase, the nurse assesses mental status (memory, attention span, perception, orientation, affect, speech/language), sensation/perception (usually the patient has decreased awareness of pain and temperature), motor control (upper and lower extremity movement), swallowing ability, nutritional and hydration status, skin integrity, activity tolerance, and bowel and bladder function. Ongoing nursing assessment continues to focus on the impairment of function in the patient's daily activities, because the quality of life after stroke is closely related to the patient's functional status.

Diagnosis

Nursing Diagnoses

Based on the assessment data, the major nursing diagnoses for a patient with a stroke may include the following:

- Impaired physical mobility related to hemiparesis, loss of balance and coordination, spasticity, and brain injury
- Pain (painful shoulder) related to hemiplegia and disuse
- Self-care deficits (hygiene, toileting, transfers, feeding) related to stroke sequelae
- Sensory/perceptual alterations
- Impaired swallowing
- Incontinence related to flaccid bladder, detrusor instability, confusion, difficulty in communicating
- Altered thought processes related to brain damage, confusion, inability to follow instructions
- Impaired verbal communication related to brain damage
- Risk for impaired skin integrity related to hemiparesis/hemiplegia, decreased mobility
- Altered family processes related to catastrophic illness and caregiving burdens
- Sexual dysfunction

Collaborative Problems/Potential Complications

Potential complications include:

- Decreased cerebral blood flow
- Inadequate oxygen delivery to the brain

Planning and Goals

The major goals for the patient (and family) may include improved mobility, avoidance of shoulder pain, achievement of self-care, continence, improved thought processes, achievement of a form of communication, skin integrity, restored family functioning, and absence of complications.

Although rehabilitation begins on the day the patient has the stroke, the process is intensified during convalescence and requires a coordinated team effort. It is helpful for the team to know what the patient was like before the stroke: his or her illnesses, abilities, mental and emotional state, behavioral characteristics, and activities of daily living.

Nursing Interventions

Improving Mobility and Preventing Joint Deformities

A hemiplegic patient has unilateral paralysis (paralysis on one side). When control of the voluntary muscles is lost, the strong flexor muscles exert control over the extensors. The arm tends to adduct (adductor muscles are stronger than abductors) and to rotate internally. The elbow and the wrist tend to flex, the affected leg tends to rotate externally at the hip joint and flex at the knee, and the foot at the ankle joint supinates and tends toward plantar flexion.

Correct positioning is important to prevent contractures; measures are used to relieve pressure, assist in maintaining good body alignment, and prevent compressive neuropathies, especially of the ulnar and peroneal nerves. Because flexor muscles are stronger than extensor muscles, a posterior splint applied at night to the affected extremity may prevent flexion and maintains correct positioning during sleep. (Refer to Chap. 10 for additional information.)

PREVENTING SHOULDER ADDUCTION

To prevent adduction of the affected shoulder, a pillow is placed in the axilla when there is limited external rotation; this keeps the arm away from the chest. A pillow is placed under the arm, and the arm is placed in a neutral (slightly flexed) position, with distal joints positioned higher than the more proximal joints. Thus, the elbow is higher than the shoulder and the wrist is higher than the elbow. This helps to prevent edema and the resultant fibrosis that will prevent normal range of motion if the patient regains control of the arm.

POSITIONING THE HAND AND FINGERS

The fingers are positioned so that they are barely flexed. The hand is placed in slight supination (palm faces upward), which is its most functional position. If the upper extremity is flaccid, a volar resting splint can be used to support the wrist and hand in a functional position. If the upper extremity is spastic, a hand roll is not used, because it stimulates the grasp reflex. In this instance a dorsal wrist splint is useful in allowing the palm to be free of pressure. Every effort is made to prevent hand edema.

CHANGING POSITIONS

The patient's position should be changed every 2 hours. To place a patient in a lateral (side-lying) position, a pillow is placed between the legs before the patient is turned. The upper thigh should not be acutely flexed. The patient may be turned from side to side, but the amount of time spent on the affected side should be limited because of impaired sensation.

If possible, the patient is placed in a prone position for 15 to 30 minutes several times a day. A small pillow or a support is placed under the pelvis, extending from the level of the umbilicus to the upper third of the thigh (Fig. 57-10). This helps to promote hyperextension of the hip joints, which is essential for normal gait and helps prevent knee and hip flexion contractures. The prone position also helps to drain bronchial secretions and prevents contractural deformities of the shoulders and knees. During positioning, it is important to reduce pressure and change position frequently to prevent the formation of pressure ulcers.

ESTABLISHING AN EXERCISE PROGRAM

The affected extremities are exercised passively and put through a full range of motion four or five times a day to maintain joint mobility, regain motor control, prevent development of a contracture in the paralyzed extremity, prevent further deterioration

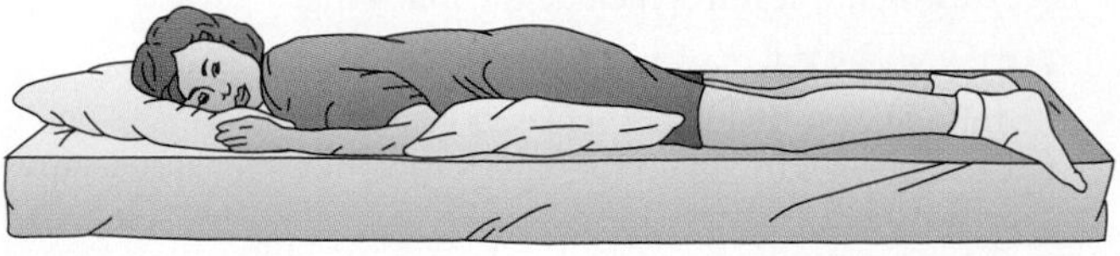

FIGURE 57•10 Prone position with pillow support helps prevent hip flexion contractures.

of the neuromuscular system, and enhance circulation. Exercise is helpful in preventing venous stasis, which may predispose the patient to thrombosis and pulmonary embolus.

Repetition of an activity forms new pathways in the central nervous system and therefore encourages new patterns of motion. At first, the extremities are usually flaccid. If tightness occurs in any area, the range-of-motion exercises should be performed more frequently. (See Chap. 10 for techniques of range-of-motion exercises.)

The patient is observed for signs and symptoms that may indicate pulmonary embolus or excessive cardiac workload during exercise; these include shortness of breath, chest pain, cyanosis, and increasing pulse rate during the exercise period. Frequent short periods of exercise always are preferable to longer periods at infrequent intervals. Regularity in exercise is most important. Improvement in muscle strength and maintenance of range of motion can be achieved only through daily exercise.

The patient is encouraged and reminded to exercise the unaffected side at intervals throughout the day. It is helpful to work out a written schedule to remind the patient of the exercise activities. The nurse has the responsibility of supervising and supporting the patient during these activities. The patient can be taught to put the unaffected leg under the affected one to move it when turning and exercising. Flexibility, strengthening, coordination, endurance, and balancing exercises prepare the patient for ambulation and provide a goal. Quadriceps muscle setting and gluteal setting exercises are started early to improve the muscle strength needed for walking; these are performed at least five times daily for 10 minutes at a time.

PREPARING FOR AMBULATION

As soon as possible, the patient is assisted out of bed. Usually, when hemiplegia has resulted from a thrombosis, an active rehabilitation program is started as soon as the patient regains consciousness; a patient who has had a cerebral hemorrhage cannot participate actively until all evidence of bleeding is gone.

The patient is first taught to maintain balance while sitting and then to learn to balance while standing. If the patient has difficulty in achieving standing balance, a tilt table, which slowly brings the patient to an upright position, can be used. Tilt tables are especially helpful for patients who have been on bed rest for prolonged periods and are having orthostatic blood pressure changes.

If the patient needs a wheelchair, the folding type with hand brakes is the most practical because it allows the patient to manipulate the chair. The chair should be low enough to allow the patient to propel it with the uninvolved foot and narrow enough to permit it to be used in the home. When the patient is transferred from the wheelchair, the brakes must be applied on both sides of the chair.

The patient is usually ready to walk as soon as standing balance is achieved. Parallel bars are useful in these first efforts. A chair or wheelchair should be readily available in case the patient suddenly becomes fatigued or feels dizzy.

The training periods for ambulation should be short and frequent. As the patient gains strength and confidence, an adjustable cane can be used for support. Generally, a three- or four-pronged cane provides a stable support in the early phases of the training program.

Preventing Shoulder Pain

Up to 70% of stroke patients suffer severe pain in the shoulder that prevents them from learning new skills, because shoulder function is essential in achieving balance and performing transfers and self-care activities. Three problems can occur: painful shoulder, subluxation of the shoulder, and shoulder–hand syndrome.

A flaccid shoulder joint may be overstretched by the use of excessive force in turning the patient or from overstrenuous arm and shoulder movement. To prevent shoulder pain, the nurse should never lift the patient by the flaccid shoulder or pull on the affected arm or shoulder. If the arm is paralyzed, subluxation (incomplete dislocation) at the shoulder can occur from overstretching the joint capsule and musculature by the force of gravity when the patient sits or stands in the early stages after a stroke. This results in severe pain. Shoulder–hand syndrome (painful shoulder and generalized swelling of the hand) can cause a frozen shoulder and ultimate atrophy of subcutaneous tissues. When a shoulder becomes stiff, it is usually more painful.

These problems can be prevented by proper patient movement and positioning. The flaccid arm is positioned on a table or pillows while the patient is seated. Some clinicians advocate the use of a properly worn sling when the patient first becomes ambulatory to prevent the paralyzed upper extremity from dangling without support. Range-of-motion exercises are important in preventing painful shoulder. Overstrenuous arm movements are avoided. The patient is instructed to interlace the fingers, place the palms together, and push the clasped hands slowly forward to bring the scapulae forward; he or she then raises both hands above the head. This is repeated throughout the day. The patient is instructed to flex the affected wrist at intervals and move all the joints of the affected fingers. He or she is encouraged to touch, stroke, rub, and look at both hands. Pushing the heel of the hand firmly down on a surface is useful. Elevation of the arm and hand is also important in preventing dependent edema of the hand. Patients with continuing pain after movement and positioning have been attempted may require the addition of analgesia to their treatment program.

Enhancing Self-Care

As soon as the patient can sit up, personal hygiene activities are encouraged. The patient is helped to set realistic goals; if feasible, a new task is added daily. The first step is to carry out all self-care activities on the unaffected side. Such activities as combing the hair, brushing the teeth, shaving with an electric razor, bathing, and eating can be carried out with one hand and are suitable for self-care. Although the patient may feel awkward at first, the various motor skills can be learned by repetition, and the unaffected side will become stronger with use. The nurse must be sure that the patient does not neglect the affected side. Assistive devices will help make up for some of the patient's deficits (Chart 57-3). A small towel is easier to control while drying after bathing, and boxed paper tissues are easier to use than a roll of toilet tissue.

The patient's morale will improve if ambulatory activities are carried out in street clothes. The family is instructed to bring in clothing that is preferably a size larger than that normally worn. Clothing fitted with front or side fasteners or Velcro closures is the most suitable. The patient has better balance if most of the dressing activities are done in a seated position.

Perceptual problems may make it difficult for the patient to dress without assistance because of an inability to match the clothing to the body parts. To assist the patient, the nurse can take steps to keep the environment organized and uncluttered, because the patient with a perceptual problem is easily distracted. The clothing is placed on the patient's affected side in the order in which the garments are to be put on. Using a large mirror while dressing promotes the patient's awareness of what he or she is

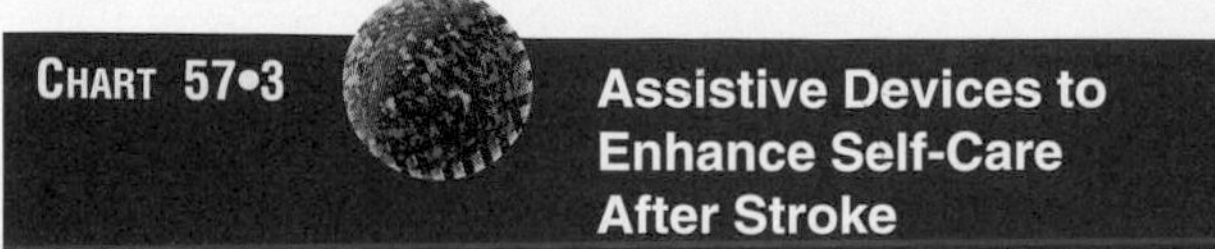
CHART 57•3
Assistive Devices to Enhance Self-Care After Stroke

The following list identifies products that may help neurologically impaired patients perform self-care more easily and safely after a stroke or other disorders.

Eating Devices
- Nonskid mats to stabilize plates
- Plate guards to prevent food from being pushed off plate
- Wide-grip utensils to accommodate a weak grasp

Bathing and Grooming Devices
- Long-handled bath sponge
- Grab bars, nonskid mats, hand-held shower heads
- Electric razors with head at 90 degrees to handle
- Shower and tub seats, stationary or on wheels

Toileting Aids
- Raised toilet seat
- Grab bars next to toilet

Dressing Aids
- Velcro closures
- Elastic shoelaces
- Long-handled shoe horn

Mobility Aids
- Canes, walkers, wheelchairs
- Transfer devices such as transfer boards and belts

putting on the affected side. Each garment is put on the affected side first. The patient has to make many compensatory movements when dressing; these can produce fatigue and painful twisting of the intercostal muscles. Support and encouragement are provided to prevent the patient from becoming overly fatigued and discouraged. Even with intensive training, not all patients can achieve independence in dressing skills.

Managing Sensory-Perceptual Difficulties

Patients with a decreased field of vision should be approached on the side where visual perception is intact. All visual stimuli (clock, calendar, television) should be placed on this side. The patient can be taught to turn the head in the direction of the defective visual field to compensate for this loss. The nurse should make eye contact with the patient and draw his or her attention to the affected side by encouraging the patient to move the head. The nurse may also want to stand at a position that encourages the patient to move or turn to visualize who is in the room. Increasing the natural or artificial lighting in the room and providing eyeglasses are important in increasing vision.

The patient with homonymous hemianopsia (loss of half of the visual field) turns away from the affected side of the body and tends to neglect that side and the space on that side; this is called amorphosynthesis. In such instances, the patient cannot see food on half of the tray, and only half of the room is visible. It is important for the nurse to constantly remind the patient of the other side of the body, to maintain alignment of the extremities, and, if possible, to place the extremities where the patient can see them.

Managing Dysphagia

Stroke can result in swallowing problems (dysphagia) due to impaired function of the mouth, tongue, palate, larynx, pharynx, or upper esophagus. Stoke patients must be observed for paroxysms of coughing, food dribbling out of or pooling in one side of the mouth, food retained for long periods in the mouth, or nasal regurgitation when swallowing liquids. Swallowing difficulties place the patient at risk for aspiration, pneumonia, dehydration, and malnutrition.

A speech therapist will evaluate the patient's gag reflexes and ability to swallow. Even if partially impaired, swallowing function may return in some patients over time, or the patient may be taught alternative swallowing techniques, advised to take smaller boluses of food, and informed of foods that are easier to swallow. The patient may initially be started on a thick liquid or puréed diet because these foods are easier to swallow than thin liquids. Having the patient sit upright, preferably out of bed in the chair, will help prevent aspiration. The patient's diet may be advanced as he or she becomes more proficient at swallowing. If the patient cannot resume oral intake, a gastrointestinal feeding tube will be placed for ongoing tube feedings.

MANAGING TUBE FEEDINGS

Enteral tubes can be either nasogastric, placed in the stomach, or nasoenteral, placed in the duodenum to reduce the risk of aspiration. Nursing responsibilities in feeding include elevating the head of the bed at least 30 degrees to prevent aspiration, checking the position of the tube before feeding, ensuring that the cuff of the tracheostomy tube (if in place) is inflated, and giving the tube feeding slowly. The feeding tube is aspirated periodically to ensure that the feedings are passing through the gastrointestinal tract. Retained or residual feedings increase the risk of aspiration. Patients with retained feedings may benefit from the placement of a gastrostomy tube or a percutaneous endoscopic gastrostomy tube. In a patient with a nasogastric tube, the feeding tube should be placed in the duodenum to reduce the risk of aspiration. For long-term feedings, a gastrostomy tube is preferred.

Attaining Bowel and Bladder Control

After a stroke, the patient may have transient urinary incontinence due to confusion, inability to communicate needs, and inability to use the urinal/bedpan because of impaired motor and postural control. Occasionally after a stroke, the bladder becomes atonic, with impaired sensation in response to bladder filling. Sometimes control of the external urinary sphincter is lost or diminished. During this period, intermittent catheterization with sterile technique is carried out. When muscle tone increases and deep tendon reflexes return, bladder tone increases and spasticity of the bladder may develop. Because the patient's sense of awareness is clouded, persistent urinary incontinence or urinary retention may be symptomatic of bilateral brain damage. The patient's voiding pattern is analyzed and the urinal/bedpan offered on this pattern or schedule. The upright posture and standing position is helpful for male patients during this aspect of rehabilitation.

Patients may also have problems with bowel control or constipation, with constipation being more common. Unless contraindicated, a high-fiber diet and adequate fluid intake (2 to 3 liters per day) should be provided, and a regular time established (usually after breakfast) for toileting. (See also Chap. 10 for bowel and bladder retraining programs.)

Improving Thought Processes

After a stroke, the patient may have problems with cognitive, behavioral, and emotional deficits related to brain damage. In many instances, however, a considerable degree of function can be recovered because not all areas of the brain are equally damaged; some remain more intact and functional than others.

After assessment procedures that delineate and describe the patient's problems, the neuropsychologist, in collaboration with the primary care physician, psychiatrist, nurse, and other professionals, structures a training program using cognitive-perceptual retraining, visual imagery, reality orientation, and cuing procedures to compensate for losses.

The role of the nurse is supportive. The nurse reviews the results of neuropsychological testing, observes the patient's performance and progress, gives positive feedback, and, most importantly, conveys an attitude of confidence and hope. Interventions capitalize on the patient's strengths and remaining abilities while attempting to improve performance of affected functions. Other interventions are similar to those for improving cognitive functioning after a head injury (see Chap. 58).

Improving Communication

Aphasia, which impairs the patient's ability to understand what is being said and to express himself or herself, may become apparent in various ways (Chart 57-4 defines terms related to aphasia). The cortical area responsible for integrating the myriad association pathways required for the comprehension and formulation of language is called Broca's area. It is located in a convolution adjoining the middle cerebral artery. This area is responsible for control of the combinations of muscular movements needed to speak each word. Broca's area is so near the left motor area that a disturbance in the motor area often affects the speech area. This is why so many patients paralyzed on the right side (due to damage or injury to the left side of the brain) cannot speak, whereas those paralyzed on the left side are less likely to have speech disturbances.

The speech pathologist assesses the communication needs of the stroke patient, describes the precise deficit, and suggests the best overall method of communication for the patient. With many language intervention strategies for the aphasic adult, the program can be individually tailored. Goals are jointly established; the patient is expected to take an active part.

An aphasic person may become depressed because of the inability to talk to others. The inability to talk on the telephone or answer a question, or exclusion from conversation causes anger, frustration, fear of the future, and hopelessness. Nursing interventions include doing everything possible to make the atmosphere conducive to communication. This includes being sensitive to the patient's reactions and needs and responding to them in an appropriate manner, always treating the patient as an adult. The nurse lends strong moral support and understanding to allay anxiety.

A common pitfall is for the nurse or other health care team member to complete the thoughts or sentences of the patient. This should be avoided because it may cause the patient to feel more frustrated at not being allowed to speak and may deter efforts to practice putting thoughts together and completing the sentence. A consistent schedule, routines, and repetitions help the patient to function despite significant deficits. A written copy of the daily schedule, a folder of personal information (birth date, address, names of relatives), checklists, and an audiotaped list help the patient's memory and concentration. The patient may also benefit from a communication board, which has pictures of commonly requested needs and phrases. The board may be translated into several languages.

CHART 57•4 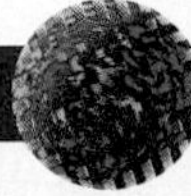 **Terms Related to Aphasia***

acalculia; dyscalculia: difficulty in dealing with mathematical processes or numeric symbols in general

agnosia: failure to recognize familiar objects perceived by the senses

- **auditory agnosia:** inability to recognize significance of sounds
- **color agnosia:** inability to recognize differences in color
- **tactile agnosia:** inability to recognize familiar objects by touch or feel
- **visual object agnosia:** inability to recognize objects; visual acuity may or may not be intact

agraphia; dysgraphia: disturbances in writing intelligible words

alexia; dyslexia: difficulty in reading

anomia; dysnomia: difficulty in selecting appropriate words particularly nouns

aphasia: loss of the ability to express oneself or to understand language

- **receptive aphasia:** inability to understand what someone else is saying; often associated with damage to the temporal lobe area
- **expressive aphasia:** inability to express oneself; often associated with the left frontal lobe area
- **paraphasia:** a frequently observed characteristic in many aphasic patients; uses wrong words, word substitutions, grammatical errors, faults in word usage, may be observed in both oral and written language

apraxia: inability to perform previously learned purposeful motor acts on a voluntary basis

- **verbal apraxia:** difficulty in forming and organizing intelligible words although the musculature is intact

dysarthria: defects of articulation due to neurologic causes

hemianopsia: blindness of one half of the field of vision in one or both eyes

perseveration: continued and automatic repetition of an activity or word or phrase that is no longer appropriate

* The prefix *a* means "without" or "absence." The prefix *dys* refers to "difficulty" or "disordered," frequently used interchangeably in these conditions.

When talking with the patient, it is important to have the patient's attention, speak slowly, and keep the language of instruction consistent. One instruction is given at a time, and time is allowed for the patient to process what has been said. The use of gestures may enhance comprehension. Speaking is thinking out loud, and the emphasis is on thinking. The patient must sort out incoming messages and formulate a response. Listening requires mental effort; the patient must struggle against mental inertia and needs time to organize an answer.

In working with the aphasic patient, the nurse must remember to talk to the patient during care activities. This provides social contact for the patient. Chart 57-5 describes points to keep in mind when communicating with the aphasic patient.

Maintaining Skin Integrity

The patient who has had a stroke may be at risk for skin and tissue breakdown because of altered sensation and inability to respond to pressure and discomfort by turning and moving. Therefore, preventing skin and tissue breakdown requires frequent

CHART 57•5 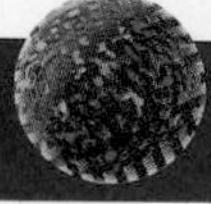 Communicating With the Aphasic Patient

- Face the patient and establish eye contact.
- Speak in a normal manner and tone.
- Use short phrases and pause between phrases to allow the patient time to understand what is being said.
- Limit conversation to practical and concrete matters.
- Use gestures, pictures, and objects.
- As the patient uses and handles an object, say what the object is. It helps to match the words with the object or action.
- Be consistent in using the same words and gestures each time you give instructions or ask a question.
- Keep extraneous noises and sounds to a minimum. Too much background noise can distract the patient or make it difficult to sort out the message being spoken.

assessment of the skin, with particular emphasis on bony areas and dependent parts of the body. During the acute phase, a specialty bed (eg, low-air-loss bed) may be used until the patient can move independently or assist in moving.

A regular turning and positioning schedule must be followed to minimize pressure and prevent skin breakdown. Pressure-relieving devices may be employed but must not be used in place of regular turning and positioning. The turning schedule (at least every 2 hours) must be adhered to even if pressure-relieving devices are used to prevent tissue and skin breakdown. When the patient is positioned or turned, care must be used to minimize shear and friction forces, which cause damage to tissues and predispose the skin to breakdown.

The patient's skin must be kept clean and dry; gentle massage of healthy (nonreddened) skin and maintenance of adequate nutrition are other factors that help to maintain normal skin and tissue integrity. (Chap. 10 provides additional information.)

Improving Family Coping

Family members play an important role in the patient's recovery. Some type of counseling and support system should be available to them to prevent the care of the patient from taking a significant toll on their health and interfering too radically with their lives. Respite care—planned short-term care to ease the burden of the family in providing continuous 24-hour care—may be available from an adult day care center. Some hospitals also offer weekend respite care. Family coping is also facilitated by involving others in the patient's care and teaching stress-management techniques and methods for maintaining personal health.

The family may have difficulty accepting the patient's disability and may be unrealistic in their expectations. They are given information about the expected outcomes and are counseled to avoid doing for the patient those things that he or she can do. They are assured that their love and interest are part of the patient's therapy.

The family needs to be informed that the rehabilitation of the hemiplegic patient requires many months; progress may be slow. The gains made by the patient in the hospital or rehabilitation unit must be maintained. All should approach the patient with a supportive and optimistic attitude, focusing on the abilities that remain. The rehabilitation team, the medical and nursing team, the patient, and the family all must be involved in developing attainable goals for the patient at home.

Most relatives of stroke patients handle the physical changes better than the emotional aspects of care. The family should be prepared to expect occasional episodes of emotional lability. The patient may laugh or cry easily and may be irritable and demanding or depressed and confused. The nurse can explain to the family that the patient's laughing does not necessarily connote happiness, nor does crying reflect sadness, and that emotional lability usually improves with time.

The nurse should recognize the potential effects of caregiving on the family. Not all families have the adaptive coping skills and psychological functioning necessary for the long-term care of another. The spouse may be elderly with health problems; in some instances the stroke patient may have been the provider of care to such a spouse. Even healthy caregivers may find it difficult to maintain a schedule that includes being available around-the-clock. Some effects of sustained caregiving include increased risk of depression and substance abuse, and increased use of health care services by the caregiver. Depressed caregivers are more likely to resort to physical or emotional abuse of the patient and are more likely to place the patient in a nursing home. Respite care can provide caregivers with needed time to themselves. Nurses should encourage families to arrange for such services and should provide information to assist them.

Helping the Patient Cope With Sexual Dysfunction

Sexual functioning can be profoundly altered by stroke. Often stroke is such a catastrophic illness that the patient experiences loss of self-esteem and value as a sexual being. Although research in this area of stroke management is limited, it appears that stroke patients consider sexual function to be important, but most have sexual dysfunction. The patient and partner may benefit from sexual counseling about alternative approaches to sexual expression.

Promoting Home and Community-Based Care

TEACHING PATIENTS SELF-CARE

Patient and family education is a fundamental component of rehabilitation, and ample opportunity for learning about stroke, its causes and prevention, and the rehabilitation process should be provided. Refer to the teaching checklist for topics to be covered. In both the acute care and rehabilitation facilities, the focus is on teaching patients to resume as much self-care as possible. This may entail the use of assistive devices or modification of the home environment to facilitate the challenge of living with a disability.

An occupational therapist may be helpful in assessing the patient's home environment and recommending modifications to help the patient become more independent. For example, a shower is more convenient than a tub for the hemiplegic patient, because most patients do not gain sufficient strength to get up and down from a tub. Sitting on a stool of medium height with rubber suction tips permits the patient to wash with greater ease. A long-handled bath brush with a soap container is helpful to the patient who has only one functional hand. If a shower is not available, a stool may be placed in the tub and a portable shower hose attached to the faucet. Handrails may be attached beside the bathtub and the toilet. Other assistive devices include special utensils and containers for eating, grooming devices, and dressing equipment (see Chart 57-3).

CONTINUING CARE

The recovery and rehabilitation process after stroke may be prolonged, requiring patience and perseverance on the part of the patient and family. Depending on the specific neurologic deficits resulting from the stroke, the patient at home may require the ser-

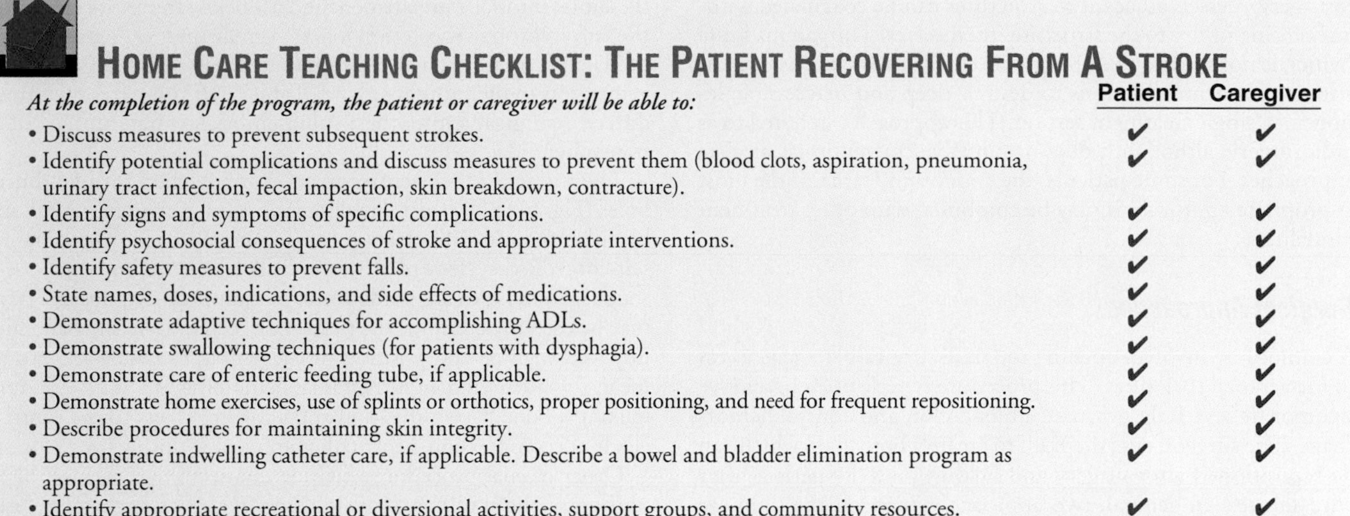

HOME CARE TEACHING CHECKLIST: THE PATIENT RECOVERING FROM A STROKE

At the completion of the program, the patient or caregiver will be able to:	Patient	Caregiver
• Discuss measures to prevent subsequent strokes.	✔	✔
• Identify potential complications and discuss measures to prevent them (blood clots, aspiration, pneumonia, urinary tract infection, fecal impaction, skin breakdown, contracture).	✔	✔
• Identify signs and symptoms of specific complications.	✔	✔
• Identify psychosocial consequences of stroke and appropriate interventions.	✔	✔
• Identify safety measures to prevent falls.	✔	✔
• State names, doses, indications, and side effects of medications.	✔	✔
• Demonstrate adaptive techniques for accomplishing ADLs.	✔	✔
• Demonstrate swallowing techniques (for patients with dysphagia).	✔	✔
• Demonstrate care of enteric feeding tube, if applicable.	✔	✔
• Demonstrate home exercises, use of splints or orthotics, proper positioning, and need for frequent repositioning.	✔	✔
• Describe procedures for maintaining skin integrity.	✔	✔
• Demonstrate indwelling catheter care, if applicable. Describe a bowel and bladder elimination program as appropriate.	✔	✔
• Identify appropriate recreational or diversional activities, support groups, and community resources.	✔	✔

vices of a number of health care professionals. The care of the patient at home is often coordinated by the nurse. The patient's family—often the patient's spouse—will require assistance in planning and providing aspects of care. Simultaneously, the caregiver often requires reminders to attend to his or her own health problems and well-being.

The family is advised that the patient often tires easily, may become irritable and upset by small events, and is likely to show less interest in things. Because a stroke frequently occurs in the later stages of life, there is the possibility of intellectual decline related to dementia.

Emotional problems associated with stroke are often related to speech dysfunction and frustrations about being unable to communicate effectively. A speech therapist who visits the home allows the family to be involved and gives the family practical instructions to help the patient between therapy sessions.

Depression is a common and serious problem in the stroke patient. Antidepressant therapy may help if depression dominates the patient's life. As progress is made in the rehabilitation program, some problems will diminish. The family can help by continuing to support the patient and by giving positive reinforcement for the progress that is being made.

Community-based stroke clubs allow the patient and family to learn from others with similar problems and to share their experiences. The patient is encouraged to continue with hobbies, recreational and leisure interests, and contact with friends to prevent social isolation. All nurses coming in contact with the patient should encourage the patient to keep active, adhere to the exercise program, and remain as self-sufficient as possible.

Evaluation

Expected Outcomes

Expected outcomes may include:

1. Achieves improved mobility
   a. Avoids deformities; absence of contractures and footdrop
   b. Participates in prescribed exercise program
   c. Achieves sitting balance
   d. Uses unaffected side to compensate for loss of function of hemiplegic side
2. Has no complaints of shoulder pain
   a. Demonstrates shoulder mobility; exercises shoulder
   b. Elevates arm and hand at intervals
3. Achieves self-care; performs hygienic care; uses adaptive equipment
4. Turns head to see people or objects
5. Demonstrates improved swallowing ability
6. Achieves normal bowel and bladder elimination
7. Participates in cognitive improvement program
8. Demonstrates improved communication
9. Maintains intact skin without breakdown
   a. Demonstrates normal skin turgor
   b. Participates in turning and positioning activities
10. Family members demonstrate a positive attitude and coping mechanisms
    a. Encourage patient in exercise program
    b. Take an active part in rehabilitation process
    c. Contact respite care program or arrange for other family members to assume some care responsibilities
11. Has positive attitude regarding alternative approaches to sexual expression

INTRACRANIAL SURGERY

Technological advances and refinement of imaging procedures and surgical techniques have made it possible for neurosurgeons to localize and treat intracranial lesions with greater precision than ever before. Improved imaging techniques, illumination, and magnification have made it possible to obtain a three-dimensional view of the surgical site. Microsurgical instruments allow delicate tissue to be separated without trauma. Ultrasonic dissecting systems permit certain brain and spinal cord tumors to be removed quickly and precisely. Probes can be placed deep into brain tissue to apply interstitial radiation, hyperthermia, or chemotherapy. Suture material smaller than a strand of human hair permits very small nerves and vessels to be sutured and anastomosed.

The use of stereotactic frames and equipment allows precise localization of a specific target point in the brain; stereotactic approaches are used with lasers and the gamma knife. Lasers enable neurosurgeons to remove tumors precisely with minimal trauma to surrounding tissue, an important consideration in neurosurgery. Vessels adjacent to structures can be coagulated without causing injury to the structures themselves. The gamma knife (which is not really a knife) is used to deliver a high level of radiation to intracranial lesions to destroy deep and inaccessible lesions in a single treatment session. This approach is referred to as radiosurgery, although it does not involve conventional surgical approaches. For some patients, the craniotomy remains the most appropriate approach; it may be combined with other treatment modalities.

Surgical Approaches

A craniotomy involves opening the skull surgically to gain access to intracranial structures. This procedure is performed to remove a tumor, relieve ICP, evacuate a blood clot, and control hemorrhage. The surgeon cuts the skull to create a bony flap, which can be repositioned after surgery and held in place by periosteal or wire sutures. In general, two approaches through the skull are used: (1) above the tentorium (supratentorial craniotomy) into the supratentorial compartment and (2) below the tentorium into the infratentorial (posterior fossa) compartment. A transsphenoidal approach through the mouth and nasal sinuses is used to gain access to the pituitary gland. Table 57-6 compares the three different surgical approaches: supratentorial, infratentorial, and transsphenoidal.

The intracranial structures may be approached through burr holes (Fig. 57-11), which are circular openings made in the skull by either a hand drill or an automatic craniotome (which has a self-controlled system to stop the drill when the bone is penetrated). Burr holes are made for exploration or diagnosis. They may be used to determine the presence of cerebral swelling and injury and the size and position of the ventricles. They are also a means of evacuating an intracranial hematoma or abscess and for making a bone flap in the skull and allowing access to the ventricles for decompression, ventriculography, or shunting procedures.

Other cranial procedures include craniectomy (excision of a portion of the skull) and cranioplasty (repair of a cranial defect by means of a plastic or metal plate).

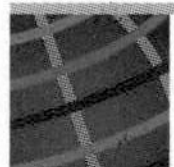

TABLE 57•6 Comparison of Cranial Surgical Approaches

SUPRATENTORIAL	INFRATENTORIAL	TRANSSPHENOIDAL
		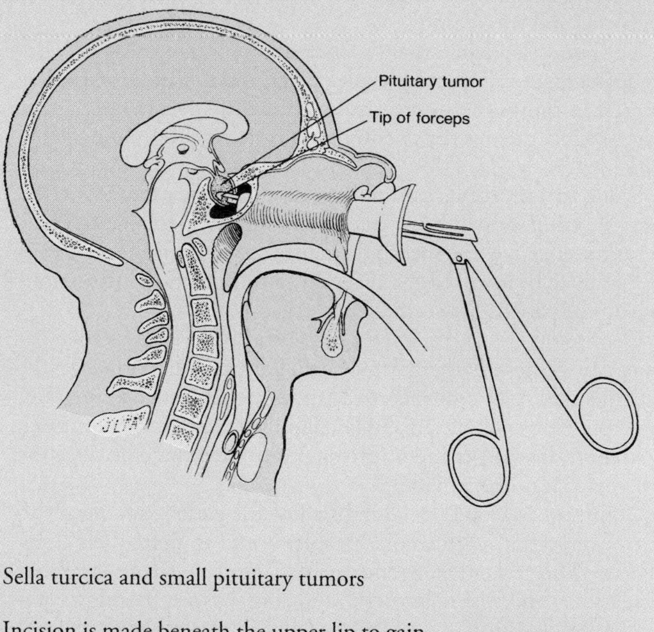 Pituitary tumor Tip of forceps
Site of Surgery		
Above the tentorium	Below the tentorium, brain stem	Sella turcica and small pituitary tumors
Incision Location		
Incision is made above the area to be operated on; is usually located behind the hairline.	Incision is made at the nape of the neck, around the occipital lobe.	Incision is made beneath the upper lip to gain access into the nasal cavity.
Selected Nursing Interventions		
Maintain head of bed elevated 30 to 45 degrees, with neck in neutral alignment. Position patient on either side or back. (Avoid positioning patient on operative side if a large tumor has been removed.)	Maintain neck in straight alignment. Avoid flexion of the neck to prevent possible tearing of the suture line. Position the patient on either side. (Check hospital's protocol for guidelines for positioning of patient.)	Maintain nasal packing in place and reinforce as needed. Instruct patient to avoid blowing the nose. Provide frequent oral care. Keep head of bed elevated to promote venous drainage and drainage from the surgical site.

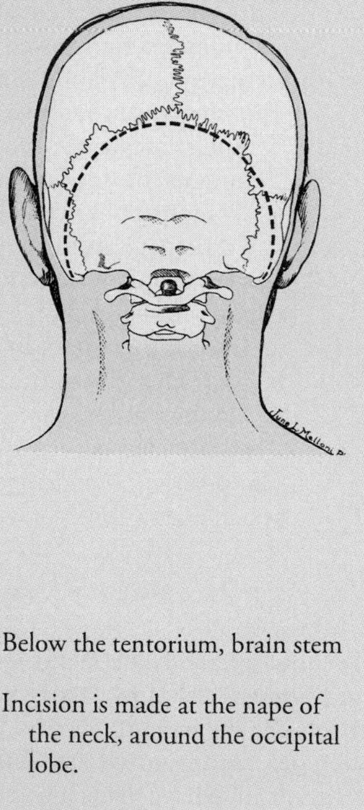

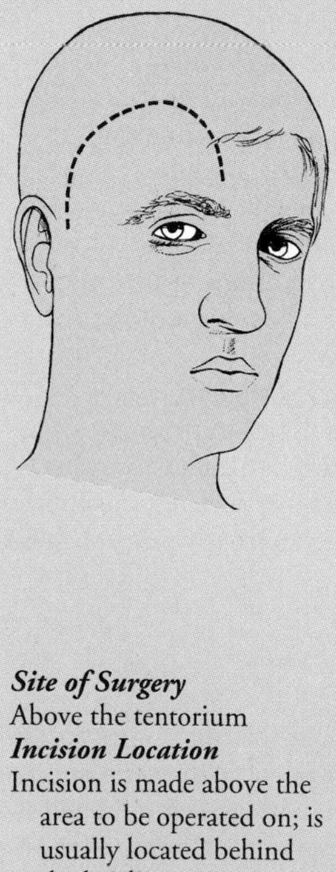

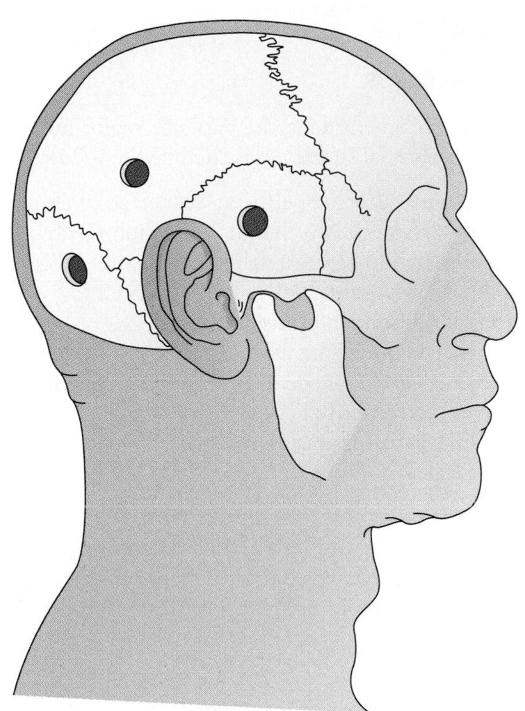

FIGURE 57•11 Burr holes may be used in neurosurgical procedures to make a bone flap in the skull, to aspirate a brain abscess, or to evacuate a hematoma.

Preoperative Evaluation

Preoperative diagnostic procedures may include CT scanning to demonstrate the lesion and show the degree of surrounding brain edema, the ventricular size, and the displacement. MRI provides information similar to that of the CT scan and examines the lesion in other planes. Cerebral angiography may be used to study the tumor's blood supply or give information about vascular lesions. Transcranial Doppler flow studies are used to evaluate the blood flow of intracranial blood vessels.

Complications

Complications of intracranial surgery include increased ICP, infection, and neurologic deficits. Increased ICP may develop as a result of cerebral edema or swelling and is treated with mannitol, an osmotic diuretic. The patient may also require intubation and use of paralyzing agents.

Infection is possible because of the open incision. The patient should receive antibiotic therapy, and the dressing and wound site should be monitored for signs of infection: increased drainage, foul odor, purulent drainage, and redness and swelling along the incision line. Neurologic deficits may result from the surgery. After surgery, the patient's neurologic status is closely monitored for any changes from the patient's preoperative baseline.

Preoperative Management

Usually patients are placed on anticonvulsant medication (phenytoin) before surgery to reduce the risk of postoperative seizures. Before surgery, steroids (dexamethasone) may be administered to reduce cerebral edema. Fluids may be restricted. A hyperosmotic agent (mannitol) and a diuretic (furosemide) may be given intravenously immediately before and sometimes during surgery if the patient tends to retain fluid, as do many who have intracranial dysfunction. An indwelling urinary catheter is inserted before the patient is taken to the operating room to drain the bladder during the administration of diuretics and to permit urinary output to be monitored. The patient may have a central line placed for fluid administration and central venous pressure monitoring after surgery. The patient may be given antibiotics if there is a chance of cerebral contamination, or diazepam before surgery to allay anxiety.

The scalp is shaved immediately before surgery (usually in the operating room) so that any resultant superficial abrasions do not have time to become infected.

Postoperative Management

An arterial line and a central venous pressure line may be in place to monitor blood pressure and central venous pressure. The patient may be intubated and may receive supplemental oxygen therapy.

REDUCING CEREBRAL EDEMA

Medication therapy to reduce cerebral edema includes the administration of mannitol, which increases serum osmolality and draws free water from areas of the brain (with an intact blood–brain barrier). The fluid is then excreted by osmotic diuresis. Dexamethasone may be administered intravenously every 6 hours for 24 to 72 hours; subsequently, the dosage is tapered.

RELIEVING PAIN AND PREVENTING SEIZURES

Acetaminophen is usually given for temperature exceeding 99.6°F (37.5°C) and for pain. Commonly, the patient has a headache after a craniotomy, usually as a result of the scalp nerves being stretched and irritated during surgery. Codeine, given parenterally, is usually sufficient to relieve headache. Anticonvulsant medication (phenytoin, diazepam) is prescribed for patients who have undergone supratentorial craniotomy, because of the high risk of epilepsy after supratentorial neurosurgical procedures. Serum levels are monitored to keep the medications within the therapeutic range.

MONITORING ICP

A ventricular catheter, or some type of drainage, is frequently inserted in patients undergoing surgery for tumors of the posterior fossa. The catheter is connected to an external drainage system. The patency of the catheter is noted by the pulsations of the fluid in the tubing. The ICP can be assessed by setting up the system with a stopcock attached to the pressure tubing and transducer. The ICP can be monitored by the turn of the stopcock. Care is required to ensure that the system is tight at all connections and that the stopcock is in the proper position to avoid drainage of CSF; collapse of the ventricles may result if excessive fluid is removed. The catheter is removed when the ventricular pressure is normal and stable. The neurosurgeon must be notified if the catheter appears to be obstructed.

Ventricular shunting is sometimes performed before certain surgical procedures to control intracranial hypertension, particularly in patients with posterior fossa tumors.

Nursing Management

The preoperative assessment serves as a baseline against which postoperative status and recovery can be judged. This assessment includes evaluating the level of consciousness and responsiveness to stimuli and identifying any neurologic deficits, such as paralysis, visual dysfunction, alterations in personality or speech, and bladder and bowel disorders. Motor function of the extremities is tested by the strength of the hand grip or pedal pushes.

The patient's and family's understanding of the anticipated surgical procedure and its possible sequelae is assessed, along with their reactions to the impending surgery. The availability of support systems for the patient and family is assessed.

In preparation for surgery, the patient's physical status and emotional status are brought to an optimal level to reduce the risk of postoperative complications. The patient's physical status is assessed for neurologic deficits and their potential impact after surgery. If the arms or legs are paralyzed, trochanter rolls are applied to the extremities and the feet are positioned against a footboard. A patient who can ambulate is encouraged to do so. If the patient is aphasic, writing materials or picture and word cards showing the bedpan, glass of water, blanket, and other frequently used items may be supplied to help improve communication.

The emotional preparation of the patient includes providing information about what to expect after surgery. The large head dressing applied after surgery may impair hearing temporarily. Vision may be limited if the eyes are swollen shut. If a tracheostomy or endotracheal tube is in place, the patient will be unable to speak until the tube is removed, so an alternative method of communication should be established.

An altered cognitive state may make the patient unaware of the impending surgery. Even so, encouragement and attention to the patient's needs are necessary. Whatever the state of awareness of the patient, the family needs reassurance and support because they recognize the seriousness of brain surgery.

NURSING PROCESS: THE PATIENT UNDERGOING INTRACRANIAL SURGERY

Assessment

After surgery, the frequency of postoperative monitoring is based on the patient's clinical status. Assessing respiratory function is essential because a small degree of hypoxia can increase cerebral ischemia. The respiratory rate and pattern are monitored, and arterial blood gas values are reviewed. Fluctuations in vital signs are carefully monitored and documented because they indicate increased ICP. The patient's temperature is measured at intervals to assess for hyperthermia secondary to damage to the hypothalamus. Neurologic checks are made frequently to detect increased ICP resulting from cerebral edema or bleeding. A change in LOC or response to stimuli may be the first sign of increasing ICP.

Assessment of neurologic status focuses on LOC, eye signs, motor response, and vital signs. The patient is observed for subtle signs of neurologic deficit, such as diminished response to stimuli, speech problems, difficulty in swallowing, weakness or paralysis of an extremity, visual changes (diplopia, blurred vision), or paresthesias. Seizures are a potential complication; any seizure activity is carefully recorded and reported. Restlessness may occur as the patient becomes more responsive or may be due to pain, confusion, hypoxia, or other stimuli.

The surgical dressing is inspected for evidence of bleeding and CSF drainage. In patients undergoing transsphenoidal surgery, the nasal packing inserted during surgery is checked for blood or CSF drainage. The nurse must be alert to the development of complications; all assessments are carried out with these problems in mind.

Diagnosis

Nursing Diagnoses

Based on the assessment data, the patient's major nursing diagnoses after intracranial surgery may include the following:

- Altered cerebral tissue perfusion related to cerebral edema
- Potential for ineffective thermoregulation related to damage to the hypothalamus, dehydration, and infection
- Potential for impaired gas exchange related to hypoventilation, aspiration, and immobility
- Sensory-perceptual alterations (visual, auditory, speech) related to periorbital edema, head dressing, endotracheal tube, and effects of ICP
- Body image disturbance related to change in appearance or physical disabilities

Other nursing diagnoses may include impaired communication (aphasia) related to insult to brain tissue and high risk for impaired skin integrity related to immobility, pressure, and incontinence. There may be impaired physical mobility related to a neurologic deficit secondary to the neurosurgical procedure.

Collaborative Problems/Potential Complications

Potential complications may include:

- Increased ICP
- Bleeding and hypovolemic shock
- Fluid and electrolyte disturbances
- Infection
- Seizures

Planning and Goals

The major goals for the patient may include adequate preparation for surgery, neurologic homeostasis to improve cerebral tissue perfusion, thermoregulation, normal ventilation and gas exchange, ability to cope with sensory deprivation, adaptation to changes in body image, and absence of complications.

Nursing Interventions

Achieving Neurologic Homeostasis

Attention to the respiratory status is essential because even slight decreases in the oxygen level (hypoxia) can cause cerebral ischemia and can affect the patient's clinical course and outcome. The endotracheal tube is left in place until the patient shows signs of awakening and has adequate spontaneous ventilation, as evaluated clinically and by arterial blood gas analysis. Secondary brain damage can result from impaired cerebral oxygenation.

Cerebral edema is an increase in the water content of brain tissue, leading to an increase in brain volume. Some degree of cerebral edema occurs after brain surgery; it tends to peak 24 to 36 hours after surgery, producing decreased responsiveness on the second postoperative day. The control of cerebral edema is discussed in the section on management of increased ICP. Nursing strategies used to control factors that may raise ICP are found earlier in this Chapter in Nursing Process: The Patient With Increased ICP. Intraventricular drainage is carefully monitored, using strict asepsis if any part of the system is handled.

The vital signs and neurologic checks (LOC and responsiveness, pupillary and motor responses) are assessed every 15 minutes to 1 hour. Extreme head rotation is avoided because this raises ICP. After supratentorial surgery, the patient is placed on the back or side (unoperated side if a large lesion was removed) with one pillow under the head. The head of the bed may be elevated 30 degrees, according to the level of the ICP and the neurosurgeon's preference. After posterior fossa (infratentorial) surgery, the patient is kept flat on one side (off the back) with the head on a small, firm pillow. The patient may be turned on either side, keeping the neck in a neutral position. When the patient is being turned, the body should be turned as a unit to prevent placing strain on the incision and possibly tearing the sutures. The head of the bed may be elevated slowly as tolerated by the patient.

The patient's position is changed every 2 hours, and skin care is given frequently. During position changes, care is taken to prevent disruption of the ICP monitoring system. A turning sheet from the head to the midthigh makes it easier to move and turn the patient.

Regulating Temperature

Moderate temperature elevation can be expected after intracranial surgery because of reaction to blood at the operative site or in the subarachnoid space. Injury to the hypothalamic centers that regulate body temperature can occur during surgery. High fever is treated vigorously to combat the effect of an elevated temperature on brain metabolism and function.

Nursing interventions include monitoring the temperature and using the following measures to reduce body temperature: removing blankets, applying ice bags to axilla and groin areas, using a hypothermia blanket as prescribed, and administering prescribed medications to reduce fever.

Conversely, hypothermia may be seen after lengthy neurosurgical procedures. Therefore, frequent measurements of rectal temperature are necessary. Rewarming should occur slowly to prevent shivering and increased cellular oxygen demand.

Improving Gas Exchange

The patient undergoing neurosurgery is at risk for impaired gas exchange and pulmonary infections because of immobility, immunosuppression, decreased levels of consciousness, and fluid restriction. Immobility compromises the respiratory system by causing pooling and stasis of secretions in dependent areas and the development of atelectasis. Patients whose fluid intake is restricted may be more vulnerable to atelectasis as a result of inability to expectorate thickened secretions. Pneumonia is frequently seen in neurosurgical patients, possibly related to aspiration.

The patient is observed for signs of respiratory infection: rise in temperature, increase in pulse rate, and changes in respirations. The lungs are auscultated for decreased breath sounds and adventitious sounds.

The patient is repositioned every 2 hours to mobilize secretions and prevent stasis. When the patient regains consciousness, additional measures are instituted, such as yawning, sighing, deep breathing, use of incentive spirometry, and coughing (unless contraindicated) to expand collapsed alveoli. Suctioning may be needed to remove secretions that cannot be raised by coughing; however, coughing and suctioning increase ICP. Increasing the humidity may help to loosen secretions. The nurse and the respiratory therapist work together to monitor the effects of chest physical therapy.

Managing Sensory Deprivation

Periorbital edema is a common consequence of intracranial surgery because fluid drains into the dependent periorbital areas when the patient has been positioned in a prone position during surgery. A hematoma may form under the scalp and spread down to the orbit, producing an area of ecchymosis (black eye). Sometimes the eyes cannot be opened for a few days because of edema of the eyelids.

Before surgery, the patient and family should be informed that one or both eyes may be edematous temporarily after surgery. After surgery, placing the patient in a head-up position and applying cold compresses over the eyes will help reduce the edema. If periorbital edema increases significantly, the surgeon is notified because it may indicate that a postoperative clot is developing or that there is increasing ICP and poor venous drainage. Health care personnel should announce their presence when entering the room to avoid startling the patient whose vision is impaired because of the periorbital edema.

Enhancing Self-Image

The patient is encouraged to verbalize feelings and frustrations about any change in appearance. Nursing support is based on the patient's reactions and feelings. Factual information may need to be provided if the patient has misconceptions about puffiness about the face, periorbital bruising, and hair loss. Attention to grooming, the use of personal clothing, and covering the head with a turban (and ultimately a wig until hair growth occurs) are encouraged. Social interaction with close friends, family, and hospital personnel may increase the patient's sense of self-worth.

As the patient assumes more responsibility for self-care and participates in more activities, a sense of control and personal competence will develop. The family and social support system can be of assistance to the patient until adaptation is fully made.

Monitoring and Managing Potential Complications

Complications that may develop within hours after surgery include increased ICP, bleeding and hypovolemic shock, altered fluid and electrolyte balance (including water intoxication), infection, and seizures. These problems require close collaboration between the nurse and the surgeon.

MONITORING FOR INCREASED ICP, BLEEDING, AND HYPOVOLEMIC SHOCK

Increased ICP, bleeding, and hypovolemic shock are life-threatening to the patient who has undergone intracranial neurosurgery. The following must be kept in mind when caring for all patients who undergo such surgery:

- An increase in blood pressure and decrease in pulse with respiratory failure may indicate increased ICP.
- A drop in blood pressure, rapid pulse and respirations, and a pale and cold body are usually manifestations of hypovolemic shock after lengthy surgical procedures. Treatment depends on the cause of the hypovolemic shock. Fluid replacement is indicated if hypovolemia is due to fluid loss or diabetes insipidus; blood component therapy is indicated if blood loss is the cause.
- An accumulation of blood under the bone flap (extradural, subdural, intracerebral) may pose a threat to life. A

clot must be suspected in any patient who does not awaken as expected or whose condition deteriorates. An intracranial hematoma is suspected if the patient has any new postoperative neurologic deficits (especially a dilated pupil on the operative side). In these events, the patient is returned to the operating room immediately for evacuation of the clot if indicated.

- Cerebral edema, infarction, metabolic disturbances, and hydrocephalus are conditions that may simulate the clinical manifestations of a clot

The patient is monitored closely for indicators of complications, and early signs and trends in clinical status are reported to the surgeon. Treatments are initiated promptly, and the nurse assists in evaluating the patient's response to treatment. The nurse also provides support to the patient and family.

Should signs and symptoms of increased ICP occur, efforts to decrease the ICP are initiated: alignment of the head in a neutral position without flexion to promote venous drainage, elevation of the head of the bed to 30 degrees, administration of mannitol (osmotic diuretic), and possible administration of pharmacologic paralyzing agents.

MANAGING FLUID AND ELECTROLYTE DISTURBANCES

Fluid and electrolyte imbalance may occur because of the patient's underlying condition and its management or as complications of surgery. Fluid and electrolyte disturbances can contribute to the development of cerebral edema.

The postoperative fluid regimen depends on the type of neurosurgical procedure and is calculated on an individual basis. The volume and composition of fluids are adjusted according to daily electrolyte determinations and intake and output.

Sodium retention may occur in the immediate postoperative period. Serum and urine electrolytes, blood urea nitrogen, blood glucose, weight, and clinical status are monitored. Intake and output are measured in view of losses associated with fever, respiration, and CSF drainage. Fluids may have to be restricted in patients with cerebral edema.

Oral fluids are usually resumed in a short period, and the body's homeostatic mechanisms regulate electrolyte balance. Some patients with posterior fossa tumors may have impaired swallowing, however, and fluids may have to be administered by alternate routes.

Patients undergoing surgery for brain tumors may be receiving large doses of corticosteroids and thus tend to develop hyperglycemia. Therefore, serum glucose levels are measured every 4 hours.

Because these patients are prone to gastric ulcers, antacids or histamine-2 receptor receptor antagonists (H_2 blockers) may be prescribed to suppress the secretion of gastric acid. The patient is monitored for bleeding and assessed for gastric pain.

After surgery in and around the pituitary gland and hypothalamus, the patient may develop symptoms of diabetes insipidus, which is characterized by excessive urinary output. The urine specific gravity is measured hourly, and fluid intake and output records are monitored. Fluid replacement must compensate for urine output, and serum potassium must be monitored.

SIADH, which results in water retention with hyponatremia and serum hypo-osmolality, occurs in a wide variety of central nervous system dysfunctions (brain tumor, head trauma) causing fluid disturbances. Nursing management of this syndrome requires careful intake and output measurements, specific gravity determinations of urine, and monitoring of serum and urine electrolyte studies, while following directives for fluid restriction. This syndrome is usually self-limiting.

PREVENTING INFECTION

The patient undergoing neurosurgery is at risk for infection related to the neurosurgical procedure (brain exposure, bone exposure, wound hematomas) and the presence of intravenous and arterial lines for fluid administration and monitoring. Risk for infection is increased in patients who undergo lengthy intracranial operations and those with external ventricular drains in place longer than 48 to 72 hours.

The incision site is monitored for evidence of redness, tenderness, bulging, separation, or foul odor. The dressing is often stained with blood in the immediate postoperative period. It is important to reinforce the dressing with sterile pads so that contamination and infection are avoided. (Blood is an excellent culture medium for bacteria.) If the dressing is heavily stained or displaced, this should be reported immediately. (A drain is sometimes placed in the craniotomy incision to facilitate drainage.)

After suboccipital surgical procedures, CSF may leak through the incision. This complication is dangerous because of the possibility of meningitis. Any sudden discharge of fluid from a cranial or spinal incision is reported at once because a massive leak requires direct surgical repair. Attention should be paid to the patient who complains of a salty taste, because this can be due to CSF trickling down the throat. The patient is advised to avoid coughing, sneezing, or nose blowing, which may cause CSF leakage by creating pressure on the operative site.

Other causes of infection in the patient undergoing intracranial surgery are similar to those in other postoperative patients: phlebitis, deep vein thrombosis, and urinary tract infections.

Aseptic technique is used when handling dressings, drainage systems, and intravenous and arterial lines. The patient is monitored carefully for signs and symptoms of infection, and cultures are obtained from the patient with suspected infection. Appropriate antibiotics are administered as prescribed.

MONITORING FOR SEIZURE ACTIVITY

Seizures and epilepsy may be complications after any intracranial neurosurgical procedure. Preventing seizures is essential to avoid further cerebral edema. Administering the prescribed anticonvulsant medication before and immediately after surgery may prevent the appearance of seizures in subsequent months and years. Status epilepticus (prolonged seizures without recovery of consciousness in the intervals between seizures) may occur after craniotomy and also may be related to the development of complications (hematoma, ischemia). The management of status epilepticus is described in Chapter 59.

MONITORING AND MANAGING OTHER COMPLICATIONS

Other complications may occur during the first 2 weeks or later and may threaten the patient's recovery. The most important of these are thromboembolic complications (deep vein thrombosis, pulmonary embolism), pulmonary and urinary infection, and pressure ulcers. Most of these complications may be avoided by frequent changes of position, adequate suctioning of secretions, assessment for pulmonary complications, observation for urinary complications, and skin care.

Promoting Home and Community-Based Care

TEACHING PATIENTS SELF-CARE

The recovery at home of a neurosurgical patient depends on the extent of the surgical procedure and its success. The patient's strengths as well as limitations are explained to the family, along with their part in promoting recovery. Because administration of anticonvulsant medication is a priority, the patient and family are encouraged to use a check-off system to make sure the medication is taken. The patient may need to be accompanied while walking if sudden attacks of dizziness or seizures occur.

Usually dietary restrictions are not required unless another health problem requiring a special diet exists. Although taking a shower or tub bath is permitted, the scalp should be kept dry until all the sutures have been removed. A clean scarf or cap may be worn until a wig or hairpiece is purchased. If skull bone has been removed, the neurosurgeon may suggest a protective helmet.

After a craniotomy, the patient is usually more sensitive to loud noises. Television noise can be irritating to the convalescing person. If the patient is aphasic, speech therapy may be necessary. This is likely to be a long-term and time-consuming process, requiring patience and continuing encouragement on the part of all who are working with the patient.

CONTINUING CARE

Barring complications, patients are discharged from the hospital as soon as possible. Patients with motor deficits require management similar to that after a stroke. Those with postoperative cognitive and speech impairments require psychological evaluation, speech therapy, and rehabilitation. The nurse works collaboratively with the physician and other health care professionals during hospitalization and home care to achieve as complete a rehabilitation as possible.

When tumor, injury, or disease makes the prognosis poor, care is directed toward making the patient as comfortable as possible. With return of the tumor or cerebral compression, the patient becomes less alert and aware. Other possible consequences include paralysis, blindness, and seizures. The home care nurse, hospice nurse, and social worker work with the family to plan for additional home health care or hospice services or placement of the patient in an extended-care facility. (See also the section on cerebral metastases in Chap. 59. The patient's end-of-life preferences should be respected.)

Evaluation

Expected Outcomes

Expected outcomes may include:

1. Achieves neurologic homeostasis/improved cerebral tissue perfusion
   a. Opens eyes on request; uses recognizable words, progressing to normal speech
   b. Obeys commands with appropriate motor responses
2. Attains thermoregulation and normal body temperature
3. Has normal gas exchange
   a. Has arterial blood gas values within normal ranges
   b. Breathes easily; lung sounds clear without adventitious sounds
   c. Takes deep breaths and changes position as directed
4. Copes with sensory deprivation
5. Demonstrates improving self-concept
   a. Pays attention to grooming
   b. Visits and interacts with others
6. Absence of complications
   a. Exhibits ICP within normal range
   b. Has minimal bleeding at surgical site; surgical incision is healing without evidence of infection
   c. Registers normal body temperature
   d. Shows fluid balance and electrolyte levels within desired ranges
   e. Exhibits no evidence of seizures

An overview of care of the patient undergoing intracranial surgery is presented in Chart 57-6.

Transsphenoidal Surgery

Tumors within the sella turcica and small adenomas of the pituitary can be removed through the transsphenoidal approach (see Table 57-6). The incision is made beneath the upper lip; entry is then gained successively into the nasal cavity, sphenoidal sinus, and sella turcica. Although the initial opening may be made by an otorhinolaryngologist, the neurosurgeon completes the opening into the sphenoidal sinus and exposes the floor of the sella. Microsurgical techniques provide improved illumination, magnification, and visualization so that nearby vital structures can be avoided.

The transsphenoidal approach offers direct access to the sella with minimal risk of trauma and hemorrhage. It avoids many of the risks of craniotomy, and the postoperative discomfort is similar to that of other transnasal surgical procedures. It may also be used for pituitary ablation (removal) in patients with disseminated breast or prostatic cancer.

Complications

Manipulation of the posterior pituitary gland during surgery may produce transient diabetes insipidus of several days' duration. It is treated with vasopressin but occasionally persists. Other complications include CSF leakage, postoperative meningitis, and SIADH.

Preoperative Evaluation

The preoperative workup includes a series of endocrine tests, rhinologic evaluation (to assess the status of the sinuses and nasal cavity), and neuroradiologic studies. Funduscopic examination and visual field determinations are performed, because the most serious effect of pituitary tumor is localized pressure on the optic nerve or chiasm. In addition, the nasopharyngeal secretions are cultured because a sinus infection is a contraindication to an intracranial procedure through this approach. Corticosteroids may be given before and after surgery (because the surgery involves removal of the pituitary, the source of adrenocorticotropic hormone [ACTH] is removed). Antibiotics may or may not be administered prophylactically.

Deep breathing is taught before surgery. The patient is instructed on the technique for avoiding vigorous coughing and sneezing, because these actions may cause a CSF leak after surgery. Instructions include applying pressure on the inner aspect of both sides of the nose to control sneezing.

Postoperative Management

Because the procedure disrupts the oral and nasal mucous membranes, management focuses on preventing infection and promoting healing. Medications include antimicrobials (which are continued until the nasal packing inserted at the time of surgery

CHART 57•6 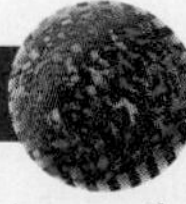 Overview of Nursing Management for the Patient After Intracranial Surgery

Postoperative Interventions

Nursing Diagnosis: Potential for ineffective breathing pattern related to postoperative cerebral edema
Goal: Achievement of adequate respiratory function

1. Establish proper respiratory exchange to eliminate systemic hypercapnia and hypoxia, which increase cerebral edema.
   a. Unless contraindicated, place the patient in a lateral or a semiprone position to facilitate respiratory gas exchange until consciousness returns.
   b. Suction trachea and pharynx *cautiously* to remove secretions; suctioning can raise ICP.
   c. Maintain patient on controlled ventilation if prescribed to maintain normal ventilatory status; monitor arterial blood gas results to determine respiratory status.
   d. Elevate the head of the bed 30.5 cm (12 in) after patient is conscious to aid venous drainage of the brain.
   e. Administer nothing by mouth until active coughing and swallowing reflexes are demonstrated, to prevent aspiration.

Nursing Diagnosis: Potential alteration in fluid volume related to intracranial pressure or diuretics
Goal: Attainment of fluid and electrolyte balance

1. Monitor for polyuria, especially during first postoperative week; diabetes insipidus may develop in patients with lesions around the pituitary or hypothalamus.
   a. Measure urinary specific gravity at intervals.
   b. Monitor serum and urinary electrolyte levels.
2. Evaluate patient's electrolyte status; patients may retain water and sodium.
   a. Early postoperative weight gain indicates fluid retention; a greater-than-estimated weight loss indicates negative water balance.
   b. Loss of sodium and chloride will produce weakness, lethargy, and coma.
   c. Low potassium levels will cause confusion and decreased level of responsiveness.
3. Weigh patient daily; keep intake and output record.
4. Administer prescribed intravenous fluids cautiously—rate and composition depend on fluid deficit, urine output, and blood loss. Fluid intake and fluid losses should remain relatively equal.

Nursing Diagnosis: Alteration in sensory perceptions (visual/auditory) related to periorbital edema and head dressings
Goal: Compensate for sensory deprivation; prevention of injury

1. Perform supportive measures until the patient can care for self.
   a. Change position as indicated; position changes can increase ICP.
   b. Administer prescribed analgesics (codeine) that do not mask the level of responsiveness.
2. Use measures prescribed to relieve signs of periocular edema.
   a. Lubricate eyelids and around eyes with petrolatum.
   b. Apply light, cold compresses over eyes at specified intervals.
   c. Observe for signs of keratitis if cornea has no sensation.
3. Put extremities through range-of-motion exercises.
4. Evaluate and support patient during episodes of restlessness.
   a. Evaluate for airway obstruction, distended bladder, meningeal irritation from bloody CSF.
   b. Pad patient's hands and bed rails to prevent injury.
5. Reinforce blood-stained dressings with sterile dressing; blood-soaked dressings act as a culture medium for bacteria.
6. Orient patient frequently to time, place, and person.

Monitor and Manage Complications

1. Cerebral edema
   a. Assess patient's level of responsiveness/consciousness; decreased level of consciousness may be the first sign of increased ICP.
      (1) Eye opening (spontaneous, to sound, to pain); pupillary reactions to light
      (2) Response to commands
      (3) Assessment of spinal motor reflexes (pinch Achilles tendon, arm, or other body site)
      (4) Observation of patient's spontaneous activity
   b. Maintain a neurologic flow sheet to assess and document neurologic status, fluid administration, laboratory data, medications, and treatments.
   c. Evaluate for signs and symptoms of increasing ICP, which can lead to ischemia and further impairment of brain function.
      (1) Assess patient minute by minute, hour by hour, for:
         - Diminished response to stimuli
         - Fluctuations of vital signs
         - Restlessness
         - Weakness and paralysis of extremities
         - Increasing headache
         - Changes or disturbances of vision; pupillary changes
      (2) Modify nursing management to prevent further increases in ICP.
   d. Control postoperative cerebral edema as prescribed.
      (1) Administer corticosteroids and osmotic diuretics as prescribed to reduce brain swelling.
      (2) Monitor fluid intake; avoid overhydration.
      (3) Maintain a normal temperature. Temperature control may be impaired in certain neurologic states, and fever increases the metabolic demands of the brain.
         - Monitor rectal temperature at specified intervals. Assess temperature of extremities, which may be cold and dry due to impaired heat-losing mechanisms (vasodilation and sweating).
         - Employ measures as prescribed to reduce fever: ice bags to axillae and groin; hypothermia blanket. Use ECG monitoring to detect dysrhythmias during hypothermia procedures.
      (4) Employ hyperventilation when prescribed (results in respiratory alkalosis, which causes cerebral vasoconstriction and reduces intracranial pressure).
      (5) Elevate head of bed to reduce ICP and facilitate respirations.
      (6) Avoid excessive stimuli.
      (7) Use ICP monitoring if patient is at risk for intracranial hypertension.
2. Intracranial hemorrhage
   a. Postoperative bleeding may be intraventricular, intracerebellar, subdural, or extradural.
   b. Observe for progressive impairment of state of consciousness and other signs of increasing ICP.
   c. Prepare deteriorating patient for return to surgery for evacuation of hematoma.
3. Seizures (greater risk with supratentorial operations)
   a. Administer prescribed anticonvulsants; monitor anticonvulsant medication blood levels.
   b. Observe for status epilepticus, which may occur after any intracranial surgery.

(*continued*)

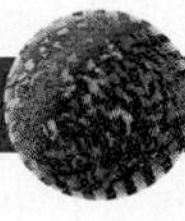

CHART 57•6 Overview of Nursing Management for the Patient After Intracranial Surgery (*continued*)

4. Infections
   a. Urinary tract infections
   b. Pulmonary infections related to aspiration secondary to depressed level of responsiveness; may result in atelectasis and aspiration pneumonia
   c. CNS infections (postoperative meningitis, CSF shunt infection)
   d. Surgical site infections/septicemia
5. Venous thrombosis
   a. Assess Homans' sign.
   b. Apply elastic pressure stockings.
   c. Administer anticoagulant therapy as prescribed.
6. Leakage of CSF
   a. Differentiate between CSF and mucus.
      (1) Collect fluid on Dextrostix; if CSF is present, the indicator will have a positive reaction, as CSF contains glucose.
      (2) Assess for moderate elevation of temperature and mild neck rigidity.
   b. Caution patient against nose blowing or sniffing.
   c. Elevate head of bed as prescribed.
   d. Assist with insertion of lumbar CSF drainage system if inserted to reduce CSF pressure.
      (1) Ventricular catheters may be inserted in the patient undergoing surgery of the posterior fossa (ventriculostomy); the catheter is connected to a closed drainage system.
      (2) Administer antibiotics as prescribed.
7. Gastrointestinal ulceration; monitor for signs and symptoms of hemorrhage, perforation, or both (probably caused by stress response).

Evaluation

Expected outcomes

1. Demonstrates normal breathing pattern
   a. Absence of crackles
   b. Demonstrates active swallowing and coughing reflexes
2. Attains/maintains fluid balance
   a. Takes fluids orally
   b. Maintains weight within expected range
3. Compensates for sensory deprivation
   a. Makes needs known
   b. Demonstrates improvement of vision
4. Exhibits absence of complications
   a. No evidence of increased ICP
   b. Opens eyes on request
   c. Obeys commands
   d. Has appropriate motor responses
   e. Shows increasing alertness
   f. No evidence of rhinorrhea, otorrhea, or CSF leakage
   g. Absence of fever
   h. No evidence of inflammation or infection at surgical site
   i. Absence of seizures

is removed), corticosteroids, analgesics for discomfort, and agents for the control of diabetes insipidus when necessary.

The nasal packing is removed in 24 hours to several days. The area around the nares is cleaned with the prescribed solution to remove crusted blood and moisten the mucous membranes.

Nursing Management

Vital signs are measured to monitor hemodynamic, cardiac, and ventilatory status. Because of the anatomic proximity of the pituitary gland to the optic chiasm, visual acuity is assessed at regular intervals. One method is to ask the patient to count the number of fingers held up by the nurse. Evidence of decreasing visual acuity suggests an expanding hematoma.

The head of the bed is raised to decrease pressure on the sella turcica and to promote normal drainage. The patient is cautioned against blowing the nose or engaging in any activity that raises ICP, such as bending over or straining during urination or defecation.

Intake and output are measured as a guide to fluid and electrolyte replacement. The urinary specific gravity is measured after each voiding. Daily weight is monitored. Fluids are generally given when nausea ceases, and the patient then progresses to a regular diet.

The major discomfort is related to the nasal packing and to mouth dryness and thirst from mouth-breathing. Oral care is provided every 4 hours or more frequently. Usually, the teeth are not brushed until the incision above the teeth has healed. The use of warm saline mouth rinses and a cool mist vaporizer is helpful. Petrolatum is soothing when applied to the lips. A room humidifier assists in keeping the mucous membranes moist.

Home care considerations include advising the patient to use a room humidifier to keep the mucous membranes moist and to soothe irritation. The head of the bed is elevated for at least 2 weeks after surgery.

NEUROLOGIC AND NEUROSURGICAL APPROACHES TO PAIN MANAGEMENT

Managing long-term pain requires a multidisciplinary approach. (See Chap. 12 for a discussion of pain, its assessment, and pharmacologic and noninvasive methods of treatment.)

Intractable pain refers to pain that cannot be relieved satisfactorily by the usual approaches, including medications. Such pain usually is the result of malignancy (especially of the cervix, bladder, prostate, and lower bowel), but it may occur in other conditions, such as postherpetic neuralgia, trigeminal neuralgia, spinal cord arachnoiditis, and uncontrollable ischemia and other forms of tissue destruction.

Neurologic and neurosurgical methods available for pain relief include (1) stimulation procedures—intermittent electric stimulation of a tract or center to inhibit the transmission of pain impulses, (2) administration of intraspinal opioids, and (3) interruption of the tracts conducting the pain impulse from the periphery to cerebral integration centers. The latter are destructive or ablative procedures.

Stimulation Procedures

Electrical stimulation, or neuromodulation, is a method of suppressing pain by applying controlled low-voltage electrical pulses to the different parts of the nervous system. Electrical stimulation is thought to relieve pain by blocking painful stimuli or by stimulating the release of endogenous opioids (natural pain-relieving peptides, or endorphins). This pain-modulating technique is administered by many modes. Transcutaneous electrical nerve stimulation (TENS) and dorsal column stimulation are the most common types of electrical stimulation used. In addition, there are also brain-stimulating techniques, in which electrodes are implanted in the periventricular area of the posterior third ventricle, allowing the patient to stimulate this area to produce analgesia.

TENS is the passage of small electrical currents through the skin to control localized pain. Electrodes are placed over the site of pain, along the course of the major peripheral nerves innervating the area, or over the peripheral plexus. The patient operates the amplitude control until stimulation, detected by a vibration, buzzing, or tapping sensation, is felt within the deeper tissue. The amplitude is increased slowly until the sensation is perceived at the site or origin of pain or along radiating pathways. The patient controls the amplitude, frequency, and duration of stimulation. TENS has been successful in well-prepared patients in the early management of acute pain as well as in patients with chronic pain. It is most effective when used as part of a comprehensive rehabilitation program for relief and elimination of pain.

In dorsal column stimulation, a technique used for the relief of chronic, intractable pain, a surgically implanted device allows the patient to apply pulsed electrical stimulation to the dorsal aspect of the spinal cord to block pain impulses. (The largest accumulation of afferent fibers is found in the dorsal column of the spinal cord.) The dorsal column stimulation unit consists of a radio frequency stimulation transmitter, a transmitter antenna, a radio frequency receiver, and a stimulation electrode. The battery-powered transmitter and antenna are worn externally; the receiver and electrode are implanted. A laminectomy is performed above the highest level of pain input, and the electrode is placed in the epidural space over the posterior column of the spinal cord. (The placement of the stimulating systems varies.) A subcutaneous pocket is constructed over the clavicular area or some other site for placement of the receiver. The two are connected by a subcutaneous tunnel.

Percutaneous epidural neurostimulation is a method of neurostimulation in which electrodes are inserted percutaneously into the spinal epidural space. It appears to be effective in treating arachnoiditis and postamputation neuroma.

Deep brain stimulation is performed for special pain problems when the patient does not respond to the usual techniques of pain control. With the patient under local anesthesia, electrodes are introduced through a burr hole in the skull and inserted into a selected site in the brain, depending on the location or type of pain. After the effectiveness of stimulation is confirmed, the implanted electrode is connected to a radiofrequency device or pulse-generator system operated by external telemetry.

Nursing Interventions

With each of these systems, the patient is provided with written and verbal instructions about its use and side effects.

With TENS, the skin is cleansed and electrode gel is applied to the electrodes, which are then placed over the nerves that innervate the painful area. The electrodes are secured with hypoallergenic tape. Skin irritation from the tape, gels, or electrodes is the most common adverse effect of TENS. The patient is instructed to keep a record evaluating the effectiveness of TENS. If there is a progression of pathology (as in advanced cancer), changes in amplitude may be necessary.

After surgery or percutaneous insertion of electrodes to establish the dorsal column stimulation, epidural neurostimulation, or deep brain stimulation system, the patient is assessed for infection or drainage (CSF) at the insertion site. Other postprocedure assessments are based on the specific procedure performed; for example, the care for the patient undergoing surgery to insert electrodes for the dorsal column stimulator is similar to that required for a laminectomy. The patient is assessed for evidence of paraplegia, quadriplegia, and urinary incontinence. Complications include infection, cord trauma, CSF leakage, and pain around the implantation site. Failure of the stimulating system and development of tolerance may occur later.

Nursing interventions include teaching the patient and family about the system, encouraging the patient to keep a record of amplitude and frequency settings and the relief obtained, and monitoring for complications.

Intraspinal Opioids

Opioid receptors exist not only in the brain but also in the substantia gelatinosa of the spinal cord. These receptors can combine with locally administered opioids (morphine) injected epidurally or intrathecally to produce long-lasting pain relief with little or no blunting of the patient's level of responsiveness and no losses of sensory, motor, or sphincter function. (Care of the patient receiving intraspinal opioids for pain relief is discussed in detail in Chap. 12.)

Numerous techniques are employed, but most include placing a catheter in the epidural or subarachnoid space with a spinal needle and inserting the catheter as near as possible to the spinal segment where the pain is projected. Small doses of morphine are injected into the system at regular intervals. If the patient requires long-term management, an implantable programmable pump is used.

After the procedure, the patient is evaluated for the degree of pain relief, which ranges from good to excellent. The catheter insertion site is inspected for evidence of infection.

This method allows the patient to be at home. The necessary dose of medication is small; the patient is alert and usually able to function at a relatively high level. The patient may complain of generalized itching and urinary retention (self-limited) for several days. With long-term use, there can be tolerance and mechanical failure (catheter obstructed, dislodged, broken) of the administration system. If the patient has rapid tumor growth, the dosage of morphine is increased, but the doses needed are low in comparison with those required for systemic administration for intractable pain.

Cordotomy

Pain-conducting fibers can be interrupted at any point from their origin to the cerebral cortex. Some part of the nervous system is destroyed, resulting in varying amounts of neurologic deficit and incapacity. In time, pain usually returns as a result of either regeneration of axonal fibers or the development of alternative pain pathways. These procedures are referred to as ablative or destructive procedures. Cordotomy is the division of certain tracts of the spinal cord. It may be performed percutaneously, by the open method after laminectomy, or by other techniques.

Percutaneous cordotomy uses radio frequency currents to produce lesions in the anterolateral surface of the spinal cord. With the patient under local anesthesia, a needle is inserted into the neck below and behind the mastoid process. It is advanced into the spinal cord under x-ray guidance, and an electrode is inserted through it. By means of radio frequency currents, a lesion is made at the desired spinal cord level. Verification of electrode placement is determined by the patient's response to stimulation. The procedure generally is well tolerated by even emaciated and debilitated patients.

Open cordotomy involves the surgical division of the anterolateral columns of the spinal pain fibers high in the thoracic or cervical region. This procedure interrupts or destroys conduction of pain and temperature sensation, whereas touch and position sense are preserved. The spinal cord is exposed by laminectomy.

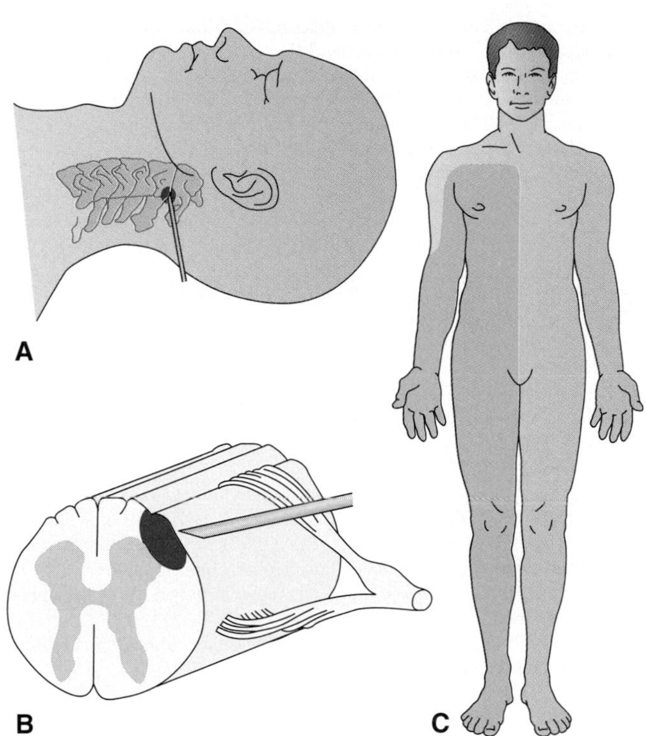

FIGURE 57•12 (**A**) Site of percutaneous C1–C2 cordotomy. (**B**) Lesion produced by percutaneous C1–C2 cordotomy. (**C**) Extent of analgesia produced by left C1–C2 percutaneous cordotomy. From Hickey, J. V. (1997). *The clinical practice of neurological and neurosurgical nursing* (4th ed.). Philadelphia: Lippincott-Raven.

Cordotomy is used most frequently in controlling the severe pain of terminal cancer, especially of the thorax, abdomen, or lower extremities. Because a significant percentage of cordotomies lose their effectiveness in 1 to 5 years, the procedure is used for pain associated with conditions in which survival time is limited. A percutaneous approach for a cordotomy is shown in Figure 57-12.

Nursing Management

The principles of nursing management after a laminectomy (see Chap. 59) apply to the postoperative and rehabilitation care of patients undergoing cordotomy. After a cordotomy, the patient may be kept flat for the prescribed time, because there is less tension on the incision in this position. A patient with a thoracic cordotomy may be turned to the prone position. In instances of a cervical incision, pillows should not be used when the patient is in a supine position. Trauma to the surgical site is reduced when the neck is kept in a neutral position. The patient is turned as a unit (log fashion) by two or more people using a turning sheet to avoid twisting the body and putting pressure on the incision.

The patient is monitored for respiratory complications as well as signs of fatigue and weakening of the voice. The patient may ventilate adequately while awake but may experience progressive hypercarbia and hypoxia while asleep. Therefore, arterial blood gas levels or pulse oximetry is monitored, and assisted mechanical ventilation is initiated if required.

Because hemorrhage may result in motor and sensory loss, the motion, strength, and sensation of each extremity must be tested every few hours, or more frequently if necessary, during the first 48 hours after surgery. If hemorrhage is suspected or detected, immediate surgical intervention is imperative. Because the patient has no sense of temperature, the skin should be palpated at intervals to ascertain any changes in temperature. Because pressure ulcers may develop without the patient realizing it, the patient is taught to inspect the skin using a hand mirror to view hard-to-see areas and to change position frequently. Urinary retention may occur. There is usually a slow return to normal voiding, but this cannot be guaranteed. If there is permanent loss of urinary control from a high cervical procedure, a bladder training program is started.

Rhizotomy

Rhizotomy, the surgical division of the spinal roots, is also an ablative procedure and is used for controlling the severe chest pain of lung cancer and for pain relief in head and neck malignancies. Rhizotomy is used for patients expected to survive for an extended time.

Because many patients with metastatic malignancies may not be able to tolerate an open rhizotomy, a percutaneous rhizotomy may be performed. In this procedure, a radiofrequency current is used to coagulate only the pain fibers, preserving the fibers concerned with touch and proprioception. A surgical approach for rhizotomy is shown in Figure 57-13.

In a chemical rhizotomy, alcohol, phenol, or a mixture of agents is injected into the subarachnoid space. The medication is maneuvered over the affected nerve roots by tilting the patient to the desired level. This renders the sensory nerve roots functionless. The patient's perception of pain is absent, but the motor nerve roots are usually not affected.

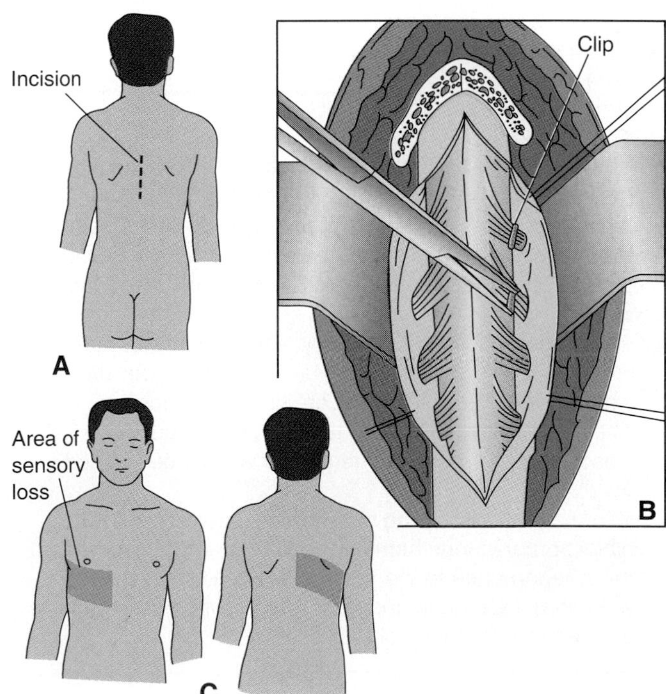

FIGURE 57•13 A rhizotomy may be performed surgically, percutaneously, or chemically depending on a patient's condition and needs. The procedure is usually done to relieve severe chest pain, for example, from lung cancer. In (**A**) a surgical rhizotomy, (**B**) the spinal roots are divided and banded with a clip to form a lesion and subsequent (**C**) loss of sensation. Adapted with permission from Bonica, J. J. (1990). *The management of pain* (2nd ed.). Philadelphia: Lea & Febiger (Lippincott Williams & Wilkins).

Psychosurgical Approaches

The purpose of psychosurgical procedures is to alter the patient's response to pain. A thalamotomy is the destruction (either unilateral or bilateral) of the specific cell groups within the thalamus. Burr holes are made in the skull, electrodes are placed in the target area by stereotactic techniques, and a radiofrequency current is then directed through the electrodes to create the lesion. This procedure represents the highest level in the central nervous system in which pain pathways can be interrupted; it is usually performed for malignancy of the head and neck. On completion of the procedure, the patient will lose temperature and pain sensation below the level that is destroyed.

Cingulotomy is a unilateral or bilateral interruption of the anterior cingulate bundle in the frontal lobe of the brain. It is accomplished by either an open or a stereotactic approach. It tends to modify the patient's affective reaction to pain.

Nursing Management

The nursing care of patients who undergo neurologic and neurosurgical procedures for the relief of chronic pain depends on the type of procedure performed, its effectiveness in relieving the pain, and the changes in neurologic function that accompany the procedure. After the procedure, the patient's pain level and neurologic function are assessed. Other nursing interventions that may be indicated include positioning, turning and skin care, bowel and bladder management, and initiation of interventions to promote patient safety. Pain management remains an important aspect of nursing care with each of these procedures.

Critical Thinking Exercises

1. Your patient had symptoms of an ischemic stroke approximately 2 hours ago and is undergoing a confirmatory CT scan in 30 minutes. You know t-PA must be administered within 3 hours of the symptoms. What actions would you take? What is your rationale for these actions?
2. After undergoing cranial surgery, your patient has had elevated ICP for 15 minutes. Mannitol, an osmotic diuretic, was administered, but the ICP remains unchanged. The patient is receiving sedation and pain medication. Describe some other interventions that may be initiated.
3. Your patient is admitted with hemorrhagic stroke and exhibits homonymous hemianopsia. How would you explain this phenomenon to the patient and family? Describe ways that the patient and family may work together to compensate for this problem.

References and Selected Readings

BOOKS

Abram, S. E., & Haddox, J. D. (Eds.). (1999). *The pain clinic manual* (2nd ed.). Philadelphia: Lippincott Williams & Wilkins.

Agency for Health Care Policy and Research, Public Health Service. U.S. Department of Health and Human Services. Panel for the Prediction and Prevention of Pressure Ulcers in Adults. (1992). *Pressure ulcers in adults: Prediction and prevention.* Clinical Practice Guideline Number 3. AHCPR Publication No. 92-0047. Rockville, MD.

Agency for Health Care Policy and Research, Public Health Service. U.S. Department of Health and Human Services. Urinary Incontinence Guideline Panel. (1992). *Urinary incontinence in adults.* Clinical Practice Guideline. AHCPR Publication No. 92-0038. Rockville, MD.

Agency for Health Care Policy and Research, Public Health Service. U.S. Department of Health and Human Services. Panel for the Prediction and Prevention of Pressure Ulcers in Adults. (1994). *Treatment of pressure ulcers.* Clinical Practical Guideline No. 15. AHCPR Publication No. 94-0652. Rockville, MD.

Agency for Health Care Policy and Research, Public Health Service. U.S. Department of Health and Human Services. (1995). *Post-stroke rehabilitation.* Clinical Practice Guideline. AHCPR Publication No. 95-0662. Rockville, MD.

Aronoff, G. M. (1999). *Evaluation and treatment of chronic pain.* Baltimore: Lippincott Williams & Wilkins.

Benzon, H. T. (1999). *Essentials of pain medicine and regional anesthesia.* New York: Churchill Livingstone.

Bickley, L. S., & Hoekelman, R. A. (1999). *Bates' guide to physical examination and history taking* (7th ed.). Philadelphia: Lippincott Williams & Wilkins.

Cousins, M. J., & Bridenbaugh, P. O. (Eds.). (1998). *Neural blockade in clinical anesthesia and management of pain.* Philadelphia: Lippincott-Raven.

Cruz, J. (Ed.). (1998). *Neurological and neurosurgical emergencies.* Philadelphia: W. B. Saunders.

Hickey, J. V. (1997). *The clinical practice of neurologic and neurosurgical nursing* (4th ed.). Philadelphia: Lippincott-Raven.

Kaye, A. (1997). *Essential neurosurgery* (2nd ed.). New York: Churchill Livingstone.

Kelley, W. N. (1997). *Textbook of internal medicine.* Philadelphia: Lippincott-Raven.

Marler, J., Jones, P. W., & Emr, M. (1997). *National symposium on rapid identification and treatment of acute stroke.* National Institutes of Health, National Institute of Neurological Disorders and Stroke. NIH Publication 97-4239.

Nolan, M. (1996). *Introduction to the neurologic examination.* Philadelphia: F. A. Davis.

Ojemann, R., Heros, R., & Crowell, R. (1995). *Surgical management of cerebrovascular disease* (2nd ed.). Baltimore: Williams & Wilkins.

Portencyt, R., & Kanner, R. (1996). *Pain management: Theory and practice.* Philadelphia: F. A. Davis.

Salerno, E., & Willens, J. (1996). *Pain management handbook.* St. Louis: Mosby–Year Book.

Strub, R. L., & Black, F. W. (1993). *The mental status examination in neurology.* Philadelphia: F. A. Davis.

Watson, C. (1995). *Basic human neuroanatomy: An introductory atlas* (5th ed.). Boston: Little, Brown.

Wiebers, D., et al. (1997). *Cerebrovascular disease in clinical practice.* Boston: Little, Brown.

Westmoreland, B. F., et al. (1994). *Medical neurosciences: An approach to Anatomy, pathology and physiology by systems and levels.* Boston: Little, Brown.

JOURNALS

Asterisks indicate nursing research articles.

General

*Cammermeyer, M., et al. (1997). Profiles of cognitive functioning in subjects with neurologic disorders. *Journal of Neuroscience Nursing, 29*(3), 163–169.

Downey, D. L., et al. (1998). Eye movements: Pathophysiology, examination and clinical importance. *Journal of Neuroscience Nursing, 30*(1), 15–22.

*Grossman, D., et al. (1995). Current nursing practices in fever management. *MedSurg Nursing, 4*(3), 193–198.

Henker, R., Kramer, D., & Rogers, S. (1997). Fever. *AACN Clinical Issues, 8*(3), 351–367.

League, D. (1995). Interactive, image-guided, stereotactic neurosurgery systems. *AORN Journal, 61*(2), 360–370.

*Leveck, M. D. (1997). Neuroscience nursing research: Challenges for the next decade. *Journal of Neuroscience Nursing, 29*(5), 338–341.

Lucke, K., et al. (1995). Continuous bedside cerebral blood flow monitoring. *Journal of Neuroscience Nursing, 17*(3), 164–173.

*Myles, G. L., et al. (1995). Quantifying nursing care in barbiturate-induced coma with the therapeutic intervention scoring system. *Journal of Neuroscience Nursing, 27*(1), 35–42.

Ozuna, J. (1996). Persistent vegetative state: Important considerations for the neuroscience nurse. *Journal of Neuroscience Nursing, 28*(3), 199–203.

*Richmond, T. (1997). Cerebral resuscitation after global brain ischemia: Linking research to practice. *AACN Clinical Issues, 8*(2), 171–181.

*Robert, I., et al. (1998). Absence of evidence for the effectiveness of five interventions routinely used in the intensive care management of severe head injury: A systematic review. *Journal of Neurologic and Neurosurgical Psychiatry, 65*(5), 729–733.

Sulkowski, J., & Judy, K. (1997). Acute mental status changes. *AACN Clinical Issues, 8*(3), 319–334.

Tolley, G., & Prevost, S. (1997). Case management of the critically ill elders: A case study. *AACN Clinical Issues, 8*(4), 635–642.

*Way, C., & Segatore, M. (1994). Development and preliminary testing of the neurological assessment instrument. *Journal of Neuroscience Nursing, 26*(5), 278–287.

Care of the Neurosurgical Patient

Campbell, P. J., et al. (1997). Hyperdynamic therapy: The nurse's role in treatment of cerebral vasospasm. *Journal of Neuroscience Nursing, 29*(5), 318–324.

Counsell, C., et al. (1995). Nimodipine: A drug therapy treatment of vasospasm. *Journal of Neuroscience Nursing, 27*(1), 53–56.

Cousins, M., et al. (1996). Postoperative pain management in the neurosurgical patient. *International Anesthesiology Clinics, 34*(4), 179–193.

Gentilello, L. M. (1995). Advances in the management of hypothermia. *Surgical Clinics of North America, 75*(2), 243–256.

Increased Intracranial Pressure

Brain Trauma Foundation. (1996). Indications for intracranial pressure monitoring. *Journal of Neurotrauma, 13*(11), 667–679.

*Brucia, J., & Rudy, E. (1996). The effect of suction catheter insertion and tracheal stimulation in adults with severe head injury. *Heart and Lung, 25*(4), 295–303.

Fortune, J., et al. (1995). Effect of hyperventilation, mannitol and ventriculostomy drainage on cerebral blood flow after head injury. *Journal of Trauma, 39*(6), 1091–1099.

Geraci, E., & Geraci, T. (1996). Hyperventilation and head injury. *Journal of Neuroscience Nursing, 28*(6), 381–387.

*Kerr, M., et al. (1997). Effect of short-duration hyperventilation during endotracheal suctioning on intracranial pressure in severe head-injured adults. *Nursing Research, 46*(4), 195–201.

*Martin, N., et al. (1997). Characterization of cerebral hemodynamic phases following severe head trauma: Hypoperfusion, hyperemia, and vasospasm. *Journal of Neurosurgery, 87*(1), 9–19.

Minahan, R., et al. (1997). Critical care monitoring for cerebrovascular disease. *New Horizons, 5*(4), 406–421.

Brain Trauma Foundation. (1996). Recommendations for intracranial pressure monitoring technology. *Journal of Neurotrauma, 13*(11), 685–692.

Schwab, S., et al. (1996). The value of intracranial pressure monitoring in acute hemispheric stroke. *Neurology, 47*(2), 393–398.

Schwab, S., et al. (1997). Barbiturate coma in severe hemispheric stroke: Useful or obsolete? *Neurology, 48*(6), 1608–1613.

*Simmons, B. J. (1997). Management of intracranial hemodynamics in the adult: A research analysis of head positioning and recommendations for clinical practice and future research. *Journal of Neuroscience Nursing, 29*(1), 44–49.

Neurologic and Neurosurgical Management of Pain

Dubuisson, D. (1995). Treatment of occipital neuralgia by partial posterior rhizotomy at C1-3. *Journal of Neurosurgery, 82*(4), 581–586.

Seres, J. (1993). The neurosurgical management of pain: A critical review. *Clinical Journal of Pain, 9*(4), 284–290.

Pain

Miaskowski, C. (1993). Current concepts in the assessment and management of acute pain. *MedSurg Nursing, 2*(1), 28–32.

North, R., & Levy R. (1994). Consensus conference on the neurosurgical management of pain. *Neurosurgery, 34*(4), 756–760.

Richardson, D. (1995). Deep brain stimulation for the relief of chronic pain. *Neurosurgery Clinics of North America, 6*(1), 135–144.

Stroke and Transient Ischemic Attacks

Barch, D., et al. (1997). Nursing management of acute complications following rt-PA in acute ischemic stroke. The NINDS rt-PA Stroke Study. *Journal of Neuroscience Nursing, 29*(6), 367–372.

Braimah, J., et al. (1997). Nursing care of acute stroke patients after receiving rt-PA therapy. The NINDS rt-PA Stroke Study Group. *Journal of Neuroscience Nursing, 29*(6), 373–383.

Bratina, P., et al. (1997). Pathophysiology and mechanisms of acute ischemic stroke. The NINDS rt-PA Stroke Study Group. *Journal of Neuroscience Nursing, 29*(6), 356–360.

Broderick, J., Brott, T., Kothari, R., et al. (1998). The greater Cincinnati/northern Kentucky stroke study: Preliminary first-ever and total incidence rates of stroke among blacks. *Stroke, 29*(2), 415–421.

Chiu, D., et al. (1998). Intravenous tissue plasminogen activator for acute ischemic stroke: Feasibility, safety, and efficacy in the first year of clinical practice. *Stroke, 29*(1), 18–22.

Hinkle, J. L. (1997). New developments in managing transient ischemic attack and acute stroke. *AACN Clinical Issues, 8*(2), 205–213.

Hinkle, J. L., & Forbes, E. (1996). Pilot project on functional outcomes in stroke. *Journal of Neuroscience Nursing, 28*(1), 13–18.

National Institute of Neurologic Disorders and Stroke (NINDS) rt-PA Stroke Study Group. (1997). A systems approach to immediate evaluation and management of hyperacute stroke: Experience at eight centers and implications for community practice and patient care. *Stroke, 28*(8), 1530–1540.

Rosier, P. K. (1998). Stroke following vertebral artery dissection: A case study. *MedSurg Nursing, 7*(4), 214–216.

Sauerbeck, L. R. (1998). Emerging drug therapies for acute cerebral ischemia. *American Journal of Nursing, 98*(10), 16AA, 16EE–16GG.

Smith-Rooker, J. L., & Hodges, L. C. (1998). Managing patients with carotid stenosis. *MedSurg Nursing, 7*(5), 280–292.

Spilker, J., et al. (1997). Using the NIH Stroke Scale to assess stroke patients. The NINDS rt-PA Stroke Study Group. *Journal of Neuroscience Nursing, 29*(6), 384–392.

Testani-Dufour, L., et al. (1997). Brain attack: Correlative anatomy. *Journal of Neuroscience Nursing, 29*(4), 213–222.

Wood, P., et al. (1997). Dysphagia: A screening tool for stroke patients. *Journal of Neuroscience Nursing, 29*(5), 325–329.

Wright, C. K. (1998). A brief update on stroke. *American Journal of Nursing, 98*(5), 62, 64, 67.

Unconsciousness and Coma

Ackerman, L. (1993). Alteration in level of responsiveness. A proposed nursing diagnosis. *Nursing Clinics of North America, 28*(4), 729–745.

*Lawrence, M. (1995). The unconscious experience. *American Journal of Critical Care, 4*(3), 227–232.

Ozuna, J. (1996). Persistent vegetative state: Important considerations for the neuroscience nurse. *Journal of Neuroscience Nursing, 28*(3), 199–203.

Sulkowski, J,. & Judy, K. (1997). Acute mental status changes. *AACN Clinical Issues, 8*(3), 319–334.

Resources

American Heart Association, 7320 Greenville Avenue, Dallas, TX 75231; 1-800-553-6321; www.americanheart.org

National Institute of Neurological Disorders and Stroke, National Institutes of Health. Bethesda, MD 20892. www.ninds.nih.gov

National Stroke Association, 96 Inverness Drive East, Suite I, Englewood, CO 80112; 1-800-787-6537 or 303-649-9299; fax: 303-649-1328; www.stroke.org

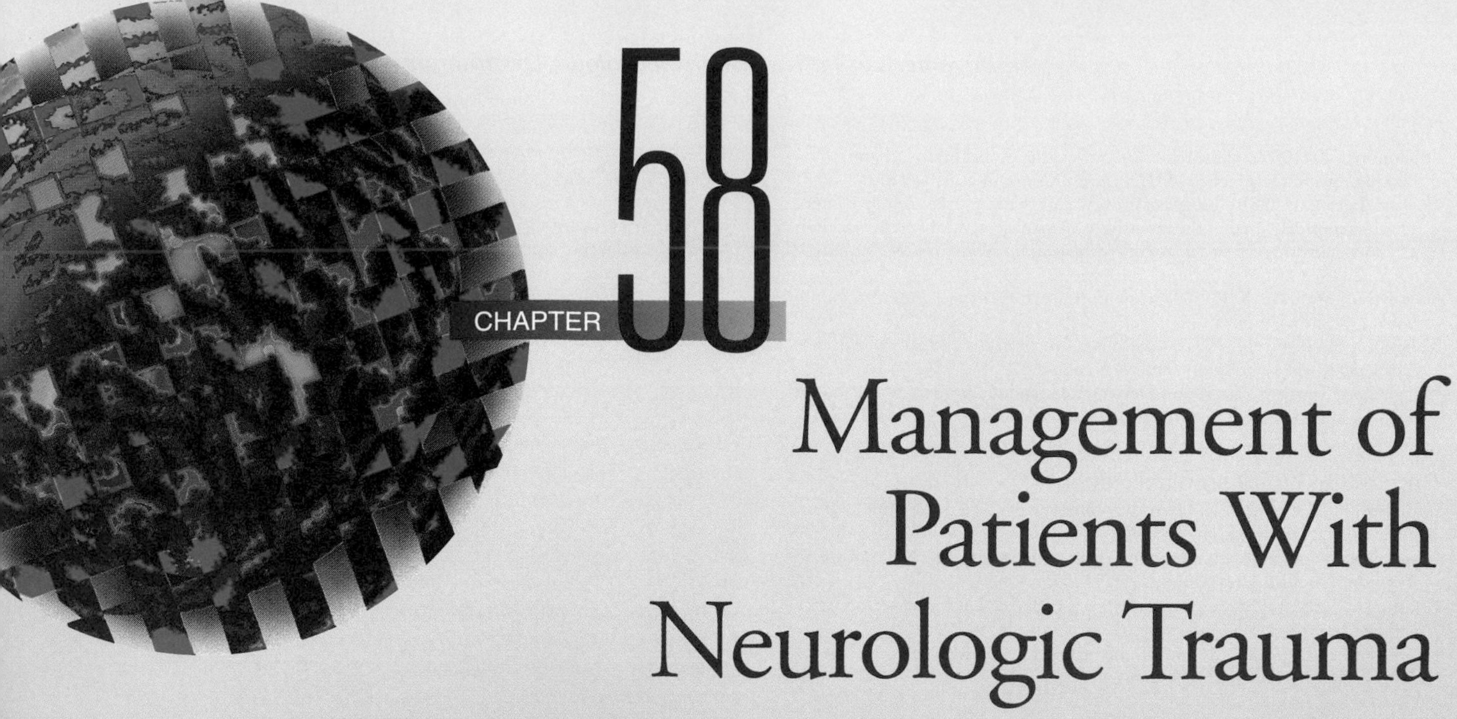

Management of Patients With Neurologic Trauma

Learning Objectives

On completion of this chapter, the learner will be able to:

1. Differentiate among head injuries by mechanism of injury, clinical signs and symptoms, diagnostic testing, and treatment options.
2. Describe the nursing management related to head injuries.
3. Develop a plan of care for the patient with traumatic brain injury.
4. Identify the population at risk for spinal cord injury.
5. Describe three clinical features of spinal shock.
6. Discuss the pathophysiology of autonomic dysreflexia and describe the appropriate nursing interventions.
7. Develop a plan of care for a patient with a cervical spinal cord injury.

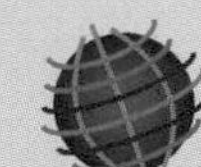

Trauma involving the central nervous system can be life-threatening. Even if not life-threatening, brain and spinal cord injury may result in major physical and psychological dysfunction and can alter the patient's life completely. Neurologic trauma affects the patient, the family, the health care system, and society as a whole because of its major sequelae and the costs of acute and long-term care of patients with trauma to the brain and spinal cord.

GLOSSARY

autonomic hyperreflexia: a life-threatening emergency in spinal cord injury patients that causes a hypertensive emergency

brain injury: an injury to the skull or brain that is severe enough to interfere with normal functioning

concussion: an injury occurring from violent shaking

contusion: bruising of the brain surface

halo vest: a lightweight vest with an attached halo that stabilizes the cervical spine

neurogenic bladder: a loss of bladder tone that places spinal cord injury patients at an increased risk for urinary tract infection

spinal cord injury (SCI): an injury to the spinal cord, vertebral column, supporting soft tissue, or intervertebral disks caused by trauma

transection: severing of the spinal cord; can be complete or incomplete

HEAD INJURIES

Types of head injuries include trauma to the scalp, skull, or brain. Approximately 2 million head injuries occur each year in the United States (NIH, 1998). They are among the most frequent and serious sources of neurologic impairment and have reached epidemic proportions as a result of motor vehicle crashes. Other causes of head injury include falls, assaults, and sports injuries. An estimated 75,000 to 100,000 people die annually from head injuries, and more than 500,000 have injuries severe enough to require hospitalization. Of this group, between 70,000 and 90,000 people a year are left with intellectual or behavioral deficits that preclude their return to normal life. Two thirds of these are younger than age 30, with males outnumbering females by 3 to 1. The second highest incidence of head injury occurs in the elderly population (Pieper et al, 1996).

A major risk to the patient with a head injury is damage to the brain from bleeding or swelling. The bleeding and swelling causes increased intracranial pressure (ICP), which is described in detail in Chapter 57.

Scalp Injury

Scalp trauma is classified as a minor head injury. Because its many blood vessels constrict poorly, the scalp bleeds profusely when injured. Trauma may result in an abrasion (brush wound), contusion, laceration, or hematoma beneath the layers of tissue of the scalp (subgaleal hematoma). Diagnosis is based on physical examination, inspection, and palpation. Scalp wounds are potential portals of entry of organisms that cause intracranial infections. Therefore, the area is irrigated before the laceration is sutured to remove foreign material and to reduce the chance of infection. Subgaleal hematomas usually absorb on their own and do not require any specific treatment.

Skull Fractures

A skull fracture is a break in the continuity of the skull caused by forceful trauma. It may occur with or without damage to the brain. Skull fractures are classified as linear, comminuted, depressed, or basilar. A fracture may be open, indicating a scalp laceration or tear in the dura, or closed, in which the dura is intact.

Clinical Manifestations

The symptoms, apart from those of the local injury, depend on the severity and the distribution of brain injury. Persistent, localized pain usually suggests that a fracture is present. Fractures of the cranial vault produce swelling in the region of the fracture; therefore, an x-ray is needed for diagnosis.

Fractures of the base of the skull tend to traverse the paranasal sinus of the frontal bone or the middle ear located in the temporal bone (Fig. 58-1). Thus, they frequently produce hemorrhage from the nose, pharynx, or ears, and blood may appear under the conjunctiva. An area of ecchymosis (bruising) may be seen over the mastoid (Battle's sign). Basal skull fractures are suspected when cerebrospinal fluid escapes from the ears (CSF otorrhea) and the nose (CSF rhinorrhea). A halo sign—a blood stain surrounded by a yellowish stain—may be seen on bed linens or the head dressing and is highly suggestive of a CSF leak. Drainage of CSF is a serious problem because meningeal infection can occur if organisms gain access to the cranial contents through the nose,

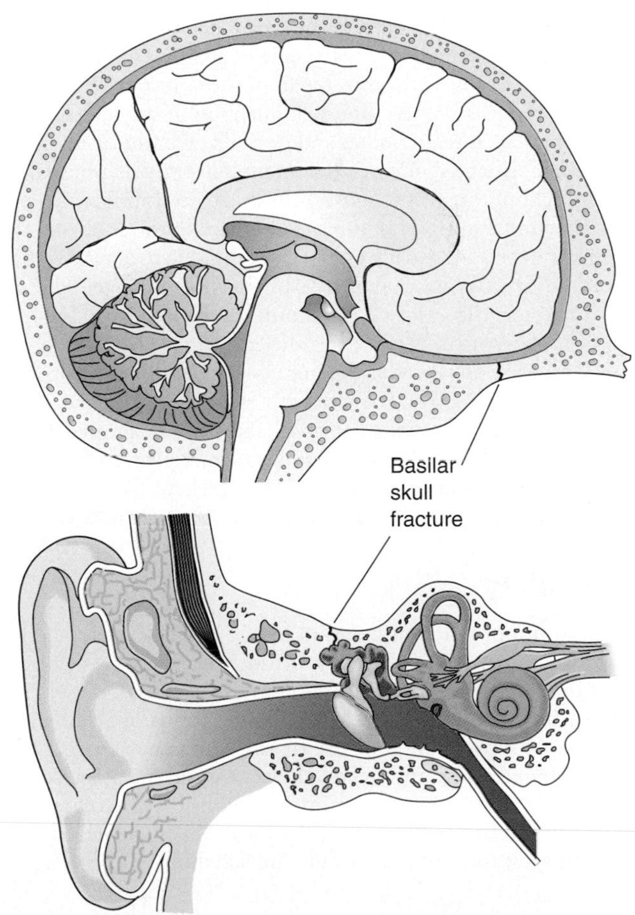

FIGURE 58•1 Basilar fractures allow cerebrospinal fluid to leak from the nose and ears. Adapted from Hickey, J. V. (1997). *The clinical practice of neurological and neurosurgical nursing* (4th ed., p. 451). Philadelphia: Lippincott-Raven.

ear, or sinus through a tear in the dura. Bloody CSF suggests brain laceration or contusion.

Assessment and Diagnostic Findings

Although a rapid physical examination and evaluation of neurologic status detects the more obvious brain injuries, a computed tomography (CT) scan can detect less apparent abnormalities by the degree to which the soft tissue absorbs the x-rays. It is accurate and safe in showing the presence, nature, location, and extent of the lesion as well as in disclosing cerebral edema, contusion, intracerebral or extracerebral hematoma, subarachnoid and intraventricular hemorrhage, and late traumatic changes (infarction, hydrocephalus). Magnetic resonance imaging (MRI) is also used to evaluate patients with head injury.

Cerebral angiography may also be used; it demonstrates the presence of supratentorial, extracerebral, and intracerebral hematomas and cerebral contusions. Lateral and anteroposterior views of the skull are obtained.

Medical Management

Nondepressed skull fractures generally do not require surgical treatment; however, close observation of the patient is essential. Many depressed skull fractures are managed conservatively; only contaminated or deforming fractures require surgery.

If surgery is necessary, the scalp is shaved and cleansed with large amounts of saline to remove debris, and the fracture is exposed. The skull fragments are elevated and the area is débrided. Large defects can be repaired immediately with bone or artificial grafts; if significant cerebral edema is present, repair of the defect can be delayed for 3 to 6 months. Penetrating wounds require surgical débridement to remove foreign bodies and devitalized brain tissue and to control hemorrhage. Antibiotic treatment is instituted immediately, and blood component therapy is administered if indicated.

As stated previously, fractures of the base of the skull are serious because they are usually open (involving the paranasal sinuses or middle or external ear) and result in CSF leakage. The nasopharynx and the external ear should be kept clean. Usually a plug of sterile cotton is placed in the ear, or a sterile cotton pad may be taped loosely under the nose or against the ear to collect the draining fluid. The patient who is conscious is cautioned against sneezing or blowing the nose. The head is elevated 30 degrees to reduce ICP and promote spontaneous closure of the leak. (Some neurosurgeons prefer that the bed be kept flat.) Persistent CSF rhinorrhea or otorrhea usually requires surgical intervention.

Brain Injury

The most important consideration in any head injury is whether or not the patient has suffered a **brain injury**. Even seemingly minor injury can cause significant brain damage secondary to obstructed blood flow and decreased tissue perfusion. The brain cannot store oxygen and glucose to any significant degree. Irreversible brain damage and cell death occur when the blood supply is interrupted for only a few minutes, because the cerebral cells need an uninterrupted blood supply for these nutrients. Clinical signs and symptoms of brain injury are listed in Chart 58-1.

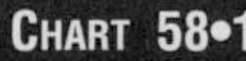
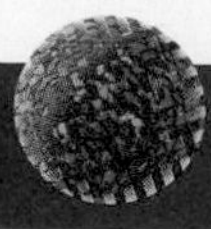

CHART 58•1 Clinical Manifestations of Brain Injury

Altered level of consciousness
Confusion
Pupillary abnormalities (changes in shape, changes in responsiveness to light)
Altered or absent gag reflex
Absent corneal reflex
Sudden onset of neurologic deficits
Changes in vital signs (altered respiratory pattern, hypertension, bradycardia, tachycardia, hypothermia or hyperthermia)
Vision and hearing impairment
Sensory dysfunction
Spasticity
Headache
Vertigo
Movement disorders
Seizures

Concussion

A cerebral **concussion** after head injury is a temporary loss of neurologic function with no apparent structural damage. A concussion generally involves a period of unconsciousness lasting from a few seconds to a few minutes. The jarring of the brain may be so slight as to cause only dizziness and spots before the eyes ("seeing stars"), or it may be severe enough to cause complete loss of consciousness for a time. If the brain tissue in the frontal lobe is affected, the patient may exhibit bizarre irrational behavior, whereas involvement of the temporal lobe can produce temporary amnesia or disorientation.

The patient may be hospitalized overnight for observation or discharged from the hospital in a relatively short time after a concussion. Treatment involves observing the patient for headache, dizziness, lethargy, irritability, and anxiety. The occurrence of these symptoms after this injury is referred to as postconcussion syndrome. Giving the patient information, explanations, and encouragement may reduce some of the problems of postconcussion syndrome. The patient is advised to resume normal activities slowly, and the family is instructed to observe for the following signs and symptoms and to notify the physician or clinic or bring the patient back to the emergency department if they occur:

- Difficulty in awakening
- Difficulty in speaking
- Confusion
- Severe headache
- Vomiting
- Weakness of one side of the body

A concussion was once thought of as a minor head injury without significant sequelae. However, studies have demonstrated that there are often disturbing and sometimes residual effects, including headache, lethargy, personality and behavior changes, attention deficits, difficulty with memory, and disruption in work habits.

GERONTOLOGIC CONSIDERATIONS

The elderly patient with confusion or behavioral disturbances should be assessed for head injury, because unrecognized "minor" head trauma may account for behavioral and confusional episodes in some elderly people. A misdiagnosed or untreated episode of confusion in an elderly patient may result in long-term disability that might have been avoided if the injury had been detected and treated promptly.

Contusion

Cerebral **contusion** is a more severe injury in which the brain is bruised, with possible surface hemorrhage. The patient is unconscious for a considerable period. Clinical signs and symptoms depend on the size of the contusion and the amount of associated cerebral edema. The patient may lie motionless, with a faint pulse, shallow respirations, and cool, pale skin. Often there is involuntary evacuation of the bowels and the bladder. The patient may be aroused with effort but soon slips back into unconsciousness. The blood pressure and the temperature are subnormal, and the picture is somewhat similar to that of shock.

In general, patients with widespread injury who have abnormal motor function, abnormal eye movements, and elevated ICP have poor outcomes—that is, brain damage, disability, or death. Conversely, the patient may recover consciousness completely and perhaps pass into a stage of cerebral irritability. In the stage of cerebral irritability, the patient is conscious and easily disturbed by any form of stimulation such as noises, light, and voices; he or she may become hyperactive at times. Gradually, the pulse, respirations, temperature, and other body functions return to normal, but full recovery is often delayed. Residual headache and vertigo are common, and impaired mental function or seizures may occur as a result of irreparable cerebral damage.

Diffuse Axonal Injury

Diffuse axonal injury involves widespread damage to axons in the cerebral hemispheres, corpus callosum, and brain stem. It can be seen in mild, moderate, or severe head trauma and results in axonal swelling and disconnection. Clinically, the patient has no lucid intervals and experiences immediate coma, decorticate and decerebrate posturing, and global cerebral edema. Diagnosis is made by clinical signs in conjunction with a CT scan or MRI. Recovery depends on the severity of the axonal injury.

Intracranial Hemorrhage

Hematomas (collections of blood) that develop within the cranial vault are the most serious brain injuries. A hematoma may be epidural, subdural, or intracerebral, depending on its location (Fig. 58-2). Major symptoms are frequently delayed until the hematoma is large enough to cause distortion and herniation of the brain and increased ICP. The signs and symptoms of cerebral ischemia resulting from the compression by a hematoma are variable and depend on the speed with which vital areas are affected and the area that is injured. In general, a rapidly developing hematoma, even if small, may be fatal, whereas a more massive but slowly developing hematoma may allow compensation for increases in ICP.

EPIDURAL HEMATOMA (EXTRADURAL HEMATOMA OR HEMORRHAGE)

After a head injury, blood may collect in the epidural (extradural) space between the skull and the dura. This can result from a skull fracture that causes a rupture or laceration of the middle meningeal artery, the artery that runs between the dura and the skull inferior to a thin portion of temporal bone. Hemorrhage from this artery causes rapid pressure on the brain.

The symptoms are caused by the expanding hematoma. Usually, there is a momentary loss of consciousness at the time of injury, followed by an interval of apparent recovery (lucid interval). Although the lucid interval is characteristic of an epidural hematoma, it does not occur in approximately 15% of patients with this lesion. During the lucid interval, compensation for the expanding hematoma takes place by rapid absorption of CSF and decreased intravascular volume, both of which help maintain a normal ICP. When these mechanisms can no longer compensate, even a small increase in the volume of the blood clot produces a marked elevation of ICP. Then, often suddenly, signs of compression appear (usually deterioration of consciousness and signs of focal neurologic deficits such as dilation and fixation of a pupil or paralysis of an extremity), and the patient deteriorates rapidly.

An epidural hematoma is considered an extreme emergency, and marked neurologic deficit or even respiratory arrest may occur within minutes. Treatment consists of making openings through the skull (burr holes) to decrease ICP emergently, removing the clot, and controlling the bleeding point. A craniotomy may be required to remove the clot and control the bleeding. A drain is usually placed after creation of burr holes or a craniotomy, to prevent reaccumulation of blood.

SUBDURAL HEMATOMA

A subdural hematoma is a collection of blood between the dura and the brain, a space normally occupied by a film of fluid. The most common cause is trauma, but it may also occur from coagulopathies and with rupture of an aneurysm. A subdural hemorrhage is more frequently venous in origin and is attributed to the rupture of small vessels that bridge the subdural space. A subdural hematoma may be acute, subacute, or chronic, depending on the size of the involved vessel and the amount of bleeding present.

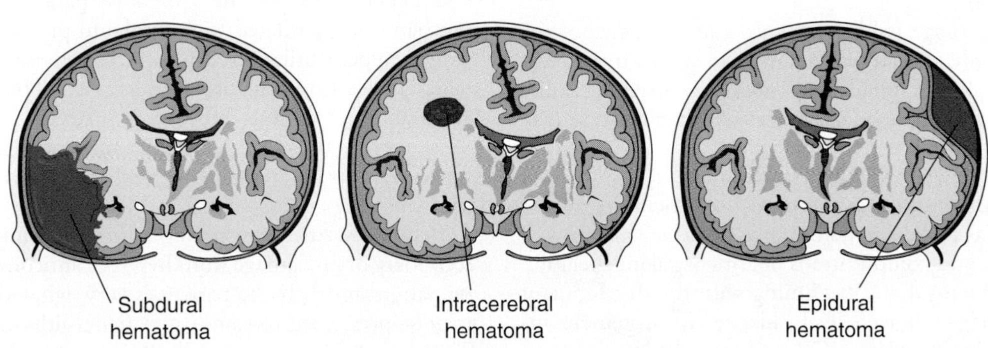

FIGURE 58•2 Locations of intracranial hemorrhages.

Acute and Subacute Subdural Hematoma.

Acute subdural hematomas are associated with major head injury involving contusion or laceration. Clinical symptoms develop over 24 to 48 hours. Signs and symptoms include changes in level of consciousness (LOC), pupillary signs, and hemiparesis. Coma, increasing blood pressure, decreasing heart rate, and slowing respiratory rate are signs of a rapidly expanding mass requiring immediate intervention.

Subacute subdural hematoma is the sequela of less severe contusions and head trauma. Clinical manifestations usually appear between 48 hours and 2 weeks after the injury. Signs and symptoms are similar to those of an acute subdural hematoma.

If the patient can be transported rapidly to the hospital, an immediate craniotomy is performed to open the dura, allowing the solid subdural clot to be evacuated. Successful outcome also depends on the control of ICP and careful monitoring of respiratory function (see "The Patient Undergoing Intracranial Surgery" in Chap. 57). The mortality rate for patients with acute and subacute subdural hematomas is high because of associated brain damage.

Chronic Subdural Hematoma.

Chronic subdural hematomas can develop from seemingly minor head injuries and are seen most frequently in the elderly. The elderly are prone to this type of head injury secondary to brain atrophy, which is an expected consequence of the aging process. Seemingly minor head trauma may result in enough impact to shift the brain contents abnormally, with negative sequelae. The time between injury and onset of symptoms may be lengthy (eg, 3 weeks to months), so the actual insult may be forgotten.

A chronic subdural hematoma resembles other conditions and may be mistaken for a stroke. The bleeding is less profuse and there is compression of the intracranial contents. The blood within the brain changes in character in 2 to 4 days, becoming thicker and darker. In a few weeks, the clot breaks down and has the color and consistency of motor oil. Eventually, calcification or ossification of the clot takes place. The brain adapts to this foreign body invasion, and the patient's clinical signs and symptoms fluctuate. There may be severe headache, which tends to come and go; alternating focal neurologic signs; personality changes; mental deterioration; and focal seizures. Unfortunately, the patient may be labeled neurotic or psychotic if the cause of the symptoms is overlooked.

The treatment of a chronic subdural hematoma consists of surgical evacuation of the clot by suction or irrigation of the area. The procedure may be carried out through multiple burr holes, or a craniotomy may be performed for a sizable subdural mass that cannot be drained through burr holes.

INTRACEREBRAL HEMORRHAGE AND HEMATOMA

Intracerebral hemorrhage is bleeding into the substance of the brain. It is commonly seen in head injuries in which force is exerted to the head over a small area (missile injuries or bullet wounds; stab injury). These hemorrhages within the brain may also result from systemic hypertension, which causes degeneration and rupture of a vessel; rupture of a saccular aneurysm; vascular anomalies; intracranial tumors; systemic causes, including bleeding disorders such as leukemia, hemophilia, aplastic anemia, and thrombocytopenia; and complications of anticoagulant therapy.

The onset may be insidious, beginning with the development of neurologic deficits followed by headache. Management includes supportive care, control of ICP, and careful administration of fluids, electrolytes, and antihypertensive medications. Surgical intervention by craniotomy or craniectomy permits removal of the blood clot and control of hemorrhage but may not be possible either because of the inaccessible location of the bleeding or the lack of a clearly circumscribed area of blood that can be removed.

Management of Brain Injuries

Assessment and diagnosis of the extent of injury are accomplished by the initial physical and neurologic examinations. CT scanning and MRI are the primary neuroimaging diagnostic tools and are useful in evaluating soft tissue injuries. Positron emission tomography (PET scan) is available in some centers; this method of scanning examines brain function rather than structure.

A person with a head injury is presumed to have a cervical spine injury until proved otherwise. From the scene of the injury, the patient is transported on a board, with head and neck maintained in alignment with the axis of the body. Slight traction should be maintained on the head, and a cervical collar should be applied and maintained until cervical spine x-rays have been obtained and the absence of cervical spinal cord injury documented.

All therapy is directed toward preserving brain homeostasis and preventing secondary brain damage. This includes stabilization of cardiovascular and respiratory function to maintain adequate cerebral perfusion. Hemorrhage is controlled, hypovolemia is corrected, and blood gas values are maintained at acceptable values.

TREATMENT OF INCREASED INTRACRANIAL PRESSURE

As the damaged brain swells with edema or blood collects within the brain, a rise in ICP occurs; this requires aggressive treatment. See Chapter 57 for discussion of the relation of ICP to cerebral perfusion pressure. If the ICP remains elevated, it can decrease the cerebral perfusion pressure.

ICP is monitored closely and, if increased, is managed by maintaining adequate oxygenation; administering mannitol, which reduces cerebral edema by osmotic dehydration; hyperventilation; elevation of the head of the bed; and possibly neurosurgical intervention. Surgery is required for evacuation of blood clots, débridement and elevation of depressed fractures of the skull, and suture of severe scalp lacerations. Devices to monitor ICP and/or drain CSF can be inserted during surgery or at the bedside using aseptic technique. The patient is cared for in the intensive care unit, where high-acuity nursing and medical care is readily available.

SUPPORTIVE MEASURES

Treatment also includes ventilatory support, seizure prevention, fluid and electrolyte maintenance, nutritional support, and pain and anxiety management. Comatose patients are intubated and mechanically ventilated to control and protect the airway. Controlled hyperventilation also induces hypocapnia (low $PaCO_2$), which prevents vasodilation, lowers cerebral blood flow, decreases cerebral blood volume, and thus reduces ICP. A $PaCO_2$ of 30 to 35 mm Hg is usually effective for most patients with head injury; however, if the ICP remains elevated, $PaCO_2$ levels may be lowered to 27 mm Hg.

Because seizures are common after head injury and can cause secondary brain damage from hypoxia, anticonvulsant agents may be administered. If the patient is very agitated, benzodiazepines may be prescribed to calm the patient without decreasing LOC. These medications do not affect ICP or cerebral perfusion pressure, making them good choices for the head-injured patient.

A nasogastric tube may be inserted because reduced gastric motility and reverse peristalsis are associated with head injury, making regurgitation common in the first few hours.

NURSING PROCESS: THE PATIENT WITH A BRAIN INJURY

Assessment

The health history may include the following questions:

- At what time did the injury occur?
- What caused the injury—a high-velocity missile? An object striking the head? A fall?
- What was the direction and force of the blow?
- Was there a loss of consciousness? What was the duration of the unconscious period? Could the patient be aroused? (A history of unconsciousness or amnesia after a head injury indicates a significant degree of brain damage. Changes that occur minutes to hours after the initial injury can reflect recovery or indicate the development of secondary brain damage.)

In addition to questions that establish the nature of the injury and the patient's condition immediately after the injury, the nurse assesses LOC, ability to respond to verbal commands (if the patient is conscious), level of responsiveness to tactile stimuli (if not conscious), pupillary response to light, corneal and gag reflexes, and motor function (Fig. 58-3). Additional detailed neurologic and systems assessments are made initially and at frequent intervals throughout the acute phase of care. This baseline and ongoing assessment is a critical nursing intervention for the brain-injured patient, whose condition can worsen dramatically and irrevocably if subtle signs are overlooked. More information on assessment is provided below.

Diagnosis

Nursing Diagnoses

Based on the assessment data, the patient's major nursing diagnoses may include the following:

- Ineffective airway clearance and ventilation related to hypoxia
- Fluid volume deficit related to disturbances of consciousness and hormonal dysfunction?
- Altered nutrition, less than body requirements, related to metabolic changes, fluid restriction, and inadequate intake
- Risk for injury (self-directed and directed at others) related to disorientation, restlessness, and brain damage
- Risk for altered body temperature, increased, related to damage to temperature-regulating mechanism
- Potential for impaired skin integrity related to bed rest, hemiparesis, hemiplegia, and immobility
- Altered thought processes (deficits in intellectual function, communication, memory, information processing) related to brain injury

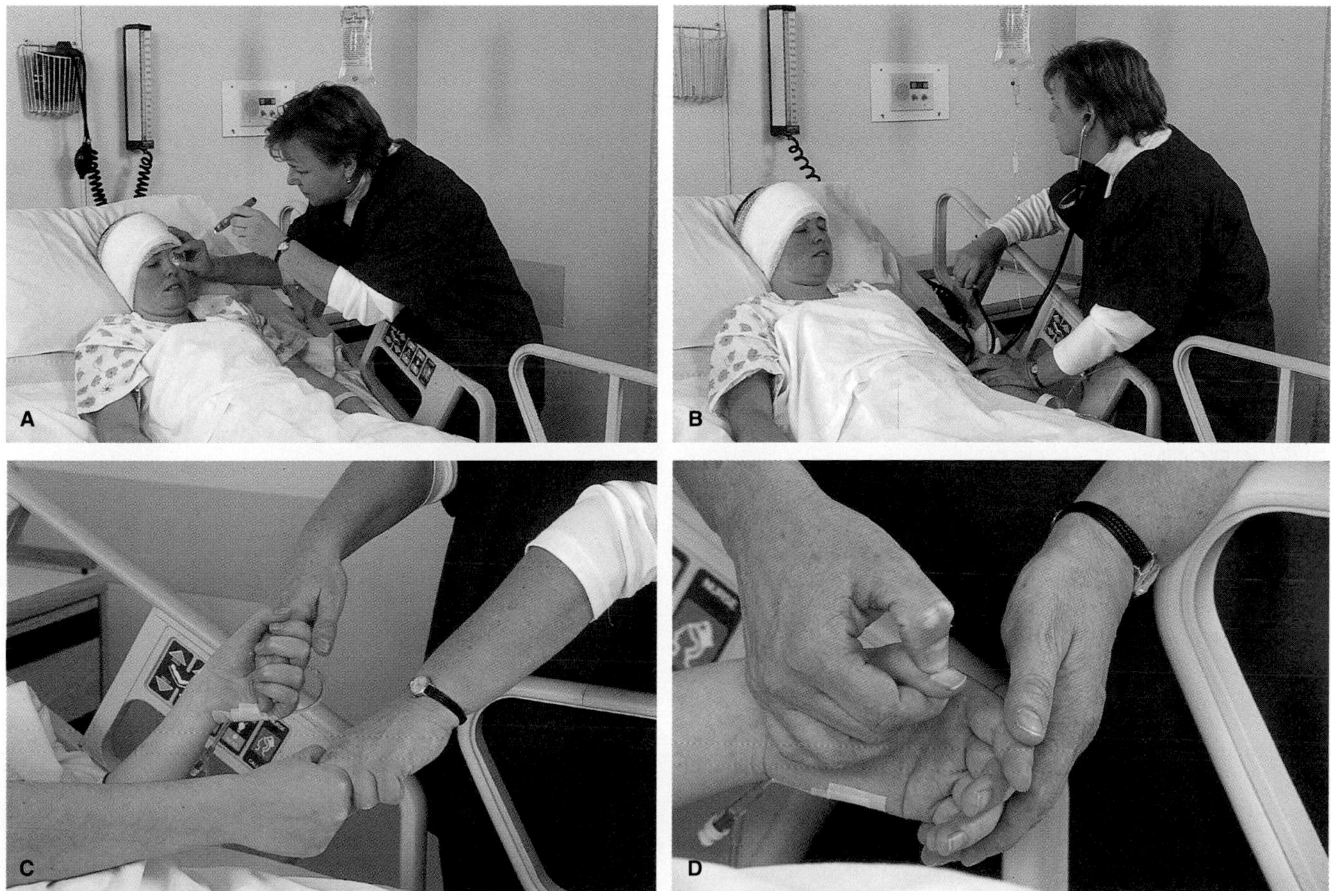

FIGURE 58•3 Assessment parameters for the patient with a head injury include (**A**) eye opening and responsiveness, (**B**) vital signs, and (**C**, **D**) motor response reflected in hand strength or response to painful stimulus. Photo © B. Proud.

- Potential for sleep pattern disturbance related to head injury and frequent neurologic checks
- Potential for ineffective family coping related to unresponsiveness of patient, unpredictability of outcome, prolonged recovery period, and the patient's residual physical and emotional deficit
- Knowledge deficit about rehabilitation process

The nursing diagnoses for the unconscious patient and the patient with increased ICP also apply (see Chap. 57).

Collaborative Problems/Potential Complications

Based on all the assessment data, the major complications include the following:

- Cerebral edema and herniation
- Decreased cerebral perfusion
- Impaired oxygenation and ventilation
- Impaired fluid, electrolyte, and nutritional balance

Planning and Goals

The goals for the patient may include maintenance of a patent airway, adequate cerebral perfusion pressure, fluid and electrolyte balance, adequate nutritional status, prevention of injury, maintenance of normal body temperature, maintenance of skin integrity, improvement of cognitive function, prevention of sleep deprivation, effective family coping, increased knowledge about the rehabilitation process, and absence of complications.

Nursing Interventions

The nursing interventions for the patient with a head injury are extensive and diverse; they include making nursing assessments, setting priorities for nursing interventions, anticipating needs and complications, and initiating rehabilitation (Table 58-1).

Assessing for Declining Neurologic Function

The importance of ongoing assessment of the brain-injured patient cannot be overstated. The following parameters are assessed initially and as frequently as the patient's condition requires. As soon as the initial assessment is made, a neurologic flow chart is started and maintained.

LEVEL OF CONSCIOUSNESS AND RESPONSIVENESS

LOC or responsiveness is regularly assessed because an alteration in LOC precedes all other changes in vital and neurologic signs. The Glasgow coma scale is used to assess LOC based on the three criteria of eye opening, verbal responses, and motor responses to verbal commands or painful stimuli. It is particularly useful for monitoring changes during the acute phase, the first few days after a head injury. It does not take the place of an in-depth neurologic assessment; rather, it evaluates the patient's motor, verbal, and eye opening responses. The patient's best responses to predetermined stimuli are recorded, as shown in Chart 58-2. Each response is given a number (high for normal and low for impaired), and the sum of these figures gives an indication of the severity of coma and a prediction of possible outcome. The lowest score is 3 (least responsive); the highest is 15 (most responsive). A score of 7 or less is generally accepted as coma (see Chart 58-2).

The Rancho Los Amigos Level of Cognitive Function is another scale frequently used to assess cognitive function and evaluate ongoing recovery from head injury. Nursing interventions for each level are identified in Table 58-2.

VITAL SIGNS

Although a change in the patient's LOC is the most sensitive neurologic indication of impending danger, vital signs are monitored at frequent intervals to assess the intracranial status. Figure 58-3 depicts the general assessment parameters for the patient with a head injury.

Signs of increasing ICP include slowing of the pulse (bradycardia), increasing systolic blood pressure, and widening pulse pressure. As brain compression increases, the vital signs tend to be reversed—respirations become rapid, the blood pressure may decrease, and the pulse slows further. This is an ominous development, as is a rapid fluctuation of vital signs. A rapid rise in body temperature is regarded as unfavorable because hyperthermia increases the metabolic demands of the brain and may indicate brain stem damage—a poor prognostic sign. The temperature is maintained at less than 38°C (100.4°F). Tachycardia and arterial hypotension may indicate that bleeding is occurring elsewhere in the body.

MOTOR FUNCTION

Motor function is assessed frequently by observing spontaneous movements, asking the patient to raise and lower the extremities, and comparing the strength and equality of the hand grasp and pedal push at periodic intervals. To assess the hand grasp, the nurse instructs the patient to squeeze the examiner's fingers tightly. The nurse assesses pedal push by placing the hands on the soles of the patient's feet and asking the patient to push down against the examiner's hands. The presence or absence of spontaneous movement of each extremity is also noted, and speech and eye signs are assessed.

If the patient does not demonstrate spontaneous movement, responses to painful stimuli are assessed. Motor response is assessed by applying a central stimulus, such as orbital pressure or pinching the pectoralis major muscle, to determine the patient's best response. Peripheral stimulation may provide inaccurate assessment data because it may result in a reflex movement rather than a voluntary motor response. Abnormal responses (lack of motor response; extension responses) carry a poorer prognosis.

The patient's ability to speak and the quality of speech are also assessed. The capacity to speak indicates a high level of brain function.

The patient's spontaneous eye opening is evaluated. The size and equality of the pupils and their reaction to light are assessed. A unilaterally dilated and poorly responding pupil may indicate a developing hematoma, with subsequent pressure on the third cranial nerve due to shifting of the brain. If both pupils become fixed and dilated, overwhelming injury and intrinsic damage to the upper brain stem usually are indicated, another poor prognostic sign.

OTHER NEUROLOGIC SIGNS

Deterioration in the patient's condition may be due to an expanding intracranial hematoma, progressive cerebral edema, and herniation of the brain.

The head-injured patient may develop focal nerve palsies such as anosmia (lack of sense of smell) or eye movement abnormalities and focal neurologic deficits such as aphasia, memory deficits, and posttraumatic seizures or epilepsy. Patients may be left with residual organic psychological deficits (impulsiveness, emotional

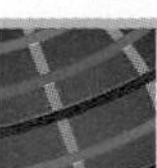

TABLE 58•1 Summary of Multisystem Assessment Measures for the Brain-Injured Patient

System-Specific Considerations	Assessment Data
Integumentary System (Skin)	
• Immobility secondary to injury and unconsciousness contributes to the development of pressure areas and skin breakdown. • Intubation causes irritation of the mucous membrane.	• Assessment of skin integrity and character of the skin
Musculoskeletal System	
• Immobility contributes to musculoskeletal changes. • Decerebrate or decorticate posturing makes proper positioning difficult.	• Assessment of range of motion of joints and development of deformities or spasticity
Gastrointestinal System	
• Administration of corticosteroids places the patient at high risk for GI hemorrhage. • Injury to the GI tract can result in paralytic ileus. • Constipation can result from bed rest, NPO status, fluid restriction, and opioids given for pain control. • Incontinence is related to the patient's unconscious state or altered mental state.	• Assessment of abdomen for bowel sounds and distention • Monitoring for decreased hemoglobin
Genitourinary System	
• Fluid restriction or use of diuretics can alter the amount of urinary output. • Urinary incontinence is related to the patient's unconscious state.	• Intake and output record
Metabolic (Nutritional) System	
• The patient receives all fluids intravenously for the first few days until the GI tract is usable. • A nutritional consultation is initiated within the first 24–48 h; total parenteral nutrition may be started.	• Assessment of fluid and electrolyte balance • Recording of weight, if possible • Hematocrit • Electrolyte studies
Neurologic System	
• Severe head injury will result in unconsciousness and will alter many neurologic functions. • All body functions must be supported. • Increased ICP and herniation syndromes are life-threatening • Institute measures to control elevated ICP.	• Assessment of neurologic signs • Assessment for signs and symptoms of ICP elevation • Calculation of cerebral perfusion pressure if ICP monitor is in place • Monitoring of anticonvulsant medication blood levels
Respiratory System	
• Complete or partial airway obstruction will compromise the oxygen supply to the brain. • An altered respiratory pattern can result in cerebral hypoxia. • A short period of apnea at the moment of impact can result in spotty atelectasis. • Systemic disturbances from head injury can cause hypoxemia. • Brain injury can alter brain stem respiratory function. • Shunting of blood to the lungs as a result of a sympathetic discharge at the time of injury can cause neurogenic pulmonary edema.	• Assessment of respiratory function —Auscultate chest for breath sounds. —Note the respiratory pattern if possible (not possible if a ventilator is being used). —Note the respiratory rate —Note whether the cough reflex is intact. • Arterial blood gas levels • Complete blood count • Chest x-ray studies • Sputum cultures • O_2 saturation using pulse oximetry
Cardiovascular System	
• The patient may develop cardiac dysrhythmias, tachycardia, or bradycardia. • The patient may develop hypotension or hypertension. • Because of immobility and unconsciousness, the patient is at high risk for deep vein thromboses and pulmonary emboli. • Fluid and electrolyte imbalance can be related to several problems, including alterations in antidiuretic hormone (ADH) secretion, the stress response, or fluid restriction. • Specific conditions may occur: —Diabetes insipidus (DI) —Syndrome of inappropriate secretion of ADH (SIADH) —Electrolyte imbalance —Hyperosmolar nonketotic hyperglycemia	• Assessment of vital signs • Monitoring for cardiac dysrhythmias • Assessment for deep vein thromboses of legs • Electrocardiogram • Electrolyte studies • Blood coagulation studies • I^{125} fibrinogen scan of legs • Glucose level • Acetone level • Osmolality
Psychological/Emotional Response	
• The severely head-injured patient is unconscious. • The family needs much support to deal with the crisis.	• Collection of information about the family and the role of the head-injured person within that unit • Assessment of the family to determine how functional it was before the injury occurred

CHART 58•2 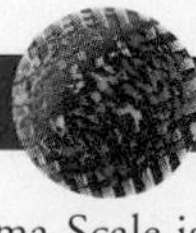 **Glasgow Coma Scale**

The Glasgow Coma Scale is a tool for assessing a patient's response to stimuli. A score of 10 or less indicates a need for emergency attention; a score of 7 or less is generally interpreted as coma.

Eye opening response	Spontaneous	4
	To voice	3
	To pain	2
	None	1
Best verbal response	Oriented	5
	Confused	4
	Inappropriate words	3
	Incomprehensible Sounds	2
	None	1
Best motor response	Obeys command	6
	Localizes pain	5
	Withdraws (pain)	4
	Flexion (pain)	3
	Extension (pain)	2
	None	1
Total		3 to 15

lability, or uninhibited, aggressive behaviors) and, as a consequence of the impairment, lack insight into their emotional responses.

Maintaining the Airway

One of the most important nursing goals in the management of the patient with a head injury is to establish and maintain an adequate airway. The brain is extremely sensitive to hypoxia, and a neurologic deficit can worsen if the patient is hypoxic. Therapy is directed toward maintaining adequately oxygenated circulation so that there is a supply of oxygenated blood to the brain to preserve cerebral function. An obstructed airway causes CO_2 retention and hypoventilation, which produces cerebral vessel dilation and increases ICP.

Therapeutic and nursing activities to ensure an adequate exchange of air are summarized in Chapter 22 and include the following:

- Keep the unconscious patient in a position that facilitates drainage of oral secretions, with the head of the bed elevated about 30 degrees to decrease intracranial venous pressure.
- Establish effective suctioning procedures. (Pulmonary secretions produce coughing and straining, which increase ICP.)
- Guard against aspiration and respiratory insufficiency.
- Monitor arterial blood gas values to assess the adequacy of ventilation. (The goal is to keep blood gas values within the normal range to ensure adequate cerebral blood flow.)
- Monitor the patient who is receiving mechanical ventilation.

Monitoring Fluid and Electrolyte Balance

Brain damage can produce metabolic and hormonal dysfunctions. The monitoring of serum electrolyte levels is important, especially in patients receiving osmotic diuretics, those with inappropriate antidiuretic hormone secretion, and those with post-traumatic diabetes insipidus.

Serial studies of blood and urine electrolytes and osmolality are carried out because head injuries may be accompanied by disorders of sodium regulation. Sodium retention may last several days, followed by sodium diuresis. Increasing lethargy, confusion, and seizures may be due to electrolyte imbalance.

Endocrine function is evaluated by monitoring serum electrolytes, blood glucose values, and intake and output. Urine is tested regularly for acetone. A record of daily weights is maintained, especially if the patient has hypothalamic involvement and is at risk for the development of diabetes insipidus.

Promoting Adequate Nutrition

Head injury results in metabolic changes that increase calorie consumption and nitrogen excretion. As soon as the patient's condition has stabilized, enteral feedings are started via a nasogastric feeding tube unless there is discharge of CSF from the nose (CSF rhinorrhea). Oral feeding tubes may be placed in patients with CSF rhinorrhea.

Elevating the head of the bed, and aspirating the enteral tube before feeding (for evidence of residual feeding) are measures used to prevent distention, regurgitation, and aspiration. A continuous-drip infusion or pump may be used to regulate the feeding. The principles and technique of enteral feedings are discussed in Chapter 33. The feeding tube usually is kept in place until the swallowing reflex returns and the patient can meet caloric requirements orally.

Preventing Injury

As the patient emerges from coma, there is often a period of lethargy and stupor followed by a period of agitation. Each phase is variable and depends on the individual, the location of the injury, the depth and duration of coma, and the patient's age. The patient emerging from a coma may become increasingly agitated toward the end of the day. Restlessness may be due to hypoxia, fever, pain, or a full bladder. It may indicate injury to the brain but may also be a sign that the patient is regaining consciousness. (Some restlessness may be beneficial because the lungs and extremities are exercised.) Agitation may also be due to annoyance from an indwelling urinary catheter, intravenous lines, restraints, and repeated neurologic checks.

- Assess the patient to ensure that the airway is adequate and the bladder is not distended. Check bandages and casts for constriction.
- To protect the patient from self-injury and dislodging of body tubes, use padded side rails or wrap the patient's hands in mitts (Fig. 58-4). Avoid restraints, because straining against them can increase ICP or cause other injury.
- Avoid opioids as a means of controlling restlessness because these medications depress respiration, constrict the pupils, and alter the patient's responsiveness.
- Minimize environmental stimuli by keeping the room quiet, limiting visitors, speaking calmly, and providing frequent orientation information (eg, explaining where the patient is and what is being done).

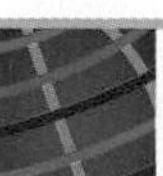

TABLE 58•2 Rancho Los Amigos Scale: Levels of Cognitive Function

Cognitive Level	Description	Nursing Management
For levels I–III, the key approach is to *provide stimulation.*		
I: No response	Completely unresponsive to all stimuli, including painful stimuli	Multiple modalities of sensory input should be used. Examples are listed below, but should be individualized and expanded based on available materials and patient preferences (determined by obtaining information from the family).
II: Generalized response	Nonpurposeful response; responds to pain, but in a nonpurposeful manner	*Olfactory:* perfumes, flowers, shaving lotion *Visual:* family pictures, card, personal items
III: Localized response	Responses more focused: withdraws to pain; turns toward sound; follows moving objects that pass within visual field; pulls on sources of discomfort (eg, tubes, restraints); may follow simple commands but inconsistently and in a delayed manner	*Auditory:* radio, television, tapes of family voices or favorite recordings, talking to patient (nurse, family members). The nurse should tell patient what is going to be done, discuss the environment, provide encouragement. *Tactile:* touching of skin, rubbing various textures on skin *Movement:* range of motion exercises, turning, repositioning, use of water mattress
For levels IV–VI, the key approach is to *provide structure.*		
IV: Confused, agitated response	Alert, hyperactive state in which patient responds to internal confusion/agitation; behavior nonpurposeful in relation to the environment; aggressive, bizarre behavior common	For level IV, which lasts 2–4 weeks, interventions are directed at decreasing agitation, increasing environmental awareness, and promoting safety. • Approach patient in a calm manner, and use a soft voice. • Screen patient from environmental stimuli (eg, sounds, sights); provide a quiet, controlled environment. • Remove devices that contribute to agitation (eg, tubes), if possible. • Functional goals cannot be set, because the patient is unable to cooperate.
V: Confused, inappropriate response	When agitation occurs, it is the result of external rather than internal stimuli; focused attention is difficult; memory is severely impaired; responses are fragmented and inappropriate to the situation; there is no carryover of learning from one situation to the other.	For levels V and VI, interventions are directed at decreasing confusion, improving cognitive function, and improving independence in performing ADLs. • Provide supervision. • Use drill method and cues to teach ADLs. Focus the patient's attention and help to increase his or her concentration.
VI: Confused, appropriate response	Follows simple directions consistently but is inconsistently oriented to time and place; short-term memory worse than long-term memory; can perform some ADLs	• Help the patient organize activity. • Clarify misinformation and reorient when confused. • Provide a consistent, predictable schedule (eg, post daily schedule on large poster board).
For levels VII and VIII, the key approach is *integration into the community.*		
VII: Automatic, appropriate response	Appropriately responsive and oriented within the hospital setting; needs little supervision in ADLs; some carryover of learning; patient has superficial insight into disabilities; has decreased judgment and problem-solving abilities; lacks realistic planning for future	For levels VII and VIII, interventions are directed at increasing the patient's ability to function with minimal or no supervision in the community. • Reduce environmental structure. • Help the patient plan for adapting ADLs for self into the home environment. • Discuss and adapt home living skills (eg, cleaning, cooking) to patient's ability.
VIII: Purposeful, appropriate response	Alert, oriented, intact memory; has realistic goals for future; judgment and problem-solving skills intact; has realistic plans for community integration	• Discuss integration into the community setting (outside home, church, social activities, possibly the work environment). • Help the patient plan, anticipate concerns, and solve problems.

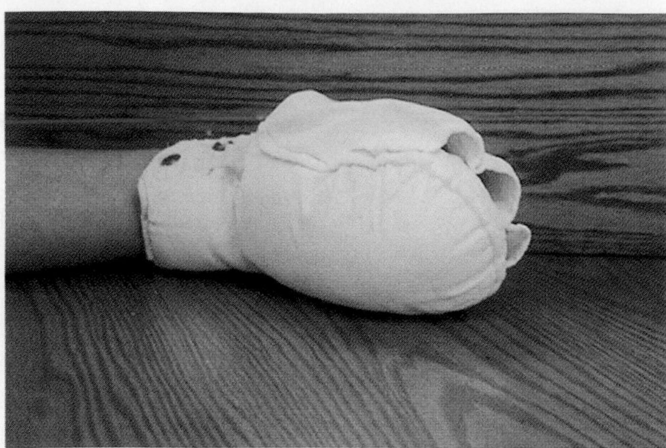

FIGURE 58•4 Hands of the patient with a head injury may be placed in a Posey mitt to prevent self-injury. This mitt has finger holes so that circulation can be assessed without removing the mitt. Photo courtesy of Sarah Trainer, RN, Roxborough Hospital, Philadelphia.

- Provide adequate lighting to prevent visual hallucinations.
- Do not disrupt the patient's sleep–wake cycles.
- Lubricate the skin with oil or emollient lotion to prevent irritation due to rubbing against the sheet.
- If incontinence occurs, consider using an external sheath catheter on a male patient. Because prolonged use of an indwelling catheter inevitably produces infection, the patient may be placed on an intermittent catheterization schedule.

Maintaining Body Temperature

An increase in body temperature in the head-injured patient can be the result of damage to the hypothalamus, cerebral irritation from hemorrhage, or infection. The nurse monitors the patient's temperature every 4 hours. If the temperature rises, efforts are undertaken to control it using acetaminophen and cooling blankets as prescribed and to identify the cause. If infection is suspected, potential sites of infection are cultured and antibiotics are prescribed and administered.

Maintaining Skin Integrity

Patients with traumatic head injury often require assistance in turning and positioning because of immobility or unconsciousness. Prolonged pressure on the tissues will decrease circulation and lead to tissue necrosis. Potential areas of breakdown need to be identified early to avoid the development of pressure ulcers.

- Assess all body surfaces and document skin integrity at least every 8 hours.
- Turn and reposition the patient every 2 to 4 hours.
- Provide skin care every 4 hours.
- Assist patient to get out of bed to a chair three times a day.

Improving Cognitive Functioning

Although many brain-damaged patients survive because of resuscitative and supportive technology, they frequently have significant cognitive sequelae that may not be detected during the acute phase of injury. Cognitive impairment includes memory deficits, decrease in ability to focus and sustain attention to a task (easily distracted), reduced ability to process information, and slowness in thinking, perceiving, communicating, reading, and writing. Psychiatric or emotional problems develop in an estimated 25% to 38% of these patients. Resulting psychosocial, behavioral, emotional, and cognitive impairments are devastating to the family as well as to the patient.

These problems require collaboration among many disciplines. A neuropsychologist (specialist in evaluating and treating cognitive problems) plans a program and initiates therapy or counseling designed to help the patient reach maximal potential. Cognitive rehabilitation activities are directed at redeveloping the patient's ability to devise new problem-solving strategies. The retraining is carried out over an extended period and may include the use of sensory stimulation and reinforcement, behavior modification, reality orientation, computer-training programs, and video games. Assistance from many disciplines is necessary during this phase of recovery. Intellectual ability may not improve after time, but social and behavioral aspects may.

There are fluctuations in the orientation and memory of such patients (see Table 58-2). They are easily distracted. If they are pushed to a level greater than their impaired cortical functioning allows, symptoms of fatigue and stress (headache, dizziness) may occur.

Preventing Sleep Pattern Disturbance

Patients who require frequent monitoring of neurologic status may experience sleep deprivation. They are awakened hourly to assess LOC and as a result are deprived of long periods of sleep and rest. In an effort to allow the patient longer times of uninterrupted sleep and rest, the nurse can group nursing care activities so that the patient is disturbed less frequently. Environmental noise is decreased and the room lights are dimmed. Back rubs and other strategies to increase patient's comfort can assist in promoting sleep and rest.

Supporting Family Coping

Serious head injury can produce a great deal of prolonged stress in the family because of the patient's physical and emotional deficits, the unpredictable outcome, and altered family relationships. Families report difficulties in dealing with changes in the patient's temperament, behavior, and personality. These are associated with disruption in family cohesion, loss of leisure pursuits, and loss of work capacity, as well as social isolation of the caretaker. The family may experience anger, grief, guilt, and denial in recurring cycles.

The family is asked how the patient is different at this time. What has been lost? What is most difficult about coping with this situation? Helpful interventions include providing family members with accurate and honest information and encouraging them to continue to set well-defined, mutual, short-term goals. Family counseling helps deal with overwhelming feelings of loss and helplessness and gives guidance for the management of inappropriate behaviors. Support groups are available to provide a forum for sharing problems, developing insight, referring information, networking, and gaining assistance in maintaining realistic expectations and hope.

CHART 58•3 Controlling ICP in Brain-Injured Patients

- Elevate the head of the bed to 30 degrees.
- Maintain the patient's head and neck in neutral alignment (no twisting).
- Initiate measures to prevent the Valsalva maneuver (ie, stool softeners).
- Administer medications prescribed to decrease ICP (ie, diuretics).
- Maintain normal body temperature.
- Hyperventilate the patient receiving mechanical ventilation, PCO_2 30–35 mm Hg; administer oxygen, PaO_2 >100 mm Hg
- Maintain fluid balance with 0.5% normal saline solution.
- Avoid noxious stimuli (suctioning, painful procedures).
- Administer sedation to reduce metabolic demands.
- Maintain cerebral perfusion pressure >70 mm Hg.

The National Head Injury Foundation serves as a clearinghouse for information and resources for patients with head injuries and their families, including specific information on coma, rehabilitation, behavioral consequences of head injury, and family issues. This organization can provide names of facilities and professionals who work with patients with head injuries and can assist families in organizing local support groups.

Monitoring and Managing Potential Complications

The patient with a head injury is at risk for many severe complications. Traumatic head injury often results in increased brain swelling. Cerebral edema is the most common cause of increased ICP in the patient with a head injury; the swelling peaks approximately 48 to 72 hours after injury. The ICP increases because of the inability of the intact skull to expand despite the increased volume of its contents with swelling of the brain resulting from trauma. As a result of the edema and increased ICP, pressure is exerted on brain tissue and the rigid internal structures of the skull. Depending on the site of the swelling, downward or lateral displacement (herniation) of the brain through or against the rigid structures occurs, producing ischemia, infarction, irreversible brain damage, and brain death.

Maintenance of adequate cerebral perfusion pressure is important to prevent serious complications of head injury due to decreased cerebral perfusion. Adequate cerebral perfusion pressure is greater than 70 mm Hg. Any decrease in brain perfusion can cause brain hypoxia and ischemia, leading to permanent damage. Therapy (ie, osmotic diuretics, elevation of the head of the bed, and hyperventilation) is directed toward decreasing cerebral edema and increasing venous outflow from the brain. Systemic hypotension causes vasoconstriction, which produces a significant decrease in perfusion pressure. Measures to control ICP are listed in Chart 58-3.

Impaired oxygen and ventilation may necessitate mechanical ventilatory support. The patient must be monitored for a patent airway, altered breathing patterns, and the occurrence of hypoxemia and pneumonia. Interventions may include endotracheal intubation, mechanical ventilation, and positive end expiratory pressure (PEEP). These topics are discussed in further detail in Chapter 22.

Fluid, electrolyte, and nutritional imbalances are common in the patient with a head injury. Common imbalances may include hyponatremia, which is often associated with the syndrome of inappropriate secretion of antidiuretic hormone (see Chap. 38), hypokalemia, and hyperglycemia. Modifications in fluid intake by tube feedings or intravenous fluids may be prescribed to treat these imbalances. Insulin administration may be prescribed to treat hyperglycemia.

Undernutrition is also a common problem in response to the increased metabolic needs associated with severe head injury. If the patient cannot eat, enteral feedings or total parenteral nutrition may be initiated within 24 hours of injury to provide adequate nutrients.

Other complications after traumatic head injuries include systemic infections (pneumonia, urinary tract infection, septicemia), neurosurgical infections (wound infection, osteomyelitis, meningitis, ventriculitis, brain abscess), and heterotrophic ossification (painful bone overgrowth in weight-bearing joints).

Promoting Home and Community-Based Care

TEACHING PATIENTS SELF-CARE

Teaching early in the course of head injury often focuses on reinforcing information given to the family about the patient's condition and prognosis. As the patient's status and expected outcome change over time, teaching of family members may focus on interpretation and explanation of changes in the patient's physical and psychological responses.

If the patient's physical status allows the patient to be discharged home, the patient and family are instructed about limitations that can be expected and complications that may occur. Monitoring for complications that merit contacting the neurosurgeon is explained to the patient and family verbally and in writing. Depending on the patient's prognosis and physical and cognitive status, the patient may be included in teaching about self-care management strategies.

Because posttraumatic seizures are common, anticonvulsant medications may be prescribed for 1 to 2 years after injury. The patient and family require instruction about the side effects of these medications and about the importance of taking them as prescribed.

CONTINUING CARE

Rehabilitation of the patient with a head injury begins at the time of injury and extends into the home and community. Depending on the degree of brain damage, the patient may be referred to a rehabilitation setting that specializes in cognitive restructuring of the brain-injured patient. The patient is encouraged to continue the rehabilitation program after discharge, because improvement in status may continue 3 or more years after injury. Changes in the head-injured patient and the effects of long-term rehabilitation on the family and their coping abilities need frequent assessment. Teaching and continued support of the patient and family are essential as their needs and the patient's status change. Aspects of teaching the family of the patient with a head injury going home are described in Home Care Teaching Checklist: The Patient with a Head Injury.

Home Care Teaching Checklist: The Patient With a Head Injury

At the completion of the program, the patient or caregiver will be able to:

	Patient	Caregiver
• Explain the need for monitoring for changes in neurologic status and for complications	✔	✔
• Identify changes in neurologic status and signs and symptoms of complications that should be reported to the neurosurgeon or nurse		✔
• Demonstrates safe techniques to assist patient with self-care, hygiene, and ambulation		✔
• Demonstrate safe technique in feeding patient or assisting patient with eating		✔
• Explain rationale for taking medications as prescribed	✔	✔
• Identify need for close monitoring of behavior due to changes in cognitive functioning		✔
• Describe household modifications needed to ensure safe environment for the patient		✔
• Describe strategies for reinforcing positive behaviors		✔
• State importance of continuing follow-up by health care team	✔	✔

Depending on his or her status, the patient is encouraged to return to normal activities gradually. Referral to support groups and the National Head Injury Foundation may be warranted.

Evaluation

Expected Outcomes

Expected outcomes may include:

1. Attains or maintains effective airway clearance, ventilation, and brain oxygenation
   a. Achieves normal blood gas values and has normal breath sounds on auscultation
   b. Mobilizes and clears secretions
2. Achieves satisfactory fluid and electrolyte balance
   a. Demonstrates serum electrolytes within normal range
   b. Has no clinical signs of dehydration or overhydration
3. Attains adequate nutritional status
   a. Has less than 50 mL of aspirate in stomach before each tube feeding
   b. Is free of gastric distention and vomiting
   c. Shows minimal weight loss
4. Avoids injury
   a. Shows lessening agitation and restlessness
   b. Is oriented to time, place, and person
5. Does not have a fever
6. Demonstrates intact skin integrity
   a. Exhibits no redness or breaks in skin integrity
   b. Exhibits no pressure ulcers
7. Shows improvement in cognitive function and improved memory
8. Demonstrates normal sleep–wake cycle
9. Demonstrates absence of complications
   a. Exhibits normal ICP, normal vital signs and body temperature, and increasing orientation to time, place, and person
   b. Demonstrates desired response to measures to reduce ICP
10. (For family members) Demonstrate adaptive coping mechanisms
   a. Join support group
   b. Share feelings with appropriate health care personnel
11. (For patient and family members) Participate in rehabilitation process as indicated
   a. Take active role in identifying rehabilitation goals and participate in recommended patient care activities
   b. Prepare for discharge of patient

Spinal Cord Injury

Spinal cord injury (SCI) is a major health problem, affecting 200,000 to 500,000 people in the United States, with an estimated 10,000 new injuries occurring each year. SCI occurs predominantly in males, with young men accounting for more than 82% of all such injuries. Half of these injuries result from motor vehicle crashes; most of the others occur from falls, sporting and industrial injuries, and gunshot wounds. Sixty percent of the victims are between 16 and 30 years old. The estimated total annual cost of these injuries exceeds $10 billion a year. There is a high frequency of associated injuries and medical complications.

The predominant risk factors for SCI include age, gender, and substance abuse, including alcohol and drug use. The frequency with which these risk factors are associated with SCI serves to emphasize the importance of primary prevention. To prevent this devastating and catastrophic injury, the following steps should be taken:

1. Drivers should slow down.
2. Drivers and passengers should use seat belts and shoulder harnesses.
3. Motorcyclists and bicyclists should wear helmets.
4. Educational programs should be directed against driving while intoxicated.
5. Water safety instruction should be provided.
6. Steps should be taken to prevent falls.
7. Athletes should use protective devices; coaches should be educated in proper coaching techniques.

Paramedical personnel are taught the importance of properly removing car-crash victims from a motor vehicle and of following proper methods in transporting the victim to a hospital emergency department to avoid further and possibly permanent damage to the spinal cord.

The vertebrae most frequently involved in SCI are the 5th, 6th, and 7th cervical (neck), the 12th thoracic, and the 1st lumbar vertebrae. These vertebrae are the most susceptible because there is a greater range of mobility in the vertebral column in these areas.

Pathophysiology

Damage to the spinal cord ranges from transient concussion (from which the patient fully recovers) to contusion, laceration, and compression of the cord substance (either alone or in combination), to complete **transection** of the cord (which renders the patient paralyzed below the level of the injury).

SCIs can be separated into two categories: primary injuries and secondary injuries. Primary injuries are the result of the initial insult or trauma and are usually permanent. Secondary injuries are usually the result of a contusion or tear injury, in which the nerve fibers begin to swell and disintegrate. A secondary chain of events produces ischemia, hypoxia, edema, and hemorrhagic lesions, which in turn result in destruction of myelin and axons (Hickey, 1997). These secondary reactions, believed to be the principal causes of spinal cord degeneration at the level of injury, are now thought to be reversible 4 to 6 hours after injury. Therefore, if the cord has not suffered irreparable damage, some method of early treatment with corticosteroids is needed to prevent partial damage from developing into total and permanent damage (see the section on management).

Clinical Manifestations

Manifestations depend on the type and level of injury (Chart 58-4). The type of injury refers to the extent of injury to the spinal cord itself. Neurologic level refers to the lowest level at which sensory and motor functions are normal. Below the neurologic level, there is total sensory and motor paralysis, loss of bladder and bowel control (usually with urinary retention and bladder distention), loss of sweating and vasomotor tone, and marked reduction of blood pressure from loss of peripheral vascular resistance. Severe SCI can result in paraplegia or quadriplegia, as described in Chart 58-5.

If conscious, the patient usually complains of acute pain in the back or neck, which may radiate along the involved nerve. Often the patient speaks of fear that the neck or back is broken.

Respiratory problems are related to the level of injury. The muscles contributing to respiration are the abdominals and intercostals (T1 to T11) and the diaphragm. In high cervical cord injury, acute respiratory failure is the leading cause of death.

Assessment and Diagnostic Findings

A detailed neurologic examination is performed. Diagnostic x-rays (lateral cervical spine x-rays) and CT scanning are performed. A search is made for other injuries, because spinal trauma often is accompanied by concomitant injuries, commonly to the head and chest. Continuous electrocardiographic monitoring may be indicated because bradycardia (slow heart rate) and asystole (cardiac standstill) are common in acute cervical injuries.

Emergency Management

The immediate management of the patient at the scene of the injury is critical, because improper handling can cause further damage and loss of neurologic function. Any victim of a motor vehicle or diving injury, a contact sport injury, a fall, or any direct trauma to the head and neck must be considered to have SCI until such an injury is ruled out. Initial care must include a rapid assessment, immobilization, extrication, stabilization or control of life-threatening injuries, and transportation to an appropriate medical facility.

At the scene of the injury, the victim must be immobilized on a spinal (back) board, with head and neck in a neutral position, to prevent an incomplete injury from becoming complete. One member of the team must assume control of the patient's head to prevent flexion, rotation, or extension. The hands are placed on both sides of the head at about the ear to maintain traction and alignment while a spinal board or cervical immobilizing device is applied. At least four people should slide the victim carefully onto a board for transfer to the hospital. Any twisting movement may irreversibly damage the spinal cord by causing a bony fragment of the vertebra to cut into, crush, or sever the cord completely.

The patient must be referred to a regional spinal injury or trauma center because of the multidisciplinary personnel and support services required to counteract destructive changes that occur in the first few hours after injury. During treatment in the emergency and radiology departments, the patient is kept on the transfer board. The patient must always be maintained in an extended position. No part of the body should be twisted or turned, nor should the patient be allowed to sit up. The patient should be placed on a Roto Rest, Stryker, or other turning frame when transfer to a bed is planned. Later, if it has been proved that there is no cord injury, the patient can always be moved to a conventional bed without harm; the reverse, however, is not true. If a Roto Rest bed, Stryker, or turning frame is not available, the patient should be placed on a firm mattress with a bedboard under it.

Management of Spinal Cord Injuries (Acute Phase)

The goals of management are to prevent further SCI and to observe for symptoms of progressive neurologic deficits. The patient is resuscitated as necessary, and oxygenation and cardiovascular stability are maintained. Many changes in the treatment of SCI have occurred during the past 20 years. Treatments such as hypothermia, corticosteroids, and naloxone were investigated and used during the 1980s; of these, high-dose corticosteroids have shown the most promise. Currently, regeneration therapy is being investigated; this involves transplanting fetal tissue into the injured spinal cord in hopes of regenerating the damaged tissue. SCI continues to be a devastating event, and new treatment methods are continually being investigated.

Pharmacologic Therapy

The administration of high-dose corticosteroids, specifically methylprednisolone, has been found to improve prognosis and reduce disability if given within 8 hours of injury. A loading dose of 30 mg/kg is given over 15 minutes. After a 45-minute period, a continuous infusion of 5.4 mg/kg is started and continued for 23 hours. This treatment has been associated with significant clinical improvement in patients with SCI.

Respiratory Therapy

Oxygen is administered to maintain a high arterial PO_2 because hypoxemia can create or worsen a neurologic deficit of the spinal cord. If endotracheal intubation is necessary, extreme care is taken to avoid flexing or extending the neck, which can result in an extension of cervical injury. Diaphragmatic pacing (electrical stimulation of the phrenic nerve) may be considered for the patient with a high cervical lesion but is usually carried out after the acute phase. In high cervical spine injuries, spinal cord innervation to the phrenic nerve, which stimulates the diaphragm, is lost. Diaphragmatic pacing attempts to stimulate the diaphragm to help the patient breathe.

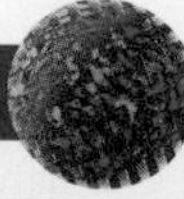

CHART 58•4 Effects of Spinal Cord Injuries

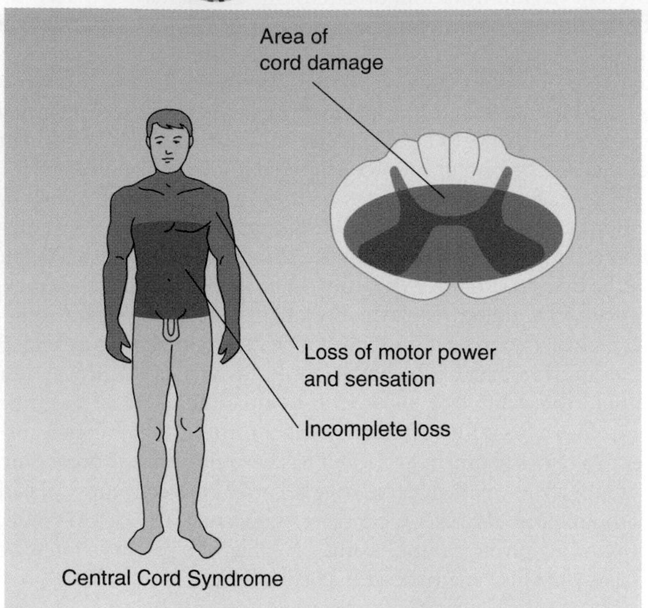

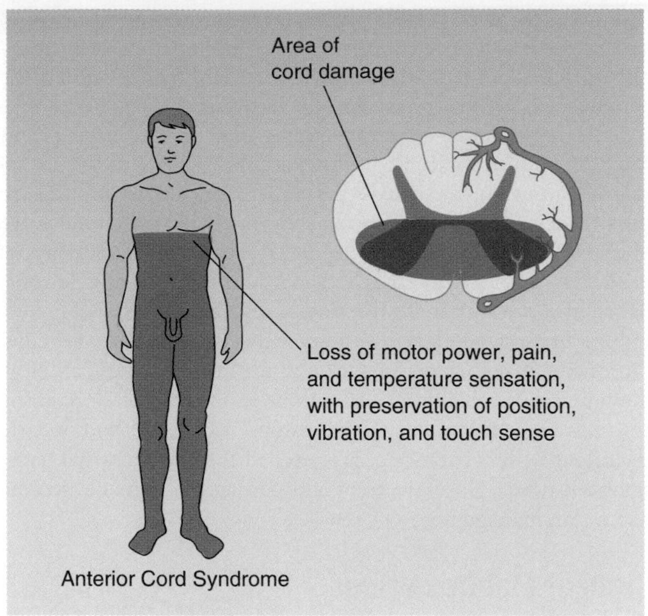

Central Cord Syndrome

- *Characteristics:* Motor deficits (in the upper extremities as compared to the lower extremities; sensory loss varies, but is more pronounced in the upper extremities); bowel/bladder dysfunction is variable, or function may be completely preserved.
- *Cause:* Injury or edema of the central cord, usually of the cervical area.

Anterior Cord Syndrome

- *Characteristics:* Loss of pain, temperature, and motor function is noted below the level of the lesion; light touch, position, and vibration sensation remain intact.
- *Cause:* The syndrome may be caused by acute disk herniation or hyperflexion injuries associated with fracture–dislocation of vertebra. It also may occur as a result of injury to the anterior spinal artery, which supplies the anterior two thirds of the spinal cord.

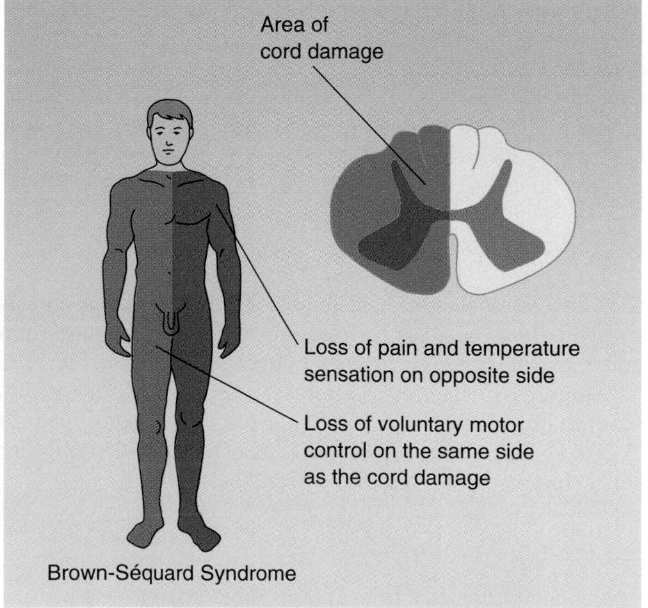

Brown-Séquard Syndrome (Lateral Cord Syndrome)

- *Characteristics:* Ipsilateral paralysis or paresis is noted, together with ipsilateral loss of touch, pressure, and vibration and contralateral loss of pain and temperature.
- *Cause:* The lesion is caused by a transverse hemisection of the cord (half of the cord is transected from north to south), usually as a result of a knife or missile injury, fracture–dislocation of a unilateral articular process, or possibly an acute ruptured disk.

Adapted from Hickey, L. (1997). *The clinical practice of neurological and neurosurgical nursing* (4th ed.). Philadelphia: Lippincott-Raven.

Skeletal Reduction and Traction

Management of SCI requires immobilization and reduction of dislocations (restoration of normal position) and stabilization of the vertebral column.

Cervical fractures are reduced and the cervical spine is aligned with some form of skeletal traction, such as skeletal tongs or calipers, or with use of the halo device. Early surgical stabilization has reduced the need for cervical traction in many patients with cervical spine injuries. A variety of skeletal tongs are available, all of which involve fixation in the skull in some manner (Fig. 58-5). The Gardner-Wells tongs require no predrilled holes in the skull. Crutchfield and Vinke tongs are inserted through holes made with a special drill under local anesthesia.

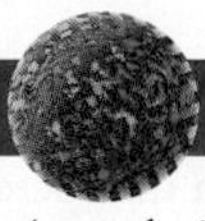

CHART 58•5 Selected Terms Related to Neurologic Lesions of the Spinal Cord

- Quadriplegia (tetraplegia) results from a lesion involving one of the cervical segments of the spinal cord with dysfunction of both arms, both legs, bowel, and bladder.
- Paraplegia results from a lesion involving the thoracic lumbar, or sacral regions of the spinal cord with dysfunction of the lower extremities, bowel, and bladder.
- Complete lesion (complete quadriplegia or complete paraplegia) implies total loss of sensation and voluntary muscle control below the injury.
- Incomplete lesion implies preservation of the sensor or motor fibers, or both, below the lesion. Incomplete lesions are classified according to the area of spinal cord damage: central, lateral, anterior, or peripheral.

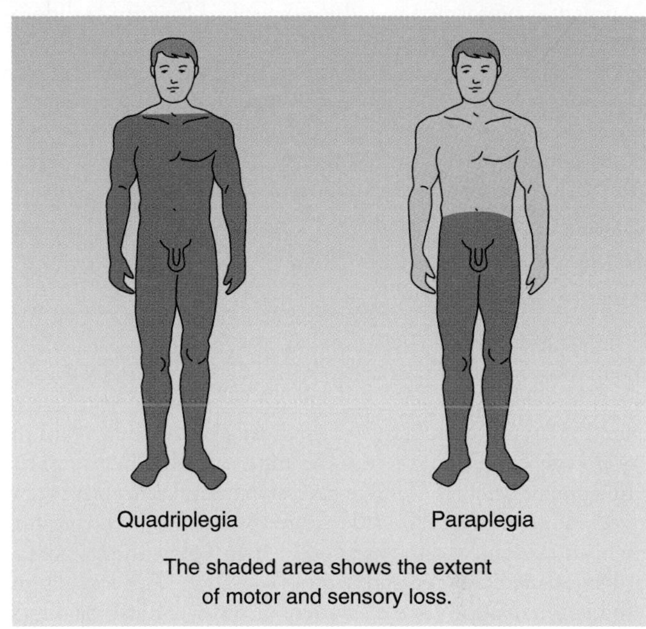
Quadriplegia
Paraplegia
The shaded area shows the extent of motor and sensory loss.

Adapted from Hickey, L. (1997). *The clinical practice of neurological and neurosurgical nursing* (4th ed.). Philadelphia: Lippincott-Raven.

Traction is applied to the tongs by weights, the amount depending on the patient's size and the degree of fracture displacement. The traction force is exerted along the longitudinal axis of the vertebral bodies, with the patient's neck in a neutral position. Then the traction is gradually increased by adding more weights. As the amount of traction is increased, the spaces between the intervertebral disks widen and the vertebrae slip back into position. Reduction usually takes place after correct alignment has been restored. Once reduction is achieved, as verified by cervical spine films and neurologic examination, the weights are gradually removed until the amount of weight needed to maintain the alignment is obtained. The weights should hang freely so as not to interfere with the traction. The patient is placed on a Stryker or other turning frame.

A halo device may be used initially with traction or may be applied after removal of the tongs (Fig. 58-6). It consists of a stainless-steel halo ring that is fixed to the skull by four pins. The ring is attached to a removable **halo vest**, which suspends the weight of the unit circumferentially around the chest. A metal frame connects the ring to the chest. Halo devices provide immobilization of the cervical spine while allowing early ambulation.

Thoracic and lumbar injuries are usually treated through surgical intervention followed by immobilization with a fitted brace. Traction is not indicated either before or after surgery.

Surgical Intervention

Surgery is indicated in any of the following instances:

1. Compression of the cord is evident.
2. The injury is a compound fracture.
3. The injury involves a wound that penetrates the cord.

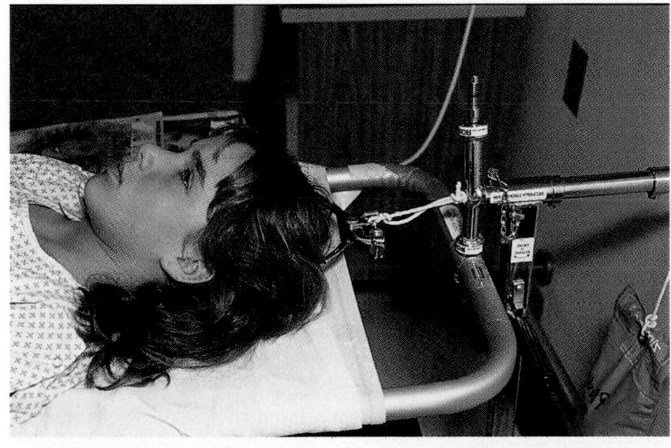

FIGURE 58•5 Traction for cervical fractures may be applied with tongs.

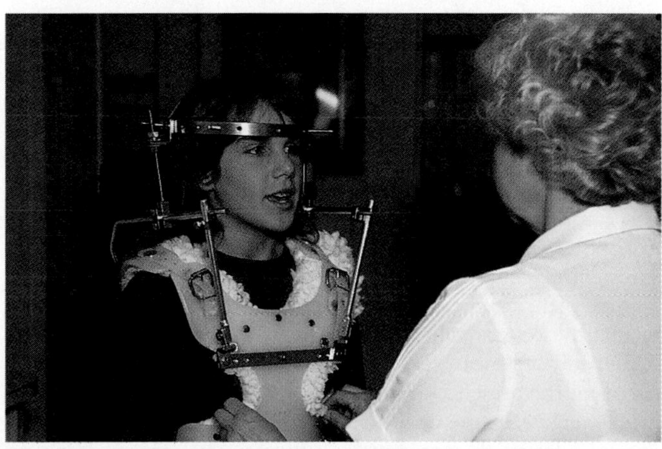

FIGURE 58•6 A halo vest may be used to maintain alignment in cervical injuries.

4. There are bony fragments in the spinal canal.
5. The patient's neurologic status is deteriorating.

Surgery is performed to reduce the spinal fracture or dislocation or to decompress the cord.

A laminectomy (excision of the posterior arches and spinous processes of a vertebra) may be indicated in the presence of progressive neurologic deficit, suspected epidural hematoma, or penetrating injuries that require surgical débridement, or to permit direct visualization and exploration of the cord.

Management of Complications of Spinal Cord Injury

SPINAL SHOCK

The neurogenic shock associated with SCI is commonly referred to as spinal shock. Spinal shock represents a sudden depression of reflex activity in the spinal cord (areflexia) below the level of injury. In this condition, the muscles innervated by the part of the cord segment below the level of the lesion become completely paralyzed and flaccid, and the reflexes are absent. The blood pressure and heart rate fall, and the parts of the body below the level of the cord lesion are paralyzed and without sensation. This loss of sympathetic innervation causes a variety of other clinical manifestations, including a decrease in cardiac output, venous pooling in the extremities, and peripheral vasodilation.

With injuries to the cervical and upper thoracic spinal cord, innervation to the major accessory muscles of respiration is lost and respiratory problems develop: decreased vital capacity, retention of secretions, increased partial pressure of carbon dioxide (PCO_2), decreased PO_2, respiratory failure, and pulmonary edema.

The reflexes that initiate bladder and bowel function also are affected. (The management of the patient with a **neurogenic bladder**—that is, a bladder disturbance due to a lesion of the central nervous system—is discussed in Chap. 10.) Bowel distention and paralytic ileus caused by depression of the reflexes may be treated with intestinal decompression. The patient does not perspire on the paralyzed portions of the body because sympathetic activity is blocked; therefore, close observation is required for early detection of an abrupt onset of fever. (A detailed discussion of shock can be found in Chap. 14.)

Nursing Alert *The patient's body defenses must be supported and maintained until spinal shock abates and the system has recovered from the traumatic insult (3 to 6 weeks). Special attention also must be directed to the respiratory system. The patient may be unable to generate sufficient intrathoracic pressure to cough effectively. Chest physical therapy and suctioning may assist in clearance of pulmonary secretions.*

DEEP VEIN THROMBOSIS

Deep vein thrombosis is a common complication of immobility and is common in patients with SCI. Patients in whom deep vein thrombosis develops are at risk for pulmonary embolism, a life-threatening complication. Manifestations of pulmonary embolism include pleuritic chest pain, anxiety, shortness of breath, and abnormal blood gas values (increased PCO_2 and decreased PO_2). Thigh and calf measurements are made daily. The patient is evaluated for the presence of deep vein thrombosis if there is a significant increase in the circumference of one extremity. Low-dose anticoagulation therapy usually is initiated to prevent deep vein thrombosis and pulmonary embolism, along with thigh-high elastic pressure stockings or pneumatic compression devices.

OTHER COMPLICATIONS

In addition to respiratory complications (respiratory failure, pneumonia) and **autonomic hyperreflexia** (characterized by pounding headache, profuse sweating, nasal congestion, piloerection [gooseflesh], bradycardia, and hypertension), other complications that may occur include pressure ulcers and infection (urinary, respiratory, and local infection at the skeletal traction pin sites).

NURSING PROCESS: THE PATIENT WITH ACUTE SPINAL CORD INJURY

Assessment

The breathing pattern is observed, the strength of the cough is assessed, and the lungs are auscultated, because paralysis of abdominal and respiratory muscles diminishes coughing and makes it difficult to clear bronchial and pharyngeal secretions. Reduced excursion of the chest also results.

The patient is monitored closely for any changes in motor or sensory function and symptoms of progressive neurologic damage. It may be impossible in the early stages of SCI to determine whether the cord has been severed, because signs and symptoms of cord edema are indistinguishable from those of cord transection. Edema of the spinal cord may occur with any severe cord injury and may further compromise spinal cord function.

Motor and sensory function are assessed through careful neurologic examination. These findings are recorded so that changes in the baseline neurologic status can be evaluated accurately.

- Motor ability is tested by asking the patient to spread the fingers, squeeze the examiner's hand, and move the toes or turn the feet.
- Sensation is evaluated by pinching the skin or pricking it with the broken end of a cotton swab, starting at shoulder level and working down both sides of the extremities. The patient should have both eyes closed so that the examination reveals true findings, not what the patient hopes to feel. The patient is asked where the sensation is felt.
- Any decrease in neurologic function is reported immediately.

The patient is also assessed for spinal shock, a complete loss of all reflex, motor, sensory, and autonomic activity below the level of the lesion that causes bladder paralysis and distention. The patient's lower abdomen is palpated for signs of urinary retention and overdistention of the bladder. Further assessment is made for gastric dilation and ileus due to an atonic bowel, a result of autonomic disruption.

Temperature is monitored because the patient may have periods of hyperthermia as a result of alteration in temperature control due to autonomic disruption.

Diagnosis

Nursing Diagnoses

Based on the assessment data, the patient's major nursing diagnoses may include the following:

- Ineffective breathing patterns related to weakness or paralysis of abdominal and intercostal muscles and inability to clear secretions
- Ineffective airway clearance related to weakness of intercostal muscles
- Impaired physical mobility related to motor and sensory impairment

- Sensual/perceptual alterations related to motor and sensory impairment
- Risk for impaired skin integrity related to immobility and sensory loss
- Urinary retention related to inability to void spontaneously
- Constipation related to presence of atonic bowel as a result of autonomic disruption
- Pain and discomfort related to treatment and prolonged immobility

Collaborative Problems/Potential Complications

Based on the assessment data, potential complications that may develop include:

- Deep vein thrombosis
- Orthostatic hypotension
- Autonomic hyperreflexia

Planning and Goals

The goals for the patient may include improved breathing pattern and airway clearance, improved mobility, improved sensory and perceptual awareness, maintenance of skin integrity, relief of urinary retention, improved bowel function, promotion of comfort, and absence of complications.

Nursing Interventions

Promoting Adequate Breathing and Airway Clearance

Possible impending respiratory failure is detected by observing the patient, measuring vital capacity, monitoring O_2 saturation through pulse oximetry, and monitoring arterial blood gas values. Early and vigorous attention to clearing bronchial and pharyngeal secretions can prevent retention of secretions and resultant atelectasis. Suctioning may be indicated, but caution must be used during suctioning because this procedure can stimulate the vagus nerve, producing bradycardia, which can result in cardiac arrest.

If the patient cannot cough effectively because of decreased inspiratory volume and inability to generate sufficient expiratory pressure, chest physical therapy and quad-assisted coughing may be indicated. Specific breathing exercises are supervised by the nurse to increase the strength and endurance of the inspiratory muscles, particularly the diaphragm. Assisted coughing provides an opportunity for the patient to clear the upper respiratory tract of secretions. It is important to ensure proper humidification and hydration to prevent secretions from becoming thick and difficult to remove even with coughing. The patient is assessed for signs of respiratory infection (cough, fever, dyspnea). Smoking is discouraged because it increases bronchial and pulmonary secretions and impairs ciliary action.

Ascending edema of the spinal cord in the acute phase may cause respiratory difficulty that requires immediate intervention. Therefore, the patient's respiratory status must be monitored frequently.

Improving Mobility

Proper body alignment is maintained at all times. The patient is repositioned frequently and is out of bed as soon as the spinal column is stabilized. The feet are prone to footdrop. High-top sneakers can help prevent footdrop. The sneakers are removed and reapplied every 2 hours. Trochanter rolls are applied from the crest of the ilium to the midthigh of both legs to prevent external rotation of the hip joints.

Patients with lesions above the midthoracic level have loss of sympathetic control of peripheral vasoconstrictor activity, leading to hypotension. These patients may tolerate changes in position poorly and require monitoring of blood pressure when positions are changed. Usually the patient is turned every 2 hours (Fig. 58-7). If not on a turning frame, the patient should not be turned unless the spine is stable and the physician has indicated that it is safe to do so. Guidelines for turning a patient not on a turning frame are found in Guideline 58-1. Adequate preparation and time must be made for turning the patient, maintaining a gentle, firm, and steady touch.

Contractures develop rapidly with immobility and muscle paralysis. A joint that is immobilized too long becomes fixed as a result of contractures of the tendon and joint capsule. Atrophy of the extremities results from disuse. Many of these complications can be prevented by range-of-motion exercises. These exercises preserve joint motion and stimulate circulation. Exercises may be prescribed and implemented within 48 to 72 hours after injury. Toes, metatarsals, ankles, knees, and hips should be put through a full range of motion at least four, and ideally five, times daily.

For most patients with a cervical fracture without neurologic deficit, reduction in traction followed by rigid immobilization for about 16 weeks restores skeletal integrity. These patients are allowed to move gradually to an erect position. A four-poster neck brace or molded collar is applied when the patient is mobilized after traction is removed.

Promoting Adaptation to Sensory and Perceptual Alterations

The nurse assists the patient to compensate for sensory and perceptual alterations that occur with SCI. The area above the level of the injury is stimulated through aromas, flavorful food and beverages, conversation, and music. Additional strategies include the following:

- Providing prism glasses to enable the patient to see from the supine position
- Encouraging use of hearing aids, if indicated, to enable the patient to hear conversations and environmental sounds

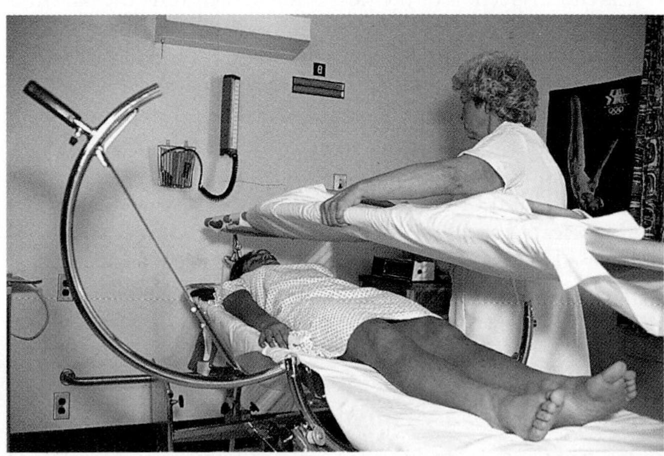

FIGURE 58•7 A patient on the Stryker frame is turned frequently to relieve pressure.

58•1 GUIDELINES FOR TURNING THE PATIENT WITH CRUTCHFIELD TONGS

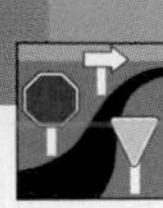

If Crutchfield tongs are used and the patient is not on a turning frame, an order from the physician must be obtained before the patient is turned. The patient's head *should never be flexed,* either forward or laterally, and at all times must be kept in a direct line with the axis of the cervical spine.

To Turn the Patient

- Three persons should turn the patient in a logrolling fashion, making sure that the shoulder turns with the head and the neck. One nurse should support the head; the second nurse or assistant, the shoulders; and the third person, the hips and the legs.
- The nurse supporting the head gives the commands for turning.
- A pillow is placed between the legs of the patient to prevent the upper leg from slipping forward and jarring the patient's head.
- A pillow is placed longitudinally on the chest, with the patient's upper arm resting on it. The pillow prevents the shoulder from sagging and pulling on the neck as the patient is turned.
- As the patient is turned in a logrolling fashion, the traction should be moved carefully to keep it in a direct line with the cervical spine. The patient's position should be adjusted so that the traction, the patient's head, and the cervical spine are in correct alignment.
- While the nurse still supports the head in the lateral position, a small pillow is placed under the head to maintain cervical alignment.

- Providing emotional support to the patient
- Teaching the patient strategies to compensate for or cope with these deficits

Maintaining Skin Integrity

Because the patient with SCI is immobilized and has loss of sensation, there is an ever-present, life-endangering threat of pressure ulcers. In areas of local tissue ischemia, where there is continuous pressure and where the peripheral circulation is inadequate as a result of the spinal shock and recumbent position, pressure ulcers have developed within 6 hours. Prolonged immobilization of the patient on a transfer board increases the risk of pressure ulcers. The most common sites are over the ischial tuberosity, the greater trochanter, and the sacrum.

The patient's position is changed at least every 2 hours. Turning not only assists in the prevention of pressure ulcers but also prevents the pooling of blood and tissue fluid in the dependent areas.

Careful inspection of the skin is made each time the patient is turned. The skin over the pressure points is assessed for redness or breaks in the skin; the perineum is checked for soilage and the catheter is observed for adequate drainage. The patient's general body alignment and comfort are assessed. Special attention should be given to pressure areas in contact with the transfer board.

Every few hours, the patient's skin is washed with a mild soap, rinsed well, and blotted dry. Pressure-sensitive areas are kept well lubricated and soft with bland cream or lotion. Massage is performed gently, using a circular motion.

The patient is informed about the danger of pressure ulcers and is encouraged to participate in preventive measures. (See Chap. 10 for other aspects of the prevention of pressure ulcers.)

Maintaining Urinary Elimination

Immediately after SCI, the urinary bladder becomes atonic and cannot contract by reflex activity. Urinary retention is the immediate result. Because the patient has no sensation of bladder distention, overstretching of the bladder and detrusor muscle may occur, delaying the return of bladder function.

Intermittent catheterization is carried out to avoid overdistention of the bladder and urinary tract infection. If this is not feasible, an indwelling catheter is inserted temporarily. At an early stage, family members are shown how to carry out intermittent catheterization and are encouraged to participate in this facet of care, because they will be involved in long-term follow-up and must be able to recognize complications so that treatment can be instituted.

The patient is taught to record fluid intake, voiding pattern, amounts of residual urine after catheterization, characteristics of urine, and any unusual sensations that may occur.

The management of a neurogenic bladder is discussed in detail in Chapter 10.

Improving Bowel Function

Immediately after SCI, a paralytic ileus usually develops due to neurogenic paralysis of the bowel; a nasogastric tube is often required to relieve distention and prevent aspiration.

Bowel activity usually returns within the first week. As soon as bowel sounds are heard on auscultation, the patient is given a high-calorie, high-protein, high-fiber diet, with the amount of food gradually increased. The nurse administers prescribed stool softeners to counteract the effects of immobility and pain medications. A bowel program is instituted as early as possible.

Providing Comfort Measures

After cervical injury, when tongs or calipers are in place, the patient's skull is assessed for signs of infection, including drainage around the tongs. The back of the head is checked periodically for signs of pressure and is massaged at intervals, with care taken not to move the neck. The hair around the tongs usually is shaved to facilitate inspection. Probing under encrusted areas is avoided.

HOME CARE TEACHING CHECKLIST: THE PATIENT WITH A HALO VEST

At the completion of the program, the patient or caregiver will be able to:	Patient	Caregiver
• Describe the rationale for use of the halo vest	✔	✔
• Demonstrate assessment of frame, traction, tongs, and pins		✔
• Describe emergency measures if respiratory or other complications develop while patient is in halo vest or if frame becomes dislodged		✔
• Demonstrate pin care using correct technique		✔
• Identify signs and symptoms of infection	✔	✔
• Assess the skin for reddened or irritated areas and breakdown		✔
• Demonstrate care of skin		✔
• Demonstrate safe techniques to assist patient with self-care, hygiene, and ambulation		✔
• Identify signs and symptoms of complications (deep venous thrombosis, respiratory impairment, urinary tract infection)	✔	✔

THE PATIENT IN HALO TRACTION

Patients who have been placed in a halo device after cervical stabilization may have a slight headache or discomfort around the skull pins for several days after the pins are inserted. The patient initially may not appreciate the rather startling appearance of this apparatus but can readily adapt to it because the device provides comfort for the unstable neck. The patient may complain of being caged in and of noise created by any object coming in contact with the steel frame, but he or she can be reassured that adaptation to such annoyances will occur.

The areas around the pin sites are cleansed daily and observed for redness, drainage, and pain. The pins are observed for loosening, which may contribute to infection. If one of the pins becomes detached, the patient's head is stabilized in a neutral position while another person notifies the neurosurgeon. A torque screwdriver should be readily available should the screws on the frame need tightening.

The skin under the halo vest is inspected for excessive perspiration, redness, and skin blistering, especially on the bony prominences. The vest is opened at the sides to allow the patient's torso to be washed. The liner of the vest is not allowed to become wet, because dampness causes skin problems. Powder is not used inside the vest, because it may contribute to the development of pressure ulcers.

Monitoring and Managing Potential Complications

THROMBOPHLEBITIS

Thrombophlebitis is a relatively common complication in patients after SCI. Deep vein thrombosis occurs in a high percentage of SCI patients; thus, they are at risk for the development of pulmonary embolism. The patient must be assessed for symptoms of thrombophlebitis and pulmonary embolism; chest pain, shortness of breath, and changes in arterial blood gas values must be reported promptly to the physician. The circumference of the thighs and calves is measured and recorded daily; further diagnostic studies will be performed if a significant increase is noted. Patients remain at risk for thrombophlebitis for up to 3 months after the initial injury. Immobilization and the associated venous stasis, as well as varying degrees of autonomic disruption, contribute to the high risk and susceptibility for deep vein thrombosis.

Anticoagulation is initiated once head and other injuries have been ruled out. Low-dose heparin may be followed by long-term oral anticoagulation (ie, warfarin). Additional measures such as range-of-motion exercises, thigh-high elastic pressure stockings, and adequate hydration are all important preventive measures. Pneumatic compression devices may also be used to reduce venous pooling and promote venous return. It is also important to avoid the external pressure on the lower extremities that may result from flexion of the knees while the patient is in bed.

ORTHOSTATIC HYPOTENSION

For the first 2 weeks after SCI, the blood pressure tends to be unstable and quite low. There is a gradual return to preinjury levels, but periodic episodes of severe orthostatic hypotension frequently interfere with efforts to mobilize the patient. Interruption in the reflex arcs that normally produce vasoconstriction in the upright position, coupled with dilation and pooling in abdominal and lower extremity vessels, can result in blood pressure readings of 40 mm Hg systolic and 0 mm Hg diastolic. Orthostatic hypotension is a particularly common problem for patients with lesions above T7. It has been found that in some quadriplegic patients, even slight elevations of the head can result in dramatic changes in blood pressure.

A number of techniques can be used to reduce the frequency of hypotensive episodes. Close monitoring of vital signs before and during position changes is essential. Vasopressor medication can be used to treat the profound vasodilation. Thigh-high elastic pressure stockings should be applied to improve venous return from the lower extremities. Activity should be planned in advance and adequate time given for a slow progression of position changes from recumbent to sitting and upright. Tilt tables frequently are helpful in assisting patients to make this transition.

AUTONOMIC HYPERREFLEXIA

Autonomic hyperreflexia (autonomic dysreflexia) is an acute emergency that occurs as a result of exaggerated autonomic responses to stimuli that are innocuous in normal people. It occurs only after spinal shock has resolved. This syndrome is characterized by a severe, pounding headache with paroxysmal hypertension, profuse diaphoresis (most often of the forehead), nausea, nasal congestion, and bradycardia. It occurs among patients with cord lesions above T6 (the sympathetic visceral outflow level), after spinal shock has subsided. The sudden rise in blood pressure may cause a rupture of one or more cerebral blood vessels or lead to increased ICP. A number of stimuli may trigger this reflex: distended bladder (the most common cause); distention or contraction of the visceral organs, especially the bowel (from constipation, impaction); or stimulation of the skin (tactile, pain, thermal stimuli, pressure ulcer). Because this is an emergency situation, the objective is to remove the triggering stimulus and to avoid the possibly serious complications.

The following measures are carried out:

- The patient is placed immediately in a sitting position to lower blood pressure.
- Rapid assessment to identify and alleviate the cause is imperative.
- The bladder is emptied immediately via a urinary catheter. If the catheter is not patent, it is irrigated or replaced with another catheter.
- The rectum is examined for a fecal mass. If one is present, a topical anesthetic is inserted 10 to 15 minutes before the mass is removed, because visceral distention or contraction can cause autonomic dysreflexia.
- The skin is examined for any areas of pressure, irritation, or broken skin.
- Any other stimulus that can be the triggering event, such as an object on the skin or a draft of cold air, must be removed.
- If these measures do not relieve the patient's hypertension and excruciating headache, a ganglionic blocking agent (hydralazine hydrochloride [Apresoline]) is prescribed and given slowly intravenously.
- The patient's medical record should be labeled with a clearly visible note about the risk for autonomic hyperreflexia.
- The patient is instructed about prevention and management measures.
- Any patient with a lesion above the T6 segment is informed that such an episode is possible and may even occur many years after the initial injury.

The rehabilitation of the patient with a permanent SCI (ie, the quadriplegic or paraplegic patient) is discussed below.

Promoting Home and Community-Based Care

TEACHING PATIENTS SELF-CARE

In most cases, SCI patients need long-term rehabilitation. The process begins during hospitalization as acute symptoms begin to abate or come under better control and the overall deficits and long-term effects of the injury become clear. The goals begin to shift from merely surviving the injury to learning strategies necessary to cope with the alterations that injury imposes on activities of daily living. The emphasis shifts from ensuring that the patient is stable and free of complications to specific assessment and planning designed to meet the patient's rehabilitation needs. Patient teaching may initially focus on the injury and its effects on mobility, dressing, and bowel, bladder, and sexual function. As the patient and family acknowledge the consequences of the injury, the focus of teaching may broaden to address issues necessary to carry out the tasks of daily living. Teaching begins in the acute phase and continues throughout the patient's rehabilitation and even throughout the patient's life as changes occur and if new problems arise.

Although maintaining function and preventing complications will remain important, goals regarding the skills necessary for self-care and preparation for discharge will assist in a smooth transition to rehabilitation and eventually to the community.

CONTINUING CARE

The ultimate goal of the rehabilitation process is independence. The nurse becomes a support to both the patient and the family, assisting them to assume responsibility for increasing aspects of patient care and management. Care for the SCI patient involves members from all the health care disciplines; these may include nursing, medicine, rehabilitation, respiratory therapy, physical and occupational therapy, case management, social services, and so forth. The nurse often serves as coordinator of the management team and as a liaison with rehabilitation centers and home care agencies. The patient and family often require assistance in dealing with the psychological impact of the injury and its consequences; referral to a psychiatric clinical nurse specialist or other mental health care professional often is helpful.

As more patients survive acute SCI, they will face the changes associated with aging. Thus, teaching in the home and community focuses on health promotion and addresses the need to minimize risk factors (eg, smoking, alcohol and drug abuse, obesity). Home care nurses and others who have contact with patients with SCI are in a position to teach patients about healthy lifestyles.

Evaluation

Expected Outcomes

Expected outcomes may include:

1. Demonstrates improvement in gas exchange and clearance of secretions, as evidenced by normal breath sounds on auscultation
   a. Breathes easily without shortness of breath
   b. Performs hourly deep-breathing exercises, coughs effectively, and clears pulmonary secretions
   c. Is free of respiratory infection (ie, has normal temperature, respiratory rate, and pulse, normal breath sounds, absence of purulent sputum)
2. Moves within limits of the dysfunction and demonstrates completion of exercises within functional limitations
3. Demonstrates adaptation to sensory and perceptual alterations
   a. Uses assistive devices (prism glasses, hearing aids) as indicated
   b. Describes sensory and perceptual alterations as a consequence of injury
4. Demonstrates optimal skin integrity
   a. Exhibits normal skin turgor; skin is free of reddened areas or breaks
   b. Participates in skin care and monitoring procedures within functional limitations
5. Regains urinary bladder function
   a. Exhibits no signs of urinary tract infection (ie, has normal temperature; voids clear, dilute urine)
   b. Has adequate fluid intake
   c. Participates in bladder training program within functional limitations
6. Regains bowel function
   a. Reports regular pattern of bowel movement
   b. Consumes adequate dietary fiber and oral fluids
   c. Participates in bowel training program within functional limitations
7. Reports absence of pain and discomfort
8. Is free of complications
   a. Demonstrates no signs of thrombophlebitis, deep vein thrombosis, or pulmonary embolus

b. Exhibits no manifestations of pulmonary embolism (eg, no chest pain or shortness of breath; arterial blood gas values are normal)
c. Maintains blood pressure within normal limits
d. Has no lightheadedness with position changes
e. Exhibits no manifestations of autonomic hyperreflexia (ie, no headache, diaphoresis, nasal congestion, bradycardia, or diaphoresis)

Management of the Quadriplegic or Paraplegic Patient

Quadriplegia refers to the loss of movement and sensation in all four extremities and the trunk, associated with injury to the cervical spinal cord. *Paraplegia* refers to loss of motion and sensation in the lower extremities and all or part of the trunk as a result of damage to the thoracic or lumbar spinal cord or to the sacral root (see Chart 58-5). Both conditions most frequently follow trauma such as falls, injuries, and gunshot wounds, but they may also be the result of spinal cord lesions (intervertebral disk, tumor, vascular lesions), multiple sclerosis, infections and abscesses of the spinal cord, and congenital disorders.

The patient faces a lifetime of great disability, requiring ongoing follow-up and care and the expertise of a number of health professionals, including physicians (specifically a physiatrist), rehabilitation nurses, occupational therapist, physical therapist, psychologist, social worker, rehabilitation engineer, and vocational counselor at different times as the need arises.

As the years go by, these patients also have the same medical problems as others in the aging population. In addition, they face the threat of complications associated with their disability. Usually the patient is encouraged to attend a spinal clinic when problems arise. Lifetime care includes assessment of the urinary tract at prescribed intervals, because there is the likelihood of continuing alteration in detrusor and sphincter function and the patient is prone to urinary tract infections.

Long-term problems and complications of SCI include autonomic dysreflexia (discussed earlier), bladder and kidney infections (discussed in Chap. 41), spasticity, pressure ulcers with complications of sepsis, osteomyelitis, fistulas, and depression. Flexor muscle spasms may be particularly disabling. Heterotopic ossification (overgrowth of bone) in the hips, knees, shoulders, and elbows occurs in 20% to 40% of SCI patients. This complication is quite painful and can produce a loss of range of motion. Management includes observing and caring for any alteration in physiologic status and psychological outlook, and the prevention and treatment of long-term complications. The nursing role is that of emphasizing the need for vigilance in self-assessment and care.

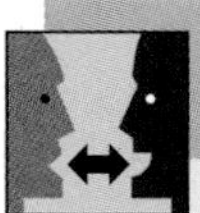

ETHICS AND RELATED ISSUES

End-of-Life Care

Situation

A 70-year-old man has been in neurologic intensive care since he suffered a complete C1–C2 cervical fracture two weeks ago, leaving him quadriplegic and ventilator dependent. Since his admission, he has asked to be allowed to die. He has a living will and his wife is his designated durable power of attorney for health. Before his injury, his health was exceptional. He played golf daily and was very active. He is awake, alert, and oriented and can communicate by letter board. He states that he does not want to spend his life unable to do the things he enjoys. He continues to request extubation so that he can die. His family and friends are with him, and he has asked his attorneys to tend to his affairs. With the loving support of his family, the decision to remove the ventilator has been made. Sedatives will be administered to help him deal with hypoxia and anoxia.

Dilemma

What is the nurse's role in caring for this patient at this time?

Discussion

Is the removal of the ventilator an act of patient-assisted suicide? Is it active or passive euthanasia?

What is the nurse's role in caring for the patient if this action conflicts with his/her personal beliefs? If no other nurse is available to provide care? If the physician writes the order for the nurse to remove the ventilator?

NURSING PROCESS: THE PATIENT WITH QUADRIPLEGIA OR PARAPLEGIA

Assessment

Assessment focuses on the patient's general condition, the presence of complications, and how the patient is managing at that particular point in time. A head-to-toe assessment and review of systems should be part of the database, with particular emphasis on the areas prone to problems in this population. Specifically, a thorough inspection of all areas of the skin for redness or breakdown is critical. It is also important to review with the patient the established bowel and bladder program, because the program must continue uninterrupted. Patients with quadriplegia or paraplegia have varying degrees of loss of motor power, deep and superficial sensation, vasomotor control, bladder and bowel control, and sexual function. They are faced with potential problems related to immobility, skin breakdown and pressure ulcers, recurring urinary tract infection, contractures, and psychosocial disruptions. Knowledge about these particular problems can further guide the assessment in any setting. Nurses in all settings, including home care, must be aware of these potential problems in the lifetime management of these patients.

An understanding of the emotional and psychological responses to quadriplegia or paraplegia is achieved by observing the responses and behaviors of the patient and family and by listening to their concerns. Documenting these assessments and reviewing the plan with the entire team on a regular basis provides insight into how both the patient and the family are coping with the changes in lifestyle and body functioning. Additional information frequently can be gathered from the social worker or psychiatric/mental health worker.

It usually takes time for the patient and the family to comprehend the magnitude of the resulting disability. They may go through stages of adjustment, including shock, disbelief, denial, depression, grief, and acceptance. During the acute phase of the injury, denial can be a protective mechanism to shield patients from the overwhelming reality of what has happened. As they realize the finality of paraplegia or quadriplegia, the grieving process may be prolonged and all-encompassing because of the recognition that long-held plans and expectations may be interrupted or permanently altered. A period of depression often follows as the patient experiences a loss of self-esteem in areas of self-identity, sexual functioning, and social and emotional roles.

Exploration and assessment of these issues can assist in developing a meaningful plan of care.

Diagnosis

Nursing Diagnoses

Based on the assessment data, the major nursing diagnoses of the patient with quadriplegia or paraplegia may include the following:

- Immobility related to inability to walk
- Impairment of skin integrity related to permanent sensory loss and immobility
- Urinary retention related to level of injury
- Constipation related to effects of spinal cord disruption
- Sexual dysfunction related to neurologic dysfunction
- Ineffective individual coping related to impact of dysfunction on daily living
- Knowledge deficit about requirements for long-term management

Collaborative Problems/Potential Complications

Based on all the assessment data, potential complications of quadriplegia or paraplegia that may develop include:

- Spasticity
- Infection and sepsis

Planning and Goals

The goals for the patient may include attainment of some form of mobility, maintenance of healthy, intact skin, achievement of bladder management without infection, achievement of bowel control, achievement of sexual expression, strengthening of coping mechanisms, and absence of complications.

Nursing Interventions

The patient requires extensive rehabilitation, which is less difficult if appropriate nursing management has been carried out during the acute phase of the injury or illness. Nursing care is one of the key factors determining the success of the rehabilitation program. The main objective is for the patient to live as independently as possible in the home and community.

Increasing Mobility

EXERCISE PROGRAM

The unaffected parts of the body are built up to optimal strength to promote maximal self-care. The muscles of the hands, arms, shoulders, chest, spine, abdomen, and neck must be strengthened in the paraplegic patient because he or she must bear full weight on these muscles to ambulate. The triceps and the latissimus dorsi are important muscles used in crutch walking. The muscles of the abdomen and the back also are necessary for balance and for maintaining the upright position.

To strengthen these muscles, the patient can do push-ups when in a prone position and sit-ups when in a sitting position. Extending the arms while holding weights (traction weights can be used) also develops muscle strength. Squeezing rubber balls or crumbling newspaper promotes hand strength.

With encouragement from all members of the rehabilitation team, the paraplegic patient can develop the increased exercise tolerance needed for gait training and ambulation activities.

MOBILIZATION

When the spine is stable enough to allow the patient to assume an upright posture, mobilization activities are initiated. A brace or vest may be used, depending on the level of the lesion. A patient whose paralysis is due to complete severance of the cord can begin weight-bearing early because no further damage can be incurred. The sooner muscles are used, the less chance of disuse atrophy. The earlier the patient is brought to a standing position, the less opportunity for osteoporotic changes to take place in the long bones. Weight-bearing also reduces the possibility of renal calculi and enhances many other metabolic processes.

Braces and crutches enable some paraplegic patients to ambulate for short distances and even to drive manually operated automobiles. Crutch ambulation in paraplegics requires high energy expenditure. Modern developments, such as motorized wheelchairs and specially equipped vans, contribute to the greater independence and mobility of patients with high-level SCI or other lesions.

Promoting Skin Integrity

Because these patients spend a great portion of their lives in wheelchairs, pressure ulcers are an ever-present threat. Contributing factors are permanent sensory loss over pressure areas; immobility, which makes relief of pressure difficult; trauma from bumps (against the wheelchair, toilet) that cause unperceived abrasions and wounds; loss of protective function of the skin from excoriation and maceration due to excessive perspiration and possible urine and fecal incontinence; and poor general health (anemia, edema, malnutrition), leading to poor tissue perfusion. The prevention and management of pressure ulcers are discussed in detail in Chapter 10.

The person with quadriplegia or paraplegia must take responsibility for monitoring his or her skin status. This involves relieving pressure and not remaining in any position for longer than 2 hours, in addition to ensuring that the skin receives meticulous attention and cleansing. The patient is taught that ulcers develop over bony prominences exposed to unrelieved pressure in the lying and sitting positions. The most vulnerable areas are identified. The paraplegic patient is instructed to use mirrors, if possible, to inspect these areas morning and night, observing for redness, slight edema, or any abrasions. While in bed, the patient should turn at 2-hour intervals and then inspect the skin again for redness that does not fade on pressure. The bottom sheet should be checked for wetness and for creases. The quadriplegic patient who cannot perform these activities is encouraged to inform others of the need to check these areas and prevent ulcers from developing.

The patient is taught to relieve pressure while in the wheelchair by doing push-ups, leaning from side to side to relieve ischial pressure, and tilting forward while leaning on a table. The caregiver for the quadriplegic patient will need to perform these activities if the patient cannot do so independently. Each person requires a wheelchair cushion prescribed to meet individual needs, which may change in time with alterations in posture, weight, and skin tolerance. A referral can be made to a rehabilitation engineer, who can measure pressure levels while the patient is sitting and then tailor the cushion and other necessary aids and assistive devices to the patient's needs.

The diet for the quadriplegic or paraplegic patient should be high in protein, vitamins, and calories to ensure minimal wasting of muscle and the maintenance of healthy skin, and high in fluids to maintain well-functioning kidneys.

Improving Bladder Management

The effect of the spinal lesion on the bladder depends on the level of the cord injury, the degree of cord damage, and the length of time after injury. A patient with quadriplegia or paraplegia usually has either a reflex or a nonreflex bladder (see Chap. 10). Both problems increase the risk of urinary tract infection.

The nurse emphasizes the importance of maintaining an adequate flow of urine by encouraging a fluid intake of about 2.5 L daily. The patient should empty the bladder frequently so there is minimal residual urine and should pay attention to personal hygiene, because infection of the bladder and kidneys almost always occurs by the ascending route. The perineum must be kept clean and dry and attention given to the perianal skin after defecation. Underwear should be cotton (more absorbent) and changed at least once a day.

If an external catheter (condom catheter) is used, the sheath is removed nightly; the penis is cleansed to remove urine and is dried carefully, because warm urine on the periurethral skin promotes the growth of bacteria. Attention also is given to the collection bag. The nurse emphasizes the importance of monitoring for indications of urinary tract infection: cloudy, foul-smelling urine or hematuria (blood in the urine), fever, or chills.

The female patient who cannot achieve reflex bladder control or self-catheterization may need to wear pads or waterproof undergarments. Surgical intervention may be necessary to perform a urinary diversion procedure.

Establishing Bowel Control

The objective of a bowel training program is to establish bowel evacuation through reflex conditioning. This technique is described in Chapter 10. If a cord injury occurs above the sacral segments or nerve roots and there is reflex activity, the anal sphincter may be massaged to stimulate defecation. If the cord lesion involves the sacral segment or nerve roots, anal massage is not performed because the anus may be relaxed and lack tone. Massage is also contraindicated if there is spasticity of the anal sphincter. The anal sphincter is massaged by inserting a gloved finger (which has been adequately lubricated) 2.5 to 3.7 cm (1 to 1.5 in) into the rectum and moving it in a circular motion or from side to side. It soon becomes apparent which area triggers the defecation response. This procedure should be performed at the same time (usually every 48 hours), after a meal, and at a time that will be convenient for the patient on returning home. The patient also is taught the symptoms of impaction (frequent loose stools; constipation) and cautioned to watch for the development of hemorrhoids. A diet with sufficient fluids and fiber is essential to a successful bowel training program.

Counseling on Sexual Expression

Many paraplegic and quadriplegic patients can have some form of meaningful sexual relationship, although some modifications will be necessary. The patient and partner benefit from counseling about the range of sexual expression possible, special techniques, positions, exploration of body sensations offering sensual feelings, and urinary and bowel hygiene as related to sexual activity. Penile prostheses are available for men with erectile failure and enable them to have and sustain an erection. Sildenafil (Viagra) is an oral smooth muscle relaxant that causes blood to flow into the penis, resulting in an erection. Although there are side effects and contraindications to sildenafil, many men report satisfaction with its use (Goldstein et al, 1998).

Sexual education and counseling services are included in the rehabilitation services at spinal centers. Small-group meetings in which the patients can share their feelings, receive information, and discuss sexual concerns and practical aspects are helpful in producing effective attitudes and adjustments (Sipski & Alexander, 1997).

Enhancing Coping Mechanisms

The impact of the disability and loss becomes marked when patients return home. Each time something new enters their life (eg, a new relationship, going to work), they are reminded anew of their limitations. Grief reactions and depression frequently are encountered.

To be able to work through this depression, patients must have some hope for relief in the future. Thus, they are guided toward a sense of confidence in their ability to achieve self-care and relative independence. The role of the nurse ranges from caretaker during the acute phase to teacher, counselor, and facilitator as patients gain mobility and independence.

Adjustment to the disability leads to the development of realistic goals for the future, making the best of the abilities that are left intact and reinvesting in other activities and relationships. Rejection of the disability causes self-destructive neglect and noncompliance with the therapeutic program, which leads to more frustration and depression. Crises for which interventions may be sought include social, psychological, marital, sexual, and psychiatric problems. The family usually requires counseling, social services, and other support systems to help them cope with the changes in their lifestyle and socioeconomic status. (The psychological implications of a disability are discussed also in Chap. 10.)

A major goal of nursing management is to help these patients overcome their sense of futility and to encourage them in the emotional adjustment that must be made before they are willing to venture into the outside world. However, an excessively sympathetic attitude on the part of the nurse may cause patients to develop an overdependence that defeats the purpose of the entire rehabilitation program. Patients are taught and assisted when necessary, but the nurse should not try to perform activities that patients can do for themselves with a little effort. This approach to care more than repays itself in the satisfaction of seeing a completely demoralized and helpless patient begin to find meaning in a newly emerging lifestyle.

Monitoring and Managing Potential Complications

SPASTICITY

Muscle spasticity is one of the most problematic complications of quadriplegia and paraplegia. These incapacitating flexor or extensor spasms, which occur below the level of the spinal cord lesion, interfere with both the rehabilitation process and activities of daily living. Spasticity results from an imbalance between the facilatory and inhibitory effects on neurons that exist normally. The area of the cord distal to the site of injury or lesion becomes disconnected from the higher inhibitory centers located in the brain. Facilatory impulses, which originate from muscles, skin, and ligaments, thus predominate.

Spasticity is defined as a condition of increased muscle tone in a muscle that is weak. Initial resistance to stretching is quickly followed by sudden relaxation. The stimulus that precipitates spasm can be either obvious, such as movement or position change, or subtle, such as a slight jarring of the wheelchair. Most patients with quadriplegia or paraplegia have some degree of spasticity. With SCI, the onset of spasticity usually occurs from a few weeks to 6 months after the injury. The same muscles that are flaccid during the period of spinal shock will develop spasticity during recovery. The intensity of spasticity tends to peak around 2 years after the injury, after which the spasms tend to regress.

Management of spasticity is based on the severity of symptoms and the degree of incapacitation. Antispamodic medications such as diazepam (Valium), baclofen (Lioresal), and dantrolene (Dantrium) are frequently effective in controlling spasm but cause drowsiness, weakness, and vertigo in some patients. Passive range-of-motion exercises and frequent turning and repositioning are helpful because stiffness tends to increase spasticity. These activities also are essential in the prevention of contractures, pressure ulcers, and bowel and bladder dysfunction. The major problems that complicate day-to-day care are the difficulty with positioning and the lack of mobility. A number of surgical procedures have been tried with varying degrees of success. These techniques are used if more conservative approaches fail.

INFECTION AND SEPSIS

Quadriplegic and paraplegic patients are at increased risk for infection and sepsis from a variety of sources: urinary tract, respiratory tract, and pressure ulcers. Sepsis remains a major cause of death and complications in these patients. Prevention of infection and sepsis is essential through maintenance of skin integrity, complete emptying of the bladder at regular intervals, and prevention of urinary and fecal incontinence. The risk of respiratory infection can be decreased by avoiding contact with people with symptoms of respiratory infection, performing coughing and deep-breathing exercises to prevent pooling of respiratory secretions, receiving yearly prophylactic influenza vaccines, and giving up smoking. A high-protein diet is important in maintaining an adequate immune system, as is avoiding factors that may reduce immune system function (eg, excessive stress, drug abuse, excessive alcohol intake).

If infection occurs, the quadriplegic or paraplegic patient requires thorough assessment and prompt treatment. Antibiotic therapy and adequate hydration, in addition to local measures (depending on the site of infection), are initiated immediately. Urinary tract infections are minimized or prevented by:

- Aseptic technique in catheter management
- Adequate hydration
- Bladder training program
- Prevention of overdistention of the bladder and stasis

Skin breakdown and infection are prevented by:

- Maintenance of a turning schedule
- Frequent back care
- Regular assessment of all skin areas
- Regular cleansing and lubrication of the skin
- Pressure relief, particularly over broken skin areas, bony prominences, and heels
- Wrinkle-free bed linen

Pulmonary infections are managed and prevented by:

- Frequent coughing, turning, and deep-breathing exercises and chest physiotherapy
- Aggressive respiratory care and suctioning of the airway if a tracheostomy is present
- Assisted coughing
- Adequate hydration

Infections of any kind can be life-threatening. Therefore, aggressive nursing interventions are key to their prevention and management.

Promoting Home and Community-Based Care

TEACHING PATIENTS SELF-CARE

Patients with quadriplegia or paraplegia are at risk for complications for the rest of their lives. Thus, a major aspect of nursing care is teaching patients and their families about these complications and about strategies to minimize this risk. Urinary tract infections, contractures, infected pressure ulcers, and sepsis may necessitate hospitalization. Other late complications that may occur include lower extremity edema, joint contractures, respiratory problems, and pain. To avoid these and other complications, the patient and a family member are taught skin care, catheter care, range-of-motion exercises, breathing exercises, and other care techniques. Teaching is initiated as soon as possible and extends into the rehabilitation or long-term care facility and home.

CONTINUING CARE

Referral for home care is often appropriate for assessment of the home setting, patient teaching, and evaluation of the patient's physical and emotional status. During visits by the home care nurse, teaching about strategies to prevent or minimize potential complications is reinforced. The home environment is assessed for adequacy for care and for safety. Environmental modifications are made and specialized equipment is obtained (ideally before the patient goes home).

The home care nurse also assesses the patient's and the family's adherence to recommendations and their use of coping strategies. The use of inappropriate coping strategies such as drug and alcohol use is assessed, and referral to counseling is made for the patient and family. Appropriate and effective coping strategies are reinforced. The nurse reviews previous teaching and determines the need for further physical or psychological assistance. The patient's self-esteem and body image may be very poor at this time. Because people with high levels of social support often report feelings of well-being despite major physical disability, it is beneficial for the nurse to assess and promote further development of the support system and effective coping strategies of each patient.

The patient requires continuing, life-long follow-up by the physician, physical therapist, and other rehabilitation team members because the neurologic deficit is usually permanent and new problems can develop. These problems require prompt attention before they take their toll in additional physical impairment, time, morale, and financial costs. The local counselor for the Office of Vocational Rehabilitation works with the patient with respect to job placement or additional educational or vocational training.

Evaluation

Expected Outcomes

Expected outcomes may include:

1. Attains some form of mobility
2. Maintains healthy, intact skin
3. Achieves bladder control, absence of urinary tract infection
4. Achieves bowel control
5. Reports sexual satisfaction
6. Shows improved adaptation to environment and others
7. Exhibits reduction in spasticity
   a. Reports understanding of the precipitating factors
   b. Reports understanding of measures to reduce spasticity
8. Describes long-term management required
9. Exhibits absence of complications

Critical Thinking Exercises

1. A patient has been brought to the emergency department after a fall on his head at work. He says he was knocked out for about 10 minutes but now seems alert and oriented. What type of injury has he most likely sustained? What discharge instructions are warranted for this patient's family? How would you modify your discharge instructions if the patient lives alone?

2. A patient with a T4 SCI has just returned to the nursing unit from physical therapy. He reports a severe, pounding headache and nausea. His blood pressure is very elevated and his pulse rate is slow. What are the possible causes of these signs and symptoms? What immediate actions should you take? What medical treatments can you anticipate? What teaching is warranted, and why?

References and Selected Readings

BOOKS

Cammermeyer, M., & Appledorn, C. (Eds.). (1996). *Core curriculum for neuroscience nurses* (4th ed.). Chicago: American Association of Neuroscience Nurses.

Cardona, V. (1994). *Trauma nursing: From resuscitation through rehabilitation.* Philadelphia: W. B. Saunders.

Consortium for Spinal Cord Medicine. (1998). *Neurogenic bowel management in adults with spinal cord injury.* Clinical Practice Guidelines, Paralyzed Veterans of America, Washington, D.C.

Greenberg, M. S. (1994). *Handbook of neurosurgery* (3rd ed.). Lakeland, FL: Greenberg Graphics.

Hickey, J. V. (1997). *The clinical practice of neurological and neurosurgical nursing* (4th ed.). Philadelphia: Lippincott-Raven.

Kaye, A. (1997). *Essential neurosurgery* (2nd ed.). New York: Churchill Livingstone.

Porth, C. M. (1998). *Pathophysiology concepts of altered health states* (5th ed.). Philadelphia: Lippincott-Raven.

Ropper, A. (Ed.). (1993). *Neurological and neurosurgical intensive care* (3rd ed.). New York: Raven.

Sipski, M. L., & Alexander, C. J. (1997). *Sexual function in people with disability and chronic illness: A health professional's guide.* Gaithersburg, MD: Aspen.

Young, G. B., Ropper, A. H., & Bolton, C. F. (1993). *Coma and impaired consciousness: A clinical perspective.* New York: McGraw-Hill.

JOURNALS

Asterisks indicate nursing research articles.

Atterbury, J. L., & Groome, L. J. (1998). Pregnancy in women with spinal cord injuries. *Nursing Clinics of North America, 33*(4), 603–613.

Bullock, R. (1995). Mannitol and other diuretics in severe neurotrauma. *New Horizons, 3*(3), 448–452.

Chesnut, R. M. (1995). Secondary brain insults after head injury: Clinical perspectives. *New Horizons, 3*(3), 366–375.

Clifton, G. L. (1995). Hypothermia and hyperbaric oxygen as treatment modalities for severe head injury. *New Horizons, 3*(3), 474–477.

Davis, A. E., & White, J. J. (1995). Innovative sensory input for the comatose brain-injured patient. *Critical Care Nursing Clinics of North America, 7*(2), 351–361.

Dibsie, L. G. (1998). Clearing cervical spine injuries: A discussion of the process and the problems. *Critical Care Nursing Quarterly, 21*(2), 36–41.

Duff, D. L., & Wells, D. L. (1997). Postcomatose unawareness/vegetative state following severe brain injury: A content methodology. *Journal of Neuroscience Nursing, 29*(5), 305–317.

*Faragi, B., & Yu, P. (1998). Serum phenytoin levels of patients on gastrostomy tube feeding. *Journal of Neuroscience Nursing, 30*(1), 55–59.

Farmer, J. C., et al. (1998). Neurologic deterioration after cervical spinal cord injury. *Journal of Spinal Disorders, 11*(3), 192–196.

Farmer, J. C., et al. (1998). The changing nature of admissions to a spinal cord injury center: Violence on the rise. *Journal of Spinal Disorders, 11*(5), 400–403.

Geraci, E. B., & Geraci, T. A. (1996). Hyperventilation and head injury: Controversies and concerns. *Journal of Neuroscience Nursing, 28*(6), 381–387.

Goldstein, I., et al. (1998). Oral sildenafil in the treatment of erectile dysfunction. *New England Journal of Medicine, 338*(20), 1397–1404.

Grzankowski, J. A. (1997). Altered thought processes related to traumatic brain injury and their nursing implications. *Rehabilitation Nursing, 22*(1), 24–31.

Halbert, L. A. (1998). Breastfeeding in the woman with a compromised nervous system. *Journal of Human Lactation, 14*(4), 327–331.

Huston, C. J. (1998). Cervical spine injury. *American Journal of Nursing, 98*(6), 33.

Johnson, R. L., et al. (1998). Secondary conditions following spinal cord injury in a population-based sample. *Spinal Cord, 36*(1), 45–50.

Kannisto, M., et al. (1998). Comparison of health-related quality of life in three subgroups of spinal cord injury patients. *Spinal Cord, 36*(3), 193–199.

Lucke, K. T. (1998). Pulmonary management following acute SCI. *Journal of Neuroscience Nursing, 30*(2), 91–104.

National Institutes of Health. (1998). Consensus statement: Rehabilitation of persons with traumatic brain injury. October 26–28, 1998.

Nolan, M., & Nolan, J. (1998). Rehabilitation following spinal injury: The nursing response. *British Journal of Nursing, 7*(2), 97–104.

Patyk, M., Gaynor, S., Kelly, J., & Ott, V. (1998). Touch screen computerized education for patients with brain injuries. *Rehabilitation Nursing, 23*(2), 34–87.

Peik, J. (1995). Medical complications in severe head injury. *New Horizons, 3*(3), 534–538.

*Prieto-Fingerhut, T., Banovac, K., & Lynne, C. M. (1997). A study comparing sterile and nonsterile urethral catheterization in patients with spinal cord injury. *Rehabilitation Nursing, 22*(6), 299–302.

Richmond, T. S. (1997). Cerebral resuscitation after global brain ischemia: Linking research to practice. *AACN Clinical Issues, 8*(2), 171–181.

Shackelford, M., Farley, T., & Vines, C. L. (1998). A comparison of women and men with spinal cord injury. *Spinal Cord, 36*(5), 337–339.

*Simmons, B. J. (1997). Management of intracranial hemodynamics in the adult: A research analysis of head positioning and recommendations for clinical practice and future research. *Journal of Neuroscience Nursing, 29*(1), 44–49.

Travers, P. L. (1999). Autonomic dysreflexia: A clinical rehabilitation problem. *Rehabilitation Nursing, 24*(1), 19–23.

Wilberger, J. E., & Cantella, D. (1995). High-dose barbiturates for intracranial pressure control. *New Horizons, 3*(3), 469–473.

Yu, D. (1998). A crash course in spinal cord injury. *Postgraduate Medicine, 104*(2), 109–110, 113–116, 119–122.

Resources

American Association of Neuroscience Nurses (AANN), 218 N. Jefferson St., #204, Chicago, IL 60606; (312) 993-0043; www.aann.org

American Association of Spinal Cord Injury Nurses (AASCIN), 75-20 Astoria Blvd., Jackson Heights, NY 11370-1177; (718) 803-3782

American Paralysis/Spinal Cord Hotline, (800) 526-3456

Association of Rehabilitation Nurses, 5700 Old Orchard Rd., Skokie, IL 60077; (708) 966-8673

The Brain Injury Association, 105 N. Alfred St., Alexandria, VA 22314; (703) 236-6000; www.biausa.org; family helpline: 800-444-6443

Independent Living for the Handicapped, 1301 Belmont St., NW, Washington, DC 20009; (202) 797-9803

Information Center for Individuals with Disabilities, Fort Point Place, 27-43 Wormwood St., Boston, MA 02210-1606; (617) 727-5540

The Library of Congress, Division of the Blind and Physically Handicapped, 1291 Taylor St., NW, Washington, DC 20542; (202) 707-5100

National Head Injury Foundation, 1776 Massachusetts Ave., NW, Suite 100, Washington, DC 20036; family helpline (800) 444-6443

National Rehabilitation Information Center, 8455 Colesville Rd., Suite 935, Silver Spring, MD 20910; (301) 588-9284

National Spinal Cord Injury Association, 8300 Colesville Rd., Silver Spring, MD 20910; (301) 588-6959; www.spinalcord.org

Paralyzed Veterans of America, 801 18th St., NW, Washington, DC 20006; (202) 872-1300; www.pva.org

Rehabilitation Services Administration Department of Human Services, Room 101M, 605 G St., NW, Washington, DC 20001; (202) 727-3211

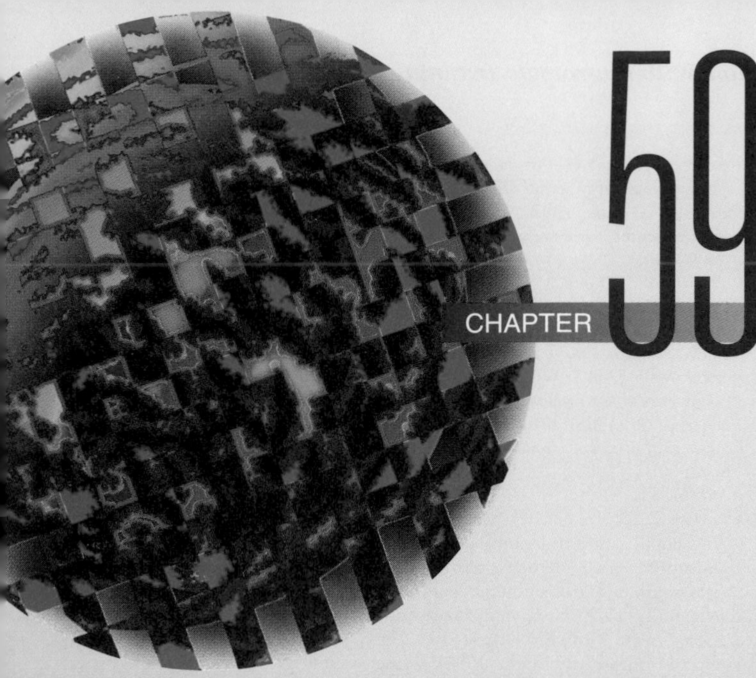

Management of Patients With Neurologic Disorders

Learning Objectives

On completion of this chapter, the learner will be able to:

1. Compare the various types and causes of headaches.
2. Use the nursing process as a framework for care of patients with migraine headaches.
3. Describe brain tumors: their classification, clinical manifestations, diagnosis, and management.
4. Use the nursing process as a framework for care of patients with cerebral metastases or inoperable brain tumors.
5. Describe subarachnoid precautions and their application to the patient with a cerebral aneurysm.
6. Use the nursing process as a framework for care of patients with multiple sclerosis.
7. Use the nursing process as a framework for care of patients with Parkinson's disease.
8. Compare myasthenia gravis, amyotrophic lateral sclerosis, and muscular dystrophy: their pathophysiology, clinical manifestations, and nursing and medical management.
9. Describe disorders of the cranial nerves, their manifestations and indicated nursing interventions.

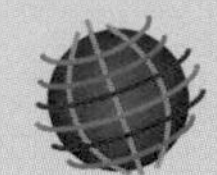

Although some neurologic disorders may be self-limiting and cause mild inconvenience, many are acute or chronic disorders that may or may not be progressive. Those that are acute may be life-threatening and may result in a variety of long-term rehabilitation needs. Neurologic disorders that have a progressive course require that the patient and family be well informed about the disorder and the requisite care that will be needed to maintain the patient's maximum level of independence and quality of life. The nurse who cares for patients with neurologic disorders must have an understanding of the neurologic system and the consequences of neurologic dysfunction to anticipate and prevent problems when possible.

GLOSSARY

akathisia: restlessness, urgent need to move around, and agitation

ataxia: impaired ability to coordinate movement, often seen as a staggering gait or postural imbalance

bradykinesia: very slow voluntary movements and speech

chorea: rapid, jerky, involuntary, purposeless movements of the extremities or facial muscles, including facial grimacing

dementia: a progressive organic mental disorder characterized by personality changes, confusion, disorientation, and deterioration of intellect associated with impaired memory and judgement

diplopia: double vision or the awareness of two images of the same object occurring in one or both eyes

dysarthria: speech that is difficult or defective and poorly articulated because of impaired muscles that control speech (content and meaning of words remain normal)

dyskinesia: impaired ability to execute voluntary movements

dysphagia: difficulty swallowing, causing the patient to be at risk for aspiration

dysphonia: abnormal voice quality caused by weakness and incoordination of muscles responsible for speech.

homonymous hemianopsia: blindness in the right or left halves of the visual fields of both eyes

Korsakoff's syndrome: personality disorder characterized by psychosis, disorientation, delirium, insomnia, and hallucinations

micrographia: very minute and often illegible handwriting

myoclonus: spasms of a single muscle or group of muscles

neurodegenerative: a disease, process, or condition that leads to deterioration of normal cells or function of the nervous system

neurotransmitter: a chemical that is released when the axon of a presynaptic neuron is excited; examples—acetylcholine, norepinephrine, dopamine

nystagmus: rhythmic, involuntary movements or oscillations of the eyes

paresthesia: a sensation of numbness, tingling, or a "pins and needles" sensation

positron emission topography (PET): a computerized radiographic technique that uses radioactive substances to examine the metabolic activity of body structures

radiculopathy: disease of a spinal nerve root often resulting in pain and extreme sensitivity to touch

sciatica: inflammation of the sciatic nerve resulting in pain and tenderness along the nerve through the thigh and leg

scotoma: a defect in vision in a specific area in one or both eyes

spasticity: muscular hypertonicity with increased resistance to stretch often associated with weakness, increased deep tendon reflexes, and diminished superficial reflexes

spondylosis: degenerative arthritis or osteoarthritis of the cervical or lumbar vertebrae resulting in stiffness of the vertebral joint

spongiform: having the appearance or quality of a sponge, as in Creutzfeldt-Jacob disease, that is characterized by small holes in the gray matter of the brain, leading to severe dementia and myoclonus

HEADACHE

Headache, or cephalgia, is one of the most common of all human physical complaints. Headache is actually a symptom rather than a disease entity and may indicate organic disease (neurologic or other disease), a stress response, vasodilation (migraine), skeletal muscle tension (tension headache), or a combination of the above. A primary headache is one for which no organic cause can be identified; these types of headache include migraine, tension-type, and cluster headaches. A secondary headache is workload associated with organic causes, such as a brain tumor or aneurysm. Most headaches do not indicate serious disease, although persistent headaches require further investigation. Serious disorders related to headache include brain tumors, severe hypertension, meningitis, and head injuries.

Diagnostic testing is not often helpful in the investigation of headache, and there are often few pathophysiologic findings. In addition, headaches may manifest differently within an individual over the course of a lifetime, and the same type of headache may present differently from patient to patient. Still in use, a classification of headaches was issued by the Headache Classification Committee of the International Headache Society in 1988; an abbreviated list is provided in Chart 59-1.

Assessment and Diagnostic Evaluation

The diagnostic evaluation includes a detailed history, a physical assessment of the head and neck, and a complete neurologic examination. The health history focuses on assessing the headache itself, with particular emphasis on the factors that precipitate or provoke the headache. Patients are asked to describe their headaches in their own words.

Because headache often can be the presenting symptom of various physiologic and psychological disturbances, a *general health history* is an essential component of the patient database. Headache may be a symptom of endocrine, hematologic, gastrointestinal, infectious, renal, cardiovascular, or psychiatric disease. Therefore, general review questions should cover major medical and surgical illness as well as a body systems review.

CHART 59•1 International Headache Society Classification of Headache

1. Migraine
2. Tension-type headache
3. Cluster headache and chronic paroxysmal hemicrania
4. Miscellaneous headaches unassociated with structural lesion
5. Headache associated with head trauma
6. Headache associated with vascular disorders
7. Headache associated with nonvascular intracranial disorder
8. Headache associated with substances or their withdrawal
9. Headache associated with noncephalic infection
10. Headache associated with metabolic disorder
11. Headache or facial pain associated with disorder of cranium, neck, eyes, ears, nose, sinuses, teeth, mouth or other facial or cranial structures
12. Cranial neuralgias, nerve trunk pain, and deafferentation pain
13. Headache not classifiable

* Headache classification committee of the International Headache Society. (1988). Classification and diagnostic criteria for headache disorders, cranial neuralgias and facial pain. *Cephalalgia, 8* (Suppl. 7), 13–17.

The patient's *medication history* can provide insight into the overall health status. Antihypertensives, such as hydralazine, diuretics, anti-inflammatory agents, and monoamine oxidase inhibitors, are a few of the categories of medications that can provoke headaches. Although sometimes exaggerated in importance, emotional factors can play a role in precipitating many headaches. Stress is thought to be a major initiating factor in migraine headaches; therefore, sleep patterns, level of stress, recreational interests, appetite, emotional problems, and family stressors are relevant. Additionally, there is a strong familial tendency for headache disorders, and a positive family history may help in making a diagnosis.

A direct relationship may exist between exposure to toxic substances and headache. Careful questioning may uncover chemicals to which a worker has been exposed. Under the Right to Know law, employees have access to the Material Safety Data Sheets for all the substances with which they come in contact in the workplace. The occupational history also includes assessment of the workplace as a possible source of stress and of whether there is an ergonomic basis for muscle strain.

A complete *description of the headache* itself is crucial. The patient's age at onset of headache; its frequency, location, and duration; the type of pain; factors that relieve and precipitate the event; and associated symptoms are reviewed. The data obtained should reflect the patient's own words about the headache as described in response to the following questions:

- What is the location? Is it unilateral or bilateral? Does it radiate?
- What is the quality—dull, aching, steady, boring, burning, intermittent, continuous, paroxysmal?
- How many headaches occur during a given time?
- What are the precipitating factors, if any (environmental, such as sunlight and weather change; foods; exertion; other)?
- What makes the headache worse (coughing, straining)?
- What time (day or night) does it occur?
- Are there any associated symptoms, such as facial pain, lacrimation (excessive tearing), or **scotomas** (blind spots in the field of vision)?
- What usually relieves the headache (aspirin, ergot preparation, food, heat, rest, neck massage)?
- Does nausea, vomiting, weakness, or numbness in the extremities accompany the headache?
- Does the headache interfere with daily activities?
- Do you have any allergies?
- Do you have insomnia, poor appetite, loss of energy?
- Is there a family history of headache? "Sick" headache?
- What is the relationship of the headache to lifestyle or physical or emotional stress?
- What medications are you taking?

For patients who demonstrate abnormalities on the neurologic examination, computed tomography (CT), cerebral angiography, or magnetic resonance imaging (MRI) may be used to detect underlying causes, such as tumor or aneurysm. Electromyography (EMG) may reveal a sustained contraction of the neck, scalp, or facial muscles. Laboratory tests may include complete blood count, erythrocyte sedimentation rate, electrolytes, glucose, creatinine, and thyroid panel.

Migraine

Migraine is a symptom complex characterized by periodic and recurrent attacks of severe headache. The cause of migraine has not been clearly demonstrated, but it is primarily a vascular disturbance that occurs more commonly in women and has a strong familial tendency. The typical time of onset is puberty, and the incidence is highest in adults 20 to 35 years of age. There are seven subtypes of migraine, including migraine with and without aura. Most patients have migraine without an aura.

Pathophysiology

The cerebral signs and symptoms of migraine result from varying degrees of cortical ischemia. Abnormal metabolism of serotonin, a vasoactive **neurotransmitter** found in platelets and cells of the brain, plays a major role. The headache is preceded by a rise in plasma serotonin, which dilates the extracranial carotid artery and constricts the intracranial carotid artery, affecting the arteries of the scalp and certain cerebral or retinal vessels. Studies suggest the dilated artery becomes hyperpermeable, and sterile local inflammatory reactions occur in the vicinity of the painful, dilated arteries. This process is followed by a fall in plasma serotonin and a pulsating, throbbing pain.

Headaches can be triggered by menstrual cycles, bright lights, stress, depression, sleep deprivation, fatigue, overuse of certain medications, and certain foods containing tyramine, monosodium glutamate, nitrites, or milk products. Foods in these categories include aged cheese and many processed foods. Oral contraceptives may be associated with increased frequency and severity of attacks in some women.

Clinical Manifestations

The headache often begins in the early hours of the morning, resulting in a headache on awakening, but it can occur at any time. The migraine with aura can be divided into four phases: prodrome, aura, the headache, and recovery (headache termination and postdrome).

PRODROME

The prodrome phase is experienced by 60% of patients with symptoms that occur hours to days before a migraine headache. Symptoms include depression, irritability, feeling cold, food cravings, anorexia, change in activity level, increased urination, diarrhea, or constipation. Patients usually experience the same prodrome with each migraine headache.

AURA PHASE

Aura occurs in about 20% of patients who have migraines. The aura usually lasts less than an hour and may provide enough time for the patient to take the prescribed medication to avert a full-blown attack (described in a later section). This period is characterized by focal neurologic symptoms. Visual disturbances (ie, light flashes and bright spots) are common and may be hemianopic (affect one half of the visual field). Other symptoms that may follow include numbness and tingling of the lips, face, or hands; mild confusion; slight weakness of an extremity; drowsiness; and dizziness.

This period of aura corresponds to the painless vasoconstriction that is the initial physiologic change characteristic of classic migraine. Cerebral blood flow studies performed during migraine headaches demonstrate that during all phases of the attack, cerebral blood flow is reduced throughout the brain, with subsequent loss of autoregulation and impaired CO_2 responsiveness.

HEADACHE PHASE

As vasodilation and a decline in serotonin levels occur, a throbbing headache (unilateral in 60% of patients) intensifies over several hours. This headache is severe and incapacitating and is often associated with photophobia, nausea, and vomiting. Its duration varies, ranging from 4 to 72 hours.

RECOVERY PHASE

In the recovery phase (termination and postdrome), the pain gradually subsides. Muscle contraction in the neck and scalp is common with associated muscle ache and localized tenderness, exhaustion, and mood changes. Any physical exertion exacerbates the headache pain. During this postheadache phase, patients may sleep for extended periods.

Prevention

Preventive medical management of migraine employs the daily use of one or more agents that are thought to block the physiologic events leading to an attack. Medication therapy is carried out at intervals of 3 to 6 months and is gradually tapered because natural remissions of migraine do occur. Treatment regimens vary greatly, as do patient responses; thus, close monitoring is indicated.

The most widely used medication for the prevention of migraine is propranolol (Inderal). Beta-blocking agents, such as propranolol, inhibit the action of beta-receptors—cells in the heart and brain that control the dilation of blood vessels. This is thought to be a major reason for their antimigraine action.

Calcium antagonists (verapamil HCl) are frequently used but may require several weeks at a therapeutic dosage before improvement is noted. Calcium-channel blockers are not as well established as beta-blockers for prevention but may be more appropriate for some patients, such as those with bradycardia, diabetes mellitus, or asthma.

Methysergide (Sansert) is an prophylactic agent effective in preventing frequent and severe migraine attacks; before the widespread use of propranolol in migraine prevention, it was the medication of choice. It is thought to inhibit or block the effects of serotonin. Troublesome side effects include abdominal discomfort, muscle cramps, edema, numbness, tingling of extremities, and depression. There should be a medication-free interval of at least 1 to 2 months after every 6-month course of treatment because of the potential complications of retroperitoneal, pleuropulmonary, and cardiac fibrosis.

Anticonvulsants, such as divalproex sodium (Depakote), are effective in treating some patients with frequent disabling migraines. Numerous side effects may occur and include, nausea, constipation, stomatitis, and hepatic failure. Liver function should be monitored regularly.

Additional pharmacotherapy includes the use of antidepressants, barbiturates, and tranquilizers. These medications should be used cautiously and only on a short-term basis because of the risk of drug dependence.

Medical Management

Therapy for migraine headache is divided into abortive (symptomatic) and preventive approaches. The abortive approach is best employed in patients who suffer frequent attacks and is aimed at relieving or limiting a headache at the onset or while it is in progress. The preventive approach is used in patients who experience frequent attacks at regular or predictable intervals and may have medical conditions that preclude the use of abortive therapies.

Serotonin receptor agonists are the most specific antimigraine agents available. These agents cause vasoconstriction, reduce inflammation, and may reduce pain transmission. Available agonists include ergotamine, sumatriptan, and dihydroergotamine (DHE). Numerous serotonin receptor agonists are under study.

Ergotamine preparations (taken orally, sublingually, subcutaneously, intramuscularly, by rectum, or by inhalation) may be effective in aborting the headache if taken early in the migraine process. Ergotamine tartrate acts on smooth muscle, causing prolonged constriction of the cranial blood vessels. Each patient's dosage is based on individual needs. Side effects include aching muscles, **paresthesias** (numbness and tingling), nausea, and vomiting. Cafergot, a combination of ergotamine and caffeine, can arrest or reduce the severity of the headache in 90% of migraine sufferers, especially if administered early.

Sumatriptan succinate (Imitrex) is available in oral, intranasal, and subcutaneous preparations and is used for the treatment of acute migraine and cluster headaches. The subcutaneous form usually relieves symptoms within an hour and is available in an autoinjector for immediate patient use. Sumatriptan has been found to be significantly more effective than oral Cafergot in relieving moderate to severe migraines in a large number of patients. Sumatriptan may cause chest pain and is contraindicated in patients with ischemic heart disease. Careful administration and dosing instruction to patients is important to prevent adverse reactions, such as increased blood pressure, drowsiness, muscle pain, sweating, and anxiety.

DHE is available in intramuscular and intravenous forms; an intranasal form is also available. Advantages of DHE include less arterial constriction and less nausea than occur with ergotamine. DHE is highly effective in prolonged migraine attacks that last more than 72 hours. DHE is contraindicated in patients with coronary and peripheral vascular disease.

Researchers have found evidence that lidocaine in nosedrop form, used to treat cluster headaches for many years, may be effective in treating migraines. Intranasal lidocaine has a rapid onset of 5 to 15 minutes. Minor side effects include irritation of the nasal passages (Maizels et al., 1996).

During the acute attack, the patient may find relief by lying quietly in a darkened room with the head slightly elevated. Drinking black coffee also may be helpful in some patients. Symptomatic therapy for migraines includes analgesics, sedatives, antianxiety agents, and antiemetics.

Nursing Management

When migraine headache has been diagnosed, the goals of nursing management are to administer medications to treat the acute event of the headache and to prevent recurrent episodes. Prevention involves patient education regarding precipitating factors, possible lifestyle or habit changes that may be helpful, and pharmacologic measures.

RELIEVING PAIN

Nursing care is directed toward treatment of the acute episode. A migraine headache in the early phase requires abortive medication therapy instituted as soon as possible. Some headaches may actually be prevented if the appropriate medications are taken before the onset of pain. Nursing care during a fully developed attack includes comfort measures, such as a quiet, dark environment and elevation of the head of the bed 30 degrees. In addition, symptomatic treatment, such as antiemetics, may be indicated.

PROMOTING HOME AND COMMUNITY-BASED CARE

Teaching Patients Self-Care. Although there is a wide variation in the personality types of those who are subject to migraine, there is some evidence that the hard-driving, somewhat compulsive perfectionist is most vulnerable to this condition. Migraine headaches are likely to occur when a person is ill, overtired, or feeling stressed. Instruction about the importance of proper diet, adequate rest, and coping strategies may help the patient deal with stress. Identifying circumstances that precipitate headaches and assisting the patient in the development of alternate means of coping should be part of the teaching plan.

Patients can be helped to develop insight into their feelings, behavior, and conflicts and to make the necessary modifications in lifestyle on the basis of these analyses. Regular periods of exercise and relaxation are suggested, and any offending or provoking factors (allergens, fatigue, foods, environmental stresses) are removed or reduced to obtain relief.

Continuing Care. The National Headache Foundation (see Resources at end of the chapter) provides a list of clinics in the United States and the names of physicians who specialize in headache and who are members of the American Association for the Study of Headache.

Cluster Headache

Cluster headaches are another severe form of vascular headache. They are seen most frequently in men between the ages of 20 and 40 years. The headaches are unilateral and come in clusters of one to eight daily, with excruciating pain localized in the eye and orbit and radiating to the facial and temporal regions. The pain is accompanied by watering of the eye and nasal congestion. Each attack lasts from 15 minutes to 3 hours and may have a crescendo–decrescendo pattern. The headache is often described as penetrating and steady.

The cause of cluster headache is not fully known. One theory is that it is due to dilation of orbital and nearby extracranial arteries. Cluster headaches may be precipitated by alcohol, nitrites, vasodilators, and histamines. Eliminating these factors helps in preventing the headaches. Medication therapy includes tricyclic antidepressants and vasoconstricting agents (ergotamine tartrate, DHE, sumatriptan). The serotonin antagonist methysergide, the beta-blocker propranolol, and calcium-channel blockers may provide relief. The use of lidocaine intranasally on the side of the headache has been reported to relieve pain immediately. It is not known whether this effect is local or a result of direct action on the splenopalatine ganglion.

Cranial Arteritis

Inflammation of the cranial arteries is characterized by a severe headache localized in the region of the temporal arteries. The inflammation may be generalized, in which cranial arteritis is part of a vascular disease, or of a focal type, in which only the cranial arteries are involved. Cranial arteritis is a cause of headache in the older population, reaching its greatest incidence in those older than 70 years of age.

The disease often begins with general manifestations, such as fatigue, malaise, weight loss, and fever. Clinical manifestations associated with inflammation (heat, redness, swelling, tenderness, or pain over the involved artery) usually are present. Sometimes, a tender, swollen, or nodular temporal artery is visible. Visual problems are caused by ischemia of the involved structures.

Cranial arteritis is thought to represent an immune vasculitis in which immune complexes are deposited within the walls of affected blood vessels, producing vascular injury and inflammation. A biopsy may be performed on the involved artery to make the diagnosis.

Treatment consists of early administration of a corticosteroid to prevent the possibility of loss of vision due to vascular occlusion or rupture of the involved artery. The patient is instructed not to stop the medication abruptly because this can lead to relapse. Analgesic agents are given for comfort.

Tension Headache (Muscle Contraction Headache)

Emotional or physical stress may cause contraction of the muscles in the neck and scalp, resulting in tension headache. Most tension headaches are caused by stress. The headache may be characterized by a steady, constant feeling of pressure that usually begins in the forehead, the temple, or the back of the neck. It is often bandlike or may be described as "a weight on top of my head." Tension headaches tend to be more chronic than severe and are probably the most common type of headache. The patient needs reassurance that the headache is not due to a brain tumor. This is a common unspoken fear. Stress reduction techniques, such as biofeedback, exercise programs, and meditation, are examples of nonpharmacologic therapies. Symptomatic relief may be obtained by local heat, massage, analgesics, antidepressants, and muscle relaxants.

HOME CARE TEACHING CHECKLIST: THE PATIENT WITH MIGRAINE HEADACHES

At the completion of the program, the patient or caregiver will be able to:	Patient	Caregiver
• Define migraine headaches and describe characteristics and manifestations.	✔	✔
• Identify triggers of migraine headaches and how to avoid such triggers as:	✔	✔
• Foods that contain tyramine, such as chocolate, cheese, coffee, dairy products		
• Dietary habits that result in long periods between meals		
• Menstruation and ovulation (causes hormone fluctuation)		
• Alcohol (causes vasodilation of blood vessels)		
• Fatigue and fluctuations in sleep patterns		
• State importance of keeping and how to develop a headache diary.	✔	✔
• State stress management and lifestyle changes to minimize the frequency of headaches.	✔	✔
• State pharmacologic management: acute therapy and prophylaxis, to include medication regimen and side effects.	✔	✔
• Identify comfort measures during headache attacks, such as resting in a quiet and dark environment, applying cold compresses to the painful area, and elevating the head.	✔	✔
• Identify resources for education and support, such as the National Headache Foundation.	✔	✔

BRAIN TUMORS

A brain tumor is a localized intracranial lesion that occupies space within the skull. Tumors usually grow as a spherical mass but can grow diffusely, infiltrating tissue. The effect of neoplasms occurs from compression and infiltration of tissue. A variety of physiologic changes result, causing any or all of the following pathophysiologic events:

- Increased intracranial pressure (ICP) and cerebral edema
- Seizure activity and focal neurologic signs
- Hydrocephalus
- Altered pituitary function

Primary brain tumors originate from cells and structures within the brain. Secondary, or metastatic, brain tumors develop from structures outside the brain and occur in 20% to 40% of all cancer patients. Brain tumors rarely metastasize outside of the central nervous system, but metastatic lesions to the brain occur commonly from the lung, breast, lower gastrointestinal tract, pancreas, kidney, and skin (melanomas). The cause of primary brain tumors is unknown. Possible causes include genetics, defective immune system, heredity, viruses, and head injury.

The incidence of brain tumors appears to have increased. Epidemiologic data, however, suggest that this is due to more aggressive and accurate diagnosis rather than an actual rise in incidence. It is estimated that there are more than 17,000 new cases of primary brain tumors and more than 17,000 cases of secondary brain tumors per year (American Cancer Society, 1999). The highest incidence of brain tumors in adults occurs in the fifth, sixth, and seventh decades, with a slightly higher incidence in men. In adults, most brain tumors originate from glial cells (glial cells make up the structure and support system of the brain and spinal cord) and are supratentorial (located above the covering of the cerebellum). Neoplastic lesions in the brain ultimately cause death by impairing vital functions, such as respiration, or by increasing ICP.

Brain tumors may be classified into several groups: those arising from the coverings of the brain (ie, dural meningioma), those developing in or on the cranial nerves (ie, acoustic neuroma), those originating within brain tissue (ie, gliomas), and metastatic lesions originating elsewhere in the body. Tumors of the pituitary and pineal glands and of cerebral blood vessels are also included in the types of brain tumors, as indicated in Chart 59-2. Relevant clinical considerations include the location and the histologic character of the tumor. Tumors may be benign or malignant. A benign tumor can occur in a vital area and can grow large enough to have effects as serious as those of a malignant tumor.

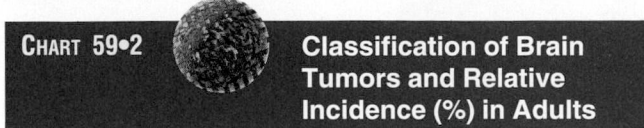

I. Intracerebral tumors
- A. Gliomas—infiltrate any portion of the brain; most common type of brain tumor
  1. Astrocytomas (grades I and II): 10%
  2. Glioblastoma multiforme (astrocytoma grades III and IV): 20%
  3. Oligodendrocytoma (grades I to IV): 5%
  4. Ependymoma (Grades I to IV): 6%
  5. Medulloblastoma: 4%

II. Tumors arising from supporting structures
- A. Meningiomas: 15%
- B. Neuromas (acoustic neuroma, schwannoma): 7%
- C. Pituitary adenomas: 7%

III. Developmental tumors
- A. Angiomas: 4%
- B. Dermoid, epidermoid, teroma, craniopharyngioma: 4%

IV. Metastatic lesions: 10%

Pathophysiology

GLIOMAS

Malignant glioma is the most common brain neoplasm, accounting for about 45% of all brain tumors. Gliomas are graded from I to IV, indicating the degree of malignancy. Grade is based on cellular density, cell mitosis, and appearance. Usually, these tumors spread by infiltrating into the surrounding neural tissue and therefore cannot be totally removed without causing considerable damage to vital structures. Astrocytomas are the most common type of glioma.

PITUITARY ADENOMAS

Pituitary tumors represent about 8% to 12% of all brain tumors and cause symptoms as a result of pressure on adjacent structures or hormonal changes (hyperfunction or hypofunction of the pituitary). The pituitary gland, also called the hypophysis, is a relatively small gland located in the sella turcica. It is attached to the hypothalamus by a short stalk (hypophyseal stalk) and is divided into two lobes: the anterior (adenohypophysis) and the posterior (neurohypophysis).

Pressure Effects of Pituitary Adenomas. Pressure from pituitary adenomas may be exerted on the optic nerves, optic chiasm, or optic tracts or on the hypothalamus or the third ventricle when the tumors invade the cavernous sinuses or expand into the sphenoid bone. These pressure effects produce headache, visual dysfunction, hypothalamic disorders (eg, disorders of sleep, appetite, temperature, emotions), increased ICP, and enlargement and erosion of the sella turcica.

Hormonal Effects of Pituitary Adenomas. Functioning pituitary tumors can produce one or more hormones normally produced by the anterior pituitary. These hormones may cause prolactin-secreting pituitary adenomas (prolactinomas), growth hormone-secreting pituitary adenomas that produce acromegaly in adults, and adrenocorticotropic hormone (ACTH)-producing pituitary adenomas that result in Cushing's disease. Adenomas that secrete thyroid-stimulating hormone or follicle-stimulating hormone and luteinizing hormone occur infrequently, whereas adenomas that produce both growth hormone and prolactin are relatively common.

The female patient whose pituitary gland is secreting excessive quantities of prolactin presents with amenorrhea or galactorrhea (excessive or spontaneous flow of milk). Male patients with prolactinomas may present with impotence and hypogonadism. Acromegaly, caused by excess growth hormone, produces enlargement of the hands and feet, distortion of the facial features, and pressure on peripheral nerves (entrapment syndromes). The clinical features of Cushing's disease, a condition associated with prolonged overproduction of cortisol, occur with excessive production of ACTH. Manifestations include a form of obesity with redistribution of fat to the facial, supraclavicular, and abdominal areas; hypertension; purple striae and ecchymoses; osteoporosis; elevated serum glucose levels; and emotional disorders.

ANGIOMAS

Brain angiomas (masses composed largely of abnormal blood vessels) are found either in or on the surface of the brain. They occur in the cerebellum in 83% of cases. Some persist throughout life without causing symptoms; others cause symptoms of brain tumor. Occasionally, the diagnosis is suggested by the presence of another angioma somewhere in the head or by a bruit (an abnormal sound) audible over the skull. Because the walls of the blood vessels in angiomas are thin, these patients are at risk for a cerebral vascular accident (stroke). In fact, cerebral hemorrhage in people younger than 40 years of age should suggest the possibility of an angioma.

ACOUSTIC NEUROMAS

An acoustic neuroma is a tumor of the eighth cranial nerve, the cranial nerve most responsible for hearing and balance. It usually arises just within the internal auditory meatus, where it frequently expands before filling the cerebellopontine recess.

An acoustic neuroma may grow slowly and attain considerable size before it is correctly diagnosed. The patient usually experiences loss of hearing, tinnitus, and episodes of vertigo and staggering gait. As the tumor becomes larger, painful sensations of the face may occur on the same side as a result of the tumor's compression of the fifth cranial nerve.

With improved imaging techniques and the use of the operating microscope and microsurgical instrumentation, even large tumors can be removed through a relatively small craniotomy. Some of these tumors may be suitable for stereotactic radiotherapy rather than surgery. See the discussion of stereotactic radiotherapy later in this chapter.

MENINGIOMAS

Meningiomas are common benign encapsulated tumors of arachnoid cells on the meninges and represent 15% to 20% of all primary brain tumors. They are slow growing and occur most often in middle-aged adults, more often in women. Meningiomas most often occur in areas proximal to the venous sinuses. Manifestations depend on the area involved and are the result of compression rather than invasion of brain tissue. Standard treatment is surgical with complete removal or partial dissection.

Clinical Manifestations

Brain tumors produce both diffuse clinical manifestations when they cause increased ICP and localized signs and symptoms as a result of the tumor interfering with specific regions of the brain. Figure 59-1 indicates common tumor sites in the brain.

SYMPTOMS OF INCREASING INTRACRANIAL PRESSURE

As discussed in Chapter 57, the skull is a rigid compartment containing essential noncompressible contents: brain matter, intravascular blood, and cerebrospinal fluid (CSF) according to the

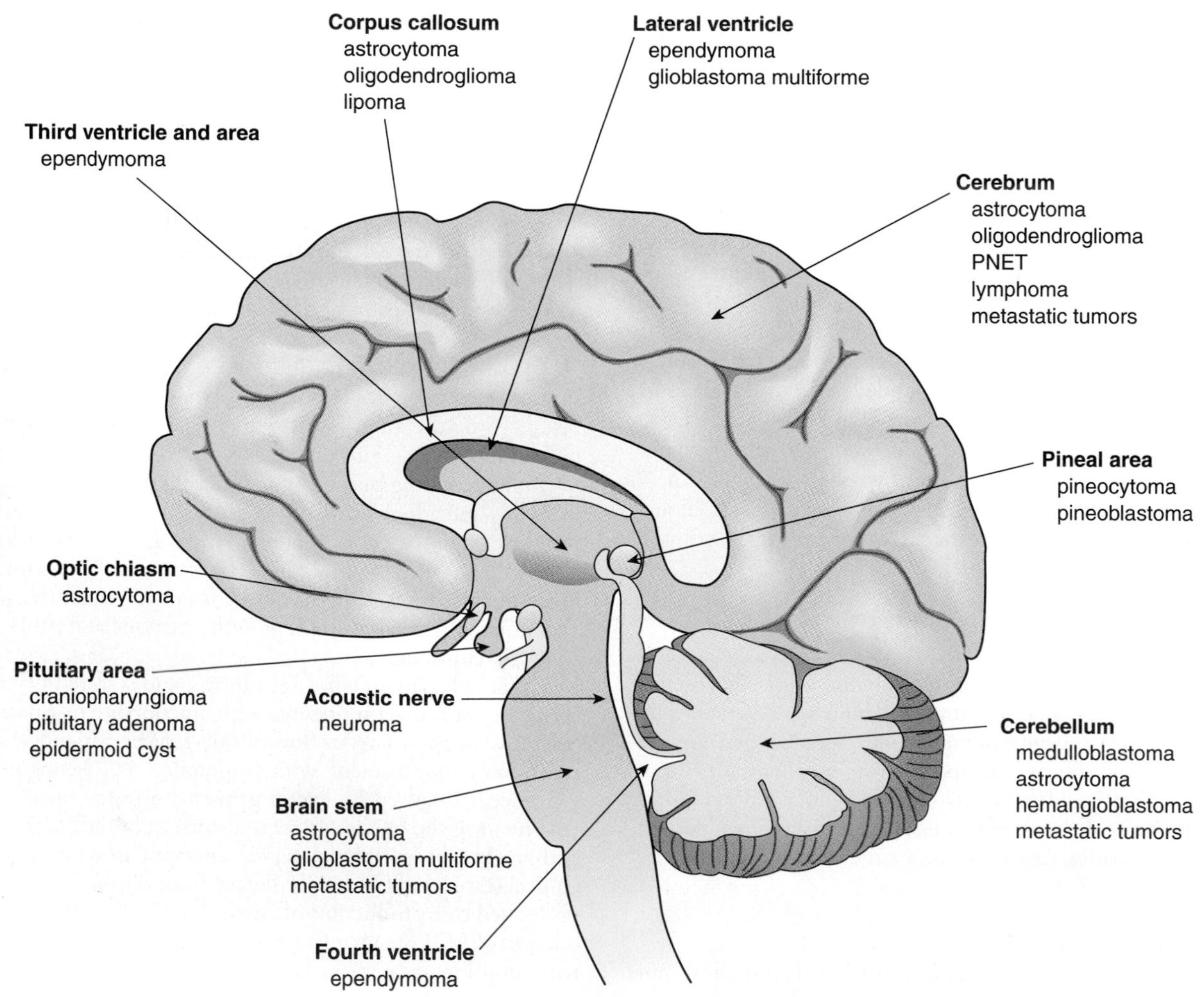

FIGURE 59•1 Common brain tumor sites.

modified Monro-Kellie hypothesis. If any one of these components of the skull increases in volume, ICP increases unless one of the other components decreases in volume. Consequently, any change in volume occupied by the brain—as occurs with disorders such as brain tumor or cerebral edema—produces signs and symptoms of increased ICP.

Symptoms of increased ICP are caused by a gradual compression of the brain by the enlarging tumor. The effect is to disrupt the equilibrium that exists between the brain, the CSF, and the cerebral blood—all located within the skull. As the tumor grows, compensatory adjustments may occur through compression of intracranial veins, through reduction of CSF volume (by increased absorption or decreased production), a modest decrease of cerebral blood flow, and reduction of intracellular and extracellular brain tissue mass. When these compensatory mechanisms fail, the patient develops signs and symptoms of increased ICP.

The three classic signs of increased ICP are headache, vomiting, and papilledema ("choked disc" or edema of the optic nerve). Personality changes and a variety of focal deficits, including motor, sensory, and cranial nerve dysfunction, are also common.

Headache, although not always present, is most common in the early morning and is made worse by coughing, straining, or sudden movement. It is thought to be caused by the tumor invading, compressing, or distorting the pain-sensitive structures or by edema that accompanies the tumor. Headaches are usually described as deep or expanding or as dull but unrelenting. Frontal tumors usually produce a bilateral frontal headache; pituitary gland tumors produce pain radiating between the two temples (bitemporal); in cerebellar tumors, the headache may be located in the suboccipital region at the back of the head.

Vomiting, seldom related to food intake, is usually due to irritation of the vagal centers in the medulla. If the vomiting is of the forceful type, it is described as projectile vomiting.

Papilledema (edema of the optic nerve) is present in 70% to 75% of patients and is associated with visual disturbances such as decreased visual acuity, **diplopia** (double vision), and visual field deficits.

LOCALIZED SYMPTOMS

When specific regions of the brain are disrupted, local signs and symptoms occur, such as sensory and motor abnormalities, visual alterations, alterations in cognition, language disturbances, and seizures. The progression of the signs and symptoms is important because it indicates tumor growth and expansion.

Although some tumors are not easily localized because they lie in so-called silent areas of the brain (ie, areas in which functions are not definitely determined), many tumors can be localized by correlating the signs and symptoms to known areas of the brain, as follows:

- A motor cortex tumor produces seizure-like movements localized on one side of the body, called Jacksonian seizures.
- An occipital lobe tumor produces visual manifestations: contralateral **homonymous hemianopsia** (visual loss in one half of the visual field on the opposite side of the tumor) and visual hallucinations.
- A cerebellar tumor causes dizziness, an ataxic or staggering gait with a tendency to fall toward the side of the lesion, marked muscle incoordination, and **nystagmus** (involuntary rhythmical eye movements), usually in the horizontal direction.
- A frontal lobe tumor frequently produces personality disorders, changes in emotional state and behavior, and a disinterested mental attitude. The patient often becomes extremely untidy and careless and may use obscene language.
- A cerebellopontine angle tumor usually originates in the sheath of the acoustic nerve and gives rise to a characteristic sequence of symptoms. Tinnitus and vertigo appear first, soon followed by progressive nerve deafness (eighth cranial nerve dysfunction). Numbness and tingling of the face and the tongue occur (due to involvement of the fifth cranial nerve). Later, weakness or paralysis of the face develops (seventh cranial nerve involvement). Finally, because the enlarging tumor presses on the cerebellum, abnormalities in motor function may be present.

Assessment and Diagnostic Findings

The history of the illness and the manner in which the symptoms evolved are important in diagnosing brain tumors. A neurologic examination indicates the areas of the central nervous system involved. To assist in the precise localization of the lesion, a battery of tests is performed. CT imaging gives specific information concerning the number, size, and density of the lesions and the extent of secondary cerebral edema. It also provides information about the ventricular system. MRI is helpful in the diagnosis of brain tumors. Its use has resulted in the detection of smaller lesions; it is particularly helpful in detecting tumors in the brain stem and pituitary regions, where bone interferes with CT (Fig. 59-2). Computer-assisted stereotactic (three-dimensional) biopsy is being used to diagnose deep-seated brain tumors and to provide a basis for treatment and prognostic information. Cerebral angiography provides visualization of cerebral blood vessels and can localize most cerebral tumors.

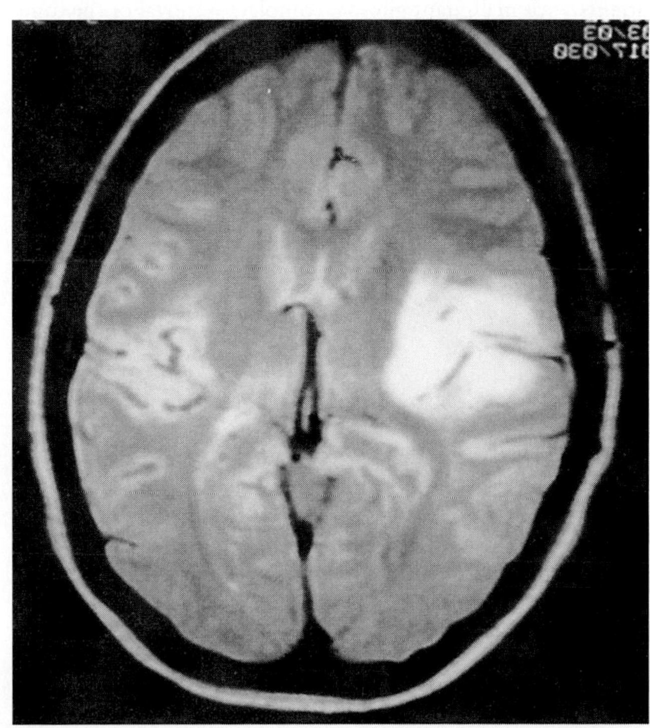

FIGURE 59•2 Low-grade glioma. MRI image of the brain shows a mass of abnormal density in the right temporal lobe. Courtesy of the Hospital of the University of Pennsylvania, Nuclear Medicine Section, Philadelphia, Pennsylvania.

An electroencephalogram (EEG) can detect abnormal brain waves in regions occupied by a tumor and is used to evaluate temporal lobe seizures and assist in ruling out other disorders.

Cytologic studies of the CSF may be performed to detect malignant cells because tumors of the central nervous system are capable of shedding cells into the CSF.

Gerontologic Considerations

Intracranial tumors can produce personality changes, confusion, speech dysfunction, or disturbances of gait, especially in elderly patients. The most frequent tumor types in the elderly are anaplastic astrocytoma, glioblastoma multiforme, and cerebral metastases from other sites. The incidence of primary brain tumors and the likelihood of malignancy increase with age.

Medical Management

The objective is to remove or destroy all of the tumor or as much as possible without increasing the neurologic deficit (paralysis, blindness) or to achieve relief of symptoms by partial removal (decompression). A variety of treatment modalities may be used; the specific approach depends on the type of tumor, its location, and accessibility. In many patients, combinations of these modalities may be used. Most pituitary adenomas are treated by transsphenoidal microsurgical removal (see Chap. 57), whereas the remainder of tumors that cannot be removed completely are treated by radiation. An untreated brain tumor ultimately leads to death, either from increasing ICP or from the brain damage it causes.

Conventional surgical approaches require an incision into the skull (craniotomy). This approach is used in general to cure patients with meningiomas, acoustic neuromas, cystic astrocytomas of the cerebellum, colloid cysts of the third ventricle, congenital tumors such as dermoid cyst, and some of the granulomas. For patients with malignant glioma, complete removal of the tumor and cure are not possible, but the rationale for resection includes relieving intracranial pressure, removing any necrotic tissue, and reducing the bulk of the tumor, which theoretically leaves behind fewer cells to become resistant to radiation or chemotherapy.

Stereotactic approaches involve use of a three-dimensional frame that allows very precise localization of the tumor; a stereotactic frame and multiple imaging studies (x-rays, CT scans) are used to localize the tumor and verify its position (Fig. 59-3). New "brain-mapping" technology helps determine how close diseased areas of the brain are to structures essential for normal brain function. Lasers or radiation can be delivered with stereotactic approaches. Radioisotopes (iodine 131 [^{131}I]) can also be implanted directly into the tumor to deliver high doses of radiation to the tumor (brachytherapy) while minimizing effects on surrounding brain tissue.

The use of the gamma knife to perform "radiosurgery" allows deep, inaccessible tumors to be treated, often in a single session. Precise localization of the tumor is accomplished using the stereotactic approach and by minute measurements and precise positioning of the patient. A very high dose of radiation is then delivered by multiple narrow beams. An advantage of this method is that no surgical incision is needed; a disadvantage is the lag time between treatment and the desired result.

Other treatment modalities include chemotherapy and external-beam radiation therapy, used by themselves or in combination with the approaches described previously. Radiation therapy, the cornerstone of treatment of many brain tumors, also decreases recurrences of incompletely resected tumors. Brachytherapy, the surgical implantation of radiation sources to deliver high doses at a short distance, has had promising results for primary malignancies. It is generally used as an adjunct to conventional radiotherapy or a rescue measure for recurrent disease. Intravenous autologous bone marrow transplantation is used in some patients who will receive chemotherapy or radiation therapy because it has the potential to "rescue" the patient from the bone marrow toxicity associated with high doses of chemotherapy and radiation. A fraction of the patient's bone marrow is aspirated, usually from the iliac crest, and

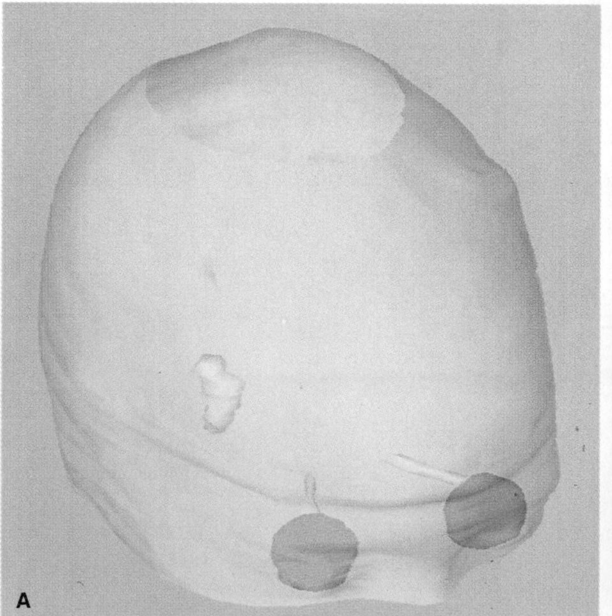

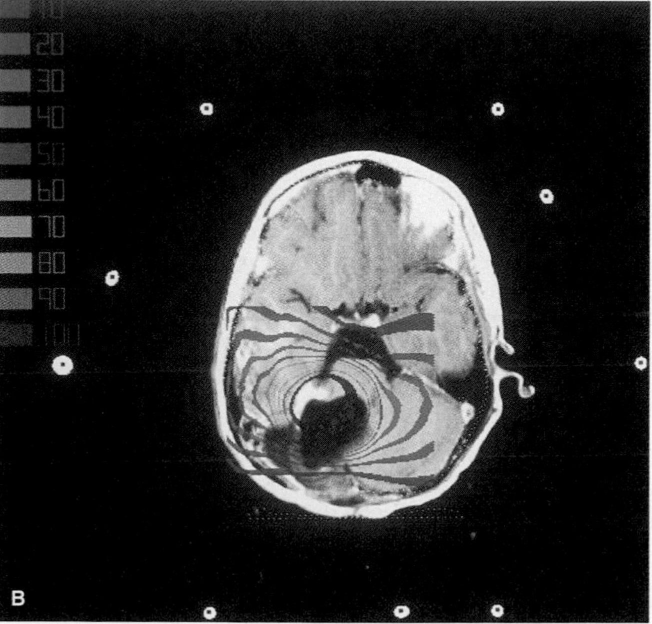

FIGURE 59•3 (**A**) Using stereotactic or "brain-mapping" guided approach, a 3-D computer image fuses the CT and MRI to pinpoint the exact location of the brain tumor. This low-grade astrocytoma is localized adjacent to the brain stem, is nonoperable, and is treated with radiation. Note the optic chasm and optic nerves. (**B**) Computerized image of the prescribed radiation dose.

stored. The patient receives large doses of chemotherapy or radiation therapy to destroy large numbers of malignant cells. The marrow is then reinfused intravenously after treatment is completed. Corticosteroids may be used before treatment to permit a thorough diagnostic evaluation and afterward to reduce cerebral edema and promote a smoother, more rapid recovery. Gene-transfer therapy uses retroviral vectors to carry genes to the tumor, reprogramming the tumor tissue for susceptibility to treatment. This approach is currently being tested.

Nursing Management

The patient with a brain tumor may have problems with aspiration related to cranial nerve dysfunction. Preoperatively, the gag reflex and ability to swallow are evaluated. If there is a diminished gag response, care includes teaching the patient to direct food and fluids toward the unaffected side, having the patient sit upright to eat, offering a semisoft diet, and having suction readily available. Function should be reassessed postoperatively because changes can occur.

The problems of increased ICP caused by the tumor mass are reviewed in Chapter 57. The nurse performs neurologic checks, monitors vital signs, maintains a neurologic flow chart, spaces nursing interventions to prevent rapid increase in ICP, and reorients the patient when necessary to person, time, and place. Patients with changes in cognition caused by the lesion require frequent reorientation and the use of orienting devices (personal possessions, photographs, lists, clock), supervision of and assistance with self-care, and ongoing monitoring and intervention for prevention of injury. Patients with seizures are carefully monitored.

Motor function is checked at intervals because specific motor deficits may be involved, depending on the tumor's location. Sensory disturbances are assessed. The patient's speech is evaluated. Eye movement and pupillary size and reaction may be affected by cranial nerve involvement.

The nursing process applied to the patient undergoing neurosurgery is found in Chapter 57.

Cerebral Metastases

A significant number of patients with cancer experience neurologic deficits caused by metastasis to the brain. Metastatic lesions to the brain constitute 10% of all intracranial tumors. Cerebral metastasis is the most common neurologic complication of systemic cancer. This fact becomes more important clinically as more patients with all forms of cancer live longer as a result of improved therapies.

Neurologic signs and symptoms include headache, gait disturbances, visual impairment, personality changes, altered mentation (memory loss and confusion), focal weakness, paralysis, aphasia, and seizures. These problems can be devastating to both patient and family.

Medical Management

The treatment of metastatic brain cancer is palliative and involves eliminating or reducing serious symptoms. Even when palliation is the goal, distressing signs and symptoms can be resolved, thereby improving the quality of life for both the patient and family. Patients with intracerebral metastases who are not treated have a steady downhill course with a limited survival time, whereas those who are treated may survive for slightly longer periods. The therapeutic approach includes radiation therapy, which is the foundation of treatment, surgery (usually for a single intracranial metastasis), and chemotherapy, with combination treatment being the optimal method. Gamma knife radiosurgery is considered when three or fewer lesions are present.

Corticosteroids are useful in relieving headache and alterations of consciousness. It is thought that corticosteroids (dexamethasone, prednisone) reduce inflammation around the metastatic deposits and decrease the edema surrounding them. Other medications used include osmotic agents (mannitol, glycerol) to decrease the fluid content of the brain, which leads to a decrease in ICP. Anticonvulsant agents (phenytoin) are used to prevent and treat seizures. Venous thromboembolic events occur in about 15% of patients and are associated with significant morbidity. Anticoagulants are generally not prescribed because of the risk for central nervous system hemorrhage; however, prophylactic therapy with low-molecular-weight heparin is currently under investigation.

Chemotherapy has played a small role in the management of brain metastasis as a result of poor penetration across the blood–brain barrier. Poor drug penetration and sensitivity of brain cells are two factors that determine the responsiveness of metastatic brain tumors to chemotherapy. Research is currently directed at multidrug regimens and drug resistance. Encouraging results have been seen with chemotherapeutic agents such as carmustine (BCNU), lomustine (CCNU), and PCV, which is a triple-drug combination of procarbazine, lomustine, and vincristine. Promising results have been seen in the use of topotecan (Hycamtin), another chemotherapy agent.

Pain is managed in a "step-ladder" progression in the doses and type of analgesic agents needed for effective relief. If the patient has severe pain, morphine can be infused into the epidural or subarachnoid space through a spinal needle and a catheter as near as possible to the spinal segment where the pain is projected. Small doses of morphine are administered at prescribed intervals (see Chap. 12).

NURSING PROCESS: THE PATIENT WITH CEREBRAL METASTASES OR INCURABLE BRAIN TUMOR

Assessment

The nursing assessment includes a baseline neurologic examination and focuses on how the patient is functioning, moving, and walking; adapting to weakness or paralysis and to visual and speech loss; and dealing with seizures. Assessment addresses symptoms that cause distress to the patient, including pain, respiratory problems, bowel and bladder problems, sleep disturbances, and impairment of skin integrity, fluid balance, and temperature regulation. These problems may be caused by tumor invasion, compression, or obstruction.

The patient's nutritional status is assessed because cachexia (weak and emaciated condition) is common in patients with metastases. The patient is assessed for changes associated with poor nutritional status: anorexia, pain, weight loss, altered metabolism, muscle weakness, malabsorption, and diarrhea. The patient is asked about altered taste sensations that may be secondary to dysphagia, weakness, and depression and about distortions and diminution of the sense of smell (anosmia).

A dietary history is taken to assess dietary intake and food intolerance and preferences. Anthropometric measurements confirm the loss of subcutaneous fat and lean body mass. Biochemical measurements (albumin, transferrin, total lymphocyte count, creatinine index, and urinary tests) are reviewed to assess the degree of malnutrition, impaired cellular immunity, and electrolyte balance. A dietitian assists in determining the caloric needs of the patient.

The nurse works with other members of the health care team to assess the impact of the patient's illness on the family in terms of home care, altered relationships, financial problems, time pressures, and intrafamily problems. This information is important in helping family members cope with the diagnosis and changes associated with it.

Diagnosis

Nursing Diagnoses

Based on the assessment data, the patient's major problems may include the following:

- Self-care deficits related to loss or impairment of motor and sensory function and decreased cognitive abilities
- Altered nutrition, less than body requirements, related to cachexia due to treatment and tumor effects, decreased nutritional intake, and malabsorption
- Anxiety related to anticipation of death, uncertainty, change in appearance, altered lifestyle
- Potential for altered family processes related to anticipatory grief and the burdens imposed by the care of the person with a terminal illness

Other nursing diagnoses of the patient with cerebral metastases may include pain related to tumor compression; impaired gas exchange related to dyspnea; constipation related to decreased fluid and dietary intake and medications; alteration in urinary elimination related to reduced fluid intake, vomiting, and reactions to medications; sleep pattern disturbances related to discomfort and fear of dying; impairment of skin integrity related to cachexia, poor tissue perfusion, and decreased mobility; potential or actual fluid volume deficit related to fever, vomiting, and low fluid intake; impaired thermal regulation related to hypothalamic involvement, fever, and chills. The reader is referred to Chapter 15 for appropriate assessment and nursing interventions for the patient with cancer.

Planning and Goals

The goals of the patient may include compensating for self-care deficits, attaining improved nutrition, reducing anxiety, and enhancing family coping skills.

Nursing Interventions

Compensating for Self-Care Deficits

The patient may have difficulty participating in goal setting as the tumor metastasizes and affects cognitive function. It is important to encourage the family to keep the patient as independent as possible for as long as possible. Increasing assistance with self-care activities is required. The patient with cerebral metastasis and the family live with uncertainty. They are encouraged to plan for each day and to make the most of each day. The tasks and challenges are to assist the patient to find useful coping mechanisms, adaptations, and compensations in solving problems that arise. This helps patients maintain some sense of control. An individualized exercise program helps maintain strength, endurance, and range of motion. Eventually, referral for home care may be necessary.

Improving Nutrition

Patients with nausea, vomiting, breathlessness, and pain are rarely interested in eating. These symptoms are managed or controlled through assessment, planning, and care.

The nurse teaches the family how to position the patient for comfort during meals. Meals are planned for the times the patient is more rested and in less distress from pain or the effects of treatment. The patient needs to be clean, comfortable, and free of pain for meals, in an environment that is as attractive as possible. Oral hygiene before meals helps to improve oral intake. Offensive sights, sounds, and odors are eliminated. Creative strategies may be required to make food more palatable, provide enough fluids, and increase opportunities for socialization during meals. The family may be asked to keep a daily weight chart and to record the quantity of food eaten to determine the daily calorie count.

Dietary supplements, if acceptable to the patient, can be provided to meet increased caloric needs. If the patient is not interested in most usual foods, those foods preferred by the patient should be offered.

When the patient shows marked deterioration as a result of tumor growth and effects, some other form of nutritional support (tube feeding, total parenteral nutrition) may be indicated if consistent with the patient's end-of-life preferences. Nursing interventions include assessing the patency of the central and intravenous line or feeding tube, monitoring the insertion site for infection, checking the infusion rate, monitoring intake and output, and changing the intravenous tubing and dressing. The patient's family members are instructed in these techniques if they will be providing care at home. Total parenteral nutrition can also be provided at home if indicated.

The quality of life for the patient may serve to guide in the selection, initiation, and maintenance of nutritional support. The patient may become weary with all the urging to eat and the discussions about food and may not desire aggressive nutritional intervention. The subsequent course of action must be congruent with the wishes and choices of the patient and family.

Relieving Anxiety

People with cerebral metastases may be restless, with changing moods that may include intense depression, euphoria, paranoia, and severe anxiety. The response of patients to terminal illness reflects their pattern of reaction to other crisis situations. Serious illness imposes additional strains that often bring other unresolved problems to light. The patient's own coping strategies can help deal with anxious and depressed feelings. Caregivers need to be sensitive to the patient's stated concerns.

Patients need the opportunity to exercise some control over their situation. A sense of mastery can be gained as they learn to understand the disease and its treatment and how to deal with their feelings. The presence of family, friends, clergy, and health professionals may be supportive. Support groups, such as the Brain Tumor Support Group, may provide a feeling of support and strength.

Spending time with patients allows them time to talk and to communicate their fears and concerns. Open communication and acknowledging fears are often therapeutic. Touch is also a form of communication. These patients need reassurance that continuing care will be provided and that they will not be abandoned. The situation becomes more endurable when others share in the experience of dying. If a patient's emotional reactions are very intense or prolonged, additional help from a member of the clergy, social worker, or mental health professional may be indicated.

Enhancing Family Coping

The family needs to be reassured that their loved one is receiving optimal care and that attention will be paid to the patient's changing symptoms and to their concerns. When the patient can no longer carry out self-care, the family, additional support systems (social worker, home health aid, home care nurse, hospice care) may be needed. A nursing goal is to keep anxiety at a manageable level.

Promoting Home and Community-Based Care

TEACHING PATIENTS SELF-CARE

The patient and family often have major responsibility for care at home. Therefore, teaching includes strategies of pain management, prevention of complications related to treatment strategies, and methods to ensure an adequate fluid and food intake. Teaching needs of the patient and family regarding that care are likely to change as the disease progresses. It is important to assess the changing needs of the patient and the family and to inform them about resources and services that may assist family members to deal with changes in the patient's condition.

CONTINUING CARE

Home care nursing and hospice services are valuable resources that should be made available to the patient and the family. Anticipating needs before they occur often can assist in smooth initiation of services. Home care needs and interventions focus on four major areas: palliation of symptoms and pain control, assistance in self-care, control of treatment complications, and administration of specific forms of treatment, such as parenteral nutrition. The home care nurse assesses the adequacy of pain management, respiratory status, occurrence of complications of the disorder and its treatment, and the patient's cognitive and emotional status. Additionally, the nurse assesses the family's ability to perform necessary care and notifies the physician about changing needs or the occurrence of complications if indicated.

The patient and family who elect to care for the patient at home as the disease progresses benefit from the care and support provided through hospice services. Steps to initiate hospice care, including discussion of hospice care as an option, should not be postponed until the patient's death is imminent. Exploration of hospice care as an option should be initiated at a time when hospice care can provide support and care to the patient and family consistent with their end-of-life decisions and assist in allowing death with dignity.

Evaluation

Expected Outcomes

Expected outcomes may include:

1. Engages in self-care activities as long as possible
   a. Uses assistive devices or accepts assistance as needed
   b. Schedules periodic rest periods to permit maximal participation in self-care
2. Maintains as optimal a nutritional status as possible
   a. Eats and accepts food within limits of condition and preferences
   b. Accepts alternative methods of providing nutrition if indicated
3. Reports being less anxious
   a. Is less restless and is sleeping better
   b. Verbalizes concerns about death
   c. Participates in activities of personal importance as long as feasible
4. Family members seek help as needed
   a. Demonstrate ability to bathe, feed, and care for the patient and participate in pain management and prevention of complications
   b. Express feelings and concerns to appropriate health professionals
   c. Discuss and seek hospice care as an option

INTRACRANIAL INFECTIONS

Meningitis

Meningitis is an inflammation of the meninges (membranes surrounding the brain and spinal cord) and is caused by a viral, bacterial, or fungal organism. Meningitis is further classified as aseptic, septic, or tuberculous. Aseptic meningitis refers to either viral

HOME CARE TEACHING CHECKLIST: THE PATIENT WITH CEREBRAL METASTASES

At the completion of the program, the patient or caregiver will be able to:	Patient	Caregiver
• State effects of the tumor according to its location in the brain and type.	✔	✔
• Describe side effects of treatment.	✔	✔
• Identify community resources, including:	✔	✔
• Home health services		
• Hospices		
• Support groups		
• Identify coping strategies, such as:	✔	✔
• Taking control, setting daily goals, and staying positive		
• Rehabilitation to improve self-care		
• Relaxation techniques		
• Family support		
• Verbalize an understanding of the medical plan for:	✔	✔
• Medications and pain control		
• Nutritional needs		
• Contacting the health care provider		

meningitis or cases of meningeal irritation from other causes, such as brain abscess, encephalitis, lymphoma, leukemia, or blood in the subarachnoid space. Septic meningitis refers to meningitis caused by bacterial organisms, such as meningococcus, staphylococcus, or influenza bacillus. Tuberculous meningitis is caused by the tubercle bacillus.

Meningeal infections generally originate in one of two ways: either through the bloodstream as a consequence of other infections, such as cellulitis, or by direct extension such as might occur after a traumatic injury to the facial bones. In a small number of cases, the cause is iatrogenic or secondary to invasive procedures (eg, lumbar puncture) or invasive devices (eg, ICP monitoring devices). Meningitis also occurs as an opportunistic infection in patients with acquired immunodeficiency syndrome (AIDS) and as a complication of Lyme disease (Chart 59-3).

By far the most significant form of meningitis is the bacterial type. The bacteria most frequently encountered in acute bacterial meningitis are *Neisseria meningitidis* (meningococcal meningitis), *Streptococcus pneumoniae* (in adults), and *Haemophilus influenzae* (in children and young adults). These three organisms account for about 75% of the cases of bacterial meningitis.

The mode of transmission is by direct contact, including droplets and discharge from the nose and throat of carriers (most often) or infected people. Of those exposed to it, most do not develop the infection but become carriers. An increased incidence of meningitis caused by enteric gram-negative bacteria has occurred in the elderly as well as in those who have had neurosurgery or who have a compromised immune response.

Bacterial meningitis is endemic in the United States and throughout the world and occurs most frequently in the winter and spring months. Overall, the incidence of bacterial meningitis has declined in the Western world, primarily as a result of sophisticated social and hygienic standards. Outbreaks are most likely to occur among those living in crowded conditions, such as in cities, crowded institutions, military installations, or prisons, although the disease also occurs in rural areas. In less-developed countries, meningitis remains a major health problem.

CHART 59•3 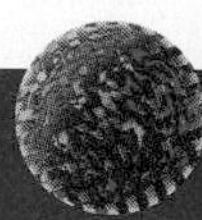 **Meningitis in Specific Populations**

Meningitis can occur as a complication of other diseases and is an opportunistic infection seen with greater frequency in patients with acquired immunodeficiency syndrome (AIDS)

Meningitis in AIDS Patients

- Aseptic, cryptococcal, and tuberculous forms of meningitis have been reported in patients with AIDS.
- Acute and chronic forms of aseptic meningitis may occur with AIDS; both are accompanied by headache, but signs of meningeal irritation generally occur with the acute form.
- Aseptic meningitis may be accompanied by cranial nerve palsies. The meningitis is thought to be related to direct infection of the central nervous system by human immunodeficiency virus (HIV) because it can be isolated from the cerebrospinal fluid (CSF).
- Cryptococcal meningitis is the most common fungal infection of the central nervous system in patients with AIDS and has a 50% to 60% relapse rate. Patients may experience headache, nausea, vomiting, seizures, confusion, and lethargy. Treatment consists of IV administration of amphotericin B followed by fluconazole. Maintenance therapy with fluconazole may be necessary to prevent relapse.
- Some immunosuppressed patients develop few if any symptoms because of blunted inflammatory responses; others develop atypical features.

Meningitis in Lyme Disease

- Lyme disease is a multisystem inflammatory process caused by the tick-transmitted spirochete *Borrelia burgdorferi.*
- Neurologic abnormalities are seen in later stages (stages 2 or 3). Stage 2 occurs either with the characteristic rash or from 1 to 6 months after it has disappeared.
- Neurologic abnormalities include aseptic meningitis, chronic lymphocytic meningitis, and encephalitis.
- Cranial nerve inflammation, including Bell's palsy and other peripheral neuropathies, is common.
- Stage 3 (the chronic form of the disease) begins years after the initial tick infection and is characterized by arthritis, skin lesions, and neurologic abnormalities.
- Most patients with stage 2 and 3 Lyme disease are treated with intravenous antibiotics, usually ceftriaxone or penicillin G.
- Meningeal and systemic symptoms begin to improve within days, although other symptoms, such as headache, may persist for weeks.

Pathophysiology

Bacterial meningitis usually starts as an infection of the nasopharynx and is followed by septicemia. Bacteria can enter from penetrating head wounds and skull fractures. The infection extends to the pia-arachnoid layers of the meninges and the subarachnoid space, including the CSF, spreading quickly to other areas of the brain and the upper region of the spinal cord.

Predisposing factors include upper respiratory tract infections, otitis media, mastoiditis, sickle cell anemia and other hemoglobinopathies, recent neurosurgical procedures, head trauma, and immunosuppressed status. The venous channels serving the posterior nasopharynx, middle ear, and mastoid drain toward the brain and are near the veins draining the meninges; these channels favor bacterial proliferation.

The organism enters the bloodstream and causes an inflammatory reaction in the meninges and underlying cortex, which may result in thromboses and reduced cerebral blood flow. The cerebral tissue is metabolically impaired as a result of meningeal exudate, vasculitis, and hypoperfusion. A purulent exudate may spread over the base of the brain and spinal cord. The inflammation also spreads to the membrane lining the cerebral ventricles. Bacterial meningitis is associated with profound alterations in intracranial physiology, including increased permeability of the blood–brain barrier, cerebral edema, and increased ICP.

In acute infections, however, the patient dies from the toxin of the bacteria before meningitis develops. In these patients, the infection is overwhelming, with adrenal damage, circulatory collapse, and associated widespread hemorrhages (Waterhouse-Friderichsen syndrome) occurring as a result of endothelial damage and vascular necrosis caused by the meningococci.

The prognosis of bacterial meningitis depends on the causative organism, the severity of the infection and illness, and the timeliness of treatment. Complications include visual impairment, deafness, seizures, paralysis, hydrocephalus, and septic shock.

Clinical Manifestations

The symptoms of meningitis result from infection and increased ICP. Headache and fever are frequently the initial symptoms. The headache associated with meningitis is usually severe and is the result of meningeal irritation. Fever is generally present and remains high throughout the course of the illness.

Changes in level of consciousness are associated with bacterial meningitis. Disorientation and memory impairment are common early in the course of the illness. The changes that occur are dependent on the severity of the infection as well as the individual response to the physiologic processes. Behavioral manifestations are also common. As the illness progresses, lethargy, unresponsiveness, and coma may develop.

Meningeal irritation results in a number of well-recognized signs commonly seen in all types of meningitis:

- Nuchal rigidity (stiff neck) is an early sign. Any attempts at flexion of the head are difficult because of the presence of spasm in the muscles of the neck. Forceful flexion causes severe pain.
- Positive Kernig's sign: When the patient is lying with the thigh flexed on the abdomen, the leg cannot be completely extended (Fig. 59-4).
- Positive Brudzinski's sign: When the patient's neck is flexed, flexion of the knees and hips is produced; when passive flexion of the lower extremity of one side is made, a similar movement is seen in the opposite extremity (see Fig. 59-4).
- Photophobia or extreme sensitivity to light is common, but the cause is unclear.

Seizures and increased ICP are also associated with meningitis. Seizures occur secondary to focal areas of cortical irritability. Signs of increasing ICP secondary to accumulation of purulent exudate or cerebral edema include the characteristic vital sign changes (widened pulse pressure and bradycardia), respiratory irregularity, headache, vomiting, and depressed levels of consciousness.

A rash is one of the striking features of meningococcal meningitis (*Neisseria meningitidis*). About half of all patients with this type of meningitis develop skin lesions ranging from a petechial rash with purpuric lesions to large areas of ecchymosis.

A fulminating infection occurs in about 10% of patients with meningococcal meningitis, with signs of overwhelming septicemia: an abrupt onset of high fever, extensive purpuric lesions (over the face and extremities), shock, and signs of disseminated intravascular coagulopathy. Death may occur within a few hours of onset of the infection.

Assessment and Diagnostic Findings

The infecting organisms usually can be identified through cultures of the CSF and blood. The latex agglutination test and counterimmunoelectrophoresis are widely used to detect bacterial antigens in body fluids, particularly CSF and urine.

Prevention

People in close contact with the patient should be considered candidates for antimicrobial prophylaxis (rifampin). Close contacts are observed and immediately examined if fever or other signs and symptoms of meningitis develop.

The available meningococcal vaccines include the polysaccharides of groups A, C, W135, and Y. The ability of the vaccines to produce immunity differs in various age groups. Group A vaccine is highly immunogenic in children 3 months of age and older. In contrast, group C vaccine is immunogenic only in adults and children 2 years of age or older. The use of this vaccine in military recruits has decreased the incidence of meningococcal meningitis by 90%. The vaccine may be of benefit to some travelers to countries with epidemic meningococcal disease. Vaccination should be considered as an adjunct to antibiotic chemoprophylaxis for anyone living with a person who develops meningococcal infection.

A polysaccharide vaccine (*Haemophilus b* polysaccharide vaccine) against invasive *H. influenzae* type b has been licensed in the United States and is now used routinely in pediatrics for the prevention of meningitis.

Pneumococcal polysaccharide vaccine contains antigens from 23 capsular types of pneumococci. The Centers for Disease Control and Prevention recommends vaccination for everyone aged 65 years or older and for those 2 years of age and older who have chronic diseases that put them at risk, absence of a spleen, or compromised immune systems and those who live in environments where risk for infection is high. Revaccination is recommended after 5 years in specific at-risk populations.

Medical Management

Successful management depends on the administration of an antibiotic that crosses the blood-brain barrier into the subarachnoid space in sufficient concentration to halt the multiplication of bacteria. Cultures of CSF and blood are obtained, and antimicrobial therapy is started immediately. Penicillin, ampicillin, or chloramphenicol or one of the cephalosporins (ceftriaxone, cefotaxime) may be used. Vancomycin alone or in combination with rifampin may be used if resistant strains of bacteria are identified. The patient is maintained on large intravenous doses of the appropriate antibiotic. Dexamethasone has been shown to be beneficial as adjunct therapy in the treatment of *H. influenzae* type b meningitis and in pneumococcal meningitis if given with or before the first dose of antibiotic. Recent studies indicate that dexamethasone reduces the incidence of deafness (a complication of meningitis), especially in children (McIntyre et al., 1997).

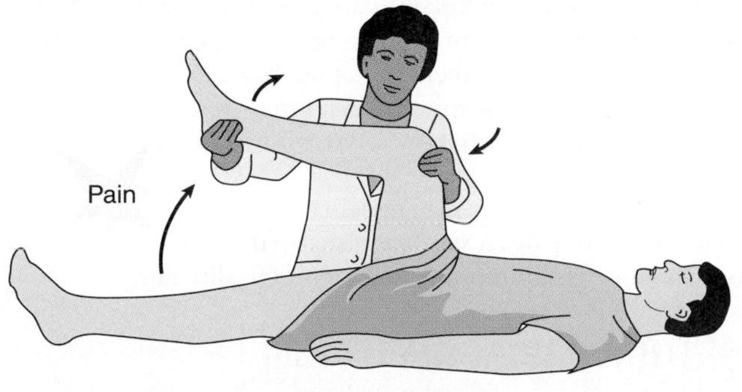

A Kernig's Sign

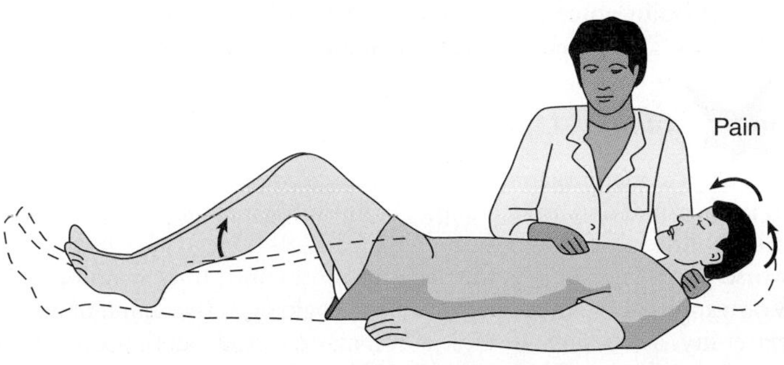

B Brudzinski's Sign

FIGURE 59•4 Testing for meningeal irritation. (**A**) Kernig's sign. (**B**) Brudzinski's sign.

Dehydration or shock is treated with fluid volume expanders. Seizures, which may occur in the early course of the disease, are controlled with diazepam or phenytoin. An osmotic diuretic (eg, mannitol) may be used to treat cerebral edema.

Nursing Management

The patient's prognosis may depend on the supportive care given. The patient may be critically ill, and the combination of fever, dehydration, alkalosis, and cerebral edema may predispose to seizures. Airway obstruction, respiratory arrest, or cardiac dysrhythmias may follow. Thus, many of the nursing interventions are collaborative with those of the physician.

In meningitis of all types, the patient's clinical status and vital signs are constantly assessed because altered consciousness may lead to airway obstruction. Arterial blood gas determinations, insertion of a cuffed endotracheal tube (or tracheostomy), and mechanical ventilation may be initiated. Oxygen may be needed to maintain the arterial partial pressure of oxygen at desired levels.

Arterial pressures are monitored to assess for incipient shock, which precedes cardiac or respiratory failure. Generalized vasoconstriction, circumoral cyanosis, and cold extremities may be noted. Efforts are made to reduce the high fever to decrease the workload on the heart and the brain's oxygen demand.

Rapid intravenous fluid replacement may be prescribed, but care is taken not to overhydrate the patient because of the risk for cerebral edema.

The body weight, serum electrolytes and urine volume, specific gravity, and osmolality are closely monitored, especially if the syndrome of inappropriate antidiuretic hormone secretion is suspected.

Continuing nursing management requires ongoing assessment of the patient's clinical status, attention to skin and oral hygiene, promotion of comfort, and protection during seizures (discussed later) and while comatose.

Discharge from the nose and mouth is considered infectious. Respiratory isolation is recommended until 24 hours after the initiation of antibiotic therapy.

Brain Abscess

A brain abscess is a collection of infectious material within the tissue of the brain. It may occur by direct invasion of the brain from intracranial trauma or surgery; by spread of infection from nearby sites, such as the sinuses, ears, and teeth (paranasal sinus infections, otitis media, dental sepsis); or by spread of infection from other organs (lung abscess, infective endocarditis). It can also be a complication associated with some forms of meningitis. Brain abscess is a complication encountered increasingly in patients whose immune systems have been suppressed through either therapy or disease. To prevent brain abscess, otitis media, mastoiditis, sinusitis, dental infections, and systemic infections should be treated promptly.

Clinical Manifestations

The clinical manifestations of a brain abscess result from alterations in intracranial dynamics (edema, brain shift), infection, or the location of the abscess as indicated in Chart 59-4. Headache, usually worse in the morning, is the patient's most continuing symptom. Vomiting is also common. Focal neurologic signs (weakness of an extremity, decreasing vision, seizures) may occur, depending on the site of the abscess. There may be a change in the patient's mental status, as reflected in lethargic, confused, irritable, or disoriented behavior. Fever may or may not be present.

Chart 59•4 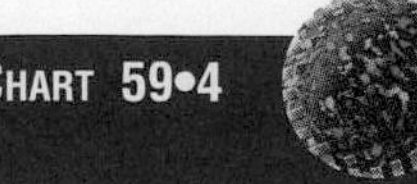 **Symptoms of Brain Abscesses**

Frontal Lobe

- Hemiparesis
- Aphasia (expressive)
- Seizures
- Frontal headache

Temporal Lobe

- Localized headache
- Changes in vision
- Facial weakness
- Aphasia

Cerebellar Abscess

- Occipital headache
- Ataxia (inability to coordinate movements)
- Nystagmus (rhythmic, involuntary movements of the eye)

Adapted from Hickey, J. V. (1997). *The clinical practice of neurological and neurosurgical nursing* (4th ed. p. 647). Philadelphia: Lippincott-Raven.

Assessment and Diagnostic Findings

Repeated neurologic examinations and continuing assessment of the patient are necessary to determine accurately the location of the abscess. CT is invaluable in locating the site of the abscess, after the evolution and resolution of suppurative lesions, and in determining the optimal time for surgical intervention. MRI is useful to obtain images of the brain stem and posterior fossa.

Management

The goal of management is to eliminate the abscess. Brain abscess is treated with antimicrobial therapy and surgical incision or aspiration. If the abscess is incapsulated, CT-guided stereotactic needle aspiration under local anesthesia may be performed. Antimicrobial treatment is given to eliminate the causative organism or reduce its virulence.

Penicillin G (20 to 24 million U) and chloramphenicol (4 to 6 g/day given intravenously in divided doses) are usually given because anaerobic streptococci and bacterioids are the most common causative organisms. Large IV doses are usually prescribed preoperatively to penetrate brain tissue and the brain abscess. The therapy is continued postoperatively. Corticosteroids may be given to help reduce the inflammatory cerebral edema if the patient shows evidence of an increasing neurologic deficit. Anticonvulsant medications (phenytoin, phenobarbital) may be given to prevent seizures. Multiple abscesses may be treated with appropriate antimicrobial therapy alone, with close monitoring by CT scans.

Neurologic deficits that may remain after treatment of brain abscess include hemiparesis, seizures, visual defects, and cranial nerve palsies. Relapse is common, with a high mortality rate.

INTRACRANIAL ANEURYSM

An intracranial (cerebral) aneurysm is a dilation of the walls of a cerebral artery that develops as a result of weakness in the arterial wall (Fig. 59-5). The cause of aneurysms is unknown, although

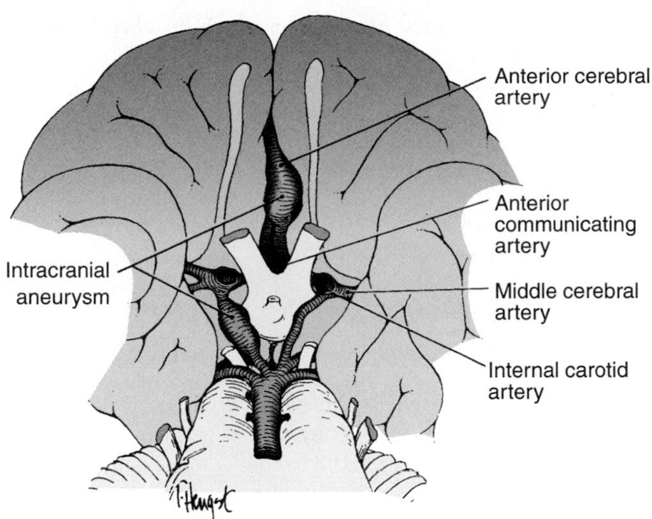

FIGURE 59•5 Intracranial aneurysm.

research is ongoing in an attempt to understand this problem. An aneurysm may be due to atherosclerosis, resulting in a defect in the vessel wall with subsequent weakness of the wall; a congenital defect of the vessel wall; hypertensive vascular disease; head trauma; or advancing age.

Cerebral aneurysms usually occur at the bifurcations of the large arteries at the circle of Willis (see Fig. 59-5). The cerebral arteries most commonly affected by an aneurysm are the internal carotid (ICA), anterior cerebral (ACA), anterior communicating (ACoA), posterior communicating (PCoA), posterior cerebral artery (PCA), and middle cerebral arteries (MCA). Multiple cerebral aneurysms are not uncommon.

Pathophysiology

Symptoms are produced when the aneurysm enlarges and presses on nearby cranial nerves or brain tissue or, more dramatically, when the aneurysm ruptures, causing subarachnoid hemorrhage (hemorrhage into the cranial subarachnoid space). Normal brain metabolism is disrupted by the brain being exposed to blood; by an increase in ICP resulting from the sudden entry of blood into the subarachnoid space, which compresses and injures brain tissue; or by ischemia of the brain resulting from the reduced perfusion pressure and vasospasm that frequently accompany subarachnoid hemorrhage.

Clinical Manifestations

Rupture of the aneurysm usually produces a sudden, unusually severe headache and often loss of consciousness for a variable period. There may be pain and rigidity of the back of the neck (nuchal rigidity) and spine due to meningeal irritation. Visual disturbances (visual loss, diplopia, ptosis) occur when the aneurysm is adjacent to the oculomotor nerve. Tinnitus, dizziness, and hemiparesis may also occur.

At times, an aneurysm "leaks" blood, leading to the formation of a clot that seals the site of rupture. In this instance, the patient may show little neurologic deficit. In other cases, severe bleeding occurs, resulting in cerebral damage followed rapidly by coma and death.

Prognosis depends on the neurologic condition of the patient, age, associated diseases, and the extent and location of the aneurysm. Subarachnoid hemorrhage from an aneurysm is a catastrophic event with up to a 50% mortality rate.

Assessment and Diagnostic Findings

The diagnosis is confirmed by CT scan and cerebral angiography, which shows the location and size of the aneurysm and gives information about the affected artery, adjoining vessels, and vascular branches. Lumbar puncture is performed if there is no evidence of increased ICP and the CT scan results are negative and subarachnoid hemorrhage must be confirmed. Lumbar puncture in the presence of increased ICP could result in brain stem herniation or rebleeding.

The Hunt-Hess classification system of clinical grades guides the physician in diagnosing the severity of subarachnoid hemorrhage after an aneurysmal bleed and in timing the surgery (Table 59-1). Morbidity and mortality from surgery are high if the patient is stuporous or comatose (grade IV or V). Classifying the patient by severity of neurologic deficit provides a baseline for further comparison.

Management

The goals of treatment are to allow the brain to recover from the initial insult (bleeding), to prevent or minimize the risk for rebleeding, and to prevent or treat other complications. Potential complications include rebleeding; cerebral vasospasm resulting in cerebral ischemia; acute hydrocephalus, which results when free blood obstructs the reabsorption of CSF by the arachnoid villi; and seizures. Management consists of bed rest with sedation to prevent agitation and stress, management of the vasospasm, and surgical or medical treatment to prevent rebleeding.

VASOSPASM

The development of cerebral vasospasm (narrowing of the lumen of the involved cranial blood vessel) is a serious complication of subarachnoid hemorrhage and accounts for 40% to 50% of the morbidity and mortality of those who survive the initial intracranial bleed. The mechanism responsible for the spasm is not clear, but the occurrence of vasospasm is associated with increasing amounts of blood in the subarachnoid cisterns and cerebral fissures, as visualized by CT scan.

Vasospasm leads to increased vascular resistance, which impedes cerebral blood flow and causes brain ischemia and infarc-

TABLE 59•1 Hunt-Hess Clinical Grades for Cerebral Aneurysms

Grade	Descriptive Criteria
I	Alert, oriented, symptom free
II	Alert, oriented, headache, stiff neck
III	Lethargic or confused; minor focal deficits, such as hemiparesis
IV	Stupor; moderate to severe focal deficits, such as hemiplegia
V	Comatose; severe neurologic deficits, such as posturing

From Hickey, J. V. (1997). *The clinical practice of neurological and neurosurgical nursing* (4th ed., p. 572). Philadelphia: Lippincott-Raven.

tion. The signs and symptoms exhibited by the patient reflect the areas of the brain involved. Vasospasm is often heralded by a worsening headache, a decrease in level of consciousness (confusion, lethargy, disorientation), or the appearance of a new focal neurologic deficit (aphasia, hemiparesis [partial paralysis affecting one side of the body]).

Vasospasm frequently occurs 4 to 14 days after initial hemorrhage when the clot undergoes lysis (dissolution), increasing the chances of rebleeding.

It is believed that early surgery to clip the aneurysm prevents rebleeding and that removal of blood from the basal cisterns around the major cerebral arteries may prevent vasospasm. The intravenous administration of the calcium-channel blocker nimodipine during the critical time in which vasospasm may occur may prevent delayed ischemic deterioration. Advances in technology have led to the introduction of interventional neuroradiology for the treatment of aneurysms. Endovascular techniques may be used in selected patients to occlude the artery supplying the aneurysm with a balloon or to occlude the aneurysm itself. As more studies on these techniques are completed, their use will increase.

Management of vasospasm remains difficult and controversial. Based on one theory that vasospasm is caused by an increased influx of calcium into the cell, medication therapy may be used to block or antagonize this action and prevent or reverse the action of vasospasm already present. Calcium-channel blockers may include nimodipine (Nimotop), verapamil (Isoptin), and nifedipine (Procardia). Other therapy for vasospasm is aimed at minimizing the deleterious effects of the associated cerebral ischemia and includes fluid volume expanders and induced arterial hypertension, normotension, or hemodilution. The use of recombinant tissue plasminogen activator (t-PA) is being investigated. Instilled into the basal cisterns at the time of aneurysm clipping, t-PA dissolves the clot so that substances causing spasm of the vessel may be removed, reducing the risk for and severity of vasospasm.

INCREASED INTRACRANIAL PRESSURE

An increase in ICP almost always follows a subarachnoid hemorrhage, usually because of disturbed circulation of CSF caused by blood in the basal cisterns. If the patient shows evidence of deterioration from increased ICP (due to cerebral edema, herniation, hydrocephalus, or vasospasm), CSF drainage may be instituted by cautious lumbar puncture or ventricular catheter drainage, and mannitol is given to reduce ICP. When mannitol is used as a long-term measure to control ICP, dehydration and disturbances in electrolyte balance (hyponatremia or hypernatremia; hypokalemia or hyperkalemia) may occur. Mannitol acts by pulling water out of the brain tissue by osmosis as well as by reducing total-body water through diuresis. The patient is monitored for signs of dehydration and for rebound elevation of ICP.

If surgery is delayed or contraindicated, antifibrinolytic agents (aminocaproic acid; tranexamic acid) may be administered to delay or prevent dissolution of the clot at the site of the aneurysmal rupture.

SYSTEMIC HYPERTENSION

Efforts are made to prevent sudden systemic hypertension. The goal of therapy is to maintain the systolic blood pressure at about 150 mm Hg. If blood pressure is elevated, antihypertensive therapy (labetolol, nicardipine, nitroprusside) may be prescribed. Hemodynamic monitoring by arterial line is carried out to detect and avoid a precipitous drop in blood pressure, which can produce brain ischemia. Because seizures cause blood pressure elevation, anticonvulsant agents are administered prophylactically. Stool softeners are used to prevent straining, which can also elevate the blood pressure.

Analgesics (codeine, acetaminophen) may be prescribed for head and neck pain. The patient is fitted with elastic stockings to prevent deep vein thrombosis (DVT), a threat to any patient on bed rest.

SURGICAL MANAGEMENT

The patient is prepared for surgical intervention as soon as the condition is considered stable. The nursing management of the patient after a craniotomy is discussed in Chapter 57.

The goal of surgery is to prevent further bleeding. This objective is accomplished by isolating the aneurysm from its circulation or by strengthening the arterial wall. An aneurysm may be excluded from the cerebral circulation by means of a ligature or a clip across its neck. If this is not anatomically possible, the aneurysm can be reinforced by wrapping it with muslin or some other substance to provide support and induce scarring.

An extracranial-intracranial arterial bypass may be performed to establish collateral blood supply to allow surgery on the aneurysm. Alternatively, an extracranial method may be used, whereby the carotid artery is gradually occluded in the neck to reduce pressure within the blood vessel. After ligation of the carotid artery, there is some risk for cerebral ischemia and sudden hemiplegia because during the surgical procedure, there is a temporary occlusion of the blood supply to the brain (unless a temporary inlying bypass shunt is used). In anticipation of these complications, cerebral blood flow and internal carotid pressure may be measured to identify those patients who are at risk for postoperative ischemic episodes.

Other postoperative complications include psychological symptoms (disorientation, amnesia, **Korsakoff's syndrome,** personality changes), intraoperative embolization, postoperative internal artery occlusion, fluid and electrolyte disturbances (from dysfunction of the neurohypophyseal system), and gastrointestinal bleeding.

NURSING PROCESS: THE PATIENT WITH A CEREBRAL ANEURYSM

Assessment

A complete neurologic assessment is performed initially and should include evaluation for the following:

- Altered level of consciousness
- Sluggish pupillary reaction
- Motor and sensory dysfunction
- Cranial nerve deficits (extraocular eye movements, facial droop, presence of ptosis)
- Speech difficulties and visual disturbance
- Headache and nuchal rigidity or other neurologic deficits

Neurologic assessment findings are documented and reported as indicated. Frequency of these assessments varies and is determined by the patient's condition. Any changes in the patient's condition require reassessment and thorough documentation; changes should be reported immediately.

Alteration in level of consciousness often is the earliest sign of deterioration in a patient with a cerebral aneurysm. Because nurses have the most frequent contact with patients, it is often the nurse who is the first to detect what may be subtle changes. Mild drowsiness and slight slurring of speech may be early signs that the patient's level of consciousness is deteriorating. Frequent nursing assessment is crucial in the patient with known or suspected cerebral aneurysm.

Diagnosis

Nursing Diagnoses

Based on the assessment data, the patient's major nursing diagnoses may include the following:

- Altered cerebral tissue perfusion due to bleeding from the aneurysm
- Sensory or perceptual alteration due to the restrictions of aneurysm precautions
- Anxiety due to illness or restrictions of subarachnoid precautions

Collaborative Problems/Potential Complications

Based on the assessment data, potential complications that may develop include the following:

- Vasospasm
- Seizures
- Hydrocephalus
- Aneurysm rebleeding

Planning and Goals

The goals for the patient may include improved cerebral tissue perfusion, relief of sensory and perceptual deprivation, relief of anxiety, and the absence of complications.

Nursing Interventions

Improving Cerebral Tissue Perfusion

The patient is closely monitored for neurologic deterioration occurring from recurrent bleeding, increasing ICP, or vasospasm. A neurologic flow record is maintained. The blood pressure, pulse, level of responsiveness (an indicator of cerebral perfusion), pupillary responses, and motor function are checked hourly. The respiratory status is monitored because reduction in oxygen in areas of the brain with impaired autoregulation increases the chances of a cerebral infarction. Any changes are reported immediately.

Aneurysm precautions are implemented to provide a nonstimulating environment and prevent increases in ICP pressure and further bleeding. The patient is placed on immediate and absolute bed rest in a quiet, nonstressful environment because activity, pain, and anxiety elevate the blood pressure, which increases the risk for bleeding. Visitors, except for family, are restricted.

The head of the bed is elevated 15 to 30 degrees to promote venous drainage and decrease ICP. Some neurologists, however, prefer that the patient remain flat to increase cerebral perfusion.

Any activity that suddenly increases the blood pressure or obstructs venous return is avoided. This includes the Valsalva maneuver, straining, forceful sneezing, pushing up in bed, acute flexion or rotation of the head and neck (which compromises the jugular veins), and cigarette smoking. Any activity requiring exertion is contraindicated. The patient is instructed to exhale through the mouth during voiding or defecation to decrease strain. No enemas are permitted, but stool softeners and mild laxatives are prescribed. Both prevent constipation, which would cause an increase in ICP, as would enemas. Dim lighting is helpful because photophobia (visual intolerance of light) is common. Coffee and tea, unless decaffeinated, are usually eliminated.

Thigh-high elastic pressure stockings or sequential compression boots may be prescribed to decrease the incidence of DVT resulting from immobility. The legs are observed for signs and symptoms of DVT (tenderness, swelling, warmth, discoloration, positive Homans' sign) and abnormal findings are reported.

All personal care is administered by the nurse. The patient is fed and bathed to prevent any exertion that might raise the blood pressure. External stimuli are kept to a minimum, including no television, no radio, no reading, and maintenance of visitor restriction. Visitors are restricted in an effort to keep the patient as quiet as possible. This precaution must be individualized based on patient condition and response to visitors. A sign indicating this restriction should be placed on the door of the room, and the restrictions should be discussed with both patient and family. The purpose of aneurysm precautions should be thoroughly explained to both the patient (if possible) and family.

Relieving Sensory Deprivation and Anxiety

Sensory stimulation is kept to a minimum. For patients who are awake, alert, and oriented, an explanation of the restrictions helps reduce the patient's sense of isolation. Reality orientation is provided to help maintain orientation.

Keeping the patient well informed of the plan of care provides reassurance and helps minimize anxiety. Appropriate reassurance also helps relieve the patient's fears and anxiety. The family also requires information and support.

Monitoring and Managing Potential Complications

VASOSPASM

The patient must be assessed for signs of possible vasospasm: intensified headaches, a decrease in level of responsiveness (confusion, disorientation, lethargy), or evidence of aphasia or partial paralysis. These signs may develop several days after surgery or on the initiation of treatment and must be reported immediately. If vasospasm is diagnosed, calcium-channel blockers or fluid volume expanders may be prescribed.

SEIZURES

Seizure precautions are maintained for every patient who may be at risk for seizure activity. Should a seizure occur, maintaining the patient's airway and preventing injury are the primary goals. Medication therapy is initiated at this time if not already prescribed. The medication of choice is phenytoin (Dilantin) because this agent usually provides adequate anticonvulsant action while causing no drowsiness at therapeutic levels.

HYDROCEPHALUS

Blood in the subarachnoid space prevents the circulation of CSF, resulting in hydrocephalus. Diagnosis is confirmed by CT scan that indicates dilated ventricles. Hydrocephalus can occur within the first 24 hours (acute) after subarachnoid hemorrhage or days (subacute) to several weeks (delayed) later. Symptoms vary according to the time of onset and may be nonspecific. Acute hydrocephalus is characterized by sudden onset of stupor or coma and is managed with a ventriculostomy drain to decrease ICP. Symptoms of subacute and delayed hydrocephalus include gradual onset of drowsiness, behavioral changes, and ataxic gait. A ventriculoperitoneal shunt is surgically placed to treat chronic hydrocephalus. Changes in patient responsiveness are reported immediately.

ANEURYSM REBLEEDING

Rebleeding occurs most frequently in the first 2 weeks after the initial hemorrhage and is considered a major complication. Symptoms of rebleeding include sudden severe headache, nausea, vomiting, decreased level of consciousness, and neurologic deficit. A CT scan is performed to confirm a rebleeding. Blood pressure is carefully maintained with medications. Antifibrinolytic medications (epsilon-aminocaproic acid) may be administered to delay the lysis of the clot surrounding the rupture. The most effective preventive treatment is early clipping of the aneurysm if the patient is a candidate for surgery.

Evaluation

Expected Outcomes

Expected outcomes may include:

1. Demonstrates intact neurologic status and normal vital signs and respiratory patterns
   a. Is alert and oriented to time, place, and person
   b. Demonstrates normal speech patterns and intact cognitive processes
   c. Demonstrates normal and equal strength, movement, and sensation of all four extremities
   d. Exhibits normal deep tendon reflexes and pupillary responses
2. Demonstrates normal sensory perceptions
   a. States rationale for subarachnoid precautions
   b. Exhibits clear thought processes
3. Exhibits reduced anxiety level
   a. Is less restless
   b. Exhibits absence of physiologic indicators of anxiety (ie, normal vital signs; normal respiratory rate; absence of excessive, fast speech)
4. Is free of complications
   a. Exhibits absence of vasospasm
   b. Exhibits normal vital signs and neuromuscular activity without seizures
   c. Verbalizes understanding of seizure precautions
   d. Exhibits normal mental status and normal motor and sensory status
   e. Reports no visual changes

DEGENERATIVE NEUROLOGIC DISORDERS

Degenerative diseases of the nervous system are fairly common and affect all age groups. Although etiologic factors differ, the overall approach to patients with degenerative disorders is similar: to maintain independent function as long as possible. Many of these patients are managed primarily in their homes and communities, and hospitalization in the acute care setting may be limited to instances of relapse or disease-related complications.

Patients with degenerative diseases benefit from a collaborative, interdisciplinary approach to care. Nursing care often focuses on helping the patient and family adapt to declining function, providing extensive patient and family education, and helping the individual maintain a high quality of life.

Multiple Sclerosis

Multiple sclerosis (MS) is a chronic, degenerative progressive disease of the central nervous system characterized by the occurrence of small patches of demyelination in the brain and spinal cord. Demyelination refers to the destruction of myelin, the fatty and protein material that surrounds certain nerve fibers in the brain and spinal cord, which results in impaired transmission of nerve impulses (Fig. 59-6).

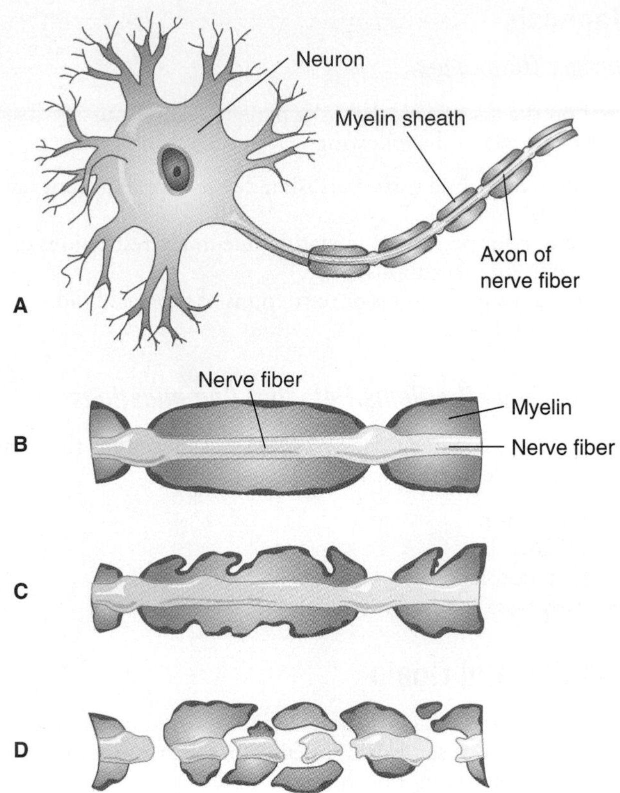

FIGURE 59•6 The process of demyelination. **A** and **B** depict a normal nerve cell and axon with myelin. **C** and **D** show the slow disintegration of myelin, resulting in a disruption in axon function.

The cause of MS is not known. Among the theories are immunologic factors, viruses, genetics, and environmental factors. Research evidence suggests that myelin damage is the primary event and that it results from a viral infection early in life that becomes apparent as an immune process later in life. Although some form of viral infection may be the initiating mechanism, a defective immune response is thought to have a major role in the pathogenesis of MS.

Patients diagnosed with MS have the presence of the HLA gene complex on chromosome 6 more frequently than those without MS (Adams, Victor, & Ropper, 1997). This supports the theory that there is a genetic contribution, but there is no conclusive evidence at this time.

MS is more common in people living in the northern temperate climate zones. It is one of the most disabling neurologic diseases of young adults (20 to 40 years of age) in the United States, affecting twice as many women as men. Its occurrence in patients who are young increases the medical, psychological, social, and economic problems encountered by both patient and family.

Pathophysiology

In MS, the demyelination is scattered irregularly throughout the central nervous system (Fig. 59-7). Myelin is lost from the axis cylinders, and the axons themselves degenerate. The plaques or patches in the involved areas become sclerosed, interrupting the flow of nerve impulses and resulting in a variety of manifestations, depending on which nerves are affected. The areas most frequently affected are the optic nerves, chiasm and tracts; the cerebrum; the brain stem and cerebellum; and the spinal cord.

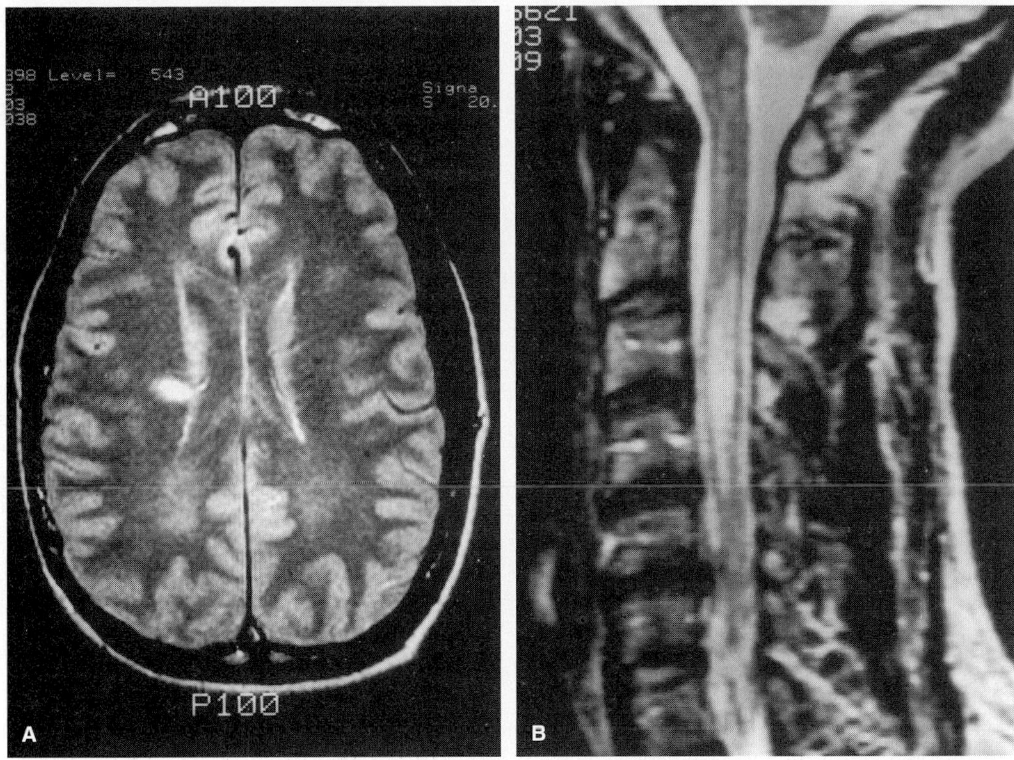

FIGURE 59•7 Multiple sclerosis. (**A**) CT scan of brain demonstrates an area of demyelination in the periventricular white matter of the right frontal lobe. The plaque is perpendicular to the lateral ventricle, a typical finding in MS. (**B**) An MRI of the spinal cord in the same patient highlights another typical finding; a flame-shaped area of demyelination within the midcervical region of the spinal cord. Courtesy of the Danbury Hospital Department of Radiology.

Clinical Manifestations

The course of MS may assume many different patterns. Most patients begin with a relapsing–remitting course, with complete recovery between clearly defined relapses. This form of the disease does not progress between relapses. Other patients have a primary progressive course from the outset with a progressive decline in function. Patients with a secondary progressive course usually begin with a relapsing–remitting pattern followed by disease progression. A progressive–relapsing course has clear acute relapses with or without full recovery. In other patients, the disease follows a benign course, with a normal life span and symptoms so mild that patients do not seek health care and treatment.

The signs and symptoms of MS are varied and multiple, reflecting the location of the lesion (plaque) or combination of lesions. The primary symptoms most commonly reported are fatigue, weakness, numbness, difficulty in coordination, and loss of balance. Visual disturbance due to lesions in the optic nerves or their connections may include blurring of vision, diplopia, patchy blindness (scotoma), and total blindness.

Spasticity of the extremities and loss of the abdominal reflexes are due to involvement of the main motor pathways (pyramidal tracts) of the spinal cord. Disruption of the sensory axons may produce sensory dysfunction (paresthesias, pain). Cognitive and psychosocial problems, including depression, may reflect frontal or parietal lobe involvement; severe cognitive changes with **dementia** are rare. Involvement of the cerebellum or basal ganglia can produce **ataxia** (impaired coordination of movements) and tremor. Loss of the control connections between the cortex and the basal ganglia may occur and cause emotional lability and euphoria in patients with MS. Bladder, bowel, and sexual problems are common.

Secondary complications of MS include urinary tract infections, constipation, pressure ulcers, contracture deformities, dependent pedal edema, pneumonia, and reactive depressions. Emotional, social, marital, economic, and vocational problems may also be a consequence of the disease.

Exacerbations and remissions are characteristic of MS. During exacerbations, new symptoms appear, and existing ones worsen; during remissions, symptoms decrease or disappear. Relapses may be associated with periods of emotional and physical stress. MRI studies demonstrate that many plaques do not produce serious symptoms, and patients with these plaques are not seriously incapacitated but have long periods of remission between episodes. There is evidence that remyelination actually occurs in some patients.

Assessment and Diagnostic Findings

MRI is the primary diagnostic tool for visualizing small plaques and for evaluating the course of the disease and effect of the treatment. Electrophoresis study of the CSF usually discloses the presence of *oligoclonal banding* (several bands of immunoglobulin G [IgG]), reflecting immunoglobulin abnormalities. In fact, abnormal IgG antibody appears in the CSF of up to 95% of patients with MS. Evoked potential studies are carried out to help define the extent of the disease process and monitor changes. Underlying bladder dysfunction is diagnosed by urodynamic studies. Neuropsychological testing may be indicated to assess cognitive impairment. A sexual history helps to identify changes in sexual function in men and women with MS.

Medical Management

No cure exists for MS. An individualized, organized, and rational treatment program is indicated to relieve the patient's symptoms and provide continuing support. The goals of treatment are to delay the progression of the disease, manage chronic symptoms, and treat acute exacerbations. Many patients with MS have stable disease and require only intermittent treatment, whereas others experience steady progression of their disease. Symptoms requiring intervention include spasticity, fatigue, bladder dysfunction, and ataxia. Management strategies target the various motor and sensory symptoms and effects of immobility that can occur.

PHARMACOLOGIC THERAPY

Immunotherapeutic medications prevent destruction of nerve tissue by suppressing the immune system and decreasing inflammation. Corticosteroids (prednisone and methylprednisolone) and ACTH (Acthar, Cortrosyn) are used as anti-inflammatory agents that may improve nerve conduction. Because immune mechanisms may be a factor in the pathogenesis of MS, a number of nonsteroidal immunosuppressive agents are being tried to modulate the immune response, reduce the rate at which the disease progresses, and decrease the frequency and severity of the exacerbations. These medications include azathioprine (Imuran), cyclophosphamide (Cytoxan), cyclosporine (Sandimmune), glatiramer acetate (Copaxone), and the interferons.

The interferons beta-1b (Betaseron) and beta-1a (Avonex) are used in relapsing–remitting MS. Both interferons have been found to be effective in significantly reducing the number and severity of acute exacerbations, with MRI scans showing fewer areas of demyelination in brain tissue.

Researchers continue to investigate other possible treatments of MS. The most intensive research involves medications intended to limit demyelination by reducing inflammation and modifying the immune response. Methods under investigation include other interferons, growth hormone (insulin-like growth factor I), colchicine, monoclonal antibodies, methotrexate, and T-cell receptor peptide.

Other medications are prescribed for specific symptom management. Baclofen, an antispasmodic agent, is the current treatment of choice for spasticity. Patients with severe spasticity and contractures may require nerve blocks and surgical intervention to prevent further disability. More than 75% of MS patients complain of fatigue that interferes with activities of daily living and may be treated with amantadine (Symmetrel), pemoline (Cylert), or fluoxetine (Prozac). Ataxia is a chronic problem most resistant to treatment. Medications used to treat ataxia include beta-adrenergic blockers (Inderal), anticonvulsants (Neurontin), and benzodiazepines (Klonopin).

Management of bladder and bowel control is often among the patient's most difficult problems. Generally, bladder symptoms fall into the following categories: (1) inability to store urine (hyperreflexic, uninhibited); (2) inability to empty the bladder (hyporeflexic, hypotonic); and (3) a mixture of both types. A variety of medications (anticholinergics, alpha-adrenergic blockers, or antispasmodic agents) may be used to treat these problems. Intermittent self-catheterization is an effective treatment of bladder dysfunction.

Urinary tract infection is often superimposed on the underlying neurologic dysfunction. Ascorbic acid may be given to acidify the urine, making bacterial growth less likely. Antibiotics are prescribed when appropriate.

NURSING PROCESS: THE PATIENT WITH MULTIPLE SCLEROSIS

Assessment

Nursing assessment addresses actual and potential problems associated with the disease, including neurologic problems, secondary complications, and the impact of the disease on the patient and family. The patient's movements and walking are observed to determine if there is danger of falling. Assessment of function is carried out both when the patient is well rested and when fatigued. The patient is assessed for weakness, spasticity, visual impairment, incontinence, and disorders of swallowing and speech. Additional areas of assessment include the following: How has MS affected the patient's lifestyle? How well is the patient coping? What would the patient like to do better?

Nursing Diagnosis

Based on the assessment data, the patient's major nursing diagnoses may include the following:

- Impaired physical mobility related to weakness, muscle paresis, spasticity
- Risk for injury related to sensory and visual impairment
- Altered urinary and bowel elimination (urgency, frequency, incontinence, constipation) related to spinal cord dysfunction
- Impaired speech and swallowing related to cranial nerve involvement
- Altered thought processes (loss of memory, dementia, euphoria) related to cerebral dysfunction
- Ineffective individual coping
- Impaired home maintenance management related to physical, psychological, and social limits imposed by MS
- Potential for sexual dysfunction related to spinal cord involvement or psychological reactions to condition

Planning and Goals

The major goals for the patient may include promotion of physical mobility, avoidance of injury, achievement of bladder and bowel continence, promotion of speech and swallowing mechanisms, improvement of cognitive function, development of coping strengths, improved self-care, and adaptation to sexual dysfunction.

Nursing Interventions

An individualized program of physical therapy, rehabilitation, and education is combined with emotional support. The nursing interventions include patient education to enable the person with MS to deal with the physiologic, social, and psychological problems that accompany chronic disease.

Promoting Physical Mobility

Relaxation and coordination exercises promote muscle efficiency for the person with MS. Progressive resistive exercises are used to strengthen weak muscles because diminishing muscle power is often a significant problem for the patient with MS.

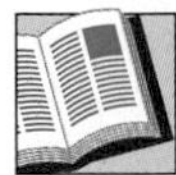

NURSING RESEARCH

Exercise Can Enhance Physical Functioning in Patients With MS

Stuifbergen, A. K. (1997). Physical activity and perceived health status in persons with multiple sclerosis. *Journal of Neuroscience Nursing, 29*(1), 238–243.

Purpose

Regular physical activity and exercise are recommended for maintaining health and fitness. In people with multiple sclerosis (MS), participation in activity and exercise may prevent deconditioning and maintain optimum function. This study was conducted to determine the relationship of participation in physical activity to social, mental, and physical health and well-being in people with MS.

Study Sample and Design

A convenience sample of 37 people with MS was included in the study. Participants completed the Human Activity Profile (HAP) and the Medical Outcomes Study Short-Form Health Survey (SF36) at home and returned the surveys by mail, representing a response rate of 59%. A Maximal Activity Score (MAS) and Adjusted Activity Score (AAS) were derived from the HAP. The MAS reflects the highest item of activity that the subject is "still doing" and is considered the best estimate of the respondent's highest level of energy expenditure. The AAS reflects usual daily activities and is an estimate of the subject's average level of energy expenditure. The SF36 provided information about limitations in physical, social, and role activities because of physical health problems; presence of pain; general medical health; limitations in role activities because of emotional problems; vitality; and general health perceptions. Demographic data and information about MS symptoms and disability were also obtained through self report.

The mean age of the sample subjects was 49.46 years (SD = 12.28 years); ages ranged from 23 to 77 years. Most participants were women.

Findings

Motor symptoms were reported by 60% and sensory symptoms by 49% of the participants. As a group, the study participants reported lower levels of participation in physical activity and exercise than previous reports of healthy people and of patients with a variety of chronic disorders. Further, when the difference between MAS and AAS scores was calculated, the average level of activity of the MS group was much lower than the maximal level they were able to accomplish. Higher activity scores (MAS and AAS) were associated with higher scores on the SF36 subscores of physical function and general health. Subjects who reported participation in regular exercise had significantly higher scores on physical functioning, as assessed by the physical function subscale of the SF36, than those who did not exercise.

Nursing Implications

The results of this study reveal that people with MS have lower average and lower maximal levels of activity than the general population. Although these findings may be due to a variety of factors (disease-related physical limitations, recommendations from health care providers, energy-conserving efforts, or deconditioning), the consequences of decreased participation in physical activity and exercise should be examined. Individualized programs to prevent deconditioning through exercise and activity within the patient's disease-related limitations should be considered in an effort to promote health and well-being of people with MS.

EXERCISES

Walking exercises improve the gait, particularly when there is loss of position sense of the legs and feet. If certain muscle groups are irreversibly affected, other muscles can be trained to take over their actions. Instruction in use of assistive devices may be needed to ensure their correct and safe use.

MINIMIZING SPASTICITY AND CONTRACTURES

Muscle spasticity is common and, in its later stages, is characterized by severe adductor spasm of the hips with flexor spasm of the hips and knees. If this is not relieved, fibrous contractures of these joints with resultant pressure ulcers over the sacrum and hips (due to inability to position the patient properly) occur. Warm packs may be beneficial, but hot baths should be avoided because of risk for burn injury secondary to sensory loss and the risk of increasing symptoms that is associated with an elevation of the body temperature.

Daily exercises for muscle stretching are prescribed to minimize joint contractures. Special attention is given to hamstrings, gastrocnemius muscles, hip adductors, biceps, and wrist and finger flexors. Muscle spasticity is common and interferes with normal function. A stretch–hold–relax routine is helpful for relaxing and treating muscle spasticity. Swimming and stationary bicycling are useful, and progressive weight-bearing can relieve spasticity in the legs. The patient should not be hurried in any of these activities because this often increases spasticity.

ACTIVITY AND REST

The patient is encouraged to work up to a point just short of fatigue. Very strenuous physical exercise is not advisable because it raises the body temperature and may aggravate symptoms. Prolonged exercise that tires an extremity may cause paresis, numbness, or incoordination. The patient is advised to take frequent short rest periods, preferably lying down. Extreme fatigue may be a contributing factor in the exacerbation of symptoms.

MINIMIZING EFFECTS OF IMMOBILITY

Because of the decreased physical activity and immobility that often occur with MS, complications associated with immobility, including pressure ulcers, expiratory muscle weakness, and accumulation of bronchial secretions, need to be considered and steps taken to prevent them. Measures to prevent such complications include assessment and maintenance of skin integrity and coughing and deep breathing exercises.

Preventing Injury

If motor dysfunction causes problems of incoordination and clumsiness, or if ataxia is apparent, the patient is at risk for falling. To overcome this disability, the patient is taught to walk with feet wide apart to widen the base of support and to increase walking stability. If there is loss of position sense, the patient is taught to watch the feet while walking. Gait training may require assistive devices (walker, cane, braces, crutches, parallel bars) and instruction about their use by a physical therapist. If the gait remains inefficient, a wheelchair or motorized scooter may be the solution. The occupational therapist is a valuable resource person in suggesting and securing aids to promote independence. If incoordination is a problem and tremor of the upper extremities occurs when voluntary movement is attempted (intention tremor), weighted bracelets or wrist cuffs are helpful. The patient is trained in transfer and activities of daily living.

Because sensory loss may occur in addition to motor loss, pressure ulcers are a continuing threat to skin integrity. Confinement to a wheelchair increases the risk. (See Chap. 10 for a discussion of the prevention and treatment of pressure ulcers.)

Enhancing Bladder and Bowel Control

The patient with urinary frequency, urgency, or incontinence requires special support. The sensation of the need to void must be heeded immediately, so the bedpan or urinal should be readily available. A voiding time schedule is set up (every 1½ to 2 hours initially, with gradual lengthening of the time intervals). The patient is instructed to drink a measured amount of fluid every 2 hours and then attempt to void 30 minutes after drinking. Using a timer or wristwatch with an alarm may be helpful for the patient who does not have enough sensation to signal the need to empty the bladder. The nurse encourages the patient to take the prescribed medications to treat bladder spasticity because this allows greater independence. Intermittent self-catheterization has been successful in maintaining bladder control in patients with MS.

If the female patient has permanent urinary incontinence, urinary diversion procedures may be considered. The male patient may wear a condom appliance for urine collection.

Bowel problems include constipation, fecal impaction, and incontinence. Adequate fluids, dietary fiber, and a bowel-training program are frequently effective in solving these problems.

Managing Speech and Swallowing Difficulties

When the cranial nerves controlling the mechanisms of speech and swallowing are involved, **dysarthrias** (defects of articulation) marked by slurring, low volume of speech, and difficulties in phonation may occur. Swallowing disturbances (**dysphagia**) may also occur. A speech therapist evaluates speech and swallowing and instructs the patient, family, and health team members about strategies to compensate for speech and swallowing problems. The nurse reinforces this instruction and encourages the patient and family to adhere to the plan. Impaired swallowing increases the patient's risk for aspiration; therefore, strategies (eg, having suction apparatus available, careful feeding, proper positioning for eating) are needed to reduce that risk.

Improving Sensory and Cognitive Function

Measures may be taken if visual defects (the cranial nerves affecting vision may be affected by MS) or changes in cognitive status occur.

VISION

An eye patch or an eyeglass occluder may be used to block visual impulses of one eye when the patient has diplopia (double vision). Prism glasses may be helpful for the bedridden patient who is having difficulty reading in the supine position. People with physical limitations preventing them from reading regular-print materials are eligible for the free talking book services of the Library of Congress or may wish to obtain large-type books available at most local libraries.

COGNITION AND EMOTIONAL RESPONSES

Cognitive impairment and emotional lability may occur early in MS in some patients and may impose numerous stresses on the patient and family. Some patients with MS are forgetful and easily distracted and may exhibit emotional lability.

Patients adapt to illness in a variety of ways, which may include denial, depression, withdrawal, and hostility. Emotional support assists patients and their families to adapt to the changes and uncertainties associated with MS and to cope with the disruption in their lives. The patient is assisted to set meaningful and realistic goals to achieve a sense of purpose, to remain as active as possible, and to keep up social interests and activities. Hobbies may help the patient's morale and provide satisfying interests if the disease progresses to the stage in which normal activities cannot be pursued.

The family should be made aware of the nature and degree of cognitive impairment. The environment is kept structured, and lists and other memory aids are used to help the patient with cognitive changes to maintain a daily routine.

STRENGTHENING COPING MECHANISMS

The diagnosis of MS is always distressing to the patient and family. They need to know that no two patients who have MS have identical symptoms or courses of illness. Although some patients do experience significant disability early, others have a near-normal life span with minimal disability. Some families, however, face overwhelming frustrations and problems. MS affects people who are often in a productive stage of life and concerned about career and family responsibilities. Family conflict, disintegration, separation, and divorce are not uncommon. Often, very young family members assume the responsibility of caring for a disabled parent. Nursing interventions in this area include alleviating stress and making appropriate referrals for counseling and support to minimize the adverse effects of dealing with chronic illness.

The nurse, mindful of these complex problems, initiates home care and coordinates a network of services, including social services, speech therapy, physical therapy, and homemaker services. To strengthen the patient's coping skills, as much information as possible is provided. People who live with chronic illness need an updated list of assistive devices, services, and resources that are available.

Coping through problem solving involves helping the patient define the problem and develop alternatives for its management. Careful planning and maintaining flexibility and a hopeful attitude are useful for psychological and physical adaptation.

Improving Self-Care Abilities

MS can affect every facet of daily living. After certain abilities are lost, they are often impossible to regain. Physical function may vary from day to day. Modifications that allow independence in self-care should be implemented (assistive eating devices, raised toilet seat, bathing aids, telephone modifications, long-handled comb, tongs, modified clothing). Physical and emotional stresses should be avoided as much as possible because these may worsen symptoms and impair performance. Exposure to heat increases fatigue and muscle weakness. Therefore, air-conditioning in at least one room is recommended. Exposure to extreme cold may increase spasticity.

Promoting Sexual Functioning

Patients with MS and their partners face problems that interfere with sexual activity, arising not only as a direct consequence of nerve damage but also from psychological reactions to the disease. Easy fatigability, conflicts arising from dependency and depression, emotional lability, loss of self-esteem, and feelings of self-worth compound the problem. Erectile and ejaculatory disorders in men and orgasmic dysfunction and adductor spasms of the thigh muscles in women can make sexual intercourse difficult or impossible. Bladder and bowel incontinence and urinary tract infections add to the difficulties.

An experienced sexual counselor helps bring into focus the patient's or partner's sexual resources and suggests relevant information and supportive therapy. Sharing and communicating feelings, planning for sexual activity (to minimize the effects of fatigue), and exploring alternative methods of sexual expression may open up a wide range of sexual enjoyment and experiences.

Promoting Home and Community-Based Care

TEACHING PATIENTS SELF-CARE

If the disease progresses, the patient and family will require assistance to deal with new disabilities and changes. Teaching of new self-care techniques may be initiated in the hospital or clinic setting and reinforced in the home. Teaching about self-care may address use of assistive devices, self-catheterization, and administration of medications that affect the course of MS or treat MS complications. Exercises that enable the patient to continue some form of activity or that maintain or improve swallowing, speech, or respiratory function may be taught to the patient and family.

CONTINUING CARE

If the disease progresses, the patient and family will require assistance to deal with new disabilities and changes. Teaching and reinforcement of these new techniques is often provided in the patient's home by the home care nurse. Nurses in the home setting assess for changes in the patient's physical and emotional status, provide physical care to the patient if required, coordinate outpatient services and resources, and encourage health promotion and adaptation. If changes in the disease or its course are noted, the home care nurse encourages the patient to contact the primary care provider because treatment of an acute exacerbation or new problem may be indicated. Continuing health care and follow-up are recommended.

The nurse who has continuing contact with the patient and the family is often in an ideal situation to assess how both the patient and the family are coping with these changes. Because the diagnosis of MS is often made when the patient is in the most productive years of life, many questions about the disease and the patient's future arise. The patient with MS is encouraged to contact the local chapter of the National Multiple Sclerosis Society for services, publications, and contact with others with MS. Local chapters also provide direct services to patients. Through group participation, the patient has an opportunity to meet others with similar problems, to share experiences, and to learn self-help methods in a social environment.

Evaluation

Expected Outcomes

Expected outcomes may include:

1. Adapts to impaired mobility and spasticity
   a. Participates in gait-training and rehabilitation program
   b. Establishes a balanced program of rest and exercise
   c. Uses assistive devices correctly and safely
2. Avoids injury
   a. Uses visual cues to compensate for decreased sense of touch or position
   b. Asks for assistance when necessary
3. Attains or maintains improved bladder and bowel control
   a. Monitors self for urine retention and employs intermittent self-catheterization technique, if indicated
   b. Identifies the signs and symptoms of urinary tract infection
   c. Maintains adequate fluid and fiber intake
4. Participates in strategies to improve speech and swallowing
   a. Practices exercises recommended by speech therapist
   b. Maintains adequate nutritional intake without aspiration
5. Compensates for cognitive dysfunction
   a. Uses lists and other aids to compensate for memory losses
   b. Discusses problems with trusted advisor or friend
   c. Substitutes new activities for those that are no longer possible
6. Demonstrates improved coping strategies
   a. Maintains sense of control
   b. Modifies lifestyle to fit goals and limitations
   c. Verbalizes desire to pursue goals and developmental tasks of adulthood
7. Adapts to changes in sexual function
   a. Is able to discuss problem with partner and appropriate health professional
   b. Identifies alternate means of sexual expression

Parkinson's Disease

Parkinson's disease is a slowly progressing neurologic movement disorder that eventually leads to disability. Among the several types of Parkinson's disease, the degenerative or idiopathic form is most common. Although the cause of Parkinson's disease is unknown, research has suggested several causative factors, including genetics, atherosclerosis, excessive accumulation of oxygen free radicals, viral infections, head trauma, chronic antipsychotic medication use, and some environmental exposures. Parkinsonian symptoms usually first appear in the fifth decade of life; however, cases have been diagnosed at the age of 30 years. It is the fourth most common

HOME CARE TEACHING CHECKLIST: THE PATIENT WITH MULTIPLE SCLEROSIS

At the completion of the program, the patient or caregiver will be able to:	Patient	Caregiver
• State how to access MS Society and available resources.	✔	✔
• Discuss the clinical course of MS.	✔	✔
• Identify strategies to manage symptoms (pain, cognitive responses, dysphagia, tremors, visual disturbances).	✔	✔
• State how to prevent complications (pressure ulcers, pneumonia, depression).	✔	✔
• Identify coping strategies.	✔	✔
• Identify ways to minimize fatigue.	✔	✔
• Explain how to prevent injury.	✔	✔
• State ways to adapt to sexual dysfunction.	✔	✔
• Discuss ways to control bowel and bladder function.	✔	✔
• Name benefits of exercise and physical activity.	✔	✔
• Identify ways to minimize immobility and spasticity.	✔	✔
• Describe medication regimen and potential adverse effects.	✔	✔

neurodegenerative disease. Parkinson's disease affects men more frequently than women and nearly 1% of the population older than 65 years of age.

Pathophysiology

Parkinson's disease is associated with decreased levels of dopamine due to destruction of pigmented neuronal cells in the substantia nigra in the basal ganglia of the brain (Fig. 59-8). The nuclei of the substantia nigra project fibers or neuronal pathways to the corpus striatum, where neurotransmitters are key to control of complex body movements. Through the neurotransmitters acetylcholine (excitatory) and dopamine (inhibitory), striatal neurons relay messages to the higher motor centers that control and refine motor movements (Fig. 59-9). The loss of dopamine stores in this area of the brain results in more excitatory neurotransmitters than inhibitory neurotransmitters, leading to an imbalance that affects voluntary movement.

Clinical symptoms do not appear until 60% of the pigmented neurons are lost and the striatal dopamine level is decreased by 80%. Cellular degeneration causes impairment of the extrapyramidal tracts that control semiautomatic functions and coordinated movements. Motor cells of the motor cortex and the pyramidal tracts are not affected by the disease.

Clinical Manifestations

Parkinson's disease has a gradual onset, a slow progression of symptoms, and a chronic, prolonged course. The three cardinal signs of Parkinson's disease are tremor, rigidity, and **bradykinesia** (abnormally slow movements). Other features include hypokinesia, flexed posture, loss of postural reflexes, and the freezing phenomenon.

TREMOR

Although symptoms are variable, a slow, unilateral, resting tremor is present in 70% of patients at the time of diagnosis. Resting tremor characteristically disappears with purposeful movement, but is evident as the extremities maintain a motionless position and increases with walking. The tremor may present as a rhythmic, slow turning motion (pronation-supination) of the forearm and the hand, and a motion of the thumb against the fingers as if rolling a pill between the fingers. It is present while the patient is at rest. It increases when the patient is concentrating or is anxious.

RIGIDITY

Muscle rigidity is characterized by resistance to passive limb movement. Passive movement of an extremity may cause it to move in jerky increments referred to as cogwheeling. Rigidity of the passive extremity increases when another extremity is engaged in voluntary active movement. Stiffness of the neck, trunk, and shoulders is common and, early in the disease, the patient may complain of shoulder pain.

BRADYKINESIA

One of the most common features of Parkinson's disease is bradykinesia. Patients take longer to complete most activities and have difficulty initiating movement, such as rising from a sitting position or turning in bed.

Hypokinesia (abnormally diminished movement) is common and may appear after the tremor. The freezing phenomenon is a transient inability to perform active movement and is thought to be an extreme form of bradykinesia. There is a tendency to shuffle and a decrease in arm swing. Patients tend to develop **micrographia** (shrinking, slow handwriting) as dexterity declines. The face becomes increasingly masklike and expressionless; there is decreased frequency of blinking. Speech becomes soft, slurred, low pitched, and less audible. Patients often develop dysphagia, begin to drool, and are at risk for choking and aspiration.

PATHOPHYSIOLOGY

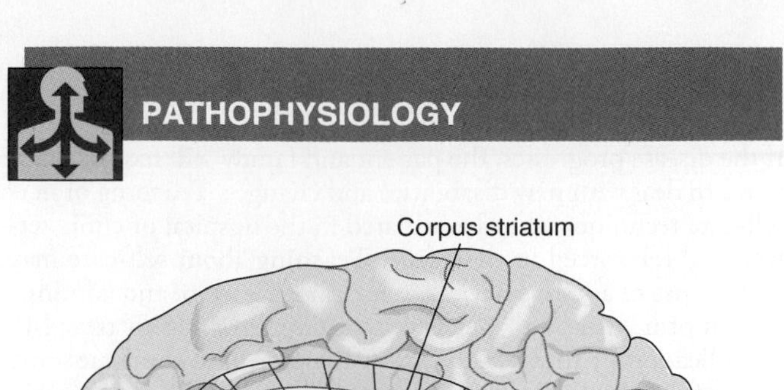

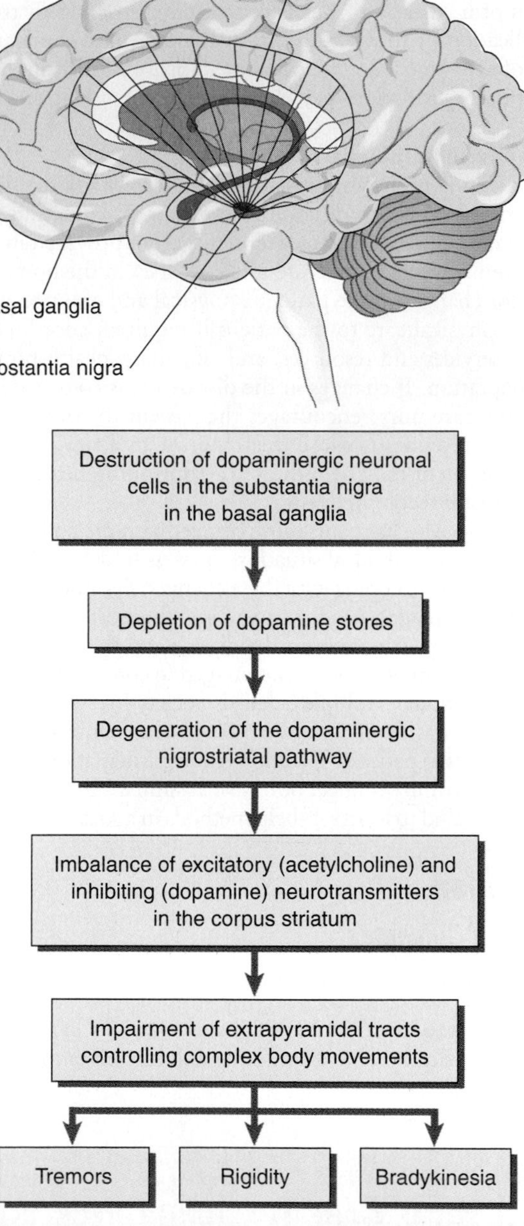

FIGURE 59•8 The nuclei in the substantia nigra project fibers to the corpus striatum. The nerve fibers carry dopamine to the corpus striatum. The loss of dopamine nerve cells from the brain's substantia nigra is thought to be responsible for the symptoms of parkinsonism.

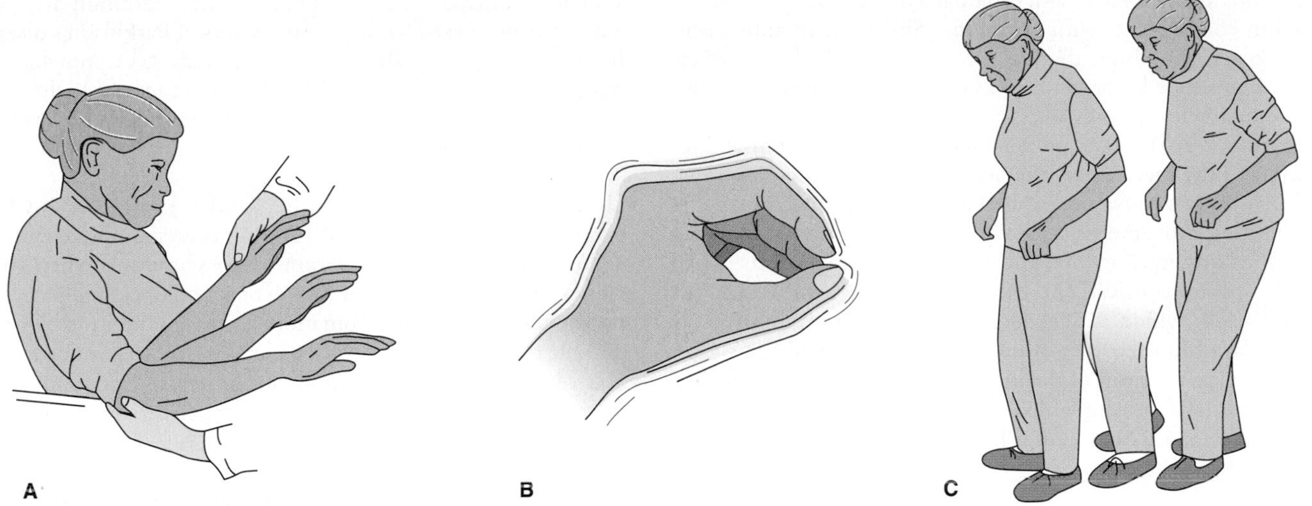

FIGURE 59•9 Parkinson's disease is manifested by (**A**) "cogwheeling" that accompanies passive extremity movement; (**B**) "pill-rolling" tremor; (**C**) postural instability, forward stoop, shuffling gait.

The patient with Parkinson's disease often develops postural and gait problems. There is a loss of postural reflexes, and the patient stands with head bent forward and walks with a propulsive gait. The posture is caused by the forward flexion of the neck, hips, knees, and elbows. The patient may walk faster and faster, trying to move the feet forward under the body's center of gravity (shuffling gait). Difficulty in pivoting and loss of balance (either forward or backward) places the patient at risk for falls.

OTHER MANIFESTATIONS

The effect of Parkinson's disease on the basal ganglia often produces autonomic symptoms that include excessive and uncontrolled sweating, orthostatic hypotension, gastric and urinary retention, and constipation. Sleep disorders are common.

Depression is common, but it has not been established whether the depression is a reaction to the disorder or is related to a biochemical abnormality. Mental changes may appear in the form of cognitive, perceptual, and memory deficits, although intellect is not usually affected. A number of psychiatric manifestations (personality changes, psychosis, dementia, acute confusion) are common among the elderly. The prevalence of dementia is about 25% to 40%, and the pattern is similar to that of patients with Alzheimer's disease.

Complications associated with Parkinson's disease are common and are typically related to disorders of movement. As the disease progresses, patients are at risk for respiratory and urinary tract infection, skin breakdown, and injury due to falls. Numerous complications are caused by the adverse effects of medications used to treat parkinsonian symptoms.

Assessment and Diagnostic Findings

Laboratory tests and imaging studies are not helpful in the diagnosis of Parkinson's disease, although **positron emission tomography** (PET) scanning has been used in the evaluation of levodopa (precursor of dopamine) uptake and conversion to dopamine in the corpus striatum. Currently, the disease is diagnosed clinically from the patient's history and the presence of two of the three cardinal manifestations: tremor, muscle rigidity, and bradykinesia.

Early diagnosis of Parkinson's disease can be difficult because the patient can rarely pinpoint when symptoms started. Often, a family member notices a change, such as stooped posture, a stiff arm, a slight limp, tremor, or slow, small handwriting. The medical history, presenting symptoms, neurologic examination, and response to pharmacologic management are carefully evaluated when making the diagnosis.

Medical Management

Treatment is directed at controlling symptoms and maintaining the patient's functional independence because there are no medical or surgical approaches that prevent disease progression. Care is individualized for each patient based on presenting symptoms and social, occupational, and emotional needs. Pharmacologic management is currently the mainstay of treatment, although advances in research have led to increased interest in surgical interventions. Patients with Parkinson's disease are usually cared for at home and admitted to the hospital only for complications of the disease, to initiate new treatment options, or for "drug holidays," a period during which medication is stopped temporarily.

PHARMACOLOGIC THERAPY

Antiparkinsonian medications act by (1) increasing striatal dopaminergic activity or (2) reducing the excessive influence of excitatory cholinergic neurons on the extrapyramidal tract, thereby restoring a balance between dopaminergic and cholinergic activities.

Levodopa Therapy. Levodopa is the most effective agent for the treatment of Parkinson's disease. Because it is thought to precipitate oxidation that further damages the substantia nigra and eventually speeds disease progression, physicians delay prescribing the medication or increasing the dosage for as long as possible. Levodopa is converted from L-dopa to dopamine in the basal ganglia, producing symptom relief. The beneficial effects of levodopa are most pronounced in the first few years of treatment. Benefits begin to wane and adverse side effects become more severe over time. Confusion, hallucinations, depression, and sleep alterations are associated with prolonged use. Levodopa is usually given in combination with carbidopa (Sinemet), an amino acid decarboxylase inhibitor that helps to maximize the beneficial effects of levodopa by preventing its breakdown outside the brain and reducing its adverse effects.

Within 5 to 10 years, most patients develop a response fluctuation to the medication characterized by **dyskinesia** (abnormal involuntary movements), including facial grimacing, rhythmic jerking movements of the hands, head bobbing, chewing and smacking movements, and involuntary movements of the trunk and extremities. The patient may experience an on–off syndrome in which sudden periods of near immobility ("off effect") are followed by a sudden return of effectiveness ("on effect"). One method of dealing with on–off fluctuations is a "drug holiday," during which the medication is stopped temporarily. This usually requires hospitalization and expert medical and nursing care.

Anticholinergic Therapy. Anticholinergic agents (trihexyphenidyl, cycrimine, procyclidine, biperiden, and benztropine mesylate) are effective in controlling the tremor and rigidity of parkinsonism. These medications may be used in combination with levodopa. They counteract the action of the neurotransmitter acetylcholine. Because the side effects include blurred vision, flushing, rash, constipation, urinary retention, and acute confusional states, these medications are often poorly tolerated in the elderly. Intraocular pressure must be closely monitored because these medications are contraindicated in patients with narrow-angle glaucoma. Patients with prostatic hyperplasia are monitored for signs of urinary retention.

Antiviral Therapy. Amantadine hydrochloride (Symmetrel) is an antiviral agent used early in the treatment of Parkinson's disease to reduce rigidity, tremor, and bradykinesia. It is thought to act by releasing dopamine from neuronal storage sites. Amantadine has a low incidence of side effects, which include psychiatric disturbances (mood changes, confusion, depression, hallucinations), lower extremity edema, nausea, epigastric distress, urinary retention, headache, and visual impairment.

Dopamine Agonists. Bromocriptine mesylate and pergolide (ergot derivatives) are dopamine receptor agonists and are useful in postponing the initiation of carbidopa or levodopa therapy. Dopamine agonists are often added to the medication regimen when carbidopa or levodopa loses effectiveness. Pergolide (Permax) is 10 times more potent than bromocriptine mesylate (Parlodel), although this provides no therapeutic advantage. Adverse reactions to these medications include nausea, vomiting, diarrhea, lightheadedness, hypotension, impotence, and psychiatric effects.

Two new dopamine agonists, ropinirole and pramipexole (nonergot derivatives), are primarily for patients in the early stages of Parkinson's disease and are not expected to have the potentially serious adverse effects of pergolide and bromocriptine mesylate. Pramipexole (Mirapex) can be used without levodopa for treatment of early disease and with levodopa in advanced stages. Cabergoline (Dostinex), an ergot alkaloid with a long duration of action, has been approved for use.

Monoamine Oxidase Inhibitors. L-Deprenyl (selegiline) is one of the most exciting and controversial developments in the pharmacotherapy of Parkinson's disease. This medication inhibits dopamine breakdown and is thought to slow the progression of the disease. Researchers believe this medication may have a neuroprotective effect in the early stages of Parkinson's disease, but this has not been shown in clinical trials. L-Deprenyl is currently used in combination with a dopamine agonist to delay the use of carbidopa or levodopa therapy. Adverse effects are similar to those of levodopa.

Catechol-O-methyltransferase (COMT) Inhibitors. Clinical trials suggest that the COMT inhibitors entacapone and tolcapone have no effect on parkinsonian symptoms when given alone, but can increase the duration of action of carbidopa or levodopa when given in combination. COMT inhibitors block an enzyme that metabolizes levodopa, making more levodopa available for conversion to dopamine in the brain. Entacapone and tolcapone reduce motor fluctuations in patients with advanced Parkinson's disease.

Antidepressants. Tricyclic antidepressants may be given to alleviate the depression that is so common in Parkinson's disease. The usual dosage is one third to one half the dose used in depressed patients without Parkinson's disease. Amitriptyline is often prescribed because of its anticholinergic and antidepressant effect. Serotonin reuptake inhibitors, such as fluoxetine and bupropion, are effective for treating depression but may aggravate parkinsonism.

Antihistamines. Diphenhydramine, orphenadrine, and phenindamine have mild central anticholinergic and sedative effects and may reduce tremors.

SURGICAL MANAGEMENT

The limitations of levodopa therapy, improvements in stereotactic surgery, and new approaches in transplantation have renewed interest in the surgical treatment of Parkinson's disease. In patients with disabling tremor, rigidity, or severe levodopa-induced dyskinesia, surgery may be considered. Although surgery provides some relief in selected patients, it has not been demonstrated to alter the course of the disease or produce permanent improvement.

Stereotactic Procedures. Thalamotomy and pallidotomy are performed under local anesthesia and are effective in relieving many of the symptoms of Parkinson's disease. Patients are usually chosen for these procedures because of an inadequate response to medical therapy and must meet strict criteria to be eligible for the procedure. Patients considered candidates for these procedures are those with idiopathic Parkinson's disease who are taking maximum doses of antiparkinsonism medications. Patients with dementia and atypical Parkinson's disease are usually excluded from consideration for stereotactic procedures. Parkinson's disease rating scales and specific neurologic testing are used to identify patients eligible for the procedures.

The intent of thalamotomy and pallidotomy is to interrupt the nerve pathways and alleviate tremor or rigidity. During thalamotomy, a stereotactic electrical stimulator destroys part of the ventrolateral portion of the thalamus in an attempt to reduce tremor. The most common complications of thalamotomy are ataxia and hemiparesis. Pallidotomy involves destroying part of the ventral aspect of the medial globus pallidus through electrical stimulation and is effective in reducing rigidity, bradykinesia, and dyskinesia. Complications include hemiparesis, stroke, and visual changes.

CT, radiography, MRI, or angiography is used to localize the appropriate surgical site in the brain. The patient's head is placed in a stereotactic frame (Fig. 59-10), an incision is made in the

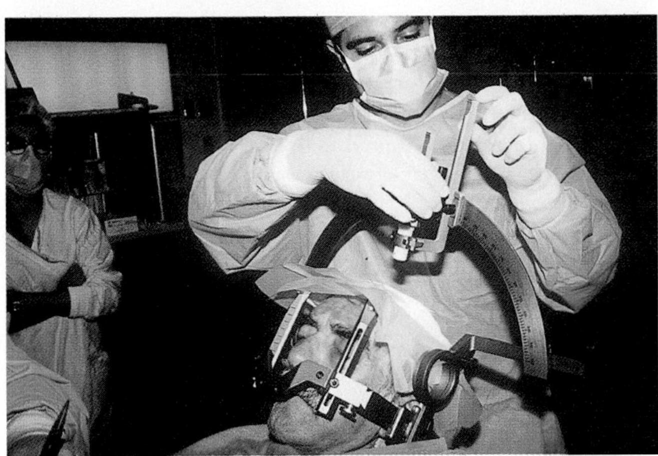

FIGURE 59•10 Patient being prepared for pallidotomy using a stereotactic frame to immobilize the head.

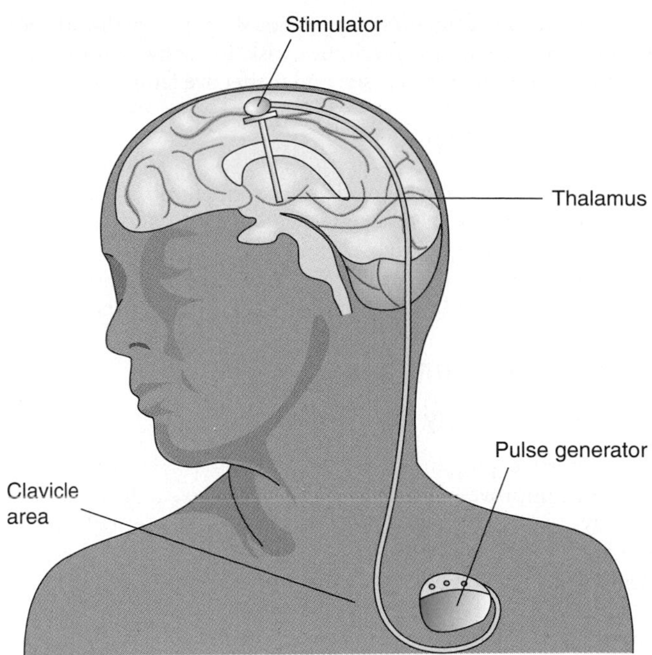

FIGURE 59•11 Deep brain stimulation. A pulse generator, surgically implanted in a pouch beneath the clavicle, sends high-frequency electrical impulses to the thalamus, thereby blocking the nerve pathways associated with tremors in Parkinson's disease.

skin, a burr hole is made, and an electrode is passed through the burr hole to the target area in the thalamus or globus pallidum. The desired response of the patient to the electrical stimulation is the basis for the final site chosen by the neurosurgeon. Stereotactic procedures are completed on one side of the brain at a time. If rigidity or tremor are bilateral, a 6-month interval is suggested between procedures.

Neural Transplantation. Surgical implantation of adrenal medullary tissue into the corpus striatum is performed in an effort to reestablish normal dopamine release. Preliminary evidence has shown high morbidity and mortality rates, and the implants appear to improve parkinsonian symptoms for only 6 months. Researchers are conducting studies to determine if transplanting human fetal brain cells into the nigrostriatal region is effective (Tapper, 1997). Recent results indicate that dosages of antiparkinson medications can be reduced after the surgery (Krauss & Jankovic, 1996). Legal and ethical issues surrounding the use of fetal brain cells have limited implementation of this procedure.

Deep Brain Stimulation. Although not yet approved by the Food and Drug Administration, pacemaker-like brain implants are showing promising results in relieving the tremors of Parkinson's disease. An electrode is placed in the thalamus and connected to a pulse generator implanted in a subcutaneous subclavical or abdominal pouch. The battery-powered pulse generator sends high frequency electrical impulses through a wire placed under the skin to a lead anchored to the skull (Fig. 59-11). The electrode blocks nerve pathways in the brain that cause tremors.

NURSING PROCESS: THE PATIENT WITH PARKINSON'S DISEASE

Assessment

Assessment focuses on how the disease has affected the patient's activities of daily living and functional abilities. Patients are observed for degree of disability and what functional changes occur throughout the day, such as responses to medication. Nearly every patient with a movement disorder has some functional alteration and may have some type of behavioral dysfunction. The following questions may be helpful:

- Do you have leg or arm stiffness?
- Have you experienced any irregular jerking of your arms or legs?
- Have you ever been "frozen" or rooted to the spot and unable to move?
- Does your mouth water excessively? Have you (or others) noticed yourself grimacing or making faces or chewing movements?
- What specific activities do you have difficulty doing?

During this assessment, the nurse observes the patient for quality of speech, loss of facial expression, swallowing deficits (drooling, poor head control, coughing), tremors, slowness of movement, weakness, forward posture, rigidity, evidence of mental slowness, and confusion.

Nursing Diagnosis

Based on the assessment data, the patient's major nursing diagnoses may include the following:

- Impaired physical mobility related to muscle rigidity and motor weakness
- Self-care deficits (eating, drinking, dressing, hygiene) related to tremor and motor disturbance
- Constipation related to medication and reduced activity
- Altered nutrition, less than body requirements, related to tremor, slowness in eating, difficulty in chewing and swallowing
- Impaired verbal communication related to decreased speech volume, slowness of speech, inability to move facial muscles
- Ineffective individual coping related to depression and dysfunction due to disease progression

Other nursing diagnoses may include sleep pattern disturbances, knowledge deficit, risk for injury, risk for activity intolerance, alteration in thought processes, and ineffective family coping.

Planning and Goals

The patient's goals may include improvement of functional mobility, maintenance of independence in activities of daily living, achievement of adequate bowel elimination, attainment and maintenance of acceptable nutritional status, achievement of effective communication, and development of positive coping mechanisms.

Nursing Interventions

Improving Mobility

A progressive program of daily exercise will increase muscle strength, improve coordination and dexterity, reduce muscular rigidity, and prevent contractures that occur when muscles are not used. Walking, riding a stationary bicycle, swimming, and gardening are all exercises that help maintain joint mobility. Stretching (stretch–hold–relax) and range-of-motion exercises help increase joint flexibility. Postural exercises are important to counter the tendency of the head and neck to be drawn forward and down. A physical therapist may be helpful in developing an individualized exercise program and can provide instruction to the patient and caregiver on exercising safely. Faithful adherence to an exercise and walking program helps to delay the progress of the disease. Warm baths and massage in addition to passive and active exercises help relax muscles and relieve painful muscle spasms that accompany rigidity.

The patient's balance may be adversely affected because of the rigidity of the arms. (Arm swinging is necessary in normal walking.) Special walking techniques must also be learned to offset the shuffling gait and the tendency to lean forward. The patient is taught to concentrate on walking erect, to watch the horizon, and to use a wide-based gait (ie, walking with the feet separated). A conscious effort must be made to swing the arms and raise the feet while walking and to use a heel-toe, heel-toe gait in fairly long strides. The patient is advised to practice walking to marching music or to the sound of a ticking metronome because this provides sensory reinforcement. Breathing exercises while walking help to move the rib cage and to aerate parts of the lungs. Frequent rest periods aid in preventing frustration and fatigue.

Enhancing Self-Care Activities

Encouraging, teaching, and supporting the patient during activities of daily living promote self-care. (See Chap. 10 for rehabilitation techniques.)

Environmental modifications are necessary to compensate for functional disabilities. These patients may have severe mobility problems that make normal activities impossible. Adaptive or assistive devices may be useful. A hospital bed at home with bedside rails, an overbed frame with a trapeze, or a rope tied to the foot of the bed can provide assistance in pulling up without help. An occupational therapist can evaluate the patient's needs in the home and make recommendations regarding adaptive devices and teach the patient and caregiver how to improvise.

Improving Bowel Elimination

A patient with parkinsonism may have severe problems with constipation. Among the factors causing constipation are weakness of the muscles used in defecation, lack of exercise, inadequate fluid intake, and decreased autonomic nervous system activity. The medications used for the treatment of the disease also inhibit normal intestinal secretions. A regular bowel routine may be established by encouraging the patient to follow a regular time pattern, consciously increase fluid intake, and eat foods with a moderate fiber content. A raised toilet seat is useful to facilitate toilet activities because the patient has difficulty in moving from a standing to a sitting position.

Improving Nutrition

Patients with parkinsonism have difficulty in maintaining their weight. Eating becomes a very slow process requiring concentration. Their mouths are dry from the medications, and they experience difficulty chewing and swallowing. They are at risk for aspiration because of impaired swallowing and the accumulation of saliva. They may not be aware that they are aspirating and may develop bronchopneumonia.

Monitoring weight on a weekly basis indicates whether caloric intake is adequate. Supplementary feedings increase caloric intake. As the disease progresses, a nasogastric tube or percutaneous endoscopic gastroscopy may be necessary to maintain adequate nutrition. A dietitian can be consulted regarding the patient's nutritional needs.

ENHANCING SWALLOWING

Swallowing disorders can be due to poor head control, tongue tremor, hesitancy in initiating swallowing, difficulty in shaping food into a bolus, and disturbances in pharyngeal motility. To offset these problems, the patient should sit in an upright position during mealtime. A semisolid diet with thick liquids is easier to swallow than solids and thin liquids. Thin liquids should be avoided. It is helpful for patients to think through the swallowing sequence. The patient is taught to place the food on the tongue, close the lips and teeth, lift the tongue up and then back, and swallow. The patient is encouraged to chew first on one side of the mouth and then on the other. To control the buildup of saliva, the patient is reminded to hold the head upright and make a conscious effort to swallow. Massaging the facial and neck muscles before meals may be beneficial.

ENCOURAGING THE USE OF ASSISTIVE DEVICES

An electric warming tray keeps food hot and permits the patient to rest during the prolonged time that it takes to eat. Special utensils also assist at mealtime. A plate that is stabilized, a nonspill cup, and eating utensils with built-up handles are useful self-help devices. The occupational therapist can assist in identifying appropriate adaptive devices.

Improving Communication

Speech disorders are present in most patients with Parkinson's disease. Their low-pitched, monotonous, soft speech requires that they make a conscious effort to speak slowly, with deliberate attention to what they are saying. Patients are reminded to face the listener, exaggerate the pronunciation of words, speak in short sentences, and take a few deep breaths before speaking.

A speech therapist may be helpful in designing speech improvement exercises and assisting the family and health care personnel to develop and use a method of communication to meet the patient's needs. A small electronic amplifier is helpful if the patient has difficulty being heard.

Supporting Coping Abilities

Support can be given by encouraging the patient and pointing out that activities are being maintained through active participation. A combination of physiotherapy, psychotherapy, medication therapy, and support group participation may help reduce the depression that often occurs.

Patients with Parkinson's disease often feel embarrassed, apathetic, inadequate, bored, and lonely. These feelings may be due, in part, to physical slowness and the great effort that even small tasks require. Patients are assisted and encouraged to set achievable goals (eg, improvement of mobility).

NURSING RESEARCH

A Sense of Hope Associated With Health Promotion Activities

Fowler, S. B. (1997). Hope and a health-promoting lifestyle in persons with Parkinson's disease. *Journal of Neuroscience Nursing, 29* (2), 111–116.

Purpose

Recognition of the importance of health promotion and health-promoting lifestyle behaviors is increasing. Parkinson's disease (PD), a chronic progressive neurologic disorder with an unpredictable course and no cure, presents challenges to those interested in health promotion. Hope has been identified as one factor that is positively related to health-promotion behaviors in patients with chronic illnesses. However, the relationship between hope and health-promoting lifestyle has not been examined in people with PD. The purpose of this study was to determine whether there is a relationship between hope and health-promoting lifestyle in adults with Parkinson's disease.

Study Sample and Design

The Herth Hope Index (HHI) was used to measure hope in a sample of people with PD. The Health-Promoting Lifestyle Profile II (HPLP II) was used to measure health-promoting actions. The six dimensions of health-promoting lifestyle addressed by the HPLP are spiritual growth, health responsibility, physical activity, nutrition, interpersonal relations, and stress management. Subscores and total scores are obtained; higher scores indicate more health-promoting behaviors. Subjects were also asked to identify the stage of Parkinson's disease they were experiencing by selecting the physical symptoms that best described their disease. Questionnaires were distributed to 89 people with PD through support groups. A return rate of 30% resulted in a sample of 42 subjects. Most subjects were male and married. Their mean age was 71 years (SD, 9.11). The average length of time with PD symptoms was about 8 years. Stages 1 through 4 of Parkinson's disease were represented in the sample; none of the participants in the study reported stage 5, that is, being bedridden or wheelchair bound.

Findings

Subjects reported a high level of hope and a moderately high level of health-promoting behaviors. The highest HPLP scores were on the interpersonal relations and nutrition subscales. A moderate, positive relationship was found between hope and a health-promoting lifestyle ($r = .40$; $p = .008$). Hope was also significantly correlated with the spiritual growth and interpersonal relations scores on the HPLP.

Nursing Implications

The findings of this study support those of other studies of hope and health promotion in chronically ill people. They emphasize the importance of maintaining and fostering hope to promotion of a healthy lifestyle. Nurses can apply these findings by promoting hope and fostering a health-promoting lifestyle by encouraging supportive relationships and participation in spiritual activities.

Because parkinsonism tends to lead to withdrawal and depression, patients must be active participants in their therapeutic program, including social and recreational events. There should be a planned program of activity throughout the day to prevent too much daytime sleeping as well as disinterest and apathy.

Every effort should be made to encourage patients to carry out the tasks involved in meeting their own daily needs and to remain independent. Doing things for the patient merely to save time is contrary to the basic goal of improving coping abilities and promoting a positive self-concept.

Promoting Home and Community-Based Care

TEACHING PATIENTS SELF-CARE

Patient and family education is important in the management of Parkinson's disease. Teaching needs depend on the severity of symptoms and the stage of the disease. The patient's and family's need for information about Parkinson's disease is ongoing as adaptations become necessary. The education plan should include a clear explanation of the disease, assisting the patient to remain as functionally independent for as long as possible. Every effort is made to explain the nature of the disease and its management to offset disabling anxieties and fears. The patient and family must be taught about the effects and side effects of medications and about the importance of reporting side effects to the physician.

CONTINUING CARE

Patients with Parkinson's disease are well managed at home in the early stages. Family members often serve as caregivers, with home care or community services available to assist in meeting health care needs as the disease progresses.

The family caregiver is under considerable stress from living with and caring for a disabled person. Providing information about treatment and care prevents many unnecessary problems. The caregiver is included in the plan and may be counseled to learn stress reduction techniques, to include others in the caregiving process, to obtain periodic relief from responsibilities, and to have a yearly health assessment. Allowing family members to express feelings of frustration, anger, and guilt is often helpful to them.

The patient should be evaluated in the home for adaptation and safety needs and compliance with the plan of care. In the advanced stages, patients are placed in long-term care facilities when family support is absent. Admission to an acute care facility may be necessary for changes in medical management or treatment of complications. Nurses provide support, education, and monitoring of patients over the course of illness.

Informational booklets and a newsletter for patient education are published by the National Parkinson's Foundation, Inc. and the American Parkinson's Disease Association.

Evaluation

Expected Outcomes

Expected outcomes may include:

1. Strives toward improved mobility
    a. Participates in exercise program daily
    b. Walks with wide base of support; exaggerates arm swinging when walking
    c. Takes medications as prescribed
2. Progresses toward self-care
    a. Allows time for self-care activities
    b. Uses self-help devices

HOME CARE TEACHING CHECKLIST: THE PATIENT WITH PARKINSON'S DISEASE

At the completion of the program, the patient and caregiver will be able to:	Patient	Caregiver
• Define Parkinson's disease and discuss its long-term effects.	✔	✔
• Identify the medication regimen and name adverse effects, and precautions.	✔	✔
• Discuss the risk for injury, prevent falls; implement adaptive measures in the home.	✔	✔
• Describe nutritional needs, dietary restrictions, dysphagia management, and ways to prevent aspiration.	✔	✔
• Manage constipation: fluid intake, bowel routine.	✔	✔
• Manage urinary problems: functional incontinence, retention (Foley catheter care, suprapubic catheter care).	✔	✔
• Explain effects of immobility and define preventive care: skin breakdown (frequent turning, pressure release, skin care), pneumonia (deep breathing, movement), contractures (range of motion exercises).	✔	✔
• Define benefits of daily exercise program.	✔	✔
• Walk and balance safely.	✔	✔
• Demonstrate speech and communication skills: speech exercises, communication techniques, breathing exercises.	✔	✔
• Name signs and symptoms of infection (urinary and respiratory) and state when health care provider should be notified.	✔ ✔	✔ ✔
• Describe strategies to promote self-care activities and independence.	✔	✔
• Identify resources: American Parkinson's Disease Association, National Parkinson's Disease Foundation, and local support groups.		

3. Maintains bowel function
   a. Consumes adequate fluid intake
   b. Increases dietary intake of fiber
   c. Reports regular pattern of bowel function
4. Attains improved nutritional status
   a. Swallows without aspiration
   b. Takes time while eating
5. Achieves a method of communication
   a. Communicates needs
   b. Practices speech exercises
6. Copes with effects of Parkinson's disease
   a. Sets realistic goals
   b. Demonstrates persistence in meaningful activities
   c. Verbalizes feelings to appropriate person

Huntington's Disease

Huntington's disease (HD) is a chronic, progressive, hereditary disease of the nervous system that results in progressive involuntary choreiform (dancelike) movement and dementia. It affects men and women of all races. Because it is transmitted as an autosomal dominant genetic disorder, each child of a parent with HD has a 50% risk of inheriting the illness.

Pathophysiology

The basic pathology involves premature death of cells in the striatum (caudate and putamen) of the basal ganglia, the region deep within the brain involved in the control of movement. There is also loss of cells in the cortex, the region of the brain associated with thinking, memory, perception, and judgment, and in the cerebellum, the area that coordinates voluntary muscle activity. Researchers now believe that a building block for protein, called glutamine, abnormally collects in the cell nucleus, causing cell death (Barinaga, 1996). Why the protein destroys only certain brain cells is unknown. The cells' destruction results in a lack of the neurotransmitters, gamma-aminobutyric acid and acetylcholine, which inhibit nerve action. Onset usually occurs between the ages of 35 and 45 years; about 10% of patients are children. The disease progresses slowly. Despite a ravenous appetite, patients usually become emaciated and exhausted. Patients succumb in 10 to 15 years to heart failure, pneumonia, or infection, or die as a result of a fall or choking.

Clinical Manifestations

The most prominent clinical features of the disease are abnormal involuntary movements (**chorea**), intellectual decline, and, often, emotional disturbance.

As the disease progresses, a constant writhing, twisting, uncontrollable movement may involve the entire body. These motions are devoid of purpose or rhythm, although patients may try to turn them into purposeful movement. All of the body musculature is involved. Facial movements produce tics and grimaces. Speech is affected, becoming slurred, hesitant, often explosive, and eventually unintelligible. Chewing and swallowing are difficult, and there is a constant danger of choking and aspiration. Choreiform movements persist but diminish during sleep.

As with speech, the gait becomes disorganized to the point that ambulation eventually is impossible. Although independent ambulation should be encouraged for as long as possible, a wheelchair usually becomes necessary at some point. (Eventually, the patient is confined to bed when the chorea interferes with walking, sitting, and all other activities.) Control of bladder and bowel is lost.

Cognitive function is usually affected, with dementia usually occurring. Initially, the patient generally is aware that the disease is responsible for the myriad dysfunctions that are occurring.

The mental and emotional changes that occur with HD may be more devastating to the patient and family than the abnormal movements. Patients may be nervous, irritable, or impatient. In the early stages of the illness, patients are particularly subject to uncontrollable fits of anger; profound, often suicidal depression; apathy; or euphoria. Judgment and memory are impaired, and dementia eventually ensues. Hallucinations, delusions, and paranoid thinking may precede the appearance of disjointed movements. Emotional symptoms often become less acute as the disease progresses.

Assessment and Diagnostic Findings

The diagnosis of HD is made on clinical presentation of characteristic symptoms, establishment of positive family history, and exclusion of other causes. Although there is no specific diagnostic test, imaging studies, such as CT and MRI, may show atrophy of the striatum once HD is well established.

A genetic marker for HD has been identified through the use of recombinant deoxyribonucleic acid (DNA) technology. As a result, researchers can now identify presymptomatic individuals who will develop this disease. Although this presymptomatic test for HD can remove the uncertainty, it offers no hope of cure or even specific determination of its onset. Researchers continue to study the genetic causes that lead to the death of brain cells.

Management

Although no treatment halts or reverses the underlying process, several methods of management have fairly good palliative results. The phenothiazines, butyrophenones, and thioxanthenes, which predominantly block dopamine receptors, improve the chorea in many patients. Chorea also is lessened by reserpine (depletes presynaptic dopamine) and tetrabenazine (reduces dopaminergic transmission). The patient's motor signs must be assessed and evaluated on an ongoing basis so that optimal therapeutic drug levels may be reached. **Akathisia** (motor restlessness) in the overmedicated patient is dangerous because it may be mistaken for the restless fidgetiness of the illness and consequently can be overlooked.

In certain types of the disease, hypokinetic motor impairment resembles parkinsonism. In patients who present with rigidity, some temporary benefit may be obtained from antiparkinsonism therapy, such as levodopa.

Patients who have emotional disturbances, particularly depression, may be helped by antidepressant medications. The threat of suicide is always present. Psychotic symptoms usually respond to antipsychotic medications. Psychotherapy aimed at allaying anxiety and reducing stress may be beneficial. It is imperative that nurses look beyond the disease to focus on the patient's needs and capabilities (Chart 59-5).

PROMOTING HOME AND COMMUNITY-BASED CARE

Patient Teaching for Self-Care Management. The needs of the patient and family for education depend on the nature and severity of physical, cognitive, and psychological changes experienced by the patient. Patients and their family members are taught about medications that are prescribed and about signs indicating a need for change in medication or its dosage. The teaching plan addresses strategies to manage symptoms, such as chorea, swallowing problems, limitations in ambulation, and loss of bowel and bladder function. Consultation with a speech therapist may be indicated to assist in identifying alternative communication strategies if the patient's speech is affected.

Individuals of childbearing age may wish information about their risk for HD when considering pregnancy and childbearing. For most people, the benefits of testing are unclear because of ethical and confidentiality issues.

Not only is genetic counseling crucial, but patients and their families also require access to long-term psychological counseling, marriage counseling, and emotional, financial, and legal support.

Continuing Care. A program combining medical, nursing, psychological, social, occupational, speech, and physical rehabilitation services is needed to help the patient and family cope with this severely disabling illness. HD exacts enormous emotional, physical, social, and financial tolls on every member of the patient's family. Entire families often live under a heavy burden of uncertainty, anxiety, and guilt. Regular follow-up helps to allay fear of abandonment.

Home care assistance, day care centers, respite care, and eventually skilled long-term care can assist the patient and family in coping with the constant strain of the illness. Although the relentless progression of the disease cannot be halted, families can benefit from supportive care.

Voluntary health organizations are major aids to families and have been largely responsible for bringing the illness to national attention. The Huntington's Disease Foundation of America is oriented toward helping patients and their families by providing information, referrals, family and public education, and support for research.

Alzheimer's Disease

Alzheimer's disease, or senile dementia of the Alzheimer's type, is a chronic, progressive, and degenerative brain disorder accompanied by profound effects on memory, cognition, and ability for self-care. About 10% of the population older than the age of 65 is affected, and the prevalence reaches 47% by 85 years of age. It is one of the most feared disorders of modern times because it has catastrophic consequences for the patient and family, who experience what has been termed an "endless funeral." (See Chap. 11 for a detailed discussion of the manifestations, management, and nursing care of the patient with Alzheimer's disease.)

Creutzfeldt-Jakob Disease

Creutzfeldt-Jakob disease (CJD) is a rare, transmissible, progressively fatal disease of the central nervous system. The mode of transmission is unknown; however, the agent has been found in transplanted organs, grafts from infected cadavers, and human growth hormone. CJD is characterized by **spongiform** (small holes) degeneration of the gray matter of the brain that results in severe dementia and **myoclonus** (spasms of a single muscle or group of muscles). CJD affects primarily adults older than 50 years of age, with an incidence estimated at 1 to 30 cases per million people, with about 15% occurring in familial groups. The long incubation period is between 10 and 40 years. Once symptoms appear, the patient deteriorates, with death occurring in 1 to 12 months. CJD is similar to bovine spongiform encephalopathy (BSE), also known as "mad cow disease." Both BSE and CJD produce similar symptoms and are always fatal.

Clinical Manifestations

Although the cause of CJD is unknown, researchers believe that the source may be a virus or a self-replicating protein called a prion (Kretzschmar, Ironside, DeArmond, & Tateishi, 1996). The neurologic changes are caused by progressive destruction of brain tissue and neuronal cells. Diagnosis is usually made on clinical presentation of motor, sensory, and language deficits. Absolute diagnosis can only be made on brain biopsy. Clinical decline is rapid and may include tremors, ataxia, myoclonus, rigidity, and confusion progressing to dementia. Fever is not present, and the white blood cell count and CSF are normal. Decorticate and decerebrate posturing may be seen during the terminal stage of the disease. An EEG can be useful in diagnosis, indicating diffuse slowing of brain waves with periods of synchronous discharges. CT and MRI may show cortical atrophy.

CHART 59•5 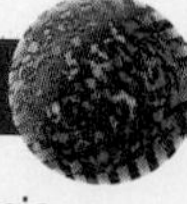 Care of the Patient With Huntington's Disease

Nursing Diagnosis

Potential for injury from falls and possible skin breakdown (pressure ulcers, abrasions), resulting from constant movement.

Nursing Interventions

Pad the sides and head of the bed; ensure that the patient can see over the sides of bed.

Use lamb's wool padding for heel and elbow protection.

Keep the skin meticulously clean.

Apply emollient cleansing agent and skin lotion frequently.

Use soft sheets and bedding.

Have patient wear football padding or other forms of padding.

Encourage ambulation with assistance to maintain muscle tone.

Secure the patient (only if absolutely necessary) in bed or chair with padded protective devices, making sure that they are loosened frequently.

Nursing Diagnosis

Inadequate nutritional intake and dehydration resulting from difficulty in swallowing or chewing and danger of choking or aspirating food.

Nursing Interventions

Administer phenothiazines as prescribed before meals (appears to calm some patients).

Use a warming tray.

Talk to the patient before mealtime to promote relaxation; use mealtime for social interaction. Provide undivided attention. Help the patient enjoy the mealtime experience.

Learn the position that is best for *this* patient. Keep patient as close to upright as possible while feeding. Stabilize patient's head gently with one hand while feeding.

Show the food and tell the patient what the foods are (eg, whether hold or cold).

Encircle the patient with one arm and get as close as possible to provide stability and support. Use pillows and wedges for additional support.

Do not interpret stiffness, turning away, or sudden turning of the head as rejection; these are uncontrollable choreiform movements.

For feeding, use a long-handled spoon (iced-tea spoon). Place spoon on middle of tongue and exert slight pressure.

Place bite-sized food between teeth. Serve stews, casseroles, thick liquids, avoid too many milk drinks (produces mucus).

Disregard messiness. Treat the person with dignity.

Wait for the patient to chew and swallow before introducing another spoonful. Make sure that bite-sized food is small.

Give between-meal feedings. Constant movement uses more calories. Patients often have voracious appetites, particularly for sweets.

Use blenderized meals if patient cannot chew; do not repeatedly give the same strained baby foods; gradually introduce increased textures and consistencies to the diet.

For swallowing difficulties:

- Apply gentle deep pressure around the patient's mouth.
- Rub fingers in circles on the patient's cheeks.
- Rub fingers simultaneously down each side of the patient's throat.

Develop skill in Heimlich maneuver (to be used in the event of choking).

Nursing Diagnosis

Psychological isolation and ineffective communication from excessive grimacing and unintelligible speech

Nursing Interventions

Read to the patient.

Employ biofeedback and relaxation therapy to reduce stress.

Consult with speech therapist to help maintain and prolong communication abilities.

Try to devise a communication system, perhaps using cards with words or pictures of familiar objects, before verbal communication becomes too difficult. Patients can indicate correct card by hitting it with hand, grunting, or blinking the eyes.

Learn how this particular patient expresses needs and wants—particularly nonverbal messages (widening of eyes, responses).

Patients can understand even if unable to speak. Do not isolate patients by ceasing to communicate with them.

Nursing Diagnosis

Intellectual impairment and emotional disturbance

Nursing Interventions

Have clock, calendar, and wall posters to view.

Interact with the patient in a creative manner.

Use every opportunity for one-to-one contact.

Use music for relaxation.

Reorient the patient after awakening.

Have the patient wear an identification bracelet with name, telephone number, and "memory impaired" on it.

Keep the patient in the social mainstream.

Recruit and train volunteers for social interaction. Role model appropriate interactions.

Do not abandon a patient because the disease is eventually terminal. Patients are *living* until the end.

Management

There is no effective treatment for CJD. The care of the patient is supportive and palliative. Goals of care include prevention of injury and complications, promotion of patient comfort, and provision of support and education for the family.

The patient is at risk for injuries related to dementia, seizures, and myoclonus. Seizure precautions should be initiated. Limited mobility necessitates frequent repositioning and meticulous skin care.

The patient may experience fear, anxiety, and discomfort but be unable to communicate or verbalize those feelings. A private room with low lights and a quiet environment help decrease stimuli that increase neurologic symptoms. Sedation and analgesics may be prescribed to control myoclonus. Music, touch, and a soft voice may be used to relax the patient.

Much time and energy are spent in providing the patient's family with support. Providing education about CJD can assist the family in coping with the inevitable outcome. Anger, anxiety, and disbelief are common feelings. Psychiatric liaison nurses, social workers, and clergy may be of assistance to the family and the staff in coping.

Prevention of disease transmission is an important part of providing nursing care. Although patient isolation is not necessary, use of standard precautions is important. Institutional protocols are followed for blood and body fluid exposure and decontamination of equipment because the agent that causes CJD is difficult to kill using conventional methods. Organ donation is not an option because of the risk for disease transmission.

Myasthenia Gravis

Myasthenia gravis is a disorder affecting the neuromuscular transmission of the voluntary muscles of the body; it is characterized by excessive weakness and fatigability, particularly of voluntary muscles and those innervated by cranial nerve function. Although onset can occur at any age, it is seen most often in women between the ages of 15 and 35 years and in men older than 40 years of age.

Pathophysiology

The basic abnormality in myasthenia gravis is a defect in the transmission of impulses from nerve to muscle cells due to loss of available or normal receptors on the postsynaptic membrane of the neuromuscular junction. Studies have shown a 70% to 90% reduction in the number of acetylcholine receptors at individual neuromuscular junctions. Myasthenia gravis is considered an autoimmune disease in which antibodies directed against acetylcholine receptors impair neuromuscular transmission (Fig. 59-12).

Clinical Manifestations

The disease is characterized by extreme skeletal muscle weakness and easy fatigability, which generally is worse after effort and is relieved by rest. The muscle groups most commonly affected are those involved in eye movements, breathing, head control, chewing, swallowing, and speech. Patients with this disease tire on slight exertion (eg, combing the hair, chewing, and talking) and must stop for rest. Symptoms vary according to the muscles affected. Symmetric muscles are involved, particularly those innervated by the cranial nerves. Because of the involvement of the ocular muscles, diplopia (double vision) and ptosis (drooping of the eyelids) are early symptoms. The patient has a sleepy, masklike expression because the facial muscles are affected.

Laryngeal involvement produces **dysphonia** (voice impairment) in the form of a nasal sound of the voice or difficulty in articulation. Weakness of the bulbar muscles presents a danger of choking and aspiration. Some 15% to 20% of patients complain of weakness of arm and hand muscles and, less commonly, of leg muscle weakness, which makes these patients subject to falls. Progressive weakness of the diaphragm and intercostal muscles may produce respiratory distress, which is an acute emergency.

Assessment and Diagnostic Findings

The signs and symptoms of myasthenia gravis are sometimes so striking that a presumptive diagnosis can be made on the basis of the patient's history and physical examination. An injection of edrophonium (Tensilon), a medication that facilitates the transmission of impulses at the myoneural junction, is used to confirm the diagnosis. Within 30 seconds of an intravenous injection of edrophonium, most patients with myasthenia gravis improve substantially but only temporarily. Improvement in muscle strength after administration of this agent represents a positive test and usually confirms the diagnosis.

The acetylcholine receptor antibodies that attack postsynaptic receptor sites are found in the serum in nearly 80% of patients with generalized myasthenia and in about 60% of those with symptoms restricted to the eye muscles (ocular form). EMG is used to measure the electrical potential of muscle cells but is not specific for myasthenia gravis.

Medical Management

Management of myasthenia gravis is directed at improving function through the administration of anticholinesterase medications and reducing and removing circulating antibodies. Therapy includes anticholinesterase agents and immunosuppressive therapy, including plasmapheresis, as well as thymectomy.

PHARMACOLOGIC THERAPY

Anticholinesterase agents act by increasing the relative concentration of available acetylcholine at the neuromuscular junction. They are given to increase the response of the muscles to nerve impulses and to improve strength. However, they provide only symptomatic relief.

Medications in current use include pyridostigmine bromide (Mestinon) and neostigmine bromide (Prostigmin).

Most patients prefer pyridostigmine because it produces fewer side effects. The dosage is increased gradually until maximal benefits are obtained (additional strength, less fatigue), although normal muscle strength may not be achieved, and the patient will likely have to adapt to some disability. The adverse effects of anticholinesterase medications involve the gastrointestinal, skeletal, and central nervous systems.

The nursing (and patient) priority is administration of the prescribed medication according to an exact time schedule to control the patient's symptoms.

Nursing Alert *Any delay in administration of medications may result in the patient's inability to swallow, making oral administration problematic.*

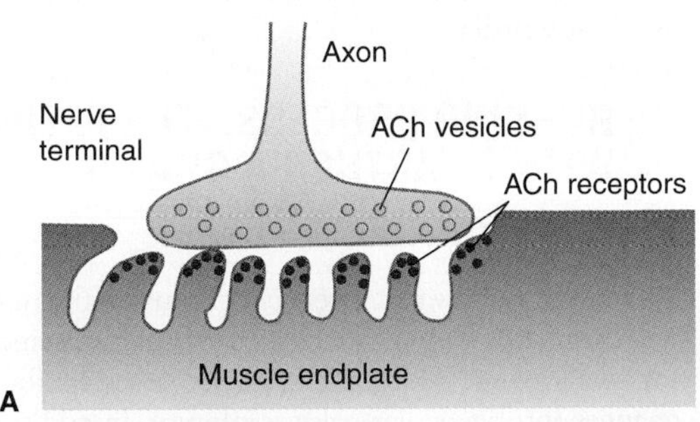

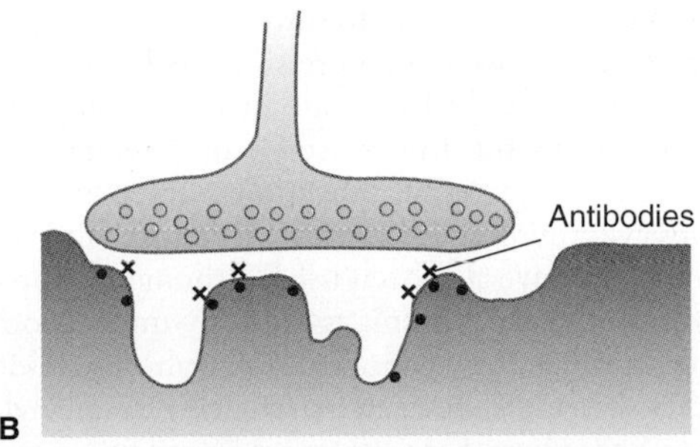

FIGURE 59•12 Myasthenia gravis. (**A**) Normal ACh receptor site. (**B**) ACh receptor site in myasthenia gravis.

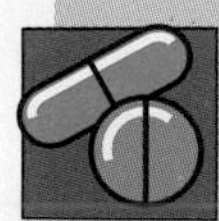

PHARMACOLOGY

Potential Adverse Effects of Anticholinesterase Medications

CNS

Irritability
Anxiety
Insomnia
Headache
Dysarthria
Syncope
Seizures
Coma
Diaphoresis

Respiratory

Bronchial relaxation
Increased bronchial secretions

Cardiovascular

Tachycardia
Hypotension

Gastrointestinal

Abdominal cramps
Nausea
Vomiting
Diarrhea
Anorexia
Increased salivation

Skeletal Muscles

Fasciculations
Spasms
Weakness

Genitourinary

Frequency
Urgency

Integumentary

Rash
Flushing

An increase in muscle strength within 1 hour after the administration of the anticholinesterase drug is expected.

After the initial medication doses have been adjusted, the patient learns to take the medication according to individual needs and time plan. Further adjustments may be necessary in the presence of physical or emotional stress and intercurrent infection. When the patient is hospitalized, it is important to determine what the patient's medication therapy schedule was while at home because this same schedule is likely to be the one of choice at the time of discharge.

Immunosuppressive therapy is directed toward reducing the production of antireceptor antibody or removing it directly by plasma exchange (described later). Immunosuppressive therapy includes corticosteroids, plasmapheresis, and thymectomy. Corticosteroid therapy may benefit the patient with severe generalized myasthenia. Corticosteroids exert their effect by suppressing the patient's immune response, thus decreasing the amount of blocking antibody. The anticholinesterase dosage is lowered while the patient's ability to maintain effective respirations and to swallow is monitored. The steroid dosage is gradually increased, and the anticholinesterase medication is slowly reduced.

Prednisone, taken on alternate days to lower the incidence of side effects, appears to be successful in suppressing the disease. The patient sometimes shows a marked decrease in muscle strength right after therapy is started, but this is usually only temporary. If hospitalized, the patient is given a call bell to use in emergency situations and is closely monitored for signs of respiratory distress.

Cytotoxic medications have also been used, although the precise mechanism of action in myasthenia is not fully understood. Medications such as azathioprine (Imuran), cyclophosphamide (Cytoxan), and cyclosporine reduce the circulating antiacetylcholine receptor antibody titers. Side effects are significant, however, and only patients with advanced disease are treated with these agents.

PLASMA EXCHANGE

Plasma exchange (plasmapheresis) is a technique that allows selective removal of the patient's plasma and plasma components. The remaining cells are reinfused. Plasma exchange produces a temporary reduction in the titer of circulating antibodies. This process has caused remarkable improvement in some patients but does not treat the underlying abnormality (production of antireceptor antibody) over the long term.

SURGICAL MANAGEMENT

In myasthenia gravis patients, the thymus seems to be involved in the process of acetylcholine receptor antibody production. Thymectomy (surgical removal of the thymus) causes substantial remission of the disease, especially in patients with tumor or hyperplasia of the thymus gland. Thymectomy is carried out through the sternum because the entire thymus must be removed.

It is thought that thymectomy early in the course of the disease prevents formation of antireceptor antibodies. After surgery, the patient is monitored in an intensive care unit with special attention given to ventilatory function. After the thymus gland is removed, it may take 2 to 10 years to benefit from the procedure, owing to the long life of circulating T cells.

DRUG INTERACTION PRECAUTIONS

A number of medications aggravate myasthenia gravis, and the patient is advised to consult with the physician before taking any new medications, including antibiotics, cardiovascular medications, anticonvulsant and psychotropic medications, morphine, quinine and related agents, beta-blockers, and nonprescription medications. Procaine (Novocain) should be avoided, and the patient's dentist is so advised.

Complications: Myasthenic Crisis Versus Cholinergic Crisis

Myasthenic crisis is the sudden onset of muscular weakness in patients with myasthenia and usually is the result of undermedication or no cholinergic medication at all. In addition, myasthenic crisis may result from progression of the disease itself, emotional upset, systemic infections, certain medications, surgery, or trauma. It is manifest by the sudden onset of acute respiratory distress and an inability to swallow or speak. Weakness of respiratory, laryngeal, and bulbar musculature can cause respiratory depression and airway obstruction if not treated promptly.

Cholinergic crisis is caused by overmedication with cholinergic or anticholinesterase agents. In addition to the muscle weakness and respiratory depression of myasthenic crisis, these patients experience a variety of gastrointestinal symptoms, including nausea, vomiting, and diarrhea, as well as sweating, increased salivation, and bradycardia.

NURSING PROCESS: THE PATIENT WITH MYASTHENIA GRAVIS

Assessment

The health history and assessment focus on the presence of muscle weakness, especially of the respiratory muscles and those required for swallowing. The patient is also assessed for visual and eye changes (ptosis, ocular palsy, diplopia). In addition, the patient's functional capability and support systems are assessed because they aid in determining discharge needs for services.

Diagnosis

Nursing Diagnoses

Based on the assessment data, the patient's potential nursing diagnoses may include the following:

- Ineffective breathing pattern related to respiratory muscle weakness
- Impaired physical mobility due to voluntary muscle weakness
- Risk for aspiration related to weakness of bulbar muscles
- Impaired verbal communication related to weakened speech muscles
- Sensory/perceptual alteration related to impaired vision

Other nursing diagnoses of the patient with myasthenia gravis may include risk for injury related to voluntary muscle weakness; activity intolerance; ineffective airway clearance; anxiety; altered nutrition, less than body requirements; and body image disturbance.

Collaborative Problems/Potential Complications

Based on the assessment data and knowledge of the disease process, potential complications that may develop include the following:

- Myasthenic crisis
- Cholinergic crisis

Planning and Goals

The patient's major goals may include improved respiratory function, increased physical mobility, avoidance of aspiration, improved ability to communicate, improved vision, and absence of complications.

Nursing Interventions

Improving Respiratory Function

The nurse assesses respiratory rate, depth, and breath sounds and monitors the results of pulmonary function tests (tidal volume, vital capacity, inspiratory force) at frequent intervals to detect pulmonary problems before changes in arterial blood gas levels occur and before symptoms become clinically apparent.

When there is severe weakness of abdominal, intercostal, and pharyngeal muscles, the patient is unable to cough and breathe deeply or clear secretions. Chest physical therapy, including postural drainage to mobilize secretions and suctioning to remove secretions, may have to be performed frequently.

The patient with insufficient gas exchange experiences anxiety sometimes bordering on panic. This is compounded by an inability to communicate verbally and by a tendency to choke. Acknowledging the patient's fears and addressing the problem promptly can give assurance that the nurse understands the concerns. The patient gains some sense of control through skilled care and the calm support of the nurse.

Increasing Physical Mobility

The patient's goal is improvement of strength and endurance. To be a participant in treatment, the patient must learn the basic facts about anticholinesterase agents—their actions, timing, dosage adjustment, symptoms of overdose, and toxic effects. The importance of taking the medication on time is emphasized. The patient is encouraged to keep a diary to determine fluctuation of symptoms and to know when the medication is wearing off.

In addition, the patient is encouraged to take the following steps:

- Time meals to coincide with peak effects of anticholinesterase medications for maximal muscle strength
- Plan adequate rest periods throughout the day
- Set a realistic schedule daily and spacing activities
- Wear appropriate shoes to minimize weakness and prevent injury

Certain factors may increase weakness and precipitate a myasthenic crisis: emotional upset, infections (particularly respiratory infections), vigorous physical activity, and exposure to heat (hot baths, sun bathing) and cold. Thus, these situations should be avoided. To avoid the risk for fatigue, it is best to rest before becoming too tired. A cervical collar can be useful for patients with weak neck muscles who are having difficulty supporting the head. Adaptive or self-help devices are useful in helping the patient handle the disease more effectively and live as full a life as possible. The patient is advised to wear a medical identification bracelet.

Improving Communication

The weakened speech muscles in patients in myasthenic crisis may interfere with communication. Techniques for improving communication include listening to patients; repeating what they have tried to communicate to clarify and verify information; and asking patients to blink their eyes or wiggle their fingers or toes for yes and no answers. After the period of myasthenic crisis has resolved, patients usually are able to make their needs known.

Providing Eye Care

Impaired vision results from ptosis of one or both eyelids, decreased eye movement, or double vision. Nursing interventions to help the patient cope include taping the eyes open for short intervals, instilling artificial tears to prevent corneal damage when eyelids do not close completely, placing a patch over one eye when double vision is a problem, and keeping the patient informed while giving care.

Applying a thin adhesive tape over the upper eyelid helps relieve ptosis. Patients who wear eyeglasses can have "crutches" attached to help keep eyelids up. Sunglasses diminish the effects of bright light that frequently increase eye problems.

Preventing Aspiration

Decreased ability to chew and swallow may result in choking and aspiration. The patient is assessed for drooling, regurgitation through the nose, and choking while attempting to swallow. Suction should be immediately available. Rest before meals is encouraged to reduce muscle fatigue. The patient is seated in an upright position with the neck slightly flexed to facilitate swallowing. Soft foods in gravy or sauces appear to be swallowed more easily than liquids. Because muscles of mastication may be stronger in the morning, calorie intake can be increased at breakfast. The patient is encouraged to rest after eating.

Mealtimes should coincide with the peak effects of anticholinesterase if the patient has difficulty swallowing. If choking occurs frequently, blenderized food may be easier to swallow. Again, suction should be available at home as well as during hospitalization and the patient and family instructed in its use. Gastrostomy feedings may be necessary in some patients to ensure adequate nutritional status.

Monitoring and Managing Potential Complications

MYASTHENIC AND CHOLINERGIC CRISES

Respiratory distress, combined with varying signs of dysphagia (difficulty swallowing), dysarthria (difficulty speaking), eyelid ptosis, diplopia, and prominent muscle weakness, is a symptom of myasthenic or cholinergic crisis.

Providing adequate ventilatory assistance takes precedence in the immediate management of the patient with myasthenic crisis. The patient is suctioned because aspiration is a common problem. Arterial blood is drawn for arterial blood gas analysis. Endotracheal intubation and mechanical ventilation may be needed (see Chap. 22). The patient is placed in an intensive care unit for constant monitoring because this condition is marked by intense and sudden fluctuations.

Intravenous edrophonium is used to differentiate the type of crisis. It improves the condition of the patient in myasthenic crisis and temporarily worsens that of the patient in cholinergic crisis. If the patient is in true myasthenic crisis, neostigmine methylsulfate is administered intramuscularly or intravenously.

If the edrophonium test is inconclusive or there is increasing respiratory weakness, all anticholinesterase medications are withdrawn, and atropine sulfate is given to reduce excessive secretions.

Other assessment strategies and supportive measures include the following:

- Arterial blood gases, serum electrolytes, input and output, and daily weight are monitored.
- If the patient is unable to swallow, nasogastric tube feedings may be prescribed (200 mL at a time). (Postural drainage should not be performed for 30 minutes after feeding.)
- Sedatives and tranquilizers are avoided because these agents aggravate hypoxia and hypercapnia and can cause respiratory and cardiac depression.

Promoting Home and Community-Based Care

PATIENT TEACHING FOR SELF-CARE MANAGEMENT

The patient with myasthenia gravis is usually managed as an outpatient unless hospitalization is required for diagnostic testing or to manage symptoms or complications. The more knowledgeable the patient and family, the less likely the patient is to develop complications. Thus, patient and family teaching is an important component of the treatment regimen. The patient and family require information to assist them in dealing with daily needs, crisis intervention, and coping with the disease process. The patient and family are carefully instructed about the importance of administering medications on the prescribed schedule; additionally, they are taught about myasthenic and cholinergic crises and how to detect and manage these complications if they occur at home. Family members are taught emergency measures that may be needed and are provided an opportunity to practice these measures.

CONTINUING CARE

Patients with myasthenia gravis are hospitalized during crisis but are otherwise managed in the outpatient setting with the help of home care nurses and other community resources. Support groups, services, and educational materials for lay and professional readers are provided by the Myasthenia Gravis Foundation of America.

Evaluation

Expected Outcomes

Expected outcomes may include:

1. Achieves adequate respiratory function
   a. Exhibits normal respiratory rate and depth and normal muscle strength
   b. Adheres to established medication schedule
   c. States that manual resuscitation bag and portable suction are available for home use
   d. Avoids situations that may predispose to colds and infections, which might exacerbate symptoms
2. Adapts to impaired mobility
   a. Establishes a balanced program of rest and exercise
   b. Identifies measures to conserve energy; paces self
   c. Uses assistive devices
   d. Establishes and adheres to a medication schedule that maximizes muscle strength
3. Experiences no aspiration
   a. Exhibits normal breath sounds
   b. Eats slowly and selects appropriate (soft) diet
   c. Establishes a medication schedule that coincides with mealtime
4. Uses communication methods
   a. Makes needs known
   b. Expresses emotions and concerns

HOME CARE TEACHING CHECKLIST: THE PATIENT WITH MYASTHENIA GRAVIS

At the completion of the program, the patient and caregiver will be able to:	Patient	Caregiver
• Describe the disease and current therapies.	✔	✔
• Discuss medications: indications, dosage, fixed-dose timing for optimal muscle strength, and adverse effects; state importance of not taking over-the-counter drugs.	✔	✔
• Prevent complications by recognizing signs and symptoms of myasthenia and cholinergic crisis and securing needed home equipment (suction equipment, manual resuscitation bag); avoid triggers that provoke exacerbation (stress, fatigue, illness, hormonal swings, excessive exposure to temperature extremes).	✔	✔
• State the importance of wearing a MedicAlert bracelet and carrying a card with the name of the patient's primary physician.	✔	✔
• Conserve energy: frequent rest periods, eating slowly, pacing activities.	✔	✔
• Wear shoes that provide support to minimize weakness and loss of balance.	✔	✔
• Contact the Myasthenia Gravis Foundation by mail or telephone for support services and educational materi-	✔	✔

5. Reports ability to see objects and people in environment
6. Recovers from myasthenic and cholinergic crises
   a. Lists signs and symptoms of crisis
   b. Adheres to medication regimen
   c. Wears MedicAlert bracelet or carries identification card at all times

Amyotrophic Lateral Sclerosis

Amyotrophic lateral sclerosis (ALS) is a disease of unknown cause in which there is a loss of motor neurons (nerve cells controlling muscles) in the anterior horns of the spinal cord and the motor nuclei of the lower brain stem. As these cells die, the muscle fibers that they supply undergo atrophic changes. The degeneration of the neurons may occur in both the upper and lower motor neuron systems. Several theories exist regarding the cause of ALS, including autoimmune disease and free radical damage. The leading theory held by researchers is that overexcitation of nerve cells by the neurotransmitter glutamate leads to cell injury and neuronal degeneration.

ALS affects more men than women, with onset occurring usually in the fifth or sixth decade. It is often referred to as Lou Gehrig's disease after the famous ballplayer who suffered from it.

Clinical Manifestations

The clinical manifestations of ALS depend on the location of the affected motor neurons because specific neurons activate specific muscle fibers. The chief symptoms are progressive muscle weakness, atrophy, and fasciculations (twitching). Loss of motor neurons in the anterior horns of the spinal cord results in progressive weakness and atrophy of the muscles of the arms, trunk, or legs. Spasticity usually is present, and the deep tendon stretch reflexes become brisk and overactive. Usually, the anal and bladder sphincters are intact because the spinal nerves that control muscles of the rectum and urinary bladder are not affected.

In about 25% of patients, weakness starts in the musculature supplied by the cranial nerves, and there is difficulty talking, swallowing, and ultimately breathing. When the patient ingests liquids, soft palate and upper esophageal weakness causes the liquid to be regurgitated through the nose. Weakness of the posterior tongue and palate impairs the ability to laugh, cough, or even blow the nose. When bulbar muscles are impaired, there is progressive difficulty in speaking and swallowing, and aspiration becomes a problem. The voice assumes a nasal sound, and speech articulation becomes so disrupted that the patient's speech is unintelligible. Some emotional lability may be present, but intellectual function is not impaired. Eventually, respiratory function is compromised.

The prognosis generally is based on the area of the central nervous system involved and the speed with which the disease progresses. Death usually occurs as a result of infection, respiratory failure, or aspiration. The average time from onset of the disease to death is about 3 years. A small number of patients may survive for longer periods.

Assessment and Diagnostic Findings

ALS is diagnosed on the basis of the signs and symptoms because no clinical or laboratory tests are specific for this disease. EMG studies of the affected muscles indicate reduction in the number of functioning motor units.

Management

There is no specific therapy for ALS. The medication riluzole (Rilutek), a glutamate antagonist, was approved by the Food and Drug Administration in 1995 after clinical trials indicated that riluzole slows the deterioration of motor neurons. How riluzole works is not clear, but its pharmacologic properties suggest that it may have a neuroprotective effect in the early stages of ALS. Symptomatic treatment and rehabilitative measures are employed to support the patient and improve the quality of life. Baclofen (Lioresal), dantrolene sodium (Dantrium), or diazepam (Valium) may be useful for patients troubled by spasticity because spasticity causes pain and interferes with self-care. Quinine therapy may be prescribed for painful muscle cramps. The effect of high doses of thyrotropin-releasing hormone, a naturally occurring hormone produced by the brain and found in the motor neurons of the spinal cord, is under investigation. Interferon, a compound that appears to stimulate the body's defense system, is another investigational medication.

A patient experiencing problems with aspiration and swallowing may require nasogastric feeding. A cervical esophagostomy (opening into the esophagus) or a gastrostomy may be performed to bypass the larynx, to prevent aspiration, and to provide for long-term nutritional support.

Mechanical ventilation (using negative-pressure ventilators) is an option when alveolar hypoventilation develops. The decision of whether to use life support measures is made by the patient and family and should be based on a thorough understanding of the disease, the prognosis, and the implications of initiating such therapy. Patients are encouraged to complete an advance directive or "living will" to preserve their autonomy in decision making.

The ALS Association has broad programs of research funding, patient and clinical services, patient information and support, and medical and public information. The *ALS Association Quarterly Newsletter* is a source of practical information.

Muscular Dystrophies

The muscular dystrophies are a group of chronic muscle disorders characterized by progressive weakening and wasting of the skeletal or voluntary muscles. Most of these diseases are inherited. The pathologic features include degeneration and loss of muscle fibers, variation in muscle fiber size, phagocytosis and regeneration, and replacement of muscle tissue by connective tissue. The common characteristics of these diseases include varying degrees of muscle wasting and weakness; abnormal elevation in serum creatine phosphokinase, indicating a leakage of muscle enzymes; and myopathic findings on EMG and muscle biopsy. The differences center around the pattern of inheritance, the muscles involved, the age of onset, and the rate of progression.

Medical Management

Treatment of the muscular dystrophies at this time focuses on supportive care and prevention of complications. Supportive management is intended to keep the patient as active and functioning as normally as possible and to minimize functional deterioration. An individualized therapeutic exercise program is prescribed to prevent muscle tightness, contractures, and disuse atrophy. Night splints and stretching exercises are used to delay contractures of the joints, especially the ankles, knees, and hips. Braces may compensate for muscle weakness.

Spinal deformity is a severe problem. Weakness of trunk muscles and spinal collapse occur almost routinely in patients with severe neuromuscular disease. In the battle against spinal deformity, the patient is fitted with an orthotic jacket to improve sitting stability and reduce trunk deformity. This measure also supports cardiovascular status. In time, spinal fusion is performed to maintain spinal stability. Other procedures may be carried out to correct deformities.

Compromised pulmonary function may be due either to progression of the disease or to deformity of the thorax secondary to severe scoliosis. Intercurrent illnesses, upper respiratory infections, and fractures from falls must be vigorously treated in a way that minimizes immobilization because joint contractures become worse when the patient's activities are restricted more than usual.

Other difficulties may be manifested in relation to the underlying disease. Dental and speech problems may result from weakness of the facial muscles, which makes it difficult to attend to dental hygiene and to speak coherently. Gastrointestinal tract problems may include gastric dilation, rectal prolapse, and fecal impaction. Finally, cardiomyopathy appears to be a common complication in all forms of muscular dystrophy.

Genetic counseling is advised for parents and siblings of the patient because of the genetic nature of this disease. The Muscular Dystrophy Association works to combat neuromuscular disease through research, programs of patient services and clinical care, and professional and public education.

Nursing Management

The goals of the patient and the nurse are to maintain function at optimal levels and to enhance the quality of life. Therefore, the patient's physical requirements, which are considerable, are addressed without losing sight of emotional and developmental needs. The patient and family are actively involved in decision making, including end-of-life decisions.

During hospitalization for treatment of complications, the knowledge and expertise of the patient and family members responsible for caregiving in the home are assessed. Because the patient and family caregivers often have developed caregiving strategies that work effectively for them, these strategies need to be acknowledged and accepted, and provisions must be made to ensure that they are maintained during hospitalization.

PROMOTING HOME AND COMMUNITY-BASED CARE

Patient Teaching for Self-Care Management. Many of the management goals are addressed in the patient's home and community. Thus, the patient and family require information and instruction about the disorder, its anticipated course, and care and management strategies that will optimize the patient's growth and development and physical and psychological status. Members of a variety of health-related disciplines are involved in patient and family teaching; recommendations are communicated to all members of the health care team, so that they may work toward common goals.

Continuing Care. Both the neuromuscular disease and the associated deformities may progress in adolescence and adulthood. Self-help and assistive devices can aid in maintaining maximum independence. Additional self-help devices, recommended by physical and occupational therapists, often become necessary as more muscle groups are affected.

The family is taught to monitor the patient for respiratory problems. As respiratory difficulties develop, patients and their families need information regarding appropriate respiratory support. Options currently exist that can provide ventilatory support (negative-pressure devices, positive-pressure ventilators) while allowing mobility. Patients can remain relatively independent in a wheelchair, for example, while being maintained on a ventilator at home for many years.

The patient is encouraged to continue with range-of-motion exercises to prevent contractures, which are particularly disabling. Practical adaptations must be made, however, to cope with the effects of chronic neuromuscular disability. The patient at various stages of the disease may require a manual or an electric wheelchair, gait aids, upper and lower extremity and spinal orthoses, seating systems, bathroom equipment, lifts, ramps, and additional assistive devices, all of which require a team approach. The home care nurse assesses how the patient and family are managing, makes referrals, and coordinates the activities of the physical therapist, occupational therapist, and social services.

Of great concern to the patient are the issues surrounding the threat of increasing disability. The patient is faced with a progressive loss of function, leading eventually to death. Feelings of helplessness and powerlessness are common. Each functional loss is accompanied by grief and mourning. The patient and family are assessed for depression, anger, or denial. The patient and family are assisted to address decisions about end-of-life options before their need arises.

A psychiatric nurse clinician or other mental health professional may assist the patient to cope and adapt to the disease. By understanding and addressing the physical and psychological needs of the patient and family, the nurse provides a hopeful, supportive, and nurturing environment.

SEIZURE DISORDERS

Seizures

Seizures are episodes of abnormal motor, sensory, autonomic, or psychic activity (or a combination of these) resulting from sudden excessive discharge from cerebral neurons. A part or all of the brain may be involved. The seizures usually are sudden and transient.

The causes are varied and can be categorized as idiopathic (genetic, developmental defects) and acquired. Among the causes of acquired seizures are hypoxemia of any cause, including vascular insufficiency, fever (childhood), head injury, hypertension, central nervous system infections, metabolic and toxic conditions (eg, renal failure, hyponatremia, hypocalcemia, hypoglycemia, pesticides), brain tumor, drug withdrawal, and allergies. Stroke and cerebral metastasis are the leading causes of seizures in the elderly.

The patient often has memory loss during the seizure and for a short time thereafter. Brain damage may occur when seizures are severe or prolonged. The patient is at risk for hypoxia, vomiting, and pulmonary aspiration or persistent metabolic abnormalities.

The immediate therapeutic goal is to control the seizure, and the long-term goal is to determine and control the cause.

Nursing Management During a Seizure

A major responsibility of the nurse is to observe and to record the sequence of symptoms. The nature of the seizure usually indicates the type of treatment that is required. Before and during a seizure, the following are assessed and documented:

1. The circumstances before the seizure (visual, auditory, or olfactory stimuli, tactile stimuli, emotional or psychological disturbances, sleep, hyperventilation)

2. The first thing the patient does in a seizure—where the movements or the stiffness starts, conjugate gaze position, and the position of the patient's head at the beginning of the seizure. This information gives clues to the location of the epileptogenic focus in the brain. (In recording, it is important to state whether or not the beginning of the seizure was observed.)
3. The type of movements in the part of the body involved
4. The areas of the body involved (turn back bedding and expose patient)
5. The size of both pupils. Are the eyes open? Did the eyes or head turn to one side?
6. The presence or absence of automatisms (involuntary motor activity, such as lip smacking or repeated swallowing)
7. Incontinence of urine or stool
8. Duration of each phase of the seizure
9. Unconsciousness, if present, and its duration
10. Any obvious paralysis or weakness of arms or legs after the seizure
11. Inability to speak after the seizure
12. Movements at the end of the seizure
13. Whether or not the patient sleeps afterward
14. Cognitive status (confused or not confused) after the seizure

In addition to providing data about the seizure, nursing care is directed at preventing injury and supporting the patient. This includes not only physical, but also psychological injury. Steps to prevent or minimize injury to the patient are presented in Guideline 59-1.

Nursing Management After a Seizure

After a patient has a seizure, the nurse's role is to observe the patient for complications (eg, aspiration, injury) and document the events leading to and occurring during the seizure. The patient is positioned in the side-lying position to facilitate drainage of oral secretions, and is suctioned if needed to prevent aspiration and maintain a patent airway as described in Guideline 59-1. The patient may be drowsy and desire to sleep after the event and may not remember events leading up to the seizure. Seizure precautions are initiated, including having available fully functioning suction equipment with suction catheter and an oral airway. The bed is placed in a "low" position with side rails up and padded if necessary to prevent patient injury.

The Epilepsies

The epilepsies are a symptom complex of several disorders of brain function characterized by recurring seizures. Thus, epilepsy is not a disease but a symptom. There may be associated loss of consciousness, excess movement or loss of muscle tone or movement, and disturbances of behavior, mood, sensation, and perception. Types of epilepsies are differentiated by how the seizure activity manifests (Chart 59-6) and by the results of neuroimaging studies and EEG findings.

The problem is an electrical disturbance (dysrhythmia) in the nerve cells in one section of the brain, causing them to emit abnormal, recurring, uncontrolled electrical discharges. The characteristic epileptic seizure is a manifestation of this excessive neuronal discharge.

An estimated 1% of the population (more than 2 million people) in the United States have epilepsy, with 100,000 new patients diagnosed each year. Epilepsy occurs before the age of 20 years in greater than 75% of patients. There has been an increasing incidence of this condition, probably due to a number of factors. Improved obstetric and neonatal care saves babies who experience respiratory, circulatory, and other distress during delivery; these infants may be predisposed to intermittent seizures. The improved treatment of head injuries, brain tumors, meningitis, and encephalitis saves those whose conditions may be associated with seizures. Also, advances in EEG use have aided in the diagnosis of epilepsy. The general public has been educated about epilepsy, which has reduced the stigma associated with it, so that more people are willing to acknowledge the diagnosis.

Although there is evidence that susceptibility to some types of epilepsy may be inherited, the cause of seizures in many people is unknown. Epilepsy can follow birth trauma, asphyxia neonatorum, head injuries, some infectious diseases (bacterial, viral, parasitic), toxicity (carbon monoxide and lead poisoning), circulatory problems, fever, metabolic and nutritional disorders, and drug or alcohol intoxication. It is also associated with brain tumors, abscesses, and congenital malformations. In most cases of epilepsy, the cause is unknown (idiopathic).

Pathophysiology

Messages from the body are carried by the neurons (nerve cells) of the brain by means of discharges of electrochemical energy that sweep along them. These impulses occur in bursts whenever a nerve cell has a task to perform. Sometimes, these cells or groups of cells continue firing after a task is finished. During the period of unwanted discharges, parts of the body controlled by the errant cells may perform erratically. Resultant dysfunction ranges from mild to incapacitating and often causes unconsciousness. When these uncontrolled, abnormal discharges occur repeatedly, a person is said to have epilepsy.

Epilepsy is not associated with intellectual level. People with epilepsy without other brain or nervous system disabilities fall within the same intelligence ranges as the overall population. Epilepsy is not synonymous with mental retardation or illness. Many who are developmentally disabled because of serious neurologic damage, however, often have epilepsy as well.

Clinical Manifestations

Depending on the location of the discharging neurons, seizures may range from a simple staring episode to prolonged convulsive movements with loss of consciousness. Seizures have been classified according to the area of the brain involved and have been identified as partial, generalized, and unclassified. Partial seizures are focal in origin and affect only part of the brain. Generalized seizures are nonspecific in origin and affect the entire brain simultaneously. Unclassified seizures are so termed because of incomplete data.

The initial pattern of the seizures indicates the region of the brain in which the seizure originates. In simple partial seizures, only a finger or hand may shake, or the mouth may jerk uncontrollably. The person may talk unintelligibly, may be dizzy, and may experience unusual or unpleasant sights, sounds, odors, or tastes, but without loss of consciousness.

In complex partial seizures, the person either remains motionless or moves automatically but inappropriately for time and place, or may experience excessive emotions of fear, anger, elation, or irritability. Whatever the manifestations, the person does not remember the episode when it is over.

59•1
GUIDELINES FOR

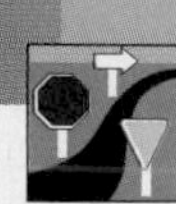

CARE OF THE PATIENT HAVING A SEIZURE

During Seizure

- Provide privacy and protect the patient from curious onlookers. (The patient who has an *aura* [warning of an impending seizure] may have time to seek a safe, private place.)
- Ease the patient to the floor, if possible.
- Protect the head with a pad to prevent injury (from striking a hard surface).
- Loosen constrictive clothing.
- Push aside any furniture that may injure the patient during the seizure.
- If the patient is in bed, remove pillows and raise siderails.
- If an aura precedes the seizure, insert an oral airway to reduce the possibility of the tongue or cheek being bitten.
- *Do not attempt to pry open jaws that are clenched in a spasm to insert anything.* Broken teeth and injury to the lips and tongue may result from such an action.
- No attempt should be made to restrain the patient during the seizure because muscular contractions are strong and restraint can produce injury.
- If possible, place the patient on one side with head flexed forward, which allows the tongue to fall forward and facilitates drainage of saliva and mucus. If suction is available, use it if necessary to clear secretions.

After the Seizure

- Keep the patient on one side to prevent aspiration. Make sure the airway is patent.
- There is usually a period of confusion after a grand mal seizure.
- A short apneic period may occur during or immediately after a generalized seizure.
- The patient, on awakening, should be reoriented to the environment.
- If the patient experiences severe excitement after a seizure (postictal), use calm persuasion and gentle restraint.

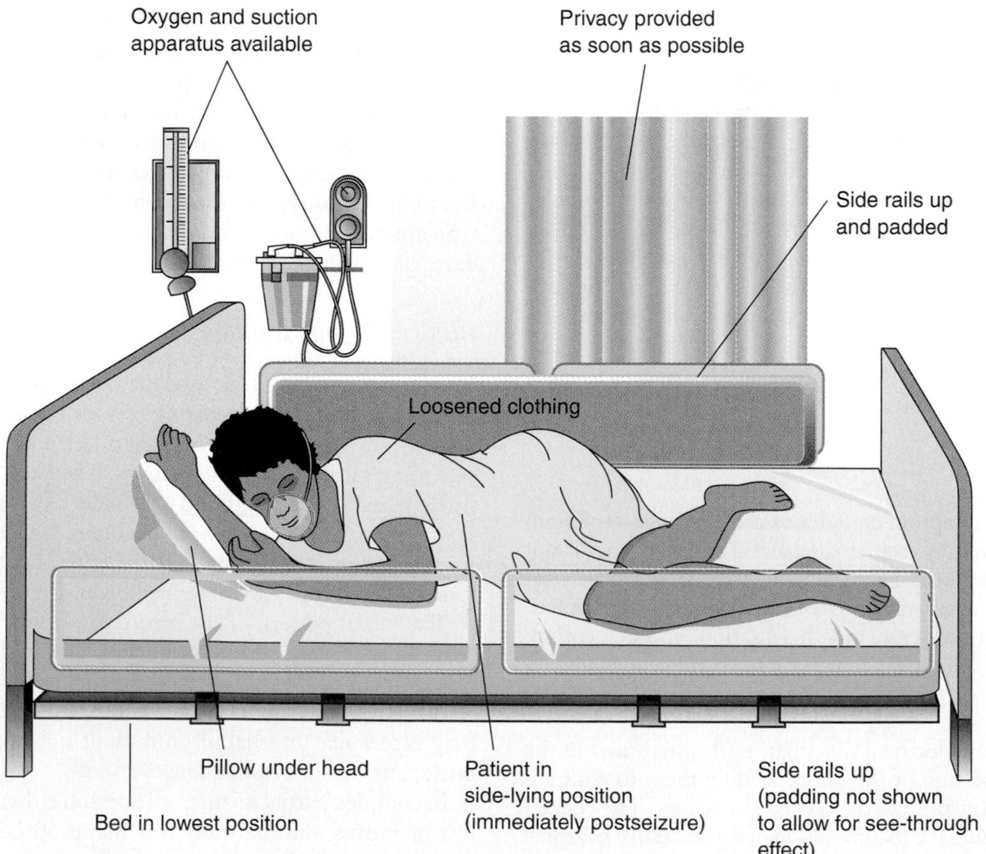

CHART 59•6 International Classification of Seizures

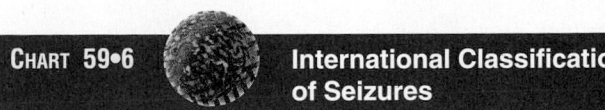

Partial Seizures (seizures beginning locally)

Simple partial seizures (with elementary symptoms, generally without impairment of consciousness)

- With motor symptoms
- With special sensory or somatosensory symptoms
- With autonomic symptoms
- Compound forms

Complex partial seizures (with complex symptoms, generally with impairment of consciousness)

- With impairment of consciousness only
- With cognitive symptoms
- With affective symptoms
- With psychosensory symptoms
- With psychomotor symptoms (automatisms)
- Compound forms

Partial seizures secondarily generalized

Generalized Seizures (convulsive or nonconvulsive, bilaterally symmetric, without local onset)

Tonic-clonic seizures

Tonic seizures

Clonic seizures

Absence seizures

Atonic seizures

Myoclonic seizures (bilaterally massive epileptic)

Generalized seizures, more commonly referred to as *grand mal seizures,* involve both hemispheres of the brain, causing both sides of the body to react. There may be intense rigidity of the entire body followed by jerky alternations of muscle relaxation and contraction (generalized tonic–clonic contraction). The simultaneous contractions of the diaphragm and chest muscles may produce a characteristic epileptic cry. The tongue is often chewed, and the patient is incontinent of urine and stool. After 1 or 2 minutes, the convulsive movements begin to subside; the patient relaxes and lies in deep coma, breathing noisily. The respirations at this point are chiefly abdominal. In the postictal state (after the seizure), the patient is often confused and hard to arouse and may sleep for hours. Many patients complain of headache or sore muscles.

Assessment and Diagnostic Findings

The diagnostic assessment is aimed at determining the *type* of seizures, their frequency and severity, and the factors that precipitate them. A developmental history is taken, including events of pregnancy and childbirth, to seek evidence of preexisting injury. A search is made for illnesses or head injuries that may have affected the brain. In addition to a physical and neurologic examination, diagnostic examinations include biochemical, hematologic, and serologic studies. CT and MRI imaging is used to detect lesions in the brain, focal abnormalities, cerebrovascular abnormalities, and cerebral degenerative changes.

The EEG furnishes diagnostic evidence in a substantial proportion of patients with epilepsy and aids in classifying the type of seizure. Abnormalities in the EEG usually continue between seizures, or, if not apparent, may be elicited by hyperventilation or during sleep. Microelectrodes can be inserted deep in the brain to probe the action of single brain cells. It should be noted, however, that some people with seizures may have normal EEGs, whereas others who have never had seizures may have abnormal EEGs. Telemetry and computerized equipment are used to obtain and store EEG readings on computer tapes while patients pursue their normal activities. Video recording of seizures taken simultaneously with EEG telemetry is useful in determining the type of seizure as well as its duration and magnitude. This type of intensive monitoring is changing the treatment of severe epilepsy.

Women With Epilepsy

Women have particular needs in the management of epilepsy. Women with epilepsy often note an increase in seizure frequency during menses; this has been linked to the increase in sex hormones that alter the excitability of neurons in the cerebral cortex. Women of childbearing age require special care and guidance before, during, and after pregnancy. Many women note a change in the pattern of seizure activity during pregnancy. Fetal malformation has been linked to the use of multiple antiepileptic medications to control seizures. The effectiveness of contraceptives is decreased by antiepileptic medications. Therefore, patients should be encouraged to discuss family planning with their physician and to obtain preconception counseling if they are considering childbearing.

Gerontologic Considerations

The elderly, 65 years of age and older, have a high incidence of new-onset epilepsy. Increased incidence is associated with stroke, head injury, dementia, infection, alcoholism, and aging. Treatment depends on the underlying cause. Because many elderly people have chronic health problems, they may be taking other medications that could interact with medications prescribed for seizure control. In addition, the absorption, distribution, metabolism, and excretion of medications are altered in the elderly as a result of age-related changes in renal and liver functions. Therefore, the elderly must be monitored closely for adverse and toxic effects of antiepileptic medications and for osteoporosis. The cost of antiepileptic medications could lead to poor compliance in adhering to the prescribed regimen in elderly patients on fixed incomes.

Prevention

Society-wide efforts are the key to the prevention of epilepsy. The risk for congenital fetal anomaly is two to three times higher in mothers with epilepsy. The effects of maternal seizures, antiepileptic medications, and genetic predisposition are all mechanisms that contribute to possible malformation. Because the unborn infants of mothers who take certain antiepileptic medications for epilepsy are at risk, these women need careful monitoring, including blood studies to detect the level of antiepileptic medications taken throughout pregnancy. High-risk mothers (teenagers, women with histories of difficult deliveries, drug use, patients with diabetes or hypertension) should be identified and monitored closely during pregnancy because damage to the fetus during pregnancy and delivery may increase the risk for epilepsy.

Childhood infections (measles, mumps, bacterial meningitis) should be prevented by appropriate vaccination. Lead poisoning is another preventable cause of epilepsy. Parents with a child who has had a febrile seizure should be instructed about methods to control fever (cool sponging, antipyretic medications).

Screening programs help to identify children with seizure disorders at an early age, and seizure prevention programs with the judicious use of anticonvulsant medications and modification of lifestyle are part of this prevention plan.

Head injury is one of the main causes of epilepsy that can be prevented. Through highway safety programs and occupational safety precautions, lives can be saved and epilepsy due to head injury prevented.

Medical Management

The management of epilepsy is individualized to meet the needs of each patient and not just to manage and prevent seizures. Management differs from patient to patient because some forms of epilepsy arise from brain damage and others are due to altered brain chemistry.

PHARMACOLOGIC THERAPY

Many antiepileptic and anticonvulsant medications are available to control seizures, although the mechanisms of their actions are still unknown. The objective is to achieve seizure control with minimal side effects. Medication therapy controls rather than cures seizures. Medications are selected on the basis of the type of seizure being treated and the effectiveness and safety of the medications. If properly prescribed and taken, medications control seizures in 50% to 60% of patients with recurring seizures and provide partial control in another 15% to 35%. The condition is not improved by any available medication in 20% and 35% of patients with generalized and partial epilepsy, respectively (DeVinsky, 1999).

Treatment is usually started with a single medication. The starting dose and the rate at which the dosage is increased depend on the occurrence of side effects. The medication levels in the blood are monitored because the rate of drug absorption varies among people. Changing to another medication may be necessary if seizure control is not achieved or if toxicity makes it impossible to increase the dosage. The medication may need to be adjusted because of concurrent illness, weight changes, or increases in stress. Sudden withdrawal of antiepileptic medication can cause seizures to occur with greater frequency or can precipitate the development of status epilepticus.

Side effects of antiepileptic agents may be divided into three groups: (1) idiosyncratic or allergic disorders, which present primarily as skin reactions; (2) acute toxicity, which may occur when the medication is initially prescribed; or (3) chronic toxicity, which occurs late in the course of therapy.

The manifestations of drug toxicity are variable, and any organ system may be involved. Periodic physical examinations and laboratory tests are performed for patients receiving medications known to have hematopoietic, genitourinary, or hepatic effects. Table 59-2 summarizes the medications in current use.

SURGICAL MANAGEMENT

Surgery is indicated for patients whose epilepsy results from intracranial tumors, abscess, cysts, or vascular anomalies. Some patients have intractable seizure disorders that do not respond to medication. There may be a focal atrophic process secondary to trauma, inflammation, stroke, or anoxia. If the seizures originate in a reasonably well-circumscribed area of the brain that can be excised without producing significant neurologic deficits, the removal of the area generating the seizures may produce long-term control and improvement.

This type of neurosurgery has been aided by several modern advances, including microsurgical techniques, depth EEGs, improved illumination and hemostasis, and the introduction of neuroleptanalgesic agents (droperidol and fentanyl). These techniques, combined with use of local anesthetic agents, enable the neurosurgeon to perform surgery on an alert and cooperative patient. With special testing devices, electrocortical mapping, and the patient's response to stimulation, the boundaries of the epileptogenic focus are determined. Any abnormal epileptogenic focus (ie, abnormal area of the brain) is then removed.

As an adjunct to medication and surgery in adolescents and adults with partial seizures, a generator may be implanted under the clavicle. The device is connected to the vagus nerve in the cervical area, where it delivers electrical signals to the brain to control and reduce seizure activity. An external programming system is used by the physician to change stimulator settings. Patients can turn the stimulator on and off with a magnet.

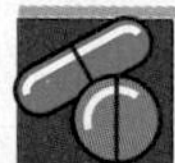

TABLE 59•2 Major Anticonvulsant/Antiepileptic Medications

Medication	Dose-Related Side Effects	Toxic Effects
clonazepam (Klonopin)	Drowsiness, behavior changes, headache, hirsutism, alopecia, palpitations	Hepatotoxicity, thrombocytopenia, bone marrow failure, ataxia
carbamazepine (Tegretol)	Dizziness, drowsiness, unsteadiness, nausea and vomiting, diplopia, mild leukopenia	Severe skin rash, blood dyscrasias, hepatitis
primidone (Mysoline)	Lethargy, irritability, diplopia, ataxia, sexual impotence	Skin rash
phenytoin (Dilantin)	Visual problems, hirsutism, gingival hyperplasia, dysrhythmias, dysarthria, nystagmus	Severe skin reaction, peripheral neuropathy, ataxia, drowsiness, blood dyscrasias
phenobarbital (Luminal)	Sedation, irritability, diplopia, ataxia	Skin rash, anemia
ethosuximide (Zarontin)	Nausea and vomiting, headache, gastric distress	Skin rash, blood dyscrasias, hepatitis, lupus erythematosus
valproate (Depakote, Depakene)	Nausea and vomiting, weight gain, hair loss, tremor, menstrual irregularities	Hepatotoxicity, skin rash, blood dyscrasias, nephritis
felbamate (Felbatol)	Cognitive impairments, insomnia, nausea, headache, fatigue	Aplastic anemia, hepatotoxicity
gabapentin (Neurontin)	Drowsiness, fatigue, dizziness, nausea, ataxia, weight gain, somnolence	Leukopenia, hepatotoxicity
lamotrigine (Lamictal)	Drowsiness, tremor, nausea, ataxia, dizziness, headache, weight gain	Severe rash (Stevens-Johnson syndrome)
topiramate (Topamax)	Fatigue, somnolence, confusion, ataxia, anorexia, depression, weight loss	Nephrolithiasis

NURSING PROCESS: THE PATIENT WITH EPILEPSY

Assessment

The nurse elicits information about the patient's seizure history. The patient is asked about the factors or events that may precipitate the seizures. Alcohol intake is documented. It is also important to determine if the patient has had an aura, a premonitory or warning sensation before an epileptic seizure, which may indicate the origin of the seizure (eg, seeing a flashing light may indicate the seizure originated in the occipital lobe). Observation and assessment during and after a seizure assist in identifying the type of seizure and its management.

The effects of epilepsy on lifestyle are assessed: What limitations are imposed by the seizure disorder? Does the patient have a recreational program? Social contacts? Is work a positive experience? What coping mechanisms are used?

Diagnosis

Nursing Diagnoses

Based on the assessment data, the patient's major nursing diagnoses may include the following:

- Fear related to the possibility of seizures
- Ineffective individual coping related to stresses imposed by epilepsy
- Knowledge deficit about epilepsy and its control

Collaborative Problems/Potential Complications

The major potential complication of patients with epilepsy is as follows:

- Status epilepticus

Planning and Goals

The major goals for the patient may include control of seizures, achievement of a satisfactory psychosocial adjustment, acquisition of knowledge and understanding about the condition, and absence of complications.

Nursing Interventions

Reducing Fear of Seizures

Fear that a seizure may occur unexpectedly can be reduced by the patient's compliance with the prescribed treatment. Cooperation of the patient and family and their confidence in the value of the prescribed regimen are essential for control of seizures. It is emphasized that the prescribed antiepileptic medication must be taken on a continuing basis without fear of drug dependence or addiction. Periodic monitoring is necessary to ensure adequacy of the treatment regimen and to prevent side effects.

In an effort to control seizures, factors that may precipitate them are identified: emotional disturbances, new environmental stressors, onset of menstruation in female patients, or fever. The patient is encouraged to follow a regular and moderate routine in lifestyle, diet (avoiding excessive stimulants), exercise, and rest. (Sleep deprivation may lower the patient's threshold to seizures.) Moderate activity is therapeutic, but excessive exercise should be avoided.

Photic stimulation (bright flickering lights, television viewing) may precipitate seizures; wearing dark glasses or covering one eye may help control this problem. Tension states (anxiety, frustration) induce seizures in some patients. Classes in stress management may be of value. Because seizures are known to occur with alcohol intake, alcoholic beverages are restricted. The patient is advised to avoid stimuli that precipitate seizures.

Improving Coping Mechanisms

It has been noted that the social, psychological, and behavioral problems frequently accompanying epilepsy can be more of a handicap than the actual seizures. Epilepsy may be accompanied by feelings of fear, alienation, depression, and uncertainty. The patient must cope with the constant fear of a seizure and its consequences. Children with epilepsy may be ostracized and excluded from school and peer activities. These problems are compounded during adolescence and add to the challenges of dating, not being able to drive, and feeling different. Adults face these problems in addition to the burden of finding employment, concerns about relationships and childbearing, noninsurability, stigma, and legal barriers. Alcohol abuse may complicate matters. Family reactions may vary from outright rejection of the person with epilepsy to overprotection. As a result, many people with epilepsy have psychological and behavioral problems.

Counseling assists the individual and family to understand the condition and the limitations imposed by it. Social and recreational opportunities are necessary for good mental health. Some people are not able to cope with epilepsy; others have psychological problems resulting from brain damage. Those with seizures originating in the temporal lobes of the brain (areas controlling thought and emotions) have particular emotional problems. Symptoms of schizophrenia and impulsive or irritable behavior may be due to brain damage associated with temporal lobe seizures. These patients require comprehensive mental health services.

Fostering a Positive Mental Outlook

Of all the care contributed by the nurse to the person with epilepsy, perhaps the most valuable efforts are those to modify the attitudes of the patient and family toward the disease itself. The person who experiences seizures may consider every seizure a potential source of humiliation and shame. This may result in anxiety, depression, hostility, and secrecy on the part of the patient and family.

Ongoing encouragement should be given to patients to enable them to overcome these feelings. The patient with epilepsy should carry an emergency medical identification card or wear a MedicAlert bracelet.

Promoting Home and Community-Based Care

TEACHING PATIENTS SELF-CARE

Thorough oral hygiene after each meal, gum massage, daily flossing, and regular dental care are essential to prevent or control gingival hyperplasia in patients receiving phenytoin (Dilantin). The patient is also counseled to inform all health care providers of the medication being taken because of the possibility of drug interactions. An individualized comprehensive teaching plan is needed to assist the patient and family to adjust to this chronic disorder.

CONTINUING CARE

Financial Considerations. Because epilepsy is a long-term disorder, the use of costly medications may create a sizable financial burden. The Epilepsy Foundation of America offers a mail-

HOME CARE TEACHING CHECKLIST: THE PATIENT WITH EPILEPSY

At the completion of the program, the patient and caregiver will be able to:

	Patient	Caregiver
• Take medications daily as prescribed to keep the blood–drug level constant to prevent seizures. Medications should *never* be discontinued by the patient, even when there is no seizure activity.	✔	
• Keep a "drug and seizure chart," noting when medications are taken and any seizure activity.	✔	
• Notify the patient's physician if patient cannot take medications due to illness.	✔	✔
• Have anticonvulsant serum levels checked regularly. When testing is prescribed, the patient should report to the laboratory for blood sampling before taking morning medication.	✔	✔
• Avoid activities that require alertness and coordination (driving, operating machinery) until after the effects of the medication have been evaluated.	✔	
• Report signs of toxicity so dosage can be adjusted. Common signs include drowsiness, lethargy, dizziness, difficulty walking, hyperactivity, confusion, inappropriate sleep, and visual disturbances.	✔	✔
• Avoid over-the counter medications unless approved by the patient's physician.	✔	
• Carry a MedicAlert bracelet or personal identification card specifying the name of the patient's anticonvulsant medication and physician.	✔	
• Avoid seizure "triggers," such as alcoholic beverages, electrical shocks, stress, caffeine, constipation, fever, hyperventilation, hypoglycemia.	✔	
• Take showers rather than tub baths to avoid drowning; never swim alone.	✔	
• Exercise in moderation in a temperature-controlled environment to avoid excessive heat.	✔	
• Develop regular sleep patterns to minimize fatigue and insomnia	✔	
• Avail oneself of the Epilepsy Foundation of America's special services, including help in obtaining medications, vocational rehabilitation, and coping with epilepsy.	✔	✔

order program to provide medications at minimal cost and access to life insurance. This organization serves as a referral source for special services for people with epilepsy.

Vocational Rehabilitation. For many, employment problems still remain the greatest handicap of epilepsy. State vocational rehabilitation agencies can provide information about job training. The Epilepsy Foundation of America has a training and placement service. If the individual's seizures are not well controlled, information about sheltered workshops or home employment programs may also be obtained.

Federal and state agencies and federal legislation may be of assistance to people with epilepsy who experience job discrimination. As a result of the Americans With Disabilities Act of 1992, the number of employers who knowingly hire people with epilepsy is increasing.

Ongoing Evaluation. People who have uncontrollable seizures and psychological and social maladaptation with other overwhelming problems can be referred to comprehensive epilepsy centers where continuous audio-video and EEG monitoring, specialized treatment, and rehabilitation services are available.

Genetic Counseling. Hereditary transmission of epilepsy has not been proved. Decisions about marriage and childbearing are made on an individual basis, and such options should not be denied to people with epilepsy. Genetic and preconception counseling is advised, however.

Monitoring and Managing Potential Complications

Status epilepticus, the major complication, is described later. Another complication is toxicity of medications. The patient and family are instructed about side effects and are given specific guidelines to assess and report signs and symptoms indicating medication overdose.

Evaluation

Expected Outcomes

Expected outcomes may include:

1. Maintains control of seizures
   a. Complies with treatment regimen and identifies the hazards of stopping the medication
   b. Identifies the side effects of medications
   c. Avoids factors or situations that may precipitate seizures (flickering lights, hyperventilation, alcohol)
   d. Follows a healthy lifestyle by getting enough sleep and eating meals at regular times to avoid hypoglycemia
2. Exhibits psychosocial adjustment
3. Exhibits knowledge and understanding of epilepsy
4. Is free of seizures and the complication of status epilepticus

Status Epilepticus

Status epilepticus (acute prolonged seizure activity) is a series of generalized seizures that occur without full recovery of consciousness between attacks. The term has been broadened to include continuous clinical or electrical seizures lasting at least 30 minutes, even without impairment of consciousness. It is considered a major medical emergency. Status epilepticus produces cumulative effects. Vigorous muscular contractions impose a heavy metabolic demand and can interfere with respirations. There is some respiratory arrest at the height of each seizure that produces venous congestion and hypoxia of the brain. Repeated episodes of cerebral anoxia and swelling may lead to irreversible and fatal brain damage. Factors that precipitate status epilepticus include withdrawal of antiepileptic medication, fever, and concurrent infection.

Medical Management

The goals of treatment are to stop the seizures as quickly as possible, to ensure adequate cerebral oxygenation, and to maintain the patient in a seizure-free state. Airway and adequate oxygenation are established. If the patient remains unconscious and unresponsive, a cuffed endotracheal tube is inserted. Intravenous diazepam (Valium), lorazepam (Ativan), or fosphenytoin (Cerebyx) is given slowly in an attempt to halt seizures immediately. Other medications (phenytoin, phenobarbital) are given later to maintain a seizure-free state.

An intravenous line is established, and blood samples are obtained to monitor serum electrolytes, urea, and glucose levels. EEG monitoring may be useful in determining the nature of epileptogenic activity. Vital signs and neurologic signs are monitored on a continuing basis. An intravenous infusion of dextrose is given if the seizure is due to hypoglycemia. If initial treatment is unsuccessful, general anesthesia with a short-acting barbiturate may be used. Serum concentration of the anticonvulsant medication is measured because a low level suggests that the patient was not taking the medication or that the dosage was too low. Cardiac involvement or respiratory depression may be severe and life-threatening. There is also the potential for postictal (after a seizure) cerebral swelling.

Nursing Management

The nurse initiates ongoing assessment and monitoring of respiratory and cardiac function because of risk for delayed depression of respiration and blood pressure secondary to administration of anticonvulsants and sedatives to halt the seizures. Nursing assessment also includes monitoring and documenting the seizure activity and the responsiveness of the patient.

The patient is turned to a side-lying position if possible, to assist in draining pharyngeal secretions. Suction equipment must be available because of the risk for aspiration. The intravenous line is closely monitored because it may become dislodged during seizures.

A person who has received long-term anticonvulsant therapy has a significant risk for fractures resulting from bone disease (osteoporosis, osteomalacia, and hyperparathyroidism), a side effect of drug therapy. Thus, during seizures, the patient should be protected from injury using seizure precautions and monitored closely. No effort should be made to restrain movements. The patient having seizures can inadvertently injure nearby people, so nurses should take care to protect themselves. Other nursing interventions for the person having seizures are presented in Guideline 59-1.

DISORDERS OF THE SPINAL CORD

Intraspinal Tumors

Tumors within the spine are classified according to their anatomic relation to the spinal cord. They include *intramedullary* lesions (within the spinal cord), *extramedullary-intradural* lesions (within or under the spinal dura), and *extramedullary-extradural* lesions (outside the dural membrane). Tumors occurring within the spinal cord or exerting pressure on it cause symptoms ranging from localized or shooting pains and weakness and loss of reflexes above the tumor level to progressive loss of motor function and paralysis. Usually, sharp pain occurs in the area innervated by the spinal roots that arise from the cord in the region of the tumor. In addition, increasing sensory deficits develop below the level of the lesion.

The diagnosis is made by neurologic examination and MRI, CT scanning, and myelography.

Medical Management

Treatment of specific intraspinal tumors depends on the type and location of the tumor and the presenting symptoms and physical status of the patient. Surgical intervention is the primary treatment for most spinal cord tumors. Other treatment modalities include partial removal of the tumor, decompression of the spinal cord, chemotherapy, and radiation therapy, particularly for intramedullary tumors and metastatic lesions. If the patient has epidural spinal cord compression resulting from metastatic cancer (from breast, prostate, or lung), high-dose dexamethasone combined with radiation therapy is effective in relieving pain.

SURGICAL MANAGEMENT

The removal of the tumor is desirable but not always possible. The goal is to remove as much tumor as possible while sparing uninvolved portions of the spinal cord. Microsurgical techniques have improved the prognosis for surgical treatment of intramedullary tumors. The prognosis is related to the degree of neurologic impairment at the time of surgery, the speed with which symptoms occurred, and the tumor's origin. Patients with large neurologic deficits before surgery usually do not make significant functional recovery even after successful tumor removal.

Nursing Management

PROVIDING PREOPERATIVE CARE

The objectives of preoperative care include recognition of neurologic changes through ongoing assessments, pain control, management of altered activities of daily living due to sensory and motor deficits and bowel and bladder dysfunction. The patient is assessed for weakness, muscle wasting, spasticity, sensory changes, bowel and bladder dysfunction, and potential pulmonary problems, especially if a cervical tumor is present. The patient is also evaluated for coagulation deficiencies. A history of aspirin intake is obtained and reported because the use of aspirin may impede hemostasis postoperatively. Breathing exercises are taught and demonstrated preoperatively. Pain management strategies to be used postoperatively are discussed with the patient before surgery.

ASSESSING THE PATIENT AFTER SURGERY

The nursing management is similar to that after disk surgery. The patient is monitored for deterioration in neurologic status. A sudden onset of neurologic deficit is an ominous sign and may be due to vertebral collapse associated with spinal cord infarction. Neurologic checks are made, with emphasis on movement, strength, and sensation of the upper and lower extremities. Sensory function is assessed by pinching the skin of the arms, legs, and trunk to determine if there is loss of feeling and, if so, at what level. Vital signs are monitored at intervals.

MANAGING PAIN

The prescribed pain medication should be given in adequate amounts and at appropriate intervals to relieve pain and prevent its recurrence. Pain is the hallmark of spinal metastasis. Patients with sensory root involvement or vertebral collapse may suffer excruciating pain and require effective pain management.

The bed is usually kept flat initially. The patient is turned as a unit, keeping shoulders and hips aligned. The back is kept straight. The side-lying position is usually the most comfortable because it avoids pressure on the surgical site. A pillow is placed between the knees of the patient in a side-lying position, and extreme knee flexion is avoided.

MONITORING AND MANAGING POTENTIAL COMPLICATIONS

If the tumor was in the cervical area, there is always the possibility of postoperative respiratory compromise. The patient is monitored for asymmetry of chest movement, abdominal breathing, and abnormal breath sounds. In the instance of a high cervical lesion, the endotracheal tube is left in place until adequate respiratory function is ensured. Deep breathing and coughing are encouraged.

The area over the patient's bladder is palpated for urinary retention. Incontinence may be present. Urinary dysfunction usually implies significant decompensation of spinal cord function. An intake and output record is maintained. Additionally, the abdomen is auscultated for bowel sounds.

Staining of the dressing may indicate leakage of CSF from the surgical site, which may lead to serious infection or to an inflammatory reaction in the surrounding tissues that can cause severe pain in the postoperative period.

PROMOTING HOME AND COMMUNITY-BASED CARE

Teaching Patients Self-Care. In preparation for discharge, patients are assessed for their ability to function independently in the home and for the availability of resources, such as family members to assist in caregiving. Patients with residual sensory involvement are cautioned about the dangers of extremes in temperature. They should be alert to the dangers of heating devices (eg, hot water bottles, heating pads, space heaters). The patient is taught to check skin integrity daily. Patients with impaired motor function related to motor weakness or paralysis may require training in activities of daily living and an assistive device, such as a cane or walker.

The patient and family member are instructed about pain management strategies, bowel and bladder management, and assessment for signs and symptoms that should be reported promptly.

Continuing Care. Referral for inpatient or outpatient rehabilitation may be warranted to improve self-care abilities. A home care referral may be indicated and provides the home care nurse with the opportunity to assess the patient's physical and psychological status and the patient's and family's ability to adhere to recommended management strategies. During the home visit, the nurse determines whether changes in neurologic function have occurred. The patient's respiratory and nutritional status is assessed. The adequacy of pain management is assessed, and modifications are made to ensure adequate pain relief. The need for hospice services or placement in an extended care facility is discussed with the patient and family if warranted, and the patient is asked about preferences for end-of-life care.

Social workers are involved to assist patients and family members in identifying support groups and agencies that can best provide help in coping with the disease process.

Herniation of an Intervertebral Disk

The intervertebral disk is a cartilaginous plate that forms a cushion between the vertebral bodies (Fig. 59-13**A**). This tough, fibrous material is incorporated in a capsule. A ball-like cushion in the center of the disk is called the *nucleus pulposus.* In herniation of the intervertebral disk (ruptured disk), the nucleus of the disk protrudes into the annulus (the fibrous ring around the disk), with subsequent nerve compression. Protrusion or rupture of the nucleus pulposus usually is preceded by degenerative changes that occur with aging. Loss of protein polysaccharides in the disk decreases the water content of the nucleus pulposus. The development of radiating cracks in the annulus weakens resistance to nucleus herniation. After trauma (falls, accidents, and repeated minor stresses, such as lifting), the cartilage may be injured.

In most patients, the immediate symptoms of trauma are short lived, and those resulting from injury to the disk do not appear for months or years. Then, with degeneration in the disk, the capsule pushes back into the spinal canal, or it may rupture and allow the nucleus pulposus to be pushed back against the dural sac or against a spinal nerve as it emerges from the spinal column (see Fig. 59-13**B**). This sequence produces pain due to pressure in the area of distribution of the involved nerve endings (**radiculopathy**). Continued pressure may produce degenerative changes in the involved nerve, such as changes in sensation and reflex action.

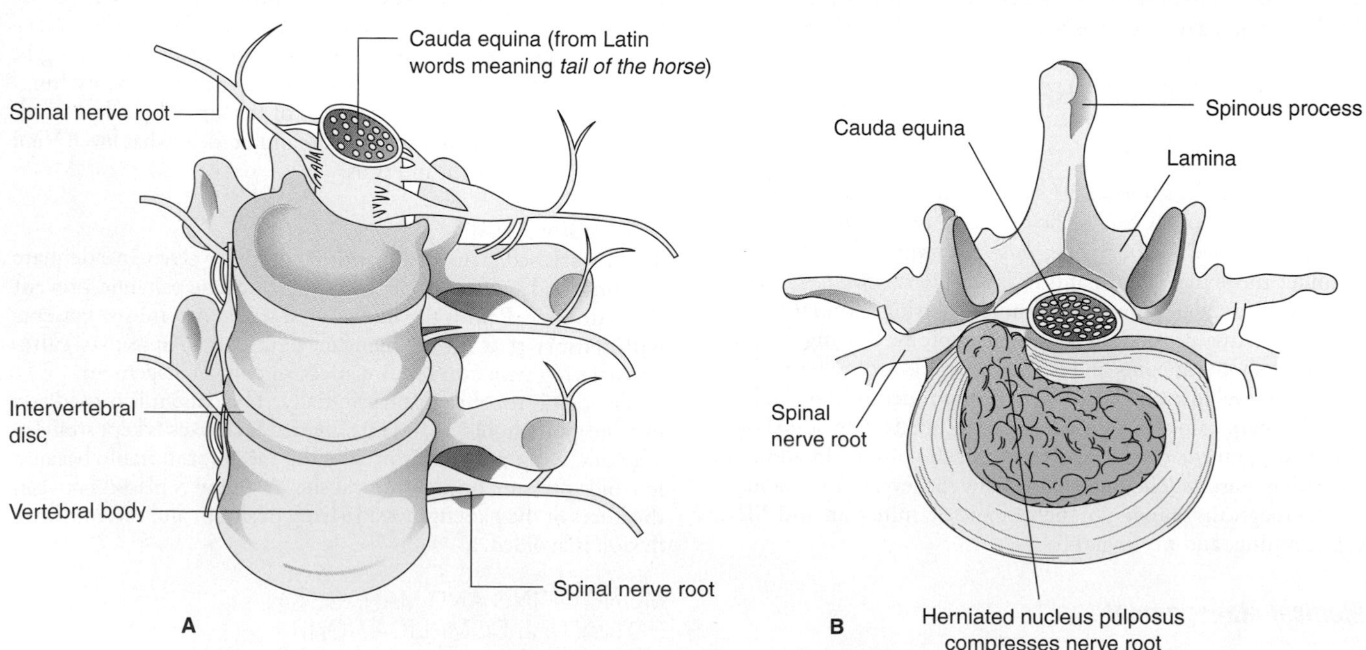

FIGURE 59•13 (**A**) Normal lumbar spine vertebrae, intervertebral disks, and spinal nerve root. (**B**) Ruptured vertebral disk.

Clinical Manifestations

A herniated disk with accompanying pain may occur in any portion of the spine: cervical, thoracic (rare), or lumbar. The clinical manifestations depend on the location, the rate of development (acute or chronic), and the effect on the surrounding structures.

Assessment and Diagnostic Findings

MRI has become the diagnostic tool of choice for localizing even small disk protrusions, particularly for lumbar spine disease. In patients in whom clinical symptoms and the pathology seen on MRI are discrepant, CT and myelogram are then be performed. A neurologic examination is carried out to determine if there is reflex, sensory, or motor impairment from root compression and to provide a baseline for future assessment. EMG may be used to localize the specific spinal nerve roots involved.

Medical Management

Herniations of the cervical and the lumbar disks occur most commonly and are usually managed conservatively with bed rest and medication. The specific conservative management strategies, along with surgical interventions for each form of herniation, are discussed next.

SURGICAL MANAGEMENT

In general, surgical excision of a herniated disk is performed when there is evidence of a progressing neurologic deficit (muscle weakness and atrophy, loss of sensory and motor function, loss of sphincter control), and continuing pain and **sciatica** that are unresponsive to conservative management. The goal of surgical treatment is to reduce the pressure on the nerve root to relieve pain and reverse neurologic deficits. Microsurgical techniques are making it possible to remove precisely that amount of tissue that is absolutely necessary. This approach better preserves the integrity of normal tissue and imposes less trauma on the body. During these procedures, spinal cord function can be monitored electrophysiologically.

To achieve the goal of pain relief, several surgical techniques are used, depending on the type of disk herniation, surgical morbidity, and overall results of surgery:

- Discectomy—removal of herniated or extruded fragments of intervertebral disk
- Laminectomy—removal of the lamina to expose the neural elements in the spinal canal; allows the surgeon to inspect the spinal canal, identify and remove pathology, and relieve compression of the cord and roots
- Hemilaminectomy—part of the lamina and part of the posterior arch of the vertebrae are removed
- Laminotomy—division of the lamina of a vertebra
- Discectomy with fusion—a bone graft (from iliac crest or bone bank) is used to fuse the vertebral spinous process; the object of spinal fusion is to bridge over the defective disk to stabilize the spine and reduce the rate of recurrence
- Foraminotomy—removal of the intervertebral foramen to increase the space for exit of a spinal nerve, resulting in reduced pain, compression, and edema

Surgical procedures for herniated cervical disk and lumbar disk are discussed in detail in the sections that follow.

Herniation of a Cervical Intervertebral Disk

The cervical spine is subjected to stresses that result from disk degeneration (from aging, occupational stresses) and **spondylosis** (degenerative changes occurring in disk and adjacent vertebral bodies). Cervical disk degeneration may lead to lesions that can cause damage to the spinal cord and its roots.

A cervical disk herniation usually occurs at the C5–C6 and C6–C7 interspaces. Pain and stiffness may occur in the neck, the top of the shoulders, and the region of the scapulae. Sometimes, patients interpret these signs as symptoms of heart trouble or bursitis. Pain may also occur in the upper extremities and head, accompanied by paresthesia and numbness of the upper extremities. The diagnosis is usually confirmed by cervical MRI.

Medical Management

The goals of treatment are (1) to rest and immobilize the cervical spine to give the soft tissues time to heal, and (2) to reduce inflammation in the supporting tissues and the affected nerve roots in the cervical spine. Bed rest (usually 2 weeks) is important because it eliminates the stress of gravity and relieves the cervical spine from the need to support the head. It also reduces inflammation and edema in soft tissues around the disk, relieving pressure on the nerve roots. Proper positioning on a firm mattress may bring dramatic relief from pain.

The cervical spine may be rested and immobilized by a cervical collar, cervical traction, or a brace. A collar allows maximal opening of the intervertebral foramina and holds the head in a neutral or slightly flexed position. The patient may have to wear the collar 24 hours a day during the acute phase. The skin under the collar is inspected for irritation. When the patient is free of pain, cervical isometric exercises are started to strengthen the muscles in the neck.

Cervical traction is accomplished by means of a head halter attached to a pulley and weight. It increases vertebral separation and thus relieves pressure on the nerve roots. The head of the bed is elevated to provide countertraction. If the skin becomes irritated, the halter can be padded. Experience has shown that a male patient may suffer more skin irritation if he shaves; the beard offers a natural form of padding.

PHARMACOLOGIC THERAPY

Analgesics (nonsteroidal anti-inflammatory drugs [NSAIDs], propoxyphene [Darvon], oxycodone [Tylox], or hydrocodone [Vicodin]) are given during the acute phase to relieve pain, and sedatives may be administered to control the anxiety often associated with cervical disk disease. Muscle relaxants (cyclobenzaprine [Flexeril], methocarbamol [Robaxin], metaxalone [Skelaxin]) are administered to interrupt the cycle of muscle spasm and to promote patient comfort. NSAIDs (aspirin, ibuprofen [Motrin, Advil], naproxen [Naprosyn, Anaprox], or corticosteroids are given to treat the inflammatory response that usually occurs in the supporting tissues and affected nerve roots. Occasionally, an injection of a corticosteroid into the epidural space may be administered for relief of radicular (spinal nerve root) pain. NSAIDs are given with food and antacids to prevent gastrointestinal irritation. Hot, moist compresses (for 10 to 20 minutes) applied to the back of the neck several times daily increase blood flow to the muscles and help to relax the spastic muscles and the patient.

SURGICAL MANAGEMENT

Surgical excision of the herniated disk may be necessary when there is a significant neurologic deficit, progression of the deficit, evidence of cord compression, or pain that either worsens or fails to improve. A cervical discectomy, with or without fusion, may be performed to alleviate symptoms. An anterior surgical approach may be used through a transverse incision to remove disk material that has herniated into the spinal canal and foramina, or a posterior approach may be used at the appropriate level of the cervical spine. Potential complications for the anterior approach include carotid or vertebral artery injury, recurrent laryngeal nerve dysfunction, esophageal perforation, and airway obstruction. Complications of the posterior approach include damage to the nerve root or to the spinal cord due to retraction or contusion of either of these structures, resulting in weakness of muscles supplied by the nerve root or cord.

Microsurgery, such as endoscopic microdiscectomy, may be performed in selected patients through a small incision and using magnification techniques. The patient who undergoes microsurgery usually has less tissue trauma and pain and consequently a shorter hospital stay than after conventional surgical approaches.

NURSING PROCESS: THE PATIENT UNDERGOING A CERVICAL DISCECTOMY

Assessment

The patient is asked about past injuries to the neck (whiplash) because unresolved trauma may cause persistent discomfort, pain and tenderness, and symptoms of arthritis in the injured joint of the cervical spine. Assessment of the patient's problems includes determining the onset, location, and radiation of pain, paresthesias, limited movement, and diminished function of the neck, shoulders, and upper extremities. It is important to determine whether or not the symptoms are bilateral because with large herniations, bilateral symptoms may be due to cord compression. The area around the cervical spine is palpated to assess muscle tone and tenderness. Range of motion in the neck and shoulders is evaluated.

The patient is asked about any health problems that may influence the postoperative course. The nurse determines the patient's need for information about the surgical procedure and reinforces what has been explained by the physician. Strategies for pain management are discussed with the patient.

Diagnosis

Nursing Diagnoses

Based on the assessment data, the patient's major nursing diagnoses may include the following:

- Pain related to the surgical procedure
- Impaired physical mobility related to postoperative surgical regimen
- Knowledge deficit about the postoperative course and home care management

Other nursing diagnoses may include preoperative anxiety, postoperative constipation, urinary retention related to surgical procedure and dehydration, self-care deficits related to neck orthosis, and sleep pattern disturbance related to disruption in lifestyle.

Collaborative Problems/Potential Complications

Based on all the assessment data, the potential complications may include the following:

- Hematoma at the surgical site, resulting in cord compression and neurologic deficit
- Recurrent or persistent pain after surgery

Planning and Goals

The goals of the patient may include relief of pain, improved mobility, increased knowledge and self-care ability, and prevention of complications.

Nursing Interventions

Assessing the Patient After Surgery

Assessment includes monitoring the blood pressure and pulse to evaluate cardiovascular status. The patient is evaluated for bleeding and hematoma formation by assessing for excessive pressure in the neck or severe pain in the incisional area. The dressing is inspected for serosanguineous drainage, which suggests a dural leak. In this event, meningitis is a threat. A complaint of headache requires careful evaluation. Neurologic checks are made for swallowing deficits and upper and lower extremity weakness because cord compression may produce rapid or delayed onset of paralysis. The patient who has had an anterior cervical discectomy is also assessed for a sudden return of radicular (spinal nerve root) pain, which may indicate instability of the spine.

Throughout the postoperative course, the patient is monitored frequently to detect any signs of respiratory difficulty because the recurrent laryngeal nerve may be injured by retractors during surgery, resulting in hoarseness and the inability to cough effectively and clear pulmonary secretions.

Relieving Pain

The patient may be kept flat in bed for 12 to 24 hours. If the patient has had a bone fusion with bone removed from the iliac crest, considerable pain may be experienced. Interventions consist of monitoring the donor site for hematoma formation, administering the prescribed postoperative analgesic, positioning for comfort, and reassuring the patient that the pain can be relieved. If the patient experiences a sudden reappearance of pain, extrusion of the graft may have occurred, requiring reoperation and surgical repositioning of the graft. Pain should be promptly reported.

The patient may experience a sore throat, hoarseness, and dysphagia due to temporary edema. These symptoms are relieved by throat lozenges, voice rest, and humidification. A pureed diet may be given if the patient has dysphagia.

Improving Mobility

Postoperatively, a cervical collar (neck orthosis) is usually worn, which contributes to limited neck motion and altered mobility. Patients are instructed to turn the body instead of the neck when looking from side to side. The neck should be kept in a neutral (midline) position. Patients are assisted during position changes, making sure that head, shoulders, and thorax are kept aligned. When assisting a patient to a sitting position, the nurse supports the patient's neck and shoulders. Patients should wear shoes when ambulating to increase stability.

Monitoring and Managing Potential Complications

Bleeding at the surgical site and subsequent hematoma formation may occur. Severe localized pain not relieved by analgesics should be reported to the surgeon. A change in neurologic status (motor or sensory function) should be reported promptly because it suggests hematoma formation that may necessitate surgery to prevent irreversible motor and sensory deficits.

Promoting Home and Community-Based Care

TEACHING PATIENTS SELF-CARE

The patient's hospital stay is likely to be short; therefore, the patient and family should understand the care that is important for a smooth recovery. A cervical collar is usually worn for about 6 weeks. The patient is instructed in care and use of the cervical collar. Patients are instructed to alternate tasks in which the body does not move (eg, reading) with tasks that require greater body movement.

The patient is instructed about strategies for pain management and about signs and symptoms that may indicate complications that should be reported to the physician. The nurse assesses the patient's understanding of these management strategies, limitations, and recommendations. Additionally, the nurse assists the patient in identifying strategies to cope with activities of daily living (ie, self-care and child care) and minimize risks to the surgical site.

A discharge teaching plan is developed collaboratively by members of the health team to decrease the risk for recurrent disk herniation. Topics include those previously discussed as well as proper body mechanics, maintenance of optimal weight, proper exercise techniques, and modifications in activity.

CONTINUING CARE

Patients are instructed to see their physician at prescribed intervals to document the disappearance of old symptoms and for assessment of range of motion of the neck. Recurrent or persistent pain may occur despite removal of the offending disk or disk fragments. Patients who undergo discectomy usually have consented to surgery after prolonged pain; they have often undergone repeated courses of ineffective conservative management and previous surgeries to relieve the pain. Therefore, the recurrence or persistence of symptoms postoperatively, including pain and sensory deficits, is often discouraging for the patient and family. The patient who experiences recurrence of symptoms requires emotional support and understanding. Additionally, the patient is assisted in modifying activities and in considering options for subsequent treatment.

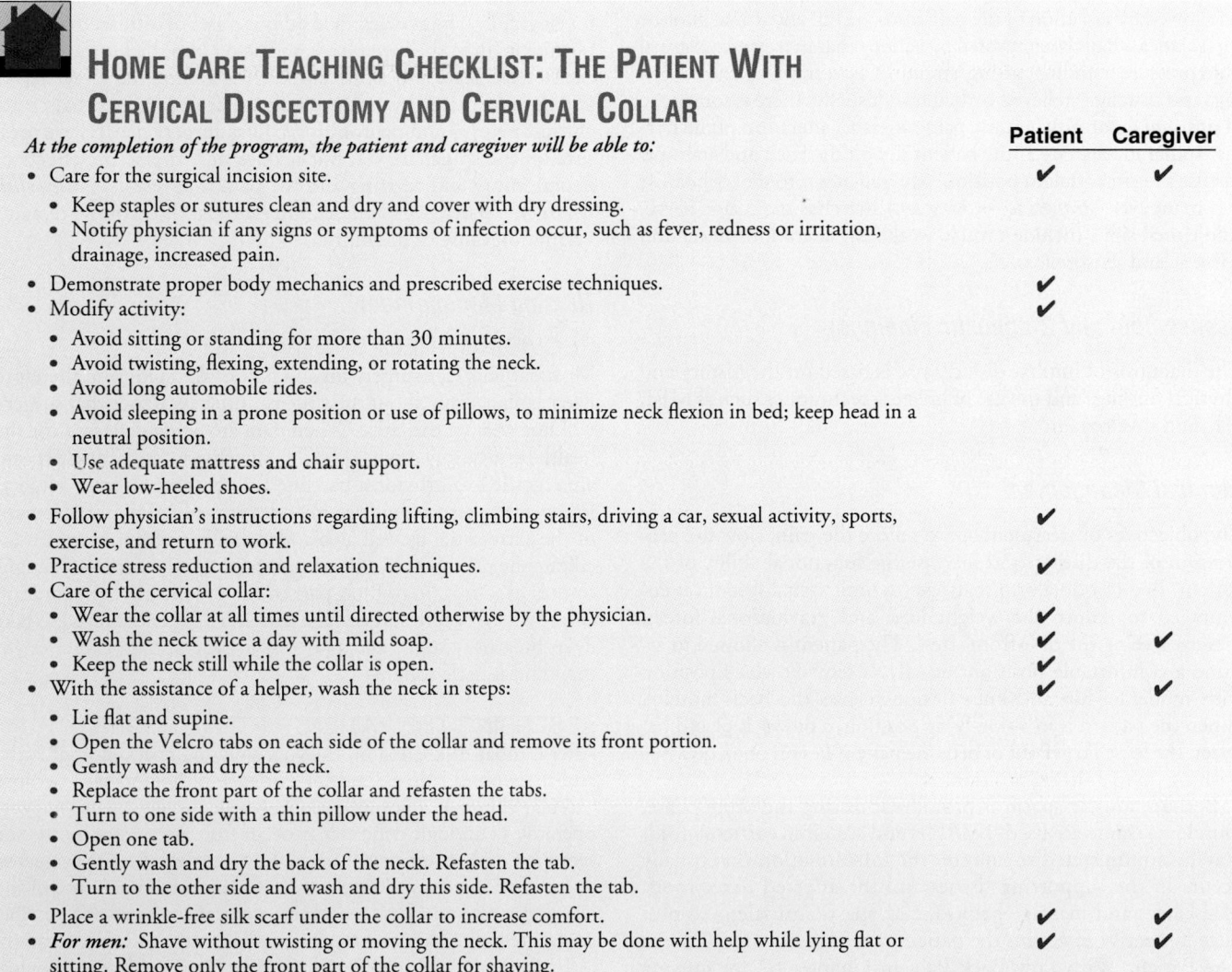

HOME CARE TEACHING CHECKLIST: THE PATIENT WITH CERVICAL DISCECTOMY AND CERVICAL COLLAR

At the completion of the program, the patient and caregiver will be able to:	Patient	Caregiver
• Care for the surgical incision site.	✔	✔
• Keep staples or sutures clean and dry and cover with dry dressing.		
• Notify physician if any signs or symptoms of infection occur, such as fever, redness or irritation, drainage, increased pain.		
• Demonstrate proper body mechanics and prescribed exercise techniques.	✔	
• Modify activity:	✔	
• Avoid sitting or standing for more than 30 minutes.		
• Avoid twisting, flexing, extending, or rotating the neck.		
• Avoid long automobile rides.		
• Avoid sleeping in a prone position or use of pillows, to minimize neck flexion in bed; keep head in a neutral position.		
• Use adequate mattress and chair support.		
• Wear low-heeled shoes.		
• Follow physician's instructions regarding lifting, climbing stairs, driving a car, sexual activity, sports, exercise, and return to work.	✔	
• Practice stress reduction and relaxation techniques.	✔	
• Care of the cervical collar:		
• Wear the collar at all times until directed otherwise by the physician.	✔	
• Wash the neck twice a day with mild soap.	✔	✔
• Keep the neck still while the collar is open.	✔	
• With the assistance of a helper, wash the neck in steps:	✔	✔
• Lie flat and supine.		
• Open the Velcro tabs on each side of the collar and remove its front portion.		
• Gently wash and dry the neck.		
• Replace the front part of the collar and refasten the tabs.		
• Turn to one side with a thin pillow under the head.		
• Open one tab.		
• Gently wash and dry the back of the neck. Refasten the tab.		
• Turn to the other side and wash and dry this side. Refasten the tab.		
• Place a wrinkle-free silk scarf under the collar to increase comfort.	✔	✔
• *For men:* Shave without twisting or moving the neck. This may be done with help while lying flat or sitting. Remove only the front part of the collar for shaving.	✔	✔

Evaluation

Expected Outcomes

Expected outcomes may include:

1. Reports increasing comfort
2. Demonstrates improved mobility
3. Demonstrates progressive participation in self-care activities
   a. Lists the signs and symptoms to be reported
   b. Identifies prescribed activity limitations and restrictions
   c. Demonstrates proper body mechanics
4. Is free of complications
   a. Reports no increase in incisional pain or sensory symptoms
   b. Demonstrates normal findings on neurologic assessment

Herniation of a Lumbar Disk

Most lumbar disk herniations occur at the L4–L5 or the L5–S1 interspaces. A lumbar disk produces low back pain accompanied by varying degrees of sensory and motor impairment.

Clinical Manifestations

The patient complains of low back pain with muscle spasms, which is followed by radiation of the pain into one hip and down into the leg (sciatica). Pain is aggravated by actions that increase intraspinal fluid pressure (bending, lifting, straining, as in sneezing and coughing) and usually is relieved by bed rest. Usually, there is some type of postural deformity because pain causes an alteration of the normal spinal mechanics. If the patient lies on the back and attempts to raise a leg in a straight position, pain radiates into the leg because this maneuver (*straight leg–raising test*) stretches the sciatic nerve. Additional signs include muscle weakness, alterations in tendon reflexes, and sensory loss.

Assessment and Diagnostic Findings

The diagnosis of lumbar disk disease is based on the history and physical findings and the use of imaging techniques such as MRI, CT, and myelogram.

Medical Management

The objectives of treatment are to relieve the pain, slow the progression of the disease, and increase the functional ability of the patient. Bed rest on a firm mattress (to limit spinal flexion) is encouraged to reduce the weight load and gravitational forces, thereby freeing the disk from stress. The patient is allowed to assume a comfortable position; usually, a semi-Fowler's position with moderate hip and knee flexion relaxes the back muscles. When the patient is in a side-lying position, a pillow is placed between the legs. To get out of bed, the patient lies on one side while pushing up to a sitting position.

Because muscle spasm is prominent during the acute phase, muscle relaxants are used. NSAIDs and systemic corticosteroids may be administered to counter the inflammation that usually occurs in the supporting tissues and the affected nerve roots. Moist heat and massage help to relax spastic muscles and produce a sedative effect on the patient. See also Nursing Process: The Patient With Low Back Pain in Chapter 62 for nursing interventions.

SURGICAL MANAGEMENT

In the lumbar region, surgical treatment includes lumbar disk excision through a posterolateral laminotomy and the newer techniques of microdiscectomy and percutaneous discectomy.

Microdiscectomy incorporates the use of the operating microscope to visualize the offending disk and compressed nerve roots; it permits a small incision (2.5 cm [1 inch]) and minimal blood loss and takes about 30 minutes of operating time. Generally, it involves a short hospital stay, and the patient makes a rapid recovery.

Percutaneous discectomy is an alternative treatment for herniated intervertebral disks of the lumbar spine at the L4–L5 level. One approach in current use is through a 2.5-cm (1-inch) incision just above the iliac crest. A tube, trocar, or cannula is inserted under x-ray guidance through the retroperitoneal space to the involved disk space. Special instruments are used to remove the disk. The operating time is about 15 minutes. Blood loss and postoperative pain are minimal, and the patient is generally discharged within 2 days after surgery. The disadvantage of this procedure involves the possibility of damage to structures located in the surgical pathway.

Complications of Disk Surgery. A person having a disk procedure at one level of the vertebral column may have degenerative process at other levels. A herniation relapse may occur at the same level or elsewhere, so that the patient may become a candidate for another disk procedure. Arachnoiditis (inflammation of the arachnoid membrane) may occur after surgery (and after myelography); it involves an insidious onset of diffuse, frequently burning pain in the lower back, radiating into the buttocks. Disk excision can leave adhesions and scarring around the spinal nerves and dura, which then produce inflammatory changes that create chronic neuritis and neurofibrosis. Disk surgery may relieve pressure on the spinal nerves, but it does not reverse the effects of neural injury and scarring and the pain that results. *Failed disk syndrome* (recurrence of sciatica after lumbar discectomy) remains a common cause of disability.

Nursing Management

PROVIDING PREOPERATIVE CARE

Most patients fear surgery on any part of the spine and therefore need explanations about the surgery and reassurance that surgery will not weaken the back. When data are being collected for the health history, any reports of pain, paresthesia, and muscle spasm are recorded to provide a baseline for comparison after surgery. Preoperative assessment also includes an evaluation of movement of the extremities as well as bladder and bowel function. To facilitate the postoperative turning procedure, the patient is taught to turn as a unit (logroll) as part of the preoperative preparation (Fig. 59-14). Before surgery, the patient is also encouraged to take deep breaths, cough, and perform muscle-setting exercises (to maintain muscle tone).

ASSESSING THE PATIENT AFTER SURGERY

After lumbar disk excision, the vital signs are checked frequently, and the wound is inspected for evidence of hemorrhage because vascular injury is a complication of disk surgery. Because postoperative neurologic deficits may occur from nerve root injury, the sensation and motor power of the lower extremities are evaluated at specified intervals, along with the color and temperature of the legs and sensation of the toes. It is important to assess for possible urinary retention, another sign of possible neurologic deterioration.

In discectomy with fusion, the patient has an additional surgical incision if bone fragments were taken from the iliac crest or fibula

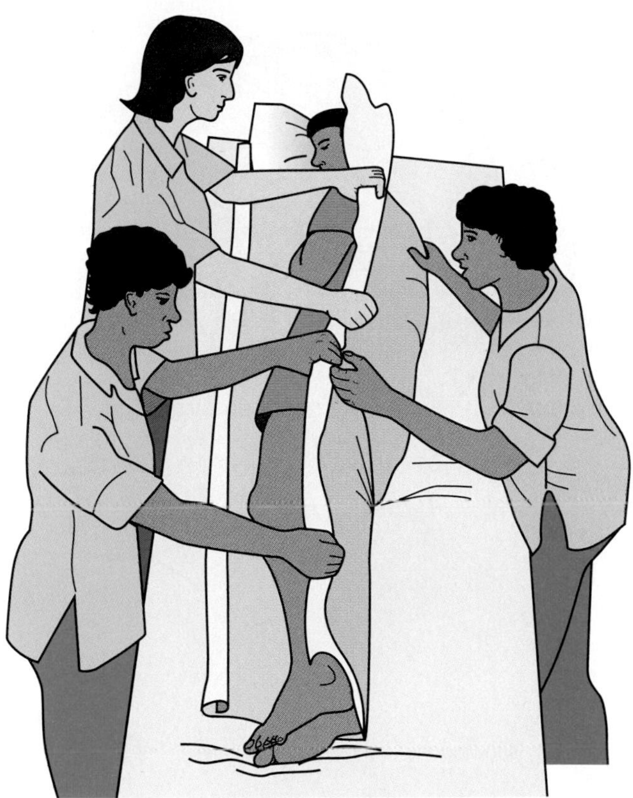

FIGURE 59•14 Before the patient undergoes laminectomy surgery, the logrolling technique that will be used for turning the patient should be demonstrated. The patient's arms will be crossed and the spine aligned. Then to avoid twisting the spine, the head, shoulders, knees and hips are turned at the same time so that the patient rolls over like a log. When in a side-lying position, the patient's back, buttocks, and legs are supported with pillows. From Taylor, C., Lillis, C., & LeMone, P. (1997). *Fundamentals of nursing: The art and science of nursing care* (3rd ed.). Philadelphia: Lippincott-Raven.

to serve as wedges in the spine. The recovery period is somewhat longer than for those patients who have undergone discectomy without spinal fusion because bony union must take place.

POSITIONING THE PATIENT

To position the patient, a pillow is placed under the head, and the knee rest is elevated slightly because slight knee flexion relaxes the muscles of the back. When the patient is lying on one side, however, extreme knee flexion must be avoided. The patient is encouraged to move from side to side to relieve pressure but is first reassured that no injury will result from moving. When the patient is ready to turn, the bed is placed in a flat position and a pillow is placed between the legs. The patient turns as a unit (logrolls), without twisting the back.

To get out of bed, the patient lies on one side while pushing up to a sitting position. At the same time, the nurse or family member eases the patient's legs over the side of the bed. Coming to a sitting or standing posture is accomplished by one long, smooth motion. Most patients walk to the bathroom the same day as surgery. Sitting is discouraged except for defecation.

PROMOTING HOME AND COMMUNITY-BASED CARE

Teaching Patients Self-Care. The patient is advised that activity is to be gradually increased up to the point of tolerance because it takes up to 6 weeks for the ligaments to heal. Excessive activity may result in spasm of the paraspinal muscles.

Activities that produce flexion strain on the spine (eg, driving a car) should be avoided until healing has taken place. Heat may be applied to the back to relax muscle spasms. Scheduled rest periods are important, and the patient is advised to avoid heavy work for 2 to 3 months after surgery. Exercises are prescribed to strengthen the abdominal and erector spinal muscles. A back brace or corset may be necessary if back pain persists.

CRANIAL NERVE DISORDERS

Because the brain stem and cranial nerves involve vital motor, sensory, or autonomic functions of the body, these nerves may be affected by conditions arising primarily within these structures or in secondary extension from adjacent disease processes. The cranial nerves (Fig. 59-15) are examined separately and in sequence (see Chap. 56). Some cranial nerve deficits can be detected by observing the patient's face, eye movements, speech, and swallowing. Electromyography is used to investigate motor and sensory dysfunction. MRI is used to obtain images of the cranial nerves and brain stem. An overview of disorders that may affect each of the cranial nerves, including clinical manifestations and nursing interventions, is presented in Table 59-3. The following discussions center on trigeminal neuralgia, a condition affecting the fifth cranial nerve, and on Bell's palsy, caused by involvement of the seventh cranial nerve.

Trigeminal Neuralgia (Tic Douloureux)

Trigeminal neuralgia is a condition of the fifth cranial nerve characterized by paroxysms of pain similar to an electric shock or a lancinating burning sensation in the area innervated by one or more branches of the trigeminal nerve. The pain ends as abruptly as it starts. Each pain episode can be described as stabbing, lasting from a few seconds to minutes, and produces contraction of some of the facial muscles, such as a sudden closing of the eye or a twitch of the mouth; hence the name *tic douloureux* (painful twitch). The cause is not certain, but chronic compression or irritation of the trigeminal nerve or degenerative changes in the gasserian ganglion are suggested causes. Vascular pressure from structural abnormalities (loop of an artery) encroaching on the trigeminal nerve, gasserian ganglion, or root entry zone has also been suggested as a cause.

Early attacks, appearing most often in the fifth decade of life, are usually mild and brief. Pain-free intervals may be measured in terms of minutes, hours, days, or longer. With advancing years, the painful episodes tend to become more and more frequent and agonizing. The patient lives in constant fear of attacks.

The pain of this neuralgia is felt in the skin, not in the deeper structures, but it is more severe at the peripheral areas of distribution of the affected nerve, notably over the lip, the chin, the nostrils, and in the teeth. Paroxysms are aroused by any stimulation of the terminals of the affected nerve branches, such as washing the face, shaving, brushing the teeth, eating, and drinking. A draft of cold air and direct pressure against the nerve trunk may also cause pain. Certain areas are called *trigger points* because the slightest touch immediately starts a paroxysm or episode. To avoid stimulating these areas, patients with trigeminal neuralgia try not to touch or wash their faces, shave, chew, or do anything else that might cause an attack. Behavior of this type is a clue to diagnosis.

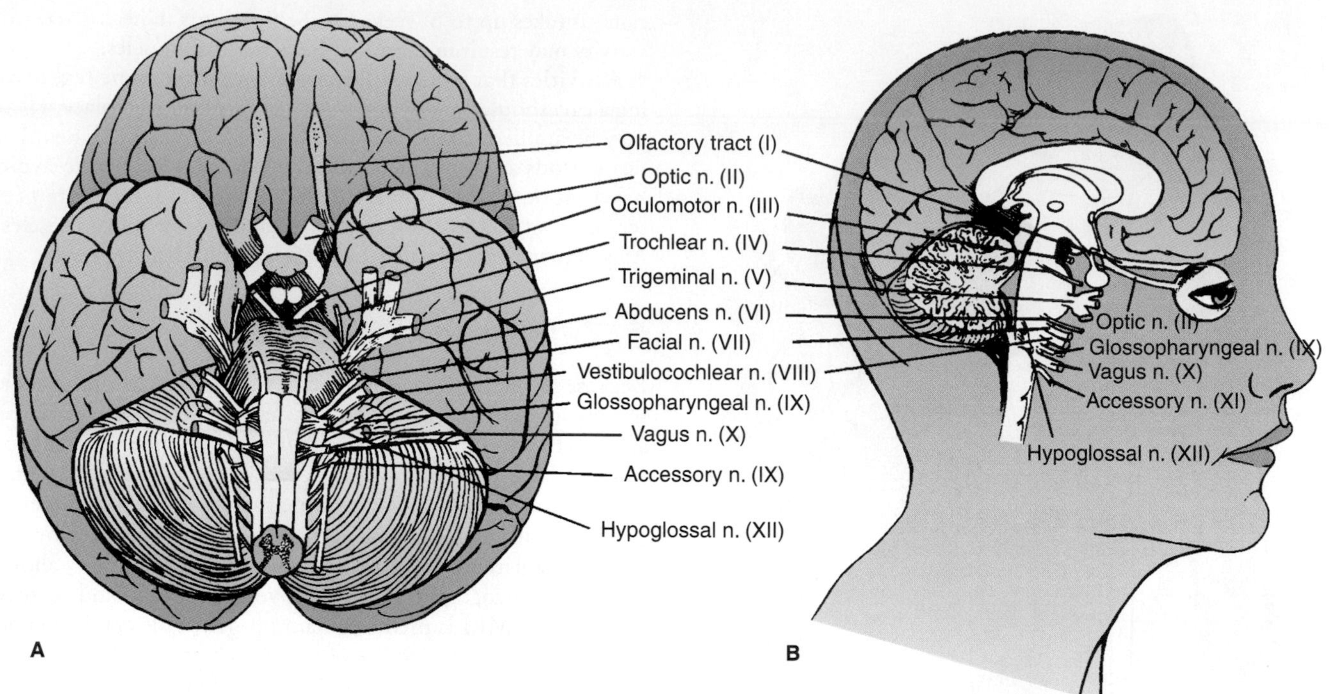

FIGURE 59•15 The cranial nerves. (**A**) Inferior view of the brain showing the cranial nerve. (**B**) Lateral view showing a schematic version of the cranial nerves.

Medical Management

PHARMOCOLOGIC THERAPY

The anticonvulsant agents carbamazepine (Tegretol) and phenytoin (Dilantin) relieve pain in most patients with trigeminal neuralgia by reducing the transmission of impulses at certain nerve terminals. Carbamazepine is taken with meals, in dosages gradually increased until relief is obtained. Side effects include nausea, dizziness, drowsiness, and hepatic dysfunction. The patient is monitored for bone marrow depression during long-term therapy. Phenytoin also produces such side effects as nausea, dizziness, nystagmus, somnolence, ataxia, gum hyperplasia, and skin rashes or eruptions.

Alcohol or phenol injection of the gasserian ganglion and peripheral branches of the trigeminal nerve relieves pain for several months. However, the pain returns with nerve regeneration.

SURGICAL MANAGEMENT

When these methods fail to relieve pain, a number of surgical options are available, as described in the following paragraphs. The choice of procedure depends on the patient's preference and health status.

Percutaneous Radiofrequency Trigeminal Gangliolysis.

Percutaneous radiofrequency interruption of the gasserian ganglion, in which the small unmyelinated and thinly myelinated fibers that conduct pain are thermally destroyed, is becoming the surgical procedure of choice for trigeminal neuralgia.

Under local anesthesia, the needle is introduced through the cheek on the affected side. Under fluoroscopic guidance, the needle electrode is guided through the foramen magnum into the gasserian ganglion. The divisions of the gasserian ganglion (mandibular, maxillary, and ophthalmic) are encountered sequentially. The nerve is stimulated with a small current while the patient is awake. The patient then reports when a tingling sensation is felt. When the electrode needle is in the desired position, the patient is anesthetized briefly, and a radiofrequency current (heating current to destroy the nerve) is passed in a controlled manner to injure the trigeminal ganglion and rootlets thermally. The patient is then awakened from the anesthetic and examined for sensory deficits. This is repeated until the desired effect is achieved. The procedure takes less than 1 hour and gives permanent pain relief in most patients. Touch and proprioceptive functions are left intact.

Microvascular Decompression of the Trigeminal Nerve.

An intracranial approach can be used to decompress the trigeminal nerve because the pain may be caused by vascular compression of the entry zone of the trigeminal root by an arterial loop and occasionally by a vein. With the aid of an operating microscope, the artery loop is lifted from the nerve to relieve the pressure, and a small prosthetic device is inserted to prevent recurrence of impingement on the nerve. This procedure relieves facial pain while preserving normal sensation. It is a major procedure, involving a craniotomy. The postoperative management is the same as for other intracranial surgeries (see Chap. 57).

Nursing Management

PREVENTING PAIN

Preoperative management of a patient with trigeminal neuralgia includes recognizing that certain factors may aggravate excruciating facial pain, such as food that is too hot or too cold or jarring the patient's bed or chair. Even washing the face, combing the hair, or brushing the teeth may produce acute pain. The nurse can prevent or reduce this pain in a variety of ways, such as providing cotton pads and room-temperature water for washing the patient's face, instructing the patient to rinse his or her mouth after eating when tooth brushing causes pain, and performing personal hygiene during pain-free intervals. The patient is advised to take food and fluids at room temperature, to chew on the unaffected side, and to in-

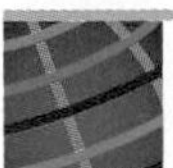

TABLE 59•3 Disorders of Cranial Nerves

Disorder	Clinical Manifestations	Nursing Interventions
Olfactory Nerve—1		
Head trauma Intracranial tumor Intracranial surgery	Unilateral or bilateral anosmia (temporary or persistent) Diminished taste for food	Assess for cerebrospinal fluid rhinorrhea if patient has sustained head trauma.
Optic Nerve—II		
Optic neuritis Increased intracranial pressure Pituitary tumor	Lesions of optic tract producing homonymous hemianopsia	Assess level of visual acuity. Restructure environment to prevent injuries. Teach patient to accommodate for visual loss.
Oculomotor Nerve—III		
Trochlear Nerve—IV		
Abducens Nerve—VI		
Vascular Brain stem ischemia Hemorrhage and infarction Neoplasm Trauma Infection	Dilation of pupil with loss of light reflex on one side Impairment of ocular movement Diplopia Gaze palsies Ptosis of eyelid	Assess extraocular movement and for non-reactive pupil.
Trigeminal Nerve—V		
Trigeminal neuralgia Head trauma Cerebellopontine lesion Sinus tract tumor and metastatic disease Compression of trigeminal root by tumor	Pain in face Diminished or loss of corneal reflex Chewing dysfunction	Assess for pain and triggering mechanisms for pain. Assess for difficulty in chewing. Discuss trigger zones and pain precipitants with patient. Protect cornea from abrasion. Ensure good oral hygiene. Educate patient about medication regimen.
Facial Nerve—VII		
Bell's palsy Facial nerve tumor Intracranial lesion Herpes zoster	Facial dysfunction; weakness and paralysis Hemifacial spasm Diminished or absent taste	Recognize facial paralysis as emergency; refer for treatment as soon as possible. Teach protective care for eyes. Select easily chewed foods; patient should eat and drink from unaffected side of mouth. Emphasize importance of oral hygiene. Provide emotional support for changed appearance of face.
Vestibulocochlear Nerve—VIII		
Tumors and acoustic neuroma Vascular compression of nerve Ménière's syndrome	Tinnitus Vertigo Hearing difficulties	Assess pattern of vertigo. Provide for safety measures to prevent falls. Ensure that patient can obtain balance before ambulating. Caution patient to change positions slowly. Assist with ambulation. Encourage use of activity of daily living aids.
Glossopharyngeal Nerve—IX		
Glossopharyngeal neuralgia from neurovascular compression of cranial nerves IX and X Trauma Inflammatory conditions Tumor Vertebral artery aneurysms	Pain at base of tongue Difficulty in swallowing Loss of gag reflex Palatal, pharyngeal, and laryngeal paralysis	Assess for paroxysmal pain in throat, decreased or absent swallowing, gag and cough reflexes. Monitor for dysphagia, aspiration, nasal dysarthric speech. Position patient upright for eating or tube feeding.
Vagus Nerve—X		
Spastic palsy of larynx; bulbar paralysis; high vagal paralysis Guillain-Barré syndrome Carotid endarterectomy Vagal body tumors Nerve paralysis from malignancy, surgical trauma	Voice changes (temporary or permanent hoarseness) Vocal paralysis Dysphagia	Assess for airway obstruction/provide airway management. Prevent aspiration. Support patient having voice reconstruction procedures.

(continued)

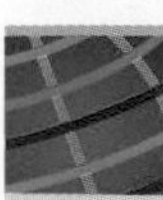

TABLE 59•3 Disorders of Cranial Nerves *(Continued)*

Disorder	Clinical Manifestations	Nursing Interventions
Spinal Accessory Nerve—XI		
Spinal cord disorder Amyotrophic lateral sclerosis Trauma Guillain-Barré syndrome	Drooping of affected shoulder with limited shoulder movement Weakness or paralysis of head rotation, flexion, extension; shoulder elevation	Support patient undergoing diagnostic tests.
Hypoglossal Nerve—XII		
Medullary lesions Amyotrophic lateral sclerosis Polio and motor system disease, which may destroy hypoglossal nuclei Multiple sclerosis Trauma	Abnormal movements of tongue Weakness or paralysis of tongue muscles Difficulty in talking, chewing, and swallowing	Observe swallowing ability. Observe speech pattern. Be aware of swallowing or vocal difficulties. Prepare for alternate feeding methods (tube feeding) to maintain nutrition.

gest soft foods. The nurse must recognize that anxiety, depression, and insomnia often accompany chronic painful conditions and use appropriate interventions and referrals.

PROVIDING POSTOPERATIVE CARE

Postoperative neurologic assessments are conducted to evaluate for facial motor and sensory deficits. If the surgery results in sensory deficits to the affected side of the face, the patient is instructed not to rub the eye because pain will not be felt in the event there is injury. The eye is assessed for irritation or redness. Artificial tears may be prescribed to prevent dryness to the affected eye. The patient is cautioned not to chew on the affected side until numbness has diminished. The patient is observed carefully for any difficulty in eating and swallowing foods of different consistency.

Bell's Palsy

Bell's palsy (facial paralysis) is due to peripheral involvement of the seventh cranial nerve on one side, which results in weakness or paralysis of the facial muscles. The cause is unknown, although possible causes may include vascular ischemia, viral disease (herpes simplex, herpes zoster), autoimmune disease, or a combination of all of these factors.

Bell's palsy is considered by some to represent a type of pressure paralysis. The inflamed, edematous nerve becomes compressed to the point of damage, or its nutrient vessel is occluded, producing ischemic necrosis of the nerve. There is distortion of the face from paralysis of the facial muscles; increased lacrimation (tearing); and painful sensations in the face, behind the ear, and in the eye. The patient may experience speech difficulties and may be unable to eat on the affected side because of weakness or paralysis of the facial muscles.

Management

The objectives of treatment are to maintain the muscle tone of the face and to prevent or minimize denervation. The patient should be reassured that no stroke has occurred and that spontaneous recovery occurs within 3 to 5 weeks in most patients.

Corticosteroid therapy (prednisone) may be given to reduce inflammation and edema which, in turn, reduces vascular compression and permits restoration of blood circulation to the nerve. Early administration of corticosteroid therapy appears to diminish the severity of the disease, relieve the pain, and prevent or minimize denervation.

Facial pain is controlled with analgesics. Heat may be applied to the involved side of the face to promote comfort and blood flow through the muscles.

Electrical stimulation may be applied to the face to prevent muscle atrophy. Although most patients recover with conservative treatment, surgical exploration of the facial nerve may be indicated in patients who are suspected of having a tumor or for surgical decompression of the facial nerve and for surgical rehabilitation of a paralyzed face.

PROMOTING HOME AND COMMUNITY-BASED CARE

Teaching Patients Self-Care. While the paralysis lasts, the involved eye must be protected. Frequently, the patient's eye does not close completely, and the blink reflex is diminished, so that the eye is vulnerable to dust and foreign particles. Corneal irritation and ulceration are potential complications that may occur if the eye is unprotected. Distortion of the lower lid alters the proper drainage of tears. To manage these problems, the eye should be covered with a protective shield at night. The eye patch may abrade the cornea, however, because there is some difficulty in keeping the partially paralyzed eyelids closed. The application of eye ointment at bedtime causes the eyelids to adhere to one another and remain closed during sleep. The patient can be taught to close the paralyzed eyelid manually before going to sleep. Wrap-around sunglasses or goggles may be worn to decrease normal evaporation from the eye.

Continuing Care. If the nerve is not too sensitive, the face may be massaged several times daily to maintain muscle tone. The technique is to massage the face with a gentle upward motion. Facial exercises, such as wrinkling the forehead, blowing out the cheeks, and whistling, may be performed with the aid of a mirror in an effort to prevent muscle atrophy. Exposure of the face to cold and drafts is avoided.

DISORDERS OF THE PERIPHERAL NERVOUS SYSTEM

Peripheral Neuropathies

A peripheral neuropathy is a disorder affecting the peripheral motor, sensory, or autonomic nerves. Peripheral nerves, by connecting the spinal cord and brain to all other organs, transmit motor impulses outward and relay sensory impulses to encode sensation in the brain. A *mononeuropathy* affects a single peripheral nerve, whereas the involvement of multiple single peripheral nerves or their branches is termed *multiple mononeuropathy* or *mononeuritis multiplex. Polyneuropathies* are characterized by bilateral and symmetric disturbance of function, usually beginning in the feet and hands. (Most nutritional, metabolic, and toxic neuropathies take this form.)

The most common causes of peripheral neuropathy are diabetes, alcoholism, and occlusive vascular disease. Many bacterial and metabolic toxins and exogenous poisons also cause peripheral neuropathy. Because of the growing use of chemicals in industry, agriculture, and medicine, the number of substances causing peripheral neuropathies and incidence of peripheral neuropathies have increased. In developing countries, leprosy is a major cause of severe nerve disease because *Mycobacterium leprae* invade the peripheral nervous system.

The major symptoms of peripheral nerve disorders are loss of sensation, muscle atrophy, weakness, diminished reflexes, pain, and paresthesia (numbness, tingling) of the extremities. The patient frequently describes some part of the extremity as numb. Autonomic features include decreased or absent sweating, orthostatic hypotension, nocturnal diarrhea, tachycardia, impotence, and atrophic skin and nail changes.

Peripheral nerve disorders are diagnosed by history, physical examination, EMG, and somatosensory evoked potentials.

Mononeuropathy

Mononeuropathy is limited to a single peripheral nerve and its branches. It arises when the trunk of the nerve is compressed or entrapped (as in carpal tunnel syndrome); traumatized, as when bruised by a blow, or overstretched, as in cases of joint dislocation; punctured by a needle used to inject a drug or damaged by the drugs thus injected; or inflamed because an adjacent infectious process extends to the nerve's trunk. Mononeuropathy frequently is seen in the patient with diabetes.

Pain is seldom a major symptom of mononeuropathy when the condition is due to trauma, but in patients with complicating inflammatory conditions, such as arthritis, this feature is prominent. Such pain is increased by all body movements that tend to stretch, strain, or cause pressure on the injured nerve and by sudden jarring of the body, such as that associated with coughing and sneezing. The skin in the areas supplied by nerves that are injured or diseased may become reddened and glossy; the subcutaneous tissue may become edematous, and the nutrition of the nails and the hair in this area become defective. Chemical injuries to a nerve trunk, such as those caused by drugs injected into or near it, are often permanent.

The objective of treatment of mononeuropathy is to remove the cause, if possible, such as by freeing the compressed nerve. Local corticosteroid injections may reduce inflammation and the pressure on the nerve. Pain may be relieved by aspirin or codeine.

Guillain-Barré Syndrome (Polyradiculoneuritis)

Guillain-Barré syndrome is a rapidly progressing clinical syndrome of unknown cause involving the cranial, spinal, and peripheral nerves. In most patients, the syndrome is preceded by an infection (respiratory or gastrointestinal) 1 to 4 weeks before the onset of neurologic deficits. In some instances, it has occurred after vaccination or surgery. It may be due to a primary viral infection, an immune reaction, some other process, or a combination of processes. One hypothesis is that a viral infection induces an autoimmune reaction that attacks the myelin of the peripheral nerves. (*Myelin* surrounds or ensheathes the axons of certain nerves and plays an important role in the transmission of nerve impulses.)

Proximal portions of the nerves tend to be affected most often, and the nerve roots within the subarachnoid space are commonly involved. Autopsy findings have shown inflammatory edema and demyelination with some lymphocytic infiltration that is especially prominent in the spinal nerve roots.

Clinical Manifestations

There is variation in the mode of onset. The initial neurologic symptoms are *paresthesia* (tingling and numbness) and muscle weakness of the legs, which may ascend to the upper extremities, trunk, and facial muscles. Muscle weakness may be followed quickly by complete paralysis. The cranial nerves frequently are affected, leading to paralysis of the ocular, facial, and oropharyngeal muscles and thus causing marked difficulty in talking, chewing, and swallowing. Autonomic dysfunction frequently occurs and takes the form of overreactivity or underreactivity of the sympathetic or parasympathetic nervous systems, as manifested by disturbances of heart rate and rhythm, blood pressure changes (transient hypertension, orthostatic hypotension), and a variety of other vasomotor disturbances. There may be severe and persistent pain in the back and calves of the legs. Frequently, the patient exhibits loss of position sense as well as diminished or absent tendon reflexes. Sensory changes are manifested by paresthesias. Cognitive function or level of consciousness is not affected.

Most patients make a full recovery over several months to a year, but about 10% are left with a residual disability.

Assessment and Diagnostic Findings

The diagnosis of Guillain-Barré syndrome is made based on the clinical presentation, history of recent viral infection, and results of laboratory and diagnostic studies. The spinal fluid shows an increased protein concentration with a normal cell count. Electrophysiologic testing demonstrates marked slowing of nerve conduction velocity.

Management

Guillain-Barré syndrome is considered a medical emergency, and the patient is managed in an intensive care unit. A patient with respiratory problems requires mechanical ventilation, sometimes for prolonged periods. Plasmapheresis (plasma exchange), which produces a temporary reduction in circulating antibodies, may be used in the severely affected and deteriorating patient to limit the deterioration and demyelination. Continuous electrocardiographic (ECG) monitoring may be required because of possible alteration in cardiac rate or rhythm. Cardiac dysrhythmias associated with autonomic abnormalities are treated with propranolol to prevent tachycardia and hypertension. Atropine may be administered to avoid episodes of bradycardia during endotracheal suctioning and physical therapy.

NURSING PROCESS: THE PATIENT WITH GUILLAIN-BARRÉ SYNDROME

Assessment

Assessment for complications of Guillain-Barré syndrome involves constant monitoring for life-threatening acute respiratory failure. Other complications include cardiac dysrhythmias, which necessitate ECG monitoring, and observing the patient for signs of DVT and pulmonary embolism, which are threats to any immobilized and paralyzed patient.

Diagnosis

Nursing Diagnoses

Based on the assessment data, the patient's major diagnoses may include the following:

- Ineffective breathing pattern and gas exchange related to rapidly progressive weakness and impending respiratory failure
- Impaired physical mobility related to paralysis
- Altered nutrition, less than body requirements, related to inability to swallow, which is secondary to cranial nerve dysfunction
- Impaired verbal communication related to cranial nerve dysfunction
- Fear and anxiety related to loss of control and paralysis

Collaborative Problems/Potential Complications

Based on the assessment data, potential complications that may develop include the following:

- Respiratory failure
- Autonomic dysfunction

Planning and Goals

The major goals of the patient may include improved respiratory function, increased mobility, improved nutritional status, effective communication, decreased fear and anxiety, and absence of complications.

Nursing Interventions

Maintaining Respiratory Function

The patient with Guillain-Barré syndrome is dependent on nursing surveillance and care for recovery. Mechanical ventilation is likely if serial measurements of the patient's vital capacity show progressive deterioration, indicating increasing respiratory muscle weakness. The nursing management of the patient requiring mechanical ventilation is discussed in Chapter 22. Patients are at particularly high risk if they have difficulty swallowing and are unable to cough effectively to clear the airway, which may cause aspiration and acute respiratory failure. Chest physical therapy and elevation of the head of the bed facilitate respirations and effective coughing. Suctioning may be needed to maintain a clear airway.

Reducing Effects of Immobility

The paralyzed extremities are supported in functional positions, and passive range-of-motion exercises are performed at least twice daily. The nurse collaborates with the physical therapist to prevent contracture deformities by using careful positioning and range-of-motion exercises. DVT and pulmonary embolism are threats to the paralyzed patient, who is unable to move the extremities. Nursing interventions include ensuring adequate hydration, assisting with physical therapy, the use of elastic stockings, and administering the prescribed anticoagulants.

A paralyzed person has the potential to develop compression neuropathies, most often of the ulnar and peroneal nerves. Padding may be placed over the elbows and head of the fibula to prevent this problem. The prevention of pressure ulcers is a major nursing challenge. For paralyzed patients, the principles of nursing management of the unconscious patient (see Chap. 57) may be applied, although cognitive function is unaffected.

When recovery begins to take place, these patients may experience orthostatic hypotension (from autonomic dysfunction) and probably require the use of a tilt table to help them assume an upright posture.

Providing Adequate Nutrition

Attention is paid to adequate nutrition and prevention of muscle wasting. Paralytic ileus may result from insufficient parasympathetic activity. In this event, the nurse administers intravenous fluids and total parenteral nutrition as prescribed and monitors the patient for return of bowel sounds. If the patient is unable to swallow, nasogastric tube feedings may be prescribed. When the patient can swallow normally, oral feeding is gradually and carefully resumed.

Improving Communication

Because of paralysis, tracheostomy, and intubation, the patient is unable to talk, laugh, or cry and thus has no outlet for emotional expression. These problems are compounded by boredom, dependency, isolation, and frustration. To establish some form of communication, lip-reading and the use of picture cards, combined with a system of blinking the eyes to indicate yes or no, may be tried. If the patient remains on the ventilator for a prolonged period, a referral to a speech therapist may be made. Diversional therapy (television, cassette tapes, visits from the family) can alleviate some of the frustrations that are encountered.

Relieving Fear and Anxiety

Involving the family and friends with selected patient care activities and diversions (eg, reading aloud) will reduce the sense of isolation of the patient. Nursing interventions that are helpful in increasing the patient's sense of control (and, hence, reducing fear) include providing information about the patient's condition, emphasizing a positive appraisal of coping resources, encouraging relaxation exercises and distraction techniques, and giving positive feedback. The attitude and atmosphere created by the nurse, physical therapist, and occupational therapist are important. Giving expert nursing care, explanations, and reassurance helps the patient gain some control over the situation.

Monitoring and Managing Potential Complications

Thorough assessment of respiratory function at regular intervals is essential because respiratory insufficiency and subsequent failure due to weakness or paralysis of the intercostal muscles and diaphragm may develop quickly. Respiratory failure is the major cause of mortality, which is reported to be as high as 10% to 20%. The patient's vital capacity is monitored frequently and at regular intervals in addition to respiratory rate and the quality of respirations, so that respiratory insufficiency can be anticipated. Decreasing vital capacity associated with weakness of the muscles used in swallowing, which causes difficulty in both coughing and swallowing, indicates impending respiratory failure. Signs and symptoms include breathlessness while speaking, shallow and irregular breathing, use of accessory muscles, tachycardia, and changes in respiratory pattern.

Parameters for determining the onset of respiratory failure are established on admission, allowing intubation and the initiation of mechanical ventilation on a nonemergent basis. This also allows the patient to be prepared for the procedure in a controlled manner that reduces anxiety and complications.

Other complications include cardiac dysrhythmias, which necessitate ECG monitoring, transient hypertension, orthostatic hypotension, DVT, pulmonary embolism, urinary retention, and other threats to any immobilized and paralyzed patient. These require monitoring and attention to prevent their occurrence and prompt treatment if indicated.

Promoting Home and Community-Based Care

TEACHING PATIENTS SELF-CARE

Patients with Guillain-Barré syndrome and their families are usually frightened by the sudden onset of life-threatening symptoms and their severity. Therefore, teaching the patient and family about the disorder and its generally favorable prognosis is important. During the acute phase of the illness, the patient and family are instructed about strategies they can implement to minimize the effects of immobility and other complications. As function begins to return, family members and other home care providers are instructed about care of the patient and their role in the rehabilitation process. Preparation for discharge is an interdisciplinary effort requiring family or caregiver education by all team members, including the nurse, physician, occupational and physical therapists, speech therapist, and respiratory therapist.

CONTINUING CARE

Most patients with Guillain-Barré syndrome experience complete recovery within weeks or months. Those patients who have experienced total or prolonged paralysis require intensive rehabilitation. The extent of such a program depends on the assessment of the patient's needs. Approaches include a comprehensive inpatient program if deficits are significant, an outpatient program if the patient is able to travel by car, or a home program of physical and occupational therapies. The recovery phase may be long and will require patience as well as involvement on the part of the patient and family.

The acute onset and dramatic progression of symptoms may not allow time for the patient to adjust to the sudden change in function. A Guillain-Barré support group offers both information and group interaction, which may be helpful during the recovery phase.

Evaluation

Expected Outcomes

Expected outcomes may include:

1. Maintains effective respirations and airway clearance
   a. Has normal breath sounds on auscultation
   b. Demonstrates gradual improvement in respiratory function
2. Shows increasing mobility
   a. Regains use of extremities
   b. Participates in rehabilitation program
3. Demonstrates ability to swallow
   a. Consumes diet adequate to meet nutritional needs
   b. Is able to swallow without risk for aspiration
4. Demonstrates recovery of speech
   a. Is able to communicate needs through alternative strategies
   b. Practices exercises recommended by the speech therapist
5. Shows lessening fear and anxiety
6. Is free of complications
   a. Breathes spontaneously
   b. Has vital capacity within normal range
   c. Exhibits normal arterial blood gases and oximetry

HOME CARE TEACHING CHECKLIST: THE PATIENT WITH GUILLAIN-BARRÉ SYNDROME

At the completion of the program, the patient and caregiver will be able to:	Patient	Caregiver
• State the disease process of Guillain-Barré syndrome.	✔	✔
• Manage respiratory needs: tracheostomy care, suctioning.	✔	✔
• Demonstrate proper body mechanics regarding lifting and transfers.	✔	✔
• Practice gait training and strength endurance.	✔	✔
• Perform range-of-motion exercises.	✔	✔
• Perform activities of daily living and manage self-care:	✔	✔
• Nutrition		
• Bowel and bladder management		
• Skin care		
• Adaptive equipment for bathing, hygiene, grooming, dressing		
• Operate and explain function of medical equipment and mobility aids: walkers, wheelchairs, bedside commodes, tub transfer benches, adaptive devices	✔	✔
• Use coping mechanisms and diversional activities appropriately.	✔	✔
• Implement safety measures in the home.	✔	✔
• Know how to contact and use community resources and the Guillain-Barré Syndrome Foundation International.	✔	✔

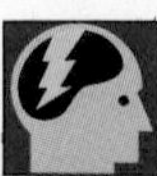

Critical Thinking Exercises

1. Your patient has been informed that she has MS. She is distraught and believes that MS is the same as ALS, which caused rapid deterioration and death in a family friend. How would you explain the differences between MS and ALS to her, and how would you devise a program to help her adjust to the diagnosis? Describe the patient behaviors that would indicate a successful outcome.
2. A patient who is experiencing frequent migraine headaches is being treated at a local clinic. She does not understand the relationship between her headaches and the recommended dietary restrictions. How would you explain this relationship and the reasons for the dietary restrictions? What assessment parameters would you expect were explored to determine other factors that would precipitate her headaches?
3. While you are in the grocery store, another shopper experiences a grand mal seizure. How would you respond to this event, and why would you take these actions? If the shopper had a 3-year-old child with her, how might you address this additional consideration?
4. You have a patient with epilepsy who develops status epilepticus. Based on your knowledge of this disorder, describe the medical management you would anticipate to control the seizures and the nursing measures that are indicated. Identify the patient outcomes that would indicate that the goals have been achieved.
5. A patient assigned to your care has been admitted to the hospital for control of myasthenic crisis. Describe the differences between myasthenic crisis and cholinergic crisis. Explain how your nursing actions would differ for myasthenic and cholinergic crisis and what the underlying rationale would be for these interventions.

References and Selected Readings

BOOKS

Adams, R., Victor, M., & Ropper, A. (1997). *Principles of neurology* (6th ed.). New York: McGraw-Hill.

Bannister, B., Begg, N., & Gillespie, S. (1997). *Infectious disease.* Cambridge, MA: Blackwell Scientific.

Hickey, J. V. (1997). *The clinical practice of neurological and neurosurgical nursing* (4th ed.). Philadelphia: Lippincott-Raven.

Hoeman, S. P. (1996). *Rehabilitation nursing: Process and application* (2nd ed.). St. Louis: C. V. Mosby.

Levin, V. A. (Ed.). (1996). *Cancer in the nervous system.* New York: Churchill Livingstone.

Rice, R. (1996). *Home health nursing practice: Concepts and application* (2nd ed.). St. Louis: C. V. Mosby.

Santilli, N. (Ed.). (1996). *Managing seizure disorders: A handbook for health care professionals.* Philadelphia: Lippincott-Raven.

Shulman, S. T., Phair, J. P., Peterson, L. R., & Warren, J. R. (1997). *The biologic and clinical basis of infectious disease* (5th ed.). Philadelphia: W. B. Saunders.

Sipski, M. L., & Alexander, C. J. (Eds.). (1997). *Sexual function in people with disability and chronic illness: A health professional's guide.* Gaithersburg, MD: Aspen.

Wiesel, S. W., Delahay, J. N. (1997). *Essentials of orthopaedic surgery* (2nd ed.). Philadelphia: W. B. Saunders.

Youmans, J. R. (Ed.). (1996). *Neurological surgery* (4th ed.). Philadelphia: W. B. Saunders.

JOURNALS

Asterisks indicate nursing research articles.

General

*Cammermeyer, M., & Prendergast, V. (1997). Profiles of cognitive functioning in subjects with neurological disorders. *Journal of Neuroscience Nursing, 29*(3), 163–169.

Crigger, N., & Forbes, W. (1997). Assessing neurologic function in older patients. *American Journal of Nursing, 97*(3), 37–39.

Lewis, K. S. (1998). Emotional adjustment to chronic illness. *Lippincott's Primary Care Practice, 2*(1), 38–51.

McCool, F. D. (1995). Inspiratory muscle training in the patient with neuromuscular disease. *Physical Therapy, 75*(11), 1006–1014.

Powers, J. H., & Scheld, W. M. (1996). Fever in neurological diseases. *Infectious Disease Clinics of North America, 10*(1), 45–66.

*Stuifbergen, A. K., & Rogers, S. (1997). Health promotion: An essential component of rehabilitation for persons with chronic disabling conditions. *Advanced Nursing Science, 19*(4), 1–20.

*Williams, J., & Schutte, D. (1997). Benefits and burdens of genetic carrier identification. *Western Journal of Nursing Research, 19*(1), 71–81.

Amyotrophic Lateral Sclerosis

McNair, N. (1996). Rilutek (riluzole) may extend survival in ALS. *Journal of Neuroscience Nursing, 28*(4), 275.

Wagner, M. L., & Landis, B. E. (1997). Riluzole: A new agent for ALS. *Annals of Pharmacology, 31*(6), 738–744.

Brain Tumors

American Cancer Society (1999). Facts and Figures, Atlanta: American Cancer Society.

Armstrong, T., & Gilbert, M. (1996). Glial neoplasms: Classification, treatment, and pathways for the future. *Oncology Nursing Forum, 23*(4), 615–627.

Batchelor, T., & DeAngelis, L. (1996). Medical management of cerebral metastases. *Neurosurgical Clinics of North America, 7*(3), 435–446.

Brady, S., Thornhill, A., & Colapinto, E. (1997). Stereotactic biopsy procedures for brain tumor diagnosis. *AORN Journal, 65*(5), 890–900.

Dennis, M. J., Beijnen, J. H., Grochaw, L. B., et al. (1997). An overview of the clinical pharmacology of topotecan. *Seminars in Oncology, 24*(1 Suppl 5), S5-12–S5-18.

Fernandez, P. M., & Brem, S. (1997). Malignant brain tumors in the elderly. *Clinics in Geriatric Medicine, 13*(2), 327–337.

O'Hanlon-Nichols, T. (1996). Intracranial tumors. *American Journal of Nursing, 96*(4), 38–39.

Page, M. S., & Rabbitt, J. E. (1995). Issues in metastatic disease. *Critical Care Nursing Clinics of North America, 7*(1), 143–149.

Ward-Smith, P. (1997). Stereotactic radiosurgery for malignant brain tumors: The patient's perspective. *Journal of Neuroscience Nursing, 29*(2), 117–122.

Cerebral Aneurysms and Intracranial Hemorrhage

Ausman, J. I. (1997). The future of neurovascular surgery. Part I: Intracranial aneurysm. *Surgical Neurology, 48*(1), 98–100.

Bader, M. K. (1997). The complexity of caring for patients with ruptured cerebral aneurysm: Case studies. *AACN Clinical Issues, 8*(2), 182–195.

Bell, T. E., & Kongable, G. L. (1996). Innovations in aneurysmal subarachnoid hemorrhage: Intracisternal t-PA for the prevention of vasospasm. *Journal of Neuroscience Nursing, 28*(2), 107–113.

Counsell, C., Gilbert, M., & Snively, C. (1995). Nimodipine: A drug therapy for treatment of vasospasm. *Journal of Neuroscience Nursing, 27*(1), 53–55.

Morrison, S. R. (1997). Gugielmi detachable coils: An alternative therapy for surgically high-risk aneurysms. *Journal of Neuroscience Nursing, 29*(4), 232–237.

Parker, C. D. (1995). Fast action for subarachnoid hemorrhage. *American Journal of Nursing, 95*(1), 47.

Rinkel, G., Prins, N., & Algra, A. (1997). Outcome of aneurysmal subarachnoid hemorrhage in patients on anticoagulant treatment. *Stroke, 28*(1), 6–9.

Stachniak, J., Layon, A., Day, A., & Gallagher, T. (1996). Craniotomy for intracranial aneurysm and subarachnoid hemorrhage. *Stroke, 27*(2), 276–281.

Wang, A., Shetty, A., Kirsch, J., Woo, H., & Wesolowski, D. (1996). Intracranial magnetic resonance angiography. *Applied Radiology, 25*(6), 28–36, 39.

Zimmer, D. L., & Martin, K. M. (1997). Giant intracranial aneurysm obliteration using deep hypothermic circulatory arrest. *AACN Clinical Issues, 8*(2), 196–204.

Cervical and Lumbar Disk Herniation

*Holmes, K. L., & Lenz, E. R. (1997). Perceived self-care information needs and information-seeking behaviors before and after elective spinal procedures. *Journal of Neuroscience Nursing, 29*(2), 79–85.

McCulloch, J. A. (1996). Focus issue on lumbar disc herniation: Macro- and microdiscectomy. *Spine, 21*(24S), 45S–56S.

Nerbay, J., Caspi, I., Levinkopf, M. et al. (1997). Percutaneous laser nucleolysis of the intervertebral lumbar disc. *Clinical Orthopaedics and Related Research, 337,* 42–44.

Regan, J. J. (1996). Percutaneous endoscopic thoracic discectomy. *Neurosurgical Clinics of North America, 7*(1), 87–97.

Woertgen, C., Holzschuh, M., Rothoerl, R., et al. (1997). Prognostic factors of posterior cervical disc surgery. *Neurosurgery, 40*(4), 724–728.

Creutzfeldt-Jakob Disease

Beardsley, T. (1996). Deadly enigma: The US wakes up to the threat of mad cow disease and its relatives. *Scientific American, 275*(6), 16–18.

Epstein, L. G., & Brown, P. (1997). Bovine spongiform encephalopathy and a new variant of Creutzfeldt-Jakob disease. *Neurology, 48,* 569–571.

Johnson, R. T., & Gibbs, C. J. (1998). Creutzfeldt-Jacob disease and related transmissible spongiform encephalopathies. *New England Journal of Medicine, 339*(27), 1994–2004.

Kretzschmar, H. A., Ironside, J. W., DeArmond, S. J., & Tateishi, J. (1996). Diagnostic criteria for sporadic Creutzfeldt-Jakob disease. *Archives of Neurology, 53,* 913–920.

Guillain-Barré Syndrome

Bakker-Hatten, B. S., Lankhorst, G. J., Kriek, L., & Slootman, J. R. (1995). Functional outcome of Guillain-Barré syndrome. *Journal of Rehabilitation Science, 8*(3), 82–86.

Barall-Inman, R. A. (1995). Question and answer: Guillain-Barré syndrome. *Journal of the American Academy of Nurse Practitioners, 7*(4), 165–169.

Bolton, C. F. (1995). The changing concepts of Guillain-Barré syndrome. *New England Journal of Medicine, 333*(21), 1415–1417.

Easton, K. L. (1995). Perspectives: When a serious illness hits home. *Rehabilitation Nursing, 20*(5), 283–284.

McMahon-Parkes, K., & Cornock, M. A. (1997). Guillain-Barré syndrome: biological basis, treatment, and care. *Intensive Critical Care Nursing, 13*(1), 42–48.

Prevots, D. R., & Sutter, R. W. (1997). Assessment of Guillain-Barré syndrome mortality and morbidity in the U.S.: Implications for acute flaccid paralysis surveillance. *Journal of Infectious Diseases, 175*(Suppl 1), S151–S155.

Headache

Berman, G. D., Saper, J. R., & Solomon, G. D. (1996). Chronic headache: Management strategies that make sense. *Patient Care, 30*(2), 54–66.

Bruckenthal, P. (1997). A guide to the diagnosis and management of migraine headaches for the nurse practitioner. *American Journal of Nurse Practitioners,* 1(3):12-18.

Dodick, D. (1997). Headache as a symptom of ominous disease. *Postgraduate Medicine, 101*(5), 46–64.

Edmeads, J. (1997). Headaches in older people: How are they different in this age group? *Postgraduate Medicine, 101*(5), 91–100.

Evers, S., Bauer, B., Suhr, B., et al. (1997). Cognitive processing in primary headache: A study on event-related potentials. *Neurology, 48*(1), 108–113.

Haan, J., Terwindt, G., & Ferrari, M. (1997). Genetics of migraine. *Neurologic Clinics, 15*(1), 43–55.

Kirk, E., Giordano, J., & Anderson, A. (1997). Serotonin receptors as targets for pharmacotherapy. *Journal of Neuroscience Nursing, 29*(3), 191–198.

Maizels, M., Scott, B., Cohen, W., & Chen, W. (1996). Intranasal licodaine for treatment of migraine. A randomized double-blind, controlled trail. *Journal of American Medical Association, 276*(4), 319–321.

Mathew, N. T. (1997). Transformed migraine, analgesic rebound, and other chronic daily headaches. *Neurologic Clinics, 15*(1), 167–185.

Mathew, N. T. (1997). Serotonin 1D (5-HT1D) agonists and other agents in acute migraine. *Neurologic Clinics, 15*(1), 61–83.

Nussbaum, E. (1996). Migraines: The latest on symptom relief and prevention. *American Journal of Nursing, 96*(10), 36–37.

Olin, J. S. (1997). Cluster headaches. *Cleveland Clinic Journal of Medicine, 63*(4), 237–244.

Pryse-Phillips, W. E., Dodick, D. W., Edmeads, J. J., et al. (1997). Guidelines for the diagnosis and management if migraine in clinical practice. *Canadian Medical Association Journal, 156*(9), 1273–1287.

Solomon, S. (1997). Diagnosis of primary headache disorders: Validity of the International Headache Society Criteria in Clinical Practice. *Neurologic Clinics, 15*(1), 15–25.

Solomon, G. D. (1997). Evolution of the measurement of quality of life in migraine. *Neurology, 48*(Suppl 3), S10–S15.

Zeigler, D. K. (1997). Opioids in headache treatment. *Neurologic Clinics, 15*(1), 199–207.

Huntington's Disease

Barinaga, M. (1996). An intriguing new lead on Huntington's disease. *Science, 271*(5269), 1233–1234.

Cummings, J. L. (1995). Behavioral and psychiatric symptoms associated with Huntington's disease. *Advances in Neurology, 65,* 179–186.

Hayden, M. R., Bloch, M., & Wiggins, S. (1995). Psychological effects of predictive testing for Huntington's disease. *Advances in Neurology, 65,* 210–210.

Mlynik-Scmid, A. (1997). Psychological consequences of presymptomatic testing for HD. *Lancet, 349*(9054), 808.

Rohs, G., & Klimek, M. L. (1996). Ethical, social, and legal issues in HD: the nurse's role. *AXON, 17*(3), 55–59.

Shulman, K., Lennox, A., & Karlinsky, H. (1996). Late-onset HD: A geriatric psychiatry perspective. *Journal of Geriatric Psychiatry and Neurology, 9*(1), 26–29.

Siemers, E., Foroud, T., Bill, D., Sorbel, J., Norton, J., Hodes, M., et al. (1996). Motor changes in presymptomatic HD gene carriers. *Archives of Neurology, 53*(6), 487–492.

Meningitis and Brain Abscess

Ashwal, S. (1995). Neurological evaluation of the patient with acute bacterial meningitis. *Neurologic Clinics, 13*(3), 549–577.

Baumann, C. K. (1997). Multiple bilateral cerebral abscesses with hemorrhage. *Journal of Neuroscience Nursing, 29*(1), 4–14.

Green, G., & Demasi, R. (1996). Case report: Penicillin-resistant pneumococcal meningitis: Navigating a therapeutic minefield. *American Journal of Nursing, 311*(4), 180–185.

McIntyre, P., Berkey, C., King, S., et al. (1997). Dexamethasone as adjunctive therapy in bacterial meningitis: A meta-analysis of randomized clinical trials since 1988. *Journal of the American Medical Association, 278*(11), 925–931.

Schuchat, A., Robinson, K., Wenger, J., et al. (1997). Bacterial meningitis in the U.S. *New England Journal of Medicine, 337*(14), 970–976.

Sigurdardottir, B., Bjornsson, O., & Jonsdottir, K. (1997). Acute bacterial meningitis in adults: A 20-year overview. *Archives of Internal Medicine, 157*(4), 425–430.

Townsend, G. C., & Scheld, W. M. (1996). The use of corticosteroids in the management of bacterial meningitis in adults. *Journal of Antimicrobial Chemotherapy, 37,* 1051–1061.

Multiple Sclerosis

Costello, K., & Conway, K. (1997). Nursing management of MS patients receiving interferon beta-1b therapy. *Rehabilitation Nursing, 22*(2), 62–72.

Halper, J., & Holland, N. (1998). Meeting the challenge of multiple sclerosis. Part I. Treating the person and the disease. *American Journal of Nursing, 98*(10), 26–31.

Halper, J., & Holland, N. (1998). Meeting the challenge of multiple sclerosis. Part II. New strategies, new hope. *American Journal of Nursing, 98*(11), 39–45.

Jacobs, L. D., Cookfair, D. L., Rudick, R. A., Herndon, R. M., Richert, J. R., Salazar, A. M., et al. (1996). Intramuscular interferon beta-Ia for disease progression in relapsing multiple sclerosis. *Annals of neurology, 39*(3), 283–284.

Keating, M. M., & Ostby, P. L. (1996). Education and self-management if interferon beta-1b therapy for multiple sclerosis. *Journal of Neuroscience Nursing, 28*(6), 350–359.

Kelley, C. L. (1996). The role of interferons in the treatment of multiple sclerosis. *Journal of Neuroscience Nursing, 28*(2), 114–120.

Miller, A. (1997). Current and investigational therapies used to alter the course of disease in multiple sclerosis. *South Medical Journal, 90*(4), 367–375.

Rudick, A., Cohen, J., Weistock-Guttman, B., et al. (1997). Management of multiple sclerosis. *New England Journal of Medicine, 337*(22), 1604.

*Smeltzer, S. C., & Lavietes, M. H. (1999). Reliability of maximal respiratory pressures in MS. *Chest, 115*(6), 1546–1552.

*Smeltzer, S. C., Lavietes, M. H., & Cook, S. D. (1996). Expiratory training in multiple sclerosis. *Archives of Physical Medicine Rehabilitation, 77*(9), 909–912.

*Stuifbergen, A. K. (1997). Physical activity and perceived health status in persons with MS. *Journal of Neuroscience Nursing, 29*(4), 238–243.

*Stuifbergen, A. K., & Rogers, S. (1997). The experience of fatigue and strategies of self-care among persons with multiple sclerosis. *Applied Nursing Research, 10*(1), 2–10.

Swain, S. E. (1996). Multiple sclerosis: Primary health care implications. *Nurse Practitioner, 21*(7), 40–54.

Myasthenia Gravis

Massey, J. M. (1997). Acquired myasthenia gravis. *Neurologic Clinics, 15*(3), 577–593.

Thomas, C. E., Mayer, S. A., Gungor, Y., et al. (1997). Myasthenia crisis: Clinical features, mortality, complications, and risk factors for prolonged intubation. *Neurology, 48*(5), 1253–1260.

Wittbrodt, E. T. (1997). Drugs and myasthenia gravis. *Archives of Internal Medicine, 157,* 399–408.

Parkinson's Disease

Aminoff, M. J., Burns, R. S., & Silverstein, P. M. (1997). Update on Parkinson's disease. *Patient Care, 31*(10), 12–25.

Chisholm, A. H. (1996). Fetal transplantation for the treatment of parkinson's disease: A review of the literature. *Journal of Neuroscience Nursing, 28*(5), 329–338.

*Fowler, S. B. (1997). Hope and a health-promoting lifestyle in persons with Parkinson's disease. *Journal of Neuroscience Nursing, 29*(2), 111–116.

Gilbert, M., Counsell, C. M., & Snively, C. (1996). Pallidotomy: A surgical intervention for control of Parkinson's Disease. *Journal of Neuroscience Nursing, 28*(1), 219–221.

Goldsmith, C. (1999). Parkinson's disease. *American Journal of Nursing, 99*(2), 46–47.

Krauss, J. K., & Jankovic, J. (1996). Surgical treatment of Parkinson's Disease. American Family Physician. 1996; 54(5):1621–1627.

Lang, A. E., & Lozano, A. M. (1998). Parkinson's Disease. First of two parts. *New England Journal of Medicine, 339*(15), 1044–1053.

Lang, A. E., & Lozano, A. M. (1998). Parkinson's Disease. Second of two parts. *New England Journal of Medicine, 339*(16), 1130–1143.

Lusis, S. A. (1997). Pathophysiology and management of idiopathic Parkinson's disease. *Journal of Neuroscience Nursing, 29*(1), 24–31.

Roberts, J. (1996). Nursing care of patients undergoing pallidotomy. *Nursing Standard, 10*(35), 44–47.

Tapper, V. (1997). Pathophysiology, assessment, and treatment of Parkinson's disease. *Nurse Practitioner, 22*(7), 76–95.

Vernon, G., & Jenkins, M. (1995). Health maintenance behaviors in advanced Parkinson's disease. *Journal of Neuroscience Nursing, 27*(4), 229–235.

Seizures

Callahan, M. (1997). Pregnancy and related issues for women with epilepsy. *Clinical Nursing Practice in Epilepsy, 4*(3), 4–7.

Brodie, M. J., & Dichter, M. A. (1996). Antiepileptic drugs. *New England Journal of Medicine, 334,* 168–175.

Devinsky, O. (1999). Patients with refractory seizures. *New England Journal of Medicine, 340*(20), 1565–1570.

Hilton, G. (1997). Seizure disorders in adults: Evaluation and management of new-onset seizures. *Nurse Practitioner, 22*(9), 42–59.

Hulihan, J. F. (1997). Seizures in special populations: Children, the elderly, and patients with coexistent medical illness. *Postgraduate Medicine, 102*(1), 165–178.

Johannessen, S. I. (1997). Pharmacokinetics and interaction profile of topiramate: Review and comparison with other newer antiepileptic drugs. *Epilepsia, 38*(Suppl 1), S18–S23.

Liporace, J. D. (1997). Women's issues in epilepsy: Menses, childbearing, and more. *Postgraduate Medicine, 102*(1), 123–138.

Lowenstein, D. H., & Alldredge, B. K. (1998). Current concepts: Status epilepticus. *New England Journal of Medicine, 338*(14), 970–976.

Ozuna, J. (1997). Pharmacologic management if epilepsy: An update. *Journal of Neuroscience Nursing, 29*(5), 330–335.

Pourmand, R. (1996). Seizures and epilepsy in older patients: Evaluation and management. *Geriatrics, 51*(3), 39–52.

Long, L., & Reeves, A. (1996). The practical aspects of epilepsy: Critical components of comprehensive patient care. *Journal of Neuroscience Nursing, 29*(4), 249–254.

Salinsky, M., Uthman, B., Ristanovic, R., et al. (1996). Vagus nerve stimulation for the treatment of medically intractable seizures. *Archives of Neurology, 53,* 1176–1180.

Shafer, P. (1997). Hormone sensitive seizures in women with epilepsy. *Clinical Nursing Practice in Epilepsy, 4*(3), 8–10.

Shafer, P., Sierzant, T., & Dean, P. (1997). Alternative and complementary therapies: Focus on epilepsy. *Clinical Nursing Practice in Epilepsy, 4*(2), 4–8.

Sirven, J. I., & Liporace, J. D. (1997). New antiepileptic drugs. *Postgraduate Medicine, 102*(1), 147–162.

Spinal Cord Tumors

Bell, G. R. (1997). Surgical treatment of spinal tumors. *Clinical Orthopaedics and Related Research, 335,* 54–63.

McKinley, W., Conti-Wyneken, A., & Vokac, C. (1996). Rehabilitative functional outcome of patients with neoplastic spinal cord compression. *Archives of Physical Medicine and Rehabilitation, 77*(9), 892–895.

Walton, P. G., & Broughton, E. L. (1997). Transoral resection of spinal cord tumor and posterior cervical spine stabilization. *AORN Journal, 65*(1), 47–48.

Trigeminal Neuralgia and Neuropathies

Bauer, C. A. (1996). Update on facial nerve disorders. *Otolaryngology Clinics of North America, 29*(3), 445–454.

Brown, J. (1997). The trigeminal complex: Anatomy and physiology. *Neurosurgery Clinics of North America, 8*(1), 1–10.

Costa, M. E. (1998). Trigeminal neuralgia. *American Journal of Nursing, 98*(6), 42–43.

Gouda, J., & Brown, J. (1997). Atypical facial pain and other syndromes: Differential diagnosis and treatment. *Neurosurgery Clinics of North America, 8*(1), 87–102.

Kondziolka, D., Lunsford, L., Habeck, M., et al. (1997). Gamma knife radiosurgery for trigeminal neuralgia. *Neurosurgery Clinics of North America, 8*(1), 79–86.

Lovely, T., & Jannetta, P. (1997). Microvascular decompression for trigeminal neuralgia:surgical technique and long-term results. *Neurosurgery Clinics of North America, 8*(1), 11–30.

Walchenbach, R., & Voormolen, J. (1996). Surgical treatment for trigeminal neuralgia. *British Medical Journal, 313*(10), 1027–1026.

Resources

American Cancer Society, 1599 Clifton Road NE, Atlanta, Georgia 30329; 1-800-227-2345; www.cancer.org

American Parkinson's Disease Association, 1250 Hyland Blvd., Staten island, NY 10310; 1-800-223-2732; www.apdaparkinson.com

Amyotrophic Lateral Sclerosis Association, 27001 Agpira Road, Suite 150, Calabasas Hills, CA 91301; 1-800-782-4747; 1-818-880-9007 (patients only); www.alsa.org

Epilepsy Foundation of America, 4351 Garden City Drive, Landover, MD 20785; 1-800-332-1000; FAX: 301-577-4941; www.efa.org

Guillain-Barré Syndrome Foundation International, P.O. Box 262, Wynnewood, PA 19096; 1-610-667-0131; FAX: 610-667-7036; E-mail: gbint@ix.netcom.com

Huntington's Disease Society of America, 140 W. 22nd Street, 6th Floor, New York, NY 10011-2420; 1-800-345-4372; 1-212-242-1968; curehd@hdsa.ttisms.com; neuro-www2.mgh.harvard.edu/hdsa/hdsadmin.nclk

Muscular Dystrophy Association, 3300 East Sunrise Drive, Tucson, AZ 85718; 1-800-572-1717; www.mdausa.org

Myasthenia Gravis Foundation of America, 222 S. Riverside Plaza, Ste. 1540, Chicago, IL 60606; 1-800-541-5454; 1-312-258-0522; FAX: 312-258-0461; www.myasthenia.org

National Headache Foundation, 428 W. St. James Place, 2nd Floor, Chicago, IL 60614-2750; 1-800-843-2256; FAX: 773-525-7357; www.headaches.org

National Multiple Sclerosis Society, 733 Third Avenue, New York, NY 10017; 1-800-344-4867; www.nmss.org

National Parkinson's Disease Foundation, Columbia Presbyterian Medical Center, Neurological Building, 710 W. 168th Street, New York, NY 10032; www.parkinsons-foundation.org

UNIT

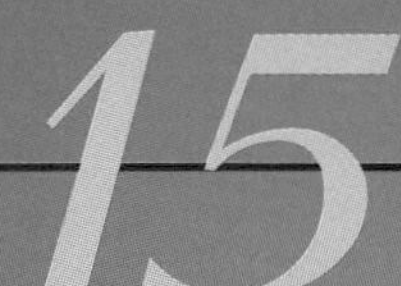

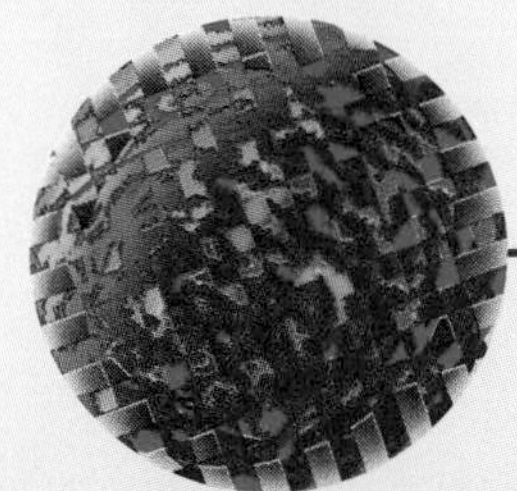

Musculoskeletal Function

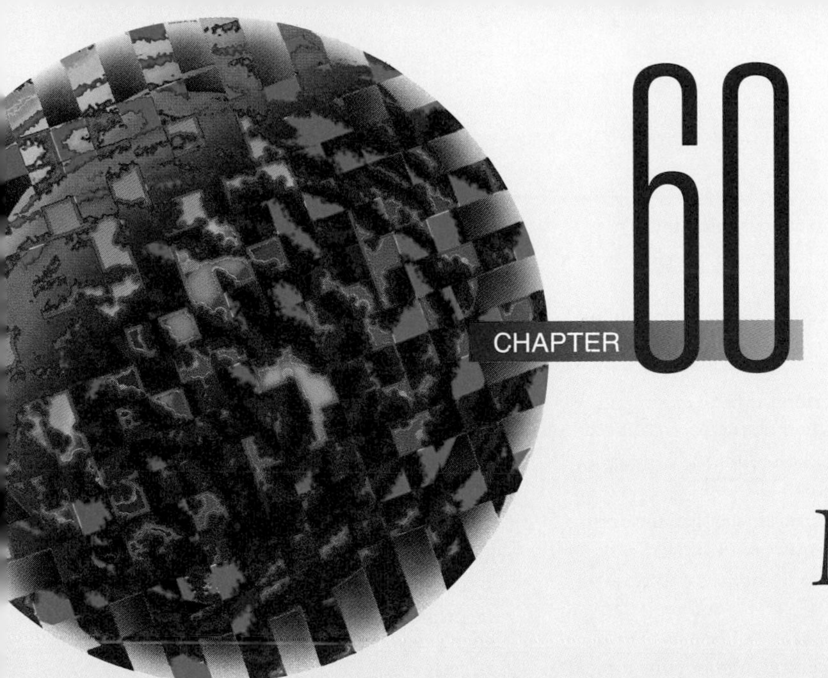

Assessment of Musculoskeletal Function

Learning Objectives

On completion of this chapter, the learner will be able to:

1. Describe the anatomy and physiology of the musculoskeletal system.
2. Discuss the significance of the health history to assessment of musculoskeletal health.
3. Describe the significance of physical assessment to the diagnosis of musculoskeletal dysfunction.
4. Specify the diagnostic tests used for assessment of musculoskeletal function.
5. Discuss nursing implications of assessing patients with musculoskeletal disorders.

The musculoskeletal system includes the bones, joints, muscles, tendons, ligaments, and bursae of the body. The problems associated with these structures are common and affect all age groups. Problems with the musculoskeletal system are generally not life-threatening, but they have a significant effect on the patient's normal activities and productivity. Nurses in all practice areas encounter patients with altered musculoskeletal function.

GLOSSARY

atonic: without tone; denervated muscle that atrophies

atrophy: shrinkage-like decrease in the size of a muscle

bursa: fluid-filled sac found in connective tissue, usually in the area of joints

callus: fibrous tissue at fracture site

cancellous bone: spongy, lattice-like bone structure; trabecular bone

cartilage: special tissue at ends of bone

clonus: rhythmic contraction of muscle

contracture: abnormal shortening of muscle and/or joint; fibrosis

cortical bone: compact bone

crepitus: grating or crackling sound or sensation; may occur with movement of ends of a broken bone or irregular joint surface

diaphysis: shaft of long bone

effusion: excess fluid in joint

endosteum: marrow cavity lining of hollow bone

epiphysis: end of long bone

fascia (epimysium): fibrous tissue that covers, supports, and separates muscles

fasciculation: involuntary twitch of muscle fibers

flaccid: limp; absence of muscle tone

hypertrophy: enlargement; muscle increases in size

isometric contraction: muscle tension increased, length unchanged, no joint motion

isotonic contraction: muscle tension unchanged, muscle shortened, joint moved

joint: area where bone ends meet; provides areas of motion and flexibility

joint capsule: fibrous tissue that encloses bone ends and other joint surfaces

kyphosis: increase in thoracic curvature of spine

lamellae: mature compact bone structures that form concentric rings of bone matrix; lamellar bone

ligament: fibrous band connecting bones

lordosis: increase in lumbar curvature of spine

ossification: process in which minerals (calcium) are deposited in bone matrix

osteoblast: bone-forming cell

osteoclast: bone resorption cell

osteocyte: mature bone cell

osteogenesis: bone formation

osteoid: pertaining to bone matrix tissue; "pre-bone"

osteon: microscopic functional bone unit

osteoporosis: abnormal loss of bone mass and strength

paralysis: absence of muscle movement suggesting nerve damage

paresthesia: abnormal sensations (eg, burning, tingling, numbness, and so forth)

periosteum: fibrous connective tissue covering bone

remodeling: process of reorganizing new bone structure according to function

resorption: removal, destruction of tissue, such as bone

scoliosis: lateral curving of the spine

spastic: having greater than normal muscle tone

synovium: membrane in joint that secretes lubricating fluid

tendon: cord of fibrous tissue connecting muscle to bone

tone: normal tension (resistance to stretch) in resting muscle

trabecula: lattice-like bone structure; trabecular bone

ANATOMIC AND PHYSIOLOGIC OVERVIEW

The health and proper functioning of the musculoskeletal system are interdependent with that of the other body systems. The bony structure provides protection for vital organs, including the brain, heart, and lungs. The bony skeleton provides a sturdy framework to support body structures. The bone matrix stores calcium, phosphorus, magnesium, and fluoride. More than 98% of the total-body calcium is present in bone. In addition, the red bone marrow located within bone cavities produces red and white blood cells in a process called hematopoiesis. A **joint** is a part of the skeleton in which two or more bones meet; joints hold the bones together while allowing the body to move. The muscles attached to the skeleton also allow the body to move, and contraction of the muscles produces heat, which helps to maintain body temperature.

Anatomy and Function of the Skeletal System

There are 206 bones in the human body, divided into four categories:

- Long bones (eg, femur)
- Short bones (eg, metacarpals)
- Flat bones (eg, sternum)
- Irregular bones (eg, vertebrae)

The shape and construction of a specific bone are determined by its function and the forces exerted on it. Bones are constructed of **cancellous** (trabecular or spongy) or **cortical** (compact) bone tissue. Long bones are shaped like rods or shafts with rounded ends (Fig. 60-1). The shaft, known as the **diaphysis**, is primarily cortical bone. The ends of the long bones, called **epiphyses**, are primarily cancellous bone. The epiphyseal plate separates the epiphyses from the diaphysis and is the center for longitudinal growth in children. In the adult, it is calcified. The ends of long bones are covered at the joints by articular **cartilage**, which is a tough, elastic, bonelike tissue. Long bones are constructed for weight bearing and movement. Short bones consist of cancellous bone covered by a layer of compact bone. Flat bones are important sites for hematopoiesis and frequently provide vital organ protection. They are made of cancellous bone layered between compact bone. Irregular bones have unique shapes related to their functions. Generally, irregular bone structure is similar to that of flat bones.

Bone is composed of cells, protein matrix, and mineral deposits. The cells are of three basic types—**osteoblasts**, **osteocytes**, and **osteoclasts**. Osteoblasts function in bone formation by secreting bone matrix. The matrix is collagen and ground substances (glycoproteins and proteoglycans). The matrix is a framework in which inorganic mineral salts are deposited. Osteocytes are mature bone cells involved in bone-maintenance functions and are located in lacunae (bone matrix units). Osteoclasts, located in shallow Howship's lacunae (small pits in bones), are multinuclear cells involved in destroying, resorbing, and remolding bone. The microscopic functioning unit of mature cortical bone is the **osteon** (haversian system). The center of the osteon, the haversian canal, contains a capillary. Around the capillary are circles of mineralized bone matrix called **lamellae**. Within the lamellae are lacunae containing osteocytes. These are nourished through tiny structures, canaliculi (canals), that communicate with adjacent blood vessels within the haversian system (see Fig. 60-1).

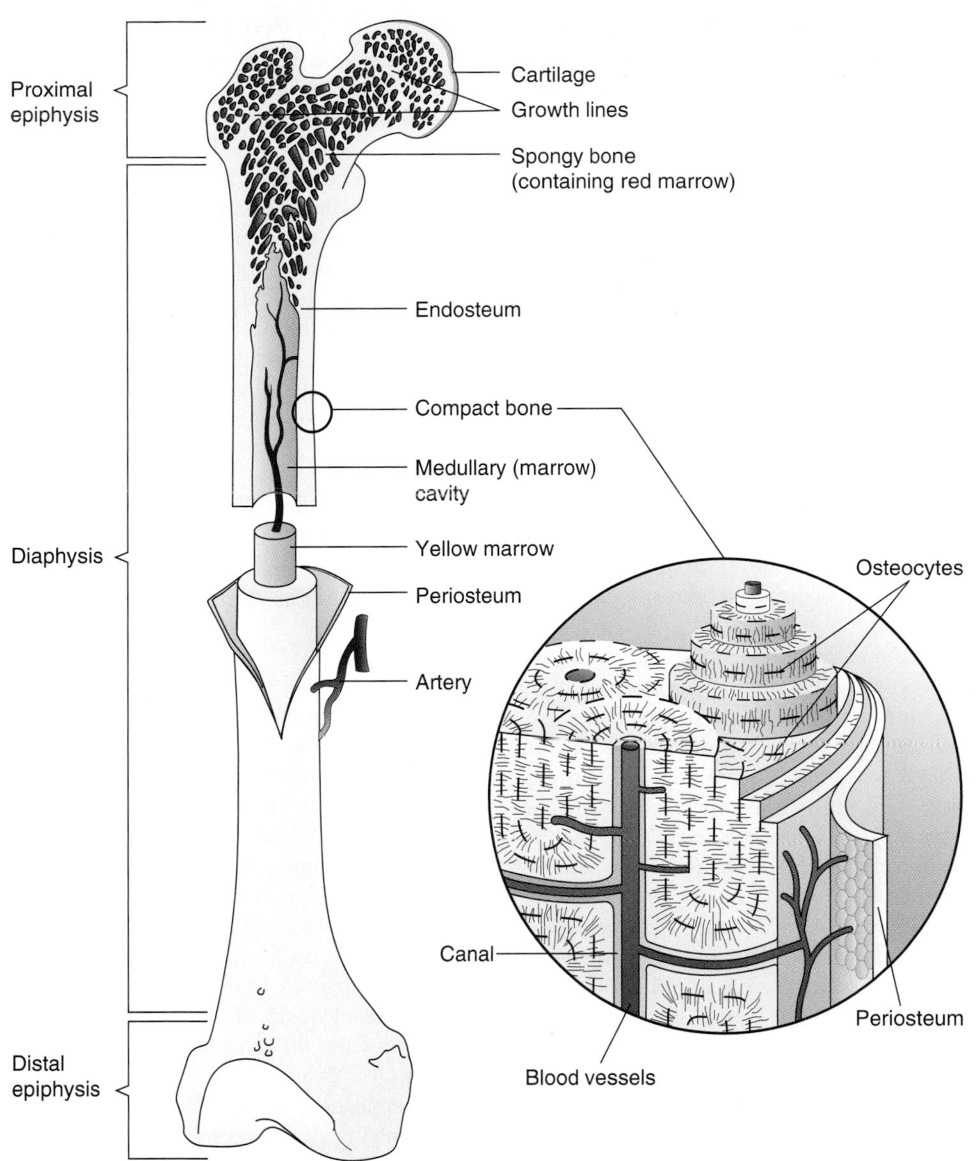

FIGURE 60•1 Structure of a long bone; composition of compact bone.

Lacunae in cancellous bone are layered in an irregular lattice network (**trabeculae**). Red bone marrow fills the lattice network. Capillaries nourish the osteocytes located in the lacunae.

Covering the bone is a dense, fibrous membrane known as the **periosteum**. The periosteum nourishes bone and allows for its growth as well as provides for the attachment of tendons and ligaments. The periosteum contains nerves, blood vessels, and lymphatics. The layer closest to the bone contains osteoblasts, which are bone-forming cells.

Endosteum is a thin, vascular membrane covering the marrow cavity of long bones and the spaces in cancellous bone. Osteoclasts, which dissolve bone to maintain the marrow cavity, are located near the endosteum in Howship's lacunae.

Bone marrow is a vascular tissue located in the medullary (shaft) cavity of long bones and in flat bones. Red bone marrow, located mainly in the sternum, ilium, vertebrae, and ribs in adults, is responsible for producing red and white blood cells. In adults, the long bone is filled with fatty, yellow marrow.

Bone tissue is well vascularized. Cancellous bone receives a rich blood supply through metaphyseal and epiphyseal vessels. Periosteal vessels carry blood to compact bone through minute Volkmann's canals. In addition, nutrient arteries penetrate the periosteum and enter the medullary cavity through foramina (small openings). Nutrient arteries supply blood to the marrow and bone. The venous system may accompany arteries or may exit independently.

Bone Formation

Bone begins to form long before birth. **Ossification** is the process by which the bone matrix (eg, collagen fibers and ground substance) is formed and hardening minerals (eg, calcium salts) are deposited on the collagen fibers in an electronegative environment. The collagen fibers give tensile strength to the bone, and the calcium provides compressional strength.

There are two basic models of ossification: intramembranous and endochondral. Intramembranous ossification, in which bone develops within membrane, occurs in the bones of the face and skull. Therefore, when the skull heals, it is by fibrous union. The other kind of bone formation is known as endochondral ossification, in which a cartilage model exists. **Osteoid** tissue, which is cartilage-like tissue, is formed, resorbed, and replaced by bone. Most bones in the body are formed and heal by endochondral ossification.

Bone Maintenance

Bone is a dynamic tissue in a constant state of reforming and **resorption**, creation, and destruction. The important regulating factors that determine the balance between bone formation and bone resorption include local stress, vitamin D, parathyroid hormone, calcitonin, and blood supply.

Local stress (weight bearing) acts to simulate bone formation and remolding. Weight-bearing bones are thick and strong. Without weight bearing or stress, as in prolonged bed rest, the bone loses calcium (resorption) and becomes osteoporotic and weak. The weak bone may fracture easily.

Vitamin D functions to increase the amount of calcium in the blood by promoting absorption of calcium from the gastrointestinal tract. A deficiency of vitamin D results in bone mineralization deficit, deformity, and fracture.

Parathyroid hormone and calcitonin are the major hormonal regulators of calcium homeostasis. Parathyroid hormone regulates the concentration of calcium in the blood, in part by promoting movement of calcium from the bone. In response to low calcium levels in the blood, increased levels of parathyroid hormone prompt the mobilization of calcium, the demineralization of bone, and the formation of bone cysts. Calcitonin, secreted by the thyroid gland in response to elevated blood calcium levels, increases the deposit of calcium in bone.

Blood supply to the bone also affects bone formation. With diminished blood supply or hyperemia (congestion), **osteogenesis**, which is the formation of bone, decreases, and bone density decreases. Bone necrosis occurs when the bone is deprived of blood.

Bone Healing

Most fractures heal through endochondral ossification. When the bone is injured, the bone fragments are not merely patched together with scar tissue. Instead, the bone regenerates itself by undergoing several stages of fracture healing:

1. Fracture hematoma
2. Inflammation with neovascularization
3. Reparative phase with callus formation and ossification
4. Remodeling into mature bone (Fig. 60-2)

FRACTURE HEMATOMA

With a fracture, the body's response is similar to that of injury elsewhere in the body. There is bleeding into the injured tissue and formation of a fracture hematoma. The fracture fragment ends become devitalized because of the interrupted blood supply.

INFLAMMATION AND REVASCULARIZATION

The injured area is invaded by macrophages (large white blood cells), which dèbride the area. Inflammation, swelling, and pain are present. The inflammatory stage lasts several days and resolves with a decrease in pain and swelling. Within about 5 days, the fracture hematoma undergoes organization. Fibrin strands form within the clot, creating a network for revascularization and invasion by fibroblasts and osteoblasts.

REPARATIVE PHASE

Fibroblasts and osteoblasts (developed from osteocytes, endosteal cells, and periosteal cells) produce collagen and proteoglycans for a collagen matrix at the fracture. Cartilage and fibrous connective (osteoid) tissue develop. The cartilage at the bone fragments grows toward the other until the fracture gap is bridged. This process is known as **callus** formation and is stimulated by minimal micromotion but is disrupted by excessive motion at the fracture site. Actively growing bone exhibits electronegative potentials. The shape of the callus and the volume of tissue required to bridge the defect are directly proportional to the amount of bone damage and displacement. Generally, it takes 3 to 4 weeks for fracture fragments to be united by cartilage or fibrous tissue. Clinically, the fragments are no longer easily moved.

OSSIFICATION

Ossification of the callus begins within 2 to 3 weeks of fracture. Minerals continue to be deposited until the bone is firmly reunited. With major adult long bone fractures, ossification takes 3 to 4 months. The callus surface continues to be electronegative.

REMODELING

The final stage of fracture repair consists of **remodeling**, or removing any remaining devitalized tissue and reorganizing the new bone into its former structural arrangement. Remodeling may take months to years, depending on the extent of bone modification needed, the function of the bone, and the functional stresses on the bone. Cancellous bone heals and remodels more rapidly than compact cortical bone, especially at points of direct contact. When remodeling is complete, the fracture surface charge is no longer electronegative.

The progress of bone healing is monitored by serial x-rays. The rate of fracture healing is influenced by the type of bone fractured, the adequacy of blood supply, the surface contact of the fragments, and the general health of the person. Adequate immobilization is essential until there is evidence of callus formation with ossification on x-ray. Progression of the therapeutic regimen (eg, applying a cast brace to a patient who has had a femur fracture reduced and immobilized by skeletal traction) is determined by evidence of healing of the fracture.

BONE HEALING WITH FRAGMENTS FIRMLY APPROXIMATED

When fractures are treated with open rigid fixation techniques, the bony fragments can be placed in direct contact. Motion at the fracture is eliminated. In this situation, the stages of bone healing are modified. Hematoma formation is not essential and does not occur. Little or no external cartilaginous callus develops. Primary bone healing occurs through cortical bone remodeling.

Immature bone develops from the endosteum. There is an intensive regeneration of new osteons, which develop in the fracture line by a process similar to normal bone maintenance. Fracture strength is obtained when the new osteons have become established.

Anatomy and Function of the Articular System

The junction of two or more bones is called a joint (articulation). There are three basic kinds of joints: synarthrosis, amphiarthrosis, and diarthrosis joints. *Synarthrosis joints* are immovable, as

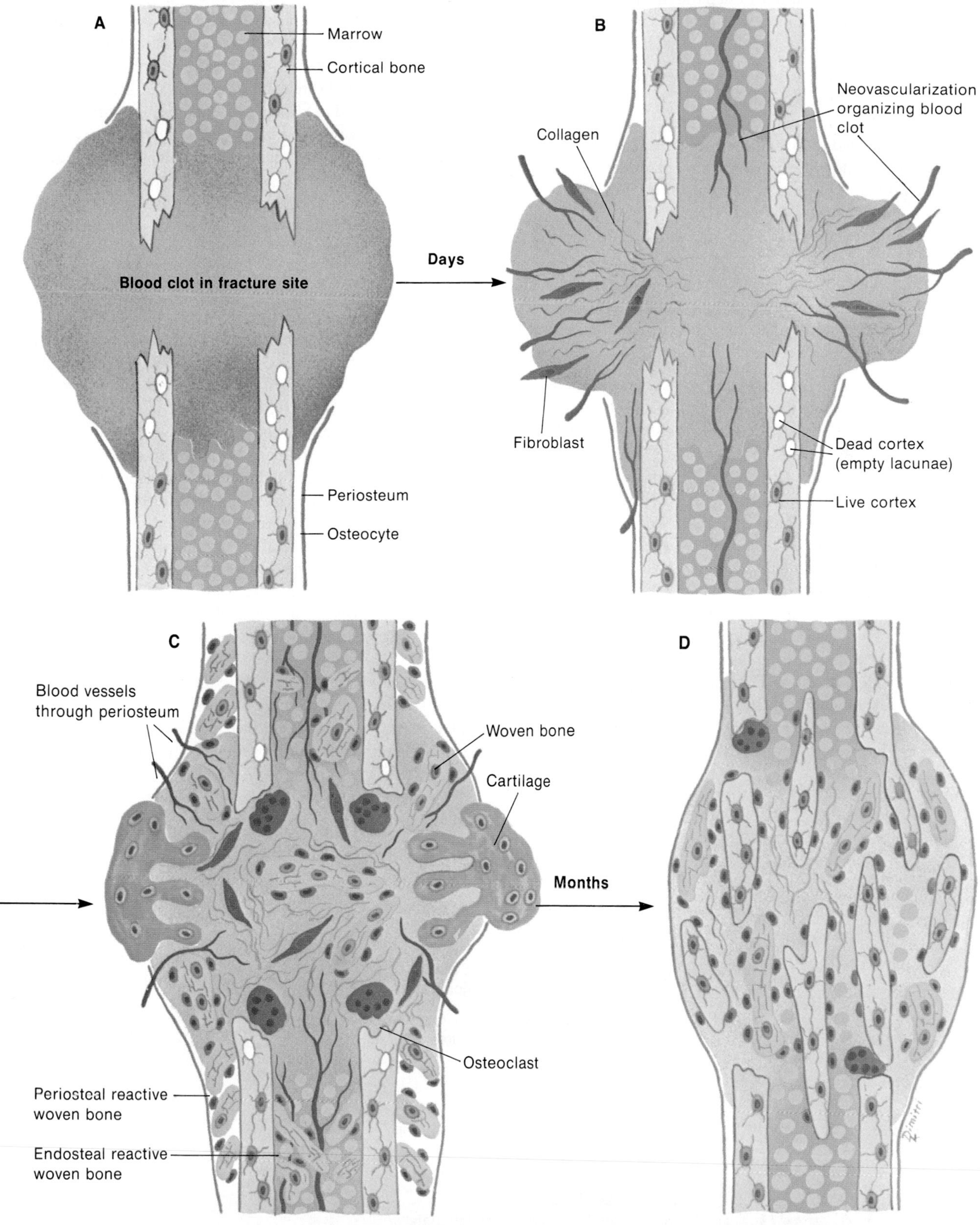

FIGURE 60•2 Healing of a fracture. (**A**) Soon after a fracture, an extensive blood clot forms in the subperiosteal and soft tissue. (**B**) Inflammatory phase: neovascularization and beginning organization of the blood clot. (**C**) Reparative phase: formation of a callus of cartilage and woven bone near the fracture site. (**D**) Remodeling phase: the cortex is revitalized.

exemplified by the skull sutures. *Amphiarthroses,* such as the vertebral joints and symphysis pubis, allow limited motion. The bones of amphiarthroses joints are separated by fibrous cartilage. *Diarthroses* are freely movable joints (Fig. 60-3).

There are several types of diarthrosis joints:

- *Ball-and-socket* joints, best exemplified by the hip and the shoulder, permit full freedom of movement.
- *Hinge* joints permit bending in one direction only and are best exemplified by the elbow and knee.
- *Saddle joints* allow movement in two planes at right angles to each other. The joint at the base of the thumb is a saddle, biaxial joint.
- *Pivot* joints are characterized by the articulation between the radius and the ulna. They permit rotation for such activities as turning a doorknob.
- *Gliding* joints allow for limited movement in all directions and are represented by the joints of the carpal bones in the wrist.

At a typical movable joint, the ends of the articulating bones are covered with smooth hyaline cartilage. The articulating bones are surrounded by a tough, fibrous sheath, which is the **joint capsule**. The capsule is lined with a membrane, the **synovium**, which secretes the lubricating and shock-absorbing **synovial fluid** into the joint capsule. Therefore, the bone surfaces are not in direct contact. In some synovial joints (eg, the knee), **fibrocartilage disks** are located between the articular cartilage surfaces. These disks provide shock absorption.

Ligaments (fibrous connective tissue bands) bind the articulating bones together. Ligaments and muscle tendons, which pass over the joint, provide joint stability. In some joints, interosseous ligaments (eg, the cruciate ligaments of the knee) are found within the capsule and add stability to the joint.

A **bursa** is a synovial fluid-filled sac that cushions the movement of tendons, ligaments, and bones at a point of friction. Bursae are generally found at the elbow, shoulder, knee, and some other joints.

Anatomy and Function of the Skeletal Muscle System

Muscles are attached by **tendons** (cords of fibrous connective tissue) or aponeuroses (broad, flat sheets of connective tissue) to bones, connective tissue, other muscles, soft tissue, or skin. The muscles of the body are composed of parallel groups of muscle cells (fasciculi) encased in fibrous tissue called epimysium, or **fascia**. The more fasciculi contained in a muscle, the more precise the movements. Muscles vary in shape and size according to the activity for which they are responsible. Skeletal (striated) muscles are involved in body movement, posture, and heat-production functions. Muscles contract to bring the two points of attachment closer together, resulting in movement.

Skeletal Muscle Contraction

Each muscle cell (also referred to as a muscle fiber) contains myofibrils, which in turn are composed of a series of sarcomeres, the actual contractile units of skeletal muscle. Sarcomeres contain thick myosin and thin actin filaments.

Muscle fibers contract in response to electrical stimulation delivered by an effector nerve cell at the **motor end plate**. When stimulated, muscle cell depolarizes and generates an action potential in a manner similar to that described for nerve cells. These action potentials propagate along the muscle cell membrane and lead to the release of calcium ions that are stored in specialized organelles called the sarcoplasmic reticulum. When there is a local increase in calcium ion concentration, the myocin and actin filaments slide across one another. Shortly after the muscle cell membrane is depolarized, it recovers its resting membrane voltage. Calcium is rapidly removed from the sarcomeres by active reaccumulation in the sarcoplasmic reticulum. When calcium concentration in the sarcomere decreases, the myosin and actin filaments cease to interact, and the sarcomere returns to its original resting length (relaxation). Actin and myosin do not interact in the absence of calcium.

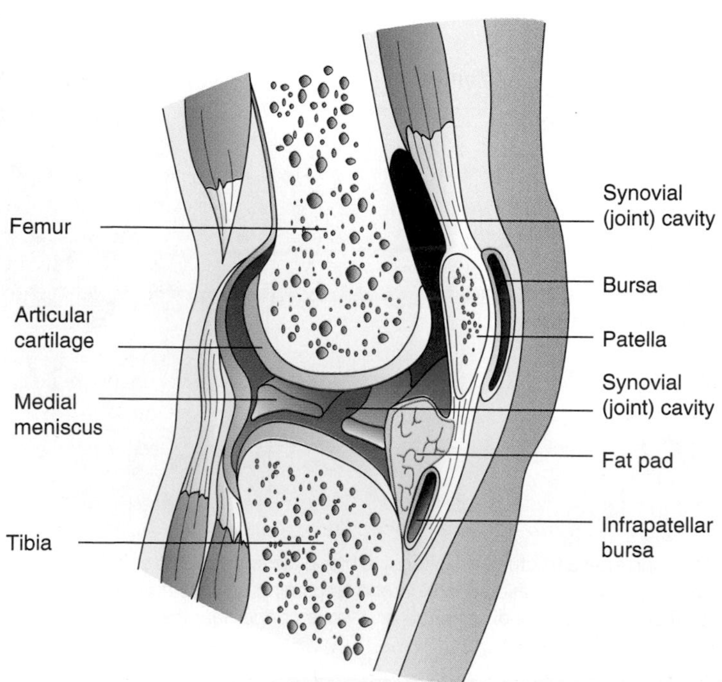

FIGURE 60•3 Hinge joint of the knee.

Energy is consumed during muscle contraction and relaxation. The primary source of energy for the muscle cells is adenosine triphosphate (ATP) that is generated through cellular oxidative metabolism. At low levels of activity (ie, sedentary activity), the skeletal muscle synthesizes ATP from the oxidation of glucose to water and carbon dioxide. During periods of strenuous activity, when sufficient oxygen may not be available, glucose is metabolized primarily to lactic acid, an inefficient process compared with that of oxidative pathways. Stored muscle glycogen is used to supply glucose during periods of activity. Muscle fatigue is thought to be caused by depletion of glycogen and accumulation of lactic acid. As a result, the cycle of muscle contraction and relaxation cannot continue.

During muscle contraction, the energy released from ATP is not completely used. This excess energy is dissipated in the form of heat. During isometric contraction, almost all the energy is released in the form of heat; during isotonic contraction, some of the energy is expended in mechanical work. In some situations, such as shivering because of cold, the need to generate heat is the primary stimulus for muscle contraction.

Types of Muscle Contractions

The contraction of muscle fibers can result in either isotonic or isometric contraction of the muscle. In **isometric contraction**, the length of the muscles remains constant but the force generated by the muscles is increased; an example of this is when one pushes against an immovable wall. **Isotonic contraction**, on the other hand, is characterized by shortening of the muscle with no increase in tension within the muscle; an example of this is flexion of the forearm. In normal activities, many muscle movements are a combination of isometric and isotonic contraction. For example, during walking, isotonic contraction results in shortening of the leg, and during isometric contraction, the stiff leg pushes against the floor.

The speed of the muscle contraction is variable. Myoglobulin is a hemoglobin-like protein pigment present in striated muscle cells that transports oxygen. Muscles containing large quantities of myoglobulin (red muscles) have been observed to contract slowly and powerfully (eg, respiratory and postural muscles). Muscles containing little myoglobulin (white muscles) contract quickly (eg, extraocular eye muscles). Most body muscles contain both red and white muscle fibers.

Muscle Tone

Relaxed muscles demonstrate a state of readiness to respond to contraction stimuli. This state of readiness is known as muscle **tone** (*tonus*) and is due to the maintenance of some of the muscle fibers in a contracted state. Muscle spindles, which are sense organs in the muscles, monitor muscle tone. Muscle tone is minimal during sleep and increased when the person is anxious. A muscle that has less than normal tone is known as **flaccid**; a muscle with greater than normal tone is described as **spastic**. In conditions characterized by lower motor neuron destruction (eg, polio), denervated muscle becomes **atonic** (soft and flabby) and atrophies.

Muscle Actions

Muscles accomplish movement by contraction. Through the coordination of muscle groups, the body is able to perform a wide variety of movements (Chart 60-1). The prime mover is the muscle that causes a particular motion. The muscles assisting the prime mover are known as synergists. The muscle causing movement opposite to that of the prime mover is known as the antagonist. The antagonist must relax to allow the prime mover to contract, producing motion. For example, when contraction of the biceps causes flexion of the elbow joint, the biceps is the prime mover, and the triceps is the antagonist. A person with muscle **paralysis**, which is a loss of movement possibly from nerve damage, may be able to retrain functioning muscles within the synergistic group to produce the needed movement. Muscles of the synergistic group then become the prime mover.

Exercise, Disuse, and Repair

Muscles need to be exercised to maintain function and strength. When a muscle repeatedly develops maximum or close to maximum tension over a long time, as in regular exercise with weights, the cross-sectional area of the muscle increases. This enlargement, known as **hypertrophy**, is due to an increase in the size of individual muscle fibers without an increase in the number of muscle fibers. Hypertrophy persists only if the exercise is continued. The opposite phenomenon occurs with disuse of muscle over a long period of time. Age and disuse cause loss of muscular function as fibrotic tissue replaces the contractile muscle tissue. The decrease in the size of a muscle is called **atrophy**. Bed rest and immobility cause loss of muscle mass and strength. When immobility is due to a treatment mode (eg, casting or traction), the patient can decrease the effects of immobility by isometric exercise of the muscles of the immobilized part. Quadriceps setting exercises (tightening the muscles of the thigh) and gluteal setting exercises (tightening of the muscles of the buttocks) help maintain the larger muscle groups that are important in ambulation. Active and weight-resistant exercises of uninjured parts of the body maintain muscle strength. When muscles are injured, they need rest and immobilization until tissue repair occurs. The healed muscle then needs progressive exercise to resume its preinjury strength and functional ability.

Gerontologic Considerations

Multiple changes in the musculoskeletal system occur with aging. Bone mass peaks at about 35 years of age, after which there is a universal gradual loss of bone. There is a loss of height due to **osteoporosis** (abnormal excessive bone loss), kyphosis, thinned intervertebral disks, and flexion of the knees and hips. Numerous metabolic changes, including menopausal withdrawal of estrogen and decreased activity, contribute to osteoporosis. Women lose more bone mass than men. Additionally, bones change in shape and have reduced strength. If a fracture occurs, fibrous tissue develops more slowly in the aged. In the elderly, collagen structures are less able to absorb energy. Ligaments become weak. The articular cartilage degenerates in weight-bearing areas and heals less readily. This contributes to the development of osteoarthritis. Joints enlarge, and range of motion decreases. Muscle mass and strength are also diminished. There is an actual loss in the size and number of muscle fibers due to myofibril atrophy with fibrous tissue replacement. Increased inactivity, diminished neuron stimulation, and nutritional deficiencies contribute to loss of muscle strength. In addition, remote musculoskeletal problems for which the patient has compensated may become new problems with age-related changes. For example, people who have recovered from polio and who have been able to function normally by using synergistic muscle groups may discover increasing incapacity because

CHART 60•1 Body Movements Produced by Muscle Contraction

Muscle contraction produces a variety of movements:

- Flexion—bending at a joint (eg, elbow)
- Extension—straightening at a joint
- Abduction—moving away from midline
- Adduction—moving toward midline
- Rotation—turning around a specific axis (eg, shoulder joint)
- Circumduction—conelike movement
- Supination—turning upward
- Pronation—turning downward
- Inversion—turning inward
- Eversion—turning outward
- Protraction—pushing forward
- Retraction—pulling backward

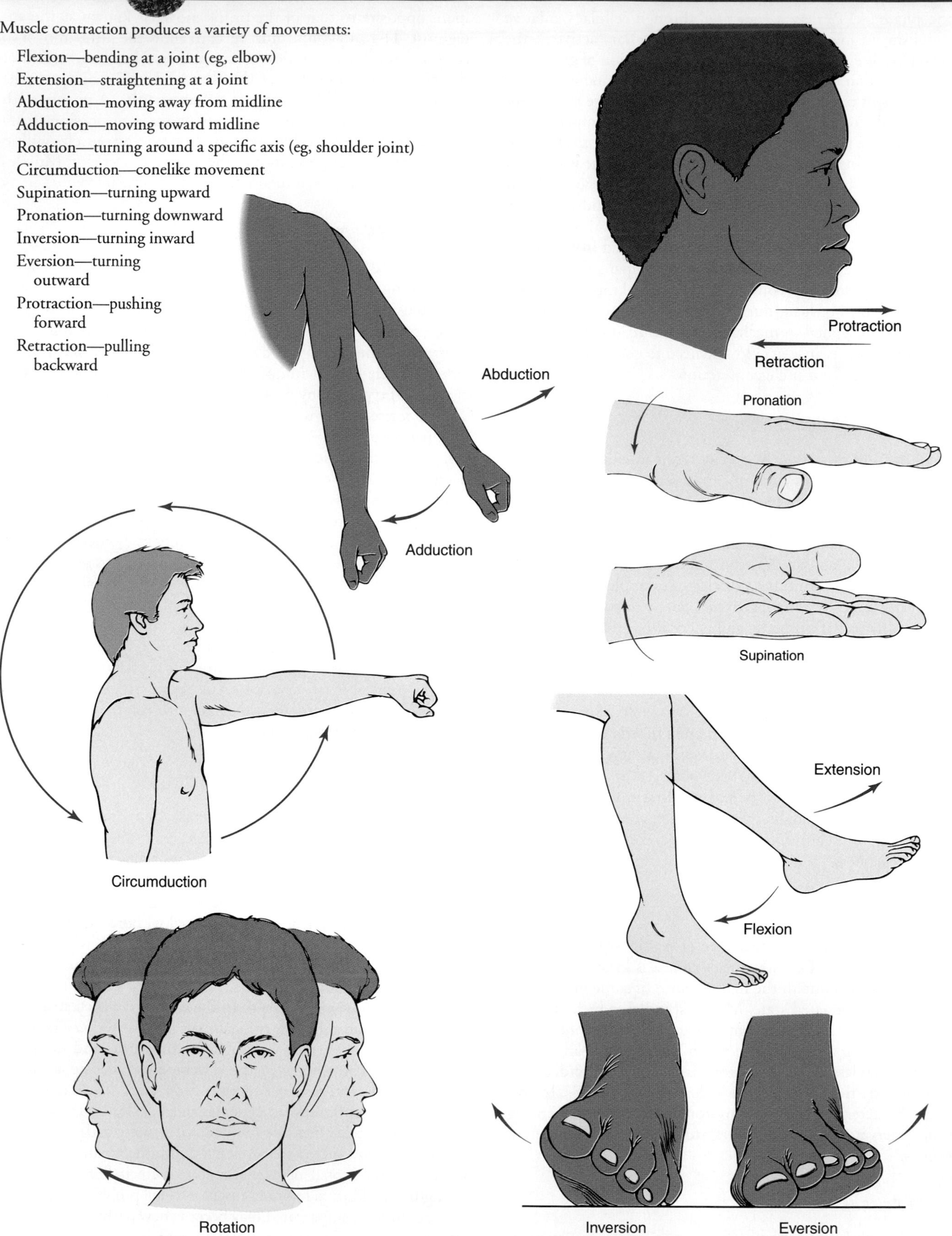

From Weber, J. W., & Kelley, J. (1998). *Health assessment in nursing.* Philadelphia: Lippincott-Raven.

of a reduced compensatory ability. Many of the effects of aging, however, can be slowed if the body is kept healthy and active through positive lifestyle behaviors.

ASSESSMENT

Health History

The nursing assessment of the patient with musculoskeletal dysfunction includes an evaluation of the effects of the musculoskeletal problem on the patient. The nurse is concerned with assisting patients with musculoskeletal problems to maintain their general health, accomplish their activities of daily living, and manage their treatment programs. The nurse ensures systemic homeostasis, encourages optimal nutrition, and prevents problems related to immobility. Through an individualized plan of nursing care, the nurse helps the patient achieve maximum health.

Initial Interview

In the initial interview, the nurse obtains a general impression of the patient's health status, obtaining subjective data from the patient concerning the onset of the problem and how it has been managed, as well as the patient's perceptions and expectations related to health. Concurrent health problems (eg, diabetes, heart disease, upper respiratory infection) need to be considered as well when developing the plan of care. A history of medication use and response to pain medication aids in designing medication management regimens.

The nurse notes allergies and describes them in terms of the reactions they produce in the patient. The nurse also assesses the patient's use of tobacco, alcohol, and other drugs to evaluate how these agents may affect patient care. Information concerning the patient's learning ability, economic status, and current occupation is needed for rehabilitation and discharge planning. Additions to the initial interview data are made as the nurse interacts with the patient. Such data assist the nurse to adjust the individualized plan of care as needed.

Subjective Assessment Data

During the interview and physical assessment, the patient may report pain, tenderness, tightness, and abnormal sensations. The nurse assesses and documents this information.

PAIN

Most patients with diseases and traumatic conditions or disorders of muscles, bones, and joints experience pain. Bone pain is characteristically described as a dull, deep ache that is boring in nature, whereas muscular pain is described as soreness or aching and is referred to as "muscle cramps." Fracture pain is sharp and piercing and is relieved by immobilization. Sharp pain may also result from bone infection with muscle spasm or pressure on a sensory nerve.

Most musculoskeletal pain is relieved by rest. Pain that increases with activity may indicate joint sprain or muscle strain, whereas steadily increasing pain points to a progression of an infectious process (osteomyelitis), a malignant tumor, or neurovascular complications. Radiating pain occurs in conditions in which pressure is exerted on a nerve root. Pain is variable, and its assessment and nursing management must be individualized.

Questions that the nurse can ask regarding pain include the following:

- What was the patient doing before the pain occurred?
- Is the body in proper alignment?
- Is there pressure from traction, bed linens, a cast, or other appliances?
- Is there tension on the skin at the pin site?
- Is the pain localized?
- How does the patient describe the pain?
- How intense is the pain on a scale of 0 to 10 (with 10 being the worst possible pain)?
- What was the manner of onset?
- Does the pain radiate? If so, in what direction?
- Is there pain in any other part of the body?
- What is the character of the pain (sharp, dull, boring, shooting, throbbing, cramping)?
- Is it constant?
- What relieves it?
- What makes it worse?
- Does the patient experience increased discomfort when overly tired from lack of sleep, exciting stimuli, or too much activity?

It is important that the patient's pain and discomfort be managed successfully. Not only is pain exhausting; if prolonged, it can force the patient to become increasingly preoccupied and dependent (see Chap. 12).

ALTERED SENSATIONS

Sensory disturbances are frequently associated with musculoskeletal problems. The patient may describe **paresthesias**, which are burning, tingling sensations or numbness. These sensations may be from pressure on nerves or circulatory impairment. Soft tissue swelling or direct trauma to these structures can impair their function. Loss of function can result from impaired nerves and circulatory structures. The nurse assesses the neurovascular status of the involved musculoskeletal area. Questions that the nurse can ask regarding altered sensations include the following:

- Is the patient experiencing any abnormal sensations or numbness?
- When did this begin? Is it getting worse?
- Does the patient also have pain?
- What is the color of the part distal to the affected area? Is it pale? Dusky? Cyanotic?
- Is a pulse palpable distal to the affected area?
- Does rapid capillary refill occur? (The nurse can gently squeeze the nail until it blanches, after which the nail pressure is released. The amount of time for the color under the nail to return to normal is noted. Color normally returns within 3 seconds. The return of color is evidence of capillary refill.)
- Is the motor component of the nerve intact? Can the patient move the innervated part?
- Is edema present?
- Is any constrictive device or clothing causing nerve or vascular compression?
- Are symptoms decreased by elevating the affected part or modifying its position?

Physical Assessment

An examination of the musculoskeletal system ranges from a basic assessment of functional capabilities to sophisticated physical examination maneuvers that facilitate diagnosis of specific bone, muscle, and joint disorders. The extent of assessment depends on the patient's physical complaints, health history, and physical clues that warrant further exploration. The nursing assessment is primarily a functional evaluation, focusing on the patient's ability to perform activities of daily living.

Techniques of inspection and palpation are employed to evaluate the patient's posture, gait, bone integrity, joint function, and muscle strength and size. In addition, assessing the skin and neurovascular status is an important part of a complete musculoskeletal assessment. The nurse also should understand and be able to perform correct assessment techniques on patients with musculoskeletal trauma. When specific symptoms or physical findings of musculoskeletal dysfunction are apparent, the nurse carefully documents the examination findings and shares the information with the physician, who may decide that more extensive examination and diagnostic workup are necessary.

Assessing Posture

The normal curvature of the spine is convex through the thoracic portion and concave through the cervical and lumbar portions. Common deformities of the spine include **kyphosis**, an increased forward curvature of the thoracic spine; **lordosis**, or swayback, an exaggerated curvature of the lumbar spine (Fig. 60-4) and **scoliosis**, a lateral curving deviation of the spine. Kyphosis is frequently seen in the elderly patient with osteoporosis and in some patients with neuromuscular diseases. Scoliosis may be congenital, idiopathic (without an identifiable cause), or a result of damage to the paraspinal muscles, as in poliomyelitis. Lordosis is frequently seen during pregnancy as the woman adjusts her posture for changes in her center of gravity.

During inspection of the spine, the entire back, buttocks, and legs are exposed. The examiner inspects the spinal curves and trunk symmetry from posterior and lateral views. Standing behind the patient, the examiner notes any differences in the height of the shoulders or iliac crests. The gluteal folds are normally symmetric. Shoulder and hip symmetry, as well as the line of the vertebral column, are inspected with the patient erect and bending forward (flexion). (Scoliosis is evidenced by an abnormal lateral curve in the spine, shoulders that are not level, asymmetric waistline, and a prominent scapula, accentuated by the bending forward test.) Older adults experience a loss in height due to loss of vertebral cartilage and osteoporosis. Therefore, an adult's height should be measured periodically.

Assessing Gait

Gait is assessed by having the patient walk away from the examiner for a short distance.

The examiner observes the patient's gait for smoothness and rhythm. Any unsteadiness or irregular movements (frequently noted in elderly patients) are considered abnormal. When a limping motion is noted, it is most frequently due to painful weight bearing. In such instances, the patient can usually pinpoint the area of discomfort, thus guiding further examination. When one extremity is shorter than another, a limp may also be observed as the patient's pelvis drops downward on the affected side with each step. Limited joint motion may affect gait. In addition, a variety of neurologic conditions are associated with abnormal gaits (eg, spastic hemiparesis gait—stroke; steppage gait—lower motor neuron disease; shuffling gait—Parkinson's disease).

Assessing Bone Integrity

The bony skeleton is assessed for deformities and alignment. Symmetric parts of the body are compared. Abnormal bony growths due to bone tumors may be observed. Shortened extremities, amputations, and body parts that are not in anatomic alignment are noted. Fracture findings may include abnormal angulation of long

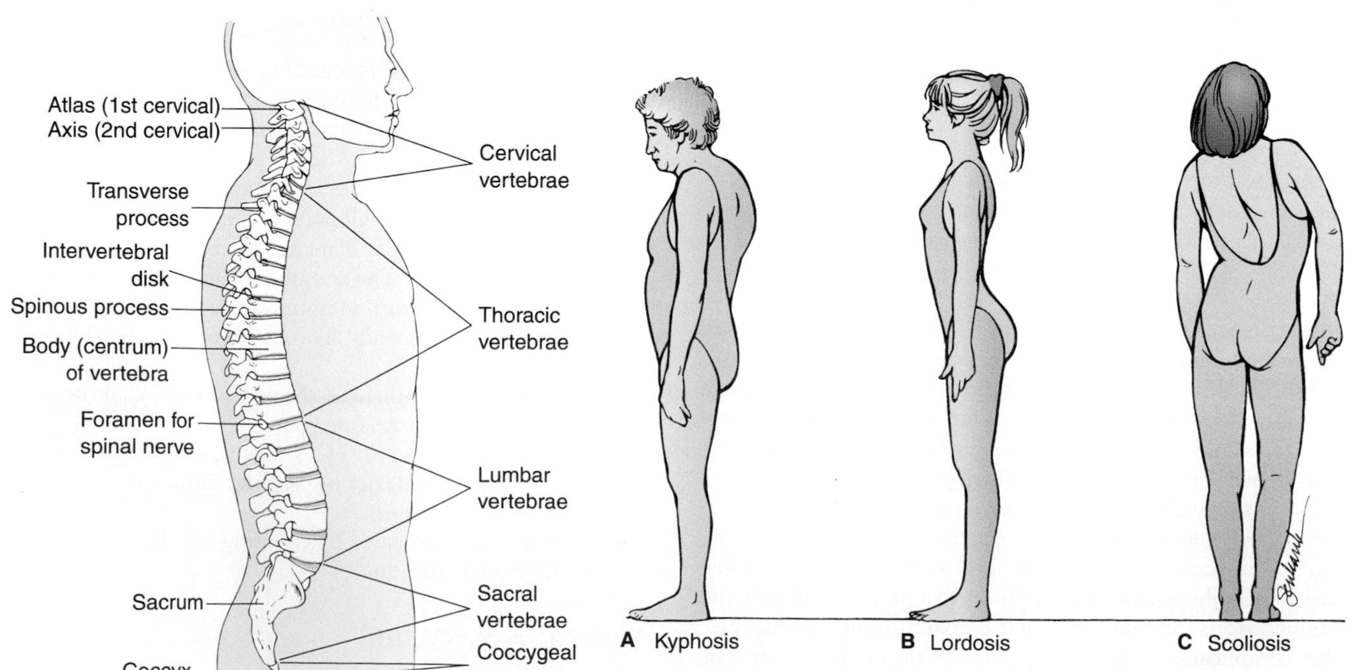

FIGURE 60•4 A normal spine and three abnormalities. (**A**) Kyphosis: an increased convexity or roundness of the spine's thoracic curve. (**B**) Lordosis: swayback; exaggeration of the lumbar spine curve. (**C**) Scoliosis: a lateral curvature of the spine.

bones, motion at points other than joints, and **crepitus** (a grating sound) at the point of abnormal motion. Movement of fracture fragments must be minimized to avoid additional injury.

Assessing Joint Function

The articular system is evaluated by noting range of motion, deformity, stability, and nodular formation. Range of motion is evaluated both actively (joint is moved by the muscles surrounding the joint) and passively (joint is moved by the examiner). The examiner is familiar with the normal range of motion of major joints. (See Chap. 10 for normal ranges of motion.) Precise measurement of range of motion can be made by a goniometer (a protractor designed for evaluating joint motion). Limited range of motion may be due to skeletal deformity, joint pathology, or **contracture** of surrounding muscles and tendons. In elderly patients, limitations of range of motion associated with degenerative joint disease may reduce their ability to perform activities of daily living.

If joint motion is compromised or the joint is painful, the joint is examined for **effusion,** which is excessive fluid within the capsule; swelling; and increased temperature that may reflect active inflammation. An effusion is suspected when the joint is swollen in size and the normal bony landmarks are obscured. The most common site for joint effusion is the knee. If a small amount of fluid is present in the joint spaces beneath the patella, it may be identified by the following maneuver: the medial and lateral aspects of the extended knee are milked firmly in a downward motion. This displaces any fluid downward. As pressure is exerted against the medial or lateral side, the examiner observes the opposite side for a bulge below the patella. When larger amounts of fluid are present, the patella becomes elevated from the femur during knee extension and the ballottement test is positive (Fig. 60-5). When inflammation or fluid is suspected in a joint, physician consultation is indicated.

Joint deformity may be due to **contracture** (shortening of surrounding joint structures), dislocation (complete separation of joint surfaces), subluxation (partial separation of articular surfaces), or disruption of structures surrounding the joint. Weakness or disruption of joint-supporting structures may result in a weak joint that requires an external supporting appliance (eg, brace).

Palpation of the joint while it is passively moved provides information about the integrity of the joint. Normally, the joint moves smoothly. A snap or a crack may indicate that a ligament is slipping over a bony prominence. Slightly roughened surfaces, as in arthritic conditions, result in **crepitus** (grating, crackling sound or sensation) as the irregular joint surfaces are moved across one another.

The tissues surrounding joints are examined for nodule formation. Rheumatoid arthritis, gout, and osteoarthritis produce characteristic nodules. The subcutaneous nodules of rheumatoid arthritis are soft and occur within and along tendons that provide extensor function to the joints. The nodules of gout are hard and lie within and immediately adjacent to the joint capsule itself. They may rupture, exuding white uric acid crystals onto the skin surface. Osteoarthritic nodules are hard and painless and represent bony overgrowth that has resulted from destruction of the cartilaginous surface of bone within the joint capsule. They are frequently seen in older adults.

Often, the size of the joint is exaggerated by the atrophy of muscles proximal and distal to that joint. This is seen in rheumatoid arthritis of the knees, in which the quadriceps muscle may atrophy dramatically. In rheumatoid arthritis, joint involvement assumes a symmetric pattern (Fig. 60-6). (See Chap. 50 for further information about rheumatoid arthritis.)

Assessing Muscle Strength and Size

The muscular system is assessed by noting the patient's ability to change position, muscular strength and coordination, and the size of individual muscles. Weakness of a group of muscles might indicate a variety of conditions, such as polyneuropathy, electrolyte disturbances (particularly potassium and calcium), myasthenia gravis, poliomyelitis, and muscular dystrophy. By palpating the muscle while passively moving the relaxed extremity, the nurse can determine the muscle tone. Muscle strength can be assessed by having the patient perform certain maneuvers with and without added resistance. For example, the biceps can be tested by requesting the patient to extend the arm fully and then flex it against resistance applied by the nurse. A simple handshake may provide an indication of grasp strength.

Muscle **clonus** (rhythmic contractions of a muscle) may be elicited in the ankle or wrist by sudden, forceful, sustained dorsiflexion of the foot or extension of the wrist. **Fasciculations** (involuntary twitching of muscle fiber groups) may be observed.

The girth of an extremity may be measured to monitor increased size due to exercise, edema, or bleeding into the muscle; also, it may be used to detect a decrease in size due to atrophy. The unaffected extremity is measured and used as the reference standard. Measurements are to be taken at the maximum circumference of the

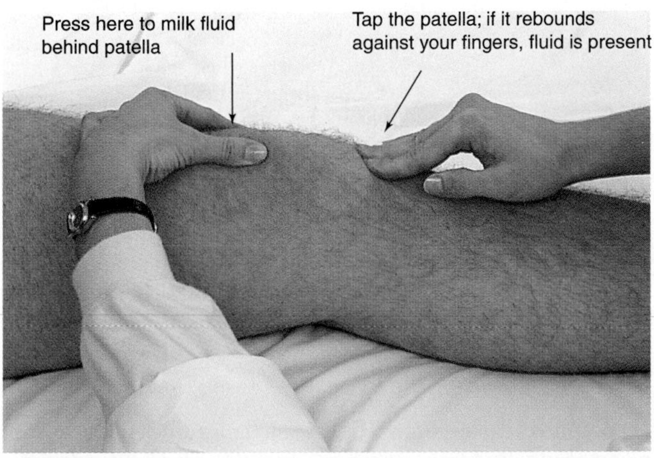
Press here to milk fluid behind patella
Tap the patella; if it rebounds against your fingers, fluid is present

FIGURE 60•5 Ballottement test to detect fluid in the knee. From Weber, J.W., & Kelley, J. (1998). *Health assessment in nursing.* Philadelphia: Lippincott-Raven.

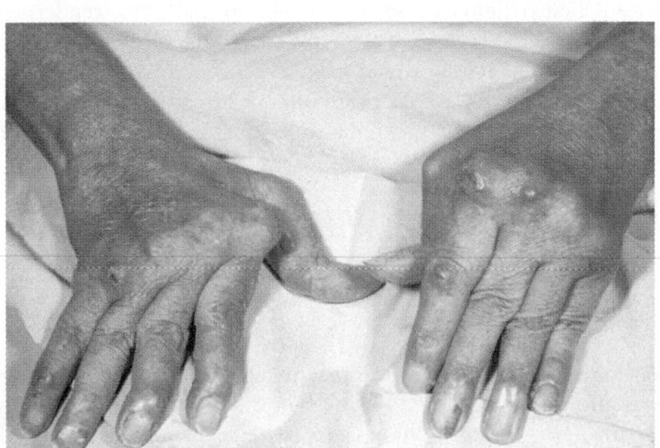

FIGURE 60•6 Rheumatoid arthritis.

extremity. It is important that the measurements be at the same location on the extremity and with the extremity in the same position with the muscle at rest. Distance from a specific anatomic landmark (eg, 10 cm below the medial aspect of the knee for measurement of the calf muscle) should be indicated in the patient's record so that subsequent measurements are made at the same point. For ease of serial assessment, the point of measurement can be indicated by marking the skin. Variations in size greater than 1 cm are considered significant.

Assessing Skin

In addition to assessing the musculoskeletal system, the nurse inspects the skin for edema, temperature, and color. Palpation of the skin can reveal whether any areas are warmer, suggesting increased perfusion or infection, or cooler, suggesting decreased perfusion, and whether edema is present. Cuts, bruises, skin color, and evidence of decreased circulation or infection can influence nursing management of musculoskeletal conditions.

Assessing Neurovascular Status

It is important for the nurse to perform frequent neurovascular assessments on the patient with a musculoskeletal disorder (especially fractures) because of the risk of tissue and nerve damage. One complication that the nurse needs to be alert for when assessing the patient is compartment syndrome. This major neurovascular problem is caused by pressure within a muscle compartment increasing to such an extent that microcirculation decreases, which leads to nerve and muscle anoxia and necrosis. Permanent function can be lost if the anoxic situation continues for more than 6 hours. Assessment of neurovascular status (Chart 60-2) is frequently referred to as assessment of CMS (circulation, motion, and sensation).

Assessing the Patient with Musculoskeletal Injury

Special precautions must be taken when assessing a trauma patient. With injury to the extremity, it is important to assess for soft tissue trauma, deformity, and neurovascular status (ie, CMS). If the patient has a possible cervical spine injury and is wearing a cervical collar, the collar must not be removed until absence of spinal cord injury is confirmed by x-ray. When the collar is removed, the cervical spine area is gently assessed for swelling, tenderness, and deformity. With pelvic injury, abdominal organ injuries may occur. The patient is assessed for abdominal pain, tenderness, hematomas, and the presence or absence of femoral pulses. When blood is present at the urinary meatus, bladder and urethral injury are suspected, and the patient should not be catheterized. Instead, such findings should be reported immediately to the primary health care provider.

ASSESSMENT
PERIPHERAL NERVE FUNCTION

Assessment of peripheral nerve function has two key elements: evaluation of sensation and evaluation of motion. One or all of the following may be performed by the nurse during a musculoskeletal assessment.

	Test of Sensation	Test of Movement	
	Peroneal nerve		
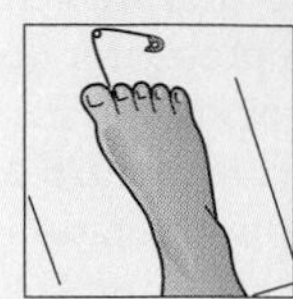	Prick the skin centered between the great and second toe.	Ask the patient to dorsiflex the ankle and extend the toes.	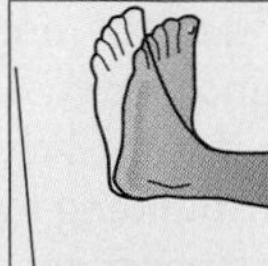
	Tibial nerve		
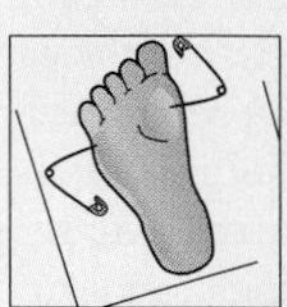	Prick the medial and lateral surface of the sole.	Ask the patient to plantar flex toes and ankle.	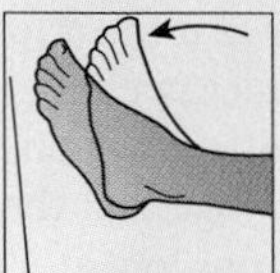
	Radial nerve		
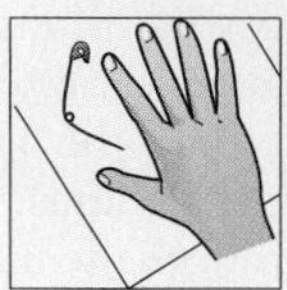	Prick the skin centered between the thumb and second finger	Ask the patient to stretch out thumb, then the wrist, and then the fingers at the metacarpal joints	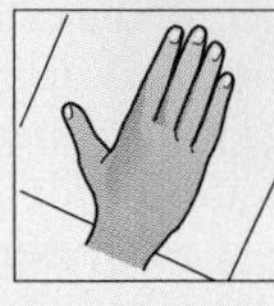
	Ulnar nerve		
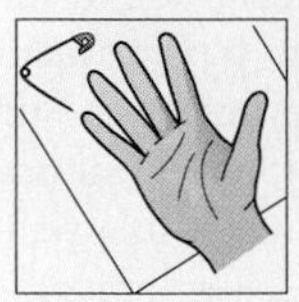	Prick the fat pad at the top of the small finger	Ask the patient to spread all fingers	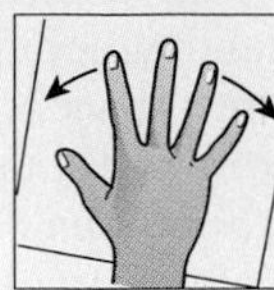
	Median nerve		
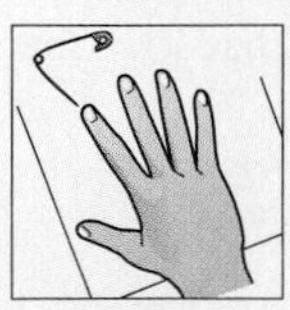	Prick the top or distal surface of the index finger	Ask the patient to touch the thumb to the little finger. Also observe whether the patient can flex the wrist.	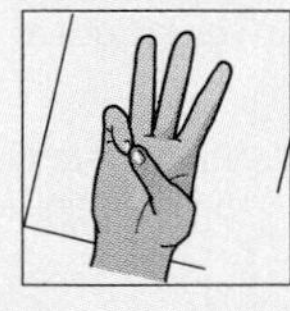

DIAGNOSTIC EVALUATION

Imaging Procedures

Radiographic Studies

Radiographic studies are important in evaluating patients with musculoskeletal disorders. Bone x-rays determine bone density, texture, erosion, and changes in bone relationships. Multiple x-rays are needed for full assessment of the structure being examined. X-ray study of the cortex of the bone reveals any widening, narrowing, and signs of irregularity. Joint x-rays reveal fluid, irregularity, spur formation, narrowing, and changes in the joint structure. When positioned for the study, the patient must remain still while the x-rays are taken.

Computed Tomography

A computed tomography (CT) scan shows in detail a specific plane of involved bone and can reveal tumors of the soft tissue or injuries to the ligaments or tendons. It is used to identify the location and extent of fractures in areas difficult to evaluate (eg, the acetabulum). CT studies, which may be performed with or

CHART 60•2 Indicators of Neurovascular Compromise

Circulation
- Color: Pale or cyanotic
- Temperature: Cool
- Capillary refill: More than 3 seconds

Motion
- Weak
- Paralysis

Sensation
- Paresthesia
- Unrelenting pain
- Pain on passive stretch
- Absence of feeling

without contrast agents, last about 1 hour. The patient must remain still during the procedure.

Magnetic Resonance Imaging

Magnetic resonance imaging (MRI) is a noninvasive, special imaging technique that uses magnetic fields, radio waves, and computers to demonstrate abnormalities (ie, tumors or narrowing of tissue pathways through bone) of soft tissue, such as muscle, tendon, cartilage, nerve, and fat. Because an electromagnet is used, patients with any metal implants, clips, or pacemakers are not candidates for MRI. Jewelry, hair clips, hearing aids, credit cards with magnetic strips, and other metal must be removed before the MRI. Patients who experience claustrophobia may be unable to tolerate the confinement of closed MRI equipment without sedation. To enhance visualization of anatomic structures, contrast media may be injected intravenously. During the procedure, the patient needs to lie still for 1 to 2 hours and will hear a rhythmic knocking sound.

Arthrography

Arthrography is useful in identifying acute or chronic tears of the joint capsule or supporting ligaments of the knee, shoulder, ankle, hip, or wrist. A radiopaque substance or air is injected into the joint cavity to outline soft tissue structures and the contour of the joint. The joint is put through its range of motion to distribute the contrast agent while a series of x-rays are obtained. If a tear is present, the contrast agent leaks out of the joint and is evident on the radiographs.

Bone Densitometry

Bone densitometry is used to estimate bone density. This can be done through the use of x-rays or ultrasound. Dual-photon absorptiometry and dual-energy x-rays determine bone mineral density at the wrist, hip, or spine to estimate the extent of osteoporosis and to monitor a patient's response to treatment for osteoporosis. Bone sonometer (ultrasound) measures heel bone quantity and quality and is used to estimate bone density and the risk of fracture for people with osteoporosis. Studies demonstrate that ultrasonic measures are comparable to those of absorptiometry in accurately diagnosing osteoporosis and predicting a person's risk for fracture.

Nursing Interventions

Before the patient undergoes an imaging study, the nurse should assess for conditions that may require special consideration during the study or that may be a contraindication to the study, for example, pregnancy; claustrophobia; inability to tolerate required positioning due to age, debility, or deformity; and metal implants. The nurse should make sure that the patient removes all jewelry, hair clips, hearing aids, and other metal before having an MRI. If contrast agents will be used for CT scan, MRI, or arthrography, the nurse should carefully assess for possible allergy.

After an arthrogram, the joint is usually rested for 12 hours, and a compression elastic bandage is applied as prescribed. In addition, the nurse provides comfort measures (mild analgesia, ice) as appropriate. The nurse should explain to the patient that it is normal to experience clicking or crackling in the joint for a day or two after the procedure while the contrast agent or air is absorbed.

Nuclear Studies

Bone Scan

A bone scan is performed to detect metastatic and primary bone tumors, osteomyelitis, certain fractures, and aseptic necrosis. A bone-seeking radioisotope is injected intravenously. The scan is performed 2 to 3 hours after the injection. At this point, distribution and concentration of the isotope in the bone are determined. The degree of nuclide uptake is related to the metabolism of the bone. An increased uptake of isotope is seen in primary skeletal disease (osteosarcoma), metastatic bone disease, inflammatory skeletal disease (osteomyelitis), and certain types of fractures.

NURSING INTERVENTIONS

Before the patient undergoes a bone scan, the nurse should assess for possible allergy to the radioisotope and for any condition that would contraindicate performing the procedure (eg, pregnancy). In addition, it is important to encourage the patient to drink plenty of fluids to help distribute and eliminate the isotope. Prior to the scan the nurse asks the patient to empty the bladder.

Endoscopic Studies

Arthroscopy

Arthroscopy is a procedure that allows direct visualization of a joint to diagnose joint disorders. Treatment of tears, defects, and disease processes may be performed through the arthroscope. The procedure is carried out in the operating room under sterile conditions; injection of a local anesthetic into the joint or general anesthesia is used. A large-bore needle is inserted, and the joint is distended with saline. The arthroscope is introduced, and joint structures, synovium, and articular surfaces are visualized. After the procedure, the puncture wound is closed with adhesive stripes or sutures and covered with a sterile dressing. Complications are rare but may include infection, hemarthrosis, neurovascular compromise, thrombophlebitis, stiffness, effusion, adhesions, and delayed wound healing.

NURSING INTERVENTIONS

The joint is wrapped with a compression dressing to control swelling. In addition, ice may be applied to control edema and discomfort. Frequently, the joint is kept extended and elevated to reduce swelling. It is important to monitor neurovascular function. The nurse administers prescribed analgesics to control discomfort. The nurse should explain when the patient can resume activity and what weight-bearing limits to follow as prescribed by the primary care provider.

Other Studies

Arthrocentesis

Arthrocentesis (joint aspiration) is carried out to obtain synovial fluid for purposes of examination or to relieve pain due to effusion. Examination of synovial fluid is helpful in the diagnosis of septic arthritis and other inflammatory arthropathies and reveals the presence of hemarthrosis (bleeding into the joint cavity), which suggests trauma or a bleeding disorder. Normally, synovial fluid is clear, pale, straw-colored, and scanty in volume. Using aseptic technique, the physician inserts a needle into the joint and aspirates fluid. Anti-inflammatory medications may be injected into the joint. A sterile dressing is applied after aspiration. There is a risk for infection after this procedure.

Electromyography

Electromyography provides information about the electrical potential of the muscles and the nerves leading to them. The test is done to evaluate muscle weakness, pain, and disability. The purpose of the procedure is to determine any abnormality of function and to differentiate muscle and nerve problems. Needle electrodes are inserted into selected muscles, and responses to electrical stimuli are recorded on an oscilloscope. Warm compresses may relieve residual discomfort after the study.

Biopsy

Biopsy may be performed to determine the structure and composition of bone marrow, muscle, and synovium to help determine specific diseases.

NURSING INTERVENTIONS

The nurse monitors the biopsy site for edema, bleeding, pain, and infection. The nurse applies ice as prescribed to control bleeding and edema. In addition, analgesics are administered as prescribed for comfort.

Laboratory Studies

Examination of the patient's blood and urine can provide information about a primary musculoskeletal problem (eg, Paget's disease), a developing complication (eg, infection), the baseline for instituting therapy (eg, anticoagulant therapy), or response to therapy. The complete blood count includes the hemoglobin level (frequently lower after bleeding associated with trauma and surgery) and the white blood cell count (elevated in acute infections, trauma, acute hemorrhage, tissue necrosis). Before surgery, coagulation studies are performed to detect bleeding tendencies (because bone is very vascular tissue).

Blood chemistry studies provide data about a wide variety of musculoskeletal conditions. Serum calcium levels are altered in patients with osteomalacia, parathyroid function, Paget's disease, metastatic bone tumors, and prolonged immobilization. Serum phosphorus levels are inversely related to calcium levels and are diminished in osteomalacia associated with malabsorption syndrome. Acid phosphatase is elevated in Paget's disease and metastatic cancer. Alkaline phosphatase is elevated during early fracture healing and in diseases with increased osteoblastic activity (eg, metastatic bone tumors). Bone metabolism may be evaluated through thyroid studies and determination of calcitonin, parathyroid hormone, and vitamin D levels. Serum enzyme levels of creatine kinase and aspartate aminotransferase (serum glutamic-oxaloacetic transaminase) become elevated with muscle damage. Aldolase is elevated in muscle diseases (eg, muscular dystrophy and skeletal muscle necrosis). Serum osteocalcin (bone GLA protein) indicates the rate of bone turnover. Urine calcium levels increase with bone destruction (eg, parathyroid dysfunction, metastatic bone tumors, multiple myeloma).

NURSING IMPLICATIONS

Determining the patient's functional status and health care needs is an integral part of the nursing assessment. Nursing diagnoses and the care plan are developed and modified according to the patient's needs.

During the period of assessment, the patient requires support and nursing care, including physical and psychological preparation for examinations and tests. Patient education before the tests (what is to be done; why it is being done; what the patient can expect to experience, including tactile, visual, and auditory sensations; and what patient participation is expected) reduce anxiety and enable the patient to be an active participant in care.

The resulting medical diagnosis and prescribed treatment regimen affect the nursing management of the patient. The nursing plan of care includes nursing measures to facilitate the resolution of the patient's health problems and promotion of health. The nursing assessment enables the nurse to identify the health problems that can be improved by nursing interventions. In collaboration with the patient, health goals and nursing strategies are formulated to resolve the identified nursing diagnoses.

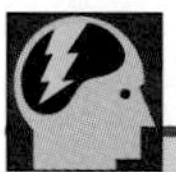

Critical Thinking Exercises

1.
A young man who has a cast applied to his fractured arm expresses concern that he will lose muscle strength because he cannot exercise his arm. How would you respond to him and address his concern? If the patient were an elderly woman who had broken her arm in a fall and now was fearful of falling again, how would your approach differ in addressing this patient's concerns?

2.
The son of an elderly patient asks why his mother is "so much shorter than she used to be." How would you explain this phenomenon to him? How might you incorporate preventive measures related to his mother's musculoskeletal condition into a teaching session?

3.
After arthroscopy, a patient complains that the dressing on his knee is too tight. He begins to loosen it. How would you react to his actions and why? If the patient had removed the dressing during the night without being detected and you discovered the fact early the next morning, how would the patient's situation have changed, and how would you respond to this different set of circumstances?

References and Selected Readings

Asterisks indicate nursing research.

BOOKS

*Bickley, L. S. & Hoekelman, R. A. (1999). *Bates' guide to physical assessment* (7th ed.). Philadelphia: Lippincott Williams & Wilkins.

Bucholz, R. (1996). *Orthopaedic decision making* (2nd ed.). St. Louis: C. V. Mosby.

Bullock, B. L. (1996). *Pathophysiology: Adaptations and alterations in function* (4th ed.). Philadelphia: Lippincott-Raven.

Carpenito, L. J. (1997). *Nursing diagnosis: Application to clinical practice* (7th ed.). Philadelphia: Lippincott-Raven.

Fischbach, F. (1996). *A manual of laboratory and diagnostic tests* (5th ed.). Philadelphia: Lippincott-Raven.

Maher, A. B., et al. (1998). *Orthopaedic nursing* (2nd ed.). Philadelphia: W. B. Saunders.

Porth, C. M. (1998). *Pathophysiology: Concepts of altered health states* (5th ed.). Philadelphia: Lippincott-Raven.

Salmond, S. W., et al. (Eds.). (1996). *Core curriculum for orthopaedic nursing* (3rd ed.). Pitman NJ: National Association of Orthopaedic Nurses.

*Seidel, H., et al. (1995). *Mosby's guide to physical examination* (3rd ed.). St. Louis: C. V. Mosby.

JOURNALS

Gallegos, S., & Michalec, D. (1996). Neurological assessment of the orthopaedic patient. *Orthopaedic Nursing, 15*(5), 23–29.

Krug, B. (1997). Rheumatoid arthritis and osteoarthritis: A basic comparison. *Orthopaedic Nursing 16*(5), 73–75.

Kunkler, C. (1999). Neurovascular assessment. *Orthopaedic Nursing 18*(3), 63–71.

*Maldonado, A., & Barger, M. (1998). Comprehensive assessment of common musculoskeletal disorders. *Journal of Nurse-Midwifery, 40*(2), 202–215.

O'Hanlon-Nichols, T. (1998). Basic assessment series: Musculoskeletal system. *American Journal of Nursing, 98*(6), 48–52.

Ross, D. (1996). Chronic compartment syndrome. *Orthopaedic Nursing, 15*(3), 23–27.

Schwappach, J., et al. (1997). Orthopedics. *Journal of the American Medical Association, 277*(23):1883–1884.

Strange, C. (1997). Muscles: Use them or lose them. *NCRR Reporter, 21*(1), 5–6, 8.

*Vonfrolio, L., & Noone, J. (1995). Understanding orthopedic emergencies. *Nursing, 25*(9), 32.

Resources

National Association of Orthopaedic Nurses (NAON), North Woodbury Road, Box 56, Pitman, NJ 08071-0056; 1-609-256-2310; naon@mail.ajj.com (E-mail); www.inurse.com/~naon

National Institute of Arthritis and Musculoskeletal and Skin Diseases, National Institutes of Health, Information Clearing House, Box AMS, 9000 Rockville Pike, Bethesda, MD 20892; 1-301-495-4484

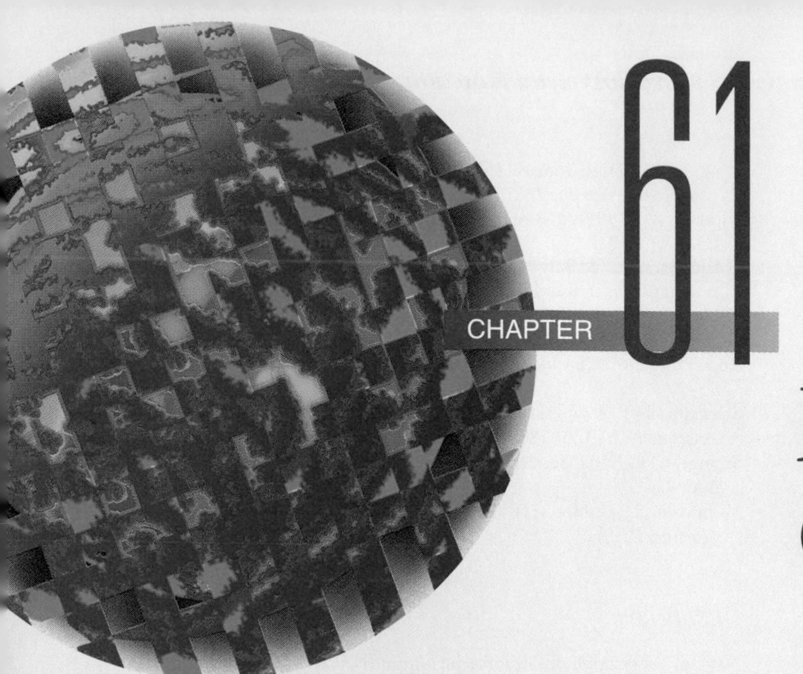

CHAPTER 61

Musculoskeletal Care Modalities

Learning Objectives

On completion of this chapter, the learner will be able to:

1. Describe the preventive and health teaching needs of the patient with a cast.
2. Use the nursing process as a framework for care of the patient with a cast.
3. Describe the various types of traction and the principles of effective traction.
4. Specify the preventive nursing care needs of the patient in traction.
5. Use the nursing process as a framework for care of the patient in traction.
6. Compare the nursing needs of the patient undergoing total hip replacement with those of the patient undergoing total knee replacement.
7. Use the nursing process as a framework for care of the patient undergoing orthopedic surgery.

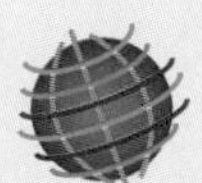

A **cast** is a rigid external immobilizing device that is molded to the contours of the body. The purposes of a cast are to immobilize a body part in a specific position and to apply uniform pressure on encased soft tissue.

GLOSSARY

abduction: movement away from the center or median line of the body

arthrodesis: surgical fusion of a joint

arthroplasty: surgical repair of a joint; joint replacement

avascular necrosis: death of tissue due to insufficient blood supply

brace: externally applied device to support body, control movement, and prevent injury

cast: rigid external immobilizing device molded to contours of body part

continuous passive motion (CPM) device: an instrument that promotes range of motion, healing, and circulation

edema: soft tissue swelling due to fluid accumulation

external fixator: external metal frame attached to and stabilizing bone fragments

fasciotomy: surgical procedure to release constricting muscle fascia to relieve muscle tissue pressure

fracture: a break in the continuity of the bone

heterotrophic ossification: formation of bone in the periprosthetic space

muscle spasm: involuntary contraction of muscle

neurovascular status: neurologic (motor and sensory components) and circulatory functioning of a body part

open reduction with **internal fixation (ORIF):** surgery to repair and stabilize a fracture

osteomyelitis: infection of the bone

osteotomy: surgical cutting of bone

sling: bandage used to support an arm

splint: device designed specifically to support and immobilize body part in desired position

traction: application of a pulling force to a part of the body

trapeze: overhead patient-helping device to promote patient mobility in bed

MANAGING CARE OF THE PATIENT IN A CAST

A cast is used specifically to immobilize a reduced **fracture**, correct a deformity, apply uniform pressure to underlying soft tissue, or support and stabilize weakened joints. Generally, casts permit mobilization of the patient while restricting movement of a body part.

The condition being treated influences the type and thickness of the cast applied. Generally speaking, the joints proximal and distal to the area to be immobilized are included in the cast. With some fractures, however, cast construction and molding may allow movement of a joint while immobilizing a fracture (eg, three-point fixation in a patellar tendon weight-bearing cast). Various types of casts include the following:

Short arm cast: Extends from below the elbow to the palmar crease, secured around the base of the thumb. If the thumb is included, it is known as a *thumb spica* or *gauntlet* cast.

Long arm cast: Extends from the upper level of the axillary fold to the proximal palmar crease. The elbow usually is immobilized at a right angle.

Short-leg cast: Extends from below the knee to the base of the toes. The foot is at a right angle in a neutral position.

Long-leg cast: Extends from the junction of the upper and middle third of the thigh to the base of the toes. The knee may be slightly flexed.

Walking cast: A short- or long-leg cast reinforced for strength.

Body cast: Encircles the trunk.

Shoulder spica cast: A body jacket that encloses the trunk and the shoulder and elbow.

Hip spica cast: Encloses the trunk and a lower extremity. A double hip spica cast includes both legs.

Figure 61-1 illustrates the long-arm and long-leg cast and areas in which pressure problems commonly occur with these casts.

Casting Materials

Plaster

The traditional cast is made of plaster. Rolls of plaster bandage are wet in cool water and applied smoothly to the body. A crystallizing reaction occurs, and heat is given off (an exothermic reaction). The heat given off during this reaction can be uncomfortable, and the nurse can inform the patient about the sensation of increasing warmth so that the patient does not become alarmed. Additionally, the nurse can explain that the cast needs to be exposed to allow maximum dissipation of the heat and that most casts cool after about 15 minutes.

The crystallization process produces a rigid dressing. The speed of the reaction varies from a few minutes to 15 to 20 minutes. The orthopedist determines the plaster setting speed appropriate for the cast being applied. After the plaster sets, the cast remains wet and somewhat soft. It does not have its full strength until dry. While damp, the cast can be dented. Therefore, it must be handled with the palms of the hand and not allowed to rest on hard surfaces or sharp edges. Cast dents may produce pressure areas on the skin under the cast, thereby promoting undesired irritation and potential skin breakdown. The cast requires 24 to 72 hours to dry completely, depending on its thickness and the environmental drying conditions. A freshly applied cast should be exposed to circulating air to dry and should not be covered with clothing or bed linens. A wet plaster cast appears dull and gray, sounds dull on percussion, feels damp, and smells musty. A dry plaster cast is white and shiny, resonant, odorless, and firm.

Nonplaster

Generally referred to as fiberglass casts, these water-activated polyurethane materials have the versatility of plaster but are lighter in weight, stronger, water resistant, and durable. They consist of an open-weave, nonabsorbent fabric impregnated with hardeners that reach full rigid strength in minutes.

Nonplaster casts are porous and therefore diminish skin problems. They do not soften when wet, which allows for hydrotherapy (use of water for treatment). When wet, they are dried with a hair drier on a cool setting. Thorough drying is important to prevent skin breakdown.

Arm Casts

The patient whose arm is immobilized in a cast must readjust to many routine tasks. The unaffected arm must assume all the upper extremity activities. The patient may experience fatigue

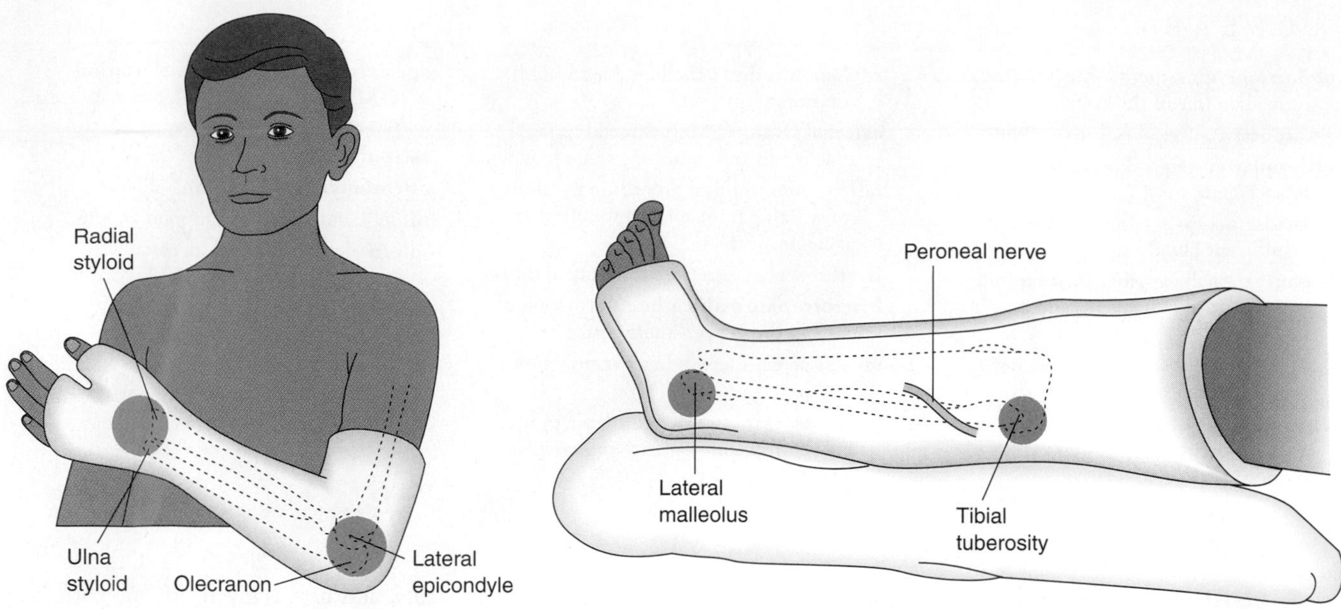

FIGURE 61•1 Pressure areas in common types of casts.

due to modified activities and the weight of the cast. Frequent rest periods are necessary.

Nursing Interventions

To control swelling, the nurse elevates the immobilized arm. When the patient is lying down, the arm is elevated so that each joint is positioned higher than the preceding proximal joint (eg, elbow higher than the shoulder, hand higher than the elbow).

A **sling** may be used when the patient ambulates. To prevent pressure on the cervical spinal nerves, the sling should distribute the supported weight over a large area and not on the back of the neck. The nurse encourages the patient to remove the arm from the sling and elevate it frequently.

Circulatory disturbances in the hand may become apparent with signs of cyanosis, swelling, and an inability to move the fingers. One serious effect of circulatory constriction in an arm cast is Volkmann's contracture, a form of compartment syndrome. Contracture of the fingers and wrist occurs as the result of obstructed arterial blood flow to the forearm and hand. The patient is unable to extend the fingers, describes abnormal sensation (eg, unrelenting pain, pain on passive stretch), and exhibits signs of diminished circulation to the hand.

This serious complication can be prevented with nursing surveillance and proper care. The nurse makes frequent neurovascular checks (see Chap. 60). Compartment syndrome is managed in part by bivalving the cast to remove constricting cast and dressings. A **fasciotomy** may be necessary to improve vascular status. Permanent damage develops within a few hours if action is not taken.

Leg Casts

The application of a leg cast imposes a degree of immobility on the patient. The cast may be a short leg cast, extending to the knee, or a long leg cast, extending to the groin. The fresh cast must be handled in a manner that will not cause denting or disruption.

Nursing Interventions

The nurse supports the patient's leg on pillows to heart level to control swelling and applies ice packs as prescribed over the fracture site for 1 or 2 days.

As with other cast applications, it is important to assess the leg for adequate circulation and normal nerve function. The nurse assesses circulation by observing the color, temperature, and capillary refill of the exposed toes. It is important to assess nerve function by observing the patient's ability to move the toes and by asking about the sensations in the foot. Numbness, tingling, and burning may be due to peroneal nerve injury from pressure at the head of the fibula.

Nursing Alert *Injury to the peroneal nerve as a result of pressure is a cause of footdrop (the inability to maintain the foot in a normally flexed position). Consequently, the patient drags the foot when ambulating.*

When the cast is hard and dry, the nurse teaches the patient how to transfer and ambulate safely with assistive devices (eg, crutches, walker). The gait to be used depends on whether the patient is permitted to bear weight. If weight-bearing is allowed, the cast is reinforced to withstand the body weight. A cast boot to wear over the casted foot provides a broad, nonskid walking surface.

When seated, the patient should elevate the casted leg. The patient should also lie down several times a day with the casted leg elevated to promote venous return.

Body or Spica Casts

Casts that encase the trunk (body cast) and portions of one or two extremities (spica cast) require special nursing strategies. Body casts are used to provide spinal immobility. Hip spicas are used for some femoral fractures and after some hip joint surgeries. Shoulder spica casts are used for some humeral neck fractures.

Nursing Interventions

Preparing and positioning the patient, assisting with skin care and hygiene, and monitoring for cast syndrome are nursing responsibilities. Explaining the procedure helps reduce the patient's apprehension about being encased in a large cast. The nurse reassures the patient that several people will provide care during the application, that support for the injured area will be adequate, and that care providers will be as gentle as possible. Medications for pain and relaxation administered before the procedure enable the patient to cooperate during the procedure.

Cracking or denting of the cast can be prevented by supporting the patient on a firm mattress and with flexible, waterproof pillows until the cast dries. The nurse positions the pillows next to each other because spaces between pillows allow the damp cast to sag, become weak, and possibly break. It is important not to place a pillow under the head and shoulders of a patient in a body cast while the cast is drying because this causes pressure on the chest.

The nurse turns the patient as a unit toward the uninjured side every 2 hours to relieve pressure and to allow the cast to dry. It is important to avoid twisting the patient's body within the cast. Sufficient personnel (at least three people) are needed when the patient is turned so that the fresh cast can be adequately supported with the palms of the hands at vulnerable points (ie, body joints) to prevent cracking. The nurse encourages the patient to assist in the repositioning, if not contraindicated, by using the **trapeze** or bed rail. A stabilizing abduction bar incorporated into a spica cast should not be used as a turning device. It is important to readjust pillows to provide support without creating areas of pressure.

The nurse turns the patient to a prone position, twice daily if tolerated, to provide postural drainage of the bronchial tree and relieve pressure on the back. A small pillow under the abdomen enhances comfort. The nurse can either place a pillow lengthwise under the dorsa of the feet or allow the toes to hang over the edge of the bed to prevent the toes from being forced into the mattress.

It is important to inspect the skin around the edges of the cast frequently for signs of irritation. Some of the area under the cast can be inspected by pulling the skin taut and using a flashlight. The skin can be bathed and massaged by reaching under the cast edges with the fingers.

The perineal opening must be large enough for hygienic care. To protect the cast from soiling, the nurse can insert clean dry plastic sheeting under the cast and over the cast edge before each elimination. Generally, fracture bedpans are easier for patients with a hip spica cast to use than regular bedpans.

Patients immobilized in large casts may develop cast syndrome, psychological and physiologic responses to the confinement. The psychological component is similar to a claustrophobic reaction. The patient exhibits an acute anxiety reaction characterized by behavioral changes and autonomic responses (eg, increased respiratory rate, diaphoresis, dilated pupils, increased heart rate, elevated blood pressure). The nurse needs to recognize the anxiety reaction and provide an environment in which the patient feels secure.

The physiologic cast syndrome responses are associated with immobility. With decreased physical activity, gastrointestinal motility decreases, intestinal gases accumulate, intestinal pressure increases, and ileus may occur. The patient exhibits abdominal distention, abdominal discomfort, nausea, and vomiting. As with other adynamic ileus situations, the patient is treated conservatively with decompression (nasogastric intubation connected to suction) and intravenous fluid therapy until gastrointestinal motility is restored. If the cast restricts the abdomen, the abdominal window must be enlarged. After the ileus resolves and bowel sounds resume, the patient gradually resumes an oral diet. Occasionally, the distention places traction on the superior mesenteric artery, reducing the blood supply to the bowel. The bowel may become gangrenous, which requires surgical intervention. The nurse monitors the patient in a large body cast for potential cast syndrome, noting bowel sounds every 4 to 8 hours, and reports distention, nausea, and vomiting.

NURSING PROCESS: THE PATIENT IN A CAST

Assessment

Before the cast is applied, the nurse completes an assessment of the patient's general health, presenting signs and symptoms, emotional status, understanding of the need for the cast, and condition of the body part to be immobilized in the cast. Physical assessment of the part to be immobilized must include assessment of the **neurovascular status**, degree and location of swelling, bruising, and skin abrasions.

Diagnosis

Nursing Diagnoses

Based on the assessment data, major nursing diagnoses for the patient with a cast may include the following:

- Knowledge deficit related to the treatment regimen
- Pain related to the musculoskeletal disorder
- Impaired physical mobility related to the cast
- Self-care deficit: bathing/hygiene, feeding, dressing/grooming, or toileting due to restricted mobility
- Impaired skin integrity related to lacerations and abrasions
- Risk for peripheral neurovascular dysfunction related to physiologic responses to injury and compression effect of cast

Collaborative Problems/Potential Complications

Based on the assessment data, potential complications that may develop include the following:

- Compartment syndrome
- Pressure ulcer
- Disuse syndrome

Planning and Goals

The major goals of the patient with a cast include knowledge of the treatment regimen, relief of pain, improved physical mobility, achievement of maximum level of self-care, healing of lacerations and abrasions, maintenance of adequate neurovascular function, and absence of complications.

Nursing Interventions

Explaining the Treatment Regimen

Before the cast is applied, the patient needs information concerning the pathologic problem and the purpose and expectations of the prescribed treatment regimen. This knowledge promotes the patient's active participation in and adherence to the treatment program. It is important to prepare the patient for the application of the cast by describing the anticipated sights, sounds, and sensations (eg, heat from hardening reaction of plaster). The patient needs to know what to expect during application and that the body part will be immobilized after casting (see Guideline 61-1).

Relieving Pain

The nurse must carefully evaluate pain associated with musculoskeletal problems, asking the patient to indicate the exact site and to describe the character and intensity of the pain to help determine its cause. Most pain can be relieved by elevating the involved part, applying cold as prescribed, and administering usual dosages of analgesics.

Nursing Alert *The nurse must immediately report unrelieved pain to the physician to avoid possible paralysis and necrosis.*

Pain associated with the disease process (eg, fracture) is frequently controlled by immobilization. Pain due to **edema** that is associated with trauma, surgery, or bleeding into the tissues can frequently be controlled by elevation and, if prescribed, intermittent application of cold. Ice bags (one-third to one-half full) or cold application devices are placed on each side of the cast, if prescribed, making sure not to indent the cast.

Pain may be indicative of complications. Pain associated with compartment syndrome is relentless and is not controlled by modalities such as elevation, application of cold if prescribed, and usual dosages of analgesics. Severe pain over a bony prominence warns of an impending pressure ulcer. Pain decreases when ulceration occurs. Discomfort due to pressure on the skin may be

61•1 GUIDELINES FOR APPLYING A CAST

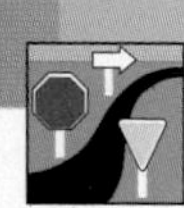

Procedure	Rationale
1. Support extremity or body part to be casted.	1. Minimizes movement; maintains reduction and alignment; increases comfort.
2. Position and maintain part to be casted in position indicated by physician during casting procedure.	2. Facilitates casting; reduces incidence of complications (eg, malunion, nonunion, contracture).
3. Drape patient.	3. Avoids undue exposure; protects other body parts from contact with casting materials.
4. Wash and dry part to be casted.	4. Reduces incidence of skin breakdown.
5. Place knitted material* (eg stockinette) over part to be casted.	5. Protects skin from casting materials.
• Apply in smooth and nonconstrictive manner.	Protects skin from pressure.
• Allow additional material.	Folds over edges of cast when finishing application; creates smooth, padded edge; protects skin from abrasion.
6. Wrap soft, nonwoven roll padding* smoothly and evenly around part.	6. Protects skin from pressure of cast.
• Use additional padding around bony prominences and at nerve grooves (eg, head of fibula, olecranon process).	Protects skin at bony prominences. Protects superficial nerves.
7. Apply plaster or nonplaster casting material evenly on body part.	7. Creates smooth, solid, well-contoured cast.
• Choose appropriate width bandage.	Facilitates smooth application.
• Overlap preceding turn by half the width of the bandage.	Creates smooth, solid, immobilizing cast.
• Use continuous motion, maintaining constant contact with body part.	Shapes cast properly for adequate support.
• Use additional casting material (splints) at joints and at points of anticipated cast stress.	Strengthens cast.
8. "Finish" cast:	
• Edges smooth.	8. Protects skin from abrasion.
• Trim and reshape with cast knife or cutter.	Assures full range of motion of adjacent joints.
9. Remove particles of casting materials from skin.	9. Prevents particles from loosening and sliding underneath cast.
10. Support cast during hardening. • Handle hardening casts with palms of hands. • Support cast on firm smooth surface. • Do not rest cast on hard surfaces or on sharp edges. • Avoid pressure on cast.	10. Casting materials harden in minutes. Maximum hardness of nonplaster cast occurs in minutes. Maximum hardness of plaster cast occurs with drying (24 to 72 hours, depending on thickness of cast and environment). Avoids denting of cast and pressure areas.
11. Promote drying of cast. • Leave cast uncovered and exposed to air. • Turn patient every 2 hours supporting major joints. • Fans may be used to increase air flow.	11. Facilitates drying.

* Nonabsorbent materials are used with nonplaster casts.

relieved by elevation that controls edema or by positioning that alters pressure. It may be necessary, however, to modify the cast or to recast.

Nursing Alert The nurse never ignores complaints of pain from the patient in a cast because of the possibility of potential problems, such as impaired tissue perfusion or pressure ulcer formation.

Improving Mobility

Every joint that is not immobilized should be exercised and moved through its range of motion to maintain function. If the patient has a leg cast, the nurse encourages toe exercises. If the patient has an arm cast, the nurse encourages finger exercises.

Promoting Healing of Skin Abrasions

Before the cast is applied, it is important to treat skin lacerations and abrasions to promote healing. The nurse thoroughly cleans the skin and treats it as prescribed. Sterile dressings are used to cover the injured skin. If the skin wounds are extensive, an alternative method (eg, external fixator) may be chosen to immobilize the body part. While the cast is on, the nurse observes the patient for systemic signs of infection, odors from the cast, and purulent drainage staining the cast. It is important to notify the physician if these occur.

Maintaining Adequate Neurovascular Function

Swelling and edema are natural responses of the tissue to trauma and surgery. The patient may complain that the cast is too tight. Vascular insufficiency and nerve compression due to unrelieved swelling can result in compartment syndrome (see Chap. 63). The nurse monitors circulation, motion, and sensation of the affected extremity, assessing the fingers or toes of the casted extremity and comparing them with those of the opposite extremity. Normal findings include minimal swelling, minimal discomfort, pink color, warm to touch, rapid capillary refill response, normal sensations, and ability to exercise fingers or toes. The nurse encourages the patient to exercise fingers or toes hourly when awake to stimulate circulation.

It is important to perform frequent, regular assessments of neurovascular status. Early recognition of diminished circulation and nerve function is essential to prevent loss of function. When data indicate potential compartment syndrome (eg, progressive unrelieved pain, pain on passive stretch, paresthesia, motor loss, sensory loss, coolness, paleness, slow capillary refill, sensation of tightness), the nurse adjusts the extremity so that it is no higher than heart level to enhance arterial perfusion and control edema and then notifies the physician at once.

Monitoring and Managing Potential Complications

COMPARTMENT SYNDROME

Compartment syndrome occurs when there is increased tissue pressure within a limited space (eg, cast, muscle compartment) that compromises the circulation and the function of the tissue within the confined area. To relieve the pressure, the cast must be bivalved (cut in half) while maintaining alignment, and the extremity must be elevated no higher than heart level (Chart 61-1). If pressure is not relieved and circulation is not restored, a fasciotomy may be necessary to relieve the pressure within the muscle compartment. The nurse closely monitors the patient's response to conservative and surgical management of compartment syndrome. The nurse records neurovascular responses and promptly reports changes to the physician.

CHART 61•1 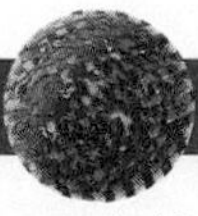 **Bivalving a Cast**

When cutting a cast in half (bivalving), the physician or nurse practitioner proceeds as follows:

1. With a cast cutter, a longitudinal cut is made to divide the cast in half.
2. The underpadding is cut with scissors.
3. The cast is spread apart with cast spreaders to relieve pressure and to inspect and treat the skin without interrupting the reduction and alignment of the bone.
4. After the pressure is relieved, the anterior and posterior parts of the cast are secured together with an elastic compression bandage to maintain immobilization.
5. To control swelling and promote circulation, the extremity is elevated (but no higher than heart level).

PRESSURE ULCERS

Pressure of the cast on soft tissues may cause tissue anoxia and pressure ulcers. Lower extremity sites most susceptible to pressure are the heel, malleoli, dorsum of the foot, head of the fibula, and anterior surface of the patella. The main pressure sites on the upper extremity are located at the medial epicondyle of the humerus and the ulnar styloid (see Fig. 61-1).

Generally, the patient with a pressure ulcer reports pain and tightness in the area. A warm area on the cast suggests underlying tissue erythema. The area may break down. The drainage may stain the cast and emit an odor. Discomfort may not occur with tissue breakdown and necrosis; however, extensive loss of tissue may occur. The nurse must monitor the patient with a cast for pressure ulcer development and report findings to the physician.

To inspect the pressure area, the physician may bivalve the cast or cut an opening (window) in the cast. If the physician elects to create a window to inspect the pressure site, a portion of the cast is cut out. The affected area is inspected and possibly treated. The portion of the cast is replaced and held in place by an elastic compression dressing or tape. This prevents the underlying tissue from swelling through the window and creating pressure areas around its margins.

DISUSE SYNDROME

While in a cast, the patient needs to learn to tense or contract muscles (eg, isometric muscle contraction) without moving the part. This helps to reduce muscle atrophy and maintain muscle strength. The nurse teaches the patient with a leg cast to "push down" the knee and teaches the patient in an arm cast to "make a fist." Muscle-setting exercises (eg, quadriceps-setting and gluteal-setting exercises) are important in maintaining muscles essential for walking (Chart 61-2). Isometric exercises should be performed hourly while the patient is awake.

At times, portable electrical muscle stimulators may be attached to the skin over large muscles before cast application. Muscle contractions are electrically stimulated for about 8 hours a day to prevent the development of disuse atrophy.

CHART 61•2 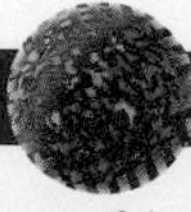 **Muscle-Setting Exercises**

Isometric contractions of the muscle maintain muscle mass and strength and prevent atrophy.

Quadriceps-Setting Exercise

- Position patient supine with leg extended.
- Instruct patient to push knee back onto the mattress by contracting the anterior thigh muscles.
- Encourage patient to hold the position for 5 to 10 seconds.
- Let patient relax.
- Have the patient repeat the exercise 10 times each hour when awake.

Gluteal-Setting Exercise

- Position the patient supine with legs extended, if possible.
- Instruct the patient to contract the muscles of the buttocks and abdomen.
- Encourage the patient to hold the contraction for 5 to 10 seconds.
- Let the patient relax.
- Have the patient repeat the exercise 10 times each hour when awake.

Promoting Home and Community-Based Care

TEACHING PATIENTS SELF-CARE

Self-care deficits occur when a portion of the body is immobilized. The nurse encourages the patient to participate actively in personal care and to use assistive devices safely. The nurse must assist the patient in identifying areas of self-care deficit and in developing strategies to assist the patient to achieve independence in activities of daily living (ADLs). (See the accompanying Home Care Teaching Checklist: The Patient With a Cast.) The patient's participation in planning and accomplishing ADLs is an important aspect of self-care, independence, maintaining control, and avoiding untoward psychological reactions, such as depression.

When the cast is dry, the nurse instructs the patient as follows:

- Move about as normally as possible but avoid excessive use of the injured extremity and avoid walking on wet, slippery floors or sidewalks.
- Perform prescribed exercises regularly, as scheduled.
- Elevate the casted extremity to heart level frequently to prevent swelling.
- Do not attempt to scratch the skin under the cast. This may cause a break in the skin and result in the formation of a skin ulcer. Cool air from a hair dryer may alleviate an itch.
- Cushion rough edges of the cast with tape.
- Keep the cast dry but do not cover it with plastic or rubber because this causes condensation, which dampens the cast and skin. Moisture softens a plaster cast. (A wet fiberglass cast must be dried thoroughly with a hair dryer on a cool setting to avoid skin problems.)
- Report the following to the physician: persistent pain, swelling that does not respond to elevation, changes in sensation, decreased ability to move exposed fingers or toes, and changes in skin color and temperature.
- Note odors around the cast, stained areas, warm spots, and pressure areas. Report them to the physician.
- Report a broken cast to the physician; do not attempt to fix it yourself.

Cast Removal. The nurse prepares the patient for cast removal or cast changes by explaining what to expect (see Guideline 61-2). The cast is cut using a cast cutter, which vibrates. The patient can feel the vibration and pressure during its use. The cutter does not penetrate deeply enough to hurt the patient's skin. The cast padding is cut with scissors.

The casted body part is weak from disuse, stiff, and may appear atrophied. Therefore, support is needed when the cast is removed. The skin, which is usually dry and scaly from accumulated dead skin, is vulnerable to injury from scratching. The skin needs to be washed gently and lubricated with an emollient lotion.

The nurse teaches the patient to resume activities gradually within the prescribed therapeutic regimen. Because the muscles are weak from disuse, the body part that has been casted cannot withstand normal stresses immediately. In addition, the nurse teaches the patient who has noticeable swelling of the affected extremity after the cast is removed to continue to elevate the extremity to control swelling until normal muscle tone and use are reestablished.

HOME CARE TEACHING CHECKLIST: THE PATIENT WITH A CAST

At the completion of the program, the patient or caregiver will be able to:	Patient	Caregiver
• Describe techniques to promote cast drying (eg, do not cover, leave exposed to circulating air; handle damp plaster cast with palms of hands, and do not rest the cast on hard surfaces or sharp edges that can dent soft cast)	✔	✔
• Describe approaches to controlling swelling and pain (eg, elevate casted extremity to heart level, apply intermittent ice bag if prescribed, take analgesics as prescribed)	✔	✔
• Report pain uncontrolled by elevating the casted limb and by analgesics (may be an indicator of impaired tissue perfusion—compartment syndrome or pressure ulcer)	✔	
• Demonstrate ability to transfer (eg, from a bed to a chair)		
• Use mobility aids safely		
• Avoid excessive use of injured extremity; observe prescribed weight-bearing limits		
• Manage minor irritations from cast (eg, for skin irritation from cast edge, pad rough edges with tape, to relieve itching, blow cool air from hair drier)	✔	✔
• Demonstrate exercises to promote circulation and minimize disuse syndrome	✔	
• State indicators of complications to report promptly to physician (eg, uncontrolled swelling and pain; cool, pale fingers or toes; paresthesia; paralysis; purulent drainage staining casts; signs of systemic infection; cast breaks)	✔	✔
• Describe care of extremity following cast removal (eg, skin care; gradual resumption of normal activities to protect limb from undue stresses; management of swelling)	✔	✔

61•2 GUIDELINES FOR REMOVING A CAST

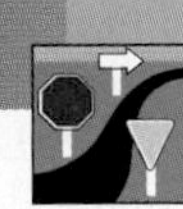

Procedure	Rationale
1. Inform the patient about the procedure.	1. Facilitates cooperation and reduces fear about the procedure.
2. Assure patient that the electric saw or cast cutter will not cut skin.	2. Reduces anxiety. (Blade oscillates to cut cast.)
3. Bivalve cast using a series of alternating pressures and linear movements of blade along the line to be cut.	3. Cuts cast in halves. Avoids burning sensation from prolonged contact of oscillating blade with padding.
4. Wear eye protection (patient and cast cutter operator).	4. Protects eyes from flying cast particles.
5. Cut padding with scissors.	5. Releases all of the casting materials.
6. Support body part as it is removed from the cast.	6. Reduces stresses on body part that has been immobilized.
7. Gently wash and dry area that has been immobilized.* Apply emollient lotion.	7. Removes dead skin that has accumulated during immobilization. Keeps skin supple.
8. Teach patient to avoid rubbing and scratching skin.	8. Prevents skin breakdown.
9. Teach patient to resume active use of body part gradually within the guidelines of prescribed therapeutic regimen.	9. Protects weakened part from excessive stress. Progressive exercises reduce stiffness, restore muscle strength and function.
10. Teach patient to control swelling by elevating the extremity or using elastic bandage if prescribed.	10. Facilitates circulation (ie, venous return) and controls fluid pooling.

* If a new cast is to be applied, follow guidelines for application of a cast and associated nursing care.

Evaluation

Expected Outcomes

Expected outcomes may include:

1. Understands the therapeutic regimen
   a. Elevates affected extremity
   b. Exercises according to instructions
   c. Keeps cast dry
   d. Reports any problems that develop
   e. Keeps follow-up clinic or physician appointments
2. Reports less pain
   a. Elevates extremity that is in the cast
   b. Repositions self
   c. Uses occasional oral analgesic
3. Demonstrates increased mobility
   a. Uses assistive devices safely
   b. Exercises to increase strength
   c. Changes position frequently
   d. Performs range-of-motion exercises of joints not in the cast
4. Exhibits healing of abrasions and lacerations
   a. Demonstrates no local signs of infection (ie, local discomfort, purulent drainage, staining, odor)
   b. Demonstrates no systemic signs or symptoms of infection
   c. Demonstrates intact skin when cast is removed
5. Maintains adequate neurovascular function of affected extremity
   a. Exhibits normal skin color and temperature
   b. Experiences minimal swelling
   c. Exhibits satisfactory capillary refill on testing
   d. Demonstrates active movement of fingers or toes
   e. Reports normal sensations in casted body part
   f. Reports that pain is controllable
6. Exhibits absence of complications
   a. Demonstrates normal neurovascular status of casted extremity
   b. Develops no pressure ulcers
   c. Exhibits minimal muscle wasting
7. Participates in self-care activities
   a. Performs hygiene and grooming activities independently or with minimal assistance
   b. Performs ADLs independently or with minimal assistance

MANAGING THE PATIENT WITH SPLINTS AND BRACES

Contoured **splints** of plaster or pliable thermoplastic materials may be used for conditions that do not require rigid immobilization, for those in which swelling may be anticipated, and for those that require special skin care. The splint needs to immobilize and support the body part in a functional position. The splint must be well padded to prevent pressure, skin abrasion, and skin breakdown. The splint is overwrapped with an elastic bandage applied in a spiral fashion and with pressure uniformly distributed so that the circulation is not restricted. The nurse frequently assesses the neurovascular status of the splinted extremity.

Soft immobilizers may be used to support an injured body part. Usually, the extremity is wrapped with an elastic bandage and then secured to a padded, contoured, canvas immobilizer. Rigid immobilization is not achieved; however, skin care and adjustments for swelling are facilitated.

For long-term use, **braces** (orthoses) are used to provide support, control movement, and prevent additional injury. They are custom fitted to various parts of the body. Braces may be constructed of plastic materials, canvas, leather, or metal. The orthotist adjusts the brace for fit, positioning, and motion.

The nurse helps the patient learn to apply the brace and to protect the skin from irritation and breakdown. The nurse also assesses neurovascular integrity and comfort when the patient is wearing the brace, encourages the patient to wear the brace as prescribed, and reassures the patient that minor adjustments of the brace by the orthotist will increase comfort and minimize problems associated with its long-term use.

MANAGING THE PATIENT WITH AN EXTERNAL FIXATOR

External fixators are used to manage open fractures with soft tissue damage. They provide stable support for severe comminuted (crushed or splintered) fractures while permitting active treatment of damaged soft tissue (Fig. 61-2). Complicated fractures of the humerus, forearm, femur, tibia, and pelvis are managed with external skeletal fixators. The fracture is reduced, aligned, and immobilized by a series of pins inserted in the bone fragments. Pin position is maintained through attachment to a portable frame. The fixator facilitates patient comfort, early mobility, and active exercise of adjacent uninvolved joints. Complications related to disuse and immobility are minimized.

Nursing Interventions

It is important to prepare the patient psychologically for application of the external fixator. The apparatus looks clumsy and foreign. Reassurance that the discomfort associated with the device is minimal and that early mobility is anticipated promotes acceptance of the device.

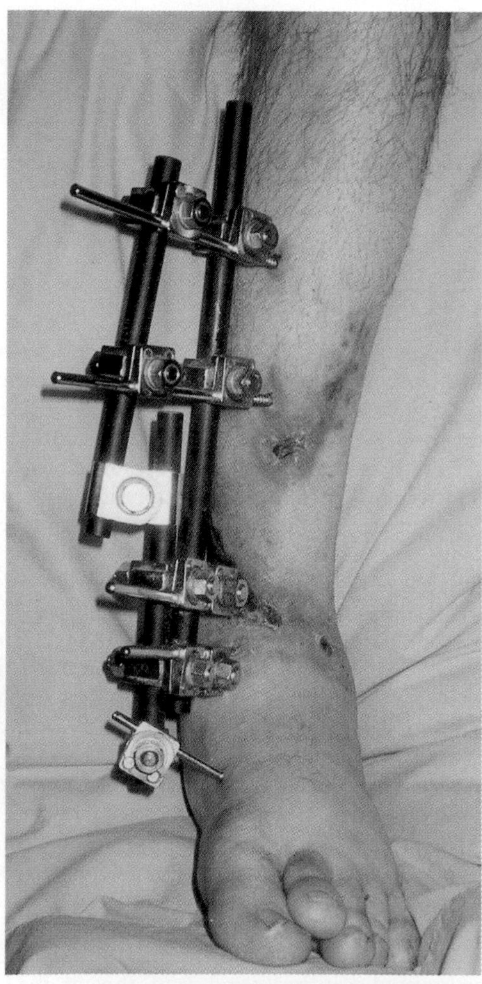

FIGURE 61•2 External fixation device. Pins are inserted into bone fragments. The fracture is reduced and aligned and then stabilized by attaching the pins to a rigid portable frame. The device facilitates treatment of soft tissue damaged in complex fractures.

After the external fixator is applied, it is important to cover sharp points on the fixator or pins to prevent device-induced injuries. The extremity is elevated to reduce swelling. The nurse monitors the neurovascular status of the extremity every 2 hours and assesses each pin site for redness, drainage, tenderness, pain, and loosening of the pin. Some serous drainage from the pin sites is to be expected. The nurse must be alert for potential problems due to pressure by the device on the skin, nerves, or blood vessels and development of compartment syndrome (see Chap. 63).

The nurse carries out pin care as prescribed to prevent pin tract infection. This typically includes cleaning each pin site separately three times a day with cotton-tipped applicators soaked with sterile saline solution. Crusts should not form at the pin site. If signs of infection are present or if the pins or clamps seem loose, the nurse notifies the physician.

Nursing Alert *The nurse never adjusts the clamps on the external fixator frame. Rather, the physician does so.*

The nurse encourages isometric and active exercises within the limits of tissue damage. When the swelling subsides, the nurse helps the patient to mobilize within the prescribed weight-bearing limits (non–weight bearing to full weight bearing). Adherence to weight bearing minimizes the chance of the pins loosening when stress is applied to the bone–pin interface. The fixator is removed when the soft tissue heals. The fracture may require additional stabilization by cast or molded orthosis while healing.

The Ilizarov external fixator is a special device used to correct angulation and rotational defects, to treat nonunion (failure of the bone fragments to heal), and to lengthen limbs. Tension wires are attached to fixator rings, which are joined by telescoping rods. Callus and bone formation is stimulated by prescribed daily adjustment of the telescoping rods. It is important to teach the patient how to adjust the telescoping rods and how to perform skin care. Generally, the nurse can encourage weight-bearing. When the desired correction has been achieved, no additional adjustments are made, and the fixator is left in place until the bone heals.

PROMOTING HOME AND COMMUNITY-BASED CARE

Teaching Patients Self-Care. The nurse teaches the patient to perform pin site care according to prescribed protocol and to report signs of pin site infection promptly (ie, redness, tenderness, increased or purulent pin site drainage, and fever). The nurse also instructs the patient and family to monitor neurovascular status and report any changes promptly. The nurse teaches the patient or family member to check the integrity of the fixator frame daily and to report loose pins or clamps. A physical therapy referral is helpful in teaching the patient how to transfer, use ambulatory aids safely, and adjust to weight bearing limits and altered gait patterns (see the Home Care Teaching Checklist: The Patient With an External Fixator).

MANAGING THE PATIENT IN TRACTION

Traction is used primarily as a short-term intervention until other modalities, such as external or internal fixation, are possible. This reduces the risk of disuse syndrome. **Traction** is the application of a pulling force to a part of the body. Traction is used to minimize muscle spasms; to reduce, align, and immobilize fractures;

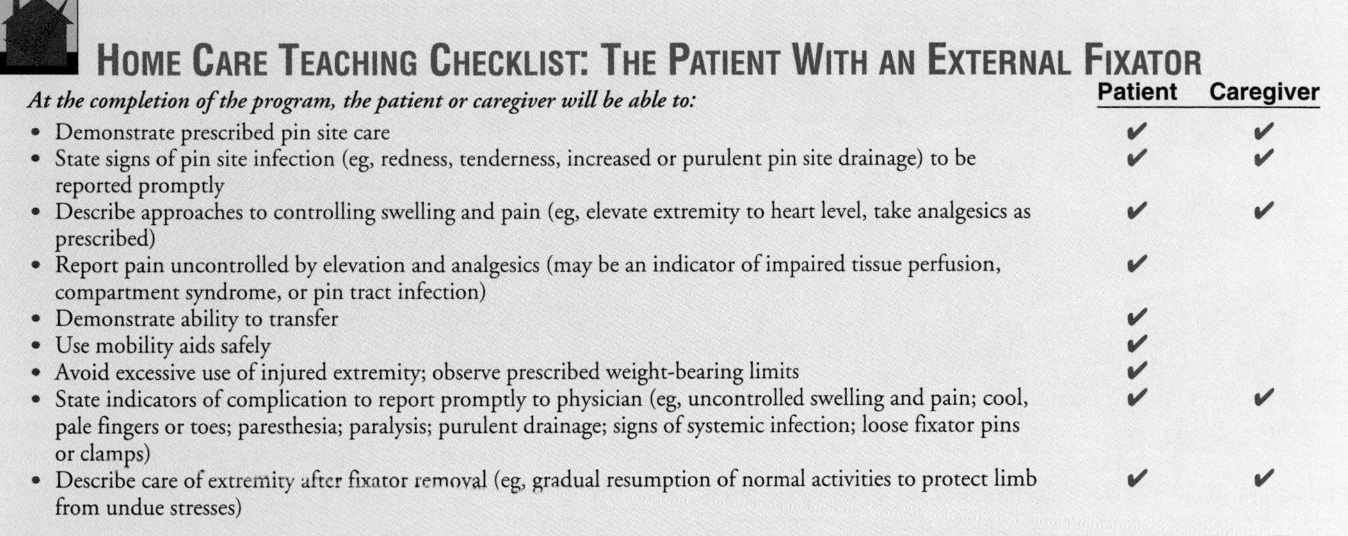

HOME CARE TEACHING CHECKLIST: THE PATIENT WITH AN EXTERNAL FIXATOR

At the completion of the program, the patient or caregiver will be able to:	Patient	Caregiver
• Demonstrate prescribed pin site care	✔	✔
• State signs of pin site infection (eg, redness, tenderness, increased or purulent pin site drainage) to be reported promptly	✔	✔
• Describe approaches to controlling swelling and pain (eg, elevate extremity to heart level, take analgesics as prescribed)	✔	✔
• Report pain uncontrolled by elevation and analgesics (may be an indicator of impaired tissue perfusion, compartment syndrome, or pin tract infection)	✔	
• Demonstrate ability to transfer	✔	
• Use mobility aids safely	✔	
• Avoid excessive use of injured extremity; observe prescribed weight-bearing limits	✔	
• State indicators of complication to report promptly to physician (eg, uncontrolled swelling and pain; cool, pale fingers or toes; paresthesia; paralysis; purulent drainage; signs of systemic infection; loose fixator pins or clamps)	✔	✔
• Describe care of extremity after fixator removal (eg, gradual resumption of normal activities to protect limb from undue stresses)	✔	✔

to reduce deformity; and to increase space between opposing surfaces. Traction must be applied in the correct direction and magnitude to obtain its therapeutic effects. As muscle and soft tissues relax, the amount of weight used may be changed to obtain the desired effect.

At times, traction needs to be applied in more than one direction to achieve the desired line of pull. When this is done, one of the lines of pull counteracts the other line of pull. These lines of pull are known as the vectors of force. The actual resultant pulling force is somewhere between the two lines of pull (Fig. 61-3). The effects of traction are evaluated with radiographic studies, and adjustments are made if necessary.

Principles of Effective Traction

Whenever traction is applied, the countertraction must be used to achieve effective traction. Countertraction is the force acting in the opposite direction. Generally, the patient's body weight and bed position adjustments supply the needed countertraction.

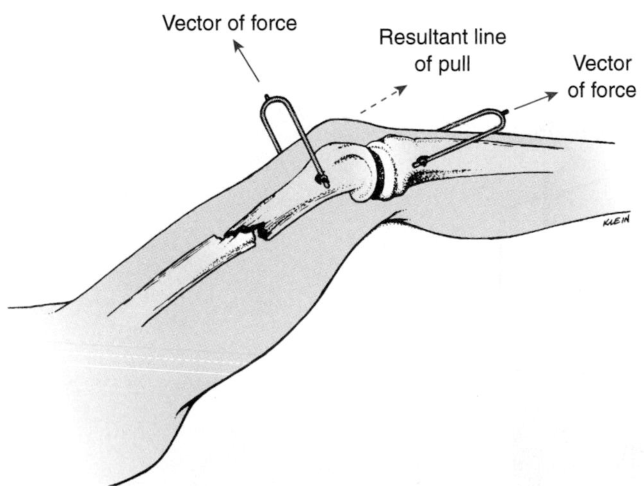

FIGURE 61•3 Traction may be applied in different directions to achieve the desired therapeutic line of pull. Adjustments in applied forces may be prescribed over the treatment period.

Nursing Alert *Countertraction must be maintained for effective traction.*

The following are additional principles to follow when caring for the patient in traction:

- Traction must be continuous to be effective in reducing and immobilizing fractures.
- Skeletal traction is *never* interrupted.
- Weights are not removed unless the traction is prescribed intermittently.
- Any factor that might reduce the effective pull or alter its resultant line of pull must be eliminated.
- The patient is in good body alignment in the center of the bed when traction is applied.
- Ropes must be unobstructed.
- Weights must hang free and not rest on the bed or floor.
- Knots in the rope or the footplate must not touch the pulley or the foot of the bed.

There are several different types of traction. *Straight* or *running traction* applies the pulling force in a straight line with the body part resting on the bed. Buck's extension traction (Fig. 61-4) and pelvic traction are examples of straight traction. *Balanced suspension traction* (Fig. 61-5) supports the affected extremity off the bed and allows for some patient movement without disruption of the line of pull.

Traction may be applied to the skin (*skin traction*) or directly to the bony skeleton (*skeletal traction*). The mode of application is determined by the purpose of the traction. Traction can be applied with the hands (*manual traction*). This is temporary traction that may be used when applying a cast, giving skin care under a Buck's extension foam boot, or adjusting the traction apparatus.

Skin Traction

Skin traction is used to control muscle spasm and to immobilize an area before surgery. Skin traction is accomplished by a weight pulling on traction tape or a foam boot attached to the skin. The amount of weight applied must not exceed the tolerance of the skin. No more than 2 to 3.5 kg (4.5 to 8 lb) of traction can be used on an extremity. Pelvic traction is generally 4.5 to 9 kg (10 to 20 lb), depending on the weight of the patient.

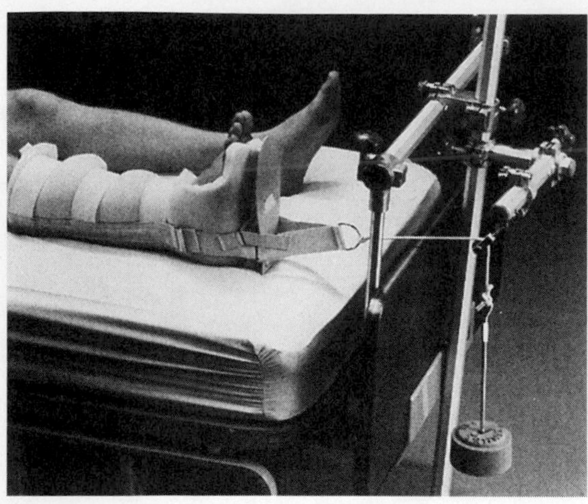

FIGURE 61•4 Buck's extension traction. Lower extremity in unilateral Buck's extension traction is aligned in a foam boot and traction applied by the free-hanging weight.

Appendicular (pertaining to the extremities) types of skin traction used for adults include **Buck's extension traction, Russell's traction**, and **Dunlop's traction.** Axial (involving the head and trunk) types of skin traction, including cervical head halter and pelvic belt, are used to treat back pain.

Buck's Extension Traction

Buck's extension (unilateral or bilateral) is skin traction to the lower leg. The pull is exerted in one plane when partial or temporary immobilization is desired (see Fig. 61-4). It is used to provide immobility and comfort after injuries to the hip before surgical fixation.

Before the traction is applied, the nurse inspects the skin for abrasions and circulatory disturbances. The skin and circulation must be in healthy condition to tolerate the traction. The extremity should be clean and dry before the foam boot or the traction tape is applied.

To apply Buck's traction, one nurse elevates and supports the extremity under the patient's heel and knee while another nurse places the foam boot under the leg, with the patient's heel in the heel of the boot. Next, the nurse secures Velcro straps around the leg. Traction tape overwrapped with elastic bandage in a spiral fashion may be used instead of the boot. Excessive pressure is avoided over the malleolus and proximal fibula during application to prevent pressure ulcers and nerve damage. The nurse then passes the rope affixed to the spreader or footplate over a pulley fastened to the end of the bed and attaches the weight—usually 5 to 8 pounds—to the rope.

Russell's Traction

Russell's traction, which may be used for fractures of the tibial plateau, supports the flexed knee in a sling and applies the horizontal pulling force using traction tape and elastic bandage to the lower leg. If prescribed, the leg may be supported by a pillow to ensure proper knee flexion and to prevent pressure on the heel.

Dunlop's Traction

Dunlop's traction is applied to the upper extremity for supracondylar fractures of the elbow and humerus. Horizontal traction is applied to the abducted humerus, and vertical traction is applied to the flexed forearm.

Complications

Complications that may develop as a result of the traction include skin breakdown, nerve pressure, and circulatory impairment. Skin breakdown results from irritation caused by contact of the skin with the tape and foam or use of shearing forces when applying traction. Older adults are at greater risk for this complication because of their sensitive, fragile skin.

Nerve pressure results from pressure on the peripheral nerves. One type of nerve pressure can cause footdrop. This occurs when pressure is applied to the peroneal nerve at the point at which it passes around the neck of the fibula just below the knee.

Circulatory impairment is manifested by cold skin temperature, decreased peripheral pulses, slow capillary refill time, and bluish skin. Deep vein thrombosis (DVT), a serious circulatory impairment, is manifested by calf tenderness, swelling, and positive Homans' sign.

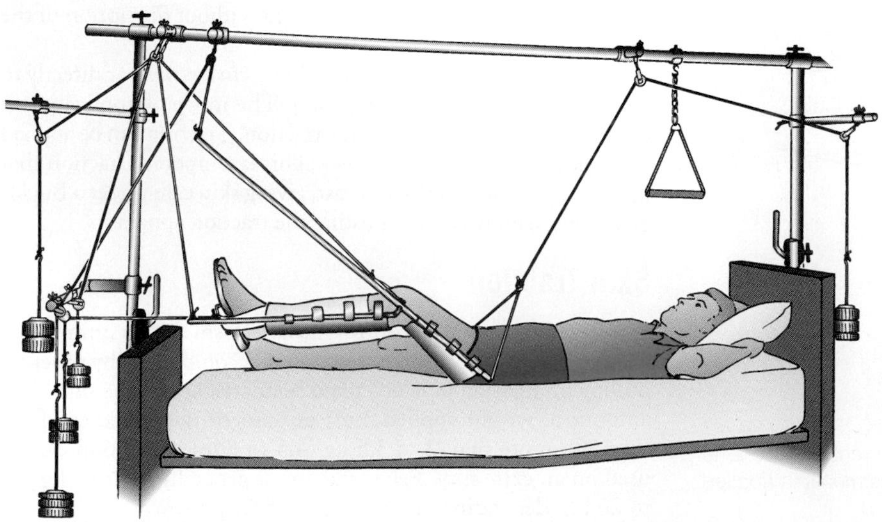

FIGURE 61•5 Balanced suspension skeletal traction with Thomas leg splint. The patient can move vertically as long as the resultant line of pull is maintained.

Nursing Interventions

ENSURING EFFECTIVE TRACTION

To ensure effective skin traction, it is important to avoid wrinkling and slipping of the traction bandage and to maintain countertraction. Proper positioning must be maintained to keep the leg or arm in a neutral position. To prevent bony fragments from moving against one another, the patient should not turn from side to side but can shift position slightly with assistance.

MONITORING AND MANAGING POTENTIAL COMPLICATIONS

Skin Breakdown. During the initial assessment, the nurse identifies sensitive, fragile skin (common in older adults). The nurse also closely monitors reaction of the skin in contact with tape and foam to ensure that shearing forces are avoided. The nurse performs the following to monitor and manage skin breakdown:

- Removes the foam boots to inspect the skin, the ankle, and the Achilles tendon three times a day. A second nurse is needed to support the extremity during the inspection and skin care.
- Palpates the area of the traction tapes daily to detect underlying tenderness.
- Provides back care at least every 2 hours to prevent pressure ulcers. The patient who must remain in a supine position is at increased risk for developing a pressure ulcer.
- Uses special mattress overlays (eg, air-filled, high-density foam) to minimize development of skin ulcers.

Nerve Pressure. Skin traction can place pressure on peripheral nerves. When traction is applied to the lower extremity, care must be taken to avoid pressure on the peroneal nerve at the point at which it passes around the neck of the fibula just below the knee. Pressure at this point can cause footdrop. The nurse questions the patient about sensation and asks the patient to move the toes and foot. Dorsiflexion of the foot demonstrates function of the peroneal nerve. Weakness of dorsiflexion or foot movement and inversion of the foot might indicate pressure on the common peroneal nerve. Plantar flexion demonstrates function of the tibial nerve.

When applying skin traction to the arm, the nurse avoids a tight wrapping at the area around the elbow where the ulnar nerve is located. Ulnar nerve function can be assessed by active abduction of the little finger and sensation on the ulnar side of the little finger. The following are important points to keep in mind when caring for the patient in traction:

- Regularly assess sensation and motion.
- Immediately investigate any complaint of burning sensation under the traction bandage or boot.
- Promptly report altered sensation and motor function.

Circulatory Impairment. After skin traction is applied, the nurse assesses circulation of the foot or hand within a few minutes and then every 1 to 2 hours. Circulatory assessment consists of the following:

- Peripheral pulses, color, capillary refill, and temperature of the fingers or toe.
- Indicators of DVT, including calf tenderness, swelling, and positive Homans' sign

The nurse also encourages the patient to perform active foot or hand exercises every hour when awake.

Skeletal Traction

Skeletal traction is applied directly to the bone. This method of traction is used most frequently to treat fractures of the femur, the tibia, the humerus, and the cervical spine. The traction is applied directly to the bone by use of a metal pin or wire (eg, Steinmann pin; Kirschner wire) that is inserted through the bone distal to the fracture, avoiding nerves, blood vessels, muscles, tendons, and joints. Tongs applied to the head (eg, Gardner-Wells or Vinke tongs) are fixed in the skull to apply traction that immobilizes cervical fractures.

Local or general anesthesia may be used for the surgical procedure. Skeletal traction is applied by the orthopedic surgeon under conditions of surgical asepsis. The insertion site is prepared with a surgical scrub agent, such as povidone-iodine solution. A local anesthetic is administered at the insertion site and periosteum. The surgeon makes a small skin incision and drills the sterile pin or wire through the bone. If the patient has not received a general anesthetic, he or she feels pressure during this procedure and possibly some pain when the periosteum is penetrated.

After insertion, the pin or wire is attached to the traction bow or caliper. The ends of the wire are covered with corks or tape to prevent injury to the patient or care givers. The weights are attached to the pin or wire bow by a rope and pulley system that exerts the appropriate amount and direction of pull for effective traction. Skeletal traction frequently uses 7 to 12 kg (15 to 25 lb) to achieve the therapeutic effect. The weights applied initially must overcome the shortening spasms of the affected muscles. As the muscles relax, the traction weight is reduced to prevent fracture dislocation and to promote healing.

Often, skeletal traction is balanced traction, which supports the affected extremity, allows for some patient movement, and facilitates patient independence and nursing care while maintaining effective traction.

The Thomas splint with a Pearson attachment is frequently used with skeletal traction in fractures of the femur (see Fig. 61-5). It may be used with skin traction and other balanced suspension apparatus. Because upward traction is required, an overbed frame is used.

When x-rays disclose callus formation, skeletal traction is discontinued. The extremity is gently supported while the weights are removed. The pin is cut close to the skin and removed by the physician. Casts or splints are then used to support the healing bone.

Nursing Interventions

MAINTAINING EFFECTIVE TRACTION

When traction is used, the nurse checks the apparatus to see that the ropes are in the wheel grooves of the pulleys, that the ropes are not frayed, that the weights hang freely, and that the knots in the rope are tied securely. The nurse also evaluates the patient's position because slipping down in bed results in ineffective traction.

Nursing Alert *The nurse must never remove weights from skeletal traction unless a life-threatening situation occurs. Removing the weights completely defeats their purpose and may result in injury.*

MAINTAINING POSITIONING

The nurse must maintain alignment of the patient's body in traction as prescribed to promote an effective line of pull. The nurse positions the foot to avoid footdrop (plantar flexion), inward rotation (inversion), or outward rotation (eversion). The patient's foot may be supported in a neutral position by orthopedic devices (eg, foot supports).

PREVENTING SKIN BREAKDOWN

The patient's elbows frequently become sore, and nerve injury may occur if most repositioning is done by the patient pushing on the elbows. In addition, patients frequently use the heel of the unaffected leg to act as a brace when they raise themselves. This digging of the heel into the mattress may injure the tissues. Therefore, the nurse should protect and inspect the elbows and heel for pressure areas. To encourage movement without using the elbows or heel, the nurse can suspend a trapeze overhead within easy reach of the patient. This apparatus helps the patient to move about in bed and on and off the bedpan.

Specific pressure points are assessed for redness and skin breakdown. Areas that are particularly vulnerable to pressure caused by traction apparatus applied to the lower extremity include the ischial tuberosity, popliteal space, Achilles tendon, and heel. When a patient is not permitted to turn on one side or the other, the nurse must make a special effort to provide back care and to keep the bed dry and free of crumbs and wrinkles. The patient can assist by holding the overhead trapeze and raising the hips off the bed. If the patient cannot do this, the nurse can push down on the mattress with one hand to relieve pressure on the back and bony prominences and to provide for some shifting of weight. Pressure-relieving air or a high-density foam mattress overlay may reduce the risk of pressure ulcer.

To change the bed linens, the patient raises the torso while nurses on both sides of the bed roll down and replace the upper mattress sheet. Then, as the patient raises the buttocks off the mattress, the nurses slide the sheets under the buttocks. Finally, they replace the lower section while the patient rests on the back. Sheets and blankets are placed over the patient in such a way that the traction is not disrupted.

MONITORING NEUROVASCULAR STATUS

The nurse assesses the neurovascular status of the immobilized extremity at least every hour initially and then several times a day. The nurse instructs the patient to report any changes in sensation or movement immediately so that they can be promptly evaluated. DVT is a significant risk for the immobilized patient. The nurse encourages the patient to do active flexion–extension ankle exercises and isometric contraction of the calf muscles (calf-pumping exercises) 10 times an hour while awake to decrease venous stasis. In addition, elastic stockings, compression devices, and anticoagulant therapy may be prescribed to help prevent thrombus formation.

Prompt recognition of a developing neurovascular problem is essential so that corrective measures can be instituted promptly.

PROVIDING PIN SITE CARE

The wound at the pin insertion site requires attention. The goal is to avoid infection and development of **osteomyelitis**. Initially, the site is covered with a sterile dressing. Subsequent care of the pin site is individually prescribed. The nurse must keep the area clean. Slight serous oozing at the pin site is expected; crusting should be prevented. The nurse assesses the drainage and pin site for signs of infection, such as inflammation, tenderness, and purulent drainage. The patient may experience discomfort at the pin site due to traction on the skin caused by an unsupported muscle.

Nursing Alert *The nurse must inspect the pin site at least every 8 hours for signs of inflammation and evidence of infection.*

PROMOTING EXERCISE

Patient exercises within the therapeutic limits of the traction assist in maintaining muscle strength and tone and in promoting circulation. Active exercises include pulling up on the trapeze, flexing and extending the feet, range-of-motion and weight-resistance exercises for noninvolved joints, and isometric exercises of the immobilized extremity (quadriceps-setting and gluteal-setting exercises) are important in maintaining strength in major ambulatory muscles (see Chart 61-2). Without exercise, the patient will lose muscle mass and strength, and rehabilitation will be greatly prolonged.

NURSING PROCESS: THE PATIENT IN TRACTION

Assessment

The nurse must consider the psychological and physiologic impact of the musculoskeletal problem, traction device, and immobility. Traction restricts one's mobility and independence. The equipment often looks threatening, and its application can be frightening. Confusion, disorientation, and behavioral problems may develop in patients who are confined in a limited space for an extended time. Therefore, the nurse must assess and monitor the patient's anxiety level and psychological responses to traction.

It is important to evaluate the body part to be placed in traction and its neurovascular status (ie, color, temperature, capillary refill, edema, pulses, ability to move, sensations) and compare it with the unaffected extremity. The nurse also assesses skin integrity along with body system functioning for baseline data. Ongoing assessment is indicated for the patient in traction. Immobility-related problems may include pressure ulcers, stasis pneumonia, constipation, loss of appetite, urinary stasis, urinary tract infections, and venous stasis. Early identification of preexisting or developing problems facilitates prompt interventions to resolve the problems.

Diagnosis

Nursing Diagnoses

Based on the nursing assessment, the patient's major nursing diagnoses related to traction may include the following:

- Knowledge deficit related to the treatment regimen
- Anxiety related to health status and traction device
- Pain and altered comfort related to musculoskeletal disorder, traction, and/or immobility
- Self-care deficit: feeding, hygiene, or toileting related to traction
- Impaired physical mobility related to musculoskeletal disorder and traction

Collaborative Problems/Potential Complications

Based on the assessment data, potential complications that may develop include the following:

- Pressure ulcer
- Pneumonia
- Constipation
- Anorexia
- Urinary stasis and infection
- Venous stasis with DVT

Planning and Goals

The major goals of the patient in traction may include understanding of the treatment regimen, reduced anxiety, maximum comfort, maximum level of self-care, maximum mobility within therapeutic limits of traction, and absence of complications.

Nursing Interventions

Promoting Understanding of the Treatment Regimen

The patient must understand the problem being treated and the rationale for the traction therapy. Frequently, the nurse may need to repeat and reinforce the information. With increased understanding of the therapy, the patient becomes an active participant in health care.

Reducing Anxiety

Before any traction is applied, the patient needs to be informed about the procedure, its purpose, and its implications. The nurse encourages the patient to participate in decisions affecting care. Increasing the patient's sense of control reduces feelings of helplessness, allays apprehension, and fosters coping.

After being in traction for a while, the patient may react to being confined to a limited space. Frequent visits by the nurse should reduce feelings of isolation and confinement. The nurse should encourage family and friends to visit frequently for the same reason. It is also a good idea to encourage diversional activities that can be performed within the limits of the traction.

Achieving Maximum Level of Comfort

Because the patient is immobilized in bed, the mattress needs to be firm. Special mattress pads designed to minimize the development of pressure ulcers may be placed on the bed before applying the traction. The nurse can relieve pressure on dependent body parts by turning and positioning the patient for comfort within the limits of the traction and by making sure the bed linens stay wrinkle-free and dry. The nurse promptly investigates every complaint of the patient in traction.

Achieving Maximum Self-Care

Initially, the patient may require assistance with self-care activities. The nurse helps the patient eat, bathe, dress, and toilet. Assistive devices, such as reachers and an overbed trapeze, may facilitate self-care. With resumption of self-care activities, the patient feels less dependent and less frustrated and experiences improved self-esteem.

Because some assistance is required throughout the period of immobility, the nurse and the patient can creatively develop routines that maximize the patient's independence.

Attaining Maximum Mobility With Traction

During traction therapy, the nurse encourages the patient to exercise muscles and joints not in traction to guard against their deterioration. The physical therapist can design bed exercises that minimize loss of muscle strength. During the patient's exercise, the nurse ensures that traction forces are maintained and that the patient is properly positioned to prevent complications resulting from poor alignment.

Monitoring and Managing Potential Complications

PRESSURE ULCERS

The nurse examines the patient's skin frequently for evidence of pressure or friction, paying special attention to bony prominences. It is helpful to reposition the patient frequently and to use protective devices (eg, elbow protectors) to relieve pressure. If the risk of skin breakdown is high, such as with a multitrauma patient or with a debilitated elderly patient, use of a specialized bed is considered to prevent skin breakdown. If a pressure ulcer develops, the nurse consults with the physician and wound care nurse specialist.

PNEUMONIA

The nurse auscultates the patient's lungs to determine respiratory status and teaches the patient deep-breathing and coughing exercises to aid in fully expanding the lungs and moving pulmonary secretions. If patient history and baseline assessment indicate that the patient is at high risk for developing respiratory complications, specific therapies (eg, incentive spirometer) may be indicated. If a respiratory problem develops, prompt institution of prescribed therapy is needed.

CONSTIPATION AND ANOREXIA

Reduced gastrointestinal motility results in constipation and anorexia. A diet high in fiber and fluids may help to stimulate gastric motility. If constipation develops, therapeutic measures might include stool softeners, laxatives, suppositories, and enemas. To improve the patient's appetite, the nurse identifies and includes the patient's food preferences, as appropriate, within the prescribed therapeutic diet.

URINARY STASIS AND INFECTION

Incomplete emptying of the bladder related to positioning in bed can result in urinary stasis and infection. In addition, the patient may find use of the bedpan uncomfortable and limit fluids to minimize frequency of urination. The nurse monitors the fluid intake and the character of the urine. The nurse also teaches the patient to consume adequate amounts of fluid and to void every 3 hours. If the patient exhibits signs or symptoms of urinary tract infection, the nurse notifies the physician.

VENOUS STASIS AND DEEP VEIN THROMBOSIS

Venous stasis occurs with immobility. The nurse teaches the patient to perform ankle and foot exercises within the limits of the traction therapy every 1 to 2 hours when awake to prevent DVT that may result from venous stasis. The patient is encouraged to drink fluids to prevent dehydration and associated hemoconcentration, which contribute to stasis. The nurse monitors the patient for signs of DVT, including calf tenderness, warmth, redness, or swelling (increased calf circumference) or a positive Homans' sign (discomfort in the calf when the foot is forcibly dorsiflexed). The nurse promptly reports findings to the physician for definitive evaluation and therapy.

Evaluation

Expected Outcomes

Expected outcomes may include:

1. Demonstrates knowledge of traction regimen
   a. Describes purpose of traction
   b. Participates in plan of care

2. Exhibits reduced anxiety
   a. Appears relaxed
   b. Uses effective coping mechanisms
   c. Expresses concerns and feelings
3. States increased level of comfort
   a. Requests occasional oral analgesia
   b. Repositions self frequently
4. Performs self-care activities
   a. Requires minimal assistance with feeding, bathing, dressing, and toileting
5. Demonstrates increased mobility
   a. Performs prescribed exercises
   b. Uses assistive devices safely
6. Experiences no complications
   a. Has intact skin
   b. Has clear lungs
   c. Does not report shortness of breath
   d. Does not have a productive cough
   e. Exhibits a regular bowel evacuation pattern
   f. Has a normal appetite
   g. Exhibits clear, yellow, nonconcentrated urine of adequate amount
   h. Does not exhibit signs or symptoms of venous stasis

MANAGING THE PATIENT UNDERGOING ORTHOPEDIC SURGERY

Many patients with musculoskeletal dysfunction undergo surgery to correct the problem. Problems that may be corrected by surgery include unstabilized fracture, deformity, joint disease, necrotic or infected tissue, and tumors. Frequent surgical procedures include **open reduction with internal fixation** (ORIF) for fractures; arthroplasty, meniscectomy, and joint replacement for joint problems; amputation for severe extremity problems (eg, gangrene, massive trauma); bone graft for joint stabilization, defect-filling, or stimulation of bone healing; and tendon transplantation for improving motion. The goals include improving function by restoring motion and stability and relieving pain and disability. See Chart 61-3 for categories of orthopedic surgery.

Joint surgery is one the most frequently performed orthopedic surgeries. Joint disease or deformity may necessitate surgical intervention to relieve pain, improve stability, and improve function. Surgical procedures include excision of damaged and diseased tissue, repair of damaged structures (eg, ruptured tendon), removal of loose bodies (débridement), **arthrodesis** (immobilizing fusion of a joint), and **arthroplasty** (replacement of all or part of the joint surfaces).

The procedure is selected according to the patient's underlying orthopedic condition, general physical health, impact of joint disability on daily activities, and age. Timing of these procedures is important to ensure maximum function. Surgery should be performed before surrounding muscles become contracted and atrophied and serious structural abnormalities occur. The patient is carefully evaluated by the physician so that the most appropriate procedure is performed.

Because these are elective procedures, many patients donate their own blood during the weeks preceding their surgery. This blood is used to replace blood lost during surgery. Autologous blood transfusions eliminate many of the risks of transfusion therapy.

CHART 61•3 Definition of Terms

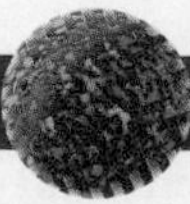

Open reduction: the correction and alignment of the fracture after surgical dissection and exposure of the fracture

Internal fixation: the stabilization of the reduced fracture by the use of metal screws, plates, nails, and pins

Arthroplasty: the repair of joint problems through the operating arthroscope (an instrument that allows the surgeon to operate within a joint without a large incision) or through open joint surgery

Hemiarthroplasty: the replacement of one of the articular surfaces (eg, in a hip hemiarthroplasty, the femoral head and neck are replaced with a femoral prosthesis—the acetabulum is not replaced)

Joint arthroplasty or *replacement:* the replacement of joint surfaces with metal or synthetic materials

Total joint arthroplasty or *replacement:* the replacement of both articular surfaces within a joint with metal or synthetic materials

Meniscectomy: the excision of damaged joint fibrocartilage

Tendon transfer: the movement of tendon insertion to improve function

Bone graft: the placement of bone tissue (autologous or homologous grafts) to promote healing, to stabilize, or to replace diseased bone

Amputation: the removal of a body part

Fasciotomy: the incision and diversion of the muscle fascia to relieve muscle constriction, as in compartment syndrome, or to reduce fascia contracture

Joint Replacement

Patients with severe joint pain and disability may undergo joint replacement. Conditions contributing to joint degeneration include osteoarthritis (degenerative joint disease), rheumatoid arthritis, trauma, and congenital deformity. Some fractures (eg, femoral neck fracture) may cause disruption of the blood supply and subsequent **avascular necrosis**; management with joint replacement may be elected over ORIF. Joints frequently replaced include the hip, knee (Fig. 61-6), and finger joints. Less frequently, more complex joints (shoulder, elbow, wrist, ankle) are replaced. The procedure is usually an elective one.

Most joint replacements consist of metal and high-density polyethylene components. Finger prostheses are generally Silastic. The joint implants may be cemented in the prepared bone with polymethyl methacrylate (PMMA), a bone-bonding agent that has properties similar to bone. Loosening of the prosthesis due to cement–bone interface failure is a common reason for prosthesis failure. Ingrowth prostheses (porous-coated, cementless artificial joint components) that allow the patient's bone to grow into and securely fix the prosthesis in the bone are being used more frequently than prostheses that are cemented. Accurate fitting and the presence of healthy bone with adequate blood supply are important in the use of cementless components. Much progress has been made in reducing prosthesis failure rate through improved techniques, improved materials, and use of bone grafts.

With joint replacement, excellent pain relief is obtained in most patients. Return of motion and function depends on preoperative soft tissue condition, soft tissue reactions, and general muscle strength. Early failure of joint replacement is associated with high levels of activity and preoperative joint pathology.

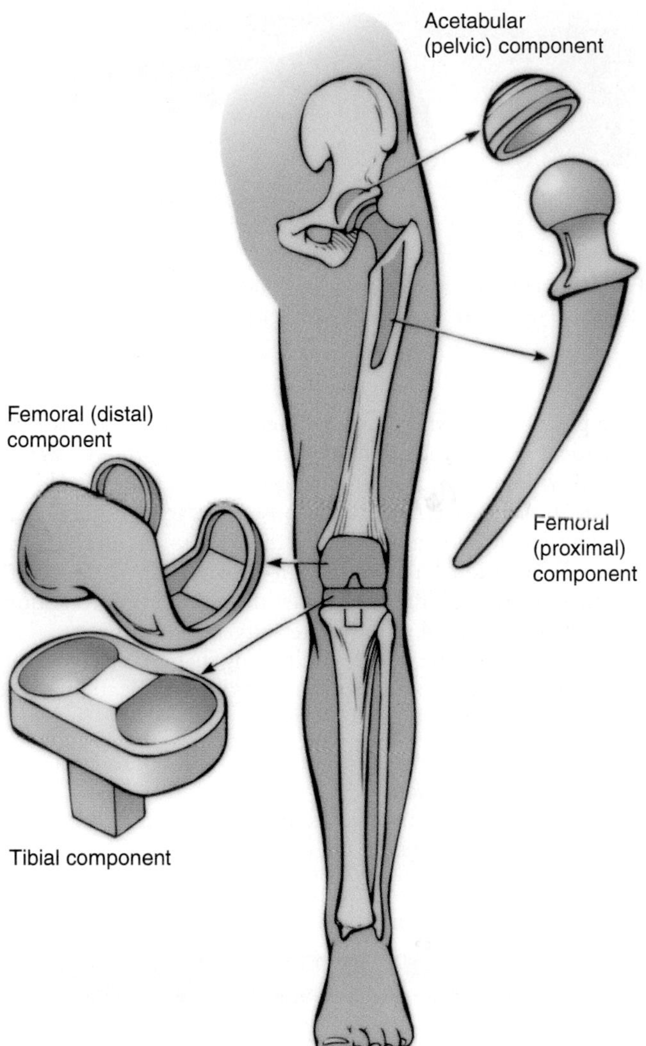

FIGURE 61•6 Hip and knee replacement.

Nursing Interventions

Assessment of the patient and preoperative management are aimed at having the patient in optimal health at the time of surgery. Preoperatively, it is important to evaluate cardiovascular, respiratory, renal, and hepatic functions. Age, obesity, preoperative leg edema, history of DVT, and varicose veins increase the risk of postoperative DVT and pulmonary embolism. These are the most common causes of postoperative mortality in patients older than 60 years of age undergoing total hip replacement. Every effort is made to prevent these complications.

Preoperatively, it is important to assess the neurovascular status of the extremity undergoing joint replacement. Postoperative assessment data are compared with preoperative assessment data to identify changes and deficits. For example, an absent pulse postoperatively is of concern unless the pulse was also absent preoperatively. Nerve palsy could occur during surgery.

PREVENTING INFECTION

Preoperative assessment of the patient for infection, including urinary tract infection, is necessary because of the risk of postoperative infection. Any infection 2 to 4 weeks before planned surgery may result in postponement of surgery. Preoperative skin preparation frequently begins 1 or 2 days before the surgery. Most deep infections are caused by bacteria, mostly from airborne sources, which contaminate the wound at the time of surgery. Therefore, as with any surgery, there is strict adherence to aseptic principles, and the operating area is controlled and made as bacteria free as possible.

Short courses of prophylactic antibiotics are administered perioperatively. Culture of the joint during surgery, before intraoperative antibiotic therapy is begun, may be important in identifying and treating subsequent infections.

If osteomyelitis develops, it is difficult to treat. Infection at the site of the prosthesis generally requires removal of the implant and joint revision, which is a complex procedure. Also, it is not always possible to achieve a functional joint when the reconstruction procedure has to be repeated.

PROMOTING AMBULATION

Patients with total hip or total knee replacement begin ambulation with a walker or crutches within 1 or 2 days after surgery. The goal is independent ambulation. At first, the patient may only be able to stand for a brief period because of orthostatic hypotension. Specific weight-bearing limits on the prosthesis are determined by the physician and are based on the patient's condition, the procedure, and the fixation method. Generally, cemented prostheses can have weight-bearing as tolerated by the patient. If the patient has a press-fit, cementless, ingrowth prosthesis, weight-bearing immediately after surgery may be limited to minimize micromotion of the prosthesis in the bone. As the patient can tolerate more activity, the nurse encourages transferring to a chair several times a day for short periods and walking progressively greater distances.

Total Hip Replacement

Total hip replacement is the replacement of a severely damaged hip with an artificial joint. Indications for this surgery include arthritis (degenerative joint disease, rheumatoid arthritis), femoral neck fractures, failure of previous reconstructive surgeries (failed prosthesis, **osteotomy**, femoral head replacement), and problems resulting from congenital hip disease. A variety of total hip prostheses are available. Most consist of a metal femoral component topped by a spherical ball fitted into a plastic acetabular socket (see Fig. 61-6). The surgeon selects the prosthesis most suited to the individual patient, considering various factors, including skeletal structure and activity level.

The patient is usually 60 years of age or older and has unremitting pain or irreversibly damaged hip joints. With the advent of improved prosthetic materials and operative techniques, the life of the prosthesis is extended, and younger patients with severely damaged and painful hip joints are undergoing total hip replacement.

NURSING INTERVENTIONS

The nurse must be aware of and monitor for specific potential complications associated with total hip replacement. Complications that may occur include dislocation of the hip prosthesis, excessive wound drainage, thromboembolism, and infection. Other complications for which the nurse must monitor include those associated with immobility, **heterotrophic ossification** (formation of bone in the periprosthetic space), avascular necrosis (bone death caused by loss of blood supply), and loosening of the prosthesis.

Preventing Dislocation of the Hip Prosthesis. Maintaining the femoral head component in the acetabular cup is essential. The nurse teaches the patient about positioning the leg in **abduc-**

tion, which helps to prevent dislocation of the prosthesis. The use of an abduction splint, wedge pillow (Fig. 61-7), or two or three pillows between the legs keeps the hip in abduction. When the nurse turns the patient in bed, it is important to keep the operative hip in abduction. Depending on the surgeon's preference, some patients are not permitted to be turned onto the affected side, whereas others may be turned side to side.

The patient's hip is never flexed more than 90 degrees. Therefore, to prevent hip flexion, the nurse does not elevate the head of the bed more than 60 degrees. When using the fracture bedpan, the nurse instructs the patient to flex the unaffected hip and to use the trapeze to lift the pelvis onto the pan. The patient is also reminded not to flex the affected hip.

Limited flexion is maintained during transfers and when sitting. When the patient is initially assisted out of bed, an abduction splint or pillows are kept between the legs. The nurse encourages the patient to keep the affected hip in extension, instructing the patient to pivot on the unaffected leg while assisted by the nurse, who protects the affected hip from adduction, flexion, internal or external rotation, and excessive weight bearing.

High-seat (orthopedic) chairs, semireclining wheelchairs, and toilet seat extenders may be used to minimize hip joint flexion. When sitting, the patient's hips should be higher than the knees. The patient's affected leg should not be elevated when sitting. The patient may flex the knee.

The nurse teaches the patient protective positioning, which includes maintaining abduction and avoiding internal and external rotation, hyperextension, and acute flexion. The patient should use a pillow between the legs when in a supine or side-lying position and when turning. Generally, the nurse instructs the patient not to sleep on the side on which the surgery was performed without consulting the surgeon. At no time should the patient cross the legs. The patient must avoid acute flexion of the hip. The patient should not bend at the waist to put on shoes and socks. Occupational therapists can provide the patient with devices to assist with dressing below the waist. Hip precautions are needed for about 4 months after surgery (Chart 61-4).

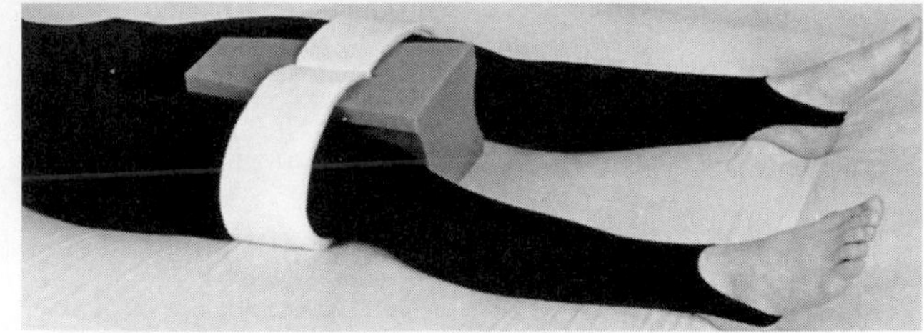

FIGURE 61•7 An abduction pillow may be used after a total hip replacement to prevent dislocation of the prosthesis.

Dislocation may occur with positioning that exceeds the limits of the prosthesis. The nurse must recognize dislocation of the prosthesis. Indicators are as follows:

- Increased pain related to the surgical procedure, swelling, and immobilization
- Acute groin pain in affected hip or increased discomfort
- Shortening of the leg

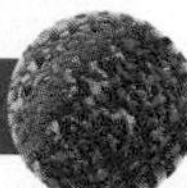

CHART 61•4 Avoiding Hip Dislocation After Replacement Surgery

Until the hip prosthesis stabilizes after hip replacement surgery, the patient needs to learn about proper positioning so that the prosthesis remains in place. Dislocation of the hip is a serious complication of surgery that causes pain and necessitates reoperation to correct the dislocation. Desirable positions include abduction, neutral rotation, and flexion of less than 90 degrees. When the patient is seated, the knees should be lower than the hip.

Guidelines for avoiding displacement include the following:

- Keep the knees apart at all times.
- Put a pillow between the legs when sleeping.
- Never cross the legs when seated.
- Avoid bending forward when seated in a chair.
- Avoid bending forward to pick up an object on the floor.
- Use a raised toilet seat.
- Do not flex the hip to put on clothing such as pants, stockings, socks or shoes.

Positions to avoid after total hip replacement are illustrated below.

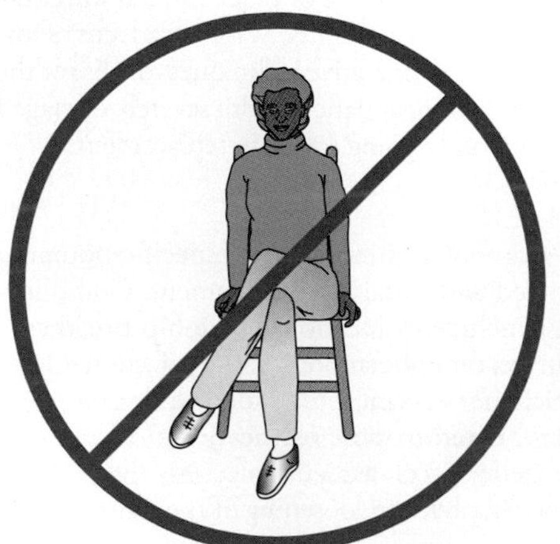

Affected leg should not cross the center of the body

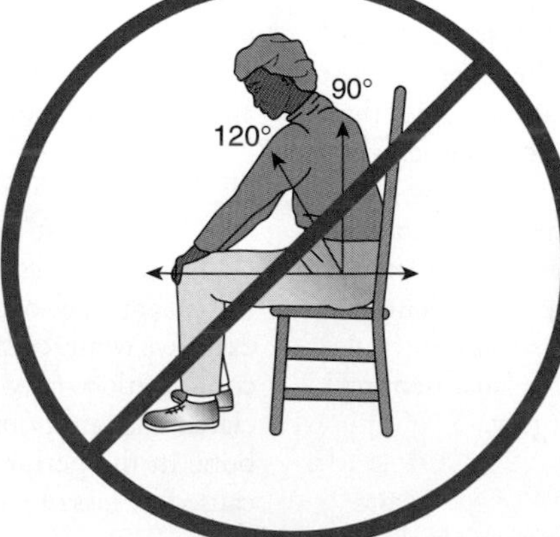

Hip should not bend more than 90 degrees

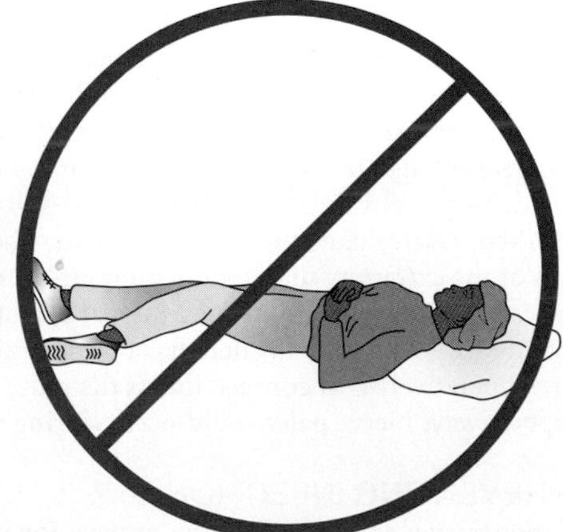

Affected leg should not turn inward

- Abnormal external or internal rotation
- Restricted ability or inability to move leg
- Reported "popping" sensation in hip

If a prosthesis becomes dislocated, the nurse (or patient if at home) immediately notifies the surgeon because the hip must be reduced and stabilized promptly so that the leg does not sustain circulatory and nerve damage. As the muscles and joint capsule heal, the chance of dislocation diminishes. Stresses to the new hip joint should be minimal for the first 3 to 6 months.

Monitoring Wound Drainage. Fluid and blood accumulating at the surgical site are generally drained with a portable suction device. This prevents accumulation of fluid, which could contribute to discomfort and provide a site for infection. Drainage of 200 to 500 mL in the first 24 hours is expected; by 48 hours postoperatively, the total drainage in 8 hours usually decreases to 30 mL or less, and the suction device is then removed. The nurse promptly notifies the physician of any drainage volumes greater than anticipated.

When extensive blood loss is anticipated after total joint replacement surgery, an autotransfusion drainage system (ie, the drained blood is filtered and reinfused into the patient during the immediate postoperative period) may be used to decrease the need for homologous blood transfusions.

Preventing Deep Vein Thrombosis. The risk for thromboembolism is particularly great after reconstructive hip surgery. The incidence of DVT is 45% to 70%. About 20% of patients with DVT develop pulmonary emboli, of which about 1% to 3% of cases are fatal. Therefore, the nurse must institute preventive measures and monitor the patient closely for the development of DVT and pulmonary emboli. Measures to promote circulation and decrease venous stasis are priorities for the patient undergoing hip reconstruction. The nurse encourages the patient to perform ankle and foot exercises hourly while awake, use elastic stockings and sequential compression devices as prescribed, and transfer out of bed and ambulate with assistance beginning the first postoperative day. Low-dose heparin or enoxaparin (Lovenox) is used as prophylaxis for DVT after hip replacement surgery.

Preventing Infection. Infection, a serious complication of total hip replacement, may necessitate removal of the implant. Patients who are elderly, obese, or poorly nourished and patients who have diabetes, rheumatoid arthritis, concurrent infections (eg, urinary tract infections, dental abscesses), or large hematomas are at high risk for infection.

Because total joint infections are so disastrous, all efforts are undertaken to minimize their occurrence. Potential sources of infection are scrupulously avoided. Prophylactic antibiotics are prescribed. If indwelling urinary catheters and portable wound suction devices are used, they are removed as soon as possible to avoid infection. Prophylactic antibiotics are recommended if the patient needs any future surgical instrumentation, such as tooth extraction or cystoscopic examination.

Acute infections may occur within 3 months of surgery and are associated with progressive superficial infections or hematomas. Delayed surgical infections may appear 4 to 24 months after surgery and may cause return of discomfort in the hip. Infections occurring more than 2 years after surgery are attributed to the spread of infection through the bloodstream from another site in the body. If an infection occurs, antibiotics are prescribed. Severe infections may require surgical débridement or removal of the prosthesis.

PROMOTING HOME AND COMMUNITY-BASED CARE

Teaching Patients Self-Care. Before the patient prepares to leave the acute care setting, the nurse provides a thorough teaching program to promote continuity of the therapeutic regimen and active participation in the rehabilitation process (see the accompanying Health Promotion and Illness Prevention chart).

The nurse advises the patient of the importance of the daily exercise program in maintaining the functional motion of the hip joint and strengthening the abductor muscles of the hip. It will take time to strengthen and reeducate the muscles.

Assistive devices (crutches, walker, or cane) are used for a time. When sufficient muscle tone has developed to permit a normal gait without discomfort, these devices are not necessary. In general, by 3 months, the patient can resume routine ADLs. Stair climbing is permitted as prescribed and kept to a minimum for 3 to 6 months. Frequent walks, swimming, and use of a high rocking chair are excellent for hip exercises. Sexual activities should be carried out with the patient in the dependent position (flat on the back) for 3 to 6 months to avoid excessive adduction and flexion of the new hip.

At no time during the first 4 to 6 months should the patient cross the legs or flex the hip more than 90 degrees. Assistance in putting on shoes and socks may be needed. The patient should avoid low chairs and sitting for more than 45 minutes at a time. These precautions minimize hip flexion, the risk for prosthetic dislocation, hip stiffness, and flexion contracture. Traveling long distances should be avoided unless frequent position changes are possible. Other activities to avoid include tub baths, overexertion, lifting heavy loads, and excessive bending and twisting (lifting, shoveling snow, forceful turning).

Continuing Care. A home visit may be necessary to make sure that there are no physical barriers to impede the patient's rehabilitation. In addition, the nurse may need to assist the patient in acquiring devices, such as reachers to help with dressing or toilet seat extenders. The nurse also may need to make a home visit to assess for potential problems (see the Health Promotion and Illness Prevention chart).

After successful surgery and rehabilitation, the patient can expect a hip joint that is free or nearly free of pain, has good motion, is stable, and permits normal or near-normal ambulation (Plan of Nursing Care 61-1).

Total Knee Replacement

Total knee replacement surgery is considered for patients who have severe pain and functional disabilities related to joint surfaces destroyed by arthritis (osteoarthritis, rheumatoid arthritis, posttraumatic arthritis), and bleeding into the joint, such as may result from hemophilia. Metal and acrylic prostheses designed to provide the patient with a functional, painless, stable joint may be used. If the patient's ligaments have weakened, a fully constrained (hinged) or semiconstrained prosthesis may be used to provide joint stability. A nonconstrained prosthesis depends on the patient's ligaments for joint stability.

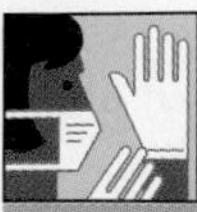

Health Promotion and Illness Prevention

Home Care After Hip Replacement

Considerations
- Pain management
- Wound care
- Mobility
- Self-care (activities of daily living)
- Potential problems

Nursing Interventions

Discuss with patient methods to reduce pain:
- Periodic rest
- Distraction and relaxation techniques
- Medication therapy (eg nonsteroidal anti-inflammatory drugs, opioid analgesics): actions of medications, administration, schedule, side effects

Instruct patient in the following:
- Keeping incision clean and dry
- Taking care of the wound and changing the dressing
- Recognizing signs of wound infection (eg pain, swelling, drainage, fever)

Explain that sutures or staples will be removed 10 to 14 days after surgery.

Teach patient about the following:
- Safe use of assistive devices
- Weight-bearing limits
- How to change positions frequently
- Limitations on hip flexion and adduction (eg avoid acute flexion and crossing legs)
- How to stand without flexing hip acutely
- Avoidance of low-seated chairs
- Sleeping with pillow between legs to prevent adduction
- Gradual increase in activities and participation in prescribed exercise regimen

Assess home environment for physical barriers.

Instruct patient to use elevated toilet seat and to use reachers to aid in dressing.

Encourage patient to accept assistance with activities of daily living during early convalescence until mobility and strength improve.

Assess patient for development of potential problems, and instruct patient to report signs of potential problems:
- Dislocation of prosthesis (eg, increased pain, shortening of leg, inability to move leg, popping sensation in hip, abnormal rotation)
- Deep vein thrombosis (eg, calf pain, swelling)
- Wound infection (eg, swelling, purulent drainage, pain, fever)

NURSING INTERVENTIONS

Postoperatively, the knee is dressed with a compression bandage. Ice may be applied to control edema and bleeding. The nurse assesses the neurovascular status of the leg. It is important to encourage active flexion of the foot every hour when the patient is awake. Efforts are directed at preventing complications (thromboembolism, peroneal nerve palsy, infection, limited range of motion).

A wound suction drain removes fluid accumulating in the joint. Drainage during the first 24 hours after surgery ranges from 200 to 400 mL and diminishes to less than 25 mL by 48 hours after surgery. The drains are then removed by the surgeon. If extensive bleeding is anticipated, an autotransfusion drainage system may be used during the immediate postoperative period.

Frequently, the patient's leg is placed on a **continuous passive motion** (CPM) device in the postanesthesia care unit. This device promotes healing by increasing circulation and movement of the knee joint. The rate and amount of extension and flexion are prescribed. Usually, 10 degrees of extension and 50 degrees of flexion are initiated, increasing to 90 degrees of flexion with full extension (0 degrees) by discharge.

The nurse encourages the patient to use the device most of the time. The physical therapist supervises exercises for strength and range of motion. If satisfactory flexion is not achieved, gentle manipulation of the knee joint under general anesthesia may be necessary about 2 weeks after surgery.

The nurse assists the patient to get out of bed the evening of the surgery or the day after surgery. The knee is usually protected with a knee immobilizer and is elevated when the patient sits in a chair. Weight-bearing limits are prescribed by the physician. Progressive ambulation, using assistive devices and within the prescribed weight-bearing limits, begins the day after the surgery.

After discharge from the hospital, the patient may continue to use the CPM device at home and undergo physical therapy on an outpatient basis. Late complications that may occur include infection and loosening and wear of prosthetic components. Generally, the patient can achieve a pain-free, functional joint and participate more fully in life activities.

NURSING PROCESS: PREOPERATIVE CARE OF THE PATIENT UNDERGOING ORTHOPEDIC SURGERY

Assessment

Assessment of the patient is focused on hydration, current medication history, and possible infection. Adequate hydration is an important goal for orthopedic patients. Immobilization and bed rest contribute to DVT, to urinary stasis and associated bladder infections, and to kidney stone formation. Adequate hydration decreases blood viscosity and venous stasis and ensures adequate urine flow. To determine preoperative hydration, the nurse assesses the skin and mucous membranes, vital signs, urinary output, and laboratory values.

The medication history provides information for perioperative management. The patient with chronic illness (eg, rheumatoid arthritis, chronic pulmonary disease) frequently has received corticosteroid medications to control symptoms. The corticosteroid should be administered preoperatively, intraoperatively, and postoperatively as prescribed to prevent the occurrence of adrenal insufficiency from suppressed adrenal function. The use of other medications, such as anticoagulants, cardiovascular agents, or

(text continues on page 1800)

61•1

Plan of Nursing Care 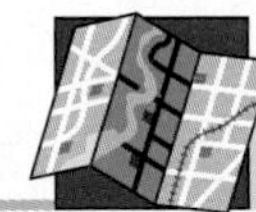 The Patient With a Total Hip Replacement

Nursing Interventions	Rationale	Expected Outcomes
Nursing Diagnosis: Pain related to total hip replacement **Goal:** Relief of pain		
1. Assess patient for pain.	1. Pain is expected after a surgical procedure because of the surgical trauma and tissue response. Muscle spasms occur after total hip replacements. Immobility causes discomfort at pressure points.	• Patient describes discomfort • Expresses confidence in efforts to control pain • States pain is reduced • Appears comfortable and relaxed • Uses physical, psychological, and pharmacologic measures to reduce discomfort
2. Ask patient to describe discomfort.	2. Pain characteristics may help to determine cause of discomfort. Pain may be due to complication (hematoma, infection, flatus). Pain is an individual experience—it means different things to different people.	
3. Acknowledge existence of pain; inform patient of available analgesics or muscle relaxants.	3. The nurse can reduce the stress experienced by patient by communicating concern and availability of assistance to help patient deal with the pain	
4. Use pain-modifying techniques.	4.	
a. Use analgesics.	a. Patient will require parenteral opioids during the first 24–48 hours, and then will progress to oral analgesics.	
b. Change position within prescribed limits.	b. Use of pillows to provide adequate support and relief of pressure on bony prominences assists in minimizing pain.	
c. Modify environment.	c. Interactions with others, distractions, and sensory overload or deprivation may affect pain experience.	
d. Notify surgeon if necessary.	d. Surgical intervention may be necessary if pain is due to hematoma or excessive edema.	
5. Evaluate and record discomfort and effectiveness of pain-modifying techniques.	5. Effectiveness of action is based on experience; notations provide data concerning pain experiences, management, and pain relief.	
Nursing Diagnosis: Impaired physical mobility related to enforced bed rest after hip replacement **Goal:** Achieves pain-free, functional, stable hip joint		
1. Maintain proper positioning of hip joint (abduction, neutral rotation, limited flexion).	1. Prevents dislocation of hip prosthesis.	• Prescribed position maintained • Patient assists in position changes • Shows increased independence in transfers • Exercises hourly • Participates in progressive ambulation program • Actively participates in exercise regimen • Uses ambulatory aids correctly and safely
2. Instruct and assist in position changes and transfers.	2. Encourages patient's active participation while preventing dislocation.	
3. Instruct and supervise isometric quadriceps- and gluteal-setting exercises.	3. Strengthens muscles needed for walking.	
4. In consultation with physical therapist, instruct and supervise progressive safe ambulation within limitations of weight-bearing prescription.	4. Amount of weight-bearing depends on patient's condition and prosthesis; ambulatory aids are used to assist the patient with non–weight-bearing and partial weight-bearing ambulation.	
5. Offer encouragement and support exercise regimen.	5. Reconditioning exercises can be uncomfortable and fatiguing; encouragement helps patient comply with exercise program.	
6. Instruct and supervise safe use of ambulatory aids.	6. Prevents injury from unsafe use.	

(continued)

61•1 **Plan of Nursing Care**

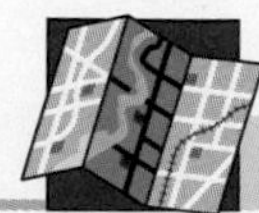

The Patient With a Total Hip Replacement (*continued*)

Nursing Interventions	Rationale	Expected Outcomes
Collaborative Problems: Hemorrhage; neurovascular compromise; dislocation of prosthesis; deep vein thrombosis; infection related to surgery **Goal:** Absence of complications		
Hemorrhage		
1. Monitor vital signs, observing for shock.	1. Changes in pulse, blood pressure, and respirations may indicate development of shock. Blood loss and stress of surgery may contribute to development of shock.	• Vital signs stabilize within normal limits • Amount of drainage decreases • No bright red bloody drainage • Hematology values are within normal limits
2. Note character and amount of drainage.	2. Within 48 hours, bloody drainage collected in portable suction device decreases to 25–30 mL per 8 hours. Excessive drainage (more than 250 mL in first 8 hours after surgery) and bright red drainage may indicate active bleeding.	
3. Notify surgeon if patient develops shock or excessive bleeding and prepare for administration of fluids, blood component therapy, and medications.	3. Corrective measures need to be instituted.	
4. Note hemoglobin and hematocrit values.	4. Anemia due to blood loss may develop. Blood replacement therapy may be needed.	
Neurovascular Compromise		
1. Assess affected extremity for color and temperature.	1. The skin becomes pale and feels cool with decreased tissue perfusion. Venous congestion may produce cyanosis.	• Color normal • Extremity warm • Normal capillary refill • Moderate edema and swelling; tissue not palpably tense • Pain controllable • No pain with passive dorsiflexion • Normal sensations • No paresthesia • Normal motor abilities • No paresis or paralysis • Pulses strong and equal
2. Assess toes for capillary refill response.	2. After compression of the nail, rapid return of pink color indicates good capillary perfusion.	
3. Assess extremity for edema and swelling. Listen to patient complaints of leg tightness.	3. The trauma of surgery will cause edema. Excessive swelling and hematoma formation can compromise circulation and function.	
4. Elevate extremity (keep lower than hip when in chair).	4. Minimizes dependent edema.	
5. Assess for deep, throbbing, unrelenting pain.	5. Surgical pain can be controlled; pain due to neurovascular compromise is refractory to treatment.	
6. Assess for pain on passive flexion of foot.	6. With nerve ischemia, there will be pain on passive stretch. Additionally, pain may indicate deep vein thrombosis—positive Homans' sign.	
7. Assess for sensations and numbness.	7. Diminished pain and paresthesia may indicate nerve damage. Sensation in web between great and second toe—peroneal nerve; sensation on sole of foot—tibial nerve.	
8. Assess ability to move foot and toes.	8. Dorsiflexion of ankle and extension of toes indicate function of peroneal nerve. Plantar flexion of ankle and flexion of toes indicate function of tibial nerve.	
9. Assess pedal pulses in both feet. Notify surgeon if diminished neurovascular status is noted.	9. Indicator of extremity circulation. Function of extremity needs to be preserved.	

(*continued*)

61•1

Plan of Nursing Care 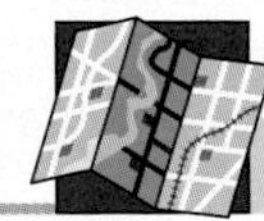 **The Patient With a Total Hip Replacement (*continued*)**

Nursing Interventions	Rationale	Expected Outcomes
Dislocation of Prosthesis		
1. Position patient as prescribed.	1. Hip component positioning (femoral component in acetabular component) needs to be maintained.	• Prosthesis not dislocated
2. Use abductor splint or pillows to maintain position and to support extremity.	2. Keep hip in abduction and in a neutral rotation to prevent dislocation.	
3. Support leg and place pillows between legs when patient is turning and side-lying; turn to the unaffected side.	3–5. Prevent dislocation.	
4. Avoid acute flexion of hip (head of bed at 60 degrees or less).		
5. Avoid crossing legs.		
6. Assess for dislocation of prosthesis (extremity shortens, internally or externally rotated, severe hip pain, patient unable to move extremity)	6. Findings may indicate dislocation of prosthesis.	
7. Notify surgeon of possible dislocation.	7. Joint dislocations compromise neurovascular status and future function of extremity.	
Deep Vein Thrombosis		
1. Use elastic stocking or sequential compression device as prescribed.	1. Aid in venous blood return and prevent stasis.	• Wears elastic stockings; uses compression device
2. Remove stocking for 20 minutes twice a day and provide skin care.	2. Skin care is necessary to avoid breakdown. Extended removal of stockings defeats purpose of stockings.	• No skin breakdown • Pulses equal and strong • Skin temperature normal
3. Assess popliteal, dorsalis pedis, and posterior tibial pulses.	3. Pulses indicate arterial perfusion of extremity.	• Negative Homans' sign • Changes position with assistance and supervision
4. Assess skin temperature of legs.	4. Local inflammation will increase local skin temperature.	• Participates in exercise regimen
5. Assess for Homans' sign every 8 hours.	5. Pain on dorsiflexion of ankle may indicate deep vein thrombosis.	• No chest pain; lungs clear to auscultation; no evidence of pulmonary emboli
6. Avoid pressure on popliteal blood vessels from appliances or pillows.	6. Compression of blood vessels diminishes blood flow.	
7. Change position and increase activity as prescribed.	7. Activity promotes circulation and diminishes venous stasis.	
8. Supervise ankle exercises hourly.	8. Muscle exercise promotes circulation.	
9. Monitor body temperature.	9. Body temperature increases with inflammation.	
Wound Infection		
1. Monitor vital signs.	1. Temperature, pulse, and respirations increase in response to infection. (Magnitude of response may be minimal in an elderly patient.)	• Vital signs normal • Well-approximated incision without drainage or excessive inflammatory response • Minimal discomfort; no hematoma
2. Use aseptic technique for dressing changes and emptying of portable drainage.	2. Avoids introducing organisms.	• Patient tolerates antibiotics
3. Assess wound appearance and character of drainage.	3. Red, swollen, draining incision is indicative of infection.	
4. Assess complaints of pain.	4. Pain may be due to wound hematoma—a possible locus of infection—that needs to be surgically evacuated.	
5. Administer prophylactic antibiotics if prescribed, and observe for side effects.	5. Infected prosthesis is avoided.	

(*continued*)

61•1

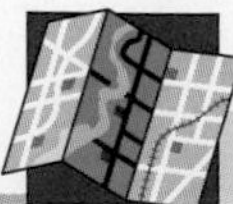

Plan of Nursing Care: The Patient With a Total Hip Replacement (*continued*)

Nursing Interventions	Rationale	Expected Outcomes
Nursing Diagnosis: Potential impaired home maintenance management related to total hip replacement **Goal:** Cares for self at home		
1. Assess home environment for discharge planning.	1. Physical barriers (especially stairs, bathrooms) may limit patient's ability to ambulate and care for self at home.	• Home is accessible for patient at time of discharge
2. Encourage patient to express concerns about care at home; explore together possible solutions to the problem.	2. Patient may have special problems that need to be identified and resolved.	• Patient appears relaxed and develops strategies to deal with identified problems • Personal assistance is available
3. Assess availability of physical assistance for health care activities.	3. Because of limitation of mobility and limited hip range of motion, patient may require some assistance in routine health care.	• Patient demonstrates ability to provide necessary assistance within therapeutic prescription • Complies with home care program • Keeps follow-up health care appointments
4. Teach caregiver home health care regimen.	4. Understanding of rehabilitative regimen is necessary for compliance.	
5. Instruct patient on posthospital care: a. Activity limitations (avoid stressing prosthesis) b. Exercise instructions c. Safe use of ambulatory aids d. Wound care e. Measures to promote healing f. Medications, if any g. Potential problems h. Continuing health care supervision and management	5. Lack of knowledge and poor preparation for care at home contribute to patient anxiety, insecurity, and nonadherence to therapeutic regimen.	

insulin, needs to be documented and discussed with the surgeon and anesthesiologist to ensure adequate management.

The nurse asks the patient specifically about the occurrence of colds, dental problems, urinary tract infections, and other infections within the 2 weeks before surgery. Osteomyelitis could develop through hematologous spread. Permanent disability can result if infection occurs within a bone or joint. Preexisting infections must be resolved before elective orthopedic surgery.

Other areas of preoperative assessment are similar to those for any patient undergoing surgery. The patient who is to receive "on-call" intramuscular preoperative medications receives them by injection into an uninvolved area because tissue absorption is better in nontraumatized tissues.

Diagnosis

Nursing Diagnoses

Based on the nursing assessment data, the patient's major preoperative nursing diagnoses related to orthopedic status may include the following:

- Pain related to fracture, orthopedic problem, swelling, or inflammation
- Risk for peripheral neurovascular dysfunction related to swelling, constricting devices, or impaired venous return
- Risk for ineffective management of therapeutic regimen related to insufficient knowledge or available support and resources
- Impaired physical mobility related to pain, swelling, and possibly an immobilization device
- Self-esteem disturbance: body image, related to impact of musculoskeletal problem

Planning and Goals

The major goals of the patient before orthopedic surgery may include relief of pain, adequate neurovascular function, health promotion, improved mobility, and positive self-esteem.

Nursing Interventions

Relieving Pain

Physical, pharmacologic, and psychological strategies to control pain are useful in the preoperative period. Specific strategies are tailored to the individual patient. Immobilization of a fractured bone or injured, inflamed joint decreases discomfort. Elevation of an edematous extremity promotes venous return and reduces associated discomfort. Ice, if prescribed, relieves swelling and directly reduces discomfort by diminishing nerve stimulation. Analgesics are frequently prescribed to control the acute pain of musculoskeletal injury and associated muscle spasm. During the immediate preoperative period, the nurse needs to discuss and coordinate the administration of analgesic medications with the anesthesiologist and surgeon. Alternative methods of pain control (eg, distraction, focusing, guided imagery, quiet environment, back rubs) may be used to decrease pain perception.

Maintaining Adequate Neurovascular Function

Trauma, edema, or immobilization devices may interrupt tissue perfusion. The nurse must frequently assess neurovascular status (ie, color, temperature, capillary refill, pulses, edema, pain, sensation, motion) of the extremity and document the findings. If circulation is compromised, the nurse institutes measures to restore adequate circulation. These include promptly notifying the physician, elevating the extremity, and releasing constricting wraps or casts as prescribed.

Promoting Health

The nurse assists the patient in activities that promote health during the perioperative and rehabilitative periods. The nurse assesses nutritional status and hydration and provides adequate diet and fluids. The preoperative fasting regimen is usually tolerated well. If the patient has diabetes, is elderly and frail, or is the victim of multiple trauma, special provisions may be necessary.

The nurse monitors fluid intake, urinary output, urinalysis findings, and complaints of burning on urination. At times, patients may limit their fluid intake to minimize the use of a bedpan. A small fracture pan may be more comfortable for the patient to use. An indwelling catheter should be used judiciously to minimize the risk of urinary tract infection. Data suggest urinary tract infection must be addressed prior to surgery.

Coughing, deep breathing, and use of the incentive spirometer are practiced preoperatively for improved respiratory function during the postoperative period. Preoperative teaching facilitates postoperative compliance. Smoking should be stopped during the preoperative period to facilitate optimum respiratory function.

The nurse provides skin care, paying special attention to pressure points. It is important to institute the use of pressure-reducing surfaces before surgery for patients at risk for skin breakdown.

To minimize the risk for infection, the nurse meticulously and gently cleans the skin with soap and water the day before surgery. If the surgery is elective, the orthopedic surgeon may instruct the patient to use a germicidal soap several days before hospitalization.

The nurse discusses with the patient and the family the need for assistance with ADLs and the therapeutic regimen during convalescence so that adequate support is available when the patient is discharged. Modification of the home environment may be necessary to accommodate the altered mobility of the patient after surgery. A referral to the social worker and the physical therapist may be needed to ensure smooth transition to home care.

Improving Mobility

Preoperatively, the patient's mobility may be impaired by pain, swelling, and immobilizing devices (eg, splints, casts, traction). The nurse should elevate and adequately support edematous extremities with pillows. It is important to control pain before an injured part is moved by administering medication in time for it to take effect and by supporting the injured part when it is moved. The nurse encourages movement within the limits of therapeutic immobility. The patient should perform active range-of-motion exercises of uninvolved joints and, unless contraindicated, isometric contraction of the calf muscles and ankle. The nurse teaches gluteal-setting and quadriceps-setting isometric exercises to maintain the muscles needed for ambulation (see Chart 61-2). The patient who will be using assistive devices postoperatively may exercise to strengthen the upper extremities and shoulders. If use of assistive devices (eg, crutches, walker, wheelchair) is anticipated, the nurse encourages the patient to practice with them preoperatively to facilitate their safe use and promote earlier independent mobility.

Helping the Patient Maintain Self-Esteem

Preoperatively, orthopedic patients may need assistance in accepting changes in body image, diminished self-esteem, or inability to perform their roles and responsibilities. The degree of assistance required in this area varies greatly, depending on the events preceding hospitalization, the surgery and rehabilitation planned, and the temporary or permanent nature of the problems. The nurse promotes a trusting relationship for patients to express concerns and anxieties and helps them examine their feelings about changes in self-concept. The nurse clarifies any misconceptions patients may have and helps them work through modifications needed to adapt to alterations in physical capacity and self-esteem.

Evaluation

Expected Outcomes

Expected outcomes may include:

1. Reports relief of pain
   a. Uses multiple approaches to reduce pain
   b. States that medication is effective in relieving pain
   c. Moves with increasing comfort
2. Exhibits adequate neurovascular function
   a. Exhibits normal skin color
   b. Has warm skin
   c. Has normal capillary refill response
   d. Demonstrates normal sensation and motion
   e. Demonstrates reduced swelling
3. Promotes health
   a. Eats balanced diet appropriate to meet nutritional needs
   b. Maintains adequate hydration
   c. Abstains from smoking
   d. Practices respiratory exercises
   e. Repositions self to relieve skin pressure
   f. Engages in strengthening and preventive exercises
   g. Plans for assistance during convalescence at home
4. Maximizes mobility within the therapeutic limits
   a. Requests assistance when moving
   b. Elevates edematous extremity after transfer
   c. Uses immobilizing devices and assistive devices as prescribed
5. Expresses positive self-esteem
   a. Acknowledges temporary or permanent changes in body image
   b. Discusses role performance changes
   c. Participates in decisions about care

NURSING PROCESS: POSTOPERATIVE CARE OF THE PATIENT UNDERGOING ORTHOPEDIC SURGERY

Assessment

After orthopedic surgery, the nurse continues the preoperative care plan, modifying it to the patient's current postoperative status. The nurse reassesses the patient's needs in relation to pain, neurovascular status, health promotion, mobility, and self-esteem. Skeletal trauma and surgery performed on bones, muscles, and joints can produce significant pain, especially during the first 1 or 2 postoperative days. Tissue perfusion must be monitored closely because edema and bleeding into the tissues may compromise circulation and result in compartment syndrome. Inactivity contributes to venous stasis and development of DVT.

Assessment of respiratory, gastrointestinal, and urinary function provides data about function of these systems. General anesthesia, analgesia, and immobility can result in altered functioning of these systems.

The nurse notes the prescribed limits on mobility and assesses the patient's understanding of the mobility restrictions. Reassessing the patient's self-esteem allows the nurse to modify the preoperative plan of care more easily.

In addition, the nurse assesses and monitors the patient for potential problems related to the surgery. Frequent assessment of vital signs, level of consciousness, neurovascular status, wound drainage, breath sounds, bowel sounds, fluid balance, and pain provides the nurse with data that may suggest the possible development of complications. The nurse reports abnormal findings to the physician promptly.

With major orthopedic surgery, there is a risk of hypovolemic shock because of blood loss. Muscle dissection frequently produces wounds in which hemostasis is poor. Wounds that are closed under tourniquet control may bleed during the postoperative period. The nurse must be alert for signs of hypovolemic shock.

Changes in the patient's pulse rate, respiratory rate, or color may indicate pulmonary or cardiovascular complications. Atelectasis and pneumonia are common and may be related to preexisting pulmonary disease, deep anesthesia, decreased activity, analgesics, and reduced respiratory reserve due to advanced age or an underlying musculoskeletal disorder (eg, restrictive lung expansion secondary to kyphosis or osteoporosis).

Voiding in unnatural positions may contribute to urinary retention. In addition, elderly men usually have some degree of prostate enlargement and may already have difficulty voiding. Therefore, it is important to monitor urinary output.

Temperature elevations within the first 48 hours are frequently related to atelectasis or other respiratory problems. Temperature elevations during the next few days are frequently associated with urinary tract infections. Superficial wound infections take about 4 to 6 days to develop. Fever from phlebitis generally occurs during the end of the first week through the second week.

Thromboembolic disease (see Deep Vein Thrombosis in Chap. 28 and Pulmonary Embolism in Chap. 21) is one of the most common and most dangerous of all complications occurring in the postoperative orthopedic patient. Advancing age, venous stasis, lower extremity orthopedic surgery, and immobilization are significant risk factors. The nurse assesses the patient daily for calf swelling, tenderness, warmth, redness, and a positive Homans' sign. The nurse promptly reports abnormal findings to the physician.

In addition, fat embolus (see Chap. 63) may occur with orthopedic surgery. The nurse must be alert to changes in respiration, behavior, and level of consciousness that suggest the development of fat embolus.

Diagnosis

Nursing Diagnoses

Based on all assessment data, the patient's major nursing diagnoses after orthopedic surgery may include the following:

- Pain related to the surgical procedure, swelling, and immobilization
- Risk for peripheral neurovascular dysfunction related to swelling, constricting devices, or impaired circulation
- Risk for ineffective adherence to therapeutic regimen related to insufficient knowledge or available support and resources
- Impaired physical mobility related to pain, edema, or an immobilizing device (eg, splint, traction, cast)
- Risk for self-esteem disturbance: body image or role performance related to impact of musculoskeletal problem

Collaborative Problems/Potential Complications

Based on the assessment data, potential complications may include the following:

- Hypovolemic shock
- Atelectasis; pneumonia
- Urinary retention
- Infection
- Venous stasis and DVT

Planning and Goals

The major goals of the patient after orthopedic surgery may include relief of pain, adequate neurovascular function, health promotion, improved mobility, positive self-esteem, and absence of complications.

Nursing Interventions

Relieving Pain

After orthopedic surgery, pain can be intense. Edema, hematomas, and muscle spasms contribute to the pain experienced. Some patients report that the pain is less than that experienced preoperatively, and only moderate amounts of analgesics are needed. The nurse closely monitors the patient's pain level and response to therapeutic measures and makes every effort to relieve the pain and discomfort.

Multiple pharmacologic approaches to pain management exist. Patient-controlled analgesia (PCA) and epidural analgesia may be prescribed to control the pain. If intramuscular and oral analgesics are prescribed on an as-needed basis (PRN), the nurse instructs the patient to request the analgesic before the pain becomes severe. The nurse rotates intramuscular injection sites, avoiding the operative hip and thigh. The nurse may administer medications on a preventive basis within the prescribed intervals if the onset of pain can be predicted (eg, 30 minutes before planned activity such as transfer or exercise).

In addition to pharmacologic approaches to controlling pain, elevation of the operative extremity and application of cold, if prescribed, help to control edema and pain. Portable suction of the wound decreases fluid accumulation and hematoma formation. The nurse may find that repositioning, relaxation, distraction, and guided imagery help in reducing the patient's pain.

The nurse should report increasing and uncontrollable pain to the orthopedic surgeon for evaluation. Pain should diminish rapidly after the initial postoperative period. After 2 to 3 days, most patients require only occasional oral analgesia for residual muscle soreness and spasm.

Maintaining Adequate Neurovascular Function

The nurse continues the preoperative plan of care. The nurse monitors the neurovascular status of the involved body part and notifies the physician promptly of indications of diminished tissue perfusion. The patient is reminded to perform muscle-setting, ankle, and calf-pumping exercises hourly while awake to enhance circulation.

Maintaining Health

The nurse continues the preoperative plan of care. It is important to encourage the patient to participate in the postoperative treatment regimen.

A well-balanced diet with adequate protein and vitamins is needed for wound healing. The patient progresses to a full and balanced diet as soon as possible. Large amounts of milk should not be given to orthopedic patients who are on bed rest, however, because this adds to the calcium pool in the body and requires that more calcium be excreted by the kidneys, which increases the risk for urinary calculi.

The nurse monitors the patient for pressure ulcers, which are a threat to any patient who must spend an extended time in bed or who is elderly, malnourished, or unable to move without assistance. Turning, washing, and drying the skin and minimizing pressure over bony prominences are necessary to avoid skin breakdown.

Improving Physical Mobility

Patients are frequently afraid to move after orthopedic surgery. Preoperative education about the planned postoperative treatment regimen promotes patient participation in physical activities. Patients often increase their mobility once they have been assured that movement within therapeutic limits is beneficial, that assistance will be provided by the nurse, and that discomfort can be controlled. Although soft tissue heals more rapidly than bone and the incision may appear healed, the underlying bone requires more time to repair and regain normal strength. This is especially important to remember in patients undergoing leg surgery.

Metal pins, screws, rods, and plates used for internal fixation are designed to maintain the position of the bone until ossification occurs. They are not designed to support the body's weight and can bend, loosen, or break if stressed. The estimated strength of the bone, the stability of the fracture, reduction and fixation, and the amount of bone healing are important considerations in determining weight-bearing limits. Some orthopedic procedures require weight-bearing restrictions. The orthopedic surgeon will prescribe the weight-bearing limits and use of protective devices (orthoses), if necessary, after surgery.

The physical therapist tailors the exercise program to the individual patient's needs. The goal is the patient's return to the highest level of function in the shortest time possible. Rehabilitation involves progressively increasing the patient's activities and exercises. Assistive devices (crutches, walker) may be used for postoperative mobility. Preoperative practice with assistive devices helps the patient use them postoperatively. The nurse makes sure that the patient uses these devices safely. (Crutch walking and using a walker are discussed in Chap. 10.)

Maintaining Self-Esteem

The nurse continues the preoperative plan of care. The nurse and the patient set realistic goals. Increasing self-care activities within the limits of the therapeutic regimen and resumption of roles facilitate recognition of abilities and promote self-esteem, personal identity, and role performance. Acceptance of altered body image is facilitated by support provided by the nurse, family, and others.

Monitoring and Managing Potential Complications

HYPOVOLEMIC SHOCK

Excessive loss of blood during or after surgery can result in shock. The nurse monitors the patient for signs and symptoms of hypovolemic shock: increased pulse rate, decreased blood pressure, urine output less than 30 mL per hour, restlessness, change in mentation, thirst, decreased hemoglobin and hematocrit. The nurse reports these findings to the orthopedic surgeon for appropriate management. (See Chap. 14 for a discussion of managing patients in shock.)

ATELECTASIS AND PNEUMONIA

The nurse monitors the patient's lung sounds and encourages deep breathing and coughing exercises. Full expansion of the lungs prevents accumulation of pulmonary secretions and development of atelectasis and pneumonia. Incentive spirometry, if prescribed, is encouraged. If signs of respiratory problems develop (eg, increased respiratory rate, productive cough, diminished or adventitious breath sounds, fever), the nurse reports the findings to the surgeon.

URINARY RETENTION

The nurse closely monitors the urinary output after surgery. The nurse encourages the patient to void every 3 to 4 hours to prevent urinary retention and bladder distention. It is important to provide privacy during toileting. Because the patient may need to void in an unusual position, the nurse assists the patient with positioning. Fracture bedpans may be more comfortable than other bedpans. Voiding in the side-lying position may be helpful to the male patient. Some male patients can void only if standing, and clarification with the surgeon of the activity prescription may be needed before assisting the patient to a standing position. If the patient is unable to void, intermittent catheterizations may be prescribed until the patient is able to void independently. Indwelling urinary catheters are to be used judiciously and removed as soon as possible.

INFECTION

Infection is a risk after any surgery, but it is of particular concern for the postoperative orthopedic patient because of the high risk for osteomyelitis. Osteomyelitis often requires prolonged courses of intravenous antibiotics. At times, the infected bone and prosthesis or internal fixation devices must be surgically removed. Therefore, prophylactic systemic antibiotics are usually prescribed during the perioperative and immediate postoperative period. The nurse assesses the patient's response to these antibiotics. When changing dressings and emptying wound drainage devices, aseptic technique is essential. The nurse monitors the patient's vital signs, incision, and drainage. The nurse monitors the patient for signs of urinary tract infection. Prompt assessment for and treatment of infection are essential.

VENOUS STASIS AND DEEP VEIN THROMBOSIS

Prevention of DVT requires use of ankle- and calf-pumping exercises, elastic stockings, and sequential compression devices. Adequate hydration and early mobilization are equally important. Prophylactic warfarin, adjusted-dose heparin, or low-molecular-weight heparin, such as enoxaparin sodium, may be prescribed. Aspirin has no apparent anti-DVT effect in the orthopedic patient. The nurse monitors the patient for signs of DVT and promptly reports findings to the physician for management.

Promoting Home and Community-Based Care

TEACHING PATIENTS SELF-CARE

The length of stay in the hospital after orthopedic surgery is usually less than a week. Convalescence and rehabilitation take place at home or in a nonacute care setting. The nurse teaches the patient and the family to recognize complications that must be reported promptly to the orthopedic surgeon. The patient must understand the prescribed medication regimen. The nurse should demonstrate proper wound care. The patient gradually resumes physical activities and adheres to weight-bearing limits. The patient must be able to perform transfers and use mobility aids safely. Specific exercises need to be taught and practiced before discharge. The nurse discusses recovery and health promotion, emphasizing a healthy lifestyle and diet.

CONTINUING CARE

If special equipment or home modifications are needed for safe care at home, they must be secured before the patient is discharged home. The nurse, physical therapist, and social worker can assist the patient and family in identifying their needs and in getting ready to care for the patient at home.

Frequently, home health nursing and home physical therapy are part of the discharge plan of care. These referrals provide resources and help the patient and the family cope with the demands of care during convalescence and rehabilitation. The nurse can explore problems that the patient and family identify during the home care visit. The nurse assesses the patient's progress and monitors for possible complications. Regular medical follow-up care after discharge needs to be arranged (see the accompanying Home Care Teaching Checklist: The Patient Who Has Had Orthopedic Surgery).

Evaluation

Expected Outcomes

Expected outcomes may include:

1. Reports decreased level of pain
   a. Uses multiple approaches to reduce pain
   b. Uses occasional oral medication to control discomfort
   c. Elevates extremity to control edema and discomfort
   d. Moves with greater comfort
2. Exhibits adequate neurovascular function
   a. Exhibits normal skin color
   b. Has warm skin
   c. Has normal capillary refill response
   d. Demonstrates intact sensory and motor function
   e. Demonstrates reduced swelling
3. Promotes health
   a. Eats balanced diet appropriate for nutritional needs
   b. Maintains adequate hydration
   c. Abstains from smoking
   d. Practices respiratory exercises
   e. Repositions self to relieve pressure on skin
   f. Engages in strengthening and preventive exercises
4. Maximizes mobility within the therapeutic limits
   a. Requests assistance when moving
   b. Elevates edematous extremity after transfer
   c. Uses immobilizing devices as prescribed
   d. Complies with prescribed weight-bearing limitation
5. Expresses positive self-esteem
   a. Discusses temporary or permanent changes in body image
   b. Discusses role performances
   c. Views self as capable of assuming responsibilities
   d. Actively participates in planning care and in the therapeutic regimen
6. Exhibits absence of complications
   a. Does not experience shock
   b. Maintains normal vital signs and blood pressure
   c. Has clear lung sounds
   d. Demonstrates wound healing without signs of infection
   e. Has wound drainage that is not purulent
   f. Does not experience urinary retention
   g. Demonstrates clear urine clear
   h. Exhibits no signs of DVT

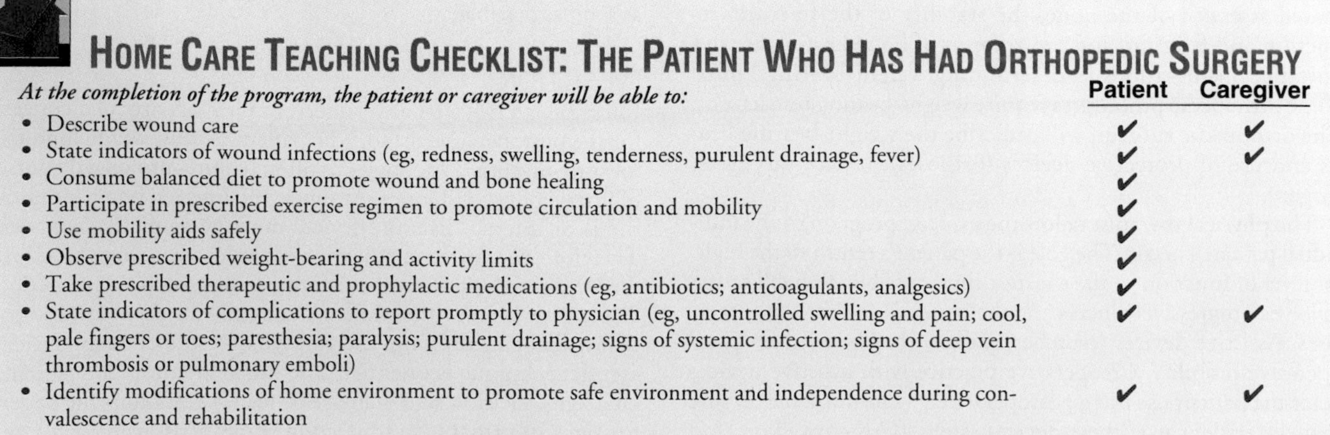

HOME CARE TEACHING CHECKLIST: THE PATIENT WHO HAS HAD ORTHOPEDIC SURGERY

At the completion of the program, the patient or caregiver will be able to:	Patient	Caregiver
• Describe wound care	✔	✔
• State indicators of wound infections (eg, redness, swelling, tenderness, purulent drainage, fever)	✔	✔
• Consume balanced diet to promote wound and bone healing	✔	
• Participate in prescribed exercise regimen to promote circulation and mobility	✔	
• Use mobility aids safely	✔	
• Observe prescribed weight-bearing and activity limits	✔	
• Take prescribed therapeutic and prophylactic medications (eg, antibiotics; anticoagulants, analgesics)	✔	
• State indicators of complications to report promptly to physician (eg, uncontrolled swelling and pain; cool, pale fingers or toes; paresthesia; paralysis; purulent drainage; signs of systemic infection; signs of deep vein thrombosis or pulmonary emboli)	✔	✔
• Identify modifications of home environment to promote safe environment and independence during convalescence and rehabilitation	✔	✔

Critical Thinking Exercises

1. You are caring for two patients in the same room. One patient has had a knee replacement. The other patient has had a hip replacement. Both patients are experiencing pain. How would you compare and contrast the pain management strategies for each patient? How would you describe the differences in general care related to their respective mobility limitations?

2. A patient who was in a motor vehicle crash has a cast on his leg. He complains that the cast feels tight and that the pain medication is not relieving his pain. What do you think is happening? What actions would you take and why?

3. A patient who has had internal fixation of the hip complains about her elastic stockings and requests that they be removed. How would you respond to this request, and how would you explain the purpose of the stockings? The patient does not understand English and keeps trying to remove the stockings. Describe two different strategies you could follow in this circumstance and the pros and cons of each intervention.

4. You are caring for two patients in the same room. One patient has skeletal traction applied to his leg, and the other has skin (Buck's) traction. The patients ask you why their traction setups are different. How would you explain the differences to them? Describe the different priorities of care for each of these patients.

5. You are making a home visit to a patient who had experienced an open fracture of the lower leg. The fracture is being managed with an external fixator. What would you include in your assessment of the fixator and the pin sites? During your assessment, the patient states that the pin in the foot is tender, and it is loose on examination. What action should you take? What is the basis for this action?

References and Selected Readings

BOOKS

Bucholz, R. W. (1996). *Orthopaedic decision making* (2nd ed.). St. Louis: C. V. Mosby.

Carpenito, L. J. (1997). *Nursing diagnosis: Application to clinical practice* (7th ed.). Philadelphia: Lippincott-Raven.

Epps, C. (1994). *Complications in orthopaedic surgery* (3rd ed.). Philadelphia: J. B. Lippincott.

Maher, A. B., et al. (1998). *Orthopaedic nursing* (2nd ed.). Philadelphia: W. B. Saunders.

Mercer, W. (1996). *Mercer's orthopaedic surgery.* London: Oxford University Press.

Salmond, S. W., et al (Eds.). (1996). *Core curriculum for orthopaedic nursing* (3rd ed.). Pitman, NJ: National Association of Orthopaedic Nurses.

JOURNALS

Asterisks indicate research articles.

Altizer, L. (1995). Total hip arthroplasty. *Orthopaedic Nursing, 14*(4), 7–18.

Anderson, L., Dale, K. (1998). Infections in total joint replacements. *Orthopaedic Nursing, 17*(1), 7–11.

*Autar, R. (1996). Nursing assessment of clients at risk of deep vein thrombosis (DVT): The Autar DVT scale. *Journal of Advanced Nursing, 23,* 763–770.

Barrows, S. (1995). Easing your patient's joint replacement. *Nursing, 25*(5), 32C–32D, 32F.

Beckles, S. (1996). Community assessment of a patient following hip replacement. *British Journal of Nursing, 5*(20), 1241–1246.

*Blake, D., et al. (1997). Oral tenoxicam for peripheral orthopaedic surgery: A pharmacokinetic study. *Anaesthesia and Intensive Care, 25*(2), 142–146.

Carlisle, D. (1996). Fresh look at rehabilitation of hip-replacement patients: Elderly care counts. *Nursing Times, 92*(44), 32–33.

*Colwell, C., & Morris, B. (1995). Patient-controlled analgesia compared with intramuscular injection of analgesics for the management of pain after an orthopaedic procedure. *Journal of Bone and Joint Surgery, 77-A*(5), 726–733.

*Crutchfield, J., et al. (1996). Preoperative and postoperative pain in total knee replacement patients. *Orthopaedic Nursing, 15*(2), 65–72.

Davis, A. (1996). Primary care management of chronic musculoskeletal pain. *Nurse Practitioner, 21*(8), 72–82, 89.

DeGeorge, P., & Dunwoody, C. (1995). Transfer techniques of the lower extremity with an external fixator. *Orthopaedic Nursing, 14*(6), 17–21.

Dickerson, R., et al. (1996). Use of compression stockings. *Nursing Standard, 10*(30), 30–31.

*Gammon, J., & Mulholland, C. (1996). Effect of preparatory information prior to elective total hip replacement on psychological coping outcomes. *Journal of Advanced Nursing, 24*(2), 303–308.

Hurst, S. (1996). Multidisciplinary discharge planning. *Professional Nurse, 12*(2), 113–116.

Knight, R., & Pellegrini, V. Jr. (1996). Bladder management after total joint arthroplasty. *Journal of Arthroplasty, 11*(8), 882–888.

*Lin, P., et al. (1997). Comparing the effectiveness of different educational programs for patients with total knee arthroplasty. *Orthopaedic Nursing, 16*(5), 43–49.

*Meyers, S., et al. (1996). Inpatient cost of primary total joint arthroplasty. *Journal of Arthroplasty, 11*(3), 281–285.

*Miller, J., et al. (1996). A study of discomfort and confusion among elderly surgical patients. *Orthopaedic Nursing, 15*(6), 27–34.

Morris, B., Colwell, C., Hardwick, M. (1998). The use of low-molecular weight heparin in the prevention of venous thrombolytic disease. *Orthopaedic Nursing, 17*(6), 23–30.

Muntz, J. (1997). Perioperative DVT and pulmonary embolism: Diagnosis, management, and treatment. *Orthopaedic Nursing March–April Supplement,* 25–29, 66.

Novy, C., & Jagmin, M. (1997). Pain management in the elderly orthopaedic patient. *Orthopaedic Nursing, 16*(1), 51–57.

*O'Brien, S., et al. (1996). A study of the factors in hip replacement dislocation: Part 1. *Nursing Standard, 11*(7), 33–38.

*O'Brien, S., et al. (1996). A study of the factors in hip replacement dislocation: Part 2. *Nursing Standard, 11*(8), 39–42.

*Ouellet, L., et al. (1996). Dietary fiber and laxation in postop orthopedic patients. *Clinical Nursing Research, 5*(4), 428+.

*Roach, J., et al. (1995). Preoperative assessment and education program: Implementation and outcomes. *Patient Education and Counseling, 25*(1), 83–88.

Santavirta, N., et al. (1994). Teaching of patients undergoing total hip replacement surgery. *International Journal of Nursing Studies, 31*(2), 135–142.

*Schilke, J., et al. (1996). Effects of muscle-strength training on the functional status of patients with osteoarthritis of the knee joint. *Nursing Research, 45*(2), 68–72.

Sims, M., & Saleh, M. (1996). Protocols for the care of external fixator pin sites. *Professional Nurse, 11*(4), 261–264.

Spica, M., & Schwab, M. (1996). Sexual expression after total joint replacement. *Orthopaedic Nursing, 15*(5), 41–44.

Sprague, J. (1998). Cast syndrome. *Orthopaedic Nursing, 17*(4), 12–15.

Styrcula, L. (1994). Traction basics. Part I: Traction. *Orthopaedic Nursing, 13*(4), 34–44.

Styrcula, L. (1994). Traction basics. Part II: Traction equipment. *Orthopaedic Nursing, 13*(3), 55–59.

Styrcula, L. (1994). Traction basics. Part IV: Traction for lower extremities. *Orthopaedic Nursing, 13*(5), 59–68.

Williamson, V. (1997). Clinical pathways for a patient with a total joint replacement. *Orthopaedic Nursing March–April Supplement,* 41–45.

*Wynd, C., et al. Factors influencing postoperative urinary retention following orthopaedic surgical procedures. *Orthopaedic Nursing, 15*(1), 43–50.

Yandrich, T. (1995). Preventing infection in total joint replacement surgery. *Orthopaedic Nursing, 14*(2), 15–19.

Yarnold, B. (1999). Hip fracture: Caring for a fragile population. *American Journal of Nursing, 99*(2), 36–41.

Zimlich, R., et al. (1996). Current status of anticoagulation therapy after total hip and total knee arthroplasty: A comprehensive review. *Journal of the American Academy of Orthopaedic Surgeons, 4*(1), 54-62.

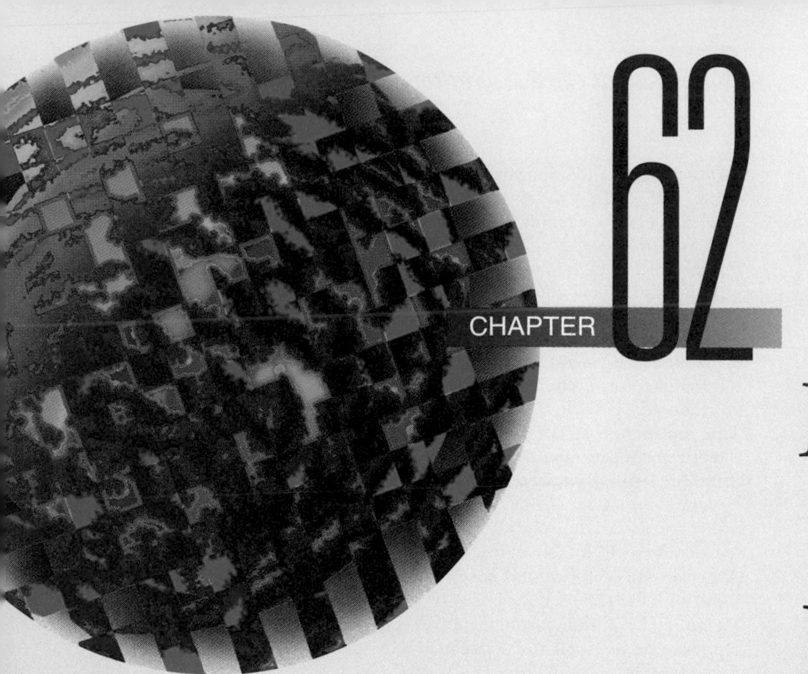

Management of Patients With Musculoskeletal Disorders

Learning Objectives

On completion of this chapter, the learner will be able to:

1. Use the nursing process as a framework for care of the patient with low back pain.
2. Describe the rehabilitation and health education needs of the patient with low back pain.
3. Describe conditions of the upper extremities and nursing care of the patient undergoing surgery of the hand or wrist.
4. Use the nursing process as a framework for care of the patient undergoing foot surgery.
5. Explain the pathophysiology, pathogenesis, prevention, and management of osteoporosis.
6. Identify the causes and related medical management of osteomalacia.
7. Describe the medication therapy program for the patient with Paget's disease.
8. Use the nursing process as a framework for care of the patient with osteomyelitis.
9. Use the nursing process as a framework for care of the patient with a bone tumor.

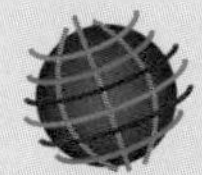

Major musculoskeletal disorders, such as impairment of the back and spine, are leading health problems and causes of disability, particularly in people during their employment years. The limitations imposed on the patient are severe, and the economic cost, in terms of loss of productivity, compensable costs, and medical expenses, is in the billions of dollars.

GLOSSARY

bursitis: inflammation of fluid-filled sac in joints
contracture: abnormal shortening of muscle or fibrosis of joint structures
involucrum: new bone growth around sequestrum
radiculopathy: disease of a nerve root
sciatica: sciatic nerve pain; pain travels down back of thigh into foot
sequestrum: dead bone in abscess cavity

COMMON MUSCULOSKELETAL PROBLEMS

Acute Low Back Pain

The number of medical visits resulting from low back pain is second only to the number of visits for upper respiratory illnesses. Most low back pain is caused by any one of a large number of musculoskeletal problems, including acute lumbosacral strain, unstable lumbosacral ligaments and weak muscles, osteoarthritis of the spine, spinal stenosis, intervertebral disk problems, and unequal leg length.

Older patients may experience back pain associated with osteoporotic vertebral fractures or bone metastasis. Other causes include kidney disorders, pelvic problems, retroperitoneal tumors, abdominal aneurysms, and psychosomatic problems.

In addition, obesity, stress, and occasionally depression may contribute to low back pain. Back pain due to musculoskeletal disturbances usually is aggravated by activity, whereas pain due to other conditions is not. Patients with chronic low back pain may develop a dependence on alcohol or analgesics.

Pathophysiology

The spinal column can be considered an elastic rod constructed of rigid units (vertebrae) and flexible units (intervertebral disks) held together by complex facet joints, multiple ligaments, and paravertebral muscles. The unique construction of the back allows for flexibility while providing maximum protection for the spinal cord. The spinal curves absorb vertical shocks from running and jumping, the trunk muscles help to stabilize the spine, and the abdominal and thoracic muscles are important in lifting activities. Disuse weakens these supporting structures. Obesity, postural problems, structural problems, and overstretching of the spinal supports may result in back pain.

The intervertebral disks change in character as the person ages. A young person's disks are mainly fibrocartilage with a gelatinous matrix. As a person ages, the disks become dense, irregular fibrocartilage. Disk degeneration is a common cause of back pain. The lower lumbar disks, L4–L5 and L5–S1, are subject to the greatest mechanical stress and the greatest degenerative changes. Disk protrusion (herniated nucleus pulposa) or facet joint changes can cause pressure on nerve roots as they leave the spinal canal, which results in pain that radiates along the nerve. (Management of intervertebral disk disease is discussed in Chap. 57.)

Clinical Manifestations

The patient complains of either acute back pain or chronic back pain (lasting more than 3 months without improvement) and fatigue. The patient may report pain radiating down the leg (**radiculopathy; sciatica**), which suggests nerve root involvement. The patient's gait, spinal mobility, reflexes, leg length, leg motor strength, and sensory perception may be altered. Physical examination may disclose paravertebral muscle spasm (greatly increased muscle tone of the back postural muscles) with a loss of the normal lumbar curve and possible spinal deformity.

Assessment and Diagnostic Findings

The Agency for Heath Care Policy and Research developed guidelines for assessment and management of acute low back pain (Bigos, et al., 1994). These safe, conservative, and cost-effective guidelines have reduced or eliminated the use of noneffective therapeutic interventions, including prolonged bed rest.

The initial evaluation of acute low back pain includes a focused history and physical examination, including general observation of the patient, back examination, neurologic testing (eg, reflexes, sensory impairment, straight-leg raising, muscle strength, and muscle atrophy). The findings suggest either nonspecific back symptoms or potentially serious problems, such as sciatica, spine fracture, cancer, infection, cauda equina, or rapidly progressing neurologic deficit. If initial examination does not suggest a serious problem, additional testing is not helpful during the first 4 weeks of symptoms.

The diagnostic procedures described in Chart 62-1 may be indicated for the patient with potentially serious or prolonged low back pain. The nurse prepares the patient for these studies, provides the necessary support during the testing period, and monitors the patient for any adverse responses to the procedures.

Medical Management

Most back pain is self-limiting and resolves within 4 weeks with analgesics, rest, stress reduction, and relaxation. Based on initial assessment findings, the patient is reassured that the assessment indicates that the back pain is not due to a serious condition. Management focuses on relief of pain and discomfort, activity modification, and patient education.

CHART 62•1 Diagnostic Procedures for Low Back Pain

X-ray of the spine—may demonstrate the presence of fracture, dislocation, infection, osteoarthritis, or scoliosis

Bone scan and blood studies—may disclose infections, tumors, and bone marrow abnormalities

Computed tomography—useful in identifying underlying problems, such as obscure soft tissue lesions adjacent to the vertebral column and problems of vertebral disks

Magnetic resonance imaging—permits visualization of the nature and location of spinal pathology

Myelogram and discogram (in which a small amount of contrast agent is injected into the intervertebral disk to allow radiographic visualization)—may be performed to demonstrate degenerative disk or disk protrusions

Epidural venograms—used to assess lumbar disk disease by demonstrating displacement of epidural veins

Electromyogram and nerve conduction studies—used to evaluate spinal nerve root disorders (radiculopathies)

Nonprescription analgesics (ie, acetaminophen, ibuprofen) are usually effective in achieving pain relief. At times, the patient requires the addition of muscle relaxants or opioids. Heat or cold therapy frequently provides temporary relief of symptoms. In the absence of radiculopathy symptoms, manipulation may be helpful.

Other physical modalities having no proven efficacy in treating acute low back pain include traction, massage, diathermy, ultrasound, cutaneous laser treatment, biofeedback, and transcutaneous electrical nerve stimulation. Likewise, acupuncture and injection procedures have no proven efficacy (Bigos, 1994).

Most patients need to alter their activity patterns to prevent aggravating the back or debilitation. Twisting, bending, lifting, and reaching, all of which stress the back, are avoided. The patient is taught to change position frequently. Sitting should be limited to 20 to 50 minutes based on level of comfort. Bed rest is recommended for 2 to 4 days only if pain is severe. A gradual return to activities and low-stress aerobic exercise is recommended. Conditioning exercises for the trunk muscles are begun in about 2 weeks.

If there is no improvement within 1 month, additional assessments for physiologic abnormalities are completed, and management is based on findings.

NURSING PROCESS: THE PATIENT WITH ACUTE LOW BACK PAIN

Assessment

The nurse encourages the patient with low back pain to describe the discomfort (eg, location, severity, duration, characteristics, radiation, associated weakness in the legs). Descriptions of how the pain occurred—with a specific action (eg, opening a garage door) or with an activity in which weak muscles were overused (eg, weekend gardening)—and how the patient has dealt with the pain often suggest areas for intervention and patient teaching. If back pain is a recurrent problem, information about previous successful pain control helps in planning current management. The nurse also may ask how the back pain affects the patient's lifestyle.

Information about work and recreational activities helps to identify areas for back health education. Because stress and anxiety can evoke muscle spasms and pain, the nurse needs insight into environmental variables, work situations, and family relationships. In addition, the nurse assesses the effect of chronic pain on the emotional well-being of the patient. Referral to a psychiatric nurse clinician for assessment and management of stressors and depression contributing to the experienced low back pain may be appropriate.

During the interview, the nurse observes the patient's posture, position changes, and gait. Often, the patient's movements are guarded, with the back kept as still as possible. The patient selects a chair of standard seat height with arms for support. The patient may sit and stand in an unusual position, leaning away from the most painful side, and may ask for assistance when undressing.

On physical examination, the nurse assesses the spinal curves, leg length discrepancy, and pelvic crest and shoulder symmetry. The nurse palpates the paraspinal muscles and notes spasm and tenderness. In a prone position, the paraspinal muscles relax, and any deformity caused by spasm subsides. The nurse asks the patient to bend forward and laterally and notes any discomfort and limitations in movement. It is important to determine the effect of these limitations in movement on activities of daily living (ADLs). The nurse evaluates nerve involvement by assessing deep tendon reflexes, sensations (eg, paresthesia), and muscle strength. Back and leg pain with straight-leg raises (eg, with the patient supine, the patient's leg is lifted upward with the knee extended) suggests nerve root involvement. Obesity can contribute to low back pain. If the patient is obese, the nurse completes a nutritional assessment.

Nursing Diagnosis

Based on the assessment data, the patient's major nursing diagnoses may include the following:

- Pain related to musculoskeletal problems
- Impaired physical mobility related to pain, muscle spasms, and decreased flexibility
- Knowledge deficit related to back-conserving body mechanics techniques
- Self-concept disturbance related to impaired mobility, chronic pain, and altered role performance
- Altered nutrition: more than body requirements, related to obesity

Planning and Goals

The major goals of the patient may include relief of pain, improved physical mobility, use of back-conserving body mechanics techniques, improved self-concept, and weight reduction.

Nursing Interventions

Relieving Pain

To relieve pain, the nurse encourages the patient to reduce stress on the back muscles and to change position frequently. Patients are taught to control and modify the perceived pain through behavioral therapies that reduce muscular and psychological tension. Diaphragmatic breathing and relaxation help reduce muscle tension contributing to low back pain. Diverting the patient's attention from the pain to another activity (eg, reading, conversation, watching television) may be helpful in some instances. Guided imagery, in which the relaxed patient learns to focus on a pleasant event, may be used along with other pain-relief strategies (see "The Patient With Low Back Pain" on the next page.)

If medication is prescribed, the nurse assesses the patient's response to each medication. As the acute pain subsides, medications are reduced as prescribed. Self-applied intermittent heat or cold may reduce the pain. The nurse evaluates and notes the patient's response to various pain management modalities.

Improving Physical Mobility

Physical mobility is monitored through continuing assessments. The nurse assesses how the patient moves and stands. As the back pain subsides, self-care activities are resumed with minimal strain on the injured structures. Position changes should be made slowly and carried out with assistance as required. Twisting and jarring motions are avoided. The nurse encourages the patient to alternate lying, sitting, and walking activities frequently and advises the patient to avoid sitting, standing, and walking for long periods. The patient may find that sitting in a chair with arm rests to support some of the body weight and a soft support at the small of the back provides comfort.

With severe pain, the patient limits activity for 2 to 4 days. Extended periods of inactivity are not effective and result in debilitation. The patient rests in bed on a firm, nonsagging mattress (a bed board may be used). The patient increases lumbar flexion by elevating the head and thorax 30 degrees using pillows or a foam wedge and slightly flexing the knees supported on a pillow (Fig. 62-1). Alternatively, the patient assumes a lateral position

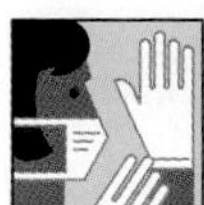

HEALTH PROMOTION AND ILLNESS PREVENTION
The Patient With Low Back Pain

Pain Management
Discuss with patient methods to reduce pain: limited bed rest with knees flexed to decrease strain on back
Nonpharmacologic approaches: distraction, relaxation, imagery, thermal interventions (eg, ice or heat), stress reduction
Pharmacologic approaches: nonsteroidal anti-inflammatory agents, analgesics, muscle relaxants

Exercise
Encourage patient to perform prescribed back exercises to increase function, emphasizing gradual increases in time and repetitions
Stretching, flexibility, strengthening

Body Mechanics
Instruct patient to:
- Practice good posture
- Avoid twisting body

When lifting:
- Keep load close to body
- Bend knees and tighten abdominal muscles
- Avoid overreaching
- Use wide base of support
- Use back brace to protect back

Work Modification
Encourage patient to:
- Adjust work area to avoid stress on back
- Adjust height of chair or work table
- Use lumbar support in chair
- Avoid prolonged standing and repetitive tasks
- Avoid bending, twisting, and lifting heavy objects
- Avoid work involving continuous vibrations

Stress Reduction
Discuss with patient the interdependence of stress and anxiety on muscle tension and pain
Explore effective coping mechanisms
Teach stress reduction techniques
Refer patient to back clinic

with knees and hips flexed (curled position) with a pillow between the knees and legs and a pillow supporting the head. A prone position is avoided because it accentuates lordosis. The nurse instructs the patient to get out of bed by rolling to one side and placing the legs down while pushing the torso up, keeping the back straight.

As the patient achieves comfort, activities are gradually resumed, and an exercise program is initiated. Initially, low-stress aerobic exercises, such as short walks or swimming, are suggested. After 2 weeks, conditioning exercises for the abdominal and trunk muscles are started. The physical therapist designs an exercise program for the individual patient to reduce lordosis, increase flexibility, and reduce strain on the back. It may include hyperextension exercises to strengthen the paravertebral muscles, flexion exercises to increase back movement and strength, and isometric flexion exercises to strengthen trunk muscles. Each exercise period begins with relaxation. Exercises are begun gradually and then increased as the patient recovers.

The nurse encourages the patient to adhere to the prescribed exercise program. Erratic exercising is ineffective. For most exercise programs, it is suggested that the person exercise twice a day, increasing the number of exercises gradually. Some patients may find it difficult to adhere to a program of prescribed exercises for a long period. These patients are encouraged to improve their posture, use good body mechanics on a regular basis, and engage in regular exercise activities, such as walking or swimming, to maintain a healthy back. Activities should not cause excessive lumbar strain, twisting, or discomfort (eg, horseback riding and weight-lifting are avoided).

Promoting Proper Body Mechanics

Good body mechanics and posture are essential to avoid recurrence of back pain. The patient must be taught how to stand, sit, lie, and lift properly (Figs. 62-2 and 62-3). Providing the patient with a list of suggestions helps in making these long-term changes (see the accompanying display, Activities to Promote a Healthy Back). The patient who wears high heels is encouraged to change to low heels.

The patient who is required to stand for long periods should shift weight frequently and should rest one foot on a low stool, which decreases lumbar lordosis. The proper posture can be verified by looking in a mirror to see if the chest is up and the abdomen is tucked in. Locking the knees when standing is avoided, as is bending forward for long periods.

When the patient is sitting, the knees and hips should be flexed, and the knees should be level with the hips or higher to

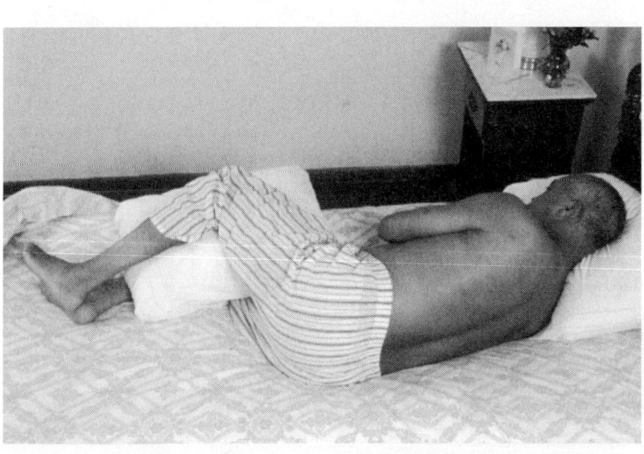

FIGURE 62•1 Positioning to promote lumbar flexion. © B. Proud.

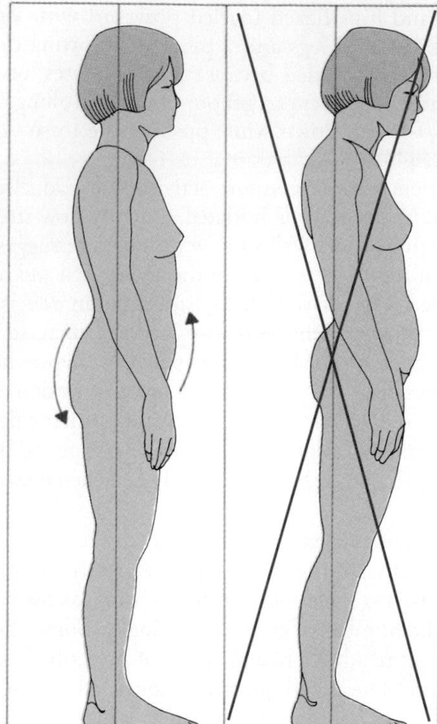

FIGURE 62•2 Proper and improper standing postures. (*Left*) Abdominal muscles contracted, giving a feeling of upward pull, and gluteal muscles contracted, giving a downward pull. (*Right*) Slouch position, showing abdominal muscles relaxed and body out of proper alignment.

minimize lordosis. The feet should be flat on the floor. The back needs to be supported. The patient should sleep on the side with knees and hips flexed, or supine with knees supported in a flexed position. Sleeping prone is to be avoided.

The nurse instructs the patient in the correct way to lift objects—using the strong quadriceps muscles of the thighs, with minimal use of weak back muscles. With feet placed to provide a wide base of support, the patient should bend the knees, tighten the abdominal muscles, and lift the object close to the body with a smooth motion, avoiding twisting and jerking. To prevent recurrence of acute low back pain, the nurse instructs the patient to wear a back brace to support the back when repeated lifting is

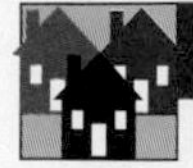

PATIENT EDUCATION AND HOME CARE
Activities to Promote a Healthy Back

Standing

Avoid prolonged standing and walking.
When standing for any length of time, rest one foot on a small stool or box to relieve lumbar lordosis.
Avoid forward flexion work positions.

Sitting

Stress on the back may be greater in the sitting position than in the standing position.
Avoid sitting for prolonged periods.
Sit in a straight-back chair with back well supported. Use a foot stool to position knees higher than hips if necessary.
Eradicate the hollow of the back by sitting with the buttocks "tucked under."
Avoid knee and hip extension. When driving a car, have the seat pushed forward as far as possible for comfort.
Maintain back support.
Guard against extension strains—reaching, pushing, sitting with legs straight out.
Alternate periods of sitting with walking.

Lying

Rest at intervals; fatigue contributes to spasm of the back muscle.
Place a firm bed board under the mattress.
Avoid sleeping in a prone position.
When lying on the side, place a pillow under the head and one between the legs, which should be flexed at the hips and knees.
When supine, use a pillow under the knees to decrease lordosis.

Lifting

When lifting, keep the back straight and hold the load as close to the body as possible.
Lift with the large leg muscles, not the back muscles.
Protect back with a back-supporting belt when lifting.
Squat while keeping the back straight when it is necessary to pick something off the floor.
Avoid twisting the trunk of the body, lifting above waist level, and reaching up for any length of time.

Exercise

Daily exercise is important in the prevention of back problems.
Walking and gradually increasing the distance and pace of walking is recommended.
Perform prescribed back exercises twice daily, increasing exercise gradually.
Avoid jumping and jarring activities.

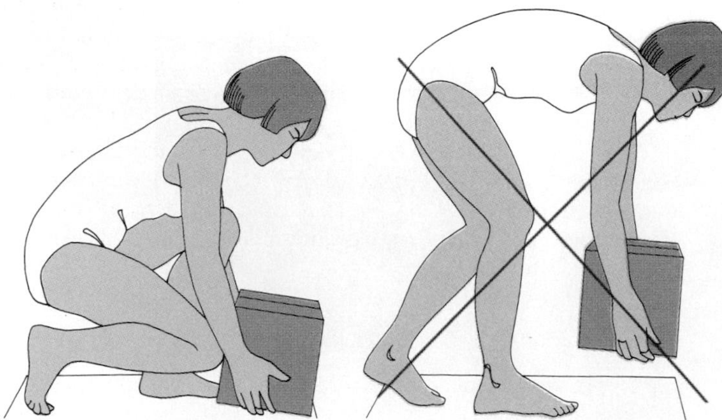

FIGURE 62•3 Proper and improper lifting techniques. (*Left*) Correct position for lifting. This person is using the long and strong muscles of the arms and legs and holding the object so that the line of gravity falls within the base of support. (*Right*) Incorrect position for lifting because pull is exerted on the back muscles and leaning causes the line of gravity to fall outside the base.

required and to avoid lifting more than one third of his or her weight without help.

It takes about 6 months for a person to readjust postural habits. Practicing these protective and defensive postures, positions, and body mechanics results in natural strengthening of the back and diminishes the chance that back pain will recur.

Improving Self-Concept

Because of the immobility associated with low back pain, the patient may depend on others to do various tasks. Dependency may continue beyond physiologic needs and become a way to fulfill psychosocial needs. Assisting both the patient and support people to recognize continued dependency helps the patient identify and cope with the underlying reason for the dependency.

Role-related responsibilities may have been modified with the onset of low back pain. As recovery from acute low back pain and immobility progresses, the patient may resume former role-related responsibilities.

If these activities contributed to the development of low back pain, however, it may be difficult to resume them without chronic low back pain syndrome, with associated disability and depression resulting. If the patient experiences secondary gains associated with low back disability (eg, workman's compensation, easier lifestyle or workload, increased emotional support), a "low back neurosis" may develop. The patient may need help in coping with specific stressors and in learning how to control stressful situations. When people successfully deal with stress, they develop confidence in their abilities to manage other stressful situations. Psychotherapy or counseling may be needed to assist the person in resuming a full, productive life.

Back clinics use multidisciplinary approaches to help the patient with pain and with resumption of role-related responsibilities. Working with these patients is a challenge because major adjustments are coupled with the cure.

Modifying Nutrition for Weight Reduction

Obesity contributes to back strain by stressing the relatively weak back muscles. Exercises are less effective and more difficult to perform when the patient is overweight. Weight reduction through diet modification may prevent recurrence of back pain. Weight reduction is based on a sound nutritional plan that includes a change in eating habits to maintain desirable weight. Monitoring weight reduction, noting achievement, and providing encouragement and positive reinforcement facilitate adherence. Frequently, back problems resolve as normal weight is achieved.

Evaluation

Expected Outcomes

Expected outcomes may include:

1. Experiences pain relief
   a. Rests comfortably
   b. Changes positions comfortably
   c. Obtains relief through use of physical modalities, psychological techniques, and medications
   d. Avoids drug dependency
2. Demonstrates resumption of physical mobility
   a. Resumes activities gradually
   b. Avoids positions that cause discomfort and muscle spasm
   c. Plans recumbent rest periods throughout day
3. Demonstrates back-conserving body mechanics
   a. Improves posture
   b. Positions self to minimize stress on the back
   c. Demonstrates use of good body mechanics
   d. Participates in exercise program
4. Resumes role-related responsibilities
   a. Uses coping techniques to deal with stressful situations
   b. Demonstrates decreased dependence on others for self-care
   c. Resumes occupation as low back pain resolves
   d. Resumes full, productive lifestyle
5. Achieves desired weight
   a. Identifies need to lose weight
   b. Sets realistic goals
   c. Participates in development of weight-reduction plan
   d. Complies with weight-reduction regimen

COMMON PROBLEMS OF THE UPPER EXTREMITY

The structures in the upper extremity are frequently the sites of painful syndromes. The structures that are most frequently affected include the shoulder, wrist, and hand.

Bursitis and Tendinitis

Bursitis and **tendinitis** are inflammatory conditions that commonly occur in the shoulder. Bursa are fluid-filled sacs that prevent friction between joint structures during joint activity. When inflamed, they are painful. Similarly, muscle tendon sheaths become inflamed with repetitive stretching. The inflammation causes proliferation of synovial membrane and pannus formation, which restricts joint movement. Conservative treatment includes rest of the extremity, intermittent ice and heat to the joint, and nonsteroidal anti-inflammatory drugs (NSAIDs) to control the inflammation and pain. Arthroscopic synovectomy may be considered if shoulder pain and weakness persist.

Loose Bodies

Loose bodies may occur in a joint due to articular cartilage wear and bone erosion. These fragments interfere with joint movement, locking the joint, and cause painful movement. Loose bodies are removed by arthroscopic surgery.

Impingement Syndrome

Overuse (microtrauma) may produce an impingement syndrome in the shoulder. The supraspinatus and biceps tendons become irritated and edematous and press against the acromion process, limiting shoulder motion. The patient experiences pain, shoulder tenderness, limited movement, muscle spasm, and atrophy. The process may progress to a rotator cuff tear. Conservative treatment includes NSAIDs, joint injections, and physical therapy (see Patient Education and Home Care: Measures to Promote Shoulder Healing). Arthroscopic débridement is used for persistent pain. Gentle joint motion is begun after surgery. (See Chap. 63 for a discussion of rotator cuff injury.)

Carpal Tunnel Syndrome

Carpal tunnel syndrome is an entrapment neuropathy that occurs when the median nerve at the wrist is compressed by a thickened

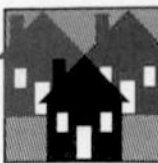

PATIENT EDUCATION AND HOME CARE
Measures to Promote Shoulder Healing

The nurse provides guidelines for general care and instructs the patient in carrying out measures that will promote shoulder healing. Patient education includes the following:

1. During the acute phase, rest the joint in a position that minimizes stress on the joint structures to prevent further damage and the development of adhesions.
2. Support the affected arm on pillows while sleeping, to keep from rolling over onto the shoulder.
3. For the first 24 to 48 hours of the acute phase, apply cold to reduce swelling and discomfort, and then, according to the treatment plan, apply heat intermittently to promote circulation and healing.
4. Gradually resume motion and use of the joint. Assistance with dressing and other activities of daily living may be needed.
5. Avoid working and lifting above shoulder level or pushing an object against a "locked" shoulder.
6. Perform the prescribed daily range-of-motion and strengthening exercises.

flexor tendon sheath, skeletal encroachment, edema, or soft tissue mass. The syndrome is commonly due to repetitive hand activities but may be associated with arthritis, hypothyroidism, or pregnancy. The patient experiences pain, numbness, paresthesia, and possibly weakness along the median nerve (thumb, first and second fingers). The Tinel's sign may be used to help identify carpal tunnel syndrome (Fig. 62-4). Night pain is common. Treatment is based on cause. Rest splints to prevent hyperextension and prolonged flexion of the wrist, avoidance of repetitive flexion of the wrist, NSAIDs, and carpal canal cortisone injections may relieve the symptoms. Surgical release of the transverse carpal ligament may be necessary. Full recovery of motor and sensory function after surgical release may take several weeks or months.

Ganglion

A ganglion, a collection of gelatinous material near the tendon sheaths and joints, appears as a round, firm, cystic swelling, usually on the dorsum of the wrist. It most frequently occurs in women younger than 50 years of age. The ganglion is locally tender and may cause an aching pain. When a tendon sheath is involved, weakness of the finger occurs. Treatment may include aspiration, corticosteroid injection, or surgical excision. A compression dressing and splint immobilization are used after treatment.

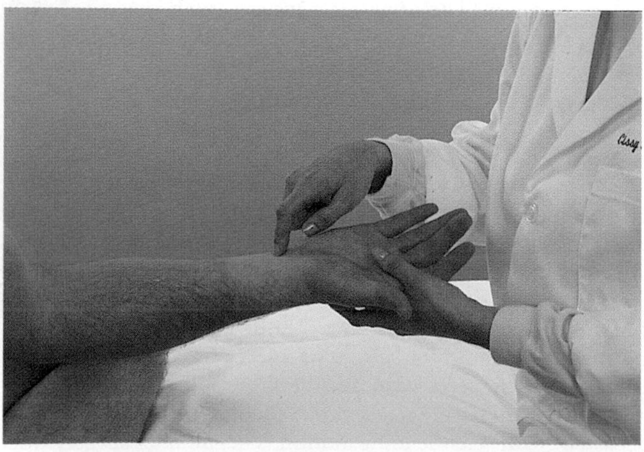

FIGURE 62•4 Tinel's sign may be elicited in patients with carpal tunnel syndrome by percussing lightly over the median nerve, located on the inner aspect of the wrist. If the patient reports tingling, numbness, and pain, the test for Tinel's sign is considered positive. From Weber, J. W., & Kelley, J. (1998). *Health assessment in nursing.* Philadelphia: Lippincott-Raven.

Dupuytren's Contracture

Dupuytren's deformity is a slowly progressive contracture of the palmar fascia, which causes flexion of the fourth and fifth fingers and frequently the middle finger. This renders the fingers more or less useless (Fig. 62-5). It is caused by an inherited autosomal dominant trait, occurring most frequently in men older than 50 years of age who are of Scandinavian or Celtic origin. It is also associated with arthritis, diabetes, gout, and alcoholism. It starts as a nodule of the palmar fascia. The nodule may not change, or it may progress so that the fibrous thickening extends to involve the skin in the distal palm and produces a contracture of the fingers. The patient may experience dull aching discomfort, morning numbness, cramping, and stiffness in the affected fingers. This condition starts in one hand, but eventually both hands are affected symmetrically. Initially, finger-stretching exercises may prevent contractures. With contracture development, palmar and digital fasciectomies are performed to improve function. Finger exercises are begun on postoperative day 1 or 2.

NURSING PROCESS: THE PATIENT UNDERGOING SURGERY OF THE HAND OR WRIST

Assessment

Surgery of the hand or wrist, unless related to major trauma, is generally an ambulatory surgery procedure. Before surgery, the nurse assesses the patient's level and type of discomfort and limitations in function caused by the ganglion, carpal tunnel syndrome, Dupuytren's contracture, or other condition of the hand.

Nursing Diagnosis

Based on the assessment data, the nursing diagnoses for the patient with surgery of the hand or wrist may include the following:

- Risk for peripheral neurovascular dysfunction related to surgical procedure
- Pain related to inflammation and swelling
- Self-care deficit related to bandaged hands
- Risk for infection related to surgical procedure

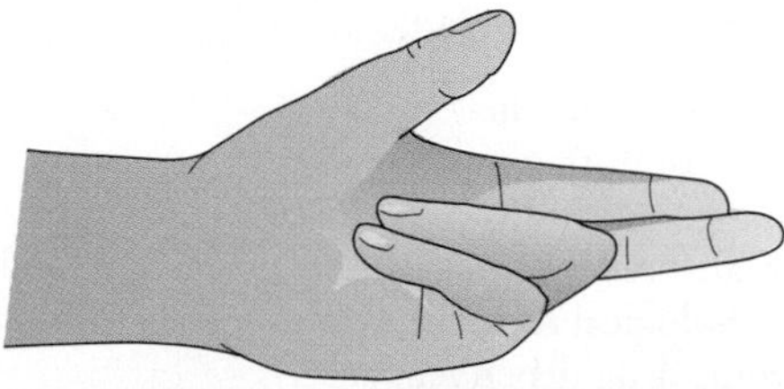

FIGURE 62•5 Dupuytren's contracture, a flexion deformity caused by an inherited trait, is a slowly progressive contracture of the palmar fascia, which severely impairs the function of the fourth, fifth, and, sometimes, the middle fingers.

Planning and Goals

The goals of the patient may include relief of pain, improved self-care, and absence of infection.

Nursing Interventions

Promoting Neurovascular Function

Neurovascular assessment of the exposed fingers every hour for the first 24 hours is essential for monitoring function of the nerves and perfusion of the hand. The nurse compares the affected hand with the unaffected hand and the postoperative status with the documented preoperative status. The nurse asks the patient to describe the sensations in the hands and to demonstrate finger mobility. With tendon repairs and nerve, vascular, or skin grafts, motor function is tested only if prescribed. The nurse assesses the temperature of the affected hand. Dressings are to be supportive but nonconstrictive. Pain uncontrolled by analgesics suggests compromised neurovascular functioning.

Relieving Pain

Pain may be related to surgery, edema, hematoma formation, or restrictive bandages. To control swelling that may increase the patient's pain and discomfort, the nurse elevates the hand to heart level with pillows. When higher elevation is prescribed, an elevating sling may be attached to an intravenous pole or overhead frame. If the patient is ambulatory, the arm is elevated in a conventional sling with the hand at heart level.

Intermittent ice packs to the surgical area during the first 24 to 48 hours may be prescribed to control swelling. Unless contraindicated, active extension and flexion of the fingers to promote circulation are encouraged, even though movement is limited by the bulky dressing.

Generally, the pain and discomfort can be controlled by oral analgesics. The nurse evaluates the patient's response to analgesics and to other pain-control measures. Patient education concerning analgesics is important.

Improving Self-Care

During the first few days after surgery, the patient needs assistance with ADLs because one hand is bandaged and independent self-care is impaired. The patient may need to arrange for assistance with feeding, bathing/hygiene, dressing, grooming, and toileting. Within a few days, the patient develops skills in one-handed ADLs and is usually able to function with minimal assistance. The nurse encourages use of the involved hand within the limits of discomfort. As rehabilitation progresses, the patient resumes use of the injured hand. Physical therapy–directed exercises may be prescribed. The nurse emphasizes adherence to the therapeutic regimen.

Preventing Infection

As with all surgery, there is a risk for infection. The nurse teaches the patient to monitor temperature and signs and symptoms that suggest an infection. It also is important to instruct the patient to keep the dressing clean and dry and to report any drainage, foul odor, or increased pain and swelling. Patient education includes aseptic wound care as well as education related to prescribed prophylactic antibiotics.

Promoting Home and Community-Based Care

TEACHING PATIENTS SELF-CARE

After the patient has hand surgery, the nurse teaches the patient how to monitor neurovascular status and the signs of complications (eg, paresthesia, paralysis, uncontrolled pain, coolness of fingers, extreme swelling, excessive bleeding, purulent drainage, temperature) that need to be reported to the surgeon. The nurse discusses prescribed medications with the patient. In addition, the nurse teaches the patient to elevate the hand above the elbow and to apply ice if prescribed to control swelling. Unless contraindicated, the nurse encourages extension and flexion exercises of fingers to promote circulation. For bathing, the nurse instructs the patient to keep the dressing dry by covering it with a secured plastic bag. Generally, the wound is not redressed until the patient's follow-up visit with the surgeon. (See the Home Care Teaching Checklist: Hand Surgery.)

Evaluation

Expected Outcomes

Expected outcomes may include:

1. Maintains peripheral tissue perfusion
   a. Demonstrates normal skin temperature and capillary refill
   b. Exhibits normal sensations
   c. Exhibits acceptable motor function

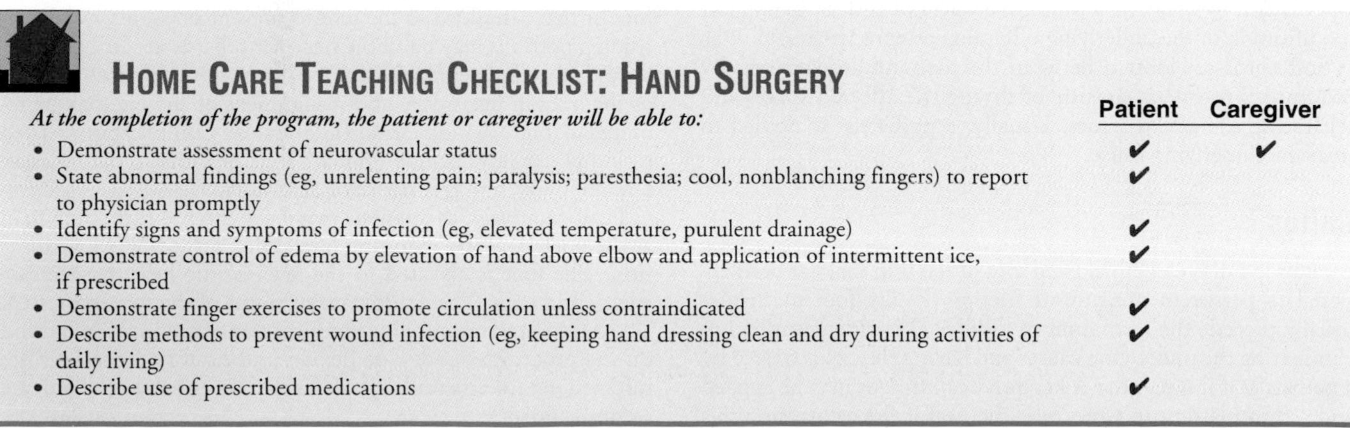

HOME CARE TEACHING CHECKLIST: HAND SURGERY

At the completion of the program, the patient or caregiver will be able to:

	Patient	Caregiver
• Demonstrate assessment of neurovascular status	✔	✔
• State abnormal findings (eg, unrelenting pain; paralysis; paresthesia; cool, nonblanching fingers) to report to physician promptly	✔	
• Identify signs and symptoms of infection (eg, elevated temperature, purulent drainage)	✔	
• Demonstrate control of edema by elevation of hand above elbow and application of intermittent ice, if prescribed	✔	
• Demonstrate finger exercises to promote circulation unless contraindicated	✔	
• Describe methods to prevent wound infection (eg, keeping hand dressing clean and dry during activities of daily living)	✔	
• Describe use of prescribed medications	✔	

2. Achieves pain relief
   a. Reports increased comfort
   b. Controls edema through elevation of the hand
   c. Experiences no discomfort with movement
3. Demonstrates independent self-care
   a. Secures assistance with ADLs during first few days postoperatively
   b. Adapts to one-handed ADLs
   c. Uses injured hand within its functional capability
4. Demonstrates absence of wound infection
   a. Complies with treatment protocol and prevention strategies
   b. Reports temperature and pulse within normal limits
   c. Experiences no purulent wound drainage
   d. Experiences no wound inflammation

COMMON FOOT PROBLEMS

Disabilities of the foot are commonly due to poorly fitting shoes. Fashion, vanity, and eye appeal, rather than function and physiology of the foot, are the determining factors in the design of footwear. Ill-fitting shoes distort normal anatomy while inducing deformity and pain.

Several systemic diseases affect the feet. Patients with diabetes are prone to develop corns and peripheral neuropathies with diminishing sensation, leading to ulcers at pressure points of the foot. Patients with peripheral vascular disease and arteriosclerosis complain of burning and itching feet with attendant scratching and skin breakdown. Foot deformities may occur with rheumatoid arthritis. Dermatologic problems commonly affect the feet in the form of fungal infections and plantar warts.

The discomforts of foot strain can be treated by rest, elevation, physiotherapy, supportive strappings, and orthotic devices. The patient must inspect the foot and skin under pads and orthotic devices for pressure and skin breakdown daily. If shoes are cut to relieve pressure over a bony deformity, the skin must be monitored daily for breakdown from the "window" area. Active foot exercises promote the circulation and help strengthen the feet. Walking in properly fitting shoes is considered the best form of exercise.

Corn

A corn is an area of hyperkeratosis (overgrowth of a horny layer of epidermis) produced by internal pressure (the underlying bone is prominent because of congenital or acquired abnormality, commonly arthritis) or external pressure (shoes). The usual sites are the small toes, mainly the fifth toe, but all toes may be involved.

Corns are treated by soaking and scraping off the horny layer by a podiatrist, by applying a protective shield or pad, or by surgical modification of the underlying offending osseous structure.

Soft corns are located between the toes and are kept soft by moisture. Treatment consists of drying the affected spaces and separating the affected toes. Usually, a podiatrist is needed to treat the underlying cause.

Callus

A callus is a discretely thickened area of the skin that has been exposed to persistent pressure or friction. Faulty foot mechanics usually precede the formation of a callus. Treatment consists of eliminating the underlying causes and having the callus treated by a podiatrist if it is painful. A keratolytic ointment may be applied and a thin plastic cup worn over the heel if the callus is on this area. Felt padding with adhesive backing is also used to prevent and relieve pressure. Orthotic devices can be made to remove the pressure from bony protuberances, or the protuberance may be excised.

Ingrown Toenail

An ingrown toenail (onychocryptosis) is a condition in which the free edge of a nail plate penetrates the surrounding skin, either laterally or anteriorly. It may be accompanied by secondary infection or granulation tissue. This painful condition is caused by improper self-treatment, external pressure (tight shoes or stockings), internal pressure (deformed toes, growth under the nail), trauma, or infection. Trimming the nails properly (clipping them straight across and filing the corners consistent with the contour of the toe) can prevent this problem. Active treatment consists of antibiotics and relieving the pain by decreasing the pressure on the surrounding soft tissue by the nail plate. Warm, wet soaks help to drain an infection. A toenail may need to be excised if there is severe infection.

Hammer Toe

Hammer toe is a flexion deformity of the interphalangeal joint, which may involve several toes (Fig. 62-6). The condition is usually an acquired deformity. Tight socks or shoes may push an overlying toe back into the line of the other toes. The toes usually are pulled upward, forcing the metatarsal joints (ball of the foot) downward. Corns develop on top of the toes, and tender calluses develop under the metatarsal area. The treatment consists of conservative measures: wearing open-toed sandals or shoes that conform to the shape of the foot, carrying out manipulative exercises, and protecting the protruding joints with pads. Surgical correction is necessary for an established deformity.

Hallux Valgus

Hallux valgus (bunion) is a deformity in which the great toe deviates laterally (see Fig. 62-6). Associated with this is a marked prominence of the medial aspect of the first metatarsal–phalangeal joint. There is also osseous enlargement (exostosis) of the medial side of the first metatarsal head, over which a bursa may form (secondary to pressure and inflammation). Acute bursitis symptoms include a reddened area, edema, and tenderness.

Factors contributing to bunion formation include heredity, narrow shoes, and gradual lengthening and widening of the foot associated with aging. Osteoarthritis is frequently associated with hallux valgus. Treatment depends on the patient's age, the degree of deformity, and the severity of symptoms. If a bunion deformity is uncomplicated, wearing a shoe that conforms to the shape of the foot or that is molded to the foot to prevent pressure on the protruding portions may be all the treatment that is needed. Corticosteroid injections control acute inflammation. Surgical removal of the bunion (exostosis) and realignment of the toe may be required to improve function and appearance. Complications related to bunionectomy include limited range of motion, paresthesias, tendon injury, and recurrence of deformity.

Postoperatively, the patient may have intense throbbing pain at the operative site, requiring liberal doses of analgesic medication. The foot is elevated to the level of the heart to decrease edema and pain. The neurovascular status of the toes is assessed. The duration of immobility and initiation of ambulation depend on the procedure used. Toe flexion and extension exercises are initiated to facilitate walking. Shoes that do not stress the foot are recommended.

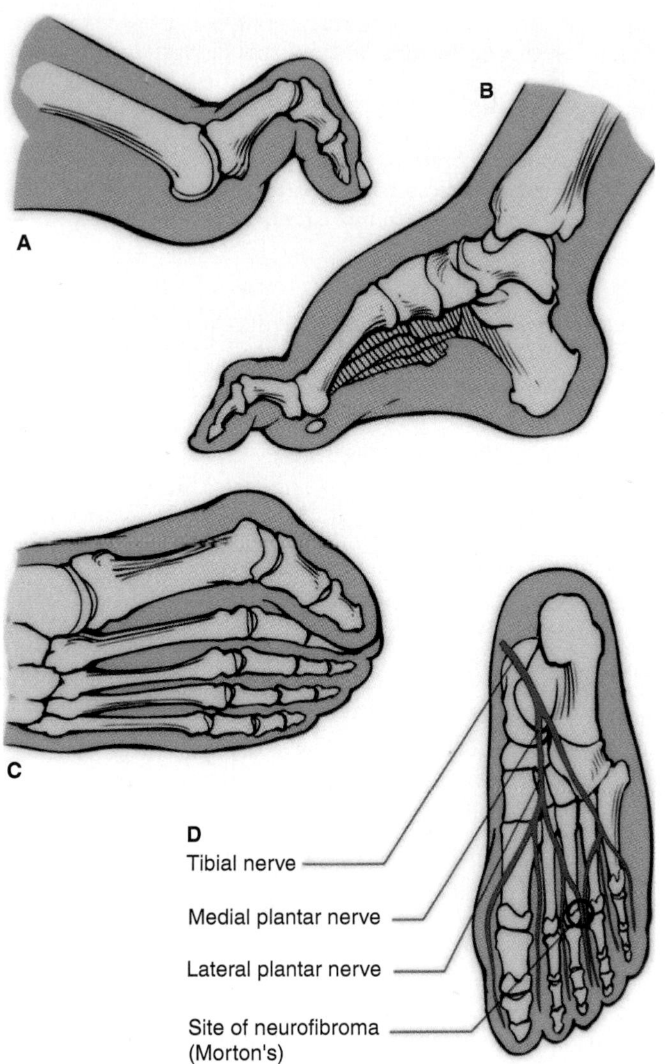

FIGURE 62•6 Common foot deformities. (**A**) Hammer toe. (**B**) Pes cavus (clawfoot). (**C**) Bunion (hallux valgus). (**D**) Site for Morton's neuroma.

Pes Cavus

Pes cavus (clawfoot) refers to a foot with an abnormally high arch and a fixed equinus deformity of the forefoot (see Fig. 62-6). The shortening of the foot and increased pressure produce calluses on the metatarsal area and on the dorsum (bottom) of the foot. Charcot-Marie-Tooth disease (a peripheral neuromuscular disorder associated with a familial degenerative disorder), diabetes mellitus, and tertiary syphilis are common causes of pes cavus. Exercises are prescribed to manipulate the forefoot into dorsiflexion and relax the toes. Bracing to protect the foot may be used. In severe cases, arthrodesis (fusion) is performed to reshape and stabilize the foot.

Morton's Neuroma

Morton's neuroma (plantar digital neuroma, neurofibroma) is a swelling of the third (lateral) branch of the median plantar nerve (see Fig. 62-6). The third digital nerve, which is located in the third intermetatarsal (web) space, is most commonly involved. Microscopically, digital artery changes cause an ischemia of the nerve.

The result is a throbbing, burning pain in the foot that is usually relieved when the patient rests. Conservative treatment consists of inserting innersoles and metatarsal pads designed to spread the metatarsal heads and balance the foot posture. Local injections of hydrocortisone and a local anesthetic may provide relief. If these fail, surgical excision of the neuroma is necessary. Pain relief and loss of sensation are immediate and permanent.

Flatfoot

Flatfoot (pes planus) is a common disorder in which the longitudinal arch of the foot is diminished. It may be due to congenital abnormalities or associated with bone or ligament injury, muscle and posture imbalances, excessive weight, muscle fatigue, poorly fitting shoes, or arthritis. Symptoms include a burning sensation, fatigue, clumsy gait, edema, and pain.

Exercises to strengthen the muscles and to improve posture and walking habits are helpful. A number of foot orthoses are available to give the foot additional support. Severe flatfoot problems are usually treated by an orthopedic surgeon or a podiatrist.

NURSING PROCESS: THE PATIENT UNDERGOING FOOT SURGERY

Assessment

Surgery of the foot may be necessary because of various conditions, including neuromas and foot deformities (bunion, hammer toe, clawfoot). Generally, foot surgery is performed on an outpatient basis. Before surgery, the nurse assesses the patient's ambulatory ability and balance and the neurovascular status of the foot. Additionally, the nurse considers availability of assistance at home after surgery and the structural characteristics of the home in planning for care during the first few days after surgery. The nurse uses these data, in addition to knowledge of the usual medical management of the problem, to formulate appropriate nursing diagnoses.

Nursing Diagnosis

Based on the assessment data, the nursing diagnoses for the patient undergoing foot surgery may include the following:

- Risk for altered peripheral tissue perfusion related to surgical procedure
- Pain related to inflammation and swelling
- Impaired physical mobility related to the foot-immobilizing device
- Risk for infection related to the surgical procedure/surgical incision

Planning and Goals

The goals of the patient may include adequate tissue perfusion, relief of pain, improved mobility, and absence of infection.

Nursing Interventions

Promoting Tissue Perfusion

Neurovascular assessment of the exposed toes every 1 to 2 hours for the first 24 hours is essential to monitor the function of the nerves and the perfusion of the tissues. If the patient is discharged within several hours of the surgery, the nurse teaches the patient and family how to assess for swelling and neurovascular status (circulation, motion, sensation). Compromised neurovascular function can increase the patient's pain.

Relieving Pain

Pain experienced by patients who undergo foot surgery is related to inflammation and edema. Formation of a hematoma may contribute to the discomfort. To control the swelling, the foot should be elevated on several pillows when the patient is sitting or lying.

Intermittent ice packs applied to the surgical area during the first 24 to 48 hours may be prescribed to control swelling and provide some pain relief. As activity increases, the patient may find that dependent positioning of the foot may be uncomfortable. Simply elevating the foot often relieves the discomfort. Oral analgesics may be used to control the pain. The nurse instructs the patient and family about appropriate use of these medications.

Improving Mobility

After surgery, the patient will have a bulky dressing on the foot, protected by a light cast or a special protective boot. Limits for weight-bearing on the foot will be prescribed by the surgeon. Some patients are allowed to walk on the heel and progress to weight-bearing as tolerated; other patients are restricted to non–weight-bearing activities. Assistive devices (eg, crutches, walker) may be needed. Choice of the devices depends on the patient's general condition and balance and on the weight-bearing prescription. Safe use of the assistive devices must be ensured through adequate patient education and practice before discharge. Problems of moving around the house safely while using assistive devices are discussed with the patient. As healing progresses, the patient gradually resumes ambulation within prescribed limits. The nurse emphasizes adherence to the therapeutic regimen.

Preventing Infection

Any surgery carries a risk for infection. In addition, percutaneous pins may be used to hold bones in position, and these pins serve as potential sites for infection. Because the foot is on or near the floor, care must be taken to protect it from dirt and moisture. When bathing, the patient can secure a plastic bag over the dressing to prevent it from getting wet. Patient instruction concerning aseptic wound care and pin care may be necessary.

The nurse teaches the patient to monitor for temperature and infection. Drainage on the dressing, foul odor, or increased pain and swelling could indicate infection. The nurse promptly reports any of these findings to the physician. If prophylactic antibiotics are prescribed, the nurse provides instruction about their correct use.

Promoting Home and Community-Based Care

TEACHING PATIENTS SELF-CARE

The nurse plans patient teaching for home care, focusing on neurovascular status, pain management, mobility, and wound care. (See Health Promotion and Illness Prevention: The Patient Who Has Had Foot Surgery.)

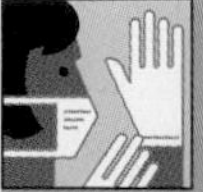

HEALTH PROMOTION AND ILLNESS PREVENTION
The Patient Who Has Had Foot Surgery

Neurovascular Status

Teach patient indicators of impaired circulation: change in sensation, inability to move toes, toes or foot cool to touch, color changes

Pain Management

Discuss with patient methods to reduce pain:
- Elevate foot to heart level
- Apply ice as prescribed
- Use analgesics as prescribed

Report pain that is not relieved

Mobility

Instruct patient in safe use of assistive devices

Reinforce prescribed weight-bearing limits

Encourage patient to wear special protective shoe over wound dressing

Wound Care

Instruct patient to keep dressing or cast clean and dry

Instruct patient about signs of wound infection (eg pain, drainage, fever)

Discuss prescribed antibiotic regimen with patient

Explain that initial dressing change will be performed by the surgeon

Evaluation

Expected Outcomes

Expected outcomes may include:

1. Maintains peripheral tissue perfusion
   a. Demonstrates normal skin temperature and capillary refill
   b. Exhibits normal sensations
   c. Exhibits acceptable motor function
2. Obtains pain relief
   a. Elevates foot to control edema
   b. Applies ice to foot as prescribed
   c. Uses oral analgesics as needed and prescribed
   d. Reports decreased pain and increased comfort
3. Demonstrates increased mobility
   a. Uses assistive devices safely
   b. Resumes weight-bearing gradually as prescribed
   c. Exhibits diminished disability associated with preoperative condition
4. Develops no infection
   a. Reports temperature and pulse within normal limits
   b. Reports no purulent drainage or signs of wound inflammation
   c. Maintains clean and dry dressing
   d. Takes prophylactic antibiotics as prescribed

METABOLIC BONE DISORDERS

Osteoporosis

Osteoporosis is a disease that threatens more than 28 million Americans (National Osteoporosis Foundation, 1997). The disorder is characterized by a reduction of total bone mass and a change in bone structure, which increases susceptibility to fracture. The normal homeostatic bone turnover changes; the rate of bone resorption is greater than the rate of bone formation, resulting in a reduced total bone mass. With osteoporosis, the bones become progressively porous, brittle, and fragile; they fracture easily under stresses that would not break normal bone. Osteoporosis frequently results in compression fractures (Fig. 62-7) of the thoracic and lumbar spine, fractures of the neck and intertrochanteric region of the femur, and Colles' fractures of the wrist. Multiple compression fractures of the vertebrae result in skeletal deformity. Osteoporosis is a costly disorder not only in terms of health care dollars but also in terms of human suffering, pain, disability, fracture, and death.

A gradual collapse of a vertebra may be asymptomatic; it is observed as progressive kyphosis. With the development of kyphosis ("dowager's hump"), there is an associated loss of height (Fig. 62-8). Frequently, postmenopausal women lose height from vertebral collapse. The postural changes result in relaxation of the abdominal muscles and a protruding abdomen. The deformity may also produce pulmonary insufficiency. Many patients complain of fatigue.

Early identification of at-risk teenagers and young adult women, increased calcium intake, participation in regular weight-bearing exercise, and modification of lifestyle (eg, reduce use of caffeine, cigarettes, and alcohol) decrease the risk for developing osteoporosis, fractures, and associated disability later in life.

Gerontologic Considerations

The prevalence of osteoporosis in women older than 80 years of age is 84% (Genant, et al., 1997). The average 75-year-old woman has lost 25% of her cortical bone and 40% of her trabecular bone. With the aging of the population, the incidence of fractures (1.5 million fractures per year), pain, and disability associated with osteoporosis is rising (Thomas, 1997). Elderly people absorb dietary calcium less efficiently and excrete it more readily through their kidneys; therefore, postmenopausal women and the elderly actually need to consume liberal amounts of calcium. As much as 1500 mg daily for postmenopausal women may be prescribed.

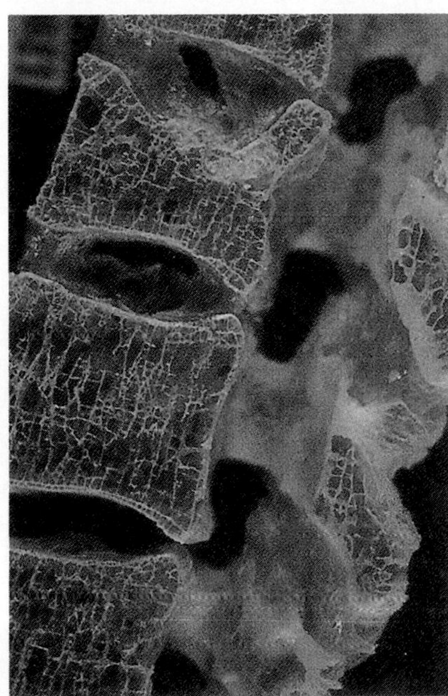

FIGURE 62•7 Progressive osteoporotic bone loss and compression fractures. From Rubin, E. & Farber, I. L. (1999). *Pathology* (3rd ed.), Philadelphia: Lippincott Williams & Wilkins.

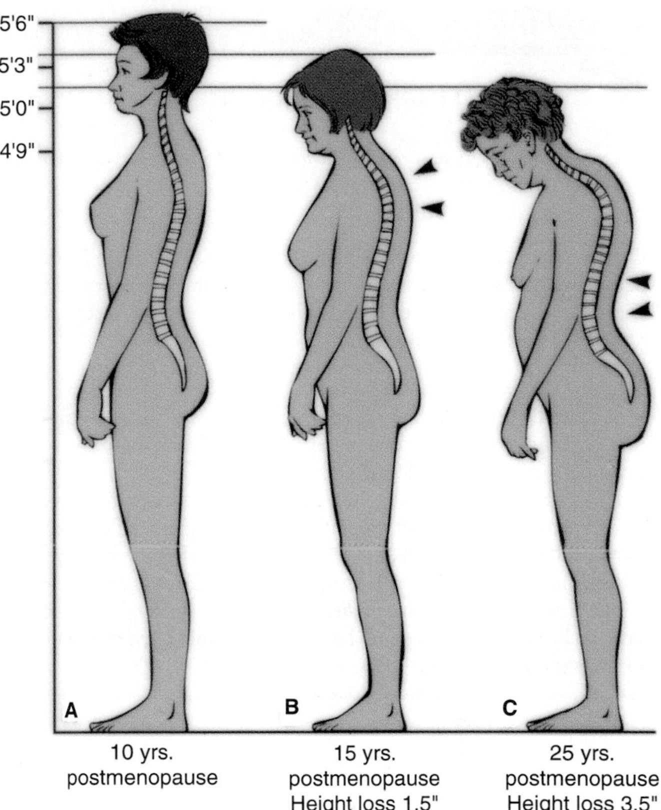

FIGURE 62•8 Typical loss of height associated with osteoporosis and aging.

Pathophysiology

Normal bone remodeling in the adult results in increased bone mass until about 35 years of age. Genetics, aging, nutrition, lifestyle choices (eg, smoking, caffeine and alcohol consumption), and physical activity influence the peak bone mass and development of osteoporosis.

Loss of bone mass is a universal phenomenon associated with aging. Age-related loss begins soon after the peak bone mass is achieved. Calcitonin, which inhibits bone resorption and promotes bone formation, is decreased. Estrogen, which inhibits bone breakdown, decreases with aging. On the other hand, parathyroid hormone increases with aging and increases bone resorption. The consequence of these changes is net bone mass loss over time.

The withdrawal of estrogens at menopause and with oophorectomy causes an accelerated bone resorption that continues during the postmenopausal years. Women develop osteoporosis more frequently and more extensively than men because of lower peak bone mass and the effect of estrogen loss during menopause. More than half of all women older than 45 years of age show evidence of osteoporosis on x-ray.

Risk Factors

Small-framed, nonobese white women are at greatest risk for osteoporosis. African American women, who have a greater bone mass than white women, are less susceptible to osteoporosis. Men have a greater peak bone mass and do not experience sudden hormonal

NURSING RESEARCH

Loss of Height and Bone Mass

Hunt, A. (1996). The relationship between height change and bone mineral density. *Orthopedic Nursing 15*(3), 57–64.

Purpose

Osteoporosis is a major health problem associated with aging. This study compares the loss of height with the loss of bone mass. This exploratory study investigates the use of excessive height loss as a low cost predictor of bone mass loss (osteoporosis).

Study Sample and Design

The basis for determining excessive height loss was based on the normal expected height loss formula of an annual loss of 0.09% of total height beginning at age 45 years.

The convenience sample of 76 subjects consisted of patients in a bone health clinic. Most of the subjects had a diagnosis of osteoporosis ($n = 61$) or Paget's disease ($n = 6$). All subjects had bone density measurements (dual-energy x-ray absorptiometry and/or quantitative computed tomography). Maximum height was determined by recall and by driver's license records. Actual height measurements were made with subjects standing without shoes.

Results

The study confirmed a high significant correlation ($r = 0.97$) between recall and driver's license maximum height. The study demonstrated a higher than expected height loss for the group (mean loss, 0.8 inches greater than expected). Those who had lower bone mass had a greater incidence of height loss. Similarly, those who had experienced documented compression fractures had greater than expected height loss, were older, and were shorter than those without fractures.

Nursing Implications

Adults older than 45 years of age should be measured during health assessments to determine height loss. Recalled maximum height or driver's license height can be used to determine maximum height. Expected height loss can be calculated based on the age-expected height loss formula. Patients who are found to be experiencing height loss greater than expected should be encouraged to have bone density studies performed and engage in preventive and/or therapeutic regimens to preserve and increase bone mass.

changes. As a result, osteoporosis occurs in men at a lower rate and at an older age. One of two white women and one of eight white men older than 50 years of age have an osteoporosis-related fracture in their lifetime (National Osteoporosis Foundation, 1998).

Nutritional factors contribute to the development of osteoporosis. Vitamin D is necessary for calcium absorption and for normal bone mineralization. Dietary calcium and vitamin D must be adequate to maintain bone remodeling and body functions. The best source of calcium and vitamin D is fortified milk. Inadequate intake of calcium or vitamin D over a period of years results in decreased bone mass and the development of osteoporosis. The 1997 recommended Adequate Intake (AI) level of calcium for the age range of puberty through young adults (9 to 19 years of age) is 1300 mg per day. The goal of this daily level of calcium is to maximize peak bone mass. The AI level for adults 19 to 50 years of age is 1000 mg per day, and the AI adults 51 years and older is 1200 mg per day. The actual estimated average daily intake is 300 to 500 mg.

Bone formation is enhanced by the stress of weight and muscle activity. Immobility contributes to the development of osteoporosis. When immobilized by casts, paralysis, or general inactivity, the bone is resorbed faster than it is formed, and osteoporosis occurs.

Coexisting medical conditions (eg, malabsorption syndromes, lactose intolerance, alcohol abuse, renal failure, liver failure, Cushing's syndrome, hyperthyroidism, and hyperparathyroidism) contribute to bone loss and the development of osteoporosis. Medications (eg, corticosteroids, isoniazid, heparin, tetracycline, aluminum-containing antacids, furosemide, anticonvulsants, and thyroid supplements) affect the body's use and metabolism of calcium. The degree of osteoporosis is related to the duration of medication therapy. When the therapy is discontinued or the metabolic problem is corrected, the progression of osteoporosis is halted, but restoration of lost bone mass usually does not occur.

Assessment and Diagnostic Findings

Osteoporosis is identified on routine x-rays when there has been 25% to 40% demineralization. There is a radiolucency to the bone. When the vertebrae collapse, the thoracic vertebrae become wedge shaped and the lumbar vertebrae become biconcave. Dual-energy x-ray absorptiometry (DEXA) provides information about bone mass at the spine and hip. These studies are useful in identifying osteoporotic bone and assessing response to therapy. Ultrasonic heel-density (bone sonometer) studies are used to diagnose osteoporosis and predict risk of fracture.

Laboratory studies (eg, serum calcium, serum phosphate, serum alkaline phosphatase, urine calcium excretion, urinary hydroxyproline excretion, hematocrit, erythrocyte sedimentation rate) and x-rays are used to exclude other possible medical diagnoses (eg, multiple myeloma, osteomalacia, hyperparathyroidism, malignancy) that contribute to bone loss.

Medical Management

An adequate, balanced diet rich in calcium and vitamin D throughout life, with an increased calcium intake during adolescence, young adulthood, and the middle years, protects against skeletal demineralization. This would include three glasses of skim or whole vitamin D milk or other foods high in calcium (eg, cheese and other dairy products, steamed broccoli, canned salmon with bones) daily. To ensure adequate calcium intake, a calcium supplement (calcium carbonate) may be prescribed and taken with meals or with a beverage high in vitamin C to promote absorption. Common side effects of calcium supplements are abdominal distention and constipation.

Regular weight-bearing exercise promotes bone formation. From 20 to 30 minutes of aerobic exercise (eg, walking) 3 days or more a week is recommended. In addition, exercise improves balance, reducing falls and fractures.

PHARMACOLOGIC THERAPY

At natural or surgical menopause, hormone replacement therapy (HRT) with estrogen and progesterone may be prescribed to retard bone loss and prevent occurrence of fractures. Estrogen replacement decreases bone resorption and increases bone mass, reducing the incidence of osteoporotic fractures. Estrogen therapy has been associated with a slightly increased incidence of breast and endometrial cancers. Using the lowest effective dose reduces the cancer risk. Also, combined estrogen and progesterone therapy diminishes the potential risk for endometrial cancer. HRT is contraindicated in patients who are pregnant or who have undiagnosed vaginal bleeding; active thrombophlebitis; endometrial, breast, and estrogen-dependent tumors; and acute liver disease. The use of hormones for long-term therapy (10 years or more) to decrease hip fracture continues to be evaluated. Therefore, during HRT, the patient must examine her breasts monthly and have a pelvic examination, including Papanicolaou's smear and endometrial biopsy (if indicated), one or two times a year. Common side effects from HRT include periodic bleeding or spotting, gastrointestinal upset, breast tenderness, mood swings, fluid retention, and weight gain. "Designer estrogens," such as raloxifene (Evista), reduce the risk for osteoporosis without increasing the risk for breast cancer.

Other medications that may be prescribed to manage osteoporosis include alendronate (Fosamax) and calcitonin. Alendronate offers an alternative to HRT and produces increased bone mass (by inhibiting osteoclast function) and decreased bone loss. Alendronate should be taken each morning with water 30 to 60 minutes before food or other medications for maximum absorption. Adequate calcium and vitamin D intake is needed for maximum effect. Side effects of alendronate include gastrointestinal symptoms (eg, dyspepsia, nausea, flatulence, diarrhea, constipation).

Calcitonin primarily suppresses bone loss through direct action on osteoclasts and reduced bone turnover. It is administered by nasal spray or by subcutaneous or intramuscular injection. Side effects include nasal irritation, flushing, gastrointestinal disturbances, and urinary frequency.

NURSING PROCESS: THE PATIENT WITH A SPONTANEOUS VERTEBRAL FRACTURE RELATED TO OSTEOPOROSIS

Assessment

Health promotion, identification of people at risk for osteoporosis, and recognition of problems associated with osteoporosis form the basis for nursing assessment. The health history includes questions concerning the occurrence of osteoporosis and focuses on family history, previous fractures, dietary consumption of calcium, exercise patterns, onset of menopause, and use of corticosteroids as well as alcohol, smoking, and caffeine intake. Any symptoms the patient is experiencing, such as back pain, constipation, or altered body image, are explored.

Physical examination may disclose a fracture, kyphosis of the thoracic spine, or shortened stature. Problems in mobility and breathing may exist as a result of changes in posture and weakened muscles.

Nursing Diagnosis

Based on the assessment data, the major nursing diagnoses for the patient who experiences a spontaneous vertebral fracture related to osteoporosis may include the following:

- Knowledge deficit about the osteoporotic process and treatment regimen
- Pain related to fracture and muscle spasm
- Constipation related to immobility or development of ileus (intestinal obstruction)
- Risk for injury: fracture related to osteoporosis

HOME CARE TEACHING CHECKLIST: OSTEOPOROSIS

At the completion of the program, the patient will be able to:	Patient	Caregiver
ADOLESCENT AND YOUNG WOMEN		
• List risk factors for osteoporosis	✔	
• Identify calcium- and vitamin D–rich foods	✔	
• Consume balanced diet with adequate calcium (1000–1300 mg/day)	✔	
• Engage in weight-bearing exercise daily	✔	
• Modify lifestyle choices—avoid smoking, alcohol, caffeine, sodas, and excessive protein	✔	
MENOPAUSAL AND POSTMENOPAUSAL WOMEN		
• List risk factors for osteoporosis	✔	
• Identify calcium- and vitamin D–rich foods	✔	
• Consume balanced diet with adequate calcium (1200–1500 mg/day)	✔	
• Discuss calcium supplements	✔	
• Engage in weight-bearing exercise daily	✔	
• Engage in exercise that improves balance to reduce the incidence of falls	✔	
• Demonstrate good body mechanics	✔	
• Modify lifestyle choices—avoid smoking, alcohol, caffeine, sodas, and excessive protein	✔	
• Discuss use of hormone replacement therapy and other pharmacologic agents to maintain and enhance bone mass	✔	
• Review concurrent medical conditions and medications with health care provider to identify factors that contribute to bone mass loss	✔	✔
• Assess home environment for hazards contributing to falls	✔	✔

Planning and Goals

The major goals of the patient may include knowledge about osteoporosis and the treatment regimen, relief of pain, improved bowel elimination, and absence of additional fracture.

Nursing Interventions

Promoting Understanding of Osteoporosis and the Treatment Regimen

Patient teaching focuses on factors influencing the development of osteoporosis, interventions to arrest or slow the process, and measures to relieve symptoms. Adequate dietary or supplemental calcium, regular weight-bearing exercise, and modification of lifestyle, if necessary (eg, cessation of smoking and reduced use of caffeine and alcohol), help to maintain bone mass. Diet, exercise, and physical activity are the primary keys to developing high-density bones that are resistant to osteoporosis. It is emphasized that elderly people continue to need sufficient calcium, vitamin D, sunshine, and exercise to minimize the progression of osteoporosis.

Patient teaching related to medication therapy is important. Because gastrointestinal symptoms and abdominal distention are frequent side effects of calcium supplements, the nurse instructs the patient to take the calcium supplements with meals. Also, it is important to teach the patient to drink adequate fluids to reduce the risk of renal calculi. If HRT is prescribed, the nurse teaches the patient about the importance of compliance and periodic screening for breast and endometrial cancer. Alendronate requires compliance with taking it on an empty stomach with water and an adequate daily intake of dietary calcium. Nasal calcitonin is administered daily, alternating the nares.

Relieving Pain

Relief of back pain resulting from compression fracture may be accomplished by resting in bed in a supine or side-lying position several times a day. The mattress should be firm and nonsagging. Knee flexion increases comfort by relaxing back muscles. Intermittent local heat and back rubs promote muscle relaxation. The nurse instructs the patient to move the trunk as a unit and to avoid twisting. The nurse encourages good posture and teaches body mechanics. When the patient is assisted out of bed, a lumbosacral corset may be worn for temporary support and immobilization, although such a device is frequently uncomfortable and poorly tolerated by many elderly patients. The patient gradually resumes activities as pain diminishes.

Improving Bowel Elimination

Constipation is a problem related to immobility, medications, and age. Early institution of a high-fiber diet, increased fluids, and the use of prescribed stool softeners help to prevent or minimize constipation. If the vertebral collapse involves T10–L2 vertebrae, the patient may develop an ileus. The nurse therefore monitors the patient's intake, bowel sounds, and bowel activity.

Preventing Injury

Physical activity is essential to strengthen muscles, prevent disuse atrophy, and retard progressive bone demineralization. Isometric exercises can strengthen trunk muscles. The nurse encourages walking, good body mechanics, and good posture. Sudden bending, jarring, and strenuous lifting are avoided. Daily weight-bearing activity, preferably outdoors in the sunshine, is necessary to enhance the body's ability to produce vitamin D.

Gerontologic Considerations

Elderly people fall frequently as a result of environmental hazards, neuromuscular disorders, diminished senses and cardiovascular responses, and responses to medications. It is important to identify and eliminate hazards. Supervision and assistance should be readily available.

The patient and family need to be included in planning for continued care and preventive management regimens. The home environment is assessed for potential hazards (eg, scatter rugs, cluttered rooms, toys on the floor, pets underfoot), and a safe environment is created (eg, well-lighted staircases with secure hand rails, grab-bars in the bathroom, properly fitting footwear).

Evaluation

Expected Outcomes

Expected outcomes may include:

1. Acquires knowledge about osteoporosis and the treatment regimen
   a. States relationship of calcium intake and exercise to bone mass
   b. Consumes adequate dietary calcium
   c. Increases level of exercise
   d. Takes prescribed hormonal or nonhormonal therapy
   e. Undergoes prescribed screening procedures
2. Achieves pain relief
   a. Experiences pain relief at rest
   b. Experiences minimal discomfort during ADLs
   c. Demonstrates diminished tenderness at fracture site
3. Demonstrates normal bowel elimination
   a. Has active bowel sounds
   b. Reports regular bowel movements
4. Experiences no new fractures
   a. Maintains good posture
   b. Uses good body mechanics
   c. Consumes balanced diet high in calcium and vitamin D
   d. Engages in weight-bearing exercises (walks daily)
   e. Rests by lying down several times a day
   f. Participates in outdoor activities
   g. Creates a safe home environment
   h. Accepts assistance and supervision as needed

Osteomalacia

Osteomalacia is a metabolic bone disease characterized by inadequate mineralization of bone. (A similar condition in children is called *rickets.*) In adults, osteomalacia is chronic, and skeletal deformities are not as severe as in children because skeletal growth has been completed. In these patients, a large amount of osteoid or remolded bone does not calcify. As a result of faulty mineralization, there is softening and weakening of the skeleton, causing pain, tenderness to touch, bowing of the bones, and pathologic fractures. The malnutrition type of osteomalacia (deficiency in vitamin D often associated with poor intake of calcium) is due to poverty, food faddism, and lack of knowledge about nutrition. It occurs most frequently in parts of the world where vitamin D is not added to food, where dietary deficiencies exist, and where sunlight is rare.

Pathophysiology

The primary defect in osteomalacia is a deficiency of activated vitamin D (calcitriol), which promotes calcium absorption from the gastrointestinal tract and facilitates mineralization of bone. The supply of calcium and phosphate in the extracellular fluid is low. Without adequate vitamin D, calcium and phosphate are not moved to calcification sites in bones.

Osteomalacia may result from failed calcium absorption (eg, malabsorption syndrome) or excessive loss of calcium from the body. Gastrointestinal disorders in which fats are inadequately absorbed are likely to produce osteomalacia through loss of vitamin D (along with other fat-soluble vitamins) and calcium, the latter being excreted in the feces with fatty acids. Such disorders include celiac disease, chronic biliary tract obstruction, chronic pancreatitis, and small bowel resections.

Severe renal insufficiency results in acidosis. The body uses available calcium to combat the acidosis, and the parathyroid hormone stimulates a release of skeletal calcium in an attempt to reestablish a physiologic pH. During this continual drain of skeletal calcium, bony fibrosis occurs, and bony cysts form. Chronic glomerulonephritis, obstructive uropathies, and heavy-metal poisoning result in a reduced serum phosphate level and demineralization of bone.

In addition, liver and kidney diseases can produce a lack of vitamin D because these are the organs that convert vitamin D to its active form. Hyperparathyroidism leads to skeletal decalcification and thus to osteomalacia by increasing phosphate excretion in the urine. Prolonged anticonvulsant therapy (phenytoin, phenobarbital) poses a risk for osteomalacia, as does insufficient vitamin D (dietary, sunlight).

Gerontologic Considerations

A nutritious diet is particularly important in elderly people. Adequate intake of calcium and vitamin D is promoted. Because sunlight is necessary, older people should be encouraged to spend some time in the sun. Prevention, identification, and management of osteomalacia in the elderly are essential to reduce the incidence of fractures. When osteomalacia is combined with osteoporosis, the incidence of fracture increases.

Clinical Manifestations

The most common and distressing symptoms of osteomalacia are bone pain and tenderness. The description of the discomfort may be vague. On physical examination, skeletal deformities are noted. Spinal kyphosis and bending deformities of the long bones (legs become bowed) give patients an unusual appearance and a waddling or limping gait. These patients may be uncomfortable with their appearance. As a result of calcium deficiency, there is usually muscle weakness. Muscle weakness and unsteadiness increase the risk for falls and fractures.

Assessment and Diagnostic Findings

On x-ray, generalized demineralization of bone is evident. Studies of the vertebrae may show a compression fracture with indistinct vertebral end-plates. Laboratory studies show low serum calcium and phosphorus levels and a moderately elevated alkaline phosphatase level. Urine calcium and creatinine excretion is low. Bone biopsy demonstrates an increased amount of osteoid.

Medical Management

The underlying cause of osteomalacia is corrected when possible. If osteomalacia is dietary in origin, a diet with adequate protein and increased calcium and vitamin D is provided. The patient is instructed about dietary sources of calcium and vitamin D (eg, fortified milk and cereals, eggs, chicken livers). The safe use of supplements is reviewed. Because high doses of vitamin D are toxic and enhance the risk of hypercalcemia, the importance of monitoring serum calcium levels is stressed. Vitamin D raises the concentration of calcium and phosphorus in the extracellular fluid and thus makes these ions available for mineralization of bone.

If osteomalacia is due to malabsorption, increased doses of vitamin D, along with supplemental calcium, are usually prescribed. Exposure to sunlight for ultraviolet radiation to transform a cholesterol substance (7-dehydrocholesterol) present in the skin into vitamin D may be recommended.

Physical, psychological, and pharmaceutical measures are used to reduce the patient's discomfort and pain. When assisting the patient to change positions, the nurse handles the patient gently, and pillows are used to support the body. As the patient responds to therapy, the skeletal discomforts diminish.

Frequently, skeletal problems associated with osteomalacia resolve themselves when the underlying nutritional deficiency or pathologic process is adequately treated. Long-term monitoring of the patient is appropriate to ensure stabilization or reversal of osteomalacia. Some persistent orthopedic deformities may need to be treated with braces or surgery (eg, osteotomy may be performed to correct long bone deformity).

Paget's Disease

Paget's disease (osteitis deformans) is a disorder of localized rapid bone turnover, most commonly affecting the skull, femur, tibia, pelvic bones, and vertebrae. There is a primary proliferation of osteoclasts, which produces bone resorption. This is followed by a compensatory increase in osteoblastic activity that replaces the bone. As bone turnover continues, a classic mosaic (disorganized) pattern of bone develops. The Paget's diseased bone is highly vascularized and structurally weak. Pathologic fractures occur. Structural bowing of the legs causes malalignment of the hip, knee, and ankle joints, which contributes to the development of arthritis and pain.

Paget's disease occurs in about 3% of the population older than 50 years of age. The incidence is slightly greater in men than women and increases with aging. A family history has been noted, with siblings developing the disease. The cause of Paget's disease is not known.

Clinical Manifestations

Paget's disease is insidious; most patients never know they have it. Some patients do not experience symptoms but have skeletal deformity. A few patients have symptomatic deformity and pain. The condition is most frequently identified on x-rays during a routine physical examination or in the course of workup for another problem. Sclerotic changes, skeletal deformities (eg, bowing of femur and tibia, enlargement of the skull), and cortical thickening of the long bones are seen.

In most patients, skeletal deformity involves the skull or long bones. The skull may thicken, and the patient may report that a hat no longer fits. In some cases of Paget's disease, the cranium, but not the face, is enlarged. This gives the face a small, triangular appearance. Most patients with skull involvement have impaired hearing from cranial nerve compression and dysfunction. Other cranial nerves may also be compressed.

The femurs and tibiae tend to bow, producing a waddling gait. The spine is bent forward and is rigid; the chin rests on the chest. The thorax is compressed and immobile on respiration. The trunk is flexed on the legs to maintain balance; the arms are bent outward and forward and appear long in relation to the shortened trunk, giving the patient an apelike posture.

Pain and tenderness of the bones may be noted. The pain is mild to moderate, deep, and aching and increases with weight-bearing if the lower extremities are involved. Pain and discomfort may precede skeletal deformities of Paget's disease by years and are often wrongly attributed by the patient to old age or arthritis.

The temperature of the skin overlying the affected bone increases because the vascularity of the bone increases. Patients with large, highly vascular lesions may develop high-output cardiac failure because of the increased vascular bed and metabolic demands.

Assessment and Diagnostic Findings

The serum alkaline phosphatase and urinary hydroxyproline excretion are usually increased, reflecting increased osteoblastic activity. The higher these values, the more active the disease. Patients with Paget's disease have normal blood calcium levels. X-rays confirm the diagnosis of Paget's disease. Local areas of demineralization and bone overgrowth produce characteristic mosaic patterns and irregularities. Bone scans demonstrate the extent of the disease. Bone biopsy may aid in the differential diagnosis.

Medical Management

Usually, no treatment is recommended for patients who do not have symptoms. Pain usually responds to administration of NSAIDs. Weight is controlled to reduce stress on weakened bones and malaligned joints.

Fractures, arthritis, and hearing loss are complications of Paget's disease. Fractures are managed according to location. Healing occurs if fracture reduction, immobilization, and stability are adequate. Severe degenerative arthritis may require total joint replacement. Loss of hearing is managed with hearing aids and communication techniques used with the hearing-impaired person (eg, lip reading, body language).

PHARMACOLOGIC THERAPY

Patients with a moderate to severe disease may benefit from suppressive therapy. At present, there are several medications that reduce bone turnover. Calcitonin, a polypeptide hormone, retards bone resorption by decreasing the number and availability of osteoclasts. Calcitonin therapy facilitates remodeling of abnormal pagetic bone into normal lamellar bone, relieves bone pain, and helps alleviate neurologic and biochemical signs and symptoms. Calcitonin is administered subcutaneously or by nasal inhalation. Side effects include flushing of the face and nausea. The effect of calcitonin therapy is evident in 3 to 6 months.

Bisphosphates, such as etidronate disodium (Didronel) and alendronate sodium (Fosamax), produce rapid reduction in bone turnover and relief of pain. They also reduce elevated serum alkaline phosphatase and urinary hydroxyproline levels. Food inhibits absorption of these medications.

Plicamycin (Mithracin), a cytotoxic antibiotic, may be used to control the disease. This medication is reserved for severely affected patients with neurologic compromise and for those who are resistant to other therapy. This medication has dramatic effects on pain reduction and on serum calcium, alkaline phosphatase, and urinary hydroxyproline levels. It is given by intravenous infusion and requires that hepatic, renal, and bone marrow function be monitored during therapy. Clinical remissions may continue for months after the medication is discontinued.

Gerontologic Considerations

Careful assessment of the patient's pain and discomfort is necessary. Patient teaching helps the patient understand the treatment regimen and compensate for altered musculoskeletal functioning. The home environment is assessed for safety to prevent falls and to reduce the risk for fracture. Coping with a chronic health problem and its effect on quality of life needs to be assessed.

MUSCULOSKELETAL INFECTIONS

Osteomyelitis

Osteomyelitis is an infection of the bone. The bone becomes infected by one of three modes:

- Extension of soft tissue infection (eg, infected pressure or vascular ulcer, incisional infection)
- Direct bone contamination from bone surgery, open fracture, or traumatic injury, such as a gunshot wound
- Hematogenous (blood-borne) spread from other sites of infection (eg, infected tonsils, boils, infected teeth, upper respiratory infections). Osteomyelitis resulting from hematogenous spread typically occurs in a bone area of trauma or lowered resistance, possibly from subclinical (nonapparent) trauma.

Patients who are at high risk for osteomyelitis include those who are poorly nourished, elderly, or obese. Also at risk are patients with impaired immune systems, with chronic illnesses (eg, diabetes, rheumatoid arthritis), or on long-term corticosteroid therapy.

Postoperative surgical wound infections occur within 30 days after surgery. They are classified as incisional (superficial), located above the deep fascia layer, or deep, involving tissue beneath the deep fascia. When an implant has been used, deep postoperative infections may occur within a year. Deep sepsis after arthroplasty may be classified as follows:

Stage 1, acute fulminating: occurring during the first 3 months after orthopedic surgery; frequently associated with hematoma, drainage, or superficial infection

Stage 2, delayed onset: occurring between 4 and 24 months after surgery

Stage 3, late onset: generally a result of hematogenous spread; occurring 2 or more years after surgery

Bone infections are more difficult to eradicate than soft tissue infections because the infected bone becomes walled off. Natural body immune responses are blocked, and there is less penetration of antibiotics. Osteomyelitis may become chronic and affect quality of life.

Pathophysiology

Staphylococcus aureus causes 70% to 80% of bone infections. Other pathogenic organisms frequently found in osteomyelitis include *Proteus* and *Pseudomonas* species and *Escherichia coli*. The incidence of penicillin-resistant, nosocomial, gram-negative, and anaerobic infections is increasing.

The initial response to infection is inflammation, increased vascularity, and edema. After 2 or 3 days, thrombosis of the blood vessels occurs in the area, resulting in ischemia with bone necrosis. The infection extends into the medullary cavity and under the periosteum and may spread into adjacent soft tissues and joints. Unless the infective process is treated promptly, a bone abscess forms. The resulting abscess cavity contains dead bone tissue (the **sequestrum**), which does not easily liquefy and drain. Therefore, the cavity cannot collapse and heal, as occurs in soft tissue abscesses. New bone growth (the **involucrum**) forms and surrounds the sequestrum. Although healing appears to take place, a chronically infected sequestrum remains and produces recurring abscesses throughout the patient's life. This is referred to as chronic osteomyelitis.

Clinical Manifestations

When the infection is carried by the blood, the onset is usually sudden, occurring often with the clinical manifestations of septicemia (eg, chills, high fever, rapid pulse, and general malaise). The systemic symptoms at first may overshadow the local signs. As the infection extends through the cortex of the bone, it involves the periosteum and the soft tissues. The infected area becomes painful, swollen, and extremely tender. The patient may describe a constant, pulsating pain that intensifies with movement as a result of the pressure of the collecting pus.

When osteomyelitis occurs from spread of adjacent infection or direct contamination, there are no symptoms of septicemia. The area is swollen, warm, painful, and tender to touch.

The patient with chronic osteomyelitis presents with a continuously draining sinus or experiences recurrent periods of pain, inflammation, swelling, and drainage. The low-grade infection thrives in scar tissue with its reduced blood supply.

Assessment and Diagnostic Findings

In acute osteomyelitis, early x-rays demonstrate soft tissue swelling. In about 2 weeks, areas of irregular decalcification, bone necrosis, periosteal elevation, and new bone formation are evident. Bone scans and magnetic resonance imaging (MRI) help with early definitive diagnosis. Blood studies reveal elevated leukocytes and an elevated sedimentation rate. Wound and blood cultures are obtained to identify appropriate antibiotic therapy.

With chronic osteomyelitis, large, irregular cavities, raised periosteum, sequestra, or dense bone formations are seen on x-rays. Bone scans may be performed to identify areas of infection. The sedimentation rate and white blood cell count are usually normal. Anemia, associated with chronic infection, may be evident. The abscess is cultured to determine the infective organism and appropriate antibiotic therapy.

Prevention

Prevention of osteomyelitis is the goal. Treatment of focal infections diminishes hematogenous spread. Elective orthopedic surgery should be postponed when a patient has a current infection (eg, urinary tract infection, sore throat) or a history of a recent infection. Prophylactic antibiotics are frequently recommended for patients who have had joint replacement surgery when they undergo dental procedures or other invasive procedures (eg, cystoscopy).

During orthopedic surgery, careful attention is paid to the surgical environment and technique to decrease direct bone contamination. Prophylactic antibiotics, administered to achieve adequate tissue levels at the time of surgery and for 24 to 48 hours after surgery, are helpful. Urinary catheters and drains are removed as soon as possible to decrease the incidence of hematogenous spread of infection.

Aseptic postoperative wound care reduces the incidence of superficial infections and osteomyelitis. Prompt management of soft tissue infections reduces extension of infection to the bone.

Medical Management

The affected area is immobilized to decrease discomfort and to prevent pathologic fracture of the weakened bone. Warm wet soaks for 20 minutes several times a day may be prescribed to increase circulation. The initial goal of therapy is to control and halt the infective process. Antibiotic therapy depends on the results of blood and wound cultures. Frequently, the infection is caused by more than one pathogen.

PHARMACOLOGIC THERAPY

As soon as the culture specimens are obtained, intravenous antibiotic therapy is begun, assuming that infection results from a staphylococcal infection that is sensitive to a semisynthetic penicillin or cephalosporin. The aim is to control the infection before the blood supply to the area diminishes as a result of thrombosis. Around-the-clock dosage is necessary to achieve a sustained high therapeutic blood level of the antibiotic. An antibiotic to which the causative organism is sensitive is prescribed when the culture and sensitivity reports are known. Intravenous antibiotic therapy is continued for 3 to 6 weeks. When the infection appears to be controlled, the antibiotic may be administered orally and continued for up to 3 months. To enhance absorption of the orally administered medication, antibiotics should not be administered with food.

SURGICAL MANAGEMENT

If the patient does not respond to antibiotic therapy, the infected bone is surgically exposed, the purulent and necrotic material removed, and the area irrigated directly with sterile saline solution. Antibiotic-impregnated beads may be placed in the wound for direct application of antibiotics for 2 to 4 weeks. Intravenous antibiotic therapy is continued.

In chronic osteomyelitis, antibiotics are adjunctive therapy to surgical débridement. A sequestrectomy (removal of enough involucrum to enable the surgeon to remove the sequestrum) is performed. Often, sufficient bone is removed to convert a deep cavity into a shallow saucer (saucerization). All dead, infected bone and cartilage must be removed before permanent healing occurs. A closed suction irrigation system may be used to remove debris. Wound irrigation using sterile physiologic saline solution may be performed for 7 to 8 days.

The wound is either closed tightly, to obliterate the dead space, or packed, to be closed later by granulation or possibly by grafting. The débrided cavity may be packed with cancellous bone graft to stimulate healing. With a large defect, the cavity may be filled with a vascularized bone transfer or muscle flap (in which a muscle is moved from an adjacent area with blood supply intact). These microsurgery techniques enhance the blood supply. The improved blood supply facilitates bone healing and eradication of the infection. These surgical procedures may be staged over time to ensure healing. Surgical débridement weakens the bone. Internal fixation or external supportive devices may be needed to stabilize or support the bone to prevent pathologic fracture.

NURSING PROCESS: THE PATIENT WITH OSTEOMYELITIS

Assessment

The patient reports an acute onset of signs and symptoms (eg, localized pain, swelling, erythema, fever) or recurrent draining of an infected sinus with associated pain, swelling, and low-grade fever. The nurse assesses the patient for risk factors (eg, older age, diabetes, or long-term corticosteroid therapy) and for history of previous injury, infection, or orthopedic surgery. The patient avoids pressure on the area and guards movement. In acute hematogenous osteomyelitis, the patient exhibits generalized weakness due to the systemic reaction to the infection.

Physical examination reveals an inflamed, markedly swollen, warm area that is tender. Purulent drainage may be noted. The patient has an elevated temperature. With chronic osteomyelitis, the temperature elevation may be minimal, occurring in the afternoon or evening.

Nursing Diagnosis

Based on the nursing assessment data, nursing diagnoses for the patient with osteomyelitis may include the following:

- Pain related to inflammation and swelling
- Impaired physical mobility related to pain, use of immobilization devices, and weight-bearing limitations
- Risk for extension of infection: bone abscess formation
- Knowledge deficit related to the treatment regimen

Planning and Goals

The goals of the patient may include relief of pain, improved physical mobility within therapeutic limitations, control and eradication of infection, and knowledge of treatment regimen.

Nursing Interventions

Relieving Pain

The affected part may be immobilized with a splint to decrease pain and muscle spasm. The joints above and below the affected part should be gently placed through the range of motion. The wounds are frequently very painful and must be handled with great care and gentleness. Elevation reduces swelling and associated discomfort. The nurse monitors neurovascular status of the affected extremity. Pain is controlled with prescribed analgesics and other pain-reducing techniques.

Improving Physical Mobility

Treatment regimens restrict activity. The bone is weakened by the infective process and must be protected by immobilization devices and avoidance of stress on the bone. The patient must understand the rationale for the activity restrictions. The nurse encourages full participation in ADLs within the physical limitations to promote general well-being.

Controlling the Infectious Process

The nurse monitors the patient's response to antibiotic therapy and observes the intravenous site for evidence of phlebitis or infiltration. With long-term, intensive antibiotic therapy, the nurse monitors the patient for signs of superinfection (eg, oral or vaginal candidiasis, loose or foul-smelling stools).

If surgery was necessary, the nurse takes measures to ensure adequate circulation (wound suction to prevent fluid accumulation, elevation of the area to promote venous drainage, avoidance of pressure on grafted area), to maintain needed immobility, and to comply with weight-bearing restrictions. The nurse changes dressings using aseptic technique to promote healing and to prevent cross-contamination.

The nurse monitors the general health and nutrition of the patient. A balanced diet high in protein and vitamin C ensures a positive nitrogen balance and promotes healing. The nurse encourages adequate hydration as well.

Promoting Home and Community-Based Care

TEACHING PATIENTS SELF-CARE

It is important that the patient and family understand the importance of strict adherence to the therapeutic regimen of antibiotics and of prevention of falls or other injuries that could result in bone fracture. The patient needs to know how to maintain and manage the intravenous access and intravenous administration equipment. Medication education includes drug name, dosage, frequency, administration rate, safe storage and handling, adverse reactions, and necessary laboratory monitoring. In addition, aseptic dressing changes and warm compress techniques are taught.

The nurse carefully monitors the patient for development of additional painful areas or sudden increases in temperature. The nurse instructs the patient to observe and report elevated temperature, drainage, odor, increased inflammation, adverse reactions, and signs of superinfection.

CONTINUING CARE

Management of osteomyelitis, including wound care and intravenous antibiotic therapy, may be performed at home. The patient must be medically stable, physically capable, and motivated to adhere strictly to the therapeutic regimen of antibiotic therapy. The home care environment needs to be conducive to promotion of health and to the requirements of the therapeutic regimen.

If warranted, the nurse completes a home assessment to determine the patient's and family's abilities regarding continuation of the therapeutic regimen. If the patient's support system is questionable or if the patient lives alone, a home care nurse may be needed to assist with administration of the antibiotics. The nurse monitors the patient for response to the treatment, signs and symptoms of superinfections, and adverse drug reactions. The nurse stresses the importance of follow-up health care appointments.

Evaluation

Expected Outcomes

Expected outcomes may include:

1. Experiences pain relief
   a. Reports decreased pain
   b. Experiences no tenderness at site of previous infection
   c. Experiences no discomfort with movement

HOME CARE TEACHING CHECKLIST: OSTEOMYELITIS

At the completion of the program, the patient or caregiver will be able to:

	Patient	Caregiver
• Describe osteomyelitis	✔	✔
• Control pain with pharmacologic and nonpharmacologic interventions	✔	
• State weight-bearing and activity restrictions	✔	
• Demonstrate safe use of ambulatory aids and assistive devices	✔	
• Describe use of prescribed medications	✔	
• Comply with antibiotic regimen	✔	
• Promote healing through aseptic dressing changes	✔	
• Demonstrate proper wound care	✔	
• Report signs and symptoms of continuing infection or superinfection	✔	

2. Increases physical mobility
   a. Participates in self-care activities
   b. Maintains full function of unimpaired extremities
   c. Demonstrates safe use of immobilizing device and assistive device
3. Shows absence of infection
   a. Takes antibiotic as prescribed
   b. Reports normal temperature
   c. Shows absence of swelling
   d. Reports absence of drainage
   e. Laboratory results indicate normal white blood cell count and sedimentation rate
   f. Wound cultures are negative
4. Complies with therapeutic plan
   a. Takes medications as prescribed
   b. Protects weakened bones
   c. Demonstrates proper wound care
   d. Reports problems promptly
   e. Eats a balanced diet that is high in protein and vitamin C
   f. Keeps follow-up health appointments
   g. Reports increased strength
   h. Reports no elevation of temperature or recurrence of pain, swelling, or other symptoms at the site

Septic (Infectious) Arthritis

Joints can become infected by spread of infection from other parts of the body (hematogenous spread) or directly by trauma or surgical instrumentation. Previous trauma to joints, coexisting arthritis, and diminished host resistance contribute to the development of an infected joint. Gonococci and staphylococci cause most adult joint infections. Prompt recognition and treatment of an infected joint are important because accumulating pus results in chondrolysis (destruction of hyaline cartilage), which heals poorly.

Clinical Manifestations

The patient with acute septic arthritis usually presents with a warm, painful, swollen joint with decreased range of motion. Systemic chills, fever, and leukocytosis are present. Elderly patients and patients taking corticosteroids or immunosuppressive medications may not exhibit typical clinical manifestations of infection.

Assessment and Diagnostic Findings

Assessment for the source of infection is performed. Diagnostic studies include aspiration, examination, and culture of the synovial fluid. Computed tomography and MRI may disclose damage to the joint lining. Radioisotope scanning may be useful in localizing the process.

Management

Prompt treatment is essential. Intravenous antibiotics, such as nafcillin, cefoperazone, and gentamicin, are started promptly. Penicillin G is used for gonococcal septic arthritis. The intravenous antibiotics are continued until symptoms disappear. The synovial fluid is monitored for sterility and decrease in white blood cells.

In addition to prescribing antibiotics, the physician may aspirate the joint with a needle to remove excessive joint fluid, exudate, and debris. This promotes comfort and decreases joint destruction due to the action of the proteolytic enzymes in the purulent fluid. Occasionally, arthrotomy or arthroscopy is used to drain the joint and remove dead tissue.

The inflamed joint is supported and immobilized in a functional position by a splint that increases the patient's comfort. Analgesics, such as codeine, may be prescribed to control pain. After the infection has responded to antibiotic therapy, NSAIDs may be prescribed. The patient's nutrition and fluid status is monitored. Progressive range-of-motion exercises are prescribed when the infection subsides.

If septic joints are treated promptly, recovery of normal function should occur. The patient is assessed periodically for recurrence. If the articular cartilage was damaged during the inflammatory reaction, joint fibrosis and diminished function may result.

The nurse describes the septic arthritis process to the patient and teaches the patient how to control pain using pharmacologic and nonpharmacologic interventions. The nurse also explains the importance of supporting the affected joint, adhering to the prescribed antibiotic regimen, and observing weight-bearing and activity restrictions. Additionally, the nurse demonstrates and encourages the patient to practice safe use of ambulatory aids and assistive devices.

The nurse teaches the patient how to promote healing through aseptic dressing changes and proper wound care. The patient is then encouraged to perform range-of-motion exercises when the infection subsides.

BONE TUMORS

Neoplasms of the musculoskeletal system are of various types, including osteogenic, chondrogenic, fibrogenic, muscle (rhabdomyogenic), and marrow (reticulum) cell tumors as well as nerve, vascular, and fatty cell tumors. They may be primary tumors or metastatic tumors from primary cancers elsewhere in the body (eg, breast, lung, prostate, kidney). Metastatic bone tumors are more common than primary bone tumors.

Benign Bone Tumors

Benign tumors of the bone and soft tissue are more common than malignant primary bone tumors. Benign bone tumors generally are slow growing and well circumscribed, present few symptoms, and are not a cause of death. Benign primary neoplasms of the musculoskeletal system include osteochondroma, enchondroma, bone cyst (eg, aneurysmal bone cyst), osteoid osteoma, rhabdomyoma, and fibroma. Some benign tumors, such as giant cell tumors, have the potential of undergoing malignant transformation.

Osteochondroma is the most common benign bone tumor, usually occurring as a large projection of bone at the end of long bones (at the knee or shoulder). It develops during growth and then becomes a static bony mass. The cartilage cap of the osteochondroma may undergo malignant transformation after trauma, and a chondrosarcoma may develop.

Enchondroma is a common tumor of the hyaline cartilage that develops in the hand, ribs, femur, tibia, humerus, or pelvis. Generally, the only symptom is a mild ache. Pathologic fractures may occur.

Bone cysts are expanding lesions within the bone. *Aneurysmal bone cysts* are seen in young adults and present with a painful, palpable mass of the long bones, vertebrae, or flat bone. *Unicameral bone cysts* occur in children and cause mild discomfort and possible pathologic fractures of the upper humerus and femur, which may heal spontaneously.

A painful tumor that occurs in children and young adults is the osteoid osteoma. The neoplastic tissue is surrounded by reactive bone formation that assists in its radiologic identification.

Giant cell tumors (osteoclastoma) are benign for long periods but may invade local tissue and cause destruction. They occur in young adults and are soft and hemorrhagic. Eventually, giant cell tumors may undergo malignant transformation and metastasize.

Malignant Bone Tumors

Primary malignant musculoskeletal tumors are relatively rare and arise from connective and supportive tissue cells (sarcomas) or bone marrow elements (myelomas). Malignant primary musculoskeletal tumors include osteosarcoma, chondrosarcoma, Ewing's sarcoma, and fibrosarcoma. Soft tissue sarcomas include liposarcoma, fibrosarcoma of soft tissue, and rhabdomyosarcoma. Bone tumor metastasis to the lungs is common.

Osteogenic sarcoma (osteosarcoma) is the most common and most often fatal primary malignant bone tumor. The tumor carries a high mortality rate because the sarcoma often has spread to the lungs by the time the patient seeks health care. Osteogenic sarcoma appears most frequently in males between the ages of 10 and 25 years (in bones that grow rapidly), in older people with Paget's disease, and as a result of radiation exposure. It is manifested by pain, swelling, limitation of motion, and weight loss (which is considered an ominous finding). The bony mass may be palpable, tender, and fixed, with an increase in skin temperature over the mass and venous distention. The primary lesion may involve any bone, but the most common sites are the distal femur, the proximal tibia, and the proximal humerus.

Malignant tumors of the hyaline cartilage are called chondrosarcomas. These tumors are the second most common primary malignant bone tumor. They are large, bulky, slow-growing tumors that affect adults (men more frequently than women). The usual tumor sites include the pelvis, ribs, femur, humerus, spine, scapula, and tibia. Metastasis to the lungs occurs in fewer than half of patients. When these tumors are well differentiated, large bloc excision or amputation of the affected extremity results in increased survival rates. These tumors may recur.

Metastatic Disease to the Bone

Metastatic bone disease (secondary bone tumor) is more common than any primary bone tumor. Tumors arising from tissues elsewhere in the body may invade the bone and produce localized bone destruction (lytic lesions) or bone overgrowth (blastic lesions). The most common primary sites of tumors that metastasize to bone include the kidney, prostate, lung, breast, ovary, and thyroid. Metastatic tumors most frequently attack the skull, spine, pelvis, femur, and humerus and involve more than one bone (polyostatic).

Pathophysiology

A tumor in the bone causes the normal bone tissue to react by osteolytic response (bone destruction) or osteoblastic response (bone formation). Primary tumors cause bone destruction, which weakens the bone, resulting in bone fractures. Adjacent normal bone responds to the tumor by altering its normal pattern of remodeling. The bone's surface changes, and the contours enlarge in the tumor area.

Malignant bone tumors invade and destroy adjacent bone tissue. Benign bone tumors, in contrast to malignant ones, have a symmetric controlled growth pattern and place pressure on adjacent bone tissue. This weakens the structure of the bone until it can no longer withstand the stress of ordinary use. Pathologic fracture commonly results.

Clinical Manifestations

Patients with bone tumor may have a wide range of associated problems. They may be symptom free or have pain (mild and occasional to constant and severe), varying degrees of disability, and, at times, obvious bone growth. Weight loss, malaise, and fever may be present. The tumor may be diagnosed only after pathologic fracture has occurred.

With spinal metastasis, spinal cord compression may occur. It can progress rapidly or slowly. Neurologic deficits (eg, progressive pain, weakness, gait abnormality, paresthesia, paraplegia, urinary retention, loss of bowel or bladder control) must be identified early and treated with decompressive laminectomy to prevent permanent spinal cord injury.

Assessment and Diagnostic Findings

The differential diagnosis is based on the history, physical examination, and diagnostic studies, including computed tomography, bone scans, myelograms, arteriography, MRI, biopsy, and biochemical assays of the blood and urine. Serum alkaline phosphatase levels are frequently elevated with osteogenic sarcoma. With metastatic carcinoma of the prostate, serum acid phosphatase levels are elevated. Hypercalcemia is present with breast, lung, and kidney cancer bone metastasis. Symptoms of hypercalcemia include muscle weakness, fatigue, anorexia, nausea, vomiting, polyuria, cardiac dysrhythmias, seizures, and coma. Hypercalcemia must be identified and treated promptly. Surgical biopsy is performed for histologic identification. Extreme care is taken during biopsy to prevent seeding and resultant recurrence after excision of the tumor.

Chest x-rays are performed to determine the presence of lung metastasis. Surgical staging of musculoskeletal tumors is based on tumor grade and site (intracompartmental or extracompartmental) as well as on metastasis. Staging is used for planning treatment.

During the diagnostic period, the nurse explains the diagnostic tests and provides psychological and emotional support to the patient and family. The nurse assesses coping behaviors and encourages use of support systems.

Medical Management

PRIMARY BONE TUMORS

The goal of primary bone tumor treatment is to destroy or remove the tumor. This may be accomplished by surgical excision (ranging from local excision to amputation and disarticulation), radiation therapy when the tumor is radiosensitive, and chemotherapy (preoperative, postoperative, and adjunctive for possible micrometastasis). Major gains are being made in using wide bloc excision with restorative grafting technique. Survival and quality of life are important considerations in procedures that attempt to save the involved extremity.

Limb-sparing (salvage) procedures remove the tumor and adjacent tissue. The resected portion is replaced by a customized prosthesis, total joint arthroplasty, or bone tissue from the patient (autograft) or a cadaver donor (allograft). Soft tissue and blood vessels may need grafting because of the extent of the excision. Complications may include infection, loosening or dislocation of the prosthesis, allograft nonunion, fracture, devitalization of the skin and soft tissues, joint fibrosis, and recurrence of the tumor. Function and rehabilitation after limb salvage depend on reducing the risk for complications and positive encouragement.

Surgical removal of the tumor may require amputation of the affected extremity, with the amputation extending well above the tumor to achieve local control of the primary lesion. (See Nursing Process: The Patient Undergoing an Amputation in Chap. 28.)

Because of the danger of metastasis with malignant bone tumors, combined chemotherapy is started before and continued after surgery in an effort to eradicate micrometastatic lesions. The goal of combined chemotherapy is greater therapeutic effect at a lower toxicity rate with reduced resistance to the medications. There is an improved long-term survival rate when a localized osteosarcoma is removed and chemotherapy is initiated. Soft tissue sarcomas are treated with radiation, limb-sparing excision, and adjuvant chemotherapy.

METASTATIC DISEASE TO THE BONE

The treatment of metastatic bone cancer is palliative. The therapeutic goal is to relieve the patient's pain and discomfort while promoting quality of life.

If metastatic disease weakens the bone, structural support and stabilization are needed to prevent pathologic fracture. At times, large bones with metastatic lesions are strengthened by prophylactic internal fixation. Internal fixation of pathologic fractures, arthroplasty, or methylmethacrylate (bone cement) reconstruction minimizes associated disability and pain. Patients with metastatic disease are at higher risk for pulmonary congestion, hypoxemia, deep vein thrombosis, and hemorrhage than are other orthopedic surgery patients.

If hypercalcemia results from breakdown of bone, treatment includes hydration with intravenous administration of normal saline solution, diuresis, mobilization, and medications such as biphosphates, mithramycin, and calcitonin. Hematopoiesis is frequently disrupted by tumor invasion of the bone marrow or treatment (chemotherapy or radiation). Blood product transfusions restore hematologic factors.

Pain can be due to multiple factors, including the osseous metastasis, surgery, chemotherapy or radiation side effects, or arthritis. Pain must be assessed accurately and managed with adequate, appropriate opioid, non-opioid, and nonpharmaceutical interventions. (See Chap. 12 for more information about pain management.)

Additional therapies are consistent with methods used to treat the original cancer. Radiation and hormonal therapy may be effective in reducing pain as well as in promoting healing of osteolytic lesions. Chemotherapy is used to control the primary disease.

NURSING PROCESS: THE PATIENT WITH A BONE TUMOR

Assessment

The nurse asks the patient about the onset and course of symptoms. During the interview, the nurse notes the patient's understanding of the disease process, how the patient and the family have been coping, and how the patient has managed the pain. On physical examination, the nurse gently palpates the mass and notes its size and associated soft tissue swelling, pain, and tenderness. Assessment of the neurovascular status and range of motion of the extremity provides baseline data for future comparisons. The nurse evaluates the patient's mobility and ability to perform ADLs.

Diagnosis

Nursing Diagnoses

Based on the nursing assessment data, the major nursing diagnoses for the patient with a bone tumor may include the following:

- Knowledge deficit related to the disease process and the therapeutic regimen
- Pain related to pathologic process and surgery
- Risk for injury: pathologic fracture related to tumor
- Ineffective coping related to fear of the unknown, perception of disease process, and inadequate support system
- Disturbance in self-esteem related to loss of body part or alteration in role performance

Collaborative Problems/Potential Complications

Potential complications may include the following:

- Delayed wound healing
- Nutritional deficiency
- Infection

Planning and Goals

The major goals of the patient include knowledge of the disease process and treatment regimen, control of pain, absence of pathologic fractures, effective patterns of coping, improved self-esteem, and absence of complications.

Nursing Interventions

The nursing care of a patient who has undergone excision of a bone tumor is similar in many respects to that of other patients who have had skeletal surgery. Vital signs are monitored; blood loss is assessed; and observations are made to assess for the development of complications, such as deep vein thrombosis, pulmonary emboli, infection, contracture, and disuse atrophy. The affected part should be elevated to control swelling and to assess the neurovascular status of the extremity.

Promoting Understanding of the Disease Process and Treatment Regimen

Patient and family teaching about the disease process and diagnostic and management regimens is essential. Explanation of diagnostic tests, treatments (eg, wound care), and expected results (eg, decreased range of motion, numbness, change of body contours) helps the patient deal with the procedures and changes. Cooperation and adherence to the therapeutic regimen are enhanced through understanding. The nurse can most effectively reinforce and clarify information provided by the physician by being present during these physician–patient discussions.

Relieving Pain

Accurate pain assessment is the foundation for pain management. Pharmacologic and nonpharmacologic pain management techniques are used to relieve pain and increase the patient's comfort level. The nurse works with the patient in designing the most effective pain management regimen, thereby increasing the patient's control over the pain. The nurse prepares the patient and gives support during painful procedures. Prescribed intravenous or epidural analgesics are used during the early postoperative period. Later, oral or transdermal opioid or nonopioid analgesics are usually adequate to relieve pain.

Preventing Pathologic Fracture

Bone tumors weaken the bone to a point at which normal activities or even position changes can result in fracture. During nursing care, the affected bones must be supported and handled gently. External supports (eg, splints) may be used for additional protection. Prescribed weight-bearing restrictions must be followed. The nurse teaches the patient how to use assistive devices safely and how to strengthen unaffected extremities.

Promoting Coping Skills

The nurse encourages the patient and family to verbalize their fears, concerns, and feelings. They need to be supported as they deal with the impact of the malignant bone tumor. Feelings of shock, despair, and grief are expected. Referral to a psychiatric nurse liaison, psychologist, counselor, or clergy may be indicated for specific psychological help.

Promoting Self-Esteem

Independence versus dependence is an issue for the patient who has a malignancy. Lifestyle is dramatically changed, at least temporarily. It is important to support the family in working through the adjustments that must be made. The nurse assists the patient in dealing with changes in body image due to surgery and possible amputation. It is helpful to provide realistic reassurance about the future and resumption of role-related activities and to encourage self-care and socialization. The patient participates in planning daily activities. The nurse encourages the patient to be as independent as possible. Involvement of the patient and family throughout treatment encourages confidence, restoration of self-concept, and a sense of being in control of one's life.

Monitoring and Managing Potential Complications

DELAYED WOUND HEALING

Wound healing may be delayed because of tissue trauma from surgery, previous radiation therapy, inadequate nutrition, or infection. The nurse minimizes pressure on the wound site to promote circulation to the tissues. An aseptic, nontraumatic wound dressing promotes healing. Monitoring and reporting of laboratory findings facilitate prescription of interventions to promote homeostasis and wound healing.

Repositioning the patient at frequent intervals reduces the incidence of skin breakdown due to pressure. Special therapeutic beds may be needed to prevent skin breakdown and to promote wound healing after extensive surgical reconstruction and skin grafting.

INADEQUATE NUTRITION

Because loss of appetite, nausea, and vomiting are frequent side effects of chemotherapy and radiation therapy, it is necessary to provide adequate nutrition for healing and health promotion. Antiemetics and relaxation techniques reduce the gastrointestinal reaction. Stomatitis is controlled with anesthetic or antifungal mouthwash. Adequate hydration is essential. Nutritional supplements or total parenteral nutrition may be prescribed to achieve adequate nutrition.

OSTEOMYELITIS AND WOUND INFECTIONS

Prophylactic antibiotics and strict aseptic dressing techniques are used to diminish the occurrence of osteomyelitis and wound infections. During healing, other infections (eg, upper respiratory infections) need to be avoided so that hematogenous spread does not result in osteomyelitis. If the patient is receiving chemotherapy, it is important to monitor the white blood cell count and to instruct the patient to avoid contact with people who have colds and infections.

Promoting Home and Community-Based Care

TEACHING PATIENTS SELF-CARE

Preparation for and coordination of continuing health care are begun early as a multidisciplinary effort. Patient teaching is directed at medication, dressing, treatment regimens, and the importance of physical and occupational therapy programs. The nurse teaches weight-bearing limitations and special handling to prevent pathologic fractures. It is important that the patient and family know the signs and symptoms of possible complications as well as resources available for continuing care.

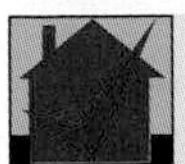

Home Care Teaching Checklist: Bone Tumor

At the completion of the program, the patient or caregiver will be able to:	Patient	Caregiver
• Describe tumor process	✔	✔
• Control pain with pharmacologic and nonpharmacologic interventions	✔	✔
• Support affected musculoskeletal area	✔	
• Describe use of prescribed medications	✔	
• Comply with medication regimen	✔	
• Consume balanced diet to promote healing and health	✔	
• State weight-bearing and activity restrictions	✔	
• Demonstrate safe use of ambulatory aids and assistive devices	✔	✔
• Protect affected bone from pathologic fracture	✔	✔
• Identify complications of tumor and therapy	✔	✔
• Report signs and symptoms of complications promptly	✔	
• Use effective coping strategies	✔	
• Maintain role performance	✔	

CONTINUING CARE

Frequently, arrangements are made with a home health care agency for home care supervision and follow-up. The home care nurse assesses the patient's and family's abilities to meet the patient's needs and determines if the services of other agencies are appropriate. The nurse advises the patient to have readily available the telephone numbers of people to contact in case problems arise.

The nurse emphasizes the need for long-term health supervision to ensure cure or to detect tumor recurrence or metastasis. If the patient has metastatic disease, end-of-life issues may need to be explored. Referral for hospice care is made when appropriate.

Evaluation

Expected Outcomes

Expected outcomes may include:

1. Describes disease process and treatment regimen
   a. Describes pathologic problem
   b. States goals of the therapeutic regimen
   c. Seeks clarification of information
2. Achieves control of pain
   a. Uses multiple pain control techniques, including prescribed medications
   b. Experiences no pain or decreased pain at rest, during ADLs, or at surgical sites
3. Experiences no pathologic fracture
   a. Avoids stress to weakened bones
   b. Uses assistive devices safely
   c. Strengthens uninvolved extremities
4. Demonstrates effective coping patterns
   a. Verbalizes feelings
   b. Identifies strengths and abilities
   c. Makes decisions
   d. Requests assistance as needed
5. Demonstrates positive self-concept
   a. Identifies home and family responsibilities that can be accomplished
   b. Exhibits confidence in own abilities
   c. Demonstrates acceptance of altered body image
   d. Demonstrates independence in ADLs
6. Exhibits absence of complications
   a. Demonstrates wound healing
   b. Experiences no skin breakdown
   c. Maintains or increases body weight
   d. Experiences no infections
   e. Manages side effects of therapies
   f. Reports symptoms of drug toxicity or complications of surgery
7. Participates in continuing health care at home
   a. Complies with prescribed regimen (ie, takes prescribed medications, continues physical and occupational therapy programs)
   b. Acknowledges need for long-term health supervision
   c. Keeps follow-up health care appointments
   d. Reports occurrence of symptoms or complications

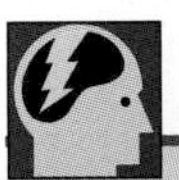

Critical Thinking Exercises

1. A classmate who has a small child states that she has been having low back pain for several months. She asks for your advice. Describe how you would assess this situation, indicate the questions you would ask, and explain the kind of information you are seeking and why. How would your thinking redirect your assessment if the woman (1) is overweight, (2) jogs regularly, and (3) is expecting another child?

2. You volunteer to help with a health fair in your community. You are asked to participate in the booth that will offer information about osteoporosis. How would your advice differ when you are talking to (1) teenagers, (2) young adults, and (3) elderly people? Explain the reasons for your modifications.

3. You are visiting with a patient in an extended-care facility. The patient's daughter states that her mother has osteoarthritis and her aunt has osteoporosis. She asks if these conditions are the same because her mother and aunt developed them late in life and both are debilitated. What explanations do you feel would be helpful to her? How would the care of people with these two disorders differ? How would the care be similar?

References and Selected Readings

BOOKS

Bigos, S., et al. (1994). *Acute low back problems in adults.* Clinical Practice Guidelines. Quick Reference Guide Number 14, AHPR Pub. No. 95-0643. Rockville MD, USHHS, PHS, AHCPR, December 1994.

Bucholz, R. (1996). *Orthopaedic decision making* (2nd ed.). St. Louis: C. V. Mosby.

Carpenito, L. J. (1997). *Nursing diagnosis: Application to clinical practice* (7th ed.). Philadelphia: J. B. Lippincott.

Epps, C. H. (Ed.) (1994). *Complications in orthopaedic surgery* (3rd ed.). Philadelphia: J. B. Lippincott.

Maher, A. B., et al. (1998). *Orthopaedic nursing* (2nd ed.). Philadelphia: W. B. Saunders.

Mercier, L. R. (1995). *Practical orthopedics* (4th ed.). St. Louis: Mosby–Year Book.

Mourad, L. (1995). *Orthopaedic nursing.* Albany, NY: Delmar.

National Osteoporosis Foundation. (1997). *1996 and 2015 osteoporosis prevalence figures. Stated by state prevalence report.* Washington, DC: National Osteoporosis Foundation.

National Osteoporosis Foundation. (1998). *Fast facts on osteoporosis.* Washington, DC: National Osteoporosis Foundation.

Porth, C. M. (1998). *Pathophysiology: Concepts of altered health states* (5th ed.). Philadelphia: Lippincott-Raven.

Salmond, S. W., et al. (Eds.). (1996). *Core curriculum for orthopaedic nursing* (3rd ed.). Pitman, NJ: National Association of Orthopaedic Nurses.

JOURNALS

Asterisks indicate research articles.

Agency for Health Care Policy and Research. (1995). Acute low back problems in adults: Assessment and treatment. *Orthopaedic Nursing, 14*(5), 37–52.

*Alman, B., et al. (1995). Massive allografts in the treatment of osteosarcoma and Ewing sarcoma in children and adolescents. *Journal of Bone and Joint Surgery, 77*(1), 54–64.

Anonymous. (1996). Fosamax approved by FDA for treatment of osteoporosis. *Orthopaedic Nursing, 15*(1), 93.

Anonymous. (1996). New treatment option for osteoporosis. *American Journal of Nursing, 96*(2), 53–54.

Berg, E. (1997). Calcific tendinitis of the shoulder. *Orthopaedic Nursing, 16*(6), 68–69.

Blue, C. (1996). Preventing back injury among nurses. *Orthopaedic Nursing, 15*(6), 9–20.

Dealy, M., et al. (1995). Care of the adolescent undergoing an allograft procedure. *Cancer Nursing, 18*(2), 130–137.

Doheny, M., et al. (1995). Reducing orthopaedic hazards of the computer work environment. *Orthopaedic Nursing, 14*(1), 7–15.

Dowd, R., & Cavalieri, R. J. (1999). Help your patient live with osteoporosis. *American Journal of Nursing, 99*(4), 55–56.

Genant, H., et al. (1997). Osteoporosis: A treatment approach to long-term care patients. *Nursing Home Medicine, 5*(Suppl. G), 1G–24G.

*Gold, D. (1996). Paget's disease of the bone and quality of life. *Journal of Bone and Mineral Research, 11*(12), 1897–1903.

Gorski, L. A. (1997). From hospital to home care: Discharge planning for the patient requiring home intravenous antimicrobial therapy. *Orthopaedic Nursing, 16*(3), 43–48.

Gray, M. A. (1995). Local application of antibiotics in orthopaedic infections. *Orthopaedic Nursing, 14*(5), 69–70.

Hooker, R. (1998). Management of established osteoporosis. *Lippincott's Primary Care Practice, 2*(1), 32–37.

*Hunt, A. (1996). The relationship between height change and bone mineral density. *Orthopaedic Nursing, 15*(3), 57–66.

Jones, A. (1997). Primary care of acute low back pain. *Nurse Practitioner, 22*(7), 50–52, 61–63, 66, 68.

Kessenich, C. (1997). Obtaining a diagnosis of postmenopausal osteoporosis. *Lippincott's Primary Care Practice, 1*(5), 474–484.

Kessenich, C. (1996). Update on pharmacologic therapies for osteoporosis. *Nurse Practitioner, 21*(8), 19–24.

*Kessenich, C., & Rosen, C. (1996). Vitamin D and bone status in elderly women. *Orthopaedic Nursing, 15*(3), 67–71.

Linsey, R. (1996). The menopause and osteoporosis. *Obstetrics and Gynecology, 87*(Suppl. 27), 16S–19S.

Long, J. (1996). Shoulder arthroscopy. *Orthopaedic Nursing, 15*(2), 21–31.

*Mankin, H., et al. (1996). Long-term results of allograft replacement in the management of bone tumors. *Clinical Orthopaedics, 324*, 86–97.

McDonald, D. (1994). Limb-salvage surgery for treatment of sarcomas of the extremities. *American Journal of Roentgenology, 163*(3), 509–516.

McGee, C. (1997). Secondary amenorrhea leading to osteoporosis: Incidence and prevention. *Nurse Practitioner, 22*(5), 38–64.

*Neal, C. (1997). The assessment of knowledge and application of proper body mechanics in the workplace. *Orthopaedic Nursing, 16*(1), 66–69.

Patel, P., & Lauerman, W. (1997). The use of magnetic resonance imaging in the diagnosis of lumbar disc disease. *Orthopaedic Nursing, 16*(1), 59–65.

Piasecki, P. (1996). Nursing care of the patient with metastatic bone disease. *Orthopaedic Nursing, 15*(4), 25–33.

Scharbo-Dehann, M. (1996). Hormone replacement therapy. *Nurse Practitioner, 21*(Suppl. 12), 1–13.

Sedlak, C. A., Doheny, M. O., & Jones, J. L. (1998). Osteoporosis prevention in young women. *Orthopaedic Nursing, 17*(3), 53–60.

*Silverman, S. L., et al. (1997). Effect of bone density information of decisions about hormone replacement therapy: A randomized trial. *Obstetrics and Gynecology, 89*(3), 321–325.

Sipos, D. (1995). Carpal tunnel syndrome. *Orthopaedic Nursing, 14*(1), 17–21.

Smith, C., et al. (1995). Telephone triage of upper extremity problems. *Orthopaedic Nursing, 14*(6), 31–36.

Steffen, K. A., & Carnes, M. (1999). Hormone replacement therapy in the aging women. Part II: HRT and osteoporosis. *Annals of Long-Term Care, 7*(7), 277–281.

Thomas, T. (1997). Lifestyle risk factors for osteoporosis. *MedSurg Nursing, 6*(5), 275–277, 287.

Winzeler, S., & Rosenstein, B. (1997). Orthopedic problems of the upper extremities: Assessment and diagnosis. *AOHN Journal, 45*(4), 188–200.

Wipf, J. E., & Deyo, R. A. (1995). Low back pain. *Medical Clinics of North America, 79*(2), 247–260.

Yasko, A., & Johnson, M. (1995). Surgical management of primary bone sarcoma. *Hematology-Oncology Clinics of North America, 9*(4), 719–731.

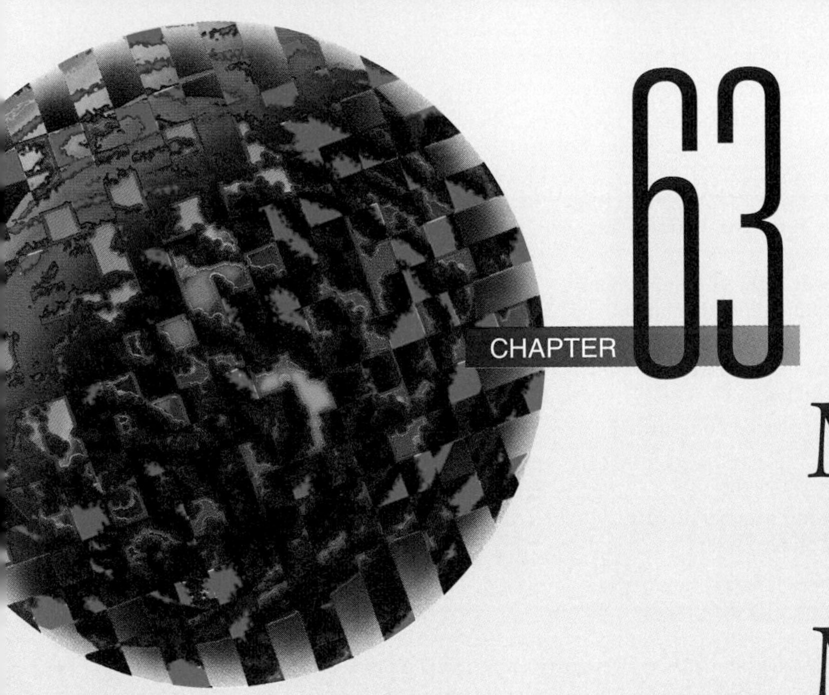

CHAPTER 63

Management of Patients With Musculoskeletal Trauma

Learning Objectives

On completion of this chapter, the learner will be able to:

1. Differentiate between contusions, strains, sprains, and dislocations.
2. Describe selected sports injuries and their nursing management.
3. Specify the clinical manifestations of a fracture and the emergency management of the patient with a fracture.
4. Describe the principles and methods of fracture reduction, fracture immobilization, and management of open fractures.
5. Use the nursing process as a framework for care of the patient with a simple fracture.
6. Describe the prevention and management of immediate and delayed complications of fractures.
7. Describe the rehabilitative needs of patients with fractures of the clavicle, upper and lower extremities, pelvis, hips, ribs, and thoracolumbar spine.
8. Use the nursing process as a framework for care of the elderly patient with fracture of the hip.
9. Describe the rehabilitative and health education needs of the patient who has had an amputation.
10. Use the nursing process as a framework for care of the patient with an amputation.

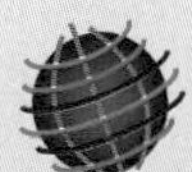

Injury to one part of the musculoskeletal system usually results in injury or dysfunction of adjacent structures and of structures enclosed or supported by them. If the bone is broken, the muscles cannot function, and blood vessels and nerves in the vicinity of the fracture may be injured. If the nerves do not send impulses to the muscles, as in paralysis, the bones cannot move. If the joint surfaces do not articulate normally, neither the bones nor the muscles can function properly.

Treatment of injury of the musculoskeletal system involves providing support for the injured part until healing is complete. Support may be provided by externally applied bandages, adhesive strapping, splints, or casts. Alternatively, support may be applied directly to the bone in the form of pins or plates. At times, traction must be applied to correct deformity or shortening.

After the immediate and the painful effects of the injury have passed, treatment efforts are focused on preventing fibrosis and stiffness in the injured muscles and joint structures. Proper exercise guards against this disability. In some cases, the support applied may permit early activity. The healing process and recovery of function may be hastened by various forms of physical therapy.

GLOSSARY

allograft: tissue harvested from a donor for use in another person

amputation: removal of a body part, usually a limb or part of a limb

arthroscope: surgical instrument used to examine internal joint structures

autograft: tissue harvested from one area of the body and used for transplantation to another area of the body

débridement: surgical removal of contaminated and devitalized tissues and foreign material

dislocation: separation of joint surfaces

fracture: a break in the continuity of a bone

fracture reduction: restoration of fracture fragments into anatomical alignment and rotation

malunion: healing of a fractured bone in a malaligned position

meniscus: crescent-shaped fibrocartilage

nonunion: failure of fragments of a fractured bone to heal together

phantom limb pain: pain perceived as being in the amputated limb

RICE: acronym for rest, ice, compression, elevation

rotator cuff: shoulder muscles (supraspinatus, subscapularis, infraspinatus, and teres minor) and their tendons

sprain: an injury to ligaments and other soft tissue at a joint

strain: a muscle pull or tear

subluxation: partial separation or dislocation of joint surfaces

tendinitis: inflammation of a tendon

CONTUSIONS, STRAINS, AND SPRAINS

A *contusion* is a soft tissue injury produced by blunt force (eg, a blow, kick, or fall). Many small blood vessels rupture and bleed into soft tissues (*ecchymosis,* bruising). A hematoma develops when the bleeding is sufficient to cause an appreciable collection of blood. Local symptoms (pain, swelling, and discoloration) are controlled with intermittent application of cold. Most contusions resolve in 1 to 2 weeks.

A **strain** is a "muscle pull" from overuse, overstretching, or excessive stress. Strains are microscopic, incomplete muscle tears with some bleeding into the tissue. The patient experiences soreness or sudden pain with local tenderness upon muscle use and isometric contraction.

A **sprain** is an injury to the ligaments surrounding a joint, caused by a wrenching or twisting motion. The function of a ligament is to maintain stability while permitting mobility. A torn ligament loses its stabilizing ability. Blood vessels rupture and edema occurs; the joint is tender and movement of the joint becomes painful. The degree of disability and pain increases during the first 2 to 3 hours after the injury because of the associated swelling and bleeding. The patient should have an x-ray to evaluate for bone injury. Avulsion fracture (a bone fragment is pulled away by a ligament or tendon) may be associated with a sprain.

Management

Treatment of contusions, strains, and sprains consists of resting and elevating the affected part, applying cold, and using a compression bandage. (The acronym **RICE**—rest, ice, compression, elevation—is helpful for remembering treatment interventions.) Rest prevents additional injury and promotes healing. Moist or dry cold applied intermittently for 20 to 30 minutes during the first 24 to 48 hours after injury produces vasoconstriction, which decreases bleeding, edema, and discomfort. Care must be taken to avoid skin and tissue damage due to excessive cold. An elastic compression bandage controls bleeding, reduces edema, and provides support for the injured tissues. Elevation controls the swelling. If the sprain is severe (torn muscle fibers and disrupted ligaments), surgical repair or cast immobilization may be necessary so that the joint will not lose its stability. The neurovascular status (circulation, motion, sensation) of the injured extremity is monitored frequently.

After the acute inflammatory stage (eg, 24 to 48 hours after injury), heat may be applied intermittently (for 15 to 30 minutes, four times a day) to relieve muscle spasm and to promote vasodilation, absorption, and repair. Depending on the severity of injury, progressive passive and active exercises may begin in 2 to 5 days. Severe sprains may require 1 to 3 weeks of immobilization before protected exercises are initiated. Excessive exercise early in the course of treatment delays recovery. Strains and sprains take weeks or months to heal. Splinting may be used to prevent reinjury.

JOINT DISLOCATIONS

A **dislocation** of a joint is a condition in which the articular surfaces of the bones forming the joint are no longer in anatomic contact. The bones are literally "out of joint." A **subluxation** is a partial dislocation of the articulating surfaces. Traumatic dislocations are orthopedic emergencies because the associated joint structures, blood supply, and nerves are distorted and severely stressed. If the dislocation is not treated promptly, *avascular necrosis* (tissue death due to anoxia and diminished blood supply) and nerve palsy may occur.

Dislocations may be congenital, present at birth (most often the hip); spontaneous or pathologic, due to disease of the articular or the periarticular structures; or traumatic, resulting from injury in which the joint is disrupted by force.

Signs and symptoms of a traumatic dislocation are pain, change in contour of the joint, change in the length of the extremity, loss of normal mobility, and change in the axis of the dislocated bones. X-rays confirm the diagnosis and demonstrate possible associated fracture.

Medical Management

The affected joint needs to be immobilized while the patient is transported to the hospital. The dislocation is promptly reduced (ie, displaced parts brought into normal position) to preserve joint function. Analgesia, muscle relaxants, and possibly anesthesia are used to facilitate closed reduction. The joint is immobilized by bandages, splints, casts, or traction and is maintained in a stable position. Neurovascular status is monitored. Several days to weeks after reduction, gentle, progressive, active and passive movement three or four times a day is begun to preserve range of motion and restore strength. The joint is supported between exercise sessions.

Nursing Management

Nursing concerns are directed at providing comfort, evaluating the patient's neurovascular status, and protecting the joint during healing. The nurse teaches the patient how to manage the immobilizing devices and how to protect the joint from reinjury.

SPORTS INJURIES

Many people participate in recreational sports. These recreational athletes may push themselves beyond the level of their physical conditioning and incur injuries. Injuries to the musculoskeletal system may be acute (sprains, strains, dislocations, fractures) or may be gradual, resulting from overuse (chondromalacia patella, tendinitis, stress fractures). Professional athletes are also susceptible to injury, even though their training is supervised closely to minimize the occurrence of injury.

Contusions result from direct falls or blows. The initial dull pain becomes greater, with edema and stiffness occurring by the next day. Sprains commonly occur in fingers, ankles, and knees. If the ligament damage is major, the joint becomes unstable, and surgical repair may be required. In addition, an avulsion fracture may exist.

Strains present with a sharp, stabbing pain from bleeding and immediate protective muscle contraction. Tennis players often suffer calf muscle strains; soccer players often experience quadriceps strains; and swimmers, weight lifters, and tennis players often suffer shoulder strains. Tendinitis (inflammation of a tendon) is due to overuse and is seen in tennis players (epicondylar tendinitis or "tennis elbow"), runners and gymnasts (Achilles tendinitis), and basketball players (infrapatellar tendinitis). Meniscal injuries of the knee occur with excessive rotational stress. Dislocations are seen with throwing and lifting sports. Fractures occur with falls. Skaters and bikers frequently suffer Colles' fractures of the wrist when they fall on outstretched arms; ballet dancers and track and field athletes may experience metatarsal fractures. Stress fractures occur with repeated bone trauma from activities such as jogging, gymnastics, basketball, and aerobics. The tibias, fibulas, and metatarsals are most vulnerable.

Patients who have experienced a sports-related injury are often highly motivated to return to their previous level of activity. Compliance with restriction of activities and gradual resumption of activities may be a significant problem for these patients. They need to be taught how to avoid further injury or new injury. With recurrence of symptoms, they need to diminish the level and intensity of activity to a comfortable level and to treat the symptoms with RICE. Recovery from sports-related injury can take a few days or more than 6 weeks.

Prevention

Sports-related injuries can be prevented by using proper equipment (eg, running shoes) and by effectively training and conditioning the body. Specific training needs to be tailored to the person and the sport. Warm-up routines generally include walking or slow jogging for about 5 minutes, followed by slow, gradual stretching. The stretch is held for 10 to 20 seconds before relaxing and repeating the stretch (Fig. 63-1). Preparing the body for sport activities increases the person's flexibility and decreases the incidence of strains and sprains.

After exercise, the body needs to cool off to prevent cardiovascular problems, such as hypotension, syncope, and dysrhythmias. Changes in activities and stresses should occur gradually. In addition, the athlete needs to be taught to "tune in" to body symptoms that indicate stress and to modify activities to minimize injury and to promote healing.

Rotator Cuff Tears

Rotator cuff tears may be due to an acute injury or to chronic joint stresses. Patients complain of pain, limited range of motion, and some joint dysfunction, including muscle weakness. In many cases, the patient with rotator cuff tear experiences night pain and is unable to sleep on the involved side. The patient is unable to perform over-the-head activities. The acromioclavicular joint is tender, and crepitus may be present. Arthrography and magnetic resonance imaging (MRI) are used to determine the extent of the rotator cuff tear.

Medical Management

Initial conservative management includes nonsteroidal anti-inflammatory drugs (NSAIDs), rest with modification of activities, injection of a corticosteroid into the shoulder joint, and progressive range-of-motion physical therapy. Some rotator cuff tears require arthroscopic débridement (removal of foreign matter and devitalized tissue) or arthroscopic or open acromioplasty with tendon repair. Postoperatively, the shoulder is immobilized for several days. An abduction splint may be used for 3 to 4 weeks. Shoulder exercises are begun in about 4 to 6 weeks and resistive exercises in about 8 weeks. Full recovery is achieved in 6 to 12 months.

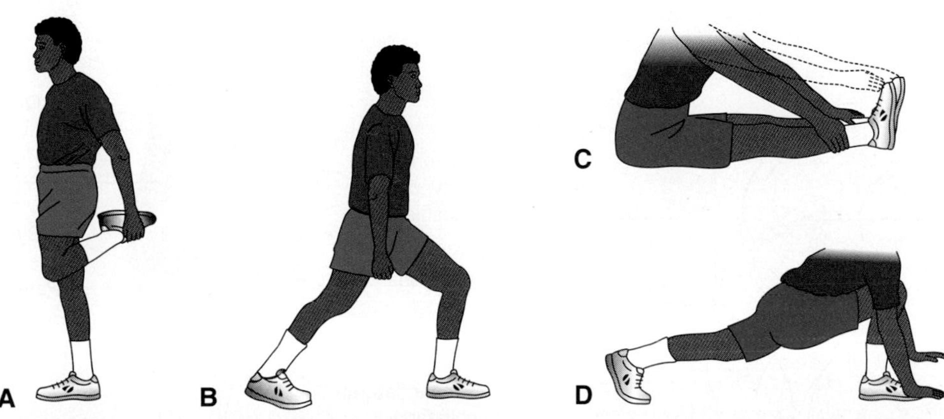

FIGURE 63•1 Stretching exercises. After walking to warm the muscles, slow, gradual stretching increases flexibility and decreases the incidence of sprains and strains. Lower extremity stretches include (**A**) quadriceps stretch; (**B** and **C**) heel cord stretch; and (**D**) hamstring and quadriceps stretch.

Epicondylitis (Tennis Elbow)

Epicondylitis is a chronic painful condition that is due to excessive, repetitive extension, flexion, pronation, and supination activities of the forearm. These excessive, repetitious activities result in inflammation (tendinitis) and minor tears in the tendons at the origin of the muscles at the medial or lateral epicondyles. Activities contributing to the development of epicondylitis include tennis, racket sports, pitching, gymnastics, and repetitive use of a screwdriver. The pain characteristically radiates down the extensor (dorsal) surface of the forearm. The patient may have a weakened grasp. Most often, relief is obtained by rest and avoiding the aggravating activity.

Medical Management

Applying ice after the activity and taking NSAIDs relieve the pain. In some instances, the arm is immobilized in a molded splint or cast. Due to its degenerative effects on tendons, local injection of a corticosteroid is reserved for patients with severe pain who do not respond to NSAIDs and immobilization. If osteophyte and loose body formation occur, joint débridement may be needed. When pain subsides, rehabilitation exercises include gentle, gradually increased stretching of the tendons. A tennis elbow counterforce strap to limit extension of the elbow may be prescribed when activity is resumed.

Lateral and Medical Collateral Ligament Injury

Lateral and medial collateral ligaments of the knee (Fig. 63-2) provide stability at the sides of the knee. Injury to these ligaments occurs when the foot is firmly planted and the knee is struck, either medially, causing stretching and tearing injury to the lateral collateral ligament, or laterally, causing stretching and tearing injury to the medial collateral ligament. The patient experiences pain, joint instability, and inability to walk without assistance.

Medical Management

Emergency management includes rest, ice, compression, and elevation (RICE). The joint is evaluated for fracture. Hemarthrosis (bleeding into the joint) may develop, contributing to the pain. The joint fluid is aspirated to relieve pressure.

The treatment depends on the severity of the sprain. Conservative management includes limited weight bearing and use of protective elastic bandaging or brace. The patient's return to full activities and sports depends on return of range of motion and muscle strength.

If needed, surgical reconstruction may be immediate or delayed. Generally, the leg is immobilized, and weight bearing is restricted for 6 to 8 weeks. A progressive rehabilitation program helps to restore the function and strength of the knee. Rehabilitation requires many months, and the patient may need to wear a derotational brace when engaging in sports.

Nursing Management

The nurse provides patient teaching about proper use of ambulatory devices, the healing process, and activity limitation to promote healing. The nurse teaches the surgical patient about pain management, medications (analgesics, antibiotics), cast care, wound care, possible complications (eg, altered neurovascular status, infection, skin breakdown), and self-care.

Anterior and Posterior Cruciate Ligament Injury

Anterior and posterior cruciate ligaments of the knee (Fig. 63-2) stabilize forward and backward motion of the femur and tibia. These ligaments crisscross in the center of the knee. Injury occurs when the foot is firmly planted, the knee is hyperextended, and the person twists the torso and femur. Usually, the anterior cruciate ligament (ACL) is torn. The patient experiences pain, joint instability, and pain with ambulation.

Medical Management

Emergency management includes rest, ice, compression, and elevation (RICE). The joint is evaluated for fracture. Joint effusion and hemarthrosis requires joint aspiration and wrapping with a compression elastic dressing.

Treatment depends on the severity of the injury and the effect of the injury on daily activities. Conservative treatment involves application of a brace and physical therapy. Surgical ACL reconstruction includes tendon repair with grafting and is performed as ambulatory arthroscopic surgery. After surgery, the patient is taught to control pain with oral opioid analgesics, NSAIDs, and cryotherapy (cooling pad incorporated in dressing). The patient is taught about monitoring neurovascular status of the leg, wound care, and signs of complications that need to be reported

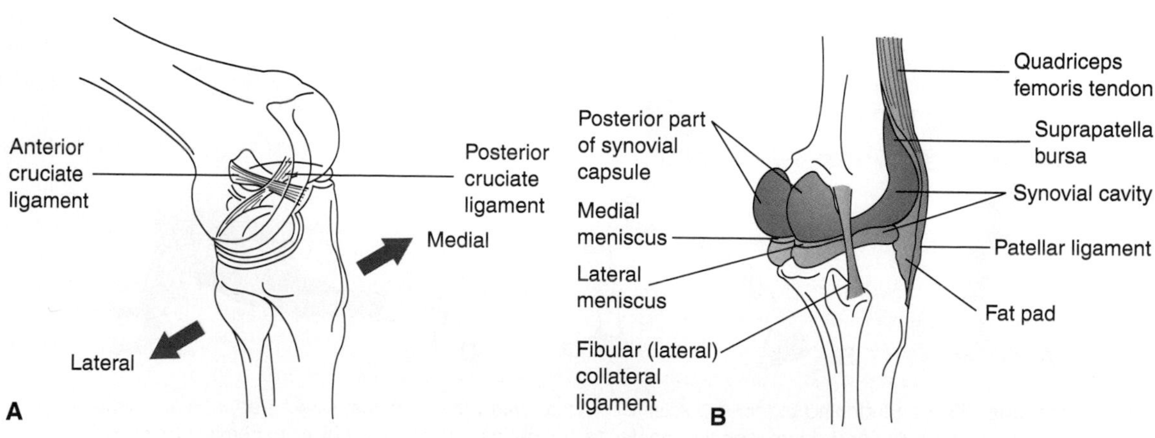

FIGURE 63•2 Knee ligaments. (**A**) Anterolateral view. (**B**) Posterolateral view.

promptly to the surgeon. Exercises (ankle pumps, quads, and hamstring sets) are encouraged during the early postoperative period. The nurse reinforces instruction about weight-bearing limits, exercise restrictions, and the use of knee brace or immobilizer. The patient must protect the graft by complying with exercise restrictions. The physical therapist supervises progressive range of motion and weight bearing (as the patient is permitted). Continuous passive motion may be helpful in restoring full range of motion. Rehabilitation after surgery typically takes 6 to 12 months.

Meniscal Injuries

In the knee (see Fig. 63-2), the two crescent-shaped (semilunar) cartilages (meniscus) attached to the edge of the shallow articulating surface of the head of the tibia move slightly backward and forward to accommodate the condyles of the femur when the leg is flexed or extended. Normally, little torsion movement is permitted in the knee joint. In sports or accidents, twisting of the knee or repetitive squatting and impact may result in either torn cartilage or tearing the cartilage from its attachment to the head of the tibia.

These injuries leave loose cartilage in the knee joint that may slip between the femur and the tibia, preventing full extension of the leg. If this happens during walking or running, patients often describe their leg as "giving way" under them. Patients may hear or feel a click in the knee when they walk, especially when they extend the leg that is bearing weight, as in going upstairs. When the cartilage is attached to the front and back of the knee, but torn loose laterally (bucket-handle tear), it may slide between the bones to lie between the condyles and prevent full flexion or extension. As a result, the knee "locks." Meniscal injuries produce disturbing disabilities because the patient never knows when the knee will malfunction. Also, the torn cartilage is an irritant in the joint, causing inflammation and chronic synovitis.

Medical Management

Usually, the damaged cartilage is surgically removed (meniscectomy) through an operation in which the surgeon uses an **arthroscope** to visualize and repair the damage. After surgery, a pressure dressing is applied, and a knee-immobilizing splint may be required. The most common complication is an effusion into the knee joint, which produces marked pain. The physician may need to aspirate the joint to remove fluid and relieve the pressure. These patients are taught quadriceps-setting and range-of-motion exercises. Additional exercises help to restore full function, stability, and strength. After arthroscopic meniscectomy, most patients resume activities in a day or two, and sports can be resumed in several weeks, as prescribed by the physician.

Rupture of the Achilles Tendon

Traumatic rupture of the Achilles tendon, generally within the tendon sheath, occurs during activities when there is a sudden contraction of the calf muscle with the foot fixed firmly to the floor. The patient experiences sharp pain and is unable to plantar flex the foot. Immediate surgical repair of complete Achilles tendon ruptures is usually recommended to obtain satisfactory results. In some situations, conservative management with a plantar-flexed cast for 6 to 8 weeks may be used.

FRACTURES

A **fracture** is a break in the continuity of bone and is defined according to type and extent. Fractures occur when the bone is subjected to stress greater than it can absorb. Fractures can be caused by a direct blow, crushing force, sudden twisting motion, and even extreme muscle contraction. When the bone is broken, adjacent structures are also affected, resulting in soft tissue edema, hemorrhage into the muscles and joints, joint dislocations, ruptured tendons, severed nerves, and damaged blood vessels. Body organs may be injured by the force that caused the fracture or by the fracture fragments.

Types of Fractures

A *complete fracture* involves a break across the entire cross-section of the bone and is frequently displaced (removed from normal position). In an *incomplete fracture* (eg, greenstick fracture), the break occurs through only part of the cross-section of the bone. A *comminuted* fracture has several bone fragments. A *closed fracture* (simple fracture) does not produce a break in the skin. An *open fracture* (compound, or complex, fracture) is one in which the skin or mucous membrane wound extends to the fractured bone. Open fractures are graded according to the following criteria:

- Grade I is a clean wound less than 1 cm long.
- Grade II is a larger wound without extensive soft tissue damage.
- Grade III is highly contaminated, has extensive soft tissue damage, and is the most severe.

Fractures may also be described according to anatomic placement of fragments, particularly if they are displaced or nondisplaced. Specific types of fractures are highlighted in Chart 63-1.

Clinical Manifestations

The clinical manifestations of a fracture are pain, loss of function, deformity, shortening of the extremity, crepitus, and local swelling and discoloration. Not all of these clinical manifestations, however, are present in every fracture. For example, many are not present with linear or fissure fractures or with impacted fractures. The diagnosis of a fracture depends on the patient's symptoms, the physical signs, and x-ray examination. Usually, the patient reports having sustained an injury to the area.

PAIN

The pain is continuous and increases in severity until the bone fragments are immobilized. The muscle spasm that accompanies fracture is a type of natural splinting designed to minimize further movement of the fracture fragments.

LOSS OF FUNCTION

After a fracture, the part cannot be used and tends to exhibit abnormal movement (false motion). The extremity cannot function properly because normal function of the muscles depends on the integrity of the bones to which they are attached.

DEFORMITY

Displacement of the fragments in a fracture of the arm or leg causes a deformity (either visible or palpable) of the extremity detectable when compared with the uninjured extremity.

CHART 63•1 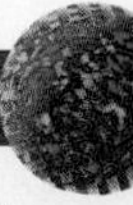 Specific Types of Fractures

Avulsion—a pulling away of a fragment of bone by a ligament or tendon and its attachment

Comminuted—a fracture in which bone has splintered into several fragments

Compound—a fracture in which damage also involves the skin or mucous membranes

Compression—a fracture in which bone has been compressed (seen in vertebral fractures)

Depressed—a fracture in which fragments are driven inward (seen frequently in fractures of skull and facial bones)

Epiphyseal—a fracture through the epiphysis

Greenstick—a fracture in which one side of a bone is broken and the other side is bent

Impacted—a fracture in which a bone fragment is driven into another bone fragment

Oblique—a fracture occurring at an angle across the bone (less stable than transverse)

Pathologic—a fracture that occurs through an area of diseased bone (bone cyst, Paget's disease, bony metastasis, tumor); can occur without trauma or a fall

Simple—a fracture that remains contained; does not break the skin

Spiral—a fracture twisting around the shaft of the bone

Transverse—a fracture that is straight across the bone

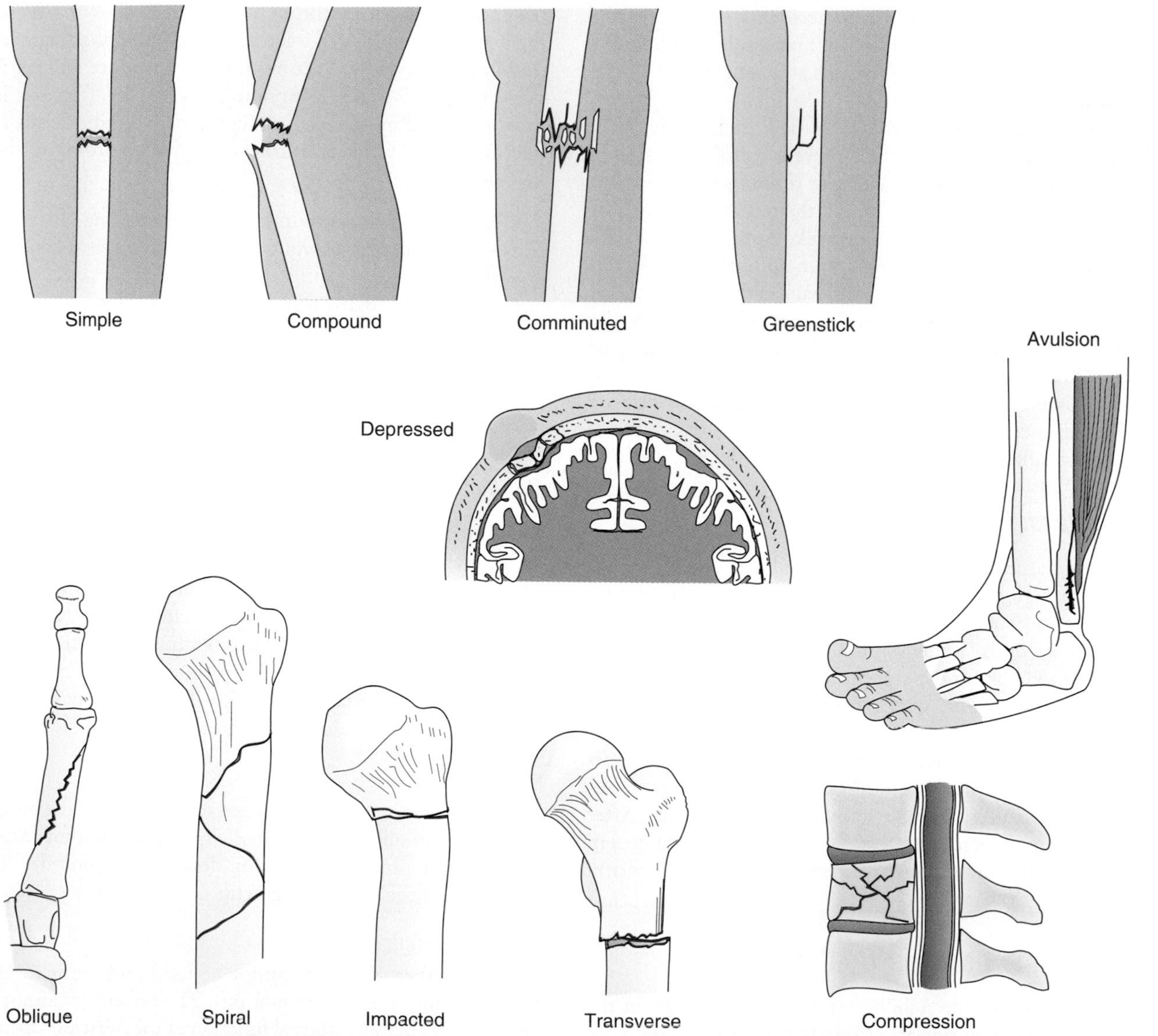

SHORTENING

In fractures of long bones, there is actual shortening of the extremity because of the contraction of the muscles that are attached above and below the site of the fracture. The fragments may often overlap by as much as 2.5 to 5 cm (1 to 2 inches).

CREPITUS

When the extremity is examined with the hands, a grating sensation called *crepitus* can be felt because of the rubbing of the fragments against each other. (Testing for crepitus can produce further tissue damage and should be avoided.)

SWELLING AND DISCOLORATION

Localized swelling and discoloration of the skin occur as a result of trauma and hemorrhage that follow a fracture. These signs may not develop for several hours or days after the injury.

Kinds of Fracture Complications

Complications of fractures fall into two categories—early and delayed. Early complications include shock, fat embolism, compartment syndrome, thromboembolism (pulmonary embolism), disseminated intravascular coagulopathy (DIC), and infection. Delayed complications include delayed union and nonunion, avascular necrosis of bone, reaction to external fixation devices, reflex sympathetic dystrophy, and heterotrophic ossification.

Shock

Hypovolemic or traumatic shock, resulting from hemorrhage (both visible and nonvisible blood loss) and loss of extracellular fluid into damaged tissues, may occur in fractures of the extremities, thorax, pelvis, and spine. This may be fatal within a few hours after injury. Because the bone is very vascular, large quantities of blood may be lost as a result of trauma, especially in fractures of the femur and pelvis. Treatment of shock consists of restoring blood volume and circulation, relieving the patient's pain, providing adequate splinting, and protecting the patient from further injury (see Chap. 14 for a discussion of shock) and other complications.

Fat Embolism Syndrome

After fracture of long bones or pelvis, multiple fractures, or crush injuries, fat emboli may develop, especially in young adult men, typically 20 to 30 years old. At the time of fracture, fat globules may move into the blood because the marrow pressure is greater than the capillary pressure or because catecholamines elevated by the patient's stress reaction mobilize fatty acids and promote the development of fat globules in the bloodstream. The fat globules combine with platelets to form emboli, which then block the small blood vessels that supply the brain, lungs, kidneys, and other organs. The onset of symptoms is rapid, usually occurring within 24 to 72 hours, but may occur up to a week after injury.

CLINICAL MANIFESTATIONS

Presenting features include hypoxia, tachypnea, tachycardia, and pyrexia. Cerebral disturbances (due to hypoxia caused by the lodging of fat emboli in the brain) are manifested by mental status changes varying from mild agitation and confusion to delirium and coma. The respiratory response includes tachypnea, dyspnea, crackles, wheezes, precordial chest pain, cough, large amounts of thick white sputum, and tachycardia. Occlusion of a large number of small vessels causes the pulmonary pressure to rise. Edema and hemorrhages in the alveoli impair oxygen transport, leading to hypoxia. Blood gas values show Po_2 below 60 mm Hg, with an early respiratory alkalosis and later respiratory acidosis. The chest x-ray exhibits a typical "snowstorm" infiltrate. Eventually, acute pulmonary edema, adult respiratory distress syndrome, and heart failure develop.

Nursing Alert *Subtle personality changes, restlessness, irritability, or confusion in a patient who has sustained a fracture are indications for immediate blood gas studies.*

With systemic embolization, the patient appears pale. Petechiae are noted in the buccal membranes and conjunctival sacs, on the hard palate, on the fundus of the eye, and over the chest and anterior axillary folds. The patient develops a temperature of more than 39.5°C (about 103°F). Free fat may be found in the urine when emboli reach the kidneys. Kidney failure may develop.

PREVENTION AND MANAGEMENT

Immediate immobilization of fractures, minimal fracture manipulation, and adequate support for fractured bones during turning and positioning are measures that may reduce the incidence of fat emboli. Monitoring high-risk patients (men between ages 20 and 30 years and patients with altered mental status) assists in the early identification of this problem. Prompt initiation of respiratory support is essential.

The objectives of management are to support the respiratory system and to correct homeostatic disturbances. Respiratory failure is the most common cause of death. Respiratory support is provided with oxygen given in high concentrations. Controlled volume ventilation with positive end-expiratory pressure may be used to prevent or treat pulmonary edema. Corticosteroids may be given to treat the inflammatory lung reaction and to control cerebral edema. Vasoactive medications to support cardiovascular function are given to prevent hypotension, shock, and interstitial pulmonary edema. Accurate fluid intake and output records facilitate adequate fluid replacement therapy. Morphine may be prescribed for pain and anxiety for the patient on a ventilator. In addition, the nurse provides calm reassurance to allay apprehension. The patient's response to therapy is closely monitored.

Because fat emboli are a major cause of death in patients with fractures, the nurse must recognize early indications of fat embolism syndrome and report them promptly to the physician. Respiratory support must be instituted early.

Compartment Syndrome

Compartment syndrome is a complication that develops when tissue perfusion in the muscles is less than that required for tissue viability. The patient complains of deep, throbbing, unrelenting pain, which is not controlled by opioids. This can be due to (1) reduction of the muscle compartment size because the enclosing muscle fascia is too tight or a cast or dressing is constrictive, or (2) an increase in muscle compartment contents because of edema or hemorrhage associated with a variety of problems (eg, fractures, crush injuries). The forearm and leg muscle compartments are involved most frequently. The pressure within a muscle compartment may increase to such an extent as to decrease microcirculation, causing nerve and muscle anoxia and necrosis. Permanent function can be lost if the anoxic situation continues for more than 6 hours.

ASSESSMENT AND DIAGNOSTIC FINDINGS

Frequent assessment of neurovascular function after fracture is essential. Peripheral circulation is evaluated by assessing color, temperature, capillary refill time, swelling, and pulses. Swelling (edema) reduces tissue perfusion. Cyanotic (blue-tinged) nail beds suggest venous congestion. Pale or dusky and cold fingers or toes suggest diminished arterial perfusion. Nail bed capillary refill time is prolonged (longer than 3 seconds). Edema may obscure the presence of arterial pulsation, and Doppler ultrasound may be used to verify a pulse. Pulselessness is a sign of arterial occlusion and *not* compartment syndrome because the tissue pressure would need to be above the systolic blood pressure for major artery occlusion to occur.

Motion is evaluated by asking the patient to move fingers or toes distal to the potential problem. Motor weakness may occur because of guarding by the patient to avoid pain or as a late sign of nerve ischemia. No movement, *paralysis,* suggests nerve damage. Sensory deficits include paresthesia, unrelenting pain, and hypoesthesia. *Paresthesia* (burning or tingling sensation) and numbness along the involved nerve are early signs of nerve involvement.

As the situation progresses, the patient complains of deep, throbbing, unrelenting pain, which is greater than expected and not controlled by opioids. Passive stretching of the muscle causes acute pain. With continued nerve ischemia and edema, the patient experiences sensations of hypoesthesia and then absence of feeling. Palpation of the muscle, if possible, reveals it to be swollen and hard. The actual tissue pressure can be measured by inserting a fluid-filled needle or wick catheter into the muscle compartment and determining the pressure with a pressure transducer monitoring setup or by using a tissue pressure measuring device (normal pressure is 8 mm Hg or less). Nerve and muscle tissues deteriorate as compartment pressure increases. Prolonged pressure of 30 to 40 mm Hg can result in compromised microcirculation. Nerve tissue is more sensitive to elevated tissue pressures than muscle. Paresthesias generally occur before paralysis.

MANAGEMENT

Prompt management of acute compartment syndrome is essential. The physician needs to be notified immediately when neurovascular compromise is suspected. Delay may result in permanent nerve and muscle damage or even necrosis, which requires amputation.

Compartment syndrome is managed by controlling swelling by elevation of the extremity to the heart level, releasing restrictive devices (dressings or cast), or both. If conservative measures do not restore tissue perfusion and relieve pain within 1 hour, a fasciotomy (surgical decompression with excision of the fibrous membrane covering and separating muscles) may be needed to relieve the constrictive muscle fascia. Elevated tissue pressure warranting fasciotomy depends on multiple factors, including systolic blood pressure and hemodynamic status. After fasciotomy, the wound is not sutured but instead is left open to permit the muscle tissues to expand and is covered with moist sterile saline dressings. The limb is splinted in a functional position and elevated, and passive range-of-motion exercises are usually prescribed every 4 to 6 hours. In 3 to 5 days, when the swelling has resolved and tissue perfusion has been restored, the wound is débrided and closed (possibly with skin grafts).

Other Early Complications

Deep vein thrombosis (DVT), thromboembolism, and pulmonary embolus are associated with reduced skeletal muscle contractions and bed rest. Patients with fractures of the lower extremities and pelvis are at high risk for thromboembolism. Pulmonary emboli may cause death several days to weeks after injury. (See Chap. 28 for discussion of DVT and Chap. 21 for discussion of pulmonary embolism).

Disseminated intravascular coagulopathy (DIC) includes a group of bleeding disorders with diverse causes, including massive tissue trauma. Manifestations of DIC include ecchymoses, unexpected bleeding after surgery, and bleeding from the mucous membranes, venipuncture sites, and gastrointestinal and urinary tracts. The treatment of DIC is discussed in Chapter 30.

All open fractures are considered contaminated. Surgical internal fixation of fractures carries the risk for infection. The nurse must monitor and teach the patient to monitor for signs of infection, including tenderness, pain, redness, swelling, local warmth, elevated temperature, and purulent drainage. Infections must be treated promptly. Antibiotic therapy must be appropriate and adequate for prophylaxis and treatment.

Delayed Union and Nonunion

Delayed union occurs when healing does not advance at a normal rate for the location and type of fracture. Delayed union may be associated with systemic infection and distraction (pulling apart) of bone fragments. Eventually, the fracture heals.

Nonunion results from failure of the ends of a fractured bone to unite. The patient complains of persistent discomfort and movement at the fracture site. Factors contributing to union problems include infection at the fracture site, interposition of tissue between the bone ends, inadequate immobilization or manipulation that disrupts callus formation, excessive space between bone fragments (bone gap), limited bone contact, and impaired blood supply resulting in avascular necrosis.

In nonunion, fibrocartilage or fibrous tissue exists between the bone fragments; no bone salts have been deposited. A false joint (pseudarthrosis) often develops at the site of the fracture. Fractures of the middle third of the humerus, the neck of the femur in elderly people, and the lower third of the tibia most frequently result in nonunion.

MEDICAL MANAGEMENT

Nonunion may be managed by bone grafting. Surgically, the fractured bone fragments are trimmed, infection (if present) is removed, and a bone graft—**autograft** (tissue harvested from the donor for the donor), frequently from the iliac crest, or **allograft** (tissue harvested from a donor other than the person who will receive it)—is placed in the bony defect. The bone graft fills the bone gap, provides a lattice work for invasion by bone cells, and actively promotes bone growth. The type of bone selected for grafting depends on function—cortical for structural strength, cancellous for osteogenesis, and corticocancellous for strength and rapid incorporation. Bone grafts may be chips, wedges, blocks, bone segments, or demineralized bone matrix. At times, autograft bone, allograft bone, and demineralized cortical matrix are combined to optimize graft incorporation and bone healing. Free vascularized bone autografts are grafted with their own blood supply, allowing for primary fracture healing.

Bone grafts provide for osteogenesis, osteoconduction, or osteoinduction. *Osteogenesis* is bone formation and is due to transplantation of bone containing osteoblasts. *Osteoconduction* is the structural matrix provided by the graft for ingrowth of blood vessels and osteoblasts. *Osteoinduction* is the stimulation of host stem cells to differentiate into osteoblasts by several growth factors, including bone morphogenic proteins. Bone transplants undergo creeping substitution, a reconstructive process in which the bone transplant is gradually replaced by new bone (Cypher & Grossman, 1996).

After grafting, immobilization and non–weight bearing are required while the bone graft becomes incorporated and the fracture or defect heals. Depending on the type of bone grafted, healing may take 6 months to more than a year. Bone grafting problems include wound or graft infection, fracture of the graft, and nonunion. Infrequent specific allograft problems include partial acceptance (lack of host and donor histocompatibility retard graft incorporation), graft rejection (graft is rapidly and completely resorbed), and transmission of disease (rare). Specific autograft problems include limited quantity of bone available for harvest, increased surgery time, increased blood loss, and donor site pain, hematoma, and infection.

Osteogenesis in nonunion may be stimulated by electrical impulses; its effectiveness is similar to that of bone grafting. It is not effective with large bone gaps or synovial pseudarthrosis. The electrical stimulation modifies the tissue environment, making it electronegative, which enhances mineral deposition and bone formation.

In some situations, pins that act as cathodes are inserted percutaneously directly into the fracture site, and electrical impulses are directed to the fracture continuously. Direct current methods cannot be used when infection is present.

Another method is noninvasive inductive coupling. Pulsing electromagnetic fields are delivered to the fracture for 3 to 10 hours a day by an electromagnetic coil over the nonunion site (Fig. 63-3). During the electrical stimulation treatment period, which takes 3 to 6 months or longer, rigid fracture fixation with adequate support is needed.

NURSING MANAGEMENT

Nursing responsibilities for the patient with bone graft include pain management, monitoring the patient for signs of infection at the donor and recipient sites, and patient education. The nurse needs to reinforce information concerning the objectives of the bone graft, immobilization, non–weight bearing, wound care, signs of infection, and follow-up care with the orthopedic surgeon.

The patient with electrical stimulation for nonunion has experienced an extended time in fracture treatment and frequently becomes frustrated with prolonged therapy. The nurse provides emotional support and encouragement to the patient and encourages compliance with the treatment regimen. Patient education includes immobilization, non–weight bearing, and daily use of the stimulator as prescribed. The orthopedist evaluates the progression of bone healing with periodic x-rays.

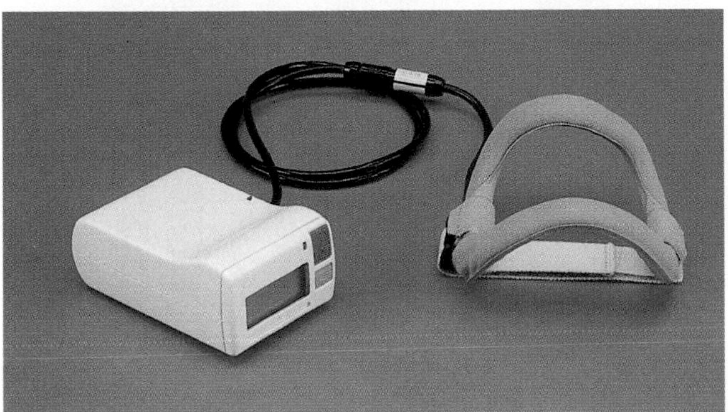

FIGURE 63•3 Bone healing stimulator. Courtesy of EBI Medical Systems.

Avascular Necrosis of Bone

Avascular necrosis occurs when the bone loses its blood supply and dies. It may follow a fracture with disruption of the blood supply (especially of the femoral neck). It is also seen with dislocations, bone transplantation, prolonged high-dosage corticosteroid therapy, chronic renal disease, sickle cell anemia, and other diseases. The devitalized bone may collapse or reabsorb. The patient develops pain and experiences limited movement. X-rays reveal calcium loss and structural collapse. Treatment generally consists of attempts to revitalize the bone with bone grafts, prosthetic replacement, or arthrodesis (joint fusion).

Reaction to Internal Fixation Devices

Internal fixation devices may be removed after bony union has taken place. In most patients, however, the device is not removed unless it produces symptoms. Pain and decreased function are the prime indicators that a problem has developed. Such problems may include mechanical failure (inadequate insertion and stabilization); material failure (faulty or damaged devices); corrosion of the device, causing local inflammation; allergic response to the metallic alloy used; and osteoporotic remodeling adjacent to the fixation device. (Stress needed for bone strength is carried by the device, causing a disuse osteoporosis.) If the device is removed, the bone needs to be protected from refracture related to osteoporosis, altered bone structure, and trauma. Bone remodeling reestablishes the bone's structural strength.

Reflex Sympathetic Dystrophy Syndrome

Reflex sympathetic dystrophy (RSD) syndrome is an uncommon, painful, sympathetic nervous system problem. It usually occurs in an extremity after trauma and is seen more often in women. Clinical manifestations of RSD include severe, burning pain, local edema, hyperesthesia, muscle spasms, vasomotor skin changes (ie, fluctuating warm, red, dry and cold, sweaty, cyanotic), and trophic changes. This syndrome is frequently chronic with extension of symptoms to other areas of the body. Disuse muscle atrophy and bone deossification occur with persistence of RSD. Patients may exhibit ineffective individual coping related to the chronic pain.

MANAGEMENT

Early effective pain relief is the focus of management. Pain may need to be controlled with physical therapy modalities, analgesics, nerve root injection of cortisone and anesthetic, or intravenous biophosphonate pamidronate (Cortet et al., 1997). Muscle relaxants and antidepressants are also used. With pain relief, the patient can participate in ROM exercises and functional use of the affected area. The nurse needs to help the patient cope with RSD manifestations and explore multiple ways to control pain (see Chap. 12). The nurse avoids using the involved extremity for blood pressures and venipunctures.

Heterotrophic Ossification (Myositis Ossificans)

Heterotrophic ossification is the abnormal formation of bone near bones or in muscle in response to soft tissue trauma after blunt trauma, fracture, or total joint replacement. The muscle is painful, and normal muscular contraction and movement are limited. The abnormal bone may be excised 6 to 12 months after the injury when the bone has matured.

Emergency Management of Fractures

Immediately after injury, when a fracture is suspected, it is important to immobilize the body part before the patient is moved. If an injured patient must be removed from a vehicle before splints can be applied, the extremity is supported above and below the fracture site to prevent rotation as well as angular motion.

Adequate splinting, including joints adjacent to the fracture, is essential to prevent damage to the soft tissue. Movement of fracture fragments causes additional pain, soft tissue damage, and bleeding. Temporary, well-padded splints, firmly bandaged over clothing, immobilize the fracture. Immobilization of the long bones of the lower extremities may be accomplished by bandaging the extremities together, with the unaffected extremity serving as a splint for the injured one. In an upper extremity injury, the arm may be bandaged to the chest, or an injured forearm may be placed in a sling. The neurovascular status distal to the injury should be assessed to determine adequacy of peripheral tissue perfusion and nerve function.

In an *open fracture,* the wound is covered with a clean (sterile) dressing to prevent contamination of deeper tissues. No attempt is made to reduce the fracture, even if one of the bone fragments is protruding through the wound. Splints are applied as described previously.

In the emergency department, the patient is evaluated completely. The clothes are gently removed, first from the uninjured side of the body and then from the injured side. The patient's clothing may be cut away. The fractured extremity is moved as little as possible to avoid more damage.

Medical Management of Fractures

The principles of fracture treatment include reduction, immobilization, and regaining of normal function and strength through rehabilitation.

REDUCTION

Reduction of a fracture ("setting" the bone) refers to restoration of the fracture fragments into anatomic alignment and rotation. *Closed reduction* or *open reduction* may be used to reduce a fracture. The specific method selected depends on the nature of the fracture; however, the underlying principles are the same. Usually, the physician reduces fractures as soon as possible to prevent tissues from losing their elasticity from infiltration by edema or hemorrhage. In most cases, fracture reduction becomes more difficult as the injury begins healing.

Before fracture reduction and immobilization, the patient is prepared for the procedure; permission for the procedure is obtained, and an analgesic is administered as prescribed. Anesthesia may be administered. The injured extremity must be handled gently to avoid additional damage.

Closed Reduction. In most instances, closed reduction is accomplished by bringing the bone fragments into apposition (ends in contact) by manipulation and manual traction. The extremity is held in the desired position while a cast, splint, or other device is applied by the physician. The immobilizing device maintains the reduction and stabilizes the extremity for bone healing. X-rays are obtained to determine that the bone fragments are correctly aligned.

Traction (ie, skin, skeletal) may be used to effect fracture reduction and immobilization. Traction may be used until the patient is physiologically stable and able to withstand surgical fixation or until the fracture begins to heal. X-rays are used to monitor the fracture reduction, approximation of the bony fragments, and callus formation. When the callus is well established, a cast or splint may be used for continued immobilization. Use of traction and the nursing management of a patient in traction are discussed more fully in Chapter 61.

Open Reduction. Some fractures require open reduction. Through a surgical approach, the fracture fragments are reduced. Internal fixation devices in the form of metallic pins, wires, screws, plates, nails, or rods may be used to hold the bone fragments in position until solid bone healing occurs. These devices may be attached to the sides of bone or inserted through the bony fragments or directly into the medullary cavity of the bone (Fig. 63-4). Internal fixation devices ensure firm approximation and fixation of the bony fragments.

IMMOBILIZATION

After the fracture has been reduced, bone fragments must be immobilized, or held in correct position and alignment until union occurs. Immobilization may be accomplished by external or internal fixation. Methods of external fixation include bandages, casts, splints, continuous traction, or external fixators. Metal implants used for internal fixation serve as internal splints to immobilize the fracture.

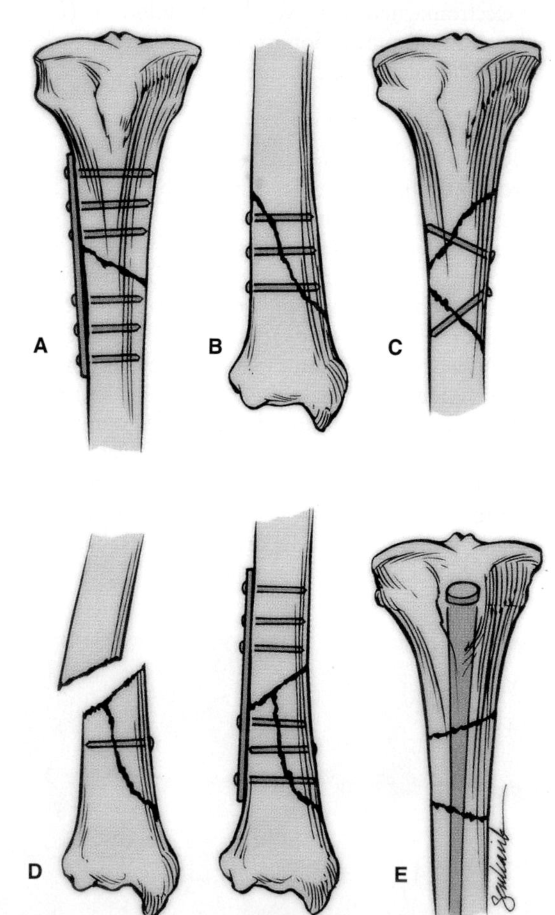

FIGURE 63•4 Techniques of internal fixation. (**A**) Plate and six screws for a transverse or short oblique fracture. (**B**) Screws for a long oblique or spiral fracture. (**C**) Screws for a long butterfly fragment. (**D**) Plate and six screws for a short butterfly fragment. (**E**) Medullary nail for a segmental fracture.

MAINTAINING AND RESTORING FUNCTION

Reduction and immobilization are maintained as prescribed to promote bone and soft tissue healing. Swelling is controlled by elevating the injured extremity and applying ice as prescribed. Neurovascular status (circulation, movement, sensation) is monitored, and the orthopedic surgeon is notified immediately if signs of neurovascular compromise are identified. Restlessness, anxiety, and discomfort are controlled with a variety of approaches (eg, reassurance; position changes; pain relief strategies, including analgesics). Isometric and muscle-setting exercises are encouraged to minimize disuse atrophy and to promote circulation. Participation in activities of daily living (ADLs) is encouraged to promote independent functioning and self-esteem. Gradual resumption of activities is promoted within the therapeutic prescription. With internal fixation, the surgeon determines the amount of movement and weight-bearing stress the extremity can withstand and prescribes the level of activity. (See Nursing Process sections in Chap. 61 for more information about caring for patients with casts, in traction, and undergoing orthopedic surgery).

Nursing Management

PATIENTS WITH CLOSED FRACTURES

The nurse encourages patients with closed (simple) fractures to return to their usual activities as rapidly as possible. The nurse teaches patients how to control swelling and pain associated with the fracture and soft tissue trauma and encourages them to be active within the limits of the fracture immobilization. It is important to teach exercises to maintain the health of unaffected muscles and to increase strength of muscles needed for transferring and for using assistive devices (eg, crutches, walker). The nurse teaches patients how to use assistive devices safely. Planning is done to help patients modify their home environment as needed and to secure personal assistance if necessary. Patient teaching includes self-care, medication information, monitoring for potential complications, and the need for continuing health care supervision. Fracture healing and restoration of full strength and mobility may take months.

PATIENTS WITH OPEN FRACTURES

In an open fracture, there is risk of osteomyelitis, tetanus, and gas gangrene. The objectives of management are to prevent infection of the wound, soft tissue, and bone and to promote healing of soft tissue and bone. The nurse administers tetanus prophylaxis. Serial irrigation and débridement remove anaerobic organisms. Intravenous antibiotics are prescribed to prevent or treat infection.

Prompt thorough wound irrigation and débridement in the operating room is necessary. The wound is cultured. Devitalized bone fragments are removed. The fracture is carefully reduced and stabilized by external fixation (see External Fixators in Chap. 61) or intramedullary nails. Any damage to blood vessels, soft tissue, muscles, nerves, and tendons is repaired.

With open fractures, primary wound closure is delayed. Heavily contaminated wounds are left unsutured and dressed with sterile gauze to permit swelling and wound drainage. Wound irrigation and débridement are repeated, removing infected and devitalized tissue and increasing vascularity in the region. When it is determined that infection is not present, the wound is closed in 5 to 7 days, and all dead space is obliterated by autogenous skin or flap graft.

The nurse elevates the extremity to minimize edema. It is important to assess neurovascular status frequently. The nurse measures the patient's temperature at regular intervals and monitors the patient for signs of infection. In 4 to 8 weeks, bone grafting may be necessary to bridge bone defects and to stimulate bone healing.

Fracture Healing

Weeks to months are required for most fractures to heal. Many factors influence the speed with which fractures heal (Chart 63-2). The reduction of fracture fragments must be accurate and maintained to ensure healing. The affected bone must have an adequate blood supply. The type of fracture also affects healing time. In general, fractures of flat bones (pelvis, scapula) heal rapidly. Fractures at the ends of long bones, where the bone is more vascular and cancellous, heal more quickly than do fractures in areas where the bone is dense and less vascular (midshaft). Weight-bearing stimulates healing of stabilized fractures of the long bones in the lower extremities.

If fracture healing is disrupted, the bone union time may be delayed or stopped completely. Factors that may interrupt fracture healing include inadequate fracture immobilization, inadequate blood supply to the fracture site or adjacent tissue,

HOME CARE TEACHING CHECKLIST: CLOSED FRACTURE

At the completion of the program, the patient or caregiver will be able to:	Patient	Caregiver
• Describe approaches to controlling swelling and pain (eg, elevate extremity to heart level; take analgesics as prescribed).	✔	✔
• Report pain uncontrolled by elevation and analgesics (may be an indicator of impaired tissue perfusion or compartment syndrome).	✔	✔
• Describe management of immobilizing device or care of incision.		
• Consume balanced diet to promote bone healing.	✔	
• Demonstrate ability to transfer.	✔	
• Use mobility aids safely.	✔	
• Avoid excessive use of injured extremity; observe prescribed weight-bearing limits.	✔	✔
• State indicators of complication to report promptly to physician (eg, uncontrolled swelling and pain; cool, pale fingers or toes; paresthesia; paralysis; signs of systemic infection; signs of thromboembolism; problems with immobilization device).		
• State possible delayed complications of fractures (ie, delayed union; nonunion; avascular necrosis; reaction to internal fixation device; reflex sympathetic dystrophy syndrome, heterotrophic ossification).		
• Describe gradual resumption of normal activities when medically cleared, and discuss how to protect fracture site from undue stresses.	✔	✔

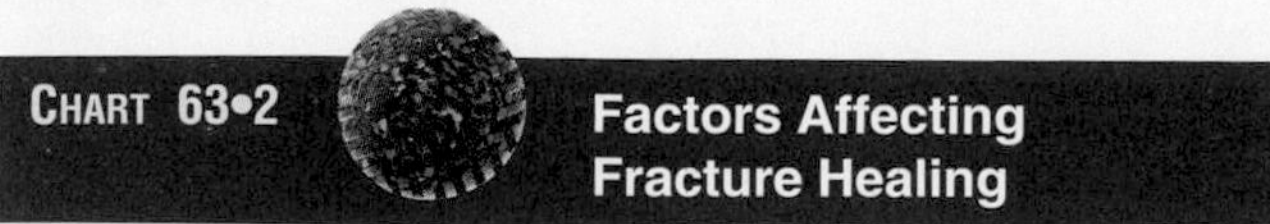

CHART 63•2 Factors Affecting Fracture Healing

Factors Enhancing Fracture Healing

- Immobilization of fracture fragments
- Maximum bone fragment contact
- Sufficient blood supply
- Proper nutrition
- Exercise: weight-bearing for long bones
- Hormones: growth hormone, thyroid, calcitonin, vitamin D, anabolic steroids
- Electric potential across fracture

Factors Inhibiting Fracture Healing

- Extensive local trauma
- Bone loss
- Inadequate immobilization
- Space/tissue between bone fragments
- Infection
- Local malignancy
- Metabolic bone diseases (e.g., Paget's disease)
- Irradiated bone (radiation necrosis)
- Avascular necrosis
- Intra-articular fracture (synovial fluid contains fibrolysins, which lyse the initial clot and retard clot formation)
- Age (elderly persons heal more slowly)
- Corticosteroids (inhibit the repair rate)

extensive space between bone fragments, interposition of soft tissue between bone ends, infection, and metabolic problems.

Fractures of Specific Sites

An injury to the skeletal structure may vary from a simple linear fracture to a severe crushing injury. Therapeutic management is determined by the type and location of the fracture and the extent of damage to surrounding structures. Maximum functional recovery is the goal of management.

Clavicle

Fracture of the clavicle (collar bone) is a common injury that results from a fall or a direct blow to the shoulder. Head or cervical spine injuries may be seen with these fractures. The clavicle helps to hold the shoulder upward, outward, and backward from the thorax. Therefore, when the clavicle is fractured, the patient assumes a protective position—slumping the shoulders and immobilizing the arm to prevent shoulder movements. The treatment goal is to align the shoulder in its normal position by means of closed reduction and immobilization.

More than 80% of these fractures occur in the medial two thirds of the clavicle. A clavicular strap, also called a *figure-of-eight bandage* (Fig. 63-5), may be used to pull the shoulders back, reducing and immobilizing the fracture. When a clavicular strap is used, the axillae are well padded to prevent a compression injury to the brachial plexus and axillary artery. Circulation and nerve function of both arms are monitored.

Fracture of the distal third of the clavicle without displacement and ligament disruption is treated with a sling and restricted motion of the arm. When a fracture in the distal third is accompanied by a disruption of the coracoclavicular ligament, there is displacement, which may be treated by open reduction and internal fixation.

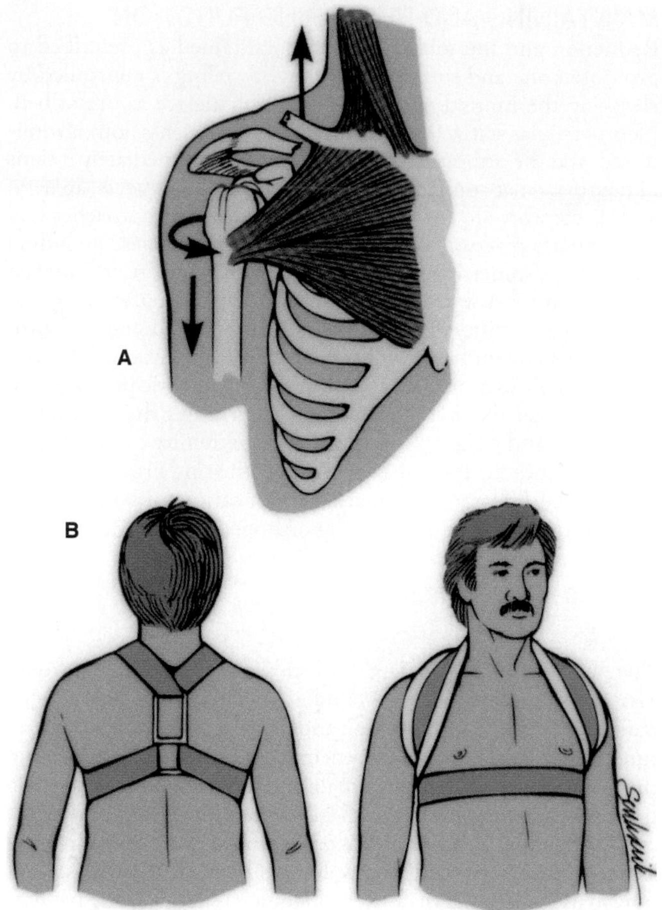

FIGURE 63•5 Fracture of the clavicle. (**A**) Anteroposterior view shows typical displacement in midclavicular fracture. (**B**) Immobilization is accomplished with a clavicular strap.

Complications of clavicular fractures include trauma to the nerves of the brachial plexus, injury to the subclavian vein or artery from a bony fragment, and **malunion** (poorly aligned healing of the fractured bone). Malunion may be a cosmetic problem, for example, when low-neckline clothing is worn.

NURSING MANAGEMENT

The nurse cautions the patient not to elevate the arm above shoulder level until the ends of the bone have united (about 6 weeks) but encourages the patient to exercise the elbow, wrist, and fingers as soon as possible. When prescribed, shoulder exercises (Fig. 63-6) are performed to obtain full shoulder motion. It is important to tell the patient that vigorous activity is limited for 3 months.

Humeral Neck

Fractures of the proximal humerus may occur through either the anatomic or the surgical neck of the humerus. The anatomic neck is located just below the humeral head. The surgical neck is the region below the tubercles. Impacted fractures of the surgical neck of the humerus are seen most frequently in older women after a fall on an outstretched arm. These are essentially nondisplaced fractures. Active middle-aged patients may suffer severely

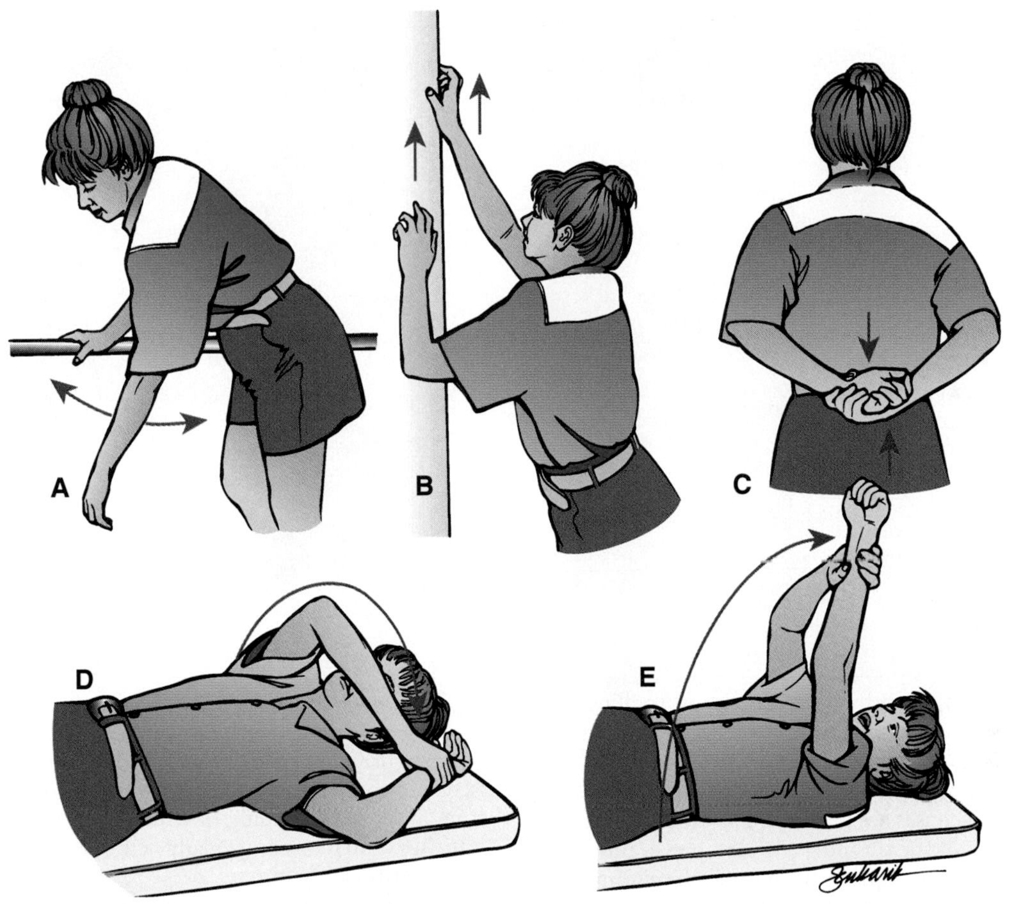

FIGURE 63•6 Exercises that develop shoulder range of motion include (**A**) pendulum exercise and (**B**) wall climbing. The unaffected arm is used to assist with (**C**) internal rotation, (**D**) external rotation, and (**E**) elevation. In C, D, and E, the unaffected arm is used for power.

displaced humeral neck fractures with associated rotator cuff damage.

The patient presents with the affected arm hanging limp at the side and supported by the uninjured hand. Neurovascular assessment of the involved extremity is essential to evaluate fully the extent of injury and possible involvement of the neurovascular bundle (nerves and blood vessels) of the arm.

MANAGEMENT

Many impacted fractures of the surgical neck of the humerus are not displaced and do not require reduction. The arm is supported and immobilized by a sling and swathe that secure the supported arm to the trunk (Fig. 63-7). A soft pad is placed in the axilla to absorb moisture and avoid skin breakdown. Limitation of motion and stiffness of the shoulder occur from disuse. Therefore, pendulum exercises are begun as soon as tolerated by the patient. (In pendulum or circumduction exercises, the patient is instructed to lean forward and allow the affected arm to abduct and rotate [see Fig. 63-6].) Early motion of the joint does not displace the fragments if motion is carried out within the limits imposed by pain.

These fractures require 6 to 10 weeks to heal, and the patient should avoid vigorous activity, such as tennis, for an additional 4 weeks. Residual stiffness, aching, and some limitation of range of motion may persist for 6 or more months.

When a humeral neck fracture is displaced, treatment consists of closed reduction, open reduction with internal fixation, or replacement of the humeral head with a prosthesis. In this type of fracture, exercises are started only after a prescribed period of immobilization.

Humeral Shaft

Fractures of the shaft of the humerus are most frequently caused by (1) direct trauma that results in a transverse, oblique, or comminuted fracture, or (2) an indirect twisting force that results in a spiral fracture. The nerves and brachial blood vessels may be injured with these fractures. Wrist drop is indicative of radial nerve injury. Initial neurovascular assessment is essential to differentiate between trauma from the injury and complications from treatment.

MANAGEMENT

Frequently, the weight of the arm helps to correct any displacement so that surgery is not required. With an oblique, spiral, or displaced fracture that has resulted in shortening of the humeral shaft, a hanging cast may be used. This cast is designed so that its weight provides traction to the arm when the patient is upright, thereby reducing and immobilizing the fracture. The hanging cast must be dependent (allowed to hang free without support) because the weight of the cast is the means by which continuous traction is applied to the long axis of the arm. The patient is advised to sleep in an upright position so that traction from the weight of the cast is maintained. Complications encountered

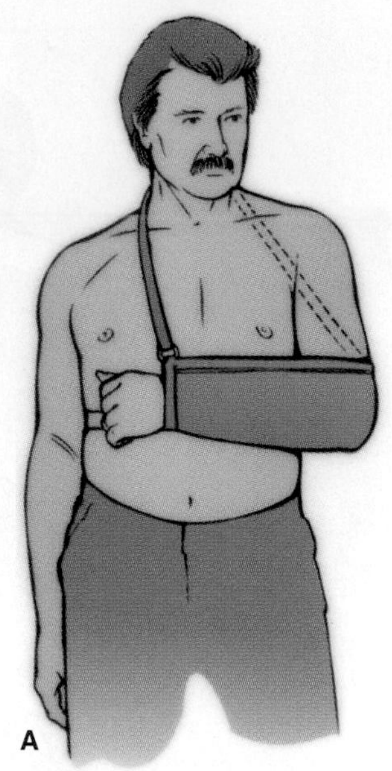

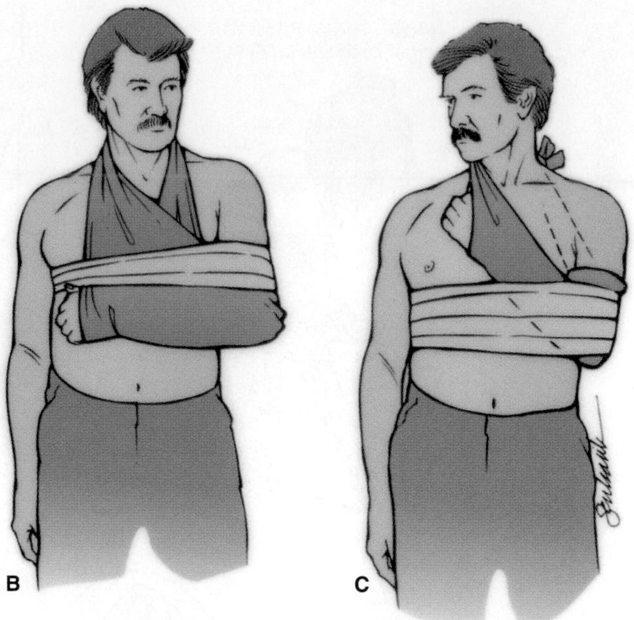

FIGURE 63•7 Immobilizers for proximal humeral fractures: (**A**) Commercial sling with immobilizing strap permits easy removal for hygiene and is comfortable on the neck; (**B**) conventional sling and swathe; (**C**) stockinette Velpeau and swathe are used when there is an unstable surgical neck component; this position relaxes the pectoralis major.

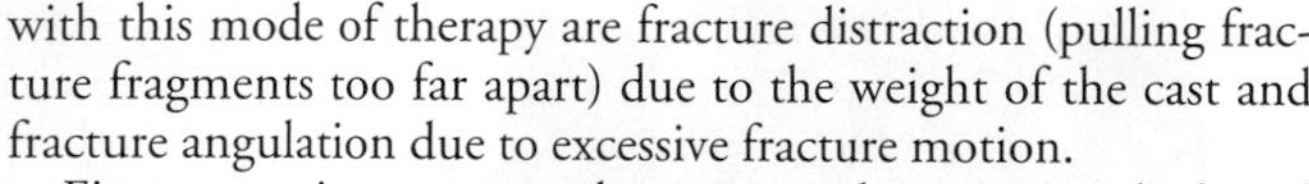

with this mode of therapy are fracture distraction (pulling fracture fragments too far apart) due to the weight of the cast and fracture angulation due to excessive fracture motion.

Finger exercises are started as soon as the cast is applied, and pendulum shoulder exercises are performed as prescribed to provide active movement of the shoulder, thereby preventing adhesions of the shoulder joint capsule. Isometric exercises may be prescribed to prevent muscle atrophy.

After the cast is removed, a sling is applied, and exercises of the shoulder, elbow, and wrist are begun. Humeral fractures require about 10 weeks to heal when treated with hanging casts.

Elderly patients may not tolerate a cast. A sling and swathe (see Fig. 63-7*B*) may provide adequate comfort and immobilization. Shoulder exercises are begun in about 3 weeks.

Functional bracing is another form of treatment being used for these fractures. A contoured thermoplastic sleeve is secured in place with interlocking fabric (Velcro) closures around the upper arm, immobilizing the reduced fracture. As swelling decreases, the sleeve is tightened, and uniform pressure and stability are applied to the fracture. Functional bracing allows active use of muscles, shoulder and elbow motion, and good approximation of fracture fragments. The callus that develops is substantial, and the sleeve can be discontinued in about 9 weeks.

A shoulder spica cast may be used during early treatment of unstable humerus fracture. Generally, the patient is uncomfortable and feels awkward. Skeletal traction (eg, over-the-face traction; balanced side-arm traction) may be appropriate for patients who must remain in bed because of other injuries (Figs. 63-8 and 63-9). The patient is encouraged to perform active exercises of the hand and wrist. Open fractures of the humeral shaft are treated by external fixators (see Chap. 61). Open reduction with internal fixation of a humerus fracture is necessary with nerve palsy or pathologic fractures.

Elbow

Fractures of the distal humerus result from motor vehicle crashes, falls on the elbow (in the extended or flexed position), or a direct blow. These fractures may result in injury to the median, radial, or ulnar nerves.

The patient is evaluated for paresthesias and signs of compromised circulation in the forearm and hand. The most serious complication of a supracondylar fracture of the humerus is Volkmann's ischemic contracture (a compartment syndrome), which results from antecubital swelling or damage to the brachial artery. The nurse needs to monitor regularly neurovascular status and for signs of compartment syndrome.

Other potential complications are damage to the joint articular surfaces and hemarthrosis (blood in the joint). With hemarthrosis, the physician may aspirate the joint to remove the blood, thereby relieving the pressure and pain.

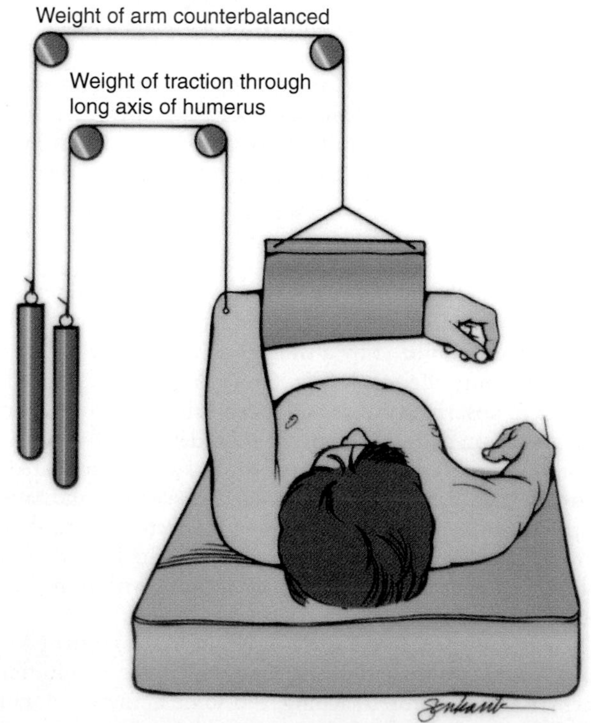

FIGURE 63•8 Over-the-face traction for supracondylar fracture reduces swelling by creating a very effective elevation of the extremity.

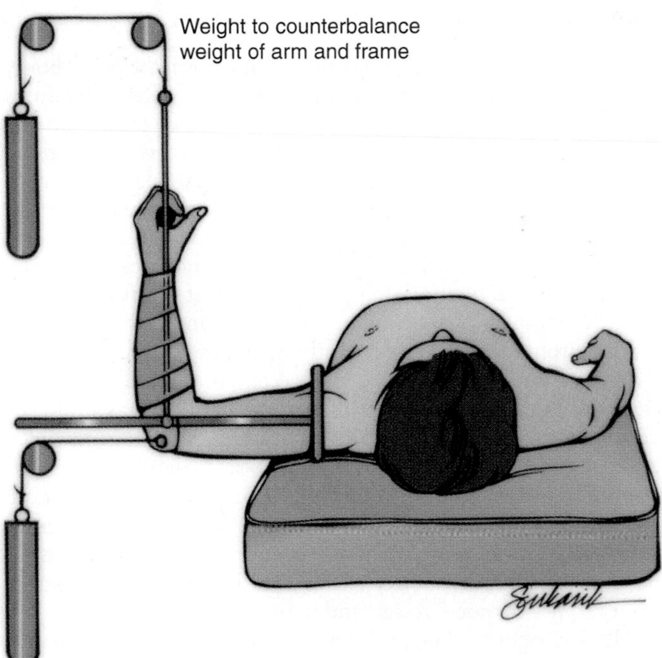

FIGURE 63•9 Balanced side-arm traction. The arm is passed through the ring, so that it encompasses the shoulder. The upright attachment for the forearm may be moved to accommodate the length of the humerus. A cloth sling is placed on the horizontal segment to provide a surface on which the arm may rest. The forearm is placed between the two upright supports and is usually held there with a circumferentially applied elastic bandage. A rope is attached to the vertical section and is passed through pulleys. A weight is attached to exactly counterbalance the weight of the arm and the frame. Skeletal traction is then applied in the desired amount through the pin in the olecranon. The entire extremity is counter-balanced so that a balanced traction system is created.

MANAGEMENT

The goal of therapy is prompt reduction and stabilization of the distal humerus fracture, followed by controlled active motion when swelling has subsided and healing has begun. If the fracture is not displaced, the arm is immobilized in a cast or posterior splint with the elbow at 45 to 90 degrees of flexion and a sling.

A displaced fracture is usually treated by traction or open reduction and internal fixation. Excision of bone fragments may be necessary. Additional external support with a splint is then applied.

Active finger exercises are encouraged. Gentle range-of-motion exercise of the injured joint is begun about 1 week after internal fixation and after 2 weeks with closed reduction. Motion promotes healing of injured joints by movement of synovial fluid into the articular cartilage. Active exercise of the elbow is carried out when prescribed residual limitation of motion may result without an intensive rehabilitation program.

Radial Head

Radial head fractures are common and are usually produced by a fall on the outstretched hand with the elbow extended.

MANAGEMENT

If blood has collected in the elbow joint (hemarthrosis), it is aspirated to relieve pain and allow early range of motion. Immobilization for these undisplaced fractures is accomplished by a splint. If the fracture is displaced, surgery is required, with excision of the radial head when necessary. Postoperatively, the arm is immobilized in a posterior plaster splint and sling. The patient is encouraged to carry out a program of active motion of the elbow and forearm when prescribed.

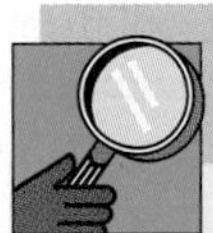

ASSESSMENT
VOLKMANN'S CONTRACTURE

- Observe the distal limb for swelling, skin color, nail bed capillary refill, and temperature. Compare affected and unaffected hands.
- Assess radial pulse.
- Assess for paresthesias (tingling and burning sensations) in the hand, because this may indicate nerve injury or impending ischemia.
- Evaluate patient's ability to move fingers.
- Explore intensity and character of pain.
- Directly measure tissue pressure as prescribed.
- Report indications of diminished nerve function or diminished circulatory perfusion promptly before irreparable damage occurs. Fasciotomy may become necessary.

Radial and Ulnar Shafts

Fractures of the shaft of the bones of the forearm occur most frequently in children. The radius or the ulna may be fractured at any level. Frequently, displacement occurs when both bones are broken. The forearm's unique functions of pronation and supination must be preserved by maintaining good anatomic position and alignment.

MANAGEMENT

If the fragments are not displaced, the fracture is treated by closed reduction with a long arm cast applied from the upper arm to the proximal palmar crease. A loop may be incorporated in the cast near the elbow and a sling pulled through it to prevent the cast from sagging against the forearm.

The circulation, motion, and sensation of the hand are assessed after the cast is applied. The arm is elevated to control edema. Frequent finger flexion and extension are encouraged to reduce edema. Active motion of the involved shoulder is essential. The reduction and alignment are monitored closely by x-rays to ensure adequate immobilization. The fracture is immobilized for about 12 weeks; during the last 6 weeks, the arm may be in a functional forearm brace that allows exercise of the wrist and elbow.

Displaced fractures are managed by open reduction with internal fixation, using a compression plate with screws, intramedullary nails, or rods. The arm is usually immobilized in a plaster splint or cast. Open fractures may be managed with external fixation devices. The arm is elevated to control swelling. Neurovascular status is monitored. Elbow, wrist, and hand exercises are begun as permitted by the immobilization device.

Wrist

Fractures of the distal radius (Colles' fracture) are common and are usually the result of a fall on an open, dorsiflexed hand. This fracture is frequently seen in elderly women with osteoporotic bones and weak soft tissues that do not dissipate the energy of the fall.

The patient presents with a deformed wrist, radial deviation, pain, swelling, weakness, limited finger range of motion, and numbness.

MANAGEMENT

Treatment usually consists of closed reduction and immobilization with a cast. For more severe fractures, a wire may be inserted to maintain reduction. The wrist and forearm are elevated for 48 hours after reduction to control swelling.

Active motion of the fingers and shoulder should begin promptly. The patient is taught to do the following exercises to reduce swelling and prevent stiffness:

- Hold the hand at the level of the heart.
- Move the fingers from full extension to flexion. Hold and release. (Repeat at least 10 times every hour when awake.)
- Use the hand in functional activities.
- Actively exercise the shoulder and elbow, including complete range of motion exercises of both joints.

Fingers may swell from diminished venous and lymphatic return. The sensory function of the median nerve is assessed by pricking the distal aspect of the index finger, and the motor function is assessed by testing the ability to touch the thumb to the little finger. Diminished circulation and nerve function must be treated promptly by release of constricting bandages.

Hand

Trauma to the hand often requires extensive reconstructive surgery. The objective of treatment is always to regain maximum function of the hand.

MANAGEMENT

For an undisplaced fracture of the distal phalanx (finger bone), the finger is splinted for 3 to 4 weeks to relieve pain and protect the fingertip from further trauma. Displaced fractures and open fractures may require open reduction with internal fixation, using wires or pins.

The neurovascular status of the injured hand is evaluated. Swelling is controlled by elevation of the hand. Functional use of the uninvolved portions of the hand is encouraged.

Pelvis

The sacrum, ilium, pubis, and ischium bones form the pelvic bone, a fused, stable, bony ring in adults (Fig. 63-10). Pelvic fractures may be caused by falls, motor vehicle crashes, or crush injuries. Pelvic fractures are serious because at least two thirds of these patients have significant and multiple injuries. Management of severe, life-threatening pelvic fractures is coordinated with the trauma team. Hemorrhage and thoracic, intra-abdominal, and cranial injuries have priority over treatment of fractures. There is a high mortality rate associated with pelvic fractures from hemorrhage, pulmonary complications, fat emboli, intravascular coagulation, thromboembolic complications, and infection.

Pelvic fracture symptoms include ecchymosis; tenderness over the symphysis pubis, anterior iliac spines, iliac crest, sacrum, or coccyx; local swelling; numbness or tingling of pubis, genitals, and proximal thighs; and inability to bear weight without discomfort. Computed tomography of the pelvis helps to determine the extent of injury by demonstrating sacroiliac joint disruption, soft tissue trauma, pelvic hematoma, and fractures. Neurovascular assessment of the lower extremities is completed to detect injury to pelvic blood vessels and nerves.

Hemorrhage and shock are two of the most serious consequences that may occur. Bleeding arises from the cancellous surfaces of the fracture fragments, from laceration of veins and arteries by bone spicules, and possibly from a torn iliac artery. The peripheral pulses of both lower extremities are palpated; absence of pulses may indicate a torn iliac artery or one of its branches. Peritoneal lavage may be performed to detect intra-abdominal hemorrhage. The patient is handled gently to minimize further bleeding and shock.

The nurse assesses for injuries to the bladder, rectum, intestines, other abdominal organs, and pelvic vessels and nerves. To assess for urinary tract injury, the patient's urine is examined for blood. A voiding cystourethrogram and an intravenous urogram may be performed. Laceration of the urethra is suspected in males with anterior fracture of the pelvis and blood at the urethral meatus. (Females rarely experience lacerated urethra.) A catheter should not be inserted until the status of the urethra is known. Abdominal pain and signs of peritonitis suggest injury to the intestines or abdominal bleeding. Paralytic ileus may accompany pelvic fractures.

Numerous classification systems have been used to describe the pelvic fracture in relation to the anatomy, stability, and mecha-

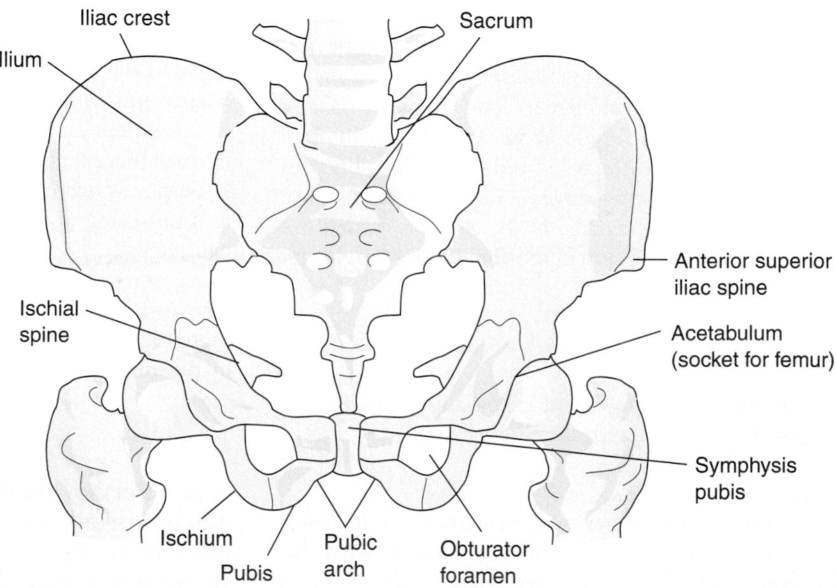

FIGURE 63•10 Pelvic bones.

nism of injury. Some fractures of the pelvis do not disrupt the pelvic ring, whereas others disrupt the ring and may be rotationally or vertically unstable. The severity of pelvic fractures varies.

During the period of immobility associated with pelvic fractures, exercises (leg, respiratory, range-of-motion, and strengthening), elastic stockings, and elevation of the foot of the bed to aid venous return are appropriate measures to help diminish the effects of bed rest. When prescribed, the patient is mobilized with progressive weight bearing, usually with crutches. Long-term complications of pelvic fractures include malunion, nonunion, residual gait disturbances, and back pain from ligament injury.

STABLE PELVIC FRACTURES

Stable fractures of the pelvis (Fig. 63-11) may include fracture of a single pubic or ischial ramus, fracture of ipsilateral pubic and ischial rami, fracture of the pelvic wing of ilium (ie, Duverney's fracture), or fracture of the sacrum or coccyx. Also, when an injury results in only a slight widening of the pubic symphysis or the anterior sacroiliac joint and the pelvic ligaments are intact, the disrupted pubic symphysis is likely to heal spontaneously with conservative management. Most fractures of the pelvis heal rapidly because the innominate bone (hip bone) is made up mostly of cancellous bone, which has a rich blood supply.

Stable pelvic fractures are treated with a few days of bed rest and symptom management until the pain and discomfort are controlled. The patient on bed rest is at risk for complications from immobility, including constipation, venous stasis, and pulmonary complications. Fluids, dietary fiber, ankle and leg exercises, log rolling, coughing and deep breathing, and skin care reduce the risk for complications and increase the patient's comfort. The patient with a fractured sacrum is at risk for paralytic ileus, and bowel sounds should be monitored.

The patient with fracture of the coccyx experiences pain on sitting and with defecation. Sitz baths may be prescribed to relieve pain, and stool softeners may be given to prevent the need to strain on defecation. As pain resolves, activity is gradually resumed using ambulatory aids for protected weight bearing. Early mobilization reduces immobility-related problems.

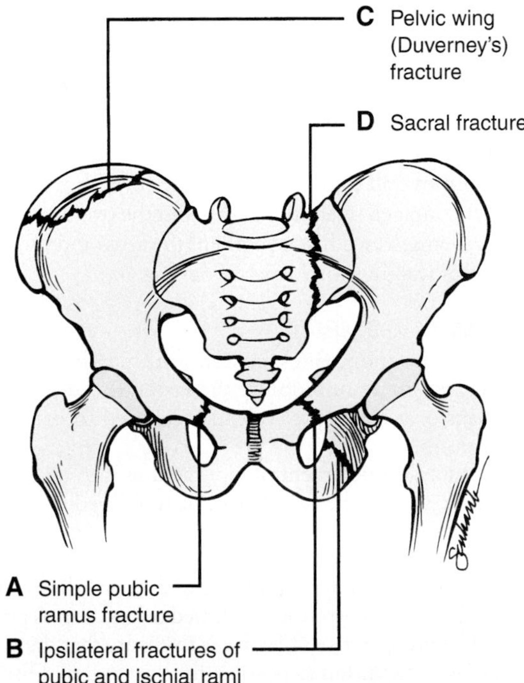

FIGURE 63•11 Stable pelvic fractures.

UNSTABLE PELVIC FRACTURES

Unstable fractures of the pelvis (Fig. 63-12) may be rotationally unstable (eg, the open book type in which a separation occurs at the symphysis pubis with some sacral ligament disruption), vertically unstable (eg, vertical shear type with superior-inferior displacement of the sides of the pelvis), or a combination of both. Lateral or anterior-posterior compression of the pelvis produces rotationally unstable pelvic fractures. Vertically unstable pelvic fractures occur when force is exerted on the pelvis vertically, such as happens to those falling from a height onto extended legs or those struck from above by a falling object. Treatment of unstable pelvic fractures generally involves external fixation or open reduction and internal fixation. This promotes hemostasis, hemodynamic stability, comfort, and early mobilization.

VERTICAL SHEAR PELVIC FRACTURES

Vertical shear pelvic fractures involve the anterior and posterior pelvic ring with vertical displacement, usually through the sacroiliac joint. There is generally complete disruption of posterior sacroiliac, sacrospinous, and sacrotuberous ligaments. Vertical displacement of the hemipelvis is usually evident. Treatment modalities may include external fixation with or without skeletal traction and open reduction internal fixation.

ACETABULUM

Fractures of the acetabulum are seen after motor vehicle crashes in which the femur is jammed into the dashboard. Treatment depends on the pattern of fracture. Some fractures are managed with traction; some are managed with protected weight bearing. Displaced and unstable acetabular fractures are treated with open reduction, joint débridement, and internal fixation or arthroplasty. Internal fixation permits early non–weight-bearing ambulation and range-of-motion exercise. Complications seen with acetabular fractures include nerve palsy, heterotopic ossification, and posttraumatic arthritis.

Hip

There is a high incidence of hip fractures among elderly people, who have brittle bones from osteoporosis (particularly women) and who tend to fall frequently. Weak quadriceps muscles, general frailty due to age, and conditions that produce decreased cerebral arterial perfusion (transient ischemic attacks, anemia, emboli, cardiovascular disease, effects of medications) contribute to the incidence of falls. The patient who has sustained a hip fracture frequently has a comorbidity (ie, cardiovascular, pulmonary, renal, endocrine). A hip fracture is often viewed by the patient and the family as a catastrophic event that will have a negative impact on the patient's lifestyle and quality of life.

There are two major types of hip fractures. *Intracapsular fractures* are fractures of the neck of the femur. *Extracapsular fractures* are fractures of the trochanteric region (between the base of the neck and the lesser trochanter of the femur) and the subtrochanteric region (Fig. 63-14A). Fractures of the neck of the femur may damage the vascular system that supplies blood to the head and the neck of the femur. The nutrient vessels within the bone may be interrupted, and the bone may die. For this reason, nonunion or aseptic necrosis is common in patients with these types of fractures.

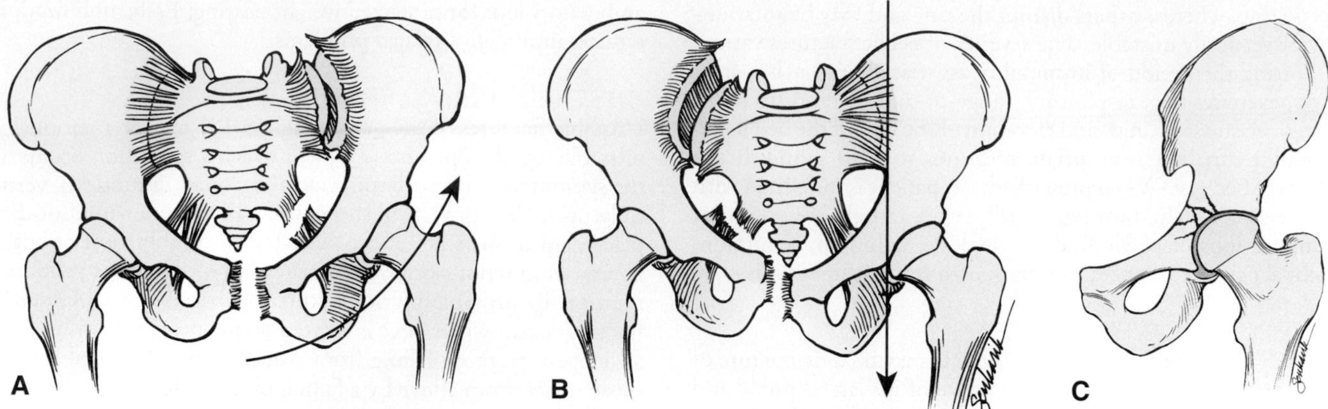

FIGURE 63•12 Unstable pelvic fracture. (**A**) Rotationally unstable fracture. Symphysis pubis separated and anterior sacroiliac, sacrotuberous, and sacrospinous ligaments disrupted. (**B**) Vertically unstable fracture. Displacement of hemipelvis anteriorly and posteriorly through symphysis pubis and sacroiliac joint ligaments disrupted. (**C**) Undisplaced fracture of the acetabulum.

Extracapsular intertrochanteric fractures have an excellent blood supply and heal readily. Extensive soft tissue damage, however, may occur at the time of injury. It is not uncommon for the fracture to be comminuted and unstable. There is a fairly high mortality rate after intertrochanteric hip fractures, mainly because the patients are usually elderly (ages 70 to 85 years) and are poor surgical candidates.

CLINICAL MANIFESTATIONS

With fractures of the femoral neck, the leg is shortened, adducted, and externally rotated. The patient may complain of slight pain in the groin or in the medial side of the knee. With most fractures of the femoral neck, the patient is unable to move the leg without significant increase in pain. The patient is most comfortable with the leg slightly flexed in external rotation. Impacted femoral neck fractures cause moderate discomfort (even with movement), may allow the patient to bear weight, and may not demonstrate obvious shortening or rotational changes. With extracapsular femoral fractures, the extremity is significantly shortened, externally rotated to a greater degree than intracapsular fractures, exhibits muscle spasm that resists positioning of the extremity in a neutral position, and has an associated large hematoma or area of ecchymosis. The diagnosis of fractured hip is confirmed on x-rays.

GERONTOLOGIC CONSIDERATIONS

Hip fractures are a frequent contributor to death after the age of 75 years. Stress and immobility related to the trauma predispose the older adult to pneumonia, sepsis, and reduced ability to cope with other health problems.

Many elderly people hospitalized with hip fracture are confused as a result of the stress of the trauma, unfamiliar surroundings, sleep deprivation, medications, and systemic illness. Preoperative predictors of postoperative delirium include age older than 70 years, alcohol abuse, poor cognitive status, poor functional status, and markedly abnormal serum sodium, potassium, or glucose (Marcantonio, et al, 1994). In addition, confusion that develops in some elderly patients may be due to mild cerebral ischemia. Other factors associated with confusion include responses to medications and anesthesia, malnutrition, dehydration, infectious processes, mood disturbances, and blood loss.

To prevent complications, the nurse must assess the elderly patient for chronic conditions that require close monitoring. Examination of the legs may reveal edema due to congestive heart failure and peripheral pulselessness from arteriosclerotic vascular disease. Similarly, chronic respiratory problems may be present and contribute to the possible development of inadequate pulmonary ventilation. Coughing and deep-breathing exercises are encouraged. Frequently, the elderly are taking cardiac, antihypertensive, or respiratory medications that need to be continued. The patient's responses to these medications should be monitored.

Dehydration and poor nutrition may be present. At times, elderly people who live alone are unable to summon help at the time of injury. A day or two may pass before assistance is provided, and as a result, dehydration occurs. Dehydration contributes to hemoconcentration and predisposes to thromboembolism problems. Therefore, the patient needs to be encouraged to consume adequate fluids and a balanced diet.

Muscle weakness and wasting may have contributed to the fall and fracture in the first place. Bed rest and immobility will cause an additional loss of muscle strength unless the nurse encourages the patient to move all joints except the involved hip and knee. Patients are encouraged to use their arms and the overhead trapeze to reposition themselves. This strengthens the arms and shoulders, which facilitates walking with assistive devices.

MEDICAL MANAGEMENT

Temporary skin traction, Buck's extension, may be applied to reduce muscle spasm, to immobilize the extremity, and to relieve pain. Sandbags or a trochanter roll may be used to control the external rotation.

The goal of surgical treatment of hip fractures is to obtain a satisfactory fixation so that the patient can be mobilized quickly and avoid secondary medical complications. Surgical treatment consists of (1) open reduction of the fracture and internal fixation (ORIF) or (2) replacement of the femoral head with a prosthesis (hemiarthroplasty). Surgical intervention is carried out as soon as possible after injury. The preoperative objective is to ensure that the patient is in as favorable a condition as possible for the surgery. Displaced femoral neck fractures may be treated as emergencies, and reduction and internal fixation are performed within 12 to 24 hours after frac-

NURSING RESEARCH

Effects of Confusion and Pain in Elderly Surgical and Trauma Patients

Miller, J., Moore, K., Schofield, A., & Ng'andu, N. (1996). A study of discomfort and confusion among elderly surgical patients. *Orthopaedic Nursing 15*(6), 27–34.

Purpose

The researchers investigated the assessment of discomfort in elderly, confused patients who had experienced trauma or surgery.

Study Sample and Design

This descriptive study focused on discomfort of older adults, more than 74 years of age, who were hospitalized in an orthopedic or trauma unit and had a NEECHAM Confusion Scale score of less than 27. Little research has included the confused patient. Acute pain may overwhelm confused patients and increase their confusion, diminishing their ability to participate in care activities.

The researchers examined the assessment and management of pain and discomfort during postoperative nursing activities (turning in bed, transfers from bed, venipunctures). Their research questions addressed (1) the relationship of an objective measure of discomfort, the Discomfort Screen–Dementia Alzheimer Type (modified) (DS-DAT), and self-report by confused elderly surgical patients of discomfort in response to direct questioning; (2) the relationship between level of acute confusion and ability of confused elderly surgical patients to self-report discomfort; and (3) identification of actions taken by nurses to manage the discomfort of acutely confused elderly adults.

Forty-seven patients older than 74 years of age were screened for acute confusion, and 36 were found to be at risk for confusion or to be acutely confused during screening. These 36 patients served as subjects for this study. The Discomfort Conditions Screen of the patient's medical record demonstrated that these subjects had acute discomfort from a fall or surgery as well as chronic pain from conditions such as arthritis or degenerative disk disease.

Findings

During nursing activities, these patients were noted to have discomfort as scored on the DS-DAT. Many of the patients who acknowledged pain were unable to rate the pain. Patients who were less confused reported more discomfort. Patients who were more severely confused were unable to quantify the amount of their discomfort on a scale of 0 to 10.

Few nursing actions to reduce pain and discomfort were observed. Usually, nursing assessments, when performed, were of the patient's physical state and only occasionally of the level of comfort. Analgesics were not given before transfers or other painful nursing interventions. Nurses did assist patients with repositioning, which could contribute to their comfort. Patient instructions for management of discomfort (eg, use of patient-controlled analgesia, deep breathing for relaxation) were infrequent.

Nursing Implications

The observations made in this study indicate that self-report is not a realistic indicator of pain and discomfort in elderly confused patients. The researchers encourage nurses to anticipate discomfort and engage in activities to modify discomfort and pain when they provide care for confused older adults.

ture. This minimizes the effects of diminished blood supply and reduces the risk for avascular necrosis.

After general or spinal anesthesia, the hip fracture is reduced under radiographic visualization using an image intensifier. A stable fracture is usually fixed with nails, a nail-and-plate combination, multiple pins, or compression screw devices (Fig. 63-13). The choice of fixation device is determined by the fracture site and the preference of the orthopedic surgeon. Adequate reduction is important for fracture healing (the better the reduction, the better the healing).

Replacement of the head of the femur with a prosthesis is usually reserved for a fracture that cannot be satisfactorily reduced or securely nailed. Some orthopedic surgeons prefer this method because nonunion and avascular necrosis of the head of the femur are common complications of internal fixation techniques. Total hip replacement (see Chap. 61) may be used in selected patients with acetabular defects.

POSTOPERATIVE NURSING MANAGEMENT

The immediate postoperative care of a patient with a hip fracture is similar to that for other patients undergoing major surgery (see Care of the Patient Undergoing Orthopedic Surgery in Chap. 61 and Unit 4). Attention is given to preventing secondary medical problems and to early mobilization of the patient so that independent functioning can be restored.

During the first 24 to 48 hours, relieving pain and preventing complications are priorities. The nurse encourages deep breathing, coughing, and foot flexion exercises every 1 to 2 hours. The nurse administers prescribed intravenous prophylactic antibiotics and monitors hydration, nutritional status, and urine output. Thigh-high elastic compression stockings and pneumatic compression devices are used to prevent venous stasis. A pillow is placed between the legs to maintain abduction and alignment and to provide needed support when turning.

Repositioning the Patient. The nurse may turn the patient on the affected or unaffected extremity as prescribed by the physician. The standard method involves placing a pillow between the legs to keep the affected leg in an abducted position. The patient is then turned onto the side while maintaining proper alignment and supported abduction.

Promoting Strengthening Exercise. The patient is encouraged to exercise as much as possible by means of the overbed trapeze. This helps strengthen the arms and shoulders in preparation for protected ambulation. On the first postoperative day, the patient transfers to a chair with assistance and begins assisted ambulation. The amount of weight bearing that can be permitted depends on the stability of the fracture reduction. The physician prescribes the amount of weight bearing permitted and the rate at which the patient can progress to full weight bearing. Physical therapists work with the patient on transfers, ambulation, and the safe use of walker and crutches.

The patient who has experienced a fractured hip can anticipate discharge with the use of an assistive device. Some modifications in the home may be needed to permit safe use of walkers and crutches and for the patient's continuing care.

Monitoring and Managing Potential Complications. Elderly people who suffer hip fractures are particularly prone to complications that may require more vigorous treatment than the fracture itself. In some instances, shock may prove fatal. Achievement of homeostasis after injury and surgery is accomplished through careful monitoring and collaborative management, including adjustment of therapeutic interventions as indicated.

Neurovascular complications may occur because of direct injury of nerves and blood vessels or from increased tissue pressure. With hip fracture, bleeding into the tissues is expected. Excessive

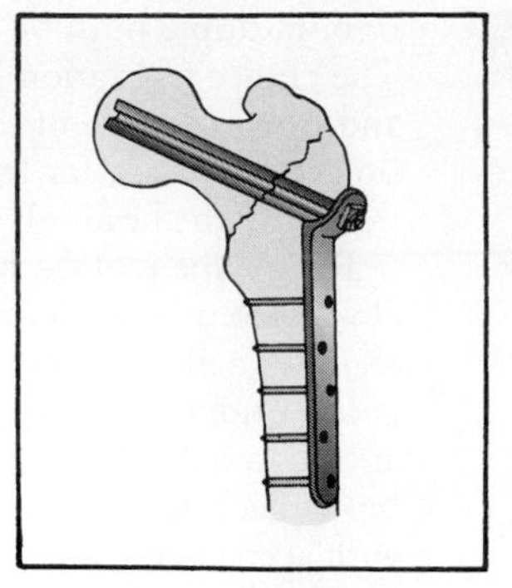
Smith-Petersen nail with McLaughlin plate

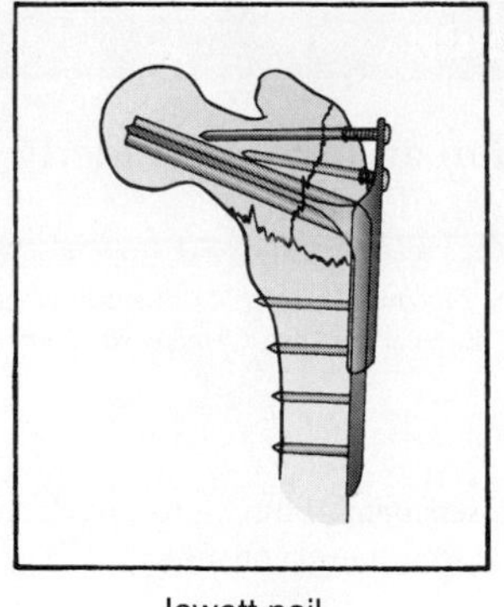
Jewett nail with overlay plate

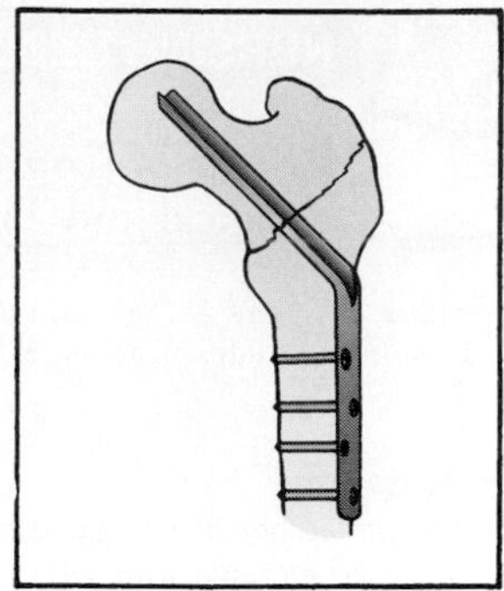
Neufeld nail

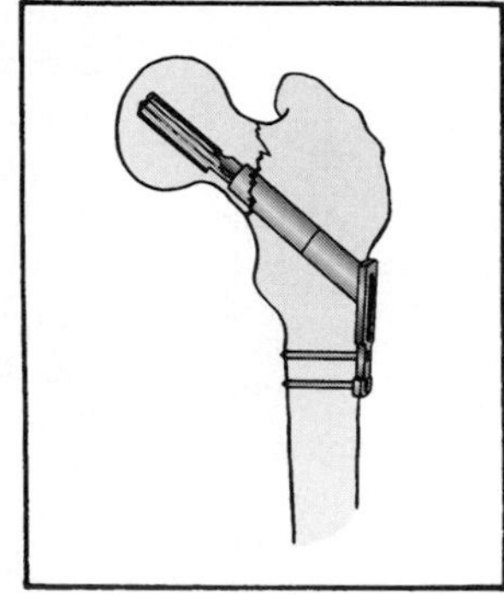
Massie nail assembly

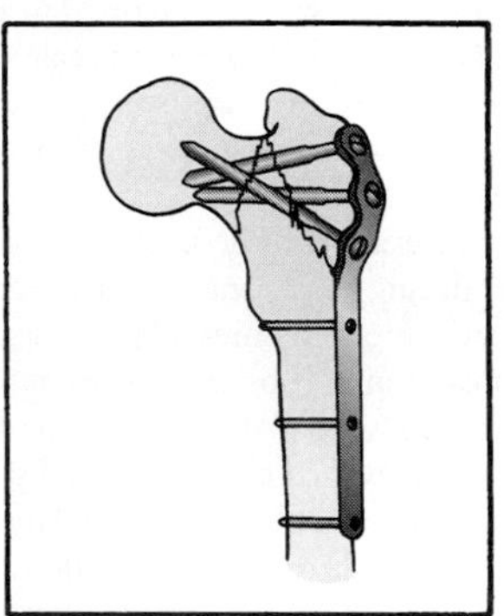
Moe intertrochanteric plate

FIGURE 63•13 Examples of internal fixation for hip fractures. Internal fixation is achieved through the use of nails and plates specifically designed for stability and fixation. Courtesy of Zimmer-USA, Warsaw, Indiana.

swelling may be observed. Therefore, the nurse must monitor the neurovascular status of the affected leg.

DVT is the most common complication. To prevent DVT, the nurse encourages fluids and ankle and foot exercises. Elastic stockings, sequential compression devices, and prophylactic anticoagulant therapy may be prescribed. The nurse assesses the patient's legs at least every 4 hours for signs of DVT.

Pulmonary complications are a threat to elderly patients undergoing hip surgery. Deep-breathing exercises, a change of position at least every 2 hours, and the use of an incentive spirometer help to prevent respiratory complications. The nurse assesses breath sounds at least every 4 to 8 hours to detect adventitious or diminished sounds.

Skin breakdown is often seen in elderly patients with fractured hips. Blisters caused by tape are related to the tension of soft tissue edema under the nonelastic tape. Elastic tape applied in a vertical fashion may reduce the incidence of tape blisters (Blaylock, et al, 1995). In addition, patients with hip fractures tend to remain in one position and may develop *pressure ulcers.* Proper skin care, especially on the heels, back, sacrum, and shoulders, helps to relieve pressure. A high-density foam, static air, or other special mattress may provide protection by distributing pressure more evenly.

Loss of bladder control (incontinence) may occur. In general, the routine use of an indwelling catheter is avoided because of the high risk for urinary tract infection. Urinary retention is common after surgery. Therefore, the nurse must assess the patient's voiding patterns. To ensure proper urinary tract function, the nurse encourages liberal fluid intake within the cardiovascular tolerance of the patient.

Delayed complications of hip fractures include *infection, nonunion, avascular necrosis* of the femoral head (particularly with femoral neck fractures), and *fixation device problems* (eg, protrusion of the fixation device through the acetabulum; loosening of hardware). Infection is suspected if the patient complains of moderate discomfort in the hip and has a mildly elevated sedimentation rate. The nursing management of the elderly patient with a hip fracture is summarized in Plan of Nursing Care 63-1.

Femoral Shaft

Considerable force is required to break the shaft of the femur in adults. Most of these fractures are seen in young men who have been involved in a motor vehicle crash or have fallen from a high place. Frequently, these patients have associated multiple trauma.

The patient presents with an enlarged, deformed, painful thigh and cannot move the hip or the knee. The fracture may be transverse, oblique, spiral, or comminuted. Frequently, the patient develops shock because the loss of 2 to 3 units of blood into the tissues is common with this fracture. An expanding diameter of the thigh may indicate continued bleeding.

ASSESSMENT AND DIAGNOSTIC FINDINGS

Assessment includes checking the neurovascular status of the extremity, especially circulatory perfusion of the foot (popliteal, posterior tibial, and pedal pulses and toe capillary refill are assessed), A Doppler ultrasound monitoring device may be needed to assess blood flow. Dislocation of the hip and knee may accompany these fractures. Knee effusion suggests ligament damage and possible instability of the knee joint.

MANAGEMENT

Continued neurovascular monitoring is needed. Treatment is begun with skin traction for comfort and immobilization of the fracture so that additional soft tissue damage does not occur.

(text continues on page 1856)

63•1

PLAN OF NURSING CARE 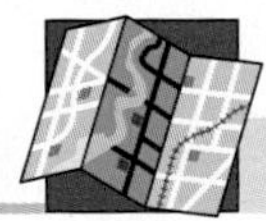 Care of the Elderly Patient With a Fractured Hip

Nursing Diagnosis: Pain related to fracture, soft tissue damage, muscle spasm, and surgery
Goal: Relief of pain

Nursing Interventions	Rationale	Expected Outcomes
1. Assess type and location of patient's pain.	1. Pain is expected after fracture; soft tissue damage and muscle spasm contribute to discomfort; pain is subjective and is evaluated through description of characteristics and location, which are important for determining cause of discomfort and for proposing interventions. Continuing pain may indicate development of neurovascular problems.	• Patient describes discomfort • Expresses confidence in efforts to control pain • Expresses little discomfort with position changes • Expresses comfort when leg is positioned and immobilized • Minimizes movement of extremity before reduction and fixation • Uses physical, psychological, and pharmacologic measures to reduce discomfort • Describes a decrease in pain in 24–48 hours after surgery • Requests pain medications and uses pain relief measures early in pain cycle • States that positioning provides comfort • Appears comfortable and relaxed • Moves with increasing comfort as healing progresses
2. Acknowledge existence of pain; inform patient of available analgesics; record patient's baseline discomfort.	2. Reduces stress experienced by the patient by communicating concern and availability of help in dealing with pain. Documentation provides baseline data.	
3. Handle the affected extremity gently, supporting it with hands or pillow.	3. Movement of bone fragments is painful; muscle spasms occur with movement; adequate support diminishes soft tissue tension.	
4. Apply Buck's traction as prescribed. Use trochanter roll.	4. Immobilizes fracture to decrease pain and additional tissue trauma; decreases muscle spasm and external rotation of hip.	
5. Use pain-modifying strategies.	5. Pain perception can be diminished by distraction and refocusing of attention.	
a. Modify the environment.	a. Interaction with others, distraction, and environmental stimuli may modify pain experiences.	
b. Administer prescribed analgesics as needed.	b. Analgesics reduce the pain; muscle relaxants may be prescribed to decrease discomfort associated with muscle spasm.	
c. Encourage patient to use pain relief measures before pain is "unbearable."	c. Mild pain is easier to control than severe pain.	
d. Evaluate patient's response to medications and other pain-reduction techniques.	d. Assessment of effectiveness of measures provides basis for future management interventions; early identification of adverse reactions is necessary for corrective measures and care plan modifications.	
e. Consult with physician if relief of pain is not obtained.	e. Change in treatment plan may be necessary.	
6. Position for comfort and function.	6. Alignment of body facilitates comfort; positioning for function diminishes stress on musculoskeletal system.	
7. Assist with frequent changes in position.	7. Change of position relieves pressure and associated discomfort.	

Nursing Diagnosis: Impaired physical mobility related to fractured hip
Goal: Achieves pain-free, functional, stable hip

Nursing Interventions	Rationale	Expected Outcomes
1. Maintain neutral positioning of hip.	1. Prevents stress on fixation.	• Patient engages in therapeutic positioning • Uses pillow between legs when turning • Assists in position changes; shows increased independence in transfers • Exercises hourly
2. Use trochanter roll.	2. Minimizes external rotation.	
3. Place pillow between legs when turning.	3. Supports leg; prevents adduction.	
4. Instruct and assist in position changes and transfers.	4. Encourages patient's active participation while preventing stress on hip fixation.	

(continued)

63•1 PLAN OF NURSING CARE

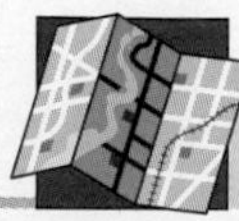

Care of the Elderly Patient With a Fractured Hip (*continued*)

Nursing Interventions	Rationale	Expected Outcomes
5. Instruct in and supervise isometric, quadriceps-setting, and gluteal-setting exercises.	5. Strengthens muscles needed for walking.	• Uses trapeze • Participates in progressive ambulation program • Actively participates in exercise regimen • Uses ambulatory aids correctly and safely
6. Encourage use of trapeze.	6. Strengthens shoulder and arm muscles necessary for use of ambulatory aids.	
7. In consultation with physical therapist, instruct in and supervise progressive safe ambulation within limitations of weight-bearing prescription.	7. Amount of weight-bearing depends on the patient's condition, fracture stability, and fixation device; ambulatory aids are used to assist the patient with non–weight-bearing and partial–weight-bearing ambulation.	
8. Offer encouragement and support exercise regimen.	8. Reconditioning exercises can be uncomfortable and fatiguing; encouragement helps patient comply with the program.	
9. Instruct in and supervise safe use of ambulatory aids.	9. Prevents injury from unsafe use.	

Nursing Diagnosis: Actual impairment of skin integrity related to surgical incision
Goal: Achieves wound healing

Nursing Interventions	Rationale	Expected Outcomes
1. Monitor vital signs.	1. Temperature, pulse, and respiration increase in response to infection. (Magnitude of response may be minimal in elderly patients.)	• Patient maintains vital signs within normal range • Exhibits well-approximated incision without drainage or excessive inflammatory response • Relates minimal discomfort; demonstrates no hematoma • Tolerates antibiotics; exhibits no evidence of osteomyelitis
2. Use aseptic dressing changes.	2. Avoids introducing infectious organisms.	
3. Assess wound appearance and character of drainage.	3. Red, swollen, draining incision is indicative of infection.	
4. Assess complaint of pain.	4. Pain may be due to wound hematoma, a possible locus of infection, which needs to be surgically evacuated.	
5. Administer prophylactic antibiotic if prescribed, and observe for side effects.	5. Osteomyelitis is to be avoided.	

Nursing Diagnosis: Potential alteration in patterns of urinary elimination related to immobility
Goal: Maintains normal urinary elimination patterns

Nursing Interventions	Rationale	Expected Outcomes
1. Monitor intake and output.	1. Adequate fluid intake ensures hydration; adequate urinary output minimizes urinary stasis.	• Intake and output are adequate; patient exhibits normal voiding patterns • Demonstrates no evidence of urinary tract infection
2. Avoid/minimize use of indwelling catheter.	2. Source of bladder infection.	

Nursing Diagnosis: Potential ineffective individual coping related to injury, anticipated surgery, and dependence
Goal: Uses effective coping mechanisms to modify stress

Nursing Interventions	Rationale	Expected Outcomes
1. Encourage patient to express concerns and to discuss the possible impact of fractured hip.	1. Verbalization helps patient deal with problems and feelings. Clarification of thoughts and feelings promotes problem-solving.	• Patient describes feelings concerning fractured hip and implications for lifestyle • Uses available resources and coping mechanisms; develops health promotion strategies • Uses community resources as needed • Participates in development of health care plan
2. Support use of coping mechanisms. Involve significant others and support services as needed.	2. Coping mechanisms modify disabling effects of stress; sharing concerns lessens the burden and facilitates necessary modification.	
3. Contact social services, if needed.	3. Anxiety may be related to financial or social problems; facilitates management of problems associated with continuing care.	
4. Explain anticipated treatment regimen and routines to facilitate positive attitude in relation to rehabilitation.	4. Understanding of plan of care helps to diminish fears of the unknown.	
5. Encourage patient to participate in planning.	5. Participating in care provides for some control of self and environment.	

(*continued*)

63•1

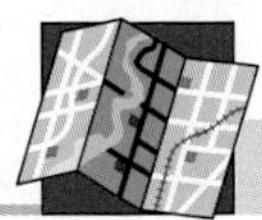

PLAN OF NURSING CARE — Care of the Elderly Patient With a Fractured Hip (*continued*)

Nursing Interventions	Rationale	Expected Outcomes
Nursing Diagnosis: Potential alteration in thought process related to age, stress of trauma, unfamiliar surroundings, and medication therapy **Goal:** Remains oriented and participates in decision making		
1. Assess orientation status.	1. Evaluate presenting orientation of patient; confusion may result from stress of fracture, unfamiliar surroundings, coexisting systemic disease, cerebral ischemia, or other factors. Baseline data are important for determining change.	• Patient establishes effective communication • Demonstrates orientation to time, place, and person • Participates in self-care activities • Remains mentally alert • Avoids episodes of confusion
2. Interview family regarding patient's orientation and cognitive abilities before injury.	2. Provides data for evaluation of current findings.	
3. Assess patient for auditory and visual deficits.	3. Diminished vision and auditory acuity frequently occur with aging; glasses and hearing aid may increase patient's ability to interact with environment.	
a. Assist patient with use of sensory aids (eg, glasses, hearing aid) b. Control environmental distractors	a. Aids must be in good working order and available for use. b. Facilitates communication.	
4. Orient to and stabilize environment a. Use orientation activities and aids (eg, clock, calendar, pictures, introduction of self). b. Minimize number of staff working with patient.	4. a. Short-term memory may be faulty in the elderly; frequent reorientation helps. b. Consistency of caregivers promotes trust.	
5. Give simple explanations of procedures and plan of care.	5. Promotes understanding and active participation.	
6. Encourage participation in hygiene and nutritional activities.	6. Participation in routine activities promotes orientation, increases awareness of self.	
7. Provide for safety. a. Keep side rails up when patient is in bed. b. Keep light on at night. c. Have call bell available. d. Provide prompt response to requests for assistance.	7. Side rails decrease chance for additional injury from falls; mechanism for securing assistance is available to patient; independent activities based on faulty judgment may result in injury.	
8. Assess mental responses to medications, especially sedatives and analgesics.	8. Elderly people tend to be more sensitive to medications; abnormal responses (eg, hallucinations, depression) may occur.	
Collaborative Problems: Hemorrhage; neurovascular compromise; deep vein thrombosis; pulmonary complications; pressure ulcers related to surgery and immobility **Goal:** Patient experiences an absence of complications		
Hemorrhage 1. Monitor vital signs, observing for shock.	1. Changes in pulse, blood pressure, and respirations may indicate development of shock; blood loss and stress may contribute to development of shock.	• Vital signs are stabilized within normal limits • Experiences no excessive or bright red drainage • Exhibits hemoglobin and hematocrit values within normal limits
2. Consider preinjury blood pressure values and management of coexisting hypertension, if present.	2. Necessary for interpretation of current blood pressure determinations.	
3. Note character and amount of drainage.	3. Excessive drainage and bright red drainage may indicate active bleeding.	
4. Notify surgeon if patient develops shock or excessive bleeding.	4. Corrective measures need to be instituted.	

(*continued*)

63•1

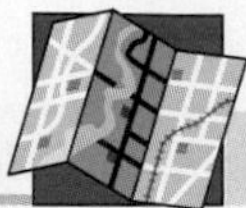

PLAN OF NURSING CARE — Care of the Elderly Patient With a Fractured Hip (*continued*)

Nursing Interventions	Rationale	Expected Outcomes
5. Note hemoglobin and hematocrit values, and report decreases in values.	5. Anemia due to blood loss may develop; bleeding into tissues after hip fracture may be extensive; blood replacement may be needed.	
Pulmonary Complications		
1. Assess lung status: respiratory rate, depth, and duration, breath sounds, sputum. Monitor temperature.	1. Anesthesia and bed rest diminish respiratory effort and cause pooling of respiratory secretions. Adventitious breath sounds, respiratory pain, shortness of breath, blood tinged sputum, cough, etc., indicate possible pulmonary emboli.	• Patient has clear breath sounds • Breath sounds present in all fields • Exhibits no shortness of breath, chest pain, or elevated temperature • Po_2 on room air within normal limits • Performs respiratory exercises; uses incentive spirometer as instructed • Changes position frequently • Consumes adequate fluids
2. Report adventitious and diminished breath sounds and elevated temperature.	2. Elevated temperature in the early postoperative period may be due to a respiratory problem.	
3. Supervise deep breathing and coughing exercises. Encourage use of incentive spirometer if prescribed.	3. Promote optimal ventilation. Coexisting respiratory conditions diminish lung expansion.	
4. Administer oxygen as prescribed.	4. Reduced ventilatory efforts may diminish Po_2 when patient is on room air.	
5. Turn and reposition patient at least every 2 hours. Mobilize patient (assist patient out of bed) as soon as possible.	5. Promotes optimal ventilation. Diminishes pooling of respiratory secretions.	
6. Ensure adequate hydration.	6. Liquefies respiratory secretions. Facilitates expectoration.	
Neurovascular Compromise		
1. Assess affected extremity for color and temperature.	1. The skin becomes pale and feels cool with decreased tissue perfusion. Venous congestion may cause cyanosis.	• Patient has normal color and the extremity is warm • Demonstrates normal capillary refill response • Exhibits moderate swelling; tissue not palpably tense • States pain is controllable • Reports no pain with passive dorsiflexion • Reports normal sensations and no paresthesia • Demonstrates normal motor abilities and no paresis or paralysis • Has strong and equal pulses
2. Assess toes for capillary refill response.	2. After compression of the nail, rapid return of pink color indicates good capillary perfusion.	
3. Assess affected extremity for edema and swelling.	3. The trauma of surgery will cause swelling; excessive swelling and hematoma formation can compromise circulation and function; edema may be due to coexisting cardiovascular disease.	
4. Elevate affected extremity.	4. Minimizes dependent edema.	
5. Assess for deep, throbbing, unrelenting pain.	5. Surgical pain can be controlled; pain due to neurovascular compromise is refractory to treatment with analgesics.	
6. Assess for pain on passive flexion of foot.	6. With nerve ischemia, there will be pain on passive stretch.	
7. Assess for sensations and numbness.	7. Diminished pain and paresthesia may indicate nerve damage. Sensation in web between great and second toe—peroneal nerve; sensation on sole of foot—tibial nerve.	
8. Assess ability to move foot and toes.	8. Dorsiflexion of ankle and extension of toes indicate function of peroneal nerve. Plantar flexion of ankle and flexion of toes indicate functioning of tibial nerve.	
9. Assess pedal pulses in both feet.	9. Indicator of circulatory status of extremities.	
10. Notify surgeon if diminished neurovascular status occurs.	10. Function of extremity needs to be preserved.	

(*continued*)

63•1 PLAN OF NURSING CARE 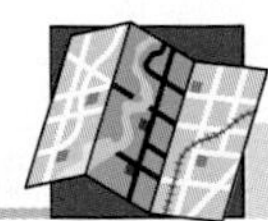

Care of the Elderly Patient With a Fractured Hip (*continued*)

Nursing Interventions	Rationale	Expected Outcomes
Deep Vein Thrombosis		
1. Apply thigh-high elastic stockings and/or sequential compression device as prescribed.	1. Compression aids venous blood return and prevents stasis.	• Wears thigh-high elastic stockings • Uses sequential compression device • Experiences no skin breakdown • Experiences no more warmth than usual in skin areas • Exhibits no increase in calf circumference • Demonstrates a negative Homans' sign • Changes position with assistance and supervision • Participates in exercise regimen • Experiences no chest pain; has lungs clear to auscultation; presents no evidence of pulmonary emboli • Exhibits no signs of dehydration; has normal hematocrit • Maintains normal body temperature
2. Remove stockings for 20 minutes twice a day, and provide skin care.	2. Skin care is necessary to avoid skin breakdown. Extended removal of stocking or device defeats purpose.	
3. Assess popliteal, dorsalis pedis, and posterior tibial pulses.	3. Pulses indicate arterial perfusion of extremity. With coexisting arteriosclerotic vascular disease, pulses may be diminished or absent.	
4. Assess skin temperature of legs.	4. Local inflammation increases local skin temperature.	
5. Assess for Homans' sign every 4 hours.	5. Pain in calf on dorsiflexion of ankle may indicate deep vein thrombosis.	
6. Measure calf circumference twice daily.	6. Increased calf circumference indicates edema or altered perfusion.	
7. Avoid pressure on popliteal blood vessels from appliances or pillows.	7. Compression of blood vessels diminishes blood flow.	
8. Change position and increase activity as prescribed.	8. Activity promotes circulation and diminishes venous stasis.	
9. Supervise ankle exercises hourly.	9. Muscle exercise promotes circulation.	
10. Ensure adequate hydration.	10. Elderly people may become dehydrated because of low fluid intake, resulting in hemoconcentration.	
11. Monitor body temperature.	11. Body temperature increases with inflammation (magnitude of response minimal in elderly people).	
Pressure Ulcers		
1. Monitor condition of skin at pressure points (eg, heels, sacrum, shoulders).	1. Elderly patients are subject to skin breakdown at points of pressure because of diminished subcutaneous tissue.	• Patient exhibits no signs of skin breakdown • Skin remains intact • Repositions self frequently • Uses protective devices
2. Reposition patient at least every 2 hours. Avoid skin shearing.	2. Avoids prolonged pressure and trauma to the skin.	
3. Administer skin care, especially to pressure points.	3. Immobility causes pressure at bony prominences; position changes relieve pressure.	
4. Use special care mattress and other protective devices (eg, heel protectors).	4. Devices minimize pressure on skin at bony pominences.	
5. Institute care according to protocol at first indication of potential skin breakdown.	5. Early interventions prevent tissue destruction and prolonged rehabilitation.	

Nursing diagnosis: Potential impaired home maintenance related to fractured hip and impaired mobility
Goal: Cares for self at home

Nursing Interventions	Rationale	Expected Outcomes
1. Assess home environment for discharge planning.	1. Physical barriers (especially stairs, bathrooms) may limit patient's ability to ambulate and care for self at home.	• Home is accessible for patient at time of discharge • Patient appears relaxed and develops strategies to deal with identified problems • Has personal assistance available • Demonstrates ability to use necessary assistance within therapeutic prescription • Complies with home care program; keeps follow-up health care appointments
2. Encourage patient to express concerns about care at home; explore with patient possible solutions to problems.	2. Patient may have special problems that need to be identified and dealt with.	
3. Assess availability of physical assistance for health care activities.	3. Because of limitation of mobility, patient may require some assistance in routine health care.	
4. Teach caregiver the home health care regimen.	4. Understanding of rehabilitative regimen is necessary for compliance.	

(*continued*)

63•1 PLAN OF NURSING CARE

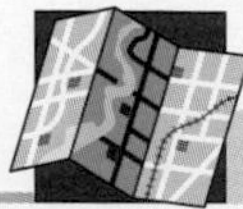

Care of the Elderly Patient With a Fractured Hip (*continued*)

Nursing Interventions	Rationale	Expected Outcomes
5. Instruct patient in posthospital care: a. Activity limitations b. Reinforce exercise instructions c. Safe use of ambulatory aids d. Wound care e. Measures to promote healing (nutrition, wound care) f. Medications, if any g. Potential problems h. Continuing health care supervision	5. Lack of knowledge and poor preparation for care at home contribute to patient anxiety, insecurity, and nonadherence to therapeutic regimen.	

Generally, skeletal traction (Fig. 63-14) is used to achieve muscle relaxation and alignment of the fracture fragments before open reduction and internal fixation procedures.

Internal fixation is generally carried out a few days after injury. Intramedullary nailing devices, interlocking nail, or compression plate and screws provide adequate internal fixation, permitting early mobilization. Active muscle movement enhances healing by increasing blood supply and electrical potentials at the fracture site. A thigh cuff orthosis may be used for external support. Compression plates may need to be removed after 18 months. When plates are being removed, a thigh cuff orthosis is used for several months to provide support while bone remodeling occurs.

Fractures of the middle and distal shaft (supracondylar) may be managed with skeletal traction. Two to 4 weeks after the injury, when pain and swelling have subsided, the patient is removed from skeletal traction and placed in a cast brace. The cast (fracture) brace is a total contact device that holds the reduced fracture. The muscle, through hydrodynamic compression, stabilizes the bone and stimulates healing. Minimal partial weight bearing is begun and is progressed to full weight bearing as tolerated. Functional ambulation stimulates fracture healing. The cast brace is worn for 12 to 14 weeks. An external fixator may be used if the patient has experienced an open grade III fracture, has extensive soft tissue trauma, has lost bone, has an infection, or has hip and tibial fractures.

A major management goal for femoral shaft fractures is rapid functional healing with sufficient strength to support the multiple stresses placed on the femur. To preserve muscle strength, the patient should exercise the lower leg, foot, and toes on a regular basis. A common complication after fracture of the femoral shaft

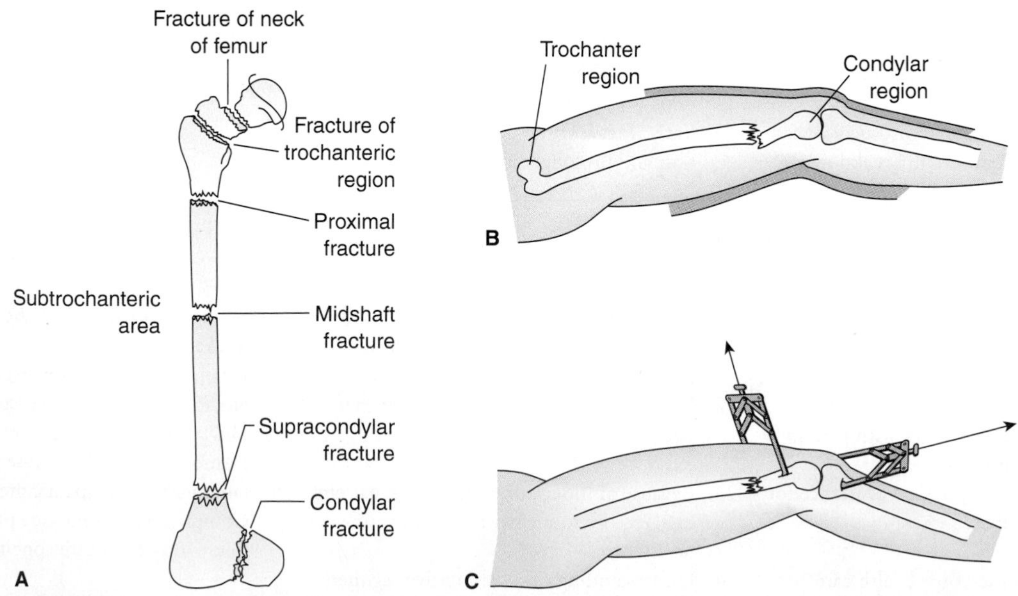

FIGURE 63•14 (**A**) Kinds of femoral fractures. One method of correction for a fracture of the femur in distal third is two-wire skeletal traction. (**B**) Example of deformity on admission to hospital. (**C**) Adequate reduction is achieved when additional wire is inserted in lower femoral fragment and vertical lift is secured.

is restriction of knee motion. Active and passive knee exercises are performed as soon as possible, depending on the management approach and the stability of the fracture and knee ligaments.

Tibia and Fibula

The most common fracture below the knee is one of the tibia (and fibula) that results from a direct blow, falls with the foot in a flexed position, or a violent twisting motion. Fractures of the tibia and fibula often occur in association with each other. The patient presents with pain, deformity, obvious hematoma, and considerable edema. Frequently, these fractures involve severe soft tissue damage because there is little subcutaneous tissue in the area.

ASSESSMENT AND DIAGNOSTIC FINDINGS

Peroneal nerve damage is assessed. If nerve function is impaired, the patient is unable to dorsiflex the great toe and has diminished sensation in the first web space. Tibial artery damage is assessed by evaluating skin temperature and color and by testing the capillary refill response. Fracture near the joint may be complicated by hemiarthroses or ligament damage.

The patient is monitored for an anterior compartment syndrome. Symptoms include pain unrelieved by medications and increasing with plantar flexion, tense and tender muscle lateral to tibial crest, and paresthesia.

MANAGEMENT

Most closed tibial fractures are treated with closed reduction and initial immobilization in a long leg-walking or patellar-tendon-bearing cast. Reduction must be relatively accurate in relation to angulation and rotation. At times, it is difficult to maintain reduction, and percutaneous pins may be placed in the bone and held in position by a plaster cast (ie, pins-in-plaster technique), or an external fixator may be used. Partial weight bearing is usually prescribed in 7 to 10 days. Activity decreases edema and increases circulation. The cast is changed to a short leg cast or brace in 3 to 4 weeks, which allows for knee motion. Fracture healing takes 6 to 10 weeks.

Comminuted fractures may be treated with skeletal traction; internal fixation with rods, plates, or nails; or external fixation. External plaster support may be used with internal fixation. Foot and knee exercises are encouraged within the limits of the immobilizing device. Weight bearing is begun when prescribed, usually in about 4 to 6 weeks. Open fractures are treated with external fixation. Distal fractures with extensive soft tissue damage heal slowly and may require bone grafting.

As with other lower-extremity fractures, the leg should be elevated to control edema. Continued neurovascular evaluation is needed. The development of compartment syndrome requires prompt recognition and resolution to prevent permanent functional deficit.

Rib

Uncomplicated fractures of the ribs occur frequently in adults and usually result in no impairment of function. Because these fractures produce painful respirations, the patient tends to decrease respiratory excursions and refrains from coughing. As a result, tracheobronchial secretions are not mobilized, aeration of the lung is diminished, and a predisposition to *pneumonia* and *atelectasis* results. To help the patient cough and take deep breaths, the nurse may splint the chest with her hands. Occasionally, intercostal nerve blocks may be administered by the physician to relieve pain and permit productive coughing.

Chest strapping to immobilize the rib fracture is *not* usually used because decreased chest expansion may result in pneumonia and atelectasis. The pain associated with rib fracture diminishes significantly in 3 or 4 days, and the fracture heals within 6 weeks. In addition to pneumonia and atelectasis, complications may include a *flail chest, pneumothorax,* and *hemothorax.* The management of patients with these conditions is discussed in Chapter 22.

Thoracolumbar Spine

Fractures of the thoracolumbar spine may involve (1) the vertebral body, (2) the lamina and articulating processes, and (3) the spinous processes or transverse processes. The T12 to L2 area of the spine is most vulnerable to fracture. Fractures are generally due to indirect trauma caused by excessive loading, sudden muscle contraction, or excessive motion beyond physiologic limits. Osteoporosis contributes to vertebral body collapse.

The patient with a spinal fracture presents with acute tenderness, swelling, paravertebral muscle spasm, and change in normal curves or gap between spinous processes. Pain is greater when moving, coughing, or weight bearing. Immobilization is essential until initial assessments have determined if there is any spinal cord injury and if the fracture is stable or unstable. Few spinal fractures are associated with neurologic deficits. If spinal cord injury with neurologic deficit does occur, it usually requires immediate surgery (laminectomy with spinal fusion) to decompress the spinal cord.

Stable spinal fractures are due to flexion, extension, lateral bending, or vertical loading. The anterior structural column (vertebral bodies and disks) or the posterior structural column (neural arch, articular processes, ligaments) has been disrupted. Unstable fractures occur with fracture-dislocations and exhibit disruption of both anterior and posterior structural columns. The potential for neural damage exists.

MEDICAL MANAGEMENT

Stable spinal fractures are treated conservatively with limited bed rest, with the head of bed elevated less than 30 degrees until the acute pain subsides (several days). Analgesics are prescribed for pain relief. The patient is monitored for a transient *paralytic* ileus due to associated retroperitoneal hemorrhage. Sitting is avoided until the pain subsides. A spinal brace or plastic thoracolumbar orthosis may be applied for support during progressive ambulation and resumption of activities.

The patient with an unstable fracture is on bed rest possibly using a special turning device (eg, Stryker frame) to maintain spinal alignment. Neurologic status is monitored closely during the preoperative and postoperative periods. Within 24 hours of fracture, open reduction, decompression, and fixation with spinal fusion and instrument stabilization are usually accomplished. Postoperatively, the patient may be cared for on the turning device or bed with firm mattress. Progressive ambulation is begun a few days after surgery with the patient using a body brace orthosis. Patient teaching emphasizes good posture, good body mechanics, and, when healing is sufficient, back-strengthening exercises.

AMPUTATION

Amputation is the removal of a body part, usually an extremity. Amputation of a lower extremity is often necessary as a result of progressive peripheral vascular disease (often a sequela of diabetes mellitus), fulminating gas gangrene, trauma (crushing injuries, burns, frostbite, electrical burns), congenital deformities, chronic osteomyelitis, or malignant tumor. Of all these causes, peripheral vascular disease accounts for most amputations of lower extremities. (See Chap. 28 for more information.)

Amputation can be considered a type of reconstructive surgery. It is used to relieve symptoms, improve function, and save or improve the patient's quality of life. If the health care team communicates a positive attitude, the patient adjusts to the amputation more readily and actively participates in the rehabilitative plan, learning how to modify activities and how to use assistive devices for ADLs and mobility.

Levels of Amputation

Amputation is performed at the most distal point that will heal successfully. The site of amputation is determined by two factors: circulation in the part, and functional usefulness (ie, meets the requirements of the prosthesis).

The circulatory status of the extremity is evaluated through physical examination and specific studies. Muscle and skin perfusion is important for healing. Doppler flowmetry, segmental blood pressure determinations, and transcutaneous partial pressure of oxygen (PaO_2) are valuable diagnostic aids. Angiography is performed if revascularization is considered an option.

The objective of surgery is to conserve as much extremity length as possible. Preservation of knee and elbow joints is desired. Figure 63-15 shows the different levels at which an extremity may be amputated. Almost any level of amputation can be fitted with a prosthesis.

The amputation of toes and portions of the foot causes minor changes in gait and balance. A Syme's amputation (modified ankle disarticulation amputation) is performed most frequently for extensive foot trauma and produces a painless, durable extremity end that can withstand full weight-bearing. Below-knee amputations are preferred to above-knee amputations because of the importance of the knee joint and the energy requirements for walking. Knee disarticulations are most successful with young, active patients who are able to develop precise control of the prosthesis. When above-knee amputations are performed, all possible length is preserved, muscles are stabilized and shaped, and hip contractures are prevented for maximum ambulatory potential. If a hip disarticulation amputation is performed, most people must rely on a wheelchair for mobility. Upper-extremity amputations are performed to preserve the maximum functional length. The prosthesis is fitted early for maximum function.

A *staged amputation* may be used when gangrene and infection exist. Initially, a guillotine amputation is performed to remove the necrotic and septic tissue. The wound is débrided and allowed to drain. The sepsis is treated with systemic antibiotics. In a few days, when the infection has been controlled and the patient has stabilized, a definitive amputation with skin closure is performed.

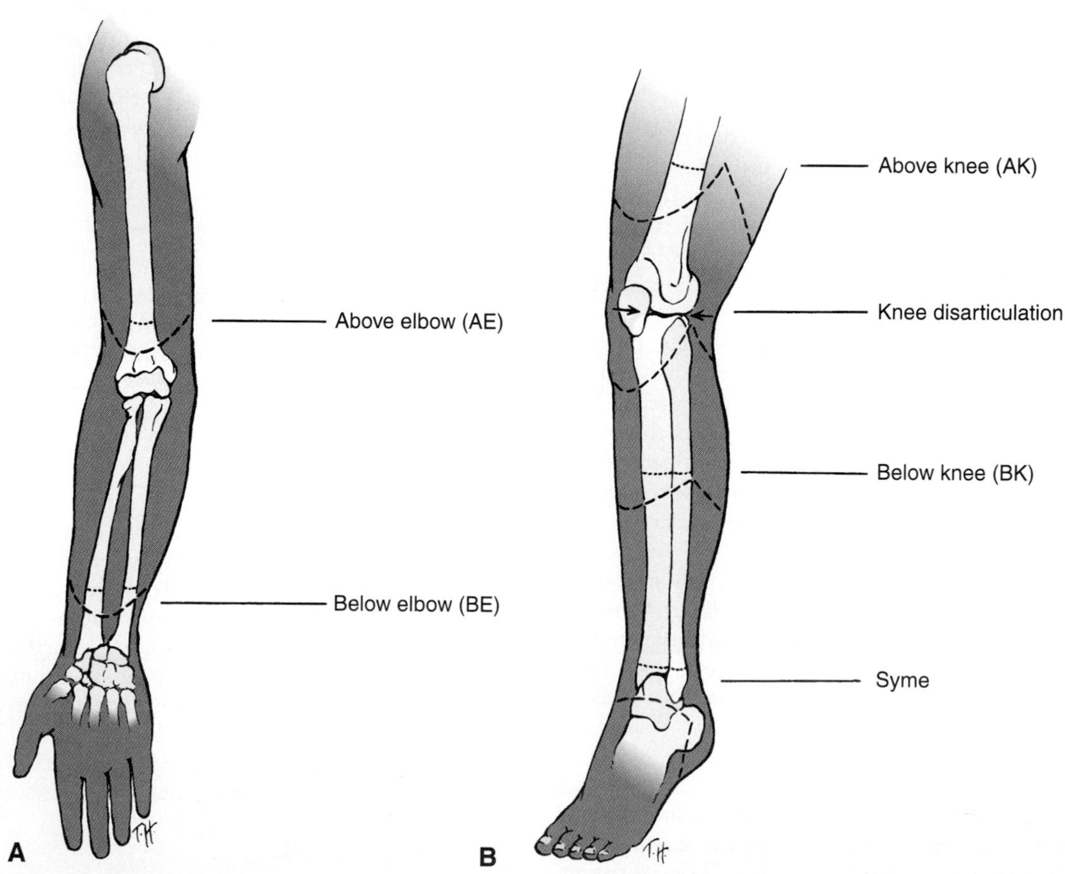

FIGURE 63•15 Levels of amputation are determined by circulatory adequacy, type of prosthesis, function of the part, and muscle balance. (**A**) Levels of amputation of upper extremity. (**B**) Levels of amputation of lower extremity.

Complications

Complications that may occur with amputation include *hemorrhage, infection, skin breakdown,* and *phantom limb pain.* Because major blood vessels have been severed, massive bleeding may occur. Infection is a risk in all surgical procedures. The risk for infection increases with contaminated wounds after traumatic amputation. Skin irritation caused by the prosthesis may result in skin breakdown. Phantom limb pain is due to the severing of peripheral nerves.

Medical Management of Lower Extremity Amputation

The objective is to achieve healing of the amputation wound, resulting in a nontender residual limb (stump) with healthy skin for prosthesis use. Healing is enhanced by gentle handling of the residual limb, controlling residual limb edema through rigid or soft compression dressings, and using aseptic technique in wound care to avoid infection.

A *closed rigid cast dressing* is frequently used to provide uniform compression, to support soft tissues to control pain, and to prevent contractures. Immediately after surgery, a sterilized residual limb sock is applied to the residual limb. Felt pads are placed over pressure-sensitive areas. The residual limb is wrapped with elastic plaster-of-paris bandages while firm, even pressure is maintained. Care is taken not to constrict circulation. The plaster cast is equipped to attach a temporary prosthetic extension (pylon) and an artificial foot. This rigid dressing technique is used as a means of creating a socket for immediate postoperative prosthetic fitting. The length of the prosthesis is tailored to the individual patient. Early minimal weight-bearing on the residual limb with rigid cast dressing and pylon attached produces little discomfort. The cast is changed in about 10 to 14 days. Elevated body temperature, severe pain, or a loose-fitting cast may require earlier replacement.

A *soft dressing* with or without compression may be used when frequent inspection of the residual limb (stump) is desired. An immobilizing splint may be incorporated in the dressing. Stump (wound) hematomas are controlled with wound drainage devices to minimize infection.

Rehabilitation Therapy

Patients who require amputation due to severe trauma are generally, but not always, young and healthy, heal rapidly, and participate in a vigorous rehabilitation program. Because the amputation is the result of an injury, the patient needs much psychological support in accepting the sudden change in body image and in dealing with the stresses of hospitalization, long-term rehabilitation, and modification of lifestyle. These patients need time to work through their feelings about their permanent loss and change in body image. Their reactions are unpredictable and can include anger, bitterness, and hostility.

The multidisciplinary rehabilitation team (patient, nurse, physician, social worker, psychologist, prosthetist, vocational rehabilitation worker) helps the patient achieve the highest possible level of function and participation in life activities (Fig. 63-16). Prosthetic clinics and amputee support groups facilitate this rehabilitation process. Vocational counseling and job retraining may be necessary to help patients return to work.

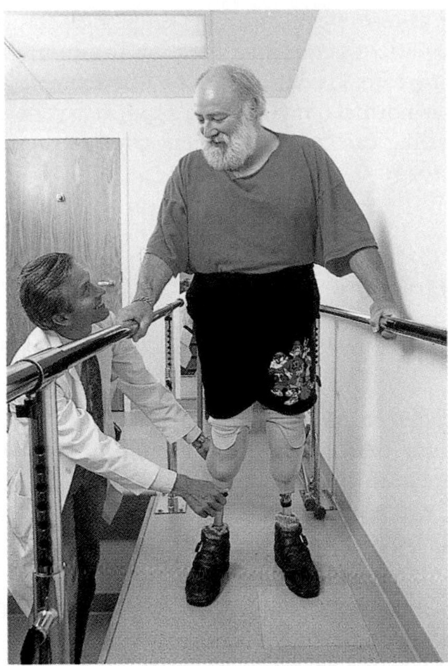

FIGURE 63•16 Many amputees receive prostheses soon after surgery and begin learning how to use them with the help and support of the rehabilitation team, which includes nurses, physicians, physical therapists and others.

Psychological problems (eg, denial, withdrawal) may be influenced by the type of support the patient receives from the rehabilitation team and by how quickly ADLs and use of the prosthesis are learned. Knowing the full options and capabilities available with the various prosthetic devices can give the patient a sense of control over the disability. The patient is not fully rehabilitated until a prosthesis has been fitted and the patient has learned how to use it. This is best accomplished in a specialized rehabilitation unit or center.

NURSING PROCESS: THE PATIENT UNDERGOING AN AMPUTATION

Assessment

Before surgery, the nurse must evaluate the neurovascular and functional status of the extremity through history and physical assessment. If the patient has experienced a traumatic amputation, the nurse assesses the function and condition of the residual limb. The nurse also assesses the circulatory status and function of the unaffected extremity. If infection or gangrene develop, the patient may have associated enlarged lymph nodes, fever, and purulent drainage. A culture is taken to determine appropriate antibiotic therapy.

The nurse evaluates the patient's nutritional status and creates a plan for nutritional care if indicated. For wound healing, a balanced diet with adequate protein and vitamins is essential.

Any concurrent health problems (eg, dehydration, anemia, cardiac insufficiency, chronic respiratory problems, diabetes mellitus) need to be identified and treated so that the patient is in the best possible condition to withstand the trauma of surgery. The use of corticosteroids, anticoagulants, vasoconstrictors, or vasodilators may influence management and wound healing.

The nurse assesses the patient's psychological status. Determination of the patient's emotional reaction to amputation is essential for nursing care. Grief response to a permanent alteration in body image is normal. An adequate support system and professional counseling can help the patient cope in the aftermath of amputation surgery.

Diagnosis

Nursing Diagnoses

Based on the assessment data, the patient's major nursing diagnoses may include the following:

- Pain related to amputation
- Sensory/perceptual alteration: phantom limb pain related to amputation
- Impaired skin integrity related to surgical amputation
- Body image disturbance related to amputation of body part
- Coping, ineffective (individual) related to failure to accept loss of body part
- Grieving related to loss of body part
- Self-care deficit: feeding, bathing, dressing, grooming, and toileting, related to loss of extremity
- Impaired physical mobility related to loss of extremity

Collaborative Problems/Potential Complications

Based on the assessment data, potential complications that may develop include the following:

- Postoperative hemorrhage
- Infection
- Skin breakdown

Planning and Goals

The major goals of the patient may include relief of pain, absence of altered sensory perceptions, wound healing, acceptance of altered body image, resolution of the grieving process, independence in self-care, restoration of physical mobility, and absence of complications.

Nursing Interventions

Relieving Pain

Surgical pain can be effectively controlled with opioid analgesics, nonpharmaceutical interventions, or evacuation of the hematoma or accumulated fluid. The pain may be an expression of grief and alteration of body image. Severe pain may be due to excessive pressure on a bony prominence or hematoma. Muscle spasms may add to the patient's discomfort. Changing the patient's position or placing a light sandbag on the residual limb to counteract the muscle spasm may improve the patient's level of comfort. Evaluation of the patient's pain and responses to interventions is an important part of the nurse's role in pain management.

Minimizing Altered Sensory Perceptions

Amputees usually experience *phantom limb* pain soon after surgery or 2 to 3 months after amputation. It occurs more frequently in above-knee amputations. The patient describes pain or unusual sensation, such as a feeling that the extremity is present and is crushed, cramped, or twisted in an abnormal position. When a patient describes phantom pains or sensations, the nurse acknowledges these feelings and helps the patient modify these perceptions.

Phantom sensation eventually disappears. The pathogenesis of the phantom limb phenomenon is unknown. Keeping the patient active helps decrease the occurrence of phantom limb pain. Early intensive rehabilitation and stump desensitization with kneading massage brings relief. Distraction techniques and activity are helpful. Transcutaneous electrical nerve stimulation, ultrasound, or local anesthetics may provide relief for some patients. In addition, β-blockers may relieve dull, burning discomfort; anticonvulsants control stabbing and cramping pain; and tricyclic antidepressants are used to improve mood and coping ability.

Promoting Wound Healing

The residual limb must be handled gently. Whenever the dressing is changed, aseptic technique is required to prevent wound infections and possible osteomyelitis.

Nursing Alert *If the cast or elastic dressing inadvertently comes off, the nurse must immediately wrap the residual limb with an elastic compression bandage. If not, excessive edema will develop in a short time, resulting in a delay in rehabilitation. The nurse notifies the surgeon if a cast dressing comes off so that another cast can be applied.*

Residual limb shaping is important for prosthesis fitting. The nurse instructs the patient in wrapping the residual limb with elastic dressings (Figs. 63-17 and 63-18). When the incision is healed, the nurse teaches the patient to care for the residual limb.

Enhancing Body Image

Amputation is a reconstructive procedure that alters the patient's body image. The nurse who has established a trusting relationship with the patient is better able to communicate acceptance of the patient who has experienced an amputation. The nurse encourages the patient to look at, feel, and then care for the residual limb. It is important to identify the patient's strength and resources to facilitate rehabilitation. The nurse assists the patient to regain the previous level of independent functioning. The patient who is accepted as a whole person is more readily able to resume responsibility for self-care; self-concept improves, and body-image changes are accepted. Even with highly motivated patients, this process may take months.

Helping the Patient Resolve Grieving

The loss of an extremity (or part of one) may come as a shock even though the patient was prepared preoperatively. The patient's behavior (eg, crying, withdrawal, apathy, anger) and expressed feelings (eg, depression, fear, helplessness) will demonstrate how the patient is coping with the loss and working through the grieving process. The nurse acknowledges the loss by listening and providing support.

The nurse creates an accepting and supportive atmosphere in which the patient and family are encouraged to express and share their feelings and work through the grief process. Support from family and friends promotes acceptance of the loss. The nurse helps the patient deal with immediate needs and become oriented to realistic rehabilitation goals and future independent functioning. Referrals to a mental health specialist and support groups may be appropriate.

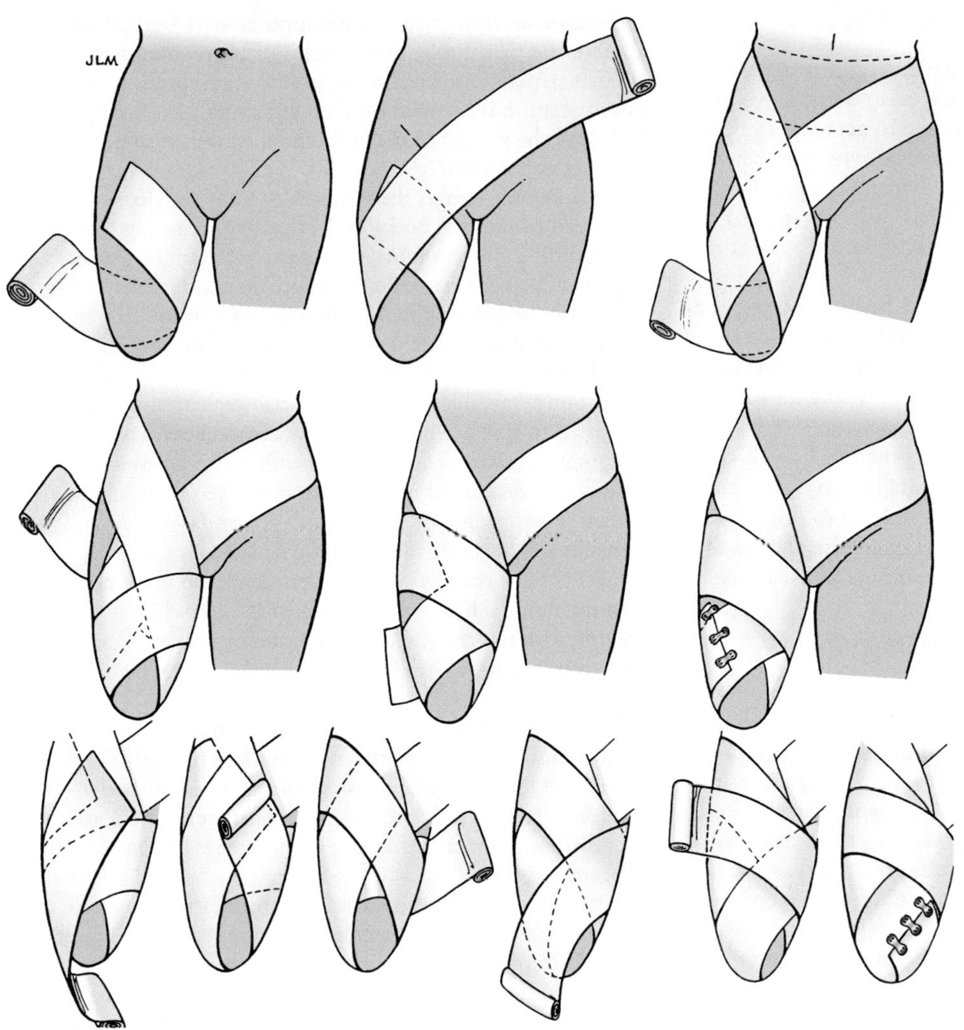

FIGURE 63•17 Wrapping the residual leg after an above-knee amputation. Elastic bandaging minimizes edema and shapes the stump in a firm conical form to fit a prosthesis.

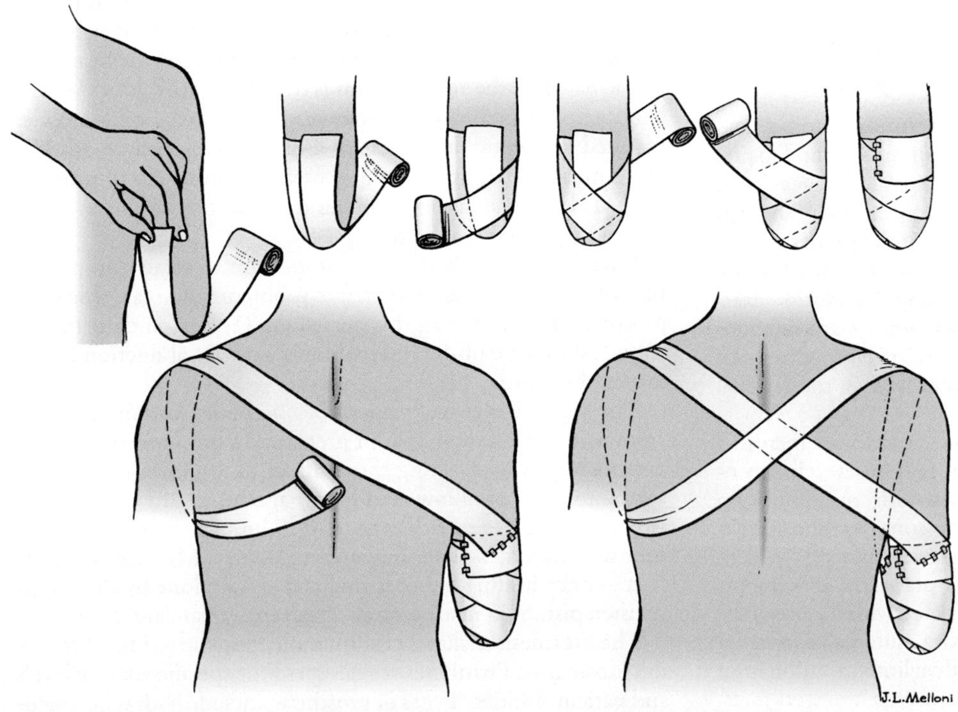

FIGURE 63•18 Wrapping the residual arm after an above-elbow amputation. Passing the bandage wrap across the back and shoulders may augment security.

Promoting Independent Self-Care

Amputation of an extremity affects the patient's ability to provide adequate self-care. The patient is encouraged to be an active participant in self-care. The patient needs time to accomplish these tasks and must not be rushed. Practicing an activity with consistent, supportive supervision in a relaxed environment enables the patient to learn self-care skills. The patient and nurse need to maintain positive attitudes and minimize fatigue and frustration during the learning process.

Independence in dressing, toileting, and bathing (shower or tub) depends on balance, transfer abilities, and physiologic tolerance of the activities. The nurse works with the physical therapist and occupational therapist in teaching and supervising the patient in these self-care activities.

The patient with an upper-extremity amputation has self-care deficits in feeding, bathing, and dressing. Assistance is provided only as needed; the nurse encourages the patient to learn to do the task using feeding and dressing aids. The nurse, therapists, and prosthetist work with the patient to achieve maximum independence.

Helping the Patient Achieve Physical Mobility

The upper extremities, trunk, and the abdominal muscles are exercised and strengthened. The extensor muscles in the arm and the depressor muscles in the shoulder play an important part in crutch walking. An overhead trapeze can be used by the patient to change position and strengthen the biceps. The patient may flex and extend the arms while holding weights. Doing push-ups while seated strengthens the triceps muscles. Exercises, such as hyperextension of the residual limb, conducted under the supervision of the physical therapist, also aid in strengthening muscles as well as increasing circulation, reducing edema, and preventing atrophy.

To prevent the development of a hip or knee contracture, abduction, external rotation, and flexion of the lower extremity are avoided. Depending on the surgeon's preference, the residual limb may be placed in an extended position or elevated for a brief period after surgery. If the residual limb is to be elevated, this should be done by raising the foot of the bed.

***Nursing Alert** The residual limb should not be placed on a pillow because a flexion contracture of the hip may result.*

The nurse encourages the patient to turn from side to side and to assume a prone position to stretch the flexor muscles and to prevent flexion contracture of the hip. The nurse discourages sitting for prolonged periods to prevent flexion contracture. The legs should remain close together to prevent an abduction deformity.

Postoperative range-of-motion exercises are started early because contracture deformities develop rapidly. Range-of-motion exercises include hip and knee exercises for below-knee amputations and hip exercises for above-knee amputations. It is important that the patient understand the importance of exercising the residual limb.

Strength and endurance are assessed and activities are increased gradually to prevent fatigue. As the patient progresses to independent use of the wheelchair, ambulation with aids, or ambulation with prosthesis, the nurse emphasizes safety considerations. Environmental barriers (eg, steps, inclines, doors, wet surfaces) are identified, and methods of managing them are practiced. It is important to identify and manage problems associated with the use of the mobility aids (eg, pressure on the axilla from crutches, skin irritation of the hands from wheelchair use, residual limb irritation from prosthesis).

Because an upper-extremity amputee uses both shoulders to operate the prosthesis, the muscles of both shoulders are exercised. A patient with an above-the-elbow amputation or shoulder disarticulation is likely to develop a postural abnormality caused by loss of the weight of the amputated extremity. Thus, postural exercises are helpful.

Amputation changes the center of gravity; therefore, the patient may need to practice position changes (eg, standing from sitting and standing on one foot). The patient is taught transfer techniques early and is reminded to maintain good posture when getting out of bed. A well-fitting shoe with a nonskid sole should be worn. During position changes, the patient should be guarded and stabilized with a transfer belt at the waist to prevent falling.

As soon as possible, the patient with lower extremity amputation is assisted to stand between parallel bars to allow extension of the temporary prosthesis to the floor with minimal weight bearing. How soon after surgery the patient is allowed to touch down the artificial foot depends on the patient's physical status. As endurance increases and balance is achieved, ambulation is started within the parallel bars or crutches. The patient learns to use a normal gait with the residual limb moving back and forth while the patient is walking with the crutches. To prevent a permanent flexion deformity from occurring, the residual limb should *not* be held up in a flexed position.

The patient with an upper extremity amputation is taught how to carry out the ADLs with one arm. The patient is started on one-handed self-care activities as soon as possible. The use of the temporary prosthesis is encouraged. The patient who learns to use the prosthesis soon after the amputation relies less on one-handed self-care activities.

A patient with an upper extremity amputation may wear a cotton T-shirt to prevent contact between the skin and shoulder harness and to promote absorption of perspiration. The prosthetist advises about cleaning the washable portions of the harness. Periodically, the prosthesis is inspected for potential problems.

The residual limb must be conditioned and shaped into a conical form to permit accurate fit, maximum comfort, and function of the prosthetic device. This is done by applying bandages, an elastic residual limb shrinker, or an air splint. The nurse teaches the patient or a member of the family the correct method of bandaging.

Bandaging supports the soft tissue and minimizes the formation of edema while the residual limb is in a dependent position. The bandage is applied in such a manner that the remaining muscles required to operate the prosthesis are as firm as possible, whereas those muscles that are no longer useful atrophy. An improperly applied elastic bandage contributes to circulatory problems and a poorly shaped residual limb.

Effective preprosthetic care is important to ensure proper fitting of the prosthesis. The major problems that can delay the prosthetic fitting during this period are (1) flexion deformities, (2) nonshrinkage of the residual limb, and (3) abduction deformities of the hip.

The physician usually prescribes activities to condition or "toughen" the residual limb in preparation for a prosthesis. The patient begins by pushing the residual limb into a soft pillow, then into a firmer pillow, and finally against a hard surface. The patient is taught to massage the residual limb to mobilize the scar, decrease tenderness, and improve vascularity. Massage is usually started once healing has occurred and is first done by the physical therapist. Skin inspection and preventive care are taught.

The prosthesis socket is custom molded to the residual limb by the prosthetist. Prostheses are designed for specific activity levels and patient abilities. Types of prostheses include hydraulic, pneumatic, biofeedback-controlled, myoelectrically controlled, and synchronized prostheses.

Adjustments of the prosthetic socket are made by the prosthetist to accommodate the residual limb changes that occur during the first 6 months to 1 year after surgery. A light plaster cast, an elastic bandage, or a shrinking sock is used to limit edema during the times the patient is not wearing the permanent prosthesis.

Some patients may not be candidates for a prosthesis and are thus *nonambulatory amputees.* If use of a prosthesis is not possible, the patient is instructed in the use of a wheelchair to achieve independence. A special wheelchair designed for patients who have had amputations is recommended. Because of the decreased weight in the front, a regular wheelchair may tip backward when the patient sits in it. In an amputee wheelchair, the rear axle is set back about 5 cm (2 inches) to compensate for the change in weight distribution.

Monitoring and Managing Potential Complications

After any surgery, efforts are made to reestablish homeostasis and prevent problems related to surgery, anesthesia, and immobility. The nurse assesses body systems (eg, respiratory, gastrointestinal, genitourinary) for problems associated with immobility (eg, pneumonia, anorexia, constipation, urinary stasis) and institutes corrective management. Avoiding problems associated with immobility and restoring physical activity are necessary for maintenance of health.

Massive *hemorrhage* due to a loosened suture is the most threatening problem. The nurse monitors the patient for any signs or symptoms of bleeding. It is also important to monitor the patient's vital signs, and observe the suction drainage.

Nursing Alert *Immediate postoperative bleeding may develop slowly or take the form of a massive hemorrhage resulting from a loosened suture. A large tourniquet should be in plain sight at the patient's bedside so that if severe bleeding occurs, it can be applied to the residual limb to control the hemorrhage. The nurse immediately notifies the surgeon in the event of excessive bleeding.*

Infection is a frequent complication of amputation. Patients who have undergone traumatic amputation have a contaminated wound. The nurse administers antibiotics as prescribed. It is important to monitor the incision, dressing, and drainage for indications of infection (eg, change in color, odor, consistency of drainage, increasing discomfort). The nurse also monitors for systemic indicators of infection (eg, elevated temperature) and promptly reports indications of infection to the surgeon.

Skin breakdown may result from immobilization and pressure from various sources. The prosthesis may cause pressure areas to develop. The nurse and the patient assess for breaks in the skin. Careful skin hygiene is essential to prevent skin irritation, infection, and breakdown. The residual limb is washed and dried (gently) at least twice daily. The skin is inspected for pressure areas, dermatitis, and blisters. If present, they must be treated before further skin breakdown occurs. Usually, a residual limb sock is worn to absorb perspiration and prevent direct contact between the skin and the prosthetic socket. The sock is changed daily and must fit smoothly to prevent irritation caused by wrinkles. The socket of the prosthesis is washed with a mild detergent, rinsed, and dried thoroughly with a clean cloth. The nurse advises the patient that the socket must be thoroughly dry before the prosthesis is applied.

Promoting Home and Community-Based Care

TEACHING PATIENTS SELF-CARE

Before discharge to the home or to a rehabilitation facility, the nurse encourages the patient and family to become active participants in care. They participate, as appropriate, in skin care and residual limb care and in the management of the prosthesis. The patient receives ongoing instructions and practice sessions in learning how to transfer and how to use mobility and ADL aids safely. The nurse explains signs and symptoms of complications that must be reported to the physician.

CONTINUING CARE

When the patient has achieved physiologic homeostasis and has demonstrated achievement of major health care goals, rehabilitation continues either in a rehabilitation facility or at home. Continued support and supervision by the home care nurse are essential.

HOME CARE TEACHING CHECKLIST: AMPUTATION

At the completion of the program, the patient or caregiver will be able to:	Patient	Caregiver
• Describe approaches to controlling pain (eg, take analgesics as prescribed; use nonpharmacologic interventions).	✔	✔
• Report pain that is uncontrolled by analgesics and other pain management techniques.	✔	
• Describe care of residual limb and conditioning for prosthesis.	✔	✔
• Consume balanced diet to promote wound healing.	✔	
• Demonstrate ability to transfer.	✔	
• Use mobility and activity aids safely.	✔	
• Participate in rehabilitation program to regain functional independence.	✔	✔
• State indicators of complication to report promptly to physician (eg, uncontrolled pain; signs of local or systemic infection; residual limb skin breakdown).	✔	✔
• Identify professionals and community agencies to help with transition to home.	✔	✔
• Identify support group to facilitate rehabilitation.	✔	
• Describe effects of amputation on self-image.	✔	
• Acknowledge grieving as part of coping process.	✔	
• Identify modifications of home environment to promote safe environment and independence during rehabilitation.	✔	✔

Before the patient's discharge to the home, the nurse should assess the home environment. Modifications are made to ensure the patient's continuing care, safety, and mobility. An overnight or weekend experience at home may be tried to identify problems that were not identified on the assessment visit. Physical therapy and occupational therapy may continue in the home or on an outpatient basis. Transportation to continuing health care appointments must be arranged. The social service department of the hospital or community agency managing continued health care may be of great assistance in securing personal assistance and transportation services.

During follow-up health visits, the nurse evaluates the patient's physical and psychosocial adjustment. Periodic preventive health assessments are necessary. Frequently, an elderly spouse is unable to provide the assistance required, and additional help at home is needed. Modifications in the plan of care are made on the basis of such findings. Often, the patient and family find involvement in an amputee support group to be of value; here, they are able to share problems, solutions, and resources. Talking with those who have successfully dealt with a similar problem may help the patient develop a satisfactory solution.

Evaluation

Expected Outcomes

Expected outcomes may include:

1. Experiences absence of pain
   a. Appears relaxed
   b. Verbalizes comfort
   c. Uses measures to increase comfort
   d. Participates in self-care and rehabilitative activities
2. Experiences absence of phantom limb pain
   a. Reports not perceiving sensations from amputated part
   b. Verbalizes absence of abnormal sensation in residual limb
3. Achieves wound healing
   a. Controls residual limb edema
   b. Achieves healed, nontender, nonadherent scar
   c. Demonstrates residual limb care
4. Demonstrates improved body image
   a. Acknowledges change in body image
   b. Participates in self-care activities
   c. Demonstrates increasing independence
   d. Projects self as a whole person
   e. Resumes role-related responsibilities
   f. Reestablishes social contacts
   g. Demonstrates confidence in abilities
5. Exhibits resolution of grieving
   a. Expresses grief
   b. Uses family and friends to work through feelings
   c. Focuses on future functioning
6. Achieves independent self-care
   a. Asks for assistance when needed
   b. Uses aids and assistive devices to facilitate self-care
   c. Verbalizes satisfaction with abilities to perform ADLs
7. Achieves maximum independent mobility
   a. Avoids positions contributing to contracture development
   b. Demonstrates full active range of motion
   c. Maintains balance when sitting and transferring
   d. Increases strength and endurance
   e. Demonstrates safe transferring technique
   f. Achieves functional use of prosthesis
   g. Overcomes environmental barriers to mobility
   h. Uses community services and resources as needed
8. Exhibits absence of complications of hemorrhage, infection, skin breakdown
   a. Does not experience excessive bleeding
   b. Maintains normal blood values
   c. Is free of local systemic signs of infection
   d. Repositions self frequently
   e. Is free of pressure-related problems
   f. Reports any skin discomfort and irritations promptly.

Critical Thinking Exercises

1.
A classmate tells you that she is going to start jogging and that her goal is to run in a marathon in several months. Describe the kind of advice you would give her and explain your rationale for making these suggestions.

2.
A middle-aged patient who has been hospitalized for 3 days with a fractured pelvis is making plans for discharge. His wife approaches you and expresses concern that he has become very irritable and that he "just doesn't seem to be himself." Analyze this information and speculate as to the possible causes for this behavior. Describe the additional kinds of information you would seek in a further assessment of the situation. What findings would confirm your initial speculation? What findings would lead to a different conclusion?

3.
You witness a person falling on a patch of ice and you offer assistance. She does not seem to be seriously injured, but she complains that her left elbow is sore and her left hand feels weak. She indicates that she thinks she can drive herself home and will then decide if she needs to seek medical attention. What conclusions would you draw from the complaints she described? Based on that conclusion, how would you advise her and why?

4.
You are visiting an elderly gentleman who is in an extended-care facility recovering from a below-knee amputation. He expresses satisfaction that he has progressed to the point that he has the stamina to sit in his wheelchair from breakfast time until after dinner. How would you advise him to modify his daily routine and why? Describe the plan of care you would devise for him and the outcomes you hope to have him achieve through this plan.

References and Selected Readings

BOOKS

Bucholz, R. W. (1996). *Orthopaedic decision making* (2nd ed.). St. Louis: C. V. Mosby.

Epps, C. (1994). *Complications in orthopaedic surgery* (3rd ed.). Philadelphia: J. B. Lippincott.

Jarvis, C. (1996). *Physical examination and health assessment.* Philadelphia: W. B. Saunders.

Maher, A. B., et al. (1998). *Orthopaedic nursing* (2nd ed.). Philadelphia: W. B. Saunders.

Malone, T. (1997). *Orthopedic and sports physical therapy* (3rd ed.). St. Louis: C. V. Mosby.

Mercier, L. R. (1995). *Practical orthopedics* (4th ed.). St. Louis: Mosby–Year Book.

Mourad, L. (1995). *Orthopaedic nursing.* Albany, NY: Delmar Publications.

Salmond, S. W., et al. (Eds.). (1996). *Core curriculum for orthopaedic nursing* (3rd ed.). Pitman, NJ: National Association of Orthopaedic Nurses.

Simon, R., & Koenigsknecht, S. (1995). *Emergency orthopedics: The extremities* (3rd ed.). Norwalk, CT: Appleton & Lang.

Turek, S., et al. (1994). *Turek's orthopaedics: Principles and their application* (5th ed.). Philadelphia: J. B. Lippincott.

JOURNALS

Asterisks indicate research articles.

Adami, S., et al. (1997). Bisphosphonate therapy of reflex sympathetic dystrophy syndrome. *Annals of Rheumatic Disease, 56*(3), 201–204.

*Anders, R., & Ornellas, E. (1997). Acute management of patient with hip fracture. *Orthopaedic Nursing, 16*(2), 31–46.

Artlet, J., & Mazieres, B. (1997). Medical treatment of refex sympathetic dystrophy. *Hand Clinics, 13*(3), 477–483.

*Blaylock, B., et al. (1995). Tape injury in the patient with total hip replacement. *Orthopaedic Nursing, 14*(3), 25–28.

Blitch, E. L., & Ricotta, P. J. (1996). Introduction to bone grafting. *Journal of Foot and Ankle Surgery, 35*(5), 458–462.

*Bradley, C., & Kozak, C. (1995). Nursing care and management of the elderly hip fractured patient. *Journal of Gerontologic Nursing, 21*(8), 15–22.

Brown, C., et al. (1996). Surgical treatment of patients with open tibial fractures. *AORN Journal, 63*(5), 875–881, 885–896.

Brown, F. (1996). Anterior cruciate ligament reconstruction as an outpatient procedure. *Orthopaedic Nursing, 15*(1), 15–20.

Cortet, R., et al. (1997). Treatment of severe, recalcitrant reflex sympathetic dystrophy: Assessment of efficacy and safety of the second generation bisphosphonate pamidronate. *Clinical Rheumatology, 16*(1), 51–56.

Cypher, T. J., & Grossman, J. P. (1996). Biological principles of bone graft healing. *Journal of Foot and Ankle Surgery, 35*(5), 413–417.

Eihorn, T. (1995). Current concepts review: Enhancement of fracture-healing. *Journal of Bone and Joint Surgery, 77-A*(6), 940–956.

Gazdag, A. R., et al. (1995). Alternatives to autogenous bone graft: Efficacy and indicators: A comprehensive review. *Journal of the American Academy of Orthopedic Surgeons, 3*(1), 1–8

*Greipp, M. E., & Thomas, A. F. (1994). Reflex sympathetic dystrophy syndrome: A longitudinal study. *MedSurg Nursing, 3*(5), 378–381.

Hager, C., Brncick, N. (1998). Fat embolism syndrome: A complication of orthopedic trauma. *Orthopaedic Nursing 17*(2): 41–46, 58.

Hofbauer, M. H., et al. (1996). Autogenous bone grafting. *Journal of Foot and Ankle Surgery, 35*(5), 386–390.

Hefti, D. (1995). Complications of trauma: The nurse's role in prevention. *Orthopaedic Nursing, 14*(6), 9–16.

Heveron, B., & Kaempffe, F. (1995). Tears of the rotator cuff. *Orthopaedic Nursing, 14*(6), 38–41.

Johnson, J., et al. (1995). Roller traction: Mobilizing patients with acetabular fractures. *Orthopaedic Nursing, 14*(1), 21–24.

Kapton, J. (1996). Life begins with a loss. *Rehabilitation Nursing, 21*(2), 98–99.

Klinger, D. (1995). Acetabular fractures. *AORN Journal, 61*(1), 157–178.

Lappe, J. (1998). Prevention of hip fractures. *Orthopaedic Nursing 17*(3): 15–26.

Larkin, B. (1997). Understanding bone banking. *Orthopaedic Nursing, 16*(4), 49–55.

Long, J. (1996). Shoulder arthroscopy. *Orthopaedic Nursing, 15*(2), 21–31.

*Lu-Yao, G., et al. (1994). Treatment and survival among elderly Americans with hip fractures: A population-based study. *American Journal of Public Health, 84*(8), 1287–1291.

*Marcantonio, E. R., et al. (1994). A clinical prediction rule for delirium after elective noncardiac surgery. *Journal of the American Medical Association, 271*(2), 134–139.

McCann, S., & Gruen, G. (1997). Fracture blisters: A review of the literature. *Orthopaedic Nursing, 16*(2), 17–22.

McConnell, E. (1997). Myths and facts . . . about amputations. *Nursing, 27*(4), 17.

McFarland, E., et al. (1997). Shoulder immobilization devices: Part 1. The sling. *Orthopaedic Nursing, 16*(4), 17–20.

McFarland, E., et al. (1997). Shoulder immobilization devices: Part 2. Shoulder immobilizers. *Orthopaedic Nursing, 16*(5), 66–71.

McFarland, E., et al. (1997). Shoulder immobilization devices: Part 3. Shoulder immobilizers. *Orthopaedic Nursing, 16*(6), 47–54.

Mendicino, S., et al. (1996). The use of bone grafts in the management of nonunions. *Journal of Foot and Ankle Surgery, 35*(5), 452–457.

Neal, L. (1996). Outpatient ACL surgery: The role of the home health nurse. *Orthopaedic Nursing, 15*(4), 9–13.

Paletta, J. (1997). Nursing care of sports-related injuries. *Orthopaedic Nursing. 16*(6), 43 46.

Savenwhite, C., & Simpson, P. (1998) Patient and family perspectives regarding early discharge and care of the older adult undergoing fractured hip rehabilitation. *Orthopaedic Nursing 17*(1):30–36.

Schott, G. (1997). Bisphosphonates for pain relief in reflex sympathetic dystrophy. *Lancet, 350*(9085), 1117.

Taffet, R. (Ed.). (1997). Trauma to the adult pelvis and hips. *Orthopedic Clinics of North America, 28*(3), 299–477.

Walsh, C., & McBride, A. Jr. (1997). A joint protocol for home skeletal traction. *Orthopaedic Nursing, 16*(3), 28–33.

*Williams, M., et al. (1994). Early outcomes after hip fracture among women discharged home and to nursing homes. *Research in Nursing & Health, 17*(3), 175–183.

Williamson, V. (1998). Management of lower extremity fractures. *Orthopaedic Nursing 17*(5): 84–87.

Yaremchuk, M., & Gan, B. (1996). Soft tissue management of open tibia fractures. *Acta Orthopaedica Belgica, 62*(Suppl. 1), 188–192.

Yetzer, E. (1996). Helping the patient through the experience of an amputation. *Orthopaedic Nursing, 15*(6), 45–49.

Zavotsky, K. E., & Banavage, A. (1995). Management of the patient with complex orthopaedic fractures. *Orthopaedic Nursing, 14*(5), 53–54, 56–57.

Resources

American Amputee Foundation, P.O. Box 250218, Hillcrest Station, Little Rock, AR 72225; 1-501-666-2523

Amputee Shoe and Glove Exchange, P.O. Box 27067, Houston, TX 77227

National Amputation Foundation, 12–45 150th Street, Whitestone, NY 11357

National Easter Seal Society, 70 E. Lake Street, Chicago, IL 60601; 1-312-726-6200

National Handicap Housing Institute, Inc., 4556 Lake Drive, Robbinsdale, MN 55422

National Institute of Arthritis and Musculoskeletal and Skin Diseases Information Clearing House, Box AMS, 9000 Rockville Pike, Bethesda, MD 20892; 1-301-495-4484

National Odd Shoe Exchange, P.O. Box 56845, Phoenix, AZ 85079

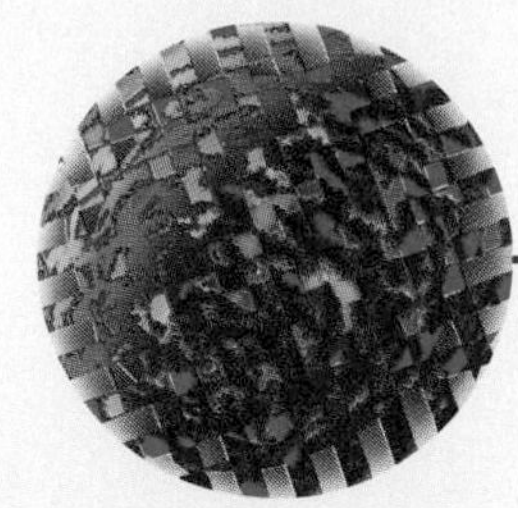

UNIT

Other Acute Problems

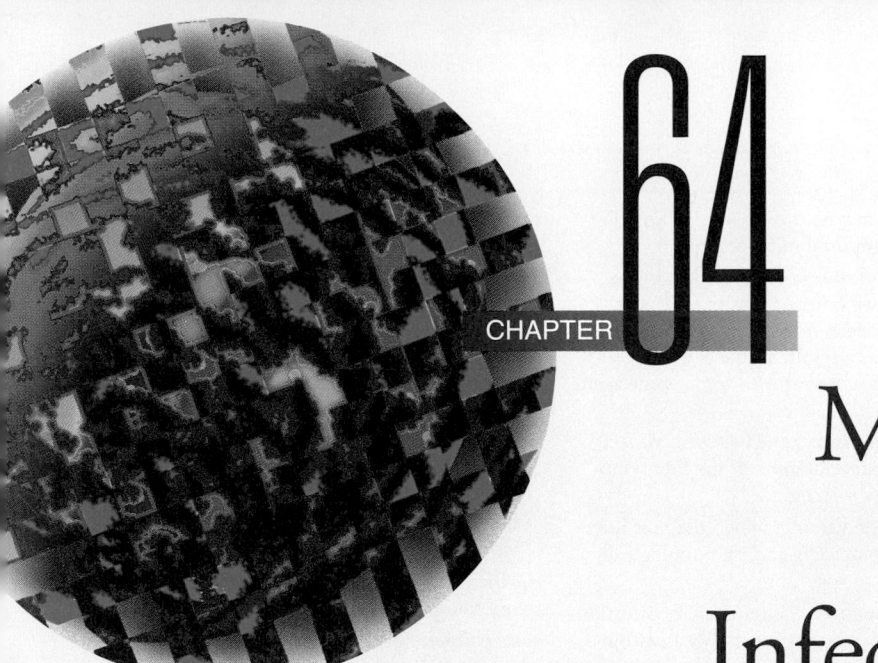

Management of Patients With Infectious Diseases

Learning Objectives

On completion of this chapter, the learner will be able to:

1. Differentiate between colonization, infection, and disease.
2. Use information obtained from the microbiology report to interpret infectious disease evidence.
3. Identify federal and local resources available to the nurse seeking information about infectious diseases.
4. Identify the merit of vaccines recommended for health care workers.
5. Identify the reasons for standard and transmission-based precautions and discuss recommended behaviors.
6. Describe the concept of emerging infectious diseases and factors that lead to the development of these diseases.
7. Use the nursing process as a framework for care of patients with sexually transmitted disease.
8. Describe home health care measures that reduce the risk for infection.
9. Use the nursing process as a framework for care of patients with infectious disease.

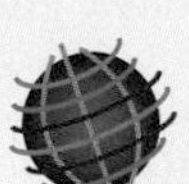

An infectious disease is characterized by two criteria:

- A physiologic interaction between a human host and a microorganism
- A degree of subsequent pathology suffered by the human

Infectious diseases may or may not be communicable (contagious). Although modern science has succeeded in controlling, decreasing the incidence of, or eradicating many infectious diseases, increases in infections caused by bacteria-resistant organisms, emerging infectious diseases (eg, Lyme disease), and sexually transmitted diseases are of great concern. Examples of these types of infectious diseases are highlighted in this chapter. Other infectious diseases are discussed in the appropriate systems chapters (eg, information on tuberculosis is found in Chap. 21: Management of Patients with Chest and Lower Respiratory Tract Disorders).

It is important to understand patterns of infection in humans and to recognize contagious, serious, and common infections. Table 64-1 presents an overview of many infectious diseases, their causative organisms, mode of transmission, and usual **incubation periods** (the time between contact and development of the first symptomatology).

Study of infectious diseases requires understanding of the routes of transmission and effective control methods. The role of the nurse has always been important in infection control. Hand washing, aseptic wound care, and promoting patient activity and nutrition are viewed as important infection-reduction strategies.

GLOSSARY

bacteremia: laboratory-proven presence of bacteria in the bloodstream

carrier: a person who carries an organism without apparent symptomatology; one who is able to transmit to others

Centers for Disease Control and Prevention (CDC): The federal agency with responsibility for conducting surveillance to measure endemic and epidemic disease; for recommending strategies to decrease infectious disease and other disease incidence; and for publishing guidelines to reduce risk to patients and health care workers

colonization: microorganisms present in or on a host, without host interference or interaction, and without symptoms to the host

disease: state in which the infected host displays a decline in wellness due to the infection

emerging infectious diseases: diseases of infectious origin of which incidence in humans has increased within the past two decades or threatens to increase in the near future

fungemia: a bloodstream infection caused by a fungal organism

high-level disinfection: removal of all microorganisms with the possible exception of spores; this level of disinfection is appropriate for instruments that come in contact with mucous membranes but that cannot be sterilized because of mechanical difficulties

host: a person who provides living conditions to support a microorganism

immune: a person with protection in the form of antibodies or sensitized T cells from a previous infection or immunization and who, as a result, is able to avoid reinfection when exposed to the same agent again

incubation period: time between contact and when development of the first symptomatology is recognized

infection: condition in which the host interacts physiologically and immunologically with a microorganism

latency: time interval after primary infection in which a microorganism dwells within the host without producing clinical evidence

methicillin-resistant *Staphylococcus aureus* (MRSA): bacterium *Staphylococcus aureus* that is not susceptible to extended-penicillin antibiotic formulas, such as methicillin, oxacillin, or nafcillin

normal flora: colonization with an organism or organisms that persists for long periods of time. In the skin, these organisms reside in low levels in the dermis layer

nosocomial infection: an infection acquired in the hospital that was not present nor incubating at the time of hospital admission

primary bloodstream infection: bacteremia or fungemia, which occurs without infection identified at another anatomic site

reservoir: any person, plant, animal, substance, or location that provides living conditions for microorganisms and that enables further dispersal of the organism

secondary bloodstream infection: bacteremia or fungemia infection of another anatomic site, which serves as a source for bloodstream contamination

Standard Precautions: strategy of considering all patients as though they may carry infectious agents and of using appropriate barrier precautions for all health care worker–patient interactions

sterilization: the complete removal of all microorganisms

susceptible: not possessing immunity to a particular pathogen

transient flora: organisms that recently have been acquired and are likely to be shed from skin or other site in a relatively short period of time

Transmission-Based Precautions: Precautions used in addition to Standard Precautions when contagious or epidemiologically significant organisms are recognized. The three types of transmission-based precautions are airborne, droplet, and contact

virulence: the degree of pathogenicity of an organism

vancomycin intermediate *Staphylococcus aureus* (VISA): bacterium *Staphylococcus aureus* that is not susceptible to vancomycin

THE INFECTIOUS PROCESS

A complete chain of events is necessary for infection to occur. Figure 64-1 illustrates the elements of the chain and points to weak links where health care workers' interventions can interrupt the chain. The necessary elements of infection include the following:

- A causative organism
- A reservoir of available organisms
- A portal or mode of exit from the reservoir
- A mode of transmission from reservoir to host
- A susceptible host
- A mode of entry to host

CAUSATIVE ORGANISM

Any microorganism can serve as a causative organism. Bacteria, rickettsiae, viruses, protozoa, fungi, and helminths can cause infections.

RESERVOIR

Reservoir is the term used for any person, plant, animal, substance, or location that both provides nourishment for microorganisms and enables further dispersal of the organism. The causative organism and the reservoir represent the source for infection.

MODE OF EXIT

The organism must have a mode of exit from the reservoir. An infected **host** (the person who provides living conditions to support a microorganism) must shed the organisms to another host or to the environment for transmission to occur. Organisms exit through the respiratory tract, the gastrointestinal tract, the genitourinary tract, and the blood.

ROUTE OF TRANSMISSION

A route of transmission is necessary to connect the infectious source with its new host. Organisms may be transmitted through sexual or parenteral fluids; through direct skin-to-skin, close contact or exposure; or through infectious particles in the air. It is important to recognize that different organisms require specific routes of transmission for infection to occur. For example, tuberculosis (TB) is almost always transmitted by the airborne route. The health care worker does not "carry" TB bacteria on their hands or clothing.

In contrast, bacteria such as *Staphylococcus aureus* are easily transmitted from patient to patient on the hands of health care workers. The knowledgeable nurse should explain routes of disease transmission to patients with infectious diseases. For example, a patient may question sharing a room with a patient with human immunodeficiency virus (HIV) infection. Concern is reduced when the patient understands that such proximity does

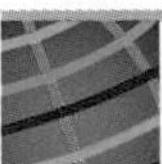

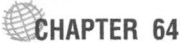

TABLE 64•1 Infectious Diseases, Causative Organisms, Modes of Transmission, and Usual Incubation Period

Disease or Condition	Organism	Usual Mode of Transmission	Usual Incubation Period (Infection to First Symptom)
Acquired immunodeficiency syndrome	Human immunodeficiency virus	Sexual; percutaneous; perinatal	Median of 10 years
Amebiasis	*Entamoeba histolytica*	Contaminated water	2–4 weeks
Chancroid	*Haemophilus ducreyi*	Sexual	3–5 days
Chickenpox	Varicella zoster	Airborne contact	About 14 days
Cholera	*Vibrio cholerae*	Ingestion of water contaminated with human waste	A few hours to 5 days
Cryptococcosis	*Cryptococcus neoformans*	Probably by inhalation	Unknown
Cryptosporidiosis	*Cryptosporidium* species	Ingestion of contaminated water; direct contact with carrier	Probably 1–12 days
Cytomegalovirus (CMV) infection	Cytomegalovirus	Transfusion and transplantation; sexual; perinatal	Highly variable: 3–8 weeks after transfusion, 3–12 weeks after delivery of newborn
Diarrheal disease (common causes)	*Campylobacter* species	Ingestion of contaminated food	3–5 days
	Clostridium difficile	Fecal–oral	Variable; in part related to the influence of antibiotics
	Salmonella species	Ingestion with contaminated food or drink	12–36 hours
	Shigella species	Ingestion of contaminated food or drink; direct contact with carrier	1–3 days
	Yersinia species	Ingestion of contaminated food or drink; direct contact with carrier	1–3 days
Gonorrhea	*Neisseria gonorrhoeae*	Sexual; perinatal	2–7 days
Hand, foot, and mouth disease	Coxsackievirus	Direct contact with nose and throat secretions and with feces of infected people	3–5 days
Hantavirus pulmonary syndrome (HPS)	Sin nombre virus	Contact (direct or indirect) with rodents	Unclear
Foodborne hepatitis	Hepatitis A virus	Ingestion of contaminated food or drink; direct contact with carrier	15–50 days
	Hepatitis E virus	Ingestion of contaminated food or drink; direct contact with carrier	Unclear
Bloodborne hepatitis	Hepatitis B virus	Sexual; perinatal; percutaneous	45–160 days
	Hepatitis C virus	Sexual; perinatal; percutaneous	6–9 months
	Hepatitis D	Sexual; perinatal; percutaneous	Unclear
	Hepatitis G	Percutaneous	Unclear
Herpangina	Coxsackievirus	Direct contact with nose and throat secretions and feces of infected people	3–5 days
Herpes simplex	Human herpesvirus 1 and 2	Contact with mucous membrane secretions	2–12 days
Histoplasmosis	*Histoplasma capsulatum*	Inhalation of airborne spores	5–18 days
Hookworm disease	*Necator americanus; Ancyclostoma duodenale*	Contact with soil contaminated with human feces	A few weeks to many months
Impetigo	*Staphylococcus aureus*	Contact with *S. aureus* carrier	4–10 days
Influenza	Influenza virus A, B, or C	Droplet spread	24–72 hours
Legionnaires' disease	*Legionella pneumophila*	Airborne from water source	2–10 days
Listeriosis	*Listeria monocytogenes*	Foodborne; perinatal	Unclear; probably 3–70 days
Lyme disease	*Borrelia burgdorferi*	Tick bite	14–23 days
Lymphogranuloma venereum	*Chlamydia inguinale*	Sexual	Weeks to years
Malaria	*Plasmodium vivax; Plasmodium malariae; Plasmodium falciparum; Plasmodium ovale*	Bite from *Anopheles* species mosquito	12–30 days
Meningococcal meningitis or bacteremia	*Neisseria meningitidis*	Contact with pharyngeal secretions; perhaps airborne	2–10 days
Mononucleosis	Epstein-Barr virus	Contact with pharyngeal secretions	4–6 weeks
Mycobacterial diseases (nontuberculosis *Mycobacterium* species)	*Mycobacterium avium; Mycobacterium kansasii; Mycobacterium fortuitum; Mycobacterium gordonae;* other *Mycobacterium* species	Variable; probably contact with soil, water, or other environmental source; none are transmissible person-to-person	Variable

(*continued*)

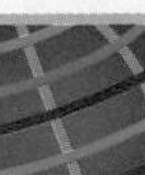

TABLE 64•1 Infectious Diseases, Causative Organisms, Modes of Transmission, and Usual Incubation Period *(Continued)*

Disease or Condition	Organism	Usual Mode of Transmission	Usual Incubation Period (Infection to First Symptom)
Mycoplasmal pneumonia	*Mycoplasma pneumoniae*	Droplet inhalation	14–21 days
Pediculosis	*Pediculus humanus capitis* (head louse); *Phthirus pubis* (crab louse)	Direct contact	1–2 weeks
Pinworm disease	*Enterobius vermicularis*	Direct contact with egg-contaminated articles	4- to 6-week life cycle; often takes months of infection before recognition
Pneumocystis carinii pneumonia	*Pneumocystis carinii*	Unknown; not transmitted person-to-person	Infants: 1–2 months; adults: unclear
Pneumococcal pneumonia	*Streptococcus pneumoniae*	Droplet spread	Probably 1–3 days
Rabies	Rabies virus	Bite from rabid animal	2–8 weeks
Respiratory synctial disease	Respiratory syncytial virus	Self-inoculation by mouth or nose after contact with infectious respiratory secretions	3–7 days
Ringworm	*Microsporum* species; *Trychophyton* species	Direct and indirect contact with lesions	4–10 days
Rocky mountain spotted fever	*Rickettsia ricketsii*	Bite from infected tick	3–14 days
Roseola infantum	Human herpes virus 6	Saliva	10–15 days
Rotavirus gastroenteritis	Rotavirus	Fecal–oral route	About 48 hours
Rubella	Rubella virus	Droplet spread; direct contact	14–21 days
Scabies	*Sarcoptes scabei*	Direct skin contact	2–6 weeks
Syphillis	*Treponema pallidum*	Sexual; perinatal	10 days to 10 weeks
Tetanus	*Clostridium tetani*	Puncture wound	4–21 days
Trichinosis	*Trichinella spiralis*	Ingestion of insufficiently cooked foods, especially pork and beef	10–14 days
Tuberculosis	*Mycobacterium tuberculosis*	Airborne	4–12 weeks to the formation of primary lesion

not represent risk because transmission requires intimate contact (sexual or parenteral).

SUSCEPTIBLE HOST

For infection to occur, the host must be **susceptible** (not possessing immunity to a particular pathogen). Previous infection or vaccine may render the host **immune** (not susceptible) to further infection with an agent. Many infections are prevented because of the powerful human immune defense. Although exposure to potentially infectious microorganisms happens essentially on a constant basis, our elaborate immune systems generally prevent infection from occurring. The immune-suppressed person has much greater susceptibility than the "normal" host.

PORTAL OF ENTRY

A portal of entry is needed because the organism must gain access to the host. For example, airborne TB does not cause disease when it settles on the skin of an exposed host. The only entry route of concern is through the respiratory system.

Colonization, Infection, and Disease

The brain, heart, and vascular system and fluids from those sites (blood and cerebral spinal) are normally sterile. Most other human tissues have microorganisms present. Most bacteria and other organisms introduce neither risk nor benefit. Others provide beneficial **normal flora** to compete with potential pathogens, to facilitate digestion, or to work in other ways symbiotically with the host.

COLONIZATION

The term **colonization** is used to describe microorganisms present without host interference or interaction. Understanding the principle of colonization facilitates interpretation of microbiologic reports. Organisms reported in microbiology results often reflect colonization rather than infection.

INFECTION

Infection indicates a host interaction with an organism. A patient colonized with *S. aureus* may have staphylococci on the skin without any skin interruption or irritation. If the patient had an incision, *S. aureus* could enter the wound, with an immune system reaction of local inflammation and a routing of of white cells to the site. The clinical evidence of redness, heat, and pain and the laboratory evidence of white cells on the wound specimen smear would suggest infection. In this example, the host identifies the staphylococci as "foreign." Infection is recognized both by host reaction and by organism identification.

DISEASE

It is also important to recognize the difference between infection and **disease**. Infectious disease is the state in which the infected host displays a decline in wellness due to the infection. Often, an infection is present in which the host interacts immunologically

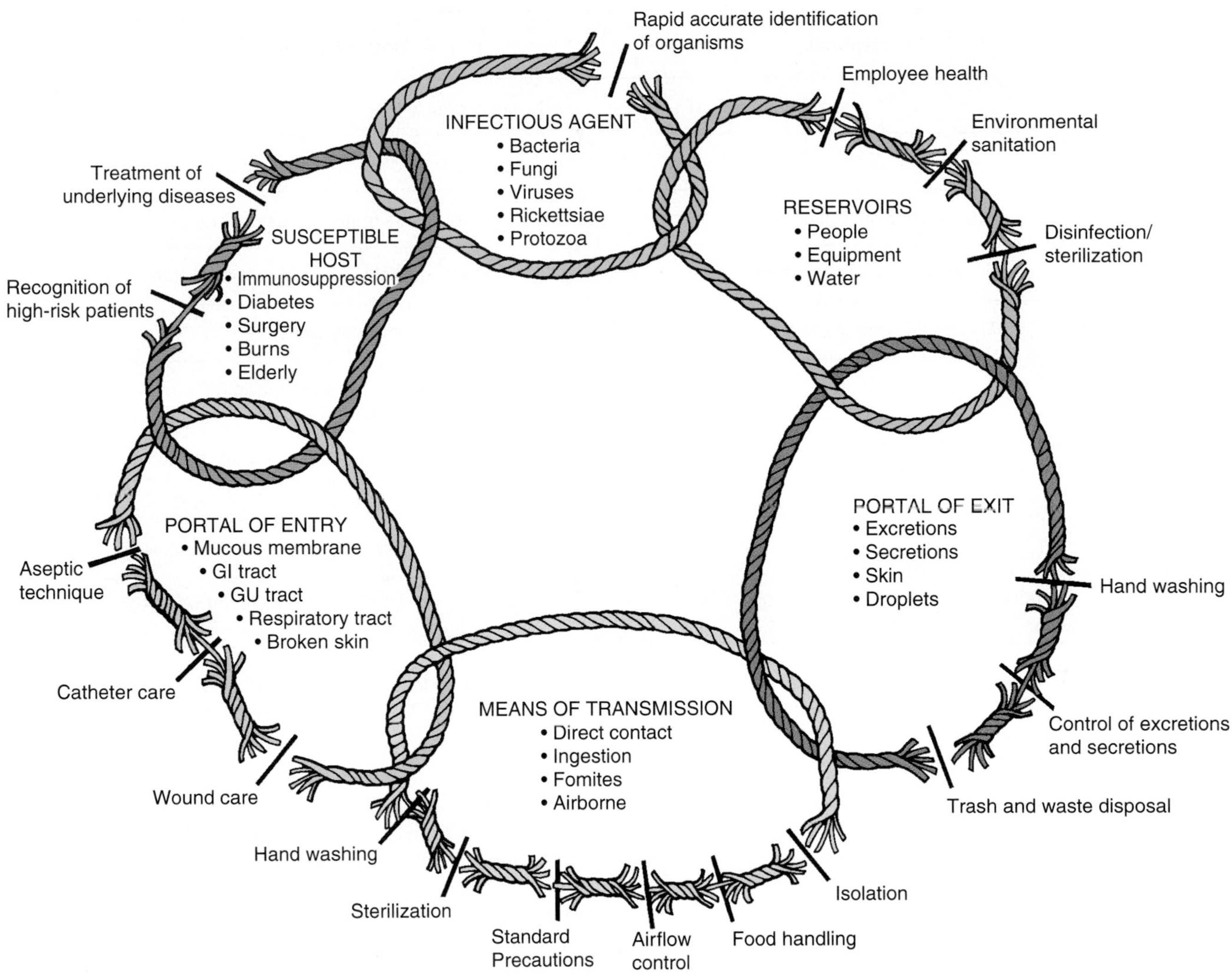

FIGURE 64•1 Health care workers' interventions used to break the chain of infection transmission.

with the organism but remains symptom free. TB is an example of an organism that often persists as infection without producing disease. The host may become infected after exposure to the tubercle bacillus. The definition of infection is met when bacteria are first detected by nonspecific recognition, and later as newly sensitized immune system T cells propagate daughter lines of TB-specific T cells. After this initial infection, the untreated host has a low probability of actually becoming ill. About 90% of infected hosts do not develop the disease of TB. Figure 64-2 depicts response to bacterial infection at the cellular level and at the host level.

The Microbiologic Report

The primary source of information about most bacterial infections is the microbiology report. The microbiology report should be viewed as a tool to be used along with clinical indicators to determine whether a patient is colonized, infected, or diseased.

When specimens are sent to the laboratory for culture, results usually show three components: the smear and stain, the culture and organism identification, and the antimicrobial susceptibility (or sensitivity). As a marker for the likelihood of infection, the smear and stain generally provides the most helpful information as it most closely represents the mix of cells present at the site at the time of specimen collection. In contrast, culture and sensitivity processes refine and broaden information obtained on the smear but may reflect distortion induced by laboratory manipulation rather than host reactions.

INFECTION CONTROL AND PREVENTION

Organizations Involved in Infection Prevention

Centers for Disease Control and Prevention

Many infectious diseases vary through time as microorganisms mutate, as human behavior patterns shift, or as therapeutic options change. The **Centers for Disease Control and Prevention** (CDC) serve an important function in providing timely scientific recommendations about many of the situations that a nurse may face when caring for or teaching a patient with an infectious disease. The CDC routinely publishes recommendations, guidelines, and summaries. The *Morbidity and Mortality Weekly Report* (MMWR) describes significant cases, outbreaks, environmental hazards, or other public health problems. Examples of important summaries that have been provided by the MMWR include (1) Guidelines for Preventing the Transmission of Tuberculosis

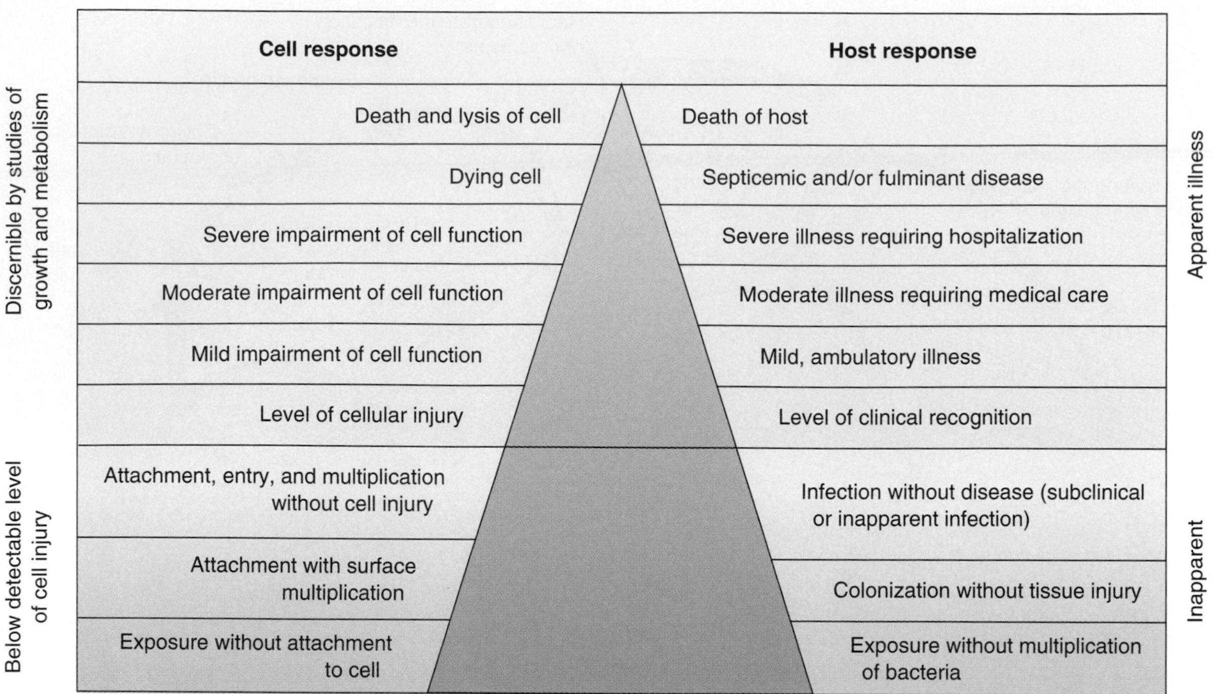

FIGURE 64•2 Biologic spectrum of response to bacterial infection at the cellular level (*left*) and of the intact host (*right*). Redrawn from Evans, A. S., & Brachman, P. S. (1991). *Bacterial infections in humans.* New York, Plenum.

in Health Care Facilities, (2) Recommendations for Prevention of HIV Transmission in Health Care Settings, (3) Sexually Transmitted Diseases Treatment Guidelines, and (4) Standards for Pediatric Immunization Practices

The CDC itself can serve as an important resource if questions arise about a specific infectious disease or risk-reduction strategy. By contacting the CDC, nurses, epidemiologists, or other specialists often can obtain needed information or guidance. (Information can be easily obtained on-line at www.cdc.gov.)

Occupational Safety and Health Administration

Whereas the goal of the CDC is *disease reduction,* the goal of the Occupational Safety and Health Administration (OSHA) is the reduction of risk *exposure.* CDC Guidelines are voluntary, whereas OSHA publishes mandatory regulations and imposes fines on those found noncompliant. OSHA requires that all health care workers have routine educational updates about prevention of bloodborne pathogens and about TB control. Because each health care institution is required to prepare and disseminate to its employees both a bloodborne exposure plan and a TB exposure plan, nurses should be familiar with the details of control in their specific institutions.

Preventing Infection in the Community

Prevention and control of infection in the community are goals that are shared by the CDC and state and local public health departments. A significant amount of emphasis is placed on prevention, so that situations will be avoided that will require control. Methods of infection prevention include sanitation techniques (eg, water purification, disposal of sewage and other potentially infectious materials), regulated health practices (eg, handling, storage, packaging, and preparation of food by institutions), and immunization programs. In the United States, the incidence of infectious diseases has been markedly decreased by immunizations. Immunization programs have proved to be one of the most effective (if not the most effective) means of preventing infection in the community.

Vaccination Programs

Vaccination programs have greatly reduced morbidity and mortality associated with a number of infectious diseases. The goal of vaccination programs is to use wide-scale efforts to prevent specific infectious diseases from occurring in a population. Public health decisions about vaccine campaign implementation efforts are complex. Risks and benefits for the individual and the community must be evaluated in terms of morbidity, mortality, and financial benefit.

The most successful vaccine programs are those for the prevention of smallpox, measles, mumps, rubella, polio, diphtheria, pertussis, and tetanus. The eradication of smallpox (certified in 1979) and discontinuation of the smallpox vaccination program serve as a model for other vaccination and eradication planning endeavors.

There are currently more than 25 vaccines licensed in the United States. Vaccines are made of antigen preparations in a suspension and are intended to produce a human antibody response to protect the host from future encounters with the organism. No vaccine is completely safe for all recipients. Some people are allergic to the antigen or the carrier substance. When live organisms are used as antigen, the actual disease (often with a modified course) may follow. It is important that contraindications on package inserts of vaccine be heeded. These guidelines detail general experience with allergy and other complications and provide crucial information about refrigeration, storage, dosage, and administration.

Variations to the recommended vaccination schedule should be made on a case-by-case basis depending on the patient's risk factors

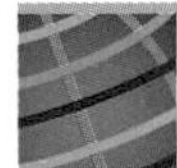

TABLE 64•2 Recommended Childhood Immunization Schedule*

Vaccine	At Birth (Before Hospital Discharge)	1–2 months	6 weeks to 2 months	4 months	6 months	6–18 months	12–15 months	15 months	4-6 years (Before School Entry)
Diphtheria-tetanus-pertussis (DTP)			DTP	DTP	DTP			DTP	
Polio; (inactivated poliovirus) (oral polio virus)			IPV	IPV			OPV		OPV
Measles-mumps-rubella (MMR)							MMR		MMR
Haemophilus influenzae type b (Hib)			Hib	Hib	Hib		Hib		
Hepatitis B (Hep B)	Hep B	Hep B				Hep B			
Varicella (Var)							Var		

* United States, January to December 1998. Approved by the Advisory Committee on Immunization Practices (ACIP), the American Academy of Pediatrics (AAP), and the American Academy of Family Physicians.

and ability to return for follow-up vaccinations at the appointed time. For example, although the first dose of measles vaccine is recommended at the age of 12 to 15 months, babies in developing countries (where measles contributes significantly to childhood morbidity and mortality) should be vaccinated at 9 months.

The standard recommended vaccination schedule for infants and children as developed by the CDC is shown in Table 64-2. The schedule is revised as epidemiologic evidence warrants, and nurses are advised to consult the CDC to determine when the most recent schedule has been published.

Vaccine recommendations for adults are designed to protect those with underlying diseases that increase their risk for infectious disease, those with potential for occupational exposure, and those who may be exposed to infectious agents during travel. Immunosuppressed adults (including those who have had splenectomy) should be vaccinated for pneumococcus, meningococcus, and *Haemophilus influenzae*. Health care workers should be immune to measles, mumps, rubella, and varicella. It is recommended that all of the above adult groups and those with asthma or other chronic respiratory conditions receive annual influenza vaccine.

The CDC provides a 24-hour telephone hotline for information about routine pediatric or adult vaccine advice (404-332-4553), and a 24-hour travelers' hotline for information about preventing specific communicable diseases while traveling abroad (404-332-4559).

The incidence of vaccine-preventable diseases, such as measles, mumps, rubella, and diphtheria, is also affected by immigration from developing countries. Vaccine campaigns in developing countries are often financially and logistically constrained. Therefore, immigrants from such areas may increase the population of those susceptible to the disease, which in turn increases disease incidence.

It is important to increase vaccine programs in all locations, to include immigrants in such programs to reduce their direct health risks, and to reduce epidemic risk to other susceptible individuals.

CONTRAINDICATIONS

Patients who have experienced previous anaphylaxis or anaphylactic-like reactions, patients who have developed an encephalopathy within 7 days of a previous diphtheria, tetanus, and pertussis (DTP) dose, and those who have developed other moderate or severe sequelae after a previous dose should not receive further doses. In addition, DTP is often deferred for the child who previously developed a fever of greater than 40°C (104°F) within 48 hours of vaccination, or who had seizure or developed a shock-like state within 3 days of previous vaccination. Live vaccines usually are not indicated for patients with severe immunosuppression such as may be seen with HIV infection, leukemia, lymphoma, generalized malignancy, significant corticosteroid use, use of immunosuppressive medications to prevent transplant rejection, or exposure to immunocompromised patients. The measles, mumps, and rubella vaccine (MMR) should not be administered to pregnant women.

MEASLES, MUMPS, AND RUBELLA VACCINE

Since the measles, mumps, and rubella vaccines were licensed, reported cases of these diseases have decreased by more than 99% in the United States. The U.S. Public Health Service has formulated goals to eliminate measles, rubella, and congenital rubella and to decrease mumps incidence to fewer than 500 cases per year by the year 2000 (CDC, 1998f). To accomplish this, all public health departments are encouraged to promote vaccination vigorously for all children and for susceptible adults unless contraindicated. Routine MMR vaccination should be given to children at 12 to 15 months of age, with repeat dosing at 4 to 6 years of age.

All people who work in health care should demonstrate evidence of immunity to these three viruses by one of the following: (1) having been born before 1957, (2) documented administration of 2 doses of vaccine, (3) laboratory evidence of immunity, or (4) documentation of physician-diagnosed measles or mumps.

Side Effects. Many different side effects have been reported after vaccination. Epidemiologic evidence supports that the risk for side effects is greater in nonimmune vaccine recipients than in those receiving repeat doses. Patients should be advised that fever, transient lymphadenopathy, or hypersensitivity reaction may occur. Antipyretics may be used to decrease the risk for fever, but aspirin should be avoided in infants and children because of the risk for Reye's syndrome.

Nurses should ask parents or adult vaccine recipients to report all side effects. The National Childhood Vaccine Injury Act of 1986 requires health care providers to report all such events by calling 1-800-822-7967 or though the internet at http:\\www. cdc.gov./nip/vaers.htm.

CHICKENPOX VACCINE

Varicella zoster is the causative viral agent of chickenpox and herpes zoster. The varicella vaccine was first recommended as part of the routine vaccine schedule in the United States in 1996. Thus, the epidemiologic experience for varicella to date has been that of natural infection. As the vaccine's use is increased, this pattern should be altered significantly. In its natural state, the varicella virus attacks most individuals as children, causing disseminated disease in the form of chickenpox. Chickenpox is a much more severe disease in adults than in children. About 3 million cases of chickenpox occur in the United States each year. Varicella is quite contagious, and humans serve as the reservoir. Transmission apparently occurs by the airborne and contact routes. With rare exception, varicella infects an individual only once. At the time of first infection (primary disease manifested as chickenpox), most hosts experience a generalized illness with rash, fever, and malaise. The incubation period is about 2 weeks (with a range from 10 to 21 days). During a prodrome with general malaise (often noted about 2 days before the rash develops), the newly infected host is capable of transmitting the virus to other susceptible contacts. Typically, the rash is vesicular and pustular and spreads rapidly from few to many lesions in a matter of hours. New lesion formation continues for 2 to 3 days, with lesions appearing at different stages throughout this time. By the fourth symptomatic day, the lesions begin to dry, and new lesions usually do not develop. Fever is common during the 4 to 6 days of rash progression. When the lesions have crusted, the patient is no longer contagious to others.

INFLUENZA VACCINE

Influenza is an acute viral disease that predictably and periodically causes worldwide epidemics. Epidemics occur every 2 to 3 years, with a highly variable degree of severity. During epidemics, an increase in the general mortality rate is probably directly attributable to influenza and its accompanying pneumonia and other chronic cardiopulmonary sequelae. It is estimated that in excess of 70,000 deaths per year were attributed to influenza or its sequelae in vulnerable groups between 1977 and 1994 (CDC, 1998g).

Immunization Practices Advisory Committee of the Public Health Service recommends annual influenza vaccinations for those at high risk for complications of influenza and for health care workers. Each year a new vaccine is available, composed of the three virus strains (usually two type A influenza and one type B influenza) considered most likely to be present in the coming season. When the presumed influenza agents have been correctly anticipated and included in that year's vaccine, vaccine effectiveness reaches 70% protection for healthy children and young adults. Although less effective in the elderly (as low as 30% to 40% in the frail elderly), it decreases the severity of illness in those who do get infected, is 50% to 70% effective in preventing pneumonia and hospitalization, and is 80% effective in preventing death. In extended care facilities, risk of transmission is greatly reduced by vaccination of all residents (CDC, 1998g).

The vaccine is recommended for the following groups at risk for influenza complications: those older than 65 years of age, residents of extended care facilities, those with chronic pulmonary or cardiovascular diseases, and those with diabetes, immunosuppression, or renal dysfunction. Vaccination is also advised for children (such as those with juvenile rheumatoid arthritis) who require long-term aspirin therapy to reduce the likelihood of developing Reye's syndrome. Health care workers and household members of those in high-risk groups are advised to become vaccinated to reduce the risk of transmission to those vulnerable to influenza sequelae. Vaccine campaigns among health care workers and patients should be intensified when there is evidence of community influenza disease.

Preventing Infection in the Hospital

Nurses specializing in infection control are responsible for agency-wide policy development and program direction. Staff nurses play an important role in risk reduction by careful attention to hand washing and careful administration of antibiotics as prescribed and by following procedures to reduce the risks associated with patient care devices. Infection risk is significantly increased as technical equipment associated with patient care becomes more complex and as more devices that disrupt naturally protective anatomic barriers are used.

Each year, an estimated 2 million patients in the United States acquire infections while hospitalized. These infections, referred to as **nosocomial,** are estimated to cost more than $4.5 billion per year and cause more than 19,000 deaths per year in the United States. In addition, nosocomial infections are a contributing factor in more than 55,000 deaths (Gaynes, 1997).

In the 1970s, the CDC conducted a massive investigation on the effectiveness of nosocomial infection reduction programs. That study, known as SONIC (Study of Nosocomial Infection Control), found that about one third of all nosocomial infections could be prevented when effective infection control programs were in place. An effective program was found to include the following four components: (1) a program of surveillance for nosocomial infections and vigorous control efforts, (2) at least one infection control practitioner for every 250 hospital beds, (3) a trained hospital epidemiologist, and (4) feedback to surgeons about individual surgical site infections. Unfortunately, many hospitals have not yet introduced all four required aspects, and thus only an estimated 9% of expected infections are prevented.

Specific Organisms With Nosocomial Infection Potential

CLOSTRIDIUM DIFFICILE

Clostridium difficile is a bacterium with significant nosocomial potential. The organism is a gram-positive, spore-forming bacterium. Spore formation facilitates the organism's ability to be spread by environmental sources and personnel. After antibiotic treatment, a person's normal intestinal flora is often disrupted. *C. difficile*, with its protective spore, is often resistant to antimicrobial therapy and thus is able to proliferate relatively unimpeded in this setting.

The organism works as a pathogen by releasing toxins into the lumen of the bowel. The toxins cause destruction at the site, rather than actual invasion by the organism. In pseudomembranous colitis, the most extreme form of *C. difficile* infection, debris from the invaded lumen and white blood cells accumulate in the form of pseudomembranes or studded areas of the colon. The destruction of such a large anatomic area can produce profound sepsis.

Because many people receive antibiotics to treat infection, the risk for *C. difficile* pathology is widely distributed. The nosocomial potential is compounded because the spore is relatively resistant to cleaning and hand-washing agents and can be spread on the hands of health care workers and by contact with equipment that has been previously contaminated with *C. difficile*. Even in environments that have been cleaned, complete assurance that *C. difficile* has been eliminated is often unrealistic.

METHICILLIN-RESISTANT *STAPHYLOCOCCUS AUREUS*

Methicillin-resistant *Staphylococcus aureus* (MRSA) is a common nosocomial infection in hospitals and extended care facilities. MRSA is the term used to describe *S. aureus* that is resistant to methicillin or its comparable pharmaceutical agents, oxacillin and nafcillin. Since the introduction of antibiotics in the 1940s, there has been concern about antibiotic-resistant *S. aureus*. When penicillin was first introduced, almost all isolates of *S. aureus* were sensitive to the drug. It was not long, however, before *S. aureus* became all but universally penicillin resistant. Fortunately, alternative therapies in the forms of cephalosporins and, more importantly, synthetic penicillin solutions such as methicillin, oxacillin, or nafcillin were introduced. It was not until the late 1970s that *S. aureus* showed resistance to the synthetic penicillin, methicillin. At that time, MRSA was seen infrequently; the prevalence of the organism was originally linked epidemiologically to the intravenous drug use community. Since the late 1970s, however, *S. aureus* has become increasingly resistant to methicillin, and transmission of MRSA within hospitals and nursing homes has become well documented. Vancomycin is usually the preferred alternative treatment for serious MRSA infection. However, the concern with using vancomycin to treat MRSA is that it too will lose its effectiveness in treating *S. aureus*. In fact, for the first time, in 1997, several patients in the United States and Japan were diagnosed with infections caused by **vancomycin intermediate *Staphylococcus aureus*** (VISA).

Health care workers easily transmit MRSA to patients because *S. aureus* frequently colonizes skin. Because colonization is seldom recognized, the health care worker must assume that *every* patient contact offers the possibility of MRSA exposure. Although there is no evidence that MRSA is more virulent than other strains of staphylococci, the colonized patient faces the likelihood of infection with MRSA when invasive procedures, such as intravenous therapy, respiratory therapy, or surgery, are performed. Additionally, the patient colonized with MRSA serves as a reservoir of resistant organisms to be transmitted to others. MRSA acquired in the hospital may persist as normal flora in the patient in the future.

VANCOMYCIN-RESISTANT ENTEROCOCCUS

Enterococcus is a gram-positive bacterium that is part of the normal flora of the gastrointestinal tract. However, it has the capability of producing significant infections in certain situations. Enterococcus is now the second most frequently isolated cause of nosocomial infection in the United States.

As a relatively resistant organism at baseline, therapy for enterococcus has been essentially limited to penicillin formulations (such as ampicillin) or vancomycin in combination with aminoglycoside (such as gentamicin). In the 1980s, initial recognition of resistance to all of these agents was reported. Between 1989 and 1993, the CDC recorded a more than 20-fold increase in the percentage of cases of vancomycin-resistant enterococcus (VRE) infection (Martone, 1998).

This rapidly growing problem has serious implications. Patients with vancomycin-resistant enterococcus are frequently resistant to all other antimicrobial therapies, leaving them with bacterial infections for which there is no pharmaceutical treatment available. Additionally, there is great concern that VRE may serve as a reservoir of genes coded for vancomycin resistance that may be transferred to the even more prevalent and virulent *S. aureus*.

Enterococcus has the following traits that make it an ideal nosocomial organism: (1) the host carries an abundance of the organism even in a noninfected state; (2) the organism is bile resistant and can withstand harsh anatomic sites, such as the intestine; (3) enterococcus has the potential for resistance to many antibiotics, so that therapeutic agents reducing local bacterial competition may leave it to replicate freely; and (4) the enterococcus endures well on the hands of health care workers and on environmental objects.

Preventing Nosocomial Bloodstream Infections (Bacteremia and Fungemia)

Preventing nosocomial bloodstream infections requires special precautions (in addition to standard and transmission-based precautions, discussed later) that must be taken to prevent their occurrence. If a nosocomial bloodstream infection occurs, early detection is essential. If left untreated, bloodstream infections may progress to sepsis and septic shock and, possibly, death,

Bacteremia is defined as laboratory-proven presence of bacteria in the bloodstream. **Fungemia** is a bloodstream infection caused by a fungal organism. There are two categories of nosocomial bloodstream infections—primary and secondary. **Primary bloodstream infections** are those in which the host has no pre-existing infection and the bloodstream becomes contaminated through mechanical manipulation (most frequently with vascular access devices). Any vascular access device (VAD) can serve as the source for a primary bloodstream infection. Contamination can occur from the patient's own flora traversing the exterior of a catheter or by contamination of internal tubing during manipulation. The intravenous fluid itself can become contaminated and serve as a source of infection. VADs are widely used for both hospitalized patients and outpatients receiving care in a clinic or home setting. In all instances, the nurse must consider the infectious potential of the VAD. Chart 64-1 identifies conditions that suggest the presence of nosocomial VAD-related bacteremia or fungemia.

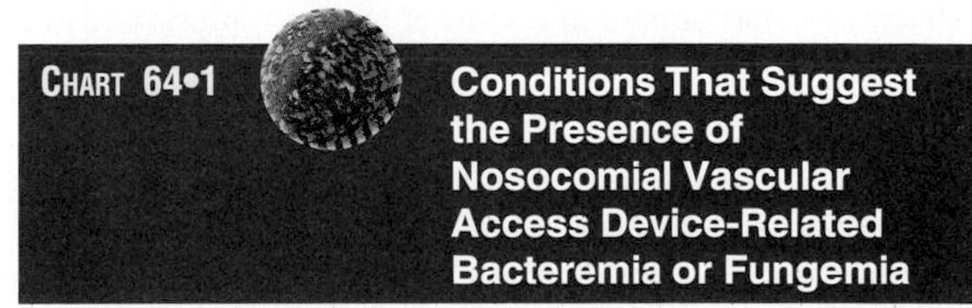

CHART 64•1 Conditions That Suggest the Presence of Nosocomial Vascular Access Device-Related Bacteremia or Fungemia

- The patient has catheter in place, appears septic, but has no obvious reason to suggest predisposition to sepsis.
- There is no infection at another body site to indicate probable source of sepsis.
- The site of vascular line insertion is red, swollen, or draining (especially purulent drainage).
- The patient has a central vascular line in place at the onset of sepsis.
- The bloodstream infection is caused by *Candida* species or by common skin organisms such as coagulase-negative staphylococci, *Bacillus* species, or *Corynebacterium* species.
- The patient remains septic after appropriate therapy without removal of the vascular access device.

Secondary bloodstream infection occurs when a host has another site of infection that can serve as a source of contamination to the bloodstream. For example, organisms present in a localized abscess can enter the bloodstream to cause disseminated bacteremia.

DISINFECTING SKIN

During the insertion of all vascular access devices, there must be strict attention to aseptic technique. Those inserting VADs must vigorously wash hands before insertion. Sterile gloves are worn for the placement of all central and arterial lines. Because the rate of bloodstream infection associated with central VADs is greater than with those peripherally placed, barrier methods such as gowns with long sleeves, masks, and a large drape over the patient are used in many settings for the insertion of such lines.

The site of insertion is disinfected with povidone iodine or alcohol (if the patient is allergic to povidone iodine). The relative benefit of topical antimicrobial ointment use at the site has not yet been conclusively studied, and its use varies among institutions.

Although there are inconclusive data about whether gauze or polyurethane transparent dressings confer greater benefit, the intended benefits of either type of dressing at the insertion site are to protect the catheter from contamination and to protect the site from trauma (Treston-Aurand, 1997; Tripepi-Bova, 1997).

USING GUIDE WIRES

Guide wires are often used when replacing central lines. They offer decreased risk for vascular injury, less manipulation (with the goal of less contamination), and less risk for pneumothorax for subclavian and internal jugular catheters. As with many strategies for bacteremia risk reduction, it is not clear whether guide wires offer infectious risk or benefit. In general, guide wires are helpful when there are limited alternative insertion sites available, when the central line requires removal because it has been in place for an extended period of time, or when the catheter is cracked or leaking. If the patient has sepsis that may be linked to catheterization, or if the insertion site is red or has purulent drainage, a new site should be chosen for catheter insertion.

CHANGING INFUSION SETS, CATHETERS, AND SOLUTIONS

Infusion sets and catheters used at peripheral sites should be changed every 24 to 72 hours unless an infusion set is used for the delivery of blood or lipid solutions, or when an infusion-related bacteremia is suspected. In these cases, the infusion set should be changed on completion of the solution or as soon as infection is suspected. Intravenous solutions are changed at least every 24 hours. Signs of sepsis in patients with indwelling vascular lines should be promptly assessed and treated.

Nurses have an important role in the prevention of bloodstream infections as they assess patients for evidence of infection, make daily VAD site inspections, and monitor the interval of line changes.

Isolation Precautions

Isolation precautions are guidelines created to prevent transmission of microorganisms in hospitals. In 1997, the Hospital Infection Control Practices Advisory Committee (HICPAC), along with the CDC, implemented two tiers of isolation precautions. The first tier, standard precautions, was designed for the care of *all* patients in the hospital and is the primary strategy for preventing nosocomial infections. The second tier, transmission-based precautions, was designed for care of patients with known or suspected infectious diseases spread by one of the following routes—airborne, droplet, or contact.

STANDARD PRECAUTIONS

Standard Precautions, a set of protective behaviors, replace the previously recommended Universal Precautions (which were designed solely to prevent bloodborne infections) and Body Substance Isolation (which was designed to prevent transmission of pathogens from moist body substances).

The tenets of Standard Precautions are that all patients are colonized or even infected with microorganisms without signs or symptoms, and that a uniform level of caution should be used in the care of all patients. The elements of standard precautions include hand washing, glove use, use of mask, eye protection, face shield, gown use, handling of patient care equipment, environmental control, handling of linen, occupational health and bloodborne pathogens, and patient placement. Hand washing, glove use, needlestick prevention, and avoidance of splash or spray of body fluids are discussed later. See Guideline 48-1 in Chapter 48: Management of Patients with HIV infection and AIDs for a detailed presentation of Standard Precautions.

Hand Washing. Many outbreaks of infections in health care facilities are preventable with proper, consistent hand washing. Normal skin flora usually consist of coagulase-negative staphylococci or diphtheroids. Only with host immune suppression or use of indwelling devices does the low quantity of colonization from these relatively nonpathogenic organisms have infectious potential.

In the health care setting, it is common for employees to temporarily carry bacteria **(transient flora)** such as *S. aureus*, *Pseudomonas aeruginosa*, and other organisms with strong pathogenic potential. Generally, these organisms are weakly attached and are shed with hand washing and skin regeneration.

Hand washing is important in the health care setting because transient bacteria can be easily removed before transfer to other patients. Effective hand washing calls for at least *10 seconds of vigorous scrubbing* with special attention to the area around nail beds and between fingers where there is high bacterial burden. Hands should be thoroughly rinsed after this washing (Fig. 64-3).

Antimicrobial hand-washing agents, such as chlorhexidine gluconate, alcohol, iodophors, chloroxylenol, or triclosan, should be used when the patient is in the intensive care unit (commonly a reservoir for virulent organisms) or when a patient is known to be colonized with antibiotic-resistant bacteria.

Glove Use. Gloves provide an effective barrier for hands from the microflora associated with patient care. Gloves should be worn whenever a health care worker has contact with secretions or excretions of any patient. Gloves must be discarded after each patient care contact. Additionally, because hospital organisms colonizing health care workers' hands can proliferate in the warm, moist environment provided by gloves, hands must be thoroughly washed after gloves are removed. As patient advocates, nurses have an important role in promoting hand washing and glove use by other hospital workers, such as laboratory personnel, technicians, and others who have contact with patients.

Latex gloves are often preferred over vinyl gloves because of greater comfort and fit and because some studies indicate that they afford greater protection from exposure. With their increased use in recent years, however, there have been accompanying increased reports of allergic reactions to latex in health care workers. Reactions range from local skin irritation to more severe

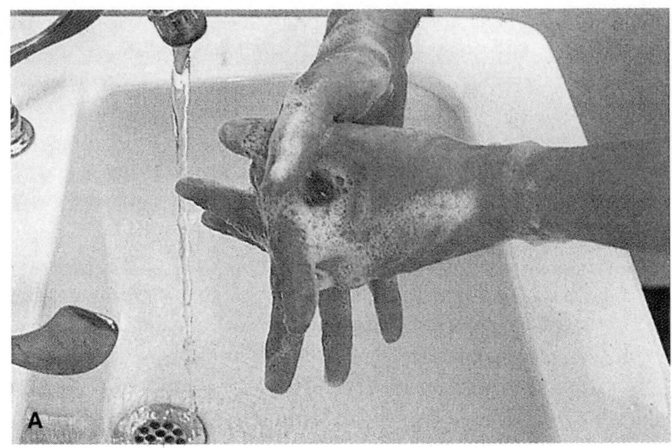
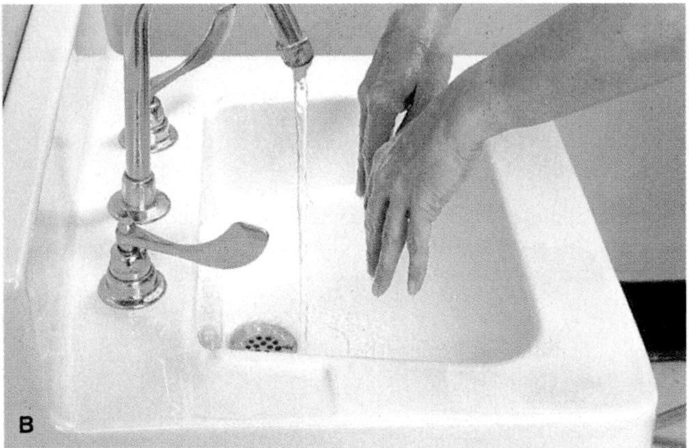

FIGURE 64•3 Effective hand washing. (**A**) Washing hands and forearms with firm rubbing and circular motions. (**B**) Rinsing thoroughly.

reactions, including generalized dermatitis, conjunctivitis, asthma, angioedema, and anaphylaxis. Reactions can be immunologic in response to the proteins from the rubber tree *(Hevea braziliensis)* or may be due to irritation from chemicals used in the manufacture of the gloves. It is often difficult for the clinician to distinguish allergy from irritation when assessing the local symptoms of erythema, scaling, and bleeding. Systemic allergic reactions occur rarely and are due to the formation of antibodies specific to latex. The response can be triggered by skin contact, as when gloves are donned, or can result from airborne exposure to the latex allergen that may be freed as the glove powder is released with handling.

The nurse who experiences irritation or allergic reaction associated with exposure to latex should report symptoms to an occupational health specialist, dermatologist, or private physician. Suggested methods for reducing the incidence of such reactions include use of vinyl gloves, powder-free gloves, or "low-protein" latex gloves.

Needlestick Prevention. The most important aspect of reducing the risk of bloodborne infection is the avoidance of percutaneous injury. Extreme care is essential in all situations in which needles, scalpels, and other sharp objects are handled. Used needles should not be recapped. Instead, they are placed directly into puncture-resistant containers in the vicinity of their use. If a situation dictates that a needle must be recapped, it is important that the nurse use a mechanical device to hold the cap, or use a one-handed approach to decrease the likelihood of skin puncture.

Avoidance of Spray and Splash Exposure. Whenever the health care worker is involved in an activity in which body fluids may be sprayed or splashed, appropriate barriers must be used. If a splash to the face may occur, goggles and face mask are warranted. If the health care worker is handling material that may soil clothing or is involved in a procedure in which clothing may be splashed with biologic material, a cover gown should be worn.

TRANSMISSION-BASED PRECAUTIONS

Some organisms are so contagious or so epidemiologically significant that precautions in addition to Standard Precautions should be used when such organisms are recognized. HICPAC and the CDC developed a second tier of precautions called **Transmission-Based Precautions**. The additional precautions are called airborne, droplet, and contact precautions.

Airborne precautions are required for patients with presumed or proven pulmonary TB, chickenpox, or measles. When hospitalized, patients should be put in rooms with negative pressure; the door should remain closed, and health care workers should wear a mask at all times while in the patient room.

Droplet precautions are used for organisms that can be transmitted by close, face-to-face contact, such as influenza or meningococcal meningitis. While taking care of a patient requiring droplet precautions, the nurse should wear a facemask, but because the risk of transmission is limited to close contact, the door may remain open.

Contact precautions are used for organisms that are spread by skin to skin contact, such as antibiotic-resistant organisms or *C. difficile.* Contact precautions are designed to emphasize cautious technique for organisms that have serious epidemiologic consequences or those easily transmitted by contact between health care worker and patient. Thus, the principles of transmission control used in Standard Precautions are accentuated. When possible, the patient requiring contact isolation is given a private room to facilitate hand washing and protection of garments from environmental contamination. Masks are not needed, and doors do not need to be closed (Chart 64-2).

EMERGING INFECTIOUS DISEASES

As defined by the CDC, **emerging infectious diseases** are diseases of infectious origin of which incidence in humans has increased within the past two decades or threatens to increase in the near future (CDC, 1994). Four examples of emerging infectious diseases are presented within this section—diarrheal diseases (although not all organisms that cause diarrhea are considered emerging infections), legionnaires' disease, Lyme disease, and Hantavirus pulmonary syndrome. (See Table 64-1 for an overview of infectious diseases, including emerging infectious diseases.) Many factors contribute to newly emerging or reemerging infectious diseases, including global travel, globalization of food supply and central processing of food, population growth and increased urban crowding, population movements (due to war, famine, disaster), ecologic changes, human behavior (eg, risky sexual behavior, intravenous drug use), antimicrobial resistance, environmental sources, or breakdown in public health measures. Although there are many reasons for the emergence or reemergence of infectious diseases, travel and immigration is one of the most historical and most obvious modes of transmission.

CHART 64•2 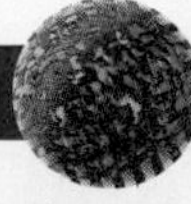 Synopsis of Types of Precautions and Patients Requiring the Precautions

Standard Precautions

Use Standard Precautions for the care of all patients.

Airborne Precautions

In addition to Standard Precautions, use Airborne Precautions for patients known or suspected to have serious illnesses transmitted by airborne droplet nuclei. Examples of such illnesses include the following:

- Measles
- Varicella (including disseminated zoster)*
- Tuberculosis

Droplet Precautions

In addition to Standard Precautions, use Droplet Precautions for patients known or suspected to have serious illnesses transmitted by large particle droplets. Examples of such illnesses include:

- Invasive *Haemophilus influenzae* type b disease, including meningitis, pneumonia, epiglottitis, and sepsis
- Invasive *Neisseria meningitidis* disease, including meningitis, pneumonia, and sepsis
- Other serious bacterial respiratory infections spread by droplet transmission, including:
  - Diphtheria (pharyngeal)
  - *Mycoplasma pneumoniae*
  - Pertussis
  - Pneumonic plague
  - Streptococcal (group A) pharyngitis, pneumonia, or scarlet fever in infants and young children
- Serious viral infections spread by droplet transmission, including:
  - Adenovirus*
  - Influenza
  - Mumps
  - Parvovirus B19
  - Rubella

Contact Precautions

In addition to Standard Precautions, use Contact Precautions for patients known or suspected to have serious illnesses easily transmitted by direct patient contact or by contact with items in the patient's environment. Examples of such illnesses include:

- Gastrointestinal, respiratory, skin, or wound infections or colonization with multidrug-resistant bacteria judged by the infection control program, based on current state, regional, or national recommendations, to be of special clinical and epidemiologic significance
- Enteric infections with a low infectious dose or prolonged environmental survival, including:
  - *Clostridium difficile*
  - For diapered or incontinent patients: enterohemorrhagic *Escherichia coli* O157:H7, *Shigella* species, hepatitis A, or rotavirus
- Respiratory syncytial virus, parainfluenza virus, or enteroviral infections in infants and young children
- Skin infections that are highly contagious or that may occur on dry skin, including:
  - Diphtheria (cutaneous)
  - Herpes simplex virus (neonatal or mucocutaneous)
  - Impetigo
  - Major (noncontained) abscesses, cellulitis, or pressure ulcers
  - Pediculosis
  - Scabies
  - Staphylococcal furunculosis in infants and young children
  - Zoster (disseminated or in the immunocompromised host)*
- Viral and hemorrhagic conjunctivitis
- Viral hemorrhagic infections (Ebola, Lassa, or Marburg)

* Certain infections require more than one type of precaution.
Source: CDC, 1997

Travel and Immigration

There is a well-founded concern that infectious diseases may be imported through travel or the influx of immigrants. Historically, migration of populations often led to epidemics of disease in immunologically naive new lands. Because of trade, immigration, and wars, yellow fever, malaria, hookworm, leprosy, smallpox, measles, mumps, syphilis, and many other infectious diseases have been brought to the Western Hemisphere.

Despite rapid travel, most of the diseases carried by travelers to the United States do not efficiently spread in our environment with enforced vaccination, clean water, and insect and rodent control.

However, the potential for disease outbreaks linked to global travel persists. The CDC maintains an active surveillance system to monitor prospectively the incidence of many diseases now rare in the United States. This vigilance has proved to be effective in halting transmission of many diseases.

The most significant infectious disease transmission impact associated with immigration is from HIV, acquired immunodeficiency syndrome (AIDS), and TB. There is a growing concern that vector-borne diseases, such as dengue, might be transmitted by mosquitoes if a reservoir of infected humans is established.

Immigration and HIV/AIDS

The fact that AIDS reached pandemic proportions in less than a decade after its recognition attests to the efficiency of world travel in spreading disease. The significance of such rapid transmission rates is especially dramatic in that HIV essentially requires intimate contact between two people either through sexual activity or sharing blood through needles.

Although the reservoir of HIV-1 in the United States is currently estimated to be greater than 1 million people, it was probably first introduced in the 1970s when asymptomatically infected travelers returned to the United States after having acquired the virus in other countries. The only cases of HIV-2 that have been identified in the United States are from people who have spent time in West Africa. Because of the long asymptomatic period associated with either HIV virus, **carriers** (people who carry an organism without apparent symptomatology and are able to transmit to others) of HIV-2 may be unrecognized and introduce a chain of infection similar to that which we have witnessed with HIV-1. Control methods to prevent this occurrence involve routine seroprevalence studies to establish any introduction of the virus and routine screening of donated blood for the virus.

Immigration and Tuberculosis

Immigration has always been an important influence in the dynamic epidemiology of TB in the United States. TB is a major cause of death in developing nations. Immigration to the United States from such countries adds to the total number of U.S. inhabitants with latent and active disease.

Transmission potential is made greater because many tourists and immigrants visit and live in large cities, which are the epicenter of the HIV epidemic. Screening effectiveness is limited because purified protein derivative (PPD) does not provide information about the infectivity of the host. The complexity of PPD interpretation is increased because of the common use of the vaccine BCG (bacillus Calmette-Guérin) in many foreign countries. BCG is a vaccine designed to protect against TB, but its effectiveness is extremely variable. After receiving BCG, individuals are often PPD positive for a prolonged time, thus decreasing the ability of the PPD to serve as a TB screen.

Immigration and Vector-Borne Diseases

Malaria, yellow fever, and dengue are diseases that cause significant morbidity and mortality throughout the developing world. These diseases are spread by infected mosquitoes. Many other vector-borne parasitic diseases in developing countries rely on mosquitoes and other organisms to complete their life cycles and transmit disease.

Dengue fever is an example of the risk of imported vector-borne disease. The disease is caused by a virus that is spread through human populations by the *Aedes aegypti* mosquitoes. The mosquitoes thrive in tropical zones and breed in stagnant water sources.

Infection from dengue produces flulike symptoms of fever, chills, eye pain, and back pain. Muscle and joint pain, along with nausea and vomiting, may be present, and patients may exhibit a hyperpigmented rash that blanches on touch. Symptoms often wax and wane and are generally self-limited. A small proportion of patients may develop hemorrhagic disease, which can be life-threatening in extreme forms.

Travelers, immigrants, and returning military personnel can serve as reservoirs of infection. There has been a recent increase in the incidence of dengue virus isolated in the Caribbean, which has caused concern about waves of infection in the United States in areas where vector mosquitoes are present. There is no specific treatment for this infection. Control efforts rely on local effective mosquito control.

Diarrheal Diseases

In developing countries of the world, infectious diarrhea kills about 4 million people per year. In the United States, it is estimated that children younger than 5 years of age experience more than 20 million episodes of diarrheal diseases each year, with about 400 deaths per year attributed to such episodes. Dehydration is the most important factor of both morbidity and mortality associated with diarrheal disease. Dehydration is largely controllable by using rehydration therapy.

Transmission

The portal of entry of all diarrheal pathogens is oral ingestion. Although the food we eat is far from sterile, the high acidity of the stomach and the antibody-producing cells of the small bowel generally serve to decrease the potential of pathogens. If the number of organisms is large enough or if the food serves as a neutralized carrier to protect the organism in the acidic environment, however, pathogenic reactions can occur. Decreased gastric acidity with disruption of normal bowel flora (as occurs after surgery), use of antimicrobial agents, and the immune dysfunction of AIDS all decrease intestinal defenses.

Specific Causes

There are many viral, bacterial, and parasitic causes for diarrheal diseases. Rotavirus is the most important viral cause of diarrhea in young children. Common causes of bacterial infection include *Escherichia coli* and *Salmonella*, *Shigella*, *Campylobacter*, and *Yersinia* species. Parasitic infections of importance include *Giardia* and *Cryptosporidium* species and *Entamoeba histolytica*.

ESCHERICHIA COLI

E. coli is the most common aerobic organism colonizing the large bowel. *E. coli* identified from fecal cultures does not usually represent pathology but rather reflects normal flora. However, certain strains of *E. coli* with increased **virulence** (degree of pathogenicity of an organism) have been responsible for significant morbidity and even a number of deaths in recent outbreaks. These stronger pathologic strains share the basic biologic properties of all *E. coli* but can be subgrouped as enterotoxigenic *E. coli* (ETEC). ETEC strains are distinguished by their production of enterotoxins. Cholera-like disease with rapid severe dehydration can follow infection with one of these strains.

During recent times, outbreaks of an *E. coli* species, 0157:H7, have often been linked to the ingestion of undercooked beef. This bacterium lives in the intestines of cattle and can be introduced into meat at the time of slaughter. Prevention of disease from this strain of *E. coli* is aimed at teaching the public to cook ground beef thoroughly (until the meat is no longer pink and the juices run clear).

SALMONELLA SPECIES INFECTION

Salmonella is a gram-negative bacillus with many species, including the very pathogenic *S. typhi* (typhoid fever). Of the nontyphi species, most organisms are prevalent in animal food sources. It is estimated that *Salmonella* species contaminate more than 50% of commercially available chicken products and are frequently found in eggs (whether or not shells are broken), raw milk, and occasionally beef. Along with contamination from food and water, person-to-person transmission can occur. Hospitals, long-term care facilities, and other institutions account for nearly one third of all reported epidemics of *Salmonella*. Routes of transmission in these settings are probably both through contaminated food and person-to-person transmission.

There is great variability of symptoms associated with *Salmonella* species infection, including asymptomatic carrier state, gastroenteritis, and systemic infection. Diarrhea with gastroenteritis is common. Disseminated disease and bacteremia, whether or not accompanied by diarrhea, is less common.

The person with *Salmonella*-caused diarrhea can be a source for transmission to others. The importance of good hygiene should be emphasized, and health care workers should use special care when handling bedpans, stool specimens, or other objects that may have fecal contamination. Hand washing is imperative after any contact with a person with *Salmonella* diarrhea. Patients with gastroenteritis generally are not treated with antibiotics. Antibiotic use may increase the period of time that the patient carries the bacteria, while not improving the clinical outcome of the patient. However, those with systemic salmonellosis require antimicrobial therapy.

SHIGELLA SPECIES INFECTION

The *Shigella* species is a gram-negative organism that invades the lumen of the intestine and causes disease and severe watery (possibly bloody) diarrhea. *Shigella* species spread through the fecal–oral route, with easy transmission from one person to another. Small numbers of organisms are needed to cause disease. Because transmission occurs easily with improper hygiene, it is not surprising that *Shigella* organisms disproportionately affect pediatric populations. Disease in the very young may infrequently be complicated by pulmonary or neurologic symptoms.

Antimicrobial therapy should be instituted early. Frequently, initial therapy choices must be altered when final microbiologic testing reveals the organism's sensitivity.

CAMPYLOBACTER SPECIES INFECTIONS

In the United States, diarrheal disease attributed to *Campylobacter* species surpasses that recorded for *Salmonella* and *Shigella* species. The organism is found abundantly in animal food sources. It is especially common in poultry but can also be found in beef and pork. Transmission appears to be almost entirely by the fecal–oral route, with food sources serving as the reservoir of infection. Direct person-to-person transmission appears to be less common than for other enteric pathogens, such as *Shigella*.

Cooking and storing food at appropriate temperatures protects against *Campylobacter*. It is important that kitchen utensils used in meat preparation be kept away from other food to prevent *Campylobacter* transmission.

After a person is infected, the organism probably directly attacks the lumen of the intestine and may cause disease through enterotoxin release. Symptoms can range from mild abdominal cramping and minimal diarrhea to severe disease with profuse watery (sometimes bloody) diarrhea and debilitating abdominal cramping. Antimicrobial therapy is recommended only for those who are seriously ill.

GIARDIA LAMBLIA

Giardia lamblia is a protozoan. Transmission occurs when food or drink is contaminated with viable cysts of the organism. People often become infected while traveling to endemic areas in both industrialized and nonindustrialized countries of the world, or by drinking contaminated water from mountain streams within the United States. The organism can be transmitted by close contact as seen in day care settings. Transmission by sexual contact has also been documented.

Frequently, the infection goes unnoticed. Infection is often recognized more easily in children than in adults. In extreme cases, the patient may experience abdominal pain and chronic diarrhea, usually described as containing mucus and fat, but not blood. Microscopic examination of stool specimens reveals the trophozoite or cyst stages of the parasitic life cycle.

The infection can usually be treated with metronidazole. Patients with *Giardia* infections should be instructed that the organism can be easily transmitted in family or group settings. Personal hygiene measures should be reinforced, and those who travel or camp where water is not treated and filtered should be advised to avoid local water supplies unless water is purified before drinking or used in cooking.

VIBRIO CHOLERA

Although in recent decades reported cases of cholera have been rare in the United States, no discussion of infectious diarrhea is complete without mention of this very serious infectious disease. Historically, epidemics of cholera have influenced all aspects of life–from medical to political–and infection rates have been significant enough to destroy governments and armies.

The *Vibrio cholera* organism is a gram-negative organism with several different serotypes. The type usually associated with epidemics is toxigenic *V. cholera* 01. The organism is transmitted by contaminated food or water. In recent years, most cases in the United States have been from contaminated shellfish found in the Gulf of Mexico.

Cholera causes disease with very rapid onset of copious diarrhea in which up to 1 L of fluid per hour can be lost. Dehydration, with subsequent cardiopulmonary collapse, may cause rapid progression from newly recognized disease to death. The principal therapy is rehydration. Rehydration efforts should be vigorous and sustained. If oral rehydration cannot be accomplished, the patient should be hospitalized for intravenous therapy support.

In the United States, cholera should be suspected in patients who have watery diarrhea after eating shellfish that have been harvested from the Gulf of Mexico. Confirmation of the causative organism can be made by stool culture. It is imperative that all cases are reported to local and state public health authorities.

NURSING PROCESS: THE PATIENT WITH INFECTIOUS DIARRHEA

Assessment

The most important element of assessment in the patient with diarrhea is to determine hydration status. The goal of rehydration is to correct the degree of dehydration. Assessment includes evaluation for thirst, oral mucous membrane dryness, sunken eyes, a weakened pulse, and loss of skin turgor. Careful observation for these signs is especially important in rapidly dehydrating diseases (most notably cholera) and in younger children.

Intake and output measurements are crucial in determining fluid balance. Liquid stool should be measured and recorded along with a record of the frequency of stools. It is important to note the consistency and appearance of stool as important indicators of the type and severity of the diarrheal disease. The presence of mucus or blood should also be noted.

When conducting a health history, it is important to determine whether the patient has recently traveled, whether the patient is currently being treated with antibiotics, whether the patient has been in contact with anyone who has recently had diarrheal disease, and what the patient has recently eaten. Frequently, patients attribute the most recent meals eaten as the cause of symptoms. However, the incubation period for most diarrheal conditions is longer than the time interval between meals. Therefore, it is important to get detailed information, not only about the meal preceding the illness, but about all food intake in the previous 3 to 4 days. When eliciting this kind of history, it is helpful to ask the patient to list every food tasted. In addition, it is important to ask patients if they are employed in a food preparation service. The local public health departments should be notified about any patient with infectious diarrhea who works in the food industry.

Diagnosis

Nursing Diagnoses

Based on the assessment data, the patient's major nursing diagnoses may include the following:

- Fluid volume deficit related to fluid lost through diarrhea
- Knowledge deficit about the infection and the risk of transmission to others

Collaborative Problems/Potential Complications

Based on the assessment data, potential complications that may develop include the following:

- Bacteremia
- Shock

Planning and Goals

The most important goals are maintenance of fluid and electrolyte balance, knowledge about the disease and risk of transmission, and the absence of complications.

Nursing Interventions

Providing Rehydration Therapy for Diarrhea

The patient is assessed to determine the degree of dehydration. This assessment helps determine the amount and route of rehydration needed. Oral therapy can rehydrate most patients. Oral rehydration therapy is a strategy used to reduce the severe complications of diarrheal disease regardless of causative agent. It is inexpensive and effective but is often underused because of sustained cultural beliefs discouraging oral intake during episodes of diarrhea. After much refinement of the formula, the World Health Organization (WHO) and the United Nation's International Children's Emergency Fund (UNICEF) agreed on the makeup of a single solution for treatment of dehydration and electrolyte imbalance associated with cholera and other forms of diarrheal disease. The solution contains (in millimoles per liter) sodium, 90; potassium, 20; chloride, 80; base, 30; and glucose 111.

MILD DEHYDRATION

The patient exhibits dry mucous membranes of the mouth and increased thirst. The rehydration goal at this level is to deliver about 50 mL/kg oral rehydration solution (ORS) over a 4-hour interval.

MODERATE DEHYDRATION

Sunken eyes, loss of skin turgor, and dry oral mucous membranes are frequent manifestations. An infant may have a sunken fontanel. The rehydration goal is about 100 mL/kg over 4 hours for the patient with moderate dehydration.

SEVERE DEHYDRATION

The patient shows signs of shock (rapid thready pulse, cyanosis, cold extremities, rapid breathing, lethargy, or coma) and should receive intravenous replacement until hemodynamic and mental status return to normal. When improvement is evident, the patient can be treated with ORS.

Administering Rehydration Therapy

Commercially available preparations in the United States, such as Pedialyte and Ricelyte, have been effective replacements for children with viral diarrheal disorders common in this country. When diarrheal losses are very high (more than 10 mL/kg/h), however, the lower sodium concentrations of these formulas make them less appropriate than the WHO formula.

For the hospitalized child, diarrheal fluid loss should be weighed, and ORS should be administered at a rate of 1 mL for each gram of diarrheal stool. Stool losses can be approximated so that the patient receives about 10 mL/kg ORS for each diarrheal stool.

It is important for children and adults suffering from acute diarrheal symptoms to maintain caloric intake. Infants who are breastfed should continue to feed on demand; those who are receiving formula should receive full-strength lactose-free or lactose-reduced formulas immediately after rehydration. Children who normally eat semisolid or solid food should have that food offered. Recommended foods include starches, cereals, yogurt, fruits, and vegetables. Foods that are high in simple sugars, such as undiluted apple juice or gelatin, should be avoided.

Because diarrheal episodes are often accompanied by vomiting, rehydration and refeeding can be difficult. Oral rehydration therapy should be delivered in small, frequent amounts. When vomiting is persistent, small children often require administration of fluids by frequent spoonfuls rather than by drinking from a bottle or a cup. Intravenous therapy is necessary for the patient who is severely dehydrated or in shock.

Increasing Knowledge and Preventing Spread of Infection

Public health nurses, school nurses, and others who are involved in patient teaching should emphasize principles of safe food preparation, with special attention to meat preparation and cooking. Ground beef should be cooked until no longer pink, and all meat should be kept at temperatures below 45°F or above 140°F. In planning events for groups of people, adequate provision for storage and reheating to meet temperature thresholds is important. When preparing food, it is important to use different surfaces, knives, and other equipment for meat and nonmeat items.

Diarrheal diseases discussed in this section must be reported to local or state health departments. The goal of reporting is to provide information that will be used to assess disease incidence trends and to identify at the earliest point if there is a restaurant or other food preparation establishment that is serving contaminated food.

The need for rehydration and refeeding should be taught to parents of children with diarrheal disease. Beliefs about illness and food patterns may have a traditional or cultural basis, and any teaching of health facts requires sensitivity.

Good hygiene in the health care delivery and home settings must be a focus when caring for patients with infectious diarrheal diseases. The principles of hand washing and glove use that are emphasized with standard precautions are important aspects of disease control.

Monitoring and Managing Potential Complications

BACTEREMIA

E. coli and *Salmonella* and *Shigella* species are all organisms that can be introduced into the bloodstream and disseminate to other organs. It is important that the acutely febrile patient with diarrhea have blood cultures done. If initial smear results reveal gram-negative organisms, antibiotic therapy is instituted.

SHOCK

Shock associated with diarrheal diseases demands accurate intake and output assessment and vigorous fluid replacement. In rare instances, patients with severe fluid imbalance require intensive care nursing support with aggressive hemodynamic monitoring.

Evaluation

Expected Outcomes

Expected outcomes may include:

1. Attains fluid balance
   a. Output approximates intake
   b. Mucous membranes appear moist
   c. Normal skin turgor
   d. Ingests adequate amounts of fluids and calories
   e. Absence of vomiting
   f. Stools of normal color and consistency
2. Acquires knowledge and understanding about infectious diarrhea and transmission potential
   a. Takes proper precautions to prevent spread of infection to others
   b. Describes principles and techniques of safe food storage, preparation, and cooking
3. Absence of complications
   a. Temperature within normal range
   b. Negative blood culture reports
   c. Achieves fluid balance

Legionnaires' Disease

Legionnaires' disease is a multisystem illness that frequently includes pneumonia and is caused by the gram-negative bacteria, *Legionella pneumophila.* Named after an outbreak of the disease among people attending a convention of the American Legion, its potential to cause outbreaks has been demonstrated numerous times in hospitals and other settings. *Legionella* organisms are found in many man-made and naturally occurring water sources. Although the organisms may initially be introduced in low numbers, growth is enhanced by water storage, scaling on the inside of water towers, temperatures ranging from 25° to 42°C, and certain amoebae frequently present in water that can support intracellular growth of legionellae.

Pathophysiology

L. pneumophila is transmitted by an aerosolized route from an environmental source to the respiratory tract of a person. It is not transmitted from person to person. In hospitals, patients may be exposed to aerosols created by cooling towers, water sources from plumbing, and respiratory therapy equipment. Because underlying medical conditions can increase host susceptibility and subsequent severity of disease, and because hospital plumbing systems are often very complex, outbreaks occur in hospitals more frequently than at other community centers. Mortality rates among hospitalized patients are about twofold greater than those for people with community acquired legionnella pneumonia.

Risk Factors

Risk factors strongly associated with *Legionella* infection include diseases that lead to severe immune suppression, such as AIDS, hematologic malignancy, end-stage renal disease, or use of immunosuppressive agents. Other factors associated with increased risk include advanced age, diabetes, alcohol abuse, smoking, and other pulmonary disease.

Clinical Manifestations

The lungs are the principal organs of infection. Other organs may be involved, however, and disease without pulmonary involvement has been reported. The incubation period ranges from 2 to 10 days. Early symptoms may include malaise, myalgias, headache, and dry cough. With disease progression, the patient develops increased pulmonary symptoms, including productive cough, dyspnea, and chest pain. Patients are usually febrile, and temperature curves may reach 103°F (39.4°C) and higher. Diarrhea and other gastrointestinal complaints commonly accompany the pulmonary array of symptoms. In severe cases, multiorgan involvement and failure may follow.

Assessment and Diagnostic Findings

Laboratory diagnostic tests available for diagnosis of *Legionella* include culture (using special microbiologic methods and media), immunofluorescent microscopy, antibody titer interpretation, and urinary antigen detection. Diagnosis of *Legionella* by antibody titer requires evidence that titers have increased at least fourfold over time. A single elevated titer is not sufficient to determine current disease. The urinary antigen (for *L. pneumophila* serotype 1, the most prevalent subspecies) test is a very helpful test because urine is easy to obtain and the test remains positive after initial antibiotic treatment. This persistent marker is very helpful because patients with community-acquired pneumonia are often treated empirically, and *Legionella* culture is not useful if an individual patient is being further diagnosed or if an epidemic is being investigated. Frequently, more than one laboratory test is used in the diagnosis of *Legionella* because no one test is 100% sensitive. The diagnostic approach generally involves accumulation of information obtained from history, physical, x-ray, and laboratory findings and assessment of therapeutic effectiveness. Chest x-ray abnormalities may vary in extensiveness and in location of diseased site.

Medical Management

Erythromycin is considered the antibiotic of choice. Other choices include rifampin, azithromycin, clarithromycin, and trimethoprim sulfa.

Nursing Management

The nursing management described for the patient with any pneumonia (see Chap. 21) should form the basis of care for the patient with legionnaires' pneumonia. Special isolation techniques are not used for these patients because there is no evidence of transmission between humans.

Lyme Disease

Lyme disease, caused by the spirochete *Borrelia burgdorferi,* is transmitted to humans by ticks. It is more common in the Northeast and Mid-Atlantic states, where the deer tick *(Ixodes dammini)* is prevalent. Ticks may feed on infected white-tailed deer or white-footed mice and then serve as a vector to transmit disease to humans. Lyme disease is less common in the Western states, where the California black-legged tick *(Ixodes pacificus),* capable of transmitting Lyme disease, prefers to feed on reptiles, which do not carry *B. burgdorferi.*

Lyme disease can be manifested by a wide range of symptoms and severity. In its early form, a rash is often present and may be accompanied by regional lymphadenopathy. In later stages, neurologic manifestations ranging from Bell's palsy to Guillain-Barré–like syndrome or dementia are possible. Other sites that may be affected include skin, joints, heart, and eyes.

Assessment and Diagnostic Findings

The diagnosis of Lyme disease is usually made by detecting a rash typical of Lyme disease and at least one late manifestation associated with the disease (musculoskeletal, neurologic, or cardiovascular system involvement) in the presence of laboratory confirmation of infection. Laboratory diagnosis alone is unreliable because of the frequency of false-negative and false-positive results and because tests are not well standardized in interpretation at this point.

Medical Management

Doxycycline, ceftriaxone, and azithromycin are among the commonly used antibiotics. Treatment regimens are usually for 3 to 4 weeks. Patients should be encouraged to complete the full course of therapy and to report changes in symptomatology during therapy because the regimen may need to be altered if treatment appears to be failing.

Hantavirus Pulmonary Syndrome

Hantavirus pulmonary syndrome (HPS), a severe cardiopulmonary illness with a case mortality rate of about 45%, is caused by the Sin Nombre virus and is transmitted to humans by direct or indirect contact with rodents. Cases occur most frequently in the Western states, but the rodents known to carry the virus are found throughout the country.

Assessment and Diagnostic Findings

The diagnosis of HPS should be suspected in patients who live in rural areas, who may have had exposure to rodents, and who report fever, aching muscles, and nausea. Laboratory evidence of thrombocytopenia and hemoconcentration are also common.

Medical Management

Although no specific treatment for Hantavirus has been approved, early treatment with ribavirin may reduce mortality. Early identification, assessment, and maintenance of respiratory status are the most important aspects of care for these patients. Intake and output measurements should be made carefully because overhydration is possible with cardiopulmonary compromise.

Prevention and Patient Education

Reduction of risk requires strategies to reduce human contact with rodents and their droppings. Public health programs and clinics in rural areas should regularly teach people to eliminate food sources to rodents in areas close to humans. Openings in walls or cabinets should be sealed. Traps should be used in areas such as sheds and barns in which rodents may enter and in which humans may work. Gloves should be worn when removing the animal from the trap, and gloves and traps should be disinfected with a 10% bleach solution. People entering such areas should be taught to avoid stirring up dust or breathing potentially contaminated dust. Brooms and vacuum cleaners should be used with caution; areas that may emit dust while being cleaned should first be dampened with a bleach solution to reduce viral contaminant and the potential for dust propulsion.

SEXUALLY TRANSMITTED DISEASES

A sexually transmitted disease (STD) is a disease acquired through sexual contact with an infected person. Table 64-3 identifies diseases that can be classified as STDs. There are other organisms that can be transmitted during sexual contact, although they are generally not considered STDs. For example, *G. lamblia*, usually associated with contaminated water, can also be transmitted through sexual exposure.

STDs are the most common infectious diseases in the United States and are epidemic in most parts of the world (see Risk Factors for Sexually Transmitted Diseases).Two of the STDs discussed here are also considered emerging infectious diseases—HIV/AIDS and chlamydial infection. The incidence of these two STDs has significantly increased during the past two decades. Portals of entry of STD microorganisms and sites of infection include the skin and mucosal linings of the urethra, cervix, vagina, rectum, and oropharynx.

Prevention

The use of a condom to provide a protective barrier from transmission of STD-related organisms has been broadly promoted, especially since the recognition of AIDS. At first referred to as a method to ensure *safe sex*, the use of condoms has been shown to reduce but not eliminate the risk of transmission of HIV and other venereal diseases. The term *safer sex* more appropriately connotes the public health message to be used when promoting the use of condoms.

Significance

STDs provide a unique set of challenges for the nurse, physician, and public health official. Because of perceived stigma and possible threat to emotional relationships, those with symptoms of

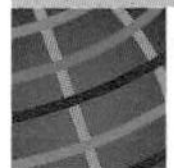

TABLE 64•3 **Conditions Classified as Sexually Transmitted Diseases (STDs) and Their Routes of Transmission**

Disease	Route(s) of Transmission
HIV infection/AIDS	Sexual, percutaneous, perinatal
Hepatitis B (HBV)	Sexual, percutaneous, perinatal
Hepatitis C (HCV)	Percutaneous, probably sexual, probably perinatal
Syphilis	Sexual, perinatal
Gonorrhea	Sexual, perinatal
Chlamydia	Sexual
Herpes simplex	Sexual
Human papillomavirus (HPV)	Sexual
Cytomegalovirus (CMV)	Sexual, less intimate contact
Chancroid, *Lymphogranuloma venereum,* and *Granuloma inguinale*	Sexual

Risk Factors for STDs

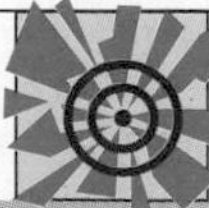

The following factors increase one's risk for acquiring STDs:

- Those at risk for acquiring STDs are sexual partners of infected people.
- One's risk of infection increases proportionately with the number of sexual partners.
- Sexual activity in adolescence accounts for an increased incidence of STD cases in that age group.
- An increase in illicit drug use and homelessness may promote prostitution, which in turn influences a wide transmission of STDs.
- Oral and anal sexual practices expose one to a potentially greater bacterial and viral load of organisms.

STDs are often reluctant to seek health care in a timely fashion. Similar to many other infectious diseases, STDs may progress without symptoms. A delay in diagnosis and treatment is potentially harmful because the risk of complications for the infected individual and the risk of transmission to others increases over time.

Infection with one STD suggests the possibility of infection with other organisms as well. Therefore, once one STD is identified, diagnostic evaluation for others should be performed. The possibility of HIV infection should be pursued whenever an STD is diagnosed.

Human Immunodeficiency Virus

HIV is the causative agent of AIDS. AIDS may occur when the immune system has been significantly weakened by the HIV virus. The definition of AIDS, as determined by the CDC, has changed several times since the syndrome was first recognized in 1981. In general, the definition sets a point in the continuum of HIV deterioration in which the host has clinically demonstrated profound immune dysfunction. A large number of opportunistic infections and neoplasms serve as markers for immune suppression severity. Since 1993, the AIDS definition has also included a CD4+ count of less than 200 as a threshold criterion. The CD4+ cell is a subset of the lymphocyte and is one of the target cells of HIV infection.

Types of HIV

HIV has two viral types identified. Almost all cases of recognized HIV infection in the United States are attributed to HIV-1. HIV-2, a similar virus with identical transmission routes and clinical course, also has the ability to cause AIDS. Since 1992, all donated blood and blood components or products have been screened for this rare virus (HIV-2). Serologic testing can distinguish between HIV-1 and HIV-2. Throughout the remainder of this section, "HIV" refers to HIV-1.

Pathophysiology

HIV is transmitted through sexual contact, percutaneous injection of contaminated blood, or perinatally from infected mother to fetus. Most people infected by the percutaneous route are intravenous drug users who share contaminated needles, but transmission is also remotely possible through contaminated blood transfusion. Since 1985, all blood transfusions have been screened, and transfusion-related transmission of HIV is now extremely unlikely.

There is strong evidence that other STDs, especially those characterized by ulceration, increase the risk of sexual transmission of HIV. Because of a failing immune system, people with HIV infection may also be more susceptible to other STDs. Factors associated with increased risk of sexual transmission are failure to use condoms, frequency of sexual contact, anal intercourse, and sexual activity during menstruation.

Risk to Health Care Workers

NEEDLESTICK INJURIES

Health care workers can be infected through the percutaneous route if needlestick or other injury from a sharp object introduces contaminated blood. Prospective studies (eg, Henderson, 1997) of this risk demonstrate that less than 1% of such occupational exposures (in which the source patient is infected with HIV) lead to transmission. Despite the rarity of transmission, standard precautions are recommended by the CDC and enforced by OSHA as a strategy to decrease this risk. Health care workers are advised to take extreme care to avoid needlestick or mucous membrane exposure to blood of all patients. Since 1996, the CDC has recommended postexposure prophylaxis for significant occupational exposures to HIV. An algorithm based on the degree of exposure and the probable degree of contagiousness in the specific patient is used to determine which combination of zidovudine and protease inhibitors should be offered to the health care worker. To be effective, the prophylaxis must be given within 2 hours of the exposure. Therefore, all health care workers should understand the urgency of reporting a needlestick or other percutaneous exposure immediately. Counseling about the advisability of prophylaxis and appropriate medication and dose selection should be made on a case-by-case basis.

Medical Management

To date, there is no cure for AIDS, although antiviral therapy (using zidovudine, protease inhibitors, or other therapies) may prolong the period of time that a patient with HIV is well. In addition, specific therapies to treat the different opportunistic infections and cancers associated with AIDS serve to increase life expectancy after diagnosis.

The impact of HIV is felt in all aspects of health care planning and delivery as well as socially and financially throughout the world. HIV and AIDS are discussed in detail in Chapter 48.

Syphilis

Syphilis is an acute and chronic infectious disease caused by the spirochete *Treponema pallidum*. It is acquired through sexual contact or may be congenital in origin.

Stages of Syphilis

In the untreated person, the course of syphilis can be divided into three stages: primary, secondary, and tertiary. These stages reflect the time from infection and the clinical manifestations observed in that period, and are the basis for treatment decisions.

Primary syphilis occurs 2 to 3 weeks after initial inoculation with the organism. A painless lesion at the site of infection is called a *chancre*. Untreated, these lesions usually resolve spontaneously within about 2 months.

Secondary syphilis occurs when the hematogenous spread of organisms from the original chancre leads to generalized infection. The rash of secondary syphilis generally occurs about 2 to 8 weeks after the chancre and involves the trunk and the extremities, including the palms of the hands and the soles of the feet. Transmission of the organism can occur through contact with these lesions. Generalized signs of infection may include lymphadenopathy, arthritis, meningitis, hair loss, fever, malaise, and weight loss.

After the secondary stage, there is a period of **latency** in which the infected person is without signs or symptoms of syphilis. Latency can be interrupted by a recurrence of secondary syphilis.

Tertiary syphilis is the final stage in the natural history of the disease. It is estimated that between 20% and 40% of those infected do not exhibit this final level of clinical findings. In this stage, syphilis presents as a slowly progressive inflammatory disease with the potential to affect multiple organs. The most common manifestations at this level are aortitis and neurosyphilis, as evidenced by dementia, psychosis, paresis, stroke, or meningitis.

Assessment and Diagnostic Findings

Because syphilis shares symptoms with many diseases, clinical history and laboratory evaluation are important. The conclusive diagnosis of syphilis can be made by direct identification of the spirochete obtained from the chancre lesions of primary syphilis. Serologic tests used in the diagnosis of secondary and tertiary syphilis require clinical correlation in interpretation. The serologic tests are summarized as follows:

- *Nontreponemal* or *reagin tests*, such as the Venereal Disease Research Laboratory (VDRL) or the rapid plasma reagin circle card test (RPR-CT), are generally used for screening and diagnosis. After adequate therapy, the test is expected to decrease quantitatively until it is read as negative, about 2 years after therapy.
- *Treponemal tests*, such as the fluorescent treponemal antibody absorption test (FTA-ABS) and the microhemagglutination test (MHA-TP), are used to verify that the screening test did not represent a false-positive result. Positive results usually are positive for life, and so are not appropriate to determine therapeutic effectiveness.

Medical Management

The current treatment of all stages of syphilis is administration of antibiotics. Penicillin G benzathine is the medication of choice for early syphilis or latent syphilis of less than 1 year's duration. It is given by intramuscular injection at a single session. The same therapy is recommended for patients with early latent syphilis. Patients with late latent or latent syphilis of unknown duration should receive three injections at 1-week intervals. Patients who are allergic to penicillin are usually treated with doxycycline. The patient treated with penicillin is monitored for 30 minutes after the injection to observe for a possible allergic reaction.

Treatment guidelines established by the CDC are updated on a regular basis. Recommendations provide special guidelines for treatment in the setting of pregnancy, allergy, HIV infection, pediatric infection, congenital infection, and neurosyphilis.

Nursing Management

Syphilis is a reportable communicable disease. In any health care facility, a mechanism should be in place to ensure that all patients who are diagnosed are reported to the state or local public health department to ensure community follow-up. The public health department is responsible for interviewing the patient to determine sexual contacts, so that contact notification and screening can be initiated.

Lesions of primary and secondary syphilis may be highly infective. Gloves are worn when having direct contact with lesions, and hands are washed after gloves are removed. Isolation in a private room is not required. (See Patient Education and Home Care: Treating and Preventing the Spread of Syphilis.)

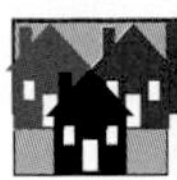

PATIENT EDUCATION AND HOME CARE

Treating and Preventing the Spread of Syphilis

- The patient is instructed to complete the full course of therapy if multiple penicillin injections are required.
- The patient with primary or secondary syphilis is assured that with proper treatment, skin lesions and other sequelae of infection will improve, and serology eventually will reflect cure.
- The patient is instructed to refrain from sexual contact with previous or current partners until they have been treated.

Gonorrhea

Neisseria gonorrhoeae is a gram-negative bacterium that is transmitted primarily through sexual contact. Infection can also occur in neonates as a result of contact during birth. *N. gonorrhoeae* can cause mucosal, local, or disseminated infection. Asymptomatic infection is somewhat common.

Clinical Manifestations

Gonorrhea most frequently presents with local manifestations. In men, urethritis and epididymitis are the most common symptoms. Gonorrhea is more likely to be asymptomatic in women than in men. The uterine cervix is the primary site of local infection, and symptoms often include urinary tract infection, increased vaginal discharge, and itching. The most common complication of localized gonococcal infection in women is pelvic inflammatory disease (PID), in which the organism infects the uterus, fallopian tubes, or peritoneal fluid. A complication of gonococcal PID is increased risk for ectopic pregnancy and bilateral tubal occlusion, which results in infertility.

In rare circumstances, the organism may disseminate in untreated, infected people. Other systemic signs, such as arthritis or dermatitis, can accompany bacteremia. In rare instances, valves of the heart can be infected with *N. gonorrhoeae*, or gonococcal meningitis can develop.

Assessment and Diagnostic Findings

The patient is assessed for fever, for urethral, vaginal, and rectal discharge, and for signs of arthritis. Culture and sensitivity studies are the usual and preferred methods of diagnosing and verifying effectiveness of therapy. In the male patient, specimens are obtained from the urethra, anal canal, and pharynx. In the female patient, cultures from the endocervix, pharynx, and anal canal are obtained. When obtaining these cultures, the nurse should wear disposable gloves and wash hands thoroughly after glove removal. Lubricating jelly is not used for the vaginal examination because it may contain substances that inhibit growth or kill some pathogens, thus decreasing the microbiologic test accuracy. Instead, water is used as the lubricant. Because *N. gonorrhoeae* are susceptible to environmental changes, specimens must be delivered to the laboratory immediately after they are obtained.

Medical Management

The CDC-recommended treatment for gonorrheal infections is administration of ceftriaxone (or cefixime, ciprofloxacin, or ofloxacin) along with doxycycline. Doxycycline is added to first-line therapy to treat presumptive *Chlamydia trachomatis*, which commonly causes coinfection in patients with gonorrhea. Patients with uncomplicated gonorrhea who are treated with CDC-recommended therapy do not routinely need to return for a proof-of-cure visit. If the patient reports a new episode of symptoms or tests reveal gonorrhea again, the most likely explanation is reinfection rather than treatment failure.

Serologic testing for syphilis and HIV should be offered to patients with gonorrhea because any STD represents increased risk for other STD infections.

Nursing Management

Gonorrhea is a reportable communicable disease. In any health care facility, a mechanism should be in place to ensure that all patients diagnosed with gonorrhea are reported to the local public health department, so that follow-up of the patient can be ensured. In addition, the public health department is responsible for interviewing the patient to determine sexual contacts, so that contact notification and screening can be initiated.

Chlamydia trachomatis

C. trachomatis is a bacterium that requires attachment to the host cell, invasion, intracellular growth, and replication. This requirement for intracellular growth, which is similar to that of viruses, has made the identification and laboratory study more difficult than for organisms that grow and replicate independently. Recent advances have made diagnosis and screening much more available.

Clinical Manifestations

In women, sexual intercourse is the usual route of transmission. The most frequent clinical manifestation is PID, but many times, symptoms are so subtle that pathologic progression can occur without detection. Long-term effects may include chronic pain, increased risk for ectopic pregnancy, postpartum endometritis, and infertility.

Transmission of infection from an infected pregnant woman to her vaginally born infant is common. About 15% to 20% of infected infants develop chlamydial conjunctivitis, and about 10% develop chlamydial pneumonia.

Although men infected with *Chlamydia* are frequently asymptomatic, they easily transmit the infection to their sexual partners. Urethritis is the most common illness associated with infection in the heterosexual man with symptoms. Among homosexual men, the rectum is the common site of infection.

Assessment and Diagnostic Findings

Chlamydia should be suspected in cases of gonorrhea, nongonorrheal urethritis, PID, and epididymitis. Diagnostic tools include cell culture techniques and a relatively wide range of nonculture techniques, including immunologic assays, DNA probes, and enzyme-sensitive tests.

Medical Management

Treatment of chlamydial infection is usually administration of either doxycycline or azithromycin. Neither of these antibiotics is recommended in pregnancy. Guidelines published by the CDC should be used to determine alternative therapy for the patient who is pregnant or allergic or who has complicated chlamydial infection. It is important that both the patient and the sexual partner be treated.

Prevention and Patient Education

The target group for preventive patient teaching about *C. trachomatis* is the adolescent and young adult population. Abstinence, postponing the age of initial sexual exposure, limiting the number of sexual partners, and use of condoms for barrier protection should be promoted. It should also be stressed that screening for *Chlamydia* and treating infection at an early stage are important to decrease disease progression common to women and to decrease the likelihood of infection in infants.

NURSING PROCESS: THE PATIENT WITH A SEXUALLY TRANSMITTED DISEASE

Assessment

Health History

The patient should be asked to describe the onset and progression of symptoms and to characterize any lesions by location and describe drainage if present. Protecting confidentiality is important when discussing sexual issues. When a detailed sexual history is necessary, it is important to respect the patient's right to privacy. Brief explanations of why the information is asked and how confidentiality is maintained are often helpful. Clarification of terms may be necessary if the patient or nurse uses words unfamiliar to the other. Asking specific information about sexual contacts should generally be done only when the nurse is part of a team that will contact the partners for follow-up. In the history-taking process, discussion about the patient's understanding of responsibility to inform sexual partners may be helpful in determining patient teaching goals.

During physical examination, the presence of rashes, lesions, drainage, discharge, or swelling is noted. Inguinal nodes are palpated to elicit tenderness and to note swelling. Women are examined for abdominal or uterine tenderness. The mouth and throat are examined for signs of inflammation or exudate.

The nurse wears gloves while examining the mucous membranes, and gloves are changed and replaced after vaginal or rectal examination.

Diagnosis

Nursing Diagnoses

Based on assessment data, the patient's major nursing diagnoses may include the following:

- Knowledge deficit about the disease and risk for spread of infection and reinfection

- Noncompliance with treatment
- Fear related to anticipated stigmatization and to prognosis and complications

Collaborative Problems/Potential Complications

Based on assessment data, potential complications that may develop include the following:

- Increased risk for ectopic pregnancy
- Infertility
- Transmission of infection to fetus resulting in congenital abnormalities and other outcomes
- Neurosyphilis
- Gonococcal meningitis
- Gonococcal arthritis
- Syphilitic aortitis
- HIV-related complications

Planning and Goals

Major goals are increased patient understanding of the natural history and treatment of the infection, increased compliance with therapeutic and preventive goals, reduction in fear, and absence of complications.

Nursing Interventions

Increasing Knowledge and Preventing Spread of Disease

Education about and prevention of the spread of STDs to others often are simultaneous activities. Discussion about risk factors should emphasize that the same behaviors that led to infection with one STD may introduce risk for any other STD, including HIV. Methods used to contact sexual partners should be discussed. The patient should understand that until the partner has been treated, continued sexual exposure to the same person may lead to reinfection. Patients may need help in planning discussion with partners. If the patient is especially apprehensive about this aspect, referral to a social worker or other specialist may be appropriate. Such support is especially important when the patient has newly diagnosed HIV infection.

The relative value of condoms in reducing the risk for infection with STDs should be addressed. When appropriate, the patient should be encouraged to discuss any reasons for resistance to condom use, so that decision making about this preventive method can be facilitated.

The infected patient should be told what the causative organism is and should receive an explanation of the usual course of the infection (including interval of potential communicability to others) and possible complications. The nurse should stress the importance of following therapy as prescribed and the need to report any therapeutic side effects or symptom progression.

Reducing Fear

When appropriate, the patient is encouraged to discuss anxieties and fear associated with the diagnosis, therapy, or prognosis. By individualizing teaching efforts, factual information applied to specific needs may offer reassurance. For example, patients with HIV should be encouraged to participate in well-coordinated programs in which support, education, counseling, and therapeutic goals are combined. Such programs are designed to offer coordinated care throughout the course of disease progression.

Increasing Compliance

In group settings (such as may be offered in an outpatient obstetric setting), or in a one-on-one setting, open discussion about STD information facilitates patient teaching. Discomfort can be reduced by factual explanation of causes, consequences, treatments, prevention, and responsibilities. Because most communities have expanded STD prevention resources, referrals to appropriate agencies can complement individual educational efforts and ensure that later questions or uncertainties can be addressed by experts. [The CDC-maintained STD National Hotline (1-800-227-8922) provides toll-free information and confidential referral services for STDs.]

Monitoring and Managing Potential Complications

INFERTILITY AND INCREASED RISK FOR ECTOPIC PREGNANCY

STDs may lead to PID and with it, increased risk for ectopic pregnancy and infertility.

CONGENITAL INFECTIONS

All STDs can be transmitted to infants in utero or at the time of birth. Complications of congenital infection can range from localized infection (eg, throat infection with *N. gonorrhea*) to congenital abnormalities (eg, stunting of growth or deafness from congenital syphilis), to life-threatening disease (eg, congenital herpes simplex virus).

NEUROSYPHILIS, GONOCOCCAL MENINGITIS, GONOCOCCAL ARTHRITIS, SYPHILITIC AORTITIS

STDs can cause disseminated infection. The central nervous system may be infected, as seen with neurosyphilis or gonococcal meningitis. Gonorrhea that infects the skeletal system may result in gonococcal arthritis. Syphilis can infect the cardiovascular system by forming vegetative lesions on the mitral or aortic valves.

HIV-RELATED COMPLICATIONS

HIV, which is primarily spread as an STD, leads to the profound immune suppression of AIDS. Complications of HIV infection include many opportunistic infections, including *Pneumocystis carinii*, *Cryptococcus neoformans*, cytomegalovirus, and *Mycobacterium avium.*

Evaluation

Expected Outcomes

Expected outcomes may include:

1. Acquires knowledge and understanding of STDs
2. Complies with treatment
   a. Achieves effective treatment
   b. Reports for follow-up examination if necessary
3. Demonstrates a less anxious demeanor
   a. Recalls signs and symptoms of the most common STDs
   b. Inspects self for lesions, rashes, and discharge

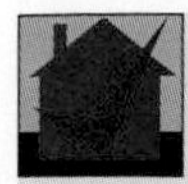

HOME CARE TEACHING CHECKLIST: PREVENTION OF INFECTION IN THE HOME CARE SETTING

At the completion of the program, the patient or caregiver will be able to:	Patient	Caregiver
• Demonstrate aseptic technique in the care of technical equipment such as intravenous catheter, indwelling urinary catheter.	✔	✔
• Demonstrate thorough hand washing after patient care.	✔	✔
• Provide assurance of compliance with antibiotic regimen or with completion of vaccination series.	✔	✔
• State the rationale for thoroughly cooking all foods and storing meat products separate from other food groups.	✔	✔

   c. Assists with sharing information about infection to sexual partners
   d. Chooses a form of risk-reduction behavior through monogamy, reduction in sexual partners, and the use of condoms
4. Experiences absence of complications
   a. When possible, infections are treated before opportunity for transmission to fetus
   b. Infection is treated before PID or sterility develops
   c. Patients with syphilis are treated in primary stage, so that progression to later stages or complications are avoided
   d. Patients with gonorrhea are treated in early stage before dissemination occurs

HOME-BASED CARE OF THE PATIENT WITH AN INFECTIOUS DISEASE

Reducing Risk

The nurse who cares for the patient in the home will need to provide infection risk prevention for the patient, the family, and the caregiver (see Home Care Teaching Checklist: Prevention of Infection in the Home Care Setting).

Reducing Risk to the Patient

Patients requiring home care are often those with immune suppression from underlying conditions, such as HIV or cancer, or those who have therapy-induced immune suppression, as may be seen with antineoplastic agents. Careful assessment for signs of infection are important.

HAND WASHING

Hand washing in the home is an important preventive strategy. Whether a treatment is performed by the nurse, the family, or the patient, hand washing reduces the risk of transient flora.

EQUIPMENT CARE

Health care equipment increases infection risk because it is complex and invasive. All caregivers must be taught to pay careful attention to disinfection, asepsis, and appropriate usage intervals. The nurse should maintain a record of the time intervals of vascular catheter insertion. Tunneled catheters, such as the Groshong, should not be routinely changed. Patients or family members who administer intravenous fluid or medication should be taught how to use aseptic technique during these procedures. The predetermined changing schedule of other vascular access devices should be followed. The nurse and the family members should be alert for any redness, swelling, or drainage around the catheter insertion site. Catheter-related sepsis should be suspected in a patient who has unexplained fever.

There is no recommended interval for the changing of indwelling urinary catheters. The nurse should promptly report to the patient's physician signs of urinary tract infection or of generalized sepsis.

PATIENT TEACHING

When assessing the immune-suppressed patient in the home environment for infectious risk, it is important to realize that intrinsic colonizing bacteria and latent viral infections present a greater risk than do extrinsic environmental contaminants. The patient and family need reassurance that their home does not need to be sterile. Common-sense approaches to cleanliness and risk reduction are helpful. The severely neutropenic patient should refrain from eating uncooked fruits and vegetables. For patients with neutropenia or with T-cell dysfunction (eg, AIDS patients) it is wise to restrict visits of people with potentially contagious illnesses.

Reducing Risk to Household Members

ESTABLISHING BARRIERS AND PRECAUTIONS

Establishing careful barriers to infection transmission in the household is an important part of home care. The route of transmission of the organism in question must first be determined. The nurse can then teach household members to reduce their risk of becoming infected. If the patient has active pulmonary TB, the public health department should be contacted to provide screening and treatment for family members. Decisions about prevention of other airborne diseases, such as chickenpox, need to be made based on the family situation. For example, precautions are not usually recommended to prevent healthy siblings from being exposed to a child with chickenpox. If one of the household members is pregnant and has no previous history of chickenpox, however, avoiding contact during the infectious period is wise.

FOOD PREPARATION AND PERSONAL HYGIENE

Organisms transmitted by the fecal–manual–oral route may be readily spread in a household setting unless careful attention to food preparation and personal hygiene is maintained. Family caregivers are vulnerable to acquiring organisms such as *Shigella* species and *C. difficile* when assisting in personal care. Hands should be washed carefully after such contact. The family should be reassured that common household disinfectants are effective in killing environmental sources of such organisms.

BLOODBORNE INFECTION RISK

Family members who assist in the care of a patient with a bloodborne infection such as HIV should be alert for the potential of transmission if sharp objects contaminated with blood are handled. Family teaching may be designed to discuss the need for caution when shaving the patient, performing dressing changes, or administering any intravenous, intramuscular, or subcutaneous medication. It is important to set up an impenetrable container for the collection of needles, syringes, and vascular access equipment.

The nurse should also teach the family about infections that do not pose a risk. With the exception of TB, the opportunistic infections associated with AIDS do not pose a risk to the healthy family member. Family members should be reassured that dishes are safe to use after being washed with hot water, and linens and clothing also are safe to use after being washed in a hot-water cycle.

Reducing Risk to the Caregiver

Recognizing that a health history may not identify all active or latent infections, the caregiver should follow careful infection control practices (including standard precautions) in the home. Setting up a work environment in which hand washing and aseptic technique can be accomplished as carefully as they are in a hospital setting is important.

Receiving hepatitis B vaccination and yearly vaccination with the influenza vaccine is a wise preventive strategy. Having a PPD test annually is an important method to verify that new infection with TB has not occurred.

NURSING PROCESS: THE PATIENT WITH AN INFECTIOUS DISEASE

Assessment

Symptoms of infectious diseases vary significantly both between and within diseases. For some infections, such as chickenpox (varicella), widely disseminated rash represents the first suggestion of infection and is present in most newly infected people. In other infections, such as TB and HIV, latency is prolonged and most of those infected do not have symptoms; instead, infection is determined through diagnostic procedures.

History taking, physical examination, and the use of diagnostic tests are important determinants of infection and infectious diseases.

The goals of eliciting history are to establish the likelihood and probable source of infection and the degree of associated pathology or pain. The patient's previous medical record is reviewed when possible. In obtaining a health history, some of the following questions may be asked:

- Does the patient have a history of previous or recurrent infections? Is the patient aware of infection with an organism associated with prolonged latency, such as HIV, herpes, or TB?
- Has there been fever? How high has the patient's temperature been? What is the fever pattern? Is the temperature constant, or does it rise and fall? Has fever been associated with chills? Has the patient taken medication to relieve fever?
- Is there cough? Is the cough chronic or acute? Is it associated with shortness of breath? Does the cough produce sputum? Is the sputum bloody? Has the patient had a PPD test performed recently? If so, what were the results? Has the patient been given isoniazid (INH) prophylaxis for TB infection? Has the patient been treated for TB in the past?
- Is there pain? Where is the pain? What is the nature of the pain? Are there sore throat, headache, myalgias, arthralgias? Is there pain on urination or other activity?
- Is there swelling? Is there drainage associated with the swelling? Is the swollen area warm to touch?
- Is there a draining site? Is the drainage associated with trauma or a previous procedure? Is the drainage purulent or clear?
- Does the patient have diarrhea, vomiting, or abdominal pain?
- Is there rash? What is the nature of the rash—is it flat, raised, red, crusted, purulent, lacelike?
- What is the vaccination history?
- Has the patient taken medications that could induce rash?
- Has there been exposure to another person who has an identified infectious disease or rash?
- Has there been an insect or animal bite? Has there been an animal scratch or other exposure to pets, farm animals, or experimental animals?
- What medications are used? Have antibiotics been taken recently or chronically? Is the patient being treated with corticosteroids, immunosuppressing agents, or chemotherapy?
- Is there a history of substance abuse?
- Has the patient been treated in the past for other infectious diseases? Has the patient been hospitalized for infectious diseases?
- If sexual history is pertinent, has there been sexual exposure to another person with a known STD? Has the patient been treated for STDs in the past? Is the patient pregnant or has she recently been pregnant? Has the patient been tested for HIV?
- Has the patient traveled to or from a developing country or abroad? What was the immunization or antimicrobial prophylaxis used for protection while traveling?
- What is the patient's occupation?

Because infection may occur in any body system, physical examination may reveal signs of infection at any body site. Generalized signs of chronic infection may include significant weight loss or pallor associated with anemia of chronic diseases. Acute infection may present with fever, chills, lymphadenopathy, or rash. Localized signs vary significantly according to the source of infection. Purulence, pain, swelling, and redness are strongly associated with localized infection. Cough and shortness of breath may be due to influenza, pneumonia, or TB as well as to many noninfectious causes.

Diagnosis

Nursing Diagnoses

Infection may cause an interruption in normal function of any affected body system. For alteration in each system, the reader should review nursing diagnoses for body systems listed in the appropriate chapters.

Based on assessment data, the patient's major nursing diagnoses that relate specifically to infection may include the following:

- Risk for infection transmission
- Knowledge deficit about the disease, cause of infection, treatment, and prevention measures
- Altered body temperature (fever) related to the presence of infection

Collaborative Problems/Potential Complications

Based on the assessment data, potential complications that may develop include the following:

- Secondary bloodstream infection
- Septic shock
- Dehydration
- Abscess formation
- Endocarditis
- Infectious disease–related cancers
- Infertility
- Congenital abnormalities

Planning and Goals

Major goals for the patient may include prevention of spread of infection, knowledge about the infection and its treatment, control of fever and related discomforts, and absence of complications.

Nursing Interventions

Preventing Infection Transmission

Preventing the spread of infection requires an understanding of the usual routes of transmission for the organism. The hospitalized patient may serve as a risk for transmission to other patients if the patient's disease was spread by the airborne route, or if infected by an organism such as *C. difficile*, which can be spread directly to others by persistence of spores in the environment. In these situations, strict adherence to isolation measures is important in reducing the opportunity for spread. Preventing transmission of organisms from patient to patient usually requires participation of the health care team. Transmission of organisms on the hands and gloves of health care workers remains a common source of cross-infection in the hospital or clinic setting.

Nurses serve an important role in prevention of transfer of organisms in two ways. First, as the health professional who often spends the greatest amount of time with patients, the opportunity for spreading organisms is great. It is imperative that nurses wash their hands before and after contact with patients and after performing a potentially hand-contaminating activity. Hands must be washed each time gloves are removed. For example, the nurse who has performed endotracheal suctioning should remove gloves and wash hands before performing wound care on the same patient.

The second way that nurses reduce hand-to-hand spread is to serve as patient advocates. With the number of health care workers involved in patient care each day, there is a significant opportunity for breaks in hand-washing technique. To the degree feasible, the nurse should observe the hand-washing activities of other professionals and discuss them when lapses in technique are observed.

Teaching About the Infectious Process

For infectious diseases, interruption of transmission requires infection recognition as well as patient understanding of the significance of the infection and a commitment to prevention. The nurse's role in this situation is to educate and, in some situations, to report the case to public health officials for contact tracing and verification of follow-up.

In educational efforts, it is also necessary to stress the importance of immunization to parents of young children and to others for whom certain vaccines are recommended. Nurses should assess their personal responsibility to receive hepatitis B and annual influenza vaccine to reduce potential transmission to self and vulnerable patient groups.

Infectious diseases often seem mysterious and frequently carry socially stigmatizing effects. Patient teaching efforts require empathy and sensitivity. For example, patients who are to receive INH prophylaxis for 6 months may be confused by the information that they are infected but not diseased, and yet need to adhere to prolonged therapy. In the past, TB was a very stigmatized disease. Some patients still feel shame when learning of this infection. Patient teaching must be directed at the details and advantages of INH prophylaxis. It should be clarified that infection is not a guilt-associated issue.

Controlling Fever and Accompanying Discomforts

Whereas infectious diseases usually cause fever, there are other noninfectious causes of fever as well. Therefore, a new fever requires investigation of its source. There is evidence that fever, as mediated by the hypothalamus, is a part of a syndrome of reactions known as *acute-phase reaction.* These reactions include changes in liver protein synthesis; alterations in serum metals, such as iron; and increased production of certain classes of white blood cells as well as other immune system cells. Fever may potentiate some beneficial functions of this acute-phase reaction. Severe fever, such as seen with meningococcal meningitis, may cause other complications in the form of heat stroke, but this is uncommon because most fevers are physiologically self-controlled to stay below 105.8°F (41°C). Even with this control, however, fever and its accompanying fatigue, chills, and diaphoresis can be very uncomfortable for the patient. Decisions regarding fever control are made by the physician. Whether or not fever is treated, adequate fluid intake is important during febrile episodes.

Nursing Alert *Because fever offers clues about infection severity and success of antibiotic therapy, outpatients with fever should be taught to obtain accurate readings. Frequently, parents will know that a child has warm skin but will not trouble the child by taking a temperature reading. Body temperature information can be very helpful in adjusting therapy or in reevaluating a preliminary diagnosis.*

Monitoring and Managing Potential Complications

The patient with a rapidly progressive infectious disease should have vital signs and level of consciousness closely monitored for signs of sepsis. Laboratory values from microbiology, immunology, hematology, cytology, and parasitology, along with x-ray findings, must be interpreted in the context of other clinical findings to assess the infectious disease course. Antibiotic therapy is frequently complex, with modifications necessary because of sensitivity test results and disease progression. It is important to initiate antibiotic therapy as soon as it is prescribed, rather than waiting until routine medication scheduling times. This ensures that therapeutic blood levels can be attained as quickly as possible. See Plan of Nursing Care 64-1 for nursing interventions for specific complications of infection.

(*text continues on page 1898*)

64•1

Plan of Nursing Care 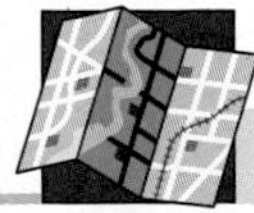 Care of the Patient With An Infectious Disease

Nursing Interventions	Rationale	Expected Outcomes
Nursing Diagnosis: Risk for infection transmission **Goal:** Preventing transmission of infectious agents		
1. Prevent patient-to-patient infection spread	1. Organisms that are spread through an airborne route or are very contagious through direct contact can be transmitted in a health care setting.	• No evidence of patient-to patient transmission of infection • No evidence of transmission via health care workers • No occupationally acquired infections in nurses and other health care workers • No evidence of transmission due to contaminated equipment • Absence of primary bloodstream infections • Absence of urinary tract infections • Absence of pneumonia
a. Provide isolation according to CDC guidelines and Standard Precautions	a. CDC isolation strategies are developed to reduce the likelihood of transmission from patient to patient.	
b. Ensure that patients with airborne infections remain in private rooms during hospital stay. If they must leave their rooms, arrangements should be made to decrease the likelihood of contact with other patients. Rooms should be ventilated according to CDC criteria. Personal protective equipment in the form of masks or respirators should be worn. In any care setting where patients may have increased risk for the sequelae of influenza, annual influenza vaccination should be encouraged for personnel and patients.	b. Engineering controls are important in the prevention of airborne diseases. Influenza vaccine safely reduces risk of illness associated with this highly communicable, and frequently virulent, organism.	
c. Ensure that patients with highly transmissible, nonairborne organisms such as *Clostridium difficile* and *Shigella* species are physically separated from other patients if hygiene or institutional policy dictates.	c. Increased prevention strategy is needed when the organism has high epidemic potential.	
2. Prevent health care workers' transfer of organisms from patient to patient	2. Transfer of organisms on the hands of health care workers is a common route of transmission. Hospital organisms colonizing the hands of health care workers may be virulent.	
a. Hand washing should be performed consistently and thoroughly—washing hands before and after each patient contact, and following procedures that offer contamination risk while caring for an individual patient	a. Hand-washing technique is important in reducing transient flora on outer epidermal layers of skin.	
b. Gloves must be used when handling any body fluid from any patient. Gloves must be changed between patient care activities, and hands must be washed after gloves are removed.	b. Gloves provide effective barrier protection. Gloves quickly become contaminated and then become a potential vehicle for the transfer of organisms between patients. Microflora on hands are likely to proliferate while gloves are worn.	
c. Nurses should monitor the hand washing and glove use behaviors of other health care professionals caring for the patient	c. Poor compliance with hand washing among health care workers has been well documented and should be anticipated. It is important for the nurse as the patient's advocate to communicate this protective behavior.	

(*continued*)

64•1

Plan of Nursing Care 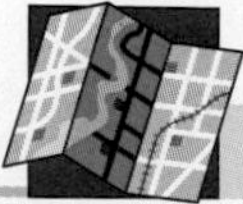 Care of the Patient With An Infectious Disease (*continued*)

Nursing Interventions	Rationale	Expected Outcomes
3. Prevent patient-to-health care worker transmission of infection.	3. Health care workers may acquire infections occupationally due to close contact with patients.	
a. Risk of infection with tuberculosis may be avoided by:	a. The most important element in the reduction of tuberculosis is early identification. Many of the symptoms of tuberculosis are subtle, and may be first observed by the nurse who has prolonged contact with the patient.	
(1) Participation in the early identification of patients with active disease. Patients will be asked about risk factors, symptoms, previous exposure, and PPD status. Diagnostic work-up with chest x-ray, sputum analysis for organisms, and PPD administration as appropriate are expedited.	(1) Confining airflow to the immediate vicinity of the patient and exhausting air to the outside reduce the likelihood of transmission to health care workers in areas outside of the patient room.	
(2) Maintain engineering controls. Keep the patient in a private room with a closed door.	(2) Masks and respirators are designed to reduce health care worker risk.	
(3) Use protection in isolation room or when participating in procedures that are likely to generate cough, such as suctioning, intubation, or administering nebulized medications.		
b. Risk of transmission of bloodborne diseases such as hepatitis B, hepatitis C, and the human immunodeficiency virus will be avoided by:	b. Health care workers can contract bloodborne diseases via percutaneous injury such as needlestick or by contact with blood or bloody body fluids to mucous membranes, such as eyes and mouth.	
(1) Vaccination with hepatitis B vaccine	(1) Hepatitis B vaccine should be used to reduce risk from this contagious bloodborne virus.	
(2) Use of Standard Precautions as defined by the CDC	(2) Standard Precautions are based on the recognition that most patients are not identified as infected by physical assessment or history taking. Health care workers must assume that all patients may be infected with bloodborne or other infection and must use barrier precautions appropriately for *all* patients.	
c. Avoid risk of airborne diseases. (1) Get influenza vaccination annually. (2) Get vaccinated or produce proof of immunity to measles, mumps, rubella, and varicella.	c. Influenza vaccine is recommended for health care workers to reduce the likelihood of transmission in health care settings where immunocompromised patients can become exposed.	
4. Prevent patient exposure to contaminated medical equipment.	4. Technologic advances offer increased opportunity for invasive procedures. Equipment may be complex and difficult to clean.	

(*continued*)

64•1

Plan of Nursing Care 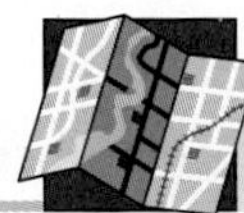 Care of the Patient With An Infectious Disease (*continued*)

Nursing Interventions	Rationale	Expected Outcomes
a. Equipment that is inserted through intact skin must be sterilized between patient uses.	a. Sterilization renders equipment free of all microorganisms.	
b. Equipment that has contact with mucous membranes must be sterilized or "high-level disinfected" between patient uses.	b. High-level disinfection with a product such as glutaraldehyde renders an object free of all microorganisms with the possible exception of spore-producing organisms.	
c. Equipment used against intact skin should be thoroughly cleaned and "low-level disinfected" between patient uses.	c. The disinfection goal for low-level disinfection is to reduce the load of microorganisms to a level that is not threatening to the host with intact skin.	
5. Follow established guidelines for the routine removal and replacement of intravenous devices.	5. Indwelling intravascular devices can serve as a conduit for organisms to migrate into the bloodstream.	
6. Remove urinary catheters at the earliest time possible.	6. The risk of urinary tract infections is directly proportional to the length of time that a urinary catheter remains in place.	
7. Remove endotracheal and nasogastric tubes at the earliest reasonable-time.	7. The risk for pneumonia is increased as the duration of indwelling equipment increases.	

Nursing Diagnosis: Knowledge deficit about disease, cause of infection, and preventive measures
Goal: Acquisition of knowledge about the infectious process

Nursing Interventions	Rationale	Expected Outcomes
1. Listen carefully to what the patient says about illness and previous treatment.	1. Listening facilitates detection of misunderstanding and misinformation and provides opportunity for education.	• Patient actively participates in treatment. • Patient complies with infection control measures
2. Provide pertinent explanations about: a. Organism and route of transmission b. Treatment goals c. Follow-up schedule d. Prevention of transmission to others	2. Knowledge about specific diagnoses and treatments may increase compliance.	
3. Allow opportunities for questions and discussions	3. The patient's questions indicate issues that need clarification.	
4. Teach the patient and family about: a. Prophylaxis or immunization, if recommended b. Community resources, if necessary c. Means of preventing transmission within the home	4. Understanding of the risks and precautions associated with an infectious disease may reduce the opportunity for further spread.	

Nursing Diagnosis: Altered body temperature (fever) related to the presence of infection
Goal: Patient comfort and return of normal temperature

Nursing Interventions	Rationale	Expected Outcomes
1. Monitor temperature, pulse, and respirations at regular intervals	1. Trends in fever can be classified as continuous, remittent, or intermittent to provide diagnostic clues. Additionally, fever curves provide a measurement of severity and duration of infectious processes.	• Body temperature within normal limits • Maintenance of fluid and electrolyte balance • Patient comfortable

(*continued*)

64•1

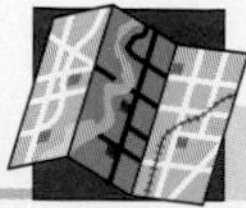

Plan of Nursing Care: Care of the Patient With An Infectious Disease (*continued*)

Nursing Interventions	Rationale	Expected Outcomes
Collaborative Problems: Different infectious agents have different potential for producing complications. Among potential complications are secondary bloodstream infection, septic shock, dehydration, abscess formation, endocarditis, infectious disease–related cancers, obstructive pathology, infertility, and congenital abnormalities.		
Goal: Absence of complications		
Secondary Bloodstream Infection		
1. Monitor patient for evidence of infection at any location.	1. Vigilance for bacterial or fungal infection at any site promotes early recognition and treatment and reduces the likelihood of secondary infections.	• No episode of secondary infection • Effective treatment of identified bacterial and fungal infections without progression to secondary bloodstream infection • Early improvement in septic course
2. Assess treatment effectiveness of all identified infections.	2. Effective control of localized infections reduces the risk of secondary bloodstream infection.	
3. Administer antibiotics as prescribed with first dose given at the earliest time possible.	3. The natural course of some infections may be rapid without prompt treatment.	
Septic Shock		
1. Routinely, and as warranted, monitor vital signs for patients with recognized infections and severely immune suppressed patients at risk for shock. In particular, be alert for signs of: a. Fever b. Tachycardia (more than 90 bpm) c. Tachypnea (more than 20 breaths/min) d. Evidence of decreased perfusion or dysfunction of vital organs in the form of (1) Change of mental status (2) Hypoxemia as measured by arterial blood gases (3) Elevated lactate levels (4) Urine output (less than 30 mL/h)	1. Early recognition of the signs of impending shock may reduce the associated severity or mortality.	• Absence of symptoms of septic shock • Hemodynamic and respiratory status within normal range
2. Administer antibiotics, fluid replacement, vasopressors, and oxygen as prescribed.	2. Therapeutic maintenance of hemodynamic and respiratory status is necessary until infection is effectively treated with antimicrobial regimen.	
Dehydration		
1. Assess for dehydration (thirst, dryness of mucous membranes, loss of skin turgor, reduced peripheral pulses, urine output less than 30 mL/h).	1. Signs of dehydration provide a basis for fluid replacement and suggest possible further complications of circulatory collapse.	• Attains fluid balance (output approximates intake: body weight unchanged) • Mucous membranes appear moist; normal skin turgor • Serum electrolytes are within normal limits
2. Monitor weight.	2. Rapid changes in weight indicate fluid volume changes.	
3. Monitor intake and output and serum electrolyte levels.	3. Dehydration produces a deficit in some electrolytes. Decreased urine production may indicate a lack of systemic hydration.	
4. Replace fluids as needed. If the patient can tolerate oral fluids, offer fluids every 2–4 hours. Administer intravenous fluids as prescribed.	4. When possible, oral hydration is preferable because the patient can select the beverage, control the rate and interval of replacement, and care for self at home. Additionally, the risks associated with vascular devices are avoided. If intravenous fluid is required, intravenous solutions are formulated to facilitate intestinal reabsorption of fluid and electrolytes.	

(*continued*)

64•1

Plan of Nursing Care 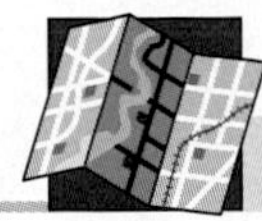

Care of the Patient With An Infectious Disease (*continued*)

Nursing Interventions	Rationale	Expected Outcomes
Abscess Formation		
1. Assess vascular access sites, wound sites, pressure ulcers, and other appropriate sites for apparent collections of purulent material.	1. Collections of purulent material often require drainage before antimicrobial therapy is effective.	• Absence of abscess • Early identification of signs of intra-abdominal sepsis to expedite surgery
2. Assess the patient who has had abdominal surgery or trauma to abdominal area for localized signs of intra-abdominal abscess. These signs include: a. Low-grade fever b. Elevated peripheral white blood cell count c. Localized pain d. Abdominal tenderness e. Visible or palpable mass f. Postoperative diarrhea g. GI bleeding	2. Intra-abdominal abscess formation is most common following traumatic or surgical disruption of the GI tract. Signs are often initially subtle.	
3. Assess patient who has had percutaneous abscess drainage to assess if drainage has been successful. Be alert for all of the above signs and symptoms.	3. After percutaneous drainage, recurrent or persistent signs of abscess may indicate the need for surgical treatment.	
4. Administer antibiotics as prescribed	4. Antibiotics, along with drainage, are the most important elements of intra-abdominal abscess management.	
Endocarditis		
Prevention		
1. Patients with the following conditions should be taught about the value of antibiotic prophylaxis for events and procedures that may introduce the risk of endocarditis: a. Valvular disease b. Congenital heart disease c. Intracardiac prosthesis d. Previous endocarditis	1. Patients with underlying valvular disease and other cardiac abnormalities are at increased risk for "seeding" of the cardiac valves during procedures that can cause bacteremia.	• Informs health care professionals of cardiac conditions that require antibiotic prophylaxis before invasive procedures • Takes prophylactic antibiotics as prescribed
Management		
1. Blood cultures should be obtained as prescribed; results should be carefully recorded. Persistent bloodstream infections with an organism should be noted.	1. A definitive diagnosis of endocarditis requires blood culture confirmation.	• Endocarditis is diagnosed, treated, and cured.
2. Obtain a detailed history about the duration of fever in the absence of well-recognized cause.	2. Endocarditis should be suspected in patients who report an unexplained fever of more than 1 week's duration	
3. Administer intravenous antibiotic therapy at prescribed time schedule.	3. Intravenous therapy is usually required for cure. The goal of therapy is complete eradication of all organisms. Careful adherence to following the scheduled administration is therefore essential.	

Infectious Disease-Related Cancers, Infertility, Congenital Abnormalities

These potential complications of infectious diseases are prevented by primary avoidance of infection. Management of them is directed toward treating each of them as a non-infectious entity. For example, the management of cancer secondary to hepatitis B is handled as an oncology issue, not as an infectious disease issue. Similarly, the care of the child with deafness will be managed from the otolaryngology and behavioral aspects of deafness, rather than the treatment of cytomegalovirus.

Evaluation

Expected Outcomes

Expected outcomes may include:

1. Uses appropriate methods to prevent the spread of infection
2. Acquires knowledge about the infectious process
3. Exhibits absence of elevated body temperature
4. Attains fluid balance

Critical Thinking Exercises

1.
A nurse who is returning to nursing after 10 years is being oriented to your nursing unit. She is assigned to take care of a patient with AIDS. She questions why the patient is not isolated. What conclusions might you draw from her comment? To ensure appropriate care for this patient, how would you explain to the nurse the best way to approach AIDS patients when giving care?

2.
You are supervising a patient care technician who is changing the bed of a postoperative patient. There is fresh blood on the patient's sheet from a venipuncture that was just performed. The technician is not wearing gloves as she disposes of the linen. How would you evaluate this situation, and what action would you take? Explain the rationale for your decision.

3.
An elderly patient with cardiac disease questions you about why her physician suggested that she receive an influenza vaccination. She states that she received the vaccination years ago and then "got the flu from the vaccine." How would you respond to her and explain the situation? Describe the line of reasoning you would follow to convince her to get the vaccine. If she rejects your explanation, examine the different courses of action you could take and the pros and cons of each strategy.

References and Selected Readings

BOOKS

Beneson, A. (1995). *Control of communicable diseases in man.* Washington, D.C.: American Public Health Association.
Cheeseman, S. H. (1998). Cytomegalovirus. In H. Gorbach, J. G. Bartlett, N. R. Blacklow (Eds.). *Infectious diseases.* Philadelphia: W. B. Saunders.
Gorbach, S. L., Bartlett, J., & Blacklow, N. R. (1998). *Infectious diseases.* Philadelphia: W. B. Saunders.
Henderson, D. K. (1997). HIV-1 In the health care setting. In G. L. Mandell, R. G. Douglas, & J. E. Bennett. (1997). Principles and Practice of Infectious Diseases. New York: Churchill Livingstone.
Long, S. S., Pickering, L. K., & Prober, C. G. (1997). *Principles and practice of pediatric infectious diseases.* New York: Churchill Livingstone, 1997.
Mandell, G. L., Douglas, R. G., & Bennett, J. E. (1997). *Principles and practice of infectious diseases.* New York: Churchill Livingstone.
Mayhall, G. (1996). *Hospital epidemiology and infection control.* Baltimore: Williams & Wilkins.
Sandford, J. (1998). *Guide to antimicrobial therapy.* Dallas: Antimicrobial Therapy.
Toosi, Z., & Elmer, J. (1998). *Mycobacterium tuberculosis* and other mycobacteria. In S. L. Gorbach, J. Bartlett, & N. R. Blacklow (Eds.). *Infectious diseases.* Philadelphia: W. B. Saunders.
Wenzel, R. (1997). *Prevention and control of nosocomial infections.* Baltimore: Williams & Wilkins.

JOURNALS

Asterisks indicate nursing research articles.
Boyce, J. M., et al. (1994). Methicillin-resistant *Staphylococcus aureus* (MRSA): A briefing for acute care hospitals and nursing facilities. *Infection Control and Hospital Epidemiology, 15*(2), 105–115.
Capriotti, T. (1997). Emerging antibiotic resistance among community-acquired and nosocomial bacterial pathogens. *MedSurg Nursing, 6*(4), 296–298.
Centers for Disease Control. (1992). The management of acute diarrhea in children: Oral rehydration, maintenance, and nutritional therapy. *MMWR CDC Surveillance Summaries, 41*(RR-16), 1–20.
Centers for Disease Control. (1993a). Hepatitis E among US travelers, 1989–1992. *MMWR CDC Surveillance Summaries, 42*(1), 1–4.
Centers for Disease Control. (1993b). Nosocomial enterococci resistant to vancomycin—United States, 1989–1993. *MMWR CDC Surveillance Summaries, 42*(30), 597–599.
Centers for Disease Control. (1994). Addressing emerging infectious disease threats: A prevention strategy for the United States. Executive Summary. *MMWR CDC Surveillance Summaries, 43*(RR-5), 1–18.
Centers for Disease Control. (1996). Prevention of hepatitis A through active or passive immunization. Recommendations of the Advisory Committee on Immunization Practices (ACIP). *MMWR CDC Surveillance Summaries, 45*(RR-15), 1–30.
Centers for Disease Control. (1997a). Measles eradication: Recommendations from a meeting co-sponsored by the World Health Organization, the Pan American Health Organization, and the CDC. *MMWR CDC Surveillance Summaries, 46*(RR-11), 1–20.
Centers for Disease Control. (1997b). Immunization of health-care workers: Recommendations of the Advisory Committee on Immunization Practices (ACIP) and the Hospital Infection Control Advisory Committee. *MMWR CDC Surveillance Summaries, 47*(RR-18), 1–42.
Centers for Disease Control. (1998a). Hantavirus pulmonary syndrome: Colorado and New Mexico 1998. *MMWR CDC Surveillance Summaries, 47*(22), 449–452.
Centers for Disease Control. (1998b). Draft guideline for the prevention of surgical site infection, 1998b. *Federal Register, 63*(116), 33167–33190.
Centers for Disease Control. (1998c). Guideline for infection control in health-care personnel, 1998c. *Infection Control and Hospital Epidemiology, 19*(6), 407–463.
Centers for Disease Control. (1998d). Public Health Service guidelines for the management of health-care worker exposures to HIV and recommendations for postexposure. *MMWR CDC Surveillance Summaries, 47*(RR-7), 1–33.
Centers for Disease Control. (1998e). 1998 Guidelines for treatment of sexually transmitted diseases. *MMWR CDC Surveillance Summaries, 47*(RR-01), 1–102.
Centers for Disease Control. (1998f). Measles, mumps, and rubella: Vaccine use and strategies for elimination of measles, rubella, congenital rubella syndrome and control of mumps. Recommendations of the Advisory Committee on Immunization Practices. *MMWR CDC Surveillance Summaries, 47*(RR-8), 1–57.
Centers for Disease Control. (1998g). Prevention and control of influenza. Recommendations of the Advisory Committee on Immunization Practices. *MMWR CDC Surveillance Summaries, 47*(RR-6), 1–26.
Cochran, A. & Wilson, B. A. (1999). Current management of AIDS and related opportunistic infections. *MedSurg Nursing, 8*(4): 257–264.
Cohen, F., & Larson, E. (1996). Emerging infectious diseases: Nursing responses. *Nursing Outlook, 44*(4), 164–168.
Doyle, T., et al. (1998). Viral hemorrhagic fevers and hantavirus infections in the Americas. *Infectious Disease Clinics of North America, 12,* 95–110.
Edmond M. B., et al. (1996). Vancomycin-resistant *Staphylococcus aureus:* Perspectives on measures needed for control. *Annals of Internal Medicine, 124*(3), 329–334.
*Fitchie, C. (1992). Central venous catheter-related infection and dressing type. *Intensive Critical Care Nursing, 8*(4), 199–202.
Force, M. V. (1999). Living with Lyme disease. *MedSurg Nursing, 8*(3):184–190.
Gaynes, R. P. (1997). Surveillance of nosocomial infections: A fundamental ingredient for quality. *Infection Control and Hospital Epidemiology, 18*(7), 475–478.
Griffith, D. E. (1998). Mycobacteria as pathogens of respiratory infection. *Infectious Disease Clinics of North America, 12*(3), 593–611.
Lange, B. J., et al. (1997). Impact of changes in catheter management on infectious complications among children with central venous catheters. *Infection Control and Hospital Epidemiology, 18*(5), 326–332.
*Larson, E. L., et al. (1997). A multifaceted approach to changing handwashing behavior. *American Journal of Infection Control, 25*(1), 3–10.
Martone, W. J. (1998). Spread of vancomycin-resistant enterococci: Why did it happen in the United States? *Infection Control and Hospital Epidemiology, 19*(8), 539–545.
McEachern, R., & Campbell, G. D. (1998). Hospital-acquired pneumonia: Epidemiology, etiology, and treatment. *Infectious Disease Clinics of North America, 12*(3), 761–779.

Russell, B. (1999). Nosocomial infections. *American Journal of Nursing, 99*(6):24J–24.

Sharts-Hopko, N. (1997). STDs in women: What you need to know. *American Journal of Nursing, 97*(4), 46–54.

Shay, L. E. & Freifeld, A. G. (1999). The current state of infectious disease: A clinical perspective on antimicrobial resistance. *Lippincott's Primary Care Practice 3*(1):1–17.

Society for Healthcare Epidemiology of America: Long Term Care Committee. (1996). Antimicrobial resistance in long term care facilities. *Infection Control and Hospital Epidemiology, 17,* 129–140.

Society for Healthcare Epidemiology of America and the Infectious Diseases Society of America Joint Committee on the Prevention of Antimicrobial Resistance. (1997). Guidelines for the prevention of antimicrobial resistance in hospitals. *Infection Control and Hospital Epidemiology, Feb,* 275–291.

Thomason, M. H., et al. (1996). Nosocomial pneumonia in ventilated trauma patients during stress ulcer prophylaxis with sucralfate, antacid, and ranitidine. *Journal of Trauma, 41*(3), 503–508.

Treston-Aurand, J., et al. (1997). Impact of dressing materials on central catheter infection rates. *Journal of Intravenous Nursing, 20*(4), 201–206.

Tripepi-Bova, K. A., et al. (1997). A comparison of transparent polyurethane and dry dressings for peripheral IV catheter sites: Rates of phlebitis, infiltration, and dislodgement by patients. *American Journal of Critical Care, 6*(5), 377–381.

*VandenBosch, T. M., et al. (1997). Research utilization: Adhesive bandage dressing regimen for peripheral venous catheters. *American Journal of Infection Control, 25*(6), 513–519.

Wilde, M. H. (1997). Long-term indwelling urinary catheter care: Conceptualizing the research base. *Journal of Advanced Nursing, 25*(6), 1252–1261.

Resources

INTERNATIONAL AGENCIES

World Health Organization Avenue, Appia, CH1211 Geneva 27, Switzerland

World Health Organization Collaborating Center on AIDS, c/o Centers for Disease Control, 1600 Clifton Road, NE, Atlanta, GA 30333; www.who.ch

GOVERNMENTAL AGENCIES

Centers for Disease Control and Prevention (Center for Prevention Services Center for Environmental Health, Center for Health Promotion and Education, Center for Infectious Diseases), 1600 Clifton Road NE, Atlanta, GA 30333; www.cdc.gov/nicdod.hip/hip.htm

National Institute of Allergy and Infectious Diseases, National Institutes of Health, 9000 Rockville Pike, Bethesda, Md 20205; www.niad.nih.gov

U.S. Department of Health and Human Services Public Health Service, 5600 Fishers Lane, Washington, DC 20201

Department of Infectious and Parasitic Disease Pathology Armed Forces Institute of Pathology, Washington DC 20306; www.afip.org

VOLUNTARY AGENCIES

American Lung Association, 1740 Broadway, New York, NY 10019; www.lungusa.org

American Public Health Association, 1015 Fifteenth Street NW, Washington DC 20005; www.apha.org

American Social Health Association, P.O. Box 13827, Research Triangle Park, North Carolina, 27709

Association for Professionals in Infection Control and Epidemiology, Inc., 1016 16th St. NW, Washington, DC 20036; www.apic.org

National Foundation for Infectious Diseases, P.O. Box 42022, Washington, DC 20015; www.nfid.org

Society for Healthcare Epidemiology of America, 875 Kings Highway, Suite 200, Woodbury, NJ 08096; www.medscape.com/Affiliates/SHEA

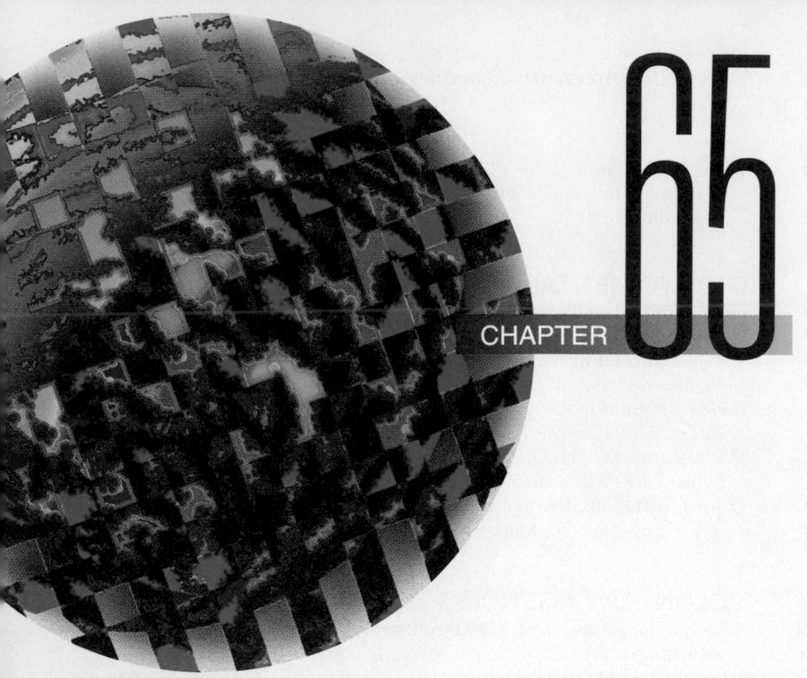

Emergency Nursing

Learning Objectives

On completion of this chapter, the learner will be able to:

1. Explain emergency care as a collaborative, holistic approach that includes the patient, the family, and significant others.
2. Discuss priority emergency measures instituted for any patient with an emergency condition.
3. Describe the emergency management of patients with intra-abdominal injuries.
4. Identify the priorities of care for the patient with multiple injuries.
5. Compare and contrast the emergency management of patients with heat stroke, frostbite, and hypothermia.
6. Specify the similarities and differences for the emergency management of patients with swallowed or inhaled poisons, skin contamination, and food poisoning.
7. Discuss the emergency management of patients with drug overdose and with acute alcohol intoxication.
8. Describe the significance of crisis intervention in the care of the rape victim.
9. Differentiate between the emergency care of patients who are overactive, violent or depressed, and suicidal.

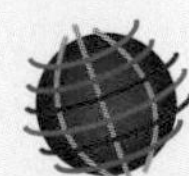

The term *emergency management* traditionally refers to care given to patients with urgent and critical needs. Because many people lack access to primary care, however, the emergency department (ED) is increasingly used for nonurgent problems. Thus, the philosophy of emergency management has broadened to include the concept that an emergency is whatever the patient or the family considers it to be.

Large numbers of people seek emergency help for serious life-threatening cardiac conditions, such as myocardial infarction, acute heart failure, pulmonary edema, and cardiac dysrhythmias. Priorities for managing these cardiac conditions are discussed in previous chapters (Chaps. 24, 25 and 27). Emergency management of trauma and other conditions not found elsewhere in this book are discussed here. *It is assumed that care and treatment are provided under the direction of a physician or emergency nurse practitioner.*

GLOSSARY

alcohol withdrawal delirium: acute toxic state due to sudden cessation of alcohol intake after prolonged intake or binge drinking

anaphylactic reaction: acute systemic hypersensitivity reaction occurring within seconds to minutes of exposure to a foreign substance

antivenin: antitoxin manufactured from venom of poisonous snakes to assist the patient's immune system response to an envenomation

café coronary: foreign body obstruction of the upper airway resulting in unconsciousness and cardiopulmonary arrest

carboxyhemoglobin: hemoglobin bound to carbon monoxide and therefore unable to bind with oxygen and resulting in hypoxemia

corrosive poison: alkaline or acidic agent exposure leading to tissue destruction after contact

cricothyroidotomy: surgical opening of the cricothyroid membrane to obtain an airway that is maintained with a tracheostomy or endotracheal tube

decompression sickness (DCS): accumulation of nitrogen bubbles in an area of the body within 24 hours of diving or high-altitude flight; results in pain or ischemia to the body area involved

diagnostic peritoneal lavage: instillation of lactated Ringer's or normal saline solutions into the abdominal cavity to detect red blood cells, white blood cells, bile, bacteria, amylase, or gastrointestinal contents indicative of abdominal injury

emergent: life-threatening or potentially life-threatening injuries or illnesses requiring immediate treatment; may include limb-threatening injuries when not in a disaster situation

fasciotomy: surgical incision of the extremity to the level of the fascia to relieve pressure and restore neurovascular function to the extremity

frostbite: exposure to freezing temperatures resulting in freezing of the tissue fluids in the cell and intercellular spaces

Hare traction: portable in-line traction applied to the lower extremity to manage femur or hip fractures or dislocations

heat stroke: failure of the heat-regulatory mechanisms of the body resulting in a medical emergency

hypothermia: core body temperature 35°C or less due to cold exposure

immediate: nonacute, non–life-threatening injuries or illnesses requiring attention and management without significant delay

near-drowning: survival after a period of submersion

posttraumatic stress disorder (PTSD): characteristic symptoms after a psychologically stressful event that was out of the range of normal human experience

shock: loss of effective circulating blood volume resulting in end-organ ischemia and cellular metabolic derangement; types include hypovolemic, septic, cardiogenic, anaphylactic, and neurogenic

trauma: intentional or unintentional wounds or injurics inflicted on the human body from a particular mechanical mechanism that exceeds the body's ability to protect itself from injury

triage: process of assessing patients who come to the emergency department to determine management priorities

urgent: minor injuries or illnesses requiring first-aid level of management but not immediate treatment

OVERVIEW OF EMERGENCY NURSING

The emergency nurse has had specialized education, training, and experience to gain expertise in assessing and identifying patients' health care problems in crisis situations. In addition, the emergency nurse establishes priorities, monitors and continuously assesses acutely ill and injured patients, supports and attends to families, supervises allied health personnel, and teaches patients and families within a time-limited, high-pressured care environment. Nursing interventions are accomplished interdependently in consultation with or under the direction of a licensed physician or nurse practitioner. The strengths of nursing and medicine are complementary in an emergency situation. Appropriate nursing and medical interventions are anticipated based on assessment data. The emergency health care staff members work as a team in performing the highly technical, hands-on skills required to care for patients in an emergency.

The nursing process provides a logical framework for problem solving in this environment. Patients in the ED have a wide variety of actual or potential problems. The patient's condition may change constantly. Therefore, nursing assessment must be continuous, and nursing diagnoses change with the patient's condition. Although a patient may have several diagnoses at a given time, the focus is on the most immediate ones often requiring both independent and interdependent nursing interventions.

Priorities and Principles of Emergency Care

Priorities

The focus of emergency care is to preserve life, prevent deterioration before definitive treatment can be given, and restore the patient to optimal function. When care is given to a patient in an emergency situation, many crucial decisions must be made. These decisions require sound judgment based on an understanding of the condition that produced the emergency and its effect on the person.

For the patient who enters the ED, care focuses on determining the extent of injury or illness and on establishing priorities for initiating treatment. These priorities are determined by any threat to the person's life. Conditions interfering with vital physiologic function (eg, obstructed airway, massive bleeding) take precedence. Usually, injuries of the face, neck, and chest that impair respiration are given the highest priorities. Emergency team members work together to provide comprehensive, individualized patient care.

Principles

The emergency care of any patient is based on the following objectives:

- Establish a patent airway and provide adequate ventilation—employing resuscitation measures when necessary—protecting the cervical spine first and assessing chest injuries with subsequent airway obstruction or ventilatory impairment.
- Evaluate and restore cardiac output by controlling hemorrhage and its consequences, preventing and treating shock, and maintaining or restoring effective circulation.
- Determine the patient's ability to follow commands, and evaluate motor skills and pupillary size and reactivity.
- Carry out a rapid initial and ongoing physical examination (the clinical course of the injured or seriously ill patient is not static).
- Start cardiac monitoring, if appropriate.
- Splint suspected fractures.

- Protect and clean wounds; apply sterile dressings.
- Identify allergies and medical history that is significant (eg, diabetes mellitus or epilepsy controlled by phenytoin).
- Document on the medical record the patient's vital signs, blood pressure, neurologic status, and intake and output to guide decision making.

Triage

The word **triage** comes from the French word *trier* meaning "to sort." In the daily routine of the ED, triage is used to determine those patients in need of immediate treatment and those who can safely wait. There are three main categories of triage: **emergent** (life-threatening or potentially life-threatening injury or illness requiring immediate treatment), **immediate** (nonacute, non–life-threatening injury or illness), and **urgent** (minor illness or injury needing first-aid–level treatment). With the increased use of the ED for primary care, the patient may also be classified into *fast track* or essentially first-aid–level management. These patients may also be referred to a primary physician's office or a clinic for treatment.

Triage is a learned skill. Emergency nurses spend many hours learning to classify different illnesses and injuries to ensure proper management of the "emergency." Emergent life-threatening or potentially life-threatening scenarios (eg, myocardial infarction, multiple trauma, airway loss, anaphylaxis, or stroke) are managed immediately in the acute care section of the ED. Immediate issues are usually dealt with in the nonacute area of the ED. Urgent and first-aid types of problems are handled in the fast-track area of the ED or in the clinic.

Nurses in the triage area collect a few crucial pieces of information: vital signs and history, neurologic assessment findings, and blood glucose level if necessary. Protocols may be followed to initiate laboratory or x-ray studies from the triage area while the patient waits for a bed in the ED. Collaborative protocols are developed and used based on the experience of the triage nurse.

Field Triage

In disasters (eg, natural events, such as tornadoes and earthquakes); in events injuring large numbers of people at once, such as train, plane, or bus crashes, explosions, or fires; or in a group of patients whose needs exceed the capabilities of the ED at the time of the event, a slightly different system of triage is used. *Field triage* is carried out by the emergency medical personnel at the scene. Patients are categorized as "red" emergent, "yellow" immediate, "green" urgent, and "blue" fast-track or psychological support needed. "Black-tagged" patients are either dead or progressing rapidly toward death. When resources are limited, only patients considered potentially survivable are "red tagged." The availability of surgeons and operating room space also affects these decisions. Such decisions are often the most difficult ones that any health care professional will ever make. Patients are triaged again at the door of the ED by the surgical staff and taken to designated areas and managed. All available personnel assist with managing these patients.

Gerontologic Considerations

By 2020, more than 64 million people will be older than 65 years of age. Each year elderly people, who make up a greater proportion of the U.S. population, are major consumers of emergency health care. In fact, this population accounts for more than 99 million visits to emergency facilities each year. Elderly patients typically arrive in the ED with one or more presenting conditions commonly involving the skin, cardiovascular system, or abdomen. Nonspecific symptoms, such as weakness and fatigue, episodes of falling, incontinence, and change in mental status, may be manifestations of acute illness in the elderly person. Many of these conditions, although not considered urgent in a younger person, can readily become life-threatening in elderly people if left untreated.

The elderly patient may perceive the emergency as a crisis signaling the end of an independent lifestyle or even resulting in death. Referrals for support services, for example, from the social service department, may be necessary.

ASSESSMENT
THE EMERGENCY SITUATION

Considering the emergent situation, the nurse keeps questions to a minimum but tries to obtain a brief history of the injury or illness from the patient or the person accompanying the patient to the emergency department. The following are some of the questions asked. Of course, all answers are documented for reference by other health care providers.

1. What were the circumstances, precipitating events, location, and time of the injury or illness?
2. When did the symptoms appear?
3. Was the patient unconscious after the injury or onset of illness?
4. How did the patient get to the hospital?
5. What was the health status of the patient before the injury or illness?
6. Is there a medical or surgical history? A history of admissions to the hospital?
7. Is the patient currently taking any medications, especially hormones, insulin, digitalis, anticoagulants?
8. Does the patient have any allergies? If so, what are they?
9. Does the patient have any bleeding tendencies?
10. When was the last meal eaten? (This is important if general anesthesia is to be given or if the patient is unconscious.)
11. Is the patient under a physician's care? What are the name and location of the physician?
12. What was the date of the patient's most recent tetanus immunization?

Special Considerations for Emergency Nursing

Data Collection

If possible, a brief history of the injury or illness is obtained from the patient or the person accompanying the patient to the ED. The questions listed in the accompanying assessment display reflect the minimum information that should be obtained.

Infection Control

Because of the increasing numbers of people infected with hepatitis B and with human immunodeficiency virus (HIV), health care providers are at an increased risk for exposure to communicable diseases through blood or other body fluids. This risk is further compounded in the ED because of the common use of invasive treatments in addition to the wide range of patient conditions. All emergency health care providers should adhere strictly to standard precautions for minimizing exposure.

The reemergence of tuberculosis, a major health problem of the 1990s, is complicated by multidrug-resistant tuberculosis and tuberculosis concomitant with HIV. Early identification and adherence to transmission-based precautions for patients who are potentially infectious are crucial. Nurses in the ED are usually fitted with a personal hepa-filter mask apparatus to use when treating patients with airborne diseases.

Discharge Planning

Most patients who receive emergency care are discharged directly from the ED to their homes. Before discharge, instructions for continuing care are given to the patient and the family or significant others. All instructions should be both verbal and written so that the patient can refer to them later. Many EDs have preprinted standard instruction sheets for more common conditions. These instructions are then individualized for each patient. In many cases, these instructions are available in a variety of languages. If instructions are not available in the language that the patient needs, an interpreter should be used. Instructions should include information about prescribed medications, treatments, diet, activity, and when to contact a health care provider or schedule follow-up appointments.

COMMUNITY SERVICES

Before discharge, some patients require the services of a social worker to help them meet continuing health care needs. For patients and families who cannot provide care at home, community agencies (eg, Home Care Nursing Services, Visiting Nurse Association) may be contacted to arrange services before discharge. This is particularly important for elderly patients who need assistance. Identifying continuing health care needs and making arrangements for meeting these needs can prevent return visits to the ED and readmission to the hospital.

For patients returning to extended care facilities or for those who already rely on community agencies for continuing health care, communication about the patient's condition and any changes that have occurred in health care needs must be provided to these facilities or agencies. This communication is essential to promote continuity of care and ensure ongoing care to meet the patient's changing health care needs.

Psychological Support

Sudden illness or trauma is an insult to physiologic and psychological homeostasis that requires physiologic and psychological healing. Patients and families experiencing sudden injury or illness are often overwhelmed by anxiety because they have not had time to mobilize their resources to adapt to the crisis. They experience real and terrifying fear of death, mutilation, immobilization, and other assaults on their personal identity and body integrity. When confronted with trauma, severe disfigurement, severe illness, or sudden death, the family experiences several stages of crisis. The stages begin with anxiety and progress through denial, remorse and guilt, anger, grief, and reconciliation. The initial goal for the patient and family is anxiety reduction, a prerequisite to recovering the ability to cope.

Assessment of the patient and family's psychological functioning includes evaluating emotional expression, degree of anxiety, and cognitive functioning (orientation to time, place, and person). A brief physical examination of the patient is also performed, focusing on the clinical problem that caused the patient to seek help. Possible nursing diagnoses may include anxiety related to uncertain potential outcomes of the illness or trauma, and ineffective individual coping related to acute situational crisis. In addition to anxiety, possible nursing diagnoses for the family may include anticipatory grieving and alterations in family processes related to acute situational crises.

PATIENT-FOCUSED INTERVENTIONS

Those caring for the patient should act confidently and competently to relieve anxiety. Reacting and responding to the patient in a warm manner promotes a sense of security. Explanations should be given on a level that the patient can understand because an informed patient is better able to cope positively with stress. Human contact and reassuring words reduce the panic of the severely injured person and aid in dispelling fear of the unknown.

The unconscious patient should be treated as if conscious. The patient should be touched, called by name, and given an explanation of every procedure that is performed. As the patient regains consciousness, the nurse should orient the patient by stating his or her name, the date, and the location. This basic information should be provided repeatedly, as needed, in a reassuring way.

FAMILY-FOCUSED INTERVENTIONS

The family is kept informed of where the patient is and that expert care is being given. The family is allowed to stay with the patient when possible. Additional interventions used are based on the assessment of the stage of crisis that the family is experiencing.

Anxiety and Denial. During these stages, family members are encouraged to recognize and talk about their feelings of anxiety. Asking questions is encouraged. Answers that are honest and at the level of the family's understanding must be provided. Although denial is an ego-defense mechanism that protects one from recognizing painful and disturbing aspects of reality, prolonged denial is not encouraged or supported. The family must be prepared for the reality of what has happened and what may come.

Remorse and Guilt. Expressions of remorse and guilt are frequently heard, with family members accusing themselves (or each other) of negligence or minor omissions. Family members are urged to express remorse until they realize that there was probably little that they could have done to prevent the injury or illness.

Anger. Expressions of anger, common in crisis situations, are a way of handling anxiety and fear. Anger is frequently directed at the patient, but it is also often expressed toward the physician, the nurse, or admitting personnel. The therapeutic approach is to allow the anger to be ventilated to help the family identify their feelings of frustration.

Grief. Grief is a complex emotional response to anticipated or actual loss. The key nursing intervention is to help family members work through their grief and to support their coping mechanisms, letting them know that it is normal and acceptable for them to cry, feel pain, and express loss (Guideline 65-1).

Documentation

Consent to examine and treat the patient is part of the ED record. The patient must consent to invasive procedures (eg, angiography, lumbar puncture) unless the patient is unconscious or in a critical condition and unable to make decisions. If the patient is unconscious and brought to the ED without family or friends, this fact should be documented. Monitoring of the patient's condition (serial parameters) and all instituted treatments and times

65•1 GUIDELINES FOR

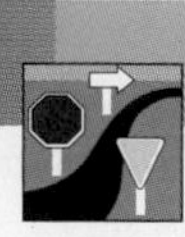

HELPING FAMILY MEMBERS COPE WITH SUDDEN DEATH

- Take the family to a private place.
- Talk to the family together, so that they can mourn together.
- Assure the family that everything possible was done; inform them of the treatment rendered.
- Avoid using euphemisms such as "passed on." Show the family that you care by touching, offering coffee, and offering the services of a chaplain.
- Encourage family members to support each other and to express emotions freely (grief, loss, anger, helplessness, tears, disbelief).
- Avoid giving sedation to family members; this may mask or delay the grieving process, which is necessary to achieve emotional equilibrium and to prevent prolonged depression.
- Encourage the family to view the body if they wish; this action helps to integrate the loss. Cover mutilated areas before the family sees the body. Go with the family to see the body. Show acceptance by touching the body to give the family "permission" to touch.
- Spend a few minutes with the family, listening to them and identifying any needs that they may have for which the nursing staff can be helpful.
- Allow the family members to talk about the deceased and what he or she meant to them; this permits ventilation of feelings of loss. Encourage the family to talk about events preceding admission to the emergency department. Do not challenge initial feelings of anger or denial.
- Avoid volunteering unnecessary information (eg, patient was drinking).

performed must be documented. After treatment, a notation is made on the record about the patient's condition on discharge or transfer and about instructions given to the patient and family for follow-up care.

PRIORITY EMERGENCY MEASURES

Establishing an Airway

The first priority in treating any patient with an emergency condition is establishing the airway. If the airway is obstructed, resulting hypoxia produces permanent brain damage or death within 3 to 5 minutes.

Establishing an airway may be as simple as repositioning the patient's head to prevent the tongue and epiglottis from obstructing the pharynx. On the other hand, additional maneuvers, such as abdominal thrusts, may be needed to remove a foreign body from the airway or insert specialized equipment to open and maintain the airway. In such a case, nursing diagnoses would include ineffective airway clearance due to obstruction of the tongue, object, or fluids (blood, saliva). The nursing diagnosis may also be ineffective breathing pattern due to obstruction or injury.

The first step in establishing an airway is to determine that the patient is truly unconscious, which is accomplished by gently shaking the victim and shouting, "Are you okay?" Doing so prevents injury from attempted resuscitation of a person who is not truly unconscious. The patient is then placed supine on a firm, flat surface. If the patient is lying face down, the body is turned as a unit so that the head, shoulders, and torso move simultaneously with no twisting. Next, the airway is opened using either the head-tilt–chin-lift or jaw-thrust maneuver. After these maneuvers are performed, the patient is assessed for breathing by watching for chest movement and listening and feeling for air movement.

Maneuvers to Open the Airway

HEAD-TILT–CHIN-LIFT MANEUVER

One hand is placed on the victim's forehead, and firm backward pressure is applied with the palm to tilt the head back. The fingers of the other hand are placed under the bony part of the lower jaw near the chin and lifted up. The chin and the teeth are brought forward almost to occlusion to support the jaw.

Nursing Alert *This maneuver, which helps to tilt the head back, should be used only if it is determined that the patient's cervical spine is not injured.*

JAW-THRUST MANEUVER

After placing one hand on each side of the patient's jaw, the angles of the victim's lower jaw are grasped and lifted, displacing the mandible forward. This is a safe approach to opening the airway of a victim with suspected neck injury because it can be accomplished without extending the neck.

Management of Airway Obstruction

Foreign bodies may cause either partial or complete airway obstruction.

Complete airway obstruction is recognized immediately: the patient suddenly stops breathing, becomes cyanotic, and loses consciousness for no apparent reason.

Partial airway obstruction interferes with air-flow, producing an apprehensive appearance, inspiratory and expiratory stridor, labored breathing, use of accessory muscles (suprasternal and intercostal retraction), flaring nostrils, increasing anxiety, restlessness, and confusion. Cyanosis of the earlobes, lips, and nail beds is a late sign. Partial obstruction of the airway can lead to progressive hypoxia, hypercarbia, respiratory and cardiac arrest.

Obstruction of the upper airway by food (**café coronary**) causes unconsciousness and can lead to cardiopulmonary arrest. In adults, a piece of meat is the most common obstructor. Factors associated with choking on food include large, poorly chewed pieces of food, alcohol consumption, and the presence of upper or lower dentures.

GERONTOLOGIC CONSIDERATIONS

For elderly patients, especially those in extended care facilities, sedatives and hypnotic medications, diseases affecting motor coordination (eg, Parkinson's disease), and mental dysfunction (eg, dementia, mental retardation) are risk factors for asphyxiation by food. Nursing staff involved in the care of elderly patients must be aware of the symptoms of upper airway obstruction and be skillful in performing the Heimlich maneuver. Typically, the victim with a foreign body airway obstruction cannot speak, breathe, or cough. The patient may clutch the neck between the thumb and fingers (*universal distress signal*). The first response is to ask this person if he or she is choking.

If the patient can breathe and cough spontaneously, a partial obstruction should be suspected. The victim is encouraged to cough forcefully and continue to persist with spontaneous coughing and breathing efforts as long as good air exchange exists. There may be some wheezing between coughs. If the patient demonstrates a weak, ineffective cough, high-pitched noise while inhaling, increased respiratory difficulty, and, possibly, cyanosis, the patient is managed as if there were complete airway obstruction. Management of a complete airway obstruction is presented in Guideline 65-2.

After the obstruction is removed, rescue breathing is initiated. If the patient has no pulse, cardiac compressions are instituted. These measures provide oxygen to the brain, heart, and other vital organs until definitive medical treatment can restore and support normal heart and ventilatory activity.

Additional Measures for Airway Management

OROPHARYNGEAL AIRWAY

An oropharyngeal airway is a semicircular tube or tubelike plastic device that is inserted over the back of the tongue into the lower posterior pharynx in a patient who is breathing spontaneously but who is unconscious (Guideline 65-3). This type of airway prevents the tongue from falling back against the posterior pharynx and obstructing the airway. It also allows health care providers to suction secretions.

ENDOTRACHEAL INTUBATION

The purpose of endotracheal intubation is to establish and maintain the airway in patients with respiratory insufficiency or hypoxia. Endotracheal intubation is indicated for the following reasons: (1) to establish an airway for patients who cannot be adequately ventilated with an oropharyngeal airway, (2) to bypass an upper airway obstruction, (3) to prevent aspiration, (4) to permit connection of the patient to a resuscitation bag or mechanical ventilator, and (5) to facilitate the removal of tracheobronchial secretions (Fig. 65-1). Because the procedure requires skill, endotracheal intubation is performed only by those who have had extensive training. These include physicians, nurse anesthetists, respiratory therapists, flight nurses, and nurse practitioners. The emergency nurse, however, is commonly called on to assist with the insertion.

Alternative Intubation Method. If the patient is outside the hospital and cannot be intubated in the field, the emergency medical personnel may insert a Combitube. The tube rapidly provides pharyngeal ventilation. When the tube is inserted into the trachea, it functions like an endotracheal tube.

The two balloons around the tube can be inflated. One balloon is large (100 mL) and occludes the oropharynx. This could effectively provide for ventilation through forced air by way of the larynx. The smaller balloon is inflated with 15 mL of air and can effectively occlude the trachea if placed there. Breath sounds are auscultated to make sure that the oropharyngeal cuff does not obstruct the glottis. Patients can be ventilated through either port of the tube, depending on its placement.

CRICOTHYROIDOTOMY (CRICOTHYROID MEMBRANE PUNCTURE)

Cricothyroidotomy is the opening of the cricothyroid membrane to establish an airway. This procedure is used in emergency situations in which endotracheal intubation is either not possible or contraindicated, as in airway obstruction from extensive maxillofacial trauma, cervical spine injuries, laryngospasm, laryngeal edema (after an allergic reaction), hemorrhage into neck tissue, or obstruction of the larynx.

Controlling Hemorrhage

Only a few conditions, such as obstructed airway or a sucking wound of the chest, take precedence over the immediate control of hemorrhage. Stopping the bleeding is essential to the care and survival of patients in an emergency or disaster situation. Hemorrhage that results in the reduction of circulating blood volume is a primary cause of shock. Minor bleeding, which is usually venous, generally stops spontaneously unless the patient has a bleeding disorder or has been taking anticoagulants.

The patient is assessed for cool, moist skin (resulting from poor peripheral perfusion), falling blood pressure, increasing heart rate, delayed capillary refill, and decreasing urine volume (a late sign). Goals of emergency management are to control the bleeding, maintain an adequately circulating blood volume for tissue oxygenation, and prevent shock. Patients who hemorrhage are at risk for cardiac arrest caused by hypovolemia with secondary anoxia. Nursing interventions are carried out collaboratively with other members of the emergency health care team.

Management

FLUID REPLACEMENT

Whenever a patient is experiencing hemorrhage—be it external or internal—a loss of circulating blood leads to a fluid volume deficit and decreased cardiac output. Therefore, fluid replacement is a must. Typically, two large-bore intravenous cannulae are inserted to provide a means for fluid and blood replacement, and blood samples are obtained for analysis, typing, and cross-matching. Replacement fluids are administered as prescribed, depending on clinical estimates of the type and volume of fluid lost. Replacement fluids may include isotonic electrolyte solutions (lactated Ringer's or normal saline) and blood component therapy.

- Packed red blood cells are infused when there is massive blood loss (O-negative for emergency use in women of childbearing age or O-positive for men and postmenopausal women).
- Additional platelets and clotting factors are given when large amounts of blood are needed because replacement blood is deficient in clotting factors.

Nursing Alert *The infusion rate is determined by the severity of the blood loss and the clinical evidence of hypovolemia. If massive blood replacement is necessary, the blood must be warmed using a commercial blood warmer because administration of large amounts of blood has a core cooling effect that may lead to cardiac arrest.*

CONTROL OF EXTERNAL HEMORRHAGE

If a patient is hemorrhaging externally, for example, from a wound, a rapid physical assessment is performed as the patient's clothing is cut away in an attempt to identify the area of hemorrhage. Direct,

65•2 Guidelines For Managing a Foreign Body Airway Obstruction

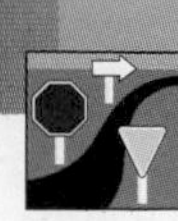

Action	Rationale/Amplification
ASSESS FOR INDICATIONS OF AIRWAY OBSTRUCTION Victim may clutch his neck between his thumb and fingers. Weak, ineffective cough; high-pitched noises on inspiration. Increased respiratory distress. Inability to speak, breathe, or cough. Collapse.	Air movement is absent in the presence of *complete airway obstruction.* Oxygen saturation in the blood decreases rapidly because the obstructed airway prevents entry of air into the lungs. Thus, oxygen deficit occurs in the brain, resulting in unconsciousness, with death following rapidly.
HEIMLICH MANEUVER (SUBDIAPHRAGMATIC ABDOMINAL THRUSTS): **For Standing or Sitting Conscious Patient** 1. Stand behind the patient; wrap your arms around the patient's waist, and proceed as follows: 2. Make a fist with one hand, placing the thumb side of the fist against the patient's abdomen, in the midline slightly above the umbilicus and well below the xiphoid process. Grasp the fist with the other hand.	The term *Heimlich maneuver* is used for the sake of uniformity. The terms *subdiaphragmatic abdominal thrusts* and *abdominal thrusts* are used interchangeably, depending on the circumstances.
3. Press your fist into the patient's abdomen with a quick upward thrust. Each new thrust should be a separate and distinct maneuver.	A subdiaphragmatic abdominal thrust, by elevating the diaphragm, can force air from the lungs to create an artificial cough intended to move and expel an obstructing foreign body from the airway.
With Patient Lying (Unconscious) 1. Position patient on the back. 2. Kneel astride the patient's thigh, facing the head. 3. Place the heel of one hand against the patient's abdomen, in the midline slightly above the umbilicus and well below the tip of the xiphoid; place the second hand directly on top of the first. 4. Press into the abdomen with a quick upward thrust.	
Finger Sweep 1. Open the adult patient's mouth by grasping both the tongue and lower jaw between the thumb and fingers and lifting the mandible (tongue–jaw lift). 2. Insert the index finger of the other hand down along the inside of the cheek and deeply into the throat to the base of the tongue.	This maneuver is to be used *only in the unconscious adult patient.* This action draws the tongue away from the back of the throat and away from the foreign body that may be lodged there.
3. Use a hooking action to dislodge the foreign body and maneuver it into the mouth for removal.	Care is used to avoid forcing the object deeper into the throat.
Chest Thrusts With Conscious Patient Standing or Sitting 1. Stand behind patient with arms under patient's axillae to encircle patient's chest. 2. Place thumb side of your fist on middle of patient's sternum, taking care to avoid xiphoid process and margins of rib cage.	This technique is to be used *only in the advanced stages of pregnancy or in the markedly obese person.*
3. Grasp your fist with the other hand and perform backward thrusts until the foreign body is expelled or patient becomes unconscious.	Each thrust should be administered with the intent of relieving the obstruction.
Chest Thrust With Patient Lying (Unconscious) 1. Place the patient on his back and kneel close to the side of his body. 2. Place the heel of your hand on the lower half of the sternum. 3. Deliver each chest thrust slowly and distinctly with the intent of relieving the obstruction.	This maneuver is used *only in the advanced stages of pregnancy or when the rescuer cannot apply the Heimlich maneuver effectively to the unconscious, markedly obese person.*

Adapted from Cardiopulmonary Resuscitation (CPR). Tulsa, CPR Publishers, 1998.

65•3 GUIDELINES FOR INSERTING AN OROPHARYNGEAL AIRWAY

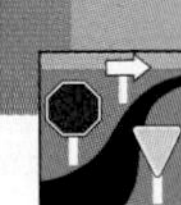

1. Measure the oral airway alongside the head. The airway should reach from lip to ear.

2. Extend the patient's head by placing one hand beneath the neck close to the occiput (*only if the cervical spine is uninjured*). Gently lift the neck; simultaneously, with other hand, tilt the head backward by applying pressure to the forehead.

3. Open the patient's mouth.

4. (**A**) Insert the oropharyngeal airway with the tip facing up toward the roof of the mouth until it passes the uvula. (**B**) Rotate the tip 180 degrees so that the tip is pointed down toward the pharynx. This displaces the tongue anteriorly, and the patient then breathes through and around the airway.

5. The distal end of the oropharyngeal airway is in the hypopharynx and the flange is approximately at the patient's lips. Make sure that the tongue has not been pushed into the airway.

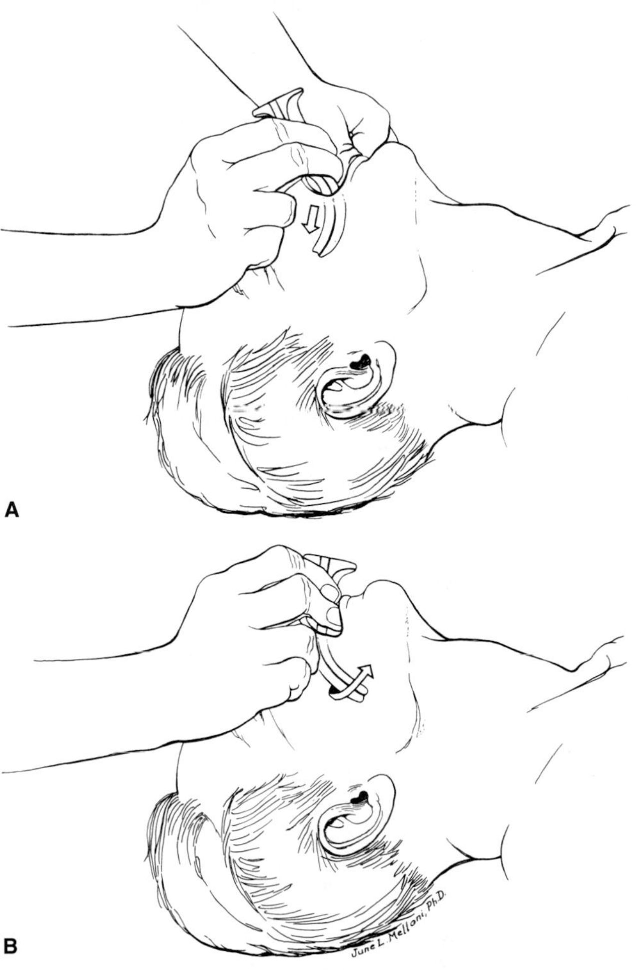

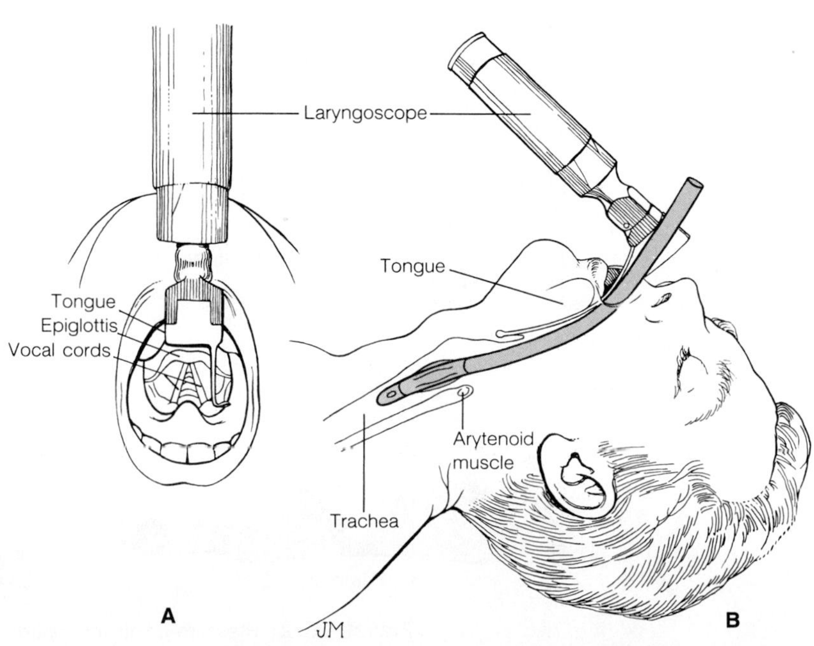

FIGURE 65•1 Endotracheal intubation in a patient without a cervical spine injury. (**A**) The primary glottic landmarks for tracheal intubation as visualized with proper placement of the laryngoscope. (**B**) Positioning the endotracheal tube.

firm pressure is applied over the bleeding area or the involved artery (Fig. 65-2). Most bleeding can be stopped by applying direct pressure, except when a major artery has been severed. Otherwise, unchecked arterial bleeding results in death. A firm pressure dressing is applied, and the injured part is elevated to stop venous and capillary bleeding if possible. If the injured area is an extremity, the extremity is immobilized to control blood loss.

Tourniquets. A tourniquet is applied to an extremity only as a *last resort* when the external hemorrhage cannot be controlled in any other way. Care must be taken when applying a tourniquet because of the risk for loss of the extremity. The tourniquet is applied just proximal to the wound and tied tightly enough to control arterial blood flow. The patient is tagged with a skin-marking pencil or on adhesive tape on the forehead with a T, stating the location of the tourniquet and the time applied. Periodically, the tourniquet is loosened to prevent irreparable vascular or neurologic damage. If there is no arterial bleeding, the tourniquet is removed and a pressure dressing applied. If the patient has suffered a traumatic amputation with uncontrollable hemorrhage, the tourniquet remains in place until the patient is in the operating room.

CONTROL OF INTERNAL BLEEDING

If the patient shows no external signs of bleeding but exhibits tachycardia, falling blood pressure, thirst, apprehension, cool and moist skin, or delayed capillary refill, internal hemorrhage is suspected. Typically, packed red blood cells (O-negative) are administered as prescribed at the rate of blood loss, and the patient is prepared for surgery. Additionally, arterial blood specimens are obtained to evaluate pulmonary function and tissue perfusion and to establish baseline hemodynamic parameters, which are then used as an index for determining the amount of fluid replacement the patient can tolerate and the response to therapy. The patient is maintained in the supine position and monitored closely until hemodynamic or circulatory parameters improve or until transport to surgery.

Controlling Hypovolemic Shock

Shock is a condition in which there is loss of effective circulating blood volume. Inadequate organ and tissue perfusion follows, resulting ultimately in cellular metabolic derangements. In any emergency situation, the onset of shock should be anticipated by assessing all injured people immediately. The underlying cause of shock (hypovolemic, cardiogenic, neurogenic, or septic shock) must be determined. Of these, hypovolemia is the most common cause (see Chap. 14).

Altered tissue perfusion related to failing circulation, impaired gas exchange related to a ventilation–perfusion imbalance, and decreased cardiac output related to decreased circulating blood volume are possible problems associated with hypovolemic shock. Thus, the goals of treatment are to restore and maintain tissue perfusion and to correct physiologic abnormalities.

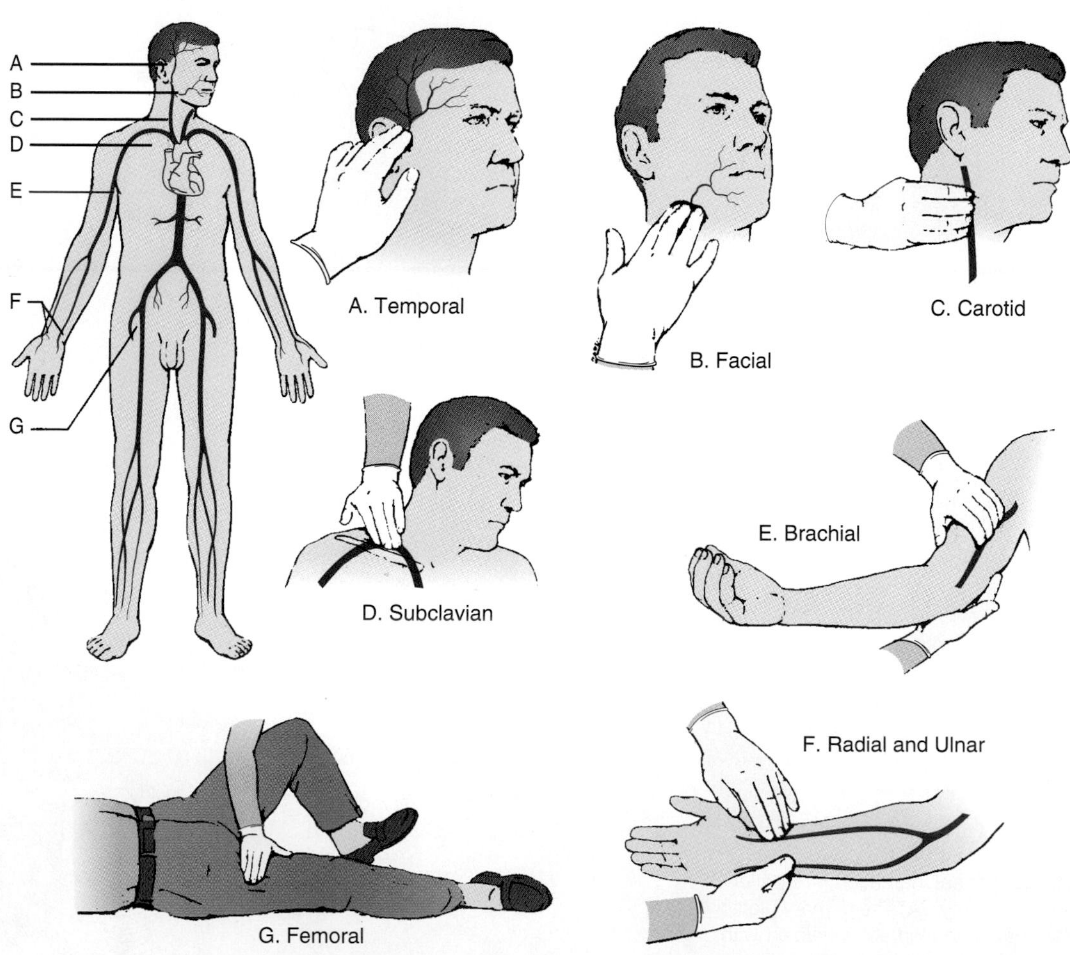

FIGURE 65•2 Pressure points for control of hemorrhage.

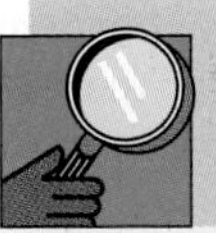

ASSESSMENT SIGNS AND SYMPTOMS OF HYPOVOLEMIC SHOCK

Decreasing arterial pressure
Increasing pulse rate
Cold, moist skin
Delayed capillary refill
Pallor
Thirst
Diaphoresis
Altered sensorium
Oliguria
Metabolic acidosis
Hyperpnea

Management

For the patient experiencing hypovolemic shock, ensuring a patent airway and maintaining breathing are crucial. Additional ventilatory assistance is given as required. A rapid physical examination is performed to determine the cause of shock.

Restoration of the circulating blood volume is accomplished with rapid fluid and blood replacement as prescribed based on test results, such as arterial blood gas levels, chemistry studies, and hemoglobin and hematocrit values. Replacements help to optimize cardiac preload, correct hypotension, and maintain tissue perfusion.

Large-gauge intravenous needles or catheters are inserted into peripheral veins. Two or more catheters are necessary for rapid fluid replacement and reversal of hemodynamic instability. The emphasis is on volume replacement. If it is suspected that a major vessel in the chest or abdomen has been disrupted, intravenous lines may be established in both upper and lower extremities.

A central venous pressure catheter also may be inserted (in or near the right atrium) to serve as a guide for fluid replacement. Continuous central venous pressure (CVP) readings give the direction and degree of change from baseline readings. The catheter is also a vehicle for emergency fluid volume replacement.

Intravenous fluids are infused at a rapid rate until systolic blood pressure or CVP rises to a satisfactory level above the baseline measurement or until there is improvement in the patient's clinical condition. Infusion of lactated Ringer's solution is useful initially because it approximates plasma electrolyte composition and osmolality, allows time for blood typing and cross-matching, restores circulation, and serves as an adjunct to blood component therapy.

Blood component therapy may also be prescribed, especially when blood loss has been severe or when the patient continues to hemorrhage. Measures to control hemorrhage are instituted because hemorrhage compounds the shock state. Serial hematocrit values are obtained if continued bleeding is suspected. Also, the feet are elevated slightly to improve cerebral circulation and promote venous return to the heart. However, this position is contraindicated for patients with head injuries. Unnecessary movement is also avoided.

An indwelling urinary catheter is inserted to record urinary output every hour. Urine volume indicates the adequacy of kidney perfusion. However, fluid replacement is not delayed by waiting to measure hourly urine output.

Ongoing nursing surveillance of the *total patient* is maintained. Blood pressure, heart and respiratory rates, skin temperature, color, pulse oximetry, CVP, arterial blood gases, electrocardiogram (ECG) recordings, hematocrit, hemoglobin, coagulation profile, electrolytes, and urinary output are monitored serially to assess patient response to treatment. Commonly, a flow sheet is used to document these parameters, providing an analysis of trends rather than single values to reveal improvement or deterioration of the patient's condition.

Additionally, the body's defense mechanisms should be supported. The patient should be reassured and comforted. Sedation may be necessary to relieve apprehension. Analgesics are used cautiously to relieve pain. Body temperature is maintained within normal limits to prevent increasing the metabolic demands that the body may be unable to meet.

WOUNDS

Wounds involving injury to soft tissues can vary from minor tears to severe crushing injuries. The types of wounds that may occur are defined in the Chart 65-1. The primary goal is to restore the physical integrity and function of the injured tissue, which is accomplished with minimal scarring and without infection. Proper documentation of the wound using precise descriptions and correct terminology is essential for identification. Such information may be needed in the future for forensic evidence. Photographs are helpful because they provide an accurate, visible description of the wound.

Assessment

Determining *when* and *how* the wound occurred is important because a treatment delay exceeding 3 hours increases infection risk. Using aseptic technique, the clinician inspects the wound to determine the extent of damage to underlying structures. Sensory, motor, and vascular function are evaluated for changes that might indicate complications.

Management

WOUND CLEANSING

If the patient has hair around the wound, the hairs may be clipped or shaved (only as directed) if it is anticipated that the hairs will interfere with wound closure. Typically, the area around the wound is cleaned with normal saline solution or a polymer agent

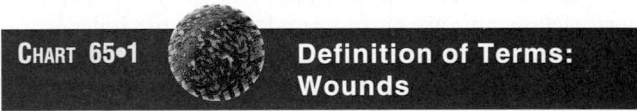

CHART 65•1 Definition of Terms: Wounds

Laceration: skin tear with irregular edges and vein bridging
Avulsion: tearing away from supporting structures
Abrasion: denuded skin
Contusion: blood trapped under the surface of the skin
Hematoma: tumorlike mass of blood trapped under the skin
Stab: incision of the skin with well-defined edges usually caused by a sharp instrument; a stab wound is typically deeper than long
Cut: incision of the skin with well-defined edges, usually longer than deep
Patterned: wound representing the outline of the object causing the wound

(eg, SureClens). Antibacterial agents, such as povidone-iodine (Betadine) or hydrogen peroxide, should not be allowed to get deep into the wound without thorough rinsing. These agents are used only for the initial cleansing because they injure exposed and healthy tissues.

If indicated, the area is infiltrated with a local intradermal anesthetic through the wound margins or by regional block. Patients with soft tissue injuries usually have localized pain at the site of injury. The nurse then assists the physician, nurse practitioner, or physician's assistant in cleaning and débriding the wound.

The wound is irrigated gently and copiously with sterile isotonic saline solution to remove surface dirt. Devitalized tissue and foreign matter are removed because these impede healing and may encourage infection. Any small bleeding vessels are clamped or tied. Alternatively, hemostasis may be achieved with cauterization. After wound treatment, a nonadherent dressing is commonly applied to protect the wound. The dressing may serve as a splint and also as a reminder to the patient that the area is injured.

PRIMARY CLOSURE

The decision to suture a wound depends on the nature of the wound, the time since the injury was sustained, the degree of contamination, and the vascularity of tissues. If primary closure is indicated, the wound is sutured, usually by the physician, with the patient receiving a form of anesthetic known as conscious sedation. Wound closure begins with subcutaneous fat being brought together loosely with a few sutures to close off the dead space. The subcuticular layer is then closed, and finally the epidermis is closed. Sutures are placed close to the wound edge with the skin edges leveled carefully to promote optimal healing. Instead of sutures, sterile strips of reinforced microporous tape or a bonding agent (skin glue) may be used to close clean, superficial wounds.

DELAYED PRIMARY CLOSURE

Delayed primary closure may be indicated in cases of tissue loss or high potential for infection.

A thin layer of gauze (to ensure drainage and prevent pooling of exudate) covered by an occlusive dressing may be used. Other options include split-thickness cadaver or porcine xenografts to simulate the function of epithelium. The wound is splinted in a functional position to prevent motion and decrease the possibility of contracture.

When there are no signs of suppuration, the wound may be sutured (with the patient receiving a local anesthetic). Use of antibiotics to prevent infection depends on factors such as how the injury occurred, the age of the wound, and the risk for contamination. If the wound is contaminated, the site is immobilized and elevated to limit accumulation of fluid in the interstitial spaces of the wound.

Tetanus prophylaxis is administered as prescribed, based on the condition of the wound and the patient's immunization status. The patient is instructed about signs and symptoms of infection and is informed to contact the health care provider or clinic if there is sudden or persistent pain, fever or chills, bleeding, rapid swelling, foul odor, drainage, or redness surrounding the wound.

TRAUMA

Trauma, the unintentional or intentional wound or injury inflicted on the body from a mechanism against which the body cannot protect itself, is the third leading cause of death in the United States, following atherosclerosis and cancer. Trauma is the leading cause of death in children and in adults younger than 44 years of age. The incidence is increasing in adults older than 44 years of age. Alcohol and drug abuse are implicated as factors in both blunt and penetrating trauma.

Collection of Forensic Evidence

In assessing and managing any patient with an emergency condition, but especially the patient experiencing trauma, documentation of all that occurs is essential. Included in documentation are descriptions of all wounds, mechanism of injury, time of events, and collection of evidence. In trauma care, the nurse must be exceedingly careful with all potential evidence, handling and documenting it properly.

The basics of managing care of patients with traumatic injury include an understanding that trauma in any patient (living or dead) has potential legal, or forensic, implications. Hence, proper patient management from both a medical and forensic perspective is essential.

When clothing is removed from the patient who has experienced trauma, the nurse must be careful not to cut through or disrupt any tears, holes, blood stains, or dirt present on the clothing. Each piece of clothing should be placed in an individual paper bag. If the clothing is wet, it should be hung to dry. Clothing should not be given to families. Valuables should be placed in the hospital safe or clearly documented to which family member they were given. If a police officer is present to collect clothing or any other items from the patient, each item is labeled. The transfer of custody to the officer, the officer's name, the date, and the time are documented.

If suicide or homicide is suspected in a deceased trauma patient, the medical examiner will examine the body on site or have the body moved to the coroner's office for autopsy. All tubes and lines must remain in place. The patient's hands must be covered with paper bags to protect evidence on the hands or under the fingernails. In the surviving patient, tissue specimens may be swabbed from the hands and the nails as potential evidence. Photographs of wounds or clothing are essential.

Documentation should also include any statements made by the patient in the patient's own words and surrounded by quotation marks. A chain of evidence is essential. Documentation must be clear; if the patient's case is adjudicated in the future, clear documentation will assist the judicial process and help to identify the activities that occurred in the ED.

Injury Prevention

Any discussion of trauma management must not overlook injury prevention. A component of the emergency nurse's daily role is to provide injury prevention information to every patient with whom there is contact. This includes patients admitted for reasons other than injury. The only way to stop the problem known as trauma is to prevent the injuries in the beginning. Everyone can benefit from injury prevention information. Using the information after leaving the ED or other health care site is the patient's responsibility. However, the information must be provided.

The key to decreasing the incidence of trauma and saving the lives of productive members of society and children is injury prevention. The emergency nurse should make injury prevention part of daily nursing practice.

There are three components of injury prevention. The first is education. Providing information and materials to help prevent violence and to maintain safety at home and in vehicles is important. Involvement in local injury prevention organizations, nursing organizations, and health fairs promotes wellness and safety. In practice, nursing and other health care professionals should avoid using the word "accident" because trauma accidents are *preventable* and should be viewed as such rather than as "fate" or "happenstance." Responsibility and accountability must be assigned to traumatic incidents, particularly because of the high rate of trauma recidivism. Those who are at risk for trauma and repeated trauma should be identified and provided with education and counseling directed toward altering risky behaviors and preventing further trauma.

The second component of injury prevention is legislation. Nurses should be actively involved in safety legislation at the local, state, and federal levels. Such legislation is meant to provide universal safety measures, not to infringe on rights. The third component is automatic protection. Airbags and automatic safety belts are in this category. These mechanisms provide for safety without requiring personal intervention.

Intra-Abdominal Injuries

Intra-abdominal traumatic injuries are categorized as penetrating and blunt trauma. *Penetrating* abdominal injuries (gunshot wounds, stab wounds) are serious and usually require surgery. Penetrating abdominal trauma results in a high incidence of injury to hollow organs, particularly the small bowel. The liver is the most frequently injured solid organ. In gunshot wounds, the most important factor is the velocity at which the missile enters the body. High-velocity missiles (bullets) create extensive tissue damage. All abdominal gunshot wounds crossing the peritoneum or associated with peritoneal signs require surgical exploration. Stab wounds may be managed nonoperatively.

Blunt trauma to the abdomen may result from motor vehicle crashes, falls, and blows. Blunt trauma is commonly associated with extra-abdominal injuries to the chest, head, or extremities. Patients with blunt trauma are a challenge because of injuries that may be hidden and difficult to detect. The incidence of delayed and trauma-related complications is greater than the incidence of complications associated with penetrating injuries. This is especially true of blunt injuries involving the liver, kidneys, spleen, or blood vessels, which can lead to substantial blood loss into the peritoneal cavity.

Assessment

A history of the injuring mechanism, such as a penetrating force from a gunshot or knife or a blunt force from a blow, is essential to determine the type of management needed. In conjunction with this history, the abdomen is inspected for obvious signs of injury, including obvious penetrating injuries, bruises, and abrasions. Abdominal assessment continues with auscultation of bowel sounds to provide baseline data from which changes can be noted. Absence of bowel sounds may be an early sign of intraperitoneal involvement, although stress can also decrease or eliminate bowel sounds. Further abdominal assessment may reveal progressive abdominal distention, involuntary guarding, tenderness, pain, muscular rigidity, or rebound tenderness along with changes in bowel sounds, all of which are signs of peritoneal irritation. Hypotension and signs and symptoms of shock may also be noted. If signs of peritoneal irritation are present, an exploratory laparotomy (surgical incision into the abdominal cavity) is usually performed. Additionally, the chest and other body systems are assessed for injuries that frequently accompany intra-abdominal injuries.

Management

As indicated by the patient's condition, resuscitation procedures (restoration of airway, breathing, circulation) are initiated. A patent airway is maintained along with attempts to stabilize the respiratory, circulatory, and nervous systems. Bleeding is controlled by applying direct pressure to any external bleeding wounds and by occlusion of any chest wounds. Circulating blood volume is maintained with intravenous fluid replacement, including blood component therapy. The patient is monitored for signs and symptoms of shock after an initial response to transfusion therapy because these are often the first signs of internal hemorrhage.

With blunt abdominal trauma, the patient is kept on a stretcher to immobilize the spine. A backboard may be used for transporting the patient to radiology or to the operating room. Cervical spine immobilization is maintained until cervical x-rays have been completed and cervical spine injury ruled out.

All wounds are located and counted but not labeled as exit or entry wounds. Hemorrhage frequently accompanies abdominal injury, especially if the liver and spleen have been traumatized. Therefore, the patient is assessed continuously for signs and symptoms of external and internal bleeding. The front of the body, flanks, and back are inspected for bluish discoloration, asymmetry, abrasion, and contusion. If abdominal viscera protrude, the area is covered with sterile, moist saline dressings to keep the viscera from drying.

The abdomen is assessed for tenderness, rebound tenderness, guarding, rigidity, spasm, increasing distention, and pain. Referred pain is a significant finding because it helps to detect intraperitoneal injury. Pain in the left shoulder may be encountered in a patient bleeding from a ruptured spleen, whereas pain in the right shoulder can result from laceration of the liver. Even though the patient complains of pain, administration of opioids is avoided during the observation period because their effect may mask the clinical picture.

Typically, oral fluids are withheld in anticipation of surgery, and the stomach contents are aspirated with a nasogastric tube to prevent complications of potential aspiration. Nasogastric aspiration also decompresses the stomach in preparation for diagnostic procedures. A rectal or vaginal examination is performed to determine injury to the pelvis, bladder, and intestinal wall. To decompress the bladder and monitor urine output, an indwelling catheter is inserted after a rectal examination (not before).

To determine whether there is intraperitoneal injury and bleeding, the patient is usually prepared for diagnostic procedures, such as peritoneal lavage, abdominal ultrasonography, or abdominal computerized tomography (CT) scan. **Diagnostic peritoneal lavage** involves instilling 1 L of warmed lactated Ringer's or normal saline solution into the abdominal cavity. After a minimum of 400 mL has been returned, the fluid is then drained and sent to the laboratory for analysis. Positive laboratory findings include red blood cells in excess of 100,000/mm^3, a white blood cell count exceeding 500/mm^3, or the presence of bile, feces, or food.

Abdominal CT scans permit detailed evaluation of abdominal contents and retroperitoneal examination. Abdominal ultrasound studies can be used to rapidly assess patients who are hemodynamically unstable for signs of intraperitoneal blood and for signs of pericardial tamponade.

In patients with stab wounds, sinography may be performed to detect peritoneal penetration. With this procedure, a purse-string suture is placed around the wound, and a small catheter is introduced through the wound. A contrast agent is then introduced through the catheter, and x-rays are taken to identify any peritoneal penetration.

Other laboratory studies include the following:

- Urinalysis to detect hematuria indicative of a urinary tract injury
- Serial hematocrit levels to evaluate trends reflecting the presence or absence of bleeding
- White blood cell count to detect elevation generally associated with trauma
- Serum amylase analysis to detect rising levels, which suggest pancreatic injury or perforations of the gastrointestinal tract

Trauma predisposes to infection by disruption of mechanical barriers, exogenous bacteria from the environment at the time of injury, and diagnostic and therapeutic maneuvers (nosocomial infection). Tetanus prophylaxis and broad-spectrum antibiotics are administered as prescribed.

Throughout the stay in the ED, the patient's condition is continuously monitored for changes. If there is continuing evidence of shock, blood loss, free air under the diaphragm, evisceration, hematuria, or suspected or known abdominal injury, the patient is rapidly transported to surgery.

Crush Injuries

Crush injuries occur when a person is caught between objects, run over by a moving vehicle, or compressed by machinery.

Assessment

The patient is observed for the following:

- Hypovolemic shock resulting from extravasation of blood and plasma into injured tissues after compression has been released
- Paralysis of a body part
- Erythema and blistering of skin
- Damaged body part (usually an extremity) appearing swollen, tense, and hard
- Renal dysfunction (prolonged hypotension causes kidney damage and acute renal insufficiency; myoglobinuria secondary to muscle damage can cause acute renal failure)

Emergency Management

In conjunction with maintaining the airway, breathing, and circulation, the patient is observed for acute renal insufficiency. Injury to the back may cause severe kidney damage. Severe muscular damage causes a significant release of myoglobin, which can result in acute tubular necrosis. Additionally, major soft tissue injuries are splinted early to control bleeding and pain.

If an extremity is involved, it is elevated to relieve swelling and pressure. To restore neurovascular function, the physician may perform a **fasciotomy** (surgical incision to the level of the fascia). Medications for pain and anxiety are then administered as prescribed, and the patient is quickly transported to the operating suite for wound débridement and fracture repair. Then, if available, a hyperbaric chamber can be used for hyperoxygenation of the crushed tissue.

Multiple Injuries

Care of the patient with multiple injuries requires a team approach, with one person responsible for coordinating the treatment. Immediately after injury, the body is hypermetabolic, hypercoagulable, and severely stressed. Mortality in patients with multiple injuries is related to the severity of the injuries and the number of systems and organs involved.

Multiple trauma potentially affects every body system. The nursing staff assumes responsibility for assessing and monitoring the patient, ensuring intravenous access, administering prescribed medications, collecting laboratory specimens, and documenting activities and the patient's response.

Assessment

Gross evidence of trauma may be slight or absent. The injury regarded as the least significant in appearance may be the most lethal.

Management

The goals of treatment are to determine the extent of injuries and to establish priorities of treatment. Any injury interfering with a vital physiologic function (eg, airway, breathing, circulation) is an immediate threat to life and has the highest priority for immediate treatment. *Imperative life-saving procedures are performed simultaneously by the emergency team.* As soon as the patient is resuscitated, clothes are usually cut off, and a rapid physical assessment is performed. Transfer from field management to ED must be orderly and controlled. Treatment in a level I trauma center is appropriate for patients experiencing major trauma.

Treatment priorities are illustrated in Figure 65-3.

Fractures

Immediate management of a fracture may determine the patient's outcome and mean the difference between recovery and disability. When examining the patient for fracture, the body part is handled gently and as little as possible. Clothing is cut off to visualize the body. Assessment is conducted for pain over or near a bone, swelling (from blood, lymph, and exudate infiltrating the tissue), and circulatory disturbance. The patient is assessed for ecchymosis, tenderness, and crepitation. *The examiner must remember that the patient may have multiple fractures accompanied by head, chest, spine, or abdominal injuries.*

Management

Immediate attention is given to the patient's general condition. Assessment of airway, breathing, and circulation (which includes pulses in the extremities) is conducted. The patient is also evaluated for neurologic or abdominal injuries before the extremity is treated unless a pulseless extremity is detected.

If a pulseless extremity is identified, repositioning of the extremity to proper alignment is required. If the pulseless extremity involves a fractured hip or femur, **Hare traction**, a portable in-line traction device, may be applied to assist with alignment. If repositioning is ineffective, a rapid total-body assessment should be completed, followed by transfer of the patient to the operating room for arteriography and possible arterial repair.

After the initial evaluation has been completed, all injuries identified are evaluated and treated. The fractured body part is inspected. Using a systematic head-to-toe approach, the entire body is inspected. The inspector looks for lacerations, swelling, and deformities, including angulation (bending), shortening, rotation, or asymmetry. All peripheral pulses, especially the pulse distal to the fractured extremity, are palpated. The extremity is also assessed for

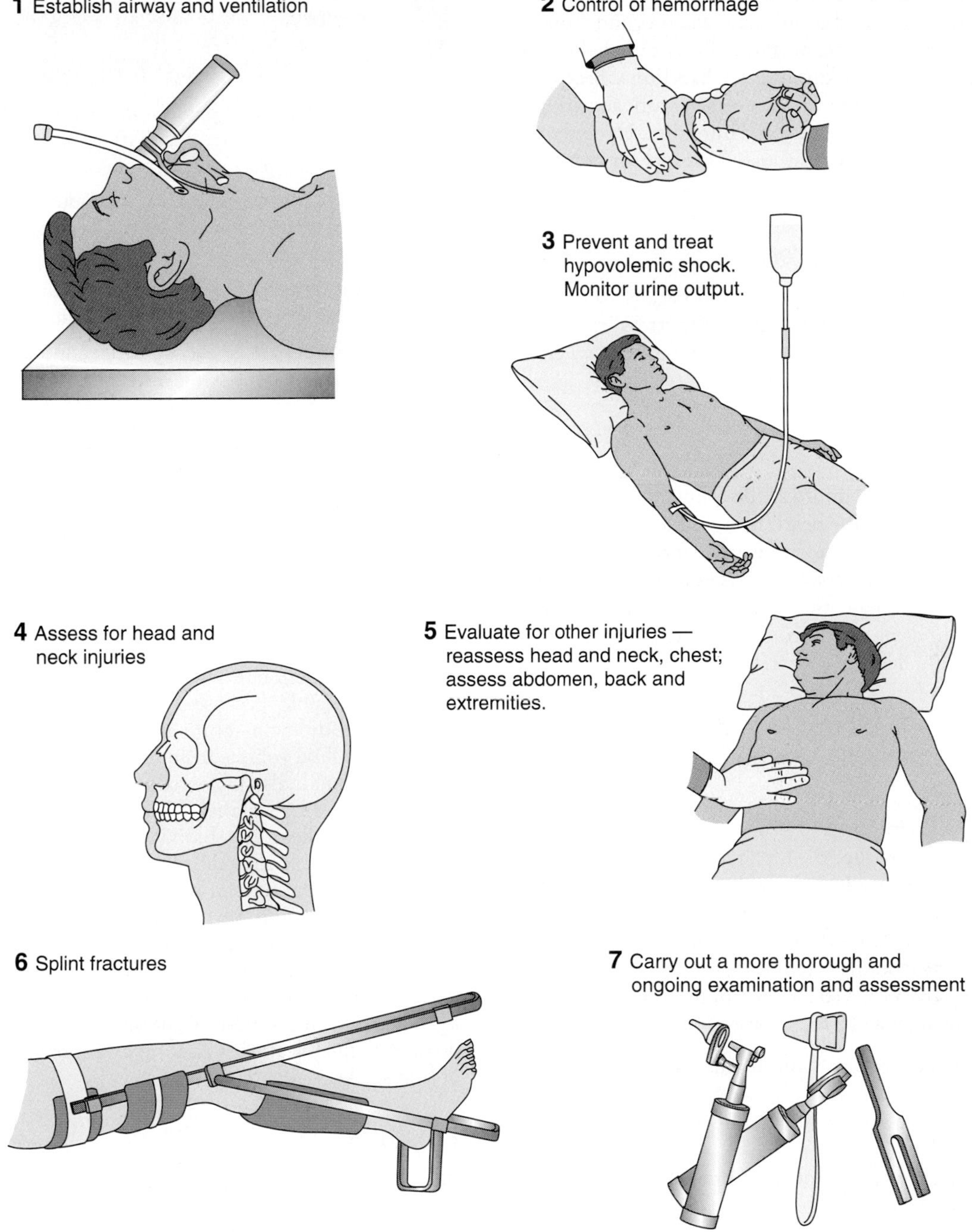
1 Establish airway and ventilation
2 Control of hemorrhage
3 Prevent and treat hypovolemic shock. Monitor urine output.
4 Assess for head and neck injuries
5 Evaluate for other injuries — reassess head and neck, chest; assess abdomen, back and extremities.
6 Splint fractures
7 Carry out a more thorough and ongoing examination and assessment

FIGURE 65•3 Management of the patient with multiple injuries.

coolness, blanching, and decreased sensation and motor function, indicative of injury to the extremity's neurovascular supply.

Before moving the patient, a splint is applied. Splinting immobilizes the joint above and below the fracture, relieves pain, restores or improves circulation, prevents further tissue injury, and prevents a closed fracture from becoming an open one. To splint an extremity, one hand is placed distal to the fracture and some traction is applied while the other hand is placed beneath the fracture for support. The splints should extend beyond the joints adjacent to the fracture. Upper extremities must be splinted in functional position. If the fracture is open, a moist sterile dressing is applied.

After splinting, the vascular status of the extremity is checked by assessing color, temperature, pulse, and blanching of the nail bed. If there is evidence of neurovascular compromise, the splint is removed and reapplied. In addition, any complaints of pain or pressure are investigated. (See Chap. 63 for a complete discussion of fracture management.)

ENVIRONMENTAL EMERGENCIES

Heat Stroke

Heat stroke is an acute medical emergency caused by failure of the heat-regulating mechanisms of the body. It usually occurs during extended heat waves, especially when accompanied by high humidity. People at risk are those not acclimatized to heat, elderly and very young people, those unable to care for themselves, those with chronic and debilitating diseases, and those taking certain medications (eg, major tranquilizers, anticholinergics, diuretics, beta-adrenergic blocking agents). **Exertional heat stroke** occurs in healthy individuals during sports or work activities, for example, exercising in extreme heat and humidity. Hyperthermia results because of inadequate heat loss. This type of heat stroke can also cause death.

Gerontologic Considerations

Most heat-related deaths occur in the aged because their circulatory systems are unable to compensate for stress imposed by heat. Elderly people have a decreased ability to sweat as well as a decreased thirst mechanism to compensate for heat.

Assessment

Heat stroke causes thermal injury at the cellular level and resulting widespread damage to the heart, liver, kidney, and blood coagulation. Recent patient history reveals exposure to elevated ambient temperature or excessive exercise during extreme heat. When assessing the patient, the examiner notes the following symptoms: profound central nervous system dysfunction (manifested by confusion, delirium, bizarre behavior, coma); elevated body temperature (40.6°C [105°F] or more); hot, dry skin; and usually anhidrosis (absence of sweating), tachypnea, and tachycardia.

Management

The primary goal is to reduce the high temperature as quickly as possible because mortality is directly related to the duration of hyperthermia. Simultaneous treatment focuses on stabilizing oxygenation using the ABCs of basic life support.

After the patient's clothing is removed, the core (internal) temperature is reduced to 39°C (102°F) as rapidly as possible. One or more of the following may be used as directed:

- Cool sheets and towels or continuous sponging with cool water
- Ice applied to the skin while spraying with tepid water
- Cooling blankets
- Iced saline lavage of the stomach or colon if the temperature does not decrease

During cooling, the patient is massaged to promote circulation and maintain cutaneous vasodilation. An electric fan is positioned so that it blows on the patient to augment heat dissipation by convection and evaporation. The patient's temperature is constantly monitored with a thermistor placed in the rectum, bladder, or esophagus to evaluate core temperature. Caution is used to avoid hypothermia and to prevent hyperthermia, which may recur spontaneously within 3 to 4 hours.

Throughout treatment, the patient's status is monitored carefully including vital signs, ECGs (for possible myocardial ischemia, myocardial infarction, and dysrhythmias), CVP, and level of responsiveness, all of which may change with rapid alterations in body temperature. A seizure may be followed by recurrence of hyperthermia. To meet tissue needs exaggerated by the hypermetabolic condition, 100% oxygen is administered. The patient may require endotracheal intubation and mechanical ventilation to support failing cardiopulmonary systems.

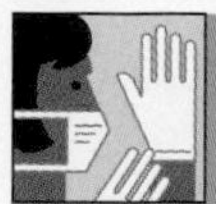

HEALTH PROMOTION AND ILLNESS PREVENTION
Prevention of Heat Stroke

Advise the patient to avoid immediate reexposure to high temperatures; hypersensitivity to high temperatures may remain for a considerable time.

Emphasize the importance of maintaining adequate fluid intake, wearing loose clothing, and reducing activity in hot weather.

Advise athletes to monitor fluid losses during work activities or exercise and replace fluids.

Advise the patient to use a gradual approach to physical conditioning, allowing sufficient time for acclimatization.

Direct frail elderly patients living in urban settings with high environmental temperatures to places where air conditioning is available (eg, shopping mall, library, church).

Intravenous infusion therapy is initiated as directed to replace fluid losses and maintain adequate circulation. These fluids are administered carefully because of the dangers of myocardial injury from high body temperature and poor renal function. Cooling redistributes fluid volume from the periphery to the core.

Urine output is also measured frequently because acute tubular necrosis is a complication of heat stroke from rhabdomyolysis (myoglobin in the urine). Blood specimens are obtained for serial testing to detect bleeding disorders, such as disseminated intravascular coagulopathy, and for serial enzyme studies to estimate thermal hypoxic injury to the liver, heart, and muscle tissue. Permanent liver, cardiac, and central nervous system damage may occur.

Additional supportive care may include dialysis for renal failure, anticonvulsant agents to control seizures, potassium for hypokalemia, and sodium bicarbonate to correct metabolic acidosis. Patient education is also important to prevent a recurrence of heat stroke.

Frostbite

Frostbite is trauma from exposure to freezing temperatures and actual freezing of the tissue fluids in the cell and intercellular spaces. It results in cellular and vascular damage. Body parts most frequently affected by frostbite include the feet, hands, nose, and ears.

Assessment

A frozen extremity may be hard, cold, and insensitive to touch and may appear white or mottled blue-white. The extent of injury from exposure to cold is not always initially known.

Management

The goal of management is to restore normal body temperature. Constrictive clothing and jewelry that could impair circulation are removed. If the lower extremities are involved, the patient should not be allowed to ambulate.

Controlled yet rapid rewarming is instituted. The extremity is usually placed in a 37° to 40°C (98.6° to 104°F) whirlpool for

30- to 40-minute spans. This is repeated until circulation is effectively restored. Early rewarming appears to decrease the amount of ultimate tissue loss. During rewarming, an analgesic for pain is administered as prescribed because the rewarming process may be very painful, and the part not handled to avoid further mechanical injury. *Massage is contraindicated.*

Once rewarmed, the part is protected from further injury and elevated to help control swelling. Sterile gauze or cotton is placed between affected fingers or toes to prevent maceration. A foot cradle may be used to prevent contact with bedclothes if the feet are involved. Blebs, which develop 1 hour to a few days after rewarming, are left intact and not ruptured.

A physical assessment is conducted with rewarming to observe for concomitant injury, such as soft tissue injury, dehydration, alcohol coma, or fat embolism. Problems such as dehydration, hyperkalemia, and hypovolemia, which occur frequently in frostbite victims, are corrected. Risk for infection is also great; therefore, strict aseptic technique is used during dressing changes, and tetanus prophylaxis is administered as indicated.

Additional measures that may be carried out when appropriate include the following:

- Whirlpool bath for the affected extremity to aid circulation, débride necrotic tissue, and help prevent infection
- Escharotomy (incision through the eschar) to prevent further tissue damage, allow for normal circulation, and permit joint motion
- Fasciotomy to treat compartment syndrome

After rewarming, hourly active motion of the affected digits is encouraged to promote maximal restoration of function and to prevent contractures. The patient is also encouraged to avoid tobacco or caffeine because of the vasoconstrictive effects, further reducing the already deficient blood supply to injured tissues.

Hypothermia

Hypothermia is a condition in which the core (internal) temperature is 35°C (95°F) or below as a result of exposure to cold. Hypothermia occurs when a patient loses the ability to maintain body temperature. Urban hypothermia (extreme exposure to cold in an urban setting) is associated with a high mortality rate; elderly people, infants, people with concurrent illnesses, and the homeless are particularly susceptible. Alcohol ingestion increases susceptibility due to systemic vasodilation. Trauma victims are also at risk for hypothermia due to treatment with cold fluids, unwarmed oxygen, and exposure during examination.

Assessment

Hypothermia leads to physiologic changes in all organ systems. There is progressive deterioration with apathy, poor judgment, ataxia, dysarthria, drowsiness, and eventual coma. Shivering may be suppressed below a temperature of 32.2°C (90°F) because the body's self-warming mechanisms become ineffective. The heartbeat and blood pressure may be so weak that peripheral pulses become undetectable. Cardiac irregularities may also occur. Other physiologic abnormalities include hypoxemia and acidosis.

Management

Management consists of continual monitoring, rewarming, and supportive care.

MONITORING

The ABCs of basic life support are a priority. The patient's vital signs, CVP, urine output, arterial blood gas levels, blood chemistry determinations (blood urea nitrogen, creatinine, glucose, electrolytes), and chest x-rays are evaluated frequently. Body temperature is monitored with an esophageal, bladder, or rectal thermistor. Continuous ECG monitoring is performed because cold-induced myocardial irritability leads to conduction disturbances, especially ventricular fibrillation. An arterial line is inserted and maintained to record blood pressure and to facilitate blood sampling.

REWARMING

Rewarming methods include active core (internal) rewarming, active external rewarming, and passive or spontaneous rewarming.

Core rewarming methods include cardiopulmonary bypass, warm fluid administration, warm humidified oxygen by ventilator, and warmed peritoneal lavage. Core rewarming is recommended for severe hypothermia. Monitoring for ventricular fibrillation as the patient passes through 31° to 32°C (88° to 90°F) is essential.

Passive external rewarming includes the use of warm blankets or over-the-bed heaters. Passive rewarming of the extremities increases blood flow to the acidotic, anaerobic extremities. The cold blood with high lactic acid levels returning to the core has significant effects on the core temperature and metabolic response, possibly causing cardiac dysrhythmias and electrolyte disturbances.

SUPPORTIVE CARE

Supportive care during rewarming includes the following as directed:

- External cardiac compression (may not be instituted in the very cold patient)
- Defibrillation of ventricular fibrillation. Patients whose temperature is less than 32°C (90°F) will experience spontaneous ventricular fibrillation if moved or touched. Defibrillation is ineffective in patients with temperatures lower than 31°C (88°F).
- Mechanical ventilation with positive end-expiratory pressure (PEEP) and heated humidified oxygen to maintain tissue oxygenation
- Administration of warmed intravenous fluids to correct hypotension and maintain urine output and core rewarming as described previously
- Administration of sodium bicarbonate to correct metabolic acidosis if necessary
- Administration of antiarrhythmic medications
- Insertion of indwelling urinary catheter to monitor fluid status

Near-Drowning

Near-drowning is survival for at least 24 hours after submersion. The most common consequence is hypoxemia. Drowning is the third most common cause of unintentional death and the leading cause of unintentional death in children under 15 years of age in 10 states. An estimated 7000 drownings and 90,000 near-drownings occur yearly in the United States. Children under 4 years of age account for 40% of drownings.

Factors associated with drowning and near-drowning include alcohol ingestion, inability to swim, diving injuries, hypothermia, and exhaustion. Efforts to save the victim should not be abandoned prematurely. Successful resuscitation with full neurologic recovery has occurred in near-drowning victims with prolonged submersion in cold water. This is due to a decrease in metabolic demands or the diving reflex.

After resuscitation, hypoxia and acidosis, the primary problems of a victim who has nearly drowned, require immediate intervention in the ED. Resultant pathophysiologic changes and pulmonary injury depend on the type of fluid (fresh or salt water) and the volume aspirated. Fresh water aspiration results in a loss of surfactant, hence an inability to expand the lungs. Salt water aspiration leads to pulmonary edema from the osmotic effects of the salt within the lung. After a person survives submersion, acute respiratory distress syndrome resulting in hypoxia, hypercarbia, and respiratory or metabolic acidosis can occur.

Management

Therapeutic aims include maintaining cerebral perfusion and adequate oxygenation to prevent further damage to vital organs. Immediate cardiopulmonary resuscitation is the factor with the greatest influence on survival. The treatment goal is prevention of hypoxia, accomplished by ensuring an adequate airway and respiration, thus improving ventilation (which helps to correct respiratory acidosis) and oxygenation. Arterial blood gas analyses are performed to evaluate oxygen, carbon dioxide, and bicarbonate levels and pH. These parameters determine the type of ventilatory support needed. Use of endotracheal intubation with positive-pressure ventilation (with PEEP) improves oxygenation, prevents aspiration, and corrects intrapulmonary shunting and ventilation-perfusion abnormalities (caused by aspiration of water). If the patient is breathing spontaneously, supplemental oxygen may be administered by mask. However, an endotracheal tube is necessary if the patient does not breathe spontaneously.

Because of submersion, the patient is usually hypothermic. A rectal probe is used to determine the degree of hypothermia. Prescribed rewarming procedures (eg, extracorporeal warming, warmed peritoneal dialysis, inhalation of warm aerosolized oxygen, torso warming) are started during resuscitation. The choice is determined by the severity and duration of hypothermia and available resources. Intrasvascular volume expansion and inotropic agents are used to manage hypotension and impaired tissue perfusion. ECG monitoring is initiated because dysrhythmias frequently occur. An indwelling urinary catheter is inserted to measure urine output. Hypothermia and accompanying metabolic acidosis may compromise renal function. Nasogastric intubation is used to decompress the stomach and to prevent the patient from aspirating gastric contents.

In case the patient appears deceptively healthy, close monitoring continues with serial vital signs, serial arterial blood gas values, ECG monitoring, intracranial pressure assessments, serum electrolyte levels, intake and output, and serial chest x-rays. After a near-drowning, the patient is at risk for complications, such as hypoxic or ischemic cerebral injury, acute respiratory distress syndrome, pulmonary damage secondary to aspiration, and life-threatening cardiac arrest.

Decompression Sickness

Decompression sickness (DCS), also called the bends, occurs in patients who have engaged in diving, high-altitude flying, or flying commercial aircraft within 24 hours of diving. Although DCS occurs in relatively few divers compared with the number of dives worldwide, its effects can be hazardous. Being aware of DCS and assessing the patient properly will ensure proper management of the patient and result in the least morbidity possible.

DCS results from nitrogen bubbles trapped in the body. They may occur in joint or muscle spaces, resulting in musculoskeletal pain, numbness, or hypesthesia. More significantly, nitrogen bubbles can become air emboli in the bloodstream and thereby produce stroke (brain), paralysis (spine), or death (heart). Taking a rapid history about the events preceding the symptoms is essential. Recompression is necessary as soon as possible, which may necessitate a low-altitude flight to the nearest hyperbaric chamber.

Assessment

To identify DCS, a detailed history is obtained from the patient or diving buddy. Evidence of rapid ascent, loss of air in the tank, buddy breathing, recent alcohol intake or loss of rest, or a flight home within 24 hours of diving suggests the potential for DCS. Note that some patients describe a perfect dive profile yet still have the signs and symptoms of DCS and must be treated as such.

Signs and symptoms include joint or extremity pain, numbness, hypesthesia, or loss of range of motion. Neurologic symptoms mimicking a stroke or spinal cord injury could indicate an air embolus. Cardiopulmonary arrest can also occur with severe cases of DCS. Because of hypoxia, these patients seldom survive. Onset of cardiopulmonary arrest can occur while the patient is still in the water. Any neurologic symptoms should be rapidly assessed. All patients with DCS need rapid transfer to a hyperbaric chamber.

Management

A patent airway and adequate ventilation are established as described previously, and 100% oxygen is administered on board the ship and throughout treatment and transport. A chest x-ray is obtained to identify aspiration, and at least one intravenous line is started with lactated Ringer's or normal saline solution.

The cardiopulmonary and neurologic systems are supported as needed. If an air embolus is suspected, the head of the bed should be lowered. The patient's wet clothing is removed, and the patient is kept warm. Transfer to the closest hyperbaric chamber capable of treating DCS is initiated. The Divers Alert Network (DAN) can be contacted by telephone (1-919-684-8111) to locate the nearest chamber. If air transport is necessary, low-altitude flight (below 8000 feet) is required. However, the patient who is awake and alert without central neurologic deficits may be able to travel by ground ambulance or car depending on the severity of symptoms. Throughout treatment, the patient is continually assessed, and changes are documented. If aspiration is suspected, antibiotics may be prescribed.

Anaphylactic Reaction

An **anaphylactic reaction** is an acute systemic hypersensitivity reaction that occurs within seconds or minutes of exposure to various foreign substances, such as medications (eg, penicillin, iodinated contrast material), and other agents, such as insects (bee, wasp, yellow jacket, hornet) or foods (eggs, peanuts). Repeated administration of parenteral or oral therapeutic agents may also precipitate an anaphylactic reaction.

An anaphylactic reaction is the result of an antigen–antibody interaction in a sensitized individual who, as a consequence of

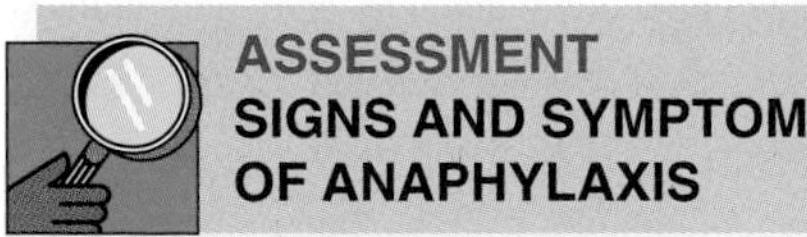

ASSESSMENT SIGNS AND SYMPTOMS OF ANAPHYLAXIS

Respiratory Signs

Nasal congestion
Itching
Sneezing and coughing
Possible respiratory distress that progresses rapidly (caused by bronchospasm or edema of the larynx)
Chest tightness
Other respiratory difficulties, such as wheezing, dyspnea, and cyanosis

Skin Manifestations

Flushing with a sense of warmth and diffuse erythema
Generalized itching over the entire body (indicates developing general systemic reaction)
Urticaria (hives)
Massive facial angioedema possible with accompanying upper respiratory edema

Cardiovascular Manifestations

Tachycardia or bradycardia
Peripheral vascular collapse as indicated by:
- Pallor
- Imperceptible pulse
- Decreasing blood pressure
- Circulatory failure, leading to coma and death

Gastrointestinal Problems

Nausea
Vomiting
Colicky abdominal pains
Diarrhea

previous exposure, has developed a special type of antibody (immunoglobulin) that is specific for this particular allergen. The antibody immunoglobulin E (IgE) is responsible for most of the immediate type of human allergic responses. The individual becomes sensitive to a particular antigen after production of IgE to this antigen. A second exposure to the same antigen results in a more severe and more rapid response (see Chap. 49).

Clinical Manifestations

Anaphylactic reaction produces a wide range of clinical manifestations.

Management

With an anaphylactic reaction, establishing a patent airway and ventilation are essential. (This is performed while another person administers epinephrine.) Early endotracheal tube intubation is essential to avoid loss of the airway, and oropharyngeal suction may be necessary to remove excessive secretions. Resuscitative measures are used, especially for patients with stridor and progressive pulmonary edema. If glottal edema occurs, a cricothyroidotomy is used to provide an airway.

Simultaneously with airway management, aqueous epinephrine is administered as prescribed to provide rapid relief of hypersensitivity reaction. Epinephrine may be given again, if necessary and as prescribed. Judgment is used in choosing the route of administration, as follows:

- Subcutaneous injection for mild, generalized symptoms
- Intramuscular injection when the reaction is more severe and progressive, and with concern that vascular collapse will inhibit absorption
- Intravenous route (aqueous epinephrine diluted in saline solution and given *slowly*), used in rare instances in which there is complete loss of consciousness and severe cardiovascular collapse. This method may precipitate cardiac dysrhythmias. ECG monitoring with a readily available defibrillator is necessary. This method is controversial and not usually recommended because it can lead to more distress than is initially present. An intravenous infusion of saline solution is initiated to provide for emergency access to a vein and to treat hypotension.

Additional treatments may include antihistamines to block further histamine binding at target cells; aminophylline by slow intravenous infusion for severe bronchospasm and wheezing that is refractory to other treatment; albuterol inhalers or humidified treatments to decrease bronchoconstriction; crystalloids, colloids, or vasopressors to treat prolonged hypotension; isoproterenol or dopamine for reduced cardiac output; oxygen to enhance tissue perfusion; intravenous benzodiazepines for control of seizures; and corticosteroids for prolonged reaction with persistent hypotension or bronchospasm. After the acute symptoms have been treated, the patient is usually admitted to the hospital for observation. The patient should be informed about ways to prevent anaphylactic reactions.

Latex Allergy

Another allergy situation with which emergency nurses are dealing on a daily basis is latex allergy. The number of products that contain latex is staggering. Nurses must be aware of latex allergy (health care providers have died from anaphylaxis related to latex allergy) and the potential for patients to react to latex.

There is an increased awareness among manufacturers of the need for products that are latex free. Latex-free gloves are often provided for nurses who have latex allergies or who have signs of allergy, such as itching, redness, or rash associated with use of a latex product. Severe anaphylaxis can occur even on the first exposure, which is why recognition of the signs and symptoms of anaphylaxis is essential. Treatment must be rapid, and the latex product should be removed promptly.

Injected Poisons: Stinging Insects

A person may have an extreme sensitivity to the venoms of the Hymenoptera (the stings of bees, hornets, yellow jackets, and wasps). Venom allergy is thought to be an IgE-mediated reaction, which constitutes an acute emergency. Although stings in any area of the body can trigger anaphylaxis, stings of the head and neck are especially serious.

Clinical Manifestations

Clinical manifestations range from generalized urticaria, itching, malaise, and anxiety due to laryngeal edema to severe bronchospasm, shock, and death. Generally, the shorter the time between the sting and the onset of severe symptoms, the worse the prognosis.

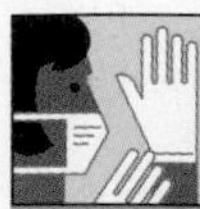

HEALTH PROMOTION AND ILLNESS PREVENTION

Preventing Anaphylactic Reactions

Be aware of the danger of anaphylactic reactions and the early signs of anaphylaxis.

Ask the patient about previous allergies to medications, foods, stings, etc.

Before giving a foreign serum or other type of antigenic agent, ask the patient or caregiver whether the agent was received at some earlier time.

Question the patient about previous allergic reactions to food or pollen.

Ask about allergies to eggs.

Avoid giving medications to patients with hay fever, asthma, and other allergic disorders unless absolutely necessary.

Avoid giving parenteral medications unless absolutely necessary because anaphylactic reactions are more likely to occur when the agent is given parenterally.

Perform a skin test before administration of certain materials known to produce anaphylactic reactions, such as horse serum. Remember that negative skin test results do not always indicate safety and that skin testing can precipitate anaphylaxis in highly sensitive individuals. Have epinephrine, IV infusions, and intubation and tracheostomy equipment available as precautionary measures.

If the patient is an outpatient, keep him or her in the office, hospital, or clinic for at least 30 minutes after injection of any agent. Caution the patient to return if symptoms develop.

Caution patients who are highly sensitive (eg, to insect bites and stings) to carry kits equipped to treat insect stings (epinephrine). Instruct the patient, the family, and significant others in the use of the emergency supplies.

Encourage patients with allergies to wear medical identification tags or bracelets.

Management

Epinephrine (aqueous) is injected subcutaneously (*not intravenously*), and the site is massaged to hasten absorption. The patient is assessed for signs and symptoms of anaphylactic reaction and treated as necessary. (See previous discussion and also Chap. 14, which discusses shock and multisystem failure.) Desensitization therapy should be given to people who have had systemic or significant local reactions.

Patient and family education is an important measure in preventing exposure to stinging insects.

Snake Bites

Venomous (poisonous) snakes cause about 3.74 bites per 100,000 population in the United States yearly and result in 9 to 15 deaths. Children between the ages of 1 and 9 years are the most likely victims. The greatest number of bites occur through the daylight hours into early evening in summer months. Venomous snake bites are medical emergencies.

PATIENT EDUCATION AND HOME CARE

Limiting Exposure to Stinging Insects

- Avoid places where stinging insects congregate, such as camp and picnic sites, and insect feeding areas, such as flower beds, ripe fruit orchards, garbage, fields of clover.
- Wear covering on the feet, and avoid going barefoot outdoors because yellow jackets nest and pollinate on the ground.
- Avoid perfumes, scented soaps, and bright colors, which attract bees.
- Keep car windows closed.
- Spray garbage cans with quick-acting insecticide.
- Secure a professional exterminator to dispose of wasp and hornet nests or beehives in the home area.
- Remain motionless if an insect is buzzing around. Motion, especially running, increases the likelihood of being stung.
- Carry a self-treatment kit containing injectable and inhalant forms of epinephrine, an oral antihistamine, and written instructions. Carry it with you at all times.
- If stung, do the following:
  1. Inject self immediately with epinephrine.
  2. Remove the stinger with one quick scrape of the fingernail. *Do not* squeeze the venom sac because this may cause injection of additional venom.
  3. Clean the area with soapy water, and apply ice.
  4. Report to the nearest health care facility for further examination.

Nineteen different species of venomous snakes are found in every part of the United States, with different parts of the country and the world having different types of snakes. Because snake bites are medical emergencies, nurses should be familiar with the types of snakes that are common to the geographic region where they practice. Snake venom consists primarily of proteins with a broad range of physiologic effects. Multiple organ systems, especially the neurologic, cardiovascular, and respiratory systems, may be affected.

Management

Initial first aid at the site of the snake bite includes having the victim lie down, removing constrictive items such as rings, providing warmth, cleansing the wound, covering the wound with a light sterile dressing, and immobilizing the injured body part below the level of the heart. Ice or a tourniquet *is not* applied. Initial evaluation in the ED is performed quickly and includes information about the following:

- Whether the snake was venomous or nonvenomous; if the snake is dead, it should be transported to the ED with the patient for identification
- Where and when the bite occurred and the circumstances of the bite
- Sequence of events, signs and symptoms (fang punctures, pain, edema, and erythema of the bite and nearby tissues)
- Severity of poisonous effects
- Vital signs
- Circumference of the bitten extremity or area at several points
- Laboratory data (complete blood count, urinalysis, and clotting studies)

The course and prognosis of snake bite injuries depend on the kind and amount of venom injected, where on the body the bite occurred, and the general health, age, and size of the victim. There is no one specific protocol for treatment of snake bites. Generally, ice, tourniquets, heparin, and corticosteroids are not used during the acute stage. Corticosteroids are contraindicated in the first 6 to 8 hours after the bite because they may depress antibody production and hinder the action of **antivenin** (antitoxin manufactured from the snake venom).

Parenteral fluids may be used to treat hypotension. If vasopressors are used to treat hypotension, their use should be short-term. Surgical exploration of the bite is rarely indicated. Typically, the patient is observed closely for at least 6 hours. The patient is *never* left unattended.

ADMINISTRATION OF ANTIVENIN (ANTITOXIN)

It is rare that envenomation (injection of a poisonous material by sting, spine, bite, or other means) occurs with snake bites. An assessment of progressive signs and symptoms is essential before considering administration of antivenin, which is most effective if administered within 12 hours of the snake bite. The dosage depends on the type of snake and the estimated severity of the bite. Children may require more antivenin than adults because their smaller bodies are more susceptible to toxic effects of venom. A skin or eye test should be performed before the initial dose to detect allergy to the antivenin. However, because even the skin test can cause an anaphylactic reaction, patients should not be tested unless antivenin is to be given.

Before administering antivenin and every 15 minutes thereafter, the circumference of the affected part is measured proximally. Premedication with diphenhydramine and cimetidine decreases the allergic response to antivenin. Antivenin is administered as an intravenous infusion whenever possible, although intramuscular administration can be used. Depending on the severity of the bite, the antivenin is diluted in 500 to 1000 mL of normal saline solution; the fluid volume may be reduced for children. The infusion is started slowly, and the rate is increased after 10 minutes if there is no reaction. The total dose should be infused during the first 4 to 6 hours after poisoning. The initial dose is repeated until symptoms decrease. After the symptoms decrease, the circumference of the affected part should be measured every 30 to 60 minutes for the next 48 hours to detect symptoms of compartment syndrome (swelling, loss of pulse, increased pain, and paresthesias).

The most common cause of allergic reaction to the antivenin is its too-rapid infusion, although about 3% of patients with negative skin test results develop reactions not related to infusion rate. Reactions may consist of a feeling of fullness in the face, urticaria, pruritus, malaise, and apprehension. These symptoms may be followed by tachycardia, shortness of breath, hypotension, and shock. In this situation, the infusion should be stopped immediately and intravenous diphenhydramine administered. Vasopressors are used for patients in shock, and resuscitation equipment must be on standby while antivenin is infusing.

POISONING

A poison is any substance that when ingested, inhaled, absorbed, applied to the skin, or produced within the body in relatively small amounts injures the body by its chemical action. Poisoning from inhalation and ingestion of toxic materials, both unintentional or by design, constitutes a major health hazard and an emergency situation. Emergency treatment is initiated with the following goals:

- To remove or inactivate the poison before it is absorbed
- To provide supportive care in maintaining vital organ systems
- To administer a specific antidote to neutralize a specific poison
- To implement treatment that hastens the elimination of the absorbed poison

Ingested (Swallowed) Poisons

Swallowed poisons may be corrosive. **Corrosive poisons** include alkaline and acid agents that can cause tissue destruction after coming in contact with mucous membranes.

Alkaline products: lye, drain cleaners, toilet bowl cleaners, bleach, nonphosphate detergents, oven cleaners, button batteries (batteries used to power watches, calculators, cameras), Clinitest tablets

Acid products: Toilet bowl cleaners, pool cleaners, metal cleaners, rust removers, battery acid

Management

Control of the airway, ventilation, and oxygenation are essential. In the absence of cerebral or renal damage, the patient's prognosis depends largely on successfully managing respiration and circulation. Measures are instituted to stabilize cardiovascular and other body functions. ECG, vital signs, and neurologic status are monitored closely for changes. Shock, which may result from the cardiodepressant action of the substance ingested, venous pooling in lower extremities, or reduced circulating blood volume resulting from increased capillary permeability, is treated. An indwelling urinary catheter is inserted to monitor renal function. Blood specimens are obtained to test for concentration of drug or poison.

Efforts are initiated to determine what substance was taken; the amount; time since ingestion; signs and symptoms, such as pain or burning sensations, any evidence of redness or burn in the mouth or throat, pain on swallowing or an inability to swallow, vomiting, or drooling; age and weight of the patient; and pertinent health history.

Nursing Alert *The area poison control center should be called if an unknown toxic agent has been taken or if it is necessary to identify an antidote for a known toxic agent.*

Measures are instituted to remove the toxin or decrease its absorption. The patient who ingested a corrosive poison is given water or milk to drink for dilution. However, dilution is not attempted in patients with acute airway edema or obstruction or in patients with clinical evidence of esophageal, gastric, or intestinal burn or perforation. The following gastric emptying procedures may be used as prescribed:

- Syrup of ipecac to induce vomiting in the alert patient. Vomiting *is not induced,* however, after ingestion of caustic substances (acid or alkaline) or petroleum distillates.
- Gastric lavage for the obtunded patient (Guideline 65-4). Gastric aspirate is saved and sent to the laboratory for testing (toxicology screens).
- Activated charcoal administration if poison is one that is absorbed by charcoal
- Cathartic, when appropriate

The specific chemical antagonist or physiologic antagonist is administered as early as possible to reverse or diminish the effects

65•4 Guidelines For Assisting With Gastric Lavage

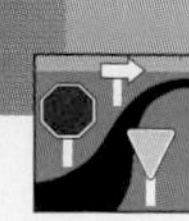

Gastric lavage is the aspiration of the stomach contents and washing out of the stomach by means of a large-bore gastric tube. Gastric lavage is contraindicated after acid or alkali ingestion, in the presence of seizures, or after ingestion of hydrocarbons or petroleum distillates. It is particularly dangerous after ingestion of strong corrosive agents.

Purposes

1. For urgent removal of ingested substance to decrease systemic absorption
2. To empty the stomach before endoscopic procedures
3. To diagnose gastric hemorrhage and to arrest hemorrhage

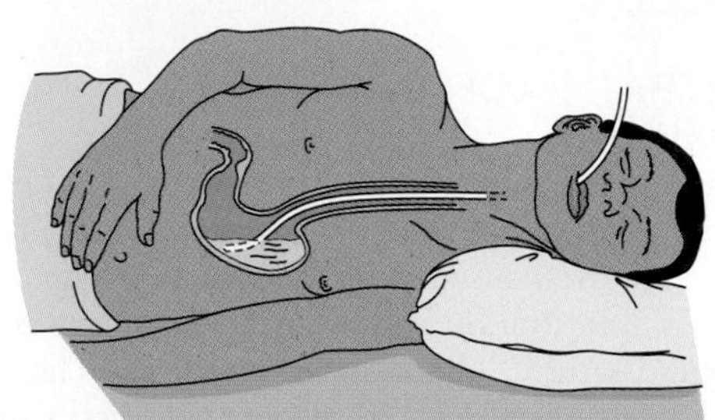

During gastric lavage, the patient is positioned on the left side, which allows the gastric contents to pool and decreases the passage of fluid into the duodenum during lavage.

Equipment

Large-bore Levin tubes or large-bore Ewald tube

Large irrigating syringe with adapter

Large plastic funnel with adapter to fit tube

Water-soluble lubricant

Tap water or appropriate antidote (milk, saline solution, sodium bicarbonate solution, fruit juice, activated charcoal)

Container for aspirate, suction

Nasotracheal or endotracheal tubes with inflatable cuffs

Containers for specimens

Procedure

Action	**Rationale/Amplification**
1. Remove dentures and inspect the oral cavity for loose teeth.	1. This will prevent accidental aspiration of teeth.
2. Measure the distance between the bridge of the nose and the xiphoid process. Mark the tube with indelible pencil or tape.	2. This distance is a rule-of-thumb measurement of the distance the tube is passed to reach the stomach. This avoids curling and kinking of excess tubing in the stomach.
3. Lubricate the tube with water-soluble lubricant.	3. Lubrication eases insertion of the tube.
4. If comatose, the patient is intubated with a cuffed nasotracheal or endotracheal tube before placement of the nasogastric tube.	4. A cuffed nasotracheal or endotracheal tube prevents aspiration of gastric contents.
5. Place the patient in a left lateral position with the head lowered about 15 degrees.	5. This position decreases passage of gastric contents into the duodenum during lavage.
6. Pass the tube orally while keeping the head in a neutral position. Pass the tube to the adhesive marking or about 50 cm (20 in). Encourage patient to swallow to assist with passage of the tube. Then lower the head of the lavage table. Have standby suction available.	6. The depth of insertion of the tube will vary with the size of the patient. If the tube enters the trachea instead of the esophagus, the patient will experience coughing, dyspnea, stridor, and cyanosis. Positive confirmation of tube placement can be accomplished by x-ray.
7. Aspirate the stomach contents with the syringe attached to the tube before instilling water or an antidote. Save the specimen for analysis. Assure placement before installation.	7. Aspiration is carried out to determine that the tube is in the stomach and to remove the stomach contents. Positive confirmation of tube placement can be accomplished by x-ray.
8. Remove the syringe. Attach the funnel to the end of the tube, or use a 50-mL syringe to inject lavage solution in the gastric tube. The volume of fluid placed in the stomach should be small.	8. Overfilling the stomach may cause regurgitation and aspiration or force the stomach contents through the pylorus.
9. Elevate the funnel above the patient's head and pour about 150 to 200 mL of solution into the funnel.	
10. Lower the funnel and siphon the gastric contents into the bucket.	10. The fluid should flow in freely and drain by gravity.
11. Save samples of the first two washings.	11. Keep the first washing sample isolated from other washings for toxicologic analysis.
12. Repeat the lavage procedure until the returns are relatively clear and no particulate matter is seen.	12. This usually requires a total volume of at least 2 L; some clinicians advocate the use of 5 to 20 L.

(continued)

65•4 GUIDELINES FOR ASSISTING WITH GASTRIC LAVAGE *(continued)*

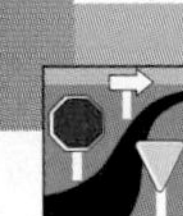

13. At the completion of lavage:
    a. The stomach may be left empty.
    b. An adsorbent (powder form of activated charcoal mixed with water to form a liquid the consistency of thick soup) may be instilled in the tube and allowed to remain in the stomach.
    c. A saline cathartic may be instilled in the tube.

13.
    b. Activated charcoal reduces absorption by adsorbing (attaching to its surface) a wide range of substances; it renders the poison inaccessible to the circulation, thereby reducing its toxicity.
    c. A cathartic may be given to hasten the elimination of remaining ingested material.

14. Pinch off the tube during removal or maintain suction while the tube is being withdrawn.

14. Pinching off the tube prevents aspiration and the initiation of the gag reflex. Keeping the patient's head lower than the body also helps to prevent initiation of the gag reflex.

15. Warn the patient that his stools will turn black from the charcoal.

---

of the toxin. If these measures are ineffective, procedures are initiated to remove the ingested substance. These procedures include administering multiple doses of charcoal, or diuresis (for substances excreted by the kidneys), dialysis, and hemoperfusion. Hemoperfusion involves detoxifying the blood by processing it through an extracorporeal circuit and an adsorbent cartridge containing charcoal or resin, after which the cleaned blood is returned to the patient.

Throughout detoxification, the patient's vital signs, CVP, and fluid and electrolyte balance are monitored closely. Hypotension and cardiac dysrhythmias are possible. Seizures are also possible because of central nervous system excitement from the poison or from oxygen deprivation. If the patient complains of pain, analgesics are given cautiously because severe pain causes vasomotor collapse and reflex inhibition of normal physiologic functions.

When the patient's condition has stabilized and discharge is imminent, written material indicating the signs and symptoms of potential problems and procedures requiring notification or evaluation should be given to the patient. If poisoning was determined to be a suicide attempt, a psychiatric consultation should be requested before discharging the patient. In cases of accidental poison ingestion, poison prevention and home poison-proofing instructions should be provided to the patient and family.

Inhaled Poisons: Carbon Monoxide Poisoning

Carbon monoxide poisoning may occur as a result of industrial or household incidents or attempted suicide. It is implicated in more deaths than any other toxin except alcohol. Carbon monoxide exerts its toxic effect by binding to circulating hemoglobin and thereby reducing the oxygen-carrying capacity of the blood. Hemoglobin absorbs carbon monoxide 200 times more readily than it absorbs oxygen. Carbon monoxide-bound hemoglobin, called **carboxyhemoglobin,** does not transport oxygen.

Clinical Manifestations

Because the central nervous system has a critical need for oxygen, central nervous system symptoms predominate with carbon monoxide toxicity. A person suffering from carbon monoxide poisoning appears intoxicated (from cerebral hypoxia). Other signs and symptoms include headache, muscular weakness, palpitation, dizziness, and mental confusion, which can progress rapidly to coma. Skin color, which can range from pink or cherry red to cyanotic and pale, is not a reliable sign. Pulse oximetry is also not valid because the hemoglobin is well saturated. It is not saturated with oxygen, but the pulse oximeter reads the saturation as such and presents false evidence that the patient is doing well. Exposure to carbon monoxide requires immediate treatment.

Management

Goals of management are to reverse cerebral and myocardial hypoxia and to hasten carbon monoxide elimination. Whenever a patient inhales a poison, the following general measures apply:

- Carry the patient to fresh air immediately; open all doors and windows.
- Loosen all tight clothing.
- Initiate cardiopulmonary resuscitation (CPR) if required. Administer oxygen.
- Prevent chilling; wrap the patient in blankets.
- Keep the patient as quiet as possible.
- Do not give alcohol in any form.

In addition, for the patient with carbon monoxide poisoning, carboxyhemoglobin levels are analyzed on arrival at the ED and before treatment with oxygen if possible. Then 100% oxygen is administered at atmospheric or hyperbaric pressures to reverse hypoxia and accelerate the elimination of carbon monoxide. Oxygen is administered until the carboxyhemoglobin level is less than 5%, and the patient is observed constantly. Psychoses, spastic paralysis, ataxia, visual disturbances, and deterioration of personality may persist after resuscitation and may be symptoms of permanent central nervous system damage.

When unintentional carbon monoxide poisoning occurs, the health department should be contacted, so that the dwelling or building in question will be inspected. A psychiatric consultation is warranted if poisoning was determined to be a suicide attempt.

Skin Contamination Poisoning (Chemical Burns)

Skin contamination injuries from exposure to chemicals are challenging because of the large number of offending agents with diverse actions and metabolic effects. The severity of a chemical burn

ASSESSMENT
FOOD POISONING

Use the following questions to elicit information about the circumstances surrounding the possibility of food poisoning:

- How soon after eating did the symptoms occur? (Immediate onset suggests chemical, plant, or animal poisoning.)
- What was eaten in the previous meal? Did the food have an unusual odor or taste? (Most foods causing bacterial poisoning *do not* have unusual odor or taste.)
- Did anyone else become ill from eating the same food?
- Did vomiting occur? What was the appearance of the vomitus?
- Did diarrhea occur? (Diarrhea is usually absent with botulism and with shellfish or other fish poisoning.)
- Are any neurologic symptoms present? (These occur in botulism and in chemical, plant, and animal poisoning.)
- Does the patient have a fever? (Fever is characteristic in salmonella, ingestion of fava beans, and some fish poisoning.)
- What is the patient's appearance?

is determined by the mechanism of action, penetrating strength and concentration, and amount and duration of exposure of the chemical to the skin.

Management

The skin should be drenched immediately with running water from a shower, hose, or faucet.

Nursing Alert *Water should not be applied to burns from lye or white phosphorus because of the potential for an explosion or for deepening the burn.*

A constant stream of water should continue as the patient's clothing is being removed. The skin of health care personnel assisting the patient should be appropriately protected if the burn is extensive or if the agent is significantly toxic or still present. Prolonged lavage with generous amounts of tepid water is important.

In the meantime, attempts to determine the identity and characteristics of the chemical agent are necessary for future treatment. The standard burn treatment appropriate for the size and location of the wound (antimicrobial treatment, débridement, tetanus prophylaxis as prescribed) is instituted. The patient may require plastic surgery for further wound management. The patient is instructed to have the affected area reexamined at 24 and 72 hours and in 7 days because of the risk for underestimating the extent and depth of these types of injuries.

Food Poisoning

Food poisoning is a sudden, explosive illness that may occur after ingestion of contaminated food or drink. Botulism is a serious form of food poisoning that requires continual surveillance.

Management

The key to treatment is determining the source and type of food poisoning. If possible, the suspected food should be brought to the medical facility and a history obtained from the patient or family.

Food, gastric contents, vomitus, serum, and feces are collected for examination. The patient's respirations, blood pressure, sensorium, CVP (if indicated), and muscular activity are monitored closely. Measures are instituted to support the respiratory system. Death from respiratory paralysis can occur with botulism, fish poisoning, and other food poisonings.

Because large volumes of electrolytes and water are lost by vomiting and diarrhea, fluid and electrolyte balance is also an important area to assess. Severe vomiting produces alkalosis, and severe diarrhea produces acidosis. Hypovolemic shock may also occur from severe fluid and electrolyte losses. The patient is assessed for signs and symptoms of fluid and electrolyte imbalances, including lethargy, rapid pulse rate, fever, oliguria, anuria, hypotension, and delirium. Weight and serum electrolyte levels are obtained for future comparisons.

Measures to control nausea are also important to prevent vomiting, which could further exacerbate fluid and electrolyte imbalances. An antiemetic medication is administered parenterally as prescribed if the patient cannot tolerate fluids or medications by mouth. For mild nausea, the patient takes sips of weak tea, carbonated drinks, or tap water. After nausea and vomiting subside, clear liquids are usually prescribed for 12 to 24 hours, and the diet gradually progresses to a low-residue, bland diet.

SUBSTANCE ABUSE

Substance abuse is the misuse of specific substances to alter mood or behavior; drug and alcohol abuse are two examples of substance abuse.

Drug Abuse and Overdose

Drug abuse is the use of drugs for other than legitimate medical purposes. People who use drugs often take a variety of drugs simultaneously (eg, alcohol, barbiturates, opioids, and tranquilizers), which may have additive effects. Intravenous drug users are at increased risk for HIV infection, AIDS, and hepatitis B and are the most frequent victims of tetanus in the United States.

Clinical manifestations vary with the drug used, but underlying principles of management are essentially the same. Table 65-1 identifies commonly abused drugs, listing their clinical manifestations and therapeutic management. Treatment goals for a patient suffering from drug overdose are to support the respiratory and cardiovascular functions, to enhance clearance of the agent, and to provide for safety of the patient and staff.

Acute Alcohol Intoxication

Alcohol is a psychotropic drug affecting mood, judgment, behavior, concentration, and consciousness. Many heavy drinkers are young adults as well as people older than 60 years of age. There is a high prevalence of alcoholism in ED patients. Because patients who abuse alcohol return frequently to the ED, they often exasperate and tax the patience of health care professionals caring for them. Their management requires patience and thoughtful, accurate, and long-term treatment.

Assessment

Alcohol, or ethanol, is a direct multisystem toxin and central nervous system depressant that causes drowsiness, incoordination, slurring of speech, sudden mood changes, aggression, belligerency, grandiosity, and uninhibited behavior. Taken in excess, it also can cause stupor, coma, and death. In the ED, the patient is assessed for head injury, hypoglycemia (which mimics intoxication), and

(*text continues on page 1925*)

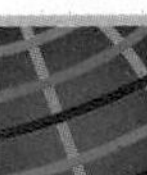

TABLE 65•1 Emergency Management of Drug Abuse Patients and Patients with Drug Overdose

Drug	Clinical Manifestations	Therapeutic Management
Narcotics		
Cocaine Intranasally ("snorting"): inhaled into nostrils through straws By smoking ("freebasing"): cocaine hydrochloride dissolved in ether to yield a pure cocaine alkaloid base (called "crack"); smoking in a small pipe delivers large quantities of cocaine to lungs Intravenously	Cocaine is a CNS stimulant that can increase heart rate and blood pressure and cause hyperpyrexia, seizures, and ventricular dysrhythmias. It produces intense euphoria, then anxiety, sadness, insomnia, and sexual indifference; cocaine hallucinations with delusions; psychosis with extreme paranoia and ideas of persecution; and hypervigilance. Chronic psychotic symptoms may persist.	1. Ensure airway and ventilation. 2. Control seizures. 3. Monitor cardiovascular effects; have lidocaine and defibrillator available. 4. Treat for hyperthermia. 5. If ingested, use charcoal to treat. 6. Refer for psychiatric evaluation and treatment in an inpatient unit that eliminates access to the drug.
Heroin Opium or paregoric Morphine, codeine, synthetic derivatives (methadone, meperidine) Fentanyl (Sublimaze)	Acute intoxication (overdose) Pinpoint pupils (may be dilated with severe hypoxia); decreased blood pressure Marked respiratory depression Stupor → coma Fresh needle marks along course of any superficial vein; skin abscesses	1. Support respiratory and cardiovascular functions. 2. Establish an IV line; withdraw blood for chemical and toxicologic analysis. Patient may be given bolus of glucose to eliminate possibility of hypoglycemia. 3. Give narcotic antagonist (naloxone hydrochloride [Narcan]) as prescribed to reverse severe respiratory depression and coma. 4. Continue to monitor level of responsiveness and respirations, pulse, and BP. Duration of action of naloxone hydrochloride is shorter than that of heroin; repeated dosages may be necessary. 5. Send urine for analysis; opiates can be detected in urine. 6. Obtain an ECG. 7. Do not leave patient unattended; he or she may lapse back into coma rapidly. Clinical status may change from minute to minute. Hemodialysis may be indicated for severe drug intoxication. 8. Monitor for pulmonary edema, which is frequently seen in patients who abuse/overdose on narcotics. 9. Refer patient for psychiatric evaluation before discharge.
Barbiturates		
Pentobarbital (Nembutal) Secobarbital (Seconal) Amobarbital (Amytal)	Acute intoxication (may mimic alcohol intoxication): Respiratory depression Flushed face Decreased pulse rate; decreased blood pressure Increasing nystagmus Depressed deep tendon reflexes Decreasing mental alertness Difficulty in speaking Poor motor coordination Coma, death	1. Maintain airway and give respiratory support. 2. Endotracheal intubation or tracheostomy is considered if there is any doubt about the adequacy of airway exchange. a. Check airway frequently. b. Perform suctioning as necessary. 3. Support cardiovascular and respiratory functions; most deaths result from respiratory depression or shock. 4. Start intravenous infusion through large-gauge needle or intravenous catheter to support blood pressure; coma and dehydration result in hypotension and respond to infusion of intravenous fluids with elevation of blood pressure. Sodium bicarbonate may be prescribed to alkalinize urine; it promotes excretion of barbiturates. 5. Evacuate stomach contents or lavage as soon as possible to prevent absorption; repeated doses of activated charcoal may be administered. 6. Assist with hemodialysis for severely overdosed patient. 7. Maintain neurologic and vital sign flow sheet. 8. Patient awakening from overdose may demonstrate combative behavior; this can stimulate automatic angry response by health care personnel. 9. Refer for psychiatric consultation to evaluate suicide potential and drug abuse.
Amphetamine-Type Drugs (Pep Pills, "Uppers," "Speed," "Crystal," "Meth")		
Amphetamine (Benzedrine) Dextroamphetamine (Dexedrine)	Nausea, vomiting, anorexia, palpitations, tachycardia, increased	1. Provide airway support, ventilation, cardiac monitoring; insert IV line.

(continued)

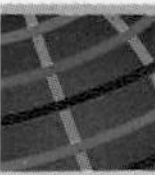

TABLE 65•1 **Emergency Management of Drug Abuse Patients and Patients with Drug Overdose** *(Continued)*

Drug	Clinical Manifestations	Therapeutic Management
Methamphetamine (Desoxyn) MDMA ("Ecstasy," "Adam") MDEA ("Eve") MDA	blood pressure, tachypnea, anxiety, nervousness, diaphoresis, mydriasis Repetitive or stereotyped behavior Irritability, insomnia, agitation Visual misperceptions, auditory hallucinations Fearful anxiety/depression, cold, distant hostility, paranoia Hyperactivity, rapid speech, euphoria Seizures, coma, hyperthermia, cardiovascular collapse, rhabdomyolysis	2. Employ gastrointestinal decontamination in cases of oral overdose; activated charcoal, gastric lavage. 3. Keep in calm, quiet environment; elevated temperature potentiates amphetamine toxicity. 4. Use small doses of diazepam (IV) or haloperidol as prescribed for CNS and muscular hyperactivity. 5. Administer appropriate pharmacologic therapy as prescribed for severe hypertension and ventricular dysrhythmias. 6. Treat seizures with benzodiazepines. 7. Treat sympathetic stimulation with beta-blocker agents. 8. Try to communicate with patient if delusions or hallucinations are present. 9. Place in a protective environment (preferably psychiatric security room with video monitoring) to observe for suicide attempt. 10. Refer for psychiatric evaluation.
Hallucinogens or Psychedelic-Type Drugs		
Lysergic acid diethylamide (LSD) Phencyclidine HCI (PCP, "angel dust") Mescaline, psilocybin Cannabinoids (marijuana)	Nystagmus, mild hypertension Marked confusion bordering on panic Incoherence, hyperactivity Withdrawn Combative behavior; delirium, mania, self-injury Hallucinations, body image distortion Hypertension, hyperthermia, renal failure *Flashback:* recurrence of LSD-like state without having taken the drug; may occur weeks or months after drug was taken Seizures, coma, circulatory collapse, death	*Emergency Management* 1. Evaluate and maintain patient's airway, breathing, and circulation. 2. Determine whether the patient has ingested hallucinogenic drug or has a toxic psychosis. by urine or serum drug screen. 3. Try to communicate with and reassure the patient. a. "Talking down" involves understanding the process through which the patient is proceeding and helping him overcome his fears while establishing contact with reality. b. Remind the patient that fear is common with this problem. c. Reassure the patient that he is not losing his mind but is experiencing the effect of drugs and that this will wear off. d. Instruct the patient to keep the eyes open; this reduces the intensity of reaction. e. Reduce sensory stimuli: minimize noise, lights, movement, tactile stimulation. 4. Sedate the patient as prescribed if hyperactivity cannot be controlled; diazepam (Valium) or a barbiturate may be prescribed. 5. Search for evidence of trauma; hallucinogen users have a tendency to "act out" their hallucinations. 6. Manage seizures. 7. Observe patient closely; patient's behavior may become hazardous. 8. Monitor for hypertensive crisis if patient has prolonged psychosis due to drug ingestion. 9. Place patient in a protected environment under proper medical supervision to prevent self-inflicted bodily harm. *Management for Phencyclidine Abusers* 1. Place patient in a calm, supportive environment to minimize stimuli; protect from self-injury. 2. Avoid talking down. 3. Do not leave patient unobserved. Treat symptoms as they occur. a. Drug effects are unpredictable and prolonged. b. Symptoms are likely to exacerbate; patient becomes out of control. 4. Refer patient for psychiatric evaluation.

(continued)

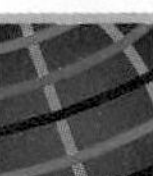

TABLE 65•1 Emergency Management of Drug Abuse Patients and Patients with Drug Overdose *(Continued)*

Drug	Clinical Manifestations	Therapeutic Management
Drugs Producing Sedation, Intoxication, or Psychological and Physical Dependence (Nonbarbiturate Sedatives)		
Diazepam (Valium) Chlordiazepoxide (Librium) Oxazepam (Serax) Lorazepam (Ativan) Midazolam (Versed)	Acute intoxication: Respiratory depression Decreasing mental alertness Confusion Slurred speech, decreased blood pressure Ataxia Pulmonary edema Coma, death	*Management* 1. Endotracheal tube is inserted as a precaution; use assisted ventilation to stabilize and correct respiratory depression. Observe for sudden apnea and laryngeal spasm (especially in patients dependent on glutethimide [Doriden]). 2. Assess for hypotension a. Insert indwelling urinary catheter for comatose patient; decreased urinary volume is an index of reduced renal flow associated with reduced intravascular volume or vascular collapse. b. Start volume expansion with saline or dextrose as prescribed. 3. Evacuate stomach contents; emesis; lavage; activated charcoal; cathartic. 4. Start ECG monitoring. Observe for dysrhythmias. 5. Administer flumazenil (Romazicon), the benzodiazepine antagonist (reversal agent)
Salicylate Poisoning		
Aspirin (present in compound analgesic tablets)	Restlessness, tinnitus, deafness, blurring of vision Hyperpnea, hyperpyrexia, sweating Epigastric pain, vomiting, dehydration Respiratory and metabolic acidosis Disorientation, coma, cardiovascular collapse	1. Treat respiratory depression. 2. Induce gastric emptying by lavage. 3. Give activated charcoal to adsorb aspirin; a cathartic may be administered with charcoal to help ensure intestinal cleansing. 4. Support patient with intravenous infusions as prescribed to establish hydration and correct electrolyte imbalances. 5. Enhance elimination of salicylates as directed by forced diuresis, alkalinization of urine, peritoneal dialysis, or hemodialysis, according to severity of intoxication. 6. Monitor serum salicylate level for efficacy of treatment. 7. Administer specific prescribed pharmacologic agent for bleeding and other problems.
Acetaminophen (present in prescription and non-prescription analgesics, antipyretics, and cold remedies)	Lethargy to encephalopathy and death GI upset, diaphoresis Right upper quadrant pain Abnormal liver function tests, prolonged PT, increased bilirubin Hepatomegaly leading to liver failure	1. Maintain airway 2. Obtain acetaminophen level. Levels ≥ 140 mg/kg are toxic. 3. Lab studies—liver function tests, PT/PTT, CBC, BUN, creatinine 4. Administer syrup of ipecac and follow emesis with activated charcoal. 5. Prepare for possible hemodialysis which will clear acetaminophen but does not halt liver damage. 6. Administer *N*-acetylcysteine (NAC, Mucomyst) as soon as possible. NAC replenishes essential liver enzymes and requires a total of 18 doses every 4 hours: Charcoal absorbs NAC—so do not administer together. Repeat NAC dose if patient vomits.

other health problems. Ineffective breathing pattern related to central nervous system depression and risk for violence (self-directed or directed at others) related to severe intoxication from alcohol are possible nursing diagnoses.

Management

Treatment involves detoxification of the acute poisoning, recovery, and rehabilitation. Commonly, the patient uses mechanisms of denial and defensiveness. The nurse should approach the patient with a nonjudgmental manner, using a firm, consistent, accepting, and reasonable attitude. Speaking in a calm and slow manner is helpful because alcohol interferes with thought processes. If the patient appears intoxicated, hypoxia, hypovolemia, or neurologic impairment must be ruled out before assuming that the patient is intoxicated. The patient is likely intoxicated even though he or she may deny alcohol intake. Typically, a blood specimen is obtained for analysis of the blood–alcohol level.

If drowsy, the patient should be allowed to sleep off the state of alcoholic intoxication. During this time, maintenance of a patent airway and observation for symptoms of central nervous system depression are essential. The patient should be undressed and kept warm with blankets. On the other hand, if the patient is noisy or belligerent, sedation may be necessary. If sedation is used, the patient should be monitored carefully for hypotension and decreased level of consciousness.

Additionally, the patient is examined for alcohol withdrawal delirium and also for injuries and organic disease, such as head injury, seizures, pulmonary infections, hypoglycemia, and nutritional deficiencies that may be masked by alcoholic intoxication. People with alcoholism suffer more injuries than the general population. Also, acute alcohol intoxication is the cause of trauma for many nonalcoholic patients. Pulmonary infections are also more common in patients with alcoholism, resulting from respiratory depression, an impaired defense system, and a tendency toward gastric aspiration. The patient may show little increase in temperature or white blood cell count. The patient may be hospitalized or admitted to a detoxification center in an effort to examine problems underlying substance abuse.

Alcohol Withdrawal Delirium (Delirium Tremens)

Alcohol withdrawal delirium is an acute toxic state that occurs as a result of sudden cessation of alcohol intake following a bout of heavy drinking or, more usually, after prolonged intake of alcohol. Severity of symptoms depends on how much alcohol was ingested and for how long. Delirium tremens may be precipitated by acute injury or infection (pneumonia, pancreatitis, hepatitis).

Clinical Manifestations

Patients suspected of alcohol withdrawal delirium show signs of anxiety, uncontrollable fear, tremor, irritability, agitation, insomnia, and incontinence. They are talkative and preoccupied and experience visual, tactile, olfactory, and auditory hallucinations that often are terrifying. Autonomic overactivity occurs and is evidenced by tachycardia, dilated pupils, and profuse perspiration. Usually, all vital signs are elevated in the alcoholic toxic state. Alcohol withdrawal delirium is life-threatening and carries a high mortality rate.

Management

Goals of management are to give adequate sedation and support to allow the patient to rest and recover without danger of injury or peripheral vascular collapse. A physical examination is performed to identify preexisting or contributing illnesses or injuries (eg, head injury, pneumonia). A drug history is obtained to elicit information that may facilitate adjustment of any sedative requirements. Baseline blood pressure is determined because the patient's subsequent treatment may depend on blood pressure changes.

Usually, the patient is sedated as directed with a sufficient dosage of medication to establish and maintain sedation, which reduces agitation, prevents exhaustion, and promotes sleep. The patient should be calm, able to respond, and able to maintain an airway safely on his or her own. A variety of medications and combinations of medications are used, for example, chlordiazepoxide (Librium), diazepam, and clonidine. Haloperidol or droperidol may be given for severe acute alcohol withdrawal delirium. Dosages are adjusted according to the patient's symptoms (agitation, anxiety) and blood pressure response.

The patient is placed in a calm, nonstressful environment (usually a private room) and observed closely. The room remains lighted to minimize potential for illusions and hallucinations. Homicidal or suicidal responses may result from hallucinations. Closet and bathroom doors are closed to eliminate shadows. Someone is designated to stay with the patient as much as possible. The presence of another person has a reassuring and calming effect, which helps the patient maintain contact with reality. Any visual misrepresentations (illusions) are explained to strengthen the the patient's link with reality.

Nursing Alert *Protective devices and restraints are used as prescribed if necessary and when other alternatives have been unsuccessful. The least restrictive device that will prevent the patient from injuring self and others is used. Caution is taken to ensure that restraints are applied properly and that they are not applied in such a way that they impair circulation to any part of the body or interfere with respirations. Physical observation (eg, skin integrity, circulatory status, respiratory status) is ongoing, and the patient's response is documented.*

Fluid losses may result from gastrointestinal losses (vomiting), profuse perspiration, and respiration (hyperventilation). In addition, the patient may be dehydrated as a result of alcohol's effect on antidiuretic hormone (decreased). The oral or intravenous route is used to restore fluid and electrolyte balance.

Temperature, pulse, respiration, and blood pressure are recorded frequently (every 30 minutes in severe forms of delirium) in anticipation of peripheral circulatory collapse or hyperthermia (the two most lethal complications). Phenytoin (Dilantin) or other anticonvulsant medications may be prescribed to prevent or control repeated withdrawal seizures.

Frequent complications include infections (eg, pneumonia), trauma, hepatic failure, hypoglycemia, and cardiovascular problems. Hypoglycemia may accompany alcohol withdrawal because alcohol depletes liver glycogen stores and impairs gluconeogenesis; many patients with alcoholism suffer from malnutrition. Parenteral dextrose may be prescribed if the liver glycogen level is depleted. Orange juice, Gatorade, or other carbohydrates are given to stabilize the blood sugar and counteract tremulousness. Supplemental vitamin therapy and a high-protein diet are provided as prescribed to counteract vitamin deficiency. The patient should be referred to an alcoholic treatment center for follow-up and rehabilitation.

VIOLENCE, ABUSE, AND NEGLECT

Family Violence, Abuse, and Neglect

EDs are often the first place where victims of family violence, abuse, or neglect go to seek help. Each year, about 3 to 4 million women are battered, 1.5 million children are seriously abused, an additional 5 million children are maltreated, and 2.5 million elders are abused or neglected. On the average, between 6% and 28% of women seen in the ED have suffered abuse, with up to 6% of these patients seeking treatment for a complaint related to a recent event. Of the ED visits, between 20% and 35% relate to continuous abuse. Elder abuse takes many forms, including physical and psychological abuse, neglect, violation of personal rights, and financial abuse.

Clinical Manifestations

When victims of abuse seek treatment, they may present with physical injuries or health problems, such as anxiety, insomnia, or gastrointestinal symptoms, that are related to stress. They usually do not identify their abuser.

The possibility of abuse should be investigated whenever a person presents with multiple injuries that are in various stages of evolution, when injuries are unexplained, or the explanation does not fit the physical picture. The possibility of neglect should be

ASSESSMENT
ABUSE, MALTREATMENT, AND NEGLECT

The following questions may be helpful when assessing the patient for abuse, maltreatment, and neglect:

- I noticed that you have a number of bruises. Can you tell me how they happened? Has anyone hurt you?
- You seem frightened. Has anyone ever hurt you?
- Sometimes patients tell me that they have been hurt by someone at home. Could this be happening to you?
- Are you afraid of anyone at home? Or of anyone with whom you come in contact?
- Has anyone failed to help you to take care of yourself when you needed help?
- Has anyone prevented you from seeing friends or other people whom you wish to see?
- Have you signed any papers that you did not understand?
- Has anyone forced you to sign papers against your will?

investigated whenever a dependent person with adequate resources and a designated care provider shows evidence of inattention to hygiene, to nutrition, or to known medical needs, such as unfilled medication prescriptions or missed appointments with health care providers. In EDs, the most common physical injuries seen are unexplained bruises, lacerations, abrasions, head injuries, or fractures. The most common clinical manifestations of neglect are malnutrition and dehydration.

Assessment

Nurses in EDs are uniquely positioned to provide early detection and interventions for victims of domestic violence. This requires an acute awareness of the signs of possible abuse, maltreatment, and neglect. They must be skilled in interviewing techniques that are likely to elicit accurate information. A careful history is crucial in the screening process. Questions asked in private—away from others—may be helpful in eliciting information about abuse, maltreatment, and neglect.

Whenever evidence leads one to suspect abuse or neglect, an evaluation with careful documentation of descriptions of events and drawings or photos of injuries is important because the medical record may be used as part of a legal document. Assessment of the patient's general appearance and interactions with significant others, an examination of the entire surface area of the body, and a mental status examination are crucial.

Management

Whenever abuse, maltreatment, or neglect are suspected, the health care worker's primary concern should be the safety and welfare of the patient. Treatment focuses on the consequences of the abuse, violence, or neglect and prevention of further injury. Protocols of most EDs indicate that a multidisciplinary approach be used. Nurses, physicians, social workers, and community agencies work collaboratively to develop and implement a plan for meeting the patient's needs.

If in immediate danger, the patient should be separated from the abusing or neglecting person whenever possible. On the basis of this danger, or on the basis of injuries or neglected medical conditions, hospitalization is justified until alternative plans are made. However, it must be remembered that third-party payers may not approve hospitalization that is based solely on abuse or neglect.

When abuse or neglect is considered to be the result of stress experienced by a caregiver who is no longer able to cope with the burden of caring for an elderly person or a person with chronic disease, respite services may be necessary. Support groups may be helpful to these caregivers. When mental illness of the abuser or neglecter is responsible for the situation, alternative living arrangements may be required.

Nurses must be mindful that competent adults are free to accept or refuse the help that is offered to them. Some patients will insist on remaining in the home environment where the abuse or neglect is occurring. The wishes of patients who are competent and not cognitively impaired should be respected. However, all possible alternatives and available resources should be explored with the patient.

Mandatory reporting laws exist in most states requiring health care workers to report *suspected* abuse to an official agency, usually Adult (or Child) Protective Services. All that is required for reporting is the suspicion of abuse. The health care worker is not required to prove anything. Likewise, health care workers who report suspected abuse are immune to civil or criminal liability if the report is made in good faith. Subsequent home visits resulting from the report of suspected abuse is part of gathering information about the patient in the home environment. In addition, many states have resource hotlines for use by health care workers and patients who seek answers to questions about abuse and neglect.

Sexual Assault

The legal definition of *rape* is carnal knowledge of a female by force or the threat of force against her will. Considered an act of violence, however, rape not only affects females. It happens to males, especially young males. The feminist movement has focused on the rights and care of rape victims, and law enforcement agencies are becoming increasingly sensitive and aggressive in managing these crimes. Rape crisis centers offer support, educate victims, and help them through the subsequent courtroom experience.

The manner in which the patient is received and treated in the ED is important to his or her future psychological well-being. Crisis intervention should begin when the patient enters the health care facility. The patient should be seen immediately. Most hospitals have a written protocol that reflects consideration for the victim's physical and emotional needs as well as forensic evidence collection that is required.

The Sexual Assault Nurse Examiner

In many states, there is now the opportunity for emergency nurses to become trained sexual assault nurse examiners (SANEs). The role allows for specific training in forensic evidence collection, history taking, documentation, and ways to approach the patient and family. Specialized training also includes proper photography and the use of colposcopy. Colposcopy increases assessment by examination for microtrauma through magnification. Evidence is collected through photography, videography, and specimens. Improved documentation of injuries has been phenomenal. Another useful tool to SANEs is the light-staining microscope, which enables the examiner to identify motile and nonmotile sperm and infection. This tool saves time and also enhances assessment. Sexual assault nurse examiners complement the ED staff and can spend more time with both the patient and police investigating the incident.

Assessment

The patient's reaction to rape has been termed *rape trauma syndrome* and is seen as an acute stress reaction to a life-threatening situation. The nurse performing the assessment is aware that the patient may go through several phases of psychological reactions:

- An acute disorganization phase, which may manifest as an expressed state in which shock, disbelief, fear, guilt, humiliation, anger, and other such emotions are encountered or as a controlled state in which feelings are masked or hidden and the victim appears composed
- A phase of denial and unwillingness to talk about the incident, followed by a phase of heightened anxiety, fear, flashbacks, sleep disturbances, hyperalertness, and psychosomatic reactions
- A phase of reorganization, in which the incident is put into perspective. Some victims never fully recover and develop chronic stress disorders and phobias.

Management

Goals of management are to give sympathetic support, to reduce the emotional trauma of the patient, and to gather available evidence for possible legal proceedings. All of the interventions have the ultimate goal of having the patient regain control over his or her life.

Throughout the patient's stay in the ED, the patient's privacy and sensitivity must be respected. The patient may exhibit a wide range of emotional reactions, such as hysteria, stoicism, or feelings of being overwhelmed. Support and caring are crucial. The patient should be reassured that anxiety is natural and asked if a support person can be called. Appropriate support is available from professional and community resources. Rape Victim Companion Program, if available in the community, can be contacted, and services of a volunteer can be requested. The patient should never be left alone.

PHYSICAL EXAMINATION

A written, witnessed informed consent must be obtained from the patient (or parent or guardian if the patient is a minor) for examination, for taking photographs, and for release of findings to police. A history is obtained only if the patient has not already talked to a police officer, social worker, or crisis intervention worker. The patient should not be asked to repeat the history. Any history of the event obtained should be recorded in the patient's own words. The patient is asked if he or she has bathed, douched, brushed teeth, changed clothes, urinated, or defecated since the attack because this may alter interpretation of subsequent findings. The time of admission, time of examination, date and time of alleged rape, and the patient's emotional state and general appearance (including any evidence of trauma, such as discoloration, bruises, lacerations, secretions, torn and bloody clothing) are documented.

For the physical examination, the patient is helped to undress and draped properly. Each item of clothing is placed in a separate paper bag. Plastic bags are not used because they retain moisture, which may promote mold and mildew formation, which can destroy evidence. The bags are labeled and given to appropriate law enforcement authorities.

The patient is examined (from head to toe) for injuries, especially to the head, neck, breast, thighs, back, and buttocks. Body diagrams and photographs aid in documenting the evidence of trauma. The physical examination focuses on the following:

- External evidence of trauma (bruises, contusions, lacerations, stab wounds)
- Dried semen stains (appearing as crusted, flaking areas) on the patient's body or clothes
- Broken fingernails and body tissue and foreign materials under nails (if found, samples are taken)
- Oral examination, including a specimen of saliva and prescribed cultures of gum and tooth areas

Pelvic and rectal examinations are also performed. The perineum and other areas are examined with a Wood lamp or other filtered ultraviolet light. Areas that appear fluorescent may indicate semen stains. The color and consistency of any discharge present is noted. A water-moistened rather than a lubricated vaginal speculum is used for the examination. Lubricant contains chemicals that may interfere with later forensic testing of specimens and acid phosphatase determinations. The rectum is examined for signs of trauma, blood, and semen. During the examination, the patient should be advised of the nature and necessity of each procedure and given the rationale for each question asked.

SPECIMEN COLLECTION

During the physical examination, numerous laboratory specimens may be collected, including the following:

- Vaginal aspirate, examined for presence or absence of motile and nonmotile sperm
- Secretions (obtained with a sterile swab) from the vaginal pool for acid phosphatase, blood group antigen of semen, and precipitin test against human sperm and blood
- Separate smears from the oral, vaginal, and anal areas
- Culture of body orifices for gonorrhea
- Blood serum for syphilis and HIV testing; a sample of serum for syphilis may be frozen and saved for future testing
- Pregnancy test if there is a possibility that the patient may be pregnant
- Any foreign material (leaves, grass, dirt), which is placed in a clean envelope
- Pubic hair samples obtained by combing or trimming. Several pubic hairs with follicles are placed in separate containers and identified as the patient's hairs.

Each specimen is labeled with the name of the patient, date, time of collection, body area from which specimen was obtained, and names of personnel collecting specimens to preserve chain of evidence. Then the specimens are given to a designated person (eg, crime laboratory technician), and an itemized receipt is obtained.

ADDITIONAL MEASURES

After the initial physical examination is completed and specimens have been obtained, any associated injuries are treated as indicated. The patient is given the option of prophylaxis against sexually transmitted disease. Ceftriaxone (Rocephin), administered intramuscularly with 1% lidocaine (Xylocaine), may be prescribed as prophylaxis for gonorrhea. Doxycycline (Vibramycin) taken for 10 days may be prescribed as prophylaxis for syphilis and chlamydia.

Antipregnancy measures may be considered if the patient is of childbearing age, is not using contraceptives, and is at high risk in her menstrual cycle. A postcoital contraceptive medication, such as Ovral, which contains estrogen ethinyl estradiol and progestin norgestrel, may be prescribed after a pregnancy test. To promote effectiveness, Ovral should be administered within 12 to 24 hours and no later than 72 hours after intercourse. The 21-day package rather than the 28-day package is prescribed, so that the patient does not take the inert tablets by mistake. An antiemetic may be given as prescribed to decrease discomfort from side effects. Cleansing douche, mouthwash, and fresh clothing are usually offered.

FOLLOW-UP

The patient is informed of counseling services to prevent long-term psychological effects. Counseling services should be made available to both the patient and the family. A referral is made to the Rape Victim Companion Program, if available. Appointments for follow-up surveillance for pregnancy, sexually transmitted disease, and HIV testing also are made.

The patient is encouraged to return to the previous level of functioning as soon as possible. When leaving the health care facility, the patient should be accompanied by a family member or friend.

Other Violence in the Emergency Department

Not only do ED staff members have to deal with patients who are violent from substance abuse, injury, or other emergencies, they also have to deal with the rest of the environment. Patients and families waiting for assistance are increasingly volatile. Often, waiting rooms are the site for dissatisfaction, fear, and anger to be acted out in violence. Not only have some EDs assigned security officers to the area, they have also installed metal detectors to identify weapons and protect patients, families, and staff. It is not unusual for a patient to come to the ED armed. Nurses and other personnel must be prepared to deal with such circumstances.

Management

Safety is the first priority. Protecting the ED on a daily basis will prevent any untoward events from occurring. Protection of the department provides protection for the patients, families, and staff. It is essential that all nurses be aware of the environment in which they are working.

Metal detectors, silent alarm systems, and secured entry into the department assist in maintaining safety. Members of gangs and feuding families need to be separated in the ED, waiting room, and later in the inpatient nursing care unit to avoid angry confrontations. Security officers should be ready to assist at all times. The department should be able to be locked against entry if security is at all in question.

Patients from prison or who are under guard need to be shackled to the bed with appropriate assessment as if restrained. The same assessment and care that is provided to patients with hand or ankle restraints is provided to patients with handcuffs. In addition, the following precautions are used:

- Never release the hand or ankle restraint (handcuff).
- Always have a guard present in the room.
- Place the patient face down on the stretcher to avoid injury from head-butting, spitting, or biting.
- Use restraints on any violent patient as needed.
- Administer medication if necessary to control violent behavior until definitive treatment can be obtained.

In the case of gunfire in the ED, self-protection is a priority. There is no use in protecting others if the caregivers are also injured. Security officers and police must gain control of the situation first and then tend to the injured.

PSYCHIATRIC EMERGENCIES

A psychiatric emergency is an urgent, serious disturbance of behavior, affect, or thought that makes the patient unable to cope with life situations and interpersonal relationships. A patient presenting with a psychiatric emergency may display overactive or violent, underactive or depressed, or suicidal behaviors.

The most important concern of the ED personnel is whether the patient is at risk for injuring self or others. The aim is to try to maintain the patient's self-esteem (and life, if necessary) while providing care. Determining whether the patient is currently under psychiatric treatment is important so that contact can be made with the therapist or physician working with the patient.

Overactive Patients

Patients who display disturbed, uncooperative, and paranoid behavior and who feel anxious and panicky may be prone to assaultive and destructive impulses and abnormal social behavior. Intense nervousness, depression, and crying are evident in some patients. Disturbed and noisy behavior may be exacerbated or compounded by alcohol or drug intoxication.

Management

A reliable source is needed to identify events leading to the crisis, and a history is obtained. Past mental illness, hospitalizations, injuries, serious illnesses, use of alcohol or drugs, crises in interpersonal relationships, or intrapsychic conflicts are explored. Because abnormal thoughts and behavior may be manifestations of an underlying physical disorder, such as hypoglycemia, stroke, epilepsy, head injury, and drug or alcohol toxicity, a physical assessment is performed when possible.

The immediate goal is to gain control of the situation. If the patient is potentially violent, security or local police should be nearby. Restraints are used as a *last* resort and as ordered. Approaching the patient with a calm, confident, and firm manner is therapeutic and has a calming effect. Helpful interventions include the following:

- Introducing yourself by name
- Telling the patient, "I am here to help you"
- Repeating the patient's name from time to time
- Speaking in one-thought sentences and being consistent
- Giving the patient space and time to slow down
- Showing interest in, listening to, and encouraging the patient to talk about personal thoughts and feelings
- Offering appropriate explanations, and telling the truth

A psychotropic (exerting an effect on the mind) agent may be prescribed for emergency management of functional psychosis. However, personality disorders cannot and should not be treated with psychotropic medications; nor are psychotropic medications used if the patient's behavior results from using hallucinogens (eg, LSD).

Agents such as chlorpromazine (Thorazine) or haloperidol (Haldol) act specifically against psychotic symptoms of thought fragmentation and perceptual and behavioral aberrations. The initial dosage depends on the patient's body weight and the severity of the symptoms. After administration of the initial dose, the patient is observed closely to determine the degree of change in psychotic behavior. Subsequent dosages depend on the patient's response.

Typically, when stabilized, the patient is admitted to a psychiatric unit, or psychiatric outpatient treatment is arranged.

Violent Behavior

Violent and aggressive behavior, usually episodic, is a means of expressing feelings of anger, fear, or hopelessness about a situation. Usually, the patient has a history of outbursts of rage, temper tantrums, or impulsive behavior. People with a tendency for violence frequently lose control when intoxicated with alcohol or drugs. Family members are the most frequent victims of their aggression. This was discussed previously in the section on family violence, abuse, and neglect. Patients with a propensity for violence include those intoxicated by drugs or alcohol; those going through drug or alcohol withdrawal; and those diagnosed with acute paranoid schizophrenic state, acute organic brain syndrome, acute psychosis, paranoid character, borderline personality, or antisocial personality disorders.

Management

The goal of treatment is to bring the violence under control. A specially designated room with at least two exits should be used for the interview. The door of the room should be kept open, and the nurse should remain in clear view of the staff, *staying between the patient and the door*. However, the patient's exit to the door must not be blocked because the patient may feel trapped and threatened. No objects that could be used as weapons should be in sight, in the room, or carried in with health care personnel. If the interviewer feels anxious or uneasy about the patient's response, security staff, a family member, or another health care worker should be asked to remain in the hall nearby in the event that additional help is needed. The patient should never be left alone because this may be interpreted as rejection or provide an opportunity for self-harm.

To bring the violence under control, a calm, noncritical approach while remaining in control of the situation is crucial. Sudden movements are avoided. External calm and structure in conjunction with providing the patient some space may help the patient gain control. If the patient is carrying a weapon, the emergency health care provider should ask that it be surrendered. If the patient is unwilling to surrender the weapon, the security staff is called. If necessary, the security staff may seek further assistance from the local police department.

The patient's violent behavior is a crisis situation for the patient and the ED. Crisis intervention, achieved by talking and listening to the patient, is best accomplished by expressing an interest in the patient's well-being while attempting to tune in to the patient and remain firm. The patient's agitated state is acknowledged by statements, for example, "I want to work with you to relieve your distress."

The patient is allowed the opportunity to ventilate anger verbally. If the patient is delusional, challenging the patient is avoided. Trying to hear what the patient is saying, conveying an expectation of appropriate behavior, and making the patient aware that help is available are key. The patient should be informed that violent behavior may be frightening others and that violence is not acceptable. Help that is available in crisis situations, for example, from a clinic, ED, or mental health facility, should be described and offered. Often, the offer of protection by hospitalization is welcomed by the patient, who fears losing control or harming self or others. If the patient does not calm down, security personnel or police intervention may be necessary.

If these measures fail to alleviate the patient's tension, medication may be prescribed (rapid tranquilization with haloperidol, diazepam, or chlorpromazine) to reduce tension, anxiety, and hyperactivity. Restraints must be ordered by a physician. They are applied with a minimum of force and only when necessary and when other alternatives have been unsuccessful.

Nursing Alert *The least restrictive device to prevent the patient from injuring self and others is used. Caution is taken to ensure that restraints are applied properly. Restraints should be used with verbal intervention to calm the patient and promote compliance. Appropriate personnel must be available when applying restraints (in such a way that they do not impair circulation to any part of the body or interfere with breathing). Physical observation (eg, skin integrity, circulatory status, respiratory status) is ongoing, and the patient's response is documented.*

After combativeness, agitation, and fear have decreased, the patient is referred for further mental health treatment.

Posttraumatic Stress Disorder

Posttraumatic stress disorder (PTSD) is the development of characteristic symptoms after a psychologically stressful event that is considered outside the range of normal human experience (eg rape, combat, motor vehicle crash, natural catastrophe). Symptoms of this disorder include intrusive thoughts and dreams, phobic avoidance reaction (avoidance of activities that arouse recollection of the traumatic event), heightened vigilance, exaggerated startle reaction, generalized anxiety, and societal withdrawal. PTSD may be acute, chronic, or delayed.

Assessment

Assessment includes an evaluation of the patient's pretrauma history, the trauma itself, and posttrauma functioning. PTSD often presents as multiple readmissions to the ED for minor or recurring complaints without evidence of injury. The patient is allowed to discuss the traumatic event and permitted to grieve.

Management

The patient's goal is to organize and begin to integrate the experience so that he or she can return to the pretrauma level of functioning as soon as possible. Emergency management focuses on the patient's presenting behaviors. A wide range of interventions are carried out, including crisis intervention strategies, establishing a trusting and sharing relationship, and educating the patient and family about stress management and support services available in the community. Psychiatric support may be useful to the patient.

Depressed Patients

In the ED, depression may be seen as the primary condition bringing the patient to the health care facility, or it may be masked by anxiety and somatic complaints. The depressed person has a mood disturbance.

Clinical Manifestations

Clinical manifestations may include sadness, apathy, feelings of worthlessness, self-blame, suicidal thoughts, desire to escape, avoidance of simple problems, anorexia and weight loss, decreased interest in sex, sleeplessness, and ceaseless activity or reduction in activity. The agitated depressed individual may exhibit motor restlessness and severe anxiety.

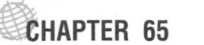

Management

The depressed patient benefits from ventilating personal feelings and should be provided an opportunity to talk about personal problems while the emergency health care personnel listen in a calm unhurried manner. Information about a perceived or real illness or a sudden worsening of depression are important clues. Any patient who is depressed may be at risk for suicide.

Attempts are made to find out if the patient has thought about or attempted suicide. Questions such as, "Have you ever thought about taking your own life?" may be helpful. Generally, the patient is relieved to have an opportunity to discuss personal feelings. If the patient is seriously depressed, relatives should be notified. The patient should never be left alone because suicide is usually committed in solitude.

The patient needs to understand that depression is treatable. Antidepressant and antianxiety agents may be prescribed. Crisis and supportive services in the community, including mental health centers, telephone counseling and referral, suicide prevention centers, group therapy, marital and family counseling, and befriending programs should be offered to the patient and family. Usually, the patient is referred for psychiatric consultation or to a psychiatric facility.

Suicidal Patients

Attempted suicide is an act that stems from depression (eg, the loss of a loved one, the loss of body integrity or status, or poor self-image) and can be viewed as a cry for help and intervention. Males are at greater risk than females. Others at risk are elderly people; young adults; people who are enduring unusual loss or stress; those who are unemployed, divorced, widowed, or living alone; those showing signs of significant depression (eg, weight loss, sleep disturbances, somatic complaints, suicidal preoccupation); and those with a history of a previous suicide attempt, suicide in the family, or psychiatric illness.

Assessment

Being aware of people at risk and assessing for specific factors that predispose a person to suicide are key management strategies. Specific signs and symptoms of potential suicide include the following:

- Communication of *suicidal intent,* such as preoccupation with death or talking of someone else's suicide (eg, "I'm tired of living. I've put my affairs in order. I'm better off dead. I'm a burden to my family")
- History of a previous suicide attempt (the risk is much greater in these cases)
- Family history of suicide
- Loss of a parent at an early age
- Specific plan for suicide
- A means to carry out the plan

Management

Emergency management focuses on treating the consequences of the suicide attempt (eg, gunshot wound, drug overdose) and preventing further self-injury. A patient who has made a suicidal gesture may do so again. Crisis intervention is employed to determine suicidal potential, to discover areas of depression and conflict, to find out about the patient's support system, and to determine whether hospitalization or psychiatric referral is necessary. Depending on the patient's potential for suicide, the patient may be admitted to the intensive care unit, referred for follow-up care, or admitted to the psychiatric unit.

Critical Thinking Exercises

1. A young man arrives at the ED by ambulance after a car crash. He is immobilized on a backboard with a cervical collar. An oxygen mask is in place. You note shallow, slow respirations and no movement of the left chest wall. His scalp is bleeding, and his left leg is angulated. How would you prioritize the patient's needs? Generate an assessment strategy and describe the patient's treatment needs.

2. A homeless man comes to the ED for treatment of frostbite of his feet. He insists that his feet be placed in a pan of hot water. Describe how you would respond and the explanation you would give to this patient. How would you proceed with managing this patient? Describe the discharge planning issues to be addressed for a homeless person.

3. A young woman with a toddler in her arms waits her turn in line at the triage desk of the ED. The child is crying and rubbing her eyes and face. You overhear the mother telling another patient that the child has had an allergic reaction to her first soft-cooked egg, which the child smeared on her face. Analyze this information and explain the conclusion you would draw and why. Then describe the action you would take and the rationale for your decision.

4. An elderly patient is brought to the ED by her son. She is complaining of pain in her hip, and the son says that she tripped over a child's toy and fell. Upon initial assessment you notice that the patient has many bruises on her body in varying stages of resolution. What conclusions might you draw from these findings, and how might you proceed to evaluate the situation to determine your course of action?

References and Selected Readings

BOOKS

Auerbach, P. S. (1995). *Wilderness medicine* (3rd ed.). St. Louis: C. V. Mosby.

Bayley, E. W., & Turcke, S. A. (1992). *A comprehensive curriculum for trauma nursing.* Boston: Jones & Bartlett.

Bove, A. A., & Davis, J. C. (1997). *Diving medicine.* Philadelphia: W. B. Saunders.

Bullock, B. L. (1996). *Pathophysiology.* Philadelphia: Lippincott-Raven.

Emergency Nurses Association. (1994). *Emergency nursing core curriculum* (4th ed.). Philadelphia: W. B. Saunders.

Handysides, G. (1996). *Triage in emergency practice.* St. Louis: C. V. Mosby.

Holleran, R. S. (1996). *Flight nursing principles and practice.* (2nd ed.). St. Louis: C. V. Mosby.

Sheehy, S. B. (1998). *Emergency nursing principles and practice* (4th ed.). St. Louis: C. V. Mosby.

JOURNALS

Berger, D. (1995). Suicide risk in the general hospital. *Psychiatry and Clinical Neurosciences, 49*(1), S85–89.

Bernstein, M. L. (1998). Latex safe emergency cart products list. *Journal of Emergency Nursing, 24*(1), 58–61.

Blank-Reid, C. (1996). The incidence, etiology, and management of anaphylaxis presenting to an accident and emergency department. *Quarterly Journal of Medicine, 89*(11), 859–864.

Borges, G., & Rosovsky, H. (1996). Suicide attempts and alcohol consumption in an emergency room sample. *Journal of Studies on Alcohol, Sept,* 543–548.

Chez, N. (1994). Helping the victim of domestic violence. *American Journal of Nursing, 94*(7), 32–37.

DeBoer, S. L. (1997). Neurological outcomes after near drowning. *Critical Care Nurse, 17*(4), 19–25.

Glow, S. D. (1997). Acutely agitated patients: A comparison of the use of haloperidol and droperidol in the emergency department. *Journal of Emergency Nursing, 23*(6), 626–628.

Gofin, R., DeLeon, D., Knishkowy, B., & Palti, H. (1995). Injury prevention program in primary care. *Injury Prevention, 1*(1), 35–39.

Goldman, B. (1994). Facing up to violent patients. *Emergency Medicine, 26*(8), 121–126.

Hansen, K. A. (1998). It's no accident. . . . it's preventable. *Journal of Emergency Nursing, 24*(1), 101–103.

Harrahil, M. (1997). Strategies for improving trauma documentation. *Journal of Emergency Nursing, 23*(2), 187–188.

Hart, B. G., & Trickett, D. (1995). Alcohol and trauma in the emergency department. *Journal of Emergency Nursing, 21*(5), 426–429.

Hoag-Apel, C. M. (1998). Violence in the emergency department. *Nursing Management, 29*(7), 60–62.

Hoak, S., & Koestner, A. (1997). Esophageal tracheal Combitube in the emergency department. *Journal of Emergency Nursing, 23*(4), 347–350.

Hollingsworth, H. (1997). Preventing insect sting anaphylaxis. *Journal of the American Medical Association, 277*(15), 1196–1197.

Hopkins, A. G. (1994). The trauma nurse's role with families in crisis. *Critical Care Nurse, 14*(2), 35–43.

Judkins, D., & Neff, J. (1995). Innovations in care: The cutting edge—fluids and blood warming systems. *Journal of Trauma Nursing, 2*(4), 105–109.

Keltie, D. (1996). Providing emergency wound care. *Community Nurse, 2*(6), 17–18.

Kinkle, S. L. (1993). Violence in the ED: How to stop it before it starts. *American Journal of Nursing, 93*(7), 22–24.

Kulig, K. (1992). Initial management of ingestions of toxic substances. *New England Journal of Medicine, 326*(25), 1677–1681.

Lachs, M. S., & Pillemer, K. (1995). Abuse and neglect of elderly people. *New England Journal of Medicine, 332*(7), 437–443.

Lenehan, G. (1995). An ED forensic kit. *Journal of Emergency Nursing, 21*(5), 440–444.

Luci, T. S., & Merrell, J. C. (1995). Perceived dangerousness of recreational drugs. *Journal of Drug Education, 25*(4), 297–306.

McCormack, J. E. (1997). Case studies: Sudden death and the tasks of mourning. *Journal of Trauma Nursing, 4*(2), 45–48.

O'Brien, C. (1997). Improved forensic documentation of genital injuries with colposcopy. *Journal of Emergency Nursing, 23*(5), 461–462.

O'Brien, C. (1998). Light staining microscope: Clinical experience in a sexual assault nurse examiner (SANE) program. *Journal of Emergency Nursing, 24*(1), 95–97.

Pakieser, R. A., Lenaghan, P. A., & Muelleman, R. L. (1998). Battered women: Where they go for help. *Journal of Emergency Nursing, 24*(1), 16–19.

Raven, C. (1993). The complicated elderly trauma patient. *Critical Care Nurse, 14*(2), 63–69.

Rice, V. (1991). Shock, a clinical syndrome: An update. Part 1. *Critical Care Nurse, 11*(4), 20–27.

Rice, V. (1991). Shock, a clinical syndrome: An update. Part 2. *Critical Care Nurse, 11*(5), 74–85.

Rice, V. (1991). Shock, a clinical syndrome: An update. Part 3. *Critical Care Nurse, 11*(6), 34–39.

Rice, V. (1991). Shock, a clinical syndrome: An update. Part 4. *Critical Care Nurse, 11*(7), 28–40.

Ringland, R., & Early, S. (1997). Conscious sedation: Documenting the procedure. *Journal of Emergency Nursing, 23*(6), 611–617.

Snyder, J. A. (1994). Emergency department protocols for domestic violence. *Journal of Emergency Nursing, 20*(1), 65–68.

Somerson, J. J., et al. (1996). Mastering emergency airway management. *American Journal of Nursing, 96*(5), 24–30.

Sommers, M. S. (1994). The near-death experience following multiple trauma. *Critical Care Nurse, 14*(2), 62–66.

Soukas, J., & Lonnqvist, J. (1995). Suicide attempts in which alcohol is involved: A special group in general hospital emergency rooms. *Acta Psychiatrica Scandinavica, 91,* 36–40.

Stamatos, C. A. (1994). Geriatric trauma patients: Initial assessment and management of shock. *Journal of Trauma Nursing, 1*(2), 45–56.

Tilden, V. P., et al. (1994). Factors that influence clinicians' assessment and management of family violence. *American Journal of Public Health, 84*(4), 628–633.

Vernon, D. D., & Gleich, M. C. (1997). Poisoning and drug overdose. *Critical Care Clinics, 13*(3), 646–677.

Wofford, J. L., et al. (1993). The role of emergency services in health care for the elderly: A review. *Journal of Emergency Nursing, 11*(3), 317–326.

Wright, J. A. (1997). Seven abdominal assessment signs every emergency nurse should know. *Journal of Emergency Nursing, 23*(5), 446–450.

Yap, H. L. (1993). Assessment of suicide risk. *Singapore Medical Journal, 34,* 164–166.

APPENDIX A Understanding Clinical Pathways

Clinical pathways (also called critical pathways) are care plans developed collaboratively by physicians, nurses, physical therapists, technicians, pharmacists, speech therapists, case managers, and other staff members involved in patient care. Nurses are instrumental in ensuring the successful use of clinical pathways and can best contribute by gaining a thorough understanding of why and how pathways are used.

Understanding and Using Clinical Pathways in Patient Care

Clinical pathways grew out of financial upheaval in the health care industry. They represent a significant change in how patient care is managed. In the past (and currently for many patients), each health care discipline developed its own plan of care and used the patient's chart (medical record) as the primary communication tool. Each care provider needed to read the notes written by other care providers of other disciplines to get a complete picture of the plan of care and the patient's progress. Although there was probably general agreement about how patient progress would be facilitated and measured, individual steps in the processes of care and outcomes to be achieved were not usually specifically articulated. The physician managed the case and most patients remained in the hospital until they required very little care or could be transferred to a convalescent center. The length of hospital stay was not an issue; 2 to 3 weeks in an acute care facility was not unusual.

Cost and Effects

Although this system worked for decades, it was expensive. Not including charges for diagnostic tests or treatments, each day in the hospital could easily cost $800 or more. The federal government and, later, insurance companies balked at paying these costs when highly skilled care was no longer needed. So they determined how many days of hospitalization a patient with a specific diagnosis required and decided to reimburse the insured parties only for that number of days. At the same time, hospitals tried to obtain meaningful financial data about the costs of hospital-based patient care—where the greatest costs were generated and how they could be reduced. Decreasing the length of stay was seen as one way to save money. As hospital stays became shorter and shorter, nurses and physicians began to express concerns about the quality of care. Patients were discharged to home or rehabilitation centers much sooner than before. They were weaker, had relatively fresh incisions, or often could not perform even minimal self-care independently. Regulatory agencies and consumers shared these concerns and demands arose for hard data demonstrating that patients were not being harmed.

This scenario compelled hospital administrators and clinicians to develop a new way to measure and manage costs, quality, and outcomes. Thoughtful examination of how patient care was provided exposed inefficiencies and highlighted the lack of face-to-face communication among disciplines. It became apparent that patient care could be managed more cost-effectively, possibly saving hundreds of thousands of dollars yearly. Hospitals adopted a system known as case management to address these issues.

Case Management

Under case management, care is planned collaboratively so that important events, such as initiation of physical therapy, home care consultation, or discontinuation of invasive treatments, occur on a schedule that clinicians, through experience or research, have identified as optimum for enhancing recovery. Care is mapped out by day or by other pivotal time intervals and goals or desired outcomes are specified for each time frame. When the patient has met all the goals, he or she is ready for discharge to home or to the next level of care. Responsibility for monitoring an individual patient's progress and tracking variance or deviation from the pathway is given to the case manager who usually but not always is a nurse. The tool on which all this information is contained is the clinical pathway. The purposes of a clinical pathway are to

- promote quality care and improve clinical outcomes
- standardize important aspects of care
- reduce unnecessary delays in care
- reduce costs

Elements of a Clinical Pathway

Clinical pathways are now used in a variety of settings and cover diverse diagnoses and conditions. They are often developed by individual organizations and, although the format varies from institution to institution, clinical pathways have major features in common.

Patient Population

The first important element of the clinical pathway is the patient population (Fig. AP-1**A**). Each pathway clearly specifies the patients appropriate for inclusion on the pathway. Pathways tend to cover patient groups in which the treatment and recovery are relatively predictable. Institutions typically use a diagnosis-related group (DRG) to identify patients, but qualifiers may be added. For example, a pathway for community-acquired pneumonia may exclude patients with *Pneumocystis carinii* pneumonia or underlying obstructive pulmonary disease because those patients require highly individualized treatment plans and may not respond as quickly to intervention as patients without these underlying disorders.

Time Frames

All pathways are divided into useful time frames (Fig. AP-1**B**). The identified time frame may be minutes, hours, days, weeks, or phases. Conditions requiring emergency treatment (myocardial infarction, head injury, stroke) might be divided into 15-minute intervals, whereas conditions requiring chronic care (chronic pain, spinal cord injury rehabilitation) may be divided into

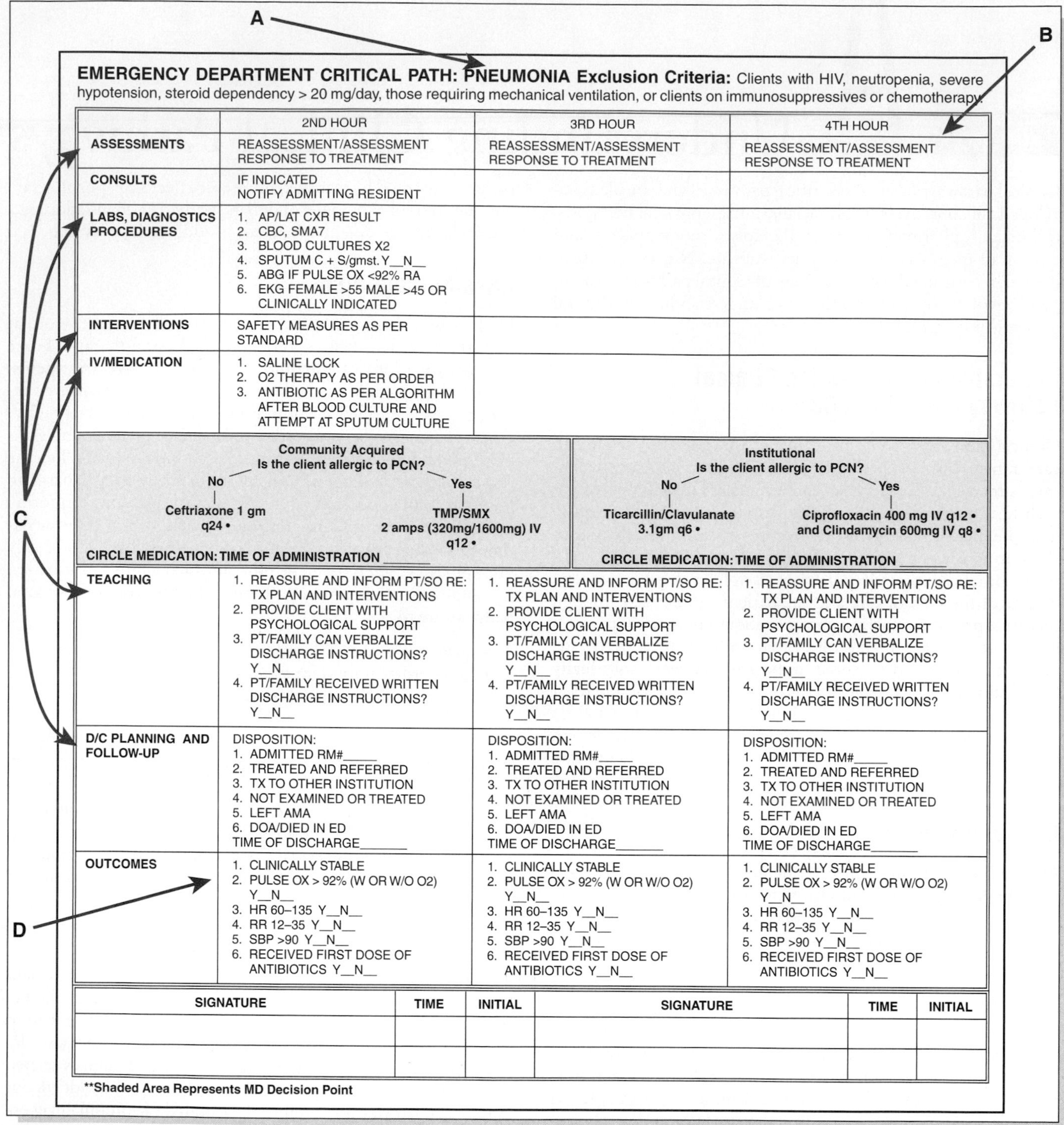

EMERGENCY DEPARTMENT CRITICAL PATH: PNEUMONIA Exclusion Criteria: Clients with HIV, neutropenia, severe hypotension, steroid dependency > 20 mg/day, those requiring mechanical ventilation, or clients on immunosuppressives or chemotherapy.

	2ND HOUR	3RD HOUR	4TH HOUR
ASSESSMENTS	REASSESSMENT/ASSESSMENT RESPONSE TO TREATMENT	REASSESSMENT/ASSESSMENT RESPONSE TO TREATMENT	REASSESSMENT/ASSESSMENT RESPONSE TO TREATMENT
CONSULTS	IF INDICATED NOTIFY ADMITTING RESIDENT		
LABS, DIAGNOSTICS PROCEDURES	1. AP/LAT CXR RESULT 2. CBC, SMA7 3. BLOOD CULTURES X2 4. SPUTUM C + S/gmst. Y__N__ 5. ABG IF PULSE OX <92% RA 6. EKG FEMALE >55 MALE >45 OR CLINICALLY INDICATED		
INTERVENTIONS	SAFETY MEASURES AS PER STANDARD		
IV/MEDICATION	1. SALINE LOCK 2. O2 THERAPY AS PER ORDER 3. ANTIBIOTIC AS PER ALGORITHM AFTER BLOOD CULTURE AND ATTEMPT AT SPUTUM CULTURE		

Community Acquired
Is the client allergic to PCN?
No — **Ceftriaxone 1 gm q24 •**
Yes — **TMP/SMX 2 amps (320mg/1600mg) IV q12 •**
CIRCLE MEDICATION: TIME OF ADMINISTRATION ______

Institutional
Is the client allergic to PCN?
No — **Ticarcillin/Clavulanate 3.1gm q6 •**
Yes — **Ciprofloxacin 400 mg IV q12 • and Clindamycin 600mg IV q8 •**
CIRCLE MEDICATION: TIME OF ADMINISTRATION ______

	2ND HOUR	3RD HOUR	4TH HOUR
TEACHING	1. REASSURE AND INFORM PT/SO RE: TX PLAN AND INTERVENTIONS 2. PROVIDE CLIENT WITH PSYCHOLOGICAL SUPPORT 3. PT/FAMILY CAN VERBALIZE DISCHARGE INSTRUCTIONS? Y__N__ 4. PT/FAMILY RECEIVED WRITTEN DISCHARGE INSTRUCTIONS? Y__N__	1. REASSURE AND INFORM PT/SO RE: TX PLAN AND INTERVENTIONS 2. PROVIDE CLIENT WITH PSYCHOLOGICAL SUPPORT 3. PT/FAMILY CAN VERBALIZE DISCHARGE INSTRUCTIONS? Y__N__ 4. PT/FAMILY RECEIVED WRITTEN DISCHARGE INSTRUCTIONS? Y__N__	1. REASSURE AND INFORM PT/SO RE: TX PLAN AND INTERVENTIONS 2. PROVIDE CLIENT WITH PSYCHOLOGICAL SUPPORT 3. PT/FAMILY CAN VERBALIZE DISCHARGE INSTRUCTIONS? Y__N__ 4. PT/FAMILY RECEIVED WRITTEN DISCHARGE INSTRUCTIONS? Y__N__
D/C PLANNING AND FOLLOW-UP	DISPOSITION: 1. ADMITTED RM#_____ 2. TREATED AND REFERRED 3. TX TO OTHER INSTITUTION 4. NOT EXAMINED OR TREATED 5. LEFT AMA 6. DOA/DIED IN ED TIME OF DISCHARGE______	DISPOSITION: 1. ADMITTED RM#_____ 2. TREATED AND REFERRED 3. TX TO OTHER INSTITUTION 4. NOT EXAMINED OR TREATED 5. LEFT AMA 6. DOA/DIED IN ED TIME OF DISCHARGE______	DISPOSITION: 1. ADMITTED RM#_____ 2. TREATED AND REFERRED 3. TX TO OTHER INSTITUTION 4. NOT EXAMINED OR TREATED 5. LEFT AMA 6. DOA/DIED IN ED TIME OF DISCHARGE______
OUTCOMES	1. CLINICALLY STABLE 2. PULSE OX > 92% (W OR W/O O2) Y__N__ 3. HR 60–135 Y__N__ 4. RR 12–35 Y__N__ 5. SBP >90 Y__N__ 6. RECEIVED FIRST DOSE OF ANTIBIOTICS Y__N__	1. CLINICALLY STABLE 2. PULSE OX > 92% (W OR W/O O2) Y__N__ 3. HR 60–135 Y__N__ 4. RR 12–35 Y__N__ 5. SBP >90 Y__N__ 6. RECEIVED FIRST DOSE OF ANTIBIOTICS Y__N__	1. CLINICALLY STABLE 2. PULSE OX > 92% (W OR W/O O2) Y__N__ 3. HR 60–135 Y__N__ 4. RR 12–35 Y__N__ 5. SBP >90 Y__N__ 6. RECEIVED FIRST DOSE OF ANTIBIOTICS Y__N__

SIGNATURE	TIME	INITIAL	SIGNATURE	TIME	INITIAL

****Shaded Area Represents MD Decision Point**

FIGURE AP•1 Key elements of a clinical pathway. (**A**) Patient population clearly defined. (**B**) Clinically meaningful time frames. (**C**) Interventional categories. (**D**) Outcomes for each time frame should be specific and measurable. Reproduced with permission from Graduate Hospital, Philadelphia, Pennsylvania.

weekly or monthly intervals. An example of interventions by phases might be seen in postanesthesia care pathways.

Interventional Categories

Interventional categories consist of the groups of activities that make up a comprehensive treatment plan and are shown in the left-hand column of the pathway (Fig. AP-1**C**). Although the order in which they are listed varies, these categories typically include

- Tests
- Treatments and nursing interventions
- Consultations
- Medications
- Diet

- Activity
- Patient and family education
- Discharge planning

Clinical pathway teams begin working with a blank grid and fill in the appropriate interventions. The discipline responsible for the intervention recommends the optimal timing.

Outcomes

Defined outcomes provide the focus for patient care activities and unify the various disciplines. All well-written pathways include outcomes identified for each time interval (Fig. AP-1**D**). They should be realistic, reflect incremental progress, and be achievable by 90% of the population. Pathway outcomes are similar in content and language to the goals or expected outcomes written into nursing plans of care; physiologic, psychological, social, and educational outcomes are included to capture all elements of complete recovery.

Variance Record

The variance record (Fig. AP-2) is an extremely important part of the pathway and represents the mechanism through which improvements in patient care can be accomplished. Variance is defined as any deviation from the pathway. Because all events on the pathway are critical to recovery, deviations can have a negative impact on outcomes. If the pathway calls for a specific test or treatment on day 2 and it is not carried out on day 2, a variance has occurred. If the patient is to ambulate 3 times a day and ambulates only once, a variance has occurred. The variance and the causes are recorded. Some variance records require a written note and others use code numbers (see Fig. AP-2). Many hospitals have developed or purchased software so that variance can be recorded electronically.

Case managers collect and analyze the variance data to identify trends in patient care and outcomes. For example, a pneumonia pathway may specify that the first dose of antibiotics be given within 3 hours of admission to the hospital (delays in administration of the first dose of an antibiotic are associated with increased morbidity and mortality). The case manager reviews the variance records and determines that only 40% of pneumonia patients are receiving the antibiotic in that time frame. Assessment of the problem reveals that delays are a result of the length of time it takes for the medication order to be taken off the chart and delivered to the pharmacy, and the length of time it takes for the medication to be delivered. The pneumonia pathway team discusses this problem and determines that the first dose of medication should be given in the emergency department since the emergency department stocks these medications. The pathway is revised to reflect this change in care. At the next review, the case manager reports that 92% of pneumonia patients on the clinical pathway received their antibiotics within 1 to 2 hours of admission. This scenario illustrates how pathway use and variance data collection provide the forum for assessing a problem, determining a plan of action, implementing the plan, and evaluating the effectiveness of the plan.

The Nurse's Role

Nurses have a key role in all aspects of clinical pathway use. Participating in the development of the pathway is the first step. Because they begin and end the chain of staff involved in delivering care, nurses possess a unique perspective in how health care systems work to enhance or impede the delivery of care. In the above example about antibiotic administration, staff nurses were able to identify the problem quickly and suggest solutions. Other staff from other disciplines, being single links in the chain, cannot supply this global view of the problem.

Nurses are also responsible for initiating the pathway on appropriate patients and ensuring that the various events occur as planned. In some care settings or conditions, case managers who are advanced practice nurses closely follow pathway patients; in others, staff nurses or community-based nurses function as case managers. In any environment, enhancing and monitoring outcome achievement is a nursing activity. Patients are often given a printed patient pathway for reference. The pathway describes the care plan in simple language and pictures. The nurse discusses the pathway with the patient and focuses on achieving specific outcomes.

Nurses are also responsible for completing required documentation. Practices vary, but well-designed pathways strive for simplicity and should not duplicate documentation required elsewhere. For example, a separate nursing plan of care is not necessary when using a clinical pathway. The outcome section of the pathway usually requires documentation; other areas may need to be checked off or initialed so that other providers can readily see what has been accomplished. Documenting variance and initiating steps to address the variance are equally important as is participating in redesigning care practices to promote the highest quality of cost-effective care.

Pathways in Practice

Several pathways are provided in the following pages to demonstrate the variety of formats the nurse may encounter. **Figure AP-3** is the clinical pathway used at Vanderbilt University Medical Center for myocardial infarction patients undergoing reperfusion intervention. The time frames are by phase of care and vary from 1 hour to 3 days in the hospital, and several months in follow-up care. The pathway includes clear outcomes and space for recording additional individualized outcomes. The authors have incorporated national standards of care into the pathway, highlighting them in bold. Variance data are entered into a computer data base. **Figures AP-4** and **AP-5** are other pathways used at Vanderbilt University Medical Center. Figure 4 is a critical care clinical pathway for hemodynamic and/or respiratory instability. This pathway is very detailed and reflects the growing use of pathways (and other guidelines) in managing serious, complex medical conditions.

Figure AP-6 is a pain management pathway used at the University of Wisconsin Hospital and Clinics. This pathway includes a documentation code. (Note: the final path day has been omitted). **Figure AP-7** is a pathway with an atypical format. Although it looks different from other pathways, it still contains all the elements of a pathway. It also functions as a physician order sheet. (Note: days 2 and 3 have been omitted).

Whatever format is used or condition treated, clinical pathways are documents in transition; they will change as research suggests better treatment strategies and as variance data are analyzed. Nurses' participation in these processes is essential for the successful implementation of clinical pathways and, ultimately, the opportunity to improve patient care.

Clinical Pathway: ____________________
(Department Name)

Patient's Name: ____________________ **MedRecNo:** _ _ _ _ _ _

(Please list each code separately)

Date	Path Day #	Variance Code	Comment / Action Taken
__/__/__			
__/__/__			
__/__/__			
__/__/__			
__/__/__			

A

VARIANCE CODES

Patient's Condition/Problem

A1. Operative
- A1a. Further surgery to control bleeding
- A1b. Further surgery for other reason
- A1c. Perioperative myocardial infarction
- A1d. Tamponade (early or late)
- A1e. Dissection

A2. Infection
- A2a. Sternum, requiring debridement
- A2b. Sternum, superficial (antibiotics and dressings only)
- A2c. Leg
- A2d. Urinary tract infection
- A2e. Sepsis

A3. Neurological
- A3a. Stroke, temporary or permanent deficit
- A3b. Delirium
- A3c. Coma
- A3d. Confusion or agitation

A4. Respiratory
- A4a. Prolonged ventilation
- A4b. Adult respiratory distress syndrome
- A4c. Respiratory failure, reintubation
- A4d. Pneumonia
- A4e. Atelectasis

A5. Renal
- A5a. Renal failure
- A5b. Dialysis

A6. Cardiac
- A6a. Atrial arrhythmia
- A6b. Ventricular arrhythmia
- A6c. Heart block with or without pacemaker implantation
- A6d. Heart failure
- A6e. Cardiac arrest
- A6f. Hemodynamic instability
- A6g. Unable to wean off inotropic agents

A7. Vascular
- A7a. Deep vein thrombosis
- A7b. Limb ischemia

Other Condition/Problem

A8. Other
- A8a. Major gastrointestinal complication requiring surgery (eg, bleeding, perforation, ileus)
- A8b. Minor gastrointestinal complication requiring bowel rest (eg, ileus, nausea, high nasogastric output)
- A8c. Large volume of chest-tube drainage
- A8d. Poor wound healing (ie, significant sterile drainage from leg or chest wound)
- A8e. Pulmonary embolism
- A8f. Anticoagulant complication
- A8g. Thromboembolism
- A8h. Activity intolerance
- A8i. Medication reaction
- A8j. Altered skin integrity

B: Practitioner Related
- B1. Practitioner unavailability
- B2. Transcription error
- B3. Incorrect sequencing of therapy
- B4. Delay in consult or referral
- B5. Incomplete discharge planning
- B6. Delay or cancel test or procedure
- B7. Discharge day delay
- B8. Other

C: Hospital/System
- C1. Bed unavailable (state issue)
- C2. Equipment or supplies not available
- C3. Results not available
- C4. Unable to schedule test, procedure, or therapy
- C5. Case, test, procedure, or therapy delayed
- C6. Preoperative teaching not documented
- C7. Follow-up after discharge not documented

D: Family/Placement
- D1. Extended care not available
- D2. Homecare not available
- D3. Patient or family delaying discharge planning
- D4. Financial issues
- D5. Other

Form used at Westchester County Medical Center for tracking variances from clinical pathway for cardiac surgery (CABG).

B

FIGURE AP•2 Variance record. (**A**) Blank pages for recording variance. (**B**) Variance codes. Reproduced with permission from *Critical Care Nurse*, 17(6) December 1997, pp. 29–30.

VANDERBILT UNIVERSITY MEDICAL CENTER

Acute MI with Primary Intervention

Adm. date ______________ Attending MD ______________________

D/C date ______________ Team ______________________

ELOS: ______________ Referring MD ______________________

	Phase 1 Initial Management ED: Hour 0–1	Phase II: Reperfusion Cath Lab	Phase III: Stabilization CCU (1–2 days)	Phase IV: Recovery 7N (2–3 days)	Phase V Discharge Day 3–4 post MI
Entrance Date/Time/ Initial	Date: ________ Time: ________ Initial: ________	Date: ________ Time: ________ Initial: ________	Date: ________ Time: ________ Initial: ________	Date: ________ Time: ________ Initial: ________	Date: ________ Time: ________ Initial: ________
Outcomes	Diagnosis of Acute MI Initiate treatment Angina score decreased Select method of reperfusion within 15 min of arrival to ED	**Time from arrival at cath lab to reperfusion 20–40 min** • Time from arrival at cath lab to groin puncture 5–10 min. • Time from groin puncture to completion of diagnostic cath 5–10 min. • Completion of diagnostic cath to reperfusion 5–10 min. • TIMI III flow	*Hemodynamics:* Stable w/ or w/o vasoactive infusions: - SBP 90–160 - DBP < 100 - HR 50–100 - Extremities warm and dry *ECG:* Stable heart rhythm *Angina* free *PTCA access site* without complications - no bleeding - no hematoma - no pseudoaneurysm *Respiratory:* Stable - SpO_2 > 93% on ≤ 6L nasal cannula O_2 - RR 12–26/min *Education:* Pt./family education tool initiated	*Hemodynamics:* Stable w/o vasoactive infusions: - SBP 90–160 - DBP < 100 - HR 50–100 - Extremities warm and dry *ECG:* Stable heart rhythm *Angina* free with ambulation *PTCA access site* without complications - no bleeding - no hematoma - no pseudoaneurysm *Respiratory:* status stable *Education:* Pt./family education tool in progress	Discharge with • PTCA access site without complication • No angina with ambulation • Diagnostic test results • Knowledge of emergency access *Education:* Pt./family demonstrates basic understanding of CAD, risk factors and DC meds
Individualized Outcomes		Re-establish patency to ______, ______, ______, ______ coronary artery(ies) via O PTCA O Stent Atherectomy O DCA (Directional Coronary Atherectomy) O TEC (transluminal extraction catheter) O Rolablater			
Assessment & Evaluation	SpO_2 monitoring Vital signs q 5 min Continuous ECG monitoring ST segment monitoring Complete MI flowsheet Assess & document payor information	Level of sedation Continuous ECG monitoring SpO_2 monitoring	Vital signs q 2° If on vasoactive infusion- VS q 5' while titrating, then q 1° I & O Daily weight SpO_2 monitoring Continuous ECG monitoring Post-intervention VS, site and distal pulse checks per protocol	Vital signs q 2°–4° ± I & O Daily weight Telemetry Bowel movement PTCA access site Distal pulses Assess affordability of discharge meds Assess functional status and ability to return to home/work activities	Vital signs q 4° Telemetry PTCA access site Distal pulses Assess functional status and ability to return to home/work activities
		Assess Cardiac Risk Factors (check all that apply): O DM O HTN O Family History O Age male > 45 y/o female > 55 y/o	O Post menopausal woman Hormone replacement yes____ no____ O Homocysteine O Dyslipidemia: LDL>100____, HDL<35____ O Sedentary life-style	O PVD or Cerebrovascular disease O Obese O Tobacco use: ____pks/day X ____ years	

Boldface words represent national standard of care. If not ordered, reason must be documented in chart.

FIGURE AP•3 Acute MI with primary intervention. Reproduced with permission from Vanderbilt University Medical Center, Nashville, Tennessee.

(*continued*)

	Phase 1 Initial Management ED: Hour 0–1	Phase II: Reperfusion Cath Lab	Phase III: Stabilization CCU (1–2 days)	Phase IV: Recovery 7N (2–3 days)	Phase V Discharge Day 3–4 post MI
Labs/Tests	Troponin I CK & MB @ _________ Chem 7 & ± Mg ± PT/PTT (if on warfarin or heparin) CBC with plts CXR 15-lead ECG @ _________ Guiaic Stool Lipid-HDL panel (Chol, TG, HDL, LDL - calc)	ACT ______sec. @ _________	1st 24 hours • CK & MB, ECG post-intervention, then 8' after ED adm. @ _________ and 16' @ _________ • 12-lead ECG on adm. to CCU 24°–48° • PCV w/ plts in AM • Chem-7 in AM • 12-lead ECG in AM	LV ejection fraction assessment before discharge • ECHO or • LV gram ± Homocysteine	12-Lead ECG day of discharge
Meds/IV	**NTG SL** **Chewable ASA 160–325 mg** **Metoprolol 5mg IV q 5min X 3 doses** **IV NTG 10 mcg/min titrated for angina relief** (caution w/ RV MI) ± Narcotic (Dilaudid) Heparin bolus 60 units/kg Heparin infusion 15 units/kg/hr O_2 2–4 L/min if O_2 Sat $\le$ 93%	ReoPro Bolus _________mg ReoPro infusion 21 cc/hr Heparin Bolus__________units Intracoronary NTG O_2 2–4 L/min if O_2 Sat $\le$ 93%	Wean NTG infusion to off ReoPro infusion 21 cc/hr DC 12' $\bar{p}$ starting@ ________ ±Half-dose Heparin infusion (Depending on angiographic results & thrombus burden in infarct CA) **No Ca-channel blocker** if EF < 50% **ASA** **H_2 blocker** **Colace** **Beta-blocker** (unless contraindicated) **ACE inhibitor** (if Ant MI, CHF, EF < 40%) **Ticlopidine if stent** NTG SL pm angina IVF's per post intervention orders PRN's: Acetominophen, MOM, Benadryl O_2 2–4 L/min if O_2 Sat $\le$ 93%	**ASA** **H_2 blocker** **Colace** **Beta blocker** (unless contraindicated) **ACE inhibitor** (if Ant MI, CHF, EF < 40%) **Ticlopidine if stent** ± Estrogen replacement ± Lipid lowering agent ± Nitrates PRN's: NTG SL, Acetominophen, MOM, Benadryl IV saline lock Consider medication cost to patient/payor formulary	Discharge meds: **NTG SL prn** **ASA** ± **Beta blocker** ± **ACE inhibitor** **Ticlopidine if stent** **Estrogen replacement in post-menopausal females** ± **Warfarin if LV thrombus or Afib** ± **Lipid lowering agent** Vit. E ± Isordil ± Folate
Activity	BR with BSC	BR	Sheath ________ Fr. removed @ _______, if Femstop, BR 6° post-sheath removal until_____ If vasoseal, BR 3° post-sheath removal until ______ Phase I Cardiac rehab BRP progressing to chair TID Assist with bath	Phase I Cardiac rehab, • Chair TID • Ambulate in room and to BR • Bathes self Progressing to: • Ambulate to tolerance, 10 min. maximum	Ambulate to tolerance, 15 min. maximum
Diet	NPO	NPO	Cardiac diet Low Na (if indicated)	Cardiac diet Low Na (if indicated)	Cardiac diet Low Na (if indicated)
Teaching/ D/C Plan	Orient pt/family to ED Discuss pain control Discuss treatment plan	Pre-procedure explanation Family/pt updated q 1°	Orient pt./family to unit Orient pt./family to "Patient Pathway" Discuss pain control Assess patient's knowledge and readiness to learn Initiative reviewing "Living the Healthy Heart Way" with pt./family	Initiate individual teaching plan ○ Address modifiable risk factors ○ Smoking cessation ○ Diet instructions ○ Exercise plan Reinforce "Living the Healthy Heart Way" with pt./family CPR video (family), EZ TV	Meds **MI warning S&S** Follow up/return appts **Chest pain mgmt** (NTG SL) **Smoking cessation** (if applicable) Diet Activity
Consults	Cath lab attending within 10 min of arrival to ED Cath lab (per Cath lab attending) CCU attending Cardiology fellow Primary MD		Finalize plans for discharge Utilize "Consultation Criteria and Guidelines" to initiate appropriate consults: • Case Manager • Cardiac Rehab • Social Worker • Nutrition Svcs • Pastoral Svcs • PT	• OT • Home Health • Subacute Unit • Skilled Nursing Facility • Other ______________	Case manager ○ Vanderbilt Heart Disease Prevention Program Referral or to ________ for cardiac rehab
Patient Flow	ED	Cath Lab	CCU	7N	Discharge

Date Time	Signature	Initial	Date Time	Signature	Initial	Date Time	Signature	Initial

THIS DOCUMENT IS INTENDED AS A GUIDELINE AND SHOULD BE ADAPTED FOR INDIVIDUAL PATIENT NEEDS.

Boldface words represent national standard of care. If not ordered, reason must be documented in chart.

Figure AP•3 *(Continued)*

	Phase VI Outpatient Follow-up 2 weeks Post-Discharge	1 month Post-MI	6 months Post-MI
Entrance Date/Time/ Initial	Date: ______ Time: ______ Initial: ______	Date: ______ Time: ______ Initial: ______	Date: ______ Time: ______ Initial: ______
Outcomes	Hemodynamically stable Angina free or stable Increasing activity	Hemodynamically stable Angina free or stable Increasing activity Risk stratification evaluated • Ideal body weight • No tobacco • Participating in a formal cardiac rehab program or exercising 20–30 min. a day	Hemodynamically stable Angina free LDL cholesterol < 100
Individualized Outcomes			
Assessment & Evaluation	V/S (sitting and standing if on anti-HTN meds) Weight H & P Risk factor modification plan	V/S Weight Focus visit H & P Risk factor modification plan follow-up	V/S Weight H & P Risk factor modification plan follow-up

	Phase VI Outpatient Follow-up 2 weeks Post-Discharge	1 month Post-MI	6 months Post-MI
Labs/Tests	CBC and plts (if Ticlid or procedure) SMA-7 (if on diuretics or ACEI)	Max ETT Fasting lipids Liver profile (if lipid tx initiated in hospital)	ECHO Fasting lipid-HDL profile
Meds/IV	**ASA** **± Beta blocker** **± ACE inhibitor** **± Lipid lowering agent** **Estrogen replacement in post menopausal females** **Ticlid if stent** ± Warfarin ± Vit. E ± Folate **NTG SL**	**ASA** **± Beta blocker** **± ACE inhibitor** **± Lipid lowering agent** **Estrogen replacement in post menopausal females** **Ticlid DC after 30 days** ± Warfarin ± Vit. E ± Folate **NTG SL**	**ASA** **± Beta blocker** **± Lipid lowering agent** **Estrogen replacement in post menopausal females** **Ticlid DC after 30 days** ± Warfarin ± Vit. E ± Folate **NTG SL** **DC ACE inhibitor if EF > 40%**
Activity			
Diet	Low fat ± Low sodium	Low fat ± Low sodium	Low fat ± Low sodium
Teaching	Medications Activity Diet Impact of disease on patient and family	Return to work/activities Diet Rehab	
Consults	If indicated: ○ Cardiac Rehab ○ Social Work ○ Case Manager ○ Nutrition	If needed: ○ Cardiac Rehab ○ Social Work ○ Case Manager ○ Nutrition	

FIGURE AP•3 *(Continued)*

VANDERBILT UNIVERSITY MEDICAL CENTER

Critical Care for Hemodynamic and/or Respiratory Instability

Inclusion criteria: (Check both if applicable)

____ Ventilator Support Required

____ Hemodynamic Instability

	Phase I Stabilization (ICU 2 days)	Phase II Chronic Respiratory Support (ICU 10 days)	Phase III Weaning (ICU 2 days)	Phase IV Post Positive Pressure Ventilation (ICU 1 day → Floor)	Phase V Discharge (Floor 3 days → Home)
Entrance Date/Time/ Initial	Date:____ Time:_____ Initial:______	Date:____ Time:_____ Initial:______	Date:____ Time:_____ Initial:______	Date:____ Time:_____ Initial:______	Date:____ Time:_____ Initial:______
Goals	**Hemodynamic status:** stable with or without vasoactive drips • HR > 60 < 140 • BPS > 90 < 150 • Evidence of adequate perfusion per clinical exam and/or high normal cardiac index **Respiratory status:** stable and meets criteria for chronic respiratory support when: • pH > 7.25–7.50 • O_2Sat ≥ 88% • RR 15–35 • Ventilatory targets achieved: - FiO_2 ≤ .80 - Plateau pressure ≤ 35 (Accept early hypercapnia to maintain plateau pressure ≤ 35, except in head injury) **Patient comfort and rest:** ensured → **Patient & Family orientation:** to unit/ hospital and communication mechanism established →	**Hemodynamic status:** stable without high dose vasoactive drips: • HR > 60 < 140 • BPS > 90 <150 **Respiratory status:** stable and meets criteria for weaning phase when: • Ventilatory target achieved: - FiO_2 ≤ .50 - PEEP ≤ 5 • Successful 5 minute CPAP trial with: - O_2Sat ≥ 88% - RR ≤ 35 - VE < 12 **Nutrition status:** needs met → **Patient comfort and rest:** ensured → **Patient & Family support:** → information and needs are met	**Hemodynamic status:** stable on no drips • HR > 60 < 140 • BPS > 90 <150 **Respiratory status:** stable and meets criteria for extubation: • Ventilatory targets achieved - FiO_2 ≤ .50 - PEEP ≤ 5 - Pressure support ≤ 5 • LOC adequate maintain airway protection • Sustains unassisted breathing for ≥ 120 minutes with: - O_2Sat ≥ 88% - RR ≤ 35 **Nutrition status:** needs met → **Patient comfort and rest:** → ensured **Patient & Family support:** → information and needs are met	**Transition status:** D/C from ICU when meets criteria: • Overnight observation • Hemodynamically stable • No upper airway obstruction • Effectively clearing secretions • Stable, spontaneous respiratory rate **Respiratory status:** tolerates extubation: • O_2Sat ≥ 88% • RR > 12 < 30 • FiO_2 < .40 • Effective cough and gag **Nutrition status:** needs met → **Patient comfort and rest:** → ensured **Patient & Family support:** → information and needs are met	**D/C status:** D/C from hospital when meets criteria: • Effectively clearing secretions • O_2Sat ≥ 88% on nasal cannula ≤ 3L/min • Home care assistance coordinated as indicated • Able to transfer from bed to chair • Patient/family teaching is completed/ documented • F/U appointment scheduled **Nutrition status:** needs met **Patient comfort and rest:** ensured **Patient & Family support:** information and needs are met
Individualized Goals					
Assessment & Evaluations	History and physical exam Nursing assessment Continuously monitor and record q 1°–2°: • VS • SaO_2 • I & O • FiO_2 Monitor and record q 3°–4°: • PIP • VE • VT • Plateau pressure	Continuously monitor and record q 2–4°: • VS • I & O • SaO_2 • FiO_2 • PIP • VE • VT • Plateau pressure Monitor for TF intolerance: N/V, tight abdomen, reflux of TF Consider: trach at 14–21 days if weaning does not seem possible	Assess q 30" to 4 hours throughout extubation process to guide ventilator support reduction • Patient comfort • LOC • O_2 Sat • RR • Secretions • HR, BP • Secretions • Respiratory muscle effort	Monitor for airway obstruction and laryngeal edema → VS continuously monitored x 30 minutes post extubation, then q 1 hour x 2 then per routine	
Tests & Labs	On admit and daily: • SMA 7 • ABG • CBC with diff, plts • CXR On admit: • SMA 12 • PT, PTT • EKG For fever of unknown origin: → • Blood culture q 3 days • Urine culture • Sputum for gram stain/culture • If w/u negative and fever persists change lines	Q 3 days: → • SMA 7 • SMA 12 • CBC with plts, diff prn • CXR ABG for sustained O_2SAT < 88%, respiratory distress (RR > 35) or change in LOC →			

SIGNATURE	INITIAL	SIGNATURE	INITIAL	SIGNATURE	INITIAL	SIGNATURE	INITIAL

THIS DOCUMENT IS INTENDED AS A GUIDELINE AND SHOULD BE ADAPTED FOR INDIVIDUAL PATIENT NEEDS.

FIGURE AP•4 Critical care for hemodynamic and/or respiratory instability. Reproduced with permission from Vanderbilt University Medical Center, Nashville, Tennessee.

	Phase I: Stabilization (ICU 2 days)	Phase II: Chronic Respiratory Support (ICU 10 days)	Phase III: Weaning (ICU 2 days)	Phase IV: Post Extubation (ICU 1 day→Floor)	Phase V: Discharge (Floor 3 days→Home)
Treatments	Orotracheal intubation and total ventilatory support → Arterial line if indicated: → • Frequent blood draws • Hemodynamic instability GI access —(OG tube preferred) → Foley catheter → Suction pm for ↑ PIP/secretions/ ↓ V_T/ adventitious breath sounds → Pulmonary artery catheter if: → • Diagnosis uncertain • Hemodynamic instability Pulse oximeter → Daily weight → Routine ICU care → Therapeutic bed if meet criteria (order) → Protective devices as per standard →	Decrease ventilatory support as tolerated → Change q 5–7 days → (If NG required, change to Dobhoff tube after 3 days) → Change q 3–5 days → Consider changing level of care to II If central line in use, change q 5–7 days → (elevate HOB 30°) →	Begin extubation maneuvers - adjust parameters by 0–50% q 30" to 4" as tolerated → extubation as appropriate Establish day/night orientation → Reassess need for therapeutic bed →	O_2 via nasal cannula (mask PRN O_2sat < 88%) Remove ventilator 2 hours post extubation if stable (Target before 12N or 12M) Cough and deep breathe D/C Pulse oximeter 6 hours post extubation if stable	
Individualized Treatments					
Diet	Feeding optional	Enteral feedings: • 30 Kcal/kg • Basic Formula: Ultracal - Standard with Fiber Perative - High Protein Needs Osmolyte HN - Standard with Lower Protein Needs TPN for failure of TF	Hold feeding 2 hours prior to extubation	Assess swallowing (nursing) Begin PO feeding with soft or pureed diet, then advance as tolerated (avoid liquids as initial diet)	Regular
Meds/IV	IV access → • NS for fluid resuscitation • Vasoactive medications if needed • Blood transfusion for PCV ≤ 25 Antibiotics as indicated for fever: • Broad spectrum AP coverage Heparin 5000 units SQ q 12° for DVT/ pulmonary embolus prophylaxis (if cannot anticoagulate, then SCD) → Analgesia: MSO_4 or Fentanyl (IV) use as indicated to lower impact on GI motility → Sedatives: Diazepam or Lorazepam (IV) → Haldol 2–5 mg TID as adjunct to sedation as needed Gastric bleeding prophylaxis: → • with gastric feeding → optional • with no feeding → H_2 blocker PO/PT Paralytic agents (Pavulon-intermittent and minimum amount needed to achieve goal) only if: • refractory ventilator dyssynchrony • short term use with selective procedures **Individualized Meds - see MAR** →	Reassess need for and response to antibiotics in 72 hours: → • D/C if no indication • Initiate appropriate antibiotics for known infections for 7–10 day intervals → When possible change to PO/PT →	Adjust analgesia and sedatives to enhance LOC and resp drive during weaning/extubation	Saline lock IV → Analgesia as indicated	
Activity	BR → Increase HOB if hemodynamically stable	ROM (active and passive) per RN	OOB as tolerated (minimum BID) Elevate HOB with weaning	OOB TID and as tolerated Ambulate q day	
Consults	Pulmonary/Critical Care Respiratory Care Case Manager Dietary	Physical Therapy (assessment and plan) OT (splints) Social services (if long term placement anticipated)		Social Services for D/C planning	
Teaching D/C Plan	Code Status written w/in 24° of admit Pt/Family assessment → Pt/Family oriented to ICU & hospital → Pt/Family support → Provide information to family regarding procedures/plan of care	Explain goals for total respiratory support phase to patient/family	Explain weaning procedure/ goals to patient/family	Prepare family for move to next level of care Coordinate transfer with floor staff Explain post extubation care/goals	Home care as indicated F/U appointment scheduled in 3 weeks
Individualized Teaching D/C Plan					
Equipment	Routine ICU set up → Pulse oximeter → Ventilator (pressure preset) → Arterial line (per criteria) → PA/ central line (per criteria) — Computation constant: ______ → GI access → Foley catheter → Bag/PEEP valve → IV pump (per criteria) → Therapeutic bed (per criteria) →		(Reassess need) → (Reassess need) → O_2 administration set up (Nasal cannula) →	D/C 6 hours post extubation D/C 2 hours post extubation Saline lock → Yankauer	

FIGURE AP•4 *(Continued)*

VANDERBILT UNIVERSITY MEDICAL CENTER

Adult Asthma Management*

* If intubated in the MICU, refer to Critical Care Pathway for Respiratory & Hemodynamic Instability

Expected Length of Stay: 2.5 days

	MICU	Stabilization/Floor	D/C Home
Entrance Date/Time/ Initial	Date ______ Time ______ Initial ______	Date ______ Time ______ Initial ______	Date ______ Time ______ Initial ______
Goals	**Hemodynamic Status: stable without vasoactive drips** • HR > 50 < 130 • SBP > 90 < 150 **Respiratory Status: stable without continuous nebulizers for 4 hours** • RR > 12 < 30 • PEFR < 50% baseline • FiO_2 < 40% / 6 LNC **Patient Comfort and Rest: ensured** • Adequate sedation to meet needs **Education Status: program implemented** • Patient/family introduced to asthma teaching plan	**Hemodynamic Status: stable** • HR > 50 < 130 • SBP >90 < 150 **Respiratory Status: stable** • Improve air flow as evidenced by minimal/no wheezing • PEFR > 70% admission baseline • FiO_2 < 2 LNC **Patient Comfort and Rest: ensured** • Pt able to sleep through night • Pt able to do ADL's with minimal distress/ SOB **Education Status: program reinforced** • Pt/family understands importance of using asthma action plan • Pt/family able to actively participate in teaching program with nursing staff and respiratory staff	**Discharge Status: ready to discharge when:** • All meds oral • Beta-agonist use < or = every four hours • Oral corticosteroid prescription written and filled • Action plan implemented and pt understands use • Appointment made with PCP within 7 days of discharge • PEFR at pt's normal baseline **Education Status: program completed**
Individualized Goals			
Assessment	• Seen by MD within 30 minutes of admission → • Detailed history (on admit) → • Physical exam → • VS q 2° • Cardiac monitoring → • Add oximetry for 24° → • MD visits 2 times daily →	VS q 4°/8°	VS q 8° Oximetry prn
Tests and Labs	• CBC (stat) → • SMA 7 prn → • ABG prn → • Theophylline level (if applicable) → • PT/PTT (once) → • UA prn → • Sputum (if produced) → • SMA 12 prn → • Chest X-ray PA and lateral (once)		

FIGURE AP•5 Adult asthma management. Reproduced with permission from Vanderbilt University Medical Center, Nashville, Tennessee.

	MICU	Stabilization/Floor	D/C Home
Treatments	• Supplemental O_2 maintain $SaO_2 > 88\%$ • Peakflow before/after each tx • CPPD only for sputum ≥ 100ml/day		• Action plan designed by MD and patient
Individualized Treatments			
Diet	NPO $\bar{x}$ meds	Clear liquids/advance as tolerated	Regular
Activity	Bedrest with BRP	As tolerated	Must walk in hall prior to discharge
Consults	Pulmonary Social Worker → Respiratory Therapy for asthma teaching →	Social worker as needed General Medicine Case Manager → (Respiratory Therapy for asthma teaching) →	Smoking cessation program PCP for follow-up and plan (General Medicine Case Manager) →
Meds/IV	If able to take po oral prednisone .5 to 1mg/kg/day If NPO, → IV solumed methylprednisolone 40–125mg IV q 6 HR Consider antibiotic therapy → Criteria: • Febrile • Purulent sputum • infiltrate on chest x-ray/pneumonia (IV antibiotics) • significant pre-steroid leukocytosis • suspected bronchitis: (p.o. Bactrim, Doxycycline, Amoxicillin, Erythromycin) Albuterol 2.5 mg/dose q 2° (Reassess need for nebulizer tx per RT protocol) Consider Atrovent Consider Theophylline/Aminophylline therapy	PO prednisone .5 to 1 mg/kg/day (If NPO) → Inhaled corticosteroids (Consider antibiotic therapy) →	PO prednisone Beta-agonist MDI with spacer ≤ q 4°
Teaching/ D/C Plan	D/C Plan: • RT to instruct on use of peak flow meter • Education packet provided by RT →	D/C Plan: • RT to instruct on use of peak flow meter and diary • Educational packet provided by RT • Nursing to go over medications	• Pt able to verbalize action plan (Follow-up in 7 days; key signs and symptoms, home plan) • Pt must demonstrate accurate use of peak flow 2 times prior to D/C home • Pt must demonstrate accurate use of MDI with spacer 2 times prior to D/C home • Inhaled anti-inflammatory meds
Equipment	Asthma teaching folder per RT → Peak flow meter → Cardiac monitoring → Oximeter → IV pump Routine ICU setup Placebo MDI and spacer → Mechanical ventilation	(Asthma teaching folder per RT) → (Peak flow meter) → (Cardiac monitoring) (Oximeter) → (Placebo MDI and spacer) →	(Asthma teaching folder per RT) → (Peak flow meter) → (Placebo MDI and spacer) →

Signature	Initial	Signature	Initial	Signature	Initial	Signature	Initial

THIS DOCUMENT IS INTENDED AS A GUIDELINE AND SHOULD BE ADAPTED FOR INDIVIDUAL PATIENT NEEDS.

Figure AP•5 *(Continued)*

PAIN MANAGEMENT ONC 004

Admitting/MD Service ____________________
Primary Nurse ____________________ Associate Nurse ____________
Allergies ____________________ Religion: ____________
Case Manager ____________________
Admitting Diagnosis: ____________________

Addressograph

History: Hospice Care? ☐Y ☐N

Pt/family support systems; special considerations include: ___
____
____

Significant Other *(Name & Phone)*: ____________________

Working Diagnosis															
Date/Time Interval	Acute Pain Management Phase/___	N	D	E	Pain Control & Titration to po/___	N	D	E	N	D	E	Pain Management Steady State/___	N	D	E
Unit/Setting															
Consults	Unit pain resource RN														
Labs	Heme survey, diff PLT's Chem 7														
Specimens (RN)															
Tests															
Activity I = Independent A = Assist (indicate amount needed) D = Dependent Indicate assistive devices	BR c̄ BRP Eating: Bathing: A Transfer Chair/amb ___x/d				Eating: Bathing Transfer Chair/amb ___x/d							Eating: Bathing Transfer Chair/amb ___x/d			
Treatments ***Call H.O. for:*** **T > 38^5** ____ **P < 55 > 120** ____ **R ≤ 8** ____ **BP** ____ ____ **Pulse ox** ____ **Sedation score=3 or persistent uncontrolled pain**	Admission Wt I & O q̄ 5" during loading dose VS Pulse ox pain rating sedation score p̄ loading dose, repeat above assessments: q̄ 1 hr x 4 q̄ 2 hr x 2 then q̄ 4 hrs & PRN See Standing Orders for Cancer Pain Management Implement nurse protocol for acute pain management Start IV infusion D5.9 NS @ TKO				VS q̄ 4° & PRN I & O Δ in order if pain rating ____ for two consecutive ratings in a 4° period							VS q̄ 8° & PRN I & O			
Diet	General Encourage fluids				General Encourage fluids							General Encourage fluids			

Pt Name: ____________________ MR# ____________________

FIGURE AP•6 Pain management oncology. Reproduced with permission from University of Wisconsin Hospital and Clinics, Madison, Wisconsin.

Discharge Planning	*Patient Health Profile:* Pt/family (Part I) completed Nursing (Part II & III) completed Residence__________ __________ Consider DC needs	Anticipated DC date:________Time:_____ Nursing Home/Other:__________ Transportation:________ Phone:_____ LMD:__________ Home services needed: RN____ HHA ____ PT____ OT ____ Other______ Provider:________ Phone______ Reason:__________	Plan DC prior to noon Referrals to:__________ Fax:________ Assess for needed equipment/supplies/additional supports DC supplies ordered Pt needs discussed at DC planning rounds on:______ __________ Referral called on:________ by:________ Pt's goal for functional status @ DC:________
Nursing Activity & Teaching	***Assess:*** • per Standing Orders for Cancer Pain Management ***Teach PT/Family:*** • unit routines/pathway • Primary RN/caregivers • procedures • medications • ongoing pain ratings ***Other Interventions:*** • document pt's goal for functional status @ D/C • response to prev. interventions • implement pain flowsheet • HFFY:________	***Assess:*** • complete systems q̄ 8° • level of pain q̄ 2° • pt/family understanding of causes/ treatment • for side effects; const, N/V, sedation, resp, depression q̄____° • DC planning needs ***Teach PT/Family:*** • disease process • pain management ***Other Interventions:*** • initiate DC plan • update activity plan & functional outcomes based on current status & anticipated DC status	***Assess:*** • complete systems q̄ 8° • level of pain q̄ 4° • pt/family understanding of causes/ treatment • for side effects; const, N/V, sedation, resp, depression q̄____° • functional status q̄____° • readiness for DC ***Teach PT/Family:*** • pain management ***Other Interventions:*** • update activity plan • consider Δ to po meds
Other Disciplines Activity & Teaching	***Clinical Nutrition:*** • nutrition screen - screened @ low risk - screened @ risk (eval to follow)		
Anticipated Variances	***Funct:*** pt's baseline	***Funct:*** ADLs c assist	
Outcomes ***(The patient/family will...)***	VS within MD parameters LBM_____ (min q̄ 48°) ***Pts Pain Goal:***______ Reports pain ≤ goal c̄ acceptable side effects ***Verbalize/Demonstrate:*** • primary RN/caregivers • plan of care • interventions, procedures	VS within MD parameters LBM_____ (min q̄ 48°) ***Pts Pain Goal:***______ Reports pain ≤ goal c̄ acceptable side effects Pain score is rated at ≤ 5 ***Verbalize/Demonstrate:*** • interventions, procedures • progress anticipated	VS within MD parameters LBM_____ (min q̄ 48°) ***Pts Pain Goal:***______ Reports pain ≤ goal c̄ acceptable side effects Pain score is rated at ≤ 5 ***Verbalize/Demonstrate:*** • pain management techniques for use @ home • understanding re: analgesic regimen, SE management, when to call RN/MD

Pt Name____________________ MR#____________________

FIGURE AP•6 *(Continued)*

CRITICAL PATHWAY
HIV WITH DIARRHEA

Doctor: Draw a line through any items you do not wish to order and fill in any blank orders. Use a separate order sheet for additional orders.

Goals: ***By the end of this pathway, the patient/family will be able to:***
1. Discuss disease process
2. State action(s) to take to maintain intact skin at peri-anal area
3. Plan diet within restrictions
4. Describe ordered GI-related diagnostic test including rationale for use, preparation, and patient participation, if applicable
5. Describe discharge drug regimen including drug name, dose, time, major side effects, if applicable

Date initiated: ________ Allergies: ________ Ht: ______ Wt: lb: ______ Kg: ______

DAY 1	SHIFT N	D	E
Admission Admit to: __________			
Pathway Criteria Diarrhea = stool output ≥ 1,500 cc/24° and/or ≥ BM's/24°			
1. Vital Signs BP/P/RR: q4° Temp: q4° (tympanic) Blood cultures q15' X 2 if T > 100.5°F			
2. Weight On admission & QD			
3. Nutrition NPO OR: if no nausea/vomiting, clear liquids Nutrition consult within 24° for diarrhea			
4. IVs ________ @ ______ cc/hr Start peripheral IV OR: use existing indwelling venous access device			
5. I & O q8° Use Stool Flow Sheet			
6. Stool Collection Use Bed Side Commode (BSC) or Speci-pan Avoid urine contamination of stool specimen Diaper, if needed-weigh after each change			
7. Infection Control Contact isolation Private room			

DAY 1	SHIFT N	D	E
8. Labs CBC w/differential Renal profile Stool for: leukocytes guaiac culture for *Salmonella, Shigella,* & *Campylobacter* Ova & parasites *Cryptosporidia* *Clostridium difficile* (toxin)			
9. Medications Patient may self-administer Imodium 2 mg cap PO after each BM; up to 16 mg/day Anusol HC Cream to rectum PRN Tuck's pads to rectum PRN			
10. Activity Bed Rest (BR) with Bed Side Commode (BSC) or BRP			
11. Psychological/Cultural Provide emotional support re: illness, altered body image, isolation Orient to unit, if applicable Orient family/significant other to unit, visiting hours, call-in times if applicable Assess, attend to & document specific cultural needs PRN			
12. Patient Teaching & Discharge Planning Begin to teach HIV with Diarrhea Patient Teaching Standard (PTS) Begin Generic PTS, if applicable			

Nurse Signature & Initials

MD Signature & Code
Your signature authorizes the implementation of orders on pages 1–4 of this pathway unless otherwise changed in writing.

FIGURE AP•7 HIV with diarrhea. Reproduced with permission from Mount Sinai Medical Center, Miami Beach, Florida. *Note:* Days 2 and 3 not illustrated.

CRITICAL PATHWAY
HIV WITH DIARRHEA

Date: ____________________

Weight: ____________________

DAY 4	SHIFT N	SHIFT D	SHIFT E	DAY 4	SHIFT N	SHIFT D	SHIFT E
1. Vital Signs Continue BP/P/RR/Temp (tympanic): q4°				**12. Medications** Patient may self-administer Imodium 2 mg cap PO after each BM; up to 16 mg/day Anusol HC Cream to rectum PRN Tuck's pads to rectum PRN If causative organism identified as: *Campylobacter jejuni:* Ciprofloxacin 500 mg PO BID *Clostridium difficile:* Metronidazole 250 mg PO QID *Cryptosporidium:* Consider paromomycin 500 mg PO QID OR: nonspecific antidiarrheal agents: ____________ *Entamoeba histolytica:* Metronidazole 750 mg PO TID followed by iodoquinol 650 mg PO TID *Giardia lamblia:* Metronidazole 750 mg PO TID followed by iodoquinol 650 mg PO TID *Isospora belli:* TMP/SMX 1 double strength tablet PO QID *Microsporidium:* Nonspecific antidiarrheal agent: ____________ *For Positive Salmonella cultures:* Ciprofloxacin 500 mg PO BID *Shigella:* Ciprofloxacin 500 mg PO BID *Strongyloides stercoralis:* Thiabendazole 22 mg/kg (______ mg) PO q 12°			
2. Weight In AM							
3. Nutrition Continue NPO OR regular diet as tolerated							
4. IVs Continue ____________ @ ______ cc/hr							
5. I & O D/C							
6. Stool Collection D/C							
7. Infection Control Continue contact isolation Continue private room							
8. Labs N/A							
9. Activity Continue BR with BSC							
10. Consults Continue Case Management Continue Home Health, if ordered Continue GI, if ordered							
11. Psychosocial Continue to provide emotional support re: illness, altered body image, isolation				**13. Patient Teaching & Discharge Planning** Continue HIV with Diarrhea PTS			

Nurse Signature & Initials

FIGURE AP•7 *(Continued)*

APPENDIX B

Nursing Outcomes Classification (NOC) and Nursing Interventions Classification (NIC)

The Nursing Outcomes Classifications (NOC) and the Nursing Interventions Classification (NIC), were developed at the Center for Nursing Classification at the University of Iowa College of Nursing, Iowa City. NOC and NIC are standardized taxonomies.

NOC identifies, codes, and organizes nearly 200 outcomes that are expected to result from nursing interventions. Each outcome is defined with indicators and measures to evaluate whether the expected outcome has been achieved. The NOC taxonomy is presented below.

NURSING OUTCOMES CLASSIFICATION (NOC)

Outcome Codes and Labels

2306 Abuse Cessation
2300 Abuse Protection
2301 Abuse Recovery: Emotional
2302 Abuse Recovery: Financial
2303 Abuse Recovery: Physical
2304 Abuse Recovery: Sexual
1400 Abusive Behavior Self-Control
1300 Acceptance: Health Status
1600 Adherence Behavior
1401 Aggression Control
0200 Ambulation: Walking
0201 Ambulation: Wheelchair
1402 Anxiety Control
0202 Balance
0700 Blood Transfusion Reaction Control
1200 Body Image
0203 Body Positioning: Self-Initiated
1104 Bone Healing
0500 Bowel Continence
0501 Bowel Elimination
1000 Breastfeeding Establishment: Infant
1001 Breastfeeding Establishment: Maternal
1002 Breastfeeding Maintenance
1003 Breastfeeding Weaning
0400 Cardiac Pump Effectiveness
2200 Caregiver Adaptation To Patient Institutionalization
2201 Caregiver Emotional Health
2202 Caregiver Home Care Readiness
2203 Caregiver Lifestyle Disruption
2204 Caregiver-Patient Relationship
2205 Caregiver Performance: Direct Care
2206 Caregiver Performance: Indirect Care
2207 Caregiver Physical Health
2208 Caregiver Stressors
2209 Caregiver Well-Being
2210 Caregiving Endurance Potential
1301 Child Adaptation To Hospitalization
0100 Child Development: 2 Months
0101 Child Development: 4 Months
0102 Child Development: 6 Months
0103 Child Development: 12 Months
0104 Child Development: 2 Years
0105 Child Development: 3 Years
0106 Child Development: 4 Years
0107 Child Development: 5 Years
0108 Child Development: Middle Childhood (6–11 Years)
0109 Child Development: Adolescence (12–17 Years)
0401 Circulation Status
0900 Cognitive Ability
0901 Cognitive Orientation
2100 Comfort Level
0902 Communication Ability
0903 Communication: Expressive Ability
0904 Communication: Receptive Ability
1601 Compliance Behavior
0905 Concentration
1302 Coping
0906 Decision Making
1303 Dignified Dying
1403 Distorted Thought Control
0600 Electrolyte & Acid/Base Balance
0001 Endurance
0002 Energy Conservation
1404 Fear Control
0601 Fluid Balance
1304 Grief Resolution
0110 Growth
1700 Health Beliefs
1701 Health Beliefs: Perceived Ability To Perform
1702 Health Beliefs: Perceived Control
1703 Health Beliefs: Perceived Resources
1704 Health Beliefs: Perceived Threat
1705 Health Orientation
1602 Health Promoting Behavior
1603 Health Seeking Behavior
1201 Hope
0602 Hydration
1202 Identity
0204 Immobility Consequences: Physiological
0205 Immobility Consequences: Psycho-Cognitive
0701 Immune Hypersensitivity Control
0702 Immune Status
1900 Immunization Behavior
1405 Impulse Control
0703 Infection Status
0907 Information Processing
0206 Joint Movement: Active
0207 Joint Movement: Passive
1800 Knowledge: Breastfeeding
1801 Knowledge: Child Safety
1802 Knowledge: Diet
1803 Knowledge: Disease Process
1804 Knowledge: Energy Conservation
1805 Knowledge: Health Behaviors
1806 Knowledge: Health Resources
1807 Knowledge: Infection Control
1808 Knowledge: Medication
1809 Knowledge: Personal Safety
1811 Knowledge: Prescribed Activity
1812 Knowledge: Substance Use Control
1814 Knowledge: Treatment Procedure(s)
1813 Knowledge: Treatment Regimen
1604 Leisure Participation
1203 Loneliness

List compiled from Iowa Outcomes Project. M. Johnson & M. Maas (Eds.). (1997). *Nursing outcomes classification (NOC)*. St. Louis: Mosby.

0908 Memory
0208 Mobility Level
1204 Mood Equilibrium
0209 Muscle Function
2305 Neglect Recovery
0909 Neurological Status
0910 Neurological Status: Autonomic
0911 Neurological Status: Central Motor Control
0912 Neurological Status: Consciousness
0913 Neurological Status: Cranial Sensory/Motor Function
0914 Neurological Status: Spinal Sensory/Motor Function
1004 Nutritional Status
1005 Nutritional Status: Biochemical Measures
1006 Nutritional Status: Body Mass
1007 Nutritional Status: Energy
1008 Nutritional Status: Food & Fluid Intake
1009 Nutritional Status: Nutrient Intake
1100 Oral Health
1605 Pain Control Behavior
2101 Pain: Disruptive Effects
2102 Pain Level
2104 Pain: Psychological Response
1500 Parent-Infant Attachment
2211 Parenting
1901 Parenting: Social Safety
1606 Participation: Health Care Decisions
0113 Physical Aging Status
0114 Physical Maturation: Female
0115 Physical Maturation: Male
0116 Play Participation
0117 Preterm Infant Organization
1305 Psychosocial Adjustment: Life Change
2000 Quality Of Life
0402 Respiratory Status: Gas Exchange
0403 Respiratory Status: Ventilation
0003 Rest
1902 Risk Control
1903 Risk Control: Alcohol Use
1904 Risk Control: Drug Use
1905 Risk Control: Sexually Transmitted Diseases (STD)
1906 Risk Control: Tobacco Use
1907 Risk Control: Unintended Pregnancy
1908 Risk Detection
1501 Role Performance
1909 Safety Behavior: Fall Prevention
1910 Safety Behavior: Home Physical Environment
1911 Safety Behavior: Personal
1912 Safety Status: Falls Occurrence
1913 Safety Status: Physical Injury
0300 Self-Care: Activities Of Daily Living (ADL)
0301 Self-Care: Bathing
0302 Self-Care: Dressing
0303 Self-Care: Eating
0304 Self-Care: Grooming
0305 Self-Care: Hygiene
0306 Self-Care: Instrumental Activities Of Daily Living (IADL)
0307 Self-Care: Non-Parenteral Medication
0308 Self-Care: Oral Hygiene
0309 Self-Care: Parenteral Medication
0310 Self-Care: Toileting
1205 Self-Esteem
1406 Self-Mutilation Restraint
0004 Sleep
1502 Social Interaction Skills
1503 Social Involvement
1504 Social Support
2001 Spiritual Well-Being
1407 Substance Addiction Consequences
1306 Suffering Level
1408 Suicide Self-Restraint
1608 Symptom Control Behavior
2103 Symptom Severity
0800 Thermoregulation
0801 Thermoregulation: Neonate
1101 Tissue Integrity: Skin & Mucous Membranes
0404 Tissue Perfusion: Abdominal Organs
0405 Tissue Perfusion: Cardiac
0406 Tissue Perfusion: Cerebral
0407 Tissue Perfusion: Peripheral
0408 Tissue Perfusion: Pulmonary
0210 Transfer Performance
1609 Treatment Behavior: Illness or Injury
0502 Urinary Continence
0503 Urinary Elimination
0802 Vital Signs Status
2002 Well-Being
1206 Will To Live
1102 Wound Healing: Primary Intention
1103 Wound Healing: Secondary Intention

Like NOC, NIC is a standardized taxonomy of nearly 450 nursing interventions performed in response to nursing diagnoses—namely those generated and standardized by the North American Nursing Diagnosis Association (NANDA). The interventions are performed to achieve desired patient outcomes. The NIC identifies nursing activities for individuals, families, or groups in various settings and specialties. The interventions are organized into 27 classes and 6 domains to facilitate planning and documentation. The standardized language helps to communicate sets of nursing activities to other nurses and to health care professionals from other disciplines. It is anticipated that these will facilitate reimbursement for services rendered.

NURSING INTERVENTIONS CLASSIFICATION (NIC)

6400 Abuse Protection
6402 Abuse Protection: Child
6404 Abuse Protection: Elder
1910 Acid-Base Management
1911 Acid-Base Management: Metabolic Acidosis
1912 Acid-Base Management: Metabolic Alkalosis
1913 Acid-Base Management: Respiratory Acidosis
1914 Acid-Base Management: Respiratory Alkalosis
1920 Acid-Base Monitoring
4920 Active Listening
4310 Activity Therapy
1320 Acupressure
7310 Admission Care
3120 Airway Insertion and Stabilization
3140 Airway Management
3160 Airway Suctioning
6410 Allergy Management
6700 Amnioinfusion
3420 Amputation Care
2210 Analgesic Administration
2214 Analgesic Administration: Intraspinal
2840 Anesthesia Administration
4640 Anger Control Assistance
4320 Animal Assisted Therapy
5210 Anticipatory Guidance
5820 Anxiety Reduction
6420 Area Restriction
4330 Art Therapy
3180 Artificial Airway Management
3200 Aspiration Precautions
4340 Assertiveness Training
6710 Attachment Promotion
5840 Autogenic Training
2860 Autotransfusion
1610 Bathing
0740 Bed Rest Care
7610 Bedside Laboratory Testing
4350 Behavior Management
4352 Behavior Management: Overactivity/Inattention
4354 Behavior Management: Self Harm
4356 Behavior Management: Sexual
4360 Behavior Modification
4362 Behavior Modification: Social Skills
4680 Bibliotherapy
5860 Biofeedback
6720 Birthing
0550 Bladder Irrigation
4010 Bleeding Precautions
4020 Bleeding Reduction
4021 Bleeding Reduction: Antepartum Uterus
4022 Bleeding Reduction: Gastrointestinal
4024 Bleeding Reduction: Nasal
4026 Bleeding Reduction: Postpartum Uterus
4028 Bleeding Reduction: Wound
4030 Blood Products Administration
5220 Body Image Enhancement
0140 Body Mechanics Promotion
1052 Bottle Feeding
0410 Bowel Incontinence Care
0412 Bowel Incontinence Care: Encopresis
0420 Bowel Irrigation
0430 Bowel Management
0440 Bowel Training
1054 Breastfeeding Assistance
5880 Calming Technique

List compiled from Iowa Intervention Project—McCloskey, J. C., & Bulechek, G. M. (Eds.). (1996). *Nursing Interventions Classification (NIC)* (2nd ed.) St. Louis: Mosby-Year Book.

4040 Cardiac Care
4044 Cardiac Care: Acute
4046 Cardiac Care: Rehabilitative
4050 Cardiac Precautions
7040 Caregiver Support
0762 Cast Care: Maintenance
0764 Cast Care: Wet
2540 Cerebral Edema Management
2550 Cerebral Perfusion Protection
6750 Section Care
2240 Chemotherapy Management
3230 Chest Physiotherapy
6760 Childbirth Preparation
4060 Circulatory Care
4064 Circulatory Care: Mechanical Assist Device
4070 Circulatory Precautions
6140 Code Management
4700 Cognitive Restructuring
4720 Cognitive Stimulation
4974 Communication Enhancement: Hearing Deficit
4976 Communication Enhancement: Speech Deficit
4978 Communication Enhancement: Visual Deficit
5000 Complex Relationship Building
2260 Conscious Sedation
0450 Constipation Infection Management
1620 Contact Lens Care
7620 Controlled Substance Checking
5230 Coping Enhancement
3250 Cough Enhancement
5240 Counseling
6160 Crisis Intervention
7640 Critical Path Development
7330 Culture Brokerage
1340 Cutaneous Stimulation
5250 Decision-Making Support
7650 Delegation
6440 Delirium Management
6450 Delusion Management
6460 Dementia Management
7050 Development Enhancement
0460 Diarrhea Management
1020 Diet Staging
7370 Discharge Planning
5900 Distraction
7920 Documentation
1630 Dressing
5260 Dying Care
2580 Dysreflexia Management
4090 Dysrhythmia Management
1640 Ear Care
1030 Eating Disorders Management
2000 Electrolyte Management
2001 Electrolyte Management: Hypercalcemia
2002 Electrolyte Management: Hyperkalemia
2003 Electrolyte Management: Hypermagnesemia
2004 Electrolyte Management: Hypernatremia
2005 Electrolyte Management: Hyperphosphalemia
2006 Electrolyte Management: Hypocalcemia
2007 Electrolyte Management: Hypokalemia
2008 Electrolyte Management: Hypomagnesemia
2009 Electrolyte Management: Hyponatremia
2010 Electrolyte Management: Hypophosphalemia
2020 Electrolyte Monitoring
6771 Electronic Fetal Monitoring: Antepartum
6772 Electronic Fetal Monitoring: Intrapartum
6470 Elopement Precautions
4104 Embolus Care: Peripheral
4106 Embolus Care: Pulmonary
4110 Embolus Precautions
6200 Emergency Care
7660 Emergency Cart Checking
5270 Emotional Support
3270 Endotracheal Extubation
0180 Energy Management
1056 Enteral Tube Feeding
6480 Environmental Management
6481 Environmental Management: Attachment Process
6482 Environmental Management: Comfort
6484 Environmental Management: Community
6486 Environmental Management: Safety
6487 Environmental Management: Violence Prevention
6489 Environmental Management: Worker Safety
7680 Examination Assistance
0200 Exercise Promotion
0202 Exercise Promotion: Stretching
0221 Exercise Therapy: Ambulation
0222 Exercise Therapy: Balance
0224 Exercise Therapy: Joint Mobility
0226 Exercise Therapy: Muscle Control
1650 Eye Care
6490 Fat Prevention
7100 Family Integrity Promotion
7104 Family Integrity Promotion: Childbearing Family
7110 Family Involvement
7120 Family Mobilization
6784 Family Planning: Contraception
6786 Family Planning: Infertility
6788 Family Planning: Unplanned Pregnancy
7130 Family Process Maintenance
7140 Family Support
7150 Family Therapy
1050 Feeding
7160 Fertility Preservation
3740 Fever Treatment
6500 Fire Setting Precautions
6240 First Aid
0470 Flatulence Reduction
4120 Fluid Management
4130 Fluid Monitoring
4140 Fluid Resuscitation
2080 Fluid/Electrolyte Management
1660 Foot Care
1080 Gastrointestinal Intubation
5242 Genetic Counseling
5290 Grief Work Facilitation
5294 Grief Work Facilitation: Perinatal Death
5300 Guilt Work Facilitation
1670 Hair Care
6510 Hallucination Management
7960 Health Care Information Exchange
5510 Health Education
7970 Health Policy Monitoring
6520 Health Screening
7400 Health System Guidance
3780 Heat Exposure Treatment
1380 Heat/Cold Application
2100 Hemodialysis Therapy
4150 Hemodynamic Regulation
4160 Hemorrhage Control
6800 High Risk Pregnancy Care
7180 Home Maintenance Assistance
5310 Hope Instillation
5320 Humor
2120 Hyperglycemia Management
4170 Hypervolemia Management
5920 Hypnosis
2130 Hypoglycemia Management
3800 Hypothermia Treatment
4180 Hypovolemia Management
6530 Immunization/Vaccination Administration
4370 Impulse Control Training
7980 Incident Reporting
3440 Incision Site Care
6820 Infant Care
6540 Infection Control
6545 Infection Control: Intraoperative
6550 Infection Protection
7410 Insurance Authorization
2590 Intracranial Pressure (ICP) Monitoring
6830 Intrapartal Care
6834 Intrapartal Care: High Risk Delivery
4190 Intravenous (IV) Insertion
4200 Intravenous (IV) Therapy
4210 Invasive Hemodynamic Monitoring
6840 Kangaroo Care
6850 Labor Induction
6860 Labor Suppression
7690 Laboratory Data Interpretation
5244 Lactation Counseling
6870 Lactation Suppression
6560 Laser Precautions
6570 Latex Precautions
5520 Learning Facilitation
5540 Learning Readiness Enhancement
3460 Leech Therapy
4380 Limit Setting
3840 Malignant Hyperthermia Precautions
3300 Mechanical Ventilation
3310 Mechanical Ventilatory Weaning
2300 Medication Administration
2301 Medication Administration: Enteral
2302 Medication Administration: Interpleural
2303 Medication Administration: Intraosseous
2304 Medication Administration: Oral
2305 Medication Administration: Parenteral
2306 Medication Administration: Topical
2307 Medication Administration: Ventricular Reservoir
2380 Medication Management
2390 Medication Prescribing
5960 Meditation
4760 Memory Training
4390 Milieu Therapy
5330 Mood Management
8020 Multidisciplinary Care Conference
4400 Music Therapy
4410 Mutual Goal Setting
1680 Nail Care
2620 Neurologic Monitoring
6880 Newborn Care
6890 Newborn Monitoring
6900 Nonnutritive Sucking
7200 Normalization Promotion
1100 Nutrition Management
1120 Nutrition Therapy
5246 Nutritional Counseling
1160 Nutritional Monitoring
1710 Oral Health Maintenance
1720 Oral Health Promotion
1730 Oral Health Restoration
8060 Order Transcription
6260 Organ Procurement
0480 Ostomy Care
3320 Oxygen Therapy
1400 Pain Management
5562 Parent Education: Adolescent
5564 Parent Education: Childbearing Family
5566 Parent Education: Childrearing Family
7440 Pass Facilitation
4420 Patient Contracting
2400 Patient Controlled Analgesia (PCA) Assistance
7450 Patient Rights Protection
7700 Peer Review
0560 Pelvic Floor Exercise
1750 Perineal Care
2660 Peripheral Sensation Management
4220 Peripherally Inserted Central (PIC) Catheter Care
2150 Peritoneal Dialysis Therapy
4232 Phlebotomy: Arterial Blood Supply
4234 Phlebotomy: Blood Unit Acquisition

4238 Phlebotomy: Venous Blood Sample
6924 Phlebotomy: Neonate
6580 Physical Restraint
7710 Physician Support
4430 Play Therapy
6590 Pneumatic Tourniquet Precautions
0840 Positioning
0842 Positioning: Intraoperative
0844 Positioning: Neurologic
0846 Positioning: Wheelchair
2870 Postanesthesia Care
1770 Postmortem Care
6930 Postpartal Care
7722 Preceptor: Employee
7726 Preceptor: Student
6247 Preconception Counseling
6950 Pregnancy Termination Care
6960 Prenatal Care
2880 Preoperative Coordination
5580 Preparatory Sensory Information
6340 Presence
3500 Pressure Management
3520 Pressure Ulcer Care
3540 Pressure Ulcer Prevention
7760 Product Evaluation
1460 Progressive Muscle Relaxation
1780 Prosthesis Care
7800 Quality Monitoring
6600 Radiation Therapy Management
6300 Rape-Trauma Treatment
4820 Reality Orientation
5360 Recreation Therapy
0490 Rectal Prolapse Management
8100 Referral
4860 Reminiscence Therapy
7886 Reproductive Techology Management
8120 Research Data Collection
3350 Respiratory Monitoring
7260 Respite Care
6320 Resuscitation
6972 Resuscitation: Fetus
6974 Resuscitation: Neonate
6610 Risk Identification
6612 Risk Identification: Childbearing Family
5370 Role Enhancement
6630 Seclusion
5380 Security Enhancement
2680 Seizure Management
2690 Seizure Precautions
5390 Self-Awareness Enhancement
1800 Self-Care Assistance
1801 Self-Care Assistance: Bathing/Hygiene
1802 Self-Care Assistance: Dressing/Grooming
1803 Self-Care Assistance: Feeding
1804 Self-Care Assistance: Toileting
5400 Self-Esteem Enhancement
4470 Self-Modification Assistance
4480 Self-Responsibility Facilitation
5248 Sexual Counseling
8140 Shift Report
4250 Shock Management
4254 Shock Management: Cardiac
4256 Shock Management: Vasogenic
4258 Shock Management: Volume
4260 Shock Prevention
7280 Sibling Support
6000 Simple Guided Imagery
1480 Simple Massage
6040 Simple Relaxation Therapy
3584 Skin Care: Topical Treatments
3590 Skin Surveillance
1850 Sleep Enhancement
4490 Smoking Cessation Assistance
5100 Socialization Enhancement
7820 Specimen Management
5420 Spiritual Support
0910 Splinting
7830 Staff Supervision
2720 Subarachnoid Hemorrhage Precautions
4500 Substance Use Prevention
4510 Substance Use Treatment
4512 Substance Use Treatment: Alcohol Withdrawal
4514 Substance Use Treatment: Drug Withdrawal
4516 Substance Use Treatment: Overdose
6340 Suicide Prevention
7840 Supply Management
5430 Support Group
5440 Support System Enhancement
2900 Surgical Assistance
2920 Surgical Precautions
2930 Surgical Preparation
6650 Surveillance
6656 Surveillance: Late Pregnancy
6654 Surveillance: Safety
7500 Sustenance Support
3620 Suturing
1860 Swallowing Therapy
5602 Teaching: Disease Process
5604 Teaching: Group
5606 Teaching: Individual
5608 Teaching: Infant Care
5610 Teaching: Preoperative
5612 Teaching: Prescribed Activity/Exercise
5614 Teaching: Prescribed Diet
5616 Teaching: Prescribed Medication
5618 Teaching: Procedure/Treatment
5620 Teaching: Psychomotor Skill
5622 Teaching: Safer Sex
5624 Teaching: Sexuality
7880 Technology Management
8180 Telephone Consultation
3900 Temperature Regulation
3902 Temperature Regulation: Intraoperative
5465 Therapeutic Touch
5450 Therapy Group
1200 Total Parenteral Nutrition (TPN) Administration
5460 Touch
0940 Traction/Immobilization Care
1540 Transcutaneous Electrical Nerve Stimulation (TENS)
0960 Transport
6360 Triage
5470 Truth Telling
1870 Tube Care
1872 Tube Care: Chest
1874 Tube Care: Gastrointestinal
1875 Tube Care: Umbilical Line
1876 Tube Care: Urinary
1878 Tube Care: Ventriculostomy Lumbar Drain
6982 Ultrasonography: Limited Obstetric
2760 Unilateral Neglect Management
0570 Urinary Bladder Training
0580 Urinary Catheterization
0582 Urinary Catheterization: Intermittent
0590 Urinary Elimination Management
0600 Urinary Habit Training
0610 Urinary Incontinence Care
0612 Urinary Incontinence Care: Enuresis
0620 Urinary Retention Care
5480 Values Clarification
2440 Venous Access Devices (VAD) Maintenance
3390 Ventilation Assistance
7560 Visitation Facilitation
6680 Vital Signs Monitoring
1240 Weight Gain Assistance
1260 Weight Management
1280 Weight Reduction Assistance
3660 Wound Care
3662 Wound Care: Closed Drainage
3680 Wound Irrigation

APPENDIX C

Diagnostic Studies and Interpretation

TEST VALUE STUDIED

Reference Ranges—Hematology
Reference Ranges—Serum, Plasma, and Whole Blood Chemistries
Reference Ranges—Immunodiagnostic Tests
Reference Ranges—Urine Chemistry
Reference Ranges—Cerebrospinal Fluid (CSF)
Miscellaneous Values

SELECTED ABBREVIATIONS USED IN REFERENCE RANGES

Conventional Units

kg = kilogram
gm = gram
mg = milligram
μg = microgram
μμg = micromicrogram
ng = nanogram
pg = picogram
dL = 100 milliliters
mL = milliliter
mm^3 = cubic millimeter
fL = femtoliter
mM = millimole
nM = nanomole
mOsm = milliosmole
mm = millimeter
μm = micron or micrometer
mm Hg = millimeters of mercury
U = unit
mU = milliunit
μU = microunit
mEq = milliequivalent
IU = International Unit
mIU = milliInternational Unit

SI Units

g = gram
L = liter
d = day
h = hour
mol = mole
mmol = millimole
μmol = micromole
nmol = nanomole
pmol = picomole

TABLE C•1 Reference Ranges—Hematology*

Determination	Reference Range: CONVENTIONAL UNITS	Reference Range: SI UNITS	CLINICAL SIGNIFICANCE
A_2 hemoglobin	1.5%–3.5% of total hemoglobin	Mass fraction: 0.015–0.035 of total hemoglobin	Increased in certain types of thalassemia
Bleeding time	1–9 min	1–9 min	Prolonged in thrombocytopenia, defective platelet function, and aspirin therapy
Factor V assay (proacceleri factor)	60%–140%		
Factor VIII assay (antihemophiliac factor)	50%–200%		Deficient in classical hemophilia
Factor IX assay (plasma thromboplastin component)	75%–125%		Deficient in Christmas disease (pseudohemophilia)
Factor X (Stuart factor)	60%–140%		Deficient in Stuart clotting defect
Fibrinogen	200–400 mg/dL	2–4 g/dL	Increased in pregnancy, infections accompanied by leukocytosis, nephrosis Decreased in severe liver disease, abruptio placentae
Fibrin split (degradation) products	Less than 10 mg/L	Less than 10 mg/L	Increased in disseminated intravascular coagulation
Fibrinolysins (whole blood clot lysis time)	No lysis in 24 h		Increased activity associated with massive hemorrhage, extensive surgery, transfusion reactions
Partial thromboplastin time (activated)	20–45 sec		Prolonged in deficiency of fibrinogen, factors II, V, VIII, IX, X, XI, and XII, and in heparin therapy
Prothrombin consumption	Over 20 sec		Impaired in deficiency of factors VIII, IX, and X
Prothrombin time	9.5–12 sec		Prolonged by deficiency of factors I, II, V, VII, and X, fat malabsorption, severe liver disease, coumarin anticoagulant therapy.
INR	1.0 2–3 for therapy in atrial fibrillation, deep vein thrombosis, and pulmonary enbolism 2.5–3.5 for therapy in prosthetic heart valves		INR used to standardize the prothrombin time and anticoagulation therapy
Erythrocyte count	Males: 4,600,000–6,200,000/cu mm Females: 4,200,000–5,400,000/cu mm	$4.6–6.2 \times 10^{12}$/L $4.2–5.4 \times 10^{12}$/L	Increased in severe diarrhea and dehydration, polycythemia, acute poisoning, pulmonary fibrosis Decreased in all anemias in leukemia, and after hemorrhage, when blood volume has been restored
Erythrocyte indices			
Mean corpuscular volume (MCV)	80–94 (cu μ)	80–94 fL	Increased in macrocytic anemias; decreased in microcytic anemia
Mean corpuscular hemoglobin (MCH)	27–32 μμg/cell	27–32 pg	Increased in macrocytic anemias; decreased in microcytic anemia
Mean corpuscular hemoglobin con centration (MCHC)	33%–38%	Concentration fraction: 0.33–0.38	Decreased in severe hypochromic anemia
Reticulocytes	0.5%–1.5% of red cells	Number fraction: 0.005–0.015	Increased with any condition stimulating increase in bone marrow activity (ie, infection, blood loss [acute and chronically following iron therapy in iron deficiency anemia], polycythemia rubra vera)

(continued)

TABLE C•1 Reference Ranges—Hematology* *(Continued)*

Determination	Reference Range: CONVENTIONAL UNITS	Reference Range: SI UNITS	CLINICAL SIGNIFICANCE
			Decreased with any condition depressing bone marrow activity, acute leukemia, late stage of severe anemias
Erythrocyte sedimentation rate (ESR)—Westergren method	Males under 50 yr: <15 mm/h Males over 50 yr: <20 mm/h Females under 50 yr: <20 mm/h Females over 50 yr: <30 mm/h	<15 mm/h <20 mm/h <20 mm/h <30 mm/h	Increased in tissue destruction, whether inflammatory or degenerative; during menstruation and pregnancy; and in acute febrile diseases
Erythrocyte sedimentation ratio—Zeta centrifuge	41%–54%	Fraction: 0.41–0.54	Significance similar to ESR
Hematocrit	Males: 42%–50% Females: 40%–48%	Volume fraction: 0.42–0.5 Volume fraction: 0.4–0.48	Decreased in severe anemias, anemia of pregnancy, acute massive blood loss Increased in erythrocytosis of any cause, and in dehydration or hemoconcentration associated with shock
Hemoglobin	Males: 13–18 gm/dL Females: 12–16 gm/dL	2.02–2.79 mmol/L 1.86–2.48 mmol/L	Decreased in various anemias, pregnancy, severe or prolonged hemorrhage, and with excessive fluid intake Increased in polycythemia, chronic obstructive pulmonary disease, failure of oxygenation because of congestive heart failure, and normally in people living at high altitudes
Hemoglobin F	Less than 2% of total hemoglobin	Mass fraction: <0.02	Increased in infants and children, and in thalassemia and many anemias
Leukocyte alkaline phosphatase	Score of 40–100		Increased in polycythemia vera, myelofibrosis, and infections Decreased in chronic granulocytic leukemia, paroxysmal nocturnal hemoglobinuria, hypoplastic marrow, and viral infections, particularly infectious mononucleosis
Leukocyte count	Total: 5,000–10,000/cu mm	$5–10 \times 10^9$/L	Elevated in acute infectious diseases, predominantly in the neutrophilic fraction with bacterial diseases, and in the lymphocytic and monocytic fractions in viral diseases Elevated in acute leukemia, following menstruation, and following surgery or trauma Depressed in aplastic anemia, agranulocytosis, and by toxic chemotherapeutic agents used in treating malignancy Eosinophils elevated in collagen disease, allergy, intestinal parasitosis
Neutrophils	60%–70%	Number fraction: 0.6–0.7	
Eosinophils	1%–4%	Number fraction: 0.01–0.04	
Basophils	0%–0.5%	Number fraction: 0.00–0.05	
Lymphocytes	20%–30%	Number fraction: 0.2–0.3	
Monocytes	2%–6%	Number fraction: 0.02–0.06	
Platelet count	100,000–400,000/cu mm	$0.1–0.4 \times 10^{12}$/L	Increased in malignancy, myeloproliferative disease, rheumatoid arthritis, and postoperatively; about 50% of patients with unexpected increase of platelet count will be found to have a malignancy Decreased in thrombocytopenic purpura, acute leukemia, aplastic anemia, and during cancer chemotherapy.

*Laboratory values may vary according to the techniques used in different laboratories.

Table C•2 Reference Ranges—Serum, Plasma, and Whole Blood Chemistries

Determination	Normal Adult Reference Range: Conventional Units	Normal Adult Reference Range: SI Units	Clinical Significance: Increased	Clinical Significance: Decreased
Acetoacetate	0.2–1.0 mg/dL	19.6–98 µmol/L	Diabetic acidosis Fasting	
Acetone	0.3–2.0 mg/dL	51.6–344.0/µmol/L	Diabetic ketoacidosis Toxemia of pregnancy Carbohydrate-free diet High-fat diet	
Acid, total phosphatase	0–11 UL	0-11 UL	Carcinoma of prostate Advanced Paget's disease Hyperparathyroidism Gaucher's disease	
Acid, phosphatase, prostatic—RLA	0–10 ng/mL Borderline: 2.5–3.3 IU/L	0–10 µg/L	Carcinoma of prostate	
Alkaline phosphatase	Adults: 30–150 mU/mL	30–150 µ/L	Conditions reflecting increased osteoblastic activity of bone Rickets Hyperparathyroidism Hepatic disease Bone disease	
Alkaline phosphatase, thermostable fraction	Thermostable fraction >35%: hepatic disease and combined disease with predominant hepatic component Thermostable fraction between 25% and 35%: combined hepatic and skeletal disease Thermostable fraction <25%: skeletal disease with increased osteoblastic activity			
Adrenocorticotropic hormone (ACTH) (plasma)—RIA*	Less than 50 pg/mL	Less than 50 mg/L	Pituitary-dependent Cushing's syndrome Ectopic ACTH syndrome Primary adrenal atrophy	Adrenocortical tumor Adrenal insufficiency secondary to hypopituitarism
Aldolase	3–8 Sibley-Lehninger U/dl at 37°C	22–59 mU/L at 37°C	Hepatic necrosis Granulocytic leukemia Myocardial infarction Skeletal muscle disease	
Aldosterone (plasma)—RIA	Supine: 3–10 ng/dL Upright: 5–30 ng/dL Adrenal vein: 200–800 ng/dL	0.08–0.30 nmol/L 0.14–0.90 nmol/L 5.54–22.16 nmol/L	Primary aldosteronism Secondary aldosteronism	Addison's disease
Alpha-1-antitrypsin	200–400 mg/dL	2–4 g/L		Certain forms of chronic lung and liver disease in young adults
Alpha-1-fetoprotein	None detected		Hepatocarcinoma Metastatic carcinoma of liver Germinal cell carcinoma of the testicle or ovary Fetal neural tube defects—elevation in maternal serum	
Alpha-hydroxybutyric dehydrogenase	Up to 140 U/mL	Up to 140 U/L	Myocardial infarction Granulocytic leukemia Hemolytic anemias Muscular dystrophy	
Ammonia (plasma)	40–80, ug/dL (enzymatic method); varies considerably with method	22.2–44.3/µmol/L	Severe liver disease Hepatic decompensation	

(continued)

* By radioimmunoassay.

TABLE C•2 Reference Ranges—Serum, Plasma, and Whole Blood Chemistries *(Continued)*

Determination	Normal Adult Reference Range: CONVENTIONAL UNITS	Normal Adult Reference Range: SI UNITS	Clinical Significance: INCREASED	Clinical Significance: DECREASED
Amylase	60–160 Somogyi U/dL	111–296U/L	Acute pancreatitis Mumps Duodenal ulcer Carcinoma of head of pancreas Prolonged elevation with pseudocyst of pancreas Increased by drugs that constrict pancreatic duct sphincters: morphine, codeine, cholinergics	Chronic pancreatitis Pancreatic fibrosis and atrophy Cirrhosis of liver Pregnancy (2nd and 3rd trimesters)
Arsenic	6–20 μg/dL; if 50 μg/dL, suspect toxicity	0.78–2.6 μmol/L	Intentional or unintentional poisoning Excessive occupational exposure	
Ascorbic acid (vitamin C)	0.4–1.5 mg/dL	23–85 μmol/L	Large doses of ascorbic acid as a prophylactic against the common cold	
ALT (alanine aminotransferase), formerly SGPT	10–40 U/mL	5–20 U/L	Same conditions as AST (SGOT), but increase is more marked in liver disease than AST (SGOT)	
AST (aspartate aminotransferase), formerly SGOT	7–40 U/mL	4–20 U/L	Myocardial infarction Skeletal muscle disease Liver disease	
Bilirubin	Total: 0.1–1.2 mg/dL Direct: 0.1–0.2 mg/dL Indirect: 0.1–1 mg/dL	1.7–20.5/μmol/L 1.7–3.4/μmol/L 1.7–17.1 μmol/L	Hemolytic anemia (indirect) Biliary obstruction and disease Hepatocellular damage (hepatitis) Pernicious anemia Hemolytic disease of newborn	
Blood gases				
Oxygen, arterial (whole blood):				
Partial pressure (PaO_2)	95–100 mm Hg	12.64–13.30kPa	Polycythemia	Anemia Cardiac or pulmonary disease
Saturation (SaO_2)	94%–100%	Volume fraction: 0.94–1	Anhydremia	Cardiac decompensation Chronic obstructive lung disease
Carbon dioxide, arterial (whole blood) partial pressure ($PaCO_2$)	35–45 mm Hg	4.66–5.99 kPa	Respiratory acidosis Metabolic alkalosis	Respiratory alkalosis Metabolic acidosis
pH (whole blood, arterial)	7.35–7.45	7.35–7.45	Vomiting Hyperventilation Fever Intestinal obstruction	Uremia Diabetic acidosis Hemorrhage Nephritis
Calcitonin	Basal: nondetectable 400 pg/mL	400 ng/L	Medullary carcinoma of the thyroid Some nonthyroid tumors Zollinger-Ellison syndrome	
Calcium	8.5–10.5 mg/dL	2.125–2.625 mmol/L	Tumor or hyperplasia of parathyroid Hypervitaminosis D Multiple myeloma Nephritis with uremia Malignant tumors Sarcoidosis Hyperthyroidism Skeletal immobilization Excess calcium intake:milk alkali syndrome	Hypoparathyroidism Diarrhea Celiac disease Vitamin D deficiency Acute pancreatitis Nephrosis After parathyroidectomy

(continued)

TABLE C•2 Reference Ranges—Serum, Plasma, and Whole Blood Chemistries *(Continued)*

Determination	Normal Adult Reference Range: CONVENTIONAL UNITS	Normal Adult Reference Range: SI UNITS	Clinical Significance: INCREASED	Clinical Significance: DECREASED
CO_2, venous	Adults 24–32 mEq/L Infants: 18–24 mEq/L	24–32 mmol/L 18–24 mmol/L	Tetany Respiratory disease Intestinal obstruction Vomiting	Acidosis Nephritis Eclampsia Diarrhea Anesthesia
Catecholamines (plasma)—RIA	Epinephrine, random: up to 90 pg/mL Norepinephrine, random 100 550 pg/mL Dopamine, random up to 130 pg/mL	Up to 490 pmol/L 590–3240 pmol/L Up to 850 pmol/L	Pheochromocytoma	
Ceruloplasmin	30–80 mg/dL	300–800 mg/L		Wilson's disease (hepatolenticular degeneration)
Chloride	95–105 mEq/L	95–105 mmol/L	Nephrosis Nephritis Urinary obstruction Cardiac decompensation Anemia	Diabetes Diarrhea Vomiting Pneumonia Heavy metal poisoning Cushing's syndrome Intestinal obstruction Febrile conditions
Cholesterol	150–200 mg/dL	3.9–5.2 mmol/L	Lipemia Obstructive jaundice Diabetes Hypothyroidism	Pernicious anemia Hemolytic anemia Hyperthyroidism Severe infection Terminal states of debilitating disease
Cholesterol esters	60%–70% of total	Fraction of total cholesterol 0.6–0.7		The esterified fraction decreases in liver diseases
Cholinesterase	Serum: 0.6–1.6 delta pH Red cells-0.6–1 delta pH	0.6–1.6 U 0.6–1 U	Nephrosis Exercise	Nerve gas intoxication (greater effect on red cell activity) Insecticide poisoning
Chorionic gonadotropin, beta subunit	0–5 IU/L	0–5 IU/L	Pregnancy Hydatidiform mole Choriocarcinoma	Threatened abortion Ectopic pregnancy
Complement, human C_3	70–150 mg/dL	880–2520 mg/L	Some inflammatory diseases, acute myocardial infarction, cancer	Acute glomerulonephritis Disseminated lupus erythematosus with renal involvement
Complement C4	16–45 mg/dL	140–510 mg/L	Some inflammatory diseases, acute myocardial infarction, cancer	Often decreased in immunologic disease, especially with active systemic lupus erythematosus Hereditary angioneurotic edema
Complement, total (hemolytic)	90%–94% complement	25–70 U/mL	Some inflammatory diseases	Acute glomerulonephritis Epidemic meningitis Subacute bacterial endocarditis
Copper	70–165 µg/dL	11–25.9 µmol/L	Cirrhosis of liver Pregnancy	Wilson's disease

(continued)

TABLE C•2 Reference Ranges—Serum, Plasma, and Whole Blood Chemistries *(Continued)*

Determination	Normal Adult Reference Range: Conventional Units	Normal Adult Reference Range: SI Units	Clinical Significance: Increased	Clinical Significance: Decreased
Cortisol-RIA	8 AM: 7–25/μg/dL 4 PM: 2–9 μg/dL	193–690 nmol/L 55–248 nmol/L	Stress: infectious disease, surgery, burns, etc. Pregnancy Cushing's syndrome Pancreatitis Eclampsia	Addison's disease Anterior pituitary hypofunction
C-peptide reactivity	1.5–10 ng/mL	1.5–10 μg/L	Insulinoma	Diabetes
Creatine	0.2–0.8 mg/mL	15.3–61 μmol/L	Pregnancy Skeletal muscle necrosis or atrophy Starvation Hyperthyroidism	
Creatine phosphokinase (CPK)	Males: 50–325 mU/mL Females: 50–250 mU/mL	50–325 U/L 50–250 U/L	Myocardial infarction Skeletal muscle diseases Intramuscular injections Crush syndrome Hypothyroidism Alcohol withdrawal delirium Alcoholic myopathy Cerebrovascular disease	
Creatine phosphokinase isoenzymes	MM band present (skeletal muscle)-MB band absent (heart muscle)		MB band increased in myocardial infarction, ischemia	
Creatinine	0.7–1.4 mg/dL	62–124 μmol/L	Nephritis Chronic renal disease	
Creatinine clearance	100–150 mL of blood cleared of creatinine per min	1.67–2.5 mL/s		Kidney diseases
Cryoglobulins, qualitative	Negative		Multiple myeloma Chronic lymphocytic leukemia Lymphosarcoma Systemic lupus erythematosus Rheumatoid arthritis Infective subacute endocarditis Some malignancies Scleroderma	
11-Deoxycortisol	1/μg/dL	<0.029 μmol/L	Hypertensive form of virilizing adrenal hyperplasia due to an 11-β-hydroxylase defect	
Dibucaine number	Normal: 70%–85% inhibition Heterozygote: 50%–65% inhibition Homozygote: 16%–25% inhibition			Important in detecting carriers of abnormal cholinesterase activity who are susceptible to succinylcholine anesthetic shock
Dihydrotestosterone	Males: 50–210 ng/dL Females: none detectable	1.72–7.22 nmol/L		Testicular feminization syndrome
Estradiol—RIA	Females: Follicular: 10–90 pg/mL Midcycle: 100–500 pg/mL Luteal: 50–240 pg/mL Follicular phase: 2–20 ng/dL Midcycle: 12–40 ng/dL Luteal phase: 10-30 ng/dL Postmenopausal: 1–5 ng/dL Males: 0.5–5 ng/dL	 37–370 pmol/L 367–1835 pmol/L 184–881 pmol/L	Pregnancy	Depressed or failure to peak—ovarian failure

(continued)

TABLE C•2 **Reference Ranges—Serum, Plasma, and Whole Blood Chemistries** *(Continued)*

Determination	Normal Adult Reference Range: CONVENTIONAL UNITS	SI UNITS	Clinical Significance: INCREASED	DECREASED
Estriol—RIA	Nonpregnant females: <0.5 ng/mL	<1.75 nmol/L	Pregnancy	Depressed or failure to peak—ovarian failure
	Pregnant females:			
	1st trimester: up to 1 ng/mL	Up to 3.5 nmol/L		
	2nd trimester: 0.8–7 ng/mL	2.8–24.3 nmol/L		
	3rd trimester: 5–25 ng/mL	17.4–86.8 nmol/L		
Estrogens, total—RIA	Females: cycle days:		Pregnancy	Fetal distress
	Day 1–10: 61–394 pg/mL	61–394 ng/L	Measured on a daily basis, can be used to evaluate response of hypogonadotrophic, hypo-estrogenic women to human menopausal or pituitary gonadotropin	Ovarian failure
	Day 11–20: 122 437 pg/mL	122–437 ng/L		
	Day 21–30: 156–350 pg/mL	156–350 ng/L		
	Males: 40–115 pg/mL	40–115 ng/L		
Estrone—RIA	Females:			Depressed or failure to peak—ovarian failure
	Day 1–10: 4.3–18 ng/dL	15.9–66.6 pmol/L		
	Day 11–20: 7.5–19.6 ng/dL	27.8–72.5 pmol/L		
	Day 21–30: 13–20 ng/dL	48.1–74 pmol/L		
	Males: 2.5–7.5 ng/dL	9.3–27.8 pmol/L		
Ferritin—RIA	Males: 29–438 ng/mL	29–438 µg/L	Nephritis	Iron deficiency
	Females: 9–219 ng/mL	9–219 µg/L	Hemochromatosis Certain neoplastic diseases Acute myelogenous leukemia Multiple myeloma	
Folic acid—RIA	2.5–20 ng/mL	6–46 nmol/L		Megaloblastic anemias of infancy and pregnancy Inadequate diet Liver disease Malabsorption syndrome Severe hemolytic anemia
Follicle stimulating hormone (FSH)—RIA	Males: 2–10 mIU/mL		Menopause and primary ovarian failure	Pituitary failure
	Females:	5–20 IU/L		
	Follicular phase: 5–20 mIU/mL			
	Peak of middle cycle: 12–30 mIU/mL	12–30 IU/L		
	Luteinic phase: 5–15 mIU/mL	5–15 IU/L		
	Menopausal females: 40–200 mIU/mL	40–200 IU/L		
Galactose	<5 mg/dL	<0.28 mmol/L		Galactosemia
Gamma glutamyl transpeptidase	Males: <45 IU/L	45 U/L	Hepatobiliary disease	
	Females: <30 IU/L	30 U/L	Drug toxicity Myocardial infarction Renal infarction Zollinger-Ellison syndrome	
Gastrin—RIA	Fasting: 50–155 pg/mL	50–155 ng/L	Peptic ulceration of the duodenum Pernicious anemia	
	Postprandial: 80–170 pg/mL	80–170 ng/L		

(continued)

TABLE C•2 Reference Ranges—Serum, Plasma, and Whole Blood Chemistries *(Continued)*

Determination	Normal Adult Reference Range: CONVENTIONAL UNITS	SI UNITS	Clinical Significance: INCREASED	DECREASED
Glucose	Fasting: 60–110 mg/dL Postprandial (2 h): 65–140 mg/dL	3.3–6.05 mmol/L 3.58–7.7 mmol/L	Diabetes Nephritis Hyperthyroidism Early hyperpituitarism Cerebral lesions Infections Pregnancy Uremia	Hyperinsulinism Hypothyroidism Late hyperpituitarism Pernicious vomiting Addison's disease Extensive hepatic damage
Glucose tolerance (oral)	Features of a normal response: 1. Normal fasting between 60–110 mg/dL 2. No sugar in urine 3. Upper limits of normal: Fasting = 125 1 hour = 190 2 hours = 140 3 hours = 125	3.3–6.05 mmol/L 6.88 mmol/L 10.45 mmol/L 7.70 mmol/L 6.88 mmol/L	Two-hour value >200 mg/dL (11.1 mmol/L) is diagnostic for diabetes	Decreased 2 and 3 hour values may occur with hypoglycemia
Glucose-6-phosphate dehydrogenase (red cells)	Screening: Decolorization in 20–100 min Quantitative: 1.86–2.5 IU/mL RBC	1860–2500 U/L		Drug-induced hemolytic anemia Hemolytic disease of newborn
Glycoprotein (alpha-1-acid)	40–110 mg/dL	400–1100 mg/L	Neoplasm Tuberculosis Diabetes complicated by degenerative vascular disease Pregnancy Rheumatoid arthritis Rheumatic fever Infectious liver disease Lupus erythematosus	
Growth hormone—RIA	< 10 ng/mL	< 10 mg/L	Acromegaly	Failure to stimulate with arginine or insulin—hypopituitarism
Haptoglobin	50–250 mg/dL	0.5–2.5 g/L	Pregnancy Estrogen therapy Chronic infections Various inflammatory conditions	Hemolytic anemia Hemolytic blood transfusion reaction
Hemoglobin (plasma)	0.5–5 mg/dL	5–50 mg/L	Transfusion reactions Paroxysmal nocturnal hemoglobinuria Intravascular hemolysis	
Glycohemoglobin (GHB, hemoglobin A_{1c}, hemoblobin A1)	Nondiabetics & diabetics with good control: 4.4%–6.4%		Suboptimal glucose control	Anemia, pregnancy, chronic renal failure
Hexosaminidase, total	Controls: 333–375 nM/mL/h	333–375 µmol/L/h	Sandhoff's disease	
Hexosaminidase A	Controls: 49%–68% of total Heterozygotes: 26%–45% of total Tay-Sachs disease: 0%–4% of total Diabetics: 39%–59% of total	Fraction of total: 0.49–0.68 0.26–0.45 0–0.04 0.39–0.59		Tay-Sachs disease and heterozygotes

(continued)

TABLE C•2 Reference Ranges—Serum, Plasma, and Whole Blood Chemistries *(Continued)*

	Normal Adult Reference Range		Clinical Significance	
Determination	CONVENTIONAL UNITS	SI UNITS	INCREASED	DECREASED
High-density lipoprotein cholesterol (HDL cholesterol)	Males: 35–70 mg/dL Females: 35 –85 mg/dL	0.91–1.81 mmol/L 0.91–220 mmol/L		HDL cholesterol is lower in patients with increased risk for coronary heart disease
17 Hydroxy-progesterone—RIA	Males: 0.4–4 ng/mL Females: 0.1–3.3 ng/mL Children: 0.1–0.5 ng/mL	1.2–12 nmol/L 0.3–10 nmol/L 0.3–1.5 nmol/L	Congenital adrenal hyperplasia Pregnancy Some cases of adrenal or ovarian adenomas	
Immunoglobulin A	Adults: 50–300 mg/dL (in children the normals are lower and vary with age)	0.5–3 g/L	Gamma A myeloma Wiskott-Aldrich syndrome Autoimmune disease Hepatic cirrhosis	Ataxia telangiectasis Agammaglobulinemia Hypogammaglobulinemia, transient Dysgammaglobulinemia Protein-losing enteropathies
Immunoglobulin D	0–30 mg/dL	0–300 mg/L	IgD multiple myeloma Some patients with chronic infectious diseases	
Immunoglobulin E	20–740 ng/mL	20–740 μg/L	Allergic patients and those with parasitic infections	
Immunoglobulin G	Adults: 565–1765 mg/dL	6.35–14 g/L	IgG myeloma Following hyperimmunization Autoimmune disease states Chronic infections	Congenital and acquired hypogammaglobulinemia IgA myelomas, Waldenstrom's (IgM) macroglobulinemia Some malabsorption syndromes Extensive protein loss
Immunoglobulin M	Adults: 55–375 mg/dL	0.4–2.8 g/L	Waldenström's macroglobulinemia Parasitic infections Hepatitis	Agammaglobulinemias Some IgG and IgA myelomas Chronic lymphatic leukemia
Insulin—RIA	5–25 μU/mL	0.2–1 μg/L	Insulinoma Acromegaly	Diabetes mellitus
Iron	50–160/μg/dL	9–29 μmol/L	Pernicious anemia Aplastic anemia Hemolytic anemia Hepatitis Hemochromatosis	Iron deficiency anemia
Iron-binding capacity	IBC: 150–235 μg/dL TIBC: 230–410 μg/dL % Saturation: 20–50	26.9–42.1 μmol/L 41–73 μmol/L Fraction of total iron-binding capacity: 0.2-0.5	Iron deficiency anemia Acute and chronic blood loss Hepatitis	Chronic infectious diseases Cirrhosis
Isocitric dehydrogenase	50–180 U	0.83–3 UIL	Hepatitis, cirrhosis Obstructive jaundice Metastatic carcinoma of the liver Megaloblastic anemia	
Lactic acid (whole blood)	Venous: 5–20 mg/dL Arterial: 3–7 mg/dL	0.6–2.2 mmol/L 0.3–0.8 mmol/L	Increased muscular activity Congestive heart failure Hemorrhage Shock Lactic acidosis Some febrile infections May be increased in severe liver disease	

(continued)

TABLE C•2 Reference Ranges—Serum, Plasma, and Whole Blood Chemistries *(Continued)*

Determination	Normal Adult Reference Range: CONVENTIONAL UNITS	Normal Adult Reference Range: SI UNITS	Clinical Significance: INCREASED	Clinical Significance: DECREASED
Lactic dehydrogenase (LDH)	100–225 mU/mL	100–225 U/L	Untreated pernicious anemia Myocardial infarction Pulmonary infarction Liver disease	
Lactic dehydrogenase isoenzymes				
Total lactic dehydrogenase	100–225 mU/mL	100–225 U/L Fraction of total LDH:	LDH-1 and LDH-2 are increased in myocardial infarction, megaloblastic anemia, and hemolytic anemia LDH-4 and LDH-5 are increased in pulmonary infarction, congestive heart failure, and liver disease	
LDH-1	20%–35%	0.2–0.35		
LDH-2	25%–40%	0.25–0.4		
LDH-3	20%–30%	0.2–0.3		
LDH-4	0–20%	0–0.2		
LDH-5	0–25%	0–0.25		
Lead (whole blood)	Up to 40 µg/dL	Up to 2 µmol/L	Lead poisoning	
Leucine aminopeptidase	80–200 U/mL	19.2–48 U/L	Liver or bilary tract diseases Pancreatic disease Metastatic carcinoma of liver and pancreas Biliary obstruction	
Lipase	0.2–1.5 U/mL	55–417 U/L	Acute and chronic pancreatitis Biliary obstruction Cirrhosis Hepatitis Peptic ulcer	
Lipids, total	400–1000 mg/dL	4–10 g/L	Hypothyroidism Diabetes Nephrosis Glomerulonephritis Hyperlipoproteinemias	Hyperthyroidism
Low-density lipoprotein cholesterol (LDL cholesterol)	mg/dL desirable levels: <160 if no coronary artery disease (CAD) and <2 risk factors <130 if no CAD and 2 or more risk factors <100 if CAD present		LDL cholesterol is higher in patients with increased risk for coronary heart disease	
Luteinizing hormone—RIA	Males: 4.9–15 MIU/mL	4.9–15 mg/L	Pituitary tumor Ovarian failure	Depressed or failure to peak—pituitary failure
	Females:			
	Follicular phase: 2–3 MIU/mL	0.5–6.9 mg/L		
	Ovulatory peak: 40–200 MIU/mL	9.2 –46 mg/L		
	Luteal phase: 0–20 MIU/mL	0–5 mg/L		
	Postmenopausal: 35–120 mIU/mL	8–27.5 mg/L		
Lysozyme (muramidase)	2.8–8 µg/mL	2.8–8 mg	Certain types of leukemia (acute monocytic leukemia) Inflammatory states and infections	Acute lymphocytic leukemia
Magnesium	1.3–2.4 mEq/L	0.7–1.2 mmol/L	Excess ingestion of magnesium-containing antacids	Chronic alcoholism Severe renal disease Diarrhea Defective growth
Manganese	0.04–1.4 µg/dL	72.9–255 nmol/L		
Mercury	Up to 10 µg/dL	Up to 0.5/µmol/L	Mercury poisoning	

(continued)

TABLE C•2 Reference Ranges—Serum, Plasma, and Whole Blood Chemistries *(Continued)*

Determination	Normal Adult Reference Range: CONVENTIONAL UNITS	SI UNITS	Clinical Significance: INCREASED	DECREASED
Myoglobin—RIA	Up to 85 ng/mL	Up to 85 μg/mL	Myocardial infarction Muscle necrosis	
5′ Nucleotidase	3.2–11.6 IU/L	3.2–11.6 U/L	Hepatobiliary disease	
Osmolality	280–300 mOsm/kg	280–300 mmol/L	Diabetes insipidus Osmotic diuresis	Inappropriate secretion of ADH Addison's disease
Parathyroid hormone	160–350 pg/mL	160–350 ng/L	Hyperparathyroidism	Chronic renal failure Hypoparathyroidism
Phenylalanine	1.2–3.5 mg/dL 1st week 0.7–3.5 mg/dL thereafter	0.07–0.21 mmol/L 0.04–0.21 mmol/L	Phenylketonuria	
Phosphohexose isomerase	20–90 IU/L	20–90 U/L	Malignancy Disease of heart, liver, and skeletal muscles	
Phospholipids	125 300 mg/dL	1.25–3 g/L	Diabetes Nephritis	
Phosphorus, inorganic	2.5–4.5 mg/dL	0.8–1.45 mmol/L	Chronic nephritis Hypoparathyroidism	Hyperparathyroidism Vitamin D deficiency
Potassium	3.8–5 mEq/L	3.8–5 mmol/L	Renal Failure Acidosis Cell lysis Tissue breakdown or hemolysis	GI losses Diuretic administration
Progesterone—RIA	Follicular phase: up to 0.8 ng/mL Luteal phase: 10–20 ng/mL End of cycle: <1 ng/mL Pregnant: up to 50 ng/mL in 20th week	2.5 nmol/L 31.8–63.6 nmol/L <3 nmol/L Up to 160 nmol/L	Useful in evaluation of menstrual disorders and infertility and in the evaluation of placental function during pregnancies complicated by toxemia, diabetes mellitus, or threatened miscarriage	
Prolactin—RIA	6–24 ng/mL	6–24 μg/L	Pregnancy Functional or structural disorders of the hypothalamus Pituitary stalk section Pituitary tumors	
Prostate-specific antigen	<4 ng/mL		Prostatic cancer, benign prostatic hyperplasia, prostatitis	
Protein, total Albumin Globulin	6–8 gm/dL 3.5–5 gm/dL 1.5–3 gm/dL	60–80 g/L 35–50 g/L 15–30 g/L	Hemoconcentration Shock Multiple myeloma (globulin fraction) Chronic infections (globulin function) Liver disease (globulin)	Malnutrition Hemorrhage Loss of plasma from burns Proteinuria
Protein Electrophoresis (cellulose acetate) Albumin Alpha-1 globulin Alpha-2 globulin Beta globulin Gamma globulin	 3.5–5 gm/dL 0.1–0.4 gm/dL 0.4–1.2 gm/dL 0.6–1.2 gm/dL 0.5–1.6 gm/dL	35–50 g/L 24 g/L 6–10 g/L 1–4 g/L 4–12 g/L 5–11 g/L 5–16 g/L		
Protoporphyrin erythrocyte (whole blood)	15–100 μg/dL	0.27–1.80 μmol/L	Lead toxicity Erythropoietic porphyria	
Pyridoxine	3.6–18 ng/mL			A wide spectrum of clinical conditions, such as mental depression, peripheral neuropathy, anemia, neonatal seizures, and reactions to certain drug therapies

(continued)

TABLE C•2 Reference Ranges—Serum, Plasma, and Whole Blood Chemistries *(Continued)*

Determination	Normal Adult Reference Range: CONVENTIONAL UNITS	SI UNITS	Clinical Significance: INCREASED	DECREASED
Pyruvic acid (whole blood)	0.3–0.7 mg/dL	34–80 μmol/L	Diabetes Severe thiamine deficiency Acute phase of some infections, possibly secondary to increased glycogenolysis and glycolysis	
Renin (plasma)—RLA	Normal diet: Supine: 0.3–1.9 ng/mL/h Upright: 0.6–3.6 ng/mL/h Low salt diet: Supine: 0.9–4.5 ng/mL/h Upright: 4.1–9.1 ng/mL/h	 0.08–0.52 ng/L/S 0.16–1.00 μg/L/S 0.25–1.25 μg/L/S 1.13–2.53 μg/L/S	Renovascular hypertension Malignant hypertension Untreated Addison's disease Primary salt-losing nephropathy Low-salt diet Diuretic therapy Hemorrhage	Frank primary aldosteronism Increased salt intake Salt-retaining steroid therapy Antidiuretic hormone therapy Blood transfusion
Sodium	135–145 mEq/L	135–145 mmol/L	Hemoconcentration Nephritis Pyloric obstruction	Alkali deficit Addison's disease Myxedema
Sulfate (inorganic)	0.5–1.5 mg/dL	0.05–0.15 mmol/L	Nephritis Nitrogen retention	
Testosterone—RIA	Females: 25–100 ng/dL Males: 300–800 ng/dL	0.9–3.5 nmol/L 10.5–28 nmol/L	Females: Polycystic ovary Virilizing tumors	Males Orchidectomy for neoplastic disease of the prostate or breast Estrogen therapy Klinefelter's syndrome Hypopituitarism Hypogonadism Hepatic cirrhosis
T_3 (triiodothyronine) uptake	25%–35%	Relative uptake fraction: 0.25–0.35	Hyperthyroidism Thyroxine-binding globulin (TBG) deficiency Androgens and anabolic steroids	Hypothyroidism Pregnancy TBG excess Estrogens and antiovulatory drugs
T_3 total circulating—RIA	75–200 ng/dL	1.15–3.1 nmol/L	Pregnancy Hyperthyroidism	Hypothyroidism
T_4 (thyroxine)—RIA	4.5–11.5 μg/dL	58.5–150 nmol/L	Hyperthyroidism Thyroiditis Elevated thyroxine-binding proteins caused by oral contraceptives Pregnancy	Primary and pituitary hypothyroidism Idiopathic involvement Cases of diminished thyroxine-binding proteins caused by androgenic and anabolic steroids Hypoproteinemia Nephrotic syndrome
T_4, free	1–2.2 ng/dL	13–30 pmol/L	Euthyroid patients with normal free thyroxine levels may have abnormal T3 and T4 levels caused by drug preparations	
Thyroid-stimulating hormone (TSH)—RIA		0.3–5 m/IU/L	Hypothyroidism	Hyperthyroidism
Thyroid-binding globulin	10–26 μg/dL	100–260/μg/L	Hypothyroidism Pregnancy Estrogen therapy Oral contraceptives Genetic and idiopathic liver disease	Use of androgens and anabolic steroids Nephrotic syndrome Marked hypoproteinemia

(continued)

TABLE C•2 Reference Ranges—Serum, Plasma, and Whole Blood Chemistries *(Continued)*

	Normal Adult Reference Range		Clinical Significance	
Determination	CONVENTIONAL UNITS	SI UNITS	INCREASED	DECREASED
Transferrin	230–320 mg/dL	2.3–3.2 g/L	Pregnancy Iron deficiency anemia due to hemorrhaging Acute hepatitis Polycythemia Oral contraceptives	Pernicious anemia in relapse Thalassemic and sickle cell anemia Chromatosis Neoplastic and hepatic diseases
Triglycerides	10–150 mg/dL	0.10–1.65 mmol/L		
Tryptophan	1.4–3 mg/dL	68.6–147 nmol/L		Tryptophan-specific malabsorption syndrome
Tyrosine	0.5–4 mg/dL	27.6–220.8 mmol/L	Tyrosinosis	
Urea nitrogen (BUN)	10–20 mg/dL	3.6–7.2 mmol/L	Acute glomerulonephritis Obstructive uropathy Mercury poisoning Nephrotic syndrome	Severe hepatic failure Pregnancy
Uric acid	2.5–8 mg/dL	0.15–0 mmol/L	Gouty arthritis Acute leukemia Lymphomas treated by chemotherapy Toxemia of pregnancy	Defective tubular reabsorption
Viscosity	1.4–1.8 relative to water at 37°C (98.6°F)		Patients with marked increases of the gamma globulins	
Vitamin A	50–220 Hg/dL	1.75–7.7 µmol/L	Hypervitaminosis A	Vitamin A deficiency Celiac disease Sprue Obstructive jaundice Giardiasis Parenchymal hepatic disease
Vitamin B, (thiamine)	1.6–4 µg/dL	47.4–135.7 nmol/L		Anorexia Beriberi Polyneuropathy Cardiomyopathies
Vitamin B6 (pyridoxal phosphate)	3.6–18 ng/mL	14.6–72.8 nmol/L		Chronic alcoholism Malnutrition Uremia Neonatal seizures Malabsorption, such as celiac syndrome
Vitamin B12—RIA	130–785 pg/mL	100–580 pmol/L	Hepatic cell damage and in association with the myeloproliferative disorders (the highest levels are encountered in myeloid leukemia)	Strict vegetarianism Alcoholism Pernicious anemia Total or partial gastrectomy Ileal resection Sprue and celiac disease Fish tapeworm infestation
Vitamin E	0.5–2 mg/dL	11.6–46.4 µmol/L		Vitamin E deficiency
Xylose absorption test	2 hr, 30–50 mg/dL	2–3.35 mmol/L		Malabsorption syndrome
Zinc	55–150/µg/dL	7.65–22.95 µmol/L	Coronary artery disease Arteriosclerosis Industrial exposure	Metastatic liver disease Tuberculosis Sprue

TABLE C•3 Reference Ranges—Immunodiagnostic Test

Determination	Normal Value	Clinical Significance
Acetylcholine receptor binding antibody	Negative or <0.03 nmol/L	Considered to be diagnostic for myasthenia gravis in patients with symptoms.
Anti-ds-DNA antibody	<70 U by enzyme-linked immunosorbent assay (ELISA) <1:20 by indirect fluorescence	Valuable in supporting diagnosis or monitoring disease activity and prognosis of systemic lupus erythematosus (SLE).
Antiglomerular basement membrane antibody	Negative or less than 10 U	Primarily used in the differential diagnosis of glomerular nephritis induced by antiglomerular basement membrane antibodies from other types of glomerular nephritis.
Anti-insulin antibody	<3% binding of labeled beef and pork insulin by patient's serum; or <9 mIU/L	Helpful in determining the best therapeutic agent in diabetics and the cause of allergic manifestations. Also used to identify insulin resistance.
Antimitochondrial antibody and anti-smooth muscle antibody	<1:5 and <1:20, respectively	Increased in cirrhosis, autoimmune disease, thyroiditis, pernicious anemia.
Antinuclear antibody	Negative, <1:20	Increased in SLE, chronic hepatitis, scleroderma, leukemia, and mononucleosis.
Anti-parietal cell antibody	Negative, <1:20	Helpful in diagnosing chronic gastric disease and differentiating autoimmune pernicious anemia from other megaloblastic anemias.
Antiribonucleoprotein antibody	Negative	Helpful in differential diagnosis of systemic rheumatic disease.
Antiscleroderma antibody	Negative	Highly diagnostic for scleroderma.
Anti-Smith antibody	Negative	Highly diagnostic of SLE.
Anti-SS-A/anti-SS-B antibody	Negative	SS-A antibodies are found in Sjögren's syndrome alone or associated with lupus. SS-B antibodies are associated with primary Sjögren's syndrome.
Antithyroglobulin and antimicrosomal antibodies	<1:100 titer by gelatin or hemagglutination	Presence and concentration is important in evaluation and treatment of various thyroid disorders, such as Hashimoto's thyroiditis and Graves' disease. May indicate previous antoimmune disorders.
CA 15-3 tumor marker	<22 IU/ml	Increased in metastatic breast cancer.
CA 19-9 tumor marker	<37 IU/ml	Increased in pancreatic, hepatobiliary, gastric, and colorectal cancer, gallstones.
CA 125	0–35 IU/ml	Increased in colon, upper gastrointestinal (GI), ovarian, and other gynecologic cancers: pregnancy, peritonitis.
Carcinoembryonic antigen (CEA)—RLK	0–2.5 11g/L (nonsmoker) 0–5/μg/L (smoker)	The repeatedly high incidence of this antigen in cancers of the colon, rectum, pancreas, and stomach suggests that CEA levels may be useful in the therapeutic monitoring of these conditions, but it is not a screening test
Cold agglutinins	<1:16	Increased in mycoplasma pneumonia, viral illness, mononucleosis, multiple myeloma, scleroderma.
C-reactive protein	<0.8 mg/dL	Increase indicates active inflammation.
Cytomegalovirus antibodies (CMV IgG)	Negative: <0.9 units/mL	Positive >1.0 unit/mL if exposed to CMV at anytime. Acute and convalescent specimens can help identify acute infection.
Cytomegalovirus antibodies (CMV IgM)	Negative: <0.79 Equivocal: 0.80–1.20	Positive >1.20 usually indicates acute infection. Repeat specimen in 1–2 weeks for equivocal result.
Epstein-Barr virus serology (viral capsid antigen IgG and IgM, early antigen IgG, and nuclear antigen IgG)	Negative is <1:20 or <20 for each individual test	Differentiation of acute from chronic or old infection by interpretation of table below.

EBV Interpretation

	VCA-IgG	VCA-IgM	EA-IgG	EBV-NA
Susceptible	–	–	–	–
Acute infection	+	+	±	–
Convalescent phase	+	±	±	+
Chronic or reactivated	+	–	+	±
Old infection	±	–	–	+

Antibody present: +
Antibody absent: –
VCA, viral capsid antigen; EA, early antigen; EBV-NA, Epstein Barr virus-nuclear antigen

(*continued*)

TABLE C•3 Reference Ranges—Immunodiagnostic Test *(Continued)*

Determination	Normal Value	Clinical Significance
Hepatitis A virus antibodies, IgM (HAV-Ab/IgM)	Negative	Positive in acute-stage hepatitis A; develops early in disease.
Hepatitis A virus antibodies, IgG (HAV-Ab/IgG)	Negative	Positive if previous exposure and immunity to hepatitis A.
Hepatitis B surface antigen (HBsAg)	Negative	Positive in acute-stage hepatitis B.
Hepatitis B surface antibody (HBsAb)	Negative	Positive if previous exposure and immunity to hepatitis B.
Hepatitis C virus antibodies	Negative	Positive in exposure to hepatitis C virus; may indicate acute, chronic, or cleared infection.
Hepatitis C virus RNA	Negative	Positive in hepatitis C infection, can be quantitative
Infectious mononucleosis tests (monospot, monotest, heterophile antigen test, Epstein-Barr virus (EBV), antiviral capsid antigen IgM and IgG)	Negative, <1:80	Positive monospot and monotest are presumptive, positive EBV IgM and IgG indicate acute and recent or past infection, respectively.
Lyme disease titer	Negative, <1:256 by indirect fluorescent antibody method <0.8 by ELISA	Positive results help diagnose Lyme disease. False positive may occur with high rheumatoid factor titers or syphilis. Positive ELISA confirmed by Western blot test.
Pyroglobulin test	Negative	These abnormal proteins may be associated with myeloma, lymphoma, polycythemia vera, and SLE.
Rheumatoid factor	Negative or less than 60 IU/mL	Elevated in rheumatoid arthritis, lupus endocarditis, tuberculosis, syphilis, sarcoidosis, cancer.
T and B cell lymphocyte surface markers T-helper/T-suppressor ratio	T and B cell lymphocyte surface markers: Percent T cells (CD2) 60–88% Percent helper cells (CD4) 34–67% Percent suppressor cells (CD8) 10–42% Percent B cells (CD19) 3–21% Absolute counts: Lymphocytes 0.66–4.60 thou/mL T cells 644–2201 cells/mL Helper cells 493–1191 cells/mL Suppressor T cells 182–785 cells/mL B cells 92–392 cells/mL Lymphocyte ratio: T_H/T_S ratio > 1	Done to evaluate immune system by identifying the specific cells involved in the immune response. Valuable in diagnosis of lymphocytic leukemia, lymphoma, and immunodeficiency diseases including acquired immunodeficiency syndrome, and in the assessment of patient response to chemotherapy and radiation.

TABLE C•4 Reference Ranges—Urine Chemistry

	Normal Adult Reference Range		Clinical Significance	
Determination	CONVENTIONAL UNITS	SI UNITS	INCREASED	DECREASED
Acetone and acetoacetate	Zero		Uncontrolled diabetes Starvation	
Aldosterone	With normal salt diet: Normal: 4–20 μg/24 h Renovascular: 10–40 μg/24 h Tumor: 20–100 μg/24 h	 11.1–55.5 nmol/24h 27.7–111 nmol/24 h 55.4–277 nmol/24 h	Primary aldosteronism (adrenocortical tumor) Secondary aldosteronism Salt depletion Potassium loading ACTH in large doses Cardiac failure Cirrhosis with ascites formation Nephrosis Pregnancy	

(continued)

TABLE C•4 Reference Ranges—Urine Chemistry *(Continued)*

	Normal Adult Reference Range		Clinical Significance	
Determination	CONVENTIONAL UNITS	SI UNITS	INCREASED	DECREASED
Alpha amino nitrogen	50–200 mg/24 h	3.6–14.3 nmol/24 h	Leukemia Phenylketonuria Other metabolic diseases	
Amylase	35–260 units excreted per h	6.5–48.1 U/h	Acute pancreatitis	
Arylsulfatase A	>2.4 U/mL			Metachromatic leukodystrophy
Bence-Jones protein	None detected		Myeloma	
Calcium	<150 mg/24 h	<3.75 mmol/24 h	Hyperparathyroidism Vitamin D intoxication Fanconi's syndrome	Hypoparathyroidism Vitamin D deficiency
Catecholamines	Total: 0–275 μg/24 h Epinephrine: 10%–40% Norepinephrine: 60%–90%	0–275 μg/24 h Fraction total: 0.10–8.4 Fraction total: 0.60–0.90	Pheochromocytoma Neuroblastoma	
Chorionic gonadotrophin, qualitative (pregnancy test)	Negative		Pregnancy Chorionepithelioma Hydatidiform mole	
Copper	20–70 μg/24 h	0.32–1.12 μmol/24 h	Wilson's diseases Cirrhosis Nephrosis	
Coproporphyrin	50–300 μg/24 h	0.075–0.45 μmol/24 h	Poliomyelitis Lead poisoning Porphyria	
Cortisol, free	20–90 Hg/24 h	55.2–248.4 mmol/d	Cushing's syndrome	
Creatinine	0–200 mg/24 h	0–1.52 mmol/24 h	Muscular dystrophy Fever Carcinoma of liver Pregnancy Hyperthyroidism Myositis	
Creatine	0.8–2 gm/24 h	7–17.6 mmol/24 h	Typhoid fever Salmonella infections Tetanus	Muscular atrophy Anemia Advanced degeneration of kidneys Leukemia
Creatinine clearance	100–150 mL of blood cleared of creatinine per mm	1.67–2.5 mL/s		Measures glomerular filtration rate Renal diseases
Cystine and cysteine	10–100 mg/24 h	0.08–0.83 mmol/24 h	Cystinuria	
Delta aminolevulimic acid	0–0.54 mg/dL	0–40/μmol/L	Lead poisoning Porphyria hepatica Hepatitis Hepatic carcinoma	
11-Desoxycortisol	20–100 μg/24 h	0.6–2.9/μmol/d	Hypertensive form of virilizing adrenal hyperplasia due to an 11-beta hydroxylase defect	
Estriol (placental)	(see below)			Decreased values occur with fetal distress of many conditions, including preeclampsia, placental insufficiency, and poorly controlled diabetes mellitus

Weeks of pregnancy	μm/24 h	mmol/24 h
12	<1	<3.5
16	2–7	7–24.5
20	4–9	14–32
24	6–13	21–45.5
28	8–22	28–77
32	12–43	42–150
36	14–45	49–158
40	19–46	66.5–160

(continued)

TABLE C•4 Reference Ranges—Urine Chemistry *(Continued)*

	Normal Adult Reference Range		Clinical Significance	
Determination	CONVENTIONAL UNITS	SI UNITS	INCREASED	DECREASED
Estrogens, total (fluorometric)	Females: Onset of menstruation: 4–25 μg/24 h Ovulation peak: 28 μg/24 h Luteal peak: 22–105 μg/24 h Menopausal: 1.4–19.6 μg/24 h Males: 5–18 μg/24 h	 4–25 μg/24 h 28 μg/24 h 22–105 μg/24 h 1.4–19.6 μg/24 h 5–18 μg/24 h	Hyperestrogenism due to gonadal or adrenal neoplasm	Primary or secondary amenorrhea
Etiocholanolone	Males: 1.9–6 mg/24 h Females: 0.5–4 mg/24 h	6.5–20.6 μmol/24 h 1.7–13.8 μmol/24 h	Adrenogenital syndrome Idiopathic hirsutism	
Follicle-stimulating hormone—RIA	Females: Follicular: 5–20 IU/24 h Luteal: 5–15 IU/24 h Midcycle: 15–60 IU/24 h Menopausal: 50–100 IU/24 h Males: 5–25 IU/24 h	 5–20 IU/d 5–15 IU/d 15–60 IU/d 50–100 IU/d 5–25 IU/d	Menopause and primary ovarian failure	Pituitary failure
Glucose	Negative		Diabetes mellitus Pituitary disorders Increased ICP Lesion in floor of 4th ventricle	
Hemoglobin and myoglobin	Negative		Extensive burns Transfusion of incompatible blood Myoglobin increased in severe crushing injuries to muscles	
Homogentistic add, qualitative	Negative		Alkaptonuria Ochronosis	
Homovanillic acid	Up to 15 mg/24 h	Up to 82 μmol/d	Neuroblastoma	
17-hydroxycorticosteroids	2–10 mg/24 h	5.5–27.5 μmol/d	Cushing's disease	Addison's disease Anterior pituitary hypofunction
5-Hydroxyindoleascetic add, qualitative	Negative		Malignant carcinoid tumors	
Hydroxyproline	15–43 mg/24 h	0.11–0.33 μmol/d	Paget disease Fibrous dysplasia Osteomalacia Neoplastic bone diseases Hyperparathyroidism	
17-ketosteroids, total	Males: 10–22 mg/24 h Females: 6–16 mg/24 h	35–76 μmol/d 21–55 μmol/d	Interstitial cell tumor of testes Simple hirsutism, occasionally Adrenal hyperplasia Cushing's syndrome Adrenal cancer, virilism Adrenoblastoma	Thyrotoxicosis Female hypogonadism Diabetes mellitus Hypertension Debilitating disease of mild to moderate severity Eunuchoidism Addison's disease Panhypopituitarism Myxedema Nephrosis
Lead	Up to 150 μg/24 h	Up to 60 μmol/24 h	Lead poisoning	
Luteinizing hormone	Males: 5–18 IU/24 h Females: Follicular phase: 2–25 IU/24 h	 2–25 IU/d	Pituitary tumor Ovarian failure	Depressed or failure to peak—pituitary failure

(continued)

TABLE C•4 Reference Ranges—Urine Chemistry *(Continued)*

Determination	Normal Adult Reference Range: Conventional Units	Normal Adult Reference Range: SI Units	Clinical Significance: Increased	Clinical Significance: Decreased
	Ovulatory peak: 30–95 IU/24 h	30–95 IU/d		
	Luteal phase: 2–20 IU/24 h	2–20 IU/d		
	Postmenopausal: 40–110 IU/24 h	40–110 IU/d		
Metanephines, total	Less than 1.3 mg/24 h	Less than 6.5 μmol/d	Pheochromocytoma, a few patients with pheochromocytoma may have elevated urinary metanephines but normal catecholamines and vanillylmandelic acid (VMA)	
Osmolality	Males: 390–1090 mM/kg Females: 300–1090 mM/kg	390–1090 mmol/kg 300–1090 mmol/kg	Useful in the study of electrolyte and water balance	
Oxalate	Up to 40 mg/24 h	Up to 456/μmol/d	Primary hyperoxaluria	
Phenylpyruvic acid qualitative	Negative		Phenylketonuria	
Phosphorus, inorganic	0.8–1.3 gm/24 h	26–24 mmol/24 h	Hypoparathyroidism Vitamin D intoxication Paget's disease Metastatic neoplasm to bone	Hypoparathyroidism Vitamin D deficiency
Porphobilinogen, qualitative	Negative		Chronic lead poisoning Acute porphyria Liver disease	
Porphobilinogen quantitative	0–1 mg/24 h	0–4.4 μmol/24 h	Acute porphyria Liver disease	
Porphyrins, qualitative	Negative		See porphyrins, quantitative	
Porphyrins, quantitative (coproporphyrin and uroporphyrin)	Coproporphyrin: 50–160 μg/24 h Uroporphyrin: up to 50 μ/24 h	0.075–0.24 μmol/24h Up to 0.06 μmol/24 h	Porphyria Lead poisoning (only coproporphyrin increased)	
Potassium	40–65 mEq/24 h	40–65 mmol/24 h	Hemolysis Chronic renal failure Acidosis Cushing's disease	Diarrhea Adrenocortical insufficiency
Pregnanediol	Females:		Corpus luteum cysts When placental tissue remains in the uterus following parturition Some cases of adrenocortical tumors	Placental dysfunction Threatened abortion Intrauterine death
	Proliferative phase: 0.5–1.5 mg/24 h	1.6–4.8 μmol/24 h		
	Luteal phase: 2–7 mg/24 h	6–22 μmol/24 h		
	Menopause: 0.2–1 mg/24 h	0.6–3.1 μmol/24 h		
	Pregnancy:			
	Weeks of gestation — mg/24 h	μmol/24 h		
	10–12 — 5–15	15.6–47		
	12–18 — 5–25	15.6–78.0		
	18–24 — 15–33	47.0–103.0		
	24–28 — 20–42	62.4–131.0		
	28–32 — 27–47	84.2–146.6		
	Males: 0.1–2 mg/24 h	0.3–6.2 μmol/24 h		
Pregnanetriol	0.4–2.4 mg/24 h	1.2–7.1 μmol/24 h	Congenital adrenal androgenic hyperplasia	
Protein	Up to 100 mg/24 h	Up to 100 mg/24 h	Nephritis Cardiac failure	

(continued)

TABLE C•4 Reference Ranges—Urine Chemistry *(Continued)*

Determination	Normal Adult Reference Range: CONVENTIONAL UNITS	Normal Adult Reference Range: SI UNITS	Clinical Significance: INCREASED	Clinical Significance: DECREASED
Sodium	130–200 mEq/24 h	130–200 mmol/24 h	Mercury poisoning Bence-Jones protein in multiple myeloma Febrile states Hematuria Useful in detecting gross changes in water and salt balance	
Titratable acidity	20–40 mEq/24 h	20–40 mmol/24 h	Metabolic acidosis	Metabolic alkalosis
Urea nitrogen	9–16 gm/24 h	0.32–0.57 mol/L	Excessive protein catabolism	Impaired kidney function
Uric add	250–750 mg/24 h	1.48–4.43 mmol/24 h	Gout	Nephritis
Urobilinogen	Random urine: <0.25 mg/dL 24-hour urine: up to 4 mg/24 h	<0.42 mol/24 h Up to 6.76 μmol/24 h	Liver and biliary tract disease Hemolytic anemias	Complete or nearly complete biliary obstruction Diarrhea Renal insufficiency
Uroporphyrins	Up to 50 μg/24 h	Up to 0.06 μmol/24 h	Porphyria	
Vanillylmandelic acid (VMA)	0.7–6.8 mg/24 h	3.5–34.3 μmol/24 h	Pheochromocytoma Neuroblastoma Ingestion of coffee, tea, aspirin, bananas, and several different drugs	
Xylose absorption test (5-hour)	16%–33% of ingested xylose	Fraction absorbed: 0.16–0.33		Malabsorption syndromes
Zinc	0.15–1.2 mg/24 h	2.3–18.4 μmol/24 h		

TABLE C•5 Reference Ranges—Cerebrospinal Fluid (CSF)

Determination	Normal Adult Reference Range: CONVENTIONAL UNITS	Normal Adult Reference Range: SI UNITS	Clinical Significance: INCREASED	Clinical Significance: DECREASED
Albumin	15–30 mg/dL	150–300 mg/L	Certain neurologic disorders Lesion in the choroid plexus or blockage of the flow of CSF Damage to the blood central nervous system (CNS) barrier	
Cell count	0–5 mononuclear cells per cu mm	$0–5 \times 10^6$/L	Bacterial meningitis Neurosyphilis Anterior poliomyelitis Encephalitis lethargica	
Chloride	100–130 mEq/L	100–300 mmol/L	Uremia	Acute generalized meningitis Tuberculous meningitis
Glucose	50–75 mg/dL	2.75–4.13 mmol/L	Diabetes mellitus Diabetic coma Epidemic encephalitis Uremia	Acute meningitides Tuberculous meningitis Insulin shock
Glutamine	6–15 mg/dL	0.41–1 mmol/L	Hepatic encephalopathies, including Reye's syndrome Hepatic coma Cirrhosis	
IgG	0–6.6 mg/dL	0–66 mg/L	Damage to the blood CNS barrier Multiple sclerosis	

(continued)

TABLE C•5 Reference Ranges—Cerebrospinal Fluid (CSF) *(Continued)*

Determination	Normal Adult Reference Range		Clinical Significance	
	CONVENTIONAL UNITS	SI UNITS	INCREASED	DECREASED
			Neurosyphilis Subacute sclerosing panencephalitis Chronic phases of CNS infections	
Lactic acid	<24 mg/dL	<2.7 mmol/L	Bacterial meningitis Hypocapnia Hydrocephalus Brain abscesses Cerebral ischemia	
Lactic dehydrogenase	1/10 that of serum	Activity fraction: 0.1 of serum	CNS disease	
Protein:			Acute meningitides	
Lumbar	15–45 mg/dL	150–450 mg/L	Tubercular meningitis	
Cisternal	15–25 mg/dL	150–250 mg/L	Neurosyphilis	
Ventricular	5–15 mg/dL	50–150 mg/L	Poliomyelitis Guillain-Barré syndrome	
Protein electrophoresis (cellulose acetate)	% of total:	Fraction:	An increase in the level of albumin alone can be the result of a lesion in the choroid plexus or a blockage of the flow of CSF. An elevated gamma globulin value with a normal albumin level has been reported in multiple sclerosis, neurosyphilis, subacute sclerosing panencephalitis, and the chronic phase of CNS infections. If the blood-CNS barrier has been damaged severely during the course of these diseases, the CSF albumin level may also be elevated.	
Prealbumin	3–7	0.03–0.07		
Albumin	56–74	0.56–0.74		
Alpha, globulin	2–6.5	0.02–0.065		
Alpha2 globulin	3–12	0.03–0.12		
Beta globulin	8–18.5	0.08–0.185		
Gamma globulin	4–14	0.04–0.14		

TABLE C•6 Miscellaneous Values

Determinations	Normal Value	Clinical Significance: CONVENTIONAL UNITS	SI UNITS
Acetaminophen	Zero	Therapeutic level = 10–20 μg/mL	10–20 mg/L
Aminophylline (theophylline)	Zero	Therapeutic level = 10–20/μg/mL	10–20 mg/L
Bromide	Zero	Therapeutic level = 5–50 mg/dL	50–500 mg/L
Carbamazepine	Zero	Therapeutic level = 8–12 μg/mL	34–51 μmol/L
Carbon monoxide	0%–2%	Symptoms with >20% saturation	
Chlordiazepoxide	Zero	Therapeutic level = 1–3 μg/mL	1–3 mg/L
Diazepam	Zero	Therapeutic level = 0.5–2.5 μg/dL	5–25 μg/L
Digitoxin	Zero	Therapeutic level = 5–30 ng/mL	5–30 μg/L
Digoxin	Zero	Therapeutic level = 0.5–2 ng/mL	0.5–2/μg/L
Ethanol	0%–0.01%	Legal intoxication level = 0.10% or above 0.3%–0.4% = marked intoxication 0.4%–0.5% = alcoholic stupor	
Gentamicin	Zero	Therapeutic level = 4–10 μg/mL	4–10 mg/L
Lithium	Zero	Therapeutic level = 0.6–1.2 mEq/L	0.6–1.2 mmol/L
Methanol	Zero	May be fatal in concentration as low as 10 mg/dL	100 mg/L
Phenobarbital	Zero	Therapeutic level = 15–40 μg/mL	10–20 mg/L
Phenytoin	Zero	Therapeutic level = 10–20 μg/mL	10–20 mg/L
Primidone	Zero	Therapeutic level = 5–12 μg/mL	5–12 mg/L
Quinidine	Zero	Therapeutic level = 0.2–0.5 mg/dL	2–5 mg/L
Salicylate	Zero	Therapeutic level = 2–25 mg/dL Toxic level = >30 mg/dL	20–250 mg/L 300 mg/L
Vancomycin	Zero	Therapeutic peak 18.0–26.0 μg/mL Therapeutic trough 5.0–10.0 μg/mL	
Amitriptyline	Zero	Therapeutic level 120–250 mg/mL	433–903 nmol/L
Doxepin	Zero	Therapeutic level 30–150 ng/mL	107–537 nmol/L
Imipramine	Zero	Therapeutic level 125–250 ng/mL	446–893 nmol/L
Lidocaine	Zero	Therapeutic level 1.5–6.0 μg/mL	6.4–25.6 μmol/L
Methotrexate	Zero	Toxic (48 hr. after high dose) 454 mg/mL	1000 mmol/L
Propranolol	Zero	Therapeutic level 50–100 ng/mL	193–386 nmol/L
Valproic acid	Zero	Therapeutic level 50–100 g/mg	347–693 μmol/L

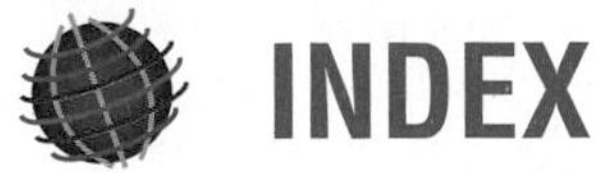

INDEX

Note: Letters following page numbers indicate the following: c – chart, f – figure, g – guideline, t – table.

A

B

H

I

J

M

N

P

Q

R

V